SO-AZS-580

Interventions Chapters

(Classification of Disorders) [included as appropriate]

    (Subclassification of Disorders) [included as appropriate]

        (Subsubclassification of Disorders) [included as appropriate]

            (Specific Disorder)

                Overview

                    Pathophysiology

                    Etiology

                    Incidence

                Prevention [included for preventable disorders]

                Collaborative Management

                Assessment

                    History

                    Physical Assessment: Clinical Manifestations

                    Psychosocial Assessment

                    Laboratory Findings

                    Radiographic Findings

                    Other Diagnostic Tests

                Analysis: Nursing Diagnosis

                  Common Diagnoses

                  Additional Diagnoses

                Planning and Implementation

                  (Specific Common Diagnosis)

                    Planning: Client Goals

                    Interventions: Nonsurgical Management [included as appropriate]

                    Interventions: Surgical Management [included as appropriate]

                ■ Discharge Planning

                  Home Care Preparation

                  Client/Family Education

                  Psychosocial Preparation

                  Health Care Resources

                Evaluation

Summary

Implications for Research

[Repeated for each specific disorder]

[Repeated for each specific common diagnosis]

Medical-Surgical Nursing

A NURSING PROCESS APPROACH

DONNA D. IGNATAVICIUS, M.S., R.N.,C.
MARILYN VARNER BAYNE, M.S., R.N.

With the Special Assistance of

Mary K. Kazanowski, M.S., R.N.,C., C.C.R.N., O.C.N., A.R.N.P.
Deitra Leonard Lowdermilk, Ph.D., R.N.,C.
M. Linda Workman, Ph.D., R.N., O.C.N.

Medical-Surgical Nursing

A NURSING PROCESS APPROACH

W.B. SAUNDERS COMPANY
Harcourt Brace Jovanovich, Inc.
Philadelphia   London   Toronto   Montreal   Sydney   Tokyo

W. B. SAUNDERS COMPANY
Harcourt Brace Jovanovich, Inc.

The Curtis Center
Independence Square West
Philadelphia, PA 19106

Library of Congress Cataloging-in-Publication Data

Ignatavicius, Donna D.
    Medical-surgical nursing: a nursing process approach/by Donna D. Ignatavicius
and Marilyn Varner Bayne.
        p.   cm.
    Includes bibliographical references.
    ISBN 0-7216-1974-6
    1. Nursing. 2. Surgical nursing. I. Bayne, Marilyn Varner. II. Title.
    [DNLM: 1. Nursing Process. 2. Surgical Nursing. WY 161 I24m]
RT41.I36 1991
610.73—dc20
DLC   90-8920

Editor: Michael J. Brown
Developmental Editor: Lee Henderson
Developmental Assistant: Michelle Davis
Designer: W. B. Saunders Staff
Production Manager: W. B. Saunders Staff
Manuscript Editors: Judith Gandy and Terry Russell
Illustrators: Sharon Iwanczuk and Elizabeth Strausbaugh
Showcase Illustrator: Drew Strawbridge
Illustration Coordinator: Cecelia Kunkle
Page Layout Artists: Dorothy Chattin and Holly McCoughian
Indexer: Alexandra Nickerson
Cover Designer: Ellen Bodner

MEDICAL-SURGICAL NURSING:
A NURSING PROCESS APPROACH   ISBN 0-7216-1974-6

Copyright © 1991 by W. B. Saunders Company

All rights reserved.   No part of this publication may be reproduced or transmitted in any form
or by any means, electronic or mechanical, including photocopy, recording, or any information
storage and retrieval system, without permission in writing from the publisher.

Printed in the United States of America.

Last digit is the print number: 9   8   7   6   5   4   3   2

To Marilyn

ABOUT THE AUTHORS

Donna D. Ignatavicius received her diploma in nursing from the Peninsula General Hospital School of Nursing in Salisbury, Maryland, in 1969. After working as a staff and charge nurse in a medical unit, she became an Instructor in Staff Development at the University of Maryland Hospital. In 1976, she received her B.S.N. from the University of Maryland School of Nursing. For 3 years she taught in a diploma school of nursing, and she completed her M.S. in nursing in 1981. Ms. Ignatavicius then taught in the baccalaureate program at the University of Maryland School of Nursing for 6 years, after which she pursued her interest in gerontology by becoming Director of Nursing at a long-term care facility. She is certified as a gerontological nurse.

Marilyn Varner Bayne received her diploma in nursing from the Wilkes-Barre General Hospital School of Nursing in Wilkes-Barre, Pennsylvania, in 1973. She then obtained her B.S.N. and M.S. in nursing from the University of Maryland School of Nursing. While completing her education, she worked as a staff and charge nurse in the Neurology Intensive Care Unit of the University of Maryland Hospital. From 1978 to 1988, the year of her death, she was Assistant Professor at the University of Maryland School of Nursing in the baccalaureate program, where she specialized in medical-surgical nursing and curriculum development.

ABOUT THEIR COLLEAGUES

Mary K. Kazanowski received her B.S. in nursing from St. Anselm College in Manchester, New Hampshire, and her M.S. in nursing from Boston University. She is a certified adult nurse practitioner. Her clinical experience includes several years as a staff nurse on medical-surgical units, with a focus on oncology, and 7 years as a staff nurse in critical care. She has also worked as a nurse practitioner on a medical inpatient unit and is currently Assistant Professor in the Nursing Department at St. Anselm College, where she teaches medical-surgical nursing. She is a staff nurse on the Oncology Unit at Elliot Hospital in Manchester, New Hampshire.

Deitra Leonard Lowdermilk received her B.S.N. from East Carolina University in Greenville, North Carolina. She received an M.Ed. in adult education with a minor focus in maternity nursing and a Ph.D. in education from the University of North Carolina at Chapel Hill. Her 20 years of teaching experience includes work in a baccalaureate nursing program, a diploma nursing program, and continuing education programs in all phases of women's reproductive health care. Her clinical practice has been in medical-surgical nursing; all areas of obstetric, gynecologic, and gynecologic oncology nursing; and community health nursing. A faculty member of the Department of Women and Children at the University of North Carolina at Chapel Hill School of Nursing, Dr. Lowdermilk teaches in a number of subject areas including biopsychosocial concepts of health care, infertility, and reproductive surgery. Her scholarly activities include several publications on women's reproductive issues and gynecologic oncology.

M. Linda Workman received her B.S.N. and M.S.N. from the College of Nursing and Health at the University of Cincinnati. She then earned a Ph.D. in developmental biology from the College of Arts and Sciences at the University of Cincinnati. Her 12 years of academic experience include teaching at the diploma, associate degree, baccalaureate, and master's levels. Areas of teaching expertise include physiology, pathophysiology, genetics, development, oncology, and immunology. Dr. Workman is Associate Professor of Nursing and Acting Chairperson of the Acute Care Nursing Department at the Frances Payne Bolton School of Nursing, Case Western Reserve University, in Cleveland, Ohio. A special talent that Dr. Workman brings to nursing education is the ability to teach complex physiologic mechanisms and processes in a manner that is both understandable and applicable to clinical nursing practice.

CONTRIBUTORS

Madalon O'Rawe Amenta, B.A., M.N., M.P.H., Dr.P.H.
Associate Professor of Nursing, The Pennsylvania State University, McKeesport, Pennsylvania
Response to Loss, Death, and Dying

Susan C. Archbold, R.N., B.S.N.
Director of Nurses and Owner of Professional Staffing Services, Newport Beach, California
Interventions for Clients in Shock

Shannon McDowell Bailey, R.N., B.S.N., M.S.
Nurse Investigator, Risk Control Coordinator and Affiliated Risk Control Administrators, Inc., St. Petersburg, Florida
Assessment of the Respiratory System; Interventions for Clients with Upper Respiratory Tract Disorders

Sally Ballenger, M.S.
Associate Professor, Department of Nursing, College of Arts and Sciences, DePaul University, Chicago, Illinois
Assessment of the Nervous System

Roxanne Aubol Batterden, R.N., B.S.N., C.C.R.N.
Nurse Educator II, Critical Care, Staff Development Department, Franklin Square Hospital Center, Baltimore, Maryland
Interventions for Clients with Biliary, Pancreatic, and Hepatic Disorders

Marilyn Varner Bayne,* M.S., R.N.
Assistant Professor, School of Nursing, University of Maryland, Baltimore, Maryland
Concepts of Health and Illness; The Nursing Profession and the Role of the Nurse; Introduction to the Nursing Process; Sensory Deprivation and Sensory Overload
* Deceased

Lindy M. Beaver, M.N., R.N., C.S.
Adjunct Faculty, University of South Carolina College of Nursing; Head Nurse (Surgical), Richland Memorial Hospital, Columbia, South Carolina
Interventions for Clients with Vascular Disorders

Suzanne C. Beyea, R.N.,C.
Professor of Nursing, New Hampshire Technical Institute, Concord, New Hampshire
Interventions for Clients with Intestinal Disorders

Anna M. Brock, R.N., Ph.D.
Dean, College of Health Sciences, Gannon University, Erie, Pennsylvania
Adult Development

Jean Ellen Cassidy, C.N.M., Dr. P.H.
Assistant Professor of Maternity Nursing, University of Maryland School of Nursing; Clinician, Planned Parenthood of Maryland, Baltimore, Maryland
Interventions for Clients with Sexually Transmitted Diseases

Jeanette K. Chambers, R.N., M.S., C.S.
Renal/Medical Clinical Nurse Specialist, Riverside Methodist Hospitals, Columbus, Ohio
Assessment of the Urinary System; Interventions for Clients with Urologic Disorders

Janice Z. Cuzzell, R.N., M.A.
Staff Nurse and Clinical Consultant, Sherman Oaks Community Hospital Burn Center, Sherman Oaks, California
Assessment of the Skin; Interventions for Clients with Skin Disorders

Ellen K. DeLuca, R.N., M.S.N.
Clinical Educator, Georgetown University Hospital, Washington, D.C.
Interventions for Clients with Lower Respiratory Tract Disorders

Mary Ann DiMola, R.N., M.A.
Adjunct Faculty, University of Florida, Gainesville, Florida; Adjunct Faculty, University of North Florida, Jacksonville, Florida; Director of Education, St. Vincent's Medical Center, Jacksonville, Florida
Interventions for Clients with Burns

Pamela Muhm Duchene, D.N.S., R.N., C.R.R.N.
Assistant Professor, Rush University; Associate Chairperson, Gerontological Nursing, Rush-Presbyterian-St. Luke's Medical Center, Chicago, Illinois
Rehabilitation for Clients with Disabling or Chronic Conditions

Anna Marie Ferrara, R.N., M.S.N., C.C.R.N.
Clinical Nurse Specialist, Research and Development, Critikow, Inc., Tampa, Florida
Interventions for Clients with Upper Respiratory Tract Disorders

Polly E. Gardner, R.N., M.N.
Clinical Instructor, Department of Physiological Nursing, University of Washington, Seattle, Washington; Critical Care Clinical Nurse Specialist, Evergreen Hospital Medical Center, Kirkland, Washington
Assessment of the Cardiovascular System; Interventions for Clients with Cardiac Disorders

Catherine D. Garofano, R.N., B.S., C.D.E.
Senior Instructor in Medicine and Nurse Specialist, Endocrinology and Diabetes, Hahnemann University School of Medicine, Philadelphia, Pennsylvania
Assessment of the Endocrine System; Interventions for Clients with Disorders

of the Pituitary and Adrenal Glands;
Interventions for Clients with Disorders
of the Thyroid and Parathyroid Glands

Barbara A. Given, R.N., Ph.D., F.A.A.N.
Professor, Michigan State University
College of Nursing, East Lansing,
Michigan
Interventions for Clients with Disorders
of the Stomach

Elizabeth F. Gloss, R.N., Ed.D.
Assistant Professor, College of
Nursing, State University of New
York Health Science Center, Brooklyn,
New York; Adjunct Assistant
Professor, Regents College Degrees,
State University of New York, Albany,
New York
Sensory Deprivation and Sensory Overload

Susan E. Goad, R.N., Ed.D.
Professor, College of Nursing, Texas
Woman's University, Dallas, Texas
Assessment of Clients with Disabling or
Chronic Conditions

Christine Grady, R.N., M.S., C.S.
Research Associate, National Center
for Nursing Research, National
Institutes of Health, Bethesda,
Maryland
Interventions for Clients with
Immunologic Disorders

Sally K. Graham, R.N.,C., M.S.N.
Adult Nurse Practitioner, Grady
Memorial Hospital, Atlanta, Georgia
Interventions for Clients with Disorders
of the Breast

Joyce P. Griffin, R.N., Ph.D.
Nurse Researcher, Portsmouth Naval
Hospital, Portsmouth, Virginia
Assessment of the Hematologic System;
Interventions for Clients with
Hematologic Disorders

Maureen Wimberly Groër, R.N., Ph.D.
Professor and Director of the Doctoral
Program, University of Tennessee
College of Nursing, Knoxville,
Tennessee
Concepts of Fluid and Electrolyte Balance

Diana W. Guthrie, R.N., Ph.D.
Professor of Pediatrics and Psychiatry,
School of Medicine, University of
Kansas Medical Center–Wichita;
Diabetes Nurse Specialist, Allied Health
Affiliate, St. Joseph Medical Center, St.
Francis Regional Medical Center, and
Wesley Medical Center, Wichita, Kansas
Interventions for Clients with Diabetes
Mellitus

Karin A. Hancher, R.N., M.S.N., C.S.
Clinical Instructor of Nursing,
Piedmont Virginia Community
College, Charlottesville, Virginia
Interventions for Clients with Disorders
of the Oral Cavity; Interventions for
Clients with Disorders of the Esophagus

Virginia Hargrave-Koertge, R.N., M.S.N., O.C.N.
University of Cincinnati Medical
Center, Cincinnati, Ohio
Interventions for Clients with
Hematologic Disorders

Kathy A. Hausman, R.N., M.S., C.N.R.N.
Director of Organization Development,
Harbor Hospital Center; Staff Nurse,
Neurologic Critical Care Unit,
University of Maryland Medical
Center, Baltimore, Maryland
Interventions for Clients with Central
Nervous System Disorders

Pamela J. Haylock, R.N., M.A.
Cancer Care Consultant, Cancer Care
Associates, Woodside, California
Concepts of Altered Cell Growth;
Interventions for Clients with Cancer

Deborah J. Henderson, R.N., B.S.N., C.I.C.
Special Assistant to the Director,
Center for Biologic Evaluation and
Research, Food and Drug
Administration, Bethesda, Maryland
Interventions for Clients with Infectious
Diseases

Gloria A. Hinderer, R.N., M.S., C.C.R.N., C.S.
Staff Nurse, Rush-Presbyterian-St.
Luke's Medical Center, Chicago, Illinois
Rehabilitation for Clients with Disabling
or Chronic Conditions; Interventions for
Clients with Peripheral Nervous System
Disorders

Sue Baird Holmes, R.N., M.S., O.N.C.
Courtesy Faculty Appointment,
Marquette University, College of
Nursing; Clinical Nurse Specialist,
Mobility, St. Joseph's Hospital,
Milwaukee, Wisconsin
Body Image

Raymond H. Hull, Ph.D.
Professor, Department of
Communication Disorders, University
of Northern Colorado, Greeley,
Colorado
Assessment of the Ear

Donna D. Ignatavicius, M.S., R.N.,C.
Director of Nursing, William Hill
Manor, Easton, Maryland
Concepts of Health and Illness; The
Nursing Profession and the Role of the
Nurse; Introduction to the Nursing
Process; Interventions for Clients with
Connective Tissue Disease; Assessment of
the Musculoskeletal System;
Interventions for Clients with
Musculoskeletal Disorders; Interventions
for Clients with Musculoskeletal Trauma

Kathleen J. Jones, R.N., M.S., O.C.N.
Oncology Clinical Nurse Specialist,
Walter Reed Army Medical Center,
Washington, D.C.
Interventions for Clients with Male
Reproductive Disorders

Mary K. Kazanowski, M.S., R.N.,C., C.C.R.N., O.C.N., A.R.N.P.
Assistant Professor, Nursing
Department, St. Anselm College; Staff
Nurse, Per Diem Pool, Oncology Unit,
Elliot Hospital, Manchester, New
Hampshire
Interventions for Clients with Intestinal
Disorders

Anne Keane, R.N., M.S.N., Ed.D.
Associate Professor of Nursing and
Chairperson, Adult Health and Illness
Nursing, University of Pennsylvania
School of Nursing, Philadelphia,
Pennsylvania
Pain

Mary Beth Kingston, R.N., M.S.N.
Head Nurse, Emergency Department,
Hospital of the University of
Pennsylvania, Philadelphia,
Pennsylvania

Assessment of the Endocrine System; Interventions for Clients with Disorders of the Pituitary and Adrenal Glands; Interventions for Clients with Disorders of the Thyroid and Parathyroid Glands

Martha Louise Larson, R.N., M.S., CDR, NC, USNR
Navy Nurse Corps Reservist, Bureau of Medicine and Surgery, Washington, D.C.
Interventions for Clients with Lower Respiratory Tract Disorders

Debra Laurent-Bopp, R.N., M.N.
Clinical Assistant Professor, Department of Physiological Nursing, University of Washington; Cardiovascular Clinical Nurse Specialist, Providence Medical Center, Seattle, Washington
Interventions for Clients with Cardiac Disorders

Deitra Leonard Lowdermilk, Ph.D., R.N.,C.
Clinical Associate Professor, University of North Carolina at Chapel Hill School of Nursing, Chapel Hill, North Carolina
Assessment of the Reproductive System; Interventions for Clients with Gynecologic Disorders; Interventions for Clients with Sexually Transmitted Diseases

Donna M. Mahrenholz, R.N., Ph.D.
Project Assistant, Center for Health Policy Research, University of Maryland, Baltimore, Maryland
Impact of the Health Care Delivery System on Medical-Surgical Nursing Practice

Judy Malkiewicz, R.N., M.S.
Assistant Professor of Nursing, School of Nursing, University of Northern Colorado, Greeley, Colorado
Assessment of the Ear

Jan Martin, R.N., M.S., G.N.P.
Assistant Professor, School of Nursing, University of Northern Colorado, Greeley, Colorado
Interventions for Clients with Ear and Hearing Disorders

Benita C. Martocchio, R.N., Ph.D.*
Associate Professor of Medical-Surgical Nursing, Director of Oncology

Nursing, and American Cancer Society Professor of Oncology Nursing, Case Western Reserve University; Clinical Associate, University Hospitals of Cleveland, Cleveland, Ohio
Response to Loss, Death, and Dying
* Deceased

Carolyn F. McCain, R.N., M.S.N.
Formerly Clinical Assistant Professor, University of North Carolina, Chapel Hill, North Carolina
Assessment of the Reproductive System

Patricia Ann Meidenbauer, B.S.N., M.S.
Instructor, Anne Arundel Community College, Arnold, Maryland
Interventions for Clients with Chronic and Acute Renal Failure

Anne Griswold Peirce, R.N., Ph.D.
Assistant Professor, Acute Care Nursing, Columbia University, New York, New York
Stress, Coping, and Adaptation

Rosemary C. Polomano, R.N., M.S.N., C.S.
Oncology/Pain Clinical Specialist, Hospital of the University of Pennsylvania, Philadelphia, Pennsylvania
Pain

Marie Rafalowski, R.N., M.S.N., C.C.R.N.
Assistant Professor, Nell Hodgson Woodruff School of Nursing, Emory University; Cardiovascular Nurse Coordinator, Emory University Hospital, Atlanta, Georgia
Interventions for Clients with Cardiac Disorders

Lynn Rew, R.N., Ed.D.
Associate Professor and Chair, Community Health Nursing Systems, The University of Texas, Austin, Texas
Human Sexuality

Judith K. Sands, R.N., Ed.D.
Assistant Professor, University of Virginia School of Nursing, Charlottesville, Virginia
Interventions for Clients with Disorders of the Esophagus

Karen S. Santmyer, R.N., M.S.
Psychiatric Liaison Clinical Specialist, The Francis Scott Key Medical Center, Baltimore, Maryland
Interventions for Clients with Eating Disorders

Pamela S. Schremp, R.N., M.S.N., C.R.N.O.
Clinical Instructor, Francis Payne Bolton School of Nursing, Case Western Reserve University; Clinical Nurse Specialist, Medical-Surgical Nursing, University Hospitals of Cleveland, Cleveland, Ohio
Assessment of the Eye; Interventions for Clients with Eye and Visual Disorders

Debra L. Spunt, R.N., M.S.
Instructor, University of Maryland School of Nursing, Baltimore, Maryland
Interventions for the Preoperative Client, Interventions for the Intraoperative Client

Thomas Szopa, R.N., M.S., O.C.N., C.E.T.N.
Adjunct Assistant Professor, Department of Nursing, University of New Hampshire, Durham, New Hampshire; Oncology Clinical Nurse Specialist/ET Nurse, Elliot Hospital, Manchester, New Hampshire
Interventions for Clients with Intestinal Disorders

Nancy L. Thayer, R.N., C.I.C.
Infection Control Consultant, Baltimore, Maryland
Interventions for Clients with Infectious Diseases

JoAnne Turner, R.N., M.N., C.S.
Adjunct Faculty Member, University of South Carolina School of Nursing; Clinical Nurse Specialist, Providence Hospital, Columbia, South Carolina
Interventions for Clients with Vascular Disorders

Kathleen M. White, R.N., M.S.
Instructor, University of Maryland School of Nursing, Baltimore, Maryland
Assessment of the Digestive System

Debra Penner Williams, R.N., M.S.
Nurse Manager, Surgical Intensive Care Unit and Post Anesthesia Care Unit, Department of Veterans Affairs–Bay Pines, Bay Pines, Florida

Interventions for Clients with Upper Respiratory Tract Disorders

James B. Winkler, R.N., M.A.
Assistant Dean of Clinical Affairs, University of Florida; Vice-President for Nursing, University Medical Center, Jacksonville, Florida
Interventions for Clients with Burns

Kathy M. Witta, R.N., M.S.N., C.C.R.N.
Pulmonary Clinical Nurse Specialist, Intermediate Medical Care Unit,

Hospital of the University of Pennsylvania, Philadelphia, Pennsylvania
Interventions for Clients with Lower Respiratory Tract Disorders

M. Linda Workman, Ph.D., R.N., O.C.N.
Associate Professor of Nursing, Frances Payne Bolton School of

Nursing, Case Western Reserve University, Cleveland, Ohio
Concepts of Fluid and Electrolyte Balance; Interventions for Clients with Fluid and Electrolyte Imbalances; Concepts of Acid-Base Balance; Interventions for Clients with Acid-Base Imbalances; Interventions for Clients in Shock; Concepts of Inflammation and the Immune Response

REVIEWERS

Ardelina Baldonado, R.N., M.S., Ph.D.
The Marcella Niehoff School of Nursing, Loyola University of Chicago, Chicago, Illinois

Roberta P. Bartee, R.N., M.S.
Formerly, Linfield College, Portland, Oregon

Patricia Bates, R.N., B.S.N., C.U.R.N.
Oregon Urology Clinic, P.C., Portland, Oregon

Nancy Benson-Shaffer, R.N., M.S.
College of Nursing, Niagara University, New York

Joyce M. Black, R.N.,C., M.S.N.
University of Nebraska Medical Center, Omaha, Nebraska

Dorothy R. Blevins, R.N., B.S.N., M.S.N.
School of Nursing, Kent State University, Kent, Ohio

Donna Zimmaro Bliss, R.N., M.S.N., C.C.R.N.
University of Pennsylvania, Philadelphia, Pennsylvania

Barbara J. Boss, R.N., Ph.D.
School of Nursing, University of Mississippi Medical Center, Jackson, Mississippi

Anne Boykin, Ph.D., R.N.
Florida Atlantic University, Boca Raton, Florida

Patricia E. Brien, R.N., M.Ed.
Berkshire Community College, Pittsfield, Massachusetts

Barbara Brillhart, R.N., Ph.D.
University of Colorado Health Sciences Center
Denver, Colorado

Nancy A. Brown, R.N., B.S.N., M.Ed.
School of Nursing, St. Margaret Memorial Hospital, Pittsburgh, Pennsylvania

Joan B. Bullas, B.S.N., M.A.
School of Nursing, University of Colorado Health Science Center, Denver, Colorado

Debra A. Byram, R.N., M.S.N., C.C.R.N.
National Institutes of Health, Bethesda, Maryland

Kay L. Carnegie, R.N., M.S.
Chemeketa Community College, Salem, Oregon

Barbara A. Cline, R.N., M.S.N.
School of Nursing, Kent State University, Kent, Ohio

Felissa L. Cohen, R.N., Ph.D., F.A.A.N.
University of Illinois at Chicago, Chicago, Illinois

Ann Coleman, M.S.N., R.N., C.S., R.N.P.
College of Nursing, University of Arkansas for Medical Sciences, Little Rock, Arkansas

Patricia A. Connor, R.N., M.S.N., C.S.
Lahey Clinic Medical Center, Burlington, Massachusetts

Marlene Croce-Burgess, R.N., B.S.N.
Wills Eye Hospital, Philadelphia, Pennsylvania

Gladys E. Deters, R.N., M.S.N.
School of Nursing, University of Virginia, Charlottesville, Virginia

Diane M. Eddy, R.N., M.S.N.
Kent State University, Kent, Ohio

Carol Jean Einhorn, B.S.N., C.U.R.N.
Northwestern Memorial Hospital, Northwestern University, Chicago, Illinois

Jo Ann Fetters, R.N., B.A., B.S.N., M.S.N.
Danville Area Community College, Danville, Illinois

Geraldine G. Flaherty, R.N., M.S.N.
College of Nursing, Wayne State University, Detroit, Michigan

Lucille Gambardella, R.N., M.S.N., C.S.
Division of Nursing, Wesley College, Dover, Delaware

Elizabeth Gloss, B.S., M.Ed., Ed.D.
College of Nursing, State University of New York, Brooklyn, New York; Regents College, Albany, New York

JoAnn Kelly Gottlieb, R.N., M.S.
School of Nursing, University of Miami, Miami, Florida

Carolyn Grous, R.N., M.S.N., C.N.O.R.
Hospital of the University of Pennsylvania, Philadelphia, Pennsylvania

Jane Hokanson Hawks, R.N.,C., M.S.N.
Bishop Clarkson College, Omaha, Nebraska

JoAnne Herman, R.N., Ph.D.
College of Nursing, University of South Carolina, Columbia, South Carolina

Frieda M. Holt, R.N., Ed.D.
School of Nursing, University of Maryland, Baltimore, Maryland

Ann H. Hunt, R.N.,C., Ph.D.
School of Nursing, Purdue University, West Lafayette, Indiana

Fred D. Jung, R.N., Ph.D.
University of North Carolina at Greensboro, Greensboro, North Carolina

Annabelle M. Keene, R.N., M.S.N.
College of Nursing, University of Nebraska, Omaha, Nebraska

Priscilla E. Kelley, R.N., M.S.
Dartmouth-Hitchcock Medical Center, Hanover, New Hampshire

Carole Ann Kenner, R.N.,C., M.S.N., D.N.S.
College of Nursing and Health, University of Cincinnati, Cincinnati, Ohio

Rose G. Kinash, R.N., B.N., B.A., M.Sc.N.
University of Saskatchewan, Saskatoon, Saskatchewan, Canada

Mary Lee S. Kirkland, R.N., M.S.N.
School of Nursing, Medical University of South Carolina, Charleston, South Carolina

Karen M. Kleeman, R.N., Ph.D., C.S.
School of Nursing, University of Maryland, Baltimore, Maryland

Jane Koeckeritz, B.S.N., M.S.N.
University of Northern Colorado, Fort Collins, Colorado

Janet G. LaMantia, R.N., M.A., C.R.R.N.
Consultant, Guilford, Connecticut

Priscilla LeMone, R.N., M.A.
School of Nursing, Southeast Missouri State University, Cape Girardeau, Missouri

Dorothy Lumb Leese, R.N., B.S.N., M.A., C.D.E.
The Medical College of Pennsylvania, Philadelphia, Pennsylvania

Marion R. Leiner, B.S.N., M.Ed.
School of Nursing, East Carolina University, Greenville, North Carolina

Linda G. Linc, R.N., Ph.D.
College of Nursing, The University of Akron, Akron, Ohio

M. Charlene Long, R.N., Ph.D.
College of Nursing, University of South Florida, St. Petersburg, Florida

Barbara Clary Martin, R.N., M.S.
University of Tulsa
Tulsa, Oklahoma

Myrna R. Mason, R.N., C.U.R.N.
St. Vincent Hospital, Portland, Oregon

Barbara J. McArthur, R.N., Ph.D., F.A.A.N.
Wayne State University, Detroit, Michigan

Margaret A. McEntree, R.N., Ph.D.
School of Nursing, University of Maryland, Baltimore, Maryland

Joanne Michener, R.N., M.S.N.
Hahnemann University Hospital, Philadelphia, Pennsylvania

Carol A. Morris, R.N., B.S.N., M.S., M.N., Ed.D.
Northeastern Oklahoma A&M College, Miami, Oklahoma

Marilyn Anne Murphy, M.S.
School of Nursing, The University of Texas Health Science Center at San Antonio, San Antonio, Texas

Geri Neuberger, R.N., Ed.D
School of Nursing, University of Kansas, Kansas City, Kansas

Collen K. Norton, R.N., M.S.N., C.C.R.N.
School of Nursing, The Catholic University of America, Washington, D.C.

Virginia Olsavsky, R.N., B.S.N., M.S.N.
Ursuline College, Pepper Pike, Ohio

Joan M. Paul, R.N., B.S.N., M.S.N.
San Antonio College, San Antonio, Texas

Elisabeth A. Pennington, R.N., Ed.D.
School of Nursing, The University of Michigan, Ann Arbor, Michigan

April E. Perry, R.N., M.Ed.
Duke University Medical Center, Durham, North Carolina

Winifred J. Pinch, R.N., B.S., M.Ed., M.S., Ed.D.
School of Nursing, Creighton University, Omaha, Nebraska

Janet A. Pitts, R.N., Ph.D.
Consultant, Seattle, Washington

Sara Lynne Roettger, R.N., M.S.N.
School of Nursing, The University of Texas Health Science Center at San Antonio, San Antonio, Texas

Patricia L. Ryan, R.N., M.A., M.S.N.
Gwynedd Mercy College, Gwynedd Valley, Pennsylvania

Carolyn E. Sabo, R.N., Ed.D.
University of Nevada, Las Vegas, Las Vegas, Nevada

Ann Sedore, R.N., Ph.D.
College of Nursing, Syracuse University, Syracuse, New York

Paula A. Shackelford, R.N., M.S.
The University of Texas M.D. Anderson Cancer Center, Houston, Texas

Mary K. Sienty, R.N., Ed.D
School of Nursing, Widener University, Chester, Pennsylvania

Gloria J. Smokvina, R.N., Ph.D.
Purdue University Calumet, Hammond, Indiana

Martha A. Spies, R.N., M.S.N.
Deaconess College of Nursing, St. Louis, Missouri

Kristan Kay Stewart, R.N., M.N., C.C.R.N., C.E.N.
University of Utah, Latter Day Saints Hospital, Salt Lake City, Utah

Carralee Ann Sueppel, R.N., C.U.R.N.
University of Iowa Hospitals and Clinics, Iowa City, Iowa

Sharon Summers, R.N., M.S.N., Ph.D.
School of Nursing, University of Kansas Medical Center, Kansas City, Kansas

Joanne Tate, R.N., B.N., M.S.Ed., M.N.Ed., Ph.D.
Shadyside Hospital School of Nursing, Pittsburgh, Pennsylvania

Janice J. Twiss, R.N., M.S.N.
College of Nursing, University of

Nebraska Medical Center, Omaha,
Nebraska

**Marie A. Whedon, R.N., M.S.,
O.C.N.**
Dartmouth-Hitchcock Medical Center,
Hanover, New Hampshire

Rosanne Wille, R.N., Ph.D.
Lehman College, City University of
New York, Bronx, New York

Paula L. Wilson, R.N., M.S.N.
College of Nursing, University of
Nebraska, Omaha, Nebraska

**Jill Winland-Brown, R.N., M.S.,
Ed.D.**
Florida Atlantic University, Boca
Raton, Florida

Frances A. Wollner, R.N., M.N.
College of Nursing, Niagara
University, New York

**Donna Jean Woodside, R.N.,C.,
M.S.N., Ed.D., C.D.E.**
University of Cincinnati, Cincinnati,
Ohio

Jonelle E. Wright, R.N., Ph.D.
School of Nursing, University of
Maryland, Baltimore, Maryland

Carolyn Zdanowicz, M.S., B.S.
Formerly, University of Massachusetts,
Boston, Massachusetts

Ulana Zinych, R.N., M.S.N.
Mattatuck Community College,
Waterbury, Connecticut

PREFACE

Why We Wrote This Textbook

The practice of medical-surgical nursing has changed dramatically over the past decade, but textbooks have not changed as quickly. To answer the need for a textbook that reflects today's realities, we have created *Medical-Surgical Nursing: A Nursing Process Approach.*

Limitations imposed today on acute care settings by prospective payment systems such as Medicare have led to clients' being admitted to hospitals only when seriously ill and being discharged quickly to home or another health care setting. Nearly two-thirds of these hospitalized people are older than 65 years of age. Most clients in this age group present with an acute episode of a chronic health problem and a multitude of secondary, often contributory, chronic diseases such as diabetes mellitus, hypertension, and arteriosclerotic cardiovascular disease. This situation creates new challenges for those providing nursing care to hospitalized adults.

Although other textbooks of medical-surgical nursing have served their readers well, they have become inadequate for preparing today's nurses. Today's medical-surgical nurse must

- Be at ease with the nursing process
- Understand the collaborative management of client problems as part of a health care team
- Have ready access to a comprehensive, current body of knowledge
- Be prepared to care for the unique problems of seriously ill adults — especially seriously ill older adults
- Know how to help clients prevent illness and maintain health
- Be prepared to teach clients and their families
- Be able to plan for clients' care after their discharge from the hospital
- Be well versed in pathophysiology, pharmacology, nutrition, diagnostic testing, physical assessment, and care planning

To meet these needs, *Medical-Surgical Nursing: A Nursing Process Approach*

- Incorporates the five-step nursing process as its central organizational framework. Although other textbooks incorporate the nursing process to some degree, we organize all interventions — without artificial distinction between nursing and medical interventions — around commonly identified NANDA-approved nursing diagnoses for each major disease or disorder likely to be encountered by a medical-surgical nurse. (Less common conditions are covered thoroughly, but — to conserve space — without specific reference to the nursing process.)
- Describes a number of conceptual approaches to client care without advocating a particular one, because no universal model or theory is appropriate for the care of the heterogeneous population found in medical-surgical nursing.
- Is accurate, up-to-date, comprehensive, and — by virtue of its unique quick-access formats for Assessment and Interventions chapters — provides readily accessible information.
- Emphasizes care of seriously ill clients and seriously ill elderly clients throughout, and highlights common assessment findings in the elderly with clear, consistent headings and special Focus on the Elderly features in each Assessment chapter.
- Integrates health promotion/maintenance information throughout, and highlights select material in easily identifiable Health Promotion/Maintenance features.
- Provides the most comprehensive, accessible coverage of discharge planning available.
- Includes client and family education in every Discharge Planning section and demonstrates client teaching in client-oriented terms in Client/Family Education features.
- Includes in-depth coverage of pathophysiology and "need-to-know" coverage of pharmacology, nutrition, diagnostic testing, physical assessment, care planning, substance abuse, emergency care, and critical care — each the subject of a book in itself. Emergency care is discussed in the text and is highlighted in Emergency Care features for appropriate instances in medical-surgical nursing.

How the Book is Organized

Medical-Surgical Nursing: A Nursing Process Approach is divided into three parts.

Part I: Perspectives for Medical-Surgical Nursing Practice provides the foundation for the framework used in the book. Chapters 1 through 3 introduce our philosophical approach to health, nursing, and the nursing process. Chapter 4 describes the health care delivery system in the United States and how that system affects the practice of medical-surgical nursing. Chapters 5 through 11 examine several key concepts in nursing practice: adult development; stress, coping, and adaptation; pain; sensory deprivation and sensory overload; body image; human sexuality; and response to loss, death, and dying. Appropriate nursing interventions are suggested.

Part II: Client Problems Affecting Multiple Body Systems consists of units on management of fluid, electrolyte, and acid-base problems; burns and shock; the surgical client; and clients with chronic illness. Because fluid, electrolyte, and acid-base problems are complex and affect virtually every body system, we have taken great pains to ensure that our coverage of these problems is clearer and more comprehensive than that in other texts.

Part III: Specific Client Problems in Medical-Surgical Nursing is the largest part of the book. It is divided into 13 units that address particular client problems, most corresponding to body systems. For example, Unit 17 is entitled Problems of Oxygenation: Management of Clients with Disruptions of the Respiratory System. Each unit typically begins with an Assessment chapter, such as Assessment of the Respiratory System, and continues with one or more Interventions chapters, such as Interventions for Clients with Upper Respiratory Tract Disorders.

Each Assessment chapter has a consistent, easy-to-follow format, beginning with an anatomy and physiology review and continuing with changes associated with aging, history taking, physical assessment, psychosocial assessment, and diagnostic assessment. A summary and list of contemporary and classic references and readings conclude each Assessment chapter. (Classic references are provided when they are regarded as the foremost primary resources in a given area.) When additional noteworthy readings are available, a list of annotated additional readings follows.

Each Interventions chapter follows a consistent, accessible format. Management of diseases and disorders that are commonly encountered by the medical-surgical nurse is described in a step-by-step fashion, beginning with an overview (a description of the pathophysiology, etiology, and incidence), a description of preventive measures (if appropriate), the five-step nursing process highlighted by Saunders' nursing process symbols, and a section on discharge planning. Interventions chapters provide at the end a summary, a list of implications for research, a list of contemporary and classic references and readings, and, when justified by the literature, a list of annotated additional readings.

Each unit concludes with a list of names, addresses, and telephone numbers of nursing and other resources.

Other Learning Aids
The illustrations included in *Medical-Surgical Nursing* were created especially to complement this text. The ideas illustrated were chosen after exhaustive review by a panel of nursing instructors with special interests in visual learning. Unique to this book are 24 "Showcase" illustrations, many of which combine art and text to convey important or difficult concepts in medical-surgical nursing. Full-color figures—located in Unit 12—illustrate subjects for which visibility of subtle variations in color is essential to learning.

In addition to the Focus on the Elderly, Health Promotion/Maintenance, Client/Family Education, and Emergency Care features mentioned previously, *Medical-Surgical Nursing* uses four other distinctively designed features to help the reader categorize and retain essential information:

■ *Key Features of Disease* highlight essential information about diseases and disorders such as risk factors and etiologies.
■ *Nursing Research* features highlight pertinent nursing research articles and include a full reference citation, a description of the research, a critique of the research, and possible nursing implications. The emphasis is on cautious use of preliminary research findings. These features are the result of extensive literature searches, which revealed a great need for nursing research in many areas. To address this need, each Interventions chapter includes implications for research.
■ *Client Care Plans* exemplify how to formulate an individualized plan of nursing care. Client Care Plans are provided for common clinical situations such as postoperative care of a client with a fractured hip. Client-oriented goals with measurable, observable outcomes are presented for each nursing diagnosis in the plan.
■ *Guidelines* features highlight nursing interventions for clients in situations not warranting treatment as Client Care Plans.

Learning Objectives and lists of Prerequisite Knowledge items (topics for student review before studying each chapter) are included in a *Student Study Guide.*

Master outlines for Assessment and Interventions chapters can be found inside the cover, as can an alphabetical list of current NANDA-approved nursing diagnoses.

The Contents in Brief and Table of Contents in the front of the book and the Guide to Special Features and the Index/Glossary at the back of the book are indicated by tabs on the edges of the pages for easy access. The Index/Glossary features defined glossary terms and boldface entries for each nursing diagnosis as part of an exhaustive index.

Part of a Complete Teaching/Learning Package
Six companion publications complement *Medical-Surgical Nursing* to form a complete teaching/learning package. A *Student Study Guide* enables the reader to pretest understanding of textbook content before formal classroom testing and helps in preparation for state boards. The *Pocket Companion to Ignatavicius & Bayne's Medical-Surgical Nursing: A Nursing Process Approach* summarizes the essentials of the textbook in an easy-to-use, pocket-sized form—an invaluable resource in the clinical setting. A 2000-item IBM-compatible computer *Test Bank* coded for pretest material, and for testing of steps of the nursing process as they relate to text content areas, is available to instructors. To complement the computer *Test Bank*, instructors may wish to use the printed *Test Manual*, which is fully indexed and includes a selection of unlabeled illustrations from the textbook

that can be photocopied and distributed to students for labeling as part of a pretest. An *Instructor's Manual* contains two versions of the Learning Objectives from the *Student Study Guide.* One version is annotated for the instructor; another appears without annotations and is printed on a separate page to be photocopied and distributed to students with or without modification. Prerequisite Knowledge items corresponding to those in the

Student Study Guide, teaching strategies, a list of instructional media, and a selection of case studies to be photocopied and assigned are also a part of the *Instructor's Manual.* A set of 100 transparencies and 200 transparency masters constitutes the *Transparencies to Accompany Medical-Surgical Nursing: A Nursing Process Approach,* which completes this comprehensive teaching/learning package.

ACKNOWLEDGMENTS

At the completion of a project of this magnitude, one can hardly begin to list all of the wonderfully supportive people who "keep authors going." Above all, thanks to Charles, Wes, and Stephanie (DI) and to Nelson and Timmy (MB) for the love and patience they consistently showed during the book's preparation.

The staff at W. B. Saunders has been great to work with. Michael Brown, Editor-in-Chief, Nursing, has been my personal motivator, supporter, and friend during the many ups and downs of this project. His developmental editors and assistants have kept us on schedule and helped us to be creative in feature and format development. Fran Mues got us started, but Lee Henderson has seen us to the finish line. Lee's gentle nature and positive reinforcement helped make the tough deadlines and frustrations bearable.

Other Saunders personnel who have done outstanding jobs include Illustration Coordinator Cecelia Kunkle, Copy Editors Judith Gandy and Terry Russell, Cover Designer Ellen Bodner, Illustrators Sharon Iwanczuk and Elizabeth Strausbaugh, and Marketing Manager David Nazaruk.

Linda Workman, Mary Kazanowski, and Dee Lowdermilk — three extremely talented and easy-to-work-with colleagues — believed in this project and made many personal and professional sacrifices for it.

Debra Spunt served as a consultant and authored Unit 5. Other nurse consultants include Verna Carson, Minerva Applegate, and Dorothy Lanuza, whose work is deeply appreciated.

CONTENTS IN BRIEF

P A R T I

PERSPECTIVES FOR MEDICAL-SURGICAL NURSING PRACTICE 1

P A R T I I

CLIENT PROBLEMS AFFECTING MULTIPLE BODY SYSTEMS 223

P A R T I I I

SPECIFIC CLIENT PROBLEMS IN MEDICAL-SURGICAL NURSING 523

CONTENTS IN BRIEF

CONTENTS

PART I

PERSPECTIVES FOR MEDICAL-SURGICAL NURSING PRACTICE 1

PART II

CLIENT PROBLEMS AFFECTING MULTIPLE SYSTEMS 223

PART III

SPECIFIC CLIENT PROBLEMS IN MEDICAL-SURGICAL NURSING   523

CONTENTS

PART I

PERSPECTIVES FOR MEDICAL-SURGICAL NURSING PRACTICE

UNIT 1

Health Promotion and Maintenance

CHAPTER 1

Concepts of Health and Illness

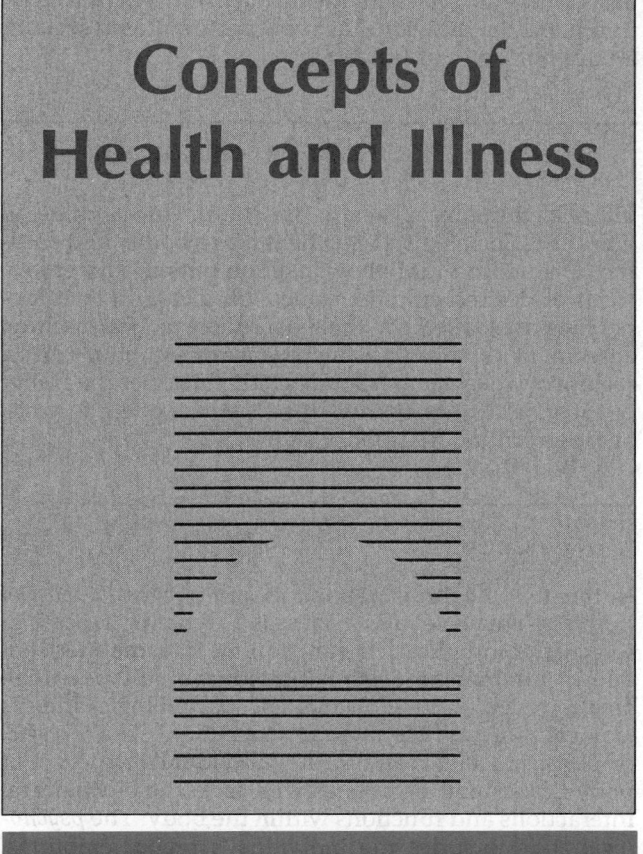

Beliefs regarding health and illness are a major feature of every known culture. How an individual views himself or herself as an entity and as part of the surrounding environment is an integral part of how health is defined. Health is often viewed as a continuum on which wellness, at one end, is the optimal level of function, and illness, at the opposite end, culminates in death (Fig. 1–1). At any point on the continuum, an individual has both positive attributes of wellness and negative attributes of illness. No one ever reaches the point of perfect existence, but there is a constant attempt to achieve as optimal a level as possible. The balance of positive and negative attributes at any time determines the individual's state of health. Health is a dynamic process that varies as interactions between individuals and their internal and external environments change.

DEFINITIONS OF HEALTH AND ILLNESS

Although the term *health* is used as part of everyday living, it is difficult to define. Many theorists and organizations have attempted to define the concept of health, but no universally accepted definition has been established. Throughout the ages, the focus and expression of health have varied depending on prevailing levels of knowledge, philosophical theories, and cultural and religious beliefs. In early times, people viewed health and disease as reward or punishment for their actions. Later, health was thought to be a soundness or wholeness of the body. A typical dictionary definition describes health in terms of an individual's ability to function normally in society. Some definitions also characterize health as a disease-free state or condition. Definitions such as these are unclear about what constitutes health and illness and seem to present an either/or situation — an individual is either healthy or ill.

WORLD HEALTH ORGANIZATION DEFINITION

As science progressed, the definition of health evolved. One of the most frequently quoted definitions is the 1947 definition presented by the World Health Organization (WHO). Health is "a state of complete physical, mental, and social well-being and not merely the absence of disease or infirmity" (WHO, 1947, p. 1). According to this definition, to be healthy, an individual must be in a state of well-being physically, mentally, and socially. Health professionals have had problems using this definition because it seems to be an unrealistic goal. This definition does not allow for degrees of health

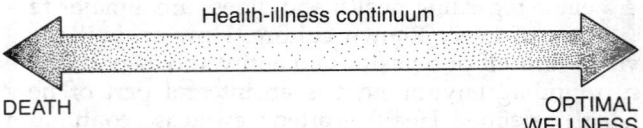

Figure 1 – 1

Common concept of health as a continuum ranging from optimal wellness at one end to illness culminating in death at the other end.

or illness, and it fails to reflect the dynamic, ever-changing nature of health.

Another concept that emerged in the search for a description of health was *homeostasis,* or internal equilibrium or balance. When a disturbance in homeostasis is experienced, the individual is considered to be unhealthy. This term is losing popularity because "stasis" implies an unchanging state, and most theorists believe that health is dynamic.

DUNN'S HIGH-LEVEL WELLNESS

In the late 1950s, Halbert Dunn presented a new concept, *high-level wellness.* Although Dunn viewed health as the absence of disease, he believed that health was active and related to the environment. Like other theorists, he advocated use of the health-illness continuum,

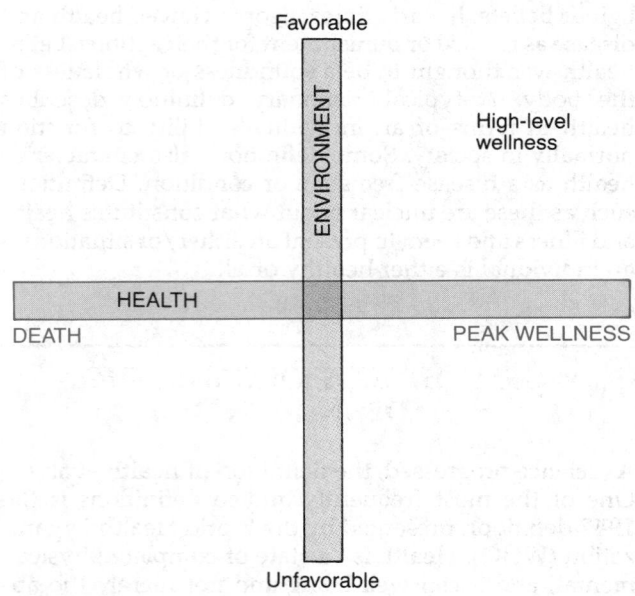

Figure 1 – 2

Dunn's theory of health and its dependence on the environment. High-level wellness occurs when peak wellness exists in a favorable environment. (Adapted from Dunn, H. [1959]. High-level wellness for man and society. *American Journal of Public Health, 49,* 786 – 792.)

but intersected by one's environment, as shown in Figure 1 – 2. The term he introduced, high-level wellness, is an action term and represents a dynamic attempt by an individual to reach his or her full potential within the environment in which he or she is functioning. On the basis of interactions with the internal and external environments, the individual actively participates in seeking an optimal level of function.

SOCIOLOGIC DEFINITIONS OF HEALTH

Other definitions of health are found throughout the literature. Sociologists view health as a bodily and emotional condition that allows for the pursuit and enjoyment of desired cultural values. Studies in which laypersons are polled for their definition of health show agreement that health is the absence of symptoms and a feeling of well-being. "Good health" includes the ability to carry out "normal" activities, such as going to work and performing household chores.

TEXTBOOK DEFINITION OF HEALTH

In this text, health is defined as *an individual's level of wellness.* This level of wellness is a dynamic process in which the individual is functioning in a manner that allows attainment of the individual's full potential. Health reflects a person's biologic, psychologic, and sociologic state, as illustrated in Figure 1 – 3. The *biologic,* or physical, state refers to the individual's structure of body tissues and organs, as well as to the biochemical interactions and functions within the body. The *psychologic* state includes the individual's mood, emotions, personality, and interaction styles. The *sociologic,* or social, state involves the interaction between the individ-

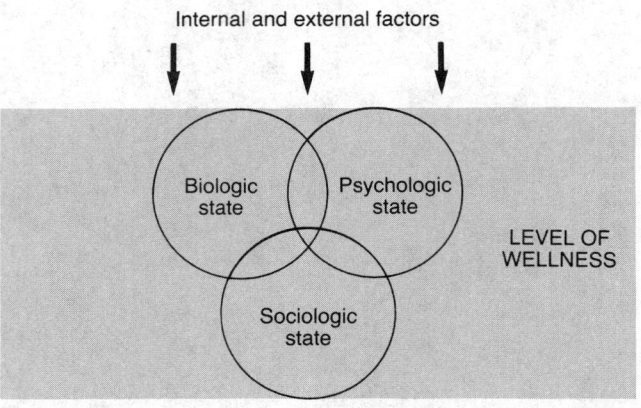

Figure 1 – 3

Textbook definition of health — the biopsychosocial state of an individual. The individual's level of wellness is affected by internal and external factors.

ual and the environment. Factors that affect the individual's biologic, psychologic, or social well-being require additional energy expenditures and thus alter the level of wellness. Therefore, a high level of wellness is achieved when the biopsychosocial needs of a person are met.

One of nursing's primary functions is to assist clients in reaching a high level of wellness. Understanding the concept of health and high-level wellness is essential. As nurses assess clients, they must be aware of factors that affect an individual's health state and must use nursing measures to promote and maintain optimal levels of wellness.

HOLISTIC HEALTH

Another frequently used term when health and wellness are discussed is *holistic health.* The holistic view of humans considers the body, mind, and spirit as dimensions of the person's being. The concept of high-level wellness, which considers the needs of the whole person, has led to the growth of holistic health care. Holistic health focuses on promoting health and preventing illness, with emphasis on the client's responsibility to achieve high-level wellness. There is also concern with bringing the person's mind, body, and spirit into harmony with the environment.

DEFINITIONS OF ILLNESS

Illness is often defined as sickness or a deviation from a healthy state. Illness has a broader meaning than disease. *Disease* refers to a biologic or psychologic alteration that results in a malfunction of a body organ or system. Disease is usually the term that is used to describe a biomedical condition and is supported by objective data, such as elevated temperature, presence of infection, or inability to move. Illness is the perception and response of the client and those around him or her to not being well. Although illness includes disturbances in normal human functioning caused by the biologic system and psychosocial changes, it also encompasses personal, interpersonal, and cultural reactions to disease. The concept of illness includes how the client interprets the origin and significance of the event, how the event affects the client's behavior and relationships with other people, and how the client tries to remedy the situation. In addition to the experience of being ill, the meaning given to that experience is a significant aspect of illness. Illness involves the whole person and is unique for each individual.

In most cases, a person is said to be ill when personal perceptions regarding impaired well-being agree with the perceptions of those around that person. For example, those near the ill person might say, "You look pale today." The process of being ill is often social in nature because it involves other people besides the client.

THEORIES OF ILLNESS CAUSATION

Disease is usually considered to be a result of the interaction of several factors. In early theories, microorganisms or factors from outside the body were thought to be the causes of illness. Although some causes of illness are known, scientists continue to explore this area to determine cause-and-effect relationships between disease-producing agents and illness in an individual. Today, theories of causation also consider the concept of stress and the individual's ability to adapt. When factors within the person's internal or external environment affect the individual's ability to maintain a biopsychosocial equilibrium, illness occurs. A person's reaction to stress and ability to adapt are further explored in Chapter 6. Various disturbances that produce illness can be classified as *mechanical, biologic,* or *normative.*

MECHANICAL DISTURBANCES

Mechanical disturbances result in structural damage to the individual. Many of these illnesses are caused by injuries sustained in an accident. This category includes acute disruptions such as trauma; the event often occurs suddenly with little or no warning. Structural disturbances are often caused by an external event over which the client has little or no control. Temperature extremes, machines, chemicals, and radiation, for example, are physical agents that may lead to such disturbances.

BIOLOGIC DISTURBANCES

This classification includes all forms of illness that have a biologic cause that affects body function. Examples of these causes include inherited genetic defects, alterations in the immune defense system, microorganisms or parasites that produce disease, excessive or deficient production of various body secretions, and biologic processes that are altered by the aging process, such as impaired sight or hearing. These illnesses often proceed at a slow rate. The body has more of an opportunity to anticipate and prepare defenses than when mechanical disturbances are encountered.

NORMATIVE DISTURBANCES

Normative disturbances are those that are psychologic and that originate in either the internal or the external environment of a person. They initially affect the mind, but physiologic changes may follow these first effects. Loss or fear of loss is a major psychologic factor that can produce disease. An example of this disturbance follows: A woman has a mastectomy. After the surgery, she may experience a loss in body image and of feelings of femininity. The psychologic results may interfere with her ability to return to the normal level of function and may lead to illness. Because individuals have different values, not all persons experience the same degree of loss in similar situations.

VARIABLES AFFECTING HEALTH AND/OR ILLNESS

Certain variables predispose an individual to illness or affect a person's level of health regardless of causation. Figure 1–4 summarizes these factors.

GENETIC INFLUENCE

The biologic make-up of an individual is predetermined by the genes present at birth. Many illnesses or chronic conditions result from the individual's genetic composition. As technology and research advance, recognition of the number of genetically influenced diseases is increasing. Examples of health problems that are related to inherent traits include diabetes mellitus, sickle cell anemia, and hemophilia.

COGNITIVE ABILITIES

The individual's cognitive abilities affect his or her view of health and illness. Educational level and cognitive abilities determine the individual's capability to reason, conceptualize, use knowledge, and make decisions. The person's definition and understanding of health and illness and the capacity to seek appropriate resources or health care depend on cognitive abilities.

DEMOGRAPHIC FACTORS

The age and sex of individuals can influence the health state. For example, many of today's elderly population will live into their 80s or 90s. The incidence of chronic disease increases with age. Men and women vary in their response to a disruption in their health. Men typically avoid seeking professional health care. Some men think that the "macho" male should never be "sick." Others worry that their families depend on them financially and thus think that the breadwinner cannot afford to be ill.

Some diseases are more predominant in one sex or the other. For example, gout and myocardial infarctions

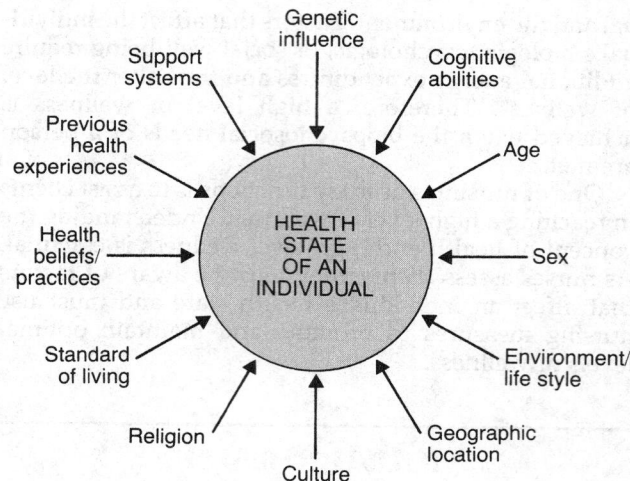

Figure 1–4

Multiple variables influence health and illness of an individual.

are more common in men, and osteoporosis and breast cancer are more common in women.

ENVIRONMENT AND LIFE STYLE

The environment in which a person lives can lead to an increased incidence of certain health problems. For instance, individuals living in inner cities around areas with heavy industry may be exposed to smog and air pollution, which negatively affect respiratory function. Persons who live in rural areas are less likely to have this type of health concern.

The amount of daily activity can also predispose individuals to certain diseases. For example, sedentary postmenopausal women are more susceptible to osteoporosis than physically active women.

Some diseases are associated with a person's occupation. Coal miners, for example, are prone to lung disease; carpet installers are likely to develop degenerative arthritis of knees. Certain recreational activities can be hazardous. Sky diving, skiing, and ice hockey are high-risk sports that frequently result in trauma.

One's dietary habits can also influence susceptibility to disease. Research in this area is expanding to relate dietary intake to certain illnesses. For example, obesity predisposes an individual to heart problems and to arthritis in weight-bearing joints.

GEOGRAPHIC LOCATION

The area of the United States or the world in which a person lives is another factor that can lead to an increased incidence of certain health problems. Persons living in the north central United States have a greater tendency to develop problems with the thyroid gland. Individuals living in the Sun Belt have a higher incidence of skin cancer. Those who live around large bodies of water (areas of high humidity) have a greater incidence of sinusitis.

CULTURE

Each culture defines health and illness in a manner that reflects its previous experience. *Culture* is the sum of traditions, practices, beliefs, and values developed by a group of people and passed on, most often by the family, from generation to generation. Cultural factors determine which signs or behaviors are perceived as abnormal. The resulting pattern of behaviors or clinical manifestations is what the culture labels as the illness. Not only does the culture influence the illness behavior, but it determines the method that the individual uses to seek help.

RELIGION

Religion can affect the individual's view of health and illness. Some religious groups regard illness as a form of punishment. The mechanisms that an individual follows to seek health care may also be influenced by religious beliefs.

STANDARD OF LIVING

Socioeconomic status may influence the individual's recognition of illness and may affect the way in which a person responds to illness. For example, individuals of upper socioeconomic status report themselves as ill more often than those of lower socioeconomic status. This difference may be related to easier affordability of health care and greater awareness of methods for receiving help.

The individual's home environment can predispose that person to various health problems. Crowded, cramped living accommodations, where cleanliness and sanitation are substandard, can lead to a higher incidence of disease and illness.

HEALTH BELIEFS AND PRACTICES

Health beliefs are the health-related opinions that the individual holds, whereas health practices are the activities that an individual carries out as a result of personal beliefs. These beliefs and practices can affect health positively or negatively. They may lead the individual to resist entry into the health care delivery system or to reject treatments that are recommended by health care professionals.

PREVIOUS HEALTH EXPERIENCES

Previous experiences of wellness or illness also contribute to the individual's reaction when ill. Persons with limited experience with illness or treatment by health care professionals may be more hesitant to admit illness and to seek treatment. Individuals who have had previous positive interactions with health care team members may be more likely to seek care when a problem first occurs. On the other hand, those who have had negative experiences with illness or health care (e.g., death of a parent or spouse, painful treatments, or unpleasant hospitalizations) may hesitate or refuse to acknowledge the problem or to seek professional care.

SUPPORT SYSTEMS

How an individual responds to illness often depends on what support systems are available, both internal and external. Some individuals cope with stress better than others, as discussed in Chapter 6. Family and significant others are often helpful as external sources of support. If these sources are not available, the person may have more difficulty adapting to the health disruption.

ASSESSMENT OF THE ILLNESS EXPERIENCE

The process of defining oneself as ill is based on the individual's perception, the perceptions of others, or both. Each person reacts differently to illness. When assessing the illness experience, the nurse considers the type of illness and the changes that may take place in the individual and the family when illness occurs.

TYPES OF ILLNESS

Acute illness usually refers to an illness or disease that has a relatively rapid onset and short duration. The condition responds to a specific treatment and is self-limiting. If no complications occur, most acute illnesses end in a full recovery, and the individual returns to the previous level of functioning.

Chronic illness is a term used to describe illnesses that include one or more of the following characteristics: permanent impairments or deviations, residual physical or cognitive disability, nonreversible pathologic changes, special rehabilitation, and long-term medical and/or nursing management. Chronic illnesses may fluctuate in intensity as acute exacerbations occur that cause physiologic instability requiring additional assistance. Causes and treatments of various chronic illnesses are discussed in greater depth throughout this text.

EFFECTS OF ILLNESS ON THE INDIVIDUAL

SUBJECTIVE CHANGES

Usually, subjective changes occur in an individual that signal the presence of illness. Examples of these changes include

1. Changes in body appearance, e.g., loss of weight, changes in skin color
2. Changes in body function, e.g., urinary frequency, increased pulse rate
3. Unusual body emissions, e.g., blood in urine or stool
4. Changes in the senses, e.g., deafness, loss of vision
5. Uncomfortable physical manifestations, e.g., headache, backache
6. Changes in emotional state, e.g., anxiety, depression
7. Changes in relationships with others, e.g., marital conflicts

Most people experience a mild form of some of these changes in their daily lives. However, when they occur to such a degree that they interfere with usual daily activities, the individual affected is often considered to be ill.

REACTION TO ILLNESS

When an individual recognizes an alteration in function related to illness, the individual's reaction to the illness may vary. Some persons seek action immediately, whereas others take no action; still others seek counter-action.

Taking Action

When an individual responds to illness by taking action, there are three overlapping sectors of health care from which to choose. The *popular sector* involves a layperson or a nonprofessional. This source of help is usually the first one sought when illness is recognized and health care activities are initiated. The health care results from self-treatment or self-medication; advice from relatives, friends, coworkers, or neighbors; activities within a church or self-help group; or consultation with another layperson who has had a similar type of problem. The main source of primary health care in most societies is the family, and therefore the family is often first consulted for assistance when illness occurs.

In some areas of the United States and in non-Western societies, another frequently used source of advice regarding health care issues is the *folk sector*, in which certain individuals specialize in forms of healing. There is a wide variation in types of folk healers, who may include herbalists, spiritual healers, and clairvoyants. Folk healers are not part of the medical system and occupy a position between the popular and professional sectors.

The third source of help that an individual can choose when seeking health care is the *professional sector*. This group includes legally licensed health professionals such as nurses, physicians, midwives, and physical therapists.

The actions sought by the person experiencing illness are influenced by several factors: availability of health care, affordability of health care, failure or success of self-prescribed treatment, the client's perception of the problem, and others' perceptions of the problem.

Availability of health care.   If the individual lives in an area with limited health care resources, the promptness with which actions are taken may be affected.

Affordability of health care.   Persons with medical insurance or adequate finances are more likely than uninsured or poorer individuals to seek health care when illness first occurs. Those with limited budgets may view health care as a less important need and either take no action or rely on self-treatment or family assistance.

Failure or success of self-prescribed treatment.   The results of self-treatment may negate the need for further professional help. However, when the problem persists despite self-care, the individual is prompted to seek outside assistance for treatment of the illness.

Client's perception of the problem.   Probably one of the greatest influences on the action of the person in seeking help is the client's perception of the situation. Clients who do not view themselves as ill are not motivated to seek health care from any source. The severity of the illness as perceived by the client may affect the source of help that is sought and the speed with which action is taken.

Others' perceptions of the problem.   The manner in which persons around the client such as the family or significant others view the problem also affects the action taken by the client. Agreement with the existence of a problem and the degree of severity may influence the actions taken by the individual to seek help.

Taking No Action

Taking no action is a response to illness. Some individuals prefer to "wait and see" whether the symptoms abate before deciding to take action. Others deny the significance of the symptoms or are unwilling to admit that they are ill. Many of the variables that influence individuals to seek action when illness occurs cause others to take no action. Unavailability of health care resources, unaffordability of health care, misperception or failure to recognize the illness, and fear are some of the major reasons that persons fail to take action.

Taking Counteraction

Some individuals respond to illness by taking counteraction. They engage in certain activities in an attempt to disprove the existence of symptoms. For example, a man with chest pain may increase his activities and workload to prove that he is not having a problem with his heart. Counteraction is an extreme form of denial and reflects deviant illness behavior. The person wants to believe that he or she is healthy when actively ill. Because the person is not open to seeking help, the condition may worsen and death may occur.

THE SICK ROLE

The concept of the *sick role* was first formulated by Talcott Parsons (1951) after he observed similar behavior patterns — regardless of the cause of the illness — in clients who were ill. People who are defined as ill are temporarily able to avoid their obligations to social groups such as the family, friends, or coworkers. These groups often feel a responsibility to care for their sick members. Therefore, the sick role provides an opportunity to withdraw from adult responsibilities and serves as a basis of eligibility for care by others. The sick role is assumed by people when they accept their illness. Although this description does not apply to every client, four aspects are typical in clients who are ill:

1. Exemption from normal social role responsibilities. This varies depending on the nature and severity of the illness. Exemption is a *right* of the sick. However, to prevent abuse of this right, society requires that this right be legitimized by others. The physician is usually the legitimizer.
2. Recognition that the sick person is not responsible for causing the condition. He or she cannot get well on his or her own accord; the individual has a condition that requires care.
3. Expectation that the state of being ill is undesirable and the client should want to get well as quickly as possible. The client should show some motivation to get well.
4. Obligation to seek competent help. The client or family must seek professional help and cooperate with health care professionals.

The sick role does not apply to all illnesses. Individuals with minor illnesses such as a cold are usually not exempted from normal social roles such as going to work or attending classes. Sick role expectations are different in clients with incurable illnesses.

STAGES OF ILLNESS

Most individuals with acute illness follow a specific sequence of behavior patterns from the onset of illness until recovery. In the stages of acute illness, behaviors seen during illness are combined with sick role behavior. Several theorists have identified a number of stages, but Suchman's (1972) classification, described as follows, is well accepted.

Experience of Symptoms

The first stage of illness involves the experience of symptoms. During this stage, there are three common occurrences: (1) physical experience of symptoms such as pain, shortness of breath, or fever; (2) cognitive awareness, that is, symptoms are interpreted in terms that have meaning; and (3) emotional response of fear or anxiety. Initially the person may deny the symptoms and continue to function as though feeling "normal." If the symptoms subside with no action, the client returns to an optimal level of wellness. Self-treatment or over-the-counter medications may cause the illness to subside. If the symptoms persist despite self-treatment, the individual moves to the next stage. If symptoms such as pain or fever are present, professional care is usually sought more rapidly than when the symptoms are mild. During this stage, people try to validate their feelings with family members or significant others in an attempt to prove that their symptoms are real.

Assumption of Sick Role

This stage of illness is referred to as the acceptance stage. The person views the problem as sufficiently severe to confirm the illness. Family, friends, and peers validate the illness, and normal duties and responsibilities are relinquished. As the sick role is assumed, a preoccupation with symptoms and other body functions occurs. The person's attention becomes inner directed, and thoughts and conversations focus on minor complaints such as variations in pulse and temperature.

At the end of this stage, there are two possible outcomes for the individual. The symptoms may change, the person feels better, and he or she no longer considers himself or herself sick. Or, symptoms may persist, and with encouragement from the family or significant others, the individual seeks professional help.

Health Care Contact

Although some individuals do not seek professional health care, most individuals do seek care in an attempt to legitimize their continuation in the sick role. They contact a physician or nurse practitioner for the diagnosis, treatment, and prognosis of their illness. If the illness is validated, they continue in the sick role. If it is not, they return to a normal role or continue seeking health care to validate the illness.

Dependent Role

When the person accepts the diagnosis and treatment plan of the health professional, he or she enters the stage of dependency. If the condition is acute, the physiologic effects of the illness decrease the energy available for independent function. Thus, the person regresses to a state of dependency. The more severe the illness, the greater the dependency of the individual. Some individuals are reluctant to assume a dependent role because it is viewed as undesirable. People vary in the ease with which they give up their independence and enter the sick role. Most persons generally accept this role of dependence on the health care professional but try to retain some control over their lives. During this time, individuals become more passive and concerned about themselves. Regressive behavior to an earlier stage in development is not uncommon.

Recovery and Rehabilitation

Although some clients may die if treatments are not successful, most people move to the final stage of recovery or rehabilitation. Although this stage begins in the hospital, it usually continues in the home. During this time, the individual gives up the sick role and resumes normal activities and responsibilities. If the illness was acute, the recovery or rehabilitation period is usually short. Individuals who have long-term illnesses may take a longer time to adjust to new life styles.

EFFECTS OF ILLNESS ON THE FAMILY

The presence of illness in a family can have dramatic effects on the function of the family as a unit. The type of effect depends on three factors: (1) which member of the family is ill, (2) the seriousness and duration of the illness, and (3) the social and cultural customs of the family. Each member of the family has a different role and performs tasks specific to that role. The type of role changes that occur vary depending on the family member affected. For instance, when the affected family member is the husband who has been the sole source of financial support, the wife or children may need to seek employment to supplement the family income. Major role adjustments are made as the man assumes a dependent role and the woman adapts to a job other than homemaker. When illness affects a woman who has normally been the person caring for the home and children, role changes also occur. The man may take on responsibilities of home care as well as those of outside employment. The woman may have a difficult time adjusting to a dependent role and feel guilty about her inability to function.

When the sick person is an elderly member of the family, the child is often forced to assume parental functions for the parent. As the population in the United States gets older, many young and middle-aged persons will be caring for their children while caring for their parents. This "sandwich generation" may experience compromised health as a result of excessive caregiver responsibilities. The elderly ill person may have dependency needs related to housing, meals, and assistance with activities of daily living. The added responsibilities on the adult child can cause conflict with personal or other role expectations. Awareness and verbalization by family members of feelings regarding role changes are important. Frustrations may occur that are destructive to effective family function.

Economic impact related to the loss of a job and the high costs of medical care and hospitalization has a significant effect on family members. A person's future ability to work and earn income may be affected, depending on the nature of the illness. Lack of medical insurance is devastating when people try to cope with expensive medical bills.

PREVENTION OF ILLNESS

In an effort to decrease the occurrence of illness, prevention is essential. Preventive health behavior is described as voluntary action taken by an individual or group to decrease the potential or actual threat of illness and its harmful consequences. Three levels of prevention are delineated in Table 1–1.

PRIMARY PREVENTION

Primary prevention is used to prevent or delay the actual occurrence of a specific disease. Strategies for health maintenance raise the general level of health and well-being of an individual, family, or community. Smoking cessation clinics, immunizations, use of seat belts, and use of helmets by motorcyclists are examples of primary prevention strategies.

SECONDARY PREVENTION

Secondary prevention begins after a disease or condition is present, although the clinical manifestations may not be evident. Intervention may lessen the complications and disability resulting from the disease. Emphasis is on early diagnosis and treatment as well as on intervention to prevent or limit permanent disability or death. Screening procedures such as the Papanicolaou smear for cervical cancer and skin tests for tuberculosis are examples. The purpose is to detect disease early and use preventive measures to avoid further complications, which occur when the disease progresses beyond the early stages.

TABLE 1–1   Behaviors Involved in the Three Levels of Illness Prevention

Level	Examples of Behaviors
Primary prevention	Wearing seat belts, helmets Eating well-balanced meals No smoking Consuming no or minimal alcohol Being immunized Maintaining ideal body weight
Secondary prevention	Having yearly Papanicolaou's smear tests Doing monthly breast and testicular self-examinations Having mammograms as recommended Getting skin test or chest x-ray for tuberculosis screening Having tonometry tests to detect glaucoma
Tertiary prevention	Following cardiac rehabilitation program Pursuing rehabilitation programs for stroke, head injury

TERTIARY PREVENTION

Tertiary prevention involves rehabilitation and begins when the disease or condition has stabilized and no further healing is expected. The goal is to return the person to the highest level of function and to prevent severe disabilities from occurring.

HEALTH PROMOTION AND MAINTENANCE

Health promotion refers to activities that are directed toward developing an individual's resources to maintain or enhance well-being as a protection against illness. Health maintenance and disease prevention are part of health promotion. Prevention involves guarding or protecting the body from a particular disease process.

Treatment of illness has often been viewed as threatening and has had negative connotations of discomfort or loss of control. Anticipation of negative consequences can result in avoidance of health care services, even when they are essential for continuing high-level wellness. Reversing the emphasis from curing the disease to promoting health provides a more positive orientation

for health care. Illness no longer needs to be the primary focus of health care relationships. Active involvement and expectations of participation by the individual have facilitated pursuit rather than avoidance of health services. Part of this new approach is reflected in the use of the term client rather than patient. Although the word *patient* is associated with a dependent position, the *client* is viewed as an active partner in the process of health care delivery and maintenance. Client is therefore the term used for the health care consumer in this text.

PRACTICES TO PROMOTE HEALTH

As more emphasis is placed on promoting health, certain health practices, which can be encouraged in individuals, have been found to have a positive correlation with high-level wellness. Some of these general health practices follow:

1. Eating three meals a day that are balanced and include foods from the four basic food groups. There should be minimal or no snacking between meals.
2. Moderate eating to maintain ideal weight and prevent obesity.
3. Moderate exercising on a routine schedule.
4. Sleeping regularly about 7 to 8 hours each day.
5. Limiting consumption of alcohol to a moderate amount.
6. No smoking.
7. Keeping exposure to the sun to a minimum.

The association of these practices with high-level wellness has been found to exist whatever the sex, age, or economic status of an individual. The greater the number of these practices followed in a consistent, routine manner, the better the health status.

As a result of some of the studies in the area of holistic health, other recommendations are suggested as effective in bringing an individual into better harmony with the environment. Health-promoting measures that are suggested by holistic health care providers include interventions such as biofeedback, therapeutic touch, imagery, massage, and meditation. These practices are described in more detail in the chapters on pain and stress.

CONSUMER EDUCATION AND AWARENESS

Consumer education and awareness have been the major focus in an attempt to influence individuals and promote wellness. Information regarding nutrition, exercise, stress management, and routine health examinations is available at schools, work sites, and community centers and in newspapers and on communication channels on radio and television. This proliferation of information and materials is a major resource for increasing public awareness of the need for health promotion.

SUMMARY

Many definitions of health exist. Although there is no universal definition of health, theorists agree that health is a dynamic process that involves the biopsychosocial aspects of the person and affects the person's ability to function within the environment. Important goals of nursing are to assess the client's health status and to develop plans to help the person achieve an optimal level of wellness. The nurse must be aware of the variables that affect the client's state of health and must explore the effects of illness on the individual as well as on the family. As more knowledge regarding factors that cause illness accumulates, increased efforts are being placed on the prevention of illness and on the promotion and maintenance of health. Chapter 4 discusses health trends and settings in which nurses function to promote health.

IMPLICATIONS FOR RESEARCH

The field of health promotion is an area in which research is actively conducted. With the escalating costs of health care delivery, much effort is placed on determining effective practices to promote a high level of wellness and to reduce the incidence of illness. Some of the current research addresses health risks such as smoking, obesity, and stress and their effects on cardiovascular disease. Nursing needs to continue research in this area. Some questions for future research are

1. Are biofeedback and therapeutic touch effective mechanisms to reduce stress and enhance wellness?
2. What additional factors can be identified as threats to an individual's health status?
3. How do health promotion interventions reduce the cost of health care delivery services?
4. How can individuals be motivated to seek primary prevention?

REFERENCES AND READINGS

Arluke, A., Kennedy, L., & Kersler, R. (1979). Re-examining the sick role concept: An empirical assessment. *Journal of Health and Social Behavior, 20,* 30.

Bergsma, J., & Thomasma, D. (1982). *Health care: Its psychosocial dimensions.* Duquesne: Duquesne University Press.

Brill, E., & Kilts, D. (1980). *Foundations for nursing.* New York: Appleton-Century-Crofts.

Dixon, J., & Dixon, J. (1984). An evolutionary based model of health and viability. *Advances in Nursing Science, 6,* 1–18.

Dunn, H. (1959). High-level wellness for man and society. *American Journal of Public Health, 49,* 786–792.

Flynn, J., & Giffin, P. (1984). Health promotion in acute care settings. *Nursing Clinics of North America, 19,* 239–250.

Fritz, W. (1984). Maintaining wellness: Yours and theirs. *Nursing Clinics of North America, 19,* 263–270.

Grasser, C., & Craft, B. (1984). The patient's approach to wellness. *Nursing Clinics of North America, 19,* 207–218.

Heckheimer, E. F. (1989). *Health promotion of the aged in the community.* Philadelphia: W. B. Saunders.

Helman, C. (1985). *Culture, health and illness.* Littleton, MA: PSG Publishing Co.

Igun, U. A. (1979). Stages in health-seeking: A descriptive model. *Social Science and Medicine, 13A,* 445–456.

Kee, C. (1984). A case for health promotion with the elderly. *Nursing Clinics of North America, 19,* 251–262.

Kozier, B., & Erb, G. (1987). *Fundamentals of nursing.* Menlo Park, CA: Addison-Wesley.

Leigh, H., & Reiser, M. (1985). *The patient: Biological, psychological, and social dimensions of medical practice* (2nd ed.). New York: Plenum.

Matteson, M. A., & McConnell, E. S. (1988). *Gerontological nursing: Concepts and practice.* Philadelphia: W. B. Saunders.

Moore, P., & Williamson, G. (1984). Health promotion: Evolution of a concept. *Nursing Clinics of North America, 19,* 195–206.

Parsons, T. (1951). *The social system.* New York: Free Press.

Pender, N. (1975). A conceptual model for preventive health behavior. *Nursing Outlook, 23,* 386.

Pender, N. (1987). *Health promotion in nursing.* Norwalk, CT: Appleton & Lange.

Schultz, C. (1984). Lifestyle assessment: A tool for practice. *Nursing Clinics of North America, 19,* 271–281.

Selye, H. (1976). *The stress of life* (rev. ed.). New York: McGraw-Hill.

Suchman, E. A. (1972). Stages of illness and medical care. In E. G. Jaco (Ed.), *Patients, physicians, and illness.* New York: Free Press.

Wolff, H. (1968). *Stress and disease* (2nd ed.). Springfield, IL: Charles C Thomas.

World Health Organization. (1947). *Constitution of the World Health Organization: Chronicle of the World Health Organization.* Geneva: Author.

Wu, R. (1973). *Behavior and illness.* Englewood Cliffs, NJ: Prentice-Hall.

CHAPTER 2

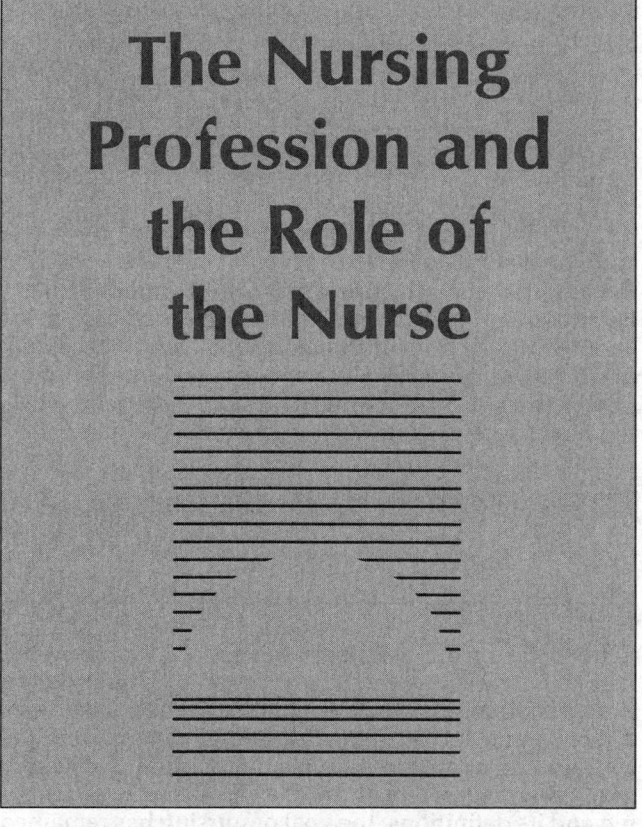

The Nursing Profession and the Role of the Nurse

Nursing today is a fast-changing profession that is influenced by increased knowledge about causes of diseases, rapid advances in science and technology, increased public awareness, and lengthening of the life span. Nursing is vital to health care and is the largest segment of the total health care delivery system. As changes occur constantly in the health field, nurses continue the processes of defining and describing their role in society and of defining their activities as a discipline and as an evolving profession.

DEFINITIONS OF NURSING

Definitions of nursing have been evolving since the time of Florence Nightingale. The question of "What is nursing?" is one that has continued to be difficult to answer. Definitions have been developed, analyzed, and reworked, but still there is controversy among nurses as to which one should be universally accepted for the profession.

Several factors contribute to the difficulty in stating a definition of nursing. First, it is hard to develop one acceptable definition because the purpose for the definition varies. Defining nursing to communicate what nursing is to other professionals requires a different emphasis from defining nursing to identify the legal scope of practice. Personal beliefs vary from one individual to another and thus affect definitions of nursing.

Another obstacle to defining nursing is the debate about the various educational levels of individuals currently entering the field. Today there are four levels: registered nurses with an associate degree, diploma, or baccalaureate degree; and licensed practical or vocational nurses with 1 to 2 years of basic educational preparation. The American Nurses' Association (ANA) recognizes only registered nursing practice and has proposed, along with several other nursing organizations, that the baccalaureate degree be the basic preparation for entry into professional nursing practice. It is thought by many nursing leaders that this controversy among nurses and nurse educators has prevented the profession from moving forward to define nursing.

Last, one definition of nursing is difficult to develop because the role of nurses is changing as technology, health consumers, and government influence its practice. Extended and expanded roles of the nurse are used by insurers, industry, and government. Independent practitioners such as nurse practitioners are employed in clinics, physicians' offices, and health maintenance organizations.

LEGAL DEFINITION

Nursing had no legal definition until the 1930s. The early laws did not define nursing; instead they included descriptions of the nurse. In the 1930s, the state nurse practice acts began to define nursing by focusing on the scope of nursing practice. Each state has a practice act that legally defines nursing at each level, as well as the scope of nursing practice; there are minor differences among the various states.

PROFESSIONAL DEFINITION

Although nursing is defined legally by means of legislation at the state level, professional organizations are also involved in developing a definition of nursing. In 1973, the ANA defined nursing in *Standards of Nursing Practice*. Nursing was defined as a "direct service, goal directed and adaptable to the needs of the individual, family and community during health and illness" (ANA, 1973, p. 2). The ANA published this definition of nursing in its Social Policy Statement of 1980: "Nursing is the diagnosis and treatment of human responses to actual or potential health problems" (ANA, 1980, p. 9).

TABLE 2–1 Theoretical Definitions of Nursing

Nurse Theorist (Date)	Definition
Peplau (1952)	Nursing is a significant, therapeutic, interpersonal process. It functions cooperatively with other human processes that make health possible for individuals.
Henderson (1960)	The unique function of the nurse is to assist clients, sick or well, in the performance of those activities contributing to health, recovery, or peaceful death.
King (1971)	Nursing is an interpersonal process of action, reaction, interaction, and transaction whereby nurse and client share information about their perceptions in the nursing situation.
Roy (1976)	As a science, nursing is a developing system of knowledge about human beings used to observe, classify, and relate the processes by which persons positively affect their health status.

THEORISTS' DEFINITIONS

Throughout nursing's history, definitions by theorists have evolved. Early definitions did not state what nursing was but provided a description of the nurse and nursing functions. A list of some prominent nursing leaders, along with the major points of their definitions, is given in Table 2–1. The changing definitions reveal that nursing is progressing from the traditional view of caring for ill individuals to a process-oriented, goal-directed service that cares for ill individuals, families, and communities and that promotes health maintenance and prevention of illness.

In addition to a definition of nursing, many nurse theorists have developed conceptual models to describe the unique role of nursing compared with that of other health care professionals. Because there is no consensus about which, if any, of the models should be accepted, this text does not embrace a specific model for application. Rather, a well-known and accepted framework, the nursing process, is used to organize the material.

GOAL OF NURSING

Differences in the definitions reflect philosophical beliefs about humans, health, and society. Most definitions of nursing also include goal statements. Goals give direction and focus to nursing care by determining the roles and functions of the nurse. Throughout the history of nursing, regardless of the changes occurring in nursing and its definitions, the goal of nursing has remained constant—promotion, maintenance, and restoration of health, with humans considered to be holistic beings.

ROLES OF THE NURSE

As professional nursing adapts to meet changing health needs, the expectations for providing client care have expanded and increased. Nurses assume various roles within the health care setting, as summarized in Figure 2–1. Although each role has specific responsibilities, some aspects of each role are interrelated and are common to all nursing positions. In assuming the following roles, theory and research are used as a basis to enhance nursing practice.

CAREGIVER

The role most commonly associated with the nurse is caregiver. In this role, nurses assess clients, analyze collected information to determine client needs, develop

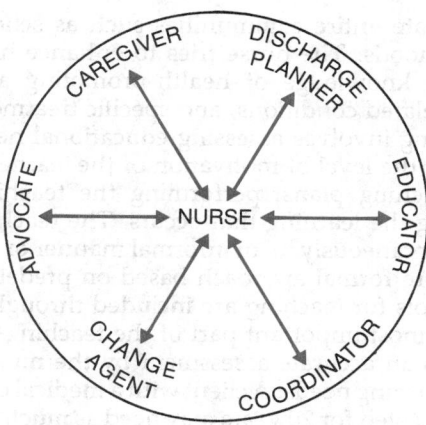

Figure 2–1

Major roles of the professional nurse.

nursing diagnoses, plan appropriate nursing care and carry out the plan, and evaluate the impact of nursing care given. This process, which is referred to as the nursing process, is described in detail in Chapter 3.

As a caregiver, the nurse provides physical care through psychomotor skills such as taking a thermometer reading, changing dressings, or administering medications (Fig. 2–2). Psychosocial interventions are also provided as the nurse encourages verbalization of the client's concerns or offers measures to allay a client's anxiety.

The functions performed by the caregiver are sometimes categorized as interdependent, or collaborative, and independent. *Interdependent* functions include those mutually determined by the nurse and the physician, e.g., activity limitations, and those directed by the physician but requiring nursing judgment to perform, e.g., administration of medication. *Independent* func-

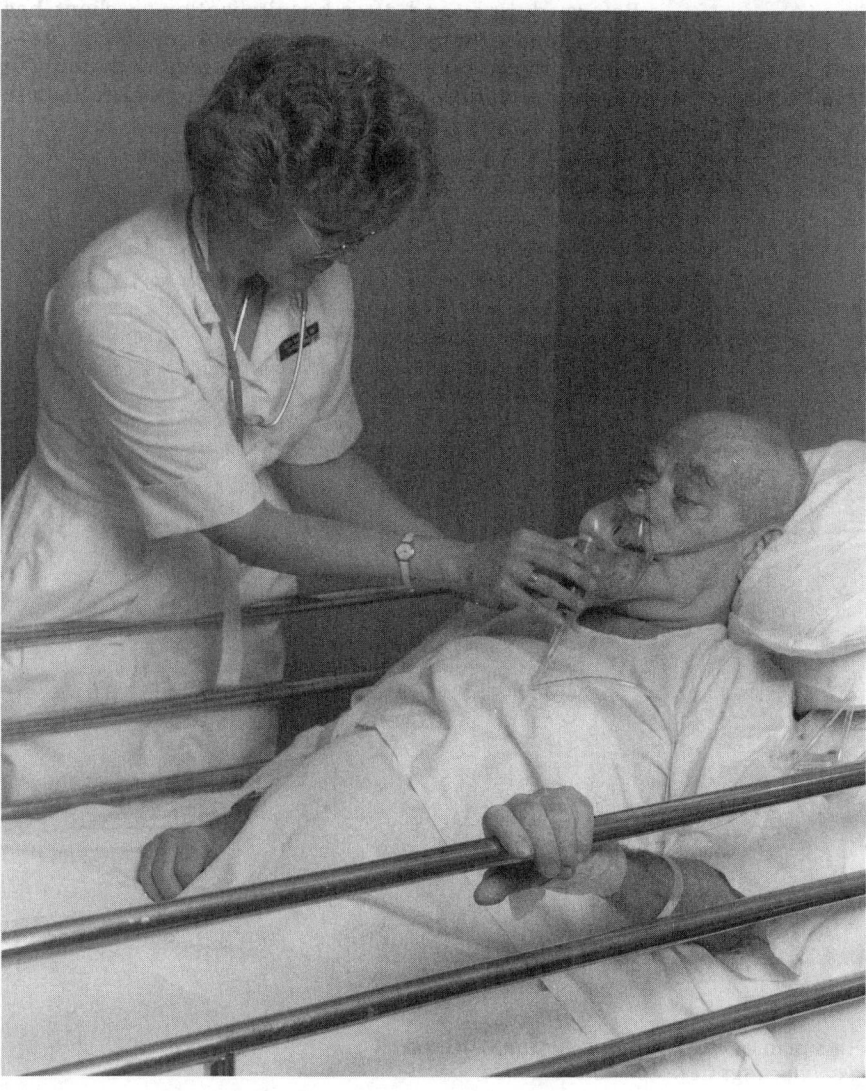

Figure 2–2

The nurse as a caregiver, monitoring client's oxygen and respiratory status. (From Matteson, M. A., & McConnell, E. S. [1988]. *Gerontological nursing: Concepts and practice.* Philadelphia: W. B. Saunders.)

tions are those initiated and carried out by the nurse without direction from another health care professional, e.g., weighing a client, listening to bowel sounds, and testing a urine specimen for glucose.

DISCHARGE PLANNER

As the focus of health care emphasizes early discharge from the acute setting to the home, the role of the nurse as discharge planner is becoming increasingly important. Discharge planning involves assessment of the client's health needs at the time of discharge, assessment of the home situation or other setting to which the client is discharged, and assessment of the resources available to the client, such as family support and equipment. Throughout this text a special section is included on discharge planning to offer guidance to the nurse while fulfilling this role.

CLIENT EDUCATOR

As educators, nurses work with individual clients as well as with family members. Community health nurses also educate entire communities such as schools and neighborhoods. The nurse tries to enhance health by providing knowledge of health-promoting activities, disease-related conditions, and specific treatments.

Teaching involves assessing educational needs, determining the level of motivation of the learner, developing teaching plans, performing the teaching, and evaluating the learning that occurs. The teaching may occur spontaneously in an informal manner or may follow a more formal approach based on predetermined plans. Tools for teaching are included throughout this text. The most important part of the teaching-learning process is an accurate assessment by the nurse of the client's learning needs. A client with a medical condition that has existed for 20 years may need as much teaching as one who is newly diagnosed. The nurse makes no assumptions but rather assesses each client individually for specific needs.

CLIENT ADVOCATE

Before, during, and after hospitalization, a client has contact with many health care team members. As a client advocate, the nurse assists the client and family in the interpretation of information from other health care

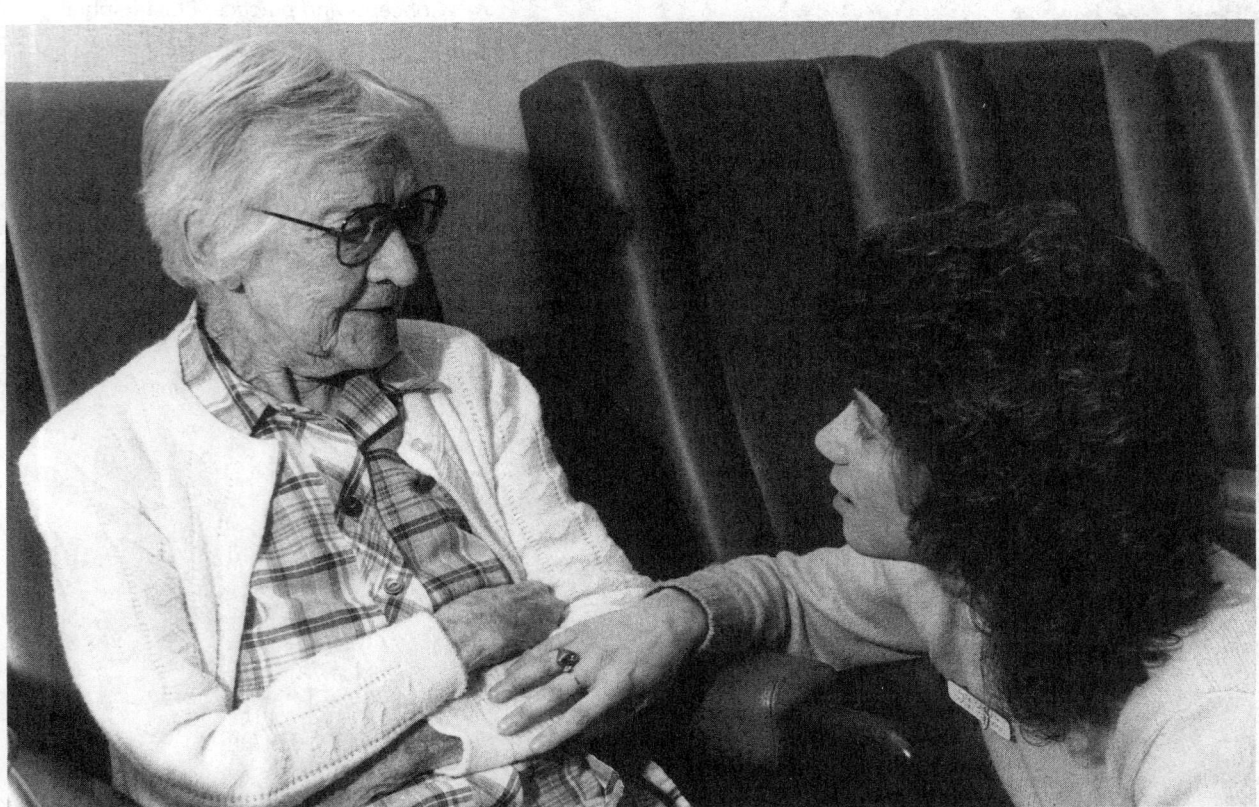

Figure 2–3
The nurse as an advocate, discussing the client's plan of care with her. (From Matteson, M. A., & McConnell, E. S. [1988]. *Gerontological nursing: Concepts and practice.* Philadelphia: W. B. Saunders.)

providers and offers additional information needed by the client to make decisions regarding health care. This assistance may include explanations about the implications of client decisions regarding health, and ensuring that clients receive adequate and appropriate care (Fig. 2–3).

COORDINATOR

Care is provided to clients by a variety of health care team members. Although the physician is usually considered to be the head of the health care team, the nurse serves an important role in coordinating the efforts of all team members in meeting the client's goals. Nurses often conduct team conferences to facilitate communication among members of the team, evaluate the services given, and plan for continued care. Management skills are used in this role to ensure the proper functioning and coordination of activities. In fact, in some health care facilities, nurses are the case managers for a group of clients from admission to discharge. Innovative nursing practice models are described in Chapter 4.

CHANGE AGENT

The professional nurse serves as a change agent within the work setting and within the profession. In the work setting the nurse assesses the client and family to identify behaviors that need altering. The role of a change agent involves planning and implementing a systematic modification in the client's health-related behaviors. The most important factor in this process is to assess the client's readiness to change. If the client is not ready, he or she will not comply with the change and the nurse will be ineffective in this role.

Within the community, nurses serve as role models and assist citizens in bringing about changes to improve the environment, work conditions, or other factors that impinge on health. Nurses work diligently to bring about change through legislation. For example, by becoming politically active, nurses provide a major thrust in supporting bills that can affect an individual's health status, such as mandatory seat belt laws. Chapter 4 discusses in detail the nurse's role in the legislative and political process.

PRACTICE SETTINGS FOR THE NURSE

Historically, nurses practiced in the homes of clients. Hospitals were seen as places to go if family members were unable to provide care or if the client was expected to die. As medical care became more organized and institutionalized, nurses began to work more in hospitals. Today, nurses have opportunities to provide health care in a variety of settings.

Hospitals are the largest employer of nurses; approximately two-thirds of all nurses work within hospitals. In this setting, the nurse collaborates with other health care providers in all phases of client care. Because of the different specialty areas within this type of institution, there are various nursing opportunities, and nurses can select the type of nursing practice that they prefer.

Critical care units are areas for intense, critically ill clients. This situation requires a nurse who thrives on crisis situations, works effectively under stress, and can care for a succession of seriously ill clients in a sensitive manner. This nurse is highly skilled in making accurate observations of clients' conditions and interprets findings correctly. The nurse-to-client ratio is typically 1 : 1 or 1 : 2.

Intermediate care units have clients who require fewer highly technical procedures. Many clients begin ambulation and by the time of discharge can perform activities of daily living with little assistance from nursing personnel. The nurse in these areas must be able to adapt to various types of illness and must be interested in health teaching and discharge planning. Medical-surgical units are typical intermediate care areas.

Long-term care (LTC) units are areas within the hospital in which clients have chronic illnesses or short-term problems requiring rehabilitation. Some clients can learn how to help themselves, whereas others are at their optimal level of wellness, which must be maintained.

The second largest practice setting for nurses is the LTC facility, or *nursing home.* Approximately 8% of nurses work in these settings. These health facilities provide long-term nursing care to clients predominantly older than age 65 years. With the increasing interest in gerontological nursing and the escalating number of clients who are elderly or chronically ill, nurses are turning to this challenge as an alternative to nursing practice in a hospital. The primary advantage of LTC nursing is the independence to make nursing decisions about client care.

Community health agencies are the third largest practice setting for nurses and employ about 6.5% of nurses. Programs offered in this setting are vast and include family planning, drug and alcohol abuse centers, mental illness care, diagnostic and preventive care, and home nursing care. The responsibility and influence of the nurse in this setting are considerable. The current trend is a movement from traditional settings to community agencies. With the increased emphasis on health and maintaining health, the number of community agencies is growing, and more nurses will be employed in these settings. The early discharge of clients from an acute setting to the home will lead to a greater need for nurses in the area of home health.

Although the three settings discussed represent the largest settings for employment, other practice settings exist. Some of these include physicians' offices, schools of nursing, student health services, occupational health, private duty practice, and self-employment. Chapter 4 describes health care settings in further detail.

PROFESSIONAL DEVELOPMENT

A critical element related to nursing as a profession is that it has its own special body of knowledge on which its skills and services are based. Nursing continually expands this body of knowledge through education, professional association activities, and research.

EDUCATION

Ongoing education in nursing is critical because of innovations occurring in the fields of science and technology. Nurses have a responsibility to expand their knowledge, update their skills, and remain aware of current changes in the health field. Workshops, seminars, and in-service programs within institutional settings are a few of the means by which nurses can continue their education. Professional journals, programmed education texts, and correspondence courses are methods by which the nurse can obtain additional knowledge within a home setting.

Formal education programs designed for registered nurses who wish to pursue a baccalaureate degree in nursing or to continue their education through graduate courses at the master's and doctoral levels are becoming more readily available. Nurses wishing to specialize in particular areas of nursing may elect to take courses in specialties such as gerontology, trauma medicine, or cardiac nursing; nurses may also become certified in these areas by the ANA or nursing specialty organizations.

PROFESSIONAL ORGANIZATIONS

While nursing was developing as a profession, organizations were formed to establish and control policies and activities of nursing practice and to ensure maintenance of professional criteria.

AMERICAN NURSES' ASSOCIATION

The ANA is the professional organization of nursing. It was founded in 1896, and its purposes are to foster high standards of nursing practice, promote professional and educational advancement of nursing, and promote the welfare of nurses to lead to better delivery of nursing care. The ANA is the official nursing organization for the entire nursing profession.

NATIONAL LEAGUE FOR NURSING

The National League for Nursing (NLN) is another organization that was formed to assist in maintaining the purposes and goals of professional nursing within the broader perspectives of health care. The membership of the NLN includes nurses, other health professionals, and laypersons from the community. Organized in 1952, the NLN promotes the improvement of nursing service and nursing education. One of its major services is the accreditation of nursing schools to ensure high standards. It also accredits community health agencies.

NATIONAL STUDENT NURSES' ASSOCIATION

The National Student Nurses' Association (NSNA) was established in 1952 with the help of the ANA to promote professional development for nursing students and to direct participation by students in the development of nursing. It has encouraged students to become interested in and aware of current issues and trends in nursing. Membership in this organization prepares the individual for membership in professional nursing organizations.

OTHER SPECIALTY ORGANIZATIONS

Organizations have proliferated to promote specific areas such as practice, education, and administration. More than 100 specialty groups offer continuing education, publications, and interactions among nurses to keep them informed of new advancements and techniques within their areas. Some of the larger specialty groups include the American Association of Critical-Care Nurses (AACN), the Association of Operating Room Nurses (AORN), and the National Association of Orthopaedic Nurses (NAON). Information on specialty organizations is found at the end of each unit of this text under the heading Nursing Resources.

RESEARCH

The primary tasks of nursing research are to promote the growth of the science of nursing and to develop nursing theories that will serve as a scientific basis for nursing practice. Each nurse has a responsibility to become involved in nursing research. Although all nurses do not have adequate preparation in research methodology, each nurse can participate by remaining alert for nursing problems and asking questions about the practice of care. Nurses who give direct care often identify such problems, which serve as a basis for research investigation. Nurses can promote nursing care by incorporating research findings into their practice and by communicating the research to others. If studies are not shared with the nursing profession through publication, for example, the impact on professional development and the resulting effects on nursing practice are greatly hampered.

MEDICAL-SURGICAL NURSING

There are numerous specialties within the nursing profession. Throughout this text, the roles and responsibilities of the medical-surgical nurse are explored. The nurse who specializes in medical-surgical nursing may be found in any of the settings described and assumes all of the roles discussed. The focus of medical-surgical nursing is on the adult client with an acute or chronic illness. Nurses who specialize in medical-surgical nursing need broad knowledge of the biologic, psychologic, and social sciences because of the range of clients for whom they care. Clients range in age from 18 to older than 100 years, and the problems with which they present are often complex. The goal is the same as that for any other specialty: the achievement of an optimal level of wellness and prevention of illness. Standards of Care for medical-surgical nursing practice have been developed by the ANA and are found in the *Student Study Guide* to accompany *Medical-Surgical Nursing.*

SUMMARY

Although there is no one accepted definition of nursing, commonalities in the definitions exist: nursing is service oriented and goal directed, clients include individuals and groups, and goals are to promote a high level of wellness and to prevent disease. Modern technology, consumer awareness, and changes in the quality and type of health care have placed new demands on the nurse and the nursing profession. The roles assumed by nurses have become more complex. New specialized units and services have emerged that require the development of new skills, definitions of practice, and delineation of professional accountability. An examination of the definitions, roles, settings, and need for continuous professional development provides a basis for beginning to understand the complexity of nursing practice.

IMPLICATIONS FOR RESEARCH

Nursing is a relatively new profession. Only through continuous research can nursing develop theories and establish a scientific basis for practice. The following questions provide areas for further research in the area:

1. Are current nursing theories valid in clinical settings?
2. Are the ANA Standards of Nursing Practice appropriate in a variety of clinical settings?
3. How does each nursing role affect the care of the medical-surgical client?

REFERENCES AND READINGS

American Nurses' Association. (1973). *Standards of nursing practice.* Kansas City: Author.

American Nurses' Association. (1980). *The nurse practice act: Suggested state legislation.* Kansas City: Author.

American Nurses' Association. (1980). *Nursing: A social policy statement.* Kansas City: Author.

Arnold, E., & Boggs, K. (1989). *Interpersonal relationships: Professional communication skills for nurses.* Philadelphia: W. B. Saunders.

Brill, E., & Kilts, D. (1980). *Foundations for nursing.* New York: Appleton-Century-Crofts.

Castles, M. R. (1987). *Primer of nursing research.* Philadelphia: W. B. Saunders.

Chinn, P. L., & Jacobs, M. K. (1983). *Theory and nursing: A systematic approach.* St. Louis: C. V. Mosby.

DeYoung, L. (1985). *Dynamics of nursing* (5th ed.). St. Louis: C. V. Mosby.

Doheny, M., Cook, C., & Stopper, M. (1982). *The discipline of nursing: An introduction.* Bowie, MD: Robert J. Brady.

Hegyvary, S. (1982). *The change to primary nursing.* St. Louis: C. V. Mosby.

Henderson, V. (1966). *The nature of nursing.* New York: Macmillan.

King, I. (1971). *Toward a theory of nursing.* New York: Wiley.

Marriner, A. (1986). *Nursing theorists and their work.* St. Louis: C. V. Mosby.

Nightingale, F. (1940). *Notes on nursing.* New York: Appleton-Century-Crofts.

Orem, D. (1971). *Nursing: Concepts of practice.* New York: McGraw-Hill.

Peplau, H. (1952). *Interpersonal relations in nursing.* New York: G. P. Putnam's Sons.

Porter-O'Grady, T. (1985). Health versus illness: Nurses can chart the course for the future. *Nursing and Health Care,* 6, 319–321.

Portman, C. (1989, May). Make your patient's family part of the team. *RN,* 23–24.

Redman B. (1980). *The process of patient teaching in nursing* (4th ed.). St. Louis: C. V. Mosby.

Rogers, M. (1970). *An introduction to the theoretical basis of nursing.* Philadelphia: F. A. Davis.

Roper, N., Logan, W., & Tierney, A. (1985). *The elements of nursing* (2nd ed.). New York: Churchill Livingstone.

Roy, C. (1976). *Introduction to nursing: An adaptation model.* Englewood Cliffs, NJ: Prentice-Hall.

Sullivan, E. J., & Decker, P. J. (1985). *Effective management in nursing.* Menlo Park, CA: Addison-Wesley.

Watson, J. (1985). *Nursing: Human science and human care.* Norwalk, CT: Appleton-Century-Crofts.

CHAPTER 3

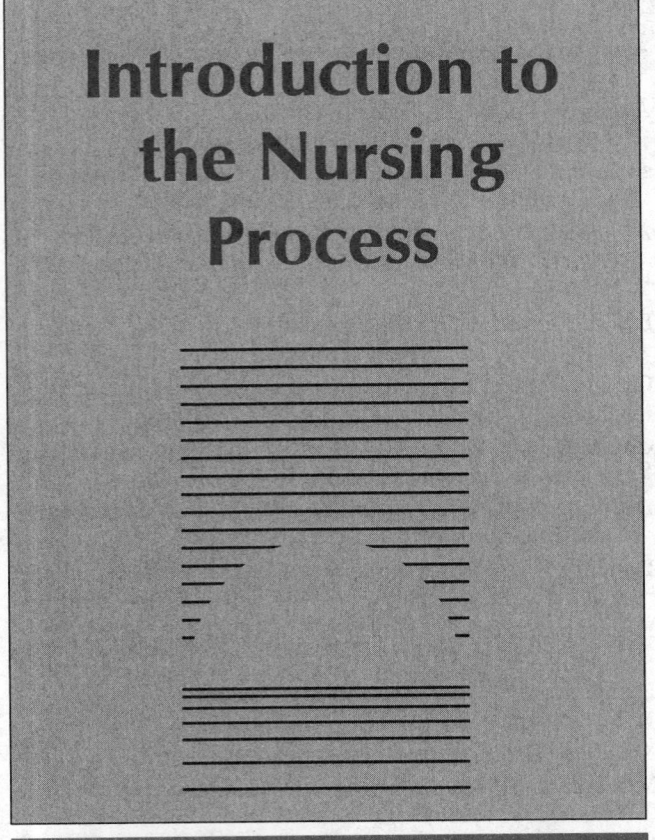

Introduction to the Nursing Process

The nursing process provides the framework for nursing and is therefore used as the organizing framework of this text. It is an organized, comprehensive, and systematic approach used by nurses to meet the health care needs of the client. The process is used to collect information about the client, identify client problems, specify plans for solutions to the problems, implement nursing actions, and evaluate the effectiveness of the actions taken to resolve the identified problems.

The nursing process can be applied in any interaction that involves a nurse and a client. There are no constraints as to who is defined as a participant in the process or where the process occurs. A client can be defined as an individual, family, group, community, or society. The process can take place in a variety of settings, such as a hospital, clinic, school, or home. Use of the nursing process enhances nursing care: individualized care is given, the specific needs are better met, and a higher level of wellness is achieved by the client.

The importance of using the nursing process in daily practice is outlined in professional documents and in legal documents for the profession. For example, state nurse practice acts require the use of each step of the nursing process by registered nurses.

THE NURSING PROCESS—A PROBLEM-SOLVING APPROACH

The term *nursing process* emerged in the mid-1960s. As nursing became more recognized and respected as a profession, there was a growing need for accountability in nursing practice and a need for evaluating the care given. The nursing process is simply a way of thinking; it qualifies the care that nurses provide for their clients. The systematic series of steps of the process have often been compared with the scientific method of solving problems. The steps are similar in the two approaches as they proceed from identification of the problem to evaluation of the solution (Table 3–1).

As the nursing process has evolved, the components have been labeled differently by various nursing leaders. The number of steps, or phases, included in the process has also varied and has ranged from three to five. Four phases were initially identified—assessment, planning, implementation, and evaluation. Today, many nurse clinicians, educators, and researchers have separated the phase of assessment into data collection and problem identification. Although the steps are known by different terms, the process accomplishes the same goals of providing structure for the delivery of nursing care and facilitating the accomplishment of client health goals. For purposes of this text, a five-step approach is followed: assessment (data collection), anal-

Scientific Method	Nursing Process
Step 1. State the problem	Step 1. Assessment: data collection
Step 2. Collect data	Step 2. Analysis: problem identification
Step 3. Formulate hypothesis	Step 3. Planning: setting of goals
Step 4. Test hypothesis	Step 4. Implementation
Step 5. Analyze and evaluate	Step 5. Evaluation

TABLE 3–1   Comparison of Scientific Method and Nursing Process

ysis (problem identification), planning, implementation, and evaluation.

Although the steps of the nursing process are discussed separately, the importance of their interrelatedness must be emphasized. The steps initially are followed in sequence; data collection is performed before problems are identified or plans are made. However, once the nursing process begins, it is continuous or cyclic, as shown in Figure 3–1. More data are obtained, additional problems are determined, and plans are altered on the basis of new findings or evaluation of previously implemented actions. There is no limit to the number of times the cycle recurs. To understand the nursing process as a whole, it is first necessary to analyze each component as a separate entity.

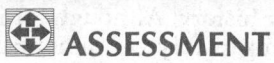 **ASSESSMENT**

Assessment is viewed as a systematic method of collecting data about the client for the purpose of identifying actual and potential problems. Because the data base

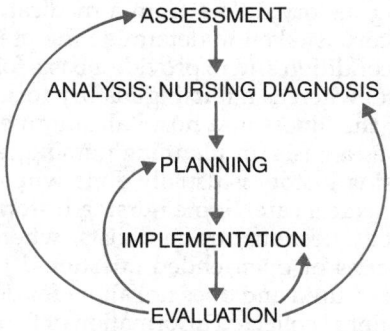

Figure 3–1

The nursing process cycle.

provides the foundation for the remaining phases of the nursing process, an adequate data base is essential. Data collection begins with the first contact made by the nurse with the client, and a baseline set of data is collected, usually within the first 24 hours after initial client contact. During all successive contacts, the nurse continues to collect information relevant to the nursing needs of the client. The additional data are compared with the initial information, or data base, to determine changes in client status.

SUBJECTIVE AND OBJECTIVE DATA

The information collected by the nurse includes both subjective and objective data. Subjective data are not directly observable or measurable by persons other than the person to whom the data relate. Subjective data include the responses, either spontaneous or after specific questions, of the client. Answers by the client to questions such as "What brings you to seek health care?" or "Can you describe your pain?" are subjective data.

Objective data are observable pieces of information about the client that are measurable and are gathered by the nurse or other members of the health team. Objective data include measurements (e.g., vital signs or laboratory findings) and information obtained using the senses (e.g., touch or smell). Feeling the warmth of a foot and observing a foul odor from a wound are also examples of objective data.

COLLECTION OF DATA

As the nurse begins the task of gathering data, three techniques are commonly used: interview, observation, and physical examination.

INTERVIEW

Interviewing is a communication skill by which the nurse can explore the thoughts, feelings, and perceptions of an individual. The nurse's approach to the client and family greatly affects the amount and quality of the information received. Establishing trust is essential to the development of a relationship in which the client feels comfortable about sharing personal data.

An interview should not be a series of routine questions and answers. Rather, it should flow in a natural progression, and cues that the client provides should be used to elicit further information.

Environment

Before the interview begins, the nurse should be aware of the surrounding environment and its effect on the interview. Privacy for the client is essential. If necessary, the nurse may need to adjust the setting to make it more conducive to sharing information. Factors such as lighting, temperature, background noise, and odors can distract the client. Full attention of both client and nurse is essential for an interaction to succeed.

Timing

The timing of the interview should be planned with consideration of the client's physical and emotional state. Clients who are experiencing pain, fatigue, hunger, or anxiety may not be able or willing to share information. Postponement of data collection until the client is more comfortable results in a more positive interaction.

OBSERVATION

The nurse gathers additional data about the client through the highly developed skill of observation. Observation involves the use of the senses of sight, hearing, smell, and touch to elicit additional information. It is an active process with mental and sensory components. To obtain meaningful data, a mental activity occurs that attaches significance to the sensory stimulus that has been perceived.

As the nurse interacts with the client, nonverbal cues as well as verbal responses are identified. General appearance, facial expressions, posture, body gestures, movements, and gait provide additional data to validate findings from the interview. Conflicting nonverbal cues and verbal responses may provide areas for further exploration by the nurse. In addition to physical observations, psychosocial interactions among the family, significant others, and the client and between the client and health team members also provide useful data for identifying problems and planning care.

Knowledge from the physical and social sciences provides a foundation for the nurse's understanding of normal behaviors. Because of this background, the nurse can recognize the significance of abnormal findings and can identify health problems. Although the keen skill of observation is essential to the collection of data, the ability to use all senses and to recognize pertinent data requires practice and experience.

PHYSICAL EXAMINATION

The nurse's qualifications and abilities to perform a physical examination vary depending on background, education, and experience. The manner by which a nurse collects data during a physical examination should be logical and organized. Some nurses perform a head-to-toe examination, whereas other nurses choose a system-by-system approach. Four techniques are usually used to collect data during a physical examination: inspection, palpation, percussion, and auscultation. *Inspection* refers to the visual examination of a client. The observations are performed systematically and focus on

one area of the body at a time. *Palpation* is the use of touch to examine the client's body and to determine characteristics of body structure under the skin. Through palpation, the nurse determines hardness, size, texture, swelling, or mobility of an internal part. *Percussion* involves the tapping of a body surface with a finger or fingers to produce sounds. The sound that results comes from the vibration of the body structures and allows the nurse to determine size, density, organ boundaries, and location. *Auscultation* is the act of listening for sounds produced by organs in the body either directly with the ear or indirectly by use of a stethoscope. It is not the intent of this chapter to teach the techniques of physical examination. For further information regarding specific physical assessment skills, the reader is referred to a textbook on those skills. The assessment chapters of this text provide a systematic review of each body system.

SOURCES OF DATA

The data base consists of specific information obtained about the client. Sources of data are classified as either primary or secondary.

CLIENT

The client is the *primary* source of data. The information provided by the client is direct and firsthand. This information is presented in the *nursing history* format.

The nursing history is the first part of the data base collected from the client. To enhance organization and completeness of data collection, a systematic plan should be used to gather information. Many guidelines and forms have been devised to assist the nurse in obtaining a nursing history. Although formats for the collection of a nursing history vary among institutions, any usable nursing history should identify the client's perception and expectations related to his or her illness, hospitalization, and care. Information such as demographic data, client's understanding of the illness, social and cultural history, usual daily patterns, ability to meet personal needs, and ability to cope with problems should also be included.

A nursing history differs from a medical history. A medical history is taken to determine the presence of a pathologic condition and to provide a basis for planning medical care, whereas a nursing history focuses on the meaning of the illness and hospitalization to the client and family as a basis for planning nursing care.

The nursing history is usually done when the client first seeks medical care. Some nursing histories contain closed-ended questions, or checklists, whereas others include a series of open-ended questions. The former format is structured and does not allow for documentation of additional collected information or further exploration of problem areas. The open-ended format provides general questions that allow the client the opportunity to elaborate on areas of concern, but it is

Closed-ended	Open-ended
Have you been hospitalized before? yes ____ no ____	Describe any previous hospitalizations. _____ _____ _____
Do you typically seek health care at a clinic? yes ____ no ____	Where do you typically go for health care? _____
Is your pain continuous or intermittent? _____	Describe the nature of your pain. _____ _____ _____

Figure 3–2

Comparison of closed- versus open-ended questions as part of a nursing history. The open-ended format facilitates comprehensive data collection.

time-consuming to administer. Most nursing history forms are a combination of the two types. Whatever the format, collection of these baseline data requires interactions between the nurse and client and family members or significant others. Figure 3–2 illustrates the difference between open-ended and closed-ended questions typically seen as part of the nursing history data base.

FAMILY AND SIGNIFICANT OTHERS

Family members or significant others of the client are *secondary* sources of data, as they may supplement or verify information provided by the client. They may be able to offer information about the client before the illness, provide family history related to health and illness, and describe the client's home environment. In instances in which the client cannot communicate, the nurse must rely solely on information supplied by these sources.

RECORDS

Medical histories, laboratory records, vital signs, and diagnostic reports provide pertinent data and validate information identified in the health history and physical examination. Initial recorded findings serve as baselines to be used as standards against which subsequent results are compared. Medical records from previous admissions to the hospital also supply additional pieces of information.

CONSULTATION

A nurse may supplement client information through consultation with other health care team members who previously had contact with the client. The physician is a key source of information, especially if the client has

sought health care previously. A social worker or community health nurse who has worked with the client can also contribute valuable information.

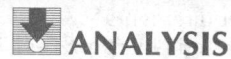ANALYSIS

SUMMARIZING DATA AND DRAWING CONCLUSIONS

The second step of the nursing process is the *analysis* of data. In this phase, the nurse summarizes the data that have been collected, organizes the data into a logical framework, and analyzes and draws conclusions from the data to determine what health problems the client may have. The client's findings are compared with normal parameters to assist in this step of the nursing process. Problems are categorized as potential problems requiring prevention, actual problems being managed, actual problems requiring interventions, or actual problems requiring further investigation. The types of problems identified may be physiologic, psychologic, or sociologic.

NURSING DIAGNOSIS

Conclusions about the client that indicate the need for nursing care are labeled *nursing diagnoses.* Many nurses have attempted to define the term nursing diagnosis. One of the most frequently cited definitions is that by Gordon, who stated that the nursing diagnosis is "a clinical diagnosis made by a professional nurse that describes actual or potential health problems which the nurse, by virtue of her education and experience, is capable and licensed to treat" (Gordon, 1987, p. 8). Unlike medical diagnoses, which identify the illness, the nursing diagnosis identifies the *response* to illness.

Nursing diagnoses examine primarily those areas identified as independent nursing functions, which involve actions instituted by the nurse without a physician's order. The functions may include preventive approaches, such as education, or corrective approaches, such as forcing fluids. However, some of the current diagnoses require nursing actions that do rely on a physician's directive. For example, "pain" is a problem that might be relieved by a nurse's intervention, such as proper positioning, but the client may need the additional help of an analgesic to achieve pain relief. Even though the physician orders the medication, the nurse must use judgment regarding when to administer the drug and must observe the client for the drug's effectiveness and possible untoward effects.

The classification of nursing diagnoses began officially in 1973 at the First National Conference for the Classification of Nursing Diagnoses. The purpose of this conference was to identify health problems that nurses could legally and independently treat. The labels or diagnostic categories were established to define and classify the scope of nursing. It was thought that such a classification system would provide standard terminology among nurses, improve communication between nurses and other health professionals, and support nursing's autonomy and independent domain.

The profession's acknowledgment and endorsement of the term nursing diagnosis began in 1973 when the American Nurses' Association published *Standards of Nursing Practice*. Standard II states: "Nursing diagnoses are derived from the data of the health status of the client" (American Nurses' Association, 1973, p. 3).

TABLE 3–2   Taxonomy I: NANDA-Approved Nursing Diagnostic Categories (as published in the Summer 1988 NANDA Nursing Diagnosis Newsletter)

Pattern 1: Exchanging

1.1.2.1	Altered Nutrition: More Than Body Requirements
1.1.2.2	Altered Nutrition: Less Than Body Requirements
1.1.2.3	Altered Nutrition: Potential for More Than Body Requirements
1.2.1.1	Potential for Infection
1.2.2.1	Potential Altered Body Temperature
**1.2.2.2	Hypothermia
1.2.2.3	Hyperthermia
1.2.2.4	Ineffective Thermoregulation
*1.2.3.1	Dysreflexia
#1.3.1.1	Constipation
*1.3.1.1.1	Perceived Constipation
*1.3.1.1.2	Colonic Constipation
#1.3.1.2	Diarrhea
#1.3.1.3	Bowel Incontinence
1.3.2	Altered Urinary Elimination
1.3.2.1.1	Stress Incontinence
1.3.2.1.2	Reflex Incontinence
1.3.2.1.3	Urge Incontinence
1.3.2.1.4	Functional Incontinence
1.3.2.1.5	Total Incontinence
1.3.2.2	Urinary Retention
#1.4.1.1	Altered (Specify Type) Tissue Perfusion (renal, cerebral, cardiopulmonary, gastrointestinal, peripheral)
1.4.1.2.1	Fluid Volume Excess
1.4.1.2.2.1	Fluid Volume Deficit
1.4.1.2.2.2	Potential Fluid Volume Deficit
#1.4.2.1	Decreased Cardiac Output
1.5.1.1	Impaired Gas Exchange
1.5.1.2	Ineffective Airway Clearance
1.5.1.3	Ineffective Breathing Pattern

1.6.1	Potential for Injury
1.6.1.1	Potential for Suffocation
1.6.1.2	Potential for Poisoning
1.6.1.3	Potential for Trauma
*1.6.1.4	Potential for Aspiration
*1.6.1.5	Potential for Disuse Syndrome
1.6.2.1	Impaired Tissue Integrity
1.6.2.1.1	Altered Oral Mucous Membrane
1.6.2.1.2.1	Impaired Skin Integrity
1.6.2.1.2.2	Potential Impaired Skin Integrity

Pattern 2: Communicating

2.1.1.1	Impaired Verbal Communication

Pattern 3: Relating

3.1.1	Impaired Social Interaction
3.1.2	Social Isolation
#3.2.1	Altered Role Performance
3.2.1.1.1	Altered Parenting
3.2.1.1.2	Potential Altered Parenting
3.2.1.2.1	Sexual Dysfunction
3.2.2	Altered Family Processes
*3.2.3.1	Parental Role Conflict
3.3	Altered Sexuality Patterns

Pattern 4: Valuing

4.1.1	Spiritual Distress (Distress of the human spirit)

Pattern 5: Choosing

5.1.1.1	Ineffective Individual Coping
5.1.1.1.1	Impaired Adjustment

Since then, many states have incorporated the term into their nurse practice acts.

The list of nursing diagnoses, better termed *diagnostic labels,* has grown during the past 20 years. Subsequent conferences since 1973 have continued to add to the identification and classification of nursing diagnoses. An organization entitled North American Nursing Diagnosis Association (NANDA) was created at the fifth nursing diagnosis conference. At the present time, 97 diagnoses have been accepted for clinical use and testing by NANDA.

Until the eighth conference, the nursing diagnostic labels were listed in alphabetic form. At that conference, Taxonomy I was officially approved. It categorizes diagnoses into nine patterns and classifies them according to their level of abstraction. This first step in formulating a well-developed classification scheme should help the profession recognize which diagnostic areas need further development and testing. The complete revised Taxonomy I appears in Table 3–2.

The list of nursing diagnoses is not exhaustive; further refinement and clinical validation are needed. The realm of nursing diagnosis is an area for further exploration. Labels that have been identified need testing and validation through research. Eventually, as research continues in the area, outcome criteria will be established and nursing interventions for each diagnosis will be supported. Other outcomes of standardized nursing diagnoses may include third-party reimbursement for nursing services, coding and computerization, and costing-out nursing services to quantify what nurses do.

Nursing diagnoses should not be confused with med-

TABLE 3–2 Taxonomy I: NANDA-Approved Nursing Diagnostic Categories (as published in the Summer 1988 NANDA Nursing Diagnosis Newsletter) *Continued*

*5.1.1.1.2	Defensive Coping		*7.1.2.1	Chronic Low Self-Esteem
*5.1.1.1.3	Ineffective Denial		*7.1.2.2	Situational Low Self-Esteem
5.1.2.1.1	Ineffective Family Coping: Disabling		#7.1.3	Personal Identity Disturbance
5.1.2.1.2	Ineffective Family Coping: Compromised		7.2	Sensory/Perceptual Alterations (Specify) (visual, auditory, kinesthetic, gustatory, tactile, olfactory)
5.1.2.2	Family Coping: Potential for Growth			
5.2.1.1	Noncompliance (Specify)		7.2.1.1	Unilateral Neglect
*5.3.1.1	Decisional Conflict (Specify)		7.3.1	Hopelessness
*5.4	Health-Seeking Behaviors (Specify)		7.3.2	Powerlessness

Pattern 6: Moving

Pattern 8: Knowing

6.1.1.1	Impaired Physical Mobility		8.1.1	Knowledge Deficit (Specify)
6.1.1.2	Activity Intolerance		8.3	Altered Thought Processes
*6.1.1.2.1	Fatigue			
6.1.1.3	Potential Activity Intolerance		**Pattern 9: Feeling**	
6.2.1	Sleep Pattern Disturbance			
6.3.1.1	Diversional Activity Deficit		#9.1.1	Pain
6.4.1.1	Impaired Home Maintenance Management		9.1.1.1	Chronic Pain
			9.2.1.1	Dysfunctional Grieving
6.4.2	Altered Health Maintenance		9.2.1.2	Anticipatory Grieving
#6.5.1	Feeding Self-Care Deficit		9.2.2	Potential for Violence: Self-directed or Directed at Others
6.5.1.1	Impaired Swallowing			
*6.5.1.2	Ineffective Breastfeeding		9.2.3	Post-Trauma Response
#6.5.2	Bathing/Hygiene Self-Care Deficit		9.2.3.1	Rape-Trauma Syndrome
#6.5.3	Dressing/Grooming Self-Care Deficit		9.2.3.1.1	Rape-Trauma Syndrome: Compound Reaction
#6.5.4	Toileting Self-Care Deficit			
6.6	Altered Growth and Development		9.2.3.1.2	Rape-Trauma Syndrome: Silent Reaction
			9.3.1	Anxiety
Pattern 7: Perceiving			9.3.2	Fear
#7.1.1	Body Image Disturbance			
#**7.1.2	Self-Esteem Disturbance			

* New diagnostic categories approved 1988.
** Revised diagnostic categories approved 1988.
# Categories with modified label terminology.

ical diagnoses. Whereas a medical diagnosis is the basis for medical interventions, a nursing diagnosis indicates a client problem within the realm of nursing practice. Nursing diagnoses are not diagnostic tests, equipment for implementation of medical therapy, or problems experienced by the nurse while caring for the client. Table 3–3 differentiates medical and nursing diagnoses.

A complete nursing diagnosis is a statement consisting of two parts joined by the phrase *related to.* The diagnostic statement begins with (1) an actual or potential *problem* of the client and identifies (2) the *probable cause* or risk factors (etiology). The problem indicates what needs to change and the etiology reflects the environmental, psychologic, sociologic, physiologic, or spiritual factors thought to be related or contributing to the problem. By including the etiology in addition to the problem statement, greater direction is given for the planning of nursing activities to prevent, correct, or alleviate the problem. An actual problem is an existing deviation from health; a potential problem is identified if risk factors are present (Gordon, 1987).

In addition to these two parts of the statement, *defining characteristics* may be included. Defining characteristics are the clinical manifestations or behaviors of the client's condition or the risk factors that make the client susceptible to a potential problem. These behaviors define certain observable and recognizable patterns that underlie the nursing diagnosis. An example of a two-part nursing diagnosis with defining characteristics is: Knowledge deficit related to diabetic foot care as characterized by <u>client history of removing corns with a razor blade</u> (defining characteristic underlined). The use of defining characteristics better enables the nurse to individualize client care and to validate the nursing diagnosis.

Throughout this text, the nursing diagnoses are given in two parts — the problem and the etiology. The classification scheme for nursing diagnoses from the eighth nursing diagnosis conference is used as a basis for stating nursing diagnoses.

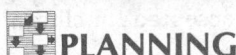

PLANNING

The *planning* phase follows the analysis and problem identification step of the nursing process. Throughout this phase, several important functions are performed: setting priorities, setting goals, planning actions, determining resources, and establishing evaluative criteria.

SETTING PRIORITIES AND GOALS

After analyzing the needs of the client and identifying nursing problems, the nurse decides on the urgency of the interventions. This step is vital, as some nursing problems are more critical than others. Problems of higher priority require more immediate intervention than problems of lower priority. Setting priorities helps the nurse organize and plan care that solves the most urgent problems. The importance of lower-priority problems is not negated; rather, a more realistic framework is simply established.

In determining the priority of the problem, the impact on the individual is considered. Several theorists have presented hierarchies to assist in determining priorities. Bower (1972) offered a three-level approach.

1. First priority — Threats to life, dignity, and integrity of the client
2. Second priority — Problems that destructively change the client
3. Third priority — Problems that affect normal growth and development

Maslow's hierarchy of needs can also serve as a useful guide for establishing priorities. The needs identified by Maslow (1970) form five levels: physiologic needs, safety or security, love and belonging, esteem, and self-actualization. The client progresses up the hierarchy when attempting to satisfy needs. As shown in Figure 3–3, physiologic needs are of greatest priority and must be met first. Once they are met, the client is more willing and able to seek fulfillment of higher-level needs.

Priorities may fluctuate as the client's level of wellness changes. Both actual and potential problems should be considered when establishing priorities. Actual problems are usually more important than potential problems. However, at times potential problems may take precedence over actual problems. For example, in a client who is asthmatic, the potential problem of alter-

TABLE 3–3   Differentiation Between Medical and Nursing Diagnoses

Medical Diagnosis	Nursing Diagnosis
Identifies pathologic basis for illness	Identifies response to illness
Focuses on physical condition of client	Focuses on physical, psychosocial, and spiritual needs of client
Addresses actual existing problems	Addresses actual and potential problems
Is not validated with the client	Is validated with the client if possible
Uses standardized goals and treatment	Uses individualized goals and interventions
May not be resolvable	Is usually resolvable

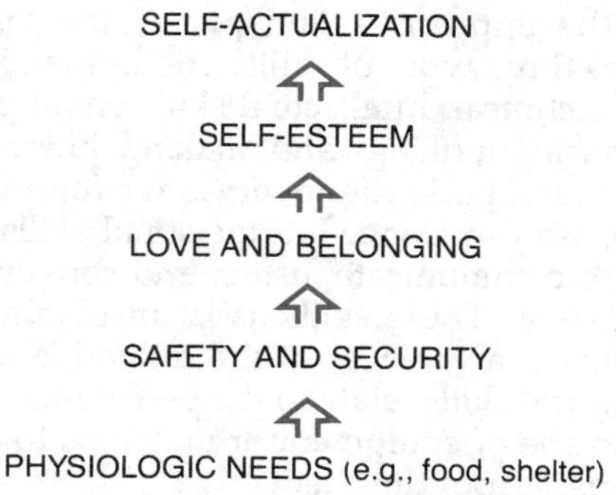

SELF-ACTUALIZATION

⇧

SELF-ESTEEM

⇧

LOVE AND BELONGING

⇧

SAFETY AND SECURITY

⇧

PHYSIOLOGIC NEEDS (e.g., food, shelter)

Figure 3-3
Maslow's needs hierarchy. Needs must be met in ascending order. For example, safety and security must be achieved before love and belonging.

ation in oxygenation may be more life-threatening than an actual problem of constipation.

The establishment of priorities reflects a mutuality between client and nurse. In addition to the guidelines for priorities that have been offered by theorists, the nurse must be aware of factors such as the client's health goals, the availability of resources, and the client's knowledge regarding the problem. The client's priorities may be more important than those outlined by theoretical guidelines.

After establishing priorities, the client and nurse mutually decide on expected goals. For the purpose of this text, a *goal* is defined as a desired client behavior to meet the individual's optimal level of wellness; it is also referred to as the *long-term goal. Expected outcomes* are interim or sequential steps needed to reach the goal. The term expected outcome may be used interchangeably with the term *short-term goal.* Projected goals serve as guides in the selection of nursing interventions and in the determination of criteria for evaluating nursing interventions. The purpose of delineating goals is to assist in the evaluation of the client's progress and to determine accomplishment, if possible, of the client's problem.

Goals should be realistic in terms of the client's potential for achievement and the nurse's ability to help the client achieve them. When writing goals, it is necessary to state them in a clear, concise manner that can be understood and measured by all health care team members. Anyone caring for the client should be able to determine whether the goals have been achieved. Using measurable, observable behaviors to identify desired outcomes and specifying the time frame for accomplishment of the goal facilitate evaluation of goal achievement. Mager (1962) listed three components of a behavioral objective or goal that should be included to enhance evaluation of goal achievement: (1) identification of the behavior act, (2) the condition under which the behavior is to occur, and (3) the criterion of acceptable performance.

An example of a goal that contains the three components follows: After health teaching by the nurse (con-

dition), the client will list (behavior) five foods high in sodium (criterion).

PLANNING ACTIONS

After the goals have been determined, strategies to accomplish these behaviors are developed. The usual format for recording these strategies is called the *client care plan.* A client care plan is a display of specific methods or proposed actions to resolve the problems that were identified by data collection and analysis.

Information about prescribed nursing actions that correspond to the client's preferences, problems, priorities, complications to be prevented, and expected outcomes is recorded. The client care plan is comprehensive and incorporates actions performed by other members of the health care team. It serves as a communication vehicle to inform health care team members about the client's problems. A well-written client care plan provides a central source of information about the client and can be an effective means to assure the client that problems will be solved and needs fulfilled. Development of a care plan is a continuous process. Revisions are made as new data indicate a need for modification. Examples of client care plans are found throughout this text.

Nursing orders are interventions, or actions, designed to assist the client in achieving outcomes. They are based on the nursing diagnosis and define activities required to promote, maintain, or restore the client's health. Independent and collaborative nursing interventions are included on the client care plan. There are four desirable characteristics of nursing orders; i.e., they must

1. Be consistent with the therapeutic plan of the health team
2. Be based on scientific rationale
3. Be specific for the individual client
4. Use the teaching-learning process

DETERMINING RESOURCES

After planning the interventions, the nurse determines what resources are necessary to implement the actions. The client is a valuable source of information about health care resources that were successful in the past. The client's family or significant others may be consulted about their abilities and desire to be involved in the plan. Inclusion of the family while planning care may promote their cooperation during the implementation phase.

Other nurses and health care team members may be valuable sources for ideas. A multidisciplinary conference during which health care team members address various aspects of the client's care and offer suggestions is one way to coordinate the health care team's available resources.

Current research and literature also serve as valuable resources in suggesting ways to achieve goals. Availability of additional resources such as equipment, time, personnel, and money is also taken into account when the feasibility of the plan is explored. The client's value system is also considered.

To save time and duplication, numerous computer programs have been developed to create standardized care plans that can be individualized as needed. Although each system is different, most programs allow the nurse to enter the client's assessment data, which then cue the computer to list the possible applicable nursing diagnoses for a given client. After the nurse selects the appropriate diagnoses, the computer offers a list of possible nursing interventions for each diagnosis, and the nurse again selects those that are suitable for the client. Expected outcomes are also available that can be modified to meet a particular client's needs. As technology advances, these programs will be more widely available to nurses in all health care settings.

ESTABLISHING EVALUATIVE CRITERIA

Before actions are implemented, mechanisms to determine goal achievement and effectiveness of nursing interventions are established. Unless criteria have been predetermined, it is difficult to know whether the goal is achieved and the problem resolved.

Another method established to guide evaluation is standards of care. Standards for medical-surgical nursing, developed by the American Nurses' Association, serve as useful guidelines for determining the implementation of nursing care. In addition, hospitals have standards, which are often unit based, to describe the care that should be provided during the planning and implementation phases of the nursing process.

 IMPLEMENTATION

The actual carrying out of a specific, individualized plan constitutes the *implementation* phase. This step is the action phase of the nursing process, as the nurse assumes the responsibility of implementing the client care plan and treating the client on the basis of the nursing diagnoses. The actions planned for the client are based on knowledge gained from the experts, suggestions from the client and other health care team members, and the nurse's creativity. Actions should be based on scientific principles and rationale, not intuition. Selection of appropriate nursing interventions is based on the following guidelines: characteristics of the nursing diagnosis, research knowledge associated with the intervention, greatest possibility of success, client's acceptance of the intervention, least amount of risk and discomfort for the client, and capability of the nurse.

During the implementation phase, the nurse frequently uses three types of skills: intellectual, interpersonal, and technical. Intellectual skills entail problem-solving, critical thinking, and making judgments. A strong theoretical background serves as a foundation for accurate decision-making. Interpersonal skills involve the ability to communicate, listen, and convey interest and compassion. These skills assist in obtaining data and in ensuring awareness of the individuality of the client. Technical skills relate to the performance of procedures and use of equipment or materials to elicit desired responses from the client.

The actions that are implemented may be independent or collaborative. Independent functions are activities performed by the nurse without a physician's order. Collaborative functions refer to carrying out the doctor's orders by using sound nursing judgment and working with other health care team members to produce a specific outcome. Some of the challenges that confront the nurse during this stage include coordination of the activities of the health care team members and delegation of responsibilities to nursing personnel, according to their backgrounds and abilities. The implementation phase concludes when the nurse's actions are completed and the results of actions and the client's reaction to them have been recorded.

DOCUMENTATION

The quality of recording (e.g., accuracy, completeness) provides evidence of the status of goal achievement and summarizes the client's reactions. Documentation of the client's status also provides guidance and direction for continued interventions. Documentation of each phase of the nursing process is essential, but it is discussed here because it is a skill that nurses perform.

Documentation is performed by various methods. Nurses' notes, flow charts, activity and treatment sheets, and the client care plan, previously discussed, are a few examples of the most frequently used methods of documentation.

There are two general methods of recording nurses' notes, although a number of specific systems have been developed. Source-oriented charting usually includes narrative notes that organize varied data that are entered into the medical record by discipline, e.g., nurses' notes and dietary notes. In the problem-oriented method of record-keeping, baseline data are collected and recorded and a master problem list is developed. Each problem is numbered, and charting refers to one of the problems identified on the list. The notes are recorded in a *SOAP* format by all disciplines on the same progress note form in the chart. The initials represent Subjective data, Objective data, Analysis, and Plan of action. This technique of documentation is systematic and limits data to only pertinent information related to the identified problem. Figure 3–4 provides an example of SOAP charting. The reader is referred to other texts that elaborate on charting systems and to specific

Problem No. 3: Activity intolerance related to joint stiffness
  S: "I'm really stiff this morning. I don't know if I'll be able to go to therapy."
  O: Grimaces when walking with cane. Moves slowly and cautiously.
  A: Joint stiffness worse in early morning — typical characteristic of rheumatoid arthritis disease.
  P: Instruct client to take warm shower before breakfast. Assist client with range-of-motion exercises.

Figure 3 – 4

Sample SOAP note. The implementation and evaluation phases of the nursing process would be documented after the plan is carried out.

agency policies and procedures for charting requirements.

Regardless of the charting system used, the nurse documents all steps of the nursing process in a logical, accurate, and complete manner. From a legal perspective, "If it was not documented, it was not done."

 # EVALUATION

Evaluation is an intellectual activity that completes the nursing process by indicating the degree to which the nursing diagnosis, plans, and actions have been successful. Through evaluation, it is possible to detect omissions that occurred during the assessment, analysis, planning, and implementation phases.

Although evaluation is given as the final step of the nursing process, evaluation is an ongoing and integral part of each step of the process (see Fig. 3 – 1). Data collection is reviewed to determine whether sufficient information was collected and whether the behaviors identified were appropriate. The diagnoses are evaluated for their accuracy and completeness. The expected outcomes and interventions are examined to determine whether they were realistic, achievable, and effective.

The outcome of evaluation may be one or a combination of the following:

1. The client responded as expected and the problem is resolved. No additional nursing actions are needed.
2. Behavioral manifestations of the client's situation indicate that the client's problem has not been resolved. Expected outcomes have been accomplished, but the overall goal has not been achieved. Re-evaluation will continue.
3. Behavioral manifestations of the client are similar to those present initially. Little or no evidence is available to show that the problem has been resolved. Reassessment and replanning are needed.
4. Behavioral manifestations indicate a new problem. Assessment, planning, and implementation of an additional plan of action are needed to resolve the problem.

The evaluation phase is vital to the nursing process. Only through deliberate appraisal and examination of each step of the nursing process can a nurse accomplish the desired goals and help the client achieve the highest possible level of wellness.

SUMMARY

The nursing process is a systematic, problem-solving method designed to fulfill the purposes of nursing, that is, to maintain and promote the client's optimal level of wellness. Collection of data, analysis of information, identification of nursing diagnoses, planning desired outcomes and nursing care, implementation of actions, and evaluation of goals achieved and problems resolved are the interrelated and dynamic steps of the nursing process. Table 3 – 4 summarizes the activities and techniques required during each phase of the process. As nurses continue to use this approach for providing nursing care, the outcomes will be twofold: a greater sense of

TABLE 3 – 4   Overview of the Nursing Process

Phase of the Nursing Process	Activities and Techniques Performed by Nurse
Assessment	Interview
	Observation
	Physical examination
Analysis	Data summary and conclusions
	Nursing diagnosis
Planning	Priority setting
	Goal formation (expected outcomes)
	Resource determination
	Client care plan
Implementation	Intellectual skills
	Interpersonal skills
	Technical skills
	Documentation*
Evaluation	Reassessment
	Restating nursing diagnosis
	Revising goals and/or action plan

* Although documentation is a part of each phase, most of it focuses on implementation.

autonomy and satisfaction for the nurse and a greater maximization of health potential for the client.

IMPLICATIONS FOR RESEARCH

Nursing diagnosis is an area in which research is increasing. Nurses are continuously proposing diagnoses to add to the growing list developed by the National Conference System. Clinical research is performed to test the validity of the nursing diagnoses, the etiologies and characteristics, the identification of critical defining characteristics, and the identification of effective treatments for each diagnosis.

Currently, emphasis is on the adoption of diagnoses that are associated with wellness rather than illness. A major objection to the previously developed list is that the majority of diagnoses focus on illness and do not consider the maintenance of a client's strengths.

As nurses continue to refine the taxonomy of nursing diagnoses through research, nursing's theory base will grow, and the resulting scientific rationale will provide a stronger foundation for decision-making and interventions. Specific questions that nursing should address include

1. What level of the taxonomy should be used in writing the diagnostic statement?
2. Are the defining characteristics of each nursing diagnosis valid?
3. What are the standardized interventions for each nursing diagnosis?
4. What other diagnoses need to be developed related to wellness?

REFERENCES AND READINGS

American Nurses' Association. (1973). *Standards of nursing practice*. Kansas City: Author.

Bates, B. (1987). *A guide to physical examination and history taking*. Philadelphia: J. B. Lippincott.

Bower, F. (1972). *The process of planning nursing care*. St. Louis: C. V. Mosby.

Bulechek, G. M., & McCloskey, J. C. (1985). *Nursing interventions: Treatments for nursing diagnoses*. Philadelphia: W. B. Saunders.

Carnevali, D. (1983). *Nursing care planning: Diagnosis and management* (3rd ed.). Philadelphia: J. B. Lippincott.

Carpenito, L. (1984). Is the problem a nursing diagnosis? *American Journal of Nursing, 84*, 1118–1119.

Carpenito, L. (1985). Nursing diagnosis: Selected dilemmas in practice. *Occupational Health Nursing, 33*, 397–400.

Carpenito, L. (1987). *Nursing diagnosis: Application to clinical practice*. Philadelphia: J. B. Lippincott.

Carroll-Johnson, R. M. (Ed.). (1989). *Classification of nursing diagnoses: Proceedings of the Eighth National Conference*. Philadelphia: J. B. Lippincott.

Cleary, M. (1985). Integration of the nursing diagnostic process within the clinical setting. *Critical Care Nurse, 5*(1), 28–29.

Davidson, S. (1984). Nursing diagnosis: Its application in the acute-care setting. *Topics in Clinical Nursing, 5*(4), 50–57.

De La Cuesta, C. (1983). The nursing process: From development to implementation. *Journal of Advanced Nursing, 8*, 365–371.

Gebbie, K. (1975). *Classification of nursing diagnoses: Proceedings of the Second National Conference*. St. Louis: Clearinghouse for Nursing Diagnosis–NANDA.

Gebbie, K. (1984). Nursing diagnosis: What is it and why does it exist? *Topics in Clinical Nursing, 5*(4), 1–9.

Gebbie, K., & Lavin, M. A. (Eds.). (1975). *Classification of nursing diagnoses: Proceedings of the First National Conference*. St. Louis: C. V. Mosby.

Gordon, M. (1987). *Nursing diagnosis: Process and application*. New York: McGraw-Hill.

Griffith, J., & Ignatavicius, D. (1986). *The writer's handbook*. Baltimore: Resource Applications.

Hurley, M. (Ed.). (1986). *Classification of nursing diagnoses: Proceedings of the Sixth National Conference*. St. Louis: C. V. Mosby.

Iyer, P. W., Taptich, B. J., & Bernocchi-Losey, D. (1986). *Nursing process and nursing diagnosis*. Philadelphia: W. B. Saunders.

Kim, M., & Moritz, D. (1982). *Classification of nursing diagnoses: Proceedings of the Third and Fourth National Conferences*. New York: McGraw-Hill.

Kritek, P. (1985). Nursing diagnosis: Theoretical foundations. *Occupational Health Nursing, 33*, 393–396.

Lillesand, K., & Korff, S. (1983). Nursing process evaluation: A quality assurance tool. *Nursing Administration Quarterly, 7*(3), 9–14.

Mager, R. (1962). *Preparing instructional objectives*. Belmont, CA: Fearon Publishers.

Marriner, A. (1983). *The nursing process* (3rd ed.). St. Louis: C. V. Mosby.

Maslow, A. (1970). *Motivation and personality*. New York: Harper & Row.

Miaskowski, C. (1985). Nursing diagnosis within the context of the nursing process. *Occupational Health Nursing, 33*, 401–404.

North American Nursing Diagnosis Association. (1989). *Taxonomy I, with official diagnostic categories*. St. Louis: Author.

Putzier, D., & Padrick, K. (1984). Nursing diagnosis: A component of nursing process and decision making. *Topics in Clinical Nursing, 5*(4), 21–29.

Rantz, M., Miller, T., & Jacobs, C. (1985). Nursing diagnosis in long-term care. *American Journal of Nursing, 85*, 916–917, 926.

Roy, C. (1984). *Classification of nursing diagnoses: Proceedings of the Fifth National Conference.* St. Louis: C. V. Mosby.

Tanner, C., & Hughes, A. (1984). Nursing diagnosis: Issues in clinical practice research. *Topics in Clinical Nursing, 5(4)*, 30–38.

Taptich, B. J., Iyer, P. W., & Bernocchi-Losey, D. (1989). *Nursing diagnosis and care planning.* Philadelphia: W. B. Saunders.

Tartaglia, M. (1985). Nursing diagnosis: Keystone of your care plan. *Nursing '85, 15(3)*, 34–37.

Ulrich, S. P., Canale, S. W., & Wendell, S. A. (1990). *Nursing care planning guides: A nursing diagnosis approach* (2nd ed.). Philadelphia: W. B. Saunders.

Young, M., & Lucas, C. (1984). Nursing diagnosis: Common problems in implementation. *Topics in Clinical Nursing, 5*, 68–77.

Yura, H., & Walsh, M. (1978). *The nursing process* (3rd ed.). New York: Appleton-Century-Crofts.

CHAPTER 4

Impact of the Health Care Delivery System on Medical-Surgical Nursing Practice

A healthy society depends on an efficient health care delivery system. Nurses are not only the largest group of health professionals in the health care system but also the most diverse in terms of education and practice. This "depth and breadth" of the nursing profession gives the nurse an extraordinary potential to influence the health care delivery system. The purpose of this chapter is to give a brief overview of the health care delivery system and the way in which changes in the system affect medical-surgical nursing. Medical-surgical nurses can influence these changes because they work directly with clients on a one-to-one basis, beginning with the client's first contact with the system. Nurses have the most knowledge about the clients and their health care needs and therefore can have the most impact.

Nurses, as individuals and as a group, can and must participate in shaping health care policies that affect the health care delivery system. Nurses as citizens should not abandon their rights to influence legislation and policies; as professionals, nurses are obligated to ensure that the public has access to quality health care at controlled costs. Because medical-surgical nurses work in a wide variety of settings, from acute care institutions to community health centers, and because they implement health care policy decisions, it is imperative—if they wish to have input into the type and quality of care delivered—that they understand how the health care delivery system is constructed and how health care policy decisions are made. Armed with this information, they can become advocates for clients and true participants in the formulation of effective health care policy. Policy decisions regarding financial resources influence the type of nursing staff, the number of nurses, the amount and type of management and support services, and supplies—all of which affect the quality of nursing care. Nurses implement numerous health care policy decisions at all levels of the health care delivery system—governmental, institutional, unit, and client.

The need to control costs of health care without diminishing its quality or access to it is becoming increasingly important. The public needs to ask continually if its monies are being well spent for health care. Nurses are well placed and well equipped to help with this analysis. Nurses cannot afford to assume that the public—even in their local community or institutions—understands how the health care system works and the nurse's role in it, unless as practicing professionals they take some responsibility for informing the public.

Because 40% of the health care spending is done by state and federal governments (Division of National Cost Estimates, 1987), the government controls spending as well as influences the quantity and quality of health care. Most of this spending involves Medicare and Medicaid programs. Governmental policies determine not only accessibility and the type of health care available but also who will deliver it, in what setting, and how much will be paid for it. This control dictates the parameters within which nursing care is delivered, the type of nursing personnel, and how much nurses are paid to deliver that care.

THE HEALTH CARE DELIVERY SYSTEM

The health care system is a highly pluralistic, complex mix of public and private organizations with multiple sources of funding, many points of decision-making, and numerous skilled personnel. This system can be divided into two broad categories: institutional care and ambulatory care. Also interacting with this system are society's values and priorities, which are manifested in the policies, laws, regulations, financing, and technologies developed for and by the health system. *Institutional care* is rendered to persons who need nursing or custodial care on a short-term or a long-term basis, whereas *ambulatory care* is for persons who can remain in their homes in the community.

This system, the *health care delivery system*, is said to provide health care, but in fact it predominantly provides illness or sick care. A common belief is that the physician, hospital, and nursing home are the main components of the health care system. In reality, the health care system encompasses more than medical and illness care; it also includes areas such as public health, health promotion, rehabilitation, and nursing care.

Although there is no agreed upon definition of health, as discussed in Chapter 1, health is more than the absence of illness or disease. Using the broad definitions of health when talking about the health care delivery system forces one to consider *all* aspects of health, not just illness care.

Before the 20th century, health care in the United States was viewed as a responsibility to be assumed by individuals or by private organizations. During the 18th and 19th centuries, the scourge of epidemics related to impure foods, contaminated water supplies, inadequate sewage disposal, and poor housing conditions impelled local governments to respond with measures to protect the health of their citizens. These recurring epidemics also led to the first public health effort by the federal government: a national port quarantine system. After the yellow fever epidemic of 1873, Congress established the Marine Hospital Services to regulate and enforce this quarantine. Thus, out of group need, the precedent of intervention by the federal government was established (Hyman, 1982).

The term *public health* has traditionally referred to the control of disease in populations by organized community actions, generally through governmental departments of public health. Today, public health includes control not only of communicable diseases but also of environmental hazards. These activities gener-

ally cannot be carried out by only private care of individuals. Public health activities include illness preventive measures and health promotion programs, ranging from nutrition programs to antismoking campaigns to automobile safety. The term has come to mean a wide range of health-related activities, especially regulation that is carried out by public agencies, i.e., governmental departments of health.

HEALTH CARE DELIVERY SETTINGS

The determination of which setting—institutional or ambulatory—is appropriate is established by how much nursing care or custodial care the individual needs, balanced with what technology is needed and who is available to care for the client.

INSTITUTIONAL CARE

Hospitals

Hospital care has become the predominant type of institutional care and constitutes approximately 40% of all health care spending. In 1986, hospital revenues were $180 billion, an increase of 7.4% from 1985 (Division of National Cost Estimates, 1987). Sixty per cent of all nurses work in hospitals (Eastaugh, 1987). Because the largest percentage of medical-surgical nurses work in the hospital, they need to be aware of how this system of care functions. Today, individuals are admitted to institutions when their illness or the treatment of their illness requires the technology or skill and knowledge of health care providers that are unavailable or inconvenient to administer on an ambulatory basis.

Development of Hospitals

The American hospital system has developed in five stages. In the *first stage*, during the colonial era, almshouses were viewed mainly as caretaking charities. Most illness care was delivered at home, and there were infrequent visits by the physician. Nursing care was given by family members. Clients went to almshouses only when they had no one to care for them or when they had no other place to go. Colonial almshouses were the forerunners of voluntary hospitals operated by charitable lay boards and public hospitals operated by cities, counties, and the federal government.

During the *second stage*, from the Civil War until the 1920s, there was a greater emphasis on medical treatment, and various religious, ethnic, and specialty hospitals evolved. During the *third stage*, from the 1920s to World War II, medical and nursing care in hospitals developed as a science as well as an art. As technology advanced, antibiotics were discovered, and aseptic techniques were used, hospitals became places to care for the ill rather than only places to go to die. Only after the 1920s was hospital care considered to be more helpful than harmful.

Nursing care in hospitals before World War II was delivered by nursing students. Students were enrolled in hospital training programs. The only licensed nurses hired by hospitals were the nurses involved in the administration of the nursing services, such as the chief nurse or head nurse, who also supervised students. Most graduate licensed nurses were hired for "cases" by families. These nurses cared for clients in the home or in the hospital and were paid on a fee-for-service basis by their clients or the clients' families. Only the poor were in hospitals without their own licensed private nurses. This type of case assignment was the forerunner of the concept of primary nursing care.

During the Great Depression and World War II, there was little hospital construction. After World War II, the *fourth stage* in hospital development occurred. To encourage hospital construction, a law—the Hospital Survey and Construction Act of 1946, popularly called the Hill-Burton Act after the two senators who introduced the legislation—was enacted. This legislation, which became Title VI of the Public Health Service Act, provided grants for the construction of hospitals. During the next 30 years, this act was amended several times to include not only hospitals but also diagnostic and treatment centers (including hospital outpatient departments), chronic disease hospitals, rehabilitation facilities, and nursing homes. Finally, in 1974, new legislation completely revised the Hill-Burton Act and incorporated it into a new Title XVI of the Public Health Service Act to become the National Health Planning and Resource Development Act of 1974. (This act was eliminated by the 99th Congress in 1986. Congress thought that it was not economical to mandate health planning on a national basis.)

Not only were more hospitals constructed during the fourth stage, but insurance coverage increased, thus encouraging the use of hospitals as the setting for delivery of health care. In general, insurance policies would pay for care only after the beneficiary had been in the hospital for 3 days. Consequently, most clients were admitted to hospitals for at least 3 days for all kinds of treatments and care. Insurance use increased to the point that in 1986 only 9.4% of all hospital revenues were paid directly by clients (Division of National Cost Estimates, 1987). Payments paid directly by clients are called out-of-pocket payments. These two factors, the Hill-Burton Act and the increased insurance coverage, encouraged the heavy use of hospitals for all types of health care until the mid-1980s. The *fifth stage* of hospital development began in 1982 when Congress enacted the hospital prospective payment plan for Medicare clients. This plan's major objectives were to halt the spiraling use of hospitals as well as to control the amount paid for hospital care. This prospective payment plan will be discussed later in this chapter.

Starting as institutions dependent on gifts from wealthy citizens to provide care for the destitute and the poor, hospitals have developed into the present-day market institutions in a competitive climate that are financed largely by insurance or other third-party payers.

Classifications of Hospitals

Today, hospitals may be classified according to type of ownership and type of services provided (Table 4–1). Type of ownership is divided into ownership by government and ownership by nongovernment agencies. *Government-owned hospitals* are identified according to the level of government—federal, state, or local. *Privately owned hospitals* are subdivided into not-for-profit (voluntary) and for-profit (proprietary) hospitals.

Private for-profit hospitals are required by law to pay taxes, whereas private not-for-profit hospitals are not required to pay taxes. The American Hospital Association is the national association representing not-for-profit hospitals, and the Federation of American Hospitals is the national association representing for-profit institutions.

Recently, the number of investor-owned hospital corporations, called hospital chains, has grown. Examples of these for-profit hospitals are the Hospital Corporation of America and Humana Corporation. These chains not only own and operate hospitals, but also own and/or manage nursing homes, health maintenance organizations (HMOs), clinical laboratories, and other such entities, not only in the United States but also in other countries. The stock of these corporations is publicly traded on the stock exchanges. These corporations usually maintain a central headquarters with experts who advise and consult with staff in the individual facilities. Controversy exists about the quality of care in these for-profit hospitals and about whether economies of scale for the purchase and delivery of services actually reduce the costs to the consumer or whether the inherent competition for clients drives the costs up. Research studies have indicated that both occur; more definitive and rigorous studies by impartial investigators need to be done.

Hospitals can also be classified according to type of care delivered: general or specialized. *General hospitals* provide care for different age groups and different illnesses. These hospitals can have specialized units (e.g., for clients with cancer), but the entire hospital delivers mixed types of services to various age groups. *Specialty hospitals* provide care for only the established specialty, such as an age group, a disease group, or a length of stay (acute versus chronic). The term *teaching hospital* refers to a hospital that has a physician residency program with interns and residents. It may not necessarily indicate affiliation with a medical school or a nursing school.

The term *tertiary hospital* is applied to institutions that have the most complex diagnostic and therapeutic treatments available and generally serve as a referral center for clients with extremely complicated problems.

TABLE 4–1 Classification of Hospitals

By Type of Ownership

Government Owned

FEDERAL

Indian health services
Military services
Veterans Administration

STATE

Psychiatric
Chronic disease
State university

LOCAL

County
City
Hospital districts

Privately Owned

NOT FOR PROFIT (VOLUNTARY)

Churches, other religious groups
Community organizations
Independent groups, e.g., Shriners

FOR PROFIT

Individual owner
Corporation
Partnership

By Type of Care

General

Community hospitals
Teaching hospitals
Tertiary hospitals

Specialty

Age group
Type of disease
Length of stay

Often community hospitals are the institutions that refer clients to a tertiary hospital, usually a university medical center.

Another type of hospital is the osteopathic institution. These hospitals are staffed by osteopathic physi-

cians (DOs). Osteopathic medicine originally held that musculoskeletal dysfunctions, especially of the spine, disrupted the body's resistance to disease. Today, osteopathic medicine has evolved into a holistic type of medicine that uses some of the same diagnostic and treatment modalities as conventional medicine.

Nursing Homes and Extended Care Facilities

Nursing Homes

There is no exact definition of a nursing home. The term is generally used to refer to a facility in which clients need primarily nursing care rather than medical care. Most nursing homes are generally thought of as homes for the aged. This may or may not be true. Nursing homes are different from chronic disease hospitals and rehabilitation facilities. Although all three types of institutions are used for longer stays than is a general acute hospital, their purposes are different. Most nursing home clients are transferred to those facilities from acute care hospitals — one aspect of the continuum of institutional care.

Before the Social Security Act of 1935, there were few nursing homes. Most clients who are currently in nursing homes would have been cared for at home by extended families or in public poorhouses. The Social Security Act made monies available to elderly beneficiaries for care in proprietary facilities. Today, 5% of persons older than age 65 years live in some type of nursing home or extended care facility.

In the past, nursing homes were classified according to the level of care provided. Two levels of care were identified: skilled nursing care and intermediate care. A *skilled nursing facility* (SNF), to be eligible for funds under the Medicare and Medicaid programs, had to provide 24-hour nursing services under the supervision of a registered nurse. This supervision was defined by the federal programs as one registered nurse available at all times. *Intermediate care facilities* (ICFs) were facilities that cared for clients with less acute illness and had a registered nurse present for 8 hours a day. In some instances, an institution could have both SNF and ICF level beds in the same physical facility. The amount of payment from the federal government's Medicare and Medicaid programs depended on the level of care identified and provided.

The definitions of SNF and ICF were revised when Public Law (PL) 100-203 was enacted in 1988. This law was based on a 1986 report from the Institute of Medicine, an arm of the National Academy of Sciences, which called for nursing home reform. One of the recommendations implemented by this legislation was the merging of SNFs and ICFs into one level of care. This law requires all nursing homes to have 24-hour licensed nurse coverage by 1990. This includes a registered nurse (RN) on duty 8 hours a day 7 days a week, with a licensed practical nurse (LPN) on duty 24 hours a day. A provision of the law allows individual states to waive the nurse staffing requirement if after a good faith effort the facility is unable to hire nurses at the prevailing wages for similar facilities. This waiver applies to the registered nurse requirement on weekends and the licensed practical nurse requirement on the night shift. The nursing home industry has stated that under the present Medicare and Medicaid reimbursement levels, the cost of requiring a registered nurse to be present at all times is prohibitive. They maintain that a *licensed* nurse is sufficient. This licensed nurse could be a registered nurse or a licensed practical nurse.

Nursing homes are licensed by states and are certified by the Health Care Financing Administration for participation in the Medicare and Medicaid programs. Accreditation is carried out by the Joint Commission on Accreditation of Healthcare Organizations. Some states require that nursing homes meet the qualifications of a certificate of need (CON) to operate in their state. These programs will be discussed under the heading Access to Care. The national nursing home association is called American Health Care Association.

Life Care or Continuing Care Facilities

The 1980s has seen the growth of *life care* or *continuing care facilities*. These facilities are a combination of retirement residences, nursing homes, and hospices. An individual or a couple, after meeting the specific requirements of the particular facility, moves into a room, an apartment, or a cottage managed by the facility. The resident pays either a large initial payment or a smaller initial payment with monthly or quarterly amount to the managing organization. The contract for the resident typically covers all health and illness care that the resident needs, including nursing home care and possibly hospice care.

Rehabilitation or Recovery Facilities

Rehabilitation facilities provide a wide spectrum of services. Although many rehabilitation centers are for clients with physical deformities or handicaps, such as spinal cord injuries, some are for clients who abuse drugs or alcohol. Clients in these centers are admitted by referring physicians or are transferred from other inpatient facilities. These centers can be freestanding entities or part of a hospital.

AMBULATORY CARE

The term *ambulatory care* refers to care delivered to clients in different settings to which they can ambulate. The term has evolved to encompass any non-inpatient care, which ranges from care in clinics to that in emergency rooms, homes, doctors' offices, and 1-day surgicenters. Ambulatory care is quickly becoming the prevalent mode of delivery because of its presumed lesser cost and the preference of clients to remain in their home and in the community.

Outpatient Clinics

Outpatient Departments

Outpatient departments (OPDs) were developed in hospitals so that clients could receive care without being hospitalized. OPDs permit follow-up care by the same staff that discharges the client from the hospital. These departments replaced freestanding dispensaries.

The population served by OPDs consists usually of clients participating in the Medicaid or Medicare programs. Some middle-income people with private insurance are also served, especially at university-related teaching hospitals. Special consultation mechanisms may be available for referring physicians. In the past, clients of OPDs were seen by the house staff (interns and resident physicians) or unpaid attending physicians (voluntary staff), but these arrangements have been changing. Private clients may be seen by physicians who have offices at the hospital under rental or other arrangements. This is done frequently by professors in medical schools and is usually distinguished from the general OPD by such terms as *private OPD*.

Health Centers

Health centers are facilities serving specific geographic areas and providing defined health care services. These community-based centers are organized in different ways. The sponsorship of the center can be purely governmental, or purely community or private organizations, or a combination of these. Examples of health centers are well-child or prenatal clinics serving a certain area of the city or county; mental health centers serving a defined area; and regional senior citizen centers.

Freestanding Centers

Freestanding centers are clinics operating independently—physically as well as organizationally—from hospitals or other institutional facilities. In the early part of the 19th century, freestanding clinics called dispensaries were established by independent charities for treatment of the poor who were ill. They were developed for the most part in parallel with hospitals and were ultimately displaced by hospital OPDs.

Today's freestanding clinics were not developed for the care of the "sick poor" but rather were developed as a means of controlling a professional practice, as a business venture, or both. Some freestanding centers have contracts with hospitals to provide emergency or inpatient services. Other freestanding clinics are one of a kind or are franchises of a national chain of centers. Hospitals have started to invade this territory by developing some creative organizational arrangements, such as establishing a satellite clinic in a neighborhood adjacent to the area from which they normally draw clients. This is done in hopes of enlarging the geographic market area to increase the number of clients. These satellite clinics are run as independent units with arrangements for hospitalization in the sponsoring hospital.

Many of these freestanding centers constitute what has come to be known as *alternative delivery systems.* Some examples of the entities that are considered to be alternative delivery centers are birthing centers, family planning clinics, surgicenters, mental health clinics, "free" clinics, abortion clinics, emergicenters, and community nursing centers.

Emergicenters

Freestanding clinics for the immediate walk-in treatment of non–life-threatening acute illnesses or injuries are called *emergicenters.* Many of these emergicenters offer low-cost, rapid care within the client's neighborhood from 7 AM to midnight. People have found them to be quick and efficient for non–life-threatening emergency episodes.

Surgicenters

Comparable to these emergicenters are the freestanding *surgicenters.* These centers provide surgical care for procedures that do not require overnight stays. Surgicenters were established to reduce the costs of surgery. Surgicenters can be specialized according to type of surgery, such as clinics for care of clients with cataracts or for plastic surgery. Hospitals have reacted to their loss of business by creating their own 1-day or short-stay surgical centers within the hospital or as satellite units.

Home Care Agencies

Care of the sick in their homes was the usual method of care until the mid-20th century explosion of hospital construction. Hospitals were generally viewed as places where people went to die. Even when clients survived hospitalization and returned home, they received home visits from the physician and the nurse.

Home care today is generally done by nursing organizations such as Visiting Nurse Associations (VNA), departments of public health, and nonprofit or for-profit home health care agencies. Home health care agencies, as defined by the federal government, are engaged primarily in providing skilled nursing services and other therapeutic services. They have policies established by a group of professional personnel, including one or more physicians and one or more registered professional nurses, and provide for supervision of these services by a physician or a registered professional nurse.

Many hospitals are now developing home care agencies to provide care to their discharged clients. This is in reaction to the prospective payment plan, which limits the amount of payment to a defined length of stay per diagnosis. Consequently, some clients are being discharged to their homes more quickly than before. Sometimes, all of the care or the education required by the clients is not accomplished in the hospital and needs to be continued at home. When hospitals have their own

home health care agencies, they do not lose clients or monies to other private freestanding home care agencies. This expansion by hospitals is reminiscent of the development of OPDs in the 19th century by hospitals in response to the success of dispensaries.

One research study that demonstrated the economic value of home care was conducted by Dorothy Brooten, a nurse, and her colleagues (Brooten, 1988). This study showed that having a clinical nurse specialist follow early discharged premature infants at home could save approximately $18,560 per infant compared with hospital care, by providing nursing care and support for the parents at home. Brooten estimated that this type of early discharge with follow-up could save between $162 million and $334 million if instituted nationally. Another nurse is attempting to replicate this study with the elderly population.

For-profit agencies, nonprofit agencies, and hospital-owned agencies have proliferated in the last 10 years until some regions in certain states are overcrowded with home care agencies. Some states require a CON for home care agencies to operate. These home care agencies have generally taken over the duties and responsibilities of the traditional public health nurse employed by the city or county. Many county or city public health nurses now do only supervisory and administrative work rather than providing home visits.

The National League for Nursing accredits freestanding home health care agencies, whereas the Joint Commission on Accreditation of Healthcare Organizations accredits hospital-based home care agencies.

Managed Care Facilities

Managed care has become a popular word of the 1980s in health policy. The federal government's philosophy has moved toward the idea that health care that is managed by a health professional is more cost-effective and has the potential to deliver quality care to a larger group of people who are eligible for the government's entitlement programs than care that is not so managed. Managed care ranges from a provider's managing one episode of an illness to an assigned case manager who oversees the health of a person for a longer period. Examples of managed care organizations are health maintenance organizations (HMOs) and preferred provider organizations (PPOs).

Health Maintenance Organizations

HMOs are the most successful of the early managed care experiments. HMOs are organizations that are responsible for the provision of relatively comprehensive health services to enrolled persons in return for a set monthly or annual fee (premium). HMOs have three characteristics: (1) a defined population of enrolled members; (2) payment by members (this is determined in advance for a specific length of time and is made periodically); and (3) services provided directly rather than on an indemnity basis.

TABLE 4 – 2 Means of Provider Payment and Location of Service for Various Types of HMOs

Type of HMO	Provider Payment	Location
Staff	Salary	HMO site
Group	Contract — per capita	HMO site
Independent practice association	Contract — per capita or fee-for-service	Provider's office site

HMOs have a variety of organizational structures (Table 4 – 2). Staff HMOs have physicians and nurse practitioners on salary and require the client to come to the HMO's physical plant for all care. The group model of HMOs has a contract with a group of physicians to provide care at the HMO site on a capitation basis. Capitation is explained later in this chapter. An IPA (independent practice association) model contracts with physicians to give care to the client at the physicians' offices. The IPA model is the fastest growing of all the HMOs because of physician acceptance of the structure.

HMOs can be owned by hospitals, HMO chains, insurance companies, or large employers, or they may be independent, solo entities. HMOs were predicted to be the delivery system of the future. Many hospitals, insurance companies, and private organizations expanded into the HMO business in the early 1980s. This expansion has not proved to be as successful as first predicted because of clients' dislike of the loss of freedom to choose their own health care provider; consequently, some consolidation and contraction of HMOs are occurring.

Preferred Provider Organizations

The next trend in health care delivery appears to be PPOs, sometimes called preferred provider arrangements (PPAs).

These new entities are now growing like the HMOs in the late 1970s and early 1980s. PPOs are groups of health care providers, such as physicians and to a lesser extent nurses, who agree to provide services to a specific group of clients on a discounted basis, generally as a fee-for-service. A PPO can be an organization, a delivery system, or an arrangement between providers and a third-party payer. They can vary by sponsorship, legal status, governance, administrative structures, method of paying providers, limitation of freedom of choice of nonproviders, and utilization review programs. These examples are a few of the many types of arrangements among providers, third-party payers, and clients.

The major advantage of PPOs and PPAs is the ability to control costs by negotiating fee schedules and the control of the use of services. These organizations are sponsored by physicians' groups, insurance companies, or hospitals. For example, an employee of a particular company can receive care at the discount rate by choosing one of the physicians, hospitals, or clinics that have contracted with their company. This arrangement allows the employee some freedom of choice in selecting a provider as well as allows the employer to get a discount rate for health care benefits. The providers also benefit by having an assured pool of clients.

PPOs are generally fee-for-service, with the provider not at risk financially. PPOs serve the employed, young to middle-aged, and healthy population. If the health care system consisted entirely of PPOs, this could lead to a three-tiered system of care: the poor, the PPO consumer, and all other consumers. Some research has been done related to client satisfaction and client outcomes in PPOs, but more needs to be done to document not only satisfaction of clients and providers but also the quality of care.

Community Nursing Centers

A managed care concept developed by the American Nurses' Association (ANA) to allow nurses to deliver care in a nurse-managed system of care to clients is called *community nursing centers*. The 100th Congress funded four demonstration projects, which began in July 1989, to investigate whether this type of health care delivery system is viable for the Medicare and Medicaid population. See LaBar and McKibbin (1986) for a more in-depth description of community nursing centers.

FACTORS AFFECTING THE HEALTH CARE DELIVERY SYSTEM

The health care delivery system has evolved incrementally. As needs arose, as technology was made available, and as personnel were trained, the system was shaped. Innovations in financing mechanisms that attempt to control costs — such as HMOs, PPOs, ambulatory surgical centers, and for-profit hospitals — are also changing the structure of this system. Brown (1985) argued that competition and the marketplace are not the stimuli for these innovations in the delivery system; rather, the stimulus is a "managerial imperative." This managerial imperative, or control over delivery of services, he predicted, would be as important in the 1980s as the "technological imperative" was in the 1970s and the "access imperative" was in the 1960s. The managerial control comes not only from the manager but also from the owner or persons who assume the financial risks of the organizations. Thus, the delivery system has been shaped by societal values, technology, costs of health care, financing mechanisms of health care, and the supply and demand of health care personnel.

PAYMENT FOR CARE

The spiraling cost of health care is a national concern and has become a dominant force in the health care delivery system. Cost has become a major factor in determining how the health care delivery system is organized, financed, and delivered. As a consequence, this system is now changing faster than at any other time in history. The shaping of the delivery system affects how nursing care is delivered, including what kind of nursing care will be delivered, who will deliver this nursing care, and how much the provider of nursing care will be paid. All of these changes determine how the medical-surgical nurse will deliver nursing care to individual clients. Therefore, medical-surgical nurses today cannot be complacent about health policy and how it is made, whether at the national, state, or hospital level.

Nursing care is the reason for the existence of nursing services in health care. Policy decisions regarding financial resources influence the type of nursing staff, the number of nurses, the amount and type of management and support services, and supplies—all of which are components of quality nursing care. Understanding how health care is financed will help the medical-surgical nurse understand the limits and the possibilities of the delivery system. How health care is paid for is the core of health care financing. It is beyond the scope of this chapter to discuss all aspects of health care financing; refer to Hawkins and Higgins' *Nursing and the American Health Care Delivery System* for more information on health care financing.

PAYMENT METHODS

Health care services are paid for by the client directly, called *self-pay or out-of-pocket* payment, or indirectly by a *third party*. A third party is someone other than the client or the provider of the service. A third party can be the government, insurance company, or charitable organization. In 1950, approximately 50% of the cost of hospital care was paid directly by the client and 50% was paid by third parties. By 1985 the share paid by the client out-of-pocket decreased by 16% (Eastaugh, 1987). The small proportion of the hospital bill paid by the client shields the client from the increasing costs of hospital care and therefore clients do not seek ways to curtail the amount, number, or price of the services they receive. Health economists and policy-makers believe that the phenomenal increases in the health care costs in the United States are due to this large proportion of costs being paid for by someone other than the person receiving the care. When costs of care are not paid by the client receiving the care, the incentive to control the amount and type of services is absent.

Payment may be made *retrospectively* or *prospectively*. Until 1983, hospital care was paid for retrospectively by all third-party payers. This type of payment is the oldest type of reimbursement. A cost is placed on each item of service, and the payer of the bill is billed for the service based on the cost plus an additional amount, which is called a charge. Cost-based reimbursement never involves the client who is covered by third-party payers; rather, the payment is negotiated between the hospital and the third-party payer. Services and care are delivered to the client with payment after the fact. Retrospective payments, especially for hospital services for Medicare clients, are based on actual costs of the services and not on the charges for the services. Consequently, under retrospective payment the more services delivered to the client, the more the hospitals will be paid. Because clients are often unaware of the actual costs of the services and care, they pay little attention to the amount of care or to the costs of the health care.

In 1983, the federal government, concerned about the increasing costs and perceived inefficiency of hospitals in controlling costs as well as the amount of services delivered to the elderly, instituted a hospital *prospective payment system* (PPS). This system was mandated as the method of payment for care delivered by hospitals to the elderly enrolled in the federal Medicare program. Prospective payment means that the third-party payer and the provider agree in advance on what amount of money will be paid for certain services and care. The federal government wanted to change the incentives in the delivery of care. By setting the amount the hospital would be paid in advance for certain diagnoses, the government anticipated that hospitals would become more cost-conscious about the services delivered.

To determine how much will be paid for what service, the Medicare program instituted a payment scheme based on *diagnosis-related groups* (DRGs). Diagnosis-related grouping is a method of classifying "related" medical diagnoses into categories based on the amount of resources consumed by a client with a certain diagnosis at discharge. In 1987, 468 DRGs were identified by Medicare. Medicare sets the amount of payment for each DRG. If the hospital delivers more services and care to the client than what is paid for by that DRG, the hospital must absorb the costs. Conversely, if the hospital can deliver services and care to the client at less cost than the payment for that DRG, the hospital gets to keep the remaining monies. Congress and proponents of the PPS believe that this will force hospitals to be more cost-conscious and efficient in their delivery of care.

DRGs are based on medical diagnoses and therefore do not always reflect the amount of nursing time or resources consumed in a particular DRG. Some nurse researchers (Halloran, 1985; Jones, 1987; Prescott, 1986) are now developing methods to measure the amount of nursing intensity within a DRG. These intensity measures take client classification one step further in the determination of nursing resource consumption.

New methods to pay for health care are being developed. The concept of DRGs is being refined so that they can be used to pay physicians and can be applied to other health care settings, such as outpatient clinics. Payment methods other than the traditional fee-for-service method are being explored.

The *fee-for-service* method refers to a fee that is charged for each service, with different fees according to the length and difficulty of the procedure. This fee is paid after the procedure has been done. This is the traditional method of payment for physicians and until World War II was the typical payment method for the majority of nurses. This method is similar to hospital retrospective reimbursement. Another method called *relative value scale* is one that uses a list of the services and procedures performed. Each task or procedure is given an index number that reflects the relative length and difficulty of the task. This index can then be multiplied by a fixed dollar amount to obtain an appropriate fee. Holmes and others (1977) developed a relative value scale for clinical nurse specialists in outpatient settings. Hsiao and others (1988) developed such a scale for the federal government in anticipation of fee schedules' being used to pay physicians for care of Medicare clients.

The *capitation* method pays a set fee for each person enrolled in a program for a certain time. The provider then supplies the services needed and either absorbs the excess costs or keeps the excess monies over the agreed set amount. HMOs and PPOs are examples of capitated delivery entities. This method of payment is the method proposed by ANA to be used in community nursing centers' demonstration projects.

The ANA was successful in getting legislation passed by the 100th Congress that mandates four demonstration projects for delivering nursing care to the elderly on a capitated basis. These projects began in July 1989. On the basis of the outcome of these projects, the federal government will determine whether nurses will be eligible to be paid providers of care to the elderly on a capitated basis. A description of these demonstration projects called community nursing centers is in the ANA publication on organizational models (1987).

SOURCES OF PAYMENT

As stated earlier, sources of payment other than the client are called third-party payers. The federal government became a large third-party payer with the advent of Medicare in 1965.

Medicare is the federal government's acute care health insurance program for people older than 65 years of age. All persons of this age group in the United States are eligible to enroll in the program, regardless of income or health status. The Medicare program, administered by the Health Care Financing Administration, is divided into two parts: Part A, which is hospital insurance (HI), and Part B, which is supplementary medical insurance (SMI) (Table 4–3). The program originally did not cover long-term nursing home care, dental care, or outpatient drugs, but in 1988, the 100th Congress passed legislation (PL 100-360, the Medicare Catastrophic Protection Act) that expanded the program to allow Medicare beneficiaries unlimited free hospitalization after payment of an annual deductible. The new program also would have phased in coverage of a percentage of outpatient drugs (see later). Under this catastrophic protection law, the number of days in a skilled nursing home would have increased to 150 days, and

---

TABLE 4–3 Summary of Federal Medicare Program Benefits

Part A: Hospital Insurance (HI)

Acute hospitalization — 60 d/per episode of illness

Nursing home — 100 d/after hospitalization

Hospice care — 210 d

Home health care — intermittent skilled nursing care

Part B: Supplemental Medical Insurance (SMI)

Physicians' services — enrollee pays first $75, then 20% of reasonable costs

Outpatient clinic services

Laboratory fees

Outpatient drugs (to start 1991)

---

payment would have been allowed even when the person was admitted for care directly from home. Custodial care in a nursing home was not covered in the catastrophic protection law, but a hospice stay would have been fully covered, with home health care covered up to 7 days a week for a maximum of 38 days per year.

From the beginning of Medicare (1965) until 1989, the elderly did not pay any premiums to Medicare for hospital care. The hospitalized enrollee paid only the required deductible amount, which was approximately equal to the cost of 1 day of hospitalization. These new benefits under the catastrophic protection law would have been financed by an amount, initially $4.00 per month, added to the deductible plus an annual income-related premium for Medicare enrollees who had incomes of more than $10,000. This addition, called a surtax, was controversial among the elderly, who started to call for repeal of this law (PL 100-360) in the summer of 1989. This taxing of the elderly users of health care services set a precedent in the United States. All other social benefits of this type have been financed in whole or in part by taxes on the general population or the working population rather than solely the users of the services.

PL 100-360 was repealed by Congress on November 22, 1989, and signed by President George Bush on December 13, 1989. Thus, the elderly were successful in their push to repeal this law. The tactics that they used with Congress, such as jeering supporting senators and representatives and writing numerous letters and making telephone calls condemning their votes, might have a backlash effect in Congress. Many members of Congress stung by this anger have voiced reluctance to address the issue of health care services for the elderly in the near future.

Part B (SMI) of Medicare is optional and requires payment of a monthly premium plus an annual deductible. In 1986, after intensive lobbying by nursing organizations, the 99th Congress added the services of nurse anesthetists to the covered services under Part B. The ANA, in conjunction with other nursing organizations, was successful in persuading the 101st Congress to pass legislation that will allow under Medicare: (1) direct payment to employers of nurse practitioners (NPs), such as clinics and physician groups, for NPs' services provided in nursing homes; and (2) for NPs and clinical nurse specialists, working in collaboration with a physician, to certify and recertify a client's need for skilled nursing care in a nursing home. The inclusion of these categories of nurses is the first time that any nurses have been classified as health care providers paid by the federal government for delivering services.

Blue Cross and Blue Shield and the commercial insurance companies have policies to cover the amounts not paid by Medicare. Sometimes there is abuse associated with these policies, known as *Medigap* policies, that are sold to the elderly. One method of abuse is preying on the elderly person's fear of costly health care and selling them policies that duplicate coverage by Medicare or other insurance.

The *Medicaid* portion of the 1965 Amendments to the Social Security Act established a single program of medical assistance for the poor and extended eligibility to include the medically indigent persons who were not receiving welfare assistance. It is a federal-state matching funding program that requires the state to administer the program and set coverage policies, and therefore it is slightly different in each state. The federal government mandated certain basic services, but left inclusion of additional services to the discretion of the individual states. The federal monetary share of the program depends on the state's per capita income. The 100th Congress expanded Medicaid to cover all pregnant women who have incomes below the poverty level, together with their infants up to 1 year of age. This addition of mandated coverage is an example of incremental policy-making.

In 1989, the 101st Congress amended the Medicaid program to allow for direct payment to certified pediatric and family NPs for the Medicaid serivces provided within the scope of state law regardless of whether the NP is supervised by or associated with a physician.

The Reagan administration encouraged the expansion of Medicare into HMOs and other capitated-type programs. Many demonstration projects are in place to investigate ways to deliver health care to the poor, the elderly, and the disabled in a cost-controlled manner. Nurses have a place in shaping these new forms of delivery settings, as well as being a paid provider in them. Only by understanding how the federal and state governments pay for care and how eligibility for coverage is determined can a nurse be ready to articulate to the government what kind of nursing services can and should be paid for by the government.

Other third-party payers are *insurance companies*. These companies are divided into two groups: the Blue Cross and Blue Shield programs and the commercial insurance companies. These payers generally follow the payment methods initiated by the federal government.

Most insurance companies now pay hospitals on a prospective basis and are watching what the federal government will do to reform the method of payment to physicians. Congress has mandated the Physician Payment Review Commission to study the possibility of changing the method of paying physicians under Medicare. Also included in this examination will be a study of how non–physician health care providers are paid. This commission will also conduct a study, due April 1, 1991, on assistants at surgery. Services of physician assistants in the operating room are reimbursed by Medicare directly to the physician, but services of nurses are not.

ACCESS TO CARE

Access to care has been defined in various ways. It is more than having a physician or a hospital within one's neighborhood. The National Academy of Sciences' Institute of Medicine has stated that access refers to the ability of a group to obtain essential health services in an appropriate manner. This ability is affected by economic, temporal, locational, architectural, cultural, racial, organizational, and informational factors, which may be either barriers or facilitators to obtaining services.

The Senate Labor and Human Resources Committee estimated that in 1987 there were 35 million uninsured or underinsured persons in the United States. These persons delay seeking health care if they do not have the money to pay for it. The necessities of life, such as shelter and food, have a higher priority until these persons' health deteriorates to the point at which they cannot function. Inability to pay for health care can be considered as a barrier to access of care.

Third-party payment influences the client's choice of health care provider. A client's freedom to choose a health care provider is thwarted when only a physician is reimbursed by third-party payers. This loss of freedom to choose is thought to add to the costs of health care. For example, if a client cannot receive nursing services and have them paid for by the third-party payer without those services first being ordered by a physician, the client loses the freedom to choose a nurse as a health care provider. These nursing services range from care in hospitals to care in nursing homes or in clients' homes. In general, to be paid for their services, a nurse must be an employee of the physician or of an institution where a physician can order nursing services. These restrictions in the payment system limit access to health care. Nineteen states have state laws permitting third-party reimbursement for some services performed by nurse practitioners. Implementation of the laws varies from state to state (Pearson, 1989).

Some states have regulations that mandate what types of health care services and how many services can operate in a defined geographic area. With the elimination of the health planning law by the 99th Congress, many states have opted to discontinue or to liberalize their *certificate of need* (CON) programs. These programs were instituted as a means to control the amount spent on facilities or services that were duplicates of existing facilities and services. In general, under a CON program, construction, renovations, and (variably) new services and equipment costing more than a set limit must be approved by a designated state agency. Evidence must be presented that the new or expanded facility or services are needed by the community. Hospitals cannot add new services or beds without meeting this needs assessment. CON can limit the amount and type of services available, thus theoretically ensuring the cost-efficient use of the services and facilities already in place by avoiding their duplication. Staff nurses are often in the best position to evaluate the effects of inadequate facilities, equipment, or technology on client care. Documentation of this need by medical-surgical nurses will aid the institution in gaining permission under the CON program to obtain the needed services or equipment.

QUALITY OF CARE

Quality of care is difficult to define. Yet, all health care providers profess their concern about it. The federal government is interested in the quality of care they pay for—"quality" has thus become a buzz word in health policy. Without defining the term, it becomes even more difficult to measure or evaluate quality. Yet, nurses are involved in delivering quality care at controlled costs. If medical-surgical nurses are unable to define, measure, or evaluate quality, how can they determine when cost-cutting measures are affecting quality?

Many health researchers are now attempting to define, measure, and evaluate quality health care. Client satisfaction and provider satisfaction are important components in this elusive concept. Established determinants of quality of care have been structure and process. Researchers and practitioners now realize that evaluating only the structure within which health care is delivered and the process of delivering health care is not enough. Outcome measures of health care, other than mortality and morbidity, need to be developed. Attempts should be made to analyze care beyond a single point in time and to look at the entire system of health care received by a client. Typically, the quality of care for one stay in a hospital is evaluated by the hospital's quality assurance program. But, clients receive care, often concurrently, from several different providers across a continuum extending from prevention through rehabilitation or chronic care.

The federal government is involved in quality as it reviews care received by beneficiaries in the Medicare program. Reductions in funds for the Medicare program by the federal government are now met with questions about how the cuts will affect the quality of care. Nurses should be able to evaluate medical-surgical nursing care so that they, realistically and with empirical data, can identify when cost-cutting policies diminish the quality of care. Nurses must be the ones who measure and evaluate the quality of the outcome of medical-surgical nursing care.

NURSING CARE PERSONNEL

Supply and Demand

The supply of qualified health care personnel is determined by policies of the government as well as the profession. The number of physicians affects the delivery of health care. Health researchers have demonstrated that the law of supply and demand does not apply to an increased supply of physicians. In economics, the law of supply and demand means that when the demand for an item exceeds its supply, the price of the item goes up. As the price increases, more people are willing to produce the item, which increases the supply. When the supply is plentiful, the price of the item decreases. However, an increase in the number of physicians does not lead to greater access to health care at a lower price. Rather, an increase in the supply of physicians leads to more tests and procedures being ordered, which results in a higher number of return visits by clients. Some researchers think that this increase in the number of tests and procedures and return visits is an attempt by physicians to meet their "target" income (Eastaugh, 1987; Feldstein, 1983).

The supply of nurses has also not followed the commonly accepted law of supply and demand, but for a different reason. Even with a shortage of nurses, salaries have not appreciably increased. Hospitals employ two-thirds of all nurses, and in most hospitals most of these nurses work on medical and surgical units. Increasing wages of hospital nurses will yield only a small increase of available nurses willing to work in a hospital. If a hospital increases salaries for the entire nursing staff, there will be a minuscule return in terms of re-entry of inactive nurses into the available hospital nurse labor pool. Therefore, it is not in the best interest of hospitals to increase nurses' salaries; rather, they purposefully control these salaries at a lower level—but not so low as to lose nurses. In the 1980s, the difference between an entry-level salary and that of an experienced nurse was approximately $7,000. This is called *wage compression.* To retain medical-surgical nurses, hospitals would be advised to spend money on creating careers for nurses within their institutions rather than losing experienced nurses because of wage compression. Hospitals need to evaluate the tradeoff between the high costs of orienting and retraining nurses and the cost of incentives to retain experienced nurses for a career within the facility.

Having only one or few hospitals in an area enables the hospitals to set the number of nurses to be hired and at what salary. If the medical-surgical nurses (sellers of medical-surgical nursing skills and knowledge) are satisfied, they will have to move to another area because the hospitals (buyers of medical-surgical nursing skills and knowledge) control the market. Economists such as Feldstein, Eastaugh, and Sorkin, who have studied the

TABLE 4–4   Cumulative Enrollment for Basic Registered Nurse Programs for 1986–1988

Year	Number of Enrollments	Percentage of Change
1986	193,712	−11.1
1987	182,642	−5.6
1988	181,363	−0.7

Data from American Nurses' Association. (1988). Data compiled by American Nurses' Association and published in Griffith, H. (1989). Capitol commentary. *Nursing Economics, 7,* 162–164.

supply and the salaries of nurses, believe that this occurs because nursing exists in an *oligopsonistic* labor market. An oligopsonistic market is the opposite of a oligopolistic market. An oligopoly occurs when there are few sellers and many buyers. The sellers can determine the price and the amount of the object they are selling. Conversely, in an oligopsonistic market, there are only few buyers and many sellers; therefore, the buyers can determine the price and amount. Hospitals are the buyers of the labor of medical-surgical nurses; medical-surgical nurses are the sellers of their time and skills.

Today, more nurses are working in United States than ever before in the history of the country. The demand for nurses has increased. An increased number of nurses per patient are needed in hospitals, and there are more settings in which a nurse can work. The future supply of nurses will diminish from the current levels because fewer individuals are entering nursing schools, although this trend appears to be stopping (Table 4–4). Thus, in the future, the increased demand for nurses will collide with the decreasing supply of nurses. Seven bills were introduced in the 100th Congress to address this issue. Congress passed and President Reagan signed the 1988 Nurse Education Act into law (PL 100-607), which called for innovative hospital nursing practice models. These demonstration models are to include testing of innovative wage structures and of restructuring of the role of the professional nurse through changes in the composition of hospital staffs so that the larger portion of nurses' time is spent in direct patient care. The Secretary of Health and Human Services mandated a Commission on Nursing to seek long-term and short-term solutions to the nursing shortage. The commission's December 1988 Final Report recommendations were in the following categories: utilization of nursing resources, nurse compensation, health care financing, nurse decision-making, development of nursing resources, and maintenance of nursing resources (Table 4–5).

Credentialing

"Credentialing exists primarily to benefit and protect the public" (Committee for the Study of Credentialing in Nursing, 1979, p. 23). A credential as defined by Webster's *New World Dictionary of the American Language* (1979) is a "certificate given to a person to show

TABLE 4–5   Recommendations of the Secretary of Health and Human Services Commission on Nursing

1. Health care delivery organizations should use the time of registered nurses (RNs) for direct patient care.
2. Health care delivery organizations should adopt innovative staffing patterns that most effectively use the different levels of education and experience of RNs.
3. Health care delivery organizations should use automated information systems and other labor-saving technologies to support nursing.
4. Health care delivery organizations, professional associations, and the government should track nurse staffing, costs, and utilization to better manage nursing resources.
5. Health care delivery organizations should provide a "targeted, one-time increase" in RN wage rates.
6. Government and private payers should reimburse at levels sufficient to recruit and retain *qualified nursing personnel.*
7. Nursing should have a more active role in policy decision-making.
8. Employers of nurses should ensure active nurse representation in administration, governance, and management of their organization.
9. Employers of nurses should foster a professionally collaborative environment among all health care providers.
10. Financial assistance to nursing students should be increased.
11. Nonfinancial barriers to nursing education should be eliminated.
12. Relevant curricula for contemporary and future nursing practices for nursing students should be developed.
13. Nursing must actively promote a positive image of the profession.
14. The Secretary's Commission on Nursing should be extended for no less than 5 years.
15. Support for research and demonstrations on the supply and demand for nursing should be increased.
16. The federal government should develop data sources needed to assess nursing resources.

that he has a right . . . to the exercise of certain position or authority." The requirements for credentialing therefore limit the entry of some individuals or entities into a profession. Types of individual credentialing include educational degrees, licensing, and certification. Accreditation and approval are types of institutional credentialing (Table 4–6).

Educational degrees are titles awarded to individuals who have successfully completed a course of learning. The degree signifies the level achieved and the area in which it was achieved. In nursing, a diploma is awarded after a person finishes a 3-year hospital program, an associate degree (AD or ADN) after a 2-year community college program, a baccalaureate degree (BS or BSN)

TABLE 4–6   Requirements for and Organizations Supplying Various Types of Credentialing

Type of Credentialing	Requirement	By Whom
Individual		
Licensure	Mandatory	Government
Certification	Voluntary	Professional organizations
Institutions		
Approval (licensure)	Mandatory	Government
Accreditation	Voluntary	Private organizations

after a 4-year university program, a master's degree after 2 or 3 years of graduate work (MS or MSN), and a doctoral degree (PhD, DNS, and others) after further graduate study.

Licensure of nurses is controlled by state governments through entities such as state boards of nursing. Licensure grants permission to individuals to engage in a profession and prohibits all others from legally doing so. The requirements for granting a license and what activities the grantee can engage in are spelled out in legislation called nurse practice acts. The first nurse practice act was passed in 1903, and by 1923 all states had nurse practice acts. These acts vary from state to state. Each state's act determines appropriate practice for nurses in that jurisdiction. Mandatory licensure protects the title of nurse and the practice of nursing by prohibiting the use of the title and the practice of nursing by anyone not possessing such a license. Registered nurse and licensed practical nurse are types of individual licenses granted by the states.

Licensure shows that an individual has met minimal standards, which protects the public. Licensure is not to protect the profession and cannot be used to keep certain people out of the profession or to control the supply of professionals.

Certification is a process by which nongovernmental agencies, generally professional organizations, recognize and attest (certify) that certain individuals have met predetermined standards and are deemed to be competent in that area. Certification shows achievement of skills and knowledge above the minimum required by law through licensure. Many nursing organizations have developed certificates for nurses. Table 4–7 gives some certifying organizations for medical-surgical nurses.

Accreditation is a process by which a nongovernmental agency approves and grants accredited status to a health care agency after it meets certain predetermined criteria. The Joint Commission on Accreditation of Healthcare Organizations is the major accrediting body for hospitals. The National League for Nursing is the accrediting body for schools of nursing. Accreditation, similar to certification, attests that the institution has met standards set by a professional organization beyond that required by law. *Approval* is the process by which a health care agency receives permission from the state government to operate after it meets minimal criteria. This is commonly referred to as *state licensure.*

TABLE 4–7   Specialty and Designation of Selected Nursing Certifying Organizations

Organization	Specialty	Designation
AACCN* Certification Corporation	Critical care	CCRN
AORN† Certification Board	Operating room	CNOR
American Board of Occupational Nurses	Occupational health	COHN
American Board of Neurosurgical Nurses	Neurosurgery	CNRN
American Nurses' Association	Medical-surgical	CS, RNC
	Community health	CS, RNC
	Family practice	CS, RNC
	Adult nurse practitioner	CS, RNC
	School nurse	CS, RNC
	Gerontology	CS, RNC
	Other specialties	CS, RNC
	Nursing administration	CNAA, CNA
Board of Nephrology Examiners	Nephrology	CHN
Emergency Nurses Association	Emergency department	CEN

* American Association of Critical-Care Nurses.
† Association of Operating Room Nurses.

IMPLICATIONS OF THE CHANGING HEALTH CARE DELIVERY SYSTEM FOR NURSES AND NURSING

HOSPITALS

Hospitals are responding to the changes in health care financing by becoming medical or hospital centers. By diversifying, hospitals can generate income from activities other than simply delivering hospital care to clients. More hospitals are developing and marketing services other than inpatient care. Some of these services are ones that other professionals or entities provide. Hospitals are acquiring HMOs, developing surgicenters, operating home health care agencies and day care centers for children and adults, or providing educational sessions for providers and support classes to the community. In some areas, hospitals are joining with other hospitals to operate medical supply companies, laundry facilities, or parking garages. This movement into noncare, but related, services enables hospitals to bring in monies from other sources.

To control costs, the trend in health care financing is to pay for care delivered in settings other than the expensive inpatient institutions. This movement out of institutions has reduced the number of clients with less acute illnesses who receive care in hospitals. It is expensive to have hospital beds available without patients in them. Increasingly, clients in hospitals have shorter lengths of stay, with an increased level of acuity of care. In other words, clients in hospitals have more severe illnesses but are staying for shorter times. This situation has become known as "quicker and sicker." These changes have a direct impact on the medical-surgical nurse in the hospital. The nurse-to-client ratio is much higher than in the past; the ratio changed from about 50 nurses to 100 clients in the 1970s to approximately 90 nurses to 100 clients today.

INNOVATIVE PRACTICE MODELS OF NURSING

Some hospital nursing service administrators are meeting this change with *innovative practice models of nursing*. By changing the mode of delivering nursing care, nursing departments are enhancing the delivery of professional medical-surgical nursing care. These models of care delivery are varied and have been adapted for the individual hospital. Most newer models are based on differentiated practice, with different nurses having different roles, and are based on the method and amount of control that the nurse has for delivery of nursing care, such as shared governance. An assessment-based approach or an education-based approach can be used to decide what role a nurse will assume. An assessment-based approach considers many criteria, including experience, preference, and ability, whereas an education-based approach uses academic preparation as the means to differentiate roles.

These new modes of delivery have various titles: collaborative practice, case management, Partners-in-Practice, and other combinations of words to indicate a different method to deliver nursing care. Mayer et al. (1990) have compiled a collection of articles describing many different models in their book *Patient Care Delivery Models*.

According to York and Fecteau (1987), one of the new models, called the *professional practice model of nursing care*, results in greater job satisfaction, decreased turnover of registered nurses, improved quality of care, and increased productivity. York and Fecteau reported that Johns Hopkins Hospital has used this practice model in three different medical-surgical nursing care units: an inpatient unit, emergency room, and operating rooms. The elements necessary for the success of the professional practice model are autonomy of nursing practice, decentralized responsibility for decision-making, and compensation practices consistent with the professional delivery of nursing care. Rather than having an established hierarchy of nursing administration, the staff nurses exercise authority in deciding among themselves who will work what hours and when. If there are many clients, the staff responds by working more hours. If the workload is light, the staff decides who will not work. If at the end of the budget year there are monies not spent because of conscious cost-effective efforts, the nurses as a group decide how to spend the funds. This expenditure can range from bonuses for the nurses to purchases of pieces of equipment for the unit that the nurses want.

The underlying principle in a professional model of practice is the assumption of authority by the professional staff nurses to make decisions about the administration of the unit and the delivery of care to clients, such as determining staffing levels and scheduling, assuring coverage, assessing performance, and disciplining peers when necessary. Primary nursing can be enhanced by group participation in the development and monitoring of standards of practice. This responsibility can be extended to home and community health agencies through outreach programs to promote continuity of care. Peer review gives staff nurses control over the level of performance of group members and a mechanism for providing feedback. York and Fecteau reported that a unit using the professional practice model consistently provided a higher number of hours of care per day than a comparable unit using a traditional model of nursing practice. Nurses are paid an annual salary rather than an hourly wage. This practice model requires the medical-surgical staff nurse delivering nursing care to be a responsible, educated professional rather than just a salaried employee of the hospital.

BILLING FOR NURSING CARE

Until recently, the cost for nursing services was included in the room rate on the client's bill, along with house-

THE UNIVERSITY OF ROCHESTER STRONG MEMORIAL HOSPITAL
601 ELMWOOD AVENUE, ROCHESTER, NEW YORK 14642
PATIENT ACCOUNTS OFFICE—OFFICE HOURS 9:30 AM–4:00 PM
Area Code—716-275-3351

PLEASE REFER TO
BILLING NUMBER
WHEN CONTACTING

THE PATIENT
ACCOUNTS OFFICE

BILLING NUMBER	ADMITTED	DISCHARGED	DAYS IN HOSPITAL	BILLING DATE	F.C.	PAGE
053158941327	06/04/86	06/12/86	8	06/19/86	20	1

PATIENT DOE, JOHN

BILL TO DOE, JOHN
25 SIMPSON AVE.
ROCHESTER, NY 14618

INSURANCE ROCH BLUE CROSS	POLICY NUMBER V 316729-10

DATE OF SERVICE	PROCEDURE CODE	DESCRIPTION	NO. OF SERVICES RENDERED	TOTAL CHARGES	INSURANCE NO. 1	INSURANCE NO. 2	PATIENT AMOUNT
		SUMMARY BY SERVICE					
		ROOM-PRIVATE	6	1326.00			
		ROOM-ICU	2	920.00			
	010	DIAGNOSTIC RADIOLOG	8	344.00			
	012	OPERATING ROOM	30	3189.94			
	014	ANESTHESIOLOGY	46	905.10			
	015	RESP. THERAPY	12	580.30			
	020	PHARMACY	08	436.45			
	022	BLOOD BANK	8	153.00			
	025	SOLUTIONS	2	28.10			
	026	SPECIAL EQUIP	1	8.00			
	027	MICROBIOLOGY	1	13.00			
	030	HEMATOLOGY LAB	16	166.60			
	038	CLINICAL LABS	26	413.20			
	39/31	SPECIAL LABS	1	28.20			
	040	HEART STATION	6	216.00			
	600	NURSING CARE	8	1434.00			
		PAYMENTS	1	217.00 −			
		TOTAL DUE		10161.89			
		TOTAL RECEIPTS		217.00 −			
		NET SUMMARY TOTALS		9944.89			

THIS IS THE ONLY DETAILED BILL YOU WILL RECEIVE WITHOUT AN ADDITIONAL CHARGE
— PLEASE SAVE FOR YOUR RECORDS —

INSURANCE BENEFITS ARE ESTIMATED
AND MAY BE ADJUSTED UPON RECEIPT OF THE FINAL INSURANCE PAYMENT

TOTAL CHARGES LESS CREDITS	10161.89	9975.89		31.00 −

DETACH AND RETURN THIS PORTION WITH YOUR PAYMENT

| DOE, JOHN

PATIENT NAME	053158941327 BILLING NUMBER	06/04/86 ADMITTED	06/12/86 DISCHARGED	06/19/86 BILLING DATE	31.00 − PATIENT BALANCE

YOU MAY RECEIVE SEPARATE BILLS FROM YOUR PHYSICIANS, INCLUDING RADIOLOGIST AND ANESTHESIOLOGIST.
THE RED CROSS SUPPLIES BLOOD WITHOUT COST. HOWEVER, THERE IS A SERVICE CHARGE FOR THE PROCESSING AND ADMINISTRATION OF BLOOD.

⬆ AMOUNT DUE WITHIN 30 DAYS

MAKE CHECKS PAYABLE TO: **STRONG MEMORIAL HOSPITAL**

Figure 4–1

See legend on opposite page.

keeping and dietary services. No one, including the hospital administrator and the nursing administrator, knew how much money was produced by delivering nursing care. Several hospitals are now *costing-out nursing services.* Edwardson and Giovannetti (1987) reviewed different cost-accounting methods used to cost-out nursing services. Costing-out requires nursing to define nursing care, to measure it, and to document when and to whom this care is given. This care then has a dollar amount attached to it, which shows up on the client's hospital bill as the price charged for nursing care. By costing-out nursing services, the hospital can then know the total amount brought into the institution for nursing care. At least 95% of the clients in a hospital are there because they need nursing care. The advantage to costing-out nursing services is the enhanced value attached to a service that brings in revenues rather than showing up solely as a cost. Figure 4-1 is a sample hospital bill illustrating costing-out of nursing care.

NONHOSPITAL CARE SETTINGS

Clients are being discharged from the hospital more rapidly, as evidenced by the decreasing length of stay, and the need for home care services is increasing. For recently discharged clients, Medicare pays for skilled nursing care in the home for a short time. Other third-party payers also pay for home care services for a defined period. Some clients discharged from the hospital still need complex technologic care. For example, clients who still require intravenous therapy for antibiotics, chemotherapy, or parenteral nutrition are being discharged. This increased use of home care services for such complex care creates an opportunity for medical-surgical nurses to work in settings other than hospitals.

The current trend is to pay for care in the least expensive setting. Some treatments and care that were traditionally administered in hospitals can now be delivered in nonhospital settings. Insurance companies are hiring nurses to assist in deciding which least expensive setting can be used. This is an excellent opportunity for medical-surgical nurses to function in an expanded role. Changes in the health care delivery system also bring changes in the traditional role of the nurse. It is limiting for a nurse to think that he or she can practice medical-surgical nursing only in an acute care hospital. The possibilities for practice settings for a medical-surgical nurse are limited only by nurses' visions and creative abilities.

HOW TO CHANGE THE HEALTH CARE DELIVERY SYSTEM

Entire books are devoted to how policies and laws are made. A few hints are given here about how a medical-surgical nurse can influence health policy. To do this, it is necessary to understand how health care policies are made and implemented. Policies can be informal or formal. *Formal policies* are those that are written, like rules, regulations, and laws. *Informal policies* are those done by custom or tradition and are usually more difficult to change. Most of the time, these informal policies are changed after a long battle and institution of a formal policy, or they are changed incrementally, a little at a time. It has become essential for nurses to become involved in the legislative process. Nurses are also becoming politically aware and are participating in the political process of elections, which helps nurses to influence elected officials. But, what happens after a law gets passed or a congressperson gets elected? Who ensures that the law or policy is implemented in the desired form? Nurses have not been vigilant about following up these activities during the phases of rules and regulations and oversight.

HOW HEALTH CARE POLICIES ARE MADE

Before any action is taken, an issue should be put on the "public agenda" (see the accompanying illustration). Placing an issue on the public agenda requires actions that bring the concern to the attention of policy-makers and the public, so that people other than those affected by the situation are aware of the issue and its consequences. The elderly have been effective in putting their concerns about costs of health care for elderly people with fixed incomes on the public agenda. They have banded together in groups, such as the American Association of Retired Persons, Gray Panthers, and even groups within their condominiums, to publicize their issues. They endorse and work for political candidates who support their concerns, give newspaper interviews, and contact legislators (local, state, and federal). In turn, other segments of the public adopt their concerns and contact policy-makers in an attempt to influence these programs. In the past, these activities produced changes

Figure 4–1

A sample itemized hospital bill illustrating costing-out of nursing care. (From Sovie, M. D., & Smith, T. C. [1986]. Pricing the nursing product: Charging for nursing care. *Nursing Economics, 4,* 224.)

in the Medicare program, and today there are attempts to amend that program to cover nursing home care and home care.

Any civics textbook will outline the legislative process to demonstrate how an idea becomes a law. It is important to know not only this process, but also what actors are involved in the process: opponents and potential opponents, as well as the proponents and those who will remain neutral on the issue. It is also necessary to identify and become familiar with the arena in which the action will take place, as well as the socioeconomic climate of the times. For example, financial support from the federal government for nursing education programs will not be a priority in congress during a stock-market crisis or a legislative battle to balance the budget by cutting funds. This assessment of the players, arena, and climate will help astute medical-surgical nurses know whether to become more active about health care policy matters or to maintain a "holding pattern." These same principles apply whether nurses want to influence federal policies, state policies, or hospital policies.

A crucial factor that is often difficult for nurses to realize is that opponents on one issue may be allies on another issue. Many times physicians and nurses are allies when pushing for health care policies but are opponents on those issues that limit direct access and payment for nursing services. This is also true of legislators and bureaucrats. Thus, one rule in policy-making is that those opposing you today may be your allies on another issue tomorrow.

After a bill is passed and signed into law, rules and regulations to implement that law are written and published for public comments. Changes in rules and regulations that implement laws are published by the executive branch of the government, at both federal and state levels. The proposed changes are published in a government document called the *Federal Register* at the national level and in a similar register at the state level. After time for public comments to be submitted, the rules and regulations are promulgated, either as published or revised. Laws are written in broad language; the rules and regulations to implement the law are written more specifically. Rules and regulations can be revised without changing the original law.

HOW MEDICAL-SURGICAL NURSES CAN INFLUENCE HEALTH CARE POLICIES

Influencing a change or a creation of a new policy begins when there is familiarity with the way laws, rules, and regulations are made. To influence a change, one should also have familiarity with the socioeconomic, political, and health care players and arena surrounding an issue. Medical-surgical nurses can influence legislators by testifying as experts on the issue, by lobbying governmental officials, and by building coalitions with other groups interested in the issue. To do this, it is important to establish personal contacts and build relationships with policy-makers. The nursing administrator, the city

council representative, the state legislator, or the congressperson will be more receptive to someone they know and respect than to a stranger. It is important for medical-surgical nurses to be skilled clinicians, but clinical skills alone will not influence policy. Nurses have expert interpersonal skills that they exercise with clients; these skills can be used in the policy arena as well.

Policies are changed incrementally rather than in one massive step. In the past, nurses have accepted these incremental changes as given, without analyzing the additive effect of all the small changes. Aware nurses will recognize the effects of the incremental changes and will support them or influence their direction. Medical-surgical nurses are responsible for the policies affecting nursing care.

SUMMARY

The term or concept of a health care delivery system was not used in the United States or elsewhere before the mid-1960s. The changes and impact of the delivery system on health care, especially medical-surgical nursing care, that have occurred in the last two decades have been tremendous.

The manner in which hospitals developed and now operate has affected the domain of medical-surgical nursing practice within them. Hospitals are reacting to new financial arrangements. Medical-surgical nurses can no longer practice to their fullest while being ignorant about who pays for care, how much and what type of care is paid for, and how to influence these arrangements.

This chapter reviewed the variety of health care delivery settings. It detailed the evolution of care settings from hospitals to the current use of the least expensive setting possible for the needed care. It also discussed the tension among quality of care, access to care, and cost of care. Nursing is responding to the changes in the health care delivery system by costing-out nursing care, creating innovative models of nursing practice, and becoming effective in influencing health care policy-making. Medical-surgical nurses have a role in health policy-making.

IMPLICATIONS FOR RESEARCH

Decision-makers are more likely to respond to an issue when empirical data are presented. Medical-surgical nurses have expert opinions about health care policies but have been slow to demonstrate factual support from empirical research for these opinions.

Selected areas within the health care delivery system

HOW FORMAL HEALTH CARE POLICIES ARE MADE

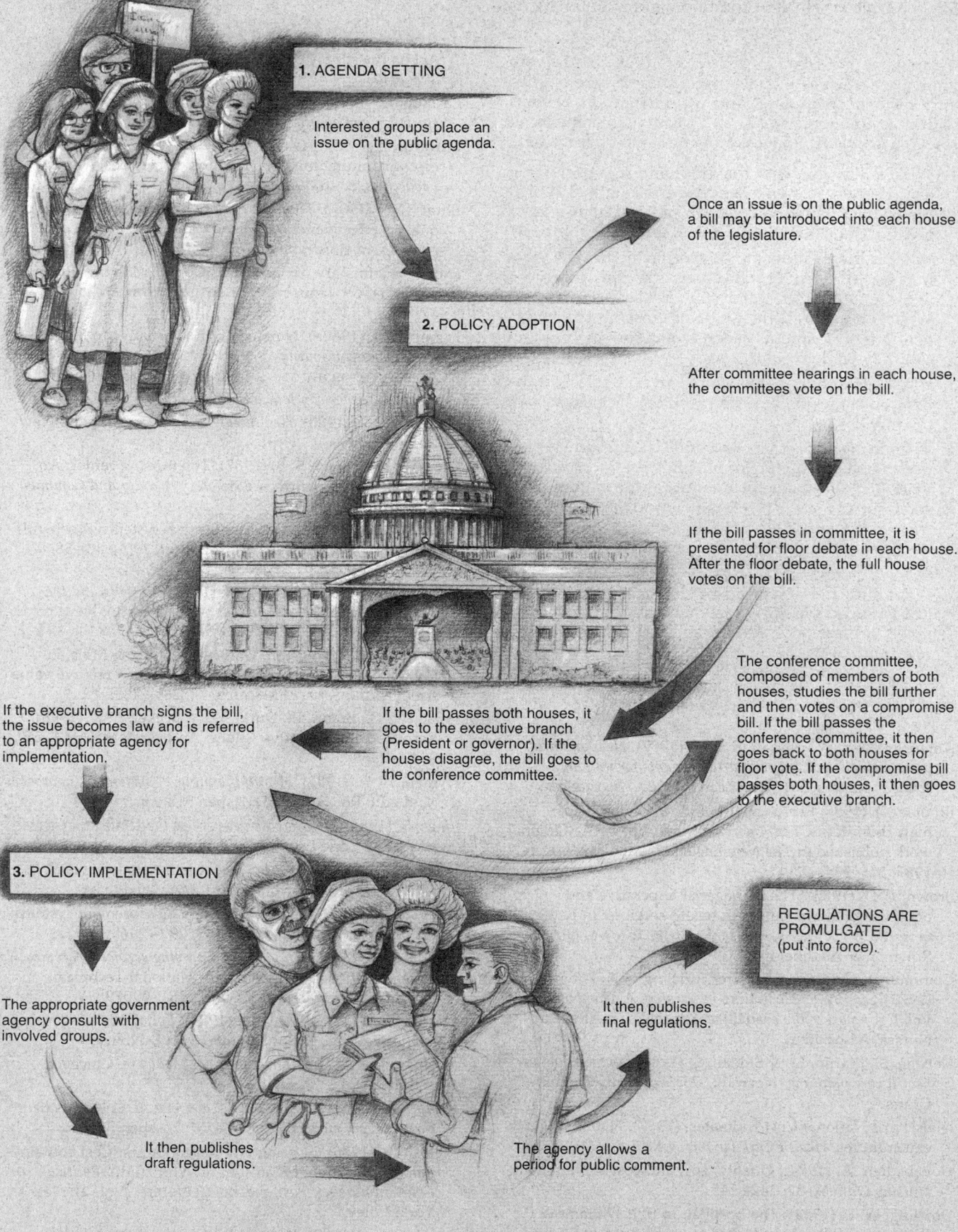

1. AGENDA SETTING

Interested groups place an issue on the public agenda.

Once an issue is on the public agenda, a bill may be introduced into each house of the legislature.

2. POLICY ADOPTION

After committee hearings in each house, the committees vote on the bill.

If the bill passes in committee, it is presented for floor debate in each house. After the floor debate, the full house votes on the bill.

The conference committee, composed of members of both houses, studies the bill further and then votes on a compromise bill. If the bill passes the conference committee, it then goes back to both houses for floor vote. If the compromise bill passes both houses, it then goes to the executive branch.

If the bill passes both houses, it goes to the executive branch (President or governor). If the houses disagree, the bill goes to the conference committee.

If the executive branch signs the bill, the issue becomes law and is referred to an appropriate agency for implementation.

3. POLICY IMPLEMENTATION

The appropriate government agency consults with involved groups.

It then publishes draft regulations.

The agency allows a period for public comment.

It then publishes final regulations.

REGULATIONS ARE PROMULGATED (put into force).

that require more data from medical-surgical nurses are innovative practice models, need for and type of support systems for nurses, and documentation systems with measurement of cost and quality inherent in all research activities. Some specific research questions are

1. What is the impact of the different types of nursing care delivery systems on cost and quality? Which model of nursing practice can provide high-quality medical-surgical nursing care at an acceptable cost?

2. What is the relationship of specific medical-surgical nursing interventions to specific patient outcomes (e.g., length of hospital stay, readmission rates)? What is the cost/benefit ratio of those nursing interventions and patient outcomes and in which setting can they be delivered?

3. What mix of nursing personnel gives the desired patient outcomes for a certain medical-surgical patient mixture?

4. What is the impact of a reduction of support personnel on cost and quality of nursing care, including the workload, use, and effectiveness of the medical-surgical nursing staff? What nonclinical support activities are being done by medical-surgical nurses and what impact does this have on nursing care and patient outcomes?

5. What is the most effective and time-conserving medical-surgical nursing documentation system that meets professional, legislative, and reimbursement requirements?

REFERENCES AND READINGS

American Nurses' Association Staff. (1987). *New organizational models and financial arrangements for nursing services.* Kansas City: American Nurses' Association.

Brooten, D. (1988, February). RN followup plan helps high-risk infants. *The American Nurse,* pp. 4, 14. (Original work published in *The New England Journal of Medicine,* 1987, *315,* 934–939)

Brown, L. D. (1985). The managerial imperative and organizational innovation in health services. In E. Ginzberg (Ed.), *The U.S. health care system.* Totowa, NJ: Rowman & Allanheld.

Committee for the Study of Credentialing in Nursing. (1979). *Study of credentialing in nursing: A new approach: Vol. I. A report of the committee.* Kansas City: American Nurses' Association.

Debella, S., Martin, L., & Siddall, S. (1986). *Nurse's role in health care planning.* Norwalk, CT: Appleton-Century-Crofts.

Division of National Cost Estimates. (1987). National health expenditures. *Health Care Financing Review, 8*(4), 1–36.

Donabedian, A. (1984). Quality, cost and cost containment. *Nursing Outlook, 32,* 142–145.

Dowling, W. L. (1984). The hospital. In S. J. Williams & P. R. Torrens (Eds.), *Introduction to health services* (2nd ed.). New York: Wiley.

Eastaugh, S. R. (1985). The impact of the Nurse Training Act on the supply of nurses, 1974–1983. *Inquiry, 22,* 404–417.

Eastaugh, S. R. (1987). *Financing health care: Economic efficiency and equity.* Dover, MA: Auburn House.

Edwardson, S. R., & Giovannetti, P. B. (1987). A review of cost-accounting methods for nursing services. *Nursing Economics, 5,* 107–117.

Ehrat, K. S. (1987). The cost-quality balance: An analysis of quality, effectiveness, efficiency, and cost. *Journal of Nursing Administration, 17*(5), 6–13.

Executive summary of Secretary's Commission on Nursing report. (1989, January–February). *Nursing Economics, 7,* 57–59.

Fagin, C. M. (1982a). Nursing as an alternative to high-cost care. *American Journal of Nursing, 82,* 56–60.

Fagin, C. M. (1982b). The economic value of nursing research. *American Journal of Nursing, 82,* 1844–1849.

Feldstein, P. J. (1983). *Health care economics* (2nd ed.). New York: Wiley.

Gloss, E. F., & Fielo, S. B. (1987). The nursing center: An alternative for health care delivery. *Family and Community Health, 10*(2), 49–58.

Haas, S. A. (1988). Patient classification systems: A self-fulfilling prophecy. *Nursing Management, 19*(5), 56–58, 60–62.

Hawkins, J. W., & Higgins, L. P. (1989). *Nursing and the American health care delivery system* (3rd ed.). New York: Tiresias Press.

Holmes, G. C., Livingston, G., Bassett, R. E., & Mills, E. (1977). Nurse clinician productivity using a relative value scale. *Health Services Research, 12,* 269–283.

Hsiao, W. C., Braun, P., Dunn, D., & Becker, E. R. (1988). Resource-based relative values: An overview. *JAMA, 260,* 2347–2360.

Hyman, H. H. (1982). *Health planning: A systematic approach* (2nd ed.). Rockville, MD: Aspen Systems.

Jonas, S. (1986). *Health care delivery in the United States* (3rd ed.). New York: Springer.

Jones, C. O. (1977). *An introduction to the study of public policy* (2nd ed.). North Scituate, MA: Duxbury.

Jones, K. R. (1987). Severity of illness measurement systems: An update. *Nursing Economics, 5,* 292–296.

Lampe, S. (1987). *Costing hospital nursing services: A review of the literature.* Springfield, VA: National Technical Information Services. (NTIS No. HRP-0907983)

MacRae, D., Jr., & Wilde, J. A. (1979). *Policy analysis for public decisions.* North Scituate, MA: Duxbury.

Marmor, T. R. (1973). *The politics of Medicare.* Chicago: Aldine.

Mayer, G. G., Madden, M. J., & Lawrenz, E. (1990). *Patient care delivery models.* Rockville, MD: Aspen Systems.

Melosh, B. (1986). Nursing and Reaganomics: Cost containment in the United States. In R. White (Ed.), *Political issues in nursing: Past, present and future:* (Vol. 2). New York: Wiley.

Pearson, L. J. (1989). How each state stands on legislative issues affecting advanced nursing practice. *Nurse Practitioner, 14*(1), 27–34.

Poulin, M. A. (1985). Configurations of nursing practice. *Issues in professional nursing practice* (Vol. 5). Kansas City: American Nurses' Association.

Sorensen, G. E. (Ed). (1985). *The economics of health care and nursing.* Kansas City: American Academy of Nursing.

Sorkin, A. L. (1984). *Health economics: An introduction* (2nd ed.). Lexington, MA: Lexington Books.

Sovie, M. D., & Smith, T. C. (1986). Pricing the nursing product: Charging for nursing care. *Nursing Economics, 4,* 216–226.

Starling, G. (1979). *The politics and economics of public policy.* Homewood, IL: Dorsey.

Werley, H. H., & Weatlake, S. K. (1985). Impact of nursing research on public policy. *Journal of Professional Nursing, 1,* 148–156.

Wilson, F. A., & Neuhauser, D. (1982). *Health services in the United States* (2nd ed.). Cambridge MA: Ballinger.

York, C., & Fecteau, D. L. (1987). Innovative models for professional nursing practice. *Nursing Economics, 5,* 162–166.

ADDITIONAL READINGS

Halloran, E. J. (1985). Nursing workload, medical diagnosis related groups, and nursing diagnoses. *Research in Nursing & Health, 8,* 421–433.

This article reports on an investigation of the amount of time nurses spent to care for clients who were classified by 37 nursing diagnoses and 383 DRGs. Halloran found that nursing work is better predicted by nursing diagnosis than by either DRG or demographic characteristics. He concluded that the client's nursing condition played a more important part in nursing decisions about various amounts of nursing care provided than did the client's medical condition. Nurses gave various amounts of nursing care to clients with the same medical condition, and most of this variation was explained by the client's nursing condition. The provision of nursing services and nurse staffing recommendations should be based on a reliable and valid measure of nursing.

McClain, J. R., & Selhart, M. S. (1984). Twenty cases: What nursing costs per DRG. *Nursing Management, 15*(10), 26–29.

This article presents the results of an examination of charts of 20 clients in two DRGs to determine the amount of time spent on direct and indirect nursing care.

Prescott, P. A. (1986). DRG prospective reimbursement: The nursing intensity factor. *Nursing Management, 17*(1), 43–44, 46, 48.

Results of a 1-year study in two DRGs at a 409-bed community hospital are reported. Prescott points out that because nursing represents such a sizable portion of the total hospital budget, if nursing costs are underestimated by prospective pricing, the hospital could be placed in such financial jeopardy that the quality of care could suffer. If prospective pricing overestimates or inaccurately distributes nursing costs, it would not accomplish its intended purpose of economizing operations to stabilize costs.

UNIT 1 RESOURCES

Nursing Resources

American Academy of Nurse Practitioners (AANP), 179 Princeton Boulevard, Lowell, MA 01851. Telephone 508-937-7343.

Promotes high standards of health care and serves as a forum to enhance the identity and continuity of nurse practitioners. Publishes the *Journal of the American Academy of Nurse Practitioners* (quarterly) and *Academy Update* (monthly newsletter).

American Association of Occupational Health Nurses (AAOHN), 50 Lenox Pointe, Atlanta, GA 30324. Telephone 404-262-1162; 800-241-8014.

Promotes occupational health nursing. Maintains its professional integrity. Enhances its professional status. Focuses on four areas to achieve those goals: professional affairs, governmental affairs, membership, and public affairs. Publishes *AAOHN Journal* (monthly) and *AAOHN News* (newsletter).

American Nurses' Association (ANA), 2420 Pershing Road, Kansas City, MO 64108. Telephone 816-474-5720.

Interacts with congressional representatives on behalf of nurses. Sets professional and educational standards on behalf of the profession. Publishes the *American Journal of Nursing* (monthly) and *The American Nurse* (newspaper, 10 times yearly).

American Nurses' Foundation (ANF), 2420 Pershing Road, Kansas City, MO 64108. Telephone 816-474-5720.

Serves as the research and trust arm of the American Nurses' Association. Receives tax-deductible contributions for nursing research from private donors. Publishes *SCAN* (newsletter) and *FOCUS* (biennial summary report).

National Association of Physician Nurses (NAPN), 900 South Washington Street, Suite G-13, Falls Church, VA 22046. Telephone 703-237-8616.

Promotes professional stature of nurses who choose to be affiliated with the medical profession through continuing education. Publishes *The Nightingale* (monthly newsletter).

National League for Nursing (NLN), 10 Columbus Circle, New York, NY 10019. Telephone 212-582-1022.

Promotes improved quality of health care through education and accreditation. Publishes *Nursing and Health Care* and many other print and video resources.

National Student Nurses' Association (NSNA), 555 West 57th Street, Suite 1325, New York, NY 10019. Telephone 212-581-2211.

Serves as a forum for student nurses at the institutional (school), state, and national levels. Fosters the development of leadership skills. Publishes *IMPRINT* (magazine, five times yearly) and *NSNA News* (newsletter).

North American Nursing Diagnosis Association (NANDA), St. Louis University School of Nursing, 3525 Caroline Street, St. Louis, MO 63104. Telephone 314-577-8954.

Develops, refines, and promotes a taxonomy of nursing diagnostic terminology of general use to professional nurses. Publishes *NANDA Newsletter* (monthly).

Visiting Nurse Associations of America (VNAA), 3801 East Florida Avenue, Suite 806, Denver, CO 80210. Telephone 303-629-8622; 800-426-2547.

Provides quality health care regardless of the client's ability to pay as an organization of community-based and community-supported nonprofit health care providers. Publishes *VNAA Voice* (biennial newsletter).

UNIT 2

Biopsychosocial Concepts Related to Health Care

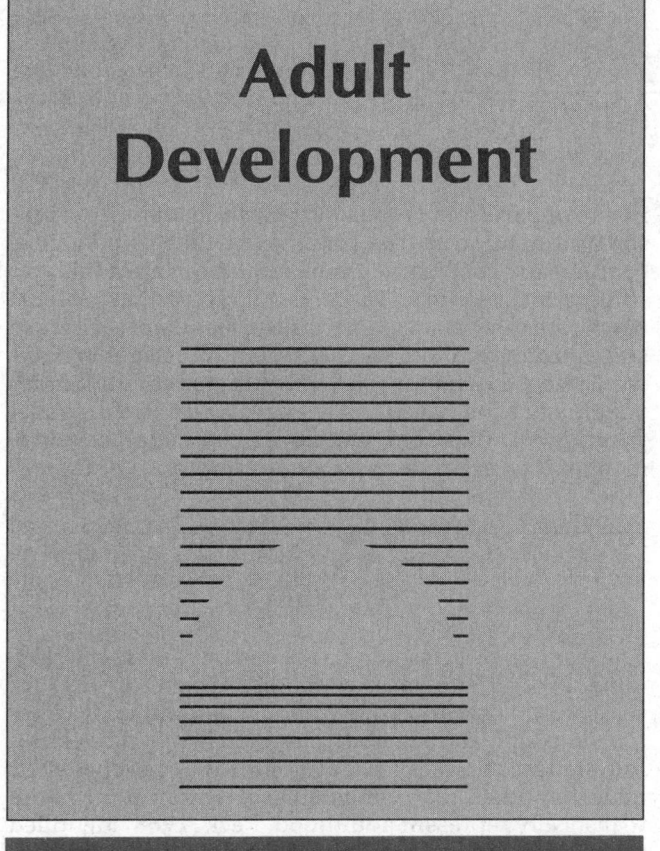

CHAPTER 5

Adult Development

Adulthood is a time of change. The many decades in the adult years do not allow a simple, linear progression toward decline, but rather are a complex setting for a myriad of changes and growth processes. Not all change need be negative, but it generally requires shifts in how one defines the situation, one's self, and one's interactions and relationships with others. The alterations in both body and mind that occur with aging require adjustments in behavior, emotional responses, and patterns of handling life's problems.

With so much change occurring, adulthood is not a time to drift; it is a time for careful self-direction. The responses that young adult people make to age changes and environmental changes largely determine in old age their way of thinking, behaving, and feeling and their outlook on life. Adverse results are the case when wise choices are not made in young adulthood. On the other hand, if people, throughout adulthood, use careful thought and patient effort to direct their responses to changes in themselves and their environments, they can have a great impact on the course of their own aging. The changes and opportunities of adulthood present a challenge to the individual to maintain health and wellness.

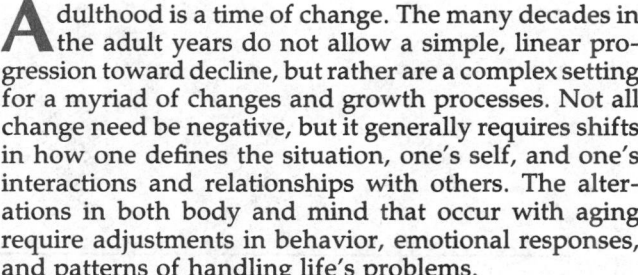

THEORIES OF ADULT DEVELOPMENT

In modern society, adolescence seems to fade gradually into adulthood. Adulthood is commonly described as having its onset at some indeterminate point after the individual achieves physical maturity. In contrast to earlier periods of the life cycle, which are clearly demarcated by specific physiologic and psychologic events, adulthood has so far defied all attempts to establish objective landmarks that would precisely characterize its onset or its stages.

It is undeniable that people share certain traits with respect to age and the rate of physical and psychologic maturation; nevertheless, many differences arise as a consequence of such factors as heredity, sex, medical history, and life experience. Accordingly, designating the arbitrary ages of 20, 40, and 60 years as the demarcations of maturity, middle age, and senescence has promoted a stereotypic view rather than a true understanding of the stages of adulthood. There is, perhaps, some merit in using chronologic age as an index for measuring change and for studying progressive and sequential transitions during the course of a human life. Age, in years, may indicate that several social milestones have passed (Fig. 5-1). Advancing age may indicate that a greater amount of wear and tear has resulted simply because a person has lived longer. Years may

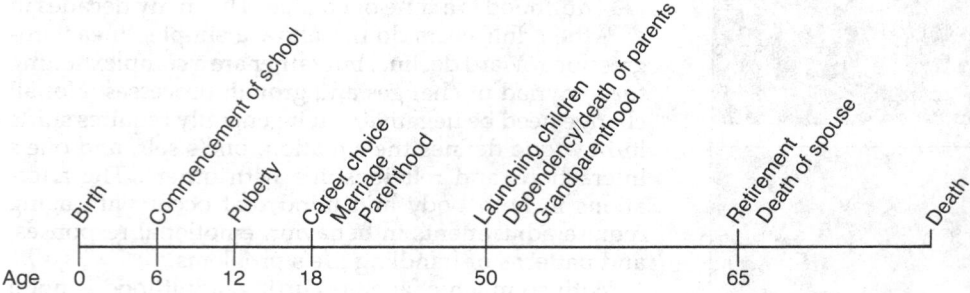

Figure 5–1

Chronologic age may indicate that several social milestones have occurred. These age demarcations are approximate because many differences may arise.

reflect an accumulation of experience, biologic change, or the evolution of different perspectives on life. As one ages, an awareness of the lengthening of past life and the shortening of future years forces a new consideration of life's meaning.

Stereotypes inevitably break down as one experiences reality, and this is no less so for groups labeled as mature, middle aged, and old. As with other age groups, there is great variability in perception and responses as a result of numerous intrinsic variables present and extrinsic influences imposed from conception and continuing throughout life. The frequent disparity among the dimensions of chronologic, psychologic, and physiologic age has led to the folkloric observation that a person is as old or as young as he/she feels. All of the foregoing considerations attest to the difficulty of establishing the origin of stages of adulthood and of identifying individual and species-specific variations. Still essentially unanswered, for example, are the fundamental questions of which events herald the beginning of the various stages of adulthood, how the rate of aging is modified by genetic and environmental factors, and, more important, what the nature of maturation is and what the mechanisms are by which aging affects the living organisms at molecular, cellular, and organismic levels. Without these answers, a single theory explaining changes during adulthood has been difficult to construct. Thus, a plethora of theories have been advanced, each representing the view of a specific discipline.

ERIKSON'S EIGHT "STAGES OF MAN"

Developmental theories imply that certain psychologic growth mechanisms can be ascribed to various ages. Most of the early theories did not delineate specific expectations for the adult person. Before Freud, little thought was given to the components of sound psychologic development at any age. The emphasis placed on early psychosocial development, by Freud and his followers, as the foundation for the later psychologic patterns has served to sensitize psychologists to the notion of an unfolding developmental process. Even though Freud viewed aging as a process restricted by early childhood development, few students of human behavior today would agree that psychologic make-up is totally fixed early in life. Erikson (1968b) was one of the

first to depart from Freud's position and attracted widespread attention to the proposition that personalities continue to evolve throughout adult life in a gradual, yet continuous, manner. Table 5–1 presents the specific developmental stages and tasks of each of Erikson's stages from birth to death. The first four stages of Erikson largely expand on Freud's stages of childhood development. The last four stages provide a useful model for understanding some general issues of adult development and changes during the adult years.

PECK'S DEVELOPMENTAL TASKS OF ADULTHOOD

The last two of Erikson's stages encompass all the middle adult and late years of the life cycle. To many researchers, this conceptualization of adulthood seems too simplistic and general. Using Erikson's model as a foundation, numerous developmental psychologists have hypothesized refinements that they think more realistically represent adulthood. Peck (1968) identified seven crucial developmental tasks for the last two periods of the life cycle (middlescence and late adulthood) (Table 5–2). Peck hypothesized that there are four crucial tasks in middlescence and three tasks in old age that must be confronted for healthy adjustment.

TABLE 5–1   Developmental Tasks of Erikson's Psychosocial Stages

Stage	Developmental Task
Infant	Basic trust versus basic mistrust
Toddler	Autonomy versus shame and doubt
Preschooler	Initiative versus guilt
School-ager	Industry versus inferiority
Adolescent	Identity versus role confusion
Young adult	Intimacy versus isolation
Middlescent	Generativity versus stagnation
Older adult	Ego integrity versus despair

TABLE 5–2   Peck's Developmental Tasks of Adulthood

Period of Life Cycle	Developmental Task
Middlescence	Valuing wisdom versus valuing physical powers
	Socializing versus sexualizing in human relationships
	Cathectic flexibility versus cathectic impoverishment
	Mental flexibility versus mental rigidity
Old age	Ego differentiation versus work-role preoccupation
	Body transcendence versus body preoccupation
	Ego transcendence versus ego preoccupation

HAVIGHURST'S THEORY OF ADULT DEVELOPMENTAL TASKS

Havighurst's (1972) ideas have contributed to the understanding of adult development in the American culture. His theory has a broad definition of successful aging that addresses social competency and flexibility of adaptation to new roles. He viewed developmental tasks as a continual discovery of new and meaningful roles. He divided the life cycle into six age periods, each containing 6 to 10 developmental tasks. The tasks for the adult periods are summarized in Table 5–3.

THEORIES OF AGING

BIOLOGIC THEORIES

Biologists exploring the phenomena of aging concluded that aging can be viewed as a progression through a continuum of events that occur from birth to death. From this developmental perspective, the aging process was defined as the sum total of all changes that occur in a living organism over the life span. On the basis of this broad definition, it was postulated that aging could best be understood by studying physiologic development. Although the perspective of viewing aging as an integral part of human development has opened many avenues of investigation of both theoretical and practical interest to the physiologist, none has explained satisfactorily all the aging processes or why people age at different rates. Over the years, many theories of physiologic aging have emerged.

TABLE 5–3   Havighurst's Developmental Tasks of the Adult

Stage	Developmental Task
Early adulthood	Selecting a mate
	Learning to live with a marriage partner
	Starting a family
	Rearing children
	Managing a home
	Getting started in an occupation
	Taking on civic responsibility
	Finding a congenial social group
Middle age	Achieving adult civic and social responsibility
	Establishing and maintaining an economic standard of living
	Assisting teen-aged children to become responsible and happy adults
	Developing leisure activities
	Accepting and adjusting to the physiologic changes of middle age
	Adjusting to the aging of parents
Later maturity	Adjusting to decreasing physical strength and health
	Adjusting to the death of a spouse
	Adjusting to retirement and reduced income
	Establishing an explicit affiliation with one's age group
	Meeting social and civic obligations
	Establishing satisfactory physical living arrangements

EXHAUSTION THEORIES

Some early theorists advanced the proposition that there is a fixed store of energy available to the body. As time passes, the energy available is depleted, and, because it cannot be restored, the organism dies.

Later, other theories emerged related to the exhaustion hypotheses. The *wear and tear theory* stated that the body is like a machine that wears out its parts with repeated use and comes to a grinding halt. The *stress theory* emphasized the physical wear and tear from sudden and unexpected stressors over which the organism has no control. This theory maintained that the organism copes with physical stressors through a three-stage process of alarm, resistance, and exhaustion. This process eventually leaves the organism weakened because of the accumulation of successive stressful events over the life span. It is maintained that, as organisms age, they are no longer capable of fighting off the various insults as a result of the accumulation of wear and tear. The concept of exhaustion and the wear and tear hypotheses are not widely accepted causal explanations of the aging process.

GENETIC THEORIES

Identification of deoxyribonucleic acid (DNA) molecules as the ultimate source of all information required by the cell for the production of essential proteins was a major breakthrough, leading to the theory that cellular death results from DNA damage. Progress in molecular genetics is expected to go a long way toward establishing or repudiating theories of aging. Molecular genetics is concerned with unraveling the genetic codes and understanding the ambiguities and subtleties, evolution, and the transformation of information stored in the code as DNA into protein.

The possibility that biologic aging results when inappropriate information is provided for normal cell function from the cell nucleus has been posed. In other words, the biologic process of aging may be related to some form of mutagenesis. Several theories suggest that aging changes occur as a result of an alteration in the genetic information.

SINGLE-ORGAN THEORIES

Physiologic theories of aging have attempted to explain aging and the life span on the basis of a single organ system or in terms of impairments in control mechanisms. One hypothesis suggested that aging results primarily from lowered oxygen supply delivered to crucial tissue, such as the *brain*. The *thyroid gland* has figured in theories of aging in which aging is assumed to be due to the slowing of metabolic processes at the cellular level because cellular metabolism is regulated by the thyroid gland. The failure of the *sexual glands* has also been postulated as a primary cause for aging, and its reversal has figured in attempts to induce rejuvenation. However, there is little evidence that aging as a biologic phenomenon can be ascribed to diminished function by any single organ.

AUTOIMMUNE THEORY

According to the autoimmune theory, as people age, mutations occur in some cells, resulting in the formation of proteins that are not recognized as part of the body. The immune system then produces antibodies against these new proteins and attempts to destroy them, causing an autoimmune disease. It is hypothesized that, with increasing age, there is a reduction in the functioning of immune systems of the body; the antibodies fail to recognize abnormal cells, allowing them to divide and multiply. Immune system failure is thought to be associated with several late-life diseases, including cancer, diabetes, and emphysema.

It is apparent from these biologic theories of aging that, although scientists are not in agreement about the

basic cause of aging, much is known concerning the effects of aging on the body. Generally, the proponents of all of these theories concluded that there is an increasing inability of the organism to adapt to the environment. Most of the principal hypotheses currently being investigated at the level of cells, organs, tissues, and systems recognize aging as the progressive deterioration of the physiologic processes necessary to sustain life, and death as the ultimate failure of the organism to sustain equilibrium.

SOCIOLOGIC THEORIES

The concept of socialization during adulthood refers to the process by which individuals, over the course of their adult lives, acquire ways to perform new roles. Several theories are relevant to how adults learn which roles bring rewards and which roles are considered undesirable and how they adjust to changing roles and role losses in society.

ROSOW'S ROLE THEORY: A CONTINUOUS AND CUMULATIVE PROCESS

Rosow (1974) maintained that socialization for roles is a continuous and cumulative process that corresponds to the developmental stages of the life cycle. Socialization for roles begins in infancy and extends through adolescence; it includes the acquisition of verbal skills; the development of a self-concept, interpersonal competency, and motivation; and the clarification of values, mores, and norms. However, the actual learning of specific role demands begins and continues as the individual moves through the stages of adulthood.

The concept of role continuity explains that role demands of the previous stage prepare the individual for the responsibilities and prerogatives associated with the next status or position that the adult assumes. Thus, role transitions through the life span progress in a coherent manner from one age level to the next.

The orderly progression holds until old age. Rosow suggested that the years at the end of the life span become increasingly nonnormative. For example, the transition to old age is marked by rites of passage, such as retirement; social losses rather than gains; declining responsibilities; increasing dependency; and sharp role discontinuity because society does not specify a role for the aged.

BRIM'S THEORY OF DIFFERENCES BETWEEN CHILDHOOD AND ADULT SOCIALIZATION

From Brim's perspective, childhood and adult socializations differ in three principal ways: (1) adult socialization is limited by the socialization that occurred during childhood, (2) the content of socialization is different, and (3) the relationships between socializing agents are different (Brim, 1968).

Adult socialization may be limited by the effects of earlier learning or lack of that learning. When this learning is absent or conflicts with the needs of the adult, later learning is much more difficult to achieve. In contrast, when earlier socialization provides a strong basis for adult development, it facilitates the process of effectively assuming new roles.

DISENGAGEMENT THEORY VERSUS ACTIVITY THEORY

It is apparent that society is rapidly changing, and this has an impact on the experience of aging as the elderly continue to grow in both numbers and population proportion. If one holds that the status of the elderly tends to decline with the acceleration of social change, it is apparent that aged persons in the United States will decline even further from their already precarious status position. Further, unless the elderly can perform useful and socially valued functions, their future may remain roleless and unmeaningful.

The disengagement theory maintains that satisfaction in old age is usually present in individuals who accept the inevitability of reduction in social and personal interactions. Activity theory, on the other hand, holds that the maintenance of activities is important to most individuals as a basis for obtaining and perpetuating satisfaction, self-esteem, and health. Further research has found that, in the aged, reduction in some activities or attitudes has resulted in compensating increases in others. Data correlating such measures as mental health, physical status, and socioeconomic status with activity level support the importance of activity as the basis for the promotion of vigor and satisfactory adjustment in the elderly. It appears that those who restrict their activities as they age tend to experience a reduction in overall life satisfaction.

PSYCHOLOGIC THEORIES

Psychologic theories are often the extension of sociologic and developmental theories. Personality theories usually consider the innate human needs and forces that motivate thought and behavior within a physical and social environment. The problem with studying personality changes throughout adulthood is that, as individuals pass through life, they become increasingly different rather than more similar. Theorists who have addressed adult personality development have primarily attended to one central issue—whether adult personality is characterized by continuity or by change.

Jung (1928/1971) was one of the first psychologists to consider that the latter half of life has a purpose of its own, quite apart from survival—the development of self-awareness through reflective activity. He strongly believed in the importance of the latter half of life. This

is characterized by inner discovery, as opposed to the first half, which is oriented toward biologic and social goals. Butler (1975) confirmed Jung's views that reflective activity is needed in adulthood. His work regarding the life review process clearly defined the growth potential for aged adults. A review of past events serves as a catalyst for personal growth, integration, and evolving identity. Neugarten (1977) hypothesized that increased reflection is characteristic of adult persons and indicated that there is a growing interest by adults in inner development during later life.

There is considerable confusion among psychologists over the definition and measurement of personality. There is a need for a personality theory that encompasses the whole life span. This theory needs to focus on the age-specific and sex-differentiated life patterns. Attention must be directed toward exploring the occurrence, duration, and timing of events within the life course and the role of the personality in adapting to these events.

STAGES OF ADULT DEVELOPMENT

YOUNG ADULTHOOD

Young adulthood is generally designated as the period between the 20th and 35th year. It seems to be an important emerging period of the life span in contemporary society. A combination of social, economic, and technologic changes has brought about this emergence and a trend toward extending the transition between childhood and adulthood.

Within the last 50 years, society has become more complex, and the demands for greater education have increased enormously. Thus, many young adults are able today, with social approval, to postpone the tasks of adulthood, to experiment, and to prolong their own transition from childhood by exploring the myriad of choices available to them. This period offers the needed time for the individual to grow and make the necessary and complex linkages with adult society.

PHYSIOLOGIC CHANGES

Musculoskeletal Changes

Even though growth essentially ceases at adolescence, minimal growth can continue. Fusion of the epiphyses of long bones occurs approximately at age 18 to 25 years. Muscular efficiency is at its peak level between ages 20 and 30 years. Thereafter, muscular strength declines. Regular exercise is important to maintain a healthy body. Individuals often become more sedentary in the postadolescent years as a result of the lack of a regular exercise plan, changes in work and leisure activities, and alterations in eating patterns. It has been generally concluded from studies that functional capacity, general health, and rate of aging are improved in more active persons. However, physical activity and its effect on physiologic age need more study.

Cardiopulmonary Changes

The developmental processes related to the heart, the blood vessels, and the lungs conclude in adolescence. Maintaining their functioning and preventing pathologic changes during the second half of life largely depend on the young adult's setting healthy life style practices that are carried into middle age and late life.

Although atherosclerotic disease becomes manifest clinically in middlescence, it represents the culmination of progressive changes in the arterial walls that began in childhood. Many of the theories about the origin, course, and eventual prevention and treatment of atherosclerosis were derived from correlating certain biologic, demographic, and social variables with the incidence of coronary artery disease in the population. From these studies have emerged a few variables that are considered definite risk factors. The major ones are hyperlipidemia, smoking, obesity, and physical inactivity.

The results of these studies on the myriad factors that predispose or aggravate atherosclerotic conditions should serve to advise young adults regarding their life styles. The literature indicates that the less sedentary the individual is, the less susceptible he/she will be to sudden death. Several insurance industry studies also indicate a relationship between the failure to maintain physical activity, ideal weight, and proper diet and the incidence of disease.

Oral contraceptives used by many woman during the childbearing years are suspected to increase the risk of disease of the cardiovascular system. Cigarette smoking is correlated with increased incidence of cardiovascular diseases, emphysema, and cancer.

Integumentary Changes

The proliferation of cosmetic products for skin care for those over 25 years of age, hair coloring products, and balding remedies attests to the aging changes that commence in young adulthood. These changes are often traumatic if a young adult has internalized society's youth-oriented value system.

Wrinkling of the skin inevitably occurs with aging and is markedly increased by exposure to the sun. Facial wrinkling becomes recognizable in the second decade in most adults and tends to be progressive thereafter. Early wrinkling is related to the habitual facial expressions, such as frowning and smiling. The skin loses its moisture and gradually dries; in later years, the atrophy of fat accentuates and increases the appearance of wrinkles.

The onset of hair graying and baldness often begins in the young adulthood period. Graying of hair results

from the inability of melanocytes to provide hair with pigment granules over time. Hair loss with aging results from a number of factors. Although it is more common in men, it also occurs in women. Early balding is a result of genetic factors and is androgen related. In the middle and later years, a slow and progressive loss of scalp and hair is often found in both sexes.

Dental Changes

The third molars, or wisdom teeth, normally erupt at the beginning of the second decade. There are four third molars, although all four may not fully develop in some adults. Wisdom teeth frequently present problems for the individual and mandate dental assistance. Their eruptions are unpredictable, and it is not uncommon for them to come in sideways or remain impacted in the gums.

PSYCHOSOCIAL DEVELOPMENT

The central issues of psychosocial development in young adulthood are related to the final working out of the identity crises begun in adolescence. These issues are worked through rather slowly. By the time the adolescent reaches young adulthood, some of these issues are nearing resolution. In adolescence, the individual is struggling to develop a coherent, unified sense of self and to determine an identity as a person and member of society.

The young adult struggles with expanding that sense of self in determining who she/he is within various social roles. In other words, in this stage of identity development, the prime concern is with the relationship between the individual and the social system. Young adults seek to resolve several major psychosocial issues in their quest for maturity.

Self-Identity

In young adulthood, the sense of self becomes sharper and clearer, more consistent, and less influenced by others. This identification is quite different from that of the adolescent, who is self-conscious and concerned with seeing the self from the viewpoint of others. This stabilization and clarification of identity result from the progressive selection and commitment to social roles that characterize adult life.

As individuals select from among the myriad choices, including acceptance or rejection of gender-based roles, selection of sexual partners, and determination of occupational roles, they become increasingly more comfortable with making decisions when faced with unexpected life events. Coping with the unexpected does not disrupt the sense of continuity and integration in the mature young adult.

As young adults participate in adult roles, they select life style patterns and role combinations that endure through later life. These decisions solidify their self-identity and enable the young adult to develop a sense of consistency in beliefs, attitudes, and behavior that will develop through their adult years.

Sexuality

The development of contraceptive pills, the fear of acquired immunodeficiency syndrome (AIDS), and changes in sexual mores have resulted in a dilemma for many young adults. Much conflict and confusion occurs when one is questioning values related to sexuality. Individuals have freedom to select their own sexual standards, but the multiplicity of choices often presents dilemmas. For example, the gay liberation movement has allowed some young adults greater freedom of personal acceptance and self-worth, yet it complicates the choice of others who may not have ever before considered homosexuality as an acceptable sexual pattern.

The AIDS epidemic is beginning to cause a re-emergence of conservative sexual behaviors and values.

Change in the sexual aspects of young adulthood relates to more than just sexual behavior. Relationships become increasingly more responsive to understanding and accepting others as they are. Interpersonal relationships depend more on appreciating others' uniqueness, and less of on a projection of one's adolescent fantasies, physiologic needs, and a search for a sense of identity. Some of the factors involved in this change include the progressive stabilization of identity, more selective choosing of relationships, and more in-depth exploration of selected relationships. The commitment of one's self to another demands a great deal of trust; many young adults find this to be an overwhelming challenge. They shrink back in fear of being hurt or rejected. This is expected when one considers that young adulthood is a time of much change and important decisions to be made. Young adults are trying to make a linkage between their identity and society, while at the same time beginning to explore others as unique, sexual human beings. This is all being done in a modern society in which there are great educational, sexual, and social changes occurring. In less complex societies, or in times of less rapid social change, these issues may well have been resolved in adolescence. In contemporary society, however, the trend seems to be toward extending the period between adolescence and the assumption of adult roles and responsibilities.

Family Structure

The major milestones of the transition from childhood to adulthood largely involve the family. These milestones, which include leaving one's family of origin, selecting a mate, marrying, and experiencing the birth of the first child, mark the entrance into adult roles and functions.

The event of marriage and the establishment phase of

the family cycle bring about many changes and crisis points in the lives of many young adults. One of the early tasks in this cycle is for the couple to work out new patterns and role relationships. Both individuals attempt to develop mutually satisfying patterns of living intimately with the other. This development calls for the resolution of conflicts, the establishment of patterns of conflict resolution, the use of decision-making and communication, and the division of family roles and responsibilities. Learning to live intimately with another individual is not as easy as many young adults initially anticipate. The high divorce rate during the early years of marriage attests to this difficulty.

The increase in divorce rates during role shift into parenthood indicates that this event is a crisis for many young adults. The birth of a child requires a major shift from a primarily spouse role, to incorporate the demands and responsibilities of a parent role. This resocialization not only requires the learning of a new role, but the ability to combine this new role into a set pattern with other roles. The addition of a dependent, demanding third person disrupts the established dyad relationship as well as one's routine patterns of living. Most texts on the family report that the birth of the first child is a severe or extensive crisis for most couples.

Often significant life changes occur simultaneously with parenthood and present emotional hazards for the new parents. Previous schedules and routines become disrupted. The parents often suddenly realize that their own childhood has ended and experience the feeling that time is passing too quickly. Young adults may feel a loss of their own identity in the press of all the responsibility. The birth of a baby often terminates social life because the couple's world centers on the baby and home. As the novelty wears off, the young adult often feels trapped and isolated because previous activities and contacts cannot be maintained.

There are many changes that the young adult experiences in making the transition from the world of childhood to adulthood. Perhaps none are perceived as being as emotionally taxing as those involved in the establishment of a family. The young adult's identity is undergoing a dramatic modification as the individual assumes the new role responsibilities and relationships as lover, companion, spouse, and parent.

Work

Entrance into the work world for the young adult involves a twofold process. The first aspect of that process is the choice of an occupation, followed by socialization in the role demands of the job. The process of selecting and maintaining an occupation in modern society presents more flexibility than in years past. The traditional factors of social class, race, intelligence, gender, aptitudes, role models, and experiences that operated to limit the range of choices have lost much of their impact. Since World War II, a number of changes have taken place in the economic and technologic spheres that affect work roles. These changes include the heightened expectations regarding standards of living, geographic mobility, the expansion of types of employment available, the disappearance of gender-defined roles, and the need for education to meet technologic advancements.

Most often, to maintain a middle-class standard of living, both spouses work outside the home. Not infrequently one spouse may need to work at two jobs. Furthermore, because of the high divorce rate in young adulthood, one of two marriages ends in a single-parent family, usually headed by the female. This has created the desire among many young adult females to ensure their earning ability. Many young adults see prolonged or continuous education as the means to obtain desired standards of living. This often means postponing marriage, or combining the roles of student, temporary worker, spouse, and parent. Balancing these responsibilities at a time when young adults are still acquiring basic knowledge and skills needed to resolve their developmental tasks creates considerable stress. To acknowledge this situation, researchers are advocating a layered model of lifelong learning, rather than a linear model of education during young adulthood, work during young adulthood and middlescence, and leisure during old age.

Leisure

Leisure in adulthood is often a difficult concept to define. This difficulty arises from the intertwining of societal values and the meaning of nonworking time. Most adults consider their work as the most meaningful activity. Work provides the necessities of life; it is also the major aspect of one's identity and status. Therefore, to many Americans, leisure is conceptualized in a negative context rather than as a potentially positive, healthful experience in its own right.

Nonrecreational use of free time in young adulthood is not surprising, given the complex social milieu in which youth struggle to lay the foundation for adulthood. Keeping pace with the economic and technologic changes of the contemporary society, coupled with young adults' gratifying their intimacy needs through marriage and parenthood, often makes time management difficult and provides multiple roles to fulfill— student, spouse, parent, and worker. Society does not foster respect for leisure in the young. Parental pressures for high achievement and success, competition for employment and difficulties in being absorbed into the labor market, and inflation serve to make the young feel guilty for spending time in recreation and relaxation rather than in studying, working, or improving one's chances for the future.

When one considers the high incidence of psychosomatic illness, suicide, early marital discord, drug and alcohol abuse, and family disruption among young adults, one has to question whether a greater acceptance for leisure might be a desirable social goal. It may be an important developmental task of early adulthood to learn to cope with free time. Young adults need to develop attitudes that permit them to be with themselves in a truly leisurely manner, rather than compulsively filling every waking minute with structured activities.

HEALTH ISSUES

The young adulthood years are the healthiest years in the life cycle. Most young adults are never seriously ill or incapacitated. As a result, young adults often feel a sense of immunity to illness and neglect health maintenance activities. The greatest potential for improving health is found to be in what people do and do not do for themselves. Young adults' decisions about diet, exercise, smoking and drug use are of critical importance to their health status in middlescence and late life.

To maintain their health status, young adults are encouraged to have annual physical examinations, with more frequent visits if there are particular problems. Young women are encouraged to have routine Papanicolaou's tests and to perform breast self-examination once a month. Routine dental examinations should be scheduled annually to avoid dental and periodontal disorders. Young adults should have regular eye examinations every 1 to 2 years. Despite a general state of good health, young adults are prone to a few major health concerns.

Accidents

In the United States, the most frequent cause of death for young adults is accidents. Injuries occur as a result of work-related incidents, thrill-seeking pleasures, gunshot wounds, automobile accidents, and war injuries. Men are consistently more frequently involved in accidents than women throughout the life cycle. Between the ages of 15 and 34 years, the male death rate is more than triple that of the female, largely because of the high rate of accidental deaths among males (American Cancer Society, 1989).

Accidents are most likely to occur when a person is under stress. Young adulthood presents much duress as the individual seeks to resolve developmental tasks. In addition, the everyday lives of young adults present stressful experiences, such as driving in city traffic, rushing to meet deadlines, or caring for small children. Excessive fatigue can easily occur in young adults who attempt to balance too many roles. Stress overload can lead to accidents, as well as other psychosomatic illnesses.

This group should be especially aware of maintaining good health care practices — prudent diets, regular exercise, and adequate sleep. Because accidents and their consequences present a major threat to the health of young adults, care must be taken when engaging in potentially hazardous activities. This includes using seat belts, following speed limits, and observing caution around machinery.

Drug and Alcohol Use and Misuse

Few issues have received as much recent attention in the United States as drug and alcohol abuse. It is evident in the professional as well as the popular literature that the use of alcohol and other psychoactive agents has increased significantly in the last decade. Even though the use of tobacco and some hard-core drugs has declined, the misuse of potentially addictive agents in young adulthood may be related to the difficulties in resolving the developmental task conflict of individuation versus alienation.

MIDDLE ADULTHOOD

Between 35 and 60 years of age is generally considered the period of middle age. These years have been described as the "best years" in the life cycle. During this span of time, adults refer to being in the "prime of life." If healthy development has occurred, the struggles of young adulthood are past and have been resolved, and middle-aged adults can enjoy the results of their labor as established, mature, social, professional, and personally valued individuals. Yet this time has its own difficulties.

Middlescence is recognized as the mid-point in the life cycle. Most individuals reflect on and evaluate their lives during this period. Evaluation is not an unusual experience, but it takes on special meaning during middle age. The accomplishments of young adulthood have shaped the life of the middlescent. At this point the individual suddenly realizes that this transitional period is the last chance to change life's direction. Many middlescents begin to examine the results of their life work against what they want to do with the rest of their lives. Most of the young adulthood years were spent in working toward achieving goals set in youth. Middlescents reassess their choices and wonder if their chosen directions will work toward realizing their mature life goals or desires. This examination may result in massive life style changes for some. This often unsettling time of life, which entails the transition to old age, is often referred to as the "mid-life crisis."

PHYSIOLOGIC CHANGES

From young adulthood through the middle years, biologic changes occur gradually. These changes are so gradual that they are hardly noticed until the fourth or fifth decade of life.

Sensory Changes

Decline in visual acuity is a progressive change that all persons eventually experience. The decreased ability of the eyes to accommodate for close and detailed work becomes evident in the fourth decade and continues throughout the rest of one's life. Pupil size becomes smaller, which affects the amount of light that reaches the retina, thus limiting the efficiency of pupillary constriction and dilation, and affecting the ability to adapt one's vision in dim light and darkness. Toward the end of middlescence, the eyes are less able to pick up the blues, violets, and greens of the color spectrum and more easily adapt to the lighter colors, such as reds, yellows, and oranges. This difficulty with color perception is linked to the yellowing of the lens with advancing age. Individuals who are in their 50s need about twice as much light to see things as they did when they were in their 20s. There is a need for more light for all visual perception with advancing age.

Hearing loss in American society is prevalent in late middlescence. Changes in the efficiency of the cochlea and the hair cells of the organ of Corti are responsible for the impaired transmission of sound waves along the nerve pathways of the brain and are considered to be the most common cause of presbycusis, which is progressive hearing loss associated with aging. Presbycusis primarily affects one's ability to hear high-pitched sounds and sibilant consonants. For example, the "s," "sh," and "ch" sounds are difficult to differentiate in conversations. Vowels that have a low pitch are more easily heard. Noise masking occurs, that is, background noise impinges on conversation so that it is difficult to hear what is being said.

The abilities to see and to hear are major contributors to communication. Losses in these abilities are not only frustrating to the individual but also threatening to security and self-esteem. Yet many middlescents are reluctant to get glasses or hearing aids, even when vision or hearing problems significantly affect functioning. Many seem to want to deny the problem rather than to admit to age-related changes. This pretense or unwillingness to wear assistive devices often has negative consequences, such as accidents.

Neuromuscular Changes

For many middlescents, sedentary life styles result in loss of muscle strength and mass. This loss of muscle tone is noticed as waistlines thicken, abdomens protrude, and facial tissue sags.

There is a gradual decline in maximal motor and sensory functioning from its peak during a person's 20s to lower levels in the middle years. Reflexes that entail responses to sudden changes in the environment may be slowed, but, for the most part, the alterations in function occur gradually and go unnoticed.

Neuromuscular changes are viewed as relatively insignificant because their progress is so gradual that most individuals have learned to compensate for them. For example, driving ability is considered to be better in middle-aged adults than in younger individuals, despite declines in coordination, increased reaction time, and sensitivity to glare. It seems that the improvement in judgment and caution compensate for the physical decrements. The same is true for manual workers. Older individuals are found to have less disabling injuries and to be more conscientious and careful than their younger counterparts.

Cardiopulmonary Changes

Coronary and pulmonary diseases are among the leading causes of morbidity and mortality in middlescence. It appears that these problems are more related to life style and genetic factors than to aging per se.

The heart function, rate, and rhythm remain unchanged in middlescence. However, when life styles become sedentary, eventually anatomic and physiologic changes occur. Lack of regular exercise over time causes the heart muscle to lose its tone, and consequently changes in rate and rhythm occur. Among the most significant factors implicated in atherosclerosis are diet, poor nutrition, lack of physical exercise, smoking, and psychologic and emotional stress.

Pulmonary changes in middlescence are largely related to whether the person is a smoker. Smoking decreases respiratory efficiency and increases the risk of lung morbidity. Smoking and chronic lung disease (recurrent colds, asthma, and bronchitis) largely account for the loss of functioning in lung tissues. These risk factors, coupled with environmental or occupational pollution, inactivity, and altered cardiac status, can result in decreased breathing capacity in the older adult.

Dental Changes

Dental problems tend to be a major concern throughout middlescence. Many persons older than 55 years of age have lost most of their teeth. Research tends to indicate that this phenomenon is related to lifelong hygienic and life style factors, rather than the aging process.

Endocrine Changes

From the research evidence, there seems to be agreement that there is a progressive decrease in the ability to metabolize glucose efficiently throughout the adult life span. In fact, this deterioration in performance is so great that nearly all older adults are thought to have abnormal glucose levels. However, there are questions and disputes about the cause of this change. Whether the change is physiologic or pathologic is yet to be determined. Even the cause, whether high glucose levels are the result of reduced ability of the pancreas to secrete insulin or a consequence of a waning insulin response, is in question.

The levels of androgenic, estrogenic, and gonadotropic hormones decrease in middlescence. Reduced hormone levels result in atrophy of the ovaries, uterus, and vaginal tissues in women and, in men, the development of firmer testes and a tendency for benign prostatic hypertrophy to occur. Women lose the ability to procreate.

PSYCHOSOCIAL DEVELOPMENT

Middlescence is an often unsettling time of questioning former goals, determining what one wants for the future, and making decisions or changes that will influence the second half of life. It is the time when most individuals acknowledge that they have begun to grow old. Although middle-aged adults recognize that they are in their prime of life, they also realize that time is limited. They know the future is finite, and many accept that they cannot achieve all that they had once hoped to. For many people, middlescence is the last chance to identify and pursue new goals and interests. For other individuals, it is merely a plateau into old age.

Self-Concept

There are common assumptions about middlescence as a critical phase in the psychosocial development of the individual. These include the following: (1) most middlescents experience an unsettling time of questioning former goals and self-concepts; (2) middlescents who attempt major changes (e.g., new careers, new marriages, and new appearances) to allow more individual fulfillment in work, marriage, and creative relaxation go through several uncomfortable years before the crisis is resolved; and (3) individuals who do not seek out new stimuli are apt to stagnate.

If the maturing years of young adulthood have been handled successfully, middlescents have the wisdom and skills to more realistically see the realities of themselves and their world. Individuals' awareness of finiteness assists them to see middlescence as a point in the life cycle when they must make changes, if they are to be made at all. Typically, the middlescent is assessing what has been achieved in the second half of life regarding their careers, marriages, children, life styles, social roles, and friendships. This reassessment can result in drastic changes in any or all of the above aspects; whereas others may elect to continue with their established patterns for the remainder of their lives.

The tasks of reassessment and acceptance of change of the middle years often result in stress and discord. This discomfort is more evident today than in years past. The rapid social and economic changes in modern society create havoc for individuals who seek stability, order, and direction. Most individuals enter into adulthood with youthful fantasies of living well, surviving into their 80s, marrying the perfect mate, having perfect children, fulfilling a rewarding career, and retiring comfortably. However, few individuals anticipate marital discord, childrearing problems, physical illnesses, death of a spouse, inflation, or diminishing job marketability. Coping with such complex issues at a time when one is more depended on by work, family, and society threatens one's confidence in the future.

For most middlescents, fulfilling the developmental tasks toward becoming a more fully functioning person is obstructed by a series of crises that arise from the need to meet new challenges. For some, these crises produce severe emotional problems that temporarily impede the restructuring of their lives. For others, continuous obstacles and prolonged stress produce stagnation and even regression to coping methods from earlier stages of living. Most middlescents, however, are able to meet the challenges, develop their potentials more fully, and discover more satisfying life styles. What seems to be apparent is that, unless one continues to change, strive, and learn in middlescence, late life becomes a vast array of problems leading to decline and despair.

Sexuality

Biologically, the most significant milestone in middlescence is the so-called change of life. This change is signaled by the climacteric, or menopause, in women, and is seen far less dramatically in men who undergo climacteric changes. Menopause refers to the process during which menses cease, ovaries stop producing ova and female sex hormones, and the genitals atrophy. Other possible signs are sweats, hot flashes, palpitations, dizziness, and emotional changes, such as irritability and depression. Investigators recently reported, however, that most women go through the menopause basically unperturbed by these changes.

Climacteric for the man involves a decrease in the levels of the male sex hormones. This decline is so gradual that most men can produce sperm until well into old age. The male climacteric is not as abrupt or intense as menopause.

Family Structure

Changes within family relationships, such as children leaving home, separation and divorce, the aging of parents, and the death of a spouse are often experienced in the middle years. Coping adequately with these changes is a major task of middlescence. Individuals must deal with these considerable changes in a manner that makes them grow toward emotional maturity and feel secure and independent, rather than depressed, ill, or dependent.

The child-launching phase begins when the first child leaves the parental home and ends when the parents face each other again as a couple. Because of their usually greater emotional and time investments in childrearing, readjustment for women tends to be more critical and profound than for men. The arrival of this change often coincides with the menopause, and, for family-oriented women, the combination of these events may result in an identity crisis, which is often labeled the empty nest syndrome. Some women seem unable, for a time, to connect with an alternative workable identity, find new ways of nurturing, or find new interests and goals to fill empty time. Reactions to child launching are dependent on individual differences and life situations. Women who have combined the work role with motherhood may find it a time of freedom from family responsibilities and financial pressures. Others may continue to find satisfaction through the

wife and grandmother roles or through work or other activities, whereas others may find their lives lonely, frustrating, and generally unsatisfying. To cope effectively, a strong sense of self-identity and an ability to shift roles are crucial.

The stage after active parenting in the family life cycle also greatly influences the marital relationship. The couple must learn to divert the energy and feelings that flowed to their children back to each other. For most couples, the happiest years of marriage are the ones before the children are born and the ones after the children are on their own. In these latter years, the couple often experiences a sense of freedom and privacy they have not had for years. This freedom provides opportunity to get to know each other as individuals. When a marriage has been shaky over the childrearing years, this is often a time when divorce occurs; however, if the relationship has been good, it is apt to improve at this time.

During middlescence, a drastic change seems to occur in the relationship between middle-aged children and their parents. Parents suddenly seem old. Aged parents begin to seek their children's help in making decisions and often become dependent for physical and financial support. Middlescents may have to make tough decisions about their parents' living arrangements. Strain is often placed on married middlescents as they weigh their responsibilities toward their parents against those toward their spouse and children. When parents move in with their children, conflict can occur because there may be competition for existing family roles, financial strains, space constraints, or anger over increased responsibilities if the aged individual is ill. If the decision to institutionalize the elder is made, the adult child often experiences guilt about the perceived abandonment of his/her parent. The sudden increase in the numbers of elders living longer life spans is a phenomenon previous generations did not have to deal with. Therefore, there are no prior role models to guide middle-aged children.

Work

The work role provides a major source of esteem, satisfaction, happiness, and identity for almost all adults. It is a frequently observed phenomenon that career-oriented men and women become increasingly preoccupied with their work as they grow older. This preoccupation with work is a common American phenomenon, tending to exclude leisure activities and other roles.

Most adults peak in their careers during middlescence and continue in their chosen fields until retirement. However, there is a new tendency toward changing occupational directions in the middle years. Seeking a second career is an emerging trend within special groups. One group comprises individuals who are forced to find new directions because of technologic or economic factors or unemployment. Another group includes women who, after devoting their young adulthood years to marriage and children, seek a career as an avenue of financial gain and personal growth and satisfaction. Similarly, many individuals who joined the work force in early adulthood and are eligible for early retirement from their jobs seek a second career rather than face retirement, which they perceive as boring, idle, and wasteful. Another group includes individuals who made career choices in young adulthood that did not succeed in providing them with a sense of satisfaction.

Leisure

During the middle adult years, most people find themselves with more time on their hands than their experience or interests can accommodate. Settling into careers, launching children, and retiring result in much unstructured time, as individuals are released from earlier responsibilities. Adjustment to this free time is largely related to the individual's attitudes toward these disengaging events. If the individual perceives these losses negatively, fears the loss of accustomed roles or friends, or is uncertain about the future, adjustment may be difficult. Negative attitudes that stem from the lack of knowledge about potential financial, health, and psychologic problems and alternatives available to use time productively and for fun can be alleviated through adult education programs. There is a need to enhance a positive self-concept through numerous pursuits and interests beyond those of the work and family roles. These alternatives can make the pending loss of roles a means for greater involvement in challenges that are equally important. It is vital for all middlescents to sustain feelings of self-worth by having several alternative life pursuits as the means for achieving a continuing sense of personal growth. Attributes such as good health, family affection, a stable social environment, and definite plans for future activity are influential in successful transition into late life.

HEALTH ISSUES

Although there are inevitable physical changes and an increasing incidence of chronic conditions as one passes through the middle years, most of the changes from young adulthood are minor ones. Few middlescents are affected by conditions or diseases that necessitate a change in their life style or that have a substantial effect on their future. In general, the health status of the older adult has rapidly improved. Today, adult men can expect to live to approximately age 70 years and women, to age 80 years. These extended life expectancies have occurred through improved nutrition, better sanitation, and discovery of cures for infectious diseases. Currently, the most common causes of death during the middle years are heart diseases, cancer, strokes, and respiratory tract diseases. Individuals who smoke, drink, are obese, have high cholesterol levels, and are inactive are at higher risk for heart disease.

General health during middlescence is better than most people expect. Yet it is important for middlescents to engage in preventive and health promotion practices

to retain optimal health. Middle-aged adults should schedule annual physical and eye examinations and biannual dental examinations to detect and treat any significant changes. Because of the relationship of smoking and cardiopulmonary diseases, smokers should limit or stop their habit. A regular exercise program and sound nutritional practices, such as reducing the intake of cholesterol and saturated fats, are effective preventive health measures. Marital state also appears to influence health maintenance, with married individuals living longer than single or widowed individuals. When roles are lost in middlescence, it is important for one's mental health to move into another life style that will be satisfying. Prolonged psychologic stress throughout these transition periods can cause injury, illness, and physical and psychologic threats.

Reactions to stress are manifested in a variety of ways by middle-aged adults. Some may endure all these changes without developing psychologic problems. For others, stress can lead to depression, drug abuse, or alcoholism.

LATE ADULTHOOD

Over the past century, the elderly population (those 60 years of age and older) has increased both relatively and absolutely at rates far higher than for other segments of the population. The proportion of elderly individuals in American society is expected to increase. In 1987 there were 29.8 million older adults, making up 12.3% of the U.S. population. By the year 2000, there will be 34.9 million Americans composing 13% of the population (AARP & AOA, 1988). Advances in health care and improved health maintenance habits have resulted in a healthier aged population, with greater numbers of elderly living longer.

The aged individual has unique attributes that can be utilized or allowed to remain dormant. Yet society often neglects or fails to activate the aged's potential because of stereotypic beliefs about old people. Gerontologic research has indicated that in the United States there is a systematic stereotyping of and discrimination against people who are old. The young are not immune to these ageisms and internalize the values and beliefs. It is clear that an accurate understanding of the aged is lacking in American society.

PHYSIOLOGIC CHANGES

As in every other age cycle, there is no arbitrary dividing line to mark when middle age ends and old age begins. Physical changes take place at different rates in different individuals. However, all the body systems are affected by the aging process. Although some changes become apparent in earlier stages, old age seems to be the time in the life cycle when the progressive changes become more readily apparent and degenerative changes occur more rapidly (see the accompanying Focus on the Elderly feature).

FOCUS ON THE ELDERLY ■ **Effects of Aging on Body Systems**

System Function	Normal Changes	Abnormal Changes
Cardiovascular	Increase in the size of the heart Increase in collagen Increase in the thickness of valves and blood vessels Decrease in cardiac output Decrease in cardiac reserve Decrease in blood flow to organs	Hypertension Coronary artery disease Congestive heart failure Peripheral vascular disease Varicose veins
Endocrine		
Pancreas	Decreased ability to metabolize glucose Reduced insulin secretion Delayed insulin response	Diabetes mellitus
Gonads	Decreased hormone levels Atrophy of ovaries, uterus, and vagina Development of firmer testes Benign prostatic hypertrophy	Cancer of the uterus, ovaries, or vagina Cancer of the prostate gland
Integumentary	Thinning of epithelial cells and subcutaneous fat layers Lines and wrinkles in the skin Age spots Roughness or dryness of the skin Thinning and loss of color of the hair Thickening and brittleness of the nails	Infections: viral, bacterial, fungal Abnormal cell growth Tumors: benign and malignant Skin ulcerations
Musculoskeletal	Loss of flexibility in joints Cartilage degeneration Bony growths at the edge of joints Decreased muscle mass	Osteoporosis Arthritis Rheumatoid arthritis Fracture Loss of height due to spinal column changes
Neurologic	General slowing of reaction time Slow response to heat and cold Changing sleep patterns Decreased cerebral blood flow	Cerebrovascular disease Parkinson's disease Senile dementia and Alzheimer's disease
Pulmonary	Increase in the diameter of the chest Decrease in coughing ability Decrease in vital capacity and tidal volume	Asthma Bronchitis Emphysema Pneumonia Tuberculosis

Continued

FOCUS ON THE ELDERLY ■ Effects of Aging on Body Systems *Continued*

System Function	Normal Changes	Abnormal Changes
	Increase in production of mucus	
	Progressive kyphosis	
	Calcification of cartilage connecting the ribs to the spinal column and sternum	
	Decreased strength of expiratory muscles	
	Thickening of the alveolar walls; decreased recoil	
Sensory		
Sight	Presbyopia	Cataracts
	Lowered acuity	Glaucoma
	Altered accommodation to light and dark	Senile ocular degeneration
	Difficulty in color discrimination	
	Decreased lens clarity	
Hearing	Decreased discrimination of pitch and acuity	Deafness
	Decreased sensitivity to higher frequency sounds	
	Excessive wax	
Touch	Decreased receptors	Total loss of feeling
	Lowered ability to distinguish temperature and feel pain	
Taste	Decreased number of taste buds	Total loss of taste
	Diminished ability to distinguish specific tastes	
Smell	Decreased olfactory function	Total loss of smell
	Diminished sensation to distinguish specific odors	
Urinary	Diminished kidney function	Urinary retention
	Decreased glomerular filtration rate	Urinary tract infection
	Decreased number of nephrons	
	Decreased muscle tone of bladder	
	Decreased bladder capacity	
	Decreased sphincter control	

Of all body tissue, the fatty tissue layer fluctuates the most throughout life and is subject to the greatest change with aging. Peripheral body parts afford the most striking examples of this alteration. For example, veins and bones of the hand become prominent under a parchment-like layer of skin, deep hollows appear in the clavicular and axillary areas of the body, breasts sag and become pendulous, and the eyes seem to sink owing to disappearance of the fat layer around the orbit. Subcutaneous tissue has a significant role in the body's adjustment to temperature change. The natural insulation that subcutaneous fat affords is lost. It is not uncommon to hear aged persons say that they are cold, nor is it uncommon to see them wearing a sweater or sitting with a lap blanket when environmental temperatures are comfortable for younger individuals.

Although subcutaneous tissue does not affect the aged person's tolerance of heat, it is important to mention that problems exist. Changes in the sweat glands, which diminish in size, number, and activity, cause a decline in the efficiency of the body's cooling mechanism. The elderly do not perspire freely, leaving them at high risk for heat exhaustion. They need to be aware of these changes and learn how to compensate. Avoidance of extreme heat conditions is important. Sudden changes in room temperature or exposure to overly heated bath water causes the blood vessels in the skin and muscles to dilate and can result in temporary slowing of blood to the brain, leading to a reversible state of confusion.

Sleep Changes

The aged take longer to move through the relaxation stages of non–rapid eye movement (non-REM) sleep. The number of awakenings and their duration increases. When asked about the quality of sleep, the aged often respond with remarks or complaints that they hardly slept all night. Their sleep is more fragmented than that of the young. These interruptions are often due to nocturnal micturition, leg cramps, and mental stimulation through worry, bereavement, or extraneous noises. It was thought at one time that the elderly needed more sleep, but this is not necessarily true. The aged seem to sleep less. If one sleeps more, it is usually because of boredom, sedation, or symptoms of disease.

The aged who are not aware that these changes are normal may worry, and the more they worry, the less they sleep. Noisy environments, unresolved fears, worries, and concerns also disrupt sleep quality and patterns. Health care providers often attempt to repair the damage by prescribing sleep medications. However, few hypnotic drugs have been found to promote the entire sleep cycle. Instead, these drugs depress the REM sleep, which is necessary for intellectual functioning and for the relief of tension and anxiety. When medications are discontinued, normal sleep patterns usually return, but not until fully re-established dreaming patterns emerge. Nightmares are sometimes increased. Some experts believe that these occur in an attempt to make up for dreams that have been repressed or obliterated by REM sleep suppression.

In one study (Zelechowski, 1977), all elderly in a health facility were weaned from routinely prescribed sleep medications and alternative actions were substituted. It was found that no one needed sleep medication if attention was given to specific bedtime needs and rituals. Backrubs have been documented to decrease the time needed to drop off to sleep. Protein foods and dairy products contain an amino acid that synthesizes serotonin — a neurotransmitter that is found to increase sleep time and reduce the time necessary to fall asleep. Therefore, warm milk, cocoa, and other ordinary food preparations that contain serotonin, if taken at bedtime, can aid the aged person to fall asleep without use of hypnotic and sedative preparations. Other interventions include playing soft music or providing wine or sherry, which supply internal warmth and relaxation. Daytime exercise has been shown to be one of the best promoters of sleep.

Neurologic and Sensory Changes

The nervous system experiences alterations related to loss of neurons, decreased blood supply, and a decrease in electrical activity. These changes may cause altered sensory perception and decreases in reaction time and movement time for the older adult. It often takes the elder a longer time to respond and initiate action in a given situation. Visual and hearing changes begun in a person's 30s become much more pronounced in old age. Vestibular functioning decreases, and the elderly person is more prone to falls and accidents.

Nutritive Changes

Loss of teeth, gum disease, and bone degeneration make eating more difficult for the elderly person. Chewing becomes more difficult and often requires a modification in the diet. Poor muscle tone, loss of digestive juices, and impaired circulation often create problems with digestion and elimination. Atrophy of the taste buds coupled with problems related to dentition and digestion diminishes the pleasure of eating for many older adults. Limited incomes and inflationary food costs often prevent the elder from eating a well-balanced diet. Changes in eating patterns often lead to anemia, malnutrition, and susceptibility to infections.

Cardiopulmonary Changes

All the body systems and organs change with age, but the most serious changes affect the heart and the lungs.

The output of the heart is decreased, and the volume of oxygen-carrying blood to all parts of the body is reduced. The continuation of the arteriosclerotic process in the blood vessels accentuates this problem. Respiratory movements of the chest decrease, altering inspiratory and expiratory volumes. Less oxygen is consumed, and lower respiratory tract infections occur more frequently in older adults.

Musculoskeletal Changes

Orthopedic disabilities are exceedingly common in old age. The most frequent conditions are hypertrophic arthritis related to degenerative joint changes; osteoporosis resulting from bone atrophy; extra-articular pathologic changes of obscure origin, including fibrositis and bursitis; and fractures caused by trauma and disease.

Urologic Changes

Neoplastic growths that involve the urologic system, infections, and calculi in the bladder are common problems in older persons. In men, hypertrophy of the prostate and carcinoma of that gland are frequently noted.

Gastrointestinal Changes

In old persons, the entire gastrointestinal tract undergoes atrophic changes that may interfere with the efficiency of its function. It has been shown, however, that, if an older person eats the right foods in the right combinations, the gastrointestinal tract can function quite effectively.

PSYCHOSOCIAL DEVELOPMENT

The last years of one's life cycle constitute the final stage of development in which adults can grow and change. It is the phase in which the individual has the opportunity to make final revisions. How well adults adapt to old age is in part predicated on how well they have resolved the tasks of the previous cycles. Individuals who enter old age with many unresolved crises from prior years experience a difficult time. For others, old age is a time to pass on the wisdom of one's experiences; continue fulfilling, productive roles; and enjoy a sense of fulfillment for a life well lived.

Self-Concept

The way people regard themselves determines their life satisfaction. Self-concept is developed by a continuous interaction between the individual and the environment. Loss of a significant other and loss of roles such as parent, spouse, and worker often erode the elder's sense of self and psychologic well-being. The need to be creative and productive is particularly important in old age to gain attention and approval from others and to compensate for a possible perception of decreased physical attractiveness and losses related to family support, work, financial resources, and social support from friends and associates.

Maintaining a positive self-concept and self-esteem depends on one's ability to satisfy one's needs and to demonstrate competence. People feel competent when they are able to control their own lives. Yet many elders are living in a state of poverty, are barely able to meet physiologic needs for food and shelter, and are without hope or motivation to tackle or seek gratification of higher-level goals. Those who have some measure of financial security are still lacking many of the resources needed to enable optimal functioning. Elders are often separated from their families, friends, and associates; work groups are no longer accessible. Physical illness or immobility makes it more difficult to socialize. For the ego to remain intact, the elder needs to have respect from others.

Older people react to these frustrations and attempt to maintain a positive self-concept in a variety of ways. These include such reactions as denial of illness, regression, hypochondria, or retreat into fantasy. It has been suggested that reminiscers use remembrance of the past as a defense against present threats to self-esteem. These reactions, while adaptive to conditions or events outside the control of the older person, do not assist individuals to develop their personal potentials. Good health, adequate income, a useful role, opportunities for social interaction, and lively interests are the main determinants of a happy old age.

Sexuality

Studies of sexual behaviors and interest in these behaviors have been limited and inconsistent in their findings. Many studies support that elders retain an interest in sexual function and are sexually active. Other studies conclude that there is a decline of sexual interest and behavior among aging individuals. Reported declines are largely the result of social, cultural, and psychologic factors, rather than biologic and physical factors. Determinants for sexual activity include present health status, past and present life satisfaction, social class, and marital status. For example, many older women are widowed or divorced and lack available sexual partners, which may account for their decline in sexual interest.

Physiologic changes associated with the aging process occur in both men and women. In women, vaginal secretions diminish and the vagina can atrophy. In men, the time required to develop an erection increases. With age, men are also able to maintain an erection for an extended period of time without ejaculation. After ejaculation, the older man often cannot have a subsequent erection for 12 to 24 hours. Despite these physiologic changes, both men and women are capable of sexual activity, including intercourse.

There are many misconceptions regarding the sexuality of elders. It is commonly believed that elders are asexual, lacking interest and/or the ability to perform sexually. It is essential that all individuals be recognized as sexual beings (Fig. 5–2) (see Chap. 10).

Family Structure

Improved health status, resulting in longer expected life spans; social changes, such as industrialization and urbanization; and normal aging processes influence family structure and functioning in late life. Most married couples see their last child launched in their middle to late 40s and can expect to live another 30 years. This long period that follows active parenting responsibilities presents a variety of problems elders have not had to deal with in previous generations.

Widowhood

Although most elderly men are married, two-thirds of all elderly women are widowed. Even when men have been widowed, their chances for remarriage are twice those of women.

A review of the literature on widowhood indicates some variables that relate to the adjustment of widowed persons to a single-life pattern (see the accompanying Focus on the Elderly feature). Ill health and poverty, coupled with the normal social losses of old age, confront the elderly widowed person with the prospect of becoming socially isolated. The ability to resist this trend

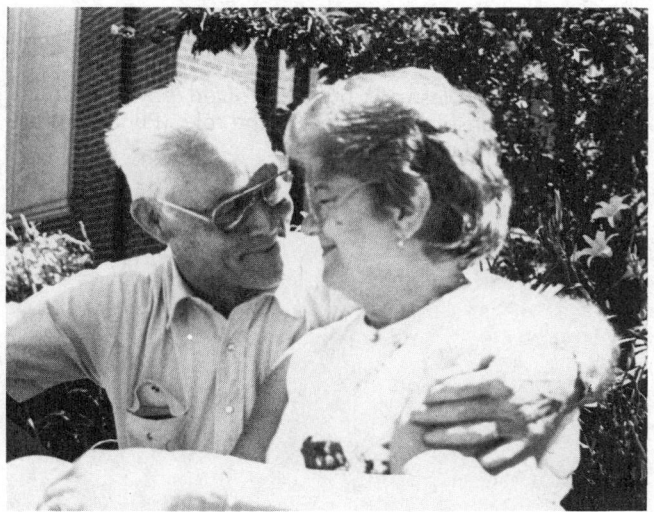

Figure 5–2

All individuals are sexual beings with individual needs. (Photographed by Marianne Matzo. Courtesy of St. Anselm College, Manchester, NH.)

FOCUS ON THE ELDERLY ■ Key Points Affecting Role Transition of Widows

Psychologic well-being in widows is significantly related to functional health status, risk factors, social readjustment, education, life style, and social participation.

Prewidowhood life style, functional health, and social readjustment are the best variables to predict psychologic well-being of widows 1 year after the death of a spouse.

Widows who have stable or increased income after the spouse's death experience significantly higher psychologic well-being than widows who have a decrease in income.

From Brock, A. M., O'Sullivan, P. (1985) From wife to widow: Role transition in the elderly. *Journal of Psychosocial Nursing and Mental Health Services, 23*(12), 6–12.

is thought to be heightened by advanced level of education, residence in a small town or a rural area, or, most important, the presence of friends and neighbors with whom one can relate. An adequate adjustment to being widowed is contingent on the social interaction of the individual before the loss and one's inner image, state of health, age, and social situation. It is asserted that older widowed persons adjust better to bereavement because of anticipatory grieving and the propensity to view death as one of the developmental tasks of old age.

Factors other than choice frequently operate to isolate the widowed person. Those who lack skills, money, health, and transportation for engaging or reengaging in society encounter more difficulties in adjusting to a change in role status. The lonely, isolated status of widows may be related to the socialization of women in past generations as dependent on men. Like any other life crisis, the loss of spouse affects people in various ways. Adjustment is related to the individual's previous life style and coping patterns.

Family Support

The relationship between adult children and their elderly parents is influenced by a variety of factors, such as distance, economics, health, and emotional health. Relationships are often taxed by a complex mixture of conflicts. Pulls between love and resentment, duty to parents and obligations for others, and wanting to do what is right and not wanting to change one's life style are not unusual in families. Yet, from the literature available, it seems that most families are able to resolve problems in a way that provides the elder with a sense of support, belonging, and love.

The majority of older people live within an hour's traveling distance of their children and manage to see them often. There are, however, some differences by social class. Upper-class and middle-class adults are likely to live greater distances from their parents than working-class adults. This difference is more a result of professional career patterns than a desire to be separated. Although patterns of aid and contact vary among the classes, there is no difference in caring. Greater distance results in fewer visits, but the quality of the visits and the frequent long-distance communication were reported to compensate for periods of absence. Distance between family members also alters the type of support exchanged. Families living close to one another tend to exchange services, such as shopping and household maintenance tasks, whereas family members who live some distance apart tend to confine their assistance to monetary supports.

Less than a third of the elderly live with their children. The results of several studies suggest that the elderly prefer this arrangement. Many elders want their privacy, independence, and freedom, rather than adjusting to their children's life style.

There is a growing proportion of frail, dependent elders. For this group there are two options available. They can live in an institution or remain in the community sustained by families, friends, and support agencies. Most elders prefer to reside in the community, but there are problems in society that make realization of this preference difficult. Families generally attempt to help but may be limited in their ability. Most adult couples are active members of the work force and still have dependent children at home or in school. Home health care services for the frail or ill elderly have not developed to the extent of the demand. The cost of long-term home health care services is frequently prohibitive. One of the greatest challenges the United States faces is to resolve the problems surrounding provision and financing of health care and social services for the rapidly expanding aged population.

Grandparenting

Grandparenting is often the most important role in the elders' life, providing them with a sense of purpose, value, and esteem. A relationship with grandparents often brings a sense of stability and perspective to their children's family. They provide the young with advice, affirmation, and a sense of roots and continuity. For their children, they can relieve some of the parenting burden by assuming actual caretaking responsibilities, especially when both parents are working.

The nature of the role assumed by the elder varies tremendously. Five major styles of grandparenting have been identified: the formal grandparent, who leaves all childrearing to the parents and confines his/her interest in the children to occasional visits and the offering of special treats; the fun seeker, who becomes a playmate and friend to the child; the surrogate parent, who assumes actual caretaking responsibility; the reservoir of family wisdom, who has an authoritarian role and dispenses special skills or resources; and the distant figure, who has remote contact with the child.

Regardless of the type of role assumed, grandparenting benefits the elder, the adult child, and the grandchild. Through the role of grandparent, the elder can maintain ego integrity and approach death with a sense of fulfillment and a feeling of extension of his/her influence into future generations. The grandchild and the adult child are provided the opportunity for anticipatory socialization into old age, as well as the emotional reward of a close and intimate relationship (Fig. 5–3).

Work and Retirement

In 1900, two of three older men were employed. In recent years, retirement has become less a matter of

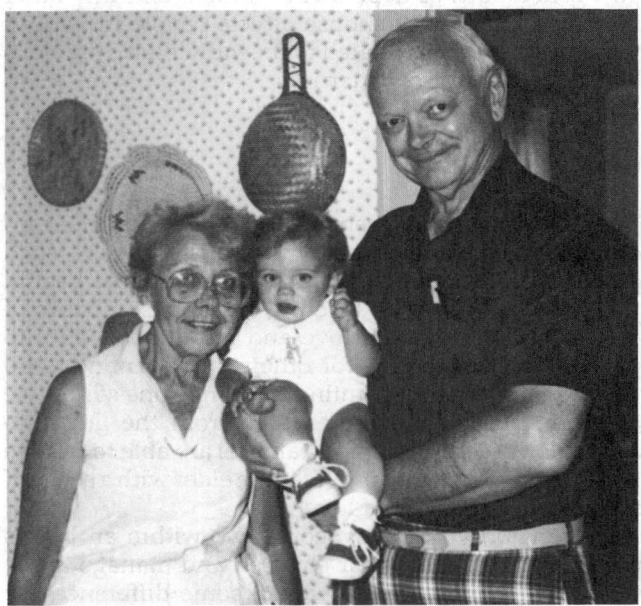

Figure 5–3

Grandparenting roles vary, but all involved may benefit from the relationship, regardless of the role. (Photographed by Susan Dolph Leach.)

choice, with only one of six older men employed (AARP & AOA, 1988). Because women were less likely to be working outside the home earlier in the century, the numbers of older female workers were less and have remained stable. This picture may change as the increased numbers of younger women who have entered the labor force age. Adjustment to retirement remains a significant crisis for a working person. One survey of retirees revealed that one-third of these retirees would prefer to work (AARP, 1988).

To most elderly people, it comes as a grim surprise that their income is less than adequate. For those who depend solely on Social Security benefits, their incomes fall below the federally established poverty levels. Therefore, one of the most serious problems retirement creates is inadequate financial resources.

Some of the developmental crises of retirement could be alleviated if adults planned their lives differently. The workaholic syndrome of the active adults years has an impact on one's aging. It is difficult for the elderly to suddenly fill their time with meaningful leisure activities. On the basis of the current evidence, it would seem that substantial social reforms regarding retirement need to take place. Preretirement counseling programs; alternative work patterns, such as second careers or shorter work weeks over longer periods; and better economic and health care provisions are being investigated.

Leisure

Adjustment to time freed from work, family, and social responsibilities in old age is dependent to a significant degree on such factors as prior attitudes toward work, aging, and retirement; health; income; geographic location; and family situation. Favorable adjustment to old age is characterized by a tendency toward substitution. To adequately adjust to the acquired status of retiree, the individual must replace or find substitutes for those satisfactions relinquished with lost roles.

Individuals tend to continue the same patterns of leisure established earlier in life. The five most popular activities before and after role losses are visiting friends, watching television, doing odd jobs at home, traveling, and reading. There do not seem to be changes in activities, but rather an increase in the frequency of customary activities.

The use of leisure is affected by sex, family status, profession, and education. The success of transitions to retirement and old age has been found to be strongly related to educational and occupational background. More highly educated persons seem able to more easily structure free time. Similarly, individuals with higher income status seem to view leisure time more positively and seem to feel that they have a greater degree of control over their life situations. A number of investigations have reported that life satisfaction in retirement is nearly always higher among professionals or among workers who manifested a positive preretirement attitude, although more professionals than other workers do continue working. Women consistently report an

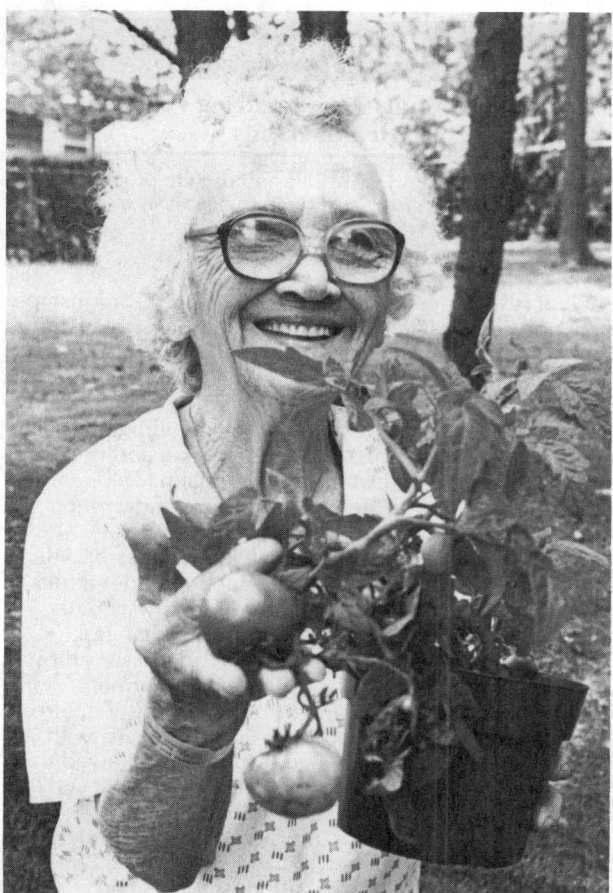

Figure 5 – 4

Elders often engage in hobbies that provide meaning and satisfaction during retirement. (Photographed by Marianne Matzo. Courtesy of St. Anselm College, Manchester, NH.)

easier adjustment to leisure time in late life than do men. Women generally have consistently developed more social relationships, been involved with their children and grandchildren, and developed more hobby interests throughout their life spans than their male counterparts have. (See Figure 5-4)

HEALTH ISSUES

Health Promotion

Health is a major concern of most elderly persons (see the accompanying Nursing Research feature). The elderly's health status can affect the ability to perform basic activities of daily living and to participate in social roles. Failure in performance of these activities increases the elder's dependence on others and tends to have a negative affect on morale and life satisfaction.

The relationship between age and morbidity and mortality is well known and well documented in life

NURSING RESEARCH

Older Adults Are Practicing Positive Health Habits.

Schafer, S. L. (1989). An aggressive approach to promoting health responsibility. *Journal of Gerontological Nursing, 15*(4), 22–27.

Several researchers have reported positive relationships between certain life style practices and physical health (Belloc & Breslow, 1972; Kaplan et al., 1987; Vallbona & Baker, 1984). Habits such as sleeping 7 to 8 hours, eating breakfast, not eating between meals, maintaining a desirable weight-to-height ratio, maintaining physical activity, avoiding excessive alcohol intake, and not smoking have been related to good health. This descriptive study was performed to determine who older adults believed were most responsible for personal health, to describe life style practices of older adults living in the community, to identify older adults' plans for change in life style, and to identify who or what would assist these adults in making changes.

A questionnaire with 18 items was administered by nursing students in a structured interview format. Complete data were obtained from 244 questionnaires. Age of respondents ranged from 60 to 88 years, with 70 years as the average. Sixty-five respondents viewed themselves most responsible for their health. Most of the adults in the study engaged in healthy life style practices (70% engaged in physical activity routinely; 69% ate breakfast routinely; 75% woke rested; 86% did not smoke; 49% of the current nonsmokers had stopped smoking; 53% visited a physician one to four times a year). Forty-eight per cent stated that they planned changes in health practices, and 48% indicated that they would not change. Forty-one per cent of the planned changes were related to diet; 36% involved exercise habits. Of the 75 persons who responded to the question about who or what would assist them in changing their habits, 40% indicated that self-reliance was important, and 16% stated that their spouse would help. No one indicated that a nurse would assist in changing health habits.

Critique. The great interest in health-promoting behaviors that was demonstrated by this population might be partially explained by the fact that all respondents were participants in a health-related screening program. The study should be replicated in settings unrelated to health care. However, the results are useful in that they give further support to the fact that many elders are independent, knowledgeable, and involved in wellness-related activities.

Possible nursing implications. A large percentage of older adults are conscious of the importance of practicing good health habits and are aware of which habits promote good health. The fact that no one considered a nurse as a resource for changing health practices suggests that nurses need to be more visible and more active in health promotion.

FOCUS ON THE ELDERLY ■ Causes of Mortality in Later Adulthood

Rank	Ages 45–64 yr	Age 65 yr and Older
1	Cancer	Heart disease
2	Heart disease	Cancer
3	Accidents	Cerebrovascular disease
4	Cerebrovascular disease	Influenza/pneumonia
5	Chronic obstructive pulmonary disease	Chronic obstructive pulmonary disease
6	Liver disease	Atherosclerosis
7	Suicide	Diabetes mellitus
8	Diabetes mellitus	Accidents
9	Pneumonia/influenza	Liver disease
10	Homicide	Kidney disease

From National Center for Health Statistics. (1985, September 26). *Monthly Vital Statistics Report, 33*(13).

expectancy tables and reports on the distribution of disease. The health problems most frequently observed among older persons tend to be chronic and are often degenerative rather than acute. Further, the health problems of the aged are frequently attributable to multiple causes, including physical, psychologic, and social components, in a complex mixture.

The Focus on the Elderly feature presents the causes of mortality in later adulthood. For both middle-aged and older adults, heart diseases and cancer are the most frequent causes of death. However, beyond the two leading causes of death, there are some interesting differences between middle-aged and older adults. Violent deaths from accidents, suicides, and homicides account for a substantial number of deaths in middlescence. For the older adult, most fatalities are due to disorders resulting from diminished physiologic defenses.

Multimorbidity and time-related physiologic changes with aging make it necessary to assess an aged person's health status differently from that of a young person. Proponents of the wellness model maintain that a focus on illness does not indicate the total health of old people. From this perspective, health is not based on absence or presence of pathologic changes, but on the level of functioning. In assessing the level of functioning, self-responsibility, nutritional awareness, physical fitness, positive stress management techniques, and environmental sensitivity are the dimensions often considered in the elderly.

Self-Responsibility

The ability to maintain a positive self-concept and self-control is often hampered by the loss of resources in the late years of life. The elderly experience a number of losses that erode their sense of effective control over their lives—deaths of significant others, loss of social and work roles, diminished finances, and loss of physical mobility.

Regardless of what the elders' situation is, it is important that they direct their life style in a manner that encourages them to feel capable and valued. The elderly need to find opportunities to be productive and take care of themselves as well as others.

To promote self-responsibility for the elder, it is crucial that society counteracts the stereotypes and myths that abound regarding the older person. Health care professionals, family, and significant others should evaluate capabilities and interests of the elders carefully, ensuring opportunities for responsibilities that are meaningful and within their ability. Older persons' self-esteem and feelings of competency can be supported by encouraging them to maintain as much control as possible over their lives, participate in decision-making, and perform as many tasks as possible.

Nutritional Awareness

The need for adequate nutrition remains constant throughout the life span, yet most elderly persons eat an inadequate diet. Inflation, reduced income, and lack of transportation are factors that frequently contribute to inadequate nutrition; reliance on inappropriate or unbalanced intake of food substances, such as an excessive proportion of high-carbohydrate foods, results in insufficient nutrition. Some elders reduce their intake of food to near-starvation levels, even with the availability of assistive programs, such as food stamps, free food, and Meals on Wheels programs. The lack of transportation, the necessity to travel a distance to obtain such services, and the inability to carry large quantities of groceries prohibit many elders from taking advantage of food programs.

Poor nutrition among the elderly may be related to loneliness. Elders often respond to loneliness, depression, and boredom by not eating, which leads to malnutrition. Many elderly who live alone have lost incentive to prepare or eat balanced diets. Others respond to stress by overeating, which leads to obesity.

The minimal nutritional requirements from youth through old age remain consistent, with a few exceptions. Increased dietary intake of calcium, vitamin C, and vitamin A is needed because alterations with age disrupt the ability to store, use, and absorb these substances. Sedentary life styles and reduced metabolic rate demand reduction in total caloric intake to maintain ideal body weight. However, other physical aging changes influence the elder's nutritional status or ability to take in needed nutritive substances. A diminished sense of taste and smell often results in a loss of appeal of food. There is a greater decline in the ability to taste sweet and salt than there is in the discrimination of bitter and sour. This phenomenon often results in overuse of table sugar and salt to compensate. Using herbs and spices to season food or varying the textures of food substances to achieve oral gratification would better serve the elderly and lessen the risk of potential problems associated with high intake of sodium and sucrose. Loss of teeth and poorly fitting dentures can cause the elderly to avoid important foodstuffs. Older people with dentition problems frequently resort to eating soft, high-calorie foods, which lack roughage and fiber. Unless the elder carefully chooses nutritious soft foods, vitamin deficiencies, constipation, and other disorders can result. The aged respond to problems associated with mobility, prescribed diuretics, and limited bladder capacity by limiting fluid intake. Fluid restrictions make the elder vulnerable to dehydration and serious electrolyte imbalances.

Physical Fitness

Exercise and activity are important to the older adult as a means of promoting and maintaining health (Fig. 5–5). Physical activity can help keep the body in shape and maintain an optimal functional level. Research indicates that regular, moderate exercise results in feelings of well-being. Numerous epidemiologic studies have indicated a lower incidence of coronary artery disease in populations engaged in regular physical activity when compared with populations that are sedentary. Without exercise, muscles, organs, and tissues tend to atrophy, and motor, sensory, and cognitive functions are impaired. The benefits and purposes of regular exercise are to improve circulation, improve blood pressure, improve respiratory function, maintain muscle tone throughout the body, reduce muscle tension, reduce muscle pain, and promote relaxation.

Stress Management

In most physiologic and psychologic theories of aging, stress and disease play significant roles. Stress can speed up the aging process over time, or it can lead to diseases that increase the rate of degeneration. Stress can impair the reserve capacity of the elderly and lessen their ability to respond and adapt to changes in their environment.

Although no period of the life cycle is free from emotional stress, the later years constitute a time of especially high risk. Frequently observed sources of stress for the older population include rapid environmental changes that require immediate reaction, changes in life style resulting from retirement or physical incapacity, acute or chronic illness, loss of significant others, financial hardships, relocation, and a general lack of purpose

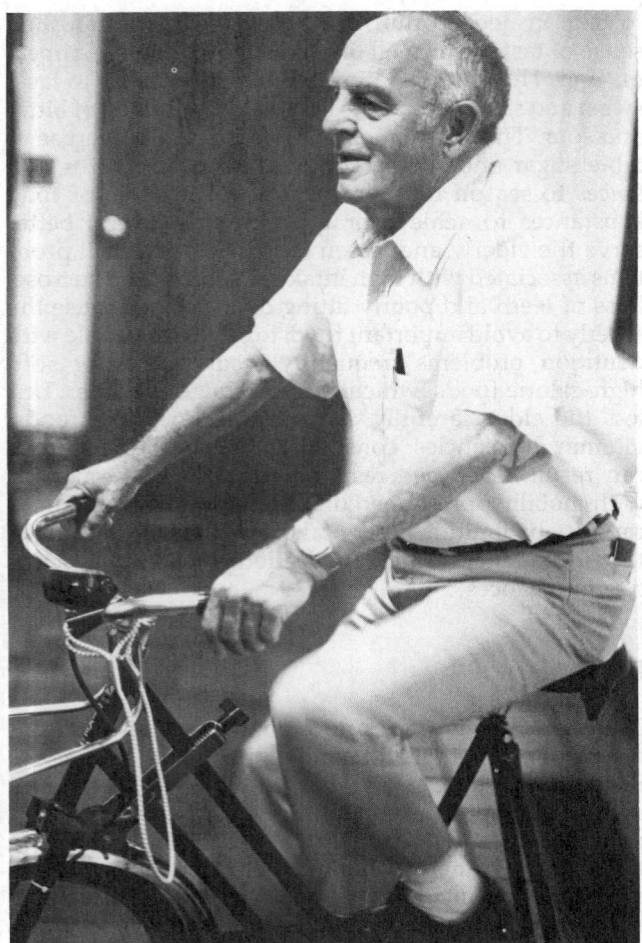

Figure 5–5

Exercise is important to elders for health promotion and maintenance. (Photographed by Marianne Matzo. Courtesy of St. Anselm College, Manchester, NH.)

in life. How people react to these stresses depends on their personal skills and support networks. The loss of roles experienced by the elderly often limits the availability of external support networks. For a number of elderly, successive role losses have left them bereft of friends and associates to whom they could turn for reaffirmation of self-concept and help. Many elderly have to rely solely on their personal resources to maintain their mental health. When poor physical health is combined with the social adversities incurred by the elderly and a lack of understanding of their plight by society, older people are susceptible to stress overload, which can result in illness and premature death.

Individuals have a responsibility to develop effective life styles and coping patterns over their life spans that will assist them in their late years. Research seems to indicate that the ways in which people adapt to old age depend less on their degree of activity and involvement in life around them than on the personality traits and habits of response that have characterized them throughout their lives. Establishing and maintaining relationships with others throughout life are important to the elder's happiness. Even more important than having friends at all is the nature of the friendships. People who have close, intimate, stable relationships with others in whom they confide are more likely to maintain integrity in times of crises.

Environmental Sensitivity

Each person's environment is formed by physical surroundings, rules, and significant others.

Physical incapacity or economic problems may force some elderly persons to relocate. If elderly persons must move to a nursing home or a long-term care facility, family members or institutional personnel need to be aware that the elder needs some personal space in the new surroundings. Older people need to participate in deciding how the space will be arranged and what they can keep in the new environment. Such participation helps to offset the feelings of powerlessness and depersonalization that often accompany relocation. The presence of personal items assists in making the new setting seem more familiar and comfortable.

The declining efficiency of the senses and decreased motor ability can create difficulties for the elderly in functioning in their environment. The less clear vision in old age, especially the poor perception of distance, makes ambulation difficult; an individual is less aware of where each step is. The reduced sense of touch gives the elder weaker awareness of body orientation (e.g., whether the foot is squarely on the step). Decreased reaction time that commonly results from age-related changes in the neurologic system also impairs the elder's ability to recognize or move from a dangerous setting or break a fall. Because of decreases in the ability to react to stimuli, elders also are prone to experience sensory overload.

Accidents

Older adults need to be aware of safety precautions that should be taken to prevent health hazards. The prevention of injury to muscles, bones, and other body parts that have grown fragile with age is not only of critical importance, but is probably the area in which aging persons can do the most to preserve their fitness. Incapacitating accidents are a primary cause of restricted physical fitness in old age.

Safeguards such as installing and holding on to handrails when using steps and getting into and out of the shower or bathtub, securing rugs with slip-proof underpads, and making sure treacherous places are well lighted are essential. Clients should be advised to concentrate on one activity at a time to minimize sensory overload. Consideration of the use of visual, hearing, or ambulatory assistive devices can be encouraged. Precautions in the environment cannot be overstressed, as serious and crippling injuries can occur from falls, strains, and other accidents.

Prohibitive costs and elderly persons' vanity and fear of overt recognition as "old" prevent them from obtaining or using hearing, visual, or ambulatory assistive devices. This could increase the risk of accidents.

Drug Use and Misuse

Drug therapy for the elderly population is another health issue that requires significant consideration. Because of multimorbidity in this age group, elderly persons account for 25% of all prescription drug expenditure (Ebert, 1989). Studies also show that elders frequently use nonprescription drugs and rarely consult a physician about such use. Analgesics, antacids, cold and cough preparations, laxatives, and vitamins are commonly used in this way. Research indicates that the occurrence of adverse drug reactions is directly related to the number and frequency of drug exposures. Elders are therefore at high risk for adverse drug reactions or interactions. Common causes and predisposing factors of adverse drug reactions in the geriatric client are summarized in the accompanying Focus on the Elderly feature.

The physiologic changes related to aging make drug therapy in elders complex. It has been recognized only recently that elders may not tolerate the standard dosage of medications traditionally prescribed for other age groups. Specific application of pharmacokinetic principles is necessary when dealing with elders. *Pharmacokinetics* is the study of the absorption, distribution, biotransformation, and excretion of drugs. The degree to which one can perform these bodily functions affects the action and concentration of drug in the body.

Age-related changes that can potentially affect drug absorption from an oral route include an increase in gastric pH, a decrease in gastric blood flow, and a decrease in gastrointestinal motility. Despite these changes, difficulty with absorption related to age-re-

lated changes alone is not a problem in most elderly. Age-related changes that do affect distribution of a drug include smaller amounts of total body water, an increased ratio of adipose tissue to lean body mass, a decreased albumin level, and a decrease in cardiac output. Increased adipose tissue in proportion to lean body mass can cause increased storage of lipid-soluble drugs. This leads to decreased concentration of drug in plasma, but increased concentration in tissue. Elimination time of the drug is prolonged. Administration of water-soluble drugs in this situation results in a high concentration of drug in the plasma and more rapid elimination. Decreased albumin level can cause an increased concentration of active drug. Biotransformation most often occurs in the liver. Age-related changes affecting biotransformation include a decrease in liver mass, a decrease in liver blood flow, and a decrease in liver enzyme activity. These changes can result in increased plasma concentrations of drug. Elimination most often involves the renal system. Age-related changes of the renal system include a decrease in renal blood flow and reduced glomerular filtration rate. These changes can result in a prolonged half-life of renally excreted drugs.

Because of these physiologic changes, elders are at risk for toxic effects from drugs. Drug reactions have a more dramatic effect and take a longer time to correct in older people. This is because elders have less reserve capacity in most organ systems. Often a lower dose of medicine is necessary to prevent adverse effects. It should be noted, however, that physiologic changes of aging are highly individual. Thus, alterations in drug therapy should always be considered for elders, but not necessarily implemented, and should be individualized.

Common adverse drug reactions in elders include nausea, vomiting, anorexia, fatigue, weakness, dizziness, urinary retention, diarrhea, constipation, and confusion. Many of these signs and symptoms could be mistakenly attributed to concurrent illness the client might be experiencing. It is imperative that all clients manifesting symptoms such as those described be thoroughly assessed for potential adverse reactions to medications.

Most people older than 65 years of age live at home and are responsible for taking their own medications. Because the risk of drug intoxication is considerably increased in the elderly population, the need to assist them assume this task responsibly is paramount. Many problems can be prevented through educating, providing clear and concise directions, and developing ways to assist the elder to overcome self-administration handicaps or difficulties.

Elders make errors in drug administration for several reasons. First, they simply forget. In the rush of daily activities, drugs may not be taken at all or may be taken too often because the person does not remember when or whether medications have been taken. Associating pill taking with daily events, such as meals, or keeping a simple chart or calendar often assists people. Pill boxes have been devised so that a daily, weekly, or monthly supply of medicine can be placed in appropriate com-

---

FOCUS ON THE ELDERLY ■ Common Causes and Predisposing Factors for Adverse Drug Reactions in the Geriatric Client

Physiologic changes of aging, including reduced vital organ capacity and function

Excessive dosage

Predisposing diseases

Polypharmacy and excessive drug prescribing

Wrong diagnosis

Noncompliance

Vitamin or mineral deficiencies

partments. Large print on the drug label assists clients with poor visual acuity. Writing the drug regimen on the top of the bottle with large letters and numbers is also helpful.

A second reason that elderly persons frequently commit errors in taking medications is poor communication with health care professionals. These difficulties stem from such sources as inadequate explanations to the elder or explanations they cannot understand because of educational limitations or language barriers. Health care professionals frequently presume that, if they told the elder about the drugs, knowledge has been acquired. Health care providers need to validate what the elders plan to do, what they think they should be doing, and why they are doing it with regard to medication schedules.

A third important reason for medication errors is one of attitude and long-ingrained feelings about taking medicine. Some people are inveterate pill takers; they think no physician can help them unless he/she prescribed medication. Conversely, others avoid taking medicine whenever they can. The fear of drug dependency may cause many to discontinue medications prematurely. Others think that two pills will be twice as effective as one; some thrifty elders take medicine that is left over from a previous illness or that has been prescribed for someone else.

The attitudes of elders toward their medication and their health problems can be influenced by health care providers. Instruction can sometimes be more effectively given by lay persons of the same socioeconomic or cultural background as the elder. A method that is being tried in some hospitals is supervised self-administration of medicine. Clients are allowed to take their own medications under supervision before they are discharged. In this manner, validation of understanding and ability are tested.

Mental Health

Some changes in cognition have been identified as age related. These changes are linked to specific functions of cognition, as opposed to intellectual capacity. They include a decreased reaction time to stimuli and an impairment of memory of recent events. It is certain, however, that gross cognitive impairment, depression, hallucinations, and delusions are not part of the normal aging process. Most elders are mentally sound.

Losses in income and physical health, lack of comprehensive health care and social services, loss of social roles, and deaths of significant others serve to deplete the resources available to the aged person for maintaining emotional stability. It is not surprising that mental illness occurs among the aged population. Depression, as a response to multiple life stresses, is one of the major disturbances in cognitive functioning in elders.

Dementia is a broad term used for a syndrome that is also characterized by a disturbance in cognition occurring in elders. It represents global impairment of intel-

lectual function and is generally chronic and progressive. There are many diseases that manifest themselves as dementia, the most common being Alzheimer's disease (senile dementia, Alzheimer type). Multi-infarct dementia is a vascular disorder, which accounts for 20% to 25% of all dementias (Gershon & Herman, 1982).

It is imperative that dementia be differentiated from delirium. *Delirium* is a state of confusion; it is different from dementia in that it is often reversible. It also has an acute onset compared with the gradual onset of dementia. There are multiple causes for delirium, including medication, metabolic disturbances, infections, circulatory and pulmonary disorders, and nutritional deficiencies.

The elder is often unaware of early symptoms of emotional or mental impairments. Symptoms may go unnoticed by family and friends and thus are allowed to progress until the elder is in crisis. The nature of the symptoms is such that their onset and development is noticed in minor behavioral or physical changes. Many elders are reluctant to admit that they need help for fear of loss of power, independence, or self-esteem. Many have mistaken ideas about psychotherapy. Others fear a lengthy and costly treatment process or institutionalization. For those older persons who are amenable to care, private treatment is expensive. Low-cost mental health care services do not exist in every community. In addition, health care practitioners who see the elderly are not always sensitive to their problems.

ECONOMIC ISSUES

Part of the American dream is the notion of economic self-reliance. Most adults hope that throughout their life cycle they can provide for their own needs. One of the greatest fears many adults have related to aging is becoming destitute and dependent on family, friends, or society. In many cases, achievement of economic self-sufficiency has not been realized successfully in recent years. One-fifth of the total population is poor, and one-fifth of the poor are more than 65 years of age. According to statistics from the U.S. Department of Commerce (1985), 83% of families headed by persons older than 65 years of age have an annual income of less than $10,000, and almost 1.1 million have incomes of less than $3,000.

Most people expect financial resources in their retirement years to decline compared with those in their working years. However, they also expect that the level of their expenditures will decline proportionately, and this has not occurred. The inflation of the 1970s reduced the value of financial assets. The elderly were especially hard hit because most rely on Social Security benefits or pension funds for the bulk of their income. These assets are usually fixed and cannot be altered by the individual. Therefore, most elders are unable to adjust their income to changing economic circumstances and hence are powerless to combat declining real income. Health care purchases are paid for in substantial part by private insurance and federal health and social programs. Yet the rising cost of these programs contributes substantially to rising government expenditures and the size of government deficits and results in more out-of-pocket costs for the aged health consumer.

Reduced inflation is especially beneficial to retired persons because it allows them to be better able to take care of themselves and affords the economy more output to share with needy nonworkers. The 1981 White House Conference on Aging suggested that action to improve the economic situation of the aged include the following components: increased labor force participation by the elderly, increased emphasis on individual savings and investment, and inflation control.

Housing

The popular conceptualization of the elderly as frail, dependent, senile individuals living out their last years in an institution has no factual basis. Only about 5% of the aged population reside in institutions providing long-term care (AARP & AOA, 1988). Many elders live in their own homes and have paid off their mortgages. Yet, living arrangements are a major problem for most individuals as they age.

It is a reality of modern times that rising energy and housing costs have joined the high costs of food and health care as factors that contribute to the economic hardship of many aging persons. In addition to the financial difficulties, housing for the aged is problematic because of a lack of environmental supports to assist them to remain residing and participating in the community.

Deterioration of property, escalation of property taxes, and maintenance service costs create many problems for elder homeowners in keeping their homes. Elderly renters are extremely vulnerable to prohibitive rent fees, real estate speculation, and loss of living quarters because of removal of substandard, low-rent apartment or hotel buildings. Physical impairments and a lack of available, affordable support services, such as household help, transportation, home health care, and assistance with meals, prohibit many aged people from being able to manage adequately in their own homes.

The need for special housing for the aged has long been recognized. Numbers of government and privately funded experiments in alternative housing for the aged have been tested. These projects incorporated such variables as the availability of a comprehensive array of personal care services, special health and safety remedies, and recreation and leisure plans. Although most of these projects provide security, improve life satisfaction, and prove cost-effective, there is no overall plan for alternative living arrangements for the elderly at present.

In part, the reluctance to expand federal support of community-based services is due to a fear that such formal programs will substitute for informal programs and hence add immeasurably to the public tax burden. However, far too little attention has been given to the current incentives for substituting home-based care for formal institutional care. Public programs pay for most living and personal care services in a nursing home, but there is little public subsidy of services in private homes that might enhance the ability of family and friends to meet the bulk of care needs at a lesser cost.

RESOURCES FOR THE ELDERLY

There is a broad range of benefits and services available from federal, state, and local sources to assist older people with problems related to health, income, or social services. It is essential that elders, their families, and health care and social service providers be aware of the types of services available to assist older people in achieving a higher quality of life. Until recently, most of these benefits and services were believed to be the responsibility of the individual rather than society. Yet, because of economic crisis, the rapid increase in the proportion of the aged in the population, and the increased incidence of chronic morbidity, problems emerged that the individual elder's effort alone could not solve. Gradually the government, in addition to providing income support and health care services, has increased its involvement in education, crime prevention, nutrition, and other programs to assist the elderly.

GOVERNMENT RESOURCES

INCOME

The major portion of federal funds supporting programs for the elderly is devoted to the Social Security programs. The Social Security Act was passed in 1935, after the Depression, when many elderly were economically impoverished. Since that time, there has been a gradual shift from a program that was intended to provide a minimal supplement to retirees' sources of income to one that is the primary source of retirement income for many people. Other provisions of this act that are significant for people less than 65 years of age are the disability and survivors' insurance provisions.

HEALTH INSURANCE

Medicare was enacted as part of the amendments to the Social Security Act of 1965. This program was created to assist older people to meet the cost of health care. Despite its deficiencies, Medicare has provided a means for elders to obtain needed health care in times of escalating costs without decimating their total personal savings.

Medicare provides health insurance to people 65 years of age and older.

Medicaid is a program designed to provide payment for medical services for the poor, inclusive of the poor elderly. For eligible individuals who are 65 years old or older, it supplements the Medicare insurance program. Eligibility is related to determination of poverty level, and each state program determines its own criteria for eligibility (see Chap. 4).

HOUSING PROGRAMS

Congress has passed a number of legislative acts designed to alleviate housing problems for older citizens. Among these programs is rental assistance of lower-income families, the elderly, and the disabled. Direct loans at low interest are available to individuals to construct special rental housing facilities for the handicapped and the elderly. The federal government supports construction and rehabilitation of nursing homes. It subsidizes rental facilities, which can be rented by the aged at rates below the existing marked price. Information related to these housing programs can be obtained in most communities by contacting the local public housing authority or the Housing and Urban Development Area Office.

SOCIAL SERVICES

The Older Americans Act of 1965 provided social services to the aged. Under this legislation, each state created an office to provide leadership in the coordination and development of services for the elderly. Some of the more significant programs and services carried out under this legislation are described in the accompanying Focus on the Elderly feature.

RESEARCH AGENCIES

The National Institute on Aging was established in 1974. Its purpose is to conduct research on the biologic, population-related, and sociologic aspects of aging at its Gerontology Research Center in Baltimore, Maryland, and to support research by others at universities and laboratories across the United States.

Within the National Institute for Mental Health, one division is devoted exclusively to problems of the aged: the Center for Studies of the Mental Health of the Aging. Its major role is to stimulate, coordinate, and support research training and to offer technical assistance relating to aging and mental health. Although it provides no monies for programs of service delivery to older people, it significantly affects the training of those working with elderly clients in community mental health centers and other service settings.

FOCUS ON THE ELDERLY ■ Social Services Provided by the Older Americans Act of 1965

Senior centers to meet the need for a central place for older people to congregate, develop new interests, and socialize.

Nutrition programs to provide nutritious meals in a centralized setting as well as to home-bound elders. Recreation, education, and health activities are incorporated in many sites as a regular part of the program.

Transportation services to accommodate elders via special fares on existing public transportation systems and the operation of specially equipped vehicles for the frail and the handicapped elderly.

Information and referral services to direct elders to the appropriate agency that provides needed services.

In-home services, such as household help, telephone reassurance, chore maintenance, and visitation by home health aides, to enable older impaired individuals to remain living in the community.

COMMUNITY RESOURCES

Over the years, it has become evident that government programs cannot provide all services needed by the aged. It has been demonstrated in many arenas that private efforts can supply the same services at lower costs and without the red tape that some government programs involve. Transportation is an area in which the private sector, state and local governments, and the federal government all have roles.

Public ownership of mass transit has expanded over the past 30 years in both municipal and regional systems. The public systems have tried to restore the services dropped by the private companies, but economic problems at city or municipal levels of government have prevented implementation. In many urban areas, governments have provided Dial-A-Ride, which provides free transportation, or similar services. These services should be continued and expanded if possible. The federal government has subsidized the development and operation of transit systems, but its aid has been focused mainly on high-use systems and routes. For occasional travel, particularly in rural areas, the best solution is probably to rely on a friend or a neighbor. Churches and community groups can help organize this approach by using sign-up sheets and recruiting volunteers to drive 1 day a week.

Neighborhood surveillance programs extend the capabilities of local police and provide a feeling of security for older people.

Education, recreation, and cultural activities are important for maintaining physical condition, mental alertness, and social contact. Education helps older people keep up with a rapidly changing world. Although advances in cable and satellite television systems promise a broad range of new educational experiences at home, the value of person-to-person discussion and the need to focus some educational activities on local issues means that community discussion groups and other informal education will remain important.

Recreation and cultural activities are best managed on a local, nongovernment basis because personal preference plays such a large role in determining individual participation. A variety of different activities run by different organizations or informal groups is likely to please more people than a large program run by a government agency. For example, in the Midwest, elders have formed square dance groups and gourmet groups, which meet frequently for socialization, as well as to compete with similar local, regional, and state groups.

Churches and other religious institutions serve the elderly in many ways. In addition to their primary role of providing organized worship, they sponsor many activities that bring elderly together with their peers as well as with younger people. Clergypersons, rabbis, and other spiritual leaders are often excellent counselors, and other members of the congregation or religious group are often willing to help older members in time of trouble.

Many communities have access to community resources books (e.g., those published by the United Way). Area agencies on aging are excellent referral centers. Some of these agencies publish directories of services that are specifically geared to the elderly.

SUMMARY

The 20th century ushered in an interest in studying what happens to the individual during the adult years. Until this time, a great deal of research has been devoted to examining how infants grew and developed into young adolescents. It was more or less accepted that if one resolved the crises of the young years, one could function effectively through adulthood. Yet, it became clear that this was not the case. Scholars from all disciplines recognized that human development is an ongoing process that continues throughout life.

This chapter attempts to describe the major concepts of biologic, social, and psychologic scientists that have contributed to the increasing understanding of the various periods of the adulthood years. Emphasis is placed on exploring the interrelationships of biologic, sociologic, and psychologic changes that affect the health and well-being of adults. Health promotion strategies,

health concerns, and appropriate measures to retard illness for each life span cycle are presented.

IMPLICATIONS FOR RESEARCH

Only comparatively recently have the fields of psychology and sociology turned their attention to the latter half of the life cycle. Various psychosocial theories of aging are in evidence in the psychology and sociology literature. The nursing literature has been conspicuously lacking in explorations of these various theories.

A large number of the clients that nurses care for are elderly; because the expected life span is increasing, these numbers are likely to increase. Geriatric medicine seems destined to be even more important in tomorrow's health care practice. Thus, the psychosocial development of the older adult is an important area of concern for the nurse.

Some major research questions that have significance for health care in the adult years and are of importance to nursing are

1. What is the impact of role transitions and stressful life events on social and psychologic states in adulthood and late life?
2. How does the family serve as a social support system and a source of social stress?
3. What impact do changes of living and household arrangements have on psychologic and social health care variables?
4. What factors relate to life satisfaction, longevity, and other measures of adaptation to aging?
5. What impact do changes in socioeconomic and marital status have on functional health status in the elderly?

REFERENCES AND READINGS

American Association of Retired Persons (AARP). (1988). *Using the experience of a lifetime* (Publication No. D13353). Washington, DC: Author.

American Association of Retired Persons (AARP), & Administration on Aging (AOA). (1988). *A profile of older Americans* (DHHS Publication No. D996). Washington, DC: U.S. Department of Health and Human Services.

American Cancer Society. (1984). *Facts and figures.* New York: Author.

American Cancer Society. (1989). Cancer statistics, 1989. *CA: A Cancer Journal for Clinicians, 39,* 3–20.

Belloc, N. B., & Breslow, L. (1972). Relationship of physical health status and health practices. *Preventive Medicine, 1,* 409–421.

Brim, O. G. (1968). Adult socialization. In J. Clausen (Ed.), *Socialization of society.* Boston: Little, Brown.

Brock, A. M. (1980). Self-administration of drugs in the elderly: Nursing responsibilities. *Journal of Gerontological Nursing, 9,* 398–418.

Brock, A. M. (1984a). Cohort influence on drug use and consumption. *Special Care in Dentistry, 4,* 160–164.

Brock, A. M. (1984b). From wife to widow: A changing lifestyle. *Journal of Gerontological Nursing, 10*(4), 8–15.

Brock, A. M. (1985). Communicating with the elderly patient. *Special Care in Dentistry, 4,* 157–159.

Brock, A. M., & O'Sullivan, P. (1985). A study to determine what variables predict institutionalization. *Journal of Advanced Nursing, 10,* 533–537.

Bunting, S. (1989). Stress on caregivers of the elderly. *Advances in Nursing Science, 11,* 63–73.

Butler, R. N. (1975). *Why survive? Being old in America.* New York: Harper & Row.

Cooley, E., & Keesey, J. (1981). Moderator variables in life stress and illness relationship. *Journal of Human Stress, 7,* 35–40.

Davis, R. L., Shapiro, M. F., & Kane, R. L. (1984). Level of care and complications among geriatric patients discharged from the medical service of a teaching hospital. *Journal of the American Geriatrics Society, 32,* 427–430.

Ebert, N. J. (1989). The nursing process applied to the aged person receiving medication. In A. G. Yurick, B. E. Spier, S. S. Robb, N. J. Ebert, & M. H. Magnussen (Eds.), *The aged person and the nursing process* (pp. 709–730). Norwalk, CT: Appleton & Lange.

Erikson, E. H. (1968a). *Childhood and society* (2nd ed.). New York: W. W. Norton.

Erikson, E. H. (1968b). *Identity: Youth and crisis.* New York: W. W. Norton.

Esberger, K. K., & Hughes, S. T. (Eds.). (1989). *Nursing care of the aged.* Norwalk, CT: Appleton & Lange.

Gershon, S., & Herman, S. P. (1982). The differential diagnosis of dementia. *Journal of the American Geriatrics Society, 30,* S58–S65.

Gress, L., & Bahr, R. (1984). *The aging person: A holistic perspective.* St. Louis: C. V. Mosby.

Hamilton, E., & Witney, E. (1979). *Nutrition: Concepts & controversies.* St. Paul, MN: West.

Havighurst, R. (1972). *Developmental tasks and education.* New York: David McKay.

Heaney, R. P. (1982). Effects of nitrogen, phosphorus, and caffeine on calcium balance in women. *Journal of Laboratory and Clinical Medicine, 99,* 46–55.

Hendricks, J., & Hendricks, C. (1981). *Aging in mass society: Myths and realities.* Cambridge, MA: Winthrop.

Jung, C. (1971). The stages of life. In J. Campbell (Ed.), *The portable Jung.* New York: Viking. (Original work published 1928)

Kane, R. L., Matthias, R., & Sampson, S. (1983). The risk of placement in a nursing home after acute hospitalization. *Medical Care, 21,* 1055–1061.

Kaplan, G. A., Seeman, T. E., Cohen, R. D., Knudsen, L. P., & Guralnik, J. (1987). Mortality among the elderly in the Alameda County Study: Behavioral and demographic risk factors. *American Journal of Public Health, 77,* 307–312.

Klein, P. (1985). Women in the labor force: The middle years. *Monthly Labor Review, 98,* 1016.

Lamy, P. (1974). Geriatric drug therapy. *Clinical Medicine, 81,* 52–57.

Larson, E. B., Reifler, B. V., & Featherstone, H. J. (1984). Dementia in the elderly outpatients: A prospective study. *Annals of Internal Medicine, 100,* 417–423.

Matteson, M. A., & McConnell, E. S. (Eds.). (1988). *Gerontological nursing.* Philadelphia: W. B. Saunders.

National Council on Alcoholism. (1981). *Facts on alcoholism and women.* New York: Author.

Neugarten, B. L. (1977). Personality and aging. In J. E. Birrin & K. W. Schaie (Eds.), *Handbook of the personality of aging.* New York: Van Nostrand Reinhold.

Neugarten, B. L., & Weinstein, K. (1964). The changing American grandparent. *Journal of Marriage and the Family, 26,* 199–204.

Olson, L., Christopher, C., & Martin, D. (1981). *The elderly and the future economy.* Lexington, MA: Lexington Books.

Peck, R. C. (1968). Psychological developments in the second half of life. In B. L. Neugarten (Ed.), *Middle age and aging.* Chicago: University of Chicago Press.

Price, J., & Andrews, P. (1982). Alcohol abuse in the elderly. *Journal of Gerontological Nursing, 8*(1), 16–18.

Riffle, K. L. (1982). Falls: Kinds, causes, and prevention. *Geriatric Nursing, 3,* 165–168.

Rosow, I. (1974). *Socialization to old age.* Berkeley: University of California Press.

Seyle, H., & Prioreschi, P. (1960). Stress theory of aging. In N. W. Shock (Ed.), *Aging: Some social and biological aspects.* Washington, DC: American Association for the Advancement of Science.

Shanas, E. (1982). The family relations of old people. *New Forum, 52,* 9.

Sheehy, G. (1976). *Passages: Predictable crises of adult life.* New York: Bantam Books.

Siegel, M. M., & Good, R. A. (Eds.). (1972). *Tolerance, autoimmunity and aging.* Springfield, IL: Charles C Thomas.

U.S. Department of Commerce, Bureau of the Census. (1985). *Statistical Abstract of the United States.* Washington, DC: U.S. Government Printing Office.

U.S. General Accounting Office. (1983). *Medicaid and nursing home care: Cost increases and the need for services are creating problems for the states and the elderly* (Publication No. IPE–84–1.13). Washington, DC: U.S. Government Printing Office.

Vallbona, C., & Baker, S. B. (1984). Physical fitness prospects in the elderly. *Archives of Physical Medicine and Rehabilitation, 65,* 194–200.

Wachtel, T. J., Derby, C., & Fulton, J. P. (1984). Predicting the outcome of hospitalization for elderly person: Home versus nursing home. *Southern Medical Journal, 77,* 1283–1285.

Wolff, M. L. (1982). Reversible intellectual impairment: An internist's perspective. *Journal of the American Geriatrics Society, 30,* 647–650.

Yurick, A. G., Spier, B. S., Robb, S. S., & Ebert, N. J. (Eds.). (1989). *The aged person and the nursing process* (3rd ed.). Norwalk, CT: Appleton & Lange.

Zelechowski, G. P. (1977). Helping your patient sleep: Planning instead of pills. *Nursing '77, 7,* 63.

ADDITIONAL READINGS

Albert, M. (1987). Health screening to promote health for the elderly. *Nurse Practitioner, 12,* 42–56.

This article provides information on significant health care problems that the elderly experience. Age-related changes are discussed to explain many of these problems, along with screening techniques and interventions.

American Association of Retired Persons (AARP). (1986). *Miles away and still caring. A guide for long-distance caregivers* (Publication No. D12748). Washington, DC: Author.

This publication provides a wealth of information for elders and their families who live far apart. Suggestions to assist families in assessing the needs of elderly relatives are provided along with multiple resources that are related to identified needs. (To obtain this publication, write AARP, 1909 K Street, NW, Washington, DC 20049.)

Brook, V. (1989, March/April). How elders adjust. *Geriatric Nursing,* pp. 66–68.

This article discusses the results of the author's research involving clients who have entered a nursing home. Verbatim notes and descriptive data were collected from 11 men and 31 women admitted to a 155-bed nursing home. Four major phases of adjusting to living in a nursing home were identified through analysis of the data. These phases included disorganization, reorganization, relationship building, and stabilization.

McKeon, V. A. (1988). Dispelling menopause myths. *Journal of Gerontological Nursing, 4*(8), 26–29.

This article provides a comprehensive discussion of myths related to menopause, their origin, and facts that dispel each myth. The author, a nurse, describes how these myths can negatively affect women and suggests that menopause be more accurately described as a normal and potentially positive event in a woman's life.

CHAPTER 6

Stress, Coping, and Adaptation

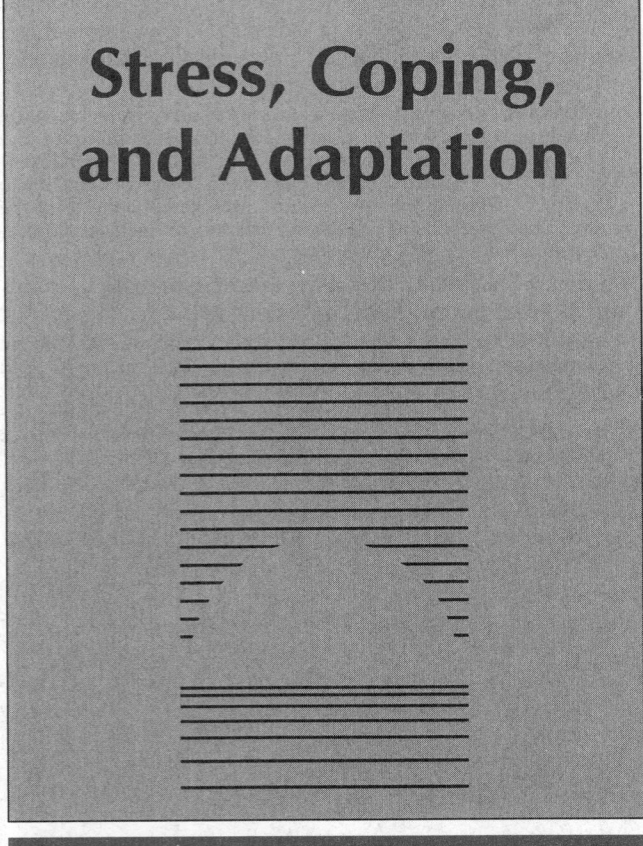

The pressures of modern American life have led to frequent manifestations of, and a resulting fascination with, stress. Stress is a familiar concept, yet there is little consensus as to its meaning. Biologists consider stress at a cellular level, whereas engineers speak of stress in structural terms. When lay individuals speak of stress, some say it is a feeling of being overwhelmed, whereas to others it is the cause of the feelings. In the social sciences, such as nursing, the concept of stress has evolved to include both the feeling and the event.

A definition of *stress* commonly used in nursing is a relationship between the individual and the environment that the individual perceives as taxing or dangerous (Lazarus & Folkman, 1984). The cognitive evaluation that an event is stressful is called an *appraisal*—of stress. The taxing or dangerous physical, psychologic, environmental, or social events that lead to the appraisal of stress are defined as *stressors*. Some examples of physiologic stressors are injuries; infectious, viral, or fungal agents; radiation; drugs; and alcohol. Psychologic stressors include frustrations, loss of control, and anger. Social stressors include losses of social support, problems in living arrangements, and the difficulties of urban living. Examples of environmental stressors are pollution, the hazards of the workplace, and extremes of temperature.

Stressors can also be classified by their duration; four classifications have been proposed by the Institute of Medicine: The first group includes acute time-limited stressors, such as diagnostic tests or school examinations. The second group comprises series of events that occur over an extended period, for example, a prolonged recovery from surgery. The third proposed grouping consists of chronic, intermittent stressors, such as weekly allergy injections. The last group includes chronic stressors such as lifelong disease and disabilities.

To deal with stress effectively, individuals use *coping strategies*. Coping strategies are the mechanisms by which the individual tries to control the causative problem or the stress-related feelings that arise. Some examples of coping strategies are denial, use of social supports, confrontation of the problem, and consideration of the positive aspects of the situation. When the stress is mastered, changed, or accepted, *adaptation* occurs. Adaptation implies that a sense of equilibrium is restored to the person disordered by stress. Adaptation is reflected in positive change in psychologic, social, or physical health.

Stress is important in the practice of medical-surgical nursing for adults, as its presence may cause, prolong, or aggravate illness. Stress can interfere with other aspects of clients' lives because it may contribute to family, spiritual, and social crises. Clients use a variety of strategies to deal with stress. Nurses are commonly in positions in which they can aid the clients' coping, either through assisting the clients' self-initiated efforts or by suggesting alternatives. Successful coping and adaptation are the goals of both the client and the nurse. All clients want stress to be reduced to manageable levels or to be eliminated. Despite the popularity of literature relating to stress, especially that which deals with how to control the effect of stressors, there are few overall assumptions that can yet be made about stress.

THEORIES RELATED TO STRESS, COPING, AND ADAPTATION

THEORIES ABOUT STRESS

Stress has been studied from three major perspectives. First, researchers have conceptualized stress as the body's physical response to threat. Second, researchers have conceptualized stress as a stimulus, or outside force, that causes a reaction. Third, stress has been examined as a transaction between the person and the event. Each of these viewpoints is discussed.

STRESS AS A RESPONSE

The biologic and medical sciences have traditionally viewed stress as the body's response to an event. That is, stress is the physiologic response or change that occurs within the body (Fig. 6–1). The idea of stress as a response gained prominence through the work of Hans Selye, who defined stress as "the nonspecific response of the body to any demand made upon it to adapt whether that demand produces pain or pleasure" (1946, p. 230). From Selye's definition, three things are immediately apparent. First, Selye thought that the *body's response to stress is nonspecific*. The body reacts as a whole organism. Second, *stress is considered a physiologic response*, not a psychologic one. Third, Selye believed that *it is not just the "bad" things in life that cause stress, but the "good" things as well*. From Selye's viewpoint, a wedding can cause the same physiologic response as a funeral. Selye called the body's generalized response to a stressor the general adaptation syndrome (GAS). The general adaptation syndrome has three distinct stages:

1. The alarm stage
2. The stage of resistance
3. The stage of exhaustion

In addition to the body's generalized response described, Selye also noted a localized response. Selye labeled the body's limited, localized response the localized adaptation syndrome (LAS). Inflammation at a surgical site is an example of the LAS.

The Alarm Stage

The physiologic response to a stressor begins with the alarm stage, in which the body prepares itself for survival. Cannon (1931) called this initial physiologic response the "fight-or-flight response." As outlined by Cannon, this response process prepares all animals, including humans, for survival. When faced with danger, the body prepares to either fight the danger or flee from it. Either reaction is thought to cause the same changes in the body.

The stress-related changes are orchestrated by the central nervous system (CNS). Within the CNS, the limbic system is the emotional response center that triggers the fight-or-flight response. The limbic system then activates the hypothalamus. The hypothalamus in turn initiates the stress response and directs the activities of the autonomic nervous system (ANS). The ANS controls the body's involuntary responses, such as hormone secretions, metabolism, and fluid regulation, and sends these control messages through the sympathetic and parasympathetic nervous systems. The sympathetic system is responsible for dynamic change, and the parasympathetic system is responsible for restoring the body to its normal resting state.

In response to stress, the sympathetic nervous system stimulates the adrenal medulla, which in turn secretes the catecholamines norepinephrine and epinephrine. The adrenal cortex is also stimulated by the pituitary gland's release of adrenocorticotropic hormone (ACTH). The circulating ACTH causes the adrenal cortex to release glucocorticoids (cortisol, corticosterone, and cortisone) and mineralocorticoids (aldosterone and deoxycorticosterone). As a result of the CNS and adrenal activity, seven major changes occur within the body.

Increase in heart rate. To prepare to fight or flee, the heart rate increases, ensuring that oxygen and nutrients are available to the muscles and the organs. The force of the heart's contraction and the volume of blood ejected with each contraction also increase. These responses are stimulated by the release of epinephrine. If it is necessary to maintain the increase in blood pressure, there is a release of mineralocorticoids in response to the pituitary gland's release of ACTH, followed by release of vasopressin by the posterior lobe of the pituitary gland, if an even more sustained reaction is called for.

Contraction of the spleen. The spleen contracts as a result of cortisol release. The spleen is a vascular organ; if there is an injury to the spleen, a great loss of blood can occur. If the spleen is in a contracted state, the possibility of injury is reduced and so is the amount of blood that will be lost. The spleen's contraction also causes the release of T lymphocytes into the blood stream. The lymphocytes are available to fight infection in case of injury.

Release of glucose. With the release of cortisol from the adrenal cortex, the body prepares itself to fuel the response to danger. Cortisol mobilizes glucose in the body for energy and creates new stores of glucose by breaking down body fats and proteins. Although the loss of fat is not usually damaging, the loss of protein is, because protein provides the essential elements for sustaining life. When continued glucose release is needed, thyroxine is released by the pituitary gland.

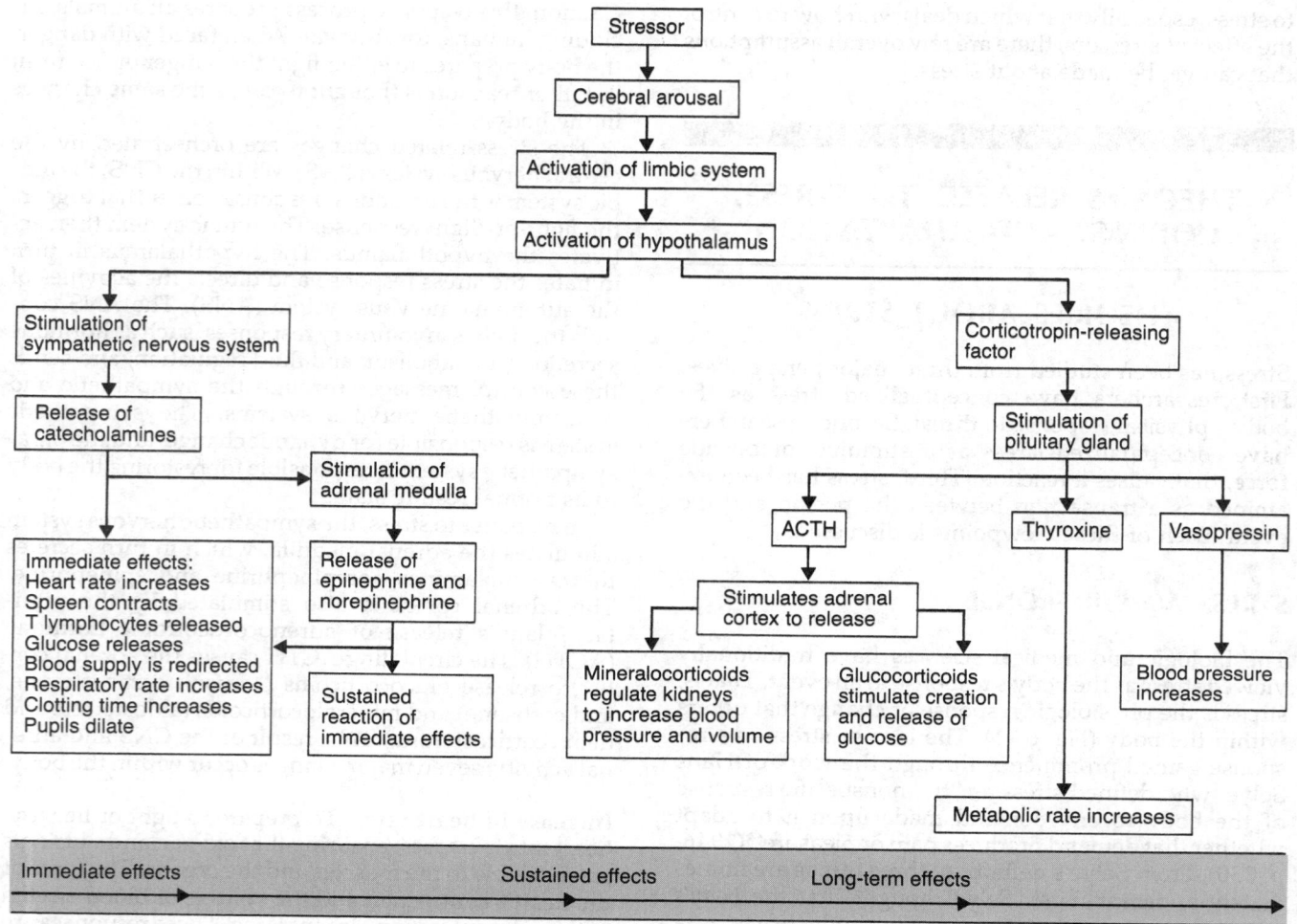

Figure 6–1

The general adaptation syndrome.

Redirection of blood supply. As part of the body's response to threat, the normal pattern of blood flow is redirected. This redirection means that some regions of the body have an increased blood flow, while others have a decreased flow. The brain's blood flow must be maintained, or increased, in times of danger. This flow to the brain is ensured by the vasodilation of the carotid arteries. The arteries supplying the deep muscles also dilate, ensuring adequate blood flow to those areas.

Other regions of the body have a decreased blood flow. The body's superficial capillaries constrict, reducing the blood flow to the skin. Although this vasoconstriction makes blood available to other more vital areas, it also provides that, if there is injury to the skin, less blood will be lost. In addition, the blood flow to the gastrointestinal system and the genitourinary system is decreased. Norepinephrine is primarily responsible for this vasoconstrictive response.

Changes in the respiratory system. To provide for effective oxygen–carbon dioxide exchange, both the respiratory rate and the depth of respiration increase. As a result, there is an increase in carbon dioxide production and in the consumption of oxygen. To provide for this exchange activity, bronchodilation occurs. Respiratory changes are brought about through the release of catecholamines.

Decrease in blood clotting time. The body also prepares for the possibility of injury by increasing the blood's coagulability and decreasing the clotting time. The faster the blood clots, the less blood is lost. Catecholamines initiate this response to threat.

Dilation of pupils. The pupils dilate in response to the release of the catecholamines, allowing for vision enhancement. Nurses who are alert to the possibility of physical stress response can assess pupillary dilation in their clients as a possible sign of the stress response.

These major changes, plus minor changes, such as increased perspiration and piloerection (hairs standing on end), appear to occur whenever the individual is threatened. Selye called these collective processes the alarm stage in the body's preparation for survival. Although these preparations may have been useful in human beings' past, they have limited utility in most of today's threat situations. It is unfortunate that these reactions persist because they result in tremendous wear and tear on the body. If these reactions occur frequently or are sustained, damage to the body's systems or illness, such as heart disease and diabetes, can occur.

The Stage of Resistance

The second stage in the GAS is called the stage of resistance. When the body recognizes continued threat, physiologic forces are mobilized to maintain an increased resistance to stressors. This resistance is hallmarked by a decrease in the production of ACTH and demonstrates the specificity of adaptation. The body concentrates its activities on those organs or organ systems that are most involved in the specific stress response. Successful adaptation implies positive growth toward a return to or improvement in physical health. The efforts can also be ineffectual, leading to a state of maladaptation in which there is deterioration in levels of physical functioning. Chronic resistance eventually causes damage to the involved systems.

The Stage of Exhaustion

When the organ or organ system shows evidence of deterioration, the body enters the third stage of the GAS, the stage of exhaustion. Selye determined that the overwhelmed body exhibits a triad of symptoms: hypertrophy of the adrenal glands, ulcerations in the gastrointestinal tract, and atrophy of the thymus gland. In this final stage, all energy for adaptation has been used, ACTH secretion increases, and a more generalized response is once again seen. This third stage can also result in what health care professionals call the diseases of adaptation, or stress-related diseases, and even death. Conditions and diseases in the accompanying Key Features of Disease represent examples of those diseases thought to be stress related or exacerbated by stress.

STRESS AS A STIMULUS

Realizing that individuals do not react to all stressors as threats, theorists and researchers began to explore the stress inherent in a stimulus. In this theory, stress is seen as the event itself or the stressor, not as the response to the event.

With the advent of the stimulus concept of stress, research efforts were directed toward determining what life events were stressful and how stressful they were. Scales were developed by researchers to quantify the stress associated with different life events. These stress scales listed events such as death, divorce, and mone-

tary and health concerns and gave each event a score that reflected its relative stressfulness. The idea behind the scales was that the accumulation of a certain number of "stress points" would result in a reaction, such as illness. Despite the popularity of these scales in both the scientific and the lay literatures, they have not proved to be valid as predictors of stress, especially in relationship to illness. No research has been able to show more than a limited predictive relationship between stressful life events and illness, hospitalization, or mortality.

According to Schroeder and Costa (1984), part of the reason why stress scales have not been able to predict illness, hospitalization, or death has to do with the scales themselves. Analysis of the stress scales has revealed that many of the events listed on the scales are related to illness and illness behavior. This means that there is no way of separating the cause of illness from the effect of illness. Thus, when people cite an illness when filling out a stress scale, they receive a higher score than they would if they filled it out before getting ill. This problem explains, in part, why stress scales have not been able to predict illness. Schroeder and Costa also noted that different personality types answered the scales in different manners, so that it was impossible to use a general stress scale and expect accurate results from the broad population.

Although the usefulness of stress scales has not proved valid, common sense would indicate that certain events can and do provoke physiologic manifestations

---

KEY FEATURES OF DISEASE ■ Some Conditions and Diseases Thought to Be Related to Stress

Cancer

Hypertension

Myocardial infarction

Cerebrovascular accident

Peripheral vascular disease

Asthma

Tuberculosis

Emphysema

Gastrointestinal ulcers

Irritable bowel syndrome

Sexual dysfunctions

Obesity

Anorexia nervosa

Bulimia

Connective tissue disease

Ulcerative colitis

Crohn syndrome

Infections

Allergic and hypersensitivity diseases

TABLE 6–1 Potential Hassles Common to Hospitalization and Illness

Eating different foods and at different times

Having a stranger for a roommate

Sleeping in a different bed

Using a different pillow

Being awakened at odd hours

Feeling too hot or too cold

Smelling hospital odors

Hearing strange hospital noises

Having movement restricted

Being unable to obtain desired objects

Having too many visitors

Having no visitors

Worrying about bills, job, or family concerns

Being uncertain of diagnosis

Not understanding medical language

Being dependent on others for bathing or toileting

Being embarrassed about revealing body parts or intimate details

Having to deal with large numbers of health care workers

---

and feelings of stress. However, it seems that the events that provoke stress symptoms may not always be life's major events, but rather the minor annoyances of everyday life. These daily stresses, or what are called hassles, have shown more relationship to illness than have the major life events (DeLongis et al., 1982). Within the hospital setting there are many potential hassles that can increase stress. Table 6–1 presents examples of environmental and psychologic hassles common to hospitalization and illness.

STRESS AS A TRANSACTION BETWEEN A PERSON AND THE ENVIRONMENT

Gradually, nurse-researchers and others have realized that all events have different meanings for different individuals. For example, a woman having a laparoscopy to retrieve an ovum for in vitro fertilization may welcome the surgical procedure. A woman having the same procedure for diagnosis of pain may find it disturbing because the outcome is uncertain. Even in these examples, the perceived stressfulness of the events may not be as it seems. The woman undergoing the ovum retrieval may have had several unsuccessful attempts to become pregnant and thus may be worried that she is facing yet another failure. The woman with the abdominal pain may welcome the possibility of finding out the cause of the pain.

The perception of stress appears to be related to the

person and event within a certain environment (see the accompanying Nursing Research feature). The view of stress as a relationship between the person and the environmental event is called the *transactional model of stress* (Lazarus & Folkman, 1984). In this model, people are more than passive recipients of stress and are not just unthinking reactors to the events around them. According to this view of stress, the person's interpretation of the event is important to consider. The meaning given to the event by the individual determines the perception of stress. Stress occurs only when the individual appraises a situation as stressful.

In the transactional model of stress, there are few universal stressors because of the differences in individual appraisal. Appraisal is the cognitive evaluation of events (primary appraisal) and available coping resources (secondary appraisal). Despite the occurrence of tornadoes, hurricanes, and other disasters that are generally thought of as stressful, no event can be considered inherently stressful. The transactional model states that there is no way of predicting how the individual will respond. Although some people experience a stress reaction to these major events, many others do not; these differences are a result of individual appraisal.

Several factors contribute to individuals' perceiving that an event is stressful by virtue of its being taxing or dangerous. These include factors specific to the person, the environment, or the event itself. Effective nursing care must include an understanding of the myriad factors that enter into the individual decision that an event is stressful.

Appraisal Factors Related to the Person

One important factor in an appraisal of stress is the *depth of feeling* that the event arouses in a person. Events about which people feel strongly are more apt to be stress producing than events that arouse little or no feeling. For example, if hospitalization interferes with an important life event, such as marriage, its appraisal may result in a perception of stress.

The strength of clients' feelings may also mean that they are more vulnerable to the threat of stress. Some research (Kasl et al., 1979) shows that when individuals are highly committed to a life experience, but unable to maintain performance, they are at a high risk for developing illness.

The *depth of commitment* is also beneficial when appraising the stress response. When an important life event is threatened, a committed individual often tries harder to cope. The athlete who undergoes knee surgery and is back playing in just a few months shows the value of commitment. The nebulous, commonly heard phrase "the will to live" probably refers to a form of commitment and can make a difference in recovery.

Along with commitments, *beliefs* are also influential in the appraisal of stress. Beliefs influence how people view the world and affect the perception of stress. For example, an individual with a strongly held religious

NURSING RESEARCH

Does Anything Make a Difference in the Way Someone Copes with the Loss of a Spouse?

Gass, K. A., & Chang, A. S. (1989). Appraisal of bereavement, coping, resources, and psychosocial health dysfunction in widows and widowers. *Nursing Research, 38*, 31–36.

Lazarus and Folkman's (1984) theory of stress, appraisal, and coping has been used to explain a variety of stress events, from college examinations to physical illness. However, this theory has not been widely applied to studies of bereavement. The authors of this study examined how appraisal of the subjects' loss of their spouses and the additional resources available to them influenced their coping methods and their psychosocial health.

The convenience sample consisted of 159 widows and widowers who stated that their bereavement was stressful to them. The sample was older (mean age > 70), bereaved 1 year or less, Catholic, and middle-class. In less than half of the sample the spouse had died suddenly. The subjects were given measures that examined appraisal of threat and coping, personal resources, appraisal of bereavement, and psychosocial health dysfunction. Validity was assessed for all the measures, and reliability was reported for the measures of coping and psychosocial health dysfunction.

The researchers found that appraisal of the event as a threat did have a major influence on the coping strategies utilized as well as the subject's psychologic health. The lower the appraisal of threat, the greater number of problem-focused coping strategies were used and the better the psychologic health of the subject was. The researchers found that, if the subject's loss of a loved one was compounded with other losses, the appraisal of stress was increased. However, the more resources (or supports) available to the subject, the more the appraisal of threat was decreased and the lower the health dysfunction score was. Sudden death and younger age resulted in the perception of fewer resources and increased appraisal of threat. The extent of resources also influenced the predominant pattern of coping strategies utilized, with more perceived resources correlating with increased use of problem-focused coping (rather than emotion focused). Men reported significantly more resource strength than did women.

Critique. This study examined bereavement within the Lazarus and Folkman Stress and Coping Model. Bereavement is a stress event that is pertinent to nurses who must provide care not only to the dying but to their families as well. That all the hypotheses were at least partially supported by the findings gives some evidence that Lazarus and Folkman's theory is appropriate to the study of bereavement. In addition, the size of the sample, the instruments and statistics used, and the use of a descriptive design were all appropriate for a first study.

The study results are limited by several factors. First, the sample was obtained from Catholic parish lists. The use of only one religious group may unnecessarily decrease the generalizability of the study. As an alternative, names could have been obtained from several religious groups or from a general source such as newspaper announcements. Second, the time of bereavement was varied and ranged from 1 month to 1 year. It can be imagined that wide differences in appraisal could exist between 1 month and 1 year of loss. Third, appraisal, which was a key element in this study, was measured with a single question. Although this is the method also employed by Lazarus and Folkman, it may restrict the findings. A more comprehensive look at appraisal may give a different view.

Possible nursing implications. Nurses who deal with the bereaved know that grieving is thought to follow a progression. However, the coping methods used to deal with grief may be influenced by individual appraisal. A sudden loss may require different coping strategies than a loss after a prolonged illness. Those who have cared for their dying spouses and those who are older, are better educated, and have higher incomes may have more resources to fall back on. Before embarking on a program to help the grieving spouse, the nurse should consider assessing the meaning of the loss to the widowed, the coping strategy in place, and the resources that can be used to facilitate the process.

belief that God can influence the course of life's events may appraise events differently from a nonreligious person.

Control is important to the stress-coping response. Many researchers have reported that most people want to maintain a sense of control over their world. For that reason, not having control can be appraised as a stressor. The key to understanding control is the recognition that control means different things to different people and in different situations. Although it is obvious that ill or hospitalized individuals cannot control situations such as the course of illness, research (Moos & Tsu, 1977) has identified a list of areas in which most people seek control even within the sick role. They include

1. Avoidance of pain and incapacitation
2. The immediate hospital environment
3. Treatments and procedures
4. Relationships with hospital personnel
5. Emotional balance
6. A satisfactory self-image
7. Relationships with family and friends
8. Preparing for an uncertain future

This list is important for several reasons. First, it alerts nurses that individuals may seek control over most aspects of their lives, whether they are ill or not. Second, it is important to realize that a loss of a sense of control can occur because of the nature of the hospital environment. A loss of the sense of control is stressful to certain individuals.

Yet there are those individuals who do not want active control. Individuals who do not desire control may experience stress when they are given control. Nurses should ascertain how much control clients want before insisting or recommending that they take control.

Because of the variability in appraisal, it is difficult to predict how people will react to events known to cause stress. One person may be devastated by the thought of having a diagnostic test, whereas another person may be less anxious. Nurses should not make generalized assumptions as to how stressful certain events may be, for a person's reaction varies tremendously from individual to individual.

Environmental Event Factors Related to Stress Appraisal

Not only are the differences in people important to accurate appraisal, but differences in the environmental events themselves are also significant. Both individual and event differences influence whether an event is perceived as stressful.

One factor that can make a difference in the appraisal of events is their *unpredictability*. People generally feel that a predictable event is less stressful than a similar unpredictable event. Part of the reason that predictability is important is that with time people can prepare. Being able to prepare for events appears to be related to a reduction in stress. Without the necessary time or information needed for preparation, events may appear more stressful than they need be. If possible, the nurse should give clients sufficient information and time to comprehend a potentially stressful event before the client experiences it.

The client's *uncertainty* about an event can also increase its potential stressfulness. It appears that most people like to know what to expect. Although this is true of life events in general, people especially like to know the odds about health-related events. The key to understanding much of the stress experienced by clients with chronic disease may lie in their uncertainty about the disease course. Not knowing how a disease will evolve or what the chances of recovery are can be stressful. Clients with cancer often provide a poignant example of the effects of uncertainty. Despite such treatments as extensive surgery, chemotherapy, and radiation, most clients can never be completely sure of a cure. Thus, the uncertainty of the event enhances its appraisal as stressful.

The *timing of events* has an impact on the level of stress. Events that are considered to be in the distant future are usually perceived as less stressful than events that are closer in time. The time that elapses between the client's hearing about an event and its occurrence can also influence appraisal. Although the stress may be manageable for a period of time, the longer a person is kept waiting, the harder it is to control the thoughts about what is to come. Thus the appraisal of threat can build up when too much time elapses. Individuals need sufficient time to prepare for events; however, too long a period of anticipation can have a detrimental effect. Unfortunately, there are no set guidelines as to timing for nurses who prepare clients for tests and procedures.

Nurses can try to limit delays and schedule events in such a way that the waiting time is reduced.

The timing of an event in relation to an individual's stage of life is also important. Having a heart attack at age 25 may be more stressful than if it occurs at age 80. Any life event that occurs at an unexpected time can be more stressful than one occurring at a time of life when it is expected.

Another factor related to timing is the *duration* of events. Chronic, long-term events can sometimes wear down an individual's ability to cope. Analogous to Selye's stage of exhaustion, constant demands over a long time can have massive psychologic as well as physical effects. However, people can also become used to, or habituated to, long-term events. The difference between the two reactions may lie in the individual's appraisal or in the coping strategies used.

Knowing what will happen, when it will happen, and how long it will last is important to the appraisal of stress. Yet, even with this information, there are always unknown elements. The unknown elements contribute to the *ambiguity* of experience. Ambiguity is important to appraisal. It is generally accepted that the more ambiguous a situation is, the more stressful it is. Ambiguity can also influence what coping strategies are used. People usually choose their coping strategies on the basis of the information that they have; however, if information is missing, the planning of specific and appropriate coping strategies is not possible.

According to Lazarus and Folkman's theory, the effectiveness of coping mechanisms depends on how accurate the appraisal of a stressful situation is. Because individuals may not correctly appraise a situation and because no one can predict the future, misappraisals cannot be avoided; they are part of life. It is the degree of difference between the appraisal of what will happen and the reality of what occurs that makes a difference in coping effectiveness. Because situations are constantly changing, coping effectiveness also depends on the individual's ability to reappraise as necessary and to change coping strategies as needed (Fig. 6–2).

THEORIES ABOUT COPING

Coping is any behavioral or cognitive activity that is used to deal with stress. If an event is perceived as taxing or dangerous, coping should occur. The concept of coping implies that most people do not remain passive and allow events to happen; rather they react. The reactions to a stress-provoking event can be either to use the problem-solving approach to change the event (problem-focused coping) or to change emotional reactions to the event (emotion-focused coping). The coping strategy or strategies used vary from person to person and event to event. It is thought that individuals generally try to use coping strategies that they have found to be successful in the past. If this coping is not successful in the current situation, other strategies may be considered.

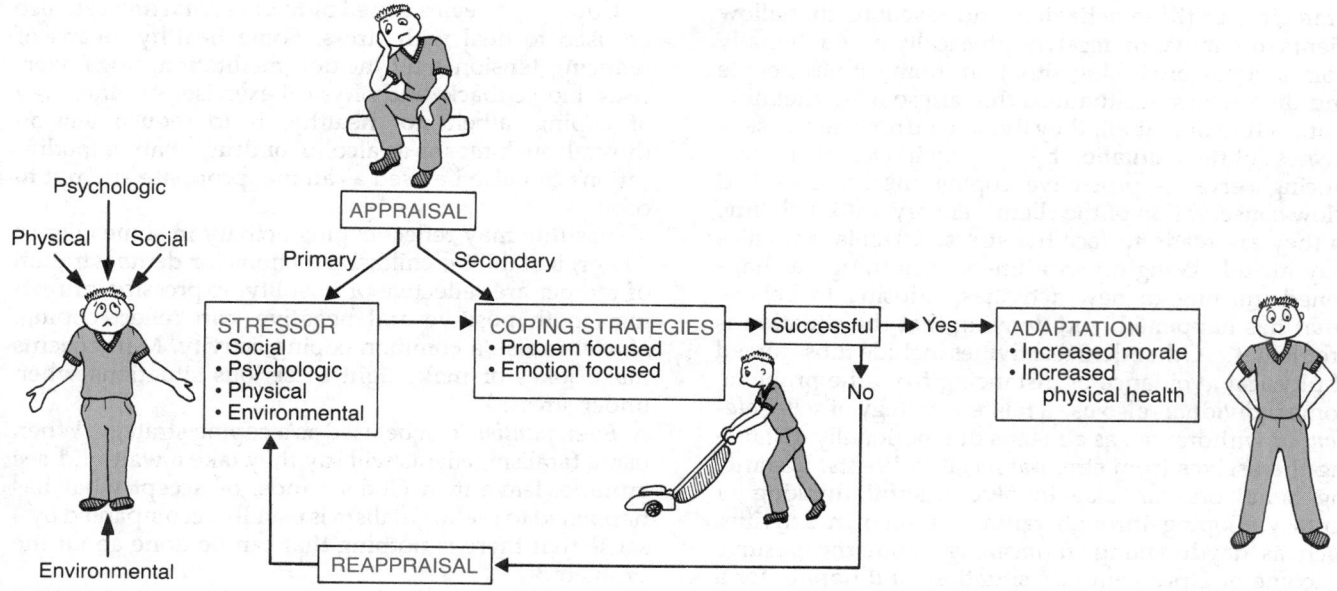

Figure 6–2

Transactional model of stress.

PROBLEM-FOCUSED COPING

In many cases the best way to deal with a causative stressor is to try to change or eliminate the problem. A major coping strategy is *problem-solving*. The inability to use problem-solving was identified by 513 clinical specialists as the major indicator of the nursing diagnosis of ineffective individual coping (Vincent, 1985). Problem-solving presented as a coping strategy involves the same skills that are seen in the nursing process. In problem-solving coping, individuals define the problem, generate alternatives, choose the best alternative, and apply it to the problem. When asked about problem-solving coping, individuals may state that they try to find out more about the problem at hand, analyze the problem, make a plan, and follow it. Effective problem-solving coping is also called *vigilance*. According to Lazarus and Folkman's theory, vigilance requires time to obtain the necessary information and sort through it to generate the best coping alternative possible. When time, information, or ability to think through the alternatives is unavailable, coping will probably be ineffective.

Some problem-solving activity is also directed inward. In this case the coping activity is directed at how the problem is faced. Inward-focused problem-solving solutions might include learning new skills, changing aspirations, or finding other avenues of gratification.

When individuals use problem-solving, they need accurate information and accurate appraisal so that their plans to deal with the stressor are based on reality. Nurses can ask clients if they have made any plans, what the plans are based on, and what is involved in these plans. When plans are unrealistic the nurse helps the client by sharing his/her expertise and information.

Many individuals cope by confronting the problem that is causing the stress. *Confrontive coping* is often used successfully in dealing with life's problems, such as those in the workplace. In addition, confrontive coping may be used when less forceful coping strategies have failed to alleviate the perception of stress. Clients in health care situations may use confrontive coping by aggressively seeking information, refusing treatments, and expressing their anger. Although not all confrontive-type coping activities reflect aggression, many times anger is the primary indicator that the individual feels stressed and is attempting to cope. The expressions of anger in confrontive coping often reflect feelings of anxiety and powerlessness in the client.

Although these problem-focused coping strategies are commonly used, they are not the only ways to cope. Nurses who are interested in supporting the client's coping need to find out how the client has coped in the past, how he/she plans to cope with the new stresses, and how other individuals with the same problem have coped.

EMOTION-FOCUSED COPING

Problem-focused coping is valuable. However, some individuals are more skilled at problem-solving than others, and some problems are more amenable to resolution. When problem-focused strategies are not appropriate, or are not sufficient, emotion-focused strategies are used. Emotion-focused strategies reduce the emotional manifestations of stress, such as anxiety or anger.

A vast array of *distancing strategies* are frequently used for coping in health-related situations. Distancing strategies are those behaviors and reactions that allow clients to remove themselves physically or emotionally from a stress-provoking situation. Many times people find themselves in situations that are so overwhelming that, to function at all, they avoid confronting the seriousness of their situation by denying it. Denial and distancing serve as protective coping mechanisms and allow conservation of the client's energy until such time as they are ready to face the stressor. Denial activities may include going on with life as if nothing has happened, turning to new activities, refusing to believe what has happened, and denying that the situation is problematic. Other denial activities include those aimed at physical avoidance or distancing from the problem. Some individuals also use a related strategy of *self-isolation*, or withdrawal, as a means of emotionally distancing themselves from stress-associated events. Distancing behaviors can also involve wishful thinking or fantasy. Coping through fantasy is seen in activities such as daydreaming, fantasizing about the positive outcome of a problem or a situation, and hoping for a miracle.

Denial appears to be a normal response to overwhelming situations. Usually, the individuals are unaware that they are in denial, although distancing, especially in the physical sense, can be a conscious act. It is only when denial is protracted, or when it seriously interferes with the client's receiving appropriate health care, that denial has negative consequences.

Blaming one's self or accepting responsibility for the problem is an effective coping mechanism in certain situations. Some individuals deny a problem or blame others, and some people accept personal responsibility for the stressor. When people accept responsibility for their contribution to the occurrence of stress, they appear to be seeking a sense of control over life events. For example, trauma patients who believe that their accident was at least in part their fault can take steps to avoid similar situations in the future. If clients think that others, fate, or external forces were the cause of the problem, they may believe that it could easily happen again and relinquish control. One study of in-hospital clients with spinal cord injuries showed that individuals who came to blame themselves for their accidents did better in the long run than those who blamed other people or circumstances (Bulman & Wortman, 1977).

A related coping strategy is seen in *drawing strength from adversity* by growing as a person, finding new faith, and rediscovering what is important in life. At other times strategies that *emphasize the positive aspects* of an event can be effective. Trying to have a positive outlook, looking on the bright side, and telling one's self that things could be worse are examples of this form of coping. Many individuals use stressful situations to foster personal growth by seeking out those aspects of the stressor that can provide an opportunity for learning. Although looking on the positive side is a form of coping, it can be ineffective if the negative aspects of a stressful situation are ignored. Nurses support this form of coping by acknowledging the clients' optimistic appraisal of events.

Coping strategies aimed at *tension reduction* can also be used to deal with stress. Some healthy means of reducing tension may include meditation, yoga exercises, biofeedback, and physical exercise. Another way of coping, albeit not healthy, is to reduce tension through such means as alcohol or drugs. Eating modifications can also be used as an inappropriate attempt to cope.

Hostility may reflect coping activity in some clients. Anger, irritability, childish reactions, or demonstration of temper are reflective of hostility. Expression of feelings, both positive and negative, can reflect coping. *Humor* is also a common coping activity. Many clients make jokes or make light of serious situations when under stress.

Even *fatalism* can be used as a coping strategy. When using fatalism, clients will say they take a wait-and-see attitude, leave it in God's hands, or accept what has happened to them. Fatalism is usually accompanied by a sense that there is nothing that can be done about the problem.

Support by family, friends, and the community can be helpful in coping. *Social support* is often a powerful aid to coping and can be extremely important to those in need of health care. By seeking support from others, people can gain information, physical help, and other forms of assistance. Both the type of help and the numbers of people willing to help can make a difference to the client's coping success. Hospital rules and regulations often interfere with clients' obtaining the social support they need. The interference with support can be especially acute within ethnic groups with large, close, and supportive families, such as Gypsies and Hispanics. Loss of social support can result when hospitalization occurs at a physical distance from the client's family, when elderly clients have outlived friends and relatives, or when the client has a socially stigmatizing illness such as acquired immunodeficiency syndrome (AIDS). The inability to use a coping strategy that one had previously depended on, such as social support, can result in further stress.

Faith in God, a deity, or an ultimate meaning of life can be an effective aid to coping. For spiritual individuals or those with a strong faith, the attitude of relinquishing control to God or believing in transcendence can be beneficial. Prayer, increased religious activity, and even a calm acceptance of God's will or an ultimate purpose are all forms of coping when they help reduce the perception of stress.

If time allows, coping often begins before the stress event occurs through *event rehearsal* (Peirce, 1987). Event rehearsal is the mental or physical preparation in anticipation of an event or practice of coping strategies before the event occurs. For example, clients who are to undergo elective surgery begin to plan their coping strategies before the actual surgery occurs. If time allows, before a potentially stressful event, clients may mentally envision how they will react or handle the situation. Some authors have called this preparatory coping the "work of worrying" (Janis, 1985). However, that term implies that clients are concerned with only the negative aspects of an upcoming experience and ignores that clients may focus on the positive aspects as well.

After a stressful event, many individuals cope by reviewing the event. This review can be mental, verbal, or both (Peirce, 1987). *Event review* probably helps people to cope by giving them the opportunity to understand what has happened to them. Often, during a stress event, there is no time to assimilate the incoming information. Review after an event occurs when there is time and energy available for assimilation. Nurses aid coping through review by encouraging clients to think or talk about their experiences.

Individuals cope with the same problem in a variety of ways. Most nurses would agree that coping in the hospital setting can be successfully accomplished through any one of a number of avenues. A listing of common coping strategies and examples of their implementation is presented in Table 6 – 2.

THEORIES ABOUT ADAPTATION

If coping is effective, the stress or the emotional reaction to stress is eliminated or managed, and a sense of equilibrium is restored. The restored equilibrium, as a result of coping, is called adaptation. Adaptation is dependent on accurate appraisal of a stressful situation and effective coping. Adaptation can have many outcomes. The two results with the most significance to nursing are psychologic and physical well-being.

PSYCHOLOGIC ADAPTATION: MORALE

It is hoped that individuals who cope adequately will be satisfied with how they coped and the outcome reached. If a client believes that the correct decision was made with regard to health care issues, such as agreeing to hospitalization, choosing medical professionals, or handling pain or discomfort, the challenge of the stress was met and coping is viewed as effective. The ability to see stress as a challenge to be overcome is important to the long-term maintenance of morale.

Morale is related to emotional equilibrium and the sense of well-being. In the past, many researchers considered well-being as the absence of depression or other signs of poor psychologic health. Recently, the approach has changed, and well-being is assessed through positive indicators, such as happiness and contentment. Healthy psychologic adaptation is reflected in the client's sense of well-being.

PHYSICAL ADAPTATION: SOMATIC HEALTH

Stress is consistently blamed for causing all illness and unhappiness. Diseases in which it can be determined that the mind influences the body's processes are called

Coping Strategy	Example
Event rehearsal	Mental and verbal preparation for an event or practice of coping strategies
Confrontation	Aggressive seeking of information, anger, refusal of treatments
Distancing or denial	Unwillingness or inability to talk about events, going on as if nothing has happened
Self-control	Stoicism, showing no feelings
Social support	Seeking out family, friends, or others in similar situations
Accepting responsibility	Verbally placing responsibility for situation on self
Faith	Praying, reading of religious material, seeking out clergy or religious guidance
Problem-solving	Making plans, verbally outlining what will be done next
Positive reappraisal	Speaking of how situation has fostered growth
Event review	Discussing situations or coping that has occurred

TABLE 6 – 2 Common Coping Strategies and Examples

psychosomatic. Stress is thought to be a major factor in psychosomatic disease. Interestingly, the link between stress and illness is far from clear. Some evidence indicates that stress may suppress the effectiveness of the immune system and thus predispose the individual to infection, cancer, and other diseases thought to be related to the immune system. Stress may also weaken the body so that any pathogens or toxic agents are more damaging than they would otherwise be. Other researchers have presented evidence that stress may precipitate damage so that it occurs at a faster rate than normal, such as in cardiovascular disease.

At one time it was hoped that a direct link could be found either between the stress event and illness or between personality type and illness. At that time, it was not uncommon to hear professionals speak of a colitis, ulcer, or stroke personality. However, none of these theories has held up under study. No research has been able to show a strong relationship among incidence of illness, personality type, and stress.

Research into the relationship between illness and personality characteristics is currently focused on *hardiness,* which is the ability to resist the effects of stress (see the accompanying Nursing Research feature). The attribute of hardiness may be one reason why some individuals are adversely affected by exposure to stress, whereas other individuals are not. Hardiness is related to three personality characteristics. The first of these characteristics is *commitment.* Commitment to work, a way of life, or ideals provides individuals with a sense of satisfaction, motivation, and possibly achievement. Second, hardy individuals look at life's occurrences as *challenges,* not as threats. These individuals welcome change for the growth it promotes. They are optimistic and curious about life. The third characteristic of hardy individuals is that they have a sense of *control* over their lives. Hardy individuals do not feel helpless in the face of what happens to them. On the other hand, people who are low in measures of hardiness usually appear bored, are hopeless, and lack enthusiasm.

Commitment, challenge, and control may be three reasons why differences exist in individuals' ability to adapt to stress. Hardiness may help buffer the effects of stress. Individuals who are hardy may be more resilient in the face of life's ups and downs. Kobasa (1979) showed that people with high stress and high illness

NURSING RESEARCH

Does a Hardy Personality Make a Difference in Whether a Nurse Experiences Stress or Burnout?

McCrane, E. W., Lambert, V. E., & Lambert, C. E. (1987). Work stress, hardiness, and burnout among hospital staff nurses. *Nursing Research, 36,* 374–378.

Kobasa (1979) and others have written about the benefits of the personality characteristics of control, commitment, and challenge. Their stress model proposed that individuals with that triad of personality characteristics are hardier when exposed to stress. The authors of the present study examined whether hardiness moderates the effect of stress on the degree of burnout in staff nurses.

The authors used a convenience sample of all 260 staff nurses from one large hospital for their study. A total of 107 nurses returned the anonymous questionnaire. They were predominantly female and married, with a mean age of 30.3 years. The sample included nurses at the diploma (18%), AD (45%), and BSN (37%) educational levels. They were almost evenly divided between those working straight and rotating shifts and between those with intensive care unit (ICU) and non-ICU work assignments. The researchers used the Tedium Scale to measure burnout, the Hardiness Scale to measure hardiness, and the Nursing Stress Scale to measure stress. The Hardiness Scale is scored so that higher scores indicate lower hardiness, whereas in the

other two instruments a higher score means higher level of stress or burnout. All the instruments had acceptable reliability and validity.

The researchers reported that they found that burnout was not associated with any of the demographic variables, except for shift work. Nurses who worked rotating shifts reported statistically significantly higher burnout scores than those who worked straight shifts. They also reported that burnout scores were statistically significantly correlated with stress scores and hardiness. Hardiness was also correlated with stress. Using multiple regression analysis, the researchers found that work shift accounted for 7% of the variance in burnout; when stress scores were added, explained variance rose to 24%; and when hardiness was added, a total of 35% of the variance was explained. The interaction of hardiness with each of the individual stress scales did not add to the burnout score. The researchers concluded that higher stress and lower hardiness contributed to burnout, but that higher hardiness did not prevent stress from leading to burnout. They contrast their findings with those of Kobasa who did find that higher hardiness was associated with less illness in the face of high stress.

Critique. Burnout is an important topic for nursing, as it is thought to contribute to loss of workers from the profession. The researchers in this study examined how hardiness and stress contribute to the problem. The question posed is thus one of importance to nursing. In addition, the instruments used were valid and reliable.

The study results are limited by several factors. The use of a sample from one hospital may provide an inadequate picture of the relationship between the variables. In addition, the sample consisted of only 41% of the target population. The 59% who did not respond may be fundamentally different from those who did, and thus results may be biased.

The results of the study are sometimes difficult to interpret. One reason for the difficulty is that in at least one instance (the mean hardiness score) the wrong number seems to have been reported. Moreover, correlational studies are designed to look at relationships between variables rather than what causes an effect. Yet the authors in their discussion appeared to assume that hardiness causes a difference first in stress and then in burnout. It could be that nurses first become burned out and then less hardy, and as a result perceive a higher level of stress. Although 35% of the burnout score was explained by stress, work pattern, and hardiness, 65% of the score is still unexplained. The authors did not speculate as to what else may contribute. Finally, the researchers' discussion of why their results differed from those of Kobasa failed to examine the differences between illness as studied by Kobasa and burnout in this study.

Possible nursing implications. Nursing is a profession whose practitioners are thought to be prone to burnout. A major contributor to burnout may be the stress of the job. If hardiness protects men from illness, as seen in the Kobasa study, it is possible that it protects nurses against burnout. However, at this point the study results on this topic are not conclusive and should be used with caution.

levels scored lower on measures of hardiness than individuals with similar levels of stress but lower incidence of illness. Because hardiness may be a personality characteristic, experts are unsure as to whether people can be taught to be hardy. However, attempts to increase hardiness may be beneficial. Table 6–3 shows a few examples of ways that clients may increase challenge, commitment, and control in everyday life.

COLLABORATIVE MANAGEMENT

 Assessment

The first step in helping clients to deal with stress is to obtain an accurate assessment of the stress situation. The problem may be in the client's appraisal of the situation, in how it is coped with, or in the inherent stressfulness of the situation, which cannot be controlled or changed. It is important that the nurse assess all three aspects of the stress response before determining what nursing interventions are appropriate.

Assessment of Stress

Physical assessment.   Within a hospital or clinic setting, many situations could serve as major stress initiators. Individuals may have illnesses brought on by or aggravated by stress. Because of the serious physical ramifications of the stress response, nurses are interested in the physiologic signs that would identify individuals under stress (see the accompanying Key Features of Disease). One of the most obvious of these signs, which is used in the literature as supporting evidence of stress, is heart rate. Although increased heart rate is a stress-related response, heart rate by itself has not proved to be a reliable indicator of the presence of stress. Among the reasons for this unpredictability is that heart rate varies with almost any stimulus, from movement to illness. Thus, heart rate is not specific enough to be a valid sign of stress. The correlation of stress and blood pressure has demonstrated the same problem.

Another sign used to indicate stress is skin conductance. Skin conductance is a measure of the skin's electrical potential and has been shown to vary with levels of stress. Although measurement of skin conductance is noninvasive, the equipment needed to measure it accurately is expensive and not practical for most settings.

Blood levels of cortisol breakdown products, such as 17-hydroxycorticosteroids, have also been examined to see how useful they might prove in diagnosing stress. However, researchers have been unable to discover a consistent pattern. Instead, researchers can only say that concentrations of these by-products in stressed individuals vary tremendously within certain ranges.

Levels of epinephrine and norepinephrine are somewhat more predictive than other laboratory values. Unlike steroid products, epinephrine and norepinephrine are released almost instantly in response to stress. Initial research has been done on athletes, astronauts, and others exposed to intense, but transient, stress-provoking episodes. Researchers have found that the norepinephrine levels almost always rise when an individual is subjected to a stressor, but that the epinephrine levels tend to stabilize with habituation. Although these results are promising, they are only preliminary findings. In addition, it is not always possible to obtain blood for laboratory analysis, and this procedure is invasive.

A variety of somatic complaints may also reflect stress in an individual. Examples of stress-related complaints are headaches, neckaches, stomachaches, muscular cramping, and other signs of muscular tension. Some individuals perspire, some get pale, and others become flushed under stress. Many people have alterations in their patterns of elimination, both bowel and urinary. Eating patterns may also reflect change, with some individuals eating more than usual and others eating less. The patterns of these changes are as different as the individuals involved.

TABLE 6–3   Techniques for Increasing Hardiness

Personality Characteristic	Techniques
Commitment	Capitalize on skills and interests to develop hobbies
	Reduce time spent watching television
	Develop a list outlining why one's work is important to the community
	Recognize and acknowledge self-worth
	Join a volunteer organization that provides services to help others
	Join political, social, or religious organizations
Challenge	Take a controlled physical risk, e.g., Outward Bound, glider flight, parachute jump, a new sport
	Take a vacation that involves little or no planning
	Take a course or attend a talk on a topic that questions one's own values
	Vary daily activities, change routines
Control	Set aside a period of time each week to do exactly what one wants
	Volunteer for leadership positions in clubs and organizations
	Become active in the political process, vote
	Seek work situations in which control is increased
	Recognize the enormous amount of control one can exercise over his/her own life

---

KEY FEATURES OF DISEASE ■ Common Signs of Stress

Physical Signs

Sleep problems

Headaches

Shaking

Inability to sit still

Muscle tenseness

Rapid speech, stuttering, or stammering

Fatigue

Increased heart rate

Digestive troubles

Increased perspiration

Light-headedness

Cold chills

Hot flashes

Palpitations

Dry mouth

Frequent urination

Menstrual cycle changes

Crying

Psychosocial Signs

Resentment toward health care workers

Anger, loss of temper

Feelings of helplessness

Resistance to treatments or tests

Overuse of drugs, including prescription and over-the-counter drugs

Withdrawal from friends and family

Overuse of alcohol

Excessive excitement

Confusion and forgetfulness

Nervousness

Irritability

Complaints of anxiety

Psychosocial assessment. There are many overt psychosocial signs that nurses use to assess stress behavior, as shown in the Key Features of Disease just cited. Many of the signs used to assess stress actually reflect coping activity. The more common signs attributed to stress include emotional excesses, such as agitation, anxiety, anger, and apathy. Other signs may include inappropriate or ineffectual coping behaviors, such as denial and blaming behaviors. Expressions of hopelessness, pow-

erlessness, or loss of control; alterations in normal communication patterns, such as a change from extreme talkativeness to silence; and changes in thought processes may signal stress, as do forgetfulness and the inability to make decisions. Even signs that are considered pathologic, such as manipulative behavior, depression, and withdrawal, may only reflect an individual's reaction to tremendous stress.

Assessment of Appraisal and Coping

The study of coping, including individual appraisal, is a new area of research, and there are many unanswered questions. Until further studies are available, nurses are best guided by the client in the perception of what is stressful and the best coping strategies to be used.

Assessment of appraisal. The nurse first tries to determine what the client perceives as stressful. The client is asked specific questions as to what aspects of hospitalization or illness are stressful. The nurse's investigation relates specifically to the appraisal process, considering such factors as perceived ambiguity, predictiveness, and uncertainty of events. The nurse can ask specific questions about how much the client knows about diagnosis, diagnostic testing, and expected length of hospitalization.

The nurse next attempts to find out from the client how stressful these items are perceived to be. Stress is an individual matter, so it is the client's perception, or appraisal, that is important (see the Nursing Research feature on p. 99). One way of determining the level of stress is to ask the client to name the most stressful thing possible and then compare the new stressor with that event.

After determining the client's appraisal of the event and the coping methods used, the nurse tries to find out what successful coping strategies the client has used in the past for similar problems.

The guide to interviewing clients regarding stress and coping in Figure 6–3 may be a helpful aid for interviewing clients.

Assessment of specific coping strategies. Nurses should remember that different individuals cope with the same problem in a variety of ways. Most nurses would agree that coping in the hospital setting can be successfully accomplished by a number of methods. If the coping strategy chosen is working, it is important that the client be supported in that effort. If the coping is ineffectual, the nurse must work with the client to develop alternatives. The following discussion covers the assessment of some, but not all, of the coping strategies available.

The nurse may note that clients are using *event rehearsal* if clients discuss or talk about the upcoming event or if, when asked, say they have been thinking about the situation. If the event rehearsal is to be effective, clients need information about the stressor. Nurses

NURSING RESEARCH

What Stressors Do Hemodialysis Patients Face and How Do They Cope?

Gurklis, J. A., & Menke, E. M. (1988). Identification of stressors and the use of coping methods in chronic hemodialysis patients. *Nursing Research, 37,* 236–239.

Chronic kidney disease is often treated with hemodialysis. Hemodialysis keeps the clients alive but does not restore them to a healthy state. Clients undergoing dialysis are thought to have to cope with loss of well-being, dietary restrictions, changes in family roles, and other stressors. The researchers in this study replicated an earlier study that had looked at the relationships between stressors, coping methods, and length of time on hemodialysis in clients receiving long-term hemodialysis. Both the earlier study and the present study used the theories of Monet and Lazarus and Folkman as the basis. The main difference between the studies was that the earlier study suggested that a larger sample size was needed, which the present authors provided.

The authors used a volunteer sample of 68 long-term clients from two hemodialysis centers. Thirty-two of the subjects were male and 36 were female; 39 were Caucasian and 28 were Black. The ages ranged from 18 to 86 years, with a mean age of 51.3 years. Nineteen of the subjects had been on dialysis for less than 1 year, 21 for 1 to 4 years, 17 for 4 to 8 years, and 11 for more than 8 years. All the subjects were given a consent form and an explanation of the study.

The instruments used were a demographic information sheet, the Hemodialysis Stress Scale, and the Jalowiec Coping Scale. The stress scale has two subscales: physiologic stressors and psychosocial stressors. The Jalowiec scale is divided into affective-oriented coping items and problem-oriented coping items. No validity measurement was reported for either of the two scales, although both had adequate reliability assessments. All the subjects completed the forms during the time they were being dialyzed.

The results of the study showed that subjects experienced a mean number of stressors of 16.41 of a possible 32. Feeling tired was the most frequently chosen stressor; the least frequently chosen items included reversal of family roles and inability to have children. The subjects found the physiologic items more stressful than the psychosocial stressors. The coping methods used most often were prayer, self-control, acceptance, and hope. The least frequently used strategies were using alcohol, taking drugs, and blaming others. The subjects said they used significantly more problem-oriented coping strategies than affective methods. To look at the relationship between coping, stress, and time on dialysis, the researchers looked at correlations between the variables. They reported that physiologic stressors were significantly related to affective coping, whereas psychosocial stressors were related to both affective and problem-oriented coping. The length of time on dialysis was related to problem-oriented coping only. The authors discussed the areas of agreement and disagreement between the earlier study and theirs.

Critique. The replication of previous studies is important to nursing, for only with replication can objectivity and validity of results be assured. The authors did a good job in replicating the previous study with a larger sample. The results provided an interesting picture of stressors and coping strategies utilized by clients receiving long-term hemodialysis. The sample size, the instruments, and the procedure were adequate for a study of this type.

Although the study was a well-done replication, future studies could perhaps improve on the results with the use of more sophisticated statistics. For example, the authors wrote that they would look at length of time on hemodialysis in relationship to stressors and coping, but the use of multiple Pearson correlation coefficients may have distorted relationships that existed. Multiple correlational analysis might have provided a clearer picture of the relationship.

Possible nursing implications. The accruing of evidence through research is the only way that nurses can build a substantive body of knowledge. This is an important study for it shows how the replication of an earlier study can result in different findings. Among the important findings of the study were that clients undergoing long-term dialysis experience a variety of stressors, but that some, such as changing family roles, may not be as important to the client as health care workers would think. Another important finding is that clients cope through prayer. Faith, prayer, and religious observances may be important coping strategies that can be facilitated by staff nurses.

---

may also make an assessment that clients are using event rehearsal when clients seek information. Many clients actively solicit information from health care providers, friends, or relatives; even comparative strangers may be consulted if they have undergone similar experiences. Nurses are often called on to supply the necessary information, for example, with preoperative teaching. Developing a plan to eliminate or reduce the effect of the stressor can be another form of coping that is reflected in information-seeking behavior. When individuals use *planned problem-solving,* they need accurate information so that the plans they make are based on reality.

If clients purposefully appear to keep their emotions or behaviors in check, they may be using *self-control* to aid their coping. Stoicism can reflect a personality type or even a culturally approved coping strategy. Other more expressive clients may not keep their emotions and feelings in check and may be using *confrontive coping strategies.* Anger, hostility, and argumentative behavior in the client may also be assessed by the nurse as coping.

Nurses may make an assessment of *denial* in clients who exhibit avoidance behavior, such as refusing to look at surgical scars or not learning self-care. Other behaviors indicative of denial are exhibited by clients who do not talk about their conditions, do not prepare for upcoming events, or appear to go on as if nothing

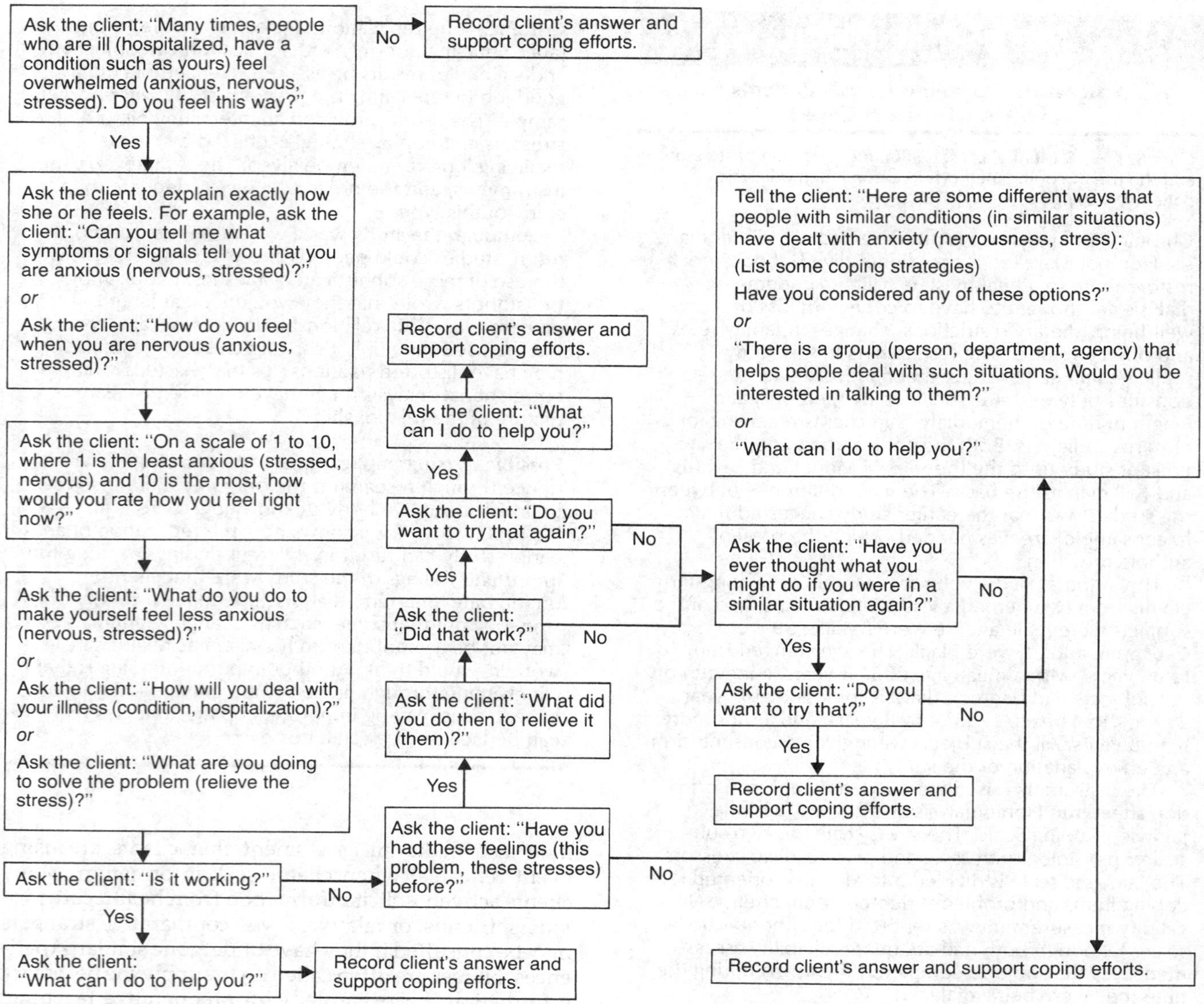

Ask the client: "Many times, people who are ill (hospitalized, have a condition such as yours) feel overwhelmed (anxious, nervous, stressed). Do you feel this way?" → No → Record client's answer and support coping efforts.

Yes ↓

Ask the client to explain exactly how she or he feels. For example, ask the client: "Can you tell me what symptoms or signals tell you that you are anxious (nervous, stressed)?"

or

Ask the client: "How do you feel when you are nervous (anxious, stressed)?"

↓

Ask the client: "On a scale of 1 to 10, where 1 is the least anxious (stressed, nervous) and 10 is the most, how would you rate how you feel right now?"

↓

Ask the client: "What do you do to make yourself feel less anxious (nervous, stressed)?"

or

Ask the client: "How will you deal with your illness (condition, hospitalization)?"

or

Ask the client: "What are you doing to solve the problem (relieve the stress)?"

↓

Ask the client: "Is it working?" → No →

Yes ↓

Ask the client: "What can I do to help you?" → Record client's answer and support coping efforts.

Tell the client: "Here are some different ways that people with similar conditions (in similar situations) have dealt with anxiety (nervousness, stress):

(List some coping strategies)

Have you considered any of these options?"

or

"There is a group (person, department, agency) that helps people deal with such situations. Would you be interested in talking to them?"

or

"What can I do to help you?"

Record client's answer and support coping efforts.

Ask the client: "What can I do to help you?"

Yes ↓

Ask the client: "Do you want to try that again?" → No →

Yes ↓

Ask the client: "Did that work?" → No →

Ask the client: "What did you do then to relieve it (them)?"

Yes ↓

Ask the client: "Have you had these feelings (this problem, these stresses) before?" → No →

Ask the client: "Have you ever thought what you might do if you were in a similar situation again?" → No →

Yes ↓

Ask the client: "Do you want to try that?" → No →

Yes ↓

Record client's answer and support coping efforts.

Record client's answer and support coping efforts.

Figure 6–3

Algorithm for interviewing clients for stress and coping.

had happened to them. Some clients may even exhibit withdrawal behavior by refusing to communicate or by communicating only minimally.

Clients who talk about only the positive aspects of their situation may not be denying, but rather using *positive reappraisal* as a coping strategy. Clients who blame themselves for their illness or hospitalization may be using the coping strategy of *self-blame*. Clients who use *faith* as a coping strategy may request clergy visits, use religious paraphernalia, and engage in prayer, which are signs that the nurse can observe.

Calling friends and family on the telephone, encouraging visitors, and socializing with others who are in the hospital may reflect *social support* as a coping strategy. Talking with others about what has occurred may reflect the use of *event review*.

 Analysis: Nursing Diagnosis

In analyzing the elements that influence stress, coping, and adaptation, the nurse may arrive at many different nursing diagnoses that could be applicable to a specific client and his/her family. The following lists provide the nurse with a few of the many diagnostic possibilities that exist.

Common Diagnoses

Two nursing diagnoses are directly related to problems of stress, appraisal, and coping.

1. Ineffective individual coping
2. Ineffective family coping

TABLE 6-4   Causes of Ineffective Coping
Fear
Isolation from friends and families
Physical dependency
Loss of control
Role changes
Lack of knowledge
Inaccurate appraisal
Stress related to hospitalization

Some examples of possible etiologic factors related to these two diagnoses are listed in Table 6-4.

Additional Diagnoses

In addition to the actual diagnoses related to coping, the client may have one or more of the following diagnoses:

1. Anxiety related to ineffective coping
2. Fear related to inaccurate stress appraisal
3. Noncompliance related to inaccurate stress appraisal
4. Powerlessness related to perceived stress
5. Self-esteem disturbance related to coping difficulty

 Planning and Implementation

Planning: Client or Family Goals

The goals related to the relevant nursing diagnoses should be mutually developed by the client or the family and the nurse. The goals in the case of ineffective individual or family coping are to (1) develop accurate appraisal of stress situations, (2) develop effective coping behaviors, and (3) experience a reduction in stress.

Interventions

Faulty appraisal or coping may lead to increased stress for the client. Stress may also be the result of the serious nature of health-related problems and hospitalization. After the nurse has assessed that there is a problem in the client's ability to appraise, or to cope, a multitude of interventions are available. Because of the individual nature of stress, coping, and appraisal, the nurse must remember that there are no universal, standard interventions.

Interventions to assist the client in appraisal. Nurses can help clients make more accurate appraisals through client education, can assist clients to recognize and correct faulty appraisal, and can provide positive reinforcement of correct appraisal. Appraisal is dependent on accurate information. For example, nurses can aid clients in appraisal by supplying information about the scheduling and the duration of events in an attempt to reduce ambiguity.

Exploring perceptions of stress and stressors to determine if appraisals are accurate is also an important step in assisting clients with appraisal. Encouraging the client to verbalize perceptions aids the nurse in identifying and correcting faulty appraisal. If appraisals are inaccurate, the nurse should intervene to supply correct information and aid the client in changing his/her perception.

The nurse may also explore different ways of thinking about stress events with clients. By encouraging clients to explore alternative appraisals, nurses can help the client redefine stress events. Clients can be taught that there are choices in what one thinks. Many events are stressful only because the client chooses to view them that way. Other situations may be inherently threatening; however, if a client can be taught to view events differently, stress may be reduced.

Interventions to assist the client in coping and reducing stress. The social support provided by friends and family is essential to coping. Nurses should encourage the involvement of these significant others to assist with the client's stress-coping response. Both the type of help and the numbers of people willing to help can make a difference to coping.

Hospital rules and regulations often interfere with the ability of clients to obtain the social support they need. Loss of social support can also occur when hospitalization occurs at a distance from the client's home or when the client has an illness such as AIDS because of social stigma associated with the illness. There are many ways that nurses can increase social support, such as obtaining special visiting passes, providing telephones, and helping friends and relatives to obtain transportation. Unfortunately, there are many times, especially with the elderly, when there are few friends or relatives. In cases of constricted social circles, nurses may try to introduce clients to others with similar problems, to obtain access to appropriate client support groups, or to contact pastoral or hospital social services.

Most adults find dependency on others stressful. To reduce the stress of dependency, nurses should allow the client as much physical independence as possible. When physical independence is not possible, sensitive care by a nurse aware of the client's feelings can be helpful in reducing stress. In most illness situations, certain role changes are expected by health care personnel. The ill individual is expected to cooperate, focus on getting well, and be dependent. Each of these role changes can be stressful. If the client finds the change in role to be stressful, the nurse should work with that client to develop a plan of care that incorporates maintenance of important role behaviors. Whenever possible, nurses should allow patients who desire it control over activities of daily living, hospital activities, and nursing actions. Control over such things as times of bathing, food choices, awake and sleep times, and scheduling of procedures can be invaluable in reducing additional stress and in maintaining self-esteem.

Although not all clients want to know about all aspects of care and hospitalization, for those who do, it is vital that they receive detailed information about those areas in which lack of knowledge is perceived as stressful. Client education is important to those who use planned problem-solving as a coping strategy. Nursing research has shown the importance of client preparation for diagnostic tests and procedures (Johnson, 1972; Johnson & Lauver, 1989). Among the content that should be included in client education are knowledge of the duration of events, expected behaviors, sensations involved, sequencing of activities, and so forth. Nurses should remember that even everyday experiences in the hospital setting, such as the administration of barium enemas, can be extremely stressful to the client.

Adequate and correct information about events is also necessary if the coping strategy of event rehearsal is to be effective. Many clients actively seek information from health care providers, friends, relatives, and even comparative strangers who have undergone similar experiences.

Time does not allow for rehearsal of all events, nor do all individuals want to rehearse. One study showed that, in a sample of coronary artery bypass clients, 60% of the clients used rehearsal-type activities before surgery to help them cope. Although 60% is a substantial number, still 40% of the clients did not use that technique. Interestingly, after surgery over 80% of the clients in the sample used rehearsal to help them to cope with their recovery and return home (King, 1985).

Some programs have been developed that utilize rehearsal as part of helping individuals with long-term stressors. One of the more well known of these programs is called *stress inoculation* (Meichenbaum & Novaco, 1985). The purpose of stress inoculation is to give sufficient information, usually in small doses, allowing the client to work through and assimilate each bit, before more is given. When a stress-producing event occurs, the individual can cope more successfully because of the practice afforded by the program. Stress inoculation has been used successfully for clients with chronic pain, phobias, and anxiety.

After a stress-provoking event, nurses can aid the client's coping through event review by encouraging clients to think or talk about their experiences. Nurses should allow clients to verbally review as much as they need to, even when the account is repetitive. The repetition of thoughts about a threatening event can facilitate coping.

When clients use positive reappraisal, nurses can support this form of coping by acknowledging the clients' appraisal of events.

Until such time that denial or distancing becomes ineffectual, the nurse should not attempt to force the client to deal with a denied stressor. Instead the nurse should concentrate on developing a positive and trusting nurse-client relationship that will be in place when the client ceases to deny or distance. When denial or distancing compromises the client, such as when it interferes with the client's seeking treatment, or when the more serious symptoms of repression or suppression occur, consultation with a colleague with expertise in mental health should be sought.

To deal with a client's hostility, nurses should not react personally because that generally only inflames the situation. Instead, reacting to the client's anger and aggression by acknowledging the client's feelings is helpful. For example, the nurse might say, "I can understand why you're angry. I would be angry too, if that had happened to me." After anger is acknowledged, it often dissipates. If the anger does not diminish, the nurse allows the client to explore his/her anger no matter how irrational it may seem. After the anger has been reduced, the nurse can explore the more logical reasons why the feelings arose. Occasionally, individuals become so angry that they become a danger to themselves or others around them. If the client loses control, the nurse should follow the institutional guidelines governing such situations.

With any of these or the many other coping strategies possible, the nurse can often best facilitate coping by supporting the clients' efforts. For example, when clients use self-controlling mechanisms they should be supported in those efforts, not forced to express their feelings. Clients should not be forced to share their feelings or to demonstrate their emotions if they are not comfortable in doing so. Nurses can aid faith as coping by contacting appropriate clergy or religious leaders, providing religious material, and allowing time and a quiet place for the client to practice religious behaviors.

Interventions to aid family coping.   Families also experience many of the same stressors that the ill or hospitalized client does. Families under stress also use coping strategies, such as seeking social support, reviewing events, and venting hostility. Nurses can aid the family in appraisal of stress and coping just as they do for the individual. In addition, the nurse can refer the family to social service agencies and other support services that are available for assistance.

Interventions to reduce the effects of stress.   When clients are facing illness, surgery, and other health-related events, they may experience a high level of stress that is not immediately reducible. The introduction of further stress can inhibit coping effectiveness. Nursing action that eliminates or reduces additional stress allows the clients to concentrate their coping activities on the major stressor and not divert their energies to coping with inconsequential annoyances.

Although it is important to recognize that many stressful aspects of illness or hospitalization can be reduced or eliminated, there are still many other aspects with which clients either cannot or will not cope, or stressors that cannot be eliminated or avoided. In such cases, effective nursing care may involve teaching the client techniques that are thought to reduce the physical impact of stress on the body as well as providing a means of physical or emotional control to the client. Examples of these techniques are biofeedback, progressive muscle relaxation (PMR), meditation, and imagery.

Biofeedback.   When outward signs of stress, such as headaches, high blood pressure, muscle tension, and

---

CLIENT/FAMILY EDUCATION ■ Sample Directions for Progressive Muscle Relaxation*

Clients should be comfortably positioned, preferably recumbent in bed. The room should be quiet and free from distractions. The following should be read to the client:

"Take a minute and feel your body's different parts. Think about what portions of your body feel tense and which parts feel relaxed."

"We are going to do an exercise that will help you to relax and remove the tension from your body. I am going to talk you through this exercise, so just relax and follow my directions."

"I am going to ask you to tense one body part at a time. When you tense the body part, try to make the muscle as tight as possible. If you feel pain or a cramp when you tighten, reduce the tightness. This tightening is called tension."

"After you hold that muscle tightness for 5 to 10 seconds, I am going to ask you to let all the tightness out of that body part, to let it go limp. This is called relaxation."

"First, point your feet and curl your toes. Feel the tension in your feet. Hold that feeling until I tell you to relax." (Have the client maintain this tightness for 5 to 10 seconds.)

"Relax—let your feet go limp. Feel the difference in going from tension to relaxation. Take a few moments to feel the relaxation."

"Now tighten the muscles in your lower legs. Feel the tension in your calves. Feel the tightness of your muscles. Hold that feeling until I say relax."

"Now relax your lower legs. Let them go limp. Feel the tightness leave and the feeling of relaxation take over."

The nurse should go through each major body part, having the client first tighten and then relax. The following sequence of body parts may be used: thighs, buttocks, stomach, chest, hands, forearms, and shoulders. The PMR ends with the neck and head as follows:

"Now tighten the muscles of your neck by clenching your lower jaw. Feel the tightness of your muscles. Feel the tenseness as you clench your jaw."

"Relax your neck and jaw. Let the tightness go, feel the relaxation take over. Feel the difference between tension and relaxation."

"Close your eyes tightly and try to tighten all the other muscles in your face. Feel how tight your face feels."

"Now relax your face and let the tenseness flow out."

"Finally, I want you to let your whole body go limp, let it all relax. Remember those feelings of relaxation and let those feelings take over. Release any feelings of tension."

"Now, it is time to end this exercise. I want you to take your time as you slowly begin to move. When you are ready, you may resume your normal activities."

*Note: The clients should be instructed in the PMR technique until they can comfortably do it themselves without prompting. If time is a problem, a tape recorder and prerecorded tape can be used after the initial instruction has occurred.

heart palpitations, occur frequently, are debilitating, or may be dangerous, biofeedback can be an effective treatment. Biofeedback works by training the individual to reverse the subtle changes that lead to a somatic response. For instance, if a headache is the result of muscle tension in the forehead, the client can be trained to relax that tension before a headache results.

Biofeedback involves using electronic instrumentation to signal the individual about selected somatic changes. The machinery used is sensitive to minute changes within a body system. For example, if the biofeedback is directed toward sampling muscle activity, the machine detects small changes in the electrical activity of the muscles. If brain wave activity is the variable considered, the machine signals the type of brain waves that are occurring at a given moment. Cardiovascular and skin surface activity can also be monitored. After the somatic clues are learned, they can be used by the client to gain control over and to reduce the undesired activity.

Many hospitals and clinics have biofeedback equipment and trained personnel available. If not, referrals can usually be made to a local practitioner.

Progressive muscle relaxation. Stress commonly causes muscle tension, which results in many of the nagging somatic symptoms of stress, such as headaches and neckaches. Control of muscle tension appears to help reduce the physical effects of such tension as well. PMR is one method used to reduce muscular tension.

PMR involves the tensing and then the relaxing of all the major muscle groups, usually in sequential steps (see the accompanying Client/Family Education feature). PMR is useful in nursing practice because it is easy to teach and can be used for a wide spectrum of clients. It is also inexpensive, unlike methods such as biofeedback that use machinery.

Meditation. Meditation is a learned process through which the individual attempts to quiet the mind. The methods used to quiet the mind involve consciously removing disturbing thoughts or filling the mind with only one thought, such as a mantra or prayer. By removing unbidden thought, it is believed that stress can be reduced. Meditation is probably best learned through a mentor, although books and other audiovisual aids are available. If clients are interested in learning meditative techniques, they should be referred to an appropriate source.

Imagery. Similar to meditation, imagery also attempts to control the mind's thoughts. Imagery seeks to fill the mind with positive and pleasant mental pictures. Usually imagery involves thinking about a peaceful scene or one in which there is total relaxation. Thinking processes are directed toward the promotion of relaxation rather than stress (see Chap. 7 for more information).

Other techniques. In addition to the popular techniques noted earlier, myriad other methods exist. For example, self-hypnosis has proved effective in reducing stress for certain individuals. Massage can be relaxing and can reduce muscle tension and its effects. Warm baths are also well known for their relaxing effects and are used in some stress clinics. Although exercise is not restful, it can be an effective means of stress reduction.

■ Discharge Planning

As discussed, stress is often the result of lack of knowledge or of inaccurate knowledge about an upcoming event. For that reason, all clients who are discharged from the hospital need to be involved in discharge planning. Every client needs to know what to expect to be able to implement effective coping strategies. For example, clients should be educated about signs and symptoms that are normal and expected as well as those that should be reported. The client should know who to call if trouble arises. Clients should always be given both verbal and written directions for home care. Having a written copy of instructions often reduces stress.

If extended care is needed after discharge, the client should be fully aware of what is needed and either who will be giving the care or how to arrange for the care. The family should understand what is involved in the recovery or convalescent period so that the client's coping efforts are supported and not sabotaged by unrealistic expectations. Nurses should remember that, although discharge is usually a positive event, it is also a stressful one for many clients; stress related to discharge can be reduced if planning starts early and actively involves the client.

If clients have received education on managing stress or improving coping, the client and the nurse can develop plans that ensure that what was learned is not discarded. Enlisting the help of family or friends may sometimes help clients in adhering to new routines. In other cases, referrals may be made to organizations that deal in stress management.

Evaluation

On the basis of the nursing diagnoses, the nurse evaluates care for the client or the family experiencing stress. The expected outcomes for the client or the family include the ability to accomplish the following:

1. Verbalize feelings related to stress, appraisal, or coping

2. Identify individual strengths to be used in coping
3. Identify when coping is effective
4. Use coping strategies that are effective in dealing with the perceived stressor
5. Use a variety of coping strategies in a stress situation
6. Use external resources to assist in coping

By achieving the above-mentioned desired outcomes, the client or the family should experience a sense of psychologic and physical well-being as a result of effective coping with perceived stress.

NURSING AND STRESS

Nurses, as well as clients, experience stress. Many nurses are affected by stress that exceeds their ability to cope. Nurses are exposed to tremendous numbers of stressors every day in their work, from exposure to death and mutilation of others to the sometimes unrealistic expectations of the work environment. The indicators of stress in clients are also indicators of stress overload in nurses.

Nurses overwhelmed by stress are sometimes referred to as being "burned out." Some of the common symptoms of burnout are resentment toward supervisors and coworkers, loss of temper at small incidents, constant fatigue, reluctance to go to work, and withdrawal from work relationships.

There are many programs available to aid the nurse in stress reduction, and there are also a variety of strategies the individual nurse may use. In addition to the strategies outlined for clients, nurses may try the following stress management techniques:

1. Learn assertiveness techniques to present feelings and thoughts in an honest, direct, and acceptable manner. Remember that hostile expression of anger and aggression usually inflame, rather than reduce, stress feelings.

2. Acknowledge the positive aspects of work and do not dwell on the negatives. Happier people have been found to be less "realistic" in their assessments of situations in that they focus on the funny and the positive aspects of life.

3. Develop alternative plans for situations known to cause stress. For example, if transportation is a problem, arrange for a friend or coworker to serve as a back-up when trouble develops.

4. Follow the same health care practices that nurses recommend to others. Remember to get adequate sleep, eat a healthy diet, reduce caffeine consumption, get regular exercise, stop smoking, and use alcohol only in moderation, if at all.

SUMMARY

Nurses are in a position to assist individuals who are stressed and having difficulty coping. By understanding that stress is an individually perceived relationship between the person and the environment, nurses can ensure that their actions are specific to the client's stress. Coping with stress involves many different physical and psychologic client responses. Some coping strategies are directed toward the problem causing the stress, whereas others are directed toward the emotions brought forth by the stress. Nurses can also assist clients by helping to identify strategies used in similar situations and by identifying new ways of coping if the old strategies are ineffective.

IMPLICATIONS FOR RESEARCH

Nursing has been at the forefront of research on stress and coping. The stress-coping response is one area where nurses can be expected to make major research contributions within the next few years. With the possible exception of technical research on the cellular aspects of the biochemical stress response, all aspects of the stress-coping response represent valid areas for nursing research. The following are possible avenues for nursing research:

1. What coping strategies are effective for clients undergoing specific tests or procedures?

2. What hospital routines contribute to the client's perception of increased stress?

3. What is the relationship between the length of waiting time for procedures and the perception of stress?

4. What nursing activities are the most effective in reducing perceived stress in selected client care situations?

REFERENCES AND READINGS

Bulman, R. J., & Wortman, C. B. (1977). Attributions of blame and coping in the "real world": Severe accident victims react to their lot. *Journal of Personality and Social Psychology, 35,* 351–363.

Cannon, W. B. (1931). *The wisdom of the body.* New York: W. W. Norton.

DeLongis, A., Coyne, J. C., Dakof, G., Folkman, S., & Lazarus, R. S. (1982). Relationship of daily hassles, uplifts and major life events to health status. *Health Psychology, 1,* 119–136.

Gurklis, J. A., & Menke, E. M. (1988). Identification of stressors and use of coping methods in chronic hemodialysis patients. *Nursing Research, 37,* 236–239.

Janis, I. L. (1985). Coping patterns among patients with life-threatening diseases. *Issues in Mental Health Nursing, 7,* 461–476.

Johnson, J. E. (1972). Effects of structuring patients' expectations on their reactions to threatening events. *Nursing Research, 21,* 499–503.

Johnson, J. E., & Lauver, D. R. (1989). Alternative explanations of coping with stressful experiences associated with physical illness. *Advances in Nursing Science, 11,* 39–52.

Kasl, S. V., Evans, A. S., & Niederman, J. C. (1979). Psychosocial risk factors in the development of infectious mononucleosis. *Psychosomatic Medicine, 41,* 445–466.

King, K. B. (1985). Measurement of coping strategies, concerns, and emotional response in patients undergoing coronary artery bypass grafting. *Heart and Lung, 14,* 579–586.

Kobasa, S. C. (1979). Stressful life events, personality, and health: An inquiry into hardiness. *Journal of Personality and Social Psychology, 37,* 1–10.

Lazarus, R. S., & Folkman, S. (1984). *Stress, appraisal and coping.* New York: Springer.

McCrae, R. R. (1984). Situational determinants of coping response: loss, threat and challenge. *Journal of Personality and Social Psychology, 46,* 919–928.

McCranie, E. W., Lambert, V. A., & Lambert, C. E. (1987). Work stress, hardiness, and burnout among hospital staff nurses. *Nursing Research, 36,* 374–377.

McNett, S. C. (1987). Social support, threat, and coping responses and effectiveness in the functionally disabled. *Nursing Research, 36,* 98–103.

Meichenbaum, D., & Novaco, R. (1985). Stress inoculation: A preventative approach. *Issues in Mental Health Nursing, 7,* 419–431.

Moos, R. H., & Tsu, V. D. (1977). The crisis of physical illness. In R. H. Moos (Ed.), *Coping with physical illness.* New York: Plenum.

Peirce, A. G. (1987). Event review in the coping process of parous women (Doctoral dissertation, University of Maryland at Baltimore, 1987). *Dissertation Abstracts International, 42,* 705B.

Pollock, S. E. (1989). The hardiness characteristic: A motivating factor in adaptation. *Advances in Nursing Science, 11,* 53–62.

Schroeder, D. H., & Costa, P. T. (1984). Influence of life events on physical illness: Substantive effects or methodological flaws? *Journal of Personality and Social Psychology, 46,* 853–863.

Selye, H. (1946). General adaptation syndrome and diseases of adaptation. *Journal of Clinical Endocrinology, 6,* 117–230.

Vincent, K. G. (1985). The validation of a nursing diagnosis: A nurse consensus survey. *Nursing Clinics of North America, 20,* 631–640.

ADDITIONAL READINGS

Hamner, M. L. (1984). Insight, reminiscence, denial, projection: Coping mechanisms of the aged. *Journal of Gerontological Nursing, 10(2),* 66–68.

Hamner presented a review of common coping strategies used by older adults to deal with the stressors that often come with old age. The article reinforced that coping mechanisms may not necessarily be influenced by age, but rather by the type of situations that different age groups deal with.

Kobasa, S. C., & Puccetti, M. C. (1983). Personality and social resources in stress resistance. *Journal of Personality and Social Psychology, 45,* 839–850.

The authors studied how different forms of social support influenced the incidence of illness in people with different levels of hardiness (high and low). Kobasa and Puccetti found that support from the boss at work was related to lower incidence of illness in both groups. However, family support was detrimental to those low in hardiness, that is, the more support reported, the more illness reported as well.

Lenehan, G. P. (1986). Emotional impact of trauma. *Nursing Clinics of North America, 21,* 729–741.

In this article the author reviewed the common responses to trauma seen in injured individuals and their families. The article stressed that there are both physical and psychosocial results of trauma. Among the recommended nursing interventions are suggestions for helping clients deal with guilt responses and maintain self-esteem. The author also suggested how to communicate with family members.

Lenz, E. R. (1984). Information seeking: A component of client decisions and health behavior. *Advances in Nursing Science, 3,* 51–72.

Lenz studied how and why people seek health-related information. The author was able to show that there are different ways of getting information and that some ways are more effective than others. The socioeconomic status of the client may make a significant difference in the type and accuracy of information obtained.

Lowery, B. J., & Jacobson, B. S. (1985). Attributional analysis of chronic illness outcomes. *Nursing Research, 34,* 82–87.

It is a common human reaction to look for a cause for perceived problems. The attribution of blame is important in understanding the different responses seen in chronic illness. People who place the blame on others, on outside forces, or on themselves may all react differently to long-term stress. The authors of this article explored the concept of attribution of blame in a research study using chronically ill clients.

CHAPTER 7

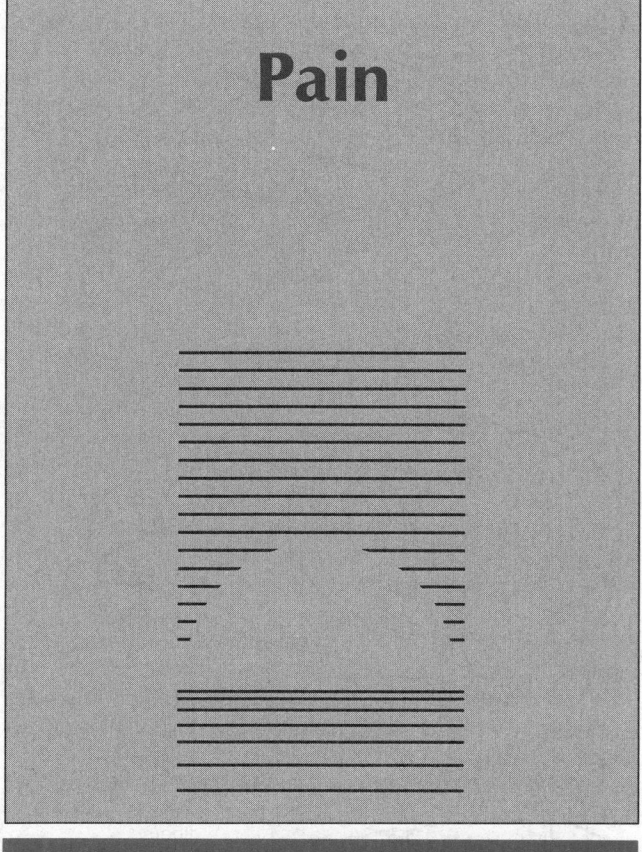

Pain

Pain is the number one symptom or complaint that causes people to seek health care. It disables or compromises the quality of life more than any other single health-related problem. Pain is a problem of great concern to nurses, who must recognize it in their clients and intervene to provide comfort and relief measures. The effective management of pain is a major challenge in the practice of nursing.

DEFINITIONS OF PAIN

Pain is experienced by everyone, but it is a complex and private experience. Because it is such an abstract phenomenon, major difficulties arise when one attempts to describe or explain it. Many factors operate to make pain hard to understand or assess. These elements include psychosocial factors, the subjectivity of the pain experience, and the lack of valid and reliable instruments to measure clinical pain. The interpretation of pain via behavioral manifestations is equally cumbersome because the magnitude of response to pain is vulnerable to individual differences.

Several attempts have been made to define pain in descriptive or measurable terms, yet no one definition is more accepted than another. Among the most popular definitions of pain are those of Sternbach, McCaffery, and the International Association on Pain. Sternbach (1968, p. 12) asserted that pain is "an abstract concept which refers to

1. a personal, private sensation of hurt
2. a harmful stimulus which signals current or impending tissue damage
3. a pattern of responses to protect the organism from harm."

This comprehensive definition serves to explain pain through a physiologic, psychologic, and social approach.

McCaffery (1979b, p. 11) offered a more personal explanation of pain when she stated that pain "is whatever the experiencing person says it is and exists whenever he says it does." This understanding of pain requires that the client is seen as the authority on the pain and as the only one who can define the experience.

Finally, the International Association on Pain (1979) described it as an unpleasant sensory and emotional experience associated with actual or potential tissue damage, or described in terms of such damage.

Regardless of the definition, most people agree that pain has both sensory and behavioral components and is strongly influenced by various physiologic, psychologic, and sociologic factors. A comprehensive understanding of pain requires knowledge of the descriptive definitions, theories, and physiology of pain. This knowledge can serve as a basis to develop an appreciation of the variety of clinical pain situations and skill in pain intervention. This understanding can also help the nurse develop a personal philosophy of pain management.

THEORETICAL BASES FOR PAIN

Several theories have been developed to explain the complex phenomenon of pain. Early theories emphasized the recognition of specific pathways of pain transmission; later ones attempted to uncover the intricate complexity of central processing of pain in specific areas of the brain. More recently, the concept of a pain-modulating network has been introduced. This concept describes the various links and connections in the spinal cord and brain, specifically the medulla and the midbrain. The identification of special chemical mediators that are involved in the pain response phenomenon, such as the endogenous opiates, has opened new horizons in understanding pain transmission and perception.

SPECIFICITY THEORY

The specificity theory was proposed in the early 1800s and was then accepted for almost 100 years as the most popular theoretical explanation for pain. This theory emphasized the highly specific structures and pathways responsible for pain transmission. Its premise is based on the existence of free nerve endings in the periphery, which act as pain receptors capable of accepting sensory input and transmitting this information along highly specific nerve fibers. In the dorsal horns of the spinal column, these fibers synapse at the *substantia gelatinosa*. The fibers then cross over to the lateral spinothalamic tract, and pain impulses ascend to the area of the thalamus. The thalamic pain impulses then travel to higher cortical areas where painful sensations are perceived (Fig. 7–1).

The general assumption of the specificity theory supports the notion that pain is as unique and specific as the other body senses, such as hearing and vision. Although this theory set the stage for further research, its major biologic orientation fails to account for the multidimensionality of the pain experience.

PATTERN THEORY

Later, in the early 1900s, an opposing pattern theory was proposed. Goldscheider (cited in Melzack, 1973), the originator of this theory, identified two major pain fibers: a rapidly conducting fiber and a slowly conducting one. Both fibers synapse in the spinal cord and relay information to the brain. The concept of central sum-

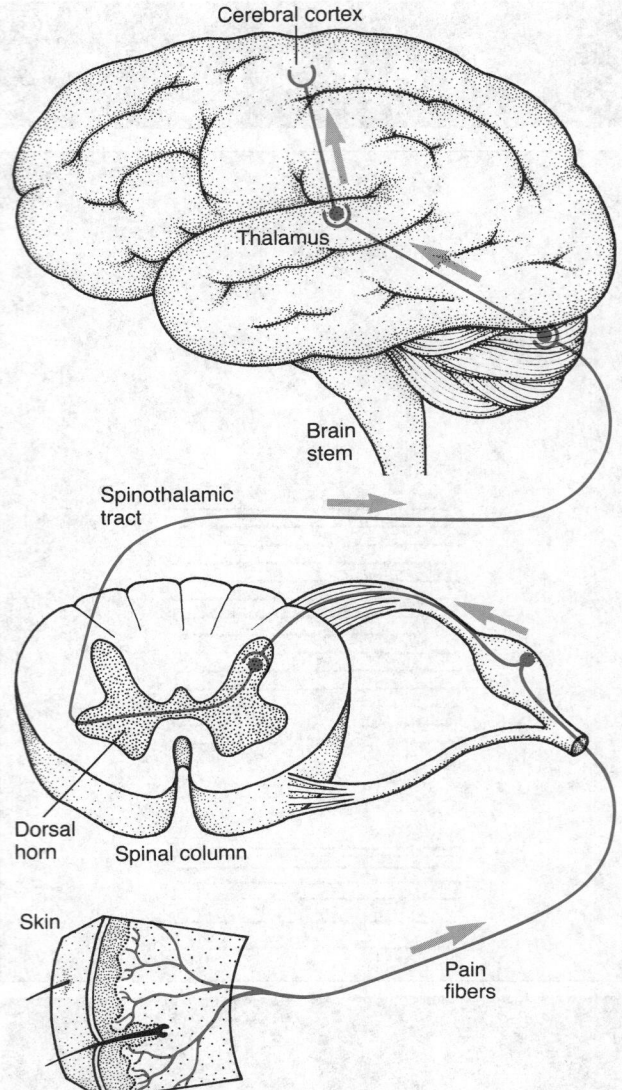

Figure 7–1

Specificity theory of pain.

mation was introduced: As small fibers converge at the level of the spinal cord, the summation of impulses from various small fibers ascends to levels of the brain. The amount, intensity, and type of sensory input to the brain allow for interpretation of the character and quantity of the noxious sensory input.

Both the pattern and the specificity theories fail to address factors that alter the perception of pain, such as anxiety, depression, and hypnosis. These theories also do not explain the failure of pain to resolve after surgical transection of the pain pathways and spinal cord.

GATE CONTROL THEORY

The gate control theory was introduced to explain the observed relationship between pain and emotion. Mel-

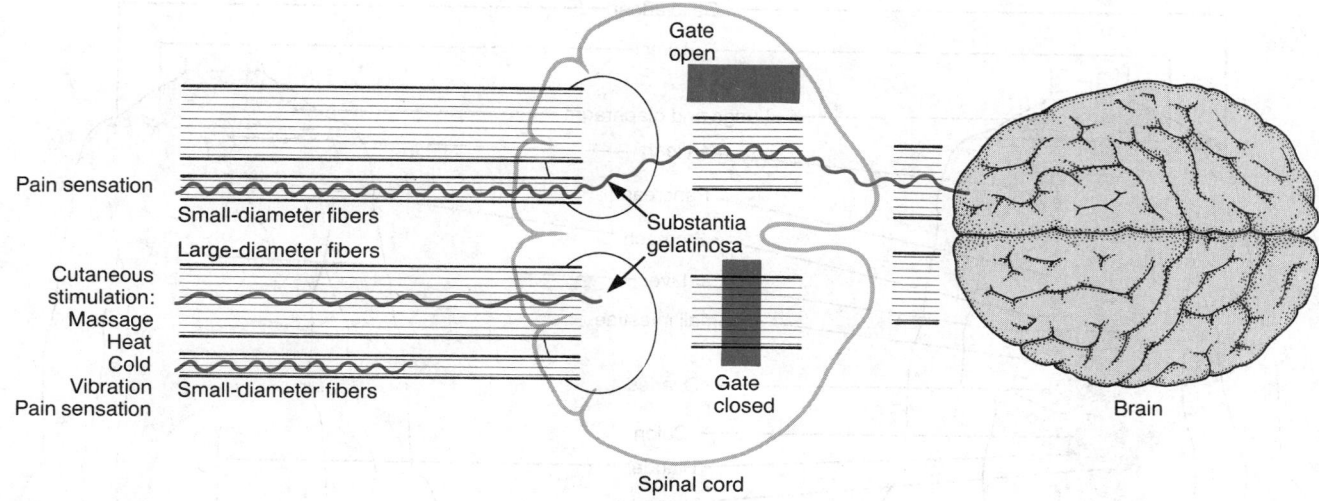

Figure 7-2

Gate control theory of pain. (Modified by permission from Potter, P. A., & Perry, A. G. *Fundamentals of nursing: Concepts, process, and practice.* St. Louis, 1989, The C. V. Mosby Co.)

zack and Wall (1982), who proposed this theory, were able to conclude that the transmission of painful stimuli is largely controlled by afferent impulses in the peripheral nerve fibers. In addition, gating mechanisms may also exist in the brain stem.

According to the gate control theory, there is a hypothetic gating mechanism, which occurs at the level of the spinal cord. Painful impulses that are transmitted by large-diameter and small-diameter fibers pass into the dorsal horns, to the area of the cord called the substantia gelatinosa. The substantia gelatinosa cells can facilitate or inhibit impulses that are transmitted to the trigger cells (T cells). When T cell activity is inhibited, the gate is closed, and impulses are less likely to be transmitted to the brain. This occurs as rapidly conducting large-diameter or facilitory fibers stimulate activity in the substantia gelatinosa area. When activity in this area is inhibited by small-diameter fibers, impulses are more likely to be transmitted to T cells and the gate is then opened, which allows painful impulses to ascend to the brain (Fig. 7-2). The gate control theory is still important today because its holistic view has encouraged a multidimensional approach to pain research.

ANATOMIC AND PHYSIOLOGIC BASES FOR PAIN

PAIN RECEPTORS

Free nerve endings or pain receptors are often referred to as *nociceptors.* These receptors are not stimulated just by pain. Thermal, mechanical, and chemical stimuli also activate them. In addition to nociceptors, other receptors in the body elicit pain with almost any type of intense stimulation.

Nociceptors are located in various parts of body tissues. Pain originates from within three major types of structures: cutaneous, deep somatic, and visceral. *Cutaneous pain* originates in the superficial structures of the skin and subcutaneous tissues. These structures are well innervated; therefore, painful stimuli are well defined and localized. Receptors in cutaneous tissues initiate two components of pain. The quick or fast component, involving A delta fibers, allows for instant recognition of sharp pain, which soon disappears when the stimulus is removed. The second component arises from deeper penetration of nerve receptors and is usually dull, achy, and poorly localized. The latter component involves pain conduction by C fibers. This phenomenon serves as the basis for transcutaneous electrical nerve stimulation, which is discussed later under the heading Physical Measures, in the section Interventions: Nonsurgical Management.

Deep somatic structures include nerve receptors originating in bone, blood vessels, nerves, muscles, and other supporting tissues. Because these structures are poorly innervated, this pain is usually dull and poorly localized. However, deep somatic structures vary in their sensitivity to noxious stimuli. Deep pain may produce nausea, associated with blood pressure changes and sweating.

Pain arising from body organs is referred to as *visceral pain.* The scarcity of nerve receptors in these structures produces poorly localized and diffuse pain. Although they are insensitive to cutting and to extremes of temperature, visceral receptors respond to stretching, inflammation, and ischemia. Visceral pain is well known for its ability to produce *referred pain,* a type of pain that is usually perceived in an area distant to the site of the

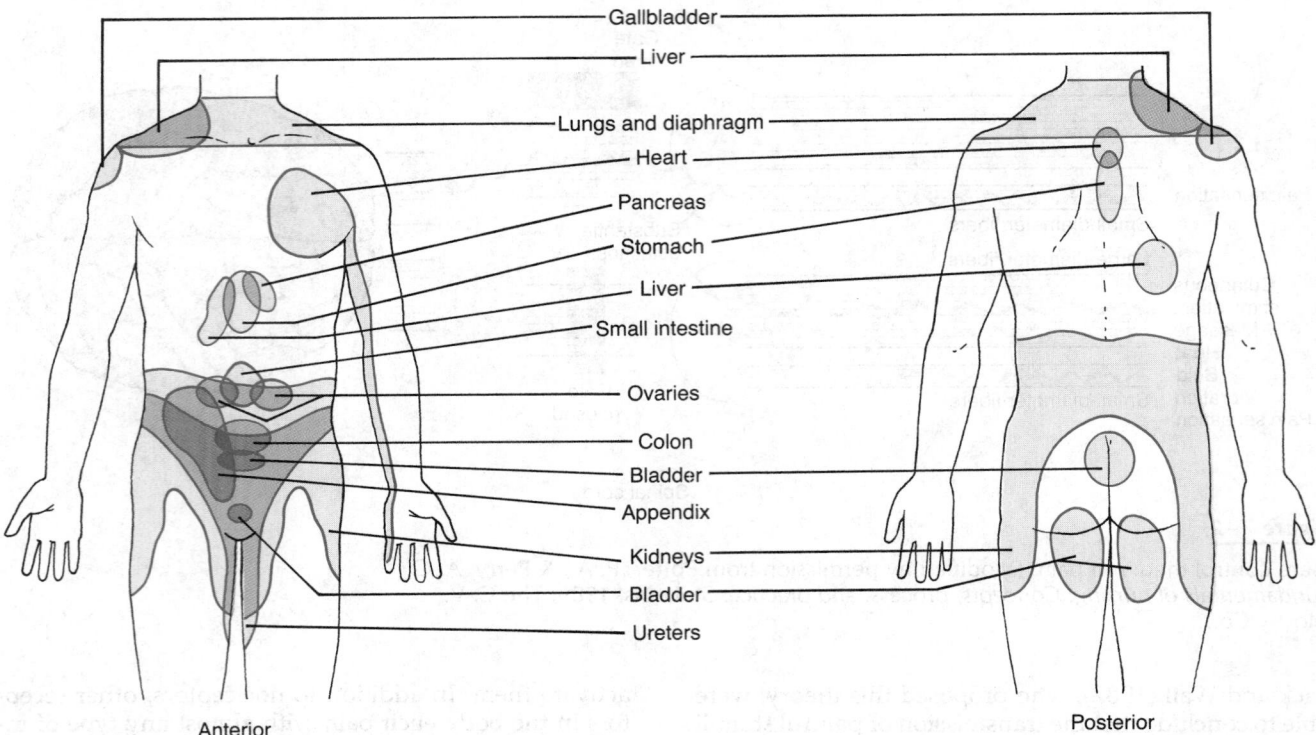

Figure 7–3
Anterior and posterior referred pain sites.

stimuli. Referred pain occurs because visceral fibers synapse at the level of the spinal cord, close to fibers innervating certain subcutaneous tissue areas of the body. A common example of referred pain is pain in the right shoulder related to gallbladder disease. This occurs because the subcutaneous tissue fibers of the scapula converge on those from the gallbladder, which are transmitting the painful stimuli. Other referred pain sites are illustrated in Figure 7–3.

PAIN STIMULI

Various types of noxious pain stimuli account for the perception of pain. Stimuli from mechanical or physical injury and from thermal and chemical sources constitute the wide range of sensory inputs capable of producing pain. In addition, vascular ischemia and muscle spasm are likely to evoke painful responses. In most circumstances, painful stimuli cause actual tissue damage, which leads to the release of certain chemical substances, such as histamine, bradykinin, serotonin, prostaglandins, and acids, that are believed to activate pain receptors. The accumulation of lactic acid is implicated in the pain related to ischemic tissue damage. Muscle contraction or spasm can also produce ischemic-type pain because oxygen demands of the muscle are increased while the blood supply is limited as a result of compression of blood vessels.

PAIN PATHWAYS

Usually, painful stimuli originate in the periphery. However, for them to be perceived, they must first be transmitted to the spinal cord and then to the central areas of the brain, their final destination. In the periphery, two specific fibers can transmit stimuli: A delta fibers that are found primarily in the skin and muscle, and C fibers that are distributed in muscle, periosteum, and viscera. *A delta fibers* are myelinated fibers that carry rapid, sharp, pricking, or piercing sensations. These sensations are generally readily localized to a fairly well-defined area. Because these fibers respond predominantly to mechanical stimuli rather than to chemical or thermal stimuli, they are called mechanical nociceptors.

The larger, unmyelinated or poorly myelinated *C fibers* conduct thermal, chemical, and strong mechanical impulses. Pain conduction from C fibers is more diffuse and dull, burning, or achy—quite different from the sensations of A delta fibers. In contrast to the intermittent nature of A delta sensations, C fibers usually produce more continuous, constant pain.

A delta and C fibers enter the spinal cord at the dorsal nerve root. The dorsal root ganglion fibers establish synapses with certain relay neurons in the dorsal horn of the spinal cord and terminate in various sections of the laminae. The substantia gelatinosa comprises sections II

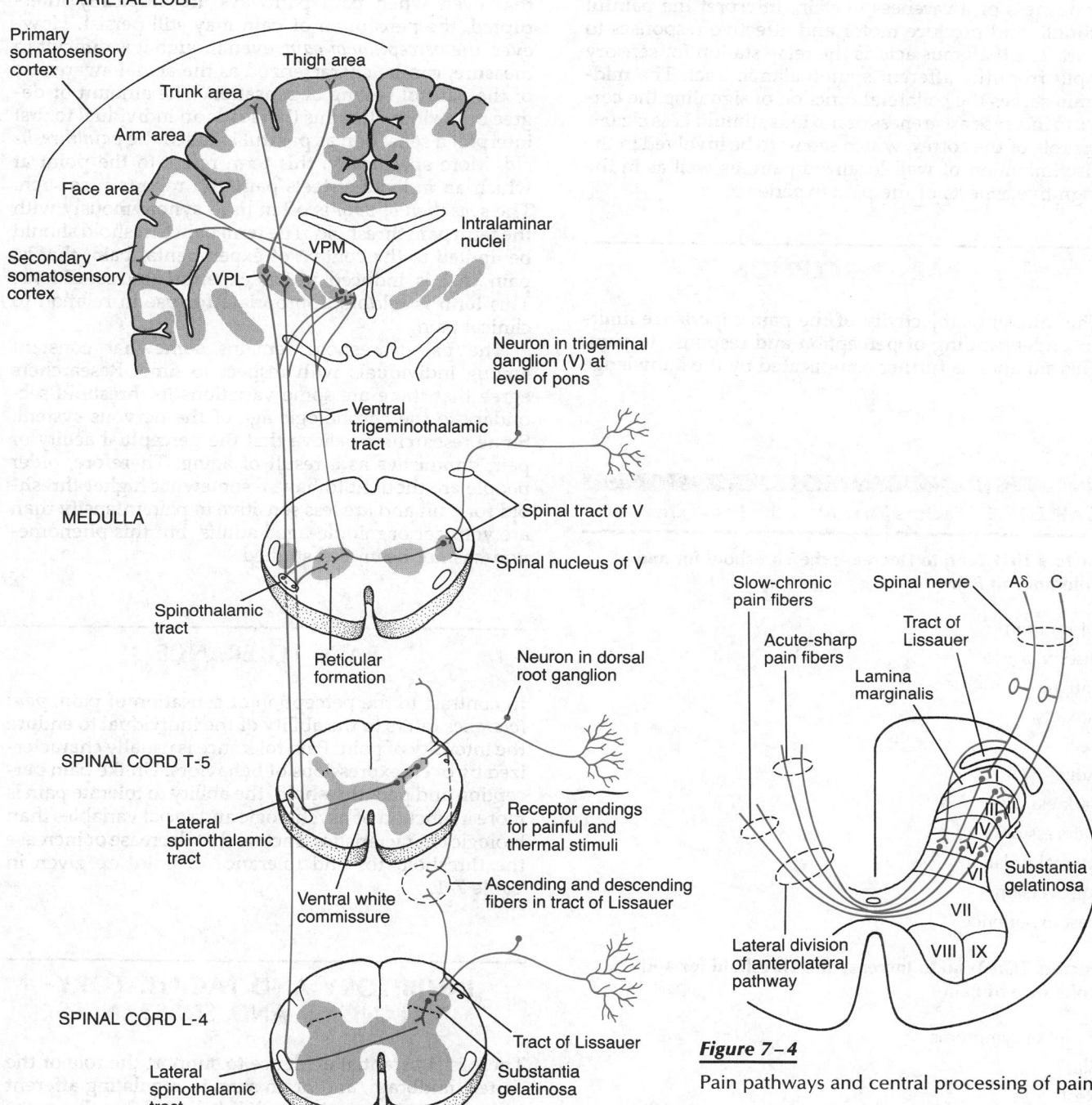

Figure 7-4

Pain pathways and central processing of pain.

and III of the laminae (Fig. 7-4). Impulses are then conveyed to neurons that transmit information to the opposite side of the spinal cord in the anterior commissure and then converge on the lateral spinothalamic tract.

The ascending spinothalamic tract can be further divided into the neospinothalamic and the paleospinothalamic pathways. The neospinothalamic tract is likely

to be responsible for relaying information about the degree and location of pain, whereas the paleospinothalamic tract deals primarily with motor emotional responses to pain without attention to the sensory components of pain.

The central processing of pain occurs at three different levels: the thalamus, midbrain, and cortex. Several parts of the central brain area cooperate to raise consciousness or awareness of pain, interpret the painful stimuli, and produce motor and affective responses to pain. The thalamus acts as the relay station for sensory input from the afferent spinothalamic tract. The midbrain serves the collateral function of signaling the cortex to increase awareness of noxious stimuli. Less clear is the role of the cortex, which seems to be involved in the discrimination of well-localized pain, as well as in the cognitive aspects of the pain experience.

PAIN PERCEPTION

The inherent subjectivity of the pain experience limits an understanding of perception and response to pain. This situation is further complicated by the knowledge

TABLE 7 – 1   Factors That Alter the Pain Experience

Factors That Tend to Decrease the Threshold for and Tolerance of Pain

Discomfort

Insomnia

Fatigue

Anxiety

Fear

Anger

Sadness

Depression

Mental isolation

Introversion

Past experience

Factors That Tend to Increase the Threshold for and Tolerance of Pain

Relief of symptoms

Sleep

Rest

Sympathy

Understanding

Diversion

Elevation of mood

Pharmacologic agents

Analgesics

Anxiolytics

Antidepressants

that even when pain pathways are surgically interrupted, the perception of pain may still persist. However, the *perception of pain*, even though it is difficult to measure, can be characterized as the actual awareness of the painful feeling or sensation. The amount or degree of noxious stimulus that leads an individual to first interpret a sensation as painful is called the *pain threshold*. More specifically, this term refers to the point at which an individual feels pain and reports it as such. The *sensation of pain* is often used synonymously with the term pain threshold. The term pain threshold should be limited to the context of experimental pain, that is, pain that is induced under experimental conditions. This term is seldom appropriate for use in relation to clinical pain.

The pain threshold remains somewhat constant among individuals with respect to time. Researchers agree that there are some variations in threshold secondary to the chronologic age of the nervous system. Some researchers believe that the perceptual acuity of pain diminishes as a result of aging. Therefore, older people are thought to have a somewhat higher threshold for pain and are less sensitive to pain intensity than are younger or middle-aged adults, but this phenomenon has not been well studied.

PAIN TOLERANCE

In contrast to the perception or sensation of pain, *pain tolerance* refers to the ability of the individual to endure the intensity of pain. Pain tolerance is usually characterized by overt expressions of behaviors. Unlike pain perception and pain threshold, the ability to tolerate pain is more a function of psychologic and social variables than biologic characteristics. Factors that decrease or increase the threshold for and tolerance of pain are given in Table 7-1.

INHIBITORY AND FACILITATORY MECHANISMS AND SUBSTANCES

There is substantial evidence to support the role of the cortex, midbrain, and brain stem in regulating afferent sensory input transmission. It is believed that the cortex and other areas of the brain inhibit or facilitate the transmission of nerve impulses by the activation of specific descending pathways. These pathways are located in the brain and transmit messages down the spinothalamic tracts to the presynaptic and postsynaptic junctions of the dorsal horn in the spinal cord. The regulatory effects of these descending pathways are not clearly understood. It is known that stimulation of certain areas of the brain leads to descending fiber activity, which in turn affects afferent nerve transmission. This means that descending messages from the brain influence ascending or afferent signals. This occurrence explains, at least partially, the cognitive or emotional influences on pain perception. In essence, the cortex serves as a feedback loop between central mechanisms of the brain and sensory pain fibers to regulate the degree of pain impulse transmission.

The conduction of pain impulses at the level of the spinal cord is inhibited or reduced by the stimulation of certain peripheral nerve fibers in the skin and subcutaneous tissues. On the basis of the gate control theory, the flow of pain impulses can be modulated by large and small nerve fibers. Stimulation of large fibers closes the hypothetic gate in the spinal cord, which diminishes the conduction of pain. Conversely, input to small fibers opens the gate, which allows more pain to travel up the spinal cord to the brain where it is perceived.

Sensory input to the spinal cord may also be influenced by chemical substances known as *neuroregulators*. These neuroregulators are classified as neurotransmitters or neuromodulators. *Neurotransmitters* are neurochemicals that exert inhibitory or excitatory activity at postsynaptic membranes. Acetylcholine, norepinephrine, epinephrine, and dopamine are documented neurotransmitters. Various other neurotransmitters possess only some characteristics of these substances and are called *putative neurotransmitters*.

More recently, *neuromodulators*, which are polypeptides found in the brain, have been implicated in the modulation of pain. These substances are composed of large amino acid peptides called alpha- and beta-*endorphins* and *enkephalins*. The analgesic effects of these substances on mammalian brains were inadvertently observed by researchers. The speculation that these natural opiate-like substances were responsible for pain relief was confirmed when induced analgesic effects were reversed with naloxone, a narcotic antagonist. Similar to morphine-like substances only more potent, these endogenous opiates are believed to play a major role in the biologic response to pain. The larger peptides, the endorphins, exert more prolonged analgesic effects than the enkephalins. Endorphins are produced by the anterior pituitary and the hypothalamus. The enkephalins, the smaller peptides, tend to be more widespread throughout the brain and dorsal horn of the spinal cord. Several types of endorphins and enkephalins have been identified. Each acts on highly specific opiate receptors in the central nervous system and spinal cord.

The production of endogenous opiates is influenced greatly by various factors. Activity of endorphins and enkephalins may be enhanced by prolonged strenuous activity, transcutaneous electrical nerve stimulators (see under the heading Interventions: Nonsurgical Management), and antidepressant therapy, which often increases serotonin levels in the body. Adequate amounts of serotonin, a neurotransmitter, have been shown to enhance analgesia through endorphin and enkephalin activity. Similarly, pain and stress are strong activators of the endogenous opiate system.

PSYCHOSOCIAL INFLUENCES ON PAIN

Several psychosocial variables affect a person's perception and response to pain. Factors such as age, sex, sociocultural background, personality characteristics, and affect or mood states, such as anxiety or depression, strongly influence the client's ability to process pain sensations and react to them. Unfortunately, studies evaluating these variables have shown conflicting and inconclusive results. For example, some investigators have demonstrated that men tolerate pain better than women, whereas others have found no sex differences. It is widely believed that it is more acceptable for women than men to express pain, and this belief may affect study results. In an earlier work, Zborowski (1969) investigated the pain behaviors of "old Americans" and compared this group to Italian Americans, American Jews, and others. He found differences among these groups and characterized the "old Americans" as more stoic and less emotive than the other groups. Zborowski's work is interesting, but the results are far from conclusive. Further information on psychosocial influences on pain can be found in Jacox (1977) and Meinhart and McCaffery (1983). For other factors that alter the pain experience, see Key Features of Disease: Factors That Alter the Pain Experience.

Even though all pain is real, it sometimes persists without any detectable physical cause. This pain is often referred to as *psychogenic* or *psychosomatic*: pain that is believed to arise from mental factors. In these situations, the lack of a physiologic or organic cause leads clients to doubt the validity of their pain. Nurses appreciate the reality of the pain experience, offer support, and intervene with appropriate pain-relieving measures. These clients are usually treated with noninvasive behavioral and cognitive techniques, which are discussed later in the Collaborative Management section. Pain that is exclusively psychogenic is rarely observed. More commonly, physiologic or organic pain resolves and leaves psychosocial components of the pain experience, which are often misinterpreted as psychogenic pain.

RESEARCH ON PAIN

Research on pain has been done by basic scientists in the laboratory and by nurses, physicians, and others in the clinical setting. Pain researchers have used both animal and human subjects and both physiologic and behavioral measures. The general purposes of the research have been to understand the pain phenomenon and its effects and to evaluate the effect of interventions designed to relieve pain.

Research generally conceptualizes pain as a complex phenomenon that is modulated by the central nervous system. Because of the complexity of the pain response, it is difficult to relate findings from animal research on pain to the human pain experience. Even studies of aspects of motivational choice or discrimination of pain stimuli in animals are not readily applied to the human situation. Although these efforts can provide some information about the sensory-discriminative aspects of the pain experience, they do not clarify the aversive or emotional aspects of pain.

Pain research done with human subjects also presents a series of problems. A major problem results from the fact that no single theory of pain is generally accepted by researchers, nor is there a unified or consistent use of pain assessment technology. Because of these problems, it is difficult to evaluate the various approaches used to measure pain in different studies. Further, no universally accepted guidelines exist to evaluate the effects of analgesic interventions. It is thus difficult to decide how meaningful or important the results of one study would be for a different group of subjects.

Clinicians have attempted to quantify or categorize behavioral data describing the activity of subjects in pain, in both inpatient and outpatient settings. Commonly reported activities have included daily activities such as moving in bed, sitting, and walking; changes in patterns of sleep or food intake; medication intake; and pain-related complaints such as moaning, groaning, facial expressions, and splinting or guarding of a body part. These data may be useful for assessing pain relief or intervention effects, but they are only indirect indicators of pain. They are also highly influenced by personal and environmental factors. Researchers need to give further attention to precisely defining the behaviors used in pain research, to understand the usefulness of this type of measure.

Many studies of pain have measured neuronal activity or the output of the autonomic nervous system. If a physiologic event can be shown to vary with reports of pain, the measure could be considered to be an effective indicator of pain. Assessments of this sort have included electromyographic measures of muscle tension; measures of pulse rate, skin conductance and resistance, and skin temperature; and electroencephalographic measures.

Neuronal or physiologic tests are thought to be valid indicators of the presence of pain, but they do not necessarily reflect the effects of emotional arousal or higher-level central nervous system processes. Emotions, previous experience, and learned reactions all contribute to the pain experience and can modify even the physiologic responses of the body to pain. Physiologic assessments of pain provide an opportunity for objective pain measurement, but these measures too may be influenced by the subjectivity of the pain experience. Many physiologic measures require sophisticated technology and laboratory situations for data collection. This requirement makes it more difficult to carry out this type of research in the clinical setting.

Nurse researchers have been concerned with the pain phenomenon, most often in relation to *measuring the effects of interventions aimed at relieving pain*. In addition to research evaluating the effectiveness of clinical interventions, nurse researchers have also investigated *the influence of nurses' attitudes on the administration of pain medication*.

A study by Wells (1982) provides an example of research designed to measure the effects of nursing interventions aimed at perceiving pain. Wells studied the postoperative effects of relaxation training in a small sample of clients who had had a cholecystectomy and found that the training reduced the psychologic discomforts related to pain, but Wells was unable to demonstrate changes on any physiologic measure.

Another evaluation of the effects of nursing intervention can be seen in the work of Keller and Bzdek (1986), who investigated the effects of therapeutic touch on tension headache pain. The McGill-Melzack Pain Questionnaire (Fig. 7–5) was used to demonstrate an average 70% pain reduction in the 4-hour postintervention period compared with a group receiving placebo touch intervention.

The introduction of patient-controlled analgesia (PCA) (see under later heading Interventions: Nonsurgical Management) into clinical settings provides a quantitative measurement instrument that avoids some of the problems related to the subjectivity of the pain experience. Guiffre et al. (1988) recommended the use of a PCA pump in research protocols in which the effects of experimental intervention on acute pain perception and the amount of narcotic required to relieve that pain are being investigated. With the PCA pump, clients can self-administer small amounts of analgesics through an indwelling intravenous catheter. This self-administration avoids the interactions and perceptions of other caregivers and also avoids many environmental effects, such as the unavailability of a nurse to administer a requested analgesic. In addition, because the use of a PCA pump provides measurement of analgesic use over time, as a research instrument it is superior to other measures such as a visual analogue scale that provide indications of the client's level of pain at discrete times.

Pain is a personal and subjective phenomenon, and the attitude of the health care provider (usually the nurse) about the pain easily influences the assessment, intervention, and evaluation of the pain experience.

Figure 7–5

The McGill-Melzack Pain Questionnaire. (From Melzack, R. [1975]. The McGill Pain Questionnaire: Major properties and scoring methods. *Pain, 1*, 272–281.)

McGill-Melzack
PAIN QUESTIONNAIRE

Patient's name _____ Age _____

File No. _____ Date _____

Clinical category (e.g., cardiac, neurologic)

Diagnosis: _____

_____

_____

Analgesic (if already administered):

1. Type _____

2. Dosage _____

3. Time given in relation to this test _____

Patient's intelligence: circle number that represents best estimate.

1 (low)   2   3   4   5 (high)

****

This questionnaire has been designed to tell us more about your pain. Four major questions we ask are

1. Where is your pain?
2. What does it feel like?
3. How does it change with time?
4. How strong is it?

It is important that you tell us how your pain feels now. Please follow the instructions at the beginning of each part.

_____

© R. Melzack, Oct. 1970

Part 1. Where Is Your Pain?

Please mark, on the drawings below, the areas where you feel pain. Put E if external, or I if internal, near the areas you mark. Put EI if both external and internal.

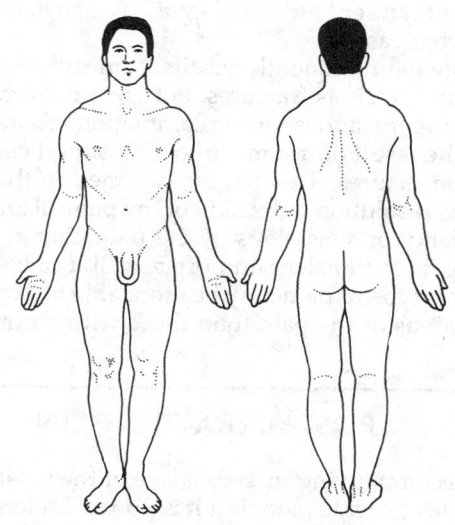

Part 2. What Does Your Pain Feel Like?

Some of the words below describe your *present* pain. Circle *ONLY* those words that best describe it. Leave out any category that is not suitable. Use only a single word in each appropriate category — the one that applies best.

1	6	11	16
Flickering	Tugging	Tiring	Annoying
Quivering	Pulling	Exhausting	Troublesome
Pulsing	Wrenching		Miserable
Throbbing		**12**	Intense
Beating	**7**	Sickening	Unbearable
Pounding	Hot	Suffocat-	
	Burning	ing	**17**
2	Scalding		Spreading
Jumping	Searing	**13**	Radiating
Flashing		Fearful	Penetrating
Shooting	**8**	Frightful	Piercing
	Tingling	Terrifying	
3	Itchy		**18**
Pricking	Smarting	**14**	Tight
Boring	Stinging	Punishing	Numb
Drilling		Grueling	Drawing
Stabbing	**9**	Cruel	Squeezing
Lancinating	Dull	Vicious	Tearing
	Sore	Killing	
4	Hurting		**19**
Sharp	Aching	**15**	Cool
Cutting	Heavy	Wretched	Cold
Lacerating		Blinding	Freezing
	10		
5	Tender		**20**
Pinching	Taut		Nagging
Pressing	Rasping		Nauseating
Gnawing	Splitting		Agonizing
Cramping			Dreadful
Crushing			Torturing

Part 3. How Does Your Pain Change With Time?

1. Which word or words would you use to describe the *pattern* of your pain?

1	2	3
Continuous	Rhythmic	Brief
Steady	Periodic	Momentary
Constant	Intermittent	Transient

2. What kind of things *relieve* your pain?

3. What kind of things *increase* your pain?

Part 4. How Strong Is Your Pain?

People agree that the following 5 words represent pain of increasing intensity. They are:

1	2	3	4	5
Mild	Discomforting	Distressing	Horrible	Excruciating

To answer each question below, write the number of the most appropriate word in the space beside the question.

1. Which word describes your pain right now? ____
2. Which word describes it at its worst? ____
3. Which word describes it when it is least? ____
4. Which word describes the worst toothache you ever had? ____
5. Which word describes the worst headache you ever had? ____
6. Which word describes the worst stomach ache you ever had? ____

Figure 7–5

See legend on opposite page.

Nurses themselves may have little personal experience with pain. They may not appreciate how painful a particular treatment or surgery may be; they may expect that persons with chronic pain will react similarly to those with acute pain and that reactions to pain, including complaints about pain, will fall within a certain norm. The more an individual with pain varies from these expected norms, the more likely it is that the attitude of the nurse toward the client is biased either positively or negatively.

Because of these issues, nurse researchers have studied clinical situations to identify ways in which the attitude of the caregiver might influence pain management in the clinical setting. The work of Beyer et al. (1983) and the work of Faherty and Grier (1984) provide examples of this. Beyer et al. studied the prescription and administration of analgesics after cardiac surgery in 50 children and 50 adults. They found significant differences in both the prescription and administration of analgesics. Children in this study received less narcotic and fewer drugs than adults.

In a study of elderly people after surgery, Faherty and Grier found that older postsurgery clients were prescribed and administered less analgesic medication than younger clients. Although smaller dosages had been prescribed for the elderly clients, nurses in this study administered a smaller percentage of the smaller dose prescribed.

Both of these studies revealed the influence of nurses' attitudes about pain management in the very young and the very old. Nurses and other caregivers frequently undermedicate these clients, and in both of these studies nurses were reluctant to administer the prescribed analgesics. Unfounded concerns about overmedication, addiction, and decreases in pain perception in these populations may contribute to this consistent undermedication. Further study in this area is needed.

TYPES OF PAIN

ACUTE PAIN

Acute pain is experienced by almost everyone at some time. Certain characteristics distinguish this type of pain from the more chronic or long-term pain, which is often associated with chronic illness. A major distinction between acute pain and chronic pain is found in the effects of pain on biologic responses. Acute pain serves a biologic purpose: it acts as a warning signal, as it can activate the sympathetic nervous system. This stimulation causes the liberation of catecholamine neurotransmitters, which give rise to various physiologic responses. As a result, clients experiencing acute pain exhibit physiologic responses similar to those found in "fight-or-flight" reactions. These responses include increased heart rate, blood pressure, and respiratory rate; dilated

TABLE 7–2 Comparison of Physiologic and Behavioral Responses to Acute and Chronic Pain

Pain Type	Physiologic Response	Behavioral Response
Acute	Increased blood pressure Increased pulse rate Increased respiratory rate Dilated pupils Perspiration	Restlessness Inability to concentrate Apprehension Distress
Chronic	Normal blood pressure Normal pulse rate Normal respiratory rate Normal pupils Dry skin	Immobility or physical inactivity Withdrawal Despair

pupils; and sweating. Behavioral signs of acute pain may include restlessness, inability to concentrate, apprehension, and overall distress (Table 7–2).

Acute pain is usually temporary, of sudden onset, and easily localized. The client can frequently describe the pain, which often subsides with or without treatment.

Health professionals do not usually have major problems in the assessment, management, or evaluation of acute pain, perhaps because acute pain, although possibly severe, is limited over time and generally can be successfully managed clinically. Both the caregiver and the client can see "an end in sight," which makes coping somewhat easier.

Acute pain frequently results from sudden, accidental trauma such as fractures, burns, and lacerations, or from surgery and acute inflammation. Acute pain is often the result of trauma involving superficial or cutaneous structures. This pain is confined to the affected area. As resolution or healing of the painful area occurs, the quality or sensations of the pain change. Because acute pain is transient and often well localized, clients with this type of pain may be more able to express their perceptions of the pain than those with chronic pain.

POSTOPERATIVE PAIN

Pain accompanying surgery is one of the most common examples of acute pain, but it is poorly understood and not always well managed. It is conservatively estimated that 20% of all patients undergoing surgery experience mild pain, 20% to 40% experience moderate pain, and 40% to 70% experience severe pain (Bonica, 1983). Even though hundreds of millions of people worldwide undergo surgery, this experience is not yet tolerable for everyone. According to some authorities, the alarmingly

TABLE 7-3 Factors Responsible for Postoperative Pain

Type of Factor	Factor
Predictable physiologic causes	Incisions, causing pain with motion and coughing Tube or drain management. Return of bowel function causing gas cramps
Unpredictable physiologic causes	Inadequate use of pain medication Serum or blood collection Tissue trauma and overly tight suture placement in wound closure Poorly stabilized tubes and drains Unstable fractures, e.g., sternum and costal margin Wound separation Wound sepsis and intra-abdominal abscesses Gastric or intestinal distention Bladder distention Phlebitis and pulmonary emboli Pancreatitis and acute cholecystitis Angina pectoris and myocardial infarction

Adapted from Wilson, R. E. (Ed.). (1979). *The management of pain in surgical practice. Postoperative pain.* Plainfield, NJ: Pfizer.

high numbers of clients experiencing pain after surgery can be attributed to inadequate analgesia. Others believe that inadequate pain control stems from societal attitudes and beliefs that those in pain should "grin and bear it." Still others identify the fear of addiction as a major factor in prescribing and administering less than optimal amounts of analgesics after surgery. Whatever the reason, people undergoing surgery suffer needlessly.

Pain is an expected outcome of surgery and has not only a sensory component related to tissue destruction, but also a major psychosocial component. Several predictable and unpredictable physiologic causes of postoperative pain are given in Table 7-3. However, several studies have indicated that the type and site of the operation are the most important predictors in determining the incidence, severity, and duration of postoperative pain. Similarly, the extent of the operative procedure, the degree of tissue trauma, and the positioning of clients during surgery contribute to the overall incidence and severity of postoperative pain.

Intrathoracic and upper intra-abdominal surgical approaches are generally associated with more severe, steady wound pain and pain on movement in the postoperative period. Conversely, approximately one-half of clients undergoing superficial surgery of the head and neck, chest wall, or limb report minimal or no pain postoperatively. Muscle splitting procedures are far more painful than muscle stretching ones. On the basis of this information, surgeons have modified their techniques in an attempt to reduce or minimize components of this type of pain.

The postoperative pain experience is not limited to the level of tissue trauma. Postoperative pain is also highly influenced by many psychosocial variables. Per-

sonal factors such as age, sociocultural group, and race are important determinants for predicting patterns of expressing and coping with postoperative pain. Older people tend to be verbal about their expression of pain; men often tend to stifle their verbal expressions of pain. Some minority groups are more or less expressive about their pain than Caucasian middle-class Americans, but these trends are probably best understood as examples of cultural differences in reporting and expressing pain. Ethnocultural differences related to pain behaviors, verbal complaints, and attitudes toward pain are believed to exist, but it is difficult to study them in a rigorous fashion. Some believe that there is enough current evidence to suggest that cultural differences, including religious and ethnic distinctions, rather than racial differences account for findings in studies of different ethnocultural groups.

Anxiety is perhaps the best-explored psychologic determinant in predicting postoperative pain. A highly anxious client may appear to be more distressed and affected by pain. Numerous studies have been done in attempts to correlate preoperative information with postoperative pain. It is generally agreed that highly anxious clients do not benefit from detailed procedural information before their surgery. However, some studies, such as Johnson and Leventhal (1974) and Johnson et al. (1978), indicate that those clients who receive preoperative procedural information (i.e., description of the expected sensation as well as techniques to enhance relaxation) seem to cope better with postoperative pain and recover more quickly than those given just factual information about the anticipated postoperative experience.

Highly anxious clients are given minimal procedural information, such as the location of the incision, the sequence of events before surgery (e.g., preoperative sedation and visits from perioperative personnel), and postoperative care regimens. Necessary postoperative information includes teaching the client how to cough, turn and deep breathe, and splint the incisional area, as well as routine postoperative care. The nurse should stress the importance of requesting analgesia when the client perceives pain. The nurse should remember that these instructions must be repeated at regular intervals if the client is highly anxious.

CHRONIC PAIN

Chronic pain represents a major health problem in our society. It has been estimated that 25% of the population is affected with a chronic illness and chronic pain. In contrast to acute pain, chronic pain does not serve a biologic purpose. After its initial warning signal, the body must learn to adapt to the persistent noxious stimuli by blocking or adjusting to the activation of the sympathetic nervous system. Because of this, many of the obvious symptoms that are associated with physiologic responses to pain are absent or are less obvious in the client with chronic pain—a point with particular relevance when assessing the client's pain or the success of nursing interventions designed to relieve chronic pain.

Chronic pain is defined as pain that persists or recurs for indefinite periods, usually for more than 6 months. It has an insidious onset, with the character and quality of the pain changing over time. Because chronic pain frequently involves deep somatic and visceral structures, the pain is usually diffuse, poorly localized, and often difficult to describe. If the underlying cause of the chronic pain is not amenable to medical treatment, controlling the long-term effects of chronic pain may be a difficult clinical challenge.

Chronic pain is associated with a variety of health problems such as cancer, arthritis, connective tissue diseases, peripheral vascular diseases, and musculoskeletal disorders, and with posttraumatic insults (phantom limb pain and low-back pain). The condition of chronic pain varies depending on the type of problem and whether it is progressive, stable, or capable of resolution. Unless the disease process is arrested or reversed, the severity of chronic pain may worsen to the point of physical and emotional debilitation. Even when the physiologic pain stimuli are eliminated or resolved, the perception of the pain may linger. Each of these chronic pain situations has its physiologic and psychosocial ramifications, which are influenced by the client's ability to cope, the availability of family support and social resources, and the severity of the physiologic and emotional consequences (see Table 7–1).

Because chronic pain persists for extended periods, it interferes with activities of daily living and personal relationships, and it causes emotional and financial burdens. Thus, the efforts of a multidisciplinary health care team are required to manage the situation effectively. If the pain is inadequately managed, it is an overwhelmingly frustrating experience for both sufferer and caregiver alike. Although many of the characteristics of chronic pain are similar in different clients, the nurse should be aware that each chronic pain situation is unique and requires a highly specialized plan of care. Included in this plan are a variety of therapeutic interventions—pharmacologic, nonpharmacologic, behavioral, and cognitive. Common pain syndromes and appropriate therapeutic interventions are summarized in the accompanying Key Features of Disease.

THE CHRONIC PAIN SYNDROME

Clients sometimes have chronic pain associated with some type of physical problem. Eventually, the physiologic alterations resolve or become less detectable. However, the perception or sensation of pain persists. The degree of pain appears to be out of proportion to the physical findings, yet the pain is a real phenomenon to the individual experiencing it. A confounding factor is that the source of the pain is unknown. Individuals in this situation frequently subject themselves to a variety of medical tests and frequent hospitalization while searching for a cause or explanation of their pain. So-called doctor shopping is common in this group of clients. Clients invest an incredible amount of time and energy in the health care system in hopes of uncovering a solution for the pain. As a result, clients with chronic pain syndrome focus on what they are not able to do rather than what they are able to do. Learned helplessness, dependency, and sick role behaviors are often evident. More important, these behaviors can be reinforced by financial incentives associated with disability payments or litigation, and by the attention, support, and compassion of family members. When the pain persists for long periods, family members are often emotionally drained, frustrated, and in dire need of help in dealing with the client. A behavioral approach, which includes family therapy coupled with emotional rehabilitation if necessary, is a useful strategy in this situation.

CANCER-RELATED PAIN

Equally as alarming as the incidence of acute postoperative pain is that of cancer-related pain. Some 40% to 60% of clients with advanced malignant disease experience severe pain (Bonica, 1983). Adequate pain control could be achieved in approximately 90% of these clients. However, even when the best pain management techniques are used, the complexity of this type of pain often limits the success of pain management efforts.

The sensory component of cancer-related pain may arise from a variety of mechanisms. As malignant tumors invade the bone, prostaglandins are released. These substances sensitize nerve receptors in the bone and increase their sensitivity to the painful stimuli. In part, this explains the extreme degree of pain associated with those suffering from bony metastases.

Arterial ischemia, venous engorgement, compression of nerves, infection, inflammation, necrosis, and ulcer-

KEY FEATURES OF DISEASE ■ Therapeutic Interventions for Common Pain Syndromes

Common Pain Syndrome	Therapeutic Interventions	Outcomes
Arthritic pain Rheumatoid arthritis: cause unknown; characterized by pain, inflammation, swelling, stiffness of involved joints Osteoarthritis, associated with degenerative changes in weight-bearing joints	Aspirin, acetaminophen, nonsteroidal anti-inflammatory agents (NSAIAs), and gold compounds (for rheumatoid arthritis) Transcutaneous electrical nerve stimulation (TENS) Physical therapy Application of heat and cold Behavioral and cognitive strategies Surgery to correct deformities or to replace joints Activity modification Weight reduction (for osteoarthritis)	Client remains as pain free as possible Client learns health care maintenance behaviors Deformities are minimized Ambulation and independence are optimized
Headache pain Migraines and cluster headaches Distention and dilation of cranial arteries often familial and affect more women than men Possibly unilateral if migraine and temporal-ocular if cluster Possibly associated with foods or personality factors	*Abortive* therapy (aimed at abolishing or minimizing headache at onset)* Ergotamine tartrate (sublingually rectally, subcutaneously, or intramuscularly) *Prophylactic* therapy (aimed at preventing onset in sufferers with frequent headaches)* Methysergide, propranolol, clonidine, amitriptyline Antiemetics for nausea Mild narcotic analgesics Biofeedback Alteration of environment: dark, quiet Elevation of head of bed Behavioral and cognitive strategies, pain clinics	Occurrence or severity will be prevented or minimized
Low-back pain Congenital defects After trauma or surgery Muscle spasm in back and radiating pain to lower extremities	Aspirin, acetaminophen, nonsteroidal anti-inflammatory agents; muscle relaxants; antidepressants Long-term management with narcotic analgesics *not* recommended unless the physiologic process is progressive or severely debilitating Surgery (laminectomy), spinal fusion if indicated Acupuncture, TENS, application of heat and cold, massage Physical therapy Instruction in proper body mechanics Bed rest, traction, brace, corset, collar Behavioral and cognitive strategies Weight reduction Vocational rehabilitation	Client remains as pain free as possible Client learns health care maintenance behaviors, especially proper use of body mechanics Client functions to optimal potential, including job and family responsibilities

Continued

KEY FEATURES OF DISEASE ■ **Therapeutic Interventions for Common Pain Syndromes** *Continued*

Common Pain Syndrome	Therapeutic Interventions	Outcomes

Pain of neuralgia
  Pain along the distribution of a
    nerve or nerves
  Trigeminal: unknown etiology;
    contributing factors: trauma,
    infection of teeth or jaw and
    flu-like illness; extreme
    sensitivity of and pain in
    cheek, lip, gum, and forehead
    related to slightest stimuli
    (touch, temperature change,
    chewing)
  Herpes zoster: varicella virus
    infection affecting dorsal
    sensory nerve roots in
    thoracic, cervical, and
    lumbosacral areas; severe,
    sharp pain along nerve
    distribution(s)
	Phenytoin, carbamazepine
	Antidepressants (amitriptyline)
	Narcotic analgesics
	Surgical nerve block, rhizotomy
	TENS
	Protect involved area from external
	    stimuli (touch, temperature
	    change, bright lights) (for
	    trigeminal pain)
		Client remains as pain free as possible
		Client maintains optimal nutrition
		    and rest

Phantom limb pain
  Related to any body part that has
    been amputated or
    traumatized
  Associated with interruption or
    denervation of sensory nerves
	Analgesic narcotics immediately
	    after operation
	Antidepressants, e.g., amitriptyline
	Phenytoin, carbamazepine
	Surgical revision of involved area
	Nerve block, rhizotomy
	TENS
	Pressure to stump
	Physical therapy with rehabilitation
	Application of prosthetic limb
		Client regains pain-free state

From Hickey, J. V. (1986). *The clinical practice of neurological and neurosurgical nursing* (pp. 549–551). Philadelphia: J. B. Lippincott.

ations are other causes of cancer-related pain. In addition, the sources of these problems are usually in deep somatic and visceral structures. These types of painful sensations, coupled with the diffuse nature of the pain, hamper the client's ability to describe and localize cancer pain. For additional information on this type of pain, see Chapter 25.

COLLABORATIVE MANAGEMENT

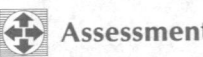 **Assessment**

History

The client's history provides information about the pain experience, including a chronology of events (precipitating and relieving factors); information about the nature of adjustments, if any, in the client's life or that of the family; and beliefs about the cause of the pain and what should be done about it (client's expectations). Clients and their families are included in this information-gathering process. Much insight can be gained from the client history, including data about drugs and other measures designed to relieve the pain. Personal characteristics such as the client's age, culture, and level of education influence attitudes about reporting a pain history and affect expectations for relief of pain and interpretations of interventions designed to interrupt the pain cycle.

Clients may still report pain in the absence of any observable or documented physiologic changes in the body. The nurse keeps in mind that all pain is real and operates from the premise that pain is "whatever the experiencing person says it is." The client's verbal and nonverbal expressions of pain are respected without making judgments or inferences about the reality of the pain. If clients perceive that health professionals doubt the existence of their pain, mistrust and other negative feelings can arise that interfere with a therapeutic client-nurse relationship.

The length of time the client has experienced pain is an important factor to assess. Clients who experience acute pain may welcome an opportunity to discuss their pain with the nurse because acute pain is a relatively short-term experience and is usually successfully localized by the clients. However, clients with chronic pain can be frustrated when they are unable to adequately describe their vague, diffuse pain experience. Repeated questioning in this situation can be nonproductive and nontherapeutic for the client.

Information about a client's pain can be quite helpful in understanding factors that are associated with the present pain or previous episodes of pain. If the client is in pain when the history is being obtained, it is important to keep the history session reasonably short. The client's family members are also included in the assessment. Data to collect include

1. *Precipitating factors* — Does the client associate any activities, ingestion of food, or other environmental factors with the onset of pain? What does the client think causes the present pain? Was the onset of pain sudden or insidious? Has the client done anything or taken anything to relieve the pain? What were the results of this intervention?

2. *Aggravating factors* — What factors make the pain worse? What influence has this pain had on the client's activity? What changes in life activity have been affected (e.g., diet, job, sleep)?

3. *Localization of pain* — Can the client localize the pain or describe where it travels or radiates?

4. *Character and quality of pain* — What words does the client use to describe the pain, its character, quality, or intensity?

5. *Duration of pain* — How long has the client experienced this pain?

Physical Assessment: Clinical Manifestations

The overt or observable manifestations of pain include the physiologic responses, motor or body movements, and affective behaviors such as crying or writhing. Although physiologic changes occur in response to acute noxious stimuli, these symptoms are usually not reliable indicators of chronic pain. Acute pain, with its property of warning an individual about harm, elicits several physiologic signs and symptoms, which are largely a function of sympathetic nervous stimulation. Clients with acute pain often manifest pronounced changes in vital body functions such as tachycardia or increased heart rate, increased respiratory rate or tachypnea, and peripheral vasoconstriction resulting in elevation of blood pressure and cold, clammy skin. In addition, clients with acute pain may become diaphoretic, restless, and apprehensive. Physiologic changes in response to chronic pain are usually masked or blunted as the body attempts to compensate for and adapt to the noxious stimuli, and the pain no longer serves as a necessary warning. Instead, the aggravating nature of the pain provokes parasympathetic nervous system responses.

Changes in vital signs related to chronic pain may be evident only when exacerbations of pre-existing pain occur or as new sites of painful stimuli arise.

Certain motor or body movements may be associated with pain. Some of these may be more exaggerated or obvious than others. Clients in pain may splint, hold painful body parts while moving, or lie listlessly because they are afraid to move. The nurse assesses the functional level and the degree of functional impairment of the client with pain.

All pain has several characteristics that must be explored. These are (1) location; (2) character and quality; (3) intensity or degree of severity; and (4) pattern.

Location. The location of pain is assessed from two dimensions: the level of pain, either deep or superficial; and the position or location of the pain. Most clients, whether they are experiencing acute or chronic pain, can usually describe the depth of pain perceived. However, the actual area or location of the pain may not be as easily identified.

Pain may be classified into four categories related to its location:

1. Localized pain — pain confined to the site of origin

2. Projected pain — pain along a specific nerve or nerves

3. Radiating pain — diffuse pain around the site of origin, not well localized

4. Referred pain — pain perceived in an area distant from the site of painful stimuli

The nurse asks the client whether the pain is superficial or deep. In general, clients having pain involving superficial or cutaneous structures describe their pain as superficial and can often localize the pain to a discrete area. These structures possess abundant nerve supplies, which contribute to ease and accuracy in localizing the pain. On the other hand, clients who perceive pain from deeper somatic or visceral structures within the body may have difficulty localizing their pain (a result of poor innervation of this area).

A client who has difficulty verbalizing the exact location of pain can be asked to point to the painful areas on his or her own body or on another person. Sometimes having the client point to or shade in the painful areas illustrated on a diagram of the front and back of the human body is helpful (see Fig. 7–5). When clients cannot identify the painful areas and state that they just "hurt all over," the nurse can encourage the client to focus on parts of the body that are not painful. The nurse has the client concentrate on different body parts, beginning with the hand and fingers of one extremity, while asking him or her to express the presence or absence of pain. As the nurse focuses attention on selected areas of the body, the client is assisted in localizing painful areas. Often clients who had stated that they hurt everywhere begin to realize that some parts of the body are not painful. As painful areas are identified, the nurse can help the client to understand the origin of the pain. This understanding is particularly important for clients with cancer because every new pain often raises the suspicion of metastasis. The pain may be caused by other reasons, such as immobility or constipation.

Character and quality. After the client is asked to locate the pain, the nurse asks the client to describe how the pain feels. Clients may use a word or group of words to convey the sensations or feelings of the pain. The nurse avoids suggesting descriptive words for the pain. Some clients who are frustrated and who are having difficulty describing their pain may benefit from use of the McGill-Melzack Pain Questionnaire (see Fig. 7–5). With this measurement tool, the client is asked to circle descriptive terms in the appropriate categories that best describe the pain. Another useful strategy includes asking the client to describe the sensation by comparing it to a situation or event that may be comparable to the feeling of pain. For example, a man with excruciating diffuse abdominal pain from advanced cancer might say that his pain felt as if a soldier were walking around inside his abdomen, with no set path or destination, stepping on mines. For this man, pain was unpredictable and never-ending and produced like a "blowing up" sensation.

Intensity. Subjective measurements of pain intensity are more reliable than the overt or observable parameters of pain. Only the client in pain can determine the amount or severity experienced. Various analogue scales are designed to quantify the degree or intensity of pain. These tools, described under the heading Tools to Measure Pain, are easier to use than other descriptive pain assessment measures.

Pattern. Pain is rarely the same at all times. It is perceived differently over time and is subjected to various precipitating and aggravating factors, which were under the heading History in the Assessment section.

Psychosocial Assessment

All pain holds significant meaning for the individual experiencing it. For clients experiencing acute pain from surgery, the pain may be interpreted as necessary and expected and may be viewed with a sign of relief that some greater problem has been resolved or alleviated with the surgery. Knowledge that the duration of the pain is limited may allow the client to deal with unpleasant or noxious sensations without too much difficulty. On the other hand, acute chest pain associated with myocardial ischemia or angina may be the beginning of a life of fear and uncertainty.

Psychosocial factors that influence chronic pain are varied. Some are similar to those found in the acute pain experience, such as anxiety or fear related to the meaning of the pain. Because pain persists in the chronic situation or is perhaps only partially relieved, the client is vulnerable to feelings of powerlessness, anger, hostility, or despair. Other reactions of people in chronic pain include depression, social withdrawal, and preoccupation with physical symptoms. The client with chronic pain is also vulnerable to pejorative labels such as ma-

lingerer or fake. Because many of the behavioral manifestations of acute pain (e.g., sweating, writhing, increased blood pressure) are absent in the client with chronic pain, the existence of the pain could be doubted by the caregiver.

If the client's pain is chronic and associated with a progressive disease such as cancer, rheumatoid arthritis, or peripheral vascular disease, the pain may be associated with worries and concerns over the consequences of the illness. Clients suffering from cancer-related pain may fear death or body mutilation. Some may think that they are being punished for some wrongdoing in life. Others may attach a religious or spiritual significance to lingering pain and may think that suffering on earth exemplifies the experience of pain so often associated with those in the Bible.

Open-ended questions, such as, "Tell me how your pain has affected your job or role as mother," can allow the client to describe personal attitudes about pain and its influence in life. This opportunity can help a client whose life has been modified by pain. Some clients will not share private information or fears related to the meaning of their pain readily, and this decision is respected by the nurse.

Tools to Measure Pain

Self-ratings. Tools are used by the nurse to measure pain in clinical settings to determine the effectiveness of relief-oriented interventions and by investigators as an outcome measure in a clinical research trial. This approach involves giving subjects a scale, which could be verbal or visual, and asking them to rate the pain stimulus by using that scale. Such scales usually indicate pain intensity, although they might also assess emotional or aversive aspects of pain. *Verbal descriptor scales* typically group words such as "none, moderate, or severe" and permit an intensity rating of pain. *Visual analogue scales* usually use a 10-cm line to represent a continuum of pain intensity and include verbal anchors that describe the intensity of the stimuli. For examples of such rating scales, see Figure 7–6.

The visual analogue scale is the most widely used scale to assess acute postoperative pain; the McGill-Melzack scale is used for clients with chronic pain. The McGill-Melzack scale is often criticized for lacking a category to indicate no pain.

Variations in the incremental, numeric, or descriptive scales are important determinants for selecting the appropriate measurement tool. Clients with chronic, nagging, diffuse pain may have difficulty using broad numeric scales ranging from 0 to 100. Some clients are better able to use word scales and prefer nominal measurements that contain descriptive words or phrases to numeric scales.

This approach to the clinical evaluation of pain is reasonably simple, economical, and understandable to most clients, and it represents an improvement from the subjective reporting of individual pain experiences. However, use of these types of scales generally allows pain to be rated only in terms of intensity. In addition,

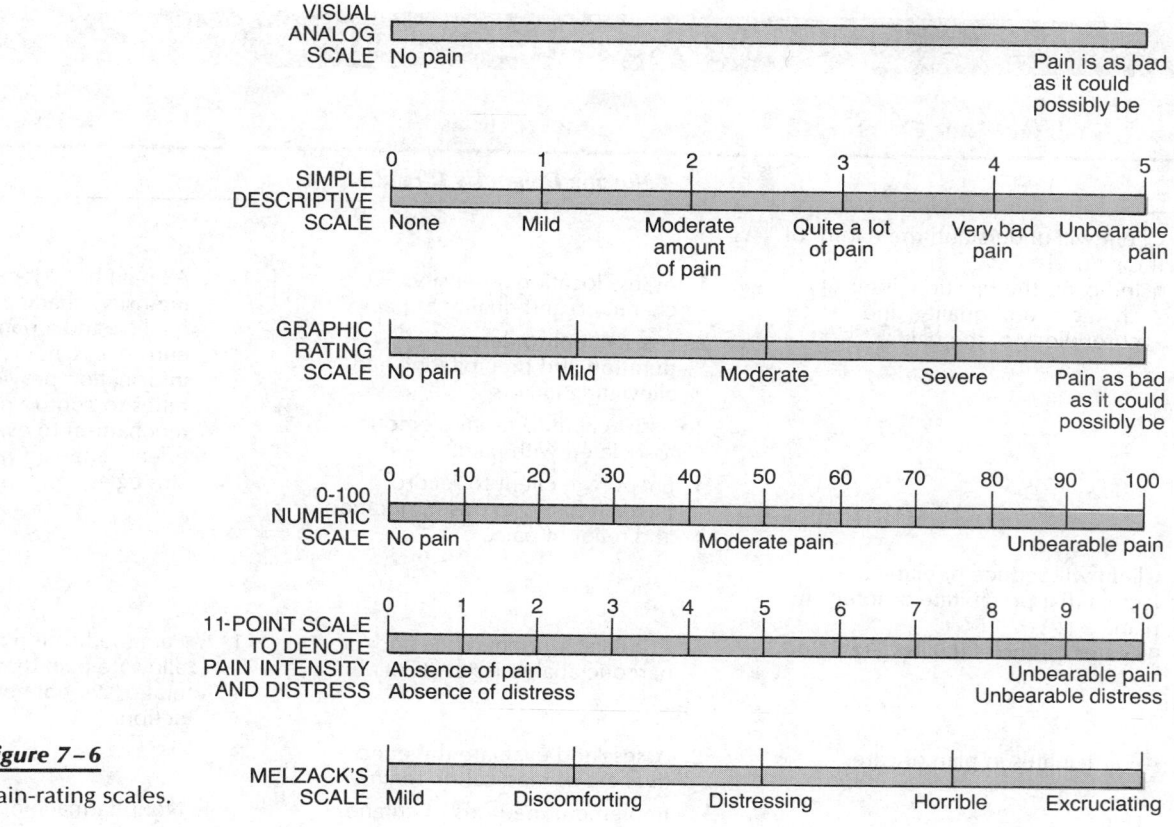

Figure 7–6

Pain-rating scales.

their use may be too difficult for subjects with poor verbal or visual discrimination skills because of lack of education or the presence of severe pain.

 Analysis: Nursing Diagnosis

The client in pain can be the hospitalized postoperative client in acute pain or the client with cancer whose chronic pain is usually controlled with pain medication. Because of the physiologic differences between acute and chronic pain and the influence of cultural and psychosocial factors, there is no typical client in pain. After gathering data and assessing the client for pain, the nurse can determine the presence of one or more of the following diagnoses.

Common Diagnoses

The actual diagnoses for a client with pain are divided into two main categories:

1. Pain
2. Chronic pain

Additional Diagnoses

The following problems may exist as either actual or potential problems:

1. Altered role performance related to inability to work
2. Ineffective individual coping related to manipulative behavior
3. Potential for injury related to decreased pain sensation
4. Knowledge deficit related to techniques for pain control
5. Self-care deficit related to pain
6. Activity intolerance related to acute pain
7. Anxiety related to ineffectiveness of pain control measures
8. Social isolation related to presence of chronic pain
9. Altered health maintenance related to inability to function because of pain
10. Altered nutrition: less than body requirements related to pain
11. Sleep pattern disturbance related to pain
12. Diversional activity deficit related to acute pain

 Planning and Implementation

See the accompanying Client Care Plan for complete nursing plans for the client with acute or chronic pain.

CLIENT CARE PLAN ■ The Client with Pain

Goal/Outcome Criteria	Interventions	Rationales
Nursing Diagnosis 1: Pain		
Client will understand the nature of the pain. ■ Indicates the location, intensity, character and quality, and chronology of the pain.	1. Assess location, intensity, character, and quality of pain. 2. Assist client to determine duration and precipitating and alleviating factors. 3. Assist client to discuss emotions associated with pain. 4. Encourage client to record factors related to onset, duration, and relief of pain.	1–4. All pain has a location, level of intensity, character and quality, and a pattern of occurrence. Understanding this information provides opportunities to control pain and a mechanism to evaluate effectiveness of pain-relieving strategies.
Client will reduce or eliminate factors that precipitate or intensify pain. ■ States methods to alleviate pain.	1. Administer nonnarcotic and/or narcotic analgesics as prescribed.	1, 2. Pain medication may act to alleviate pain through peripheral or central nervous system actions.
■ Participates in plan of care.	2. Assess and evaluate the effectiveness of medication regimen. 3. Implement methods of cutaneous stimulation, i.e., transcutaneous electrical nerve stimulation (TENS), hot and cold compresses when appropriate. 4. Educate client about alternative methods to relieve pain. 5. Involve client in care planning.	3, 4. Nonpharmacologic approaches are effective in managing acute pain. 5. Client involvement assists the nurse in establishing realistic goals and helps the client to maintain a sense of control.
Nursing Diagnosis 2: Chronic Pain		
Client will understand the nature of pain. ■ Indicates location (if possible), intensity, character and quality, and chronology of the pain.	1. Assess location (if possible), intensity, character, and quality of the pain. 2. Assist client to determine duration and precipitating and alleviating factors. 3. Assist client to discuss emotions associated with pain. 4. Encourage client to record factors related to onset, duration, and relief of pain. 5. Appreciate that chronic pain is often poorly localized, related to a variety of affective factors, and sometimes difficult for client to describe.	1–5. Because chronic pain often arises from poorly innervated body structures, localization is often difficult. The intensity, character and quality, and pattern of occurrence of pain provide useful information necessary to understand opportunities to control the pain and evaluate the effectiveness of pain-relieving strategies.

Goal/Outcome Criteria	Interventions	Rationales
Client will implement treatment plan to ensure an adequate level of analgesia. ■ Follows prescribed medication plan. ■ Recognizes side effects of analgesics.	1. Administer nonnarcotic or narcotic analgesics. 2. Administer narcotic analgesics in a convenient form (preferably oral). 3. Recommend the use of long-acting narcotics for management of cancer-related pain and other progressive pain syndromes. 4. Monitor for side effects of narcotic analgesics (i.e., sedation, nausea, constipation, respiratory depression, urinary retention, and hypotension). 5. Identify client at risk for adverse reactions to narcotic analgesics (i.e., elderly persons; those with reduced blood volume, liver impairment, or decreased respiratory reserve). Remember that central nervous system effects of sedation are potentiated by other central nervous system depressants. 6. Reassure clients that frequent administration of narcotics rarely leads to addiction. 7. Educate the client and family that physical dependence does occur with continued use of narcotics; however, tapering schedules are devised to wean clients from narcotics when appropriate.	1, 2. The use of nonnarcotic and narcotic analgesics in chronic pain management is aimed at preventing the recurrence or worsening of the pain. This requires administration of an adequate dosage on a continuous basis. 3. Frequent dosing with medication may disrupt the client's ability to maintain regular body rhythms. 4, 5. Side effects from narcotic analgesics may occur when doses are not safely escalated or when client sensitivity is evident. 6, 7. Addiction rarely occurs in clients who use narcotics for medicinal purposes. Physical dependence is a biologic adaptation of the tissues that requires continued use for normal function. Careful decrease in dosages provides safe tapering to prevent physiologic withdrawal.
Client will not develop complications related to using narcotic analgesics. ■ Manifests no or minimal side effects of analgesics.	1. Assess for signs and symptoms of constipation (i.e., decreased bowel movements, abdominal fullness, dullness on percussion, hemorrhoids, no or minimal bowel sounds). 2. Encourage diet high in fiber; increase fluid intake; maintain or increase activity level. 3. Observe for urinary retention, which may be increased if clients are taking other anticholinergic drugs (i.e., antidepressants). 4. Continue to monitor for other side effects such as nausea, respiratory depression, and hypotension.	1, 2. Narcotic analgesics act on the smooth muscle of the intestinal tract to cause hypomotility of the bowels. This problem usually persists while clients continue to take narcotics. 3. Urinary retention may occur from the anticholinergic effects of narcotics.

continued

CLIENT CARE PLAN ■ The Client with Pain *continued*

Goal/Outcome Criteria	Interventions	Rationales
Nursing Diagnosis 3: Diversional Activity Deficit		
Client will identify potential use of diversional activities. ■ Considers appropriateness of diversional activities to alleviate pain and associated stress.	1. Assess past methods of relaxation, hobbies, and interests that might aid in coping with present stress. 2. Assess causes of decreased concentration, insomnia, depression, or pain. 3. Encourage and facilitate verbalization of feelings. 4. Mutually develop and schedule activities with the patient and allow for relaxation and rest periods.	1–3. Diversional interventions require a capacity for cognitive concentration. 4. Participation in setting goals fosters increased motivation and compliance with care regimen.
Client will participate in diversional activities. ■ Engages in diversional activities to alleviate pain and accompanying stress.	1. Encourage progressive concentration exercises from listening to music, watching television, and reading. 2. Teach client relaxation techniques. 3. Encourage client to practice or use relaxation techniques at set times during the day.	1. A certain level of mental concentration is necessary for effective use of diversional activities. 2, 3. Relaxation techniques reduce anxiety associated with pain or with stressful situations. Freedom from mental and physical stress is important in relieving ongoing pain.
Client will implement noninvasive methods of pain control. ■ Uses techniques to decrease or modify pain.	1. Inform the client of pain control options (i.e., TENS, relaxation therapy, distraction, and biofeedback). 2. Assess client's willingness to assume responsibility for use of pain control techniques. 3. Implement diversional activities and relaxation techniques. 4. Consult physical therapist for evaluation of cutaneous stimulation techniques. 5. Implement the use of TENS unit if appropriate. 6. Use heat or cold packs to provide muscular relaxation.	1–4. Nonpharmacologic pain control techniques need to be explored for their effectiveness for the client to achieve optimal control of pain. 5, 6. Cutaneous stimulation provides a method of pain relief that the client can control.

CLIENT CARE PLAN ■ The Client with Pain *continued*

Goal/Outcome Criteria	Interventions	Rationales
	*Nursing Diagnosis 4: Ineffective Individual Coping*	

Nursing Diagnosis 4: Ineffective Individual Coping

Goal/Outcome Criteria	Interventions	Rationales
Client will understand the need for effective coping activities. ■ States alternative ways of coping.	1. Evaluate the client's ability to adapt to the limitations imposed by pain. 2. Encourage the client to verbalize potential to participate in activities of daily living. 3. Consider physical alterations and psychosocial factors that may affect coping. 4. Assess client and family interactions and sources of strength and support.	1–4. To improve the quality of life and optimal level of functioning in activities of daily living, clients must be aware of their existing coping patterns and sources of support when needed.
Client will improve communication channels in family and caregiving groups. ■ Openly discusses perceptions of both successful and problematic situations.	1. Encourage client participation in all aspects of care. 2. Openly discuss expectations of client involvement in care. 3. Construct mutually formulated goals. 4. Reinforce consistent setting of limits to maintain goal-oriented behaviors. 5. Collaborate with other members of health care team to provide consistency. 6. Assist client to recognize incentives and rewards necessary to achieve an optimal state of health.	1–3. The client must assume responsibility for participating in behaviors that foster control and self-care activities. 4, 5. A consistent and supportive plan of care ensures that all members maintain a unified approach. 6. Client awareness of motivating factors assists in maintaining goal-oriented change.
Client will mobilize family, community, and health care resources. ■ Uses appropriate resources.	1. Educate client and family regarding options in dealing with pain (i.e., counseling [individual and family], TENS, relaxation therapy, biofeedback). 2. Involve other health professionals, i.e., social worker, psychologist, and physical therapist. 3. Discuss the option of pain clinics and plan appropriate referrals acceptable to client and family. 4. Refer to visiting nurse for community follow-up related to medication and activity supervision, use of assistive devices, TENS, and counseling.	1. The client must be informed about available options. 2–4. Referral and coordination can ensure optimal delivery of care.

Pain

Planning: client goals. The major goal in the management of acute pain is that the client will experience pain relief.

Interventions: nonsurgical management

Drug therapy. Pharmacologic measures are the major means used to relieve acute pain. Physical measures such as the use of a pillow for splinting an incision are also effective in the relief of acute pain, but these measures are usually used in conjunction with drug therapy. An alarming number of clients experience moderate to severe pain after surgery even though optimal pain relief can often be achieved through the use of pharmacologic agents. However, physicians are reluctant to prescribe certain drugs, particularly narcotics,

and nurses are reluctant to administer these drugs. It is estimated that clients receive less than 25% of the pain medication necessary for adequate pain relief (Bonica, 1983).

Narcotic analgesics are often withheld or administered in less than optimal doses because health professionals fear that they will impair respirations or mental status and produce other unfavorable symptoms in clients who are physiologically unstable as a result of surgery. Yet the stressors pain, anxiety, and insomnia are equally as detrimental to the body's homeostatic mechanisms.

Clients who achieve adequate analgesia during the postoperative phase experience fewer complications and have shorter recuperative periods than those who have a significant degree of pain. It is a nursing responsibility to ensure that clients receive adequate amounts of analgesics after surgery. Physical measures can also be

---

TABLE 7–4   Narcotic Analgesics Used in the Management of Pain

Drug	Indications	Usual Daily Dosage*	Interventions	Rationales
Codeine	Mild to moderate pain	30–60 mg PO q 4–6 h. Tablets: 15 and 30 mg; combinations: Empirin #3 (aspirin 325 mg + codeine 30 mg); Tylenol #3 (acetaminophen 325 mg + codeine 30 mg)	1. Observe for nausea and constipation. 2. Institute measures to prevent constipation (e.g., force fluids, add fiber or bulk to diet, encourage ambulation, administer laxatives as ordered). 3. Avoid administration of codeine preparations containing aspirin and acetaminophen if assessing for elevations in temperature.	1. Doses higher than 60 mg PO q 4 h generally increase the incidence of gastrointestinal side effects. 2. Decreased bowel motility is a common side effect of narcotic analgesics. 3. Aspirin and acetaminophen may suppress the signs of a fever.
Hydromorphone (Dilaudid)	Moderate to severe pain	2–4 mg PO q 3–5 h, 1–4 mg IM/SC q 3–5 h. Tablets: 1, 2, 3, 4 mg; suppositories: 3 mg; injectable: 2 mg/ml, q 3–5 h as ordered.	1. Observe for nausea and constipation, especially with doses higher than 10 mg PO. 2. Use extreme caution if administered IV; monitor blood pressure q 2–4 h if administered IV. 3. Escalate doses carefully as ordered by physician. If	1. Less sedation, nausea, and constipation compared with morphine; severe constipation may occur with doses higher than 10 mg q 4 h. 2. Caution should be used with IV dosing because of increased incidence of hypotension.

used to alleviate pain. Techniques such as transcutaneous electrical nerve stimulation (TENS), touch, and the application of heat and cold are frequently effective in controlling pain.

Nonnarcotic analgesics. Many people underestimate the effectiveness of nonnarcotic agents. Aspirin (ASA, acetylsalicylic acid), 650 mg, and acetaminophen (Datril, Tylenol), 650 mg, produce pain relief comparable to that of codeine, 32 mg orally, and meperidine (Demerol), 50 mg orally, for mild to moderate pain. Over-the-counter medications are rarely prescribed alone for the treatment of acute pain in the hospital setting. They are usually administered in conjunction with narcotic analgesics. Aspirin must be used with caution after surgery because it can irritate the gastrointestinal tract and interfere with platelet aggregation.

Because nonsteroidal anti-inflammatory agents (NSAIAs) possess anti-inflammatory properties via in-hibition of prostaglandins, they are particularly useful in the management of acute inflammation caused by tissue destruction.

Narcotic analgesics. Immediately after surgery or traumatic injuries, small, frequent doses of parenteral narcotics, intravenous, subcutaneous, or intramuscular, are given on a continuous time schedule or on an intermittent, on demand (prn) schedule. (See Table 7–4 for information about commercially available narcotics, indications for use, usual dosages, and appropriate interventions.)

Careful monitoring of the client's vital signs and level of consciousness is required after surgery because of the relative instability of the body. The administration of narcotics may also affect the client and may cause a lowering of blood pressure, tachycardia, and depressed respirations. However, these effects are generally associated with the blood level of the medication. Therefore,

---

TABLE 7–4   Narcotic Analgesics Used in the Management of Pain *Continued*

Drug	Indications	Usual Daily Dosage*	Interventions	Rationales
			patient requires increase in dosage, low-dosage form may necessitate ingestion of many pills.	
Oxycodone (Percodan, Tylox, Percocet)	Mild to moderate pain	1–2 tablets q 4–6 h. Percocet (approximately 5 mg of oxycodone + 325 mg of acetaminophen). Percodan (approximately 5 mg of oxycodone + 325 mg of aspirin). Tylox (approximately 5 mg of oxycodone + 500 mg of acetaminophen).	1. Observe for nausea and constipation. 2. Institute measures to prevent constipation: force fluids; add bulk to diet; encourage ambulation; record frequency of bowel movements; administer laxatives as ordered. 3. Do not exceed more than 1000 mg of acetaminophen (two Tylox tablets or three Percocet tablets) more frequently than q 4 h. Do not exceed more than 3 Percodan tablets q 4 h because of aspirin content. 4. Avoid use of Percodan in clients with bleeding problems.	1. Can produce less nausea and constipation at equianalgesic doses to codeine. 2. Decreased bowel motility is a common side effect of narcotic analgesics. 3. Doses of aspirin exceeding the normal range of 650 mg PO q 4 h can cause gastritis, gastric ulceration, and bleeding. Doses of acetaminophen higher than 1000 mg q 4 h can lead to hepatotoxicity. 4. Aspirin exerts an anticoagulant effect by interfering with platelet aggregation.

* PO, by mouth; q, every; IM, intramuscularly; SC, subcutaneously.

small intermittent doses are administered to avoid peaks of drug action. The nurse remembers that pain and the accompanying stress and anxiety are potent respiratory stimulants. When narcotics are administered and a level of pain relief is achieved, a decrease in the respiratory rate is expected, and this decrease may not be an untoward effect of the narcotic. If respirations fall below 10 to 12 per minute, the client is observed frequently for signs of narcotic overdose (including sudden decrease in blood pressure and changes in mentation). Respiratory depression is reversed with naloxone (Narcan), a narcotic antagonist.

The nurse also keeps in mind that the effect from narcotic analgesics may be potentiated in a client who is elderly, has reduced blood volume, or has received anesthetic agents.

Constipation is an expected side effect of narcotic administration. Careful attention to the presence of bowel sounds, abdominal distention, and frequency of bowel movements is necessary after anesthesia, especially after abdominal surgery that requires manipulation of the bowel. For further information regarding the classification of narcotics, their actions, and adverse effects, see under the heading Drug Therapy in the later section Chronic Pain.

Intraspinal analgesics. Epidural analgesia refers to the instillation of a pain-blocking agent, usually a local anesthetic or narcotic, into the epidural space (the space between the dura mater and the vertebral column). It is far more popular than *intrathecal analgesia,* in which a pain-blocking agent is introduced into the space between the arachnoid mater and pia mater of the spinal cord. The goal with both types of analgesia is the interruption of pain conduction at the point where the sensory fibers exit from the spinal cord. Epidural analgesia has been used since the 1950s, but it has recently become more popular as newer and more innovative approaches to acute pain control are explored. Epidural analgesia is used with clients who are predisposed to respiratory complications, including those undergoing thoracic surgery, clients with pre-existing respiratory disease, and obese clients.

Complications associated with epidural analgesia are directly related to catheter placement, catheter maintenance, and the type of analgesic used. Infection results from failure to maintain aseptic technique during catheter placement and drug instillation. It also results from failure to maintain aseptic conditions for indwelling catheters at the site of insertion or at the site of tube junctions. To prevent infections, the nurse ensures that all catheter line connections are secure and that an occlusive sterile dressing is maintained over the catheter site. To avoid infections or dislodging, the catheter is usually left in place for about 48 hours. The accompanying illustration demonstrates placement of an epidural catheter.

Clients receiving epidural analgesics are at risk for respiratory depression resulting from high plasma and cerebrospinal fluid concentrations of the instilled drug. The nurse monitors respirations frequently and immediately reports to the physician respiration rates below 10 per minute during the period of administration and during the 24-hour period after the administration of epidural analgesia. Narcotic-induced respiratory depression is managed by the administration of naloxone either intravenously or intramuscularly.

Other side effects of intraspinal analgesics include pruritus secondary to histamine release (usually related to epidural narcotics), allergic reactions, and urinary retention. Expected outcomes of epidural analgesia with local anesthetics include altered levels of sensation (paresthesia) and altered motor function (muscle weakness and paralysis). These effects are rarely seen with epidural narcotics unless the catheter connects with neural tissues or narcotic toxicity has occurred.

Placebos. Placebos have been shown to be effective in the treatment of pain. McCaffery's (1979b, p. 160) definition of a placebo is: "any medical treatment (medication or procedure, including surgery) or nursing care that produces an effect in a patient because of its implicit or explicit or nursing care therapeutic intent and not because of its specific nature (physical or chemical properties)." Placebos are substances or actions that produce an effect regardless of their known value. When a client responds favorably to a placebo, this is known as the *placebo effect.*

Approximately 30% of all clients who receive placebos report pain relief (McCaffery, 1979b). Evidence has shown that these clients release endogenous opiates because of the power of suggestion, trust in the caregiver's interventions, or belief that something, regardless of what it is, will help the pain. A favorable response to a placebo does not mean that the pain "was not real" or was imaginary or faked. Placebos should never be used to determine whether a client's pain is "real." Even clients with documented physiologic causes for pain can favorably respond to placebos.

Placebos are sometimes used incorrectly and unethically. Placebos such as intramuscular saline are administered, and the client is informed that the injection contains a pain medication. This practice deceives the client and perpetuates mistrust in the caregivers and the health care system.

Patient-controlled analgesia. PCA is one way to combat the problem of inadequate analgesia in the management of acute pain. This procedure allows the client to control the dosage of analgesia received. This approach to pain control can improve pain relief and increase client satisfaction. It can also decrease the amount of narcotic consumption per day compared with that for clients dosed with conventional methods. Clients receiving conventional prn medication for postoperative pain must sense the pain, report it to the nurse, and wait until the nurse is aware of the client's need and has the time to administer the analgesic. Considerable time may pass in this sequence because the client may have waited too long before asking for the medication or the nurse may not understand the need to respond promptly to the request or may have other equally pressing responsibilities. Whatever the reasons, the

HOW COMMON TYPES OF INTRASPINAL ANALGESIA (ANESTHESIA) ARE ADMINISTERED

Epidural analgesia (also called epidural block) and intrathecal analgesia (also called spinal or subarachnoid analgesia or spinal or subarachnoid block) are administered by inserting a spinal needle between the second and third or the third and fourth lumbar vertebrae (L2-3 or L3-4). For both techniques, the client is positioned in the flexed lateral (fetal) position shown here or seated on the edge of the operating table with the back arched and the chin tucked to the chest.

For epidural analgesia, the needle is inserted to the surface of the dura mater, and a pain-blocking agent is injected—sometimes through an indwelling catheter—into the epidural space.

For intrathecal analgesia, a large spinal needle is inserted to the surface of the dura mater, and a second, smaller needle is passed through the first to penetrate the dura mater and arachnoid mater. A pain-blocking agent is injected—sometimes through an indwelling catheter—directly into the cerebrospinal fluid in the subarachnoid space.

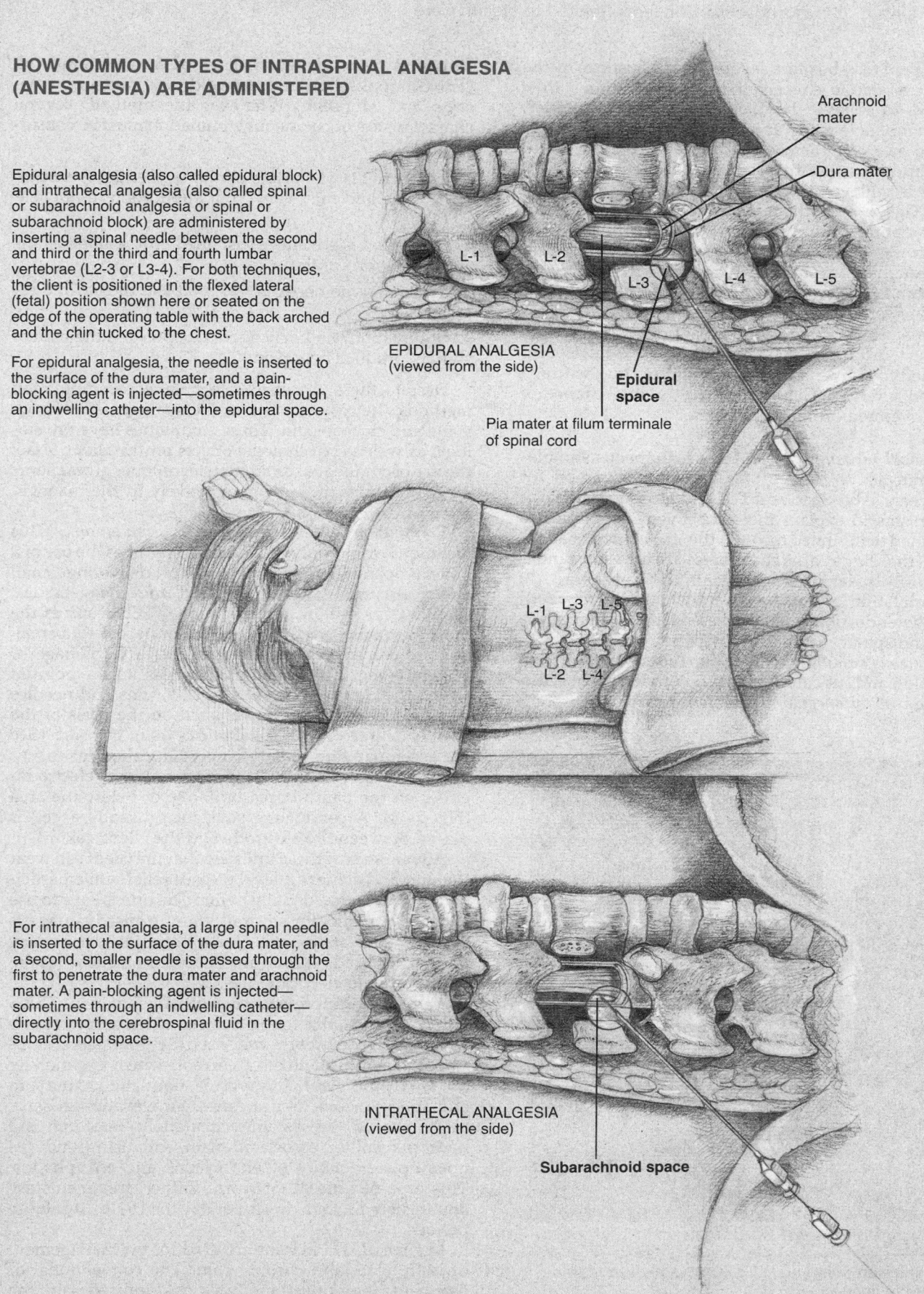

Arachnoid mater

Dura mater

L-1   L-2   L-3   L-4   L-5

EPIDURAL ANALGESIA
(viewed from the side)

Epidural space

Pia mater at filum terminale of spinal cord

L-1   L-3   L-5
L-2   L-4

INTRATHECAL ANALGESIA
(viewed from the side)

Subarachnoid space

client's pain may be more severe or out of control by the time the analgesic is received. More medication is then required to relieve the pain adequately. However, clients who have ready access to an analgesic are more likely to medicate themselves before the pain becomes severe and thus require a reduced amount.

PCA is achieved through the use of a PCA infusion pump (Fig. 7–7). Both stationary pole pumps and ambulatory pumps are available with PCA modes. The infusion pump delivers the desired amount of medication through a conventional intravenous route or via an implantable intravenous catheter inserted in subcutaneous tissue. Drug security (to avoid inadvertent overdosing) is achieved through a locked syringe pump system or locked drug reservoir system. The device is programmed to deliver a certain amount of drug within a specified interval. Therefore, there is little chance of clients overmedicating themselves.

Physical measures. The use of cutaneous stimulation strategies to relieve pain has been common for many years. Abu-Saad and Tesler (1986) suggested two mechanisms to explain their effectiveness: (1) pain is modulated or inhibited through the stimulation or activity of the large afferent fibers at the substantia-gelatinosa–thalamic (SG-T) gate in the dorsal horn; (2) the stimulation of small pain-transmitting fibers activates the endorphin-mediated analgesia system in the brain and spinal cord, thus minimizing the pain.

Cutaneous stimulation. Various types of stimulation to the skin and subcutaneous tissue produce pain relief. Methods of *cutaneous stimulation* include such techniques as transcutaneous electrical nerve stimulation (TENS); application of heat, cold, and pressure; massage; and vibration. Whatever the method, several characteristics of cutaneous stimulation must be considered:

1. The benefits of these techniques are highly unpredictable and may vary from application to application.
2. Pain relief is generally sustained only as long as the stimulation continues.
3. Trials may be necessary to establish the desired effects.
4. Stimulation itself may aggravate pre-existing pain or may produce new pain.

Despite these drawbacks to cutaneous stimulation methods, they are effective in the management of both acute and chronic pain. These techniques have physiologic as well as psychologic effects on the client. Also, the use of cutaneous stimulation techniques gives clients an opportunity to participate actively in the management of their pain.

Transcutaneous electrical nerve stimulation. This technique, commonly called TENS, involves the use of a battery-operated device capable of delivering small electrical currents to the skin and underlying tissues. The first-generation or conventional TENS unit is the most frequently used. Electrodes connected to a small box are placed over the painful sites. The voltage or current is regulated by adjusting a dial to the point at which the client perceives a prickly, pins and needles sensation. The current is adjusted on the basis of the client's degree of pain relief and level of comfort. (See the accompanying Client/Family Education feature.)

The nurse assists the client in applying the electrodes either on the painful area or above or below the area (Fig. 7–8). A conducting substance (usually a gel) is placed between the electrode and the client's skin.

Advantages of these units are that the client can wear the unit and achieve a level of pain relief while participating in activities of daily living. The unit is easy to use and can be worn for several hours. A disadvantage is that the skin at the site of electrode placement may become irritated. To prevent this, the nurse teaches the client to rotate electrode sites.

The Pain Suppressor or second-generation TENS unit is also available for pain control. This unit works by using electrodes, with water as the conducting substance. The unit delivers a current, which is generally not felt by the client. This type of stimulation to the skin and subcutaneous tissues causes an elevation in serotonin level in the systemic circulation. Serotonin is a neurotransmitter associated with enhancing endogenous opiate activity of endorphins and enkephalins. This type of unit is not worn. Rather, treatments are administered several times per day for 10- to 20-minute periods.

In general, TENS units are used for the management of both acute and chronic pain. The conventional or first-generation unit is indicated for localized pain; the

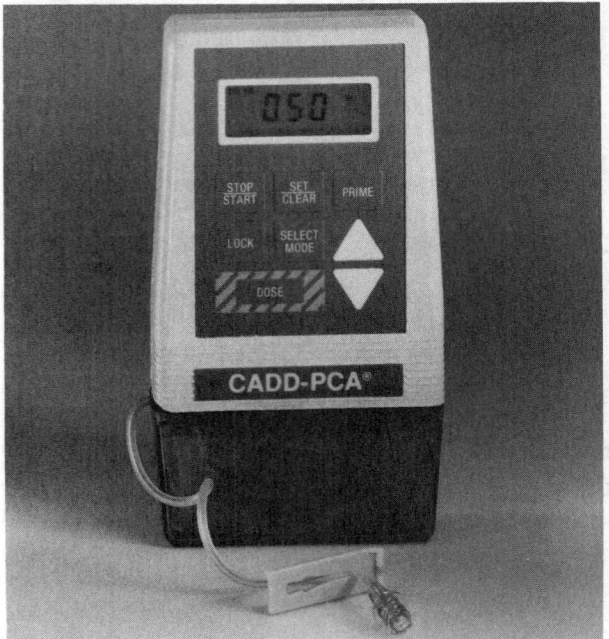

Figure 7–7

A PCA infusion pump. (CADD-PCA is a registered trademark of Pharmacia Deltec.)

second-generation unit, because of its systemic effects, can be used for diffuse pain syndromes such as those related to cancer. There has recently been an increase in the use of TENS immediately after surgery (see the Nursing Research feature on p. 132).

Other techniques.   Additional cutaneous stimulation techniques such as the use of touch, pressure, massage, and vibration, and the application of heat and cold all stimulate the skin and somehow interrupt the pain pathway. These interventions are relatively easy to learn and are fairly economical. Table 7–5 summarizes these techniques.

Cognitive and behavioral strategies.   Similar to the use of cutaneous measures, cognitive and behavioral strategies to relieve pain have been popular for years either as adjuncts to drug therapy or as alternative interventions. Theoretical explanations for the effectiveness of these measures reflect the beliefs of the gate control theory, which stresses the interaction between cognitive, motivation-affective, and sensory stimuli and the resultant perception of pain (Abu-Saad & Tesler, 1986). If any one of these interacting components is altered, the perception of pain is somehow modified.

Distraction can be an effective method of acute pain relief. Simple measures such as holding a client's hand, taking him or her for a walk, or encouraging deep breathing exercises can divert attention from the pain. Nurses often observe that clients request less pain medi-

CLIENT/FAMILY EDUCATION ■ Answers to Common Questions About TENS Units

Question	Answer
"How expensive are TENS units?"	"Comparable to a regimen of prescription drugs or surgery."
"Does insurance cover the cost of buying or leasing a TENS unit?"	"Usually."
"How long will I have to use the TENS unit?"	"Depending on the nature and severity of the pain, use varies from minimal/intermittent to long-term/nearly constant."
"How do I get a TENS device?"	"Through the prescribing physician. TENS units are available by prescription only."
"Will a TENS unit work for me?"	"It depends on the type of pain. TENS units have been used successfully on back pain, arm and leg pain, neuralgia, arthritis pain, and other types of pain. A trial period under a physician's care is generally advised."
"How difficult are TENS units to operate?"	"Relatively simple. Depending on the level of pain, the client makes day-to-day adjustments. Color-coded electrodes are attached by the client to the skin overlying the painful area."

Data from *Pain relief without drugs: Questions most frequently asked about pain.* (Publication No. 32883). (1983). (Pamphlet available from Empi, Inc., 261 South Commerce Circle, Fridley, MN 55432)

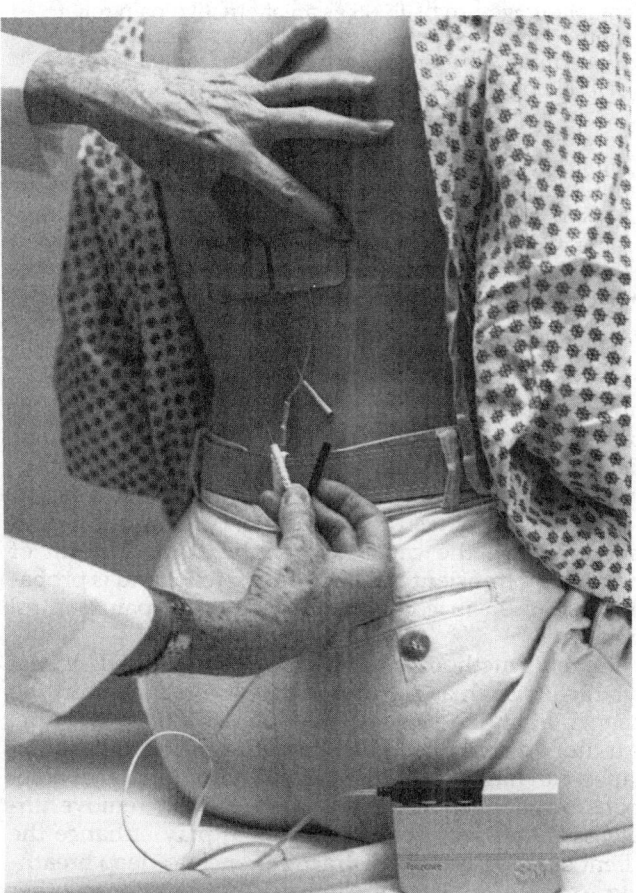

Figure 7–8
Application of a TENS unit.

NURSING RESEARCH

Use of TENS Alleviates Pain During Wound Care Procedures.

Hargreaves, A., & Lander, J. (1989). Use of transcutaneous electrical nerve stimulation for postoperative pain. *Nursing Research, 38,* 159–161.

Transcutaneous electrical nerve stimulation (TENS) has been used to control pain for a variety of clinical pain syndromes. Pain-relieving effects of TENS are related to the gate control theory, as electrical stimulation decreases the transmission of painful stimuli.

This study examined effects of TENS on incisional pain caused by cleaning and repacking the wound. Seventy subjects were randomly assigned to one of three treatment groups: no treatment (control), placebo-TENS, and TENS. The treatments were implemented during the routine dressing change on the second postoperative day. An 11-point visual analogue pain scale was used by subjects to rate their pain during the procedure. Subjects who received TENS reported significantly lower levels of pain.

Critique. This was a well-designed study that was implemented in only one setting. Although one may not generalize from these results, nurses can use the results to encourage use of TENS as an alternative pain relief method for clients undergoing painful postoperative procedures. Further research is needed on the effects of TENS on other pain induced by procedures.

Possible nursing implications. Possible nursing implications include increasing the practitioner's and other health care providers' awareness of this method of pain relief. Use of TENS can be encouraged as a safe and easy to administer alternative method of pain relief during postoperative procedures.

cation when family members are present. After visiting hours are over, many clients request something for pain. Instead of viewing distraction as a therapeutic pain relief measure, some nurses question the presence of severity of the pain if a client is easily distracted from it.

Distraction alters the perception of pain but it does not influence the cause or peripheral mechanism of pain. It is a transient method of pain relief and is probably best used in conjunction with other pain control measures.

Several methods of distraction can be used. Visual distractors such as pictures or television can divert the client's attention to something pleasant or interesting. Auditory distractors, which include music or relaxation tapes, can have a calming effect. Environmental distractions or changes in the environment can remove unpleasant stressors or reminders that may enhance the client's pain. Physical distractions such as deep breathing exercises assist the client to concentrate on other physiologic sensations.

Distraction is used for exacerbations of pain, for painful procedures (e.g., dressing changes or invasive procedures), and when the client needs a break from the constant perception of pain.

Chronic Pain

Planning: client goals. The major goal in managing chronic pain is pain relief or modification or the prevention of the recurrence or worsening of the pain. This goal is accomplished by interrupting the relentless cycle of pain, anxiety, and depression. Specific client goals for common pain syndromes are given in Key Features of Disease: Common Pain Syndromes and Their Management.

Interventions: nonsurgical management

Drug therapy. A pharmacologic approach to the treatment of chronic pain is the most effective and reliable method of pain management. General principles of management of cancer-related pain, a common example of chronic pain, are presented in Table 7–6. In general, these principles can be used as a guide in the management of severe chronic pain not of cancer origin. However, when the physiologic origin of severe chronic pain is in question, continuous narcotic treatment may not be appropriate. In this case, treatments aimed at behavior modification and at fostering adaptation may be used.

Nonnarcotic analgesics. Acetylsalicylic acid (aspirin), acetaminophen (Tylenol), and NSAIAs such as ibuprofen (Motrin) are effective in the management of mild chronic pain. They are also effective as adjunctive drugs in combination with narcotic analgesics. Aspirin and NSAIAs possess anti-inflammatory properties as they peripherally inhibit prostaglandins. This property makes them particularly useful in treating the inflammation associated with cancer and malignant tumor invasion. As noted earlier, cancer invasion of bony structures causes a hyperalgesic response resulting from the release of prostaglandins. Aspirin and NSAIAs can reduce the requirements of the client with chronic pain for narcotic analgesics. However, both aspirin and the NSAIAs can cause gastric disturbances and can have an effect on platelets or thrombocytes, which results in a tendency for bleeding. Therefore, these agents are used with caution.

Acetaminophen exerts its analgesic action by blocking peripheral pain receptors, thus increasing the threshold of these receptors to painful stimuli. Although acetaminophen has fewer side effects than aspirin and the NSAIAs, reports of liver toxicity have been associated with higher doses of this drug (1000 mg) taken more frequently than every 4 hours.

Other nonnarcotic agents that are used to control the pain of certain neuralgias (pain along the distribution of nerves) include carbamazepine (Tegretol) and phenytoin (Dilantin). The exact mechanism of action of these drugs is unknown, but it is believed that they inhibit the transmission of pain impulses. Both carbamazepine and phenytoin are associated with a wide variety of side effects (including hematopoietic, hepatic, and pulmonary effects and central nervous system toxicity). Therefore, these drugs are used with extreme caution.

TABLE 7–5 Cutaneous Stimulation Techniques Used to Interrupt the Pain Pathway

Technique	Method of Application	Comments
Touch or "laying on of hands"	The hands of the caregiver are placed on or close to the client's body.	The intent to help on the part of the caregiver may contribute to the success of this technique. This technique may extend the nurse-client relationship.
Pressure	A hand or other object is placed firmly over or around the painful area.	Pressure seems to relieve pain, decrease bleeding, and prevent swelling. Release of pressure is associated with increased blood flow and return of pain.
Massage	The hands or fingers are moved slowly or briskly over a body part. A lubricant or other substance is sometimes used.	Effects include muscle relaxation and sedation.
Vibration	Electrical and battery-operated vibrators produce a massage effect.	Vibration may decrease the intensity of the noxious (pain) stimuli.
Application of heat and cold	Heat may be applied in a variety of ways, including short-wave diathermy, microwave diathermy, ultrasound, use of melted paraffin and Hubbard tank, use of hot water bottle or heating pad, use of heat cradle and lamp, application of moist pads or towels, use of hot tub or shower, or use of gel packs. Cold may be applied in a dry or moist way, similar to heat applications. Ice chips, cold towels and packs, and chilled gel packs are commonly used.	Both heat and cold may reduce muscle spasm and decrease pain. Cold probably slows the conduction velocity of nerves. Heat increases the tendency for bleeding and therefore should not be used after trauma. Heat may also increase edema and is not indicated if circulation is poor. Both heat and cold should be used cautiously if clients have impaired sensation or cannot communicate.

Data from McCaffery, M. (1979). *Nursing management of the patient in pain* (2nd ed., pp. 117–126). Philadelphia: J. B. Lippincott.

Narcotic analgesics. Narcotic analgesics are drugs capable of relieving pain by binding to various opiate receptors located in the central nervous system. (See Table 7–4 for information about commercially available narcotics, indications for use, usual dosages, and appropriate interventions.) The term *narcotic agonist* refers to those drugs that are similar to morphine (generally considered the standard narcotic for comparative purposes) in their ability to interact with the opiate receptors and produce analgesia or pain relief. There are three categories of narcotic agonists: morphine and congeners; meperidine-like drugs; and methadone.

The equianalgesic guide (Table 7–7) can help determine the dose and route of one narcotic agonist compared with those of another. *Equianalgesic* refers to the dose and route of administration of one drug that produces approximately the same degree of analgesia as the given dosage and route of another drug. Equianalgesic drug lists should serve only as a guide in determining the comparative analgesic potencies among these drugs. Dose modifications may be necessary based on individual responses to the drugs.

Narcotic antagonists are drugs capable of reversing or blocking the effects of morphine. One group of narcotic antagonists is the *pure antagonists*. This group reverses the effects of narcotics without enhancing pain relief. Naloxone (Narcan) is the most popular narcotic antagonist of this type. Another group of narcotic antagonists not only reverses the action of morphine but also possesses analgesic properties. Drugs in this group selectively block the action of morphine agonists on certain opiate receptors while exerting a pain-relieving effect on other types of receptors. Table 7–8 identifies selected narcotic agonists and antagonists.

The use of narcotic analgesics is associated with a variety of physiologic sequelae. *Physical dependency* is associated with the administration of long-term narcotics. Physical dependency is *not* synonymous with addiction. Rather, it is a physiologic adaptation of the body tissues so that continued administration of the drug is necessary for normal tissue function. Abrupt cessation of the use of narcotic agents by a client who has become physically dependent results in so-called withdrawal symptoms. These symptoms include nau-

---

TABLE 7–6 Principles of Cancer-Related Pain Management

1. Treatment of cancer pain should begin with use of nonnarcotic agents.
2. Mild narcotics may be indicated for moderately severe pain or discomfort.
3. Narcotic analgesia should be used for severe pain.
4. Pain medication should be given frequently to keep the client comfortable in accordance with the pharmacologic action and duration of the drug. On demand (prn) methods of administration are not recommended. Round-the-clock administration is preferred.
5. All pain medication should be administered in a convenient dosage form, preferably by the oral route. Intramuscular injections should be avoided, as they are painful and provide little or no advantage over the oral route of administration.
6. An equianalgesic chart should be used when changing the route or type of narcotic analgesics (see Table 7–7).
7. A degree of physiologic tolerance to narcotic analgesics may occur, resulting in the need to adjust the dose or frequency of dosing.
8. Longer-acting medications such as methadone, levorphanol (Levo-Dromoran), and controlled-released oral morphine (MS contin R) may be required.

---

sea and vomiting, abdominal cramping, muscle twitching, profuse diaphoresis, delirium, and convulsions. When it is necessary to discontinue narcotic analgesic therapy in such a client, a slow tapering or weaning of the drug dosage lessens or alleviates withdrawal symptoms.

Drug tolerance may also result from narcotic analgesic therapy. Tolerance is characterized by a gradual resistance of the body to the effects of a narcotic, including its pain-relieving properties. When tolerance has occurred, clients usually require more of the drug to produce the same analgesic effects. Some believe that clients with malignant disease gradually require more pain medication because their pain worsens rather than because they develop physiologic resistance to the drug. Tolerance to narcotic analgesia is measured not only by the analgesic effects, but also by the body's ability to adjust to the adverse reactions of nausea and vomiting, sedation, hypotension, and respiratory depression.

Addiction is a common fear of health professionals who administer or prescribe narcotics and of clients who receive narcotics. However, if treatment is properly managed, addiction should not occur in patients with nonmalignant causes for their pain, and it rarely occurs in clients with malignant disease. In fact, addiction is a minor concern in the latter group because it occurs in less than 1% of clients with cancer. Addiction is a term used to describe persistent drug craving and abuse of a drug for recreational purpose. While this rarely occurs in clients using narcotics for medicinal relief of pain, fear of addiction is a major factor leading to the inadequate prescription and administration of narcotic analgesics.

Clients also worry about becoming addicted to the analgesics. They may be concerned about the possibility of drug withdrawal symptoms, which are often seen in the "street addict." The nurse clarifies the term addiction with clients while stressing the concept of physical dependency, which is usually not problematic and is readily managed through appropriate tapering or lessening of the drug dosage.

While caring for clients receiving narcotics, the nurse recognizes that narcotics produce effects other than analgesia. The most frequently observed adverse effects result from actions on the central nervous system. They include changes in mental status (such as altered consciousness and sedation) and mood changes (such as euphoria, dysphoria, or depression, and respiratory de-

---

TABLE 7–7 Equianalgesic Guide for Narcotics, with Dose Equivalents for Control of Chronic Pain

Analgesic	Oral (PO) Dose (mg)*	Intramuscular (IM) Dose (mg)*
Meperidine (Demerol)†	150	50
Codeine†	100	60
Pentazocine (Talwin)†	90	30
Morphine‡,§	15	5
Oxycodone (Percodan, Tylox)§	10	7.5
Methadone‖	10	5
Diacetylmorphine (heroin)	10	2.5
Oxymorphone (Numorphan)¶	5	1
Hydromorphone (Dilaudid)§	4	2
Levorphanol (Levo-Dromoran)	2	1

* Equianalgesic doses listed are obtained from a variety of sometimes conflicting studies. They are meant only as guidelines for "by-the-clock" standing-order analgesic therapy of chronic pain. No analgesic listed is superior PO to its equianalgesic dose of PO morphine. The dose interval is q 3–4 h for all except the following: meperidine, q 2–3 h, levorphanol, q 4–6 h, and methadone, q 6–8 h.

† Of little value in severe pain.

‡ Equianalgesic intravenous dosage, 3–4 mg q 3–4 h.

§ Rectal suppositories are available or preparable. The per rectum dose is equal to the PO dose.

‖ Caution: sedative side effects often accumulate despite inadequate analgesic effect.

¶ Available for nonparenteral use in rectal suppository form only.

From Levy, M. H. (1982). Symptom control manual. In B. R. Cassileth & P. A. Cassileth (Eds.), *Clinical care of the terminal cancer patient* (p. 214–262). Philadelphia: Lea & Febiger.

TABLE 7–8   Narcotic Agonists and Antagonists

Narcotic Agonists

Morphine and congeners
   Morphine
   Heroin
   Hydromorphone (Dilaudid)
   Codeine
   Oxycodone
   Levorphanol (Levo-Dromoran)
Meperidine and congeners
   Meperidine (Demerol)
Methadone (Dolophine)

Narcotic Antagonists

Morphine type
   Profadol
   Propiram
   Buprenophine
Nalorphine type
   Pentazocine (Talwin)
   Nalbuphine (Nubain)
   Butorphanol (Stadol)

From Foley, K. M. (1982). The practical use of narcotic analgesics. Symposium on clinical pharmacology of symptom control. *Medical Clinics of North America, 66,* 1092.

---

pression). The severity of central nervous system effects is related to the type of narcotic agent, dose, route, and frequency of administration. The higher the blood level of the drug, the more likely that adverse side effects will be seen. Bolus administration of narcotics (i.e., intramuscular injections or rapid intravenous infusions) are more likely to produce central nervous system changes than are equianalgesic doses administered orally or subcutaneously. Because of their selective opiate receptor actions, narcotic antagonist analgesics produce less respiratory depression than narcotic agonists. As tolerance develops from long-term use of narcotics, the occurrence of central nervous system effects diminishes. Clinically significant respiratory depression is rarely seen in clients with chronic pain who have doses of narcotic titrated to the level of producing adequate analgesia without producing untoward side effects. The nurse assesses clients receiving narcotics for mental status changes. In addition, respirations are monitored, while keeping in mind that pain and the accompanying emotional distress in clients with cancer and chronic pain from other sources are potent respiratory stimulants. As pain relief ensues, the respiratory rate may decrease as a result of comfort and relaxation.

Narcotic analgesics also affect the cardiovascular and gastrointestinal systems. Narcotic-induced vasodilation may lower the blood pressure. Nausea, vomiting, and constipation are common gastrointestinal effects. Mea-

sures to prevent constipation include the use of stool softeners, increased intake of fluids, bowel checks, and dietary modifications. Further information about specific narcotic agonist analgesics, including indications for use, dosages, route of administration, and other general information, can be found in Table 7–4.

Adjuvant therapy.   Certain cancer-related pain syndromes and some chronic pain syndromes of nonmalignant origin are managed not only with narcotic analgesics but also with adjuvant therapies such as cutaneous stimulation and cognitive-behavioral strategies. In addition, co-analgesics (drugs used in conjunction with other analgesics) are used. Table 7–9 summarizes these measures.

Narcotic potentiators.   A relatively common practice in the treatment of chronic pain is the administration of narcotic potentiators — drugs that potentiate the action or effects of narcotics. The most frequently used are hydroxyzine (Vistaril) and promethazine (Phenergan).

Evidence has shown that promethazine enhances the sedating effects of the narcotic and not the actual pain-relieving effects. However, some analgesic effects have been demonstrated with hydroxyzine alone in the treatment of postoperative pain. Several studies have documented the ability of this drug to increase the analgesic potency of narcotics, particularly morphine. These narcotic potentiators probably have an additive effect on the narcotic analgesics. Their ability to relieve anxiety and to calm the client is likely to potentiate analgesia in clients who receive them. Clients receiving promethazine and hydroxyzine in addition to narcotics are observed for sedation. These drugs should be used with caution in chronic pain situations, as the overall goal of drug therapy is to promote pain relief without dulling mental or physical capacity.

Antidepressants.   Antidepressants, such as amitriptyline (Elavil), imipramine (Tofranil), doxepin (Sinequan), and trazodone (Desyrel), are beneficial in the treatment of chronic pain. These drugs help in treating the depression that can accompany cancer. They also stimulate the activity of endogenous opiates, endorphins, and enkephalins by increasing levels of serotonin, a neurotransmitter. In some situations, antidepressants aid in the control of neuropathic or nerve pain associated with cancer. Perhaps the greatest advantage of this group of drugs is the sedative effect, which occurs when they are administered at bedtime.

Cognitive and behavioral strategies.   Cognitive and behavioral strategies, including imagery, relaxation, hypnosis, biofeedback, and acupuncture, are effective measures in the relief of chronic pain.

Imagery.   Imagery is a form of distraction in which the client is encouraged to visualize or think about some pleasant or desirable feeling, sensation, or event. *Guided imagery* takes place when a facilitator, frequently a nurse, assists the client in sustaining a sequence of thoughts aimed at diverting the client's attention away from the pain. *Mental imagery* requires concentration. Clients who are extremely anxious, agitated, or unable to concentrate, as evidenced by a short attention span,

TABLE 7–9   Typical Adjuvant Therapy Combinations for Various Types of Pain

Type of Pain	Co-analgesic	Nondrug Measures
Bone pain	Aspirin 600 mg 4 hourly, or ibuprofen, 400 mg qid	Irradiation
Raised intracranial pressure	Dexamethasone, 2–4 mg tid; diuretic (?)	Elevate head of bed, avoid lying flat
Postherpetic neuralgia, superficial dysesthetic pain	Amitriptyline, 25–100 mg; HS L-dopa (?)	
Nerve pressure pain	Prednisolone, 5–10 mg tid	Nerve block; irradiation
Intermittent stabbing pain	Valproate, 200 mg bid or tid, or carbamazepine, 200 mg tid or qid	
Gastric tenesmoid pain/bladder tenesmoid pain	Chlorpromazine, 10–25 mg 8–4 hourly	
Gastric distention pain	Metoclopromide, 10 mg 4 hourly	
Muscle spasm pain	Diazepam, 5 mg bid, or baclofen, 10 mg tid	Massage
Lymphedema	Diuretic and corticosteroid (?)	Elevate foot of bed; use elastic stocking, compression cuff
Infected malignant ulcer	Metronidazole, 400 mg tid, or alternative antibiotic	
Activity precipitated pain		Modify way of life (if possible)

From Catalano, R. (1987). Pharmacologic management in the treatment of cancer pain. In D. McGuire & C. Yarbro (Eds.), *Cancer pain management* (p. 196). Orlando, FL: Grune & Stratton.

restlessness, or inability to follow simple commands, may benefit first from mild distraction. Guided imagery is particularly useful with clients who are experiencing chronic pain. Clients who practice this technique can mentally experience sights, sounds, smells, and events or other sensations vividly. First the nurse assesses the client's level of concentration to determine if the client can sustain a particular thought or thoughts for a desired time. The time interval for mental imagery can vary from 5 to 60 minutes. Behaviors helpful in assessing capacity for imagery include the following: reading and comprehending the newspaper, listening to music or other auditory stimuli, ability to follow and participate in sustained conversation, and interest in environmental surroundings. When it is determined that the client has some ability to concentrate, the nurse assists the client in identifying a pleasant or favorable thought. The client is then encouraged to focus on this thought in sequence to divert attention from the noxious painful stimuli. Audio tapes may help the client in forming and maintaining images. The nurse, client, or family may wish to create such tapes for individual use or to use commercially available tapes. An example of guided imagery instructions follows: Imagine yourself on the beach on some deserted island. You can hear the rushing sound of waves onto the shore, the cry of the sea gulls flying high above, and the rustling of the trees as they are brushed gently by the winds. You can feel the warmth of the sun over your body and the cooling of the breeze.

Relaxation techniques. These techniques are used to reduce anxiety, tension, and emotional stress, which may aggravate pain. Measures to assist clients to relax can be both physical and psychologic. Physical measures include a body massage, back rub, warm or hot bath, modifications in the environment to reduce distractions, or moving into a comfortable position. Psychologic interventions are the use of pleasant conversation, music, and relaxation tapes. Relaxation tapes are available to assist clients with progressive relaxing of body muscles. Relaxation exercises can be effectively coupled with guided imagery, distraction, and hypnosis.

Hypnosis. Hypnosis is defined as an altered state of consciousness in which an individual falls into a trance and loses an overall sense of reality. Even though the individual is in a trance, there is some sense of awareness and contact with reality and an understanding of what is actually happening. Most researchers agree that a large majority of the population could successfully undergo hypnosis. Yet, many persons reject the idea of hypnosis because of prevailing misconceptions that those who are hypnotized lose control, say things they normally would not disclose to others, or do things against their will. People who are hypnotized actually experience more control, gain insights, and can accomplish tasks or goals as a result of posthypnotic suggestions.

Hypnosis gained scientific acceptance in the medical community when the American Medical Association recognized this technique in 1958. Today, hypnosis is used in the treatment of a variety of pain syndromes, particularly chronic pain. It is used to help clients overcome the emotional consequences of pain, as well as to promote a positive state of mind. Although nurses do not usually teach clients hypnosis, they are in a key position to help clarify misconceptions, instruct clients about relaxation and distraction, and encourage clients to practice self-hypnosis, while creating the appropriate environment. All of these interventions assist both the client and the hypnotist when hypnosis is used for pain management.

Biofeedback. This technique is used for the treatment of chronic pain, anxiety, and other stress conditions. Biofeedback involves the monitoring of various physiologic responses by an electric device capable of sensing changes in the body and reporting this information to the client (Fig. 7–9). Certain physiologic signals are transmitted to the feedback unit by electrode sensors, which are placed on the client's skin. The biofeedback unit amplifies and transforms physiologic information into visual signals (usually meter readings or colored lights). The client is first alerted to stress-related responses such as increased muscle tension or elevation in blood pressure. He or she is then taught to regulate these responses through a combination of techniques, which include deep breathing exercises, progressive relaxation exercises, distraction, and visual imagery.

Biofeedback units vary. Some measure muscle contraction via electromyography, brain activity via electroencephalography, galvanic skin response, and skin temperature reflecting changes in blood flow, heart rate, or blood pressure. Whatever the technique, physiologic responses that tend to worsen or prolong the client's pain are voluntarily controlled.

The client who is interested in learning biofeedback techniques to control pain is usually trained by a skilled therapist. The client is taught to observe the feedback information, report sensations or feelings that become apparent, and practice stress- or pain-reducing techniques. Several sessions are usually required before the client can recognize and control these responses. The client eventually becomes aware of even the most subtle

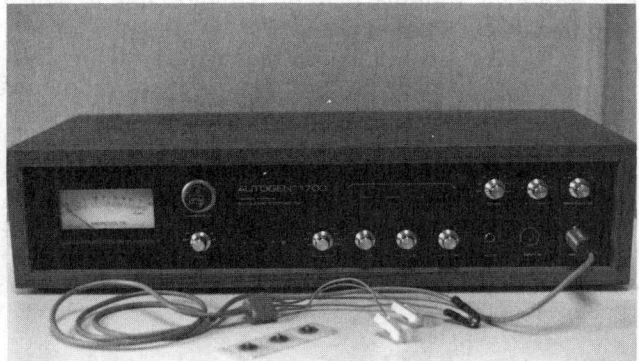

Figure 7–9

A biofeedback unit. (Courtesy of Autogenic Systems, Inc.)

changes in body function that indicate the onset or worsening of pain and automatically responds without the help of the biofeedback unit.

Biofeedback training assists the client to gain control over the pain. Biofeedback and all other cognitive therapy strategies require training and self-discipline if they are to be effectively used. For further discussion, refer to Chapter 6.

Acupuncture. The practice of acupuncture originated in China. According to ancient beliefs, the body is divided into 12 hypothetic sections by parasagittal lines or meridians. Specific acupuncture points are located within these meridians. Tiny needles are inserted into the skin and subcutaneous tissues at these points, and manual vibration or electrical stimulation is delivered. This technique is used to relieve pain and is thought to cure certain diseases.

Acupuncture is still widely acclaimed in China, but it is less popular in the United States. Because the physiologic basis for this technique is unclear, many Western health professionals are skeptical about its usefulness. Few physicians in the United States are trained to perform acupuncture. Nonetheless, acupuncture is practiced for anesthetic purposes during diagnostic and labor and delivery procedures, during surgery, and for the treatment of pain. More than 1000 acupuncture sites have been identified and 14 lines exist as meridians (Fig. 7–10).

Interventions: surgical management. The purpose of surgical interventions is to interrupt the pain pathways in situations in which pain is intractable or severely debilitating. With surgical interruption, there is tissue destruction and some degree of neurologic deficit. Because there may be axonal regeneration or the development of alternative pain pathways, relief from pain may not be permanent. When chronic or persistent pain can no longer be adequately controlled with pharmacologic agents or other pain-reducing methods, various surgical techniques are used (Fig. 7–11).

Nerve blocks are usually indicated for pain that is confined to a specific area or nerve distribution. This procedure involves the destruction of a nerve root or roots by the use of a chemical agent such as phenol or alcohol. Complications associated with this technique vary. Injections into peripheral nerve roots generally lead to decreased sensation in the area, with no effect on motor function. Injections into the lumbosacral area of the spinal cord may damage motor nerve roots, resulting in lost or impaired bowel, bladder, or sexual function. Although the intent of such procedures is to permanently destroy nerve transmission, pain relief from these nerve blocks may be only transient.

Other techniques aimed at surgically interrupting the transmission of pain include *rhizotomy* and *chordotomy*. A rhizotomy involves the destruction of sensory nerve roots where they enter the spinal cord. A *closed rhizotomy* is done by inserting a percutaneous catheter into the area and destroying the sensory nerve roots with neurolytic chemicals, coagulation, or cryodestruction. An *open*

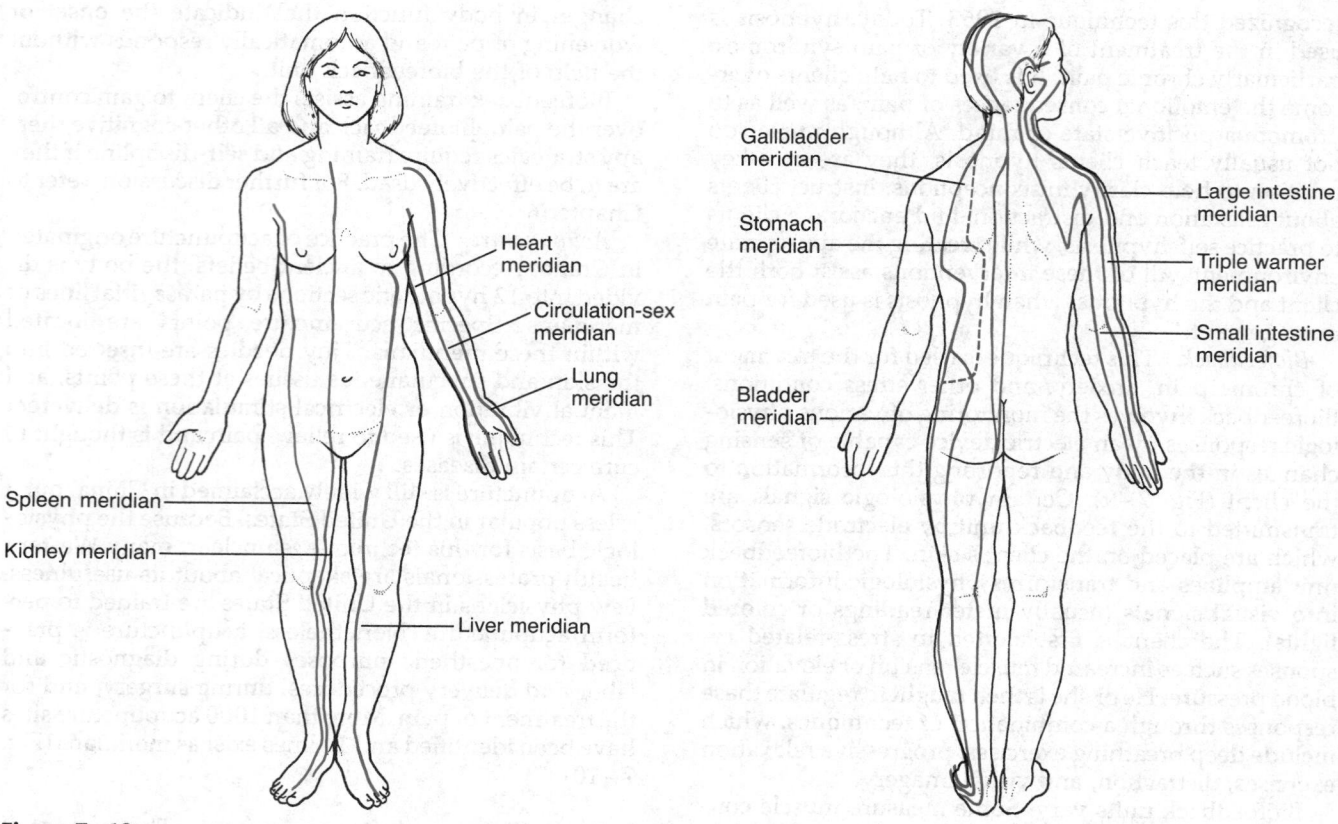

Figure 7–10
Acupuncture meridians.

Labels (front view): Heart meridian, Circulation-sex meridian, Lung meridian, Spleen meridian, Kidney meridian, Liver meridian

Labels (back view): Gallbladder meridian, Stomach meridian, Bladder meridian, Large intestine meridian, Triple warmer meridian, Small intestine meridian

rhizotomy requires a laminectomy. During this surgery, the nerve roots are isolated and then destroyed. With a chordotomy, the pain pathways are transected at the midline portion of the spinal cord before nerve impulses ascend to the spinothalamic tract. As with the other procedures, bowel, bladder, or sexual function may be impaired. Because of the complexity of the pain experience, interruption of nerve conduction and pain pathways may not totally interrupt the sensation of pain.

Nursing responsibilities after surgical intervention include assessing the nature of the neurologic deficits, if any, and teaching the client how to adapt to them. If the client is unaware that a body area is painful, he or she will need to learn how to protect that area from harm. The nurse will also assess the client's expectations related to the surgical interruption of painful sensations and help the client to express realistic expectations.

■ Discharge Planning

For some clients, the pain experience extends beyond hospitalization. Efforts to minimize the pain are not successful, and pain management must continue after discharge from the hospital. It is the nurse's responsibility to mobilize client, family, and community resources to implement plans for continuation of treatment at home.

Home Care Preparation

Preparation for home care is done with the client and family. The nurse assesses the physical layout of the home and related environs and together with the client and family identifies whether modifications are necessary, so that a reasonably pain-free regimen can be maintained after discharge. If physical modifications (e.g., installing a downstairs bathroom) are unrealistic (too expensive or unacceptable to client or family), suggestions about changes in schedules, role responsibilities, and daily routines may help avoid fatigue, which heightens awareness of pain.

Home care preparation may require referral for physical therapy, especially to continue the use of cutaneous stimulation, TENS, or heat or cold as treatment modalities. A psychiatric clinical nurse specialist or social worker may be needed to assist patients to develop coping strategies or maintain adequate family dynamics. In the management of terminally ill patients, hospice referral (hospital based or within the community) can help to maintain continuity of care.

Client/Family Education

Client education is directed toward involving clients and their families in continuing health care behaviors

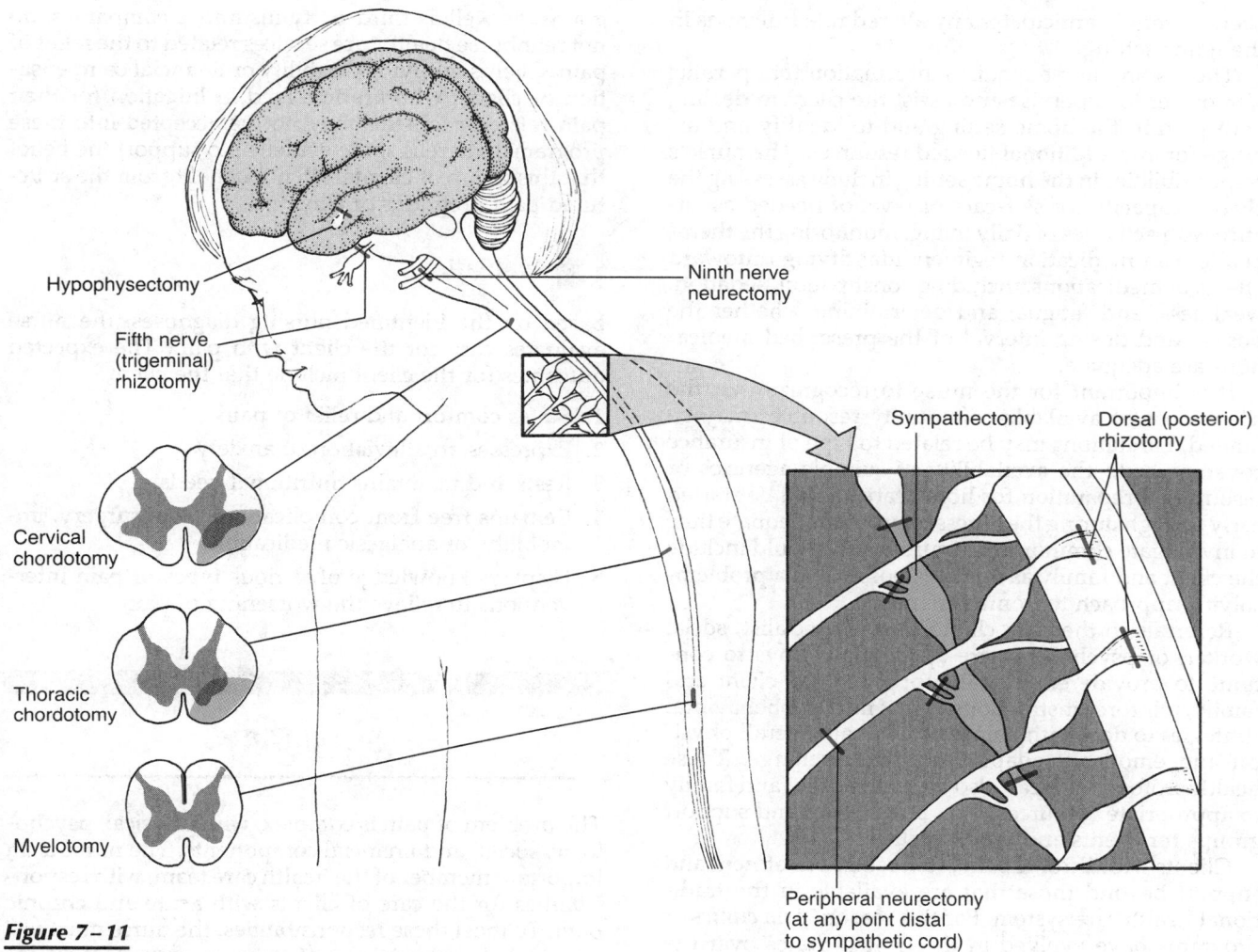

Hypophysectomy

Fifth nerve
(trigeminal)
rhizotomy

Ninth nerve
neurectomy

Cervical
chordotomy

Thoracic
chordotomy

Myelotomy

Sympathectomy

Dorsal (posterior)
rhizotomy

Peripheral neurectomy
(at any point distal
to sympathetic cord)

Figure 7–11

Surgical procedures designed to alleviate pain.

that will relieve the pain and improve psychologic well-being and overall functional status. This education is accomplished in part by teaching about analgesic regimens, the purpose and action of medications, side effects or adverse reactions, and the importance of dosage intervals.

The nurse teaches that ideally the analgesic regimen should not interfere with the client's sleep, rest, appetite, or level of physical mobility. If such interference occurs, the family is taught that consultation with the physician or visiting nurse is needed.

Psychosocial Preparation

The nurse evaluates family support systems to assist the client in adhering to and continuing the proposed medical and nursing plans. Family members are informed about and included in activities during and after hospitalization.

Ideally, the client and family have realistic expectations in the home setting. To achieve a reasonable level

of expectation for the client, the nurse suggests ways to continue participation in household, social, sexual, and work-oriented activities after discharge. The nurse can help the client to identify important activities and plan them around adequate rest schedules.

Health Care Resources

A visiting nurse referral is made when it is anticipated that clients will require assistance or supervision with their pain relief regimen in the home setting. This referral should include specific information from the hospital-based nurse about the client's overall physical condition, general level of sedation, weakness or fatigue, possible constipation or nutritional problems, and sleep patterns (e.g., sleeping through the night).

In addition to information about the client's physical status, the hospital-based nurse also describes the client's level of anxiety, depression, and general expectations about pain status after discharge. The nurse describes family interactions and determines whether the client or family anticipates any altered role functions in the home setting.

The visiting nurse requires information that permits him or her to supervise and assist the client in dealing with pain in the home setting and to identify and arrange for any additional needed resources. The nurse's responsibilities in the home setting include assessing the client's capacity for self-care or level of needed assistance with activities of daily living; monitoring the therapeutic pain medication regimen; identifying untoward effects of medications, including constipation, sedation, weakness, and fatigue; and determining whether the dosage and dosing interval of the prescribed medications are adequate.

It is important for the nurse to recognize that the client's use of available community resources may be limited. Limitations may be related to type of insurance coverage or to the availability of suitable agencies or resources. Preparation for home care should be started early enough during the illness to provide adequate time to investigate community resources and should include the client and family as much as possible in a problem-solving approach to home care needs.

Referrals to the pain clinical nurse specialist, social worker, or psychologist are appropriate ways to continue to provide emotional support to the client and family, reinforce instructions for cognitive or behavioral strategies to deal with pain, and evaluate overall physical and emotional adaptation after discharge. These health professionals can also direct the client and family to appropriate resources (e.g., pain clinics and support groups for clients and their families).

Clients with chronic pain often require treatment and support beyond those that are available in the traditional health care system. For this reason, *pain clinics* or programs have evolved in the United States over the past 10 years. The underlying premise or intent of these clinics is to foster independence and self-care behaviors while promoting pain control and maximizing the client's quality of life. These programs use physical measures, cognitive and behavioral strategies, and surgical interventions, as well as individual and group counseling for clients and family. Emphasis on many of the measures will differ, depending on the program's orientation. For example, pain clinics or programs that are organized through physical medicine or rehabilitation departments promote physical intervention measures. Those organized by psychologists or psychiatrists focus on the use of cognitive or behavioral strategies to relieve pain; those organized by anesthesiologists favor surgical interventions. Most programs discourage the use of narcotic analgesics for pain, and if pharmacologic intervention is necessary, antianxiety, antidepressant, or nonnarcotic analgesics are used.

There are strict eligibility criteria for admission into an inpatient or outpatient pain program or clinic. Usually, clients with nonprogressive pain associated with a known or unknown cause are selected. Clients must be motivated to help themselves. Even if clients desire this type of care, there may be a problem with the health care insurance coverage. Many state medical assistance pro-

grams, as well as third-party insurance companies, do not reimburse health care services related to the relief of pain. Clients receiving disability or financial compensation or clients who are involved in litigation for their pain-related problems may not be accepted into these programs. There is some evidence to support the belief that this group of clients will not benefit from the structured pain programs or clinics.

 Evaluation

Based on the identified nursing diagnoses, the nurse evaluates care for the client with pain. The expected outcomes for the client include that the client

1. States comfort and relief of pain
2. Expresses an alleviation of anxiety
3. Rests and maintains nutritional needs
4. Remains free from complications from surgery, immobility, or analgesic medications
5. Displays knowledge of various types of pain interventions to relieve the worsening of pain

SUMMARY

The problem of pain is complex, with physical, psychologic, social, and financial components. The nurse is an important member of the health care team, with responsibilities for the care of clients with acute and chronic pain. To meet these responsibilities, the nurse must understand the physiology of pain, current methods of treating pain, and appropriate ways to evaluate interventions. The goals of the pain relief interventions, whether curative or palliative, must be understood by the nurse, the client, the family, and other health care team members. Knowledge of pain and relief measures is not enough. The nurse must also develop a philosophy or belief about pain management that is caring and respectful of the client in pain.

IMPLICATIONS FOR RESEARCH

A review of nursing care of the client in pain and an understanding of the current pain literature reveal numerous implications for pain research. For example, there is need to improve objective measures of pain, to further evaluate the use of PCA, to more rigorously evaluate nonpharmacologic interventions for pain, and to study the influence of anxiety and other psychosocial characteristics on pain management. Improvement of research designs, especially the development of measurement tools and the replication of well-conceived existing investigations, could contribute greatly to knowledge in this area. Continuing investigations of nurse characteristics or attitudes about the client in pain may help in efforts to modify or control the caregiver's pain management behavior.

Some specific research questions reflecting these concerns are

1. What is the relationship between physiologic and psychologic measures of pain?

2. What is the nature of overall narcotic consumption in situations in which clients with acute pain control their analgesic intake?

3. How does advanced age affect the need for analgesia in a chronic pain situation?

4. What personal characteristics of the caregiver influence the medication of clients in acute and chronic pain situations?

REFERENCES AND READINGS

Abu-Saad, H., & Tesler, M. (1986). Pain. In V. Carrieri, A. Lindsey, & C. West (Eds.), *Pathophysiological phenomena in nursing: Human responses to illness* (pp. 235–269). Philadelphia: W. B. Saunders.

Ahles, T. A., Blanchard, E. B., & Ruckdeschel, J. C. (1983). The multidimensional nature of cancer-related pain. *Pain, 17,* 277–288.

Ahles, T. (1985). Psychological approaches to the management of cancer-related pain. *Seminar in Oncology Nursing, 1,* 141–146.

Alberico, J. G. (1984). Breaking the chronic pain cycle. *American Journal of Nursing, 87,* 1222–1225.

Ali, N. M., Hanna, N., & Hoffman J. S. (1989). Percutaneous epidural catheterization for intractable pain in terminal cancer patients. *Gynecologic Oncology, 32,* 22–25.

Anderson, K., & Poole, C. (1983). Self-administered medications on a post-partum unit. *American Journal of Nursing, 83,* 1178–1180.

Bailey, C. J., Gulczynski, B., Racky, D., & Vehrs, K. (1984). Epidural morphine infusion. Continuous pain relief. *AORN Journal, 39,* 997, 1000–1005, 1008.

Barker, E. (1987). Pain. *Journal of Neurosurgical Nursing, 19,* 233–234.

Bates, J., & Nathan, P. (1980). Transcutaneous electrical nerve stimulation for chronic pain. *Anesthesia, 35,* 817–822.

Benedetti, C., Bonica, J., & Bellucci, G. (1984). Pathophysiology and therapy of postoperative pain. In C. Benedetti, C. Chapman, & C. Moricca (Eds.), *Advances in pain research and therapy* (Vol. 7, pp. 373–407). New York: Raven.

Beyer, J., DeGood, D., Ashley, L., & Russell, G. (1983). Patterns of postoperative analgesic use with adults and children following cardiac surgery. *Pain, 17,* 71–81.

Blendis, L. (1984). Abdominal pain. In P. Wall & R. Melzack (Eds.), *Textbook of pain* (pp. 350–358). Edinburgh: Churchill Livingstone.

Bondestam, E., Hovgren, F., Johansson, F., Jern, S., Herlitz, J., & Holmberg, S. (1987). Pain assessment by patients and nurses in the early phase of acute M.I. *Journal of Advanced Nursing, 12,* 677–682.

Bonica, J. (1980). Postoperative pain. In R. Condon & J. DeCosse (Eds.), *Surgical care: A physiological approach to clinical management* (pp. 394–414). Philadelphia: Lea & Febiger.

Bonica, J. (1983). The importance of education and training in pain diagnosis and therapy: The role of continuing education courses. In R. Rizzi & M. Visentin (Eds.), *Pain therapy* (pp. 1–10). Amsterdam: Elsevier Biomedical.

Bonica, J. (1984). Local anesthesia and regional blocks. In P. Wall & R. Melzack (Eds.), *Textbook of pain* (pp. 541–557). Edinburgh: Churchill Livingstone.

Brenneis, C., Michaud, M., Bruera, E., & MacDonald, R. N. (1987). Local toxicity during the subcutaneous infusion of narcotics (SCIN). A prospective study. *Cancer Nursing, 10,* 172–176.

Brescia, F. J. (1987). A study of controlled-release oral morphine (MS Contin) in an advanced cancer hospital. *Journal of Pain Symptom Management, 2,* 193–198.

Bullingham, R. E. S. (1985). Optimum management of postoperative pain. *Pain, 29,* 376–386.

Burckhardt, C. (1984). The use of the McGill Pain Questionnaire in assessing arthritis pain. *Pain, 19,* 305–314.

Butler, R., & Gastel, B. (1980). Care of the aged. Perspectives on pain and discomfort. In L. Ng & J. Bonica (Eds.), *Pain, discomfort and humanitarian care* (pp. 297–311). New York: Elsevier.

Camp, L. D., & O'Sullivan, P. (1987). Comparison of medical, surgical and oncology patients' descriptions of pain and nurses' documentation of pain assessments. *Journal of Advanced Nursing, 12,* 593–598.

Chapman, C., & Bonica, J. (1983). *Current concepts TM: Acute pain.* Kalamazoo, MI: Upjohn.

Cohen, F. (1980). Postsurgical pain relief: Patients, status and nurses, medication choices. *Pain, 9,* 265–274.

Copp, L. (Ed.). (1985). *Perspectives of pain (Recent advances in nursing series).* Edinburgh: Churchill Livingstone.

Coyle, N. (1985). Symptom management: Pain—an overview of current concepts. *Cancer Nursing, 8*(Suppl. 1), 44–49.

Coyle, N., & Foley, K. (1985). Pain in patients with cancer: Profile of patients and common pain syndromes. *Seminar in Oncology Nursing, 1,* 93–99.

Cuschieri, R. J., Morran, C. G., Howie, J. C., & McArdle, C. S. (1985). Postoperative pain and pulmonary complications: Comparison of three analgesic regimes. *British Journal of Surgery, 72,* 495–498.

Daut, R., Cleeland, C., & Flanery, R. (1983). Development of the Wisconsin Brief Pain Questionnaire to assess pain in cancer and other diseases. *Pain, 17,* 197–210.

Donovan, M. (1982). Cancer pain: You can help! Symposium on oncologic nursing practice. *Nursing Clinics of North America, 17,* 718.

Donovan, M. (1985). Nursing assessment of cancer pain. *Seminar in Oncology Nursing, 1,* 109–115.

Faherty, B., & Grier, M. R. (1984). Analgesic medication for elderly people post-surgery. *Nursing Research, 33,* 369–372.

Flannery, R., Sos, J., & McGovern, P. (1981). Ethnicity as a factor in the expression of pain. *Psychosomatics, 22,* 39–50.

Foley, K. (1982). The practical use of narcotic analgesics. Symposium on clinical pharmacology of symptom control. *Medical Clinics of North America, 66,* 1091–1104.

Foley, K. (1985). The treatment of cancer pain. *New England Journal of Medicine, 313,* 84–95.

France, R. D. (1987). Chronic pain and depression. *Journal of Pain Symptom Management, 2,* 234–236.

Geden, E. A., Lower, M., Beattie, S., & Beck, N. (1989). Effects of music and imagery on physiologic and self report of analogued labor pain. *Nursing Research, 38,* 37–41.

Gjessing, J., & Tomlin, P. (1981). Postoperative pain control with intrathecal morphine. *Anaesthesia, 36,* 268–276.

Goldberg-Sklar, C. (1984). Chronic pain management: A research focus. *Journal of Neurosurgical Nursing, 16,* 10–14.

Grevert, P., Albert, L., & Goldstein, A. (1983). Partial antagonism of placebo analgesia by naloxone. *Pain, 16,* 129–143.

Grinde, J. W., Grina, R., & Gellatly, T. (1984). Pain management by epidural analgesia: The challenge for nursing. *Heart and Lung, 13,* 105–110.

Guiffre, M., Keane, A., Hatfield, S., & Korevaar, W. (1988). A methodology for clinical pain research measurement: Patient controlled analgesia. *Nursing Research, 37,* 254–255.

Halpern, L. (1984). Drugs in the management of pain: Pharmacology and appropriate strategies for clinical utilization. In C. Benedetti, C. Chapman, & G. Moricca (Eds.), *Advances in pain research and therapy* (Vol. 7, pp. 147–172). New York: Raven.

Harkins, S., Kwentus, J., & Price, D. (1984). Pain and the elderly. In C. Benedetti, C. Chapman, & G. Moricca (Eds.), *Advances in pain research and therapy* (Vol. 7, pp. 103–121). New York: Raven.

Hendler, N. (1981). *Diagnosis and nonsurgical management of chronic pain.* New York: Raven.

Hill, C. (1984). Pain control in cancer rehabilitation. In A. Gunn (Ed.), *Cancer rehabilitation* (pp. 137–154). New York: Raven.

Huskisson, E. (1984). Non-narcotic analgesia. In P. Wall & R. Melzack (Eds.), *Textbook of pain* (pp. 505–513). Edinburgh: Churchill Livingstone.

International Association on Pain, Mersky, H. (Chairman), Subcommittee on Taxonomy. (1979). Pain terms: A list with definitions and notes on usage. *Pain, 6,* 249.

Jacox, A. K. (1977). Sociocultural and psychological aspects of pain. In A. K. Jacox (Ed.), *Pain: A source book for nurses and other health professionals* (pp. 57–87). Boston: Little, Brown.

Johnson, J., & Leventhal, H. (1974). Effects of accurate expectations and behavioral instructions on reactions during a noxious medical examination. *Journal of Personality and Social Psychology, 29,* 710–718.

Johnson, J., Rice, V., Fuller, S., & Endress, M. (1978). Sensory information, information in a coping strategy, and recovery from surgery. *Research in Nursing and Health, 1,* 4–17.

Kaiko, R., Wallenstein, S., Rogers, A., Brabinski, P., & Houda, R. (1982). Narcotics in the elderly. *Medical Clinics of North America, 66,* 1079–1089.

Keller, E., & Bzdek, V. (1986). Effects of therapeutic touch on tension headache pain. *Nursing Research, 35,* 101–105.

Kerns, R. D., & Haythornthwaite, J. A. (1988). Depression among chronic pain patients: Cognitive-behavioral analysis on rehabilitation outcome. *Journal of Consulting and Clinical Psychology, 56,* 870–876.

Ketovvori, H. (1987). Nurses' and patients' conceptions of wound pain and the administration of analgesics. *Journal of Pain Symptom Management, 2,* 213–218.

Kim, S. (1980). Pain: Theory, research and nursing practice. *Advances in Nursing Science, 2,* 43–59.

Levin, F. F., Malloy, G., & Hyman, R. (1987). Nursing management of postoperative pain: Use of relaxation techniques with female cholecystectomy patients. *Journal of Advanced Nursing, 12,* 463–472.

Mannheimer, J., & Lampe, G. (1984). Differential evaluation for the determination of T.E.N.S. effectiveness in specific pain syndromes. In J. Mannheimer & G. Lampe (Eds.), *Clinical transcutaneous electrical nerve stimulation* (pp. 63–197). Philadelphia: F. A. Davis.

Mather, L., & Mackie, J. (1983). The incidence of postoperative pain in children. *Pain, 15,* 271–282.

McCaffery, M. (1979a). Current misconceptions about the relief of acute pain. In B. Crue (Ed.), *Chronic pain* (pp. 274–285). Jamaica, NY: Spectrum.

McCaffery, M. (1979b). *Nursing management of the patient with pain.* Philadelphia: J. B. Lippincott.

McCaffery, M. (1980). Relieving pain with noninvasive techniques. *Nursing '80, 10*(12), 54–57.

McCaffery, M. (1984). Pain in the critical care patient. *Dimensions in Critical Care Nursing, 3,* 323–325.

McCauley, K., & Polomano, R. (1980). Acute pain: A nursing perspective with cardiac surgical patients. *Topics in Clinical Nursing, 2,* 45.

McGuire, D. B. (1984). The measurement of clinical pain. *Nursing Research, 33,* 152–156.

McGuire, L., & Wright, A. (1984). Continuous narcotic infusion. It's not just for cancer patients. *Nursing '84, 14*(12), 50–55.

Meinhart, N. T., & McCaffery, M. (1983). *Pain: A nursing approach to assessment and analysis.* Norwalk, CT: Appleton-Century-Crofts.

Melzack, R. (1973). *The puzzle of pain.* New York: Basic Books.

Melzack, R. (1975). The McGill Pain Questionnaire: Major properties and scoring methods. *Pain, 1,* 277–299.

Melzack, R. (1983). The McGill Pain Questionnaire. In R. Melzack (Ed.), *Pain assessment and management* (pp. 41–47). New York: Raven.

Melzack, R., & Wall, P. D. (1982). *The challenge of pain.* New York: Basic Books.

Ottoson, D. (1988). *Pain treatment by TENS.* Berlin: Springer-Verlag.

Ozuna, J. (1987). An experience with epidural morphine in lumbar surgery patients. *Journal of Neuroscience Nursing, 19,* 235–239.

Panfilli, R., Brunckhorst, L., & Dundon, R. (1988). Nursing implications of patient controlled analgesia. *Journal of Intravenous Nursing, 11*(2), 75–77.

Relieving pain: An analgesia guide. (1988). *American Journal of Nursing, 88,* 815–826.

Schofferman, J. (1988). Pain diagnosis and management in the palliative care of AIDS. *Journal of Palliative Care, 4*(4), 46–49.

Scott, L., Glum, G., & Peoples, J. (1983). Preoperative predictors of postoperative pain. *Pain, 15,* 283–293.

Sternbach, R. A. (1968). *Pain: A psychophysiological analysis.* New York: Academic.

Sternbach, R. (1984). Acute versus chronic pain. In P. Wall & R. Melzack (Eds.), *Textbook of pain* (pp. 173–177). Edinburgh: Churchill Livingstone.

Taylor, A. G., West, B. A., Simon, B., Skelton, J., & Rowlingson, J. C. (1983). How effective is TENS for acute pain? *American Journal of Nursing, 83,* 1171–1174.

Turner, J., & Romano, J. (1984). Evaluating psychological interventions for chronic pain: Issues and recent developments. In C. Benedetti, C. Chapman, & G. Moricca (Eds.), *Advances in pain research and therapy* (Vol. 7, pp. 257–296). New York: Raven.

Venning, M., & Rogers, J. (1988). Continuous subcutaneous infusion: Flexible option in symptom control. *Australian Nurses Journal, 17*(7), 34–37.

Vessels, R. A. (1988). Sedation and pain management for the critically ill. *Critical Care Clinics, 4,* 167–181.

Wachter-Shikora, N. (1983). The elderly patient in pain and the acute care setting. *Nursing Clinics of North America, 18,* 395–401.

Wall, P. (1984). Neurophysiology of acute pain and chronic pain. In C. Benedetti, C. Chapman, & R. Moricca (Eds.), *Advances in pain research and therapy: Recent advances in the management of pain* (Vol. 7, pp. 13–25). New York: Raven.

Watt-Watson, J. H. (1987a). Nurses knowledge of pain issues: A survey. *Journal of Pain Symptom Management, 2,* 207–211.

Watt-Watson, J. H. (1987b). What do we need to know about pain? *American Journal of Nursing, 87,* 1217–1218.

Wells, N. (1982). The effect of relaxation on postoperative muscle tension and pain. *Nursing Research, 31,* 236–238.

Wells, N. (1984). Responses to acute pain and the nursing implications. *Journal of Advanced Nursing, 9,* 51–58.

West, B. (1981). Understanding endorphins: Our natural pain relief system. *Nursing '81, 11*(2), 50–53.

Whipple, B. (1987). State of the science: Methods of pain control: Review of research and literature. *Image: Journal of Nursing Scholarship, 19*(3), 142–146.

Woolf, C. (1984). Transcutaneous and implanted nerve stimulation. In P. Wall & R. Melzack (Eds.), *Textbook of pain* (pp. 679–690). Edinburgh: Churchill Livingstone.

Zborowski, M. (1969). *People in pain.* San Francisco: Jossey-Bass.

Ziga, S., & Yasko, J. (1983). Chronic pain. In J. Yasko (Ed.), *Guidelines for cancer care: Symptom management* (pp. 73–93). Reston, VA: Reston Publishing.

ADDITIONAL READINGS

Broome, M. E., Lillis, P. P., & Smith, M. C. (1989). Pain interventions with children: A meta-analysis of research. *Nursing Research, 38,* 155–158.

A meta-analysis of 27 studies on pain management with children was conducted to determine children's psychologic, behavioral, and self-report responses to a painful procedure and to describe interventions and their effectiveness in pain management. More than one-half of the studies did not report pain estimates of the reliability or validity of measures used. Highly significant relationships were found between pain management interventions and the three outcome responses of children. At least a 30% decrease in distress responses resulted from pain management interventions.

King, K., Norsen, L., Robertson, R., & Hicks, G. (1987). Patient management of pain medication after cardiac surgery. *Nursing Research, 36,* 145–150.

The effects of self-administered versus nurse-administered pain medication after cardiac surgery were studied, along with patients' desire for control, disruption in daily activities, emotional responses, and the use of pain medication over time. No differences were found between the groups, although the experimental group (self-dosing) reported higher levels of pain intensity in the immediate postoperative period.

Levin, R., Malloy, G., & Hyman, R. (1987). Nursing management of postoperative pain: Use of relaxation techniques with female cholecystectomy patients. *Journal of Advanced Nursing, 12,* 463–472.

The effectiveness of two types of relaxation techniques (rhythmic breathing and Benson's relaxation technique) in the management of postoperative pain was studied. The two treatment groups were compared with two control groups. The Benson relaxation group was different on measures of sensation and distress, but no differences between groups were found on measures of analgesic use or number of postoperative hospital days.

Manderino, M., & Bzdek, V. (1984). Effects of modeling and information on reactions to pain: A childbirth-preparation analogue. *Nursing Research, 33,* 9–14.

The efficacy of videotaping and modeling as pain reduction techniques for women during labor and delivery was studied. Three groups received videotaped information, videotaped modeling, or a combination of the two, and these groups were compared with a control group. The group receiving both the information and modeling reported less pain, but physiologic measures indicated no differences between groups.

McGuire, D. (1984). The measurement of clinical pain. *Nursing Research, 33,* 152–156.

The author describes problems associated with measuring pain in the clinical setting and in the research setting. Problems identified include the subjectivity of the pain experience, the lack of reliable and valid measuring instruments, and problematic clinical issues such as the type of pain and the personal characteristics of those in pain. Critical information is given about the type of measure available to the nurse. The use of PCA as a measure is not discussed.

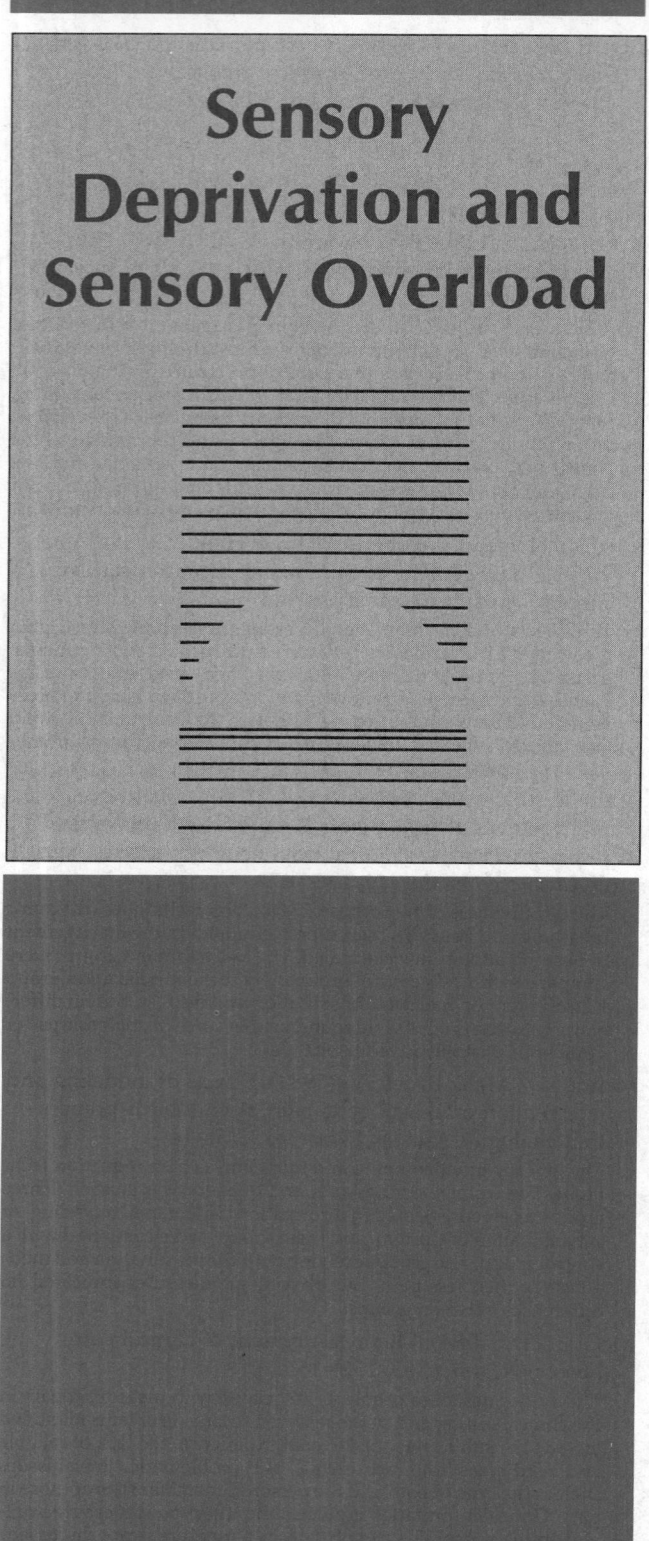

CHAPTER 8

Sensory Deprivation and Sensory Overload

The sensory process allows an individual to initiate and maintain contact and communication with others and the environment. Sight, hearing, touch, taste, and smell are the components of the sensory process that promote an awareness of the external environment. Kinesthetic and visceral sensations also are included in the process. Kinesthetic sensations arise from muscles, and visceral sensations originate from the internal organs of the body. An environment that is responsive to and compatible with the sensory process supports a state of equilibrium.

Normal sensory loss over time is not detrimental to the individual as long as the stimuli remain familiar and controllable and adaptation can be achieved. When the balance is disrupted between the stimuli and adaptation, the individual begins to demonstrate behavioral manifestations that are related to sensory deprivation or sensory overload.

The individual who enters a health care system and assumes the role of client can encounter factors that individually and collectively contribute to sensory deprivation or sensory overload. The nurse as a care provider can use strategies to prevent and interventions to manage these behavioral manifestations.

THE SENSORY PROCESS

RECEPTION AND PERCEPTION

Two aspects of the sensory process assist humans in maintaining day-to-day contact with the environment. *Reception* is the biologic component of the sensory process and involves the function of the sensory organs. *Perception* is the psychologic aspect of the process and refers to the ability to choose, organize, and give meaning to incoming sensory stimuli, which results in overt behavior. Both reception and perception are essential for humans to remain in a state of equilibrium with themselves and the environment. Alterations in the sensory process occur as a result of an increase or a reduction in the variety, patterns, and intensity of sensory input or a lack of meaningful interpretation of stimuli and may lead to major behavioral manifestations (Fig. 8–1).

THE AROUSAL MECHANISM

The concept of arousal is important in understanding how a person copes with changes in the environment. Because of different personalities, inner resources, and life styles, an identical environment is perceived differently by each individual; also, the same stimulus can be monotonous one minute and overwhelming the next.

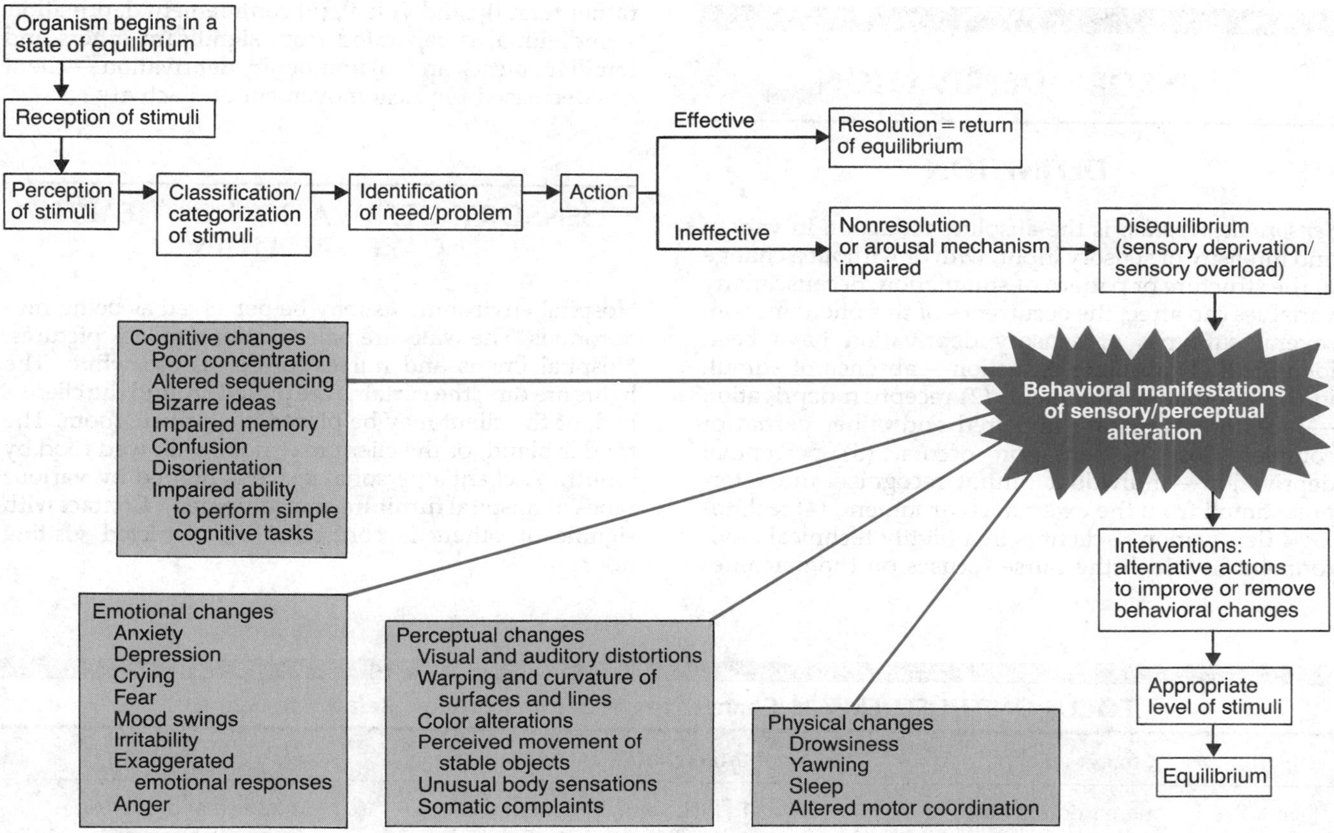

Organism begins in a state of equilibrium
Reception of stimuli
Perception of stimuli
Classification/ categorization of stimuli
Identification of need/problem
Action
Effective
Resolution = return of equilibrium
Ineffective
Nonresolution or arousal mechanism impaired
Disequilibrium (sensory deprivation/ sensory overload)
Behavioral manifestations of sensory/perceptual alteration
Interventions: alternative actions to improve or remove behavioral changes
Appropriate level of stimuli
Equilibrium
Cognitive changes
Poor concentration
Altered sequencing
Bizarre ideas
Impaired memory
Confusion
Disorientation
Impaired ability to perform simple cognitive tasks
Emotional changes
Anxiety
Depression
Crying
Fear
Mood swings
Irritability
Exaggerated emotional responses
Anger
Perceptual changes
Visual and auditory distortions
Warping and curvature of surfaces and lines
Color alterations
Perceived movement of stable objects
Unusual body sensations
Somatic complaints
Physical changes
Drowsiness
Yawning
Sleep
Altered motor coordination

Figure 8–1

The results of sensory deprivation and sensory overload.

To maintain an optimal level of functioning, it is necessary to have an optimal level of sensory stimulation. *Sensoristasis* is the term used to describe the drive state of cortical arousal that impels the individual to strive to maintain an optimal level of sensory variation. It is a mechanism that attempts to restore sensory equilibrium by limiting incoming stimuli when there is already a high level of arousal present and by enhancing incoming stimuli when the arousal level is low.

The reticular activating system (RAS) has the primary responsibility for activating the central nervous system (CNS). The RAS is stimulated by nerve impulses from visual, auditory, olfactory, cutaneous, muscular, and visceral receptors. General sensory input plays an important role in maintaining arousal. The RAS, located in the core of the brain stem, is composed of ascending and descending pathways that travel to and from the cerebral cortex. Ascending RAS fibers feed the cortex to alert the brain, and descending fibers travel from the cortex to stimulate the RAS.

All sensory input stimulates the cerebral cortex through this mechanism, and with experience the system learns to discriminate in its responses. Disorders in the arousal mechanism occur when the RAS is bombarded with input or when the RAS fails to recognize input because the stimulus lacks relevant meaning or is of low intensity and below the threshold. When stimuli are overwhelming, the cortical system is unable to regulate incoming stimuli, and individuals experience sensory overload. If the individual is in an environment that has a low level of stimulation, cortical stimulation is reduced and sensory deprivation will occur (Fig. 8–2).

Sensory overload
Overstimulation
Reception
RAS
Perception
Sensory input
Optimal stimulation
Sensoristasis
Reduced stimulation
Sensory deprivation

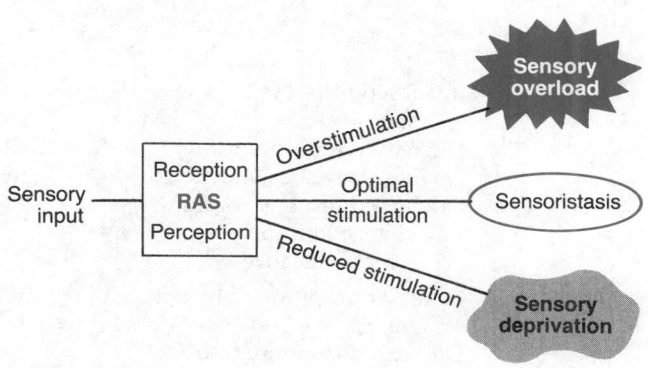

Figure 8–2

Relationship among sensory input, the reticular activating system (RAS), and response.

SENSORY DEPRIVATION

DEFINITION

Sensory deprivation is the absolute reduction in variety and intensity of sensory input, with or without a change in the structure or pattern of stimulation. Because many variables can affect the occurrence of this phenomenon, several subtypes of sensory deprivation have been identified: (1) absolute reduction—absence of stimuli in the external environment, (2) reception deprivation—receptor organs are impaired and either partial or complete loss of sensation occurs, (3) perceptual deprivation—individual cannot recognize and interpret stimuli from the external environment, (4) technologic deprivation—client is in a highly technical environment in which the nurse focuses on the machines rather than the individual, (5) confinement deprivation—individual is separated from significant others and familiar objects, and (6) immobility deprivation—client has decreased physical movement and activity.

SENSORY DEPRIVATION IN HEALTH CARE FACILITIES

Hospital environments may be perceived as being monotonous. The walls are pale in color and lack pictures. Hospital linens and nurses' uniforms are white. The lights are dim; the curtains are pulled around the client's bed, or the client may be placed in a private room. The food is bland, or the client may not be allowed food by mouth. A client's personal space is limited by various types of hospital furniture and equipment. Contact with significant others is controlled by restricted visiting hours.

FOCUS ON THE ELDERLY ■ Changes in the Sensory Process Related to Aging

Function	Changes	Interventions	Rationales
Sight	Increased response to darkness, size of objects, colors (especially green and blue).	1. Place a night light in the client's sleeping area. 2. Select large print for teaching materials. 3. Place frequently used objects within client's reach.	1–3. Abuse and overuse of the eyes can be prevented in the elderly.
Hearing	Increased response to high-frequency sounds.	1. Use light signal to indicate ringing of the telephone. 2. Avoid having mechanical equipment touch walls.	1. Visual cues assist the hearing-impaired elderly. 2. Sound distortions produce behavioral reactions in the elderly.
Touch	Decreased response to pain and different temperatures.	1. Discuss with client factors contributing to pain. 2. Keep client out of drafts.	1, 2. The environment of the elderly can be manipulated to decrease stimuli contributing to sensory alterations.
Taste	Increased response to bitter substances. Decreased response to sour and salty substances. Decreased response or no change in response to sweet substances.	1. Assess dietary intake with client. 2. Clean dentures and rinse mouth daily and after eating.	1, 2. A sense of security can be promoted in the elderly when eating is a pleasurable experience.
Smell	Increased response to noxious odors. Decreased response to fruity odors.	1. Use antibacterial soap for personal hygiene. 2. Open window in client's room daily for a minimum of ½ h.	1, 2. Elimination of unpleasant odors can enhance the environment of the elderly.

In addition to these common environmental findings in a hospital, the *age* of the client may have an impact on the sensory stimuli received (see the accompanying Focus on the Elderly feature). The elderly are particularly at high risk for developing sensory deprivation because they may have decreases in visual, hearing, and taste abilities. Because of the aging process, they are typically less able to process incoming stimuli as rapidly as a younger adult.

Illness may reduce sensory input, for example, when one of the senses is affected or when there is a metabolic condition affecting the CNS. Clients who have had eye surgery are at high risk of becoming deprived if an eye patch is used, which reduces visual ability and causes limitations in activity levels. The individual with a spinal cord injury who is placed on a Stryker frame is immobile and has limited visual stimulation because the eyes focus on the floor and ceiling. Confinement as a result of traction, body casts, bed rest, or restraints also enhances development of sensory deprivation. Clients with long-term chronic or terminal illnesses and those who are institutionalized for extended periods can develop sensory deprivation.

Treatment procedures used during an illness can result in a change or reduction in contact with the environment and cause functional behavioral changes. Isolation rooms are used if the client has an infection that can be spread to others or has a low resistance that places the client at risk of developing infections. While the client is in isolation, there is limited contact with the staff. Those who enter the room often wear gowns, masks, and gloves, which reduce visual and tactile inputs to the client. Clients who are unable to swallow may have nasogastric tubes, which affect the ability to taste or chew food. The presence of other tubes such as intravenous lines or a renal dialysis shunt or fistula causes restricted movement of one of the extremities.

Behaviors seen during sensory deprivation are separated into several categories: cognitive, emotional, perceptual, and physical (see Fig. 8–1).

FEATURES

COGNITIVE CHANGES

Some cognitive changes reported vary from poor concentration, altered sequencing of thoughts, or unusual ideas to bizarre thinking. Impaired memory, confusion, and disorientation may occur. There is also impairment in performing simple cognitive tasks such as adding a list of numbers.

EMOTIONAL CHANGES

Emotional disturbances include anxiety, depression, crying, fear, mood swings, irritability and annoyance over trivial matters, exaggerated emotional responses, and anger. The intensity of emotions observed varies from mild discomfort to panic.

PERCEPTUAL CHANGES

Changes in perception include visual and auditory distortions, warping and curvature of surfaces and lines, alterations in color, and perceived movement of stable objects. Certain individuals have reported unusual body sensations such as numbness. Some persons show a preoccupation with internal sensations and somatic complaints including dry mouth, heart palpitations, difficulty in breathing, and nausea. Olfactory sensory distortions, such as the smell of frying eggs, have also occurred in some individuals with sensory alteration.

PHYSICAL CHANGES

Physical behaviors observed include drowsiness, excessive yawning, and sleep. Sleep is used as a mechanism to escape the monotony of sensory deprivation. Motor coordination is affected, as seen in alterations of dexterity, hand-eye coordination movements, and balance.

RESEARCH

Research in the field of sensory deprivation has historically consisted of the effects of long-term sensory and/or social deprivation; deprived individuals such as prisoners in isolation, shipwrecked sailors, or explorers were studied. Individuals who were in an unchanging environment or who were placed in isolation or confinement all reported similar findings of oppressive monotony, which led to behavioral changes such as lack of affect, confusion, and depression.

During the last 25 years, studies have examined the effects on human behavior of a reduction in the level and variability of stimulation from the visual, auditory, and tactile modalities. The research has been conducted on relatively healthy individuals who were placed in environments where they could be isolated from sensory input such as patterned visual or auditory stimuli. These studies found that when people are deprived of sensory stimulation, they develop behavioral changes such as confusion, inaccurate perception, faulty reasoning, impaired memory, and hallucinations. The problem with many of these studies is the fact that healthy, young individuals were the subjects; adding variables of illness or aging, with their effects on the sensory process, may cause more drastic alterations in behavior.

Studies of sensory alterations after surgical proce-

NURSING RESEARCH

Some Sensory Alterations Are Present up to 1 Year After Mastectomy.

Lierman, L. M. (1988). Sensory and physical alterations after mastectomy. *Health Care Women International, 9*(40), 263–269.

This longitudinal descriptive study was conducted to identify sensory alterations and physical changes present after mastectomy. A total of 20 women referred from a Reach to Recovery program in one city agreed to participate. Interviews consisting of open-ended questions about alterations were conducted at five intervals (1, 4, 7, 10, and 12 months) during the first year after surgery. A total of 84 alterations were reported at the first interview; 36 were reported at the 12-month interview. The most significant decrease (71 to 50) was reported between the fourth- and seventh-month interviews. Painful and nonpainful sensory alterations were the main categories of changes, with numbness and tightness the most frequent nonpainful alterations reported.

Critique.   This is one of a few research studies to examine sensory and physical alterations of women after mastectomy that compares the subjects' responses over time as well as responses among subjects. The sample size is small, and further studies with larger groups in multiple sites are needed to address the issue of generalizability. Rating scales for measuring the magnitude of alterations could be used to provide more specific information about changes.

Nursing implications.   Nurses can use this information to teach women who have mastectomies what to expect (physical symptoms) after surgery. Nurses can also provide opportunities for women to ventilate feelings about alterations, especially pain, that they may not feel like sharing with family and friends. This intervention can reduce feelings of isolation and loneliness.

dures have also been reported (see the accompanying Nursing Research feature).

SENSORY OVERLOAD

DEFINITION

Sensory overload results from an increase in environmental stimuli—when there is multisensory bombardment of stimuli or when there is an increase in the pattern and intensity of stimuli so that the input is meaningless. The stimuli are too many, too rapid, and too diverse, and alterations or changes take place in the individual. The

behavioral manifestations of sensory overload can have a health-threatening effect on the individual.

SENSORY OVERLOAD IN HEALTH CARE FACILITIES

Hospital environments present risks of overstimulation of the client's senses. Noise associated with people and equipment can produce a steady stream of irritating sounds. Various noxious odors mingle with body odors. Invasive and noninvasive tests and examinations occur frequently and can be done repeatedly and by many different health professionals, thus producing sensory overload during a client's hospitalization.

Some clinical conditions also promote the occurrence of sensory overload. Clients with intense pain or those with dressing changes that involve discomfort may experience increased intensity of sensations above their normal threshold.

Hospital areas such as the recovery room, emergency room, and critical care units are filled with a multitude of stimuli that are foreign and lack meaning to the client. Bright continuous lights, increased noise levels, monitors or respirators with alarms, constant interventions by different members of the health care team, lack of privacy, and restrictive equipment are a few of the many unusual sensations surrounding the client. The suddenness with which the client is placed in an acute situation is another factor that affects the client's response. Often there is no time to prepare for the adjustment process required for responding to stimuli.

The literature is filled with reports of altered behaviors that are observed as a result of sensory overload in critical care areas such as burn units and coronary care units. These behaviors are often referred to as the syndrome of *ICU psychosis*. Alterations in cognitive function, confusion, disorientation, and inability to maintain attention are a few of the behaviors noted in various studies occurring on the third to seventh day of the critical care unit stay.

FEATURES

There are no clear differences between behaviors observed in sensory deprivation and those observed in sensory overload. Most of the clinical findings for sensory overload are similar to those cognitive, emotional, perceptual, and physical alterations discussed for sensory deprivation (see Fig. 8–1).

A distinguishing feature of sensory overload is that the client cannot use sleep as an escape mechanism. Sleep is a vital and basic need. Sensory overload alters the client's specific sleep pattern, and sleep integrity becomes disrupted. Sleep deprivation can contribute to sensory overload.

COLLABORATIVE MANAGEMENT

Assessment

Because both individual and environmental variables affect the function of sensation, the nurse must assess the client as well as the setting to determine whether there is an increased or decreased amount of sensory input.

History

When obtaining a client's history, the following data help to identify the client who is at risk of developing an alteration in the sensory process:

1. Age
2. Developmental level
3. Alterations in reception, e.g., decreased sight, hearing, taste, smell
4. Corrective devices required for sensory impairments
5. Alteration in mobility
6. Neurologic impairment
7. Cognitive status
8. Ability to communicate
9. Previous hospital experience
10. Recent surgery
11. Duration of hospital admission
12. Use of medications
13. Substance abuse
14. Physical environment and surroundings before admission
15. Psychologic status

Data concerning the client's status before hospitalization are important. However, it is crucial that the nurse continue to assess the client in an ongoing manner. Throughout the hospitalization, changes resulting from interventions such as surgery, activity restrictions, medications, or treatments may precipitate the occurrence of or changes in some of these conditions and thus greatly affect the sensory status.

Physical Assessment: Clinical Manifestations

The client whose sensory input is affected displays alterations in activities such as increased restlessness, drowsiness, increased sleep, and incoordination. Somatic complaints such as a dry mouth, heart palpitations, difficulty in breathing, and lack of appetite may be present. Other individuals may report auditory or visual distortions and state a feeling of numbness.

The type of medication the client is receiving is reviewed to determine side effects or toxic levels. The nurse monitors fluid, electrolyte, or nutritional imbalances through laboratory studies.

Psychosocial Assessment

Many clients do not admit to alterations such as bizarre thoughts, delusions, or hallucinations. They fear that expression of such feelings is unusual and might prejudice the caregiver. Some of these alterations in thought processes may be detected through conversations with the client. Effects on emotional responses are seen as clients display increased irritability, frequent mood swings, crying, fear, anger, and depression. Cognitive function is often impaired, and the client reports an increased incidence of daydreaming. Reduced attention spans are observed, and the client may exhibit noncompliant behaviors.

Laboratory Findings

Clients with sensory alterations have increased levels of catecholamines, 17-ketosteroids, and luteinizing hormone in the urine. An increase in thyroid-stimulating hormone levels in plasma has been identified. The existence of specific pathologic conditions needs to be determined before the laboratory findings can be considered to be conclusive for sensory disruptions.

Environmental Assessment

Several characteristics of the setting are assessed to determine the type of sensory alteration present. The nurse checks the amount and intensity of stimulation present. Imagining one's self in the client's position helps the nurse to better understand the level of stimulation present and the changes or variability that occurs. Stimuli are assessed for their pattern and meaningfulness. The degree of social isolation imposed by the environment and familiarity of surroundings to the client are two other factors that the nurse should consider.

 ## Analysis: Nursing Diagnosis

After assessing the client and the environmental factors, the nurse can draw conclusions and make a decision about the nursing diagnosis.

Common Diagnoses

Three major diagnoses are related to alterations in the sensory-perceptual process.

1. Sensory/perceptual alterations related to sensory deprivation
2. Sensory/perceptual alterations related to sensory overload

3. Sensory/perceptual alterations (sight, hearing, taste, touch, smell) related to sensory deficit

Additional Diagnoses

Along with the common nursing diagnoses, several potential nursing problems that result from alterations in the sensory/perceptual process might include the following:

1. Anxiety related to social isolation
2. Ineffective individual coping related to unfamiliar environment
3. Fear related to placement in an emergency room
4. Noncompliance related to lack of understanding of treatments
5. Powerlessness related to limited activity level
6. Sleep pattern disturbance related to noise level of a critical care unit
7. Social isolation related to lack of visitors
8. Altered thought processes related to protective isolation environment
9. Potential for injury related to decreased or increased sensations
10. Self-care deficit related to sensory impairment

 Planning and Implementation

Nursing plans and interventions are provided for the client with an actual diagnosis of sensory/perceptual alterations related to sensory deprivation, sensory overload, or sensory deficit (see the accompanying Client Care Plan and Health Promotion/Maintenance feature).

Sensory/Perceptual Alterations Related to Sensory Deprivation

Planning: client goals. The major goals for the nursing diagnosis are that the client will have (1) meaningful interpretation of sensory input and (2) orientation to time, person, and place.

Interventions. After assessing and analyzing the situation, the nurse identifies factors that contribute to sensory/perceptual deprivation. The nursing interventions are focused on preventing sensory monotony by increasing the level of intensity of stimulation and increasing the variety of patterns of incoming stimuli. The nurse should try to create an environment that resembles familiar surroundings for the client and restores meaningful stimulation.

Placing pictures on the walls of hospital rooms, putting cards on display on the bedside table, and encouraging family members to bring in personal objects or photographs of significant others from the home setting are a few suggestions for increasing familiarity of the hospital room. Colorful pillowcases, pajamas, and washcloths are other items from home that can reduce the monotony of the hospital room. The use of radio and television can help to increase stimulation through sound but require monitoring for content and volume to decrease monotony. Clocks, calendars, wrist watches, and windows to the outside are effective means of orienting the client to time. Name pins worn by staff members assist in orienting the client to persons.

Assistive devices such as hearing aids, eyeglasses, or contact lenses should be used by the client, as they can enhance reception of sensory input and help the client to feel more in control of the environment. If the client can perform any self-care measures, encouragement should be given for participation in these activities be-

---

CLIENT CARE PLAN ■ The Client with Sensory Deficit

Goal/Outcome Criteria	Interventions	Rationales
Nursing Diagnosis 1: Sensory/Perceptual Alterations (Auditory)		
Client will demonstrate self-care behaviors for hearing impairment. ■ Verbalizes acceptance of hearing loss. ■ Has no evidence of injury secondary to impaired hearing.	1. Teach client to converse face to face. 2. Facilitate use of alternative communication techniques: pantomime, sign language, writing, lip reading. 3. Encourage client to express feelings and concerns about loss. 4. Maintain safe environment for client. 5. Provide information about assistive devices (hearing aids, loud ringers for doorbells and telephones as appropriate).	1. Facing person directly allows client to position ear that hears best near the voice. 2. Use of these techniques can facilitate client's ability to compensate for deficit. 3. Such expression promotes acceptance of loss. 4, 5. Safe environment and assistive devices promote security and facilitate coping.

cause physical movement serves as a source of stimulation.

Smelling the aroma of food, providing foods of different textures, and including warm and cool foods in the diet stimulate the gustatory sense. Oral hygiene and properly fitting dentures promote the sense of taste and chewing ability. Using tactile stimulation through touch, back rubs, massage, and passive range-of-motion exercises is essential for the client with a limited level of activity.

The nurse acts as a source of stimulation by talking with the client, explaining tests and procedures, and asking simple questions to promote cognitive function. The client is also encouraged to find methods of self-stimulation such as singing and reading. Placing an individual in a lounge or hallway where social interactions occur with other clients or visitors is another means of increasing stimulation.

Sensory/Perceptual Alterations Related to Sensory Overload

Planning: client goals. The major goals of this diagnosis are the same as those for the previous diagnosis: the meaningful interpretation of sensory input and orientation to time, person, and place.

Interventions. Critical care units or emergency rooms are frequent sites for the occurrence of sensory overload. Nurses working in these units have a responsibility to reduce the intensity of incoming stimuli and to increase the meaningfulness of the stimuli. Providing a consistent, predictable pattern of stimulation helps the client to have a sense of control over the environment. Without control, stimuli are perceived as disorganized, irrelevant, and overwhelming.

The noise level in a critical care unit is great. Many of

HEALTH PROMOTION/MAINTENANCE ■ Suggestions for Preventing Sensory Alterations and for Stimulating the Senses

Preventive Measures	Stimulative Measures
Sight	
Protect eyes from injury.	Use calendars, television, newspapers to keep oriented.
Avoid eyestrain.	Have different colors in the environment.
Avoid rubbing eyes.	
Visit eye doctor as needed if client already has problems.	Be a "people watcher."
Hearing	
Avoid loud, excessive noises.	Use the telephone to maintain contacts.
Avoid putting sharp objects into the ears.	Use radio, television, tapes to stimulate mental activities.
Avoid excessive cleaning of the ears.	Develop sensitivity to different sounds.
Taste	
Practice oral hygiene.	Try different kinds of seasonings and food textures.
Avoid extreme temperatures in foods and drinks.	Think about favorite foods.
Avoid very spicy foods.	
Smell	
Avoid heavy-smelling perfumes or aftershave lotions.	Enjoy pleasant odors; avoid unpleasant smells.
Keep environment (home, room) well ventilated.	Think about pleasant or familiar smells.
Touch	
Avoid extreme temperatures on skin.	Ask for a hug or give one.
	Touch articles of different textures.

Based on McFarland, G. K., & McFarlane, E. A. (1989). *Nursing diagnosis and intervention: Planning for patient care.* St. Louis: C. V. Mosby.

the machines have controls that allow the volume of the alarm signals to be lowered. If this is possible it may be valuable, especially during the night when sleep is frequently interrupted. The avoidance of health care team members' standing in groups by the client's bedside and engaging in simultaneous conversations can reduce the number of voices and conversations heard by the client. Some critical care units provide ear plugs to the client in an attempt to reduce the sound level.

Visual stimulation in a critical care unit is usually also great. Bright lights often remain on 24 hours a day, lights blink on some pieces of equipment, cardiac patterns on monitors are visible, and there is much movement as nurses provide care to the critically ill. Dimming the lights when possible, use of eye shields, and drawing the curtain around the client may help to reduce visual stimulation.

Excessive pain is a source of overstimulation for clients who are institutionalized in any health care facility. Use of medications or other pain-relieving techniques as discussed in Chapter 7 is beneficial.

Explanation of machines, tubes, and monitors in simple terms can help to provide meaning to the vast array of unfamiliar items seen in a hospital environment.

When interacting with the client, the nurse should remain calm, use an unhurried approach, and speak in a low, modulated voice. Nurses must remember to acknowledge the client when coming to the bedside to check on equipment. Scheduling the same nurse to give care to the client each day promotes consistency and reduces the number of different caregivers or strangers whom the client meets. In addition, it is valuable to develop a routine plan of care that establishes times for activities such as eating, bathing, turning, coughing, and doing range-of-motion exercises. In this schedule there should be time allowed for uninterrupted periods of rest. Other ways to regulate sensory input include suggesting that staff and significant others increase tactile stimulation while decreasing auditory stimulation, and continuing to orient the client to reality. Limiting telephone calls and visitors may reduce some stimuli that contribute to distress.

■ Discharge Planning

The changes in hospital treatment modalities and interventions are extending to include changes in home care needs and services. The behavioral changes in hospitalized clients are expected and sometimes accepted because of the arenas for care and the sick role. Sensory deprivation and sensory overload in the home environment need to be considered in the context of the client's "real world."

The client with a known sensory/perceptual alteration is most vulnerable to sensory deprivation and sensory overload, but other clients should be identified as being at risk for these problems. Family members or significant others should be asked to assess the home

before the client's discharge for stimuli that are potential sources of difficulties for the client. Home visits by the community health nurse after the client is discharged should include ongoing assessment and should provide continuity in care for effective and compatible interventions related to stimuli and behaviors.

Clients and care providers may need to be taught skills related to home treatment with new technology or may need to relearn previously known skills that have been forgotten or changed because of hospitalization. Use of medications, monitoring health status, and maintaining activities of daily living become the responsibility of the client who may be overwhelmed by change and new tasks. Resources for care need to be mobilized and their use maximized to prevent or manage sensory deprivation and sensory overload in the home setting.

 Evaluation

To evaluate nursing care, the nurse considers the subjective and objective data and the goals for the client with alterations in the sensory/perceptual process related to sensory deprivation or sensory overload. The expected outcomes include that the client

1. Is receiving an optimal level of stimulation
2. Interprets sensory stimuli meaningfully
3. Is oriented to time, person, and place
4. Displays appropriate cognitive function
5. Maximizes use of nonaltered senses

Ongoing evaluation is required as responses and adaptations take place, stimuli and the environment change, and new goals are established by the client and the nurse.

SUMMARY

The sensory process is essential in maintaining self-awareness as well as awareness of others and the surrounding environment. Nurses should be knowledgeable about the behavioral manifestations that may occur when the sensory input levels are altered or when changes in perception occur. Nurses must continually assess the environment and the client for clues that sensory/perceptual changes are occurring. With ongoing assessment and related interventions, nurses can implement care that will provide optimal levels of sensory stimulation and enhance the meaning of incoming stimuli. Prevention, however, remains a major focus in planning client care for sensory deprivation and sensory overload.

IMPLICATIONS FOR RESEARCH

In the 1970s there was an abundance of research, and many articles were written about the alterations in behaviors that occur when an individual has sensory deprivation or sensory overload. Since that time, current research and literature in the field have been limited. As clients' needs and problems grow, both in hospitals and in home settings, the occurrence of sensory overload also may increase. While nurses become increasingly occupied with technologic aspects of care, interactions with the client as a person may be limited and may lead to feelings of deprivation in the client. Other areas for research could include sensory alterations in specific at-risk populations, which include clients with acquired immunodeficiency syndrome (AIDS), the homeless, and individuals undergoing same-day outpatient surgery. It is essential to continue research about sensory deprivation and sensory overload in individuals, groups, and communities to generate new ideas to promote health care.

The following questions are possible areas for further nursing research related to sensory alterations:

1. What input from nurses could help architects and decorators of health care facilities reduce sensory stimulation and sensory overload?

2. What questions could the nurse ask the client on admission to help identify clients who are more susceptible to sensory deprivation or sensory overload?

3. Which communication patterns are most helpful for the nurse to use when working with a client in an environment that is either overstimulating or understimulating?

4. How can intensive care unit procedures be modified to reduce the incidence of ICU psychosis?

5. Is there a relationship between the home environment of clients with sensory/perceptual alterations and sensory deprivation or sensory overload?

REFERENCES AND READINGS

Ball, C., & Barrie-Shevlin, L. (1985). Sensory deprivation. In D. O'Brian & S. Alexander (Eds.), *High dependency nursing care* (pp. 75–92). New York: Churchill Livingstone.

Ballard, K. (1981). Identification of environmental stressors in a surgical intensive care unit. *Issues in Mental Health Nursing, 3,* 89–108.

Bernardini, L. (1985). Effective communication as an intervention in the elderly client. *Topics in Clinical Nursing, 6,* 72–81.

Bolin, R. (1974). Sensory deprivation: An overview. *Nursing Forum, 13,* 240–258.

Chodil, J., & Williams, B. (1970). The concept of sensory deprivation. *Nursing Clinics of North America, 5,* 453–465.

Downs, F. (1974). Bed rest and sensory disturbances. *American Journal of Nursing, 74,* 434–438.

Gates, S. (1984). Helping your patient on bedrest cope with perceptual/sensory deprivation. *Orthopaedic Nursing, 3,* 35–38.

Gowan, N. (1979). The perceptual world of the intensive care unit: An overview of some environmental considerations in the helping relationship. *Heart and Lung, 8,* 340–344.

Hahn, K. (1989). Think twice about sensory loss. *Nursing '89, 19*(2), 97–99.

Jackson, C., & Ellis, R. (1971). Sensory deprivation as a field of study. *Nursing Research, 20,* 46–54.

Jurgens, A., Meehan, T. C., Wilson, H. L. (1987). Therapeutic touch as a nursing intervention. *Holistic Nursing Practice, 2*(1), 1–14.

Kopac, C. (1983). Sensory loss in the aged: The role of the nurse and the family. *Nursing Clinics of North America, 18,* 373–383.

MacKinnon-Kesler, S. (1983). Maximizing your ICU patient's sensory and perceptual environment. *Canadian Nurse, 79*(5), 41–45.

McFarland, G. K., & McFarlane, E. A. (1989). *Nursing diagnosis and intervention: Planning for patient care.* St. Louis: C. V. Mosby.

Moeller, T. P. (1988). Sensory changes in the elderly. *Dental Clinics of North America, 33*(1), 23–31.

Narrow, B., & Buschle, K. (1982). *Fundamentals of nursing practice.* New York: Wiley.

Neistadt, M. E. (1988). Occupational therapy for adults with perceptual deficits. *American Journal of Occupational Therapy, 42,* 434–440.

Noble, M. A. (1979). Communication in the ICU: Therapeutic or disturbing? *Nursing Outlook, 27,* 195–198.

Peduzzi, T. (Ed.). (1985). Alterations in sensory perception: Nursing implications [special issue]. *Topics in Clinical Nursing, 6*(4).

Roberts, S. (1976). *Behavioral concepts and the critically ill patient.* Englewood Cliffs, NJ: Prentice-Hall.

Roberts, S. (1978). *Behavioral concepts and nursing throughout the life span.* Englewood Cliffs, NJ: Prentice-Hall.

Taylor, C., Lellis, C., & LeMone, P. (1989). *Fundamentals of nursing; The art and science of nursing care.* Philadelphia: J. B. Lippincott.

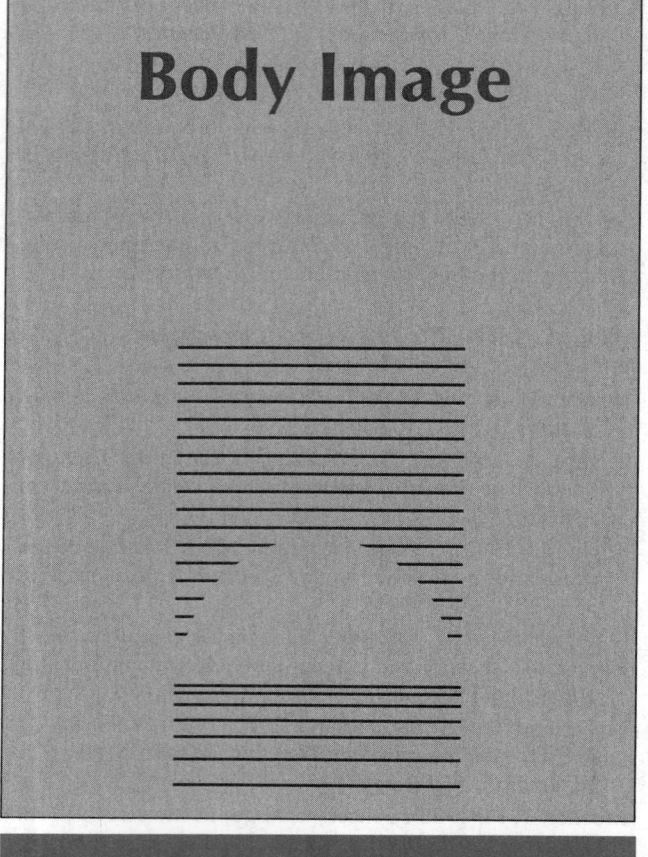

CHAPTER 9

Body Image

Self-concept is defined as the total collection of feelings a person has about himself or herself. Self-concept is the sum of self-esteem, role performance, and body image (Fig. 9–1). The concept of body image concerns both conscious and unconscious information, perceptions, and feelings about the body. Body image can also be influenced by the opinions of others. If the body image is definite and consistent with reality, the person is likely to feel satisfied with the self. When illness or chronic disability is present, it is a challenge for the physical body changes to be reintegrated into the new "image." Nursing, by diagnosing and treating responses to health problems in a holistic manner, is concerned about the total experience of body image development. Therefore, to assess client responses accurately, nursing must understand how illness can change the body image and its implications for practice. Nurses often care for clients during periods of illness that alter self-concept and body image. The nurse needs to be familiar with the concept of body image to enhance or facilitate the client's adjustment to body changes.

DEFINITIONS OF BODY IMAGE

Body image not only includes perceptions of shape, size, mass, function, structure, and significance of the physical, living body in relation to its parts, but also may include inanimate objects that are part of daily intimate contact with the body (e.g., make-up, jewelry, eyeglasses, clothing, wheelchair, crutches, or appliances). Body image is the internalized picture of all these factors (Hart, 1981). It is a complex concept that is difficult to assess in nursing practice and is influenced by many factors.

FACTORS AFFECTING BODY IMAGE

The perception of body image is influenced by several variables, including aging, culture, sex roles, and technology. American culture continues to place a major emphasis on the "ideal body"—youth, beauty, and agility. If one does not "fit" this social image, as the older adult often does not, a negative, unvalued message can be internalized. Therefore, the *normal aging process* can influence body image.

The role of *cultural influence* can also be significant in that through socialization, people learn to judge themselves in terms of how well they live up to the expectations and demands of the culture. It has been estab-

SHARING

THE HEART OF NURSING

This new nurse couldn't see beyond the technical aspects of nursing—until she uncovered the heart of her profession.

BY EVELYN A. OLYARNIK, RN
Staff Nurse
Metrohealth St. Luke's Medical Center
Cleveland, Ohio

WHEN I STARTED nursing, I was overwhelmed by all the tubes, drains, and machines. Each one seemed more complicated than the one I'd mastered the day before. *Nursing school didn't prepare me for this,* I thought. *Maybe a course in engineering would have served me better.* My frustration had nearly reached its peak when one of my co-workers put things into perspective for me.

We were caring for Mr. Bain, an 82-year-old patient who'd been admitted to our unit from a nursing home. He had coffee-ground residuals in his gastrostomy tube, and his doctor suspected a slow gastrointestinal bleed. Because he'd been admitted previously for a lengthy hospitalization, we knew him well.

During his first admission, Mr. Bain appeared healthy. His rosy cheeks and blue eyes belied any traces of ill health. Although a previous stroke had left him unable to speak, he had a special smile reserved for his wife's daily visits.

But this time, he was thinner, tired, and even his eyes were pale. "I don't think he'd want to go on like this," said his wife. She asked that no heroic measures be taken to save him.

One Friday, our staff learned that Mr. Bain wasn't expected to live past the weekend. He was my patient that day, so during late rounds my co-worker Barb and I checked him. He was dead.

We knew that Mrs. Bain was scheduled to arrive for her daily visit. So we discontinued the I.V. lines, urinary catheter, gastrostomy tube, and oxygen. Then I opened the nightstand drawer to gather Mr. Bain's few belongings—two pairs of socks, a hairbrush, and a bottle of after-shave lotion.

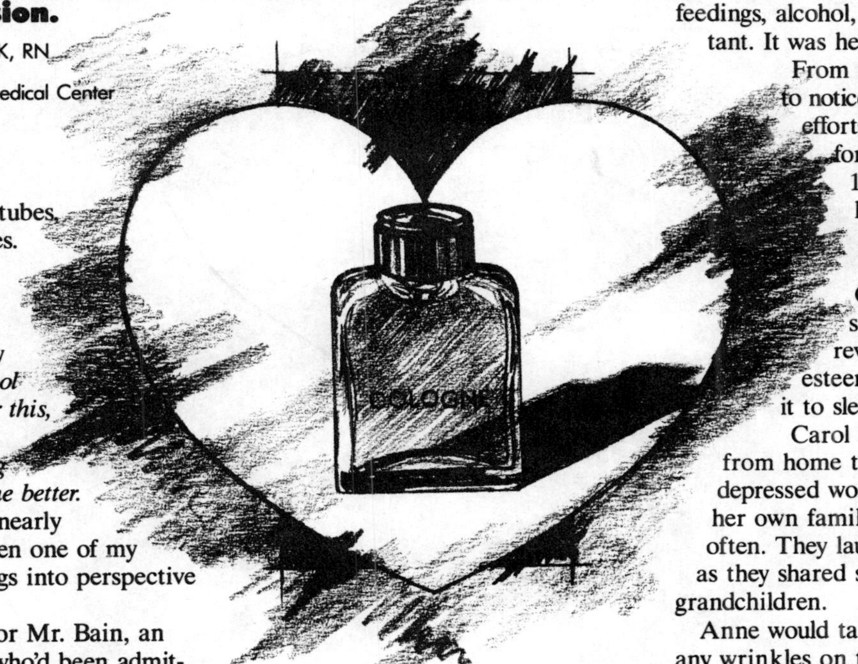

When Barb saw the after-shave lotion, she asked for it, then put some on Mr. Bain's face and neck. I didn't think it made much difference now that he was dead, but I didn't say anything.

A few moments later, Mrs. Bain arrived. When she saw her husband, she knew he was gone. She walked to his side and leaned toward his cheek to kiss him good-bye. But before she did, she closed her eyes and sniffed the air. Then she smiled.

When the moment passed, Mrs. Bain opened her eyes, and kissed her husband gently. "Thank you for every day you've given me," she said to him.

Watching this elderly woman part with the man she'd loved for more than 60 years, I knew why Barb had put the after-shave on Mr. Bain's neck. She wanted to leave Mrs. Bain with the memory of her husband's special smell—not the smell of tube feedings, alcohol, soap, or disinfectant. It was her gift to Mrs. Bain.

From that day on, I began to notice more of the special efforts nurses were making for their patients. The 19-year old man who'd had a craniotomy and was so ashamed of his bald head? Gail gave him a sports cap, instantly reviving his self-esteem. (He even wore it to sleep.)

Carol brought in pictures from home to encourage a depressed woman to talk about her own family, who couldn't visit often. They laughed together as they shared stories of their grandchildren.

Anne would take pains to remove any wrinkles on the beds and even rearrange her patients' rooms for them so they could feel special.

And where did the unusual variety of magazines in the patient and visitor lounges come from? Nurses—they'd brought them from home.

Yes, I discovered quickly that nursing is more than monitoring equipment and administering medications. It's the special empathy and caring each nurse brings to work with her—the willingness to do more for her patients than what's expected.

So machines no longer worry me. I'm too busy trying to do something extra for my patients. ∎

DO YOU HAVE A NURSING EXPERIENCE YOU'D LIKE TO SHARE? We'll award $100 for each manuscript selected for publication, and where suitable, we'll change circumstances to protect the anonymity of those concerned. Submit entries in typewritten form and allow 8 weeks for the Editorial Board's decision.

TOM MILLER

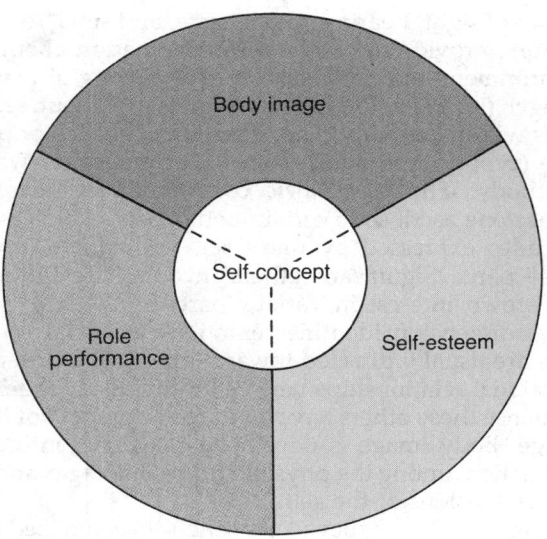

Figure 9–1

Relationship of self-concept to its components. Self-concept is the sum of self-esteem, role performance, and body image.

lished that American culture is notorious for placing a high value on physical appearance and individual popularity with peers. If one does not meet these expectations, one is perceived less favorably. For example, the obese adult may be the brunt of cruel jokes from those seated close by at a baseball game. Therefore, negative attitudes of others can contribute to the creation of a poor body image.

Societal sex roles play a major role in body image and how it develops. Even though the women's movement has had a tremendous impact on increased awareness and appreciation of the female role, a definite process remains in place for the socialization of boys and girls. Young girls continue to be dressed in pink and young boys are dressed in blue. Definite sex role messages continue to be prevalent that also influence body image

and its development. Even at young ages, children mimic sex-typed behaviors.

In the last decade, there have been an unbelievable number of *technological developments* in health care. Heart, kidney, and liver transplants are common; the artificial heart is becoming more accepted. Never before has there been such replacement of the parts of the human body! These advances have implications for the perception and reintegration of body image; however, these implications are not clearly understood.

THEORIES OF BODY IMAGE DEVELOPMENT

The image one has of the body develops and changes continuously throughout the life span. This development is related to how the body changes physically and emotionally. Body image development is also the result of integration of both internal and external stimuli, and it progresses chronologically.

People harbor many different conceptions of self, which are each weighed and may change over time and within situations, depending on a variety of factors, such as hospitalization, immobilization, or amputation. These factors can play an important part in the development of body image.

THEORIES OF SELF-CONCEPT

There are several theoretical bases for the development of the self-concept. Sullivan (1947) interpreted an individual's uniqueness as resulting from interpersonal influences. These unique characteristics, "good-me," "bad-me," and "not-me," are organized in approximately the middle of the infancy period and begin the

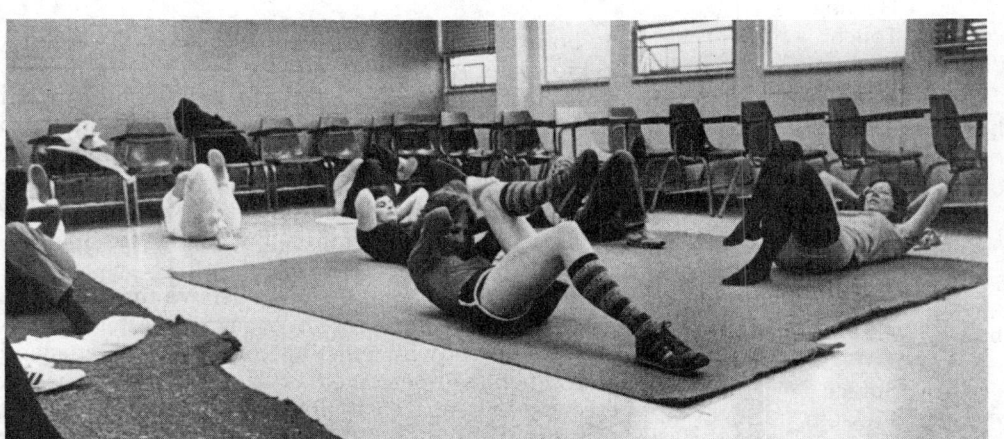

Figure 9–2

Society's emphasis on the ideal body encourages people to get into shape. Aerobics classes are popular for all ages. (Courtesy of the University of North Carolina at Chapel Hill School of Nursing.)

personality development. The concept of "good-me," or "I am good," in the infant becomes entangled with a growing awareness of the physical body. As a result, the self develops as an interaction of good-me with positive experiences of the infant. An example of a positive experience is consistent parental love being provided to the infant. Therefore, life experiences contribute to the development of a positive self-concept. Because body image is a component of self-concept, body image is also affected in a positive way.

Self theory has evolved further through the work of Maslow. Maslow's (1954) self-actualization theory organized human needs into a hierarchy in which physiologic or survival needs take precedence over esteem and self-actualization. Furthermore, a self-actualized person has high regard for others, therefore exhibiting self-acceptance. Self-actualized individuals accept their shortcomings and live comfortably with them. In this respect, one is comfortable with one's own body image and exhibits a sense of oneness, and thereby cares about others. Maslow confirmed that satisfaction of the self-esteem need leads to feelings of self-confidence, worth, strength, capability, and adequacy. If the self-esteem need is not satisfied, feelings of inferiority, weakness, and helplessness are produced. If body image and self are given negative feedback, self-esteem needs are not met, thereby creating a negative perception of both.

The concept of body image in relation to self was also clarified by Schilder (1950). Schilder interpreted body image as composed of three separate dimensions: physiologic, psychologic, and social. The *physiologic* dimension involves the central nervous system and sensory receptors (Table 9–1). Sensory receptors allow one to accumulate knowledge about the relationships of different parts of the surface of the body to each other. The senses of sight, hearing, touch, taste, and smell (exteroceptors) provide the body with information about the environment and body surface. The feeling of pain or hunger (interoceptors) sends a message about sensations within the body. The sensation of stretch or pressure (proprioceptors) identifies deep messages within the body. The *psychologic* component includes the values one ascribes to certain body parts as well as the attitudes expressed by one's self and others toward these parts. Significant others in one's life influence one's own interest in various parts of the body. The *social* dimension identifies emotions as social in that they are usually directed toward others. The closer the emotional relationships between individuals, the more influence these others have on the development of body image. Body image is developed through continuous interaction among the physiologic, psychologic, and social dimensions of the self.

Rogers (1961) believed that the self-actualized person demonstrates an openness to experience in which reality is seen without distortion. The self is comfortably discovered through life experiences. This open approach to life develops trust. By trusting one's self, an individual becomes self-accepting and looks less to others for approval or disapproval. However, in cases of negative life experiences, one might develop less trust, become less self-accepting, and therefore develop problems with body image and self.

Fischer and Cleveland (1968) identified body image in terms of *body boundary*. This concept refers to the perception of the boundary between the body and the rest of the world. Adults, by virtue of more life experiences, have a clearly delineated body boundary, although this boundary does not end precisely where the body ends and is likely to include inanimate objects. Fischer and Cleveland found that the more definite one's body boundary is, the more likely one is able to function independently, have high achievement motivation, and be goal directed, active, and communicative with others.

TABLE 9–1 Schilder's Physiologic Dimension of Concept of Body Image in Relation to Self

Receptor	Source	Sensations
Exteroceptors	Environment or body surface	Sight Hearing Touch Taste Smell
Interoceptors	Within the body	Pain Hunger Nausea Excretion/ voiding Sexual excitement
Proprioceptors	Within the body	Position of body in space Stretch Pressure

THE LIFE CYCLE OF BODY IMAGE

The body attempts to achieve consistency throughout the life cycle. Any life experience or change that does not meet or match this established, consistent life model creates increasing anxiety, which results in resistance to change. However, body image does readjust and adapt through interaction with significant others and the environment. Body image development is an ongoing process of learning and maturation that changes as one progresses through the cycle of life.

Most developmental theorists believe that development of self-concept does not occur until after birth. A baby has no body image at birth; that is, the fetus and environment are perceived as one, and the self is not perceived as a separate entity. Therefore, body image is not present. Kolb (1959) presented an opposing view that sensory feedback from the environment is perceived by the fetus in the uterus. It is known that the fetus reacts to sounds and music before birth. However, the actual development of body image in the fetus has not been clearly determined by research.

INFANCY (BIRTH TO 1 YEAR OF AGE)

The infant at birth does not distinguish between different internal stimuli, e.g., pain and hunger. Gradually, the infant begins to identify feelings of discomfort and to distinguish them from other feelings. The same process of identification occurs with regard to all internal stimuli, and as a result the infant learns to trust the body and begins to understand its signals.

The kinesthetic and tactile senses are the first to complete myelinization and therefore are important to the development of body perception. Infants touch not only themselves but also many other things and people in their environment. Touch verifies the infant's own existence and assists in defining the body image and differentiating self from nonself. The mouth is usually the first area that is stimulated, by sucking and feeding. In essence, body image is born or originates at the oral area.

Differentiation occurs during the first year of life when infants begin to see themselves as separate from the environment. Rocking and crawling behaviors provide stimuli and feedback to the infant to help form a body image that is separate from the environment.

TODDLERHOOD (1 TO 3 YEARS OF AGE)

The infant matures to toddlerhood. Language begins the identification of specific body parts and further developing body image. Through various activities (e.g., toilet training, dressing), the toddler learns that certain body parts are valued differently. In addition, the toddler can distinguish self from nonself and has learned to trust feelings. These values are acquired primarily from significant others surrounding the child, as well as from experiences of pleasure or pain derived from body parts. However, the toddler perceives larger body limits: Feces, urine, fingernails, and hair are considered to be parts of the body, and their removal can cause great distress. The conditioning process can strongly influence the child at this age, but little research has been conducted on body image development in the toddler.

PRESCHOOL YEARS (3 TO 6 YEARS OF AGE)

As the young child develops physically, body image changes. This is the age at which development of sexual identity occurs. Children can identify their sex and are aware of how different they are from each other. Attitudes and responses of significant others can again contribute to body image at this stage.

Preschoolers may begin to form the ideal image of how they would like to look as adults. Through various sensorimotor activities, body concepts are learned. The preschooler enjoys dressing up as a beautiful princess or an ugly monster, or playing the roles of mommy and daddy. These activities provide more structure for the concepts of pretty, ugly, normal, and different.

MIDDLE CHILDHOOD (6 TO 12 YEARS OF AGE)

Children of elementary school age have a considerable amount of knowledge about the function and structure of their bodies. Young children imagine their bodies as hollow containers for blood, food, and wastes. Seven-year-old children should be able to draw a recognizable human figure, but individual body parts are drawn according to the child's knowledge and understanding of the body part. Arms and hands may not be integrated into body image as consistently as are the head, trunk, and legs.

Research has identified three body types or configurations and the personality traits most often associated with them. These types are *endomorph* — heavyset, sociable, friendly, relaxed; *mesomorph* — sturdy, well-developed bone and muscle, vigorous, energetic, assertive; *ectomorph* — thin, slender, inhibited, private. The stereotyping of these three types begins during the elementary school age period. Young children rate the mesomorph most positively and the endomorph most negatively. However, this rating changes as children age.

During these years, peer relationships and adherence to social group norms are emphasized. This peer pressure centers on physical appearance. Children use as models parents, peers, and television and movie stars. Anyone who is different from these models (e.g., heavy, thin, wears glasses or braces) is criticized and teased. This teasing may be detrimental to body image development. Children who are teased may be less satisfied with their bodies as adults. However, no connection has been found between life satisfaction and childhood beauty.

ADOLESCENCE (12 TO 18 YEARS OF AGE)

The adolescent undergoes many physical changes, both external and internal. By late adolescence, all body parts have reached their final form and size. The physical changes associated with sexual development give rise to an intense awareness of and preoccupation with the body. Adolescents often compare themselves with others, exhibit concern about whether they are normal, and exhibit exaggerated modesty. Slimness and the "perfect body" can become an obsession. Any amount of excess weight is considered to be undesirable and ugly. Clothes become an important social statement and can reveal one's view of self. It is common for adolescents to feel dissatisfied with a particular facial feature, often the nose, which becomes more pronounced as adult features emerge. Acne, for some adolescents, may be quite distressing and can result in withdrawal from social contacts.

Adolescents are often confused by their sexual feelings. There is considerable pressure on American adolescents to act on these feelings. Those who do not may question whether they are sexually normal. Menstruation, seminal emissions, and erections at inopportune times can cause adolescents to feel that their bodies are unreliable. In addition, if adolescents are conditioned by their external environments to feel disgust for their bodies, body image development may be negatively influenced. Body image, at this stage, can be quite troublesome.

YOUNG ADULTHOOD (18 TO 40 YEARS OF AGE)

As body image becomes more stable over time and positive, with a view of liking one's self, young adults are concerned mainly with developing intimate relationships with others. Without these, one experiences a feeling of isolation. It is necessary for adults to have a firm sense of identity at this point. Young adulthood continues to be a time for change, although the biologic changes of adolescence are completed. A healthy and realistic body image requires positive social reinforcement. Individuals become what others tell them they are. Young adults not only need to define the self but also need to be defined by others. Stereotyping is common. People generally believe that different temperaments go with different body physiques. For example, the man with graying hair and sturdy figure may be seen as distinguished. Height is often associated with leadership ability in men, and heaviness sometimes connotes joviality. This social reinforcement can strongly influence body image development.

Certain personal characteristics seem to be more crucial to body image than others. Sexual identification is central to self-concept, and any circumstance that alters this identification can affect body image. For example, the client who experiences a mastectomy may begin to question her sexuality and femininity. Am I still desirable and attractive? Am I still a woman? Who am I? How individuals view their bodies can be strongly influenced by sexuality concerns and changes. Body image develops and changes as the physical body changes.

The kind of work in which the adult engages is another characteristic that influences body image. One's essence may center on a career as nurse, artist, musician, or farmer. Injury, illness, or early retirement may require total readjustment of the body image. The musician who no longer is able to play an instrument because of amputation must readjust and adapt to the "new" image of the body. The artist who becomes blind is also challenged with the developmental task of body image readjustment.

Women seem to have clearer and more accurate images of their bodies than men. Women tend to equate body more with self and are more aware of physical changes, especially around the face. The role of women as nurturer and mother is more closely identified with the body. Men tend to be much less specific in how they view their bodies because their role relates more to life accomplishments and attaining power and position in their careers than to their bodies (Fischer, 1964).

THE MIDDLE YEARS (40 TO 65 YEARS OF AGE)

During the middle years, because of the psychologic and physical changes of normal aging, the body image has a potential for becoming more negative. The extent of these negative feelings depends on one's personality and level of satisfaction with life up to that point. Many adults view these changes as evidence of maturity, experience, and knowledge, and thus these changes may not cause a negative body image. However, normal aging requires ongoing readjustment of body image. This readjustment can be adaptive or maladaptive.

The current interest in the United States in health maintenance and "keeping in shape" may influence body image development. Many adults participate in regular exercise programs, which may slow the normal physical aging process that results in loss of tissue collagen and rearrangement of adipose tissue.

The adult who lacks confidence and cannot reintegrate the aging, changing body may attempt to capture or mimic youth by the use of cosmetics, clothes, or hair styles. If the physical appearance continues to be perceived negatively, despite the use of cosmetics, the negative body image may result in depression, irritability, and anxiety. The middle years adult who has successfully developed a realistic body image accepts the self and the body, while realizing that acceptance from others cannot be expected unless self-acceptance is present. For the middle years adult, body image continues to develop as interaction with the environment becomes more complex.

THE LATER YEARS (MORE THAN 65 YEARS OF AGE)

No matter when older adults begin to consider themselves elderly, they tend to undergo a marked change in self-concept and body image. This change is due to thinking of self as dependent and declining instead of independent and aspiring. It is often thought that older adults are not valued members of society. Historically, the social context of aging has been negative in the United States.

Sensory deficits resulting from normal aging are common in the older adult and may decrease the ability to participate in social functions or to enjoy hobbies such as reading or listening to music. Decreased strength and increased fatigue may reduce the ability to remain a productive, active worker. These lost abilities may lead to feelings of worthlessness and despair, which influ-

Janelli, L. M. (1988). The impact of health status on body image in older women. *Rehabilitation Nursing, 13*(4), 178–180.

NURSING RESEARCH

Chronic Health Problems Can Negatively Affect the Older Woman's Perception of Body Image.

Normal aging changes may affect the older person's body image, but chronic illness may be a major threat. This exploratory study was conducted to examine the relationship between health status and body image perception in older women. Subjects were selected from long-term care, intermediate care, and adult day care facilities. A total of 150 women, aged 60 to 98 years, participated.

Three instruments were used: the Body-cathexis-Self-cathexis Scale (BcSc) and Draw a Person (DAP) were used to measure body image perception; the Physical Health Spectrum was used to measure physical health. Analysis of variance was used to analyze the relationship between body image perception and physical health. A significant difference was found in women who had no physical problems, as they were more satisfied with their body parts.

Critique. There was no strong support for the relationship between health status and body image perception as measured by these scales. The small sample size limits generalizability. Only women were studied.

Possible nursing implications. Nurses working with older women should be aware of the signs of rejection of body image—withdrawal or depression. Nurses can actively listen to clients and provide support for older women to help them realistically accept their body image.

ence the body image. In addition, events that can affect body image and self-concept are retirement, loss of a spouse, and loss of other close family members and friends (for further discussion, see Chap. 5).

Many older adults decide to retain the behavior patterns of and identification with the middle-aged adult. These older adults may become conscious of aging and intentionally avoid assuming the social and emotional characteristics of the aged (e.g., frailty, immobility, isolation). For these elderly persons, an effort is made to maintain previous roles and activities, and the body image does not require readjustment.

ALTERATIONS IN BODY IMAGE

Illness, whether chronic or acute, can change external body appearance and function. These changes can be devastating to body image development. Chronic illness is more disabling, as it requires continuous body image reintegration as the disease process continues. Stimuli

associated with illness or injury promote continual awareness of body image. For example, a client suffering from a stroke is reminded daily of the mobility and/or communication deficits that the illness has caused. As a result, the client continuously attempts to reintegrate not only the current body changes into the body image, but also the ever-present fear of future immobility or communication losses that can result from further strokes (see the accompanying Nursing Research feature).

Two major types of boundary or image disturbances are most commonly exhibited in illness (McCloskey, 1976): (1) the body wall changes either through accident or surgery but the client retains the previous body boundary, and (2) even though the client's body wall remains intact and whole, the client changes the body boundary, such as with the occurrence of a stroke. For example, body boundary disturbances are demonstrated by phantom limb pain or maladjustment to a mastectomy. The client still extends the boundary of the body to where the limb or breast used to be. The body wall includes the actual physical interpretation of body parts. The body boundary consists of the mental interpretation and placement of body parts. These two portions must be integrated to consolidate a new body image in response to a change. If they are not, body image disturbances occur.

THEORIES RELATED TO READJUSTMENT TO BODY IMAGE DISTURBANCE

The process that occurs during body image readjustment is a lengthy transition that evolves over time and does not occur at the time of injury or illness. Stages of this adaptation process include (1) psychologic shock, (2) withdrawal, (3) acknowledgment, and (4) integration (Fig. 9–3).

Psychologic shock is often the initial emotional reaction to the impact of the life change when one first becomes aware of a problem. This shock may occur at the time of the injury or illness or at a later date when body changes are seen or experienced more readily. Psychologic shock is a defense mechanism that is used in reaction to anxiety. Information is filtered and reality is distorted to the point that change can be handled. For some individuals, this reaction takes the form of selective deafness, and only so much information is filtered in so that coping remains effective. For example, the client who is a newly diagnosed diabetic may be noncompliant with the diet but may administer to herself or himself daily insulin injections. The client selects adherence to a daily insulin injection program but is unable to give up daily desserts or large meals. This is what the client at this stage is able to cope with. For others, discouragement and despair are projected to others as anger and hostility. Projection produces less anxiety than directing the anger inward.

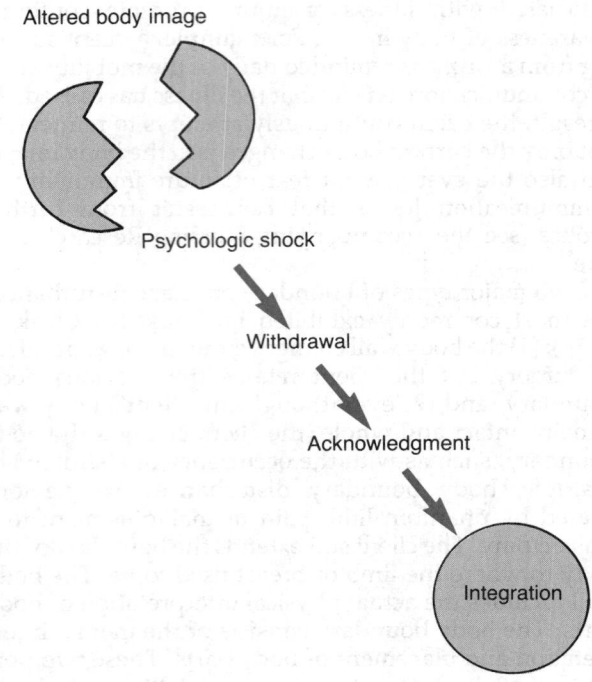

Altered body image

Psychologic shock

Withdrawal

Acknowledgment

Integration

Figure 9-3

Readjustment to altered body image. Stages of the adaptation process include psychologic shock, withdrawal, acknowledgment, and integration.

Withdrawal is the next stage in the readjustment process. Once the client becomes aware of the injury or illness and begins to think about the future, he or she may feel an overwhelming desire to run away from the reality of the situation. Because this is not physically possible, emotional retreat serves as a coping mechanism. This withdrawal provides an opportunity for the client to replenish physical and psychologic energies used during the emotional shock phase. The client may become passive and dependent and lack motivation or interest in becoming involved in the plan of care.

Gradually, *acknowledgment* occurs when the client recognizes the change in body image. Once the loss or change is acknowledged, the client can begin mourning (see Chap. 11). The client may contemplate the meaning of the change and its implications for his or her future. This acknowledgment allows the client to view the body change itself to begin reintegration of the body image.

Integration is the long and difficult process of adapting to changes in body image. The client thinks about future life changes and experiences that will be different as a result of the body change and identifies ways to manage or deal with these. Many times the stage of integration can create a new meaning about the loss of the body part for the client, and emotional growth occurs. As a result of integration of the body changes into a new image, the client will regain a sense of fulfillment. However, the total process of change, from initial impact to adaptation, can be long and painful and is different for each individual.

RESEARCH

The experience of altered body image is one that is most commonly associated with loss of body parts. It is known that any type of loss (of mobility, independence, or body part) necessitates some body image readjustment. However, research has not clarified how a client perceives the body image after a loss and how this perception relates to the emotional component of body image.

The normal human condition centers on the ability and drive to be mobile. Mobility is of such fundamental importance that healthy adults, even during resting periods, turn or change position frequently. Mobility enables the client to exert control over or influence his or her environment, and this control is threatened when mobility is restricted or lost.

The degree of immobilization can vary from minor loss or decrease in range of motion of a limited body area to a more complete loss of mobility, when the body is capable of little or no purposeful movement. Immobility, whether temporary or permanent, is viewed by the client as a loss and can influence body image. This loss and the life style changes incurred as a result can threaten the survival of the immobilized client. In this respect, body image in relation to immobility can have a considerable impact on nursing practice. (Refer to Chap. 21 for further information.)

Illness is also associated with the experience of pain. Pain can play a role in body image development (refer to Chap. 7 on pain). The impact of illness and pain on body image reintegration can be overwhelming for the client who is attempting to cope with these changes. If severe pain continues, the painful body part can become isolated from the rest of the body to the point that it becomes alienated from the body image (Schilder, 1950).

Researchers have studied how individuals with cancer view their bodies. Cancer can change the way people feel about their personal appearance. Alopecia, or hair loss, that occurs during the treatment of disease is an important factor. Baxley et al. (1984) showed that cancer clients with alopecia have a lower self-image than cancer clients without alopecia. For these clients, alopecia is seen as a constant reminder of their disease. Therefore, the experience of cancer and resulting hair loss can affect the body image.

For any client, the anticipation of surgery, whether as treatment for cancer or for another illness, can create a fear of mutilation, anxiety, and an unrealistic image about the body. Facial disfigurement resulting from surgical treatment of head and neck cancer causes severe body image disturbances. Body image alterations also develop after mastectomy (Gillies, 1984). For most women, a mastectomy results in a loss of a body part that is viewed as essential for maintaining femininity, attractiveness, and self-esteem. This loss is based on the belief that the female breast is an idealized symbol that connotes a feminine, mothering image.

Body image alterations are also common after the

surgical creation of an ostomy. These alterations can result from the client's perception about the appearance of the stoma, as well as from the reaction to the stoma by the client's significant others. The stoma is equated with the genital region and the exposure and direct handling of the stoma can be especially damaging to a healthy body image (Gillies, 1984). For body image to remain healthy, its readjustment must be realistic in terms of the actual physical changes that resulted from surgery. There must be an acceptance of the body as it is or has become. For example, the client with an ostomy needs to recognize that the stoma is present, that it was probably lifesaving, and that it serves the same purpose as the bowel tract and rectum. This recognition is realistic. The client may experience many feelings about this body change but is not denying that it has occurred.

Limb amputation or any type of paralysis also requires body image reintegration. Phantom limb pain and paraplegia create different body perceptions, which necessitate body image reintegration (Evans, 1977). There are contradictory perceptual images of the body—that is, the limb is gone but pain continues, or the limb remains but no feeling is present. Deformity is a physical change that requires adaptation of the body image because of the changed physical appearance. A deformity may also not have a socially acceptable appearance. Reintegration of these body changes presents a challenge to healthy body image development.

Obesity and other eating disorders commonly reflect body image disturbances. Obese clients have a tendency to overestimate their body size, both during and after weight loss, which results in the perception of themselves as having lost no weight even after dieting has produced a significant weight loss (Glucksman & Hirsch, 1969). In addition, negative social connotations of obesity contribute to feelings that create a negative body image.

Anorectic clients may also experience confused feelings about body image. For example, the adolescent focused on a "perfect body" may go to extremes with dieting to achieve it. However, even after becoming extremely underweight, clients may not view themselves as thin.

COLLABORATIVE MANAGEMENT

 Assessment

History

To assess and understand body image, the nurse must collect data about how the client has adapted to a body change (Table 9–2). Nursing assessment focuses on obtaining data that identify the *client's view of self*. As the client shares information about body image, the nurse is better able to diagnose body image disturbance and its cause. The nurse gathers these data by inquiring about the client's recent physical body change. Is this

---

TABLE 9–2   Assessment Guidelines for History Related to Body Image

Specific factors to include when taking a history are

The client's view of self: "How would you describe your body to another person?"

The client's and/or family's perceived body change

The client's developmental level

The client's and/or family's past successful coping strategies

The client's current occupation or work history

The client's past experience with pain

The client's environment

---

perceived positively or negatively? What feelings does this change create? Are current feelings a change from feelings before this illness? Does the client describe herself or himself as hopeful or helpless?

After the assessment of the client's view of self, the nurse must identify the *client's and/or family's perception of the body change*. It is important to assess both client and family perceptions because they may conflict and lend insight into further assessment and intervention. For example, do the client and family understand the actual physiologic surgical alteration? Is the body change perceived a certain way (lifesaving, positive, or negative)? What does this mean to them?

When assessing body image disturbance, it is also necessary to take into account the *client's developmental level*. An adult client may be functioning only as a young child. Therefore, the client's body image may not be developed to the level of an adult, and certain expectations will not be appropriate. Developmental level may be assessed by evaluating previous responses of the client to questions and the client's affect during the interview, body language, and maturity of responses. For example, does the client give inconsistent verbal responses to questions? Does the client have poor eye contact? Is the client unable to answer some questions because he or she does not understand?

Identification of the *client's and/or family's past successful coping strategies* is also necessary to establish baseline data regarding coping behaviors. These strategies can be assessed by asking: "How have you dealt with hard times in your life in the past?" "What did you do in the past that helped you get through them?" "Have you been doing some of these same things this time?" "Do you think that these things might help you now?"

The *client's current occupation or work history* can lend further insight into his or her image of self and the body. For example, is the client currently employed, laid off, fired, or retired? Does this work situation create any negative feelings or problems? Does the client anticipate return to work, or is he or she not currently working? Does the client feel useful?

Body image assessment must also include data about the *client's past experience with pain.* Has the client ever experienced pain before? Was this pain chronic or acute? Did this pain control the client's life? What caused the pain? How did the client deal with the pain? Were friends and/or family supportive about the pain? Did the pain change the client's life in any way? The nurse assesses the client's pain experience regardless of whether it is a past or current problem.

As well as assessing the client and family, the nurse must also collect data regarding the *client's immediate environment.* The environment includes immediate physical environment at home, social supports, and community. Does the client have easy access to follow-up care? Is the home environment conducive to self-care needs (e.g., one-level versus two-level home, steps into home, bathroom and bedroom locations)? Is the community supportive of this client's needs (e.g., are there wheelchair ramps, easy transportation)? By collecting all this information, the nurse can assess body image disturbances more accurately.

Physical Assessment: Clinical Manifestations

The nurse completes a collection of data concerning body changes. The North American Nursing Diagnosis Association (NANDA) identifies the following objective clinical manifestations for assessment of body image disturbance. Although they have not been clinically validated by research, they provide direction for nursing assessment (Hurley, 1986).

1. Missing body part
2. Actual change in structure or function
3. Not looking at body part
4. Not touching body part
5. Hiding or overexposing body part (intentional or unintentional)
6. Trauma to nonfunctioning part
7. Change in social involvement
8. Change in ability to estimate spatial relationship of body to environment

An obvious client characteristic that the nurse considers when assessing body image disturbance is *missing body parts.* The experience of a loss of any body part can pose definite challenges to the client attempting to redefine the new image of the body. Therefore, this characteristic may predispose the client to the development of body image disturbance. It is also important to be aware that a client born without a specific body part has not experienced this loss and may not demonstrate a body image disturbance. However, the physical body loss may not always be obvious to the nurse. In this case, the nurse inquires about past surgery experienced and prosthesis used and observes the physical body for scars, disfigurement, or extremity loss. For all clients, the nurse must include an assessment of religious practices because a certain religion may dictate special management

of the removed body part. Following this practice can be crucial to the client in the process of readjustment to a new body image.

Specific *changes in body structure or function* are also major physical losses that the nurse must assess. Any changes in mobility, self-care, or previous level of independence can create difficulty for body image reintegration. The client experiencing recent confinement to a wheelchair or permanent dependence on a walker or cane for mobility purposes may need specific nursing intervention to understand the new body image. It is important for the nurse to ask about the client's perception of this change in function, as it may not be perceived as a loss by the client. Is this a recent change for the client? Is this a significant change from previous function before this illness?

Objective data that the nurse collects concern the clients and how they may view their body. *Not looking at or not touching the body or body part* may indicate an altered body image. However, this characteristic alone is not enough to verify the existence of body image disturbance. The client may avoid viewing the surgical site of an amputation for a postoperative period because of discomfort related to observing any surgical incision or drainage. As the surgical area becomes more healed, the client may have no difficulty viewing or touching the amputation area. This clinical manifestation must be interpreted carefully.

Another example of these clinical manifestations is the client who has experienced a stroke with paralysis of the right arm. The client may ignore the right arm to the extreme that he or she hits it on door frames when entering rooms because of the loss of sensation. This form of ignoring a body part is called *neglect* and indicates other cognitive or perceptual deficits that may or may not affect body image. Again, these data are reviewed carefully by the nurse.

Hiding or overexposing any body part, whether it be intentional or unintentional, may also indicate difficulty with body image readjustment. The client recovering from a mastectomy or limb amputation may experience shame, guilt, anger, or disgust about the body alteration. As a result, the client may hide or even overexpose the changed body area in attempts to deal with this change.

The nurse must also assess the client for any *trauma that may have occurred to a nonfunctioning body part.* For example, an injury or trauma to a flaccid extremity, originally caused by a past stroke, may cause old or new feelings to surface as a result of the need to adapt to the new body image. The client struggles with these thoughts: Is my paralyzed arm worse now? Has it become more useless? The past body changes may have been successfully reintegrated into a new body image. However, the new injury to the past nonfunctioning extremity may pose a new threat to the body image, resulting in a need for further body image adaptation.

Changes in past social involvement and activities may demonstrate a potential body image disturbance. As the client may fail to reintegrate the body changes into a new image, feelings of helplessness, nonvalue, or shame may surface. As a result, the client may choose to

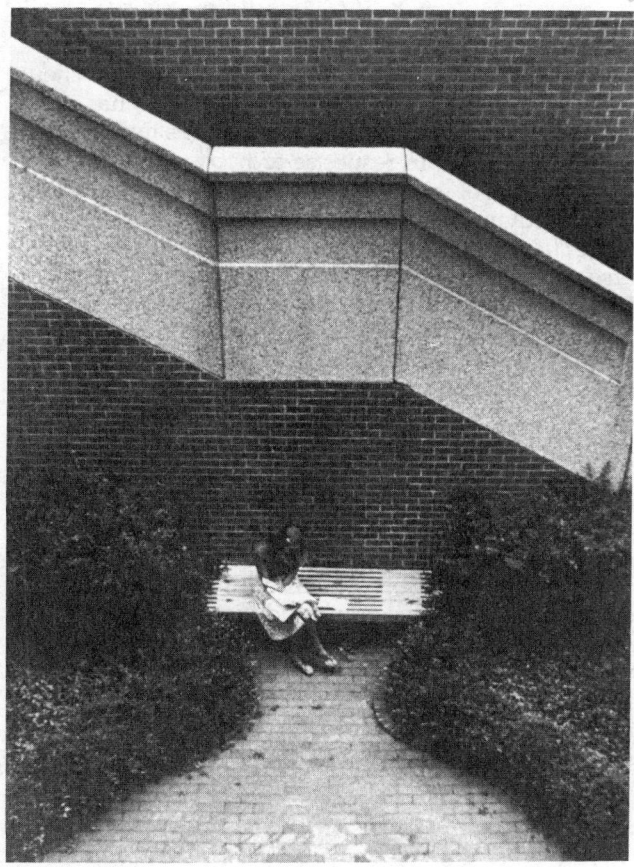

Figure 9–4

The client may choose not to interact socially if he or she fails to integrate body changes into a new image. (Courtesy of the University of North Carolina at Chapel Hill School of Nursing.)

reduce social interactions. In addition, the client's ability or access to attend social functions needs to be assessed. If the client is confined to a wheelchair, are there both public transportation and building access for these needs? What are the limitations to wheelchair access in the client's home?

In cases of body image disturbance, the client may be *unable to estimate the spatial relationships of the body to the rest of the environment.* This inability to separate body from environment is a change from a previous ability and is not due to the disease process (e.g., cognitive changes resulting from a stroke). Clients may become so confused about their body boundary, e.g., because of loss of an extremity, that they are unable to identify where the body ends and the surrounding environment begins. For example, the client who has experienced a severe stroke with resulting right-sided paralysis and cognitive and visual disturbances may attempt to move from a bed to a chair. In this attempt, the client misses the chair completely because his or her right visual field is blocked. In addition, the client cannot perceive his or her right side as separate from the rest of the

environment (e.g., chair, bed, or commode). These disturbances also influence the client's coping abilities because cognition is also affected.

Although NANDA does not identify an additional objective characteristic for body image assessment, the *presence of pain* is important to include in data collection. Pain may become incorporated into the body as a normal, day-to-day experience, such as in the case of chronic pain. By objectively assessing the client's pain, the nurse is better able to clearly understand the individual client's body image development and the possible impact of illness or injury. The nurse objectively records the client's pain behavior, such as moaning; rubbing the painful body part; tossing; making fatigued facial expressions; and refusing to participate in the treatment regimen because of pain.

Psychosocial Assessment

By establishing a trusting, therapeutic relationship, the nurse can thoroughly assess potential body image changes through observation and discussion. A purposeful interview is conducted during which open-ended questions are asked.

These defining characteristics or signs and symptoms (Hurley, 1986) need to be assessed to understand the client's emotional reaction to and perception of body change. The client may value certain habits or patterns, as well as certain body organs. The nurse must perform a thorough psychosocial assessment to ascertain an altered body image.

The nurse encourages the client to talk about *any changes in current life style* that have occurred as a result of the changes in the body. If usual life style patterns have been interrupted because of physical body changes, there may be difficulties in body image adaptation. For example, the amputee who is no longer able to perform his or her job or daily morning jogging period may experience body image disturbance.

The nurse also discusses with the client *any fears related to rejection by or reaction of significant others.* The client's perceptions about her family's reaction to the mastectomy may not be accurate. These fears need to be expressed and assessed to cope with this change successfully. In addition, fear itself may interrupt healthy body image adaptation in that the fear may be unrealistic. Clients also need to *talk about their past strengths, function, or appearance.* This focus on past abilities may not be healthy, even though the identification of remaining strengths can be an effective coping strategy. For example, the athlete who had bilateral leg amputation and who continually focuses on past running ability may be experiencing difficulty with body image readjustment.

Verbalization of negative feelings regarding the body may also indicate alteration in body image. Anger is commonly experienced by clients. The nurse can facilitate discussion of these feelings by helping the client to recognize his or her anger and then identifying the anger as a common reaction to loss. However, continually focused anger about the body and any physical changes can become destructive to healthy body image adaptation. Therefore, the nurse must also assist the client to resolve angry feelings to progress through the process of adaptation.

In addition, *feelings of helplessness, hopelessness, or powerlessness* are a common immediate response to body changes. However, if these feelings continue, body image disturbance can develop. The nurse inquires: "Do you feel as if you have control over what is happening to you?" "Are you hopeful about the future?" "Has the body change left you feeling helpless?"

Any *preoccupation with the body change or loss* may be characteristic of body image disturbance. The client may become so focused on the loss of a breast that she plans activities of a whole day around concealing this physical change. This extreme behavior does not facilitate healthy body image adaptation to the loss. This behavior can be noted unobtrusively by the nurse without threatening, invasive questioning.

As stated earlier, identifying remaining strengths can assist the client to healthy body image development. However, *specific emphasis on all remaining strengths and a sense of heightened achievement* may not be healthy behavior. For example, the client may avoid the emotional issue of dealing with an extremity loss by focusing on developing the strength and endurance necessary to walk with a prosthesis, without paying attention to other assistive devices that may be needed or without learning how to put on the prosthesis correctly. An unrealistic belief about continuing to achieve previous life goals may be destructive. The nurse must assist the client to develop realistic goals for the future.

NANDA has also identified client *extension of the body boundary to incorporate environmental objects* and *personalization of the body part or loss by name* as indicative of body image disturbance. However, research has not established these characteristics as unhealthy behavior. For example, could it be that the client who envisions the body and wheelchair as one has successfully adapted to the new body image? Has the client who calls the colostomy "Sam" also successfully incorporated this body change into a healthy image of the body? Future research may clarify these questions, but the nurse must attempt to collect data regarding these characteristics to clearly assess body image changes.

The client who *depersonalizes the body part or loss by the use of impersonal pronouns* (e.g., "it") may exhibit difficulty with adapting to the body change. The use of an impersonal pronoun to refer to a mastectomy, colostomy, or stump demonstrates an inability to perceive the body change as part of self. This reference keeps the body change impersonal and may facilitate denial of the change. By using denial, the client may demonstrate a *refusal to verify the actual body change.* This refusal then prolongs the grieving/coping process and can interrupt body image reintegration. The client may be so adamant in denying the loss of a leg that reality is threatened. These data are crucial in attempting to diagnose body image disturbance.

Data concerning the client's current coping behavior are important for the nurse to assess a particular stage of coping and the client's attempts at body image adaptation to the change. Current coping behaviors can also be compared with *past coping behaviors* to assist the client with body image changes. The client who has used anger to cope with past stressful life events may need to demonstrate anger in response to body changes. With the knowledge of these data, the nurse is better prepared to treat body image disturbance.

The *client's current family role* is also evaluated by the nurse to gain an understanding about communication patterns, support systems, and family dynamics. The client's role in the family may be a significant part of who the client is. If this image of self is interrupted by a body change, major problems with body image may occur. In addition, family members may be significantly influenced by the client's body change and inability to perform previous family roles.

The nurse must also assess *client and family support systems.* The success or failure of a client and family to deal with physical body changes can depend greatly on the existence of support systems. Support systems may be individual people, groups, communities, financial plans, or assistive devices. The nurse begins this assessment on initial contact with the client. However, much of this data collection is ongoing. Knowledge of client and family support systems is necessary for the nurse to develop an effective plan of care.

Assessment Tools

Various tools have been developed primarily through the efforts of psychology researchers who study self-concept and body image. However, these tests are time-consuming for clients to complete and difficult to evaluate. A clinically useful nursing assessment tool is needed to assist the nurse to identify body image disturbances. An attempt to clarify this body image assessment for nursing has been made (Table 9–3). The Baird Body Image Assessment Tool (BBIAT) attempts to clarify potential versus actual body image disturbances. The subjective portion is a Likert Scale format, with each question being answered by strongly agree (SA), agree (A), undecided (U), disagree (D), or strongly disagree (SD). The nurse asks clients to respond to questions 1 through 6. Points are then assigned to each answer as follows: SA = five points, A = four points, U = three points, D = two points, SD = one point. The total possible score for the subjective portion of the BBIAT is 30. Reliability and validity of this nursing tool are currently being established. A score of 23 to 30 points may indicate a serious need for nursing intervention; 19 to 22 points, a potential need that requires nursing intervention; and 18 or less, no need for nursing intervention or the client has adapted to body changes. The BBIAT is meant to be used only as a guide or tool to clarify for nurses, in daily practice, the assessment of body image alterations. The objective portion is used by the nurse to identify other physical evidence that may have an impact on body image reintegration. No score is given for this portion. However, if many objective variables exist

TABLE 9–3   Baird Body Image Assessment Tool*

Subjective Interview
Points

___ 1. I will be undergoing a major change in my job status as a result of this experience.
___ SA ___ A ___ U ___ D ___ SD
If so, what?
___ Decrease in job status   ___ Job loss
___ Change in job   ___ Other (specify)
                            _____

___ 2. I do not have someone available to help me or talk to.
___ SA ___ A ___ U ___ D ___ SD
If someone is available, who?
___ Spouse   ___ Close friend   ___ Significant other (relative)
___ Parents   ___ Children   ___ Nurse

___ 3. I think of myself differently as a result of this experience.
___ SA ___ A ___ U ___ D ___ SD
If so, how?
___ Negatively   ___ Increased physical complaints
                  ___ Other (specify) _____

___ 4. My ability to move around by myself has changed as a result of this experience.
___ SA ___ A ___ U ___ D ___ SD
If so, how?
___ Less mobile   ___ No change
                   ___ Other (specify) _____

___ 5. I have definite feelings about specific parts of my body.
___ SA ___ A ___ U ___ D ___ SD
If so, what?
___ Hate   ___ Fear
___ Disgust   ___ Other (specify)
              _____

___ 6. I am more fearful now than before this experience.
___ SA ___ A ___ U ___ D ___ SD
If so, why?
___ Fear of falling   ___ Fear of inability to care for self
___ Fear of recurrence of problem
___ Fear of others' reactions
___ Fear of pain   ___ Other (specify)
                          _____

Objective Interview

7. Does the patient display any prominent body feature?
___ Obesity   ___ Disfigurement
___ Limb loss   ___ Other (specify) _____
___ Paralysis

8. Does the patient exhibit evidence of or complain of pain?
___ Facial expression
___ Physical strain or fatigue
___ Body language (immobile, purposeless, protective, rubbing)
___ Sleep disturbances
___ Other (specify) _____

9. Does the patient exhibit any major change in affect?
___ Withdrawal ___ Crying ___ Other (specify)
___ Hostility   _____

10. Is there any equipment present?
___ Foley's catheter   ___ IV
___ NG or other tubes
___ Walker or crutches ___ Cardiac monitor
___ Cast   ___ Traction   ___ Side rails up
___ Tracheotomy
___ Other (specify) _____

* SA, strongly agree; A, agree; U, undecided; D, disagree; SD, strongly disagree; IV, intravenous; NG, nasogastric.

so that the nurse is unsure if a body image disturbance exists, this portion of the tool may help the nurse clarify the nursing diagnosis and/or etiology.

 ## Analysis: Nursing Diagnosis

Common Diagnoses

The following nursing diagnoses are related to the primary diagnosis of body image disturbance:

1. Anxiety or fear
2. Ineffective individual coping
3. Ineffective family coping: compromised
4. Anticipatory grieving

Additional Diagnoses

The client may also demonstrate other problems that may be related to a number of changes in the body. These less common diagnoses may include

1. Sexual dysfunction
2. Impaired physical mobility
3. Impaired home maintenance management
4. Pain

KEY FEATURES OF DISEASE ■ Risk Factors for Developing Body Image Disturbance

Missing body parts

Dependence on machinery

Significance of body part or function with regard to age, sex, developmental level, or basic human needs

Physiologic change caused by biochemical agents (drugs)

Physical trauma or mutilation

Pregnancy and/or maturational changes

Data from Kim, M. J., McFarland, G. K., & McLane, A. M. (1984). *Pocket guide to nursing diagnoses.* St. Louis: C. V. Mosby.

 Planning and Implementation

Anxiety; Fear

Planning: client goals.   Major goals or outcomes for these nursing diagnoses are that the client will (1) verbalize decreased anxiety or fear, and (2) demonstrate decreased anxiety or fear by participation in the plan of care.

Interventions.   Research has established the role of teaching in providing reassurance to clients who are about to undergo surgical body alterations. Preoperative teaching has been shown to decrease anxiety before and after surgery. In addition, clients may be hospitalized for shorter periods because of less anxiety (Bulecheck & McCloskey, 1985). Visits to clients by similarly affected individuals have also been effective in assisting to identify remaining strengths. The use of light touch to an extremity during discussion is effective in assisting clients with the re-establishment of changed body boundaries. This conveys to the client that the nurse values him or her and also that the physical body is still present. A review of the literature has not identified the effect of talking to the clients at equal eye level, but it can be especially helpful in establishing an open, trusting relationship with the client who is feeling anxious or fearful. The nurse encourages client verbalization and active thinking by providing for and facilitating client participation in planning for the client's own needs. Self-initiated activity also enhances a client's sense of independence and responsibility.

Ineffective Individual Coping; Anticipatory Grieving

Planning: client goals.   The major goal of the nursing management of ineffective individual coping is that the client will accept the changed body structure. It is hoped that eventually the client will establish a new body image or reintegrate and resume a fulfilling life. This does not mean that the client prefers this new image to the old, but that the reality of the situation is acknowledged and the growth process throughout life can continue. The client goal for anticipatory grieving is that the client will be able to identify and understand the grief process.

Interventions.   The nurse teaches the client the components of the healthy grieving process. This teaching begins by increasing client and family awareness of the various stages of grieving, as well as understanding coping behaviors that are used in response to loss. For example, the client or family member who denies the body change that has occurred or responds with anger may not be aware of this response. The nurse specifically helps the client and family to discuss their feelings, realize current behaviors, and possibly identify other therapeutic coping and/or grieving strategies. Through discussion, it is also important for the nurse to create an understanding of healthy body image development throughout the life span. By developing an awareness about body image development, clients and families will be better prepared to understand their fears and concerns, and coping will be more effective.

Nursing interventions also focus on setting small, achievable goals, which the nurse does together with the client and/or family. The goals are to be met during hospitalization to provide positive reinforcement about remaining strengths, as well as effective coping strategies. For example, imagine the client who is convinced that the mastectomy site is noticeable, even under clothing, finds this quite distressing, and refuses to leave the hospital room. The nurse assists the client to set a goal to dress in personal clothes of her choice and visit the gift shop on the main floor of the hospital. The client meets the goal within 3 days and by the end of the week is in the visitors' lounge every afternoon meeting new people and enjoying social interaction. It is important to note that meeting the public for the first time after surgery can be threatening and that clients become progressively desensitized to physical body changes. The nurse assists the client to be aware of his or her feelings about the public's stares and to plan coping strategies to deal with these feelings.

Clients need to realize their remaining strengths and capabilities. In addition, the nurse can provide validation for realistic concerns and fears to assist the client and/or family with identification of long-term effective coping mechanisms. For example, the amputee who has coped with past life events by jogging daily needs assistance to identify and to practice new coping behaviors. In addition, the nurse may arrange for a client who had experienced similar body changes and successfully reintegrated these changes into a new body image to visit the client and to discuss concerns. For more detailed coping and grieving nursing interventions, refer to Chapter 11, which discusses the concept of loss.

Ineffective Family Coping: Compromised

Planning: client (family) goals.   The primary goal for this nursing diagnosis is that the family will accept the client's body changes with readjustment into the family unit.

Interventions. Family members and significant others need the same kind of assistance as the client in coping with these changes. Family members need support so that they in turn can support the client. The family must be able to deal with any feelings about previous problems concerning the client, as well as new feelings related to the kind and extent of body changes incurred by the client. For example, family members may feel guilty about a belief that their mother's leg might have been saved if they had gotten the mother to the doctor sooner. The nurse serves as the client's and family's most consistent health caregiver. This consistency establishes a caring rapport, which increases comfort in discussing these sensitive issues. Providing empathy, *not* sympathy, can be the single most important intervention when treating body image disturbance. For example, an empathic supporting statement to a client might be, "This must be very difficult for you." A sympathetic statement to a client might be, "I'm so sorry for you." The nurse may convey sensitivity and empathy more clearly to the client and family by the use of light touch to the arm or hand during these discussions. In addition, the nurse's sitting at eye level with the client may facilitate even more open verbalization of concerns.

The nurse may also actively attempt to involve the family in the client's care during hospitalization, but only as they desire. This intervention may increase both the client's and family's sense of control over the situation and decrease feelings of powerlessness. In addition, with this involvement in care, family members are impressed with the importance for the client to gradually increase responsibility for self-care and other activities. For example, teaching family members how to care for the stump at home provides the client with positive reinforcement about the physical change as well as assists the family in recognizing that the client is still their loved one.

The client and family may need to restructure their relationships depending on the extent and impact of the body change. The nurse can assist with this restructuring by serving as a buffer between client and family, if this is needed, to facilitate this discussion. The nurse may also provide knowledge about community or hospital resources if family roles have changed as a result of the body change. For example, if the client is unable to maintain the family role as breadwinner, community resources may assist with financial needs. By helping the client and family to share concerns or fears and to solve problems together, the nurse can alleviate miscommunication problems and can enhance existing support systems.

Readjustment to body changes is a long-term process that requires continued evaluation and monitoring. The nurse must brainstorm and be creative in developing interventions to treat body image disturbance successfully. For example, a client with an amputation might feel useless. The nurse is aware that the client is a successful commercial artist and that the nursing unit is in serious need of artwork for a client education brochure. The nurse involves the client in sketching for the brochure. As a result, the client is given feedback about his or her remaining strengths.

The grieving process for loss of body parts, chronic disability, or deformity may never reach total resolution. This possibility poses a special nursing challenge. Problems may recur with reminders of the loss. Monitoring the adjustment process after discharge from the hospital is important.

■ Discharge Planning

Home Care Preparation

The client returning home faces many challenges concerning continued adaptation to body image changes. The community health nurse can be most effective in helping the client and family cope with these challenges. The nurse can assist with follow-up care necessary to treat the body change. For example, after discharge from the hospital, the amputee client will require future fittings for a prosthesis and continued assessment of the stump. The mastectomy client may desire future contact with mastectomy support groups. The community health nurse can effectively assist these clients with their long-term needs.

Client/Family Education

The nurse provides continued follow-up home care also by informing and updating the client and family about new improvements or changes in treatment, medication, and rehabilitation devices or programs (e.g., new prostheses or new treatment procedures). Education concerning long-term care because of a body change is also presented and reinforced. As hospital stays continue to shorten, it is even more crucial for the nurse to present education in the home and to ensure client and family understanding with follow-up visits. For example, clients with terminal illnesses are now managing parenteral intravenous drug therapy successfully at home. Clients who undergo ostomy procedures are experiencing trial-and-error periods at home with various appliances. The success of these clients' home management abilities can lie with effective teaching by the nurse about these self-care activities. The nurse teaches and promotes client independence, as this assists the body image change to stabilize.

Psychosocial Preparation

Psychosocial needs may become even more highlighted as the client returns to the previous environment, and actual losses may become more readily apparent to both the client and family. For example, the client with an ostomy becomes discouraged as the ostomy appliance he or she had been using successfully in the hospital has begun to have problems at home and as family members also find this change difficult to cope with. The nurse must continue to assess these psychosocial needs as well as to anticipate future client and family experiences in an attempt to help the client and family cope with new feelings. The client who first performs ostomy care at home must not have the unrealistic expectation that the care will always go smoothly. The family welcoming the paraplegic client home, after months of hospitalization, must also be aware of potential client reactions to returning to the previous environment. The nurse plays a major role in preparing the client and family for the emotional reactions and long-term adaptation to body changes. The client may tend to focus on and re-examine his or her changed body more closely after returning home. Activities of daily living may be completed in a new way. In addition, the familiar home environment may cause the client to remember past activities that he or she can no longer perform. Therefore, the nurse can help prepare the client and family for possible feelings of depression or anger that can occur after discharge.

Health Care Resources

Many community support groups and societies are specially geared to meet the needs of clients with specific body image problems. The nurse can direct the client and/or family to these agencies for additional help with working through the adjustment process (e.g., Arthritis Foundation, American Cancer Society, National Spinal Cord Association, Alzheimer's support groups, Multiple Sclerosis Society). The nurse can also refer the client and family to community mental health services to provide more in-depth assistance. Individuals must know what resources are available and what to expect from these resources. The nurse serves as the link between clients and families and additional resources. Also, an awareness of assistive devices or various prostheses that are available can help the client. Walkers, crutches, wheelchairs, artificial limbs, and commodes increase the client's independence in self-care and help to de-emphasize the sense of long-term or permanent disability. Nurses must provide this information to clients to assist with long-term body image adaptation.

 Evaluation

Nurses are effective in treating clients with body image disturbances. Continued awareness of the impact of body changes on well-being and health is crucial for the nurse to plan optimal health care management. The outcome criteria for the client experiencing body image disturbance include that the client

1. Verbalizes feelings indicative of self-acceptance to family or significant others or nursing staff consistently
2. Identifies and uses successful coping strategies to deal with the perceived body change
3. Attends to self-care needs of body parts or function
4. Initiates discussion with others indicating the beginning of successful coping

By achievement of these outcomes, the client and family will adjust to body changes, and anxiety or fear will be alleviated. However, this adjustment will probably occur over time. It is not realistic for nurses to expect successful coping and adaptation to be complete by the time the client is discharged from the hospital. The nurse prepares the client and family to achieve adaptation after discharge.

SUMMARY

Changes in body image caused by trauma, surgery, or illness can be a devastating experience for clients and families. Nurses are in a prime position to effectively treat clients with these responses. As new health care delivery systems continue to evolve, the nurse will be even more challenged to provide effective care. In response to these new challenges, nursing practice must be knowledgeable about the concept and experience of body image adaptation, development, and maladjustment. In addition, nurses must consistently reassess this concept in their practice to effect positive outcomes of health care.

IMPLICATIONS FOR RESEARCH

Body image disturbance is a complex phenomenon that could potentially develop for every individual who must deal with a body function loss that results in a permanent change. Because illness creates many changes in the body and requires reintegration of the body image, the nurse must develop skill in treating this nursing diagnosis. Body image disturbances can potentially affect many other components of the illness experience and require ongoing assessment and treatment.

However, because of the complexity of this human response, it has been difficult to clarify this area for nursing practice. Nursing research needs to continue to focus energies on clarifying the concept of self and its variables. Questions needing further clarification and research are

1. Is body image disturbance really a component of self-concept alteration and not a separate diagnosis?
2. What are the most measurably effective nursing interventions for treating body image disturbance?
3. What are the most reliable defining characteristics, or signs and symptoms, that indicate body image disturbance?
4. How frequently does body image disturbance occur?

REFERENCES AND READINGS

Baird, S. E. (1985). Development of a nursing assessment tool to diagnose altered body image in immobilized patients. *Orthopedic Nursing, 4,* 47–54.

Baxley, K. O., Erdman, L. K., Henry, E. B., & Roof, B. J. (1984, December). Alopecia: Effect on cancer patients' body image. *Cancer Nursing, 7,* 499–503.

Bonham, P. A., & Cheney, A. M. (1983). Concept of self: A framework for nursing assessment. In P. L. Chinn (Ed.), *Advances in nursing theory development* (pp. 173–190). Rockville, MD: Aspen Systems.

Broncatells, K. F. (1980). Auger in action: Application of the model. *Advances in Nursing Science, 3,* 13–23.

Christian, B. J. (1982). Immobilization: Psychological aspects. In C. Norris (Ed.), *Concept clarification in nursing.* Rockville, MD: Aspen Systems.

Cleveland, S. (1976). The place of the head in the body image concept. *Research and Clinical Studies in Headache, 4,* 1–7.

Corbeil, M. (1971). Nursing process for a patient with a body image disturbance. *Nursing Clinics of North America, 6,* 155–163.

Culp, R., Packard, V., & Humphrey, R. (1980). Sensorimotor versus cognitive-perceptual training effects on the body concepts of preschoolers. *American Journal of Occupational Therapy, 34,* 259–262.

Evans, J. (1977). On disturbance of the body image in paraplegia. In J. Stubbins (Ed.), *Social and psychological aspects of disability* (pp. 409–421). Baltimore: University Park.

Fischer, S. (1964). Sex differences in body perception. *Psychological Monographs,* 1–22.

Fischer, S., & Cleveland, S. (1968). *Body image and personality.* New York: Dell.

Fraiberg, S. (1959). *The magic years.* New York: Charles Scribner's Sons.

Friesen, D. (1969). *The urban teenager.* Edmonton, Alberta, Canada: University of Alberta, Department of Educational Administration.

Gellert, E. (1975). Children's constructions of their self images. *Perceptual Motor Skills, 40,* 307–324.

Gergen, K. J. (1971). *The concept of self.* New York: Holt, Rinehart, & Winston.

Gillies, O. A. (1984, September/October). Body image changes following illness and injury. *Journal of Enterostomal Therapy, 11,* 186–189.

Glucksman, M., & Hirsch, J. (1969). The response of obese patients to weight reduction: The perception of body size. *Psychosomatic Medicine, 31,* 1–7.

Gruendemann, B. J. (1975). The impact of surgery on body image. *Nursing Clinics of North America, 10,* 635–643.

Harris, M. (1986). Helping the person with an altered self image. *Geriatric Nursing, 7*(2), 90–92.

Hart, L. K. (1981). *Concepts common to acute illness: Identification and management.* St. Louis: C. V. Mosby.

Jourard, S. M. (1971). *The transparent self.* New York: Van Nostrand Reinhold.

Kim, M. J., McFarland, G. K., & McLane, A. M. (1984). *Pocket guide to nursing diagnoses.* St. Louis: C. V. Mosby.

Kirkpatrick, S., & Sanders, D. (1978). Body image stereotypes: A developmental comparison. *The Journal of Genetic Psychology, 132,* 87–95.

Koehler, M. L. (1989). Relationship between self-concept and successful rehabilitation. *Rehabilitation Nursing, 14*(1), 9–12.

Kolb, L. (1959). Disturbances of the body-image. In S. Arieti (Ed.), *American handbook of psychiatry.* New York: Basic Books.

Leonard, B. J. (1972). Body image changes in chronic illness. *Nursing Clinics of North America, 7,* 687–695.

Lowerfeld, V., & Brittain, W. (1970). *Creative and mental growth.* London: Macmillan.

Marten, L. (1978). Self-care nursing model for patients experiencing radical change in body image. *JOGNN, 7*(6), 9–13.

Maslow, A. H. (1954). *Motivation and personality.* New York: Harper.

McCloskey, J. C. (1976). How to make the most of body image theory in nursing practice. *Nursing '76, 6*(5), 68–72.

Morris, C. A. (1985). Self-concept as altered by the diagnosis of cancer. *Nursing Clinics of North America, 20,* 611–630.

Murray, R. (1972). Body image development in adulthood. *Nursing Clinics of North America, 7,* 617–629.

Murray, R. L. (1972). Principles of nursing intervention for the adult patient with body image changes. *Nursing Clinics of North America, 7,* 697–707.

Neugarten, B. L. (1979). Time, age, and the life cycle. *The American Journal of Psychiatry, 136,* 887–894.

Orr, D. P., Wilbrandt, M. L., Brack, C. J., Rauch, S. P., & Ingersoll, G. M. (1989). Reported sexual behaviors and self-esteem among young adolescents. *American Journal of Diseases of Children, 143,* 86–90.

Rice, M. A., Tate, R.C., Grossberg, G.T., Handal, D.J., Brandeberry, L., & Nakra, R. (1988). Group intervention for reinforcing self-worth following mastectomy. *Oncology Nursing Forum, 15*(1), 33–37.

Rogers, C. (1961). *On becoming a person.* Boston: Houghton Mifflin.

Ross, M. J., Tait, R. C., Grossberg, G. T., Handal, P. J., Brandenberry, L., & Nakra, R. (1989). Age differences in body consciousness. *Journals of Gerontology, 44,* 23–24.

Selekman, J. (1983, April). The development of body image in the child: A learned response. *Topics in Clinical Nursing, 5*(1), 12–21.

Sheldon, M., & Stevens, S. (1942). *The varieties of temperament.* New York: Harper.

Strange, V. R., & Sullivan, P. L. (1985). Body image attitudes during pregnancy and the postpartum period. *JOGNN, 14,* 332–337.

Sullivan, H. S. (1947). *Conceptions of modern psychiatry.*

Washington, DC: William Alanson White Psychiatric Foundation.

Wells, R. W. (1975). Body image and surgical alterations. *AORN Journal, 21,* 812–815.

ADDITIONAL READINGS

Bulecheck, G. M., & McCloskey, J. C. (1985). *Nursing interventions: Treatments for nursing diagnoses.* Philadelphia: W. B. Saunders.

This reference is excellent to consult for specific research-based nursing interventions. Literature reviews are discussed, as well as techniques for individual nursing interventions. The nursing diagnosis format is used, and case studies are also presented.

Hurley, M. E. (1986). *Classification of nursing diagnosis: Proceedings of the Sixth Conference.* St. Louis: C. V. Mosby.

This research-based reference is excellent for definition and clinical application of nursing diagnoses. Specific diagnoses, computer application, and most recent research results are discussed.

Miller, J. F. (1983). *Coping with chronic illness: Overcoming powerlessness.* Philadelphia: F. A. Davis.

This book discusses the complex concept of powerlessness as it relates to the experience of hospitalization and illness. Current research concerning various patient populations and effective nursing interventions is presented. This is a useful clinical nursing reference for better understanding and treatment of chronic illness states and the nursing diagnosis of powerlessness.

Norris, C. M. (1978). Body image: Its relevance to professional nursing. In C. E. Carlson & B. Blackwell (Eds.), *Behavioral concepts and nursing intervention* (pp. 39–65). New York: J. B. Lippincott.

This chapter presents a classic discussion of the concept of body image as it relates to nursing practice. Body image development and specific kinds of influences that require body image adaptation are discussed.

Schilder, P. (1950). *The image and appearance of the human body.* New York: International Universities Press.

This book is a classic that discusses the theory of body image related to self-concept. Specific components of body image, such as pain, are also addressed.

CHAPTER 10

Human Sexuality

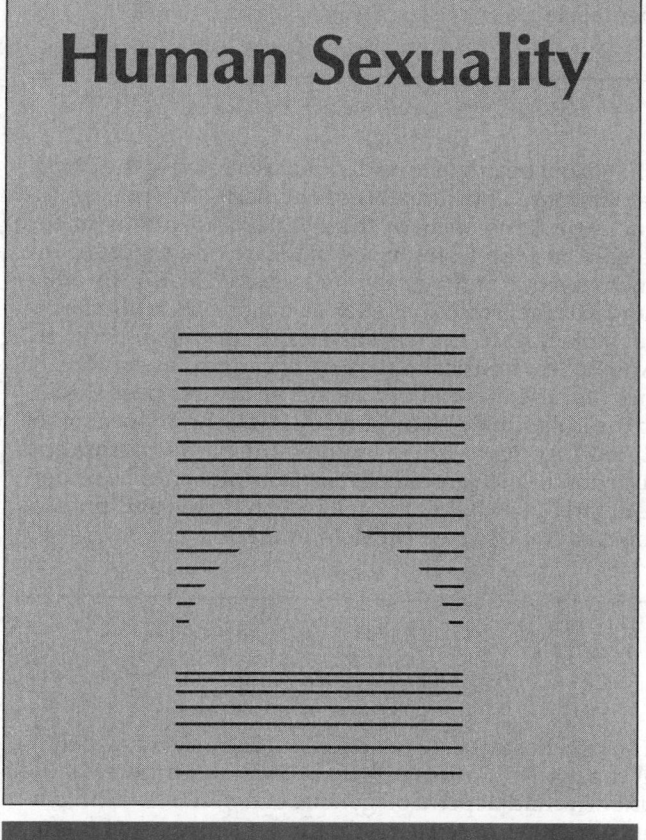

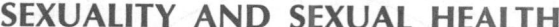

SEXUALITY AND SEXUAL HEALTH

Human *sexuality* is characterized by physical, social, psychologic, and spiritual attributes that are associated with one's gender. One's sexuality is expressed in terms of physical structure, physiologic functioning, attitudes and values, knowledge, and behaviors that result from inherited characteristics and social learning. The relationships among these factors comprise the status of an individual's sexual health. *Sexual health* includes one's freedom from physical and psychologic impairment; the awareness of open and positive attitudes toward sexual functioning; accurate knowledge of sexuality; and congruency among gender assignment, identity, and role. Nursing is concerned with issues of sexual health. Through the nursing process, the professional recognizes the importance of human sexuality and encourages growth and development of clients as sexual beings. The nurse also intervenes in a variety of situations to promote sexual health and prevent sexual dysfunctions related to illness and injury throughout the life cycle.

THEORETICAL PERSPECTIVES

Nurses, as the largest body of health care providers, are expected to assess, diagnose, and intervene in situations in which clients have actual or potential sexual problems related to altered physiologic function, loss of body parts, or deficits in coping skills and/or knowledge (Carpenito, 1987). Consequently, nurses must be adequately prepared with a broad knowledge base of the following factors that contribute to the sexual health of the individual:

1. Anatomy and physiology
2. Psychosexual development throughout the life cycle
3. Sexual response cycle of the adult
4. Effects of aging on sexual functioning
5. Effects of illness on sexuality: hospitalization, acute and chronic illness
6. Effects of drug (including alcohol) use and abuse on human sexual functioning
7. Attitudes and values of individuals and societies toward human sexuality
8. Effective interpersonal skills
9. Appropriate nursing interventions and community referral resources for the promotion of sexual health

A conceptual model of sexual health, Figure 10–1, consists of a circle that represents the life span of the

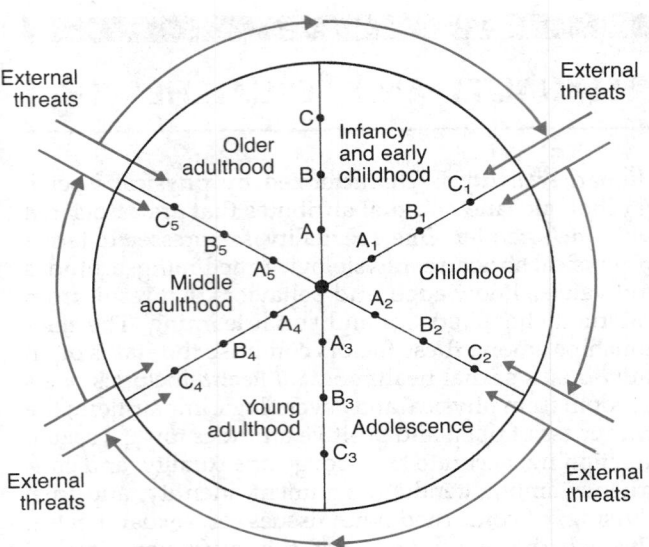

Figure 10-1

Conceptual model of sexual health throughout the life span. The desired outcome is optimal sexual health. A, physical factors; B, psychologic factors; C, sociocultural factors; A_{1-5}, physical changes over time; B_{1-5}, psychologic changes over time; C_{1-5}, sociocultural changes over time; sexual health $= A + B + C$, $A_1 + B_1 + C_1$, $A_2 + B_2 + C_2$, $A_3 + B_3 + C_3$, $A_4 + B_4 + C_4$, $A_5 + B_5 + C_5$.

individual. As a person develops, various physical, psychologic, and social factors determine his or her optimal status of sexual health at a particular moment in time. External threats in the form of physical illness, injury, or medical and surgical interventions may lead to alterations in these factors that reduce the individual's level of sexual health. Similarly, threats in the psychologic and social domains of the individual, such as changes in family composition or family violence, may result in alterations that reduce sexual health.

The point at the center of the model represents the gender of an individual, which remains stable over time. This is based on an assumption of accurate gender assignment at birth. The outcome or goal of sexual health at any moment in time is related to a synthesis of and congruity among the physical, psychologic, and sociocultural attributes of the individual that develop over the life span. Physical attributes are characteristics associated with changes in the body and include age, reproductive history, level of sexual functioning, past and present illnesses and injuries, use of medications, and specific sexual behaviors. Psychologic attributes consist of characteristics of the mind and include body image, self-esteem, knowledge of sexuality, attitudes toward gender roles, and preference for sexual partners. Sociocultural attributes include race or ethnicity, marital status, family and social support groups, occupation, and level of education.

To promote optimal sexual health in clients, nurses must assess these various attributes of the individual and compare current findings with past patterns re-

ported by the individual. The nurse must also evaluate the impact of external threats on these attributes and provide nursing interventions that reduce or prevent the negative effects of these threats. Specific strategies for coping with external threats to sexual health change as the individual progresses through different developmental stages.

ANATOMY AND PHYSIOLOGY

The sexual health of an individual is related to the physical structure and function of the body. Internal reproductive organs such as the ovaries and uterus in the female and the testes in the male are one aspect of the anatomy that influences one's sexual health. In addition, external structures such as the breasts and external genitalia affect the sexual health of the individual. Anomalies, injuries, diseases, or surgical alterations of any of these internal or external structures pose threats to the individual's sexual health. Also, the importance of the endocrine system in maintaining both structure and function of the reproductive organs must not be underestimated. For further details on anatomic and physiologic alterations, see Units 14 and 15.

PSYCHOSEXUAL DEVELOPMENT

CHILDHOOD

The psychosexual development of the individual begins at the moment of conception. Physical attributes of the unborn child depend on genetic material from both parents and the presence or absence of sex hormones after the seventh week of gestation. Genetic or chromosomal anomalies may result in one of several syndromes that affect the sexual health of the individual. Klinefelter's syndrome results when an ovum with 24 chromosomes is fertilized by a sperm bearing a Y chromosome. The result is an XXY karyotype. Males with this chromosomal abnormality develop small testes that are unable to produce mature sperm. Libido is low, and there may be additional feminine characteristics. Turner's syndrome in females occurs when an abnormal ovum with only 22 chromosomes is fertilized by a sperm bearing an X chromosome. The result of this union is an XO karyotype. Females with this abnormality have no ovaries, may be short, and experience additional defects of the kidney and heart. Pseudohermaphroditism occurs as often as 1 in 1000 births and results in individuals who have both male and female genitalia. In some cases, it may be difficult to determine the sex of these infants at birth. For further details about these disorders, the reader is directed to a text on human sexuality.

In addition to the physical development that takes place before birth, the psychosocial climate begins its subtle influence on the sexuality of the unborn. After birth, during the first 18 months of life, or infancy, the physical and psychosocial attributes of the child change rapidly. An infant experiences tactile, auditory, olfactory, and gustatory sensations, which communicate basic elements of sexuality and are critical to the development of trust. Exploration of the infant's own body begins soon after birth, and the child learns to associate pleasurable sensations with touch. Acceptance by the parents of this behavior as normal is crucial to the development of healthy gender identity and sexual satisfaction throughout the life cycle.

Gender identity and *gender role* are learned during the toddler and preschool periods. Gender identity refers to the child's knowledge of self as belonging to the female or male gender, whereas gender role refers to specific behaviors associated with gender. This social learning is reinforced by adults who directly or indirectly approve of the child's identifying self and others as boy or girl and acting in ways appropriate for the child's gender. Issues of sexuality during the preschool years may be confused with those of toilet training. It is important for parents and health professionals who work with young children to separate the functions of body orifices associated with toileting from those associated with sexual activity. The belief of some individuals that the genitalia are "dirty" does not contribute to healthy attitudes about sexuality.

Sex play among preschool children is common and crucial to development. Some of this play is associated with gender roles ("I'll be the mommy because I am a girl"), whereas other play may be more sexually explicit. The latter may take the form of individual self-stimulation or mutual exploration, as when playing doctor. Limits need to be set so that such play is not harmful or exploitive, as can be the case when the preschooler plays with much older children or siblings. The young child's learning to say "no" is essential in gaining mastery over his or her sexuality and in learning to respect the privacy of others. However, it is important for adults to avoid instilling guilt when setting limits and to teach the young child to be assertive.

Once in school, the child from 6 to 12 years of age continues to engage in social learning about gender roles as well as in purposive sex play alone or with other children. Physical development proceeds more rapidly in school-aged girls than in boys. Whereas parental attitudes and values were significant in the development of the child's gender identity at earlier ages, the peer group begins to influence the psychosexual development of the school-aged child. Children of this age express more interest in sex-linked clothing and accessories, toys, hobbies, and clubs. Formation of close friendships with members of the same sex is necessary for consolidation of gender identity.

ADOLESCENCE

At the beginning of adolescence, internal hormonal changes account for external development of secondary sexual characteristics and accompanying swings of mood. This transitional period from child to adult is an important step in the physiologic and psychosocial de-velopment of sexuality. While the body is physically maturing and becoming capable of reproduction, society demands more responsibility from the individual. The adolescent has outgrown the fantasy play of the young child and now lives as though performing in front of an audience of peers. Capable of engaging in adult sexual activity, the adolescent is urged by peers to "use it or lose it." Conflicts and fluctuations in self-confidence make this an especially difficult time for the individual to master the task of developing an identity.

Attraction to members of the same or opposite sex leads to experimentation with explicit sexual activity. This activity leads to an increased risk of an unwanted pregnancy or of acquiring a sexually transmitted disease (STD). Conforming to societal norms of heterosexuality and of saving sexual activity for marriage may be particularly difficult for the homosexual adolescent, as well as for the young person who is physically and psychologically mature and ready for a full sexual relationship with another person.

ADULTHOOD

Physiologic attributes of the adult vary throughout the life cycle. The physical maturity of the female is generally completed by the late teen years, whereas the male may continue to mature in terms of secondary sexual characteristics into the early or late 20s. Sexually explicit behaviors are pursued by adults of all ages. Factors such as age, illness or injury, and life experiences have major impacts on the sexuality of the adult. Attitudes and values are generally more firmly established in the adult than in the adolescent and influence sexually explicit behavior. Although the man may reach his peak of sexual urgency in the 20s, the woman may not reach this peak until the 30s or 40s. This mismatch may lead to conflicts within marriage or other intimate relationships.

SEXUAL RESPONSE CYCLE OF THE ADULT

The sexual response cycle of the adult is well documented as a result of the research of Masters and Johnson in the 1960s. This cycle is described as consisting of four phases: excitement, plateau, orgasm, and resolution (Table 10–1). The underlying physiology of this response cycle consists of vasocongestion and myotonia. *Vasocongestion* is the term that describes blood trapped in tissues of the breast, vulva, and penis. This congestion results in erection of the nipples, clitoris, and penis. *Myotonia* refers to tension of both voluntary and involuntary muscles that occurs during sexual excitement and orgasm. Problems of sexual dysfunction among adults are related to the phases of this cycle.

The following physiologic changes take place during the sexual response cycle. In the *excitement* phase, which results from physical and/or psychologic stimulation, noticeable physical changes occur because of the

TABLE 10-1 The Adult Sexual Response Cycle

Phase	Male Response	Female Response
Excitement	Flushed skin begins on abdomen, spreads to neck and face.	Flushed skin begins on abdomen and throat, spreads to breasts.
	Nipples become erect.	Nipples become erect, veins distend, areolae darken, and breasts enlarge by 25%.
	Myotonia of legs and arms occurs.	Myotonia of entire body occurs.
	Erection of penis may subside and return.	Clitoris becomes erect.
	Testes become elevated.	Vagina is lubricated.
	Pulse and blood pressure increase.	Pulse and blood pressure increase.
Plateau	Myotonia increases, with carpopedal spasms and facial grimaces.	Myotonia increases, with carpopedal spasms, flared nostrils, arched back.
	Penis remains erect and darkens in color.	Clitoris retracts under hood.
	Testes continue to swell and elevate toward perineum.	Vaginal barrel distends and contractions begin.
	Pulse, respirations, and blood pressure increase.	Pulse, respirations, and blood pressure increase.
Orgasm	Skin flush is maximal.	Skin flush is maximal.
	Myotonia of entire body occurs; rectal sphincter contracts.	Myotonia of entire body occurs.
	Semen is ejaculated through penis.	Clitoris remains retracted.
	Pulse and blood pressure increase.	Pulse and blood pressure increase.
	Respiratory rate doubles.	Respiratory rate doubles.
Resolution	Skin flush disappears within 5 min in most persons, followed by perspiration.	Skin flush disappears and may be followed by perspiration.
	Muscles relax.	Muscles relax.
	Nipples return to normal.	Nipples and breasts return to normal color and size.
	Penis returns to normal size in two stages.	Clitoris returns to normal position within 10 s.
	Testes return to normal size and position.	Vagina collapses and loses dark color.
	Pulse, respirations, and blood pressure return to normal rates.	Pulse, respirations, and blood pressure return to normal rates.

process of vasocongestion. Vaginal lubrication, expansion of the vaginal space, increase in the size of the clitoris and inner labia, and erection of the nipples occur in the woman. Erection of the penis, increase in size and elevation of the testes, and erection of the nipples occur in the man. A "sex flush," or rash resembling measles, may occur late in the excitement phase or in the plateau phase in both women and men.

In the *plateau* phase, the major changes in the woman include elevation of the uterus, swelling in the outer one-third of the vagina, retraction of the clitoris under its hood, and increase in size of the breasts and swelling of the areolae. The sex flush is most intense and Bartholin's glands secrete small amounts of fluid in this phase. The major changes in the man include swelling of the testes, deepening of the color of the penis, and elevation and rotation of the testes. The size of the testes may increase by 50% to 100%. During the plateau phase, the pre-ejaculatory fluid produced by Cowper's glands is secreted. Both women and men experience an increase

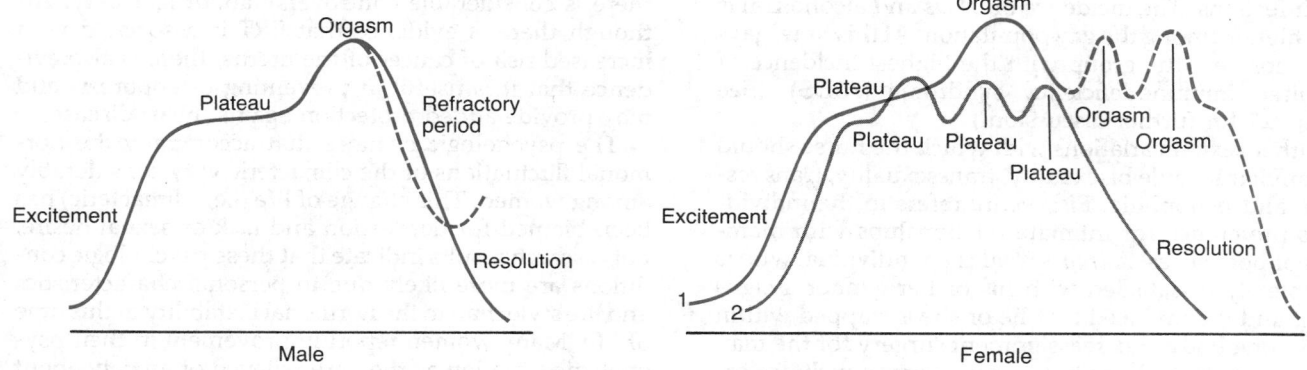

Figure 10–2

Male and female adult sexual response cycles. In the male sexual response cycle, a refractory period usually follows orgasm before another erection occurs. Women respond in various ways to sexual stimulation: Pattern 1 depicts single or multiple orgasms. Pattern 2 shows some peaks but no orgasm.

in myotonia and in vital signs during these two phases. Late in the plateau phase, spastic contractions of the hands and feet, carpopedal spasms, may occur. The heart rate may rise to 100 to 170 beats per minute, and blood pressure rises to 180/110 or higher.

Discharge of the accumulated tensions occurs in the *orgasmic* phase in both women and men. This is the shortest phase of the sexual response cycle and results in rhythmic contractions of the uterus, vagina, and anal sphincter in the woman. Orgasm is a total body response and occurs with great variation among women. The intensity of this phase is congruent with the intensity of sex flush and myotonia. In some women, orgasm is related to stimulation of the anterior wall of the vagina in an area identified as the Grafenberg spot, or G spot. Research findings concerning the existence of such an identifiable landmark and its relationship to female orgasm remain controversial at this time.

In the man, orgasm occurs in two stages. The first stage is the result of contractions in the vas deferens, prostate, and seminal vesicles and is known as ejaculatory inevitability. As a result of these contractions, semen is forced into the urethra. In the second stage, contractions of the urethra and the penis result in the ejaculation of semen from the glans of the penis. Simultaneously, the neck of the bladder closes to prevent retrograde ejaculation, or forcing of the ejaculate into the bladder (see discussion later in this chapter). Myotonia increases in this phase for both women and men and may result in carpopedal spasms.

The final phase, *resolution*, refers to the return of the individual to a state of prearousal. In general, all the physiologic responses that occurred during the excitement, plateau, and orgasm phases are reversed. In men, the resolution phase consists of an initial refractory period during which further ejaculation and orgasm are not possible. After this period, the man may be aroused again or complete resolution proceeds. Figure 10–2 depicts adult male and female sexual response cycles.

SEXUAL VARIATIONS

Sexual behavior and preference for partners may change over the life span of the individual. Although most children and many adolescents engage in some types of explicit homosexual activities, only about 10% of adults identify themselves as *homosexual* in their sexual orientation. This variation is the most common of the sexual minorities and is defined as the individual's erotic attraction to persons of the same sex. Many myths remain about stereotypic gay men and lesbian women. However, the nurse equipped with an appropriate knowledge base can do much to dispel these myths and provide nursing care that includes attention to the individual's sexual preference or orientation.

Although nursing care of the homosexual client does not differ greatly from that of the heterosexual, certain similarities and differences should be noted. Women may experience the same concerns about gynecologic and breast problems but do not have the same needs for contraception, nor are they likely to become pregnant. However, many women have a history of sexual abuse or family violence. Also, because of widespread homophobia, or fear of homosexuality, within the society, many approach the health care system cautiously. Because of the individual's fear and suspicions about the type of care that she may receive, there may be incomplete attention to minor problems that become serious.

Similarly, the gay man may avoid traditional health care systems and receive inadequate preventive or primary health care. Again, gay men may have the same concerns about genitourinary problems as heterosexual men. Because of the high incidence of anal intercourse among gay men, these clients may seek treatment more frequently for injuries of the rectum and for gastrointestinal infections known as the gay bowel syndrome. In this syndrome, the gay man is infected and reinfected with microorganisms causing one or more gastrointestinal infections. The incidence of STDs and alcoholism is also higher among the gay population. At this time, gays also represent the group with the highest incidence of acquired immunodeficiency syndrome (AIDS). (See Chap. 27 for further discussion.)

Other sexual variations with which the nurse should be familiar include bisexuality, transsexuality, transvestism, and pedophilia. *Bisexuality* refers to the individual's preference for intimate relationships with members of both sexes. A *transsexual* is an individual who is completely dissatisfied with his or her gender assignment and is convinced that he or she is trapped within the wrong body. Sex reassignment surgery for the man who has a strong urge to live as a woman includes orchiectomy, penectomy, and vaginoplasty; hormone replacement treatment is also given. For the woman who is reassigned as a man, hysterectomy, oophorectomy, and mastectomy may be done along with hormone replacement therapy.

Transvestism, or cross-dressing, occurs more frequently in men than in women and consists of wearing clothes associated with the opposite sex for the sake of sexual arousal. Unlike the transsexual, the transvestite does not have a conflict about his or her gender; many are married men, and most engage in this activity in private. *Pedophilia* refers to sexual preference for children and is a psychiatric disorder whose discussion is beyond the scope of this chapter.

CHANGES IN SEXUAL FUNCTION ASSOCIATED WITH AGING

The woman in mid-life experiences a sharp decline in estrogen production and gradually ceases menstruating. This period is known as the *climacteric*, occurring between ages 46 and 50 years. Although there is much variation in the experience of individual women, there is generally a gradual irregularity in the occurrence of menstrual periods after age 35 years. This irregularity results as the ovarian tissue becomes less responsive to the follicle-stimulating hormone and luteinizing hormone produced by the pituitary gland. The frequency of ovulation gradually diminishes, and the ovaries finally cease to produce progesterone. Physiologic changes in the lining of the vagina occur as estrogen levels drop and may lead to *dyspareunia*, or painful intercourse.

Although most women experience some symptoms of the aforementioned hormonal changes, only a few are actually treated for relief of symptoms. Approximately 80% of women experiencing the climacteric complain of hot flashes, which occur suddenly and last from a few seconds to several minutes. These flashes may be accompanied by symptoms of sweating and dizziness or may occur during sleep, which leads to fitful rest. Because estrogen deficiency is associated with these symptoms, estrogen replacement therapy (ERT) is often provided to alleviate the discomforts. However,

there is considerable controversy about its safety. Although there is evidence that ERT is associated with increased risk of cancer of the uterus, there is also evidence that it is useful in preventing osteoporosis and may provide added protection against heart disease.

The psychologic changes that accompany the hormonal fluctuations of the climacteric vary considerably among women. This change of life (i.e., climacteric) has been blamed for depression and lack of sexual desire, but research results indicate that these psychologic conditions are more likely due to personal characteristics and life style than to the hormonal instability of this time of life. Many women report improvement in their psychologic situation as they are relieved of anxiety about possible pregnancy and may be less inhibited in their sexual desire and orgasmic experiences. There are discrepant findings in the research literature concerning the relationship between physical and psychologic

NURSING RESEARCH

Sex and Sex Education Are Not Just for the Young.

Steinke, E. E. (1988). Older adults' knowledge and attitudes about sexuality. *Image Journal of Nursing Scholarship, 20*(2), 93–95.

This study is one of a few that have been conducted to identify older adults' knowledge and attitudes about sexuality and aging. A quasi-experimental design was used. A convenience sample of 24 subjects over the age of 60 years were randomly assigned to experimental and control groups. Both groups were given a pretest; the experimental group then received educational intervention (four 1-hour sessions on sexuality and aging). Both groups were retested 4–6 weeks after the intervention. Demographic data and data about sexual activity and satisfaction were also collected.

The test, ASKAS, contained 61 items—35 true and false or "don't know" items to assess knowledge about sexual and age-related changes and 26 Likert Scale items to assess attitudes. Reliability and validity of the tool have been established.

The experimental group made a significant gain in knowledge, whereas the control group showed no significant change. Neither group had a significant change in attitude, sexual behavior, or sexual satisfaction. Women were more likely to report sexual satisfaction, and more satisfaction was reported with increased age.

Critique. This study has limited generalizability because of the small sample size. Also, the subjects were volunteers, mostly women who were well educated and of middle to upper socioeconomic status.

Possible nursing implications. Nurses need to change their own negative stereotypes of sexuality and the elderly. They can use knowledge about sexuality and aging to teach older adults about the changes that accompany aging and the benefits of sexual activities.

changes during climacteric, and much remains that is unknown at this time.

As individuals age, physiologic responses continue to gradually diminish in intensity (Table 10–2). In the woman, muscle tension and breast enlargement during arousal may decrease. The reduction in muscle tension may result in reduced intensity of orgasm. The clitoral sensitivity of the female is not usually affected by the aging process, but vaginal tissues change in two important ways. First, there is a reduced elasticity of the vaginal walls, and second, there is a decrease in vaginal lubrication. Consequently, the woman may experience dyspareunia on penetration of the penis and may experience less sensitivity of the vaginal tissues during plateau and orgasm. There is research evidence to indicate that discomfort may be relieved through ERT and application of a water-soluble lubricant such as K-Y Jelly. Research findings also show a positive correlation between those women remaining sexually active and the experience of fewer physiologic limitations in sexual functioning. The woman who has enjoyed an active sex life in earlier years and who is in good health may anticipate a continuation of this functioning into later adulthood.

Men in middle adulthood usually experience some changes in sexual functioning also. They may find that arousal is prolonged and that it takes longer for an erection to occur. The resolution stage is also prolonged, and it takes more time to become aroused again. These normal physiologic changes may lead to "performance anxiety" in the man who is particularly vulnerable to the crisis of mid-life. The American man, filled with dreams of grandeur in early adulthood, may be facing harsh realities in mid-life when many of these dreams may have gone unfulfilled.

A decrease in sperm count, increase in size of the prostate gland, decrease in intensity of ejaculation, and decrease in sensitivity of the penis may lead to difficulties in arousal and potency in the older man. Such changes usually do not occur abruptly, as they accompany the normal aging process. Approximately 5% of men over the age of 60 years experience a *male climacteric*, which includes symptoms of irritability, fatigue, anorexia, reduction in potency, decreased sexual desire, and lack of concentration related to a decrease in testosterone production. This syndrome may be successfully reversed with injections of the male hormone. Although most older men do not experience a well-defined syndrome of sexual changes, some difficulties in sexual functioning are to be expected, and the nurse may assist the client in setting realistic goals in this area during this phase of life.

Sexual burnout is a problem frequently encountered by the middle-aged man or woman and should be differentiated from a lack of sexual interest, which may accompany both alcoholism and depression. Sexual burnout is recognized by a sense of fatigue, emotional emptiness, and negative sexual self-concept. It is accompanied by feelings of helplessness and hopelessness that erotic pleasure may never be rekindled. The feelings are linked directly to the sexual feelings of the individual and are more than simple boredom. With counseling and an open attitude toward change, most individuals are successfully treated for this condition. However, a small percentage of individuals choose to remain celibate for the remainder of their lives and may need assist-

TABLE 10–2 Sexual Changes During the Adult Life Span

Factor	Young Adult	Middle-Aged Adult	Older Adult
Physical	Maturation of secondary sexual characteristics.	Cessation of menses in women, with thinning of vaginal mucosa.	Gradual atrophy of vaginal tissue in women.
	Capable of fertilization. Women may bear children.	Men remain fertile. Female fertility varies.	Women are infertile. Male fertility varies.
	Sexual arousal peaks for men.	Sexual arousal may diminish in men, peak in women. Increase in size of prostate in some.	Sexual arousal takes longer. Decrease in sperm count and force of ejaculation.
Social	Form intimate relationships.	Career peaks. Relationships often strained.	Heightened need for human contact and intimacy.
Psychologic	Strong sense of gender identity and gender roles.	May experience mid-life crisis of identity and roles.	Life review. Desire to be useful. May experience low self-esteem.

ance in accepting a life style contrary to the American stereotype.

Ageism, or the attitude of prejudice against older adults, may contribute to the belief by many elderly individuals, as well as that of their health care providers, that elderly persons are no longer capable of or interested in sexual activity. This prejudice has prevented many older adults from enjoying sexual activity and from pursuing solutions to sexual problems. Although chronic health problems may have adverse effects on sexual functioning of the aging adult, ageism has by far a greater impact. In a comprehensive report of the sexual attitudes and activities of more than 4000 Americans 50 years of age or older, Consumers Union provided evidence that the stereotype of this prejudice is unfounded and is deleterious to the sexual enjoyment of individuals in this stage of life (Brecher, 1984). Some suggestions for dealing with changes associated with aging included the use of vibrators and sexually explicit reading materials to increase stimulation, and an alteration in positions and timing of sexual activity to take maximal advantage of energy levels (see the Nursing Research feature on p. 178).

EFFECTS OF ILLNESS ON SEXUALITY

HOSPITALIZATION

The process of hospitalization or institutionalization is often perceived as characterized by depersonalization. Elements of sexual identity and behaviors associated with gender roles are frequently denied or seriously curtailed by the social settings that exist in most hospitals, nursing homes, and rehabilitation centers. These settings provide little privacy, and they are places where symbols of sexual identity, such as wearing certain clothing and jewelry, are removed, and where behaviors associated with sexual arousal and satisfaction are overtly or covertly discouraged.

ACUTE ILLNESS

When an individual is hospitalized for acute illness or injury, elements of sexual health may be impaired. Not only is the social climate not conducive to sexual health for the reasons just identified, but the physical and psychologic conditions of the individual may not be congruent with sexual health. Acute medical conditions for which an individual may be hospitalized may render the person physically unable to engage in sexual activity because of anxiety, fatigue, pain, malaise, or direct tissue damage or surgical removal.

Specific acute disorders such as STDs or complications secondary to these disorders may have implications for the sexuality of the hospitalized person. Although discussion of the various STDs is beyond the scope of this chapter, nursing care that includes assessment of risk factors and sexual contacts must be consid-

ered when caring for the client with an acute condition requiring hospitalization. Because of the social stigma associated with the diagnosis of STDs, the hospitalized client may also suffer from guilt and low self-esteem, which may impair his or her pursuit of behaviors that would lead to sexual health.

Specific acute bacterial or viral infections such as pneumonia, hepatitis, gastroenteritis, and prostatitis have implications for the sexual health of the individual. In addition to fatigue and malaise that are associated with these conditions, specific alterations in body function may threaten the body image and self-esteem of the ill person.

CHRONIC ILLNESS

Sexual health of the individual with a chronic illness or impairment may be threatened in various ways (see the accompanying Key Features of Disease). Individuals with hypertension, arthritis, cancer, cardiovascular disease, diabetes, end-stage renal disease, chronic liver disease, or chronic respiratory disease face limitations of previous sexual behavior patterns. These individuals must deal with changes in body structure and/or function in addition to psychologic variables such as uncertainty, fear, and depression. The body image of the individual is threatened, and tissue damage may result in impairment of the sexual response cycle or may render the individual unable to engage in preferred sexual activities.

Adults who experience hypertension are at risk for problems in sexual functioning at mid-life. Antihypertensive drugs such as guanethidine (Ismelin), reserpine (Serpasil), and methyldopa (Aldomet) have been associated with decreased libido in both men and women. In addition, men may experience erectile and ejaculatory failure, whereas women may experience galactorrhea, the presence of milk in the breasts. These adverse effects usually disappear within 2 weeks after medication is discontinued. Clonidine (Catapres), another antihypertensive agent, may lead to urinary retention and gynecomastia (breast engorgement) in men, thus affecting the sexual response cycle. It is important for the nurse to assess the effects of such drugs in both men and women so that changes in dosages or types of medication may be considered if needed.

Individuals with arthritic disease face a chronic disabling condition that is characterized by problems with mobility, pain, and weakness. Although research is lacking concerning the specific incidence of sexual dysfunction among individuals with arthritis, there are obvious physical barriers to the usual sexual activities of persons with this condition. Limited joint movement, weakness, fatigue, pain, swelling, and stiffness of extremities make activities of daily living difficult. In addition to the often deforming nature of arthritis, large dosages of corticosteroid drugs may alter physical appearance, which results in lowered self-esteem and altered body image. Depression and anxiety about the unrelenting course of arthritic conditions may interfere

KEY FEATURES OF DISEASE ■ Effects of Illness on Adult Sexuality

Illness	Effects on Men	Effects on Women
Arthritis	Decreased libido Low self-esteem Altered body image Depression, anxiety	Dyspareunia Low self-esteem Altered body image Depression, anxiety
Cancer	Altered body image Erectile dysfunction Decreased libido Depression, anxiety Low self-esteem	Altered body image Dyspareunia Decreased libido Depression, anxiety Low self-esteem
Cardiovascular disease	Erectile dysfunction Low self-esteem Depression, anxiety	Decreased libido Low self-esteem Depression, anxiety
Diabetes	Erectile dysfunction Retrograde ejaculation Decreased fertility	Decreased libido Orgasmic dysfunction Decreased fertility Dyspareunia Chronic vaginitis Decreased vaginal lubrication
Hepatic disease	Loss of libido Sexual unresponsiveness Erectile dysfunction	Decreased libido Orgasmic dysfunction Amenorrhea
Hypertension	Decreased libido Erectile failure Ejaculatory failure Gynecomastia	Decreased libido Galactorrhea
Renal disease	Low self-esteem Altered body image Loss of libido Erectile dysfunction Decreased fertility Depression, fatigue	Low self-esteem Altered body image Loss of libido Orgasmic dysfunction Decreased fertility Depression, fatigue
Respiratory disease	Low self-esteem Decreased libido Erectile dysfunction	Low self-esteem Decreased libido Orgasmic dysfunction
Spinal cord injury	Erectile dysfunction Possible infertility Retrograde ejaculation Ejaculatory dysfunction Orgasmic dysfunction Low self-esteem Impaired body image Loss of libido	Orgasmic dysfunction Amenorrhea Low self-esteem Impaired body image Loss of libido

with interpersonal communication and result in sexual problems of decreased libido and inhibited sexual desire. Dyspareunia may result from alterations in secretory function of the vagina, as seen in clients with Sjögren's syndrome (see Chap. 28).

Various types of cancer may directly affect sexual functioning and body image. Cervical or uterine cancer resulting in hysterectomy and breast cancer resulting in mastectomy are among the obvious malignancies that affect both sexual functioning and body image in women. In men, testicular and prostatic cancer may result in radical surgeries that alter both sexual functioning and body image. Many other primary malignant tumors also contribute to decline of the individual's sexual health, including cancers of the gastrointestinal tract, urinary system, and larynx that result in surgical diversions and radical neck dissections. In addition to the damaging effects of malignant growths and surgical ablative procedures, radiation and chemotherapy affect the sexual functioning and self-esteem of the individual with cancer. Alopecia (loss of hair), fatigue, anorexia, malaise, decline in libido, and secondary ovarian or testicular failure are but a few of the side effects of these therapies. Persistence of myths about cancer as being contagious or "unclean" has also led to an increase in sexual problems among those who do not understand the nature of the illness.

The effects of cardiovascular disease on the sexuality of the individual are related to the relationship between sexual activity and demands on the cardiopulmonary system, the self-concept and self-esteem of the individual, role function, and interdependence. Resumption of sexual activity after a myocardial infarction can be planned and implemented on an individual basis. The conditions under which the activity is pursued (relaxing versus anxiety-provoking conditions) and the amount of physical stress that the heart can handle must be considered. Guidelines for planning this resumption are provided later in this chapter. The severity of tissue damage and the effects of medications may limit the degree to which sexual activity is pursued by the individual with chronic cardiovascular disease. With physical conditioning programs and regulation of drug therapy, expressions of sexuality may be continued.

Diabetes has long been associated with sexual problems. Secondary erectile dysfunction (impotence) in men is frequently associated with microvascular changes and neuropathy and occurs in approximately 50% of men with diabetes. Another 1% of men may experience retrograde ejaculation in which the ejaculate is released into the urinary bladder instead of through the urinary meatus. The latter difficulty and the presence of disease of long duration may contribute to sterility or to problems with fertility in diabetic men. Comparable changes in women lead to decreased libido and orgasmic dysfunctions. A decrease in vaginal lubrication and increased risk of infection contribute to chronic vaginitis in women. There is an increased incidence of sexual problems in those who have had diabetes for longer periods. Fertility problems in both men and women are not uncommon. Microvascular changes and neuropathy are generally cited as etiologic factors for the high incidence of secondary erectile dysfunction in men and for the decrease in vaginal lubrication in women that contributes to chronic vaginal infections.

The effects of end-stage renal disease are monumental. Every system in the body is affected by the impairment of the metabolism and regulation of electrolytes. In addition to physical limitations resulting from fatigue, pruritus, anorexia, lethargy, and muscle cramping, the individual with end-stage renal disease faces overwhelming psychosocial changes. Self-concept, body image, and self-esteem suffer as a result of the gradual deterioration of body functions and structures. Role functions and issues of dependency are altered as the individual may be forced to stop working or managing usual responsibilities in the home and the community. The financial burdens of lost income and expensive treatments add to the stressors for the person with chronic renal disease. As a result of these multiple factors, the individual may experience depression, loss of libido, decreased frequency of sexual activity, and impotence, as well as sterility. Although the interventions for individuals with end-stage renal disease must be individualized, to date the prognosis is poor, and most of these individuals are unable to resume the level of sexual functioning that they enjoyed before their illness.

Respiratory impairment can lead to increased levels of fatigue with accompanying threats to self-esteem. Individuals with chronic obstructive pulmonary disease or chronic asthma report difficulty in continuing sexual intercourse. A review of the adult sexual response cycle indicates that respiratory rates double during plateau and orgasmic phases, which makes coitus difficult for both sexes. Alternative methods of sexual pleasuring may be suggested.

Chronic conditions affecting the liver and immune system frequently lead to impairment of sexual health. Anorexia, fatigue, joint pain, nausea, fever, and jaundice associated with chronic hepatitis render the individual uninterested in sexually explicit behavior and may result in complications such as erectile dysfunction or sexual unresponsiveness. Similarly, cirrhosis of the liver related to malnutrition, infection with parasites, or alcohol abuse may lead to loss of libido and specific pathologic conditions including gynecomastia and erectile dysfunctions in men and amenorrhea in women.

Spinal cord injury leads to various sexual dysfunctions related to altered physical functioning and to psychosocial changes. Sexual dysfunctions are related to the extent and location of the injury and differ for men and women. Men with injury to the cervical cord (C1–7) are quadriplegic and usually continue to have reflexive erections of the penis; those with injury at lower levels experience erectile dysfunction because the neural pathways are damaged or destroyed. Incomplete injury of the spinal cord permits some sensation and motor function of the genitalia, whereas complete transection results in loss of libido in both men and women, loss of erection and ejaculation in men, and orgasmic dysfunction in women. Men with complete transection of the lumbosacral cord are infertile because of retrograde ejaculation or damaged sperm. Women, however, may experience temporary amenorrhea, retain fertility, and be capable of term pregnancy. Psychosocial problems may contribute to a decline in sexual health for the person with spinal cord injury because of the accompanying change in body image and loss of self-esteem. However, many persons with spinal cord injuries report satisfying sexual activity when their physical, psychologic, and social problems are addressed.

EFFECTS OF DRUG AND ALCOHOL USE AND ABUSE ON SEXUALITY

The possibility of drug abuse and alcoholism as factors in sexual functioning of both men and women in middle adulthood should not be overlooked as a central factor when sexual problems are suspected or validated. As the harsh realities of mid-life mount, many adults turn

KEY FEATURES OF DISEASE ■ Effects of Alcohol and Drugs on Sexual Functioning

Drug	Effects on Men	Effects on Women
Alcohol	Decreased libido	Decreased libido
	Increased aggression, possibly leading to sexual abuse	Increased passivity, possibly leading to sexual abuse
	Erectile dysfunction	Orgasmic dysfunction
	Decreased fertility	Amenorrhea, sterility
	Low sexual satisfaction	Low sexual satisfaction
Antidepressants	Erectile dysfunction	Delayed orgasm
	Delayed ejaculation	
Antihypertensives	Decreased libido	Decreased libido
	Erectile dysfunction	Anovulation, amenorrhea
	Ejaculatory dysfunction	Galactorrhea
	Retrograde ejaculation	Impaired orgasm
Cocaine and amphetamines	Delayed orgasm	Orgasmic dysfunction
	Delayed ejaculation	Decreased libido
Narcotics	Decreased libido	Decreased libido
	Erectile dysfunction	Spontaneous abortion
	Delayed ejaculation	Amenorrhea
Tranquilizers	Retrograde ejaculation	Galactorrhea
	Erectile dysfunction	Amenorrhea, anovulation

to drugs or alcohol to ease their anxieties, including specific anxieties related to diminished sexual functioning (see the accompanying Key Features of Disease). The primary effects of limited alcohol intake are often stimulating, and both men and women may experience release of inhibitions, relief of anxiety, and an increase in libido. However, as alcohol intake increases or as alcohol is consumed with increasing frequency, several deleterious effects occur.

In the woman, desire for sexual activity gradually decreases until there is no interest. There is a gradual decrease in vaginal lubrication and sensitivity in late alcoholism. It takes more time for the woman to have an orgasm, and fewer orgasms are experienced.

In the man, decreased desire is often accompanied by an increase in aggression and finally a total loss of desire and profound aggression in the late stage of alcoholism. Delay in erection leads to inability to attain an erection with maximum stimulation, and orgasm may be tentative or may not exist under any circumstances. The man also experiences diminished pleasurable sensations associated with sexual arousal. While erection is still possible, the resolution stage is prolonged, and the man experiences a loss of sexual satisfaction.

EFFECTS OF ATTITUDES AND VALUES ON SEXUALITY

Sexual health and behaviors are related to the attitudes and values of the individual. The psychosexual devel-

opment discussed earlier in this chapter provides a general guideline to the psychosexual tasks encountered by the individual at various stages of the life cycle. As a result of this development, the individual acquires attitudes that, through clarification and practice, become values that guide behavior. The culture of the family and community are important in shaping values. The importance of sexual health and socially appropriate sexual behavior within the family and community influences the way in which the individual views herself or himself as sexual. The presence of these attitudes and values becomes quite important in influencing the development of sexual dysfunctions and is addressed later in more detail under the heading Psychosocial Assessment.

EFFECTS OF INTERPERSONAL SKILLS ON SEXUALITY

Much of an individual's sexual behavior occurs in relationship to other individuals. Throughout the life span, individuals interact with each other in ways that may be either explicitly or implicitly sexual. Skills in verbal and nonverbal communication are essential for developing this element of sexual health. Sensitivity to one's own, as well as another's, needs and desires and the ability to communicate this sensitivity are learned through social interactions. The abilities to trust another person, to give and receive affection, and to listen openly to another are essential skills for building healthy sexual relationships.

Lack of these skills is important in contributing to sexual dysfunctions and is addressed in more detail under the heading Psychosocial Assessment.

RESEARCH

Recent interest in sexuality has resulted in a variety of scientific studies designed to describe problems in sexual functioning, to identify psychosocial factors related to these problems, and to test interventions originating in the disciplines of nursing, psychology, education, and medicine. These studies deal with problems arising from psychosocial situations as well as those with physiologic bases, such as sexual impairment resulting from the effects of sexual abuse or other psychosocial trauma and sexual dysfunctions directly related to physical development and illness. Subjects from children through older adults have been studied.

The history of research in human sexuality is fairly short. Before Alfred Kinsey's surveys of human sexual behavior in the 1930s, most research had been based on persons with deviant or criminal behavior, and little was known about the average or typical sexual behavior of individuals. Kinsey trained interviewers who questioned some 18,000 individuals in the United States about their sexual histories. Some of the findings led to new understandings about the sexual activities of women and of persons with a homosexual orientation. In addition, the findings of these studies enabled the American public to redefine the social code of acceptable sexual activities and to acknowledge more openly the reality of human sexual characteristics.

In the late 1950s and 1960s, the team of Masters and Johnson began to observe couples engaging in sexual activity and used various instruments to measure responses of both men and women. In addition to using case studies and clinical and experimental research designs to increase the knowledge base of human sexual response and behavior, this team developed and tested various interventions for use with couples who had recognizable sexual dysfunctions. Their contributions to the field of sexology as well as to the enlightenment of the general public are well documented.

In addition to the research findings available today, new questions concerning the ethics of such research have emerged. Consequently, guidelines have been established to prevent sexual problems as a result of clinical or experimental investigation. The following factors were suggested by Kolodny (1978) as essential in the planning of further studies of human sexuality:

1. Proposals must reflect a potential benefit/risk ratio that is relatively high.
2. Dignity of the individual must be preserved through informed consent and assurance of confidentiality.
3. A mechanism for peer and/or community review must be in place.
4. Interventions must be based on complete and accurate research data that describe the etiology and incidence of the problem.

Current research efforts focus on the dramatic rise in the incidence of AIDS. Although most attention has been given to the outbreak of this syndrome among the homosexual population, there is mounting evidence that the heterosexual population is also at risk. AIDS among children is another reality, and although a discussion of this entity is beyond the scope of this chapter, it is important for nurses to remain abreast of this syndrome as a rapidly developing threat to sexual health. The need for research in the physical and psychosocial domains is also great.

NURSES' COMFORT WITH SEXUALITY

The increased knowledge and awareness of human sexuality throughout the life cycle that have resulted from these research endeavors have led to an increased demand, on the part of the consumer of health care services, for solutions to problems in sexual functioning. Nursing, as a major provider of health care services, has had to respond to this demand by developing strategies to prevent the development of sexual problems and to promote sexual health.

Several factors are important to consider as nurses prepare to meet this need. Nurses must develop skills in physical and psychosocial assessment, possess open attitudes and positive values toward sexuality, develop an accurate knowledge base of the complex factors that affect sexual health, and demonstrate skills in educating and counseling clients with diverse needs.

In addition to having an adequate knowledge base in human sexuality, the nurse must feel comfortable with application of the nursing process to sexual health needs of clients. An attitude of openness and of willingness to approach the subject is prerequisite to assessment and intervention that address the goal of the client's sexual health.

To apply the nursing process to matters of sexual health in clients, one must first be aware of the elements of one's own sexuality, and clarification of one's own values and of one's own sexual health is also needed. In her discussion of human sexuality and the nursing process, Lion (1982) identified several of the aforementioned characteristics of sexually healthy persons and provided a comprehensive overview of clarification exercises related to sexual issues and values for nurses in a variety of settings. The use of values clarification exercises, such as the one in Table 10–3, enables nurses to "acknowledge

---

TABLE 10-3   Values Clarification Exercise

Situation: Mary is a 26-year-old single woman hospitalized for a radical hysterectomy. She has a malignancy. Which of the following responses by nurses is most like your response to assessing, diagnosing, and intervening with regard to her actual and potential sexual problems?

Nurse A: "I hope she doesn't ask about having sexual relations or I'll just die of embarassment!"

Nurse B: "I know how I'll handle any questions about sex. I'll just refer her to the head nurse. She can handle that stuff."

Nurse C: "It's ok if she asks about sex, but I'm not sure I know all the answers. I know I can listen and try to help her find answers if I don't know them."

Nurse D: "It's just fine if she asks about how this will affect her sexually. In fact, even if she doesn't bring it up, I will. I really believe it's an important aspect of her health."

Clarification of values in responses: If you answered that you feel most like one of the nurses above, check below to clarify what this means.

Nurse A: This nurse feels uncomfortable handling concerns about sexual health and needs to do more reading and talking about her feelings with other health professionals.

Nurse B: This nurse also feels uncomfortable and is willing to shirk responsibility, passing it on to one with more authority. Again, more learning and exploration of his or her attitudes are needed.

Nurse C: This nurse feels comfortable. Being able and willing to look for additional information is essential to helping the client.

Nurse D: This nurse also feels comfortable and is willing to take more responsibility for including sexual health in client care.

---

their feelings and thoughts, examine their attitudes and beliefs, consider their convictions and behaviors, and clarify the content and power of their sexual value system" (Lion, 1982, p. 1).

COLLABORATIVE MANAGEMENT

 Assessment

History

In managing the sexual health of individuals who are hospitalized or of those who interact with nurses in various other professional settings such as schools, clinics, or home environments, a brief sexual history is integrated with the general health history. Three areas are addressed: physical development and situational changes in sexual functioning; alterations in body image, sex role, and self-esteem; and sociocultural factors such as ritualistic practices. Examples of questions that can be asked while obtaining a history include

1. "Have you ever experienced any injury or disease of the genitourinary system? Is there any history of STDs?"

2. "What is your past experience with contraceptives? Is there any history of problems related to infertility?"

3. "What was the pattern of development of secondary sexual characteristics (e.g., menstruation)? Have there been any changes in these characteristics (e.g., hirsutism [excessive hair growth in females] or gynecomastia [breast development in males])? What changes do you attribute to your age?"

4. "Have you experienced any unwanted or traumatic sexual events such as incest or rape?"

5. "Have you noticed any changes in sexual functioning in the past related to the use of alcohol or other drugs?"

6. "Have you experienced any changes in sexual functioning or desire for sexual activity since your current illness, injury, or surgery?"

7. "Has this physical problem (illness, injury, or surgical treatment) changed the way you view your body or feel about yourself as a woman or man?"

8. "As a result of this physical problem, have you noticed changes in your usual activities as a woman or man, or changes in your usual roles, such as those of wife or mother, or husband or father?"

9. "What are some of your beliefs and practices about sexual functioning? Have any of these been affected by your current illness, injury, or surgery?"

Although some of these questions may be answered easily with "yes" or "no," they may also be posed in such a way as to invite the client to discuss her or his sexual identity, roles, or activity. Beginning each phrase with, "Tell me how" may encourage further disclosure. Additional information about the person's level of knowledge and understanding about sexual development and functioning may be obtained indirectly. Taking a sexual history is one way to identify misinformation that should be corrected as part of the nursing intervention. Table 10-4 summarizes the information contained in a brief sexual history and assessment.

Physical Assessment: Clinical Manifestations

Assessment of the various elements of sexual health may be incorporated into a general physical assessment. Subjective data concerning body image may be gathered as the nurse palpates various parts of the body,

TABLE 10-4 Brief Sexual History and Assessment Guide

Assessment Factor	History	Current Assessment
Physical	Development of secondary sexual characteristics (onset and pattern of menses in woman).	Observe and palpate. Note changes over time.
	Use of contraceptives; problems with fertility or pregnancy.	Note current use and problems with contraception; issues of fertility or pregnancy.
	Episodes of STDs.	Note recent changes in sexual activity level or pattern.
	Past genitourinary disease, injury, or surgery.	Note thickening or discharge from breast or genitalia.
	Past use of drugs and alcohol.	Note current drug use.
	Past patterns of sexual function.	Note changes in levels of sexual arousal or function.
Psychologic	Past sexual dysfunction.	Identify knowledge of sexual function.
	Past problems with body image, gender role, or self-esteem.	Note current feelings about body parts and functions and self-esteem, and current values.
	History of incest, rape, or other unwanted sexual experiences.	Identify recent unwanted sexual experiences.
Social	Cultural rituals, beliefs, and inhibitions (e.g., circumcision, menses, marriage).	Note cultural expectations for sexual behavior.
	Family composition and roles.	Note changes in composition of family or peers.
	Pattern of marital or sexual status and living arrangements.	Note change in living arrangements or marital status.
	Past sexual orientation and preference (e.g., homosexuality, bisexuality, heterosexuality, transsexuality).	Identify current sexual preference and patterns of sexual activity.

moving from relatively neutral areas such as face and extremities to the external genitalia and breasts. Concern for the individual's dignity should always be considered when assessing these more private areas. An explanation of what is to be examined, in what manner, and for what reason should be included. As in other physical assessments, attention must be given to external appearance, palpation of internal structures, and examination of any discharges (which may also need to be further scrutinized by use of laboratory tests). While the genitalia and breasts are assessed, additional information about sexual activity, knowledge, and attitudes

may be elicited. For example, when inspecting the external genitalia, the nurse might ask the client to describe her or his usual sexual activities and ask if there is any discomfort or anxiety related to these activities. A detailed description of the physical assessment of genitalia and breasts is found in Chapter 52. The clinical manifestations described in this section relate specifically to sexual functioning.

Dyspareunia, or painful intercourse, in the woman may be related to factors such as an intact hymen; scarring from episiotomy; infections of the vagina or vulva including venereal warts or other STDs; insufficient vaginal lubrication; and irritation from chemical products such as contraceptives, douches, and feminine deodorants. Pathologic conditions of the uterus, cervix, ovaries, and fallopian tubes may also result in dyspareunia, and such conditions should be ruled out through referral to a gynecologist or other physician. Dyspareunia may also be related to psychogenic factors such as trauma from rape, incest, or other unwanted sexual experiences; or previous experience with an inconsiderate partner.

In the man, dyspareunia may be related to inflammation or infection of the penis, prostate, urinary bladder, urethra, or testes. Men infrequently experience pain related to exposure to vaginal contraceptive creams or foams, or to irritation from the tail of the partner's intrauterine device (IUD). Other factors contributing to complaints of dyspareunia in the man are psychosocial.

Inhibited sexual desire is a loss of interest in sexual activity or decline in libido. In the woman it may be related to hormonal replacement therapy, use of oral contraceptives, eating disorders such as anorexia or bulimia, weight gain or loss, drug use or abuse (including alcohol), or chronic illnesses such as cancer or end-stage renal disease. Psychosocial factors such as abuse, marital discord, depression, anxiety, fear, or other environmental stressors may constitute the major contributing factor to this problem.

In the man, inhibited sexual desire may be related to the use of antihypertensive drugs, other drug use or abuse (including alcohol), or chronic illnesses affecting energy levels. The same psychosocial factors that result in inhibited sexual desire in the woman may contribute to this problem in the man.

Vaginismus is a condition in which the muscles of the outer third of the vaginal barrel contract powerfully and prevent insertion of a tampon or other object. This condition may be related to physical factors such as sexual activity during the healing phase after obstetric trauma, infections of the vagina and vulva, abnormalities of the hymen, and atrophy of the vagina. Other contributing factors include lack of information, anxiety, and fear. Vaginismus is more likely to be related to psychogenic causes including strong religious teachings, rape trauma, physical or psychosocial abuse, or homosexual experimentation. Accurate diagnosis of vaginismus cannot be made without direct pelvic examination in which the involuntary muscle spasm is evident with the simple suggestion of penetration of the vagina. If the situation is complex with multiple factors contributing to the condition, assessment may be beyond the scope of the nurse-generalist, and referral to a psychiatrist, psychologist, or sex therapist may be necessary for further evaluation of the problem.

Orgasmic dysfunction is defined as the inability to achieve orgasm (primary dysfunction) or the inability to achieve orgasm with intercourse or at an appropriate time during intercourse (secondary dysfunction). These dysfunctions are the most common sexual complaint of adult women. Orgasmic dysfunctions are related to physical factors such as adhesions of the clitoris that interfere with stimulation, lack of strength in the pubo-

coccygeal muscles, and diminished contractions of the uterus. These factors all require referral to a physician for confirmation. Other contributing factors are psychogenic and include feelings of anxiety, guilt, lack of knowledge, poor communication skills, and marital discord. Fear of rejection and conscious withholding of orgasm may lead to secondary orgasmic dysfunctions; general expectations of the culture or society may also be contributing factors. Assessment of the history and environmental circumstances under which orgasmic difficulties are experienced leads to a differentiation of the dysfunction as primary (orgasm never being experienced by the woman), secondary (history of orgasm, but lack of it at present time), or situational (orgasm with manual stimulation but not with penetration of the vagina).

Erectile dysfunction is the inability of the man to attain or maintain an erection of the penis of sufficient firmness to permit penetration. This problem may be referred to as primary if the man has never been able to sustain such an erection, or secondary if the man has experienced at least one erection of sufficient firmness to permit penetration. Erectile dysfunction is the term preferred to *impotence* in this condition. Organic causes of this disorder include spinal cord injury, diabetes mellitus, alcoholism, neurologic disease such as multiple sclerosis, endocrine disorders, various infections of the genitourinary system, and specific drug use and abuse (antihypertensives, barbiturates, sedatives, and amphetamines). Psychosocial factors contributing to erectile dysfunctions include marital discord, anxiety, depression, excessive weight gain or loss, insomnia, and fatigue.

Ejaculatory dysfunction, premature, is a condition in which the man ejaculates after penetration but sooner than either partner desires. Although there are no established norms for the timing of ejaculation during intercourse, this timing is important to the satisfaction of both partners in sexual activity. If the man is unable to exercise any voluntary control over the timing of this learned response, premature ejaculation may become a problem. Organic causes are rare, if they exist at all; psychosocial factors contribute to the learning of this response. Feelings of anxiety, guilt, and fear combined with situations in which the man may hurry toward a climax may result in this type of dysfunction.

Ejaculatory dysfunction, delayed (also referred to as ejaculatory incompetence or ejaculatory overcontrol), is a relatively rare sexual problem in men. It results in the inability to ejaculate with vaginal intercourse or in the ability to ejaculate only after a prolonged series of thrusts and to the point of discomfort in the partner. The man may be able to ejaculate at an earlier point during masturbation, with a homosexual partner, or with a casual encounter. The contributing factors are psychosocial and may include marital conflicts, resentment of the partner, fear of interruption, fear of impregnating the partner, or earlier psychologic trauma.

Retrograde ejaculation, or dry orgasm, may sometimes be confused with ejaculatory incompetence because of the lack of external evidence of the ejaculate. In this condition, the semen is discharged in a retrograde manner into the urinary bladder rather than forward through the penis. This may result from prostatic surgery, diabetes, multiple sclerosis, structural defects of the urethra and bladder neck, or use of tranquilizers. During orgasm, the bladder neck does not close and the semen is forced directly into this organ. The man experiences the sensation of orgasm but is infertile as a result of this phenomenon.

Sexual aversion in both women and men is an irrational fear or phobic reaction to the thought of sexual activity or to the actual activity. Physical symptoms such as nausea, diarrhea, profound sweating, dry mouth, chills, and tachycardia may accompany feelings of disgust and dread. Contributing factors are psychogenic and include a history of trauma from rape or incest, marital conflict, negative parental and religious attitudes, and confusion about gender identity.

Psychosocial Assessment

A more comprehensive and specific sexual health history is needed once a sexual problem is identified or suspected. Although the general sexual history described earlier is an essential part of a nursing assessment, additional information about the psychologic and social factors related to past and present sexual functioning is required when making a nursing diagnosis of sexual dysfunction. Subjective responses of the individual include the way in which the client perceives the problem, as well as how the client feels, thinks, and acts. The following questions may guide a more complete assessment of past and present factors related to sexual dysfunction:

1. How does the client describe the problem? What specific behaviors, thoughts, feelings, or attitudes are problematic?
2. What is the client's perception of what caused or what continues to contribute to the problem?
3. What environmental or situational factors were present at the onset of the problem?
4. How has the problem changed over time? Has it become more severe or less severe? Does it occur in more than one setting?
5. What has the client previously done to seek help from others, both professionals and peers, and what forms of self-help has she or he tried?
6. What are the client's expectations and goals, both realistic and ideal, for therapeutic intervention and resolution of the problem?

In addition to direct assessment of the individual's sexual health, problems of sexuality may be brought to the nurse's attention through the client's "acting-out" behaviors. In this situation, the client exhibits inappropriate behaviors such as exposing genitalia or overtly soliciting sexual favors from the nurse. It is important for the nurse to realize that this represents a coping mechanism on the part of the client, who may be overwhelmed by actual or potential threats to body image, gender identity, gender role, and sexual functioning.

Further assessment of the psychosocial factors that contribute to this inappropriate behavior is essential to helping this individual regain control over the perceived or actual threats. Affirmation of the person's gender identity and willingness to explore the meaning of the situation to him or her are essential to further assessment. Once a climate of trust has been established, the nurse might ask the following questions:

1. "How has this illness, injury, or surgery changed the way you feel about yourself?"
2. "How has this illness, injury, or surgery affected the way you act as a sexual partner?"
3. "How will this illness, injury, or surgery change your sexual activity? What specific changes do you anticipate or fear in the near future?"
4. "What medications or treatments do you believe may be contributing to these changes in your sexual activity?"

 Analysis: Nursing Diagnosis

After completion of a physical and psychosocial assessment with a sexual health history, the next step of the nursing process consists of formulating nursing diagnoses. Actual or potential problems in sexual functioning related to impairment of the adult sexual response cycle (specifically arousal and orgasm or potency), deficits in coping skills, knowledge deficits, changes in or loss of body parts, or physiologic limitations may be identified.

Common Diagnoses

The major sexual problems addressed through the nursing process are sexual dysfunctions. Common problems related to sexual dysfunctions may affect both sexes or either sex.

1. Sexual dysfunction (male and female) related to
   a. Dyspareunia
   b. Inhibited sexual desire
   c. Sexual aversion
2. Sexual dysfunction (female) related to
   a. Vaginismus
   b. Orgasmic dysfunction
3. Sexual dysfunction (male) related to
   a. Erectile dysfunction
   b. Ejaculatory dysfunction, premature
   c. Ejaculatory dysfunction, delayed
   d. Retrograde ejaculation

In addition to the common diagnoses identified, the following problems may also be identified in some clients:

1. Anxiety related to conflict about essential values or goals of life such as pregnancy or change in marital status

2. Ineffective individual coping related to situational crisis such as rape trauma
3. Ineffective individual coping related to developmental crisis such as new marriage
4. Ineffective individual coping related to personal vulnerability such as divorce
5. Sexual dysfunction related to ineffectual or absent role models such as divorce or family, single parent
6. Sexual dysfunction related to physical abuse such as rape trauma or sexual abuse
7. Sexual dysfunction related to psychosocial abuse such as divorce, impotence, or change in marital status
8. Sexual dysfunction related to misinformation or lack of knowledge such as reproductive problems, endocrine or metabolic disease, or paralysis
9. Sexual dysfunction related to lack of privacy secondary to hospitalization
10. Sexual dysfunction related to altered body structure or function secondary to amputation, mastectomy, or vasectomy

 Planning and Implementation: Common Sexual Problems in Women and Men

Sexual Dysfunction Related to Dyspareunia

Planning: client goals. The client goals are directly related to the stated sexual problem of the individual. For the individual who has an identified sexual problem of dyspareunia, the goal is that the client will be free from pain or discomfort during sexual intercourse (see the accompanying Client Care Plan).

Interventions: nonsurgical management. Nursing interventions for the woman who has a sexual problem of dyspareunia depend on the contributing factors. When pain results from physiologic factors such as an intact hymen, scarring from an episiotomy, or pathologic conditions of the reproductive organs, referral to a gynecologist is made. Infections of the vagina or vulva also require medical diagnosis and supervision. In addition, the nurse administers antibiotics, provides for increased fluid intake, and encourages rest and avoidance of sexual activity. Therapeutic communication and edu-

---

CLIENT CARE PLAN ■ The Client with an Alteration in Sexuality

Goal/Outcome Criteria	Interventions	Rationales
Nursing Diagnosis 1: Sexual Dysfunction Related to Dyspareunia: Woman		
Client will express no pain or discomfort associated with sexual intercourse or usual sexual activities.	1. Instruct client to use water-soluble lubricant before sexual intercourse or usual sexual activities.	1. Water-soluble lubricants do not dry mucosa as do petroleum products.
	2. Describe to the client the importance of erotic stimulation for vaginal lubrication; provide examples of visual, auditory, or olfactory sensations associated with sexual arousal.	2. Adequate arousal and stimulation are prerequisites to adequate lubrication.
	3. Explain the relationship between use of feminine hygiene products and destruction of the natural cleaning function of vaginal flora and secretions. Encourage use of products such as feminine deodorant sprays, vaginal douches, and scented perineal pads in moderation.	3. Overuse of feminine hygiene products destroys the natural flora and secretions of the vaginal walls.
Nursing Diagnosis 2: Sexual Dysfunction Related to Dyspareunia: Man		
Client will express no pain or discomfort associated with sexual intercourse or usual sexual activities.	1. Instruct client about possible irritation from exposure to vaginal contraceptive cream, jelly, foam, or string from IUD.	1. Skin of external genitalia may be hypersensitive to chemicals in these products.
	2. Encourage the client to clean the foreskin if client is uncircumcised.	2. Adequate hygiene of foreskin reduces mechanical irritation.
	3. Refer to physician or urologist if symptoms indicate inflammation of the urethra, prostate, or testes.	3. Treatment with an antibiotic or anti-inflammatory drug may be indicated.

cation to reduce further episodes of infection include listening with a nonjudgmental attitude and providing information about the risk of multiple partners, if this is a factor. The nurse also explains the risks involved with the person's usual sexual activities. For example, chronic irritations may result from the use of foreign objects placed into the vagina without adequate lubrication.

When the major contributing factors include inadequate vaginal lubrication or irritation from excessive use of chemical contraceptives, douches, or feminine deodorants, the nurse provides accurate information and specific suggestions for behavioral changes. The nurse reviews anatomy and physiology and emphasizes the ability of the vagina to clean itself. The nurse describes alternative methods of contraception or selection of those without scents and encourages the use of unscented tampons or sanitary pads. The nurse also suggests increasing vaginal lubrication through the use of over-the-counter water-soluble gels.

When dyspareunia results from inflammation or infection of organs within the genitourinary system of the man, the nurse intervenes through administration of antibiotics ordered by the physician and encourages the client to drink fluids, rest, and avoid foods that are irritants. The man with acute inflammation or infection is encouraged to avoid sexual intercourse with his partner until the acute condition has abated. Alternative sexual activities that avoid intercourse are suggested and explored with both partners.

When the major contributing factor for dyspareunia in the man is exposure to vaginal contraceptive creams and foams or to the presence of an IUD in the sexual partner, providing information and alternatives to the man and his sexual partner is essential. Alternatives such as mutual body massage and caressing may be suggested. Careful assessment of the nature of the man's exposure to such irritants is made before this step if the man has multiple partners.

Psychosocial factors resulting in dyspareunia in the man or woman are often of early origin (from childhood or adolescence) and require the specialized skills of a clinician with advanced education and experience in psychotherapy or counseling. However, the nurse-generalist can intervene through therapeutic communication, by acknowledging the reality of these contributing factors through empathic responses and by referring the individual and his partner to a competent therapist who may be a nurse with special preparation, a psychologist, or a psychiatrist.

The nurse-specialist with advanced education and experience intervenes with intensive therapy directed at resolving the underlying conflicts or blocks to sexual pleasure. Therapy with the family of origin may also be necessary. Behavior modification and systematic desensitization may be used as specific approaches to intervention. Specific problematic sexual behaviors, such as mild cases of sexual aversion, may be treated through modification of behaviors. Systematic desensitization is one method of modifying the client's behavior through application of a principle known as *reciprocal inhibition*. The client is assisted by the nurse in identifying a hierar-

chy of anxiety-provoking situations related to the sexual activity to which the person feels aversive. The client is then taught a progressive muscle relaxation technique. Finally, the nurse-therapist presents the client, who is in a relaxed state, with an imagined representation of the least anxiety-provoking stimulus on the hierarchical list. If the client is relaxed, the stimulus may be provided without the client's experiencing the physical symptoms of anxiety previously associated with this dysfunction. As the client becomes comfortable and stays relaxed with low-anxiety stimuli, the nurse presents additional stimuli. Such an intervention is administered over several weeks until the most anxiety-producing stimulus is presented while the client is relaxed. If the client can maintain physical and psychologic comfort in the presence of suggested stimuli, she or he is ready to practice the new relaxed behavior with actual stimuli.

Sexual Dysfunction Related to Inhibited Sexual Desire

Planning: client goals. For the individual who has an identified problem of inhibited sexual desire, the goal is that the client will have a return of libido or increased interest in engaging in sexual activity.

Interventions. If inhibited sexual desire in the woman is related to hormonal replacement therapy or oral contraceptive use, the nurse may present alternatives or refer the client to a gynecologist. The nurse may discuss with the client other methods of coping with the symptoms of menopause if this is the reason for the hormonal replacement therapy. Other methods of increasing the client's interest and arousal include suggestions that the client use erotic reading materials or change the time and setting of usual sexual activities.

When drug or alcohol abuse or chronic illness such as cancer or end-stage renal disease is the major contributing factor in clients with inhibited sexual desire, medical management of the underlying factor is a prerequisite to other interventions. If the prognosis for any of these conditions is poor, the outcome for the sexual problem is often poor. The nurse provides information about the relationship between the underlying causes and the resulting sexual dysfunction.

Psychosocial factors that have an impact on the development of inhibited sexual desire are comparable in both men and women. Marital discord, depression, anxiety, and fear may be sufficiently severe to require the specialized education and experience of a nurse-specialist or clinician with expertise in the area of psychology or psychiatry. Nursing interventions include therapeutic communication, encouragement to pursue intensive therapy, and referral to a competent professional. Often the process will involve the client, his or her sexual partner or parents, or all of these individuals.

Sexual Dysfunction Related to Sexual Aversion

Planning: client goals. For the individual who has an identified problem of sexual aversion, the goal is that the client will be free from autonomic symptoms and experience relief of irrational fear when thinking about or engaging in sexual activity.

Interventions. Because the major etiologic factors in sexual aversion are psychogenic, therapeutic interventions are aimed at resolving the underlying psychologic trauma, conflicts, attitudes, or confusions. Most of these interventions involve intensive therapies provided by a nurse-specialist with advanced education and experience or by a psychotherapist. The nurse-generalist, however, can intervene by giving the client permission to ventilate his or her aversion. Nurses can use relaxation techniques, diversionary measures, or other comfort measures to minimize the client's physical autonomic responses of nausea, diarrhea, sweating, dry mouth, chills, or tachycardia. The nurse may also encourage the client to seek the professional help of a competent nurse-specialist or psychotherapist, as this type of sexual problem can be resolved through cognitive therapies and systematic desensitization.

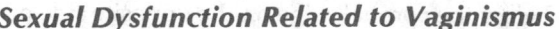
Planning and Implementation: Common Sexual Problems in Women

Sexual Dysfunction Related to Vaginismus

Planning: client goals. The goal in planning interventions for the woman with vaginismus is that the client will be able to relieve or prevent the involuntary spasms of the outer one-third of the vaginal barrel.

Interventions. The nursing interventions for an actual problem of vaginismus are directed at relieving the underlying contributing factors. The interventions for a potential problem of vaginismus are directed at educating the woman who is at risk of developing this response and thus preventing its occurrence. If the major contributing factor is psychogenic, including such situations as trauma from rape, conflicts surrounding homosexual experimentation, or strong religious teachings, the interventions are similar to those already discussed and range from giving permission to express anxiety and conflict to providing intensive therapy. On the other hand, if the major contributing factor is a physical one — such as sexual activity too soon after obstetric trauma, infection, abnormality of the hymen, or atrophy of the vagina — referral to a gynecologist may be indicated. Nursing interventions that include encouragement to explore alternatives to vaginal intercourse during the healing process and education of the woman and her sexual partner concerning the relationship between the physical factors and the involuntary muscular response are also effective.

Sexual Dysfunction Related to Orgasmic Dysfunction

Planning: client goals. The client goal when the nursing diagnosis is primary orgasmic dysfunction is that the client will be able to experience an orgasm by any means. When the nursing diagnosis is secondary orgas-

mic dysfunction, the client goal reflects an alteration of the situation in which orgasm occurs. In this case, the client will be able to experience orgasm as desired during specified sexual activity.

Interventions. When the major contributing factors in primary or secondary orgasmic dysfunction are psychogenic, the nursing interventions include giving the client permission to talk about this situation, providing education about the relationship between stressors and the physical response of orgasm, teaching the client Kegel's exercises to strengthen the pubococcygeal muscles, and encouraging general exercise to strengthen the pelvic musculature. Kegel's exercises are described here:

1. The woman is instructed to practice tightening the muscles as she would when stopping the flow of urine or tightening the vagina after insertion of a tampon.
2. The muscles should be contracted firmly and held for 2 to 3 seconds, then released.
3. The alternate contracting and relaxing of these muscles should be repeated 10 to 12 times, and this series repeated several times daily.

More intensive therapies such as marriage counseling and in-depth counseling concerning issues of anxiety and guilt may be warranted. The client may be referred to a nurse-specialist or other professional in this area. If adhesions of the clitoris result in orgasmic dysfunction, the nurse must refer the client to a physician for possible surgical intervention and provide encouragement that the condition may be corrected.

Planning and Implementation: Common Sexual Problems in Men

Sexual Dysfunction Related to Erectile Dysfunction

Planning: client goals. The goal for the male client who has a nursing diagnosis of erectile dysfunction is that he will be able to either attain or maintain an erection of the penis of sufficient firmness to permit vaginal penetration.

Interventions. Underlying disease such as diabetes mellitus, alcoholism, multiple sclerosis, endocrine disorders, and infections of the genitourinary system must be under current medical supervision for nursing interventions to influence the client's symptoms of erectile dysfunction. Appropriate nursing interventions include education, specific suggestions such as the "sensate focus" technique, and offers of alternative suggestions for satisfying sexual activities. The sensate focus is a technique that may also be used when the underlying factors are psychogenic and consists of the following steps, which the client and his partner are instructed to follow:

1. Mutual body touching and pleasuring without contact in the area of the genitalia

2. Genital stimulation resulting in penile erection, but not followed by intercourse

3. Orgasm and ejaculation through manual or oral stimulation (not vaginal penetration)

4. Vaginal penetration without orgasm or ejaculation (simple containment)

5. Vaginal penetration with orgasm and ejaculation

6. Dialogue between partners throughout steps

As with all sexual problems where the major contributing factors are psychogenic, therapeutic communication and intensive therapy are indicated. Psychotherapy directed at alleviating underlying marital discord, anxiety, or depression may be provided by the nurse-specialist or other psychotherapist, and appropriate referrals may be made.

In the absence of underlying disease or obvious psychologic factors, the use or abuse of various drugs may be the major etiologic factor in a sexual problem of erectile dysfunction. The nurse-generalist provides information to the client relating the action of drugs such as antihypertensives, barbiturates, sedatives, and amphetamines to changes in the sexual response cycle. Referral to the client's physician may be indicated so that an alternative drug, dosage, or therapy may be considered.

Sexual Dysfunction Related to Ejaculatory Dysfunction

Planning: client goals. When the nursing diagnosis is premature ejaculatory dysfunction, the goal is that the client will be able to exercise voluntary control and delay ejaculation until both sexual partners are satisfied. When the sexual problem of the client is ejaculatory incompetence or delayed ejaculation, the goal is that the client will be able to exercise voluntary control and allow ejaculation to occur with the partner during sexual activity. For the client with retrograde ejaculation, the goal is that the client will be able to reverse this process if physically possible or, if not, to accept this alteration in sexual functioning and adjust to the resulting sterility.

Interventions. Nursing interventions for premature and delayed ejaculatory dysfunctions include educating the client and sexual partner about the relationship between emotions and the sexual response cycle. The client, partner, or both may be taught systematic relaxation exercises to alleviate anxiety as a major contributing factor. The inclusion of the client's sexual partner is especially important in the treatment of ejaculatory dysfunctions because communication of their desires and expressions of distress become an integral part of maintenance of the dysfunction. With appropriate preparation, the nurse may instruct the client and his partner in the "squeeze technique" for the learning of voluntary control for premature ejaculatory dysfunction. Figure 10–3 illustrates two types of squeezes provided by the client's partner. In the traditional method, the partner places her thumb on the frenulum of the penis and with her first and second fingers just above

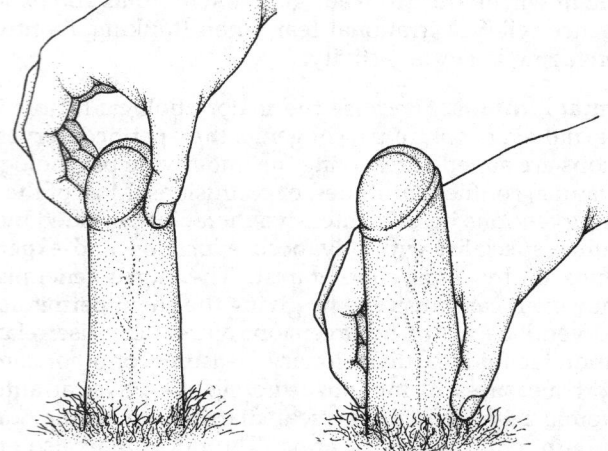

Traditional method: pressure applied front to back, below coronal ridge.

Basilar method: pressure applied front to back, base of shaft.

Figure 10–3

Traditional and basilar methods of the squeeze technique for treatment of ejaculatory dysfunction.

and below the coronal ridge on the opposite side of the penis applies a squeezing pressure. In the basilar method, the thumb and fingers are placed at the base of the penis rather than at the coronal ridge. Either position is held firmly for approximately 4 seconds, then released. The partner is instructed to always apply the pressure from the front to back of the shaft of the penis and never from side to side because this may result in tissue injury. The importance of avoiding injury from the fingernails should also be stressed. The squeeze is applied shortly after erection occurs, and periodically thereafter, until both partners are ready for penetration to take place. Once the man has been aroused to the point of ejaculatory inevitability, this technique should not be used, but ejaculation should be allowed to continue.

If ejaculatory incompetence is directly related to serious conflict between the client and his partner, intensive psychotherapy is indicated. The nurse-specialist who is prepared in counseling may provide this intervention. The nurse-generalist may make an appropriate referral and encourage the couple to seek treatment because this dysfunction may be corrected with such an intervention.

When the client's problem is one of retrograde ejaculation, the underlying cause is physiologic. Males with diabetes, prostatic disease, multiple sclerosis, and abnormalities of the bladder and urethra must be referred to a urologist for further evaluation and medical or surgical intervention. With the exception of physical abnormality, clients with diabetes, multiple sclerosis, and prostatic disease have an irreversible condition, and nursing interventions are thus directed at assisting them with coping skills. These men have an altered sensation from previous ejaculations and are rendered sterile. Education and counseling of the client and his sexual partner constitute the nursing interventions. The nurse can reassure both individuals that there are no harmful effects to the ejaculate's being deposited in the bladder. Some young diabetics who wish to have children are referred to an infertility clinic. It is possible for semen to be centrifuged from the urine and prepared for in vitro fertilization.

■ Discharge Planning

When preparing clients to return home after hospitalization for illness, injury, or surgery, plans for follow-up care and sexual counseling should be anticipated. Information about the relationship between the illness, injury, or surgery and the sexual functioning should be provided to the client and to the client's sexual partner when appropriate. For example, when clients receive surgical or chemotherapeutic treatments for cancer, they may experience temporary alterations in sexual desire. Providing information about this situation and offering suggestions for less strenuous expressions of intimacy are appropriate nursing interventions. Similarly, counseling the client who had a myocardial infarction about his or her anxiety related to resuming sexual intercourse is also appropriate.

Anticipatory guidance is provided by encouraging clients to report any adverse effects of medications on their sexual functioning. Nurses must be aware of the ways in which specific drugs affect sexual functioning and provide appropriate information to clients who will continue to receive these medications after discharge.

When clients are discharged to home health care, additional follow-up may be directed at the family caregiver. The family caregiver who takes primary responsibility for care of a client in the absence of professional home health caregivers is often a spouse whose own health needs must also be considered. Nursing interventions in the form of counseling about sexual functioning are sometimes needed in these situations. Providing nursing care and being a sexual partner of the client may present conflicts for a spouse who accepts the role of family caregiver. This conflict should be anticipated and prevented through adequate discussion of these roles for the family caregiver.

 Evaluation

The final step in the nursing process is that of evaluation. Evaluation includes consideration of the client's goals being met and of the effectiveness of the nursing interventions. The expected outcomes for the client with common sexual dysfunction problems include that the client

1. Does not experience pain or discomfort associated with intercourse.
2. Describes restored levels of libido and interest in sexual activity.
3. Expresses a rational process and positive attitude toward sexual activity.

4. Describes sexual activity that is no longer accompanied by painful involuntary spasms of the vaginal wall.
5. Experiences orgasm as desired.
6. Resolves underlying psychologic conflicts so that enjoyment of orgasm results.
7. Attains or maintains erections of the penis of sufficient firmness to permit vaginal penetration in at least 50% of attempts.
8. Learns voluntary control over the ejaculatory response. In addition, the client who previously experienced premature ejaculation will experience a delay in ejaculation that is mutually satisfying to him and his sexual partner most of the time. The client who previously experienced delayed ejaculation will experience an advance in ejaculation that is mutually satisfying to him and his sexual partner most of the time.

Clients with retrograde ejaculation may not be able to entertain a realistic goal of a return to normal ejaculation. In this situation, psychosocial adjustment to this limitation and to the possibility of sterility would become the goal, and outcome criteria would be related to the client's subjective description that he is able to cope with these limitations.

In evaluating the process of nursing interventions, the client will be able to identify interventions that were most influential in helping him or her achieve expected outcomes and to provide constructive criticism or alternative suggestions for interventions that were not useful.

SUMMARY

Sexuality is currently recognized as a natural function of human beings, and sexual health must be addressed by the professional nurse. Nursing interventions for sexual dysfunctions are based on affirmation of sexuality as a valued component of the individual's total health. Teaching clients about the anatomy and physiology of sexual functioning constitutes a major aspect of interventions for those with actual or potential sexual problems. Specific suggestions such as Kegel's exercises, sensate focus, and the squeeze technique may be appropriate for individuals or couples. If a client's sexual problem cannot be alleviated through interventions directed at teaching or making specific suggestions, counseling or referral to another health professional is the intervention of choice. If problems are related to underlying physical pathology, such as clitoral adhesions or diabetes, referral to a physician is indicated. If problems are related to serious underlying psychopathology, referral to a psychotherapist, psychiatrist, or clinical nurse-specialist is in order.

IMPLICATIONS FOR RESEARCH

Research is needed to predict clients who are at risk of developing sexual problems and to prescribe nursing interventions that are most appropriate for specific dysfunctions. Because of the sensitive nature of research in the area of human sexuality, special attention to measures for the protection of human subjects must be given. Factors identified by Kolodny that appeared earlier in this chapter must be followed.

Nurses in a variety of settings may develop preventive programs for high-risk populations such as those with diabetes and cancer. Research based on the incidence of potential problems in sexual functioning will add to the interventions that nursing can apply to these at-risk populations. Further research will also be needed to improve current nursing interventions for clients with actual problems in sexual dysfunction.

Specific questions to be answered in future nursing research include

1. What demographic variables are the best predictors of individuals who are likely to develop sexual dysfunction problems?
2. What nursing interventions offer the most relief for clients with specified sexual dysfunction problems?
3. What nursing interventions are most useful for preventing the occurrence of specified sexual dysfunction problems?
4. What educational methods enhance the comfort level of nurses in application of the nursing process to clients with sexual dysfunction problems?

Answers to these and related questions will increase the knowledge base of nursing and help to alleviate sexual dysfunction problems in a variety of client populations. Variations in sexual behaviors and roles may be found in other cultures, and research questions specific to those cultures should also be addressed.

REFERENCES AND READINGS

Annon, J. S. (1975). *The behavioral treatment of sexual problems: Vol. I. Brief therapy.* Honolulu: Enabling Systems.

Brecher, E. M. (1984). *Love, sex, and aging.* Boston: Little, Brown.

Cardin, S. (1987). Nursing's role in the sexual counseling of critical care patients. *Dimensions of Critical Care Nursing, 6*(2), 67–68.

Carpenito, L. J. (1987). *Nursing diagnosis* (2nd ed.). Philadelphia: J. B. Lippincott.

Collier, P. (1986). Education for sexual self-awareness. In V. Littlefield (Ed.), *Health education for women* (pp. 160–195). Norwalk, CT: Appleton-Century-Crofts.

Constantine, L. L., & Martinson, F. M. (1981). *Children and sex: New findings, new perspectives.* Boston: Little, Brown.

Duespohl, T. A. (1986). *Nursing diagnosis manual for the well and ill client.* Philadelphia: W. B. Saunders.

Engel, N. S. (1987). Menopausal stage, current life change, attitude towards women's roles and perceived health status. *Nursing Research, 36,* 353–357.

Gilliss, C. L., & Rankin, S. M. (1988). Social and sexual activity after cardiac surgery: A report of the first 6 months. *Progress in Cardiovascular Nursing, 3*(3), 93–97.

Haas, K., & Haas, A. (1987). *Understanding sexuality.* St. Louis: C. V. Mosby.

Higgins, L. P., & Hawkins, J. W. (1984). *Human sexuality across the life span.* Monterey, CA: Wadsworth Health Sciences Division.

Hogan, R. (1985). *Human sexuality: A nursing perspective.* Norwalk, CT: Appleton-Century-Crofts.

Kaplan, H. S. (1974). *The new sex therapy: Active treatment of sexual dysfunctioning.* New York: Brunner-Mazel.

Kilmann, P. R. (1984). *Human sexuality in contemporary life.* Boston: Allyn and Bacon.

Kolodny, R. C. (1978). Ethical issues in the prevention of sexual problems. In C. B. Qualls, J. P. Winczl, & D. H. Barlow (Eds.), *The prevention of sexual disorders: Issues and approaches* (pp. 183–196). New York: Plenum.

Kolodny, R. C., Masters, W. M., & Johnson, V. E. (1979). *Textbook of sexual medicine.* Boston: Little, Brown.

Lion, E. M. (1982). *Human sexuality in nursing process.* New York: Wiley.

Lo-Biondo-Wood, G. (1986). Health education for the homosexual female. In V. Littlefield (Ed.), *Health education for women* (pp. 252–267). Norwalk, CT: Appleton-Century-Crofts.

Masters, W. M., & Johnson, V. E. (1970). *Human sexual inadequacy.* Boston: Little, Brown.

Masters, W. M., Johnson, V. E., & Kolodny, R. C. (1985). *Human sexuality* (2nd ed.). Boston: Little, Brown.

McCracken, H. L. (1988). Sexual practice of elders: The forgotten aspect of functional health. *Journal of Gerontological Nursing, 14*(10), 13–18.

Metcalfe, M. C., & Fischman, S. H. (1985). Factors affecting the sexuality of patients with head and neck cancer. *Oncology Nursing Forum, 12*(2), 21–25.

Muscari, M. E. (1987). Obtaining the adolescent sexual history. *Pediatric Nursing, 13,* 307–310.

Northouse, L. L., & Swain, M. A. (1987). Adjustment of patients and husbands to the initial impact of breast cancer. *Nursing Research, 36,* 221–225.

Rew, L. (1989). Promoting healthy sexuality. In R. L. R. Foster, M. M. Hunsberger, & J. T. Anderson (Eds.), *Family-centered nursing care of children* (pp. 687–699). Philadelphia: W. B. Saunders.

Schover, L. R. (1984). *Prime time: Sexual health for men over 50.* New York: Holt, Rinehart, & Winston.

Smith, D. B. (1989). Discussing sexuality. *Oncology Nursing Forum, 16*(1), 106.

Stewart, R. S. (1983). Psychiatric issues in renal dialysis and transplantation. *Hospital and Community Psychiatry, 34,* 623–628.

Woods, N. F. (1984). *Human sexuality in health and illness* (3rd ed.). St. Louis: C. V. Mosby.

ADDITIONAL READINGS

Baggs, J. C., & Karch, A. M. (1987). Sexual counseling of women with coronary heart disease. *Heart and Lung, 16,* 154–159.

This is a report of a survey of 58 women who had been admitted to a coronary care unit. When asked if they wished to receive a copy of the American Heart Association booklet about resuming sexual activity, 79% replied in the affirmative and 76% stated that health professionals should routinely discuss sexual functioning with them. The authors urged nurses to become comfortable with and knowledgeable enough to provide this necessary intervention for their female clients.

Campbell, M. L. (1987). Sexual dysfunction in the COPD patient. *Dimensions of Critical Care Nursing, 6*(2), 70–74.

The effects of chronic obstructive pulmonary disease (COPD) on male sexual function are described. Physical and psychologic effects of COPD are identified, and an elaboration of the nursing process in treating the male client and his sexual partner is provided. Many practical strategies for enhancing sexual ability are presented.

Chapman, J., & Sughrue, J. (1987). A model for sexual assessment and intervention. *Health Care for Women International, 8,* 87–99.

This article is useful to prepare the professional nurse to work with individuals who may have sexual problems. Common sexual problems such as difficulty in sexual arousal, dyspareunia, and ejaculatory dysfunction are identified. Several suggestions are made for beginning to take a sexual history, and the PLISSIT model (P: permission; LI: limited information; SS: specific suggestions; IT: intensive therapy) is presented for intervention.

Cooley, M. E., & Cobb, S. C. (1986). Sexual and reproductive issues for women with Hodgkin's disease. *Cancer Nursing, 9,* 188–193.

The incidence and characteristics of Hodgkin disease in women were discussed. The various effects of treatment modalities on the sexual health of these women were described. The authors concluded that further research is needed to clarify the relationship among cancer therapies, quality of life, and the development of sexual problems.

Cooley, M. E., Yeomans, A. C., & Cobb, S. C. (1986). Sexual and reproductive issues for women with Hodgkin's disease. II. Application of PLISSIT model. *Cancer Nursing, 9,* 248–255.

This article is a companion to the article just cited. The nurse is identified as being in a key position to address the quality of life and how cancer therapies affect it. The authors provided a case study and care plan based on the PLISSIT model of intervention. A sexual assessment tool for use with patients with Hodgkin disease is delineated.

Crowther, M. (1986). Sex questions a cardiac patient may be too scared to ask. *RN, 49*(11), 44–46.

This brief article identifies the difficulty expressed by many clients who recover from acute myocardial infarction. Specific questions and answers about sexual functioning are provided in an easy-to-read format that may be used directly with a client and his or her sexual partner.

Dougherty, M. C., Abrams, R., & McKey, P. L. (1986). An instrument to assess the dynamic characteristics of the circumvaginal musculature. *Nursing Research, 35,* 202–206.

In this report the authors described an intravaginal balloon device (IVBD) that was constructed for use in research on women's health problems related to the musculature of the pelvic floor. Development of the device was prompted by the need to test nursing interventions for improving integrity of the pelvic floor in women.

Hassey, K. M. (1987). Radiation therapy for rectal cancer and the implications for nursing. *Cancer Nursing, 10,* 311–318.

Radiation is identified as an adjuvant to surgery as well as a primary treatment for some rectal cancers. Nursing assessment and interventions are offered for various client problems including alterations in sexuality and reproductive capacity. The author emphasized the importance of anticipatory guidance, support, and education for the client.

Lilley, L. L. (1987). Human need fulfillment alteration in the client with uterine cancer. *Cancer Nursing, 10,* 327–337.

This is a report of a research study comparing nurses' and clients' perceptions of need fulfillment alterations in clients with uterine cancer. The author identified many of the emotional feelings expressed by clients and found no significant differences between nurses and their clients. However, nurses tended to rate physical needs as most important, whereas clients rated psychosocial needs (including sexual integrity) higher.

Lovejoy, N. C. (1987). Precancerous lesions of the cervix. *Cancer Nursing, 10,* 2–14.

This comprehensive review of risk factors related to precancerous lesions of the cervix provides an excellent reference for nurses working with women, including adolescents. The author provided a reference list of 89 sources for reading and a list of selected audiovisual resources for increasing knowledge about this important aspect of sexuality. She also provided implications for further research and clinical practice.

Poorman, S. G. (1988). *Human sexuality and the nursing process.* Norwalk, CT: Appleton & Lange.

This brief textbook was written to specifically assist clinical nurses in applying theoretical concepts of human sexuality and sexual health to clients in various settings. Sexual functioning throughout the life span, infancy to older adulthood, is discussed. Useful information about homosexuality, bisexuality, transsexuality, and transvestism is presented.

Schover, L. R., & Fife, M. (1985). Sexual counseling of patients undergoing radical surgery for pelvic or genital cancer. *Journal of Psychosocial Oncology, 3*(3), 21–41.

This article outlines a team approach, including the clinical nurse-specialist, for providing sexual rehabilitation for persons undergoing radical prostatectomy, radical vulvectomy or hysterectomy, and penectomy. Guidelines for postoperative sexual activities are provided.

Shipes, E. (1987). Sexual function following ostomy surgery. *Nursing Clinics of North America, 22,* 303–310.

After a description of the sexual response cycle, the author identified alterations in sexual function that are both directly and indirectly related to surgical intervention resulting in ostomies. She also briefly discussed changes related to chemotherapy and radiation. She provided a nursing care plan that included using the PLISSIT model or brief counseling for the individual with an ostomy.

Shuman, N. A. (1987). Nurses' attitudes towards sexual counseling. *Dimensions of Critical Care Nursing, 6*(2), 75–81.

A report is given of 50 cardiac nurses' level of sexual knowledge, attitudes, comfort, preparation, and responsibility for counseling patients about sexuality after myocardial infarction. Although more conservative in attitudes than nurses in general, 82% of the cardiac nurses in the sample believed that nurses should provide sexual counseling. Only 52% stated that they included this in their care, and 50% reported that they were not comfortable with and did not have sufficient knowledge to provide clients with sexual counseling after myocardial infarction.

CHAPTER 11

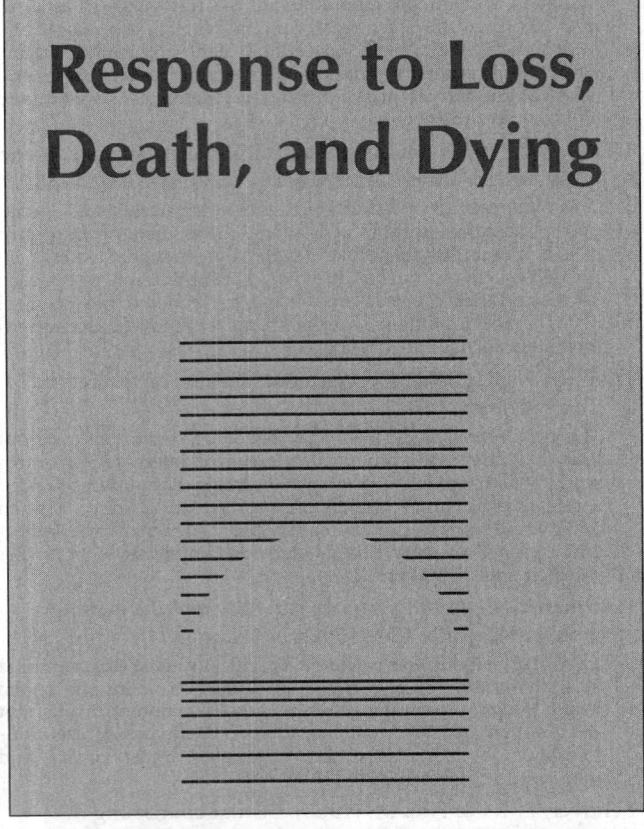

Response to Loss, Death, and Dying

Loss, dying, and death are integral parts of living, yet we give them little thought in the ordinary course of everyday events. As human beings we can intellectualize about death, but we cannot emotionally apprehend our own personal annihilation. We recognize death as inevitable, yet at the same time we preserve a belief in our own immortality.

Despite this innate need to keep loss, dying, and death removed from everyday life, we cannot escape thinking about them when we confront illness. Diseases such as cancer or myocardial infarction more readily give rise to connotations of death than do others such as cholecystitis or bronchitis. However, these too can cause feelings of deficit, if in nothing else, in our sense of hardiness and resistance.

Feelings of loss, thoughts of death, and fears of dying also accompany the normal developmental stages of adulthood. Many of the alterations in well-being associated with aging — decreasing energy levels, slower recall, aching joints — are all harbingers of senescence and eventual nonbeing.

The ultimate loss is the loss from death — a universal (we all die) and unique experience (we each die but once). Although there may be supportive and caring persons present at the moment of death, each of us must go alone in her or his characteristic way into the unknown of dying and death.

Loss, whatever the cause, can contribute to personality growth if it is accompanied by adaptive coping. *Coping* is the sum of the cognitive and behavioral strategies used to deal with threatening or challenging situations when normal or routine responses are either unavailable or ineffective. A successful coping process results in the achievement of mastery over the stress, or *resolution*, and the resumption of equilibrium.

Nurses face loss and death daily in the course of their work and must constantly deal with their own reactions along with those of clients, families, and other caregivers. Knowledge of professional theories, principles, and practices helps them to understand, to predict, and to manage these reactions and to develop sound nursing strategies. Although there are no prescriptive rules for caring for dying persons or those suffering loss, there are helpful guidelines. In this chapter, some of these theories and guidelines are presented.

LOSS

DEFINITION

Loss is the state of being deprived of or being without something valued that one once had. Synonyms are detriment, impairment, injury, and incapacitation. Some losses, such as male pattern baldness, are routine and predictable. Others, such as the loss of a limb because of an accident, are random and unforeseeable.

Losses, then, may occur gradually or suddenly; they may be nonviolent or traumatic, anticipated or unexpected, partial and minor or total and devastating.

TYPES OF LOSS

LOSS OF A LOVED ONE

The loss to any degree of a significant loved or valued person is the most stressful and disruptive loss we can endure. Such losses occur through divorce, alienation, or other kinds of emotional detachment or through geographic separation. Partial losses can also occur when a loved one is incapacitated by acute or chronic illnesses such as mental illness or Alzheimer's disease, especially when that illness results in the loss of some gratifying special attribute of the person. Change, then, no matter what the reason for the change, can engender loss in any valued relationship.

Death brings about permanent loss of loved ones. Because of the intimacy, intensity, and interdependency of the bonds, the death of a spouse or of a child carries the most profound emotional impact.

LOSS OF SELF

Another common form of loss is loss of self. By self we mean the overall mental representation each of us has of his or her body and personality. This mental image includes feelings about attractiveness, self-worth, physical and mental abilities, roles in life, and impact on the world. Loss of some aspect of self may be temporary or permanent, partial or complete.

Loss of health is an example of the loss of an aspect of self. The loss of a limb may affect not only the capacity to move normally but also the feeling of attractiveness to others. Other aspects of self that may be lost include hearing, sight, memory, intellectual powers, youth, or body functions like bowel and bladder control. Reduced libido is almost always interpreted as a partial loss of self.

LOSS OF OBJECTS

Another significant form of loss is object loss, or loss of possessions or associations—jewelry, money, furniture, house, job, homeland. Robberies precipitate a sense of personal injury that is tantamount to violation. These types of losses result in the same impairments and the same need to cope to achieve a state of restitution, but to a lesser degree, as do losses of valued parts of the self or of valued loved ones.

INTERRELATIONSHIP OF LOSSES

As may be inferred from the above-mentioned examples, losses of some aspect of self, although different in kind and degree, generally do not come one at a time. "When sorrows come, they come not single . . . but in battalions" (*Hamlet* IV, v. 78). A loss in one aspect of life is usually associated with losses in other domains. Loss of attractiveness through the mutilation caused by extensive surgery is likely to lead to loss of self-esteem. When a person loses a leg, there are forced changes in life style, at least until the person develops the skill to walk, run, dance, and perhaps ski either with or without a prosthesis. In addition, there may be permanent loss of previous social roles, such as in the worlds of work or family.

When a spouse dies, the survivor almost always loses the couple's style of living, and it takes time to become part of the world of single persons again. When couples divorce, not only do they lose each other, but one or both persons risk losing their children, who may become angry, confused, and alienated. Extended family networks of in-laws become disrupted as well. Everyone involved loses the dream of being part of the ideal or "solid" family.

LOSS AND THE LIFE CYCLE

Loss has consequences in our lives from birth until death. As we mature and assume adult responsibilities and gain fulfillment, we give up some of the dependencies and self-indulgent gratifications of childhood. These changes are seen by some persons as losses and by others as gains; still other persons take no notice. Such differences in awareness may be related in part to our innate sense of loss both as a real event and as a symbolic interpretation of the event. For instance, some individuals look forward to retirement as an earned and deserved goal. They perceive a gain. Others see retirement as a punishment for having aged, an affront to their value as persons. They perceive a loss.

It is easier to cope with loss in some of life's stages than in others such as old age, which is a time of great vulnerability. In the aged, biologic defenses and adaptive skills are diminished, and persons may react physiologically to a loss, with resulting dysfunction or disease. At any time of life, the period of bereavement after the death of a loved or valued person is a time of great risk for the precipitation of illness and even death.

DYING AND DEATH

Dying and death in contemporary American society are fraught with dilemmas and questions. The dilemmas come partly from our cultural ambivalence toward dying. The questions are rooted in our uncertainties about what constitutes death and what constitutes avoidable death. We ask, "Who should die?" "Under what circumstances?" "What comprises an appropriate or a good death?"

TWENTIETH-CENTURY VIEWS OF DEATH

DEATH AS CATASTROPHE

The ascendence of the philosophy of materialism that accompanied technologic advancement in the 20th century affected societal views about death. Progress and meaningfulness became counted in terms of accumulation of wealth and expansion of material frontiers, and death became viewed as the antithesis — a catastrophe. Modern science, in its effort to annihilate the "enemy," has succeeded in only delaying its arrival and in sequestering its course. Death the destroyer — subtle, elusive, perplexing — endures.

OBSERVING DEATH

Some assert that our pronounced discomfort with both the idea and the reality of death is due to our seldom having seen anyone die. In fact, in the United States in the late 20th century, not many people directly witness either the dying process or death.

The converse, on the other hand, has also been noted. Investigators (Baker & Sorenson, 1963; Quint & Strauss, 1964) have reported that first-hand experiences with dying and death do not necessarily lead to decreased feelings of tension in the presence of these events. Many health professionals (e.g., nurses, but more notably, physicians, because their education has not prepared them) avoid interaction with dying persons as much as laypersons. These avoidance behaviors include limiting direct contact with the client and family, evading conversations about the status of the client's condition, focusing only on the physical components of care, and giving scientific, often complex explanations of the expected effects of treatment.

CHANGES IN THE NATURE OF DYING

While medical and scientific advances have extended the length of time we live, they have also extended the length of time it takes for us to die. With control of most of the infectious diseases that were the scourges of the past, greater numbers of people now live long enough to develop the slow, chronic killers such as cancer and Alzheimer's disease. Trauma and stroke (cerebrovascular accident) victims can be maintained functionally on mechanical life support systems indefinitely. Thus greater numbers of people are living with dying for prolonged periods. This situation has given rise to many new biomedical ethical dilemmas. Among them are the criteria used to determine death, definition of extraordi-

nary treatments, and the most fitting and appropriate ways to care for dying persons.

DEFINITIONS

Dying and death are such closely associated phenomena that it is difficult to think of one without the other. Dying is a process. Death is the termination of life.

There was a time when there was little controversy about what was meant by death. Most people accepted that irreversible cessation of respiration, heartbeat, and lack of corneal reflexes were sufficient signs of death. This is no longer the case. It is now possible to maintain respiration and circulation through the use of drugs, machines, and artificial and transplanted organs.

Determination of death is important because it has far-reaching consequences. Definitions of death establish a basis for offering clients nursing and medical care options. For example, a clear definition of clinical death is the theoretical rationale for determining what is considered to be ordinary or extraordinary treatment. Many courses of action could be classified as either, depending on the circumstance. Among the more common treatments are the use of experimental drugs, life-sustaining equipment, bone marrow transplants, oxygen, antibiotics, and, in some cases, food and fluids.

The definition of *death* as cessation of brain function rather than cessation of heartbeat is critical to maintaining the viability of donor organs for use as transplants. The term *brain dead* was introduced into clinical medicine in the 1960s. Brain dead describes a client whose heart and lungs can be maintained functionally by mechanical life-support apparatus but whose respiratory centers in the brain stem no longer function. If the respirator were removed, the person would not resume spontaneous breathing.

Different organizations have published various criteria to establish brain death. The apnea test is commonly used to establish brain death in a client who has been in a coma for at least 6 hours with loss of all brain stem reflexes, including loss of response to external stimuli, loss of pupillary response to light, loss of corneal reflex, loss of eye movement with doll's eye maneuver or caloric testing, and loss of gag and cough reflexes. The presence of spinal reflexes does not exclude the diagnosis of brain death.

The apnea test is performed by assessing the presence or absence of respirations with a PCO_2 of at least 60 mmHg.

The person is dead also in the sense that the brain as the physical center of personal identity no longer operates. This same criterion applies to a persistent vegetative state. In a persistent vegetative state, a person shows no evidence of cortical functioning but has the sustained capacity for spontaneous breathing and heartbeat. This condition has been referred to as *cortical death* or *cerebral death*.

Although the cessation of respirations and heartbeat

as a definition of death is still sanctioned by Anglo-American common law, many states have passed brain death statutes. These laws, no matter how stated, are consistent in allowing death to be defined as the irreversible cessation of brain function, as determined by the use of the most reliable clinical method available.

The nursing student needs to know the legal definition of death in his or her state, as well as the policy for defining death used in relevant clinical practicum sites. In most states, it is still not legal for a nurse to pronounce a client dead; therefore, the nurse should be aware of the procedure to follow when there is no physician in attendance. She or he should be particularly aware of the correct charting procedure.

CONCEPTUALIZATIONS OF LOSS, DYING, AND DEATH

The conceptual systems that we use in discussing loss, dying, and death have been derived through research. These formulations are not meant to be prescriptive. Rather, they serve as general guides to sensitize the nurse to what may occur and, therefore, what to look for and how to proceed when a response is indicated. Using these findings to help guide care is similar to using the systematic protocols of signs and symptoms of disease that help guide all nursing observations. For example, not all persons with a myocardial infarction show all of its possible clinical manifestations, nor do they all follow the same clinical course. Knowing what can occur helps us make observations and devise early interventions to prevent complications.

RESPONSES TO DYING

In 1969, Elisabeth Kübler-Ross, a psychiatrist, described a series of stages through which people pass in response to their living through the dying process. She described the first stage as *shock and disbelief*. People could not believe that they were dying. The second stage was described as *denial*. People might say, "Yes, most people with this disease are dying, but not me!" The third stage was called *anger*, often characterized by the questions "Why me?" or "What did I do to deserve this?" The fourth stage was termed *bargaining*. In this stage, characteristic responses were, "I'll do anything if . . . " or "Just let me live until my son gets married . . . or my daughter graduates." The next stage, when the person's deteriorating physical condition led to the realization that death was inevitable, was identified as *depression*. The final stage was termed *acceptance*. Acceptance according to Kübler-Ross was a stage of self-actualization,

of feeling at peace with one's self, with one's imminent death, and with the cosmos.

PATTERNS OF LIVING-DYING

When death from a known fatal illness is preceded by several years of life, the use of the term dying from the time of diagnosis until the moment of death is paradoxical. These people frequently not only look robust, but enjoy full activity for prolonged periods. We say that they are living yet dying, and in these cases the living-dying period has the characteristics of a chronic illness.

Nursing research (Martocchio, 1982) has described four patterns of living-dying that are useful for understanding the uncertainties of living with life-threatening illness. These patterns (Table 11–1), all having a general downward course concluding in death, reflect the natural history of various diseases, such as some cancers and many cardiovascular, renal, and hepatic conditions. They also describe the effects of specific therapeutic regimens. The categories remain consistent regardless of type of disease or treatment. The patterns are termed peaks and valleys, descending plateaus, downward slopes, and gradual slants.

The *peaks and valleys* pattern is characterized by a series of peaks and valleys, or remissions and exacerbations. The peaks represent periods of well-being and the valleys, loss of well-being. Clients describe "hopeful highs" and "terrible lows." They see past highs as indicators of hope that they can rally one more time. They see the lows as threats to any hope of recovery.

The *descending plateaus* pattern is a series of steps. Each downward step represents a tangible reduction in functional ability and each plateau, a leveling-off or stable period. The plateaus and drop-offs can last for an indeterminate period and may occur any number of times. This pattern creates marked frustration as dying people and their families try, again and again, to take part in rehabilitation programs to maintain a level of function that is relentlessly but unpredictably declining.

The third pattern of living-dying is the *downward slope*. This pattern, frequently seen in intensive care

TABLE 11–1   Characteristics of the Four Patterns of Living-Dying

Pattern	Main Characteristics
Peaks and valleys	Hopeful highs/terrible lows
Descending plateaus	Rehabilitation/loss/ rehabilitation
Downward slope	No time to prepare
Gradual slant	Barely living/placement problems

units, is represented by a continuous and usually rapid downward course. In these cases, when there are relatively short-term illnesses or unexpected deaths, clients and family members have little time to prepare for the death.

The *gradual slant* pattern is characterized by a gradual decline over time. Toward the end, it is difficult to know whether these people are alive or dead. In this dying pattern, difficulties regarding quality of life and definitions of death become issues of concern. Family members and caregivers begin to see the unresponsive individual as a biologically living creature but also as a nonexistent person. As there is less meaningful interaction, the client is considered to be socially dead.

Regardless of the pattern, the direction is down. As the dying person declines and draws nearer to death, all involved with him or her undergo losses. For each person, the loss is different: The mother loses her son; the wife, her husband; the children, their father; the business partner, his colleague. Each person manifests the loss both in a universally recognized pattern and in his or her unique way.

THE GRIEF RESPONSE

Grieving is the psychologic, social, and somatic reaction to the perception of significant loss. Although a grief reaction can result from the loss of any precious element in a person's life, loss through death of a close loved one is used as the major example in the rest of this chapter.

There are two goals of grieving. The first is to be able to remember the lost loved one without undue pain. The second is to be able to reinvest emotional energy in life without losing the capacity to love. Effective grieving is achieved by facing the pain of the loss and by living through its full range of feelings and their expression.

The responses to loss include familiar and expected behaviors and also a wide range of feelings and behaviors that are unanticipated and confusing. Understanding the various processes and behaviors that are normally associated with grieving is essential for nurses to develop professional strategies to deal with them.

Since Lindemann's (1944) classic account of grieving, many authors have described the general pattern of the grieving process. Most agree that there is a universal grief response (Table 11–2) that has a more or less predictable course. The course begins with shock and disbelief and progresses to somatic distress; feelings of guilt, anger, and hostility; interruption of life's usual activities; preoccupation with thoughts of the deceased; and, finally, a state of healthy integration.

There is no fixed timetable by which a person passes through the grieving process, nor are the stages discrete. There is no rigid order to the progression, nor must each person go through all stages. Manifestations of grief vary widely, and individuals may take one step forward and two steps back, then half steps from side to side, as they cycle through their healing journey. Despite this

TABLE 11–2 Common Responses to Loss
Shock and disbelief
Yearning and protest
Anguish, disorganization, and despair
Reorganization and restitution

nonlinearity there are — as in the Kübler-Ross stages of dying — identifiable clusters, or phases, of feelings and behaviors that serve as guides for observation and a description for survivors.

SHOCK AND DISBELIEF

Shock, numbness, and disbelief are the first responses to actual or anticipated loss. People describe a sense of unreality, even though they know intellectually that the person is dead. They may appear outwardly to be accepting the loss. They continue with routine tasks and obligations as if nothing had happened. They are "on automatic pilot."

Some persons engage in searching behaviors. They search for the lost treasured person. They dream that he or she is still alive, or they may have hallucinations about the person. They may see him or her in familiar places, hear him or her at the door or on the stairs, or feel his or her touch on waking. These experiences are frightening, and survivors often interpret them as indications of emotional illness.

Grief hurts not only emotionally, but also physically. There may be muscular weakness, tremors, chest pain, tightness in the throat, diaphoresis, deep sighing, sensations of hot and cold, anorexia, nausea, fatigue, insomnia, and exhaustion. Because the immune system is temporarily impaired, clients should be observed closely because of the real risk of developing serious illness.

YEARNING AND PROTEST, ANGER AND GUILT

In most instances, in a short time, soon after the funeral, the feelings of numbness and disbelief give way to feelings of pain and distress at the separation and a powerful sense of longing. During this period, the bereaved may have extreme mood swings and erratic behavior. They may become either hyperactive or hypoactive. Depression, which is common, contributes to difficulty in concentrating and fuels excesses of anger, guilt, and extreme sadness. The bereaved may focus exclusively on the deceased and reject all offers of comfort.

Parkes and Weiss, in their research on widows, found

that feelings of yearning for the return of the relationship and protest at its loss can last for an indeterminate period. Clinging and pining behavior may be mild and gradually vanish or can be intense and persist for weeks to months. Survivors may be angry at the deceased for leaving them, at God or fate for allowing the death, and at caregivers for not saving the person's life. The anger can be mild to moderate, severe enough to destroy relationships, or so extreme and bitter that it becomes crippling.

Survivors also feel guilty because they resent others who still have their loved ones, or they envy the deceased because they themselves did not die instead. They may feel extreme self-reproach about not having done enough for the deceased. Their transgressions can range from minor omissions—"Why didn't I start a low-cholesterol diet for the whole family much sooner?"—to important perceived errors in decision-making—"Why didn't I insist on that last course of chemotherapy?"

Many survivors do not express these feelings because they question their own mental stability and worry about what others will think of them. When they discover that others have gone through similar sequences and intensities of emotion, they are more apt to share their feelings, and thus to gain some comfort from others.

ANGUISH, DISORGANIZATION, AND DESPAIR

As time goes on and the rage exhausts itself, the permanence of the loss begins to be recognized more realistically. Crying and tearfulness become common. The bereaved individuals describe feelings of confusion, aimlessness, and loss of motivation. They worry about their inability to make decisions and their lack of self-confidence. Some persons become markedly depressed and apathetic and have a feeling of loss of interest and meaning in life. Many isolate themselves socially. They may not even participate in activities such as hobbies that they had never shared with the lost loved one. Many see life as a weighty burden and describe an absence of pleasure. They cannot believe that life will ever hold meaning and joy again. They may talk of suicide during the first year of bereavement and express a strong desire for reunion with the deceased through death.

The intensity of these negative feelings can be frightening. Individuals who have had relatively stable or calm personalities may have a horror of losing emotional control. Their fears are intensified by memory lapses and difficulty in concentrating. In an attempt to gain control, they center on themselves, which can be interpreted as selfishness by themselves as well as by others.

As time passes, bereaved persons develop a new awareness of the preciousness of existence. They see life

as fragile, and they may display intense fears of being physically or emotionally hurt, or they may worry excessively about the welfare of family members. At the same time, they may engage in health-compromising behaviors, such as driving in an unsafe manner or substance abuse (excessive smoking, drinking, or using psychoactive drugs).

The need to cry is still strong but erratic. The tears burst through fiercely and unexpectedly. A song, a sunset, the smell of food or flowers, putting on the lights at dusk, or turning a corner into a certain street may start the crying. Bereaved individuals describe this startling experience as similar to being struck by lightning. They realize each time anew that they will never again see the deceased, that the loss is final, irrevocable. There was a "golden time" that is forever gone.

Bereaved persons spend much time reminiscing, thinking about the deceased, and sharing memories with others. During these reminiscences, idealization takes place. In this process, all images and anecdotes about the deceased reveal him or her in only the best light. It is also common for feelings of guilt to resurface during the process of idealization.

IDENTIFICATION WITH THE DECEASED

Identification with the deceased is also to be expected during grieving. Bereaved individuals sometimes assume the lost one's characteristics. They may adopt his or her behavior, mannerisms, values, goals, or admired qualities. Some take on the physical symptoms of the deceased's final illness or last days. Family and friends may be alarmed by the appearance of chest pain, shortness of breath, nausea, or joint pain. Although it is always prudent to investigate such physical symptoms, it may be helpful to distinguish symptoms that mimic the deceased's from those that are related to a true organic condition. Symptoms that are associated with loss abate as the loss approaches resolution.

REORGANIZATION AND RESTITUTION

There are no time limits for the length of the grieving process. Although the reorganization and restitution associated with integration of the grief can begin within 6 months of the loss, it may take a year or longer for such signs to emerge. Indeed, grieving may not end within 1 or even 2 years of the precipitating event. The feelings and symptoms of grief do not simply stop completely and forever. Sadness decreases only gradually, and a new life emerges incrementally as time passes.

Although life eventually stabilizes, the bereaved person never completely recovers from the loss of a parent, spouse, child, or other loved one. Memories persist. Some of the pain of loss may last for life and resurface with each new loss. The pain of loss can also be precipitated by circumstances that are poignant reminders of the deceased—a special place or activity, a usually shared important event, music, jokes, birthdays, anniversaries, and holidays. These responses, unlike those of early grief, are commonly transitory and mild.

EVALUATION—A CAVEAT

We should use caution when evaluating the outcome of grief in any particular case. What appears to be healthy behavior in one person may really be deleterious or diversionary in another. Readiness to invest in a new intimate relationship may indicate true recovery from grief, but it may also be an evasion of the struggle with loss. For example, early remarriage may reflect a solid sense of hope for the future for one person; for another, it may be an escape from the pain of loneliness.

Creative activities like new projects at work, painting, and writing are often taken as a sign of healthy progress in grieving. Creativity in and of itself, however, does not always reflect the realization of successful grieving. It might be yet another attempt at withdrawal from the confrontation with pain. Similarly, an active social life may in reality be a compulsive distraction, like substance abuse, and not the solid reconstitution of a healthy support network.

Mourners gradually develop new identities that reveal their changed circumstances. Movement toward the new identity is slow and frequently unsteady. The important thing for nurses as caregivers to monitor is not the speed or the regularity of the growth toward a new identity, but the consistency of the progress.

ATYPICAL GRIEF

There are people who are not able to resolve a particular loss. Between 10% and 20% (Martocchio, 1982) of newly bereaved persons have serious emotional problems. They develop atypical or abnormal grief patterns, and the nurse should be aware of the signs of this condition to be able to refer the client who will need special counseling.

When the survivor goes on with life for more than a few weeks after a major loss as if nothing serious has happened, it is termed *delayed grief*. These people do not seem to be affected. Quite remarkably, they do not talk about the death as a loss, nor do they express grief, sadness, or regret. This prolonged denial prevents the necessary realization of the pain that precedes a true coming to terms with reality. If the family warns visitors not to talk to the survivor about the death or allude to the deceased, or if the survivor shows extreme discomfort when the death or the deceased is inadvertently mentioned, the nurse should take note. Conversely, the nurse should be alert to the possible pathology of delayed grief in families in which uncontrollable weeping

and other expressions of sadness occur more than two years after a death.

Exaggerated expressions of guilt and self-reproach that continue for more than 1 year or 18 months are another indicator of abnormal grief. In these cases, people have a seemingly endless need to discuss the "If only's" and the "I should have's."

Prolonged anger and hostility are still other signs of abnormal grief. The anger may be expressed not only in conversation as accusations, but also in real or fantasized lawsuits against the health care institutions and health care providers during the final stage of illness, or against undertakers, insurance companies, and alienated relatives and friends. At the least, these people have difficulty getting along with individuals in their preloss social circle and are not likely to have an easy time developing new relationships.

Successive physical illnesses or complaints for more than 2 years after the loss might be another indication of atypical grief. The same may be true for those who drink too much or who rely heavily on medications for inducing sleep or on tranquilizers.

Death from suicide is a real danger for the abnormally bereaved. Because almost all persons who commit suicide talk about it beforehand and because not all those who talk about it really want to succeed, the alert nurse takes any talk of suicide seriously.

COLLABORATIVE MANAGEMENT

 Assessment

Effective nursing interventions are based on nursing assessments that are tailored to specific grief reactions. The severity and duration of each person's response are determined by a unique combination of factors: the circumstances of the death, and the demographic, socioeconomic, psychologic, cultural, family, physiologic, and spiritual characteristics of the survivor (see the accompanying Nursing Research feature).

History

The nurse assesses a variety of factors when working with clients who have experienced the death of a loved one. Guidelines for the nursing assessment are presented in Table 11–3. Circumstances surrounding the death and characteristics of the survivor and the deceased have an impact on the client's emotional response.

Timeliness or "fairness." The *timeliness* of a death refers to the psychologic acceptability of the death to the survivors. Conventional wisdom has it that the loss of parents represents the loss of the past; the loss of a

NURSING RESEARCH

Assessment May Help to Predict Courses of Bereavement.

Gass, K. A., & Chang, A. S. (1989). Appraisals of bereavement, coping, resources, and psychosocial health dysfunction in widows and widowers. *Nursing Research, 38,* 31–37.

One hundred widows and 59 widowers bereaved from between 1 month and 1 year who characterized their bereavements as troublesome to some degree were interviewed with the Folkman and Lazarus Ways of Coping Checklist, a psychosocial health dysfunction scale, a self-appraisal of the extent of threat to the bereavement, and a measure of resource strength.

The Ways of Coping Checklist distinguished between problem-focused and emotion-focused coping strategies. The problem-focused strategies manage or modify a problem that is causing distress, and the emotion-focused strategies manage or reduce emotional stress that is a response to the problem. Denial, evasion, and guilt are components of emotion-focused response. The self-appraisal of the extent of threat rated the bereavement as harmful but with no additional losses; as harmful with other anticipated losses and problems difficult to manage; or as a challenge and an opportunity for growth. The elements of strength in relation to dealing with loss were culled from the literature, and resource strength was measured along the following dimensions: social support; religious orientation offering an acceptance or an understanding of death; knowledge about the grieving process; sufficient time and opportunity for anticipatory grieving; belief that the death was not preventable; capacity to express grief openly; belief in own capacity to control stress; good mental health; no other concurrent losses; adequate finances; and relationship with deceased spouse characterized by sufficient intimacy, minimal dependency, and no more than normal ambivalence and conflict.

Path analysis indicated that lower threat appraisal, more problem-focused and less emotion-focused coping, and greater resource strength had direct effects on reducing psychosocial health dysfunction. Greater resource strength also directly influenced lower threat appraisal.

Critique.   This study is comprehensive with its inclusion of multiple variables and extensive analysis of the data. Replication of the study with other populations (i.e., persons without religious affiliation) might be considered.

Possible nursing implications.   Nurses are often in the best position of health care providers to predict the course of a bereavement. To perform adequate assessments, nurses need to develop tools that incorporate the major elements in a client's life situation and the emotional patterns that have been associated through research with outcome. The more the nurse knows about these elements and the client, the better she or he will be able to plan appropriate support and therapy with the client and family.

spouse that of the present; and the loss of children that of the future.

Timeliness, however, also refers to other circumstances leading to a feeling that the death is unfair. Examples are the person who retires and dies shortly thereafter, and the family that has successfully lived through an especially hard time only to have one member die before they all can share a long-anticipated satisfaction.

Suddenness or expectedness.   When death or loss is expected, there usually is time to prepare for it and to start to identify and to marshall the survivors' coping capacities. When the loss is completely unexpected, however, the grievers are grossly shocked. The sudden loss of a sense of security, reliability, and predictability in life and the feeling of being completely overwhelmed frequently contribute to severe grieving complications, which may develop into a state of chronic apprehension.

On the other hand, if the period preceding a death is excessively long, a poor adjustment after the death is also likely. During this extended period of a client's dying, the exhausted and confused family may become worn out caring for the loved one and waiting for the death. They may become isolated from relatives, friends, and work. They often partially grieve long before the actual death, and this, in turn, produces guilt and anger at the dying person that complicates post-death grieving.

Demographic and socioeconomic factors.   Maturity, both in years and in character, and intelligence have been found to be consistently and positively related to the favorable resolution of loss. The older and more intelligent the survivors, the more likely they are to have a larger repertoire of effective coping techniques and resources. In addition, they are more likely to comprehend the loss than their less intelligent or less mature counterparts. They are also apt to be well educated, employed full-time, and financially comfortable — all acknowledged advantages in dealing with grief. Finally, the older people are, the less likely they are to have dependent children under the age of 14 years, another demonstrated impediment to uncomplicated grief (Parkes & Weiss, 1983).

Psychologic factors.   The client's enduring personality traits and habitual coping behaviors for crises will indicate how he or she may be expected to deal with the present stress. People die and grieve in much the same way that they have lived. The person who has faced crises realistically and with a matter-of-fact problem-solving approach faces dying and grieving directly. The person who has coped by using cover-up and retreat will probably evade and deny grief. The client will automatically use the strategies, conscious and unconscious, functional and dysfunctional, that have worked for him or her in the past.

TABLE 11-3 Guidelines for Assessing the Client Undergoing the Loss of a Loved One Through Death

1. What was the last illness of the deceased like?
2. Was the death timely?
3. How long was the preparation for the death?
4. What was the age of the deceased?
5. What was the relationship of the deceased to the survivor?
   a. Spouse.
   b. Parent.
   c. Sibling.
   d. Grandparent.
   e. Child.
   f. Other.
6. What are the survivor's characteristics?
   a. Age.
   b. Education.
   c. Employment.
   d. Economic status.
   e. Ages of dependent children.
   f. Past depressions or personality problems.
   g. Diagnosed mental health problems.
   h. Substance abuse history.
   i. Past major losses
      ▪ Number recalled.
      ▪ When?
      ▪ Were they resolved?
7. What coping strategies has the client used with previous losses and setbacks?
8. What are characteristics of the relationship with the deceased?
   a. Degree of intimacy.
   b. Dependence (who depended on whom?).
   c. Intensity.
   d. Ambivalence.
9. What are the relevant cultural and family factors?
   a. Ethnic background.
   b. Family structure (list close members)
      ▪ Are they geographically close?
      ▪ Are they warm and supportive?
      ▪ How often are these close family members seen? talked with?
10. What are the physical factors that the client associates with responses to previous losses or stressful events? What physical symptoms has the client had since the most recent loss? Suggested list of signs and symptoms:
    a. Headache.
    b. Appetite: loss, increase.
    c. Bowel habit changes.
    d. Bladder habit changes.
    e. Sleeping and dreaming.
    f. Tightness in throat or chest.
    g. Breathlessness.
    h. Sighing: heavy, frequent.
    i. Dry mouth.
    j. Muscle weakness.
    k. General malaise.
11. What are the spiritual aspects of the client's life?
    a. Is the client a congregant of a formally organized religious group? If yes, document relevant data.

TABLE 11–3   Guidelines for Assessing the Client Undergoing the Loss of a Loved One Through Death *Continued*

b. What helps the client when frightened or in need of extra support?
c. What is the client's source of strength and hope in times of crisis?
d. What are the client's ties to the wider community? Beliefs in a hereafter?
e. What is the client's source of a sense of meaning and purpose in life?
f. Is there an unconditional love in the client's life?
g. What does the client hope for now?

12. On the basis of this assessment interview, how would the nurse evaluate the client's level of
   a. Clinging and pining?
   b. Anger and hostility?
   c. Guilt and self-reproach?

Individuals who have had anxious and worrying reactions to crisis are at higher risk of a poor outcome of the grieving process, as are those who have a history of diagnosed mental or emotional health problems and/or a history of substance abuse.

The meaning and nature of the relationship. The meaning of the loss and the nature of the relationship influence the temper of the grief. The loss of a young person is more tragic and will evoke more grief than that of an elderly person. The loss of a child, regardless of the age of the parent and child, almost always provokes the most intense and persistent reactions.

The more mutually dependent the survivor and the deceased had been and the closer the relationship, the stronger will be the feelings of yearning and insecurity. The loss of a pet, although sad for many persons, may be traumatic to an elderly person for whom the pet has meant companionship and security. The death of a grandparent may be more significant than the death of a parent if the child has had a more intimate relationship with the grandparent. The death of a spouse is universally acknowledged as one of the most emotionally devastating losses.

The depth and intensity of the relationship. The depth and intensity of the relationship also have a bearing on the character and the course of the bereavement. The intensity of the grief reaction correlates directly with the intensity of the attachment. If the attachment was strong and the survivor relied on the deceased for a sense of identity, the course of grief may be particularly difficult, just as it may be if there have been more than usual levels of ambivalence in the relationship. Bereavements after markedly ambivalent, highly mutually dependent close relationships are frequently marked by severe and prolonged guilt, as well as anger at feeling abandoned.

Unresolved losses. Unresolved losses of the past also impede coming to terms with losses of the present, as do a number of losses occurring in a relatively short time. The emotional overload created by repeated unresolved losses can render the strongest, most resilient person helpless.

Cultural and family factors. Norms, values, and sociocultural orientation have a strong effect on bereavement behavior. "Keeping a stiff upper lip," or silently and privately grieving, is as effective for some as weeping or sobbing openly and uninhibitedly may be for others. What is important is not the mode of expression, but that the person be emotionally aware of his or her feelings. The grieving process is more likely to succeed when the bereaved person has close intimate relationships and has a warm and supportive family nearby.

Physiologic factors. People also have characteristic physiologic responses to life crises. A history should gather data about headaches, loss of or increase in appetite, bowel and bladder changes, and sleeping patterns and dreaming patterns after previous stresses as well as during the present crisis. In addition, the nurse will collect data about all other physical manifestations occurring since the recent loss, such as tightness in the throat or chest, breathlessness, heavy and frequent sighing, dry mouth, and muscle weakness. The person may not associate these changes with the loss, but they may, in fact, be related to it.

Spiritual factors. Individuals who have clear, firm spiritual beliefs (whether or not they are conventionally religious), who have a secure sense of meaning and purpose in life, or who have strong ties to a community or to a world of thought, action, or history that is larger than the self are all predictably better able to integrate their grief. For specific beliefs and customs of various religious groups about death and dying, see Table 11–4.

Cautionary note. The nurse should understand that while eliciting the material for a thorough assessment, she or he will also be engaged in a therapeutic encounter. In all likelihood, the grieving client will not be able to supply all information in a businesslike and

TABLE 11-4 Concepts and Practices of Major American Religious Groups Surrounding the Event of Death

Religious Group	Afterlife	Rituals Around Dying/Funeral Services	Autopsy	Organ and Body Donation	Cremation	"Extraordinary" Life-Prolonging Measures
Eastern Orthodox (including Greek and Russian Orthodox)	Yes; soul blends into the spiritual cosmos.	Arms are crossed after death; fingers are set in a cross; special prayers are said for blessing of the sick and dying for those eligible through baptism; last rites must be delivered while person is still conscious; Holy Communion is obligatory.	Discouraged; embalming is also discouraged.	Discouraged.	Discouraged.	Encouraged.
Judaism	Dead will be resurrected with coming of Messiah; person lives on through survival of memory; for Reform, no concept of eternal punishment.	Dying and dead are not left unattended; soul should depart in the presence of people; body is ritually washed, sometimes by members of a ritual burial society; body should never be left alone until burial; burial is within 24 hours or as soon as possible after death in a wooden casket; five stages of mourning extend over a year; funerals are very simple; for Orthodox, no embalming is allowed; no flowers are at funeral because flowers are a symbol of life.	Orthodox prohibit, and no body parts are removed; Conservative and Reform permit.	Beliefs vary. Orthodox generally prohibit but may agree with rabbinical consent.	Largely prohibited; beliefs vary. Reform allow but recommend burial of ashes in a Jewish cemetery.	Generally discouraged after irreversible brain damage is determined. Orthodox advocate life support without "heroic measures."

Religion	Beliefs	Rites / Services				
Roman Catholicism	Faithful go to heaven; those who reject God's grace go to hell. Purgatory for a time; soul is released by prayers and masses; resurrection with second coming of Christ.	Family and priest choose prayers; rites for anointing the sick are mandatory; receiving Holy Communion is mandatory; may want Confession—not mandatory, but penance recommended.	Permitted, but all body parts must be given appropriate burial.	No restriction as long as donor is not harmed.	No restriction.	Discouraged.
Protestantism	Varies with sect; a firm yes with Episcopalians, Presbyterians, and Lutherans; an outright no with Quakers.	Varies; anointing rites, confession, and communion may be available but not mandatory; "healing" services may be available; there are no official sacraments; client and family may have large role in creating services and prayer; clergy may minister through prayer, scripture reading, and counseling; services range from traditional funerals to memorial services.	Varies from no restriction, to individual choice, to preferred.			Discouraged.
Nonaffiliated	Varies.	Spontaneous, individualized; possibly original or traditional or reading of prayers, e.g., Psalm 23; traditional secular funeral or memorial services used.	Individual preference.	Individual preference.	Individual preference.	Individual preference.

straightforward manner. There will be pauses at certain items for either the control of or expression of feeling. Because it is difficult to predict which parts of the assessment will affect individual clients and in what ways, the nurse should move from topic to topic not necessarily in the order given, but guided by the client's response. The key is to keep the information flowing while conferring as much comfort as possible.

Because most newly bereaved people have a need to repeat the circumstances of the terminal episode and the death, we have placed these items at the beginning of the assessment. Often by retelling the story to an empathic listener and possibly discharging tears, guilt, or anger, the client will feel accepted and understood and will not react to the more factual and sensitive assessment items as intrusive or callous.

The items about physical signs and symptoms are placed near the end because many people do not like to emphasize the psychosomatic associations in their lives. For those in whom denial is an important defense strategy, this information may be difficult to obtain on a first interview. On the other hand, for those who feel most comfortable talking to health care workers about physical matters, this section of the assessment might be used as the most effective introduction.

The items about spiritual matters are placed last. This is because the spiritual domain is not simply sensitive, it is often volatile. The spiritual layer of our lives is the one closest to the center of our identities, and it is thus most difficult, especially in crisis situations, to discuss with those whom we do not know and trust. The nurse who understands this will proceed with subtlety and delicacy. If possible, the more sensitive areas of the assessment can be dealt with later.

During the assessment interview, the nurse will get a sense of the degree of clinging and pining, anger and/or guilt, and self-reproach that the client feels. Any of these normal reactions to the loss of a loved one that appear to be extreme are predictors of poor outcome of grieving. The nurse should indicate this impression at assessment so that appropriate follow-through or referral can take place.

 Analysis: Nursing Diagnosis

From the nursing assessment, nurses derive the nursing diagnoses that are the bases of clinical interventions as well as of care plans.

Common Diagnoses

The following nursing diagnoses are common to clients experiencing loss, death, or grief:

1. Dysfunctional grieving related to an actual or perceived loss
2. Anticipatory grieving related to potential loss
3. Fear related to known and unknown factors

Additional Diagnoses

In addition to the generic or common diagnoses, the individual may have symptoms for many of the following diagnoses:

1. Self-esteem disturbance related to the loss
2. Ineffective individual coping related to impending and actual death
3. Ineffective family coping related to death and dying
4. Sleep pattern disturbance related to fear
5. Family coping: potential for growth related to actual or potential loss of family member
6. Social isolation related to dying
7. Altered thought processes related to fear of death
8. Spiritual distress related to unacceptance of death
9. Sexual dysfunction related to ineffective coping

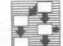 **Planning and Implementation**

The plan of care for the person undergoing loss is derived from the nursing assessment and is directed toward the achievement of specific goals. The following goals and nursing interventions are described according to the most common actual nursing diagnoses with the understanding that they do not necessarily apply to all individuals and that they need to be tailored to the situation.

Dysfunctional Grieving

Planning: client goals. The major goals are that the client will (1) accept the reality of the loss; (2) experience the pain of loss; (3) share grief with others; and (4) adjust to the environment changed by the loss.

Interventions

Teaching the family about the physical signs of death. Witnessing the death is one of the most effective experiences in helping the family begin to accept the reality of the loss. If the person has died an anticipated death at home, the family should have been supplied information about the signs of death. The nurse can discuss this during a home visit and/or she or he may leave written material with the family. Lay language should be used and technical terms avoided. The physical signs should be described in detail realistic enough to be unmistakable, yet not so graphic as to alarm.

Clients who are awake yet near death may be nauseated and gradually refuse food and fluid. This is a sign that the work of the intestines has stopped. Although the client may still complain of thirst, there may be difficulty in swallowing. The family should be taught that it is not wise to offer food and fluids in the customary manner. The food or fluids might be regurgitated or aspirated, or both. Clear fluids may be given but only in small amounts. With poor or no fluid intake, the client's mouth will become uncomfortably dry, so the caretakers should moisten, clear, and rinse it with applicators and saturated gauzes. Ice chips may be given, but only if the client is awake. Petrolatum or some other emollient may be applied to the lips.

The client may have difficulty in speaking and may lie still much of the time. He or she will sleep deeply for increasingly longer periods and may become difficult to arouse. There will be periods when the client does not appear to be breathing or is breathing irregularly. Breathing may become labored, with rapid respirations alternating with very slow and deep ones (Cheyne-Stokes). The breathing may become noisy because of the accumulation of mucus in the large bronchi. This noise is known as the death rattle. The client may be made more comfortable at any time by a change of position. Breathing discomfort may be relieved somewhat by placing the client on his or her side, with the head slightly elevated and firmly supported on a pillow.

The client's skin may be damp with cold perspiration even though he or she complains of feeling overly warm. The client should be kept dry by frequent sponging if his or her temperature is high. Only light covering is necessary.

Sensation and strength in the arms and legs gradually diminish. As peripheral circulation lessens, the hands, feet, ears, and nose become cold to the touch. The hands and feet may become mottled and blue (cyanotic). If the caretakers have been monitoring blood pressure, they will notice that it becomes lower until it disappears. The pulse, also, weakens and gradually slows, then stops. Meanwhile, respirations become shallow and they too stop. The pupils become fixed and dilated. Bladder and bowels may be emptied because of relaxation of the sphincters. When there is no breath or heartbeat for a few minutes, the attendants can assume death has taken place.

The family and, if death takes place in an institution, the nurse should be aware that the sense of hearing may remain intact when it appears that no other stimuli can be perceived. Conversation in the room and near the client should be carried on at all times as if she or he were alert. Caretakers should be encouraged to talk softly to the client, and to touch and gently stroke him or her. The client may not respond, but the family will feel better maintaining a semblance of normal interchange. This activity fosters a sense of active, reciprocal communication for everyone right up to the end. Soft music might also be played on a tape recorder.

After the death at home, the family can say their last words and perform their farewell gestures freely and naturally around the bed. They may want to remove tubings themselves before calling the hospice nurse, the physician, or the funeral director. They may wish to bathe the body as a final gesture of loving care. They can perform any religious or cultural customs they wish. The nurse will have given the family instructions about preparation of the body and communication with the proper authorities to comply with agency policy and state law.

The nurse attending a dying person in an institution uses more technical language and makes more precise observations when he or she communicates with other staff. He or she will also need to do accurate charting.

With an anticipated death in the institutional setting, the nurse frequently prepares the body for immediate postmortem viewing. All tubes and lines are removed or cut according to institutional policy, the eyes closed, dentures replaced, the bed leveled, and the body straightened and all pillows removed except for one supporting the head, which should be kept in place to delay discoloration of the face. Pads should be placed under the hips and around the perineum to absorb fecal material and fluid. The body should be washed as necessary and the hair combed and arranged. The nurse takes care that all dirty linen, apparatus, other clutter, and, if possible, odors are removed from the room.

The family may then, in private, join the newly deceased in the room. The nurse should let the family know that she or he will be near, should they have a need. If the family wish to see clergy, the nurse will do everything possible to find the hospital chaplain or appropriate community religious leader. She or he may also participate in or initiate generic spiritual expression such as touch, spontaneous prayer, or acknowledgment of the special qualities of the deceased.

Unanticipated deaths present a different set of circumstances for survivors than expected deaths. Unexpected deaths in the hospital, and possibly at home, are usually preceded by resuscitation attempts. Survivors who are not present during resuscitation may not have seen the client when he or she was obviously ill. Survivors of clients who die unexpectedly also have not had time to experience anticipatory grief. The shocking news of the death may be overwhelming. These survivors may not have had the opportunity to interact with nurses or physicians who assisted the dying client at home, in the emergency department, or in a unit of a hospital. Trust, which ideally becomes a part of the nurse-client-family and physician-client-family relationships, may not have had time to develop. For these reasons it has recently been suggested that survivors of clients who experience unexpected death view the client's body in the setting where death occurred before the area and the client are cleaned. It is recommended that tubes, medications, the "crash cart," and other supplies be left at the scene. When survivors view the deceased client, they see that efforts were made to save their loved one. Survivors also get a more realistic image of how severely ill the client was. Those who advocate this experience for survivors believe that it assists survivors in accepting the death and eventually resolving the grief.

There will be an institutional procedure to follow for preparing the body for transfer to either the hospital morgue or a funeral home. The necessary materials, such as a shroud and identification tags, are usually supplied in a packet.

Reaching out to the bereaved. A nurse's reaching out to the bereaved means more than a hasty, if heartfelt, "Call me if you need something." The nurse begins by helping the family adjust to the death from the moment it occurs. The well-prepared family at home have had instructions and are free to manage these moments in their own way. In the institution, the nurse encourages the family to visit briefly after the body has been prepared (just described).

By spending some time with the body immediately after death, the survivors are provided with a reference point in reality. When during the long period of bereavement they have times of disbelief, there is the indisputable knowledge that they either were with the dead person as he or she died or soon after the moment of death. This memory serves to counter the detachment and alienation that are frequently felt when embalming produces an effigy-like image or cremation leaves only the ashes behind.

Hospice nurses frequently, and nurses in other settings occasionally, attend the funerals of clients, which is a way of continuing the support begun at the death bed. This practice also helps the nurse, if she has known the patient and family well, to develop a sense of closure, not just for them but for herself as well. The nurse who attends the funeral or memorial service or visits the funeral parlor is a great comfort for the family. This gives them enormous satisfaction, as they perceive it as compassionate concern and the most that they could ask for. It contributes to the feeling that they gave their loved one everything possible and provides a realistic way to lessen the guilt of the bereavement period.

Telling the family about bereavement groups is another way of the nurse's reaching out. All hospices have some bereavement support activity, and nurses in other settings can supply the bereaved family with literature about grief and lists of local agencies and groups that may help. It is especially effective if the nurse can personally manage a referral.

Extended family members can be encouraged to keep reaching out to those closest to the deceased. They should be warned that they may be angrily rejected at first and that they should not take this rejection as a personal affront. Empathic, caring family, friends, and caregivers will reach out again and again.

Offering physical and emotional support. The simple presence of the caregiver offers a sense of security. Physical support such as being within sound or reach, gentle touching, holding hands, and hugging is especially important during the first phases of grief. Lending presence remains important as the weeks or months pass and the funeral crisis supports dissipate. The out-of-town relatives return home, and friends and local relatives resume activities of their own lives.

Physical and emotional support can be given by helping with meals and by encouraging the bereaved to eat, drink, rest, and stay as physically active as possible. Exercise to tolerance levels is a wonderful psychic as well as physical energizer.

Facilitating the expression of emotion. At the same time that nurses help the bereaved family to cope in practical ways, nurses must give them permission to express their grief. When necessary, nurses should facilitate its expression. Nurses do this by making themselves available to listen and to respond in nonjudgmental ways. The nurses' manner and words show that the expression of grief is not only acceptable and expected, but healthy. Acceptance is shown by moving physically closer. A gentle hand is placed on the arm, or an arm is placed around the shoulder when eyes flood with tears or voices crack. Nurses can say something such as, "Just let the tears come. Don't try to hold them back."

Preventing isolation of the bereaved. Research has demonstrated that through bereavement, those with the most and strongest ties to others have the easiest time and the soundest outcomes (Raphael, 1983). The value in social support is that bereaved individuals are constantly reassured of the possibility of re-creating a satisfactory life even though an important part of the fabric of life has been lost. It cannot be emphasized too strongly: nothing is more helpful throughout the grieving process than social support from nonjudgmental, caring persons.

An important task for nurses who plan grief therapy is identifying the real and potential sources of support in the client's environment. Family members and close friends can comfort the client as well as each other. Self-help or bereavement support groups managed by hospice organizations, clergy, or mental health therapists are also effective for certain clients.

Being realistic. The pain of loss cannot be—nor should it be—taken away no matter how committed to the client's comfort the nurse may be. To expect to make the experience anything but relatively better in incremental steps is to invite failure. Nurses must recognize the therapeutic value of the "gift of presence." Nurses must avoid pat stereotypic assurances such as "Things will be fine. Don't cry" and "Don't be upset. She wouldn't want it that way" or "In a year you will have forgotten." These sorts of comments comfort the nurse, not the client. The nurse accepts whatever the griever says about himself or herself and the situation and remains present, ready to listen attentively and guide gently. In this way nurses help her or him to prepare for the necessary reminiscence and integration of the loss.

Viewing the loss from the perspective of the bereaved. The bereaved person's, not the nurse's, perspective of the loss is crucial and will be instrumental in healing. The nurse must help the bereaved individuals define and decide for themselves what is most important for them to discuss, to explore, and to ruminate on.

Maintaining compassionate concern. It is appropriate for nurses to show that they are moved by the sadness of the griever. It is therapeutic to grievers to know that nurses care enough about them to be touched by their situation. At the same time, it is important for the nurse to not succumb to or to allow himself or herself to be overcome by the griever's despair. When professional perspective is lost, so is much of the value of the support that the nurse may have offered. Such loss of professional perspective may also encourage dependence rather than growth toward autonomy.

Avoiding explanations of the loss. The nurse should not try soon after the death to explain the loss in philosophical or religious terms. Statements like, "Everything happens for the best" or "God sends us only as much as we can bear" are not helpful when the bereaved person has yet to express feelings of anguish or anger. Telling someone too soon that they have other children to rely on, or that there are other family members who need them, does not diminish the intensity of the grief. In fact, it will probably create feelings of anger and resentment toward the nurse because it reflects an insensitivity to the acute initial pain.

Being honest, planting seeds of hope, allowing for time. Confirm for the client that the situation is difficult. Respond to and validate the client's feelings while quietly and unobtrusively planting seeds of hope that things may improve over time. Be careful not to imply a schedule. "Time" may be plus or minus 1 year for one person, 4 years or more for another. Such comments as "It is so painful right now" or "You are right, it doesn't make sense" reflect an understanding and acknowledgment of the griever's view of the situation. Reassurance that the pain will indeed decrease sometime and that no one can tolerate the current intensity and distress forever often helps grievers to go on. Some gain hope by seeing or knowing others who have survived their grief. Still others gain hope and comfort through believing that they will be reunited with the deceased in heaven or eternity, or some other concept of "beyond." In this world, hope per se lies in the expectation that the griever will successfully complete the tasks of grieving, that the pain will subside, and that life will once again have both meaning and equilibrium.

The grief of the person who is dying is similar to that of her or his survivors and is influenced by the same factors. The dying, however, grieve not only for the loss of the past and the present, but also for the future. They grieve for the loss of all that can be hoped for in human experience. They struggle with feelings of being cheated. They envy anyone who is healthy. Just beneath the surface is anger. They need to identify their losses, to talk about them, and to express their feelings. They need permission to grieve from caregivers, family members, and all those who are significant in their lives. Kübler-Ross observed that as long as a listener remains genuinely receptive, the client will talk openly about his or her concerns.

As previously discussed, there are people who cannot resolve losses. Dysfunctional grieving is the nursing diagnosis made when an individual remains in one phase of grieving and demonstrates excessive or prolonged emotional response to the loss. It is important that the nurse assess all clients dealing with death and dying for manifestations of dysfunctional grieving. These manifestations may include inhibition, suppression, or absence of emotional reactions; prolongation of normal grieving; excessive emotional reactions; or somatic expression of fear.

Anticipatory grieving over a loss such as death takes place before the actual death. When discussing the topics of death and dying, it is difficult to separate this type of grieving from the actual grieving process that occurs in response to a loss. Anticipatory grieving has been discussed throughout this care plan. Assessment, goals, and interventions for this diagnosis are similar to those identified earlier.

Fear

Many fears surround dying. The following goals and interventions address some of the most common ones.

Planning: client goals. The goals related to the nursing diagnosis of fear are that the client will (1) identify real reasons for fear and if necessary differentiate them from imagined ones, (2) gain control over fears, and (3) increase psychologic and physiologic comfort.

Interventions

Fear of the unknown. Fear of the unknown is a basic fear of all human beings. Humans fear what is unfamiliar or not understood. Throughout life, all people have some fear of dying and death.

This fear, amplified when a person is terminally ill, often surfaces in the form of questions. Some of them may be philosophical or religious, such as, "Where will I be in the hereafter?" Others are more practical. They concern the welfare of those who are left behind, how the survivors will manage, and what will happen to life plans and projects. Many questions revolve around the dying process itself: "What will happen to me?" "Will I lose control of myself?" "How will I react?" "Will I have pain?" "What will happen to my body after death?"

Nurses can help the dying by distinguishing the questions that have answers from those that do not. For the ones that have immediate answers, nurses get the information. For those that can be answered in the future, nurses begin to draw together the pertinent resources. For those that may never have an answer, nurses encourage expression of feeling. The aim is to provide comfort by eliminating as much uncertainty as is realistically possible.

When the client questions what will happen to the survivors after his or her death, it might be appropriate to assist with funeral plans and arrangements for religious observations or memorial services. This might also be the time to make sure that such things as wills and advance directives are in order.

Fear of loneliness, isolation, and abandonment. All people, and especially dying people, gain reassurance in feeling accepted by others. All persons who are involved in care can supply this reassurance by simply being with the dying. Yet, visiting a sick person often produces fear for the visitor. Nurses can prompt family and friends during their visits. Nurses can show them how to participate in the dying client's care and can help them communicate with the client. Nurses can also suggest options such as dying at home, if that is possible, either with or without the support of a participating hospice program. In this way, some of the feeling of abandonment that results from having been removed from home, family, and community to an institution can be relieved.

Fear of loss of family and friends. This fear is closely related to fear of abandonment. Dying people grieve the loss of family and friends just as the family and friends grieve the loss of the client.

Fear of loss of self-control and dependency. Self-reliance and independence are closely associated with positive self-image and the sense of human dignity. Fear of loss of control and of encroaching dependency, therefore, is a major worry of persons who are becoming progressively more debilitated. Nursing strategies to help in this area include encouraging dying persons to make as many decisions as possible about the details of their lives, such as nursing care and concerns about the future.

The client and family may also wish to think about advance directives. If they do not ask about such instructions, the nurse might introduce the idea of the living will or durable power of attorney.

Fear of suffering and pain. Many people fear dying in unbearable pain. This may or may not be a realistic concern. Nurses can help by providing information about pain in a way that mitigates fears. Clients can be reassured that there are now sophisticated combinations of invasive and noninvasive treatments for pain control that were not available 25 years ago. They can assure clients and families that if pain becomes a problem, the most effective pain relief regimen possible will be devised. Finally, they can assure nonabandonment, or an attentive presence, if pain proves to be a problem.

Evaluation

The nurse evaluates the care of the client and family undergoing loss on the basis of identified nursing diagnoses. The expected outcomes for the client and family include that they

1. Accept the reality of the loss
2. Be able to share their grief with each other
3. Adjust to the environment changed by the loss
4. Recognize specific fears and coping resources
5. Use safe and effective coping mechanisms
6. Experience psychologic and physiologic comfort
7. Gain confidence in the ability to perform new role-related responsibilities
8. Achieve a sense of renewed identity after the loss

By achieving the desired outcomes, the client and family demonstrate an ability to adapt to a loss or death. Acceptance of the loss and successful adjustment after the crisis better enable them to respond to future losses.

COMMUNITY RESOURCES

Nurses play a role in acquainting and linking the bereaved individuals with helpful community organizations, such as Widow-to-Widow and Compassionate Friends, and other resources such as bereavement discussion groups, mental health nurses, psychologists, counselors, social workers, and clergy or religious leaders involved in bereavement counseling.

Nurses can also participate in community and religious educational programs that are designed to assist people to understand grief and that reach out to the bereaved. Hospice programs are excellent sources of information and referral.

HOSPICE

Hospice is not a building or a place or an institution. It is a concept of care expressed in a centrally coordinated array of services. The aim of hospice care is to enable a dying person to live until she or he dies to the limit of his or her potential in physical strength; in mental, emotional, and spiritual capacity; and in social relationships. When appropriate, hospice care offers an alternative to the acute care of a general hospital or the custodial care of a nursing home. Although one of the prominent aspects of hospice care in the United States is the variety of organizational types and sponsoring agencies, a consistent philosophy and a set of core services are common to all accredited and certified or licensed programs.

GENERAL FEATURES

Hospice care is holistic. The interrelationship of the physical and the psychologic is acknowledged and attended to. Care, provided by an interdisciplinary team, is given to a dying person and his or her family, however defined. The care is directed at symptoms and circumstances surrounding the physical, the emotional, the spiritual, the social, and the financial spheres. Hospice care is comprehensive and nonfragmented, providing

---

TABLE 11-5 A Model Bill of Rights for Hospice Clients

The hospice's intention is to protect and support the human and legal rights of all in its care by guaranteeing patients and families the right to

- Access to care, regardless of race, religion, ethnicity, sex, age, handicap
- Be treated with dignity and respect at all times
- Full disclosure of the benefits and limitations of the program, including other options for care and costs
- Give (or withhold) informed consent for care; for being treated by others besides program staff, such as students; for being observed by other than staff; for being used as a research subject
- Confidentiality and privacy both in relation to the hospice health care team and the patient's family and attending physician
- Know the truth about diagnosis and prognosis
- Participate in the development and updating of the individualized plan of care
- Continuity of care from home to inpatient facility and through bereavement care

- State-of-the-art management of symptom and pain control
- Know the rules and regulations of the program as well as channels of communication with management and grievance procedures
- Know the program's policies with regard to resuscitation and other ''heroic'' procedures
- Know the program's usual procedures followed at the time of death
- Choose the place of death: home, inpatient setting
- Choose the time of death, if that becomes necessary
- Determine the disposition of his or her own body both at and after death
- Call on the support of any belief system or cultural practices that will help
- Have sufficient numbers of qualified, competent, compassionate staff to realize these rights

---

From Amenta, M. O., & Bohnet, N. (1986). *Nursing care of the terminally ill.* Boston: Little, Brown. Reprinted by permission of Scott, Foresman and Company.

---

continuity from one service level to another as the dying person's changes in condition and family circumstances call for changes in levels of care.

The four key features of hospice programs are

1. Symptom control or palliation for the dying person
2. The dying person and family, however defined, as the unit of care
3. Care planned and delivered by a multidisciplinary team
4. Care supervised and coordinated by the hospice program in a variety of settings

For a model bill of rights for hospice clients, see Table 11-5.

Symptom Control or Palliation

The key clinical feature of hospice care is that it is directed primarily at symptom control or palliation rather than disease control or cure. Invasive diagnostic or therapeutic procedures are seldom used. Because a diagnosis of terminal illness with prognosis of less than 6 months is an almost universally required criterion for admission to a hospice program, and because the psychosocial as well as the physical dimension is emphasized in care, there is a far greater need for intensive personal care than for intensive technical care.

This is not to say that there is never specific technologic intervention or curative treatment of the underlying disease. It means that, no matter what the treatment, relief of symptoms is the overriding goal. Active intervention in the cancer process with chemotherapy or radiation, for instance, is used only to the extent that it can be expected to contribute to the dying person's quality of life.

In certain instances, reduction of the size of a tumor can relieve an intestinal obstruction or make respiration easier. Chemotherapy can sometimes shrink tumors that are bearing on pain-sensitive tissue such as nerves or periosteum. Mild doses of radiation can relieve the pain of bone metastasis. These curative methods applied with palliative purposes may then give several weeks or months of special time to the dying person and his or her loved ones. A wedding might be planned, a will drawn up, or the reconciliation of a long estrangement realized.

As a practical matter, the problem of considering the use of sophisticated technologic procedures in hospice care arises rarely. When it does become an issue, the best decision will be an individualized one, made in light of all that is known of the client, family, and natural history of the disease.

Palliation of pain. The clinical innovation for which the hospice movement is best known is the palliative treatment of pain. Developed from experimental methods used in the pioneer hospices of the 1960s in England and the United States, this new philosophy of pain management is now spreading to many areas of clinical practice. The operative principle is that pain is whatever the client says it is, that it is as mild or severe as the client says it is, and that it responds to treatment in whatever way the client says it does.

Another fundamental principle of palliative pain control is the regular giving of medication doses in intervals that prevent the re-emergence of the pain. In this way, the client does not have to feel the pain break through the analgesic barrier before he or she gets relief. Hence, anticipation anxiety, a known potentiator of pain, is eliminated. With this type of self-controlled or self-administered regimen, clients frequently use less pain medication overall than with traditional 4-hour dosage schedules.

Many pain treatment methods are applied in hospice care. They include use of battery-operated infusion pumps, guided imagery tapes or other forms of relaxation therapy and distraction, heat or cold, massage, and transcutaneous stimulation. Medications may include nonsteroidal anti-inflammatory drugs, steroids, oral analgesics, tranquilizers, psychic energizers, and short-acting or long-acting opiates. These medications may be in the form of suppositories, injections, tablets, liquids, or continuous intravenous drips delivered via surgically implanted catheters or "lines" either with or without pumps.

All these methods are used singly or in combination. The client's response is the measure of efficacy. Side effects of various regimens are studied and counteracted. In general, the desired route of drug administration will be oral, rectal, or through a venous access catheter because the dying person usually has too little muscle or accessible vasculature to repeatedly inject medication successfully and comfortably.

The Dying Person and Family as the Unit of Care

Family involvement is important in all aspects of health care, but it takes on major significance in caring for the dying. It should be understood that *family* in the cosmos of hospice care means anyone deeply attached to the dying person—spouse, blood relation, close friend, lover, neighbor—who will take the responsibility of caring for him or her. Most hospices must identify a primary care person in each family who acts as the coordinator of care at the program/family nexus.

Those close to the dying person face problems that may seem insurmountable. Some problems develop from feelings about the impending loss, but more are related to practical responsibilities as caregivers, to living arrangements, or to financial considerations.

When the family's or primary care person's confidence in ability to manage some of these matters crumbles, the overall care of the dying person can be profoundly affected. As nurses carefully assess families and support and teach them the needed knowledge and skills and as the family's understanding of the illness and its care demands grows, the family becomes an important part of the therapeutic and coordinating team.

Hospice involvement with the family does not end with the death of the patient. Bereavement follow-up to provide reassurance and support during grieving is a component of most hospice programs. The functions of bereavement care are to assess the coping ability of the survivors; encourage and facilitate the expression of feelings related to the loss; reassure the survivors that the grieving process, although painful, is normal; identify possibly pathologic reactions; and make referrals if needed.

A Multidisciplinary Approach

Because problems in hospice care management arise from a variety of sources—physical, emotional, social, spiritual, and financial—a team approach is essential. With the client and family ideally at the center of decision-making, the interdisciplinary team also includes physicians, nurses, social workers, clergy or religious or spiritual leaders, and volunteers as key members.

The lack of sharp distinctions or blurring of roles among the functions and decision-making authority of the members of the team is an important characteristic of multidisciplinary care. Although each member has an area of expertise in which she or he has primary responsibility and authority, all members must be alert and open to problems and needs in other areas of care. Each member must be prepared to undertake care tasks that are normally in the purview of another. The better welded the team, the more role overlap is tolerated, the better the care of the client and family.

Coordination of all these caregiving participants and levels of care demands leadership and communication. By having the interdisciplinary team meet regularly on an established schedule, continuity of care is maintained.

Coordinated Care in Multiple Settings

The dying person must be in the setting most appropriate to his or her needs, and there must be continuity of care as the client shifts from one setting or level of care to another as dictated by his or her changing condition. The most usual settings are home, acute care hospital, and intermediate care facility.

The most suitable setting for a dying person at any particular time depends on many factors. These factors include the client's physical and emotional condition, home situation, attitude toward the illness and impending death, and attitude toward the family. A not insignificant factor is the family's capacity to manage care. The input of the dying person and family as well as that of the multidisciplinary team is important in making decisions about where the dying person can best receive care. Financial considerations must also be taken into account.

In addition to coordinating care in various settings, the hospice program must make services available on a 24-hour basis 7 days a week because problems arise unexpectedly at all hours of the day and night and on the weekends. A prompt response is one of the key elements of successful continuity for palliative care. The best pain and symptom control protocols can be useless if they are not maintained without interruption from home to hospital and back to home or nursing home. The accompanying resurgence of pain, anxiety, distorted relationships, and general chaos can undo weeks of careful attention and care.

HOSPICE HOME CARE

Most dying persons and their families who choose hospice care prefer the home to other caregiving environments during the final episodes of the illness. They also wish for death to take place at home, if possible. Although there are exceptions to these preferences, being surrounded by familiar people and things, the ready access to friends and relatives, and the freedom from institutional restriction, no matter how liberal, make the home setting more comfortable and give the client and family more control.

Families who choose home care supported by a Medicare-certified hospice program may also have the advantage of continuous nursing care in the home if the client's condition warrants. Inpatient respite care of the client for a short time may also be available if caregivers need a few days of rest. Home care is much less costly for the family and the overall health care system than any sort of inpatient care. In many cases, hospice home care is reimbursable either in part or totally by a third-party payer.

There are, however, some disadvantages to home care of the dying client. Families may not be able to manage the physically and psychologically demanding burden of round-the-clock care 7 days a week. Some family members may have crippling anxiety about what to do in a medical crisis. These families may become rapidly exhausted.

Families may be less fearful of attempting home care if they know they will have the support of the hospice team for physical crises and the assurance of respite time for themselves if they need it. In preparation for home care, there should be meetings between hospice staff and the family to explain such things as the roles of nurses, volunteers, and other workers; the on-call system; options for readmission to in-service hospice or for respite care; use of emergency staff visits; continuous care possibilities; and other available supports. The home must be readied with supplies and equipment such as disposable pads, hospital bed, water or alternating pressure mattress, bed pan and/or urinal, commode, dressings, intravenous poles, and irrigation sets if needed. The family should be assisted in arranging the home for caregiving comfort, convenience, and privacy.

OTHER ISSUES

EUTHANASIA

Under some conditions, especially those of high uncertainty, to keep someone alive through technologic life support rather than to actively and arbitrarily end his or her life can provide time—time to try an experimental new therapy or perhaps time for a remission. Unfortunately, an interval like this is not always good or quality time. It may be time fraught with pain, suffering, and confusion rather than peace and growth. The agonizing question emerges, "Is this kind of life worth staying alive for?" It is then that the issue of euthanasia moves to the forefront.

Euthanasia, derived from a Greek word meaning "easy or pleasant death," implies that under some circumstances death is preferable to life. Our notion of euthanasia, or "mercy killing," as it is commonly known, is surrounded with controversy. The only area of consensus would seem to be that the referent is dying or debilitated with no expected hope of recovery.

We use certain agreed upon distinctions and definitions when discussing euthanasia (Table 11–6): active, passive, voluntary, and involuntary. *Active euthanasia* refers to an act of *commission* that directly and *intentionally* shortens a person's life. In comparison, *passive euthanasia* is an act of *omission*. It usually refers to letting the person die by either withdrawing or withholding a treatment that might prolong life. The distinction between active and passive euthanasia is at best blurred because both are the result of intentional choice. Is it more moral to let someone die than to take measures specifically aimed at ending her or his life? Deciding not to act is a decision. Not acting is an action.

Voluntary euthanasia and involuntary euthanasia refer to the amount of involvement of a person in procedures and decisions leading to his or her death. In *invol-*

TABLE 11–6   Classification of Euthanasia

Person's Choice	Type of Action	
	Direct (Active)	Indirect (Passive)
Voluntary	Suicide (legal)	"Living will" (legal)
Involuntary	Murder "mercy killing" (illegal)	Letting nature take its course (possibly legal)

From Amenta, M. O., & Bohnet, N. (1986). *Nursing care of the terminally ill.* Boston: Little, Brown. Reprinted by permission of Scott, Foresman and Company.

untary euthanasia, the decisions are made by someone other than the dying person, either with or without his or her knowledge. In voluntary euthanasia, the client may actively participate in decision-making or may leave instructions to loved ones about the circumstances under which extraordinary means would or would not be desired.

Open discussions that are held when a person is mentally competent about his or her wishes regarding therapies should death be imminent is one way to ensure some participation in decision-making. The formalizations or documentations of these projected wishes are called advance directives. They help eliminate some of the nettlesome ambiguities surrounding the termination of a life by anything other than natural causes.

Two commonly used vehicles for implementing advance directives are living wills (Fig. 11–1) and durable powers of attorney (Fig. 11–2). These instruments, when executed in good faith, can safeguard a dying person's right of self-determination while freeing health care professionals from criminal liability for honoring their clients' wishes.

SUICIDE

The practice of active euthanasia may take the form of providing a dying person the means for ending her or his own life. When people take their own lives, it can be termed active voluntary euthanasia or suicide.

Individual and societal views about suicide range from opposition to suicide under all circumstances, to suicide viewed as justifiable under certain conditions, to suicide seen as a fundamental human right. Individuals who oppose suicide in all circumstances usually base their argument on the sanctity of life: Life is a gift from God, and no mere human has the right to take it away. Those at the other end of the continuum favor the quality of life argument: Life is characterized by humanness, or our potential for enjoyment and relationships with other people. In this view, human need takes precedence, death is not the worst thing that can befall a person, and each person has the right to determine his or her fate even if it means destroying his or her own life.

Some persons believe that suicide is a crime against our common humanity, an act of cowardice. Others see it as the ultimate in honor or courage. Of great interpersonal significance is the profound and enduring negative impact suicide has on survivors, especially if the survivors were not involved in the plans.

Health professionals are concerned about suicide because they are often in a position to offer alternatives. In severely ill or debilitated persons, it is sometimes difficult to know what suicidal behavior is. Is it the refusal to eat or to continue therapy? Or must it be something more overt, such as taking an overdose of a medication? Is the suicide attempt a truly voluntary act? Or might not a person have been driven to suicide by intolerable suffering, loneliness, rejection, or abandonment?

What do nurses do when a person is dying too slowly but death is inevitable and the client asks for help in ending the misery? In these cases, nurses think not only of client autonomy and self-determination but also of the entire spectrum of biomedical ethical decision-making options to which health professionals are committed. Another important biomedical ethical imperative is to never abandon care. Never abandoning care means ensuring that a dying person is not alone, that others are aware of his or her terminal condition, and that he or she is as free as possible from discomfort, pain, and anxiety. Nurses do not have a professional obligation to help people end their lives. Indeed, in strictest terms, assisting a suicide is illegal.

In many situations, suicidal behavior is a cry for help rather than the expression of definitive intent. Nurses thus have an obligation to acknowledge the suicidal inclinations of dying persons and to try to help them identify what in the current situation is contributing to such intense suffering that death seems preferable to life. Often suicide is not a rational choice but rather an attempt to cope with emotional conflict or extreme physical discomfort.

Suicide may also be a form of external control or a form of escape. Some people have carefully planned, and thus controlled, almost everything in their lives and characteristically they would like to plan and control the time and manner of their dying. Others seek escape from the uncertainties attendant to dying. Still others simply seek an end to suffering. In almost all cases, it can be inferred that poor quality of life contributes to the desire to be dead.

Improvements in the quality of life for terminally ill clients can be brought about by nurses' helping families maintain a sense of control. Nurses can teach families how to assist with the client's physical functions such as bowel and bladder regulation and how to help maintain adequate pain control. Nurses can also minimize uncertainties as much as possible by sharing what is known about the illness and the treatment, what will be known at a future time, and what is impossible to predict. Helping people know what to expect and how to develop strategies for coping offers them the perception of power—a potent tool for increasing the sense of meaning in living.

QUALITY OF LIFE

The usual scales and protocols by which we assess quality of life in most clinical situations are not applicable to the dying person. In fact, if our commonly used instruments were used to measure the quality of life of dying persons, their scores would be extremely low because the tools focus more on physical and social dimensions and less on a general sense of well-being or satisfaction with life. Dying persons perceive the quality of living from a vastly different perspective than do persons who are well or those who are chronically or acutely ill.

To My Family, My Physician, My Lawyer
And All Others Whom It May Concern

Death is as much a reality as birth, growth, and aging—it is the one certainty of life. In anticipation of decisions that may have to be made about my own dying and as an expression of my right to refuse treatment, I _____ , being of sound mind, make this statement of my wishes and instructions concerning treatment.
(print name)

By means of this document, which I intend to be legally binding, I direct my physician and other care providers, my family, and any surrogate designated by me or appointed by a court, to carry out my wishes. If I become unable, by reason of physical or mental incapacity, to make decisions about my medical care, let this document provide the guidance and authority needed to make any and all such decisions.

If I am permanently unconscious or there is no reasonable expectation of my recovery from a seriously incapacitating or lethal illness or condition, I do not wish to be kept alive by artificial means. I request that I be given all care necessary to keep me comfortable and free of pain, even if pain-relieving medications may hasten my death, and I direct that no life-sustaining treatment be provided except as I or my surrogate specifically authorize.

This request may appear to place a heavy responsibility upon you, but by making this decision according to my strong convictions, I intend to ease that burden. I am acting after careful consideration and with understanding of the consequences of your carrying out my wishes. *List optional specific provisions in the space below. (See other side)*

Durable Power of Attorney for Health Care Decisions (Cross out if you do not wish to use this section)

To effect my wishes, I designate _____ ,
residing at _____ (Phone #) _____ ,
(or if he or she shall for any reason fail to act, _____ (Phone #) _____ ,
residing at _____) as my health care surrogate—
that is, my attorney-in-fact regarding any and all health care decisions to be made for me, including the decision to refuse life-sustaining treatment—if I am unable to make such decisions myself. This power shall remain effective during and not be affected by my subsequent illness, disability or incapacity. My surrogate shall have authority to interpret my Living Will, and shall make decisions about my health care as specified in my instructions or, when my wishes are not clear, as the surrogate believes to be in my best interests. I release and agree to hold harmless my health care surrogate from any and all claims whatsoever arising from decisions made in good faith in the exercise of this power.

I sign this document knowingly, voluntarily, and after careful deliberation, this _____ day of _____, 19_____.

_____
(signature)

Address _____

_____

I do hereby certify that the within document was executed and acknowledged before me by the principal this_____ day of _____, 19 _____.

_____
Notary Public

Witness_____

Printed Name _____

Address _____

_____

Witness_____

Printed Name _____

Address _____

_____

Copies of this document have been given to:

(Optional) My Living Will is registered with Concern for Dying (No. _____)
Distributed by Concern for Dying, 250 West 57th Street, New York, NY 10107 (212) 246-6962

Figure 11–1

A living will.

Power of Attorney for
Decisions Regarding Health Care

Know all men by these presents that I, _____, the undersigned, being of sound mind, do hereby make, constitute and appoint my (wife, son, etc.) _____, (name) _____, of (address) _____, as my true and lawful attorney-in-fact for me and in my name, place, and stead for the purpose of making decisions regarding my health care at any time that I may be, by reason of physical or mental disability, incapable of making decisions on my own behalf.

If he or she is unable or unwilling to serve as my attorney at the time decisions regarding my health care must be made, I designate my (daughter, close friend, etc.) _____, (name) _____, of (address) _____, as alternate attorney-in-fact for me and in my name, place and stead for the purpose of making decisions regarding my health care.

1. I grant to said attorney-in-fact full power and authority to do and perform all and every act and thing whatsoever requisite, proper, or necessary to be done, in the exercise of the rights herein granted, as fully to all intents and purposes as I might or could do if personally present and able, with full power of substitution or revocation, hereby ratifying and confirming all that said attorney-in-fact shall lawfully do or cause to be done by virtue of this power of attorney and the rights and powers granted herein.

2. If, at any time, I am unable or unwilling to make decisions concerning my medical care and treatment, by virtue of physical, mental or emotional disability, illness or otherwise, my said attorney-in-fact shall have the authority to make all health care decisions for me and on my behalf, including consenting, refusing to consent or withdrawing consent to any care, treatment, service or procedure to maintain, diagnose or treat my mental or physical condition, subject to the provisions of paragraphs 3 and 4 hereof if I am suffering from a terminal condition.

3. If, at any time, I should have an incurable injury, disease, illness or disability, certified to be a terminal condition, and two physicians who have personally examined me (one of whom shall be my attending physician), have determined that my death will occur whether or not life-sustaining procedures are utilized, and that application of life-sustaining procedures would serve only to prolong the dying process, I specifically direct my said attorney-in-fact to authorize the withholding or withdrawal of such procedures. It is my intention that I be permitted to die naturally, with only the medication and nursing procedures necessary to alleviate pain and to provide me with comfort, dignity, and supportive care.

Figure 11-2

A power of attorney form for decisions regarding health care. (From Mishkin, B. [1985]. *Decisions in hospice*. NHO Monograph. Arlington, VA: National Hospice Organization.)

4. I also direct my said attorney-in-fact to make arrangements for the treatment of my terminal illness under the auspices of a hospice, if I should qualify for such care. I understand that acceptance into hospice care entails foregoing curative treatment and life-sustaining procedures that might otherwise be performed, such as resuscitation in case of cardiac arrest, and that foregoing such procedures might hasten my dying. I hereby consent to hospice care under such conditions, and direct my attorney-in-fact to make any and all necessary arrangements for me to receive such care, including the signing of such consent forms as may be required by the hospice, any third-party payor, and the federal government.

5. In the absence of my ability to give directions regarding my health care, it is my intention that my said attorney-in-fact shall exercise this specific grant of authority and that such exercise shall be honored by my family, physicians, nurses, and any health care facilities in which I may be treated (including ambulances by which I may be conveyed between my residence and a health care facility), as the final expression of my legal right to refuse medical or surgical treatment. I understand and accept the consequences of such refusal.

6. This instrument is to be construed and interpreted as a limited power of attorney.

7. This power of attorney shall not terminate on my disability or incompetence.

The rights, powers, and authority of said attorney-in-fact herein granted shall commence and be

in full force and effect on this _____ day of _____,

19 _____, and such rights, powers and authority shall remain in full force and effect thereafter until this power of attorney or any part thereof is revoked by means sufficient under applicable state law to cause revocation.

Dated _____, 19 _____

_____
signature

_____
address

_____

Caution: A few states require signing before a judge or notary. Check state statute.

The undersigned hereby attest to their belief that _____ was of sound

mind this _____ day of _____, 19 _____,

at _____ AM/PM when said principal signed this power of attorney.

We further attest that we are not related to the principal by blood or marriage, neither are we financially nor professionally responsible for his/her care, or employed by any institution so responsible. To the best of our knowledge, we are not entitled to any portion of the principal's estate either under the laws of intestate succession of this jurisdiction or under the terms of any will or codicil thereto.

_____   _____
(print or type name)   (print or type name)

_____   _____
(address)   (address)

_____   _____

_____   _____
signature   signature

More pertinent questions to explore with the dying are, What gives meaning to life now? What detracts from meaning in life now? Terminally ill clients give different responses to these questions on different days, but so do persons whose death is not imminent. The important thing for nurses to remember is to accept what the dying person says is contributing to or detracting from the meaningfulness of her or his life. Physical suffering might, depending on the person, contribute as much to growth and peace as to despair. The freedom to choose something, no matter how small or seemingly insignificant, confers meaning. Dying persons may realistically hope to choose the manner and setting of their dying. Nurses play a paramount role in helping them to fulfill that hope.

SUMMARY

Loss, dying, and death are universal experiences that are unique for each individual. As members of the health care team, nurses are in a prominent position to assist the individual as well as his or her significant others throughout the dying process and during the grief process. Although societal views about death have changed throughout the ages, research has found common stages or patterns of response that occur in some form and to some degree in all people who face a loss. Fear and ineffective coping are two common problems. Through assessment skills, nurses must identify the individual's reactions and plan appropriate nursing interventions during the time of bereavement. Hospice programs and community resources provide options for care during the dying process.

Issues regarding death are fraught with ethical dilemmas. As modern medicine and technology have lengthened the life span, nurses are often faced with questions regarding euthanasia and the quality of life of dying clients.

IMPLICATIONS FOR RESEARCH

Continued research in the area of loss and death is needed to identify methods to help meet the needs of clients and their families, as well as to provide support for members of the health care team, principally nurses. Additional theory development is needed to extend nursing's knowledge base of loss, dying, and death. Some questions for future research include

1. What nursing interventions are most helpful in encouraging individuals to express their feelings?

2. What type of environment provides the best care for the dying person?
3. What types of social service support are most useful to persons undergoing loss?
4. What environmental factors provide effective support to nurses who are working with dying clients?
5. What client behaviors and attitudes predict atypical grief?
6. What family coping patterns predict the course of bereavement?
7. What factors amenable to nursing intervention contribute to quality of life for dying persons and bereaved survivors?
8. What theoretical and clinical content should be included in nursing education programs to prepare nurses to work with the dying and the bereaved?
9. What factors in the domain of nursing care contribute to the expression of spiritual needs?

REFERENCES AND READINGS

Amenta, M., & Bohnet, N. (1986). *Nursing care of the terminally ill.* Boston: Little, Brown.

American Nurses' Association. (1987). *Standards and scope of hospice nursing practice.* Kansas City: Author.

Aminoff, M. J. (1988). Nervous system. In S. A. Schroeder, M. A. Krupp, & L. M. Tierney (Eds.), *Current medical diagnosis and treatment* (pp. 571–620). Norwalk, CT: Appleton & Lange.

Baker, J. M., & Sorenson, K. C. (1963). A patient's concern with death. *American Journal of Nursing, 63,* 90–92.

Hudak, C. M., Gallo, B. M., & Benz, J. J. (1990). *Critical care nursing: A holistic approach.* Philadelphia: J. B. Lippincott.

Kübler-Ross, E. (1969). *On death and dying.* New York: Macmillan.

Lindemann, E. (1944). Symptomatology and management of acute grief. *American Journal of Psychiatry, 101,* 141–149.

Lindstrom, B. (1984, November). *Issues of suicide in hospice care.* Audiotape of paper presented at Annual Meeting and Symposium of the National Hospice Organization, Hartford, CT.

Martocchio, B. C. (1982). *Living while dying.* Bowie, MD: Robert J. Brady.

McFarland, G. K., & McFarlane, E. A. (1989). *Nursing diagnosis & intervention.* St. Louis: C. V. Mosby.

National Hospice Nurses' Association (1988). *Quality assurance for hospice patient care.* Escondido, CA: Author.

National Hospice Organization. (1982). *Standards of a hospice program of care.* Arlington, VA: Author.

Osterweiss, M., Solomen, S., & Green, M. (Eds.). (1984). *Bereavement, reactions, consequences and care.* Washington, DC: National Academy Press.

Parkes, C. M., & Weiss, R. S. (1983). *Recovery from bereavement.* New York: Basic Books.

President's Commission for the Study of Ethical Problems in Medicine and Biomedical and Behavioral Research. (1981). *Defining death.* Washington, DC: U.S. Government Printing Office.

Quint, J. C. & Strauss, A. L. (1964). Nursing students, assignments, and dying patients. *Nursing Outlook, 12,* 24–27.

Raphael B. (1983). *The anatomy of bereavement.* New York: Basic Books.

Report of the Ad Hoc Committee of the Harvard Medical School to Examine the Definition of Brain Death. (1968). A definition of irreversible coma. *JAMA, 205,* 85–88.

Schraff, S. (1984). *Hospice: The nursing perspective.* New York: National League for Nursing.

Worden, W. (1982). *Grief counseling and grief therapy: A handbook for the mental health practitioner.* New York: Springer.

ADDITIONAL READINGS

Berman, H., Cragg, C. E., & Kuenzig, L. (1988). Having a parent die of cancer: Adolescents' reactions. *Oncology Nursing Forum, 15,* 159–167.

This is a descriptive study on the reactions of 10 adolescents to the death of a parent from cancer. The adolescents identified family friends, relatives, and peers as their greatest supports. These adolescents also reported that they did not receive much support from health care professionals and that they often felt isolated. The nurse authors discussed these and other results of this study as related to previous research on families and their dealings with death.

Constantino, R. E. (1988). Comparison of two group interventions for the bereaved. *Image, 20,* 83–87.

This study was undertaken to assess the effect of bereavement crisis intervention and group socialization in a sample of widows over age 50 years. Depression levels were measured in the women, who were split into three groups. The group involved in bereavement crisis intervention had an initial drop in depression scores and an increase in social activity, which later stabilized.

Moseley, J. R., Logan, S. J., Tolle, S. W., & Bentley, J. H. (1988). Developing a bereavement program in a university hospital setting. *Oncology Nursing Forum, 15,* 151–155.

This article discussed the development of a multidisciplinary program to assist survivors and staff in the bereavement process. Program activities were developed based on the unmet needs identified by survivors and nurses at the setting where the program was implemented. The nurse authors discussed the components of this program, which has gained impressive support from families, staff, administrators, and physicians.

Oerlemans-Bunn, M. (1988). On being gay, single, and bereaved. *American Journal of Nursing, 88,* 472–476.

The emotions and concerns of survivors of AIDS victims were discussed, as expressed by seven male survivors in a support group. The author pointed out that this group of individuals constitutes a new population of grievers who have few bereavement guidelines.

UNIT 2 RESOURCES

Nursing Resources

American Academy of Pain Management, 1320 Standiford, Suite 136, Modesto, CA 95350. Telephone 209-545-0754.
Certifies nurses with experience in pain management.

American Holistic Nurses' Association, 1100 Raleigh Building, 5 West Hargett Street, Raleigh, NC 27601. Telephone 919-821-0071 or 919-821-1435.
Promotes education of nurses and the public in the concepts and practice of health care of the whole person. Publishes the *Journal of Holistic Nursing* (annually) and *Beginnings* (monthly newsletter).

National Gerontological Nursing Association (NGNA), 1818 Newton Street NW, Washington, DC 20010. Telephone 202-667-NGNA.
Interested in the delivery of health care to the elderly. Publishes *New Horizons* (monthly newsletter).

National Hospice Nurses' Association, PO Box 27322, Escondido, CA 82027. Telephone 818-248-5006.

Other Resources

ACTION, 806 Connecticut Avenue NW, Washington, DC 20525. Telephone 202-254-7310.

Sponsors the following organizations: Foster Grandparents; Retired Senior Volunteer Program; Service Corps of Retired Executives and Active Corps of Executives (SCORE/ACE).

Administration on Aging, Department of Health and Human Services, 200 Independence Avenue SW, Washington, DC 20201. Telephone 202-245-0724.

American Association of Homes for the Aging, 1050 17th Street NW, Washington, DC 20036. Telephone 202-296-5960.

American Association of Retired Persons (AARP), 1909 K Street NW, Washington, DC 20005. Telephone 202-872-4700.

American Cancer Society, 1599 Clifton Road NE, Atlanta, GA 30329. Telephone 404-320-3333.

American Pain Society, PO Box 186, Skokie, IL 60076. Telephone 312-475-7300.

Association for Death Education and Counseling, 638 Prospect Avenue, Hartford, CT 06105. Telephone 203-232-4825.

Commission on Accreditation of Rehabilitation Facilities, 2500 North Pantano Road, Suite 226, Tucson, AZ 85715.
Publishes a list of approximately 70 accredited pain clinics in 25 states.

Concern for Dying, 250 West 57th Street, New York, NY 10107. Telephone 212-246-6962.

Gray Panthers, 3700 Chestnut Street, Philadelphia, PA 19104. Telephone 215-382-6644.

Fosters the concept of aging as growth throughout the life span. Works toward achieving social changes to benefit the elderly.

Hospice Association of America, 519 C Street NE, Washington, DC 20002. Telephone 202-547-5277.

House Select Committee on Aging, House Office Building, Washington, DC 20515.

Legal Research and Services for the Elderly, 1511 K Street NW, Washington, DC 20005. Telephone 202-638-4351.

National Chronic Pain Outreach Association, 4922 Hampden Lane, Bethesda, MD 20814. Telephone 301-652-4948.

National Council on the Aging, 600 Maryland Avenue SW, Washington, DC 20024. Telephone 202-479-1200.

National Hospice Organization, 1901 North Fort Myer Drive, Suite 901, Arlington, VA 22209. Telephone 703-243-5900.

Provides information on various state hospice organizations.

National Institute on Aging, Department of Health and Human Services, Public Health Service, National Institutes of Health, Building 31, Bethesda, MD 20892. Telephone 301-496-4000.

Oryx Press, 2214 North Central Avenue, Phoenix, AZ 85004. Telephone 800-457-ORYX.

Publishes *Directory of Pain Treatment Centers in the U.S. and Canada.*

Pain Resources, Ltd., 1940 South Greeley Street, Suite 122, Stillwater, MN 55082. Telephone 612-430-3892.

PART II

CLIENT PROBLEMS AFFECTING MULTIPLE BODY SYSTEMS

UNIT 3

Management of Clients with Fluid, Electrolyte, and Acid-Base Problems

CHAPTER 12

Concepts of Fluid and Electrolyte Balance

Nurses are constantly required to assess the integrity of clients' fluid and electrolyte status in both health and disease. For true homeostasis to be possible, maintaining fluid and electrolyte balances within normal limits is critical. The proper functioning of many body systems depends on normal fluid and electrolyte balance. For example, adequate cardiovascular function requires not only a healthy myocardium and an intact vascular system, but also a specific blood volume. Blood volume is well regulated, but this regulation can be disrupted by states of fluid volume excess or deficit. With either fluid volume excess or deficit, optimal function of the cardiovascular system is disturbed. In addition, many of the ions that bathe the myocardium and the smooth muscles of the vascular system influence how well myocardial muscles contract or relax and to what degree the blood vessels within the myocardium and other tissues constrict or dilate (Guyton, 1987). Such influences of ions directly and indirectly affect the health and function of almost all body tissues and organs (Chenevey, 1987).

Assessment of fluid and electrolyte status involves examining the function of every physiologic system of the body. To accomplish this large task, both psychomotor skills and cognitive understanding of the physiologic foundations of fluid and electrolyte balance are required. If nurses completely understand the physiology involved in maintaining this balance, the clinical manifestations of imbalances will be understandable, predictable, and more accurately assessed.

ANATOMY AND PHYSIOLOGY REVIEW

PHYSICAL AND BIOLOGIC INFLUENCES ON FLUID AND ELECTROLYTE BALANCE

Several important physical phenomena and active biologic processes govern the proper balance of body fluids and electrolytes. These processes work together to regulate homeostasis so that even if the external environment undergoes dramatic changes, the body's internal environment remains relatively unchanged.

Understanding the specific terminology related to solutions is necessary for comprehension of processes. Solutions are composed of a dissolving fluid which is called a *solvent* (the solvent for human body fluids is always water), and the particles that are dissolved or suspended in the solution, which are called *solutes* (Nave & Nave, 1985). The solutes vary in nature and composition from one body fluid compartment to another. The essential processes and phenomena involved in fluid and electrolyte balance include diffusion, filtration, osmosis, active transport, and capillary dynamics.

All of the above-mentioned actions influence movement of fluids and particles within fluids across biologic membranes.

FILTRATION

Filtration is the movement of fluid through a biologic membrane as a result of hydrostatic pressure differences on both sides of the membrane (Ganong, 1985). Because filtration depends on hydrostatic pressure, a clear understanding of the factors influencing hydrostatic pressure is necessary.

All fluid has weight — the result of the force of gravity. Fluid in a confined space exerts pressure — *hydrostatic pressure* — against the confining walls of the space because of the weight (mass) of the fluid against the walls. The weight of the fluid is also related to the amount of fluid present in the confined space. In addition, the physical properties of water molecules are such that the molecules seek to be a specific, organized distance apart from each other. When water molecules are in a confined space, they constantly press outward against the confining boundaries. Thus, hydrostatic pressure may be thought of as "water-pushing" pressure because this pressure is a major force in moving water out from a confined space. For example, the hydrostatic pressure of fluid in the stems of house plants is the primary factor that influences whether the plant stem is soft and droopy or firm and upright. When too little fluid (water) is present in the plant, the hydrostatic pressure exerted by the fluid is small. Thus, the stem is soft and cannot maintain the plant in the upright position. When water is added to the soil, the water is transferred via the roots to all parts of the plant including the stem, and the hydrostatic pressure exerted by the confined water molecules increases. As a result, the stem is firm and can support the plant in the upright position.

Within the human body, water is the largest component of body fluid. The amount of water in any fluid compartment is a main factor in determining the hydrostatic pressure of that fluid. The blood, a viscous fluid (one that is "thicker" than water), is confined within the blood vessels of the vascular system. Blood has hydrostatic pressure not only because of its weight and volume but also because of the pressure exerted by the heart muscle as it forcefully and dynamically ejects blood from the heart into the arterial vascular tree.

Whenever a permeable membrane separates two fluid compartments, it is possible to compare and contrast the two compartments in terms of such factors as pressures (hydrostatic and osmotic), concentrations of various solute particles, and overall electrical charges. If a factor (such as hydrostatic pressure) is the same in both fluid compartments, a state of *equilibrium* is said to exist for that factor. In biologic systems, the state of equilibrium characterizes homeostasis.

If the hydrostatic pressure, for example, is not the same in both compartments, a state of *disequilibrium* is said to exist. By definition, this disequilibrium means that the compartments have a graded difference, or a *gradient* of hydrostatic pressure. One compartment has a higher hydrostatic pressure than does the other compartment. Because the human body is a dynamic biologic system and constantly seeks equilibrium, whenever a gradient exists across a membrane, net forces act to rearrange the distribution of substances on both sides of the membrane until an equilibrium is reached. In most instances, substances are moved or rearranged in the direction from the greatest amount to the least. Thus, when a hydrostatic pressure gradient exists between two fluid compartments, fluid from the compartment with the higher pressure moves through the membrane into the fluid compartment with the lower pressure.

This net filtration force is present only as long as the hydrostatic pressure gradient exists. When enough fluid has moved into the second compartment so that the hydrostatic pressure in the second compartment equals the hydrostatic pressure in the first compartment, an equilibrium is present, a hydrostatic pressure gradient no longer exists between the two compartments, and no net filtration of fluid will occur (see the accompanying illustration).

Net movement of any substance from one side of a membrane to the other by either filtration or diffusion indicates that one side is actually losing some of the substance and the other side is actually gaining some of the substance. When an equilibrium is reached, both sides have an equal amount of this substance. Movement still occurs after an equilibrium is reached. However, the movement of the substance is now *dynamically equal*, a one-for-one exchange, so that neither side experiences a net loss or a net gain and the state of equilibrium is maintained.

Blood pressure is a hydrostatic filtering force that is measured in millimeters of mercury (mmHg). Filtration is an important factor for exchange of water, nutrients, and waste products when blood arrives at the tissue capillaries. One factor that determines if fluid can leave the vascular tree and enter the tissue spaces is the difference between hydrostatic pressure within the capillaries and that in the interstitial tissue spaces.

The endothelial lining of capillaries is only one cell layer thick, which makes the wall that holds the blood in the capillaries quite thin. In addition, large spaces or pores exist between the endothelial cells in the capillary membrane. Water can filter freely through this membrane in either direction if a hydrostatic pressure gradient is present. The arterial end of tissue capillaries usually has a blood pressure of about 32 mmHg. Because interstitial hydrostatic pressure in a tissue is only a small positive force (or may even be a negative or vacuum-like force), there is a steep downhill gradient for filtration at the arterial end of tissue capillaries. If hydrostatic pressure differences were the only pressure forces at work in the entire cardiovascular system, all of the fluid portion of the blood would be forced out (filtered) through the walls of the capillaries into the tissue spaces (Guyton, 1987). This situation exists and is critically important for function in only some special organ areas.

A clinical example of filtration that is due primarily to

THE PROCESS OF FILTRATION

The inside has more water and greater hydrostatic pressure—the pressure exerted by fluid in a confined space—than does the outside.

Water molecules move down the hydrostatic pressure gradient from inside (with a higher or greater hydrostatic pressure) through the permeable membrane to the outside (which has a lower hydrostatic pressure).

Enough water has moved from inside to outside that both sides now have the same amount of water and the same hydrostatic pressure. An equilibrium of hydrostatic pressure now exists between the two compartments, and no further *net* movement of water will occur.

hydrostatic pressure differences is the formation of urine and subsequent diuresis. In the glomerulus of the kidney, the afferent arteriole carries whole blood to the glomerular capillaries (see Chap. 57). Some diuretics dilate the afferent arteriole and constrict the efferent arteriole so that the blood flow to the glomerulus is increased and the hydrostatic pressure within the glomerular capillaries is high. The normal hydrostatic pressure in the Bowman capsule is low, and thus an extreme pressure gradient exists. Fluid from the blood moves down the pressure gradient from the glomerular capillaries into the Bowman capsule, and urinary output is ultimately increased.

A clinical situation that can develop as a result of alterations in normal hydrostatic pressure gradients is the edema that is observed in patients with right-sided congestive heart failure. Because the heart cannot pump blood into the arterial vascular system adequately, the volume of blood (and consequently the hydrostatic pressure) in the right side of the heart increases greatly. As this volume continues to accumulate in the venous system, the venous hydrostatic pressure rises. The increased venous pressure eventually causes capillary hydrostatic pressures to increase to the point that they are higher than the pressures in the interstitial spaces. Net filtration of fluid from the capillaries into the interstitial tissue spaces then occurs and results in the formation of visible edema. Fortunately, in most tissues and organs, pressures in addition to hydrostatic pressure influence the filtration of fluid from the capillaries.

The other pressure that most profoundly counterbalances hydrostatic pressure in determining whether net filtration occurs at any given point is *osmotic pressure*. A general definition of osmotic pressure is the force exerted by solute particles within a solution that tend to pull water molecules across a membrane *into* a confined space, a "water-pulling" pressure. The factors contributing to the development and maintenance of osmotic pressures are discussed later in this chapter.

DIFFUSION

Diffusion is the most important physical phenomenon that governs the movement of substances across various body membranes. In general, movement by diffusion is much more rapid than movement by other forces such as filtration. Diffusion of electrolytes into and out of cells and fluid compartments occurs via the kinetic energy of molecular motion known as *brownian motion*. Brownian motion is the oscillation or vibration of individual atoms and molecules as a result of their internuclear forces. This motion stops only when temperatures reach absolute zero. Brownian motion does not require the expenditure of energy and does cause totally random movement. This motion tends to cause atoms and molecules in a confined space (whether that space is liquid or gaseous) to disperse at relatively equal distances from each other within that space.

In addition, this random movement causes molecules to move and collide with each other within the confined space. The collisions usually cause a temporary increase in the speed of the movement. Whenever possible, atoms and molecules tend to spread out evenly through whatever space is available. They will thus move from an area of higher concentration (of atoms and molecules) to an area of lower concentration until a relative equality of concentrations is achieved in both areas.

A concentration gradient exists when two areas have different concentrations of molecules. The random motion causes the molecules to move down the concentration gradient from the area of the higher concentration to the area of the lower concentration of the same molecules. Any membrane that separates two areas will be struck repeatedly by atoms and molecules as a result of the brownian motion. When the molecule strikes a pore in the membrane that is large enough for the molecule to pass through, diffusion occurs. The likelihood of any solute molecule's colliding with the membrane and going through a pore is much greater on the side of the membrane that has a higher concentration of solute.

The speed of diffusion is directly related to the degree of concentration difference between the two sides of the membrane. The degree of concentration difference is usually refered to as the *steepness* of the gradient. The larger the concentration difference between the two sides, the steeper the gradient. Diffusion occurs more rapidly when the concentration gradient is steeper — as when a ball rolls downhill: the steeper the hill, the faster the ball rolls. The greater the difference in concentration, the more rapidly diffusion occurs from the area of higher concentration to the area of lower concentration. Diffusion of solute particles continues through the membrane as long as there is a concentration gradient between the two sides of the membrane. When the concentration of solute is the same on both sides of the membrane, an equilibrium exists and equal diffusion of solute continues.

Diffusion is important in the transport of gases and in the movement of most ions, atoms, and molecules through biologic membranes. Unlike capillary membranes, which permit diffusion of all substances down a concentration gradient, most cell membranes are selective. Some ions and molecules cannot move across a cell membrane, even when a very steep downhill gradient exists, because the membrane is *impermeable* to that ion or molecule. Thus, the concentration gradient is maintained across the membrane. This impermeability, along with special transport mechanisms, accounts for differences in concentrations of specific ions from one fluid compartment to another. For instance, the extracellular fluid (ECF) contains almost 10 times more sodium ions than does the intracellular fluid (ICF). The relative impermeability of the cell membrane to sodium, coupled with a system of active transport that moves any extra sodium out of the cell uphill against its concentration gradient and back into the ECF, accounts for this extreme concentration difference.

A clinical example illustrating that diffusion cannot always occur without assistance, even down steep concentration gradients, because of membrane selectivity is type I diabetes mellitus. In this disease, there is an absence or a profound decrease in the hormone insulin. Insulin normally binds to cell membranes and acts to facilitate the diffusion of glucose from the ECF across the cell membrane into the ICF. If there is no insulin, glucose cannot cross the membranes of most cells and the concentration of glucose in the ECF increases to the point of hyperglycemia. Even though the concentration gradient is quite steep, with a large concentration of glucose in the ECF and a low concentration or no glucose present in the ICF, glucose will not diffuse into some cell types except in the presence of insulin.

When diffusion across a cell membrane requires a transport system or carrier (such as insulin, which is a carrier for glucose), the process is called *facilitated diffusion* or transport. Because this type of transport occurs down a concentration gradient and requires no energy expenditure by the cell, it is still considered to be a form of diffusion, a purely physical phenomenon.

OSMOSIS

Osmosis is the process by which the solvent, e.g., water molecules (rather than the solute molecules) diffuses through a selectively permeable membrane (Groer, 1981). For osmosis to occur, a membrane must separate two solutions. At least one of these solutions must contain a solute that cannot move through the membrane (the membrane is therefore impermeable to this solute). A concentration gradient of this solute must also exist. If the membrane were permeable to this solute, the solute would diffuse through the membrane down its concentration gradient until the concentrations of solute were equal on both sides of the membrane. However, the membrane is impermeable to the solute, so the solute cannot cross the membrane. For the solutions to have equal concentrations of solute, the water molecules must diffuse down their concentration gradient from the side with the higher concentration of water molecules (and thus a lower concentration of solute molecules) to the side with the lower concentration of water molecules (and thus a higher concentration of solute molecules) (see the illustration on p. 233). In the less concentrated solution, there are proportionately fewer solute molecules and more water molecules than in the concentrated solution. Water therefore moves by osmosis down its concentration gradient from the area of more dilute solute to the area of more concentrated solute until a new equilibrium is achieved. At this point, the concentrations of the solute in the solutions on both sides of the membrane are the same, even though the total numbers of solute and water molecules may be different. This equilibrium is achieved by movement of water molecules rather than movement of solute molecules.

The factors that determine whether osmosis occurs and how rapidly it occurs include the overall concentration of osmotically active particles (solute) in solution,

solubility of the solute, temperature of the solution, and the amount of membrane available for osmosis. The following paragraphs provide in-depth discussions of each factor.

Concentration of solute. The concentration of osmotically active particles in solution is the primary determinant of osmosis and *osmotic pressure*. Solute concentration is directly related to osmotic pressure: the greater the solute concentration within a solution, the higher the osmotic pressure (water-pulling pressure) of that solution.

Solute concentration is determined by measuring the exact amount of all substances present in fluid or a solution. In laboratory settings, this concentration is expressed as *moles*—the molecular weight of a specific substance in grams per liter. However, because human body fluids contain relatively little solute in relation to the amount of water, expression of solute concentration in terms of moles is not useful. The concentration of solutes in human body fluids is instead expressed as *milliequivalents per liter* (mEq/L) and *milliosmoles per liter* (mOsm/L).

Milliequivalents are used to express the exact concentration of individual charged particles (ions or electrolytes) in a liter of solution. Each milliequivalent is equal to $\frac{1}{1000}$th of the gram molecular weight of the substance divided by its valence (overall number of charges) (Ganong, 1985). For example, the molecular weight of sodium (Na^+) is 23 daltons and it has a valence of one, which means that sodium has an equivalency of 23 g/L or a milliequivalency of 0.0023 g/L. The molecular weight of calcium (Ca^{2+}) is 40 and it has a valence of two, which means that calcium has the electrical equivalency of 20 g/L and the milliequivalency of 0.0020 g/L (Ganong, 1985). The concentration of an individual electrolyte in serum or plasma is most often expressed in milliequivalents per liter.

Osmole and *milliosmole* are used to express the overall or total concentration of solute particles (including electrolytes) contained within a solution. The number of osmoles in a solution is calculated by dividing the total molecular weight of the substances present in the solution by the number of freely moving particles (Ganong, 1985). The number of osmoles (actually milliosmoles because the solute concentrations in normal body fluids tend to be small) present in body fluids can be expressed as either *osmolarity* or *osmolality*. Osmolarity is defined as the number of milliosmoles present in a liter of solution; osmolality is defined as the number of milliosmoles present in a kilogram of solution (Bishop et al., 1985; Ganong, 1985; Hinchliff & Montague, 1988).

The more correct term is osmolality, although in discussions of solute concentrations in human body fluids the two terms are used interchangeably because (1) the total solute concentration is relatively small; (2) the physiologic solvent is water; and (3) 1 L of water weighs nearly 1 kg. In addition, most laboratories measure solute concentration in terms of numbers per liter rather than per kilogram. The normal osmolarity value for plasma and other body fluids ranges between 270 and 300 mOsm/L (Guyton, 1986), and the normal osmolality value (corrected) for plasma and other body fluids ranges between 275 and 295 mOsm/kg (Bishop et al., 1985).

Because the body functions most efficiently when the osmolarity of the fluids in all compartments is about 300 mOsm/L, many mechanisms function to maintain solute concentration homeostasis at this level. When all body fluids have this solute concentration, the osmotic pressures (water pulling) of the various fluid compartments are essentially the same, and no *net* water movement occurs. In such a situation, body fluids are said to be *isosmotic* to each other, or *isotonic* (sometimes called normotonic). Examples of solutions with solute concentrations equal to 270 to 300 mOsm/L include 0.9% sodium chloride in water, 5% dextrose in water, and the complex formula of Ringer's lactate in water (Trissel, 1988). Because these substances are isotonic or isosmotic to plasma, their addition to plasma does not change plasma osmolarity or plasma osmotic pressure (see Chap. 13).

In contrast to isosmotic fluids, fluids that have osmolarity values (solute concentrations) higher than 300 mOsm/L are said to be *hyperosmotic* or *hypertonic*. Hyperosmotic fluids have a greater osmotic pressure than isosmotic fluids and tend to pull water from the isosmotic fluid compartment into the hyperosmotic fluid compartment until an osmotic balance is achieved. Fluids that have osmolarity values (solute concentrations) less than 270 mOsm/L are said to be *hyposmotic* or *hypotonic*. Hyposmotic fluids have a lower osmotic pressure than isosmotic fluids. As a result, water tends to be pulled from the hyposmotic fluid compartment into the isosmotic fluid compartment until an osmotic balance is achieved (Gennari, 1984; Metheny & Snively, 1983; Urrows, 1980).

Solubility of solute. *Solubility* of solute refers to the degree to which a solute dissolves or dissociates completely in water. Solubility is directly related to osmotic pressure. The greater the solubility of the solutes in a fluid, the higher the osmotic pressure of that fluid (Groer, 1981; Guyton, 1987).

The more completely a solute compound or particle dissociates, the more osmotically active individual particles are in the solution. If a *mole* (molecular weight in grams) of a particular solute is completely dissolved in solution but the single molecules do not separate into ions or atoms, it exerts certain measurable osmotic pressure. Such is the case for glucose, which dissolves in water but does not dissociate. A mole of a different solute that both dissolves completely and dissociates into two or more ions exerts greater osmotic pressure because more osmotically active particles are present. If a milliosmole of a substance is present and does not dissociate into ions, the osmolarity is the same as the molarity. However, if a substance does dissociate into ions when dissolved in a solution (e.g., sodium chloride), a millimole is equivalent to 2 mOsm (because sodium chloride dissociates into two separate ions, sodium ions and chloride ions).

Temperature. The factor of temperature of the solution is directly related to osmosis. The kinetic motion of molecules increases as temperature increases. Thus, the number of collisions increases. This greater motion and speed increase the chances that water molecules will move through the semipermeable membrane. Because human body temperature has a rather narrow range of normal, temperature changes influence osmosis in living systems only minimally (Guyton, 1987; Nave & Nave, 1985).

Amount of available membrane. The greater the amount of membrane available through which osmosis can occur, the faster the rate of osmosis. This phenomenon is the result of increasing the chances that random motion allows water molecules to strike the membrane at a point where penetration is possible (Guyton, 1987; Nave & Nave, 1985).

Clinical Implications of Osmology in ECF and ICF

Osmolarity of the ECF is almost entirely due to sodium because this ion is the major ECF cation and cells are relatively impermeable to sodium. However, osmolarity of the ICF is nearly the same as the osmolarity of the ECF because the overall concentration and dissociation of intracellular solutes are equal to those of the ECF, even though the specific solute particles are different in the two fluid compartments. The major determinant of ICF osmotic pressure is the high protein content of the ICF (Ganong, 1985; Guyton, 1987).

In healthy individuals, minimal net osmosis occurs across cell membranes. The reason for this stability is that the ECF and ICF are isotonic to each other. Any osmotic pressure changes between the ICF and the ECF results in osmosis (water movement) into the area with the higher osmotic pressure. If cells develop an increased osmotic pressure (as a result of a higher concentration of intracellular solutes), the fluid in the cell is hypertonic compared with the ECF. Water then moves from the ECF into the cell to dilute the solute concentration. Therefore, osmotic pressure is a water-drawing or water-pulling pressure. Compartments with a high osmotic pressure draw or pull water across the membrane from a compartment that has a lower osmotic pressure.

Osmotic pressure is directly related to solute concentration and inversely related to water concentration. Solutions with a high osmotic pressure have a higher solute concentration and a lower water concentration than solutions with a low osmotic pressure. This situation favors the movement of water both down its concentration gradient and toward the higher osmotic pressure. Intravenous fluids that are given to hospitalized clients as part of therapy are frequently isotonic to body fluids so that no cellular volume changes occur. However, in

THE PROCESS OF OSMOSIS

Side 2 has more solute molecules than does side 1 even though the number of water molecules is the same on both sides. Thus side 2 has a greater osmotic (water-pulling) pressure than does side 1.

DISEQUILIBRIUM

Side 1
3.5:1 ratio of water to solute

Side 2
1.4:1 ratio of water to solute

Movement of water occurs by osmosis toward side 2 because it has greater osmotic (water-pulling) pressure. The membrane is not permeable to the solute molecules, so the actual number of solute molecules in side 1 and side 2 does not change.

Only water molecules move because the membrane is not permeable to the solute molecules.

Enough water has moved from side 1 to side 2 that the actual concentration of solutes is now the same on both sides, with a ratio of water to solute of 2:1. An equilibrium of osmotic pressure now exists between the two compartments, and no further net movement of water molecules (or solute molecules) will occur.

EQUILIBRIUM

Side 1
2:1 ratio of water to solute

Side 2
2:1 ratio of water to solute

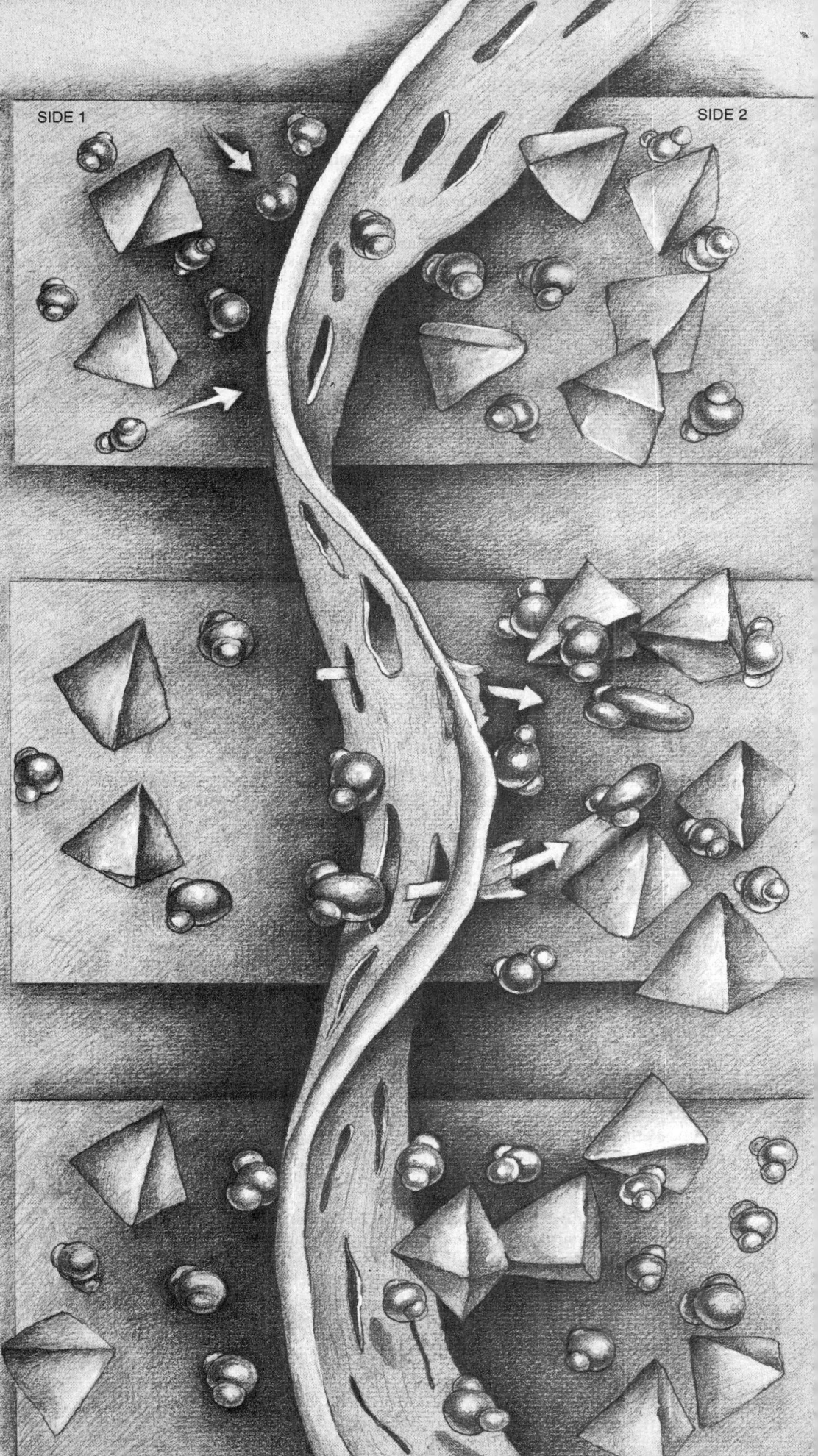

SIDE 1

SIDE 2

some situations either hypertonic or hypotonic fluids are administered intravenously, and a water shift between compartments can be expected.

The process of osmosis is an important regulator of cell volume and participates with the process of filtration in capillary fluid dynamics to regulate ECF and ICF volumes. A clinical example that illustrates the importance of osmosis in the maintenance of homeostasis is the thirst mechanism. Thirst is the result of activation of supraoptic and paraventricular nuclei in the hypothalamus of the brain that respond to changes in ECF volume and osmolarity. These cells are so sensitive to changes in ECF osmolarity that they are called *osmoreceptors*. When a person experiences a loss of body fluids, such as that seen with excessive sweating during prolonged heavy exercise, the ECF volume is somewhat decreased and the osmolarity is increased (hypertonic or hyperosmotic conditions exist). The cells in the thirst center shrink as water moves from the cells into the hypertonic ECF. Shrinking of these cells stimulates the awareness of the sensation of thirst and its resultant behavioral responses. The affected individual usually drinks enough fluid (or perhaps a little extra) to replace what was lost through sweating and restore the ECF osmolarity to its normal value. After the ECF volume and osmolarity return to normal, the osmoreceptors are also normal and no longer send stimulatory messages.

ACTIVE TRANSPORT

When a substance is moved across a cell membrane against a concentration gradient, or uphill, the cell must work and expend energy to accomplish this task. Such movement is called *active transport* because the cell must make active efforts for the net movement to occur. In most situations, the cellular energy used for this process is derived from breaking a high-energy bond in the form of a high-energy phosphate ($\sim$P). A phosphate group is split off from an adenosine triphosphate (ATP) molecule. The releasing of the energy from ATP is accomplished by the enzyme ATPase. Active transport mechanisms are complex and appear to involve carriers within the cell membrane, ATP, ATPase, and other molecules such as certain phospholipids that provide an optimal membrane environment for active transport.

Because of its energy demands, active transport is sometimes called *pumping*, and the mechanisms are known as *membrane pumps*. Some active transport pumps can carry more than one substance across the membrane at one time. In these instances, the pump usually moves one substance into a cell and a different substance out of the cell at the same time. Both transports are uphill against individual concentration gradients and require energy. The sodium-potassium pump is an example of such a linked active transport system. Because sodium has such a high ECF concentration compared with its ICF concentration, it tends to diffuse slightly down its concentration gradient into the ICF.

Similarly, because potassium has such a high ICF concentration compared with its ECF concentration, it tends to diffuse slightly down its concentration gradient into the ECF. The action of the sodium-potassium pump moves the extra sodium out of the cell while returning the lost potassium to the cell.

Optimal function of active transport pumps depends on having adequate amounts of ATP generated through the cellular metabolic processes of glycolysis, the Krebs cycle, and oxidative phosphorylation. ATP is generated most efficiently in the presence of oxygen. If either oxygen or fuel for the specific ATP-generating pathways decreases, ATP production also decreases. Inadequate amounts of ATP cause a reduction of the efficiency of the active membrane pump.

A clinical example illustrating failure of active transport is the sequelae to hypoxia. Without adequate oxygen present, ATP is no longer generated in sufficient amounts by the cell's metabolic machinery. Without ATP, the sodium-potassium pump cannot remove the sodium ions that have diffused into the ICF. The increased concentration of sodium within the ICF increases the osmolarity of the ICF, and the osmotic pressure is raised. Water moves into the cell in response to the increased osmotic pressure, which causes the cell to swell. The swelling further interrupts function and causes cells to become ischemic and perhaps to lyse and die if oxygen is not provided. Cell swelling is one of the earliest signs of cellular hypoxia.

The process of active transport is an essential mechanism by which cells can control the intracellular concentration of many substances and can regulate cell volume. Active transport does require cellular energy expenditure. Other processes that require cellular work and energy expenditure include types of endocytosis (phagocytosis and pinocytosis) and exocytosis (see Chap. 24).

CAPILLARY DYNAMICS

Because most cells are located in areas of the body that are remote from the actual entrance sites for nutrients and the exit sites for metabolic waste products, the circulatory system is the dynamic mechanism for distribution of nutrients and removal of wastes at the tissue level. The most functionally important blood vessels for this purpose are the thin-walled, porous *capillaries*. Nutrient distribution and waste removal depend on capillary fluid movement. An understanding of the processes of filtration, diffusion, and osmosis is essential before the dynamics of capillary fluid movement can be appreciated. Active transport does not play a role in movement of either solute or water at the capillary level, and the diffusion that occurs is somewhat independent of both filtration and osmosis.

Fluid movement at the capillary level is dynamic not only because it is continuous but also because relative homeostasis of vascular and interstitial fluid volumes must be maintained. Opposing processes must occur to accomplish the tasks of nutrient distribution, waste removal, and maintenance of vascular and interstitial fluid volumes. In these processes, some fluid with nutrients must leave the capillary and enter the interstitial fluid compartment for a short period, which temporarily expands the interstitial fluid volume. The nutrients now in the interstitial fluid are taken up by the cells through various membrane level transport processes. Water may be exchanged between the intracellular compartment and the interstitial compartment, but under normal circumstances no net change in water volume should occur. Metabolic wastes created in the cells are moved into the interstitial fluid. Now, the extra fluid in the interstitial space together with the excreted metabolic waste products must be returned via the capillary to systemic circulation. Without provision for return of the fluid originally lost to the interstitial compartment, the vascular volume would become progressively depleted to the point of circulatory failure, and the interstitial fluid compartment would become greatly expanded.

More than a century ago, Ernest Starling examined and defined the forces at the capillary level that permit capillary fluid loss followed by return of fluid to the capillary so that a near-equilibrium of fluid distribution is maintained at the capillary-tissue level. These forces are now called *Starling's forces* and are outlined in Figure 12–1. The basis for the near-equilibrium is that the forces that tend to move fluid out from the capillary at the arterial end are nearly equal to the forces that tend to move fluid from the interstitial compartment back into the capillary at the venous end (Guyton, 1987).

Blood flowing from one end of the capillary (usually the arterial end) to the other end (venous) is controlled by the following factors: pressure of blood, the dynamic ejection of blood from the left ventricle of the heart, patency of blood vessels, and the state of constriction of precapillary sphincters. The blood entering the arterial end of the capillary has a blood pressure, or *plasma hydrostatic pressure* (PHP), of about 32 mmHg. The capillary membrane, as described earlier, is thin and permeable. The usual tissue hydrostatic pressure is low. These factors create a natural tendency for filtration to occur from the blood outward into the tissue spaces: The fluid portion of the blood, along with most of the smaller substances dissolved in the blood, filters through the capillary membrane into the tissue spaces. By this process, nutrients and essential blood-borne substances can reach the cells.

If net filtration, as a result of plasma hydrostatic pressure, were the only force or factor involved at this level, blood volume would be progressively lost from the vascular space and would reappear in the tissues. Fortunately, other mechanisms that favor the reabsorption of tissue fluid into the capillaries are also part of capillary dynamics. Osmosis (of water) through the capillary membrane (in either direction) occurs in response to differences in the concentrations of osmotically active substances in the capillary blood and tissue fluid. It should be remembered that osmotic pressure draws or pulls water toward the area with higher osmotic pressure, or osmolarity. Few osmotically active particles are normally trapped in tissue fluid. The capillary membrane does not allow blood proteins to pass freely through it and filter into the tissue space (the capillary membrane is highly impermeable to proteins). The major blood protein is albumin, which tends to remain in the capillary blood and thus exerts significant osmotic pressure. The specific type of osmotic pressure that is exerted by plasma proteins is called *colloidal osmotic pressure* because it is due to the presence of proteins (colloidal substances) rather than dissociated ions such as sodium (crystalloid substances). The average colloidal osmotic pressure in capillary blood is about 22 mmHg.

Blood pressure (hydrostatic pressure) is greater than colloidal osmotic pressure at the arterial end of the capillary. Capillary hydrostatic pressure favors filtration into the tissue spaces and colloidal osmotic pressure favors reabsorption into the capillary, and thus the difference between these two capillary pressures at the arterial end of the capillary indicates that there is a greater filtering force outward than a reabsorbing force inward.

Two additional forces are also present and influence the movement of solutions at the capillary level. These forces are *tissue hydrostatic pressure* (THP) and *tissue osmotic pressure* (TOP). Under normal circumstances, both are relatively small forces. However, in specific pathophysiologic states, these forces can increase greatly and can significantly alter capillary dynamics.

To determine the direction of fluid movement in any one area of the capillary, it is necessary to compare the forces that tend to move fluid out of the capillary with forces that tend to move fluid into the capillary. As shown in Figure 12–1, the two forces at the arterial end that tend to move fluid out of the capillary are the plasma hydrostatic pressure (32 mmHg) and the tissue osmotic pressure (4 mmHg). These two pressures total 36 mmHg. The pressures at the arterial end that tend to return fluid to the capillary are the plasma colloidal oncotic pressure (22 mmHg) and the tissue hydrostatic pressure (4 mmHg)—a total of 26 mmHg. Because the outward filtration force is 10 mmHg higher than the inward reabsorbing force, the overall result at the arterial end of the capillary is the outward filtration of fluid and small solute particles into the tissue spaces.

Only one pressure changes along the length of the capillary as blood flows through it—the plasma hydrostatic pressure. As filtration proceeds along the capillary, water is lost from the capillary (and as the distance from the left ventricle increases), and the plasma hydrostatic pressure gradually decreases. Therefore, the pressures that create the outward filtration force become smaller while the pressures that create the inward reabsorption force remain the same. A point is eventually reached when the outward filtration pressures and the inward reabsorption pressures are the same. Finally, at the venous end of the capillary, the inward reabsorption forces exceed the outward filtration forces. The result of

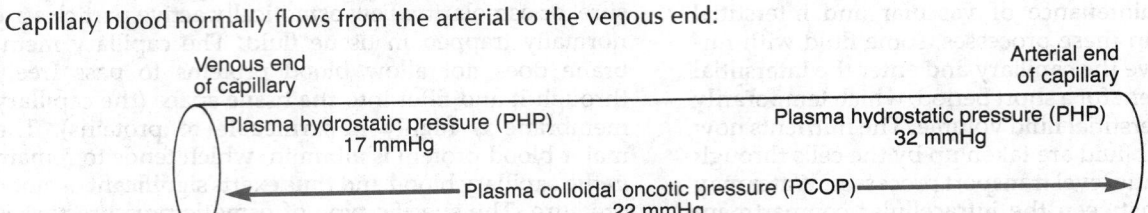

Capillary blood normally flows from the arterial to the venous end:

Venous end of capillary

Arterial end of capillary

Plasma hydrostatic pressure (PHP) 17 mmHg

Plasma hydrostatic pressure (PHP) 32 mmHg

Plasma colloidal oncotic pressure (PCOP) 22 mmHg

Tissue hydrostatic pressure (THP) 6 mmHg
Tissue osmotic pressure (TOP) 4 mmHg

Tissue hydrostatic pressure (THP) 4 mmHg
Tissue osmotic pressure (TOP) 4 mmHg

At the arterial end, the forces that tend to move fluid from the capillary into the tissue space are

Plasma hydrostatic pressure 32 mmHg
+
Tissue osmotic pressure 4 mmHg
Total forces moving fluid out = 36 mmHg

At the arterial end, the forces that tend to move fluid from the tissue spaces into the capillary are

Tissue hydrostatic pressure 4 mmHg
+
Plasma colloidal oncotic pressure 22 mmHg
Total forces moving fluid in = 26 mmHg

The total forces tending to move fluid out at the arterial end are 10 mmHg higher than the total forces tending to move fluid in at the arterial end (36 − 26 = 10). Thus, at the arterial end, fluid leaks out of the capillary into the tissue (interstitial) spaces.

At the venous end of the same capillary, the forces that tend to move fluid from the capillary into the tissue space are

Plasma hydrostatic pressure 17 mmHg
+
Tissue osmotic pressure 4 mmHg
Total forces moving fluid out = 21 mmHg

At the venous end of the capillary, the forces that tend to move fluid from the tissue spaces back into the capillary are

Tissue hydrostatic pressure 6 mmHg
+
Plasma colloidal oncotic pressure 22 mmHg
Total forces moving fluid in = 28 mmHg

The total forces tending to move fluid out at the venous end are 7 mmHg lower than the total forces tending to move fluid into the capillary at the venous end (28 − 21 = 7). Thus, at the venous end, fluid moves from the tissue spaces back into the capillary.

Because the pressures tending to move fluid out of the capillary at the arterial end (10 mmHg) are greater than the pressures that tend to move fluid back into the capillary at the venous end (7 mmHg), more fluid is lost from the capillary than is returned to it. Lymph drainage eventually returns this extra lost fluid.

Figure 12–1
Capillary dynamics.

these pressure differences is that tissue fluid (including the plasma fluid that entered the tissue space) returns to the capillary blood.

The example cited in Figure 12–1 shows the venous capillary plasma hydrostatic pressure to be only 17 mmHg, so the total outward filtration force is only 21 mmHg (17 + 4) and the total inward reabsorption force is 28 mmHg (22 + 6). Thus, at the venous end, the net force is an inward reabsorption force of 7 mmHg (28 − 21). Note that this reabsorption force is smaller than the net outward filtration force of 10 mmHg at the arterial end of the capillary. Because of this difference in net

force between the two ends of the capillary, less fluid is returned through reabsorption at the venous end than was filtered out at the arterial end. Thus, some fluid is lost from the capillary at the arterial end that does not get returned to systemic circulation at the venous end of the capillary. This fluid temporarily remains in the tissue (interstitial) space.

If more fluid were continuously lost from the arterial end of the capillary than is returned at the venous end of the capillary, a serious imbalance of fluid between the vascular space and the interstitial space would result. The vascular volume would be reduced while the interstitial volume would increase, and fluid volume homeo-stasis would be disrupted. However, another physiologic mechanism functions to return this lost fluid. The fluid that is not reabsorbed at the venous end of the capillary is normally returned to the circulatory system through the *lymphatic drainage system*. This drainage system functions well enough under normal conditions to prevent excessive interstitial fluid build-up and the formation of visible edema.

Within the tissue spaces, the filtered plasma fluid (without protein) circulates, distributing nutrients to the cells of the tissues. For capillary dynamics to function optimally, allowing for nutrient exchange at the tissue level while maintaining proper volume within the vascular system, hydrostatic pressure and osmotic pressure values must remain normal. Whenever these values are beyond the normal range, net filtration, net reabsorption, or both are altered. For example, the colloidal osmotic pressure is influenced by the number of osmotically active particles present. If the concentration of serum albumin decreases, less plasma colloidal osmotic pressure is exerted, and, therefore, less reabsorptive forces are present, which results in a greater net loss of fluid into the tissue spaces. This loss overwhelms the capacity of the lymphatic drainage system to return the extra fluid to systemic circulation, and visible edema occurs.

HORMONAL INFLUENCES ON FLUID AND ELECTROLYTE BALANCE

Many endocrine mechanisms exist that assist in the regulation of fluid and electrolyte balance. Two hormones that play important roles in these critical balances are *aldosterone* and *antidiuretic hormone* (ADH). An additional hormone-like substance that appears to influence fluid and electrolyte balance is *natriuretic factor*.

ALDOSTERONE

Aldosterone is a mineralocorticoid that is secreted by the adrenal cortex. This hormone directly regulates sodium balance. Because sodium in solution exerts osmotic pressure (water-pulling pressure), water attempts to follow sodium, in physiologic proportionate amounts (Guyton, 1987). As a result of this sodium-water relationship, aldosterone secretion also indirectly regulates water balance. The primary target tissue for this hormone is renal tubular epithelium. Aldosterone secretion is stimulated by a series of events that occur in response either to decreased levels of sodium in the ECF or to an increased load of sodium in renal tubular fluid.

Blood is supplied to the glomerulus of nephrons via afferent arterioles. Specialized cells, known as *juxtaglomerular cells*, inside the afferent arteriole near the glomerulus are sensitive to changes in serum concentrations of sodium. This area of the afferent arteriole comes into direct contact with a specialized area of the distal convoluted tubule known as the *macula densa*. Together, the juxtaglomerular cells and the macula densa form a functional group called the *juxtaglomerular complex*. When this complex senses that actual serum sodium concentrations are lower than normal or that the total blood volume is reduced, the macula densa appears to stimulate special juxtaglomerular cells to secrete the enzyme *renin*.

Renin can catalyze intrarenal and/or systemic reactions, depending on the body's needs. Renin acts enzymatically on the inactive plasma protein *angiotensinogen* (also known as renin substrate) and converts it to a smaller substance termed *angiotensin I*. Angiotensin I does cause some vasoconstriction, but these effects are minimal because this substance is almost immediately further degraded by *angiotensin-converting enzyme*, which seems to be produced in the lung and secreted into the blood. Converting enzyme catalyzes the reaction in which angiotensin I is changed into *angiotensin II*.

Angiotensin II causes massive vasoconstriction of many blood vessels and increases selective blood flow to the kidney. In addition, it causes selective constriction of either the afferent arteriole or the efferent arteriole of the nephron, depending on the overall state of hydration. If serum sodium concentration is low and blood volume is above normal, the efferent arteriole is constricted. Efferent arteriolar constriction causes the effective filtration pressure in the glomerulus to be raised, which increases glomerular filtration and urinary output. If serum sodium levels are low and blood volume is normal or low, angiotensin II causes constriction of the afferent arteriole. Blood flow to the glomerulus is thus diminished, and effective filtration pressure is low, which decreases glomerular filtration and urinary output (Guyton, 1987). This action preserves vascular volume while restoring the sodium concentration. At the same time, angiotensin II stimulates the release of aldosterone from the adrenal cortex. The role of these substances in regulation of fluid volume is summarized in Figure 12–2.

Aldosterone exerts its effects primarily on the distal convoluted tubule of the nephrons. The major effect is the reabsorption of filtered sodium in exchange for excretion of filtered potassium (and sometimes hydrogen ions). This effect appears to be mediated via indirect activation of special sodium-potassium pumps in the tubular epithelial membranes. Osmotic water reabsorption passively occurs at the same time in response to sodium reabsorption. This response constitutes a physiologic coping mechanism during volume depletion and/or sodium depletion states. The same response can occur as a result of renal hypoxia, even when the hypoxia is not related to volume depletion. In cardiac failure, for example, venous stasis without loss of blood volume occurs because of ineffective myocardial activity. The stasis leads to hypoxia, which triggers the events leading to increased reabsorption of sodium and water. In this situation, the excess water reabsorption is pathologic because the increased plasma volume is unnecessary and only further burdens the heart.

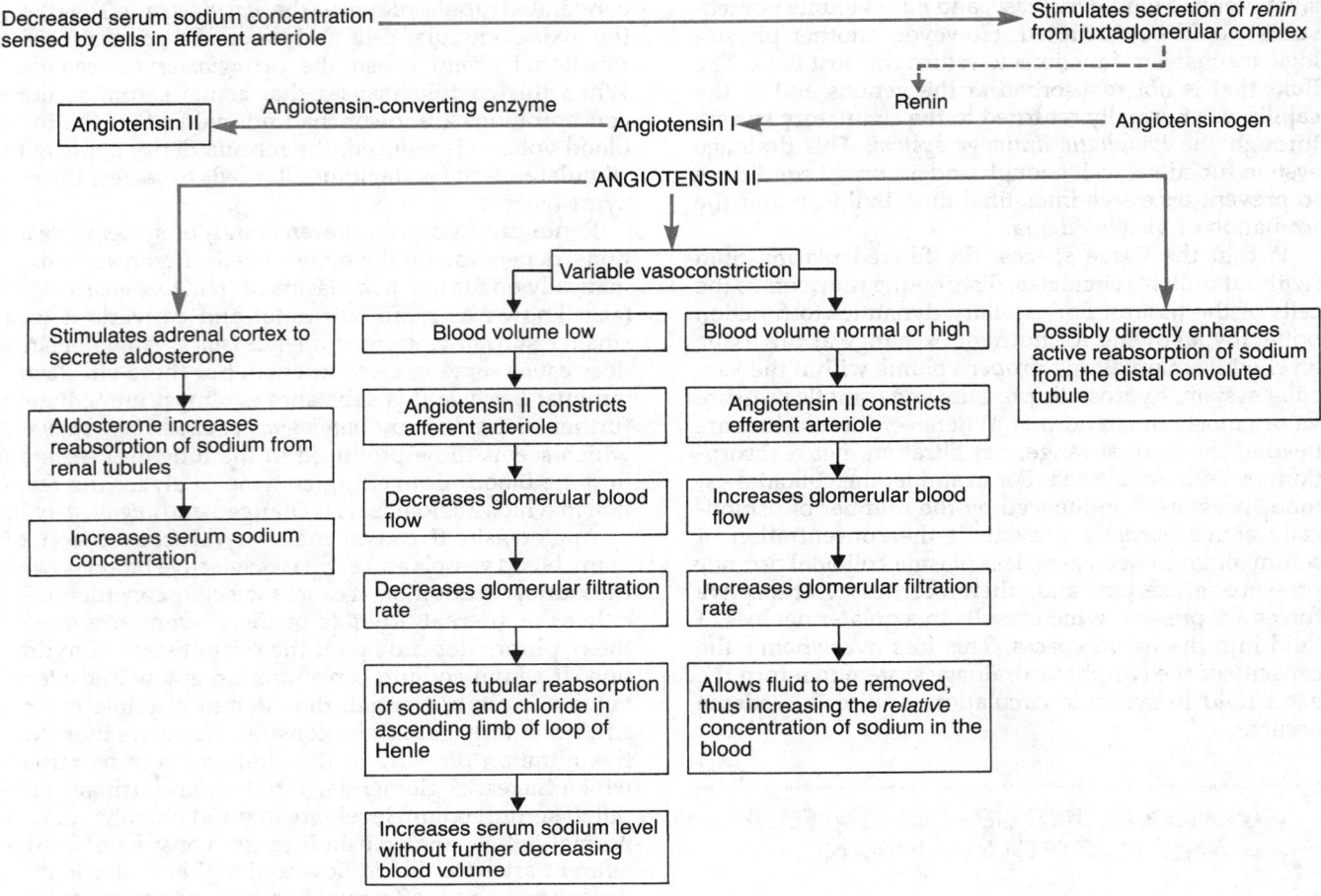

Figure 12–2

Role of angiotensinogen, angiotensin I, and angiotensin II in renal regulation of sodium and fluid volume.

ANTIDIURETIC HORMONE

ADH is released from the posterior pituitary gland in response to stimulation from the hypothalamus. The hypothalamus contains specialized cells (osmoreceptors) that are sensitive to changes in ECF osmolarity. Increased ECF osmolarity results in slight shrinkage of these cells and causes the hypothalamus to stimulate the posterior pituitary gland to secrete ADH. When osmolarity of the ECF is decreased, these osmoreceptors swell slightly and inhibit hypothalamic stimulation of the posterior pituitary gland (Groer, 1981).

ADH exerts effects on the membranes of the distal convoluted tubules and the collecting ducts of nephrons. In the presence of ADH, these membranes become thinner and more permeable to water. The tissues surrounding these tubules and ducts are hyperosmolar and thus exert a great osmotic pressure. When the membranes are made more permeable to water through the action of ADH, water in the tubular filtrate moves rapidly through the membrane by osmosis and is reabsorbed by the tubular capillary network into the systemic circulation. Thus, ADH does not directly regulate sodium absorption or excretion but influences ECF sodium concentration through the reabsorption or excretion of water.

NATRIURETIC FACTOR

Natriuretic factor is currently under investigation to determine its exact mechanism of action and characteristics. This substance is believed to be secreted by special cells lining the atria of the heart in response to increased blood volume, blood pressure, and blood osmolarity. Natriuretic factor has effects that are opposite to those of aldosterone. In the presence of natriuretic factor, glomerular filtration is greatly increased and tubular reabsorption of sodium is inhibited. The outcome is increased output of urine that has a high sodium content, which results in a decreased circulating blood volume and a decreased blood osmolarity. It is thought that natriuretic factor may play an important role in the long-term regulation of blood volume and mean arterial pressure, but the exact mechanisms of action of this substance are yet to be determined (Guyton, 1986).

BODY FLUIDS

Fluids constitute approximately 55% to 60% of adult weight and consist of the ECF, ICF, and a small amount of transcellular water. The ECF compartment constitutes about 42.5% of total body water and is composed of the following fluids: tissue, or interstitial, fluid; blood plasma; lymph; and bone and connective tissue water. The transcellular water makes up about 2.5% of total body water and constitutes mostly cell membrane water. The remaining 55% of total body water is ICF.

Age, sex, and lean-to-fat ratio influence the amounts and distribution of body fluids. The infant's body water is proportionately more of the body weight than that of the older child and adult, and a larger proportion of the water is intracellular water. Men have proportionately more body water weight than do women. Obesity is a factor in total body water, with obese individuals having proportionately less water than a lean individual of the same body weight.

Body fluids are solvents and transport media; they allow for normal nutrition of cells and transport biologic molecules (such as hormones) that are important in the regulation of normal physiologic functions. Most biochemical reactions take place in an aqueous medium and require proper pH, temperature, substrates, enzymes, coenzymes, and cofactors. Most transport processes require a fluid medium. The body fluids are constantly renewed, purified, and replaced as fluid balance is maintained through intake and output.

SOURCES OF FLUID INTAKE

Intake of fluid is normally regulated through the thirst drive. Fluids enter the body as the liquids we drink and in much of the food we ingest. In addition, water is a by-product of cellular metabolism. This by-product is called the *water of oxidation* (approximately 10% of daily water requirements are met by water of oxidation). A rising plasma osmolarity or a decreasing plasma volume stimulates the sensation of thirst. Other afferent sensory inputs to the hypothalamus, such as dryness of the oral mucosa and sensorimotor input from higher cortical centers, are also important. On the average, an adult consumes 1500 mL of fluid per day and obtains an additional 800 mL of fluid from the water of ingested foods. Most fluids consumed are hypotonic to the ECF. The water of oxidation is usually about 300 mL/day, although this amount varies directly with the overall metabolic state.

ROUTES OF FLUID LOSS

Output processes and routes are carefully regulated so that the composition and volume of fluids lost from the body do not change the proper chemistry and osmolarity of remaining body fluids.

TABLE 12–1   Routes for Removal of Water and Fluid Wastes

Route	Body Fluid*
Skin	Perspiration
Lungs	Pulmonary secretions
Kidney	Urine
Gastrointestinal	
Normal	Fecal fluid
	Saliva
Abnormal	Gastric juice
	Pancreatic juices
	Bile

* Except for urine, the body fluids are hypotonic to plasma for electrolyte solute concentrations. However, many of these body fluids contain other elements and compounds (e.g., glucose, proteins) that increase the actual osmolarity.

The body has several routes by which excess water and waste products are removed (Table 12–1). Of all the water loss routes, the kidneys are by far the most important and most sensitive, serving as the major adjustment mechanism to preserve fluid and electrolyte balance. The renal route is the route that is variable, closely regulated, and extraordinarily adjustable. The volume of urine can vary depending on the amount of fluid intake and the body's need to conserve fluids. The minimum amount of urine per day needed to dissolve and excrete the toxic waste products of metabolism ranges between 400 and 600 mL. This minimal volume is called the *obligatory urinary output*. If the volume falls below the obligatory output amount, metabolic wastes are retained and homeostasis can be disrupted. This urine is maximally concentrated, with a specific gravity of 1.032 or higher, and an osmolarity of at least 1200 mOsm/L. The relationship between specific gravity and osmolarity is demonstrated in Table 12–2.

TABLE 12–2   Relationship Between Specific Gravity and Osmolarity

Specific Gravity	Osmolarity (mOsm/L)
1.005	200
1.007	300
1.010	400
1.020	800
1.030	1200
1.035	1400

From Groer, M. (1981). *Physiology and pathophysiology of the body fluids*. St. Louis: C.V. Mosby. Copyright M. Groer.

The urine also can become maximally dilute, with a specific gravity of 1.005 and an osmolarity of 200 mOsm/L. This urine osmolarity would be the result of a large fluid intake and would be reflected in a large volume of urinary output. The concentrating and diluting abilities of the renal tubules are responses to the changes in the osmolarity of the ECF, the volumes and pressures of the ECF compartments, and variation in secretion of ADH and aldosterone.

Other normal water loss routes are the skin, lungs, and gastrointestinal tract. Additional water losses can occur by salivation, fistulas, drains, and gastrointestinal suction. Water loss through these routes is variable and consists of loss of hypotonic fluid.

Water loss from the skin and lungs, termed *insensible water loss* (IWL), can be significant. In the healthy adult, IWL is about 15 to 20 mL/kg per day. IWL can increase dramatically in hypermetabolic states such as thyroid crisis, trauma, burns, states of extreme stress, and fever. For every degree Celsius, IWL increases by 10%. When atmospheric conditions are hot and quite dry, the vapor pressure gradient is increased and IWL is also increased. Examples of clients at risk for increased IWL include individuals with assisted ventilation and those with tachypnea. IWL (not including sweat) is pure water and does not contain electrolytes. Therefore, excessive amounts of IWL result in a more hypertonic ECF of a smaller volume. If this loss is not balanced by intake, the hypertonic ECF and accompanying dehydration can lead to the pathophysiologic state of *hypernatremia* (elevated serum sodium level) (Groer, 1981).

Loss by sweating is variable but can reach a maximal rate of about 2 L/hour. Sweat is slightly hypotonic to the ECF. The amount of sweating is usually regulated by the autonomic nervous system, body temperature, and skin blood flow, with some minimal regulation provided by aldosterone. Sweating is stimulated by physical exercise, sympathetic nervous system arousal (fear, anxiety), heat, and increased metabolism.

Water loss through stool is normally minimal; however, in severe diarrhea or excessive fistula drainage, this loss can increase significantly. Clients with ulcerative colitis can have diarrheal fluid loss that amounts to several liters per day. Diarrheal fluid has basically the same composition as ileal fluid, with an osmolarity slightly less than the ECF and a pH of about 8. It contains potassium, sodium, bicarbonate, and chloride. Thus, with diarrhea there tends to be loss of hypotonic fluid containing electrolytes and bicarbonate base.

ELECTROLYTES

Electrolytes are atoms or molecules that carry an electrical charge; they are present in body fluids. *Cations* are positively charged ions, and *anions* are negatively charged ions. The body fluids are electrochemically neutral: positive ions are balanced by negative ions.

However, as discussed earlier, the composition and distribution of ions differ in the ECF and the ICF.

The separation of different ions into the ECF and ICF compartments is an important physical phenomenon that is responsible for establishing and maintaining membrane excitability and transmission of impulses, along with other specific cellular functions. The electrolyte concentration ranges in the ICF and the ECF are extremely narrow. Even small changes in these concentrations can lead to major pathologic alterations. Table 12–3 gives the major body fluid electrolytes together with their normal serum concentrations and primary functions.

Electrolyte balance is controlled via dietary intake and renal excretion or reabsorption. For example, the ECF potassium concentration is kept within tight limits of 3.5 to 5.0 mEq/L (Herlihy & Herlihy, 1987; Rice, 1982). Potassium in common foods that are ingested theoretically could increase the ECF potassium concentration dramatically and pathologically. However, renal excretion of potassium, by the processes of renal tubular secretion and excretion of urine, efficiently prevents major changes in potassium concentration.

Tables 12–4 through 12–8 provide major food sources of the electrolytes of greatest importance to normal physiology. The physiologic concentration of most electrolytes is reported in terms of milliequivalents per liter; however, the physiologic concentration of calcium may be reported as milligrams per deciliter.

SODIUM

Sodium (Na$^+$) is the *major cation in the ECF* and is the main factor responsible for maintaining ECF osmolarity. The activity of the electrogenic sodium-potassium pump keeps the sodium concentration of the ICF low (about 14 mEq/L) while maintaining high sodium concentrations in the ECF. This difference in sodium concentrations is extremely important for normal functioning of many physiologic activities, especially activities related to resting membrane potential, action potential, and impulse transmission. The concentration of sodium in the ECF primarily determines how and where water is retained or moved from one body compartment to another. In addition, because sodium is a cation, its concentration within a body fluid must be matched by an equal concentration of associated anions to maintain electrical balance. Each cation in the ECF must be balanced by an anion so that the fluid does not carry either a positive or a negative charge. When such a balance is maintained, a state of *electroneutrality* exists in that fluid. Therefore, sodium concentration influences the total solute concentration. Any alteration (increases or decreases) in ECF sodium concentration profoundly affects fluid volume and the distribution and/or concentration of other electrolytes.

In health, the normal concentration of ECF sodium (as measured by its concentration in serum) ranges be-

TABLE 12-3 Normal Serum Electrolyte Concentrations and Functions

Electrolyte	Serum Concentration (mEq/L)	Functions
Sodium (Na^+)	136-145	Maintenance of plasma osmolarity Generation and transmission of action potentials Maintenance of acid-base balance Maintenance of electroneutrality
Potassium (K^+)	3.5-5.0	Regulation of intracellular osmolarity Maintenance of electrical membrane excitability Maintenance of plasma acid-base balance
Calcium (Ca^{2+})	4.5-5.5 8.0-10.5 mg/dL	Cofactor in blood-clotting cascade Excitable membrane stabilizer Provision of strength and density to teeth and bones Essential element in contractile processes in cardiac, skeletal, and smooth muscle
Chloride (Cl^-)	96-106	Maintenance of plasma acid-base balance Maintenance of plasma electroneutrality Formation of hydrochloric acid

Data from Keyes, J. (1985). Fluid, electrolyte, and acid-base regulation. Belmont, CA: Wadsworth.

TABLE 12-4 Common Food Sources of Sodium*

Food Source	Amount (mg)
Table salt (1 tsp)	2000
Cheddar cheese (1 oz)	176
Cottage cheese (4 oz)	457
American cheese (1 oz)	439
Whole milk (8 oz)	120
Skim milk (8 oz)	126
Butter (1 tsp)	123
White bread (1 slice)	123
Whole-wheat bread (1 slice)	159
Soy sauce (1 tbsp)	1029
Ketchup (1 tbsp)	156
Mustard (1 tbsp)	188
Beef, lean (4 oz)	60
Pork, lean, fresh (4 oz)	60
Pork, cured (4 oz)	850
Chicken, light meat (4 oz)	70
Chicken, dark meat (4 oz)	70

* Adult recommended daily allowance: 1100-3300 mg.

Data from Pennington, J., & Church, H. (1985). *Bowe's and Church's food values of portions commonly used.* Philadelphia: J. B. Lippincott.

tween 136 and 145 mEq/L (see Table 12-3). Sodium enters the body via ingestion of most foods and fluids (see Table 12-4 for common food sources of sodium). The average dietary intake of sodium is about 6 to 12 g/day, although under normal circumstances an intake of only 0.5 to 1 g/day is necessary to maintain proper fluid and electrolyte balance (Keyes, 1985). In addition, sodium is stored in special interstitial fluid areas deep within the kidney medulla and can be released to the ECF as needed. Despite a great variation in sodium intake, the serum concentration of sodium usually remains within the normal range. ECF sodium balance is regulated primarily by the kidney under the influence of ADH and aldosterone.

When the ECF sodium concentration approaches low-normal ranges, the osmolarity of the blood decreases. Special osmoreceptors in the brain (hypothalamus) interpret the decreased osmolarity to mean that too much water is present in the ECF compared with the amount of solute present, which causes a dilution of the solutes (especially sodium). In response to the decreased osmolarity, the hypothalamus stops stimulating the posterior pituitary gland, which then drastically reduces ADH secretion. Without sufficient quantities of ADH, the distal convoluted tubule and collecting duct of the nephrons become less permeable to water. As a result,

TABLE 12–5   Common Food Sources of Potassium*

Food Source	Amount (mg)
Corn flakes (1¼ c)	26
Cooked oatmeal (¾ c)	99
Egg (1 large)	66
Codfish, raw (4 oz)	400
Salmon, pink, raw (3½ oz)	306
Tuna fish (4 oz)	375
Apple, raw with skin (1 medium)	159
Banana (1 medium)	451
Cantaloupe (1 c pieces)	494
Grapefruit (½ med)	175
Orange (1 medium)	250
Raisins (½ c)	700
Strawberries, raw (1 c)	247
Watermelon (1 c pieces)	186
White bread (1 slice)	27
Whole-wheat bread (1 slice)	44
Beef (4 oz)	480
Beef liver (3½ oz)	281
Pork, fresh (4 oz)	525
Pork, cured (4 oz)	325
Chicken (4 oz)	225
Veal cutlet (3½ oz)	448
Whole milk (8 oz)	370
Skim milk (8 oz)	406
Avocado (1 medium)	1097
Carrot (1 large)	341
Corn (4-in ear)	196
Cauliflower (1 c pieces)	295
Celery (1 stalk)	170
Green beans (1 c)	189
Mushrooms (10 small)	410
Onion (1 medium)	157
Peas (¾ c)	316
Potato, white (1 medium)	407
Spinach, raw (3½ oz)	470
Tomato (1 medium)	366

* Adult recommended daily allowance: 1875–5625 mg.

Data from Pennington, J., & Church, H. (1985). *Bowe's and Church's food values of portions commonly used.* Philadelphia: J. B. Lippincott.

TABLE 12–6   Common Food Sources of Calcium*

Food Source	Amount (mg)
Cheddar cheese (1 oz)	204
Cottage cheese (4 oz)	68
American cheese (1 oz)	174
Whole milk (8 oz)	288
Skim milk (8 oz)	302
Yogurt, low-fat (1 c)	415
Broccoli, raw (½ c)	75
Carrot (1 large)	37
Collard greens, raw (3 oz)	200
Green beans (1 c)	62
Rhubarb (1 c)	266
Spinach, raw (3½ oz)	93
Tofu (3 oz)	100

* Adult recommended daily allowance: 800–1200 mg.

Data from Pennington, J., & Church, H. (1985). *Bowe's and Church's food values of portions commonly used.* Philadelphia: J. B. Lippincott.

renin-angiotensinogen cascade reaction, eventually cause an increase in aldosterone secretion by the adrenal cortex. In the presence of aldosterone, the kidney tubules reabsorb more sodium and water, and return them to systemic circulation, thus assisting to increase the ECF sodium concentration.

When the ECF sodium concentration approaches high-normal levels, the osmolarity of the blood increases. The osmoreceptors in the hypothalamus interpret the increased osmolarity to mean that too little solvent (water) is present compared with the amount of solute. The hypothalamus directly stimulates the posterior pituitary gland to make and secrete increased amounts of ADH. The ADH exerts its effects directly on the distal convoluted tubules and collecting ducts of the nephrons in the kidney. More water is reabsorbed by kidney capillaries and less is lost from the body in the form of urine. The absorbed water is returned to systemic circulation, which helps to decrease the ECF sodium concentration. In addition, when the ECF sodium concentration is relatively high, less sodium is reabsorbed through the kidney tubules so that more sodium is lost from the body in the excreted urine.

POTASSIUM

In contrast with sodium, potassium (K^+) is the *major intracellular cation*. The normal serum concentration of potassium ranges between 3.5 and 5.0 mEq/L (see Table 12–3); the normal intracellular concentration of potassium is about 140 mEq/L. Because of its high ICF concentration, potassium has some control over ICF osmolarity and volume, although the major factor influencing ICF volume and osmolarity is the intracellular protein concentration. The maintenance of this large

less water is reabsorbed by kidney capillaries and more water is excreted via the urine and is thus removed from the body. The overall effect is a decrease in ECF water so that the relative concentration of all solutes (especially sodium) is increased.

As described earlier, an additional mechanism to prevent ECF sodium concentrations from becoming too low is the secretion and action of aldosterone. Special sensors located in specific kidney capillaries (afferent arterioles) are sensitive to alterations in serum sodium concentrations. When serum sodium concentrations are low-normal, these cells, through a series of reactions involving kidney tubule cells and the activation of the

TABLE 12–7 Common Food Sources of Phosphorus*

Food Source	Amount (mg)
Rolled oats, cooked (¾ c)	133
Egg (1 large)	90
Codfish (3 oz)	175
Tuna fish, white, canned (6½ oz)	405
Raisins (½ c)	75
White bread (1 slice)	26
Whole-wheat bread (1 slice)	23
Cheddar cheese (1 oz)	145
American cheese (1 oz)	211
Whole milk (8 oz)	228
Skim milk (8 oz)	247
Yogurt, low-fat (8 oz)	326
Beef (4 oz)	215
Beef liver (4 oz)	375
Pork, fresh (4 oz)	325
Chicken (4 oz)	200
Almonds (1 oz)	141
Peanuts (1 oz)	110

* Adult recommended daily allowance: 800 mg.

Data from Pennington, J., & Church, H. (1985). *Bowe's and Church's food values of portions commonly used.* Philadelphia: J. B. Lippincott.

difference in ECF and ICF potassium concentrations is critical to the ability of excitable tissues to generate action potentials and to transmit impulses. ECF potassium levels are so low that any alteration in ECF potassium

TABLE 12–8 Common Food Sources of Magnesium*

Food Source	Amount (mg)
Rolled oats (¾ c)	42
Tuna fish, white, canned (6½ oz)	59
Raisins (½ c)	25
Beef (4 oz)	24
Pork (4 oz)	30
Chicken (4 oz)	26
Whole milk (8 oz)	33
Skim milk (8 oz)	28
Yogurt, low-fat (8 oz)	40
Peanut butter (1 tbsp)	22
Avocado (1 medium)	70
Broccoli (1 stalk)	24
Cauliflower (1 c pieces)	24
Peas (¾ c)	35
Potato (1 medium)	34
Spinach, raw (3½ oz)	88

* Adult recommended daily allowance: 300–350 mg.

Data from Pennington, J., & Church, H. (1985). *Bowe's and Church's food values of portions commonly used.* Philadelphia: J. B. Lippincott.

concentration is poorly tolerated by the body and more profoundly influences physiologic activities than do alterations in ECF sodium concentrations. For example, a decrease in serum potassium level of only 1 mEq/L (e.g., from 4.0 to 3.0 mEq/L) represents a significant difference (25%) in the total ECF potassium concentration, whereas a decrease in serum sodium level of 1 mEq/L (e.g., from 140 to 139 mEq/L) is a much smaller change (less than 1%).

Potassium tends to move out of cells down its concentration gradient into the ECF. In addition, almost all ingested foods contain potassium. The average potassium intake is about 60 to 100 mEq/day. Despite heavy potassium ingestion and the tendency of potassium to move from the ICF to the ECF, the healthy body manages to keep ECF potassium within the narrow ranges of normal that are required for optimal physiologic function (Cox, 1981).

The primary controller of ECF potassium concentration is the efficiency of the sodium-potassium pumps that lie within the membranes of all body cells. The cells of excitable tissues have greater numbers of these membrane-bound pumps. When potassium leaks out of the cells and sodium leaks into the cells to the extent that the concentration differences for each ion between the ECF and the ICF decrease, the sodium-potassium pump becomes activated. The pump removes three sodium ions from the ICF for every two potassium ions it returns to the ICF. In this manner, the concentration differences for both ions can be maintained.

Some potassium regulation also occurs through kidney function. The kidney is the primary excretory route for ridding the body of ECF potassium (80% of potassium removal from the body occurs via the kidney). Unlike the situation with sodium, no hormone has been identified that directly regulates renal reabsorption and excretion of potassium, although when sodium is reabsorbed by the kidney under the influence of aldosterone, potassium is usually excreted. The kidney cannot conserve potassium directly. Rather, potassium ions and hydrogen ions are exchanged (either reabsorbed or excreted) for sodium ions in the kidney to help maintain electroneutrality.

CALCIUM

Calcium (Ca^{2+}) is a mineral whose presence and functions are closely related to the activities of phosphorus and magnesium. Calcium is a divalent cation that exists in the body in two forms, bound and ionized (or unbound, free). Bound calcium is usually conjugated to specific serum proteins, especially albumin. Ionized calcium is present in the serum and other extracellular fluids as free calcium. The free calcium is physiologically active; this form must be regulated. The body functions best when ECF calcium levels are maintained within a narrow range of normal. The normal concentration for ECF calcium is 5 mEq/L (it may also be calculated as 8.0 to 10.5 mg/dL). The ICF concentration of calcium is quite low, so a downhill gradient exists for calcium from the ECF to the ICF.

Calcium functions in many important ways and in many specialized body systems. Cardiac and neuromuscular function depends on ECF calcium levels and the release of calcium from specific intracellular storage sites into the ICF. Calcium is required for normal contraction of skeletal, smooth, and cardiac muscle. Much of the calcium needed for contraction of various types of muscle is stored intracellularly in the sarcoplasmic reticulum. Excitation of the sarcoplasmic reticulum releases calcium into the area of the myofilaments so that the filaments can bind properly and slide past each other, which causes muscle contraction. The intracellular reservoirs of calcium in the sarcoplasmic reticulum are replenished as needed from ECF calcium.

Contraction of cardiac and smooth muscle depends not only on the calcium released from the sarcoplasmic reticulum, but also on ECF calcium that moves through special membrane channels (called *calcium slow channels*) into the ICF. Calcium is also a membrane stabilizer and acts to reduce both the fluidity and the excitability of the membrane. Calcium in the membrane is believed to oppose or inhibit the influx of sodium in excitable tissues. Because the influx of sodium (through *fast channels*) is the precipitating event for the initiation of depolarization, the presence of excess calcium would delay or inhibit membrane depolarization, decrease excitability, and interfere with the generation of action potentials. In addition, calcium participates in many membrane-bound enzymatic reactions that influence cellular activity and productivity.

Calcium is also a cofactor for many steps in the process of blood coagulation. Although the presence of calcium is an absolute requirement for these processes, only relatively small quantities are needed for normal coagulation.

The body functions best when serum calcium levels are maintained within a narrow range of normal (4.5 to 5.5 mEq/L). Even small excesses or deficits of serum calcium levels can profoundly affect health and homeostasis. Therefore, the body has several well-controlled mechanisms to guard against rapid or wide alterations in ionized calcium levels in the ECF.

Calcium enters the body by dietary intake and absorption through the intestinal tract. For dietary calcium to be absorbed by the intestines, the active form of vitamin D also must be present. Once in the body, calcium is stored largely in the bones. When both ECF calcium levels and stored calcium levels are adequate, gastrointestinal absorption of dietary calcium is inhibited and urinary excretion of excess calcium increases. When more ECF calcium is needed, *parathyroid hormone* (PTH or parathormone) secretion and release from the parathyroid glands increase. PTH causes ECF calcium levels to increase through the following processes:

1. Release of free calcium from bone storage sites directly into the ECF (resorption)
2. Inhibition of renal excretion of calcium and stimulation of renal tubular reabsorption of calcium

3. Stimulation of vitamin D activation, thus increasing intestinal absorption of dietary calcium

When excesses of calcium are present in the ECF, secretion of PTH is inhibited, and secretion of *calcitonin* (a hormone secreted by the thyroid gland) is increased. Calcitonin causes the ECF calcium level to decrease through the following processes:

1. Inhibition of bone resorption of calcium
2. Increase of renal excretion of calcium in the urine
3. Inhibition of activation of vitamin D

In addition, a membrane-bound calcium pump helps to keep the ICF relatively free of calcium ions.

PHOSPHORUS

Phosphorus (P) is present in the body in both inorganic and organic forms. The vast majority of phosphorus (80%) can be found in the bones. Little phosphorus is present in the ECF, and it usually exists as HPO_4^{2-} or $H_2PO_4^-$ in a 4 : 1 ratio. Normal ECF levels of phosphorus range between 2.5 and 4.5 mg/dL. Phosphorus is the major anion in the ICF, and its concentration in the ICF is considerably higher than its ECF concentration. Physiologically, phosphorus has more ICF functions than ECF functions. Phosphorus functions intracellularly as a *cofactor*—a substance that is required to enhance the activity of other enzymes or reactions. ICF phosphorus participates in the following reactions and/or activities:

1. Activation of B complex vitamins
2. Formation and activation of high-energy substances including ATP
3. Cell division
4. Carbohydrate metabolism
5. Protein metabolism
6. Lipid metabolism

ECF phosphorus functions include acid-base buffering and calcium homeostasis. Phosphorus is contained in a wide variety of foods (nuts, legumes, dairy products, red meats, organ meats, bran, and whole grains), and the average American diet is high in phosphorus (1 to 2 g/day) (Metheny & Snively, 1983).

Phosphorus balance and calcium balance are closely intertwined. Under most conditions, ECF concentrations of calcium and phosphorus appear to exist in a balanced, reciprocal relationship to the extent that the product of the ECF concentrations remains a constant. Therefore, a change in the concentration of one should result in an equal change in the concentration of the other but in the opposite direction. However, this reciprocal relationship does not hold true in all situations (Keyes, 1985).

Dietary phosphorus is absorbed in the intestinal tract. Phosphorus is more readily absorbed than calcium, although increased calcium ingestion can inhibit phosphorus absorption because insoluble compounds of calcium and phosphorus form that are excreted in the feces. Activated vitamin D enhances intestinal absorption of phosphorus.

Regulation of ECF phosphorus occurs through the activity of PTH although the effects of this hormone on ECF phosphorus conservation and excretion are somewhat unclear. Overall, increased secretion of PTH results in a net loss of phosphorus. PTH causes phosphorus to be resorbed from bone storage sites and also increases intestinal absorption of phosphorus. However, at the same time, PTH significantly increases renal excretion of phosphorus to the extent that the combination of these actions results in reduced ECF phosphorus concentration. Reduced PTH levels enhance renal reabsorption of phosphorus, which results in increased ECF concentrations.

MAGNESIUM

Magnesium (Mg^{2+}) is another mineral that forms a divalent cation when it is dissolved in water. The average adult human body possesses an average of 25 g of magnesium, most of which (60%) is stored in bones and cartilage. Little magnesium is present in the ECF, and more than 25% of that is bound to albumin. ECF levels of unbound, or ionized, magnesium range between 1.5 and 2.5 mEq/L (Metheny & Snively, 1983). Much more magnesium is present in the ICF, which makes it the second most common cation in the ICF. Physiologically, magnesium has many more functions in the ICF than in the ECF.

Most of magnesium's ICF functions center on its role as a cofactor. The presence of ICF magnesium is critical for the proper progression of the following reactions or activities:

1. Muscle contraction
2. Carbohydrate metabolism
3. Activation and use of ATP
4. Activation of many B complex vitamins
5. DNA synthesis
6. Protein synthesis

ECF magnesium appears to be important for blood coagulation and in the regulation of neuromuscular irritability. Magnesium acts at the neuromuscular synapse, possibly by inhibiting the release of acetylcholine, thus depressing synaptic transmission and reducing skeletal muscle contractility. Magnesium is abundant in a wide variety of natural foods (nuts, vegetables, fish, and whole grains), and ingestion constitutes the primary source of this mineral. The usual daily magnesium requirement for adults is about 250 mg.

Although magnesium is similar to calcium in many respects and its presence in the ECF must be maintained within a narrow range of normal, its regulation does not appear to be tightly controlled. Little is known about the precise mechanisms for the regulation of magnesium. Magnesium is absorbed from the intestinal tract at the same point at which calcium is absorbed. Although some competition between calcium and magnesium exists for absorption at this site, both cations can be absorbed here simultaneously. The absorption of phosphorus inhibits or interferes with magnesium absorption to the same degree that it inhibits calcium absorption. PTH stimulates the release of magnesium from bone in much the same way that it stimulates the release of calcium. The kidney tubule is important for the regulation of ECF magnesium levels.

When ECF magnesium levels approach low-normal, renal reabsorption of magnesium occurs, thus conserving this ion for extracellular use. When ECF magnesium levels approach high-normal, renal excretion of magnesium increases. An additional mechanism assists in magnesium regulation by maintaining a large magnesium gradient between the ECF and the ICF. This mechanism is the membrane-bound active transport system that links movement of calcium and magnesium. This pump (plus energy in the form of ATP) moves calcium through the membrane out from the cell into the ECF while simultaneously moving magnesium from the ECF through the cell membrane into the ICF.

CHLORIDE

Chloride (Cl^-) is the major anion of the ECF. Its primary function is to cooperate with sodium in maintaining osmotic pressure in the ECF. Chloride is also important in the formation of hydrochloric acid in the stomach. The normal ECF concentration of chloride ranges between 96 and 106 mEq/L.

Because it is present in such large quantities in the ECF and because it is an anion, another major function of chloride is preservation of electroneutrality within the ECF. As a naturally occurring crystalline substance, chloride is associated with a positively charged molecule, which is frequently sodium. Sodium chloride dissociates in water into sodium ions and chloride ions. However, in the ECF the ratio of sodium to chloride ions is not 1:1 because other ions are also present in varying concentrations (as are plasma proteins, which tend to carry negative charges). Thus, the normal ratio of sodium ions to chloride ions in the ECF is 3:2.

Only a small quantity of chloride is usually present in the ICF because negatively charged particles repel its traversing of cell membranes. However, under specific circumstances chloride in the ECF can enter cells when it is exchanged for another anion that is leaving the cell. This situation is called a *chloride shift* and results in a decrease in the ECF chloride concentration but no net loss of chloride. The anion most commonly exchanged for chloride in this way is bicarbonate (HCO_3^-). Chloride enters the body through dietary intake. Because chloride exists as part of a salt, not only with sodium but also with potassium and a wide variety of other minerals, in natural and preserved foods, most diets contain more than adequate amounts of chloride to meet body needs in health.

Although the ECF concentration of chloride varies

with both sodium concentration and the state of hydration, chloride concentration can be decreased independently of these factors. Most membranes are permeable to chloride, and it diffuses freely down its concentration *and electrical* gradients. Aldosterone indirectly regulates chloride homeostasis: When aldosterone causes sodium to be actively reabsorbed by the renal tubular epithelium, chloride follows passively because of the electrical attraction of cations and anions.

Changes in chloride concentration occur most frequently in conjunction with changes in bicarbonate concentration. These two anions exist in the ECF in a constant and reciprocal relationship: If the concentration of one increases, the concentration of the other must decrease to the same degree.

FLUID AND ELECTROLYTE CHANGES ASSOCIATED WITH AGING

The elderly individual has only 45% to 50% of his or her body weight in the form of water compared with the younger adult, who has 55% to 60% of body weight as water. This decrease represents a loss of muscle mass in the elderly individual and thus a reduced ratio of overall lean body weight to total body weight. The decrease in percentage of total body water places the elderly individual at greater risk for developing water deficit states. Skin turgor is not always an accurate assessment of ECF volume deficit in the elderly individual because the natural aging process is associated with decreased turgor (see also under the heading Physical Assessment). Furthermore, the elderly individual may have a diminished thirst sensation along with decreased renal function, both of which contribute to risk and make assessment more difficult. Accurate documentation of intake and output and accurate weight measurement become extremely important when working with the elderly, as these parameters more accurately reflect hydration status in this population. In addition, the very old person may be confused or forgetful and unable to give a reliable history.

Electrolyte balance may be more difficult in the elderly individual. The normal ECF and ICF electrolyte ranges may be maintained in the elderly individual, but the electrolyte balance state is more fragile and easily disturbed. Part of the fragility in balance is related to enzymatic deficiencies that occur with aging, which result in malfunctioning physiologic regulatory mechanisms. Also contributing to the ease with which electrolyte balance may be disrupted is the phenomenon of renal aging, which manifests with disturbances in renal blood flow, glomerular filtration rate, the numbers of functional nephrons, sensitivity to ADH, and general renal tubular secretory and absorptive function. Renal and membrane changes that are associated with hypertension may be present in the elderly individual. Variation in the responses of excitable membranes to electrical changes may also influence fluid and electrolyte balance in the elderly individual. Small changes in the concentrations of potassium and calcium may produce unexpectedly large or profound results.

HISTORY

The data that the nurse collects to assess the status of fluid and electrolyte balance include a thorough and detailed history. The nature of the history depends on whether the client is newly admitted to the hospital and acutely ill, in which case a complete history is important, or whether the client is being evaluated on a daily basis, in which case an update of the history is required. Because fluid and electrolyte imbalances can develop rapidly and by a variety of alterations, the nurse needs to ask pertinent questions to elicit information that the client may not know has critical relevance to the situation. For example, a client with hyperosmolar dehydration might have either diabetes or renal disease. Because the hyperosmolar state may have been caused by excessive ingestion of cola soft drinks and snack cakes that lead to hyperglycemia, the nutritional history can often provide important clues to the underlying pathophysiologic processes influencing the condition. The client may not understand the connection between dietary intake and the onset of fluid and electrolyte imbalances and may not volunteer this important information.

The guidelines for obtaining a thorough fluid and electrolyte history do not differ from those usually used for assessing any other system; however, the kind of information collected tends to be more quantitative. For example, intake and output volumes are often extremely important. Clients may need to be guided in making an accurate subjective assessment of the amount of fluid ingested and of changes in voiding patterns. The nurse should also assess what types of fluids and foods have been ingested to determine osmolarity as well as amount. In addition, many clients do not consider any solid food to be a liquid. Because some solid foods, such as ice cream, gelatin, ices, and Popsicles, are liquids at body temperature, these items should be included when calculating fluid intake.

Output fluids should include not only urine but also fluid losses through significant diaphoresis, diarrhea, and insensible loss during fevers. The nurse also should ask specific questions about medications (both prescription and over-the-counter medications) that have been taken and should ascertain dosage, length of time taken, and compliance with the medication regimen. A client taking diuretics can easily become hypokalemic, acidotic, or volume depleted if additional threats to water balance, such as vomiting and excessive sweating, occur while the diuretic is used.

Medications that are frequently used by elderly individuals and that have the potential for disturbing fluid and electrolyte balance are laxatives. Misuse and over-use of these drugs can lead to serious imbalance states. Elderly clients often have difficulty in producing a numeric estimate of fluid loss, which makes this information less reliable. For example, a client who states that vomiting occurred all night long until the stomach was empty may overestimate or underestimate the amount vomited.

The nurse may need to question carefully and probe deeply during history and assessment so that appropriate information is collected. Common manifestations of electrolyte imbalance states include alterations in neuromuscular functions. Clients may not associate such symptoms as heart palpitations or muscle weakness with the current health problem. Such symptoms are often vague or have an insidious onset; thus, the client needs to be asked specific questions by the nurse during the review of systems to determine changes in these functions. Important information regarding these symptoms includes when the symptom first appeared and if the problem has become more severe or noticeable.

Other areas of the history that are pertinent include body weight changes, thirst or excessive drinking, exposure to environmental heat, and the presence of other pre-existing disorders such as renal or endocrine diseases (Cushing's disease, Addison's disease, diabetes mellitus, diabetes insipidus). A general assessment of the client's level of consciousness and mental status is important so that the accuracy of the historical data can be determined.

PHYSICAL ASSESSMENT

Hydration is defined as the normal state of fluid balance (Metheny & Snively, 1983). A normally hydrated adult is alert, has moist eyes and mucous membranes, has a urinary output appropriate for the amount of fluid ingested (with a specific gravity of urine of around 1.010), and has an adequate state of skin hydration as measured by *skin turgor.*

Turgor is the normal resiliency of a pinched fold of skin. This pinched fold should return immediately to its original shape after it is released. Decreased turgor, a sign of dehydration, is present when the fold remains in a pinched shape after being released and rebounds slowly *(tenting).* Skin turgor is best assessed in body areas that contain little adipose tissue, such as over the sternum or on the back of the hand. The elderly individual may have poor skin turgor because of the loss of tissue fluids that is related to the aging process; thus, a true state of hydration may be more difficult to assess than in a younger adult.

Skin hydration assessment also includes examination for dryness. Mucous membranes and eye conjunctiva are usually visibly moist. Assessment of fluid balance should therefore always include examination of the eyes, nose, and oral mucous membranes. A dry, sticky, "cottony" mouth, the absence of tearing, the presence of weight loss, and a decreased urinary output indicate the presence of an actual fluid volume deficit or of dehydration.

Several types of dehydration can occur, and their clinical findings differ (see Chap. 13). Dehydration may be isotonic, hypertonic (usually hypernatremic), or hypotonic (hyponatremic). Nursing assessment techniques for dehydration are generally related to ECF volume. When ECF volume decreases, the client demonstrates the signs and symptoms previously described. Assessment can also focus on signs of plasma volume deficits that can occur without deficits in the tissue fluid spaces. Signs of plasma volume deficit include changes in pulse volume, pulse deficit, heart rate, blood pressure, venous filling, and peripheral perfusion, and symptoms of generalized nervous system arousal as the serum concentration of sodium and other electrolytes that regulate excitable membranes rises.

Other methods of assessing hydration include evaluation of blood chemistry studies. Serum sodium level is an important indicator for assisting to determine whether the state of dehydration is hypertonic or hypotonic. Serum sodium concentration is directly related to ECF osmolarity. An approximate method of estimating osmolarity is to multiply the serum sodium value by 2 (Groer, 1981). For example, the normal serum sodium value is about 141 mEq/L, and a normal ECF osmolarity value is 285 mOsm/L. Other important laboratory values include the hematocrit and hemoglobin concentration. These values increase when the ECF deficit is either hypotonic or hypertonic and decrease if the ECF deficit is isotonic (such as is seen with hemorrhage). The increase in hematocrit and hemoglobin values in states of dehydration is artificial, being related to the concentrating effect of the fluid loss. This concentration effect can also produce increases in other serum chemistry assays, such as glucose and blood urea nitrogen, and in measures of cellular components such as the white blood cell count and the platelet count.

Volume and specific gravity of urine are also important to assess. Specific gravity is actually a measurement of density, but in physiologic fluids in which water is the solvent, density is directly related to solute concentration (osmolarity) (see Table 12–2 for the relation between specific gravity and osmolarity). In general, in dehydrated states, water is conserved and reabsorbed at the renal tubules by the action of ADH so that the volume of urinary output decreases and the specific gravity rises. The specific gravity of urine increases with a rise in any urine solute concentration, so that conditions that result in hematuria, proteinuria, or glycosuria also are reflected by an increased specific gravity value.

Behavioral and neurologic assessment should be included as part of fluid assessment because changes in fluid balance can result in alteration of neurologic function. In hypertonic states, neuronal cell shrinkage may induce serious nervous system excitability and hyperactivity, and convulsions may occur. Another parameter to assess is the degree of thirst. With an elderly, comatose client, thirst may be difficult to determine accurately. Unless responsiveness is severely limited, the offering of fluids to a dehydrated individual may evoke a response. Body temperature, a function of neural regulation, may also be an index of the state of hydration. Body temperature usually rises in response to hypertonic dehydration and is relatively unaffected by hypotonic or isotonic dehydration (Metheny & Snively, 1983).

The nurse should assess IWL in every client. In addition, special situations require assessment of fluid loss from other routes. These situations and routes include fluid losses from wounds, gastric or intestinal drainage, blood loss from hemorrhage, and surgical fistulas draining body secretions such as bile or pancreatic juices.

Most electrolytes profoundly influence the activity of various excitable membranes, and thus electrolyte imbalances are often associated with alterations in function of these membranes. Electrolyte balance assessment should include a complete neuromuscular assessment for tone, strength, movement, coordination, and tremors. Other systems to be assessed that may indicate alterations of excitable membrane function include cardiac (assess heart rate, strength of contractions, presence of arrhythmias) and gastrointestinal (assess activity of peristalsis).

Part of the nurse's assessment should always focus on changes from previous findings (including mental status, physical examination data, and laboratory data). Fluid and electrolyte imbalances can arise quickly; therefore, familiarity with the client's baseline assessment data to determine what changes have occurred is an essential component of nursing responsibility.

PSYCHOSOCIAL ASSESSMENT

The psychosocial assessment of fluid and electrolyte status includes both psychologic and cultural factors that might influence balance. For example, clients who are confused, violent, angry, or hypochondriacal are usually not completely reliable when giving history data. Psychiatric clients have been known to engage in obsessive fluid ingestion that leads to fluid volume excess states. Depressed clients may refuse fluids or forget to drink adequate amounts of fluid. Bulimic and/or anorectic clients may use laxatives to excess, which results in fluid and electrolyte imbalances.

Social and cultural practices also are important to assess. Excessive alcohol or drug use or abuse may lead to fluid or electrolyte imbalance. Cultural influences may interfere with accurate history or physical examination. For example, a Hispanic male client may not allow the female nurse to examine him, and he may give inaccurate information in response to a female questioner.

DIAGNOSTIC ASSESSMENT

Laboratory results are necessary data that, along with the physical examination and the history, allow for the diagnosis of fluid or electrolyte imbalances and assist in the implementation of an appropriate plan of care for the client with such an imbalance. Serum electrolyte values are presented in Table 12–3. The nurse should be aware of these data and should know if current information deviates from normal or previously obtained results. Other serum values that may assist assessing a client's fluid and electrolyte status include glucose, blood urea nitrogen, creatinine, pH, bicarbonate, osmolarity, and anion gap. The urinalysis results are usually of great importance in assessing fluid status. Even if a full laboratory report is not available, the nurse can perform various dipstick-type tests to help determine renal function, water and electrolyte handling by the kidney, and hyperosmolar or hyposmolar states. These tests include quantification of glucose, acetone, protein, and blood in the urine, as well as pH and specific gravity of the urine. In addition, the nurse's visual inspection of the urine provides important data about the presence of sediment, abnormal color, turbidity, and frothing.

Complete urinalysis results from the laboratory provide more information that the nurse can use to assess the client's condition. For example, a dehydrated client would be expected to have a low volume of urine with a high specific gravity and a low urine sodium concentration (indicating aldosterone stimulation, and thus renal sodium and water reabsorption). The presence of cells, blood, casts, or protein in the urine might indicate renal disease that could be causing or contributing to fluid and electrolyte imbalances. Osmolarity of the urine can provide some information about renal function or overall hydration status.

SUMMARY

This chapter has presented the physiologic foundations for the assessment of fluid and electrolyte balance. In health, a constantly maintained dynamic balance of fluids and electrolytes exists. Many physiologic mechanisms contribute to this balance, and pathophysiologic states occur only when these mechanisms become ineffective. The next chapter describes the most common alterations in fluid and electrolyte balance.

REFERENCES AND READINGS

Bishop, M., Duben-Von Laufen, J., & Fody, E. (1985). *Clinical chemistry: Principles, procedures, correlations.* Philadelphia: J. B. Lippincott.

Chenevey, B. (1987). Overview of fluids and electrolytes. *Nursing Clinics of North America, 22,* 749.

Cox, M. (1981). Potassium homeostasis. *Medical Clinics of North America, 65,* 363.

Ganong, W. (1985). Review of medical physiology (12th ed.). Los Altos, CA: Lange Medical.

Gennari, F. (1984). Serum osmolarity: Uses and limitations. *New England Journal of Medicine, 310,* 102.

Groer, M. (1981). *Physiology and pathophysiology of body fluids.* St. Louis: C. V. Mosby.

Guyton, A. C. (1986). *Textbook of medical physiology* (7th ed.). Philadelphia: W. B. Saunders.

Guyton, A. C. (1987). *Human physiology and mechanisms of disease* (4th ed.). Philadelphia: W. B. Saunders.

Herlihy, B., & Herlihy, J. (1987). Physiologic role and regulation of potassium. *Critical Care Nurse, 7*(5), 10.

Hinchliff, S., & Montague, S. (1988). *Physiology for nursing practice.* London: Baillière Tindall.

Keyes, J. (1985). *Fluid, electrolyte, and acid-base regulation.* Belmont, CA: Wadsworth.

Lancaster, L. (1987). Renal and endocrine regulation of water and electrolyte balance. *Nursing Clinics of North America, 22,* 761.

Metheny, N., & Snively, W. (1983). *Nurses' handbook of fluid balance* (4th ed.). Philadelphia: J. B. Lippincott.

Nave, C. R., & Nave, B. C. (1985). *Physics for the health sciences* (3rd ed.). Philadelphia: W. B. Saunders.

Pennington, J., & Church, H. (1985). *Bowe's and Church's food values of portions commonly used* (14th ed.). Philadelphia: J. B. Lippincott.

Rice, V. (1982). The role of potassium in health and disease. *Critical Care Nurse, 2*(3), 54.

Trissel, L. (1988). *Handbook on injectable drugs* (5th ed.). Bethesda: American Society of Hospital Pharmacists.

Urrows, S. (1980). Physiology of body fluids. *Nursing Clinics of North America, 15,* 537.

CHAPTER 13

Interventions for Clients with Fluid and Electrolyte Imbalances

FLUID AND ELECTROLYTE IMBALANCES

Fluid and electrolyte imbalances are common problems for a majority of clients in all settings. Physiologic homeostasis is heavily dependent on normal fluid and electrolyte balance. Because any physiologic derangement can upset fluid and electrolyte balance to some degree, virtually every client is at some risk. Specific imbalances are discussed separately in this chapter, although fluid levels and the concentrations of most electrolytes are so interrelated that rarely does a fluid imbalance occur without an accompanying electrolyte imbalance.

As discussed in Chapter 12, extracellular ion concentrations must be maintained within narrow limits to allow normal physiologic function, especially the generation and transmission of electrical impulses, which are referred to as cellular action potentials. Consequently, ion imbalances change the excitability of cells throughout the body and thus alter physiologic function. Not only do electrolyte imbalances affect cellular function directly, but they also may affect body fluid balance.

The following discussion considers imbalances in fluid levels and potassium, sodium, calcium, chloride, magnesium, and phosphate ion concentrations. Because problems with fluid, sodium, potassium, and calcium balance are the more common of the electrolyte-related disorders, these are discussed in depth. Imbalances of magnesium and phosphorus levels are less common, and the focus of presentation regarding these imbalances is primarily on pathophysiology and etiologic factors.

DEHYDRATION

OVERVIEW

Dehydration is a state in which the body's fluid intake is not sufficient to meet the fluid needs of the body, resulting in a fluid volume deficit (Groer, 1981). Dehydration may be *isotonic, hypotonic,* or *hypertonic* in nature, depending on whether the fluid deficit is accompanied by alterations in extracellular fluid (ECF) sodium concentrations (Metheny & Snively, 1983). Dehydration may represent an actual decrease in total body water (as seen when dehydration is caused by either an inadequate fluid intake or an excessive fluid loss). Dehydration also can be present without an actual decrease in total body water, such as when water shifts from the vascular space (plasma volume) into the interstitial space. Dehydration is actually a clinical state or condition rather than a disease. This condition is caused by one or more underlying pathologic changes.

Pathophysiology

The majority of problems associated with dehydration are related to fluid deficits in the vascular space and alterations in the serum sodium levels. The exact nature of dehydration-related problems varies with the type of dehydration, the degree of dehydration, and the speed with which the imbalance occurred (Folk-Lighty, 1984).

Isotonic Dehydration

Isotonic dehydration is the most common type of dehydration and involves general depletion of isotonic fluids from the ECF compartment (both the vascular space and the interstitial space). Because isotonic fluid is lost, ECF osmolarity remains normal, so that this type of dehydration usually does not result in an intracellular fluid (ICF) shift. The usual overall result of isotonic dehydration is an inadequate circulating volume. Compensatory mechanisms (Fig. 13–1) attempt to maintain adequate tissue perfusion to vital organs in spite of this loss in vascular volume.

When isotonic fluid is lost from the plasma volume, but the plasma proteins and cells remain, the plasma oncotic pressure is increased (Keyes, 1985). This in-

crease pulls water from the interstitial space in an attempt to help maintain vascular volume. At the same time, the decreased vascular volume results in a decreased mean arterial pressure (MAP) that is sensed by special cells in the juxtaglomerular complex of the nephrons in the kidney (Chap. 12). The low MAP results in stimulation of the secretion of renin and initiates the renin-angiotensinogen cascade, which causes the formation of angiotensin II and the release of aldosterone from the adrenal cortex. The angiotensin II causes vasoconstriction, and the aldosterone increases renal reabsorption of water and sodium. These two mechanisms together can increase plasma volume and MAP, thus assisting to maintain adequate tissue perfusion (Guyton, 1986).

When dehydration involves a 3% loss of vascular volume, the sympathetic nervous system (SNS) also is activated by the subsequent drop in the MAP in the aortic arch and the carotid sinuses. Activation of the SNS inhibits the parasympathetic division and releases catecholamines (epinephrine and norepinephrine), which increase cardiac output by increasing heart rate and contractility. At the same time, SNS stimulation causes selective systemic vasoconstriction. This action shunts blood away from the skin, the gastrointestinal (GI) tract, and the kidneys, making more blood available

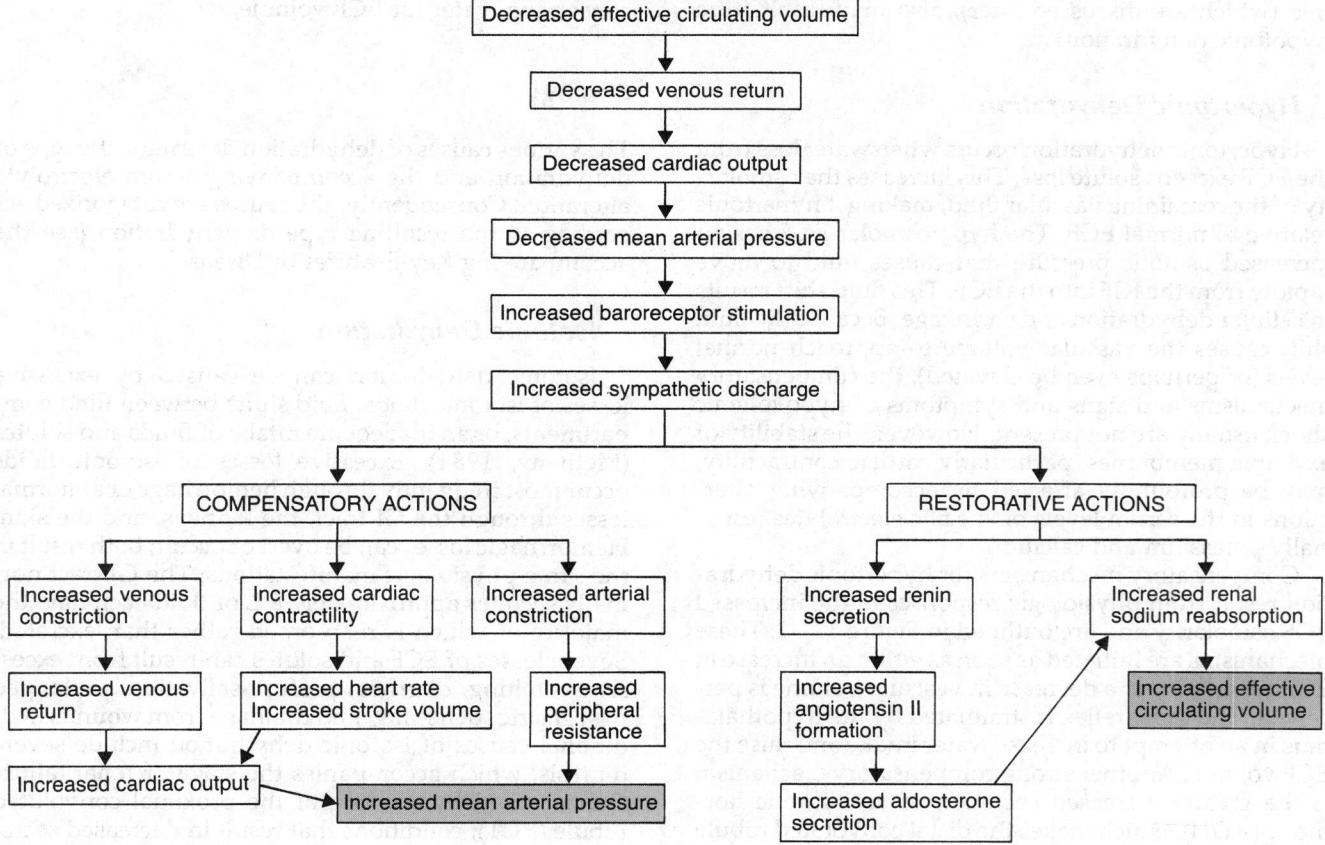

Figure 13–1

Compensatory mechanisms associated with isotonic dehydration.

to the central vascular space. These compensatory mechanisms are adequate to maintain a near-normal MAP until 25% to 30% of the vascular volume is lost. At that point, compensatory mechanisms are inadequate to maintain perfusion even to vital organs, and symptoms of severe hypovolemic shock are manifested.

Hypotonic Dehydration

Hypotonic dehydration involves the loss of solutes from the ECF in excess of water loss. This results in decreased osmolarity of the remaining ECF, making it hypotonic relative to normal ECF. The decreased ECF osmolarity causes the ECF to have a lower osmotic pressure than the ICF. As a result, water moves from the ECF into the ICF, creating a simultaneous vascular volume deficit and swelling of the cells. The vascular volume deficit results in the initiation of the same cardiovascular and SNS responses seen in isotonic dehydration.

The intracellular swelling can cause a variety of problems and symptoms, depending on which tissues sustain the influx of fluid. Generally, cells in specific areas of the brain are more sensitive to ICF changes than are the cells of other tissues and organs. Neurologic dysfunction may accompany hypotonic dehydration if swelling of brain cells occurs. In addition, specific electrolyte disorders, such as hyponatremia and hypokalemia (which are discussed later), also may result from hypotonic dehydration.

Hypertonic Dehydration

Hypertonic dehydration occurs when water loss from the ECF exceeds solute loss. This increases the osmolarity of the remaining vascular fluid, making it hypertonic relative to normal ECF. The hyperosmolar ECF has an increased osmotic pressure that causes fluid to move rapidly from the ICF into the ECF. This fluid shift results in cellular dehydration and shrinkage. Because the fluid shift causes the vascular volume to approach normal levels (or perhaps even be elevated), the compensatory mechanisms and signs and symptoms of hypovolemic shock usually are not present. However, the stability of excitable membranes, particularly cardiac contractility, may be profoundly affected by accompanying alterations in the serum levels of specific electrolytes (especially potassium and calcium).

Compensatory mechanisms for hypertonic dehydration result from physiologic responses to the increased ECF osmolarity and are outlined in Figure 13–2. These mechanisms are initiated as soon as either an increase in ECF osmolarity or a decrease in vascular volume is perceived. The thirst reflex is stimulated by the hypothalamus in an attempt to increase water intake and raise the ECF volume. Another strong compensatory mechanism is the greatly increased secretion of antidiuretic hormone (ADH), which makes the distal convoluted tubule (DCT) and the collecting duct of the nephron much more permeable to water and enhances renal reabsorp-

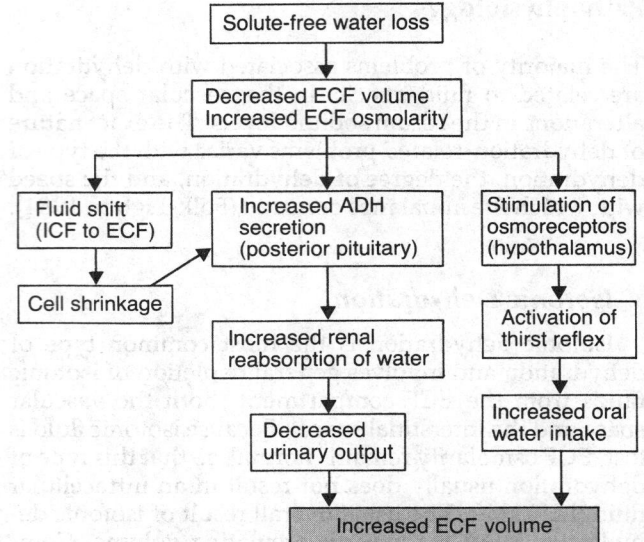

Figure 13–2

Compensatory mechanisms associated with hypertonic dehydration.

tion of water. This action decreases urinary output, thus conserving water for ECF volume.

Etiology

The various causes of dehydration determine the type of dehydration and the accompanying serum electrolyte alteration. Consequently, the causes are categorized according to the resulting type of dehydration (see the accompanying Key Features of Disease).

Isotonic Dehydration

Isotonic dehydration can be caused by excessive losses of isotonic fluids, fluid shifts between fluid compartments, or an inadequate intake of fluids and solutes (Metheny, 1984). Excessive losses of isotonic fluids occur most frequently through hemorrhage or abnormal losses through the GI tract, the kidneys, and the skin. Hemorrhagic losses can be overt or occult; both result in the same physiologic manifestations. The GI tract normally secretes approximately 8 L of fluid each day, the majority of which is reabsorbed rather than excreted. Severe losses of ECF and solutes can result from excessive vomiting, diarrhea, profuse salivation, prolonged nasogastric suctioning, and drainage from wounds. Additional causes of isotonic dehydration include severe diuresis, which accompanies the stage of renal failure characterized by scarring of the proximal convoluted tubule (PCT); conditions that result in decreased secretion of aldosterone (such as Addison disease's or adrenalectomy); and diuretic therapy.

KEY FEATURES OF DISEASE ■ Common Causes of Dehydration

Isotonic Dehydration

Hemorrhage
Vomiting
Diarrhea
Profuse salivation
Fistulas
Abscesses
Ileostomy
Cecostomy
Frequent enemas
Profuse diaphoresis
Burns
Severe wounds
Long-term NPO
Diuretic therapy
GI suction

Hypotonic Dehydration

Chronic illness
Excessive fluid replacement (hypotonic)
Renal failure
Chronic or severe malnutrition

Hypertonic Dehydration

Hyperventilation
Watery diarrhea
Renal failure
Ketoacidosis
Diabetes insipidus
Excessive fluid replacement (hypertonic)
Excessive NaHCO₃ administration
Tube feedings
Dysphagia
Impaired thirst
Unconsciousness
Fever
Impaired motor function
Systemic infection

Decreased intake of fluids and electrolytes also can result in the development of isotonic dehydration. This cause is most common among clients with motor impairments, those with a decreased level of consciousness, and those clients who receive nothing by mouth (NPO) for several days (Kennedy-Caldwell, 1986). This risk increases among clients who also have conditions such as infection or fever.

Fluid shifts from the vascular space to the interstitial space account for specific incidences of isotonic dehydration. These shifts most commonly occur as a result of increased capillary permeability or increased capillary hydrostatic pressure, which is often associated with the release of vasoactive amines, such as histamines, kinins, and serotonin (Guyton, 1987). Specific conditions that are associated with fluid shifts include extensive trauma, burns, sepsis, peritonitis, intestinal obstruction, and cirrhosis of the liver.

Hypotonic Dehydration

Hypotonic dehydration is relatively rare and is usually associated with chronic illness. Chronic renal failure, in which the kidneys are unable to concentrate solutes and specifically waste sodium, may lead to a loss of solute in excess of fluids (Leaf & Cotran, 1985). Chronic malnutrition and excessive administration of hypotonic fluids also are possible causes of hypotonic dehydration.

Hypertonic Dehydration

Hypertonic dehydration results from the loss of any body fluid that is hypotonic (lower osmolarity or fewer solute particles than isotonic body fluids). The most common cause of hypertonic dehydration is related to conditions that greatly increase insensible fluid loss. These conditions include excessive loss from the respiratory system during hyperventilation, ketoacidosis, and excessive skin water evaporation during high or prolonged fevers. The fluid lost from the skin when fever is present is not the same as normal perspiration or diaphoretic fluid. Normal perspiration is nearly isotonic, containing a variety of solutes, including sodium and chloride. This fluid is visible on the skin as it is lost from the body. The fluid lost from the skin during fever is hypotonic (almost pure water). This water evaporates so quickly that it usually cannot be detected visually on the skin. Other instances of hypotonic body fluid loss that contribute to the development of hypertonic dehydration include drainage of copious secretions from tracheostomies, watery diarrhea, renal failure in which water reabsorption is impaired, diabetes insipidus, and ketoacidosis in the diuretic phase.

In addition to these obvious mechanisms of hypotonic water loss, any condition that increases the body's metabolic rate also increases the body's need for water in oxidation reactions. Other causes of hypertonic dehydration include excessive intravenous (IV) infusions of hypertonic fluids (especially those containing sodium bicarbonate [NaHCO₃]), and long-term intake of high-osmolarity feeding solutions via tube without additional water intake (Metheny & Snively, 1983). Conditions that impair the awareness of thirst or interfere with the ability to obtain water or swallow also can contribute to the development of hypertonic dehydration.

Incidence

Illness can be defined as an abnormal biologic functioning of the body's organs or systems. The biologic func-

KEY FEATURES OF DISEASE ■ Risk Factors for Dehydration

Illnesses

Vomiting
Diarrhea
Burns
Large draining wounds
Liver dysfunction
Diabetes mellitus
Diabetes insipidus
Renal disease
Hemorrhage
Major venous obstruction
Prolonged febrile state

Other Situations

Extremes of age
Elderly, infants
Unconsciousness
Motor limitations

Therapies

Surgery
Diuretics
NPO
Excessive hypertonic enemas
Nasogastric suction

tion of most organs and systems influences fluid and electrolyte balance. Although the actual incidence of dehydration is not known, virtually every client who is ill is at risk (see the accompanying Key Features of Disease).

PREVENTION

Prevention of dehydration is aimed at identifying clients at risk so that appropriate interventions can be instituted early. After the clients at risk are identified, the nurse's responsibilities include educating the client and assisting the client to maintain an adequate intake of fluid and electrolytes to meet the body's needs. Fluid needs vary, depending on the client's age, body size, and metabolic rate and the degree of fluid loss experienced by the individual client. Although formulas exist for calculating average fluid needs, these are based on fixed physical dimensions and do not take into consideration fluctuations in metabolism and the presence of fluid loss conditions that also influence the body's fluid needs. Therefore, the best indicators of an individual client's state of hydration and fluid needs are the physical assessment findings. Because conditions can change rap-

idly in individuals at risk for dehydration, a major nursing responsibility for prevention of dehydration in susceptible clients is *frequent assessment* of those measures that indicate the state of hydration.

The clients most obviously at risk for dehydration are those with acute or chronic illnesses involving fluid losses, increased rates of metabolism, temperature elevations greater than 102° F for longer than 6 hours, or hyperventilation. Elderly clients are always at risk for dehydration. With age, the kidney loses its ability to concentrate urine, predisposing the elderly to increased fluid loss and requiring increased fluid intake. The average fluid requirement of the well elderly client is 1500 to 2000 mL of hypotonic fluid per day. Conditions that contribute to an inadequate fluid intake among the elderly include a diminished sensation of thirst and difficulty with ambulation or other motor activities involved in fluid intake (Porth, 1986).

COLLABORATIVE MANAGEMENT

 Assessment

History

The nurse collects data regarding risk factors, as well as causative factors, related to dehydration. *Age* is an important consideration, as both the very young and the elderly are prone to develop dehydration in response to relatively small fluid losses. In addition, the elderly are more likely to have chronic illnesses or to be taking medications that can lead to fluid and electrolyte imbalances. *Height* and *weight* are important measurements for calculating approximate fluid needs. If these data are not known or if the client is confused, the nurse obtains these measurements directly. Because weight and liquid measurements are related, changes in weight are good indicators of fluid losses or excesses. One liter of water weighs approximately 1 kg. Therefore, a weight change of 1 lb corresponds to a fluid volume change of 475 to 500 mL.

The nurse questions the client regarding changes in the degree of tightness of clothing, rings, and shoes. A sudden decrease in the tightness may well indicate dehydration, although an increase in the tightness may reflect a fluid shift to the interstitial space with an accompanying deficit in the vascular space. Other information relevant to cardiovascular changes associated with dehydration includes the presence of palpitations or a feeling of lightheadedness on moving from a lying or a sitting position to a standing position.

The nurse also obtains data regarding any *abnormal or excessive fluid losses*, such as perspiration, diarrhea, bleeding, vomiting, urination, salivation, and wound drainage. The nurse questions clients regarding *chronic illnesses, recent acute illnesses, recent surgery,* and *medication usage*. Not only does this information indicate potential risk for or possible causes of dehydration, but it also may indicate the presence of specific problems that have an impact on how the state of dehydration should be corrected. If the client is uncertain about this information or is confused, the nurse collects this information from recent or updated inpatient or outpatient records. An additional reliable source for such information is the client's significant other or a close family member.

Clients are asked specific questions concerning *urinary output,* including the frequency and amount of voidings. The nurse asks questions about the client's usual fluid intake and the intake during the previous 24 hours. Information about the types of fluids ingested is just as important to obtain as the amount of fluids ingested. The nurse inquires about the amount of *strenuous physical activity* the client may have engaged in recently and collects information regarding whether the activity took place under environmental conditions that included high temperatures or low humidity.

Physical Assessment: Clinical Manifestations

The clinical manifestations of dehydration are dependent on which fluid compartments sustain fluid losses, although all body systems are affected to some degree (see the accompanying Key Features of Disease). The most obvious and life-threatening clinical manifestations are seen when the dehydration involves significant fluid deficits from the vascular (plasma) portion of the extracellular space.

Cardiovascular changes are the most reliable indicators of changes in the plasma volume, although electrocardiographic (ECG) changes usually are noted only when dehydration is accompanied by an electrolyte imbalance. The heart rate increases with vascular or plasma volume deficits. The peripheral pulses are weaker, are difficult to find, and are easily obliterated with light pressure. If interstitial edema accompanies the vascular dehydration, the peripheral pulses may not be palpable. Blood pressure decreases, as does the pulse pressure, with a greater decrease being present in the systolic blood pressure. Hypotension is more profound in the standing position than in the sitting or the lying position. This type of unstable blood pressure is called *postural hypotension,* or *orthostatic hypotension.* Because the blood pressure in the standing position may be significantly lower than that in other positions, blood pressure is first measured with the client in the lying position, then in the sitting position, and lastly in the standing position.

Another cardiovascular indicator of hydration status is the degree of *neck and hand veins filling.* Normally, hand veins fill and become engorged when the hands are lower than the level of the heart. As the hand is raised above the level of the heart, the veins flatten or collapse. Neck veins are normally distended when a client is in the supine position. These veins tend to flatten as a sitting position is approached. When dehydration involves a plasma volume deficit, neck and hand veins are flat, even when these structures are dependent

---

KEY FEATURES OF DISEASE ■ Clinical Manifestations of Dehydration

Manifestations of Dehydration in General*

Cardiovascular

Increased pulse rate
Thready pulse quality
Decreased blood pressure
Postural hypotension
Flat neck and hand veins in dependent positions
Diminished peripheral pulses

Respiratory

Increased respiratory rate
Increased depth of respirations

Neuromuscular

Decreased central nervous system activity (lethargy to coma)
Fever

Renal

Decreased urinary output
Increased specific gravity

Integumentary

Skin dry and scaly
Turgor poor, tenting present
Mouth dry and fissured, paste-like coating present

Gastrointestinal

Decreased motility
Diminished bowel sounds
Constipation
Thirst

Manifestations of Hypotonic Dehydration

Skeletal muscle weakness

Manifestations of Hypertonic Dehydration

Hyperactive deep tendon reflexes
Increased sensation of thirst
Pitting edema

*These manifestations are most severe with hypotonic dehydration.

---

to the heart. The cardiovascular changes listed earlier are not seen in states of dehydration in which plasma volume is normal or above normal, such as hypertonic dehydration.

Respiratory rate increases directly with the degree of

fluid loss from the plasma volume. When ketoacidosis causes or accompanies the dehydration, the respirations become deep and rapid. This type of respiratory pattern is called Kussmaul's breathing.

Integumentary changes may be useful indicators of the state of hydration. The nurse assesses the integumentary system for changes in the skin and mucous membranes that may indicate dehydration. Specific factors to assess include skin color, the degree of moisture, turgor, and the presence of edema. In the elderly, this information may be less reliable because this population may have poor skin turgor as a result of the loss of elastic tissue and the loss of tissue fluids related to the aging process.

The nurse assesses skin turgor by noting (1) how easily the skin (over the back of the hand and over the sternum) can be gently pinched between the thumb and the forefinger (this maneuver is called tenting); (2) how soon the pinched skin resumes its normal position after release; (3) whether depressions (pits) remain in the skin after a finger is pressed firmly but gently (over the shin, over the sternum, and over the sacrum); (4) how deep the depression is (in millimeters); and (5) how long the depression remains. In generalized dehydration, skin turgor is poor, with the "tent" remaining for minutes after pinching up the skin, and skin depressions do not occur with gentle pressure. The skin has a dry or scaly appearance. Mucous membranes are not moist. They may be covered with a thick, sticky, paste-like coating or even have cracks and fissures. The surface of the tongue may have deep furrows.

When interstitial edema accompanies dehydration, the skin may be so firm that pinching the skin between the thumb and the forefinger is difficult or impossible. Another integumentary indication of an accompanying interstitial edema is that gentle pressure results in the formation of pits or depressions that require minutes to resume normal shape. When edema is present, skin color usually is pale.

Renal system indicators of the state of hydration primarily are concerned with the volume and the composition of urinary output. The nurse closely monitors *urinary output,* comparing the total output with the total fluid intake and daily weight. Accurate measurements of intake and output are a major nursing responsibility. A urinary output below 500 mL/day for any client without renal disease is cause for concern. Clients with fluid imbalance are weighed daily, at the same time and with the same scales each day. For the sake of accuracy, the client should be wearing the same amount and type of clothing for each weigh-in. Usually, catabolic tissue loss (even in starvation) only accounts for about 0.5 lb of weight loss each day. Therefore, any weight loss in excess of this amount is considered fluid loss.

Psychosocial Assessment

The nurse observes the client for behavioral changes that accompany dehydration. Initially, the client may have a flat affect and seem unconcerned or indifferent about the state of health and possible treatment regimens. As dehydration becomes more severe the client's psychosocial activities reflect abnormal functioning of the central nervous system (CNS). The client may experience apprehension, restlessness, lethargy, and confusion. These behavioral changes are more obvious with hypertonic and hypotonic dehydration because of the ICF shifts occurring directly in the brain cells, resulting in shrinkage or swelling. If the conditions causing the dehydration continue, circulation to cerebral tissues becomes so impaired that delirium and coma can result.

Laboratory Findings

No single laboratory test result confirms or rules out the state of dehydration. Instead, a diagnosis of dehydration must be interpreted from a variety of laboratory data in conjunction with the presenting signs and symptoms. Changes in serum laboratory values depend on the type of dehydration present (see the accompanying Key Features of Disease). Isotonic dehydration and hypotonic dehydration states that have an accompanying plasma volume deficit usually are manifested both as hemoconcentration, with elevated levels of hemoglobin and increased hematocrit, and as increased serum osmolarity, with increased levels of glucose, protein, blood urea nitrogen (BUN), and various electrolytes. Hemoconcentration is not evident in situations in which dehydration is the result of hemorrhage, because there is loss of all vascular products (Keyes, 1985).

Specific urine laboratory values may be of some assistance in diagnosing dehydration if the client does not have associated renal disease or if alterations in renal function have not contributed to the development of dehydration. Usually the urine of clients experiencing dehydration is highly concentrated, with a specific gravity greater than 1.030. The volume is decreased, and the osmolarity is greatly increased. Usually the color is dark amber, and a strong odor is evident.

 ### Analysis: Nursing Diagnosis

Many clients are at risk for dehydration as a result of illness or specific treatments. Age and socioeconomic factors also can increase a particular client's risk. The typical client with dehydration is a 75-year-old man receiving diuretic therapy for a hypertensive condition. The following nursing diagnoses are derived from these data (Atkinson & Murray, 1986; Kim & Moritz, 1982).

Common Diagnoses

The following nursing diagnoses are common among hospitalized clients with dehydration:

1. Fluid volume deficit related to excessive fluid loss or inadequate fluid intake
2. Altered oral mucous membrane related to inadequate oral secretions

KEY FEATURES OF DISEASE ■ Laboratory Values in Dehydration*

Values	Isotonic Dehydration	Hypotonic Dehydration	Hypertonic Dehydration
Blood Values†			
BUN	Normal or increased	Increased	Increased
Creatinine	Normal or increased	Increased	Increased
Sodium	Normal	<120 mEq	>150 mEq
Osmolarity	Normal	Decreased	Increased
Hematocrit	Increased	Increased	Normal or decreased
Hemoglobin	Increased	Increased	Normal or decreased
WBC	Increased	Increased	Normal or decreased
Protein	Increased	Increased	Increased
Urine Values			
Specific gravity	>1.010	<1.010	>1.010
Osmolarity	Increased	Decreased	Increased
Volume	Decreased	Increased	Decreased

*All values reflect dehydration states alone and not the underlying organ pathologic changes or disease states contributing to the development of the dehydration.
†BUN, blood urea nitrogen; WBC, white blood cell count.

Additional Diagnoses

In addition to the common diagnoses, one or more of the following nursing diagnoses may be applicable to the client with dehydration:

1. Constipation related to decreased body fluids
2. Potential for injury (fall) related to postural hypotension
3. Decreased cardiac output related to insufficient plasma volume
4. Knowledge deficit related to medication regimen and preventive measures
5. Potential impaired skin integrity related to deficiencies of interstitial fluid and inadequate tissue perfusion
6. Ineffective airway clearance related to thick, tenacious secretions
7. Activity intolerance related to hypotension

Planning and Implementation

The following plan of care for the client experiencing dehydration focuses on the common nursing diagnoses associated with general fluid volume deficit and plasma volume deficit. This plan is aimed at restoration of normal fluid balance, prevention of future fluid imbalances, supportive care until the current imbalance is resolved, and improvement in the client's comfort level.

Fluid Volume Deficit

Planning: client goals. The major goals for this nursing diagnosis are that the client will (1) have body fluid levels restored to normal and (2) comply with the prescribed medical regimen.

Interventions: nonsurgical management. Interventions are aimed at preventing further excessive fluid losses and increasing the body fluid compartment volumes to within normal ranges. Drugs and diet therapy are the methods of choice for this problem.

Drug therapy. Drug therapy for dehydration focuses on directly restoring the fluid balance, along with controlling the factors and conditions contributing to the development of dehydration. Whenever possible, fluids are replaced by the oral route (see later discussion of diet therapy). When dehydration is severe and complications are life-threatening, IV fluid replacement may be necessary in addition to or in place of oral fluid replacement. Calculation of the volume of replacement fluids needed is based on both the weight loss and the presenting symptoms. The rate of fluid replacement is dependent on the client's present degree of dehydration and the presence of pre-existing cardiac, pulmonary, or renal problems.

The type of fluid administered varies with the type of dehydration present and the cardiovascular status of the client. The desired outcome of the therapy is both appropriate fluid replacement and normal volumes in all body fluid compartments. Usually this therapy involves administering IV infusions of water with whatever solutes (especially electrolytes) are determined necessary, based on laboratory values. Table 13–1 lists the electrolyte content of common IV fluids. Generally, isotonic dehydration is treated with isotonic fluid solutions, hypertonic dehydration is treated with hypotonic fluid solutions, and hypotonic dehydration is treated with hypertonic fluid solutions. Clients who have lost proteins (colloids) from the vascular space (such as can occur with hemorrhage or in conditions that permit movement of proteins and fluid from the vascular space into the interstitial space) may require protein replacement either before or along with the replacement of fluids.

Drug therapy for dehydration includes the use of medications to ameliorate or correct the underlying cause of the dehydration. Antidiarrheal medications are appropriate when excessive diarrhea contributes to the development of dehydration. Antiemetics to control vomiting may be necessary when excessive vomiting produces dehydration. Antipyretics to reduce body temperature can be of value when high or prolonged fever contributes to the development of dehydration.

Diet therapy. Mild to moderate dehydration may be successfully treated with oral fluid replacement, provided that the client is alert enough to swallow and can tolerate oral fluids. Any substance that is liquid at body temperature is considered in measuring the fluid intake (gelatin, ice pops, ice cream, and so forth). The specific type of fluid needed for replacement varies with the type of dehydration present.

Client compliance with the ingestion of oral replacement fluids can be enhanced by using fluids the client enjoys at fluid temperatures that the client is comfortable with, as well as by carefully timing the intake schedule. Dividing the total amount of fluids needed by shifts helps to more evenly meet fluid needs with less danger of overhydration. Offering the client small volumes of fluids every hour may increase client compliance by eliminating the uncomfortable feeling of fullness. Usually, alert clients with dehydration have the sensation of thirst and require minimal encouragement to meet fluid needs appropriately.

Clients who ingest solid foods also are obtaining some fluid from these foods; however, the amount of fluid in solid food is not enough to increase the client's fluid volume to normal when dehydration is present. In addition, restriction of specific foods, because of their electrolyte content, may be necessary, depending on the specific type of dehydration present as well as on whether an electrolyte imbalance also is present. For example, hypernatremia often accompanies hypertonic dehydration. In this situation the client needs to avoid foods and fluids with a high sodium content. Table 12–4 in Chapter 12 provides a list of the measured amount of sodium in common foods.

Altered Oral Mucous Membrane

Planning: client goals. The major goals for this nursing diagnosis are that the client will (1) experience less discomfort and (2) not experience complications, such as infections or altered nutrition, related to dry oral mucosa.

Interventions: nonsurgical management. The major interventions useful in achieving these client goals are

---

TABLE 13–1 Characteristics of Common Intravenous Therapy Solutions

Solution	Osmolarity (mOsm/L)	pH	Calories* (kcal)	Tonicity
0.9% saline	308	5	0	Isotonic
0.45% saline	154	5	0	Hypotonic
5% dextrose in water (D_5W)	272	3.5–6.5	170	Isotonic†
10% dextrose in water ($D_{10}W$)	500	3.5–6.5	340	Hypertonic†
5% dextrose in 0.9% saline	560	3.5–6.5	170	Hypertonic†
5% dextrose in 0.45% saline	406	4	170	Hypertonic†
5% dextrose in 0.225% saline	321	4	170	Isotonic†
Ringer's lactate	273	6.5	9	Isotonic
5% dextrose in Ringer's lactate	525	4.0–6.5	179	Hypertonic†

* Calories are calculated on the basis of a volume of 1000 mL.

† *Solution tonicity at the time of administration.* Within a short period of time after administration, the dextrose is metabolized and the tonicity of the infused solution decreases in proportion to the osmolarity or tonicity of the nondextrose components (electrolytes) within the water.

From Trissel L. (1988). *Handbook on injectable drugs* (5th ed.). Bethesda: American Society of Hospital Pharmacists.

associated with the restoration of normal fluid volume, the delivery of good oral hygiene, and an early diagnosis of complications. Even before the underlying cause of decreased mucosal secretions is identified or treated, the degree of discomfort caused by this condition can be diminished with appropriate nursing care.

Drug therapy.   Drug therapy to increase body fluids is the same as that discussed earlier for fluid volume deficit. Drug therapy for decreasing oral mucosal dryness is available but of dubious effectiveness. Commercial preparations of artificial saliva are available and can be used to relieve dry mouth sensations. However, the texture and consistency of many of these preparations is aesthetically unacceptable to some clients. In addition, these preparations should not be used for clients who have altered levels of consciousness.

Diet therapy.   The role of diet therapy as an intervention for mouth dryness is to stimulate oral mucosal cells to secrete normal lubricants and saliva by increasing fluid intake to an adequate level. Nursing actions to increase fluid intake are the same as those discussed earlier for fluid volume deficit.

Oral hygiene.   Nursing actions related to oral hygiene can directly increase client comfort. Lips should be kept clean and moistened with a petrolatum-based lubricant. The thick, sticky coating present in the oral cavity during episodes of dehydration increases the client's discomfort. This coating can be removed with frequent, good oral hygiene measures. Mouth care can include brushing and flossing, but is not limited to these activities. Brushing and flossing should be done gently so as not to damage tender oral tissues. The use of focused water pressure to clean the mouth is controversial because some dentists believe that the pressure can force debris into tissues and under the gums where decay can occur undetected. Another technique to clean the mouth is simply rinsing the mouth every hour. Commercial mouthwashes that contain alcohol should be avoided, as should glycerin-containing washes and swabs, because these products tend to dry the oral mucosa further and may cause increased discomfort by stinging or burning open fissures in the mucosa. Rinsing the mouth with dilute solutions of hydrogen peroxide two or three times per day is a good form of oral hygiene; however, when used more frequently, this treatment can increase oral dryness. Other solutions that can be safely used as frequently as the client wishes are tap water and normal saline. Clients may experience increased relief if these solutions are room temperature or lukewarm rather than cold.

Prevention of complications.   Mouth dryness contributes to the development of sores and fissures in the mucosa, providing a portal of entry for a multitude of pathogens. In addition, the thick, sticky coating is an excellent breeding ground for microorganisms. A major complication of mouth dryness is the development of a wide variety of oral infections. Nursing management of oral hygiene includes assessment of the integrity of the oral mucosa during every shift. The nurse reports the presence of any suspicious open lesion and obtains a physician's order for a culture.

A dry mouth can interfere with adequate nutrition. Not only do fissures and sores cause pain and discomfort during chewing and swallowing, but the coating may alter taste sensation and decrease appetite. To help maintain the client's nutrition at an appropriate level, the nurse offers oral hygiene right before meals or snacks. The nurse assists the client in menu selection to avoid foods that are highly spiced or mechanically hard. Bland, soft, cool foods are most easily tolerated when mouth dryness is present.

■ Discharge Planning

Home Care Preparation

No extensive home care preparations are necessary for clients with mild fluid and electrolyte imbalances and for those with fluid and/or electrolyte imbalances of sudden onset secondary to improper treatment or secondary to temporary conditions that promote loss or retention of fluid and/or specific electrolytes. The imbalance is corrected before discharge and, with minimal precautions, is unlikely to recur. Clients who are most likely to be discharged before the imbalance is completely corrected and who are prone to recurrent episodes of imbalance are those with other chronic pathologic conditions, such as renal insufficiency, diabetes, malignancy, adrenal insufficiency, and specific endocrine disorders. These clients often require long-term diet and drug therapy.

Client/Family Education

Education is a key factor in the prevention and early detection of fluid and electrolyte imbalances. The teaching plan for any client at risk for a specific fluid or electrolyte imbalance includes diet therapy, specific food and fluid restrictions, drug therapy, and the signs and symptoms of the specific imbalance. Education about diet includes a list of foods to avoid and a list of permissible foods. The nurse teaches clients to determine the electrolyte content of prepared foods and medications by carefully reading the labels. The nurse consults with the dietitian for assistance in providing information on the planning and preparation of palatable meals whenever a specific electrolyte restriction is necessary. An important consideration is to teach, whenever possible, the person who actually purchases and/or prepares the meals, as well as the client.

The nurse instructs the client and family about the signs and symptoms of the specific imbalance for which the client is at risk, as well as what specific information should be reported immediately to the primary health care provider. The nurse assesses the client's understanding of the schedule for taking prescribed medications and reinforces how often the client should have serum electrolyte levels assessed. The need for follow-up care and for adherence to prescribed medical regimens is stressed.

Psychosocial Preparation

For clients whose fluid and/or electrolyte imbalance is caused by acute illness or alterations in fluid volumes, psychosocial preparation is usually minimal. The client may be concerned about the degree of vulnerability to recurrent episodes. The nurse reassures the client that such a recurrence is unlikely unless the precipitating conditions and events are repeated. In addition, the nurse instructs the client in appropriate actions to take to prevent an imbalance when specific precipitating conditions exist.

Clients who are newly diagnosed with serious chronic health problems that increase the risk of developing specific fluid and/or electrolyte imbalances may have great difficulty in accepting such a diagnosis. Extensive counseling by experienced professionals is often necessary before acceptance and participation in self-care can begin. The nurse initiates this process by contacting the clinical nurse specialist with experience in the specific health problems of the client.

Clients whose fluid and/or electrolyte imbalance episodes are the result of long-term chronic health problems may have learned to cope well and may require less extensive psychosocial support. However, this situation cannot be assumed automatically. The nurse assesses each client's psychosocial needs individually for new factors, established support patterns, changes in life style, previous and current coping patterns, and stability of the chronic disease or underlying pathologic condition.

A major psychosocial issue for clients at risk of developing specific imbalances as a result of chronic illness is that of compliance. A difficult but necessary concept that the nurse must convey to the client is that quality of life depends to a great extent on the client's compliance with the planned medical regimen. Some aspects of the regimen may be unpleasant or may require significant self-control on the part of the client. Assisting the client and family to understand fully the disease process may increase the client's sense of control, self-worth, and willingness to cooperate. In conveying this information, the nurse focuses on the potential positive outcomes of good compliance rather than on the deleterious effects of poor control and noncompliance.

Health Care Resources

Clients with severe chronic health problems may be discharged to a nursing home or extended care facility on a permanent or a temporary basis. The hospital nurse assumes responsibility for communicating on the transfer chart all important information about the client's individualized needs and special care problems.

The client with chronic health problems frequently requires some assistance with or supervision of self-care at home. A home care nurse may be needed for such follow-up. The home care nurse is contacted before the client's discharge to assist in discharge planning and to assess the need for special equipment and/or supplies in the home. The home care nurse is given a copy of the client's individualized teaching plan to enable him or her to reinforce health care education initiated in the acute care setting.

Evaluation

Based on the identified nursing diagnoses, the nurse evaluates the care for the client experiencing dehydration. The expected outcomes for the client with dehydration include that the client

1. Ingests at least 1500 mL of hypotonic fluids each day
2. Maintains a fluid output that is approximately equal to fluid intake
3. Identifies the following signs and symptoms as indications of dehydration and the need for intervention:
   a. Urinary output less than half of fluid intake
   b. Weight loss of 2 lb or more in 24 hours
   c. Persistent rapid, thready pulse
   d. Dryness of mouth and mucous membranes
   e. Poor skin turgor
   f. Dizziness, lightheadedness, or the presence of bright spots in visual fields with rapid changes in position
4. Maintains skin integrity
5. Achieves an acceptable level of oral mucosal comfort
6. Avoids falls related to postural hypotension
7. Maintains blood pressure within a range identified as normal for the client's age, weight, and general state of health
8. States correctly the prescribed medical regimen with regard to dosage and administration schedule for medications and dietary restrictions

OVERHYDRATION

OVERVIEW

Overhydration is a state of body fluid excess. It is not an actual disease, rather overhydration is a clinical state or manifestation of a physiologic problem in which fluid intake exceeds fluid loss. The state of overhydration may be characterized as either an actual excess of total body fluid or a relative fluid excess in one or more fluid compartments. Three basic types of fluid volume excess are possible. These types are *isotonic overhydration,* in which isotonic fluids are ingested or retained, resulting in expansion of the ECF compartment only; *hypotonic overhydration* (water intoxication), in which hypotonic fluids are ingested or retained, resulting in expansion of both the ECF and the ICF compartments; and *hypertonic overhydration*, in which hypertonic fluids are ingested, resulting in expansion of the ECF compartment with contraction of the ICF compartment (Keyes, 1985). This chapter limits discussion of overhydration to the two most common types, isotonic overhydration and water intoxication.

Pathophysiology

The majority of problems associated with overhydration are related to fluid volume excesses in the vascular space or dilution of specific electrolytes and blood components. The exact nature and symptoms of the problems vary with the type of overhydration and the degree of overhydration.

Isotonic Overhydration

This type of overhydration also may be called *hypervolemia*, because the problems associated with it are purely a result of excess fluid in the ECF compartment. Electrolyte dilution is not a factor, although serum protein and cellular component concentrations may be altered. In isotonic overhydration, water and solutes (especially sodium) are increased proportionately, so that osmolarity remains normal. Under these conditions, fluid does not shift between the extracellular and the intracellular compartments. The primary effects of isotonic overhydration are *circulatory overload* and *interstitial edema* (Rossi & Cadnapaphornchai, 1987).

Mild to moderate acute overhydration among healthy individuals rarely has serious consequences, because the body has several compensatory mechanisms to handle the extra fluid so that major organs are neither compromised nor overburdened. As shown in Figure 13–3, when the vascular volume increases and osmolarity remains normal, MAP and vascular hydrostatic pressure both increase. The increased volume coupled with an increased MAP results in an increased venous return and stretching of the myocardium. According to Starling's law of the heart, the greater the stretch of the myocardium is, the more forceful the ventricular contraction and the greater the cardiac output are (Guyton, 1987). The effects of this principle are evident during the early stages of isotonic overhydration or when the client has normal cardiac and renal function. In addition, the increased MAP stimulates an increase in renal blood flow and glomerular filtration. This reaction causes both water and sodium to be excreted, assisting in the resolution of overhydration (Lancaster, 1987). The increased hydrostatic pressure also compensates for the overhydration both by increasing the capacitance of the venous system and by causing the formation of visible edema as fluid is forced from the vascular space into the interstitial space.

When isotonic overhydration becomes severe or prolonged, or when it occurs in an individual with a poor cardiac status, overhydration results in congestive heart failure and pulmonary edema, with inadequate oxygenation of many tissues. Cardiac output actually decreases as the myocardium stretches beyond the optimal point, and recoil is minimal. The left ventricle then is unable to eject blood efficiently. More blood remains in the left ventricle than is ejected from it, causing a pressure increase in the left ventricle. Pressure in the left ventricle builds, forcing blood to dam up first in the left atrium and then in the pulmonary blood vessels. As the hydrostatic pressure in the pulmonary vessels increases, fluid is forced into the pulmonary interstitial spaces and into the alveoli, creating pulmonary edema (Price & Wilson, 1986).

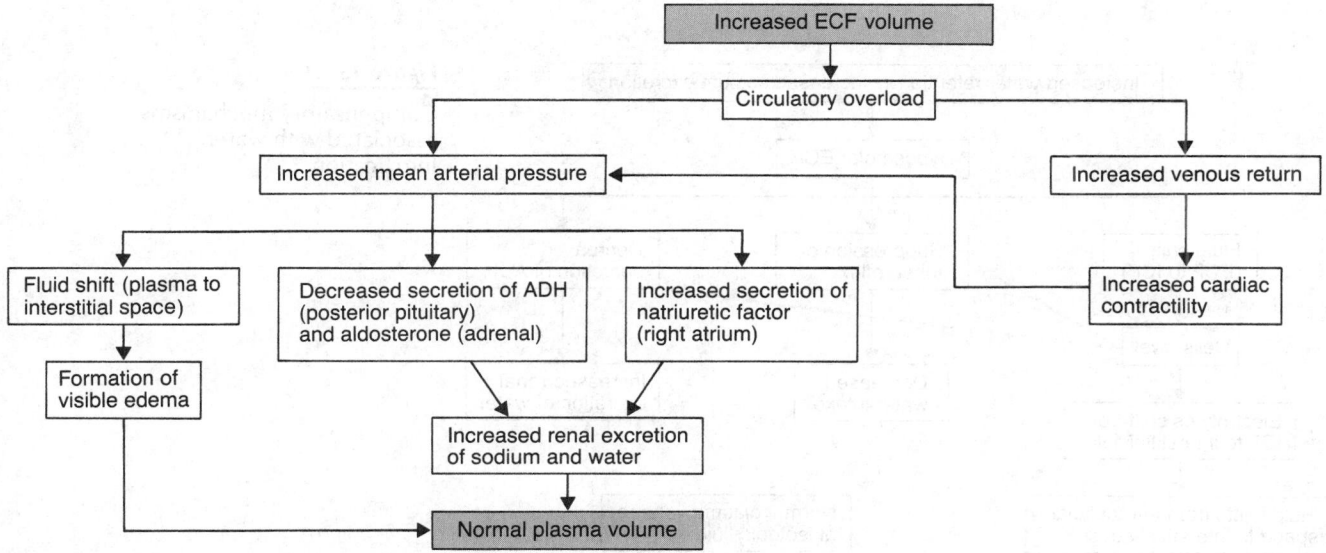

Figure 13–3

Compensatory mechanisms associated with hypervolemia.

Hypotonic Overhydration (Water Intoxication)

In this type of overhydration, the excess fluid is hypotonic to normal body fluids, so that the osmolarity of the ECF is decreased as the hydrostatic pressure is increased. Because osmotic pressure is directly related to osmolarity, the decreased vascular osmolarity causes a decrease in the vascular osmotic pressure (Fig. 13–4). In this situation, the excess fluid moves into the intracellular space as a result of the decreased vascular osmotic pressure. Thus, with hypotonic overhydration, all body fluid compartments experience expansion. Because the excess fluid is hypotonic, electrolyte imbalances as a result of dilution usually accompany hypotonic overhydration. The effects of hypotonic overhydration are related to *circulatory overload, interstitial edema, cellular edema,* and specific *electrolyte dilution.*

Etiology

The conditions leading to the development of overhydration usually are related to excessive intake or inadequate excretion of fluid. Conditions or situations that result in excessive fluid intake include excessive oral ingestion of water, poorly controlled IV therapy, excessive irrigation of any body cavity with hypotonic fluids, and the replacement of isotonic fluid losses with hypotonic fluids (Price & Wilson, 1986). Conditions in which inadequate excretion of fluid leads to hypotonic overhydration include some types of renal failure, any condition in which cardiac output and MAP are inadequate to maintain renal perfusion (such as congestive heart failure), and conditions that cause ADH to be secreted inappropriately. Such conditions include severe stress, trauma, surgery, intense pain, inflammation, and malignant states, as well as the use of certain drugs (morphine sulfate and cyclophosphamide [Cytoxan]) and excessive use of corticosteroids. Hypotonic overhydration also can occur when fluid shifts either from the interstitial fluid compartment or from the intracellular fluid compartment into the vascular space. In this situation, the client experiences many of the problems of overhydration without an actual increase in the amount of total body water.

Incidence

Because the body has several well-regulated compensatory mechanisms for handling fluid volume excesses, physiologic problems associated with overhydration rarely occur among healthy individuals. For overhydration to cause problems among healthy individuals, the fluid excess must be both acute and severe. Overhydration occurs most frequently among individuals with cardiac or renal problems that interfere with normal compensatory mechanisms for handling excess fluids. The serious complications of overhydration occur more quickly among individuals who are elderly, malnourished, or debilitated or those who have chronic illness. Other clients at risk include anyone with excessive secretion of ADH, such as can be seen as a response to severe physical or emotional stress.

Any client receiving IV fluids is at risk for overhydration as a result of improperly managed IV therapy. Although this situation occurs too frequently among hospitalized clients, it is the type that is most easily prevented by good nursing care.

PREVENTION

Prevention of overhydration is aimed at identifying clients at risk so that appropriate interventions can be

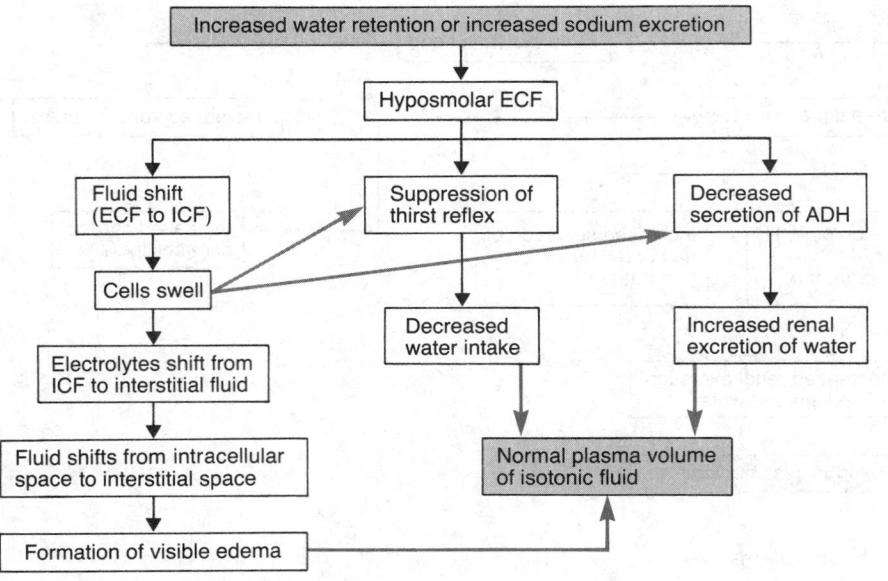

Figure 13–4

Compensatory mechanisms associated with water intoxication.

instituted early. Careful calculation of fluid needs and rigorous regulation of IV therapy can eliminate accidental overhydration of the hospitalized client. Not only should fluid losses be replaced with the appropriate amount of fluids, but also the composition and osmolarity of the replacement fluid should match those of the fluid lost. For example, all too often isotonic fluid losses are replaced with solutions of water containing 5% dextrose (D_5W). Although this solution has an osmolarity of about 300 mOsm at the time of administration, the dextrose is metabolized rapidly, and only the hypotonic water remains in the vascular space.

Because water can enter the body by osmosis through special tissues, whenever possible only isosmotic solutions should come into contact with these tissues. Solutions of 0.9% sodium chloride should be used in place of tap water or distilled water for enemas, nasogastric tube irrigations, and wound irrigations. Clients who are allowed ice chips should be given ice chips made from an oral electrolyte-balanced solution instead of tap water.

COLLABORATIVE MANAGEMENT

 Assessment

History

In obtaining a history from the client, the nurse collects data regarding risk factors, as well as causative factors, related to the development of fluid imbalances, including overhydration. *Age* is an important factor, as both the very young and the elderly are more prone to fluid disturbances. Not only are the elderly more likely to have other chronic conditions that can lead to fluid imbalances (especially renal dysfunction and cardiac decompensation), but they are also more likely to be taking medications that influence fluid and electrolyte balance. In addition, the elderly client may experience transient or continuous neurologic impairment that interferes with judgment and self-care activities. *Height* and *weight* are measured accurately on admission, not only because fluid increases are reflected in weight increases, but also because smaller-statured individuals are at greater risk of experiencing fluid imbalances than are larger-statured individuals. The total body fluid volume of a small individual is less, and any increase or decrease of fluid volume represents a greater proportional disturbance than the same increase or decrease in a larger individual. The nurse inquires about recent changes in weight, especially sudden weight gain. Clients are asked about noticeable swelling or tightness of rings, shoes, and clothing.

The nurse asks specific questions regarding *urinary output,* including the frequency and amount of voidings. The nurse asks questions regarding actual fluid intake and output in general and specifically during the previous 24 hours. The nurse inquires about the use of over-the-counter (OTC) and prescribed *medications,* especially diuretics, antacids, laxatives, and morphine. If the client is unable to recall exactly what medications are being taken, the nurse obtains this information from the client's family and from the client's most recent inpatient and outpatient records. The nurse questions the client about the presence of *disease states* and recent *therapeutic interventions.* Common interventions that may lead to overhydration include IV therapy, enemas, irrigations, and surgery (Metheny & Snively, 1978).

The nurse obtains a detailed *diet history* to determine approximate levels of sodium, protein, and sugar intake. Obtaining a dietary recall, including snacks and beverages, of the previous 24 hours is helpful in determining fluid intake and the intake of specific substances that stimulate thirst.

The nurse also collects data that may indicate the presence of actual symptoms associated with overhydration. When the client's responses are limited or not reliable, these questions are directed to a close family member. Positive answers to questions regarding the presence of the following symptoms may indicate overhydration. The client is asked whether headaches, behavior changes, increased somnolence, decreased alertness, decreased attention span, anorexia, diarrhea, or increasing fatigue have been experienced. Information about the presence of edema or changes in skin turgor is obtained. The nurse asks the client or a responsible family member to relate the client's activity during the previous 24 hours to disclose additional information about activity intolerance, unusual behavior, and the presence of increasing or unexplained fatigue. The nurse directly asks whether the client has a history of any *psychiatric disorder* involving compulsive behavior and excessive fluid intake.

Physical Assessment: Clinical Manifestations

Clinical manifestations of overhydration vary with the specific type of overhydration present, the fluid compartments that are expanded, and the degree of overhydration present (see the accompanying Key Features of Disease). The client experiencing isotonic overhydration primarily manifests problems and symptoms associated with circulatory overload and the formation of interstitial edema. The client experiencing hypotonic overhydration may have some problems associated with circulatory overload, but primarily manifests problems and symptoms associated with intracellular volume expansion and electrolyte dilution imbalances.

Isotonic overhydration. Because the primary symptoms of isotonic overhydration (hypervolemia) are related to circulatory overload and the formation of visible edema, the nurse assesses these variables first. In the compensatory stages of hypervolemia, cardiac output is increased. Pulse rate is increased, and the pulse has a bounding quality. Peripheral pulses are difficult to obliterate. Systolic and diastolic blood pressures are elevated. As the condition continues, the diastolic pressure continues to increase at a faster rate than the systolic

KEY FEATURES OF DISEASE ■ Common Clinical Manifestations of Overhydration

Manifestations of Overhydration in General

Cardiovascular

Increased pulse rate
Bounding pulse quality
Peripheral pulses full
Elevated blood pressure
Decreased pulse pressure
Elevated central venous pressure
Distended neck and hand veins
Engorged venous varicosities

Respiratory

Respiratory rate increased
Shallow respirations
Dyspnea increases with exertion or in supine position
Moist rales (crackles) present on auscultation

Integumentary

Pitting edema in dependent areas
Skin pale and cool to touch

Neuromuscular

Altered level of consciousness
Headache
Visual disturbances
Skeletal muscle weakness
Paresthesias

Gastrointestinal

Increased motility

Manifestations of Isotonic Overhydration

Liver enlargement
Ascites formation

Manifestations of Hypotonic Overhydration

Polyuria
Diarrhea
Nonpitting edema
Cardiac arrhythmias associated with electrolyte dilution
Projectile vomiting

pressure, so that the pulse pressure decreases. Venous pressure increases, and veins become distended. Distention is most noticeable in the neck veins, and these may remain distended even when the client is in the fully upright position. Hand veins are distended in the dependent position and may remain distended for more than 5 seconds after the hand is elevated above the level of the heart. Central venous pressure also becomes elevated as the condition continues or worsens. The client may complain that any pre-existing varicosity is increased at this time. Hemorrhoids may become greatly enlarged and cause the client considerable discomfort. In cases of severe isotonic overhydration, the liver becomes enlarged (it is easily palpated below the right anterior rib cage) and fluid collects in the abdominal cavity (ascites is present) (Robbins & Kumar, 1987; Watson, 1987).

As pressure in the left ventricle increases and ejection fraction decreases, less blood leaves the left ventricle. Venous return to the cardiac system, coupled with decreased left ventricular output, causes blood to back up in the pulmonary blood vessels and increases pulmonary hydrostatic pressure. The increased hydrostatic pressure causes fluid to move into the pulmonary interstitial spaces and the alveoli. The presence of fluid in these areas increases the diffusing distance for gas exchange and makes oxygenation more difficult. Pulmonary edema can be detected on auscultation as moist rales (crackles) on inhalation. The respiratory rate may increase, and the client becomes noticeably short of breath.

The greatly increased hydrostatic pressure contributes to the formation of visible edema. The edema is first noted in dependent areas and characteristically forms pits when pressure is applied to displace the fluid. The nurses assesses the hands, feet, and lower legs for the presence of pitting edema in the client who spends more time in the sitting or standing positions. The nurse assesses the sacral area, the back, and the lower arms for pitting edema in the client who spends more time in the supine position. When edema is present, the nurse notes how extensive the edema is, how deep the pits are, and how long it takes pits to disappear after pressure is released. Edema formation progresses as the overhydration continues and compensatory mechanisms fail. The edema becomes generalized and may progress so that fluid "weeps" through the skin (Robbins & Kumar, 1987). The skin is pale, is cool to the touch, and may feel clammy.

Hypotonic overhydration. Because the fluid in hypotonic overhydration affects all body fluid compartments down a concentration gradient, the fluid is distributed relatively evenly throughout the body, and a dilution effect is present. Overhydration is not confined to the extracellular space with subsequent hypervolemia. Therefore, the clinical manifestations associated with hypotonic overhydration (water intoxication) are a result of intracellular edema (especially of the brain cells) and dilution of specific ECF electrolytes.

Alterations in cerebral and upper neural functions are obvious consequences of hypotonic overhydration. The nurse assesses the client's neurologic status by first determining the client's level of consciousness and orientation to time, place, and person. Notations are made regarding whether the client is asleep or awake. If the client is asleep, the nurse gently awakens him/her and documents the ease with which the client is aroused. When the client is awake, the nurse establishes whether or not the client is oriented. The nurse avoids asking questions that can be answered with a "yes" or "no" response and documents the manner in which the client responds to the questions. Is it necessary to repeat questions to obtain a response? Does the response answer the question asked? Does the client have difficulty with word choices in forming responses? Is the client irritated or upset by the questions? Can the client concentrate on a question long enough to provide an appropriate response, or is the attention span short?

The nurse observes the client closely and documents the client's behavior. The nurse describes the behavior without interpreting it. The nurse questions family members regarding whether the behavior exhibited and the mental status are typical for this client.

The nurse assesses the client's neurologic status for other changes from baseline. Clinical manifestations of cerebral edema – associated neurologic dysfunction include the presence of headache and visual disturbances. In assessing the client's vision, the nurse makes certain that the client is wearing or using whatever devices the client normally uses to increase visual acuity. The nurse asks the client specific questions regarding blurring of vision and the presence of unusual light patterns within the field of vision. The client also may experience disturbances in hearing when cerebral edema is present. Another neurologic manifestation of hypotonic overhydration is projectile vomiting, which occurs in response to increased intracranial pressure. Additional symptoms of muscle cramps, skeletal muscle weakness, and paresthesias also may be present in response to electrolyte imbalances that develop as a result of hypotonic overhydration.

Other clinical manifestations of hypotonic overhydration are associated with either the dilution of specific electrolytes or the direct effects of fluid compartment expansion. These manifestations include watery diarrhea, polyuria, and generalized edema formation. This edema is not confined to dependent areas and is usually first noticed in the face as periorbital edema. This edema does not tend to produce pitting in response to pressure. Rather, the tissues have a firm, almost "rubbery" texture, and the skin may appear stretched and shiny (Metheny & Snively, 1983).

Overhydration may have specific renal manifestations. In addition, renal pathologic changes can contribute to the development of overhydration, especially in conditions that are characterized by diminished glomerular filtration. The nurse assesses renal perfusion by accurately measuring fluid intake and output. The color, character, and specific gravity of the urine are noted. Daily weight gain may also reflect alterations in renal function. When urine formation is decreased because of an inability to filter blood at the level of the glomerulus, ingested fluids are retained. One manifestation of water

retention is weight gain. The nurse weighs the client daily at the same time using the same scales. Whenever possible the client should be wearing the same type of clothing at each weigh-in.

Psychosocial Assessment

A careful psychosocial assessment not only provides data regarding presenting behavior, but also may help determine whether psychogenic polydipsia or alcoholism contributed to the development of overhydration. The assessment includes the components of the mental status assessment just discussed under the heading Hypotonic Overhydration. Abnormal findings of the psychologic assessment may be reflective of the actual fluid imbalance or they may be causative factors.

Laboratory Findings

No single laboratory test specifically determines the presence of overhydration. Instead, a diagnosis of overhydration is based on physical findings coupled with extrapolation and interpretation of a variety of laboratory data. In isotonic overhydration, serum electrolyte values are normal, but hemodilution results in decreased hemoglobin, hematocrit, BUN, and serum protein values. Elevated levels of most serum electrolytes (except calcium), along with elevations of BUN and serum creatinine levels, are associated with overhydration caused by renal failure (Robbins & Kumar, 1987). Hypotonic overhydration is associated with decreased serum values for blood cellular components, proteins, and electrolytes. Urine laboratory data usually are of limited value in determining the presence, type, and cause of overhydration, except when renal impairment is associated with the fluid imbalance.

 ### Analysis: Nursing Diagnosis

Many clients are at risk for developing overhydration as a result of chronic illness or in response to specific treatments. Age and socioeconomic factors also can increase a particular client's risk. The typical client with overhydration is a 70-year-old woman with diabetes, mild congestive heart failure from a previous myocardial infarction, and renal insufficiency. The following nursing diagnoses are derived from these data.

Common Diagnoses

The following nursing diagnoses are common for hospitalized clients with overhydration:

1. Fluid volume excess related to excessive fluid intake or inadequate fluid excretion
2. Ineffective breathing pattern related to pulmonary edema

Additional Diagnoses

In addition to the common diagnoses, one or more of the following nursing diagnoses may be applicable to the client with overhydration:

1. Knowledge deficit related to treatment regimen

2. Activity intolerance related to fatigue secondary to impaired gas exchange

3. Potential impaired skin integrity related to edema formation

4. Pain (headache) related to increased intracranial pressure

5. Diarrhea related to fluid volume excess and hyponatremia

6. Altered thought processes related to changes in CNS activity

7. Ineffective individual coping related to lack of effective behaviors to deal with chronic disease progression

8. Potential body image disturbance related to negative feelings about weight gain

9. Altered nutrition: less than body requirements related to fatigue

 Planning and Implementation

The following plan of care for the hospitalized client with overhydration focuses on the common nursing diagnoses associated with specific side effects that frequently accompany extracellular volume excesses. This plan of care has three aims. The primary aim is to restore normal fluid balance. The second aim is to provide supportive care for altered physiologic function and prevent associated complications until the overhydration is resolved. The final aim is to prevent future fluid volume excesses.

Fluid Volume Excess

Planning: client goals. The major goals for this nursing diagnosis are that the client will achieve and maintain normal fluid balance through (1) avoiding excessive fluid intake or (2) increasing fluid excretion.

Interventions: nonsurgical management. Diet and drug therapy are useful modalities to restore normal fluid balance. These therapies may be aimed at alleviation of the immediate existing condition, elimination or control of causative factors, and prevention of complications.

Drug therapy. Drug therapy for overhydration consists of specific treatments to rid the body of excess fluids and to support normal physiologic function of major organ systems to minimize or prevent complications. Diuretics are commonly used in situations of overhydration, provided that renal failure is not the cause of the overhydration. Osmotic diuretics (mannitol, urea) should be used first to avoid initiating or exacerbating electrolyte disturbances. Osmotic diuretics primarily enhance renal excretion of water, rather than renal excretion of sodium or potassium. If osmotic diuretics are not effective in promoting water loss, high-ceiling (loop) diuretics may be used, but the client needs to be closely monitored for signs and symptoms of electrolyte imbalances. Administration of specific electrolytes is not recommended, because the serum concentration of these ions is usually only diluted and they are not really lost from the body.

Drug therapy for overhydration as a result of inappropriate or excessive secretion of ADH may include agents that antagonize ADH (demeclocycline, lithium) or agents that block ADH receptors. Both of these categories of drugs are relatively new agents for the treatment of overhydration. Before administration, the nurse becomes familiar with the actions of the drug, the expected side effects, and potential adverse reactions. The nurse keeps antidotes to these drugs on the unit during the time the client is receiving them.

When overhydration is a result of another pathologic condition and not solely a function of direct fluid disturbance, drug therapy also focuses on the treatment of the underlying condition. For example, poor cardiac output and low MAP associated with severe congestive heart failure can cause overhydration through fluid retention as a result of inadequate renal perfusion and decreased glomerular filtration. This situation occurs because urine is formed from blood through the process of filtration at the level of the glomerulus in the nephron (Chap. 12). For glomerular filtration and urine formation to occur, the MAP usually must be at least 70 mmHg to deliver blood to the kidneys at a pressure high enough for effective filtration. When the MAP is too low for effective filtration, urine formation does not occur, and ingested fluids are retained. Treating the condition with drugs that improve cardiac output (digoxin, amrinone, deslanoside) and renal perfusion (dopamine) as well as diuretics can help restore normal fluid balance. These drugs also may be used when the overhydration causes decreased cardiac function.

Drug therapy to reduce cerebral edema is aimed at promoting CNS fluid loss. Drugs that are specific remedies for this problem include dexamethasone (Decadron) and urea. The nurse administers these agents with care and assesses the client every 2 hours for signs and symptoms indicative of excessive fluid loss or electrolyte imbalances.

Diet therapy. For mild or chronic overhydration, long-term diet therapy may be of value in controlling fluid volume through restrictions of both fluid and sodium. The factor of sodium concentration must be considered whenever overhydration is present. As discussed in Chapter 12, sodium in solution is the major determinant of osmotic pressure (water-pulling pressure) in the ECF. As a result, wherever sodium is present, a physiologically proportionate amount of water tends to remain. Thus, individuals with serum sodium levels greater than normal tend to retain water in an attempt to dilute the sodium concentration to a normal level. For these reasons, the client experiencing overhydration may need to restrict the intake of sodium.

The nurse accurately measures fluid intake and output and reinforces the reasons for the fluid restriction so that clients and families do not view the regimen as punishment. In addition to regulating the total amount of fluid to be ingested in a 24-hour period, the nurse carefully schedules fluid offerings so that some fluid is ingested throughout the 24 hours, with more fluid intake being allotted to times when the client is awake and active.

Prevention of complications. The two most common causes of death for clients experiencing overhydration are pulmonary edema and depression of vital functions as a result of cerebral edema. When overhydration is severe or life-threatening, fluid loss may be rapidly obtained through hemodialysis. This treatment is quite invasive and is not frequently used for overhydration, unless renal failure is a causative factor and death from circulatory overload is likely. Another treatment that can reduce fluid volume is rapid ultrafiltration of the ECF. This method is somewhat faster than standard hemodialysis and appears to carry less risk to the client.

Ineffective Breathing Pattern

Planning: client goals. The major client goals for this nursing diagnosis include that the client will (1) experience reduction of pulmonary edema and (2) increase the effectiveness of respiratory efforts.

Interventions: nonsurgical management. The interventions for this problem are aimed at restoring normal fluid balance in the interstitial compartment, enhancing gas exchange, and preventing respiratory arrest. The interventions directed toward restoring normal fluid balance are the same as the drug therapy and diet therapy interventions discussed earlier for fluid volume excess. The additional interventions for the ineffective breathing pattern focus on means other than restoration of fluid balance. Specific drug therapy has some value for this problem, but diet therapy does not play a role in the management of pulmonary edema.

Drug therapy. The underlying pathologic change in pulmonary edema is that fluid accumulates in the alveoli and interstitial spaces of the lungs, making gas diffusion more difficult. As a result, poor gas exchange occurs and hypoxemia develops. The hypoxemia causes tissues to be inadequately oxygenated. Clients become short of breath as the hypoxic tissues demand more oxygen and low serum oxygen levels stimulate the respiratory centers of the brain. Any condition that interferes

with respiratory effort increases the hypoxia and compounds the problem. Drug therapy to enhance respiratory effort may be of some benefit during episodes of pulmonary edema.

Bronchodilators do not diminish the edema, but can enhance respiratory effort by dilating the upper and lower airways so that ventilation is not impeded. Many of these drugs are sympathomimetic and tend to stimulate the CNS, so that further respiratory depression as a result of CNS depression does not occur. *Drugs that induce drowsiness or depress the CNS are avoided at this time.* Such drugs (diphenhydramine [Benadryl], diazepam [Valium]) may compound respiratory problems by making clients so sleepy that they do not put forth as much effort in the voluntary contraction of the skeletal muscles of respiration.

Oxygen administration may be useful in enhancing gas exchange during episodes of pulmonary edema. By increasing the oxygen concentration of inhaled air, more oxygen can diffuse through the limited alveolar surfaces and decrease the hypoxemia.

Oxygen can be administered by mask, hood, nasal cannula, nasopharyngeal tube, endotracheal tube, and tracheostomy tube. Most commonly, nasal cannulas are used to administer oxygen continuously. The nurse administers the oxygen to the client in amounts calculated by liters per minute (for cannula and nasopharyngeal tube administration) or in a concentration by percentage (for administration by mask, hood, endotracheal tube, and tracheostomy tube); these are specified by the physician's prescription. When the client has a chronic obstructive lung condition in addition to the pulmonary edema, oxygen is administered at low flow rates. Whenever oxygen is administered , it should be nebulized to prevent drying of the airway tissues. This nebulizing should occur even when pulmonary edema is present.

Promotion of gas exchange. Dyspnea with pulmonary edema increases in the supine position. The nurse assists the client to a Fowler's or a high-Fowler's position to increase ventilation to the available alveolar surfaces. Any physical activity increases metabolism and tissue demand for oxygen. Therefore, the client is restricted to bed rest, and the nurse performs all necessary care activities.

Prevention of respiratory complications. The prevention of respiratory complications in clients with impaired gas exchange as a result of overhydration is a nursing and a medical responsibility. Assessment of respiratory function is an important action in the primary and secondary prevention of respiratory complications. The nurse assesses the respiratory function of the client experiencing impairment of gas exchange as a result of overhydration at least every 2 hours.

In addition to an evaluation of the rate and depth of respiration, respiratory assessment includes auscultation of breath sounds for the presence or absence of air movement within all lung fields as well as for the presence of abnormal sounds within the lungs or airways. If abnormal sounds are heard, the nurse documents exactly a description of the sounds (for example, crackles or wheezes), where the sounds are heard, at what point in the respiratory cycle the sounds are noted, and whether the sounds remain after the client takes a deep breath or coughs. The nurse notes the ease with which the client moves air into and out of the lungs, including the presence of any retractions, and whether respiratory effort produces a sound audible without a stethoscope. Nail beds and mucous membranes are examined for color. The nurse documents the observed color, avoiding the use of the term "normal." Specific adjectives, such as pale, gray, pink, red, white, or cyanotic, are used to describe color.

Gas exchange is increased when greater numbers of alveoli are involved in respiration. Bedridden clients tend to have some degree of atelectasis from inactivity and alveolar fluid build-up. To prevent this complication the nurse encourages the client to perform sustained maximal inhalations for 3 minutes every hour while the client is awake. The client inhales to the maximal extent, holds the inhalation for 5 to 10 seconds, and then releases the air slowly through pursed lips.

■ Discharge Planning

Discharge planning for clients with overhydration is the same as that for clients with dehydration (see earlier).

 Evaluation

The nurse evaluates the care of the client experiencing problems as a result of overhydration. Care is evaluated on the basis of identified nursing diagnoses associated with this condition. The expected outcomes for the client with overhydration include that the client

1. Restores and maintains normal fluid volumes in all body fluid compartments
2. Is able to breathe effectively, with no dyspnea on mild exertion
3. Maintains or increases the current level of participation in self-care activities
4. Interprets environmental stimuli accurately
5. Maintains skin integrity
6. Identifies signs and symptoms of overhydration
7. Avoids injury
8. Maintains normal bowel elimination patterns
9. Achieves an acceptable level of relief from headache pain
10. Verbalizes understanding of the prescribed medical regimen
11. Complies with the prescribed medical regimen

POTASSIUM IMBALANCES

HYPOKALEMIA

OVERVIEW

Hypokalemia exists when the serum potassium ion (K^+) level falls below 3.5 mEq/L. Because 98% of the total body potassium is intracellular, small variations in extracellular potassium cause major changes in cell membrane excitability, as well as in other intracellular processes, such as the synthesis of proteins and glycogen. Hypokalemia is a relatively common electrolyte imbalance and a potentially life-threatening one, as the symptoms affect virtually every body system.

Pathophysiology

When extracellular potassium levels decrease, there is an increased potassium concentration gradient between the ICF and the ECF. This increased gradient causes the resting membrane potential to increase, thus reducing the excitability. Consequently, the cell membranes of all excitable tissues are less responsive to normal stimuli (Keyes, 1985). The return to resting membrane potential after depolarization is slower during hypokalemia because the permeability of the membrane to potassium is decreased. This situation results in slower impulse transmission across excitable membranes. Direct effects of hypokalemia are evident as slowed neural responses and decreased contractility of skeletal muscle, cardiac muscle, and smooth muscle. Indirect effects of hypokalemia result from alterations of both neural and muscular function and include respiratory and GI problems. Renal regulation of urine filtration and concentration during periods of hypokalemia is altered indirectly as a result of decreased protein synthesis in the kidney's tubular epithelium.

The degree of pathologic changes associated with hypokalemia is directly related to how rapidly ECF potassium levels decrease (Brenner et al., 1987; Metheny & Snively, 1983). When ECF potassium loss is slow or gradual, intracellular potassium also decreases in proportion to the ECF potassium level. In this situation, the potassium concentration gradient between the ICF and the ECF is essentially unchanged and symptoms of hypokalemia may not appear until potassium loss is extreme. Rapid changes in ECF potassium levels (representing a more rapid loss of potassium) are not compensated readily or quickly by adjustments in intracellular potassium concentrations. Thus the increased concentration gradient as a result of relatively small decreases in ECF potassium concentration leads to dramatic alterations of function. As discussed in Chapter 12, fewer control mechanisms for ECF potassium balance exist compared with those for sodium or calcium. Often potassium is preferentially lost to maintain sodium hydrogen ion balances.

Etiology

Hypokalemia may occur as a result of actual total body potassium depletion or as a result of abnormal movement of potassium from the ECF to the ICF, causing a *relative* decrease in the ECF potassium level (see the accompanying Key Features of Disease). Total body potassium may be lost as a result of excessive renal excretion of potassium or excessive potassium loss through the GI tract and skin. Potassium-wasting diuretics (such as acetazolamide, ethacrynic acid, furosemide, bumetanide, and the thiazides) or any state in which aldosterone secretion is increased promotes excessive renal excretion of potassium. Early stages of renal failure in which the kidneys have an impaired ability to concentrate urine can also cause increased or excessive potassium losses. Excessive potassium losses occur through the GI tract during periods of diarrhea, vomiting, and excessive drainage from ostomies. Specific disease processes associated directly or indirectly with potassium wasting include Cushing's disease, hyperaldosteronism, renovascular hypertension, and Bartter's syndrome (Zeluff et al., 1978).

Hypokalemia can also occur without the actual loss of potassium from the body. Some conditions cause potassium to be moved from the ECF into the ICF. This increased cellular uptake of potassium results in the same effects on excitable membranes that an actual loss of total body potassium produces. Conditions that tend to increase the cellular uptake of potassium, leading to hypokalemia, include metabolic alkalosis and the presence of excess amounts of insulin in the blood, such as during hyperalimentation infusions or during treatment of uncontrolled diabetes (Halperin & Goldstein, 1988).

Hypokalemia rarely occurs as a result of dietary deficiency among individuals who are ingesting solid foods, because potassium is present in many different food types. Clients taking nothing by mouth for several days or those receiving large amounts of parenteral fluids without potassium supplements are at risk for hypokalemia.

Incidence

Although exact statistics regarding the incidence of hypokalemia are not available, this imbalance occurs with great frequency among both hospitalized clients and those receiving outpatient care. Hypokalemia may be associated with virtually all illnesses. The degree of imbalance is usually determined by the severity of the illness, but the illness need not be severe for the imbalance to occur.

PREVENTION

Prevention of hypokalemia is aimed at identifying clients at risk so that appropriate intervention can be instituted early. Hypokalemia can occur quickly in response to illnesses, misuse of prescribed and OTC medications, and changes in dietary or health care habits. The nurse must instruct the client at risk (especially those receiving diuretics or corticosteroids) in what the proper use of medications and the signs and symptoms of hypokalemia are, when medical help should be sought, and which food sources are rich in potassium. Excessive use of enemas (more than three per 24 hours) and the misuse of laxatives should be discouraged. Good habits for bowel control, such as increased intake of dietary fiber and fruit along with adequate fluid intake, should be encouraged. Hospitalized clients also need to be provided with food sources high in potassium. Potassium should be added to intravenous (IV) fluids when a client's NPO status is prolonged. Clients may require different electrolyte solutions for maintenance and replacement needs, depending on the underlying medical problem. Fluids used to replace GI losses should be higher in potassium and titrated according to the volume of GI secretions lost.

KEY FEATURES OF DISEASE ■ Common Causes of Hypokalemia

Actual Potassium Deficits

Excess loss of potassium
    Inappropriate or excessive use of drugs
        Diuretics
        Digitalis
        Corticosteroids
    Increased secretion of aldosterone
        Cushing's syndrome
    Diarrhea
    Vomiting
    Wound drainage (especially gastrointestinal)
    Prolonged nasogastric suction
    Heat-induced excessive diaphoresis
    Renal disease impairing reabsorption of potassium
Inadequate potassium intake
    NPO

Relative Potassium Deficits

Movement of potassium from ECF to ICF
    Alkalosis
    Hyperinsulinism
    Hyperalimentation
    TPN
Dilution of serum potassium
    Water intoxication
    IV therapy with potassium-poor solutions

COLLABORATIVE MANAGEMENT

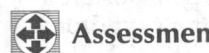 **Assessment**

History

The nurse collects data from clients at risk as well as those with actual hypokalemia. *Age* is an important factor in predisposition to hypokalemia, as the concentrating ability of the kidney diminishes gradually with age. Elderly clients are more likely to be using medications and engaging in health care practices that promote renal or GI loss of potassium. It is critical to obtain information about *medication use* (prescribed or OTC). Clients should be questioned carefully about the use of diuretics and corticosteroids, as these drugs increase renal potassium excretion. The most common cause of hypokalemia is the use and misuse of diuretics (Zeluff et al., 1978). Hypokalemia increases myocardial sensitivity to *digitalis*, making toxicity a greater risk even when the dosage is maintained within normal ranges.

The presence of any *disease state*, acute or chronic, may predispose the client to hypokalemia. Knowledge of recent illnesses and medical or surgical interventions helps the nurse to identify clients at risk for hypokalemia, as well as indicating possible causes of actual hypokalemia. A thorough diet history, including recall of a typical day's food and beverage intake at home, helps the nurse to identify clients at risk for hypokalemia whose diets also are deficient in potassium-containing substances. This information is particularly important for clients who are experiencing disorders that result in excessive potassium losses. The methods of food preparation also are important for the nurse to discern because boiling vegetables can leach out potassium along with specific vitamins.

Physical Assessment: Clinical Manifestations

Clinical manifestations of hypokalemia are associated with an alteration in the function of many systems (see the accompanying Key Features of Disease).

The *respiratory system* is profoundly affected by hypokalemia through depression of neural and muscular excitable membranes. Contraction of specific muscle groups causes respiratory movement and permits pulmonary ventilation. Weakness of the skeletal muscles of respiration results in shallow and ineffective respirations. This situation can be lethal, thus the respiratory system should be the first to be assessed. The nurse must assess the breath sounds, the ease of respiratory effort, and the color of nail beds and mucous membranes, as well as the rate and depth of respiration. The nurse assesses the client's respiratory status at least every 2 hours, because respiratory insufficiency frequently accompanies hypokalemia and is a major cause of death for clients experiencing this imbalance.

Cardiovascular changes can also accompany hypokalemia. The nurse assesses the status of the cardiovascu-

---

KEY FEATURES OF DISEASE ■ **Clinical Manifestations of Hypokalemia**

Cardiovascular

Variable pulse rate, more often rapid
Pulse quality thready and weak
Peripheral pulses difficult to palpate
Postural hypotension
ECG abnormalities
   ST depression
   Inverted T wave
   Prominent U wave
   Heart block

Respiratory

Shallow, ineffective respirations due to profound
   weakness of the skeletal muscles of respiration
Diminished breath sounds

Neuromuscular

Anxiety, lethargy, confusion, coma
Loss of tactile discrimination
General skeletal muscle weakness
Deep tendon hyporeflexia
Eventual flaccid paralysis

Gastrointestinal

Decreased motility
Hypoactive to absent bowel sounds
Nausea
Vomiting
Abdominal distention
Paralytic ileus
Constipation

Renal

Decreased ability to concentrate urine
Polyuria
Decreased specific gravity

---

lar system by palpating the *peripheral pulses*. With hypokalemia, the pulse is usually thready and weak. Palpation may be difficult, and the pulse may be easily obliterated with pressure. The pulse rate may range from excessively slow to excessively rapid, depending on what specific type of arrhythmia is present. *Blood pressure* should be measured with the client in lying, sitting, and standing positions, as postural hypotensive changes occur first and a general hypotensive state occurs later. A baseline *ECG* should be obtained followed by continuous *cardiac monitoring* for evidence of electrical conduction abnormalities that include ST depression, flattening or inversions of T waves, and increased or prominent U waves. Profound *bradycardia* and *heart block* are possible causes of death for clients with hypokalemia who are also on a digitalis regimen (Schwartz, 1987; Zeluff et al., 1978).

Neural manifestations of hypokalemia include changes in mental status. The client may experience transient irritability and anxiety followed by lethargy that progresses to confusion and coma as hypokalemia worsens. Impulse transmission in peripheral nerves is depressed; therefore, alterations in the function of some organs or systems may actually be a manifestation of depressed neural activity as a result of hypokalemia. Severe hypokalemia affects sensory nerves by decreasing the awareness of sensitivity changes. Clients may not be able to discern mild sensations of pain, touch, heat, and cold.

Skeletal muscles become weak in response to hypokalemia. This weakness has two causes. Because the resting membrane potential is greater, a stronger stimulus is needed to initiate muscle contraction. In addition, because the nerves that usually provide this stimulus are depressed during hypokalemia, skeletal muscle weakness is also a result of inadequate nervous stimulation. Clients may be unable to stand. Handgrasps will be weak (bilaterally). The response to deep tendon reflex stimulation indicates hyporeflexia. Severe hypokalemia leads to profound flaccid paralysis.

GI function is altered during hypokalemia directly by the effects on smooth muscle contraction and indirectly by depression of neural activity, influencing smooth muscle contraction. Hypokalemia results in decreased smooth muscle contractility, leading to decreased peristalsis. Clients have hypoactive bowel sounds and may experience nausea, vomiting, constipation, and abdominal distention. The nurse assesses distention by measuring abdominal girth. Bowel sounds are assessed in all four abdominal quadrants with a stethoscope before touching the abdomen for any other reason. Severe hypokalemia can result in the development of a paralytic ileus.

Renal function impairment as a result of hypokalemia includes decreased glomerular filtration and decreased ability to concentrate urine through reabsorption of water (Brenner et al., 1987; Zeluff et al., 1978). The client experiences polyuria, even though filtration is diminished, because less fluid is reabsorbed in the proximal convoluted tubule, allowing more fluid to be excreted as urine. The urine is dilute and light in color and has a low specific gravity.

Psychosocial Assessment

Hypokalemia is seldom a long-term process, so that the behavioral changes associated with hypokalemia usually occur within a short period of time. Knowledge of the client's usual mental status and mood is useful in assessing changes that may be related to hypokalemia. This information may need to be obtained from close

family members or friends, depending on the client's condition. Data regarding the onset and duration of behavioral changes as well as their association with any other physical signs and symptoms are important and need to be as accurate as possible. The client may be lethargic and unable to perform simple problem-solving tasks that require concentration, such as counting backward from 100 by threes. As hypokalemia progresses, the client may become increasingly confused, especially with regard to time and place. In severe hypokalemia coma may develop, although death as a result of cardiac arrhythmias or respiratory depression usually occurs first.

Laboratory Findings

The definitive laboratory test result that confirms the condition of hypokalemia is a serum potassium value of less than 3.5 mEq/L. However, this value does not indicate whether a true potassium deficit exists or if the low serum potassium level is a result of a shift of potassium from the ECF to the ICF. Other abnormal laboratory data that frequently accompany hypokalemia include elevated blood pH, elevated blood glucose levels, and an arterial PCO_2 greater than 45 mmHg (Brenner et al., 1987; Metheny & Snively, 1983). Hypokalemia increases renal formation and excretion of ammonia, thus contributing to the development of metabolic alkalosis (Brenner et al., 1987). Urine laboratory values may not be of much assistance in determining potassium loss, because the kidneys do not normally conserve potassium. If the hypokalemia is caused by hyperaldosteronism, however, the normal urine sodium/potassium ratio of 2 : 1 may be reversed. Occasionally a low serum potassium level may be determined by laboratory testing when no other signs or symptoms of hypokalemia are evident. This situation may result if blood for electrolyte measurement is drawn from a vein in which IV fluid infuses distal to the site of the venipuncture. Such false laboratory values also reflect the content of the IV fluid (elevated glucose level if the fluid is D_5W; elevated serum sodium and chloride levels if the fluid, or some portion of the fluid, is normal saline).

 ### Analysis: Nursing Diagnosis

Hypokalemia is a frequent occurrence among hospitalized clients because many conditions and treatments contribute to the problem. The typical client is elderly and is receiving long-term diuretic and digitalis-type treatment for the management of cardiovascular problems. The client may or may not be on a regimen of potassium replacement. The most common form of potassium supplement or replacement is potassium chloride (KCl). Most preparations of KCl have an unpleasant taste, which may contribute to a lack of client compliance. The following nursing diagnoses are derived from these data.

Common Diagnoses

The following nursing diagnoses are commonly applicable to clients with hypokalemia:

1. Potential for injury related to skeletal muscle weakness
2. Constipation related to smooth muscle atony and decreased peristalsis
3. Knowledge deficit related to treatment regimen

Additional Diagnoses

In addition to the common diagnoses, one or more of the following diagnoses may be pertinent:

1. Impaired physical mobility related to skeletal muscle weakness
2. Decreased cardiac output related to arrhythmias
3. Impaired gas exchange related to weakness of respiratory muscle contractions
4. Total self-care deficit related to weak skeletal muscle contractions

 Planning and Implementation

The following plan of care for the client with hypokalemia focuses on the common diagnoses related to decreased impulse transmission in excitable tissues and knowledge deficits concerning the impact on potassium balance of treatment regimens prescribed for other chronic conditions. The nurse must remember that the plan of care is aimed at prevention of potassium imbalances, restoration of normal potassium balance, and provision of supportive care for altered body functions until the hypokalemia is resolved.

Potential for Injury

Planning: client goals. The major goals for this nursing diagnosis are that the client will (1) not fall and (2) have serum potassium levels return to normal.

Interventions: nonsurgical management. Diet and drug therapy are useful to restore normal serum potassium levels. Increasing serum potassium levels reduces the potential for falls by increasing the contractile responsiveness of skeletal muscles to normal stimuli.

Drug therapy. Potassium supplements (oral or parenteral) commonly are given for the treatment and prevention of hypokalemia. Most potassium supplements are in the form of KCl. Parenteral potassium should be administered with extreme caution. Because potassium is a profound tissue irritant, it is not administered by either intramuscular (IM) or subcutaneous (SC) injection. IV potassium solutions irritate veins and cause a chemical phlebitis (Ledbetter, 1988). Therefore, IV potassium solutions should be well diluted and should not be administered rapidly. Moreover, IV administration of potassium can be extremely dangerous because rapid increases of serum potassium level depress cardiac muscle contractility and can lead to serious arrhythmias and cardiac arrest. For these reasons, IV potassium solutions should never be given as a bolus, and all IV solutions containing potassium should be administered through a controller or a pump device. To avoid accidental rapid infusion of potassium and to increase client comfort, 1 L of IV fluid usually contains no more than 60 mEq of potassium.

Oral preparations of potassium usually have a KCl base. These preparations may be administered as liquids or in a solid salt–like form. KCl has a strong, unpleasant taste that is difficult to mask. In addition, potassium should not be taken on an empty stomach, as the client may experience nausea or vomiting.

Diuretics that increase the renal excretion of potassium are common causes of hypokalemia. Therefore, the use of these drugs for clients with actual hypokalemia or those who are prone to hypokalemia should be avoided. Some diuretics are specifically potassium sparing in that they induce diuresis without enhancing potassium excretion. Diuretics with this action include spironolactone (Aldactone), triamterene (Dyrenium), and amiloride (Midamor). When the client with hypokalemia requires concurrent diuretic therapy, a potassium-sparing diuretic may be appropriate.

Diet therapy. Administering foods high in potassium will help restore normal potassium levels as well as prevent further loss (see Chap. 12, Table 12–5). Food preparation as well as food choice is important for increasing dietary intake of potassium. Long cooking of vegetables and fruits in water tends to increase both potassium loss and vitamin loss. Dietary potassium intake may be poor as a result of fatigue and weakness. The client may require assistance with the mechanical process of eating. Foods containing potassium may need to be finely chopped or puréed to ease chewing and swallowing efforts for fatigued clients. The nurse provides small, frequent meals and appropriate amounts of liquids.

Prevention of complications. The client must be careful to prevent falls and to avoid activities that could result in falls. Maintaining a hazard-free environment and ensuring that the client is aware of limitations and problems are necessary to meet this goal.

While the client is hospitalized, the nurse employs safety measures and eliminates hazards. The nurse assists the client in all ambulatory activities. Before ambulation, the nurse ensures that the ambulatory path is free of obstacles or slippery areas and that the client is wearing nonslip footgear. During ambulation with assistance, the client should wear a safety belt. Personal articles and the nurse call light are positioned within easy reach to reduce the need for the client to get out of bed unassisted. The side rails at the head of the bed should be in the up position whenever the client is alone.

Constipation

Planning: client goals. The primary goal for this diagnosis is that the client maintains individualized normal bowel elimination patterns.

Interventions: nonsurgical management. Interventions include restoring serum potassium levels to normal (discussed earlier as drug and diet therapies for potential for trauma), stimulating intestinal peristalsis, and avoiding conditions and actions that contribute to constipation.

Drug therapy. Laxatives that add bulk or fiber may be used to stimulate peristalsis, although caution should be taken to avoid the use of laxatives that increase potassium loss. Other drugs, such as metoclopramide (Reglan, Maxeran), that decrease gastric emptying time and stimulate GI motility can be used to prevent or treat the constipation associated with hypokalemia.

Diet therapy. Because bowel elimination is a personal care activity, the nurse questions the client about normal bowel functions and specific interventions that have worked well for the client in the past to prevent or alleviate constipation. Whenever possible the nurse uses these familiar techniques for the client experiencing constipation associated with hypokalemia. The nurse provides meals that contain high-fiber foods and plenty of liquids for clients who do not require fluid restrictions for other health problems. To ensure client cooperation, the nurse prepares a list of foods that contain high concentrations of fiber and asks the client to select favorite items from that list. The nurse helps the client to avoid food selections that tend to increase constipation, flatus formation, and abdominal distention.

Comfort measures. The nurse can assist the client to maintain normal bowel elimination patterns in a variety of ways. During times when the client is using the toilet or bedpan, the nurse provides the greatest degree of privacy possible. The nurse closes the door, pulls privacy curtains, and asks visitors to step out of the room. Physical activity and exercise promote gastric motility. The nurse encourages the client to ambulate whenever the client's condition permits. For clients restricted to bed rest, the nurse assists the client with frequent position changes and mild bed exercises to the degree that this activity is tolerated.

Knowledge Deficit

Planning: client goals. The major goal for this diagnosis is that the client will understand the causes, signs and symptoms, and treatment regimen of hypokalemia.

Interventions: nonsurgical management. The nurse assumes the responsibility for teaching the client what hypokalemia is and why conditions that contribute to potassium loss should be avoided. Instructions should focus on (1) the maintenance of an adequate dietary intake of potassium, (2) actions that avoid or prevent excessive potassium loss, and (3) the recognition of early signs and symptoms of hypokalemia.

Adequate dietary intake. The nurse consults and collaborates with a registered dietitian to ensure accurate teaching of how to maintain an adequate dietary intake of potassium. Table 12–5 in Chapter 12 indicates common foods that are rich in potassium.

Prevention of excessive potassium loss. The nurse teaches the client the importance of taking all prescribed medications correctly and seeing the attending physician on a regular basis. Clients are instructed to take potassium supplements either with meals or on a full stomach. Because normal renal excretion of potassium occurs continuously, serum potassium levels are maintained more consistently when potassium supplement doses are administered evenly three to four times per day.

Early recognition of hypokalemia. The nurse teaches the client the following signs and symptoms that may indicate the presence of hypokalemia:

1. Slow or irregular heart rate
2. Numbness or tingling sensations in the hands and feet
3. Cramping of large leg muscles
4. Sensations of weakness
5. Difficulty in maintaining mental concentration; slight confusion or forgetfulness
6. Constipation, abdominal distention, and nausea

When any of the symptoms are present, the client should have a snack that is high in potassium content. If the symptoms do not subside within an hour, the client should seek medical attention.

■ Discharge Planning

Discharge planning for clients with hypokalemia is the same as that for clients with dehydration (see earlier).

Evaluation

On the basis of the identified nursing diagnoses, the nurse evaluates the care for the client experiencing hypokalemia. The expected outcomes for the client with hypokalemia include that the client

1. Restores and maintains normal serum potassium levels
2. Uses assistance and safety devices as needed
3. Complies with diet and drug therapy
4. Identifies actions to take when signs and symptoms of hypokalemia occur

5. States to whom health care problems associated with hypokalemia should be addressed
6. Maintains normal bowel elimination patterns

By meeting the stated desired outcomes, the client is more likely to maintain a normal potassium balance. If hypokalemia occurs, the client can recognize the imbalance and take appropriate steps to prevent a mild potassium imbalance from becoming severe and life-threatening.

HYPERKALEMIA

OVERVIEW

A state of hyperkalemia exists when the serum potassium level is greater than 5.0 mEq/L. Because the range of normal serum potassium values is so narrow, even slight increases above normal can have serious, adverse effects on the physiologic function of excitable membranes. Hyperkalemia occurs less frequently than hypokalemia, but the consequences are just as life-threatening.

Pathophysiology

When extracellular potassium levels increase, there is a decreased potassium concentration gradient between the ICF and the ECF. This decreased gradient causes the resting membrane potential to decrease, thus increasing excitability. As a result, the cell membranes of all excitable tissues are more responsive to normal stimuli and may even be able to fire spontaneously. However, the function of excitable membranes is dependent on both depolarization and repolarization. When hyperkalemia is present, depolarization initially occurs more easily, but repolarization is slow. Eventually, because repolarization is necessary to return the membrane to its original resting membrane state to be able to respond again to a stimulus, depolarization also is first slowed and then blocked (Brenner et al., 1987). Therefore, some of the clinical manifestations of severe or prolonged hyperkalemia are similar to those seen in hypokalemia, although the underlying pathologic change is different. Hyperkalemia alters the function of all excitable membranes to some degree. However, cardiac muscle excitable membrane is more sensitive to increases in serum potassium levels than are other excitable membranes, so that the more serious complications of hyperkalemia are associated with alterations of cardiac function.

The degree of pathologic changes associated with hyperkalemia is directly related to how rapidly ECF potassium levels increase. Sudden increases in serum potassium levels cause profound function changes at lower potassium levels (between 6 and 7 mEq/L). When increases in serum potassium levels occur slowly or chronically, problems with excitable membrane func-

tion may not be obvious until potassium levels reach 8 to 9 mEq/L.

Etiology

As discussed in Chapter 12, no known mechanisms exist for the conservation of potassium. Thus the condition of hyperkalemia does not occur easily among healthy individuals. Hyperkalemia may occur as a result of an actual increase in the amount of total body potassium or as a result of abnormal movement of potassium from the ICF to the ECF, causing a relative increase in the serum potassium concentration. Hyperkalemia as a result of either mechanism is significant and must be treated, although the treatment varies with the exact cause (see the accompanying Key Features of Disease).

The kidneys are responsible for 80% to 90% of normal potassium excretion, with another 10% to 20% being lost through sweat and feces. Normally great variation in potassium intake is well tolerated, because renal excretion of potassium adjusts to maintain serum potassium levels within the normal range. Although the kidneys are unable to truly conserve potassium when intake is low, the kidneys can increase potassium excretion when intake is high. Renal excretion of potassium is affected by acid-base and other electrolyte balances. When renal insufficiency is present, the kidneys may not be able to excrete enough potassium to keep serum potassium levels within normal limits, and hyperkalemia results. The mineralocorticoid aldosterone en-

---

KEY FEATURES OF DISEASE ■ **Common Causes of Hyperkalemia**

Actual Potassium Excesses

Excess potassium intake
  Overingestion of potassium-containing foods or medications
    Salt substitutes
    KCl
  Rapid infusion of potassium-containing IV solution
  Bolus IV potassium injections
Decreased potassium excretion
  Adrenal insufficiency (Addison's disease, adrenalectomy)
  Renal failure
  Potassium-sparing diuretics

Relative Potassium Excesses

Movement of potassium from ICF to ECF
  Tissue damage
  Acidosis
  Hyperuricemia
  Hypercatabolism

hances renal excretion of potassium. Conditions that decrease or inhibit secretion of aldosterone may cause hyperkalemia by inhibiting renal excretion of potassium, even when kidney function is normal. Such conditions include adrenalectomy, adrenal insufficiency, and Addison's disease. Potassium-sparing diuretics also may contribute to the development of hyperkalemia.

Hyperkalemia can occur as a result of excessive potassium intake. For the healthy individual, excessive oral intake of potassium to the extent that hyperkalemia can develop is difficult, but possible. Intentional overdoses of oral potassium for suicidal purposes have been documented. Individuals with renal dysfunction (temporary or chronic) may have to carefully limit their intake of oral potassium to prevent hyperkalemia. Excessive parenteral potassium intake is too commonly a cause of hyperkalemia. Excessive parenteral potassium intake most frequently is a result of rapid administration of potassium-containing IV solutions.

Hyperkalemia also can result from movement of intracellular potassium to the ECF. This movement can occur by release of potassium either as a result of cellular destruction or as a result of cellular ion exchange mechanisms to compensate for specific ion imbalances. Acidosis, an increase in the serum hydrogen ion (H^+) concentration, causes hydrogen ions to be taken up by cells and potassium to be released by cells to decrease the serum concentration of hydrogen ions. However, this exchange can cause hyperkalemia. Common conditions that lead to acidosis and a secondary hyperkalemia include diabetic ketoacidosis, starvation, infection, and dehydration. Common conditions of cellular destruction that release potassium into the ECF include burns, crushing injuries, tumor lysis syndrome, hypercatabolism, and infusions of blood that has been stored for longer than 48 hours (Kopec & Groeger, 1988; Weisberg et al., 1987).

Incidence

Hyperkalemia is rare in persons with normally functioning kidneys. Therefore, most cases of hyperkalemia occur among hospitalized clients or those who are on medical treatment regimens. Individuals at greatest risk for hyperkalemia are those who are chronically ill, debilitated, old, or young. Also at risk are clients who receive potassium-sparing diuretics and mercurial diuretics. A concept to remember when treating clients with hypokalemia is that even relatively small amounts of potassium can overcorrect hypokalemia and push the client into a hyperkalemic state, especially if the renal system is compromised.

PREVENTION

Prevention of hyperkalemia is aimed at identifying clients at risk so that appropriate interventions can be instituted early. Clients receiving oral or IV potassium

supplements and those with chronic diseases (especially renal disorders) predisposing to hyperkalemia need to have their serum potassium levels monitored regularly. Although the ordering of laboratory tests, such as the measurement of serum electrolytes, is the physician's responsibility in most institutions, the nurse generally receives these reports first. Therefore, the nurse is in an ideal position to be cognizant of significant changes in electrolyte levels and can alert the medical staff to an impending problem. Concern is necessary for any client who shows a steadily increasing potassium level, so that interventions can begin before the onset of hyperkalemia.

A common cause of hyperkalemia in the hospitalized client is the too rapid administration of potassium-containing IV solutions. The prevention of such instances is a primary nursing responsibility. Any IV solution containing potassium should be administered using an infusion controller or a pump. This rule should apply to "piggy-backed" potassium-containing fluids, such as potassium penicillin, as well as main bag solutions. The nurse cautions clients not to self-adjust the drip rate of IV solutions. Care should be taken whenever adding potassium to bottles or bags of IV fluids currently being infused. The infusion should be slowed to a keep open rate while the potassium is being added. The bottle or bag should be gently but thoroughly agitated to evenly distribute the added potassium throughout the solution and not have it concentrated in one area (Motz-Harding & Good, 1985). No more than 60 mEq of potassium should be added to a liter of IV fluid, and solutions containing potassium should not be infused faster than 20 mEq/hour. The nurse never administers potassium-containing IV fluids by push infusion, and extreme caution should be exercised during any IV bolus administration of potassium (Burman & Berkowitz, 1986).

Another potential cause of hyperkalemia that the nurse can prevent is the improper transfusion of whole blood and packed red blood cells (Rao et al., 1980). All cells contain large concentrations of potassium. When cell membranes are damaged, intracellular potassium quickly leaks out of the cell. Therefore, when administering blood, the nurse must take precautions to avoid damaging the cells being infused. The drip chamber of the transfusion set should be filled above the level of the filter or ball. When blood cells drop directly on the ball or filter apparatus, some of the cells break and release potassium. Ideally, blood should not be transfused through any needle or IV access device smaller than 18 gauge. The longer blood is stored, the more red blood cell membranes deteriorate and release potassium into the blood fluid. Therefore, clients who are already hyperkalemic should not receive blood that has been stored longer than 48 hours.

Strict adherence to potassium-limited diets is critically important for clients with renal insufficiency and chronic hyperkalemia. Knowledge of food preparation and food sources of potassium is important because cooking methods can alter the potassium level of a particular food.

COLLABORATIVE MANAGEMENT

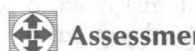 **Assessment**

History

When documenting a history for any client, the nurse collects data regarding risk factors, as well as causative factors, related to hyperkalemia. *Age* is important, primarily because of the altered renal function that occurs in the elderly client. The nurse inquires about risk factors, such as debilitating or chronic illnesses, particularly renal disease (Poyss, 1987). The nurse also asks questions concerning recent *medical or surgical interventions.* Clients who state that they do not have a medical diagnosis of renal failure or insufficiency are questioned specifically regarding *urinary output,* such as the frequency and amount of voidings. The nurse also inquires about *medication use,* particularly potassium-sparing diuretics. If the client is unable to recall this information, the nurse may need to obtain previous medical records if possible or obtain this information from the client's significant other or a close family member.

The nurse obtains a *diet history* to pinpoint possible causative factors, such as intake of potassium-containing foods, especially those eaten raw. Food preparation methods also must be determined because steaming or baking foods tends to preserve potassium. The nurse specifically asks the client about the use of salt substitutes; many of these condiments are at least partially composed of potassium salts (Sopko & Freeman, 1977; Zeluff et al., 1978).

The nurse also collects data that may indicate the presence of symptoms related specifically to hyperkalemia. The client is asked if any episodes of palpitations, skipped heartbeats, or other cardiac irregularities have been experienced. Information regarding the presence of muscle twitching, weakness in leg muscles, and unusual sensations of tingling followed by numbness in the hands, feet, or face is obtained. The nurse inquires about recent changes in bowel habits, especially the presence of diarrhea, colic, or explosive bowel movements. Having the client relate a typical day's activities may disclose additional information on recent decreases in activity level or the presence of unexplained fatigue and weakness.

Physical Assessment: Clinical Manifestations

Clinical manifestations of hyperkalemia are associated with alterations of excitable membrane activity, primarily in the cardiac and neuromuscular systems (see the accompanying Key Features of Disease).

Cardiovascular changes are the most profound and are the most common cause of death among clients experiencing hyperkalemia; therefore, cardiac status should be assessed first. The nurse assesses the cardiac status of all clients with hyperkalemia through careful observation and cardiac monitors. ECG changes indicative of

---

KEY FEATURES OF DISEASE ■ Clinical Manifestations of Hyperkalemia

Cardiovascular

Irregular heart rate, usually slow
Decreased blood pressure
ECG abnormalities
  Tall T waves
  Widened QRS complexes
  Prolonged PR intervals
  Flat P waves
Ectopic beats
Late: arrhythmias, ventricular fibrillation, cardiac arrest in diastole

Respiratory

Unaffected until late, when profound weakness of skeletal muscles causes respiratory failure

Neuromuscular

Early phase or mild hyperkalemia
  Muscle twitches, cramps
  Paresthesias
Late phase or severe hyperkalemia
  Profound weakness
  Ascending flaccid paralysis in distal to proximal direction involving arms and legs

Gastrointestinal

Increased motility
Hyperactive bowel sounds
Diarrhea

---

the presence of hyperkalemia are the presence of tall, peaked T waves; prolonged PR intervals; flattening or disappearance of P waves; and widening of QRS complexes. If the hyperkalemia has a sudden onset, these ECG changes may be observed when serum potassium levels range from 6 to 7 mEq/L. However, if the hyperkalemia is chronic or is gradual in onset, these specific changes may not occur until serum potassium levels reach 8 to 9 mEq/L. As serum potassium levels rise, impulse conduction through the cardiac Purkinje system slows and may even be blocked at the atrioventricular (AV) node. The heart muscle dilates and becomes flaccid, unable to respond to nodal depolarization. As conduction is blocked at the AV node, ectopic beats generated from outside the conduction system in the ventricles may appear. Complete heart block, ventricular standstill, or ventricular fibrillation are major life-threatening complications of severe hyperkalemia. In addition to specific ECG changes, the nurse also assesses cardiac status through peripheral pulse and blood pressure measurements. Findings consistent with hyperkalemia are a slow, weak pulse and low blood pressure, with decreased MAP as a result of weak ventricular contractility and prolonged diastole.

Neuromuscular symptoms are associated with hyperkalemia, although these are not as pronounced or severe as those seen with hypokalemia. The neuromuscular responses to hyperkalemia have a two-phase manifestation. Because hyperkalemia decreases the resting membrane potential, both nerves and muscles may depolarize spontaneously during the early stages of hyperkalemia. Skeletal muscles twitch, and the client may be aware of unusual nerve sensations (paresthesias), such as tingling and burning, followed by numbness in the hands, in the feet, and around the mouth. As hyperkalemia progresses, muscle twitching changes to weakness followed by flaccid paralysis. The weakness or paralysis ascends from distal to proximal areas and primarily affects the muscles of the arms and legs. Usually trunk, head, and respiratory muscles are not affected until serum potassium levels reach the cardiolethal levels. Although respiratory movements are not directly affected by hyperkalemia, the respiratory rate may be increased as the respiratory system attempts to maintain adequate tissue oxygenation in the presence of cardiac insufficiency.

The *smooth muscle system* of the GI tract responds to hyperkalemia by increasing peristaltic movement. The nurse assesses the GI system by listening to bowel sounds and observing elimination products. The client may experience diarrhea and spastic colonic activity. Bowel sounds are hyperactive, with frequent audible rushes and gurgles, especially over the splenic flexure and in the left lower abdominal quadrant. Bowel movements may be frequent, watery, and explosive in nature.

Psychosocial Assessment

Unlike the case with hypokalemia, behavioral changes are not usually associated with hyperkalemia, because cardiac manifestations are usually apparent and cause the client to seek medical assistance before serum potassium levels become high enough to produce CNS manifestations. Because hyperkalemia is associated with chronic renal failure, client compliance with prescribed dietary restrictions or limitations needs to be assessed. The nurse assesses the client's knowledge concerning foods to avoid and the correct use of prescribed medications. Data concerning how food is prepared and who is responsible for food preparation also are important to obtain.

Laboratory Findings

The definitive laboratory test result that confirms the condition of hyperkalemia is a serum potassium value greater than 5.0 mEq/L. If the hyperkalemia is a result of dehydration, levels of other serum electrolytes may be elevated, as will the hematocrit and hemoglobin

levels. Hyperkalemia associated with renal failure usually is accompanied by elevations of serum creatinine and blood urea nitrogen levels, a decreased blood pH, and normal or low hematocrit and hemoglobin levels. If renal function is normal, urine potassium levels are elevated. If renal disease or other oliguric conditions are the cause of the hyperkalemia, the urine potassium levels will be low (Leaf & Cotran, 1985).

 Analysis: Nursing Diagnosis

Hyperkalemia generally is easier to anticipate and prevent than hypokalemia because it most frequently results from oliguria or severe tissue injury. However, hyperkalemia can occur in response to medical treatment of other conditions, especially in clients with chronic illnesses or renal problems. The monitoring of serum potassium levels is critically important, as the detection of slowly rising potassium levels may alert the nurse to an impending hyperkalemic state before the manifestation of significant problems related to the imbalance. An example of a clinical situation in which a client is likely to experience an acute episode of hyperkalemia is within the first 24 hours after a severe traumatic injury in which large tissue areas sustain mechanical damage. A typical client is a 21-year-old man who had both legs pinned from mid-thigh down between a truck and the wall of a building. The following diagnoses are derived from these data.

Common Diagnoses

The following nursing diagnoses are commonly noted for clients with hyperkalemia:

1. Decreased cardiac output related to arrhythmias
2. Diarrhea related to smooth muscle hyperactivity and increased peristalsis

Additional Diagnoses

In addition to the common diagnoses, one or more of the following diagnoses may be appropriate:

1. Knowledge deficit related to treatment regimen
2. Total self-care deficit related to skeletal muscle weakness
3. Pain related to muscle twitching

 Planning and Implementation

The following plan of care for the client with hyperkalemia focuses on the common diagnoses related to alterations of impulse transmission in cardiac muscle and GI smooth muscle. The nurse must remember that the plan of care is aimed at prevention of potassium imbalances, restoration of normal potassium balance, prevention of complications, and provision of supportive care for altered body functions until the hyperkalemia is resolved.

Decreased Cardiac Output

Planning: client goals. The major goals for this nursing diagnosis are that the client will (1) have serum potassium levels restored to normal and (2) not experience lethal cardiac arrhythmias.

Interventions: nonsurgical management. Drug therapy can be useful for restoring normal potassium balance. Decreasing the excessive serum potassium levels reduces the chances of lethal cardiac arrhythmias by increasing the resting membrane potential of cardiac excitable membranes.

Drug therapy. Drug therapy for the treatment of hyperkalemia has three focuses: (1) to prevent further increases in serum potassium levels by eliminating additional potassium administration; (2) to enhance potassium excretion from the body; and (3) to enhance the movement of potassium from the ECF into the ICF.

Under conditions of hyperkalemia, it is necessary to eliminate parenteral potassium administration. Infusions of IV solutions containing potassium should be stopped immediately (but the IV line is kept open). Identical solutions that do not contain potassium should be substituted. Sodium penicillin can be substituted for potassium penicillin if the client's sodium tolerance is acceptable. Clients with hyperkalemia should not receive transfusions of whole blood or packed red blood cells unless absolutely necessary. Any blood products that are administered should be less than 48 hours old. Oral potassium supplements are withheld. The client should be placed on a potassium-restricted diet.

Potassium movement from the ECF to the ICF is influenced by the movement of glucose from the blood into the cell. Therefore, the administration of IV fluids that contain substantial amounts of glucose and insulin helps to decrease the serum potassium levels (usually 250 mL of 10% to 20% glucose with 10 to 20 units of regular insulin). When hyperkalemia is accompanied by or caused by metabolic acidosis, small amounts of sodium bicarbonate also may be added to the treatment solution (Schwartz, 1987). These IV solutions are hypertonic and should be administered through a central line with a high blood flow to avoid local vein inflammation (Ledbetter, 1988). Close observation and care are needed to make certain that neither hypokalemia nor hypoglycemia occur during this therapy.

Drug therapy to increase the excretion of potassium includes the use of substances known as cation exchange resins (such as sodium polystyrene sulfonate [Kayexalate]). These resins are composed of nondigestible substances (polystyrene); in the intestinal tract they release sodium (a cation) and, in exchange, absorb potassium (another cation). The potassium remains bound to the resin and is excreted through the feces. This treatment can be administered orally or rectally. If the client is able to retain the polystyrene enema for the required amount of time, the rectal route is preferred, because the action of polystyrene is more pronounced in the large intestine. Although these resins do reduce overall potassium levels, the effect can take many hours. Therefore, if potassium levels are dangerously high, additional means to reduce potassium also are necessary. When serum potassium levels approach lethal levels, reduction through dialysis (hemodialysis or peritoneal dialysis) or ultrafiltration may be necessary to rapidly reduce serum potassium to safer levels.

Cardiac monitoring. Prevention of lethal arrhythmias depends not only on reducing potassium levels, but also on recognizing early signs and symptoms that indicate the adverse response of cardiac muscle excitable membranes to the presence of increased potassium levels. The nurse compares recent ECG tracings with the client's baseline tracings or tracings obtained at a time when the client's serum potassium level was close to normal range. Changes in tracing patterns are more reliably detected when chest leads are consistently placed in the same position. Marking the chest positions with a nonerasable pen allows for consistent placement and standard tracings. Specific areas that the nurse examines for changes are the T waves, P waves, and the QRS complex on the ECG, as well as changes in rate and rhythm. The nurse is responsible for reporting and recording these findings. In some institutions or on some units the nurse may initiate medical interventions according to standard medical orders or established protocols when serious life-threatening arrhythmias are present.

Diet therapy. Dietary manipulation of potassium intake is a useful intervention when hyperkalemia is chronic or is related to inappropriate renal handling of potassium. However, when hyperkalemia is severe or sudden in onset, diet therapy is of minimal benefit.

Diarrhea

Plannings: client goals. The major client goals for this nursing diagnosis are that the client will (1) maintain bowel elimination patterns that are individually normal and (2) experience minimal abdominal discomfort.

Interventions: nonsurgical management. Interventions include restoring serum potassium levels to normal (discussed earlier as drug therapy for decreased cardiac output), decreasing intestinal irritability and peristalsis, and avoiding substances that promote GI motility.

Drug therapy. Many preparations are available that directly decrease intestinal motility and peristalsis. In addition, drugs that depress neural activity (such as narcotic analgesics) also reduce motility and peristalsis indirectly by depressing parasympathetic autonomic stimulation to the GI tract. The nurse needs to exercise caution regarding the amount and frequency of administration of any drug that decreases motility and peristalsis. Often, administration of many of these medications is ordered either as necessary (prn) or after each bowel movement. Overmedication can result in the development of constipation or even a paralytic ileus.

Diet therapy.   The nurse assists the client in menu selection to avoid foods that generally promote or stimulate peristalsis (high-fiber and high residue foods). In addition, the nurse asks questions regarding specific food items that cause the client to experience diarrhea or excessive flatus. Although adequate fluid intake is desirable and necessary to help prevent dehydration from the fluid lost in diarrheal stools, care must be taken to prevent excessive oral fluid intake that could increase peristalsis and diarrhea. The nurse maintains strict intake and output records to assist in assessing the client's actual fluid needs.

■ Discharge Planning

Discharge planning for clients with hyperkalemia is the same as that for clients with dehydration (see earlier).

Evaluation

On the basis of the identified nursing diagnoses, the nurse evaluates the care of the client experiencing hyperkalemia. The expected outcomes for the client with hyperkalemia include that the client

1. Restores and maintains normal serum potassium levels
2. Identifies interventions to take when the signs and symptoms of hyperkalemia occur
3. Maintains a regular, steady heart rate within the normal range
4. Accurately measures his/her own pulse rate and rhythm
5. Describes and complies with prescribed drug and diet therapy
6. Differentiates correctly foods to be avoided from foods permitted on the basis of potassium content
7. States to whom health care problems associated with hyperkalemia should be addressed
8. Restores and maintains normal elimination patterns

By meeting the stated outcomes, the client is more likely to remain in normal potassium balance. As a result, life-threatening complications can be avoided and the quality of life can be maintained.

SODIUM IMBALANCES

HYPONATREMIA

OVERVIEW

The condition of hyponatremia exists when the serum sodium ion (Na^+) level is less than 136 mEq/L. Because sodium is the major cation of the ECF and the primary determinant of ECF osmolarity (see Chap. 12), imbalances of sodium usually are associated with imbalances of fluid volume. Not only does hyponatremia often cause variations in fluid volume, but actual changes in fluid volume may be directly responsible for the decreased serum sodium levels.

Hyponatremia is one of the most common electrolyte imbalances that occurs among hospitalized clients. In spite of its frequency of occurrence, many aspects of hyponatremia are contradictory and confusing to health care professionals. Clients whose serum sodium levels are only 10 to 20 mEq/L below normal may exhibit side effects that are more severe and life-threatening than do clients whose serum sodium levels are more than 35 mEq/L below normal. Some of the symptoms observed with hyponatremia are identical to those seen with hypernatremia, whereas others are basically opposite from those symptoms associated with hypernatremia. Because sodium movement from the ECF across excitable membranes into the ICF is responsible for depolarization in many excitable tissues, the effects of hyponatremia are most noticeable in body systems that depend on membrane excitability for physiologic activity.

Pathophysiology

The underlying pathophysiologic changes associated with hyponatremia appear to have two general origins or mechanisms. One mechanism is related to changes in membrane excitability or responsiveness, and the other mechanism is related to the movement of water between intracellular and extracellular spaces. For the most part, as the ECF concentration of sodium decreases, the sodium concentration gradient between the ECF and the ICF also decreases. Less sodium is available to move across the excitable membrane, and this situation usually results in delayed and slower membrane depolarization. Although decreased sodium concentrations on the outside of excitable membranes normally decrease the resting membrane potential (RMP) to the extent that hypopolarization is present with increased membrane irritability and smaller stimuli are needed for depolarization, such is not usually the case in generalized hyponatremia. Rather, many excitable membranes are *less* responsive to stimuli during hyponatremia. One proposed mechanism for this apparent contradictory phenomenon is that when hyponatremia is present other disturbances in homeostasis also are present, and the body's homeostatic defenses are responding primarily (and correctly) to these other perceived disturbances.

Excitable tissues vary in their sensitivity to hyponatremia. Those excitable tissues that are inherently "leaky" to sodium or possess self-initiated depolarization mechanisms (such as specific areas of cardiac muscle tissue) are affected little by hyponatremia. The excitable tissues that are most sensitive to decreases in ECF sodium concentration are those located within the CNS. As with other electrolyte imbalances, the severity of the signs and symptoms associated with hyponatremia is dependent on the speed with which the imbalance occurs rather than solely on the severity of the imbalance.

Generally the signs and symptoms associated with mild to moderate hyponatremia reflect decreased excitability or irritability of the membranes. However, as ECF sodium concentrations decrease, the osmolarity and osmotic pressure of the ECF also decrease (and in some instances the hydrostatic pressure of the ECF increases). This situation causes extracellular water to move (by osmosis) into the cells, resulting in intracellular swelling. This swelling may interfere with the functional capacity of the cells within a given tissue. When such intracellular swelling occurs within the brain, increased cranial pressure results. This increased pressure can depress or stimulate nerve centers, depending on (1) the severity of the edema, (2) how quickly the edema forms, (3) the sensitivity of the cells to changes in size, and (4) the specific distribution of the edema within the brain. Thus, CNS symptoms of hyponatremia occur more frequently as depressed activity (drowsiness, lethargy, stupor, and coma), although occasionally symptoms of overactivity (agitation, psychoses, and seizures) are manifested.

As discussed in Chapter 12, maintaining serum sodium levels within the normal range is critical for normal physiologic function of many body systems. The body has several well-regulated mechanisms for conserving sodium and maintaining sodium balance. The presence of measurable, persistent hyponatremia accompanied by observable signs and symptoms indicates a significant physiologic problem.

Etiology

A variety of conditions can lead to hyponatremia by causing either an actual or a relative decrease in sodium content (see the accompanying Key Features of Disease). Hyponatremia can represent a loss of total body sodium, movement of sodium from the serum to other fluid spaces, or dilution of serum sodium by the presence of excessive water in the plasma volume (Adlard & George, 1978). More than one of the above processes can occur simultaneously. In addition, total body fluid volumes, as well as individual fluid compartment volumes, can be low, normal, or excessive during periods of hyponatremia. Common causes of hyponatremia are categorized on the basis of their associated ECF volumes. Causes of hyponatremia associated with increased ECF volumes include cardiac failure, hepatic failure, renal failure (nephrotic syndrome), near-drowning in freshwater, psychogenic polydipsia, and excessive irrigation with water or other hypotonic fluids (e.g., tap water enemas). Causes of hyponatremia associated with decreased ECF volumes include blood loss, excessive wound drainage, vomiting, diarrhea, administration of diuretics, and adrenal insufficiency (Addison's disease). Causes of hyponatremia associated with normal ECF volumes include excessive diaphoresis

---

KEY FEATURES OF DISEASE ■ Common Causes of Hyponatremia

Actual Sodium Deficits

Increased sodium excretion
  Excessive diaphoresis
  Diuretics (high-ceiling diuretics)
  Wound drainage (especially gastrointestinal)
  Decreased secretion of aldosterone
  Hyperlipidemia
  Renal disease (impaired DCT)
Inadequate sodium intake
  NPO
  Low-salt diet

Relative Sodium Deficits

Dilution of serum sodium
  Excessive ingestion of hypotonic fluids
  Psychogenic polydipsia
  Freshwater drowning
  Renal failure (nephrotic syndrome)
  Irrigation with hypotonic fluids
  SIADH (syndrome of inappropriate antidiuretic hormone secretion)
  Hyperglycemia
  Congestive heart failure

---

replaced only with water, hyperglycemia, hyperlipidemia, and the syndrome of inappropriate antidiuretic hormone secretion (SIADH) (Goldberg, 1981; Keyes, 1985).

Incidence

Mild hyponatremia as a result of moderate sodium loss and water dilution or sodium and fluid loss occurs frequently among the healthy population. Clients most at risk for developing this type of hyponatremia are the very young and the elderly. Such conditions may cause observable signs and symptoms because the imbalance occurs rapidly, but these conditions usually are temporary and are easily compensated through adequate oral intake of sodium. Hyponatremia among hospitalized clients also is a frequent occurrence and may be treatment induced or illness related. When the hyponatremia is a result of treatment, appropriate medical interventions can restore normal sodium balance relatively quickly. Clients at risk for treatment-induced hyponatremia include clients during the early postoperative period, clients who are NPO and receiving fluid intravenously (especially elderly, unconscious clients), and clients receiving potent diuretics without adequate sodium replacement. The most difficult hyponatremic conditions to correct or to control are those associated with serious chronic illnesses. In such instances restoration of normal sodium balance may not be possible unless the underlying chronic illness improves. Rather, management focuses on preventing the sodium imbalance from becoming worse.

The risk of serious, chronic hyponatremia is related to other illnesses, including Addison's disease, cirrhosis, renal failure (nephrotic syndrome), and profound congestive heart failure (Morrison & Murray, 1981). In addition, clients with conditions such as lung cancer, tuberculosis, head trauma, and cerebrovascular accident (CVA) are also at risk for chronic hyponatremia as a result of SIADH. Clients receiving the following drugs over extended periods of time also are at risk for hyponatremia secondary to SIADH: morphine sulfate, vincristine, and cyclophosphamide (Adlard & George, 1978).

PREVENTION

Strategies for prevention of hyponatremia vary according to the individual client and the probable cause of the imbalance. All strategies involve identification of clients at risk. When appropriate, preventive strategies include client education about measures to prevent hyponatremia. Another important aspect of prevention is the education of health care professionals in the physiology of fluid and electrolyte balance, specifically regarding sodium and water.

Among healthy individuals, hyponatremia frequently occurs when sodium and fluids are lost through excessive perspiration and fluid volume is restored by the ingestion of only hypotonic, non–sodium-containing fluids (especially water). Clients at risk for this type of hyponatremia include athletes, individuals who perform heavy labor or strenuous physical activities, and individuals exposed to high environmental temperatures for long periods of time. These clients should be taught to replace fluids frequently, before deficits become pronounced, and to drink fluids containing sodium and other electrolytes. Such beverages include common carbonated drinks, some fruit and vegetable juices, and premixed electrolyte-balanced solutions, such as Gatorade. Education also includes the signs and symptoms of mild hyponatremia (nausea, abdominal cramps, muscle weakness, and behavioral changes) so that the sodium-losing activity can be stopped and appropriate fluid replacement initiated before the imbalance worsens.

Treatment-induced hyponatremia is a common occurrence among hospitalized clients. In this situation the nurse assumes responsibility for secondary prevention (early detection) as well as primary prevention. Prevention involves identification of clients at risk and monitoring their fluid and electrolyte status. All clients receiving continuous IV fluid therapy need to have serum electrolyte levels evaluated on a daily basis. Although the ordering of laboratory tests, such as serum electrolyte measurements, is the physician's responsibility in most institutions, the nurse generally receives these reports first. Therefore, the nurse is in an ideal position to be aware of significant changes or persistent trends in the client's serum sodium levels and can alert the medical staff to an impending problem. Although the sodium balance of all clients is important, particular attention is required for clients receiving IV fluid therapy; those who are NPO or on continuous gastric suction; clients receiving potent, natriuretic diuretics; clients receiving low-sodium diets; and individuals prone to other fluid and electrolyte disturbances. In addition to daily monitoring of serum sodium levels, the nurse also assesses the client at risk during each shift for changes that indicate sodium imbalance. Clients prone to hyponatremia who also are receiving continuous IV fluid therapy should have the fluids administered through an infusion controller or a pump to reduce the risk of an inadvertent increase in the drip rate.

When mild hyponatremia is identified early, measures can be taken to prevent the imbalance from becoming more severe. Depending on the cause and whether other chronic pathologic changes also are present, the following interventions can assist in preventing a more profound hyponatremia: increasing sodium intake (oral or parenteral), restricting hypotonic fluid intake (especially water), discontinuing natriuretic diuretics, and administering osmotic diuretics.

COLLABORATIVE MANAGEMENT

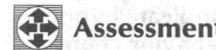 **Assessment**

History

When documenting a history from any client, the nurse collects data regarding risk factors, as well as causative factors, related to hyponatremia. *Age* is an important factor, as both young children and the elderly are more prone to fluid and electrolyte disturbances. Not only are the elderly more likely to have other chronic conditions that can lead to sodium imbalances (renal failure, cardiac failure, hepatic failure, and CVAs), they also are more likely to be taking prescribed or OTC medications that interfere with sodium balance. The nurse inquires about specific risk factors, such as renal dysfunction, including nephrotic syndrome; liver disease; and congestive heart failure. Clients are asked specific questions regarding recent illnesses or surgical treatments that promote sodium and fluid losses, such as vomiting, diarrhea, fevers, and wound drainage (for example, a T tube in place after cholecystectomy).

Clients are asked specific questions concerning *urinary output,* including the frequency and amount of voidings. The nurse asks questions regarding the actual fluid intake in general and specifically during the previous 24 hours. Information about the types of fluids ingested is just as important to obtain as information about the amounts of fluids ingested.

Information about the client's *height* and *usual weight* is important to obtain. Smaller-statured, thinner individuals respond more dramatically to fluid and electrolyte fluctuations than do larger individuals. *Recent changes in weight* (increases and decreases) also are noted.

The nurse inquires about the use of OTC and prescribed *medications,* especially diuretics, morphine, and chemotherapeutic agents. If the client is unable to recall exactly what medications are being taken, the nurse may obtain this information from the client's inpatient and outpatient records.

The nurse obtains a detailed *diet history* to determine approximate levels of sodium intake. Because many individuals are on self-prescribed dietary limitations of sodium, the nurse specifically asks the client if he/she uses table salt or salt substitutes or makes any attempt to limit or eliminate dietary sodium. Questions regarding general food intake and use of seasonings, as well as 24-hour dietary recall, are helpful.

The nurse inquires about the amount of *strenuous physical activity* the client may have engaged in recently, along with collecting information regarding environmental *temperature and humidity* conditions present during the activity.

The nurse also collects data that may indicate the presence of symptoms specifically associated with hyponatremia. Often these questions must be directed to a close family member, as the client's responses may be limited or not reliable. Although the signs and symptoms associated with hyponatremia may be vague or have such an insidious onset that they are hardly noticed by the client, positive responses to questions regarding the following symptoms may indicate hyponatremia. The client is asked whether behavior changes, headaches, increased somnolence, decreased alertness, decreased attention span, difficulty in awakening, muscle weakness, anorexia, abdominal cramping, or increasing fatigue have been experienced. Information about the presence of edema or changes in skin turgor is obtained. Having the client or a responsible family member relate the client's activity during the previous 24 hours may disclose additional information about activity intolerance, unusual behavior, and the presence of unexplained fatigue.

Physical Assessment: Clinical Manifestations

Clinical manifestations of hyponatremia vary with the degree of imbalance and whether a fluid imbalance accompanies the decrease in serum sodium levels. Another determinant of whether symptoms are manifested is how rapidly the imbalance is experienced. Rapid decreases in serum sodium levels generally produce more obvious and severe signs and symptoms. Gradual decreases in serum sodium levels are tolerated better (or compensated better) and may produce no obvious physiologic changes even when serum sodium levels drop 30 mEq/L or more below the normal range. Clinical manifestations of hyponatremia primarily are associated with alterations of excitable membrane activity, especially among the excitable tissues involved in cerebral,

neuromuscular, and gastric smooth muscle functions (see the accompanying Key Features of Disease). Other physiologic systems may either indirectly experience changes in function as a result of hyponatremia or have chronic pathologic alterations that contribute to the development of hyponatremia. These systems also should be assessed and include the *circulatory, respiratory, integumentary,* and *renal systems.*

KEY FEATURES OF DISEASE ■ Clinical Manifestations of Hyponatremia

Cardiovascular*

Normovolemic
   Rapid pulse rate
   Normal blood pressure
Hypovolemic
   Rapid pulse rate
   Pulse quality thready and weak
   Hypotensive
   Central venous pressure normal or low
   Flat neck veins
Hypervolemic
   Rapid, bounding pulse
   Central venous pressure normal or elevated
   Blood pressure normal or elevated

Respiratory

Late manifestations related to
   Skeletal muscle weakness
      Shallow, ineffective respiratory movements
   Hypervolemia
   Pulmonary edema
      Rapid, shallow respiration
      Moist rales

Neuromuscular

Generalized skeletal muscle weakness
Diminished deep tendon reflexes
Personality changes
Headache

Renal

Increased urinary output
Decreased specific gravity

Gastrointestinal

Increased motility
Nausea
Hyperactive bowel sounds
Diarrhea

* Symptoms vary with changes in vascular volume.

Alterations in cerebral and upper neural functions are the most obvious consequences of hyponatremia. Because these alterations may be manifested as either depressed activity or excessive activity (and sometimes both), establishing the normal (usual) CNS function and behavior patterns for each client is crucial to detect changes associated with hyponatremia.

The nurse observes the client closely and documents the client's behavior. The nurse describes the behavior without interpreting it. For example, the nurse may observe and document that the client is tearful, is slow to respond to questions, and has a flat affect, but the nurse does not state that the client is depressed. The nurse assesses the client's current mental status, starting with the level of consciousness. Notations are made regarding whether the client is asleep or awake. If the client is asleep, the nurse gently awakens him/her and documents the ease with which the client is aroused. If the client is awake, the nurse establishes whether the client is oriented to time, place, and person. The nurse avoids asking questions that can be answered with a "yes" or a "no" response and pays close attention to the manner in which the client responds to questions. Is it necessary to repeat questions to obtain a response? Does the response answer the question asked? Does the client have difficulty with word choices in forming responses? Is the client irritated or upset by the questions? Can the client concentrate on a question long enough to provide an appropriate response, or is the attention span short? When assessing mental status, the nurse avoids asking nonsense questions, such as "Do helicopters eat their young?" because this type of question may confuse a client or make the client doubtful about the competency of the health care professional. When asking questions to determine past memory or rational thought, the nurse asks questions about subjects that the client could be expected to know and avoids obscure trivia, such as "Who was vice president under Truman?" Other useful techniques to assess mental status and the presence of increased intracranial pressure can be found in Chapter 32. The nurse questions the family members regarding whether the behavior and the mental status are typical for this client.

The nurse assesses the client's neuromuscular status during each shift for changes from baseline values. The usual neuromuscular response to frank hyponatremia is generalized muscle weakness. Muscle tone diminishes, as do deep tendon reflex responses. The nurse assesses muscle strength by having the client (1) squeeze the nurse's hands, (2) attempt to keep the arms flexed while the nurse pulls downward on the lower arms, and (3) push both feet against a flat surface (a box or a board) while the nurse applies resistance. Muscle weakness associated with hyponatremia occurs bilaterally and is more pronounced among the muscle groups in the extremities. The nurse assesses peripheral nerve responsiveness by lightly tapping the patellar tendons and Achilles tendons with a reflex hammer and documenting the degree of reflex movement elicited.

The smooth muscle of the GI system is relatively sensitive to decreases in serum sodium levels. The usual response to hyponatremia is increased GI motility accompanied by nausea, diarrhea, and abdominal cramping. The nurse assesses the GI system by listening to bowel sounds and observing elimination products. Bowel sounds are assessed with a stethoscope before any palpation of the abdomen is undertaken. Bowel sounds are hyperactive, with frequent audible rushes and gurgles, especially over the splenic flexure and in the lower left quadrant. Bowel movements are frequent, watery, and explosive in nature. Peristaltic movements may be palpated through the abdominal wall and may even be visible on the abdominal surface.

Hyponatremia has little direct effect on cardiac muscle contractility; however, alterations in cardiac output are associated with hyponatremia. In some instances, cardiac pathologic changes (such as profound congestive heart failure with generalized edema formation) actually cause the hyponatremia. When hyponatremia is accompanied by changes in the plasma volume, these fluid changes alter cardiac function. The nurse assesses cardiac and circulatory status by measuring the central pulse rate, the central venous pressure, blood pressure, the quality of peripheral pulses, and venous filling capacity. Generally, the cardiac responses to hyponatremia with hypovolemia are manifested as a rapid, weak, thready pulse. Peripheral pulses may be difficult to palpate and are easily obliterated with light pressure. Neck veins are flat in the upright position and also may be flat in the supine position. Blood pressure is decreased, especially diastolic pressure. The client may experience profound hypotension when moving from a lying or sitting position to a standing position. The central venous pressure is normal or low. When hyponatremia is accompanied by plasma hypervolemia, cardiac manifestations include a rapid, full pulse. Blood pressure is normal or elevated. The central venous pressure is normal or elevated, depending on how well the left ventricle is handling the extra fluid. Peripheral pulses are full and difficult to obliterate (although, if significant edema is present, peripheral pulses may not be palpable).

The respiratory system is not affected directly by hyponatremia, but the influence of low serum sodium levels on cerebral function and circulatory status may be reflected as alterations in respiration. The nurse assesses the client's respiratory status by observing the rate, depth, and ease of respirations. In addition, the nurse auscultates the lung fields to determine the presence of abnormal or adventitious breath sounds. If cerebral edema and increased intracranial pressure accompany hyponatremia, respirations may be shallow and below the normal rate. If hypervolemia and congestive heart failure accompany the hyponatremic condition, the respiratory rate may be greatly increased and shallow, with moist rales or rhonchi audible on auscultation.

Changes in the integumentary system associated with hyponatremia may be confusing and are not reliable indicators of low serum sodium levels. Visible edema may not be detected easily, because extra fluids often are distributed equally between the extracellular spaces and the intracellular spaces. With some specific hyponatremic conditions, such as cirrhosis of the liver or congestive heart failure, dependent edema is profound. Even when significant fluid loss is responsible for the hyponatremia, the typical picture of dehydration with poor skin turgor may not be present. Although alterations in the integumentary system may not be reliable diagnostic indicators, the nurse assesses the integumentary system to obtain baseline data and to prevent cutaneous complications. The nurse assesses the integumentary system for skin color, temperature, degree of moisture, and presence of edema (see the discussion of integumentary assessment for hypernatremia).

Any condition that alters electrolyte and fluid balance usually has specific renal manifestations. In addition, renal pathologic changes can contribute to the development of hyponatremia (renal failure with nephrotic syndrome). The nurse primarily assesses renal perfusion by accurately measuring fluid intake and output. The nurse also notes the color and the specific gravity of the urine. Daily weights also reflect renal function. The nurse weighs the client daily at the same time of day using the same scales. Whenever possible, the client should be wearing the same amount and type of clothing at each weigh-in. The renal manifestations associated with hyponatremia vary according to the cause of the low serum sodium level and changes in ECF volume.

Psychosocial Assessment

Psychosocial assessment is critically important because behavioral changes may be the only obvious clinical manifestation of the hyponatremic condition. The nurse performs a careful mental status examination and complete neurologic assessment (see earlier discussion of physical assessment and Chap. 32). If the nurse does not have expertise in this area, consultation with a clinical nurse specializing in neuropsychiatry is appropriate.

Laboratory Findings

The most definitive laboratory test result to confirm the presence of hyponatremia is a serum sodium level less than 136 mEq/L. Usually the serum sodium value is much lower before clinical manifestations are evident. When the hyponatremia is caused by hyperglycemia or hyperlipidemia, this serum sodium value may be falsely low, indicating a sodium imbalance that does not truly exist. Other laboratory data change in association with the hyponatremia, depending on the cause and the ECF volume. If the hyponatremia is caused by water intoxication (dilution), levels of other serum electrolytes are low, as are the hematocrit, hemoglobin, and total protein levels. Hyponatremia caused by fluid and sodium shifts from the vascular space to other fluid spaces show an increase in hematocrit, hemoglobin, potassium, and blood urea nitrogen levels. Hyponatremia caused by SIADH rarely is associated with any other electrolyte imbalance. Variations in urinary output and composition are not reliable indicators of hyponatremia, because etiology, fluid volumes, and renal disease influence these factors more than the actual hyponatremia does.

The anion chloride (Cl^-) is the major electrical balance to the cation sodium in the ECF. Therefore, imbalances of sodium usually result in a corresponding imbalance of chloride (Keyes, 1985). When hyponatremia is present, hypochloremia (serum chloride less than 94 mEq/L) also is present. A few specific common conditions can lead to greater decreases in serum chloride than in serum sodium levels. These conditions include excessive vomiting or prolonged gastric suctioning. These conditions result in an actual chloride loss in excess of sodium loss. Actual losses of chloride contribute to the development of metabolic alkalosis, as serum bicarbonate levels increase to provide anion balance. During periods of metabolic acidosis a relative decrease in serum chloride levels is seen as chloride enters red blood cells in exchange for the anion buffer bicarbonate.

 ### Analysis: Nursing Diagnosis

Hyponatremia as a result of sodium and fluid loss with hypotonic fluid replacement occurs frequently among otherwise healthy individuals. Usually this condition is rectified without intervention by health care professionals. In the acute care setting, two categories of hyponatremia are found. Treatment-induced hyponatremia composes one category. The hyponatremia develops in response to various medical treatments for other conditions. This category of hyponatremia is easily corrected and requires nursing intervention; however, once corrected, the hyponatremia is seldom a recurrent problem for the client. The remaining category of hyponatremia is more persistent and difficult to treat. This form of hyponatremia is a result of some chronic pathologic change or illness. Often, complete restoration of normal sodium levels is not possible unless the underlying chronic pathologic change can be alleviated or corrected. A typical client at risk for actual hyponatremia is a 40-year-old woman who has undergone cholecystectomy with common bile duct exploration 3 days previously. She is NPO and has a nasogastric tube to intermittent low suction. A T tube is in place for gravity drainage. For fluid replacement during the 72 hours since surgery, the client has received 1 L of 5% dextrose in 0.45 normal saline, 4 L of D_5W, and 4 L of D_5W, with 20 mEq of KCl. The following diagnoses are derived from these data (Aspinall, 1978).

Common Diagnoses

The following diagnoses are commonly applicable to hospitalized clients with hyponatremia:

1. Altered thought processes related to changes in CNS activity
2. Pain (headache) related to increased intracranial pressure

Additional Diagnoses

In addition to the common diagnoses, one or more of the following nursing diagnoses may be noted:

1. Fluid volume excess related to excessive water intake
2. Altered nutrition: less than body requirements related to inadequate sodium intake
3. Potential for injury related to postural hypotension or skeletal muscle weakness
4. Total self-care deficit related to muscle weakness
5. Pain related to abdominal cramping secondary to increased GI peristalsis
6. Potential impaired skin integrity related to excesses or deficiencies of interstitial fluid
7. Body image disturbance related to weight gain
8. Knowledge deficit related to treatment regimen
9. Impaired physical mobility related to muscle weakness

 Planning and Implementation

The following plan of care for the hospitalized client with hyponatremia focuses on the common nursing diagnoses associated with specific side effects that usually accompany ECF sodium deficits. This plan of care has three distinct aims. The primary aim is to restore normal sodium and fluid balance whenever possible. The second aim is to provide supportive care for altered physiologic function and to prevent associated complications until the hyponatremia is resolved. The final aim is to prevent future sodium imbalances.

Altered Thought Processes

Planning: client goals. The major client goals for this nursing diagnosis are that the client will (1) have serum sodium levels restored to normal, (2) accurately interpret environmental stimuli, and (3) remain in a safe environment.

Interventions: nonsurgical management. Interventions are aimed at preventing further decreases in serum sodium levels, increasing below-normal serum sodium levels, and providing a safe environment. An accurate assessment of CNS activity changes from normal or from baseline is the basis for the institution of specific interventions and, therefore, constitutes a major nursing responsibility. Drug and diet therapy can play major roles in restoring normal sodium balance.

Mental status assessment. The nurse assesses the client's CNS functional activity at least during every shift to evaluate the effectiveness of current interventions and to determine whether a sodium imbalance continues to exist. Variables to be assessed include the level of consciousness; orientation to time, place, and person; past and recent memory; the ability to concentrate; and cognitive function.

Drug therapy. Drug therapy for hyponatremia primarily focuses on restoration of normal serum sodium levels. Depending on the cause of the hyponatremia, this intervention can include either the addition or the retention of sodium. (When sodium has not been lost from the body, the addition of sodium may not be appropriate.) IV saline infusions are useful in restoring both sodium content and fluid volume. Depending on the severity of the hyponatremia, IV saline solutions may be isotonic (0.9%) or hypertonic (3% to 5%) (Goldberg, 1981; Rossi & Cadnapaphornchai, 1987). Caution must be exercised in the speed with which ECF sodium and fluid are restored to normal levels. In general, the rate of infusion should be regulated by the rate of the sodium or fluid loss. When sodium is replaced too rapidly, excitable membranes, especially those in the CNS, may overrespond to the fluid and electrolyte changes with severe adverse reactions. The nurse carefully monitors infusion rates and client responses. Whenever possible, the infusions are delivered through a controller or a pump to prevent accidental alterations in infusion rates. Other substances may be added to the infusing solution, depending on the presence of other electrolyte imbalances or chronic conditions. If the physician's order is to deliver sodium by IV push, the nurse administers the solution slowly, preferably through a central line.

When hyponatremia is accompanied by fluid excess, drug therapy includes the administration of diuretics that are primarily hydrouretic (water excreting) in nature rather than natriuretic (sodium excreting). These drugs include osmotic diuretics, such as mannitol (Beck, 1981). When cerebral edema is profound, drugs that specifically promote CNS fluid loss may be prescribed (urea, dexamethasone). The nurse administers these agents with care and assesses the client every 2 to 3 hours for signs that indicate excessive loss of fluids or potassium or dramatic increases in sodium levels.

Drug therapy for hyponatremia as a result of inappropriate or excessive secretion of ADH may include agents that antagonize ADH (demeclocycline, lithium) or agents that block ADH receptors. Both of these categories of drugs are in relatively new use for the treatment of hyponatremia. Before administration of the drugs, the nurse becomes familiar with their actions, expected side effects, and potential adverse reactions. The nurse keeps antidotes to these agents on hand during the time when any client is receiving them (antidotes are amiloride for demeclocycline and acetazolamide for lithium).

When hyponatremia is a result of underlying pathologic change and not a direct disturbance of sodium balance, drug therapy focuses primarily on treatment of the underlying condition. For example, fluid retention caused by poor cardiac output and low MAP associated with severe congestive heart failure can dilute serum sodium levels to below-normal values, although there is no actual deficit in total body sodium. Treating the condition with drugs that improve cardiac output (digoxin, amrinone, deslanoside) and renal circulation (dopamine) results in restoration of normal serum sodium levels without the addition of sodium.

Diet therapy. For mild hyponatremia, diet therapy can be of benefit in restoring normal sodium balance. Table 12-4 in Chapter 12 provides the sodium content of common foods. The therapy usually consists of increasing oral sodium intake and restricting oral intake of fluids to some degree. When overhydration with oral hypotonic fluids is the underlying cause of the hyponatremia or when renal fluid excretion is impaired, fluid restriction may be a long-term regimen. The nurse accurately measures fluid intake and output. The nurse also reinforces the reasons for the fluid restriction, so that clients and families do not view the regimen as punishment. In situations in which the client either cannot or does not comply with the restriction, it may be necessary to restrict visitors and remove the handles from water faucets in the client's room. Dietary manipulation of sodium has little effect on severe hyponatremia or hyponatremia due to nonrenal chronic pathologic conditions.

Maintaining a safe environment. Changes in CNS functions and responses are expected in the client with hyponatremia. These changes vary from mild anxiety to psychosis and from drowsiness to coma or convulsions. Behavior changes are frequently manifested by the client's misinterpreting environmental stimuli. Maintaining a safe environment for the client with CNS changes is an important nursing function. This function includes assisting the client to process information correctly. The nurse orients the client to time and place at every interaction. The nurse reminds the client of who the nurse is and what the nurse is doing for the client. It may be helpful to place large calendars and clocks where the client can see them. If the client needs glasses to see properly, the nurse makes certain that the client wears the glasses whenever he/she is awake. The nurse makes certain that the client's call light is within easy reach at all times.

The nurse reduces extraneous environmental stimuli to keep the client from becoming confused. Whenever possible the client should be assigned to a private room. If a private room is not available, the nurse makes certain that the roommate does not have a personality or condition that would be inconsistent with a quiet environment. For example, clients who require ventilators or other pieces of noisy equipment that operate continuously would not be appropriate as roommates. Lighting is kept to the minimum needed for safety. The telephone is removed or the bell adjusted so that it does not ring. Radio and television programs that vary in loudness and excitement are avoided. Young children and hysterical or confused individuals should not be permitted to visit.

Care must be taken to prevent clients who are experiencing alterations in thought processes and CNS activity from becoming injured. Clients who are confused require close observation, especially when they are out of bed. The nurse anticipates the client's needs for ambulation and, when ambulation is permitted, accompanies the client (e.g., to the bathroom). The upper side rails of the client's bed are in the up position at all times. Whenever the client is alone, the bed is kept in the low position. At times it may be necessary for the nurse to prevent the client from reaching the electronic bed controls. If the client continues to remain confused and continues to get out of bed unassisted, the nurse may request an order to restrain the client with a vest or jacket-style restraint. Such devices should only be used when the client represents a clear danger to self. Ideally, having another responsible person in the room with the client at all times eliminates the need for the use of restraining devices.

When the client's condition indicates that seizure activity is likely to occur, the nurse additionally prepares the immediate environment to prevent injury to the client. Side rails are padded. The emergency cart or a box with appropriate anticonvulsive drugs is either in the room or just outside the door. The nurse checks that suction equipment and an oxygen administration set-up are available within the room and are in good working order.

Pain (Headache)

Planning: client goals. The major client goal for this nursing diagnosis is that the client will achieve an acceptable level of headache relief.

Interventions: nonsurgical management. The interventions for this problem are aimed at restoring normal sodium balance, preventing further increases in intracranial pressure, and altering the client's perception of discomfort. The interventions directed toward restoring normal sodium balance for clients with this nursing diagnosis are the same as the drug therapy and diet therapy interventions for altered thought processes (discussed earlier). The additional interventions for the specific problem of headache focus on means other than the restoration of sodium and fluid balance to prevent further increases in intracranial pressure and means to alter the client's perception of discomfort.

Drug therapy. Intracranial pressure can be increased through position changes and other body pressure changes within the client's voluntary control. The Valsalva maneuver (holding one's breath and forcefully contracting specific muscle groups) increases intracranial pressure and is used during a wide variety of normal activities, including defecating, urinating, coughing, nose blowing, lifting, and intercourse. Drug therapy is aimed at decreasing the frequency and intensity of the Valsalva maneuver for these clients. If the client has difficulty defecating, stool softeners and laxatives may be used so that bowel movements can be accomplished with minimal straining. If the client has an upper respiratory tract problem in which nose blowing, coughing, or sneezing are common occurrences, antihistamine or decongestant medications can be administered to control these symptoms and to reduce the frequency with which the client would be performing the Valsalva maneuver. The side effects of some antihistamines and decongestants include increased intracranial pressure. The nurse checks the action and side effects of all prescribed medications before administration to be certain that the medication will not contribute to the problem of increased intracranial pressure.

Drug therapy can be of benefit in helping to reduce the client's perception of pain. Analgesic medications are commonly used to decrease the perception of pain and discomfort. For clients whose hyponatremia is a result of SIADH, the nurse ensures that morphine-based derivatives are not administered to the client, because these drugs tend to worsen the SIADH.

Activity and positioning. Specific positions and position changes can increase intracranial pressure. Any time the head is on the same gravitational level as the heart or is lower than the heart, intracranial pressure is increased owing to reduced venous return. The nurse explains this phenomenon to the client and cautions the client to avoid activities that involve bending over (such as lifting objects, hair washing at a sink, retrieving items from the floor, and putting on shoes). The head of the bed is placed at a minimum of a 15-degree angle, and the client is never permitted to be in a flat or Trendelenburg's position. The nurse also makes certain that venous return from the head is not mechanically obstructed by tight collars or dressings on the neck.

Additional comfort measures. Nursing actions that may help to relieve discomfort due to headache and increase client comfort include reduction of environmental stimuli, the use of ice caps, and avoidance of activities and procedures that upset the client physically or emotionally. Actions to reduce environmental stimuli are those discussed earlier for maintaining a safe environment for clients with a nursing diagnosis of altered thought processes.

Some, but not all, clients obtain headache relief from the use of ice caps. The nurse ensures that the ice cap is not too heavy, which could increase the client's discomfort. Ice chips, rather than large ice cubes, are used to fill the cap to avoid uncomfortable edges and decrease the rigidity of the ice cap. The ice cap is covered with cloth so that extremely cold or wet surfaces do not come into direct contact with the client's skin. When the client is using an ice cap, the nurse evaluates the effectiveness in terms of pain relief every half hour. If the client states that the pain is the same or worse, the ice cap is removed. The skin under the ice cap is examined for changes that indicate adverse reactions.

The nurse examines the hospitalized client's schedule of prescribed and routine activities. Those activities that do not have a direct, positive effect on the client's condition are assessed in terms of their usefulness to the client. If the benefit (actual or potential) of the activity does not outweigh its actual or potential aggravation of the client's condition, the nurse consults with other members of the health care team about eliminating or postponing the activity. Some activities that might be candidates for cancellation or temporary postponement include hair washing, taking blood pressure more than once per day, taking rectal temperatures, engaging in respiratory therapy treatments or physical therapy, and undergoing specific invasive diagnostic tests that are not required for assessment or treatment and that may increase discomfort.

■ Discharge Planning

Discharge planning for clients with hyponatremia is the same as that for clients with dehydration (see earlier).

 ## Evaluation

The nurse evaluates the care for the client experiencing hyponatremia on the basis of the identified nursing diagnoses associated with this condition. The expected outcomes for the client with hyponatremia include that the client

1. Restores and maintains normal serum sodium levels
2. Identifies actions to take when the signs and symptoms of hyponatremia occur
3. Achieves an acceptable level of comfort related to decrease in headache and abdominal cramping
4. Maintains or increases the current level of participation in self-care activities
5. Interprets accurately environmental stimuli, as evidenced by correct orientation to time, place, and person
6. Avoids injury
7. Maintains an adequate intake of foods and fluids
8. Maintains skin integrity
9. Verbalizes knowledge of the prescribed medical regimen
10. Complies with the prescribed medical regimen

HYPERNATREMIA

OVERVIEW

A state of hypernatremia exists when the serum sodium ion level exceeds 145 mEq/L. Although some of the physiologic consequences of hypernatremia are basically opposite from those associated with hyponatremia, such is not always the case. Approximately 60% of the body's total sodium content is present in the ECF, with the medullary interstitial fluid of kidney tissue containing the highest concentration of sodium. Increases in ECF sodium levels can be caused by variations in fluid volumes and also can cause variations in fluid volumes. In addition, because the movement of sodium across excitable membranes from the ECF into the ICF is responsible for depolarization, hypernatremia from all causes profoundly influences body systems that depend on membrane excitability.

Pathophysiology

As the extracellular sodium level rises, there is a steeper sodium concentration gradient between the ECF and the ICF. More sodium is available to move more rapidly across the excitable membranes, and this situation results in earlier membrane depolarization, even in the presence of a smaller stimulus. With mild hypernatremia almost all excitable tissues are excited more easily and are said to be irritable. This irritability generally causes them to overrespond to stimuli. The signs and symptoms associated with mild hypernatremia reflect the excess excitability of the membranes. However, as the ECF sodium concentration increases, the osmolarity and the osmotic pressure of the ECF also increase. This situation causes osmosis of water from the ICF into the ECF as a compensatory action in an effort to dilute the hyperosmolar ECF. When hypernatremia persists or becomes more severe, the compensatory water osmosis causes such profound intracellular dehydration that the excitable tissues may no longer be able to respond to depolarization. Excitable tissues vary in their sensitivity to hypernatremia. Excitable tissues in the brain are the most sensitive to changes in ECF sodium concentration, followed by skeletal muscle, cardiac muscle, and smooth muscle. As with other electrolyte imbalances, the type and severity of the signs and symptoms associated with hypernatremia are dependent on both the speed with which the imbalance occurs and the severity of the imbalance.

Depending on the underlying cause, the body has several mechanisms to assist either in preventing the sodium concentration from rising or in decreasing the hypernatremia. Generally, hypernatremia suppresses the release of aldosterone. Aldosterone suppression results in an increased renal excretion of sodium. Hypernatremia also stimulates specific areas of the hypothalamus. This stimulation both triggers the thirst reflex and causes the posterior pituitary gland to release ADH. These two mechanisms together assist to dilute the ECF sodium concentration by decreasing renal water loss and increasing water intake (Chap. 12). Therefore, the presence of measurable hypernatremia that results in obvious signs and symptoms represents a real or relative sodium load beyond that which can be handled effec-

tively by the body's sodium- and water-regulating mechanisms.

Etiology

Hypernatremia may occur as a result of an actual increase in the total body sodium content or as a result of a relative sodium concentration increase in response to water depletion (see the accompanying Key Features of Disease). Both types of problems leading to hypernatremia can occur simultaneously, resulting in a more profound hypernatremia. Conditions that can cause an *actual increase* in total body sodium content include those that inhibit or impair renal excretion of sodium and those conditions that result in excessive sodium intake. Conditions that inhibit or impair renal sodium excretion include renal failure, neurologic lesions, hyperaldosteronism, Cushing's syndrome, and the use of corticosteroids. Conditions that cause hypernatremia as a result of excessive sodium intake include excessive ingestion of oral sodium chloride- or sodium bicarbonate-containing substances and excessive or inappropriate administration of sodium-containing parenteral fluids. *Relative hypernatremia* occurs as a result of conditions that directly decrease the total body water content, rather than increase the total body sodium content. Any condition that causes excessive water loss (heavy diaphoresis, ineffective ADH response, diarrhea, and os-

---

KEY FEATURES OF DISEASE ■ Common Causes of Hypernatremia

Actual Sodium Excesses

Decreased sodium excretion
 Hyperaldosteronism
 Renal failure
 Corticosteroids
 Cushing's syndrome
Increased sodium intake
 Excessive oral sodium ingestion
 Excessive administration of sodium-containing IV fluids

Relative Sodium Excesses

Decreased water intake
 NPO
Increased water loss
 Increased rate of metabolism
 Fever
 Hyperventilation
 Infection
 Excessive diaphoresis
 Watery diarrhea
 Dehydration

motic diuresis) or inadequate water intake (impaired neural function, impaired motor function, and no water available) can lead to a relative hypernatremia.

Incidence

Mild hypernatremia due to excessive water loss occurs frequently among the healthy population, but is temporary and is easily compensated through response to the thirst mechanism. Hypernatremia associated with an actual increase in total body sodium content rarely occurs in healthy individuals because the ADH and aldosterone regulatory mechanisms are so responsive to even minute changes in ECF osmolarity (Geheb, 1987). "Hypernatremia as a result of excessive sodium intake is rare, catastrophic and most frequently caused by inappropriate medical care and/or poor management of clients' fluid and electrolyte needs" (Brenner et al., 1987). Persons at highest risk for hypernatremia are clients who are unable to manage their own oral intake (very young, elderly, neuroimpaired, and motor-impaired individuals), clients with acute water-losing illnesses, and those with renal problems.

PREVENTION

Measures to assist in the prevention of hypernatremia vary according to the cause and the associated fluid volume changes. In outpatient or nonacute situations, prevention is aimed at identification of clients at risk and individual client education regarding specific risks and prophylactic measures. In acute care settings and emergency situations, prevention is aimed at (1) accurately assessing clients' fluid and electrolyte needs and (2) moderating health care reactions to conditions associated with electrolyte and acid-base imbalances.

Hypernatremia that results from inadequate water volumes (either increased pure water loss or inadequate water intake) without an actual change in the total body sodium concentration is most easily prevented (Cadnapaphornchai, 1987). This type of hypernatremia is most commonly found among clients who have lost the thirst sensation, are physically unable to obtain oral fluids for themselves, are feverish, or have prolonged deep and rapid respirations. Prevention involves maintaining a water intake (oral or parenteral) appropriate for the individual client's metabolic needs.

Hypernatremia that results from excessive fluid losses in which both water and sodium are lost (with proportionately more water being lost than sodium) usually is associated with an actual *decrease* in the total body sodium (the decrease is masked by the water volume loss). This type of hypernatremia can develop quickly in clients who are otherwise healthy but are experiencing acute episodes of severe vomiting, excessive diarrhea, or excessive diaphoresis (Geheb, 1987). Clients with renal disease specifically affecting the functional capacity of the proximal convoluted tubule

(PCT) also are at risk for developing this type of hypernatremia. Primary prevention for this type of hypernatremia is somewhat more difficult, because many of these conditions have an acute onset. For secondary prevention, clients must be taught to seek medical intervention before the imbalances become severe.

Hypernatremia that results from excessive sodium intake (to the degree that the body's sodium excretion mechanisms cannot keep pace) is generally of two types. The first category is found in clients whose renal handling of sodium is impaired. Such conditions include renal failure and primary hyperaldosteronism. Prevention for this type of hypernatremia is aimed at client education and compliance regarding strict limitations on sodium intake. The second category is the rapid administration or prolonged continuous administration of sodium-containing solutions as medical treatment for specific conditions. A classic example of hypernatremia's resulting from medical treatment is the electrolyte imbalances that may occur after resuscitation efforts for cardiac arrest. The administration of excessive IV sodium bicarbonate leads to a profound and frequently life-threatening hypernatremia (Geheb, 1987). Moreover, sodium bicarbonate administration has been found to be of little or no value in correcting the acidosis that develops during cardiac arrest. Thus, prevention is aimed at the education of health care professionals regarding proper administration of agents during resuscitation efforts or other similar acute or emergency situations.

COLLABORATIVE MANAGEMENT

 Assessment

History

Because some causes of hypernatremia are preventable, the nurse collects data regarding risk factors associated with hypernatremia, as well as causative factors. *Age* is an important factor not only because altered renal function occurs among the elderly, but also because the elderly client is more likely to be taking prescription and OTC medications that influence fluid and electrolyte balance. The nurse inquires about specific risk factors, such as the presence of renal disease and the recent occurrence of conditions that promote excessive water loss, such as feverish states, vomiting, diarrhea, and heavy diaphoresis. Clients who state that they do not have a medical diagnosis of renal failure or insufficiency are asked specific questions regarding *urinary output*, including the frequency and amount of voiding. The nurse asks specific questions regarding *actual fluid intake* during the previous 24 hours. Information about the type of fluid ingested is just as important to obtain as information regarding the amount of fluid ingested. *Recent changes in weight* are also noted.

The nurse also inquires about the *use of medication*, especially antacids. The nurse takes a *diet history* to determine approximate levels of sodium intake. Questions concerning the consumption of high-sodium foods, such as canned foods, processed and packaged foods, snack foods, crackers, cheese, and smoked meats, are asked specifically. The nurse asks the client about the use of sodium-containing condiments, such as table salt, soy-based sauces, ketchup, steak sauces, meat tenderizers (such as Accent and other brands containing monosodium glutamate), and other flavor enhancers. The nurse inquires about the amount of *strenuous physical activity* the client may have engaged in recently, along with environmental *temperature and humidity* conditions present during the activity.

The nurse also collects data that may indicate the presence of symptoms related specifically to hypernatremia. This task is difficult because, unlike many other electrolyte imbalances, hypernatremia does not have symptoms that clearly indicate the presence of an imbalance. Rather, symptoms are vague and may change with the intensity of the imbalance. The client is asked if insomnia or mental irritability have been experienced. Information regarding the presence of edema or changes in skin texture or turgor is obtained. Having the client relate the activities of the previous 24 hours may disclose additional information about changes in activity level, mental status, and the presence of unexplained weakness or fatigue.

Physical Assessment: Clinical Manifestations

Clinical manifestations of hypernatremia vary with the degree of imbalance and whether a fluid imbalance coexists with the increase in the serum sodium level. Another determinant of whether symptoms are obvious is how rapidly the imbalance is experienced. Rapid increases in serum sodium level generally produce more obvious and severe symptoms. Gradual increases in serum sodium levels may produce no observable physiologic changes, even when sodium levels are increased 25% above normal ranges. Clinical manifestations of hypernatremia primarily are associated with alterations of excitable membrane activity, especially among excitable tissues involved in cerebral, neuromuscular, and cardiac functions (see the accompanying Key Features of Disease). Other physiologic systems that experience changes in conjunction with hypernatremia and should be assessed include the integumentary and renal systems.

Cerebral and other upper neural functions are the most likely to be altered during episodes of hypernatremia (Feig, 1981). If ECF fluid volumes are near normal or decreased, upper neural activity usually is increased. The nurse assesses the client's mental status in terms of attention span, recall of recent events, and the ability to perform cognitive functions. In the presence of hypernatremia with normal or decreased fluid volumes, the client may be agitated and somewhat confused about the sequence of recent events. The attention span is short, and the client may not be able to concentrate on

---

KEY FEATURES OF DISEASE ■ Clinical Manifestations of Hypernatremia

Cardiovascular

Decreased myocardial contractility
Diminished cardiac output
Heart rate and blood pressure respond to vascular volume

Respiratory

Problems associated with pulmonary edema when hypernatremia is accompanied by hypervolemia

Neuromuscular*

Hypernatremia and normovolemia or hypovolemia
  Increased neural activity
  Agitation, confusion, seizures
Hypernatremia and hypervolemia
  Decreased neural activity
  Lethargy, stupor, coma
Mild or early hypernatremia
  Spontaneous muscle twitches
  Irregular contractions
Severe or late hypernatremia
  Skeletal muscle weakness
  Deep tendon reflexes diminished or absent

Renal

Decreased urinary output
Increased specific gravity

Integumentary

Dry, flaky skin
Presence or absence of edema related to accompanying fluid volume changes

* Upper neural function changes are related to volume changes as well as sodium increases.

---

simple tasks, such as counting backward from 100 by threes. The client's perception of noise and other environmental stimuli may be increased. If the serum sodium concentration continues to increase, the client may become manic or even experience convulsions. When hypernatremia is accompanied by an ECF volume overload, interstitial hydrostatic pressure is increased. This increased interstitial hydrostatic pressure in the brain depresses neural activity and function, and the client may exhibit symptoms of lethargy, drowsiness, stupor, and coma.

Skeletal muscles respond differently to various intensities of hypernatremia. Mild hypernatremia may induce sporadic, spontaneous muscle twitches and irregular contractions. As the degree of hypernatremia increases, the ability of skeletal muscle cells (and nerves) to respond to a stimulus diminishes. Muscles become progressively weaker and may demonstrate rigid paralysis. Deep tendon reflexes are diminished or absent. The nurse assesses neuromuscular status by observing for the presence of isolated twitching among muscle groups. The nurse also measures muscle strength by having the client (1) squeeze the nurse's hands, (2) attempt to keep the arms flexed while the nurse pulls downward on the lower arms, and (3) push both feet against a flat surface (a box or board) while the nurse applies resistance. Muscle weaknesses associated with hypernatremia occur bilaterally and have no specific progressive pattern. The nurse assesses peripheral nerve responsiveness by lightly tapping the patellar tendons and Achilles tendons with a reflex hammer and measuring the degree of reflexive movement.

The *cardiac system* is sensitive to increased ECF sodium concentrations. Hypernatremia has an overall depressive influence on myocardial contractility, even though depolarization of the myocardial membrane occurs more easily with increased serum sodium levels. Sodium ions compete with calcium ions for entrance into the myocardial cells through calcium channels (slow channels). Movement of calcium into the myocardium is an absolute requirement for cardiac muscle contraction. Increases in ECF sodium levels inhibit calcium movement into the myocardium, thus decreasing myocardial contractility. The nurse assesses the cardiac status by taking the blood pressure and measuring the rate and quality of the apical and peripheral pulses. Pulse rate and blood pressure may be at normal, above normal, or below normal levels during hypernatremic episodes, depending on the fluid volume and the speed with which the imbalance occurs. Rapid increases in ECF sodium concentrations cause rapid and dramatic changes from normal in cardiac function. Clients with normal ECF volumes during hypernatremia usually have normal pulse rates and blood pressures that do not change significantly with position changes. In clients whose hypernatremia is accompanied by plasma volume depletion, the pulse rate is increased. Peripheral pulses may be difficult to palpate and are easily obliterated with mild pressure. The client is hypotensive with pronounced postural hypotension, and the pulse pressure is greatly diminished. Clients with hypernatremia that is accompanied by increased ECF volumes may have slow to normal bounding pulses. Peripheral pulses are full and difficult to obliterate. Neck veins may be distended, even in the upright position. Blood pressure, especially diastolic pressure, is increased.

The *respiratory system* usually is not affected directly, unless the hypernatremia is accompanied by ECF volume excesses. The nurse assesses pulmonary status by observing the rate, depth, and ease of respiratory effort. The nurse auscultates the lungs for the presence of abnormal breath sounds that may indicate the presence of atelectasis or pulmonary edema.

Integumentary system changes often are good indicators of what specific type of ECF volume change accompanies the hypernatremia. The nurse assesses the integumentary system for integrity, the degree of moisture, turgor, and the presence of edema. The nurse assesses skin turgor by noting (1) how easily the skin (over the back of the hand and over the sternum) can be gently pinched up between the thumb and the forefinger (sometimes called tenting); (2) how soon the pinched-up skin resumes its normal position after release; (3) whether depressions remain in the skin after a finger is pressed firmly but gently (over the shin, over the sternum, and over the sacrum); (4) how deep the depressions are (in millimeters) and (5) how long the depressions remain. Hypernatremia as a result of pure water loss usually is accompanied by flushing of the skin and normal skin turgor. The skin is described as having a firm or rubbery texture. No depressions remain in the skin after pressure has been applied. The skin over the back of the hand is easily pinched up between the thumb and the forefinger and immediately resumes its normal position after being released. When excessive ECF volume losses accompany hypernatremia, the skin is pale and turgor is poor. Pinched-up skin remains in this position for seconds to minutes after being released. Depressions do not form when pressure is applied. When hypernatremia is accompanied by ECF volume excesses, skin color ranges from pale to flushed. Skin turgor is increased. It may be difficult or impossible to pinch the skin up to form a tent. Depressions appear in the skin in response to relatively light pressure and remain for many minutes after pressure is removed. During hypernatremia, cutaneous moisture secretion diminishes, and the skin and mucous membranes become relatively dry. The nurse assesses the skin for the presence of dry or flaking areas. This condition usually is first apparent on the extremities, but can progress to all body surfaces. The nurse assesses the oral mucosa for moisture content. The presence of a thick, sticky coating on the teeth (and gums) and tongue, along with an inability to make and excrete saliva, indicates an oral mucosa moisture deficit. In addition, fissures may be present on the lips or tongue, and the skin covering the lips may slough.

Renal function impairments may have contributed to the development of hypernatremia, and alterations in urinary output are expected manifestations of actual hypernatremia, even among clients who have no renal problems. One of the most common renal clinical manifestations of hypernatremia is greatly decreased urinary output. The urine is concentrated, is dark in color, and has a strong odor. The nurse assesses renal perfusion by comparing urinary output with fluid intake. Accurate measurements of these volumes is an essential nursing responsibility.

Psychosocial Assessment

A typical client who experiences repeated episodes of hypernatremia is a middle-aged woman with poorly controlled diabetes and renal disease. Psychosocial issues during the hypernatremic episodes primarily are related to behavior changes in response to alterations in the osmolarity of cerebral tissues. Agitation and manic excitement are not uncommon in the presence of hypernatremia. In addition to directly assessing the behavior of the client, the nurse consults with family members regarding recent changes in the client's mood and behavior patterns. Because hypernatremia is associated most frequently with chronic renal insufficiency, client compliance with the prescribed dietary limitations and medical regimen needs to be assessed. The nurse assesses the client's knowledge of the specific disease process causing the hypernatremia, as well as the client's knowledge regarding the sodium content of individual food items. In addition, the nurse assesses how accurately the client measures fluid intake.

Laboratory Findings

The definitive laboratory test result that confirms the presence of hypernatremia is a serum sodium value greater than 145 mEq/L (and frequently this value is *much* higher). Because the chloride ion is the major ECF anion that provides an electrical balance to sodium ions, any increase in ECF sodium concentration causes a proportionate increase in the serum chloride concentration (Brenner et al., 1987; Keyes, 1985).

If the hypernatremia is associated with excessive fluid loss, the levels of other serum electrolytes may be elevated, as will the hematocrit and hemoglobin values. Hypernatremia associated with renal disease usually is accompanied by elevations of serum potassium, creatinine, and blood urea nitrogen levels; a decreased blood pH; and low hematocrit and hemoglobin levels. Hypernatremia may also be associated with elevated serum protein levels. If renal function is normal, hypernatremia is associated with elevated urine sodium levels. If renal disease caused the hypernatremia, urine sodium levels are below normal.

 ### Analysis: Nursing Diagnosis

Hypernatremia as a result of pure water loss is a common imbalance among otherwise healthy individuals. Generally the condition is mild and is easily corrected when the individual can respond appropriately to the thirst reflex. Hypernatremia that requires nursing intervention generally is more severe and frequently is associated with some form of chronic illness or disability. Although such instances of electrolyte imbalance are easier to correct than hyponatremia, treatment in many cases requires long-term client adherence to strict medical regimens.

The following clinical example describes a client experiencing hypernatremia as a result of excessive sodium intake and fluid loss. The client is a 38-year-old male executive who has been under severe job-related stress for the previous month and has had indigestion and colitis continuously for 2 weeks. During this time he limited his food intake to cola soft drinks and carbohydrates. Additionally he self-medicated by drinking a solution of 1 tsp of baking soda (sodium bicarbonate) mixed in 4 oz of water. He drank this solution after every meal and before going to bed.

The nursing diagnoses and plan of care are derived from these data.

Common Diagnoses

The following nursing diagnoses are commonly applicable to clients with hypernatremia:

1. Altered nutrition: greater than body requirements related to excessive sodium intake
2. Altered oral mucous membrane related to inadequate oral secretions
3. Anxiety related to increased CNS irritability

Additional Diagnoses

In addition to the common diagnoses, one or more of the following diagnoses may be appropriate for the client with hypernatremia:

1. Potential for injury (fall) related to postural hypotension and neuromuscular changes
2. Decreased cardiac output related to decreased ventricular contractility
3. Potential impaired skin integrity related to excesses or deficiencies of interstitial fluid
4. Knowledge deficit related to treatment regimen
5. Impaired physical mobility related to skeletal muscle weakness
6. Total self-care deficit related to generalized skeletal muscle weakness

 Planning and Implementation

The following plan of care for the client with hypernatremia focuses on the common nursing diagnoses associated with specific tissue side effects of sodium excesses. The nurse must remember that the plan of care is aimed at restoration of normal sodium and fluid balances, prevention of future sodium imbalances, and provision of supportive care for altered body functions until the hypernatremia is resolved.

Altered Nutrition: Greater Than Body Requirements for Sodium

Planning: client goals. The major goals for this nursing diagnosis are that client will (1) have serum sodium levels restored to normal and (2) comply with prescribed sodium restrictions.

Interventions: nonsurgical management. Interventions are aimed at preventing further increases in serum sodium levels and decreasing elevated serum sodium levels. Drugs and diet therapy play important roles in restoring normal sodium balance. Other interventions that are more invasive, but may be necessary when hypernatremia becomes life-threatening, include hemodialysis, peritoneal dialysis, and blood ultrafiltration techniques.

Drug therapy. Drug therapy for the treatment of hypernatremia focuses on restoring fluid balance when hypernatremia is caused by fluid loss. Usually this therapy involves administering IV infusions of glucose and water (e.g., D_5W). Other substances may be added to the solution, depending on the presence of other electrolyte imbalances. When hypernatremia is caused by fluid and sodium losses, it may be necessary to replace the fluid with IV administration of isotonic NaCl solutions. When hypernatremia is caused by inadequate renal excretion of sodium, drug therapy may include the use of diuretics that are primarily natriuretic (i.e., enhance sodium loss), if sufficient renal function is present. Most of these diuretics are loop diuretics, rather than osmotic diuretics, and include such drugs as furosemide (Lasix, Furoside, Neo-Renal, Novosemide, Uritol), bumetanide (Bumex), and ethacrynic acid (Edecrin). The nurse administers these agents with care, assessing the client frequently for symptoms that indicate excessive loss of fluids, sodium, or potassium.

Diet therapy. Dietary restrictions of sodium are most useful in preventing hypernatremia and in preventing an existing hypernatremic condition from becoming worse. Dietary manipulation of sodium intake is relatively ineffective for rapid reduction of excess serum sodium levels. Clients with impaired renal handling of sodium must have their intake of sodium rigidly restricted to from 200 mg to 2000 mg/day, depending on the degree of renal impairment. Often, fluids must be restricted as well. Compliance with such a prescribed regimen requires the client's understanding of the specific disease process; knowledge of the sodium content of foods, beverages, and medications; and familiarity with appropriate ways to make a sodium-restricted diet palatable.

Altered Oral Mucous Membrane

Planning: client goals. The major planning goals for this nursing diagnosis are that the client will (1) experience less discomfort, (2) maintain a normal oral mucosal integrity, and (3) maintain an adequate nutritional intake.

Interventions: nonsurgical management. The major interventions employed for these client goals are associated with oral hygiene and early diagnosis of complications. Although the underlying problem of decreased mucosal secretions cannot be changed until the imbalance is resolved, the degree of discomfort caused by this condition can be diminished with appropriate nursing care. Drug therapy, diet therapy, oral hygiene, and measures to prevent complications are the same as those

for dehydrated clients with altered oral mucous membranes (see earlier).

Anxiety

Planning: client goals. The major client goal for this nursing diagnosis is that the client does not experience injury as a result of increased CNS irritability.

Interventions: nonsurgical management. The primary interventions for this nursing diagnosis include restoring serum sodium levels to normal (as discussed earlier for altered nutrition: greater than body requirements) and avoiding exposure of the client to excessive environmental stimuli.

Drug therapy. In addition to the drugs previously mentioned for direct treatment of hypernatremia, drugs that decrease nerve and muscle responsiveness to stimuli may also be prescribed. Drugs that reduce membrane excitability or result in skeletal muscle relaxation are used frequently. Such drugs include diazepam (Valium, Neo-Calme, E-Pam), chlordiazepoxide (Librium, Solium), lorazepam (Ativan), methocarbamol (Robaxin, Delaxin), and orphenadrine (Banflex, Myolin, and Norflex). In severe cases, anticonvulsant drugs also may be used.

Reduction of environmental stimulation. The nurse minimizes environmental stimulation of the client. Keeping the client in a quiet, relatively dark room decreases stimulation. Whenever possible, the client should be in a private room. If a private room is not available, the nurse selects a roommate whose personality and medical condition are consistent with the goal of keeping environmental stimuli to a minimum. The telephone should be removed or the bell adjusted so that it does not ring. Television viewing is avoided at this time. A major nursing responsibility is to limit visitors to those individuals who understand why these interventions are necessary and will comply with them. Young children or confused individuals should not be permitted to visit.

■ Discharge Planning

Discharge planning for clients with hypernatremia is the same as that for clients with dehydration (see earlier).

Evaluation

On the basis of the identified nursing diagnoses, the nurse evaluates the care for the client experiencing hypernatremia. The expected outcomes for the client with hypernatremia include that the client

1. Restores and maintains normal serum sodium levels
2. Identifies actions to take when signs and symptoms of hypernatremia occur

3. Achieves an acceptable level of oral mucosal comfort
4. Maintains an adequate oral intake of food and fluids
5. Differentiates correctly foods to be avoided from foods permitted based on sodium content
6. Maintains skin integrity
7. Verbalizes knowledge of the prescribed medical regimen
8. Complies with the prescribed medical regimen

In meeting the stated outcomes, sodium balance is maintained. Complications are minimized, enabling the client to achieve and maintain an individualized optimal functional status.

CALCIUM IMBALANCES

HYPOCALCEMIA

OVERVIEW

Hypocalcemia exists when the serum calcium ion (Ca^{2+}) level is less than 8 mg/dL or 4.5 mEq/L. Calcium ions, together with phosphorus and magnesium, are the primary mineral components of the body, providing density and strength to the bones of the skeleton. Only a small fraction of the total body calcium is present in either the ECF or the ICF. Relatively small fluctuations in serum calcium levels have profound effects on physiologic function. Therefore, the body has several, tightly regulated mechanisms for maintaining serum calcium levels within the narrow ranges of normal (see Chap. 12). In addition to providing bone density, calcium ions play important roles in regulating the activity of excitable membranes and in initiating the blood-clotting cascade. The immediate effects of hypocalcemia are most noticeable in body systems that are dependent on membrane excitability, although all body systems are affected to some degree.

Pathophysiology

The presence of measurable hypocalcemia indicates either that the normal protective and regulatory mechanisms are not functioning properly or that the conditions causing the hypocalcemia have been present so long that compensatory mechanisms are exhausted and are no longer adequate to maintain homeostasis. Calcium ions decrease excitable membrane permeability to sodium ions. Thus, calcium is considered a membrane stabilizer, regulating depolarization and the generation of action potentials. Low serum calcium levels increase the permeability of excitable membranes to sodium so that depolarization and the generation of action poten-

tials occur more easily, at inappropriate times, and even when a threshold level stimulus is not present.

Excitable tissues vary in their sensitivity to low serum calcium levels. The excitable tissues that demonstrate the most obvious responses to decreased serum calcium levels are peripheral nerves, skeletal muscles, GI smooth muscle, and cardiac muscle. The severity of the signs and symptoms associated with hypocalcemia is more dependent on the degree of the imbalance, although the speed with which the imbalance occurs also influences severity.

Responses of excitable tissues to hypocalcemia are also influenced by whether ECF calcium is required to enter the cell to initiate or assist with physiologic function. Hypocalcemia increases the excitability of peripheral nerves and skeletal muscles, as ECF calcium plays little or no role inside these cells (Chap. 12). Because cardiac muscle requires movement of ECF calcium into the cell to assist with muscle contraction, the hypocalcemic state has an overall depressive influence on cardiac contractility. Although GI smooth muscle does require that ECF calcium move inside the cell for proper physiologic function, hypocalcemia increases intestinal motility.

Calcium is a critical component at many points in the pathways for hemostasis and clot formation. Calcium acts as a cofactor in most of the enzymatic reactions in both the intrinsic and extrinsic pathways and in stabilization of the fibrin clot. However, because only small amounts of calcium are required for these processes, the clotting mechanism is affected by hypocalcemia only when the serum level of calcium is low or the hypocalcemic condition is prolonged.

Hypocalcemia can cause pathologic or deleterious effects on the skeletal system. Bone is the primary storage site for calcium and can release calcium into the ECF when needed; thus, prolongation of the calcium-releasing process can cause the bones to lose enough calcium to weaken their supporting structure. Chronic hypocalcemia leads to progressive osteoporosis, resulting in bones that are less dense and more prone to fracture or deformity (see Chap. 30 for a discussion of osteoporosis).

Etiology

Hypocalcemia can result from a variety of chronic and acute pathologic states, as well as from specific medical or surgical treatment (see the accompanying Key Features of Disease). The underlying causes of hypocalcemia generally can be classified as follows.

Conditions That Inhibit Calcium Absorption from the Gastrointestinal Tract

Any condition that either limits the amount of available dietary calcium or interferes with intestinal absorption falls into this category (Agus & Goldfarb, 1981).

KEY FEATURES OF DISEASE ■ Common Causes of Hypocalcemia

Actual Calcium Deficits

Inhibition of calcium absorption from the GI tract
  Inadequate oral intake or calcium
  Lactose intolerance
  Malabsorption syndromes
    Celiac sprue
    Crohn's disease
  Inadequate intake of vitamin D
Increased calcium excretion
  Renal failure — polyuric phase
  Diarrhea
  Steatorrhea
  Wound drainage (especially gastrointestinal)

Relative Calcium Deficits

Conditions that decrease the ionized fraction of calcium
  hyperproteinemia
  Alkalosis
  Calcium chelators or binders
    Citrate
    Mithramycin
    Penicillamine
    Sodium cellulose phosphate (Calcibind)
  Acute pancreatitis
  Hyperphosphatemia
  Immobility
Endocrine disturbances
  Removal or destruction of parathyroid glands
    Thyroidectomy
    Radiation to thyroid
    Strangulation
    Neck injuries

These conditions may contribute directly or indirectly to the development of hypocalcemia. Such conditions include inadequate intake of calcium-containing foods; lactose intolerance due to enzyme (lactase) deficiencies that reduce or prevent the intestinal absorption of milk products (which are rich sources of calcium); general small intestinal malabsorption syndromes (celiac, sprue, Crohn's disease, and so forth); and inadequate amounts of active vitamin D (through dietary lack or diseases that disrupt complete vitamin D synthesis).

Conditions That Decrease the Ionized Fraction of Calcium

Because it is the "free," or ionized (unbound), calcium that is physiologically active, any condition that causes ionized serum calcium to become bound contributes to the development of hypocalcemia, even though the total amount of calcium remains adequate. Because most calcium ions are bound to serum protein, any condition that increases the amount of serum proteins available for calcium binding contributes to hypocalcemia. Such conditions include actual increases in the total concentration of serum proteins and the state of alkalosis (either metabolic or respiratory, as long as the alkalosis causes the blood pH to be above normal). Alkalosis causes the proteins that act as blood pH buffers to release their hydrogen ions (H^+) in an attempt to compensate for the acid-base disorder. Proteins that release their hydrogen ions are then in a negatively charged ionized form and can easily bind with any free calcium ions present in the serum. This increased binding results in decreased amounts of unbound serum calcium.

Some drugs and chemicals are capable of binding several ions of serum calcium together through a process called *chelation*. These substances are called *calcium chelators*, or chelating agents. This chelation of calcium can occur in the GI tract or in the blood. Some of the more common chelating agents include citrate (used to keep donated blood from clotting while being stored or administered), mithramycin (used in antineoplastic treatment), and penicillamine (frequently used to reduce the risk of renal calculi in susceptible clients). Additionally, cellulose sodium phosphate (Calcibind), an ion exchange resin specific for calcium, releases sodium, preferentially binds calcium, and can contribute to the development of hypocalcemia.

Endocrine Disturbances That Decrease Serum Calcium Levels

The primary hormone for maintaining adequate amounts of ionized serum calcium is parathyroid hormone (PTH); therefore, conditions or diseases that interfere with either the synthesis or the release of PTH can cause hypocalcemia. Generally, these conditions are related to *removal or destruction of parathyroid tissue.* Thyroid surgery or radiation to the neck area can involve removal or destruction of parathyroid tissues embedded within the thyroid gland. Severe neck injuries (such as incomplete strangulation or neck injury incurred by being thrown through the windshield of a car) also can cause hypocalcemia (Desai et al., 1987). Increases in amounts of calcitonin do not appear to reduce serum calcium levels below normal. Other causes of hypocalcemia are the renal osteodystrophies associated with chronic renal failure (Robbins & Kumar, 1987). This association creates a disturbance in both the synthesis of vitamin D and the secretion of PTH. These problems are more fully discussed in Chapter 59.

Miscellaneous Conditions That Decrease Serum Calcium Levels

Acute pancreatitis (frequently associated with chronic alcoholism) appears to cause hypocalcemia. The increase in lipolytic enzymes as a result of the pancreatic inflammation causes an increase in the circulation of free fatty acids. It is thought that the fatty acids combine with ionized calcium in the serum. Another condition associated with hypocalcemia is *hyperphosphatemia.* Excess amounts of phosphates in the blood stimulate bone formation, which tends to move the ionized calcium from the ECF into the growing bone.

Hypocalcemia also can result from excessive loss of calcium through abnormal losses of ECF. Urinary loss of calcium can occur during the chronic acidosis that can accompany chronic renal failure (Leaf & Cotran, 1985). Fecal loss of calcium occurs during diarrhea and steatorrhea. Large amounts of calcium also can be lost through excessively draining wounds or intestinal fistulas.

Incidence

Hypocalcemia usually is not a primary disease or condition, but actually is a result of other diseases or conditions. Although all individuals can develop hypocalcemia, this condition is more likely to occur among the elderly, Blacks, and women. The elderly are more at risk for most electrolyte imbalances for a variety of reasons. The incidence of major organ pathologic changes increases with age. The elderly have a generally smaller fluid volume per body weight than do younger individuals, so that any variation in fluid volumes or electrolyte levels leads to imbalances more quickly. In addition, the elderly client is more likely to be taking prescription or OTC medications that disrupt fluid or electrolyte balance. Frequently, the elderly individual has serious nutritional deficits related to economic conditions or general problems with obtaining, preparing, or eating food. Because diet constitutes the primary source of calcium and vitamin D, nutritional deficits contribute to the development of hypocalcemia.

Many Black clients have a lactose intolerance related to a genetic deficiency of the enzyme lactase (Porth, 1986). Clients with this problem are unable to use the nutrients present in milk and usually experience cramping, diarrhea, and abdominal pain after ingestion of dairy products, which are a common, rich, and relatively inexpensive source of both calcium and vitamin D. These clients may have difficulty obtaining enough calcium and vitamin D from other sources to maintain normal calcium levels in the blood and storage sites.

Women are more prone to hypocalcemia than are men. The reasons for this phenomenon appear to be related to weight bearing and sex hormone action. Osteoporosis occurs when weight-bearing activity decreases or is limited. Women generally are smaller statured than men so that the female skeleton does not experience as much intrinsic weight bearing as the male skeleton. In addition, many women decrease weight-bearing activities, such as running, walking, and playing tennis, as they age. As women age, the estrogen protection against osteoporosis diminishes in direct proportion to the decrease in estrogen secretion. All of these factors increase the risk of hypocalcemia among women clients.

PREVENTION

Some of the conditions that lead to hypocalcemia cannot be prevented. However, when individuals with conditions that put them at increased risk for hypocalcemia can be identified and monitored, appropriate medical and nursing actions can be instituted early, when the potential for effectiveness is greater. Primary responsibility for identification of individuals at risk for hypocalcemia and early detection of associated signs and symptoms rests with the nurse.

Clients at risk for hypocalcemia related to a specific disease state or therapy, such as thyroidectomy or parathyroidectomy, are observed carefully for symptoms. Serum calcium levels are monitored, as well as serum phosphorus and serum albumin levels. Measures to increase serum calcium levels, such as administration of calcium-containing IV fluids (e.g., Ringer's lactate) should be instituted before the hypocalcemia becomes severe enough to induce serious or life-threatening complications. In situations in which the client receives multiple transfusions of blood or blood products, supplemental calcium is given to replace the serum calcium bound by the citrates present in the transfusion products.

Clients who have generally poor nutrition, healing bones, or lactose intolerance need to increase both calcium and vitamin D intake. Increased calcium intake also is recommended for all postmenopausal women, especially if they are not receiving estrogen therapy. For most of the at-risk clients, a daily intake of 1000 to 2000 mg of calcium is needed. If diet alone cannot supply this need (especially in the case of clients with lactose intolerance who are unable to make use of the calcium present in dairy products), supplemental calcium may be necessary. Calcium appears to be absorbed better from the GI tract when the dose is spread out through the day, rather than concentrated in one or two daily doses. Public awareness of the need for calcium has resulted in the addition of calcium to many common food and beverage items. In addition, the use of powdered milk in cooking and exposure of skin to sunlight are low-cost ways to increase intake and utilization of calcium. Many people choose to take calcium-based antacids as a means of supplementing their calcium intake. Chapter 30 describes in detail preventive measures to limit calcium loss and prevent osteoporosis.

COLLABORATIVE MANAGEMENT

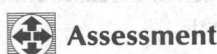 Assessment

History

The nurse collects data from clients at risk, as well as those with actual hypocalcemia. *Age* is an important factor, as the incidence of hypocalcemia tends to increase with age. *Sex* is another important factor in identifying the client at risk, because hypocalcemia is much more prevalent among women than men. Women are at an even greater risk during pregnancy, lactation, and the postmenopausal years. *Race* proves to be a significant risk factor; 50% to 70% of American Blacks are estimated to have some degree of lactose intolerance. In addition, individuals with darker complexions do not gain as much vitamin D from exposure to sunlight as do individuals with lighter complexions. *Activity level*, especially the amount of weight-bearing activity, is an important risk factor. Clients who are bedridden or who lead sedentary lives are at an increased risk for hypocalcemia. The nurse asks specific questions regarding weight bearing, such as the number of hours each day that the client engages in walking, running, lifting or carrying objects that weigh more than 10 lb, and playing force sports, such as tennis, volleyball, and dancing.

The most critical factor in assessing the risk of actual or potential hypocalcemia is the *diet history*, coupled with whether the client uses a calcium supplement on a regular basis. The nurse questions clients carefully regarding the inclusion of adequate amounts of calcium-containing foods, such as dairy products, legumes, broccoli, and tofu (Pennington & Church, 1985). In addition, the nurse asks the client how much time is spent outdoors with the skin being exposed to sunlight.

A valid historical indicator of actual hypocalcemia is the report of frequent painful muscle spasms (charley horses) in the calf or foot during periods of inactivity or sleep. Other information that can alert the nurse to the possibility that the client is at risk for hypocalcemia is a history of recent orthopedic surgery or bone healing. Although the concurrent presence of any disease state is important to note, diseases that are related to endocrine disturbances may be of significance for hypocalcemia. A history of previous thyroid surgery, therapeutic radiation to the mediastinal or neck area, or a recent anterior neck injury may predispose the client to hypocalcemia.

Physical Assessment: Clinical Manifestations

The most common clinical manifestations of hypocalcemia are related to overstimulation of nerves and muscles (see the accompanying Key Features of Disease). Although all nerves and muscles are affected to some degree, symptoms usually are noted first in the limbs, with distal to proximal ascension from the hands and feet. At first, paresthesia may be noted, with sensations of tingling alternating with sensations of numbness. If hypocalcemia continues or worsens, these sensations may progress to actual muscle twitchings or painful cramps and spasms. These symptoms are more pronounced when tissue hypoxia is also present. Progression is seen as the paresthesias include areas of the lips, nose, and ears. These symptoms may herald the approach of more serious neuromuscular overstimulation, or muscle *tetany* (McFadden et al., 1983; Quinlin, 1982).

Reliable physical indicators of hypocalcemia that nurses use in assessing the client include the elicitation

---

KEY FEATURES OF DISEASE ■ Clinical Manifestations of Hypocalcemia

Cardiovascular

Increased heart rate
Decreased myocardial contractility
Diminished peripheral pulses
Hypotension
ECG abnormalities
   Prolonged ST interval
   Prolonged QT interval

Respiratory

Not affected directly
Respiratory failure or arrest can occur as a result of decreased respiratory movement secondary to muscle tetany or seizure activity

Neuromuscular*

Anxiety, irritability, psychosis
Paresthesias followed by numbness
Irritable skeletal muscles—twitches, cramps, tetany, seizures
Hyperactive deep tendon reflexes
Positive Trousseau's sign
Positive Chvostek's sign

Gastrointestinal

Increased gastric motility
Hyperactive bowel sounds
Abdominal cramping
Diarrhea

* The neuromuscular system is most profoundly affected by hypocalcemia.

---

of a positive *Trousseau's sign* or a positive *Chvostek's sign*. Testing for *Trousseau's sign* is accomplished by placing a blood pressure cuff around the upper arm, inflating the cuff to greater than systolic pressure, and keeping it inflated for 1 to 4 minutes. Under these hypoxic conditions, the hand and fingers spasm in palmar flexion. These spasms will continue for 20 to 30 seconds after the pressure in the cuff has been released. A positive *Chvostek's sign* also may indicate the presence of hypocalcemia. Tapping on the face just below and anterior to the ear (over the facial nerve) triggers facial twitching that includes one side of the mouth, nose, and cheek. Tetany of isolated muscle groups is painful and indicates a rapidly worsening condition. This tetany can progress to convulsions. Respirations are impaired during seizure activity and even during tetany if the specific skeletal muscle contractions involve the respiratory muscles. Such involvement may lead to life-threatening complications, including respiratory failure and arrest.

Nervous system responses to hypocalcemia generally are seen in relation to the muscular system. Deep tendon reflexes are hyperactive. This sign is particularly significant if it represents a change from baseline or if tapping with a reflex hammer stimulates a persistent muscle response in addition to a tendon reflex. The level of consciousness usually is unchanged, except when seizure activity also is present. The client may show some vague symptoms of restlessness and inability to concentrate. Normal background noise or visual stimulation may increase irritability.

Hypocalcemic effects on smooth muscle activity is assessed most easily in the GI system. Overstimulation associated with hypocalcemia manifests as increased peristaltic activity. The nurse auscultates the abdomen for hyperactive bowel sounds. The client may verbalize that intestinal motion is accompanied by painful abdominal cramping and diarrhea.

The cardiovascular system also manifests signs of hypocalcemia. The heartbeat may be slightly faster than normal, but the cardiac contractility is weaker, resulting in a diminished pulse quality. Transient, mild to moderate hypocalcemia appears to alter cardiac function little. For hypocalcemia to produce significant changes in cardiac activity and function, the degree of hypocalcemia must be either severe or chronic. Under these conditions, the MAP usually drops considerably, resulting in profound hypotension and the following ECG changes: prolonging of the ST interval, leading to a prolonging of the QT interval (Chambers, 1987; Metheny and Snively, 1983). The nurse obtains the client's blood pressure in the lying, sitting, and standing positions, as postural changes make the hypotension more pronounced. If hypocalcemia continues to be present as a severe or chronic condition, the client also may experience congestive heart failure, manifested by weak peripheral pulses and the formation of visible edema. However, these cardiac manifestations of hypocalcemia are rare, because the neuromuscular problems associated with hypocalcemia generally prove to be more life-threatening than the cardiac problems, unless the client has pre-existing cardiac problems. Clients who are taking calcium channel–blocking agents, such as nifedipine (Procardia, Adalat) and verapamil (Calan, Isoptin), are at greater risk for experiencing cardiac problems in the presence of hypocalcemia.

Psychosocial Assessment

The psychosocial assessment initially may show few, rather subtle behavior changes. The individual usually remains alert and oriented unless seizure activity also occurs. Clients may appear slightly anxious at first, with increasing sensitivity to extraneous environmental noise and activity. This situation can progress to excessive irritability, irrational thinking, and even frank psychosis. A close family member may be of assistance in determining if the behavior represents a change in behavior pattern for the client.

Social assessment may reveal a lack of understanding about the use of medications and the importance of dietary calcium. Limited income or other financial problems also may be factors in the inadequate intake of calcium-containing foods or vitamin supplements. The nurse correlates the data obtained from the diet history with information concerning the financial conditions of the client and family.

Laboratory Findings

The most definitive laboratory test result to confirm the presence of hypocalcemia is a serum calcium level less than 8 mg/dL or 4.5 mEq/L. If the hypocalcemia has a rapid onset, the expected clinical manifestations are present with relatively small decreases in serum calcium levels. Other laboratory data also may be abnormal during periods of hypocalcemia, depending on the cause and the severity of the hypocalcemia. Because calcium and phosphorus usually have an inverse relationship in serum, when hypocalcemia is present, the serum phosphorus level may be *elevated* (>2.6 mEq/L). Two other abnormalities that may accompany hypocalcemia are increased total serum protein levels and an elevated arterial pH (>7.45). As discussed earlier, both these conditions can cause hypocalcemia by increasing calcium binding, resulting in less free calcium available in the serum.

Radiographic Findings

When hypocalcemia is chronic or is accompanied by osteoporosis, bone density changes can be manifested through radiographic examination. X-ray films of the spine and long bones in particular show loss of bone density. However, bone density changes are evident on x-ray examination only after a 25% to 40% bone density loss has occurred. Other radiographic indications of prolonged hypocalcemia include the presence of stress fractures and compression fractures.

Because x-ray examination is not sensitive enough to detect early bone density changes, another helpful radiographic imaging technique is computed tomography (CT) scanning. This technique is used extensively to visualize changes in the density of the cancellous bone of the spine as an indicator of early osteoporosis. A newer imaging technique that does not use radiation, but is extremely sensitive and shows great promise in detecting changes in all tissue densities (even soft tissue), is magnetic resonance imaging (MRI). The usefulness of MRI in diagnosing early bone density changes has not yet been determined and may be limited by the cost of the procedure.

Analysis: Nursing Diagnosis

Although hypocalcemia can result from a variety of chronic and acute pathologic states and specific medical or surgical treatment, hypocalcemia most frequently occurs as a chronic condition among clients at home as well as those requiring inpatient care. The typical client is an elderly, small-statured woman who has a sedentary life style and has a diet deficient in calcium or vitamin D. The following nursing diagnoses are derived from these data.

Common Diagnoses

The following diagnoses are common in clients with hypocalcemia:

1. Altered nutrition: less than body requirements related to inadequate calcium intake
2. Diarrhea related to overstimulation of gastric smooth muscle
3. Potential for injury related to tetany or seizure activity and loss of bone density

Additional Diagnoses

In addition to the common diagnoses, one or more of the following diagnoses may be noted in the client with hypocalcemia.

1. Decreased cardiac output related to decreased ventricular contractility
2. Impaired gas exchange related to ineffective respiratory movements secondary to tetany or seizure activity
3. Activity intolerance related to tetany
4. Pain related to muscle spasm and tetany
5. Sensory/perceptual alterations (tactile) related to paresthesia
6. Anxiety related to pain and irritability
7. Potential for injury related to altered thought processes
8. Knowledge deficit related to food sources of calcium
9. Total self-care deficit related to neuromuscular alterations

 Planning and Implementation

The following plan of care for the client experiencing hypocalcemia focuses on the common diagnoses related to alterations in nutrition, bowel elimination, and safety. The nurse must remember that this plan of care is aimed at restoring normal calcium balance and preventing serious complications.

Altered Nutrition: Less Than Body Requirements

When the cause of hypocalcemia is related directly to an inadequate intake of calcium, rather than to a specific disease process, the decreased serum calcium levels reflect that the normal compensatory mechanisms are no longer adequate. Thus, the nurse infers that the inadequate intake of calcium is chronic, although the clinical manifestations of hypocalcemia may have an acute onset. Generally, inadequate intake of calcium is a result of a combination of the following factors: (1) insufficient knowledge of daily dietary requirements for calcium and vitamin D; (2) insufficient knowledge of dietary sources of calcium and vitamin D; (3) intolerance of foods rich in calcium; and (4) lack of financial resources. The nurse in the inpatient setting not only is in a position to assist the client in returning to a state of normal calcium balance, but also can be instrumental through client education in preventing hypocalcemia from recurring.

Planning: client goals.   The major client goals for this nursing diagnosis are that the client will (1) restore serum calcium levels to normal and (2) have a sufficient knowledge of calcium needs and availability to plan a diet containing appropriate amounts of calcium to meet individual daily needs.

Interventions: nonsurgical management.   Primary interventions are aimed at preventing further decreases in serum calcium levels and restoring normal serum calcium levels. The interventions appropriate for this situation include drug therapy and diet therapy, including parenteral nutrition.

Drug therapy.   Oral supplements of calcium carbonate, calcium gluconate, and calcium lactate are commonly used for clients with mild hypocalcemia. Some preparations of calcium supplements are derived from oyster shell. This type of calcium supplement is more expensive, and no hard evidence exists that indicates that either the quality of the calcium or its systemic absorption is any better than with other calcium compounds. These oral supplements should be administered 30 minutes before meals to ensure maximal intestinal absorption. Many multivitamin preparations contain large amounts of calcium (500 to 1000 mg) and also contain vitamin D. Usually multivitamins should be administered only once a day. Although these preparations are adequate for the individual who has no overt vitamin or mineral deficiencies, they may not be adequate for the client with hypocalcemia. Calcium is poorly absorbed from the intestinal tract, and absorption is better when calcium intake occurs throughout the day.

Parenteral calcium is administered when the hypocalcemia is severe (as evidenced by the presence of tetany or cardiovascular complications) or when intestinal absorption is altered. The preferred route of administration is by slow IV drip unless the hypocalcemia is life-threatening. Rapid IV calcium administration can result in hypercalcemia, a condition that can be equally life-threatening. The most common agents used are solutions containing either calcium chloride or calcium gluconate. Nursing responsibilities during IV administration of calcium include continuous assessment of cardiovascular status (ideally the client should be evaluated via a cardiac monitor), assessments of Chvostek's and Trousseau's signs every 15 minutes, hourly drawing of blood for determination of serum calcium levels, and assessment of the infusion site at least every 15 minutes.

Infiltration or extravasation of fluids containing large concentrations of calcium is a serious problem, because these solutions can cause tissue hypoxia and necrosis. Poor blood return, pain at the infusion site, edema, or any other indication of infiltration warrants stopping the infusion and changing the IV site. IM injections and infusion by hypodermoclysis of these agents are contraindicated because these methods can cause severe tissue damage.

Other drugs can be used to correct hypocalcemia. These therapeutic agents do not directly add calcium to the serum, but rather indirectly increase extracellular calcium concentrations by altering the concentrations of other electrolytes that influence serum calcium regulation. Administration of vitamin D assists to increase the serum calcium levels by enhancing the intestinal absorption of calcium. Aluminum hydroxide can increase serum calcium levels by reducing serum phosphorus levels (calcium and phosphorus are present in the serum in a reciprocal but proportionate ratio). Because serum calcium and serum magnesium levels are related to each other directly (when the serum concentration of one increases, so does the serum concentration of the other), the administration of magnesium chloride or magnesium sulfate can help increase serum calcium levels.

Diet therapy.   A high-calcium, low-phosphorus diet is indicated for clients with mild hypocalcemia and for those with chronic pathologic conditions that cause them to be at continuous risk for hypocalcemia. The nurse assists the hospitalized client in selecting foods that are calcium rich (common sources of calcium are listed in Table 12–6 in Chap. 12). Whenever possible, the nurse also provides snacks or supplemental feedings that are high in calcium (dairy products can compose many of these supplemental feedings). Providing foods and food flavors that the client enjoys increases the likelihood of compliance with the regimen. When diet intake is affected by fatigue or weakness, the nurse assists the client with the mechanical process of eating. In addition, providing small meals more frequently and selecting foods that require minimal chewing also may help alleviate this problem.

Hypocalcemia can occur when the client is knowledgeable about the need for calcium, but is unable to obtain calcium supplements or specific foods rich in calcium owing to inadequate financial resources. In this situation the nurse collaborates with the social services department and dietary consultants. The social services department can assess financial needs and can assist the client with obtaining food or food resources (e.g., food stamps). Dietary consultants can help the nurse formulate an appropriate teaching plan for the client that involves supplementing food during preparation with low-cost calcium-containing substances (such as adding powdered skim milk to soups, potatoes, or puddings).

Vitamin D intake must also be adequate for dietary calcium to be beneficial. Skin exposure to sunlight enhances the body's synthesis of active vitamin D. Thus, increasing skin exposure to sunlight is an inexpensive way to increase vitamin D content. However, environmental or personal health conditions may make increased skin exposure to sunlight impractical or dangerous. Other sources of vitamin D include fortified milk, liver, eggs, fatty fish, and butterfat. Dairy products other than milk, such as cheese and yogurt, usually are *not* fortified with vitamin D.

Diarrhea

Planning: client goals.   The major client goals for this nursing diagnosis include that the client will (1) maintain bowel elimination patterns that are normal for him/her and (2) experience minimal abdominal discomfort.

Interventions: nonsurgical management.   Interventions for these client goals include restoring the serum calcium levels to normal (as described earlier for drug and diet therapy for altered nutrition: less than body requirements), decreasing intestinal irritability and peristalsis, and avoiding substances that promote GI motility. Drug therapy and diet therapy for diarrhea causing hypocalcemia are the same as those for diarrhea causing hyperkalemia (see earlier).

Potential for Injury

When the severity of the hypocalcemia is such that extensive muscle tetany or seizure activity occurs, the client is at severe risk for injury. In addition, gas exchange at the pulmonary and tissue levels may be impaired, causing a state of hypoxia or anoxia. This state can produce cellular and organ injury. The nursing interventions for this diagnosis are aimed at restoring normal calcium levels, identifying clients at risk for tetany or seizure activity, and preventing injury and hypoxic complications.

Planning: client goals.   Goals for this nursing diagnosis include that the client will (1) have serum calcium levels restored to normal, (2) experience a decrease in ectopic skeletal muscle activity, and (3) not experience hypoxic or anoxic tissue injuries from respiratory involvement.

Interventions: nonsurgical management.   Primary interventions are aimed at reducing neural irritability and overstimulation of skeletal muscles (especially respiratory muscles) while continuing with efforts to increase the serum calcium level. Diet and drug therapies to increase serum calcium levels are discussed earlier.

Drug therapy.   In addition to the drugs previously mentioned for treatment of hypocalcemia, some drugs may be prescribed to decrease the degree of nerve and muscle responsiveness and overstimulation. Drugs that reduce membrane excitability and result in skeletal muscle relaxation are sometimes used. These drugs include methocarbamol (Robaxin, Skelaxin, Delaxin), orphenadrine (Banflex, Flexoject, Myolin), carisoprodol (Soma, Rela), and diazepam (Valium, Rival, E-Pam). Magnesium sulfate also may be given to decrease the responsiveness of skeletal muscles to nervous stimulation or extraneous stimulation. Less commonly used are the standard anticonvulsant drugs, although these drugs may be of benefit if seizure activity is persistent. Anticonvulsant drugs include paramethadione (Paradione), trimethadione (Tridione), phenytoin (Dilantin), mephenytoin (Mesantoin), and carbamazepine (Tegretol, Mazepine).

Reduction of environmental stimuli. The excitable membranes of both the nervous system and the skeletal system are overstimulated in hypocalcemia. Therefore, in addition to increasing serum calcium levels, it is important to provide an environment that reduces extraneous stimulation of these systems. Activity should be minimal, as any nerve or muscle stimulation can increase muscular twitching, cramps, and tetany. If Chvostek's sign or Trousseau's sign is positive, the client must be completely restricted to bed rest, with total care being provided by the nurse. Because prolonged or intermittent physical contact that allows stimulation of the deeper tissues (such as rubbing the back) or unexpected touching of the patient can stimulate muscle tetany or even seizure activity, direct contact during nursing care must be limited to the minimum necessary to maintain safety and hygiene. The nurse avoids having the client make rapid position changes, as this activity can also stimulate unwanted nerve and muscle responses. The nurse minimizes environmental stimulation of the client by providing a quiet, relatively dark, private room for the client. Quiet radio music may be soothing, but, in general, television viewing provides too much sensory stimulation. Diagnostic and therapeutic activities not critically essential to the immediate well-being of the client are postponed. The telephone is removed from the room, or its bell is adjusted so that it does not ring. The nurse providing direct care to this client speaks softly and no more frequently than necessary. Care is taken to avoid bumping the bed and other furniture. The nurse avoids shining a light into the client's face. Visitors are restricted to those individuals who understand why these precautions are necessary and will comply with them. Babies, young children, and confused individuals are not permitted to visit.

Prevention of complications. While interventions are ongoing to correct the condition of hypocalcemia, the nurse prepares to take action to prevent complications if the condition remains unresponsive or worsens. A primary nursing responsibility is continuous assessment to identify whether the condition is improving or deteriorating. The nurse also keeps appropriate emergency or protective equipment nearby in anticipation of complications. Such equipment includes oxygen and suction equipment, along with a sterile tracheostomy tray and Ambu bag. The emergency cart, equipped with the necessary emergency drugs, endotracheal equip-

ment, and Ambu bag, is positioned near the client's room. The nurse also institutes other standard safety precautions for seizures. Such precautions include maintaining the side rails in the up position and padding them and keeping the bed in the lowest possible position.

■ Discharge Planning

Discharge planning for clients with hypocalcemia is the same as that for clients with dehydration (see earlier).

 ### Evaluation

On the basis of the identified nursing diagnoses, the nurse evaluates the care for the client experiencing hypocalcemia. The expected outcomes for the client with hypocalcemia include that the client

1. Restores and maintains normal serum calcium levels
2. Identifies actions to take when signs and symptoms of hypocalcemia occur
3. Selects foods that are rich in calcium and vitamin D
4. Describes and complies with prescribed drug and diet therapy
5. Maintains an adequate cardiac output
6. Achieves an acceptable level of muscular comfort
7. Avoids injury related to altered skeletal muscle function
8. Restores and maintains normal bowel elimination patterns

By meeting the stated outcomes, the client is more likely to remain in normal calcium balance. As a result, uncomfortable and serious complications are avoided.

HYPERCALCEMIA

OVERVIEW

Hypercalcemia exists when the serum calcium ion level is greater than 10.5 mg/dL or 5.5 mEq/L. Most of the body's calcium is stored in bone, and the amount of free calcium found in the serum represents a minute fraction of the total body calcium content. Because the normal range for serum calcium values is extremely narrow, even small increases can have profound effects on physiologic function. Calcium, as a primary body mineral, influences bone density, membrane excitability, enzymatic activity, and the effectiveness of the blood-clotting cascade. Although the effects of hypercalcemia are most noticeable in body systems dependent on membrane excitability, all body systems are affected to some degree. As discussed in Chapter 12, the body has several tightly controlled mechanisms to regulate serum calcium levels during normal fluctuations in calcium intake and loss.

Pathophysiology

The presence of hypercalcemia indicates either that the free calcium load is so great that the normal calcium-regulating mechanisms are overburdened or that at least one calcium-regulating mechanism is not functioning properly. Although hypercalcemia is an excess of ECF levels of calcium, this excess may not be reflected in the total body calcium concentration. Hypercalcemia may be present even when the total body concentration of calcium is significantly below normal.

ECF calcium ions function as "stabilizers" of excitable membranes. Calcium ions decrease the permeability of the membrane to movement of sodium from the ECF into the ICF. Because sodium movement across the membrane is the stimulus for depolarization, an excess of ECF calcium ions depresses depolarization and the generation of action potentials in excitable tissues. Thus, excitable tissues are less irritable and may require a much stronger stimulus than is normally required for physiologic function.

Excitable tissues vary in their sensitivity to excess serum calcium levels. The excitable tissues that demonstrate the most obvious and serious immediate responses to hypercalcemia are cardiac muscle tissue, peripheral and central nerve tissue, skeletal muscle, and GI smooth muscle. The degree of excitable tissue depression and the severity of the signs and symptoms associated with hypercalcemia are dependent on both the degree of the imbalance and the rapidity with which the imbalance occurs.

When hypercalcemia occurs as a result of increased bone resorption of calcium, the density of the bone is decreased. This condition weakens bones and makes them more susceptible to fractures.

Calcium is a critical cofactor for many of the enzymes involved in the blood-clotting cascade. Hypercalcemia usually results in decreased clotting times. This condition may cause clots to form at inappropriate times and places. Excessive clotting related to hypercalcemia is more likely to occur in vessels or organs in which blood flow is slow or impeded.

Etiology

The presence of hypercalcemia indicates either that the free calcium load is so great that the normal calcium-regulating mechanisms are overburdened or that one or more regulating mechanism is not functioning properly. The underlying causes of hypercalcemia generally can be explained in terms of increased absorption of calcium, decreased excretion of calcium, and increased bone resorption of calcium (see the accompanying Key Features of Disease).

KEY FEATURES OF DISEASE ■ Common Causes of Hypercalcemia

Actual Calcium Excesses

Increased absorption of calcium
  Excessive oral intake of calcium
  Excessive oral intake of vitamin D
Decreased excretion of calcium
  Renal failure
  Use of thiazide diuretics

Relative Calcium Excesses

Increased bone resorption of calcium
  Hyperparathyroidism
  Malignancy
    Direct invasion (cancers of breast, lung, prostate, and osteoclastic bone and multiple myeloma)
    Indirect resorption (liver cancer, small cell lung cancer, and cancer of the adrenal gland)
  Hyperthyroidism
  Immobility
  Use of glucocorticoids
Hemoconcentration
  Dehydration
  Use of lithium
  Adrenal insufficiency

Conditions That Decrease Renal Excretion of Calcium

Although the kidney is not the primary regulator of the body's calcium content, the kidney plays a role in calcium homeostasis at the level of the distal convoluted tubule (DCT). At this location in the nephron, calcium in the filtrate can be reabsorbed through the tubular epithelium and returned to systemic circulation, or the calcium can be excreted in the urine and removed from the body. In *renal failure*, the nephron may not be able to effectively excrete excess calcium ions, thus contributing to the development of hypercalcemia, although renal failure usually is associated with hypocalcemia.

Many diuretics exert their effects within the tubular system of the nephron. *Thiazide diuretics*, such as chlorothiazide (Diuril) and hydrochlorothiazide (Esidrix, Hydro-Diuril, Oretic, Mictrin), alter the function of the DCT. These diuretics *enhance* the reabsorption of calcium in the DCT (usually at the expense of some other electrolytes). Prolonged or excessive use of thiazide diuretics may cause hypercalcemia.

Conditions That Increase Bone Resorption of Calcium

The bones form a large storage site for calcium. Any condition or factor that directly or indirectly causes calcium to be removed from the bone into systemic circulation has the potential to cause hypercalcemia. The process of calcium movement from the bones into the ECF is called *bone resorption of calcium*. Usually when hypercalcemia is caused by increased bone resorption, the total body calcium content is *below* normal, although the serum level is above normal.

The most common cause of hypercalcemia through excessive bone resorption is *hyperparathyroidism*. Hyperparathyroidism has many causes. Whenever hyperparathyroidism is present, the parathyroid glands oversecrete PTH. This hormone directly stimulates bone resorption of calcium.

Another common cause of hypercalcemia as a result of increased bone resorption is the presence of a *malignancy* or neoplasm (Coward, 1986; Cunningham, 1982; Elbaum, 1984; Stewart, 1980). Malignancies can increase bone resorption directly or indirectly. The malignancies that invade the bone and cause physical demineralization directly include lung, breast, and prostate cancers; osteoclastic bone cancer; and multiple myeloma. Other malignancies stimulate increased bone resorption of calcium by indirect mechanisms (small cell lung cancer, liver cancers, and cancers of the adrenal gland). These malignancies, located at remote areas from bone sites, secrete substances into the circulatory system that stimulate bone resorption of calcium. Some of these substances include prostaglandins and PTH.

Another condition that stimulates bone resorption of calcium is *immobility*. Bone density is directly related to the amount of weight-bearing activity accomplished by the larger bones. When a person is immobilized, these bones are not participating in weight-bearing activity and demineralization with resorption of calcium can occur.

Excessive concentrations of *glucocorticoids* stimulate bone resorption of calcium. The exact mechanism of this phenomenon is not known.

Hyperthyroidism also can stimulate increased bone resorption of calcium. When hyperthyroidism is present, excessive amounts of thyroid hormone (TH) are secreted and released. TH directly enhances bone resorption of calcium.

Conditions That Increase Absorption of Calcium

Excessive intake of calcium can lead to hypercalcemia. Individuals who ingest large amounts of antacids are at an increased risk for hypercalcemia. Individuals who ingest large quantities of milk and other dairy products may develop hypercalcemia and are also at risk of other electrolyte imbalances through the *milk-alkali syndrome*.

The GI absorption of calcium is highly dependent on the presence of the active form of vitamin D. Hypercalcemia associated with an increased absorption of calcium can occur when an individual ingests normal amounts of calcium and *excessive amounts of vitamin D*. This condition is sometimes called *hypervitaminosis D*.

Miscellaneous Conditions That Increase the Serum Calcium Level

As in many electrolyte disorders, imbalances of fluid volume can lead to an imbalance of serum electrolyte levels. *Dehydration* with an actual fluid volume deficit can cause a relative hypercalcemia. The drug *lithium* also is associated with the development of hypercalcemia, although the exact mechanism of the imbalance is not known. *Adrenal insufficiency* also is associated with hypercalcemia. This condition is thought to increase serum calcium levels indirectly through the processes of dehydration and alterations in the serum protein levels, as well as through increasing the tubular reabsorption of calcium.

Incidence

Overt hypercalcemia rarely occurs as a primary disorder among individuals without other pathologic conditions. Therefore, most cases of hypercalcemia occur among hospitalized clients or those who are on treatment regimens for other conditions. Individuals at greatest risk for hypercalcemia are those with malignancies, other fluid and electrolyte disorders, abnormal thyroid function, and hyperparathyroidism. Hypercalcemia occurs more frequently among the very young and the elderly, especially those who are taking thiazide diuretics. Also at risk are individuals who self-prescribe excessive vitamin and mineral supplements and those clients receiving IV fluids that contain calcium in excess of physiologic concentrations.

PREVENTION

Prevention of hypercalcemia is aimed at identifying clients at risk so that appropriate medical and nursing actions can be instituted early, when the potential for effectiveness is greater. Because increases in serum calcium levels can be life-threatening, hospitalized clients at risk should have serum electrolyte levels measured on a regular schedule and whenever the signs and symptoms of imbalance are present. Prevention includes actions to avoid the addition of exogenous calcium and to limit bone resorption of calcium.

Clients at risk should not be taking drugs that increase serum calcium levels (calcium-containing antacids, calcium supplements, vitamin D supplements, thiazide diuretics, IV fluids containing calcium chloride or calcium gluconate, and aluminum hydroxide). Restriction of dietary calcium in clients at risk is controversial. Because increased serum calcium levels inhibit calcium uptake from the GI tract, it is not necessary to restrict normal amounts of calcium-containing food items, although excessive ingestion of calcium-containing foods should be avoided.

Immobility enhances the process of bone resorption in susceptible individuals and should be avoided or limited. Whenever the client's condition permits, clients should be out of bed, walking or standing to increase weight-bearing on the long bones. Even clients who are immobile as a result of neuromuscular or other abnormalities can be assisted to a partial weight-bearing position with the use of a tilt table.

COLLABORATIVE MANAGEMENT

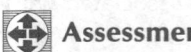 **Assessment**

History

Because hypercalcemia usually is associated with other pre-existing health problems, the nurse collects data regarding specific risk factors for hypercalcemia, as well as causative factors. Hypercalcemia occurs with equal frequency among males and females, and gender is not considered a risk factor. *Age* is an important factor, not only because chronic illness and altered organ function occur more frequently among elderly clients, but also because the elderly client is more likely to be taking prescription and OTC medications that influence fluid and electrolyte balance. The nurse inquires about specific risk factors, including the presence of a pre-existing acute or chronic illness, such as *malignancy, heart disease,* and *parathyroid or other endocrine problems.* Of particular significance is *medication use.* The nurse asks the client what medications (both prescribed and OTC) are taken on a regular basis. Specific questions regarding the use of *antacids, thiazide diuretics, glucocorticoids, thyroid replacement drugs, calcium supplements,* and *vitamin D supplements* are asked. The nurse may need to assist the client in recalling drug information by providing a list of proprietary names or pictures of actual medications. If the client is unable to recall exactly what medications are being taken, the nurse may be able to obtain this information from family members or the client's inpatient and outpatient records. *Activity level,* especially the amount of weight-bearing activity, is an important and sometimes neglected risk factor. Clients who are immobilized, are bedridden, or lead sedentary lives are at an increased risk for hypercalcemia through increased bone resorption. The nurse asks specific questions regarding weight-bearing activities, such as the number of hours each day that the client engages in walking, running, lifting or carrying objects that weigh more than 10 lb, and participating in sports such as tennis, volleyball, and dancing. The association of hypercalcemia with decreased activity and immobility can be difficult to comprehend, because these factors also lead to hypocalcemia. It is important to remember that increased bone resorption *temporarily* causes hypercalcemia, even though the total body calcium content may be *below* normal. Eventually, as the bone become increasingly demineralized, the client experiences *hypocalcemia* with bone resorption.

Another important factor to assess for risk of hypercalcemia is the *diet history.* The nurse questions the client carefully regarding the ingestion of excessive amounts of calcium-containing foods, such as dairy products, legumes, broccoli, salmon, sardines, and tofu. Brand names of specific food items may be important to obtain because many food items that contain little or no natural calcium may have calcium added (for example, certain brands of orange juice and wheat flour). When obtaining the diet history, the nurse repeats specific questions regarding calcium and vitamin D supplements; many clients who take calcium or vitamin D supplements consider these items food rather than medications.

Physical Assessment: Clinical Manifestations

The onset of clinical manifestations associated with hypercalcemia is related to both the severity of the imbalance and how quickly the imbalance occurred. Thus, it is not unusual for clients with relatively mild excesses of serum calcium levels that occurred rapidly to experience more severe signs and symptoms than do clients whose hypercalcemic states are severe but developed slowly over a long period of time. Clinical manifestations of hypercalcemia primarily are associated with alterations of excitable membrane activity (see the accompanying Key Features of Disease). Other physiologic systems that experience functional changes associated with hypercalcemia include the renal system and blood-clotting mechanisms.

The most serious and life-threatening clinical manifestations of hypercalcemia are involved with alterations of cardiac function (Tripp, 1976). Increased ECF calcium levels disturb both cardiac muscle function and electrical conduction through the heart. Mild hypercalcemia initially causes an increased heart rate and blood pressure. More severe or prolonged hypercalcemia affects conduction by shortening the plateau phase of the action potential and increases ventricular irritability (Desai et al., 1987; Zeluff et al., 1980). Bradycardia and full peripheral pulses are frequent manifestations of hypercalcemia. ECG changes associated with hypercalcemia include a shortened ST segment (as a result of a shortened QT interval) and a widened T wave. Discernible arrhythmias are present more frequently in clients receiving digitalis who are hypercalcemic, and hypercalcemia potentiates digitalis toxicities. When the condition of hypercalcemia has a rapid onset or becomes severe, cardiac arrest with sinus arrest in systole may occur.

Because increased ECF calcium levels stabilize nerve and skeletal muscle excitable membranes, depolarization is more difficult to induce. The clinical manifestations of this condition include profound muscle weakness, without accompanying paresthesia, and greatly diminished deep tendon reflexes. CNS manifestations of hypercalcemia include an altered level of consciousness that ranges from disorientation and lethargy to coma.

Changes in GI motility frequently are an early manifestation of hypercalcemia. The peristaltic action decreases, resulting in significantly slower intestinal transit times. The nurse assesses the GI tract by auscultating

---

KEY FEATURES OF DISEASE ■ Clinical Manifestations of Hypercalcemia

Cardiovascular

- Increased heart rate
- Increased blood pressure
- Bounding, full peripheral pulses
- ECG abnormalities
  - Shortened ST segment
  - Widened T wave
- Potentiation of digitalis-associated toxicities
- Decreased clotting time
- Late phase
  - Bradycardia
  - Cardiac arrest, sinus arrest

Respiratory

- Ineffective respiratory movement related to profound skeletal muscle weakness

Neuromuscular

- Disorientation, lethargy, coma
- Profound muscle weakness
- Diminished or absent deep tendon reflexes

Renal

- Increased urinary output
- Dehydration
- Formation of renal calculi

Gastrointestinal

- Decreased motility
- Hypoactive bowel sounds
- Anorexia, nausea
- Abdominal distention
- Constipation

---

for bowel sounds in all four abdominal quadrants. Bowel sounds are hypoactive or absent. The abdomen increases in size, as intestinal contents and flatus remain in the GI tract instead of being propelled to the outside. The nurse assesses abdominal size by measuring abdominal girth with a soft tape measure in a line that circles the abdomen at the level of the umbilicus. Subjective symptoms of hypercalcemic effects on the GI system include constipation, anorexia, nausea, vomiting, and abdominal pain.

Although alterations in renal function can contribute to the development of hypercalcemia, the presence of excessive serum calcium levels also influences renal function. Hypercalcemia can cause increased urinary output and lead to serious dehydration. A common result of chronic hypercalcemia is the formation of "stones," or renal calculi, in the kidney tubular system as the excess calcium precipitates out of solution into a solid form. These stones can block the flow of filtrate and urine through different parts of the renal system. When these stones reach the ureter, bladder, and urethra, they can cause considerable pain. The nurse assesses the renal system for changes associated with hypercalcemia by accurately measuring intake and output, assessing the appearance of voided urine, and straining the urine for the presence of renal calculi.

Calcium is an important cofactor for many of the enzymes and proteins necessary in the blood-clotting cascade. Although hypercalcemia does not directly cause blood clots to form, the condition of hypercalcemia permits clot formation to occur more easily whenever normal precipitating conditions are present. Thus, the client with hypercalcemia may be at an increased risk for thrombus formation in locations where blood vessel or tissue damage have occurred and in vessels or organs in which blood flow is impeded. In hospitalized clients or in those whose mobility is decreased, blood clotting is more likely to occur in the lower legs, pelvic regions, anywhere that blood flow is impeded by internal or external constrictions, and places where internal blood vessel obstructions are present.

The nurse assesses each client at risk for hypercalcemia for indications of slow or impeded blood flow. Each day the calf circumference should be measured with a soft tape measure and recorded. The nurse asks the client to alternate dorsiflexion with plantar flexion and to state whether pain is present with either position. The nurse assesses the lower legs for color and capillary refill to determine the adequacy of blood flow to and from the area.

Psychosocial Assessment

Psychosocial issues during episodes of hypercalcemia are associated largely with changes of mental status as a direct result of decreased nerve impulse conduction within the brain. To determine changes in mental status, the nurse must first know the normal behavior, or baseline, for each client. In addition to directly assessing the behavior of the client, the nurse consults with family members regarding recent changes in the client's mood and behavior patterns. The most common CNS clinical manifestations of hypercalcemia include increasing lethargy and drowsiness that can lead to stupor and coma. The client is difficult to arouse and may be disoriented to time and place. The clients' short- and long-term memory may be impaired, and they may have difficulty keeping their thought processes in order long enough to answer questions.

Laboratory Findings

The definitive laboratory test result that confirms the presence of hypercalcemia is a serum calcium value greater than 10.5 mg/dL or 5.5 mEq/L. This value alone does not assist in determining whether an actual or a relative excess of calcium is present in the ECF. If the hypercalcemia is associated with dehydration or renal disease, concentrations of other serum electrolytes are elevated as are the hematocrit and hemoglobin levels. When the hypercalcemia has an extrarenal cause, concentrations of these other electrolytes are normal. Decreased clotting times also are associated with hypercalcemia. Urine calcium levels may be increased or decreased, depending on the underlying cause of the hypercalcemia. If increased renal reabsorption of calcium is present, the urine calcium level is low. If renal reabsorption of calcium is unaffected, hypercalcemia is accompanied by high urine calcium levels.

Radiographic Findings

When hypercalcemia is not caused by increased bone resorption of calcium, radiographic studies usually are not diagnostically helpful. However, when hypercalcemia is caused, at least in part, by increased bone resorption of calcium, radiographic studies may show losses of bone density and subperiosteal resorption. In addition, these studies may reveal hairline and compression fractures resulting from slight injury to thinning bone. However, bone density changes are evident on x-ray examination only after a 25% to 40% bone density loss has occurred. Certain malignancies with specific osteoclastic activity (multiple myeloma) are associated with characteristic bone x-ray patterns that resemble "holes," or "punched-out" areas of bone.

 Analysis: Nursing Diagnosis

Hypercalcemia most frequently occurs in conjunction with or as a result of the presence of other acute or chronic pathologic conditions. For this reason, hypercalcemia is most frequently seen among hospitalized clients or clients actively under treatment for specific conditions. The typical client with hypercalcemia is a 60-year-old woman under treatment for metastatic breast cancer. The following nursing diagnoses are derived from these data.

Common Diagnoses

The following diagnoses are commonly applicable to clients with hypercalcemia:

1. Potential for decreased cardiac output related to decreased electrical conduction through cardiac muscle
2. Constipation related to decreased intestinal motility
3. Potential altered tissue perfusion related to decreased clotting time and impeded blood flow
4. Potential for injury (fracture) related to decreased bone density

Additional Diagnoses

In addition to the common diagnoses, one or more of the following diagnoses may be pertinent:

1. Pain related to bone fractures

2. Fluid volume deficit related to increased urinary output
3. Altered patterns of urinary elimination related to the formation of renal calculi
4. Altered thought processes related to decreased CNS nerve impulse transmission
5. Total self-care deficit related to muscle weakness
6. Potential for injury related to muscle weakness
7. Altered nutrition: less than body requirements related to inability to ingest food secondary to nausea and vomiting

 Planning and Implementation

The following plan of care for the client experiencing hypercalcemia focuses on the common diagnoses related to alterations in cardiac output, bowel elimination, blood clotting, and safety. The prescribed plan of care is aimed at restoring normal calcium balance, preventing serious complications, and providing supportive care for altered body functions until the hypercalcemia is resolved.

Decreased Cardiac Output

Planning: client goals. The major goals for this nursing diagnosis include that the client will (1) have serum calcium levels restored to normal and (2) not experience lethal cardiac dysfunction.

Interventions: nonsurgical management. Interventions are aimed at preventing further increases in serum calcium levels and decreasing current serum calcium levels. Although restoration of serum calcium levels to normal is a goal of therapy, care must be taken to avoid complications that can be caused by changing serum calcium levels too rapidly. In general, hypercalcemia should be reduced at the same approximate rate at which the imbalance occurred. Drug therapy plays a critical role in restoring normal calcium balance. Other interventions that are more invasive but may be necessary when hypercalcemia is causing life-threatening disturbances in cardiac function include hemodialysis, peritoneal dialysis, and blood ultrafiltration techniques.

Drug therapy. Drug therapy for the treatment of hypercalcemia focuses on restoring normal calcium balance by preventing additional calcium administration and enhancing calcium excretion.

Under conditions of hypercalcemia it is necessary to eliminate parenteral calcium administration. Infusions of IV solutions containing calcium should be stopped. Often, fluid volume replacement alone can help significantly to restore normal serum calcium levels. This therapy is appropriate when renal function is normal and the cardiopulmonary status can handle the extra fluid load. Normal saline (isotonic NaCl) is a useful solution in this situation, because it does not contain calcium and because the administration of sodium inhibits tubular reabsorption of calcium, so that saline infusions promote calcium excretion.

Administration of thiazide diuretics should be stopped. Diuretics that enhance the excretion of calcium should be administered. The most useful diuretic for this purpose is furosemide (Lasix).

Agents that act as calcium chelators or binders can be useful in lowering the serum calcium levels. Such drugs include mithramycin (Plicamycin) and penicillamine (Stewart, 1983). Drugs that inhibit calcium absorption in the GI tract may be of limited benefit in treating hypercalcemia. One such oral drug is cellulose sodium phosphate, a cation exchange resin specific for calcium that releases sodium and preferentially binds calcium in the intestinal tract.

Other agents that may be useful in treating hypercalcemia include those that inhibit calcium resorption from the bone, such as phosphorus, calcitonin (Calcimar), and prostaglandin synthesis inhibitors (aspirin, nonsteroidal anti-inflammatory drugs).

Other manipulations of drug therapy to assist in the reduction of serum calcium levels include stopping the administration of any oral agent that contains calcium or vitamin D. Many antacids have a calcium base and should be avoided during periods of hypercalcemia. Multiple vitamins and calcium supplements also should be stopped at this time.

Diet therapy. Diet therapy has a minimal beneficial effect in controlling or alleviating hypercalcemia. Generally, hypercalcemia directly inhibits intestinal absorption of calcium. Excessive administration of concentrated calcium-containing substances should be avoided, but it is not necessary to restrict all dietary intake of dairy products and other foods rich in calcium.

Dialysis. When hypercalcemia is severe enough that life-threatening cardiac dysfunction is present, drug therapy may not accomplish a reduction of the serum calcium level quickly enough to prevent death. In this situation dialysis (either hemodialysis or peritoneal dialysis) or blood ultrafiltration may be necessary. The dialyzing fluid should contain little if any calcium, so that the ECF calcium can move down its concentration gradient across the dialyzing membrane until an acceptable level of serum calcium is achieved. Further discussion of nursing responsibilities during dialysis is found in Chapter 59.

Cardiac monitoring. Prevention of lethal cardiac dysfunction depends not only on reducing serum calcium levels, but also on recognizing early signs and symptoms, including the adverse responses of cardiac excitable membranes to the presence of increased calcium levels. Such action permits the appropriate timing of aggressive therapies for reduction of serum calcium levels. The nurse compares recently obtained ECG tracings with the client's baseline tracings or tracings obtained at a time when the client's serum calcium level was close to normal range. The nurse examines the ECG for changes in the T waves and the QT interval, as well

as changes in rate and rhythm. The nurse is responsible for reporting and recording these findings.

Constipation

Planning: client goals. The primary goal for this diagnosis is that the client will maintain bowel elimination patterns that are normal for him/her.

Interventions: nonsurgical management. Interventions include restoring serum calcium levels to normal (as discussed earlier for decreased cardiac output), stimulating intestinal peristalsis, and avoiding conditions and actions that contribute to constipation. Drug therapy, diet therapy, and comfort measures for constipation causing hypercalcemia are the same as those for constipation causing hyperkalemia (see earlier).

Prevention of complications. A major complication of decreased GI motility is the development of a paralytic ileus. In this situation peristalsis in at least one intestinal segment is absent and movement is "paralyzed." As a result, when intestinal contents enter the paralyzed intestinal segment, they are not propelled further. The contents build up, increasing discomfort and distention, and may lead to intestinal blockage. To prevent such an occurrence, the nurse assesses the bowel activity of the client with hypercalcemia before the administration of oral food or liquids. If intestinal motility cannot be discerned, food and liquids are withheld pending the results of more definitive diagnostic tests.

Potential Altered Tissue Perfusion

Planning: client goals. The major client goal for this diagnosis is that the client will maintain good venous return from all body areas.

Interventions: nonsurgical management. Interventions include restoring serum calcium levels to normal (as discussed earlier for decreased cardiac output), promoting venous return, and avoiding conditions and actions that may impede blood flow.

Drug therapy. For the client at risk for thrombus formation, drug therapy includes agents that interfere with specific components of the blood-clotting cascade. If the client can tolerate oral medications and has no other conditions that contraindicate aspirin use, aspirin can effectively increase clotting time by interfering with the ability of platelets to aggregate. Heparin, a parenteral drug that inhibits the action of thrombin and prevents the conversion of fibrinogen to fibrin, frequently is used to prevent thrombus formation. Because aspirin and heparin exert their effects on different components and areas of the blood-clotting cascade, they should not be used together. A third drug that can be used to increase clotting time is warfarin (Coumadin). This drug inhibits the action of vitamin K in the liver on the synthesis of four separate factors necessary to the clotting cascade. The action of warfarin is not immediate and administration for a number of days is necessary to achieve an increase in clotting time. All of these drugs carry the inherent risk of prolonging bleeding time to such an extent that the client may be at risk for hemorrhage.

Diet therapy. Diet therapy can be useful in prevention of thrombus formation. An important cofactor in the blood-clotting cascade is vitamin K. Green leafy vegetables contain relatively large amounts of vitamin K. The nurse encourages the client to restrict the amount of fresh green leafy vegetables (especially salads) consumed during the hypercalcemic episode. In addition, the nurse encourages the client to maintain an adequate oral fluid intake to keep blood osmolarity within normal limits and to decrease resistance in peripheral vessels.

Promotion of venous return. Thrombus formation is more likely to occur in body locations where blood flow is slow or impeded. Specific activities and devices can assist in promoting venous return and preventing venous stasis. The nurse assesses the client for external factors that may impede blood flow. Constrictive clothing is loosened or removed. Antiembolism stockings are applied to all clients at increased risk for thrombus formation. The nurse ensures that the client is measured properly for good fit of the stockings (according to the manufacturer's directions). Stockings that are too tight impede blood flow, and stockings that are too large do not assist with venous return. The nurse orders two pairs of stockings for each client so that a fresh pair can be applied daily.

A major factor in the physiology of venous return is the contraction of skeletal muscles surrounding deep and superficial veins. The nurse teaches the client to perform calf-pumping exercises for 5 minutes every hour while awake. In addition, the nurse teaches the client the importance of preventing veins with sluggish flow from unnecessary restriction at bending points. Clients are encouraged to keep leg joints straight when in bed. The knee gatch of the bed is not elevated, and the client spends minimal time with the bed bent at the client's hips. Whenever possible the client is encouraged to ambulate and to avoid standing or keeping the legs in a static dependent position. If the client has a large abdomen (because of pregnancy, tumor, ascites, or fat), the nurse assists the client to assume a side-lying position, rather than a supine position, to prevent partial obstruction of the vena cava. Respiratory movements and pressure changes within the abdominal and thoracic cavities also promote venous return through these areas. The nurse encourages the client to perform deep breathing and sustained maximal inhalations for 5 minutes every hour while awake.

Prevention of complications. A major complication of thrombus formation is the breaking off and movement of the thrombus within the systemic circulation (embolus formation). The nurse assesses the client during every shift for changes in peripheral circulatory status that indicate the possible presence of a thrombus. When a thrombus is present, activity should be curtailed, as extraneous movements may cause the thrombus to move. The nurse assists the client to avoid activities that may cause a small thrombus to become an embolus. Thrombosed areas are not massaged nor kept in a dependent position.

Potential for Injury (Fracture)

Planning: client goals. The two major goals for this nursing diagnosis are that the client will (1) prevent falls and fractures resulting from falls and (2) avoid activities that could result in a fracture.

Interventions: nonsurgical management. Because the client is prone to fractures related to decreased bone density as a result of excessive bone resorption of calcium, drug therapy aimed at inhibiting bone resorption processes is of benefit in this situation. (These drugs are discussed earlier for interventions in decreased cardiac output.) Diet therapy for this situation is of limited benefit.

Prevention of complications. The client must be careful to prevent falls and to avoid activities that could cause a fracture. A hazard-free environment is necessary to meet this goal, and the nurse must teach the client about its importance.

While the client is hospitalized, the nurse employs safety measures and eliminates potential hazards. Accidents in the hospital occur most frequently between 6 and 9 PM and during peak activity times, such as meal times. The nurse assesses the client for the need for assistance during ambulation-related activities. Clients requiring assistance must feel confident that needed assistance is readily available and should avoid getting up on their own. The nurse makes certain that the client's call light is within easy reach. Keeping the upper side rails in the up position helps to prevent the client from falling and also may be used as an assistive device by the client for facilitating position changes while in bed. The nurse ensures that the immediate environment has appropriate lighting for the client's vision needs.

Because clients with hypercalcemia as a result of excessive bone resorption or destruction may have thin bones, they are at an increased risk for fractures as a result of pressure. When touching and moving these clients, the nurse takes care to avoid excessive pressure or pulling and pushing motions on any area of the client. The nurse communicates this client care problem to all individuals involved in the administration of direct care to the client. The use of a lift sheet and the assistance of at least two nurses for position changes are helpful in evenly distributing pressure and avoiding potentially traumatic actions. Clients are discouraged from moving themselves, as even the pressure caused by self-assisted position changes can result in fractures.

■ Discharge Planning

Discharge planning for clients with hypercalcemia is the same as that for clients with dehydration (see earlier).

Evaluation

On the basis of the identified nursing diagnoses, the nurse evaluates the care for the client experiencing hypercalcemia. The expected outcomes for the client experiencing hypercalcemia include that the client

1. Restores and maintains normal serum calcium levels
2. Identifies actions to take when the signs and symptoms of hypercalcemia occur
3. Complies with the prescribed drug and diet therapy
4. Maintains an adequate cardiac output
5. States that pain is reduced or alleviated
6. Restores and maintains normal bowel elimination patterns
7. States that nausea is reduced or alleviated
8. Maintains an oral intake to meet nutritional needs
9. Participates in self-care
10. Maintains good venous return from all body areas
11. Remains oriented to time, place, and person

PHOSPHORUS IMBALANCES

The absorption, function, and regulation of the three minerals calcium, phosphorus, and magnesium are interrelated and complex, making the discussion of individual imbalances somewhat difficult. An additional confusing factor is that serum calcium and serum phosphorus levels appear generally to exist in a balanced reciprocal relationship. Thus, the product of the two serum ion concentrations (serum calcium concentration $\times$ serum phosphorus concentration) should always remain a constant. For this constant to exist, when one serum ion level is out of balance, the other serum ion level must be equally out of balance *in the opposite direction.* Although this balanced reciprocal relationship is present during normal physiologic function, pathologic conditions can disrupt this reciprocal relationship.

Most of the total body phosphorus content is located in the bones. The vast majority of the phosphorus present in body fluid is located in the ICF compartment. Phosphorus is the primary anion of the ICF and functions in a variety of important roles. Intracellular phosphorus is necessary for membrane synthesis, is involved in the synthesis of high-energy substances (such as adenosine triphosphate [ATP]), and serves as a cofactor for many important enzymatic reactions (Keyes, 1985).

Only a small percentage of the total body phosphorus is located in the ECF. Measurable phosphorus exists in the serum as both HPO_4^{2-} and $H_2PO_4^-$ in a 4:1 ratio. ECF phosphorus functions as a buffer to maintain the normal pH of body fluids and as an additional source of phosphate necessary for energetics of biochemical reactions.

HYPOPHOSPHATEMIA

OVERVIEW

The state of hypophosphatemia exists when the measurable serum phosphorus level is less than 2.5 mg/dL. Although hypophosphatemia can be present when total body phosphorus concentrations are normal, decreased, or increased, its deleterious effects are most obvious when accompanied by a decrease in the total body phosphorus concentration (Keyes, 1985; Zeluff et al., 1977). Even though the serum concentration of phosphorus has a narrow range of normal values (2.5 to 4.0 mg/dL), body functions are not significantly impaired as a result of rapid, wide fluctuations in serum phosphorus levels. Alterations in function are more obvious when the hypophosphatemia is chronic. Most of the effects of hypophosphatemia are related to decreased energy metabolism and accompanying alterations of the levels of other electrolytes and body fluids.

Etiology

The underlying causes of decreased serum phosphorus levels are grouped into the three main processes of decreased absorption of phosphorus, increased excretion of phosphorus, and intracellular phosphorus shift (Zeluff et al., 1977). Specific conditions associated with each process are discussed separately.

Conditions That Decrease the Intestinal Absorption of Phosphorus

Most high-protein foods contain large amounts of phosphorus. Ingested phosphorus generally is well absorbed in the jejunum and is absorbed to some degree in the duodenum. Intestinal absorption of phosphorus is enhanced by the presence of vitamin D, although, unlike calcium absorption, phosphorus absorption is not dependent on vitamin D.

Intestinal absorption of phosphorus is decreased indirectly by *malnutrition* or *starvation.* In addition, poor nutrition with inadequate phosphorus intake also is seen in clients with severe *alcoholism. Inadequate vitamin D* synthesis or intake can also contribute to poor intestinal absorption of phosphorus (Metheny & Snively, 1983).

Certain conditions and medications cause ingested phosphorus to bind to substances within the GI tract and be eliminated in the feces, rather than absorbed through the intestinal mucosa. Antacids containing either aluminum hydroxide (Alternagel, Amphojel) or magnesium (Bisodol, milk of magnesia) bind phosphorus in the intestinal tract and inhibit its absorption (Baker, 1985). In addition, when large concentrations of calcium are present in the intestinal tract, the calcium combines with the phosphorus to form an insoluble calcium-phosphate compound that cannot cross the intestinal mucosa.

Any condition that decreases intestinal transit time can interfere with intestinal absorption of calcium. Such conditions include diarrhea, excessive use of laxatives, and loss or destruction of intestinal tissue.

Conditions That Increase the Excretion of Phosphorus

Under normal conditions, the renal system excretes phosphorus at the same rate that the intestinal tract absorbs it. In this way a balance is maintained. When phosphorus is present in the serum at or below threshold levels, the kidney reabsorbs phosphorus and returns it to the systemic circulation so that less is excreted. When serum levels of phosphorus are above threshold levels, none of the phosphorus in the filtrate is reabsorbed and all of it is excreted. The specific area of the kidney involved in reabsorption and excretion of phosphorus is the proximal convoluted tubule (PCT).

PTH acts to regulate serum phosphorus levels (Keyes, 1985). PTH causes phosphorus to be resorbed from the bones and, at the same time, greatly increases renal excretion of phosphorus. Phosphorus excretion occurs more efficiently than bone resorption of phosphorus; thus, when PTH is present, phosphorus is lost from the body. Conditions that increase the amount of PTH include *hyperparathyroidism* and *hypocalcemia.*

Other conditions can increase the renal excretion of phosphorus independently of PTH. Any condition that increases the flow rate of filtrate through the renal tubular system increases phosphate excretion by decreasing the time available for reabsorption. *Osmotic diuresis,* as a result of the administration of osmotic diuretics or ECF hyperosmolarity, stimulates renal phosphorus excretion by increasing the flow rate. In addition, *ethanol* appears to inhibit phosphorus reabsorption in the PCT.

Conditions That Shift Extracellular Fluid Phosphorus to the Intracellular Space

Because ECF phosphorus is a source for the inorganic phosphorus needed to make high-energy substances (such as ATP), whenever the demand for intracellular ATP is high, ECF phosphorus shifts to the intracellular space. Although the serum phosphorus levels are below normal under these conditions, the total body phosphorus level usually is normal. Any condition that increases the amount of glucose or glucose precursors present in the blood so that intracellular glycolysis is increased results in shifting of ECF phosphorus into the intracellular space. These conditions include *hyperglycemia,* rapid or constant *administration of total parenteral nutrition (TPN) or hyperalimentation fluids, excessive carbohydrate ingestion* ("carbohydrate loading"), and *insulin administration.* An additional condition that results in a shift of ECF phosphorus to the intracellular space is

respiratory alkalosis. The mechanism for this shift is thought to be the presence of increased amounts of oxygen, which tend to stimulate intracellular glycolysis.

COLLABORATIVE MANAGEMENT

Physical Assessment: Clinical Manifestations

The onset of clinical manifestations of hypophosphatemia usually does not occur until the decrease in serum phosphate levels is severe or prolonged (Baker, 1985). The clinical manifestations of hypophosphatemia can be categorized as acute and chronic. The acute manifestations are functional in nature, whereas the chronic manifestations are structural.

The majority of acute clinical manifestations of hypophosphatemia are related to the decreased availability of high-energy compounds necessary to perform normal cellular metabolic functions. These clinical manifestations include alterations in the function of the cardiac system, the skeletal muscle system, blood cells, and the CNS.

The cardiac manifestations of hypophosphatemia include decreased stroke volume and decreased cardiac output. Peripheral pulses are slow, difficult to find, and easy to obliterate. The myocardial depression appears to be caused by low intracellular stores of ATP. Without sufficient quantities of ATP present in myocardial cells, contractions are weak and ineffective.

The pathologic change of hypophosphatemia that weakens cardiac muscles also appears to be responsible for weakening the contractility of skeletal muscles. The weakness is generalized and unaccompanied by paresthesias (unless other electrolyte imbalances also are present). When the skeletal muscle weakness becomes profound, respiratory movements become ineffective, and this situation can lead to respiratory failure.

The metabolic activity of all blood cells is greatly diminished in the presence of hypophosphatemia. Erythrocytes are less able to release oxygen at the tissue level (this situation pushes the oxygen dissociation curve to the left), causing generalized tissue hypoxia. Leukocytes are unable to perform their specific differentiated functions of phagocytosis, synthesis and release of antibodies, and synthesis and release of specific agents that increase the numbers and activity of all cells involved in inflammation and immunity. As a result, even though the numbers of leukocytes may be within the normal range, the client is somewhat immunosuppressed and at an increased risk for infection. The effect of hypophosphatemia on platelets is a reduction in their ability to aggregate and secrete substances important in the initiation of the blood-clotting cascade. As a result, the client is more prone to episodes of prolonged bleeding in response to relatively slight trauma or tissue injury. Bruises may be evident, as may overt bleeding of the gums.

CNS manifestations usually are not apparent until the hypophosphatemia is severe. The manifestations are a result of deranged energy metabolism related to insufficient amounts of phosphate present to make enough intracellular ATP. The CNS manifestations first occur as increased irritability and progress to seizure activity followed by coma.

The chronic clinical manifestations of hypophosphatemia are most evident in the skeletal system. Bone density is considerably decreased, and fractures and alterations in bone shape are apparent.

The renal system also can manifest chronic clinical problems associated with hypophosphatemia. The most common problem is the formation of renal calculi, as the urine (or filtrate) in the tubules contains more phosphorus (because less is reabsorbed) that can precipitate.

Interventions: Nonsurgical Management

Many of the interventions for hypophosphatemia are aimed at the specific conditions that caused the phosphorus imbalance. These interventions vary, depending on the underlying pathologic change. In addition, some interventions are aimed directly at increasing the serum phosphorus level when total body phosphorus levels are decreased (Lentz et al., 1978).

Drug therapy.   The administration of drugs that contribute to the development of hypophosphatemia is stopped (antacids, osmotic diuretics, and calcium supplements). Generally, oral replacement of phosphates along with a vitamin D supplement is sufficient to correct the hypophosphatemia. Rarely is it necessary to administer phosphorus parenterally. Parenteral phosphorus administration should be initiated only when serum phosphorus levels are less than 1 mg/dL and the client is experiencing serious clinical manifestations. Even under these circumstances, parenteral (IV) phosphorus is administered slowly, because the problems associated with hyperphosphatemia can be equally serious.

Diet therapy.   Diet therapy for hypophosphatemia primarily consists of increasing the intake of food items that contain high concentrations of phosphorus and decreasing the intake of food items that contain high concentrations of calcium. Foods rich in phosphorus include beef, pork, beans, and other legumes (Grant and Kennedy-Caldwell, 1988; Pennington & Church, 1985).

HYPERPHOSPHATEMIA

OVERVIEW

The state of hyperphosphatemia exists when the measurable serum phosphorus level is greater than 4.5 mg/dL. Usually, hyperphosphatemia is present only when total body phosphorus concentrations are increased. Elevations of serum phosphorus levels above normal are tolerated well by most body systems. The health problems associated with hyperphosphatemia

center around the hypocalcemia induced as a result of the increase in serum phosphorus levels.

Etiology

The underlying causes of increased serum phosphorus levels largely fall into four categories: renal insufficiency, aggressive treatment of neoplastic conditions, increased intake of phosphorus, and hypoparathyroidism.

Renal Insufficiency

The kidney (specifically the PCT) is the primary site of phosphorus excretion from the body when the serum concentration of phosphorus is greater than threshold levels. In renal insufficiency, the primary impairments occur at the level of the glomerulus (so that filtration is impaired) and at the level of the tubule (so that reabsorption is impaired). Most renal insufficiency involves filtration impairment to the extent that phosphorus in the blood is not filtered into the urine. Thus, the phosphorus that is ingested does not have an adequate route to leave the body, and the serum level becomes excessive.

Aggressive Treatment of Neoplastic Conditions

The vast majority of the total body phosphorus not present in the bones is found in the ICF. Phosphorus is the primary anion of the intracellular fluid of *all cells*, including cancer, or neoplastic, cells. Whenever cells are damaged or killed, the membranes break down and the ICF and intracellular substances are released into the ECF. Aggressive treatment of neoplastic conditions that involve a large tumor volume (or a large number of cancer cells) results in a rapid destruction of tumor cells, which release their intracellular products into the blood and other extracellular fluids. This process is known as the *tumor lysis syndrome*, and the intracellular products include phosphorus (Kopec & Groeger, 1988). The neoplasms most likely to respond to treatment rapidly enough to significantly increase the serum phosphorus concentration include the leukemias, the lymphomas, and occasionally breast cancer.

Increased Intake of Phosphorus

Phosphorus is present in many foods; however, unless renal insufficiency is present, dietary ingestion of phosphorus is not a common cause of hyperphosphatemia for adults. Many laxatives have a phosphorus base. Clients who excessively use or abuse phosphate-containing laxatives are likely to develop hyperphosphatemia. In addition, many commercial enema solutions have a phosphorus base. Clients who frequently use these enema solutions (in large amounts) and retain them for longer than 20 minutes may greatly increase their intestinal absorption of phosphorus and cause a corresponding increase in the serum phosphorus level.

Among hospitalized clients, hyperphosphatemia can occur as a result of the IV administration of phosphorus-containing fluids, especially when these are administered to correct the condition of hypophosphatemia.

Hypoparathyroidism

When the condition of hypoparathyroidism is present, insufficient quantities of PTH are synthesized. Although PTH causes an increase in the bone resorption of phosphorus, it also produces an even greater increase in the renal excretion of phosphorus. Thus, when hypoparathyroidism is present, less phosphorus is excreted in the urine and more is reabsorbed into the systemic circulation. Conditions that lead to hypoparathyroidism include thyroid surgery, thyroid radiation, partial parathyroidectomy, and neoplasia.

COLLABORATIVE MANAGEMENT

Hyperphosphatemia produces few direct alterations in body systems. However, when hyperphosphatemia is present, a corresponding hypocalcemia also is present, because the calcium and phosphorus ions exist in the blood in a balanced reciprocal relationship. It is the accompanying hypocalcemia that dramatically alters the physiologic functioning of many body systems and has the potential for causing serious and life-threatening side effects. Thus, the management of hyperphosphatemia entails the management of hypocalcemia.

MAGNESIUM IMBALANCES

Magnesium is another important mineral component of the body, which is primarily stored in bone and cartilage. The functions and regulatory mechanisms of magnesium are related to those of calcium and phosphorus, although less is known about the exact mechanisms of magnesium regulation. As discussed in Chapter 12, only a relatively small amount of the body's total magnesium concentration is present in the ECF. Magnesium is present to a greater extent in the ICF, especially in muscle cells.

In the cell, the role of magnesium primarily is to serve as a cofactor for many enzymes and proteins involved in critical biochemical reactions. In addition, intracellular magnesium is an absolute requirement for muscle contraction.

ECF magnesium has at least three identified roles. First, magnesium is a necessary cofactor at several points in the blood-clotting cascade. Second, magnesium modifies transmission of action potentials at some neuron-to-neuron synaptic points and at neuromuscular synaptic points. Lastly, ECF magnesium appears to serve as a buffer or pool of magnesium that can be readily accessible to help meet intracellular needs for magnesium under specific metabolic conditions.

HYPOMAGNESEMIA

OVERVIEW

The state of hypomagnesemia exists when the serum magnesium ion (Mg^{2+}) level is less than 1.5 mEq/L. Because the vast majority of conditions that lead to hypomagnesemia are related to either a decreased magnesium intake or an increased magnesium loss, measurable hypomagnesemia usually reflects a decrease in the total body magnesium concentration. The primary direct physiologic effects of hypomagnesemia are related to alterations in the function of excitable membranes and accompanying imbalances of serum calcium and potassium levels.

Etiology

The major causes of hypomagnesemia usually are related to either a decreased absorption of dietary magnesium or an increase in the renal excretion of magnesium. The conditions associated with each mechanism leading to hypomagnesemia are discussed individually.

Conditions That Decrease the Intestinal Absorption of Magnesium

Magnesium is abundantly present in foods such as meats, nuts, whole-grain cereals, vegetables, legumes, and fish, and dietary intake usually supplies normal magnesium needs. In the GI tract dietary magnesium is absorbed from the same segments of the small intestine in which calcium absorption occurs, and absorption of calcium and magnesium can occur simultaneously from these segments.

Insufficient intake of magnesium can account for some instances of hypomagnesemia. Situations that contribute to this condition include *malnutrition, starvation,* and *prolonged nasogastric suctioning.*

Other situations decrease intestinal absorption of magnesium by interfering with the selective uptake of magnesium by the intestinal villi. Any condition that decreases intestinal transit time decreases intestinal absorption of magnesium by not allowing sufficient time for selective uptake to occur. Such conditions include *diarrhea, steatorrhea,* and *loss or destruction of the intestinal mucosa. Alcoholism,* especially when accompanied by *liver disease,* decreases intestinal absorption by decreasing the amount of necessary enzymes involved in the absorption process. *Excess amounts of phosphorus* in the intestinal tract at the same time that magnesium is present inhibits magnesium (and calcium) uptake by the intestinal villi.

Conditions That Increase the Renal Excretion of Magnesium

The site of renal handling of magnesium is the nephron. Magnesium is either reabsorbed or excreted by the tubular epithelium along the entire nephron. Normally, renal excretion of magnesium occurs at the same rate as intestinal absorption of magnesium, so that a constant serum level of magnesium is maintained. Specific conditions or factors can lead to hypomagnesemia by causing the renal system to decrease magnesium reabsorption or increase magnesium excretion.

Specific *drugs* interfere with renal handling of magnesium as either a primary action or a side effect (Halperin & Goldstein, 1988; Swales, 1982). These drugs include loop (high-ceiling) diuretics, such as furosemide (Lasix, Uritol) and bumetadine (Bumex); osmotic diuretics, such as mannitol and urea; aminoglycosides, such as kanamycin (Kantrex), gentamicin (Garamycin), and tobramycin (Nebcin); and some antineoplastic agents, such as cisplatin (Platinol).

Hypomagnesemia secondary to increased renal excretion occurs in response to rapid or continuous *ECF volume expansion*. Other conditions that contribute to the development of hypomagnesemia through increased renal magnesium excretion include *hypoparathyroidism* and *primary hyperaldosteronism*.

COLLABORATIVE MANAGEMENT

Physical Assessment: Clinical Manifestations

The majority of the clinical manifestations associated with hypomagnesemia occur as a result of alterations in the activity of excitable membranes. The most frequent clinical manifestations are seen in the neuromuscular system, the CNS, and the GI system.

The neuromuscular manifestations associated with hypomagnesemia are a result of increased impulse transmission at some synaptic areas (Brenner et al., 1987). The presence of magnesium inhibits the release of the neurotransmitter acetylcholine from the presynaptic membrane. Decreased levels of ECF magnesium allow greater release of acetylcholine, which increases the transmission of action potentials from nerve to nerve or nerve to skeletal muscle. Clients with hypomagnesemia generally have hyperactive deep tendon reflexes (+4) accompanied by painful paresthesia and tetanic muscle contractions. Positive Chvostek's and Trousseau's signs may be present, especially because hypomagnesemia may be accompanied by hypocalcemia. At the same time, if the intracellular magnesium also is decreased in an attempt to restore normal ECF magnesium balance, skeletal muscle weakness may be present. As the hypomagnesemia progresses, the client may develop tetany and seizures.

The CNS manifestations of hypomagnesemia also are related to a general increase in the transmission of action potentials. The client experiences an increase in CNS irritability that may be manifest as psychologic depression, frank psychosis, and confusion.

GI manifestations are associated with weakness and decreased contractility of the intestinal smooth muscle. Clients have decreased gastric motility, with anorexia, nausea, and abdominal distention. If the hypomagnesemia is severe or prolonged, a paralytic ileus may occur.

Interventions: Nonsurgical Management

The interventions for hypomagnesemia are aimed at correction of the electrolyte imbalance and management of the specific conditions that caused the hypomagnesemia. In addition, because hypocalcemia frequently accompanies hypomagnesemia, some interventions are aimed at restoration of normal serum calcium levels.

Drug therapy. Drugs that contribute to the development of hypomagnesemia are stopped (loop diuretics, osmotic diuretics, aminoglycosides, and cisplatin), as are drugs containing phosphorus. Generally, when hypomagnesemia is severe, the magnesium is replaced intravenously in the form of magnesium sulfate ($MgSO_4$). The IV route is selected, because this substance can cause pain and severe tissue damage when injected intramuscularly. In addition, oral preparations of $MgSO_4$ frequently cause diarrhea and increased magnesium loss. If hypocalcemia also is present, drug therapy to increase the serum calcium concentration is initiated.

Diet therapy. Diet therapy for hypomagnesemia usually consists of increasing the intake of food items that contain high concentrations of magnesium. Foods rich in magnesium include meats, nuts, legumes, fish, and vegetables (Pennington & Church, 1985).

HYPERMAGNESEMIA

OVERVIEW

The state of hypermagnesemia exists when the serum magnesium level is greater than 2.5 mEq/L (Keyes, 1985). In a state of health it is difficult for an individual to develop hypermagnesemia. This condition usually is related to an increased intake of magnesium coupled with decreased renal excretion of magnesium.

Etiology

Increased Magnesium Intake

Many antacids and laxatives have a high concentration of magnesium (Maalox, milk of magnesia, magnesium sulfate). Individuals who overuse or misuse these agents are at risk of hypermagnesemia related to an increased magnesium intake. Other clients at risk of hypermagnesemia are those who are receiving parenteral magnesium as a treatment for hypomagnesemia.

Conditions That Decrease the Excretion of Magnesium

The most common condition that results in decreased excretion of magnesium is *renal insufficiency* (Leaf & Cotran, 1987). Any condition that decreases the synthesis and release of aldosterone also decreases the renal excretion of magnesium. Such conditions include *Addison's disease* and *adrenalectomy*.

COLLABORATIVE MANAGEMENT

Physical Assessment: Clinical Manifestations

The majority of clinical manifestations associated with hypermagnesemia occur as a result of alterations in the activity of excitable membranes. Usually, clinical manifestations are not apparent until serum magnesium levels are greater than 4.0 mEq/L. The most frequent clinical manifestations are seen in the cardiac, central nervous, and neuromuscular systems.

Cardiac manifestations of hypermagnesemia are related to bradycardia, peripheral vasodilation, and hypotension. Manifestations are progressive and become more severe as the concentration of serum magnesium increases. ECG changes include a prolonged PR interval with a widened QRS complex (Leaf & Cotran, 1985). Bradycardia can be severe, with cardiac arrest occurring during diastole of the cardiac cycle. Hypotension is severe, with the diastolic pressure much lower than normal. A widening of the pulse pressure also is a common clinical manifestation of hypermagnesemia.

CNS clinical manifestations of hypermagnesemia are related to depression of the transmission of action potentials at specific synaptic points. As a result, the client is drowsy to the point of lethargy. Coma may ensue if the hypermagnesemic condition is prolonged or becomes severe.

Neuromuscular clinical manifestations of hypermagnesemia also are related to a decreased ability to transmit impulses at the neuromuscular junction. Deep tendon reflexes are greatly diminished or even absent. As a result, voluntary skeletal muscle contractions become progressively weaker and finally stop. When the skeletal muscles of respiration are involved, respiratory insufficiency may occur, leading to respiratory failure and death from anoxia.

Interventions: Nonsurgical Management

Interventions are aimed at both reducing the serum magnesium level and correcting the underlying pathologic change that initiated or contributed to the development of hypermagnesemia. All oral and parenteral administration of magnesium is discontinued.

Drug therapy. When renal failure is not a contributing factor to the development of hypermagnesemia, the administration of IV fluids in the form of magnesium-free solutions can assist in reducing serum magnesium levels. Further reduction in serum magnesium levels can be brought about through the administration of loop diuretics. When cardiac manifestations are severe, administration of calcium can reverse the cardiac effects of hypermagnesmia (Leaf & Cotran, 1985).

Diet therapy. Diet therapy is most effective in the prevention of hypermagnesemia when other chronic pathologic conditions are present that predispose the client to the development of excess serum magnesium levels. Dietary restrictions involve limiting the ingestion of meat, nuts, legumes, fish, vegetables, and whole-grain cereal products. When the client's condition permits, an increase in oral phosphorus intake helps to inhibit intestinal absorption of magnesium (Leaf & Cotran, 1985).

PRINCIPLES OF COLLABORATIVE MANAGEMENT FOR INTRAVENOUS THERAPY

OVERVIEW

A broad definition of IV therapy is the technique of directly placing various liquids and solids from the external environment into the ECF of a client for the benefit of the client's health. Most commonly, this technique involves the transfusion of specific, sterile solutions into the venous circulation. IV therapy is a major aspect of nursing care and has a direct impact on the well-being of the client. No one has more direct influence on the fluid and electrolyte balance of any client than the nurse who administers that client's IV therapy.

HISTORY

Today, IV therapy is a major component of medical treatment and the most common invasive procedure experienced by hospitalized clients. Additionally, IV therapy is performed routinely in outpatient and home care settings. Although it is a common procedure, IV therapy presents significant potential hazards to the health and well-being of clients. These hazards are preventable when appropriate techniques are used and follow-up care is provided. Primary responsibility for the prevention of hazards leading to complications rests with the nurse. Thus, understanding of the physiologic principles regarding safe administration of IV therapy is essential for all nurses regardless of whether they start infusions or not.

COMPLICATIONS

Most clients who receive IV therapy develop at least one mild complication directly related to the therapy. These complications can be severe enough to cause significant morbidity and even death. Complications of IV therapy are of three types: (1) infection, (2) tissue damage, and (3) rapid adverse changes in ECF volume, composition, and electrolyte balance.

Infection

Because IV therapy disrupts the integrity of the skin and provides a direct entrance point into the internal environment for as long as administration is in progress, infection by microorganisms is always possible (Crow, 1987). The skin remains "open," with a needle or cannula penetrating from the outer surface through the skin into subcutaneous tissues and a blood vessel. Under these conditions, microorganisms can enter the internal environment directly through the skin at the penetration site. Another factor that increases the risk of infection during IV therapy administration is that most IV therapy systems are open systems. Access to solution containers, lines, and needles is achieved in the external environment. The risk of introducing microorganisms into the internal environment increases in direct proportion to the number of times that access to the system is obtained, even when proper aseptic technique is used during the procedure.

The solutions used for IV therapy also increase the risk of infection. Although the solutions are sterile when administration is initiated, the basic composition can enhance growth of microorganisms. Microorganisms proliferate better in a liquid environment than in a solid or a dry environment. In addition, many IV therapy solutions contain substances such as sugars and proteins that provide nourishment to microorganisms as well as to clients. These substances allow any microorganisms that enter the system to flourish more easily.

Time is a critical factor influencing the risk of developing an infection as a result of IV therapy. The longer the therapy is continued, the greater is the risk for infection to occur.

Tissue Damage

Various aspects of the initiation and administration of IV therapy have the potential to damage tissues. The tissues most commonly damaged as a result of IV therapy include skin, blood vessels, and subcutaneous tissues. Tissue damage may be temporary or permanent. All tissue damage causes the client to experience some degree of discomfort, and most tissue damage can be avoided through the use of proper technique and adequate follow-up.

Skin. The superficial skin can be damaged at the time of initiation of IV therapy by the tourniquet application, skin preparation, needle stick, and anchoring techniques. When the tourniquet used to fill the vein is too narrow, is applied too tightly, or is left in place for too long, hematomas, contusions and abrasions can result. In addition, some nurses attempt to "bring up" a vein by slapping the skin over the vein site. This slapping can damage both the skin and the vein, especially in areas where there is little soft tissue beneath the skin to absorb the blow. The use of excessive pressure to clean the skin site, especially in combination with the use of harsh chemicals, can abrade or burn the skin. The skin also is traumatized when the needle penetrates it. The larger the needle and the more pressure applied during the penetration, the greater is the chance of causing skin damage. Skin also is susceptible to damage by anchoring materials. Many people are allergic to tape adhesives or react to adhesives when these agents are present on the skin for hours or days. Skin reactions include erythema and blister formation. Removal of adhesives also can result in skin abrasion.

Veins. Tissue damage to veins usually is the result of either mechanical or chemical trauma. Mechanical trauma is encountered during the initiation of IV therapy when full veins are slapped and broken. The insertion of the needle not only punctures the vein, but also can tear away several membrane layers. After the needle is in place, it damages the innermost endothelial lining of the vein (tunica intima) by continuously exerting mechanical pressure against blood vessel walls.

Tissue damage to veins as a result of chemical trauma is related to the type and concentrations of IV therapy solutions, as well as to the rate of the infusion. Agents capable of causing chemical trauma to veins irritate the endothelium and set up an intravascular inflammatory reaction (phlebitis or vasculitis). When the response is great enough, the signs are visible externally. This type of damage can result in permanent scarring and thickening of the endothelium. In addition, the inflammatory reaction can narrow the blood vessel lumen to the degree that blood flow is impeded, leading to the serious complications of thrombus formation and insufficient oxygenation distal to the site of the inflammation. Common agents administered intravenously that are capable of inflicting chemical trauma to veins include hypertonic solutions, potassium chloride, antibiotics, calcium, magnesium, ethyl alcohol, and chemotherapeutic agents. Nursing actions to minimize chemical trauma to veins include diluting the agents administered intravenously and infusing the agent slowly into a large vein with a high-volume blood flow.

Subcutaneous tissues. Subcutaneous tissues sustain damage during IV therapy by two different probable mechanisms. One mechanism is indirectly mediated through hypoxia, and the other mechanism is directly attributable to the tissue-damaging actions of chemical irritants and vesicants.

Specific problems occurring during IV therapy can result in diminished oxygenation to local subcutaneous tissues (hypoxia). Improper anchoring techniques that involve taping or the entire circumference of the limb at the infusion site can lead to restriction of blood flow into and out of the area distal to the infusion site. Another situation that leads to local tissue hypoxia is the leakage of IV fluids into the interstitial space, causing the formation of edema. The edema increases the diffusing distance for oxygen and other essential nutrients at the tissue and capillary levels to the degree that tissue hypoxia develops.

When IV solutions are composed of substances that are vesicants and the solutions escape into the subcutaneous tissues, severe tissue-damaging reactions can occur. These vesicants can cause tissue necrosis and sloughing wherever they contact healthy tissue. Usually, the problem is discovered early enough to confine the damage to superficial, local subcutaneous tissues. This damage is painful and may require grafting for complete and functional healing. When vesicants penetrate into deeper tissues, such as muscles, nerves, and even bones, these tissues can be permanently damaged, with significant loss of function.

Fluid and Electrolyte Imbalances

Because IV therapy involves infusion of fluids directly into the plasma volume of the ECF space, the potential risk for rapid changes in ECF volume and composition is great. The overall physiologic effects of these changes depends on what degree of change is present, how rapidly the change occurs, and what specific electrolytes are out of balance.

Fluid volume excess is the most common imbalance that occurs among clients receiving IV therapy. Often this situation occurs because the infusion proceeds too rapidly. Clients have been known to receive 1000 mL of fluid in less than 30 minutes when rapid infusion is neither prescribed nor therapeutic. Factors contributing to rapid infusion include position changes of the client or the solution container, administration of solutions without the use of a controller or a pump, and the alteration of infusion rate (accidentally or intentionally) by clients, ancillary personnel, or visitors. A wide variety of complications are associated with the rapid infusion of IV therapy solutions.

Rapid infusion can result in circulatory overload when the client's cardiopulmonary or renal status is compromised to the extent that he/she cannot adequately handle the fluid load. In addition, this situation also can result in dilution of ECF electrolytes. Some of these electrolyte imbalances have serious sequelae and can be life-threatening.

If the rapidly infused solution contains specific electrolytes in concentrations greater than normal physiologic amounts (for example, 40 mEq of KCl in 1000 mL of 0.9% saline), the rapid infusion can greatly increase the serum electrolyte concentration to dangerous or even lethal levels. Earlier discussions in this chapter address specific problems associated with individual electrolyte imbalances.

Another less frequent but possible complication of rapid infusion of IV therapy solutions is hypothermia. Most solutions are administered at ambient, or environmental, temperatures. Usually indoor environmental temperatures range from 20° to 30°F lower than body temperature. Rapid infusion of cool IV fluids can lower core body temperature to the point that the client experiences the physiologic alterations caused by hypothermia.

ADMINISTRATION OF INTRAVENOUS THERAPY

The role of nursing in managing IV therapy has changed significantly during the past 20 years. This change reflects the increasing responsibility of the nurse for managing complex client care in highly technologic environments. Nursing responsibilities in regard to IV therapy now extend from initiation (after prescription by the physician) through termination of therapy. The following discussion provides a direction and rationale for nursing actions associated with the administration of IV therapy.

Initiation of Intravenous Therapy

Processes involved in the initiation of IV therapy include site selection, equipment selection, fluid selection, site preparation, venipuncture, and anchoring techniques. All of these processes are influenced to some degree by the purposes of the prescribed therapy.

Prescription. The prescribing of IV therapy is the responsibility of the physician. Before initiating IV therapy, the nurse first ascertains that a physician's prescription, or order, for this procedure exists. In some instances this order is formal, is specific for each individual client, and includes the exact type of needle desired as well as specific fluid and administration rate. At other times and in certain areas of the hospital, "standing orders" for IV therapy administration are developed on the basis of expected client problems and routine procedures. Often, the nurse determines the site, the equipment, the site preparation, the venipuncture technique, and the anchoring method.

Purpose. The purpose of the prescribed therapy, together with the length of time the therapy is expected to be maintained, has an impact on other factors in the initiation of IV therapy. The purposes of therapy vary and include one-time medication administration, correction of an actual fluid or electrolyte imbalance, provision of long-term nutritional support, and precautionary safety measures. For example, a large-bore needle may be placed in the antecubital area of a client's dominant arm during an emergency or during acute situations or emergency procedures when danger of major vascular collapse is possible. Such site and equipment selections would be inappropriate for long-term or intermittent therapy.

Site selection. The purpose and duration of the prescribed therapy, as well as the specific anatomic or physical problems of the client, determine whether a particular site is appropriate for initiation of IV therapy. The nurse exercises judgment and considers the following principles when selecting a site for IV therapy (Plumer & Cosentino, 1987).

Initiating intravenous therapy over a joint is avoided. Although veins and other blood vessels may be more superficially located and more easily discerned over a joint, such a site is both impractical and dangerous, except for short-term therapy. For the needle or cannula to remain safely within the vessel, immobility at the site of penetration and for the length of the needle is required. When IV therapy is initiated over a joint, the joint must be immobilized externally. External immobilization is difficult to achieve and is uncomfortable for the client. Any motion can dislodge the needle and potentially cause harm to surrounding tissues. Joint immobilization not only diminishes the client's range of motion and ability to participate in self-care, but also may be the source of other complications for some clients.

Intravenous therapy is initiated only in upper extremities. In most clients, venous return is better in the upper extremities, compared with that in the lower extremities. Gravity and distance from the heart contribute to the decreased flow rate in the superficial and deeper veins of the legs. This decreased flow rate impedes venous return, diminishes nutrient exchange at the tissue level, and increases the risk of thrombus formation. Cannulation of veins in the lower extremities greatly increases the risk of these problems. Unless no other veins can be used, the veins of the lower extremities of an adult are never used for IV therapy.

Intravenous therapy is initiated through intact skin. When skin is broken, its barrier function is no longer effective. Microorganisms easily penetrate the area and can overwhelm the body's defenses against disease. Because IV therapy involves penetrating the skin and the vein with the same needle, it provides a direct portal for microorganisms on the skin to invade the circulatory system. For this reason, IV lines should never be started through breaks in the skin, such as burns, excoriations, and abrasions. Skin that is inflamed, is edematous, or has a rash also should be avoided.

Intravenous therapy is initiated in the nondominant arm. Whenever possible client comfort is considered in the selection of a site for IV therapy. The nurse always asks the client which hand is dominant before initiating IV therapy. Whenever possible, the client's nondominant arm should be used so that the client has better motor control in activities using the dominant side.

Intravenous therapy should be initiated in arm veins — not hand veins. Because the veins of the hand tend to be more visible than the veins of the arm (often evident without a tourniquet), many health care professionals select hand veins for IV therapy. Hand veins are a poor choice unless IV therapy is extremely short term. The dorsal surface of the hand has little subcutaneous

supportive tissue, thus the veins are more prominent. However, these veins are small and thin walled. The lack of subcutaneous tissues also makes institution of IV therapy at this site more painful and increases the risk of serious tissue damage if extravasation or infiltration occur. In addition, the use of this site for IV therapy limits the client's use of the hand during therapy administration. Because clients tend to change hand positions frequently, IV lines in the hand are dislodged more frequently and are prone to other problems associated with variation in administration rate. For the above reasons, the arm should be used instead of the hand. When the arm is used, the site should be located as distally as possible, while still avoiding the wrist joint area. Using the most distal sites first or earlier in IV therapy allows preservation of proximal sites for later use if necessary. Dorsal veins are used in preference to ventral veins for their size, straightness, and decreased susceptibility to mechanical damage.

Intravenous therapy should be initiated in the arm with the better venous and lymphatic return. Because cannulation impedes blood flow to some degree through a vein, the nurse takes precautions to avoid using a vein or a limb that is already experiencing venous or lymphatic flow problems. Sites to be avoided include arms on the same side on which a mastectomy or lymph node resection has been performed. Arms that have had veins removed, had shunt procedures performed, have large varicosities, or have thrombosed or sclerosed veins also should be avoided.

Equipment selection. Equipment selection includes the type and size of needle or cannula, the type of tubing, and the composition of the fluid. The specific type of fluid to be used is prescribed by the physician. The fluid composition and the expected purposes of the therapy determine the selection of tubing style and needle.

Tubing should always have at least one access site in addition to the connection site. Additional access sites may be necessary if the client is to receive different types of solutions or intermittent therapy. If blood or blood products are to be administered, the proper tubing for this purpose is used. Depending on the nature of the solution to be administered and the policy of the agency, tubing with an in-line filter may be needed for administration of specific solutions. Other solutions, such as some antibiotics and chemotherapeutic agents, should not be administered through tubing with an in-line filter (this information is available on the package insert for the medication). Tubing and solution containers are labeled with the date and time of initiation. Solution labels also include the client's name, the exact contents of the solution, the prescribed administration rate, and the name of the individual who prepared the solution. Tubing labels also include the date and time that the line should be changed.

The selection of needle type and size is largely dependent on the expected purpose and duration of the IV therapy. Always select the *smallest* needle size appropriate for the purpose of the therapy. In some situations, the size of the needle is limited by the function. For instance, blood and blood products should not be administered through a needle that is small, because the needle itself can cause mechanical destruction of the blood cells. Therefore, for an adult, an IV for the purpose of blood administration should not be smaller than a 20-gauge needle (and some agencies may mandate an even larger needle for this purpose). The higher the osmolarity or viscosity of the solution ordered, the larger the needle will have to be for adequate infusion.

Another item of equipment to select at this time is a controller or pump. Not all IV therapy situations require the use of such equipment. Pumps and controllers should always be used in the following situations:

1. When IV solutions contain substances that can cause deleterious side effects, if administered too rapidly (for example, 40 mEq of KCl)

2. When the client's cardiopulmonary system is compromised to the extent that small fluid excesses are not tolerated well

3. When the client's fluid intake is rigidly restricted

Other types of equipment that are less expensive and can limit the rate or the amount of the infusion are volume-controlled infusion devices (such as Vol-U-Trol and Sol-U-Set) and infusion tubing sets with "microdrip" chambers. Volume-controlled infusion devices are small containers in which limited volumes of solution (usually 50 to 100 mL) are placed from a larger container so that not more than the limited volume can be administered during a given time, even by accident. The normal drop regulator of a drip chamber delivers fluid at the rate of 10, 15, or 20 gt/mL. Microdrip drop-regulator drip chambers deliver fluid at rates of 60 or 100 gt/mL. These equipment items are more commonly used in pediatric and neonatal settings, but also can provide inexpensive solutions to adult IV therapy volume problems.

Site preparation. After an appropriate site is selected and the proper equipment is assembled and prepared, the nurse prepares the skin area to reduce the risk of tissue damage, client discomfort, and infection as a result of IV therapy. Jewelry and restrictive clothing are removed from the area. If the site has a lot of hair that would either interfere with proper anchoring or make tape and needle removal painful, the nurse shaves the area immediately before initiation. The nurse gently cleans the area, following the established procedure of the hospital. If chemical cleaners are specified, the nurse questions the client regarding allergies or sensitivities to these agents. Bactericidal soap and water can be used to prepare a skin site adequately for IV therapy. Care is taken to avoid abrading the skin during cleaning. The skin is allowed to dry before needle insertion.

Another component of site preparation is that of increasing the accessibility of the vein. Well-filled veins are most prominent and allow easy access. These veins bulge through or displace subcutaneous tissues and are more easily palpated or viewed through the skin. Vein filling is dependent on circulatory pressures, environmental and skin temperatures, gravity, and skeletal muscle movement (Guyton, 1986).

Superficial veins fill better when blood is not shunted away to the deeper veins. Keeping the environment warm or warming the skin for several minutes with warm towels or a hair dryer helps to prevent shunting of blood to deeper veins.

All veins fill better when venous blood flow is obstructed proximal to the selected site. Venous blood flow is diminished to some degree by the force of gravity, thus placing the arm in a position dependent to the heart increases venous filling by slightly diminishing venous return to the heart.

The use of a tourniquet proximal to the site causes partial obstruction of venous flow and allows backfilling or overfilling of the veins distal to the tourniquet. If the tourniquet is applied so tightly that arterial flow also is obstructed, venous filling is absent or diminished. Alternately contracting and relaxing the skeletal muscles distal to the tourniquet also assists in venous filling by moving blood from muscle tissues into the veins. To decrease the risk of tissue damage, the tourniquet should be at least 1 in wide, should be applied only tightly enough to interfere with venous flow, and should not remain in place for more than 3 minutes.

Venipuncture. The technique of performing successful venipuncture varies with the type and purpose of the needle, the accessibility of the vein, the cooperativeness of the client during the procedure, and the skill of the person performing the venipuncture. This purpose of this discussion is to provide the learner with principles that are appropriate to all or most situations involving IV therapy and not to provide a step-by-step description of venipuncture technique. Skill in venipuncture technique is acquired as a result of instruction and practice. Early practice should occur using venous access models. Clients should not be subjected to *repeated* venipunctures by an unskilled or ill-prepared health care professional if this situation can be prevented.

In compliance with universal precautions, the health care professional should wear disposable gloves during the venipunctures. The wearing of eye protection also is recommended. The nurse uses aseptic technique to keep the needle and the prepared skin site sterile during the procedure. The needle or cannula is placed into the vein going with the direction of blood flow (Plumer & Cosentino, 1987). If it is necessary to stick the client more than once, a new needle is used each time. After the needle is placed properly in the vein (as evidenced by backflow of blood without tissue swelling at the site), the tourniquet is removed and solution flow is established.

Anchoring method. Because successful IV therapy involves maintaining the needle in position, proper anchoring of the equipment after needle insertion is important. The most commonly used recommendations for anchoring include that the nurse

1. Does not elevate the hub of the needle of cannula
2. Never tapes or anchors the entire circumference of a limb used during IV therapy
3. Places a strip of 0.5-in tape, adhesive side up, under the hub of the needle or cannula, and folds over the top, forming a chevron, or V, on the skin
4. Places a sterile, transparent dressing (such as Op Site or Tegaderm) over the skin entrance site
5. Tapes the hub of the tubing connection to the skin
6. Makes a loop and secures the tubing to the skin, avoiding the insertion site (commercial loops also are available)
7. Marks the tape or dressing with the needle type and gauge, the insertion date, and the initials of the inserter
8. Uses armboards only when necessary
   a. If the site is over a joint
   b. Client is confused or disoriented

Maintenance of Intravenous Therapy

Clients may receive IV therapy for hours, days, weeks, or even longer. IV therapy may be administered continuously or intermittently. The nurse often is responsible for maintaining IV therapy. Safe practice in maintaining IV therapy involves adherence to established principles.

When a hospitalized client is receiving IV therapy, the nurse assesses the flow rate, equipment function, and site condition at least every hour. Assessment may need to be more frequent, depending on the client's condition and the nature of the infusion solution. The nurse determines how much solution has been infused since the last assessment. The nurse maintains the flow rate and volume delivered within the limits of the prescription.

The site is assessed for evidence of edema, fluid leakage, discoloration, skin temperature changes, and discomfort to the client. For accuracy, the nurse compares the appearance of the IV site with the same area on the client's opposite arm. A helpful technique to determine whether edema and infiltration are present is to transilluminate the tissue at the site with a penlight. In a darkened room the nurse places the bulb end of the penlight over the tissue at the site and measures how large an area of transillumination is present. Edematous and infiltrated tissues have a larger area of transillumination.

Needle placement is ascertained by lowering the solution container below the level of the heart, allowing venous pressure to force blood back up into the tubing. This technique is not possible when tubing with a backcheck valve is used. Additionally, this technique may fail to ascertain that a needle is partially out of a vein. Therefore, careful observation of the site and questioning of the client for sensation changes at the site should

always be used in conjunction with observing backflow of blood to determine needle placement.

When blood return is not obtained as a result of this maneuver, improper needle placement or clot formation within the needle sheath is suspected. Both of these conditions require discontinuing IV therapy at the current site and re-initiating therapy at a new site. Clotted needles are never irrigated to force blood or tissue from the needle into the venous circulation. The nurse always documents in writing the condition of the site at each assessment.

Some sites require specific dressing changes. Sites for central lines provide great potential access for microorganisms directly to the circulatory system. To diminish the risk of microbial infection, some central lines that are expected to serve as long-term access sites are tunneled under the skin so that the skin site is somewhat remote from the venous entrance site. All central lines with external skin penetration sites are covered with sterile dressings that are changed on a regularly scheduled basis and when needed. Most agencies have strict policies regarding the scheduling of dressing changes, techniques used for the changes, and the preparation of health care providers designated as able to change these dressings.

The care required for maintenance of sites designed for intermittent IV therapy varies with the specific site and the type of cannulation device. The most common equipment used among hospitalized clients for intermittent IV therapy is the heparin lock or well. These capped needles are placed in peripheral veins, and patency is maintained by regularly flushing the needle with a sterile heparin solution. The volume and concentration of heparin used in flushing as well as the frequency of flushing varies with agency policy, unless otherwise specified by the physician's prescription. Central lines that are used intermittently usually are flushed daily to maintain patency. Implanted devices (such as Portacaths and Mediports) usually do not require daily flushing with heparin to maintain patency. Policies for the use of these devices vary with the agency, the physician, and the manufacturer's recommendations.

Equipment is assessed in terms of patency and integrity. Leaks indicate a breach of line and sterility integrity and require changing to new sterile equipment. Some equipment requires changing on a regular basis (such as tubing, solution containers, and extenders). All equipment changes are performed using aseptic technique. New solution containers are added or superimposed according to the prescription and when the previous container is empty. In some agencies, tubing is changed when a new solution container is supplied. Other agencies have established policies for scheduled tubing changes (usually after 24 hours or 48 hours of use). It may be necessary to change the tubing more frequently when specific solutions are used and when problems arise. The nurse follows the agency's policy manual and the pharmacy's recommendations for tubing changes. New equipment is labeled with the date and time, the contents (when appropriate), and the time of the next scheduled change. Whenever equipment is changed, care is taken to maintain sterility and to avoid getting air into the lines.

Most IV therapy equipment is designed to permit independent system access when necessary on intermittent or continuous infusion systems. Such access is used for medication administration, nutritional support, and withdrawal of blood for analysis purposes. To reduce the risk of introducing microorganisms into the internal environment and the IV therapy system, the nurse prepares the access site at the time of each access. Recommended preparation of the access site varies from agency to agency and often from nurse to nurse. Access sites to peripheral lines usually are swabbed for 1 minute with a sterile alcohol-, iodine-, or zephryn-based agent before needle penetration. Most agencies have more rigid preparation policies for obtaining access to central lines and implanted venous access devices. Regardless of policy variation, absolute adherence to asepsis is a major nursing responsibility for prevention of infectious complications when obtaining access to IV therapy systems.

Termination of Intravenous Therapy

IV therapy is terminated when the purpose of the therapy is accomplished or when specific problems surrounding infusion arise. Because IV therapy is an invasive procedure, the nurse checks the physician's order for terminating (discontinuing) therapy before removing the needle. In situations in which the nurse determines that a problem with the infusion exists (such as infiltration, extravasation, clotted needle, or phlebitis at site), a physician's order for termination is not needed.

The nurse performing the termination wears gloves during the procedure. Lines are closed, and pumps or controllers are turned off. The nurse gently removes the tape and other anchoring materials from the site. A dry, sterile gauze pad is held over the needle site, and the needle or cannula is withdrawn. After withdrawal of the needle, the nurse applies firm pressure to the site for at least 1 to 3 minutes. While applying pressure, the nurse inspects the needle or cannula to determine whether it is intact. When the site is no longer bleeding or leaking fluid, the nurse assesses the site for any abnormalities of skin color or temperature and the presence of edema. After assessment, the site area is dressed. The nurse disposes of the needle or cannula in an appropriate container, determines the amount of solution infused, and discards all tubing and containers in the specified containers for biohazards.

SUMMARY

IV therapy has proved beneficial for many clients, but is not without risk. Appropriate nursing care can significantly reduce the risk of health hazards to clients receiving IV therapy. In addition, adherence to proper precautions can prevent occupational hazards associated with IV therapy to health care workers.

FLUID AND ELECTROLYTE ALTERATIONS ASSOCIATED WITH NUTRITIONAL SUPPORT

OVERVIEW

Many clients refer to IV therapy as being "fed through the veins." This concept in relation to standard IV therapy is totally in error. Commonly used solutions for IV therapy are designed to replace or add fluid volume and specific electrolytes (see Table 13-1). Even though some of these fluids contain a minimal percentage of sugar (in the form of dextrose or glucose), these solutions are not primarily intended to provide caloric needs. These fluids are profoundly deficient in all nutrients, as well as vitamins and minerals, and prolonged maintenance on these fluids alone constitutes a starvation diet.

Many body cells are always metabolically active and require a *continuous* supply of energy to maintain vital metabolic functions. The element hydrogen is the basic fuel, or energy source, for the human cellular engine. This energy is measured in terms of calories. Much of this energy is derived from carbohydrate (CHO) sources, such as sugars (dextrose and glucose) and starches. Each person requires a certain number of calories each day to maintain metabolic function. This value differs from person to person, depending on body size, activity level, and rate of metabolism. Although the body generally utilizes carbohydrates as the energy source, the body also requires other food nutrients, such as proteins and fats. Proteins provide the nitrogen source necessary for maintenance of specific body structures (such as muscle) and for synthesis of a wide variety of active hormones, enzymes, and other essential substances. Fats, in the form of fatty acids and cholesterol, also are needed to maintain plasma membranes and to synthesize steroid and lipid-based hormones and other essential chemical substances (Guyton, 1986).

Because the body primarily uses carbohydrate sources for fuel and energy, the body has reserve carbohydrates stored for use when the individual is either not eating at all or not taking in sufficient quantities of carbohydrates. The amount of these reserves is limited, and, when the individual is not ingesting nutrients at all, can last about 12 hours. When the carbohydrate reserves are gone, the body begins to utilize body proteins and fats for fuel. Fats can be broken down and directly used as an energy source, although the body does not handle fat catabolism for energy well over extended periods of time. Proteins must first be converted into carbohydrates before they are used as fuel. The body catabolizes free proteins and the formed proteins in muscle to make carbohydrates to use as fuel. Whenever individuals are using body protein as a fuel source, rather than ingested proteins and carbohydrates, healthy tissue is being destroyed through catabolism (Guyton, 1986; Price & Wilson, 1986). These individuals are said to be in a state of *negative nitrogen balance* or *negative protein balance* because more protein is being destroyed than is being ingested or replaced. Negative balance situations lead to loss of essential tissues and substances. With any loss, the individual heals more slowly (if at all) and is susceptible to the development of serious illnesses. If the loss is extreme, the individual cannot maintain homeostasis well enough to survive. A major responsibility for the health care team is to prevent any client from entering or maintaining a state of negative nitrogen balance.

Because most clients only receive 3 to 4 L of IV fluid each day and 1 L of fluid containing 5% dextrose only provides 170 kcal, standard IV therapy alone usually only provides 500 to 700 kcal each day (Trissel, 1988). Such therapy maintains adequate fluid volume (and probably appropriate electrolyte replacement), but does not provide even the minimal adult caloric requirement. When clients are well-nourished, they can tolerate several days of standard IV therapy alone without sustaining long-term or deleterious effects. However, if clients are nutritionally deficient or are not able to ingest foods in the proper amounts for prolonged periods of time, other means of providing nutritional support are necessary.

ENTERAL NUTRITION

Broadly interpreted, enteral nutrition refers to the substances ingested through the GI system that are properly catabolized for the body's use in maintaining metabolism. This method of obtaining nutrients is best because the healthy human GI tract processes ingested foods most properly for human nutritional use. Therefore, whenever possible, all nutrients (carbohydrates, proteins, fats, vitamins, minerals, trace elements, and water) are obtained through dietary intake. In other words, use of the GI tract if it is functional is physiologically nutritionally sound.

In today's health care environment the term *enteral nutrition* generally refers to the type of nutrition provided by artificially processing an appropriate combination of carbohydrates, protein, fat, vitamins, minerals, and trace elements into a liquid form and regularly administering this preparation to a client through the client's GI tract. These liquids can be ingested orally when the client is able to swallow or can be administered through specific GI access devices when the client cannot or should not swallow. Because enteral nutrition methods make use of the GI tract and are considered less invasive than IV administration, the effectiveness of enteral nutrition methods in maintaining or enhancing the client's nutritional status usually is superior to parenteral nutrition therapy.

Table 13–2 summarizes the major components of commonly used, commercially prepared enteral nutrition products. These products vary in osmolarity, total calories, and the concentration of specific electrolytes, as well as in the specific sources of carbohydrates, proteins, and fats. This variance, together with the individual client's problems and idiosyncrasies, is responsible for differences in how well clients tolerate or respond to enteral nutrition methods.

Candidates

Clients who are appropriate candidates for enteral nutritional therapy or support are those clients who are unable to maintain an adequate nutritional status through their dietary intake. Such clients include individuals whose nutritional needs increase above their capacities for dietary intake (clients with large burn injuries, extensive trauma, or prolonged generalized infections) and those individuals whose oral intake is limited by specific problems to the extent that they are unable to ingest adequate amounts of nutrients (clients who are unconscious, unable to swallow, or too fatigued to manage the activities of chewing and swallowing). Enteral nutrition can be administered as a supplement to dietary intake or may take the place of dietary intake, depending on the client's needs and abilities.

Methods of Administration

Clients who are using enteral nutrition to supplement dietary intake to maintain or enhance nutritional status usually drink the preparation as an additional beverage or snack. Some clients prefer to have the preparation partially frozen to be eaten as a custard or "slush" style dessert. Most preparations are available in several flavors to increase client acceptance.

Enteral nutrition is frequently administered as "tube feedings" through GI access devices. Differences in the types of tubes, techniques for insertion, and care required for clients with tubes in place are discussed in detail in Chapter 33. These devices may be placed in any one of several areas of the GI tract. Tubes are positioned in nasogastric, orogastric, cervical, esophageal, gastric, duodenal, or jejunal locations (Grant & Kennedy-Caldwell, 1988; Phillips & Odgers, 1986). Nasogastric and orogastric locations are used for temporary, nonsurgical tube insertions that may stay in place continuously throughout the period of time the client is on enteral nutrition or may be inserted at each feeding. Cervical, esophageal, gastric, duodenal, and jejunal access devices usually are surgically placed for long-term enteral nutritional therapy. Cervical tube placement through the piriform sinus, most commonly used for temporary but longer-term nutritional support access for clients after head and neck surgery, is rapidly being replaced by the percutaneous gastrostomy technique (PEG).

Tube feedings usually are administered as either a bolus feeding or a continuous feeding. Bolus feeding is

TABLE 13–2 Components of Common Products for Enteral Nutrition*

Product	Manufacturer	Osmolarity (mOsm/L)	Calories (kcal/mL)	Fat (g/L)	Protein (g/L)	CHO† (g/L)	Sodium mg/L	Sodium mEq/L	Potassium mg/L	Potassium mEq/L	Chloride mg/L	Chloride mEq/L	Calcium (mg/L)	Iron (mg/L)
Compleat Modified	Sandoz	300	1.07	37	43	141	670	29.1	1400	35.9	470	13.3	670	12
Compleat Regular Form	Sandoz	405	1.07	43	43	128	1300	56.5	1400	35.9	870	24.5	670	12
Criticare HN	Mead Johnson	640	1.06	3.4	38	222	634	27.6	1310	33.5	1057	29.8	528	9.5
Enrich	Ross	480	1.10	37	40	160	845	36.8	1564	40.0	1437	40.5	719	12.9
Ensure HN	Ross	470	1.06	35.3	44.4	141	930	40.5	1564	40.0	1437	40.5	757	13.6
Ensure Plus	Ross	690	1.50	53.3	55	200	1141	49.6	2113	54.1	1987	56.0	706	12.7
Entri-pak	Biosearch	300	1.0	35.0	35.0	136	700	30.5	1200	30.7	1000	28.2	500	9.0
Isocal	Mead Johnson	300	1.06	44.4	34.2	133	528	23.0	1310	33.5	1057	29.8	634	9.5
Isocal HCN	Mead Johnson	690	2.0	102.3	74.8	200	803	34.9	1691	43.2	1185	33.4	1000	18.2
Magnacal	Biosearch	590	2.0	80	70	250	1000	43.5	1252	32.0	952	26.9	1000	18.0
Meritene Liquid	Sandoz	505	0.96	32.0	57.6	110	880	38.3	1600	41.0	1600	45.1	1200	14.4
Osmolite	Ross	300	1.06	38.5	37.2	145	634	27.6	1014	25.9	845	23.8	528	9.5
Osmolite HN	Ross	300	1.06	36.8	44.4	141	930	40.5	1564	40.0	1437	40.5	757	13.6
Pulmocare	Ross	490	1.5	92.1	62.6	106	1310	57.0	1902	48.6	1691	47.7	1057	19.0
Sustacal	Mead Johnson	620	1.0	23.3	61.3	140	940	41.0	2100	54.0	1564	44.1	1010	16.9
Sustacal HC	Mead Johnson	650	1.5	57.5	60.9	190	845	36.8	1479	37.8	1268	35.8	850	15.2
TraumaCal	Mead Johnson	490	1.5	68.5	82.4	142	1184	51.5	1395	35.7	1606	45.3	748	8.9
Travasorb	Travenol	420	1.5	50.4	75.0	187	531	23.1	1521	38.9	1839	51.8	759	13.7

* Values obtained from The Ross Medical Nutrition System, August, 1986, Ross Laboratories, Columbus, OH 43216.
† CHO, carbohydrate.

an intermittent feeding of a specified amount of enteral preparation at specified times during a 24-hour period. This method can be accomplished manually or through infusion via a mechanical pump or controller device. Continuous feeding is similar to IV therapy, in that small amounts are continuously infused (by gravity drip or via a pump or controller device) throughout a specified period of time. Infusion rates for continuous feeding (and to some extent for intermittent feeding) vary with the total amount of solution to be infused, the specific composition of the preparation, and the responses (tolerance) of the client to the procedure.

Complications

A wide variety of complications can be experienced by clients receiving enteral nutrition therapy (Grant & Todd, 1982; Moghissi & Boore, 1983). For the purposes of this discussion, enteral nutrition complications are limited to those problems associated with fluid or electrolyte disturbances.

Fluid imbalances.   Clients receiving enteral nutrition therapy are at an increased risk for the development of fluid imbalances. Often, clients who receive this therapy are elderly or debilitated and may have coexisting pathologic alterations of the cardiac or renal system. In addition, tube feeding preparations and specific circumstances surrounding administration also influence whether a fluid imbalance can or will develop during enteral nutrition therapy. Fluid imbalances associated with enteral nutrition usually are related to physiologic responses of increased ECF osmolarity.

As discussed in Chapter 12, osmolarity is the amount or concentration of particles dissolved in solution. This concentration exerts a specific amount of osmotic pressure within the solution. Normal osmolarity of the ECF ranges between 270 and 300 mOsm. Although the substance that is present in the greatest concentration in the ECF is NaCl, ECF osmolarity is determined by the overall concentration of *all* particles dissolved in the plasma.

As indicated in Table 13–2, tube feeding preparations range in osmolarity from isotonic (about 300 mOsm) to extremely hypertonic (>600 mOsm). Electrolytes (including sodium) contribute to this hypertonicity, but more of the osmolarity is determined by the concentration of proteins and sugar molecules in the enteral preparation. Even when the preparation is isotonic, unless some hypotonic fluids also are administered to the client, the ECF can become hyperosmolar. This situation is most likely to develop in clients who are unconscious, unable to respond to the thirst reflex, on fluid restrictions, or receiving hyperosmotic enteral preparations.

An increase in the osmolarity of the plasma increases the osmotic pressure of the plasma. Because this increased osmolarity largely is a result of extra glucose and proteins (which tend to remain in the plasma volume rather than move to interstitial spaces), the plasma osmotic pressure (water-pulling pressure) is increased. In this situation, intracellular and interstitial water move into the plasma volume, expanding the plasma volume. This volume expansion results in an increased renal excretion of water (among clients with normal renal function) and leads to osmotic dehydration. If clients do not have normal renal and cardiac function, the expansion of the plasma volume can lead to circulatory overload and the formation of pulmonary edema.

When hyperosmolar enteral preparations are delivered quickly, the client may develop excessive diarrhea. This situation also can lead to dehydration through excessive water loss. Another cause of diarrhea-related fluid imbalances among clients receiving enteral feeding preparations is lactose intolerance. Clients receiving milk-based enteral feeding preparations may develop this problem.

Electrolyte imbalances.   Clients with pre-existing pathologic states that predispose them to specific electrolyte imbalances are at the same risk for developing these imbalances during enteral nutrition therapy as they are during standard diet therapy. Some electrolyte disturbances can be avoided by administering enteral preparations with lower concentrations of the electrolytes that the client cannot handle well. In addition to specific electrolyte imbalances related to individual client problems, the two most common electrolyte imbalances associated with enteral nutrition therapy are hyperkalemia and hypernatremia. Both of these conditions appear to be related to hyperglycemia-induced hyperosmolarity of the plasma and the resulting osmotic diuresis.

PARENTERAL NUTRITION

When a client is unable to utilize effectively the GI tract for nutritional purposes, parenteral nutritional therapy may be used to maintain or enhance the client's nutritional status. This relatively new form of treatment (developed within the last 20 years) differs from standard or traditional IV therapy in that *all* nutrients (carbohydrates, proteins, fats, vitamins, minerals, and trace elements) are delivered to the client intravenously. Parenteral nutrition is subdivided into two categories: *partial parenteral nutrition* (PPN), or peripheral parenteral nutrition, and *total parenteral nutrition* (TPN), or central parenteral nutrition. As suggested by the names, these two categories differ by site of administration and content of solutions administered. This therapy sometimes is referred to as *hyperalimentation.*

Candidates

Clients who are NPO or who are unable to ingest adequate amounts of food through the oral route for at least 5 days are candidates for parenteral nutrition. Such clients include those with severe trauma (especially burn injuries and injuries to the GI tract), malabsorptive GI dysfunction (Crohn's disease, paralytic ileus, short-gut syndrome, and pancreatitis), and any condition that greatly increases nutritional demand and simultaneously diminishes the client's capacity to ingest sufficient nutrients to meet these demands.

Methods of Administration

Parenteral nutrition can be administered peripherally or centrally. The choice of administration depends on the client's needs and condition, the expected duration of the therapy, and the components of the solutions to be administered. Clients who need less intensive (daily caloric requirements between 2000 and 2500 kcal), short-term nutritional support and have adequate peripheral veins may be served best by peripheral parenteral therapy. In addition, peripherally delivered parenteral nutrition eliminates two potential hazards associated with central delivery: air embolism and pneumothorax.

Usually PPN is delivered through an 18- or 20-gauge catheter in a large distal vein of the arm (Rutherford, 1986). Two types of solutions are commonly used in various combinations for PPN. These solutions are fat emulsions (usually derived from either soybean oil or safflower oil) and amino acid–dextrose solutions. Most fat emulsions are isotonic, whereas the tonicity of commercially prepared amino acid–dextrose solutions ranges from 300 mOsm to nearly 1200 mOsm. The amino acid–dextrose solutions are considered more stable than the fat emulsions, so that additives, such as vitamins, minerals, electrolytes, and trace elements, are administered with the amino acid–dextrose solutions. The amino acid–dextrose solution must be delivered through an in-line filter, and both fat emulsions and amino acid–dextrose solutions are administered via a pump or a controller to ensure accuracy and constancy in delivery rate.

When the client requires intensive nutritional support (in excess of 2500 kcal/day) for an extended period of time, centrally administered TPN is appropriate. TPN delivery is accomplished through access to central veins, usually the subclavian, innominate, and jugular veins. Use of these veins is necessary owing to the high osmolarity and quantity of the parenteral solutions used for TPN. Access to these veins is accomplished with large-bore, dimethicone (Silastic) catheters that remain in place for prolonged periods of time. These catheters may be tunneled under the skin so that the skin penetration site is remote from the venous penetration site, possibly reducing the risk of septicemia.

Solutions used for TPN contain high concentrations of dextrose (up to 25%) and proteins, usually in the form of synthetic amino acids or protein hydrolysates (3% to 5%). These solutions are hyperosmotic (three to six times the osmolarity of normal blood). The base solutions are available as commercially prepared solutions. Additional components (specific electrolytes, minerals, trace elements, and insulin) are added on the basis of the individual nutritional needs of the client. The purpose of this therapy is to provide needed calories and to spare body protein from catabolism for energy requirements.

The formulas are designed to promote some ketogenesis and mobilization of fatty acids to meet energy demands.

TPN solutions usually are not administered without a pump or an infusion controller device. The osmolarity of the fluid and the concentrations of the specific components make controlled delivery imperative. Currently, debate continues about whether any other solutions or medications should be administered through lines delivering TPN.

Complications

Clients receiving nutritional support by either PPN or TPN are at risk for a wide variety of serious and potentially life-threatening complications (Grant & Kennedy-Caldwell, 1988). This discussion is limited to the complications of PPN and TPN that involve fluid or electrolyte balance.

Fluid imbalances. Clients receiving PPN or TPN are at increased risk of fluid imbalance. Not only is fluid being delivered directly into the venous system, but the extreme hyperosmolarity of the solutions stimulates fluid shifts between body fluid compartments.

The hyperosmolarity of these solutions is a function of their amino acid and dextrose concentrations. The dextrose causes a hyperglycemia in the plasma volume. Some of the dextrose moves into the interstitial and intracellular spaces, where it is metabolized. However, when the solutions are administered too rapidly, without enough insulin coverage, or in the face of hyponatremia and hypokalemia, the dextrose remains in the plasma volume, causing a shift of water from the interstitial and intracellular spaces into the plasma volume. Expansion of the plasma volume together with the hyperglycemia can cause an osmotic diuresis and lead to serious dehydration and hypovolemic shock. If the client has an accompanying cardiac or renal dysfunction, the situation can lead to overhydration, congestive heart failure, and pulmonary edema.

Electrolyte imbalances. Clients receiving either PPN or TPN are at an increased risk for the development of many different electrolyte imbalances, depending on what the electrolyte composition of the solution is and whether a fluid imbalance occurs. Therefore, any client receiving parenteral nutrition therapy should have serum electrolyte levels analyzed at least daily to determine the presence of imbalances. The risk of metabolic and electrolyte complications is reduced when the rate of administration is carefully controlled and clients are closely monitored for individual responses to treatment. Potassium and sodium imbalances are common among clients receiving PPN or TPN, especially when insulin also is administered as part of the therapy. Calcium imbalances, especially hypercalcemia, are associated with PPN and TPN, although immobility may play more of a role in the development of this imbalance than the actual parenteral therapy.

SUMMARY

All hospitalized clients are at risk for the development of fluid and electrolyte imbalances. The imbalance may be related to a specific pathologic condition, may be a result of environmental conditions, or may be directly or indirectly induced in response to therapy. The elderly and individuals with renal, cardiac, or endocrine pathologic changes are at the greatest risk for fluid and electrolyte imbalances. For many of these conditions, primary prevention is not possible; however, secondary prevention (early detection) is possible and constitutes a major nursing responsibility. Because the consequences of some imbalances are life-threatening, treatment is most effective if it is instituted early and is aimed at both the actual imbalance and the underlying cause.

IMPLICATIONS FOR RESEARCH

Because fluids and electrolytes can move between compartments, the presenting signs and symptoms are associated with deficits or excesses in the plasma volume and may not truly reflect whole-body deficits or excesses. Traditional treatment of various imbalances is undergoing close scrutiny and study. A key element in treating or preventing complications of fluid and electrolyte imbalances remains the early recognition of the signs and symptoms associated with specific imbalances. Many of these clinical manifestations are vague and vary with the degree of imbalance present. More clinically descriptive data are needed to establish specific clinical manifestation patterns associated with specific imbalances.

Nursing research needs to be conducted to answer the following questions regarding the care of clients at risk for imbalances of fluid and electrolytes:

1. What effect does health care teaching have on the prevention of specific fluid and electrolyte imbalances among individual at risk?

2. What effect does health care teaching have on the early detection of specific fluid and electrolyte imbalances among individuals at risk?

3. What nursing actions are most helpful in symptom management of side effects associated with specific fluid and electrolyte imbalances?

4. How can the nurse help promote an acceptance of chronic illness by clients experiencing chronic pathologic conditions?

5. How can the nurse promote compliance with special treatment regimens among clients with chronic illnesses?

6. What assessment tool is best in determining the presence of skeletal muscle weakness?

7. What site preparation techniques are best for reducing skin flora for the initiation of IV therapy?

8. What assessment criteria are best for determining the client's hydration status?

REFERENCES AND READINGS

Adinaro, D. (1987). Liver failure and pancreatitis: Fluid and electrolyte concerns. *Nursing Clinics of North America, 22,* 843.

Adlard, J., & George, J. (1978). Hyponatremia. *Heart and Lung, 7,* 587.

Agus, Z., & Goldfarb, S. (1981). Clinical disorders of calcium and phosphorus. *Medical Clinics of North America, 65,* 385.

Aspinall, M. (1987). A simplified guide to managing patients with hyponatremia. *Nursing '87, 17*(12), 32.

Atkinson, L., & Murray, M. (1986). *Understanding the nursing process* (3rd ed.). New York: Macmillan.

Baker, W. (1985). Hypophosphatemia. *American Journal of Nursing, 85,* 999.

Beck, L. (1981). Edema states and the use of diuretics. *Medical Clinics of North America, 65,* 291.

Brenner, B., Coe, F. L., & Rector, F. C., Jr. (1987). *Renal physiology in health and disease.* Philadelphia: W. B. Saunders.

Burman, R., & Berkowitz, H. (1986). IV bolus: Effective but potentially hazardous. *Critical Care Nurse, 6*(1), 22.

Cadnapaphornchai, P. (1987). Disordered sodium metabolism: Sodium retention states. *Critical Care Clinics, 5,* 779.

Chambers, J. (1987). Metabolic bone disorders: Imbalances of calcium and phosphorus. *Nursing Clinics of North America, 22,* 861.

Coward, D. (1986). Cancer-induced hypercalcemia. *Cancer Nursing, 9,* 125.

Crow, S. (1987). Infection risks in IV therapy. *National Intravenous Therapy Association, 10,* 101.

Cunningham, S. (1982). Fluid and electrolyte disturbances associated with cancer. *Nursing Clinics of North America, 17,* 579.

Desai, T., Carlson, R., & Geheb, M. (1987). Hypocalcemia and hypophosphatemia in acutely ill patients. *Critical Care Clinics, 5,* 927.

Elbaum, N. (1984). With cancer patients, be alert for hypercalcemia. *Nursing '84, 14*(8), 58.

Feig, P. (1981). Hypernatremia and hypertonic syndromes. *Medical Clinics of North America, 65,* 271.

Folk-Lighty, M. (1984). Solving the puzzles of patients' fluid imbalance. *Nursing '84, 14*(2), 34.

Frey, A. (1986). Taking the confusion out of multiple infusion: I.V. medications and TPN. *National Intravenous Therapy Association, 9,* 460.

Geheb, M. (1987). Clinical approach to the hyperosmolar patient. *Critical Care Clinics, 5,* 797.

Goldberg, M. (1981). Hyponatremia. *Medical Clinics of North America, 65,* 251.

Grant, A., & Todd, E. (Eds.). (1982). *Enteral and parenteral nutrition: A clinical handbook.* Boston: Blackwell Scientific.

Grant, J., & Kennedy-Caldwell, C. (1988). *Nutritional support in nursing.* Philadelphia: Grune & Stratton.

Groer, M. (1981). *Physiology and pathophysiology of body fluids.* St. Louis: C. V. Mosby.

Guyton, A. C. (1986). *Textbook of medical physiology* (7th ed.). Philadelphia: W. B. Saunders.

Guyton, A. C. (1987). *Human physiology and mechanisms of disease* (4th ed.). Philadelphia: W. B. Saunders.

Halperin, M. L., & Goldstein, M. B. (1988). *Fluid, electrolyte, and acid-base emergencies.* Philadelphia: W. B. Saunders.

Kennedy-Caldwell, C. (1986). Clinical triads: Water metabolism, the NPO patient and parenteral nutrition. *Critical Care Nurse, 6*(3), 63.

Keyes, J. (1985). *Fluid, electrolyte, and acid-base regulation.* Belmont, CA: Wadsworth.

Kim, M., & Moritz, D. (Eds.). (1982). *Classification of nursing diagnoses: Proceedings of the third and fourth national conferences.* New York: McGraw-Hill.

Kopec, I., & Groeger, J. (1988). Life-threatening fluid and electrolyte abnormalities associated with cancer. *Critical Care Clinics, 4,* 81.

Lancaster, L. (1987). Renal and endocrine regulation of water and electrolyte balance. *Nursing Clinics of North America, 22,* 761.

Leaf, A., & Cotran, R. (1985). *Renal pathophysiology* (3rd ed.). New York: Oxford University Press.

Ledbetter, C. (1988). Infusion phlebitis. *Critical Care Nurse, 8*(4), 10.

Lentz, R., Brown, D., & Kjellstrand, C. (1978). Treatment of severe hypophosphatemia. *Annals of Internal Medicine, 89,* 941.

McFadden, E., Azloga, G., & Chernow, B. (1983). Hypocalcemia: A medical emergency. *American Journal of Nursing, 83,* 226.

Metheny, N. (1984). *Quick reference to fluid balance.* Philadelphia: J. B. Lippincott.

Metheny, N., & Snively, W. (1978). Perioperative fluids and electrolytes. *American Journal of Nursing, 78,* 840.

Metheny, N., & Snively, W. (1983). *Nurses' handbook of fluid balance* (4th ed.). Philadelphia: J. B. Lippincott.

Moghissi, K., & Boore, J. (1983). *Parenteral and enteral nutrition for nurses.* Rockville, MD: Aspen Systems.

Morrison, G., & Murray, T. (1981). Electrolyte, acid-base, and fluid homeostasis in chronic renal failure. *Medical Clinics of North America, 65,* 429.

Motz-Harding, E., & Good, F. (1985). The right solution—mixing I.V. drugs thoroughly. *Nursing '85, 15*(2), 62.

Pennington, J., & Church, H. (1985). *Bowe's and Church's food values of portions commonly used* (14th ed.). Philadelphia: J. B. Lippincott.

Phillips, G., & Odgers, C. (1986). *Parenteral and enteral nutrition: A practical guide* (3rd ed.). New York: Churchill Livingstone.

Plumer, A., & Cosentino, F. (1987). *Principles and practice of intravenous therapy* (4th ed.). Boston: Little, Brown.

Porth, C. (1986). *Pathophysiology: Concepts of altered health states* (2nd ed.). Philadelphia: J. B. Lippincott.

Poyss, A. (1987). Assessment and nursing diagnosis in fluid and electrolyte disorders. *Nursing Clinics of North America, 22,* 773.

Price, S., & Wilson, L. (1986). *Pathophysiology* (3rd ed.). New York: McGraw-Hill.

Quinlin, M. (1982). Solving the mysteries of calcium imbalance: An action guide. *RN, 11,* 50.

Rao, T., Mathru, M., Salem, M., & El-Etr, A. (1980). Serum potassium levels following transfusion of frozen erythrocytes. *Anesthesiology, 52,* 170.

Robbins, S. L., & Kumar, V. (1987). *Basic pathology* (4th ed.). Philadelphia: W. B. Saunders.

Rossi, N., & Cadnapaphornchai, P. (1987). Disordered water metabolism. *Critical Care Clinics, 5,* 759.

Rutherford, C. (1986). Peripheral parenteral nutrition. *National Intravenous Therapy Association, 9,* 232.

Schwartz, M. (1987). Potassium imbalances. *American Journal of Nursing, 87,* 1292.

Sopko, J., & Freeman, R. (1977). Salt substitutes as a source of potassium. *JAMA, 238,* 608.

Stewart, A. (1980). Biochemical evaluation of patients with cancer-associated hypercalcemia. *New England Journal of Medicine, 303,* 1377.

Stewart, A. (1983). Therapy of malignancy-associated hypercalcemia. *American Journal of Medicine, 74,* 475.

Swales, J. (1982). Magnesium deficiency and diuretics. *British Medical Journal, 285,* 1377.

Tripp, A. (1976). Hyper and hypocalcemia. *American Journal of Nursing, 76,* 1142.

Trissel, L. (1988). *Handbook of injectable drugs* (5th ed.). Bethesda: American Society of Hospital Pharmacists.

Watson, J. (1987). Fluid and electrolyte disorders in cardiovascular patients. *Nursing Clinics of North America, 22,* 797.

Weisberg, L., Szerlip, H., & Cox, M. (1987). Disorders of potassium homeostasis in critically ill patients. *Critical Care Clinics, 5,* 835.

Zeluff, G., Suki, W., & Jackson, D. (1977). Depletion of body phosphate—ubiquitous, subtle, dangerous. *Heart and Lung, 6,* 519.

Zeluff, G., Suki, W., & Jackson, D. (1978). Hypokalemia—cause and treatment. *Heart and Lung, 7,* 854.

Zeluff, G., Suki, W., & Jackson, D. (1980). Hypercalcemia—etiology, manifestations, and management. *Heart and Lung, 9,* 146.

C H A P T E R   1 4

Concepts of Acid-Base Balance

The physiologic functions of the body operate best when the fluids of the internal environment are maintained within specific narrow parameters for composition, temperature, and location (Bishop et al., 1985). Chapter 12 discusses normal mechanisms that maintain fluid homeostasis related to overall solute and solvent composition. This chapter discusses the normal physiologic mechanisms for maintaining body fluid homeostasis related to the specific parameter of *hydrogen ion* (H^+) concentration, as indicated by pH. Hydrogen ions have an overall positive charge and are also called *protons*. Because one factor that determines the overall concentration of free hydrogen ions is the total number and strength of acid components in body fluids compared with the total number and strength of base components in body fluids, hydrogen ion homeostasis also is called *acid-base balance.*

The normal pH of extracellular body fluids ranges from 7.35 to 7.45 (Guyton, 1986), which is slightly alkaline (basic). Important enzyme complexes on the membrane surfaces of cells operate most efficiently at this pH (Keyes, 1985). Although most electrolytes have relatively narrow ranges of normal for intracellular fluid (ICF) and extracellular fluid (ECF) concentrations, the concentration of hydrogen ions in body fluids has the most narrow range of normal (Ganong, 1985). The body poorly tolerates ECF pH levels outside this normal range, and even relatively small changes in pH for short periods can disrupt major life-sustaining physiologic processes (see Chap. 13). Maintaining homeostasis of hydrogen ion concentration in the blood and other body fluids is critical because changes in this concentration result directly in

1. Alterations of the structure and function of many proteins

2. Changes in the distribution of other electrolytes in the ICF and ECF, causing fluid and electrolyte imbalances while the body attempts to maintain electroneutrality

3. Alterations of excitable membrane activity

4. Changes in the uptake, activity, and distribution of many hormones and drugs

Because optimal physiologic function depends on pH homeostasis, or acid-base balance, the body has many well-regulated mechanisms to ensure minimal fluctuation in hydrogen ion concentration.

ANATOMY AND PHYSIOLOGY REVIEW

As discussed in Chapters 12 and 13, body fluids are electrically neutral even though they contain many different ions that have an overall positive charge (cations) and many different ions that have an overall negative charge (anions). Electroneutrality is maintained by having these fluids contain an equal number of positive and negative charges. Maintaining homeostasis of body fluid pH is accomplished by a similar process in which the numbers of acid and base components are relatively balanced and the total concentration of *free hydrogen ions* is severely limited. Acid-base balance is actually concerned with the rigid regulation of free hydrogen ions.

DEFINITIONS

An *acid* is any substance that liberates or donates (sets free) a hydrogen ion (proton) when the substance is dissolved in water (Shrout, 1985). Thus, an acid in a solution increases the concentration of free hydrogen ions in that solution. The strength of an acid is determined by how easily it gives up a hydrogen ion in solution. A strong acid, like hydrochloric acid (HCl), dissociates completely in water and readily gives up all its hydrogen ions:

$$HCl + H_2O \longrightarrow H^+ + Cl^- + H_2O$$

A weak acid does not completely dissociate in water and donates only a small number of its hydrogen ions. In the following example, each molecule of acetic acid (CH_3COOH) (a weak acid) contains a total of four hydrogen ions. When acetic acid combines with water, it liberates only *one* of its four hydrogens while the other three remain bound to the original compound:

$$CH_3COOH + H_2O \longrightarrow H^+ + CH_3COO^- + H_2O$$

A *base* is a substance that binds free hydrogen ions in solution. Thus, bases are *proton acceptors* and reduce the concentration of free hydrogen ions in solution. Strong bases bind hydrogen ions easily and may bind more than one hydrogen ion to one molecule of base. Examples of relatively strong bases are sodium hydroxide (NaOH) and ammonia (NH_3). Weak bases bind hydrogen ions less readily. An example of a weak base is bicarbonate (HCO_3^-).

Neutralization is a process in which an acid combines with a base (through proton exchange) and forms one or more new substances that are usually neither acids nor bases. One example of such a reaction is the combining of hydrochloric acid (a strong acid) with sodium hydroxide (a strong base). This combination reacts to form salt (NaCl) and water (H_2O), two neutral substances:

$$HCl + NaOH \longrightarrow NaCl + H_2O$$

The hydrochloric acid is the hydrogen donor; it gives up a hydrogen, which then binds to the hydroxyl (OH^-) group of the sodium hydroxide (the hydrogen acceptor).

This action allows the freed chloride (Cl^-) to combine with the sodium (Na^+) from the sodium hydroxide. Another example of acid-base neutralization is the combination of hydrochloric acid with sodium bicarbonate:

$$HCl + NaHCO_3 \longrightarrow NaCl + H_2CO_3$$

The result of this reaction is the formation of the neutral substance salt (NaCl) and the weak carbonic acid (H_2CO_3).

Some substances when dissolved in water have a variable dissociation and can (1) remain electrically neutral; (2) donate a hydrogen ion (act as an acid) and carry an overall negative charge; or (3) accept a hydrogen ion (act as a base) and carry an overall positive charge. These substances are said to be *amphoteric* and act as either an acid or a base depending on conditions and the body's needs.

FREE HYDROGEN ION CONCENTRATION AND pH

The pH of any solution is a calculation of the concentration of hydrogen ions. This is a *calculated* measurement for body fluids because the actual number or percentage of hydrogen ions in these fluids cannot be measured directly.

The pH calculations for any fluid are derived from the *Henderson-Hasselbalch equation*. This equation is a mathematic formula expressing the interrelatedness of three factors: the concentration of free hydrogen ions, the concentration of bases, and the concentration of acids in a solution. When other influences (such as temperature and pressures) remain constant, if two of the three factors are known it is possible to calculate the third factor. The final derivation of the Henderson-Hasselbalch equation is the following formula:

$$pH = pK + \log\frac{[A^-]}{[HA]}$$

or

$$pH = pK + \log\frac{[HCO_3^-]}{[H_2CO_3 + CO_2]}$$

pK = the point at which the protonated and unprotonated forms of an acid are present in equal concentrations. For normal human body fluids, the standard for this value is based on the dissociation tendency for *carbonic acid* (H_2CO_3), which is 6.1 (Keyes, 1985; Shrout, 1985).

A^- = the concentration of the major proton acceptor in the solution. For normal human body fluids, this factor is always considered to be the concentration of bicarbonate (HCO_3^-) (Keyes, 1985; Shrout, 1985).

HA = the concentration of the major proton donors in the solution. For normal human body fluids, this factor is always considered to be the combined concentrations of carbonic acid and carbon dioxide (Keyes, 1985; Shrout, 1985).

Because under normal physiologic conditions, the concentrations of carbonic acid and bicarbonate in the ECF are in a ratio of 1:20, the major factor in the equation just given that tends to fluctuate is the concentration of carbon dioxide. As a result, a change in the concentration of carbon dioxide leads to a corresponding change in the pH.

In the Henderson-Hasselbalch formula, the concentration of carbon dioxide is the divisor (in the denominator of the equation), which makes the concentration of carbon dioxide *inversely* related to pH. However, it is *directly* related to the hydrogen ion concentration. Thus, when the carbon dioxide concentration of a solution increases, the pH *drops*, which indicates an *increase* in the hydrogen ion concentration. Conversely, when the carbon dioxide concentration of a solution decreases, the pH *rises*, which indicates a *decrease* in the hydrogen ion concentration. The actual chemical relationship between hydrogen ions and carbon dioxide is discussed later in this chapter.

Because pH is measured in negative logarithm (log) units, the pH value is *inversely* related to the concentration of hydrogen ions. The pH scale is a 14-point scale with the following hydrogen ion concentration values (Keyes, 1985):

pH 1 = 100.0 mEq of H^+ per liter

pH 2 = 10.0 mEq of H^+ per liter

pH 3 = 1.0 mEq of H^+ per liter

pH 4 = 0.1 mEq of H^+ per liter

pH 5 = 0.01 mEq of H^+ per liter

pH 6 = 0.001 mEq of H^+ per liter

pH 7 = 0.0001 mEq of H^+ per liter

pH 8 = 0.00001 mEq of H^+ per liter

pH 9 = 0.000001 mEq of H^+ per liter

pH 10 = 0.0000001 mEq of H^+ per liter

pH 11 = 0.00000001 mEq of H^+ per liter

pH 12 = 0.000000001 mEq of H^+ per liter

pH 13 = 0.0000000001 mEq of H^+ per liter

pH 14 = 0.00000000001 mEq of H^+ per liter

With this scale, *a change of one pH unit represents a tenfold difference in the hydrogen ion concentration.* Therefore, even a one-tenth pH unit change (e.g., from pH 7.4 to pH 7.3) represents a dramatic increase in the hydrogen ion concentration of a given solution.

Solutions with a pH of 7.0 are considered to be *neu-*

tral and contain an a equilibrium of the number and strength of acid and base components. The following schematic representation provides an artificial yet concrete means to understand the concept of neutral pH. The representation artificially indicates that the *strength* as well as the amount of all acid components is equal to strength as well as the amount of all the base components in a given solution. Although such is never the actual case in human physiology, if there is acid-base homeostasis, the relative amounts and strengths of acids (A) and bases (B) are approximately equal:

Equal Acids and Bases

A	A	A	B	B	B
A	A	A	B	B	B
A	A	A	B	B	B

Solutions with a pH from 1.0 to 6.99 contain an excess in the amount and/or strength of the acid components compared with the amount and/or strength of the base components. This situation results in the formation of free hydrogen ions. Comparison of the following schematic with the representation just given illustrates this concept visually:

Actual Acid Excess							**Relative Acid Excess (Base Deficit)**				
A	A	A	A	B	B	B	A	A	A	B
A	A	A	A	B	B	B	A	A	A	B
A	A	A	A	B	B	B	A	A	A	B

Solutions with a pH ranging between 7.01 and 14.0 have an excess in the amount and/or strength of the base components compared with the amount and/or strength of the acid components. This situation results in a deficit of hydrogen ions. The following schematic represents this concept visually:

Actual Base Excess							**Relative Base Excess (Acid Deficit)**				
A	A	A	B	B	B	B	A	A	B	B	B
A	A	A	B	B	B	B	A	A	B	B	B
A	A	A	B	B	B	B	A	A	B	B	B

SOURCES OF HYDROGEN IONS

Acids are formed in the body as by-products of normal metabolism. Some common sources and mechanisms of hydrogen ion production are given here.

1. Carbon dioxide (CO_2) is a by-product of glycolysis and many oxidation-reduction reactions. When carbon dioxide is combined with water (as it is for transport in the blood and other body fluids), the follow-

ing reaction (known as the *carbonic anhydrase equation*) occurs:

$$CO_2 + H_2O \longleftrightarrow H_2CO_3 \longleftrightarrow HCO_3^- + H^+$$

Therefore, any increase in the concentration of carbon dioxide in body fluids always leads to the formation of increased numbers of hydrogen ions in those fluids, with a resulting decrease in pH value. Carbon dioxide leaves the body in the air exhaled during pulmonary ventilation. Therefore, the one determinant of pH in body fluids is how much carbon dioxide is produced by body cells during metabolism versus how fast carbon dioxide is removed from the body by the pulmonary system.

2. The catabolism of food to make products for energy results in the formation of *fixed acids*. Catabolism of protein creates sulfuric acid. Catabolism of fat creates fatty acids. These acids are usually either further degraded to form other needed substances in the body or removed from the body by the excretory system (kidney).

3. *Incomplete oxidation* (which occurs whenever cells continue to metabolize substances under anaerobic conditions) of glucose or any other carbohydrate leads to the formation of lactic acid and other organic acids.

4. Incomplete oxidation of fatty acids results in the formation of ketoacids.

5. Whenever cells are damaged or destroyed, plasma membranes are broken and lysosomal fluids are released. Most lysosomes contain acidic fluids (pH about 4), so that their release into the ECF increases the hydrogen ion concentration of the ECF.

From the above-described activities, it is clear that the production of various acids, carbon dioxide, and hydrogen ions is a continuous process as long as any cells in the body are capable of metabolism. Despite this pro-

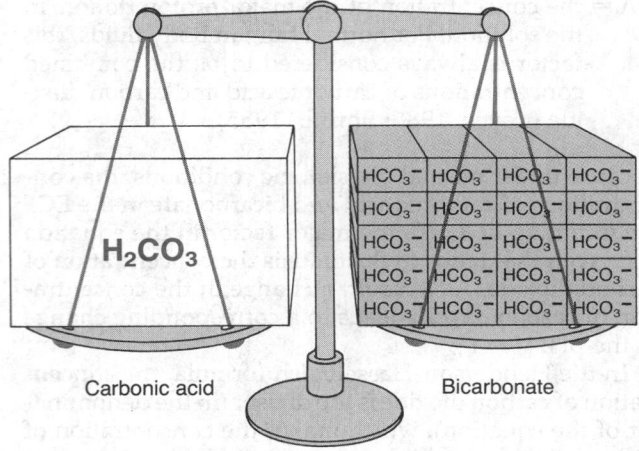

Figure 14–1

The normal ratio of carbonic acid to bicarbonate is 1:20.

duction, homeostasis of body fluids with regard to pH, bicarbonate, oxygen, and carbon dioxide concentrations is maintained under normal physiologic conditions. Table 14–1 gives normal values for these substances in arterial and venous blood. This homeostasis depends on three factors. First, hydrogen ion production must occur at consistent and normal rates. Second, carbon dioxide loss from the body through ventilation and respiration occurs at a rate that keeps pace with hydrogen ion production. Third, the ratio between carbonic acid and bicarbonate must be maintained at 1:20 (Fig. 14–1).

Bicarbonate is the principal buffer base of the ECF because of its relatively high concentration. Major sources of bicarbonate in the ECF include catalysis of carbonic acid (the carbonic anhydrase equation), gastrointestinal absorption or synthesis and secretion of bicarbonate, movement of intracellular bicarbonate into the ECF, and renal reabsorption of filtered bicarbonate (Guyton, 1987). Regardless of how bicarbonate enters ECF, once there it must be maintained at a concentration that is 20 times higher than the ECF concentration of carbonic acid for proper acid-base balance.

ACID-BASE REGULATORY MECHANISMS

To maintain the pH of the ECF within the previously described narrow ranges of normal during periods of both normal and abnormal metabolism, the body has three well-regulated mechanisms for acid-base balance. These mechanisms involve the blood, lungs, and kidneys directly, and also indirectly via neural control of the function of these organs.

CHEMICAL MECHANISMS

Chemical buffers in the ECF, especially in the plasma, constitute the first line of defense against marked fluctuations in hydrogen ion concentration and pH. Because

TABLE 14–1 Normal Arterial and Venous Blood Gas Values

Parameter*	Normal Values	
	Arterial	*Venous*
pH	7.34–7.45	7.31–7.42
PO₂ (mmHg)	> 80	30–50
PCO₂ (mmHg)	32–45	39–52
HCO₃⁻ (mEq/L)	20–26	22–28
Anion gap (mEq/L)	10–18	8–16

*PO₂, oxygen tension; PCO₂, carbon dioxide partial pressure.
Data from Shrout, J. (1985). Blood gases, pH, and buffering system. In M. Bishop, J. Duben-Von Laufen, & E. Fody (Eds.), *Clinical chemistry: Principles, procedures, correlations* (p. 258). Philadelphia: J. B. Lippincott.

they are constantly present in body fluids, buffers can engage in *immediate* actions to reduce or raise the hydrogen ion concentration to normal. Buffers convert strong acids or bases that can profoundly change the hydrogen ion concentration into much weaker acids or bases that have minimal effects on the total concentration of free hydrogen. Buffers are a mixture of two or more amphoteric substances. They function as chemical sponges to absorb or bind hydrogen ions when excess acids are present in body fluids. Because of their amphoteric nature, these same buffers can release hydrogen ions into the ECF when the pH increases to above normal. Examples of buffers include proteins and acid-base buffering pairs.

Acid-base buffering pairs are present in body fluids to cushion the effects of rapid changes in the hydrogen ion concentration. These buffering pairs are usually composed of a weak acid or a weak base and the conjugate salt of that acid or base. In the ECF, the two most important acid-base buffering pairs are the bicarbonate and the phosphate buffering systems. The bicarbonate system is the more active system in the ECF. The phosphate system does have some effect in the ECF, but it plays a more important role in buffering the ICF, especially in the renal tubular system.

Proteins constitute the largest buffer store. Although most proteins in solution in the human body tend to carry an overall negative charge, they are still amphoteric and can either bind or release hydrogen ions as needed. Both intracellular and extracellular proteins serve as buffers.

The major intracellular protein buffer is hemoglobin (Laski, 1983). Hemoglobin buffers hydrogen ions directly and the volatile acids formed during synthesis and transport of carbon dioxide (Keyes, 1985). When the hydrogen ion concentration of the blood increases, some of the excess hydrogen ions cross the plasma membrane of red blood cells. This movement of hydrogen ions from the ECF to the ICF of red blood cells has several consequences. To maintain electroneutrality of both the ECF and the ICF, as the cation hydrogen enters a cell another cation (usually potassium) leaves the cell. Once in the cell, the excess hydrogen ion can be bound by hemoglobin so that the number of free hydrogen ions is reduced. After the free hydrogen ion binds to hemoglobin, the number of positive charges in the ICF drops, and potassium re-enters the cell.

Extracellular buffering proteins include albumins and globulins. These proteins buffer both carbonic acid and the fixed acids that are present in the ECF as a result of catabolic processes (Keyes, 1985).

RESPIRATORY MECHANISMS

The respiratory system assists in control of acid-base balance by regulating the concentration of a volatile acid, carbon dioxide, in arterial blood. A major physiologic mechanism for ridding the body of carbon dioxide, which is created as a by-product of metabolism, is pulmonary ventilation (Metheny & Snively, 1983).

The concentration of carbon dioxide in venous blood increases during normal metabolism. This carbon dioxide is transported (usually by the hemoglobin transport mechanism or as bicarbonate) to the capillaries of the pulmonary tree. Because the partial pressure of carbon dioxide is far higher in the capillary blood than in the atmospheric air in the alveoli, carbon dioxide diffuses freely from the blood into the alveolar air. Once in the alveoli, carbon dioxide is exhaled during pulmonary ventilation and is lost from the body. Because the partial pressure of carbon dioxide in atmospheric air is so low as to be nearly zero, carbon dioxide usually continues to be exhaled at an appropriate rate even when alveolar gaseous exchange is impaired to some degree.

The concentration of carbon dioxide is directly related to the concentration of free hydrogen ions (the carbonic anhydrase equation). Because the respiratory system removes excess carbon dioxide so effectively and thus also indirectly reduces the hydrogen ion concentration, this system is the second line of defense against fluctuations in body fluid pH when the chemical buffers alone cannot prevent changes.

Respiratory regulation of acid-base balance is controlled by neural influences (Fig. 14–2). Special chemoreceptors in the areas of the brain that directly regulate the rate and depth of respiration are extremely sensitive to the concentration of carbon dioxide in the cerebral ECF (which is directly related to the concentration of carbon dioxide in the ECF of the body). As the concentration of ECF carbon dioxide begins to rise, these central chemoreceptors provide excitatory stimulation, in direct proportion to the excess amount of carbon dioxide, to the neurons that control the rate and depth of respiration. Under these excitatory influences, both the rate and the depth of respiration increase so that the rate at which carbon dioxide is exhaled from the alveoli increases proportionately. As a result, the ECF carbon dioxide concentration diminishes. When the arterial carbon dioxide concentration returns to normal, the rate and depth of respiration return to basal levels (Guyton, 1987).

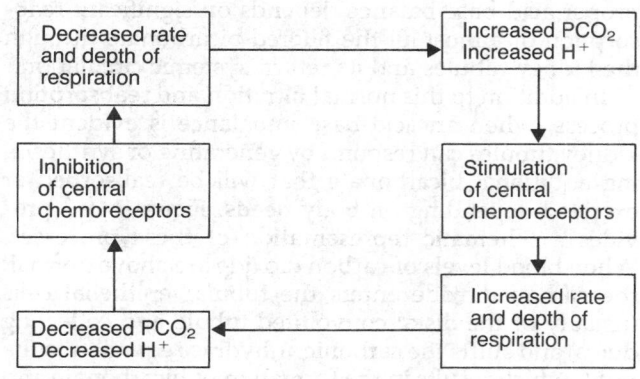

Figure 14–2

Neural regulation of respiration and hydrogen ion concentration.

If the hydrogen ion concentration of the ECF is too low, the carbon dioxide concentration is also too low. The low carbon dioxide levels are sensed by the central chemoreceptors, which inhibit stimulation of these respiratory control centers. As a result of this lack of stimulation, the rate and depth of respiration dramatically diminish so that less carbon dioxide is lost through alveolar ventilation and more carbon dioxide is retained in arterial blood. This retention, coupled with the normal carbon dioxide–generating metabolic reactions, gradually results in a return of the arterial carbon dioxide concentration (and hydrogen ion concentration) to normal levels. When these levels are normal, the rate and depth of respiration are also returned to basal levels (Guyton, 1987).

The response of the respiratory system in regulation of acid-base balance is quite fast. Changes in the rate and depth of respiration occur within seconds after changes in the hydrogen ion concentration and/or carbon dioxide concentration of the ECF are perceived.

RENAL MECHANISMS

The kidneys provide the third line of defense against fluctuations in body fluid pH. Under normal circumstances, the selective filtration and reabsorption processes of the kidney assist in maintaining fluid, electrolyte, and acid-base balance. In addition, when there are persistent changes in body fluid pH, powerful kidney mechanisms begin to operate that increase rates of excretion and reabsorption of acids or bases (depending on the direction of the pH changes). These mechanisms include renal tubular movement of bicarbonate, formation of titratable acids, and formation of ammonium (Brenner et al., 1987; Keyes, 1985).

Tubular movement of bicarbonate is accomplished in the kidney tubules in two different ways. First, much of the bicarbonate that is synthesized in other body areas is absorbed into the blood and is freely filtered into early urine at the level of the glomerulus (Chap. 12). If this filtered bicarbonate were to remain in the filtrate (early urine), it would be lost from the body through urinary excretion, which would lead to an excess of acid. Thus, proper acid-base balance depends on significant reabsorption of almost all the filtered bicarbonate through the kidney tubules and its return systemic circulation.

In addition to this normal filtration and reabsorption process, when an acid-base imbalance is evident the kidney tubules can respond by generating or synthesizing additional bicarbonate that will be reabsorbed or excreted depending on body needs. Figure 14–3 provides a schematic representation of these processes. When blood levels of carbon dioxide are above normal, the carbon dioxide enters the tubular epithelial cells (usually of the distal convoluted tubule and collecting ducts) and shifts the carbonic anhydrase equation to the right, which results in the formation of bicarbonate and hydrogen ions. The bicarbonate is secreted into capillary blood and returned to systemic circulation. The hydro-

gen ion is secreted into the tubular urine in exchange for sodium (which is actively transported through the tubular epithelial cell into renal capillary blood and systemic circulation). The overall result of this set of actions is the loss of hydrogen ions, which increases the ECF pH while maintaining electroneutrality. Once hydrogen ions are present in the final tubular urine, they must combine with another substance. If the hydrogen ions were to remain free in the urine, they would inhibit further movement of other hydrogen ions into the urine by causing the concentration of hydrogen ions in the urine to be higher than that in the tubular epithelium (Halperin & Goldstein, 1988). This situation would actually favor movement of hydrogen ions from the tubular urine into tubular epithelium (remember that most substances diffuse *down* their concentration gradient, and high concentrations of hydrogen ions in the urine would slow diffusion of hydrogen ions in that direction). The renal mechanisms of formation of a titratable acid and formation of ammonium prevent this situation from compounding an acid excess problem.

If carbon dioxide levels in the ECF are below normal (acid deficit or base excess), hydrogen ions from the tubular filtrate are reabsorbed in exchange for sodium. These hydrogen ions may be transferred directly into the blood or may force the carbonic anhydrase equation to the left in the tubular epithelium so that carbon dioxide is reabsorbed into systemic circulation. The result of these actions is a retention of acids and excretion of bases, which reduces the ECF pH.

Titratable acids are also generated at the same time that new bicarbonate is generated in the kidney tubules through the action of the phosphate buffering mechanism. Figure 14–3 schematically represents this process. When the newly generated bicarbonate is reabsorbed into systemic circulation along with the cation sodium, the tubular filtrate has an excess of anions, including phosphate (HPO_4^{2-}), which has a relatively high pK (Leaf & Cotran, 1985). This negatively charged environment strongly favors the movement of the cation hydrogen into the tubular filtrate (Brenner et al., 1987). Once in the filtrate, the hydrogen ion combines with the phosphate ion to form the titratable acid $H_2PO_4^-$, which is lost from the body as final urine. The overall results of this action are a loss of acids, a retention of bases, and an increase in the ECF pH.

Formation of ammonium (NH_4^+) from ammonia (NH_3) is the third renal mechanism for resolving the problem of ECF acid excess or base deficit. Ammonia is a by-product of normal amino acid catabolism, especially glutamine catabolism (Halperin & Goldstein, 1988). Ammonia is excreted into the tubular urine where it can combine with free hydrogen ions and form ammonium, and after which it is excreted from the body in the final urine, as illustrated in Figure 14–3. This trapping of free hydrogen ions in ammonium prevents the tubular urine hydrogen ion concentration from becoming so high that it inhibits diffusion or transport of free hydrogen ions from the ECF or tubular epithelium into the urine. The overall results of this process are a loss of acids, a reten-

1. TUBULAR MOVEMENT OF BICARBONATE

Method A: Movement of Pre-existing Bicarbonate   **Method B:** Movement of New Bicarbonate

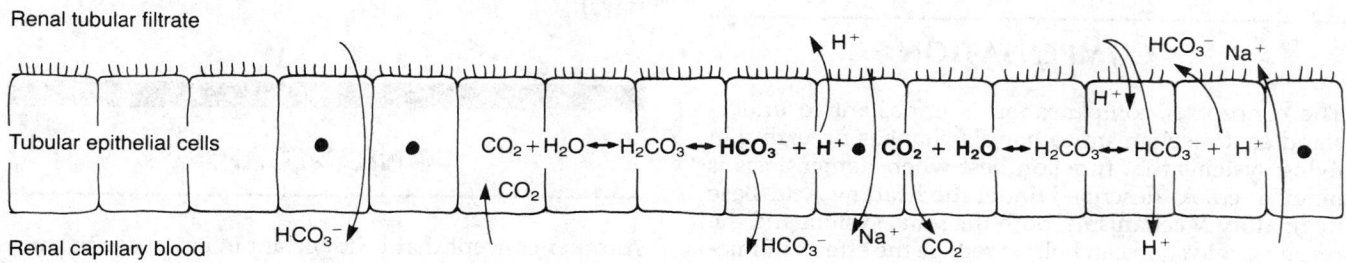

Renal tubular filtrate

Tubular epithelial cells

Renal capillary blood

Bicarbonate filtered at the glomerulus into the filtrate ("early urine") is reabsorbed across the renal tubular epithelium into the renal capillaries and returned to the systemic circulation. This movement of bicarbonate into the systemic circulation increases blood pH (makes blood less acidic).

If Blood CO₂ Levels Are High
Carbon dioxide enters the tubular epithelium, shifting the carbonic anhydrase equation to the right to form bicarbonate and hydrogen ions. Bicarbonate moves into the renal capillaries. Hydrogen moves into the tubular filtrate in exchange for sodium. The loss of hydrogen ions from blood reduces its pH (makes it less acidic).

To prevent excess hydrogen in the renal tubular filtrate, hydrogen ions must combine with other substances. The second and third renal mechanisms of acid-base balance now come into play.

If Blood CO₂ Levels Are Low
Hydrogen ions from the tubular filtrate are reabsorbed into the renal capillaries in exchange for sodium. This flow of hydrogen may be direct, or it may shift the carbonic anhydrase equation to the left so that carbon dioxide is reabsorbed into the systemic circulation and bicarbonate moves into the renal tubular filtrate. Retention of acids and excretion of bases reduce blood pH (makes blood more acidic).

2. FORMATION OF TITRATABLE ACIDS

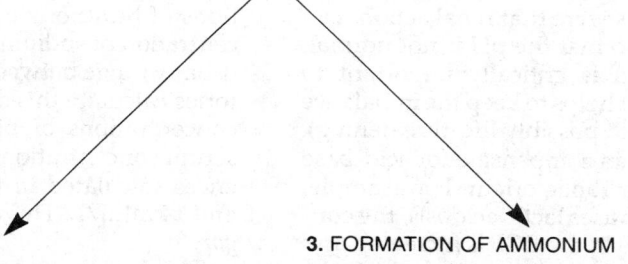

After the newly generated bicarbonate and the cation sodium are passed into the systemic circulation, the renal tubular filtrate has an excess of anions, including phosphate. The cation hydrogen is attracted to the negatively charged environment of the renal tubular filtrate. There, hydrogen binds with phosphate to form the titratable acid H_2PO_4, which is excreted in urine.

3. FORMATION OF AMMONIUM

Ammonia produced by amino acid (glutamine) catabolism is excreted into the renal tubular filtrate. There, ammonia combines with hydrogen cations to form ammonium, which is excreted in urine.

Figure 14–3

Renal mechanisms of acid–base balance.

tion of bases, and an increase in the ECF pH (Tannen, 1983).

COMPENSATION

The concept of compensation is important to understand as a mechanism to handle changes occurring in living systems that function best when homeostasis is maintained. As described under the heading Acid-Base Regulatory Mechanisms, both the renal system and the respiratory system can help to reduce the effects of fluctuations in body fluid pH when chemical buffering alone is not sufficient.

The healthy renal system can correct or *compensate* for changes in pH when the respiratory system is either overwhelmed or is actually a cause of the imbalance. For example, in chronic obstructive lung disease the respiratory system cannot exchange gases adequately. Carbon dioxide is thus retained, and the pH of the ECF falls. To counteract this process, the renal system increases excretion of hydrogen ions and reabsorption of bicarbonate. As a result, the pH of body fluids remains either within or closer to the normal range. When these back-up mechanisms are completely effective, the respiratory problems are *fully compensated* and the ECF pH is normal, even though the concentration of other substances (such as oxygen and bicarbonate) may be abnormal. Sometimes the respiratory factors contributing to the acid-base imbalance are so severe that renal actions can only *partially compensate*, so that the pH is not normal. Even partial compensation is critically important to acid-base balance because it helps to keep the imbalance from being more severe (and possibly life-threatening).

The respiratory system can compensate for acid-base imbalances that have a metabolic origin. For example, when prolonged running causes lactic acidosis, the concentration of hydrogen ions in the ECF is increased and the pH drops. The increase in hydrogen ions shifts the carbonic anhydrase equation to the left so that there is a corresponding increase in the carbon dioxide concentration. To bring the pH back to normal, the healthy respiratory system would be stimulated by the increased carbon dioxide concentration to increase both the rate and depth of respiration. These respiratory efforts cause the blood to lose carbon dioxide with each exhalation so that gradually the ECF carbon dioxide and hydrogen ion concentrations decrease. The pH returns to normal when this mechanism is capable of full or complete compensation.

Although both the renal system and the respiratory system can provide compensation for acid-base imbalances, it is important to remember that these two systems are not equal in their compensatory actions and reactions. The respiratory system is much more sensitive to acid-base changes and can begin compensation efforts within seconds to minutes of changes in ECF pH. However, these efforts are limited and can be overwhelmed easily. The renal compensatory mechanisms are much more powerful and result in dramatic changes in ECF composition. However, these more powerful mechanisms are not stimulated fully until the acid-base imbalance is sustained for a significant time (hours to days).

ANION GAP

Another concept that is important in acid-base balance is that of anion gap. Its definition is: "difference in concentration between the unmeasured cations and the unmeasured anions and is equal to the difference in concentrations of measured cations and measured anions" (Keyes, 1985).

Normal human body fluids are electrically neutral even though they contain large numbers of positively charged substances (cations) and negatively charged substances (anions). The fact that the body fluids are electrically neutral implies that there must be an equal number of positive and negative charges in these fluids. However, comparison of the numbers of positive and negative charges of the measurable substances in body fluids indicates the presence of more positive charges than negative charges. This number is calculated two different ways (Blosser, 1985). Some laboratories calculate this difference by subtracting the serum concentrations of bicarbonate and chloride from the serum concentration of sodium. Differences calculated in this way usually range between 10 and 18 mEq/L. Other laboratories calculate this difference by subtracting the serum concentrations of bicarbonate and chloride from the serum concentrations of sodium and potassium. Differences calculated in this way usually range between 7 and 14 mEq/L. This charge difference is called the *anion gap*.

The fact that a charge difference can be calculated does not truly reflect the normal neutral electrical situation in the fluids. Some substances in body fluids with variable charges cannot be measured by available methods. These substances include plasma proteins (largely albumins), organic acids, phosphates, and sulfates. For these unmeasurable charges, it is assumed that the number of negatively charged particles must outnumber the number of positively charged molecules. In addition, for the fluids to be electrically neutral overall, the net negative charges of the unmeasurable substances must be equal to the net positive charges of the measured substances.

The average normal value for the anion gap is 14 mEq/L in arterial blood and 12 mEq/L in venous blood (the concentration of bicarbonate is higher in venous blood). Changes in the anion gap, along with changes in concentrations of other substances (bicarbonate, oxygen, carbon dioxide, and other electrolytes), can help determine the type and origin of specific acid-base imbalance (Goodkin et al., 1984), which are necessary data for initiating appropriate interventions.

SUMMARY

Proper acid-base balance is critical for the normal function of most physiologic processes. The normal pH range for human ECF is 7.35 to 7.45. Fluctuations of pH between 6.8 and 7.7 can be tolerated during pathologic conditions for very short periods, although many physiologic processes are impaired to some degree by these pH levels. ECF pH values below 6.8 and above 7.7 are considered to be incompatible with life and are associated with serious pathologic conditions (see Chap. 15). The body has many well-regulated mechanisms to maintain acid-base homeostasis. These mechanisms involve chemical buffers, respiratory compensation, and renal compensation. Disturbances in these compensatory mechanisms result in either an inability to appropriately handle normal metabolic acid-base by-products or an induction of abnormal metabolic states that are characterized by increased production or losses of acids and bases.

REFERENCES AND READINGS

Bishop, M., Duben-Von Laufen, J., & Fody, E. (Eds.). (1985). *Clinical chemistry: Principles, procedures, correlations.* Philadelphia: J. B. Lippincott.

Blosser, N. (1985). Electrolytes. In M. Bishop, J. Duben-Von Laufen, & E. Fody (Eds.). *Clinical chemistry: Principles, procedures, correlations* (p. 263). Philadelphia: J. B. Lippincott.

Brenner, B., Coe, F. L., & Rector, F. C., Jr. (1987). *Renal physiology in health and disease.* Philadelphia: W. B. Saunders.

Ganong, W. (1985). *Review of medical physiology* (12th ed.). Los Altos, CA: Lange Medical.

Goodkin, D. A., Krishna, G. G., & Narins, R. G. (1984). The role of the anion gap in detecting and managing mixed metabolic acid-base disorders. *Clinics in Endocrinology and Metabolism, 13,* 333.

Guyton, A. C. (1986). *Textbook of medical physiology* (7th ed.). Philadelphia: W. B. Saunders.

Guyton, A. C. (1987). *Human physiology and mechanisms of disease* (4th ed.). Philadelphia: W. B. Saunders.

Halperin, M. L., & Goldstein, M. B. (1988). *Fluid, electrolyte, and acid-base emergencies.* Philadelphia: W. B. Saunders.

Keyes, J. (1985). *Fluid, electrolyte, and acid-base regulation.* Belmont, CA: Wadsworth.

Laski, M. (1983). Normal regulation of acid-base balance. *Medical Clinics of North America, 67,* 771.

Leaf, A., & Cotran, R. (1985). *Renal pathophysiology* (3rd ed.). New York: Oxford University Press.

Metheny, N., & Snively, W. (1983). *Nurses handbook of fluid balance* (4th ed.). Philadelphia: J. B. Lippincott.

Shrout, J. (1985). Blood gases, pH, and buffering system. In M. Bishop, J. Duben-Von Laufen, & E. Fody (Eds.). *Clinical chemistry: Principles, procedures, correlations* (p. 242). Philadelphia: J. B. Lippincott.

Tannen, R. (1983). Ammonia and acid-base homeostasis. *Medical Clinics of North America, 67,* 781.

CHAPTER 15

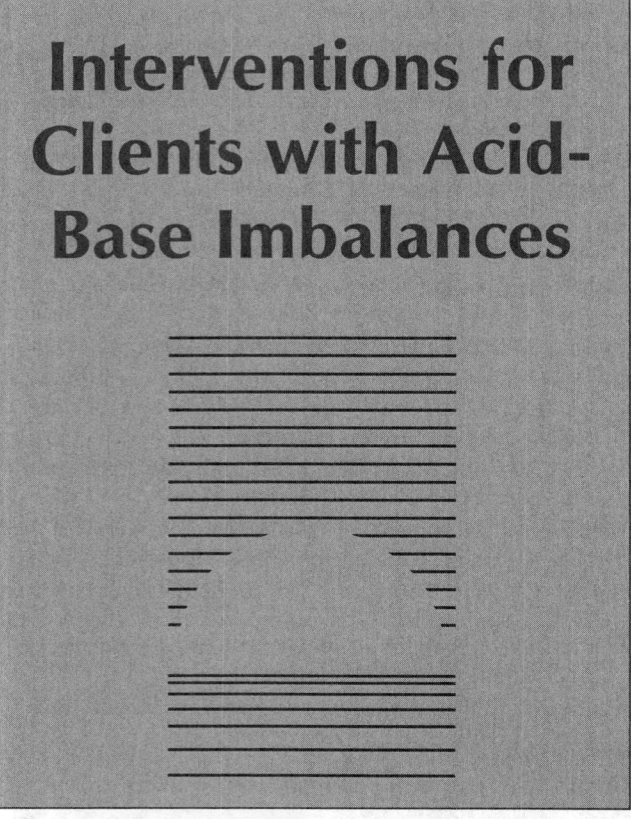

Interventions for Clients with Acid-Base Imbalances

The most carefully regulated component of human body fluids is the acid-base balance, or hydrogen ion concentration as measured as pH. The normal range for pH of body fluids is 7.34 to 7.45. Because maintaining the pH within this narrow range of normal is critical for proper functioning of many physiologic processes, the body has several highly regulated mechanisms or systems that rapidly adjust the retention or excretion of acids and bases. Thus, a proper acid-base balance is ensured regardless of the intake of acids or bases (see Chap. 14).

Disturbances in this balance usually occur as a consequence of two different types of actions. One type is indirect: conditions are present that dramatically change the concentrations of acids or bases at a rate that exceeds the body's normal capacity for regulation. The second type is direct: pathologic conditions directly impair the actions of specific regulatory mechanisms. The consequence of either type of action is an acid-base imbalance that can alter many physiologic functions and result in serious or even lethal side effects. Acid-base imbalances can be either an excess of acids compared with bases, such as in acidemia, or an excess of bases compared with acids, such as in alkalemia.

ACIDEMIA

OVERVIEW

Acidemia is a condition in which the acid-base balance of the extracellular fluid (ECF) is disturbed, with the concentration and/or strength of acid components being proportionately higher than normal compared with the concentration and/or strength of the base components (Shrout, 1985). This condition is characterized by an increase in the hydrogen ion concentration of the blood (because acids are substances that release hydrogen ions when they dissociate in water) and is reflected by an arterial blood pH below 7.34. Many people confuse the terms acidemia and acidosis. These two terms are related but not synonymous. *Acidemia* indicates the presence of too many hydrogen ions in the blood and a pH that is lower than normal. *Acidosis* is the *process* that caused the blood pH to decrease (Halperin & Goldstein, 1988; Narins & Emmett, 1980). It is important to remember that acidemia is not actually a specific disease or pathologic process; it is rather a symptom of a disease or pathologic process (Guyton, 1987; Keyes, 1985).

As discussed in Chapter 14, when the ECF pH is normal the concentration and strength of the acid components are approximately equal to the concentration and strength of the base components, as shown in the following schematic representation:

```
A   A   A   B   B   B
A   A   A   B   B   B
A   A   A   B   B   B
```

Acidemia can result from an *actual* increase in the concentration and/or strength of acid components, an *acid excess*. The following schematic displays this concept visually:

```
A  A  A  A  B  B  B
A  A  A  A  B  B  B
A  A  A  A  B  B  B
```

As an actual acid excess, acidemia is the result of processes that cause either (1) an overproduction of acids (and release of hydrogen ions) or (2) an underelimination of normally produced acids. Acidemia can also result from a *relative* increase in the concentration and/or strength of acid components, a *base deficit*. The following schematic represents this concept visually:

```
A  A  A  B  B
A  A  A  B  B
A  A  A  B  B
```

The actual amount or strength of acid components has not increased. Instead, the concentration, strength, or both of the base components have decreased, which makes the fluid relatively more acidic than basic. A relative acid excess acidemia (actual base deficit) occurs as a result of processes that cause either (1) an overelimination of base components (usually in the form of bicarbonate ions, HCO_3^-) or (2) an underproduction of base components.

The processes capable of causing acidemia include disturbances in metabolism and disturbances in pulmonary respiration. When it is caused by problems in metabolic processes, the resulting acidemia is said to have a metabolic acidosis origin. When it is caused by problems in respiratory processes, the resulting acidemia is said to have a respiratory acidosis origin. Acidemia has consequences that are serious and life-threatening. Because acidemia is the manifestation of another abnormal process, it is treated most effectively by treating the underlying abnormal process. Treatment techniques and modalities that are effective for metabolic acidosis are different from those that are effective for respiratory acidosis. Therefore, the ability to distinguish between metabolic and respiratory acidosis is important for proper treatment, as well as for prevention.

Pathophysiology

Acidemia, manifested as a pH less than 7.34, has profound effects on physiologic function regardless of whether its origin is metabolic, respiratory, or both. The primary pathologic effects of acidemia are related to the fact that hydrogen ions are cation electrolytes, and an increase in their concentration creates imbalances of other electrolytes, especially potassium, that disrupt functions of excitable membranes. Therefore, many of the early and detrimental signs and symptoms associated with acidemia are related to alterations in body systems that depend on the generation and propagation of action potentials. Physical manifestations of acidemia are associated with alterations in the neuromuscular, cardiac, respiratory, and gastrointestinal systems (Guyton, 1986; Robbins & Kumar, 1987; Taylor, 1984a).

In addition, even slight increases in the hydrogen ion concentration denature many proteins by changing their configurations and associations (tertiary and quaternary structures). Denaturing renders these proteins inactive. All naturally occurring hormones and enzymes consist of proteins, and many are absolutely essential to stimulate, catalyze, or maintain specific life-sustaining physiologic processes. Therefore, inactivation of many of these proteins for even a short period is incompatible with life.

Etiology

Acidemia can be caused by metabolic disturbances, respiratory disturbances, or combined metabolic and respiratory disturbances. The causes of metabolic and respiratory acidosis are given in the Key Features of Disease on pages 338 and 339. The general mechanisms that are involved in the various disturbances are described completely in the following paragraphs.

Metabolic Acidosis

The processes leading to metabolic acidosis are subdivided into four categories: (1) overproduction of hydrogen ions; (2) underelimination of hydrogen ions; (3) underproduction of bicarbonate ions; and (4) overelimination of bicarbonate ions.

Overproduction of hydrogen ions. Metabolic processes that increase the presence of hydrogen ions beyond the normal buffering or compensating capabilities of the body include excessive oxidation of fatty acids, hypermetabolism (anaerobic lactic acidosis), and excessive ingestion of acidic substances.

Excessive oxidation of fatty acids is usually a result of diabetic ketoacidosis or starvation. In diabetic ketoacidosis, the individual does not have sufficient amounts of insulin available to transport glucose from ECF into cells to use as fuel for generating energy. Instead, fatty tissues release fatty acids into the blood and other ECFs. The fuel-starved cells take up these fatty acids and synthesize high-energy substances from them. However, the metabolites from fatty acid oxidation form strong acids called *ketoacids*, including acetoacetic acid and hydroxybutyric acid. Each molecule of ketoacid leaves the cell and readily donates a hydrogen ion. Large amounts of ketoacids (such as would be present in a client who has poorly controlled diabetes with a high blood glucose level) release such large numbers of hydrogen ions that the normal buffering and renal acid-eliminating processes are not sufficient to control the hydrogen ion concentration, and a profound acidemia results (Kreisberg, 1987).

KEY FEATURES OF DISEASE ■ Common Causes of Metabolic Acidosis

Pathology	Conditions
Overproduction of H^+	Excessive oxidation of fatty acids
	Diabetic ketoacidosis
	Starvation
	Hypermetabolism (lactic acidosis)
	Heavy skeletal muscle exercise
	Seizure activity
	Fever
	Hypoxia, ischemia
	Excessive ingestion of acids
	Ethanol intoxication
	Methanol intoxication
	Ethylene glycol intoxication
	Salicylate intoxication
Underelimination of H^+	Renal failure
Underproduction of HCO_3^-	Renal failure
	Decreased pancreatic and hepatic functions
Overelimination of HCO_3^-	Diarrhea
	Dehydration
	Buffering of organic acids

In situations of starvation, the normal fuel substances are not taken into the body as food. During the first 12 to 24 hours of the fasting state, the body uses glycogen stores to make blood glucose. In addition, the body converts some muscle protein into glucose through a process called *gluconeogenesis*. Because of these stored sources of glucose, acidemia is usually not evident during the first day of starvation. However, after 24 hours the stored forms of glucose are depleted, and the body begins to catabolize body fat to fatty acids for fuel so that muscle mass can be conserved. Whenever fatty acids are used as the primary fuel source, ketoacids are formed and excessive numbers of hydrogen ions are released into the ECF, which causes acidemia (Brenner et al., 1987). Acidemia can also occur with weight reduction diets that stress excessive intake of dietary fats coupled with minimal intake of dietary carbohydrates.

Hypermetabolism (anaerobic lactic acidosis) occurs whenever intracellular glucose is not completely catabolized to carbon dioxide, water, and adenosine triphosphate (ATP). The presence of intracellular oxygen is needed for the most efficient and complete catabolism of glucose. This process is known as *aerobic metabolism*

(see the illustration on p. 341). When cells are forced to catabolize glucose without adequate oxygen (*anaerobic metabolism*), glucose is incompletely catabolized to a substance called *lactic acid*. Lactic acid leaves the cell and enters the ECF where it readily donates a hydrogen ion and causes acidemia. Anaerobic metabolism leading to lactic acidosis can occur either when the metabolic rate of a tissue (or larger area of the body) has increased so that the normal amount of intracellular oxygen is not adequate (a condition called hypermetabolism) or when the metabolic rate is normal but the amount of intracellular oxygen is low (Riley et al., 1987). Common conditions leading to lactic acidosis include heavy exercise of skeletal muscles, seizure activity, fever, and hypoxia.

During heavy exercise such as running or speed skating, especially for prolonged periods, some groups of muscles require excessively large amounts of energy. The extra energy production forces these tissues into a state of hypermetabolism. These muscles catabolize glucose faster than adequate amounts of oxygen can reach them. As a result, these rapidly metabolizing muscles produce large amounts of lactic acid (as evidenced by the pain in those muscles) that enter the ECF and cause acidemia.

A generalized seizure is characterized by the rapid and intense simultaneous contraction of many or all groups of skeletal muscles. This extreme activity is much greater than normal and creates a hypermetabolic state that overwhelms the normal cellular oxygen content and causes a severe lactic acidosis. At the same time, most individuals cannot breathe effectively during a grand mal seizure so that a respiratory acidosis compounds the initial metabolic problem.

The condition of fever (body temperature higher than 101° F) results in a systemic metabolic increase (Price & Wilson, 1986). Prolonged periods of fever cause a sustained hypermetabolic state in which cellular metabolism occurs at such a rapid rate that normal cellular oxygen levels cannot maintain aerobic conditions. These anaerobic conditions lead to lactic acid production and acidemia.

Lactic acid is produced whenever metabolism occurs under anaerobic conditions. Therefore, prolonged decreased blood supply to any organ or body part results in lactic acid formation in that area. If enough lactic acid is produced and released into systemic circulation, acidemia results. Nonrespiratory causes of cellular hypoxia leading to acidemia include arterial insufficiency, cardiac insufficiency, trauma, thrombus formation, and vascular and extravascular obstruction.

Excessive intake of acidic substances (poisoning) not only floods the body directly with hydrogen ions but also contributes to acidemia in two other ways. First, most acidic substances ingested in excessive amounts disrupt normal cellular processes to some degree and result in hypoxia, hypermetabolism, or both. In addition, some acidic substances directly inhibit the respiratory centers of the brain, thereby contributing to a simultaneous respiratory acidosis (Guyton, 1986; Robbins & Kumar, 1987). Some of the most common

KEY FEATURES OF DISEASE ■ Common Causes of Respiratory Acidosis

Pathology	Conditions	Pathology	Conditions

Respiratory depression (central nervous system)	Chemical depression
	  Anesthetics
	  Drugs/narcotics
	  Inhibitors of depolarization
	    Poisons
	    Blocking agents
	    Electrolyte imbalances
	Physical depression
	  Direct center depression
	    Trauma
	    Hypoxia, ischemia
	  Indirect center depression
	    Cerebral edema
	    Cerebral hypoxia
	    Increased intracranial
	      pressure
	Respiratory nerve paralysis
	  Spinal cord injuries
	  Neuritic diseases
	    Guillain-Barré
	    Infantile paralysis
	    Myasthenia gravis
			Abdominal organ displacement
			  Ascites
			  Tumor
			  Pregnancy
			  Organ enlargement

		Airway obstruction	Lower airway obstruction
			  Bronchiolitis
			  Trapping of particulate matter
			Upper airway obstruction
			  External pressure
			  Internal obstruction
			    Asthma
			    Bronchitis

Inadequate chest expansion	Skeletal deformities and trauma
	  Congenital malformations
	  Injury
	  Scoliosis
	  Osteoporosis
	Muscular weakness
	  Electrolyte imbalances
	  Muscular dystrophy
	Nonpulmonary restriction of
	  expansion
	  Obesity
	  Thoracic organ displacement
	    Pleural effusion
	    Thoracic tumor
	    Mediastinal structure
	      enlargement
		Alveolar-capillary block	Capillary problems
			  Thrombus or embolus forma-
			    tion
			  Vascular occlusive disease
			Alveolar membrane problems
			  Increased diffusion distance
			    Pneumonia
			    Pulmonary edema
			    Alveolar fibrosis
			      Tuberculosis
			      Cystic fibrosis
			      Arthus reactions
			      Pulmonary Kaposi's disease
			  Collapse of alveoli
			    Atelectasis
			    Adult respiratory distress
			      syndrome
			Destruction or loss of lung tissue
			  Pneumonectomy
			  Traumatic destruction
			  Tissue destructive diseases
			    Emphysema
			    Tuberculosis
			    Cancer

substances that cause acidemia when ingested in excess include ethanol, methanol, ethylene glycol, and acetylsalicylic acid.

Underelimination of hydrogen ions. The major routes for hydrogen ion elimination are respiratory and renal. Renal failure causes an acidosis leading to acidemia through two closely related faulty mechanisms (Leaf & Cotran, 1985). Impaired renal tubules have a diminished capacity to excrete hydrogen ions into the filtrate. This impairment allows hydrogen ions to be retained or reabsorbed into systemic circulation, which

creates an acidemia. At the same time, the impaired tubules are frequently unable to either reabsorb filtered bicarbonate or generate new bicarbonate to be returned to systemic circulation. This failure causes an ECF base deficit, and thus acidemia.

Underproduction of bicarbonate ions. Base deficit acidemia can occur when hydrogen ion production and elimination are normal but too few molecules of bases in the form of bicarbonate ions are present to balance the positive electrical charges. Such a base deficit occurs when bicarbonate ions are not produced at the normal rate. In addition to renal failure, conditions that involve decreased pancreatic and/or hepatic function are accompanied by base deficits.

The pancreas normally secretes large amounts of bicarbonate in the form of sodium bicarbonate from the epithelial cells of the small ductules that drain pancreatic acini. This bicarbonate is part of the pancreatic juice that neutralizes the contents of the duodenum. Much of this bicarbonate is absorbed from the intestine into systemic circulation. Conditions that are associated with reduced pancreatic secretion of bicarbonate into the duodenum are chronic pancreatitis and hepatic problems that block either the common bile duct or the sphincter of Oddi (Guyton, 1986). In addition, conditions that cause inhibition of the hormone secretin through scarring or fibrosis of the duodenum inhibit pancreatic secretion of bicarbonate.

Overelimination of bicarbonate ions. A base deficit acidemia can also occur when hydrogen ion production and elimination are normal but there is overelimination of bicarbonate ions. The most common cause of this type of base deficit is diarrhea. The increased intestinal motility that accompanies diarrhea causes the bicarbonate-containing intestinal fluid to be lost from the body rather than absorbed.

Base deficit acidemia is associated with dehydration, although the exact mechanism of bicarbonate loss in this situation is not clear. Because dehydration may result from conditions that contribute to the loss of bicarbonate (such as diarrhea), the acidemia may be more a result of the other condition than the dehydration. In addition, when dehydration is severe, not enough fluid is available to carry the bicarbonate made by pancreatic ductile cells into the duodenum. As a result, less bicarbonate is absorbed.

Base deficit acidemia can also occur when bicarbonate is produced and eliminated in normal amounts but is combined with other substances rather than being freely available. Bicarbonate buffers other organic acids in addition to carbonic acid (Keyes, 1985). When significant amounts of bicarbonate buffer substances other than carbonic acid, a base deficit acidemia may result.

Respiratory Acidosis

Respiratory acidosis is an alteration in some area of respiratory function that results in an inadequate exchange of oxygen and carbon dioxide. The alteration essentially causes retention of carbon dioxide to such an extent that the carbonic anhydrase equation is forced to the *right*, which causes a proportional increase in the concentration of hydrogen ions:

$$CO_2 + H_2O \longleftrightarrow H_2CO_3 \longleftrightarrow HCO_3^- + H^+$$

This increase in the free hydrogen ion concentration of the blood is acidemia. Unlike metabolic acidosis, respiratory acidosis has only one primary mechanism for acidemia: the underelimination of hydrogen ions

through the retention of carbon dioxide. Virtually all causes of pure respiratory acidosis result in an acid excess acidemia. Base deficits do not play a role in causing pure respiratory acidosis.

Pulmonary respiration begins with central nervous system stimulation of respiratory neurons. Impulses from these neurons move down the spinal cord and then into the peripheral nervous system to terminate at the myoneural junction of the respiratory skeletal muscles. These muscles are stimulated to contract and relax, which changes the size of and pressures within the thoracic cavity. Atmospheric air moves into and out of the lungs and alveoli in response to thoracic pressure changes. Actual gas exchange occurs at the level of the alveolar membrane, where the alveolar membrane comes into contact with the capillary membrane. Any problem along this pathway from the brain to the alveolar-capillary membrane can result in an inadequate exchange of oxygen and carbon dioxide, thus leading to acidemia of respiratory origin. These respiratory problems are divided into those that cause (1) respiratory depression, (2) inadequate chest expansion, (3) airway obstruction, or (4) interference with alveolar-capillary diffusion.

Respiratory depression. True respiratory depression involves altering the function of the neurons stimulating inhalation and exhalation. These neurons can be depressed at the level of the cell body, by chemical agents and physical damage, as well as at the level of the axon. The overall result of respiratory depression is a reduction in both the rate and the depth of respiration, which causes inadequate gas exchange and a retention of carbon dioxide.

Chemical depression of the respiratory neurons can occur as a result of the action of anesthetic agents, drugs (narcotics), and poisons that cross the blood-brain barrier and directly inhibit depolarization. In addition, specific electrolyte imbalances (hyponatremia, hypercalcemia, and hyperkalemia) also slow or inhibit neuronal depolarization.

The activity of respiratory neurons can also be depressed physically. Trauma that results in direct physical damage to the respiratory neurons or that creates hypoxic to ischemic conditions can interrupt or destroy the ability of these neurons to generate and transmit impulses to the skeletal muscles that are involved in respiration. Respiratory neurons can be damaged or destroyed indirectly when problems in other areas of the brain cause an increase in intracranial pressure. Increases in intracranial pressure cause edema of brain tissues, which then press the respiratory centers (located in the brain stem) against the bony sides of the foramen magnum. This action can destroy some respiratory neurons directly and also creates hypoxic or ischemic conditions in this area, which then result in destruction of respiratory neurons—an indirect effect.

Damage or paralysis of the axons of respiratory neurons inhibits impulse transmission from the central nervous system to the skeletal muscles of respiration. In

GLUCOSE METABOLISM UNDER AEROBIC CONDITIONS

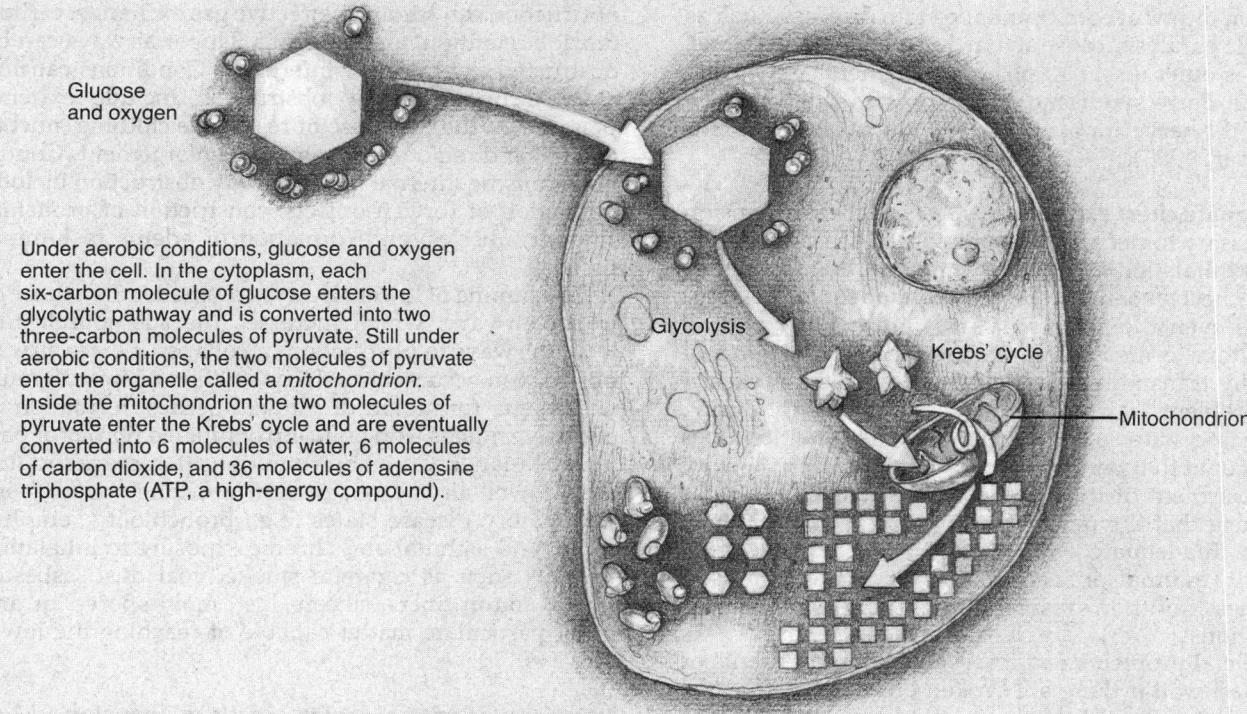

Glucose and oxygen

Under aerobic conditions, glucose and oxygen enter the cell. In the cytoplasm, each six-carbon molecule of glucose enters the glycolytic pathway and is converted into two three-carbon molecules of pyruvate. Still under aerobic conditions, the two molecules of pyruvate enter the organelle called a *mitochondrion*. Inside the mitochondrion the two molecules of pyruvate enter the Krebs' cycle and are eventually converted into 6 molecules of water, 6 molecules of carbon dioxide, and 36 molecules of adenosine triphosphate (ATP, a high-energy compound).

Glycolysis

Krebs' cycle

Mitochondrion

GLUCOSE METABOLISM UNDER ANAEROBIC CONDITIONS

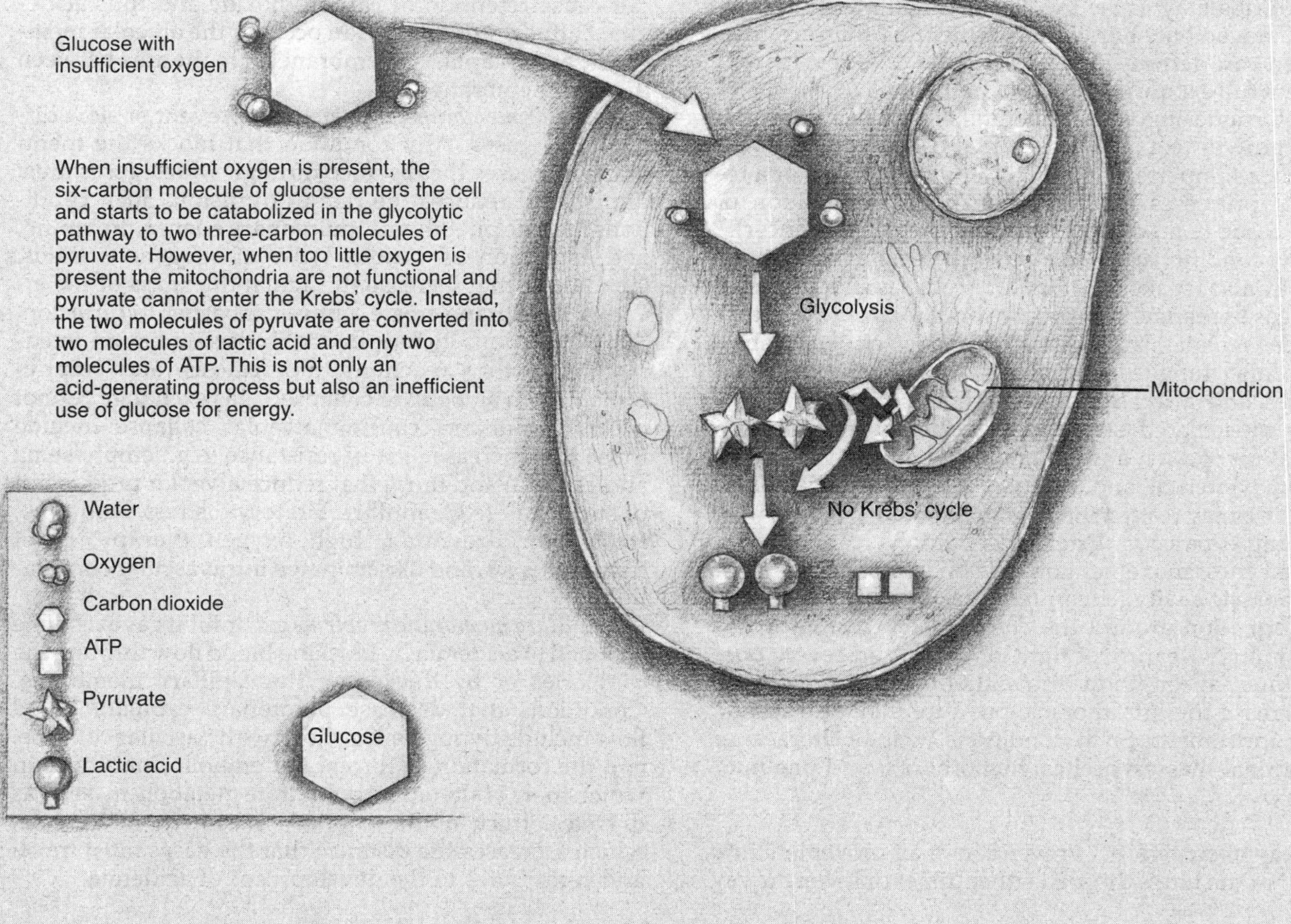

Glucose with insufficient oxygen

When insufficient oxygen is present, the six-carbon molecule of glucose enters the cell and starts to be catabolized in the glycolytic pathway to two three-carbon molecules of pyruvate. However, when too little oxygen is present the mitochondria are not functional and pyruvate cannot enter the Krebs' cycle. Instead, the two molecules of pyruvate are converted into two molecules of lactic acid and only two molecules of ATP. This is not only an acid-generating process but also an inefficient use of glucose for energy.

Glycolysis

Mitochondrion

No Krebs' cycle

Water
Oxygen
Carbon dioxide
ATP
Pyruvate
Lactic acid

Glucose

addition to spinal cord trauma, certain diseases, such as infantile paralysis, cause actual destruction of the axons, whereas other diseases, such as myasthenia gravis and Guillain-Barré syndrome, interfere with the transmission of the nerve impulse to the skeletal muscle (Robbins & Kumar, 1987).

Inadequate chest expansion. Because chest expansion is necessary to decrease the pressure in the chest cavity so that inhalation occurs, any condition that restricts or limits chest expansion results in inadequate gas exchange even though lung tissues are healthy and all respiratory center messages are being initiated and properly transmitted. Some people with chest expansion problems can exchange gases sufficiently during the resting state so that carbon dioxide retention does not occur at that time. However, any increase in activity or impairment of lung tissue creates demands for gas exchange that the person cannot meet; thus, acidemia results. Inadequate chest expansion can result from skeletal trauma or deformities, respiratory muscle weakness, or non–respiratory-associated movement restrictions.

Skeletal problems restrict respiratory movements of the chest wall if there are broken bones or malformed bones that cause a distortion in the functional shape of the chest. Broken ribs restrict chest movement by failing to provide the rigid structure needed for pressure changes to occur (flail chest). In addition, pain from broken ribs may cause the client to voluntarily restrict chest movement. Bony chest structures that are misshapen can deform the shape of the chest cavity and prevent full expansion of one or both lungs. These skeletal deformities may be congenital, a result of improper bone growth (e.g., scoliosis, renal osteodystrophy, osteogenesis imperfecta, and Hurler's syndrome), or a result of processes that cause uneven degeneration of bony tissue (e.g., osteoporosis and metastatic cancer).

Any condition causing a general weakness of skeletal muscles also weakens respiratory muscles and interferes with gas exchange. Temporary conditions of respiratory muscle weakness are associated with electrolyte imbalances and fatigue. Conditions that have protracted courses and affect respiratory function over time include muscular dystrophy, rhabdomyosarcoma, congenital myopathy, and inflammatory myositis.

Some internal and external nonrespiratory conditions also may restrict the chest movement necessary for full lung expansion. External conditions leading to restricted chest movement include body cast enclosure of the thoracic cavity, circumferential eschar and scar tissue formation around the chest, heavy taping of ribs after injury, wearing of tight clothing, and severe obesity. Internal conditions that either displace lung tissue or increase the intrathoracic pressure may also restrict chest movement. Such conditions include thoracic or abdominal masses, ascites, hemothorax, and pneumothorax.

Airway obstruction. Prevention of air movement into or out of the lungs through either upper or lower airway obstruction can lead to ineffective gas exchange, carbon dioxide retention, and acidemia. Upper airways can be obstructed externally or internally. Conditions causing external upper airway obstruction include extreme pressure on the neck, use of restrictive clothing, nuchal edema, and regional lymph node enlargement. Conditions causing internal upper airway obstruction include inhalation of foreign objects, constriction of bronchial smooth muscles, and formation of edema in luminal tissues.

The lumina of lower airways are smaller than those of upper airways, which increases the susceptibility of lower airways to obstruction or collapse. Lower airway obstruction occurs through constriction of smooth muscle, edema formation of luminal tissues, formation of excessive mucus, and build-up of inhaled fibrous or particulate matter. Common conditions that are associated with lower airway obstruction are long-standing inflammatory disease states (e.g., bronchiolitis, emphysema, and asthma) and chronic exposure to inhalation irritants such as cigarette smoke, coal dust, asbestos fibers, cotton fibers, silicon dust, mold spores, or any other particulate matter capable of reaching the lower airways.

Interference with alveolar-capillary diffusion. Most pulmonary gas exchange occurs by diffusion at the junction of the alveolar and capillary membranes. Any condition that prevents or slows this diffusion process can cause retention of carbon dioxide and thus acidemia. Diffusion problems can occur at the alveolar membrane, at the capillary membrane, or in the area between the two membranes.

Alveolar membrane problems can prevent or slow diffusion of gases. Any condition that blocks the membrane increases the distance through which gases must diffuse and reduces the rate of diffusion. Such conditions include pneumonia, pulmonary edema, drowning, and aspiration of various types of exogenous fluids. Conditions that increase the actual thickness of the alveolar membrane create a physical barrier to diffusion. Such conditions include cystic fibrosis, radiation pneumonitis, Arthus reactions, tuberculosis, and emphysema. When alveoli are collapsed, gas exchange cannot occur. Conditions causing alveolar collapse include those that increase airway resistance (e.g., emphysema and asthma) and those that reduce alveolar production of surfactant (e.g., adult respiratory distress syndrome, freshwater drowning, high oxygen therapy, chest trauma, sepsis, and disseminated intravascular coagulation).

Capillary membrane problems can inhibit gas exchange and lead to acidemia by blocking blood flow through the capillaries or by thickening the capillary membrane. Conditions that decrease pulmonary capillary blood flow include hypovolemic shock with vascular collapse, and the formation of thrombi or emboli. Conditions in which there is altered carbohydrate metabolism, such as diabetes, thicken the capillary basement membrane, which increases the distance that the gases must travel and contributes to the development of acidemia.

Combined Metabolic and Respiratory Acidosis

Metabolic and respiratory acidosis processes can occur at the same time. An uncorrected acute respiratory acidosis always leads to anaerobic metabolism and lactic acidosis. The resulting acidemia usually is more profound than either metabolic acidosis or respiratory acidosis alone. Examples of conditions leading to combined metabolic and respiratory acidosis include cardiac arrest, grand mal seizures lasting 90 seconds or longer, and development of severe diarrhea in a client with chronic obstructive lung disease.

Incidence

Because acidemia is a symptom rather than a disease state, its actual incidence is not known. However, mild metabolic acidosis as a result of lactic acidosis is common among healthy individuals. Normal respiratory compensation usually prevents this problem from becoming severe or prolonged, and no intervention is necessary. Virtually all hospitalized clients are at some risk for developing an acidosis process, either as a response to a specific disease or condition or as a response to treatment. Clients especially at risk for developing acidemia are those whose conditions impair any aspect of respiratory function to any degree.

PREVENTION

Strategies for prevention of acidemia vary according to the individual client and the probable etiology of the acid-base disorder. All strategies involve identification of clients at risk. When appropriate, preventive strategies include client education concerning measures to prevent acidosis. In addition, secondary prevention, or early detection, involves teaching health care professionals to interpret laboratory data and to recognize signs and symptoms of acidemia so that corrective interventions can be instituted early and serious complications can be prevented.

COLLABORATIVE MANAGEMENT

 Assessment

History

When obtaining a history from any client, the nurse collects data regarding risk factors as well as causative factors related to the development of acidemia. *Age* is an important factor, as the elderly are more prone to conditions that may cause an acid-base imbalance. Such conditions include impairments of cardiac, renal, and pulmonary function. In addition, elderly persons are more likely to be taking prescribed or over-the-counter *medications* that interfere with acid-base, fluid, and electrolyte balance. The nurse inquires about specific risk factors such as the presence of any type of respiratory problem, renal failure, diabetes mellitus, persistent diarrhea, pancreatitis, or fever.

Clients are asked specific questions concerning *urinary output,* including frequency and quantity of voiding. The nurse asks questions regarding actual fluid intake in general, as well as specifically during the previous 24 hours.

The nurse inquires about the use of over-the-counter and prescribed *medications,* especially products containing aspirin or alcohol. If the client cannot recall exactly what medications are being taken, this information may be obtained from the client's family, significant other, or recently updated medical records.

The nurse obtains a detailed *diet history* to determine total caloric intake as well as the approximate proportions of carbohydrates, fats, and proteins of the foods ingested. The nurse specifically asks the client if fasting has occurred during the preceding week. Questions regarding general food and alcoholic beverage intake, as well as the previous 24-hour dietary recall, are helpful.

The nurse also collects historical data that may indicate the presence of symptoms that are specifically associated with acidemia. Because the central nervous system is frequently depressed with acidemia, questions may be directed to the client's significant other or close family member, as the client's responses may be limited or not reliable. The client is asked whether headaches, behavior changes, increased somnolence, reduced alertness, reduced attention span, lethargy, anorexia, abdominal distention, nausea or vomiting, muscle weakness, or increased fatigue has been experienced. Having the client relate activities of the previous 24 hours may disclose additional information about activity intolerance, changes in behavior, and the presence of unexplained fatigue.

Physical Assessment: Clinical Manifestations

The clinical manifestations of acidemia are usually similar regardless of whether the origin of the acidemia is metabolic or respiratory (see the Key Features of Disease on p. 344). Some clinical manifestations are direct results of the acidemia, whereas others are related to the specific fluid and electrolyte imbalances that generally accompany acidemia. Clinical manifestations of acidemia are primarily associated with alterations in activity of excitable membranes that are involved in cerebral, neuromuscular, and gastric smooth muscle functions.

Central nervous system manifestations. Depression of central nervous system functions is commonly associated with acidemia and may manifest as lethargy that progresses to confusion. As the acidemia becomes worse or if it is accompanied by hyperkalemia, the client may become stuporous and unresponsive.

The nurse assesses the client's level of consciousness. Notations are made regarding whether the client is awake or asleep. If the client is asleep, the nurse makes gentle attempts to waken the client and documents the

KEY FEATURES OF DISEASE ■ Some Clinical Manifestations of Acidemia

System	Manifestations
Central nervous	Depressed activity 　Lethargy, confusion, stupor, coma
Neuromuscular	Hyporeflexia Skeletal muscle weakness Flaccid paralysis
Cardiac	Delayed electrical conduction 　Bradycardia to block 　Tall T waves 　Widened QRS complex 　Prolonged PR interval Hypotension Thready peripheral pulses
Respiratory	Kussmaul's respirations (in metabolic acidosis with respiratory compensation) Variable respirations (generally ineffective in respiratory acidosis)
Integumentary	Metabolic acidosis 　Warm, flushed, dry Respiratory acidosis 　Pale to cyanotic, dry

ease with which the client arouses. If the client does not awaken in response to gentle, normal stimuli, the nurse increases the loudness of verbal attempts. The nurse may also attempt to awaken the client by using more painful stimulation techniques such as pulling a skin hair. Failure of the client to respond to such stimuli is significant and must be documented.

If the client is awake, the nurse establishes whether the client is oriented to time, place, and person. The nurse avoids asking questions that can be answered with a "yes" or "no" response and pays close attention to the manner in which the client responds to questions. Is it necessary to repeat questions to obtain a response? Does the response answer the question asked? Does the client have difficulty with word choices in forming responses? Is the client irritated or upset by the questions? Can the client concentrate on a question long enough to provide an appropriate response or is the client's attention span short?

Neuromuscular manifestations. The actual increase in the ECF hydrogen ion concentration as well as any accompanying hyperkalemia decreases the rate of depolarization of excitable membranes of nerve and skeletal muscle. Muscle tone and deep tendon reflexes diminish. The nurse assesses muscle strength by having the client (1) squeeze the nurse's hand, (2) attempt to keep arms flexed while the nurse pulls downward on the lower arms, and (3) pushes both feet against a flat surface (board or box) while the nurse applies resistance. Muscle weakness associated with acidemia is bilateral and progresses to flaccid paralysis. Respiratory movements diminish when skeletal muscles are too weak to assist in ventilation.

Cardiac manifestations. Early cardiac manifestations of acidemia include increased heart rate and cardiac output. However, as acidemia worsens or if it is accompanied by hyperkalemia, electrical conduction through the myocardium is reduced, and bradycardia ensues. Specific electrocardiographic changes include the presence of tall T waves, widened QRS complex, and a prolonged PR interval. These cardiac problems can be life-threatening. Peripheral pulses are hard to find and easily obliterated with light pressure. Vasodilation causes hypotension.

Respiratory manifestations. The nurse assesses the respiratory system by observing the rate, depth, and ease of respirations. When the acidemia has a metabolic origin, the rate and depth of respiration increase in proportion to the increase in the hydrogen ion concentration. Respirations are deep, rapid, and not under voluntary control. This respiratory pattern is called *Kussmaul's respiration.* The client may have great difficulty in talking or eating because of the energy expended on these respiratory efforts. The increased gas exchange, coupled with a vasodilation, makes the client's skin and mucous membranes warm, dry, and pink.

When the acidemia has a respiratory origin, the effectiveness of respiratory efforts is greatly diminished. Respirations are usually shallow and may range from quite rapid to absent. Skin and mucous membranes are pale to cyanotic.

Psychosocial Assessment

Psychosocial assessment is critically important because behavioral changes may be the first observable clinical manifestations of acidemia. The nurse observes the client closely and documents presenting behavior by description rather than by interpretation. The nurse questions family members and significant others to determine whether the presenting behavior and mental status are typical for this client.

Laboratory Findings

The most definitive laboratory test to confirm the presence of acidemia is an arterial blood pH value of less than 7.34. However, this test alone gives no indication of the underlying pathologic condition or the origin of the acidemia. Because the clinical manifestations of metabolic acidosis and respiratory acidosis are similar and the effective treatments are different, additional laboratory data are critical to obtain and must be interpreted. These data should include arterial blood gas values and measurements of serum potassium level, serum chloride level, and the anion gap (see the Key Features of Disease on p. 345).

KEY FEATURES OF DISEASE ■ Laboratory Values Common to Acid-Base Imbalances

Imbalance	Laboratory Value Changes*						
	pH	HCO_3^-	PO_2	PCO_2	K^+	Ca^{2+}	Cl^-
Metabolic acidosis	↓	↓	∅	∅	↑	∅	↑
Respiratory acidosis	↓	↑	↓	↑	↑	∅	↓↑
Combined acidosis	↓	↑	↓	↑	↑	∅	↑
Metabolic alkalosis	↑	↑	∅	↑	↓	↓	↓
Respiratory alkalosis	↑	↓	∅	↓	↓	↓	↑
Combined alkalosis	↑	↑	∅	↓	↓	↓	↓

* ↑ indicates above normal; ↓, below normal; ∅, normal.

Metabolic acidosis. The laboratory data that indicate the presence of a pure metabolic acidosis causing the acidemia include a low pH, low bicarbonate level, normal PCO_2, normal PO_2, elevated serum potassium level, elevated serum chloride level, and elevated anion gap (Narins & Emmett, 1980). The pH is low because buffering and respiratory compensation are not adequate to maintain the hydrogen ion concentration at a normal level.

The reduced bicarbonate level coupled with the normal carbon dioxide level is the actual indicator that the acidosis is metabolic (Janusek, 1984a). The bicarbonate level is below normal for any one (or all) of the following reasons: Bicarbonate has been lost from the body, which leads to the actual base deficit acidemia (Metheny & Snively, 1983), or it has not been produced in sufficient quantities, which creates the actual base deficit acidemia (Guyton, 1986). In addition, bicarbonate may be bound to other substances during the buffering of organic acid-stimulated acidosis (Riley et al., 1987).

The carbon dioxide level is normal (or even slightly reduced) because gas exchange is adequate and carbon dioxide is not retained. The oxygen level is normal also because gas exchange is adequate (Romanski, 1986).

The serum potassium level is frequently elevated in metabolic acidosis as a result of the body's attempt to maintain electroneutrality during buffering (Laski, 1983). The illustration on page 347 demonstrates movement of potassium ions that is associated with changes in ECF pH. As the hydrogen ion (cation) concentration of the ECF increases, some of the excess hydrogen ions enter cells (especially red blood cells), where intracellular buffering mechanisms are located. The movement of hydrogen ions into the cells creates an intracellular excess of cations. To prevent intracellular charge imbalances, an equal number of potassium ions (cations) move from the cells into the ECF, which increases the extracellular potassium concentration and contributes to the development of an associated hyperkalemia. This hyperkalemia is usually seen in metabolic acidosis situations caused by acute renal failure, lactic acidosis, or ingestion of acidic substances (Narins & Emmett, 1980;

Riley et al., 1987). Normal to low serum potassium levels are associated with metabolic acidosis situations caused by diabetic ketoacidosis or chronic renal failure (Kreisberg, 1987; Morrison & Murray, 1981; Riley et al., 1987).

The serum chloride level is usually elevated during metabolic acidosis as a result of the body's attempt to maintain electroneutrality, especially during conditions of lactic acidosis and base deficit acidosis. Because the serum concentration of bicarbonate (anion) is low during metabolic acidosis, movement of chloride (anion) from the intracellular fluid ICF to the ECF usually occurs to compensate for the decreased numbers of anions in relation to the increased numbers of cations. Normal or low levels of serum chloride are associated with metabolic acidosis conditions accompanied by volume deficits (Kreisberg, 1987).

The anion gap usually is increased in metabolic acidosis conditions in which bicarbonate is actually depleted. These conditions include renal failure, lactic acidosis, ketoacidosis, and acidosis produced as a result of excessive ingestion of acidic substances (Goodkin et al., 1984; Riley et al., 1987). Increased anion gap values indicate the increase in nonmeasured anions present in the serum as the body attempts to maintain electroneutrality (Keyes, 1985). The acidoses that are characterized by large increases in serum chloride levels usually are associated with anion values in the normal range. These conditions generally include diarrhea and renal tubular acidoses (Riley et al., 1987).

Respiratory acidosis. The laboratory data indicating the presence of respiratory acidosis–induced acidemia include a low pH, elevated PCO_2, and decreased PO_2. Changes in bicarbonate, serum potassium, serum chloride, and anion gap levels vary with the duration of the acidosis and the degree of renal compensation.

The pH is low because of an increase in the ECF hydrogen ion concentration. If the renal system partially compensates for this acidosis, the pH is low but not as reduced as might be expected in view of the degree of derangement in the retention of carbon dioxide.

The PCO_2 is elevated and the PO_2 is reduced because the etiology of this acid-base disturbance is an impairment of gas exchange. The impairment causes retention of carbon dioxide and an inability to take in adequate amounts of oxygen (Taylor, 1984a).

When the respiratory acidosis has an acute onset, the bicarbonate level is normal because none has been lost from the body and it is buffering only carbonic acid. When the respiratory acidosis persists for at least 24 hours or longer, renal compensation for the acidosis results in increased generation and reabsorption of bicarbonate. Thus, an elevated bicarbonate level, coupled with the increased PCO_2, is an indication of the presence of chronic respiratory acidosis (Kaehny, 1983).

Other electrolyte values change when respiratory acidosis is chronic. During acute respiratory acidosis, the serum potassium level is elevated, the serum chloride level is normal or elevated, and the anion gap is normal. When respiratory acidosis is chronic and renal compensation is present, the serum potassium level is normal or low, the serum chloride level is low, and the anion gap is increased (Kaehny, 1983; Narins & Emmett, 1980).

 ### Analysis: Nursing Diagnosis

Acute episodes of acidemia require immediate and intensive intervention. Clients with acute acidemia, such as those with cardiac arrest or severe diabetic ketoacidosis, are seen and treated in emergency departments and intensive care units of hospitals. More commonly seen are the clients with health problems that result in chronic acidemia. The typical client is a middle-aged man with progressive chronic obstructive pulmonary disease. The following nursing diagnoses are derived from these data.

Common Diagnoses

The following diagnoses are common for clients experiencing acidemia as a result of chronic respiratory acidosis:

1. Ineffective breathing pattern related to ineffective gas exchange and ineffective airway clearance
2. Activity intolerance related to fatigue
3. Altered thought processes related to cerebral hypoxia and central nervous system depression

Additional Diagnoses

In addition to the common diagnoses, the client experiencing chronic acidemia may present with one or more of the following diagnoses:

1. Altered nutrition: less than body requirements related to fatigue and increased metabolic needs
2. Potential for injury related to altered thought processes
3. Impaired skin integrity related to inadequate cellular oxygenation

4. Total self-care deficit related to fatigue
5. Knowledge deficit related to pathology of chronic illness and treatment regimen
6. Potential for infection related to increased pulmonary secretions
7. Body image disturbance related to changes associated with progression of chronic disease
8. Decreased cardiac output related to decreased ventricular contractility
9. Anxiety related to altered thought processes

 ### Planning and Implementation

The following plan of care for the client experiencing acidemia as a result of chronic respiratory acidosis focuses on the common diagnoses of ineffective breathing patterns, altered thought processes, and activity intolerance. This plan of care is aimed at restoring acid-base balance and at preventing serious complications.

Ineffective Breathing Pattern

Planning: client goals. The major client goals for this nursing diagnosis include that the client will (1) have a patent airway, (2) increase the effectiveness of respiratory efforts, and (3) not experience respiratory complications.

Interventions: nonsurgical management. The interventions for this problem are aimed at maintaining a patent airway and enhancing gas exchange so that the degree of acidemia diminishes. Interventions include drug therapy, diet therapy, oxygen therapy, positioning, breathing techniques, and prevention of complications.

Drug therapy. Drug therapy includes the use of agents that improve gas exchange by increasing the diameter of upper and lower airways through relaxation of bronchial smooth muscles and agents that promote excretion of pulmonary secretions by decreasing the tenacity of the secretions. Drug therapy is not aimed directly at altering the ECF pH. Bases in the form of bicarbonate are not administered for acidosis conditions that do not include bicarbonate loss. Administration of bases under such conditions could produce a base excess alkalemia (Kaehny, 1983; Rice, 1987; Ryder, 1984).

Drugs that induce relaxation of bronchial smooth muscle generally include adrenergic agonists or sympathomimetic agents. These drugs include aminophylline (Amoline, Lixaminol, Somophyllin), theophylline (Bronkodyl, Theo-Dur), ephedrine, fenoterol (Berotec), isoproterenol (Aerolone, Isuprel), metaproterenol (Alupent), and terbutaline (Brethaire, Brethine, Bricanyl). Some of these drugs can be administered parenterally (aminophylline, isoproterenol, ephedrine, theophylline, terbutaline), as well as orally or in an inhalant form. Inhalant bronchodilators are administered before inhalant cortisol agents or inhalant mucolytic agents are given.

HOW POTASSIUM IONS BEHAVE IN ACID-BASE IMBALANCES

Under normal conditions
The extracellular fluid has a high concentration of sodium, a low concentration of potassium, and a very low concentration of hydrogen. The intracellular fluid has a high concentration of potassium.

In acidemia
The hydrogen ion concentration of the extracellular fluid increases. Some of the excess hydrogen ions move into the intracellular fluid for buffering by proteins and buffering pairs. Because these ions have a positive charge, their entry into the cell disturbs the electroneutrality of the intracellular fluid. To keep the intracellular fluid electrically neutral, a proportional number of positively charged potassium ions move from the intracellular fluid into the extracellular fluid, and hyperkalemia results.

In alkalemia
The hydrogen ion concentration in the extracellular fluid is below normal. Compensatory mechanisms (buffers in the intracellular fluid and catalysis of carbonic acid in the cell) generate hydrogen ions, which move from the intracellular fluid into the extracellular fluid. There they disturb the electroneutrality of the extracellular fluid by increasing the number of positive charges. To compensate and reduce this excess of positive charges in the extracellular fluid, potassium moves from the extracellular fluid into the intracellular fluid, and hypokalemia results.

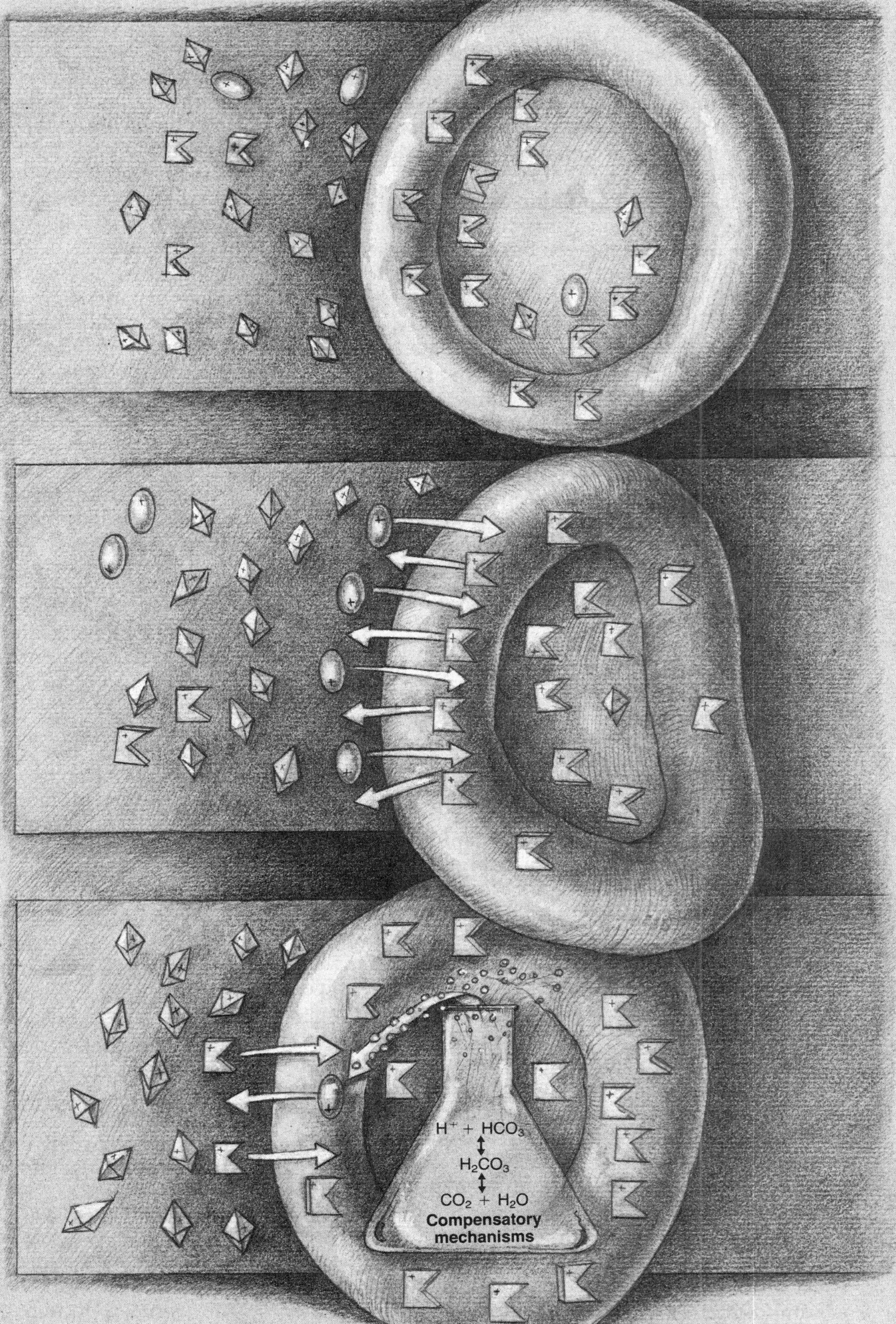

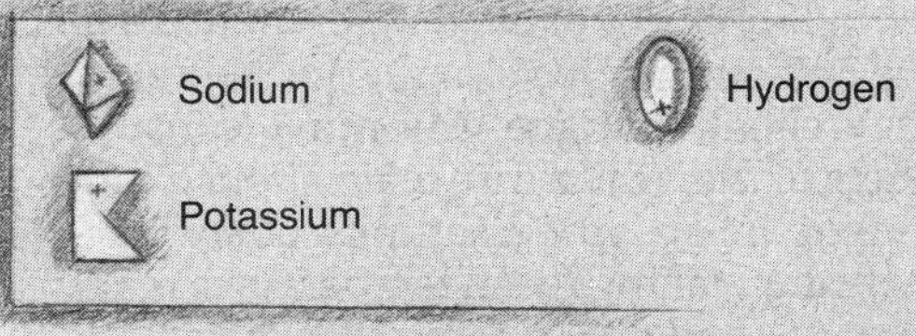

$$H^+ + HCO_3^-$$
$$\updownarrow$$
$$H_2CO_3$$
$$\updownarrow$$
$$CO_2 + H_2O$$
Compensatory mechanisms

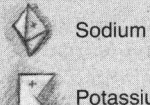 Sodium

 Hydrogen

Potassium

For chronic respiratory acidosis, some agents that increase bronchodilation by reducing inflammation of bronchial luminal tissues are used. These agents are primarily cortisol based and include beclomethasone (Vanceril, Beclovent), dexamethasone (Decadron Respihaler), and triamcinolone (Azmacort).

When thick, tenacious pulmonary secretions contribute to airway obstruction, agents that thin the secretions by breaking up mucus may be beneficial. These agents are classified as mucolytic; an example is acetylcysteine (Airbron, Mucomyst).

Diet therapy. Diet therapy is of limited value for increasing gas exchange, except for ensuring adequate hydration to maintain vascular volume and to assist in reducing the thickness of pulmonary secretions.

Oxygen therapy. Oxygen therapy may be useful in enhancing gas exchange during periods of acidemia. However, caution is necessary whenever oxygen is administered to clients with chronic obstructive pulmonary disease and carbon dioxide narcosis. In healthy individuals, the primary regulators of respiration are the central chemoreceptors, which are sensitive to changes in ECF carbon dioxide concentration. An increase in the carbon dioxide concentration triggers an increase in the rate and depth of respiration.

Clients with chronic respiratory acidosis, however, have PCO_2 levels that are chronically elevated. Over time, the central chemoreceptors adjust to these chronically high levels of carbon dioxide and no longer respond to variations in PCO_2 levels with appropriate changes in respiration. Instead, the stimulus for breathing is a decrease in arterial oxygen content that is sensed by the peripheral chemoreceptors located in the aortic arch and the carotid sinus areas. Because oxygen deprivation is the only stimulus that excites the respiratory centers of clients with carbon dioxide narcosis, it is important not to raise the arterial oxygen concentration of these clients too rapidly. Such an increase would cause the peripheral chemoreceptors to inhibit respiration and gas exchange, which would thus increase the acidemia.

Oxygen can be administered by mask, hood, nasal cannula, nasopharyngeal tube, endotracheal tube, and tracheostomy tube. Most often, nasal cannulas are used to administer oxygen continuously. The nurse administers oxygen to the client in the amount specified by the physician's prescription, as liters per minute (for cannula and nasopharyngeal tube administration) or as a percentage (for administration by mask, hood, endotracheal tube, and tracheostomy tube). Whenever oxygen is administered, it should be nebulized to prevent the drying of airway tissues.

Nursing measures to promote gas exchange. Nursing measures to promote gas exchange include positioning, techniques to enhance excretion of pulmonary secretions, and specific breathing techniques to change airway resistance and maintain inflated alveoli. The nurse assists the client to a Fowler or semi-Fowler position to enhance pulmonary ventilation. Techniques to enhance excretion of pulmonary secretions include "cupping" (patting techniques over the lung fields) and the use of hand-held vibrators over the lung fields to help loosen secretions. For clients who can tolerate supine, prone, and lateral positions, once during each shift the nurse positions the client for gravity-assisted postural drainage (see Chap. 62). The nurse encourages the client to exhale slowly through pursed lips to prevent alveolar collapse.

The nurse assesses the respiratory status of the client who is experiencing respiratory acidosis at least every 2 hours. In addition to the rate and depth of respiration, assessment includes auscultation of breath sounds. The nurse notes the ease with which the client moves air in and out of the lungs, including the presence of any retractions, and whether respiratory effort produces a sound audible without a stethoscope. Nail beds and mucous membranes are examined for color. The nurse documents the observed color and avoids using the term normal. Specific adjectives such as pale, gray, pink, red, white, and cyanotic are used to describe color.

Activity Intolerance

Planning: client goals. The major client goals for this nursing diagnosis include that the client will (1) not experience an increase in fatigue and (2) increase baseline activity.

Interventions: nonsurgical management. Interventions are aimed at preventing greater acidemia as a result of respiratory problems and at conserving the client's energy. Drug therapies and oxygen therapy are associated with enhancing gas exchange and are described under the ineffective breathing pattern nursing diagnosis.

Diet therapy. Diet therapy is indirectly related to activity intolerance and fatigue. When specific electrolyte imbalances accompany the acidemia, dietary intake of those electrolytes must be adjusted. The client must ingest enough calories to meet at least basal energy requirements. This action can be difficult when the client is extremely fatigued. The nurse provides small, frequent meals that have a high protein and carbohydrate content. Food items that are liquid in form or easy to chew require less effort to consume.

Nursing interventions to promote conservation of the client's energy. The nurse examines the hospitalized client's schedule of prescribed and routine activities. Activities that do not have a direct positive effect on the client's condition are assessed in terms of their usefulness to the client. If the benefit (actual or potential) of the activity does not outweigh its actual or potential aggravation of the client's fatigue, the nurse consults with other members of the health care team about eliminating or postponing the activity. Examples of such activities are hair washing, taking rectal temperature readings, physical therapy, and specific invasive diagnostic tests that are not required for assessment or treatment of presenting problems.

Altered Thought Processes

Planning client goals. The major client goals for this nursing diagnosis are that the client will (1) accurately interpret environmental stimuli and (2) remain in a safe environment.

Interventions: nonsurgical management. Interventions are aimed at preventing greater acidemia as a result of respiratory problems and at providing a safe environment. Accurate assessment of central nervous system activity changes from normal or from baseline serves as a basis for the institution of specific interventions and, therefore, constitutes a major nursing responsibility. Drug therapies are associated with enhancing gas exchange and are described under the ineffective breathing patterns nursing diagnosis.

Mental status assessment. The nurse assesses the client's central nervous system functional activity at least every 4 hours to evaluate the effectiveness of current interventions and to determine whether the acid-base imbalance continues to exist. Parameters to assess include level of consciousness; orientation to time, place, and person; past and recent memory; ability to concentrate; and cognitive function.

Maintenance of a safe environment. Changes in central nervous system activity and responses are expected in the client with acidemia. These changes are usually depressive, with the client first experiencing lethargy that progresses to somnolence and coma. Behavioral changes may be noted early as the client misinterprets environmental stimuli, but as acidemia increases the client usually becomes unaware of environmental stimuli.

A nursing function in maintaining a safe environment includes assisting the client to process information correctly. The nurse orients the client to time and place at every interaction. The nurse reminds the client who the nurse is and what the nurse is doing for the client. Placing large calendars and clocks where the client can see them may also help. If the client needs glasses to see properly and/or requires an assistive device for hearing, the nurse ensures that the client uses these devices while awake. The nurse makes certain that the client's call light is within easy reach at all times.

The nurse reduces extraneous environmental stimuli to keep the client from becoming confused. Lighting is kept to the minimum that is necessary for safety. The telephone is removed or the bell is adjusted so that it does not ring. Radio and television programming that varies in loudness and level of excitement is avoided.

Care is taken to prevent clients who are experiencing altered thought processes from becoming injured. Clients who are confused or somnolent require close observation, especially when they are out of bed. The nurse anticipates the client's need for ambulation and, when ambulation is permitted, accompanies the client, for example, to the bathroom. The upper side rails of the client's bed are kept raised at all times. Whenever the client is alone, the bed is kept in the low position. At times, it may be necessary for the nurse to prevent the client from reaching the electronic bed controls. If the client remains confused and continues to get out of bed unassisted, the nurse requests an order to restrain the client with a vest or jacket-style restraint. Such devices should be used only when the client represents a clear danger to himself or herself.

■ Discharge Planning

Home Care Preparation

Acidemia that occurs as a consequence of chronic respiratory acidosis may be resolved before the client's discharge from the hospital, but the underlying factors contributing to the development of the acidemia remain problematic and usually become more severe with time. Usually, the severity of the pathologic condition increases the chances that the acidemia will recur. Many clients who have chronic obstructive pulmonary disease with chronic respiratory acidosis cannot work or live alone. They require considerable assistance with activities of daily living.

If the client is being discharged to home, the hospital nurse contacts a public health nurse to assess the adequacy of the physical home environment to meet the client's needs for safety and activities of daily living. Special equipment such as an electric hospital bed and portable oxygen device is often needed. Because these illnesses are chronic, clients may already be participating in a long-term follow-up program. In this case, the primary nurse contacts the follow-up team to update the team about the client's current health status.

Client/Family Education

Education is a key factor in assisting the client to manage the chronic illness so as to slow progression of the illness and to reduce the incidence of acidemia and other complications. The educational plan for the client at risk for developing acidemia as a result of chronic obstructive pulmonary disease includes providing information about drug therapy and about signs and symptoms of acidemia, and teaching techniques for conserving energy while actively participating in self-care activities.

The prescribed medical regimen for clients with chronic obstructive pulmonary disease focuses on maintaining an adequate airway by bronchodilation and on enhancing excretion of pulmonary secretions. The nurse assesses the client's understanding of the need and the schedule for taking prescribed medications. It may be necessary for the nurse to make a detailed daily schedule chart or list of medications (including times and amounts) for the client's use at home. Included in this instruction is the appropriate use of oxygen and oxygen-administering equipment.

The nurse instructs the client and family in the signs and symptoms of acidemia. In addition, the client and family are asked to pay close attention to symptoms indicative of central nervous system depression. The client should not dismiss the presence of any headache without considering the possibility of its association with acidemia. Family members are instructed to regard as significant any persistent behavior change or lethargy of the client.

Activity intolerance is responsible for many of the changes that clients with chronic obstructive pulmonary disease must make in life style. Although chronic fatigue and some degree of activity intolerance may always be problems, it is possible for clients to conserve energy in some areas so that other activities can still be enjoyed. The nurse instructs the client in the scheduling and pacing of activities. More strenuous activities should be undertaken in the morning, after a full night's rest. Naps are planned before and after strenuous activities. Some clients increase their activity tolerance by using oxygen during a specific activity. The nurse teaches the client and family to arrange the home environment to minimize the amount of energy the client must expend during particular activities or tasks. If possible, the client should spend most of the waking period on the same floor level as the bathroom. Objects needed frequently should be placed within easy reach of the client. The client can learn to operate special devices for reaching and carrying objects.

Psychosocial Preparation

Clients whose episodes of acidemia are related to long-standing chronic obstructive pulmonary disease may have learned to cope with their health problems and require little intensive support. However, this situation cannot be assumed. The nurse reassesses each client's psychosocial needs in terms of new factors, established support systems, previous and current coping patterns, and the progression of the chronic disease. Most clients with long-standing chronic obstructive pulmonary disease have changed their life style considerably because of activity intolerance. As a result, many of these clients lack significant social interactions, and many fear being alone during a sudden exacerbation of the illness.

Another difficult but necessary concept that the nurse must convey to the client and family is the fact that the quality of life depends greatly on the client's compliance with the planned treatment regimen. Assisting the client and family to understand fully the disease process may increase the client's sense of control and willingness to cooperate. In conveying this information, the nurse focuses on the potential outcomes of good compliance rather than on the deleterious effects of negative compliance.

Health Care Resources

For the client with chronic respiratory acidosis who is discharged to home, the appropriate health care resources include the physician, pharmacist, respiratory therapist, nutritionist, and home health care nurse. So-

cial services personnel are useful if it is determined that the client cannot obtain the necessary medication and oxygen support. Such is often the case for clients with severe chronic obstructive pulmonary disease, as the illness is so debilitating that most are unable to work or maintain health insurance, and the cost of needed medications and supplies may be prohibitive. Agencies such as the American Cancer Society and the American Lung Association may be able to provide assistance in obtaining equipment.

Many clients who have chronic respiratory acidosis cannot return to home after discharge. In these situations, temporary or long-term placement in a nursing home or extended care facility may be necessary. When the client is to be discharged to another health care agency, before discharge the hospital nurse assumes responsibility for communicating all pertinent information regarding the client's specific needs and special care problems. Copies of the care plan and teaching plan that were developed for this client are included in the transfer chart.

 Evaluation

On the basis of identified nursing diagnoses, the nurse evaluates the care for the client experiencing acidemia. The expected outcomes for the client with acidemia include that the client

1. Has a breathing pattern with rate and depth within the normal range
2. Maintains a patent airway
3. Restores ECF pH to within the normal range
4. Increases activity tolerance to include participation in self-care activities
5. Is correctly oriented to time, place, and person
6. Correctly interprets environmental stimuli
7. Avoids injury
8. Identifies actions to take when signs and symptoms of acidemia occur
9. Describes and complies with prescribed drug therapy
10. Maintains appropriate nutritional status as evidenced by no loss of weight

ALKALEMIA

OVERVIEW

Alkalemia is a condition in which the acid-base balance of the ECF is disturbed, with the concentration and/or strength of base components being proportionately higher than normal compared with the concentration and/or strength of the acid components (Blosser, 1985;

Shrout, 1985). This condition is characterized by a decrease in the hydrogen ion concentration of the blood, which is reflected by an arterial blood pH above 7.45. Many people confuse the terms alkalemia and alkalosis, which are related but not synonymous. *Alkalemia* indicates a condition of too few hydrogen ions in the blood and a pH that is higher than normal. *Alkalosis* is the *process* that caused the blood pH to increase (Halperin & Goldstein, 1988). Alkalemia is not an actual disease or process; instead, it is a symptom of a disease or pathologic process.

Alkalemia can result from an *actual* increase in the concentration and/or strength of base components, a *base excess.* The following representation displays this concept visually:

```
A  A  A  B  B  B  B
A  A  A  B  B  B  B
A  A  A  B  B  B  B
```

An actual base excess alkalemia is the result of processes that cause either (1) an overproduction of base components or (2) an underelimination of normally produced base components (usually bicarbonate). Alkalemia also can result from a *relative* increase in the concentration and/or strength of base components, an *acid deficit.* The following schematic shows this concept visually:

```
A  A  B  B  B
A  A  B  B  B
A  A  B  B  B
```

The actual amount or strength of base components has not increased. Instead, the concentration, strength, or both of the acid components have decreased, which makes the fluid relatively more basic than acidic. A relative base excess alkalemia (actual acid deficit) occurs as a result of processes that cause either (1) an overelimination of acid components (usually as hydrogen ions) or (2) an underproduction of acid components.

The processes that cause alkalemia include disturbances in metabolism and disturbances in pulmonary respiration. When problems in metabolic processes cause the alkalemia, it is said to have a metabolic alkalosis origin. When problems in respiratory processes cause the alkalemia, it is said to have a respiratory alkalosis origin. Alkalemia has serious and life-threatening consequences. Because alkalemia is the manifestation of another abnormal process or processes, it is treated most effectively by treating the underlying abnormal processes. Treatment techniques and modalities that are effective for metabolic alkalosis are different from those that are effective for respiratory alkalosis. Therefore, the ability to distinguish between metabolic and respiratory origin alkalemia is important for prevention and treatment.

Pathophysiology

Alkalemia, manifested as an arterial blood pH higher than 7.45, has profound effects on specific physiologic functions regardless of whether its origin is metabolic, respiratory, or both. The primary pathologic effects of alkalemia are related to the fact that both hydrogen ions and bicarbonate ions are electrolytes. A decrease in hydrogen ion (cation) concentration or an increase in the bicarbonate ion (anion) concentration of the ECF creates other electrolyte disturbances that greatly reduce the stability of excitable membranes. Therefore, many signs and symptoms that are associated with alkalemia are related to alterations of body systems that depend on the generation and propagation of action potentials. The most common and profound manifestations of alkalemia are associated with increased excitability of the central nervous, neuromuscular, and cardiac systems (Cogan et al., 1983; Guyton, 1986).

Etiology

Alkalemia can be caused by metabolic disturbances, respiratory disturbances, or combined metabolic and respiratory disturbances (see the Key Features of Disease on pp. 351 and 352).

Metabolic Alkalosis

Most conditions leading to metabolic alkalosis create the acid-base disturbance through two mechanisms: either an actual increase of base components or an actual decrease of acid components.

Increases in base components occur as a result of oral or parenteral ingestion of bicarbonates, carbonates, acetates, citrates, and lactates. Excessive use of oral antacids

---

KEY FEATURES OF DISEASE ■ Common Causes of Metabolic Alkalosis

Pathology	Conditions

Increase of base components	Oral ingestion of bases
	  Antacids
	  Milk-alkali syndrome
	Parenteral base administration
	  Blood transfusion
	  Sodium bicarbonate correction of metabolic acidosis
	  Total parenteral nutrition
	  Excess Ringer's lactate

Decrease of acid components	Prolonged vomiting Nasogastric suctioning Cushing's syndrome Bartter's syndrome Hyperaldosteronism Use of thiazide diuretics

KEY FEATURES OF DISEASE ■ Common Causes of
Respiratory Alkalosis

Pathology
Excessive loss of carbon dioxide

Conditions
Hyperventilation
  Anxiety
  Fear
  Improperly set ventilators
Central chemoreceptor stimulation
  Compensation for metabolic acidosis
  Central nervous system lesions
  Drugs
    Salicylates
    Catecholamines
    Progesterone
Peripheral chemoreceptor stimulation
  Hypoxemia
  Asphyxiation
  High altitudes
  Shock
    Vasogenic
    Neurogenic
    Cardiogenic
    Hypovolemic
    Septic
  Early stage pulmonary
      problems
  Pneumonia
  Asthma
  Pulmonary emboli

composed of sodium bicarbonate or calcium carbonate
can cause a metabolic alkalosis (Janusek, 1984b), as can
the milk-alkali syndrome (Metheny & Snively, 1983).
Other base excesses can occur as a result of medical
treatment, such as citrate excesses during rapid and/or
massive blood transfusions, acetate and lactate excesses
during hyperalimentation, and intravenous sodium bicarbonate administration for correction of lactic acidosis
or ketoacidosis (Cogan et al., 1983; Narins & Emmett,
1980).

Metabolic aklalosis as a result of acid loss can occur in
response to specific disease processes or as a side effect
of specific medical treatment. Disease processes or conditions that are associated with metabolic alkalosis include prolonged vomiting, Cushing's syndrome, Bartter's syndrome, hyperaldosteronism, and possibly
hypoparathyroid-induced hypocalcemia (Cogan et al.,
1983; Riley et al., 1987). Specific medical treatments
that promote acid loss and can cause a metabolic alkalosis include the use of thiazide diuretics, prolonged
nasogastric suctioning, and the administration of carbenicillin and penicillin (Narins & Emmett, 1980; Riley
et al., 1987).

Respiratory Alkalosis

The mechanism responsible for respiratory alkalosis
is the excessive loss of carbon dioxide through hyperventilation, which may be seen in response to anxiety,
fear, and improper settings on mechanical ventilators
(Taylor, 1984b). Excessive ventilation can be caused
through direct stimulation of the central chemoreceptors. Conditions that stimulate the central chemoreceptors directly include fever, respiratory compensation for
metabolic acidosis, central nervous system lesions, and
drugs (e.g., salicylates, catecholamines, and progesterone). Excessive ventilation can also be caused by stimulation of the peripheral chemoreceptors, which are sensitive to decreases in arterial oxygen levels (hypoxemia).
Hypotension is also interpreted by peripheral chemoreceptors as hypoxemia. Conditions that cause excessive
ventilation by this mechanism include low concentrations of oxygen in environmental air (e.g., high altitudes
or tightly enclosed spaces), shock (e.g., vasogenic, cardiogenic, hypovolemic, and septic) and early stages of
pulmonary problems that interfere with gas exchange,
such as pneumonia, asthma, and pulmonary emboli.

Early stages of these last conditions cause a respiratory alkalosis by increasing ventilation and respiratory
loss of carbon dioxide, although gas exchange is impaired to some degree and hypoxemia is present. Carbon dioxide is lost even though inadequate amounts of
oxygen are being taken in because the rate of diffusion
for carbon dioxide from the pulmonary capillary into
the alveoli is much greater than the rate of diffusion of
oxygen from alveolar air into the pulmonary capillary.
This unequal gas exchange phenomenon is related to
the differences in partial pressure gradients for these
two gases. Atmospheric air contains practically no carbon dioxide. Therefore, the partial pressure of carbon
dioxide in the atmosphere is extremely low compared
with that in pulmonary capillary blood. As a result, the
partial pressure gradient for carbon dioxide is great, and
diffusion of carbon dioxide from capillary blood into
atmospheric air is quite rapid. On the other hand, the
concentration of oxygen in atmospheric air is only about
20% to 21%, which means that it has a moderate partial
pressure. The partial pressure of oxygen in the blood at
the venous end of pulmonary capillaries is a significant
40 mmHg. The partial pressure gradient for oxygen between atmospheric air in the alveoli and that in pulmonary capillary blood is not as great as the gradient for
carbon dioxide, and the rate of oxygen diffusion is significantly slower than that for carbon dioxide. Therefore, under normal atmospheric conditions, it is always
easier to remove carbon dioxide than it is to take in
oxygen. Even when pulmonary problems inhibit gas
exchange, more carbon dioxide is lost than oxygen is
taken in, which results in an alkalosis. However, when
these conditions persist, the reduced oxygen levels
cause cellular metabolism to be anaerobic, and organic
acids build up and the carbonic anhydrase equation
shifts to the *left*. Eventually, carbon dioxide is generated
faster than it is lost, and the conditions that originally

created a respiratory alkalosis produce a respiratory acidosis (Ganong, 1985; Guyton, 1987).

Incidence

Alkalemia is a symptom rather than an actual disease state, and its actual incidence is unknown. Among hospitalized clients, alkalemia is the most commonly seen acid-base disorder, especially among critically ill clients. Reports concerning the prevalence of metabolic alkalosis compared with respiratory alkalosis give conflicting information, although more investigators suggest that respiratory alkalosis is more common (Kaehny, 1983; Narins & Emmett, 1980; Riley et al., 1987).

PREVENTION

Strategies for prevention of alkalemia vary according to the individual client and the probable etiology of the imbalance. All strategies require identification of clients at risk. It is especially important to identify such hospitalized clients because many instances of alkalemia are treatment induced. Secondary prevention through early detection involves teaching health care professionals to interpret laboratory data and to recognize signs and symptoms associated with alkalemia so that appropriate interventions can be instituted early and serious complications can be averted.

COLLABORATIVE MANAGEMENT

 Assessment

History

For any client, the nurse collects data about risk factors as well as causative factors related to the development of alkalemia. *Age* is important, as the elderly are more prone to respiratory and renal dysfunctions that may cause an acid-base imbalance. The nurse inquires about specific risk factors such as a recent history of prolonged vomiting, fever, severe pain, excessive licorice ingestion, or any problem with respiration.

The nurse inquires about the use of over-the-counter and prescribed *medications*, especially antacids, thiazide diuretics, antihypertensive agents, and products containing aspirin or other salicylates. If the client cannot recall exactly what medications are being taken, this information may be obtained from other sources.

Because ECF fluid volume depletion is associated with many conditions leading to metabolic alkalosis, clients are asked specific questions regarding *urinary output,* including voiding frequency and quantity. The nurse asks questions about actual fluid intake in general and about intake specifically during the previous 24 hours. Clients are asked if recent losses of *weight* (associated with fluid loss) have been noted.

The nurse collects historical data that may indicate the actual presence of alkalemia. Symptoms of alkalemia are often first noted as increased excitability of the central nervous system and the neuromuscular system. Clients are asked if muscle cramping or twitching is present and if changes in memory or the ability to concentrate have been noted. Disturbances in sleep patterns or insomnia may indicate alkalemia. Having the client relate the previous 24 hours activities may reveal information about the presence of anxiety, changes in behavior, and muscle weakness associated with actual alkalemia.

Physical Assessment: Clinical Manifestations

Clinical manifestations of alkalemia are consistent whether its origin is metabolic or respiratory. Many symptoms are results of the fluid and electrolyte imbalances that usually accompany alkalemia. These manifestations are primarily associated with modifications in activities of excitable membranes that are involved in cerebral, neuromuscular, and cardiac muscle functions (see the accompanying Key Features of Disease).

Central nervous system manifestations. Overexcitement of the central and peripheral nervous systems is the major cause of symptoms that are associated with alkalemia. Clients experience lightheadedness, agitation, confusion, and hyperreflexia that may progress to seizure activity. Paresthesias may be present as tingling or numbness around the mouth and in the toes (Kaehny,

KEY FEATURES OF DISEASE ■ Common Clinical Manifestations of Alkalemia

System	Manifestations

Central nervous	Increased activity
	    Anxiety, irritability, tetany,
	      seizures
	    Positive Chvostek's sign
	    Positive Trousseau's sign
	    Paresthesias

Neuromuscular	Hyperreflexia Muscle cramping and twitching Skeletal muscle weakness
Cardiac	Increased heart rate Normal or low blood pressure Increased digitalis toxicity

Respiratory	Respiratory alkalosis
	    Increased rate and depth of
	      ventilation
	Metabolic alkalosis
	    Decreased respiratory effort
	      associated with skeletal
	      muscle weakness

1983). Another reliable indicator of alkalemia with accompanying hypocalcemia are a positive *Chvostek's sign and Trousseau's sign*. The nurse tests for Chvostek's sign by tapping on the client's face just below and anterior to the ear (over the facial nerve). If the reaction is positive, this tapping triggers facial twitching that involves one side of the mouth, nose, and cheek. The nurse tests for Trousseau's sign by placing a blood pressure cuff around the upper arm, inflating the cuff to above the systolic pressure, and keeping it inflated for 1 to 4 minutes. Under this hypoxic condition, the hand and fingers spasm in palmar flexion. The spasms continue for 20 to 30 seconds after the pressure in the cuff is released.

Neuromuscular manifestations. Alkalemia is associated with hypocalcemia and hypokalemia. Both of these states increase the ease with which nerve membranes depolarize. Nerve stimulation results in nonvoluntary skeletal muscle contractions that are manifested as cramps, twitches, and charley horses. Deep tendon reflexes are hyperactive. Tetany of isolated muscle groups may be present, is painful, and indicates a rapidly worsening condition. It is important to remember that although skeletal muscles may contract as a result of overstimulation by the nerves, the skeletal muscles themselves become weaker because of the alkalemia and hypokalemia. Hand grasp strength diminishes, and the client may be unable to walk or support his or her own weight. Respiratory efforts become less effective as the skeletal muscles of respiration become weaker.

Cardiac manifestations. Alkalemia increases the irritability of the myocardium, especially in the presence of an accompanying hypokalemia. Heart rate increases, although no corresponding increase in blood pressure is seen. When hypovolemia is also present, the client may experience profound hypotension. The myocardium has increased sensitivity to digitalis derivatives, and clients may experience problems with digitalis toxicity.

Respiratory manifestations. Alterations in the rate and depth of respiration are the underlying cause for respiratory alkalosis leading to alkalemia. Tidal volume is nearly normal, but minute respiratory volume is increased in proportion to the increase in rate. The increase in minute respiratory volume may result from other physiologic changes or may have a psychogenic basis.

Psychosocial Assessment

The initially psychosocial assessment may show few, rather subtle behavioral changes, except in episodes of respiratory alkalosis related to extreme anxiety and hyperventilation. The client usually remains alert but possibly disoriented, unless seizure activity also occurs. Clients may appear anxious and may have increasing sensitivity to extraneous environmental noise and activity. This situation can progress to excessive irritability, belligerence, irrational behavior, and even frank psychosis.

Laboratory Findings

The definitive laboratory test to confirm the presence of alkalemia is an arterial blood pH value above 7.45. However, this test alone does not identify the underlying pathologic condition or origin of the alkalemia. Because clinical manifestations of metabolic alkalosis and respiratory alkalosis are similar and the effective treatments are different, it is critical to obtain and interpret additional laboratory data. These data should include arterial blood gas values and measurements of serum potassium, serum calcium, and serum chloride levels (see the Key Features of Disease on page 345).

Metabolic alkalosis. Laboratory data that show the presence of a metabolic alkalosis causing alkalemia include a high pH, elevated bicarbonate level (above 28 mEq/L), normal PO_2, rising PCO_2, reduced serum potassium level, reduced serum calcium level, and reduced serum chloride level (Riley et al., 1987). The pH is high because buffering and respiratory compensation are not adequate to maintain a normal hydrogen ion concentration.

The increased bicarbonate level coupled with a rising PCO_2 is the hallmark of metabolic alkalosis. The rising PCO_2 is compensation for the reduced hydrogen ion concentration.

The serum potassium level is reduced as a result of the body's attempt to maintain electroneutrality during acid-base imbalances. The illustration on page 347 demonstrates movement of potassium ions that is associated with changes in ECF pH. As the hydrogen ion concentration of the ECF decreases, intracellular buffers generate hydrogen ions, which move into the ECF. To prevent an extracellular cation excess, potassium ions move from the ECF into the ICF, which causes a hypokalemic condition. Research is not clear as to whether hypokalemia can actually cause alkalemia or whether the hypokalemia present with alkalemia is a result of the alkalotic process.

As the pH increases, calcium binding increases and the concentration of serum calcium decreases, which creates an accompanying state of hypocalcemia. Most of the serious clinical manifestations of alkalemia are attributed to this accompanying hypocalcemia.

Serum chloride levels are reduced during alkalemia of metabolic origin. This hypochloremia is proposed to have two mechanisms. The first mechanism is a shift of chloride from the ECF to the ICF to maintain electroneutrality as the ECF bicarbonate ion concentration increases. The other proposed mechanism is an actual urinary excretion of chloride in response to the reduced serum concentration of potassium.

Respiratory alkalosis. Laboratory data that demonstrate the presence of a respiratory alkalosis leading to alkalemia include a high pH, reduced bicarbonate level, reduced PCO_2, reduced serum potassium level, reduced serum calcium level, and elevated serum chloride level (Kaehny, 1983). The pH is high because buffering and renal compensation cannot maintain the hydrogen ion concentration at a normal level.

The hallmarks of respiratory alkalosis are the reduced bicarbonate level (not usually below 15 mEq/L) coupled with a very low PCO_2. The carbon dioxide level is low because it is being exhaled through hyperventilation more rapidly than it is being generated. The bicarbonate level is reduced in response to the pH increase. A variety of blood and intracellular buffers generate hydrogen ions, which immediately combine with the ECF bicarbonate ions and form carbonic acid, thus reducing the ECF concentration of bicarbonate (Kaehny, 1983).

As in metabolic alkalosis, in respiratory alkalosis the serum potassium level is reduced as a result of the body's attempt to maintain electroneutrality during acid-base imbalances. Again, as the pH increases, calcium binding increases and the concentration of serum calcium decreases, and hypocalcemia results.

The increase in serum chloride levels seen with respiratory alkalosis is presumed to occur as a compensatory mechanism to maintain ECF electroneutrality. Decreases in ECF bicarbonate ions reduce the number of ECF anions. As a result of this anion loss, chloride ions are retained in the ECF and may also be reabsorbed in the kidney.

 ## Analysis: Nursing Diagnosis

Alkalemia is a common acid-base disorder among hospitalized clients, either as a complication of a specific pathologic condition and disease process or as a result of certain treatments. The body tolerates the state of alkalemia poorly, and serious, life-threatening side effects can ensue if corrective measures are not taken. One example of a client at risk for development of alkalemia is a postmenopausal woman who has been taking thiazide diuretics to control hypertension and who has also been vomiting for 2 days because of a viral infection. The following nursing diagnoses are derived from these data.

Common Diagnoses

The following diagnoses are common for clients experiencing alkalemia as a result of a metabolic alkalosis:

1. Altered thought processes related to central nervous system overexcitation
2. Potential for injury related to muscle weakness, tetany, or seizure activity

Additional Diagnoses

In addition to the common diagnoses, the client experiencing alkalemia may present with one or more of the following diagnoses:

1. Altered nutrition: less than body requirements related to nausea and vomiting
2. Pain related to muscle spasms and tetany
3. Sensory/perceptual alterations (tactile) related to paresthesia

4. Anxiety related to cerebral hypoxia
5. Impaired physical mobility related to muscle weakness
6. Fluid volume deficit related to vomiting or decreased fluid intake
7. Decreased cardiac output related to presence of arrhythmias

 ## Planning and Implementation

The following plan of care for the client experiencing alkalemia focuses on common diagnoses related to alterations in central and peripheral nervous system activity. This plan of care is aimed at restoring fluid, electrolyte, and acid-base balance and at preventing serious complications.

Altered Thought Processes

Planning client goals.   The major client goals for this nursing diagnosis include that the client will (1) have normal fluid, electrolyte, and acid-base balance, (2) accurately interpret environmental stimuli, and (3) remain in a safe environment.

Interventions: nonsurgical management.   Interventions are aimed at preventing further losses of hydrogen, potassium, calcium, and chloride ions and at providing a safe environment. A major nursing responsibility is accurate assessment of central nervous system activity changes from baseline and from normal. This assessment serves as a basis for the institution of specific interventions. Drug therapy can play a major role in restoring the fluid, electrolyte, and acid-base balances that are affected by alkalemia. Diet therapy is of limited value for the problems associated with alkalemia.

Mental status assessment.   The nurse assesses the client's central nervous system function at least every 2 hours to evaluate whether current interventions are effective and to determine whether the acid-base imbalance still exists. Parameters to be assessed include level of consciousness; orientation to time, place, and person; past and recent memory; ability to concentrate; and cognitive function.

Drug therapy.   Drug therapy for alkalemia focuses both on ameliorating the underlying problems causing the alkalosis and on restoring normal fluid, electrolyte, and acid-base balance. For the example cited, the client developed a metabolic alkalosis–induced alkalemia as a result of acid losses from diuretic therapy and prolonged vomiting. Drug therapy for these alkalotic processes includes discontinuing the diuretic therapy until the alkalemia is resolved, administering antiemetics to halt or decrease vomiting, and administering specific agents to restore fluid, electrolyte, and acid-base balance.

The client has an accompanying fluid volume deficit as a result of fluid losses through diuresis and vomiting.

In addition, she has low serum potassium, low serum calcium, and low serum chloride concentrations. Intravenous infusions of 0.9% saline are useful to restore fluid volume and chloride levels. Saline administration usually assists in also restoring potassium levels. In addition, oral potassium supplements are beneficial when the client can tolerate oral intake. If oral intake is not feasible, potassium chloride may be added to the intravenous fluids at a concentration of 20 to 40 mEq/L.

Because the hypocalcemia is a result of increased calcium binding rather than a result of calcium loss, normal calcium balance returns when the ECF pH drops to normal, and calcium administration is not necessary. These therapies are usually sufficient to restore fluid, potassium, calcium, chloride, and acid-base balance.

If the client continues to have excessive bicarbonate levels or hydrogen ion deficits, other potentially dangerous but therapeutic drugs may be used. Intravenous acetazolamide (Diamox) administration can result in rapid renal loss of bicarbonate. However, this therapy also seriously increases potassium excretion, which intensifies the existing hypokalemia (Cogan et al., 1983). Intravenous infusions of 0.15 N HCl (150 mEq/L) administered through a central line can reduce the ECF pH to normal levels. However, serious cardiac arrhythmias have been reported during this treatment (Riley et al., 1987).

Maintenance of a safe environment. Overexcitation of the central nervous system is expected in the client with alkalemia. These manifestations progress from anxiety and irritability to intensive seizure activity. Behavioral changes are frequently manifested as the client misinterprets environmental stimuli. Maintaining a safe environment for the client with overexcitation of the central and peripheral nervous systems is an important nursing function. Part of this function includes assisting the client to process information correctly. The nurse orients the client to person, time, and place at every interaction. The nurse also reminds the client what the nurse is doing for the client. It may be helpful to place large calendars and clocks where the client can see them. If the client needs glasses to see properly, the nurse makes certain that the client wears the glasses during wakeful periods. The nurse makes certain that the client's call light is always within reach.

The nurse reduces extraneous environmental stimuli to diminish the client's confusion. Whenever possible, the client should be assigned to a private room. If a private room is not available, the nurse makes certain that the roommate does not have a personality or condition that would be inconsistent with a quiet environment. For example, clients who require ventilators or other pieces of noisy equipment that operate continuously would not be appropriate roommates. Lighting is kept to the minimal safe level. The telephone is removed or the bell is turned off. Radio and television programs that vary in loudness and excitement level are avoided. Young children and uncontrolled or confused individuals should not be permitted to visit.

Care must be taken to prevent clients who are experiencing altered thought processes and central nervous system activity from injury. Confused clients require careful observation, especially when they are not in bed. The nurse anticipates the client's need for ambulation and accompanies the ambulatory client. The upper side rails of the client's bed are raised. If the client is alone, the bed is kept in a low position. The nurse may sometimes need to prevent the client from using the electronic bed controls or to restrain the client with a vest or jacket-type restraint. Ideally, having another responsible person in the room with the client at all times eliminates the need for the use of restraining devices.

When the client's condition indicates that seizure activity is likely to occur, the nurse prepares the immediate environment to prevent injury to the client. Side rails are padded. The emergency cart or box with appropriate anticonvulsive drugs is either in the room or just outside the door. The nurse checks to see that suction equipment and an oxygen administration set-up are available within the room and are in good working order.

Potential for Injury

Planning: client goals. The major client goals for this nursing diagnosis include that the client will (1) have normal fluid, electrolyte, and acid-base balance and (2) not experience injury.

Interventions: nonsurgical management. The interventions, including drug therapy and maintenance of safe environment, for this nursing diagnosis are the same as those under the nursing diagnosis Altered Thought Processes for clients experiencing alkalemia.

■ Discharge Planning

Home Care Preparation

Most clients with alkalemia as a result of acute metabolic alkalosis are discharged to home with the acid-base imbalance resolved. However, the underlying conditions leading to the alkalotic processes may be chronic, which increases the client's risk for recurrent episodes of alkalemia. Therefore, the primary focus of discharge planning is client and family education.

Client/Family Education

The focus of client and family education is aimed at prevention of recurrent episodes of alkalemia through careful adherence to the prescribed medical regimen, recognition of risk factors for the development of alkalemia, and understanding of the need for regular follow-up care. The nurse instructs the client and family about the pathologic condition and the treatment for the chronic underlying problem that can lead to the development of alkalemia. The nurse also teaches the client and family about signs and symptoms of alkalemia so that medical assistance can be sought before serious complications develop.

Psychosocial Preparation

Psychosocial preparation needs vary not only because of an individual client's background but also because of the different underlying pathologic conditions contributing to the risk of developing alkalemia. Clients who are newly diagnosed with serious chronic health problems may require extensive counseling before acceptance of and participation in self-care. Local support groups for clients and/or families can ease the process of adjustment to living with a chronic illness. The nurse provides the client with initial information about specific support groups (including local telephone numbers and names of contact people). Such information is usually available in telephone directories and through hospital social services departments.

Clients whose hyperkalemic episodes are the result of long-term chronic health problems may have learned to cope with these problems and need less psychosocial support. However, the nurse reassesses each client's needs in view of new factors, established support systems, previous and current coping patterns, and stability of the chronic disease.

A major psychosocial issue for clients at risk for developing hyperkalemia as a result of a chronic condition is that of compliance. The nurse must convince the client that compliance with the planned treatment regimen affects quality of life. Some aspects of the regimen may be unpleasant or require significant self-control on the part of the client. The nurse helps the client and family to understand the disease process. In conveying this information, the nurse focuses on the potential positive outcome of good compliance rather than on the deleterious effects of noncompliance.

Health Care Resources

The main health care resource for the client with alkalemia is the primary care physician. Some clients with chronic disease processes require assistance with home care. A home care nurse may be needed for delivery of actual care or for supervision of care provided by others in the home environment. The home care nurse is contacted before the client's discharge from the hospital to participate in discharge planning for the client and to assess the need for special equipment, supplies, or skilled care in the home. The home care nurse is given copies of the teaching plan and care plan used for the individual client in the hospital to ensure continuity of care in the home.

 Evaluation

The nurse evaluates the care for the client experiencing alkalemia on the basis of the identified nursing diagnoses associated with this condition. The expected outcomes of care for the client with alkalemia include that the client

1. Restores ECF pH to within the normal range
2. Is correctly oriented to time, place, and person

3. Correctly interprets environmental stimuli
4. Avoids injury
5. Maintains an intake of food and fluid appropriate for existing metabolic needs
6. Describes and complies with prescribed treatment regimen
7. Identifies actions to take when signs and symptoms of alkalemia or electrolyte imbalances occur

SUMMARY

Acid-base imbalances are common complications of disease states and treatments among hospitalized clients, especially those with pulmonary, renal, and/or cardiac problems. Many physiologic mechanisms cannot function properly when the pH of ECF is not within the normal range, and death ensues when pH changes are profound. The body appears to tolerate imbalances leading to acidemia better than imbalances leading to alkalemia, and more mechanisms for increasing the loss of acids have been identified than mechanisms for increasing the loss of bases.

Acidemia is present when the pH drops below 7.34, and the primary pathologic conditions that are associated with acidemia stem from depression of excitable membrane activity. Physiologic dysfunctions are seen when the pH drops below 7.2, although these dysfunctions are reversible if the imbalance is corrected. Severe impairment of physiologic function occurs when the pH of ECF is between 6.8 and 7.15, and aggressive interventions to correct the acid-base imbalance must be instituted immediately to prevent irreversible tissue damage. An ECF pH of less than 6.8 is considered to be incompatible with life.

Alkalemia is present when the pH increases above 7.45, and the primary pathologic conditions involve overstimulation of the central nervous system. Slight increases in the pH are reflected in severe physiologic dysfunction, and ECF pH above 7.8 is not compatible with life.

IMPLICATIONS FOR RESEARCH

Nursing research is needed to answer the following questions about the care of clients with an actual or potential acid-base imbalance:

1. What effect does health care teaching have on prevention of specific acid-base imbalances among individuals at risk for developing an imbalance?

2. What nursing actions help most in symptom management of side effects associated with acidemia and alkalemia?

3. What techniques are most effective for promoting client compliance with special regimens among clients with chronic illnesses predisposing to acid-base imbalance?

4. How can the nurse promote acceptance of chronic illness by clients experiencing chronic pathologic conditions?

5. What effect does a regular exercise regimen have on the activity tolerance of clients with chronic obstructive pulmonary disease?

REFERENCES AND READINGS

Blosser, N. (1985). Electrolytes. In M. Bishop, J. Duben-Von Laufen, & E. Fody (Eds.), *Clinical chemistry: Principles, procedures, correlations* (p. 263). Philadelphia: J. B. Lippincott.

Brenner, B., Coe, F. L., & Rector, F. C. (1987). *Renal physiology in health and disease.* Philadelphia: W. B. Saunders.

Cogan, M., Liu, F., Berger, B., Sebastian, A., & Rector, F. (1983). Metabolic alkalosis. *Medical Clinics of North America, 67,* 903.

Ganong, W. (1985). *Review of medical physiology* (12th ed.). Los Altos, CA: Lange Medical.

Goodkin, D. A., Krishna, G. G., & Narins, R. G. (1984). The role of the anion gap in detecting and managing mixed metabolic acid-base disorders. *Clinics in Endocrinology and Metabolism, 13,* 333.

Guyton, A. C. (1986). *Textbook of medical physiology* (7th ed.). Philadelphia: W. B. Saunders.

Guyton, A. C. (1987). *Human physiology and mechanisms of disease* (4th ed.). Philadelphia: W. B. Saunders.

Halperin, M. L., & Goldstein, M. B. (1988). *Fluid, electrolyte, and acid-base emergencies.* Philadelphia: W. B. Saunders.

Janusek, L. (1984a). Metabolic acidosis: Physiology, signs, and symptoms. *Nursing '84, 14*(7), 44.

Janusek, L. (1984b). Metabolic alkalosis: Physiology, signs, and symptoms. *Nursing '84, 14*(8), 60.

Kaehny, W. (1983). Respiratory acid-base disorders. *Medical Clinics of North America, 67,* 915.

Keyes, J. (1985). *Fluid, electrolyte, and acid-base regulation.* Belmont, CA: Wadsworth.

Kreisberg, R. (1980). Lactate homeostasis and lactic acidosis. *Annals of Internal Medicine, 92,* 227.

Kreisberg, R. (1987). Diabetic ketoacidosis: An update. *Critical Care Clinics, 5,* 817.

Laski, M. (1983). Normal regulation of acid-base balance. *Medical Clinics of North America, 67,* 771.

Leaf, A., & Cotran, R. (1985). *Renal pathophysiology* (3rd ed.). New York: Oxford University Press.

Metheny, N., & Snively, W. (1983). *Nurses' handbook of fluid balance* (4th ed.). Philadelphia: J. B. Lippincott.

Morrison, G., & Murray, T. (1981). Electrolyte, acid-base, and fluid homeostasis in chronic renal failure. *Medical Clinics of North America, 65,* 429.

Narins, R., & Emmett, M. (1980). Simple and mixed acid-base disorders: A practical approach. *Medicine, 59,* 161.

Price, S., & Wilson, L. (1986). *Pathophysiology* (3rd ed.). New York: McGraw-Hill.

Rice, V. (1987). Acid-base derangements in the patient with cardiac arrest. *Focus on Critical Care, 14*(6), 53.

Riley, L., Ilson, B., & Narins, R. (1987). Acute metabolic acid-base disorders. *Critical Care Clinics, 5,* 699.

Robbins, S. L., & Kumar, V. (1987). *Basic pathology* (4th ed.). Philadelphia: W. B. Saunders.

Romanski, S. (1986). Interpreting ABGs in four easy steps. *Nursing '86, 16*(9), 59.

Ryder, R. (1984). Lactic acidosis: High-dose or low-dose bicarbonate therapy? *Diabetes Care, 7,* 99.

Shrout, J. (1985). Blood gases, pH, and buffering system. In M. Bishop, J. Duben-Von Laufen, & E. Fody (Eds.), *Clinical chemistry: Principles, procedures, correlations* (p. 242). Philadelphia: J. B. Lippincott.

Taylor, D. (1984a). Respiratory acidosis: Physiology, signs, and symptoms. *Nursing '84, 14*(10), 44.

Taylor, D. (1984b). Respiratory alkalosis: Physiology, signs, and symptoms. *Nursing '84, 14*(11), 44.

UNIT 3 RESOURCES

Nursing Resources

Intravenous Nurses Society (INS), Two Brighton Street, Belmont, MA 02178. Telephone 617-489-5205.

Promotes delivery of quality intravenous therapy to clients. Enhances the specialty through stringent standards of practice and professional ethics. Promotes research and education in intravenous therapy. Publishes the *Journal of Intravenous Nursing* (bimonthly), *INS NEWSLINE* (bimonthly newsletter), *CRNI News* (biannual publication with an emphasis on certification), and *INS Standards of Practice.*

Intravenous Nurses Society Certification Corporation, Two Brighton Street, Suite 200, Belmont, MA 02178. Telephone 617-489-5205.

Certifies nurses specializing in intravenous therapy.

UNIT 4

Management of Clients with Special Problems

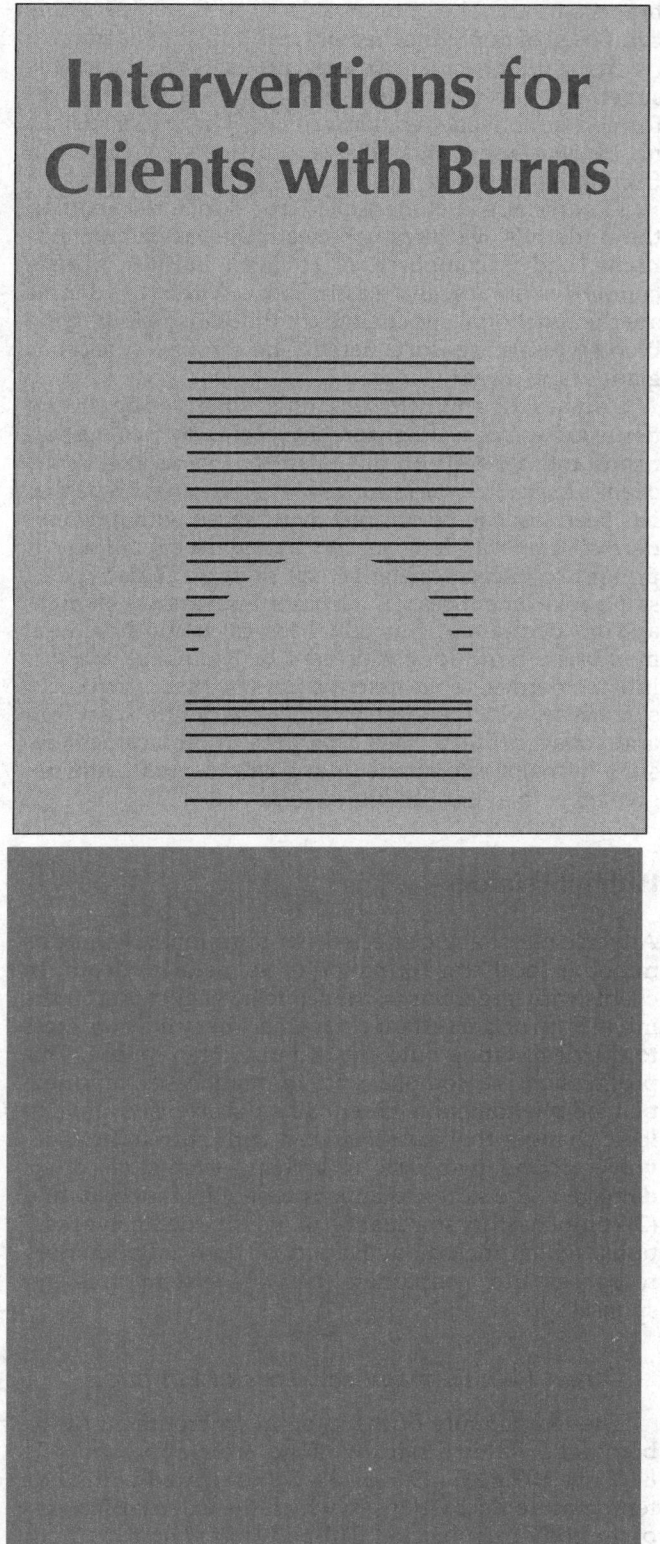

CHAPTER 16

Interventions for Clients with Burns

Burns are manifestations of injuries that are typically inflicted on the skin and other epithelial tissues. Various types of physical insults to epithelial tissues result in the formation of burns. These insults include exposure to temperature extremes, radiation, electrical current, mechanical abrasion, and chemical abrasion. Although these insults have different mechanisms of action, the final outcome — the burn — is essentially the same.

OVERVIEW

Burn injuries result in complex problems that extend well beyond the obvious physical damage evident in tissues that are traumatized directly. These complex problems affect all body systems, and many are life-threatening. Twenty years ago, an adult with a burn injury involving 50% of the total body surface area (TBSA) had less than a 50% chance of survival. In addition, complications of the injury and/or treatment usually resulted in some degree of functional impairment. Today, an adult with a 75% TBSA burn has a 50% chance of survival, and it is not unusual for specialized burn centers to discharge clients who have survived 95% TBSA burns (Feller & Jones, 1987). Reduced healing time, anticipation of and early intervention for complications, the focus on preservation of function early in the course of burn care, and more effective rehabilitation techniques all have led to the increased survival rate among clients with serious burn injuries, as well as to an increase in the ultimate functional capacity of those clients. The complex problems of clients, coupled with the advances made in survival of burn clients, present an exciting challenge for the nursing practitioner who cares for these clients.

Many unique characteristics of a burn injury result in the need for different specific interventions. These characteristics include extent of the burn injury, etiology of the injury, and anatomic location of the injury. Burns that involve a larger TBSA or that extend deeper into tissue layers require more intensive interventions than do smaller or superficial burn injuries. Burns that are caused by hot liquids, which are known as scald burns, can have a significantly different prognosis and final outcome than burns of a similar size caused by flames or exposure to ionizing radiation. Chemical burns require initial treatment that is different from that for electrical burns or burns caused by flames. A burn involving the genitalia causes a greater risk of infection than does a similar-sized burn elsewhere on the body. Burns of the hands or feet can affect the overall functional capacity of the client and require different treatment techniques from burns of other body locations (Sherif & Sato, 1989). An understanding of the general pathophysiology of burns is necessary to recognize the subtle differences that certain burns can present and to anticipate the expected, multiorgan complications that are associated with specific burn injuries.

The prognosis for clients experiencing a burn injury is directly related to the size and location of the burn. Other factors such as age, pre-existing state of wellness, and smoke inhalation can influence the severity of the injury and its accompanying effects. Clients experiencing burn injuries also often experience devastating concomitant events such as injury or death to a significant other, loss of home, or loss of the ability to earn a living.

The burned client should be referred to a facility that is best equipped to handle the immediate and long-term problems that are associated with these special injuries. Even small burns can overtax a surgical nursing unit that is not prepared to handle burn clients. In addition, burn clients and their families often require specialized assistance with many psychosocial problems related to these injuries. The American Burn Association recommends that clients with third-degree burns of more than 15% to 20% TBSA be referred to a specialized burn unit or burn center. If clients are at risk for developing complications because of age, pre-existing illness, or burns located on the face, hands, feet, or genitals, a burn center referral should also be made. When it is suspected that the client may have been a victim of abuse or may have some other unusual problem, a referral to a burn unit or center that has a specialized team of experts who are best able to assist the client is appropriate.

Transfers to other facilities are most successful when members from the sending hospital communicate with the staff of the receiving hospital. Although basic burn care is relatively consistent in the United States, sufficient variation in treatment protocols occur from agency to agency to warrant this exchange of information.

Anatomy and Physiology Review

The skin is the largest single organ of the human body and has many roles in homeostasis. The skin forms a barrier between the external world and the internal environment. This barrier helps to maintain the internal constancy for fluid, electrolyte, and temperature homeostasis and also prevents invasion of the internal environment by potentially harmful microorganisms. In addition, the skin serves as a sensory input channel and permits the individual to be aware of pain, pressure, heat, cold, touch, and other cutaneous sensations. The skin also provides identity through variations in form and character that are unique to the individual. Chapter 39 provides a more in-depth discussion of the features of this special organ.

As shown in Figure 39–1 in Chapter 39, skin is divided into two basic sections, the epidermis and the dermis. The *epidermis* is a multilayered tissue that is built on a thin, noncellular protein surface called a *basement membrane*, which separates the epidermis from the dermis. Epithelial cells in direct contact with the basement membrane are the young, less-differentiated skin cells (*keratinocytes*), which increase in number by cell division to replace the older, no longer living, differentiated cells that are lost from the outer skin surfaces through injury and normal abrasive contact. This cell division occurs only in areas where the basement membrane is intact. The outermost layer of the epidermis is composed of nonliving, heavily keratinized cells that are fused together to create a horny, protective surface. This superficial layer continuously sloughs off and is reformed from deeper epidermal cells. The epidermis has no blood vessels and receives nutrients by diffusion from fluids in the dermis.

The *dermis,* sometimes called true skin, is thicker than the epidermis, lies directly beneath the basement membrane, and is composed of collagen meshes, fibrous connective tissues, and elastic fibers. Within the dermis are the functional appendages of the skin, including the blood vessels, sensory nerves, hair roots, sebaceous glands, and sweat glands.

Skin has the ability to regenerate when cell death and tissue losses occur. Regeneration occurs by two mechanisms and depends on the extent of loss as well as the client's overall physical condition. Epidermal tissue that has been lost can be completely replaced with new epidermal tissue as long as the basement membrane is present to induce epithelial cell division. This type of skin replacement results in minor appearance changes and no permanent functional losses. If the basement membrane is no longer present or if damage extends into the dermis, replacement occurs by the formation of scar tissue, which is largely composed of fibroblast cells and collagen fibers. This type of skin replacement results in major alterations in appearance and some degree of permanent functional loss.

Pathophysiology

Adverse physiologic effects from burn injury can be as minor as local scar formation or as major as death. In clients with larger burns, the sequelae of events after the initial burn and resultant cutaneous injury may progress to the devastating outcome of multiorgan failure. This progression is a complex and, in many cases, an unexplained phenomenon. Essentially, the extensive physiologic changes that are associated with burn injuries revolve around two basic underlying events: (1) direct damage to the skin and impairment of its functions and (2) compensatory stimulation of massive defensive reactions, which include activation of both inflammatory responses and sympathetic nervous system stress responses.

Direct Skin Damage and Loss of Function

The temperature of the internal environment of the body falls within a narrow range, from approximately 84.2° to 109.4° F (29° to 43° C), compared with wide temperature fluctuations to which the external surfaces of the body are subjected. The body has several methods to compensate for the wide variations in external temperature (Guyton, 1986). Circulating blood acts as both a provider and a dissipator of heat. Dissipation of heat is efficient under normal conditions. When heat is applied to the skin, the temperature of the immediate subdermal layer rises rapidly. As soon as the heat source is removed, the body can return the area to a normal temperature within seconds. If the heat source is not removed or if it is applied at a rate or level that exceeds the capacity of the skin to dissipate it, cell destruction occurs.

As illustrated in Figure 16–1, prolonged exposure of several hours leads to tissue damage at temperatures as low as 113° F (45° C). At 158° F (70° C), cellular destruction is so rapid that only brief periods of exposure are necessary for total tissue destruction down to and including the subcutaneous level. Once cell destruction has taken place, regardless of the cause or time frame, the physical responses are similar.

Long exposure to relatively low heat or short exposure to higher temperatures can cause cell destruction at progressively deeper levels. Most burn injuries of significant size cause cell damage through all layers of the skin, although not necessarily evenly in all areas. As a result, a smooth plane of burn injury rarely occurs. When heat is applied to the external surface of the skin, the resultant damage is proportional to the degree of heat applied and the duration of exposure. Skin destruc-

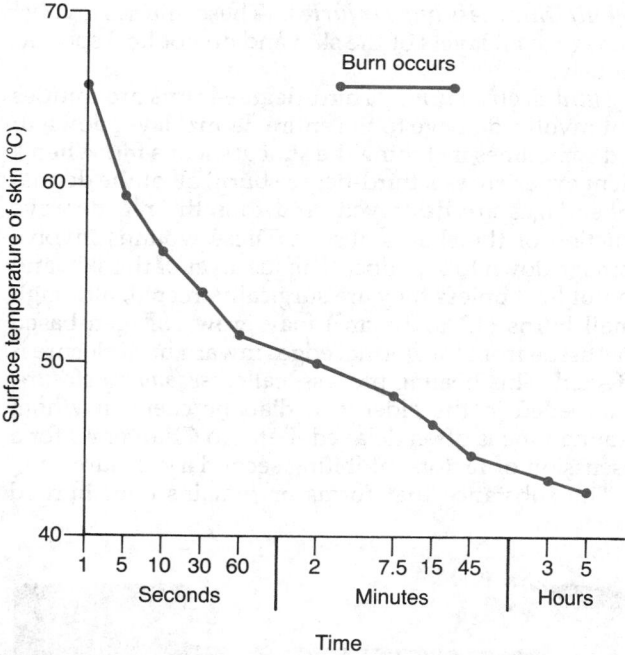

Figure 16–1

Relationship between intensity of heat and duration of exposure. Exposure for prolonged periods causes burns, even with milder temperatures. At more extreme temperatures, tissue damage results after only seconds. (Modified from Moritz, A. R. [1947]. Studies of thermal injuries II: The relative importance of time and surface temperature in and causation of cutaneous burns. *American Journal of Pathology, 23*, 695.)

tion that is caused by heat is classified according to the depth of tissue damage.

The thickness of the skin involved has an effect on the tissue damage caused by heat. Less heat and less time are needed to do similar damage in areas of the body covered with thin skin compared with areas where the skin is thicker. Skin is thickest over the back and thighs and thinnest around the medial arm, bridge of the nose, and face. Skin is generally thinner in young children and in elderly persons than in middle-aged adults. Elderly persons also have reduced layers of subcutaneous material, loss of elastic fibers, and an overall reduced ability to respond to trauma. Consequently, burns of a similar size have a more serious effect in the aged person.

Classification of burn depth. Burn wounds are classified by depth of tissue injury as defined by appearance and associated characteristics. The accompanying Key Features of Disease and the illustration on page 365 summarize the usual characteristics of burn injuries of various depths.

Partial-thickness burn injuries. *Partial-thickness* injuries damage only part of the skin, with remaining tissue capable of stimulating regeneration and successful wound healing. These injuries are further classified as superficial or deep.

First-degree burns. First-degree burns are also termed *superficial partial-thickness* injuries. First-degree burns have the least destruction of all burn types because the epidermis is the only portion of the skin that is injured or destroyed. The dermis is unharmed, and all structures that are necessary for total replacement by regrowth of epithelial cells are present. A familiar first-degree burn is a sunburn. This burn is characterized by pain, redness, increased sensitivity to heat, and some degree of swelling. Healing of this injury among healthy adults occurs within 3 to 5 days and is usually uncomplicated. First-degree burns over large portions of the body or moderate portions of the body in very young children or elderly persons can have more unpleasant effects, such as severe pain, nausea, vomiting, and, in some cases, minor blistering.

Second-degree burns. Second-degree burns are also termed *deep partial-thickness* injuries. Second-degree burns that reach only the upper layers of the dermis are called *superficial second-degree* burns. A more serious second-degree burn is one that reaches the deeper layers of the dermis and destroys structures within the dermis such as nerves and hair follicles. These burns are classified as *deep second-degree* or deep dermal burns.

Superficial second-degree burns involving the epidermis and the upper portion of the dermis are characteristically pink to red and are moist or weepy (Fig. 16–2). Because of exposed nerve endings, these burn areas are painful to touch and have increased sensitivity to heat. Swelling and blistering are usually present. Spontaneous regeneration of epithelium occurs in 2 to 3 weeks because the appendages of the skin, such as hair

KEY FEATURES OF DISEASE ■ Characteristics of Burn Injuries of Various Depths

	Partial-Thickness Burns			Full-Thickness Burns	
Characteristic	First Degree	Superficial Second Degree	Deep Second Degree	Third Degree	Fourth Degree
Color	Pink to red	Pale to red	Cherry red	Can be gray, black, brown, yellow, red, or white	Charred
Pain	Yes	Yes	Yes	Usually considered anesthetic	Usually considered anesthetic
Blisters	No	Yes, with much weeping	Can occur with much weeping	Usually no	Usually no
Eschar	No	No	Can develop—soft, dry, insensitive	Yes—dry, hard, inelastic	Yes—dry, hard, inelastic
Healing time	3–5 d	2–3 wk	3–6 wk	Depends on treatment	Depends on treatment
Grafts required	No	No	No, but usually applied	Yes	Yes

follicles, which are lined with epidermal cells, are not destroyed.

Deep second-degree burns involve injury to deeper dermal layers and some destruction of skin appendages. These wounds may or may not have blisters and are cherry red or white, as shown in Figure 16–3. Circulation to the injured area is temporarily disrupted but usually resumes within 48 hours. These wounds can heal spontaneously in 3 to 6 weeks if complications do not occur. Because of the increased length of hospital stay, susceptibility to infection, and the large amount of scarring that may occur, these wounds are often surgically treated like full-thickness burns.

Full-thickness burn injuries. These injuries involve damage to all layers of the skin and do not heal spontaneously.

Third-degree burns. Third-degree burns are injuries that involve damage to the entire dermal layer down to and sometimes including the subcutaneous fat. When a client experiences a third-degree burn, all of the dermal appendages are destroyed, and thus the regenerative function of the skin is absent. These wounds involve damage down to the subcutaneous layer of the skin and do not heal unless they are surgically treated, although small burns (12 to 16 cm^2) may grow collagen-based scar tissue from the normal edges inward until closure is effected. This healing process, called *secondary closure*, is impeded in the elderly or diabetic client in whom healing time is often delayed. Refer to Chapter 40 for a discussion of factors inhibiting secondary closure.

The substance that forms or remains over burned

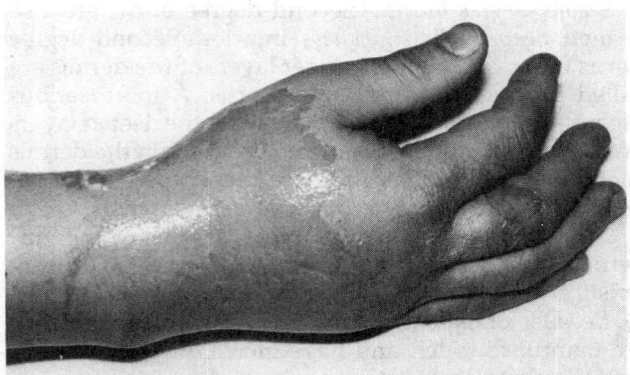

Figure 16–2.
Typical appearance of superficial second-degree burn injury.

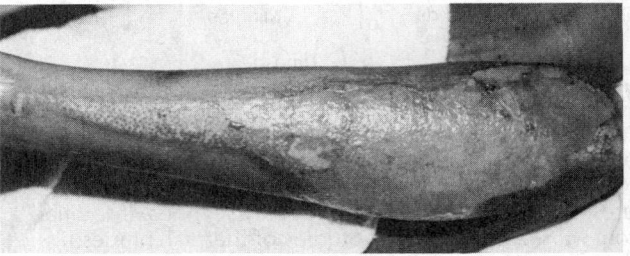

Figure 16–3.
Typical appearance of deep partial-thickness burn injury.

CLASSIFICATION OF BURN DEPTH

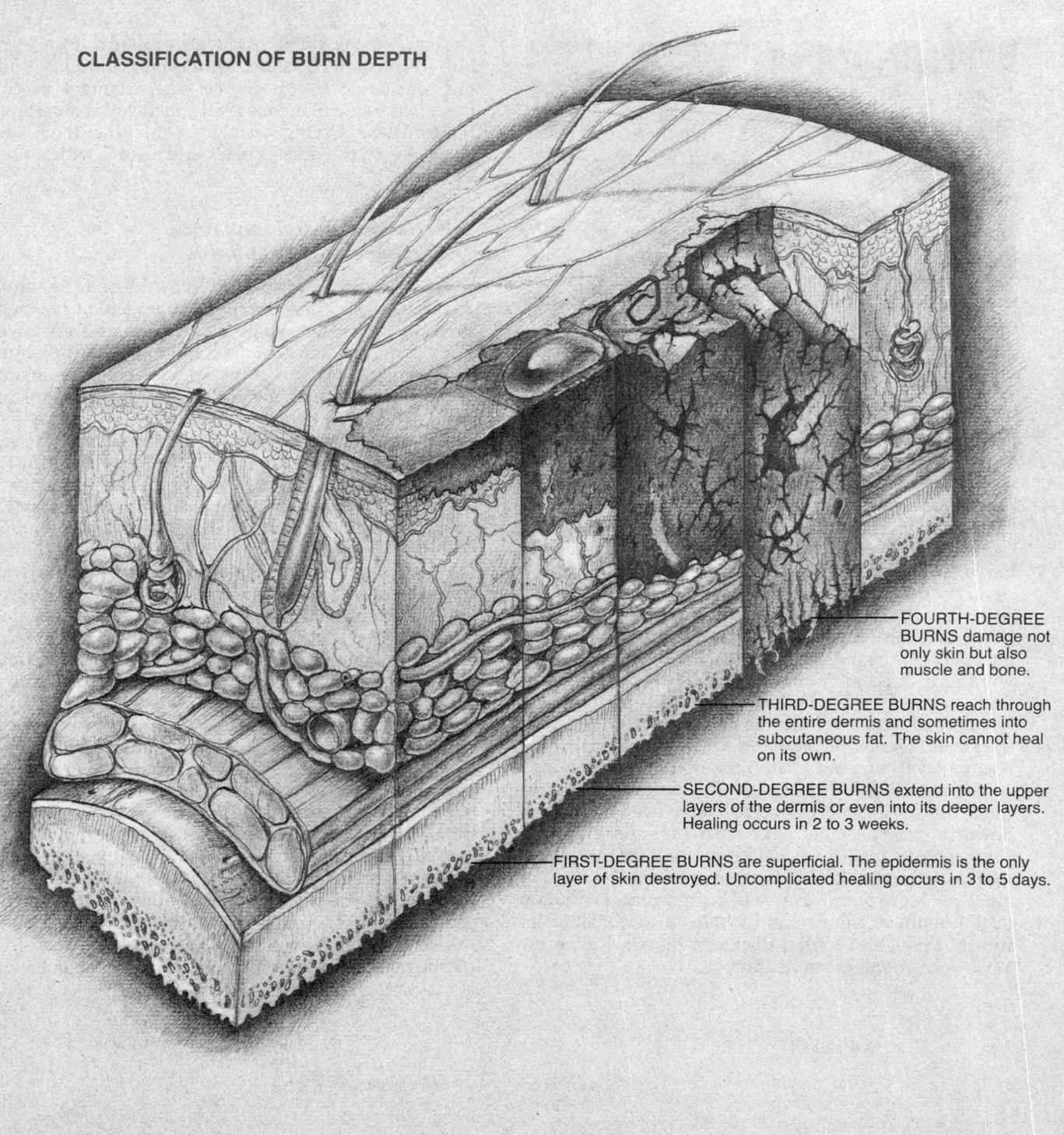

FOURTH-DEGREE BURNS damage not only skin but also muscle and bone.

THIRD-DEGREE BURNS reach through the entire dermis and sometimes into subcutaneous fat. The skin cannot heal on its own.

SECOND-DEGREE BURNS extend into the upper layers of the dermis or even into its deeper layers. Healing occurs in 2 to 3 weeks.

FIRST-DEGREE BURNS are superficial. The epidermis is the only layer of skin destroyed. Uncomplicated healing occurs in 3 to 5 days.

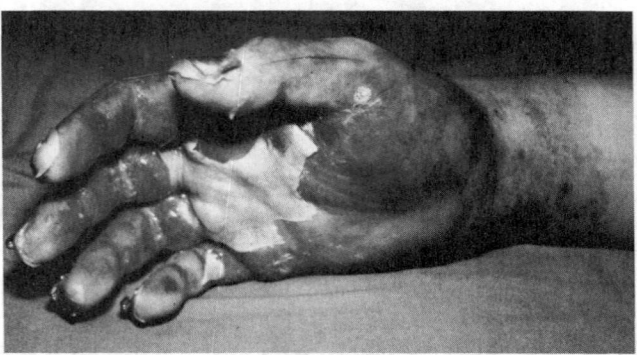

Figure 16-4

Typical appearance of third-degree burn injury.

tissue is called *eschar.* Eschar is a sloughing layer of necrotic (sometimes charred) tissue, collagen, and protein exudates. In full-thickness burns, the eschar typically is firm, thick, and leathery. The color can be ivory white, brown, gray, black, or cherry red, as seen in Figure 16-4. There are usually no blisters in third-degree burns, and the eschar is dry and cold to the touch. Eschar is nonelastic and can cause serious problems in the presence of tissue swelling or circumferential chest burns that can restrict circulation or respiratory movement. Third-degree burns damage the blood vessels within the affected tissues to such an extent that blood flow is absent or impeded, and thrombosed blood vessels may be visible within the eschar. Healing for full-thickness injuries depends on re-establishment of an adequate vascular bed within the injured area.

Theoretically, full-thickness burns are anesthetic because the sensory nerve endings have been destroyed; however, many clients who experience these injuries complain of pain. The most likely reason for this pain is that an entire area of skin is rarely affected to a consistent level. More often, an area of burn contains variation in the depth of injury and includes a combination of full-thickness and partial-thickness burns; thus, some areas contain intact nerve endings.

Fourth-degree burns. A category called fourth-degree burns is included by some authors and clinicians. Burns are considered fourth-degree when damage extends beyond the subcutaneous level and includes muscle and bone. These wounds usually contain a thick, dry, charred eschar, which is black and always without sensation.

Activation of Inflammatory Compensatory Responses

Any tissue injury is perceived by the body as a threat to homeostasis. One compensatory reaction that functions to limit physiologic disruptions and return the body to normal homeostatic conditions is the inflammatory response. Although initiation of the inflammatory response is stimulated by a variety of conditions and insults (Chap. 23), the sequence of the actual responses is always the same. The extent of the response depends on the intensity and duration of the initiating insult. An important point to remember is that the inflammatory response is a compensatory mechanism that is immediately helpful to the body when invasion or injury occurs. These actions are intended to function on a relatively local and short-term basis. When these actions are widespread and/or persistent, they may result in other physiologic complications that adversely affect the maintenance of homeostasis.

The inflammatory responses to injury occur primarily at the vascular level. Damaged tissues and macrophages within the tissues release chemical substances (histamine, bradykinin, serotonin, and other vasoactive amines) that induce vasodilation and increase capillary permeability (Fig. 16-5). When tissue damage is extensive, these substances are secreted in large amounts, are circulated systemically, and induce the vascular changes in all tissues, not just those directly involved in the injury. These vascular changes are responsible for the early clinical cardiovascular manifestations and complications that are associated with burn injuries. In addition to the substances that have effects on the blood and blood vessels, chemotactic substances are secreted by tissue macrophages, which attract specific leukocytes to

NORMAL BLOOD CAPILLARY

Water molecule

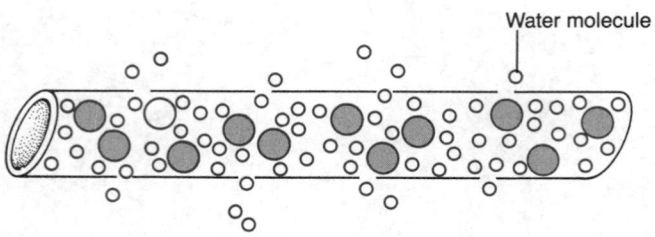

Water is the smallest molecule that can pass through the capillary pores.

POSTBURN BLOOD CAPILLARY

Protein molecule

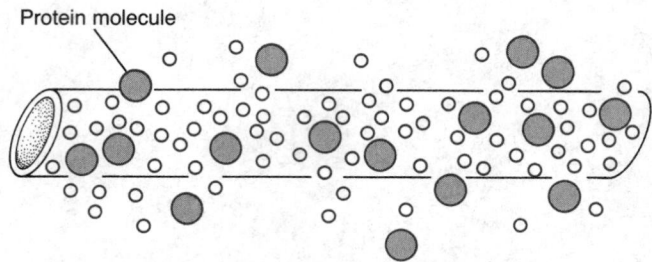

Permeability is drastically increased, which allows large molecules such as proteins to pass through the capillary pores easily.

Figure 16-5.

Vascular capillary response to burn injury.

the site of injury and alter bone marrow production and maturation of leukocytes. These alterations have profound immediate and later effects on immune function.

Activation of Sympathetic Nervous System Compensatory Responses

The sympathetic nervous system stress responses are generated by the sympathetic division of the autonomic nervous system in conjunction with the endocrine system as internal reactions to conditions that threaten to disrupt internal homeostasis. These reactions are sometimes termed the *general adaptive syndrome* or the *fight-or-flight* reactions because they prepare the body for activities that allow alteration or removal of the initiating conditions. The stress responses generate immediate physiologic changes (adaptations) that excite or enhance those functions necessary for fight or flight and inhibit those functions that do not immediately contribute to flight or flight. Figure 16–6 summarizes compensatory changes of the autonomic nervous system.

The excitatory physiologic changes include increased rate and depth of respiration; increased heart rate; se-

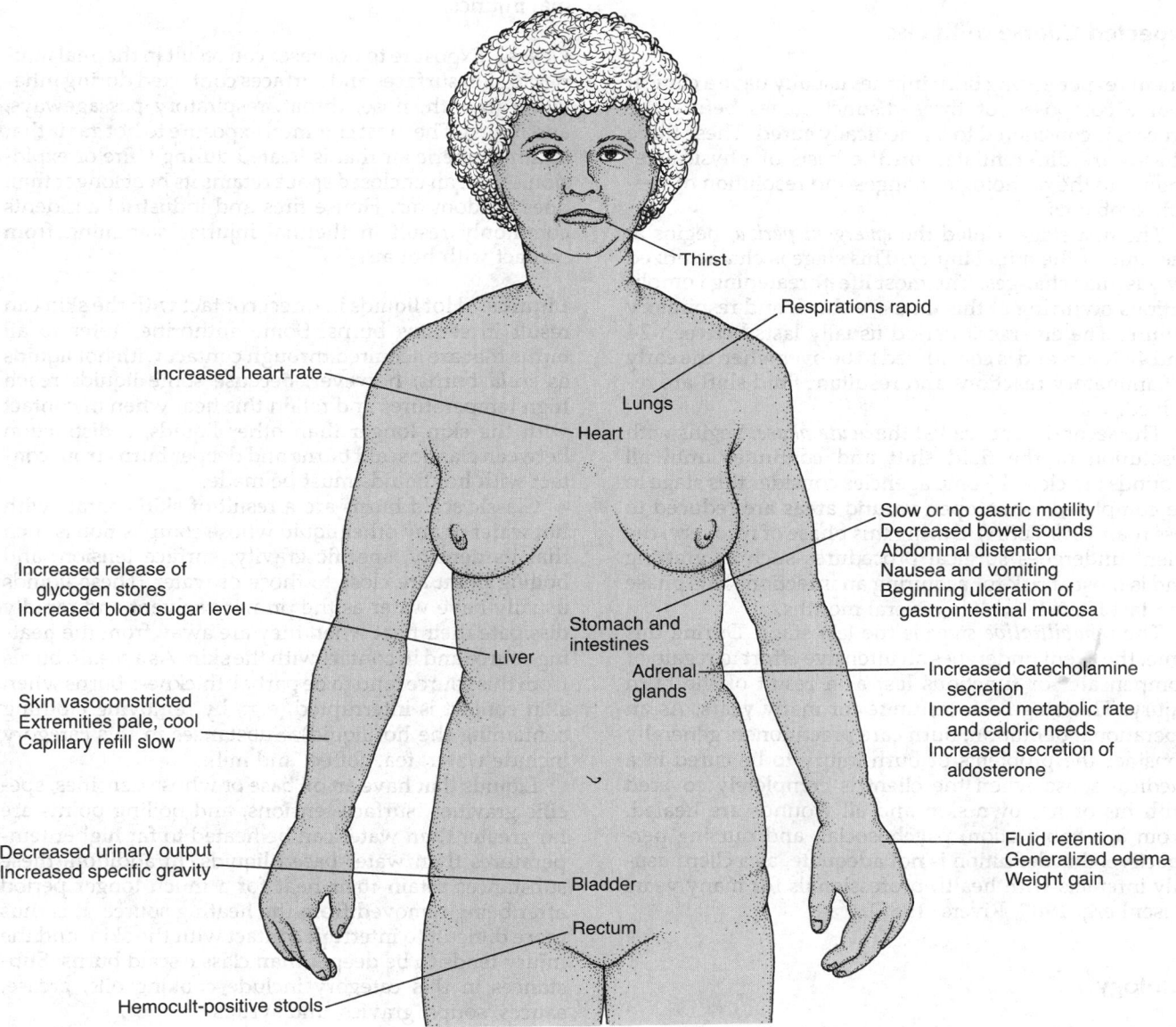

Figure 16–6.

Physiologic reactions of autonomic nervous system compensatory responses to burn injury (emergent phase).

lective vasoconstriction; increased blood flow to brain, liver, skeletal muscles, and myocardium; increased rate of metabolism and formation of high-energy substances; and release of stored glycogen and fatty fuel sources. The inhibitory physiologic changes include decreased blood flow to the skin, kidney, and gastrointestinal tract; and decreased gastrointestinal motility and secretions. These responses are beneficial to the body for short periods and assist in maintenance of proper function of vital organs under adverse conditions. However, when the sympathetic stress responses continue for prolonged periods without external intervention, the responses become more stressful than beneficial to the individual and create pathologic conditions, leading to exhaustion of adaptive resources.

Expected Course of Illness

Clients experiencing burn injuries usually have a clinical course composed of three distinct stages before the process is considered to be medically cured. These three phases are differentiated on the basis of physical response to the pathologic changes and resolution of specific problems.

The first stage, called the *emergent period,* begins at the time of the initial injury. This stage is characterized by vascular changes. The most life-threatening complications occurring at this time are shock and respiratory failure. The emergent period usually lasts between 24 and 48 hours and is considered to be over when the early inflammatory reactions and resultant fluid shift are resolved.

The second stage, called the *acute phase,* begins with resolution of the fluid shift and continues until all wounds are closed (some agencies consider this stage to be completed when open wound areas are reduced to less than 10% TBSA). During this phase of recovery, the client undergoes surgical procedures such as grafting and is most at risk for acquiring an infection. This phase can last from 1 week to several months.

The *rehabilitative stage* is the last stage. During this time, the client undergoes an intensive effort to regain or compensate for functions lost as a result of the burn injury. This stage can continue for many years. As an operational definition, burn care practitioners generally consider the problems of burn injury to be cured in a medical sense when the client is completely covered with his or her own skin and all wounds are healed. From a rehabilitation, psychosocial, and nursing perspective, this definition is not adequate, as a client usually interacts with health professionals for many years (Eisenberg, 1987; Rivers, 1987).

Etiology

Most burn injuries are acquired accidentally. Conditions or sources that are responsible for burn injuries include exposure to temperature extremes, especially heat (sun, flames, hot liquids, hot air, contact with hot solid surfaces); chemicals; high-voltage electricity; and ionizing radiation.

Thermal Burns

Thermal burn injuries involve contact of the skin with hot substances. The substances can be gases, liquids, or solids. For all hot substances, the degree of thermal injury inflicted depends on the intensity of the heat in the substance and the duration of contact with the skin and epithelial surfaces. The nature of the substances commonly causing thermal injuries changes with technology and availability. For example, during the last 20 years curling irons and foods heated rapidly in microwave ovens have been common causes of thermal injuries.

Gases.   Exposure to hot gases can result in thermal injuries to skin surfaces and surfaces contacted during inhalation (mouth, nose, throat, respiratory passageways, and lungs). The most common exposure to hot gas is that to atmospheric air that is heated during a fire or explosion. Air in an enclosed space retains its heat longer than does outdoor air. House fires and industrial accidents commonly result in thermal injuries stemming from contact with hot air.

Liquids.   Hot liquids in direct contact with the skin can result in serious burns. Some authorities refer to all burns that are acquired through contact with hot liquids as *scald* burns; however, because some liquids reach high temperatures and retain this heat when in contact with the skin longer than other liquids, a distinction between classic scald burns and deeper burns from contact with hot liquids must be made.

Classic scald burns are a result of skin contact with hot water or any other liquid whose composition is such that its density, specific gravity, surface tension, and boiling point are close to those of water. These liquids usually have water as the primary solvent and rapidly dissipate their heat when they are away from the heating source and in contact with the skin. As a result, burns from this source tend to be partial-thickness burns when skin contact is interrupted (e.g., by removing clothing containing the hot liquid). Substances in this category include water, tea, coffee, and milk.

Liquids that have an oil base or whose densities, specific gravities, surface tensions, and boiling points are far greater than water can be heated to far higher temperatures than water-based liquids. In addition, these substances retain their heat for a much longer period after being removed from the heating source. It is thus more difficult to interrupt contact with the skin, and the injury tends to be deeper than classic scald burns. Substances in this category include cooking oils, grease, sauces, soups, gravies, and syrups.

Solids.   How easily heat can be transferred from a hot solid surface to the skin depends on how much heat the solid can hold and how it conducts or dissipates heat. Solids that retain high temperatures and rapidly transfer this heat to contacted skin include metals, ceramics, some plastics, glass, concrete, and stone.

Chemical Burns

Chemical burns occur when specific chemicals (in gaseous, liquid, or solid form) come into direct contact with skin and epithelial surfaces. Although some chemical reactions produce and release heat, chemical heat production is not a requirement for a burn injury to tissues. Chemicals capable of causing burn injuries are usually strong acids, such as hydrochloric acid, chromic acid, or sulfuric acid, or strong bases, such as sodium hydroxide. Burns from these sources are most frequently encountered in industrial settings.

In addition to strong chemicals, almost any chemical can result in a burn injury if it remains in direct contact with the skin for a long enough period. Such relatively innocuous substances include soaps and soap solutions, concentrated salt solutions, and urine.

Electrical Burns

Electricity is present in American society in several forms and various strengths. Electrical current is delivered as alternating current or direct current. Alternating current, which is most prevalent in the United States, can cause more severe injuries than direct current. A volt is the measurement of electrical potential and an ampere is the measurement of electrical strength. Most severe electrical injuries are attributed to high-voltage (>7000 volts) accidents, although house current of 155 volts can also cause considerable damage.

True electrical injury causes tissue destruction as the current flows from the point of contact to the point of grounding (Fig. 16–7). It is difficult to track the path of electricity by external visualization, and often surgical exploration is needed to evaluate damage to subdermal tissue.

Electricity travels through the body moving with least resistance along the nerves; with increasing resistance along the blood vessels, muscles, skin, tendons, and fat; and with the greatest resistance through bone. As resistance increases, electrical energy is converted to heat. Therefore, the muscles surrounding the long bones of the body, where resistance is the greatest, are usually subjected to great amounts of heat and sustain the most damage. Recent studies suggest that beneath the skin, all tissues act as volume conductors and allow current to be dispersed throughout the entire mass, such as an arm or a leg, which results in severe injury. In large areas where the current can diffuse, such as the thorax, the resultant damage is usually less severe.

Electrical injuries are often masked by healthy viable surface tissues because the greatest damage generally occurs in deep muscle close to the bone. This phenomenon is called the *iceberg effect*, which alludes to the fact that most actual tissue damage is beneath the surface. In

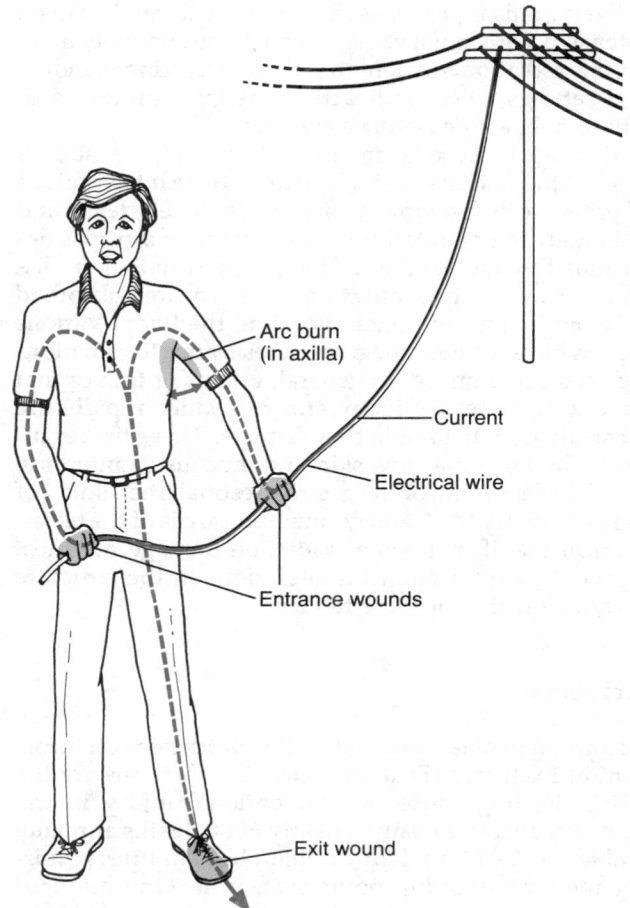

Figure 16–7.

Mechanism of electrical injury. Current travels along the path of least resistance. Nerves are the least resistant tissue, followed by blood vessels, skin, muscle, and bone.

addition to soft-tissue damage, electricity can cause bone fractures and joint dislocations as a result of tetanic contracture. The electrical current can also cause cardiac changes as minor as a skipped beat and as major as ventricular fibrillation.

Other injuries that are not directly related to the movement of current through the tissue include arc burns and flame burns. Arc burns are most often found in wet areas of the body near the junction of two surfaces, such as the axilla or the commissure of the lips. The damage is usually deep and runs from the surface downward. In addition, in an arc burn the clothing may catch fire or a flash-type injury may occur.

Radiation Burns

Radiation injuries are caused when clients are exposed to high doses of radioactive material. The most common type of radiation exposure leading to tissue injury occurs in conjunction with therapeutic radiation delivery. This injury is usually minor and rarely causes extensive skin damage. Less frequent but possibly more serious radiation accidents are those occurring in industrial settings where radioactive energy is produced or where radioactive isotopes are used.

Damage is caused primarily at the cellular level: particles in the nucleus are ionized and create interruptions of critical cell function, which leads to cell death and ultimately to organ failure. The severity of injury is determined by factors that include type of radiation, distance from source, duration of exposure, absorbed dose, and depth of penetration into the body. Various organs have different degrees of resistance to radiation-induced cell damage. In general, organs or tissues that have a high mitotic index and reproduce rapidly are most susceptible to radiation damage. These tissues include the bone marrow, skin and mucous membranes, hair follicles, lining of the gastrointestinal tract, lining of the pulmonary tract, and germinating areas of the testes. Clinical manifestations of radiation damage are most frequently associated with alterations in the structure and/or function of these tissues.

Incidence

According to data compiled by the National Burn Information Exchange (Feller & Jones, 1987), burns are the fourth leading cause of unintentional injury in the United States and result in nearly 6000 deaths annually (Table 16–1). More than 1 million burn injuries requiring medical attention occur each year. One hundred thousand of those persons injured are admitted to hospitals, with an average stay in the hospital being 12 days. Causes of burn injury in rank order of hospital admission are (1) scald burns, (2) clothing ignition, (3) gasoline accidents, (4) car fires, and (5) chemical burns. Within the home, the kitchen remains the most common

site of burn injuries. Burn injuries occur most frequently among children younger than 5 years old, adults between the ages of 18 and 30 years, and adults older than 70 years of age (Trier & Spaabaek, 1987). After early childhood, males experience burn injuries at more than twice the rate of females. More burn injuries occur among non-Caucasians and among the socioeconomically disadvantaged than among Caucasian, middle-income Americans.

PREVENTION

The vast majority of burn injuries occur as a result of an accident. Some of the changes to the individual that are caused by a burn may never be eradicated. Scars, contractures, and other disfiguring effects of burns may always remain with the client.

An estimated 50% to 70% of all burns are preventable though education or legislation (Silverstein & Lack, 1987; Varas & Hammond, 1989). Burn prevention approaches involve manipulation of either the potential victim or the causative agent. Nurses play major roles in both approaches.

In the area of education, clients in the community must be made aware of safety measures that they can take to reduce the risk of accidental burns. Before presenting information about burn prevention, the nurse assesses the needs and specific risk factors of the target audience so that the presentation is meaningful and appropriate. For example, many older people are burned in kitchen accidents or by ignition of clothing as a result of falling asleep while smoking. Therefore, information about kitchen safety is pertinent for this group, as is the recommendation not to smoke in bed, late at night, or after taking medications that induce drowsiness.

Scald burns are common injuries to children and the elderly. Recommended safety measures to avoid scalds include (1) reducing the temperature of hot-water heaters to lower than 120° F (49° C), (2) installing a special adjustable water mixing valve on showers and wash basins that does not allow water higher than a certain temperature to be dispensed, and (3) supervising children, elderly persons, and disabled adults during baths and showers.

Legislation that has helped to increase public awareness of fire safety and prevention includes the Flammable Fabric Act of 1952 (amended in 1971). This act mandates clothing manufacturers to make all children's sleepwear out of fire-retardant material. Some communities have enacted legislation for the installation and maintenance of smoke alarms in apartment buildings, public housing, schools, hotels, motels, and restaurants. Similar actions, such as legislation forcing hot-water heater manufacturers to limit the maximal temperature setting on water heaters and laws requiring cigarette manufacturers to produce a cigarette that is self-extinguishing, are currently being considered.

TABLE 16–1 Deaths Occurring from Unintentional Injury in 1986

Rank/Cause	Number of Deaths
1. Motor vehicle crashes (traffic)	47,865
2. Falls	11,444
3. Poisoning	5,740
4. Fires and burns	5,689
5. Drowning	4,777
6. Complications from medical procedures	3,069
7. Firearms	1,452

From U.S. National Center for Health Statistics. *Vital Statistics of the United States, Annual 1986.*

EMERGENCY CARE

Burn injuries can occur almost anywhere. Emergency care at the scene of injury for any burned client focuses on limiting the extent of the injury and maintaining the function of vital organs.

Emergency Interventions Limiting Extent of Injury

Thermal Injuries

For thermal injuries, prolonged contact with the source of heat increases the depth of injury. Emergency care involves removing the source of heat from the client. Clients should *Stop, Drop,* and *Roll* to smother the flames. Rescuers try to prevent the client from running because this motion tends to fan the flames and increase the risk of sustaining serious injury. Clothes that are on fire or saturated with hot liquids are removed. As simple as this instruction may seem, it is often overlooked in emergency situations, and clients have been admitted to emergency departments wearing clothes that are still smoldering. Burn wounds that are caused by flames or hot liquids are cooled with the use of tepid water. This rapid cooling prevents additional damage to the tissues. If dry, sterile dressings are available, they are applied before the client is transferred to an acute care facility. Although wet dressings are more comfortable for the client, these are avoided with large burn wounds to prevent hypothermia.

Chemical Injuries

The emergency treatment of most chemical burns usually starts with brushing the dry form of the chemicals from skin surfaces and then flushing the affected area with copious amounts of water or normal saline. Water serves to neutralize most chemicals while simultaneously dissipating any heat reaction. Some chemical burns are flushed with other specific solutions to prevent further injury. Standard flushes are listed in the accompanying Emergency Care feature. Chemical agents containing sodium or potassium may continue to burn in the presence of water. Injuries caused by these substances are covered with mineral oil before transfer of the client to a burn center. Neutralization of one chemical substance with another should be undertaken

EMERGENCY CARE ■ Early Treatment of Chemical Burns

Chemicals Causing the Burn	Specific Early Treatment	Rationale
Clorox	Flush with copious amounts of water or normal saline.	To mechanically remove surface chemicals and cool skin (saline inhibits fluid uptake and electrolyte loss from open areas).
Lye		
Phenol		
Chromic acid		
Potassium permanganate		
Cantharides		
Dimethyl sulfoxide		
Dichromic salts		
Tungstic acid		
Acetic acid		
Formic acid		
Sulfosalicylic acid		
Tannic acid		
Trichloroacetic acid		
Hydrofluoric acid	Administer topical calcium salts.	To buffer the acid and limit injury.
Sodium metal	Coat affected area with mineral oil.	To inhibit caustic action.
Cresol		
White phosphorus		
Nitrogen mustard		

only by health care practitioners who are familiar with the specific chemicals involved.

Electrical Injuries

For electrical burns, emergency treatment starts with separating the client from the electrical current. This action involves either shutting off the electric current source or carefully removing clients from the source by using nonconductive implements such as wooden poles and ropes made of plant fiber.

Radiation Injuries

Clients who are burned by exposure to radiation may require more extensive emergency care than can be administered at the site of the injury. If the radiation source is fixed or sealed, the client may be removed from the area by personnel wearing lead-lined shielding. Once removed from such a source, the client is not radioactive and does not pose a danger to others. If the radiation source is not sealed and involves particulate matter that may actually cling to the client, the client is radioactive and is a danger to others. Industries that use such radioactive materials usually have decontamination facilities and teams on site so that the decontamination process can begin there. If such facilities are not available, the client is transferred to the hospital.

Hospitals that have the potential for radiation accidents in their catchment area should have a policy and procedure for handling admission of clients who are affected by such accidents. This protocol identifies a location that is external or somewhat detached from the main hospital as an area for triage and decontamination. Staff members working to decontaminate clients take precautions similar to those used by operating room personnel. Caps, masks, plastic shoe covers, and waterproof cover gowns are worn. Double gloving is recommended when handling contaminated equipment, clothing, or wounds. Once decontamination is complete, the client is transferred to the main hospital area by transport personnel who have not been in the decontamination zone.

Emergency Interventions Supporting Vital Organ Function

The most common problems associated with burn injuries are shock, cardiac arrest, and airway obstruction. Shock is usually seen when forms of trauma in addition to the burn injury are present. Assessment of clinical manifestations and emergency management of shock are described in Chapter 17. A common complication that is associated with electrical burns is cardiac arrest, which necessitates immediate initiation of external cardiopulmonary resuscitation.

Upper airway obstruction is also possible as a result of direct injury to pulmonary epithelium or as a result of the presence of toxic substances in the inhaled air. Moving the client to an area that is free from smoke and other respiratory irritants helps to limit pulmonary damage. Any foreign objects in the mouth or upper airway are removed. If oxygen is available at the scene of the injury, it is administered to the client by mask or nasal cannula.

COLLABORATIVE MANAGEMENT

 Assessment

History

In the case of a burn client, the history must be obtained immediately on arrival of the client to the health care facility. Shortly after admission, the client frequently is intubated, is sedated, or becomes disoriented because of shock, and it may be impossible to obtain an accurate history. Information to obtain includes standard demographic data, health history, and specific data surrounding the injurious event.

In obtaining a history from a client who is burned, the nurse keeps in mind the potential complications associated with burn injuries. Pertinent information to obtain regarding the history of the accident includes (1) time of injury, (2) source of heat or injurious agent, (3) detailed description of how the burn occurred, (4) whether the influence of alcohol or drugs may have been a factor, (5) the physical surroundings of the immediate area where the burn was sustained, (6) the events occurring from the time of burn to admission to health care facility, and (7) any other events or circumstances contributing to the injury.

Burns often are associated with concomitant traumatic injuries and pre-existing disease or illness. These problems may have contributed in some way to the circumstances causing the burn and may drastically affect morbidity. *Age* is an important factor, as is the presence of *chronic illnesses, physical disabilities,* or *pathologic conditions of organs* because elderly clients experience systems alterations more commonly than do younger individuals. For example, diabetes and congestive heart failure may be present, and these processes may interfere with wound healing and fluid resuscitation during treatment. The nurse obtains information about *specific medications* (prescribed and over-the-counter), including time and dosage, that the client may have taken during the preceding 24 hours. It is important to ascertain if the client smokes or uses excessive amounts of alcohol or other chemical substances because these factors can influence treatment and physical responses.

A preburn weight, if it is known by the client, is also

of immediate importance, as is the client's height. This "dry" weight is used to calculate TBSA, extent of injury, fluid rates, energy requirements, and drug dosages. As a back-up to this reported weight, an in-hospital weight is also obtained as early in the course of treatment as possible. After treatment is initiated, an accurate estimation of preburn weight is difficult.

Other pertinent information that can be valuable in providing psychosocial support to the client and family as well as in forming a basis for rehabilitation and discharge planning includes sex, race, religion, dietary habits, cultural background, occupation, family history, social history, and financial history. Obtaining much of this information, however, can be deferred until the client's physical condition is stable.

Physical Assessment: Clinical Manifestations

Initial physical assessment findings may vary greatly from findings made later in the course of the illness. Expected assessment findings are discussed by using a systems approach. The areas or systems that are assessed first are those that can have immediate, life-threatening alterations in function.

Respiratory system. All clients with burn injuries are at risk for developing some respiratory complications related to direct heat injury, carbon monoxide toxicity, smoke poisoning, edema, or fluid therapy. Respiratory manifestations that are commonly associated with a burn injury are presented in the accompanying Key Features of Disease.

Direct airway injury. The nurse initially assesses the client's respiratory system by paying close attention to the appearance and function of the mouth, nose, pharynx, trachea, and pulmonary mechanics. Burns of the head, face, neck, and upper thorax increase the possibility of an inhalation injury. The nurse observes the client for the presence of any facial injury or singed hair on the head, eyebrows, eyelids, and nasal mucosa. The lips and oral mucosa are inspected for the presence of blisters and soot. Sputum is examined for carbonaceous particles.

Other indicators of possible impending pulmonary complications are alterations in breathing patterns. The client may become progressively hoarse, and expiratory sounds may include grossly audible wheezes, crowing, and stridor. Upper airway edema and inhalation burn damage are most notable in the trachea and mainstem bronchi. The nurse auscultates these areas, first listening for wheezes as a sign of obstruction. Clients with severe inhalation injuries may sustain such progressive obstruction that in a short time it is not possible to force air through the narrowed airways. As a result, the wheezing sounds disappear. The disappearance of wheezing sounds in such a client indicates pathologic progression and not improvement. This situation demands prompt

KEY FEATURES OF DISEASE ■ Diagnosis and Signs and Symptoms of Upper Airway Obstruction and Inhalation Injury

Upper Airway Obstruction	Inhalation Injury
Medical Diagnostic Approaches	
History taking (peak incidence — the period of peak burn edema — is 12 to 24 h after injury)	History taking (smoke exposure)
Direct laryngoscopy (mucosal changes and degree of laryngeal edema)	Confinement in an enclosed space
	Elevated carboxyhemoglobin level
Spirometry to detect early airway changes	Fiberoptic bronchoscopy to indicate the presence of injury
Fiberoptic bronchoscopy to detect mucosal injury	Ventilation-perfusion lung scanning by using ^{135}Xe to detect changes in small airways
	Measurement of extravascular lung water (of minimal benefit)
Clinical Signs and Symptoms	
Edema, erythema, and ulceration of airway mucosa, especially posterior pharynx	Airway injury
	Carbonaceous sputum
	Singed nasal hairs
Increased hoarseness	Bronchorrhea
Stridor	Wheezing
Any face or neck burn with edema formation	Pulmonary vasoconstriction
	Reduced cardiac output
Heat-induced intraoral injury	Bronchospasm

recognition and initiation of appropriate emergency interventions.

Carbon monoxide poisoning. Carbon monoxide is a gas that is a by-product of combustion. Clients with any degree of inhalation injury are at risk for concomitant carbon monoxide poisoning. Once this gas is inhaled, it easily diffuses into the blood where it binds tightly to the hemoglobin molecule at the same site where oxygen usually binds. As a result of this tight binding, carbon monoxide prevents the binding and transporting of adequate amounts of oxygen to the tissues, and severe hypoxia can occur. The accompanying Key Features of Disease summarizes the physiologic effects of carbon monoxide poisoning. The first indicators of carbon monoxide poisoning are associated with cerebral hypoxia and include headache, nausea, drowsiness, confusion, and stupor, which may progress to coma. These symptoms may be present with or without other associated respiratory alterations.

Smoke poisoning. Damage to the epithelial tissue in the lower respiratory tract can occur as a result of inhaling smoke that contains incomplete products of combustion (such as oxides) from the burning of sulfur, ni-

trogen, aldehydes, and hydrochloric acid. The exact local effect of each agent varies slightly, but these substances also produce generalized pulmonary effects. The most significant effects include atelectasis and the formation of pulmonary edema in response to decreased surfactant production and loss of epithelial cilia. Pulmonary edema is enhanced by the local and generalized increased capillary permeability and the increased fluid load resulting from treatment during the emergent phase. Six to 72 hours after the burn, pulmonary epithelial sloughing occurs, which contributes to a hemorrhagic bronchitis and pulmonary parenchymal failure.

Pulmonary parenchymal failure. Pulmonary parenchymal failure occurs when alveolar exchange becomes irreversibly impaired because of destruction of type I and type II alveolar cells. Damage can occur as a result of the burn injury, infection, immunosuppression, or treatment. Figure 16–8 shows the interrelated events contributing to pulmonary failure. Clients cannot maintain sufficient surfactant production for adequate alveolar compliance, and bronchopneumonia develops. Clients are short of breath and hypoxic. Breath sounds are moist with crackles present. Overall, the outlook for clients with this type of pulmonary problem is poor.

Pulmonary fluid overload. The condition of pulmonary edema occurs when the lung tissues have not sustained any direct damage. Instead, other damaged tissues release such large quantities of vasoactive amines, which increase capillary permeability, that even pulmonary capillaries leak fluid into pulmonary inter-

KEY FEATURES OF DISEASE ■ Effects of Carbon Monoxide Poisoning

Carbon Monoxide Level	Physiologic Effects
1–10% (normal)	Increased threshold to visual stimuli
	Increased blood flow to vital organs
11–20% (mild poisoning)	Headache
	Decreased cerebral function
	Decreased visual acuity
	Slight breathlessness
21–40% (moderate poisoning)	Headache
	Tinnitus
	Nausea
	Drowsiness
	Vertigo
	Altered mental state
	Confusion
	Stupor
	Irritability
	Decreased blood pressure and heart rate
	Depressed ST segment on electrocardiogram and arrhythmias on palpation
	Pale to reddish-purple skin
41–60% (severe poisoning)	Coma
	Convulsions
	Cardiopulmonary instability
61–80% (fatal poisoning)	Death

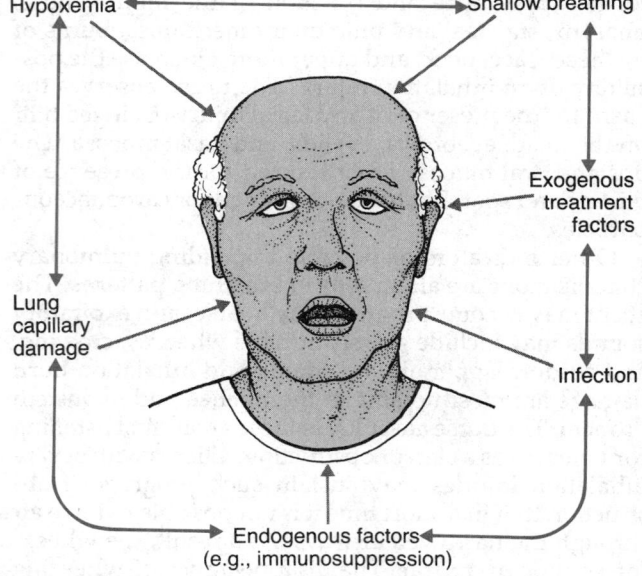

Figure 16–8.

Interactions of factors leading to pulmonary failure in clients with burn injuries.

stitial spaces. In addition, circulatory overload that is associated with fluid resuscitation causes left-sided congestive heart failure. This overload creates such high hydrostatic pressures within pulmonary vessels that even more fluid is lost from the pulmonary vascular space into the interstitial space. This excess interstitial fluid increases the diffusing distance for both oxygen and carbon dioxide between the alveoli and the capillaries. As a result, the rate and efficiency of alveolar gas exchange diminish. These clients are extremely short of breath and experience increased dyspnea in the supine position.

External factors.   Clients with burn injuries may have respiratory difficulties as a result of external factors in addition to problems associated with the pulmonary system. The most common external factor affecting respiration is the presence of tight eschar, which either restricts chest movement or compresses anatomic structures in the neck and throat to such an extent that ventilation is impaired. The nurse visually assesses the ease of respiration and the amount of chest movement that the client achieves during inhalation and exhalation.

Cardiovascular system.   Changes in the cardiovascular system begin immediately after the burn injury and include shock of various etiologies. Shock is the most common cause of death in the immediate postburn period among clients with burn injuries. Chapter 17 provides a complete discussion of the pathophysiology and compensatory mechanisms for all types of shock. The initial cardiovascular changes in clients experiencing a burn injury appear to be related to the inflammatory processes that stimulate vasogenic and hypovolemic shock.

Tissues that are damaged during the burn injury release substances (histamine, serotonin, and kinins) that cause vasodilation and increase capillary permeability (Chap. 23). With small burns (<20% TBSA), this increased capillary permeability is confined to the injured area, with resulting blister formation, formation of local edema, or both. With larger burns, the amount of substances released is so great that these vasoactive amines enter the circulatory system and cause systemic effects. The capillary pores, or fenestrations, become larger, so that even relatively low capillary hydrostatic pressures force plasma, electrolytes, and protein molecules into the interstitial space, which creates a vascular fluid volume deficit and decreased mean arterial pressure (Lund et al., 1988). These conditions cause hypovolemic shock, which, if it is allowed to progress, leads to cardiogenic shock (Chap. 17).

The initial cardiovascular clinical manifestations reflect hypovolemia and decreased cardiac output. The nurse assesses the client's cardiovascular status by measuring the central and peripheral pulses, blood pressure, and capillary refill, and by noting the presence of edema. Heart rate is rapid and thready. Blood pressure is below normal, with a wide pulse pressure. The hypotension is more acute in the upright and standing posi-

tions. Peripheral pulses are difficult to discern, especially as edema increases, and are easily obliterated. As tissue perfusion decreases, peripheral capillary refill is slow or absent. When fluid resuscitation efforts are initiated during the capillary leak phase, edema increases, as does the client's weight.

The initial phase of inflammatory response and capillary leaking usually resolves in about 48 hours. At this time, the excess interstitial fluid is returned to systemic circulation. The clinical cardiovascular manifestations that are associated with this event include rapid "bounding" pulses, elevated blood pressure (especially diastolic), diminished edema, and improved capillary refill. Clients are at risk for developing circulatory overload, heart failure, and pulmonary edema during this phase.

Electrocardiographic changes indicative of electrical damage to the heart are frequently associated with electrical burn injuries or with situational stress that induces a myocardial infarction. Cardiac function assessment includes obtaining electrocardiographic tracings at the time of the client's admission to the hospital or burn center and daily throughout the emergent period. Some burn centers maintain cardiac monitoring of all burn clients until resolution of the fluid shift is complete.

Renal system.   The renal system is seldom directly affected by a burn injury. Rather, changes in renal function associated with burn injuries are related to the secondary alterations of renal perfusion and the presence of cellular debris. During the fluid shift of the emergent period, adequate perfusion to allow glomerular filtration may be difficult to achieve. As a result, urinary output is greatly diminished compared with intravenous fluid intake. The urine is highly concentrated and has a high specific gravity.

Other substances may be present in the blood that perfuses the kidney as a result of specific tissue damage. Destroyed red blood cells release hemoglobin and potassium. When injury to muscle occurs with the burn injury, a large oxygen-carrying protein called myoglobin is released from damaged muscle and circulates to the kidney. Most damaged cells release protein products that form uric acid. All of these large molecules in the blood may precipitate in the kidney tubular system. This precipitation blocks filtrate flow and may contribute to severe renal dysfunction.

The nurse assesses renal function by accurately measuring urinary output and comparing this value to fluid intake. In addition, the nurse measures the specific gravity and the hemoglobin content of the urine. Urine is examined visually for color, odor, and the presence of particulate matter and foam.

Integumentary system.   The skin is assessed to determine the size and depth of the injury. Estimations of the size of the injury are first made in comparison to the TBSA. The size of the injury is important not only for diagnosis and prognosis but also for calculating specific therapeutic parameters such as drug dosage, fluid replacement volumes, and caloric needs. The nurse inspects the skin visually for changes in color and appearance to delineate which areas are actually injured. Except for electrical burns, this initial size assessment can usually be made accurately by using specific assessment tools and charts.

The most rapid method used to calculate the size of a burn injury in adult clients whose weights are in normal proportion to their heights is the *rule of nines*. This method, as outlined in Figure 16–9, divides the body into areas that are multiples of 9%. This method, although useful at the site of injury and in emergency departments, is not accurate for estimating percentage of TBSA for children or for adults who are of small stature, extremely thin, or obese.

Other more accurate but more time-consuming methods used to calculate the size of injury are the Lund and Browder comparison chart and the Berkow method. These methods include factors such as age and disproportionate weight-to-height conditions in the calculation equation. Figure 16–10 shows how the Berkow method is used to estimate size of injury.

Because specific treatments of burn injuries are related to depth of injury, initial assessment of the integumentary system includes estimations of burn depth.

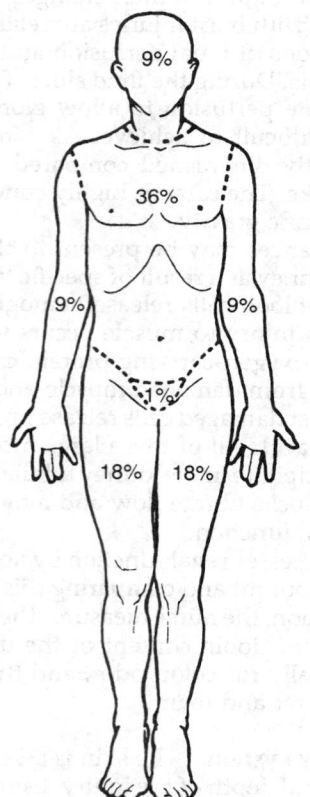

Figure 16–9.
Estimation of extent of injury by the rule of nines method.

Criteria for establishing depth of injury based on appearance and associated characteristics were discussed under the heading Classification of Burn Depth. During the course of illness, reassessments of burn size and depth are made to evaluate treatment outcomes and to plan additional interventions. Usually, these assessments are made weekly during the client's hospitalization by individuals with extensive experience in assessing wound healing and skin growth.

Gastrointestinal system. Although no direct injury occurs to the gastrointestinal tract in most burn patients, alterations in gastrointestinal function are expected after these injuries. Most of these changes occur as a result of the inflammatory and autonomic compensatory mechanisms.

In the emergent period, the profound sympathetic nervous system discharge inhibits gastric motility and secretions as the energy and resources necessary for these functions are shunted to more vital structures. Total cessation of peristalsis is common and is known as *paralytic ileus.* Food and fluids that are present in the stomach are not moved further along the tract for processing. As a result, the client cannot obtain nutrients by the oral route. In addition, gastric dilation and vomiting may occur, which increases the possibility of aspiration.

The nurse assesses gastrointestinal motility by auscultating the abdomen for bowel sounds. These sounds are diminished or absent in the client with severe burns. Associated clinical manifestations include nausea, vomiting, and abdominal distention.

The inflammatory compensatory reactions permit the release of increased amounts of histamine to all areas, including the gastrointestinal mucosa. This action, coupled with the stress response, causes ulcer formation within the gastrointestinal mucosa. These ulcerated areas can become quite large and can be responsible for blood loss. Although the conditions that initiate these responses begin in the emergent period, ulcerations may persist throughout the emergent and acute phases. The nurse examines the stool and vomitus for the presence of gross blood or material indicative of partially digested blood. In addition, rapid tests (e.g., Hemoccult) for the presence of occult blood are also performed with these specimens.

Neuroendocrine system. Many clinical manifestations that are associated with burn injuries result from compensatory responses by the neuroendocrine system. These manifestations are primarily caused by altered metabolism.

One purpose of metabolism is to provide energy in the form of heat to maintain a nearly constant core body temperature. Loss of significant amounts of skin reduces the body's ability to retain the heat that is produced by metabolism. Core body temperature is initially below normal, and some hypothermic complications may be present. As a compensatory mechanism, the metabolic rate increases dramatically (through catabolic reactions)

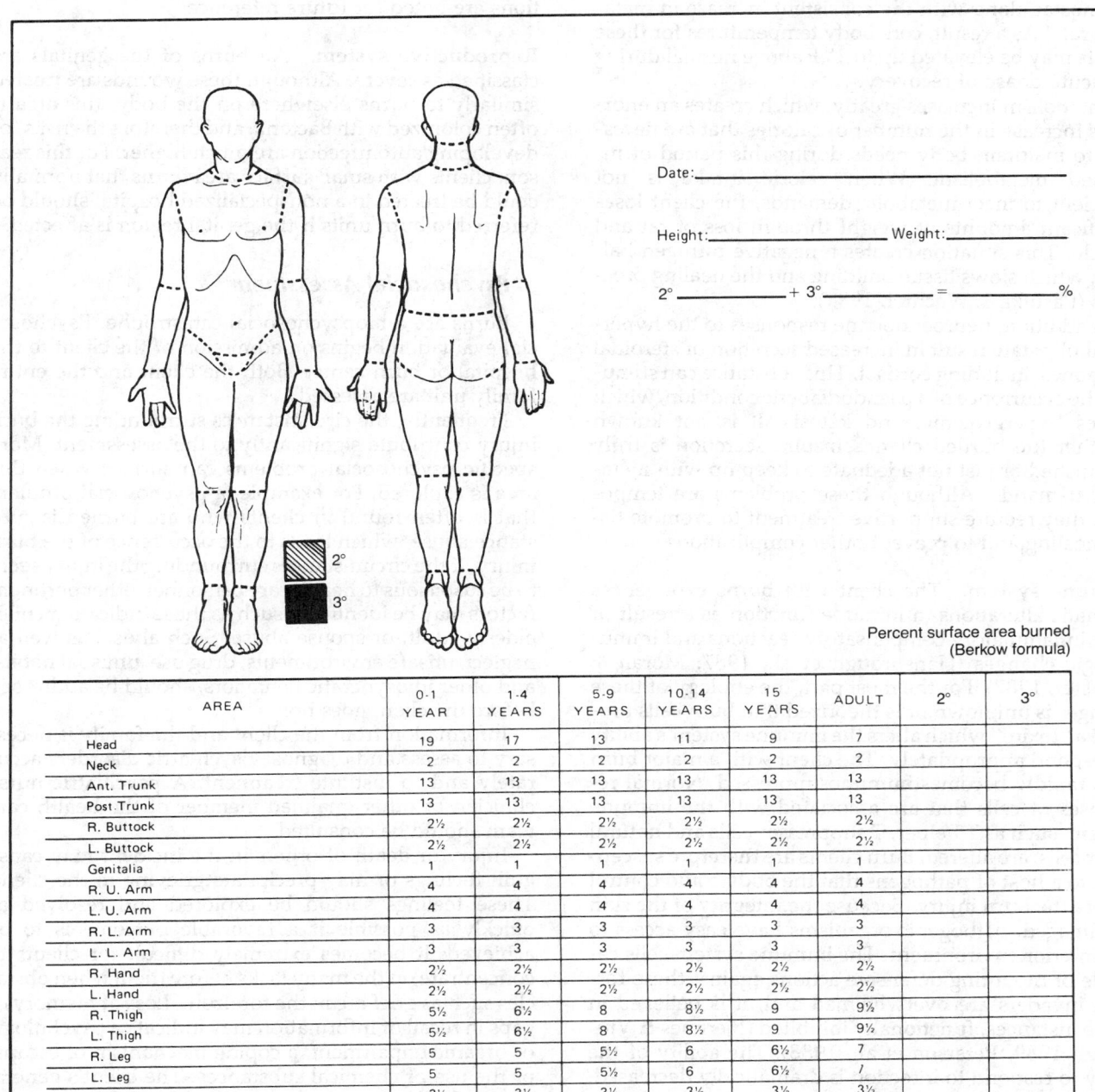

Date:_____

Height:_____   Weight:_____

2° _____ + 3° _____ = _____%

Percent surface area burned
(Berkow formula)

AREA	0-1 YEAR	1-4 YEARS	5-9 YEARS	10-14 YEARS	15 YEARS	ADULT	2°	3°
Head	19	17	13	11	9	7		
Neck	2	2	2	2	2	2		
Ant. Trunk	13	13	13	13	13	13		
Post. Trunk	13	13	13	13	13	13		
R. Buttock	2½	2½	2½	2½	2½	2½		
L. Buttock	2½	2½	2½	2½	2½	2½		
Genitalia	1	1	1	1	1	1		
R. U. Arm	4	4	4	4	4	4		
L. U. Arm	4	4	4	4	4	4		
R. L. Arm	3	3	3	3	3	3		
L. L. Arm	3	3	3	3	3	3		
R. Hand	2½	2½	2½	2½	2½	2½		
L. Hand	2½	2½	2½	2½	2½	2½		
R. Thigh	5½	6½	8	8½	9	9½		
L. Thigh	5½	6½	8	8½	9	9½		
R. Leg	5	5	5½	6	6½	7		
L. Leg	5	5	5½	6	6½	7		
R. Foot	3½	3½	3½	3½	3½	3½		
L. Foot	3½	3½	3½	3½	3½	3½		
TOTAL								

Figure 16–10.

Estimation of extent of injury by the Berkow method. Ant., anterior; Post., posterior; R., right; L., left; R. U., right upper; R. L., right lower; L. U., left upper; L. L., left lower.

to raise the rate of heat production. Eventually, most clients experience a "resetting" of the hypothalamic thermostat along with the consistent increase in metabolic rate. As a result, core body temperatures for these clients may be elevated up to 2° F above normal during the acute phase of recovery.

Catabolism increases greatly, which creates an enormous increase in the number of calories that are necessary to maintain body needs during this period of increased metabolism. When caloric intake is not sufficient to meet metabolic demands, the client loses significant amounts of weight through loss of fat and muscle. This situation creates a negative nitrogen balance, which slows tissue building and the healing processes (Pasulka & Wachtel, 1987).

In addition, neuroendocrine responses to the hypermetabolic state result in increased secretion of steroidal hormones, including cortisol. This substance can stimulate the occurrence of a pseudodiabetic condition, which causes hyperglycemia and ketosis. It is not known whether the burned client's insulin secretion is truly diminished or just not adequate to keep up with metabolic demands. Although these problems are temporary, they require supportive treatment to promote tissue healing and to prevent other complications.

Immune system. The client with burns experiences dramatic alterations in immune function as a result of both inflammatory compensatory reactions and immunologic changes (Hansbrough et al., 1987; Moran & Munster, 1987). For the most part, the etiology of these changes is unknown. It is theorized that burn cells produce a "toxin," which alters the immune system's ability to respond appropriately. The client with a major burn thus rapidly becomes immunosuppressed. Normal responses of cells that are associated with the immune system, such as T helper, T suppressor cells and natural killer cells, are altered. Burn clients are therefore susceptible to a host of pathogens that the body could control before the burn injury. Because the integrity of the skin is damaged, pathogenic organisms have easy access to the interior environment. The immune system cells capable of mounting defensive actions against these foreign invaders are overwhelmed and, it is believed in some instances, functionally inhibited (Bjerknes & Vindenes, 1989; Peterson et al., 1988). The ability of the body to respond to infection is dramatically decreased. This alteration can result in massive infection, sepsis, and death (Barber, 1986; Gurevich & Tafuro, 1986).

Musculoskeletal system. In most clients with burn injuries, the musculoskeletal system does not sustain direct damage. However, burned clients are at risk for developing musculoskeletal problems as a result of other injuries, immobility, healing processes, and treatment. An initial evaluation of the client's musculoskeletal status is necessary within the first few hours after admission to the hospital or burn center. The nurse assesses the client's active and passive range of motion for all joints, including the neck. Special attention is given to joints within the actual burn area. Ranges and limitations are noted for future reference.

Reproductive system. All burns of the genitals are classified as severe. Although these wounds are treated similarly to burns elsewhere on the body, this area is often colonized with bacteria, and therefore the risks for developing autoinfection are much higher. For this reason, clients with small surface area burns that normally could be treated in a nonspecialized hospital should be referred to burn units if the genital region is affected.

Psychosocial Assessment

Burns are a biopsychosocial catastrophe. Psychosocial evaluation begins on admission of the client to the hospital or burn center. Both the client and the entire family unit are assessed.

Frequently, the circumstances surrounding the burn injury contribute significantly to the assessment. More specific psychosocial problems can surface when this area is explored. For example, a psychosocial problem that is often found in clients who are burned is substance abuse, which leads to the occurrence of the burn injury. If the circumstances surrounding the injury seem to be suspicious to health care personnel, other pertinent factors may be identified, such as those indicating child, elderly adult, or spouse abuse. Such abuse, as well as neglect, unsafe environments, drug use, unusual habits, and other idiosyncratic behaviors, should be addressed before the client goes home.

Information from the client and the family is necessary to assess and diagnose psychiatric disorders accurately and to institute treatment. A psychiatric nurse clinician or other qualified member of the health care team should be consulted.

Injury or death of others in the incident may cause guilt feelings or may precipitate grieving in the client. These feelings should be explored and resolved as quickly as possible if a favorable outcome is to be achieved. It becomes extremely difficult for clients to concentrate on the many tasks before them when obstacles such as grief are in the forefront. Loss of memory or gaps in recall of information may indicate a psychologic or organic impairment, a coping mechanism of escape, or the use of chemical substances. The client's general physical affect may be in conflict with the words he or she is speaking. An experienced history taker notes these differences for future reference. For instance, the client may have no facial expression when relating the details of the accident, whereas most clients would show emotion at this time.

Medical conditions may be the underlying cause of psychologic conditions or vice versa. Medical history, especially acute or chronic conditions such as diabetes, organic brain syndrome, alcohol abuse, or physical handicaps, often affects the client's treatment and prognosis. For example, a client who has had chronic back pain for 10 years may not respond in the expected way to pain treatments.

Many psychosocial changes occur after a severe burn, so the client's preburn coping strategies should be identified. Without adequate psychosocial evaluation and intervention, serious changes in behavior and aberrations in social interaction occur, even in the healthiest clients. Emphasis is placed on support and development of trust to aid the client in dealing with the changes that will occur in the client's life.

Current or previously used coping mechanisms of the family members may indicate how they may be expected to cope in the present crisis. If the nurse can encourage clients to recall past ways of successfully dealing with stress and change, a plan that encompasses these previously successful mechanisms can be devised. Knowledge of support structures that are used by clients is necessary because successful coping in this crisis depends on existing support structures. If there are no existing support structures, substitute support structures may be necessary, and the nurse must try to include these in the client's care plan.

Alcohol or drug use may be the cause of the accident or may be the coping mechanism that is used to deal with other problems. If this is the case, the nurse must attempt to redirect the client in a more positive direction because use of drugs and alcohol is not possible for the hospitalized client. In addition, the nurse must be prepared for signs and symptoms of physical withdrawal from these chemicals.

Financial and employment history may be an additional stressor. If the client already has financial or employment difficulties, the accident and hospitalization may exacerbate these problems. Social support needs to be included in the care plan.

Family unit history and the disposition of significant others may have a dramatic impact on the client. It is important for the nurse who assesses the client to understand the dynamics of the family unit to better assist the family in maintaining this unit during this critical time. Cultural mores vary, and different ethnic groups deal with crisis and pain in various ways. What is a normal reaction for one group may appear to be an odd response to a person from a different culture. Strong likes and dislikes often have a cultural basis and should be explored by the nurse.

In the elderly person, senility, which may have contributed to the burn, may indicate the need for more support services in the home. The nurse should attempt to construct a discharge plan that provides for the client's periods of mental inadequacy so a similar accident or other event does not recur.

Most severely burned clients and their families express initially fears of death, and for the first 24 to 48 hours they concentrate on survival. Once survival seems assured, fears start to encompass areas more associated with the quality of life. Fears of disfigurement, loss of function, loss of identity, separation, pain, and guilt begin to emerge. Clients begin a grieving process and cope in ways that are unique to their situations. Destructive coping mechanisms must be identified, and treatment and support throughout all phases of the illness are often necessary (see Chaps. 6, 9, and 11 for further discussion of assessment).

Laboratory Findings

Alterations in laboratory test values are found in different phases of postburn recovery and usually indicate direct tissue damage and expected compensatory mechanisms. Certain alterations in specific laboratory findings indicate the presence of complications.

During the emergent phase, before the initiation of fluid resuscitation, laboratory findings for venous blood samples reflect the fluid shift and direct tissue damage. Baseline laboratory test values and early postburn variations are presented in the accompanying Key Features of Disease. Usually, hemoconcentration is present with elevations of the *hematocrit* and *hemoglobin* levels, along with a decrease in the serum protein concentration. Most serum electrolyte values are elevated at this time. Hyperkalemia and hyperuricemia may be present as potassium and uric acid precursors are released from dead and damaged cells. The composition of the administered replacement fluids may result in reductions in all of the above-mentioned values and serum osmolarity to below normal, as a result of dilution.

Burn clients — even those who have not experienced an actual blood loss — often experience a marked decrease in red blood cell counts during the acute period. This decrease is proportional to the size of the burn and often requires blood cell transfusions.

Values for arterial blood gases provide information about the client's fluid status, efficiency of gas exchange, and the functioning of other cardiovascular parameters. Ineffective gas exchange as a result of any complication associated with burn injuries is usually manifested with a decreased PO_2 and a slightly to moderately increased PCO_2. If the client was burned in an enclosed area, carbon monoxide levels are elevated.

Immune function responses to the trauma of burn injury are reflected in changes of the total white blood cell count and differential count. The burn client's total white blood cell count, especially of neutrophils, initially rises and then drops precipitously with a "left shift" (Chap. 23) as the immune system becomes unable to sustain its defenses. If sepsis occurs, the total white blood cell count may be as low as 2000 cells/mm³. Concurrent with this profound leukopenia, the platelet count falls.

Other abnormal laboratory findings that are associated with physiologic changes occurring in response to burn injuries include hyperglycemia and elevated blood urea nitrogen and serum creatinine levels. The hyperglycemia may result from the stress response or from hyperalimentation. The elevated blood urea nitrogen and creatinine levels are seen among clients who sustain

KEY FEATURES OF DISEASE ■ Baseline Laboratory Test Values and Postburn Variations

Laboratory Test	Normal Value	Postburn Variation	Cause
Serum Studies			
Hemoglobin	12–15 g/dL (women) 14–16.5 g/dL (men)	Elevated	Fluid volume loss
Hematocrit	37–45% (women) 42–50% (men)	Elevated	Fluid volume loss
Urea nitrogen	5–15 mg/dL	Elevated	Fluid volume loss
Glucose	60–100 mg/dL	Elevated	Stress response
Electrolytes			
Sodium	136–145 mEq/L	Elevated	Fluid volume loss and disruption of sodium-potassium pump
Potassium	3.5–5.0 mEq/L	Elevated	Disruption of sodium-potassium pump, tissue destruction, and red blood cell hemolysis
Chloride	96–106 mEq/L	Elevated	Fluid volume loss and resorption of chlorides in urine
Arterial Blood Gas Studies			
PO_2	80–100 mmHg	Normal	
PCO_2	32–45 mmHg		
pH	7.34–7.45	Low	Metabolic acidosis
Carboxyhemoglobin	0	Elevated	Inhalation of smoke and carbon monoxide
Total protein	6.0–8.0 g/dL	Low	Loss of protein exudate through wound
Albumin	3.5–5.0 g/dL	Low	Loss of protein through wounds and through vascular membranes because of increased permeability

some degree of acute tubular necrosis because of inadequate renal perfusion during the emergent phase.

Additional laboratory tests that provide useful information about the burn client's status include urine electrolyte assays, urine cultures, liver enzyme studies, and clotting studies. For Black clients, a sickle cell preparation is appropriate because trauma often triggers a sickle cell crisis in clients who have the disease and in those who carry the sickle cell trait. Drug and alcohol screens should be obtained if drug or alcohol intoxication is suspected.

Other Diagnostic Tests

In addition to routine laboratory tests and examinations, specific tests are given for the involved organs. For example, when burn injuries involve the eye, ophthalmic evaluation to detect corneal damage is necessary. Chapters 35 and 36 describe specific ophthalmic evaluation procedures. When visceral organ trauma is sus-

pected, specific diagnostic examinations are performed, such as intravenous pyelogram, computed tomography scan, or bronchoscopy. In addition, magnetic resonance imaging can be used to ascertain the depth of burn injuries such as electrical burns and to assess tissue deep in the muscle compartments that may have been damaged by electricity's passing through long bones.

 Analysis: Nursing Diagnosis

The client who is burned experiences dramatic changes not only in the directly damaged tissues but also in every body system. Although certain manifestations of injury can be expected in all clients who are burned, a variety of events can induce complications. The nursing diagnosis discussed in this chapter addresses several actual and numerous additional problems. Most burn clients experience all of the common and many of the additional diagnoses during the course of the illness.

Common Diagnoses

The following nursing diagnoses are common to hospitalized clients who have sustained a burn injury greater than 25% TBSA:

1. Decreased cardiac output related to increase in capillary permeability
2. Fluid volume deficit related to electrolyte imbalance and loss of plasma volume from vascular space
3. Altered (cerebral, cardiopulmonary, renal, gastrointestinal, peripheral) tissue perfusion related to decreases in cardiac output and to edema
4. Ineffective breathing pattern related to respiratory distress from inhalation injury, airway obstruction, or pneumonia
5. Pain related to exposed nerve endings in damaged dermis
6. Impaired skin integrity related to burn injury
7. Potential for infection related to impaired skin integrity
8. Altered nutrition: less than body requirements related to increases in metabolic rate
9. Impaired physical mobility related to open burn wounds, and to scar and contracture formation
10. Body image disturbance related to change in physical appearance

Additional Diagnoses

In addition to the common diagnoses, the client with burn injuries may present with one or more of the following nursing diagnoses:

1. Bowel incontinence related to drugs, nasogastric feedings, and altered mobility
2. Ineffective family coping related to loss of home, family, or significant other(s)
3. Ineffective individual coping related to situational crises
4. Anxiety related to threat of death, situational crises, and loss of control
5. Fear related to pain, unknown future, therapeutic procedures, and social re-entry
6. Fluid volume excess related to massive intravenous fluid administration
7. Anticipatory grieving related to loss of significant other(s) and health status
8. Powerlessness related to illness-related treatment regimen and immobility
9. Total self-care deficit related to pain, contractures, and loss of function in hands, other extremities, and other body parts
10. Sensory/perceptual alterations (visual) related to periorbital edema, auditory related to hospital environmental noises, tactile related to effects of burns

11. Sexual dysfunction related to perineal, genital, and breast burns; immobility; fatigue; depression; and disturbance in body image
12. Sleep pattern disturbance related to pain, treatment regimen, and environmental noise
13. Social isolation related to protective isolation treatment regimen and alterations in physical appearance
14. Altered patterns of urinary elimination related to renal failure and drug therapy
15. Altered health maintenance related to effects of burn injury
16. Knowledge deficit related to treatment regimen

 Planning and Implementation

The following plan of care focuses on the actual nursing diagnoses for most clients with burns. Specific interventions are addressed in the Client Care Plan on pages 382 to 384 for a 35-year-old male client with 10% partial-thickness and full-thickness chemical burns on the left arm and hand.

Decreased Cardiac Output; Fluid Volume Deficit; Altered Tissue Perfusion

Because the underlying pathologic conditions and eventual interventions for all three of these nursing diagnoses are the same for the client who has a burn injury, the three diagnoses are discussed together.

Planning: client goals. The major goals for these nursing diagnoses are that the client will (1) restore cardiac output to normal and (2) maintain adequate oxygenation to all vital organs.

Interventions: nonsurgical management. Interventions are aimed at increasing vascular fluid volume, supporting compensatory mechanisms, and preventing complications.

Extensive infusion of intravenous fluids is necessary to maintain a circulating volume that is sufficient for normal cardiac output, mean arterial pressure, and tissue oxygenation. The physician uses many formulas for calculating the amount of fluid needed after a severe burn. Table 16–2 summarizes the most common formulas used in burn therapy. Although the formulas vary as to type and amount of electrolytes, crystalloids, and colloid solutions used (described in Chap. 17), the ultimate purpose of all of these formulas is to prevent shock by maintaining an adequate circulating fluid volume.

Controversy persists among physicians who treat burn clients with regard to the optimal fluid formula. Many combinations of solutions, with added buffers or electrolytes, have been tried. The use of colloid and the appropriate time for its administration are also controversial.

CLIENT CARE PLAN ■ The Client with Partial-Thickness and Full-Thickness Chemical Burns

Goal/Outcome Criteria	Interventions	Rationales
Nursing Diagnosis 1: Impaired Skin Integrity Related to Injury and Treatment		

Client will have restored skin integrity.
■ Area of partial-thickness wound decreases by at least 2 mm border per week.
■ Accepts autograft.
■ Does not lose integrity in areas not involved in either the initial injury or the donor sites.
	1. Partial-thickness wound site: wound care.
	  a. Remove old dressings at least twice per day.
	  b. With aseptic technique, wash area with prescribed solutions to remove eschar, exudates, and necrotic tissue debris.
	  c. Use forceful irrigation over areas with adherent eschar to mechanically separate the eschar.
	  d. Observe wound area for bleeding, presence of small blood vessels, and a pink, shiny appearance.
	  e. Gently apply prescribed topical creams, ointments, or other agents.
		a. Access for inspection and treatment is allowed.
		b. Presence of eschar, exudates, and debris inhibits cell proliferation and delays healing.
		c. Eschar inhibits cell proliferation and delays healing.
		d. Bleeding, blood vessels, and appearance indicate wound healing.
		e. Gentleness avoids disruption of new tissues and capillaries. Topical agents allow wound areas to retain the natural moisture necessary to promote cell proliferation. Antimicrobial topical agents control microbial proliferation and prevent infection.

	f. Apply gauze dressings to cover wound.	f. Dressings prevent moisture loss, decrease exposure of wound to environmental contaminants, and provide a protective cushion over the wound.

	g. Position client so that wound areas are not dependent and have no restrictions to circulation.
	2. Partial-thickness wound site: supportive measures.
	  a. Ensure that the client has a dietary intake adequate for metabolic needs.
	  b. Encourage the client to perform isometric exercises in all voluntary muscles that are not directly under grafted areas.
	3. Graft sites
	  a. Maintain pressure dressings in place over grafts for 3–5 d (or according to physician's prescription).
		g. Free circulation of well-oxygenated blood to wound area promotes cell proliferation.
		
		a. Increased cell proliferation raises energy demands and caloric requirements.
		b. Exercises enhance blood flow to the areas and give the client a sense of active participation in the healing process.
		
		a. Dressings physically increase contact between graft and granulation bed, which aids the likelihood of establishing vascular and epithelial connections.

	b. Keep graft site elevated. c. Position client so that graft site is not next to the bed or in contact with other body surfaces.	b. Elevation prevents venous stasis and increases circulation to the area. c. Positioning enhances circulation to graft area and prevents potential damage related to shearing forces.

CLIENT CARE PLAN ■ **The Client with Partial-Thickness and Full-Thickness Chemical Burns** *continued*

Goal/Outcome Criteria	Interventions	Rationales
	d. Have client placed in Clinitron-style bed or other bed devices that reduce pressure on skin contact surfaces.	d. These devices prevent circulatory restriction and shearing forces.
	e. Observe graft site every shift after occlusive or pressure dressings are removed.	e. Observation is used to determine graft acceptance and whether necrosis or infection is present.
	f. With aseptic technique, apply topical agents and dressings as prescribed.	f. Topical agents and dressings protect graft site.
	4. Donor sites: closed method a. Observe wound area for inflammation at margins and the presence of purulent exudates under transparent film dressings.	a. Complications are identified early so that appropriate interventions can be initiated when they will be effective.
	b. Change transparent film dressing as necessary or as prescribed.	b. Loose or disrupted dressings are not effective.
	5. Donor sites: dry exposure method a. Position client off donor site.	a. Position prevents circulatory restriction and pressure-generated pain.
	b. Apply heat lamp, hair dryer, or fan to donor site while taking care to avoid heating the site or damaging the tissues. This technique requires that the nurse either remain in the room with the client during the procedure or examine the site every 10 min during the procedure.	b. Drying of fine mesh gauze and dry scab formation are enhanced.
	c. Avoid direct contact with the site by tenting or cradling sheets.	c. Tenting or cradling prevents pressure pain and reduces the risk of mechanically injuring site.
	d. As scab dries and lifts, trim the edges down to where scab is tightly adherent.	d. Trimming prevents edges of scab from catching on objects and pulling off before healing is complete. Area for sequestering microorganisms is reduced. A visible measure of healing is provided to the client.

Nursing Diagnosis 2: Potential for Infection Related to Altered Skin Integrity

Client will be free from infection. ■ Results of wound cultures are negative. ■ Results of blood cultures are negative. ■ Wound areas are free from purulent drainage or foul odor. ■ Wound areas are free from edema and redness.	1. Use clean or aseptic technique during dressing changes. a. Nurse washes hands before and after all contact with client. b. Gloves are changed between dressing different wound sites. 2. Clean burn wound with prescribed solutions.	1. Infection from cross-contamination is prevented. a. Cross-contamination is prevented. b. Autocontamination is prevented 2. Cleaning keeps microbial count as low as possible.

continued

CLIENT CARE PLAN ■ The Client with Partial-Thickness and Full-Thickness Chemical Burns continued

Goal/Outcome Criteria	Interventions	Rationales
	Nursing Diagnosis 2: Potential for Infection Related to Altered Skin Integrity	
■ White blood cell count remains below 10,000 cells/mm³ of blood with no left shift of neutrophils. ■ There is no temperature reading above 101° F.	3. Apply topical antimicrobial agents as prescribed. 4. Monitor wound for redness, purulent exudates, or foul odors. 5. Culture wound every week or when indications of infection are present. 6. Maintain a safe environment. 　a. Place client in an area of low traffic. 　b. Do not use equipment on different clients without appropriate decontamination procedures. 　c. Use masks when changing burn dressings. 　d. Clean client's room daily. 　e. Do not engage in extraneous activities such as bed making, water changing, mail delivering, or room cleaning when client's dressings are off and wounds are exposed. 　f. Assist the client with general hygiene activities, especially hand, mouth, and perineal care, every shift. 　g. Prevent skin surfaces from touching each other.	3. Agents reduce microbial proliferation. 4. Monitoring identifies the presence of infection early so that appropriate interventions can be initiated. 5. Cultures are used to identify the presence of infection early so that appropriate specific interventions can be initiated. 6. A safe environment prevents risk of infection. 　a. An area with little traffic reduces microbial influx. 　b. Microbial influx and risk of cross-contamination are reduced. 　c. Use of masks reduces risk of cross-contamination. 　d. Cleaning reduces microbial influx. 　e. Microbial influx and risk of cross-contamination are reduced. 　f. Proper care reduces risk of autocontamination. 　g. Risk of autocontamination is reduced.

TABLE 16–2 Overview of Fluid Resuscitation Formulas for the First 24 Hours of Burn Treatment

Formula	Electrolyte	Colloid	Glucose in Water
Parkland (Baxter)	Ringer's lactate, 4 mL/kg per % burn		
Brooke	Ringer's lactate, 1.5 mL/kg per % burn	0.5 mL/kg per % burn	200 mL
Modified Brooke	Ringer's lactate, 2 mL/kg per % burn		
Evans	Normal saline, 1 mL/kg per % burn	1 mL/kg per % burn	2000 mL
Hypertonic sodium solution (two ampules of NaHCO₃ in 1 L of Ringer's lactate	Volume to maintain urinary output at 30 mL/h (fluid contains 250 mEq sodium/L), approximately 2 mL/kg per % burn		

The client being resuscitated from a severe burn receives large fluid loads in a short time (Baxter & Waeckerle, 1988; Demling, 1987). For the most popular of the resuscitation formulas, the Parkland formula, it is suggested that one-half of the calculated fluid be given in the first 8 hours after the burn. The other half is then administered over the next 16-hour period, for a total of 24 hours. Colloids, such as albumin, may be given in the third or fourth 8-hour period after the burn if the clinical assessment indicates such a need. Most fluid replacement formulas recommend the practice of "catching up" on fluids. If, for example, a client was burned at 8:00 AM but was admitted to the hospital at 10:00 AM, the client's first 8-hour period would be at 4:00 PM, or 8 hours after the injury. Thus, if resuscitation were delayed until admission to the hospital, calculated fluids would need to be administered over a 6-hour period rather than an 8-hour period.

For clients with extensive burns, a large-bore central venous catheter must be placed so that these massive fluid loads can be administered. In the second 24-hour period, 5% dextrose in water replaces Ringer lactate as the crystalloid solution of choice.

The nurse monitors specific vital signs to determine adequate fluid resuscitation. These signs include clear mentation, a blood pressure that is within the normal limits for the client's age and weight, a central venous pressure between 6 and 9 mmHg and a normal pulse, and urinary output equal to 1 mL of urine per kilogram of body weight (or 30 to 100 mL) per hour. These parameters are indicators of adequate tissue perfusion to the brain, heart, and kidneys, respectively, which is the ultimate goal of this therapy. During resuscitation, the waning of any one of these parameters usually suggests a decrease in tissue perfusion to that specific organ, which indicates a deficit in fluid volume and a diminished cardiac output.

Urinary output is the most common and most sensitive noninvasive assessment parameter for cardiac output and tissue perfusion (Chaps. 12 and 17). Regardless of the total amount of fluid calculated as appropriate to meet the fluid needs for an individual client, the actual amount of fluid administered depends on how much intravenous fluid per hour is required to maintain the client's urinary output between 30 and 100 mL/hour. Adjustment of the rate of administration of intravenous fluid on the basis of urinary output plus serum electrolyte values is known as *titration* of fluid to meet perfusion needs of the client.

A frequent mistake in treatment is to administer diuretics so that urinary output increases rather than to change the amount and rate of fluids that are administered to this client. Diuretics do not increase cardiac output; they actually decrease circulating volume and cardiac output by pulling fluid from the circulating blood volume to enhance diuresis. This effect can cause a dangerous reduction in perfusion to other vital organs, especially the heart, lungs, and brain, and greatly increases the risk of shock. Therefore, diuretics are not generally used to improve urinary output for burn clients. An exception to this restricted use of diuretics is

for the client with a burn injury caused by electrical energy. In these clients, muscle and deep tissue damage can often cause the release of large protein molecules (myoglobin), which precipitate in and obstruct the renal tubules. Although the diuretic mannitol is often used in these situations, it should always be given after adequate urinary output has been established.

In some clients, particularly elderly clients or clients with a history of cardiac disease, a complicating factor in reduced cardiac output may be congestive heart failure or myocardial infarction. Drugs such as dopamine (Intropin) to increase cardiac output or digoxin (Lanoxin) to strengthen the force of myocardial contraction may be used in conjunction with fluid therapy.

Often, burn clients are in severe shock and require invasive cardiac monitoring. Nurses must be prepared to monitor vital parameters such as central venous pressure, pulmonary artery pressures, and cardiac output by using modern electronic equipment.

Cardiac arrhythmias are not common occurrences in many burn injuries. However, because the presence of an adequately functioning cardiovascular system is imperative, electrocardiographic monitoring should be done in clients who have sustained large burns. Often, rhythms that affect the mechanics of the heart, such as atrial fibrillation, are present in the elderly client. When dealing with this population, it is not unusual to use digitalis or other treatment regimens to improve cardiac function.

Interventions: surgical management.   The primary surgical procedure that is performed as treatment of inadequate tissue perfusion is *escharotomy*. This procedure incises but does not remove eschar. The burned tissue that forms the eschar is thick and inelastic. When the eschar completely surrounds a body part (such as a limb, the thorax, or the abdomen), the lack of elasticity does not allow expansion to accommodate tissue swelling or respiratory movements. As a result, tissue swelling beneath the eschar can compress blood vessels to such an extent that no blood flows through the vessels, and tissue hypoxia and ischemia occur. Under these circumstances, the eschar is cut along both sides (as when bivalving a cast) to relieve the pressures beneath the eschar (Fig. 16–11).

Escharotomies are frequently performed at the bedside or in the hydrotherapy area and require no anesthesia. The client is prepared preoperatively by removal of dressings and thorough cleaning of the operative site. Blood loss is minimal because eschar is avascular and trauma to viable tissues is avoided. After the procedure, the nurse applies topical antimicrobial agents and dressings to the site.

Ineffective Breathing Pattern

Planning: client goals.   Regardless of the underlying pathologic cause of the ineffective breathing patterns, the goals for this diagnosis are that the client will (1) maintain a patent airway and (2) have adequate gas exchange (Larson & Parks, 1988).

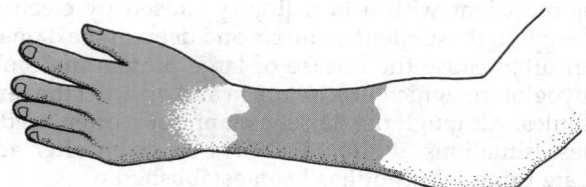

Tight, circumferential eschar restricting outward swelling as edema forms in the tissues beneath the eschar. Edema compresses blood vessels, which inhibits blood flow to the distal extremity.

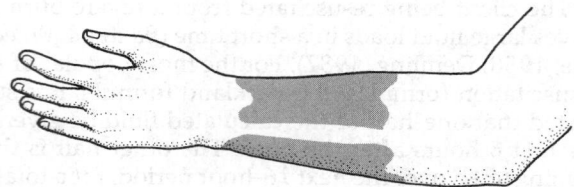

An escharotomy incision allows outward swelling of edematous tissues. Restricted blood flow through the vessels to the distal extremity is relieved.

Figure 16–11.

Escharotomy to release circumferential burn eschar and to improve circulation to a distal extremity.

Interventions: nonsurgical management. Interventions are aimed at supporting normal pulmonary mechanisms, secondary prevention of pulmonary problems, and prevention of complications. Specific plans for pulmonary management depend on the cause of the insult and the status of the respiratory tract.

Assessment. At least once per hour during the emergent phase, the nurse assesses the general respiratory status of all burn clients as described under the heading Physical Assessment: Clinical Manifestations: Respiratory System. Clients with possible pulmonary injuries are assessed more frequently. Emergency respiratory equipment, including oxygen, masks, cannulas, Ambu bags, laryngoscope, endotracheal tubes, and materials for performing a tracheostomy, are located at or near the client's bedside.

Airway. Maintenance of the airway begins at the accident scene and may involve only a chin lift or head tilt maneuver in an unconscious victim. Frequently, 8 to 16 hours after the initiation of fluid resuscitation efforts, upper airway edema becomes pronounced. These clients require immediate nasal or oral intubation once signs of crowing, stridor, and dyspnea are present. Hesitation to intubate the clients often leads to an emergency situation in which the airway becomes completely obstructed and surgical intervention is needed. A laryngoscopy is performed by the physician to visualize vocal chords of clients who are at risk for developing an obstruction; this procedure is done during admission of the client to the hospital and as needed to prevent a crisis situation from occurring. Clients with severe smoke poisoning may require bronchoscopy when they are admitted to the hospital and routinely thereafter for visualization of the respiratory tract, accurate diagnoses, deep suctioning of the lungs, and removal of sloughing necrotic tissue. The nurse assesses the patency of the tubes and ensures that proper positioning is maintained during respiratory assessment of intubated clients.

Other causes of airway obstruction are secretions and sloughed lung tissue that result from pulmonary injury or pneumonia. The nurse or respiratory therapist performs vigorous endotracheal, nasotracheal, or bronchial suctioning; chest physiotherapy; and aerosol treatments as ordered.

Ventilation. Respiration depends on skeletal muscle contractions and movement of the thoracic cavity for ventilation. This movement can be restricted by tight dressings that cover the neck, thorax, and abdomen. The nurse observes the client for ease and effectiveness of respiratory movements. Tight dressings are removed or loosened.

Gas exchange. The nurse monitors the effectiveness of gas exchange by using laboratory tests, such as arterial blood gas and carboxyhemoglobin levels, as well as by noting physical signs, such as cyanosis, disorientation, and increased pulse rate. Chest x-ray films provide information about the presence and resolution of atelectasis. Sputum cultures are obtained to determine whether a pulmonary infection is contributing to the ineffective breathing pattern. In critically ill clients, lung water catheters are inserted for measurement of extravascular lung water, which may interfere with gas exchange. This measurement indicates trends in pulmonary fluid status. Swan-Ganz catheters, which are used to measure pulmonary artery pressure, are adjunctive aids in identifying pulmonary and circulatory dysfunctions. Measurement of central venous pressure, along with that of daily weight, helps to outline a pattern that may be consistent with fluid overload.

Oxygen therapy. Management of ineffective breathing patterns may involve administering humidified oxygen via face mask, cannula, or hood. When arterial oxygenation is less than 60 ($PO_2 < 60$ mmHg), intubation is indicated and mechanical ventilation is instituted. Chapter 62 discusses specific nursing actions for clients during mechanical ventilation.

Drug therapy. When pneumonia or other pulmonary infections lead to greater pulmonary difficulties, antibiotics are prescribed. Respiratory problems that result from cardiac failure and increased pulmonary pressures may be treated with drugs that improve cardiac output and enhance renal excretion. In situations in which a client's activity severely compromises the respiratory mechanics, the use of mechanical ventilation, and the administration of sedatives, it may be necessary to use a paralytic drug such as pancuronium bromide (Pavulon). The use of paralytic agents removes all ventilatory control from the client and allows uninterrupted administration of artificial ventilation. However, these drugs do not prevent the client from seeing, hearing, or experiencing fear, pain, and loss of control. The nurse ensures that all alarms are operative because the patient cannot call for help.

Positioning — deep breathing. To assist in adequate pulmonary function, the nurse turns the client frequently, assists the client out of bed, and encourages movement as much as possible. The nurse teaches the use of incentive spirometry, coughing, and deep breathing and performs chest physiotherapy according to the client's need and the physician's prescription.

Interventions: surgical management. A tracheostomy may be necessary in clients for whom long-term intubation is expected. Tracheostomy in burn clients carries with it a greater risk of infection than that in nonburned individuals. Emergency tracheostomies are performed when an airway becomes occluded and oral or nasal intubation cannot be achieved. Other common surgical procedures to improve the burn client's respiratory status include insertion of chest tubes and use of escharotomy. Chest tubes are used to re-expand the lung when a pneumothorax or hemothorax has occurred. Chapter 62 provides specific nursing actions for clients with chest tubes. Tight eschar on the neck, chest, or abdomen can restrict respiratory movement. Escharotomies can relieve this restriction and permit greater respiratory movement.

Extracorporeal membrane oxygenation (ECMO), although still in the experimental stages, has the potential to provide dramatic improvement in clients with severely impaired lungs and bleak prognoses. Studies with this technique on sheep that have been given a pulmonary injury from smoke show promise for the use of this technique in human subjects. The procedure involves accessing a major artery or vein and removing blood from the body. The blood is oxygenated and returned via another vessel. It is suggested that this treatment performs the lung's function of oxygenation and thus allows the lungs time to heal.

Pain

Pain that is associated with burn injuries is both chronic and acute and can contribute to various complications. Many factors contribute to burn pain, and these factors are manipulated to alter the response to pain.

Planning: client goals. The primary goal is that the client will experience alleviation or reduction of pain that is associated with burn injury and its treatment.

Interventions: nonsurgical management. The plan for pain management is individualized to the client's tolerance for pain, coping mechanisms, and physical status. Interventions include drug therapy and nonpharmacologic techniques (Marvin, 1987).

Drug therapy. Narcotic and nonnarcotic analgesics, such as morphine sulfate, merperidine (Demerol, Pethadol), and pentazocine (Talwin), are given with relative frequency for the duration of hospitalization. These drugs, however, rarely offer more than moderate relief during acutely painful procedures and have such side effects as respiratory depression and diminished gastrointestinal motility. During the emergent postburn phase, these agents are administered intravenously because the fluid shift significantly limits absorption from the subcutaneous and intramuscular spaces, and thus agents administered by these routes remain in the spaces and do not provide the client with pain relief. In addition, cumulative doses administered subcutaneously or intramuscularly when edema is present are rapidly reabsorbed when the fluid shift is resolving. This delayed reabsorption can result in lethal blood levels of analgesics.

Anesthetic agents such as ketamine (Ketalar), pentobarbital sodium (Nembutal), and nitrous oxide are also used effectively for pain relief. Extreme care must be taken during their administration, and the presence of an anesthesiologist or nurse anesthetist is required.

Nonpharmacologic measures. Nonpharmacologic measures include the use of relaxation techniques, meditative breathing, guided imagery, and music therapy. Hypnosis and autohypnosis of lucid, cooperative clients can be attempted by trained individuals. Therapeutic touch, acupuncture, and acupressure are used to a limited extent with burn clients with variable results. These nontraditional types of pain interventions are discussed more thoroughly in Chapter 7.

Environmental manipulation. Client comfort can be increased by manipulations that include providing a quiet environment, using nonpainful tactile stimulation, and increasing client control.

Increasing the client's sleep or rest time helps to reduce the adverse effects of sleep deprivation, replenishes catecholamine stores, helps to prevent critical care unit psychosis, and restores diurnal effects of endorphins. The nurse attempts to perform as many procedures as possible during waking hours.

Tactile stimulation can help reduce pain. The nurse changes the client's position routinely to reduce pressure on any one specific area, which improves circulation to painful areas and reduces pain. Massaging nonburn areas may reduce pain transmission on thick pain-sensory nerve fibers by stimulating an increased release of endorphins. Applying heat and maintaining warm room temperatures prevent the client from shivering and stimulate the production of serotonin, which has been associated with triggering the relaxation response.

Allowing client participation in pain control measures reduces anxiety and increases feelings of confidence and independence. For example, the use of contracts with clients that specifies how long a painful procedure will last helps clients deal with the pain for that particular period. Patient-controlled analgesia is also an effective pain-reducing measure for burn clients.

Interventions: surgical management. In many burn centers, a technique of early surgical excision is used on the burn wound, as described under the heading Surgical Débridement in the next section. Early excision can reduce much of the pain that is associated with daily débridement at the bedside or during hydrotherapy. Treatment of burns in the operating room with the client under general anesthesia reduces the amount of pain experienced during acute procedures, but some painful procedures and dressing changes are still performed at the bedside.

Impaired Skin Integrity

Planning: client goals. The major goals for this nursing diagnosis are that the client will (1) not experience further loss of skin integrity and (2) have skin integrity restored.

Interventions: nonsurgical management. Interventions are aimed at preserving the integrity of nonburned skin, enhancing wound healing of burned skin, and preventing complications. All nursing interventions for this problem include in-depth assessment of burned and nonburned skin areas to determine the degree of skin integrity, adequacy of circulation, presence of infection, and effectiveness of therapy. Chapter 38 describes proper techniques for assessment of the skin. Nursing actions focus on caring for the burn wound.

Nonsurgical burn wound management, called *conservative treatment,* involves removing exudates and necrotic tissue, cleaning the area, stimulating granulation and revascularization, and applying dressings. Restoration of skin, whether by natural healing or by grafting, starts with removal of eschar and other cellular debris from the burn wound. This removal is called *débridement* and can be done by various techniques. Conservative treatment allows noninvasive débriding of the wound through mechanical, bacterial, and enzymatic action that stimulates the separation of eschar over time. The goal of conservative treatment is to have the wound slowly prepare itself for grafting and wound closure by a natural process.

Mechanical débridement. Burn wounds are débrided and cleaned a minimum of once each day during *hydrotherapy* (the application of water for treatment). Hydrotherapy is performed daily by nursing personnel to débride necrotic tissue and to visualize the wounds. Hydrotherapy can be accomplished by immersing the client in a tub, by showering the client on a specially designed table, or by successively washing only small areas of the wound. Showering enhances visualization of the wounds and allows water temperature to be kept constant. Figure 16–12 shows a shower table that is used in hydrotherapy. Immersion of clients in large tubs of water or antiseptic solutions has been associated with autocontamination and with increased losses of sodium

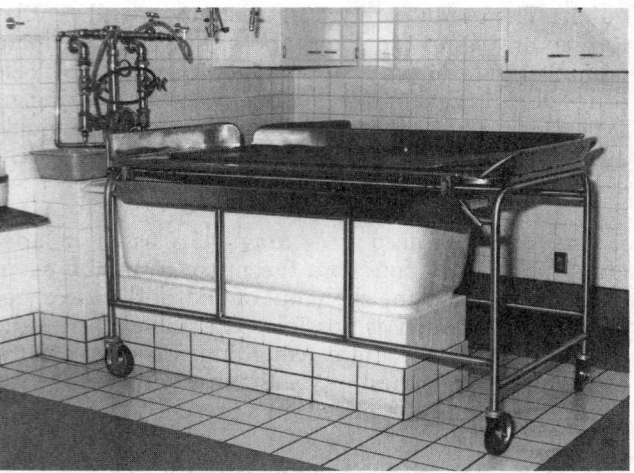

Figure 16–12.
Shower table used for wound cleaning and débridement.

through the burn wound. Nurses and skilled technicians use forceps and scissors to remove loose, nonviable tissue during this water cleaning. Occasionally, soft foam or gauze sponges can be used to facilitate débridement of "cheesy" or pseudoeschar. During hydrotherapy, in addition to eschar, old topical agents are removed, and the remaining adherent eschar is softened.

Enzymatic débridement. Enzymatic débridement can occur naturally by autolysis or artificially by application of proteolytic agents. *Autolysis* is the spontaneous disintegration of tissue by the action of the client's own cellular enzymes. Topical enzymatic agents are used with limited success to débride the burn wound chemically. One such agent is sutilains (Travase). The proteolytic enzymes in this agent selectively digest necrotic tissues when applied in a wet dressing to the burn wound. Careful observation is necessary to ensure that such agents do not penetrate and degrade viable tissue.

Dressing the burn wound. After burn wounds are cleaned and débrided, they are treated with topical antibiotics to prevent infection, as described under the heading Potential for Infection. Some type of dressing is then usually applied to the burn wound. Burn dressings include standard wound dressings, biologic dressings, and synthetic dressings.

Standard wound dressings involve the sterile application of multiple layers of gauze over the topical antibiotic on the burn wound. The number of gauze layers used depends on the depth of the injury, the amount of drainage expected, the client's mobility, and the frequency of dressing changes. The gauze layers are held in place with roller-style bandages (Kerlix) that are applied distal to proximal, or with circular net fabrics. On extremities, these dressings may also be covered with elastic (Ace) wraps, especially if the client is ambulatory. These dressings are usually changed every 8 to 12 hours. *Biologic dressings* contain some amount of viable tis-

---

TABLE 16-3   Uses, Advantages, and Disadvantages of Biologic Dressings

Uses

Débridement of untidy wounds after eschar separation

Promotion of re-epithelialization of deep second-degree wounds

Temporary coverage after burn wound excision

Protection of granulation tissue between autografts

Test graft before autograft

Advantages

Reduction of evaporative heat

Reduction of evaporative water losses

Prevention of desiccation of granulation tissue

Reduction of exudate protein losses

Reduction of pain

Assisting in wound débridement

Enhancement of healing of second-degree burns

Protection of exposed neurovascular tissue

Inhibition of bacterial proliferation

Disadvantages

Expensive

Rejection responses

Possible burn wound sepsis if applied over eschar

Availability

Storage

Refrigeration required

Possible transmission of diseases such as hepatitis

---

sue or are derived from once-living tissue. Such dressings are used on partial-thickness injuries to promote healing, protect granulation beds, and débride untidy wound areas. In addition, biologic dressings are frequently used on full-thickness burn areas to prevent fluid loss and to stimulate granulation and revascularization. Table 16-3 outlines the advantages and disadvantages of biologic dressings.

Biologic dressings are usually heterograft or homograft material. *Heterograft* is skin from another species. The most commonly used type of heterograft is pigskin because of its availability and its relative compatibility with human skin. Rejection usually occurs within 24 to 72 hours, and the pigskin is replaced on a continual basis until the wound heals naturally or until closure with an autograft is complete. *Homograft* is the skin from another human, which is usually obtained from a cadaver and is provided through a skin bank. Homograft is available fresh or frozen and is applied and cared for in

the same manner as autograft. Rejection can occur within 24 hours, but in some instances the graft has remained adherent for more than 90 days. Another natural substance that is used to dress burn wounds is *sterile amniotic membrane*. This substance, which is sometimes impregnated with a topical antimicrobial agent, is used in the same manner as is pigskin (Haberal et al., 1987).

Synthetic and *biosynthetic dressings* such as Op Site, Vigilon, Biobrane, and Tegaderm, may be used as substitutes for antimicrobial, standard, or biologic dressings. Synthetic dressings are applied directly to the surface of a clean or surgically prepared wound area and remain in place for 2 to 5 days. Because many of these dressings are transparent or translucent, visual inspection of the wound is possible without removing the dressing. Also, because these agents prevent contact of the wound with air, the client experiences pain reduction at the site. These dressings have the additional advantages of being more cost-effective than biologic dressings and rarely stimulating any allergic or adverse reactions.

Interventions: surgical management.   Surgical management of burn wounds focuses on débridement and on wound covering through *autografting,* which is the transplantation of viable skin from an intact, healthy skin area to the full-thickness burn wound. Surgical débridement usually occurs early in the postburn period. Grafting procedures for skin covering may occur throughout the acute phase as burn wounds are made ready and donor sites are available. In addition, grafting may be performed in the rehabilitative phase to improve function or appearance.

Surgical débridement.   Surgical débridement is also called the *early excision method.* This method exemplifies the recent trend toward operative management of the wound (Heimbach, 1987). Clients are taken to the operating room as early as possible within the first 5 days after injury. The burn wound is excised by either a tangential or a fascial excision technique. A skin graft or temporary covering is placed over the excised wound. Additional operative débridement and grafting procedures, if necessary, are then done every 5 to 7 days until complete, permanent coverage is achieved.

The method of early excision of burn wound eschar reduces the number of hydrotherapy treatments that are needed by the client. The risks of this difficult surgical technique include massive blood loss and complications associated with the use of anesthesia. Also, when a fascial excision technique is indicated, large amounts of body fat are removed. The long-term effects of this insult to the body are currently being evaluated.

Wound covering.   Permanent skin coverage for extensive full-thickness injuries is achieved only through the application of an autograft. *Autograft* is skin taken from one's own body. The surgeon usually removes a piece of skin from a remote area of the body that is unburned and transplants it to cover the burn wound.

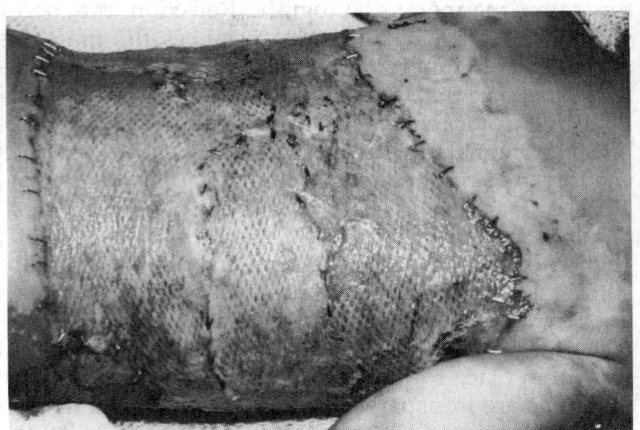

Figure 16–13.

Typical appearance of meshed autografts in the early postoperative period.

Skin grafts are generally of split thickness (0.015 in) and form a partial-thickness injury at the site of surgical removal, the *donor site* (DiMola & Winkler, 1986a). Grafts are placed either on a clean granulated bed or over a surgically excised area of burn. Detailed descriptions of grafts and of preoperative and postoperative nursing care needs are found in Chapter 40.

As the burn size increases, the availability of donor sites decreases. Clients with large surface area burns may have a mere 5% to 25% of the skin surface available to cover the 80% to 95% area that has been burned. Whether the burn is excised or treated conservatively, the available skin is used to accomplish total body coverage. Coverage is accomplished by successive reharvesting of the available donor site (allowing time for re-epithelialization and healing) and by large-mesh split-thickness skin grafts (Fig. 16–13). When this technique is used, sufficient coverage over the large interstices must be provided because their closure time is prolonged (DiMola & Winkler, 1986b). When the burn is excised, a temporary covering is used before grafting to supplement the small amount of autograft available. Biologic and biosynthetic dressings are used to supplement the autograft and to cover large-mesh grafts.

Interventions: experimental management. Research on techniques to enhance skin growth, expansion, and early coverage has resulted in successful autografts. By using the client's own skin under ideal, artificial tissue culture conditions with application of growth factors, significant rapid skin growth has been achieved. This method, although promising, is labor-intensive, and its use is currently restricted by cost and availability.

Potential for Infection

With the integrity of the skin barrier disrupted and immune function suppressed, infection is a major complication of burn injuries and is the leading cause of death among clients in the acute phase of recovery (Sittig & Deitch, 1988). Burn wound infection occurs through *autocontamination,* in which the client's own normal flora overgrows and penetrates the internal environment, and through *cross-contamination,* in which microorganisms from another person or environment are transferred to the burn client.

Planning: client goals. The major client goals for this nursing diagnosis are that the client will (1) remain free from cross-contamination–induced infection and (2) not experience septicemia.

Interventions: nonsurgical management. Interventions are aimed at minimizing exposure of the burn client to exogenous microorganisms, reducing the risk of autocontamination, and recognizing signs and symptoms of infection early.

Drug therapy. Drug therapy is appropriate for prevention as well as for early intervention of infectious processes.

Drugs for prevention of infection. Clostridium tetani grows on necrotic tissue and is a strict anaerobe. Burn wound conditions favor the growth of this organism, and all burn clients are considered at risk for developing this often-fatal infectious complication. Prophylaxis with tetanus toxoid, 0.5 mL, administered intramuscularly to all burn clients to enhance previously acquired immunity to *C. tetani,* is routine procedure when the client is admitted to the hospital. The additional administration of tetanus immune globulin (human) (Hyper-Tet) is recommended when the history of tetanus immunization is questionable.

Another strategy for infection prevention during burn care includes the use of topical antibiotics on burn wounds (Monafo & Freedman, 1987). The primary goal of topical antibiotic therapy (topical antimicrobial therapy) is to reduce bacterial proliferation in the wound to a minimal level. Most antimicrobial agents can be used before and after eschar separation. Topical antibiotics are applied by either the closed or the open technique. The *open technique* involves direct application of the agent to the burn wound, using either aseptic or clean methods, without further dressing the wound. The wound is cleaned every 8 to 12 hours, and fresh antimicrobial agents are applied. The *closed technique* includes dressing the burn wound after application of the topical agents. These drugs are not applied to freshly grafted areas because many antimicrobial agents inhibit cell growth. Table 16–4 summarizes characteristics of various topical antimicrobial agents. Three of the most commonly used topical antimicrobial agents are silver sulfadiazine (Silvadene) (Gordon, 1987), mafenide acetate (Sulfamylon), and silver nitrate.

Silver sulfadiazine is currently the most widely used topical antimicrobial agent. This broad-spectrum, water-soluble cream is effective against a wide variety of organisms present on the surfaces of partial-thickness injuries. Common adverse side effects include local allergic reactions and transient leukopenia.

Mafenide acetate is a topical antimicrobial agent that was developed in the 1960s. It has an excellent ability to penetrate eschar, continues to be effective against *Pseu-*

domonas aeruginosa, and causes great pain when used on partial-thickness injuries. These qualities make it the agent of choice for full-thickness injuries. The major dose-limiting adverse reaction for this agent is the development of a metabolic acidosis. This reaction may be avoided if each application is limited to 15% to 20% of TBSA.

Silver nitrate in a 0.5% solution is one of the oldest effective, broad-spectrum topical agents used in burn care. This agent is applied with the use of wet dressings that are time-consuming to use, bulky, and uncomfortable and that restrict the client's mobility. Major adverse reactions include electrolyte imbalance and difficulty with core body temperature maintenance.

Drugs for treatment of infection. When burn clients experience symptoms of an actual infection, antibiotics are used extensively, especially the aminoglycoside class, which includes amikacin (Amikin), gentamicin (Apogen, Cidomycin, Garamycin), and tobramycin (Nebcin) (Dacso et al., 1987). Burn clients require a higher than normal dosage of these drugs to maintain therapeutic serum levels, and appropriate dosages are determined by examination of peak and trough serum levels.

These drugs, although helpful for combating severe infections, are associated with a wide range of serious adverse effects. The most significant effects include ototoxicity and nephrotoxicity. The nurse carefully monitors clients who are treated with aminoglycosides and other powerful antibiotics, such as vancomycin and amphotericin B, for signs of renal insufficiency and hearing impairment. Dosages of these antibiotics are altered when clients exhibit any signs or symptoms of renal dysfunction and/or hearing impairment.

Isolation therapy. Isolation therapy is thought by some clinicians to reduce the incidence of cross-contamination significantly; however, methods of isolation that are used in burn care are varied and controversial. In some burn care units, virtually no isolation is practiced; in others, total sterile conditions preside. All isolation methods for the client with burns emphasize proper and consistent hand washing as the single most effective technique to prevent the transmission of infection. In addition, clients are isolated according to the specific disease or microorganism involved.

Burn clients are immunologically suppressed during the early stage of the injury. This immunosuppression can allow expression of a previously controlled viral infection, such as herpes simplex or herpes zoster. This immunosuppressed condition, coupled with the fact that antibiotic therapy can result in resistant organisms, often leads to infections that warrant isolation techniques different from those used for burn injury alone. In these instances, isolation techniques recommended by the Centers for Disease Control are used. For instance, if a client develops a pan-resistant organism, total isolation—a separate geographic location—is warranted. With such cases, the nurse consults the hospital's Infection Control Committee or infection control practitioner.

Environmental manipulation. The nurse uses gloves during all contact with open wounds. Institution policy concerning the use of sterile versus clean gloves for noninvasive, routine wound care procedures varies and is a matter of debate. Regardless of sterility, gloves are changed between handling of wounds on different areas of the body.

Equipment on burn units is not shared among clients. Disposable items (e.g., pillows, syringes, and dishes) are used as much as possible. The nurse assigns to each client equipment used in daily routine care (e.g., thermometers, blood pressure cuffs, and stethoscopes). Daily equipment cleaning and general housekeeping are essential to environmental infection control. All equipment must be cleaned after use on one client and before use on another. Because *Pseudomonas* has been shown to sequester in plants, the presence of plants and/or

NURSING RESEARCH

Use of Nonsterile Gloves for Dressing Changes and Other Routine Noninvasive Procedures Does Not Increase the Risk of Sepsis Among Burn Clients.

Sadowski, D., Pohlman, S., Maley, M., & Warden, G. (1988). Use of nonsterile gloves for routine noninvasive procedures in thermally injured patients. *Journal of Burn Care and Rehabilitation, 9,* 613–615.

This study examined whether the use of nonsterile gloves in routine noninvasive procedures (including dressing changes) contributed to the development of infection and sepsis among 13 burn clients. Cultures obtained from boxes of nonsterile gloves (as soon as they were opened and after use) and from burn wounds indicated that nonsterile gloves contained no pathogens at the time the boxes were opened. Therefore, these gloves did not contribute to infection or sepsis among the burn clients in this study. However, cultures obtained on the empty nonsterile glove boxes after use showed that the gloves had been contaminated with organisms from the clients. This finding suggested that cross-contamination of organisms from one client to another could be accomplished by using a common box of nonsterile gloves for two or more clients.

Critique. The results of this study most strongly implicate poor hand-washing technique and use of common bulk supplies among clients as a major source of cross-contamination–induced infection and/or sepsis among burn clients. Although the results also support the hypothesis that clean, nonsterile gloves may be used safely for dressing changes and other routine noninvasive procedures among burn clients, the sample size was small and no statistical analyses were presented to indicate the significance of the findings.

Possible nursing implications. The methods in this study can be used to examine other bulk items (such as paper cups or straws) as potential sources of cross-contamination among burn clients.

Text continued on page 396

TABLE 16–4 Topical Agents Commonly Used in the Treatment of Burns

Drug	Description	Action	Advantages	Disadvantages	Interventions
Antibiotics					
Silver sulfadiazine (Silvadene)	Nontoxic salt of silver sulfadiazine in water-based cream.	Binds to bacterial cell membranes and interferes with DNA synthesis.	Does not cause hypochloremia, hyponatremia, electrolyte imbalance, or kidney disease. Has wide-spectrum antimicrobial action against both gram-negative and gram-positive organisms. Has long shelf life. Delays eschar separation less than many other topical agents.	Absorbed into eschar less than mafenide acetate. May cause rash, pruritus, and burning. Is not consistently effective for burns covering more than 60% of client's body or against some bacteria and yeasts. Depresses granulocyte formation.	Watch for signs of infection such as soupiness of wound area. Watch for allergic reaction causing drop in white blood cell count.
Mafenide acetate (Sulfamylon)	Soft, white, nonstaining water-based cream.	Exerts a bacteriostatic action against many gram-negative and gram-positive organisms.	Is effective against *Pseudomonas*. Has long shelf life. Is excellent for treating electrical burns. Penetrates thick eschar.	May lead to superinfection. May cause metabolic acidosis, hyperpnea, and rash. Causes pain when applied. (Pain usually lasts 30–40 min.) Slows eschar separation.	Premedicate client for pain before application. Monitor blood gas and serum electrolyte levels if client develops hyperpnea in response to metabolic acidosis. Do not use in clients with sulfa drug allergy or respiratory or kidney disease.
Sodium hypochlorite solution (Modified Dakin's)	Aqueous sodium hypochlorite solution (percentage varies)	Is bactericidal.	Helps dry wounds that have become soupy. Aids débridement.	Dissolves blood clots and may inhibit clotting. May irritate skin. May cause electrolyte imbalances.	Change dressings every 4–12 h. Observe site carefully for signs of irritation. Keep dressings moist.

Povidone-iodine (Betadine)	Iodine complex. Available as solution, ointment, and foam.	Is microbicidal against gram-positive and gram-negative organisms.	Is effective against many infections not well controlled by silver sulfadiazine. Is available in a wide assortment of forms.	May cause metabolic acidosis and elevated serum iodine levels. May form crusts if burns are not cleaned properly. Causes rash and burning in some clients. Stains clothing and linen. Is deactivated by wound proteins.	Check serum electrolyte and serum iodine levels frequently.
Nitrofurazone (Furacin)	Antibiotic available as cream, solution, and water-soluble powder.	Is wide-spectrum antibacterial.	Is effective against *Staphylococcus aureus* and some antibiotic-resistant organisms. Causes neither pain nor maceration. Is available in a wide assortment of forms.	May cause contact dermatitis (rare). Is messy to apply in cream form. May cause renal problems if used in clients with exensive burns.	Observe client carefully for signs of allergic reaction and for evidence of superinfection.
Silver nitrate	10% silver salt solution, diluted to 0.5% for application.	Has antimicrobial action.	Is inexpensive. Applies easily.	Penetrates wound only 1–2 mm, so acts only on surface organisms. Stains and stings. May cause hyponatremia, hypochloremia, and hypocalcemia. Must be applied as constant soaks.	Keep dressings wet with solution. Check serum electrolyte levels daily.
Gentamicin sulfate (Garamycin)	Wide-spectrum antibiotic, available as a cream or solution for topical use.	Exerts antibiotic action against many organisms that do not respond to other topical antibiotics.	Effective against many organisms, including *Pseudomonas*. Does not cause pain.	May cause ototoxicity and nephrotoxicity. May result in resistance in organisms.	Use with caution in clients with decreased renal function because of possible nephrotoxicity. Order serum and urine creatinine clearance studies before treatment and weekly during treatment to monitor renal function.

Table continued on following page

TABLE 16–4 Topical Agents Commonly Used in the Treatment of Burns *Continued*

Drug	Description	Action	Advantages	Disadvantages	Interventions
Neomycin sulfate (Myciguent)	Wide-spectrum antibiotic in 0.1% to 0.5% aqueous solution.	Is bactericide used to reduce numbers of organisms before débriding and grafting wound.	Effectively combats most organisms. Can be applied easily. Is inexpensive.	May cause ototoxicity and nephrotoxicity. Is absorbed systemically.	Remove from wound after 24 h to reduce systemic absorption. Monitor client's temperature after application of cold solution. Order serum and urine creatinine tests to watch for signs of nephrotoxicity.
Bacitracin with polymyxin B sulfate (Polysporin)	Combination bactericidal ointment effective on small burn areas.	Is bactericidal for gram-positive and gram-negative organisms.	Is capable of minimal systemic absorption. Is aesthetically suitable for use on face. Does not cause pain.	May cause itching, burning, or inflammation. Cannot be used for full-thickness burns.	Observe client closely for signs of sensitivity, e.g., rash. Wash ointment off and reapply it every 8 h.
Enzymatic Débriding Agents					
Sutilains ointment (Travase)	Proteolytic enzymes developed from *Bacillus subtilis* in a petrolatum base.	Digests necrotic tissue, aiding escharotomies and débridement.	Aids initial débridement before client can tolerate surgical débridement. Can be easily applied.	Increases fluid loss. Requires refrigeration. May cause bleeding. Irritates wound and sometimes surrounding skin. Is not bactericidal.	Client must be stable enough for surgery after a few days so that digested wounds can be covered with membranes or grafted. Use with silver sulfadiazine, mafenide acetate, bacitracin, neomycin, or gentamicin. Do not use with hexachlorophene, iodine, nitrofurazone, or silver nitrate.

Agent	Preparation	Action	Advantages	Disadvantages	Nursing Considerations
					Observe client for infection. Change dressing every 18 h. Use on no more than 15% total burn surface at one time.
Fibrinolysin and desoxyribonuclease, combined (bovine) (Elase)	Two lytic enzymes combined in a petrolatum base.	Digests necrotic tissue, aiding escharotomies and débridement.	Does not require refrigeration. Has long shelf life.	Causes sensitivity in clients allergic to bovine materials. Causes itching and burning. Requires preparation immediately before application.	Wait for physician to remove any thick, dry eschar before applying. Observe client for infection. Change dressings daily.

Miscellaneous Agents

Agent	Preparation	Action	Advantages	Disadvantages	Nursing Considerations
Bismuth tribromophenate (Xeroform)	A yellow substance on gauze.	Débrides and protects donor sites and grafts.	Conforms to wound. Is nontoxic and nonsensitizing. Has long shelf life.	Sticks to wound so that removal is painful. Is neither antiseptic nor antibacterial.	Apply carefully so that sheets do not overlap. Observe client for signs of infection.
Scarlet red	A red dye in an oil base on gauze.	Promotes healing of wound.	Protects donor site. Has long shelf life. Promotes re-epithelialization.	Stains clothing and temporarily stains skin. Irritates skin. Causes pain when client moves.	Apply to donor sites at time of harvest. Leave until site heals and scarlet red gauze sloughs. Observe for infection beneath gauze. If needed, use heat lamp for a few minutes every hour to dry site.
Third's	Solution of one-third hydrogen peroxide, one-third 0.25% acetic acid, and one-third normal saline.	Inhibits bacterial growth by oxidation and changing environmental pH. Effervescence cleans wound.	Provides good cleaning action. Causes no known side effects. Is inexpensive.	Decomposes quickly and is short acting. Exerts limited antimicrobial action.	Add new solution to the dressing or change dressing every 4–6 h.
Mercurochrome (Merbromin)	Organic mercurial compound available as solution or tincture.	Acts as desiccating agent that promotes epithelialization.	Is inexpensive. Aids epithelialization of small areas. Dries wound.	Causes stains. Is not antibacterial or antiseptic.	Cover wound with nonadherent dressing to prevent sticking.

KEY FEATURES OF DISEASE ■ Signs of Sepsis

Clinical Data

Altered sensorium
Increased respiratory rate
Hypothermia or hyperthermia
Oliguria

Laboratory Data

Elevated blood glucose levels
Glycosuria
Decreased platelet counts
Increased white blood cell counts with a left shift

flowers is prohibited. Some burn units do not permit clients to eat raw foods, such as salads and fruit, to minimize exposure to exogenous microorganisms. Rugs and upholstered articles are difficult to clean and may harbor organisms; their use is thus also restricted.

Visitors are restricted when the client is immunosuppressed. Ill persons, small children, and other clients should not come into direct contact with the burn client. Some burn units recommend that all visitors wear protective clothing (gowns, gloves, masks, and shoe and hair covers) when in the client's room.

Secondary prevention—early detection. Careful monitoring of burn wounds is done on a daily basis. The nurse examines the wounds for the following signs of infection: a pervasive odor, color changes, change in texture, purulent drainage, exudate, and redness at the wound edges. Laboratory cultures and biopsies are recommended. Quantitative biopsies of the eschar and granulation tissue should be done three times per week to monitor proliferation of organisms. The signs of sepsis are outlined in the accompanying Key Features of Disease.

Interventions: surgical management. Surgical interventions may be indicated to reduce the risk for developing infectious complications. Infected burn wounds with colony counts of or approaching 105 colonies/g of tissue are life-threatening, even with antibiotic therapy. For these conditions, aggressive surgical débridement or excision of the burn wound may be necessary.

Altered Nutrition: Less Than Body Requirements

Planning: client goals. Because metabolic needs frequently double or triple caloric requirements in clients with severe burns, complications such as negative nitrogen balances, body wasting, delayed healing, and death by slow starvation can occur unless nutritional needs are

met. The goal for this nursing diagnosis is that the client will maintain a nutritional intake that is adequate to meet the body's caloric requirements as evidenced by maintaining body weight, normal serum protein levels, and expected rate of wound healing.

Interventions: nonsurgical management. Interventions are aimed at calculating the client's individualized caloric needs and providing an adequate daily source of calories and nutrients that the client can ingest and metabolize.

Diet therapy. Diet therapy begins by calculating the client's current daily metabolic needs and caloric requirements. A variety of formulas and charts are used for this calculation. Nutritional requirements for clients with a relatively large burn area can exceed 5000 kcal/day. In addition to a high-calorie intake, the burn client also requires a diet high in protein. The nurse collaborates with the dietitian and the client to plan alternatives to conventional nutritional patterns. Oral diet therapy may be delayed for several days after the injury until the client has sufficient gastrointestinal motility.

Clients who can eat solid foods are encouraged to ingest as many calories as possible by this route. Client preferences are taken into consideration for diet planning and food selection. Clients are encouraged to request food whenever they feel they can eat, not just according to the hospital's standard meal schedule. The nurse also offers frequent high-calorie, high-protein supplemental feedings. Care is taken to keep an accurate calorie count for foods and beverages that are actually ingested by the client.

Clients who are unable to swallow but who have adequate gastric motility may meet caloric and nutritional needs through enteral nutrition, or tube feedings (Chap. 13). Prepared formulas or blender feedings are administered via nasogastric tubes, gastric tubes, or duodenal or jejunal catheters. Feedings are administered by bolus or by continuous infusion. The amount and frequency of feedings are determined by the client's nutritional requirements and reactions to the feedings (Jacobs et al., 1987). Complications of these methods include aspiration, diarrhea, electrolyte imbalances, and hyperglycemia.

Drug therapy. When the gastrointestinal tract of the client is not functional or when the client's nutritional requirements cannot be met by oral feeding and enteral nutrition alone, the intravenous route or parenteral nutrition is used (Chap. 13). This method is used as a last resort because it is invasive and can have many complications, and research suggests that critically ill clients may not be able to properly metabolize calories that are given by the intravenous route.

Impaired Physical Mobility

Planning: client goals. The major client goals for this nursing diagnosis are that the client will regain and maintain optimal physical mobility.

GUIDELINES ■ How to Position a Client with Burns to Prevent Contractures

Affected Body Part	Position of Function	Interventions
Head and neck	Hyperextension	Place towel roll under client's neck or shoulder under spine or use a double mattress.
Posterior neck	Flexion	Have client turn head side to side.
Upper chest and chest	Shoulder retraction	Place client supine. Do not allow pillows. Place folded towel under spine between scapulae.
Lateral trunk burns	Flexion to uninvolved side	Place client to lie on back with arm on affected side up over head.
Anterior shoulder	Abduction and external rotation	Maintain upper arm at 90-degree abduction from lateral aspect of trunk.
Posterior shoulder	Slight flexion and interior rotation	Keep arm slightly behind midline.
Elbow	Extension and supination	Keep joint in extended position.

Interventions: nonsurgical management. Interventions are aimed at maintaining the client's preburn range of joint motion and at preventing contracture formation (Kraemer et al., 1988). The following interventions are appropriate for any burn in which a joint is involved, no matter how small the burn wound may be.

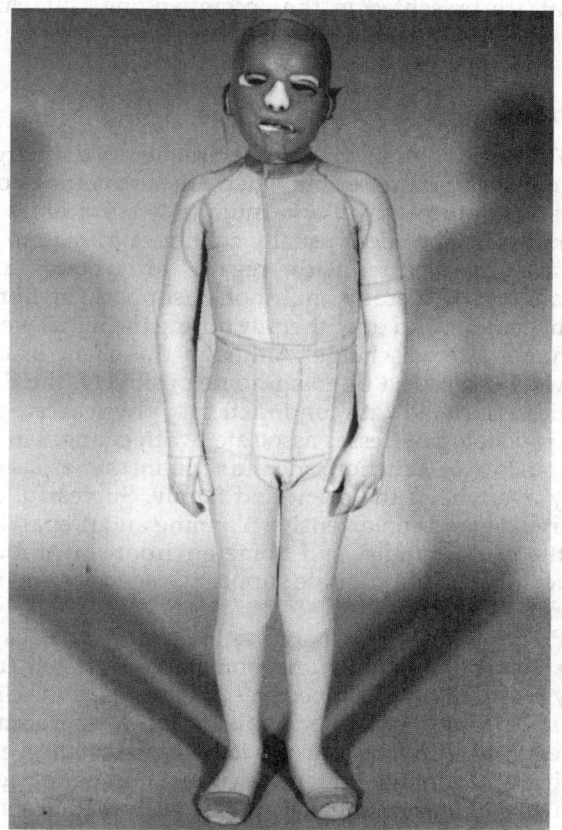

Figure 16–14.
Client wearing pressure garments.

Positioning is critically important for clients with burn injuries because many times the position of comfort for the client is one of joint flexion, which predisposes to the development of contractures. Care is taken to maintain the client in a neutral body position with minimal flexion. Recommended positions for prevention of contracture are illustrated in the accompanying Guidelines feature. Splints and other conforming devices may be used to assist in maintaining position. These devices are used most frequently on joints involving the hands, elbows, knees, neck, and axillae.

Range-of-motion exercises are performed actively at least three times per day. If the client cannot move a joint actively, the nurse performs passive range-of-motion exercises with this joint. Burned hands are given special attention, and the nurse encourages the client to perform active range-of-motion exercises for the hand, thumb, and fingers every hour while awake.

Ambulation is started as soon as possible after the fluid shift has resolved for clients who have not sustained fractures or other serious injuries to the legs and feet. Clients with a variety of attached equipment (such as intravenous catheters, nasogastric tubes, electrocardiographic leads, and extensive dressings) can ambulate with preparation and assistance. Ambulation is performed two or three times per day and progresses in length with each occurrence. This activity inhibits loss of bone density, strengthens muscles, stimulates immune function, promotes ventilation, and prevents a wide variety of complications (Hartigan et al., 1989).

Pressure dressings are used to prevent the formation of contractures and tight hypertrophic scars, which can inhibit mobility. These dressings may be elastic (Ace) wraps or specially designed, custom-fitted, elasticized clothing items (such as Jobst garments), which provide continuous and uniform pressure over burned surfaces. Figure 16–14 illustrates such garments. For maximum effectiveness, these garments must be worn 23 hours per day, every day until the scar tissue is mature. This process takes 12 to 24 months. Wearing such items has been demonstrated to be extremely beneficial in maintaining mobility and reducing the incidence of hypertrophic scarring. However, these garments cause some discomfort to the client (heat and itchiness), and compliance is usually an issue that nurses need to address.

Interventions: surgical management. Surgical management is restorative rather than preventive. Surgical techniques for contracture release are most commonly performed in the neck, axilla, and elbow flexion areas. Specific surgical procedures to improve movement are varied and individualized for the client.

Postoperative nursing responsibilities include the nonsurgical interventions described earlier to prevent contractures from re-forming, as well as care of new grafts and suture lines. The nurse constantly reinforces the need for client compliance with exercise and splinting regimens to prevent recurrence of joint immobility.

Body Image Disturbance

Planning: client goals. The major client goals for this nursing diagnosis are that the client will (1) progress through the grieving process, (2) use support systems, and (3) function independently.

Interventions: nonsurgical management. Understanding of the stages of grief is helpful for the client, family, and nurse. The nurse assesses which stage of grief the client is currently experiencing and helps to interpret client behaviors. Frequently, clients are unaware of or confused by their feelings. The nurse reassures the client that feelings of grief, loss, anxiety, anger, fear, and guilt are normal. The client may be grieving for losses of body parts, appearance, role identity, and social identity. The nurse seeks the help of other health care team members (e.g., psychologist, psychiatrist, social worker, or clergy or religious leader) in addressing these problems.

The nurse accepts the physical and psychologic characteristics of the client. Clients and families are presented with realistic expected physical outcomes for the client in terms of functional capacity and appearance. Sessions for providing information and counseling for the family or significant others are productive for identifying previous and current effective patterns of support for the client and family. The use of these systems and the development of new support systems are facilitated by the nurse. Referrals to specific support groups are made. Continuous evaluation of support resources for the client and family throughout the course of illness is necessary to identify ineffectiveness of and possible gaps in such assistance.

Engaging in decision-making and independent activities usually fosters feelings of self-worth, which are closely linked to body image. To this end, the nurse plans and encourages client participation in self-care activities. The nurse assists family members to understand that it is more beneficial for the client to perform these activities than to have them done for him or her. Families are encouraged to include the client in family decision-making to the same degree that the client participated in this process before the injury.

Interventions: surgical management. Reconstructive and cosmetic surgery can be performed for many years after the burn injury. Restoration of function and improvement of physical appearance through surgical techniques often increase the client's feelings of self-worth and promote a positive body image. Many clients may have unrealistic expectations of such surgery and envision reconstructed areas to appear identical or equal in quality to the preburn state. The nurse educates the client and family about expected cosmetic outcomes.

■ Discharge Planning

Discharge planning for the client who has a burn injury starts at the time of the client's initial admission to the hospital or burn center. In most burn centers, the multidisciplinary team meets regularly to plan for the client's discharge by evaluating the progress of each discipline toward assisting the client to reach mutually established discharge goals. Probable and possible interventions that are important to discharge planning for the burn client are presented in the accompanying Guidelines feature.

Home Care Preparation

The client with severe burns is frequently discharged from the acute care setting when life-threatening complications are resolved and minimal wound areas remain open. The client usually continues to require extensive daily care with regard to wound care, rehabilitative therapy, nutritional support, symptom management, and drug therapy during the initial weeks at home after discharge. Although the client usually views the prospect of going home positively, the difficulties associated with continuation of physical care and the psychologic stresses associated with changes in appearance, role, function, and life style are numerous and may overwhelm the client and family. Successful discharge depends on extensive planning and preparation of the client, family, and home environment through education and appropriate supportive agencies and services.

Preparation for discharge to the home includes assessment of the family and home care situation from physical and social perspectives. The needs of the client must be considered when evaluating the environment in terms of cleanliness; access to bathing facilities, electricity, and running water; stairways; number of occupants; temperature control; and safety. If the burn injuries are a result of a fire at home, a new residence may need to be established.

GUIDELINES ■ Interventions for Discharge Planning for Clients with Burns

Early patient assessment

Financial assessment

Evaluation of family resources

Weekly discharge planning meeting

Psychologic referral

Patient and family teaching (home care)

Designation of principal learners (specific family members or significant others who will help with care)

Development of teaching plan

Training for wound care

Rehabilitation referral

Home assessment (on-site visit)

Medical equipment

Public health nursing referral

Evaluation of community resources

Visit to referral agency

Re-entry programs for school or work environment

Nursing home placement

Environmental interventions

Auditory testing

Speech therapy

Prosthetic rehabilitation

Client/Family Education

Client and family education regarding burn care and living with the consequences of burn injuries begins when the client is admitted to the hospital or burn center. A weekly plan for client education is outlined, with the goal being progression toward client and family independence. Critical for this goal is the teaching of clients, family members, and/or significant others to perform specific care tasks, such as dressing changes. Clients and family members first observe the process of changing the dressings, then assist the nurse or technician in performing the changes, and finally change the dressings independently under the supervision of the burn care nurse.

Before the client's discharge from the hospital, all individuals who will be involved in the client's home care participate in discharge planning and teaching sessions. In addition to details about dressing changes, information is provided about signs and symptoms of infection, medication regimens, the proper use of prosthetic and positioning devices, and correct application and care of pressure garments.

Psychosocial Preparation

Clients with severe burn injuries are likely to experience psychologic problems during the recovery period and for some time after discharge from the hospital and may require psychologic assistance. Problems include posttraumatic stress disorder, sexual dysfunction, and severe depression (Courtemanche & Robinow, 1989). Assistance is coordinated with the client, family, and health care team. This type of assistance is best provided by a professional counselor with previous experience in helping burn clients.

One specific area to address with the client who has been burned is the reaction of others to the sight of healing wounds and disfiguring scars. Clients with facial burns are especially subjected to stares and other forms of disquieting behavior on the part of the general public. Having friends visit and having the client make short public appearances before discharge from the hospital may help the client begin adjusting to this problem.

Health Care Resources

The family is evaluated in terms of capacity and willingness to assist in providing care to the client at home. A visiting nurse referral is beneficial for helping the family with care problems that arise at home. In addition, this nurse can help the family determine what special equipment, supplies, or services will be needed to care for the client. The frequency of home visits depends on the condition of the client and the ability of family members to function as care providers.

Home care of a client after an extensive burn frequently involves daily physical therapy and rehabilitation sessions at special centers. Transportation problems are addressed and resolved before the client is discharged. In some instances, the burn center has arrangements for transportation. Some community volunteer agencies provide transportation by private car. Clients receiving public assistance may be eligible for free bus tokens or for reimbursement of cab fare.

When rehabilitation is expected to be prolonged, the client may be discharged to a special rehabilitation facility. Some facilities are private institutions, whereas others are supported by state or local tax systems. Before the client is discharged to such care, the burn care nurse consults with the rehabilitation nurse or team and provides them with copies of the care and teaching plans that have been used with the client.

 Evaluation

On the basis of the nursing diagnoses that have been identified, the expected outcomes for the client with burn injuries include that the client

1. Restores normal circulating fluid volume

2. Maintains adequate cardiac output
3. Maintains urinary output of at least 30 mL/hour
4. Remains oriented to time, place, and person
5. Is free of dyspnea
6. Has pain reduced to an acceptable level
8. Maintains integrity of nonburned skin
9. Experiences closure of all burn wounds
10. Is able to obtain a normal sleep pattern
11. Maintains an oral intake sufficient to meet nutritional demands and prevent excessive weight loss
12. Lists signs and symptoms of infection
13. Verbalizes appropriate actions to take when signs and symptoms of infection are present
14. Remains free from sepsis
15. Complies with treatment regimen regarding medications and use of pressure garments
16. Maintains normal range of joint motion
17. Can discuss permanent alterations in physical appearance
18. Participates in self-care
19. Takes an active role in family decision-making
20. Maintains social contacts
21. Resumes preburn social and professional activities
22. Resumes sexual relationship with partner
23. Accepts illness-imposed restrictions on life style
24. Uses appropriate support systems and available resources
25. Progressively increases independent functioning
26. Uses coping mechanisms to deal with anxiety-provoking circumstances

SUMMARY

Effective care for the client with burns requires a multidisciplinary and specialized approach because the effects of the burn injury extend well beyond direct trauma to epithelial tissues and beyond the time frame during which acute care is needed. Nursing care in the emergent phase focuses on supporting the client's circulatory and respiratory efforts. During the acute phase of recovery, nursing care focuses on wound care, prevention of infection, maintenance of mobility, and nutritional support. Nursing care during the rehabilitative phase focuses on restoring the client emotionally and physically to maximal functional capacity.

Because nursing care of the burn client includes surgical, medical, social, psychologic, spiritual, and rehabilitative aspects of care, the nurse caring for these clients experiences many professional and technical challenges. Critical to successful burn nursing is the concept that burn care requires a cooperative team effort.

IMPLICATIONS FOR RESEARCH

Because the nursing care problems that are associated with burn injuries are so varied and include the psychosocial as well as the physical, the areas for nursing research are virtually unlimited. Specific topics for nursing research include strategies for prevention, assessment tools, symptom management, rehabilitation, and quality of life issues. Some examples of questions to be answered by nursing research include

1. How effective are public awareness programs for fire prevention and safety?
2. What type of dressing is most suitable for a donor site?
3. What are the long-term psychosocial effects of burn injury?
4. What are the major specific sources of nosocomial infections among hospitalized burn clients?
5. Do pressure dressings on healed burn areas reduce scar formation on all skin types?

REFERENCES AND READINGS

Barber, J. (1986). Immunologic responses to trauma. *Critical Care Quarterly, 9*(1), 57–67.

Baxter, C., & Waeckerle, J. (1988). Emergency treatment of burn injury. *Annals of Emergency Medicine, 17*, 1305–1314.

Bjerknes, R., & Vindenes, H. (1989). Neutrophil dysfunction after thermal injury: Alteration of phagolysosomal acidification in patients with large burns. *Burns, 15*, 77–81.

Boswick, J. (1987). Comprehensive rehabilitation after burn injury. *Surgical Clinics of North America, 67*, 159–166.

Courtemanche, D., & Robinow, O. (1989). Recognition and treatment of the post-traumatic stress disorder in the burn victim. *Journal of Burn Care and Rehabilitation, 10*, 247–250.

Dacso, C., Luterman, A., & Curreri, P. (1987). Systemic antibiotic treatment in burned patients. *Surgical Clinics of North America, 67*, 57–68.

Demling, R. (1987). Fluid replacement in burned patients. *Surgical Clinics of North America, 67*, 15–30.

DiMola, M., & Winkler, J. (1986a). Burn care protocols: Donor site care. *Journal of Burn Care and Rehabilitation, 7*, 154–159.

DiMola, M., & Winkler, J. (1986b). Burn care protocols: Post operative management of sheet and meshed autografts. *Journal of Burn Care and Rehabilitation, 7*, 60–64.

DiMola, M., Winkler, J., & Acres, C. (1987). Burns. In M. R. Kinney, et al. (Eds.), *AACN's clinical reference for critical-care nursing* (2nd ed.). New York: McGraw-Hill.

Eisenberg, M. (1987). Burn rehabilitation. *Advances in Clinical Rehabilitation, 1,* 175–176.

Feller, I., & Jones, C. (1987). The national burn information exchange: The use of a national burn registry to evaluate and address the burn problem. *Surgical Clinics of North America, 67,* 167–189.

Gordon, M. (1987). Burn wound care: Silver sulfadiazine application. *Journal of Burn Care and Rehabilitation, 8,* 429–433.

Gurevich, I., & Tafuro, P. (1986). The compromised host: Deficit-specific infection and the spectrum of prevention. *Cancer Nursing, 9,* 263–275.

Guyton, A. C. (1986). *Textbook of medical physiology.* Philadelphia: W. B. Saunders.

Haberal, M., Oner, Z., Bayraktar, U., & Bilgin, N. (1987). The use of silver nitrate–incorporated amniotic membrane as a temporary dressing. *Burns, 13,* 159–163.

Haberal, M., Oner, Z., Gulay, H., Bayraktar, U., & Bilgin, N. (1989). Severe electrical injury. *Burns, 15,* 42–44.

Hammond, J., & Ward, C. (1988). High-voltage electrical injuries: Management and outcome of 60 cases. *Southern Medical Journal, 81,* 1351–1352.

Hansbrough, J., Zapata-Sirvent, R., & Peterson, V. (1987). Immunomodulation following burn injury. *Surgical Clinics of North America, 67,* 69–92.

Hartigan, C., Persing, J., Williamson, C., Morgan, R., Muir, A., & Edlich, R. (1989). An overview of muscle strengthening. *Journal of Burn Care and Rehabilitation, 10,* 251–257.

Heimbach, D. (1987). Early burn excision and grafting. *Surgical Clinics of North America, 67,* 93–107.

Herndon, D., Langner, F., Thompson, P., Linares, H., Stein, M., & Traber, D. (1987). Pulmonary injury in burned patients. *Surgical Clinics of North America, 67,* 31–46.

Jacobs, L., de Kock, M., & van der Merwe, A. (1987). Oral hyperalimentation and the prevention of severe weight loss in burned patients. *Burns, 13,* 154–158.

Kraemer, M., Jones, T., & Deitch, E. (1988). Burn contractures: Incidence, predisposing factors and results of surgical therapy. *Journal of Burn Care and Rehabilitation, 9,* 261–265.

Kuehn, C., Ahrenholz, D., & Solem, L. (1989). Care of the burn wound. *Trauma Quarterly, 5*(4), 33–43.

Larson, S., & Parks, D. (1988). Managing the difficult airway in patients with burns of the head and neck. *Journal of Burn Care and Rehabilitation, 9,* 55–56.

Lund, T., Wiig, H., & Reed, R. (1988). Acute postburn edema: Role of strongly negative interstitial fluid pressure. *American Journal of Physiology, 255,* H1069–H1074.

Marvin, J. (1987). Pain Management in the burn patient. *Journal of Burn Care and Rehabilitation, 8,* 307–318.

Monafo, W., & Freedman, B. (1987). Topical therapy for burns. *Surgical Clinics of North America, 67,* 133–145.

Moran, K., & Munster, A. (1987). Alterations of the host defense mechanism in burned patients. *Surgical Clinics of North America, 67,* 47–56.

Pasulka, P., & Wachtel, T. (1987). Nutritional considerations for the burned patient. *Surgical Clinics of North America, 67,* 109–131.

Peterson, V., Ambruso, D., Emmett, M., & Bartle, E. (1988). Inhibition of colony-stimulating factor (CSF) production by postburn serum: Negative feedback inhibition mediated by lactoferrin. *Journal of Trauma, 28,* 1533–1540.

Rivers, E. (1987). Rehabilitation management of the burn patient. *Advances in Clinical Rehabilitation, 1,* 177–214.

Sherif, M., & Sato, R. (1989). Severe thermal hand burns—factors affecting progress. *Burns, 15,* 42–46.

Silverstein, P., & Lack, B. (1987). Fire prevention in the United States: Are the home fires still burning?. *Surgical Clinics of North America, 67,* 1–14.

Sittig, K., & Deitch, E. (1988). Effect of bacteremia on mortality after thermal injury. *Archives of Surgery, 123,* 1367–1370.

Trier, H., & Spaabaek, J. (1987). The nursing home patient—a burn-prone person. *Burns, 13,* 483–487.

Varas, R., & Hammond, J. (1989). Burn prevention begins at home. *Journal of Burn Care and Rehabilitation, 10,* 88–89.

ADDITIONAL READINGS

Helvig, E., & Herndon, D. (1989). Airway and pulmonary management of burn patients. *Trauma Quarterly, 5*(4), 19–32.

This comprehensive article describes the significance of airway complications among clients with burn injuries. Information is presented on the incidence and pathophysiology of actual inhalation burns, as well as many indirect pulmonary complications that also are associated with burns. Nursing management of burned clients with pulmonary problems is presented in conjunction with the medical management.

Lee, J. J., Marvin, J. A., & Heimback, D. M. (1989). Effectiveness of nalbuphine for relief of burn débridement pain. *Journal of Burn Care and Rehabilitation, 10,* 241–246.

The authors used a double-blind method to compare the effectiveness of nalbuphine against that of morphine in controlling pain related to burn débridement. Parameters included vital signs, level of sedation, adverse effects, and patient evaluation of pain intensity and relief by use of an adjective and visual analogue scale. There were no significant differences in the variables measured; nalbuphine was as effective as morphine sulfate. However, the respiratory depression that often accompanies morphine therapy was not a problem with nalbuphine.

Mancusi-Ungaro, S. (1989). Psychosocial issues in burn care. *Trauma Quarterly, 5*(4), 67–70.

The author succinctly describes the expected psychosocial issues commonly experienced by many burn clients and their family members during the immediate and long-term care period after a burn injury. The information presented is free from specialty jargon and provides the burn care nurse with concrete examples of behaviors associated with specific psychosocial alterations. Emphasis is placed on assisting the nurse to view the changes that the client experiences from the client's perspective rather than on directing the nurse to engage in specific psychotherapeutic interventions.

CHAPTER 17

Interventions for Clients in Shock

OVERVIEW

Tissues and cells within the human body require a continuous supply of oxygen to maintain metabolic homeostasis. The cardiovascular system, under neural regulation and working in conjunction with the pulmonary system, supplies oxygen and other nutrients to all tissues and removes wastes that arise from normal cellular metabolism. The components of the cardiovascular system important for this homeostatic function are the *blood*, the *blood vessels*, and the *heart*. The blood is the liquid carrier medium of these nutrients, which are transported to cells and tissues through the blood vessels. Blood vessels control blood flow to specific areas and, at the level of the capillaries, are responsible for the exchange of nutrients and wastes within the tissues. The heart supplies the pumping force that initiates and maintains circulation. When any component of the cardiovascular system does not function properly for any reason, the syndrome of *shock* can result.

Shock is a pathologic condition, rather than a disease state. It is characterized by generalized abnormal cellular metabolism that occurs as a direct result of inadequate delivery of oxygen to body tissues or inadequate usage of oxygen by body tissues (Robbins & Kumar, 1987). Shock generally is classified by the site or origin of dysfunction as *hypovolemic, cardiogenic, vasogenic,* and *septic*. Many clinical manifestations of shock are similar, regardless of the site of origin or the initiating factors. These manifestations are due to physiologic compensatory mechanisms as well as specific tissue dysfunction. The common clinical manifestations of shock are summarized in the accompanying Key Features of Disease.

PHYSIOLOGY REVIEW

Cardiovascular oxygenation of any organ or tissue is dependent on the degree of arterial perfusion the organ receives. Organ perfusion is directly related to mean arterial pressure (MAP). Because the cardiovascular system is a closed but continuous circuit, the factors that determine MAP include total blood volume, cardiac output, and the size of the vascular bed. Total blood volume and cardiac output are *directly* related to MAP, so that increases in either total blood volume or cardiac output usually increase MAP. Decreases in either total blood volume or cardiac output usually decrease MAP.

The size of the vascular bed is *inversely* related to MAP, so that increases in the size of the vascular bed decrease MAP and decreases in the size of the vascular bed increase MAP. The blood vessels, especially the vessels located adjacent to capillaries (arterioles and venules), can increase in size through relaxation of smooth muscle in vessel walls or decrease in size through constriction of smooth muscle in vessel walls.

KEY FEATURES OF DISEASE ■ Clinical Manifestations of Shock

Cardiovascular

Decreased cardiac output

Increased pulse rate

Thready pulse quality

Decreased blood pressure

Narrowed pulse pressure

Postural hypotension

Low central venous pressure

Flat neck and hand veins in dependent positions

Slow capillary refill in nail beds

Diminished peripheral pulses

Respiratory

Increased respiratory rate

Shallow depth of respirations

Decreased arterial PCO_2

Decreased arterial PO_2

Cyanosis, especially around lips and nail beds

Neuromuscular

Early
    Anxiety
    Restlessness

Late
    Decreased CNS activity (lethargy to coma)
    Generalized muscle weakness
    Diminished or absent deep tendon reflexes
    Sluggish pupillary response to light

Renal

Decreased urinary output

Increased specific gravity

Sugar and acetone present in urine

Integumentary

Cool to cold

Pale to mottled to cyanotic

Moist, clammy

Mouth dry, paste-like coating present

Gastrointestinal

Decreased motility

Diminished or absent bowel sounds

Nausea and vomiting

Constipation

Increased thirst

When blood vessels dilate, but the total volume of blood remains the same, pressure within the vessels is decreased and blood flow is slower. When blood vessels constrict, but the total volume of blood remains the same, pressure within the vessels is increased and blood flow is faster.

Blood vessels are innervated by the sympathetic division of the autonomic nervous system. Usually, some of these nerves continuously stimulate vascular smooth muscle, so that blood vessels normally are partially contracted. This state of partial contraction is called *sympathetic tone*. An increase in sympathetic nerve discharge (stimulation) causes the vascular smooth muscle to constrict, increasing MAP; a decrease in sympathetic discharge causes the vascular smooth muscle to dilate, decreasing MAP.

Blood flow to body organs varies from minute to minute to accommodate local and systemic metabolic needs. The body can selectively increase blood flow to some areas and diminish blood flow to other areas. Some regulation of regional blood flow occurs locally, but the most influential control is generated from the central nervous system (CNS). Some organs, such as the skin, can tolerate low blood flow and low levels of oxygenation for relatively long periods of time without sustaining damage. Other organs, such as the heart, brain, and liver, tolerate hypoxic conditions poorly, and even just a few minutes without adequate blood flow results in serious or permanent damage.

PATHOPHYSIOLOGY

The underlying pathophysiologic feature of all types of shock, regardless of etiology, is the effects of anaerobic cellular metabolism, which result from inadequate tissue oxygenation (Shoemaker, 1987). These effects dramatically alter the balanced composition of intracellular and extracellular fluids. Because these imbalances can profoundly disturb physiologic function, the body institutes compensatory mechanisms to restore physiologic homeostasis even while the triggering events of shock are still present. When the conditions that cause shock remain unresolved, shock progresses in a predictable sequence. Although shock is a dynamic condition, stages of shock can be identified on the basis of the effectiveness of the client's compensatory mechanisms, the severity of the clinical manifestations, and the reversibility of tissue damage.

Sequence of Shock

Figure 17–1 shows the interactions of different types of shock, physiologic compensation, and the dynamic progression of shock. The primary triggering event leading to shock is a sustained decrease in MAP that occurs as a result of decreased cardiac output, decreased circulating blood volume, or expansion of the vascular bed. A decrease in MAP of 5 to 10 mmHg from the baseline is

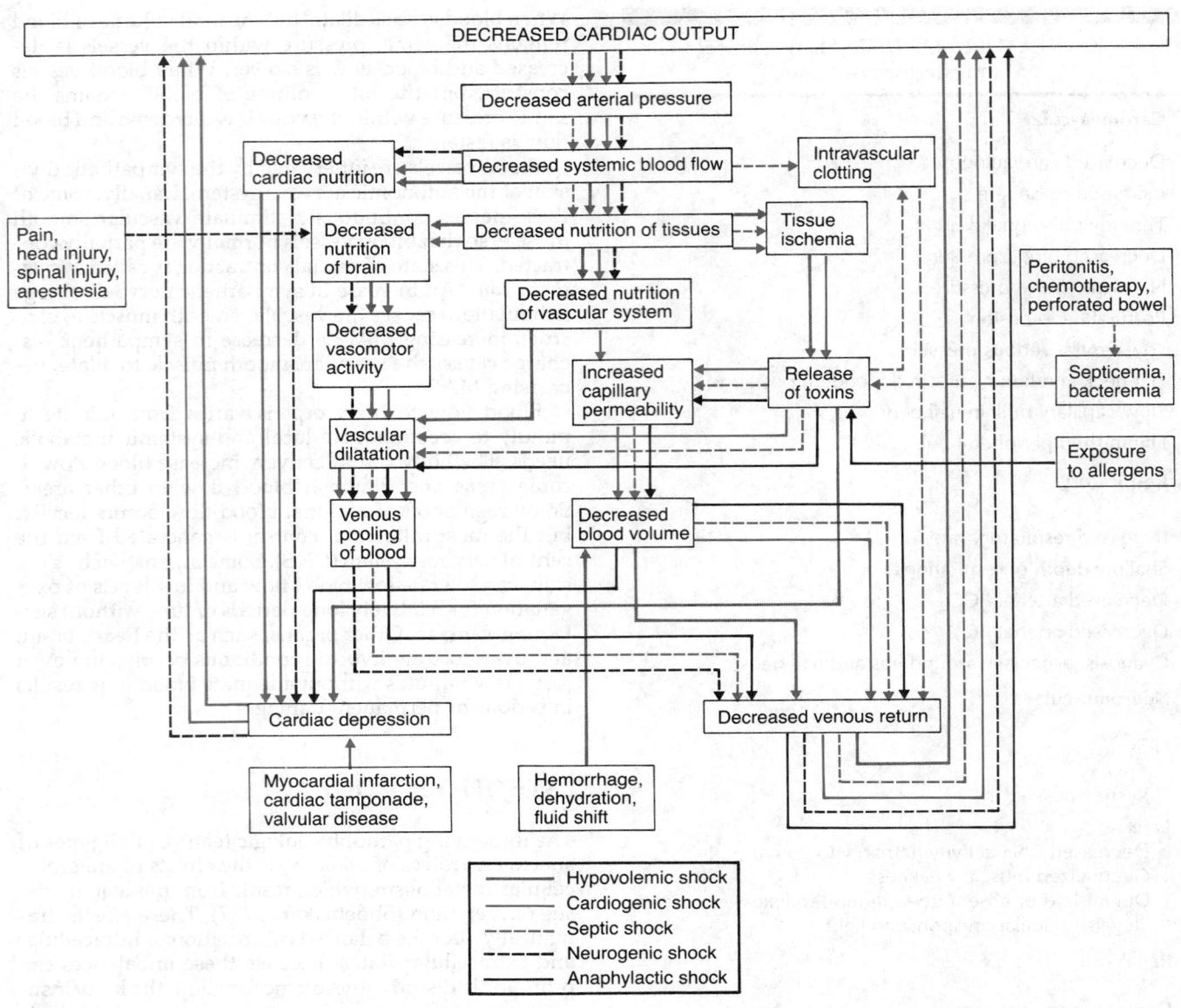

Figure 17-1

Initiators of shock and the futile cycles of physiologic compensation. (Modified from Guyton, A. C. [1986]. *Textbook of medical physiology* [7th ed.]. Philadelphia: W. B. Saunders.)

immediately detected by pressure-sensitive, afferent nerve receptors (baroreceptors) located in the aortic arch and the carotid sinus (Guyton, 1986). This information is transmitted to an integration center in the brain, which then stimulates compensatory mechanisms to ensure continued perfusion and oxygenation to vital organs, leading to the physiologic changes associated with various stages of shock.

If the events that caused the initial decrease in MAP are halted at this point, the compensatory mechanisms can return the body to a homeostatic state even without outside intervention. If the initiating events continue and MAP further decreases, some tissues will be operat-

ing under anaerobic conditions, creating an increase in lactic acid and other harmful metabolites. These substances cause electrolyte and acid-base imbalances that can exert generalized, tissue-damaging effects and depress myocardial activity (Horton, 1989). These effects are temporary and reversible if shock is corrected within a relatively short period of time. When shock-creating conditions continue for longer periods of time without the institution of supportive interventions, the resulting acid-base and electrolyte imbalances as well as the increased levels of toxic metabolites inflict such extensive damage to critical cells within vital organs that full recovery from shock is no longer possible.

The Early Stage

The early stage of shock is present when the initiating factors have caused MAP to decrease by less than 10 mmHg. This stage of shock is sometimes called nonprogressive shock, as adaptive and compensatory mechanisms are activated and are so effective at returning MAP to normal levels that perfusion to all vital organs is maintained and overall cellular metabolism is aerobic. Compensation, mediated through vascular constriction and cardiac rate changes, is relatively complete, and both cardiac output and MAP are maintained within the normal range. Because vital organ function is not disrupted during this stage, the signs and symptoms of this stage of shock are subtle and difficult to detect. Heart rate increases from baseline may be the only discernible manifestation of this stage of shock.

The Compensatory Stage

The compensatory stage of shock is observed when initiating conditions have caused a 10- to 15-mmHg drop in MAP. Renal and chemical compensatory mechanisms are activated because cardiovascular compensation alone is not sufficient to maintain MAP and supply metabolic needs for oxygen.

Sustained decreased MAP is sensed by the kidneys and the baroreceptors, resulting in the release of renin, antidiuretic hormone (ADH), aldosterone, and the catecholamines epinephrine and norepinephrine. Renal compensation is regulated through the actions of renin, aldosterone, and ADH (Chap. 12). Renin is secreted by the kidney and initiates the angiotensinogen reactions (see Chap. 12, Fig. 12–2), which eventually cause decreased glomerular filtration, decreased urinary output, increased reabsorption of sodium, and systemic vasoconstriction. ADH is secreted by the posterior pituitary gland, and its activity both increases renal reabsorption of water and causes peripheral vasoconstriction. These actions together attempt to compensate for shock by increasing central vascular volume.

Tissue hypoxia is present in nonvital organs and in the kidney, but is not great enough to cause severe symptoms or permanent damage. Because some metabolism is anaerobic, acid-base and electrolyte changes occur in response to the build-up of metabolites and compensatory mechanisms. These changes include acidemia and hyperkalemia, which alter the function of excitable tissues and are responsible for many of the clinical manifestations exhibited by clients in this stage of shock (Chaps. 13 and 15).

If this stage of shock is relatively stable and compensatory mechanisms are supported by medical and nursing interventions, the individual can remain in this stage for hours without sustaining permanent damage. Halting the conditions that initiated shock or providing supportive interventions are necessary to prevent the progression of shock. When interventions are appropriately instituted, the effects of this stage of shock are reversible.

The Intermediate Stage

The intermediate stage of shock is characterized by a sustained decrease in MAP of greater than 20 mmHg from baseline. Compensatory mechanisms are functioning, but are no longer adequate to maintain sufficient oxygen supply, even to vital organs. The hypermetabolism of tissues participating in compensatory mechanisms contributes to the problem of inadequate oxygenation. Hypoxia is present in vital organs, whereas other organs are experiencing anoxia and ischemia. As a result of inadequate oxygenation and a build-up of toxic metabolites, some tissues have extensive cell damage and cell death.

This stage of shock is a life-threatening emergency. Cells of vital organs can tolerate this situation for only a short period of time before sustaining extensive permanent damage. Immediate interventions are required to reverse the effects of this stage of shock. Tolerance of this stage is highly individual and depends to a large extent on the client's pre-existing state of health. In general, the client's life can be saved if this stage of shock is corrected within an hour. This time reference is sometimes called the "golden hour" for trauma care and is the rationale for the development of centralized trauma centers and the use of helicopter transport of trauma victims.

The Irreversible Stage

In the progression of shock, there is a point at which such widespread tissue anoxia and cell death are present that overwhelming functional changes occur in vital organs. The remaining cells are metabolizing anaerobically. Therapy is ineffective in saving the life of the client, even if the underlying cause of the shock is corrected and if MAP temporarily returns to normal. So much tissue damage has occurred and has resulted in the systemic release of toxic metabolites and degradative enzymes that cellular deterioration of vital organs continues (Border & Hassett, 1988). The most profound change that continues to occur is deterioration of the myocardium.

ETIOLOGY

Because shock is a manifestation of a pathologic condition rather than a separate disease state, the cause of shock varies, depending on the site and the type of the underlying problem. Shock is classified according to its causes as hypovolemic, cardiogenic, vasogenic, and septic (see the accompanying Key Features of Disease). It is important to remember that some pathologic conditions stimulate events that can trigger more than one type of shock simultaneously.

Hypovolemic Shock

Hypovolemic shock occurs when there is a loss of circulating fluid volume from the central vascular space

KEY FEATURES OF DISEASE ■ Causes and Clinical Manifestations Unique to Various Types of Shock

Mechanism	Etiology	Clinical Manifestations
Hypovolemic Shock		
Diminished circulating plasma volume.	External or internal hemorrhage from surgical or traumatic wounds, GI ulcers, and conditions in which blood clotting is inhibited. Fluid volume losses, such as with vomiting, diarrhea, excessive wound drainage, prolonged nasogastric suctioning, excessive perspiration, administration of diuretics, diabetes insipidus, and inadequate fluid intake. Loss of fluid from vascular space to interstitial space as seen with burns, liver disorders, malnutrition, and stress response.	*Integumentary* When caused by an actual fluid loss from the body, the skin has poor turgor and tenting may be evident. When caused by a fluid shift into the interstitial space, edema is present. The skin is stretched and shiny in appearance. Pits may be formed in response to light pressure. The skin is difficult to pinch up.
Cardiogenic Shock		
Direct or indirect failure of the heart to provide the necessary pumping force to eject a sufficient volume of blood from the left ventricle at a pressure great enough to maintain MAP.	Direct pump failure: myocardial infarction, cardiac arrest, arrhythmias, valvular disease, and myocardial degeneration. Indirect pump failure: cardiac tamponade, hyperkalemia, hypocalcemia, head trauma, and drug overdoses.	*Cardiovascular* Central venous pressure is elevated. Neck and hand veins are distended. Edema is present, first in dependent areas. *Respiratory* Pulmonary edema is present. Respiration is labored, especially in the supine position. Crackles and wheezes are present on auscultation.
Vasogenic Shock of Neural Origin		
Diminished sympathetic nerve discharge to blood vessel smooth muscle, resulting in relaxation of the smooth muscle and dilation of the blood vessels.	Spinal cord injury, spinal anesthesia, head trauma, drug or anesthetic overdose, pain, and psychogenic syncope.	*Integumentary* The skin is warm and pink.
Vasogenic Shock of Chemical Origin		
This shock is produced by a type I hypersensitivity reaction (anaphylaxis) in which the individual is exposed to an allergen and the individual's antibodies (IgE) bind to that allergen, forming a complex that causes degranulation of basophils, eosinophils, and mast cells, and releasing large amounts of heparin, histamine, other vasoactive amines. These	Exposure (repeated) of a sensitive individual to an allergen, such as penicillin, dyes, aspirin, bisulfites, blood components, vaccines, venom, eggs, shellfish, and soybeans.	*Onset and progression* are rapid. *Integumentary* The skin is warm and pink, with some edema present. *Respiratory* Breathing occurs with great difficulty—there is upper and lower airway obstruction. Stridor and wheezes are audible. Loss of consciousness occurs quickly.

KEY FEATURES OF DISEASE ■ Causes and Clinical Manifestations Unique to Various Types of Shock *Continued*		
Mechanism	Etiology	Clinical Manifestations
substances cause massive vasodilation and increased capillary permeability. The same substances cause edema of the respiratory epithelium and possibly interfere with myocardial contractility.		
Septic Shock		
Bacterial endotoxins released into the blood react with leukocytes and cell membranes, stimulating a variety of inflammatory and immune responses, which activate complement, alter microcirculation, and stimulate widespread microthrombus formation in vital organs. Inflammation causes the release of substances that produce generalized vasodilation and increased capillary permeability.	Septicemia—usually with gram-negative bacteria (*Pseudomonas aeruginosa, Escherichia coli, Klebsiella pneumoniae*), staphylococcus, streptococcus, yeast, and viruses. The gram-negative infections are most commonly associated with conditions that involve fecal contamination of the blood, such as perforated bowel and bowel surgery. Infection with other organisms is most commonly associated with conditions involving significant immunosuppression, such as cancer chemotherapy and acquired immunodeficiency syndrome (AIDS).	Usually fever is present. Neutrophilia is present. The differential leukocyte count shows a left shift. In the early stages, the cardiac output is enhanced and is normal or high. As shock progresses, the cardiac output and MAP decrease.

to the extent that MAP decreases and the body's total need for tissue oxygenation is not adequately met (Ledingham & Ramsay, 1986). This reduction in the volume of blood or blood components can be an actual loss, as with hemorrhage (external or internal) and dehydration, or can be a relative loss as a result of the shifting of fluid from the central vascular space to the interstitial space.

External hemorrhage is associated with soft-tissue trauma, wounds, and surgery. Internal, or occult, hemorrhage is associated with blunt trauma, gastrointestinal (GI) ulcers, and poor surgical hemostasis. In addition, external and internal hemorrhage can be caused by any health problem that results in inadequate levels of substances needed for coagulation. These health problems include hemophilia, malnutrition, bone marrow suppression, anemia, chronic liver dysfunction, leukemia, and anticoagulation therapy.

Hypovolemia as a result of dehydration can be caused by any condition that decreases fluid intake or increases renal and insensible fluid loss. Such conditions include altered levels of consciousness, musculoskeletal immobility, heavy exercise, excessive wound drainage, nasogastric suction, vomiting, diarrhea, hyperglycemia, diuretic therapy, and diabetes insipidus.

Hypovolemia also can occur as a result of a shift of fluid from the vascular space to the interstitial space. Such shifts are caused by increased capillary permeability, loss of plasma osmolarity, and increased vascular hydrostatic pressure. Specific conditions associated with fluid shifts include severe burns, hepatic dysfunction or enlargement, severe malnutrition, sodium-wasting renal disease, and hypoproteinemia (Carter et al., 1988).

Cardiogenic Shock

Cardiogenic shock occurs when the pumping ability of the heart is impaired either directly or indirectly. Direct pump failure can result from myocardial infarction (MI), cardiac arrest, serious arrhythmias (fibrillation or ventricular tachycardia), valvular pathologic changes, and myocardial degeneration associated with inadequate myocardial circulation, systemic infection, or exposure to chemical toxins (Jeffries & Whelan, 1988). These conditions decrease cardiac output and afterload, thus reducing MAP (Chap. 63 provides a complete discussion of preload and afterload).

Other conditions can interfere with the contractility of a healthy heart and cause cardiogenic shock indirectly. Such conditions include cardiac tamponade, electrolyte imbalances (especially hyperkalemia and hypocalcemia), administration of drugs that decrease the rate and vigor of cardiac contractility, and injuries to the cardioregulatory areas of the brain.

Vasogenic Shock

Vasogenic shock is characterized by a loss of sympathetic tone, vasodilation, pooling of blood in venous and capillary beds, and increased vascular permeability, which all contribute to decreased MAP. The origin of this set of reactions is neural (neurogenic shock) or chemical. The most commonly identified chemical origin is related to agents inducing anaphylaxis.

Neurogenically induced loss of MAP occurs when sympathetic stimulation of nerves regulating the vascular smooth muscle is inhibited and the smooth muscle relaxes, causing vasodilation. This vasodilation can be a local response to injury, but shock can result when the vasodilation is systemic. Common conditions that can cause a systemic loss of sympathetic tone include severe pain, prolonged exposure to heat, psychologic stress, neurologic damage, spinal cord injuries, and injection of nerve block anesthetics over a large area (spinal, epidural, and caudal anesthesia). Cholinergic drugs and alpha-adrenergic blocking agents also can contribute to neurogenic shock.

Vasogenic shock of chemical origin is associated with the type I delayed hypersensitivity immune reaction known as anaphylaxis. This reaction is termed delayed, although it usually begins within seconds to minutes after exposure to a specific allergen, because the individual rarely has this type of reaction the first time he/she encounters the allergen. Rather, this reaction occurs on subsequent exposure to the same allergen (Guyton, 1987). Some common allergens associated with anaphylaxis among susceptible individuals include drugs or chemicals (penicillin, radiopaque dyes, aspirin, bisulfites, vaccines, and blood components), venom (snake, bee, and wasp), and food (eggs, seafood, shellfish, and soybeans) (Dickerson, 1988).

Anaphylaxis is due to an antigen-antibody reaction occurring systemically in response to contact with a substance to which the individual has a severe hypersensitivity (allergy). The widespread antigen-antibody reaction, involving the interaction of the allergen, immunoglobulin E (IgE), basophils, and mast cells, occurs within the walls of blood vessels, myocardial cells, and bronchial epithelium. This reaction damages cells and causes the release of massive amounts of histamine and other vasoactive amines. These substances are distributed rapidly throughout the circulatory system, causing massive vasodilation and increased capillary permeability, which result in profound hypovolemia and vascular collapse (Taylor, 1984). Decreased myocardial contractility and arrhythmias can be seen during anaphylaxis, but it is not known if these symptoms are direct results of myocardial changes induced by the antigen-antibody reaction or are attributable to the profound hypovolemia. Additionally, this action in bronchial tissues causes severe edema and pulmonary obstruction, which greatly reduces pulmonary gas exchange. As a result of these pulmonary problems in combination with inadequate circulation, the individual experiences extreme hypoxia; without intervention, this condition leads to death.

Septic Shock

Septic shock shares some features with all other types of shock and has some unique features related to origin, pathologic changes, associated clinical manifestations, sequelae, and treatment. Although septic shock has been reported among clients with viral and yeast sepsis, it is associated more commonly with bacteremia. Organisms implicated in the origin of septic shock include gram-negative bacteria (Pseudomonas aeruginosa, Escherichia coli, and Klebsiella pneumoniae), staphylococcus, and streptococcus (Barry, 1989; Gilliam & Polk, 1988; Littleton, 1988). Conditions that predispose the client to septic shock include malnutrition, immunosuppression, the presence of large open wounds, mucous membrane fissures in prolonged contact with bloody or drainage-soaked packing, GI ischemia, and loss of GI integrity.

The initiation of the syndrome of septic shock is thought to occur as a result of the large amounts of metabolites and toxins, including endotoxin, produced by the bacteria and secreted into the client's blood. These bacteria-produced toxins react with cell membranes and, through leukocyte recognition, stimulate a variety of inflammatory and immune responses (Chap. 23). These toxin-host interactions stimulate systemic complement activation, alteration of microcirculation within vascular organs (including selective coagulation and thrombus formation), increased capillary permeability, cellular injury, and increased cellular metabolism (in combination with an inability of some cells to take up necessary oxygen). Metabolism becomes anaerobic as a function of decreased MAP, thrombus formation in capillaries, and poor cellular uptake of oxygen. Although bacterial toxins are generally implicated in initiating these events, some evidence indicates that the bacteria in the extracellular fluid as well as the toxins can directly initiate septic shock (Hinshaw, 1985; Lucas & Ledgerwood, 1988).

INCIDENCE

The exact incidence of all types of shock is not known because shock is a manifestation of a pathologic condition rather than a separate disease entity. However, some degree of shock is a common manifestation or complication among hospitalized clients and frequently is the reason clients seek health care assistance initially. Hypovolemic shock is the most common type of shock experienced by clients in emergency departments and after surgery or procedures that involve invasion of a major artery (Meyers & Hickey, 1988; Perkins & Kennally, 1989). Cardiogenic shock is the most frequent complication of MI and is present in an estimated 12% of clients who experience damage to 40% or more of the myocardium (Clowes, 1988; Jeffries & Whelan, 1988; Robbins & Kumar, 1987). Mild vasogenic shock of neural origin appears to be the most frequent type among otherwise healthy clients and usually resolves without medical intervention. The frequency of septic shock is increasing among clients who are immunocompromised (Barry, 1989) or who have infections (Littleton, 1988; Teplitz, 1988). Although anaphylactic shock is relatively rare, it is the most common type of hypersensitivity reaction requiring hospitalization in emergency departments and critical care units (Dickerson, 1988).

PREVENTION

Primary prevention is possible for some types of shock by identifying clients at risk for conditions and complications leading to shock and preventing the development of those complications. Clients with known allergies to drugs, chemicals, or foods should not be exposed to those allergens. Preventive measures include having the allergic person wear or carry medical alert (Medic Alert) identification and encouraging all health care professionals to search for such identification on all clients and to include specific questions regarding allergies when obtaining health histories. Hemorrhage and other conditions entailing rapid fluid loss should be treated or corrected before shock ensues. Fluid replacement for clients experiencing conditions that predispose to hypovolemic shock should be sufficient to maintain circulating volume and MAP. Strict adherence to aseptic technique during invasive procedures and during manipulation of nonintact skin and mucous membranes of clients who are immunocompromised to any degree can help to prevent septic shock.

Secondary prevention (early detection) of the clinical manifestations of shock is a major nursing responsibility. Because shock is a common complication of many conditions found in hospitalized clients, the nurse always considers the possibility and probability of shock development. Early detection requires continuous assessment of measurements indicative of impending shock for specific changes from normal values or from baseline. After shock is recognized, the nurse rapidly takes appropriate actions to halt or change the conditions contributing to shock and to support the client's physiologic compensatory mechanisms, so that life-threatening complications can be prevented.

EMERGENCY CARE

Conditions initiating shock can occur at any time, and thus clients may experience shock in almost any setting. The nurse should be prepared to assess the situation and implement appropriate emergency care whenever and wherever conditions dictate. Specific emergency care measures are presented in the accompanying Emergency Care feature.

The nurse attempts to gather information regarding the client's usual state of health and any precipitating factors leading to the development of shock. Professional emergency assistance is summoned as soon as possible. The nurse begins to care for the client in shock by keeping the client warm and loosening constrictive clothing to enhance circulation. Assessing the client's pulses provides data regarding the status and effectiveness of the client's circulation.

After trained supportive personnel have arrived, the client is prepared for transport to the nearest acute care facility. The following actions are taken during preparation and transport. Vital signs are obtained and used as a guide for the institution of appropriate treatment. An IV line is established for the administration of fluids and medications. Oxygen therapy and cardiac monitoring are initiated. A pneumatic garment (military anti-shock trousers [MAST]) may be used if the shock has a hypovolemic origin. This device is wrapped around the client's torso and lower extremities and then is inflated using a pump. The resulting pressure exerted on the body may aid in preventing stasis and promoting venous return. These actions help to maintain MAP and ensure blood flow to the vital organs.

COLLABORATIVE MANAGEMENT

 Assessment

History

The nurse collects data regarding risk factors, as well as causative factors, related to the development of shock. *Age* is an important factor for some types of shock. Hypovolemic shock associated with trauma is more frequently seen in young adults, whereas the elderly experience cardiogenic shock more frequently. The nurse questions clients specifically about cardiovascular health, such as whether known heart defects or diseases are present and whether there has been recent onset of chest pain. Clients are asked specific questions about the presence of *recent illness, trauma, or procedures or chronic conditions* that may lead to the development of

EMERGENCY CARE ■ The Client in Shock

Interventions	Rationales
All Types of Shock	
1. Assess for consciousness and an open airway.	1. Airway may be occluded by a foreign body, head position, or laryngeal spasm.
2. Ask the client for her/his name, age, and health history and about events leading to the present illness.	2. Information may assist in identifying the cause of the present event (e.g., recent MI).
3. Keep the client warm and in a supine position.	3. Body temperature often falls below normal in shock, causing further vasoconstriction. A supine position enhances blood flow to the brain.
4. Feel for the presence of pulses in the carotid areas.	4. Carotid pulses are good indicators of circulatory status.
5. Reassure the client.	5. Anxiety and restlessness are commonly seen with shock.
6. Stay with the client and have someone summon professional health care.	6. The condition of a client in shock may worsen rapidly and require life support measures (such as cardiopulmonary resuscitation).
7. On arrival of trained emergency personnel, assist with the placement of an IV line, oxygen therapy, and initiation of cardiac monitoring.	7. Fluids and medications can be administered through the IV line. Oxygen assists with gas exchange, and cardiac monitoring enables personnel to detect the presence of cardiac arrhythmias.
Hypovolemic Shock	
1. Assess the client for evidence of injury or apparent bleeding. If injury has occurred, do not attempt to move the client.	1. If a client with bone fractures is moved without the proper splinting, further damage can be caused, such as a fractured rib puncturing a lung and causing a pneumothorax or a fractured vertebra severing the spinal cord and causing paralysis.
2. Cover any wounds with a clean cloth if possible. Apply pressure to a wound if bleeding appears to be originating from an artery (large amount of bright red blood with a pulsating force).	2. Covering a wound helps to prevent further contamination. Pressure applied to an arterial bleeding site often slows the rate of blood loss.
3. After an IV line has been initiated, a solution of Ringer's lactate or normal saline is infused quickly.	3. Infusion of fluids helps to expand the circulatory blood volume and therefore increases the blood pressure while the client is being transported to the hospital.
4. If indicated by the client's blood pressure and rate of blood loss, MAST may be applied.	4. Device increases blood pressure by either decreasing arterial circulation to the lower extremities or enhancing venous return from lower extremities.
Cardiogenic Shock	
1. Inquire as to the presence, severity, and location of chest pain.	1. Sharp or pressure-type left-sided chest pain is frequently cardiac in nature.
2. Loosen any restrictive or tight clothing, such as belts, ties, shirt collars, or shoes.	2. Restrictive articles of clothing further deter circulation.
3. If strong carotid pulses are palpable, and the client is short of breath, a semi-Fowler position will assist with breathing.	3. Chest pain is often associated with shortness of breath and pulmonary congestion. If pulses are weak, indicating a low blood pressure, a supine position should be maintained.
4. Observe the client for nausea or vomiting, which frequently occurs during an MI. Prevent aspiration if vomiting occurs.	4. Vomiting is associated with an MI involving the inferior cardiac wall, low blood pressure, and cardiac arrhythmias.
5. IV morphine may be administered by emergency personnel to relieve chest pain. Lidocaine may also be administered if cardiac arrhythmias occur.	5. Morphine helps to relieve pain while also having a vasodilatory effect on the coronary arteries, thus enhancing coronary blood flow. Lidocaine is an antiarrhythmic agent and is given early to prevent lethal arrhythmias.

EMERGENCY CARE ■ The Client in Shock *Continued*

Interventions	Rationales
Vasogenic Shock	
1. Assess the client for neurologic deficits that may indicate head injury or spinal cord injury.	1. Obvious injury may not be apparent, but a neurologic assessment may reveal deficits, indicating injury.
2. If the client is conscious, inquire as to the events leading to the onset of the illness. Carefully question the client regarding exposure to any known allergens or recent infection.	2. This information gives clues as to the type of illness the client is experiencing and the appropriate emergency measures, should they become necessary.
3. Obtain information about any medications or chemical substances ingested by the client recently, as well as recent anesthesia for surgery or dental work.	3. Same as 2.
4. Carefully monitor the client's respiratory rate and effort for signs of airway obstruction (stridor, tachypnea, or sudden inability to speak). The client needs to be encouraged to breathe as easily as possible and to be reassured that help is coming. Mouth-to-mouth resuscitation may become necessary. Emergency intubation or tracheostomy may be performed by trained personnel.	4. Respiratory distress is commonly due to laryngeal spasm or bronchospasm.
5. If the client appears to be having an allergic reaction, the emergency personnel usually administer a subcutaneous injection of epinephrine.	5. Subcutaneous administration of epinephrine is effective in counteracting the histamine reactions seen with an allergic reaction.

shock. Such conditions include severe allergies, GI ulcers, GI surgery, previous MI, surgery involving the nasal mucosa, hemophilia, liver disease or dysfunction, malignancies, acquired immunodeficiency syndrome (AIDS), malnutrition, trauma to the head or the spine, prolonged vomiting or diarrhea, and urinary tract or other infections.

Use of some *medications* may directly cause changes leading to the development of shock or may indicate the presence of a disease or a problem that can contribute to the development of shock. Such medications include aspirin and aspirin-containing drugs, diuretics, alpha-adrenergic blocking agents, antacids, antibiotics, antihistamines, barbiturates, narcotics, cardiac glycosides, and chemotherapeutic agents.

The nurse inquires about the client's *fluid intake and output* during the previous 24 hours. Information regarding urinary output is especially critical because the early stage of shock is characterized by a diminished urinary output, even when fluid intake is normal. The client's *height and weight* are obtained because weight and liquid measures are related and a decrease in weight is an indicator of fluid loss.

The nurse assesses the client and the immediate environment for obvious evidence of factors leading to shock. Areas to examine for possible hemorrhage include gums, wounds, and sites of dressings, drains, and vascular access. The nurse also looks *under* the client for evidence of external bleeding. The client is observed for the presence of any swelling, skin discoloration, or visi-

ble manifestations of pain that may indicate the presence of significant internal hemorrhage (Perkins & Kennally, 1989).

Physical Assessment: Clinical Manifestations

Some clinical manifestations are common to all types of shock; other manifestations are associated with specific types of shock (see Key Features of Disease, pp. 406 and 407). Most of the observable manifestations of the syndrome of shock are a result of the physiologic changes associated with accompanying compensatory efforts. Manifestations of shock are first evident as changes in cardiovascular function. As shock progresses, functional changes in the renal, pulmonary, integumentary, musculoskeletal, and central nervous systems become evident.

Cardiovascular manifestations

Pulse. Because the pathologic changes of shock involve a decrease of MAP and the resulting early compensatory mechanisms are cardiovascular in nature, the earliest clinical manifestations of shock are associated with the cardiovascular system. The nurse assesses the central and peripheral pulses for rate and quality. In the early stage of shock, the pulse rate increases to maintain cardiac output and MAP at normal levels, although the actual stroke volume per beat usually is decreased. Because the cardiac output is decreased, the distal peripheral pulses are more difficult to palpate and are easily obliterated with minimal pressure. As shock progresses, superficial peripheral pulses may be absent.

Early-stage septic shock is the exception, as the released toxins are at first *stimulatory* to the cardiac system, causing an increase in both heart rate and stroke volume so that cardiac output actually is increased above baseline. This situation is temporary, and eventually the cardiac output greatly diminishes in clients experiencing septic shock (Spitzer et al., 1985).

Blood pressure.   Changes in blood pressure are not always present in the early stages of shock. An important concept to consider when assessing the blood pressure of a client at risk for shock is what the baseline blood pressure level for this client is. Although a blood pressure measurement of 90/50 may well indicate the presence of severe shock in one individual, it may represent the normal blood pressure value for a healthy but slightly built adult.

When compensatory efforts include vasoconstriction, the result is an increased diastolic pressure level, while the systolic pressure level remains the same. As a result, the *pulse pressure*, or the difference between the systolic and diastolic pressure measurements, is diminished. The nurse monitors the client's blood pressure for changes from baseline and changes from the previous measurement. For accuracy, the nurse uses the same equipment on the same extremity. When the client's condition permits, the nurse measures the blood pressure with the client in the lying, sitting, and standing positions. Some debate exists as to whether the bell or the diaphragm of the stethoscope is more sensitive to changes in the Korotkoff sounds reflecting blood pressure (see the accompanying Nursing Research feature).

As shock progresses and cardiac output changes, the systolic pressure level decreases, diminishing the pulse pressure even further. When the condition of shock continues and interventions are not adequate, compensatory mechanisms fail and both the systolic and diastolic pressures decrease. At this stage, only a systolic pressure may be heard.

Skin.   In shock, the skin is affected indirectly by alterations in perfusion and not as a result of pathologic changes in the skin per se. The skin is a tissue that tolerates prolonged hypoxic conditions without sustaining permanent damage, although external injury inflicted on the skin is more likely to result in damage during hypoxic episodes. Because the skin can tolerate low oxygen levels and other vital organs cannot, early compensatory mechanisms involve profound vasoconstriction in the skin and superficial tissues to the extent that perfusion to these tissues is minimal or absent. As a result, the skin feels cool or cold to the touch, and the color is pale to cyanotic. Color changes are first evident in mucous membranes and in the skin around the mouth. As shock progresses, color changes are noted in

NURSING RESEARCH

Indirect Blood Pressure Measurement May Vary Depending on the Arterial Site and Stethoscope Soundpiece Used.

Mauro, A. (1988). Effects of bell versus diaphragm on indirect blood pressure measurement. *Heart and Lung, 17,* 489–494.

Indirect blood pressure measurement using a sphygmomanometer and a stethoscope has long been used as one method of determining cardiovascular function. The American Heart Association recommends the use of the bell portion of the stethoscope to obtain blood pressure measurements because the bell is designed to auscultate low-pitched sounds and the Korotkoff sounds reflecting blood pressure are of low pitch.

This study sought to determine if blood pressure readings obtained using the bell portion of the stethoscope were significantly different from those obtained using the diaphragm portion of the stethoscope.

All measurements were obtained by one individual using the same stethoscope and mercury sphygmomanometer on the right arms over the brachial arteries of 56 individuals. The blood pressure reading for each individual was obtained twice, once each with the bell and the diaphragm, with sufficient recovery time allowed between each reading.

The results of the study indicated that, in general, the bell of the stethoscope allowed higher systolic blood pressure values and lower phase five diastolic blood pressure values to be obtained than did the diaphragm portion of the stethoscope on the same individuals. The differences in readings between bell and diaphragm ranged from 1 to 2 mmHg. These findings suggest that indirect blood pressure measurements are more accurate when the bell portion of the stethoscope is used to measure blood pressure over the brachial artery.

Critique.   The results of this study reached statistical significance, although the actual sample size was small. The investigators were able to control for many variables, increasing the validity of the study. The human ear must perceive and interpret differences in sound levels between the two portions of the stethoscope, which is a possible threat to validity. These findings were interesting and warrant further study.

Possible Nursing Implications.   Because decisions regarding the treatment of clients in shock are based on data such as indirect blood pressure measurement, it is important that such measurements be made as accurately as possible, especially when more than one nurse or other health care professional may be obtaining the measurements. The amount of difference in pressures heard between the two stethoscope heads was small, but indicated that differences probably do exist. Therefore, each unit or institution should establish guidelines for which stethoscope head should be used to measure blood pressure so that measurement techniques are consistent and differences are actual rather than an artefact of equipment.

the extremities and then in the central trunk area. The skin also feels clammy or moist to the touch. This manifestation is not the result of increased perspiration, but is present because the normal fluid lost through the skin does not evaporate quickly on cold skin.

Respiratory manifestations.   The nurses assesses the rate, depth, and ease of respiration and auscultates the lungs for the presence of any abnormal breath sounds. Unless a head injury is associated with the shock condition, the clinical manifestations of shock include an increased respiratory rate. This manifestation is a compensatory mechanism to assist in providing adequate oxygenation to critical tissues. When shock has progressed to the stage at which lactic acidosis is present, the depth of respirations increases with the rate. Pooling of blood in pulmonary tissues and the formation of pulmonary edema occur when shock is accompanied by left ventricular failure. This fluid increases the effort of respiration and may be heard as crackles on auscultation.

A possible life-threatening pulmonary complication of shock is adult respiratory distress syndrome (ARDS), also known as shock lung and wet lung (Border & Hassett, 1988). Although this complication has many causes, its association with shock is thought to be related to the formation of oxygen free radicals, which exert destructive actions on the type I and type II pulmonary epithelial cells (Robbins & Kumar, 1987). Oxygen free radicals can form as a result of oxygen therapy and in response to cellular destruction and subsequent release of oxidizing enzymes.

Renal manifestations.   The renal system compensates for the decreased MAP associated with shock by conserving body water through decreasing glomerular filtration and increasing reabsorption of filtrate. Urinary output is diminished (compared with fluid intake) or even absent in severe shock. When shock is severe and pressure in the renal artery is low, the afferent arterioles of the nephrons constrict to the extent that nephron perfusion does not occur. Of the four vital organs (heart, brain, liver, and kidney), only the kidney can tolerate hypoxia and anoxia for up to an hour without permanent damage to tubular epithelial cells. When hypoxic or anoxic conditions persist beyond this time, the client is at grave risk for ischemic acute tubular necrosis and subsequent renal failure (Perry, 1988). Whether the renal failure is permanent depends on the extent of damage to the renal tubules. If the tubular basement membrane is intact and the client receives appropriate medical and nursing support when the fluid and electrolyte imbalances of renal failure occur, the tubular epithelium can regenerate completely and provide normal kidney function (Robbins & Kumar, 1987). If the tubular basement membrane also is destroyed, renal tubular epithelium cannot regenerate and the renal failure is chronic.

Clients in shock or at great risk for shock should have an indwelling urinary catheter in place. The nurse measures the urinary output every hour and assesses the urine for such variables as color, specific gravity, and the presence of blood or protein. If septic shock is suspected, a sample of urine is sent for microscopic examination and culture.

Central nervous system manifestations.   The nurse assesses the client's level of consciousness and orientation to time, place, and person. Most causes of shock do not interfere with the generation and maintenance of nerve impulse transmission. Rather, CNS manifestations of shock are associated with cerebral hypoxia. In the early and compensatory stages of shock, the client may be restless or agitated and may experience anxiety or a feeling of impending doom that has no obvious cause. As hypoxia progresses, the client becomes confused and lethargic. Lethargy progresses to somnolence and loss of consciousness as cerebral hypoxia intensifies.

Musculoskeletal manifestations.   Although musculoskeletal manifestations are not an early or a cardinal symptom of shock, they may be present and cause discomfort for the client and motor dysfunction (Blum et al., 1988). Tissue hypoxia, anaerobic metabolism, and lactic acidosis cause skeletal muscle weakness and pain. This weakness is generalized, with no specific pattern of presentation. The accompanying electrolyte disturbances in intermediate and irreversible stages of shock compound this muscle weakness by interfering with the generation and transmission of action potentials. In this situation, deep tendon reflexes are diminished or absent.

The nurse assesses the client's muscle strength by having the client (1) squeeze the nurse's hand, (2) attempt to keep the arms flexed while the nurse pulls downward on the lower arms, and (3) push both feet against a flat surface (a board or a box) while the nurse applies resistance. The nurse assesses deep tendon reflexes by lightly tapping the patellar tendons and Achilles tendons with a reflex hammer and observing the degree of reflexive movement elicited. All assessment findings are compared with baseline measurements to determine the presence and direction of changes.

Psychosocial Assessment

Changes in mental status and behavior may be indicators of the presence of shock. Although psychosocial assessment is always important, the information obtained may be critical for treatment if shock is the result of physical abuse.

The nurse observes the client closely and documents the client's behavior. This behavior is described rather than interpreted. The nurse assesses the client's current mental status by evaluating the level of consciousness. Notations are made regarding whether the client is asleep or awake. If the client is asleep, the nurse attempts to awaken the client and documents the ease with which the client is aroused. If the client is awake, the nurse establishes whether the client is oriented to time, place, and person. Questions that can be answered with a "yes" or a "no" response are avoided. The nurse documents the manner in which the client responds to the questions. The following points are considered during evaluation. Is it necessary to repeat questions to obtain a response? Does the response answer the question asked? Does the client have difficulty with word choices during the responses? Is the client irritated or upset by the questions? Can the client concentrate on a question long enough to provide an appropriate response, or is his/her attention span limited? The nurse questions family members or a significant other to determine whether the behavior and mental status are typical for this client.

The majority of clients actually experiencing shock have some degree of anxiety associated with cerebral hypoxia. When shock is the result of trauma, postsurgical hemorrhage, drug abuse, or MI, the client and the family may experience fear concerning actual or potential pain, procedures to be performed, and the possible outcome of this situation.

Laboratory Findings

No single laboratory finding confirms or rules out the presence of shock, although changes in laboratory data may support the diagnosis of different types of shock. As shock progresses, the combination of an increase in anaerobic metabolism, cellular damage, and the presence of specific compensatory mechanisms causes physiologic changes that are reflected as abnormal arterial blood gas values. Most commonly, the pH decreases, the partial pressure of oxygen (PO_2) decreases, and the PCO_2 increases. Changes in other laboratory values may be associated with specific types of shock.

Changes in *hematocrit* and *hemoglobin* concentrations are associated with some types of hypovolemic shock. In hemorrhagic shock, hematocrit and hemoglobin concentrations are less than normal. When hypovolemic shock is the result of dehydration or plasma volume shift, the hematocrit and hemoglobin concentrations are elevated. These measurements usually are normal in cardiogenic, neurogenic, anaphylactic, and septic shock.

The presence of bacteria in blood and other extracellular fluids supports the diagnosis of septic shock. Cultures are obtained to identify the causative organisms for both diagnostic and therapeutic purposes. Other abnormal laboratory findings associated with septic shock include changes in the white blood cell count; the differential leukocyte count may demonstrate a *left shift* (Chap. 23).

Cardiogenic shock is associated with elevations of the following enzymes: lactate dehydrogenase, creatine phosphokinase (CPK), and serum glutamic-oxaloacetic transaminase (SGOT) (aspartate aminotransferase).

Electrolyte imbalances, especially alterations in serum potassium and serum calcium concentrations, may result from or may cause cardiogenic shock.

Specific laboratory findings associated with anaphylactic shock include elevated eosinophil and basophil levels in the differential white blood cell count. Even though blood analysis for the presence of specific allergens is possible, this procedure is not commonly performed.

Other Diagnostic Tests

Radiographic and other imaging techniques, such as computed tomography scanning, ultrasonography, and magnetic resonance imaging, may be useful in detecting the presence of internal hemorrhage sites. Echocardiograms can indicate the presence of cardiac valve pathologic changes or congestive heart failure with enlarged chamber size associated with cardiogenic shock. Electrocardiographic changes can be indicators of MI. Other, more invasive procedures that can assist in determining the presence of conditions leading to shock include angiography, GI endoscopy, and exploratory surgery.

 Analysis: Nursing Diagnosis

Many clients are at risk for shock as a result of trauma, sepsis, hypersensitivity, medical procedures or treatment, and MI. A typical client who is experiencing shock when admitted to an acute care facility is a 35-year-old man with multiple fractures and soft-tissue damage as a result of a motorcycle accident. The following nursing diagnoses are derived from these data (Taptich et al., 1989).

Common Diagnoses

The following nursing diagnoses are commonly noted in hospitalized clients with hypovolemic shock:

1. Fluid volume deficit related to blood loss
2. Decreased cardiac output related to decreased venous return
3. Altered thought processes related to decreased cerebral perfusion

Additional Diagnoses

In addition to the common diagnoses, one or more of the following nursing diagnoses may apply to the client experiencing hypovolemic shock:

1. Altered urinary elimination related to patterns of decreased cardiac output
2. Fluid volume excess related to replacement therapy and cardiac failure

3. Altered cardiopulmonary tissue perfusion related to inadequate circulating volume
4. Pain related to decreased tissue oxygenation
5. Knowledge deficit related to treatment
6. Sleep pattern disturbances related to anxiety and hospital routines
7. Altered family processes related to changes in life style
8. Altered nutrition: less than body requirements related to nausea and decreased GI perfusion
9. Anxiety related to decreased cerebral perfusion and outcome of diagnostic studies
10. Fear related to the possibility of death
11. Fatigue related to increased metabolic demands
12. Impaired skin integrity related to poor tissue perfusion and immobility

 Planning and Implementation

The accompanying Client Care Plan for the client experiencing shock focuses on the common nursing diagnoses associated with hemorrhagic hypovolemia. This plan is aimed at supporting the physiologic compensatory mechanisms and correcting the conditions contributing to the development of shock (see the accompanying Guidelines feature) (Meyers & Hickey, 1988).

Fluid Volume Deficit

Planning client goals. The major client goals for this nursing diagnosis are that the client will have (1) decreased blood loss and (2) body fluid levels restored to normal.

Interventions: nonsurgical management. Interventions are aimed at increasing the body fluid compartment volumes to within normal ranges and supporting the client's operating compensatory mechanisms. IV and drug therapies are the management choices for this problem.

Intravenous therapy. The two different categories of substances commonly used for fluid volume replacement during hemorrhagic hypovolemia are *colloids* and *crystalloids*. Colloids contain large molecules (usually composed of proteins or starches); IV colloid solutions are used to restore plasma volume and colloidal osmotic pressure. Crystalloid solutions are administered intravenously for fluid and electrolyte replacement; they contain nonprotein substances, such as minerals, salts, and sugars. These fluids may be used individually or together as therapy for hypovolemic shock.

Colloid fluid replacement. Protein-containing colloid fluids are good for restoring vascular osmotic pressure

as well as fluid volume. Blood and blood products are frequently used for this purpose and are the treatment of choice when hypovolemia is caused by blood loss. These products include *whole blood, packed red blood cells,* and *plasma.*

Whole blood and packed red blood cells increase the hematocrit and hemoglobin concentrations as well as vascular fluid volume. Whole blood is used to replace large volumes of blood loss because it provides increased intravascular volume while improving the oxygen-carrying capacity of the blood. Packed red blood cells are given for moderate blood loss because they replenish the red blood cell deficit and improve the oxygen-carrying capacity without giving excess fluid volume.

Blood is a liquid connective tissue, and blood cells contain cell surface antigens specific to a blood type. To prevent incompatibility reactions, only a compatible blood type is given to a client. In preparation for blood administration, two nurses check each unit of blood for proper client identification and compatibility. During and immediately after administration, the client is

GUIDELINES ■ Interventions for Problems of the Client with Hypovolemic Shock

Skin Breakdown

Maintain good body alignment while easing pressure areas with the use of pillows.
Plan nursing care to include turning of the client, skin care, and massage of pressure areas every 2 h.
Assess the skin for signs of breakdown every 4 h and monitor the response to skin care.

Fluid Volume Excess

Monitor the client's hourly and cumulative fluid input and output.
Assess the client's lungs for signs of fluid excess, such as the presence of crackles or wheezes.
Report abnormal findings to the physician and set up a plan of care to prevent further excess through fluid restriction.
Monitor the client's response to prescribed therapies.

Sleep/Rest Deprivation

Assess the client's ability to sleep during times of inactivity at the bedside.
Schedule nursing care to provide the client with undisturbed periods of rest.
Provide a quiet, darkened environment to promote rest.
Reassure the patient that she/he will not be left unobserved during periods of sleep.

CLIENT CARE PLAN ■ The Client with Hypovolemic Shock

Goal/Outcome Criteria	Interventions	Rationales
Nursing Diagnosis 1: Fluid Volume Deficit Related to Blood Loss		

Client will maintain adequate fluid volume.
■ Maintains an IV or PO fluid intake of at least 1000 mL per shift (8 h).
■ Maintains an hourly fluid intake within 30 mL of the hourly fluid output from urine, wound drainage, or blood loss.
■ Avoids weight fluctuations of greater than 5%.
	1. Administer fluid and electrolytes as well as blood and blood products as ordered.
	  a. Fluids and electrolyte solutions are given for the replacement of fluid and plasma loss.
	  b. Blood is given for replacement of blood loss.
	  c. Blood products, such as plasma protein fraction (Plasmanate), are given to replace blood and fluid loss.
		1. Replacement therapy with the appropriate solution or blood product usually resolves the fluid deficit quickly.

	2. Evaluate the client's response to therapy.	2. Evaluation helps determine which interventions are effective and should be continued.
	3. Obtain daily weights and maintain a day-to-day comparison chart.	3. Daily weight changes reflect fluid volume changes.
	4. Monitor fluid intake and output, including loss from GI tract, wounds, drains, or bleeding.	4. Fluid intake should equal fluid loss; output volume is needed to calculate appropriate fluid intake volume.

Client will demonstrate adequate oxygen-carrying capability.
■ Says he/she feels well and exhibits signs of adequate oxygen carrying capabilities, as evidenced by pink skin with adequate turgor and capillary refill.
■ Maintains a hemoglobin level of 12–14 g/100 mL and a hematocrit of 30% or greater.
	1. Assess the client for signs of fluid and electrolyte imbalance.
	  a. Poor skin turgor.
	  b. Weakness.
	  c. Irritability or confusion.
	  d. Nausea or vomiting.
		1. Dry skin, weakness, and changes in neurologic status are common findings in hypovolemia.

	2. Monitor hemoglobin and hematocrit levels daily.	2. Hemoglobin and hematocrit levels frequently show an unexplained increase if there is a fluid deficit, as the blood becomes increasingly concentrated.

Client will maintain hemodynamic stability.
■ Maintains a blood pressure of 90–120/60–80 and a heart rate of 70–110 beats/min.
■ Maintains a urinary output of at least 30 mL/h.
	1. Monitor the client's vital signs and fluid status.
	  a. Evaluate blood pressure, pulse, and urinary output.
	  b. Monitor cumulative fluid intake and output.
	  c. Note and report variations from baseline.
		1. Fluctuations in these variables, associated with changes in the client's weight, are excellent indicators of fluid balance.

Nursing Diagnosis 2: Decreased Cardiac Output Related to Decreased Venous Return		

Client will re-establish hemodynamic stability.
■ Maintains a blood pressure of 90–120/60–80.
■ Has a regular heart rate of 70–110 beats/min.
	1. Obtain and monitor the client's vital signs.
	  a. Monitor the blood pressure level for declining trends.
	  b. Monitor the pulse for increasing rate and irregularity.
		1. Documenting and comparing vital signs enhances the early detection of declining blood pressure and the compensatory increase in the heart rate.

CLIENT CARE PLAN ■ The Client with Hypovolemic Shock *continued*

Goal/Outcome Criteria	Interventions	Rationales
Nursing Diagnosis 2: Decreased Cardiac Output Related to Decreased Venous Return		

■ Has warm and dry skin and is free of discomforts associated with diminished venous return to the heart.
Client will have increased cardiac output.
■ States that he/she is feeling well.
■ Reports a sense of feeling rested and calm.
	c. Assess all body systems for the effects of diminished cardiac output.
	1. Reduce the workload of the heart by
	  a. Restricting the client to bed rest in a Fowler position.
	  b. Providing a calm, quiet atmosphere conducive to rest.
		1. Limiting the client's activity decreases the workload of the heart while also providing needed rest during illness.

Client will take medications prescribed for improving cardiac output and decreasing the workload of the heart.	1. Administer medications that increase the contractility of the heart and document their effects on the client's blood pressure and heart rate.	1. Medications that increase the contractility of the heart decrease the heart's workload and help to increase cardiac output. These effects are measurable by an improvement in the blood pressure level and heart rate.
Nursing Diagnosis 3: Altered Thought Processes Related to Decreased Cerebral Perfusion		

Client will experience improved cerebral circulation.
■ States that she/he feels alert and well oriented to the environment.
■ Communicates needs.
	1. Assess each client for baseline behavior patterns.
	  a. Response to verbal and tactile stimuli.
	  b. State of orientation.
	2. Note changes in the client's behavior indicative of cerebral hypoperfusion.
	  a. Restlessness.
	  b. Confusion.
	  c. Lethargy.
	  d. Somnolence.
	  e. Unresponsiveness.
	  f. Seizures.
	3. Notify the physician of significant findings.
		1–3. A baseline assessment of each client's behavior patterns allows the nurse to identify changes early. A client exhibits diminished alertness early in the presence of decreased cerebral perfusion and progresses to more serious manifestations if left untreated.

Client will experience decreased vasoconstriction. ■ Reports warm extremities without tingling or pain. ■ Maintains full active range of movement.	1. Assess the client for the presence of cool, moist extremities often associated with pain. 2. Assess the client for spontaneous and equal movement of all extremities.	1, 2. Same as 1–3.

Client will experience no hypoxia.
■ Remains alert and exhibits equal pupillary responses to light.
■ Is free from abnormal neurologic manifestations, such as seizures.
■ Maintains all protective reflexes.
	1. Assess each client for baseline neurologic status and document deficits. Evaluate
	  a. Level of consciousness.
	  b. Pupillary response to light.
	  c. Presence of protective reflexes, such as a blink and cough reflex.
	  d. Presence of tremors or seizures.
		1. Same as 1–3.

closely observed for signs of any adverse reactions to the blood. Common indications of a transfusion reaction include elevated temperature, chills, flushed skin, hypotension, pain, and respiratory distress. If a transfusion reaction is suspected, the administration of the unit of blood is discontinued, and it is returned to the blood bank for further study. Chapter 67 discusses nursing care issues surrounding blood administration.

Human plasma, an acellular blood product containing some clotting factors, is administered to correct plasma deficits and restore osmotic pressure when the hematocrit and hemoglobin levels are within normal ranges. Plasma protein fractions (such as Plasmanate) and synthetic plasma expanders (such as hydroxyethyl starch [Hespan]) effectively increase plasma volume and frequently are used as an early treatment of shock before a cause is established.

Crystalloid fluid replacement. These solutions are commonly administered to help establish and maintain an adequate fluid and electrolyte balance. Two common crystalloid solutions are *Ringer's lactate* and *normal saline.* Ringer's lactate contains physiologic concentrations of sodium, chloride, calcium, potassium, and lactate in water. This isotonic solution is an effective volume expander, and the lactate is an effective buffer in the presence of acidemia. Normal saline (0.9% sodium chloride in water) is a fluid replacement that can increase the plasma volume; it is used most frequently when there has been no loss of red blood cells.

Drug therapy. If the volume deficit is severe and the client does not respond sufficiently to the replacement of fluid volume and blood products, the administration of medications that cause vasoconstriction or improve myocardial contractility may be necessary. The client requires transfer to a critical care unit for close monitoring and probable insertion of central vascular access lines. Table 17–1 cites the drugs commonly used to treat shock.

Interventions: surgical management. The nurse monitors the client's fluid loss and uses the nonsurgical interventions described earlier to stabilize the client's hemodynamic status. After a definitive diagnosis is established, surgical intervention may be necessary to correct the underlying cause of shock. Such interventions include vascular repair and surgical hemostasis of major wounds, oversewing of bleeding ulcers, chemical scarring (chemosclerosis) of esophageal varicosities, and skull decompression to decrease intracranial pressure.

Decreased Cardiac Output

Planning: client goals. The major client goals for this nursing diagnosis include that the client will (1) maintain adequate oxygenation to vital organs and (2) have cardiac output restored to normal.

Interventions: nonsurgical management. Interventions are aimed at increasing the vascular fluid volume (as discussed for IV therapy of a fluid volume deficit), supporting the client's compensatory mechanisms, and preventing ischemic complications.

Drug therapy. Drug therapy is aimed at increasing venous return, improving myocardial contractility, and ensuring adequate myocardial perfusion through dilation of coronary vessels.

Vasoconstricting agents. A variety of drugs stimulate venous return by causing vasoconstriction and decreasing venous pooling of blood. These actions increase cardiac output and MAP, helping to improve tissue perfusion and oxygenation. Most of these drugs have serious side effects, and their dosages must be carefully calculated (sometimes titrated) on the basis of the size of the client and the degree of response. Drugs with systemic peripheral vasoconstricting activity include dopamine (Dopastat, Intropin, Revimine), epinephrine (Adrenalin), mephentermine (Wyamine), metaraminol (Aramine), methoxamine (Vasoxyl), norepinephrine (Levophed), phenylephrine (Neo-Synephrine), and vasopressin (Pitressin).

Agents enhancing myocardial contractility. Some drugs directly stimulate adrenergic receptor sites on the myocardium (especially beta$_1$-receptors) and increase the contractile response of the cardiac muscle cells. Such agents include dobutamine (Dobutrex), dopamine, amrinone (Inocor), epinephrine, and isoproterenol (Isuprel). Other agents enhance myocardial contractility by slowing the heart rate through altering electrical conduction and allowing the left ventricle a longer filling time. By increasing the filling time, more blood enters the left ventricle and stretches the myocardial fibers, so that greater recoil is achieved and more blood leaves the left ventricle during contraction. Some of these drugs also stimulate the ventricles at the same time. Agents with these types of actions include digoxin (Lanoxin, Purodigin) and deslanoside (Cedilanid-D).

Agents enhancing myocardial perfusion. Although the treatment of shock includes the administration of agents that produce systemic vasoconstriction to help enhance venous return and increase MAP, it is important to ensure that the myocardium is adequately perfused so that aerobic metabolism is maintained in the heart and maximum contractility can be achieved. Agents that selectively dilate coronary blood vessels while causing minimal systemic vasodilation are used for this purpose. These agents are most beneficial in cardiogenic shock and should not be used when shock results from head trauma. Care must be taken, as higher dosages can cause some systemic vasodilation. Such agents include nitroglycerin (Ang-O-Span, Klavikordal, Nitrostat, Trates, Tridil), nitroprusside (Nipride, Nitropress), erythrityl tetranitrate (Cardilate), isosorbide dinitrate (Coronex, Iso-Bid, Isonate, Sorbitrate), and pentaerythritol tetranitrate (Duotrate, Pentol, Vaso-80).

Oxygen therapy. Oxygen therapy is useful whenever conditions are such that inadequate tissue perfusion and inadequate oxygenation are present. Oxygen

TABLE 17–1 Drugs Used in the Treatment of Shock

Drug	Usual Dosage	Disadvantages	Advantages
Atropine sulfate	IV push of 0.5–1 mg every 5 min, up to a total of 2 mg	May cause rebound tachycardia. Increases workload of the heart and may cause anginal pain. May cause urinary retention. Contraindicated in clients with glaucoma or asthma.	Used for bradycardia, blocks vagal tone to the heart (which causes a slowing of the heart rate): results in an increase in heart rate.
Calcium chloride	IV push of 250–500 mg; may repeat every 10 min	Rapid administration may cause sustained contraction of the ventricles. May potentiate digitalis toxicity. Not compatible with sodium bicarbonate precipitates.	Increases cardiac contractility and tone. Increases conduction through the ventricles. Used for asystole.
Dopamine HCl (Intropin)	5–30 μg/kg per min for hypotension 2–5 μg/kg per min for renal hypoperfusion	May cause myocardial irritability and arrhythmias. May increase myocardial oxygen consumption. Not compatible with sodium bicarbonate precipitates. Peripheral infiltration may cause tissue necrosis. High doses may cause renal shutdown.	Produces sympathetic stimulation of the heart, causing an increase in cardiac output and blood pressure. Low doses increase renal blood flow, increasing urinary output.
Epinephrine HCl (Adrenalin)	IV push of 0.5–1.0 mg; follow with 0.5 mg every 5 min May also be given by intracardiac injection	May produce tachyarrhythmias, including premature ventricular contractions or ventricular fibrillation. May increase myocardial workload resulting in pain from ischemia. Not compatible with sodium bicarbonate precipitates.	Increases heart rate and myocardial contractility. Increases blood pressure. Used for cardiac arrest.
Isoproterenol (Isuprel)	Continuous IV infusion at 2–20 μg/min	May potentiate digitalis toxicity. May cause pain due to myocardial ischemia. May cause ventricular arrhythmias.	Increases heart rate and myocardial contractility. Increases venous return to the heart. Increases cardiac output.
Norepinephrine (levarterenol, Levophed)	Continuous IV infusion at 0.1–0.2 μg/kg per min; increase to maintain blood pressure of 90–100 mmHg	May cause hypertensive crisis. May increase vagal tone, resulting in bradycardia. Peripheral infiltration may cause tissue necrosis.	Produces peripheral vasoconstriction, assisting in raising the blood pressure and widening the pulse pressure.
Lidocaine HCl (Xylocaine)	IV bolus of 50–100 mg every 5 min; then infusion of 1–4 mg/min	May be toxic in clients with liver failure. Lethargy, nausea, or paresthesia require discontinuation of drug.	Slows conduction in the ventricles, supressing arrhythmia.

can be administered by mask, hood, nasal cannula, nasopharyngeal tube, endotracheal tube, and tracheostomy tube. Most commonly, masks and nasal cannulas are used to administer oxygen to clients experiencing shock. The nurse administers water-nebulized oxygen to the client in the amount of liters per minute (for administration via cannula) or concentration by percentage (for administration by mask) specified by the physician's prescription.

Altered Thought Processes

Planning: client goals. The major client goals for this nursing diagnosis are that the client will (1) accurately interpret environmental stimuli and (2) remain in a safe environment.

Interventions: nonsurgical management. Interventions are aimed at improving cerebral perfusion and providing a safe environment. Accurate assessment of CNS activity changes from normal or from baseline is the criterion for the institution of specific interventions and constitutes a major nursing responsibility. The IV, drug, and oxygen therapies described earlier for fluid volume deficit and decreased cardiac output are appropriate for this nursing diagnosis.

Mental status assessment. The nurse assesses the CNS functional activity of the client experiencing shock at least every 15 minutes to evaluate the effectiveness of current interventions and to determine whether shock is progressing. Variables to assess include the level of consciousness; pupillary responses to light; the presence of protective reflexes (cough and blink); the presence of spontaneous movement in all extremities; orientation to time, place, and person; past and recent memory; the ability to concentrate; and cognitive function.

Maintaining a safe environment. Changes in CNS activity and responses are expected in the client experiencing shock. In the early stage of shock, clients may show symptoms of increased CNS activity; as shock progresses, symptoms consistent with depressed CNS activity may be noted.

A nursing function in maintaining a safe environment includes assessing the client's ability to process information correctly. The nurse orients the client to time and place at every interaction. The nurse reminds the client of who the nurse is and what the nurse is doing for the client. If the client needs assistive devices, such as glasses or a hearing aid to see or hear properly, the nurse ensures that the client is using these devices while awake. The nurse makes certain that the client's call light is within easy reach at all times.

Care is taken to prevent injury in clients who are experiencing altered thought processes. Clients who are confused require close observation. The upper side rails of the client's bed are in the up position at all times. Whenever the client is alone, the bed is kept in the low

position. Occasionally, it may be necessary for the nurse to prevent the client from reaching the electronic bed controls. If the client remains confused and continues to attempt to get out of bed unassisted or to remove IV lines or other necessary attached equipment, the nurse requests an order to restrain the client with a vest or jacket-style restraint. Such devices should be used only when the client presents a clear danger to self or others.

■ Discharge Planning

Shock is usually a short-term occurrence. If the outcome of treatment is favorable and any complications have been resolved, the client is discharged to home after recovery.

Home Care Preparation

The history obtained when the client is admitted to the hospital usually includes essential information regarding the family composition and the home environment. The client may require minimal to moderate assistance at home for a short period after discharge from the hospital. Such assistance usually revolves around meal preparation and personal hygiene. If the client is too weak to use stairs, arrangements need to be made to have the client situated on a single level with easy access to bedroom, bathroom, walking area, and a fresh air source. If such arrangements present a problem to the client and the family, the social services department is consulted for assistance.

Client/Family Education

The client and the family should be able to identify the etiologic factors involved in the type of shock the client experienced. They should be alerted to the clinical manifestations they need to watch for during the first few days after discharge from the hospital and ways to avoid a possible recurrence. Explicit instructions are given by the nurse regarding proper method for dressing changes, including the frequency and any special techniques indicated by the type of wound.

A conference with the client and the family is held to discuss and plan activity, diet, and medication schedules. If available from the manufacturer, information sheets on newly prescribed medications are supplied. Activity progression and warning signs of overexertion should be discussed. Sexual activity is an important topic, especially for the client who has experienced cardiogenic shock attributable to an MI. Literature regarding sexual activity progression is helpful. The importance of follow-up care is emphasized.

Telephone numbers of health care resource persons are provided. The client and the family may feel anxious and reluctant when the client is discharged from the hospital after an acute illness such as shock. Reassurance as to the client's readiness for discharge assists in the transition from hospital to home.

Psychosocial Preparation

The client who has experienced shock may be from any age, race, and socioeconomic group, but the common factor is that each has experienced a life crisis requiring examination of the causes of its occurrence. The nurse assists the client and the family to deal with the aftermath of shock by encouraging questions and the verbalization of fears, which are often associated with the potential for recurrence of shock or even death.

The client frequently does not remember the acute phase of the illness and seeks answers from the nurse regarding what has occurred. The nurse can assist the client by helping to identify factors that have contributed to the onset of illness, the medical and nursing interventions prescribed, and the client's response. This information needs to be tailored to meet the individual's level of understanding and perception of her/his illness. As assessment of the coping mechanisms that the client and the family exhibit, such as denial, suppression, or anger, assists the nurse in deciding the appropriate approach to be taken for the preparation for discharge. It is essential that the client be made aware of any limitations that may be necessary, while also being encouraged to return to a normal home life and activities of daily living (ADL) as tolerated, without an overwhelming fear of recurrence.

Family members also experience a variety of feelings in response to the illness of a relative. As they prepare for the discharge of the client, family members begin to express fears about a recurrence of shock at home. Explicit instructions as to schedules for medication administration and medication side effects, activity levels, and early recognition of warning signs of complications or recurrence will assist in making the family feel more confident in the care of the client. Reassurance of the client's readiness for discharge and a period of recuperation at home is given by the nurse. A review of resources available to the client and family will help to instill a confidence that they will continue to have access to a support system even after discharge.

Health Care Resources

The client returning to the home environment may need special equipment to assist in ADL, such as a walker to prevent falls, until her/his strength returns. The client may need a bedside commode or blood pressure equipment. If the client's insurance carrier or financial resources do not cover the costs, rental of equipment should be explored.

A social services consultation to evaluate the client's eligibility for further assistance should be sought. If home care nurses are needed, it is preferable to make arrangements before the client is discharged from the hospital. A thorough summary of the client's needs should be prepared by the nurse and submitted to the home care agency to assist in maintaining the continuity of the client's care.

 Evaluation

On the basis of the nursing diagnoses identified, the expected outcomes for the client experiencing shock include that the client

1. Reduces blood and fluid loss
2. Restores normal circulating fluid volume
3. Maintains an adequate cardiac output
4. Maintains a urinary output of at least 30 mL/hour
5. Remains oriented to time, place, and person
6. Maintains good venous return from all body parts
7. Experiences reduced anxiety
8. Is free from pain
9. Is able to obtain normal patterns of sleep
10. Maintains an oral intake sufficient to meet nutritional needs
11. Participates in self-care activities
12. Maintains skin integrity
13. Lists specific factors that predispose this client to the development of shock
14. Lists clinical manifestations of shock
15. Identifies actions to take when signs and symptoms of shock occur
16. Describes the drug, diet, and activity regimen to be followed at home

SUMMARY

The nursing care of a client experiencing shock is challenging and fast paced. The onset of shock often is insidious, requiring careful evaluation of clinical data and client risk factors for its prevention, diagnosis, and treatment. More than one type of shock may be present simultaneously and contribute to the client's rapidly deteriorating condition. For example, hypovolemia as a result of blood loss from a traumatic wound may be the apparent cause of shock; however, this client may also be experiencing cardiogenic shock as a result of an MI precipitated by the traumatic event. A knowledge of this client's medical history of significant cardiac disease would enhance the diagnosis and hasten the treatment of the additional cause of shock.

IMPLICATIONS FOR RESEARCH

A review of current nursing literature reveals the need for nursing research regarding the hospitalized client who is in the early stage of shock, especially of septic shock. In addition, the development of assessment tools to be utilized by the nurse for the client at risk for shock to enhance early detection is clearly needed. Guidelines for psychosocial assessment and crisis intervention for the client and the family experiencing shock are needed, as are guidelines for the preparation of the home environment.

Nursing research is needed to answer the following questions related to the care of clients in shock:

1. How effective are nursing measures in preventing septic shock?
2. What effect does early recognition of signs and symptoms have on preventing the progression and complications of hypovolemic shock?
3. What are the effects of nursing measures on perfusion in the presence of shock?
4. Which noninvasive delivery method of oxygen therapy (nasal cannula or mask) is more effective in maintaining adequate PO_2 levels?
5. How do hospital infection control reports influence the incidence of nosocomial infections?
6. Which specific nursing care procedures are most closely associated with the development of septic shock?
7. How effective are urgent care outpatient centers in the early detection of shock?

REFERENCES AND READINGS

Barry, S. (1989). Septic shock: Special needs of patients with cancer. *Oncology Nursing Forum, 16*(1), 31–35.

Bitterman, H., Triolo, J., & Lefer, A. (1987). Use of hypertonic saline in the treatment of hemorrhagic shock. *Circulatory Shock, 21,* 271–283.

Blum, H., Schnall, M., Renshaw, P., & Buzby, G. (1988). Metabolic and ionic changes in muscle during hemorrhagic shock. *Circulatory Shock, 26,* 341–351.

Border, J., & Hassett, J. (1988). Multiple systems organ failure: History, pathophysiology, prevention and support. In G. Clowes (Ed.), *Trauma, sepsis, and shock* (pp. 335–356). New York: Marcel Dekker.

Carter, E., Tompkins, R., Yarmush, M., Walker, A., & Burke, J. (1988). Redistribution of blood flow after thermal injury and hemorrhagic shock. *Journal of Applied Physiology, 65,* 1782–1788.

Clowes, G. (Ed.). (1988). *Trauma, sepsis, and shock.* New York: Marcel Dekker.

Dickerson, M. (1988). Anaphylaxis and anaphylactic shock. *Critical Care Nursing Quarterly, 11*(1), 68–74.

Gilliam, G., & Polk, H. (1988). Factors predisposing to bacterial invasion. In G. Clowes (Ed.), *Trauma, sepsis, and shock* (pp. 55–69). New York: Marcel Dekker.

Guyton, A. C. (1986). *Textbook of medical physiology* (7th ed.). Philadelphia: W. B. Saunders.

Guyton, A. C. (1987). *Human physiology and mechanisms of disease* (4th ed.). Philadelphia: W. B. Saunders.

Halfman-Franey, M. (1988). Current trends in hemodynamic monitoring of patients in shock. *Critical Care Nursing Quarterly, 11*(1), 9–18.

Hinshaw, L. (1985). Cardiovascular dysfunction in shock: An overview with emphasis on septic shock. In H. Janssen & C. Barnes (Eds.), *Circulatory shock: Basic and clinical implications* (pp. 1–22). New York: Academic.

Horton, J. (1989). Hemorrhagic shock depresses myocardial contractile function in the guinea pig. *Circulatory Shock, 28,* 23–36.

Janssen, H., & Barnes, C. (Eds.). (1985). *Circulatory shock: Basic and clinical implications.* New York: Academic.

Jeffries, P., & Whelan, S. (1988). Cardiogenic shock: Current management. *Critical Care Nursing Quarterly, 11*(1), 48–56.

Ledingham, I., & Ramsay, G. (1986). Hypovolemic shock. *British Journal of Anesthesia, 58,* 169–189.

Littleton, M. (1988). Pathophysiology and assessment of sepsis and septic shock. *Critical Care Nursing Quarterly, 11*(1), 30–47.

Lucas, C., & Ledgerwood, A. (1988). Cardiovascular and renal response to hemorrhagic and septic shock. In G. Clowes (Ed.), *Trauma, sepsis, and shock* (pp. 187–215). New York: Marcel Dekker.

Meyers, K., & Hickey, M. (1988). Nursing management of hypovolemic shock. *Critical Care Nursing Quarterly, 11*(1), 57–67.

Perkins, S., & Kennally, K. (1989). The hidden danger of internal hemorrhage. *Nursing '89, 19*(7), 34–41.

Perry, A. (1988). Shock complications: Recognition and management. *Critical Care Nursing Quarterly, 11*(1), 1–8.

Rice, V. (1984). Shock management: Part I. Fluid volume replacement. *Critical Care Nurse, 4*(6), 69–82.

Rice, V. (1985). Shock management: Part II. Pharmacologic intervention. *Critical Care Nurse, 5*(1), 42–56.

Robbins, S., & Kumar, V. (1987). *Basic pathology* (4th ed.). Philadelphia: W. B. Saunders.

Shoemaker, W. (1987). Circulatory mechanisms of shock and their mediators. *Critical Care Medicine, 15,* 787–794.

Spitzer, J., Lang, C., McDonough, K., Burns, A., Romansky, A., & Shepherd, R. (1985). Myocardial metabolism and function in shock. In H. Janssen & C. Barnes (Eds.), *Circulatory shock: Basic and clinical implications* (pp. 47–74). New York: Academic.

Suskind, J. (1984). Handling hemorrhage wisely. *Nursing '84, 14*(1), 34–41.

Taptich, B., Iyer, P., & Bernocchi-Losey, D. (1989). *Nursing diagnosis and care planning.* Philadelphia: W. B. Saunders.

Taylor, D. (1984). Anaphylaxis: Physiology, signs, and symptoms. *Nursing '84, 14*(6), 44–45.

Teplitz, C. (1988). The pathology and ultrastructure of cellular injury and inflammation in the progression and outcome of trauma, sepsis, and shock. In G. Clowes (Ed.), *Trauma, sepsis, and shock* (pp. 71–120). New York: Marcel Dekker.

ADDITIONAL READINGS

Hancock, B., & Eberhard, N. (1988). The pharmacologic management of shock. *Critical Care Nursing Quarterly, 11*(1), 19–29.

This article presents a thorough review of the types and actions of various agents used in the general treatment of hemorrhagic and cardiogenic shock. For discussion, these agents are divided into categories of volume expanders, crystalloid therapy, colloid therapy, sympathomimetic agents, vasodilating agents, and miscellaneous agents. Presented information includes mechanisms of action, usual adult and pediatric dosages, and possible adverse reactions.

Littleton, M. (1988). Pathophysiology and assessment of sepsis and septic shock. *Critical Care Nursing Quarterly, 11*(1), 30–47.

The outstanding features of this article are the in-depth assessment guide for identifying clients with or at risk for septic shock and the complete explanations of the physiology and pathophysiology of septic shock. The assessment guide includes rationales for the clinical manifestations observed during early, intermediate, and late stages of septic shock. A description of specific nursing measures is provided to serve as a foundation for the plan of care appropriate for most clients with septic shock.

Perkins, S., & Kennally, K. (1989). The hidden danger of internal hemorrhage. *Nursing '89, 19*(7), 34–41.

Using a case presentation approach, this article describes the features of insidious shock resulting from internal hemorrhage. Stages of shock and compensatory mechanisms are well described, as are the expected changes in laboratory data and the IV agents usually used as volume expanders in the treatment of shock. The primary focus is on the implementation of nursing interventions specific for the client experiencing internal hemorrhage and shock.

UNIT 4 RESOURCES

Nursing Resources

American Society of Plastic and Reconstructive Surgical Nurses (ASPRSN), North Woodbury Road, PO Box 56, Pitman, NJ 08071. Telephone 609-589-6247.
See Unit 12 Resources for more information.
Plastic Surgical Nursing Certification Board, North Woodbury Road, PO Box 56, Pitman, NJ 08071. Telephone 609-589-6247.
Certifies nurses in plastic surgical nursing.

Other Resources

American Burn Association, Shriners Burn Institute, University of Cincinnati, 202 Goodman Street, Cincinnati, OH 45219. Telephone 513-751-3900 (extension 202).
Phoenix Society, 11 Rust Hill Road, Levittown, PA 19056. Telephone 215-946-BURN; 800-888-BURN.
Offers assistance to clients recovering from burns.

UNIT 5

Management of Surgical Clients

CHAPTER 18

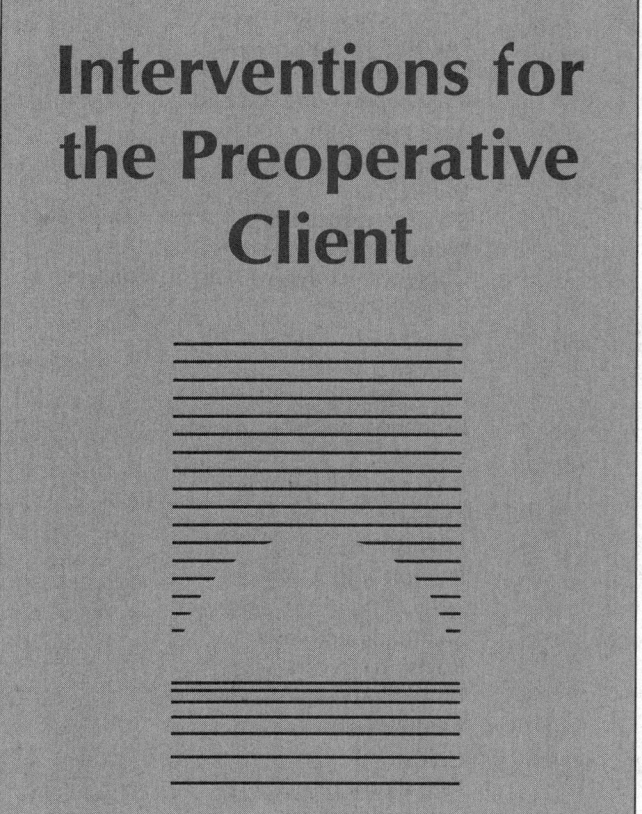

Interventions for the Preoperative Client

The role of the surgical nurse has changed in response to emerging trends in health care. With increased emphasis on reducing the length of stay in the hospital and cost and on ambulatory care, the role of the nurse has expanded to include the concept of total client care. Today, *perioperative,* or surgical, nursing focuses on the depth and scope of client care before, during, and after surgery. The nursing process serves as a major component in the implementation of the perioperative role. The perioperative period focuses on the client before surgery (*preoperative* period), during surgery (*intraoperative* period), and after surgery (*postoperative* period).

The adult who is about to undergo a surgical procedure, whether it is elective or emergency, is subject to many stressors that have an effect on physical and psychosocial equilibrium. The surgical experience, with its complex, highly technical procedures, is mysterious to most clients. The nurse plays a major role in demystifying this experience, reducing anxiety, and promoting an uncomplicated perioperative period for the client and family.

The primary role of the nurse before surgery is *educator* and *advocate.* An assessment of the client and family serves as the basis to develop an individualized teaching plan to help the client better understand the perioperative experience. Perioperative care and education begin before the client enters the surgical suite. Often, the nurse in the physician's office provides written instructions and literature to assist the client in preparing for the upcoming surgery. The nurse begins preoperative teaching and validates and clarifies information provided by the physician about the surgery and admission policies of the surgical setting.

To provide the client with comprehensive information about the surgical procedure, the nurse needs to understand how and why surgical procedures are classified. Surgical procedures are usually classified according to degree of risk, reason for the procedure, location, and extent of surgery required. Selected classifications are presented in Table 18–1, with examples of surgical procedures commonly performed.

SURGICAL SETTINGS

In response to government regulations on the length of hospital stay and to pressure to reduce costs from third-party insurance companies, changing trends in surgical settings have begun to emerge. Surgery continues to be performed under aseptic conditions, although the setting may not be the classic hospital operating room. Fifty per cent of all clients who are admitted to the hospital undergo some type of surgical procedure, whether it be diagnostic or curative. Surgical settings such as hospital-based ambulatory surgical centers, freestanding sur-

TABLE 18–1 Selected Classification of Surgical Procedures

Classification	Characteristics	Condition or Surgical Procedure
Emergency	Requires immediate interventions because of life-threatening consequences	Abdominal aortic aneurysm Gunshot or stab wound Severe bleeding Major open bone fracture Appendectomy
Urgent	Requires prompt interventions; is potentially life-threatening if treatment is delayed more than 24–48 hours	Intestinal obstruction Eye injury Bladder obstruction Kidney or ureteral stones Cholecystectomy with acute inflammation Bone fracture
Diagnostic	Requires intervention to determine origin, cause, and cell type	Cancer Endoscopy Colonoscopy Bronchoscopy Biopsy Exploratory laparotomy
Elective	Is planned for correction of nonacute problem	Cataracts Hernia repair Hemorrhoidectomy Total joint arthroplasty
Cosmetic	Is intervention primarily for alteration of personal appearance	Suction lipectomy Revision of scars Rhinoplasty Blephoplasty
Palliative	Is performed to relieve symptoms of a disease process but is not curative	Colostomy Nerve root resection Tumor debulking

gical centers, and physicians' offices are becoming increasingly more common. *Inpatient* refers to a client who is admitted to a hospital the day before or the same day of surgery and who requires hospitalization after surgery. In contrast, the *outpatient* goes to the surgical area (a surgical center or ambulatory care center) the day of the surgery and returns home on the same day. One of the many advantages of this alternative surgical experience is that clients are not separated from the comfort and security of their home and family. Research has noted that there is, along with reduced client stress, a decrease in the postoperative infection rate of the ambulatory surgical client. With the continuous improvements in surgical techniques and administration of anesthesia, more procedures are being safely performed on an outpatient basis.

In October 1983, the government mandated and compiled a list of surgical procedures that must be performed in an outpatient setting. The Health Care Financing Administration published a list of 100 procedures that are reimbursed by Medicare if they are done on an outpatient basis. The list is constantly changing and includes such procedures as cataract extraction, hernioplasty, cryosurgery, arthroscopy, and hemorrhoidectomy. This mandate has had the greatest impact on the adult and elderly population and the role of the nurse. The presence of chronic illness and the lack of a support system to assist in postoperative care increase elderly clients' stress and fears about returning home immediately after surgery.

The prospective payment system that was adopted by the federal government for Medicare clients is based on diagnosis-related groups (see Chap. 4 for a complete explanation of these groups). Reimbursement policies have changed from the traditional retrospective system to a prospective system. These changes specify who may be hospitalized for surgery and how long they may remain in the hospital after surgery. Because of these cost-containment measures and the emphasis on reducing the length of stay in the hospital, an increasing number of same-day surgical procedures are being seen. These trends are introducing a new challenge to nurses, especially in assessing, educating, and preparing the client for postoperative self-care.

COLLABORATIVE MANAGEMENT

 Assessment

History

When taking a history on a preoperative client, the nurse keeps in mind clients at risk for potential postoperative complications (Table 18–2). Data collected from the client include *age, allergies, tobacco use, medical problems, medication taken,* and *previous surgical procedures.* Today, surgery on the elderly client is less dangerous because of advances in medicine. Elderly clients are at increased risk for developing postoperative complications because of the presence of chronic illnesses. The normal aging process affects clients' physical and emotional ability to withstand the stress of surgery and anesthesia. The use of tobacco products increases the risk of pulmonary complications because of pre-existing changes to the lungs and thoracic cavity. Smokers and elderly persons have decreased oxygen diffusion and elasticity of the lungs, and the thoracic cavity, or rib cage, increases in rigidity as a result of inefficient air exchange. Medication that is routinely taken may affect how the client reacts to the perioperative experience. The potential effects of medication noted in Table 18–3 are taken into account by the health care team while completing the preoperative assessment and planning care. The number and type of previous surgeries and previous surgical history, including wound healing and complications, affect the client's recovery and potential fears and readiness for surgery. Each of these factors contributes to and increases the client's risk of developing postoperative complications.

The nurse takes a thorough surgical history to determine the client's *experience with anesthetic agents* and *allergies.* These data provide the nurse with information about tolerance and possible fears related to the use of anesthesia. The client who is sensitive or allergic to certain substances alerts the nurse to a possible reaction to anesthetic agents or substances that are used for preoperative skin preparation such as povidone-iodine, which contains some of the same components as those

TABLE 18–2   Important Points in the Preoperative Nursing History

Age
Allergies to medication and food
Current medication (prescription and over-the-counter)
History of medical and surgical problems
Previous surgical experiences
Previous experience with anesthesia
Tobacco, alcohol, and drug use

found in shellfish. Family medical history and problems with anesthetics may indicate possible intraoperative needs and reactions to anesthesia, such as malignant hyperthermia.

In addition to information about the client's history, the nurse assesses the client's environment, self-care capabilities, and support systems. Postoperative needs and discharge referrals can also be assessed at this time. It is important for all clients, especially elderly persons and dependent adults, to have discharge planning. These special groups may need referrals for transportation to and from the doctor's office, as well as the help of a home care nurse to monitor postoperative status and to instruct the client on wound care.

Physical Assessment: Clinical Manifestations

The preoperative client may be of any age with a health status that varies from healthy to debilitated. Basic preoperative assessment is performed on all clients before surgery to determine baseline data, hidden medical problems, potential complications related to the administration of anesthesia, and potential postoperative complications.

When beginning the assessment, the nurse obtains a complete set of vital signs (temperature, pulse, respiration, and blood pressure readings) to assist in determining the client's risk of postoperative complications. Table 18–4 gives interpretations of alterations in vital signs and clinical implications related to the client's care. Abnormal vital signs may cause the postponement of surgery until the underlying problem is treated and the client's condition is stable.

A complete physical assessment is performed and focuses on problem areas that have been identified from the client's history and on all body systems that are affected directly or indirectly by the surgical procedure. The elderly or chronically ill client is at increased risk for intraoperative and postoperative complications related to potential alterations in preoperative physical condition and to the aging process (see the Focus on the Elderly feature on p. 433).

Cardiovascular system. The condition of the cardiovascular system is assessed to determine the strength of the heart and its ability to tolerate surgery and anesthesia. The cardiovascular assessment includes palpation of peripheral pulses and auscultation of heart sounds for rate, regularity, and abnormalities (see Chap. 63 for details on cardiovascular assessment).

Alterations in cardiac status are responsible for approximately 30% of perioperative deaths (Wolcott, 1988). Especially important in the elderly client is the deterioration of cardiovascular function, which results in decreased cardiac output and increased diastolic blood pressure. The nurse evaluates the client for hypertension, which is a common and often undiagnosed health problem of adults and can have an impact on surgery. Medical problems such as arteriosclerosis usu-

TABLE 18–3   Effects of Medication Taken Routinely on the Perioperative Experience

Drug	Implications for the Perioperative Experience	Interventions	Rationales
Antibiotics			
Gentamicin (Garamycin)	Produces mild respiratory depression (as do other aminoglycoside antibiotics).	1. Monitor respiratory status. 2. Assess for signs of infection. 3. Make the anesthesiologist aware of antibiotics taken and document same in client's record.	1. To detect deviations 2. To detect infections. 3. To avoid respiratory complications during surgery.
Penicillin	Masks infection.		
Erythromycin	During surgery, may potentiate anesthetics that act as neuromuscular blockers. Used prophylactically to prevent complications for clients with cardiac valve disease.		
Antiarrhythmics			
Propranolol hydrochloride (Inderal)	Affects client's tolerance of anesthesia.	1. Monitor vital signs. 2. Obtain baseline electrocardiogram. 3. Assess peripheral circulation. 4. Communicate use and type of antiarrhythmics to the health care team to ensure ongoing use and monitoring.	1. To detect deviations. 2–4. To avoid cardiac complications during surgery.
Quinidine gluconate (Quinaglute)	Depresses cardiac function by decreasing cardiac output and slowing pulse rate.		
Procainamide hydrochloride (Pronestyl)	May cause peripheral vasodilation. Potentiates anesthetics that are neuromuscular blockers.		
Antihypertensives			
Methyldopa (Aldomet)	Alters response to muscle relaxants and narcotic analgesics by inhibiting synthesis and storage of norepinephrine.	1. Monitor blood pressure and pulse. 2. Assess for hypotension during transfer and turning.	1. To detect deviations. 2. To prevent hypotensive crisis.
Captopril (Capoten)			
Clonidine hydrochloride (Catapres)	May cause hypotensive crisis intra- and postoperatively.		
Corticosteroids			
Dexamethasone (Decadron)	Delays wound healing because of blockage of collagen formation.	1. Continue steroid therapy during perioperative experience. 2. Monitor vital signs. 3. Assess for signs of hyperglycemia. 4. Assess for signs of infection and bleeding. 5. Monitor wound healing, support incisional area with the use of binders, and splint wound when client is turning, coughing, and deep breathing.	1. To avoid problems associated with abrupt withdrawal. 2, 3. To detect deviations. 4. To detect signs of infection. 5. To prevent complications.
Desoxycorticosterone acetate (Percorten)	Surgery increases demand of corticosteroids in the client with no adrenal function.		
Hydrocortisone sodium (Solu-Cortef)	Increases serum glucose level, blocks fibroblast formation.		
Prednisone (Deltasone)	Increases risk of hemorrhage. Masks infection.		

TABLE 18–3   Effects of Medication Taken Routinely on the Perioperative Experience *Continued*

Drug	Implications for the Perioperative Experience	Interventions	Rationales
Anticoagulants			
Warfarin sodium (Coumadin) Heparin sodium (Lipo-Hepin) Aspirin (acetylsalicylic acid)	Increases risk of hemorrhage intra- and postoperatively.	1. Monitor coagulation time (PTT,* PT). 2. Monitor for signs of bleeding. 3. Gradually discontinue anticoagulants 48 h before surgery. 4. Have antidote (protamine sulfate for heparin and vitamin K [Mephyton] for warfarin sodium) available to reverse effects of anticoagulant.	1, 2. To detect bleeding disorders. 3. To avoid hemorrhage. 4. To prevent complications of bleeding.
Anticonvulsants			
Phenobarbital (Eskabarb) Phenytoin sodium (Dilantin)	Seizure activity could cause injury to surgical wound. Alters metabolism of anesthetics.	1. Maintain use of drug. 2. Inform anesthesiologist to allow for adjustment of dosage of anesthetic. 3. Assess for seizure activity. 4. Pad bed side rails. 5. Place padded tongue blade and suction equipment at bedside.	1–3. To prevent seizures. 4, 5. To prevent injury.
Glaucoma Medications			
Demecarium bromide (Humorsol) Echothiophate (Phospholine Iodide) Pilocarpine hydrochloride (Isopto-Carpine; Pilocar) Timolol maleate (Timoptic)	Has cumulative systemic effect. Causes respiratory and cardiovascular collapse, especially during surgery.	1. Stop drug at least 2 wk. 2. Monitor respiratory status and cardiac output. 3. Assess for increased intraocular pressure.	1. To avoid complications. 2, 3. To detect complications.
Antidiabetic Agent			
Insulin	Insulin needs decrease preoperatively when client is taking nothing by mouth. Postoperative insulin demands increase because of IV administration of dextrose and water. Insulin levels may fluctuate during healing because of dietary and activity restrictions.	1. Monitor serum and urinary glucose levels. 2. Administer antibiotics in normal saline instead of dextrose when possible.	1. To detect increased or decreased need for insulin. 2. To avoid complications.

*PTT, partial thromboplastin time; PT, prothrombin time; IV, intravenous.

TABLE 18-4 Effect of Vital Signs on the Perioperative Experience

Vital Sign	Abnormal Finding	Possible Indication	Possible Postoperative Complication
Temperature	Fever (temperature > 101° F [38.3° C] in an adult)	Infection Dehydration (when accompanied by decreased skin turgor)	Systemic infection Wound infection, dehiscence, or evisceration Fluid imbalance Shock
Pulse	Tachycardia (>100 beats per minute)	Pain Fever Dehydration Anemia Hypoxia Shock	Poor tissue perfusion Vascular collapse Cardiac arrhythmias Renal failure Anesthetic complications
	Bradycardia (<60 beats per minute)	Drug effects (for example, of digitalis) Spinal injury Head injury	Spinal shock Increased intracranial pressure (see also complications for tachycardia)
Respiration	Tachypnea (>24 breaths per minute)	Atelectasis Pneumonia Pain or anxiety Pleurisy Infection Renal failure	Tissue hypoxia Anesthetic complications Pneumonia Atelectasis
	Bradypnea (<10 breaths per minute)	Brain lesion Respiratory center depression	See complications for tachypnea
Blood pressure	Hypotension (<90 mmHg systolic)	Shock Myocardial infarction Hemorrhage Spinal injury	Poor tissue perfusion Renal failure Vasodilation Shock
	Hypertension (>140 mmHg systolic and/or 90 mmHg diastolic)	Anxiety or pain Renal disease Coronary artery disease	Stroke Hemorrhage Myocardial infarction

Reprinted with permission from Carey, K. W. (Ed.). (1983). *Nursing photobook: Caring for surgical patients.* Copyright 1983 Springhouse Corporation. All rights reserved.

ally cause decreased peripheral perfusion, which is exacerbated by the perioperative experience. Other cardiac disorders that increase risks associated with surgery are angina pectoris, myocardial infarction within the past 6 months, congestive heart failure, and arrhythmias. These disorders impair the client's ability to withstand and respond to hemodynamic changes during an operation (e.g., hypotension). The risk of intraoperative myocardial infarction is also higher in clients with preexistent heart disorders.

Respiratory system. In assessing the client's respiratory status, the nurse takes into account the client's age, history of smoking, and presence of chronic illness.

Elderly persons, smokers, and adults with chronic respiratory problems are at increased risk of *atelectasis*, or collapse of lung tissue, which prevents exchange of oxygen and carbon dioxide and causes intolerance of

anesthesia because of changes in the chest and lungs. These changes cause decreased oxygen diffusion to and oxygenation of the tissues. Increased rigidity of the thoracic cavity and loss of lung elasticity reduce the efficiency of anesthesia excretion or *blow off*. Chronic pulmonary conditions such as asthma, emphysema, and chronic obstructive pulmonary disease also reduce the elasticity of the lungs, which causes an ineffective exchange of carbon dioxide and oxygen. Baseline arterial blood gas values are assessed before surgery. Smoking increases the level of circulating carboxyhemoglobin, which, in turn, decreases oxygen delivery to organs. Concurrently, mucociliary transport decreases, which leads to increased secretions and predisposes the client to pulmonary infection and atelectasis.

In assessing pulmonary status, the nurse observes the client's posture; fingers (for clubbing); respiratory rate, depth, and rhythm; and lung expansion. Auscultation is

FOCUS ON THE ELDERLY ■ Physiologic Changes of Aging as Surgical Risk Factors

Structure	Change	Interventions	Rationales
Cardiovascular system	Decreased cardiac output. Increased diastolic blood pressure. Decreased peripheral circulation.	1. Determine normal activity levels and when client tires. 2. Monitor vital signs. 3. Teach leg exercises and turning in bed.	1. To prevent fatigue. 2. To establish baseline data and to detect deviations. 3. To promote circulation.
Respiratory system	Reduced vital capacity. Loss of lung elasticity. Decreased oxygenation of blood.	1. Teach coughing and deep breathing. 2. Monitor respirations.	1. To prevent respiratory complications. 2. To establish baseline data.
Renal system	Decreased blood flow to kidneys. Reduced ability to excrete waste products.	1. Monitor intake and output 2. Monitor electrolyte status.	1. To detect dehydration, fluid overload, and decreased renal function. 2. To detect imbalances.
Neurologic system	Sensory deficits. Slower reaction time.	1. Orient client to surroundings. 2. Allow extra time for client teaching.	1, 2. Client's orientation and presence of sensory deficits call for individualized preoperative teaching plan.
Musculoskeletal system	Increased incidence of deformities related to osteoporosis or arthritis.	1. Assess level of mobility. 2. Teach turning, positioning. 3. Encourage ambulation.	1–3. To prevent complications of immobility.

performed to determine the quality and presence of adventitious sounds and congestion, which may be evident preoperatively (see Chap. 60 for more information on respiratory assessment).

Renal system. Renal function affects the filtration and excretion of waste products, which can alter fluid and electrolyte balance, especially in the elderly client. In assessing the client's renal status, the nurse observes for clinical manifestations such as frequency urination, dysuria, anuria, and appearance and odor of the urine (see Chap. 57 for further discussion of urinary assessment). The simplest laboratory test, a urinalysis, is done preoperatively to assess for the presence of protein, glucose, blood, and bacteria in the urine. If renal disease is suspected, serum blood urea nitrogen and creatinine levels are measured to determine the degree of disease present.

Abnormal renal function can decrease the excretion rate of preoperative medications and anesthetic agents and therefore can alter their effectiveness. Scopolamine, morphine, meperidine (Demerol), and barbiturates frequently cause confusion, disorientation, apprehension, and restlessness when administered to clients with decreased renal function.

Neurologic system. Assessment of the client's level of consciousness, orientation, and ability to follow commands is an important part of preoperative teaching and postoperative care. A deficit in any of these areas affects

the type of care that is required during the perioperative experience; the presence of paralysis has a similar effect. The client's ability to ambulate and steadiness of gait are noted preoperatively as baseline data, for use in analysis of postoperative and discharge goal attainment (see Chap. 32 for complete nervous system assessment).

Musculoskeletal system. Deformities of the musculoskeletal system, such as those found in osteoporosis or caused by joint replacement, may interfere with intraoperative and postoperative positioning of the client. Clients with arthritis may be able to assume conventional intraoperative positions but suffer unnecessary discomfort postoperatively from prolonged immobilization of joints. Other anatomic characteristics, such as the shape and length of the client's neck and shape of the thoracic cavity, may interfere with respiratory and cardiac function.

Nutritional status. Malnutrition and obesity can cause increased surgical risks. Many elderly clients are prone to nutritional imbalances because of chronic illness, use of diuretics, poor dietary planning, anorexia, lack of motivation, and financial limitations. Surgery usually increases the body's metabolic rate and consequently depletes potassium, ascorbic acid, and B vitamins, which are needed for wound healing and fibrin formation. In malnourished clients, hypoproteinemia affects postoperative recovery. Negative nitrogen balance may develop because of depleted protein, thus increasing the risk of perioperative mortality.

The obese client is often malnourished because of poor eating habits and an imbalanced diet. These clients have an increased chance of poor or incomplete wound healing related to excess adipose tissue. The fatty tissue lacks nutrients, is not vascular, and has little collagen, all of which are important for wound healing. Obesity causes increased stress on the heart and reduces the available lung volume, which then affect the client's perioperative experience.

Clinical indications of alterations in the fluid and nutritional status of the preoperative client include brittle nails; wasting muscles; dry, flaky skin; and dull, sparse, dry hair. Decreased skin turgor, postural hypotension, decreased serum albumin levels, and abnormal serum electrolyte values also indicate imbalance. Hypokalemia should be reported before surgery. Potassium imbalances will increase the risk of digitalis toxicity, will slow recovery from anesthesia, and will increase cardiac irritability.

Psychosocial Assessment

An individual who is scheduled for surgery experiences some level of perioperative anxiety and fear. The extent and type of these reactions vary for each client according to the kind of surgery, the perceived effects of the surgery, and its potential outcome. Surgery may be seen as a threat to the client's biologic integrity, body image, self-esteem, self-concept, or life style. These potential threats, whether real or not, cause increased anxiety and fear for the client. A disturbance in or uneasiness about the client's psychosocial status has an effect on the client's ability to learn, cope, and cooperate with preoperative teaching and perioperative procedures. Anxiety and fear affect the amount of anesthesia that is needed and postoperative recovery. Research has noted that many clients frequently verbalize similar fears about the perioperative experience. Clients fear death, a diagnosis of life-threatening conditions, pain, helplessness, decrease in socioeconomic status, possible disabling or crippling effects, changes in body image, and the unknown. The nurse keeps these fears in mind while interviewing the client and planning preoperative teaching.

The purposes of psychosocial assessment and preparation of the client are to determine the client's coping ability, provide information, and offer support. The nurse assesses the coping mechanisms used by the client under similar situations or in the past when the client had been confronted with a stressful situation. Factors that are assessed and that influence coping are age, previous surgical and sick role experiences, emotional and physical signs of fear and anxiety (e.g., anger, crying, restlessness, increased pulse rate, diarrhea, and urinary frequency), and discomfort. The nurse's assessment reveals successful coping mechanisms and support systems to help the client reduce the stress that is related to the surgical experience.

Laboratory Findings

Preoperative laboratory tests are performed to provide baseline data regarding the client's health and to predict potential complications. The client who is scheduled for surgery in a surgical center or who is admitted to the hospital on the morning of surgery usually has preadmission testing performed at least 48 hours before the scheduled surgery. The hospitalized client usually has testing done 24 hours before surgery. The choice of laboratory tests varies from institution to institution and depends on the client's age and medical history. The most common tests are urinalysis, complete blood count, coagulation studies (prothrombin time, partial thromboplastin time), and electrolytes (SMA-6 [6/60] or Profile 7). Table 18–5 presents abnormal findings, implications for nursing care, and potential postoperative complications for each laboratory test.

Radiographic Findings

A chest x-ray is commonly taken to determine the size and contour of the heart, lungs, and major vessels. This information is added to the client's baseline data for a comprehensive assessment. Positive x-ray film results may indicate potential pulmonary complications. The presence of an infiltrate or pneumonia may cause the cancellation or delay of elective surgery. In emergency surgery, this information assists the anesthesiologist in the selection of an alternative type of anesthetic. Other radiographic studies are based on the individual client's needs, depending on the client's medical history and nature of the surgical procedure. For example, a client with back pain may have a myelogram done before a diskectomy to identify the source of pain.

Other Diagnostic Tests

An electrocardiogram (ECG) is analyzed routinely for all clients older than 40 years who are to have general anesthesia, those who have a history of cardiac disease, and those at high risk of cardiovascular complications. A client with a known cardiac condition may require a consultation with a cardiologist and the administration of a prophylactic medication such as nitroglycerine paste during the perioperative experience to reduce or prevent stress on the cardiovascular system. An ECG provides baseline information on new or existing cardiac problems. Pre-existing conditions, such as an old anterior wall myocardial infarction, can be detected on an ECG. Abnormal or potentially life-threatening ECG results may cause the cancellation of surgery until the client's cardiac status is stable.

 Analysis: Nursing Diagnosis

Common Diagnoses

Two nursing diagnoses are common in the client preparing for the perioperative experience:

TABLE 18–5   Normal Findings and Significance of Abnormal Findings in Common Blood Tests Used in Perioperative Assessment

Test	Normal Range	Abnormal Findings Increase	Abnormal Findings Decrease	Interventions	Rationales
Potassium (K+)	3.5–5.0 mEq/L	Dehydration Renal failure	Excessive use of diuretics Nausea, vomiting, hypotension, malnutrition, cardiac arrhythmias	1. Monitor serum K+ level. 2. Keep strict intake and output records. 3. Assess blood pressure and pulse. 4. Assess hydration status.	1, 3. To detect deficiencies (hypokalemia) and excesses (hyperkalemia). 2,4. To prevent dehydration and over-hydration.
Sodium (Na+)	136–145 mEq/L	Cardiac or renal failure Hypertension Excess amounts of intravenous fluids containing normal saline Edema	Nasogastric drainage Vomiting, diarrhea Excessive use of laxatives and/or diuretics	1. Monitor vital signs (pulse and blood pressure). 2. Keep strict intake and output records. 3. Monitor serum Na+ level. 4. Assess for peripheral edema and circulation.	1–4. To detect hyponatremia and hypernatremia and to prevent dehydration and over-hydration.
Chloride (Cl−)	96–106 mEq/L	Alkalosis Dehydration Renal failure	Excessive nasogastric drainage Vomiting Excessive use of diuretics	1. Monitor hydration status. 2. Keep strict intake and output records. 3. Assess use and amount of diuretics administered intra- and postoperatively.	1–3. To detect hypochloremia and hyperchloremia and to prevent dehydration and over-hydration.
Carbon dioxide (CO$_2$)	22–34 mEq/L	Chronic obstructive pulmonary disease Respiratory acidosis Intestinal obstruction Vomiting or nasogastric suctioning	Hyperventilation Diabetic acidosis Diarrhea	1. Monitor respiratory status. 2. Keep intake and output records.	1, 2. To detect metabolic acidosis and alkalosis.
Glucose (fasting)	60–100 mg/dL	Hyperglycemia Excess amounts of intravenous fluids containing glucose	Hypoglycemia	1. Monitor serum and/or urinary glucose level. 2. Monitor dietary intake.	1, 2. To detect hypoglycemia, and hyperglycemia.

(Table continued on following page)

TABLE 18–5 **Normal Findings and Significance of Abnormal Findings in Common Blood Tests Used in Perioperative Assessment** *Continued*

Test	Normal Range	Abnormal Findings		Interventions	Rationales
		Increase	*Decrease*		
		Pancreatic and/or hepatic disease			
Creatinine	0.6–1.0 mg/dL (women) 0.8–1.7 mg/dL (men)	Renal damage with destruction of large number of nephrons	Atrophy of muscle tissue	1. Monitor intake and output, especially urinary output. 2. Monitor serum creatinine levels.	1. To assess urinary excretion. 2. To detect increases, which can signal renal disease.
Blood urea nitrogen (BUN)	5–15 mg/dL	Dehydration Renal failure Excessive protein in diet	Overhydration Liver failure Malnutrition	1. Monitor intake and output. 2. Monitor BUN levels. 3. Assess hydration status. 4. Assess for signs of hepatic failure (jaundice, portal hypertension, and elevated serum Na^+ level).	1. To assess urinary excretion. 2. To detect increases, which can signal renal disease. 3, 4. To detect renal disease.
Prothrombin time (PT)	12–14 s (2–2.5 × the normal is a therapeutic range)	Coagulation defect Increased chance of hemorrhage Too high a dose of anticoagulant (aspirin, heparin, warfarin)	Increased chance of embolus (thrombo-plebitis, pulmonary emboli)	1. Assess for signs of bleeding from operative site, drains, hematoma, mucous membranes. 2. Monitor PT and PTT values. 3. Assess for thrombus formation. 4. Assess chemical composition of medications for presence of anticoagulants.	1. To evaluate the need for anticoagulant theory to be decreased. 2, 3. To detect clotting problems. 4. To prevent compli-cations.
Partial thrombo-plastin time (PTT)	28–44 s (results are compared with aging laboratory control)				

TABLE 18–5   Normal Findings and Significance of Abnormal Findings in Common Blood Tests Used in Perioperative Assessment *Continued*

| Test | Normal Range | Abnormal Findings | | Interventions | Rationales |
		Increase	*Decrease*		
White blood cell count	4500–11,000 cells/mm³	Infection	Immune deficit	1. Use strict hand washing. 2. Prevent drafts and damp dressings and/or linens. 3. Bag and discard all dressing material in sealed receptacle. 4. Monitor for temperature elevation and signs of infection.	1–3. To prevent infection. 4. To detect infection.
Hemoglobin	12–15 g/dL (women) 14–16.5 g/dL (men)	Fluid overload	Dehydration Excessive blood loss Anemia	1. Monitor hydration status. 2. Monitor administration of intravenous fluids to prevent error in amount received. 3. Assess for signs of bleeding. 4. Monitor vital signs.	1, 2. To prevent dehydration and over-hydration. 3, 4. To detect signs of shock and anemia.
Hematocrit	37–45% (women) 42–50% (men)				

1. Knowledge deficit related to the perioperative experience
2. Anxiety and fear related to the perioperative experience

Additional Diagnoses

In addition to the common diagnoses, the client may present with the following diagnoses:

1. Sleep pattern disturbance related to fear of impending surgery
2. Ineffective individual coping related to stress of impending surgery
3. Anticipatory grieving related to effect of surgery
4. Body image disturbance related to anticipated changes in body appearance or function
5. Ineffective family coping: disabling related to surgery and surgical outcome of a loved one

 ## Planning and Implementation

The following plan of care for the preoperative client focuses on the actual diagnoses. The differences between interventions for the hospitalized client and modifications for the outpatient are delineated.

Knowledge Deficit

Planning: client goals. The two major goals for this diagnosis are that the client will (1) verbalize and comply with preoperative procedures and (2) demonstrate techniques to prevent postoperative complications.

Interventions. Because the perioperative experience is usually foreign to most clients, the nurse focuses on preoperative education interventions that provide information to the client and family. Information about

Preoperative Education Program

At the completion of the preoperative teaching session(s), the client and/or the family will verbalize understanding of the following:

Education	Date	Nurse to Initial		Comments
		Yes	No (explain)	
1. View preoperative film.				
2. Preoperative regulations (dentures, jewelry, valuables).				
3. NPO				
a. Meanings				
b. Purpose				
4. Invasive procedures				
a. IVs, drains, catheters				
b. Purpose				
5. Preoperative medications				
a. Purpose				
b. Administration times				
6. Operating room				
a. Transportation				
b. Skin preparation				
c. Recovery room				
7. Postoperative monitoring				
a. Vital signs				
b. Equipment/dressing check				
8. Respiratory procedures				
a. Turning, coughing, and deep breathing				
b. Splinting				
c. Return demonstration				
d. Respiratory therapy				
9. Activity/ROM				
a. Range of motion				
b. Return demonstration				
c. Ambulation				

Figure 18–1

Preoperative educational checklist. (Courtesy of Baltimore County General Hospital, Randallstown, MD.)

Preoperative Education Program *Continued*

Education	Date	Nurse to Initial		Comments
		Yes	No (explain)	
10. Pain management				
a. Positioning				
b. Medication				
11. Visiting policies				
a. Preoperative				
b. Postoperative				
12. Critical care unit				
a. Give copy of critical care booklet				
b. Reason for transfer				
c. Critical care regulations (waiting room and visiting hours)				

Figure 18–1 Continued

informed consent, dietary restrictions, preoperative preparation (bowel and skin preparations), and postoperative exercises and procedures is important to understand to promote the client's participation in health care. Figure 18–1 is a sample comprehensive preoperative educational checklist.

Informed consent. Surgery of any type involves invasion of the body and requires informed consent from the client or legal guardian (Fig. 18–2). Consent implies that one has been provided with information necessary to understand the

1. Nature of and reason for surgery
2. All available options and risks associated with each option
3. Risks of surgical procedure and potential outcomes
4. Risks associated with administration of anesthesia

Signed permission protects the client from any unwanted procedures and the physician and institution from lawsuit claims related to unauthorized surgery or uninformed clients.

The physician is usually responsible for having the consent form signed before preoperative sedation is given and surgery is performed. It is not the responsibility of the nurse to provide detailed information about the surgical procedure, but the nurse does clarify facts that have been presented by the physician and myths

that the client and family may believe about the perioperative experience. The nurse ensures that the consent form is signed and serves as a witness to the signature, not to the fact that the client is informed. If the nurse, as the client's advocate, believes that the client has not been adequately informed, the surgeon is contacted and requested to see the client for clarification of the surgical procedure.

Clients who cannot write may sign with a "mark," which must be witnessed by two persons. In an emergency, telephone or telegram authorization is acceptable and should be followed with written consent as soon as possible. The number of witnesses (usually two) and type of documentation vary according to institutional policy. In a life-threatening situation in which every effort has been made to contact the family, consent is desired but not essential. In lieu of written or oral consent, a written consultation by at least two physicians who are not associated with the case legally suffices until a relative or guardian can sign a consent form. If the client has no family or is thought to be incapable of giving consent, the court appoints a legal guardian to represent the client's best interests.

Some surgical procedures require a special permit in addition to the standard consent. Each hospital and state determine which procedure requires this permit. Intraocular lens implants, sterilization, and experimental procedures are examples of procedures for which this extra form is usually required.

REQUEST AND AUTHORIZATION FOR
MEDICAL AND/OR SURGICAL TREATMENT

1. I hereby request and authorize Dr. _____ and/or his/her associates and whomever they may designate as their assistants to administer such treatment as is necessary to perform the following operation _____ _____ and such additional operations or procedures as are considered necessary on the basis of conditions that may be revealed during the course of said operation or treatment.

2. I request and authorize the administration of such anesthetics and/or other medications as are necessary.

3. Final disposition of any tissues or parts surgically removed is to be handled in accordance with the customary practices of the hospital.

4. Reasons why the above-named surgery and/or treatment is considered necessary, its advantages, probability of success, possible complications, and risks, as well as possible alternative modes of treatment, were explained to me by Dr. _____.

5. I am aware that the practice of medicine and surgery is not an exact science and I acknowledge that no guarantees have been made to me concerning the results of the operation or procedure.

6. I hereby acknowledge that I have read and fully understand the above request and authorization for medical and/or surgical treatment.

Date: _____   Time: _____

Signed: _____
                                                                        Client

OR: _____
                                                            Legal Representative

Witness _____   Relationship (if any)

Figure 18–2

Surgical consent form. (Courtesy of Baltimore County General Hospital, Randallstown, MD.)

Dietary restrictions. For any type of surgery and regardless of whether the client is to receive any kind of anesthetic, he or she is kept on *NPO* status (nothing by mouth) for 6 to 8 hours before surgery. NPO means no eating of food, drinking (including water), or smoking of any kind (nicotine stimulates gastric secretions). It is common practice to begin NPO status for all preoperative clients at midnight on the night before surgery. This extra precaution ensures that the stomach is free from gastric secretions, which increase the possibility of aspiration. Outpatients and clients who are scheduled for admission to the hospital on the same day that surgery will be performed must receive written and oral instructions about remaining NPO after midnight. The nurse emphasizes the importance of compliance; failure to comply can result in cancellation of surgery or an increased risk of intraoperative aspiration.

There may need to be some alterations in the client's usual medication schedule on the day of surgery. The nurse consults the client's personal physician for instructions about administration of medications such as those used for hypoglycemia, cardiac disease, or glaucoma, as well as anticonvulsants, antihypertensives, and corticosteroids. Some medications may be stopped until after surgery or may be given intravenously to maintain the client's blood level of the medication, thus not interfering with the administration schedule. Medications for cardiac disease and hypertension are commonly allowed with a sip of water if taken at least 2 hours before surgery. The diabetic client who is taking insulin may be given a reduced dose of intermediate- or long-acting insulin based on serum or urine glucose level, or the client may be given regular insulin subcutaneously or intravenously (see Chap. 51 for information on medication for diabetes). Another alternative treatment is an intravenous infusion of 5% dextrose in water, which is given along with the insulin to prevent hypoglycemia intraoperatively.

Gastrointestinal preparation. Bowel or gastrointestinal preparations are done to prevent injury to the colon, provide clear visualization of the area, and reduce the number of intestinal bacteria. Evacuation of the gastrointestinal tract is done on a client having major abdominal, pelvic, perineal, or perianal surgery. Similar bowel preparation is conducted on clients who are scheduled for diagnostic examination of the colon, such as a colonoscopy. Surgeon preference and type of surgical procedure will determine whether a single or a combination bowel preparation is done. Table 18–6 shows

TABLE 18-6   Common Bowel Preparations for the Surgical Client and Their Complications

Surgical Site	Preparation	Complications
Stomach, duodenum, and proximal jejunum	Oral laxative (e.g., castor oil preparation or bisacodyl [Dulcolax]) Clear liquid diet the evening before surgery NPO after midnight	Abdominal cramping Dehydration Electrolyte imbalance Fatigue
Small intestine	Oral laxative (e.g., magnesium citrate) Clear liquid diet the evening before surgery Multiple-position enema the evening before surgery NPO after midnight	Dehydration Electrolyte imbalance Fatigue
Large intestine to rectum	Multiple or combination of oral laxatives 12-24 h before surgery Multiple-position tap water or antibiotic (neomycin) enemas (three times) or until return flow is clear the evening and morning before surgery Oral antibiotics to sterilize bowel (e.g., neomycin and erythromycin) 24 h before surgery Clear liquid diet the day before surgery NPO after midnight	Fatigue and weakness Fluid excess or deficit Potassium and/or sodium deficit Decreased cardiac output from vagal stimulation Irritation of bowel and rectal mucosa from enemas

typical gastrointestinal preparation regimens for common surgical procedures and complications of the regimens. An enema ordered to be given until return flow is "clear" is a stressful procedure for anyone, but especially for the elderly client. Repeated enemas can cause electrolyte imbalance (especially potassium depletion), fluid deficit, vagal stimulation, and postural hypotension.

Skin preparation. The skin is the body's first line of defense against infection. A break in this protective mechanism, such as a surgical incision, increases the risk of infection to the client, especially the elderly client. Preoperative skin preparation is the first step in the prevention of wound infection. The skin preparation may be embarrassing to or uncomfortable for the client if the surgical site is in a sensitive area. If able, the client should be encouraged to participate in or perform the skin preparation during a bath or shower. The surgeon may require the client to shower using povidone-iodine (Betadine) or hexachlorophene on and around the proposed surgical site before transfer to the surgical suite. No matter who performs the preparation, the client is provided with a warm, comfortable, private, and safe environment during the procedure.

The preparation is usually done the night before and/or the day of surgery. The skin preparation begins by cleaning a wide area above and below the surgical site (Fig. 18-3) with an antiseptic like povidone-iodine. This cleaning reduces contamination of and the number of microorganisms on the surgical field.

The second and controversial step in preoperative

skin preparation is the shave. Many health care practitioners believe that shaving the skin is a possible source of contamination of the surgical area and trauma to the skin around the incisional area (Association of Operating Room Nurses, 1989). Bacteria have been found in hair follicles, and shaving disrupts the normal protective mechanisms of the skin and predisposes the client to wound contamination. The Centers for Disease Control recommends that if shaving is necessary, the hair is removed by using individual disposable sterile supplies and aseptic principles immediately before the start of the surgical procedure. In light of these recommendations, shave preparations are performed in the treatment room, holding area of the operating suite, or operating room. Besides the potential for infection, the shaving of hair, especially from the head or genital area, can be emotionally upsetting to the client and regrowth of this hair can be uncomfortable.

Tubes, drains, and intravenous lines. Preparing the client for the possibility of the insertion of *tubes, drains, and intravenous lines* reduces postoperative fear. Care is taken not to scare the client while providing information about the purpose of each tube as it relates to surgery.

Tubes. The client may require an indwelling catheter (Foley's) before, during, and/or after surgery to keep the bladder empty and to provide a means of monitoring renal function. For example, clients having genitourinary, orthopedic, or major abdominal surgery may need this catheter.

The other common tube is a nasogastric tube, which may be inserted preoperatively before emergency sur-

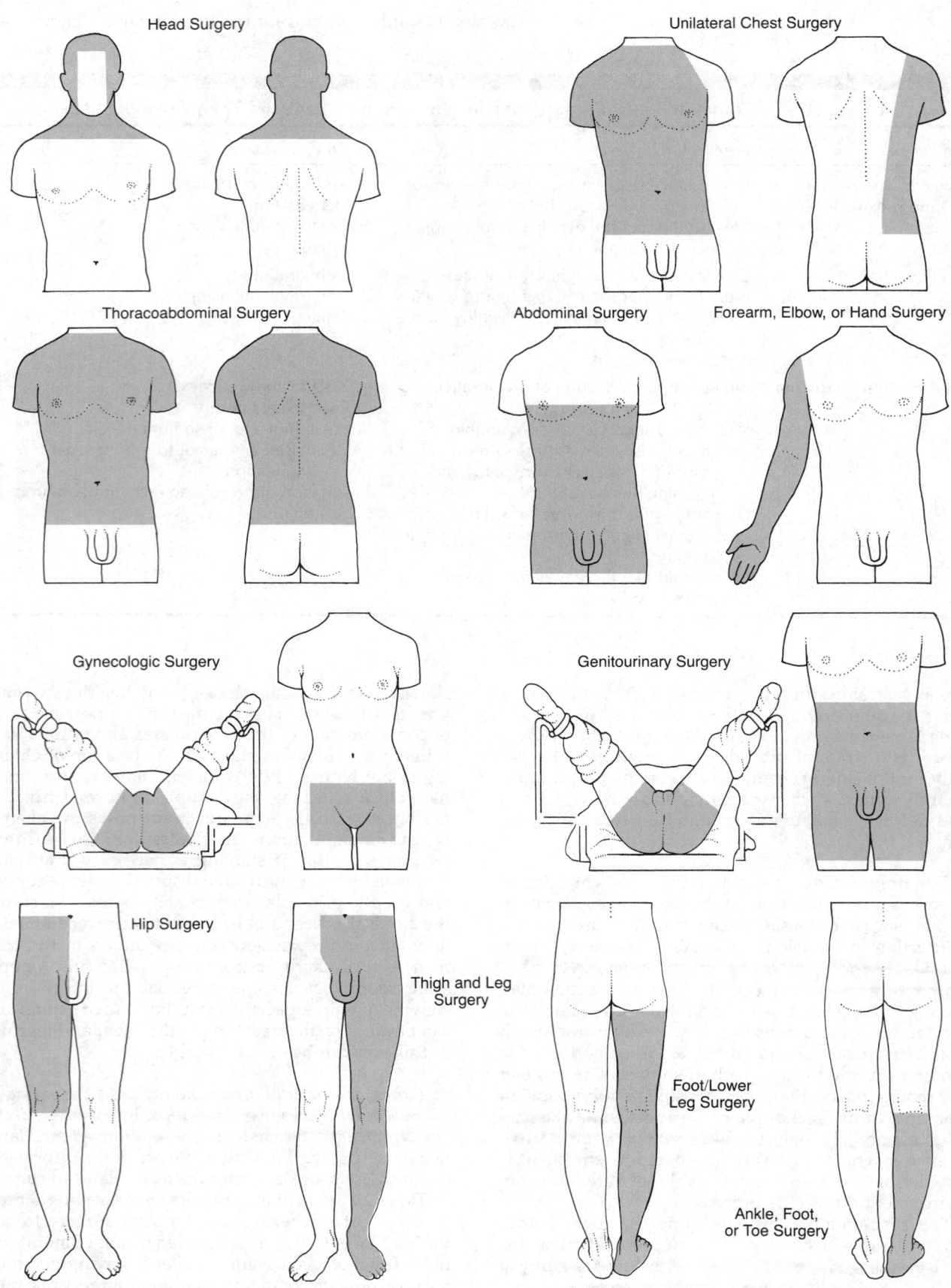

Head Surgery

Unilateral Chest Surgery

Thoracoabdominal Surgery

Abdominal Surgery

Forearm, Elbow, or Hand Surgery

Gynecologic Surgery

Genitourinary Surgery

Hip Surgery

Thigh and Leg Surgery

Foot/Lower Leg Surgery

Ankle, Foot, or Toe Surgery

Figure 18–3

Skin preparation of common surgical sites. Shaded areas indicate areas of hair removal.

gery or major abdominal surgery to decompress or empty the stomach and upper bowel. However, it is more often inserted after induction of anesthesia, when insertion is less traumatic to the client and is easier to perform (see Chap. 44 on the care and insertion of these tubes).

Drains. Drains are frequently inserted during surgery to promote the evacuation of fluid from the surgical wound. Some drains are under the dressing, whereas others are visible and require emptying. Drains come in various shapes and sizes (see Chap. 20 for a discussion and pictures of drains). The client is informed that drains are used routinely and are not painful. The client should not kink or pull on the drain.

Intravenous lines. An intravenous infusion is started for all clients receiving general anesthesia. It is started before surgery in the client's room, the holding or admission area of the surgical suite, or the operating room. The exact location depends on the individual client's need for fluid and on institutional policy.

Clients who are dehydrated, who are at risk of dehydration, or who require intravenous medication (e.g., antibiotics or corticosteroids) receive fluids before surgery. Elderly clients are more prone to dehydration because their fluid reserves are lower than those of a young or middle-aged adult.

The intravenous infusion is usually started in the arm or posterior aspect of the hand. The purpose of the infusion is to administer needed medication and fluids before, during, and after surgery. The intravenous access is usually retained for clients having any major surgical procedure. Special monitoring is required for the elderly and cardiac client with an intravenous catheter (see Chap. 13 for information on intravenous therapy).

Postoperative exercises and procedures. Instructing the client and family preoperatively about postoperative exercises and procedures reduces apprehension, increases cooperation and participation in postoperative care, and decreases the incidence and severity of postoperative complications. Discussion, demonstration, and practice aid in the performance of leg and arm exercises during the recovery phase. Along with exercises during the postoperative period, the client is often helped into a chair and/or ambulated the evening after the surgery or the next day depending on the type of surgery and the physician's preference. If clients must remain in bed, it is important for them to turn, cough, and deep breathe every 2 hours.

Diaphragmatic breathing. In *deep,* or diaphragmatic, *breathing,* the diaphragm flattens during inspiration and results in the enlargement of the upper abdominal cavity. During expiration, the abdominal muscles and diaphragm contract, which completely expands the lungs. After the nurse demonstrates and explains the technique, the client is encouraged to practice the five steps of deep breathing, which are given in the accompanying Guidelines feature. For clients with chronic obstructive pulmonary disease or limited upper chest expansion, as seen in the elderly as a result of the aging process, expansion breathing exercises (see Guidelines feature) are

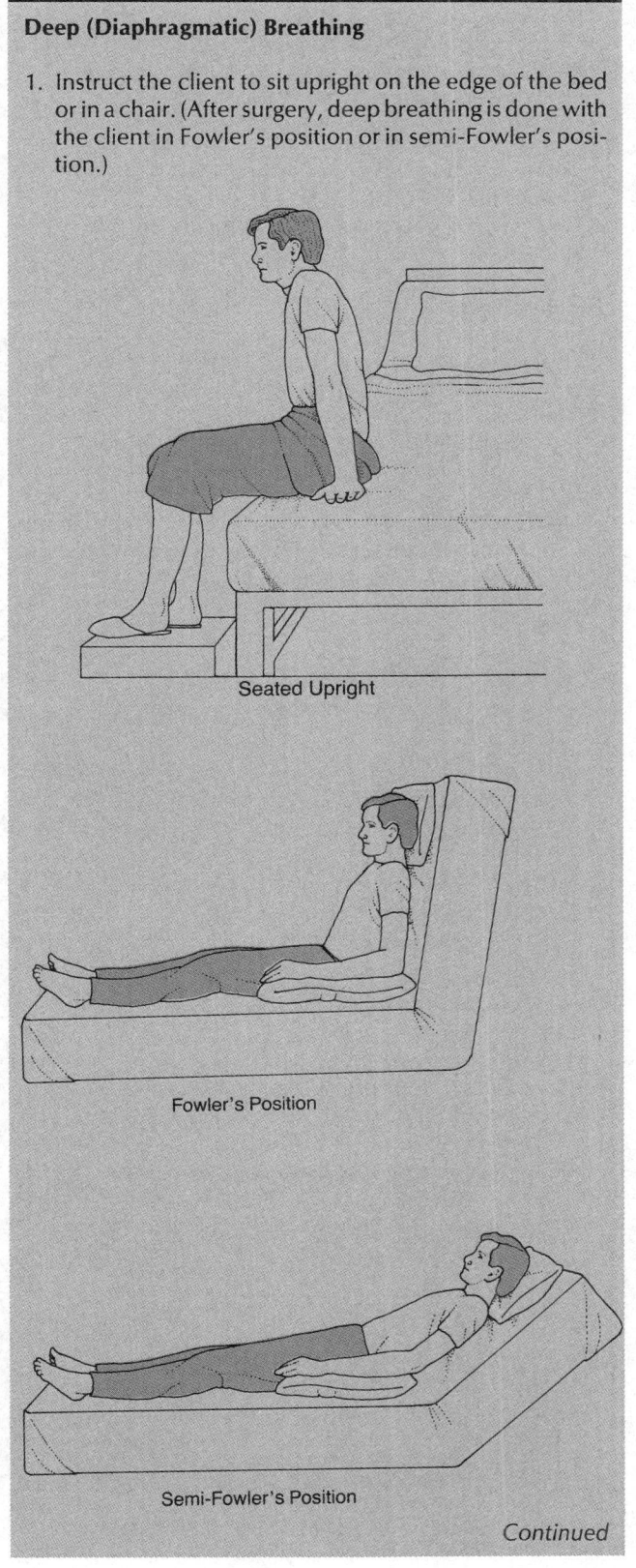

GUIDELINES ■ Perioperative Respiratory Care

Deep (Diaphragmatic) Breathing

1. Instruct the client to sit upright on the edge of the bed or in a chair. (After surgery, deep breathing is done with the client in Fowler's position or in semi-Fowler's position.)

Seated Upright

Fowler's Position

Semi-Fowler's Position

Continued

GUIDELINES ■ Perioperative Respiratory Care *Continued*

2. Instruct the client to take a gentle breath through the mouth.
3. Instruct the client to breathe out gently and completely.
4. Instruct the client to take a deep breath through the nose and mouth. The client holds this breath to the count of 5.
5. Instruct the client to exhale through the nose and mouth.

Expansion Breathing

1. Place the client in a comfortable upright position, with the client's knees slightly bent. (Bending the knees decreases tension on the abdominal muscles and decreases respiratory resistance and discomfort.)
2. Have the client place his or her hands on each side of the lower rib cage, just above the waist.
3. Instruct the client to take a deep breath through the nose, using the shoulder muscles to expand the lower rib cage outward during inhalation.

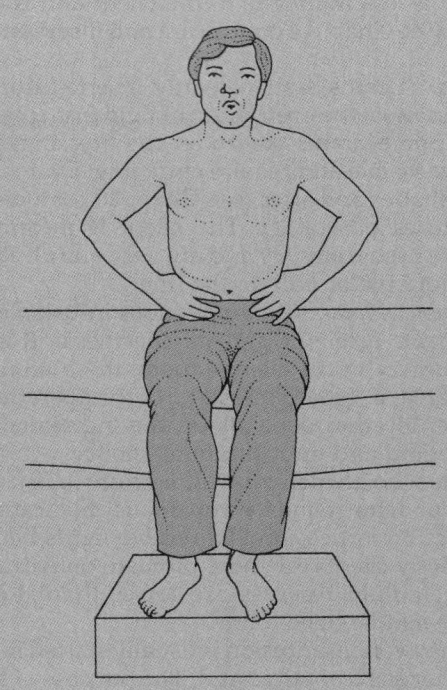

Splinting of Surgical Site and Coughing

1. Place a pillow, towel, or folded blanket over the surgical area and have the client hold it firmly in place.

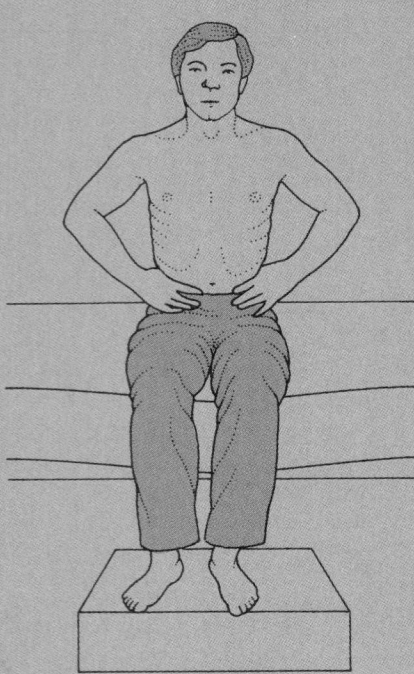

4. Instruct the client to exhale and to concentrate on the inward movement of first the chest and then the lower ribs while gently squeezing the rib cage and forcing air out of the base of the lungs.

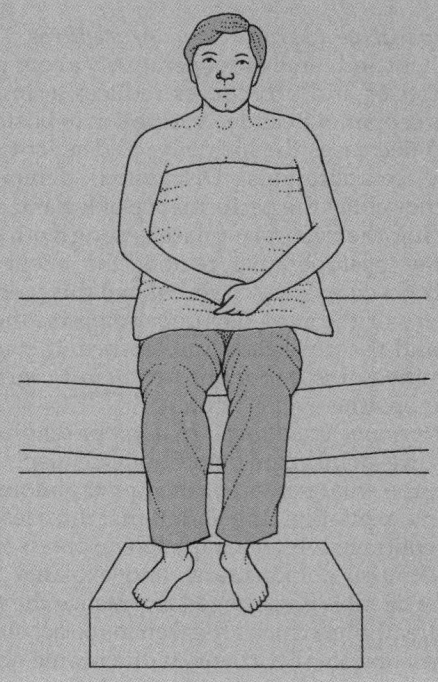

GUIDELINES ■ Perioperative Respiratory Care *Continued*

2. Have the client stimulate the cough reflex by taking three slow, deep breaths.
3. Instruct the client to inhale through the nose and exhale through the mouth.
4. On the third deep breath, instruct the client to cough to clear secretions from the lungs.

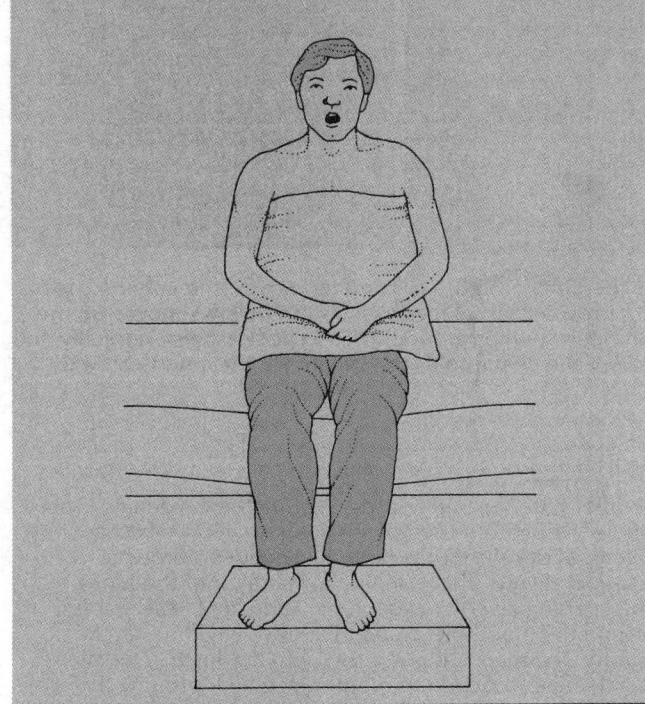

useful. If the client is scheduled for thoracic surgery, these exercises strengthen the accessory muscles preoperatively. Expansion breathing is used postoperatively during postural drainage, percussion, and vibration to loosen secretions and maintain adequate air exchange. For example, the client who has a lung lobectomy can use expansion exercises to strengthen the affected area. Regardless of which type of breathing is used, the nurse emphasizes the need to begin exercises early in the recovery phase and to continue them 5 to 10 times every 1 to 2 hours after surgery for at least the first 48 hours.

Incentive spirometry. *Incentive spirometry* and *intermittent positive-pressure breathing* are two other ways to encourage the client to take deep breaths. The purpose for both is to promote complete lung expansion and to prevent respiratory complications. Two types of incentive spirometers are commonly used in hospitals and surgical centers, as shown in Figure 18–4. The underlying principles are the same for both. The client must be able to inhale spontaneously and hold the breath for 5 seconds to achieve effective lung expansion. Visualization in the form of seeing a light move up a column or a

bellows expand often serves as a reinforcement and motivation for the client to continue performance.

In contrast, the intermittent positive-pressure breathing machine is used for a client who is unable to or refuses to voluntarily take a deep breath. The machine sends humidified air into the client's mouth and forces the lungs to expand for 3 to 5 seconds before the pressure is released (Fig. 18–5).

Coughing and splinting the surgical wound. Coughing is performed in conjunction with deep breathing every 1 to 2 hours postoperatively. The purposes of coughing are to promote expectoration of secretions, keep the lungs clear, allow full aeration, and prevent pneumonia and atelectasis. Coughing may be uncomfortable for the client, but when performed correctly it does not harm the surgical area. The proper technique for coughing and splinting the incisional site is given in the Guidelines feature. *Splinting,* or holding the incisional area, provides support and a feeling of security and reduces pain during coughing. Preoperative instruction and practice reduce postoperative fears of coughing and respiratory complications. If coughing is contraindicated for a client, the physician should write a "do not cough" order.

Turning and leg exercises. Antiembolism stockings (TED or Jobst hose) or elastic (Ace) bandages on the lower limbs are used preoperatively and postoperatively in combination with exercises to help prevent circulatory stasis, which could lead to thrombophlebitis or embolus formation. The client should be turned or should be reminded to turn every 2 hours after surgery while confined to bed. To aid the client in participating in this activity, the nurse teaches the client how to use side rails safely for turning and to protect the surgical wound when turning. Special attention is paid to aligning the body and supporting joints and extremities in elderly or disabled clients. Mobility soon after surgery stimulates gastrointestinal function by promoting postoperative flatus, and respiratory function is facilitated through mobilization of secretions.

Postoperative exercises may not be necessary for all clients, especially the outpatient who is ambulating at home within several hours of surgery. However, the client who is weak or debilitated, has had extensive surgery, or is restricted to bed is at increased risk of developing complications and needs to exercise. The tightening and relaxing of muscles or isometric exercises promote venous circulation and prevent venous stasis, which can contribute to thrombophlebitis. The Guidelines feature on page 447 describes how to perform these exercises. In addition, passive or active range-of-motion exercises to prevent rigidity of joints are appropriate postoperative exercises. The client should do these exercises three to five times each, three to four times a day while bedridden. Guidelines for range-of-motion exercises are found in Chapter 22.

Anxiety; Fear

Planning: client goals. The two goals for clients having these nursing diagnoses are that the client will (1)

Figure 18–4

Respiratory assistive devices for lung expansion. *A*, Volume incentive spirometer. It is a lightweight machine that provides feedback to the client and encourages effective deep breathing. Some of these devices are battery powered; others operate on electric current. The machine is set at a volume goal ranging from 125 to 500 mL. The range determines the expansion volume that is required to trigger the machine to reward the client with a point for a successful deep breath. The client places the mouthpiece in the mouth, forming a tight seal, and then exhales normally. After a normal exhalation, the client takes a deep breath and observes the lights on the spirometer as the lungs expand. When the goal is met, the client holds the breath for the count of 5 and exhales. *B*, Volume or flow incentive spirometer. It is lightweight, portable, and disposable. As the bellows in the spirometer moves, the volume can be measured. However, no volume can be set. This type of spirometer provides visual feedback as the bellows moves up the column. The client places the mouthpiece in the mouth and tightly seals the lips around it. The client exhales normally and then takes a deep breath. When the bellows no longer moves upward, the client holds the breath for the count of 5 and then exhales.

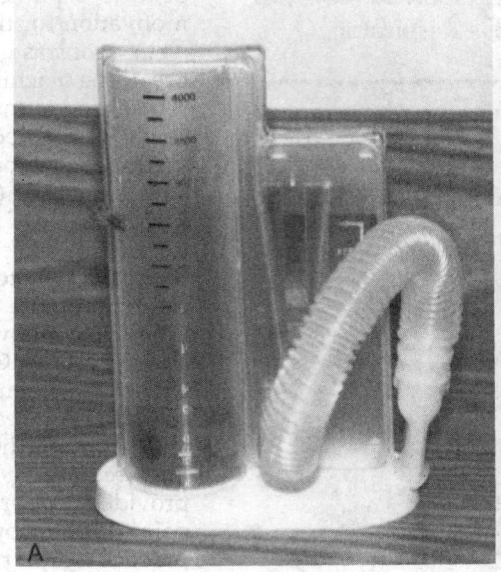
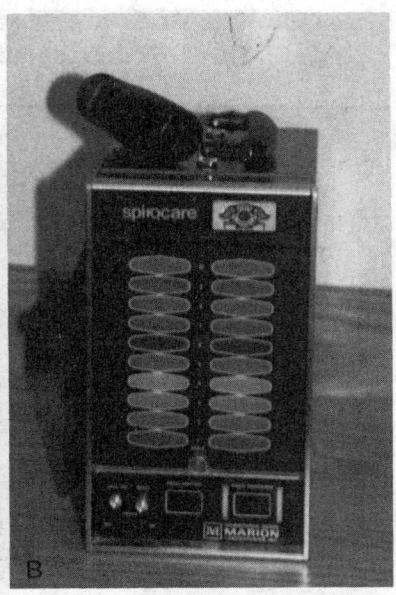

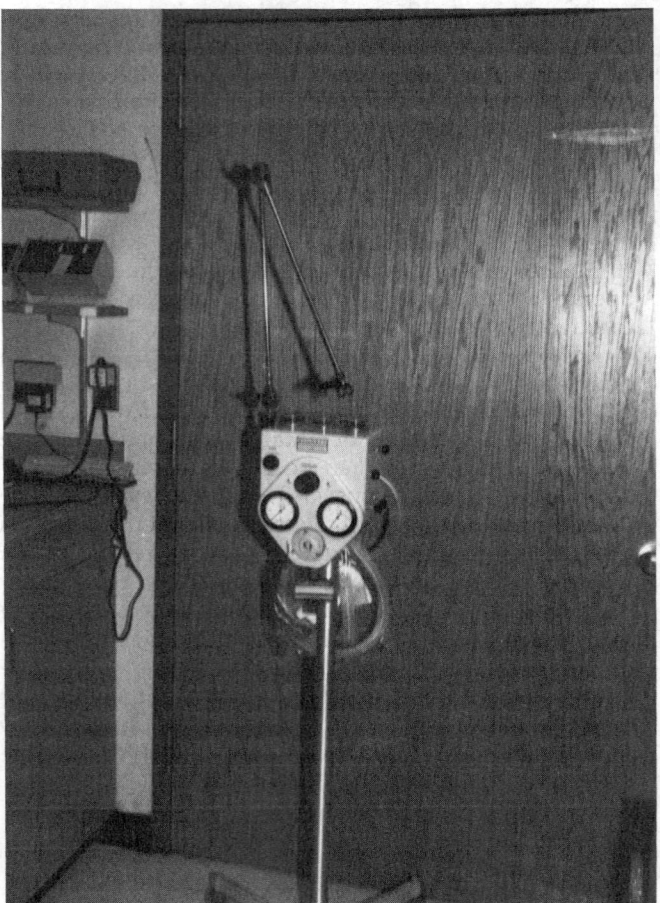

Figure 18–5

An intermittent positive-pressure breathing machine. This type of respiratory therapy is used for clients who are unable to or refuse to voluntarily take deep breaths postoperatively. This machine forces air into the lungs, thus causing alveolar expansion. The client seals the lips around the mouthpiece and inhales slowly through the mouth. The machine pushes air into the lungs. The client then exhales around the mouthpiece by loosening the seal.

GUIDELINES ■ Postoperative Leg Exercises

1. Have the client lie in semi-Fowler's position when performing leg exercises to improve peripheral circulation, prevent thrombus formation, and strengthen muscles.
2. Instruct the client to bend the knee, raise the foot, and hold this position for a few seconds. The client then extends the leg and lowers it to the bed. The client should repeat this sequence five times with each leg.

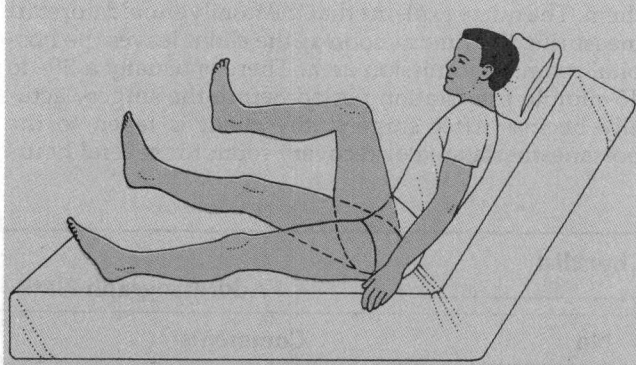

3. Instruct the client to extend the foot toward the bottom of the bed, then flex it toward the face. The client should repeat this exercise several times.

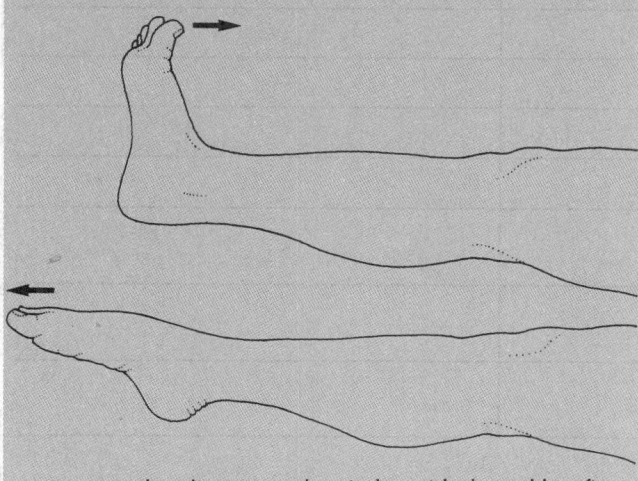

4. Instruct the client to make circles with the ankles, first to the left, then to the right. The client should repeat this exercise several times.

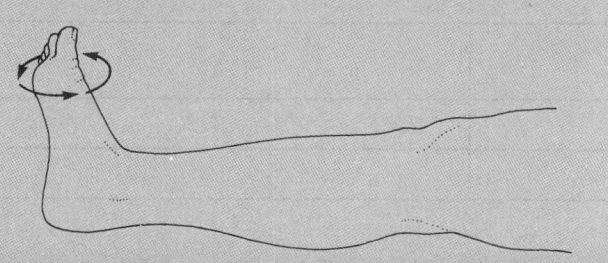

relate decreased preoperative anxiety and (2) demonstrate evidence of relaxation when at rest.

Interventions. Preoperative anxiety frequently causes the client to exhibit physical symptoms such as restlessness and sleeplessness. The surgical client perceives the perioperative experience as a threat to biopsychosocial integrity. Preoperative education, communication, and sedation help to reduce the anxiety and subsequent complications.

Preoperative teaching. The nurse assesses the client's learning level and previous knowledge related to the surgical procedure and experience. Factual information is provided to promote the client's understanding. The client can thus identify and cope with preoperative and postoperative expectations that he or she and the health care team have. Research has found that an informed, educated client is less anxious, as documented by a pen and pencil test and lower preoperative systolic blood pressure measurement (Spunt, 1983). The informed client is able to maintain self-control and is thus less anxious. The increase in same-day surgery and outpatient surgery has added a new challenge for the nurse related to educating this population. Preoperative teaching for this population can be delivered in many ways: the nurse in the physician's office may teach the client, pamphlets and written instructions may be sent to the client, and the client may be taught at the time of presurgical testing and on the day of surgery.

Communication. Verbalization of feelings, fears, and concerns is an appropriate way to reduce anxiety. The client is encouraged to show feelings freely without fear of ridicule or judgment. Clients are often uneasy about sharing personal feelings with a stranger, so the nurse must develop a trusting relationship with the client. To help the client begin, the nurse asks open-ended questions concerning feelings about the perioperative experience. As a result of the communication process, the nurse can clarify information, answer questions, and allay some of the client's apprehensions about surgery.

Rest. The stress and anxiety of impending surgery frequently interfere with the client's ability to rest and sleep the night before surgery. The perioperative experience is physically and emotionally stressful. To assist the client in relaxing, the nurse determines what the client usually does to help relax and fall asleep. Some clients enjoy reading, walking, a warm bath, or a warm drink. If permitted and able, the client is encouraged to continue these methods of relaxation. A back rub is a relaxing and therapeutic measure that should be offered to all clients. A sedative may be prescribed to ensure that the client is well rested for surgery. The nurse encourages but does not force the client to take the sedative. If the client refuses, he or she is informed that the sedative is available anytime before midnight.

Family Education

During the perioperative period, the family is kept informed about and is encouraged to assist in the client's care. The family's readiness and desire to be an active part of the health care team are assessed when the client is admitted to the hospital. A positive sign of interest is asking questions about the perioperative experience. Once the family members' readiness is determined, they are encouraged to participate in all aspects of preoperative education with the client. The inclusion of the family provides support for the client, and information for the family helps to reduce anxiety. Family members participate in discussions and practice sessions; they are not allowed to dominate the discussion. The nurse elicits the client's participation by asking direct questions. The family practices postoperative exercises with the client and encourages practice after the session with the nurse. The nurse emphasizes the important role of the family preoperatively. The family is a valuable asset to the client and health care team by reminding and motivating the client to turn, cough, and deep breathe.

The nurse informs the family of the scheduled time for surgery and of any changes. The family is encouraged to visit the client at least 1 hour before the scheduled time. The nurse reminds the family that the client may be anxious and has received preoperative sedation. The preoperative visit is usually short and limited to family only.

Most families are anxious about their loved one having surgery. To aid in reducing anxiety, the nurse explains the intraoperative and postoperative routine to them. The nurse explains that the family should not start measuring the time as soon as the client leaves the hospital room or admission area. There is usually a 30- to 45-minute preparation period before the surgery actually begins. After surgery, the client is taken to the postanesthesia area or recovery room for several hours

Preoperative Checklist			
Allergies: Date of Surgery _____			Addressograph Plate
CLINICAL DATA:	**Yes**	**No**	**Comments**
Authorization for surgical treatment completed			
Height and weight charted			
History and physical			
Chest x-ray			
ECG report			
Urine report			
Blood sugar within acceptable range (50–300 mg/dL)			
Hematocrit within acceptable range (30–50 mL/dL)			
Potassium within acceptable range (3.5–6 mEq/L)			
Unacceptable test results reported to Dr. Time By			
CLIENT PREPARATION:	**Yes**	**No**	**Comments**
Jewelry removed			
Hairpiece, wig, hairpins, barrettes, beads, rubber bands removed			
Loose teeth or caps noted			
Dentures removed			

Figure 18–6

One example of a preoperative checklist. (Courtesy of Baltimore County General Hospital, Randallstown, MD.)

before returning to the room or discharge area. The family is instructed by the nurse about the best place to wait for the client, according to institutional policy and the physician's preference.

Client Transfer to the Surgical Suite

Immediate preoperative preparation involves the review and update of the client's chart, reinforcement of preoperative teaching, assurance that the client is appropriately dressed for surgery, and administration of preoperative medication. The nurse uses a preoperative checklist to assist in the smooth, efficient transfer of the client to the surgical suite (Fig. 18–6).

Chart Review

The chart is reviewed to ensure that all documentation, preoperative procedures, and orders are completed. The surgical permit or informed consent form is checked to see that it is signed and dated, and contains the witness's signature. Height and weight must be on the chart; the accuracy of this information is important for the proper calculation of anesthetic. The results of all laboratory, radiographic, and diagnostic tests are on the chart, and any abnormal results are documented and reported to the physician and/or anesthesiologist. The nurse takes and records a current set of vital signs, and any significant physical or psychosocial observations are documented. Special needs and concerns of the

---

Preoperative Checklist *Continued*

Allergies: _____ Date of Surgery _____ Addressograph Plate

CLINICAL DATA:	Yes	No	Comments
Artificial eye, contact lenses, glasses removed			
Any prosthetic appliance removed			
Voided or catheterized—I&O sheet on chart			
Identification bracelet in place			
Parenteral fluids patent and infusing at ___ mL/h			
B/P, T.P.R. charted			
Premedication given as ordered			
Side rails up—care data and care plan on chart			

COMMUNICATION ASSESSMENT:	Normal	Abnormal	Comments
Vision			
Hearing			
Mental			
Speech			
Other			
Client's preferred name:			

NURSE TO NURSE REFERRAL

Limb for burial _____ Yes _____ No   at _____ Funeral home

Figure 18–6 *Continued*

client should be shared with the surgical team through documentation, such as if the client is a member of Jehovah's Witnesses and does not accept blood products. This information and the care plan assist the surgical team in providing continuity of care while the client is in the surgical area.

Client Preparation

Hospitals and most surgical centers require that the client remove all clothing, including underwear, and wear a hospital gown into the operating room. Antiembolism stockings or Ace bandages are applied at this time, if ordered by the surgeon, and are used for clients at risk of developing postoperative vascular complications such as thrombophlebitis. The gown prevents the possible introduction of contaminants and provides easy access to the operative area. The client's valuables, including jewelry, money, and clothes, are locked in a safe place, according to the facility's policy. Wedding rings and rings that cannot be removed are taped in place by the nurse and noted on the preoperative checklist. The tape prevents the ring from falling off or becoming damaged during the perioperative period. Religious emblems may be pinned or securely fastened to the client's gown; in some facilities paper emblems are available from a religious leader. The client wears an identification band that clearly gives first and last names, which helps to identify the sedated client.

Dentures, including partial dental plates, are removed and placed in a labeled denture cup. The removal of dentures is a safety measure to prevent aspiration and obstruction of the airway. All prosthetic devices, such as artificial eyes and limbs, are removed and safely stored. Some facilities allow hearing aids in the surgical suite to facilitate communication before and after surgery. If the client is sent to surgery with the hearing aid, the nurse communicates this to the surgical nurse to prevent accidental loss or damage to the aid. Hairpins and clips, if not removed, can conduct electrical current used during surgery and cause scalp burns. Wigs and toupees are removed to prevent loss of the item or injury to the client's scalp during surgery. The need for removal of fingernail polish is controversial; the policy of the facility is followed in this regard (Atkinson & Kohn, 1986). Removal of polish permits assessment of the nail bed color as an indicator of oxygenation and circulation during surgery.

Once the client is prepared for surgery, the nurse asks the client to empty his or her bladder to prevent incontinence or overdistention, which may prevent exposure of the surgical site. Measurement of vital signs is the final procedure to be performed before the administration of preoperative medication and transfer of the client to the surgical suite.

Preoperative Medication

Preoperative medication may be ordered for clients receiving general intravenous, spinal, or inhalation anesthesia during surgery. Preoperative medication may be omitted or the dosage decreased if the client is to receive balanced anesthesia intraoperatively. Preoperative medication reduces anxiety, promotes relaxation, reduces pharyngeal secretions, inhibits gastric secretions, and decreases the amount of anesthetic that is required for induction and maintenance of anesthesia. The selection of medication is based on the client's age, physical and psychologic condition, medical history, medications taken routinely, results of preoperative tests, height and weight, and type and extensiveness of the surgical procedure. If more than one response is required, combination therapy is usually ordered. A typical combination consists of a sedative or tranquilizer, narcotic, and anticholinergic. Table 18–7 gives important information about several common drugs of each category.

The medication is usually administered intramuscularly 1 hour before the scheduled surgical time or when the client is "on call" to the surgical suite. After administration, the nurse raises the side rails of the bed or stretcher, places the call system in easy reach while reminding the client not to get out of bed, and places the bed in a low position. The client becomes drowsy but can be easily aroused. Research has shown that without psychologic preparation (in the form of education), the client may become drowsy but remain anxious, which defeats the primary purpose of the preoperative medication (Bartlett, 1985).

Transfer

Most clients are transferred to the surgical suite on a stretcher with the side rails up. In special circumstances, the client is transferred in bed, for example, clients requiring traction; those having major vascular, thoracic, abdominal, or orthopedic surgery; and those who should be moved as little as possible immediately after surgery. Other factors that influence the nurse's decision to transfer the client in a bed are the client's age, size, and condition. The client, along with the signed consent form, completed preoperative checklist, and chart are transported to the surgical suite.

Evaluation

The nurse evaluates the care of the preoperative client according to the identified nursing diagnoses. The expected outcomes for the client in the preoperative phase of the perioperative experience include that the client

1. Verbalizes understanding of informed consent as it applies to surgery
2. States an understanding of the preoperative dietary restriction
3. Verbalizes understanding of and reason for bowel preparation
4. States the purpose of skin preparation

TABLE 18–7   Common Preoperative Medications

Drug	Usual Preoperative Dosage*	Interventions	Rationales
Sedatives and Hypnotics			
Pentobarbital sodium (Nembutal Sodium)	50–200 mg PO	1. Monitor respiratory status.	1. Sedatives and hypnotics cause respiratory depression.
Secobarbital sodium (Seconal Sodium)	200–300 mg PO	2. Monitor level of anxiety; encourage verbalization and relaxation.	2. Reduced anxiety and fear increase effectiveness of medication and lower the amount of anesthesia needed.
Chloral hydrate	0.5–1.0 g PO		
Tranquilizers			
Chloropromazine hydrochloride (Thorazine)	25–50 mg PO 12.5–25 mg IM	1. Maintain NPO status and assess for gastrointestinal upset or nausea.	1. NPO status prevents postoperative nausea, decreases intra- and postoperative vomiting, and reduces need for postoperative antiemetics.
Hydroxyzine hydrochloride (Vistaril)	50–100 mg PO 25–100 mg IM		
Diazepam (Valium)	5–10 mg PO/IM		
Promethazine hydrochloride (Phenergan)	50 mg PO 25–50 mg IM	2. Promote relaxation by dimming lights and instructing client on the importance of relaxation.	2. Relaxation allows easier intubation and visualization of surgical wound.
Narcotics (Opiates)			
Meperidine hydrochloride (Demerol)	50–100 mg IM/SC	1. Give deep intramuscular injection with 1- or 1½-in needle.	1. Narcotics can be irritating to subcutaneous tissue, and deep injection provides increased effectiveness.
Morphine sulfate	5–15 mg IM/SC		
Hydromorphone hydrochloride (Dilaudid)	2–4 mg PO/IM	2. Monitor blood pressure and respiratory status.	2. Narcotics cause respiratory and circulatory depression. Reduced doses may be used in elderly or debilitated clients.
Anticholinergics			
Atropine sulfate	0.4–0.6 mg PO/SC/IM/IV	1. Monitor blood pressure and heart rate.	1. Palpitation or bradycardia can occur with low doses; tachycardia can occur with higher doses.
Glycopyrrolate (Robinul)	0.002 mg/lb (0.004 mg/kg) of body weight IM		
Scopolamine (hyoscine)	0.3–0.6 mg/IM/SC	2. Monitor hydration and maintain NPO status.	2. Anticholinergics inhibit secretions before and during surgery, which could cause aspiration, nausea, and vomiting postoperatively.

* PO, by mouth; IM, intramuscularly; SC, subcutaneously; IV, intravenously.

5. Verbalizes understanding of potential tubes, drains, and intravenous catheters used during the perioperative experience
6. Demonstrates postoperative exercises: turning, deep breathing, splinting, coughing, and isometric exercises
7. Demonstrates use of incentive spirometer
8. Describes methods to decrease preoperative anxiety
9. States rationale for rest and ways to promote rest preoperatively

By meeting the stated desired outcomes, the likelihood of a complication-free perioperative experience is increased. As a result, anxiety and fears are diminished.

SUMMARY

The preoperative period begins when the client is scheduled for surgery and ends at the time of transfer to the surgical suite. During this phase of the perioperative experience, the nurse obtains the client's history through interview and performs a physical assessment; data are collected to form a comprehensive data base. On the basis of the collected data, the nurse identifies nursing diagnoses appropriate for the client and formulates a plan of care that is directly related to the needs of the client. Preoperative care consists primarily of client and family education that is directed at reduction of anxiety and of reduction of postoperative complications while increasing client cooperation in postoperative procedures.

IMPLICATIONS FOR RESEARCH

Changing trends, government mandates, increased average age of the population, and increased consumer awareness are providing nurses with new challenges. Questions regarding these topics need investigation by nurses. Improving the modalities of reducing anxiety, increasing cost-effectiveness without sacrificing client care, and increasing awareness of the special needs of the elderly are areas requiring research and interventions to improve client care. The following nursing research questions are appropriate to investigate when considering the needs of the client during the preoperative period:

1. Is there a difference between the anxiety level of clients admitted on the day before surgery, on the day of surgery, and to an ambulatory surgical center?

2. What effects do diagnosis-related groups have on the frequency and severity of postoperative complications on the inpatient and outpatient surgical client?
3. Do age, sex, socioeconomic status, occupation, and educational preparation affect the client's preoperative anxiety?
4. What effect does preoperative education have on length of postoperative stay in the hospital?

REFERENCES AND READINGS

Alexander, J. W. (1983). The influence of hair-removal methods on wound infection. *Archives of Surgery, 118,* 347.

Alverson, E. (1987). The preoperative interview: Its effect on perioperative nurses' empathy. *AORN Journal, 45,* 1150–1159, 1162–1164.

Association of Operating Room Nurses. (1989). *Standards of nursing practice.* Denver: Author.

Atkinson, L. J., & Kohn, M. L. (1986). *Berry and Kohn's introduction to operating room techniques.* New York: McGraw-Hill.

Blackwood, S. (1986). Back to basics: The preop exam. *American Journal of Nursing, 86,* 39–44.

Bray, C. A. (1986). Postop pain: Altering the patients' experience through education. *AORN Journal, 43,* 672, 674–675, 677.

Brent, N. J. (1987). How informed are you about consents? *Nursing Life, 6,* 37–39.

Brock, A. M. (1984). How do the aged cope with surgery? *Today's OR Nurse, 6*(9), 16, 20–22, 25.

Cerrato, P. L. (1985). Is your patient really ready for surgery? *RN, 48*(6), 69–70.

Crawford, F. J. (1985). Ambulatory surgery: The elderly patient. *AORN Journal, 41,* 356–359.

Devine, E., & Cook, T. (1983). A meta-analytic analysis of effects of psychoeducational interventions on length of postsurgical hospital stay. *Nursing Research, 32,* 267–274.

Does pre-op medication promote stress? (1984). *American Journal of Nursing, 84,* 1202.

Domar, A., Noe, J., & Benson, H. (1987). The preoperative use of the relaxation response with ambulatory surgery patients. *Journal of Human Stress, 13,* 101–107.

Evaluating the usefulness of routine preoperative tests. (1987). *AORN Journal, 45,* 696.

Fraulini, K. E. (1983). Coping mechanisms and recovery from surgery. *AORN Journal, 37,* 1198.

Gamino, L. A., Hunter, R. B., & Brandon, R. A. (1985). Psychiatric complications associated with geriatric surgery. *Geriatric Clinics of North America, 1,* 417–422.

Gorton, D. (1987a). Holistic health techniques to increase individual coping and wellness. *Perioperative Nursing Quarterly, 3*(3), 41–50.

Gorton, D. (1987b). Preoperative teaching for surgical patients. *Perioperative Nursing Quarterly, 3*(2), 8–13.

Goulart, A. E. (1987). Preoperative teaching for surgical patients. *Perioperative Nursing Quarterly, 3*(2), 8–13.

Gruendenemann, B. J., & Meeker, M. H. (1987). *Alexander's care of the patient in surgery.* St. Louis: C. V. Mosby.

Hamer, B. A. (1985). Managing OR patients' fears. *Today's OR Nurse, 7*(5), 28–30.

Hathaway, D. (1986). Effects of preoperative instruction on postop outcomes: A meta-analysis. *Nursing Research, 35,* 269–275.

Iscenheur, M. L. (1988). Quality of interpersonal care: A study of ambulatory surgery patient's perspective. *AORN Journal, 47,* 1414–1419.

Jackson, M. F. (1988). High risk surgical patients. *Journal of Gerontological Nursing, 14,* 8–15.

Jennings, B. M., & Sherman, R. A. (1987). Anxiety, locus of control, and satisfaction in patients undergoing ambulatory surgery. *Military Medicine, 152,* 206–208.

Johnson, J. (1984). Coping with elective surgery. *Annual Review of Nursing Research, 2,* 107–132.

Kapnoullas, J. (1988). Nursing interventions for relief of preoperative anxiety. *Australian Journal of Advanced Nursing, 5*(2), 8–15.

Kathal, D. K. (1984). Anxiety in surgical patients' families. *AORN Journal, 40,* 131.

Kempe, A. R. (1987). Patient education for the ambulatory surgery patient. *AORN Journal, 45,* 500–507.

Kempe, A. R., & Gelazis, R. (1985). Patient anxiety levels: An ambulatory surgery study. *AORN Journal, 41,* 390–396.

Kneedler, J. A., & Dodge, G. H. (1983). *Perioperative patient care: The nursing perspective.* Boston: Blackwell Scientific.

Knight, C. G., & Donnelly, M. K. (1988). Assessing the preoperative adult. *Nurse Practitioner, 13,* 6, 8, 13.

Kosik, S. L., & Reynolds, P. J. (1986). A nursing contribution to cost containment: A group preoperative teaching program that shortens hospital stay. *Journal of Nursing Staff Development, 2,* 18–22.

Levesque, L., Grenier, R., Kerovac, S., & Reidy, M. (1984). Evaluation of a presurgical program given at two different times. *Research in Nursing, 7,* 227–336.

Lindeman, C. A. (1988). Patient education. *Annual Review of Nursing Research, 6,* 29–60.

Luczun, M. E. (1987). Reviewing the literature: A treasure hunt . . . pre and postoperative visits do contribute to patient satisfaction. *Journal of Post Anesthesia Nursing, 2,* 120–122.

Meckes, P. F. (1984). Perioperative care of the elderly patient. *Today's OR Nurse, 6*(9), 8–11, 14–15.

A model for perioperative nursing practice. (1985). *AORN Journal, 41,* 188–194.

Nyamathi, A., & Kashiwabara, A. (1988). Preoperative anxiety: Its effects on cognitive thinking. *AORN Journal, 47,* 164–170.

Poland, V. (1985). Ambulatory surgery: Freestanding centers look beyond the early years. *AORN Journal, 42,* 105–108.

Pomorski, M. E. (1983). Surgical care for the aged patient: The decision-making process. *Nursing Clinics of North America, 18,* 365–372.

Preoperative education can cut LOS and cost, aid PPs delivery. (1985). *Hospitals, 59*(4), 78, 80, 82.

Rothrock, J. C. (1989). Perioperative nursing research. Part I. Preoperative psychoeducational interventions. *AORN Journal, 49,* 597–614.

Smallwood, S. B. (1988). Preparing children for surgery. Learning through play. *AORN Journal, 47,* 177–185.

Spearing, C., & Cornell, D. J. (1988). Incentive spirometry: Inspiring your patients to breathe deeply. *Nursing '88, 17*(9), 50–51.

Spunt, D. L. (1983). *How preoperative teaching affects patient's level of anxiety.* Unpublished master's thesis, University of Maryland, College Park, MD.

Walker, M. L. (1986). Growing old: Increased surgical risks in the elderly. *AORN Journal, 43,* 887–890.

Weaver, T. E. (1981). New life for lungs . . . through incentive spirometers. *Nursing '81, 11*(2), 54–58.

Wetcher, B. V. (1987). Patient selection criteria for 1987 . . . ambulatory surgery. *AORN Journal, 45,* 30, 32, 34–36.

Wolcott, M. W. (1988). *Ambulatory surgery and the basics of surgical care* (2nd ed.). Philadelphia: J. B. Lippincott.

Worley, B. (1986). Pre-admission testing and teaching: More satisfaction. *Nurse Manager, 17*(2), 32–33.

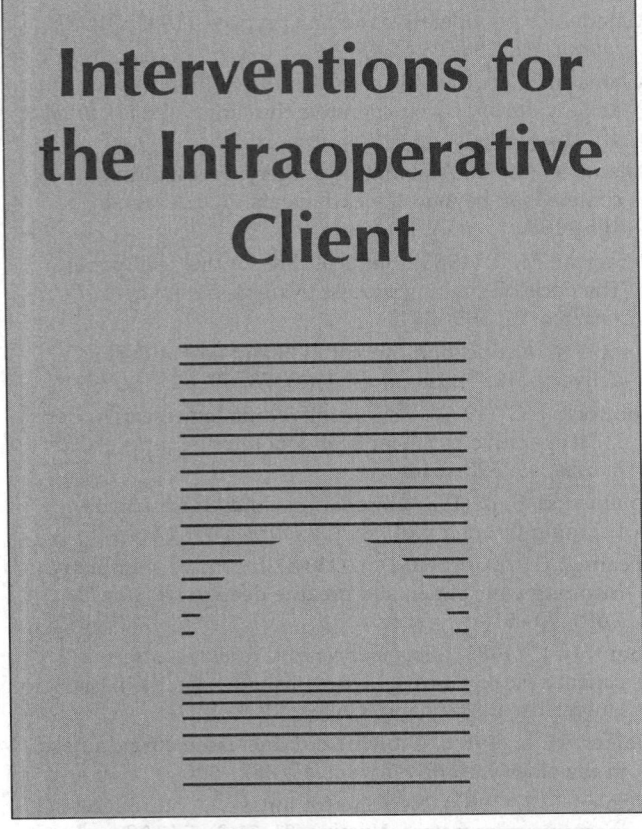

CHAPTER 19

Interventions for the Intraoperative Client

The intraoperative phase of the perioperative experience begins as the client enters the surgical suite. The circulating nurse, or operating room nurse, as a member of the surgical team, assumes the responsibility for and coordinates the client's care while the client is in the surgical suite. This is an anxious time for the client, as he/she enters a strange and threatening environment. Nursing care during the intraoperative period addresses all of the needs of the client while focusing on the client's comfort, safety, dignity, and psychologic status. Specific procedures and policies may differ among hospitals, but similarities are evident and reflect the *Standards of Nursing Practice* (Association of Operating Room Nurses [AORN], 1989).

OVERVIEW

Members of the Surgical Team

The surgical team consists of the surgeon, one or more surgical assistants, the anesthesiologist or nurse anesthetist, the circulating nurse, and the scrub nurse or the surgical technologist. The number of assistants, circulating nurses, and scrub nurses varies, depending on the complexity and projected length of the surgical procedure. Some limited, diagnostic, and outpatient procedures are considered minor and may only require a scrub nurse or a circulating nurse in addition to the surgeon.

The surgical team is headed by the senior surgeon or the surgeon who is performing the operation. The surgeon assumes complete responsibility for all medical acts and judgments regarding the client. The surgeon's assistant may be a physician, a resident, an intern, a physician's assistant, or a nurse. According to the *Standards of Nursing Practice* (AORN, 1989), in the absence of an assisting physician, a registered nurse with appropriate knowledge is the best qualified nonphysician to serve as first assistant. Under the direction of the surgeon, the assistant holds retractors and suctions the wound to provide visualization of the operative site.

The *anesthesiologist* is a physician who specializes in the administration of anesthetics. A *nurse anesthetist* is a qualified registered nurse who administers anesthetics under the direct supervision of an anesthesiologist or a surgeon. The anesthetist administers anesthetic drugs and other medication to maintain the client's physical status during the procedure. The client's vital signs and cardiopulmonary function and the administration of intravenous (IV) fluids, including blood and blood components, are monitored to maintain physiologic homeostasis.

The *circulating nurse's* role is vital to the smooth flow of events before, during, and after the operation. The circulating nurse, sets up the room, maintains the necessary supplies, checks that all equipment is safe and functional before the surgery, and positions the client and cleans the surgical field before draping. He/she meets the client on admission to the surgical suite and reviews the chart, assesses the client's physical and emotional status, provides emotional support, and orients the client to the area. During the intraoperative phase, the circulating nurse coordinates the activities in the operating room, implements the client care plan, and serves as the client's advocate. Throughout the surgery, the circulating nurse assists the anesthetist with the induction of anesthesia, monitors the traffic in the room, assesses the amount of urine and blood loss, and ensures that sterile technique is maintained by the surgical team. All medications, blood, and blood components are obtained and recorded by the circulating nurse. Before the completion of the surgical procedure, the circulating nurse completes documentation, which includes notation of drains or catheters in place, the length of surgery, and the count of all sponges, needles, and instruments. The recovery room is notified of the client's estimated time of arrival and any special needs of the client (e.g., ventilator).

When the procedure is performed under local anesthesia, the circulating nurse provides continuous emotional support and information for the client. Because the administration of local anesthesia does not require an anesthesiologist or nurse anesthetist, the nurse monitors vital signs and administers IV fluids and narcotics at the surgeon's request.

The *scrub nurse* or *the surgical technologist* is responsible for setting up and handing sterile supplies and instruments to the surgeon and the assistant. Throughout the surgical procedure, the scrub nurse maintains an accurate account of sponges, needles, and instruments. Knowledge of anatomy and physiology and familiarity with the surgical procedure allows the scrub nurse to anticipate what instruments the surgeon will need. This anticipation reduces the amount of time that the client is anesthetized.

Preparation of the Surgical Suite and Team

During the intraoperative phase, client safety is a primary concern of the nurse. Client safety is ensured by using safety straps for the client and securely locking the surgical table in place before transferring the client to or from the table. The two most important factors related to safety in the surgical suite are the operating room layout, which enables easy and quick access to the client and emergency equipment, and the prevention of infection by limiting the sources of contaminants. Other potential safety hazards may be the result of equipment defects, including the improper placement of grounding pads, or an incorrect count of equipment or sponges before, during, and after the surgical procedure.

Layout

The surgical suite should be located out of the mainstream of the hospital and adjacent to the recovery room and support services (e.g., blood bank, pathology and radiology departments, and central supply department). The flow of traffic should be such that contamination from outside the suite is minimal, and within the suite there is separation of clean and contaminated. The complications related to traffic flow can be minimized if the surgical suite is designed utilizing a four-zone plan, which includes areas designated as protective, clean, sterile, and dirty.

The size of a surgical suite is dependent on the size and surgical capabilities of the hospital. The average suite contains an admission, or preoperative holding, area; utility rooms for clean and soiled equipment; a clean linen room; a changing room; a general workroom for the cleaning and sterilizing of instruments; and a scrub area. A typical operating room contains a stretcher or operating table, a mounted ceiling light, an anesthesia station, instrument tables and stands, suction equipment, and a communication system. The exact number of tables and specialized equipment used are based on individual case needs. A reliable communication system provides the vital link between the operating room and the main desk of the surgical unit or suite. The system should include an intercom and the capability to differentiate between routine and emergency calls.

Health and Hygiene of the Surgical Team

The main sources of bacterial contamination from the surgical team are poor health and hygiene. A large number of potentially pathogenic bacteria are present on the skin and hair and in the respiratory tract of all persons. All members of the surgical team and other support personnel in the surgical suite should be free of communicable bacterial infections. Frequent washing of hands is the most effective means of controlling the spread of infection. It must be carried out by all personnel before and after client contact, even when gloves are used.

Personal hygiene aids in the control of infection. Bathing is recommended daily for all surgical suite personnel. However, because the shedding of microorganisms and skin debris is greatest immediately after showering, it is recommended that bathing be done a few hours before changing into operating room attire. Jewelry, which carries multiple microorganisms, is not permitted to be worn for personnel who are scrubbed and is encouraged to be kept to a minimum for all other surgical team members.

Surgical Attire

Surgical or scrub attire must be worn by all members of the surgical team and operating room personnel. Scrub attire is clean, not sterile, and is worn to decrease the contamination from microorganisms. It consists of a cap or hood, a mask, a pantsuit or dress, and shoe coverings (Fig. 19–1). The cap or hood is put on first to prevent hair from collecting on the attire. The hair of each member of the surgical team must be covered; this includes sideburns and facial hair, as they can also be the source of contaminants resulting in wound infection. Members of the surgical team who are not scrubbed

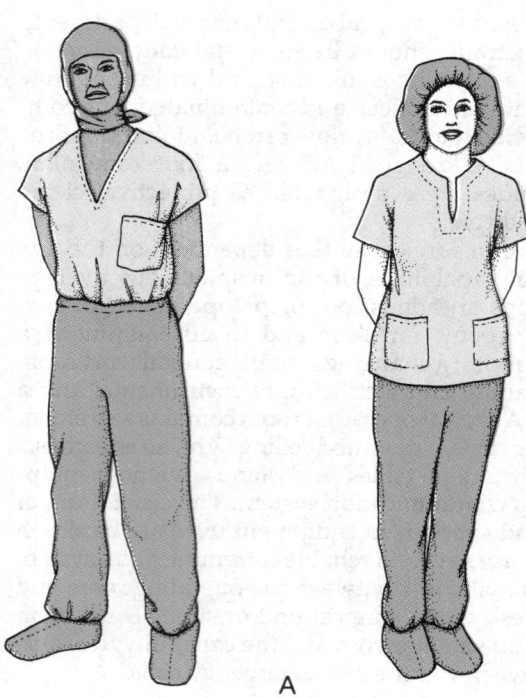

A

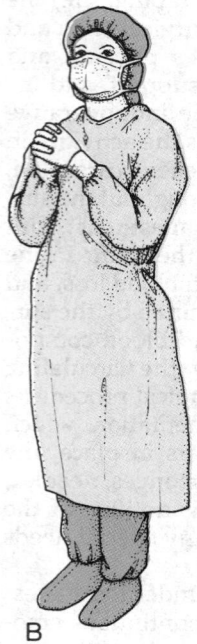

B

Figure 19–1

Proper operating room attire. *A,* Scrub tops should be tucked into pants or conform to the waist. *B,* The surgical mask should be tied securely in place, and sterile gloves should extend over the cuffs of the gown when sterile attire is worn over a scrub suit.

(e.g., anesthesiologist and circulating nurse) should wear jackets to prevent shedding from bare arms. Scrub attire should be changed daily, when it becomes wet or soiled, and when personnel leave the surgical suite without a cover gown. Shoe covers, masks, and clean attire should be changed between surgical procedures.

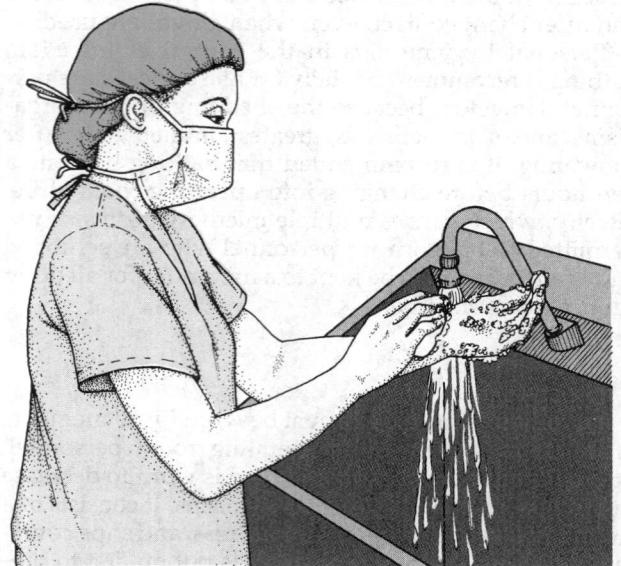

Figure 19–2

For the surgical scrub, hands are held above the level of the elbows so that contaminated water runs away from the hands.

Surgical Scrub

The surgical scrub is performed by the surgeon, all assistants, and the scrub nurse before donning (putting on) a sterile gown and gloves. The scrub does not make the hands and forearms sterile; when effectively carried out, however, it reduces the number of microorganisms. The surgical scrub is accomplished with the use of a reusable or disposable scrub brush or sponge impregnated with an antimicrobial solution, preferably iodophor (Betadine), and a nail cleaner. As with hand washing, the effectiveness of the scrub depends on the application of friction from the elbow to the fingertips. The surgical scrub takes 5 to 10 minutes, and the hands are held higher than the elbows for scrubbing and rinsing (Fig. 19–2). The hands and arms must be thoroughly dried with a sterile towel to prevent contamination of the sterile gown.

Gowns, gloves, and materials that are used within the operating room must be sterile. The sterile areas of the surgical gown are the front of the gown above the waist and 2 to 3 in distal from the elbow. Sterile drapes and equipment are handled only by properly attired members of the surgical team.

Anesthesia

The word anesthesia comes from the Greek word *anesthesis* meaning "negative sensation." Today the administration of anesthesia is an exact and sophisticated science requiring the skill of a licensed anesthesiologist or a certified nurse anesthetist. Anesthesia is an artificially induced state of partial or total loss of sensation, occurring with or without loss of consciousness. The purpose of anesthesia is to block the transmission of nerve impulses, suppress reflexes, promote muscular relaxation, and, in some cases, achieve a controlled level of unconsciousness.

The choice of anesthesia is determined primarily by the anesthesiologist on the basis of consultation with the surgeon and consideration of other specific client-related factors. The nurse or the client communicates the client's preference and fears related to a particular type of anesthesia to the anesthesiologist. Specific problems noted in the client history and the client's physical and mental status play a major role in the selection of anesthesia (as noted under the heading Assessment). Selection is also influenced by the type and duration of the procedure, the surgical site, and the client's position during the surgical procedure. The administration of anesthesia begins with the selection and administration of preoperative medication as discussed in Chapter 18.

Types of Anesthesia

The nurse needs to be cognizant of the pharmacologic characteristics of the most commonly used agents and their effects on the client during and after surgery. Anesthesia produces multiple systemic effects, which can affect the client's care and other coexisting problems. For example, most anesthetics are metabolized by the liver and excreted by the kidneys. Hepatic or renal dysfunction can significantly enhance anesthetic effects and toxicity. The state of anesthesia may be produced in a number of ways: general anesthesia, balanced anesthesia, and local or regional anesthesia (Table 19–1). Hypnoanesthesia or hypnosis (a passive trance-like state) and cryothermia (use of cold [e.g., ice] to lower the surface temperature of the surgical site, thus reducing the amount of anesthesia needed) are rarely used, and acupuncture, although commonly used in Far Eastern countries, is seldom used in the United States at this time.

General anesthesia. General anesthesia is a reversible state in which the client loses consciousness owing to the inhibition of neuronal impulses in the brain; it is achieved by the administration of a single agent or a combination of chemical agents. This type of anesthesia is appropriately used for surgery of the head, neck, and upper torso, which is of long duration and invasive, and for clients who are unable to cooperate. The anesthetic agents used induce depression of the central nervous system (CNS), which is characterized by analgesia, amnesia, and unconsciousness, with loss of muscle tone and reflexes.

Stages of general anesthesia. Four stages of general anesthesia are classically described. Table 19–2

TABLE 19–1   Advantages and Disadvantages of Various Types of Anesthesia

Method of Induction	Advantages	Disadvantages
General Anesthesia		
Inhalation	Most controlled method Induction and reversal of effects accomplished via pulmonary ventilation Few side effects (headache, vertigo)	Vapors easily contaminated Explosive Poor relaxant Must be used in combination with other agents for painful or prolonged procedures
Intravenous	Rapid and pleasant induction Requires little equipment Low incidence of postoperative nausea and vomiting	Must be metabolized and excreted from the body for complete reversal Contraindicated in the presence of hepatic or renal disease Increased cardiac and respiratory depression
Regional or Local Anesthesia		
	Simple localized administration Less disruption of physical and emotional body functions Decreased chance of sensitivity to agent	Difficult to administer to uncooperative or upset client No control of agent after administration Increased nervous system stimulation (overdose) Absorbs rapidly into the blood and causes cardiac depression (hypertension) or overdose Not practical for extensive procedures because of the amount of drug that would be required to maintain anesthesia

TABLE 19–2 Interventions for the Four Stages of General Anesthesia

Stage	Physiologic Result	Client's Response	Interventions	Rationales
1. Relaxation	Amnesia Analgesia	Feels drowsy and dizzy. Exaggerated hearing. Decreased sensation of pain.	1. Avoid external stimuli by closing the doors, dimming the lights, and controlling traffic in operating room. 2. Position and secure safety belts. 3. Provide emotional support.	1. To promote relaxation. 2. To prevent injury. 3. To decrease anxiety.
2. Excitement	Delirium	Irregular breathing. Increased muscle tone, involuntary motor activity. May vomit, hold breath, or struggle. Susceptible to external stimuli.	1. Avoid stimulating the client by noise and touch. 2. Protect extremities. 3. Assist the anesthesiologist with suctioning.	1–3. To prevent injury.
3. Operative or surgical anesthesia	Partial to complete sensory loss Progression to complete intercostal paralysis	Quiet, regular thoracoabdominal breathing. Jaw relaxed. Auditory and pain sensations lost. Moderate to maximum decrease in muscle tone. Eyelid reflex absent.	1. Assist the anesthesiologist with intubation. 2. Check the client's position.	1. To decrease the incidence of injury during intubation. 2. To ascertain appropriate alignment and prevent circulatory occlusion.
4. Danger	Medullary paralysis and respiratory distress	Respiratory muscles paralyzed. Pupils fixed and dilated. Pulse rapid and thready. Respirations cease.	1. Assist in the treatment of cardiac or respiratory arrest. 2. Provide emergency medications and defibrillation equipment. 3. Document the administration of drugs.	1–3. To decrease the incidence of injury, complication, or death related to respiratory or circulatory failure.

Adapted from Groah, L. K. (1983). *Operating room nursing: The perioperative role.* Reston, VA: Reston Publishing.

presents the client's physiologic responses and nursing interventions for each stage. *Stage 1*, or *relaxation*, begins with the client's being awake and includes the gradual loss of consciousness during which time analgesia occurs. *Stage 2*, or *excitement*, begins with total loss of consciousness to the point at which excitement occurs, with irregular breathing and involuntary limb movements. *Stage 3*, or *surgical anesthesia*, is marked by com-

plete relaxation of the jaw, regular respiration, and loss of auditory and pain sensation. *Stage 4*, or *danger*, is characterized by apnea, leading to cardiopulmonary arrest and death. The speed of *emergence*, or the reversal of anesthesia, is dependent on the type of anesthetic agent and the length of time the client is anesthetized. Retching, vomiting, and restlessness may be seen during emergence, and the nurse must have suction equipment available to prevent aspiration. During reversal, shivering, rigidity, or slight cyanosis are not uncommon and are thought to reflect a temporary disturbance in the body's temperature control. The nurse provides the client with warm blankets and oxygen to decrease the effects of emergence.

Methods of administration. The three methods of administering general anesthesia are inhalation, IV injection, and rectal instillation. The last method is generally considered obsolete because absorption in the colon is unpredictable. Table 19–3 presents some of the commonly used anesthetic agents according to method of administration.

Inhalation is the most controllable method of administering anesthesia because intake and elimination are accomplished primarily by respirations. The lungs act as a passageway for entrance and exit of the anesthesic agent. The anesthetic vapor of a volatile liquid or the anesthetic gas is inhaled and passes across the alveolar membrane to the general circulation; it is transported via the blood stream to the various tissues where it is metabolized. Respirations may be assisted or controlled to improve ventilation and control of anesthesia. This can be easily accomplished by the anesthesiologist's applying manual pressure on the reservoir (breathing) bag of the anesthesia machine, which signals the client's own respiratory effort to initiate the cycle. Controlled respiration occurs with the use of a mechanical device that automatically and rhythmically inflates the lungs with intermittent positive pressure, requiring no participation by the client. Controlled ventilation is initiated after the anesthesiologist has produced apnea by hyperventilation or the administration of respiratory depressant drugs or a neuromuscular blocker—succinylcholine (Anectine, Sucostrin) is usually the drug of choice. An endotracheal tube (ET) is then inserted by the anesthesiologist with the assistance of the circulating nurse.

A laryngoscope is used to visualize the vocal cords, and an ET is placed in the trachea. The cuff (balloon) of the tube is placed just below the vocal cords so as not to damage them (Fig. 19–3). It is then inflated to seal off the airway. Placement of the ET causes some degree of irritation and edema of the trachea. After the effects of the neuromuscular relaxant wear off, the client is maintained via ventilator or allowed to breath spontaneously. With the ET tube safely in place, the client has an open airway for the safe administration of inhalation anesthesia.

Inhalation anesthetic agents are divided into two categories: gases and volatile agents. Gaseous agents are inorganic and explosive in nature. Their combustibility increases when they are combined with oxygen for administration as an anesthetic. *Nitrous oxide* (N_2O) is the most commonly used gaseous anesthetic. It is a colorless, odorless, and nonirritating gas with rapid induction and recovery period. It is a relatively weak anesthetic and, except for short procedures, requires the addition of other agents. As an adjunct to thiopental (an IV anesthetic), narcotics, and other agents, nitrous oxide re-

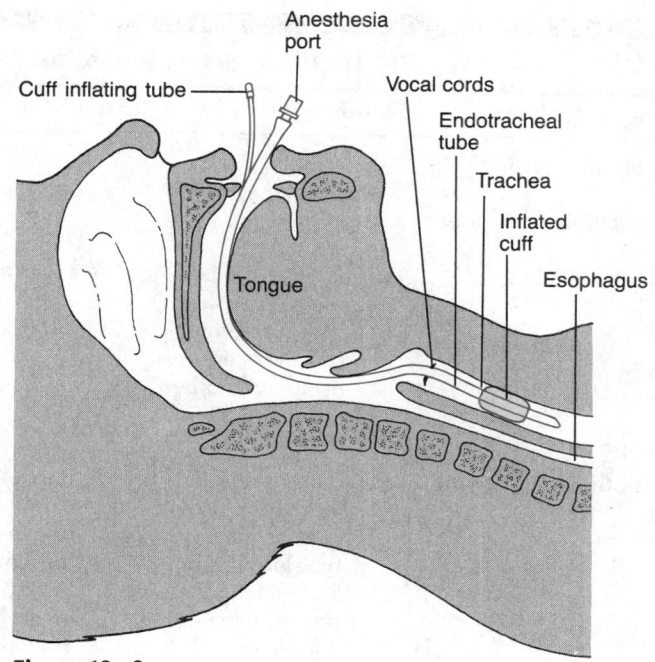

Figure 19–3

An endotracheal tube in position.

duces the required concentration of other anesthetic agents, thereby reducing circulatory and respiratory depression. Nitrous oxide can produce hypoxia if the concentration of the gas is too high.

Volatile agents are liquids that are vaporized for inhalation. Oxygen acts as a carrier, flowing over or bubbling through the liquid in the vaporizer system on the anesthesia machine. This gas mixes with nitrous oxide in a process called halogenation, producing a nonflammable agent. The most common volatile agents are halothane (Fluothane), enflurane (Ethrane), methoxyflurane (Penthrane), and isoflurane (Forane).

Halothane is nonirritating to the respiratory tract and produces minimal nausea and vomiting postoperatively. Nasopharyngeal suction equipment is assembled by the nurse or the anesthesiologist for use in preventing aspiration in case of vomiting. The nurse monitors the client's pulse and blood pressure closely, because halothane depresses the cardiovascular system, resulting in hypotension and bradycardia. It can sensitize the myocardium to arrhythmias, and the use of epinephrine for vasoconstriction may aggravate or precipitate arrhythmias. Because halothane affects the hypothalamus, the nurse covers the client with warmed blankets to prevent shivering postoperatively.

Ethrane is an inhalation anesthetic that produces adequate muscle relaxation for intra-abdominal procedures. The nurse monitors the client's respiratory function and blood pressure intraoperatively and postoperatively. Ethrane reduces the client's ventilations and decreases blood pressure as the depth of anesthesia increases, while the pulse rate and rhythm remain stable.

TABLE 19–3 Interventions for Clients Receiving Anesthetic Agents

Anesthetic	Advantages	Disadvantages	Interventions	Rationales
General Anesthetics				
Inhalation Anesthetics				
Nitrous oxide	Rapid induction of recovery, useful with oxygen for short procedures, useful with other agents for all types.	Poor relaxant, weak anesthetic; may produce hypoxia.	1. Follow precautions for combination agents.	1. To promote safety and prevent injury.
Halothane (Fluothane)	Rapid and smooth induction, useful in almost every type of surgery, low incidence of postoperative nausea or vomiting.	Requires skillful administration to prevent overdosage; may cause liver damage; may depress cardiovascular system; provides limited relaxation; expensive.	1. Monitor pulse, respirations, and blood pressure; client may shiver with prolonged use.	1. To detect deviations from normal.
Enflurane (Ethrane)	Rapid induction and recovery, potent analgesic.	Respiratory depression may develop rapidly along with electroencephalographic abnormalities.	1. Monitor respirations.	1. To detect respiratory depression.
Methoxyflurane (Penthrane)	Seldom causes postoperative nausea and vomiting, analgesic action continues for several hours after surgery, excellent muscle relaxant.	Renal damage may occur, unpleasant odor.	1. Careful observation needed because of prolonged depressant action. 2. Monitor vital signs. 3. Suction as necessary.	1. To detect return to normal level of consiousness. 2. To detect deviations from normal. 3. To prevent aspiration.
Isoflurane (Forane)	Rapid induction and recovery, enhances effects of muscle relaxants.	Respiratory depressant.	1. Monitor respirations closely.	1. To detect respiratory depression.
Diethyl ether	Excellent relaxant, wide margin of safety, inexpensive, relatively nontoxic; used for all types of surgery.	Explosive, slow induction (10 min), long recovery period; irritating to skin and eyes; may cause metabolic acidosis, causes nausea and vomiting.	1. Keep eyes closed. 2. Turn head to side.	1. To protect from irritation. 2. To prevent aspiration.

TABLE 19–3   Interventions for Clients Receiving Anesthetic Agents *Continued*

Anesthetic	Advantages	Disadvantages	Interventions	Rationales
Intravenous Anesthetics				
Thiopental sodium (Pentothal)	Rapid and pleasant induction and recovery, low incidence of postoperative nausea or vomiting.	Strong respiratory depressant, poor relaxant; may cause coughing, sneezing, and laryngospasms.	1. Monitor blood pressure, pulse, and respirations. 2. Watch for circulatory and respiratory depression, be prepared for possible laryngospasm.	1. To detect deviations from normal. 2. To prevent complications.
Fentanyl citrate (Sublimaze)	Little effect on cardiovascular system.	In high dosage acts as an alpha-adrenergic blocking agent.	1. After large doses, must be artifically ventilated.	1. To provide life support until drug no longer effective.
Fentanyl citrate with droperidol (Innovar)	Long duration of action, excellent analgesia effect postoperatively.	May lead to extrapyramidal rigidity, as in parkinsonism, because of inhibition of dopamine.	1. Keep IV and vasopressors available in case of hypotension. 2. Monitor vital signs.	1. To prevent complications. 2. To detect deviations from normal.
Ketamine (Ketalar, Ketaject)	Rapid induction, short action with nitrous oxide, can be administered as analgesic or anesthetic.	Elevated blood pressure; depressed respiration; vomiting and aspiration; may experience hallucinations; poor relaxant.	1. Avoid unnecessary stimulation, observe for signs of respiratory depression, keep resuscitative equipment nearby. 2. Monitor blood pressure and pulse.	1. To protect from injury. 2. To detect deviations from normal.
Local or Regional Anesthetics				
Procaine (Novocain) Tetracaine (Pontocaine) Lidocaine (Xylocaine) Mepivacaine (Carbocaine)	Easily administered, rapid onset; can be administered topically or by injection; excellent relaxant.	Absorbs into blood stream and can cause systemic cardiac depression; difficult to control dosage.	1. Assess for return of sensation and movement to administration area. 2. Monitor blood pressure and pulse. 3. Assess administration site for changes in pallor and drainage.	1. To assess for complications related to loss of sensation. 2. To detect deviations from normal. 3. To protect from injury related to sensory loss.

Penthrane is an effective muscle relaxant and provides an analgesic effect at low concentrations. This anesthetic is toxic to the kidneys and should only be used for short surgical procedures. The nurse monitors the client's renal function by determining if urinary output is adequate (30 to 50 mL/hour).

Forane is a relatively new halogenated compound and appears to be the ideal inhalation agent. The cardiovascular system remains stable, while the drug provides appropriate muscle relaxation, but no renal or hepatic damage. The nurse assesses the client for signs of respiratory depression when Forane is used.

IV injection of anesthetics provides a pleasant, rapid, and smooth dissipation of the anesthetic agent. The anesthesia is injected into the circulation usually via a peripheral IV line. The drug is diluted by the blood in the heart and lungs, passing in high concentration to the organs of high blood flow (brain, liver, and kidneys). The reversal and removal of the agent from circulation is not possible with this method of anesthesia, and the safety of the agent is directly related to the client's metabolism. (See Table 19–3 for an overview of IV agents.)

Barbiturates are often used for IV inductions. They act directly on the CNS, producing a reaction ranging from mild sedation to unconsciousness, but providing little relief of pain. The principal barbiturate used is the short-acting thiopental sodium (Pentothal). In addition to being used for induction, thiopental is used to supplement nitrous oxide during short procedures and as a hypnotic with regional anesthesia. It acts rapidly, resulting in unconsciousness in 30 seconds. Thiopental is a potent respiratory and cardiovascular system depressant, requiring continuous monitoring of the client's vital signs during administration.

Narcotics are used to supplement inhalation anesthesia. The most commonly used narcotics are morphine sulfate, meperidine hydrochloride (Demerol), and fentanyl citrate (Sublimaze). The use of narcotics during surgery results in adequate postoperative analgesia. Morphine and meperidine decrease alveolar ventilation and are respiratory depressants, which may be a major problem for the client and may necessitate intervention by the nurse during the recovery phase. Reduced dosages are prescribed for the elderly; the client with a circulatory problem, such as congestive heart failure; and the debilitated client because of an increased incidence of side effects in these clients related to respiratory and circulatory insufficiency.

Fentanyl citrate is a synthetic narcotic with a potency 80 to 100 times greater than that of morphine. Its duration of action is shorter than that of other narcotics; therefore, it does not have the prolonged period of impaired ventilation associated with other drugs and is often used for ambulatory clients, the elderly, or those with respiratory diseases. When fentanyl citrate is administered in large dosages, the nurse assesses the client for the return of spontaneous respiration and maintains an open airway with the use of a plastic airway or an ET tube.

Innovar is a combination of the narcotic fentanyl citrate and the tranquilizer droperidol (Inapsine). It is used in small dosages to supplement nitrous oxide or regional anesthesia. Innovar has a long duration, requiring close observation of the client for respiratory depression, hypoventilation, apnea, and hypotension during the postoperative period. The nurse maintains a patent IV access and has vasopressors available to counteract anesthetic side effects, especially hypotension, if these occur. Usually the initial dose of postoperative narcotic is reduced.

Ketamine is a dissociative anesthetic agent. This drug acts by selectively interrupting associative pathways in the brain. Given intravenously or intramuscularly, ketamine results in a rapid onset of a trance-like, analgesic state without respiratory depression or the loss of muscle tone, thus protecting the airway. The cardiovascular system is stimulated, with an increase in heart rate and blood pressure occurring. This agent is commonly used for diagnostic and short surgical procedures or to supplement weaker agents, such as nitrous oxide. During the recovery from ketamine, the client may experience unpleasant dreams, hallucinations, or distorted images and act irrationally. The use of the drug should be reported to the postanesthesia recovery (PAR) or recovery room nurse so that safety precautions are implemented during transfer from the operating room and in the recovery room. If the client is combative or restless, the side rails of the bed are padded to prevent injury. The nurse minimizes external stimuli, such as light, noise, touch, and movement, until the client awakens naturally. For severe reactions during the recovery phase, a small dose of diazepam (Valium) may be given before transfer to or in the recovery room.

Neuromuscular blockers are used to provide muscle relaxation during surgery and to facilitate passage of an ET tube. These drugs act on the striated muscles of the body by interfering with the impulses that occur at the motor end plate, the place where the motor nerve fiber joins with a muscle fiber. The drugs are administered intravenously in small amounts and may cause circulatory alterations and decreased respirations.

There are two types of muscle relaxants: depolarizers and nondepolarizers. *Depolarizing* agents produce a neuromuscular blockade by acting like acetylcholine to depolarize the membrane of the motor end plate. When these drugs are administered, the muscle fiber acts as if acetylcholine were released and the muscle contracts or twitches. The drug remains attached to the muscle fibers and prevents the repolarization required for another contracture from occurring; thus, the muscle remains relaxed. The most frequently used depolarizing agent is succinylcholine chloride. It is a rapidly acting drug with a duration of 3 to 5 minutes and is frequently used for intubation. When depolarizing agents are used, the nurse ensures the client's safety by securing the client on the operating table with safety straps and assists the anesthesiologist with intubation.

Nondepolarizing muscle relaxants act to inhibit the effects of acetylcholine at the neuromuscular junction, but they do not cause depolarization at the motor end plate. Tubocurarine (curare), pancuronium bromide (Pavulon), and gallamine triethiodide (Flaxedil) are common nondepolarizing agents.

Complications of general anesthesia. Complications from anesthesia are rare, but may be life-threatening. Most complications are minor, including those from intubation technique, such as broken or injured teeth and caps, or trauma to the vocal cords resulting from a difficult introduction of the ET tube into the trachea. Difficult intubation may be due to improper hyperextension of the neck, a small oral cavity, or a tight mandibular joint. As the client's advocate, the nurse assists the anesthesiologist with the intubations and recommends that another person should attempt the procedure if difficulties occur.

Anesthesia overdose may occur in the elderly or debilitated client because of an intolerance of the agent or decreased metabolism. More commonly, anesthesia overdose occurs because the client's height and weight are incorrectly assessed or documented, or this information is missing from the preoperative record. This information is vital in the calculation of anesthetic dosage.

Malignant hyperthermia is a rare and life-threatening complication of general anesthesia. A biochemical reaction occurs as a result of a defect in the muscle cell membrane, causing a rise in the circulating calcium level and resulting in an increase in metabolic rate and body temperature up to 46° C. This occurs most commonly with the use of halothane, Penthrane, or succinylcholine in clients susceptible to this defect. Symptoms of malignant hyperthermia include tachycardia, continual increase in body temperature (which can reoccur during the postoperative period), cyanosis, hypotension, muscle rigidity, darker color of blood at the surgical wound, and arrhythmias. Treatment and survival of the client depend on early diagnosis and cooperation of the entire surgical team. Treatment begins with immediate discontinuation of surgery and cooling of the client by the administration of iced IV solutions, iced nasogastric lavage, and packing the client in ice. Simultaneously, dantrolene sodium (Dantrium), steroids, diuretics, and 100% oxygen (to induce hyperventilation) are administered.

Balanced anesthesia.   Balanced anesthesia is one of the most widely used methods of administration; it provides a safe and controlled anesthetic experience, especially for elderly and high-risk clients. A combination of agents is used to provide hypnosis, amnesia, analgesia, muscle relaxation, and relaxation of reflexes with minimal disturbance of the client's physiologic function. Many combinations are possible, and selection reflects individual results of client assessment and the surgical procedure. An example of balanced anesthesia is the use of a barbiturate administered intravenously for induction, nitrous oxide and morphine for analgesia, and a muscle relaxant to provide additional relaxation of the muscles.

Local or regional anesthesia.   Local or regional anesthesia temporarily interrupts the transmission of nerve impulses to and from a specific area or region. Motor function may or may not be involved. The extent of the anesthetized field depends on the site of application, the total volume of anesthetic administered, and the concentration and penetrating ability of the drug. The client does not lose consciousness with this type of anesthesia. This type of anesthesia is indicated for diagnostic procedures in which the client's participation is important and for minor invasive procedures (e.g., breast biopsy, removal of superficial growths, or cataract extraction). The nurse provides the client with information, directions, and support during the procedure.

Regional anesthetics may be used when general anesthesia is contraindicated because of the presence of medical problems (e.g., arrhythmias and respiratory disease), when the client has experienced previous adverse reactions to general anesthetic agents, or when the client has a preference and a choice is possible. It can also be used in conjunction with general anesthesia to decrease operative stimuli, thereby diminishing the general stress response to surgical trauma. Table 19–3 describes the commonly used regional and local anesthesic agents and associated nursing interventions.

Complications of local or regional anesthesia are usually attributable to overdose, incorrect administration technique, or client sensitization to the anesthetic. The nurse observes for signs of a systemic toxic reaction related to an overdose of regional anesthetic, which is manifested by CNS stimulation followed by CNS and cardiovascular depression. The initial behaviors the nurse assesses for are restlessness, excitement, incoherent speech, headache, blurred vision, metallic taste, nausea, vomiting, tremors, convulsions, and increased pulse, respirations, and blood pressure. Nursing interventions include the establishment of an open airway, administration of oxygen, and notification of the surgeon for the administration of sedation using a fast- and short-acting barbiturate. If the toxic reaction remains untreated, unconsciousness, hypotension, apnea, and cardiac arrest result.

Localized complications include edema, inflammation, abscess, necrosis, and gangrene. Inflammation and abscess are usually a result of a break in sterile technique occurring at the time of anesthetic injection. Necrosis and gangrene are rare, but may occur as a result of vasoconstriction in the area of the injection.

The techniques used to administer an anesthetic agent to the nerve include topical anesthesia, local infiltration, field block, nerve block, spinal anesthesia, and caudal and epidural blocks. The nurse's role in the administration of regional anesthesia is to assist the anesthesiologist, observe for breaks in sterile technique, and provide physical and emotional support for the client. The nurse stays with the client, providing the client a chance to verbalize feelings; offers information and encouragement; and positions the client comfortably and safely, especially for a regional nerve block. The use of touch by the nurse is important during regional anesthesia to reassure the client that the nurse is present and concerned for the client as an individual.

Topical anesthesia occurs when a regional anesthetic is applied directly to the surface of the area to be anesthetized. The anesthetic is most frequently in the form of an ointment or spray. This method is often used for respiratory intubation or for diagnostic procedures, such as laryngoscopy, bronchoscopy, or cystoscopy. The onset of action is 1 minute, and the duration is 20 to 30 minutes. Collapse or depression of the cardiovascular system may occur after the application of the topical anesthetic to the respiratory tract.

Local infiltration is the injection of an anesthetic agent intracutaneously and subcutaneously into the tissue surrounding an incision, a wound, or a lesion. The anesthesia blocks peripheral nerve stimulation at its origin.

Local infiltration is commonly used during the suturing of superficial lacerations.

Field block is the term for regional anesthesia produced by a series of injections around the operative field. Injecting around a specific nerve or group of nerves depresses the entire sensory nervous system of a localized area. This type of blocking is used for herniorrhaphy, dental procedures, and plastic surgery.

A *nerve block* is achieved by injecting the local anesthetic agent into or around a nerve or nerves supplying the involved area. Nerve blocks interrupt sensory, motor, or sympathetic transmission. They are used surgically to prevent pain during a procedure, diagnostically to identify the cause of pain, and therapeutically to relieve chronic pain and increase circulation in some vascular diseases.

Figure 19–4 shows the most common sites of nerve block during operative procedures: cervical plexus (between the jaw and the clavicle), intercostal nerves (chest and abdominal wall), brachial plexus (upper arm), and radial, ulnar, and digital nerves (elbow, wrist, hand, or fingers). Lidocaine (Xylocaine) and bupivacaine (Marcaine) are commonly used for nerve blocks. A nerve block takes effect within minutes after the injection, and the anesthesia lasts longer than that achieved with local infiltration. Epinephrine added to the anesthetic potentiates the drug, causing a prolonged effect. The major complication arises if the nerve-blocking agent is injected into the blood stream. The nurse observes for signs of sensitivity or overdose: excitability, twitching or convulsions, changes in pulse or blood pressure, and respiratory distress.

Spinal anesthesia is administered in an emergency, to clients with trauma who may have eaten or who have recently been drinking alcoholic beverages, and for clients with active or unstable cardiac disease, because it causes the least amount of stress on the body. Spinal anesthesia or intrathecal block is achieved by injection of the anesthetic agent into the subarachnoid space at the level of L2-3 or L3-4 (as shown in the illustration on page 131 in Chap. 7). The drug acts on the nerves as they emerge from the spinal cord and before they leave the spinal canal through the intervertebral foramen, thereby inhibiting conduction in the autonomic, sensory, and motor systems. Absorption into the nerve fibers occurs rapidly and produces analgesia with relaxation, which is effective for abdominal and pelvic surgical procedures.

Spinal anesthesia is administered by an anesthesiologist with the assistance of the circulating nurse. The nurse assists the client into a flexed lateral (fetal) position or a sitting position on the edge of the operating table with the arms resting on the thighs and the chin resting on the chest. Both of these positions straighten the natural curvature of the spine and widen the intervertebral spaces to facilitate insertion of the spinal needle (see the illustration on page 131 in Chap. 7). The nurse holds the client securely in position, provides emotional support, and instructs the client not to move. The spread of the anesthetic agent is influenced by the specific gravity of the solution and the position of the client immediately after the injection. After the injection, the client is placed in a supine position and the operating table is positioned to facilitate movement of the anesthetic solution. For example, a client undergoing a cholecystectomy is placed in a 5-degree Trendelenburg position to move the anesthetic toward the head. The level of analgesia is fixed in 10 to 20 minutes and after that time is no longer influenced by changes in the client's position. The nurse then positions the client for the surgical procedure, paying attention to joint and body alignment of the anesthetized areas.

The two most common side effects of spinal anesthesia are *hypotension* and *spinal headache*. Hypotension is

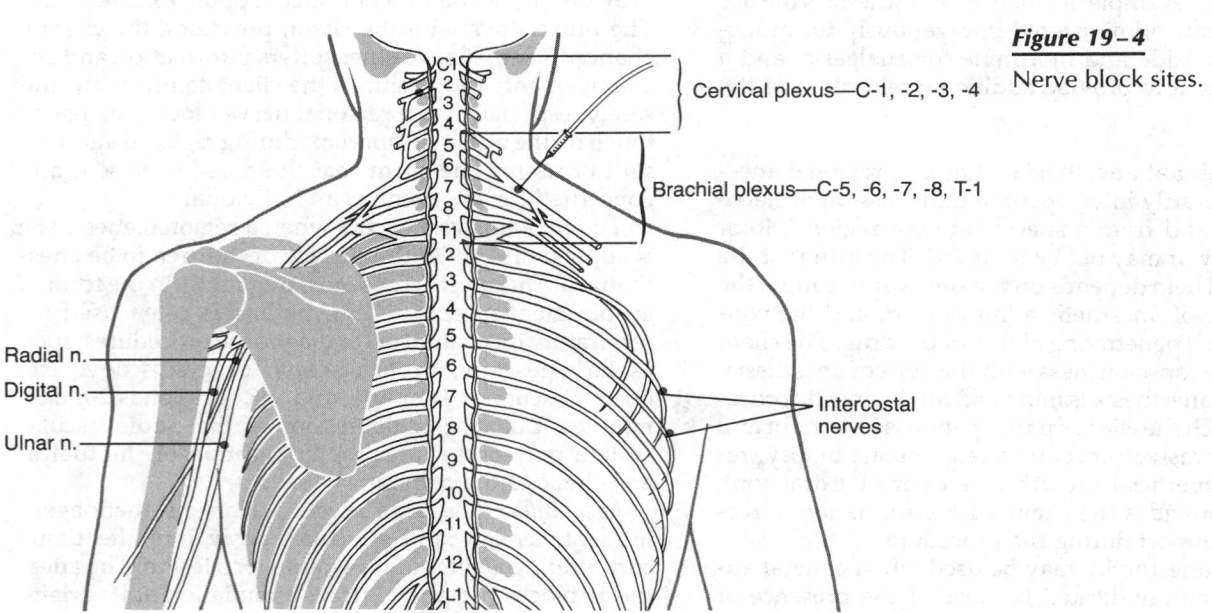

Figure 19–4

Nerve block sites.

Cervical plexus—C-1, -2, -3, -4

Brachial plexus—C-5, -6, -7, -8, T-1

Radial n.

Digital n.

Ulnar n.

Intercostal nerves

the result of a preganglionic block of the sympathetic fibers, causing vasodilation and reduction of venous return to the heart. Nursing interventions for the client consist of monitoring vital signs and peripheral circulation and administering oxygen and IV vasopressors.

Spinal headache usually occurs during the first 24 to 48 hours after the administration of the anesthetic. The headache is a result of an incomplete seal of the dura mater after removal of the needle and leakage of cerebrospinal fluid into the epidural space, decreasing cerebrospinal pressure. Prevention of a spinal headache includes having the client lie flat in bed for 6 to 12 hours postoperatively and achieving adequate hydration. Nursing interventions for the client with a headache include restricting the client to bed rest; providing a quiet, dark room; maintaining hydration, orally or via IV fluids; and administering sedatives or analgesics as needed. A spinal headache may last 3 to 5 days after receiving spinal anesthesia. If the headache persists after these measures, the anesthesiologist may perform an epidural blood patch.

Caudal and epidural anesthesia are the same in that the anesthetic is injected into the epidural space. When the injection is into the epidural space through the sacral hiatus and the caudal canal, the technique is termed caudal block. Injection of the anesthetic solution into the epidural space through the interspaces of the vertebrae is called an epidural block. (See the illustration on page 131 in Chap. 7.) Caudal and epidural blocks differ from spinal anesthesia in that the spinal needle does not penetrate the dura and subarachnoid space. The client is positioned in the same manner as for spinal anesthesia. These blocks are useful for anorectal, vaginal, and perineal procedures.

COLLABORATIVE MANAGEMENT

 Assessment

On arrival in the surgical suite, the client is placed in a holding area. The circulating nurse meets the client identifying himself/herself as the nurse who will be with the client during surgery. The nurse stands next to the midsection of the stretcher to allow clear visualization of the nurse by the client. The nurse then verifies the client's identity by asking, "What is your name?" This prevents errors that may occur, for example, when a client is asked, "Are you Mr. James?" Clients who are disoriented and those who have received preoperative sedation may be drowsy and respond inappropriately to this form of questioning. The nurse always validates the identification by checking the client's hospital identification bracelet and chart using the client's name and hospital-assigned number. Correct client identification

is the responsibility of every member of the health care team.

After the identification process is completed, the nurse validates that the surgical consent has been signed and witnessed. The nurse asks the client, "What kind of operation are you having today?" This is done to ascertain that the client's perception of the procedure, the operative permit, and the operative schedule coincide. This is especially important when validating the side on which a procedure is to be performed (e.g., for amputation, cataract extraction, or hernia repair).

Chart Review

A review of the client's chart is done in the holding area by the circulating nurse. The chart provides information needed to identify potential and actual needs of the client during the intraoperative period and allows the circulating nurse to assess and plan for the client's needs during and after surgery. A check of the chart ensures that all required data are present in the record before the procedure commences.

In reviewing the chart, the nurse questions the client about *allergies* and *previous reactions to anesthesia or blood transfusions.* Allergies or sensitivity to iodine products or shellfish may indicate the potential for a reaction to the antimicrobial agents used to clean the surgical area. The nurse clearly indicates the allergies on the chart and notifies the surgeon. The client's previous experience with anesthesia helps the nurse and the anesthesiologist plan and anticipate the client's needs. For example, some clients are restless or agitated as a reaction to anesthesia; the nurse should have padding for the stretcher's side rails and protective restraints readily available. The use of blood and blood products during surgery may be influenced by the client's history, religious beliefs, and type of reaction during transfusions in the past. *Autologous blood transfusion* (reinfusing the client's own blood) is being used increasingly for elective surgery. Nurses need to be familiar with autotransfusion procedures to provide effective care for clients undergoing surgery who choose this method of blood transfusion (see the accompanying Guidelines feature).

Reports of preoperative *laboratory and diagnostic test results* are checked by the nurse for completeness. The most recent laboratory results (usually obtained within 24 to 48 hours before surgery) are assessed to provide information for the surgical team regarding the client's medical condition and alert them to potential intraoperative and postoperative interventions. The nurse reports all abnormalities to the surgeon and the anesthesiologist. Laboratory values that are greater than or less than the normal range are potentially life-threatening for any client, but especially for the client undergoing surgery. If the hemoglobin concentration is less than 10 g/dL, the client's oxygen transport is lessened; this has an effect on the amount and type of anesthesia used and the potential for blood loss during surgery. The presence of acetone in the urine may indicate dehydration, especially in the elderly client. Serum and urine glucose

GUIDELINES ■ Perioperative Nursing Considerations for Autologous Blood Transfusion

Methods of Reinfusing in the Operating Room

Use of autologous blood collected preoperatively.

Intraoperative "salvage" of client's blood via specialized reservoirs followed by cell washings before reinfusion.

Criteria for Client Selection

Client's hemoglobin level should be at least 11 g/dL.

Client should be at risk for losing more than 1 pint of blood during surgery.

Procedure is contraindicated for clients with most malignancies.

Elderly clients, those with cardiovascular compromise, and clients with existing blood-transmitted disease (hepatitis) are poor risks for autotransfusion.

Client Benefits

Decreased risk of fatal transfusion reactions and transmission of blood-borne diseases.

May be more acceptable to clients who have religious objections to receiving blood transfusions from others.

Interventions

Preoperative

Be prepared to reinforce and clarify the physician's information to the client.

Intraoperative

Be aware of the cell-processing method to be used.
Make sure collection containers are labeled for client.
Assist with sterile set-up as necessary.
Assist with processing and reinfusion procedures as needed.
Document the transfusion process.
Monitor the client's vital signs during the transfusion procedure.

NURSING RESEARCH

Elevated Blood Glucose Levels Can Delay Wound Healing and Cause Postoperative Complications.

Keith, K. S., & Pieper, B. (1989). Perioperative blood glucose levels: A study to determine the effect of surgery. *AORN Journal, 50*, 103–110.

Surgery can lead to transient hyperglycemia and blood glucose levels greater than 180 mg/dL can cause electrolyte imbalances, delay wound healing, and lead to conditions that promote infection, especially in diabetic clients (who have a 50% chance of having surgery in their lifetime). The purpose of this study was to compare perioperative changes in blood glucose levels of insulin-dependent diabetics, non–insulin-dependent diabetics, and nondiabetics who were having elective surgery.

Thirty-six subjects participated; 28 were matched for type of surgery and anesthesia. Blood specimens were drawn (by fingerstick) five times: before surgery, in the preoperative holding area, 15 minutes after the start of surgery, hourly throughout the surgery, and 15 minutes after the client was moved to the recovery area. Specimens were checked with a blood glucose monitor (Accu-Check).

Analysis of variance was used to compare the three groups. The nondiabetic group had significantly lower blood glucose levels preoperatively than did the two groups of diabetics; intraoperatively, there were no differences among the three groups; and postoperatively, all groups had increased blood glucose levels. Clients who had general anesthesia had significantly higher blood glucose levels.

Critique. Results from this small convenience sample are not generalizable to other surgical clients without more research. Only four individuals had spinal anesthesia, so the significance of higher blood glucose levels with general anesthesia must be interpreted with caution.

Possible nursing implications. Careful preoperative monitoring of the blood glucose levels of all diabetic clients may identify those at risk for complications during surgery and postoperatively. Intraoperative blood glucose monitoring can be used to assess the need for insulin in diabetic clients and to prevent complications.

---

levels provide the nurse with important information about the status of diabetes control in the diabetic client (see the accompanying Nursing Research feature).

As well as reviewing the laboratory testing results, the nurse checks that the *medical history and physical examination findings,* including normal pulse and blood pressure for the client, are recorded. This information provides the circulating nurse, the surgeon, the anesthe-

siologist, and the PAR room nurse with baseline data to assess the client's reaction to the surgical procedure and anesthesia. Knowledge of the client's medical history and age allows the nurse to take special precautions and plan appropriate interventions for the care and safety of high-risk clients. Arthritic and osteoporotic clients need special padding and extra protection of joints during surgery. The nurse monitors elderly clients and those with cardiac disease for potential fluid overload, which can be life-threatening. The medications routinely taken by the client before surgery may have an effect on the client's reaction to surgery and wound healing. Anticoagulant therapy, including aspirin, causes decreased clotting time and a danger of hemorrhage and should be discontinued before surgery as directed by the physician.

The client's attire is checked in the holding area to ensure compliance with hospital policy. The nurse checks to see that dentures and dental prostheses (e.g., bridges and retainers), jewelry, contact lenses, wigs, and prostheses are removed for the client's safety during surgery. Special attention is paid to the removal of dentures, as the denture plate could become loose and obstruct the client's airway during surgery. Occasionally, the anesthesiology team may request that the dentures be left in place to ensure a snug fit of the anesthesia mask.

After the nurse concludes the chart review in the holding area, the client may have an IV catheter inserted, a surgical shave performed, or a cast bivalved (split lengthwise on either side) or removed. The circulating nurse provides support and explanation of procedures to the client. The client is never left unattended and is transferred to the operating room on completion of the preoperative routine.

 Analysis: Nursing Diagnosis

The intraoperative client is admitted to a hospital or an ambulatory (outpatient) surgical center for surgery. The ambulatory client is usually healthy and is scheduled for a minor procedure. The inpatient client is usually scheduled for major surgery and is at greater risk for postoperative complications. Regardless of the type of surgery, the following nursing diagnoses apply to the intraoperative client.

Common Diagnoses

Two nursing diagnoses are commonly applicable to intraoperative clients:

1. Potential for injury related to anesthesia, intraoperative positioning, and other hazards of the intraoperative environment
2. Impaired skin integrity related to the surgical wound

Additional Diagnoses

In addition to the common diagnoses, one or more of the following diagnoses may be appropriate for the intraoperative client:

1. Impaired gas exchange related to anesthesia
2. Fluid volume deficit related to loss of blood and body fluids during surgery
3. Potential for infection related to surgical wound
4. Fear related to anesthesia
5. Powerlessness related to anesthesia

 Planning and Implementation

The following plan of care for the intraoperative client focuses on the common diagnoses. Intraoperative care consists of a multidisciplinary team approach, with the circulating nurse coordinating the operating room staff and ensuring the client's safety at all times.

Potential for Injury

Planning: client goals. The primary goals for this nursing diagnosis are that the client will (1) be maintained in a safe anesthetized state during the surgical procedure and (2) be free of injury resulting from positioning or operating room equipment use.

Interventions

Anesthesia. Appropriate preparation for and use of anesthesia are necessary (see earlier discussion of anesthesia).

Positioning. Proper positioning, including the padding of joints and the placement of grounding pads, is as important to the client's care as the administration of anesthesia. The circulating nurse is responsible for coordinating the team in transferring the client to the operating room table and positioning the client for surgery. Because of the preoperative medication, anesthetic agents, and narrowness of the table, the client's normal defense mechanisms cannot guard against joint damage and muscle stretch and strain. In addition, the nurse protects the client's skin and assesses for bruising, especially if the client is on or was taking aspirin or any type of anticoagulants preoperatively. The nurse's knowledge of anatomy and physiologic functioning is imperative to ensure the client's safety and comfort. Positioning is determined by the surgical procedure and modified by the nurse on the basis of the special needs and safety for the client.

The nurse ensures proper client positioning by assessing for (1) physiologic alignment, (2) minimal interference with circulation, (3) protection of skeletal and neuromuscular structures, (4) optimal exposure of the operative site and IV line, (5) access for the anesthesiologist, (6) the client's comfort and safety, and (6) preservation of the client's dignity. Using the data gathered in the holding area, the nurse develops a care plan with attention to the client's size and respiratory, skeletal, or neuromuscular limitations, such as rheumatoid arthritis, joint replacements, or emphysema. Table 19–4 presents possible complications related to prolonged surgical immobility and preventive nursing actions.

The client is usually in a dorsal recumbent (supine) position after transfer to the operating table. Anesthesia may be administered in this position and then the client can be repositioned for the operation, or the client may be positioned and then anesthetized. Factors influencing the time of positioning are surgical site, the age and

TABLE 19–4 **Interventions to Prevent Complications Related to Intraoperative Positioning**

Anatomic Area	Complications	Interventions
Brachial plexus	Paralysis Loss of sensation in the arm and shoulder	Avoid excessive abduction. Secure the arm firmly on an arm board, positioned at shoulder level.
Radial nerve	Wrist drop	Support the wrist with padding. Do not overtighten wrist straps.
Medial or ulnar nerves	Hand deformities	Place a safety strap above or below area.
Peroneal nerve	Foot drop	Place pillow or padding under knees. Support lower extremities. Do not overtighten leg straps.
Tibial nerve	Loss of sensation on the plantar surface of the foot	Place a safety strap above the ankle. Do not place equipment on lower extremities.
Joints	Stiffness Pain Inflammation	Place pillow or foam padding under bony prominences. Maintain good body alignment. Slightly flex joints and support with pillows, trochanter rolls, or pads.

size of client, anesthetic administration technique, and pain experienced on movement of the conscious client. The dorsal recumbent, prone, and lateral positions are the most frequently used positions for surgery. Modifications of these positions may be necessary owing to the client's age, size, and weight and the type of surgery. Figure 19–5 illustrates common surgical positions and the use of protective padding. When positioning the client and throughout the intraoperative period, the nurse prevents obstruction of circulatory, respiratory, or neurologic systems caused by tight straps, improperly placed pads and pillows, or position of the table.

Use of electrical equipment. After the client is positioned and securely strapped on the table, the nurse ensures that all grounding plates are evenly covered with a conductive gel, placed on a part of the body not subject to pressure, and positioned as close to the operative site as possible. The presence of metal prostheses, such as hip replacements and metal plates, is taken into account when placing grounding plates to prevent electrocution of the client and the surgical team. Proper grounding plate placement, as well as a careful check of the control setting, prevents burns and surgical wound injury from the electrosurgical equipment (e.g., cautery equipment).

Impaired Skin Integrity

Planning: client goals. The primary goal for this nursing diagnosis is that the client will experience minimal skin impairment and contamination as a result of surgery.

Interventions. Surgery is an invasive procedure that places the client at risk for complications related to the surgical wound, such as incisional tears and lacerations, bacterial contamination, and loss of body fluids from the wound during and after surgery. Sterile surgical technique and the use of protective drapes, skin closures, and dressings help to minimize complications and promote wound healing.

Plastic adhesive drape. The scrub nurse helps the surgical assistant apply a sterile plastic adhesive drape after the surgical site has been cleaned and dried. The plastic drape is applied directly to dry skin to prevent tearing of the surgical incision. The surgeon makes the incision through the plastic drape; the cut edge remains adherent to the skin and keeps the surgical incision sealed from tears and the migration of bacteria into the wound. After closure of the surgical incision, the drape is carefully removed by the nurse and the surgical assist-

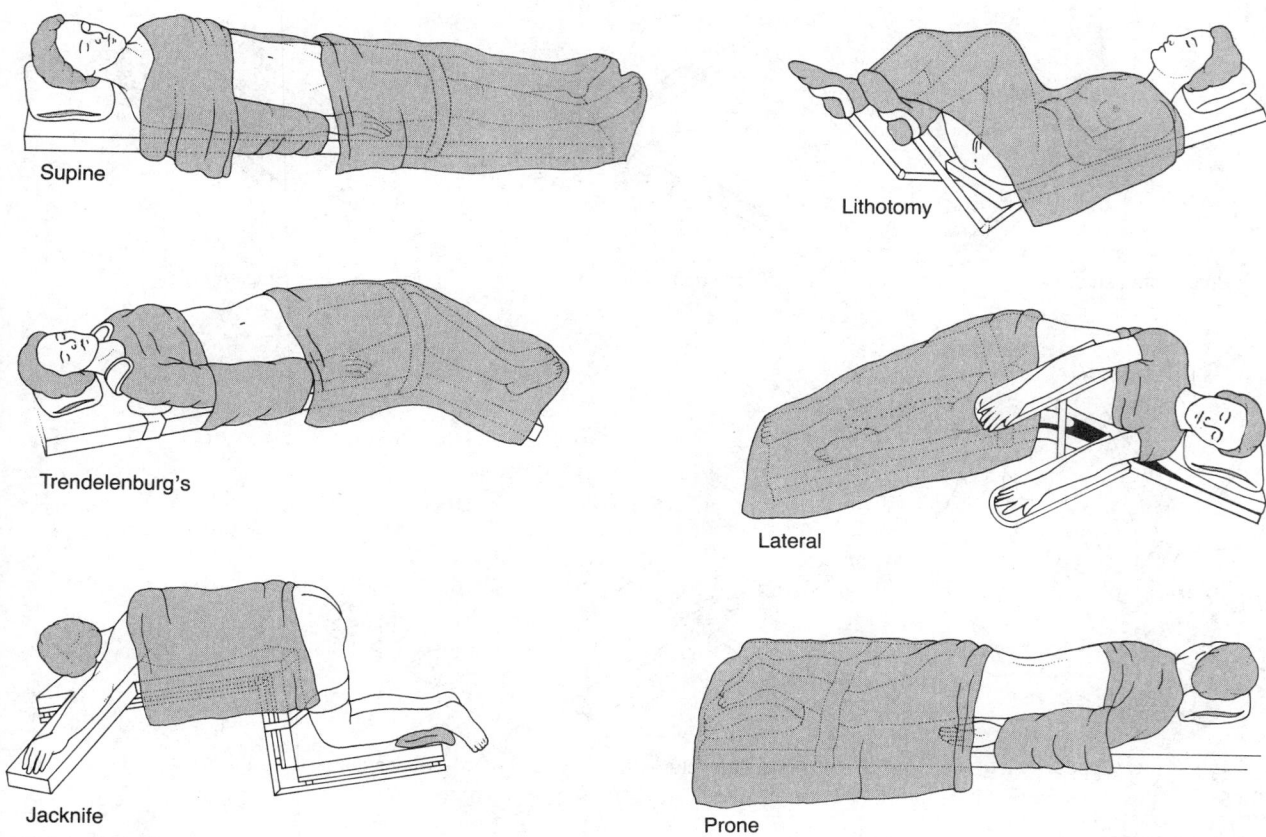

Figure 19–5

Common surgical positions. Note the use of padding for client comfort and draping for client privacy.

ant. The nurse pays special attention to the elderly and clients with fragile skin to prevent denuding of the skin during removal of the adhesive drape.

Skin closures.   Skin closures, such as sutures and clamps, are used to approximate wound edges until wound healing is complete; occlude the lumen of blood vessels, preventing hemorrhage and loss of body fluids; and prevent wound contamination (see Chap. 20 for detailed discussion of wound healing, dressings, and drains). The quality of the approximated tissue and the type of closure material are two factors that determine the strength of the closure. Suture material, when used, ensures wound integrity immediately after closure. To facilitate proper healing, the wound is usually closed in layers to maintain tissue integrity and promote healing with minimal scarring. The surgeon selects the method and type of closures to be used on the basis of the surgical site, the size and depth of the surgical wound, and the age and medical history of the client. A combination of sutures and clamps is commonly used for closure of internal layers of the wound. Staples, stay and retention sutures, and skin closure tapes (Steri-Strips) are used for

closure of superficial wounds or the epidermis. Figure 19–6 illustrates commonly used wound closures.

There are two classifications of suture material: absorbable and nonabsorbable. These are categorized according to diameter and tensile strength. A suture consists of one or more strands of material that are designated by size or gauge of the suture material. The designation sequence is in descending order from number 5 to 0, then 2-0, 3-0, and so forth, to 11-0. Size 5 is the heaviest material and is used to close the deep layers of an abdominal wound; 11-0 is the smallest-diameter suture and is used for plastic surgery.

Absorbable sutures are digested by body enzymes. These sutures first lose strength and then gradually disappear from the tissue. Catgut is a common type of absorbable suture material. The rate of absorption is influenced by the client's physical status, the presence of inflammation, and the type of catgut used.

Nonabsorbable sutures are not affected by enzymes or inflammation. Nonabsorbable sutures become encapsulated in the tissue during the healing process and remain embedded in the tissue unless they are removed. Nonabsorbable sutures are used to secure orthopedic

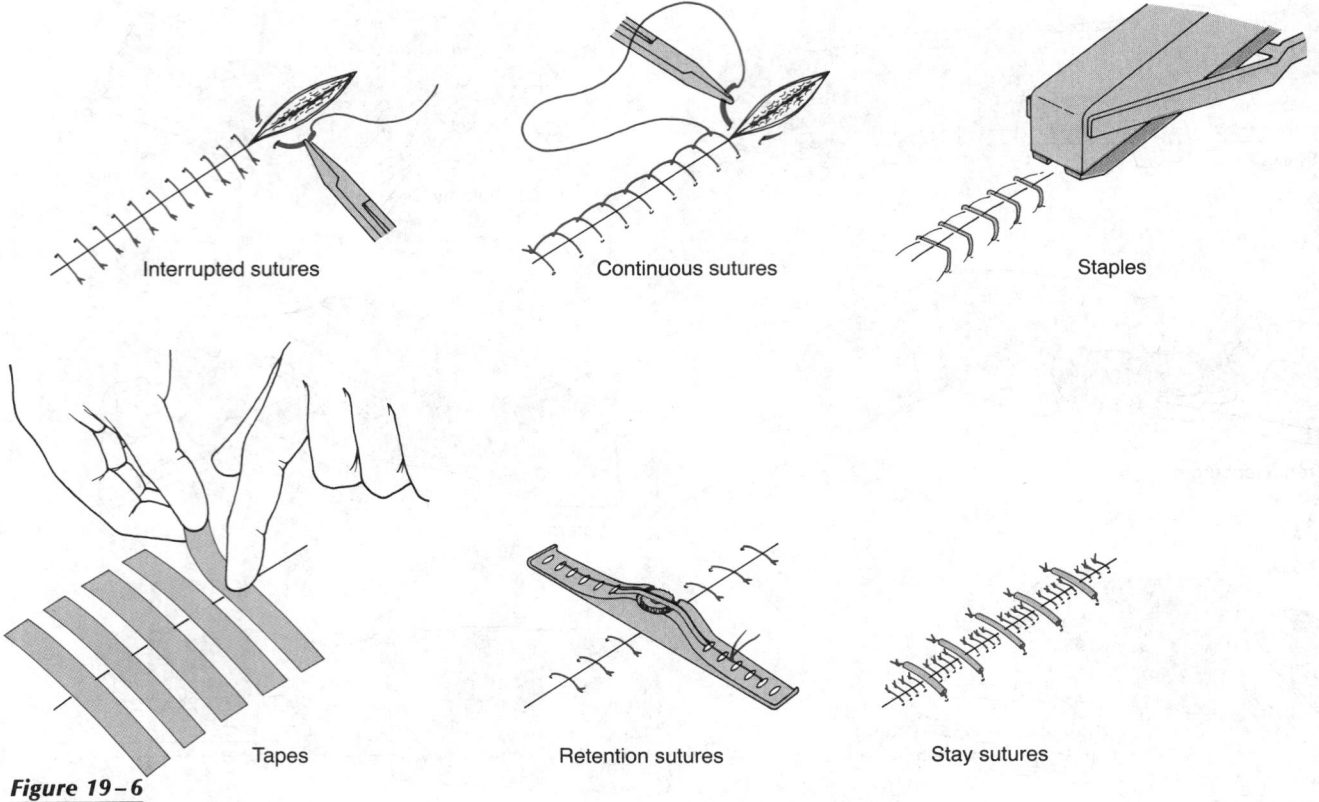

Interrupted sutures

Continuous sutures

Staples

Tapes

Retention sutures

Stay sutures

Figure 19–6

Common skin closures.

prosthetic devices in place and to close external wounds. The surgeon may use a double or interlocking stitch to increase the integrity of the closure. Figure 19–6 shows retention and stay sutures, which are frequently used in addition to standard suture material for high-risk clients, such as those having major abdominal surgery, obese clients, diabetic individuals, and clients taking steroids that inhibit wound healing.

After the incision is closed, a dressing is applied to protect it from contamination, absorb drainage, and provide support to the incision. A pressure dressing may be applied to prevent or stop a vascular area from bleeding postoperatively.

After the dressing is secure, the nurse coordinates the surgical team in repositioning and transferring the client. A roller board or a lift sheet is used to transfer the client safely from the operating room table to a stretcher or bed. The circulating nurse accompanies the client and anesthesiologist to the postanesthesia area or recovery room and gives a report of the client's intraoperative experience to the PAR nurse. Important information to be relayed includes the client's level of anxiety before anesthesia, the type and length of the surgical procedure, the location of incisions, previous reactions to anesthesia, respiratory dysfunctions, joint or limb immobility, primary language, and any special requests the client may have verbalized.

Evaluation

On the basis of the identified common nursing diagnoses, the nurse evaluates the care of the intraoperative client. Expected outcomes for the client in the intraoperative phase of the perioperative experience include that the client

1. Describes the anesthesia to be used
2. Is safely anesthetized
3. Does not experience any injury related to positioning or electrical equipment

SUMMARY

Care planning for the intraoperative client presents a unique challenge to the nurse. The intraoperative phase of the perioperative experience involves an ongoing assessment of the client's physical and psychologic status by the nurse. The nurse's knowledge of the different types of anesthetic agents, the stages of general anesthesia, and client positioning during surgery helps in planning individualized care during the intraoperative period and prevention of complications postoperatively.

IMPLICATIONS FOR RESEARCH

Changing technology, increased frequency of ambulatory surgical procedures, and increasing numbers of elderly clients are providing the nurse with new challenges related to the intraoperative client. Improvements in the effectiveness of care during the intraoperative phase and the ability to meet the special or complex needs of clients and the elderly are areas that require nursing research and interventions to improve client care. In considering these areas for research, the following questions are appropriate:

1. What effect does ambulatory surgery have on the selection of anesthetic agents, and how does the method of administration affect the client's perioperative experience?
2. What are the special needs of the elderly client, and how can the nurse best meet them?
3. How can intraoperative positioning be modified to decrease postoperative discomfort?

REFERENCES AND READINGS

Aimino, P. A. (1987). Perioperative nursing documentation. Developing the record and using care plans. *AORN Journal, 46,* 73–86.

American Society of Anesthesiologists. (1982). Technical bulletin for malignant hyperthermia. *American Society of Anesthesiologist Newsletter, Anesthesia Technical Bulletin, 1,* 5.

Association of Operating Room Nurses. (1987). Patient outcome standards for perioperative nursing. In AORN, *Standards and recommended practices for perioperative nursing* (pp. 1–4). Denver: Author.

Association of Operating Room Nurses. (1989). *Standards of nursing practice.* Denver: Author.

Atkinsson, L. J., & Kohn, M. L. (1986). *Berry and Kohn's introduction to operating room techniques.* New York: McGraw-Hill.

Baida, M. R. (1978). Nursing care in use of local anesthesia. *AORN Journal, 28,* 855–858.

Bailes, B. K. (1989). Perioperative nursing research part IV: Intraoperative phase. *AORN Journal, 49,* 1397–1409.

Baptist, G. (1985). Perioperative nursing roles for the aesthetic surgical patient. *Plastic Surgical Nursing, 5*(3), 86–93.

Barone, J. G., Qaasim, S., & Barone, J. E. (1988). Predeposited autologous blood. *American Family Physician, 37*(5), 98–102.

Birdsall, C., Carpenter, K., & Considine, R. (1988). How is autotransfusion done? *American Journal of Nursing, 88,* 108–111.

Boucher, B. A. (1986). The postoperative adverse effects of inhalation anesthetics. *Heart and Lung, 15,* 63–69.

Brown, D. G. (1985). Anesthetic gas exposure. *AORN Journal, 41,* 590–608.

Burden, N., & Iyer, J. (1987). Local anesthesia: Not always benign. *Journal of Post Anesthesia Nursing, 2,* 45–50.

Chitwood, L. B. (1987). Unveiling the mysteries of anesthesia. *Nursing '87, 17*(2), 52–55.

Churchill-Davidson, H. C. (1984). *A practice of anesthesia.* Chicago: Year Book Medical.

Copp, G., Mailhot, C. B., Zalar, M., Slezak, L., & Copp, A. (1986). Covergowns and the control of operating room contamination. *Nursing Research, 35,* 263–267.

Copp, G., Slezak, L., Dudley, N., & Mailhot, C. B. (1987). Footwear practices and operating room contamination. *Nursing Research, 36,* 366–369.

Cramer, C., & Ring, V. (1987). Preoperative care unit: An alternative to the holding room. *AORN Journal, 46,* 464–472.

Davis, N. B. (1987). Scrubbing and circulating: Both are essential for professional perioperative nursing practice. *AORN Journal, 46,* 9–11.

Dripps, R. D., Eckenhoff, J. E., & Vandam, L. D. (1988). *Introduction to anesthesia* (7th ed.). Philadelphia: W. B. Saunders.

Erbostoesser, M. (1989). Care of the patient with malignant hyperthermia. *Journal of Post Anesthesia Nursing, 4,* 71–74.

Felver, L., & Pendarvis, J. H. (1989). Electrolyte imbalances: Intraoperative risk factors. *AORN Journal, 49,* 992–1008.

French, M. M., & Phillips, K. (1984). When seconds count: Treating malignant hyperthermia. *RN, 47*(11), 26–31.

Foster, C. G. (1979). Effects of surgical positioning. *AORN Journal, 30,* 219–232.

Gibson, J. R., Mendenhall, M. K., & Axel, N. J. (1985). Geriatric anesthesia: Minimizing the risk. *Geriatric Clinics of North America, 1,* 313–320.

Girard, N. J., Morgan, R. G., & Orr, M. D. (1988). Autologous salvage of blood: Perioperative nursing considerations. *AORN Journal, 47,* 492–502.

Groah, L. K. (1983). *Operating room nursing: The perioperative role.* Reston, VA: Reston Publishing.

Gruendemann, B. J., & Meeker, M. H. (1983). *Alexander's care of the patient in surgery.* St. Louis: C. V. Mosby.

Harvey, C. (1984). OR nurse responsibility for safety in the holding area. *AORN Journal, 39,* 20.

In style: Staples, clips, zippers. (1983). *Nursing Life, 3*(12), 4.

Ivey, D. F. (1987). Local anesthesia: Implications for the perioperative nurse. *AORN Journal, 45,* 682–689.

Kneedler, J. A., & Dodge, G. H. (1983). *Perioperative patient care: The nursing perspective.* Boston: Blackwell Scientific.

Kneedler, J. A., & Purcell, S. K. (1989). Perioperative nursing research part II: Intraoperative chemical and physical hazards to personnel. *AORN Journal, 49,* 829–854.

Kneedler, J. A., & Purcell, S. K. (1989). Perioperative nursing research part III: Potential intraoperative biological hazards to personnel. *AORN Journal, 49,* 1066–1079.

Latz, P. A., & Wyble, S. J. (1987). Elderly patients: Perioperative nursing implications. *AORN Journal, 46,* 238–253.

Lichtiger, M., & Moya, F. (1978). *Introduction to the practice of anesthesia.* Hagerstown, MD: Harper & Row.

McNeal, P., & Duncan, M. L. (1984). Assessing patients in the holding area. *Today's OR Nurse, 7*(3), 16–19.

Miner, D. (1987). Patient positioning: Applying the nursing process . . . home study program. *AORN Journal, 45,* 1117–1127.

Moran-Higgins, M. E. (1985). Perioperative concerns for the patient with osteoporosis. *Orthopedic Nursing, 4*(3), 68.

Nelson, J. C. (1984). Intraoperative nursing. *AORN Journal, 40,* 564–565.

Norheim, C. (1986). Spinal anesthesia: As bad as it sounds? *Nursing '86, 16*(4), 42–44.

Phippen, M. (1984). OR nurses' guide to preventing pressure sores. *AORN Journal, 36,* 205–212.

Pomorski, M. E. (1983). Surgical care of the aged patient: The decision-making process. *Nursing Clinics of North America, 18,* 365–372.

Proposed recommended practices: Basic aseptic technique. (1985). *AORN Journal, 42,* 566–571.

Proposed recommended practice: Documentation of perioperative nursing care. (1985). *AORN Journal, 42,* 579–584.

Rogers, A. L. (1985). Malignant hyperthermia: A perioperative emergency . . . home study program. *AORN Journal, 41,* 369–379.

Silo, H. M. S. (1989). Perioperative nursing research part V: Intraoperative recommended practices. *AORN Journal, 49,* 1627–1635.

Simmons, B. P. (1983). CDC guidelines for the prevention and control of nosocomial infections: Guidelines for prevention of surgical wound infections. *American Journal of Infection Control, 11*(8), 133.

Sullivan, D. (1985). Complications from intraoperative positioning. *Orthopaedic Nursing, 4*(4), 56–59.

Tovar, M. K., & Cassmeyer, V. L. (1989). Touch: The beneficial effects for the surgical patient. *AORN Journal, 49,* 1356–1361.

Wise, R. P. (1978). Spinal and regional anesthesia. In Churchill-Davidson, H. C. (ed.), Wylie and Churchill-Davidson: *A practice of anesthesia* (4th ed.). Philadelphia: W. B. Saunders.

Wolcott, M. W. (1988). *Ambulatory surgery and the basics of emergency surgical care* (2nd ed.). Philadelphia: J. B. Lippincott.

CHAPTER 20

Interventions for the Postoperative Client

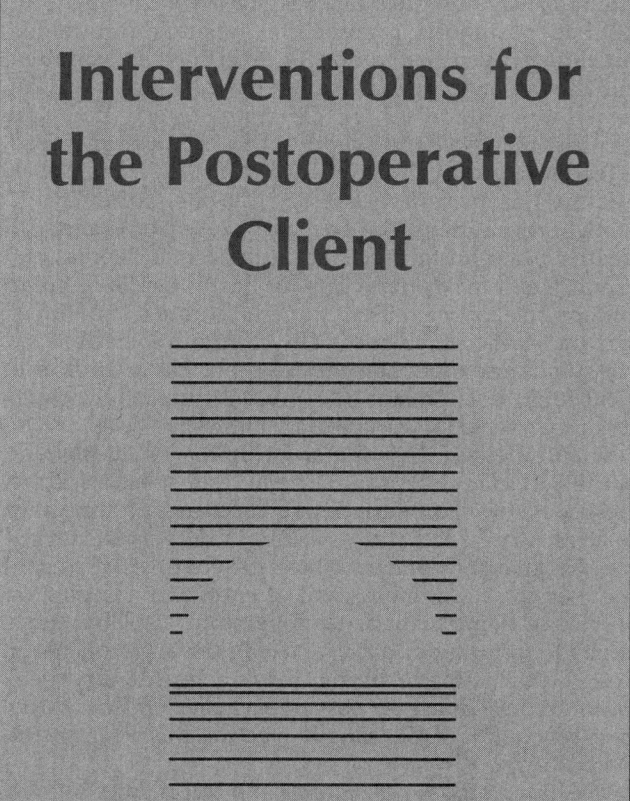

The third and final stage of the perioperative experience begins when the client is admitted to the recovery room, postanesthesia recovery (PAR) room, or postanesthesia care unit (PACU) and extends through discharge from the hospital or ambulatory care facility. During the postoperative period, the client is cared for by nurses in the PAR and on the hospital unit or floor after transfer from the recovery area. The actual time spent in the recovery area and/or hospital after surgery varies according to the client's age and physical health, type of procedure, anesthesia, and postoperative complications.

The PACU or recovery room is usually located close to the surgical suite. The room is large and provides maximal visibility of clients, appropriate ventilation and illumination, and easy access to supplies and emergency equipment. The room is often divided into individual cubicles by a curtain for privacy. Each cubicle is stocked with equipment and supplies commonly used by the nurse to monitor and care for clients, such as oxygen, suction equipment, cardiac monitors, and airways.

The circulating nurse and anesthesiologist or the nurse anesthetist and surgeon accompany the client to the recovery area, which marks the beginning of the postoperative period (Fig. 20–1). The surgeon or anesthesiologist reviews the client's record with the PACU nurse and explains the type and extent of the surgical procedure; type of anesthesia; pathologic condition;

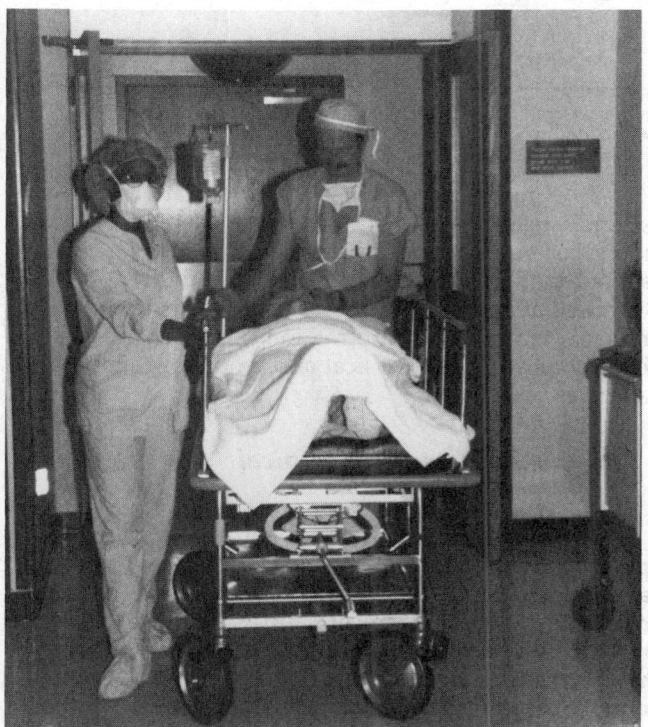

Figure 20–1

A client is transferred from the operating suite to the PACU by the anesthesiologist and a circulating nurse.

blood, intravenous solutions, and medications administered; estimated blood loss; and any complication such as traumatic intubation. The circulating nurse includes information related to the client's level of anxiety before the induction of anesthetic; joint or limb immobility, especially in the elderly client; preoperative and intraoperative respiratory dysfunction, including smoking-related problems, asthma, and chronic obstructive pulmonary disease; primary language (if other than English); special requests that were verbalized preoperatively; location and type of dressing, catheters, drains, or packing; intravenous fluids; tolerance of anesthesia and procedure; and any other important intraoperative occurrences.

The postanesthesia nurse is a specialist who is skilled in the care of clients immediately after surgery. Postanesthesia nursing requires clinical competence in caring for clients of all ages with multiple medical problems, and the ability to make quick decisions based on sound judgment. These nurses have in-depth knowledge of anesthetic agents, analgesics, and their clinical actions; physical and psychosocial assessment skills; and understanding of interventions that are required in emergencies or in case of complications. The nurse monitors the client closely and consults with the anesthesiologist and surgeon as needed during the recovery or postoperative phase.

COLLABORATIVE MANAGEMENT

 Assessment

The PAR nurse incorporates the information from the surgical team's report into the care of the client and identifies potential postoperative complications as presented in Table 20–1. After receiving the report from the circulating nurse and assessing the client, the nurse reviews the chart for information related to the client's history, presurgical physical and emotional status, and allergies.

Physical Assessment: Clinical Manifestations

The data assessed by the nurse in the PACU are compiled systematically on a postanesthesia scoring record, as shown in Figure 20–2. This type of chart is a permanent part of the client's record and assists the health care team in determining the client's readiness for transfer or discharge from the recovery room or PACU. The combination of a postanesthesia scoring and satisfactory confirmation to the facility's criteria for client discharge, such as stable vital signs, no overt bleeding, and return of gag reflex, aids the nurse in determining the client's readiness for transfer. After the PAR nurse has determined that all criteria have been met, the client is discharged by the anesthesiologist to the hospital unit or home.

Respiratory system. When the client is admitted to the PACU, the nurse immediately assesses the client for a patent airway and adequate respiratory exchange. The client is positioned to promote maximal respiratory function, prevent aspiration of secretions or vomitus, and allow maximal visualization during assessment, as shown in Figure 20–3. To determine airway patency, the nurse places a hand over the client's mouth and nose to feel exhalation. The adequacy of the air exchange is measured as the nurse assesses the rate, pattern, and depth of respirations. A respiratory rate of fewer than 10 breaths per minute may indicate narcotic depression. Rapid, shallow respirations indicate cardiovascular compromise or increased metabolic rate. The nurse auscultates the lungs bilaterally to determine adequate and symmetric expansion. If the client has an endotracheal tube, it could slip into the right main bronchus, thus preventing left lung expansion.

The immediate and ongoing respiratory assessment by the PACU and floor nurse includes inspection of the chest wall for symmetric movement, use of accessory muscles, diaphragmatic breathing, and sternal retraction, which indicate an excessive anesthetic effect, respiratory obstruction, movement of endotracheal tube, or neurologic complications such as paralysis. The nurse listens for snoring or stridor, which are signs of upper airway obstruction resulting from tracheal or laryngeal spasm, mucus in the airway, or occlusion of the airway from relaxation of the tongue (see the Key Features of Disease on p. 476).

The floor nurses auscultates the lungs for effective expansion when the client is admitted to the unit and every 4 hours during the first 24 hours postoperatively. Elderly clients, smokers, and clients with a history of respiratory disease are prone to developing postoperative complications such as atelectasis (collapse of alveoli) and pneumonia (inflammation of the lungs). For these clients and for those having cardiac or thoracic surgery, the nurse assesses respiratory effectiveness every shift for a minimum of 48 hours after the initial 24-hour period.

Chest tubes are commonly inserted intraoperatively when the pleura of the thoracic cavity has been entered to re-expand the lung and to promote drainage of fluid. The chest tube drains into a water-sealed system that prevents air from entering the thoracic cavity. The nurse assesses the chest tube dressing for bleeding and air leakage around the tube and the breath sounds for adequate lung expansion (Chap. 62 discusses assessment and care of clients with chest tubes).

Cardiovascular system. The client's circulation, blood pressure, pulse, and heart sounds are assessed at admission to the unit and every 15 minutes while in the recovery room until the client's condition is stable. Postoperative vital signs are assessed by the floor nurse according to the hospital's procedure and or the surgeon's orders. These vital signs usually include the client's tempera-

TABLE 20–1   **Interventions to Prevent Postoperative Complications**

Complication	When Seen Postoperatively	Interventions
Urinary retention	8–12 h	Monitor hydration status and encourage oral intake if permitted. Offer bedpan or help client ambulate to commode.
Pulmonary: atelectasis, pneumonia, embolus	1–2 d	Help client to turn, cough, and deep breathe every 2 h. Keep client well hydrated. Encourage frequent early ambulation.
Alterations in wound healing: dehiscence, evisceration	5–6 d	Splint incision when client coughs. Monitor client for signs of infection, malnutrition, and dehydration. Encourage high-protein diet.
Urinary tract infection	5–8 d	Encourage oral fluid intake. Encourage evacuation of bladder every 4–6 h. Monitor intake and output for urinary retention.
Thrombophlebitis	6–14 d	Assist client to exercise legs 8–10 times each hour while in bed. Encourage early ambulation and leg exercises. Apply antiembolism stockings or Ace bandages as ordered by the physician. Avoid pressure that may obstruct venous flow beyond popliteal space by not raising knee gatch of bed, placing pillows behind the knee, or crossing the legs. For prophylaxis, use low-dose heparin administered subcutaneously every 8–12 h.

POSTANESTHESIA RECOVERY SCORE		IN	15	30	45	HR	OUT
ACTIVITY ABLE TO MOVE VOLUNTARILY OR ON COMMAND	4 EXTREMITIES	2	2	2	2	2	2
	2 EXTREMITIES	1	1	1	1	1	1
	0 EXTREMITIES	0	0	0	0	0	0
RESPIRATION	ABLE TO DEEP BREATHE AND COUGH FREELY	2	2	2	2	2	2
	DYSPNEA SHALLOW OR LIMITED BREATHING	1	1	1	1	1	1
	APNEIC	0	0	0	0	0	0
CIRCULATION PREOP BP ___	BP ± 20 mm OF PREANESTHESIA LEVEL	2	2	2	2	2	2
	BP ± 20–50 mm OF PREANESTHESIA LEVEL	1	1	1	1	1	1
	BP ± 50 mm OF PREANESTHESIA LEVEL	0	0	0	0	0	0
CONSCIOUSNESS	FULLY AWAKE	2	2	2	2	2	2
	AROUSABLE ON CALLING	1	1	1	1	1	1
	NOT RESPONDING	0	0	0	0	0	0
COLOR	NORMAL	2	2	2	2	2	2
	PALE, DUSKY, BLOTCHY, JAUNDICED, OTHER	1	1	1	1	1	1
	CYANOTIC	0	0	0	0	0	0
DISMISSAL CRITERIA: TOTAL SCORE OF 10 PLUS STABLE VITAL SIGNS A DOCTOR'S ORDER IS REQUIRED FOR DISCHARGE WITH LOWER SCORE						TOTAL	

Figure 20–2

The Aldrete postanesthesia recovery scoring system. Preop BP, preoperative blood pressure. (Reprinted with permission from *AORN Journal,* Vol. 41, p. 383, February 1985. Copyright © AORN Inc., 10170 East Mississippi Avenue, Denver, CO 80231.)

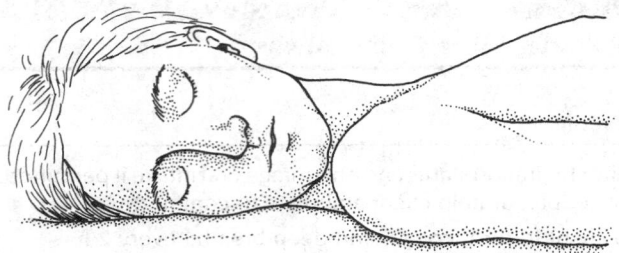

Figure 20–3

Position of the client in the PACU to promote an open airway and to prevent aspiration of secretions or vomitus.

ture, pulse, respirations, and blood pressure and the condition of the surgical dressing. These observations are usually recorded every 15 minutes for four times, every 30 minutes for four times, every 2 hours for four times, and then every 4 hours for 2 days if the client's condition is stable. After 2 days, vital signs are assessed according to the hospital's policy and nursing judgment. The nurse reports blood pressure fluctuations of more than or less than 25% of preoperative values (15- to 20-point difference, systolic or diastolic) to the anesthesiologist or surgeon. A decrease in the client's blood pressure, pulse, and heart sounds indicates possible myocardial depression, shock, hemorrhage, or oversedation. In assessing vital signs, the nurse determines the rate, rhythm, and quality of the client's apical pulse compared with a peripheral pulse such as the radial. A pulse deficit (a difference between the apical and peripheral pulse) could indicate an arrhythmia. An increased pulse rate could indicate shock, pain, or hypothermia.

Anesthesia and positioning during surgery (e.g., the lithotomy position that is used during genitourinary procedures) may compromise the client's peripheral circulation during and after surgery. The nurse assesses peripheral circulation by palpating and comparing the distal pulses bilaterally for the presence and quality of pulsation, color and temperature of extremities, sensation, and size of extremities. Palpable dorsalis pedis pulses indicate adequate circulation and tissue perfusion of distal lower extremities. The nurse tests for Homans' sign for the presence of thrombophlebitis in the lower extremities every shift while the client is in bed and once daily during the first 10 to 14 postoperative days. The presence of edema, redness, and pain in a limb also indicates thrombophlebitis (see Chap. 65 for further information).

Fluid and electrolyte balance. Extended fasting before and during surgery, loss of fluid during the procedure, and the type and amount of intravenous fluid administered affect the client's postoperative blood pressure and fluid and fluid and electrolyte balance. Complications of imbalance occur most often in elderly and debilitated clients or in clients who have medical problems such as diabetes mellitus, Crohn's disease (especially after major intestinal surgery), or severe hypertension that is being controlled by diuretics. Hydration

KEY FEATURES OF DISEASE ■ Significance of Abnormal Postoperative Respiratory Assessment Findings

Abnormal Findings	Possible Significance
Inspection	
Loud snoring, grunting, or stridor	Narrowing of airway
Unequal chest wall movement	Obstruction in one side of the bronchi
Irregular depth, rate, or rhythm	
Cyanosis of lips, ears or extremities	Ineffective respirations
Palpation	
Crepitation	Leakage of air into the subcutaneous tissue
Unequal tactile fremitus	Obstruction or narrowing of the bronchi
Percussion	
Dullness over lung fields	Pulmonary edema
	Pleural effusion
	Pneumonia
Auscultation	
Rales or crackles	Pulmonary edema
	Pneumonia
Rhonchi or gurgles	Narrowing of large airways during expirations
Wheezes	Narrowing of airways
	Bronchospasm
Pleural friction rub	Obstruction of the upper airway

status is assessed by inspecting mucous membranes for color and moist appearance, skin turgor for "tenting" and texture, and dressings for amount of drainage. Nasogastric tube drainage, urinary output, and wound drainage are measured and compared with intake to identify possible fluid imbalance. The nurse continues to assess intake and output for the first 24 hours and for as long as the client receives intravenous fluids or has a catheter, drains, or nasogastric tube, and then as needed.

The nurse administers and closely monitors intravenous fluids and blood to promote fluid and electrolyte balance. Isotonic solutions such as Ringer's lactate and 5% dextrose plus Ringer's lactate are standard intravenous fluids that are used for fluid replacement and maintenance in the PACU. After the client returns to the surgical unit, the type and rate of administration of intravenous solutions are based on individual client need (see Chap. 13 for further discussion of intravenous fluids and assessment of hydration).

Neurologic system. Regardless of the type of surgical procedure, the nurse assesses cerebral function and level of consciousness or awareness of all clients who have received general anesthesia or any type of sedation. The return to consciousness occurs in the following order: muscular irritability, restlessness and delirium, recognition of pain, and ability to reason and control behavior. To assess the level of consciousness, the nurse combines observations of the client's lethargy, restlessness, or irritability with tests of coherence and orientation to person, place, and time. The nurse determines awareness by calling the client's name, touching the face, and giving simple commands such as, "Open your eyes" or "Take a deep breath." Eye opening indicates wakefulness or arousability but not necessarily awareness. The degree of orientation is determined by asking the conscious client to answer simple questions such as, "What is your name?" "What day is it?" "Where are you?"

In clients who had surgical procedures involving the head or neck, the neurologic assessment also includes pupillary responses to light, muscle strength, and bilateral coordination. Motor function is assessed for all clients receiving general and regional anesthesia. General anesthesia depresses voluntary motor function, and regional anesthesia renders only part of the body without sensory and motor function. This assessment is especially important after the client has had spinal anesthesia. The nurse evaluates motor function by instructing the client to move each extremity. The client who had spinal anesthesia remains in the recovery area until sensation and voluntary movement of the lower extremities are re-established. In addition, the nurse assesses the strength of each limb and compares the results bilaterally.

Genitourinary system. Voluntary control of urinary function does not return for 6 to 8 hours after inhalation, intravenous, and spinal anesthesia. The anesthetic, continuous intravenous infusion, and trauma of manipulation during surgery—in combination or alone—can cause urinary retention. To prevent this complication, the nurse inspects, palpates, and percusses the client's lower abdomen for bladder distention. If the client has an indwelling urinary catheter (Foley's), the nurse assesses urine for color and amount. Urinary output should correlate with total input for a 24-hour period. Output of less than 30 mL/hour may indicate renal complications and should be reported to the physician by the nurse. Urinary output is one of many measurements that are used to determine the reversal of anesthesia. The monitoring of the client's urinary function is continued by the floor nurse, especially during the first 8 hours postoperatively when urinary retention is common and requires appropriate assessment and intervention. Chapter 57 describes the assessment of genitourinary function, including interpretation of specific gravity, electrolyte values, and osmolality of urine.

Gastrointestinal system. One of the most common postoperative reactions is nausea and vomiting. Approximately 40% of clients receiving general anesthesia have some form of gastrointestinal upset within the first 24 hours after surgery. Postoperative nausea and vomiting cause stress and irritation to abdominal and gastrointestinal wounds and can increase intracranial pressure in clients who had neck and head surgery and intraocular pressure in clients who had eye surgery. In addition to general anesthesia, abdominal surgery and narcotics reduce intestinal peristalsis during the first day after surgery and predispose the client to nausea and vomiting.

The nurse in the PACU and later on the surgical unit assesses the client's gastrointestinal function by auscultating for bowel sounds until normal peristaltic function is noted in all abdominal quadrants. Decreased peristalsis leads to *constipation* or *paralytic ileus*, which is a potential postoperative complication in which the walls of the intestine are distended and there is no movement of the intestinal wall (aperistalsis). The nurse assesses the postoperative client for clinical manifestations of paralytic ileus, which include fewer or absent bowel sounds, distended abdomen, and no excretion of stool or flatus.

A nasogastric tube may be inserted intraoperatively to prevent postoperative complications by decompressing and draining the stomach, promoting rest, and allowing the lower gastrointestinal tract to heal. It may also be used to monitor bleeding, prevent intestinal obstruction, and irrigate or instill medication. The Levin tube and the Salem sump are the two most common tubes used. The Salem sump is a double-lumen tube and has an air vent that keeps the tube from adhering to the gastric mucosa, which allows easy drainage of the stomach. The Levin tube is a single-lumen tube and has no air vent. To promote drainage, suction is applied to the tube in either a continuous or an intermittent fashion based on surgeon preference and tube type. The amount, color, and consistency of drained material are recorded by the nurse every 6 to 8 hours. Normal nasogastric drainage fluid is green-yellow; red drainage fluid indicates active bleeding and brown liquid indicates the possibility of old bleeding. The nurses assesses the client for possible complications related to nasogastric tube use, which include fluid and electrolyte imbalance and aspiration. To prevent aspiration, the nurse checks tube placement every 4 to 8 hours and before the instillation of irrigation solution or medication into the tube (see Chap. 44 for information on tube placement). After gastric surgery, the nasogastric tube should not be manipulated without an order from the physician. Fluid and electrolyte imbalances resulting from prolonged use of the nasogastric tube and from excessive drainage include dehydration, hypokalemia, hyponatremia, and metabolic alkalosis, as discussed in Chapter 13.

Integumentary system. The surgical, or clean, wound heals itself at skin level in approximately 2 weeks in the absence of infection, trauma, connective tissue disease, malnutrition, and the use of some medications such as steroids. Complete healing of underlying tissue and return to presurgical integrity may take 6 months to 1 year. The physical condition and age of the client, size and location of the wound, and stress placed on the surgical wound also affect the length of time it takes for wound healing. Wounds of the face and head heal more quickly than abdominal and leg wounds. The nurse's knowledge of wound healing is used as care and protection of the incisional area are planned. During the first few days of wound healing, the incised tissue regains blood supply and begins to bind together. After 3 to 4 days, the connective tissue cells give strength to the wound. By the 9th or 10th day, the wound appears to be healed; however, healing is not complete until the scar is strengthened (see Chap. 39 for discussion of wound healing at the cellular level).

Wound healing occurs by *first intention, second intention (granulation), or third intention,* as shown in detail in the illustration on page 479.

Ineffective wound healing may be caused by wound infection, distention from edema or paralytic ileus, or stress at the surgical site. Wound *dehiscence* is partial or complete separation of the upper layers of the wound (Fig. 20–4). *Evisceration* is the total separation of the layers and extrusion of internal organs or viscera through an open wound (see Fig. 20–4). Both of these alterations in wound healing are seen most often between the 5th and 10th postoperative day, possibly because of suture removal. Wound dehiscence or evisceration may be preceded by excessive coughing, not

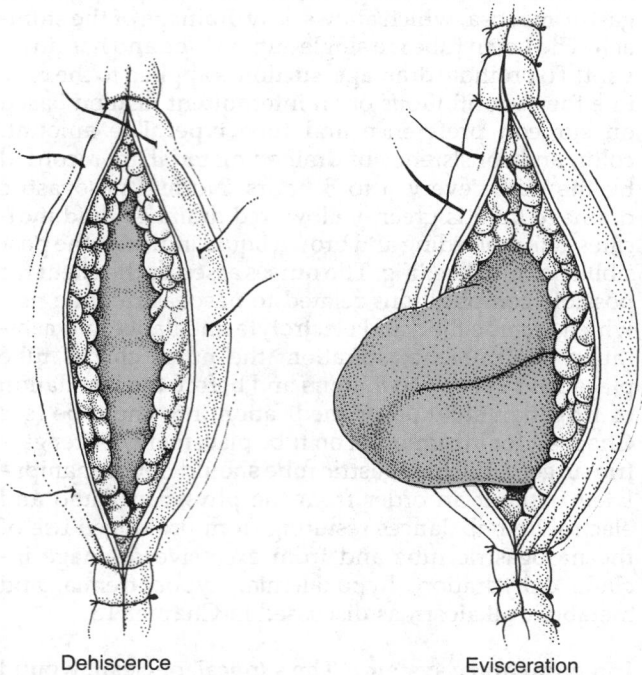

Dehiscence   Evisceration

Figure 20–4

Complications of wound healing.

splinting the surgical site, vomiting, or straining and may be reported by the client stating, "Something gave way" or "I feel as if I just split open." The nurse emphasizes to the client the importance of early coughing and deep breathing to prevent respiratory complications that will cause forceful coughing and increased incisional stress after the sutures are removed and thus an increased chance of wound dehiscence or evisceration. The client's knees should be flexed when the client is in the supine position to reduce tension on the wound.

Dressings and drains.   All dressings including casts and elastic (Ace) bandages are assessed for drainage when the client is admitted and every 15 minutes while in the PAR. The floor nurse assesses the client's dressing each time vital signs are taken. When inspecting the dressing, the nurse checks for drainage and notes the amount, color, consistency, and odor of the drainage fluid and the date and time of the observations on the client's chart. The dressing should not restrict circulation or sensation. The nurse also checks underneath the client for drainage when the dressing is assessed.

The presence of a Penrose drain (single-lumen, soft latex tube inserted into or close to the surgical wound), which is a gravity drain under the dressing, may account for the drainage. Closed suction drains such as Hemovac, VacuDrain, and Jackson-Pratt are assessed to ensure maintenance of compression and thus suction. Large amounts of sanguinous (bloody) drainage may indicate internal bleeding. All drains are assessed by the nurse for patency when the client is admitted to the PAR and every time vital signs are taken during the postoperative period. Figure 20–5 shows the drains commonly used postoperatively. The amount, color, and consistency of the drainage are monitored by the nurse while the client is in the PAR and at least every 8 hours after the client is transferred to the floor.

Pain assessment.   The surgical client in the PACU almost always reports of pain. Postoperative pain is related to the surgical wound, drains, and intraoperative positioning of the client. Agency policy determines whether pain medication is held until the client is returned to the nursing unit or administered in small dosages in the PAR. The use of narcotics or analgesics may mask or increase the number and the severity of symptoms of a reaction to anesthesia. In assessing the client's pain and need for medication, the type, extent, and length of the surgical procedure are considered. The nurse assesses for physical and emotional signs of pain such as increased pulse and blood pressure, increased respiratory rate or hyperventilation, diaphoresis, restlessness, wincing, moaning, and crying. If possible, the nurse should ask the client to quantify the pain before and after medication is given on a scale of 1 to 10, with 1 being least intense and 10 being extreme pain. When the medication is given in the PAR or on return of the client to the nursing unit, the nurse assesses for side effects, as presented in Table 20–2. Approximately 45 to 60 minutes after intramuscular injection or 5 to 10 minutes

THREE TYPES OF WOUND HEALING

HEALING BY FIRST INTENTION

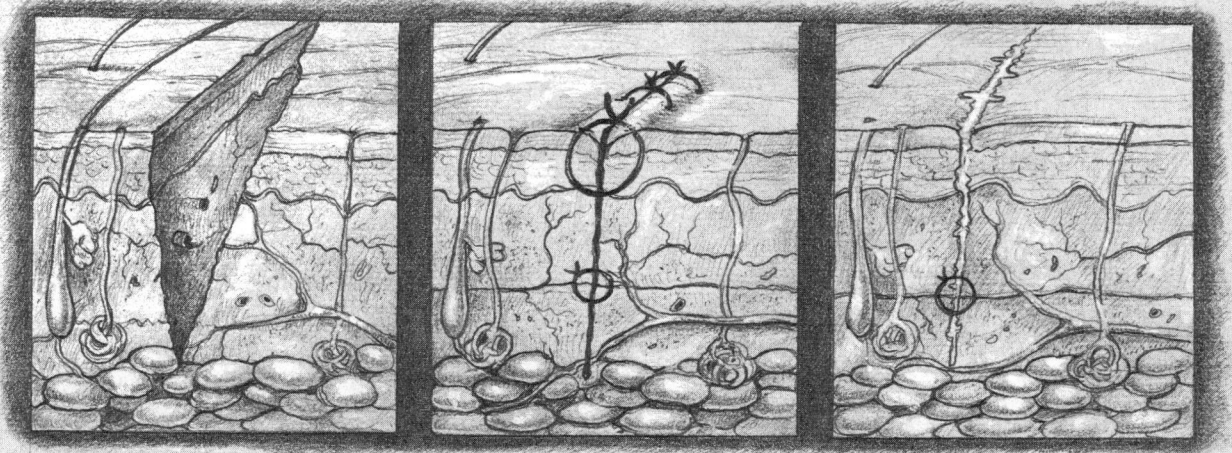

Clean incision   Early suture   "Hairline" scar

An aseptically made wound with minimal tissue destruction and minimal tissue reaction begins to heal as the edges are approximated by close sutures or staples. No open areas or dead spaces are left to serve as potential sites of infection.

HEALING BY SECOND INTENTION (GRANULATION)

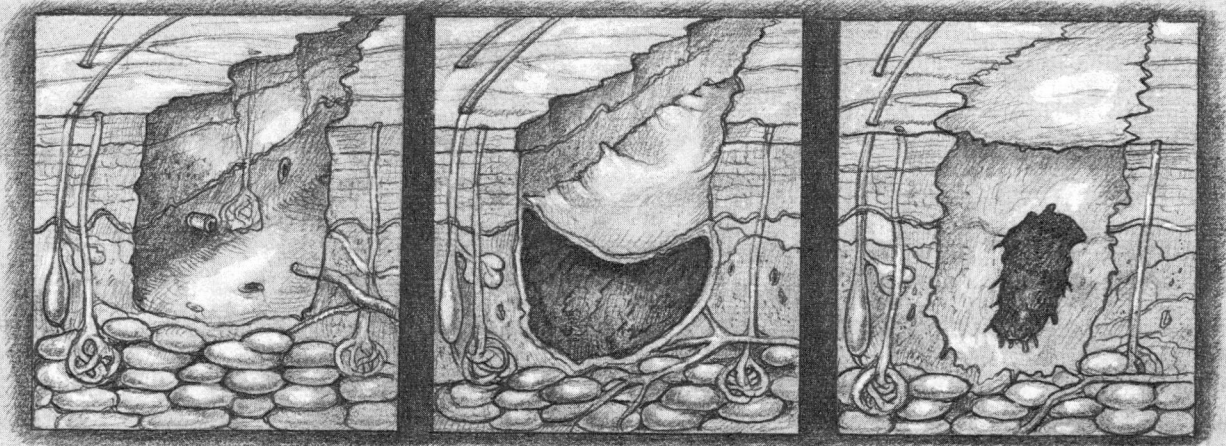

Gaping, irregular wound   Granulation   Growth of epithelium over scar

An infected wound or one with tissue damage so extensive that the edges cannot be smoothly approximated is usually left open and allowed to heal from the inside out. The nurse periodically cleans and assesses the infected wound for healthy tissue production. Scar tissue is extensive, and healing is prolonged.

HEALING BY THIRD INTENTION (DELAYED CLOSURE)

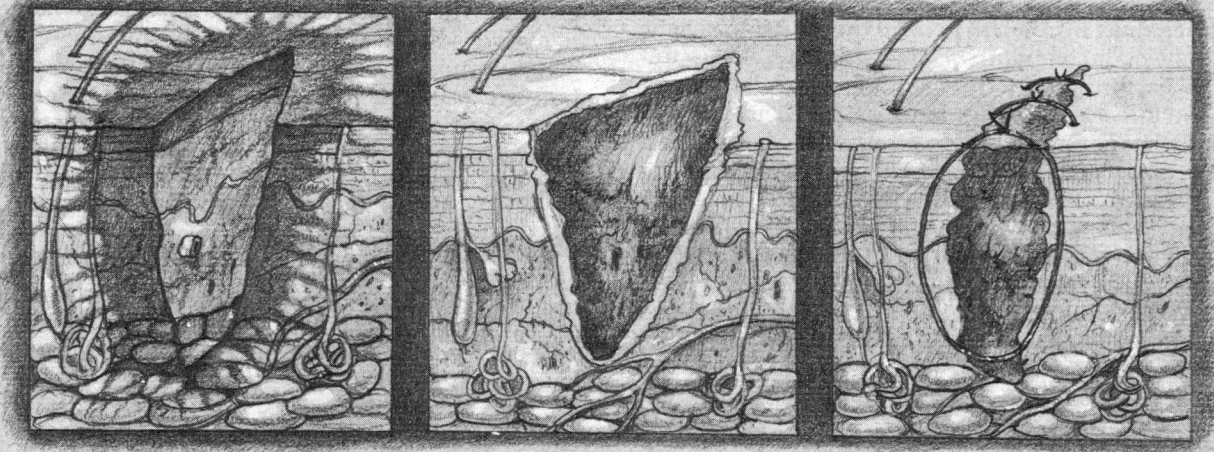

Infected wound   Granulation   Closure with wide scar

An infected wound may be left open until all evidence of infection has subsided. The wound is then closed surgically.

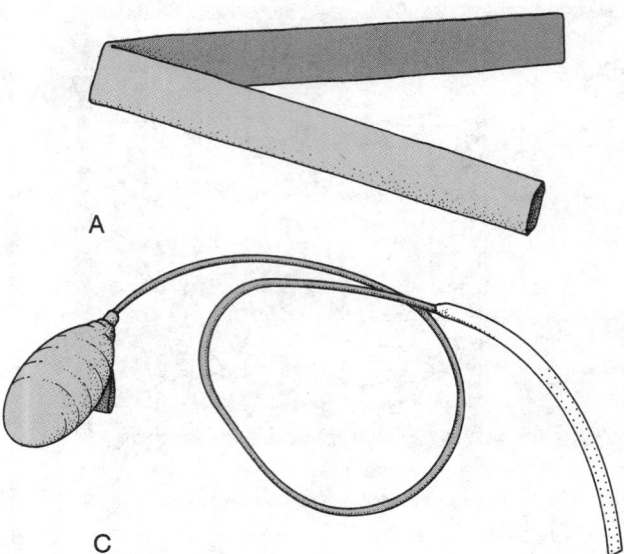
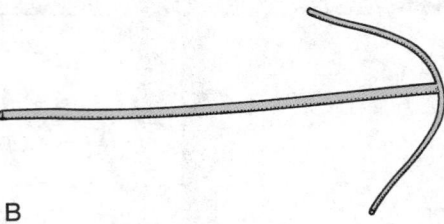
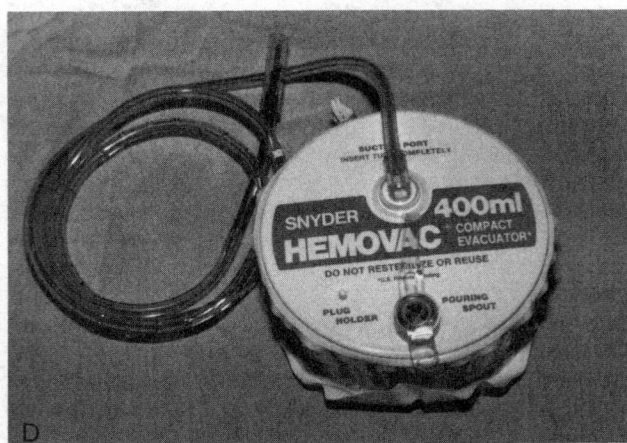

SNYDER HEMOVAC 400ml COMPACT EVACUATOR
DO NOT RESTERILIZE OR REUSE
SUCTION PORT INSERT TUBE COMPLETELY
PLUG HOLDER   POURING SPOUT

Figure 20–5

Types of surgical drains. Gravity drains, such as the Penrose (A) and the T tube (B), drain directly through a tube from the surgical area. In closed wound drainage systems, such as the Jackson-Pratt (C) and Hemovac (D), drainage is into a collecting vessel by means of compression and re-expansion of the system.

after intravenous injection, the nurse assesses the effectiveness of the medication and observes the return of physical behaviors to the client's baseline (see Chap. 7 for further discussion on pain assessment).

Psychosocial Assessment

As the nurse completes the physical aspects of postoperative assessment, the psychologic, social, and cultural characteristics of the client are considered. This assessment may be difficult to do in the PAR if the client is drowsy or incoherent. In assessing the client, the nurse takes into account the client's age, surgical procedure, and impact of the procedure on the client's recovery, body image, and life style. Physical signs that may indicate anxiety include restlessness; increased pulse, blood pressure, and respiratory rate; and crying. The client may be anxious and asking questions related to the results or findings of the surgical procedure. The nurse reassures the client that the surgeon will speak with him/her after the client is fully awake. If the surgeon has already spoken with the client, the nurse reinforces what was said.

Laboratory Findings

Postoperative laboratory tests are performed to monitor the client for complications. Tests are based on the client's surgical procedure, medical history, and postoperative clinical manifestations. Common postoperative tests include serum analysis of electrolytes, glucose, and complete blood count. The frequency and tests performed are individualized according to the client's condition intra- and postoperatively and the surgical procedure. It is not uncommon to see a change in laboratory results (e.g., electrolytes, hematocrit, and hemoglobin) during the first 24 to 48 hours postoperatively as a result of blood loss and the body's reaction to the surgical process. The blood loss will be seen as an increased hematocrit because of plasma concentration. Another common postoperative alteration in laboratory values that is expected is an elevation in the white blood cell count. This change is a direct result of the inflammatory process. Assays of arterial blood gases are performed for clients with a history of respiratory disease, those maintained on a ventilator for a prolonged time postoperatively, and those having had surgery involving the thoracic cavity (see Chaps. 14 and 15 for discussion of arterial blood gases). Urine specific gravity is also assessed postoperatively about every 4 hours for clients at risk of developing dehydration and renal insufficiency.

 Analysis: Nursing Diagnosis

The postoperative period is the longest and most variable of those in the perioperative experience. This pe-

TABLE 20–2   Drugs Used for Pain Management in the Postoperative Client

Drug	Usual Daily Dosage*	Interventions*	Rationales
Merperidine hydrochloride (Demerol)	50–150 mg q 3–4 h PO or IM Maximum 6–8 doses	1. Monitor blood pressure. 2. Move and ambulate client slowly. 3. Monitor pulse rate. 4. Assess for decreased GI motility	1. Causes decreased blood pressure. 2. Causes orthostatic hypotention. 3. Causes bradycardia. 4. Increases incidence of constipation.
Morphine sulfate	5–15 mg IM or IV 30–60 mg q 4 h PO Maximum 6 doses	1. Monitor respiratory status. 2. Monitor blood pressure. 3. Assess for GI motility and urinary output.	1. Causes respiratory depression. 2. Causes hypotension. 3. Increases constipation and urinary retention.
Codeine sulfate	15–60 mg q 4 h IM or PO Maximum 6 doses	1. Monitor respiratory status. 2. Monitor for diet intolerance. 3. Monitor fluid and electrolyte balance. 4. Assess GI motility.	1. Causes respiratory depression. 2, 3. Causes nausea and vomiting. 4. May cause constipation.
Butorphanol tartrate (Stadol)	1–4 mg q 3–4 h IM 0.5–2 mg IV Maximum 6–8 doses	1. Monitor neurologic status and changes in level of consciousness. 2. Monitor respiratory status.	1. May cause increased intracranial pressure. 2. Causes respiratory depression.
Oxycodone hydrochloride and aspirin (Percodan)	1–2 tablets (5–10 mg) q 3–4 h PO Maximum 80 mg	1. Assess GI tolerance of medication. 2. Assess for GI bleeding. 3. Monitor GI motility. 4. Monitor respiratory status. 5. Monitor coagulation studies (PT, PTT).	1. Is irritating to the stomach. 2. May increase bleeding time. 3. Increases chance of constipation. 4. May cause respiratory depression. 5. Acts as a mild anticoagulant.
Oxycodone hydrochloride and acetaminophen (Tylox)	1–2 tablets q 3–4 h PO Maximum 16 tablets	1. Monitor blood pressure and respiratory status. 2. Assess for GI motility.	1. Causes hypotension and respiratory depression. 2. Causes constipation.
Ibuprofen (Motrin)	300–600 mg q 4–6 h PO Maximum 2400 mg daily	1. Monitor upper GI tolerance of medication. 2. Monitor coagulation studies (PT, PTT). 3. Assess for signs of bleeding or delayed clotting.	1. Is irritating to stomach. 2. May increase bleeding time. 3. Has a mild anticoagulant effect.

* GI, gastrointestinal; PT, prothrombin time; PTT, partial thromboplastin time; PO, orally; IM, intramuscularly; IV, intravenously.

riod begins with the client's admission to the PACU and concludes with the client's discharge from the health care facility. The following nursing diagnoses are derived from assessment data with the goal of providing a smooth, complication-free recovery and discharge.

Common Diagnoses

Four nursing diagnoses are common in postoperative clients:

1. Impaired gas exchange related to residual effects of anesthesia, immobility, and pain
2. Impaired skin integrity related to surgical wound healing, drains and drainage, and wound infection
3. Pain related to surgical incision and position during surgery

Additional Diagnoses

In addition to the common diagnoses, the client may present with one or more of the following diagnoses:

1. Fluid volume deficit related to intra- and postoperative fluid loss
2. Ineffective airway clearance related to increased secretions
3. Altered patterns of urinary elimination (decreased) related to anesthetic agents and immobility
4. Bowel incontinence related to anesthesia, surgical manipulation of bowel, and lack of oral intake
5. Activity intolerance related to surgery and prolonged bed rest
6. Potential total self-care deficit related to surgical wound, pain, and/or treatment regimen
7. Knowledge deficit related to lack of information about treatment regimen

 Planning and Implementation ➡

The following plan for the care of the postoperative client focuses on the common nursing diagnoses and prevention of postoperative complications. General concepts of postoperative care are outlined; specific surgical procedures and appropriate care are presented in related chapters of this text.

Impaired Gas Exchange

Planning: client goals. The goal for this diagnosis is that the client will maintain adequate lung expansion and respiratory function.

Interventions. Immediate care by the nurse in the PACU includes positioning the client in a side-lying position or turning the head to the side to prevent aspiration while the client is still anesthetized. The nurse inserts an airway, which pulls and holds the tongue forward to prevent obstruction, and applies suction to prevent blockage of the airway by mucus and/or vomitus. The head of the stretcher or bed is kept flat until the client regains a voluntary gag reflex and to prevent hypotension and possible shock, unless this position is contraindicated by the client's condition or surgical procedure. After head and neck surgery, the head of the bed or stretcher is elevated to promote respiratory function and prevent postoperative edema. Oxygen is administered by the nurse via nasal cannula or mask to facilitate the excretion of inhalation anesthetic agents, increase arterial oxygen levels, and raise the level of consciousness.

After the client regains the voluntary gag reflex, the airway or endotracheal tube is removed. The PACU and floor nurses encourage the client to cough and deep breathe to expand the lungs, promote gas exchange, and hasten the elimination of inhalation anesthesia. The perioperative respiratory care Guidelines Feature in Chapter 18 reviews postoperative breathing exercises and splinting of the surgical wound area as taught to the client. As soon as the client is awake enough to follow commands and throughout the postoperative period, the nurse encourages the client to cough and take deep breaths. The floor nurse instructs the client to perform these respiratory exercises at least 5 to 10 times every 2 hours while awake, especially during the first 72 hours postoperatively. During this time, the client is at greatest risk of developing respiratory complications such as atelectasis and pneumonia. Clients who are at increased risk of developing pulmonary complications, such as those with respiratory disease, elderly clients, and smokers, are encouraged to use an incentive spirometer 5 to 10 times per hour for 48 to 72 hours postoperatively. The use of an incentive spirometer, flow incentive spirometer, "blow bottles," chest physiotherapy, mist inhalation, or intermittent positive-pressure breathing therapy promotes full expansion of the lungs (see Chap. 18, Figs. 18-4 and 18-5). The client who is unable to expectorate mucus or sputum voluntarily requires the help of a nurse or self-suction equipment. The nurse assesses the nasal passages and throat for swelling and irritation that could obstruct the trachea and cause respiratory distress.

Impaired Skin Integrity

Planning: client goals. The goal for this diagnosis is that the client's wound will heal without postoperative wound complications.

Interventions

Nonsurgical management. Postoperative nonsurgical wound care usually includes changing and care of the dressing, assessment of the wound for signs of infection, and care of drains including emptying, measuring, and documenting characteristics of the drainage.

Drug therapy.   Wound infection is a major postoperative complication that results from contamination during surgery, preoperative infection, a break in aseptic technique, or the debilitated state of the client. A client at risk for developing a wound infection is administered prophylactic antibiotic therapy with a broad-spectrum antibiotic or one that is effective in fighting organisms common to the surgical site. These antibiotics are usually given for 24 to 72 hours postoperatively to ensure that adequate antibiotic levels are reached before infection occurs.

Wounds that are infected and left open to heal or wounds that become infected are frequently treated with an antibiotic packing and prolonged systemic antibiotics. The nurse cleans the edges of the wound, loosely packs it with an antibiotic-saturated gauze, and covers the wound with a dry, sterile dressing. The packing promotes healing and débridement of the infected tissue as the wound heals.

Dressings.   In most cases, the first dressing is changed by the surgeon with the assistance of the nurse. The surgeon thus has the opportunity to assess the wound and remove packing and drains from the incision. Before the first dressing change, the nurse reinforces the dressing if it becomes wet from drainage and documents the reinforcement, as well as the color, type, amount, and odor of drainage fluid and time of observation in the client's chart. Dressing changes are ordered by the surgeon. A wet and/or damp dressing is a source of infection if it is not changed. Dressing changes by the nurse are done under aseptic conditions.

Dressings vary depending on the surgical procedure and the surgeon's preference. The standard postoperative dressing consists of gauze or nonadherent pads covered with a larger absorbent pad held in place by tape or Montgomery straps, as seen in Figure 20–6. Wound or suture care usually consists of cleaning the area with povidone-iodine (Betadine), saline, or hydrogen peroxide (H_2O_2). A clean wound may be covered with a transparent plastic surgical dressing or spray, which lasts 3 to 6 days and allows visualization of the wound while preventing contamination. After the first 24 hours, the surgeon may wish to leave the suture or staple line open to the air, which allows for easy assessment of the wound and early detection of poor approximation, drainage, swelling, or redness. Skin sutures or staples are usually removed 6 to 8 days postoperatively, and the incision is secured with Steri-Strips (see Chap. 19, Fig. 19–6).

Drains.   Drains are inserted into the wound or a separate small incision known as a *stab wound* close to the operative site during surgery. The drain provides an exit through which air and fluids such as serum, blood, and bile can be evacuated. See Figure 20–5 for commonly used drains. Drains also prevent deep wound infections and abscess formation within the surgical wound during healing.

The Penrose drain is one type of superficial device that is placed into the external aspect of the incision and drains directly onto the client's dressing and *perisurgical area* (skin around the incision). In caring for a client with a Penrose drain, the nurse changes a damp dressing by cleaning under and around the drain and pads the area distal to the drain with absorbent pads, which prevents skin irritation and contamination of the surgical wound. Care must be taken when cleaning around a drain: it is not sutured in place and can easily be dislodged or accidentally pulled out during a dressing change. The surgeon shortens the drain by pulling it out and removing the excess external portion until drainage stops.

Jackson-Pratt and Hemovac are two commonly used self-contained drainage systems by which the wound drains directly through a tube via gravity, suction, or vacuum. These drains are commonly sutured in place with a pursestring suture that seals the area when the drain is removed. The nurse empties the reservoir of the drain and records the amount and color of drainage every shift or more frequently if ordered by the surgeon. After emptying the reservoir, the nurse secures the drain to the client's gown or pajamas to prevent pulling and stress on the surgical wound.

Surgical management.   If dehiscence occurs, the nurse applies a sterile nonadherent or saline dressing and binder to the wound and notifies the surgeon. In the event of evisceration, the nurse covers the wound with a sterile towel or nonadherent dressing moistened with normal saline. The nurse does not attempt to reinsert the protruding organ or viscera. The nurse monitors the client's vital signs and assesses for possible signs of shock. The client is kept in a supine position with the knees bent and in a quiet area to reduce anxiety. Emotional support is provided by explaining what happened

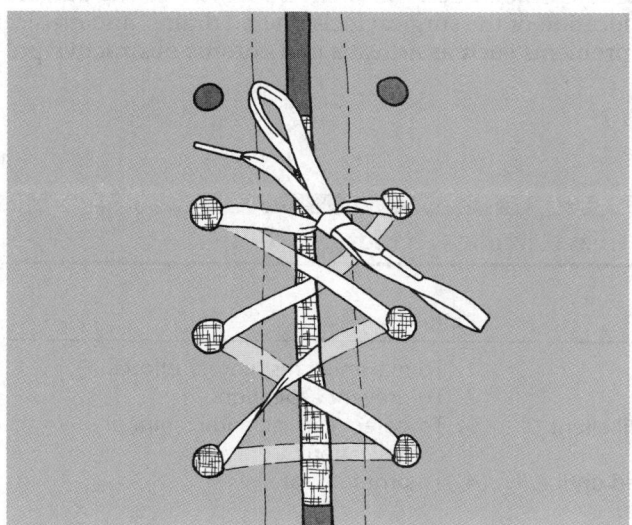

Figure 20–6

Montgomery straps may be used when frequent dressing changes are anticipated. They help to prevent skin irritation from frequent removal of tape.

while reassuring the client that he or she has done nothing wrong to cause the incisional wound to open. The nurse prepares the client for surgery to close the wound. If the client has not been prohibited from taking food and fluids by mouth and the wound is not in the thoracic cavity, spinal anesthesia or local anesthetic is used to prevent postoperative nausea and vomiting, which place undue stress on the already fragile incision. To increase incisional integrity, stay or retention sutures, which are large plastic or metal clamps, are used over the standard suture or staple line (see Chap. 19, Fig. 19-6).

Pain

Planning: client goals. The goal is that the postoperative client will experience alleviation or reduction of pain associated with the surgical wound and positioning during surgery.

Interventions. Postoperative pain management usually includes drug therapy, positioning, relaxation techniques, and distraction. Chapter 7 provides a comprehensive discussion of pain assessment and management.

Drug therapy. Narcotics and nonnarcotics are given immediately postoperatively for acute pain. Narcotics are routinely given during the first 24 to 48 hours after surgery to control pain. Drugs commonly used include meperidine hydrochloride (Demerol), morphine sulfate, codeine sulfate, butorphanol tartrate (Stadol), and oxycodone hydrochloride with aspirin (Percodan) or oxycodone with acetaminophen (Tylox or Percocet). The nurse assesses the type, location, and intensity of the pain before administration of medication. The client's vital signs are monitored closely after administration of narcotics. After extensive surgery (e.g., thoracotomy or amputation) and for clients with low pain tolerance levels, the use of patient-controlled analgesia (PCA) via intravenous or internal pump (the catheter is sutured into or proximal to the surgical area) is being tried as a means of pain control. In patient-controlled analgesia, the rate or dosage of infusion of a narcotic analgesic is adjusted by the client on the basis of the client's pain level and physical response to the drug.

The nurse should use care not to overmedicate or undermedicate the client, especially the elderly client. Elderly or debilitated clients do not tolerate pain medication well because of slower metabolism. In assessing for overmedication, the nurse monitors the client's vital signs, especially blood pressure and respiratory rate, and the level of consciousness. Complications from the use of narcotics include respiratory depression, hypotension, nausea, and vomiting. A narcotic antagonist may be administered to reverse acute effects of narcotic depression (Table 20-3).

As recovery progresses, pain medications are administered in reduced dosages and frequency. Nonnarcotics, such as acetylsalicylic acid (aspirin, Ecotrin), acetaminophen (Tylenol), and nonsteroidal anti-inflammatory drugs such as ibuprofen (Motrin), are used during convalescence or can be given with a narcotic to potentiate the effect of the narcotic (see Table 20-2 on postoperative pain medications). Pain medication administered in the PACU by the nurse is usually given at a low dosage intramuscularly or orally for the ambulatory client.

Other methods of pain control. Comfort measures provided by the nurse may lower the amount of pain medication needed. These measures reduce anxiety and allow the client to relax and rest.

Positioning. In positioning the client, the nurse takes into consideration the client's position during surgery, location of the surgical incision and drains, and medical problems such as arthritis and chronic obstructive pul-

---

TABLE 20-3 Drugs Used to Treat Narcotic Overdose

Drug	Usual Daily Dosage	Interventions	Rationales
Levallorphan tartrate (Lorfan)	0.01 mg/kg IV*	1. Maintain free airway. 2. Have suction available. 3. Monitor vital signs closely until client responds.	1. To maximize respiratory efforts. 2. To prevent aspiration. 3. To detect cardiac and respiratory complications.
Nalorphine (Nalline)	0.1 mg/kg IV	4. Do not leave client unattended until fully responsive.	4. To promote safety.
Naloxone hydrochloride (Narcan)	0.01 mg/kg IV	5. Observe for significant reversal of analgesia.	5. To avoid circulatory stress, nausea, and vomiting, which may be caused by too rapid a reversal.

* Repeat doses as necessary every 2-3 min on the basis of the client's response.

monary disease. The nurse assists the client into a position of comfort in which the client's extremities are supported with pillows or trochanter rolls. No pillows are placed under the client's knees, and the knee gatch of the bed is not raised as this could restrict circulation and increase the risk of thrombophlebitis. The nurse turns or helps the client turn at least every 2 hours while the client is bedridden to prevent stiffness and pulmonary complications of immobility.

On the basis of the surgeon's orders and the nurse's assessment of the client's tolerance, progressively increased activity is initiated to decrease stiffness and promote lung expansion. The nurse assists the client to the side of the bed and into a chair while splinting the surgical wound for support and comfort during transfer.

Massage.   Gentle massage of stiff joints or a sore back by the nurse is a therapeutic measure that is used successfully to decrease postoperative discomfort. Positioning the client in a lateral side-lying position or on the stomach and applying lotion with smooth, gentle strokes increase blood flow to the area and promote general relaxation. The legs, especially the calves, are not massaged because of the increased risk of loosening a thrombus and causing the client to develop a pulmonary embolus, which is a life-threatening situation.

Other measures.   Relaxation and distraction are used to control acute episodes of pain (see the accompanying Nursing Research feature). These techniques are used effectively by the client during painful procedures such as dressing changes and injections. Chapter 7 discusses how the nurse instructs and guides the client through these pain control methods.

■ Discharge Planning

Today, many clients are discharged after a brief hospital stay or directly from the PACU to home. Because of the shortened length of stay, discharge planning, teaching, and referral begin preoperatively and are followed through postoperatively.

Home Care Preparation

If the client is discharged directly to home, the setting must be assessed for safety, cleanliness, and availability of caregivers. The nurse uses the data base that was completed when the client was admitted to the hospital or ambulatory surgical unit to ascertain the client's needs. If, for example, the client is unable or not allowed to walk stairs and lives in a two-story house with only one bathroom located on the second floor, the nurse advises the client to rent a bedside commode. The social worker, in collaboration with the nurse, helps the client identify needs related to postoperative care, including meal preparation, dressing changes, and personal hygiene.

Client/Family Education

The teaching plan for the postoperative client includes (1) prevention of infection, (2) care of surgical

---

NURSING RESEARCH

Listening to Guided Imagery Relaxation Tapes Can Help Reduce Postoperative Anxiety.

Holden-Lund, C. (1988). Effects of relaxation with guided imagery on surgical stress and wound healing. *Research in Nursing and Health, 11,* 235–244.

This experimental study was conducted to determine effects of relaxation with guided imagery audiotapes on the psychophysiologic stress response and wound healing in clients who had a cholecystectomy. The 24 surgical clients were randomly assigned to control and experimental groups (the latter group listened to four tapes, one preoperatively and one on the first three postoperative days). Three indexes of recovery were measured four times: state anxiety, urinary cortisol level, and wound inflammatory response.

The instruments used for data collection were reported as being reliable and valid.

Analysis of variance for repeated measures showed that the experimental group had a significant reduction in state anxiety levels throughout the test periods and at the end of the study. Although differences in urinary cortisol levels and wound inflammatory response were not significant, findings suggested that relaxation with guided imagery may offer benefits in the early postoperative period.

Critique.   The sample was one of convenience and too small to make generalizations to other populations. All but two of the subjects were female.

Possible nursing implications.   Clients should be informed about the potential benefits, especially decreased anxiety, of listening to relaxation tapes. Tapes should be available for clients who desire to use them.

---

wound, (3) diet therapy, (4) drug therapy, and (5) progressive activity. If dressing changes are needed, the client and family are instructed on the importance of proper hand washing to prevent infection. A thorough explanation and demonstration of wound care by the nurse for the client and family, with a subsequent demonstration by the client and family, are necessary to evaluate learning and facilitate compliance after discharge.

After the client is allowed to take food or fluids by mouth, the nurse begins with the introduction of clear liquids as a trial to determine the client's tolerance. The nurse changes the diet slowly toward a regular diet of solid foods according to the client's tolerance.

A diet that is high in protein and calories promotes wound healing. A dietary consultation before the client is discharged can help the client to select a balanced diet plan to promote healing (see the accompanying Health Promotion/Maintenance feature). Vitamin C, iron, and multivitamins are often prescribed after surgery for

---

HEALTH PROMOTION/MAINTENANCE ■ Postoperative Dietary Progression

Diet	Approximate Time Started Postoperatively	Food Permitted
Sips	Immediate	Ice chips, sips of water
Clear liquid	4–24 h	Gelatin, broth, clear juices, tea
Full liquid	8–48 h	Creamed soup, milk, custard, ice cream
Soft	1–3 d	Breads, cereal, chicken, lean meat, fruit without skin
Regular	1–4 d	All foods including pork, cheese, and raw vegetables
Convalescence	After discharge	All foods, but especially foods high in protein and calories and sources of vitamin C and iron

---

wound healing and should be taken for 10 to 14 days postoperatively. The nurse instructs clients with dietary restrictions because of surgery or previous medical problems about the importance of following the prescribed diet during convalescence. Elderly or debilitated clients are encouraged to continue using dietary supplements between meals until the wound is completely healed and the client's energy level is restored.

The nurse instructs clients about taking pain medication, with special attention to proper dose and frequency of administration. The nurse instructs the client to notify the surgeon if the medication does not control the pain or if the pain suddenly increases. If antibiotics or other medications are prescribed the client is instructed to take the entire prescription as ordered by the surgeon.

Surgery stresses the body, and time and rest are required for healing. The nurse instructs the client to increase the activity level slowly, plan rest periods, and avoid placing a strain on or around the surgical wound. Depending on the type of surgery and the client's occupation, the surgeon decides when the client may return to work. A client whose work involves a moderate amount of physical labor may be allowed back to work 6 weeks after abdominal surgery.

Psychosocial Preparation

Clients are usually apprehensive about postoperative complications and pain; thus, it is important that the nurse allay their fears. The more extensive the surgical procedure, the more afraid clients are of assuming self-care. The nurse provides support to the client and family as they make discharge plans. The client whose surgical procedure has left visible scars requires more emotional support from the family for acceptance (see Chap. 9 for further discussion of body image). The client may express anger related to the surgical outcome or to the temporary or permanent role change and concern about financial matters and work.

Health Care Resources

After returning home, the client may need equipment and assistance with dressing changes, activities of daily living, and meal preparation. Referral to a home care agency is made and paid for by most third-party insurance payers and Medicare as long as the client is homebound and requires skilled care. The home care nurse provides dressing supplies, education in self-care, and referrals for services as needed by the client. Such referrals include Meals on Wheels, support groups, and homemaker services (e.g., house cleaning and food shopping).

 Evaluation

On the basis of the identified nursing diagnoses, the nurse evaluates the care for the postoperative client. The expected outcomes for the postoperative client include that the client

1. Maintains adequate lung expansion and respiratory function as evidenced by clear breath sounds
2. Complies with a high-protein and high-caloric diet
3. Describes and demonstrates care of dressings and drains
4. Has complete wound healing without complications
5. States that pain is reduced or alleviated

By meeting the stated desired outcomes, the recovery period of the postoperative client should reduce the likelihood of postoperative complications. As a result, anxiety and fear are decreased, and a smooth recovery with return to the client's normal life style is likely.

SUMMARY

The perioperative experience subjects the client to psychologic and physiologic stress regardless of the surgical procedure. Close monitoring of the client in the PACU and early implementation of preoperative education (turning, coughing, and deep breathing) by the nurse facilitate a complication-free recovery. The plan of care for the postoperative client includes ongoing assessment and education of the client about his or her surgical procedure, medication, diet, and activity during the recovery period.

IMPLICATIONS FOR RESEARCH

A reduced length of postoperative hospital stay and an increased number of ambulatory surgical procedures provide a challenge for the PACU and floor nurse in planning and implementing client care. Questions about the effects of shortened postoperative stay and older and sicker clients are areas requiring nursing research and interventions to maintain quality care in all clinical settings. In considering these areas for research, the following questions are appropriate:

1. How have ambulatory surgery and reduced length of stay affected readmission for postoperative complications?
2. How do the client and family perceive governmental mandates about surgical procedures and length of postoperative stay?
3. What nursing interventions are most effective for promoting wound healing in elderly or debilitated clients?
4. What is the most effective postoperative respiratory regimen for the prevention of pulmonary complications in the high-risk client?
5. What is the most effective noninvasive pain control technique for the postoperative client?

REFERENCES AND READINGS

Andrews, D. R., & Taylor, C. (1985). Documenting post-anesthesia recovery. *American Journal of Nursing, 85,* 290–291.

Ashby, D. M. (1987). Balancing fluids and electrolytes in the PACU. *Journal of Post Anesthesia Nursing, 2,* 114–116.

Barrett, J. E. (1985). Helping your post-op patient breathe easier with incentive spirometry. *Nursing '85, 15*(10), 64.

Brown, S. L. (1986). Pulmonary aspiration in the postanesthetic period. *Journal of Post Anesthesia Nursing, 1,* 87–91.

Brozenec, S. (1985). Caring for the postoperative patient with an abdominal drain. *Nursing '85, 15*(4), 54–57.

Burge, S. (1986). How painful are postop incisions? *American Journal of Nursing, 86,* 1263A, 1266D, 1266H.

Burton, F. (1984). Back to basics: Controlling postoperative infection. *Nursing '84, 14*(9), 43.

Cerrato, P. L. (1988). What diet does for wound healing. *RN, 51*(6), 73–76.

Coleman, L. G. (1983). Noise and pain in the immediate post-op period. *American Journal of Nursing, 83,* 1021.

Croushorn, T. M. (1979). Postoperative assessment: The key to avoiding the most common nursing mistakes. *Nursing '79, 9*(4), 47–50.

Curtin, L. (1984). Wound management: Care and cost—an overview. *Nursing Management, 15,* 22–25.

Cuzzell, J. Z. (1988). The new RYB color code. *American Journal of Nursing, 88,* 1342–1346.

Deters, G. E. (1987). Managing complications after abdominal surgery. *RN, 50*(3), 27–32.

Drain, C. B. (1984). Managing postoperative pain: It's a matter of signs. *Nursing '84, 14*(8), 52–55.

Drain, C. B., & Christoph, S. S. (1987). *The recovery room: A critical care approach to post anesthesia nursing* (2nd ed.). Philadelphia: W. B. Saunders.

Faherty, B. S., & Grier, M. R. (1982). Analgesic medication for elderly people post-surgery. *Nursing Research, 33,* 369–372.

Farr, L. A., Campbell-Grossman, C., & Mack, J. M. (1988). Circadian disruption and surgical recovery. *Nursing Research, 37,* 170–175.

Fay, M. F. (1987). Drainage systems: Their role in wound healing. *AORN Journal, 46,* 442–455.

Feeley, T. W. (1985). The design and staffing of a modern recovery room. *Current Review of Recovery Room Nurses, 7*(18), 143–146, 148.

Feldman, M. E. (1988). Inadvertent hypothermia: A threat to homeostasis in the postanesthetic patient. *Journal of Post Anesthesia Nursing, 3,* 82–87.

Fraulini, K. E., & Borchardt, A. C. (1988). Guide to solving postanesthesia problems. *Nursing '88, 18*(5), 66–86.

Fraulini, K. E., & Murphy, P. (1984). R.E.A.C.T., a new system for measuring postanesthesia recovery. *Nursing '84, 14*(4), 101.

Frost, E. A. M. (1985). *Recovery room practice.* Boston: Blackwell Scientific.

Gioella, E. C., & Bevil, C. W. (1985). *Nursing care of the aging client: Promoting healthy adaptation.* Norwalk, CT: Appleton-Century-Crofts.

Gould, D. (1985). Measuring recovery. *Nursing Mirror, 160*(13), 17–18.

Gray-Vickrey, M. (1987). Color them special: A sensible, sensitive guide to caring for elderly patients. *Nursing '87, 17*(5), 59–62.

Grennan, A. J. (1987). Helping your patient get his strength back . . . first few days at home. *RN, 50*(3), 70, 72.

Hardy, E. B., Cirillo, B. C., & Gutzeit, N. M. (1988). Rewarming patients in the PACU: Can we make a difference? *Journal of Post Anesthesia Nursing, 3,* 313–316.

Hogan, P., & Bell, S. (1986). How to handle postanesthetic hypertension. *Nursing '86, 16*(5), 58–63.

Kneedler, J. A., & Dodge, G. H. (1983). *Perioperative patient care: The nursing perspective.* Boston: Blackwell Scientific.

Latz, P. A., & Wyble, S. J. (1987). Elderly patients: Perioperative nursing implications. *AORN Journal, 46,* 238–253.

Leyder, B. L., & Pieper, B. (1986). Identifying discharge concerns: A study. *AORN Journal, 43,* 1298–1302.

Litwack, K., & Parnass, S. (1988). Practical points in the management of postoperative nausea and vomiting. *Journal of Post Anesthesia Nursing, 3,* 275–277.

Luce, J. M. (1984). Clinical risk factors for postoperative pulmonary complications. *Respiratory Care, 29,* 484–495.

Luczun, M. E. (1984). *Postanesthesia nursing: A comprehensive guide.* Rockville, MD: Aspen Systems.

McCaffery, M. (1985). Narcotic analgesia for the elderly. *American Journal of Nursing, 85,* 296–298.

Meckes, P. F. (1984). Perioperative care of the elderly patient. *Today's OR Nurse, 6,* 8–15.

Montanari, J. (1985). Documenting your postop assessment findings: A new form you can use. *Nursing'85, 15*(8), 31–35.

Montanari, J. (1986). Action STAT! wound dehiscence. *Nursing '86, 16*(2), 33.

Neuberger, G. B. (1987). Wound care: What's clear, what's not. *Nursing '85, 17*(2), 34–37.

Neuberger, G. B., & Reckling, J. B. (1985). A new look at wound care. *Nursing '85, 15*(2), 34–42.

O'Connor, F. W. (1987). Increasing surgical teaching. *Community Nursing Research, 20,* 23–28.

Patras A. Z., & Brozenec, S. A. (1984). Gastrointestinal assessment: Identifying significant problems. *AORN Journal, 40,* 726–731.

Pierce, S. F., & Campbell, M. (1988). Return of bladder function: A research study. *AORN Journal, 47,* 702–703, 706–712.

Podjasek, J. H. (1985). Which postop patient faces the greatest respiratory risk? *RN, 48*(9), 44–53.

Seidman, C. B. (1986). Action STAT: Malignant hyperthermia. *Nursing '86, 16*(9), 33.

Sherman, M. (1985). Thrombophylaxis with antiembolism stockings. *Orthopedic Nursing, 4*(4), 33–37.

Stickley, M., Jenkins, P. M., & Stebbins, K. (1988). Postoperative blood pressure patterns in people 12 to 30 years old. *Journal of Post Anesthesia Nursing, 3,* 332–335.

Stroud, M. D. (1986). Assessing the elderly PACU patient. *Journal of Post Anesthesia Nursing, 1,* 107–111.

Taylor, D. L. (1988). The healing process: From the inside out. *Nursing '88, 18*(6), 36–67.

Treloar, D. M. (1984). When a surgical wound bursts. *RN, 47*(6), 26–30.

Vogelsang, J. (1987). Nursing interventions to reduce patient anxiety: Visitors in the PACU. *Journal of Post Anesthesia Nursing, 2,* 25–31.

Wetchler, B. V. (1985). Postanesthesia scoring system: Discharging ambulatory surgery patients. *AORN Journal, 41,* 382–384.

Young, M. E. (1987). Fever in the postoperative patient. *Focus on Critical Care, 14*(2), 13–18.

UNIT 5 RESOURCES

Nursing Resources

American Association of Nurse Anesthetists (AANA), 216 Higgins Road, Park Ridge, IL 60068. Telephone 312-692-7050.

Represents Certified Registered Nurse Anesthetists (CRNAs) nationally. Offers educational workshops at conventions and regional meetings. Represents CRNAs before Congress. Promotes public education about anesthesia. Publishes *AANA Journal.*

American Board of Post-Anesthesia Nursing Certification, c/o Professional Examination Service, 475 Riverside Drive, New York, NY 10115.

Certifies nurses with experience in postanesthesia nursing.

American Society of Plastic and Reconstructive Surgical Nurses (ASPRSN), North Woodbury Road, PO Box 56, Pitman, NJ 08071. Telephone 609-589-6247.

See Unit 12 Resources for more information.

American Society of Post Anesthesia Nurses (ASPAN), 11508 Allecingie Parkway, Suite C, Richmond, VA 23235. Telephone 804-379-5516.

Represents nurses involved in all phases of postanesthesia care. Promotes high standards for the specialty and professional growth for its members. Publishes the *Journal of Post Anesthesia Nursing* (bimonthly), *Breathline* (bimonthly), *Standards of Nursing Practice,* a certification review text, and other materials.

Association of Operating Room Nurses (AORN), 10170 East Mississippi Avenue, Denver, CO 80231. Telephone 303-755-6300.

Promotes the concept of perioperative nursing as the role of the nurse practicing in the operating room. Enhances knowledge, skills, and performance of perioperative nurses. Promotes increased awareness of socioeconomic and governmental influences in nursing. Maintains cooperative relationships with other professional organizations. Evaluates existing practices and new developments in operating room nursing and education.

Council on Certification of Nurse Anesthetists, 216 Higgins Road, Park Ridge, IL 60068. Telephone 312-692-7050.

Certifies and recertifies nurse anesthetists.

National Certification Board, Perioperative Nursing, 1151 South Galena Street, Denver, CO 80231. Telephone 303-369-9566.

Certifies perioperative nurses.

Plastic Surgical Nursing Certification Board, North Woodbury Road, PO Box 56, Pitman, NJ 08071. Telephone 609-589-6247.

Certifies nurses in plastic surgical nursing.

UNIT 6

Management of Clients with Chronic Illnesses

CHAPTER 21

Assessment of Clients with Disabling or Chronic Conditions

OVERVIEW

The health care industry is driven by market demands. Thus, the professional nurse must prepare to respond to social changes attributable to demographic, socioeconomic, scientific, and political factors. These developments result in changes in the health care delivery system, and nursing, as a major component of every health care system, must be ready to adjust as needed.

The clientele for rehabilitation nursing is changing and expanding. For example, because of advancements in technology, a person who sustains extensive multiple-system injuries has a better chance of survival and thus a need for rehabilitation. For the nurse as well as the individual client, the issue becomes the functional abilities of the individual. After experiencing a brain or spinal cord injury, the client initially is dependent on the nurse for almost all aspects of his/her life. The nurse's role is to assist clients to resume physical and psychosocial control of their lives. The nurse also facilitates clients' reintegration into their families and communities.

All members of our society, regardless of age, physical or cognitive ability, and socioeconomic level, have the right and responsibility to remain within the mainstream of society. The presence of a chronic or disabling condition should not limit social participation. Nurses must facilitate the process of allowing these clients to remain in (or rejoin) the social mainstream and maintain an optimal standard of living.

WHO ARE THE DISABLED?

The term *illness* implies an actual or threatened imbalance or disruption in a person's ability to carry out usual activities. Acute illness is of sudden onset and may require urgent attention to prevent grave or long-term consequences. A condition lasting longer than 6 months or with frequent recurrence may be considered chronic. Chronic diseases include all impairments or pathologic deviations characterized by one or more of the following:

1. Duration for longer than 6 months
2. Residual disability
3. Nonreversible pathologic alteration as cause
4. Need for special training of the patient in rehabilitation
5. Expectation that a long period of supervision, observation, or care will be required (Mayo, 1956)

Chronic disease is America's primary health problem. Approximately 50% of the population (110 million people) have one or more chronic illnesses, and nearly 32.4 million people have limitations in performing self-care activities (U.S. Bureau of the Census, 1986). Coronary artery disease, cancer, arthritis, and spinal cord injury are among the common chronic conditions that may result in varying degrees of disability.

Miller (1983) described two general attributes of chronic illness: (1) impaired function in more than one system and (2) related demands or consequences for the individual or family that may not be completely eliminated. The duration of altered function depends on the nature of the illness and the systems affected. Alterations may be related to mobility, sensory perception, cognition, social skills, and self-care activity.

Accidents are the leading cause of death among Americans under the age of 45 years and the third leading cause of death in those 45 to 54 years of age (National Center for Health Statistics, 1985). There are, however, increasing numbers of survivors of accidents today. Those survivors are often faced with chronic or disabling conditions; thus, the need for rehabilitative programs, as well as possibly months to years of follow-up after the individual returns to the community, is on the rise.

Rehabilitation is the process of learning to live with disability. The term rehabilitation is commonly associated with disabilities related to trauma. However, rehabilitation is not limited to the restoration of function in posttraumatic situations. It can be applied to education and therapy for any chronic illness characterized by altered system function or structure. Rehabilitation related to respiratory, cardiac, or oncologic disorders represents common rehabilitation programs that do not involve trauma. All of these programs involve the restoration of the client to the fullest physical, mental, social, vocational, and economic capacity.

In any discussion of rehabilitation it is important to define and differentiate among the terms impairment, disability, and handicap. These terms have been used interchangeably in some settings; however, for this chapter, the terms are defined according to the *International Classifications of Impairments, Disabilities and Handicaps* (World Health Organization, 1980).

Impairment is an abnormality of a body structure or structures or an alteration in a system function resulting from any cause. Impairments can be temporary or permanent and may or may not be associated with an active pathologic condition. *Disability* is the consequence of an impairment. It is usually described in terms of altered functional ability of the client. A variety of disease conditions impair mobility (see the accompanying Key Features of Disease). The clinical consequences of motor impairment vary with the disease process. Many diseases result in several types of malfunction.

A *handicap* is the disadvantage experienced by an individual as a result of impairments and disabilities. This disadvantage is based on interactions that the client experiences with the environment. Handicaps are associated with the values that an individual or society ascribes to the individual's situation or experience. Handicaps reflect a disturbance between performance and expectations. Although impairments caused by pathologic changes in a body organ and the resulting disabilities are often unpreventable or irreversible, handicaps are both preventable and reversible. The nurse works with the client to assess the client's value systems, roles, and needs, and to plan and develop goals to facilitate the client's re-integration into the family and the community after trauma or disease.

PROBLEMS OF LIVING WITH A CHRONIC ILLNESS

Strauss et al. (1984) described a model for the study of chronic illness. This interactional model analyzed how well the chronically ill client adjusts and interacts with family members. The model included biologic, social, emotional, and economic aspects of illness. Strauss et al. (1984) identified seven problems of living with chronic illness: (1) managing crises, (2) managing regimens, (3) controlling symptoms, (4) dealing with the lack of money to pay for treatments, (5) managing the trajectory, (6) managing social isolation, and (7) normalizing.

Managing crises involves almost total delegation of control to others. This can be damaging to the client's self-concept.

Managing regimens involves the nurse in teaching clients the regimens for care. The timing of interventions (such as when to irrigate a colostomy), mechanisms for coping with side effects of drugs, pain management, and use of equipment for treatment must be considered.

Controlling symptoms may include redesigning the approach to activities. The client will have to discover the limitations that disease symptoms impose on certain activities to accept the consequences of the disease.

Treatments for any illness can be costly, and clients often have limited financial resources to pay for them.

Managing the trajectory involves coping with the general pattern of the chronic condition. The progression of some illnesses is predictable, but that of diseases such as multiple sclerosis cannot be anticipated. The trajectory is not merely a reflection of what is happening physiologically for the client, but is linked with the course of the disease.

Managing social isolation refers to how the client deals with the tendency to withdraw from society, and the tendency of society to withdraw from the chronically ill person.

Normalizing occurs when clients accept their new identity and when the impairment is not intrinsic to relationships with others. The new identities and relationships are based on interactional experiences that result in realistic role expectations and new rules of conduct. Strauss et al. (1984) asserted that each of the problems of living with chronic illness relates to established interaction patterns. Normalization involves maintaining normal behavior and an optimal level of functioning within the limits imposed by the chronic condition. Clients with a chronic condition do not focus on the illness; the emphasis is on whether they are con-

KEY FEATURES OF DISEASE ■ Pathophysiology and Clinical Consequences of Selected Conditions That Impair Mobility

Condition	Pathophysiology	Clinical Consequences
Cranial Lesions or Diseases		
Cerebrovascular accident	Cerebral thrombosis embolus, intracerebral hemorrhage, or subarachnoid hemorrhage.	Depending on site of lesion—hemiparesis; loss of sensation, loss of consciousness; aphasia; paralysis of contralateral face, arm, and leg; vertigo; apraxia; agnosia; or cerebral edema.
Tumor	Invasion and destruction of cranial tissue or secondary effects of increased intracranial pressure.	Increased intracranial pressure, seizures, and endocrine abnormalities.
Degenerative Central Nervous System Disorders		
Multiple sclerosis	Progressive disease of unknown cause, resulting from myelin degeneration of the white matter in the brain and spinal cord.	Depending on part of CNS attacked, weakness of extremity, incoordination, nystagmus, ataxia, or spastic paralysis.
Parkinsonism	Extrapyramidal tract disease of unknown cause; it may be caused by a virus or metabolic disorder and results in nerve cell loss.	Tremor, dyskinesia (impaired voluntary movement), bradykinesia (slowed voluntary movement), muscular rigidity, and accelerated gait (festination).
Traumatic Disorders		
Spinal cord injury	Partial or complete spinal cord injury.	For 1–6 wk, spinal shock with loss of somatic sensation, visceral sensation, motor function, and reflex activity from the level of injury downward. Flaccid paralysis at this time is due to decreased neuronal activity within the cord. After 3–6 wk, reflex activity usually returns, with an increase in tone and reflexes that evolve into a spastic paralysis. The person with quadriplegia also has great potential for life-threatening respiratory problems.
Neuromuscular Disorders		
Myasthenia gravis	Failure of the transmission of nerve impulses to second-order neurons because of blockages or destruction. Cause unknown; believed to be autoimmune disease.	Depends on the muscles involved. If oscular, ptosis and diplopia occur. Possible dysarthria, nasal voice, and weakening of facial musculature. Weakness of trunk and extremities.
Muscular dystrophy	Types vary in age of onset and muscles affected. All are hereditary. The muscle fibers of dystrophic muscles vary from small to large. Internal structure of individual fibers is deranged.	Weakness of affected muscles; certain types have a mental retardation component.

Data from Wilson, S. F. (1979). *Neuronursing*. New York: Springer.

sidered well or disabled. The disabled person is not exempted from ordinary social responsibilities and should not be insulated from the well population.

THEORIES AND PHILOSOPHIES OF REHABILITATION

POWERLESSNESS THEORY

Powerlessness is a perception that one's own action will not and cannot affect an outcome. The client perceives a lack of control over a situation. Miller (1983) applied the concept of powerlessness to clients with chronic conditions. Powerlessness can be thought of as the client's perceived inability to be involved in or influence self-care and quality of life. Because complete alleviation of symptoms and cure may not be realistic goals for the chronically ill client, the focus on alleviating powerlessness and enhancing quality of life is an appropriate nursing goal.

Miller (1983) suggested that chronically ill persons have deficits in one or several power resources (Fig.

21–1). When one or more power resources are compromised, the client has difficulty coping with problems. If nurses can aid the client in restoring power resources, the quality of life for the client can be enhanced and powerlessness can be alleviated.

In Figure 21–1, physical strength and reserve refers both to the individual's ability for optimal physical functioning and to endurance. Psychologic stamina refers to a unique resiliency present in human beings. Positive self-concept refers to positive thoughts and feelings about one's self. Energy is an active force that enables one to be capable of doing work, or it can be stored. Energy sources include nutrients and water, rest, and motivation. Knowledge (insight) is the ability to use information to learn about what is happening to one's self and is an enabling factor for the client to control his/her destiny. Motivation is the development of the client's sense of control over self and environment. The belief system entails the presence of faith and hope, which may have therapeutic results.

The nurse modifies the environment to facilitate the client's functioning, helps the client set realistic goals, and increases the client's knowledge. The nurse also assists the client in developing the power resources of physical strength, stamina (including establishing or relying on a support network), positive self-concept, knowledge, and motivation to alleviate powerlessness in the client.

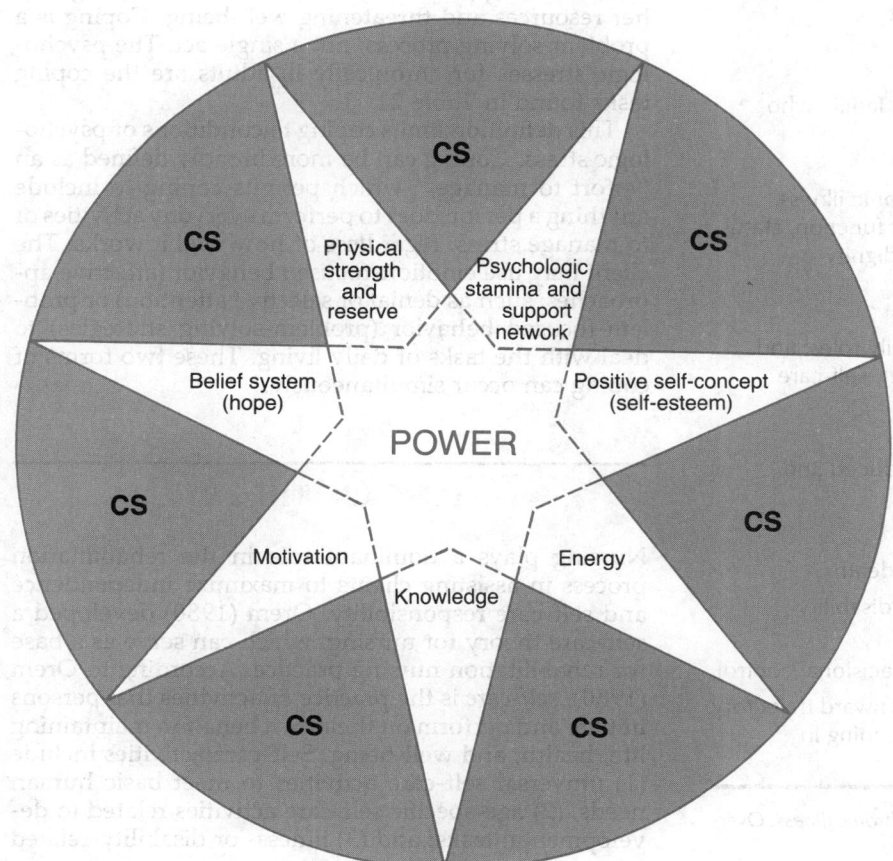

Figure 21–1

Client power resources. CS indicates an individual's unique coping strategies, which are used when resources are compromised. (From Miller, J. M. [1983]. *Coping with chronic illness: Overcoming powerlessness.* Philadelphia: F. A. Davis.)

ADAPTATION THEORY

Adaptation is defined as the ability to accommodate to change. Human beings demonstrate this ability constantly. This accommodation requires energy, motivation, and psychologic support. When assessing the adaptation potential of a client, the nurse should be aware of several factors, including previous experiences of the client in adapting to significant change, the meaning that change holds for the client as an individual, the inner energy the client has at his/her disposal at this

TABLE 21-1 **Coping Tasks of Chronically Ill Adults**

Maintaining a sense of normalcy
    Hiding or minimizing the illness and responding to the
      curious inquiries of others
    Living as normally as possible, despite daily therapy and
      obvious symptoms

Modifying daily routine and adjusting one's life style
    Including therapy and symptom control in daily routine
    Providing for safety

Obtaining knowledge and skill for continuing self-care
    Developing internal awareness
    Monitoring the effects of therapy

Maintaining a positive concept of self
    Integrating illness into one's self-concept
    Maintaining or enhancing self-esteem

Adjusting to altered social relationships
    Preserving relationships with friends and family who
      satisfy dependency needs
    Maintaining family solidarity

Grieving over losses concomitant with chronic illness
    Adjusting to the loss of physical abilities, function, status,
      income, social relationships, roles, or dignity
    Dealing with financial losses

Dealing with role change
    Adjusting to losing social, work, and family roles; and
      gaining roles as dependent help-seeker, self-care
      agent, and chronically ill client

Handling physical discomfort
    Dealing with discomfort that is illness induced and
      therapy induced

Complying with prescribed regimen

Confronting the inevitability of one's own death

Dealing with the social stigma of illness or disability

Maintaining a feeling of being in control
    Maintaining cognitive, behavioral, and decisional control

Maintaining hope despite uncertain or downward trajectory
    Looking at the effects of hope and its meaning in
      physical changes

Adapted from Miller, J. M. (1983). *Coping with chronic illness: Overcoming powerlessness.* Philadelphia: F. A. Davis.

particular time, and the willingness of the client to initiate or implement the change in behavior or beliefs that may accompany the adaptation process. The nurse must determine if the client possesses the ability to adjust as a first step in the assessment. This may indicate to the nurse the need for more sensitive listening and interpretation of client statements.

The nurse must be aware that major adaptive tasks may include coping with pain and becoming comfortable in the environment of the rehabilitation setting. Establishing a trusting nurse-client relationship during rehabilitation can be stressful for the client. In addition to developing new relationships with staff, the client also has to work on maintaining relationships with family and friends and preparing for an uncertain future.

COPING THEORY

The client with a chronic illness relies on the nurse for assistance in facing the problems of living with chronic disease. Chronically ill adults confront many coping tasks (Table 21-1).

The more coping tasks confronting the client, the greater is the likelihood that powerlessness will occur. Lazarus and Folkman (1984) defined *coping* in terms of psychologic stress theory. Psychologic stress is a particular relationship between the person and the environment that is appraised by the person as exceeding his/her resources and threatening well-being. Coping is a problem-solving process, not a single act. The psychologic stresses for chronically ill adults are the coping tasks found in Table 21-1.

This definition limits coping to conditions of psychologic stress. Coping can be more broadly defined as an "effort to manage," which permits coping to include anything a person does to perform everyday activities or to manage stress, regardless of how well it works. The client may use emotion-focused behavior (affective approaches, such as denial or selective attention) or problem-focused behavior (problem-solving strategies) to deal with the tasks of daily living. These two forms of coping can occur simultaneously.

SELF-CARE THEORY

Nursing plays a dominant role in the rehabilitation process in assisting clients to maximize independence and self-care responsibility. Orem (1980) developed a self-care theory for nursing, which can serve as a base for rehabilitation nursing practice. According to Orem (1980), *self-care* is the practice of activities that persons initiate and perform on their own behalf in maintaining life, health, and well-being. Self-care activities include (1) universal self-care activities to meet basic human needs, (2) age-specific self-care activities related to developmental tasks; and (3) illness- or disability-related self-care activities to prevent or regulate the effects of deviation from normal body structure or healthy functioning.

The role of the nurse involves assisting clients to maximize their performance of self-care activities. The nurse assesses the self-care deficits of the client to apply appropriate nursing interventions. The nurse also determines the client's self-care demands and abilities. A deviation between demand and ability indicates that nursing interventions are needed. The nurse calculates the self-care deficit and intervenes by acting directly or by guiding, supporting, or teaching the client. The nurse then evaluates the client's movement toward health.

BODY IMAGE THEORY

Body image is a term used in many different ways. Body image has been linked with self-esteem and self-concept. Schilder (1935) defined body image as the picture of one's own body that is formed in that individual's mind. This image results from the interaction of the perception and experience pool. Perceptions consist of a person's past and present sensory impressions, and the experience includes past and present memories, events, and activities.

Individuals are continually modifying their body images as new perceptions and experiences are encountered. In addition, one's body image is influenced by how others react to one's appearance. For example, if a disabled person is subjected to job discrimination, he/she may acquire a negative body image.

Body image is part of self-concept, although the terms can be used synonymously. How well defined a person's body image has become, including the foundation of self-identity established in early childhood, affects the positiveness of the self-concept. Body image develops over time, but is altered by a debilitating illness.

The nurse must assess alterations in the body image of the chronically ill client. Factors that should be considered when assessing the client include the client's developmental level, effects of treatment, the visibility of the affected body part, the functional significance of the body part involved, and the feasibility of rehabilitation. A change in body image attributable to illness or disability represents a loss for the client undergoing rehabilitation. After assessing the body image changes resulting from a chronic or disabling condition, the nurse can design interventions to help the client cope with the alteration.

FAMILY THEORY

The concept of family theory asserts that the individual is a member of a dynamic family unit. The nurse can use the systems approach to family evaluation. The systems approach considers that a group is greater than the sum of its parts and that the parts are interrelated. Any change in any of the individual members or in the family's environment has an impact on all of the members and the family as a whole. Families, like all living beings, have life cycles and are affected by situational crises. This theory has great significance for the nurse, reinforcing the concept that nursing actions affect not only the individual, but also the family. It further suggests that the family as a unit may also need professional nursing care.

The family system has interactions with the health care system that facilitate input and output to the health care system. When a family member becomes chronically ill, the family system must become open to nursing interventions. The nurse's ability to communicate with the family determines whether the interventions are successful and therapeutic. The family system is also viewed as part of the health care team.

The nurse should assess the client and family as a unit. The manner in which the family responds to the disability affects the adjustment of the client. Basic assessment and observations of the family should include whether the family is functional or dysfunctional. The nurse determines how decisions are made in the family, who is the spokesperson, and how the family usually copes with crises. The nurse analyzes family structure and roles. Structural assessment includes determining the communication patterns and the problem-solving skills of the family. Family assessment for long-term planning focuses on the status and role of the disabled person in the family and the family's economic status.

REHABILITATION AS PART OF THE HEALTH CARE DELIVERY SYSTEM

Chapter 4 presents an overview of the health care delivery system in the United States and assesses its impact on medical-surgical nursing practice. How does rehabilitation fit into the system?

The typical client hospitalized in an acute care facility remains hospitalized for up to 7 days. After an acute condition has been stabilized or reversed, the client is discharged to continue the healing process outside the hospital, generally under the follow-up care of a non-hospital health care provider, such as a family physician. The nurse uses home care preparation, client and family education, psychosocial preparation, and various health care resources to help the client resume her/his normal role in society.

However, some conditions require the intermediate step of rehabilitation, which can take place in a number of settings. The nurse's coordination of care from the acute care setting through the extended care period and the continuity of care are critical to the success of rehabilitation.

SETTINGS FOR REHABILITATION

Freestanding rehabilitation hospitals, in which the client is usually hospitalized for 2 to 3 months, and *outpatient hospital rehabilitation departments* are the most common settings for the delivery of rehabilitation services. Although it appears that the government will continue to support such traditional rehabilitation institutions, efforts to contain soaring medical costs may reduce funding for these facilities. As an alternative, support for such model programs as treatment in burn centers, spinal cord injury centers, and independent living centers, may be established. Funding of these specialized facilities will depend on their effectiveness.

Independent living centers are facilities in which clients live independently, but together with other disabled adults. Each client usually has a care provider, such as an aide, to assist with activities of daily living (ADL). The client may or may not be employed. The goal of these centers is to provide for independent living arrangements outside an institution. Their success will be determined in the future by the magnitude of funds appropriated and the enactment of legislation mandating the financial support of such services.

Vocational rehabilitation is becoming as important as physical rehabilitation, and it will soon become a priority by law. Legislation regarding worker's compensation, Social Security, and disability compensation has a major impact on vocational rehabilitation programs.

Home care with assistance to the client is also an option during rehabilitation.

THE REHABILITATION TEAM

The personnel involved in the care of a client desiring rehabilitation must consider the client as a whole person, rather than treating a specific illness or disability. Thus, successful rehabilitation is dependent on the coordinated effort of a group of health care professionals and the involvement of the client in planning and implementing care.

The rehabilitation team is concerned with two basic aims: prevention of injury and restoration of function.

Prevention includes maintaining activity levels to forestall deterioration of an unaffected organ or part and eliminating possible hazards or factors that may contribute to further injury. Prevention is a continuous aspect of care for the chronically ill patient. For example, meticulous skin care is necessary to prevent pressure ulcer formation.

The other major aim of the rehabilitation team is *restoration* of as much function as possible to the injured or diseased part.

The interdisciplinary team members in the rehabilitation setting include physicians, nurses, physical therapists, occupational therapists, speech pathologists, recreational therapists, aides, social workers, psychologists, vocational counselors, the clients themselves, and family members.

Collaboration is the basis for the team effort. The team works together toward the goal of rehabilitating the client to her/his highest functional level and preventing regression or injury. This collaboration results in a greater level of professional satisfaction for all team members. More importantly, it increases the potential for successful rehabilitation. Although the *physician* is the team leader, the *client* has final authority regarding treatment plans and interventions.

The *nurse* is a pivotal member of the team, especially in the coordination of the efforts of team members. Nursing is the diagnosis and treatment of human responses to actual or potential health problems. In clients undergoing rehabilitation, these health problems are characterized by an altered functional ability and a diminished quality of life. The goal of rehabilitation nursing is to assist the client in the restoration and maintenance of maximal health. The rehabilitation nurse must be innovative and exhibit perseverance in helping the client regain independence.

Depending on the needs of the client and the resources available, the nurse may assume an independent or an interdependent role. In the independent role, the nurse has the responsibility for the provision and coordination of all services (e.g., client education, discharge planning, client and family counseling, and referrals for support services). When functioning in an interdependent role, the nurse practices as part of an interdisciplinary team and collaborates with other health care professionals. In this model, the nurse takes a health history when the client is admitted to the rehabilitation facility, works with physicians to coordinate the information from and actions of various therapists and to implement care, makes daily rounds with the physician, and monitors the client's health status. The nurse also establishes and ensures the continuity of the client's daily care.

Physical therapists deal with interventions to achieve mobility for the client, such as facilitating ambulation and teaching the client to move with braces. ADL techniques taught by physical therapists include transferring (such as moving in and out of bed) and toileting activities.

Occupational therapists work to develop the clients' fine motor skills used for ADL, such as those required for eating, maintaining hygiene, dressing, and driving. Occupational therapists may also teach clients skills related to coordination, such as hand movements.

Speech pathologists retrain patients with language or hearing problems and swallowing or feeding disorders.

Recreational therapists work to continue or develop hobbies or interests for clients.

Aides work in the nursing or the therapy departments to assist in client care.

Various counselors are helpful in promoting community reintegration of the client and acceptance of the disability or chronic illness. *Social workers* work with clients to help them identify support services and resources. *Psychologists* also counsel clients and families on their psychologic problems and on strategies to cope with disability. *Vocational counselors* assist clients with job placement, training, or further education. Work-related skills are taught if the client needs to switch careers because of the disability.

Interdisciplinary team conferences are held with the client and family members on a regular basis for the exchange of ideas among team members. Written notes on the chart are also shared and should be read by all team members.

SUPPORT AFTER REHABILITATION DISCHARGE

There are many self-help groups that can provide continued support after the client is discharged from a rehabilitation facility. The disabled are taking up their own cause with Mainstream, Inc., a national nonprofit agency to promote affirmative action for the handicapped.

As health care professionals, nurses must know of the options available for the client after discharge from the rehabilitation facility, must communicate these options to the client, and must teach the client the value of self-worth. The nurse can serve as a client advocate and a mobilizer to help the client obtain continuing assistance through support groups.

The nurse initiates appropriate discharge planning to prepare for an orderly transition from the rehabilitation setting to another setting, whether that is another institution or back to the community. To assure the client that health care services will not be interrupted, the nurse coordinates community referrals. The client who does not have a private physician may be referred to a public health department or health maintenance organization for continued medical care. Nursing agencies that provide home health care can arrange for nursing visits to the home as needed. In addition, the client may qualify for the services of social and counseling agencies with government funding. Discharge planning coordi-

nators, public health nurses, and staff social workers are helpful resources for the nurse preparing a client for discharge from a rehabilitation facility.

ASSESSMENT OF THE CLIENT UNDERGOING REHABILITATION

For rehabilitation assessment, the data collected by the nurse focus on function rather than physiology. What individuals can do determines their health status. The nurse needs to know not only how well an individual can function physically, but also the extent of a client's psychosocial functioning. Data are collected through a health history interview and a physical assessment. A thorough nursing assessment is essential to identifying appropriate nursing diagnoses and formulating a comprehensive nursing care plan.

GENERAL BASELINE DATA

General baseline data include the client's medical status, with particular attention to any neurophysiologic factors or conditions, such as neurogenic bladder, that can be aided by restorative programs, such as retraining.

HEALTH HISTORY WITH A REHABILITATION FOCUS

The health history collected by the nurse includes the history of the present condition, any medications being used, and any treatment programs in progress.

General background data are collected regarding the client and the family. These data include the client's and the family's financial status, occupations, educational levels, and home situation. Family assessment data include the factors discussed earlier under the heading Family Theory. Architectural features of the environment must be considered, such as the layout of the home. The nurse determines if the home layout, such as the presence of stairs, will present a problem to the client. The nurse also gathers data on the type of neighborhood in which the client resides, such as the proximity of shopping centers and what transportation is available. The nurse ascertains who does the client's shopping, cooking, and housework. This information will be useful for discharge planning.

The nurse also assesses the client's *schedule and habits of normal living*. These include ADL, such as hygiene practices, eating, elimination, sexual activity, and sleep. The patient's preferred method and time of bathing and hygiene practices are assessed. In assessing dietary patterns, food likes and dislikes should be noted. The nurse ascertains if the client has any food allergies. The nurse also elicits information concerning bowel and bladder function and the client's normal pattern of elimination. Assessment of sexuality patterns elicits information on changes in sexual function since the onset of the disability (Chap. 10). The client's sleep habits are assessed with regard to the usual number of hours of sleep before the illness or injury, the use of hypnotics, and any changes in sleep pattern since the onset of the illness or injury. It is important to assess whether clients feel well rested after sleep. Sleep patterns have a significant impact on activity patterns. Assessment of activity patterns focuses on work, exercise, and recreational activities.

GENERAL ASSESSMENT OF THE CLIENT'S PHYSICAL ABILITIES AND LIMITATIONS

The physical assessment data are collected systematically by the nurse according to major body systems. The focus of assessment related to rehabilitation and chronic disease is on the functional abilities of the client. The client's ability to use self-help devices is identified during this portion of the assessment.

CARDIOVASCULAR SYSTEM

An alteration in cardiac status may affect the client's cardiac output or cause activity intolerance. The nurse assesses the manifestations of decreased cardiac output, such as chest pain, diuresis, diaphoresis, and a drop in systolic blood pressure of more than 10 mmHg from the client's normal level with activity. The nurse determines when the client experiences these symptoms and what relieves them. The nurse seeks medical consultation before the client continues activities that provoke these symptoms. The physician may order a change in medications or may prescribe a prophylactic dose of nitroglycerin to be taken before resumption of the activities. The nurse ascertains whether activities can be modified to be accomplished without these symptoms.

Manifestations of activity intolerance include fatigue at rest or with activity and diuresis with activity. The nurse assesses when and during which activities these manifestations occur. If there is no drop in the systolic blood pressure when diuresis occurs, the nurse suggests that the client try standing up more slowly. The goal is to prevent diuresis. For clients manifesting fatigue, the nurse and the client mutually plan methods of using limited energy resources. The client could, for example, incorporate frequent rest periods throughout the day, especially before undertaking activities. Major tasks could be performed in the morning, because most people have the most energy at that time. Clients who are

employed might need to address these issues with employers.

The nurse assesses the client's knowledge of the disease and compliance with the medication and rehabilitation regimen. This includes the client's awareness of any side effects from the medications or regimen. The nurse determines the client's knowledge of risk factors and signs and symptoms must be reported to health care providers.

A great hindrance to rehabilitation for clients with cardiac disorders may be fear. A client may have survived a life-threatening experience, but now is so afraid of recurrence (and death) that he/she is incapable, or unwilling, to resume *any* activity. This is a serious and complex problem that challenges the nurse. Clients manifesting fear benefit from participation in a structured cardiac rehabilitation program. The nurse discusses available programs with the client and the family. These programs focus on how clients can monitor themselves during activity and how to evaluate physical problems when they arise.

RESPIRATORY SYSTEM

The nurse assesses whether there is shortness of breath associated with activity. It is important to determine the *level of activity* that the client can accomplish without experiencing shortness of breath. For example, can the client climb one flight of stairs without shortness of breath, or does the client experience shortness of breath after climbing only two steps?

The fear associated with any inability to breathe normally can render an individual dependent in many facets of his/her life. Some of these problems related to disorders of the respiratory system can be resolved, and others can be diminished, but some breathing difficulties must be endured. It is within the scope of professional nursing to help the client determine in which category each respiratory problem belongs. This is based on physiology as well as the client's perception of the situation and values associated with disability. This information is compiled to formulate a reasonable assessment of the client's respiratory status from which a treatment plan evolves.

GASTROINTESTINAL SYSTEM

The client who has experienced any serious disease or injury may have primary or secondary changes associated with treatment resulting in alterations in ingestion or elimination patterns. A balanced diet and a fluid intake of at least 1500 mL daily are essential to successful rehabilitation.

Exceptions to the fluid requirement of 1500 mL daily might be made for clients with decreased cardiac output related to cardiac or respiratory disorders or for clients with decreased renal function. These clients might be on fluid restrictions. Specific alterations in diet might also be necessary, depending on the primary disease or injury, but balanced diets are always essential.

The nurse assesses the client's oral intake and pattern for eating. The client is also assessed for the presence of anorexia, dysphagia, nausea, vomiting, or discomfort related to or interfering with oral intake. Height, weight, hemoglobin and hematocrit levels, and serum albumin and blood glucose concentrations are assessed as needed. Weight loss or gain is particularly significant and may be related to secondary disease processes or to the illness that caused disability.

It may be difficult to assess elimination habits, as many nurses are hesitant to request — and many clients afraid to volunteer — information pertaining to elimination. When assessing the client's elimination status, the nurse first ascertains what the normal elimination patterns were for that individual before the injury or illness occurred. Elimination habits vary from person to person; they are often related to daily job or activity schedules, dietary patterns, and family or cultural background.

The nurse should be attuned to any changes in the client's bowel routine or the consistency of the stool. If the client is experiencing any alteration in elimination pattern, the nurse tries to determine if this alteration can be attributed to a change in diet, activity patterns, or the use of medications that could cause hypermotility or hypomotility of the gastrointestinal tract. It is important to determine whether any dietary modifications deemed necessary by the health care providers can be implemented and accepted by the client (and the family). Bowel habits are evaluated on the basis of what is normal for that individual. Satisfactory bowel habits consist of one bowel movement every 3 days or three or fewer bowel movements in 24 hours. The client with poor bowel habits has no stool for 3 or more days or four or more bowel movements in 24 hours. Often these habits cause discomfort, social inconvenience, and an incapacity for work.

The nurse determines whether the client is physically capable of being independent in bowel elimination. Independence in bowel elimination requires cognition, manual dexterity, sensation, muscle control, and mobility. If the client does require assistance, the nurse determines whether there is someone available at home to provide the assistance. The client's (and family's) ability to cope with any dependency in bowel elimination needs to be assessed. The nurse must be able to work with the client and the family to develop and implement a satisfactory bowel management program.

URINARY SYSTEM

Clients may experience difficulty in urinary elimination with or without any actual urologic pathologic change. The nurse's goal is to establish an effective and efficient means of urinary elimination that is acceptable to the client.

When assessing the client's urinary system, the nurse determines the client's baseline urinary patterns. Assessment of an individual's urinary elimination includes more than output measurements. The nurse gathers data regarding the number of times the client usually voids and whether the client routinely awakens in the middle of the night to empty the bladder or has uninterrupted sleep. The nurse determines the client's fluid intake patterns and volume including the type of fluids ingested and the timing of fluid consumption throughout the day. The nurse ascertains if the client has ever experienced any problems with incontinence or retention in the past. Nursing assessment includes describing the extent of neurologic involvement. If the client is voiding independently, the nurse may need to catheterize the client to measure residual urine. The nurse also monitors laboratory reports of urine culture and urinalysis.

NEUROLOGIC SYSTEM

In rehabilitation, the neurologic assessment includes identification of the functional aspects of cognition, pain, comfort, sensation, strength, and dexterity. The nurse assesses the client's pre-existing problems, general physical condition, and communication abilities.

Motor function of an extremity is compared with the function of the contralateral extremity to identify paresis (weakness) or paralysis (absence of strength).

Identification of sensory/perceptual alterations is important in assessing the client's potential for injury. Response to light touch, hot or cold temperature, and position change is assessed in each extremity and on the trunk. Levels of decreased sensation are identified. Other senses assessed include smell, vision, hearing, and taste. Perceptual assessment includes evaluating the client's ability to receive and understand what is heard and seen, and to express appropriate motor and verbal responses. During this portion of the assessment, it is important to assess short- and long-term memory.

The client's mental and cognitive abilities are determined, especially for the client with a head injury. Two assessment scales that are commonly used in rehabilitation settings are the Glasgow Assessment Scales and the Rancho Los Amigos Scale of Cognitive Levels and Expected Behavior.

Glasgow Assessment Scales

Interest in measures of the severity of head injury and the correlation with immediate prognosis and long-term outcome have influenced the development of scales to measure or predict outcome. The Glasgow Assessment Scales serve this purpose. Developed by Teasdale and Jennett (1974), the Glasgow Coma Scale enables the clinician to define coma objectively (Chap. 33). It has become the standard means of assessing the client's level of consciousness. Scores are determined by separate observations of eye opening, motor response, and verbal performance. Scores range from 3 to 15 points, with conscious clients receiving the highest scores. Scores of 8 or less indicate severe injury; 9, moderate injury; and more than 12, minor injury.

The Glasgow Outcome Scale was designed to utilize the evaluation of overall social capability of the brain-damaged person, taking into account the combined effect of specific cognitive and neurologic deficits. Four categories of survival are recognized—vegetative state, severe disability, moderate disability, and good recovery.

Rancho Los Amigos Scale of Cognitive Levels and Expected Behavior

The Rancho Los Amigos Scale of Cognitive Levels and Expected Behavior (Hagen & Malkmus, 1979) is an eight-level hierarchic scale designed to describe cognitive and behavioral characteristics of the brain-injured person. Levels range from no response to purposeful and appropriate behavior, as follows:

1. No response
2. Generalized response
3. Localized response
4. Confused, agitated
5. Confused, inappropriate
6. Confused, appropriate
7. Automatic, appropriate
8. Purposeful, appropriate

MUSCULOSKELETAL SYSTEM

As for other body systems, the rehabilitation nursing assessment of the musculoskeletal system focuses on function. The nurse assesses the client's musculoskeletal status; the client's response to the impairment; and the demands of the home, work, or school environment. The nurse emphasizes the limits of the musculoskeletal impairment, the potential for adaptation, and the meaning of the impairment. The nurse explores the endurance level of the client and measures both active and passive range of joint motion.

The nurse reviews the results of manual muscle testing, which identifies range of motion (ROM) and resistance against gravity. In this procedure an examiner ascertains the degree of muscle strength present in each body segment. The grading system usually ranges from 0 (no evidence of contractility) to 5 (normal, or complete ROM).

Advancements in the treatment of musculoskeletal impairments have been no less dramatic than those for any other organ system. Many conditions that would have had a less than promising outcome previously are now treated successfully, and those that required extended periods of immobilization are now treated on an ambulatory (outpatient) basis or during short-term hospitalization.

INTEGUMENTARY SYSTEM

The nurse's role in assessing a client's integumentary system is to identify actual or potential interruptions in the integrity of the skin. To maintain healthy skin, the body must have adequate food, water, and oxygen intake; intact waste removal mechanisms; the presence of sensation; and functional mobility. Changes in any of these variables could lead to a rapid and extensive skin breakdown. If the client is not able to protect or maintain the skin, the nurse must be able to assess and plan for client needs. The client is monitored to determine the risk of skin breakdown before it occurs.

Several assessment tools have been designed to predict the risk of skin breakdown. The assessment tool developed by Norton and colleagues has been used extensively (Frank-Stromborg, 1988). It measures five variables: physical condition, mental state, activity, mobility, and incontinence.

Pressure ulcers and disruption can be prevented if good nursing care, client instruction, and client participation are effective. If a client does develop an alteration in skin integrity, the nurse must be able to assess the problem and its possible cause. The client's skin is inspected twice daily. The depth and diameter of the problem area are described in centimeters. The pressure sore is graded clinically in four or five stages (the Key Features of Disease in Chap. 22, p. 510, describes a widely used classification system for grading). The nurse also assesses the client's understanding of the cause and treatment of skin breakdown, as well as his/her ability to self-inspect and participate in maintaining skin integrity.

FUNCTIONAL ASSESSMENT

Interdisciplinary health care team members prescribe or modify the treatment programs to address the individual needs of a client. Functional assessment tools serve as a mechanism to assess a person's abilities within the context of a predetermined evaluation process. Functional assessment is a systematic attempt to measure objectively the level at which a person is performing in any of a variety of areas, such as physical health, quality of self-maintenance, quality of role activity, intellectual status, attitude toward the world and toward self, and emotional status. Functional ability is the client's ability to perform ADL independently. Nurses are frequently responsible for assisting clients with improving or maintaining their functional status. Therefore, functional assessment includes a determination of the client's capacity for personal care, communication abilities, and perception of needs.

As today's issues in health care focus on cost containment, accountability, and appropriateness of service, it is standard practice for rehabilitation programs to include a system to measure outcome. These systems not only serve as an indicator of changes in function, in terms of client progress, but can also be a vital component of program evaluation measures. During the past 30 years, comprehensive tools have been developed and used by rehabilitation centers throughout the country. Many of these tools have been evaluated and modified, as they have been used on a long-term basis.

One of the earliest tools used was the PULSES Profile, developed in 1957 and adapted in 1975 for the purpose of evaluating and classifying functional capacity in the chronically ill and aging client population (Granger et al., 1979). The six categories included for evaluation are physical condition (basic health status), upper limb function (self-care), lower limb function (mobility), sensory components (sight, communication), excretory function, and support factors. Scoring for this tool uses four numeric grades for each category, with scores increasing as functional ability is diminished. The maximum score is 24. Higher scores indicate greater levels of dependency for the client. The adapted form of PULSES has been a useful tool in a broad range of rehabilitation programs and has served to reflect the level of independence in life-functioning skills necessary for an individual to make adaptations to community living.

One of the best known and most widely used instruments was developed during the 1950s from observations of clients with fractured hips. The Katz Index of ADL addresses six functional activities: bathing, dressing, toileting, achieving transfers, continence, and feeding (Katz et al., 1970). Each of the six areas is scored as either dependent or independent on the basis of the client's need for assistance to perform the task. The overall functional status is then assigned a grade from A (independent in feeding, continence, transferring, toileting, dressing, and bathing) through G (dependent in all six functions) from total scores. The Katz Index of ADL has been used for clients with many types of chronic illnesses. It has been used to evaluate care and develop data about the course of an illness over time.

The Barthel Index (Mahoney & Barthel, 1965) was designed to measure functional levels and mobility in the physically impaired individual. This tool consists of 10 variables in which the individuals are scored by their degree of independence in performance. Categories include feeding, bathing, and mobility. The scoring system consists of two descriptive areas: doing an activity with help or performing an activity independently. Scores range from 0, indicating total dependence, to 100, indicating complete independence. Use of this tool was intended for both immediate and long-term care restorative programs.

Granger et al. (1977) adapted the Barthel Index to measure a greater range of functional activities related to daily living skills. Categories for responses included "can do by myself," "can do with help of someone else," and "cannot do at all." Scoring ranged from 0 to 100.

The Level of Rehabilitation Scale (LORS) was developed by Carey and Posavec (1978) to provide a general assessment of the client's functioning for the purpose of program evaluation rather than clinical assessment. Use of the tool provides an overview through measurement of function pertaining to ADL, cognition, home activi-

ties, outside activities, and social interactions. Use of the tool was then expanded to serve as a means to document inpatient improvement as a support to the accreditation process. The revised tool, referred to as LORS-II, includes 11 items related to ADL, mobility, and communication (Posavec & Carey, 1982). These items receive a score of 0 to 4, determined through the use of a coding manual ascribing numeric values to behavioral terms.

Assessment tools have also been designed for use on a national level; thus, uniform outcome data can be obtained from numerous rehabilitation programs. An example of this kind of system, referred to as a uniform data system, is the Functional Independence Measure (FIM) developed by Granger and Gresham (1984). The FIM, as a basic indicator of the severity of a disability, is intended to quantify what the person actually does, whatever the diagnosis or impairment. It is important to note that it does not measure what a person should do or how the person would perform under a different set of circumstances. To eliminate the bias of a particular discipline, the assessment may be done by trained clinicians: the entire assessment may be done by one person, or certain categories may be performed by representatives of various disciplines. Categories for assessment are self-care, sphincter control, mobility and locomotion, communication, and social cognition. Scoring is done on a numeric basis using a predetermined criteria for measurement. The evaluation is done when the client is admitted to and discharged from a rehabilitation institution and at a specified follow-up time.

PSYCHOLOGIC ASSESSMENT

To adequately assess the client's psychologic needs, the nurse must have a clear understanding of the theories of body image and self-esteem. These concepts serve as a basis for understanding psychologic responses to chronic illness and resulting disability. The nurse assesses both verbal indicators and behaviors related to these concepts. The client's self-esteem and body image are assessed through verbal indicators and descriptions of self-care that the client gives. Body image can also be assessed by self-administered instruments such as the Self-Attitude Questionnaire. This is a 40-item multiple-choice tool, which includes questions about the parts of the body liked the most or the least, social life, and whether clients view themselves as fat or thin.

The nurse assesses the client's use of defense mechanisms and manifestations of anxiety, such as those noted in facial expressions and communication patterns. To assess the client's response to loss, the client's feelings concerning the loss of body part or function should be described. Stress-related physical problems are noted. The client may manifest symptoms of depression, such as fatigue, change in appetite, or feelings of lack of power.

The availability of support systems for the client is also assessed. The major support system for the client is the family (see earlier discussion of family theory).

Therefore, the family interaction and coping patterns should be assessed.

VOCATIONAL ASSESSMENT

The rehabilitation nurse assists the client to maximize his/her functional status, allowing the client to resume many normal activities. The nurse needs to be aware of appropriate resources for each client in compiling a vocational data base. The nurse works with vocational counselors to help the client find meaningful training, education, or employment after discharge from the hospital. The nurse compiles data on the client's educational and employment history, including jobs held by the client. The assessment of employers' attitudes toward the disabled client and information on the client's performance on the job, such as absenteeism and work record, are obtained. The nurse needs to obtain information on the cognitive and physical demands of the jobs held and to ascertain if the client can return to the former job or if the client will need retraining in another field. Physical demands of jobs range from light in sedentary occupations (0 to 10 lb frequently lifted) to heavy (over 100 lb frequently lifted). The nurse must also consider other aspects of the job, such as strength, mobility, or senses required in the job (e.g., hearing).

Job analysis also involves assessing the work environment of the client's former job. The nurse works with the counselor to determine if the environment is conducive to the client's return. Union contracts must also be considered, and any job modifications must be noted. If the injured worker requires vocational rehabilitation, the nurse refers the client to vocational rehabilitation personnel and works with the counselors on skill evaluation and learning of new skills for employment. The nurse may also help with job placement in the community.

SUMMARY

Any illness characterized by altered system function or body structure that lasts longer than 6 months is considered chronic. Rehabilitation is the process of learning to live with disability related to chronic illness.

Rehabilitation of the chronically ill client requires an interdisciplinary approach to care. Interventions take place in a variety of rehabilitation settings. The nurse plays a pivotal role in the functioning of this team in all settings. The nurse acts as a catalyst, assisting clients to restore and maintain optimal function. Theories and philosophies of rehabilitation are the basis for assessments and interventions with these clients. Assessment of each body system is particularly important, and several instruments have been developed to assess functional status.

IMPLICATIONS FOR RESEARCH

Rehabilitation of the client with a chronic condition is important to enable the client to maximize his/her potential. Nurses continue to research both theoretical concepts and assessment methods to improve rehabilitation nursing practice. The major problems of living with a chronic illness are areas of future investigation for nurses.

Nursing research should be conducted to answer the following questions related to the care of clients desiring rehabilitation:

1. What are the major problems of living with a chronic illness?
2. What methods do clients employ to cope with chronic illness?
3. Are the power resources illustrated in the power model (Fig. 21–1) validated by empirical testing?
4. Do nursing diagnoses and consequent nursing interventions improve the disabled client's ability to perform self-care?
5. How effective are various self-care practices?
6. What are the strengths and weaknesses of the functional assessment tools described in this chapter?
7. Which functional assessment tools are more valid for the chronically ill adult?
8. What are the strengths and weaknesses of functional assessment tools in comparison with psychologic measurements?

REFERENCES AND READINGS

Carey, R. G., & Posavac, E. J. (1978). Program evaluation of a physical medicine and rehabilitation unit: A new approach. *Archives of Physical Medicine and Rehabilitation, 59,* 330–337.

Conway-Rutkowski, B. L. (1982). *Carini and Owens' neurological and neurosurgical nursing.* St. Louis: C. V. Mosby.

Ducanis, A. J., & Golin, A. K. (1979). *The interdisciplinary health care team.* Germantown, MD: Aspen Systems.

Frank-Stromborg, M. (1988). *Instruments for clinical nursing research.* Norwalk, CT: Appleton & Lange.

Goad, S. (1983). Clinical application of the motor impairment concept. *Rehabilitation Nursing, 8*(4), 30–32.

Granger, C. V., Albrecht, G. L., & Hamilton, B. B. (1979). Outcome of comprehensive medical rehabilitation:

Measurement of PULSES Profile and the Barthel Index. *Archives of Physical Medicine and Rehabilitation, 60,* 145–154.

Granger, C. V., & Gresham, G. E. (1984). *Functional assessment in rehabilitation medicine.* Baltimore: Williams & Wilkins.

Granger, C. V., & Hamilton, B. (1986). *Guide for the use of the uniform data system for medical rehabilitation.* Buffalo: State University of Buffalo.

Granger, C. V., Sherwood, C. C., & Greer, D. S. (1977). Functional status measures in a comprehensive stroke care program. *Archives of Physical Medicine and Rehabilitation, 58,* 555–561.

Hagen, C., & Malkmus, D. (1979). *Intervention strategies for language disorders secondary to head trauma.* Short courses conducted for the American Speech-Language-Hearing Association, Atlanta.

Jennett, B., & Teasdale, G. (1981). *Management of head injuries.* Philadelphia: F. A. Davis.

Katz, S., Downs, T. D., Cash, H. R., & Grotz, R. C. (1970). Progress in development of the index of ADL. *Gerontologist, 10*(1, Pt. 1), 20–22.

Lawton, M. P. (1971). The functional assessment of elderly people. *Journal of the American Geriatrics Society, 19,* 465.

Lazarus, R. S., & Folkman, S. (1984). *Stress, appraisal and coping.* New York: Springer.

Mahoney, F. I., & Barthel, D. W. (1965). Functional evaluation: The Barthel Index. *Maryland State Medical Journal, 14,* 61–65.

Martin, N., Holt, N., & Hicks, D. (1981). *Comprehensive rehabilitation.* New York: McGraw-Hill.

Mayo, L. (1956). Problem and challenge. In National Health Council, *Guides to action on chronic illness* (pp. 9–13, 35, 55). New York: Author.

Miller, J. M. (1983). *Coping with chronic illness: Overcoming powerlessness.* Philadelphia: F. A. Davis.

Mumma, C. M. (Ed.). (1987). *Rehabilitation nursing: Concepts and practice. A core curriculum* (2nd ed.). Evanston, IL: Rehabilitation Nursing Foundation.

National Center for Health Statistics. (1985, September 26). *Monthly Vital Statistics Report, 33*(13).

Norton, D., McLaren, F., & Exton-Smith, A. (1975). An investigation of geriatric nursing problems in hospitals. Edinburgh: Churchill Livingstone.

Orem, D. (1980). *Nursing concepts of practice.* New York: McGraw-Hill.

Posavec, E. J., & Carey, R. G. (1982). Using a level of function scale (LORS-II) to evaluate the success of inpa-tient rehabilitation programs. *Rehabilitation Nursing 7*(6), 17–19.

Schilder, P. (1935). *The image and appearance of the human body.* London: Kegan Paul, Trency, Trubrer.

Strauss, A. L., Corbin, J., Fagerhaugh, S., Glaser, B., Maines, D., Suczek, B., & Weiner, C. L. (1984). *Chronic illness and the quality of life.* St. Louis: C. V. Mosby.

Teasdale, G., & Jennett, B. (1974). Assessment of coma and impaired consciousness: A practical scale. *Lancet, 2,* 81–84.

World Health Organization. (1980). *International classifications of impairments, disabilities and handicaps.* Geneva: Author.

U.S. Bureau of the Census. (1986). *Statistical abstracts of the United States.* Washington, DC: U.S. Government Printing Office.

Wilson, S. F. (1979). *Neuronursing.* New York: Springer.

ADDITIONAL READINGS

Brown, M. D. (1988). Functional assessment of the elderly. *Journal of Gerontological Nursing, 14*(5), 13–17.

Because of degenerative changes, reduced physical reserve, and a high incidence of chronic illness in the elderly population, elders should be assessed from a specific perspective. A comprehensive functional assessment of an elder integrates biologic, psychologic, and functional domains and includes an interdisciplinary approach. This article provides one assessment protocol, and it discusses several tools to assess specific functional abilities.

Gillies, D. A. (1987). Family assessment and counseling by the rehabilitation nurse. *Rehabilitation Nursing, 12*(2), 65–69.

This article discusses several classification systems used to categorize dysfunctional families with reference to their primary structural or functional problem. The rehabilitation nurse should assist key family members to make necessary role transitions when a member becomes disabled. Suggestions for interventions are given to ameliorate common functional problems.

Jacelon, C. S. (1986). The Barthel Index and other indices of functional ability. *Rehabilitation Nursing, 11*(4), 9–11.

The Barthel Index was developed in 1965 by Mahoney and Barthel to measure functional ability in daily activities. This article presents a review of the literature pertaining to the studies using the Barthel Index.

Watson, P. G. (1988). Rehabilitation legislation of the 1980s: Implications for nurses as healthcare providers. *Rehabilitation Nursing, 13*(3), 136–141.

This article discusses federal legislation of the 1980s regarding rehabilitation and compares it with that of the 1970s. The nurse-author points out the importance of nurses' being familiar with existing legislation and the political process. By monitoring legislative issues and influencing future legislation, nurses can assist disabled clients in attaining maximum resources.

CHAPTER 22

Rehabilitation for Clients with Disabling or Chronic Conditions

OVERVIEW

Rehabilitation nursing is a specialty practice focusing on promoting independence for individuals with disabling conditions or illnesses. Rehabilitation nurses work in a variety of institutional settings, but usually serve as members of an interdisciplinary team.

The concept of rehabilitation has traditionally been linked to clients with neurologic deficits related to trauma. However, rehabilitation can and should be implemented for clients with any chronic illness characterized by altered system function or structure, such as generalized weakness or debilitation related to cancer. Just as clients with neurologic trauma should be rehabilitated to achieve their fullest potential, so should clients with cardiac or respiratory disease, cancer, or other disabling conditions.

Critical aspects of the rehabilitation nurses' role are teaching and promoting self-care skills. One of the primary ways in which the specialty of rehabilitation nursing differs from other nursing specialties is in the use of functional assessment, rather than an emphasis on physical assessment. Rehabilitation nurses look specifically at the client's ability to function and perform activities of daily living (ADL), including self-care and home management skills. Functional assessment tools, such as the PULSES Profile, the Barthel Index, and the Functional Independence Measures (FIM), enable clinicians to evaluate disability and predict rehabilitation outcome (Chap. 21). Rehabilitation entails involvement of the client in planning and goal setting and facilitation of the client's abilities to return to as much functional independence as possible.

COLLABORATIVE MANAGEMENT

 Analysis: Nursing Diagnosis

The client with a chronic illness or disability may be admitted to a hospital or a rehabilitation facility for the initial occurrence of a disabling illness or injury or for continuation or an exacerbation of a chronic problem.

Common Diagnoses

Regardless of the client's age or specific disability, the following nursing diagnoses are commonly applicable to clients with chronic illness or disability:

1. Impaired physical mobility related to denervation, muscle atrophy, tissue degeneration, or activity intolerance

2. Total self-care deficit related to impaired mobility
3. Potential for impaired skin integrity related to impaired sensation or immobility
4. Constipation related to impaired sensation or immobility
5. Bowel incontinence related to impaired central nervous system or impaired mobility
6. Diarrhea related to impaired central nervous system
7. Altered patterns of urinary elimination related to impaired sensation of bladder fullness or immobility
8. Reflex incontinence related to impaired sensation of bladder fullness
9. Total incontinence related to impaired sensation of bladder fullness
10. Urinary retention (chronic) related to inhibition of reflex arc

Additional Diagnoses

Other nursing diagnoses that may be applicable to individuals with chronic illness and disability include the following:

1. Ineffective airway clearance related to musculoskeletal impairment or decreased lung expansion
2. Sexual dysfunction related to altered body structure
3. Chronic pain related to altered sensation or tissue damage
4. Ineffective individual coping related to a change in body image and life style alterations
5. Potential for injury related to cognitive and perceptual impairments
6. Sensory/perceptual alterations (kinesthetic) related to cognitive deficits regarding position of body in space or body part location

Planning and Implementation ➡

The nursing care plan for clients with chronic illness or disability focuses on the common nursing diagnoses.

Impaired Physical Mobility

The majority of problems requiring rehabilitation relate to immobility. Muscular atrophy may result. Denervation studies involving skeletal muscles have shown that changes occur within weeks. After 2 months of immobility, the muscle fibers may be less than half of their original size. Without use, muscles decrease in size and in ability to function.

Planning: client goals. The primary client goals for this diagnosis are that the client will (1) achieve the maximal physical mobility possible with the least restriction of activity and (2) prevent complications resulting from immobility.

Interventions: nonsurgical management

Prevention of complications. Table 22–1 reviews some complications of immobility and strategies to prevent them. The complications of immobility occurring frequently include contractures, pneumonia, and pressure ulcers. Implementing range-of-motion (ROM) routines, adhering to schedules for turning and repositioning the client, and maintaining skin care should be constant components of rehabilitation nursing care to forestall such complications. The mainstay of prevention of the numerous and systemic complications of inactivity is increasing the client's mobility. One way in which this can be done, even with clients who are bedridden, is through ROM exercises. ROM techniques are beneficial for any client with decreased mobility (Table 22–2). Although basic ROM techniques are presented in textbooks of nursing fundamentals, a few key principles are pertinent for rehabilitation nursing care. First, the human body contains more joints than simply the knees, hips, elbows, and shoulders. For ROM techniques to be effective in the prevention of musculoskeletal contractures, *all* joints must be exercised, including each joint of the fingers, hands, toes, and so forth. Second, in performing ROM activities, the nurse completes full-range movement of each joint *five* or more times and completes the entire process *at least* three times daily. Finally, the nurse does not move joints beyond points at which the client expresses pain or the nurse perceives stiffness or difficulty. Clients with decreased mobility who are able to follow directions are taught by the nurse to perform active ROM exercises.

Transfer techniques. Clients with decreased mobility may require assistance with transfers, for example, from bed to chair, commode, or wheelchair. The degree of assistance required varies with the client and the specific disability, so the nurse must perform a careful assessment of the client's mobility status before attempting a transfer. When information on the client's ability to transfer is not available, the nurse assumes that the client is not able to assist during the transfer. The nurse always remembers to plan the transfer before initiating it. Basic techniques for the nurse to use in assisting in the transfers of clients from bed to chair or wheelchair, and vice versa, are identified in the Guidelines feature on page 507 for transfer techniques.

Gait training. In the process of regaining the ability to ambulate, clients may need to use canes or walkers (Fig. 22–1). When working with clients who are using such assistive devices, the nurse ensures that the client has a level surface on which to walk. See the Guidelines feature on page 507 on gait training techniques for information on using assistive devices for ambulation.

TABLE 22–1　Prevention of Some Common Hazards of Immobility

Body System	Complication	Prevention
Musculoskeletal	Contractures	ROM exercises
	Foot drop	Foot support while in bed, ROM activities
	Osteoporosis	ROM exercises
	Susceptibility to fractures	Weight-bearing exercises
	Muscular atrophy	Passive or active ROM exercises
Gastrointestinal	Constipation	Increased activity level
	Decreased motility	Diet high in fiber
Circulatory	Decreased cardiac output	ROM exercises
	Increased venous stasis	Exercise, support hose
	Thrombus formation	Exercise, support hose
	Embolism	Avoidance of leg massage
Neurologic	Disorientation	Sleep-wake schedule in accord with light-dark pattern
		Reorientation (to person, place, and time)
		Control of sensory stimulation
	Postural hypotension	Avoidance of sudden position changes
Renal	Calculi	Decreased dietary calcium level
		Increased fluid intake
		Maintenance of acidic urine
Respiratory	Pneumonia	Frequent repositioning
		Respiratory exercises
Integumentary	Pressure ulcers	Frequent repositioning
		Pressure relief devices

TABLE 22–2　Types of Range-of-Motion Exercises

Type	Description	Indications
Passive	Exercises are performed by the nurse for the client.	Client is too weak to participate actively.
Active	Exercises are performed by the client.	Client is able to complete ROM movements.
Assisted	Exercises are performed by the client but are guided by the nurse.	Client is weak and needs assistance.
Resistive	Actions of the client are in opposition to those performed by the nurse.	Client has full ROM, and an increase in strength is desired.

Total Self-Care Deficit

ADL, or self-care skills, include bathing, dressing, grooming, eating, and toileting. The nurse assesses the client's ability to perform these activities through the use of an ADL assessment scale (refer to Chap. 21 for specific information on assessment of ADL tools).

Planning: client goals.　The primary goal for this diagnosis is that the client will achieve personally acceptable means for completing ADL.

Interventions: nonsurgical management.　Self-care activities include personal hygiene and grooming. Bathing, mouth care, fingernail care, hair care, and dressing are components of self-care. The nurse encourages clients to perform as much self-care as possible and works with the client and occupational therapist to identify ways in which self-care activities can be modified to facilitate independence. For example, the nurse and occupational therapist teach a hemiplegic client to put a shirt on by placing the affected (weak) arm in the sleeve first and putting the unaffected (strong) arm in the appropriate sleeve next (Fig. 22–2).

A variety of assistive devices are available for clients

GUIDELINES ■ Transfer Techniques

Bed to Wheelchair or Chair

1. Place chair at an angle to the bed on the client's strong side.
2. Lock wheelchair brakes or secure chair position.
3. Assist the client to stand and move his/her strong hand to the armrest.
4. Keep the client's body weight forward and pivot.
5. When the client's legs touch the chair edge, assist the client in sitting.

Wheelchair or Chair to Bed

1. Place chair with client's strong side next to bed.
2. Lock wheelchair brakes or secure.
3. Assist client to stand and move the client's strong hand to the armrest.
4. Keep the client's body weight forward and pivot.
5. When the client's legs touch the bed edge, assist the client in sitting and then reclining.

Use of a Sliding Board

1. Place the chair or wheelchair as close to the bed as possible.
2. Remove the armrest from the chair or (if removable) wheelchair.
3. Powder the sliding board.
4. Place the sliding board under the client's buttocks.
5. Instruct the client to reach toward the client's side.
6. Assist the client in sliding gently to the bed.

GUIDELINES ■ Gait Training Techniques

Walker Assisted

1. Apply a gait belt around the client's waist.
2. Assist the client to a standing position.
3. Assist the client in placing both hands on the walker.
4. Ensure that the client is well balanced.
5. Assist the client repeatedly to perform the following sequence:
   a. Lift the walker.
   b. Move the walker 2 ft forward and set it down on all legs.
   c. While resting on the walker, take small steps.
   d. Check balance.

Cane Assisted

1. Apply a gait belt around the client's waist.
2. Assist the client to a standing position.
3. Assist the client in placing his/her strong hand on the cane.
4. Ensure that the client is well balanced.
5. Assist the client repeatedly to perform the following sequence:
   a. Move the cane forward.
   b. Move the weaker leg one step forward.
   c. Move the stronger leg one step forward.
   d. Check balance.

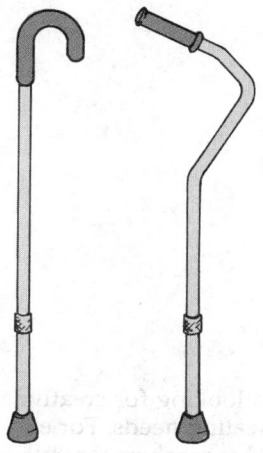
Straight canes

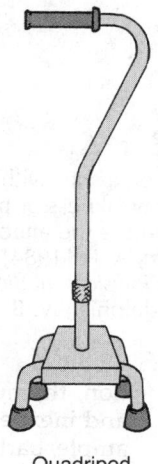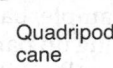
Quadripod cane

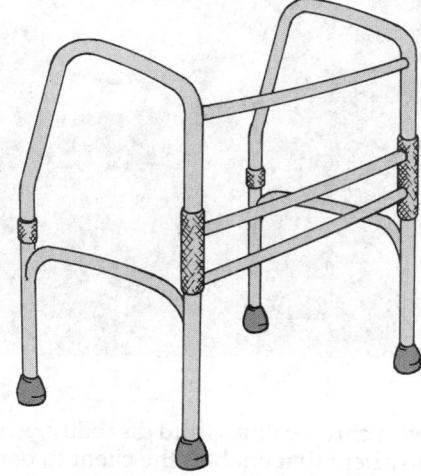
Standard walker

Figure 22–1

Assistive devices for ambulation. Assistive devices vary in the amount of support they provide. A straight cane provides less support than a quadripod cane or a walker.

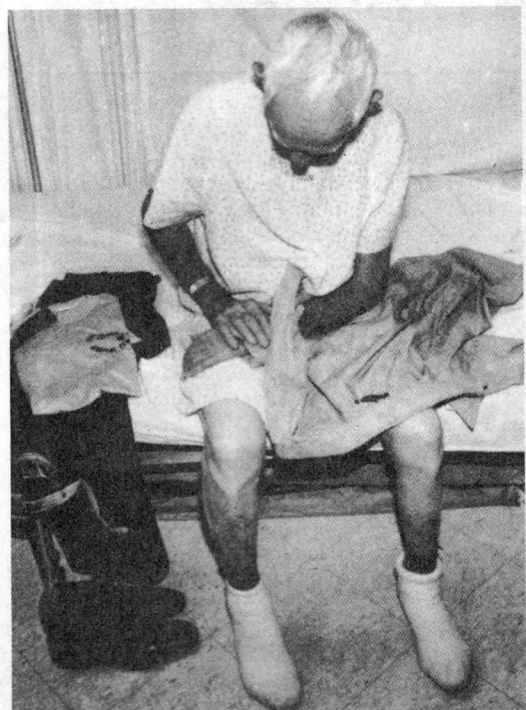
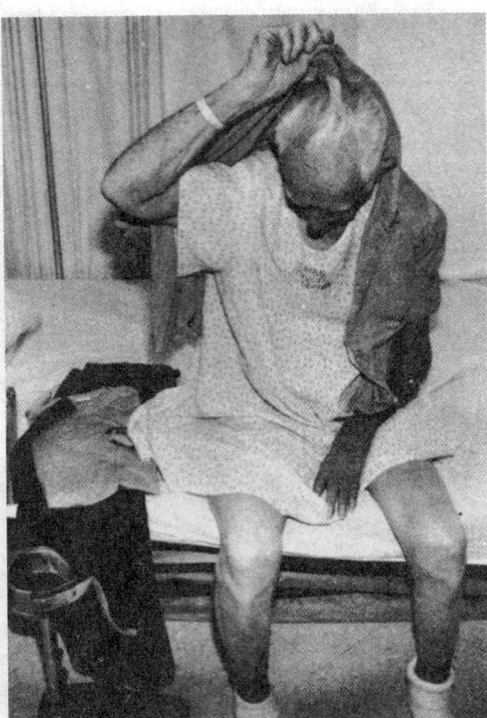
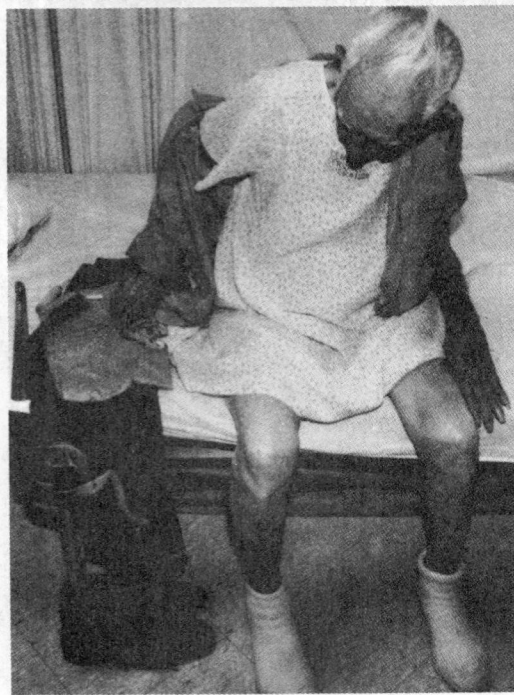

Figure 22–2

How to put on a shirt with one weak arm. Clients with weakness or paralysis of one side should dress the affected side first. (From Ruskin, A. P. [1984]. *Current therapy in physiatry: Physical medicine and rehabilitation.* Philadelphia: W. B. Saunders.)

with chronic illness and disability. An assistive device is any item that enables the client to perform all or part of an activity independently. Table 22–3 identifies common self-care support devices and describes their use. Many department stores now carry clothing and assistive devices designed for clients with disabilities. The nurse works with the client to determine the client's specific needs with regard to such equipment. In addi-

tion, the nurse assists the client in looking for creative and inexpensive alternatives to meeting needs. For example, barbecue tongs may be used as reachers for pulling up pants or obtaining items on high shelves. A foam curler with the plastic insert removed may be placed over a pencil or eating utensil to make a built-up device. An extended shoe horn may be used to operate light switches from wheelchair height.

TABLE 22-3   Use of Self-Care Support Devices

Device	Use
Buttonhook	Threaded through the buttonhole to enable clients with weak finger mobility to button shirts.
	Alternate uses include serving as a pencil holder or a cigarette holder.
Extended shoe horn	Assists in the application of shoes for clients with decreased mobility.
	Alternate uses include turning light switches off or on while in a wheelchair.
Plate guard	Applied to plate to assist clients with weak hand and arm mobility to self-feed.
Gel pad	Placed under a plate or a glass to prevent dishes from slipping and moving.
	Alternate uses include placement under bathing and grooming items to prevent moving.
Foam build-ups	Applied to eating utensils to assist clients with weak handgrasps to self-feed.
	Alternate uses include application to pens and pencils to assist with writing or over a buttonhook to assist with grasping the device.
Hook and loop fastener (Velcro) straps	Applied to utensils, buttonhook, or pencil to slip over hand and provide a method of stabilizing the device when the client's handgrasp is weak.
Long-handled reacher	Assists in obtaining items located on high shelves or at ground level for clients who are not able to change positions easily.

Energy conservation techniques. Nurses work with occupational therapists to assess the client's self-care abilities and to determine possible ways of achieving energy conservation. Strategies for energy conservation are developed after evaluating the client's self-care routines. Preparation for ADL can be helpful in reducing the client's effort and energy expenditure, for example, teaching the client to gather all needed equipment before starting grooming routines. Assessing the client's

energy level pattern may be of assistance. Clients with high energy levels in the morning are taught to schedule energy-intensive activities in the morning, rather than later in the day or evening. Spacing activities is helpful in terms of energy conservation. Allowing time to rest before and after eating and toileting will decrease the strain on the client's energy level.

Diet therapy. The key principle of diet therapy for clients with self-care deficits is maintenance of adequate nutritional balance, specifically a diet containing the proper proportions and amounts of foods from the four basic food groups. Clients with inadequate nutrition will be weaker and less effective at attempts to perform self-care activities.

Prevention of complications. The nurse should plan appropriate interventions for the client with self-care deficits. The most likely problem is designing a self-care, or ADL, program that is too complex for the client to follow. The nurse prevents such an occurrence by assessing the client's life style and working with the client and members of the interdisciplinary health care team in determining the self-care program most apt to work effectively for the client and significant others.

Potential for Impaired Skin Integrity

Chronic illness and disability frequently result in immobility. Possibly the most common, yet least understood, complication of immobility is pressure ulcers. Even the terminology is misunderstood. Pressure ulcers are sometimes referred to as decubitus or bed sores. Decubitus is derived from the Latin *decumbere* meaning "lying down," which implies that the pressure ulcer is the result of being bedridden. The terms decubitus ulcer and bed sore do not reflect the actual source of the pathologic condition, which is pressure. Therefore, *pressure ulcer* is preferred, as this term includes the causative factor.

Pressure ulcers are areas of cellular necrosis, usually occurring over bony prominences that have been subjected to pressure from the weight of the body or an extremity in excess of capillary pressure for a period of time sufficient to cause cell death. When skin and layers of subjacent tissue are compressed between bone and an external firm surface, ischemia of the affected area may occur. When pressure is released from the area, vasodilation occurs, with reactive hyperemia, which is demonstrated by localized flushing or redness and warmth. As blood flow returns to the ischemic area, it removes toxic materials and restores nutrition. Normally, one experiences discomfort when pressure becomes excessive, and one shifts position, relieving the pressure and resulting in healthy return of blood flow to the ischemic area. However, any situation that interferes with the sensation of pressure or the ability to move places the individual at risk for cellular damage. For cellular damage to occur, pressure must exceed capillary pressure (the force of blood flow through the capillary system), which is 12 to 32 mmHg. The normal pressure experienced over the bony prominences when a person has been sitting for 1 hour is 60 to 70 mmHg. When pressure is relieved after a long interval, there is a leakage of cells from damaged vessels, resulting in an accumulation of fluid, in addition to a dilation of local blood vessels and migration of inflammatory cells. Continued pressure interferes with cellular metabolism and results in necrosis of fat, fibrous tissue, muscle, and bone.

The best intervention for pressure ulcers is prevention. To prevent the formation of pressure ulcers, the nurse assesses clients for their level of risk for ulcer development. Clients with sensory or mobility deficits are at a high risk for pressure ulcer development, as they rely on the nurse or caregiver for pressure relief and proper positioning. Sometimes, however, even if a client is repositioned correctly every 1 to 2 hours, a pressure ulcer develops. Pressure ulcer development may occur with low amounts of pressure if cellular nutrition is inadequate or healing is compromised. Therefore, clients with inadequate nutrition are at greater risk for pressure ulcer development.

Because pressure ulcers vary extensively in appearance and depth, it is essential that common criteria be used for accurate documentation. The classification system given in the accompanying Key Features of Disease is widely used for documentation and description of pressure ulcers.

Planning: client goals.   The primary goals for this nursing diagnosis are that the client will (1) experience prevention of skin impairment through pressure relief or (2) promote the healing of impaired skin.

Interventions: nonsurgical management.   An enormous variety of topical and mechanical remedies have been developed for the prevention and treatment of pressure ulcers; these measures have had varying success rates.

Preventive measures.   The cornerstone of prevention of pressure ulcers is frequent position changes in combination with adequate skin care and sufficient nutritional intake. In general, the nurse should turn and reposition the client every 2 hours; however, this may not be sufficient for individuals who are frail and emaciated. Therefore, the nurse assesses the client's skin condition each time the client is turned and repositioned to determine the best turning schedule. For example, if the client has been sleeping soundly for 2 hours, and the nurse decides to postpone turning for 1 hour, reddened areas over the client's bony prominences may be found. If such reddened areas do not fade within 30 minutes after pressure relief, they may be classified as preulcer areas. Some clients need to be turned and repositioned every hour to prevent development of pressure ulcers; others may tolerate 2 to 3 hours between turnings (see Chap. 40).

Adequate skin care is an essential component of pressure ulcer prevention. The nurse performs or assists the client in completing skin care each time the client is turned, repositioned, or bathed. Skin care includes the cleaning of soiled areas, followed by careful drying, massage, and application of body lotion. If preulcer areas are noted, the nurse does not rub these areas, as this causes more extensive damage to the already fragile capillary system. Rather, the nurse maintains careful observation of the preulcer areas for further breakdown and relieves pressure on the areas as much as possible.

Sufficient nutrition is required for both wound repair and pressure ulcer prevention. The nurse works with the dietitian to assess the client's diet and ensure that it contains adequate protein and carbohydrates.

Mechanical devices.   Pressure-relieving devices include water beds, foam mattresses, air mattresses, alternating-pressure mattresses, and air-fluidized devices (Fig. 22–3). Pressure-relieving devices are effective, but do not eliminate the need for turning and repositioning. Water beds, foam mattresses, and air mattresses eliminate limited amounts of pressure from the bony prominences and reduce the risk of skin breakdown. It is essential that frequent turning and repositioning schedules be maintained while such mattresses are used.

Air-fluidized therapy provides highly effective pressure relief, whereby the client is maintained in a nearly pressure-free environment. If optimal nutritional status and healing conditions are maintained, skin breakdowns that have occurred should heal with continued use of air-fluidized therapy. The primary disadvantage of such treatment is its expense, which may exceed several hundred dollars for each day of use. The cost of air-fluidized therapy may be reimbursed by some health insurance providers or by Medicare, in some cases.

Topical treatment.   Numerous topical agents have been used for the prevention and treatment of pressure

KEY FEATURES OF DISEASE ■ Classification of Pressure Ulcers

Type of Ulcer	Characteristics
Preulcer	The skin remains unbroken, and there is an area of redness or discoloration that does not fade for 30 min or more after the removal of pressure.
Grade 1 ulcer	The ulcerated area is limited to superficial epidermal and dermal layers.
Grade 2 ulcer	The ulcerated area involves the subcutaneous adipose tissue.
Grade 3 ulcer	The ulcerated area involves the muscle tissue.
Grade 4 ulcer	The ulcerated area involves the muscle, bone, and joint structures.

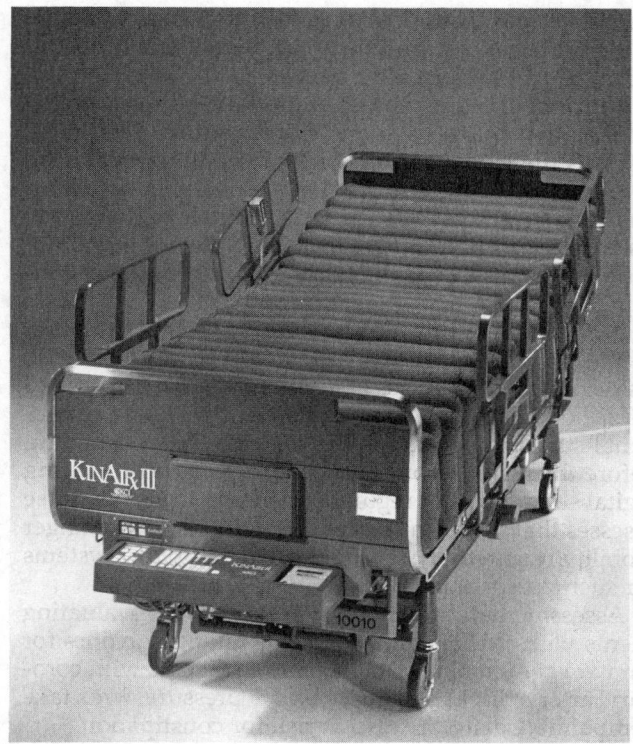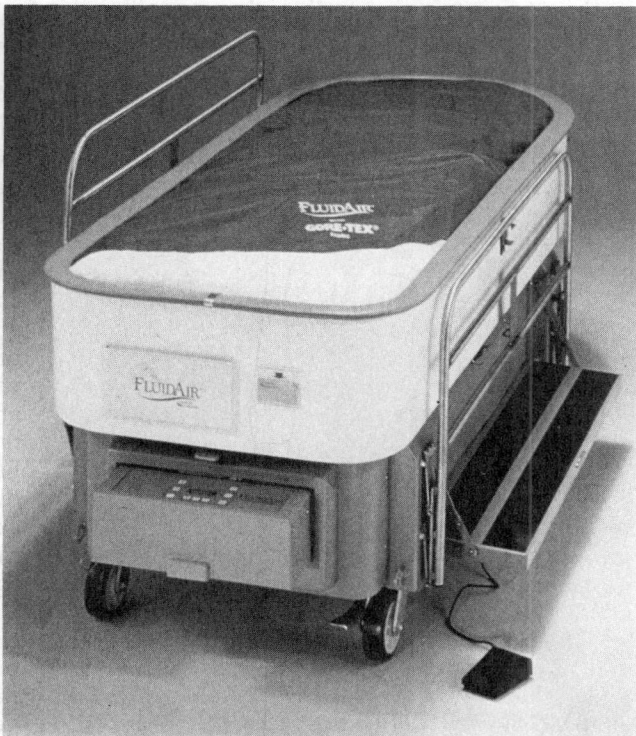

Figure 22 – 3

Pressure relief devices. *Left*, KinAir beds provide controlled air suspension to redistribute body weight away from bony prominences. *Right*, FluidAir beds use airflow and bead fluidization. Both of these beds are covered with Gore-Tex fabric, which resists tearing. This fabric is also waterproof and acts as a barrier for bacteria. (Courtesy of Kinetic Concepts, Inc., San Antonio, TX.)

ulcers, including sugar, absorbable gelatin (Gelfoam), dried blood, honey, insulin, antibiotic cream, hydrogen peroxide, povidone-iodine preparations (Betadine), acetic acid, and soaps. Although some of these treatments may seem odd, each is based on correcting a deficiency of the pressure ulcer. The use of sugar, honey, and blood is based on the belief that the pressure ulcer is due to a lack of nutrition. There is some truth in this, in that the cause of a pressure ulcer is the deprivation of blood supply to the ulcerated area. Treatments such as hydrogen peroxide and povidone-iodine are believed to clean the ulcer area, thus preventing infection. Insulin is used to increase protein synthesis. Each of the agents used has been documented to have some degree of success in the treatment of pressure ulcers, but studies to confirm the effectiveness of such agents are limited. Chapter 40 describes pressure ulcer care in detail.

Constipation; Bowel Incontinence; Diarrhea

Bowel control problems commonly result from various chronic disorders. These problems can be caused by the disease or the treatment of the disease. Specific nursing diagnoses have been developed for particular elimination problems; these include but are not limited to constipation, bowel incontinence, and diarrhea.

The specific type of elimination problem that develops depends on the underlying cause of the illness or disability. For example, a client with a neurologic structural defect, such as spinal cord injury, may manifest bowel incontinence. A client with chronic cardiac or respiratory disease or cancer is more likely to have a problem related to drug therapy, immobility, or poor nutrition. Because different bowel elimination problems occur with chronic illness, and because all are assessed similarly, they are discussed together.

The structures of the gastrointestinal (GI) system are composed of smooth muscle. The external anal sphincter remains contracted while in a resting state. Either the forceful movement of feces or the pressure created with abdominal muscles by means of Valsalva maneuver is needed to overcome the contraction of the external anal sphincter. GI motility is the result of two actions: peristalsis (or wave-like contractions) in the small intestine and mass movement in the large intestine. In the absence of a structural defect, mass movement occurs two or three times per day, usually after meals, and leads to the urge to defecate. Defecation usually occurs every 24 to 48 hours, but may occur more or less frequently. The defecation reflex occurs in the following manner: As mass movement occurs, feces are propelled into the rectum. As the rectum becomes distended, stretch receptors located within the rectum are stimulated and an impulse is relayed to the spinal cord at the level of S2-4, where it is simultaneously transmitted to the cortical region of the brain and interpreted as the

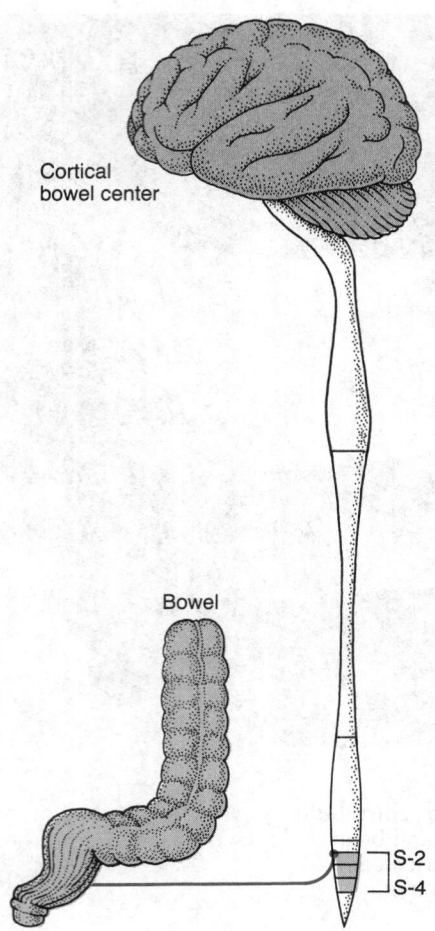

Figure 22–4

The defecation reflex. Normal defecation involves impulses that travel from the rectum to the spinal cord at the level of S2-4, then upward to the cortical region of the brain. An upper motor neuron disease or defect may result in a reflex bowel pattern because impulses are not transmitted to the cortical center. Lower motor neuron defects interfere with nerve transmission across the reflex arc.

defecation urge (Fig. 22–4). The individual may suppress or allow the reflex. Defecation requires abdominal and pelvic strength and the Valsalva maneuver.

While assessing clients for impaired bowel function, the nurse takes a careful history of bowel function, nutritional status, functional and physical status, and drug therapy. The nurse assesses current and previous bowel habits. Assessment includes a determination of the normal stool frequency and characteristics before the illness or injury occurred. Did the client use enemas or laxatives frequently before the injury or illness? Consistent use of laxatives and enemas leads to decreased bowel tone and laxative or enema dependence. Of additional importance is any routine the client had regarding defecation. The nurse assesses individual defecation patterns to determine the elements of bowel retraining that will have a high likelihood of success. An elderly man who before

his stroke rose every morning, had two cups of coffee and a big breakfast, and then had a stool will probably return to this pattern after stroke.

Nutritional status is also important because of the interrelationship of diet and bowel habits. The nurse assesses the client's nutritional habits, in particular, to determine if the client regularly eats foods or drinks fluids that promote constipation, diarrhea, or flatulence. Assessment of fluid intake includes a determination of the quantity as well as the types of fluids routinely consumed.

Assessment of physical status includes an evaluation of the client's injury and a determination of possible ways in which the illness or injury may be anticipated to affect bowel habits. The nurse assesses the client's functional status to determine the optimal bowel program. Before the nurse recommends a program incorporating digital stimulation or regular suppository use, the nurse assesses that the client is capable of the hand and finger mobility required or that the client has support systems for such personal care.

Assessment of drug therapy is essential in evaluating clients with chronic illness. Clients taking narcotics for pain are at high risk for constipation. Clients with coronary artery disease or high blood pressure who take verapamil (Calan) are also at risk for constipation.

Planning: client goals. The primary client goals for these diagnoses are that the client will (1) achieve a personally acceptable form of bowel elimination and (2) prevent bowel elimination complications.

Interventions: nonsurgical management. An overview of nonsurgical management of bowel elimination problems is given in the accompanying Key Features of Disease (refer to Chaps. 33 and 45 for additional information). In many cases, clients are not able to regain control over their bowel function in the manner previously possible. The nurse assists the client in designing a bowel elimination program that accommodates the current disability.

Neurologic problems often affect the client's bowel pattern in one of three ways. Upper motor neuron diseases and injuries, such as a high-level spinal cord injury, may result in a *reflex* bowel pattern, with defecation occurring suddenly and without warning. With a reflex pattern, any facilitation or triggering mechanism may lead to defecation if the lower colon contains stool. The nurse can suggest numerous techniques, including facilitation or triggering mechanisms, to stimulate defecation; these may be incorporated into a bowel training program. If there is an upper motor neuron problem, and the reflex arc is intact (reflex bladder pattern), any stimulus that sends the message to the spinal cord level S2-4 that the lower bowel might be distended can initiate the defecation response. Examples of facilitation or triggering techniques include providing anal stimulation (by inserting a finger [using either a finger cot or rubber glove and lubrication] to the first joint), gently pinching the anus, and pulling pubic hair.

KEY FEATURES OF DISEASE ▪ Types of Bowel Dysfunction and How They Are Managed

Functional Type	Neurologic Disability	Dysfunction	Re-establishing Defecation Patterns
Reflex	Upper motor neuron spinal cord injury above T-12	Defecation without warning	Triggering mechanisms Facilitation techniques High-fiber diet Suppository (glycerin) use Consistent toileting schedule
Flaccid	Lower motor neuron spinal cord injury below T-12	Frequent stools	Triggering or facilitating techniques High-fiber diet Suppository (glycerin) use Consistent toileting schedule
Uninhibited	Brain damage, hemiplegia	Frequency, urgency, and constipation	Consistent toileting schedule High-fiber diet Stool softener use

Data from Martin, N., Holt, N. B., & Hicks, D. (1981). *Comprehensive rehabilitation nursing.* New York: McGraw-Hill.

Lower motor neuron diseases and injuries interfere with transmission of the nervous impulse across the reflex arc and may result in a *flaccid* bowel pattern, with defecation occurring frequently and in small amounts. Although a flaccid bowel pattern is more difficult to control successfully, the use of facilitation and triggering mechanisms in combination with toilet use scheduling and suppository use yields the best results.

Neurologic injuries affecting the brain may cause an *uninhibited* bowel pattern, with frequent defecation, urgency, and complaints of constipation. Uninhibited bowel patterns may be managed through consistent scheduling, a high-fiber diet, and the use of stool softeners.

First-line management for clients with neurologic bowel dysfunction should include dietary modification (discussed later). In addition, the nurse works with the client to schedule bowel elimination as close to the client's previous routine as possible. A client who had stools at noon, every other day, before the illness or injury, should have the bowel program scheduled likewise. Methods to facilitate the defecation response may include digital stimulation and glycerin or bisacodyl (Dulcolax) suppository use. Digital stimulation is most frequently employed for clients with primary neurologic disorders. This method should not be used for clients with cardiac disease because of the risk of inducing a vagal response (a drop in heart rate). Laxatives are often used for clients with chronic cardiac and cancer-related illness. Should these methods be unsuccessful in assisting the client to achieve a regular defecation pattern, the nurse incorporates enemas into the client's bowel program.

Drug therapy. Bowel programs for clients with neurologic defects frequently are designed to include the combination of suppository use and a consistent toilet-ing schedule (Table 22-4). Although medications should not be a first resort when determining a bowel program, the nurse routinely considers the need for a glycerin or bisacodyl suppository if the client does not re-establish defecation habits through consistent scheduling of toileting, dietary modification, and anal stimulation. The most common agents given as suppositories in bowel programs are bisacodyl and glycerin. Both agents are equivalent in effect, with results occurring in 10 to 15 minutes. The suppository should be administered at the time at which the client would expect to defecate. For example, if a client had a previous bowel habit of defecating every other day after breakfast, the suppository should be administered every other day after breakfast. Ordinarily, administering the suppository every second or third day is effective in re-establishing defecation patterns. Depending on individual need, other medications may be indicated for bowel programs (see Table 22-4) such as laxatives.

Diet therapy. Factors affecting bowel elimination are directly related to the type and quality of food and fluid ingested. The accompanying Health Promotion/Maintenance feature lists some foods affecting motility. A high-fiber diet is a mainstay of most bowel programs and includes whole-grain foods, bran, and fresh and dried fruits. Increasing dietary fiber is effective in facilitating defecation only if fat intake is reduced. In the case of a flaccid bowel pattern, occurring with lower motor neuron involvement, the frequency of stools may be increased and a diet high in fiber should be avoided.

Prevention of complications. Common complications of any bowel program are constipation, diarrhea, and flatulence. The nurse assesses clients for these complications and modifies the bowel program accordingly. One infrequent complication occurring primarily in

TABLE 22–4 Drugs Used for Clients in Bowel Programs

Drug	Usual Daily Dosage	Interventions	Rationales
Suppositories			
Bisacodyl (Dulcolax)	10 mg	Encourage defecation within 10–15 min.	Effects usually occur in 15–20 min.
Vacuetts	1 suppository	Do not use with petrolatum lubricants.	Petrolatum negates the efficacy.
Glycerin	1 suppository	Encourage defecation within 15–20 min.	Effects usually occur in 30 min.
Bulk-Forming Laxatives			
Psyllium hydrophilic mucilloid (Metamucil, Hydrocil)	1 tsp in one to three doses	Give with 8 oz of fluids.	Action is dependent on sufficient water intake.
Lubricant Laxatives			
Mineral oil	1–2 tbsp	Give h.s. at least 2 h p.c.	Reflux aspiration can occur.
Fleet mineral oil enema	160 mL	Long-term use is not recommended.	
Saline Laxatives			
Magnesium hydroxide (milk of magnesia)	2–4 tbsp	Give with glass of water. Use for less than 1 wk is recommended.	Acts by drawing water into the gut. Complications with long-term use include magnesium retention.
Lactulose (Cephulac)	15–30 mL	Give with breakfast. Long-term use is not recommended.	Effects occur in 24 h or more. Use is expensive and promotes dependence.

HEATLH PROMOTION/MAINTENANCE ■ Foods That Affect Gastrointestinal Motility

Foods That Increase Motility

Whole grains
Coarse bran
Oranges
Apples
Carrots
Brussels sprouts
Dried fruits
Coffee
Alcohol

Foods That Decrease Motility

Milk
Cheese
High-fat foods

clients with high-level spinal cord injuries is autonomic hyperreflexia. (See the discussion regarding the prevention of complications of altered patterns of urinary elimination later for information on the pathophysiology of autonomic hyperreflexia.) For clients with quadriplegia who are susceptible to autonomic hyperreflexia, the nurse applies dibucaine (Nupercainal) ointment to the anus at least 10 minutes before digital stimulation, suppository administration, or rectal checks.

Altered Patterns of Urinary Elimination; Reflex Incontinence; Total Incontinence; Urinary Retention

The most frequent type of urinary problem is incontinence. The incidence of incontinence has been estimated to range from 16% to 42% (Martin et al., 1981). Those especially troubled with incontinence are the elderly and individuals with muscular and neurologic problems. Bladder function should be controlled for rehabilitation to be successful. Incontinence disrupts and limits all activity. Individuals who are incontinent are

TABLE 22 – 4 Drugs Used for Clients in Bowel Programs Continued

Drug	Usual Daily Dosage	Interventions	Rationales
Fleet enema	160 mL	Give near commode or toilet. Long-term use is not recommended.	Effects occur in 2 – 5 min. Use promotes dependence.
Stimulant Laxatives			
Cascara	5 mL	Long-term use is not recommended.	Agent is habit forming and may cause mucosal irritation.
Danthron (Modane)	1 tablet (75 mg) or 1 – 2 tsp liquid	Long-term use is not recommended.	Agent is habit forming and may cause mucosal irritation.
Senna (Senokot)	2 tablets or 1 tsp granules	Give at h.s. Long-term use is not recommended.	Agent is habit forming and may cause mucosal irritation.
Castor oil	15 – 60 mL	Long-term use is not recommended.	Agent is habit forming and may cause mucosal irritation.
Bisacodyl (Dulcolax)	10 – 15 mg	Give with evening meal. Long-term use is not recommended.	Effect occurs in 6 h. Agent is habit forming and may cause mucosal irritation.
Stool Softeners			
Docusate sodium (Colace, Modane Soft)	50 – 200 mg	Do not use with mineral oil.	Use may increase intestinal absorption of mineral oil.
Docusate calcium (Surfak)	240 mg	Do not use with mineral oil.	Use may increase intestinal absorption of mineral oil.

unable to work or travel; even short trips or errands (e.g., to the grocery store) may be problematic. Incontinence results in social isolation from family and friends and disrupts ADL. Incontinent individuals may fear causing offense or receiving complaints regarding body and urine odors from others at home, school, and work. A primary goal of rehabilitation is for the client to achieve and maintain acceptable forms of urinary bladder emptying. In determining interventions and components of a bladder program, the nurse considers the client's personality and individual desires regarding methods and routines for bladder management.

To be able to assess bladder function, the nurse must understand the voiding reflex. When the bladder fills with urine, the nerves lining the bladder or detrusor muscles are stimulated. The impulse travels through the afferent fibers to the spinal cord at the S2-4 level and is transmitted to the frontal lobe (cortical bladder center) (Fig. 22 – 5).

Planning: client goals. The primary client goals for these diagnoses are that the client will (1) achieve a personally acceptable form of urinary elimination and (2) prevent urinary elimination complications.

Interventions: nonsurgical management. An overview of nonsurgical management of urinary elimination problems is given in the accompanying Key Features of Disease (for additional information, see Chaps. 33 and 58).

Three basic types of neurologic problems may interfere with successful bladder control. Injuries that cause damage to the lower motor neuron at the spinal level of S2-4 (e.g., multiple sclerosis and paraplegia) may directly interfere with the reflex arc and result in inappropriate interpretation of the efferent and afferent impulses. The bladder fills, and afferent impulses conduct the message via the spinal cord to the cortical region of the brain; but, because of the injury, the impulse is not interpreted correctly by the cortical bladder center, with a failure to respond with a message for the bladder to empty. A *flaccid bladder* occurs, with urinary retention.

Neurologic problems affecting the upper motor neuron may occur with high-level spinal cord injuries

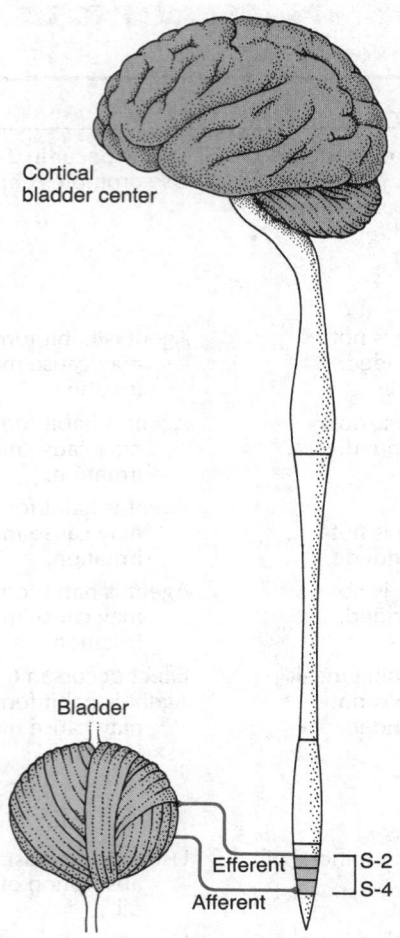

Figure 22–5

The voiding reflex. Normal urination involves nerve transmission from a filled bladder to the spinal cord at level S2-4 and upward toward the cortical bladder center in the brain. Upper motor neuron defects result in the failure of impulse transmission to the cortical center. Clients with this problem do not sense a full bladder. If the reflex arc is intact, a reflex bladder results, leading to incontinence. Lower motor neuron defects interfere with function of the reflex arc. A flaccid bladder results, leading to urinary retention.

(e.g., quadriplegia), resulting in a failure of impulse transmission to or from the lower spinal cord areas to the cortex. Therefore, the bladder fills and transmits impulses to the spinal cord, but the individual is not conscious of the filling sensation. However, if there is no injury at the lower spinal cord level, and the voiding reflex arc is intact, the efferent impulse is relayed that the bladder should empty. A *reflex bladder* occurs, with incontinence characterized by sudden gushing voids.

A third type of bladder problem is an *uninhibited bladder*, which may occur with neurologic problems that affect the cortical bladder center of the brain (frontal lobe), such as stroke or brain injury.

There are numerous techniques, including facilitating or triggering techniques, that the nurse uses to stimulate voiding, and these may be incorporated into a bladder training program. If there is an upper motor neuron problem, and the reflex arc is intact (reflex bladder pattern), any stimulus that sends the message to the spinal cord level S2-4 that the bladder might be full can initiate the voiding response. Examples of such techniques include stroking the medial aspect of the thigh, pinching the area above the inguinal ligament, pulling pubic hair, massaging the penoscrotal area, pinching the posterior aspect of the glans penis, and providing anal stimulation.

When the client has a lower motor neuron problem, the voiding reflex arc may not be intact (flaccid bladder pattern), and additional stimulation may be needed to initiate voiding. Two types of techniques used to facilitate voiding include the *Valsalva maneuver* and the *Credé maneuver*. The Valsalva maneuver is implemented by the nurse's instructing the client to hold his/her breath and bear down as if trying to urinate. The nurse assists the client in performing the Credé maneuver by placing the client's hand in a cupped position directly over the bladder area, and pushing inward and downward as if massaging the bladder to empty.

Bladder training. The techniques used by the nurse to assist the client in "repatterning" voiding, or bladder training, include intermittent catheterization, intermittent clamping of an indwelling urinary catheter, and consistent scheduling of toileting routines.

KEY FEATURES OF DISEASE ■ Types of Urinary Elimination Dysfunction and How They Are Managed

Functional Type	Neurologic Disability	Dysfunction	Re-establishing Voiding Patterns
Reflex	Upper motor neuron spinal cord injury above T-12	Urinary frequency, urgency	Triggering or facilitating techniques Medications
Flaccid	Lower motor neuron spinal cord injury below T-12	Dribbling, overflow, stress incontinence	Valsalva's and Credé's maneuvers Medications
Uninhibited	Brain damage, hemiplegia	Frequency, urgency, voiding in small amounts	Consistent toileting schedule Regulation of fluid intake

Intermittent catheterization is a method of bladder training frequently used for problems involving a flaccid bladder pattern, often caused by a lower motor neuron problem. In assisting the client with intermittent catheterization, the nurse inserts a urinary catheter every 2 to 3 hours initially, after the client has attempted voiding and has used Valsalva's and Credé's maneuvers. If less than 150 mL of residual urine is obtained, the nurse increases the interval between catheterizations to 3 to 4 hours. The interval may be increased to a maximum of 4 to 6 hours, but the client should not go beyond 6 hours between catheterizations, unless the residual urine volume is less than 150 mL each time, with an adequate intake of fluids (see discussion of diet therapy later). If the client will be performing intermittent self-catheterization at home after discharge from the hospital, the nurse instructs the client on clean (not sterile) technique. The nurse instructs the client on proper hand washing and perineal cleaning before catheterization. The female client is instructed in the use of a mirror for catheter insertion. The nurse instructs the client that a catheter should be washed in hot soapy water after each use and should be kept in a clean plastic bag or glass jar between uses. The catheter should be discarded when it is no longer soft and flexible. If the client becomes rehospitalized, the nurse instructs the client to use a sterile catheter with each catheterization to prevent nosocomial infections (infections related to the hospital environment).

Intermittent clamping of the indwelling catheter is seldom used because of insufficient documentation as to the technique's effectiveness with regard to regaining bladder capacity and tone. However, the nurse needs to be aware of the technique and its safe performance, as the risks of complication include bladder rupture, vesicoureteral reflux, and kidney damage. Intermittent clamping of the indwelling catheter is done on a regular basis, usually by clamping the catheter for 2 to 3 hours initially, with release for 15 minutes and then reclamping. The clamping intervals are gradually increased, up to 4 hours, with release for 15 minutes. After catheter removal, the nurse assesses the client for re-establishment of an acceptable voiding pattern, incontinence, or urinary retention. If at all possible, the practice of intermittent clamping of the indwelling catheter should be avoided, as the use of an indwelling catheter increases the client's risk of urinary tract infection. Intermittent catheterization and bladder training through establishing a consistent toileting schedule are the preferred techniques.

Consistent toileting routines may be the optimal way of re-establishing voiding continence when an uninhibited bladder pattern (associated with brain damage or head injury) is displayed. The nurse assesses the client's previous voiding pattern and determines the client's daily routine. At a minimum, the nurse assists the client with voiding in the morning, after rising, before and after meals, before and after physical activity, and at bedtime. The nurse considers the client's bladder capacity, which may range from 100 to 500 mL, in addition to

the client's mobility and clothing that may be restrictive. The nurse determines the client's bladder capacity by measuring the urinary output. In addition, the nurse ensures that the client is aware of nearby bathrooms at all times or has a call system to contact the nurse for assistance.

Drug therapy. Medications that may be used for urinary elimination problems include cholinergics, antispasmodics, anticholinergics, and skeletal muscle relaxants (Table 22–5). Medications are not usually the initial management for bladder problems, but may be used to augment a bladder program. In general, anticholinergics, antispasmodics, and skeletal muscle relaxants may promote continence in clients with a reflex bladder. Cholinergics may decrease urinary retention problems in clients with a flaccid bladder. Clients with uninhibited bladder do not routinely require medications for bladder programs, unless the urinary function is affected by additional pathologic changes.

Diet therapy. The nurse instructs the client to maintain an adequate intake of fluids, at least 3000 mL/day. This amount of fluid intake should be modified to prevent complications in clients with congestive heart disease or renal problems. The nurse encourages the client to drink fluids that *promote an acidic urine,* including cranberry juice, prune juice, bouillon, tomato juice, plum juice, and water. Fluids that promote an *alkaline urine are discouraged,* including citrus juices, excessive milk and milk products, and carbonated beverages. An acidic urine is preferred to minimize risks of urinary tract infection and calculi formation. In addition, fluids high in caloric content are discouraged, as these promote weight gain.

Prevention of complications. Autonomic hyperreflexia or dysreflexia may occur with upper motor neuron problems when there is a noxious stimulus occurring below the level of the injury, for example, urinary retention, constipation, or pressure ulcer. The stimulation causes sympathetic nervous system hyperactivity, with release of norepinephrine, leading to arteriolar spasm and to vasoconstriction below the level of injury. The client experiences hypertension, blurred vision, redness of the skin, diaphoresis, and vasodilation above the level of the injury. The client's blood pressure level may rise to greater than 300/175. The client may experience headache and seizures. Autonomic hyperreflexia is considered a medical emergency and may result in cerebrovascular accident (CVA), respiratory arrest, and myocardial failure if not treated rapidly. Initial treatment should include raising the head of the bed by 45 degrees to create orthostatic hypotension. The nurse identifies and removes the noxious stimulus, monitors the client's blood pressure every 3 to 5 minutes, gives oxygen, and monitors the client's cardiac condition. Catheterization may be necessary, as urinary retention is a frequent cause of autonomic hyperreflexia. Other common causes include kinking of the urinary catheter and im-

TABLE 22–5 Drugs Used for Clients in Bladder Programs

Drug	Usual Daily Dosage	Interventions	Rationales
Cholinergics			
Bethanechol chloride (Urecholine)	10–50 mg bid–qid PO	1. Give 1 h before or 2 h after meals. 2. Instruct clients to change positions slowly.	1. This agent may cause nausea and vomiting. 2. Orthostatic hypotension is a possible side effect.
Antispasmodics			
Oxybutynin chloride (Ditropan)	5 mg bid or tid PO	1. Instruct the client to avoid driving. 2. Instruct the client to avoid hot environmental temperatures. 3. Assess for urinary retention.	1. Vertigo, drowsiness, and blurred vision may occur. 2. Sweating is suppressed. 3. Retention may be a side effect of drug.
Flavoxate hydrochloride (Urispas)	100–200 mg tid or qid PO	1. Instruct the client to avoid driving. 2. Instruct the client to avoid hot environmental temperatures. 3. Assess for urinary retention.	1. Drowsiness, mental confusion, and blurred vision may occur. 2. Sweating is suppressed. 3. Retention may be a side effect of drug.
Anticholinergics			
Propantheline bromide (Pro-Banthine)	7.5 mg tid PO for elderly or clients of small stature; 15 mg qid for other clients	1. Give 30 min before meals and at h.s. 2. Assess for urinary retention and constipation. 3. Instruct clients to change positions slowly during early therapy. 4. Assess for confusion, agitation, drowsiness.	1. Drugs are better absorbed at these times. 2. These may occur as side effects of drug. 3. Orthostatic hypotension may occur. 4. These symptoms can occur in elderly or debilitated clients.
Skeletal Muscle Relaxants			
Dantrolene (Dantrium)	25 mg once daily PO initially; increase to 25 mg bid–qid, then by 25-mg increments up to 100 mg	1. Instruct the client to avoid driving. 2. Instruct the client to avoid prolonged sun exposure.	1. Fatigue, dizziness, and muscular weakness are side effects. 2. Photosensitivity may occur.
Baclofen (Lioresal)	5 mg tid PO, may increase by 5 mg daily until desired effect attained to maximum of 80 mg	1. Instruct the client to avoid alcohol. 2. Instruct the client to avoid driving.	1. Alcohol potentiates drug effects. 2. Drowsiness and dizziness may occur.

Data from Dittmar, S. (1989). *Rehabilitation nursing. Process and application.* St. Louis: C. V. Mosby; and from Govani L. E., & Hayes, J. E. (1988). *Drugs and nursing implications.* Norwalk, CT: Appleton & Lange.

paction (the nurse *must* apply dibucaine ointment to the anus before checking for fecal impaction when autonomic hyperreflexia is suspected).

Other complications of urinary elimination problems include bladder overdistention and increased urinary residual volume. The nurse monitors the client for urinary problems and adjusts the bladder program to ensure effectiveness.

■ Discharge Planning

The focus of medical-surgical nursing care of clients with rehabilitation needs is on education and preparation for discharge. As such, the nurse begins discharge planning at or before admission. If the client is being transferred from a hospital to a rehabilitation unit or facility, the nurse orients the client to the change in routine and emphasizes self-care. When the client is admitted to the rehabilitation unit or facility, the nurse assesses the client's current living situation at home. The nurse determines, with the client and significant others, the adequacy of the client's current situation and potential needs after discharge to home. Clients with chronic illness and disability who are discharged to home may require home care, assistance with ADL, nursing care, or physical or vocational therapy. The nurse assesses these needs and plans with the client, the family, the social worker, the physical or vocational therapist, and the physician ways to best meet identified needs.

Home Care Preparation

Before the client's return home, the client's readiness for discharge from the hospital must be assessed. The client's home may be assessed in multiple ways. A common method is through a predischarge visit to the home by the nurse or the occupational therapist to assess the home's layout and accessibility. Because of the stress of hospitalization, a client with a fractured hip, who is ambulating well with a walker, may neglect to explain to the nurse that the home has three steps at the entrance and that the bathroom is accessible by stairway only. The client may not consider it important to mention to the nurse that throw rugs are scattered throughout the apartment, which do not provide a completely level surface on which to use a cane. During a predischarge visit to the home, the nurse and occupational therapist inspect the accessibility of the home in general and of the bathrooms, bedrooms, and kitchen. If the client will be wheelchair dependent after discharge, ramps will be needed to replace steps, and doorways need to be checked for adequate width. Usually, a doorway width of 36 to 38 in is sufficient for a standard-sized wheelchair. Any room that the client needs to use is checked. In the bedroom, there needs to be sufficient room for the client to maneuver transfers to and from wheelchair to bed. Space requirements vary, depending on the client's

need to use a wheelchair, a walker, or a cane. In the bathroom, grab bars may need to be installed before the client is discharged from the hospital or rehabilitation facility. Bathtub benches provide support to clients who have difficulty with mobility and, when used in combination with a hand-held showerhead, can provide easily accessible bathing facilities. Assessment of the kitchen may or may not be critical, depending on whether the client has assistance with cooking and preparing meals. If the client will be responsible for cooking after discharge, the kitchen is assessed for wheelchair or walker accessibility, appliance accessibility, and the need for adaptive equipment.

A second method for assessing the client's home is through a brief home visit by the client before discharge. The nurse prepares the client by explaining the need for the trial home visit and by assessing the client's comfort level with this idea. Clients who have been hospitalized for a lengthy period may feel intense anxiety about returning home. Careful preparation by the nurse may allay such anxieties. Before the visit, the nurse meets with the client and significant others to set goals for the experience and to identify specific tasks that the client should attempt during the time at home. After the client has been home, the nurse interviews the client to determine the success of the visit and additional education or training needs before final discharge.

Client/Family Education

Education of the client and the family is the cornerstone of nursing care. Every component of the client's care is assessed by the nurse to determine how the client can be taught to perform ADL independently or to direct self-care activities. The nurse assesses the client's learning potential and cognitive deficits. As care is provided, the nurse explains the procedure and rationale. The client is encouraged to perform or direct the technique independently to verify understanding. Written material explaining the steps in the procedure is given to the client to reinforce learning and to provide support with the technique after discharge from the hospital. However, before giving the client written material, the nurse assesses the reading level of the material and determines whether it is appropriate for the client's reading ability and language skills.

Psychosocial Preparation

Any chronic illness or disability necessitates changes in a client's life style and body image. The nurse assists the client in dealing with such changes by encouraging the client to verbalize feelings and emotions and by helping the client to focus on existing capabilities instead of disabilities. The nurse assists the client with psychosocial preparation for discharge by assessing the client's ability to deal with the chronic illness or disabil-

NURSING RESEARCH

When Clients with Spinal Cord Injury Believe That Skin Care Is Important, They Comply with Skin Care Regimens.

Dai, Y-T., & Catanzaro, M. (1987). Health beliefs and compliance with a skin care regimen. *Rehabilitation Nursing, 12*(1), 13–16.

The Health Belief Model by Rosenstock (1974) has been proposed to examine variables related to compliance with health care regimens. Studies have demonstrated that the variables related to compliance with preventive regimens include (1) perceived susceptibility to the disease, (2) perceived severity of the disease, (3) perceived efficacy of the preventive regimens, (4) perceived barriers to performing preventive regimens, (5) cues to action, and (6) modifying factors. This descriptive study surveyed a convenience sample of 20 paraplegic men, ranging in age from 23 to 59 years. The mean age was 37.6 years. The clients were able to independently carry out routine skin care, and their mean educational level was 7.6 years. They had been injured 0.5 to 8.1 years before the study.

The investigators developed a questionnaire to assess the participants' health beliefs. A Likert-type scale was utilized to score the responses. The validity and the reliability of the questionnaire were not evaluated. Compliance was measured by both the participants' knowledge of skin care strategies and actual behavioral performance and compliance with skin care regimens. A multiple-choice questionnaire was used to measure knowledge. No validity or reliability data were reported for this instrument.

The mean scores for perceived susceptibility, perceived seriousness, perceived efficiency, and perceived barriers were 5.95, 7.70, 7.50, and 6.35, with maximal possible scores of 9, 9, 8, and 8, respectively. The researchers found that the perceived severity of pressure sores, the perceived efficacy of skin care, and the sum of the participants' beliefs about skin care were positively related to compliance with skin care. Perceived barriers to skin care and perceived susceptibility to pressure sores were not found to be significantly correlated with skin care compliance.

Critique. Results of this study are supported by other studies of client education. Therefore, nurses should implement these findings in their practice. There are, however, limitations to the study, including a small sample size, a sample that was not randomly selected, and a lack of validity and reliability of instruments.

Possible nursing implications. In teaching paraplegic clients, nurses need to emphasize the following: (1) information concerning the severity of pressure sores, (2) knowledge and appropriate techniques of skin care, and (3) evidence of benefits of efficient skin care. The nurse should utilize the clients' health beliefs as motivational factors to influence compliance with skin care. The nurse should point out to clients when they are performing skin care correctly and efficiently. The nurse can also help the client relate the importance of correct skin care regimens to the prevention of skin breakdown.

ity. A right-handed client who has left-sided weakness from a CVA may not recognize that there is any disability. Such a client may fail to relate psychologically to the disability during hospitalization, in spite of the efforts of the nurse toward preparation, and will be a safety risk after discharge to home. The client may display anger or frustration in attempting to perform self-care routines before discharge from the hospital. The nurse encourages the client to be open about such feelings and to talk about ways to prevent worries from becoming realities after discharge. The predischarge home visit assists the client and significant others in psychosocial preparation for discharge, as it allows the client to experience the home situation while being able to return to the hospital environment after a few hours. Clients often find that their fears were not realized during the home visit and, not infrequently, find new problems in the home that must be addressed before discharge from the hospital. The nurse reviews this information with the client in furthering the preparation for discharge.

Health Care Resources

Various health care resources (such as physical therapy and vocational therapy) are available to clients with chronic illness and disability after discharge from the hospital or rehabilitation facilities. The nurse assesses the client's need for additional care and support throughout the client's hospitalization and works with the social worker and the physician in arranging for services.

Postdischarge Follow-up

An essential component of nursing care of clients with chronic illness and disability is evaluation and follow-up. Nursing interventions with such clients are directed toward anticipating and meeting the client's needs after discharge. The nurse contacts the client after discharge to determine how well the client feels things are going. The nurse notifies the client before discharge that the client will be contacted at a specified time after discharge and inquires as to the best telephone number and time of day to call. During the telephone call, the nurse assesses the client's functional abilities as self-reported by the client to determine the success of predischarge planning. If problems are detected, the nurse contacts the physician or the home care nurse, as indicated. Information obtained during the follow-up contact is used by the nurse in revision of the client's ongoing home plan of care and is used in the determination of care plans for clients with similar problems.

Evaluation

On the basis of the identified nursing diagnoses, the client and the nurse evaluate the rehabilitative interventions for the client with disabling or chronic conditions. Expected outcomes include that the client

1. Demonstrates the ability to perform ADL with minimal or no assistance
2. Shows maximal physical mobility
3. Has intact skin
4. Demonstrates effective bowel elimination
5. Demonstrates effective urinary elimination

SUMMARY

The nurse cares for clients with chronic illness or disability during continuation or exacerbation of a chronic problem or after the initial occurrence of the disabling illness or injury. The rehabilitation process is not limited to care of the client with neurologic defects, such as spinal cord injury. Instead, it is applicable to clients with any chronic illness that has an associated alteration in functional ability (impairment).

The goal of rehabilitation is to restore clients to the fullest functional level possible. Nursing intervention focuses on teaching self-care skills and aiding the client in the development of these skills. All interventions are implemented in preparation for discharge from the hospital.

IMPLICATIONS FOR RESEARCH

Diverse research is affecting the care of clients with chronic illness and disability. Clinical investigation and inquiry regarding methods to promote mobilization, elimination, comfort, and coping behaviors are occurring actively and will result in improved client care.

Nursing research needs to be conducted to answer the following questions related to the care of clients with chronic illness and disability:

1. What effect does nursing care have on the outcome for clients with chronic illness and disability?
2. How should the role of nursing within the interdisciplinary health care team be defined and made operational?

3. What are the most efficient and cost-effective methods of reducing the incidence of pressure ulcers?
4. What effect does health teaching have on successful client outcome after discharge?

REFERENCES AND READINGS

American Nurses' Association and Association of Rehabilitation Nurses. (1988). *Standards of rehabilitation nursing practice.* Kansas City: American Nurses' Association.

Brillhart, B. (1986). Predictors of self-acceptance. *Rehabilitation Nursing, 11*(2), 8–12.

Carlson, C. (1980). Psychological aspects of neurologic disability. *Nursing Clinics of North America, 15*, 309–320.

Dittmar, S. (1989). *Rehabilitation nursing: Process and application.* St. Louis: C. V. Mosby.

Falvo, D. R. (1985). *Effective patient education.* Rockville, MD: Aspen Systems.

Grunewald, J. (1986). Wheelchair selection from a nursing perspective. *Rehabilitation Nursing, 11*(6), 31–32.

Martin, N., Holt, N. B., & Hicks, D. (1981). *Comprehensive rehabilitation nursing.* New York: McGraw-Hill.

Norman, V., & Snyder, M. (1982). Assessment of self-care readiness. *Rehabilitation Nursing, 7*(3), 17–21.

ADDITIONAL READINGS

Dudas, S., & Carlson, C. E. (1988). Cancer rehabilitation. *Oncology Nursing Forum, 15*(2), 183–188.

This article discusses the importance of emphasizing rehabilitation for clients with cancer. Functional disabilities common among clients with cancer are addressed as they relate to physical, psychologic, and social functions. Goals and interventions for these clients are also discussed.

Nelson, A. K., & Kelley, B. (1983). Patient and family workshops: A new teaching approach for spinal cord injury. *Rehabilitation Nursing, 8*(6), 13–16.

This article presents a format used for a 2-day client and family training workshop at a Veterans Administration Hospital. A client-family group approach was used for teaching. Sample goals, objectives, and a discharge skills check list are included.

Parchert, M. A., & Simon, J. M. (1988). The role of exercise in cardiac rehabilitation: A nursing perspective. *Rehabilitation Nursing, 13*(1), 11–14.

This article describes the physiologic and psychologic benefits of exercise in the rehabilitation of clients with cardiac disease. Rehabilitation programs should be individualized to maximize benefits. Nursing assessment and the development of nursing diagnoses pertinent to each client's situation were recommended to achieve this goal.

Voith, A. M. (1988). Alterations in urinary elimination: Concepts, research, and practice. *Rehabilitation Nursing, 13*(3), 122–131.

This three-part article demonstrates how nursing diagnoses are developed and confirmed. The diagnosis of altered patterns of urinary elimination is presented. The article describes several ways in which a systematic application of the findings could occur.

UNIT 6 RESOURCES

Nursing Resources

American Association of Spinal Cord Injury Nurses (AASCIN), 75-20 Astoria Boulevard, Jackson Heights, NY 11370. Telephone 718-803-3782.
See Unit 10 Resources for more information.

Association of Rehabilitation Nurses, 2506 Gross Point Road, Evanston, IL 60201. Telephone 312-475-1000.

Association of Rehabilitation Nurses Certification Board, 2506 Gross Point Road, Evanston, IL 60201. Telephone 312-475-1000.
Certifies rehabilitation nurses.

Other Resources

American Association on Mental Deficiency, PO Box 96, Willimantic, CT 06226.

American Cancer Society, 1599 Clifton Road NE, Atlanta, GA 30329. Telephone 404-320-3333.

American Diabetes Association, National Service Center, 1600 Duke Street, Alexandria, VA 22314. Telephone 800-232-3472.

American Lung Association, 1740 Broadway, New York, NY 10019. Telephone 212-315-8700.

Arthritis Foundation, 1314 Spring Street NW, Atlanta, GA 30309. Telephone 404-872-7100.

Mainstream (national office), 1030 15th Street NW, Suite 1010, Washington, DC 20005. Telephone 202-898-1400.

National Association for Retarded Citizens, 2501 Avenue J, Arlington, TX 76011.

National Center for American Heart Association, 7320 Greenville Avenue, Dallas, TX 75231. Telephone 214-373-6300.

National Easter Seal Society, 2023 West Ogden Avenue, Chicago, IL 60612. Telephone 312-243-8400.

National Head Injury Foundation, 333 Turnpike Road, Southborough, MA 01722. Telephone 508-485-9950.

National Rehabilitation Association, 633 South Washington, Alexandria, VA 22314. Telephone 703-836-0850.

National Spinal Cord Injury Association, 600 West Cumming Park 3200, Woburn, MA 01801. Telephone 800-962-9629.

Office for Handicapped Individuals, Department of Education, 400 Maryland Avenue SW, Room 3106 Switzer Building, Washington, DC 20202. Telephone 202-245-0080.

PART III

SPECIFIC CLIENT PROBLEMS IN MEDICAL-SURGICAL NURSING

UNIT 7

Management of Clients with Disruptions in Cell Growth and Structure

CHAPTER 23

Concepts of Inflammation and the Immune Response

GENERAL CONCEPTS

Immunity is composed of functions that protect humans against the side effects that can accompany invasion of or injury to the body. People interact with many other living organisms in the environment. The size of these organisms varies from quite large (other humans and animals) to microscopic and submicroscopic (bacteria, viruses, molds, spores, pollens, protozoa, and cells from other people or animals). Humans usually exist in harmony with many of these organisms as long as the organisms do not enter the human body's internal environment. The human body has many defenses to prevent such organisms from gaining access to the internal environment. However, these defenses do not work perfectly, and invasion of the body's internal environment by microorganisms occurs relatively often. The fact that invasion occurs much more frequently than does overt expression of an actual disease or illness is directly related to the immune system's proper functioning.

The ultimate purpose of the cells that compose the immune system is to neutralize, eliminate, or destroy microorganisms that penetrate or invade the internal environment before the invaders have a chance to multiply and overwhelm body defenses. To accomplish this purpose without harming the body, immune system cells mount defensive actions only against *nonself* cells. Therefore, immune system cells can differentiate between the body's own, healthy *self* cells and other *nonself* cells. Nonself cells include infected or debilitated body cells, self cells that have undergone malignant transformation into cancer cells, and all foreign cells (Gallucci, 1987; Groenwald, 1980; Workman, 1989). This ability to recognize self versus nonself, which is necessary so that healthy body cells are not destroyed along with the invaders, is called *self-tolerance*. Recognition and self-tolerance are possible because immune system cells can examine and interpret the surface proteins that are present on any cell that is directly contacted.

SELF VERSUS NONSELF

All organisms are made up of cells. Each cell is surrounded by a plasma membrane (Fig. 23–1). Various different proteins protrude through the membranes of all cells. For example, liver cells have many different proteins present on the cell surface (protruding through the membrane). The amino acid sequence of each protein type differs from that of all other protein types. Some of these proteins are found on the liver cells of all animals (including humans) that have livers because these protein types are specific to the liver and actually serve as a *marker* for liver tissues. Other protein types are found only on the liver cells of human beings because

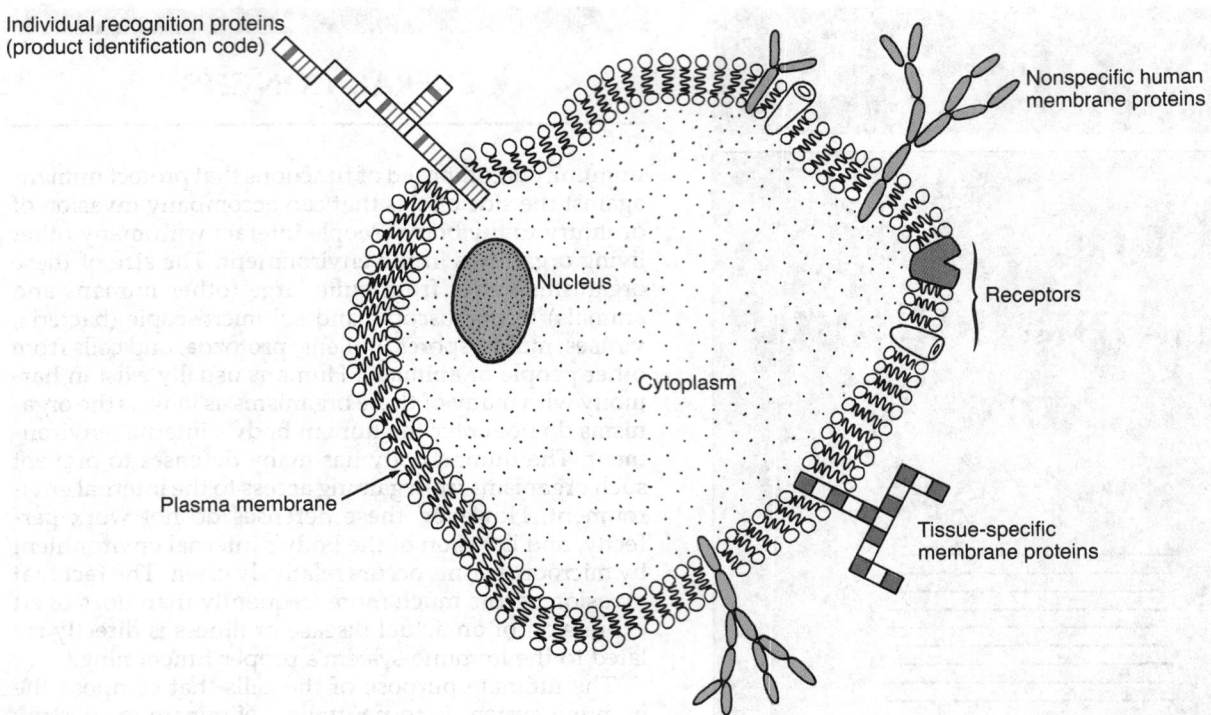

Figure 23 – 1

Properties of human cell membrane proteins.

these protein types are specific markers for humans. Still other protein types are found only on the liver cells of humans with a specific blood type. In addition, each human's liver cells have surface protein types that are specific to that human. These proteins are unique to the individual and would be identical only to the same proteins of an identical twin. These unique proteins, which are found on the surface of all body cells of that individual, serve as a "product identification code" for that person (Guyton, 1986; Roitt, 1984). The proteins that make up the product identification code for one person are recognized as foreign by the immune system of another person, and these proteins are called *antigens.*

This unique product identification code for each person is composed of the *human leukocyte antigens* (HLAs). The term leukocyte antigen is not actually correct because these antigens are also present on the surfaces of all cells containing a nucleus, not just on leukocytes. These antigens specify the *tissue type* of an individual. Humans express about 40 *major* leukocyte antigens (known as histocompatibility antigens determined by a series of genes collectively called the *major histocompatibility complex* [MHC], but the exact number of human leukocyte antigens that any individual has is not known. It is thought that the number of *minor* antigens far exceeds the number of major antigens. The specific 40 major antigens that an individual has (out of a large number of possible major antigens) are genetically determined. These major antigens must be closely matched between donor and recipient for the best outcome of organ transplantation.

This product identification code is a key feature for recognition and self-tolerance. The immune system cells constantly come into contact with other body cells and with any invader that happens to enter the body's internal environment. At each encounter, the immune system cells attempt to compare the surface protein product identification codes to determine whether the encountered cell belongs in the body's internal environment (Fig. 23 – 2). If the encountered cell's product identification code perfectly matches the code of the immune system cell, the encountered cell is considered to be self and is not further molested by the immune system cell.

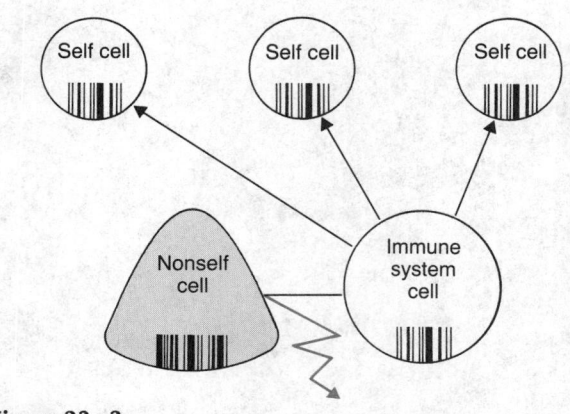

Figure 23 – 2

Determination of self versus nonself.

If the encountered cell's product identification code does not perfectly match the code of the immune system cell, the encountered cell is considered to be nonself or foreign, and the immune system cell will take steps to neutralize, destroy, or eliminate the foreign invader.

GENERAL ORGANIZATION OF THE IMMUNE SYSTEM

The immune system does not reside in any one organ or area of the body. Instead, the cells of the immune system originate in the bone marrow. Some of these cells mature in the bone marrow, whereas others mature in different specific body sites. After maturation, most immune system cells are released into the blood, after which they circulate to most areas of the body and exert specific effects.

The bone marrow is the source of all blood cells and platelets. The bone marrow produces an immature, undifferentiated cell called a *stem cell* (Kemp, 1986). This immature stem cell is also referred to by such adjectives as *pluripotential, multipotential, totipotential,* and even *omnipotential.* These adjectives actually describe the potential of the stem cell. When the stem cell is first created in the bone marrow, it is undifferentiated. The cell is not yet committed to differentiating into a specific cell type. At this stage, the stem cell is flexible and has the potential to become any one of a variety of mature blood cells. Figure 23–3 presents a scheme showing the major possible maturational outcomes for the stem cell. The specific cell type of the mature stem cell depends on which maturational pathway it follows.

The selection of or commitment to a maturational pathway appears to be an irreversible event. For instance, if a stem cell is committed to the platelet pathway and becomes a megakaryocyte, it does not appear to be able to revert to the pluripotent state and later become a T lymphocyte. The cell may stop in the maturational process and never completely mature, but once commitment to a specific maturational pathway occurs the cell continues to follow that path. The maturational pathway of any stem cell depends, to some extent, on body needs at the time and also on the presence of specific chemicals (termed *factors* or *poietins*) that stimulate specific commitment and induce maturation. For example, erythropoietin is synthesized in the kidney. When immature stem cells are exposed to erythropoietin, the immature stem cells are committed to the erythrocyte maturational pathway and eventually become mature red blood cells.

White blood cells (leukocytes) are the cells that protect the body from the effects of invasion by foreign microorganisms. These cells are the immune system cells. The leukocytes can provide protection through a variety of defensive actions (Abernathy, 1987; Grady, 1988; Smith, 1986). These actions include

1. Recognition of self versus nonself

2. Phagocytic destruction of foreign invaders, cellular debris, and unhealthy or abnormal self cells

3. Lytic destruction of foreign invaders and unhealthy self cells

4. Production of antibodies directed against foreign invaders

5. Activation of complement

6. Production of substances that stimulate increased formation of leukocytes in bone marrow

7. Production of substances that increase specific leukocyte growth and activity

Not all leukocytes perform every defensive action in this list. Leukocytes are separated into different categories based on appearance, structure, and specific activity. Table 23–1 summarizes the categories and functions of leukocytes.

GRANULAR LEUKOCYTES

Some leukocytes have many small granules and vesicles within the cytoplasm, which gives the cells a rough or granular appearance under the microscope. These cells are called *granulocytes,* and most of the granules are called *lysosomes.* Lysosomes are intracellular bags of enzymes that can digest or degrade proteins and cellular debris. These enzymes are contained within the lysosomes so that the enzymes do not digest essential parts of the immune system cell. Granulocytes include eosinophils, basophils, and neutrophils.

Eosinophils normally make up a small percentage of the total white blood cell count (about 1% to 2%), except during allergic reactions. These cells are relatively weak phagocytes and function most prominently in reactions that destroy or remove parasitic larvae from humans. In addition, eosinophils participate in allergy-related inflammatory reactions in sensitive individuals.

Basophils are the rarest of the granulocytes. These cells make up less than 0.5% of the total white blood cell count. Basophils release histamine and heparin in areas of tissue damage and pathogenic invasion. They appear to be most important in the generation of acute inflammatory reactions.

The cell type that is thought to be the most functionally important granulocyte is the *neutrophil.* Other names for neutrophils are derived from the unusual shape of the nucleus and include polymorphonuclear cells ("polys"), banded neutrophils ("bands" or "stabs"), and segmented neutrophils ("segs"). Neutrophils are the most numerous of the leukocytes and are efficient phagocytic cells.

NONGRANULAR LEUKOCYTES

The leukocytes that have smooth-appearing cytoplasm under low-power microscopic examination were previously called *agranulocytes,* although this term is inac-

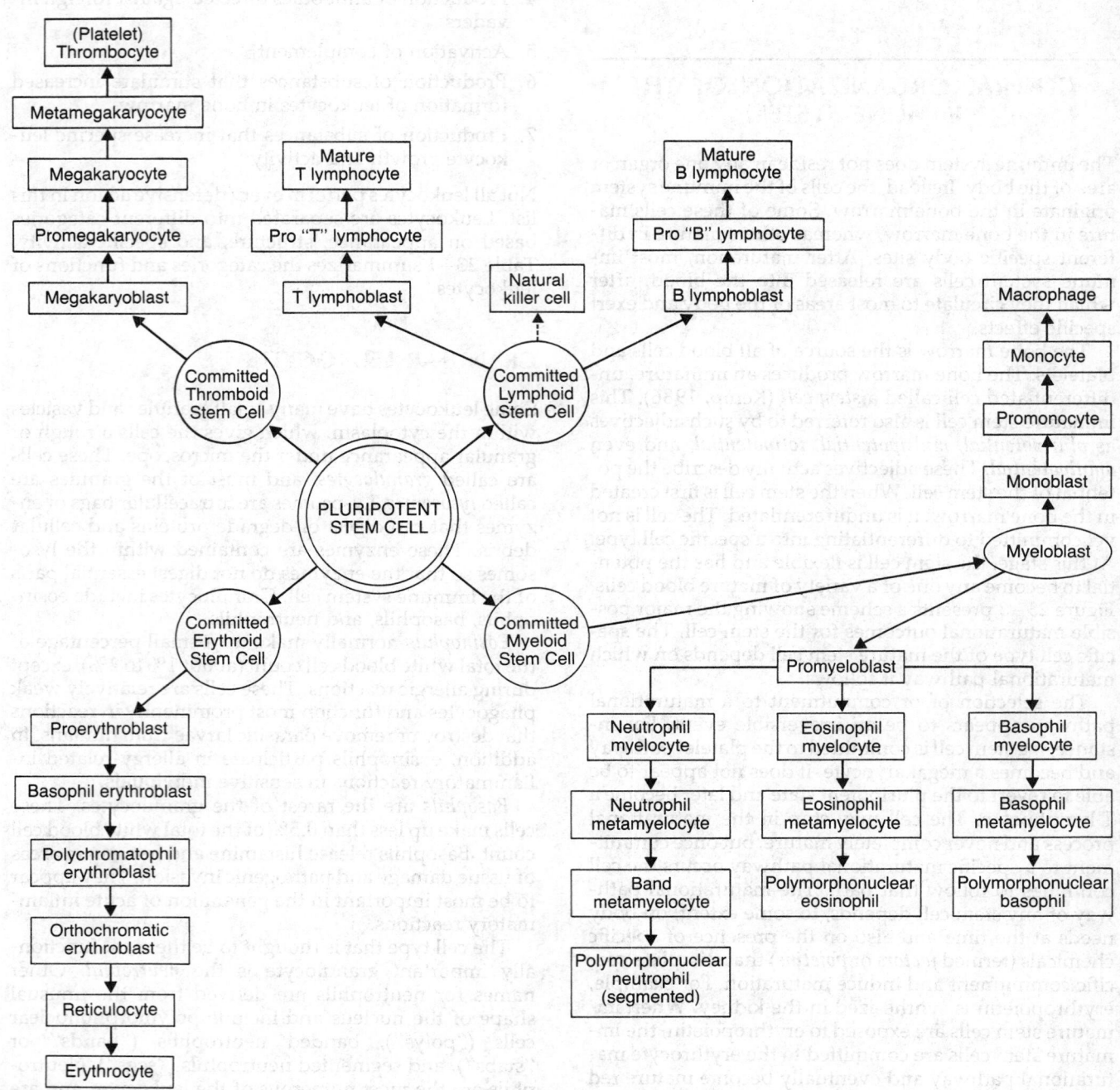

Figure 23–3

Stem cell differentiation and maturational pathways.

TABLE 23–1   Immune Functions of Specific Leukocytes

Immune Division	Leukocyte	Function
Inflammation	Neutrophil	Nonspecific ingestion and phagocytosis of microorganisms and foreign protein
	Macrophage	Nonspecific recognition of foreign proteins and microorganisms; ingestion and phagocytosis
	Monocyte	Destruction of bacteria and cellular debris; matures into macrophage
	Eosinophil	Weak phagocytic action; releases vasoactive amines during allergic reactions
	Basophil	Releases histamine and heparin in areas of tissue damage
Antibody-mediated immunity	B lymphocyte	Becomes sensitized to foreign cells and proteins
	Plasma cell	Secretes immunoglobulins in response to the presence of a specific antigen
	Memory cell	Remains sensitized to a specific antigen and can secrete increased amounts of immunoglobulins specific to the antigen
Cell-mediated immunity	T lymphocyte helper cell	Enhances immune activity through secretion of various factors, cytokines, and lymphokines
	Cytotoxic T cell	Selectively attacks and destroys nonself cells, including virally infected cells, grafts, and transplanted organs
	Natural killer cell	Nonselectively attacks nonself cells, especially body cells that have undergone mutation and have become malignant; also attacks grafts and transplanted organs

curate and rarely used today. Most textbooks include the lymphocytes, monocytes, and macrophages as nongranular leukocytes, even though monocytes and macrophages contain relatively large amounts of fine lysosomal granules in the cytoplasm.

Lymphocytes are divided into *B lymphocytes* and *T lymphocytes*. These cells are critical for providing sustained, long-lasting protection against a vast array of microorganisms that invade the human body. Lymphocytes usually make up about 25% to 30% of the total white blood cell count. B lymphocytes secrete antibodies and participate in antibody-mediated immunity (see under later heading Antibody-Mediated Immunity). T lymphocytes function in a wide variety of activities to provide cell-mediated immunity.

Monocytes are an intermediate type of cell that is released into the circulation from the bone marrow before functional maturation is complete. Monocytes usually make up only 2% to 4% of the total white blood cell count. These cells are committed to maturation and differentiation into macrophages. Until they mature, monocytes are not functionally active components of the immune system. The name monocyte is derived from the appearance of these cells as relatively large entities with a single, large nucleus.

Macrophages are the final maturation stage of monocytes. Macrophages are large, efficient at recognition of self versus nonself, and exceptionally competent phagocytic cells. Maturation of monocytes into macrophages usually occurs when the monocytes migrate into the tissues. Therefore, the circulating population of white blood cells usually has few macrophages, but this value does not reflect the enormous number of noncirculating, active macrophages that are present in many body tissues.

The processes that are necessary for immunity and the cells that are involved in these processes can be divided into the following three categories: inflamma-

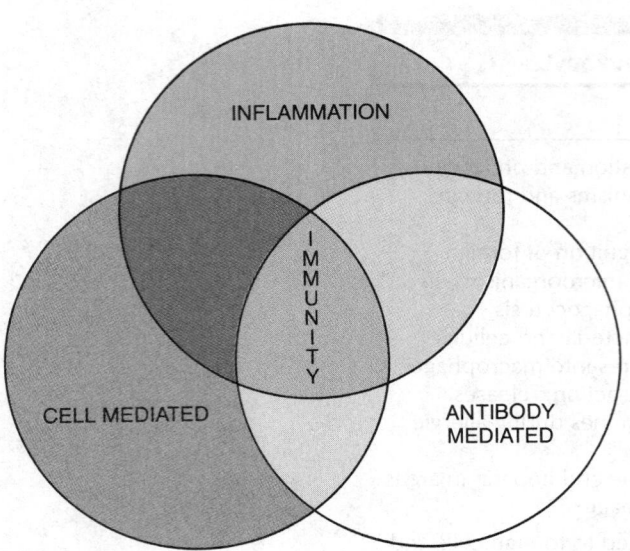

Figure 23–4

The three divisions of immunity. Each of the three divisions of immunity (inflammation, antibody-mediated immunity, and cell-mediated immunity) has an important independent function. In addition, the function of each division of immunity is profoundly influenced by the other two divisions. Most important, optimal function of all three divisions is necessary for complete immunity.

tion, antibody-mediated immunity (humoral immunity), and cell-mediated immunity (Fig. 23–4). These three divisions represent diverse defensive actions and processes. Some of these defensive actions are nonspecific and provide immediate but short-term protection against the side effects of tissue injury or invasion by foreign proteins. Other defensive actions are specific and provide long-lasting immunity. *Full immunity*, or *immunocompetence*, requires the adequate function and interaction of all three divisions, even though some functions of each division appear to overlap with functions of the other divisions.

SPECIFIC CONCEPTS

INFLAMMATION

OVERVIEW

Inflammation or the inflammatory response is not always considered to be a true part of the immune system. Differences in mechanisms of action and in duration of action between inflammation and the other two divisions are responsible for the inconsistent classification of inflammatory responses. Inflammation differs

somewhat from antibody-mediated immunity and cell-mediated immunity in two important ways. First, inflammation is a *nonspecific* response to invasion or injury. Second, inflammatory responses provide immediate but short-term protection against the effects of injury or foreign invaders rather than sustained, long-term immunity on repeated exposures to the same foreign invaders.

Inflammatory responses also result in actions in tissues that generate observable and frequently uncomfortable symptoms in individuals experiencing inflammation. Despite the discomfort, these inflammatory reactions benefit the individual and are also crucial for the neutralization, destruction, and elimination of microorganisms. Moreover, interaction of inflammatory responses with both antibody-mediated and cell-mediated actions appears to be necessary to initiate the more specific immune processes that are provided by these other two divisions of immunity. Without proper function of the inflammatory processes, individuals are at grave risk of succumbing to the side effects of tissue injury or of invasion by microorganisms.

A confusing issue that surrounds inflammation is that this process occurs in response to tissue injury as well as to invasion by microorganisms or other foreign proteins. Under normal conditions, infection is always accompanied by inflammation; however inflammation can occur without the accompanying presence of foreign proteins or microorganisms. For example, inflammatory responses that are not associated with infection occur with sprain injuries to joints, myocardial infarction, sterile surgical incisions, thrombophlebitis, and blister formation as a result of either temperature extremes or mechanical trauma. Examples of inflammatory responses that are associated with noninfectious invasion by foreign proteins include allergic rhinitis, some types of contact dermatitis, and other immediate-type allergic reactions. Inflammatory responses that are associated with invasion by pathogenic (disease-causing) microorganisms include otitis media, appendicitis, bronchitis, bacterial peritonitis, viral hepatitis, and bacterial myocarditis, among others. These clinical examples of inflammation may also involve concurrent stimulation of either cell-mediated or antibody-mediated immunity.

Inflammation is considered to be a *nonspecific* body defense against the side effects of injury or invasion. This defense is nonspecific because the same tissue responses occur as a result of any type of injury or invasion, regardless of the location on the body or the specific initiating agent (Dawson, 1988a; Price & Wilson, 1986). Therefore, the inflammatory processes that are stimulated by a scald burn to the hand are virtually the same as the inflammatory processes that are stimulated by either the reflux of stomach contents into the esophagus or the presence of bacteria in the middle ear. How widespread the physical reactions to inflammation are in the body depends on the intensity, severity, duration, and extent of exposure to the initiating injury or invasion.

CELLULAR COMPONENTS

The leukocytes that are responsible for the generation of inflammatory responses are neutrophils, macrophages, eosinophils, and basophils. Neutrophils and macrophages primarily participate in phagocytosis, with destruction and elimination of foreign invaders. Eosinophils and basophils usually act on specific cells within the vascular system to initiate tissue-level inflammatory responses.

Neutrophils

Mature neutrophils (polymorphonuclear cells) usually constitute between 55% and 70% of the total white blood cell count. Neutrophils originate from the stem cells and complete the maturation process in the bone marrow (Fig. 23–5). Under normal conditions, maturation from the undifferentiated stem cell to the functional segmented neutrophil requires 12 to 14 days. This time can be shortened considerably by certain conditions that stimulate the body to synthesize and release specific chemical factors such as granulocyte-macrophage colony-stimulating factor (GM-CSF) and granulocyte colony-stimulating factor (G-CSF). In the immunocompetent, healthy individual, more than 100 billion fresh, mature neutrophils are released from the bone marrow into the systemic circulation daily. This massive generation of neutrophils is necessary because the life span of a circulating neutrophil is extremely short, averaging only about 12 to 18 *hours*. Once in the blood, neutrophils move by ameboid motion. They are capable of penetrating the endothelial lining of small blood vessels, especially capillaries, and thus can also exert their effects in interstitial fluid.

Although the neutrophils as a group compose the largest number of circulating leukocytes, the individual cell is quite small. This army of powerful little cells provides the first line of defense, via phagocytosis, against foreign invaders, particularly bacteria, in blood and extracellular fluid. The specific structures of the neutrophil that allow successful completion of the phagocytic process are the granules. The cytoplasm of the mature neutrophil is filled with large numbers of two different types of granules, which contain a variety of enzymes (Tizard, 1984). Each of these specific enzymes and enzyme groups helps to degrade different components of foreign invaders that are ingested by neutrophils.

Neutrophils have a finite energy supply and no internal mechanism for replenishing either energy-making substances or the enzymes used in degradation. For this reason, each neutrophil is capable of only one episode of phagocytic destruction before its supplies are exhausted and its death ensues.

It is important for understanding the protection provided by inflammation to note that the mature, segmented neutrophil is the only neutrophil stage that is capable of immediate, effective phagocytosis. Because this cell is responsible for providing continuous, instant, nonspecific protection against invasion by microorganisms, the percentage and actual number of circulating white blood cells that are mature neutrophils are a reliable measure of a client's susceptibility to infection: the higher the numbers, the greater the resistance to infection. This measurement is the *absolute neutrophil count* (sometimes called the absolute granulocyte count [AGC] or total granulocyte count and is calculated by adding the percentages of segmented neutrophils and banded neutrophils together and multiplying the total white blood cell count by this number. For example, if a client has a total white blood cell count of 8000 cells/mm³ of blood with a differential that includes 60% segmented neutrophils and 2% banded neutrophils, the absolute neutrophil count is 62% of 8000 (0.62 × 8000) or 4960 cells/mm³. The percentage of circulating banded neutrophils is included in this count because, even though they are not capable of phagocytic action, they will mature rapidly (within a few hours) into segmented neutrophils. The absolute neutrophil count is important because it represents the number of fighting cells that are ready and able to mount a defense against an invading microorganism.

The differential of a white blood cell count usually indicates that most of the neutrophils that are released into the blood from the bone marrow are segmented

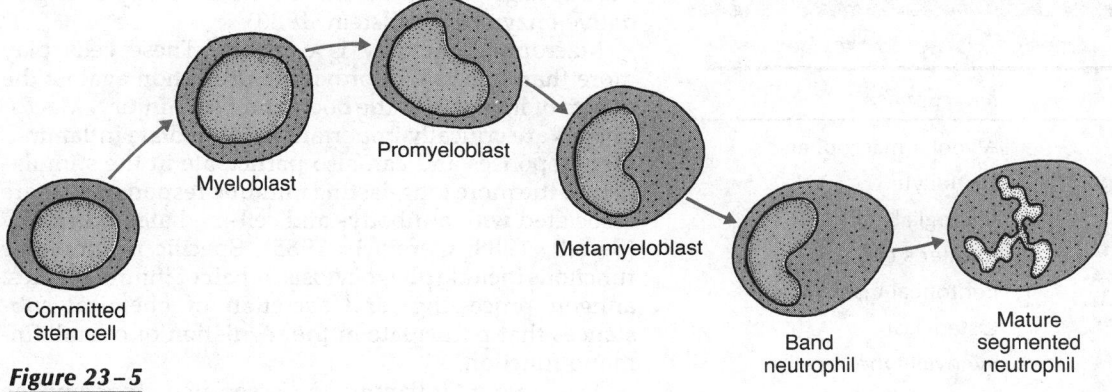

Figure 23–5

Neutrophil maturation.

neutrophils, with only a small percentage being banded neutrophils. The less mature neutrophil forms should not be present in the blood. Some infectious conditions cause the major population of neutrophils in the blood to change from being mostly segmented neutrophils to being mostly a less mature form. This situation is termed a *left shift* because the greatest number of circulating neutrophils is no longer the segmented neutrophil, which is seen at the far right of the neutrophil maturational pathway (see Fig. 23–5). Instead, the major population is one of the cell types that is found further left on the neutrophil maturational pathway. This situation is an ominous clinical sign, as it indicates that the client's bone marrow production of mature neutrophils cannot keep pace with the continuing presence of infectious microorganisms and must release immature neutrophils into the blood. Unfortunately, most of these immature neutrophils are of no benefit to the client, as they are not functional phagocytic cells and cannot continue to mature in the blood.

Macrophages

These interesting and multifunctional cells originate from the committed myeloid stem cell in the bone marrow. Under the influence of specific factors, this cell begins to differentiate into a monocyte and is released into the blood at this stage. Most monocytes migrate into various tissues, where they complete the maturation process into macrophages. Macrophages in various tissues have slightly different appearances (morphologies) and different names. Table 23–2 summarizes the names of the different tissue macrophages. Figure 23–6 shows the distribution of tissue macrophages throughout the body. The liver and spleen contain the greatest concentration of these cells.

At one time, the tissue macrophage system was referred to as the reticuloendothelial system and was thought to be a new body system. Later, this name was deemed to be inappropriate and was replaced by the term *mononuclear phagocytic system*.

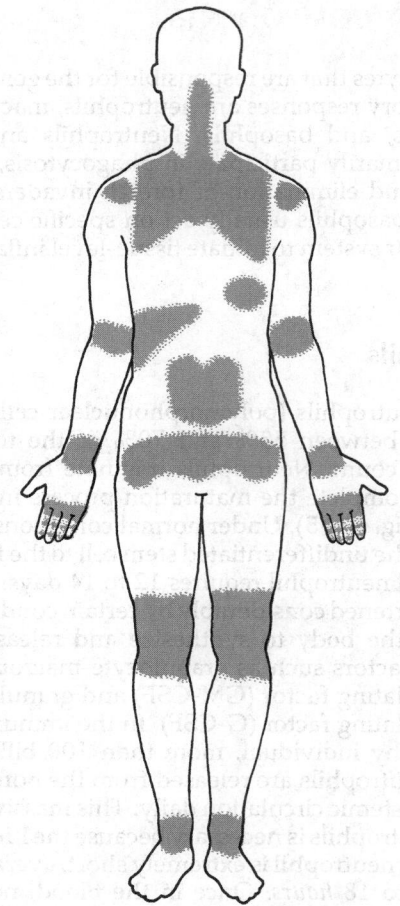

Figure 23–6

Areas of highest concentration of tissue macrophages.

TABLE 23–2   Names of Tissue Macrophages

Tissue	Macrophage
Lung	Alveolar macrophage
Connective tissue	Histiocyte
Brain	Microglial cell
Liver	Kupffer's cell
Peritoneum	Peritoneal macrophage
Bone	Osteoclast
Joints	Synovial type A cell
Kidney	Mesangial cell

The life span of the macrophage depends primarily on the nature of the substances that are taken in during phagocytosis. Tissue macrophages usually have relatively long life spans, lasting from months to years, compared with other leukocytes. Macrophages are the largest of all the leukocytes, contain large amounts of cytoplasm, and have a single nonlobulated nucleus. Macrophage granules contain a wide variety of degradative enzymes (Goldstein, 1983).

Macrophage activity is complex. These cells play more than one role in providing protection against the effects of invasion of the body and tissue injury. Macrophages are critically important in immediate inflammatory responses and can also participate in the stimulation of the more long-lasting immune responses that are associated with antibody- and cell-mediated immunity (Barrett, 1988; Gurevich, 1985). Specific macrophage functions include phagocytosis, repair of injured tissues, antigen processing, and secretion of chemical substances that participate in the regulation of overall immune function.

The major inflammation-associated macrophage function is phagocytosis. Macrophages are efficient at distinguishing between self and nonself. Many tissue macrophages have large cytoplasmic extensions to assist in physically trapping foreign proteins. Unlike neutrophils, macrophages have the intracellular machinery that is necessary to regenerate chemical energy supplies in the form of adenosine triphosphate (ATP) and all of the enzymes that are needed to degrade foreign protein. Therefore, each macrophage is quite capable of participating in many phagocytic events during its life span.

Basophils

Basophils are the smallest of all the leukocytes and the most rare. They are derived from myeloid stem cells and are released from the bone marrow after a short maturation period. Even though they are rare, basophils are associated with the obvious signs and symptoms that often accompany inflammation. Basophils do not have the capacity for ameboid movement and cannot engage in phagocytic action (Barrett, 1988). These cells contain enormous numbers of cytoplasmic granules and have the immunoglobulin (Ig) E attached to their membrane surfaces. It is thought that the attached IgE molecules assist the basophils in recognizing nonself cells.

Basophilic granules contain heparin and a variety of different vasoactive amines, including histamine, serotonin, kinins, and leukotrienes. The actions of most of these vasoactive amines, when they are released into the blood, affect the integrity and function of many types of smooth muscle and vascular endothelium. Heparin inhibits coagulation of blood and other protein-containing extracellular fluids. Histamine constricts the smooth muscles of the respiratory system and venules. Constriction of respiratory smooth muscle narrows the lumen of airways and restricts pulmonary ventilation. Constriction of venular smooth muscle inhibits blood flow through small veins and diminishes venous return. This effect causes blood to collect in capillaries and small arterioles, which increases the hydrostatic pressure within these vessels. Kinins cause slow vasodilation of arterioles. Together, kinins and serotonin dramatically enhance capillary permeability, which permits the plasma portion of the blood to leak into the interstitial space.

Eosinophils

Eosinophils are not efficient phagocytes, although they can act against infestations of parasitic larvae. Cytoplasmic granules of eosinophils contain a wide variety of substances with vastly different actions. Some of these substances are vasoactive amines, which produce inflammatory and often severe tissue-damaging reactions when released. This action may be responsible for some of the uncomfortable and damaging side effects that are associated with exposure to allergens in sensitive individuals. Another function of eosinophils is to modulate and regulate tissue-level inflammatory reactions. In ad-

dition, eosinophilic granules contain special enzymes to degrade the vasoactive amines and other agents that are released by basophils and mast cells. These enzymes limit the activity of the vasoactive amines and thus may serve to control or modulate the extent of inflammatory reactions that are generated in response to invasion of the body and tissue injury.

PHAGOCYTOSIS

The key mechanism for the successful outcome of inflammation—the destruction of nonself cells—is phagocytosis. *Phagocytosis* is the process by which leukocytes engulf cellular debris or foreign proteins and destroy them via a series of intracellular degradative events. When inflammation is initiated purely by tissue injury, leukocyte phagocytic action removes cellular debris. When inflammation is initiated purely by invasion by foreign proteins, leukocyte phagocytic action destroys and removes the invaders. Although all mature leukocytes except for basophils can perform phagocytic actions to some extent, neutrophils and macrophages are most efficient. Phagocytosis occurs in a predictable manner and involves the following seven steps (see the illustration on p. 537):

1. Exposure/invasion
2. Attraction
3. Adherence
4. Recognition
5. Cellular ingestion
6. Phagosome formation
7. Degradation

Exposure/Invasion

Leukocytes that are capable of engaging in phagocytosis and stimulating inflammation are present in extracellular fluids. For the initiation of phagocytosis, these leukocytes must first be exposed to substances that are released because of internal tissue damage or the presence of foreign proteins.

External or internal events can cause tissue damage. Tissue damage occurs as a result of direct mechanical and chemical disruption of cellular integrity. Such events include wounds created by pressure or by temperature extremes and movement of chemicals that are usually confined to a specific body area into a different body area. Some tissue-damaging events allow simultaneous penetration of foreign proteins into the body's internal environment. Such events include cuts, puncture wounds, abrasions, and any tissue injury that results in loss of integrity of the skin or mucous membranes.

Foreign proteins can also enter the body's internal environment through routes that do not involve tissue damage. Some "internal" body areas come into direct contact with the external environment. These areas include the entire oral and gastrointestinal tract, the nasorespiratory tract, and the genitourinary tract. When these areas are exposed to excessive amounts of foreign proteins, the normal surface defenses may be overwhelmed and the foreign proteins gain entry into the body's internal environment.

Attraction

Phagocytosis is effective only when the phagocytic cell comes into direct contact with the target or victim cell. Because tissue injury or invasion by foreign proteins can occur at sites that are somewhat remote from the presence of either neutrophils or macrophages, mechanisms to unite phagocytic cells with their intended targets are necessary.

Special chemical substances can act as chemical magnets that attract a variety of leukocytes, including neutrophils and macrophages (Werb & Goldstein, 1987). These substances are called *chemotaxins* or *leukotaxins*. Damaged tissues excrete chemotaxins. In addition, substances that are present in plasma and other extracellular fluids as a result of blood vessel injury also attract neutrophils and macrophages. These substances include fibrin, collagen, and plasminogen activator. Bacterial endotoxins are often powerful chemotaxins. In addition, substances that combine with surface components of invading foreign proteins serve as chemotaxins. This combining (and attracting) mechanism is described more completely in the section on opsonins and opsonization.

Adherence

Because phagocytosis requires direct contact of the phagocyte with its intended target, the phagocytic cell must first bind to the surface of the target. In living systems, many substances that are suspended in the blood cannot come into direct contact with each other because the surfaces of these substances carry an overall negative charge. Because like charges repel each other, two particles or cells that both have negative surface charges would have great difficulty in coming into direct contact. Because opposite charges attract each other, direct contact is enhanced when the surface charge of one cell is changed to neutral or to an overall positive charge. Adherence of phagocytic cells to targets is enhanced by a process called *opsonization*, which changes the surface charge of target cells to neutral or positive.

The word *opsonin* is derived from the Greek and literally means "to cover food with a sauce in preparation for eating." In biology, opsonins coat a target cell, which changes its surface charge, in preparation for eating by phagocytic cells. A variety of substances can act as opsonins and change the surface charge of cellular debris and foreign proteins so that they are more easily trapped and adhered to by phagocytic cells (Tizard, 1984). Some

of these substances are residual particles from dead neutrophils, antibodies, and activated (fixated) complement components.

Neutrophils, by sheer virtue of their numbers, more easily bind to many foreign proteins than do macrophages. However, neutrophils are small and are usually destroyed during the phagocytic process. On destruction of the neutrophil, particles of the cell can remain attached to the surface of a target foreign protein, change the protein's charge, and enhance subsequent macrophage adherence to that target foreign protein.

Antibodies do not carry an overall positive or negative charge and thus are electrically neutral. When antibodies surround and bind to a target foreign protein, they change the foreign protein's surface charge and directly enhance adherence of phagocytic cells to it. In addition, binding of some antibodies indirectly assists with adherence by activation of the complement cascade.

A well-characterized mechanism of opsonization and enhancement of phagocytic adherence to target cellular debris or foreign proteins is *complement activation and fixation* (Colten, 1985; Cooper, 1987). Approximately 20 different inactive protein components of the complement system are present in the blood. The major complement proteins are labeled C1 through C9. Some of these major proteins have subsets (e.g., the C1 protein complex can be separated into C1q, C1r, and C1s), so that the number of currently identified complement components is approximately 20. These components are synthesized by the liver. With the correct stimulation, these individual complement proteins become activated rapidly and then act in concert to cause dramatic biologic actions as a result of fixation to specific tissues. Because the biologic effects of complement fixation are usually needed quickly but can have devastating consequences if exerted at the wrong time or in the wrong place, the complement system functions as a cascade reaction, with multiple sites of activation and control through various feedback integration points.

Cascade reactions are chain reactions in which events must occur in a specific sequence. In the case of the complement cascade for complement activation and fixation, a specific component of complement must be activated first. Activation of this component leads to activation of the next component, which leads to activation of the next component, and so on. When all components of complement are activated and bound or fixed to the surface of the target foreign protein, the surface charge is changed and phagocytic cells adhere more easily.

Recognition

When the phagocytic cell is adhering to the surface of the target cell, recognition of self versus nonself occurs. The mechanism for recognition at this point is identical to the mechanism described earlier in this chapter for self-tolerance and involves examination of product

THE STEPS OF PHAGOCYTOSIS

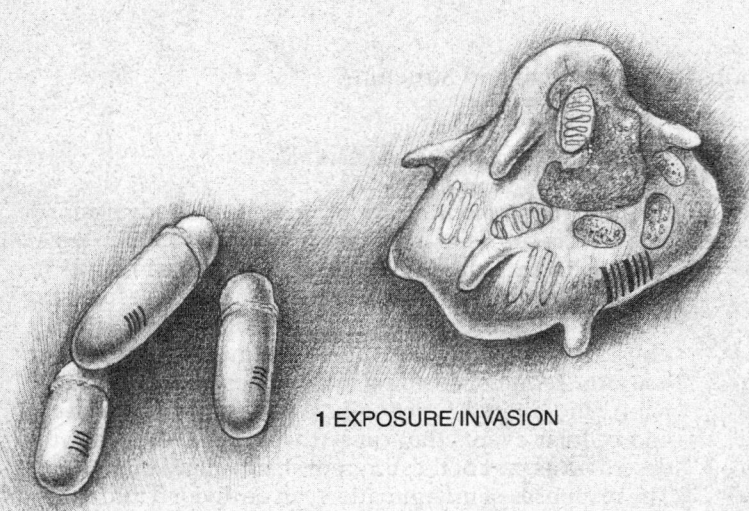

1 EXPOSURE/INVASION

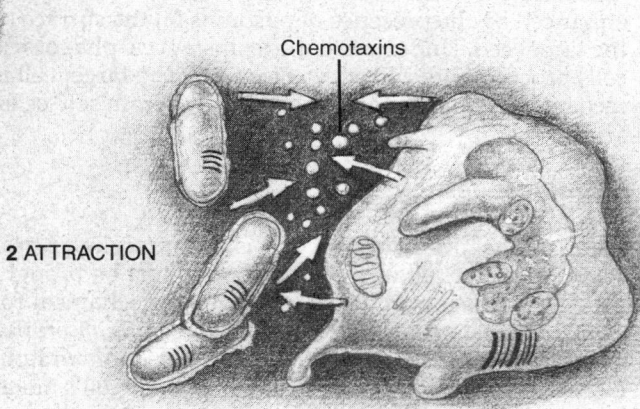

Chemotaxins

2 ATTRACTION

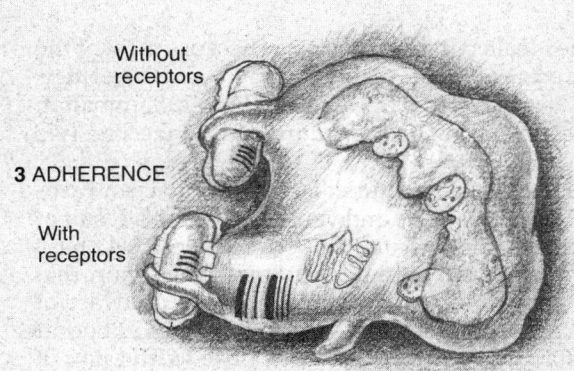

Without receptors

3 ADHERENCE

With receptors

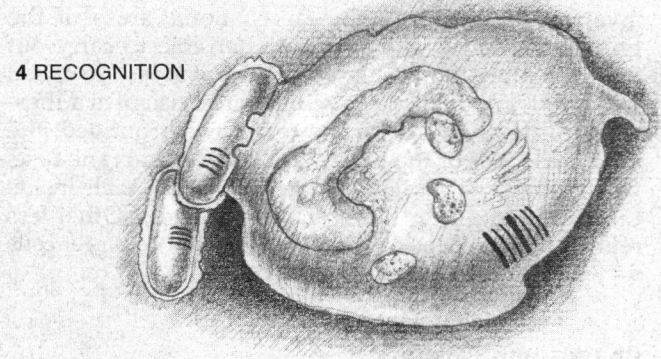

4 RECOGNITION

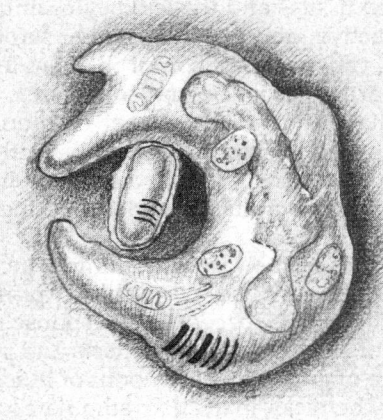

5 CELLULAR INGESTION

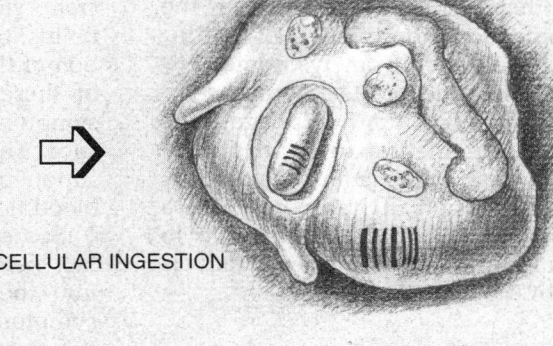

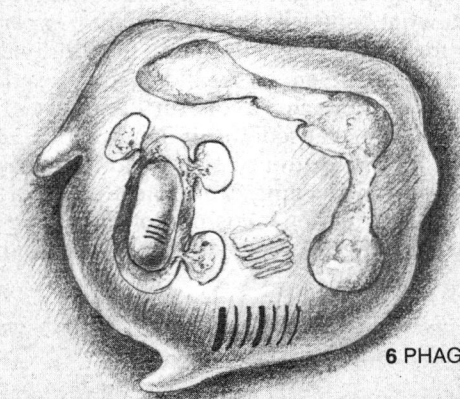

6 PHAGOSOME FORMATION

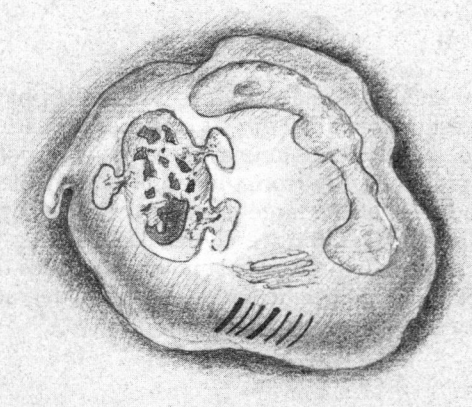

7 DEGRADATION

identification codes. Recognition of nonself is slightly enhanced by the presence of opsonins on the surface of the target cell. Under normal circumstances, phagocytic cells proceed with phagocytosis only if the target cell is recognized either as foreign or as debris from self-cells.

Cellular Ingestion

Because phagocytic destruction is an intracellular process, the target cell or foreign protein must be brought inside the phagocytic cell. The primary mechanism for cellular ingestion of target cells or debris is *absorptive endocytosis.* This mechanism permits ingestion without disruption of the integrity of the phagocytic cell's membrane.

After adherence to and recognition of the target cell, the phagocytic cell changes shape and its membrane invaginates to enclose the target. Some areas of the phagocytic membrane appear better able to carry out this maneuver than other areas. These areas are called *coated pits,* and they may also be more efficient at adherence to the target. Once the target is surrounded, the touching edges of the phagocytic cell's membrane fuse, which effectively seals the target within a vesicle inside the phagocytic cell, thus forming a vacuole. Other less refined mechanisms for cellular ingestion of target cells may also operate in phagocytic cells.

Phagosome Formation

If some of the phagocyte's cytoplasmic granules are inside the vacuole, the structure is called a *phagosome.* When these cytoplasmic granules degranulate and release enzymes and other lytic substances within the fluid of the phagosome, some destruction of the ingested target begins. Assistance from lysosomes enhances this intracellular destruction. Lysosomal membranes have the same composition as phagosomal membranes. Therefore, lysosomes can fuse with phagosomes to form a special destructive organelle, which is termed a *phagolysosome.* Fusion of lysosomes with a phagosome allows lysosomal degradative products to be incorporated within the phagosome. These products enhance destruction of the target.

Degradation

The granular and lysosomal enzymes within the phagolysosome exert their specific effects on different parts of the ingested target. Some enzymes remove carbohydrate and lipid molecules from the target, which allows easier degradation of the target by enzymes that digest proteins. Protein-degrading enzymes first break the large target molecule into many smaller molecules that are more sensitive to specific and nonspecific degradation by other enzymes.

INFLAMMATORY RESPONSES

Inflammatory responses for protecting the body against side effects of tissue injury or invasion by foreign proteins occur in a predictable sequence. The sequence is the same regardless of the initiating stimulus. Responses at the tissue level are responsible for the five cardinal physical manifestations of inflammation: increased warmth, redness, swelling, altered sensations (usually pain), and altered function (usually decreased). Tissue and cellular events that cause these manifestations are described as part of the different stages of inflammation. The responses of inflammation can be divided into three distinct functional stages, although the timing of the stages may overlap.

Stage I

This stage is called the *vascular stage* because most of the early effects of this response involve physiologic changes at the vascular level. When inflammation occurs as a result of tissue injury, this stage has two phases.

The first phase is an immediate but short-term vasoconstriction of arterioles and venules as a direct result of physical trauma to vascular smooth muscle. This phase lasts only seconds to minutes and may be so short that the individual undergoing the response is unaware of the vasoconstriction. Usually, this phase does not occur when inflammation is purely a response to invasion of the body.

The second phase is characterized by hyperemia and swelling (edema formation) at the site of injury or invasion. Injured tissues and the leukocytes in this area secrete vasoactive amines (histamine, serotonin, and kinins) that cause constriction of the venules and dilation of the arterioles in the immediate area. The effects of these changes in blood vessel dilation cause the symptoms of redness and increased warmth of the tissues. The purpose of this response is to increase the supply of nutrients at the tissue level by increasing the blood flow.

Some of these same vasoactive amines increase capillary permeability, which allows blood plasma to leak into the interstitial space. This response causes the symptoms of swelling as fluid collects and pain as both the pressure of an increased amount of fluid in the area and caustic chemicals in the fluid stimulate local sensory nerve endings. Pain, although an uncomfortable sensation, is somewhat beneficial to the individual experiencing inflammation. Pain increases the individual's awareness that a problem exists and encourages the individual to take actions that avoid further injury or alter the conditions that caused the inflammation. Edema formation at the site of injury or invasion is an overall helpful event. This swelling can protect the area from further injury by creating a cushion of fluid. The extra fluid can also dilute the concentration of any toxins or microorganisms that entered the area. The plasma that leaked into the interstitial space contains fibrin and other protein factors that can cause the interstitial fluid in the area of injury or invasion to clot, which isolates the site and confines the effects largely to the immediate area. The duration of these responses depends on the severity of the initiating event.

The major leukocyte that is involved in this stage of inflammation is the tissue macrophage. The response of the tissue macrophages is immediate because they are already in place at the site of injury or invasion. However, this response is limited because the number of such macrophages is so small. In addition to functioning in phagocytosis, the tissue macrophages secrete several substances to enhance the inflammatory response. One substance is colony-stimulating factor, which stimulates the bone marrow to reduce leukocyte production time from 14 days to a matter of hours. In addition, tissue macrophages secrete substances that increase the release of neutrophils from the bone marrow and attract them to the site of injury or invasion, which leads to the next stage of inflammation.

Stage II

This stage of inflammation is also called the *cellular exudate stage*. It is characterized by neutrophilia (increase in the percentage and number of circulating neutrophils), secretion of many factors into the interstitial fluid, and formation of exudate.

The most prominent leukocyte in this stage is the neutrophil. Under the influence of chemotactic agents and substances that increase the number and rate of maturation of neutrophils, the actual neutrophil count can increase up to fivefold within 12 hours of the onset of inflammation. The purposes of the neutrophils at the site of inflammation are to (1) attack and destroy foreign materials and (2) remove dead and dying tissue. Both of these functions are accomplished through phagocytosis.

During acute inflammatory responses that are short, the otherwise healthy individual can synthesize enough mature neutrophils to keep pace with the side effects of injury and invasion and to eventually overcome the ability of invaders to multiply. At the same time, these leukocytes secrete factors that permit reproduction of tissue macrophages and increase bone marrow production of monocytes. Although this reaction is slower to start, its effects are relatively long-lasting.

When infectious processes stimulating inflammation are longer or chronic, the bone marrow cannot synthesize and release enough mature neutrophils into the blood to keep pace with the ability of microorganisms to multiply. In this situation, the bone marrow begins to release immature neutrophils, many of which cannot phagocytose or complete maturation. Such a reduction in the number of functional phagocytic neutrophils limits the effectiveness of the inflammatory response

and dramatically increases the susceptibility of the individual to new and recurring microbial infections.

Stage III

This stage of inflammation is also called the *tissue repair and replacement stage*. Although this stage is completed last, it begins at the time of injury and is critical to the ultimate function of the inflamed area.

Some of the leukocytes involved in inflammation are capable of stimulating repair of lost or damaged tissues by inducing the remaining healthy tissue to divide. In tissues that are not mitotically active (nondividing tissues), leukocytes stimulate revascularization and the laying down of different types of collagen to form scar tissue. Because scar tissue does not behave in the same manner as normal differentiated tissue, some functional loss occurs in areas where damaged tissues are replaced with scar tissue. The extent of the functional loss is determined by the percentage of tissue that is replaced by scar tissue.

Inflammation provides immediate protection against the side effects of tissue injury and invading foreign proteins. Although inflammatory responses are usually beneficial, some are accompanied by unpleasant and even tissue-damaging actions. The capacity of an individual to generate an inflammatory response is a critical component to the overall health and well-being of an individual. Alone, inflammation cannot confer immunity; however, the interaction of specific components of inflammation with other leukocytes and tissues assists in providing long-lasting immunity against re-exposure to the same microorganisms.

ANTIBODY-MEDIATED IMMUNITY

OVERVIEW

Antibody-mediated immunity (AMI), which is also known as humoral immunity, primarily involves antigen-antibody actions to neutralize, eliminate, or destroy foreign proteins. These actions are accomplished directly by populations of B lymphocytes, although they are assisted by several other leukocytes. The primary function of B lymphocytes is to become sensitized to a specific foreign protein, or *antigen*, and synthesize an antibody directed specifically against that protein. The antibody (rather than the actual B lymphocyte) then participates in one of a variety of actions to neutralize, eliminate, or destroy that antigen.

CELLULAR COMPONENTS

The leukocytes that play the most direct role in antibody-mediated immunity are the B lymphocytes. Because B lymphocytes have limited specific functions and are not efficient at recognition of self versus nonself, major interactions with cells that are responsible for inflammation (especially macrophages) are required to initiate and complete antigen-antibody actions. In addition, special T lymphocytes (helper T cells) secrete products that regulate the activity of B lymphocytes and assist with recognition of nonself. Therefore, for antibody-mediated immunity to be optimal, the entire immune system must function adequately.

B lymphocytes start life as pluripotent stem cells in the bone marrow. The pluripotent stem cells that are destined to become B lymphocytes commit early to the lymphocyte maturational pathway (see Fig. 23–3), possibly under the influence of a specific lymphopoietic factor. At the point of commitment, these stem cells are no longer pluripotent but are limited to differentiation into lymphocytes. The committed lymphocyte stem cells are released from the bone marrow into the blood, and they then migrate into various lymphoid tissues.

In birds, the maturation and differentiation of committed lymphocyte stem cells into B lymphocytes occur in a special area of lymphoid tissue called the bursa of Fabricius (hence the designation *B*). Humans do not have any one tissue or organ that is analogous to the bursa of Fabricius. Instead, in humans these committed lymphocyte stem cells must first migrate into germinal centers of lymph nodes, tonsils, Peyer's patches of the intestinal tract, the white pulp of the spleen, and possibly other lymphoid areas (Vogler & Lawton, 1985). Once maturation has occurred in these areas, the B lymphocytes are released into the general circulation.

ANTIGEN-ANTIBODY INTERACTIONS

Generating sufficient quantities of specific antibody to provide an individual with long-lasting immunity against the specific microorganisms or toxins that are responsible for causing a disease requires time and a series of special interactions. These interactions center on the actions of B lymphocytes but also include specific and nonspecific activities of other leukocytes. Developing the capacity to secrete a unique and specific antibody that is directed against a unique and specific antigen whenever the individual is exposed to that antigen involves seven steps (see the accompanying illustration):

1. Exposure/invasion
2. Antigen recognition
3. Lymphocyte sensitization
4. Antibody production and release
5. Antigen-antibody binding
6. Antibody-binding reactions
7. Sustained immunity/memory

Exposure/Invasion

Antigen-antibody interactions occur in the body's internal environment. To make an antibody that can exert its effects on a specific antigen, the body must first be exposed to that antigen to the degree that the antigen penetrates the body's external defensive barriers (primarily the skin and mucous membranes). Even when exposure includes penetration and invasion of the body's internal environment, not all exposures result in the stimulation of antibody production. Invasion by the antigen must occur in such large numbers that some of the antigen either evades detection by the normal nonspecific defenses or overwhelms the abilities of the inflammatory responses to neutralize, eliminate, or destroy the invador (Tami, 1986).

For example, an individual has never contracted or even been exposed to the childhood viral disease chickenpox. This person baby-sits for three children who show chickenpox lesions within the next 10 hours. These children, in the pre-eruption stage, shed many millions of live chickenpox virus particles via the droplets from the upper respiratory tract. Because small children are often unconcerned about the finer points of infection control, these children drink out of the baby sitter's soft drink can, kiss her directly (and wetly) on the lips, and both sneeze and cough directly into her face. After spending 5 hours with the children at close range, the baby sitter has been overwhelmingly invaded by the chickenpox virus (varicella-zoster) and will become sick with this disease within 14 to 21 days. While this individual is incubating the virus and developing the disease, her leukocytes are participating in the next steps in the series of antigen-antibody interactions to prevent her from developing chickenpox more than once.

Antigen Recognition

To begin to make antibodies against an antigen, the "virgin" or previously unsensitized B lymphocyte must first recognize the antigen as nonself. B lymphocytes are the least efficient of all the leukocytes in recognizing self and nonself, and, in fact, may not be able to carry out this important function alone. For this reason, antigen recognition by B lymphocytes requires the assistance of macrophages and helper T cells.

This cooperative effort appears to be initiated by the macrophages. After the membrane of the antigen has been altered somewhat by opsonization (discussed earlier under the heading Adherence), the macrophage recognizes the invading foreign protein (antigen) as nonself and physically attaches itself to the antigen. This particular macrophage attachment to the antigen does not result in phagocytosis or in immediate destruction of the antigen. Instead, the macrophage brings the attached antigen into contact with a helper T cell. At this time, the helper T cell and the macrophage process the antigen in some way to expose the antigen's recognition

INITIATION OF ANTIBODY-MEDIATED IMMUNITY

1 EXPOSURE/INVASION
Invasion of the body by new antigens in sufficient numbers to overwhelm the inflammatory responses.

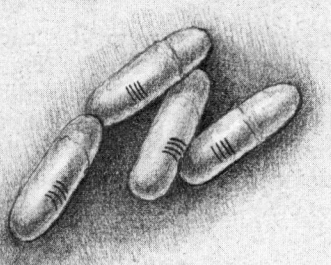

2 ANTIGEN RECOGNITION
Recognition by a "virgin" B lymphocyte that this antigen is foreign.

3 LYMPHOCYTE SENSITIZATION
Engulfment of the antigen by a B lymphocyte and sensitization of the B lymphocyte to this specific antigen.

7 SUSTAINED IMMUNITY/MEMORY
On re-exposure to the same antigen, the sensitized lymphocytes begin to make large amounts of antibody specific to the antigen. In addition, new virgin lymphocytes become sensitized.

4 ANTIBODY PRODUCTION AND RELEASE
Antibodies produced by the B lymphocyte are directed specifically against the initiating antigen. The antibodies are released from the B lymphocyte and float freely in the blood and some other extracellular fluids.

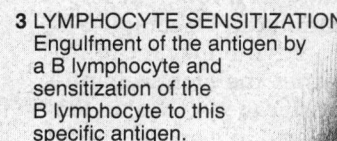

5 ANTIGEN-ANTIBODY BINDING

6 ANTIBODY-BINDING REACTIONS
Antibody binding causes cellular events and attraction of other leukocytes to the complex. The result is neutralization, elimination, or destruction of the antigen.

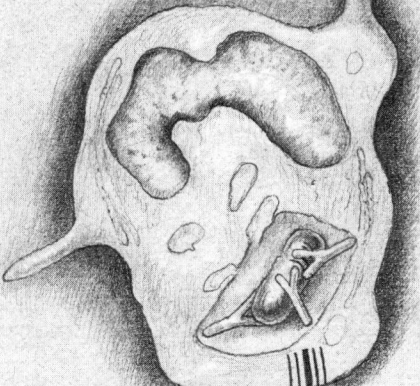

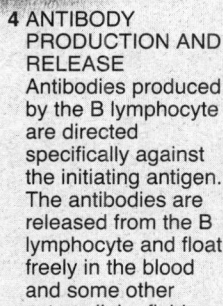

sites (product identification code). After processing the antigen, the helper T cell brings the antigen into contact with the B lymphocyte so that the B lymphocyte can recognize the antigen as nonself. In addition, the helper T cell appears to secrete special substances that enable the B lymphocyte to initiate and continue the processes that result in antibody production.

Lymphocyte Sensitization

Once the B lymphocyte recognizes the antigen as nonself, the cell carries out special steps to become sensitized to this antigen. An individual virgin B lymphocyte can undergo sensitization only once. Therefore, in theory, each B lymphocyte can be sensitized to only one antigen.

The exact mechanisms of the extracellular and intracellular events that result in B lymphocyte sensitization are not precisely known, although it appears that the B lymphocyte must ingest the antigen through absorptive endocytosis before sensitization can be completed. As a result of sensitization, this B lymphocyte can respond to any substance that carries the identical antigenic determinants (product identification codes) as the original antigen. Once it is sensitized to a specific antigen, the B lymphocyte remains sensitized to that specific antigen. In addition, all progeny of that sensitized B lymphocyte are also sensitized to that specific antigen.

Immediately after it is sensitized, the B lymphocyte (or B blast) divides and forms two different types of lymphocytes, each one remaining sensitized to that specific antigen (Fig. 23–7). One new cell becomes a *plasma cell* and immediately starts to produce antibody that is directed specifically against the antigen that originally sensitized the B lymphocyte. The other new cell becomes a *memory cell*. The plasma cell functions immediately and has a rather short life span. The memory cell remains sensitized but functionally dormant until the next exposure to the same antigen (discussed under the later heading Sustained Immunity/Memory).

Antibody Production and Release

Antibody production is the responsibility of the plasma cell. When it is fully stimulated, each plasma cell can produce as much as 300 molecules of antibody per second. Each plasma cell produces antibody specific only to the antigen that originally sensitized the parent B lymphocyte. For example, in the case of the baby sitter who was exposed to and invaded by chickenpox viruses, the plasma cells derived from the B lymphocytes that were sensitized to the chickenpox virus can produce only antichickenpox antibodies. The exact antibody type that the plasma cell can produce (e.g., IgG or IgM) may vary with time and circumstances, but the specificity of that antibody remains forever directed against chickenpox virus. Individual plasma cells have life spans of approximately 1 week.

Most of the antibody molecules that are produced by the plasma cells are secreted into the blood and other

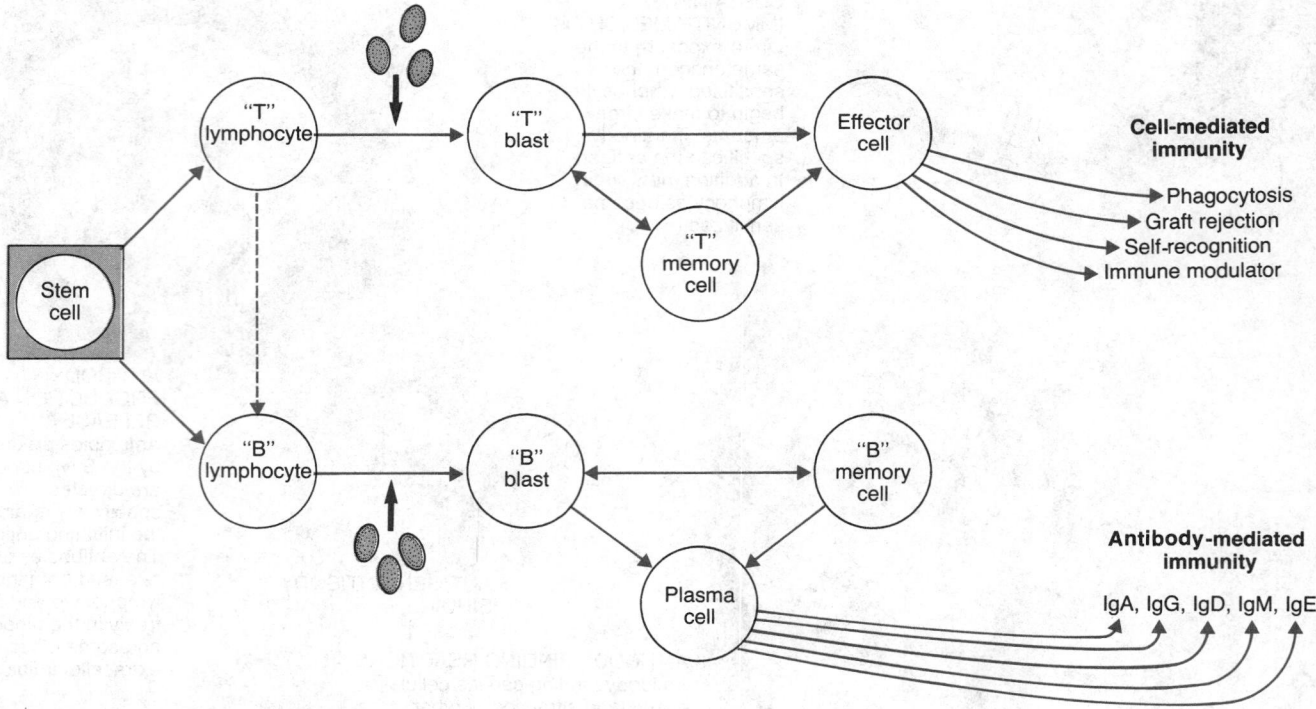

Figure 23–7

B cell differentiation into plasma cells and memory cells and T cell differentiation.

extracellular fluids as free antibody by the process of exocytosis. The life span of free antibody varies with the type of antibody that is generated. IgG has the longest life span (a half-life of approximately 30 days), and IgD has the shortest (a half-life of 2 to 3 days). Because the antibody circulates in body fluids (or body "humors") and is separate from the B lymphocytes, the immunity provided is called *humoral immunity*. Circulating antibodies can be transferred from one person to another to provide immediate artificial passive immunity of short duration.

Antigen-Antibody Binding

An antibody is basically a bilaterally symmetric Y-shaped molecule (Fig. 23–8). The tips of the short arms of the Y are the areas that actually recognize the specific antigen and bind to it. Because each individual antibody molecule has two Fab fragments, antibody molecules are bivalent and can bind to either two separate antigen molecules or two areas of the same antigen molecule.

In most instances, the actual binding of the antibody to the antigen is not directly lethal to the antigen. Instead, the physical binding of the antibody to the antigen has both permissive and catalytic roles in initiating other actions that ultimately result in the neutralization, elimination, or destruction of the antigen.

Antibody-Binding Reactions

The action of binding antibody to antigen allows or initiates specific reactions to cause the neutralization, elimination, or destruction of the antigen. The characteristics

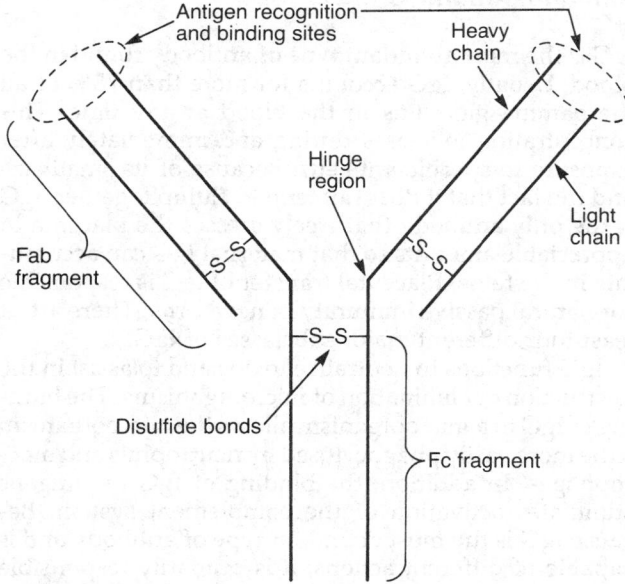

Figure 23-8

Basic antibody structure.

of the major reactions are fully described here. Simultaneous occurrence of all types of major reactions is likely during any one episode of antigen-antibody interactions.

Agglutination

This antibody action is a result of the bivalency of antibody molecules. In agglutination, the binding of multiple antigen molecules to each antibody unit does not directly destroy the antigen. Agglutination permits defensive effects by at least two mechanisms. First, this type of interaction slows the movement of the antigen through the extracellular fluids. Second, the highly irregular shape of the antigen-antibody complex increases the likelihood that this complex will be attacked by other leukocytes, including macrophages, neutrophils, and cytotoxic T cells.

Lysis

The action of lysis occurs as a physical result of antibody's binding to membrane-bound antigens of some foreign invaders. The actual binding causes a disruption of the invading foreign protein's membrane surface. Such disruption permits rapid and lethal changes of the intracellular environment of the invader. Critical substances may be lost from the invader, or other harmful substances may gain easy access to the invader, or both events may occur. The nonself cells that are most susceptible to damage through lysis that is mediated by the binding of antibody to membrane surface antigens are bacteria and viruses.

Complement Fixation

Specific classes of antibodies can cause the neutralization, elimination, or destruction of nonself antigen through activation of the complement cascade and complement fixation. The mechanism by which complement assists in immunity is discussed earlier in detail under the heading Adherence. The two classes of antibody that are frequently associated with stimulating the complement system are IgG and IgM. Binding of antibody from either of these classes to the appropriate antigen provides a recognition or binding site for the first component of complement (C1q). Once C1q is activated, the other components of the entire complement system are activated in a cascade, which greatly amplifies the effectiveness of opsonization.

Precipitation

Precipitation is similar to agglutination. However, in precipitation, antibody closely binds so much antigen that large, insoluble antibody-antigen complexes are formed. These complexes are unable to stay in suspension in the blood. They instead form a large, nonmoving precipitate, which can be acted on and removed by other nonspecific leukocytes.

Inactivation/Neutralization

This antibody action is unique in that it does not result in the immediate destruction of the antigen. Usually, an antigen has a relatively small area that is actually responsible for exerting harmful and unpleasant effects. The rest of the antigen performs duties and activities that are important to the antigen but not harmful to the host. Binding of antibody can interfere with the function of the active site by directly covering it up or by inducing a change in the active site's physical configuration. Either mechanism inhibits the activity of the antigen and renders it harmless without destroying or eliminating it.

Sustained Immunity/Memory

This function or action of antibody-mediated immunity provides humans with long-lasting or sustained immunity to a specific antigen. Sustained immunity is provided via the action of the B lymphocyte *memory* cells that are generated during the lymphocyte sensitization stage. These memory cells remain sensitized to the specific antigen to which they were originally exposed. On re-exposure to the same antigen, the memory cells are stimulated into rapid response. First, the cells divide and form new sensitized blast cells and new sensitized plasma cells. The blast cells continue to divide to generate even more sensitized plasma cells. The sensitized plasma cells begin to rapidly secrete large amounts of the antibody specific for the sensitizing antigen.

This ability of the sensitized memory cells to initiate events on a second or subsequent exposure to the antigen that originally sensitized the B lymphocyte allows a much more rapid and widespread immune response to the antigen. Usually, this response completely eliminates or neutralizes the invading antigen so that the individual does not become ill or experience side effects of antigen exposure. Because of this process, most individuals do not get chickenpox or many other viral diseases more than once, even though they are exposed many times to the causative organism. Without the process or action of memory, individuals would remain susceptible to specific diseases on subsequent exposure to the antigen and no sustained immunity would be generated.

GENERAL ANTIBODY CLASSIFICATION

All antibodies are referred to as *immunoglobulins* and *gamma globulins*. These names are based on the structure, location, and function of antibodies. A globulin is a type of protein structure that is globular. Antibodies are composed of this type of protein, and thus they are globulins. The name immunoglobulin is appropriate for antibodies because they are globular proteins that assist in immune function. Antibodies are called gamma globulins because during the process of electrophoresis, different groups of proteins in blood plasma separate out at

different times depending on how they move in response to the electrical charge. The different protein groups are named based on when they emerge. The first group to emerge are the plasma albumins, which make up a rather large group. Three smaller groups emerge at specific times after the albumins. The fourth group or protein fraction (gamma fraction) contains all five different types of antibody proteins. For this reason, antibodies are called gamma globulins. The five antibody types or classifications are based on differences in antibody structure, molecular weight, and patterns of association (Goodman, 1987).

Immunoglobulin A

IgA is also known as the *secretory* Ig. This antibody is made by B lymphocytes in the blood but is not stored in the blood or serum to any appreciable extent. Instead, IgA moves from the blood into other body fluids and secretions such as tears, urine, saliva, milk, and mucus of the respiratory, genitourinary, and gastrointestinal tracts. Because IgA does not remain in the blood, serum levels of IgA are normally quite low.

The purpose of IgA is to participate in actions on the outer body surfaces to prevent antigens (foreign invaders) from entering the body's internal environment. IgA accomplishes this purpose primarily by inhibiting bacteria and viruses (through some unknown mechanism) from adhering to the surfaces of skin and mucous membranes. This inhibition makes it more difficult for foreign invaders to penetrate and enter the body's internal environment.

Immunoglobulin G

IgG is the most abundant type of antibody found in the blood. Usually, IgG accounts for more than 75% of all the gamma globulins in the blood at any time. This concentration increases during and immediately after exposure to specific antigens. Because of its small size and the fact that it does not tend to clump together, IgG is the only antibody that freely crosses the placenta in appreciable amounts so that maternal IgG can accumulate in the fetus. Placental transfer of IgG is responsible for natural passive immunity in newborns. There are at least four different major subclasses of IgG.

IgG functions to neutralize toxins and to assist in the destruction or elimination of microorganisms. The binding of IgG to a microorganism allows the microorganism to be more easily phagocytosed by neutrophils and macrophages. In addition, the binding of IgG to antigens stimulates activation of the complement system. Because IgG is the most abundant type of antibody and is capable of different actions, it is primarily responsible for providing most of the naturally and artificially acquired sustained immunity.

Immunoglobulin M

IgM is sometimes called a macroglobulin because of its large size and tendency to self-associate. This antibody constitutes approximately 10% of the total serum concentration of Igs. Under some conditions (autoimmune responses), significant amounts of IgM can be found in certain extracellular body fluids.

IgM responds to the presence of bacteria in the blood and is especially efficient at the antibody actions of agglutination and precipitation. Binding of IgM to an antigen stimulates activation of the complement system.

IgM is the primary Ig protein type forming anti-A and anti-B antibodies in individuals of different blood groups. Individuals with type A blood have anti-B antibodies. Individuals with type B blood have anti-A antibodies. Individuals with type O blood have both anti-A and anti-B antibodies. These antibodies are useful for laboratory determination of an individual's blood type.

IgM is thought to be involved in the initiation of autoimmune responses, although the mechanisms and relationships of IgM to autoimmunity are not clear. Elevation of IgM is frequently a diagnostic indicator for the presence of specific autoimmune diseases.

Immunoglobulin E

The serum concentration of IgE is low, although it varies from individual to individual and is determined genetically. The IgE molecule tends to associate closely with basophils and mast cells and is responsible for the manifestations of most immediate hypersensitivity reactions. The binding of IgE to antigen results in degranulation of the basophilic and mast cell membranes. This membrane degranulation allows large amounts of histamine, kinins, serotonin, and other vasoactive amines to be released from basophils and mast cells. The vasoactive amines stimulate an inflammatory response on contact with tissues and blood vessels. These reactions are responsible for most of the uncomfortable (and sometimes life-threatening) symptoms that clients experience during allergic reactions.

The actual purpose of IgE is unclear, although this antibody is immunologically useful during parasitic infestations. In addition, individuals with IgE deficiency are at a significantly increased risk for development of respiratory infections. Some immunologists suggest that IgE may have had a more important function for humans during earlier evolutionary periods, and now this antibody appears to have limited beneficial value.

Immunoglobulin D

IgD is found in plasma in low concentrations, usually far less than 1%. Its actual function is not clear. Because IgD is frequently found on the surface of B lymphocytes, usually close to molecules of IgM, it is thought that IgD may modify the activity of IgM in some way. Because information about the function and features of IgD is limited, it is sometimes called the mystery protein.

ACQUIRING ANTIBODY-MEDIATED IMMUNITY

Two broad categories of immunity are innate immunity and acquired immunity. *Innate immunity* is a genetically determined characteristic of an individual, group, or species. An individual either has or does not have innate immunity. This type of immunity cannot be developed or bought and is not an adaptive response to exposure or invasion by foreign proteins.

Acquired immunity is the immunity that every individual's body makes (or can receive) as an adaptive response to invasion by foreign proteins. Antibody-mediated immunity is an acquired immunity. Acquired immunity occurs either naturally or artificially and is characterized as either active or passive.

Active Immunity

Active immunity occurs when antigens enter the body and the body responds by making specific antibodies against the antigen. This type of immunity is active because the body takes an active part in making the antibodies. Active immunity can occur under conditions that are either natural or artificial.

Natural active immunity occurs when an antigen enters the body, without human assistance, and the body responds by actively making antibodies against that antigen (e.g., chickenpox virus). Most of the time, the first invasion of the body by this antigen results in the individual's manifesting signs and symptoms of the disease. However, processes occurring in the body at the same time allow the individual to acquire immunity to that antigen so that he/she will not become ill after a second exposure to the same antigen. This type of immunity is best and the most long-lasting.

Artificial active immunity is a type of protection that has been developed against certain illnesses that have the potential for such serious side effects that total avoidance of the disease is most desirable. In this situation, small amounts of specific antigens are deliberately placed in the body so that the body will respond by actively making antibodies against the antigen. The antigens that are used for this procedure have been specially processed to make them less likely to proliferate within the body so that this exposure does not in itself cause the disease.

Examples of diseases for which artificially acquired active immunity is provided include tetanus, diphtheria, measles, smallpox, mumps, and rubella, among others.

This type of immunity lasts many years, although to maintain complete protection against the antigen repeated but smaller doses of the original antigen are required as a booster. The following classes of agents are used for stimulating artificially acquired active immunity:

1. Toxoids
2. Vaccines
   a. Killed
   b. Attenuated

Passive Immunity

Passive immunity occurs when antibodies against a specific antigen are in a specific body but that body did not actively participate in the generation of these antibodies. Instead, these antibodies are generated in the body of another person or animal and then are transferred to the body of a specific individual. Because these antibodies are foreign to the individual, the body recognizes the antibodies as nonself and takes steps to eliminate them relatively quickly. For this reason, passive immunity can provide only immediate, very short-term protection against a specific antigen.

Natural passive immunity occurs when antibodies are passed from the mother to the fetus via the placenta or to the infant through colostrum and breast milk. These antibodies are not artificially or deliberately placed in the body of another human.

Artificial passive immunity involves deliberately injecting one person with antibodies that were produced in another person or animal. This type of immunity is usually used in situations in which a person is exposed to a serious disease or illness for which he/she has little or no known actively acquired immunity. Instead, the injected antibodies are expected to inactivate the antigen. This type of immunity provides only temporary protection for only days to a few weeks. The following classes of agents are used to provide artificially acquired passive immunity.

1. Antitoxins and antivenins
2. Human immune serum
   a. Specific
   b. Nonspecific

FACTORS INFLUENCING ANTIBODY-MEDIATED IMMUNITY

A number of factors influence the effectiveness of antibody-mediated immunity. The degree of effectiveness or activity of the other two components of immunity, inflammation and cell-mediated immunity, profoundly affects antibody-mediated immune function because B lymphocytes require assistance from other leukocytes for B lymphocyte proliferation and activation, recogni-

tion of self versus nonself, antigen processing, and antibody-dependent cytotoxic actions.

In addition, non–immune-associated factors influence the general function and effectiveness of antibody-mediated immunity. Major factors include metabolic rate, oxygenation, general nutrition, and protein balance. Functional B lymphocytes are metabolically active and require energy-generating substrates such as oxygen, glucose, and ATP. Proteins are needed for synthesis of Igs and for synthesis of the multitude of enzymes necessary to catalyze immune biochemical reactions.

CELL-MEDIATED IMMUNITY

OVERVIEW

Cell-mediated immunity (or cellular immunity) (CMI) involves a variety of leukocyte actions, reactions, and interactions that range from the simple to the complex. This type of immunity is provided by leukocytes that quickly recognize nonself cells and respond to them either by exerting direct cytotoxic action or by assisting the cytotoxic activities of other cells. Some responses and characteristics of cell-mediated immunity influence and regulate the activities of antibody-mediated immunity and inflammation. Therefore, optimal function of cell-mediated immunity is needed for total immunocompetence. Alterations in this function profoundly affect the function of antibody-mediated immunity and inflammation.

CELLULAR COMPONENTS

The leukocytes that appear to play the most important roles in cell-mediated immunity include several specific T lymphocyte subsets, along with a special population of cells known as natural killer cells. T lymphocytes start life as pluripotent stem cells in the bone marrow (see Fig. 23–3). As described earlier, the pluripotent stem cell is an immature cell that has the potential to mature into any one type of differentiated blood cell depending on which maturational pathway the cell enters. The committed lymphocyte stem cells are released from the bone marrow into the blood, and they migrate into the thymus gland and/or differentiate into T lymphocytes. The committed lymphocyte stem cells that migrate to other lymphoid tissues mature into B lymphocytes.

Although B and T lymphocytes have a common origin and similar appearances, their functional characteristics are quite different. Moreover, T lymphocytes further differentiate into a variety of subsets, each with different functions (Stutman, 1985). One way to identify different T lymphocyte subsets is by determining the presence or absence of certain *marker proteins* (antigens) on the cell membrane surface. Fifty different T cell marker proteins have been identified, and 11 of these (named T1 through T11) are commonly used in clinical situations to determine the efficacy of immune components (Stites et al., 1987). Antibodies have been made for each of these 11 proteins so that each T lymphocyte subset can be identified by its reaction to the monoclonal antibodies. Most T lymphocytes have more than one antigen on the cell membrane. For example, all mature T lymphocytes contain T1, T3, T10, and T11 proteins. The T3 antigen reacting specifically to a synthetic T3 antibody is often used in clinical situations to distinguish T lymphocytes from all other leukocytes. Certain T lymphocyte subsets also contain other specific T lymphocyte membrane antigens.

The nomenclature that is used to identify specific T lymphocyte subsets includes the specific membrane antigen and the overall functional activities of the cells in a subset. The three subsets that are critically important for the development and continuation of cell-mediated immunity are helper T cells, cytotoxic T cells, and suppressor T cells.

Mechanisms of Action and Specific Protection

The cells that are involved in cell-mediated immunity generate the immunity through a wide variety of mechanisms of action. Some actions are quite specific, whereas others are general or nonspecific.

Helper T Cells

The cell membranes of these T lymphocytes contain the T4 protein, and, most commonly in clinical situations, these cells are called T4 cells or T_H cells. The most accurate name for the helper T cells is CD4, an abbreviation for cluster of differentiation 4.

Helper T cells function efficiently in the processes that are involved in the recognition of self versus nonself. Although helper T cells can act as phagocytes, phagocytosis against nonself cells is not their primary function. Rather, these T cells participate indirectly in cell-mediated immunity by stimulating the activity of many other leukocytes. In response to the recognition of nonself, helper T cells secrete special chemical substances, called *lymphokines*, that can regulate the activity of other leukocytes.

The major lymphokine that assists in cell-mediated immunity is interleukin-2 (IL-2). This lymphokine helps to increase the proliferation of a variety of leukocytes. Interleukin-2 also appears to enhance the activity of natural killer cells. In addition, helper T cells secrete macrophage-activating factor (MAF), so that cell-mediated immunity responses usually also trigger nonspecific inflammatory responses. Helper T cells also secrete interferon when these cells are infected with viruses. One function of interferon is to assist in protecting other noninfected leukocytes from becoming infected with viral particles.

Other important chemical substances that helper T cells secrete include interleukin-3 and colony-stimulating factor. The activities of these chemicals and their roles in cell-mediated immunity are the objects of much current research.

Cytotoxic T Cells

These special T lymphocytes also are called T_c cells. Cytotoxic T cells function in cell-mediated immunity by forming an antibody-like substance in response to a foreign protein (antigen) present on the surface of a nonself cell. This process requires that the cytotoxic T cell become sensitized against the antigen(s) of the nonself cell in much the same way that B lymphocytes become sensitized to foreign protein antigens. In addition, the nonself cell must share at least one major histocompatibility protein (tissue type) with the cytotoxic T cell for the cytotoxic T cell to mount an immune action against the nonself cell. The antibody-like substance that is formed by the cytotoxic T cell is not released into the blood as free antibody but instead remains attached to the surface of the cytotoxic T cell. This attached structure increases the effectiveness of the cytotoxic T cell's defensive actions against foreign invaders.

The binding of the antibody-like substance to the membrane antigen of the target nonself cell also results in the binding of the cytotoxic T cell to the nonself cell. This binding results in the direct lysis and death of the nonself cell.

Suppressor T Cells

The cell membranes of suppressor T lymphocytes contain the T8 lymphocyte antigen and the CD11 antigen. These cells are commonly called T8 cells, CD8 cells, or T_s cells. Suppressor T cells participate in the regulation of cell-mediated immunity.

The primary function of these cells is to prevent continuous overreaction or hypersensitivity reactions from occurring in response to exposure to nonself cells or proteins. The suppressor T cells secrete substances that have an overall inhibitory action on most, and perhaps on all, cells of the immune system. These substances inhibit both proliferation and activation of immune system cells.

In general, suppressor T cells directly oppose the activity of helper T cells. Therefore, optimal functioning of cell-mediated immunity requires that a balance be maintained between helper T cell activity and suppressor T cell activity. This balance is usually provided when the helper T cells outnumber the suppressor T cells by a ratio of 2 : 1. When this ratio increases, hypersensitivity reactions can be expected to occur (some of these hypersensitivity reactions are tissue damaging as well as unpleasant). When the ratio of helper to suppressor cells decreases, immune function is suppressed profoundly, and the individual is much more vulnerable to invasion by nonself cells or protein and to infections of all types.

This immune defect is the primary pathology associated with the acquired immunodeficiency syndrome (AIDS).

Natural Killer Cells

This interesting leukocyte population is extremely important for cell-mediated immunity. The actual site of differentiation and maturation of natural killer cells is unknown and currently the subject of much controversy. Although this cell population has some T lymphocyte characteristics, it does not appear to be a true T lymphocyte subset.

The primary function of natural killer cells is to exert direct cytotoxic or cytolytic effects on targeted nonself cells. Unlike cytotoxic T cells, natural killer cells can exert these effects without first undergoing a period of sensitization to the nonself cell membrane. In addition, natural killer cells do not need to have any major histocompatibility proteins in common with the nonself cell to initiate defensive actions against the nonself cell. The defensive actions of these cells appear to be totally unrelated to either antigen sensitivity or the interactions of other leukocytes.

Natural killer cells appear to be most effective in destroying unhealthy or abnormal self cells. The nonself cells that are most susceptible to the actions of these cells are self cells that are infected by organisms that live within host cells (virally infected cells) and self cells that have mutated at the DNA level and are no longer totally normal (cancer cells).

Natural killer cells and cytotoxic T cells have actions that result in the destruction of cells from other individuals or animals. Although these defensive actions usually benefit the individual, they are also responsible for rejection of grafts and transplanted organs. Therefore, cell-mediated immunity must be deliberately suppressed in individuals who receive grafts or organ transplants to prevent the destruction of these lifesaving transplanted tissues.

INTERACTIONS

Cell-mediated immunity regulates and works with antibody-mediated immunity and the inflammatory responses to provide full immunity or immunocompetence. Although some of the characteristics of cell-mediated immunity resemble a combination of both inflammation and antibody-mediated immunity, most of the functions of cell-mediated immunity are unique to this division of immunity. The actions in cell-mediated immunity different from the nonspecific inflammatory response in two ways. First, phagocytosis, the most critical feature of inflammation, is at best only a minor function of the cells that participate in cell-mediated immunity. Second, some of the leukocytes that are involved in cell-mediated immunity require prior sensitization to the nonself cells before being able to exert cytotoxic or cytolytic effects. This process requires specificity and is

an adaptive response rather than a general, nonspecific response. Because certain cells and aspects of cell-mediated immunity actually regulate the activity of the other two divisions of immunity, whenever the functions of cell-mediated immunity are less than optimal, the functions of inflammation and antibody-mediated immunity are also less than optimal.

SUMMARY

The processes that are involved in immunity are divided into three distinct functional areas that overlap and interact. These divisions include inflammation, antibody-mediated immunity, and cell-mediated immunity. All three divisions must be functional for individuals to have adequate protection against the effects of invasion of the internal environment by foreign proteins or organisms.

The phagocytic cells that are involved in inflammation are neutrophils and macrophages. These cells provide the individual with immediate and dramatic, although short-term, protection that is nonspecific and can be triggered by most invaders.

Antibody-mediated immunity is generated by B lymphocytes and provides specific, long-term protection against the effects of *repeated* invasion by specific antigens. This protection is most effective against viruses.

Cell-mediated immunity is generated by T lymphocytes and natural killer cells. This division regulates the activity of the entire immune system as well as provides specific and nonspecific protection against the effects of foreign invaders and unhealthy self cells. This division of immunity, in addition to protecting against the effects of invasion by foreign proteins, is especially important in providing protection against the development of cancer.

Less than optimal functioning of inflammation and immunity reduces the individual's protective responses and increases the individual's risk for developing an infectious disease. Excessive activity of the immune system may initiate tissue-damaging reactions against the host's own healthy cells or tissues. Such reactions are undesirable and can have life-threatening results.

REFERENCES AND READINGS

Abernathy, E. (1987). How the immune system works. *American Journal of Nursing, 87,* 456.

Barber, J. (1986). Immunologic responses to trauma. *Critical Care Quarterly, 9*(1), 57.

Barrett, J. (1988). *Textbook of immunology* (5th ed.). St. Louis: C. V. Mosby.

Colten, H. (1985). Complement biosynthesis. *Clinics in Immunology and Allergy, 5*, 287.

Cooper, N. (1987). The complement system. In D. Stites, J. Stobo, & J. Wells (Eds.), *Basic and clinical immunology* (6th ed.). Norwalk, CT: Appleton & Lange.

Dawson, M. (1988a). Immunology: Non-specific immunity. *Nursing Times, 84*(17), 75.

Dawson, M. (1988b). Specific immunity: 1. *Nursing Times, 84*(18), 73.

Dawson, M. (1988c). Specific immunity: 2. *Nursing Times, 84*(19), 69.

Epersen, S. (1986). Nursing support of host defenses. *Critical Care Quarterly, 9*(1), 51.

Gallucci, B. (1987). The immune system and cancer. *Oncology Nursing Forum, 14*(Suppl.), 3.

Goldstein, E. (1983). Hydrolytic enzymes of alveolar macrophages. *Review of Infectious Diseases, 5*, 1078.

Goodman, J. (1987). Immunoglobulins I: Structure and function. In D. Stites, J. Stobo, & J. Wells (Eds.), *Basic and clinical immunology* (6th ed.). Norwalk, CT: Appleton & Lange.

Grady, C. (1988). Host defense mechanisms: An overview. *Seminars in Oncology Nursing, 4*(2), 86.

Groenwald, S. (1980). Physiology of the immune system. *Heart and Lung, 9*, 645.

Gurevich, I. (1985). The competent internal immune system. *Nursing Clinics of North America, 20*, 151.

Gurevich, I., & Tafuro, P. (1986). The compromised host. *Cancer Nursing, 9*, 263.

Guyton, A. C. (1986). *Textbook of medical physiology* (7th ed.). Philadelphia: W. B. Saunders.

Huffer, T., Kanapa, D., & Stevenson, G. (1986). *Introduction to human immunology*. Boston: Jones & Bartlett.

Jett, M., & Lancaster, L. (1983, September/October). The inflammatory-immune response: The body's defense against invasion. *Critical Care Nurse*, pp. 64–83.

Kemp, D. (1986). Development of the immune system. *Critical Care Quarterly, 9*(1), 1.

Price, S., & Wilson, L. (1986). *Pathophysiology* (3rd ed.). New York: McGraw-Hill.

Roitt, I. (1984). *Essential immunology* (5th ed.). Boston: Blackwell Scientific.

Smith, S. (1986). Physiology of the immune system. *Critical Care Quarterly, 9*(1), 7.

Stites, D. (1987). Clinical laboratory methods for detection of cellular immune function. In D. Stites, J. Stobo, & J. Wells (Eds.), *Basic and clinical immunology* (6th ed.). Norwalk, CT: Appleton & Lange.

Stites, D., Stobo, J., & Wells, J. (Eds.). (1987). *Basic and clinical immunology* (6th ed.). Norwalk, CT: Appleton & Lange.

Stutman, O. (1985). Ontogeny of T cells. *Clinics in Immunology and Allergy, 5*, 191.

Tami, J., Parr, M., & Thompson, J. (1986). The immune system. *American Journal of Hospital Pharmacy, 43*, 2483.

Taylor, D. (1984a). Anaphylaxis: Physiology, signs and symptoms. *Nursing '84, 14*(6), 44.

Taylor, D. (1984b). Immune response: Physiology, signs and symptoms. *Nursing '84, 14*(5), 52.

Tizard, I. (1984). *Immunology: An introduction*. Philadelphia: Saunders College Publishing.

Tizard, I. (1987). *Veterinary immunology: An introduction* (3rd ed.). Philadelphia: W. B. Saunders.

Vogler, L., & Lawton, A. (1985). Ontogeny of B cells and humoral immune functions. *Clinics in Immunology and Allergy, 5*, 235.

Werb, Z., & Goldstein, I. (1987). Phagocytic cells: Chemotaxis and effector functions of macrophages and granulocytes. In D. Stites, J. Stobo, & J. Wells (Eds.), *Basic and clinical immunology* (6th ed.). Norwalk, CT: Appleton & Lange.

Workman, M. (1989). Immunologic late effects in children and adults. *Seminars in Oncology Nursing, 5*(1), 36.

CHAPTER 24

Concepts of Altered Cell Growth

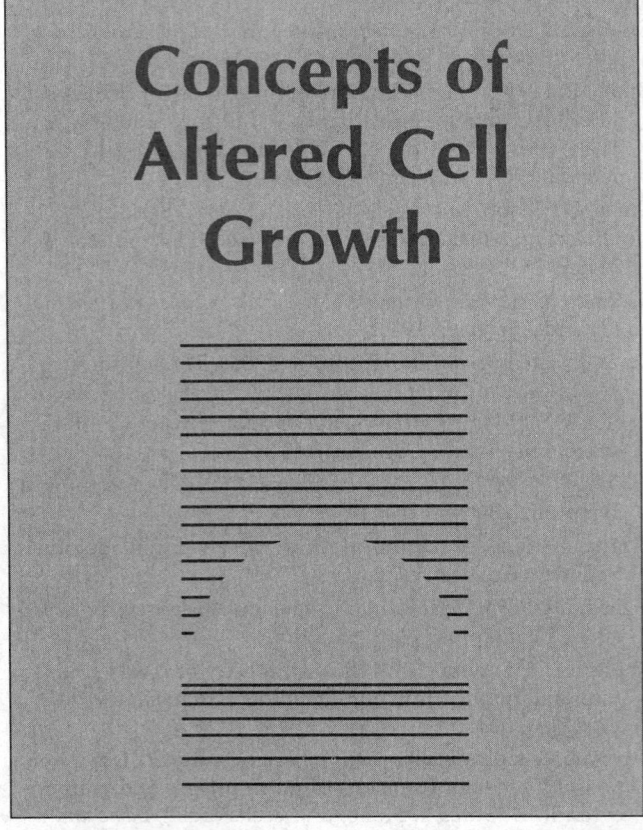

Individuals with cancer exhibit changes or disruptions in body function that are directly or indirectly related to altered cell development and proliferation. Although alterations in the growth of individual cells cannot be observed clinically, care of individuals who are affected by cancer is based on understanding of the process of altered cell growth and the effect of this process on the client and family. A major responsibility of each member of the health care team is to monitor the client's unique responses to altered cell growth.

WHAT IS CANCER?

Cancer is characterized by an increased number of abnormal cells arising from normal tissues. It may invade surrounding tissues, with possible lymphatic or blood-borne spread of malignant cells to regional lymph nodes and to distant sites. Although there is no universally accepted definition of cancer, that offered by the American Cancer Society (ACS) (1989, p. 3) is at least a generic summarization of major concepts incorporated into most modern definitions: "Cancer is a large group of diseases characterized by uncontrolled growth and spread of abnormal cells."

There are approximately 100 different types of cancer. They are generally divided into two major categories: solid tumors and hematologic malignancies. Solid tumors are associated with the organs from which they develop, e.g., breast cancer or lung cancer. Hematologic malignancies originate from hematopoietic tissue, which communicates with all organs. Hematologic malignancies include the leukemias and lymphomas.

Terminology related to cancer is summarized in Table 24–1. The term *neoplasia* is often used interchangeably with the term cancer. Neoplasia simply means growth of new and abnormal cells. In some instances, neoplastic growth may form a lump and is called a *tumor* — a word derived from the Latin *tumere*, meaning "to swell." There are two main categories of neoplastic growth: benign and malignant.

Neoplasia results from disruptions in the normal controls over cell reproduction and differentiation. Changes in the immune system of the individual with cancer seem to reduce the body's ability to recognize cancer cells as nonself or the immune system's ability to destroy cancer cells even when they are recognized (see p. 548).

Because normal controls over reproduction and differentiation are absent, neoplastic cells often have a longer life span and fail to develop a specialized function compared with their normal counterparts. It is significant that not all transformed cells lead to the disease known as cancer. In addition to abnormal reproduction and loss of specialization, a major characteristic of

---

TABLE 24–1   Terminology Related to Cancer

Anaplasia:	a total loss of differentiation
Cancer:	a large group of diseases that are characterized by uncontrolled growth and spread of abnormal cells
Differentiation:	the degree of similarity of cells to their tissue of origin
Doubling time:	the time needed for a tumor to double in size
Dysplasia:	a process in which cellular appearance is abnormal but cellular function continues to be normal
Grading:	the pathologic evaluation of differentiation
Hyperplasia:	an increase in the number of cells
Metastasis:	the way in which cancer spreads
Neoplasia:	growth of new abnormal cells, often used interchangeably with the term cancer; not specifically malignant growth
Oncology:	the study of tumors
Primary tumor:	tumor at site of origination
Solid tumors:	tumors associated with organs of origin
Staging:	the method used to describe the extent of cancer spread
Tumor:	a mass of cells that may be malignant or benign

---

cancer cells is their capacity to spread or *metastasize* to other parts of the body.

Benign neoplastic cells have been transformed but do not metastasize. Instead, they form solid tumors that are surrounded by a fibrous capsule. Some benign tumors stop growing spontaneously, whereas others may become quite large. However, benign tumors are not harmless. The impact of the presence of benign neoplasia depends greatly on the location of the tumor. Benign tumors located in a body space or compartment that is expandable may not cause significant symptoms, whereas benign tumors in the cranium not only may present devastating symptoms, but may also be inaccessible for surgical resection. In many instances, benign tumors can be removed surgically, and no further treatment is required.

The accompanying Key Features of Disease compares characteristics of benign and malignant tumors. *Differentiation* refers to the similarity of cellular function compared with the function of tissues of origin or parent tissues. The more differentiated a tumor is, the more similar it is to its tissue of origin. As tumors lose their differentiation, they become less like the parent tissue. Loss of differentiation in tissue indicates that tissue is more malignant. *Anaplasia* is total loss of differentiation.

Terminology for neoplasia has been developed to describe the tissue of origin for neoplastic cells and the classification of benign or malignant. Prefixes include *fibro-* (originating from fibrous or connective tissues), *adeno-* (originating from glandular tissues), and *lipo-* (originating from fat cells).

Benign tumor names are derived from these prefixes and the suffix *-oma.* Malignant neoplasia terminology incorporates the roots *sarc-* and *carcino-.* Sarcomas are malignancies of connective tissues, bone, and cartilage. Other roots are derived from the embryonic origin of the involved neoplastic cells. Neoplasias originating from endoderm and ectoderm give rise to *carcinomas.* Other characteristics that are used for neoplasia nomenclature and classification include biologic behavior, anatomic site, and degree of differentiation. Examples of neoplasms and their classification are given in the Key Features of Disease on page 552.

KEY FEATURES OF DISEASE ■ Differential Features of Benign and Malignant Tumors

Characteristic	Benign Tumors	Malignant Tumors
Differentiation/anaplasia	Well differentiated; structure may be typical of tissue of origin.	Some lack of differentiation with anaplasia; structure is often atypical.
Rate of growth	Usually progressive and slow; may come to a standstill or regress; mitotic figures are rare and normal.	Erratic and may be slow to rapid; mitotic figures may be numerous and abnormal.
Local invasion	Usually cohesive and expansile well-demarcated masses that do not invade or infiltrate the surrounding normal tissues.	Locally invasive, infiltrating the surrounding normal tissues.
Metastasis	Absent.	Frequently present; the larger and more undifferentiated the primary, the more likely are metastases.

From Cotran, R. S., Kumar, V., & Robbins, S. L. (1989). *Robbin's pathologic basis of disease* (4th ed., p. 250). Philadelphia: W. B. Saunders.

KEY FEATURES OF DISEASE ■ Classification of Neoplasms

Tissue Origin	Benign Tumors	Malignant Tumors
Epithelial tissue		
Glandular	Adenoma (e.g., thyroid follicular adenoma)	Adenocarcinoma (e. g., adenocarcinoma of lung)
Squamous and transitional	Polyp, papilloma (e.g., squamous papilloma of skin)	Squamous cell carcinoma (e.g., squamous cell carcinoma of skin), transitional cell carcinoma
Connective tissue	Tissue type plus suffix *-oma* (e.g., osteoma, hemangioma)	Sarcoma (e.g., osteosarcoma, hemangiosarcoma)
Hematopoietic and lymphoreticular tissue		Lymphoma (e.g., large cell lymphoma, Hodgkin's disease), leukemia (e.g., myelocytic leukemia)
Neural tissue	Neuroma, neurofibroma	Sarcoma (e.g., neurofibrosarcoma), blastoma (e.g., glioblastoma multiforme)
Mixed tissue	Teratoma (e.g., teratoma of ovary)	Teratocarcinoma (e.g., teratocarcinoma of testis)

From Bonfiglio, T. A., & Terry, R. (1983). The pathology of cancer. In P. Rubin (Ed.), *Clinical oncology: A multidisciplinary approach* (6th ed., p. 22). New York: American Cancer Society.

A malignant tumor is a large collection of cancer cells, all descendants of a single cell. This ancestor was once a normal cell with a normal function in a particular tissue, which somehow underwent a fundamental change. As a result of that change, this ancestor cell began to divide and proliferate in response to directions other than stimuli that result in normal cell reproduction. Eventually, the cell parented billions of similarly altered cells composing the tumor mass.

cancer has been identified. However, many factors are associated with the development of cancer.

Today, more than 5 million Americans are alive who have a history of cancer, nearly 3 million of whom can be considered to be cured (ACS, 1989). In 1989, more than 1 million people will have been newly diagnosed as having cancer. Cancer occurs at any age, but it does strike more frequently with advancing age. Cancer will occur in approximately three of every four families in the United States (ACS, 1989).

HISTORICAL PERSPECTIVE

Cancer is not a new phenomenon. There is evidence that prehistoric humans experienced cancer. Ancient Egyptian papyri dating to at least 3400 BC describe various tumors. Hippocrates is credited with designating the process as *karkinos* or, in Latin, "cancer," meaning "crab-like." It was not until 1951 that the normal cell cycle and its role in cancer development was introduced.

Since 1951, progress in understanding cancer has accelerated. A theory of carcinogenesis has evolved, along with the identification of multiple factors that can stimulate its development. The theory of immune surveillance has also been developed to assist in explaining cancer development. At the present time, a complete understanding of what happens to a normal cell to cause it to become a cancer cell is lacking. No one cause for

NORMAL CELL REPRODUCTION

A basic understanding of the physiology of normal cell reproduction is necessary to understand both the development of cancer and the rationale for various therapeutic options.

All humans begin life as a single cell. At conception, the fertilized egg contains cells that are undifferentiated, that is, they have no specialized function. These embryonic cells divide rapidly without specialized function. Eight days after conception, these cells become committed as specific tissue types with their own functions. They are now differentiated cells. There are differentiated cardiac cells, differentiated gastrointestinal cells, and so on. Most cells in the body contain the same genes. At commitment, all cells express certain genes for dif-

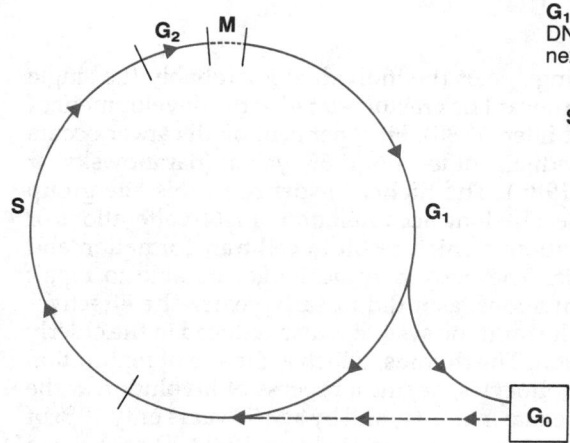

G_1 is the period from the end of mitosis to DNA synthesis. The cell is preparing for the next cell division.

S is the period of DNA synthesis.

G_2 is the period from the end of DNA synthesis to the beginning of mitosis.

In M phase, mitosis, the cell divides, producing two daughter cells.

G_0 is the resting state. Cells can exit from G_1 or G_2 to enter the resting state. Most cells are in this phase at any given time.

Figure 24–1

The cell cycle.

ferentiation and repress others. Genes that are repressed at commitment are normally inactivated for life.

Unlike embryonic cells, normal differentiated cells have slow or absent cellular division, are tightly adherent and nonmigratory, and have contact inhibition (i.e., they will not divide unless space and resources are available for division).

Normal cell reproduction involves the orderly movement of cells through a cycle comprising four distinct phases (Fig. 24–1). The phases are

1. Gap 1 (G_1), the time from the end of mitosis to DNA synthesis
2. Synthesis (S), the period of DNA synthesis
3. Gap 2 (G_2), the time from the end of DNA synthesis to the beginning of mitosis
4. Mitosis (M), the time the cell is in division with production of two daughter cells

A fifth phase, G_0, refers to a resting phase; cells exit from either G_1 or G_2 to enter G_0. At any given time, only 15% to 30% of cells in tissues are actively cycling; thus, the G_0 cells make up the largest population of cells. *Cell cycle time* is defined as the time from the end of one mitotic event to the end of the next mitotic event. Cell cycle time is 24 hours for most cells. Both daughter cells should have the exact amount of deoxyribonucleic acid (DNA), which is identical to the parent DNA.

CARCINOGENESIS

Carcinogenesis is the process by which normal cells become malignant cells. This process, which is also referred to as *malignant transformation*, occurs in many steps over time. The major steps are identified as *initiation* and *promotion*. Both of these events depend on car-

cinogens to stimulate the malignant transformation of a cell.

Thousands of carcinogens have been identified in the environment. They are classified as physical, chemical, or viral and are discussed in more detail later in this chapter. *Complete carcinogens* are agents that are capable of inducing both initiation and promotion. *Incomplete carcinogens* can induce only initiation. *Promoters* are capable of stimulating only promotion. Carcinogens that cause initiation may be chemical, viral, or physical. Initiation is a process in which a carcinogen causes damage to the genetic make-up of a cell, which leads to a permanently altered gene. Promotion has two stages. The first stage, *fixation*, results in proliferation of initiated cells that have altered DNA. The second stage involves a process called *derepression*. In this stage, genes in the cell that were meant to be inactive or shut off are activated or *expressed*. Carcinogens that can cause promotion include specific or certain chemicals and viral agents. However, these carcinogens cannot cause malignant transformation unless initiation has occurred.

In 1983, oncogenes were identified as a critical component of carcinogenesis. *Oncogenes* are genes that were meant to be repressed but are expressed after being stimulated by a promoter. When inactive, these genes are referred to as *proto-oncogenes*.

More than 40 different oncogenes have been identified. It is not known whether the activation of several oncogenes or specific oncogenes is needed for malignant transformation to take place.

The process of carcinogenesis takes years. It is not simple and predictable. Instead, it is multifactorial, dependent on a number of intrinsic and extrinsic factors.

INTRINSIC FACTORS RELATED TO DEVELOPMENT OF CANCER

In addition to an individual's expression of oncogenes, other intrinsic factors affect whether that individual develops cancer. Intrinsic factors include the function of the immune system, age, and genetic predisposition.

IMMUNE SURVEILLANCE

The function of the immune system is to protect the body from foreign invaders and nonself cells (see Chap. 23). Nonself cells include cells that are made in the body but that are altered, i.e., cancer cells. The segment of the immune system that is most responsible for protecting against cancer is cell-mediated immunity. Of the cells that are involved in cell-mediated immunity, natural killer (NK) cells are most important for immune surveillance. When an NK cell recognizes a nonself cell, it binds to the membrane of that cell and releases a series of lysosomal enzymes into the nonself cell. The NK cell then releases the nonself cell. Enzymes inside the target digest critical components of the cell, and the cell quickly self-destructs. It has also been suggested that NK cells release a substance called natural killer cytotoxic factor, which is directly cytotoxic to target cells.

The fact that the immune system is instrumental in protecting the body from cancer is well supported by cancer incidence statistics in immunosuppressed individuals. Children younger than 2 years and adults older than 60 years have an immune system that functions at a less than optimal level. These individuals also have a higher incidence of cancer compared with the general population. Organ recipients who are taking immunosuppressive drugs to reduce the risk of organ rejection also have a higher incidence of cancer. In clients with acquired immunodeficiency syndrome, the incidence of cancer may be as high as 70% (Moran, 1988).

In the past, the theory that the immune system was involved in carcinogenesis (immune surveillance) was rejected partly because it did not explain how cancer develops in an individual with a competent immune system. In fact, many individuals with cancer have intact immune systems. It is now thought that cancer cells can outmaneuver the immune surveillance system of the body by a variety of mechanisms. Cancer cells may retain surface characteristics of normal cells, which may help them to evade NK cells or other cells in the immune system. Cancer cells may be coated with fibrin or platelets, which similarly protects them from being recognized as nonself. Cancer cells may shed surface proteins that identify them as nonself into the circulatory system. NK cells may attack the surface proteins in the blood and leave the residual cancer cells alone so that they can proliferate. Cancer cells are known to sequester in sanctuaries that the immune system does not easily enter, such as the central nervous system and the eyes. These are considered to be immunoprivileged sites.

Another possible reason for the immune system's lack of total control is that the early burden of cancer cells may be so small that the immune system does not recognize the cells until rapid division occurs. At the point of recognition, the cell burden might be too large for NK cells to eliminate it.

AGE

Advancing age of the individual is probably the single most significant risk factor related to the development of cancer (Miller, 1980). Fifty per cent of all cancer occurs in individuals older than 65 years (Baranowsky & Myers, 1986). The higher incidence in this age group may reflect lifelong accumulation of DNA alterations or cell mutations, which result in cell transformation and neoplasia. The body may no longer be able to repair these mutations, as it did in early years. The effectiveness of the immune system is also reduced in the elderly population. The thymus, which is the site of maturation of T lymphocytes, begins a process of involution at the time of sexual maturity, and by age 50 years only 10% of the thymus mass remains (Weksler, 1985). The result is a loss of thymic capacity to differentiate T cells, a subsequent increase of immature T cells in circulation, and a reduced response of the immune system to altered cells.

Manifestations of a malignancy in elderly persons may get overlooked and attributed to changes that coincide with normal aging. It is essential that elders be aware of and report symptoms such as the seven warning signs of cancer to health care providers. Health care providers must treat these reports with respect and thoroughly investigate all manifestations suggesting disease.

GENETIC PREDISPOSITION

As previously discussed, oncogenes are primary intrinsic factors related to carcinogenesis. Proto-oncogenes, precursors of oncogenes, are passed on from generation to generation. The development of cancer, however, depends on more than the presence of these genes. For a cancer to develop, the proto-oncogene needs to be damaged or altered to allow expression of the oncogene. Patterns of genetic predisposition for cancer other than oncogenes have also been identified. These patterns include inherited predisposition for specific cancers, inherited conditions associated with malignancies, and familial clustering.

Inherited Predisposition for Specific Cancers

A few cancers occur because a defective gene is inherited from one parent. In these situations, the individual who receives the dominant defective gene is initiated at the time of conception. Malignancy develops at a later time when the gene is exposed to a promoting agent. Cancers that are considered to be inheritable are retinoblastoma and Wilms' tumor.

Inherited Conditions Associated with Malignancies

Malignancies in this category occur secondary to the primary disease, which is inherited. The inherited disease puts the individual at risk for developing cancer. Inherited diseases that are associated with specific malignancies include Down's syndrome, which is associated with leukemia, and familial polyposis, which is associated with colon cancer.

Familial Clustering

Several malignancies appear to occur with greater frequency among relatives but lack an identifiable genetic link. Breast cancer occurs at rates that are higher than expected in daughters and siblings of women who have been diagnosed with breast cancer before menopause. Some families are also known to have higher rates of different types of cancer than would be expected. The role of extrinsic factors in the development of cancer in these families is difficult to determine. Environmental carcinogens can modify genetic messages. Even though breast cancer has a higher than expected incidence in first-generation relatives, less than 8% of women with breast cancer have breast cancer in their family (Workman & Ellerhorst-Ryan, 1989).

CHROMOSOMAL ABERRATIONS

In addition to these genetic patterns that predispose an individual to cancer, a number of chromosomal aberrations have been identified and linked to specific malignancies. Of individuals who are afflicted with chronic myelocytic leukemia, more than 95% carry the Philadelphia chromosome (Adamson, 1987). Aberrations have also been identified in individuals with other leukemias, lymphomas, and solid tumors. The significance of these aberrations is unclear. For example, it is not certain whether the aberration is a cause or a result of the malignancy.

RACE

The incidence of cancer varies among races. ACS data demonstrate that Black Americans have a higher incidence of cancer than Caucasian, and the death rate is higher for Black persons. The overall cancer incidence rate for Black persons has increased 27% since 1960 (Newell, 1985), whereas it increased 12% for Caucasians in that same period. Cancer sites and cancer-related mortality vary along racial lines as well. Sites that are affected in the Black population more frequently include the lung, prostate, colon, rectum, esophagus, and uterine cervix.

When assessing risks for the development of cancer, however, race and genetic predisposition cannot be considered in a vacuum. Behavior that is related to culture or ethnic group, geographic location, diet, and socioeconomic factors also need to be assessed. The ACS has reported that cancer incidence and survival are often related to socioeconomic factors such as availability of health care services (ACS, 1986).

It is difficult if not impossible to separate geographic and racial factors from other demographic and epidemiologic factors for the simple reason that human populations and individuals are mobile — they migrate from one location to another, and one group mixes with another group, and cultural, social, and ethnic influences are mingled. For example, the Chinese population in San Francisco, California, especially the first generation of immigrant families, has a high incidence of nasopharyngeal cancer. The incidence is similar to that found in various provinces of the People's Republic of China. The incidence drops in later generations in the United States. It is unclear if the incidence is related to social or environmental factors (the nitrite content of prepared foods has been implicated) or to the Epstein-Barr virus, which is also prevalent in individuals with nasopharyngeal cancer.

EXTRINSIC FACTORS RELATED TO DEVELOPMENT OF CANCER

It is estimated that up to 80% of cancer in the United States may be the result of environmental or extrinsic factors. However, the actual role of these factors is not totally understood (Li, 1987). The term *carcinogen* designates agents that elicit neoplastic changes in any tissue type. Environmental carcinogens are physical, chemical, or biologic agents that have been identified as causing cancer. The accompanying Key Features of Disease lists established environmental causes of human cancer. The lack of clarity related to environmental causation of cancer is primarily the result of the delay between exposure to carcinogens and diagnosis of disease, which is usually years or even decades. An additional complication is related to the lack of a definitive relationship between dose or exposure and the fact that only a small proportion of people who are exposed to agents actually develop cancer. It is also recognized that specific exposures rarely occur unrelated to other factors.

If it is true that 80% of cancers are related to environmental exposures, it follows that environmental factors can be controlled in an effort to prevent cancer to reduce risks of developing cancer.

CHEMICAL CARCINOGENS

The study of chemical carcinogenesis began with findings of a high incidence of certain cancers in individuals who are exposed to large amounts of tobacco snuff, coal tar, and aromatic amines. The relationship of nasal cancers to the use of snuff was noted in 1761, and lip cancer was linked to clay pipe smoking in 1794. Scrotal cancer was the first designated occupational cancer for chimney sweeps in 1775. This revelation stimulated the first known attempts to prevent cancer when the Danish Chimney Sweeper's Guild urged members to take daily baths. This action decreased the incidence of scrotal

KEY FEATURES OF DISEASE ■ Established Environmental Causes of Human Cancer

Carcinogen	Cancer Site or Associated Neoplasm
Alcoholic beverages	Liver, esophagus, mouth, pharynx, larynx
Alkylating agents (melphalan, cyclophosphamide, chlorambucil, nitrosoureas)	Acute myelocytic leukemia, bladder (cyclophosphamide)
Androgenic steroids	Liver
Aromatic amines	Bladder
Arsenic (inorganic)	Lung, skin
Asbestos	Lung, pleura, peritoneum, pericardium
Benzene	Acute myelocytic leukemia
bis-Chloromethyl ether	Lung
Chromium	Lung
Chronic hepatitis B infection	Liver
Cyclosporine	Non-Hodgkin's lymphoma
Diethylstilbestrol (prenatal exposure)	Vagina (adenocarcinoma)
HTLV-I	Adult T cell leukemia/lymphoma
Immunosuppressive drugs (azathioprine, cyclosporine)	Non-Hodgkin's lymphoma
Ionizing radiation	Almost all organs
Isopropyl alocohol production	Nasal sinuses
Mustard gas	Lung, larynx, nasal sinuses
Nickel dust	Lung, nasal sinuses
Phenacetin	Renal pelvis, bladder
Polycyclic hydrocarbons	Lung, scrotum, skin (squamous carcinoma)
Sunlight (ultraviolet)	Skin, intraocular melanoma
Synthetic estrogens	Endometrium
Tobacco	Lung, mouth, pharynx, larynx, esophagus, pancreas, bladder, kidney, renal pelvis
Vinyl chloride	Liver (angiosarcoma)
Wood dust	Nasal sinuses

From Li, F. P. (1989). Cancer epidemiology and prevention. In E. Rubenstein & D. D. Federman (Eds.). SCIENTIFIC AMERICAN Medicine, Section 12, Subsection 1. © 1989 Scientific American, Inc. All rights reserved.

cancer among Northern European sweeps (Miller & Miller, 1979). The list of chemicals that are known to be carcinogenic to humans now includes more than 20 organic and inorganic industrial chemicals, drugs, and others products used in everyday life. Some chemicals in and of themselves are capable of causing initiation or promotion, or both. Other chemicals may not be harmful in their original state but can stimulate changes in the cell after they are metabolized. Some chemicals are complete carcinogens that can cause both initiation and promotion. Others are pure initiating agents, or incomplete carcinogens. Still others are only promoting agents.

RADIATION

Radiation is a physical agent that is capable of causing carcinogenesis. Even low-dose radiation affects cells. Some effects are temporary and reparable, whereas other effects are irreversible and may be lethal to the affected cell. The two types of radiation that are associated with carcinogenesis are ionizing and ultraviolet. Both ionizing radiation and ultraviolet radiation produce gene mutations and chromosomal damage.

Doses of ionizing radiation have been described in terms of roentgen and rad. *Roentgen* is a quantity of x-radiation or gamma radiation, and *rad* is a unit of absorbed dose of radiation.

Sources of ionizing radiation occur naturally in the environment in minerals such as radon, uranium, and radium. Most rocks and soil contain various concentrations of uranium and radium. The decay of radium results in the release of radon into the air and water. It is thought that many homes might be the major source of exposure to radon for the general population.

The two most important routes of entry for ionizing radiation are ingestion and inhalation. Ingestion is most likely to occur with contaminated foods or water. Either the radionuclide is absorbed through the gastrointestinal tract or the tract itself is irradiated during passage of the radionuclide. Inhaled radionuclides can be deposited in any compartment of the respiratory tract, but they may also exert toxic effects on other structures including the pulmonary lymph nodes, gastrointestinal tract, blood, and tissue compartments like skeleton, liver, and kidneys.

Other sources of ionizing radiation include diagnostic and therapeutic x-rays, synthetic radioactive materials such as radioisotopes, and cosmic radiation. More than 90% of the annual dose received from synthetic sources is from medical diagnostic procedures (National Council on Radiation Protection and Measurements, 1987). The risk of developing cancer from a diagnostic test is estimated to be 1 in 1 million per year (Harwood & Yaffe, 1982). Even though this risk is low, there has been concern in the medical community about the risk of radiation. Emphasis is now on careful selection of clients for diagnostic x-rays, and a limitation or elimination of routine diagnostic procedures for which the risk might outweigh the benefit.

Cancers that have been related to exposure to ionizing radiation include cancers of the breast, thyroid, and hematopoietic tissues. Certain leukemias have been related to radiation, with peak incidence occurring within 2 to 4 years after exposure. It is well-known that the incidence of certain solid tumors and hematopoietic malignancies increased considerably after the use of the atomic bomb in Japan near the end of World War II. Experts predict a similarly increased incidence of radiation-related malignancies in the future as a result of

the 1986 nuclear accident in Chernobyl in the Soviet Union.

Factors that are known to modify the body's response to a given exposure to radiation include dose rate, type of radiation, geometry of the exposure, portion of the body exposed, species, age, sex, oxygen tension, and the body's metabolic status (Hobbs & McClellan, 1986). Cell or tissue sensitivity to the damaging effects of radiation — *radiosensitivity* — is related to how often the cells undergo mitosis. Cells that go through mitosis frequently, or tissues composed of these cells, are the most radiosensitive. Cells (or tissues) with no mitosis are the most *radioresistant.* Rubin and Casarett (1968) developed a working classification of cells and their radiosensitivity (Table 24–2). Cells can and do repair some amount of radiation damage depending on the cell's position in the cell cycle and the time between exposures to subsequent radiation doses.

Ultraviolet radiation sources include the sun and industrial equipment such as welding arcs and germicidal lights. It is thought that this radiation causes DNA damage leading to skin cancer. Multiple exposures to high doses are probably necessary for this to occur. Basal cell carcinoma, squamous cell carcinoma, and malignant melanoma are three types of skin cancer that occur in the United States. The incidence of all three types is increasing.

VIRAL CARCINOGENS

Evidence of viral carcinogenesis has been found that relates hepatitis B virus to liver cancer, Epstein-Barr virus to Burkitt's lymphoma, human T cell lymphotrophic virus to adult T cell leukemia and lymphoma, and human papillomavirus to cervical carcinoma.

Overall, few viruses that are carcinogenic in humans have been identified. As with other carcinogens, the actual carcinogenic agent or event is difficult to pinpoint, but it is thought that viruses become part of the DNA of the cells, which results in cell mutation.

DIET

Epidemiologic data relate development of neoplasia to many dietary practices or combinations of dietary practices and environmental exposures. However, the relationship of diet to carcinogenesis is poorly understood. Dietary factors that are suspected of being related to cancers of the large bowel include ingestion of a small amount of fiber, associated with slow bowel transit time and high intake of fat and calories. The prevailing theory is that metabolic end products of fats are carcinogenic, and the slow bowel transit time increases the exposure time of these carcinogens to the bowel lining.

Preservatives, contaminants, preparation methods, and additives (dyes, flavorings, and sweeteners) are being assessed for possible carcinogenic effects. Conversely, certain food types and components — green

TABLE 24–2 Classification of Radiosensitivity

Cell Type	Radiosensitivity
Vegetative intermitotic cells are short-lived cells, primitive, and dividing regularly to produce daughter cells.	Most radiosensitive (hematopoietic stem cells; dividing cells of intestines; type A spermatogonia; granulosa cells of ovarian follicles; germinal cells of epidermis and gastric and holocrine glands; large and medium lymphocytes).
Differentiating intermitotic cells are short-lived cells, divide for a limited number of divisions, and differentiate somewhat between divisions.	Slightly less radiosensitive (differentiating hematopoietic cells in bone marrow, more differentiated spermatogonia and spermatocytes, oocytes).
Multipotent connective tissue cells divide irregularly or sporadically in response to special stimuli.	Of intermediate radiosensitivity (endothelial cells, fibroblasts, mesenchymal cells).
Reverting postmitotic cells have long lives and do not divide at high rate except with special stimuli.	Radioresistant (epithelial parenchymal cells, duct and glandular cells).
Fixed postmitotic cells normally do not divide or have lost ability to divide and are well differentiated and specialized.	Most radioresistant (neurons, some muscle cells, neutrophils, erythrocytes, spermatids, spermatozoa, superficial cells of alimentary tract, epithelial cells of sebaceous glands).

Data from Rubin, P., & Casarett, G. W. (1968). *Clinical radiation pathology* (pp. 34–35). Philadelphia: W. B. Saunders.

vegetables, fruits, vitamins (A, C, D, and E), calcium, and selenium — are among substances that appear to be protective (Ames, 1983; Greenwald, 1984; Li, 1987).

Incidence rates of certain gastrointestinal tract cancers have changed as people migrate, modify diets, and possibly modify other environmental exposures. Populations that consume fewer meat products, e.g., Mormons and Seventh-Day Adventists, have lower rates of cancer of the large bowel. The association of cigarette smoking and intake of alcohol is accepted as etiologic for development of cancers of the respiratory tract, oral cavity, larynx, and gastrointestinal tract.

Because dietary considerations are rarely independent of other possible carcinogenic stimuli or promoters, evidence of dietary contributions to development of cancer is clouded. Many experts regard existing evidence as insufficient to recommend specific dietary alterations, whereas others advocate dietary modifications. Such recommended measures include controlling caloric intake, with fats composing less 30% of total caloric intake; increasing intake of fresh fruits, vegetables, and other high-fiber foods and foods rich in vitamins A and C; and limiting ingestion of salt-cured, smoked, and nitrite-cured foods, alcohol, and chewing tobacco.

NEOPLASTIC PATHOLOGY

CHARACTERISTICS OF CANCER CELLS

To understand how cancer affects so many physiologic functions, characteristics of the altered, malignant cell needs to be clarified. Unlike normal cells, cancer cells have the following properties:

1. Cell division is rapid.
2. Partial or complete differentiated function of parent cells is lost.
3. Cells are able to migrate.
4. Cells are loosely adherent.
5. Cells do not recognize or respect tissue borders.
6. Cells are not contact inhibited.
7. Growth rate is not well regulated.
8. There is a large nucleus-to-cytoplasm ratio.

Cancer cells multiply under conditions in which the reproduction of normal cells would be restrained. In a way, cancer cells have achieved the prerequisites for cell immortality. Cancer cells have escaped mechanisms that control growth, and this condition is associated with a loss of ability to achieve specialized structure and function. If the cells function at all, the function is not regulated and does not relate to the true needs of the rest of the tissue, organ, or body.

PROGRESSION

Progression is the name of the stage of cellular development of cancer cells. In this stage, these cancer cells continue to grow, invade, metastasize, and alter their gene number and arrangement. The cancer cell progresses from being low grade, well differentiated to being high grade, poorly differentiated (see under later heading Cancer Stage and Grade). The DNA content of cells becomes unstable during progression. Many tumors have extra chromosomal material and are called *aneuploid*. Other malignant tumors retain the normal number of chromosomes and are termed *diploid*. Aneuploid tumor cells are thought to be more aggressive.

As cancer genes change in number and arrangement, they produce subpopulations of tumor cells that are heterogeneous to the original cancer cell. Heterogeneous tumors are often able to survive regardless of the environmental conditions.

METASTASIS

The sequence of metastatic spread can be summarized by these eight events:

1. Extension of the primary tumor into surrounding tissues
2. Penetration of the primary tumor into body cavities and vessels
3. Release of cancer cells into cavities, lymph, and blood
4. Transport of cancer cells to secondary sites
5. Implantation or arrest of cancer cells at secondary sites
6. Invasion of tissues at secondary sites
7. Evasion of host responses attempting to inhibit survival or growth of cancer cells
8. Establishment of microenvironment conducive to continued neoplastic cell reproduction

Cancer cells' ability to metastasize depends on important characteristics of the cancer cells and interactions of the cells with host factors.

Anatomy of the lymphatic system influences metastatic spread. Primary sites that are rich in lymphatics are more prone to early metastatic spread than areas with few lymphatics. The position of lymphatics around a primary site is also a significant factor in the distribution of metastases. For example, lymphatics of the large bowel are circumferential, as opposed to lying longitudinally along the bowel. As a result, metastases are likely to spread circumferentially around the bowel and result in obstruction at that site.

LOCAL SEEDING

Local seeding is a form of metastatic spread that involves distribution of shed cancer cells in the local area of the primary tumor. Local seeding is typified by ovarian cancer, in which cells often spill from the primary tumor into the peritoneal cavity and set up multiple seeding sites there. Ovarian cancers tend to remain in the peritoneal cavity, not spreading to distant sites until late in the course of the disease.

BLOOD-BORNE METASTASES

Release of tumor cells into the blood is the most significant step in the process of neoplasia. Combined with seeding, distribution via the blood stream determines the area of metastases, and metastatic disease is the major cause of cancer-related death. In general, factors that promote the release of tumor cells in the blood stream increase as the size of primary tumor increases and the cells are less differentiated.

The vast majority of circulating tumor cells are destroyed by mechanical factors in the circulation, immune responses, or unsuitable environments in various organs where the cells stop. The ability of cancer cells to produce metastases is enhanced if they are able to form clumps of cells. Clumps of tumor cells produce micrometastases as they become trapped in capillaries. Platelets adhere to capillary endothelial junctions and expose basement membrane. The basement membrane is destroyed, which allows tumor cells to enter the surrounding connective tissue matrix. A metastatic tumor site is thus created (Freil, 1988).

CANCER STAGE AND GRADE

STAGE

Confirmation of malignant neoplasia is the first step in clinical evaluation of the client with cancer. Staging and classification of the specific cancer are necessary to determine appropriate treatment, to reliably evaluate the results of management, and to confidently compare statistics reported from local, regional, national, and international sources.

The anatomic extent of cancer is the primary basis of *staging*. There are some site-specific staging systems such as the Dukes staging of colon and rectal cancer. The Dukes system was first developed in 1932 and is still in use in some areas of clinical practice (see Chap. 45). It describes malignancy on the basis of depth of anatomic spread and lymph node metastases.

More recently, the American Joint Committee on Cancer (AJCC) developed the *TNM* (tumor, node, metastasis) system for use in describing the anatomic extent of cancers. The stages described are useful as guides to treatment, prognosis, and comparison of the end results of treatment. The TNM staging system is based on the premise that histologically similar cancers share similar patterns of growth and extension. According to the AJCC *Manual for Staging of Cancer* (Beahrs et al., 1988, p. 3): "The size of the untreated primary cancer or tumor

(T) increases progressively and at some point in time regional lymph node involvement (N) and, finally, distant metastases (M) occur." The presence of tumor growth, spread to primary lymph nodes, and metastases is used as these characteristics appear (or do not appear) during clinical examination and indicate the degree of extension or spread of the cancer. Therapeutic procedures alter the course and history of cancer, and therefore accurate staging is significant during various points in the course of disease.

TNM staging systems are specific to each solid tumor site. Table 24-3 gives basic definitions for the specific staging systems. However, TNM staging is not applicable to several types of cancers.

Malignancies of the lymphatic system — lymphomas — and hematologic malignancies — leukemias — do not lend themselves to the TNM system, which is useful for classification of solid tumors. Numerous classification systems have evolved during the past 85 years and continue to present challenges related to useful and consistent classification. Lymphomas are classified as *Hodgkin's disease* or *non-Hodgkin's lymphoma*. Clinical presentation in Hodgkin's disease usually involves lymphatic enlargement in areas *above the diaphragm* (especially enlarged cervical nodes). Clinical presentation of non-Hodgkin's lymphoma is similar to that for Hodgkin's disease with certain exceptions, including a greater number of enlarged lymphatics below the diaphragm, with frequent involvement of the gastrointestinal tract and bone.

The staging system for Hodgkin's disease involves a numeric classification that ranges from I through IV.

TABLE 24-3   TNM Clinical Classification

Primary Tumor (T)

TX	Primary tumor cannot be assessed.
T0	No evidence of primary tumor.
Tis	Carcinoma in situ.
T1, T2, T3, T4	Increasing size and/or local extent of the primary tumor.

Regional Lymph Nodes (N)

NX	Regional lymph nodes cannot be assessed.
N0	No regional lymph node metastasis.
N1, N2, N3	Increasing involvement of regional lymph nodes.

Distant Metastasis (M)

MX	Presence of distant metastasis cannot be assessed.
M0	No distant metastasis.
M1	Distant metastasis

Modified from American Joint Committee on Cancer. (1988). Beahrs, O. H., Henson, D. E., Hutter, R. V., & Myers, M. H. (Eds.). *Manual for staging of cancer* (3rd ed., p. 7). Philadelphia: J. B. Lippincott.

Stage designations are based on disease involvement above and/or below the diaphragm, with lower numeric classifications carrying a better prognosis. Non-Hodgkin's lymphomas are classified by cell type and biologic behavior, i.e., indolent (low grade), intermediate grade, or aggressive (high grade).

The *leukemias* are neoplasias of the hematopoietic system originating in the bone marrow. Although clinical manifestations are similar (decrease in number of red blood cells, granulocytes, and platelets), various categories define different leukemias in terms of morphologic, histochemical, and immunologic characteristics. Anatomic classification is not applicable in this disease.

Multiple myeloma is neoplastic proliferation of plasma cells. Diagnosis of multiple myeloma is made on determination of excess plasma cells in the blood, in combination with clinical signs and symptoms that are characteristic of this form of neoplasia. Multiple myeloma is associated with bone lesions and rising concentration of serum or urinary globulins, and some forms of anemia. Because of the nature of this disease, it is also not compatible with current staging systems.

GRADE

It is known that various histologic types of cancer, even though arising from the same organ, behave differently and cannot be considered together in meaningful classification systems. The *grade* is a pathologic evaluation of the degree of differentiation, which usually relates to the cancer's potential for spread. Two systems are currently used. One system uses a numeric grade of 1 to 4, and the other uses descriptive gradients ranging from *well-* to *moderately* to *poorly differentiated* to describe cell behavior. Low numeric grades, which correspond to the well-differentiated classification, designate cancer cells that deviate only slightly from their tissues of origin or power tissues. Higher numeric designation, and therefore poorly differentiated, cells least resemble normal cell or tissue patterns. Table 24–4 gives descriptions of each cancer grade.

THE EVOLUTION OF A CANCER

Three general factors determine the development of cancer. The first is genetic make-up. All individuals have proto-oncogenes, which are normally repressed. If these become damaged (e.g., through initiation), they may be expressed as oncogenes. Other genetic traits may also predispose an individual to cancer, but alone they do not determine that cancer will occur. They depend on other factors that are involved in the evolution of the malignancy.

The second factor—multiple carcinogens in the environment—can promote carcinogenesis if the right set of circumstances exists. The third factor that determines the development of cancer is the immune system. If cells that have undergone initiation and promotion escape the surveillance of NK cells, the malignancy remains. Cancer cells group, proliferate, and become tumors.

Growth of tumors is discussed in terms of doubling time, i.e., the amount of time it takes for a tumor to double in size. The smallest tumor that is likely to be detected by a physical examination or diagnostic test is 1 cm in diameter. At this size, it contains 10^8 or 10^9 (one billion) tumor cells. To reach this size, a tumor will have undergone 30 doublings (Tannock, 1989).

Tumors have a wide range of growth rates. Fast-growing tumors, such as lymphomas, may double in 4 weeks, whereas an adenocarcinoma of the lung doubles in 21 weeks. Given these rates and the fact that 30 doublings are required for clinical detection of a tumor, one can appreciate the long latency period for cancer. Before an adenocarcinoma of the lung is detected, it often has been growing for 12 years. During that time, it may have invaded surrounding tissue and metastasized to different sites. Chromosomal changes and formation of heterogeneous subpopulations may have occurred. All of these malignant changes make treatment of the cancer more difficult.

Because diagnosis of cancer often occurs late in the life of the malignancy, avoidance of exposure to carcinogens is considered to be a prime strategy in the war against cancer. A great deal of information has been dispersed to the public about carcinogenic agents in the environment, yet exposure continues. In 1982, the surgeon general of the United States reported, "There is no single action an individual can take to reduce the risk of cancer more effectively than quitting smoking, particularly cigarettes" (U.S. Department of Health and Human Services [DHHS], 1982). Despite this, 50 million Americans continue to smoke (DHHS, 1985).

Tobacco smoking. Tobacco is a complete carcinogen capable of inducing both initiation and promotion. It is estimated that tobacco smoke contains more than 3600 individual compounds. The major contributor to carci-

---

TABLE 24–4 Grading of Cancer

GX	Grade cannot be determined.
G1	Tumor cells are well differentiated and closely resemble parent tissue or tissue of origin.
G2	Tumor cells are moderately differentiated; they retain some characteristics of parent tissue.
G3	Tumor cells are poorly differentiated; identity of parent tissue can usually be established.
G4	Tumor cells are very poorly differentiated, often called anaplastic. Determination of tissue of origin is difficult and perhaps impossible.

Modified from American Joint Committee on Cancer. (1988). Beahrs, O. H., Henson, D. E., Hutter, R. V., & Myers, M. H. (Eds.). *Manual for staging of cancer* (3rd ed., p. 7). Philadelphia: J. B. Lippincott, and from Workman, M. D., & Ellerhorst-Ryan, J. M. (1989, May 17). The biology of cancer and metastasis. Pre-Congress Workshop, 14th Annual Congress of the Oncology Nursing Society, San Francisco.

TABLE 24–5   Total Mortality and Smoking-Attributable Mortality (SAM), by Disease, Cancer Site, and Sex — United States, 1984 (Adults ≥ 20 Years Old)

Cancer Site	Men Deaths	SAM	Women Deaths	SAM	Total SAM*
Lip, oral cavity, pharynx	5,754	3,958	2,689	1,110	5,068
Esophagus	6,310	3,717	2,345	1,257	4,974
Stomach	8,463	1,455	5,772	1,467	2,922
Pancreas	11,513	3,459	11,634	1,653	5,112
Larynx	2,959	2,385	664	274	2,660
Trachea, lung, bronchus	82,459	65.659	36,227	27,170	92,829
Cervix uteri	0	0	4,562	1,685	1,685
Urinary bladder	6,597	2,447	3,114	853	3,299
Kidney, other urinary	5,424	1,319	3,403	403	1,722

* Sums may not equal total because of rounding.
From Centers for Disease Control. (1987). Smoking-attributable mortality and years of potential life lost — United States. *Morbidity and Mortality Weekly Report, 30,* 42.

nogenesis in tobacco is tar, which is itself a mixture of many compounds. Polynuclear aromatic hydrocarbons, which are prime components of tar, act as initiators. In addition to the multiple promoters in cigarette smoke, there are multiple cocarcinogens. Cocarcinogens are not initiators or promoters but are chemicals that enhance carcinogenesis when given with initiators.

The risk that an individual who smokes cigarettes has for developing cancer depends on the immune system, duration of exposure to cigarettes, amount of exposure, depth and mode of exposure, and tar content of the tobacco. The type of cancer that develops depends on the susceptibility of specific sites to various concentrations of tobacco, its constituents, and its metabolites.

The organs with the greatest risk for developing cancer are those that have direct contact with the tobacco smoke. Cigarette smoking is a major cause of cancer of the lungs, larynx, oral cavity, and esophagus, and it contributes to the development of bladder, pancreas, and kidney cancer. There is also a link between smoking and cancer of the stomach and uterine cervix (DHHS, 1982).

For smoking to be considered a major cause of disease, rigorous criteria must be met. Other environmental carcinogens can induce carcinogenesis in these same organs. However, the significant impact that smoking alone has on the development of cancer cannot be minimized. Table 24–5 summarizes cancer deaths that are attributable to tobacco.

tumor and beyond. The process of malignant transformation is multifactorial, dependent on genetic predisposition, exposure to environmental carcinogens, and immune surveillance. Multiple agents have been identified as carcinogens. Despite the fact that no one agent can take the blame for the development of all cancers, some carcinogens, such as tobacco, have been identified as being the major cause of many malignancies.

Nurses have established themselves in caring for clients afflicted with malignant disease. They now need to take a greater role in educating individuals about carcinogenesis and carcinogenic agents to assist in the prevention of cancer.

REFERENCES AND READINGS

Adamson, J. W. (1987). The myeloproliferative diseases. In E. Brunwald, K. J. Iscelbacher, R. G. Petersdorf, J. D. Wilson, J. B. Martin, & A. S. Fauci (Eds.), *Harrison's principles of internal medicine* (11th ed., pp. 1527–1533). New York: McGraw-Hill.

American Cancer Society. (1986). *Special report. Cancer in the economically disadvantaged.* New York: Author.

American Cancer Society. (1989). *Cancer facts and figures— 1989.* Atlanta: Author.

Ames, B. N. (1983). Dietary carcinogens and anticarcinogens: Oxygen radicals and degenerative diseases. *Science, 221,* 1256–1262.

Baranovsky, A., & Myers, M. H. (1986). Cancer incidence and survival in patients 65 years of age and older. *CA: A Cancer Journal for Clinicians, 36,* 22–37.

American Joint Committee on Cancer. (1988). Beahrs, O. H., Henson, D. E., Hutter, R. V. P., & Myers, M. H. (Eds.). *Manual for staging of cancer* (3rd ed.). Philadelphia: J. B. Lippincott.

Benditt, E. P., & Benditt, J. M. (1973). Evidence for a monoclonal origin of human atherosclerotic plaques.

SUMMARY

This chapter described the biologic development of cancer from its origin as a normal cell to a malignant

Proceedings of the National Academy of Sciences USA, 70, 1753–1756.

Birkeland, S. A., Kemp, E., & Hauge, M. (1975). Renal transplantation and cancer: The Scandia transplant material. *Tissue Antigens, 6,* 28–36.

Bonfiglio, T. A., & Terry, R. (1983). The pathology of cancer. In P. Rubin (Ed.), *Clinical oncology: A multidisciplinary approach* (6th ed.). New York: American Cancer Society.

Bressler, R. (1985). Drug use in elderly patients. *Annals of Internal Medicine, 102,* 218–228.

Cannon, W. B. (1932). *The wisdom of the body.* New York: W. W. Norton.

Cullen, J. W. (1989). Principles of cancer prevention: Tobacco. In V. T. DeVita, Jr., S. Hellman, & S. A. Rosenberg (Eds.), *Cancer: Principles and practice of oncology* (3rd ed., pp. 181–195). Philadelphia: J. B. Lippincott.

Doull, J., & Bruce, M. C. (1986). The origin and scope of toxicology. In C. D. Klaasen, M. O. Amdur, & J. Doull (Eds.), *Casarett and Doull's toxicology: The basic science of poisons* (3rd ed., pp. 3–10). New York: Macmillan.

Dyer, A. R., Stamler, J., Berkson, A.M., Lindberg, H. A., & Stevens, E. (1975). High blood pressure: A risk factor for cancer mortality? *Lancet 1,* 1051–1056.

Farber, E. (1984). The multistep nature of cancer development. *Cancer Research, 44,* 4217–4223.

Fisher, E. R., & Hermann, C. M. (1979). Historic milestones in cancer pathology. *Seminars in Oncology, 6,* 428–432.

Frei, E. (1988). Pathobiology of cancer. In E. Rubenstein & D. D. Federman (Eds.), *Medicine* (Vol. 2, Section 12, pp. 1–18). New York: Scientific American.

Fry, R. J. M. (1989). Principles of carcinogenesis: Physical. In V. T. DeVita, Jr., S. Hellman, & S. A. Rosenberg (Eds.), *Cancer: Principles and practice of oncology* (3rd ed., pp. 136–148). Philadelphia: J. B. Lippincott.

Goldstein, S., & Reis, R. (1985). Mechanisms of cellular aging. *Annals of Internal Medicine, 102,* 218–228.

Green, M. I., Fujimoto, S., & Sehon, A. W. (1977). Regulation of the immune response to tumor antigens: Characterization of thymic suppressor factor(s) produced by tumor-bearing hosts. *Journal of Immunology, 119,* 757–764.

Greenwald, P. (1984). Manipulation of nutrients to prevent cancer. *Hospital Practice, 19*(5), 119–134.

Ham, A. W., & Cormack, D. H. (1979). *Histology* (8th ed.). Philadelphia: J. B. Lippincott

Harwood, A. R., & Yaffe, M. (1982). Cancer in man after diagnostic or therapeutic irradiation. In I. Penn (Ed.), *Cancer surveys* (Vol. 1, pp. 703–731). Oxford: Oxford University Press.

Henderson, B. E., Louie, E., SooHoo Jing, J., Buell, P., & Gardner, M. B. (1976). Risk factors associated with nasopharyngeal cancer. *New England Journal of Medicine, 295,* 1101–1106.

Heppner, G. H., & Miller, B. E. (1989). Therapeutic implications of tumor heterogeneity. *Seminars in Oncology, 16,* 92–105.

Heyward, W. L., Lanier, A. P., McMahon, B. J., Fitzgerald, M. A., Kilkenny, S., & Paprocki, T. R. (1985). Early detection of primary hepatocellular carcinoma: Screening for primary hepatocellular carcinoma among persons infected with hepatitis B virus. *JAMA, 254,* 3052–3054.

Hobbs, C. H., & McClellan, R. O. (1986). Toxic effects of radiation and radioactive materials. In C. D. Klaasen, M. O. Amdur, & J. Doull (Eds.), *Casarett and Doull's toxicology: The basic science of poisons* (3rd ed., pp. 669–705). New York: Macmillan.

Ihde, D. C. (1987, August). Paraneoplastic syndromes. *Hospital Practice, 15,* 105–124.

Jones, S. E. (1989). Status of adjuvant therapy for node negative breast cancer and new risk factors. *Cope 3*(6), 35–36.

Judson, S. C., Henle, W., & Henle, G. (1977). A cluster of Epstein-Barr virus–associated American Burkitt's lymphoma. *New England Journal of Medicine 297,* 464–488.

Kardinal, C. G., & Yarbro, J. W. (1979). A conceptual history of cancer. *Seminars in Oncology, 6,* 396–408.

Killion, J. J., & Fidler, I. J. (1989). The biology of tumor metastasis. *Seminars in Oncology, 16,* 106–115.

Lewis, J. P., & Heidecker, G. (1984). Oncogenes, proto-oncogenes and cytogenetics—the evolution of a new discipline: Molecular cytogenetics. *Karyogram, 10,* 37–41.

Lewis, J. P., Jenks, H., & Lazerson, J. (1983). Philadelphia chromosome-negative chronic myelogenous leukemia in a child with t(8:9) (p11 or 12: q34). *American Journal of Pediatric Hematology/Oncology, 5,* 262–269.

Li, F. P. (1987). Cancer epidemiology and prevention. In E. Rubenstein & D. D. Federman (Eds.), *Medicine* (Vol. 2, Section 12, pp. 2–10). New York: Scientific American.

Linker, C. (1988). Blood. In S. A. Schroeder, M. A. Krupp, & L. M. Tierney (Eds.), *Current medical diagnosis and treatment* (pp. 294–342). Norwalk, CT: Appleton & Lange.

Longman, A. J., & Rogers, B. P. (1984). Altered cell growth in cancer and the nursing implications. *Cancer Nursing, 7,* 405–412.

Matthews, M. J., & Linnoila, R. I. (1988). Pathology of lung cancer—an update. In J. D. Bitran, H. M. Golomb, A. G. Little, & R. R. Weichselbaum (Eds.), *Lung cancer: A comprehensive treatise.* Orlando, FL: Grune & Stratton.

Mettlin, C. (1989). Trends in years of life lost to cancer: 1970 to 1985. *CA: A Cancer Journal for Clinicians, 39,* 33–39.

Miller, D. G. (1980). On the nature of susceptibility to cancer. *Cancer, 46,* 1307–1318.

Miller, E. C., & Miller, J. A. (1979). Milestones in chemical carcinogenesis. *Seminars in Oncology, 6,* 445–460.

Moran, T. A. (1988). Cancers in HIV infection. In G. Gee & T. Moran (Eds.), *AIDS concepts in nursing practice* (pp. 123–140). Baltimore: Williams & Wilkins.

National Council on Radiation Protection and Measurement (NCRP). (1987). *Ionizing radiation exposure of the population of the United States* (NCRP Report No. 93). Bethesda, MD: Author.

Newell, G. R. (1985). Epidemiology of cancer. In V. T. De Vita, Jr., S. Hellman, & S. A. Rosenberg (Eds.), *Cancer: Principles and practice of oncology* (2nd ed., pp. 151–195). Philadelphia: J. B. Lippincott.

Nicolson, G. L., & Poste, G. (1976). The cancer cell. Dynamic aspects and modifications in cell-surface organization (parts 1 and 2). *New England Journal of Medicine, 295,* 197–203, 253–258.

Pariza, M. W. (1984). A perspective on diet, nutrition, and cancer. *JAMA, 251,* 455.

Penn, I. (1970). *Malignant tumors in organ transplant recipients.* New York: Springer-Verlag.

Pitot, H. (1986). *Fundamentals of oncology* (2nd ed.). New York: Marcel Dekker.

Pitot, H. C. (1989). Principles of carcinogenesis: Chemical. In V. T. DeVita, Jr., S. Hellman, & S. A. Rosenberg (Eds.), *Cancer: Principles and practice of oncology* (3rd ed., pp. 116–135). Philadelphia: J. B. Lippincott.

Prescott, D. M., & Flexer, A. S. (1986). *Cancer: The misguided cell* (2nd ed.). Sunderland, MA: Sinauer Associates.

Rodenhuis, S., Van De Wetering, M. L., Mooi, W. J., Evers, S. G., Zandwijk, N. V., Bos, J. L. (1987). Mutational activation of the K-ras oncogene: A possible pathogenetic factor in adenocarcinoma of the lung. *New England Journal of Medicine, 317,* 929–935.

Rubin, P., & Casarett, G. W. (1968). *Clinical radiation pathology* (p. 33). Philadelphia: W. B. Saunders.

Sachs, L. (1986). Growth, differentiation and the reversal of malignancy. *Scientific American, 254*(1), 40–47.

Seifter, E. J., & Ihde, D. C. (1988). Small cell lung cancer: a distinct clinicopathologic entity. In J. D. Bitran, H. M. Golomb, A. G. Little, & R. R. Weichselbaum (Eds.), *Lung cancer: A comprehensive treatise.* Orlando, FL: Grune & Stratton.

Selye, H. (1956). *The stress of life.* New York: McGraw-Hill.

Selye H. (1974). *Stress without distress.* Philadelphia: J. B. Lippincott.

Steinfeld, J. L. (1986). Smoking and cancer. In A. I. Holleb (Ed.), *The American Cancer Society cancer book.* New York: American Cancer Society.

Sutherland, D. J. (1987). Hormones and cancer. In I. F. Tannock & R. P. Hill (Eds.), *The basic science of oncology* (pp. 204–222). New York: Pergamon.

Sutherland, R. M. (1988). Cell and environment interactions in tumor microregions: The multicell spheroid model. *Science, 240,* 177–184.

Tannock, I. F. (1989). Principles of cell proliferation: Cell kinetics. In V. T. DeVita, Jr., S. Hellman, & S. A. Rosenberg (Eds.), *Cancer: Principles and practice of oncology* (3rd ed., pp. 3–13). Philadelphia: J. B. Lippincott.

U. S. Department of Health and Human Services. (1985). *National Center for Health Statistics: National health interview survey.* Washington, DC: U.S. Government Printing Office.

U.S. Department of Health and Human Services, Office on Smoking and Health. (1982). *The health consequence of smoking: Cancer. A report of the surgeon general* (DHHS Publication No. PHS 82-50179). Washington, DC: U.S. Government Printing Office.

Velu, T. J., Beguinot, L., Vass, W. C., Willingham, M. C., Merlino, G. T., Pastan, I., & Lowy, D. R. (1987). Epidermal-growth-factor–dependent transformation by a human EGF receptor proto-oncogene. *Science, 238,* 1408–1410.

Weinberg, R. A. (1983). A molecular basis of cancer. *Scientific American, 249*(5), 126–142.

Weksler, M. (1985). The immune system during aging. *Annals of Internal Medicine, 102,* 218–228.

Williams, G. M., & Weisburger, J. H. (1986). Chemical carcinogens. In C. D. Klaasen, M. O. Amdur, & J. Doull (Eds.), *Casarett and Doull's toxicology: The basic science of poisons* (3rd. ed., pp. 99–173). New York: Macmillan.

Wong, A. J., Ruppert, J. M., Eggleston, J., Hamilton, S. R., Baylin, S. B., & Vogelstein, B. (1986). Gene amplification of the c-myc and N-myc in small cell carcinoma of the lung. *Science, 233,* 461–464.

Workman, M. S., & Ellerhorst-Ryan, J. M. (1989, May 17). The biology of cancer and metastasis. Pre-Congress Workshop, 14th Annual Congress of the Oncology Nursing Society, San Francisco.

Wynder, E. L., & Hoffman, D. (1982). Tobacco. In D. Schottenfield & J. F. Fraumeni (Eds.), *Cancer epidemiology and prevention* (pp. 277–292). Philadelphia: W. B. Saunders.

ADDITIONAL READINGS

Gallucci, B. (1987). The immune system and cancer. *Oncology Nursing Forum, 14*(6), 3–12.

This article provides a detailed description of the human immune system as it relates to malignant tumors. The author, a nurse, discusses recent developments in biotechnology related to cancer and states that current research is focused on differentiating immune responses that protect the client from those that enhance tumor growth.

Hammond, E. C., & Horn, D. (1988). Classics in oncology: Smoking and death rates—report on forty-four months of follow-up of 187,783 men. *CA: A Cancer Journal for Clinicians, 38,* 28–58.

This article, which was originally printed in 1958, reports on a study of the relationship between smoking and death. Results of the study showed that death rates were higher among cigarette smokers than among men who never smoked, that mortality rates increased with the number of cigarettes smoked per day, and that death rates were higher among pipe and cigar smokers than among men who never smoked. Although the majority of deaths were reported to be caused by heart and circulatory disease, 2326 of the 11,870 individuals who died had cancer. The authors describe the cancer deaths by site and relationship to smoking.

Loescher, L. J. (1987). Cancer: The nurse's role in primary prevention. *Innovations in Oncology Nursing, 4*(3), 3–5, 9.

This article discusses life style risks that are related to the development of cancer and the role of the nurse in primary cancer prevention. Tobacco use, diet, and sexual factors are described as they relate to specific sites of malignancy.

Lyman, G. H. (1987). Groundwater radium and indoor radon as causes of cancer. *Innovations in Oncology, 3*(2), 13–14.

Radium-contaminated groundwater is being investigated as a possible cause of leukemia, and radon-contaminated indoor air has been associated with an increased risk for developing lung cancer. Although environmental exposure to radon has not been established as a cause of cancer, these data should guide public safety efforts toward cancer prevention.

CHAPTER 25

Interventions for Clients with Cancer

Cancer is a chronic disease that has historically been poorly understood. It is one of the diseases most feared by both clients and health care professionals.

The role of the nurse caring for the client with cancer has changed drastically since Rose Hawthorne Lathrop (1851–1926) initiated a campaign to provide care for persons with cancer in New York City. She was appalled by the poor care, anguish, total lack of emotional support, and absence of love experienced by these people throughout their illness. Unlike Rose Hawthorne Lathrop, nurses today have more than gifts, kindness, and comfort to offer persons with cancer. Contemporary nurses have an increasingly large scientific knowledge base from which to develop technologic, physiologic, and psychosocial interventions. Nurses are able to define and provide optimal care to persons affected by cancer. Major advances in prevention, detection, diagnosis, and treatment of cancer have also improved survival rates and the quality of life for clients with cancer.

Pathophysiology

Any organ or tissue can be involved in malignant transformation. The danger of cancer is that it invades and destroys normal tissue, compromising physiologic function in that tissue. Cancerous tumors produce disease when they cause obstruction, pressure, hemorrhage, infection, or ulceration. Tumors that have grown to be 1 kg in size with 10^{12} cells are potentially lethal (Tannock, 1989).

In addition to these primary tumor effects, pathophysiologic changes can occur as a result of treatment regimens for cancer. Pathologic alterations that occur as a result of treatment are considered secondary effects.

Physiologic dysfunction related to cancer and its treatment can lead to impaired immune and hematopoietic function, malnutrition, alterations in the structure and function of the gastrointestinal (GI) tract, and motor and sensory deficits. Multiple symptoms may accompany these changes, including (but not limited to) pain, fatigue, anorexia, nausea, vomiting, and dyspnea.

Altered immune and hematopoietic functions occur most often in clients with hematologic malignancies and clients who undergo immunosuppressive therapy. In hematologic malignancies, tumor cells invade bone marrow. These clients also have defects in cell-mediated immunity and diminished levels of circulating immunoglobulins. Clients with solid tumors have primary immunologic defects less frequently, but other factors may affect their immune and hematopoietic functions. Advanced age, stress, and malnutrition hinder the production of red and white blood cells, which are necessary for maintaining normal function in these systems. Secondary immunosuppressive effects include granulocytopenia, thrombocytopenia, and anemia. Each of these may occur as a result of bone marrow suppression related to chemotherapy or radiation involving long bones or a large body surface area.

Anemia can also occur after blood is lost during surgical procedures to remove tumors or when tumors press against blood vessels, causing them to erode and bleed. Anemia can lead to respiratory or circulatory complications. These result from the decreased oxygen-carrying capacity of the blood. Thrombocytopenia can cause bleeding, which may be extensive.

In addition to being immunosuppressed, clients with cancer often have altered mechanical and chemical defense mechanisms to guard against other organisms in the environment. Intact skin and mucous membranes normally provide a physical barrier to prevent entry and colonization of microorganisms. The chemical composition of body fluids provides defense against outside invaders. Surgical and percutaneous procedures disrupt the barrier provided by intact skin. Chemotherapy and radiation can also affect the skin and mucous membrane barriers. The chemical composition of body fluids can be altered by medications or by procedures that interfere with their actions or effects.

Granulocytopenia and impaired chemical and physical barriers put the client at risk for infection. Infections in clients with cancer generally originate in one of five sites: the lower respiratory tract, the perianal area, the pharynx, the genitourinary tract, and the skin and subcutaneous tissue. Pneumonia, cutaneous cellulitis, cutaneous abscesses, furunculosis, and septicemia are the most common types of infection in this population.

The majority of infections arise from the client's normal microflora. The most common pathogens in granulocytopenic clients are gram-negative bacilli (*Pseudomonas aeruginosa, Escherichia coli, Klebsiella pneumoniae,* and *Enterobacter agglomerans*), *Staphylococcus aureus,* and *Staphylococcus epidermidis.* Fungal (*Candida albicans, Aspergillus*) and mycobacterial infections can also occur readily in granulocytopenic clients.

If infection is not recognized or identified early, or if it does not respond to treatment, septicemia may occur with or without septic shock. Septicemia is a condition in which microorganisms invade the blood stream. Septic shock (Chap. 17) is a life-threatening consequence of septicemia with mortality between 30% and 80% (Barry, 1989).

Multiple primary and secondary effects of cancer can alter GI function and nutritional patterns. Tumors may cause obstruction or compression anywhere along the GI tract. This can interfere with the client's ability to take in and digest adequate nutrients. Tumors can also produce substances that react with receptors in the GI tract to produce early satiety and decreased appetite stimulation. Basal metabolic rates can be altered by tumors, thus increasing the client's requirements for protein, carbohydrates, and fat. The satiety and anorexia that the client experiences, along with GI effects resulting from treatment, often interfere with the client's ability to meet energy requirements. Cachexia develops from the negative balance between intake and expenditure. Cachexia may occur in spite of what appears to be adequate nutritional intake. Malnutrition may result from a variety of cancer-related factors (see the accompanying Key Features of Disease).

GI function may be altered by chemotherapy or radiation. Secondary effects of these treatments include mucositis, stomatitis, nausea, vomiting, and diarrhea. The mucous membrane tissue lining the GI tract is composed of cells that proliferate at a rapid rate and, as such, are susceptible to the deleterious effects of chemotherapy and radiation.

Systemic distribution of antineoplastic agents makes the entire GI tract susceptible to the effects of these agents. Inflammation and denudation of the GI tract lining (manifested by stomatitis, esophagitis, mucositis, nausea, vomiting, and diarrhea) interfere with the digestion and absorption of glucose, fat, and other nutrients.

Inflammation of the small and large intestines may be a consequence of local radiation to a field encompassing portions of these organs. This may create increased flatulence. Intestinal motility increases, resulting in an increased number of bowel movements and possibly diarrhea.

Nausea and vomiting are two of the most distressing side effects associated with cancer and cancer therapy. Nausea is experienced by many clients receiving chemotherapy, steroids, analgesics, and other medications. Radiation-related nausea occurs if the treatment field encompasses the brain, stomach, or small intestine.

Vomiting occurs in many clients soon after the administration of some antineoplastic agents. It is important to acknowledge the variations in emetic potential of common chemotherapeutic agents (Table 25-1). Anticipatory nausea and vomiting is a learned response stimulated by thoughts, sights, tastes, and odors related to previous treatment experiences. Vomiting may also occur in clients undergoing radiation therapy of the brain, stomach, or small intestine.

Nausea and vomiting result from the stimulation of a complex reflex coordinated by the vomiting center located in the medullary lateral reticular formation. Pathways involved include the chemoreceptor trigger zone in the floor of the fourth ventricle and vagal visceral afferents, which carry stimuli related to GI inflammation, ischemia, and irritation. The vestibulocerebellar afferents relay information in response to body motion, and the cerebral cortex and limbic system respond to anxiety, pain, and other sensory stimuli with increases in intracranial pressure. Incoming stimuli converge on the vomiting center and are mediated by neurotransmitters.

Alterations in taste sensations can be related to the disease process itself or to the treatment of disease. Clients often have decreased sensitivity to tasting sweets, an increased sensitivity to bitterness, and an aversion for various foods, especially red meat. The degree of taste abnormality usually directly correlates with the extent of disease. Changes affecting the oropharynx

KEY FEATURES OF DISEASE ■ Causes of Malnutrition in Clients with Cancer

Anorexia

Local causes
  Pelvic or abdominal tumors
  Hepatic metastases
  Intestinal compression or obstruction
  Others
Remote causes
  Food aversions
  Early satiety
Treatment-related causes
  Postsurgical small stomach or stasis
  Drugs, including chemotherapy
  Radiation—local and systemic effects
Systemic illness
  Infection
  Hepatitis or pancreatitis
  Endocrinopathies
Taste disorders
  Drugs (e.g., metronidazole)
  Remote effects of neoplasm and its treatment
  Local disease and its treatment (e.g., stomatitis, naso-
    pharyngeal tumor, radiation, and surgery)
  Nausea and vomiting
Psychogenic causes
  Depression
  Anxiety
  Conditioned aversions
Intolerance of institutional food

Difficulty in Eating

Head and neck tumors and their treatment
Xerostomia
Stomatitis

Difficulty in Eating

Loss of teeth and dental problems
Dysphagia and odynophagia

Maldigestion or Malabsorption

Pancreatitic insufficiency
Bile salt deficiency
Hypersecretory states
  Zollinger-Ellison syndrome
  Pancreatic cholera
  Bowel infiltration
  Diffuse invasion (e.g., lymphoma)
  Local blockage
  Fistula
Postsurgical causes
  Esophageal surgery (with vagotomy, gastric stasis,
    diarrhea, and steatorrhea)
  Gastrectomy—dumping, achlorhydria, or afferent loop
    syndrome
  Small intestine resections
Postirradiation causes
  Enteritis (may occur as late sequela)
  Fistula
  Stenosis
  Obstruction

Protein-Losing Enteropathy

Malutilization

Cancer cachexia
Steroids
  Nitrogen wasting
  Hyperglycemia
  Calcium loss

(e.g., surgical intervention, mucosal changes, and decreased salivation) cause a loss of functional taste and smell receptors.

Some antineoplastic drugs also contribute to changes in taste. Agents such as methotrexate and doxorubicin can alter taste acuity, and others such as cyclophosphamide and vincristine can be tasted after injection. Radiation therapy fields that include the head, neck, or oral cavity; salivary glands; or oral mucous membranes can affect taste buds directly or alter taste sensation indirectly. Radiation to the head and neck not only damages taste buds, but also may injure or totally destroy salivary glands if they are exposed to more than 4000 to 5000 rad. Oral mucous membrane effects of radiation may alter the client's ability to chew and swallow.

Constipation is commonly caused by narcotic analgesics, immobility, and poor nutrition. Constipation and adynamic ileus are major side effects of the chemotherapeutic agent vincristine.

Motor or sensory deficits occur when primary or metastatic tumors invade bone. Most clients who develop bone metastases have primary cancers in the prostate, breast, or lung. Bone sites most affected include vertebral bodies, ribs, the pelvis, and the femur, but the humerus, the scapula, the sternum, the skull, and the clavicle are also common metastatic sites. Blood-borne spread of tumor cells to bone accounts for the initial appearance of metastatic lesions in the marrow. Bone metastases can cause further complications, including pathologic fractures, spinal cord compression, and hy-

---

TABLE 25–1 Chemotherapeutic Agents with the Potential to Induce Emesis

High Potential

Cisplatin
Dacarbazine
Dactinomycin
Mechlorethamine
Cyclophosphamide

Moderate Potential

Carmustine
Lomustine
Doxorubicin
Cytarabine
Procarbazine

Low Potential

Etoposide
Mitomycin C
Methotrexate
5-Fluorouracil
Hydroxyurea
Bleomycin
Vinca alkaloids
Chlorambucil

From Clark, R. A., Tyson, L. B., Gralla, R. J., & Kris, M. G. (1989). Antiemetic therapy: Management of chemotherapy-induced nausea and vomiting. *Seminars in Oncology Nursing, 5*(Suppl. 1), 53–57.

percalcemia. Immobility results if pain occurs with movement and motor function is impaired. In the case of pathologic fractures and spinal cord compression, immobility is the prescribed treatment.

The respiratory system can be affected by cancer in a variety of ways. Primary or metastatic tumors involving airways can induce symptoms of direct airway obstruction. If lung tissue is involved, pulmonary capacity is compromised. Tumor growth can compress vascular and lymphatic structures; this is manifested by edema, effusions, and obstruction of the superior vena cava (SVC).

Limited mobility imposed by debility interferes with normal muscular activity, in turn slowing venous and lymphatic return. Malnutrition, malabsorption, and protein losses from exudates or drainage may induce hypoalbuminemia, altering osmotic forces and allowing fluid to escape from vessels. Ascites and pleural and peritoneal effusions exemplify clinical manifestations of alterations in circulatory system performance and subsequent fluid accumulation, which interfere with ventilatory processes. Malnutrition affects lung structure, ventilatory drive, lung defense mechanisms, and the structure and function of respiratory muscles.

Pain is not an inevitable consequence of cancer, but it is a significant problem. Physical causes of pain can be related to cancer or cancer treatment (see the Key Features of Disease on p. 568).

Clients undergoing certain cancer treatments have physiologic changes that may cause organic sexual dysfunction. Surgery involving the genitals, urinary tract, colon, and rectum may cause permanent organic dysfunction. Surgical procedures that create urinary and fecal diversions may disturb innervation, causing erectile impotence and ejaculatory dysfunction in male clients and dyspareunia in female clients.

Radiation can result in loss of ovarian and testicular function and other changes in sexual functions. Radiation to gonadal tissues in excess of 400 to 500 rad produces permanent sterility. Below these thresholds, sterility is temporary.

Chemotherapy can be implicated in ovarian suppression in adult women and testicular dysfunction in adult men. The alkylating agents are most toxic to testicular germ cells. Up to a certain dose, and depending on the drug, germinal cell changes are reversible with the alkylating agents. Other antineoplastic drug classifications produce irreversible damage in men older than 40 years of age.

Alkylating agents can cause ovarian suppression and failure. Ovarian activity after chemotherapy is classified in three categories: primary failure (failed ovary), irregular ovarian activity (failing ovary), and normal cyclic ovarian activity (functioning ovary). Women older than 35 to 40 years are more susceptible to chemotherapy-induced ovarian failure.

Many treatments are also associated with changes that affect sexuality by causing discomfort to body parts often involved with sexual expression. Intracavitary radiation used in endometrial, cervical, and vaginal cancers can cause vaginal dryness, inflammation, ulceration, fibrosis, and stenosis. Chemotherapy-induced mucositis and vaginitis produce dryness, inflammation, and ulceration, resulting in discomfort and dyspareunia associated with coitus.

Etiology

All cancers begin as a normal cell. Damage to that cell occurs through exposure to a carcinogen, and carcinogenesis is stimulated. Further carcinogen exposure over time is necessary for malignant transformation to occur. In the absence of effective immune surveillance by the host, a malignant cell is allowed to survive and proliferate to become a tumor.

Many environmental carcinogens and other risk factors for cancer, such as age and heredity, have been identified (Chap. 24).

Incidence

More than 5 million Americans alive today have a history of cancer (American Cancer Society [ACS], 1989).

KEY FEATURES OF DISEASE ■ Causes of Pain in Clients with Cancer

Effects of Cancer

Bone infiltration by primary or metastatic tumor (most common cause of pain)

Nerve infiltration involving peripheral nerves, nerve plexus, or spinal cord

Nerve compression

Soft-tissue infiltration

Visceral involvement

Muscle spasm

Lymphedema

Increased intracranial pressure

Myopathy

Treatment

Surgery, especially thoracotomy, mastectomy, radical neck dissection; phantom limb

Chemotherapy

Peripheral neuropathy

Postherpetic neuralgia

Extravasation

Dysesthesias

Aseptic necrosis of the humeral head

Nerve block

Treatment (Continued)

Postoperative adhesions

Postirradiation fibrosis, especially when fields include plexus

Postirradiation myopathy

Mucositis

Debility or Immobility

Constipation

Capsulitis of shoulder

Pressure ulcer

Pulmonary embolus

Penile spasm or urinary catheterization

Concurrent Disorders

Musculoskeletal disease
　　Myofascial
　　Lumbar disk disease
　　Osteoporosis
　　Osteoarthritis
　　Others

Migraine

Miscellaneous

Data from Foley, K. M. (1984). A review of pain syndrome in patients with cancer. *The Management of Cancer Pain Symposium*. Nutley, NJ: Roche Laboratories; and Twycross, R. G. (1988). The management of pain in cancer: A guide to drugs and dosages. *Oncology, 2*(4), 35–44.

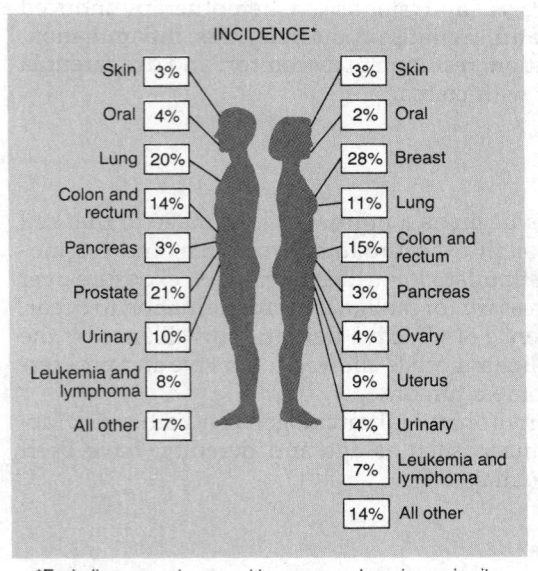

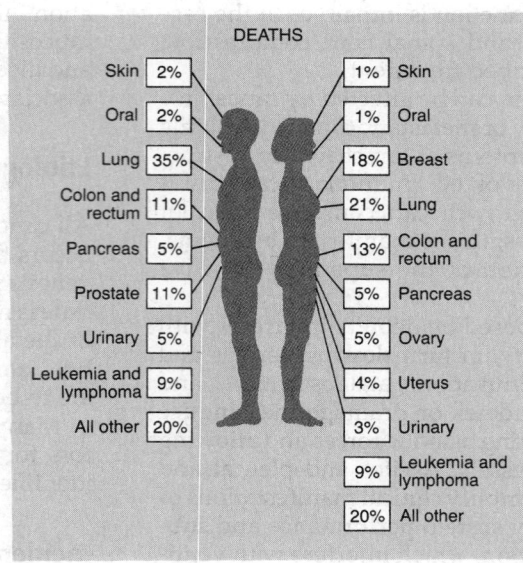

*Excluding nonmelanoma skin cancer and carcinoma in situ.

Figure 25–1

Cancer incidence and deaths by site and sex—1990 estimates. (From American Cancer Society. [1990]. *Cancer facts and figures—1990*. Atlanta: Author.)

More than 1 million new cases are diagnosed each year, affecting three of four families in the United States. Although nearly 1500 people die *each day* from cancer, it is estimated that at least 35% of these people might have been saved by earlier diagnosis and treatment (ACS, 1989).

Cancer occurs in both sexes, although some types of cancer are either sex specific or occur more frequently in one sex. Figure 25–1 describes cancer incidence and deaths by site and sex in the United States.

PREVENTION

Many forms of cancer have known causes, and steps have been identified that might be taken to prevent these types of cancer. Primary prevention refers to the avoidance of factors associated with cancer. This takes place *before* the development of cancer. Factors that should be avoided include tobacco smoking, alcohol consumption, and excessive sunlight exposure. Chemical carcinogens, such as asbestos, vinyl chloride, nickel, and chromate, should also be avoided. Radiation exposure should be limited, and the use of medications such as estrogen in postmenopausal women should be reserved for those who will receive more benefit than risk. Nutritional practices recommended to avoid cancer include avoidance of high-fat, salt-cured, and smoked or nitrite-cured foods. Diets should be high in fiber, cruciferous vegetables, and foods rich in vitamins A and C.

Secondary prevention (early detection) refers to steps taken to identify cancer or a precancerous state after it has occurred. Early detection is crucial to increased survival rates. The ACS has developed a useful mnemonic outlining general, nonspecific early signs and symptoms of cancer, toward the goal of discovering cancers at early, more treatable stages (see the accompanying Key Features of Disease). The ACS has also established secondary prevention screening guidelines for individuals without symptoms or special risk factors (Table 25–2).

KEY FEATURES OF DISEASE ■ CAUTION: Cancer's Seven Warning Signals

Change in bowel or bladder habits

A sore that does not heal

Unusual bleeding or discharge

Thickening or a lump in the breast or elsewhere

Indigestion or difficulty in swallowing

Obvious change in a wart or a mole

Nagging cough or hoarseness

TABLE 25–2 Protocol for Early Detection of Cancer in People Without Symptoms

General

A cancer-related check-up
Every 3 yr for those 20–40 yr of age
Every year for those 40 yr and older
Should include health counseling (such as tips on quitting smoking) and examinations for cancer of the thyroid, testes, the prostate, the mouth, ovaries, the skin, and lymph nodes

Breast

Ages 20–40 years
Breast examination by a physician every 3 yr
Breast self-examination every month
Baseline mammogram between 35 and 39 yr of age

Ages 40 years and older
Breast examination by a physician every year
Breast self-examination every month
Mammography
Every 1–2 yr for ages 40–49 yr
Every year for ages 50 yr and older

Uterine Cervix

For sexually active people or those aged 18 yr and older: Papanicolaou (Pap) stain test and pelvic examination yearly (after three or more consecutive normal annual test results, Pap test may be performed less frequently at the discretion of the woman's physician)

Colon and Rectum

Ages 40 years and older
Digital rectal examination every year

Ages 50 years and older
Digital rectal examination every year
Stool blood test every year
Proctoscopic examination every 3–5 yr after normal results obtained from two initial examinations 1 yr apart

---

From American Cancer Society. (1989). *Cancer facts and figures—1989*. Atlanta: Author.

COLLABORATIVE MANAGEMENT

 Assessment

History

When assessing an individual's risk of cancer, *personal history and family history* are significant. Knowledge of risk factors also allows the establishment of guidelines for early detection. Many cancers are associated with inherited traits. For example, sisters and daughters of women who have had breast cancer are at increased risk for breast cancer. Thus, assessment of women with known breast cancer should include questions about daughters and sisters—regarding past history of disease or the client's ability to encourage screening for these family members.

Determination of whether *exposure to known carcinogens* has occurred also contributes to the assessment of risks. A history of smoking and inhalation of other carcinogens is significant to an individual's risk for development of many types of cancer (Chap. 24). *Dietary habits*, in addition to family and personal history, might indicate risk factors for colon or rectal cancer.

Physical Assessment: Clinical Manifestations

When a diagnosis of cancer is suspected or confirmed, the nurse performs a complete examination of all organ systems to assess for dysfunction directly or indirectly related to cancer. The nurse focuses on the organ system associated with the primary tumor and possible sites of metastases. If the tumor has not metastasized, or metastatic sites have not been diagnosed, the nurse assesses those sites of selected metastases known to be associated with the primary tumor. For example, breast cancer most commonly spreads to lymph nodes (76%), bone (71%), lung (69%), liver (65%), pleura (51%), adrenal glands (49%), and skin (30%) (Entrekin, 1987). The most common sites of metastases for all malignancies include lung, liver, bone, bone marrow, adrenal glands, and brain.

Because clients with cancer frequently have suppressed immune systems and altered physical and mechanical barriers, the nurse is vigilant for manifestations of *infection.* The clinical presentation of infection varies, and diagnosis may be difficult. The inflammatory response and immune reaction may be diminished or absent if the client is granulocytopenic. Physical findings of edema, exudate, local heat, and regional adenopathy may be subtle or absent. Erythema and pain at local sites of infection are usually present. Steroids and other anti-inflammatory agents may suppress fever, although only rarely is fever totally absent, even if the client exhibits neutropenia and granulocytopenia. Slight elevation of temperature may be the only manifestation of infection.

Thrombocytopenic clients are at increased risk for *bleeding,* which might be manifested by petechiae, ecchymoses, and hematomas. The nurse assesses for bleeding from the nose and gums, bleeding from venipuncture or other sites of invasive procedures, hematuria, hemoptysis, vaginal bleeding, rectal bleeding, hematemesis, or coffee-ground vomitus. More covert signs of bleeding, such as headache or a change in orientation or level of consciousness, are also assessed. These signs could indicate increased intracranial pressure from bleeding.

Clients with or at risk for *anemia* are assessed for shortness of breath, tachycardia, and chest pain, which could indicate respiratory or cardiac deficiencies. These clients are also assessed for symptoms of fatigue and the relationship of fatigue to daily activities is determined. The onset, duration, and intensity of fatigue are assessed, as well as sleep-rest patterns and the need for sleep aids. Symptoms that affect sleep or rest, such as pain or nausea, also are identified.

The client's *nutritional status* is assessed. The client's

TABLE 25–3   Karnofsky's Performance Scale

Able to carry on normal activity; no special care is needed	100 Normal; no complaints; no evidence of disease
	90 Able to carry on normal activity; minor signs or symptoms of disease
	80 Able to carry on normal activity with effort; some signs of symptoms of disease
Unable to work; able to live at home and care for most personal needs; a varying amount of assistance is needed	70 Cares for self; unable to carry on normal activity or to do active work
	60 Requires occasional assistance, but is able to care for most of own needs
	50 Requires considerable assistance and frequent medical care
Unable to care for self; requires equivalent of institutional or hospital care; disease may be progressing rapidly	40 Disabled; requires special care and assistance
	30 Severely disabled; hospitalization is indicated, although death not imminent
	20 Very sick; hospitalization necessary; active supportive treatment necessary
	10 Moribund; fatal processes progressing rapidly
	0 Dead

weight is measured and compared with the ideal or the normal weight for that client. Previous and current dietary patterns, the presence of satiety, the time of day of greatest appetite, and food preferences and aversions are also noted.

Oral assessment for white or cream-colored particles or lesions is crucial because of the high incidence of thrush and herpes in immunosuppressed clients. All clients are assessed for changes in taste, dry mouth, nausea, vomiting, abdominal distention, and altered patterns of bowel elimination. A *neurologic assessment,* including mental status determination and motor and sensory examination of the client, is imperative. The overall ability of the clients to perform activities of daily living (ADL) independently is also assessed. The Karnofsky Performance Scale is frequently used to describe the client's level of disability and dependence (Table 25–3).

All clients with cancer are assessed for *pain* and discomfort throughout the course of their disease. Accurate assessment of pain is crucial to its successful management. Variables related to pain are outlined in Table 25–4. The nurse should always ask whether the pain is "new" or "different" from chronic pain the client may have been experiencing. Recent onset of pain or a change in its character requires a work-up to identify the cause. Pain in the back or extremities is particularly important to identify early, as it might indicate a pathologic fracture or spinal cord compression.

Changes potentially or actually affecting a client's sexual function are assessed by the nurse. Components of the sexual assessment are found in Chapter 10.

Psychosocial Assessment

Cancer has different implications for different people, which are based on individual, group, or cultural values. The person with cancer is more than a "vessel for a neoplastic process" (Weisman, 1979). Jobs are lost; family ties and friendships are challenged and may falter. Conflicts are aggravated. Goals are put aside during the pursuit of a cure that may never come, and new diseases can arise as a result of treatment. Despite these obstacles, the great majority of people with cancer cope quite well with illness, treatment and related problems, and the uncertainty imposed by this illness (Friedman, 1980; Weisman, 1979).

Periods of emotional distress for clients with cancer include the initial diagnostic work-up, the actual diagnosis of malignancy, the initial treatment, a recurrence, and a minimal response to treatment. Stressors are related to life style, body image, roles, self-concept, and self-esteem. All of these are assessed as they relate to physiologic changes accompanying cancer and its treatment. Significant others who have changes imposed on them by another's disease process or treatment are also subject to distress.

Assessment of the client's specific stressors includes client perception of the stressors and beliefs about the causes. The individual's available resources, patterns of communication, efficacy of coping strategies, problem-

solving abilities, and physical and emotional liabilities and strengths provide a basis for planning interventions to promote successful coping. The coping capabilities of caregivers or significant others are also considered.

TABLE 25–4   Important Points in the Assessment of Pain

Evaluation of Pain

Location

Have client mark the location of pain on an outline of the body.

Ask the client to indicate whether the pain is "internal" or "external."

Ask the client to point with one finger to the site of pain. (If the client can precisely indicate the site, it is superficial and localized and local or regional interventions are appropriate. If the site cannot be precisely located or there are many sites, systemic, cortical, or thalamic interventions are indicated.)

Quantity (Severity and Duration)

Visual analogue scales can be used.

Ask the client to quantify pain on a numeric scale (0 = no pain and 10 = the worst pain imaginable).
  "What number represents your pain at its worst?"
  "What number represents your pain at its least?"
  "What number represents the level of pain you are willing to tolerate?"

Influencing Factors

Determine what factors affect pain.
  Increased mobility or change in position
  Certain foods
  Weather changes
  Visitors
  Time of day

Observation

Evaluate the following:
  Client's behavior
  Client's ability to interact
  Others' ability to interact with the client
  Pattern of use of pain relief methods
  Client's use and efficacy of distraction techniques
  Social, attitudinal, situational, psychologic, and physiologic variables
Obtain vital signs.
  These are useful *only* as a baseline from which to judge the onset of relaxation or the side effects of medications.
Review previous therapy and its effects.
Determine established patterns of coping.

Laboratory Findings

White blood cell count. The client with leukemia may have an elevated leukocyte count (leukocytosis), which can range from 100,000 to 400,000/mm^3. The client with bone marrow depression resulting from chemotherapy or radiation has a decreased leukocyte count.

Differential leukocyte count. The client with bone marrow suppression may have a decreased neutrophil (granulocyte) count (granulocytopenia) with normal or elevated levels of band neutrophils. Calculation of the absolute neutrophil count (ANC) or absolute granulocyte count (AGC) is obtained by multiplying the fraction of granulocytes by the total number of white blood cells. An ANC from 500 to 1000 signifies increased risk of infection.

Platelet count. Leukemias and tumors metastasizing to bone may cause a decrease in the number of platelets (thrombocytopenia). This can also occur if there is bone marrow depression after chemotherapy or radiation therapy to long bones or a large body surface area.

Red blood cell count. Anemia occurs in leukemias and tumors that metastasize to the bone. Anemias also occur when tumors erode blood vessels or when blood is lost through surgical resection of a tumor.

Serum calcium level. This is commonly elevated in clients with bone metastases from breast, lung, and kidney cancer.

Uric acid levels. Rapid neoplastic cell growth accompanies some leukemias and lymphomas. Rapid cell destruction also occurs with chemotherapeutic treatment of some malignancies, such as leukemia. Both of these situations lead to elevated uric acid levels.

Tumor markers. Tumor markers are substances secreted in association with specific cancers. They include oncofetal proteins, ectopic hormones, and enzymes. The production of these substances is stimulated by tumor cells or cells associated with tumors.

Tumor markers are generally not used for diagnosis, as they are not consistently specific for cancer. They are often not measurable until cancers are advanced. Thus, at this time, they are not useful for early detection. Tumor markers are often used to follow a client's response to treatment and to check for recurrence of tumors.

Acid phosphatase levels are often elevated in the client with prostate, primary bone, or metastatic bone cancer.

Alkaline phosphatase levels are elevated in clients with metastatic cancer to bone and liver, osteogenic sarcoma, and myeloma.

Alpha-fetoprotein (AFP) concentration is frequently elevated with hepatocellular cancers and teratocarcinoma and is occasionally elevated in gastric carcinoma.

Carcinoembryonic antigen levels are frequently increased with colon cancer. They may also be elevated in recurrent breast cancer.

Chorionic gonadotropin-beta levels are increased in choriocarcinoma, testicular teratoma, and some other cancers.

CA 15-3 is elevated in clients with breast cancer.

Ovarian carcinoma antigen (CA 125) concentration is elevated in ovarian cancer.

Pancreatic oncofetal antigen is present in a large percentage of clients with pancreatic tumors.

Prostate-specific antigen is elevated in clients with cancer of the prostate. *Prostatic acid phosphatase* (PAP) is elevated in many clients with prostate cancer that has metastasized.

Other laboratory tests. In addition to the measurement of these markers, a more thorough evaluation of renal and hepatic function, including an SMA-12, is performed to stage the disease and determine how the client will tolerate treatment.

Radiographic Findings

Chest radiography visualizes masses or lesions in the lung or chest that require further diagnostic work-up, if no primary site has been identified. Computed tomography (CT) has a significant role in evaluating the size and location of a wide variety of primary tumors and metastatic sites.

Other Diagnostic Tests

Magnetic resonance imaging (MRI) is considered the best noninvasive means of evaluating brain and spinal cord tumors, but is also used to assess other sites for tumors.

Biopsy of the tumor is crucial to establishing a diagnosis of cancer. The major types are incisional, excisional, and needle. Incisional biopsy involves removing a portion of tumor tissue. Excisional biopsy involves removing the complete tumor with little or no margin of surrounding normal tissue. Needle biopsy involves withdrawing or aspirating fluid or tissue with a needle. Procedures to obtain the biopsy vary with the site of the suspected disease. A bronchoscopy is done under local anesthesia to obtain a biopsy specimen of the bronchus of the lung. An endoscopy allows a biopsy specimen to be obtained from the esophagus or stomach. Sigmoidoscopy facilitates tissue biopsy of the anus and sigmoid colon. Colonoscopy allows biopsy of the colon. Liver biopsy is performed via a percutaneous approach. Exploratory laparotomy of the abdominal cavity and thoracotomy of the chest cavity may be performed to obtain biopsy of lesions that cannot be assessed with other approaches.

After biopsy, staging of a malignant tumor is performed to assess tumor size, nodal involvement, and evidence of metastasis. Depending on the type of cancer, staging might be done surgically (e.g., by exploratory lymphotomy for Hodgkin's disease) or medically by CT scan or MRI.

Ultrasonography is commonly used early in the diagnostic process and is especially useful for pelvic tumors.

Bone scans are commonly done as part of the staging process for breast, prostate, or lung cancer to rule out metastases.

 ## Analysis: Nursing Diagnosis

Cancer is a concern of all individuals, whether or not a diagnosis of malignancy has been made. Prevention and early detection are essential components in the fight against cancer, and these need to be addressed in the care of all clients.

Common Diagnoses

The most common nursing diagnosis applicable to clients with cancer is

1. Knowledge deficit related to prevention or early detection of cancer

Other nursing diagnoses in clients who have been diagnosed with cancer include

2. Potential for injury related to tumor proliferation and metastasis
3. Potential for infection related to immunosuppressive effects of cancer or its treatment
4. Potential for altered (cardiopulmonary) tissue perfusion related to thrombocytopenia
5. Activity intolerance related to anemia, poor nutritional status, and disruption of activity-rest patterns
6. Altered nutrition: less than body requirements related to tumor effect on GI system or side effects of treatment
7. Diarrhea related to chemotherapy or abdominal radiation therapy
8. Constipation related to narcotic analgesics, immobility, and altered nutrition
9. Impaired physical mobility related to pain, pathologic fracture, fatigue, or treatment
10. Pain related to nerve compression by tumor or bone metastases and side effects of treatment
11. Potential for impaired skin integrity related to chemotherapy and radiation
12. Impaired gas exchange related to pleural effusions or obstruction
13. Sexual dysfunction related to physiologic changes or psychologic responses to cancer and/or its treatment
14. Ineffective individual coping related to diagnosis of cancer and its treatment.

Additional Diagnoses

The following diagnoses may also be applicable to clients with cancer:

1. Fear related to the disease process and the risk of recurrence
2. Body image disturbance related to the effects of cancer and its treatment
3. Altered patterns of urinary elimination related to chemotherapy's effect on kidneys and bladder
4. Sensory/perceptual alterations (tactile) related to chemotherapy or complications of spinal cord compression
5. Powerlessness related to the disease process
6. Altered oral mucous membrane related to chemotherapy

 ## Planning and Implementation

The following plan for care is based on the common nursing diagnoses.

Knowledge Deficit

Planning: client goals. The goal is for all clients to state and identify individual risks, methods to avoid, and practices to detect cancer.

Interventions: nonsurgical management. The nurse assesses all clients for their knowledge and personal risk for cancer. The nurse gives all clients oral and written information regarding prevention (e.g., ACS primary and secondary prevention recommendations). Clients with high risk for developing cancer (e.g., women whose mothers or sisters had premenopausal breast cancer) are referred to their primary health care providers for additional or more frequent examinations. The nurse is prepared to teach breast self-examination (BSE) to all female clients and testicular self-examination (TSE) to all male clients (see the accompanying Client/Family Education features). Although TSE is not part of the ACS guidelines, it is a potentially lifesaving practice that all men should be familiar with.

In addition to educating individual clients, the nurse has the role of advocate to promote the implementation of prevention and early detection programs. In some states, fees for various screening procedures are not covered or reimbursed by insurance policies or state and federal health care programs. Nurses have been instrumental in changing reimbursement schedules for mammography. Nurse-advocates have promoted low-cost screening, education, and smoking cessation programs in many communities. Nurses' political and advocacy activities are expanding and have the potential to markedly influence health care policy.

CLIENT/FAMILY EDUCATION ■ **Instructions for Breast Self-Examination**

1. "If you have a regular menstrual cycle, you should examine your breasts at the end of your monthly period. If you do not have menstrual periods, BSE should be done on the same day of every month."

2. "Lie down. Flatten your right breast by placing a pillow under your right shoulder. If your breasts are large, use your right hand to hold your right breast while you do the examination with your left hand. Feel for lumps or thickening, using a rubbing motion. Press firmly enough to feel different breast tissues."

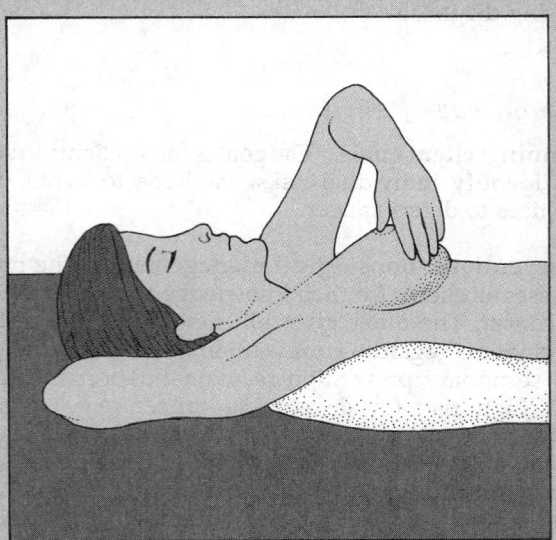

3. "Completely feel all of the breast and chest area. Be sure to examine the breast tissue that extends toward the shoulder. Allow enough time for a complete examination. Women with small breasts will need at least 2 min to examine each breast. Larger breasts will take longer."

4. "Use the same routine or pattern to feel every part of the breast tissue. Choose the method easiest for you." [The accompanying figure shows the clock or oval pattern.]

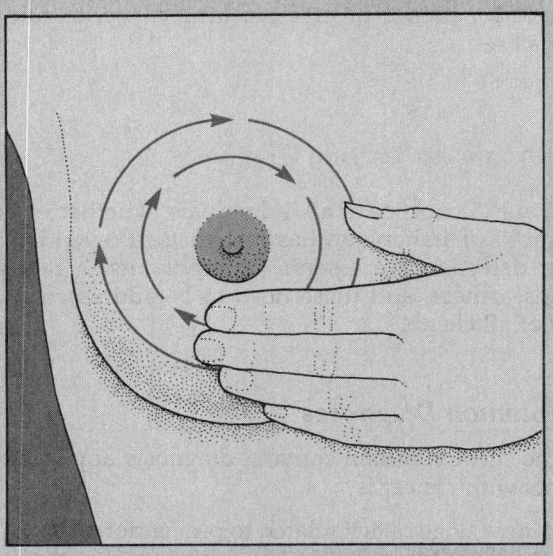

5. "After you have completely examined your right breast, examine your left breast with the same method. Compare what you have felt in one breast with the other."

6. "You may want to examine your breasts while bathing, when your skin is wet and lumps may be easier to feel."

7. "You can also check your breasts in a mirror by raising your arms and looking for an unusual shape, dimpling, or changes in the nipple." [see p. 575]

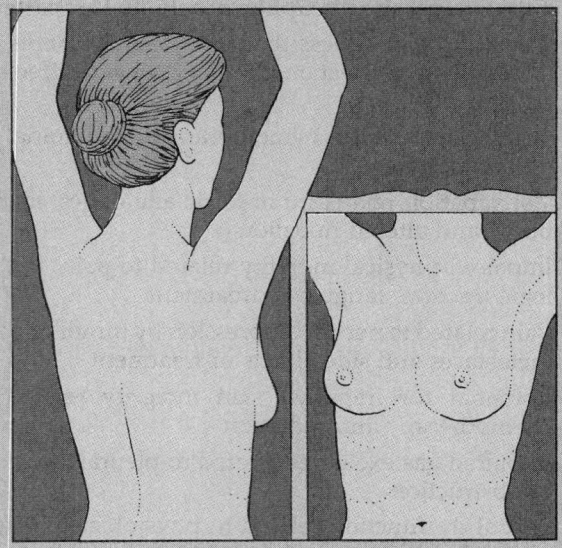

8. "If you notice any changes, see your doctor without delay. Further investigation of the abnormality may be necessary."

CLIENT/FAMILY EDUCATION ■ Instructions for Breast Self-Examination *Continued*

Swelling or elevated area

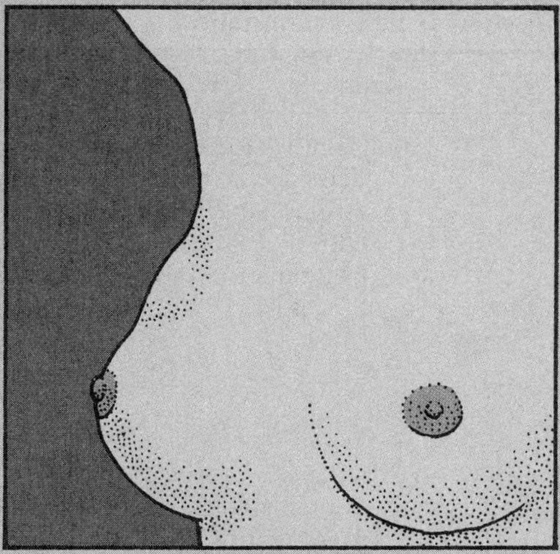

Redness or inflammation

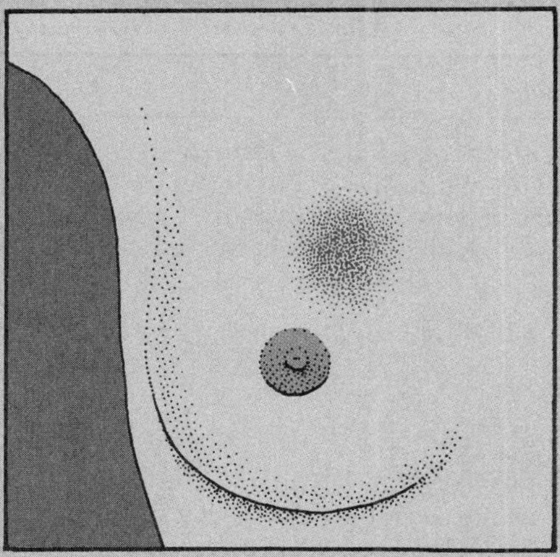

Puckering or dimpling

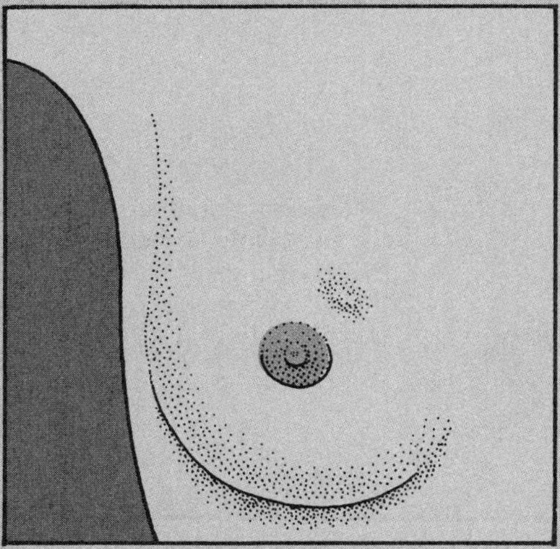

Nipple pulled inward

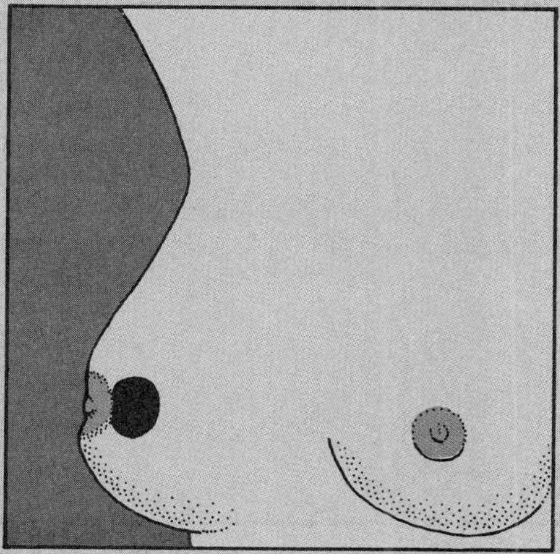

Depression or sunken area

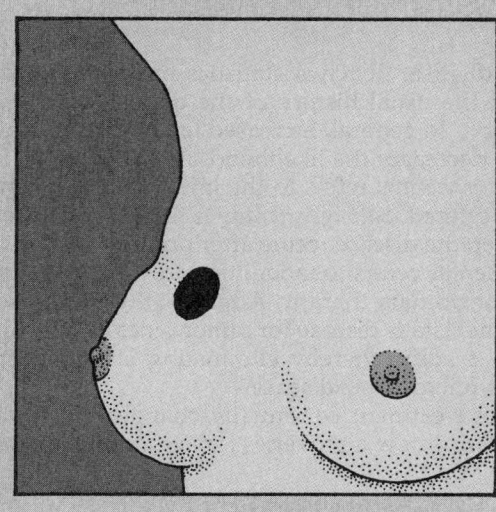

Nipple pulled askew compared with the other nipple

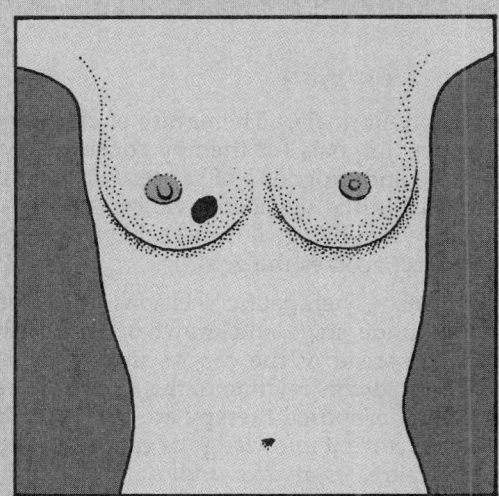

Modified from American Cancer Society. (1987). *Special touch facilitator's guide.* Atlanta: Author.

CLIENT/FAMILY EDUCATION ■ Instructions for Testicular Self-Examination

Instructions	Rationales
1. "It is important that you learn to perform testicular self-examination and do it monthly, right after a bath or a shower."	1. Monthly TSE facilitates early detection of malignancies. The scrotal skin is most relaxed after a bath or a shower, so this is the best time to examine the testes.
2. "Examine each testicle by gently rolling it between the thumbs and fingers of both hands."	2. Thumb stabilizes the scrotal skin to facilitate sensation of an abnormality by the finger pads.
3. "Report any lump or swelling to your doctor."	3. Not all swellings are malignant. If caught early, testicular malignancies are highly curable. Incidentally, it is unusual for tumors to occur in both testicles.

Vas deferens, Epididymis, Testis, Scrotum, Tumor

Modified from *How to examine your testes.* (1979). Madison, WI: Wisconsin Clinical Cancer Center; and American Cancer Society. (1982). *For men only.* Atlanta: Author.

Potential for Injury

Planning: client goals. The nature of cancer requires modifications of goals for therapy consistent with the type, extent, and prognosis of cancer and the host factors. The goal is that the client's cancer will be cured or controlled. When this goal is not achievable, palliation of symptoms becomes the goal.

Interventions. Therapeutic decisions are determined by the type, grade, stage, and known or usual patterns of growth and spread of the cancer and by the goal of therapy. Host factors relating to the ability of the client to tolerate the proposed therapy are also considered.

Given the current knowledge of cancer, the achievement of a "cure" is always under close scrutiny. The time from the initial curative therapy to the time of maximum risk for recurrence is determined by the growth rate of the type of tumor. The growth rate varies considerably, even among individuals with the same

type of disease. Survival statistics must be viewed in terms of the usual history of the disease over a wide population. In general, increased length of disease-free survival decreases the likelihood of recurrence.

Primary therapy refers to the initial or major form of therapy offered. *Salvage therapy* is initiated to cure disease when the disease recurs after primary therapy. *Adjuvant therapy* refers to modalities provided as an addition to the primary therapy. Adjuvant therapy is used to control metastatic disease for tumor types known to metastasize readily, thereby eliminating clinically undetected or microscopic disease.

Cancer treatment continually changes. Each day is likely to bring new discoveries for agents that kill cancer cells.

Surgical management. Surgery is the oldest and perhaps the classic treatment for cancer. Surgical treatment of cancer was historically undertaken because cancer was considered a localized disease: if the cancer was diagnosed early, it could be removed and cured by surgical intervention. It has become increasingly clear that cancer is *not* a localized disease and often has become a systemic disease by the time of diagnosis.

Surgery is frequently the primary mode of therapy in many major cancers. As with all treatment modalities, surgery may be a treatment option with curative, control, palliative, and prophylactic goals. Surgery is often offered as definitive treatment — meant to totally eradicate tumor cells. Skin cancers are often treated by local and wide excisions alone. Total removal of tumor and surrounding structures or tissues with nodal drainage is termed *en bloc* dissection. Other surgical procedures remove as much tumor and surrounding structures as possible, or remove the major bulk of tumor cells, leaving what is suspected to be microscopic disease behind. In this debulking procedure, minimal tumor remains to be controlled by adjuvant treatment modalities. Often, normal tissue surrounding the tumor is removed with the tumor, to ensure that all the tumor was removed with clean, disease-free margins. The extent of surgery is determined by the type of cancer and its growth pattern. Metastases to regional lymph nodes occur with most carcinomas and some sarcomas. Removal of the tumor-bearing organ with its adjacent nodes is preferably done without disfigurement. Some cancers may be cured by aggressive surgery involving resection of multiple organs.

Surgical interventions applied to less invasive types of cancer (e.g., carcinoma in situ) include electrosurgery, cryosurgery, chemosurgery, and carbon dioxide (CO_2) laser surgery. Electrosurgery involves application of electrical current directly to cancer cells. Cryosurgery involves application of liquid nitrogen directly to tumor tissue. This freezes and destroys cancer cells. Chemosurgery combines the application of cytotoxic chemicals and surgical excision of tissue. CO_2 laser is used for local excision of cancer cells.

Palliative surgical procedures are performed to remove tumors, either primary or metastatic, that cause distressing symptoms, such as organ obstruction, hemorrhage, and abscesses. Surgical intervention is often selected to eliminate complications related to hormones — ablative surgery prevents hormonal influence by removing the hormone-producing organ (Chaps. 54 and 55).

Prophylactic surgery removes nonvital organs associated with a high incidence of cancer that may occur at some point during the person's life span. Decisions in favor of prophylactic surgery are based on the presence or absence of symptoms, the assessment of risk, the probability of early detection, the effectiveness of treatment should cancer occur, and the effects of surgery on the client's appearance and ability to function.

Reconstructive surgery attempts reconstruction of defects, resulting in improved function or appearance. The most publicized example is probably breast reconstruction, but head and neck reconstruction, ostomy revision, and implantation of prostheses add immeasurably to the quality of life for many individuals.

Surgical skill is also necessary to insert equipment useful in providing treatment and managing side effects of disease. Gastrostomy tubes, right atrial catheters and arterial catheters, ventricular (Ommaya) reservoirs, and implanted venous access devices are examples of equipment that has become standard in state-of-the-art cancer care (Chaps. 13, 33, and 64).

Nursing management associated with surgical oncologic practice may not appear to be vastly different from that related to other surgical subspecialties (Chap. 20). Probably the major difference is that nursing care for clients undergoing cancer surgery must consider all the physical and psychosocial factors related to this individual's ability (or the ability of family and significant others) to cope. This surgery is performed because cancer, a disease that is greatly feared, is a distinct possibility or reality for this client. All nursing care is planned in this light.

Nonsurgical management

Radiation. Radiation is used as a primary, adjuvant, or palliative modality. It involves the therapeutic application of high-energy rays to tumors. It is estimated that more than 50% of people who are diagnosed with cancer receive radiotherapy at some point during the course of their disease.

Clients may have fears and anxieties regarding the use of radiation. The nurse needs to be knowledgeable about radiation sources to explain their effects to clients and families.

When high voltage is applied to an electronic vacuum tube, high-speed electrons are produced. These electrons hit a target and, although most of the energy is transformed into heat, some electrons form a beam of energy. Cobalt machines commonly used in radiotherapy contain a radioactive cobalt source. Linear accelerator units accelerate electrons, producing high-energy radiation. As the energy increases, so does the penetration ability of the radiation, which allows the beams to reach deeper levels of tissue.

Different sources for ionizing radiation produce various wavelengths and forms and therefore offer a variety of therapeutic applications for radiation. Electromagnetic waves (x-rays and gamma rays) used in therapy include electrons, protons, heavy ions, and neutrons. Naturally occurring or artificially produced radioactive particles used therapeutically include beta particles and neutrons.

Radiation works by causing damage to deoxyribonucleic acid (DNA) of cells. The degree of injury to the cell is dependent on the amount of DNA damage. Cell death may occur immediately, at the time of cellular division, or later as a result of cellular degeneration. The potential for cell injury or cell radiosensitivity relates to the rate of cell division, the cell cycle phase, oxygenation of the cell, and the degree of cell differentiation.

The action of ionizing radiation is essentially the same on both normal and malignant cells, although normal cells have greater reparative ability than do cancer cells. Normal cells that survive an initial, sublethal dose usually recover within 24 hours. Interruption of exposure to radiation promotes repair of normal cells and is the rationale for fractionation of therapeutic exposure to radiation. *Fractionation* is the administration of fractions of a prescribed total dose of radiation over a given period of time. This allows for maximal cancer cell kill with tolerable side effects for the client. Malignant cells cannot recover, and when they are again exposed to radiation and further injury, cell death ultimately results.

The radiation absorbed dose (rad) is a measurement of the amount of radiation absorbed by the tissues. In attempts to facilitate international communication, the term centigray (cGy) is gradually replacing the term rad. In some instances, gray is the measurement of choice and is equal to 100 cGy, or 100 rad.

Biologic effects of radiation can be modified, which expands the range of therapeutic approaches. The presence of oxygen enhances the cell-killing effects of radiation. Agents called hypoxic sensitizers are being developed to eliminate hypoxic cells. There are also efforts to develop compounds that could protect normal tissues against radiation injury.

Some cytotoxic chemicals interact with radiation and are incorporated into combined-modality treatment protocols. Combined-modality therapy is designed to maximize the interaction between radiation and chemotherapy for enhanced therapeutic success.

Application of heat alters the tumor's environment, potentiating the effects of radiation and certain antineoplastic drugs. To date, the integration of heat and radiation is the most effective application of hyperthermia, although the use of hyperthermia alone continues to be explored.

The type and method of delivery of radiation is determined by the location, depth, and stage of the cancer; the field size needed; the radiosensitivity of the cancer; and the client's history and physical condition. With the exception of total body irradiation, most therapeutic irradiation is delivered to a specified field, which includes the tumor and a limited volume of surrounding tissue. Localized radiation *affects only the tissue within the treatment field.*

Radiation can be delivered from an external source or from an internal source. External therapy is most often provided in an ambulatory setting but clients may receive it while they are hospitalized. External radiation most often involves the use of gamma rays, which have maximal penetrating power, and occasionally beta particles, with less penetrating power. Tissues most affected by external radiation are hematopoietic, epithelial (including mucous membranes and hair follicles), and gonadal tissues.

Tissues composed of cells with high proliferation rates, whether normal or neoplastic in nature, are most susceptible to damage from radiation. Damage to normal cells is the primary cause of side effects and toxicities associated with radiation. Side effects of radiation therapy and appropriate nursing interventions are outlined in Table 25–5.

Skin reactions commonly occur and can range from erythema to dry desquamation or wet desquamation. Since the development of linear accelerator units, skin reactions have become less significant. In the past, skin reactions from radiation therapy were referred to as burns. This is no longer appropriate, because burn implies an accidental or unexpected damage, neither of which accurately explains the occurrence of the reaction.

Radiation effects may be considered acute (occurring during treatment and up to 6 months), subacute (after 6 months), and chronic (with a variable time to expression). Acute side effects are those involving cell lines that have high reproductive rates (skin, mucous membranes, and hair follicles) and eventually might involve cell lines that divide more slowly (muscles and vascular system). Early effects, which are often reparable, involve changes such as parenchymal cell loss. Late effects, which are more likely to be permanent, may relate to vascular changes exemplified by arteriocapillary fibrosis. The process of inflammation and repair is responsible for fibrotic changes and atrophy of normal tissues within the treated area (the treatment field).

Some centers provide intraoperative irradiation—delivering irradiation directly to the tumor site during a surgical procedure—for selected tumor sites. Internal, or brachytherapy, techniques use various radioisotopes to deliver concentrated doses of radiation in or near tumor sites.

Intracavitary implants involve the temporary insertion of a sealed source into a body cavity, such as the vagina or uterus. In general, radium, radon, or cesium, sealed in an applicator adapted for the site, is inserted and left in place for several hours or days, depending on the prescribed dose. The client is, for the most part, immobilized throughout the treatment period to prevent displacement of the implant. The position of the source is crucial to the accurate execution of the treatment plan. Position is initially verified by radiography and is closely monitored throughout the course of treatment.

Radioactive isotopes that are "sealed" are placed inside wires, needles, catheters, or seeds in interstitial implants to position the radioactive source directly into the tumor and surrounding tissues. Interstitial implants can be temporary or permanent. Temporary implants can become dislodged, and positioning needs to be closely monitored. Interstitial techniques are useful in treating cancers of the head and neck, breast, and prostate and are being explored as a treatment modality in lung, brain, and liver cancers. Permanent implants, using radioactive gold seeds, are most often used for prostate cancer.

^{131}I, as an unsealed radioactive source, is used to treat thyroid cancer and hyperthyroidism. ^{131}I ablates residual normal thyroid tissue after surgery or treatment of metastatic or recurrent thyroid tumors. All body fluids should be considered contaminated, because the unsealed radioisotope circulates freely throughout the body. The client is a source of external radiation to persons who come near her/him. The radioactivity of the

TABLE 25-5 Side Effects and Related Interventions for Clients Receiving Radiation Therapy

Site	Acute Effect	Chronic Effect	Interventions
Skin	Erythema (3000–4000 rad), dry desquamation, moist desquamation (4500–6000 rad)	Fibrosis, atrophy, telangiectasia, permanent darkening of the skin	Avoid trauma to skin, extremes of temperature, and use of harsh chemicals or soaps.
Oral cavity	Change and loss of taste, dryness, mucositis (3000–4000 rad)	Permanent xerostomia, permanent taste alterations, dental caries	Monitor weight. Provide artificial saliva, viscous lidocaine, preventive dental care with fluoride, and nutritional counseling to maintain dietary status.
Esophagus	Pain, esophagitis	Fibrosis	Give antacids and viscous lidocaine.
Stomach	Nausea and vomiting (125 rad)	Obstruction, ulceration, fibrosis	Administer antiemetics 1 h before treatment.
Intestines	Diarrhea (2000–3000 rad)	Malabsorption, strictures, necrosis (6000–7000 rad)	Supply medication for diarrhea. Institute dietary modifications (e.g., low-residue diet), and good skin care and perineal hygiene.
Kidney		Radiation nephritis	
Bladder	Cystitis (3000 rad)	Fibrosis, contracted bladder (6500–7000 rad)	Increase fluid intake. May administer prophylactic urinary antiseptics.
Bone marrow	WBC and platelets may be diminished	Possibility of chronic anemia, especially with combined-modality treatment	Initiate bleeding precautions and measures to prevent infection as indicated.
Respiratory system	Pneumonitis (2500–3000 rad)	Fibrosis	Institute pulmonary hygiene measures to alleviate cough and dyspnea.
Cardiovascular system	Rare reports of pericarditis, myocarditis	Fibrosis	
Central nervous system (brain and spinal cord, peripheral nerves)	Edema and inflammation	Infarction, occlusion, necrosis	Monitor sequelae of steroid administration, assess neurologic status, and monitor for headaches.
Eyes		Cataracts	
Bone and cartilage of child		Growth disturbances if growth plate of bone is in field (2000–3000 rad)	
Gonads			
Spermatogonia	Decreased sperm count after 90–120 d; temporary sterility (100–300 rad)		Counsel patient regarding the effect of radiation on fertility.
Ovary	Sterility (500–1000 rad), depends on age		

From Strohl, R. A. (1988). The nursing role in radiation oncology: Symptom management of acute and chronic reactions. *Oncology Nursing Forum, 15*(4), 429–434.

isotope is monitored, and the client remains hospitalized until radioactivity is diminished by excretion or decay — usually 24 to 48 hours after administration.

The total dose and fractionation schedule prescribed are individualized for each client and are determined according to the client's ability to tolerate treatment; the tumor size, stage, and grade; previous treatment (including chemotherapy as well as radiation); and documented experience with the tumors being targeted. Maximal tolerated doses have been determined for various organ systems, including normal and neoplastic tissues. Accurate and individualized treatment planning ensures that maximal doses are not exceeded and that killing of tumor cells is maximized, with minimal exposure to normal tissue.

Nurses and other health care professionals are concerned about occupational exposure to radiation. This fear can be communicated to clients and may affect the care they receive. Health care professionals and clients need to know that external radiotherapy does *not* render the client radioactive. Brachytherapy techniques do require modifications of care because of the presence of a radioactive source, but safe care can be provided with basic precautions and techniques (see the accompanying Guidelines feature).

The National Council on Radiation Protection

(NCRP) (1976) established guidelines for dose limits of radiation exposure. Dose limits are based on postulated amounts of radiation exposure that would damage ovaries and testes. The intent is to keep radiation exposure as low as is reasonably achievable. Regulations stipulate that the maximal permissible dose for whole-body exposure to radiation is 5000 mrem/year or 3000 mrem in a 3-month period. Exposure of radiation oncologists working with implants rarely exceeds 1000 mrem/year; most staff nurses receive less than 50 mrem/year (Hassey, 1985; NCRP, 1976).

Guidelines for protection are based on three concepts: time, distance, and shielding. Exposure to radiation is minimized by limiting the overall exposure time. This requires organization of tasks and, to the extent possible, encouraging clients to perform self-care. Care providers should rotate client assignments to minimize exposure. In general, clients undergoing brachytherapy are capable of self-care, and direct nursing care can be limited to ½ hour per provider per shift (Bucholtz, 1987; Hassey, 1985).

The intensity of radiation decreases with distance from the source (Fig. 25–2). It is important to stay as far as possible from the radioactive source. Direct care can be provided from the head, foot, or side of the bed, depending on the location of the source. When the nurse is not providing direct care, communicating with the client from a distance is preferable.

Lead shields, although cumbersome, provide additional protection from radioactive sources when used appropriately. Lead aprons do not shield against gamma rays. Time limitations and distance precautions are easier to implement and provide appropriate levels of protection.

Chemotherapeutic agents. Chemotherapy has made significant contributions to improved survival rates. It is used as primary, adjuvant, or palliative therapy.

Before the institution of chemotherapy, surgery and radiation cured about one-third of all people with cancer. Most clients with cancer receive more than one therapeutic modality.

The first antineoplastic drug was probably colchicine, which was used in the first century AD. However, there were few chemotherapeutic agents used until nitrogen mustard was demonstrated to have antitumor activity in 1942.

From 1942 on, the development of chemotherapeutic agents accelerated. This resulted in cures for certain cancers and increased survival for others. More recent research on chemotherapy has focused on the development of analogues to current agents with fewer side effects and on the development of different protocols for optimal effect.

Antineoplastic chemicals interfere with cellular activities. Some agents are cell cycle nonspecific (CCNS), or equally toxic to cells in any phase of the cell cycle. The ability these agents have to kill cells and cause toxicities is proportional to the total dose given.

Other agents are cell cycle specific (CCS), damaging cells during a specific phase of the cell cycle. The effects

---

GUIDELINES ■ Care of the Client with Sealed Implants of Radioactive Sources

Assign the client to a private room with a private bath.

Place a "Caution: Radioactive Material" sign on the door of the client's room.

Wear a dosimeter film badge at all times while caring for clients with radioactive implants. The badge offers no protection, but measures an individual's exposure to radiation and should be used by only one individual.

Pregnant nurses should not care for these clients; do not allow children under 16 years of age or pregnant women to visit.

Limit each visitor to one-half hour per day. Be sure visitors are at least 6 ft from the source.

Never touch the radioactive source with bare hands. In the rare instance that it is dislodged, use a long-handled forceps to retrieve it. Deposit the radioactive source in the lead container kept in the client's room.

Save all dressings and bed linens until after the radioactive source is removed. After the source is removed, dispose of dressings and linens in the usual manner. Other equipment can be removed from the room at any time.

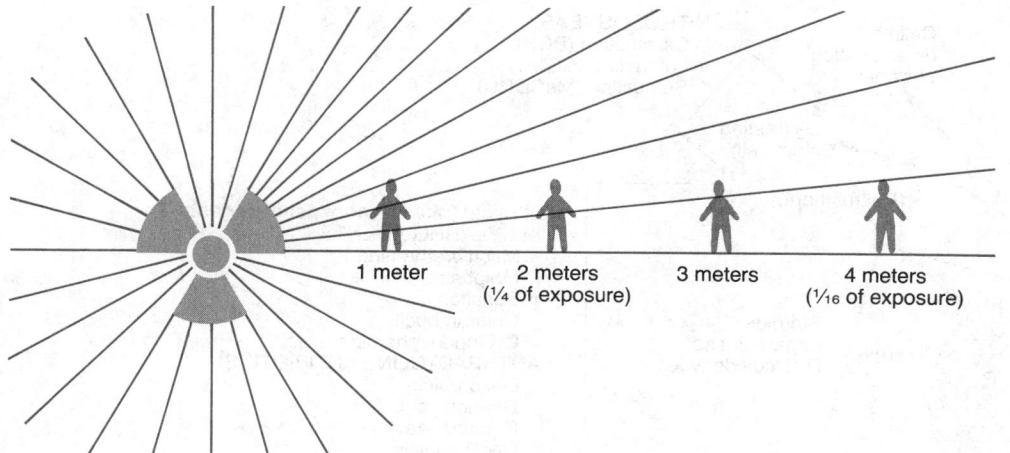

Figure 25–2

The inverse law of radiation exposure: the intensity of radiation decreases with the distance from the source. (From Sedhom, L. N., & Yann, M. I. Y. [1985]. Radiation therapy and nurses' fears of radiation exposure. *Cancer Nursing, 8,* 129–134.)

of these agents are dependent on a schedule: the cell must be in a specific phase and cytotoxic levels of the drug must occur during that phase for the therapeutic effect to be achieved. Most CCS drugs affect the cell during the DNA synthesis (S) phase and interfere with DNA and ribonucleic acid (RNA) synthesis (Fig. 25–3). Combination chemotherapy protocols integrate agents with a variety of cell injury targets; this strategy minimizes the severity of toxicities to single agents.

Antimetabolites are CCS, specific to the S phase, and include methotrexate, cytarabine, 5-fluorouracil, mercaptopurine and thioguanine. Vinca alkaloids (vincristine and vinblastine) are CCS, acting during the mitotic phase and blocking metaphase.

Many CCNS drugs are alkylating agents and are believed to bond alkyl groups to cellular enzymes and DNA, causing cross-linking of DNA strands. Cross-linking of DNA strands is associated with RNA imbalance and eventual death of the cell. Common alkylating agents are cyclophosphamide and melphalan.

Antineoplastic antibiotics are CCNS and interfere with nucleic acid synthesis and block DNA and RNA transcription. Commonly used antineoplastic antibiotics include doxorubicin, daunomycin, dactinomycin, and bleomycin.

Some hormonal agents possess antineoplastic activity and are usually classified as CCNS. Hormonal agents are thought either to block the cytoplasmic receptors regulating cell growth or to interfere with nuclear processes. Tamoxifen is a nonsteroidal antiestrogen agent, which competes for estrogen receptors to interfere with nuclear functions and cell reproduction.

The cytotoxic effects of antineoplastic agents are not specific to cancer cells. Like radiation, antineoplastic chemicals target actively proliferating cells. The difference between doses offering maximal tumor cell kill and doses that can be overwhelmingly toxic to the entire body is slight. For maximal effectiveness, an antineoplastic agent must be the right drug delivered to the right cells in the right concentration at the right time.

The normal cells most susceptible to the effects of chemotherapy include hematopoietic cells, epithelial cells of the GI tract, hair follicles, and cells of the gonads. Damage to normal cells is the basis of the most common side effects of chemotherapy. These include bone marrow suppression, stomatitis, mucositis, nausea, vomiting, anorexia, and alopecia. Stomatitis is the inflammation of mucous membranes of the oral cavity. Mucositis is inflammation of any mucous membranes, but commonly refers to the GI and genitourinary tracts. Alopecia involves loss of hair, which can involve any part of the body, but most often involves the scalp.

Cutaneous (skin) reactions can occur with specific chemotherapeutic agents. Some alkylating agents produce alterations in pigmentation. Topical application of antineoplastic agents, whether intentional or accidental, can result in contact dermatitis. Antimetabolites have been reported to reactivate ultraviolet injury, as well as cause hyperpigmentation, erythema, and desquamation of the palms of the hands and the soles of the feet. Methotrexate is frequently associated with photosensitivity and hyperpigmentation of skin, of nails, and along injected veins.

The antineoplastic antibiotic dactinomycin (Actinomycin D) produces lesions resembling acne: erythema followed by papules, pustules, and occluded follicles. Doxorubicin increases melanin pigmentation in nails, skin, and mucous membranes and causes generalized urticaria. A unique reaction associated with doxorubicin is radiation recall phenomenon — in which skin reactions associated with previous radiation exposure can be reactivated.

Extravasation (infiltration of irritating agents into cutaneous and subcutaneous tissues) creates an insult to skin integrity, which has serious sequelae of pain, infection, and skin loss, sometimes necessitating surgical intervention. Chemotherapeutic agents that are capable of causing extravasation are called *vesicants*. Actinomycin, daunomycin, doxorubicin, mithramycin, mitomycin, vinblastine, and vincristine are the most commonly

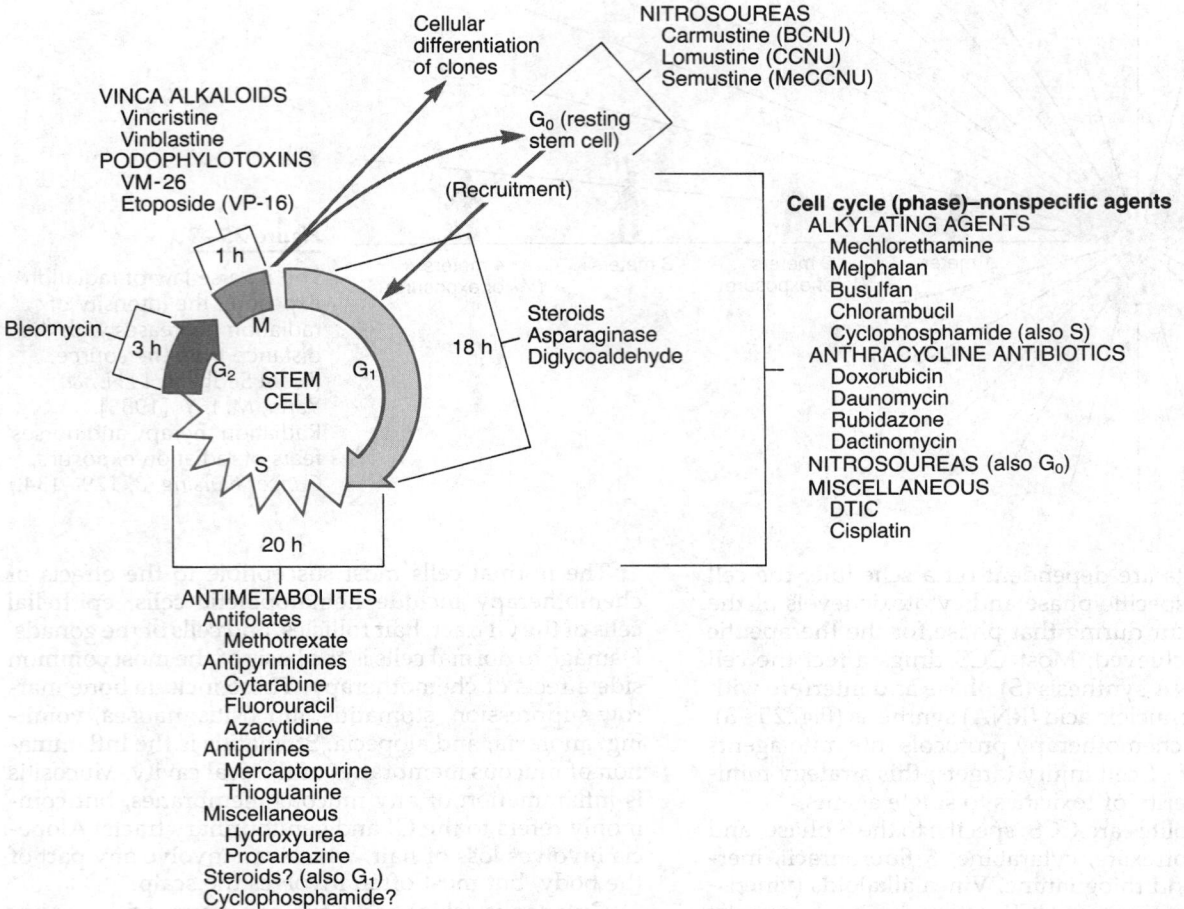

Figure 25–3

Cell cycle phases affected by chemotherapeutic agents. In phase G_1, enzymes necessary for DNA production are produced. In S phase, DNA is synthesized. In G_2, specialized proteins and RNA are synthesized. In M phase, mitosis occurs. G_0 is a resting phase in which the cell is not committed to division. (Reprinted by permission of the publisher from *Cancer chemotherapy handbook*, by Dorr, R. T., & Fritz, W. L., p. 5. Copyright 1980 by Elsevier Science Publishing Co., Inc.)

used vesicant agents associated with extravasation and subsequent local necrosis.

Other adverse effects of chemotherapy include those that affect the cardiac, pulmonary, renal, and neurologic systems. Cardiotoxicity is associated with the chemotherapeutic agents doxorubicin (Adriamycin) and daunomycin. It can lead to cardiomyopathy, manifested by congestive heart failure.

Pulmonary toxicity is a high risk for clients receiving bleomycin, busulphan, and carmustine. It can lead to pneumonitis and interstitial fibrosis. Cyclophosphamide (Cytoxan) can cause toxicity in the urinary bladder, resulting in hemorrhagic cystitis. Cisplatin is associated with renal toxicity and can cause acute tubular necrosis.

Neurotoxicity may occur with the administration of vincristine and is manifested by paresthesias of the hands or feet, constipation, weakness, or impotence. L-Asparaginase may cause cerebral dysfunction. Cis-

platin can also cause paresthesias, which may be painful.

Dosages of these and other drugs capable of causing adverse effects are limited to decrease the risk of toxicities. To rule out cardiac, respiratory, or renal deficits, clients are screened through laboratory and other tests specific to the organ system at risk before receiving these drugs. For example, clients who are to receive bleomycin are given pulmonary function tests, and chest x-ray films are obtained to evaluate pulmonary function before receiving this agent. Clients receiving cisplatin have creatinine clearance or serum creatinine measurements before and during therapy. Before cisplatin administration, clients are hydrated with intravenous (IV) fluid followed by the administration of diuretics, to keep the kidneys flushed and to prevent the accumulation of the drug in the renal tubules. Neurotoxicities associated with cisplatin may result from the hypomagnesemia induced by this drug. Serum magnesium levels are measured, and magnesium sulfate is administered to avoid neuropathy.

The nurse monitors the specific organ system known to be at high risk for toxicity by frequent physical assessment and assessment of pertinent laboratory data. Clients and families are taught specific signs and symptoms that should be watched for and reported. In addition to causing serious morbidity to clients, the toxic effects of chemotherapeutic agents are a significant concern because their presence may require decreased dosing or cessation of treatment. Such changes in treatment could affect treatment goals and reduce the chance for cure.

Measures to control chemotherapy-related alopecia have been attempted (Keller & Blausey, 1988). These measures, such as soft rubber tourniquets around the scalp and scalp hypothermia via ice or cold air devices, are undertaken to vasoconstrict superficial scalp blood vessels to inhibit drug uptake by hair follicles. Despite some success, prevention or control of alopecia cannot be guaranteed, and the risk of not effectively treating a possible scalp metastasis may be unacceptable. Methods to prevent alopecia are therefore often not employed.

A few drugs are being used in conjunction with chemotherapeutic agents to protect normal tissue against the effects of chemotherapy without decreasing their effect against tumors. Mesna (Mesnex) is used with ifosfamide (Ifex) to protect against renal toxicity. Leucovorin (Citrovorum) is a folinic acid given in conjunction with the antimetabolite methotrexate to prevent bone marrow toxicity. Timing of administration of chemoprotective agents is crucial to avoid toxicities. These agents allow higher doses of chemotherapy to be given for a greater antitumor effect.

The nurse has the final responsibility for confirming the accuracy and appropriateness of a drug prescription and ensuring that no contraindications exist for use of that drug before its administration. The functions of the nurse relative to chemotherapy include assessment of clinical and psychosocial status, assessment of client's knowledge level regarding treatment options, evaluation of the consistency of prescribed treatment with relevant research or standard therapy guidelines, and skillful administration of prescribed agents. The nurse is aware of complications associated with drug administration and appropriate interventions. The client's response to treatment and complications are assessed and communicated to other members of the health care team to facilitate provision of optimal care.

Important factors in determining the route of administration of various agents include the pharmacokinetics of the drug, therapeutic goals, specific tumor factors, and the client's clinical status. Oral and IV routes are most commonly used. Venous access devices, right atrial catheters, and implantable devices are frequently used for IV administration. They facilitate long-term systemic therapy. Implantable ports are illustrated in Figure 25–4. Intra-arterial delivery is occasionally used for the treatment of certain cancers. It provides high concentrations of agent directly to tumor sites while decreasing systemic effects. Intraperitoneal administration is also used for certain site-specific cancers. It is modeled after peritoneal dialysis techniques and involves bathing intraperitoneal tumor sites with high concentrations of selected drugs. As with intra-arterial administration, this method spares the client many toxic side effects that would be associated with equivalent systemic doses.

Some agents are delivered into the pleural spaces via a thoracotomy tube. Intrapleural chemotherapy causes sclerosis of the pleural lining with the goal of preventing reinvasion of the pleural cavity with fluid.

Intrathecal drug administration (chemotherapy delivered to the central nervous system [CNS] via the spinal canal through a lumbar puncture or ventricular reservoirs) is used for potential or diagnosed CNS involvement with tumor cells. Many chemotherapeutic agents do not pass through the blood-brain barrier, necessitating direct access to the CNS.

Public opinion of chemotherapy is often focused on its adverse side effects. The nurse assesses the client and the family for attitudes and knowledge of chemotherapy and the basis for attitudes. Clients need to be taught that there are various types of drugs with different side effects and that not all individuals react the same way to medications. The nurse confers with the medical oncologist regarding each individual's potential for side effects. Plans for prophylactic therapy to minimize side effects are made with the client on the basis of an individualized assessment of the client and past experience with the chemotherapy protocol being implemented.

It is known that exposure to cytotoxic drugs is related to various symptoms, including mucous membrane, eye, and skin irritation; dizziness; nausea; and headache. There are reports of mutagenesis and fetal deaths related to occupational exposures of unprotected workers (Bingham, 1985; Cloak et al., 1985; Selevan et al., 1985; Stellman et al., 1984). These findings may not be entirely conclusive, but they do highlight the importance of safe handling and worker protection in association with neoplastic agents.

Exposure to cytotoxic drugs occurs through three major routes: inhalation of drug aerosols or droplets, absorption of the drug through the skin, and ingestion through contact with contaminated food or cigarettes. Occupational exposures occur during drug preparation and administration and during disposal of contaminated materials. General protective guidelines include wearing surgical latex gloves and nonabsorbent gowns during preparation and administration. Biologic safety cabinets and vertical, laminar airflow are used during preparation to protect from drug aerosolization.

Because most cytotoxic agents are excreted in body fluids, proper handling and disposal of body fluids by personnel caring for these clients is important. Surgical latex gloves and gowns should be worn when handling blood, vomitus, or body excreta of clients who have received cytotoxic drugs within the previous 48 hours.

Gowns and surgical latex gloves and eye protection are recommended for personnel involved in cleaning

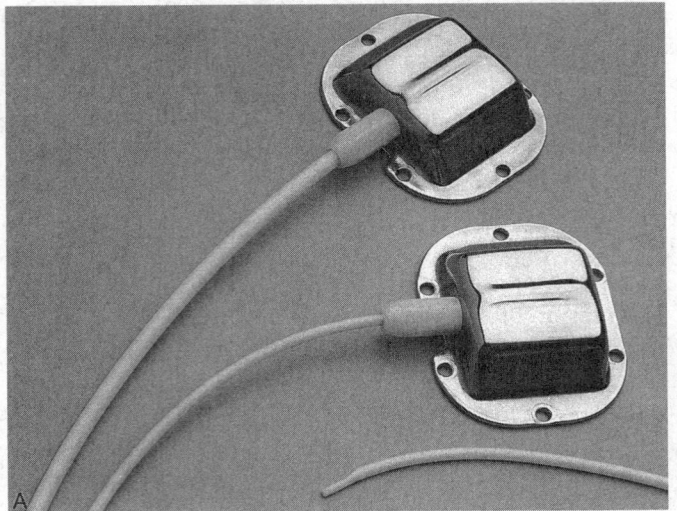

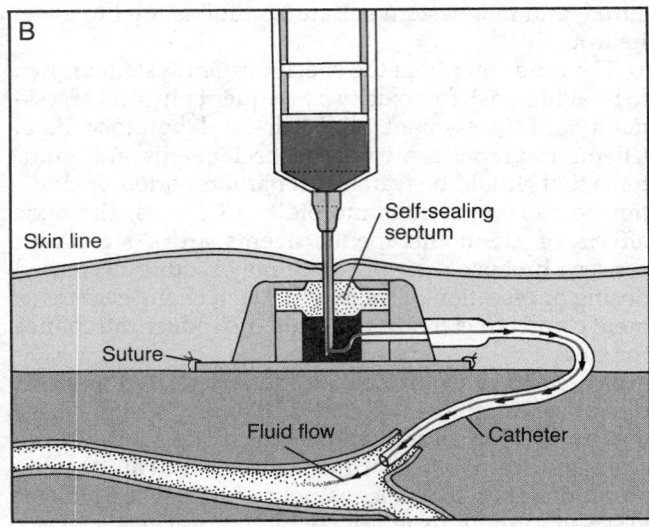

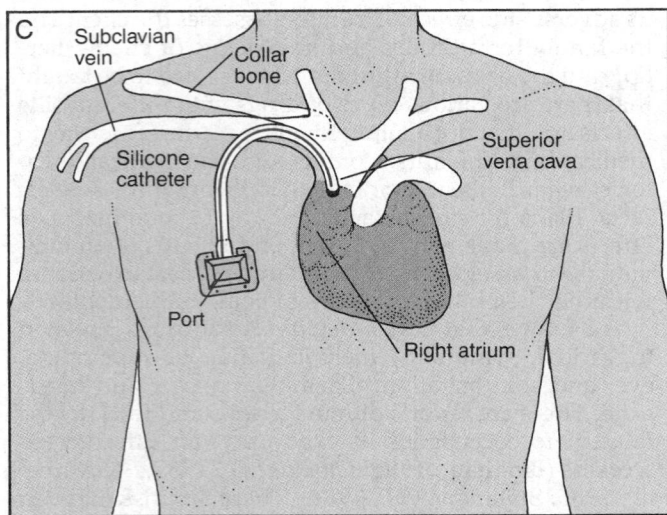

Figure 25–4

Implantable ports for venous access. *A,* The dual-access implantable port. *B,* A needle puncture through the skin into the port allows drugs, fluids, and blood to be administered. *C,* For systemic drug and fluid delivery, the catheter is placed in the subclavian vein. (*A,* Courtesy of Harbor Medical Devices, Inc., Boston, MA. *B and C,* redrawn from Winters, V. [1984]. Implantable vascular access devices. *Oncology Nursing Forum, 11*[6], 25–30.)

cytotoxic drug spills. Respiratory masks are recommended in the case of spills of more than 5 mL or 5 g of cytotoxic drugs. Disposal of cytotoxic wastes incorporates protective handling guidelines in conjunction with specially designated waste disposal bags, storage facilities, and final disposal.

Employers must provide employees with information related to potential hazards of exposure to cytotoxic agents. Many facilities have implemented health monitoring and surveillance programs for employees at risk for exposure. Institutional policies should address protection of pregnant or breastfeeding female employees or those trying to conceive. Practice guidelines have been developed by individual institutions, and others have been published (Occupational Safety and Health Administration, 1986; Oncology Nursing Society, 1988).

Biologic response modifiers. Biologic response modifiers (BRMs) are considered the fourth treatment modality for cancer. Most of the agents are still in the experimental stage. However, they hold promise for more widespread use in the future.

BRMs are agents or approaches that modify the host's biologic responses to tumor cells. The basis of this approach is the belief that the human immune system can be manipulated to restore or enhance a normal function that has become ineffective.

Biologicals and BRMs act in several ways in the biotherapy of cancer. They augment the host's defenses, increase differentiation of tumor cells, and increase the host's ability to tolerate damage from other cytotoxic modalities of cancer treatment. Major classifications include immunomodulating agents, interferons and interferon inducers, thymosins, lymphokines and cytokines, antigens, effector cells, and monoclonal antibodies.

Nurses involved with administration of biologicals must be familiar with symptom patterns expected with specific BRMs. Nurses need to have an in-depth knowledge of the immune system, knowledge of the activity and rationale for use of BRMs, and the technical skills to

TABLE 25-6   **Risk Factors and Interventions for Clients Receiving Biologic Response Modifiers**

Side Effects	Risk Factors	Usual Time Frame	Interventions*
Constitutional			
Headache, fever, chills, myalgias, and influenza-like symptoms	Age Poor performance status	Acute	Observe for presence and severity of symptoms (acute symptoms generally abate with repeated dosing).
Fatigue, malaise, and weakness	Age Poor performance status Malnutrition Anemia Other medications Inadequate social support system	Chronic	Monitor use of other medications (e.g., propranolol can contribute to fatigue). Monitor nutritional status (e.g., weight change) and hematologic status.
Cardiovascular	History of cardiac disease Unstable hypertension Dehydration Age	Acute and chronic	Observe orthostatic blood pressure changes and vital signs. Monitor for potential cardiac symptoms.
Neurologic	History of seizures, mood swings, and depression Age	Acute and chronic	Observe for cognitive and mood alterations. Educate family to report subtle changes.
Gastrointestinal	History of GI disorders	Acute	Observe for symptoms.
Hematologic	History of coagulation disorders Leukemia Multiple myeloma Bone marrow suppression	Chronic	Routinely monitor CBC, differential and platelet counts, PT, and PTT.
Renal or metabolic	Renal diseases	Acute and chronic	Routinely monitor BUN, creatinine, and electrolyte levels. Monitor for proteinuria in high-risk patients.
Hepatic	History of alcohol abuse Other hepatotoxic drugs Malnutrition Pre-existent liver disease	Chronic	Obtain baseline liver function tests. Routinely monitor LDH, ALP, ALT, AST, and bilirubin levels. Assess nutritional status. Monitor alcohol and other drug intake.

* ALP, alkaline phosphatase; ALT, alanine aminotransferase; AST, aspartate aminotransferase; BUN, blood urea nitrogen; CBC, complete blood count; LDH, lactate dehydrogenase; PT, prothrombin time; PTT, partial thromboplastin time.
From Irwin, M. M. (1987). Patients receiving biological response modifiers: Overview of nursing care. *Oncology Nursing Forum, 14*(Suppl.), 32–37.

administer these agents. Nurses also play a crucial role in developing and implementing administration protocols, client-monitoring procedures, and strategies to manage side effects.

Because most biologicals are still in various phases of clinical trials, knowledge of side effects for the various agents, preparations, doses, and routes of administration is far from complete. There are unique toxicities associated with specific biologicals, but most have a similarly broad range of potential organ and system side effects manifested as acute or chronic symptoms. Table 25–6 lists side effects, risk factors, time frame, and suggested interventions. The most common side effects include fatigue and influenza-like symptoms (fever, chills or rigors, myalgias, and headache) (Table 25–7).

Biologicals are administered orally, directly into the lesion, intradermally, intravenously, or intravesically.

Potential for Infection

Planning: client goals. The goal is that the client will not develop an infection or septicemia.

TABLE 25–7 Influenza-like Signs and Symptoms Associated with the Use of Biologic Response Modifiers

Agent	Fever	Chills or Rigor	Myalgias	Headache	Is Response Dose Dependent?
Interferons	Almost universal Rapid onset Monophasic Tolerance may develop	Common	Common May be moderately severe	Common	Yes
Interleukin-2	Almost universal Delayed onset	Common	Uncommon	Uncommon	Yes
Tissue necrosis factor	Common Rapid onset Biphasic patterns Tolerance may develop	Common	Common	Common	Yes
Monoclonal antibodies	Common Various patterns Antigen-antibody reaction	Common	Arthralgias	Common	Not clearly
Colony-stimulating factors	Depends on agent Low grade	Uncommon	Common May be severe	Common	Not clearly

From Haeuber, D. (1989, May). Recent advances in the management of biotherapy-related side effects: Flu-like syndrome. *Symposium: The Biotherapy of Cancer—III*, San Francisco. Nutley, NJ: Roche Laboratories.

Interventions: nonsurgical management. The most important step in control of infection in clients with cancer is prevention. Exposures to pathogens are anticipated, and care is provided in consideration of sites known to be at high risk for infection. Clients receiving chemotherapy should avoid contact with large crowds or individuals with upper respiratory tract infections when they are susceptible to infection. This period, which is referred to as the client's *nadir*, occurs when leukocyte and granulocyte levels are lowest, generally between 7 and 14 days after the administration of chemotherapeutic agents. Invasive procedures, such as insertion of a Foley catheter or a surgical procedure, are avoided for all immunosuppressed clients, especially when an individual is most susceptible.

Highly compromised hospitalized clients, with absolute granulocyte counts between 500 and 1000/mm³, are placed on neutropenic precautions. These generally involve a private room with strict hand washing required for all staff and visitors who enter the room. Fresh flowers, fruits, and vegetables are also prohibited, as are visitors with upper respiratory tract infections. Reverse or protective isolation has not been shown by research to reduce the risk of infection any more than consistent hand washing by staff. The greatest risk of infection is thought to be from endogenous colonization within the client. Good hygiene and nutrition are essential preventive interventions. To limit organisms in the oral cavity, clients are instructed to rinse their mouth after each meal and at bedtime with a normal saline solution. A typical solution is 1 tsp of baking soda and 1 tsp of salt added to 1 qt of water.

The nurse has a high index of suspicion for the development of infection in all immunosuppressed clients. Any subtle change in physical assessment findings is reported at once. Clients who are febrile, with or without other symptoms of infection, have sputum, urine, blood, and, if applicable, wound cultures obtained along with chest radiography. Broad-spectrum antibiotics, such as a cephalosporin, a synthetic penicillin, and an aminoglycoside, are administered after culture specimens are obtained. Antibiotic administration is altered on the basis of culture reports and sensitivities. Clients are closely monitored for their response to antibiotics, manifested by a reduction in fever or the resolution or development of other signs of infection. If fevers do not decrease with appropriate antibiotic administration, further cultures are obtained and a fungal source of infection is considered.

The nurse closely monitors all immunosuppressed clients for early (warm) septic shock (Table 25–8), which may occur with septicemia. Early recognition and management of this common complication of infection are essential to avoid morbidity and mortality (Chap. 17).

Potential for Altered (Cardiopulmonary) Tissue Perfusion

Planning: client goals. The goal is that the client will not experience bleeding from any internal or external tissue. Thrombocytopenia secondary to bone marrow

---

TABLE 25–8 Assessment Findings in Early Septic Shock

Assessment	Findings
General	
Assess mental status and level of consciousness.	Irritability, restlessness, lethargy, disorientation, and inappropriate euphoria
Check oral temperature.	Normal, subnormal, or elevated temperature
Integumentary System	
Inspect and palpate skin. Note color, vascularity, moisture, temperature, texture, thickness, mobility, and turgor. Assess oral mucosa.	Warm flushed skin and peripheral edema
Respiratory System	
Observe rate, rhythm, and effort of breathing. Observe symmetry of chest expansion.	Tachypnea, hyperventilation
Percuss and auscultate lungs. Note onset of adventitious sounds.	Rales and decreased breath sounds
Check blood gas levels.	Respiratory alkalosis
Cardiovascular System	
Check pulse and blood pressure. Document pulse pressure with each blood pressure reading.	Tachycardia: normal mean arterial blood pressure; widening pulse pressure
Check peripheral pulses.	Bounding peripheral pulses
Auscultate heart sounds at four valvular sites and record the onset of murmur or gallop.	No murmur or gallop

From Barry, S. A. (1989). Septic shock: Special needs of patients with cancer. *Oncology Nursing Forum, 16*(1), 31–35.

depression after chemotherapy is a common risk factor for altered tissue perfusion in clients with cancer.

Interventions: nonsurgical management. Nursing management related to the client with actual or potential thrombocytopenia is directed toward minimizing potential for injury that might initiate bleeding. The nurse teaches the client assessment skills and recognition of signs of bleeding, risk factors, implications of bleeding, self-care measures, and appropriate actions, should bleeding occur. Other nursing measures provide data to quantify and qualify actual bleeding and provision of psychosocial and emotional support during this time. Transfusion of platelets if platelet counts are less than 20,000/mm³ is often prescribed (Sanford, 1985; Wroblewski and Wroblewski, 1981).

Bleeding precautions are instituted that involve avoiding or minimizing invasive or traumatic procedures, including venipuncture; injections; suctioning; the use of rectal thermometers; and the administration of suppositories, enemas, and douches. If necessary, the nurse should apply pressure to venipuncture and injection sites for 5 minutes. Oral care should incorporate a soft-bristle toothbrush or sponged tooth swabs and avoid the use of floss or toothpicks. A bowel program should be implemented to avoid constipation and straining at bowel movements. The client should use an electric razor for shaving and in general avoid or use particular caution with sharp instruments.

Activity Intolerance

Planning: client goals. The goal is that the client will manage activity intolerance in a way that will enable participation in valued activities.

Interventions: nonsurgical management. Interventions that are effective in reducing fatigue incorporate teaching and implementation of planned rest periods, general stress management, energy conservation techniques, and aerobic exercise. Figure 25–5 provides a framework for the management of activity intolerance in clients with cancer. Optimal nutritional intake is crucial to improving activity tolerance, particularly for clients with anemia. These clients may also require oxygen therapy or red blood cell transfusions to correct poor oxygenation of vital organs such as the heart and the lungs.

Altered Nutrition: Less Than Body Requirements

Planning: client goals. The goal is that the client will manage nutrition in a way that facilitates health and comfort.

Interventions: nonsurgical management
Food intake. Nursing interventions promote the intake of foods high in protein and calories. The DeWys

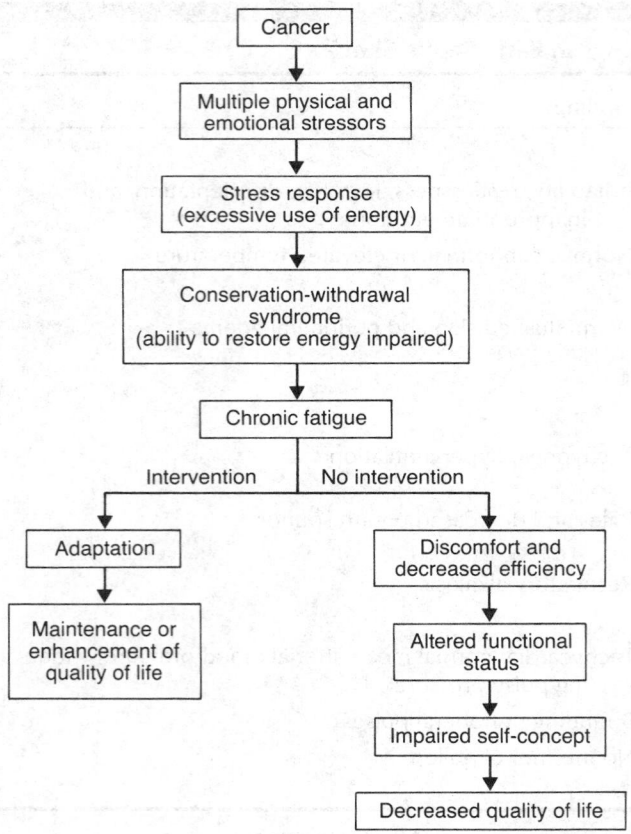

Figure 25 – 5

Framework for management of activity intolerance in clients with cancer. (From Aistars, J. [1987]. Fatigue in the cancer patient: A conceptual approach to a clinical problem. *Oncology Nursing Forum, 14*[6], 25 – 30.)

formula used to calculate minimal daily caloric requirements is simple and useful in setting dietary goals to maintain present body weight.

Body weight (in kilograms) $\times$ 20 + 1100
= minimum calories/day

According to this formula, a client weighing 56.8 kg might use 2236 kcal as a daily intake goal. Protein requirements for clients with cancer range from 1.5 to 4 g/day, depending on the level of stress.

Oral feedings. Many clients have discovered that one particular meal is tolerated better than others. This is most often breakfast. Incorporating as much as one-third of daily nutrients into the best-tolerated meal might be helpful in reaching daily intake goals. The addition of nonfat dry milk and egg whites to baked goods, the use of cream and ice cream with milk beverages, and the addition of whole eggs, egg whites, or yolks to fruit beverages can bolster nutrient intake. Vitamin supplementation might be prescribed. Small, frequent meals as opposed to the traditional two or three major meals can be helpful for clients who experience early satiety.

Taste changes can be countered by varying the spices used in cooking and marinating meats in sweet sauces, sweet wines, or fruit juice. Cooking odors can be noxious and, if possible, are avoided.

Oral hygiene before and after meals is particularly important for the promotion of adequate intake as well as the integrity of the oral cavity. Although there are many oral hygiene products marketed, the most important action of any product is fostered by consistent use as opposed to individual ingredients. Controversy exists as to oral care solutions. Normal saline solutions (1 tsp of baking soda and 1 tsp of salt in 1 qt of water) are favored. Solutions of hydrogen peroxide, usually mixed as half hydrogen peroxide and half water, are sometimes used, but the caustic action of peroxide makes this particular remedy subject to criticism. Commercially available mouthwashes are usually alcohol based and damage the oral mucosa.

Probably the most frequently found bedside care item is the lemon-glycerin swab, which is erroneously used for oral care and dry mouth. Most providers of cancer care believe that this particular item should be banned from use in the care of people with cancer, if not totally eliminated from the health care market. Glycerin is a great bacterial medium, encouraging dental caries and other oral problems. Lemon flavor and citric acid are astringent and therefore defeat the intent of providing anything but transient relief. New mouth-moistening agents are available that simulate human saliva and are the preferred intervention for dry mouth or xerostomia.

The National Cancer Institute (NCI) has published *Eating Hints: Recipes and Tips for Better Nutrition During Cancer Treatment* (NCI, 1987). This booklet is available free of charge through the NCI. It provides eating hints based on interviews with people with cancer dealing with nausea and vomiting, anorexia, stomatitis and xerostomia, GI symptoms, and fatigue. This booklet should be made available to all clients with cancer.

Enteral feedings. If the client is unable to take in adequate nutrients, but the digestive system is functional, enteral support may be beneficial. High-calorie, high-protein, high-fiber supplements are commercially available and can be offered in addition to whatever the client is able to take in or can be administered by nasogastric, gastrostomy, or jejunostomy tube feeding. In addition to energy needs, clients receiving complete enteral support require at least 1500 to 2000 mL of free water per day. Actual fluid recommendations may be altered on the basis of renal function studies (Chap. 13).

Parenteral nutrition. If the digestive system is *not* functional, total parenteral nutrition (TPN) may be considered for clients with treatable cancer or other conditions that result in anatomic or functional loss of the gut. TPN solutions provide total caloric, fluid, protein, electrolyte, vitamin, and trace mineral requirements. TPN also incorporates intermittent administration of IV fat emulsions (Chap. 13).

Drug therapy. Nausea, vomiting, and pain often require pharmacologic interventions to control their effects on altered nutrition. Pain occurring with stomatitis can be treated with local therapy, such as application of lidocaine (Xylocaine) before meals. Round-the-clock systemic therapy might also be needed.

Nausea and vomiting are treated with different classes of antiemetic agents. These agents interrupt different pathways involved in nausea and vomiting. Drug classes commonly incorporated in antiemetic protocols include anticholinergics, antihistamines, phenothiazines, substituted benzamides, butyrophenones, cannabinoids, and benzodiazepines. Protocols using drugs of several types combine actions to enhance antiemetic effects. Antiemetic regimens should be started before the administration of chemotherapeutic drugs with the potential to cause nausea and vomiting or before the initiation of radiation therapy involving fields encompassing the stomach or small bowel. Antiemetic drugs are administered 30 to 60 minutes before chemotherapy and then at appropriate intervals throughout the expected duration of nausea and vomiting.

Many of the antiemetic drugs have significant side effects, which may be cumulative. Phenothiazines and benzodiazepines are often given together, and both groups of drugs can cause sedation. Theoretically, sedation could put the client who is nauseated and vomiting at risk for aspiration. Clinically, this is not a major problem in clients receiving chemotherapy, but the nurse monitors the level of sedation for all clients.

The cholinergic metoclopramide (Reglan) is a commonly used drug; it is capable of causing extrapyramidal side effects, such as restlessness, involuntary movements, rigidity, or tremors. The nurse reports the occurrence of these side effects immediately and obtains an order to administer diphenhydramine hydrochloride (Benadryl), which reverses these effects.

Diarrhea

Clients who receive radiation therapy to the bowel, or who receive certain types of chemotherapy, may experience diarrhea.

Planning: client goals. The goal is that the client's diarrhea will resolve.

Interventions: nonsurgical management. A low-residue diet and fluid intakes of at least 2000 mL are encouraged unless these measures are contraindicated by the presence of congestive heart failure (Chap. 45). Clients are asked to keep track of the number of loose, watery stools daily and report them. Clients experiencing diarrhea as a result of abdominal radiation often require antidiarrheal drugs, such as loperamide (Imodium) or diphenoxylate with atropine (Lomotil), two to four times per day until the diarrhea stops. See Chapter 45 for other interventions for diarrhea.

Constipation

Constipation is a common problem for clients with cancer because of impaired mobility, poor nutrition, or the use of narcotic analgesics.

Planning: client goals. The goal is that the client will have a bowel movement without discomfort at least every 3 days.

Interventions: nonsurgical management. Interventions depend on the frequency of constipation, which is related to the cause. Clients who experience minimal impaired mobility or poor nutrition might control constipation with high-fiber diets or occasional laxatives. Clients who require narcotic analgesics, especially those who take them on a round-the-clock basis, often require a laxative such as senna (Senokot) prophylactically with additional laxatives such as milk of magnesia as needed. If clients do not respond to this treatment, a more potent laxative, such as mineral oil or magnesium citrate, is given with or without a phospho-soda (Fleet) enema.

Impaired Physical Mobility

Planning: client goals. The goal is that the client will demonstrate the maximal physical mobility that is consistent with her/his disease and therapy.

Interventions: nonsurgical management. In the absence of pain, pathologic fracture, or spinal cord compression, clients are encouraged to avoid bed rest and ambulate as much as possible. Clients may require the assistance of another individual, a cane, or a walker, depending on their motor strength. Clients not able to ambulate are encouraged to be out of bed by being lifted or pivoting to a chair. This will help decrease calcium resorption from bone, avoiding hypercalcemia.

If bone metastasis is present, treatment decisions are related to symptom management and prevention of complications. Radiation therapy offers most clients partial or complete relief of pain.

Interventions: surgical management. If a pathologic fracture occurs, internal fixation of the bone is sometimes required. Internal fixation or joint replacement may be performed prophylactically for major weight-bearing structures, such as the femur or acetabulum.

All clients with bone metastases are taught signs and symptoms of hypercalcemia, as described on page 595. Clients are also taught to report pain, weakness, or change of sensation in extremities, which might indicate spinal cord compression.

Pain

Many clients remain pain free in the early stages of cancer. Eventually, half experience pain. In terminal cancer, pain is a problem for 75% of all clients, and 25% of all clients with cancer die without adequate pain control (Foley, 1985). It is estimated that of all clients with cancer, only 10% should have pain that is difficult (although not impossible) to control (Billings, 1985).

Planning: client goals. The goal is that the client will verbalize consistent relief, control, or absence of pain.

A well-designed, thorough, multidisciplinary pain management program is an integral part of each client's overall plan of care. An important aspect of a pain management program is for the client to learn that pain management is usually an achievable goal and that trusted resources are available to assist in accomplishing that goal.

Pain management allows the client to tolerate diagnostic and therapeutic approaches required to treat the cancer. For those with advanced cancer, appropriate pain management allows the client to function at the comfort level he/she chooses and to die relatively pain free.

The management of cancer pain may be directed at control of the pathologic events causing the pain or at symptomatic control of the perception of pain. Symptomatic control is achieved by elevating the pain threshold. Attempts to achieve this goal pharmacologically involve the use of analgesics.

Interventions: nonsurgical management

Analgesics. Analgesics are an integral part of the multidisciplinary approach to pain management. Principles of analgesic therapy for clients with cancer are outlined in Table 25–9. Peripheral and central pain perception and electrical and neurochemical substances regulating pain are involved in a series of complex interactions resulting in the perception of pain. The interaction of factors forms the basis for the efficacy of a wide variety of analgesic interventions aimed at minimizing undesirable effects and maximizing pain relief.

Oral analgesics afford the client the most normal and mobile life style and are therefore preferable to other routes of administration. Parenteral therapy is reserved for clients who are unable to take medication via oral or rectal routes.

Analgesics that are often selected for mild to moderate pain include salicylates, acetaminophen, or nonsteroidal anti-inflammatory drugs.

As pain becomes more severe, narcotic analgesics are given in addition to nonnarcotic analgesics. Weak narcotic agents, exemplified by codeine, are used with aspirin or acetaminophen for additive effects. Weak narcotic agents and nonnarcotics have a clinical ceiling. If pain control is not achieved with two or three incremental increases, morphine or equivalent agents (hydromorphine hydrochloride, levorphanol tartrate, or methadone hydrochloride) are used.

Morphine is available in solutions of varying concentrations, tablets, and sustained-release tablets for oral administration; rectal suppositories; and parenteral solutions. Clients receive more effective pain control if they adhere to a regular administration schedule consistent with the preparation, route of administration, and duration of action of the drug. Each dose of the analgesic should be delivered before the effects of the previous dose are diminished. Dosing increments are increased by 50% after 24 to 48 hours of suboptimal pain relief.

Morphine dosage is increased as needed because, unlike weaker narcotic and nonnarcotic analgesics, morphine does not appear to have a ceiling (Twycross, 1982).

New preparations and routes of administration are constantly being developed to maximize analgesic effects, minimize side effects, and promote optimal levels of activity for the client. Some analgesics are available for sublingual administration, which can be useful when the client has GI obstruction, limited venous access, or reduced muscle mass.

Continuous IV and subcutaneous infusions of narcotic analgesics use various systems to deliver small amounts of drugs at a constant rate, providing consistent plasma levels of analgesic and lower daily requirements. Infusions are titrated to the individual needs of the client. Reported dosages for morphine in adults range from 1 to 750 mg/hour (Foley, 1984). Hospital or institutional policies guide the nurse in monitoring continual narcotic infusions. The nurse assesses the respiratory rate and level of consciousness of the client, titrating the continuous narcotic infusion according to hospital policy. Respiratory depression is a potential side effect of all narcotics. However, it occurs infrequently in clients taking narcotics for chronic pain. As clients develop a tolerance to the analgesic effects of narcotics, they also develop a tolerance to the respiratory depressant effect. Other side effects of narcotic analgesics include nausea, vomiting, constipation, and lethargy. The client's metabolic function, especially hepatic and renal functions, which are largely responsible for the excretion of analgesics, should be monitored. Slow excretion could result in toxicities or overdosing. Some nonsteroidal agents have been associated with renal failure, proteinuria, and increased blood urea nitrogen (BUN) and creatinine levels.

Nutritional and hydration status is important. Hypoalbuminemia requires adjustment of the dosage of analgesics that bind with protein (e.g., aspirin). The free concentration of aspirin is directly related to the serum albumin level.

Adjuvant analgesics. Several categories of drugs produce analgesia by mechanisms that are not clear.

TABLE 25–9   Principles of Analgesic Therapy for Clients with Cancer

Establish an etiologic diagnosis for each pain.

Remember not all cancer pain is responsive to analgesia.

Use adequate analgesic doses.

Use oral preparations whenever possible.

Administer analgesics prophylactically to prevent pain — no prn orders.

Titrate analgesic doses individually for adequate control.

Anticipate side effects (e.g., constipation or nausea).

Never use placebos.

Reproduced by permission of *The Western Journal of Medicine* (Brigden, M. L., & Barnett, J. B., A practical approach to improving pain control in cancer patients, 1987, *146*[5], pp. 580–584).

NURSING RESEARCH

Controlled-Release Analgesia Is More Effective Than Short-Acting Analgesia for Cancer Pain, but It Is Not Without Side Effects.

Ferrell, B., Wisdom, C., Wenzl, C., & Brown, J. (1989). Effects of controlled-release morphine on quality of life for cancer pain. *Oncology Nursing Forum, 16*(4), 521–525.*

Recent attention has been given to the use of quality of life as an outcome measure in cancer research. Quality-of-life assessment is considered critical in drug trials or intervention studies.

The purposes of this study were to apply the concept of quality of life as an outcome measure in a clinical trial of analgesics and to compare the effectiveness of controlled-release analgesia with that of short-acting analgesia. Specific questions addressed whether there is a significant difference in pain and quality of life between clients receiving controlled-release analgesia and those receiving short-acting analgesia. The investigation also continued the development of the quality-of-life concept and demonstrated the reliability and the validity of the quality-of-life tool.

Five instruments were used to evaluate quality of life outcomes. A Demographic Data Tool was used to describe the study subjects. The second tool, the Pain Experience Measure, is an interview guide to obtain information regarding the client's descriptions of pain, as well as drug and nondrug pain relief methods. The third instrument was the Present Pain Intensity Scale from the McGill-Melzack Pain Questionnaire. The Karnofsky Performance Scale provided an additional measure of function. The fifth instrument, the City of Hope Medical Center Quality of Life Survey, represented areas of psychologic well-being, general symptom control, specific symptom control, and social support.

Subjects were 83 adult clients with chronic cancer pain. The setting was the oncology units of two mid-western hospitals. Subjects were randomly assigned to one of two experimental groups. Group I consisted of clients receiving short-acting analgesics who remained on those drugs. Group II consisted of clients who changed from short-acting analgesics to controlled-release analgesics. A third group provided a control and consisted of clients who had been receiving controlled-release analgesia for at least 2 wk and who remained on that drug.

Results of the study indicate that pain and quality of life are related and that controlled-release analgesia has an impact on many indicators of quality of life. Outcomes of successful pain management may be that the client maintains social and psychosocial adjustment and maintains physical strength, all previously demonstrated to relate to clients' perceptions of quality of life. Study results also indicated that clients receiving controlled-release analgesics experienced more distress related to nausea and bowel disturbances than did clients receiving short-acting analgesics.

Critique. This study expanded on previous studies designed to explore the relationship of pain and quality of life, to develop tools to define these concepts, and to contribute to the art of providing comfort to people in pain. This paper did not define a baseline level of pain nor differentiate pain syndromes, but instead data were based only on the site of primary disease and current treatment status. The study results seemed to assert that controlled-release analgesia is a more effective pain management strategy than the use of short-acting analgesics, but this might be confusing in that the clients continuing to receive short-acting analgesics were less compliant with their pain control regimen. The success of the pain management strategy is dependent on compliance and self-care strategies, which might be more significant than the type of drug preparation offered. Compliance factors, including self-care abilities, caregiver abilities, and level of understanding, were not incorporated into the study design and could be significant variables.

Overall, the study provided valuable data for consideration in designing plans of care for clients at risk for experiencing pain. The study represented a relatively new area of exploration, in that it is an attempt to define factors relating to quality of life, which is an abstract concept. The study was not intended to be definitive regarding pain management strategies, but instead provided support for consideration of an option in pain management strategies.

Possible nursing implications. Nurses have the opportunity to influence quality of life by making advances in developing and implementing pain management strategies. The issue of compliance is critical in pain management, and continued exploration is needed in this area. Clients and their families need to comprehend dosage schedules and regimens to achieve optimal effect of the pain management strategy. The role of the nurse is to educate, support, and follow up with clients to ensure compliance. The issue of distressing GI symptoms related to the more successful pain control strategy is important as well. Clients should not have to sacrifice pain control to avoid other side effects. Continued research in pain intervention strategies and quality-of-life outcomes will contribute to the nursing art of providing comfort and enhancing quality of life.

* This paper received the Oncology Nursing Society/Upjohn Company–sponsored Quality of Life Award, 1989.

Anticonvulsant agents, phenothiazines, butyrophenones, tricyclic antidepressants, antihistamines, amphetamines, steroids, and levodopa have provided analgesic effects according to anecdotal reports.

Anesthetics. Short-acting and long-acting anesthetics are used for temporary and diagnostic nerve blocks. Phenol, alcohol, and cryoanalgesia (freezing) are agents used for permanent nerve blocks. These agents demyelinate the nerve, producing secondary nerve degeneration. Permanent nerve blocks are used when a temporary block has demonstrated efficacy in relieving pain. These procedures are undertaken only after consideration of the loss of sensory function effected by the block of several nerves to achieve the desired anesthesia. Epidural and intrathecal nerve blocks can produce motor weakness and autonomic dysfunction associated with urinary or rectal incontinence, motor weakness, or paresthesias.

Chemical hypophysectomy and intermittent inhalation of nitrous oxide have provided pain relief, particularly in the terminal stages of disease or for widespread bone metastases.

Behavioral approaches. Relaxation techniques (progressive muscle relaxation and guided imagery), biofeedback, hypnosis, music, art, and recreation promote a sense of control for clients and serve as a diversion. Clients can learn these skills and use them independently. Other methods of pain control cited by clients include use of heat, massage, exercise, positional changes, limited activity, and distraction techniques.

Cutaneous stimulation. Transcutaneous electrical nerve stimulation (TENS) utilizes an impulse generator and skin surface electrodes to provide an electrical stimulus. The cutaneous stimulus is believed to excite myelinated afferents, which in turn inhibit the transmission of nociceptive information. TENS may be helpful in management of phantom limb pain, postherpetic neuralgia, and other types of pain associated with peripheral nerve damage.

Heat or cold applications may also be tried and continued if effective (Chap. 7).

Interventions: surgical management. Neurosurgical management of pain is one of many interventions that must be considered in designing care for the client with pain. Nerve blocks involve the injection of an anesthetic into specific nerve tracts. Cordotomy, either in conjunction with a laminectomy (open technique) or percutaneous (without an incision, but rather via a needle under radiographic guidance), can be a useful palliative measure. A cordotomy involves the surgical interruption of the anterior lateral spinothalamic tract in the cervical or thoracic region. It is useful in managing unilateral pain sensations below the waist. Cordotomy successfully relieves pain initially, but, by the end of 1 year, many clients report return of the pain. Other neurosurgical techniques involve the placement of epidural, intrathecal, and intraventricular catheters for drug delivery.

Reasons for inadequate management of pain include failure to recognize and implement established methods for cancer pain management and a "lack of systematic teaching of health-care students and professionals about pain" (Twycross, 1982). It is reported that physicians as well as nurses with flexible medication orders undermedicate for pain at least 50% of the time. Responsibility for poor pain management can have many origins, including health care professionals who exhibit ignorance and apathy, pharmacists who do not stock or release analgesics, physicians who refuse to order them, or nurses who falsely assume that only a few clients really experience pain. In addition, nurses, physicians, and clients fear that the client may become addicted. Some responsibility for inadequate pain relief may belong to the persons experiencing the pain — their inability to identify or communicate their own needs or simply their desire not to impose on the nursing staff. Systematic teaching must include skills in determining the cause of pain, assessment of pain, and knowledge of analgesic pharmacology as well as the influences of cultural and attitudinal biases.

Potential for Impaired Skin Integrity

Clients who receive certain types of chemotherapy or radiation are at risk for developing skin reactions.

Planning: client goals. The goal is that the client will not experience skin reactions that result in discomfort or necessitate modification of treatment regimens.

Interventions: nonsurgical management. Many of the cutaneous problems related to chemotherapy are self-limiting and do not require intervention. Extravasation is a serious problem, which needs to be anticipated. It can usually be prevented by nursing measures. These include assessing for good blood return in the IV catheter before and intermittently throughout the administration of chemotherapeutic agents.

Management of extravasation is a subject for ongoing research. General management is directed at removing excess vesicant from the tissue and inhibiting further drug distribution, minimizing the inflammatory reaction, and neutralizing the vesicant agent. Specific interventions are sometimes employed for certain vesicants that have extravasated. For example, after removal of the IV tubing, hyaluronidase (Wydase) dissolved in saline has been shown to be effective when injected into the extravasation site caused by vincristine or vinblastine. More often however, there is no known antidote. Frequently, intervention is limited to terminating the infusion and removing IV tubing immediately after extravasation is recognized.

Clients who are receiving external radiation are taught to avoid or reduce irritation, friction, temperature extremes, chemical irritants, tapes, and dressings on treatment sites to prevent skin reactions. Agents or factors that should be avoided include warm packs, heat lamps, mentholated rubs, metallic talcs, antiperspirants, and exposure to sunlight or sun lamps.

Interventions for clients who experience skin reactions are directed toward promoting skin integrity and minimizing morbidity associated with the reaction. There is no consensus on the best method to accomplish these goals. Substances recommended to manage erythema and dry desquamation include cornstarch, baby powder, baby oil, Eucerin, xiphamide (Aquaphor), anhydrous lanolin, and other alcohol- and menthol-free moisturizers.

Interventions for moist desquamation include application of moisture vapor–permeable and hydrocolloid dressings. Other occlusive, nonadherent materials are also used. Topical antibiotics should be used only in the presence of proven infection. Topical steroids can relieve itching associated with dry desquamation, but reduce blood flow to the skin, resulting in increased susceptibility to injury.

Skin reactions can be *dose-limiting toxicities* (side effects that limit the body's ability to tolerate the full, prescribed treatment). Inadequate treatment may be a factor in insufficient response to treatment and treatment failure. Prevention of morbidity associated with skin reactions is essential, not only for comfort but also to avoid compromising treatment.

Interventions: surgical management. Severe necrosis may occur after an extravasation. Débridement and skin grafting may be required as long-term treatment for necrosis.

Impaired Gas Exchange

Clients with primary or metastatic lung cancer often experience impaired gas exchange as a result of tumor cells or pleural effusions.

Planning: client goals. The goal is that the client will experience improved gas exchange and relief of dyspnea.

Interventions: nonsurgical management. Interventions are dependent on the location or the effects of the tumor. The primary concern in the treatment of malignant pleural effusions is the palliation of symptoms. Some malignant pleural effusions, such as those that occur with metastatic breast cancer or lymphoma, may respond to systemic chemotherapy, hormonal treatment, or irradiation. If this therapy is ineffective in resolving the effusion or if the disease is advanced, local therapy is indicated. Local therapy is directed toward evacuating pleural fluid, re-expanding the lung, and obliterating the pleural space. Chest tubes are inserted and connected to water seal drainage and suction. Sclerosing agents are added to the pleural cavity through the chest tube immediately or after a period of drainage. Agents used to sclerose the pleural surfaces include antineoplastic agents (nitrogen mustard, 5-fluorouracil, bleomycin, and triethylenethiophosphoramide [thioTEPA]), radioisotopes of gold or phosphorus, and tetracycline. The chest tube is clamped for varying lengths of time, depending on the sclerosing agent used. After the release of the chest tube clamp, water seal drainage and mild suction is continued until pleural drainage is less than 60 mL/24 hours.

For malignant lung tumors without pleural effusions, external radiation is often used to relieve dyspnea. Tumors within the bronchi may be treated with intraluminal radiation or brachytherapy.

Interventions: surgical management. Surgical pleurectomy is infrequently performed for malignant pleural effusions. Tumors obstructing the bronchi can often be treated with bronchoscopic laser photocoagulation.

Sexual Dysfunction

Certain cancer treatments risk sexual dysfunction.

Planning: client goals. The goal for this diagnosis is that the client will (1) adapt to changes in sexual function and (2) express himself/herself sexually in a satisfying way.

Interventions: nonsurgical management. The potential for sexual dysfunction resulting from surgery, radiation, or chemotherapy is discussed with the client before the treatment is instituted. Many clients for whom infertility is a concern may wish to consider depositing sperm in a sperm bank or making embryo or egg donations before undergoing therapy. In vitro fertilization and embryo transfer provide alternatives for suitable candidates.

Many clinicians recommend the use of birth control during and for 2 years after cancer chemotherapy because of the mutagenic potential of these agents on ovarian and gonadal cells. Diaphragms and condoms are recommended methods. Oral contraceptives are often contraindicated because of the hormonal dependence of some tumors and the increased susceptibility to yeast infections associated with progesterone. Intrauterine devices may cause bleeding and infection and should be avoided.

For clients experiencing discomfort during sexual expression, lubricants may help to alleviate discomfort. Vaginal stenosis may be relieved by progressive dilation using a vaginal obturator.

Interventions appropriate for sexual dysfunction from any cause include giving the client permission to have sexual thoughts and feelings, providing information that may assist in changing or adding approaches to sexual expression, and referring clients to an appropriate resource for specific interventions.

Interventions: surgical management. Ovariopexy, the surgical displacement of ovaries, may prevent ovarian exposure to irradiation by moving the ovaries outside the anticipated treatment field.

Ineffective Individual Coping

The client's perception of the disease and its treatment may cause ineffective coping, as may the possibility of rejection, disfigurement, treatment failure, and death.

Planning: client goals. The goal is that the client will use coping strategies to assist in adapting to the disease and its treatment.

Interventions: nonsurgical management. Coping involves discovering how to balance acceptance and resist the constraints and changes imposed by cancer. The nurse plays a vital role in the lives of clients by helping them learn coping techniques and strategies. Nurses help the client and significant others manage stress by promoting the coping abilities that the client is using or those that were described by Friedman (1980) (see the accompanying Guidelines feature). The nurse needs to remember that each individual will cope in his/her own way, depending on perceptions of the situation, personality, and past experience. Interventions specific to other coping strategies, body image disturbance, and loss, death, and dying are discussed in Chapters 6, 9, and 11.

GUIDELINES ■ Interventions to Promote Client Use of Friedman's 10 Coping Strategies

1. Seeking Information

Share information consistent with the needs of the client.

Facilitate open communication with health care professionals and significant others.

Provide a gentle exposure to reality.

Encourage clients to participate in the decision-making process.

Promote knowledge of choices that can be made.

Promote acknowledgment of possible outcomes of the cancer.

2. Turning to Others for Support

Provide opportunities for one-to-one and group contacts with other clients with cancer.

Facilitate verbalization of fears and anxieties and sharing of these feelings.

Facilitate support from other resources: physician, nurses, clergy or spiritual leader, relatives, friends, and social workers.

3. Following Orders, Having Faith in Professionals

Encourage self-care to the extent possible.

Promote relief of distressing physical and emotional symptoms.

Promote the client's dignity and privacy.

4. Denying, Escaping

Avoid forcing details on the client.

Encourage sharing of anxieties and fears.

Encourage verbalization and use of the word "cancer."

5. Finding Meaning for the Disease and Making the Most of Life

Promote the client's involvement in work and activity.

Promote the quality of life, as well as the prolongation of life.

5. Finding Meaning for the Disease and Making the Most of Life (Continued)

Emphasize what the client "has" instead of what he/she has "lost."

Encourage ways the client may assist others with cancer.

6. Preparing for Death

Facilitate acceptance of the limitations imposed by cancer.

Assist or facilitate preparation for death if there is little hope for survival.

7. Returning to Employment

Facilitate resumption of accustomed roles: arrange for physical and occupational therapy, ensure assistance from community resources, facilitate rehabilitation processes, and so forth.

Promote understanding and knowledge among coworkers.

8. Relying on Past Coping Strategies

Assess past experiences and coping strategies or skills that might be implemented.

9. Tension-Reducing Strategies: Smoking, Drinking, Overeating, and Focusing on Physical Symptoms

Facilitate implementation of relaxation and meditation techniques.

Promote new activities.

Facilitate meeting new people.

Provide opportunities to express fears, anxieties, and feelings.

10. Blaming One's Self, Someone, or Something Else

Explore with the client possible inaccuracies associated with the belief that someone or something is to blame.

Promote freedom of expression.

From Friedman, B. D. (1980). Coping with cancer: A guide for health care professionals. *Cancer Nursing, 3,* 105–110.

Oncologic Emergencies

Cancer has historically been considered a chronic disease. However, a number of acute conditions associated with cancer result in significant morbidity and mortality. These conditions often require immediate intervention and thus are termed oncologic emergencies. Early recognition of these conditions is essential to avoid devastating consequences.

Paraneoplastic syndromes are conditions associated with cancer that occur as a result of (1) a tumor product, (2) destruction of normal tissue by tumor, or (3) unknown mechanisms associated with the tumor. Some paraneoplastic syndromes, such as hypercalcemia and syndrome of inappropriate antidiuretic hormone (SIADH), are also considered oncologic emergencies.

Sepsis. Sepsis (septicemia) is a condition in which microorganisms (bacteria, viruses, fungi, rickettsia, or protozoa) invade the blood stream. Septic shock is a life-threatening consequence of sepsis and a frequent cause of death in clients with cancer. Clients with cancer are at increased risk for infection and sepsis because they frequently are granulocytopenic, may have altered hematopoietic function, and often have impaired defense mechanisms (see page 564). Early recognition and treatment of infection or sepsis are essential for client survival. See page 586 and Chapter 17 for assessment and management of clients with sepsis and septic shock.

Hypercalcemia. Hypercalcemia occurs in approximately 10% of all clients with cancer, most frequently in those with breast cancer, lung cancer, or multiple myeloma (Bunn & Ridgway, 1989). Immobilization is also related to the development of this condition. Early signs include lethargy, anorexia, nausea, vomiting, constipation, polyuria, nocturia, and dehydration. Total serum calcium levels exceed 10.5 mg/dL, and the severity of symptoms is dependent on the serum calcium level.

Emergency treatment consists of hydrating the client with IV fluid, followed by IV administration of a diuretic such as furosemide (Lasix). Mithramycin (Mithracin) may be administered intravenously in clients with severe hypercalcemia. Diphosphanates, such as etidronate (Didronel), have recently been given with good effect. For long-term maintenance, treatment of the malignancy is necessary.

Syndrome of inappropriate antidiuretic hormone. SIADH is most often associated with small cell lung cancer, but can also occur with other primary neoplasms. It is manifested by hyponatremia, serum hyposmolality, and urinary hyperosmolality characterized by continued sodium excretion. The usual clinical presentation is one of water retention progressing to water intoxication. Mild symptoms, including weakness, muscle cramps, anorexia, and fatigue, occur with serum sodium levels ranging from 115 to 120 mEq/L. Progression of symptoms is related to water retention and is characterized by alterations in mentation, such as irritability, disorientation, confusion, combativeness, lethargy, psychotic behavior, and extrapyramidal signs. As sodium levels approach 110 mEq/L, seizure, coma, and death may follow unless the condition is quickly reversed.

Diagnostic criteria for SIADH include hyponatremia and hyposmolality; urine osmolality greater than 11 mOsm/kg of water; and urinary sodium concentration greater than 20 mEq/24 hours.

Initial treatment involves fluid restriction, which may be successful if the syndrome has been recognized early. Diuretics, such as furosemide, may be tried. In cases of severe hyponatremia, hypertonic saline, such as 3% saline, might be cautiously administered intravenously. Demeclocycline and lithium are other agents for the treatment of SIADH. Careful measurement of fluid intake and output and daily weights is essential. Long-term fluid restriction may be necessary to prevent recurrence.

Spinal cord compression. Spinal cord compression resulting from metastatic tumors is an emergency situation requiring prompt diagnosis and treatment if permanent neurologic sequelae are to be prevented.

Spinal cord compression occurs with direct tumor invasion of the spinal canal or vertebral collapse from tumor invasion. Tumors may be primary, but are more commonly metastatic. Spinal cord compression is associated with lung, prostate, breast, and colon cancers; lymphoma; or multiple myeloma. Back pain at the level of the tumor occurs in most cases and usually precedes neurologic changes. Neurologic deficits are related to the level of compression and include numbness; tingling; loss of urethral, vaginal, and rectal sensation; and motor weakness. If paralysis develops, it is usually irreversible. Ten per cent of cord compression is cervical; 50%, thoracic; 20%, lumbar; and 20%, sacral or coccygeal (cauda equina). Myelography or MRI is done to assess blockage. Interventions most commonly include radiation therapy with IV corticosteroids. Emergency decompression laminectomy may be indicated in clients with rapidly progressing signs and symptoms.

Disseminated intravascular coagulation. Disseminated intravascular coagulation (DIC) is an abnormal activation of coagulation and fibrinolysis involving destruction of coagulation factors and platelets. It occurs in many severe illnesses, including neoplastic disease. DIC is observed in cancer of all cell types, but is most often associated with leukemia; adenocarcinomas of lung, pancreas, stomach, and prostate; and metastatic neoplasms, particularly those with metastases involving the liver.

It is thought that tissue thromboplastin from tumors triggers DIC. DIC is commonly associated with gram-negative sepsis, but the initiating mechanism in that situation is different.

DIC is characterized by concurrent bleeding and thrombosis. Bleeding from multiple sites is the most common symptom, and it ranges in degree from mild bleeding to fatal hemorrhage. Thrombotic vascular occlusion and organ ischemia are manifested by pain, neurologic alterations (syncope, hemiplegia, cerebrovascular accident–like symptoms, and paresthesias), dyspnea, tachycardia, oliguria, and bowel necrosis.

A clotting profile reveals prolonged prothrombin time and partial thromboplastin time, decreased fibrinogen and platelet levels, and elevated fibrin split products.

Interventions are focused on treating the underlying cause. Sepsis is commonly associated with DIC in clients with cancer, and possible sources for infection should be assessed. Broad-spectrum antibiotics may be administered pending results of an infection work-up. Supportive treatment for DIC may include the administration of fresh frozen plasma, platelets, or red blood cells (Chap. 67).

Hyperuricemia. Clients with cancer are at risk for elevated serum uric acid from tumor breakdown. Although this can occur spontaneously, it is more commonly seen in clients receiving chemotherapy for rapidly proliferating hematologic malignancies, such as leukemia, lymphoma, and myeloma. Hyperuricemia after chemotherapy is called tumor lysis syndrome.

The danger of hyperuricemia is that it can lead to acute urate nephropathy, a form of renal failure characterized by uric acid crystallization in the distal tubules of the kidneys. Acute urate nephropathy is a danger when the serum uric acid level is greater than 15 mg/dL.

Prophylactic treatment of clients receiving chemotherapy for rapidly proliferating tumors can prevent this oncologic emergency. Allopurinol (Zyloprim) is given to inhibit uric acid formation in clients with hematologic malignancies on the day of, or 1 day prior to, initiation of chemotherapy. Serum uric acid and creatinine are assessed prior to and following chemotherapy. If hyperuricemia develops, intravenous fluids, sodium bicarbonate, and allopurinol are administered. Individuals with uric acid levels greater than 25 to 30 mg/dL may require hemodialysis.

Superior vena cava syndrome. Compression of the superior vena cava (SVC) can lead to a painful and life-threatening emergency. SVC compression is usually related to bronchogenic cancers (primarily small cell cancer), but lymphoma, metastatic breast, and GI cancers can also cause this syndrome (Fig. 25–6). The rapidity with which symptoms appear is related to the cancer cells' proliferative rate: cancers with high growth rates cause rapid onset of symptoms. SVC syndrome, however, often develops gradually, with early symptoms being only slightly noticeable as distended neck veins, venous engorgement of the anterior chest wall, or cough.

If compression increases, collateral vessels cannot provide adequate blood return from the upper body. Vascular congestion may lead to edema of the face and the hands, severe dyspnea, cerebral anoxia, hemorrhage, and strangulation from edema of the glottis and

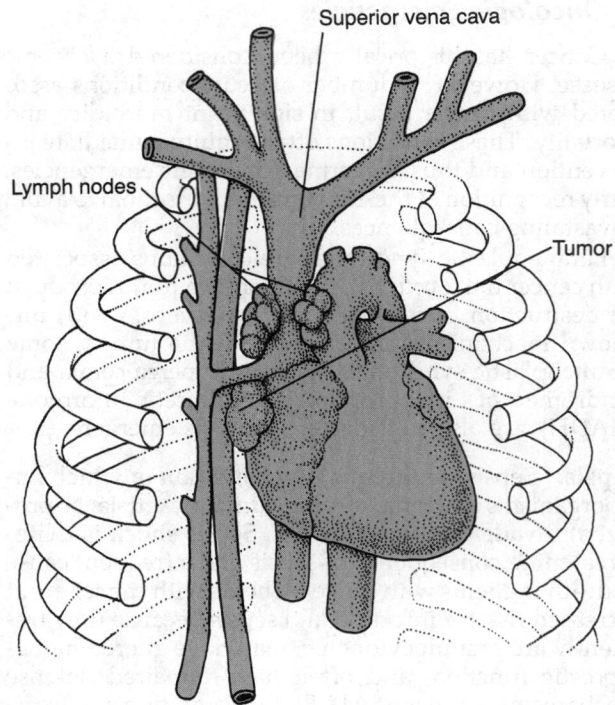

Figure 25–6

Compression of the superior vena cava in SVC syndrome. (From Varricchio, C. [1985]. Clinical management of superior vena cava syndrome. *Heart and Lung, 14,* 411.)

the airways. Death can result if compression is not relieved.

Radiation to the site of the compression is standard therapy for SVC syndrome. Compression related to rapidly dividing tumors (e.g., small cell lung cancer and lymphoma) may also respond well to chemotherapy. The nurse assists the client in keeping the upper body upright to facilitate breathing and venous drainage. Oxygen and diuretics may also be administered for temporary relief of symptoms until radiation or chemotherapy takes effect.

Pericardial effusion and cardiac tamponade. Pericardial effusion and cardiac tamponade can occur in traumatic and other nonmalignant situations, but the most common cause of pericardial effusion is cancer. Malignant pericardial disease can be caused by direct extension of a thoracic tumor or hematogenous metastasis from a distant primary site. Lung and breast cancers are most often associated with malignant pericardial effusion. Lymphoma, leukemia, and melanoma have tendencies to metastasize to the heart in general and the pericardium in particular.

Pericarditis can also be a complication of direct irradiation to the heart in doses exceeding 4000 rad. Radiation-induced pericarditis may develop months or years after completion of the course of radiation. However, with modern treatment planning and delivery of radiation therapy, radiation-induced pericarditis is extremely rare. Pericardial effusion occurs when the volume of pericardial fluid exceeds 20 mL. Chronic accumulation allows gradual stretching and adaptation. If there is gradual accumulation, the pericardium may accommodate as much as 2500 mL before tamponade occurs. Rapid accumulation does not allow adaptation. Accumulation in a short period of time of even 100 mL of fluid causes sudden increases in intrapericardial pressure associated with profound circulatory derangement. Fluid accumulation prevents full expansion of the heart during diastole, resulting in increased and nearly equal intracardiac pressures in all chambers of the heart, with decreased cardiac output and systolic blood pressure.

The classic signs of cardiac tamponade include high central venous pressure, arterial hypotension, and distant, muffled heart sounds. However, all three signs are exhibited in less than 50% of clients experiencing tamponade. Other signs and symptoms include shortness of breath with normal breath sounds, weakness, diaphoresis, and alterations in mental status. As tamponade progresses, blood pressure is unobtainable by cuff and pulses are not palpable. Without immediate intervention, cardiac arrest is imminent.

Pericardial effusion can be visualized and monitored on echocardiograms, providing a sensitive indicator of impending cardiac tamponade. The immediate therapeutic goal is to support compensatory responses while definite treatment is planned. Effusion and mild tamponade may be relieved with corticosteroids and diuretics. Definitive treatment for severe tamponade with impending circulatory collapse is removal of pericardial fluid, most often by pericardiocentesis. Alternative measures for long-term control may be achieved with drainage and instillation of a sclerosing agent, insertion of a pericardial window, or pericardiectomy.

■ Discharge Planning

Clients with cancer are often hospitalized for diagnostic work-ups and primary surgical treatment of the cancer. Radiation therapy and chemotherapy are most often administered on an ambulatory (outpatient) basis. Exceptions to this include individuals who are extremely ill or those experiencing complications of cancer, such as spinal cord compression. Clients with hematologic malignancies are usually hospitalized for their chemotherapy because of the high risk of infection after immunosuppression. Clients on complicated chemotherapy protocols or complicated antiemetic protocols might also be hospitalized for their therapy. Aside from these brief interludes in the hospital, and outpatient treatment, clients optimally manage their care at home.

Clients being treated with external radiation therapy commonly receive outpatient therapy every Monday through Friday, for up to 6 weeks, depending on the site of cancer and the treatment protocol. Clients being treated with chemotherapy commonly receive their medications every 28 days in the outpatient setting, with visits at 2-week intervals for laboratory evaluation.

Clients with advanced cancers are commonly hospitalized before being discharged for hospice care in an extended care facility or at home.

Home Care Preparation

The nurse assesses the home environment for safety and nutritional resources in terms of the client's performance status (see Table 25-3). The availability of transportation to health care facilities is assessed because these clients have frequent interactions with health care providers. If the client is receiving narcotic analgesics for pain, the nurse notifies the pharmacy about the client's prescription needs. Many pharmacies are reluctant to stock narcotics and special arrangements might need to be made to meet these needs.

Client/Family Education

Clients with cancer and their families often require information about malignant transformation and factors known to be associated with the development of cancer. The nurse stresses that the development of cancer is a multifactorial process and there are many different types of cancer. Educational needs are specific to the client's particular type of cancer and treatment modalities for that cancer. Clients who have undergone surgical tumor resections require teaching about wound care. Education for clients receiving chemotherapy is based on the known adverse effects related to the chemotherapy being administered and the client's white blood cell, platelet, hemoglobin, and hematocrit counts. If granulocytopenia is an expected adverse effect, clients are taught to avoid crowds, practice good hygiene, and rinse their mouths after meals and at bedtime with a salt-and-water or normal saline solution. Clients at risk for thrombocytopenia are instructed regarding bleeding precautions. Clients with low hemoglobin and hematocrit levels are instructed to report any shortness of breath or chest pain and to practice energy conservation techniques. Clients who are expected to experience alopecia (hair loss) are advised to obtain a wig before the hair loss occurs. Clients are encouraged to consult with their insurance company regarding possible reimbursement for wigs. The nurse informs clients that hair will grow back after all chemotherapy is complete but that color and texture might be slightly different.

Clients experiencing external radiation on an outpatient basis are taught that the effects of treatment are generally localized to the treatment site but that fatigue is common. The client and the family are told that external radiation does not make the client radioactive.

For clients experiencing pain, continuity of care is essential to maintain pain control. The clients and the family are given written schedules for medications that have proved effective in controlling the pain during hospitalization. If continuous infusion devices are being used, clients and their families are taught how to load and operate them before discharge from the hospital. Follow-up nursing care is arranged for clients receiving continuous narcotic infusions to ensure continuity of medication administration. These clients and others often have long-term vascular access devices, which require insertion site care and flushing as recommended by the manufacturer.

All clients are taught to report any new or changed symptoms, such as pain, change in motor or sensory function, nausea, vomiting, diarrhea, constipation, fever, or chills. Because nutrition is an area of concern for clients with cancer, all clients are taught the importance of eating a well-balanced diet.

Psychosocial Preparation

Clients with cancer often fear that malignancies will return after treatment. The nurse consults with the health care team and the client regarding expected responses to treatment. Clients' concerns and fears are acknowledged by the nurses, who also reinforce the possibility of a response to treatment if this is realistic. Most often clients are encouraged to resume a functional life style, with continued participation or reintegration into the community. Clients with advanced metastatic disease who do not respond to treatment are supported in their preparation for death.

Health Care Resources

Resources for clients and families affected by cancer are well established. The ACS sponsors the programs such as I Can Cope and Cansurmount, which provide information and emotional support to clients and their families. Other support programs focus on specific types of cancer (e.g., those of the Leukemia Society of America) or specific physiologic needs for clients with cancer (e.g., Reach to Recovery). Many support groups and services are available for clients with advanced disease, including inpatient or outpatient hospice care (Chap. 11). The nurse provides the client and the family with written information regarding available resources. Follow-up care, including nursing care, physical therapy, or nutritional support, is arranged by the nurse when indicated.

 Evaluation

On the basis of the identified nursing diagnoses, the nurse evaluates the care provided for the client at risk for or with cancer. The expected outcomes include that the client

1. Identifies risk factors for cancer development, methods to avoid these risk factors, and practices to detect cancer
2. Demonstrates total or partial response to treatment

3. Demonstrates absence of infection
4. Demonstrates absence of bleeding
5. Demonstrates tolerance to valued activities
6. Maintains weight and nutritional status
7. Demonstrates formed bowel movements at least every 3 days without discomfort
8. Participates in all ADL independently
9. Verbalizes consistent relief from, control of, or absence of pain
10. Demonstrates intact skin integrity
11. Demonstrates PO_2 of 70 mmHg or greater and PCO_2 of less than 45 mmHg without dyspnea
12. States that he/she is able to meet sexuality needs
13. Demonstrates and states effective coping strategies

SUMMARY

Nursing care of the client experiencing cancer incorporates a variety of traditional and nontraditional nursing care methods. Cancer can occur in any age group, involving single or multiple organ systems or physiologic functions. Cancer elicits psychologic and emotional responses and is a threat to human relationships, values, financial security, and role responsibilities. Cancer also affects the family and friends of the individual who has cancer. Given these variables, it is impossible to include all cancer-related nursing interventions in this discussion. Instead, general concepts and guidelines for dealing with the more common issues and problems have provided the focus for this chapter.

Knowing what to look for (what to suspect) when caring for people with cancer may avert a crisis, hospitalization, and death. Nurses must maintain a high index of suspicion and be aware of and prepared to treat the multiple physiologic and psychologic responses to malignant disease. Constant vigilance and readiness on the part of nurses affords many people with cancer opportunities to live longer and have a better quality of life.

IMPLICATIONS FOR RESEARCH

Cancer is the second leading cause of death in the United States, and some speculate that it will surpass heart disease in death toll by the year 2000 (Greenwald & Sondik, 1986; Silverberg & Lubera, 1989). The National Cancer Institute has set a goal to reduce cancer mortality 50% by the year 2000 (Greenwald & Sondik, 1986). Three approaches have been identified to meet this goal: that health care providers induce individuals to stop smoking, that health care providers induce individuals to eat properly, and that state-of-the-art cancer treatment be implemented throughout the country.

To help achieve these goals, nursing research needs to be conducted to answer the following questions:

1. What methods are most effective in teaching clients the risks of smoking and improper diet related to cancer?
2. What tactics lead clients to stop smoking and change diets to decrease cancer risks?
3. How effective are nurse screening programs in decreasing cancer mortality?
4. How cost efficient are screening programs when compared with treatment of advanced disease?
5. How accessible is state-of-the-art cancer treatment to clients?

REFERENCES AND READINGS

Ahles, T. A. (1985). Psychological approaches to the management of cancer-related pain. *Seminars in Oncology Nursing, 1*, 141–146.

Aistars, J. (1987). Fatigue in the cancer patient: A conceptual approach to a clinical problem. *Oncology Nursing Forum, 14*(6), 25–30.

Amenta, M. O., & Bohnet, N. L. (1986). *Nursing care of the terminally ill.* Boston: Little, Brown.

American Cancer Society. (1989). *Cancer facts and figures— 1989.* Atlanta: Author.

American Cancer Society (1990). *Cancer facts and figures— 1990.* Atlanta: Author.

American Nurses' Association and Oncology Nursing Society. (1987). *Standards of oncology nursing practice.* Kansas City: Author.

Andejeski, J. (1985). Injury potential for, related to anemia. In J. C. McNally, J. C. Stair, & E. T. Somerville (Eds.), *Guidelines for cancer nursing practice* (pp. 152–158). Orlando, FL: Grune & Stratton.

Baldwin, P. D. (1983). Epidural spinal cord compression secondary to metastatic disease: A review of the literature. *Cancer Nursing, 6*, 441–446.

Barbour, L. A., McGuire, D. B., & Kirchhoff, K. T. (1986). Nonanalgesic methods of pain control used by cancer outpatients. *Oncology Nursing Forum, 13*(6), 56–60.

Barry, S. A. (1989). Septic shock: Special needs of patients with cancer. *Oncology Nursing Forum, 16*(1), 31–35.

Bayuk, L. (1985). Relaxation techniques: An adjunct therapy for cancer patients. *Seminars in Oncology Nursing, 1*, 147–150.

Bender, C. M. (1987). Chemotherapy. In C. R. Ziegfeld (Ed.), *Core curriculum for oncology nursing* (pp. 225–235). Philadelphia: W. B. Saunders.

Benedict, S. (1989). The suffering associated with lung cancer. *Cancer Nursing, 12*, 34–49.

Berdjis, C. C. (1971). *Pathology of irradiation.* Baltimore: Williams & Wilkins.

Billings, A. J. (1985). *Outpatient management of advanced cancer.* Philadelphia: J. B. Lippincott.

Bingham, E. (1985). Hazards to health workers from antineoplastic drugs [Letter]. *New England Journal of Medicine, 313*, 1220–1221.

Blank, J. J., Longman, A. J., & Atwood, J. R. (1989). Perceived home care needs of cancer patients and their caregivers. *Cancer Nursing, 12*, 78–84.

Bloomer, W. D., & Hellman, S. (1975). Normal tissue responses to radiation therapy. *New England Journal of Medicine, 293*, 80–83.

Boyd, J. D. (Ed). (1989). *The Cancer Letter, 15*(25), 4–5.

Brandt, B. A. (1984). A nursing protocol for the client with neutropenia. *Oncology Nursing Forum, 11*(2), 24–28.

Brigden, M. L., & Barnett, J. B. (1987). A practical approach to improving pain control in cancer patients. *Western Journal of Medicine, 146*, 580–584.

Brown, J. (1987). Chemotherapy. In S. L. Groenwald (Ed.), *Cancer nursing principles and practices* (pp. 320–344). Boston: Jones & Bartlett.

Brown, M. L., Carrieri, V., Janson-Bjerklie, S., & Dodd, M. J. (1986). Lung cancer and dyspnea: The patient's perception. *Oncology Nursing Forum, 13*(5), 19–24.

Brown, S. J. (1986). Assessing albumin levels with hypercalcemia [Letter]. *Oncology Nursing Forum, 13*(3), 16.

Bucholtz, J. (1987). Radiation therapy. In C. R. Ziegfeld (Ed.), *Core curriculum for oncology nursing* (pp. 207–224). Philadelphia: W. B. Saunders.

Bunn, P. A., & Ridgway, E. C. (1989). Paraneoplastic syndromes. In V. T. DeVita, Jr., S. Hellman, & S. A. Rosenberg (Eds.), *Cancer: Principles and practice of oncology* (3rd ed., pp. 1896–1940). Philadelphia: J. B. Lippincott.

Butler, J. H. (1980). Nutrition and cancer: A review of the literature. *Cancer Nursing, 3*, 131–136.

Cairns, J. (1978). *Cancer: Science and society.* San Francisco: W. H. Freeman.

Carlson, A. C. (1985). Infection prophylaxis in the patient with cancer. *Oncology Nursing Forum, 12*(3), 56–64.

Catalano, R. B. (1985). Pharmacology of analgesic agents used to treat cancer pain. *Seminars in Oncology Nursing, 1*, 126–140.

Clark, R. A., Tyson, L. B., Gralla, R. J., & Kris, M. G. (1989). Antiemetic therapy: Management of chemotherapy-induced nausea and vomiting. *Seminars in Oncology Nursing, 5*(Suppl. 1), 53–57.

Clarke, D. E., & Sandler, L. S. (1989). Factors involved in nurses' teaching breast self-examination. *Cancer Nursing, 12*, 41–46.

Cloak, M. M., Connor, T. H., Stevens, K. R., Theiss, J. C., Alt, J. M., Matney, T. S., & Anderson, R. W. (1985). Occupational exposure of nursing personnel to antineoplastic agents. *Oncology Nursing Forum, 12*(5), 33–39.

Coleman, C. N. (1989). Modification of radiotherapy by radiosensitizers and cancer chemotherapy agents. I. *Radiosensitizers, 16*, 169–175.

Concilus, E. M., & Bohachick, P. A. (1984). Cancer: Pericardial effusion and tamponade. *Cancer Nursing, 7*, 391–398.

Dalton, J. A. (1989). Nurses' perceptions of their pain assessment skills, pain management practices, and attitudes toward pain. *Oncology Nursing Forum, 16*(2), 225–231.

Dalton, J. A., Toomey, T., & Workman, M. R. (1988). Pain relief for cancer patients. *Cancer Nursing, 11*, 322–328.

Dirksen, S. R. (1989). Perceived well-being in malignant melanoma survivors. *Oncology Nursing Forum, 16*(3), 413–416.

Dolan, J. A., Fitzpatrick, M. L., & Herrmann, E. K. (1983). *Nursing in society: A historical perspective* (15th ed.). Philadelphia: W. B. Saunders.

Dolan, L., Kennelly, L., Manigan, M., Murphy, P. P., & Yurkovic, C. (1985). Mobility, impaired physical, related to lymphedema. In J. C. McNally, J. C. Stair, & E. T. Somerville (Eds.), *Guidelines for cancer nursing practice* (pp. 195–199). Orlando, FL: Grune & Stratton.

Donovan, M. I. (1985). Nursing assessment of cancer pain. *Seminars in Oncology Nursing, 1*, 109–115.

Entrekin, N. (1987). Breast cancer. In C. R. Ziegfeld (Ed.), *Core curriculum for oncology nursing*. Philadelphia: W. B. Saunders.

Fisher, S. G. (1983). The psychosocial effects of cancer and cancer treatment. *Oncology Nursing Forum, 10*(22), 63–68.

Foley, K. M. (1984). A review of pain syndromes in patients with cancer. *The Management of Cancer Pain Symposium.* Nutley, NJ: Roche Laboratories.

Foley, K. M. (1985). The treatment of cancer pain. *New England Journal of Medicine, 313*, 84–95.

Foote, M., Sexton, D. L., & Pawlik, L. (1986). Dyspnea: A distressing sensation in lung cancer. *Oncology Nursing Forum, 13*(5), 25–31.

Friedman, B. D. (1980). Coping with cancer: A guide for health care professionals. *Cancer Nursing, 3*, 105–110.

Galvin, J. M. (1981). The physics of radiation therapy equipment. *Seminars in Oncology, 8*, 18–37.

Gentzsch, P. (1985). Mobility, impaired physical, related to spinal cord compression. In J. C. McNally, J. C. Stair, & E. T. Somerville (Eds.), *Guidelines for cancer nursing practice* (pp. 202–206). Orlando, FL: Grune & Stratton.

Gentzsch, P. (1988). Patient controlled analgesia: An effective form of pain control with cancer patients [Abstract]. *Oncology Nursing Society, 13th Annual Congress Proceedings.*

Goodman, M. (1989). Managing the side effects of chemotherapy. *Seminars in Oncology Nursing, 5*(Suppl. 1), 29–52.

Grant, M. (1987). Nausea, vomiting, and anorexia. *Seminars in Oncology Nursing, 3*, 227–286.

Greenfield, L. D., Herman, M. W., & Patrick, J. (1978). Radiation safety precautions with 131-iodine therapy. *Cancer Nursing, 1*, 279–384.

Greenwald, P., & Sondik, E. J. (Eds.). (1986). Cancer control objectives for the nation: 1985–2000. *National Cancer Institute Monograph, 2.*

Haeuber, D. (1989, May). Recent advances in the management of biotherapy-related side effects: Flu-like syndrome. *Symposium: The Biotherapy of Cancer—III,* San Francisco. Nutley, NJ: Roche Laboratories.

Hanucharurnkul, S. (1989). Predictors of self-care in cancer patients receiving radiotherapy. *Cancer Nursing, 12*, 21–27.

Hassey, K. M. (1985). Demystifying care of patients with radioactive implants. *American Journal of Nursing, 85*, 788–792.

Hassey, K. M. (1988). Pregnancy and parenthood after treatment for breast cancer. *Oncology Nursing Forum, 15*(4), 439–444.

Haylock, P. J. (1987). Breathing difficulty: Changes in respiratory function. *Seminars in Oncology Nursing, 3*, 293–298.

Haylock, P. J., & Hart, L. K. (1979). Fatigue in patients receiving localized radiation. *Cancer Nursing, 2*, 461–467.

Hellman, K. (1987). Introduction. In K. Hellman & S. K. Carter (Eds.), *Fundamentals of cancer chemotherapy* (pp. 1–7). New York: McGraw-Hill.

Herberth, L., & Gosnell, D. J. (1987). Nursing diagnosis of oncology nursing practice. *Cancer Nursing, 10*, 41–51.

Hilderley, L. J. (1987). Radiotherapy. In S. L. Groenwald (Ed.), *Cancer nursing principles and practices* (pp. 320–344). Boston: Jones & Bartlett.

Howard-Ruben, J. (1985). Sexual dysfunction related to disease process and treatment. In J. C. McNally, J. C. Stair, & E. T. Somerville (Eds.), *Guidelines for cancer nursing practice* (pp. 268–273). Orlando, FL: Grune & Stratton.

Irwin, M. M. (1987). Patients receiving biological response modifiers: Overview of nursing care. *Oncology Nursing Forum, 14*(Suppl.), 32–37.

Johnson, J. (1982). Call me healthy. The Mara Mogensen Flaherty Memorial Lecture. *Oncology Nursing Forum, 9*(3), 73–76.

Jones, L. A. (1987). Superior vena cava syndrome. An oncologic complication. *Seminars in Oncology Nursing, 3*, 211–215.

Kaplan, M. (1989). Investigation of age as a prognostic factor in early stage invasive cancer of the cervix: Implications for nursing. *Cancer Nursing, 12*, 177–182.

Keller, J. F., & Blausey, L. A. (1988). Nursing issues and management in chemotherapy-induced alopecia. *Oncology Nursing Forum, 15*, 603–607.

Knobf, M. K., Mullen, J. C., Xistris, D., & Mortiz, D. A. (1983). Weight gain in women with breast cancer receiving adjuvant chemotherapy. *Oncology Nursing Forum, 10*(2), 28–33.

Lamb, M. A. (1985). Sexual dysfunction in the gynecologic oncology patient. *Seminars in Oncology Nursing, 1*, 9–17.

Loescher, L. J. (1988). Cancer: The nurse's role in primary prevention. *Innovations in Oncology Nursing, 4*(3), 3–9.

Looney, W. B., & Hopkins, H. A. (1989). Modification of radiotherapy by radiosensitizers and cancer chemotherapeutic agents. 11. Cancer chemotherapeutic agents. *Seminars in Oncology, 16*, 176–179.

Lydon, J. (1986). Nephrotoxicity of cancer treatment. *Oncology Nursing Forum, 13*(2), 68–76.

McMillan, S. C. (1989). The relationship between age and intensity of cancer-related symptoms. *Oncology Nursing Forum, 16*(2), 237–241.

McNally, J. C., Stair, J. C., & Somerville, E. T. (Eds.). (1985). *Guidelines for cancer nursing practice.* Orlando, FL: Grune & Stratton.

Moore, C. L. (1984). Hyperthermia: A modern experiment in cancer treatment. *Oncology Nursing Forum, 11*(2), 31–35.

Moore, C. L. (1984). Nursing management of the patient receiving local or regional hyperthermia. *Oncology Nursing Forum, 11*(3), 40–43.

Nail, L. M., & King, K. B. (1987). Fatigue. *Seminars in Oncology Nursing, 3,* 257–262.

National Cancer Institute. (1987). Eating hints: Recipes and tips for better nutrition during cancer treatment (Publication No. 87–2079). Bethesda: Author.

National Council on Radiation Protection. (1976). Radiation protection for medical and allied personnel (Report No. 48). Washington, DC: U.S. Government Printing Office.

Nurses Clinical Library. (1985). *Neoplastic disorders.* Springhouse, PA: Springhouse Corp.

Occupational Safety and Health Administration. (1986). *Work practice guidelines for personnel dealing with cytotoxic (antineoplastic) drugs* (OSHA Instructional Publication 8-1.1). Washington, DC: Office of Occupational Medicine.

Oldham, R. K. (1984). Biologicals and biologic response modifiers. Fourth modality of cancer treatment. *Cancer Treatment Reports, 68,* 221–231.

Oncology Nursing Society. (1988). *Cancer chemotherapy guidelines* (Modules I–V). Pittsburgh, PA: Author.

Oncology Nursing Society. (1989a). *Biological response modifier guidelines: Recommendations for nursing education and practice.* Pittsburgh, PA: Author.

Oncology Nursing Society. (1989b). *Standards of oncology nursing education.* Pittsburgh, PA: Author.

Patterson, W. B. (1983). Principles of surgical oncology. In P. Rubin (Ed.), *Clinical oncology: A multidisciplinary approach* (6th ed., pp. 30–38). New York: American Cancer Society.

Petrelli, N. J. (1982). *Malignant pleural effusions: An overview. What's new in cancer care.* San Francisco: West Coast Cancer Foundation.

Piper, B. F. (1989, May). Recent advances in the management of biotherapy-related side effects: Fatigue. *Symposium: The Biotherapy of Cancer—III,* San Francisco. Nutley, NJ: Roche Laboratories.

Piper, B. F., Lindsey, A. M., & Dodd, M. J. (1987). Fatigue mechanisms in cancer patients: Developing nursing theory. *Oncology Nursing Forum, 14,* 17–23.

Poe, C. M., & Radford, A. I. (1985). The challenge of hypercalcemia in cancer. *Oncology Nursing Forum, 12*(6), 29–34.

Poe, C. M., & Taylor, L. M. (1989). Syndrome of inappropriate antidiuretic hormone: Assessment and nursing implications. *Oncology Nursing Forum, 16*(3), 373–381.

Poland, J. M. (1987). Comparing Moi-Stir to lemon-glycerin swabs. *American Journal of Nursing, 87,* 422, 424.

Reheis, C. E. (1985). Neutropenia: Causes, complications, treatment, and resulting nursing care. *Nursing Clinics of North America, 20,* 219–225.

Ritter, M. A. (1981). The radiobiology of mammalian cells. *Seminars in Oncology, 8,* 3–17.

Root, R. (1985). Infectious diseases: pathogenetic mechanisms and host responses. In L. Smith & S. Their (Eds.), *Pathophysiology—the biochemical principles of disease* (pp. 164–172). Philadelphia: W. B. Saunders.

Rubin, P., & Casarette, G. W. (1968). *Clinical radiation pathology.* Philadelphia: W. B. Saunders.

Salmon, S. E. (1988). Malignant disorders. In S. A. Schroeder, M. A. Krupp, & L. M. Tierney (Eds.), *Current medical diagnosis and treatment.* Norwalk, CT: Appleton & Lange.

Sanford, A. C. (1985). Injury, potential for, related to thrombocytopenia. In J. C. McNally, J. C. Stair, & E. T. Somerville (Eds.), *Guidelines for cancer nursing practice* (pp. 147–151). Orlando, FL: Grune & Stratton.

Schag, C. C., Heinrich, R. L., & Ganz, P. A. (1984). Karnofsky performance status revisited: Reliability, validity, and guidelines. *Journal of Clinical Oncology, 2,* 187–193.

Schain, W. S. (1988). A sexual interview is a sexual intervention. *Innovations in Oncology Nursing, 3*(4), pp. 2, 3, 15.

Schwab, C. W., Phillips, K. F., Royer, M. G., & Worthen, D. B. (1986). The cost-effectiveness of enteral nutritional support in the DRG era. *Contemporary Orthopaedics, 13*(2), 31–39.

Scogna, D. M., & Schoenberger, C. S. (1982). Biological response modifiers: An overview and nursing implications. *Oncology Nursing Forum, 9*(1), 45–49.

Sedhom, L. N., & Yanni, M. I. Y. (1985). Radiation therapy and nurses' fears of radiation exposure. *Cancer Nursing, 8,* 129–134.

Selevan, G., Lindbohm, M., Hornung, R., & Hemminki, K. (1985). A study of occupational exposure to antineoplastic drugs and fetal loss in nurses. *New England Journal of Medicine, 313,* 1173–1178.

Shell, J. A., Stanutz, F., & Grim, J. (1986). Comparison of moisture vapor permeable (MVP) dressings to conventional dressings for management of radiation skin reactions. *Oncology Nursing Forum, 13*(1), 11–16.

Sheppard, K. C. (1986). Care of the patient with superior vena cava syndrome. *Heart and Lung, 15,* 636–641.

Silverberg, E., & Lubera, J. (1989). Cancer statistics, 1989. *CA: A Cancer Journal for Clinicians, 39,* 3–20.

Stellman, J. M., Aufiero, B. M., & Taub, R. N. (1984). Assessment of potential exposure to antineoplastic agents in the health care setting. *Preventive Medicine, 13,* 245–255.

Strauman, J. J. (1988). The nurse's role in the biotherapy of cancer: Nursing research of side effects. *Oncology Nursing Forum, 15*(Suppl.), 35–39.

Strohl, R. A. (1983). Nursing management of the patient

with cancer experiencing taste changes. *Cancer Nursing,* 6, 353–359.

Strohl, R. A. (1984). Understanding taste changes. *Oncology Nursing Forum, 11*(3), 81–84.

Strohl, R. A. (1987). Goals and principles of treatment. In C. R. Ziegfeld (Ed.), *Core curriculum for oncology nursing* (pp. 195–198). Philadelphia: W. B. Saunders.

Strohl, R. A. (1988). The nursing role in radiation oncology: Symptom management of acute and chronic reactions. *Oncology Nursing Forum, 15*(4), 429–434.

Suppers, V. J., & McClamrock, E. A. (1985). Biologicals in cancer treatment: Future effects on nursing practice. *Oncology Nursing Forum, 12*(3), 27–32.

Szopa, T. J. (1987). Surgery. In C. R. Ziegfeld (Ed.), *Core curriculum for oncology nursing* (pp. 199–206). Philadelphia: W. B. Saunders.

Tait, N., & Aisner, J. (1989). Nutritional concerns in cancer patients. *Seminars in Oncology Nursing, 5*(Suppl. 1), 58–62.

Tannock, I. F. (1987). Cell kinetics and cancer chemotherapy. In K. Hellman & S. K. Carter (Eds.), *Fundamentals of cancer chemotherapy* (pp. 7–18). New York: McGraw-Hill.

Tannock, I. F. (1989). Principles of cell proliferation: Cell kinetics. In V. T. DeVita, Jr., S. Hellman, & S. A. Rosenberg (Eds.), *Cancer: Principles and practice of oncology* (3rd ed., pp. 3–13). Philadelphia: J. B. Lippincott.

Tenenbaum, L. (1989). *Cancer chemotherapy: A reference guide.* Philadelphia: W. B. Saunders.

Twycross, R. G. (1982). Morpine and diamorphine in the terminally ill patient. *Acta Anaesthesiologica Scandinavica, 74*(Suppl.), 128–134.

Valentine, A. S., & Stewart, J. A. (1983). Oncologic emergencies. *American Journal of Nursing, 83,* 1282–1285.

Vitello-Cicciu, J., & Eagan, J. S. (1988). Data acquisition from the cardiovascular system. In M. R. Kinney, D. R. Racka, & S. B. Dunbar (Eds.), *AACN's clinical reference for critical-care nursing* (2nd ed., pp. 530–570). New York: McGraw-Hill.

Walligora-Serafin, B. (1988, March). Prediction of emotional distress in newly diagnosed cancer patients [Abstract]. *Association of Community Cancer Centers 14th National Meeting.* Rockville, MD: Association of Community Cancer Centers.

Walters, P. (1990, February). Chemo: A nurse's guide to action, administration, and side effects. *RN,* pp. 52–66.

Weisman, A. D. (1979). *Coping with cancer.* New York: McGraw-Hill.

Welch-McCaffrey, D. (1988a). Metastatic bone cancer. *Cancer Nursing, 11,* 103–111.

Welch-McCaffrey, D. (1988b). Preventing cancer: New concerns for an old disease. *Innovations in Oncology Nursing, 4*(3), pp. 1, 10–11.

West, J. B. (1985). *Respiratory physiology—the essentials* (3rd ed.). Baltimore: Williams & Wilkins.

Wilson, M. E., & Williams, H. A. (1988). Oncology nurses' attitudes and behaviors related to sexuality of patients with cancer. *Oncology Nursing Forum, 15*(1), 49–53.

Winningham, M. L., & MacVicar, M. G. (1988). The effect of aerobic exercise on patient reports of nausea. *Oncology Nursing Forum, 15*(4), 447–450.

Woods, N. F., Lewis, F. M., & Ellison, E. S. (1989). Living with cancer: Family experiences. *Cancer Nursing, 12,* 28–33.

Wroblewski, S. S., & Wroblewski, S. H. (1981). Caring for the patient with chemotherapy-induced thrombocytopenia. *American Journal of Nursing, 81,* 746–749.

Yarbro, C. H. (1987). The role of the oncology nurse in cancer chemotherapy practice. In K. Hellman & S. K. Carter (Eds.), *Fundamentals of cancer chemotherapy* (pp. 379–386). New York: McGraw-Hill.

Yarbro, C. H., & Perry, M. C. (1985). The effect of cancer therapy on gonadal function. *Seminars in Oncology Nursing, 1,* 3–8.

Yasko, J. M. (1982). *Care of the client receiving external radiation therapy.* Reston, VA: Reston Publishing.

ADDITIONAL READINGS

Bram, P. J., & Katz, L. F. (1989). A study of burnout in nurses working in hospice and hospital oncology settings. *Oncology Nursing Forum, 16*(4), 555–560.

This study explored work-related variables hypothesized to contribute to burnout in nurses providing care for terminally ill patients. Variations in degree of burnout were identified as related to the perceptions of support in the work setting, nurse-client staffing ratios, the amount of direct nursing care time provided for these clients, and demographic characteristics of the nurses in the study population. The caregivers in the hospital setting experienced more burnout than did those in the hospice setting. The degree of burnout was negatively correlated with the amount of direct care time—negating the notion that burnout is related to providing care to these clients. This study could provide significant data related to administration-staff communication practices and policies, staffing practices, and exploration of the perception of dissonance between nurses' values and the work environment.

Jordan, L. N. (1989). Effects of fluid manipulation on the incidence of vomiting during outpatient cisplatin infusion. *Oncology Nursing Forum, 16*(2), 213–218.

Management of chemotherapy-related side effects, nausea and vomiting in particular, relates to many client problems—diminished nutritional intake, metabolic disturbances, physical and mental deterioration, and loss of self-care ability. The techniques in this study are representative of nursing management directed at diminishing chemotherapy-related nausea and vomiting. By manipulating oral and IV fluid intake, symptoms of vomiting were reduced in this study population, suggesting a relationship between hydration and the incidence of vomiting. Nursing interventions could be established to reduce the client's distress through identification and manipulation of hydration variables that prevent vomiting.

Northouse, L. (1989). A longitudinal study of the adjustment of patients and husbands to breast cancer. *Oncology Nursing Forum, 16*(4), 511–516.

This study describes the psychosocial adjustment of clients and husbands 3 days to 18 months after mastectomy for breast cancer. Many clients and husbands reported moderate to severe distress levels 18 months after surgery, even though role functions were not significantly altered. These results imply that psychosocial adjustment to breast cancer is an ongoing process associated with varying levels of distress for clients and their husbands. Interestingly, stress levels at 18 months were comparable with those at 3 and 30 days postoperatively. The study results also suggest the existence of a group of clients and husbands at higher risk for long-term adjustment problems. Study implications support viewing the impact of cancer from a family systems framework and suggest that nursing concerns need to be ongoing, extending over time. Other studies might be undertaken to identify high-risk characteristics of clients and family members to intervene appropriately and expediently to prevent morbidity associated with high levels of client and family distress.

Oberst, M. T., Thomas, S. E., Gass, K. A., & Ward, S. E. (1989). Caregiving demands and appraisal of stress among family caregivers. *Cancer Nursing, 12,* 209–215.

This exploratory study assessed the demands placed on ambulatory clients and families managing illness and treatment-related side effects at home. Cognitive appraisal models of stress and coping provided the conceptual framework for this study. Study results indicate that considerable time and effort is expended on the part of caregivers, which intensifies and becomes increasingly stressful over time. The possibility of escalating patterns of distress indicates a necessity for periodic reassessment of family coping. Further study is required to evaluate appraisal patterns in longer treatment protocols and to document associated emotional and physical outcomes.

CHAPTER 26

Interventions for Clients with Infectious Diseases

An infectious disease is caused by invasion by a biologic agent. Infectious diseases include those that are considered communicable (e.g., measles, hepatitis, and influenza) and infections that are not contagious (not spread from person to person; e.g., nephritis, pancreatitis, and trichinosis).

Infectious diseases account for about 20% of all acute and chronic clinical diseases seen in ambulatory care settings, with 70% of these being acute respiratory tract illnesses. Infectious diseases that must be reported to the Centers for Disease Control (CDC) are listed in the accompanying Key Features of Disease.

Although effective vaccines and increasingly efficacious antibiotic therapy have made many infectious diseases among the most easily preventable and treatable illnesses, new organisms continue to emerge as causes of human disease. In addition, as people live longer and as improvements in medical technology occur, more invasive procedures are performed and immunosuppressive therapies are increasingly used. Thus, organisms that previously caused no harm can gain access to the body and can cause infection.

THE INFECTIOUS DISEASE PROCESS

DEFINITIONS

A few basic definitions are necessary to provide a framework for the discussion of the infectious disease process. The process of infection requires a *pathogen,* or causative agent, and a susceptible *host,* or recipient of infection. A pathogen is any microorganism that is capable of producing disease in a human. People are surrounded by countless numbers of microorganisms that possess different degrees of *pathogenicity* (ability to cause disease). *Virulence* is often used as a synonym for pathogenicity, but it is related more to the frequency with which disease occurs in persons exposed to the organism (degree of communicability) and the ability to invade and damage a host; it can also be related to the severity of the disease. Attenuated vaccines are made from strains of microorganisms with low virulence. A highly virulent pathogen is one that requires few organisms to be present in a host to cause disease. Another important characteristic of pathogens is *invasiveness,* the ability to spread and grow in the tissues of a host after entrance has occurred.

The vast majority of microorganisms commonly reside in or on the human host without causing disease. Some bacteria are actually beneficial. For example, each body location harbors its own characteristic bacteria, or *normal flora.* One important function of normal flora is to compete with and prevent infection with unfamiliar organisms that attempt to invade a body site. In some instances, microorganisms may be present in the tissues

KEY FEATURES OF DISEASE ■ Infectious Diseases That Must Be Reported to the Centers for Disease Control

Acquired immunodeficiency syndrome (AIDS)

Amebiasis

Anthrax

Aseptic meningitis

Botulism

Brucellosis

Cholera

Diphtheria

Encephalitis, primary infections

Encephalitis, postinfectious

Gonorrhea

Hepatitis A

Hepatitis B

Hepatitis, non-A, non-B

Hepatitis, unspecified

Legionellosis

Leprosy

Leptospirosis

Malaria

Measles (rubeola)

Meningococcal infections

Mumps

Pertussis

Plague

Poliomyelitis, paralytic

Psittacosis

Rabies, human

Rheumatic fever

Rubella (German measles)

Rubella congenital syndrome

Salmonellosis

Shigellosis

Syphilis, primary and secondary

Tetanus

Toxic shock syndrome

Trichinosis

Tuberculosis

Tularemia

Typhoid fever

Typhus fever (Rocky Mountain spotted)

Varicella (chickenpox)

of the host, yet cause neither symptomatic nor subclinical disease. This process is known as *colonization.*

Unfortunately, in many instances, microorganisms behave as *parasites,* that is, the microorganisms live at the expense of their human hosts. In the process of this interaction with its host, the microbe gains some advantage and infection occurs. *Infection* is the establishment of a host-parasite interaction. Infection may be *subclinical,* causing no apparent reaction in the host and thus eliciting no detectable symptoms. Most often, the occurrence of subclinical infection can only be identified by the immune response of the host, demonstrated by a rise in the titer of antibody directed against the infecting agent. Clinically apparent infection in which the host-parasite interaction causes overt injury is accompanied by a myriad of clinical manifestations and is known as *infectious disease.* Disease caused by an infectious agent may range from mild to fatal.

CHAIN OF INFECTION

The development of an infectious disease is dependent on the interplay of a variety of factors, frequently referred to as the chain of infection (Fig. 26–1). Factors that must be present for transmission of infection are the host, pathogen, portal of entry, mode of transmission, and portal of exit. Prevention of the spread of infection is dependent on breaking the chain of infection. This is accomplished by eliminating the organism, providing the host with immunity, or, most often, interrupting the mode of transmission. In the hospital setting this is accomplished by scrupulous hand washing, implementing isolation barriers, using antimicrobial agents, and wearing gloves when handling blood and body fluids.

HOST FACTORS

Several host factors influence the development of infection (see the Key Features of Disease on p. 607). The human body has an efficient system for self-protection from pathogens known as host defense (see later discussion). Breakdown of any of these defense mechanisms may increase the susceptibility of the host to infection.

The client's immune status plays the largest role in determining her/his risk for infection. Congenital abnormalities as well as acquired defects (such as acquired immunodeficiency syndrome [AIDS]) can result in numerous immunologic deficiencies. Such depression of the immune system may render the host particularly susceptible to infection or cripple the host's ability to combat organisms that have gained entry.

Natural immunity is resistance to infection that occurs without previous exposure to an infecting organism. Several host factors influence natural immunity. Age has been frequently cited as a risk factor for the development of infection. Infants and elderly clients are clearly at increased risk. In both these populations, increased

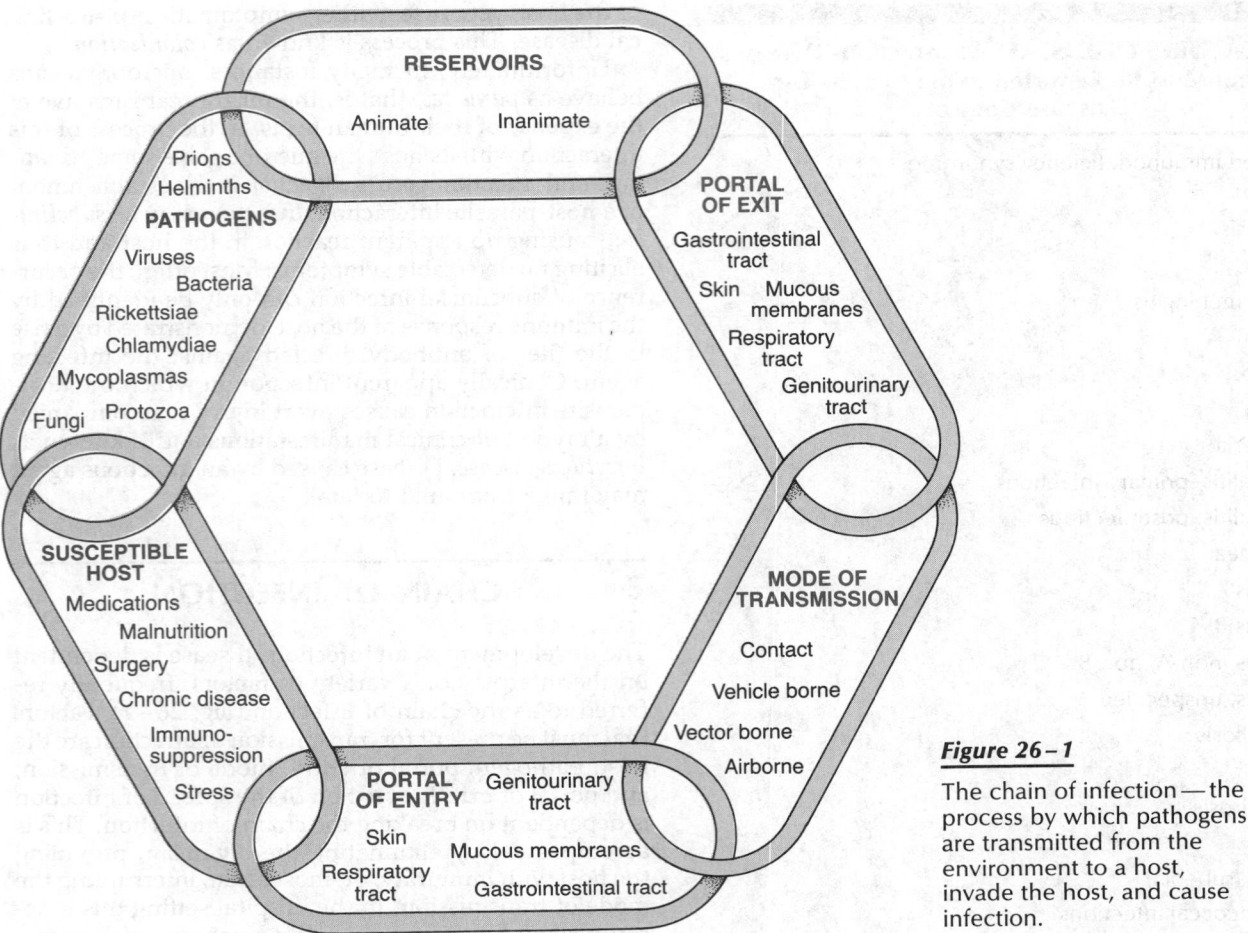

Figure 26–1

The chain of infection — the process by which pathogens are transmitted from the environment to a host, invade the host, and cause infection.

risk for infection probably relates to the decreased ability to mount an adequate immune response. The infant's immune system is immature and is marked by inadequate phagocytic function. Immunity declines in the elderly, especially manifested by decreasing T cell response and diminished primary antibody response. Ethnicity may have some influence on host susceptibility to infection. For example, the mortality rate from tuberculosis in native Americans is three to four times greater than that in Caucasians. Whether genetic differences influence disease resistance or whether apparent differences in immunity are due to other factors, such as nutrition, is still unclear. (See Chap. 23 for general information about the immune system.)

Hormonal factors play a role in the incidence and mortality rate of many infectious diseases. Persons with diabetes mellitus and adrenal insufficiency experience increased numbers of acute and chronic bacterial infections. In addition, during pregnancy, cellular immunity is weakened. This decrease in cellular immunity renders the pregnant woman particularly susceptible to severe complications if infection with any of a number of pathogens occurs, among them influenza virus, group A beta-hemolytic streptococcus, or *Neisseria gonorrhoeae*.

Certain environmental factors may influence an indi-

vidual client's immune status and thus susceptibility to or ability to fight infection. Examples include alcohol consumption, inhalation of toxic chemicals that may suppress bone marrow function, and certain vitamin deficiencies. Malnutrition, especially protein-calorie malnutrition (which may result from chronic illnesses such as end-stage renal disease, hepatic or gastrointestinal [GI] disease, or alcoholism), has clearly been identified as placing a client at increased risk for infection.

Finally, certain types of medical interventions may suppress the immune response. Percutaneous intravascular catheters, urethral catheters, and endotracheal tubes are examples of medical devices that impair or violate normal host defense mechanisms. Also, corticosteroid therapy, chemotherapy for malignancies, and cytotoxic therapy specifically intended to suppress the immune response (e.g., cytoxan for lupus nephritis and cyclosporine in organ transplant recipients) increase the client's risk for infection.

PORTAL OF ENTRY

Organisms may enter the body in a variety of ways (see the Key Features of Disease, p. 608). A number of pathogens enter the body through the *respiratory tract*. Orga-

KEY FEATURES OF DISEASE ■ Host Factors That
Influence Risk of Infection

Host Factor	Increased Risk of Infection
Natural immunity	Congenital or acquired immunodeficiencies
Normal flora	Alteration of normal flora by antibiotic therapy
Age	Infants and elderly clients
Hormonal factors	Pregnancy, diabetes, corticosteroid therapy, and adrenal insufficiency
Phagocytosis	Defective phagocytic function, circulatory disturbances, and neutropenia
Skin/mucous membranes/normal excretory secretions	Break in skin or mucous membrane integrity; interference with flow of urine, tears, or saliva, cough reflex, or ciliary action; changes in gastric secretions
Nutrition	Malnutrition
Environmental factors	Smoking, alcohol consumption, and inhalation of toxic chemicals
Medical interventions	Invasive therapy, chemotherapy, radiation therapy, and steroid therapy; surgery

nisms are contained in contaminated droplets and are sprayed into the air by the talking, coughing, or sneezing of persons with infected oral, nasal, or throat tissues. These droplets are then inhaled by a susceptible host and either localize in the lung or disseminate via the lymphatics or the blood stream to other areas of the body. Examples of organisms that enter the body by the respiratory tract, but often produce distant infection include *Mycobacterium tuberculosis*, influenza virus, and *Neisseria meningitidis* (the organism most commonly responsible for epidemic meningitis).

Some pathogens enter the body through the *gastrointestinal tract*. Of these, some stay in the GI tract and produce disease, for example, enteroviruses, *Giardia*, and the organisms that cause self-limited food poisoning. Others invade the GI tract to produce local, then distant, infection (e.g., *Salmonella enteriditis*); still others produce limited GI symptoms only to disseminate, producing either a systemic infection (e.g., *Salmonella typhi*) or profound involvement of another organ (e.g., hepatitis A virus).

A third portal of entry for microorganisms is the *geni-*

tourinary tract. Urinary tract infection is one of the most common infectious diseases treated in the United States each year. Especially in females, microorganisms (usually normal bacterial flora from the colon) colonize the perineal area, the urethral meatus, and finally the bladder.

Some pathogens, such as *Treponema pallidum*, are able to enter the body through intact *skin* or *mucous membranes*, but most enter through breaks in these normally effective surface barriers. Access is also gained as a result of a medical procedure that creates a break in the normal cutaneous or mucocutaneous barriers. Such medically induced infections are *iatrogenic*; examples include surgical wound infections and catheter-acquired bacteremia.

Finally, microorganisms can gain access to the blood stream. Insects can inject organisms into the blood stream by biting the host, causing infections such as malaria, yellow fever, and Rocky Mountain spotted fever.

PATHOGEN-RELATED FACTORS

Microbial invaders have evolved over time to become more pathogenic. Certain bacterial strains produce materials or structures that facilitate attachment to and invasion of human cells. Bacterial *fimbriae*, or *pili*, are examples of specialized structures that facilitate adherence of microorganisms to the host cell (Fig. 26–2). In several infections, including viral, bacterial, fungal, and parasitic infections, adherence has been shown to correlate with pathogenicity.

Many bacterial and fungal pathogens produce polysaccharide capsular material, which prevents phagocytosis of the organism by host cells. This smooth capsule that surrounds a microorganism, such as the pneumo-

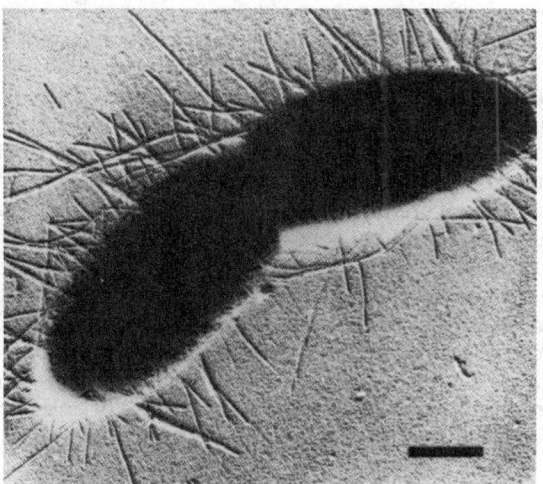

Figure 26–2

Bacterial pili (fimbriae). (From Clegg, D. C., & Old, S. [1979]. Fimbriae of *Escherichia coli* K-12 strain AW405 and related bacteria. *Journal of Bacteriology, 137,* 1010.)

KEY FEATURES OF DISEASE ■ Portals of Entry of Selected Disease-Producing Organisms

Portal of Entry	Infecting Organisms	Resulting Diseases
Respiratory tract	*Neisseria meningitidis*	Meningococcal pneumonia, meningococcal meningitis, meningococcemia
	Cryptococcus neoformans	Cryptococcal meningitis, cryptococcal pneumonia
	Mycobacterium tuberculosis	Tuberculosis
	Influenza A virus	Influenza
	Streptococcus pneumoniae	Pneumococcal pneumonia
	Measles virus (rubeola)	Measles
	Legionella pneumophilia	Legionnaires' disease
	Varicella-zoster virus	Chickenpox
Gastrointestinal tract	*Salmonella enteritidis*	Gastroenteritis
	Salmonella typhi	Typhoid fever
	Giardia lamblia	Diarrhea
	Clostridium botulinum	Botulism
	Poliovirus	Poliomyelitis
	Hepatitis A virus	Hepatitis A
Genitourinary tract	*Neisseria gonorrhoeae*	Gonorrhea
	Chlamydia trachomatis	Lymphgranuloma venereum, cervicitis, urethritis, endometritis
	Enterobacteriaceae (*Escherichia coli*, *Klebsiella* sp., *Serratia* sp., *Proteus* sp.)	Urinary tract infections
Intact skin or mucous membranes	Rhinovirus	Common cold
	Respiratory syncytial virus	Pneumonia, bronchiolitis, tracheobronchitis
	Schistosoma sp.	Schistosome dermatitis (swimmer's disease)
	Herpes simplex virus	Oral or genital herpes
Blood stream	Hepatitis B virus	Hepatitis B
	Plasmodium	Malaria
	Clostridium tetani	Tetanus
	Human immunodeficiency virus (HIV)	AIDS

coccus, essentially enables the organism to "slip away" from the process of phagocytosis.

Survival and continued multiplication of an infecting organism are often accompanied by the production of toxins. *Toxins* are protein molecules that are released by bacteria to affect host cells at a distant site. *Exotoxins* are produced and released by certain bacteria into the surrounding environment. Botulism, tetanus, and diphtheria are examples of diseases attributed to exotoxins. *Endotoxins* are produced in the cell walls of certain bacteria and are released only when cell lysis occurs. Typhoid and meningococcal diseases are examples of endotoxin-caused diseases.

CAUSATIVE AGENTS

Several different classes or groups of organisms produce infection (see the Key Features of Disease, p. 609). Until recently, viruses were thought to be the simplest pathogens producing infection in humans. Recently, however, tiny agents called *prions* have been identified as the pathogens responsible for certain degenerative neurologic diseases in humans and other animals. These agents appear to have no nucleic acids and, as such, are unique.

Other than the prions, *viruses* are the only microbes that have only one type of nucleic acid and lack ribosomes. Viruses are obligate intracellular parasites. They are entirely dependent on the host cell for energy and for the ability to produce proteins and additional nucleic acids, critical elements for the continued production of viral progeny.

Viral illnesses range from those that are little more than nuisances, such as rhinovirus infection producing the common cold, to those that are nearly universally fatal, such as rabies. Infection rates also vary widely,

KEY FEATURES OF DISEASE ■ Organisms That Produce Infection in Humans*

Organism Class	Common Examples	Common Disease Manifestations
Prions		Creutzfeldt-Jakob disease, kuru
Viruses	Poliovirus	Poliomyelitis
	Hepatitis A virus	Hepatitis
	Rhinovirus	Common cold
	Influenza A virus	Influenza
	Mumps virus	Mumps
Chlamydiae	*Chlamydia trachomatis*	Trachoma, lymphogranuloma venereum, conjunctivitis
	C. psittaci	Psittacosis (parrot fever)
Mycoplasmas	*Mycoplasma pneumoniae*	Pneumonia
	Ureoplasma urealyticum	Urethritis
	Mycoplasma hominis	Pyelonephritis, pelvic inflammatory disease
Rickettsiae	*Rickettsia rickettsii*	Rocky Mountain spotted fever
	R. prowazekii	Typhus
	Coxiella burnetii	Q fever
Bacteria	*Staphylococcus* sp.	Superficial skin infections, osteomyelitis, pneumonia, bacteremia
	Streptococcus sp.	Pharyngitis, skin infections, pneumonia
	Neisseria meningitidis	Meningitis
	Escherichia coli	Urinary tract infection
	Pseudomonas aeruginosa	Skin infection, otitis, urinary tract infection
Fungi	*Candida albicans*	Thrush, vaginitis
	Aspergillus sp.	Sinusitis, brain abscess
	Cryptococcus neoformans	Meningitis, pneumonia
	Histoplasma capsulatum	Pneumonia
	Coccidioides immitis	Pneumonia
Protozoa	*Entamoeba histolytica*	Diarrhea, colitis
	Plasmodium sp.	Malaria
	Leishmania sp.	Fever, weight loss, cutaneous lesions
	Toxoplasma gondii	Chorioretinitis, encephalitis
	Pneumocystis carinii	Pneumonia
Helminths	*Ancylostoma duodenale* (hookworm)	Anemia
	Ascaris lumbricoides (roundworm)	Intestinal obstruction
	Enterobius vermicularis (pinworm)	Anal pruritus
	Schistosoma sp. (blood flukes)	Hydronephrosis
	Taenia solium (pork tapeworm)	Epilepsy from cysticercosis

* Organisms are presented in order of increasing complexity.

although nearly all viruses cause some subclinical, or inapparent, infection.

Many, if not most, viral pathogens are capable of infecting hosts with normal defense mechanisms. However, certain viruses, particularly members of the herpesvirus group, produce more frequent recurrences and more severe infections in clients with underlying defects in cell-mediated immunity, including those receiving immunosuppressive chemotherapy and those with AIDS.

Viral infections have been historically considered to be almost entirely community acquired. Recently, it has become apparent that certain viral pathogens are associated with a substantial risk for nosocomial transmis-

sion. Among the viral pathogens with a definite role in nosocomial infection are hepatitis B virus, cytomegalovirus (transfusion related), respiratory syncytial virus, and enteroviruses.

Chlamydiae are intermediate in complexity between viruses and bacteria. These organisms contain both deoxyribonucleic acid (DNA) and ribonucleic acid (RNA), have a cell wall, and contain ribosomes. Unlike bacteria, however, chlamydiae are obligate intracellular parasites in that they are unable to synthesize compounds that can be used as an energy source.

Chlamydiae produce a spectrum of illnesses, including trachoma, urethritis, proctitis, endometritis, pneumonitis, and epididymitis. Infections caused by chlamydiae are primarily sexually transmitted. These organisms are easily engulfed by human phagocytes. However, the organisms possess the unusual ability to continue to proliferate within the phagosome. Chlamydial antigens prevent phagosome-lysosome fusion. The organism is thereby protected from normal host defenses. Through a long developmental cycle, the chlamydiae develop inclusion bodies, which nearly fill entire host cells. In the inclusion bodies, reproduction occurs, and new organisms are able to infect susceptible hosts cells continually.

Mycoplasmas lack cell walls, but are able to grow and divide on a cell-free medium. As such, the mycoplasmas are the smallest and least complex free-living microbes. They are, therefore, capable of producing substances that serve as an energy source. This group of organisms includes pathogens that produce pneumonitis, pharyngitis, pyelonephritis, and nongonococcal urethritis and that contribute to the development of some cases of pelvic inflammatory disease.

Rickettsiae are obligate intracellular pathogens that contain both RNA and DNA. Although these organisms are parasites, they clearly share many common features of bacteria, including similar membrane characteristics. Culture of these organisms is virtually impossible, except in reference laboratories, and great care must be taken in the handling of specimens that are processed for tissue culture. For this reason, the diagnosis of rickettsial infection is most often based on serologic tests. Only one rickettsial pathogen, *Coxiella burnetii*, the agent responsible for Q fever, is capable of surviving outside of host cells. Rickettsiae produce a group of illnesses characterized by fever, headache, and rash. Because most of these illnesses are transmitted by an insect vector (usually ticks), they are frequently limited by climate (they are seasonal) and, to a lesser extent, by the geographic distribution of the vector. In the United States, *Rickettsia rickettsii* is the causative agent for Rocky Mountain spotted fever and lives in the dog tick and the wood tick.

Bacteria represent a widely diverse group of organisms; all have both DNA and RNA. The DNA is present in a double-stranded loop, which is not surrounded by a nuclear membrane. This absence of a nuclear membrane makes the genetic material of bacteria more accessible to environmental agents. Bacteria also contain ribosomes that are responsible for protein synthesis of the cell.

Several factors determine bacterial pathogenicity. The presence of flagella (most common on gram-negative, rod-shaped bacteria) allows cell motility. Pili, or fimbriae (also common in gram-negative rods), appear to aid in bacterial adherence to host tissues. Some bacteria produce a gelatinous capsule, which enables the cell to escape phagocytosis. Finally, some bacteria (e.g., *Clostridium* and *Bacillus* species) possess the ability to form spores under the adverse condition of inadequate nutritional supply. These spores are resistant to destruction by temperature or chemicals and allow the bacterial cells to survive until conditions become more favorable.

Bacteria can cause disease in virtually every organ system. Bacterial infection may range from simple invasion of intact skin, causing a subcutaneous abscess, to localized visceral infection, involving an organ such as the lung, spleen, kidney, or heart. At any time, widespread blood stream invasion may occur via the lymphatic channels when local phagocytic mechanisms are overcome. Bacterial seeding may lead to endotoxemia, septicemia, and even death.

Fungi are divided into two groups: yeasts and molds. The cell walls of fungi are primarily composed of polysaccharide, which permits cell synthesis even in the presence of antibacterial agents. Inside the fungal cell wall is a cytoplasmic membrane that is rich in sterols; this is the site of action of the antifungal agents amphotericin B and nystatin.

Fungal diseases are known as *mycoses* and are classified as systemic or cutaneous. Fungi causing serious systemic disease include *Blastomyces, Coccidioides, Histoplasma,* and *Cryptococcus. Candida* sp., frequently encountered fungal pathogens, may cause deep infection in immunocompromised hosts, but more often cause infection of the skin or mucous membranes. *Aspergillus,* a common mold, may also cause deep and widespread infection in a client with diminished host defenses. Dermatophytoses (e.g., ringworm [tinea]), preferentially involve structures that are rich in keratin, such as the hair, nails, and epidermis.

More than 65,000 species of protozoa have been recognized, although only a few are human pathogens (Atlas, 1984). *Protozoa* can cause localized GI illness (amebiasis and giardiasis), genitourinary tract infection (trichomoniasis), or widespread infection of the blood stream and hematopoietic system (malaria).

The largest and most complex of human pathogens is the *helminth,* or worm. Helminths are visible to the naked eye and are most easily divided into three categories: flukes (trematodes), tapeworms (cestodes), and roundworms (nematodes). Worms infect humans via ingestion, penetration of the skin, or injection by an insect vector. Manifestations of helminth infection vary widely, from the local pruritus of pinworm infestation (enterobiasis), to diarrhea associated with trichinosis, to life-threatening bladder, intestinal, or liver disease that may be associated with schistosomiasis.

RESERVOIRS

Reservoirs, or sources of infectious agents, are numerous. A reservoir is any place where the pathogen is found; it can be *animate* or *inanimate.* Animate reservoirs include humans, animals, and insects. Inanimate reservoirs include soil, water, other environmental sources, and medical equipment, such as intravenous (IV) solutions and urine collection devices. The host's own body can be a reservoir, because pathogens can colonize in skin and body substances, such as feces, sputum, saliva, and wound drainage. Human reservoirs can be people with an active infection or asymptomatic *carriers* who do not have a disease but harbor the infectious agent. Carriers can be *incubating* the pathogen before the development of signs and symptoms, have a *subclinical* (unrecognized) infection, be *convalescing* from an infection, or be a *chronic* carrier of the pathogen. Examples of community reservoirs are sewage or stagnant water and certain improperly cooked foods.

MODE OF TRANSMISSION

For infection to be transmitted, a mechanism must exist for transport of the invading organism from the infected source to a susceptible host. Microorganisms are transmitted by several routes, and the same microorganism may be transmitted by more than one route.

Contact Transmission

Many infections are spread by contact, which may be direct or indirect, or by droplet.

With *direct contact*, the source and host come into physical contact and microorganisms are transferred directly. Often called person-to-person transmission, direct contact is best illustrated by sexual spread of venereal disease.

Indirect contact leading to transmission of infectious agents involves transfer of microorganisms from a source to a host via passive transfer from an intermediate object, most often inanimate, also called a *fomite*. Contaminated articles, especially those that may contact nonintact skin or mucous membranes, may serve as sources of infection. One example of transmission via indirect contact is transfer of hepatitis B virus from a contaminated source to a susceptible host via a poorly cleaned razor.

Droplet spread involves transmission of infection through contact with infective secretions. Such droplets are relatively large, usually greater than 5 μm in size. These droplets are most often produced by talking or sneezing and travel through the air only a short distance (usually less than 3 ft). Susceptible hosts may acquire infection via contact with droplets that are deposited on the membranes of the nose, mouth, or conjunctivae. A common example of droplet-spread infection is measles. Susceptible individuals who are closest to the infected source have the highest risk for infection with a droplet-spread organism.

Airborne Transmission

Airborne transmission occurs when small, airborne, infected particles leave the infected source and travel a distance of greater than 1 m in the air. These particles are usually contained in droplet nuclei or dust and are most often propelled from the respiratory tract by coughing or sneezing. Particles are then inhaled directly into the respiratory tract of a susceptible individual. Tu-

berculosis, legionnaires' disease, and chickenpox are transmitted via the airborne route.

Common Vehicle Transmission

Common vehicle transmission or source of spread occurs when infectious agents are transmitted through a common source such as contaminated food, water, or IV fluid. Salmonellosis is an example of common vehicle–transmitted disease.

Vector-Borne Transmission

Vector-borne transmission of infection involves insects and animals that act as intermediaries between two or more hosts. For example, ticks can transmit Rocky Mountain spotted fever, and mosquitoes can spread malaria.

PORTAL OF EXIT

To complete the chain of infection, an infecting organism exits from the once-susceptible individual who has become a reservoir for infection. Exit from the host most often occurs via the portal of entry. An organism such as *M. tuberculosis* enters the susceptible client via the respiratory route and exits via the respiratory route as the infected host coughs the organism into the air. However, some organisms may travel via several routes of exit from the infected host. For example, varicella-zoster virus can spread through direct contact with infective fluid present in the chickenpox vesicles and by droplet contact.

DEFENSE AGAINST INFECTION

NONSPECIFIC DEFENSES

Several host factors influence the development of infection. Strong and intact host defenses can prevent a microbial invader from entering the host or destroy a pathogen that has gained entry. Conversely, impaired host defenses may be unable to defend against microbial invasion, allowing entry of microorganisms that can destroy host cells and cause infection.

Host defense mechanisms may be classified as nonspecific or specific. Nonspecific mechanisms, most often representing the first encounter an invading pathogen has with its human host, include physical barriers, such as the skin and mucous membranes; chemical barriers, often present in various body secretions; phagocytosis; and inflammation.

Intact skin forms the first and most important physical barrier to the entry of microorganisms into the body. In addition to providing a mechanical barrier, the skin's slightly acidic pH (resulting from the breakdown of lipids into fatty acids) works in conjunction with the normal skin flora to create a hostile environment for pathogenic bacteria.

Mucous membranes, by their mucociliary action, provide some mechanical protection against pathogenic invasion. More importantly, however, mucous membranes are bathed in secretions that are able to inactivate many microorganisms. *Lysozyme,* an enzyme that dissolves the cell walls of some bacteria, is present in large quantities in many body secretions, particularly in nasal mucus and in tears.

Other body systems provide natural barriers to infection. The *respiratory tract* has mechanisms that are able to clear about 90% of all inhaled material by filtration in the upper airways, humidification, mucociliary transport, and expulsion by coughing. The *gastrointestinal tract* provides peristaltic action to mechanically empty pathogenic organisms. Additionally, the acid pH of the stomach, intestinal secretions, pancreatic enzymes, and bile together with normal bowel flora competition provide an environment that protects the GI tract from invasion by harmful organisms. In the *genitourinary tract,* the flushing action of urine acts to eliminate pathogenic organisms. The low pH of urine also serves to maintain a sterile environment.

Whenever a foreign substance evades the first-line mechanical barriers and enters the body, the process of *phagocytosis* occurs. Various types of leukocytes function differently in the immune reaction, but neutrophils bear the primary responsibility for phagocytosis. This process of engulfing, ingesting, killing, and disposing of an invading organism is an essential mechanism in host defense. Phagocytic dysfunction dramatically increases a client's risk for infection and recurrent infections.

A nonspecific defense mechanism that is important in preventing the spread of infection is *inflammation.* The process of inflammation occurs when tissue becomes damaged. The release of enzymes from the damaged cells results. Polymorphonuclear leukocytes are attracted to the infected site from the blood stream. One important enzyme, *histamine,* increases the permeability of the capillaries in the inflamed tissues, thus allowing fluid, proteins, and white blood cells to enter the inflamed area. Still other enzymes activate *fibrinogen,* causing the leaked fluid to clot and prevent its flow away from the damaged site into unaffected tissue, essentially "walling off" the inflamed tissue. The process of phagocytosis then disposes of the invading microorganism and often the dead tissue. If the inflammation is caused by infection, the end products of inflammation form the substance commonly known as *pus,* which is subsequently absorbed or exits the body through a break in the skin. Further discussion of the inflammatory response is found in Chapter 23.

SPECIFIC DEFENSES

Specific defense against infection, that is, specific responses to specific microorganisms, is provided by the humoral and cellular immune systems. The *humoral immune system* produces *antibodies* directed against certain pathogens. These antibodies serve to inactivate or eradicate the invading organism, as well as to protect against future infection with that organism. Resistance to other microorganisms is mediated by the action of specifically sensitized T lymphocytes and is therefore called *cell-mediated immunity.* The various components of the immune system work both independently and together to protect against infection and are discussed in much greater detail in Chapter 23.

PREVENTION OF INFECTION

Spread of infection requires three major elements: (1) a source for an infecting organism; (2) a host, susceptible to infection with the organism; and (3) a mechanism for transmission of the organism from the source to the host. Factors that relate to the source of infection are often difficult to control or modify.

Attempts to interrupt the chain of infection are most often directed at transmission. Mechanisms utilized to block the transmission of a microorganism from an infected source to a susceptible host depend on the way in which the organism may spread.

INFECTION CONTROL IN HEALTH CARE FACILITIES

HAND WASHING

Hand washing is the single most effective mechanism for preventing the spread of infection. Effective hand washing consists of wetting, soaping, lathering, applying friction, rinsing, and drying adequately. Friction in cleaning the hands may be supplied by soft brushes or simply by rubbing the skin surfaces together. Friction is essential to emulsify the oils that are present on the skin and to disperse such substances as transient bacteria and soil from the skin surface. To avoid chapped or cracked skin, hands should be thoroughly rinsed and dried.

Medical personnel should always wash their hands before and after direct contact with a client and immediately after contact with blood, secretions, or excretions. The use of gloves does not preclude hand washing. The CDC recommends the use of *antiseptic solutions,* such as chlorhexadine or povidone-iodine, for hand washing when caring for clients who are at high risk (e.g., newborns and immunocompromised persons). The use of these solutions is widely accepted when caring for persons who are colonized or infected with virulent or multiply-resistant organisms.

The client in an intensive care unit (ICU) is often a uniquely susceptible host for infection. This client is usually seriously ill, is often poorly nourished, and is frequently experiencing complications of an immunosuppressive disease or therapy. Widespread use of antimicrobial therapy in this setting, both prophylactic and therapeutic, inhibits the growth of normal flora. Multiple invasive devises, which are frequently manipulated by numerous health care providers, allow ready access for invading microorganisms against which the client can mount only a weak defense. The ICU also often houses a number of clients, in proximity, which facilitates the transmission of organisms from one client to another. Hand washing with an antibacterial solution is thus also recommended before and after care of clients in the ICU setting (see the accompanying Nursing Research feature).

NURSING RESEARCH

Plain Soap Removes Dirt but Has Little Effect on Colonizing Flora.

Larson, E., Mayur, K., & Laughon, B. A. (1989). Influence of two handwashing frequencies on reduction in colonizing flora with three handwashing products used by health care personnel. *American Journal of Infection Control, 17*, 83–88.

This experimental study compared the effectiveness of three antimicrobial hand washing products with that of a non-antimicrobial control product in reducing colonizing hand flora. Block randomization was used to assign 80 adult volunteers to 10 groups. The volunteers were taught a standardized hand washing procedure and were supervised during hand washing for 5 consecutive days. Half of the groups washed 6 times a day, whereas the other half washed 18 times a day. Microorganisms were harvested three times—before beginning the study, after the first wash, and after the last wash. There was no significant difference among the products at 6 times a day. At 18 times a day, all three products were significantly better than the control.

Critique. This was a well-controlled study that used a standardized hand washing procedure. Variables that could have been examined are the amount of soap used and the duration of hand washing.

Possible nursing implications. Antimicrobial soaps are recommended when hand washing frequency is high and when long-term reduction of flora colonization is desired. For example, antimicrobial soaps are suggested for use in clinical settings in which clients are at high risk for infection (e.g., surgical suites, neonatal care units, and critical care units).

NOSOCOMIAL INFECTION CONTROL

Infection acquired in the hospital (*not* present or incubating at the time of admission) is termed *nosocomial.* Of the estimated 40 million people hospitalized yearly, about 5.7% will develop a nosocomial infection (Garner & Faverno, 1985). Nosocomial infections can be *endogenous* (from the client's own flora) or *exogenous* (from outside the client, usually from the hospital environment or the hands of health care workers). The increased hospital stay of 5 to 10 days required for treatment of a nosocomial infection costs approximately $4 billion annually. The costs associated with the additional morbidity and mortality cannot be measured. However, one study determined that approximately 25% of all clients with bacteremia died as a result of the infection (Wenzel, 1981). Infection control within a health care facility is designed to reduce the risk of nosocomial infection and thus reduce morbidity and mortality and their associated costs.

ISOLATION PRECAUTIONS

Meticulous hand washing is essential within a health care facility. In some instances, however, hand washing alone may be insufficient for infection control. *Isolation precautions* are designed to prevent transmission in these circumstances.

The CDC issued guidelines for isolation precautions for use in hospitals in 1983. However, these recommendations are based entirely on information that was available in 1983 regarding the transmission of infectious organisms. The latest guidelines recommended by the CDC should be reviewed by each institution's infection control committee and then tailored to meet the specific needs of that institution.

The CDC isolation guidelines describe two alternative systems (Garner & Simmons, 1983). *Category-specific isolation precautions* involve grouping isolation procedures into seven distinct categories on the basis of the disease's modes of transmission and similar indicated precautions (see the accompanying Guidelines feature). Category-specific isolation instruction cards are frequently posted outside the client's room.

Strict isolation is designed to prevent transmission of organisms that may be spread by direct contact and by the airborne route. Various barriers are used to prevent contact with the infectious agents (e.g., masks to prevent inhalation and gloves and gowns to prevent direct contact). This category is rarely encountered in hospitals today.

Contact isolation is designed to prevent transmission of organisms that are spread primarily by close or direct contact. This category was created specifically to prevent the spread of organisms that are highly resistant to antibiotic therapy, for example, methicillin-resistant *Staphylococcus aureus.* Masks, gowns, and gloves are required for anyone working in proximity to the client or

GUIDELINES ■ Category-Specific Isolation Precautions

Isolation Category	Private Room*	Masks	Gowns	Gloves	Common Diseases Placed into Isolation Category
Strict isolation	Always	Always	Always	Always	Varicella-zoster (chickenpox); pharyngeal diphtheria; shingles (zoster), localized in an immunocompromised client or disseminated
Contact isolation	Always	For close contact	If soiling with infective material is likely	If contact with infective material is likely	Acute respiratory tract infection in infants and young children; disseminated herpes simplex; methicillin-resistant *Staphylococcus aureus*; pediculosis; scabies
Respiratory isolation	Always	For close contact	No	No	Measles; meningococcal meningitis, pneumonia, or meningococcemia; mumps; pertussis
Acid-fast bacteria isolation	Always	If client is coughing	Only to prevent gross contamination	No	Tuberculosis (primary pulmonary or pharyngeal)
Enteric precautions	Only if the client's hygiene is poor	No	If soiling with infective material is likely	If contact with infective material is likely	Enteroviral infection, including meningitis; infectious gastroenteritis (e.g., giardiasis, salmonellosis, shigellosis); hepatitis A, *Clostridium difficile* enterocolitis
Drainage and secretion precautions	No	No	If soiling with infective material is likely	If contact with infective material is likely	Minor or limited abscess, wound, burn, or skin infection; conjunctivitis
Blood and body fluid precautions	Only if the client's hygiene is poor	If contact with blood or body fluids is likely	If contact with splashes of blood or body fluids is likely	If contact with blood or body fluids is likely	AIDS; hepatitis B; non-A, non-B hepatitis; malaria

* In most instances when a private room is required, clients infected with the same organism may share a room.

GUIDELINES ■ Blood and Body Fluid Precautions

These precautions are to be used with all clients to protect health care providers from blood-borne communicable diseases.

Gloves should be worn for contact with blood and body fluids, nonintact skin, and mucous membranes of all clients; for handling surfaces or items that are soiled with blood and body fluids; and for performing venipuncture and other vascular access procedures. Gloves should be changed after each client contact.

Masks or protective goggles should be worn during procedures that are likely to cause splashes of blood or body fluids.

Gowns or aprons should be worn during procedures that are likely to result in splashes of blood or body fluids.

Hand washing should be done immediately on contact with blood or other body fluids. One should wash hands as soon as gloves are removed.

Needles and sharp instruments should be placed in puncture-resistant containers for disposal to prevent injuries from needles or other sharp items. Needles should not be recapped, bent, or removed from the syringe.

Mouth-to-mouth resuscitation should be performed using mouthpieces or other ventilation devices.

Based on Centers for Disease Control. (1987). Recommendations for prevention of HIV transmission in health-care settings. *Morbidity and Mortality Weekly Report, 36*(2S), 3–17.

anyone having direct contact with infective material. Hand washing is paramount.

Respiratory isolation precautions are recommended to prevent the transmission of infectious diseases spread by large droplets that travel only a short distance through the air. Thus, the barrier mechanism required in this category is masks for all who come close to an infected client.

Acid-fast bacteria (AFB) isolation is recommended to prevent the spread of laryngeal and pulmonary tuberculosis. The recommended procedure for this category is for health care personnel and visitors to wear a mask at all times if the client is coughing. This category is called AFB isolation to protect the client's privacy.

Enteric precautions have been formulated to prevent infections that are transmitted by contact with feces. Barrier mechanisms (gowns and gloves) are recommended to prevent contact with feces of such clients, thus preventing transmission of infection. Although most clients with infections that require this type of isolation manifest GI symptoms, some do not. For example, some types of encephalitis and meningitis are caused by enteroviruses that, although causing neuro-

logic symptoms, are transmitted via contact with infectious feces.

The category of *drainage and secretion precautions* includes procedures to prevent the transmission of infections that are spread by direct or indirect contact with infectious material from an infected body site. Diseases included in this category are primarily limited skin or wound infections that produce purulent drainage and can be adequately contained in a dressing.

Blood and body fluid precautions are designed to prevent infections that are spread via direct or indirect contact with infectious blood or body fluids (see the accompanying Guidelines feature). This category includes diseases such as malaria, AIDS, and hepatitis B. These precautions should be used for all clients because those who are infected with blood-borne pathogens cannot always be identified.

Category-specific isolation has several advantages. The system is relatively simple, convenient, and familiar in most health care institutions. However, because of the grouping of many diseases into a few broad categories, some unnecessary techniques are used for some infections. Thus, in some instances, overisolation occurs. As a mechanism to avoid this problem, the CDC recommended *disease-specific* isolation.

Disease-specific isolation involves the use of a single instruction card for all clients with a transmissible infection. This instruction card lists all possible isolation specifications (e.g., masks, gowns, gloves, and private room) and requires that a health care professional indicate which are appropriate for a specific disease. Using only those particular precautions needed to interrupt the transmission of a specific disease eliminates overisolation and the costs of unnecessary precautions. However, the disease-specific system requires more training and attention on the part of health care personnel.

The CDC (1987) published universal precaution guidelines. Although infection control professionals have advocated the concept that *all patients' blood and body fluids are potentially infectious and should be handled accordingly,* it has not been widely accepted by health care workers until recently. One would expect the practice of employing isolation barriers to be changing over the next few years. If health care workers truly avoid exposure to all clients' blood and body fluids, this will obviate the need for several categories of isolation.

Whichever system of isolation is used within a health care facility, care must be taken to prevent client solitude and to promote quality care, despite the need for extra precautions. Institution of isolation precautions may be associated with a number of untoward psychosocial effects. Even if the client is not confined to his/her room, the presence of an isolation placard on the door may produce anxiety. For clients who must be confined to their rooms, the constant environment of the hospital room may be difficult to tolerate. Family members may also express fear or anxiety because the client is isolated. Clients in strict isolation, visited only by persons wearing masks, gowns, and gloves, may actually experience sensory deprivation (see Chap. 8). Finally, the need for isolation precautions may present a barrier to good client care. Donning isolation garb is time-consuming and uncomfortable. The health care provider may be less inclined to deliver frequent care when the additional task of utilizing precautions is required. The need for preventing the transmission of infection within a health care facility must be balanced against the disadvantages to the isolated client.

INFECTION CONTROL IN THE HOME SETTING

The Medicare reimbursement plan based on various diagnosis-related groups (DRGs) is putting pressure on hospitals to minimize expenses. One outcome of such pressure is that clients are being discharged from hospitals earlier, perhaps with transmissible infectious diseases. In addition, the rapid growth of ambulatory (outpatient) services such as chemotherapy and radiation therapy for malignancies results in a large number of clients with increased susceptibility to infection who are living at home. Finally, medical procedures that previously were limited to hospitalized clients, such as IV antibiotic therapy or total parenteral nutrition are increasingly becoming components of home care. Thus, infection control has become an integral part of the care of clients not only within health care institutions but in the home environment as well.

In most cases, the same principles of *asepsis* (the use of techniques that exclude infection-causing microorganisms) apply in homes and in hospitals. Common sense indicates the necessity for the preservation of a clean environment. Meticulous hand washing to prevent the transmission of any infection within the home cannot be overemphasized. The same types of barrier mechanisms that are used as isolation precautions in the hospital may be used in the home. Appropriate gloves, gowns, and masks, as well as sterilized equipment, such as IV catheters and surgical dressings, should be provided by the home health care team. Because the client's home is not likely to harbor the virulent organisms often found in the hospital, when appropriate and practical, some procedures that are performed only under sterile conditions in the hospital may be practiced as clean procedures in the home. For example, intermittent bladder catheterization is often taught to be self-administered as a clean procedure, although it is performed using sterile technique in the hospital.

Economic considerations may also determine that some items designated for single use only in the hospital may be resterilized by boiling at home to permit multiple use. Disposable respiratory therapy equipment is often boiled and reused in the home.

INFECTION CONTROL IN THE COMMUNITY

Prevention of community-wide infection is in the realm of public health care and is administered primarily through local and state health departments and the Department of Health and Human Services, especially the CDC.

Primary prevention, prevention of the occurrence of disease, involves immunization, food and water sanitization, and proper waste disposal.

Secondary prevention, the early detection and treatment of infectious diseases to prevent their spread to others, is accomplished through screening programs and outbreak investigation. Routine tuberculosis screening within a hospital is an example of secondary prevention. The goal of routine screening is to identify infected personnel early and initiate therapy before transmission to others can occur. Outbreak investigation identifies individuals who may have had contact with an infected source to institute timely treatment and prevent further spread of infection.

COMPLICATIONS OF INFECTION

Most complications of infection are related to inadequate therapy, attributable either to inappropriate choice of antimicrobials or to poor compliance by clients receiving anti-infective treatment. Perhaps the most obvious complication of inadequate therapy is *relapse*. Relapse of the infection may be a serious problem for many reasons. First, some infections may become active again in a more subtle fashion. Thus, the client may think that the infection is getting better slowly on its own, whereas, in fact, the infection is not under control. Second, incomplete compliance with the regimen (e.g., taking the medication sporadically) may expose the bacterial flora to subinhibitory concentrations of antimicrobial agents, thereby facilitating the emergence of strains resistant to the antimicrobial.

Other serious infectious complications may occur as a result of incomplete anti-infective therapy. Local infections, such as cellulitis and pneumonia, which could be cured without complications, may progress to *abscess formation* in the absence of continued appropriate antimicrobial therapy. Although adequate antimicrobial therapy does not always prevent abscess development, early appropriate therapy may prevent, or at least limit the size of, an individual abscess.

In addition to abscess formation, the client may also develop *systemic complications* as a result of inadequate therapy. If a client's infection is incompletely eradicated or if the infection is being treated with antimicrobial agents that are not effective against the offending organism, the pathogen may seed the blood stream, resulting in *systemic sepsis*. Even small local infections, if left untreated or treated inadequately, may spread locally or via the blood stream to produce significant complications such as leukocytosis or leukopenia and disseminated intravascular coagulation. After pathogens invade the blood stream, virtually no site is protected from metastatic invasion.

The fundamental defect in persons with sepsis is insufficient cardiac output compounded by hypovolemia, causing inadequate blood supply to vital organs and leading to hypoxia and metabolic failure. Therapy for sepsis must be prompt. If metabolic acidosis occurs, the prognosis is poor. Basic life support, ensuring pulmonary gas exchange, is paramount. This is followed by restoration of adequate tissue perfusion and then treatment of the infection. (For additional information on sepsis, see Chap. 17.)

COLLABORATIVE MANAGEMENT

 Assessment

History

Careful attention to the history of a client with a possible infectious disease helps the nurse to determine the presence of risk factors for infection. The *age* of a client, history of *cigarette smoking* or *alcohol* use, past and current *medication* use, *familial predisposition,* and poor *nutritional status* may all place the client at increased risk for a number of infectious diseases.

The nurse also determines whether exposure to infectious agents has occurred. A history of *recent exposure to someone with similar clinical symptoms or to contaminated food or water,* as well as the time of exposure, assists in identifying a possible source for infection. This information may also help determine the incubation period for the disease and thus provide a clue to its cause.

Contact with animals, including pets, may facilitate exposure to infection. The nurse questions the client about recent contact with animals at home, at work, or in the course of leisure activities such as hunting. The nurse also asks the client about recent *contact with insects.*

The nurse obtains a *travel history* from the client. Travel to areas both within and outside the United States may expose a susceptible individual to infectious organisms that she/he may not encounter in the local community.

A thorough *sexual history* may reveal sexual behavior that is associated with increased risk of sexually transmitted diseases. The nurse should obtain additional history concerning *IV drug use* and *transfusion history* to assess the client's risk for hepatitis B, non-A, non-B hepatitis, and human immunodeficiency virus (HIV) infection.

Eliciting the *type and location of symptoms* may provide a key to the affected organ system. The *order of onset of symptoms* may also provide clues to the client's diagnosis.

Physical Assessment: Clinical Manifestations

Disorders caused by infectious agents are extremely variable, depending on the cause and the site of infec-

---

KEY FEATURES OF DISEASE ■ Clinical Manifestations Associated with Specific Sites of Infection

Gastrointestinal Tract	Skin
Fever	Redness
Nausea and vomiting	Warmth
Diarrhea	Swelling
Abdominal distention	Drainage
	Pain
Genitourinary Tract	
	Generalized Infection
Dysuria	
Frequency	Fever
Urgency	Malaise
Hematuria	Fatigue
Fever	Muscle aches
Purulent discharge	Joint pain
Pelvic or flank pain	
Respiratory tract	
Cough	
Congestion	
Rhinitis	
Sore throat	
Sputum	
Fever	
Chest pain	

tion. Common clinical manifestations are associated with specific sites of infection (see the accompanying Key Features of Disease). A number of clinical manifestations are highly suggestive of an infectious process. Symptoms of infection at any site include *pain, swelling, heat, redness,* and the presence of *pus.* The nurse should carefully inspect any visible lesions for these symptoms.

Fever (body temperature greater than 101° F [38° C]), *chills,* and *malaise* are primary indicators of an infectious process, although fever may also accompany other noninfectious disorders and infection can certainly be present in the absence of fever. The nurse assesses the client for the presence of these symptoms and carefully questions the client concerning the history and patterns of symptoms.

Lymphadenopathy, photophobia, pharyngitis, and GI disturbance are often associated with the presence of infection. In the elderly, a change in mental status may be the first, if not the only, presenting symptom. The careful nursing assessment should include palpation of the cervical and axillary lymph nodes to detect enlargement and direct examination of the throat for redness or exudate.

Laboratory Findings

The definitive diagnosis of an infectious disease requires identification of a microorganism that is present in the tissues of an infected client. Direct examination of blood, body fluids, and tissues under a microscope may not yield positive identification of an organism, but usually provides helpful information about the microorganism, such as its shape, motility, and reaction to various staining agents. Even when direct microscopy does not prove diagnostic, enough information often is gathered to initiate appropriate antimicrobial therapy.

The most definitive procedure for organism identification is *culture,* or isolation of the agent by cultivation in tissue cultures or various artificial media. Culture may be performed on almost any body fluid or tissue. Proper collection and handling of specimens for culture is essential to obtain accurate results. The specimen collected must be appropriate for the suspected infection. Material must be in sufficient quantity, freshly obtained, and placed in a sterile container that adequately preserves the specimen and organism to be examined (see the accompanying Guidelines feature).

After an organism has been isolated in culture, antimicrobial sensitivity testing is often performed to determine in a qualitative or quantitative way the effects of various antibiotics on that particular microorganism. An organism that is killed by acceptable levels of an antimicrobial is considered *sensitive* to that agent. An organism that is not killed by tolerable levels of an antimicrobial agent is considered *resistant* to that agent.

A less specific laboratory test to determine the presence of an infectious organism is a *serologic* test, a blood test performed to look for antibodies that react with a certain antigen. Serologic tests are available for virtually all classes of organisms. Examples of diseases for which serologic studies commonly aid diagnosis include syphilis, mononucleosis, Rocky Mountain spotted fever, and cryptococcosis. A positive serologic test result does not necessarily indicate active infection, but merely signifies that the client has had previous exposure to the antigen in question. Two serum specimens should be obtained from a client to examine for antibody titers, the first during the acute phase of illness and the second 7 to 10 days later. A fourfold or greater rise in antibody titer in the second specimen is likely to indicate recent infection.

Complete blood count (CBC) is nearly always performed on the client with a suspected infectious disease. Five types of leukocytes have been identified: neutrophils, lymphocytes, monocytes, eosinophils, and basophils. In most cases of active infection, especially those caused by bacteria, the total leukocyte count is elevated. Various diseases are characterized by changes in the percentages of the different types of leukocytes. Most often, the differential count shows an increased number of immature neutrophils. A few infectious diseases, however, are associated with neutropenia, such as malaria and infectious mononucleosis (see Chaps. 66 and 67 for further discussion of CBC).

The *erythrocyte sedimentation rate* (ESR) is a measurement of the rate at which red blood cells fall through plasma. This rate is most significantly affected by an increased number of acute phase reactants, which occurs with inflammation. Thus, an elevated ESR

(>15 mm/hour) indicates the presence of inflammation. Chronic infection, most notably osteomyelitis, and the presence of chronic abscesses are commonly associated with an elevated ESR, and the effectiveness of therapy is often monitored by a fall in this value.

Radiographic Findings

X-ray films are often obtained to determine infectious activity or destruction by an infectious agent. Radiologic studies such as chest films, sinus films, joint films, GI roentgenographic studies, and IV pyelograms are typically obtained to diagnose infection in a specific body site.

A more sophisticated technique for diagnosis of an infection is computed tomography. This method is particularly helpful in assessing the presence and location of abscesses.

Other Diagnostic Tests

Another noninvasive diagnostic tool for the evaluation of a client with an infectious disease is ultrasonography. This procedure is helpful in detecting infection that has caused vegetations on the heart valves.

Scanning techniques using radioactive substances, such as gallium, are employed to determine the presence of inflammation. Inflammatory tissue is identified by its increased uptake of the injected radioactive material.

Because isolation of a causative agent may be essential for effective treatment of an infectious disease, biopsy of the infected site may become necessary to obtain tissue for culture. Biopsy sites may include the liver, the bone marrow, the skin, the pleura, lymph nodes, the kidney, bone, or even the brain. Invasive procedures, such as bronchoscopy or endoscopy, or even surgery, such as open lung biopsy or laparotomy, may be necessary to obtain specimens for examination.

Psychosocial Assessment

The client with an infectious disease often has a unique constellation of psychosocial concerns. Typically, a number of diagnostic tests must be performed, and definitive identification of the microorganism responsible for the client's symptoms may involve a prolonged interval of time. This delay produces frustration and anxiety for the client. The nurse assesses the client's level of understanding about various diagnostic procedures and the time that may be required to obtain accurate results.

Frequently noted symptoms of infection are prolonged feelings of malaise and easy fatiguability. The nurse assesses the client's psychologic and sociologic adjustment to a decreased energy level. The nurse evaluates the client's current level of activity and the impact of these symptoms on normal family, occupational, and recreational activities.

An additional stress associated with diagnosis of an infection is the potential transmissibility of infection to others. The client may curtail family and social interac-

GUIDELINES ■ Collection Techniques for Commonly Cultured Specimens

Specimen	Collection Method	Comments
Blood	1. Decontaminate skin with 70% alcohol followed by 2% tincture of iodine, allowed to dry. 2. Perform venipuncture and collect 10 mL of blood (2 mL in infants). 3. Inject into sterile culture bottles — usually one vented and one unvented for anaerobic culture.	Usually three separate specimens are collected over a 24-hr period to ensure isolation of the causative organism.
Urine Clean void	1. Clean urethral meatus with tincture of iodine or other antiseptic solution. 2. Have client void small amount and then collect approximately 2 mL of midstream urine specimen into a sterile container.	Specimen may be refrigerated. If not, the specimen must be delivered to the laboratory within 30 min to be useful for quantitative studies.
Indwelling catheter	1. Clean aspiration site on catheter with iodine. 2. Collect 2-mL specimen into a sterile container.	
Wound	1. Decontaminate the skin with 70% alcohol. 2. Swab an active margin of the wound with a sterile swab and place the swab into sterile tube.	
Throat	1. Swab an inflamed area of throat, especially areas of exudate. 2. Place the swab into sterile media for transport.	Inform the laboratory of any suspected organism other than group A streptococcus.
Sputum	1. Collect first morning expectorated sputum into sterile container.	Production of adequate specimen may be aided by saline aerosol administration or by postural drainage. Sputum specimens may also be collected via tracheal or transtracheal aspiration.
Pus (abscesses)	1. Decontaminate the skin with alcohol. 2. Coat a sterile swab rapidly with pus. 3. Insert the swab immediately into a specially prepared anaerobic transport tube.	Deliver the specimen to the laboratory immediately.
Vagina	1. Wipe the vagina clean of secretions with dry gauze. 2. Swab the exudate with a sterile swab. 3. Insert into sterile container or into specially prepared media.	If trichomoniasis is suspected, place the swab in a small amount sterile saline and send to the laboratory immediately.
Rectal swab	1. Insert the swab into the rectum approximately 1 in and rotate once. 2. Place into transport media.	Specimen is usually sent on 3 consecutive days. Swab should show obvious soiling.
Stool	1. Collect stool in a clean waxed cardboard container.	Deliver to the laboratory immediately. Specimen is often collected on 3 consecutive days.
Intravenous catheters	1. Clean catheter insertion site with alcohol. 2. Withdraw catheter and cut off approximately 5-cm tip with sterile scissors. 3. Place into sterile container.	In general, catheter tips that are contaminated during removal will grow only a few colonies, whereas infected catheters usually show heavy growth.

tions as a result of fear of spreading the illness. The nurse assesses the client's and the family's levels of understanding of the infection, its mode of transmission, and mechanisms that may limit or prevent transmission. The nurse assesses the effects of the client's illness on usual interpersonal interactions.

Finally, a number of transmissible infectious diseases, especially those associated with socially unacceptable life style (such as promiscuous sexual activity and IV drug abuse), are associated with some degree of social stigmatization. As a result, the client may feel socially isolated and may experience guilt related to behavior that increases the risk for infection. The nurse observes carefully for signs of the client's reaction to stigmatization and how these feelings further affect socialization.

 Analysis: Nursing Diagnoses

Most often, the client with an infectious disease is admitted to the hospital for either diagnosis or therapy. The client commonly has fever and malaise. Anxiety is extremely common for the client with an infection and is related to the delayed or prolonged period of diagnosis, the potential for transmission of infection to others, and social isolation caused by fear of transmission.

Common Diagnoses

Three nursing diagnoses are commonly applicable to the client with an infectious disease.

1. Potential altered body temperature related to infection
2. Activity intolerance related to malaise and easy fatiguability secondary to infection
3. Social isolation related to potential for disease transmission to others

Additional Diagnoses

Clients with infectious diseases may have a variety of other nursing diagnoses, depending on the location and cause of their infection. These include the following:

1. Ineffective airway clearance related to infection and inflammation of pulmonary system
2. Diarrhea related to infection involving the GI tract
3. Decreased cardiac output related to sepsis
4. Ineffective individual coping related to chronic disease progression
5. Altered family processes related to fear of disease transmission
6. Knowledge deficit related to treatment regimen
7. Noncompliance related to prolonged antimicrobial therapy
8. Altered sexuality patterns related to fear of transmission of infection

9. Impaired tissue integrity related to inflammation and infectious destruction

 Planning and Implementation

The following plan of care for the client with an infectious disease focuses on the common nursing diagnoses.

Potential Altered Body Temperature

Planning: client goals. The primary goal is that the client will have a return to normal body temperature.

Interventions: nonsurgical management. Several mechanisms exist for the control of body temperature. It is important, however, to eliminate the underlying cause of hyperthermia—to eradicate the causative microorganism. Measures are implemented to reduce fever, such as antipyretic drug therapy, external cooling techniques, and fluid administration.

Antimicrobial therapy. The cornerstone of therapy for infectious diseases is antimicrobial chemotherapy. The first antibiotic group, the sulfonamides, were used in the mid-1930s. Shortly thereafter, in the 1940s, penicillin became the first antibiotic to be used systemically. Since these early days, a wide variety of antimicrobial drugs have been developed to treat as well as prevent infection associated with virtually every class of organism. Table 26-1 presents important information on the most commonly used classes of antimicrobial chemotherapeutic agents. Effective antimicrobial agents are available to treat nearly all bacterial infections. However, fewer effective antifungal agents have been developed, and these drugs generally exhibit more toxicity than do antibacterial agents. Few effective chemotherapeutic agents are currently available to treat infections caused by viruses.

Effective antimicrobial therapy requires (1) delivery of the appropriate agent, (2) sufficient dosage, (3) proper route of administration, and (4) sufficient duration of therapy. Fulfilling these four requirements ensures that a concentration of drug is delivered in excess of that needed to inhibit or kill the infecting organism at the site of infection.

Antimicrobial drugs act on susceptible pathogens by inhibiting cell wall synthesis (penicillins and cephalosporins), injuring the cytoplasmic membrane (antifungal agents), inhibiting biosynthesis (erythromycin, tetracycline, and gentamicin), and inhibiting nucleic acid synthesis (actinomycin).

Antipyretic therapy. Antipyretic drugs, such as aspirin and acetaminophen, are often used to decrease hyperthermia. However, by masking fever, antipyretics may create difficulty in monitoring the course of the client's disease. Therefore, unless the client is extremely uncomfortable or if hyperthermia presents a significant risk (e.g., in clients with heart failure, febrile seizures,

TABLE 26–1   Commonly Used Antimicrobial Agents

Drug	Usual Daily Dosage	Comments
Penicillins		
Penicillin G	5–30 million units IM, IV, PO	Allergic reactions are common; anaphylaxis may occur. Watch for central nervous system toxicity, especially in high doses or in clients with renal failure. Penicillins are primarily useful for gram-positive infections, such as *Streptococcus pyogenes* and *Streptococcus pneumoniae,* and are the drugs of choice for syphilis and gonorrhea.
Procaine penicillin	600,000–1.2 million IM, IV, PO	
Benzathine penicillin	1.6–2.4 million units IM, IV, PO	
Semisynthetic penicillins (antistaphylococcal penicillins)		
Methicillin	4–6 g IM, IV, PO	These agents cannot be used if the client is allergic to penicillin. Nephritis is common with methicillin. Hepatitis occurs with oxacillin. High-dose nafcillin is associated with neutropenia. These drugs used primarily for *Staphylococcus aureus* infections.
Oxacillin	2–3 g IM, IV, PO	
Nafcillin	2–3 g IM, IV, PO	
Cloxacillin	1–3 g IM, IV, PO	
Dicloxacillin	0.5–1 g IM, IV, PO	
Extended-spectrum penicillins		
Ampicillin	1–2 g IV, PO	High sodium content in carbenicillin may cause congestive heart failure. Rash is common with ampicillin. Ampicillin has good cerebrospinal fluid penetration and is useful for sensitive *Haemophilus influenzae* and *Streptococcus faecalis* infections. Others provide broad gram-negative coverage, except for *Klebsiella* spp.
Carbenicillin	15–40 g IV, PO	
Ticarcillin	12–18 g IV, PO	
Azlocillin	12–18 g IV, PO	
Mezlocillin	24 g IV, PO	
Piperacillin	12–18 g IV, PO	
Cephalosporins		
First generation		
Cephalothin	2–6 g IM, IV, PO	Thrombophlebitis occurs commonly. Allergic reactions are common. Allergy occurs in 5%–10% of clients allergic to penicillin. These agents are useful primarily against gram-positive organisms, especially *Staphylococcus aureus.*
Cefazolin	1–6 g IM, IV, PO	
Cephapirin	2–6 g IM, IV, PO	
Cephalexin	1–4 g IM, IV, PO	
Second generation		
Cefoxitin	4–8 g IV, IM	These agents are similar to first-generation cephalosporins. They are somewhat less effective against gram-positive organisms. These agents offer better gram-negative coverage and some anaerobic gram-negative coverage.
Cefamandole	1.5–6 g IV, IM	
Cefuroxime	2–4.5 g IV, IM	
Cefaclor	4 g PO	
Cefotetan	1–2 g IV, IM	
Cefonicid	1–2 g IV, IM	
Third generation		
Cefotaxime	4–8 g IM, IV	These agents are similar to first- and second-generation cephalosporins. Significant bleeding may occur with moxalactam.
Ceftizoxime	2–6 g IM, IV	
Ceftriaxone	2–6 g IM, IV	
Moxalactam	2–6 g IM, IV	

Table continued on following page

TABLE 26–1 **Commonly Used Antimicrobial Agents** *Continued*

Drug	Usual Daily Dosage	Comments
		Third-generation cephalosporins provide a markedly extended spectrum, good gram-negative coverage, and somewhat decreased gram-positive coverage. They are not generally useful for *Pseudomonas* spp.
Third generation with anti-*Pseudomonas* activity		
Ceftazidime	2–4 g IM, IV	These agents are similar to other cephalosporins. There is some loss of activity against gram-positive organisms and good activity against *P. aeruginosa*.
Cefsulodin	2–4 g IM, IV	
Cefoperazone	2–4 g IM, IV	
Other beta-lactam agents		
Monobactams		Allergic reactions occur.
Aztreonam	500 mg–2 g bid–tid IM, IV	Mild liver toxicity may be noted.
Penems		Leukopenia and liver toxicity may occur.
Imipenem	250 mg–1 g tid–qid IV	These agents have a broad spectrum of activity. These agents provide good gram-positive, gram-negative, anti-*Pseudomonas,* and anaerobic coverage.
Tetracyclines		
Tetracycline	1–2 g PO, IV	Hypersensitivity reactions are common.
Doxycycline	100–200 mg PO, IV	Toxic reactions (photosensitivity) can occur.
Minocycline	100–200 mg PO, IV	Discoloration of teeth in children results. These agents should not be administered with milk, food, or other medications. They are useful in rickettsial infections, borreliosis, plague, cholera, and chlamydial infections.
Chloramphenicol	1 g IM, IV, PO	Dose-related bone marrow suppression occurs. Rarely, aplastic anemia results. Chloramphenicol should not be given to neonates. It is useful for some cases of meningitis (especially in penicillin-allergic clients). It is used for typhoid fever and rickettsioses.
Macrolides and lincosamides		
Erythromycin	1–4 g IM, IV, PO	GI upset is common with erythromycin, including nausea, vomiting, and abdominal cramping.
Lincomycin	1500–2000 mg IM, IV, PO	Clindamycin may predispose to pseudomembranous colitis (*C. difficile* colitis).
Clindamycin	150–1200 mg IM, IV, PO	Erythromycin is useful as alternative therapy for penicillin-allergic patients, mycoplasma, legionellosis, diphtheria, and pertussis. Clindamycin is highly effective against intestinal anaerobes, including *B. fragilis*.
Vancomycin	2 g IV	Vancomycin may cause sudden hypotension if infused too rapidly.

TABLE 26–1   Commonly Used Antimicrobial Agents *Continued*

Drug	Usual Daily Dosage	Comments
		Vancomycin is ototoxic and nephrotoxic. It is useful for penicillin- and methicillin-resistant gram-positive infections. It is administered orally (though not absorbed) to treat *C. difficile*–associated colitis.
Antituberculous agents		Hepatitis occurs with INH and rifampin.
Isoniazid (INH)	300 mg PO	Neuropathy occurs with INH.
Rifampin	600 mg PO	Loss of color vision occurs with ethambutol.
Ethambutol	900–1500 mg PO	The usual course of treatment includes at least two agents.
Antifungal agents		Nephrotoxicity occurs with amphotericin.
Amphotericin B	15 mg IV	Rapid infusion of amphotericin may be associated with high fever, shaking chills, severe malaise, and occasionally sudden death. A 1-mg test dose should be administered before the first full dose.
Miconazole	200–3600 mg IV	
Ketoconazole	200 mg PO	Ketoconazole has been associated with hepatitis and interference with steroidogenesis.
Flucytosine (5-fluorocytosine; 5-FC)	3–9 g PO	5-FC may cause diarrhea and bone marrow suppression. For most systemic fungal infections, the drug of choice is amphotericin B.
Antiviral agents		Most parenteral agents are toxic drugs and are usually given only to seriously ill clients.
Acyclovir	900 mg IV, PO	
Vidarabine (adenine arabinoside; Ara-A)	900 mg topically in sufficient quantities to cover lesion	Oral acyclovir may hasten healing of genital herpes lesions. These agents generally treat only symptoms (lesions) and do not cure infection. Acyclovir is useful in herpes simplex encephalitis, local and disseminated herpes zoster, genital herpes, and mucocutaneous herpes simplex.

head injury, or pregnancy), antipyretics should not be given. In cases of viral illness, specifically chickenpox and influenza, aspirin should not be used because of the association with Reye's syndrome. If antipyretics are employed, the nurse must be alert for waves of sweating after each dose, which may be accompanied by a fall in blood pressure and subsequent return of fever. These unpleasant side effects of antipyretic therapy can often be alleviated by liberal fluid administration and by regular scheduling of drug administration.

External cooling.   Cooling or hypothermia blankets or ice bags and packs are highly effective external mechanisms to reduce fever. The nurse sponges the client's body with tepid water or saline solution or applies cool compresses to the skin and pulse points to reduce body temperature. Although alcohol sponging has often been recommended for rapid body cooling because of its rapid evaporation rate, the pungent odor of alcohol may cause nausea in some clients. Additionally, the rapid cooling associated with the application of alcohol may lead to shivering, which may, in fact, increase body temperature. Use of alcohol is therefore somewhat controversial.

Severe, life-threatening hyperthermia that requires immersion in ice water, intragastric cooling, or cooling of arterial blood by hemodialysis rarely occurs as a symptom of an infectious process.

Fluid administration. The client with fever has increased volume loss attributable to rapid evaporation of body fluids as well as increased perspiration. As body temperature increases, this fluid volume loss increases as well. The nurse carefully monitors signs of dehydration, such as increased thirst, decreased skin turgor, and dry mucous membranes. The nurse encourages increased oral fluid intake and administers IV fluids as prescribed.

Activity Intolerance

Planning: client goals. The primary goal for this nursing diagnosis is that the client will progress to the previous level of activity. Achievement of this goal is dependent on recognition and correction of factors that contribute to activity intolerance.

Interventions: nonsurgical management. Malaise and easy fatiguability are classic clinical manifestations of an infectious process. Fever accelerates many metabolic processes, accentuating weight loss and nitrogen wasting. The heart rate is increased and water loss may be excessive, both contributing to a feeling of general malaise.

Diet management. The nurse observes the client for causative factors of malaise and easy fatiguability, such as nutritional deficiencies or fluid and electrolyte imbalances. The nurse works with the client and dietitian to establish a dietary program that is tolerable for the client and meets calorie and protein requirements.

Activity management. The nurse encourages bed rest during the acute phase of the clients's illness while therapy for the underlying infection is initiated. The nurse works closely with the client to develop a progressive program for return to his/her normal level of activity. The program depends on the client's response to anti-infective therapy, as evidenced by diminished clinical manifestations of infection. Frequent rest periods are encouraged. Throughout the course of the client's illness, the nurse encourages the client to verbalize feelings of frustration and discouragement related to chronic fatigue and decreased ability to perform activities of daily living.

Social Isolation

Planning: client goals. The primary goal for this diagnosis is that the client will not experience feelings of social isolation.

Interventions: nonsurgical management. Education is the major intervention employed to meet this goal. The nurse develops an educational program to instruct the client and the client's family about the mode of transmission of infection and mechanisms that prevent the spread of the organism from the client to others. The nurse also initiates appropriate isolation precautions.

The nurse ensures that the client and the family understand the client's disease process and its cause. Specifically, the nurse explains the mode of transmission of the infecting organism, the risk for transmission to others, and mechanisms that may be employed to prevent transmission. The nurse ensures that the client and the family are able to state specific ways in which precautions will be instituted in the home after discharge from the hospital.

Because the client requiring isolation precautions may feel secluded, the nurse encourages health care personnel as well as family members and friends to maintain contact with the client. The nurse reminds all individuals caring for the client that the disease requires isolation—not the client. The nurse encourages family members and friends to visit the client, utilizing the appropriate barrier precautions when needed. Communication via the telephone is often an effective means for continuing contact with loved ones. Television and radio help bring the outside world into the life of the client who is confined to his/her room. (For other suggestions for the care of a client experiencing sensory deprivation, the reader is referred to Chap. 8).

If the client is in isolation, the nurse emphasizes the importance of preventing the spread of infection without compromising the quality of care of the client. Special effort must be expended to be certain that isolation precautions do not impose unnecessary restrictions on the client and seem punitive.

■ Discharge Planning

Home Care Preparation

The client with an infectious disease who is discharged from the hospital to home may require continued, long-term antimicrobial therapy. The nurse emphasizes the importance of a clean home environment, especially for the client who continues to be immunocompromised or who is uniquely susceptible to superinfection (i.e., reinfection or second infection of the same kind) because of antimicrobial drug administration. Particularly if therapy is to be given via the IV or the intramuscular route, medications often require refrigeration. The nurse ensures that the client has access to proper storage facilities and instructs the client to observe medication for signs of improper storage, such as discoloration.

The nurse questions the client to be certain that hand washing facilities are available in the home and provides supplies and instructions as needed.

Client/Family Education

The teaching plan for the client who has an infectious disease includes several important issues. First, the nurse explains the disease and makes certain that the client understands what is causing the illness. Next, the nurse explains whether the pathogen causing the client's infection can be spread to family members, social contacts, or other community contacts. In instances in which the client has an infectious disease caused by a transmissible agent, the nurse then explains how the pathogen causing the client's infection is transmitted. Finally, if the client has an infectious disease that is potentially transmissible, the nurse teaches the client, the family, or home caregivers the precautions to prevent transmission of infection. Often general household cleaning measures are sufficient (e.g., washing dishes in a dishwasher and clothing in a washer and dryer). If those are not available, dishes can be sanitized with weak bleach solution (100 parts per million available chlorine), attained by adding 1 oz of bleach to 4 gal of water. Clothing that is soiled with blood or other body fluids can be washed with bleach or disinfectant (e.g., Lysol). Recommended cleaning measures should be based on actual equipment or facilities that are available.

For clients who are discharged to the home setting to complete a course of anti-infective therapy, the nurse also explains the importance of compliance with the planned antimicrobial regimen, in terms of both the timing of doses and the completion of the planned number of days of therapy. The nurse also teaches the client how the agents should be taken (e.g., before meals, with meals, and without other agents). The nurse teaches the client and the family about the side effects of medications to be taken at home—those that are expected, such as GI upset after the oral administration of erythromycin, as well as more severe adverse reactions, such as rash, fever, or other systemic signs and symptoms of an acute adverse drug reaction (Table 26–2).

In the past, a client who had a deep-seated infection often was hospitalized for several weeks simply to receive IV antimicrobial therapy. In the past few years, many clients have been discharged with an IV device in place and continue to receive IV anti-infective agents at home. The antimicrobials are administered by the client, a family member, or a home care nurse. In situations in which a client is discharged with an indwelling intravascular device in place, the nurse teaches the client or family members who are assisting the client how to care for the intravascular device. The nurse also instructs the client to be alert for malfunction of the device as well as signs of inflammation resulting from infection at the

TABLE 26–2   Allergic Reactions to Antimicrobial Agents
Flushing
Wheezing
Sneezing
Pruritus
Urticaria
Rashes
Maculopapular to exfoliative dermatitis
Vascular eruptions
Erythema multiforme (Stevens-Johnson syndrome)
Angioneurotic edema
Serum sickness (headache, fever, chills, hives, malaise, and conjunctivitis)
Anaphylaxis (laryngeal edema, bronchospasm, hypotension, vascular collapse, and cardiac arrest)
Death

catheter insertion site (i.e., redness, heat, pain, swelling, and purulent discharge).

In clients who receive parenteral antimicrobial therapy for an extended period, peripheral venous access may become extremely difficult. In the past several years, this problem has been at least in part circumvented by the use of implanted central venous vascular access devices, such as Hickman catheters, Broviac catheters, and Port-a-Caths. If clients are discharged to home to continue antimicrobial therapy through such a device, the nurse teaches the client appropriate techniques to enter the system, administer the antimicrobial agent, flush the device, dress the insertion site if appropriate, and deal with emergencies. In addition, the nurse describes the signs and symptoms of the major complications associated with the use of these intravascular devices: infection, thrombosis, and mechanical malfunction. The nurse instructs the client to return to a health care facility if any of these problems arise (see Chap. 3 for detailed discussion of venous access catheters). Similar information is provided by the nurse to family members, friends, or home care personnel who will be caring for the client at home.

Psychosocial Preparation

The client with an infectious disease is often anxious and fearful that the infection will be transmitted to family members or friends. The nurse must allay these fears by teaching the client and the family mechanisms that block the spread of disease. Careful attention is paid to the client's concerns, and the nurse makes concrete suggestions (e.g., "Your wife can wear gloves when changing your dressing") to address those specific concerns.

The client with an infectious disease associated with life style behaviors, such as sexual activity, homosexuality, or IV drug abuse, may experience guilt related to the disease. Social stigmatization is also a possibility for clients with these illnesses. The nurse encourages the client to verbalize feelings associated with the illness. The nurse assists the client in locating psychosocial support mechanisms that may help alleviate these problems. Supportive family members, friends, or groups are often helpful in easing the client's adjustment to illness.

Health Care Resources

In unusual instances, a client who has been hospitalized for an infectious disease may be unable to return immediately to the home setting. In such circumstances, temporary placement in a long-term care facility may be advantageous. The nurse from the hospital carefully notes the client's care requirements, medication schedules, and personal needs and preferences on the transfer documents. When possible, the nurse communicates directly with a nurse at the receiving facility to facilitate a smooth transition from the hospital to the intermediate care setting.

Because of funding dependent on DRGs, clients who have deep-seated infections are often discharged to home before completion of long-term antimicrobial therapy for their infections. Often, clients may continue to receive IV anti-infective agents at home. Clients who are ambulatory may be asked to return to an outpatient facility every third day to have a new peripheral venous catheter placed for use as a heparin lock. The client's primary nurse communicates with the outpatient facility staff, again with the intent of effecting a smooth transition from the hospital to the outpatient setting.

In other instances, a home health service may be used to ensure appropriate administration of antimicrobials at the client's home. These home care services have proved efficient, effective, and much less expensive than hospitalization or intermediate care facilities. Occasional visits from a home care nurse may also facilitate detection of early antimicrobial failures, toxicity, or other side effects of therapy.

Evaluation

On the basis of the identified common nursing diagnoses, the nurse evaluates the care of the client with an infectious disease. Expected outcomes for the client with an infectious disease include that the client

1. Describes and complies with the antimicrobial regimen as ordered
2. Maintains normal body temperature
3. Exhibits no symptoms of fluid or electrolyte imbalance
4. States that he/she has returned to a normal level of activity

5. Describes and implements precautions so that infection is not transmitted to others
6. Exhibits no clinical manifestations of recurrence, relapse, or reinfection

By achieving the desired outcomes, the client comprehends the importance of meticulous compliance with antimicrobial therapy and thus eliminates the microorganism responsible for infection. The client is able to progressively return to normal activities in a disease-free state. The client who understands the chain of infection from infected source to susceptible host is also able to institute measures that prevent the transmission of infection to others. A thorough understanding of the mechanisms of transmission enables the client to employ precautions that are appropriate and to eliminate precautions that are inappropriate and unnecessary. Thus, with effective nursing interventions, which are heavily dependent on effective client and family teaching, the client achieves wellness and others are protected, with minimal social isolation of the client.

SUMMARY

Care planning and implementation for the client with an infectious disease present a unique challenge to the nurse. Infection can involve virtually any organ system and has a variety of clinical manifestations, depending on the system affected. Diagnosis is often a prolonged process, and therapy is often extensive.

Because of increasing economic demands on health care resources, clients are being discharged from acute care facilities much sooner, often before therapy is completed. Thus, infection control has moved rapidly outside the realm of the acute care facility, and the importance of meticulous attention to control of infection must be emphasized in all settings. As medical technology advances, clients are living longer, undergoing more invasive therapies, and becoming increasingly susceptible to infection. With the current emphasis on containment of health care costs, health care personnel must assume increasing responsibility for the prevention of infection. All members of the health care team need to understand the routes of transmission of infection and utilize the appropriate means to prevent the spread of microorganisms.

IMPLICATIONS FOR RESEARCH

Little scientific evidence exists to support many of the commonly employed infection control procedures. Many issues regarding the care and management of clients with infectious diseases remain unresolved.

Most, if not all, of these issues are appropriate topics for nursing research. Among the questions for which there is limited scientific information are the following:

1. Should antimicrobial ointment be applied to peripheral IV catheter insertion sites?

2. How should a peripheral IV catheter be anchored and dressed? Are semipermeable dressings associated with lower, similar, or higher rates of catheter-acquired infection?

3. What are the psychosocial effects of isolation on the hospitalized client? Does intervention (explanation of isolation, perhaps providing written materials) by the infection control staff decrease anxiety associated with isolation?

4. Do various antimicrobial agents inserted into the collection bags of indwelling urinary drainage devices decrease the incidence of urinary tract infection in clients with these devices?

REFERENCES AND READINGS

General

Allen, J. C. (1976). *Infections and the compromised host.* Baltimore: Williams & Wilkins.

Bennett, J. V., & Brachman, P. S. (Eds.). (1986). *Hospital infections* (2nd ed.). Boston: Little, Brown.

Centers for Disease Control. (1987). Recommendations for prevention of HIV transmission in health-care settings. *Morbidity and Mortality Weekly Report, 36*(2S), 3–17.

Hoeprich, P. D. (Ed.). (1983). *Infectious diseases* (3rd ed.). Hagerstown, MD: Harper & Row.

Larson, E. L. (Ed.). (1984). *Clinical microbiology and infection control.* Boston: Blackwell Scientific.

Mandell, G. L., Douglas, R. G., & Bennett, J. E. (Eds.). (1985). *Principles and practices of infectious diseases* (2nd ed.). New York: Wiley.

Petersdorf, R. G., Adams, R. D., Braunwald, E. A., Isselbacher, K. J., Martin, J. D., & Wilson, J. D. (Eds.). (1983). *Harrison's principles of internal medicine* (10th ed.). New York: McGraw-Hill.

Schurman, L. M. (1981). *Principles of epidemiology* (DHHS Publication No. 00–038). Atlanta: Centers for Disease Control.

Wenzel, R. P. (1987). *Prevention and control of nosocomial infections.* Baltimore: Williams & Wilkins.

Epidemiology and Infection Control

Centers for Disease Control. (1982). *National nosocomial infections study report (annual summary 1979).* Atlanta: Author.

Coleman, D. (1987). The when and how of isolation. *RN, 50*(10), 5–8.

Garner, J. S., & Faverno, M. S. (1985). *Guidelines for handwashing and hospital environmental control. Hospital infections program.* Atlanta: Centers for Disease Control.

Eickhoff, T. C. (1980). General comments on the study of the efficacy of nosocomial infection control. *American Journal of Epidemiology, 111,* 465–469.

Garner, J. D., & Simmons, B. P. (1983). Guideline for isolation precautions in hospitals. *Infection Control, 4,* 247–325.

Maki, D. G. (1981). Epidemic nosocomial bacteremias. In R. P. Wenzel (Ed.), *Handbook of hospital acquired infections* (p. 371). Boca Raton, FL: CRC Press.

Maki, D. G. (1981). Nosocomial bacteremia: An epidemiologic overview. *American Journal of Medicine, 70,* 719–732.

Nauseef, W. M., & Maki, D. G. (1981). A study of the value of simple protective isolation in patients with granulocytopenia. *New England Journal of Medicine, 304,* 448–451.

Pizzo, P. A. (1981). The value of protective isolation in preventing nosocomial infections in high risk patients. *American Journal of Medicine, 70,* 631–635.

Rose, R., Hunting, K. J., & Townsend, T. R. (1977). The morbidity, mortality and economics of hospital-acquired blood stream infections. A controlled study. *Southern Medical Journal, 70,* 1267–1270.

Steere, A. C., & Mallison, G. F. (1975). Handwashing practices for the prevention of nosocomial infections. *Annals of Internal Medicine, 83,* 683–686.

Turck, M., & Stamm, W. E. (1981). Infections of the urinary tract. *American Journal of Medicine, 70,* 651–654.

Wong, E. S. (1983). Guidelines for prevention of catheter-associated urinary tract infections. *American Journal of Infection Control, 11,* 28–33.

Pathogenesis and Host Defense

Barrett, J. T. (1980). *Basic immunology and its medical application* (2nd ed.). St. Louis: C. V. Mosby.

Berheim, H. A., Block, L. H., & Atkins, E. (1979). Fever: Pathogenesis, pathophysiology, and purpose. *Annals of Internal Medicine, 91,* 261–270.

Maki, D. G. (1978). Control of colonization and transmission of pathogenic bacteria in the hospital. *Annals of Internal Medicine, 89*(5 Pt. 2 Suppl.), 777–780.

Mermel, L., & Maki, D. (1988). Epidemic bloodstream infections from hemodynamic pressure monitoring: Sign of the times. *Infection Control and Hospital Epidemiology, 10,* 47–53.

Rose, N. R., & Friedman, H. (Eds.). (1980). *Manual of clinical immunology* (2nd ed.). Washington, DC: American Society for Microbiology.

Stamm, W. E. (1978). Infections related to medical devices. *Annals of Internal Medicine, 89*(5 Pt. 2 Suppl.), 764–769.

Turck, M., & Stamm, W. E. (1981). Infections of the urinary tract. *American Journal of Medicine, 70,* 651–654.

Microbiology and Antimicrobial Therapy

Atlas, R. M. (1984). *Microbiology: Fundamentals and applications* (p. 435). New York: Macmillan.

Brown, R. B. (1988). Prescribing antibiotics in home healthcare: Problems and prospects. *Geriatrics, 43*(12), 43–49.

Burton, S. M. (1988). Drug update: Antibacterial agents. *Professional Nurse, 3*(5), 171–173.

Calderwood, S. B., & Mollering, R. C. (1980). Common adverse effects of antibacterial agents on major organ systems. *Surgical Clinics of North America, 60,* 65–81.

Larson, E. (1988). Guidelines for use of antimicrobial agents. *American Journal of Infection Control, 16,* 253–263.

Mollering, R. C., Jr. (1985). Principles of anti-infective therapy. In G. L. Mandell, R. G. Douglas, & J. E. Bennett (Eds.), *Principles and practices of infectious diseases* (2nd ed., pp. 153–162). New York: Wiley.

Plorde, J. J. (1983). The diagnosis of infectious diseases. In R. G. Petersdorf, R. D. Adams, E. Braunwald, K. J. Isselbacher, J. B. Martin, & J. D. Wilson (Eds.), *Harrison's principles of internal medicine* (pp. 843–850). New York: McGraw-Hill.

Pritchard, V. (1988). Preventing and treating geriatric infections. *RN, 51*(3), 36–38.

William, T. W., & Jackson, D. (1980). New antibiotics—uses and dangers. *Heart and Lung, 9,* 1089–1095.

Nursing Care

Arking, L., & Saravolatz, L. (1980). Antimicrobial treatment: A coordination challenge for nursing. *Nursing Clinics of North America, 15,* 689–702.

Dixon, R. E. (1978). Effect of infections on hospital care. *Annals of Internal Medicine, 89*(5 Pt. 2 Suppl.), 749–753.

Farber, B. (1988). The multi-lumen catheter: Proposed guidelines for its use. *Infection Control and Hospital Epidemiology, 9,* 206–208.

Griffin, J. P. (1986). Nursing care of the immunosuppressed patient in an intensive care unit. *Heart and Lung, 15,* 179–186.

Gurevich, I., & Tafuro, P. (1985). Nursing measures for the prevention of infection in the compromised host. *Nursing Clinics of North America, 20,* 257–260.

Hargiss, C. O. (1980). The patient's environment: Haven or hazard. *Nursing Clinics of North America, 15,* 671–688.

Hoyt, N. J. (1988). Infection and infection control. In V. D. Cardona, P. D. Hurn, P. J. Bastnagel Mason, A. M. Scanlon-Schilipp, & S. W. Veise-Berrg (Eds.), *Trauma nursing: From resuscitation through rehabilitation* (pp. 224–262). Philadelphia: W. B. Saunders.

Lind, M. (1980). The immunologic assessment: A nursing focus. *Heart and Lung, 9,* 658–661.

Preston, G. A., Larson, E. L., & Stamm, W. E. (1981). The effect of private isolation rooms on patient care practices, colonization, and infection in an intensive care unit. *American Journal of Medicine, 70,* 641–645.

ADDITIONAL READINGS

LeClair, S. M., Schicker, J. M., Duthie, E. H., Hoffman, R. G., & Franson, T. R. (1988). Survey of nursing personnel attitudes towards infections and their control in the elderly. *American Journal of Infection Control, 16,* 159–166.

This article reports a survey of nursing attitudes about infection control issues in four different geriatric care settings. Attitudes about infection control practices, approaches to fever treatment, ranking of infections, client and health care worker vaccinations, and the need for educational programs about infections were reported and discussed. Recommendations for infection control in long-term facilities are suggested.

Mooney, B. R., & Armington, L. C. (1987). Infection control: How to prevent nosocomial infections. *RN, 50*(9), 21–23.

This article identifies clients who are at high risk for acquiring an infection, specifically clients who have had surgery, IV therapy, or urinary catheters. Measures that health care providers can implement to reduce the client's risk of nosocomial infection are also discussed.

UNIT 7 RESOURCES

Nursing Resourses

American Radiological Nurses Association (ARNA), 2462 Stantonsburg Road, Suite 162, Greenville, NC 27834.
Promotes quality care in diagnostic and therapeutic radiology departments. Publishes *ARNA IMAGES* (quarterly newsletter).

Association for Practitioners in Infection Control, 505 East Hawley Street, Mundelein, IL 60060. Telephone 312-949-6052.
Promotes improved client care through monitoring and reduction of infectious risks. Serves as a forum for infection control practitioners. Provides education regarding infection control practices and the development of practice criteria. Supports certification of infection control practitioners through the Certification Board of Infection Control. Publishes *American Journal of Infection Control, APIC News,* an AIDS educational packet, and other materials.

Oncology Nursing Certification Corporation, 1016 Greentree Road, Pittsburgh, PA 15220. Telephone 412-921-7373.
Certifies nurses with experience in oncology.

Oncology Nursing Society (ONS), 1016 Greentree Road, Pittsburgh, PA 15220. Telephone 412-921-7373.

Other Resources

American Cancer Society, 1599 Clifton Road NE, Atlanta, GA 30329. Telephone 404-320-3333.

Centers for Disease Control, Department of Health and Human Services, U.S. Public Health Service, Atlanta, GA 30333. Telephone 404-639-3534.

Leukemia Society of America, 31 St. James Avenue, Boston, MA 02116. Telephone 617-482-2256.

National Coalition for Cancer Survivorship, 323 Eighth Street SW, Albuquerque, NM 87102. Telephone 505-764-9956.

National Institute of Allergy and Infectious Diseases (NIAID), Building 10, Bethesda, MD 20892. Telephone 301-496-4000.

Office of Cancer Communications, National Cancer Institute, Building 31, Room 10A24, Bethesda, MD 20892. Telephone 800-4-CANCER.

UNIT 8

Problems of Protection: Management of Clients with Disruptions of the Immune System

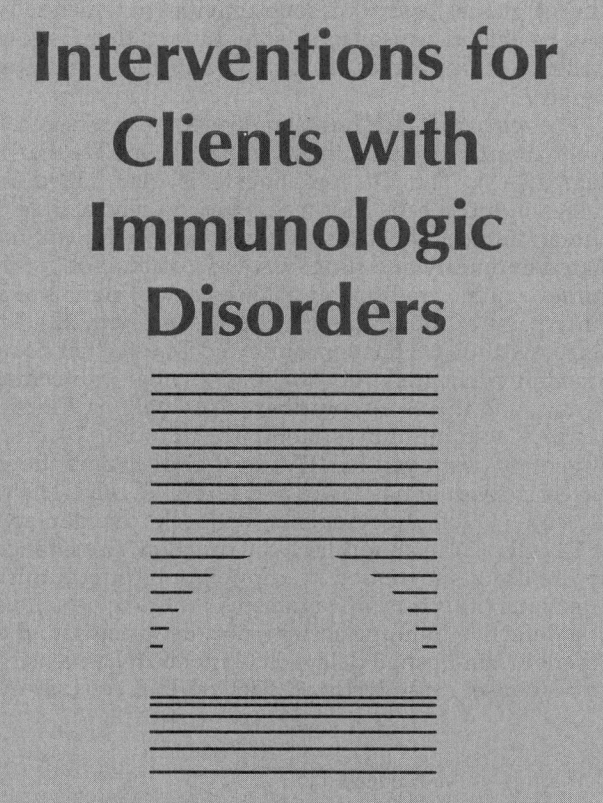

CHAPTER 27

Interventions for Clients with Immunologic Disorders

The highly complex and integrative immune system of the body is constantly at work and usually goes unnoticed. Occasionally, however, the immune system malfunctions. The malfunction may take the form of inadequate or deficient function, excess or exaggerated function, and/or inappropriate function. The result is a host who is susceptible to damage and disease. For some clients, malfunction of the immune system is the cause of disease; for others, it is the result. In this chapter, malfunctions of the immune system are discussed by focusing on four categories of disorders that result: immunodeficiencies, hypersensitivities, gammopathies, and autoimmunities.

IMMUNODEFICIENCIES

A deficient response of the immune system that is due to a missing immune component, a damaged immune component, or a missing step in the process of cell-mediated or antibody-mediated (humoral) immunity is known as an *immunodeficiency*. The immunodeficient person is unable to adequately resist or combat potentially harmful substances that an immunocompetent person can handle well. The immunodeficient person is unable to recognize and eliminate antigens normally and is therefore susceptible to infections, malignancies, and other diseases.

Some people are born lacking a specific substance or function that is essential to normal immune function. They are said to have a *congenital* or *primary* immunodeficiency. Others are born with a normally functioning immune system, and later, as a consequence of another disease, injury, or unknown cause, *acquire* an immunodeficiency. These individuals are sometimes referred to as *immunocompromised* because their immune system has surrendered to or has been compromised by some overwhelming influence that leaves their immune resistance impaired. An acquired immunodeficiency is sometimes referred to as a *secondary* immunodeficiency.

The immunodeficient client poses a major challenge to health care providers. The client manifests clinical symptoms that vary in severity and occur in multiple systems of the body. For many immunodeficiencies, the cause is unknown or uncontrollable, and the pathophysiology is often not well understood. Effective treatment for many immunodeficiencies is currently not available. The complications can often be treated, but not the immune defect itself. Immunodeficiencies are chronic conditions; often substantial periods of wellness are interspersed with the occurrence of infections, malignancies, or other clinical problems. Sometimes the clinical problems are severe and life-threatening. The immunodeficient individual lives under the cloud of knowing that the next infection could be an infection from which he or she will not recover. Normal environmental exposures to people, objects, and microorganisms pose potential and significant danger to the immunodeficient client. Nurses can be instrumental in teaching the immunodeficient person what to do to avoid infection, as well as what signs and symptoms to monitor. The nurse is also crucial in assessing the client for subtle changes, in being alert for signs of early infection, and in treating the client thoroughly and quickly according to physician's orders. Supporting the client and family is an essential part of nursing care.

Acquired Immunodeficiencies

ACQUIRED IMMUNODEFICIENCY SYNDROME

OVERVIEW

The *acquired immunodeficiency syndrome* (AIDS) is a relatively new disease, the first cases being described in the United States in the early 1980s, with several cases of *Pneumocystis carinii* pneumonia and Kaposi's sarcoma (KS) reported in young, otherwise healthy men in New York City and Los Angeles, California. Although it is uncertain how AIDS began, there are several theories. Many researchers believe that the source was the African green monkey, which serves as a host for a virus that is quite similar to the one that causes AIDS, but in the monkey the virus does not cause disease. Sometime in the last 15 years or so, this virus may have undergone random mutations and crossed the boundary from animal to human.

AIDS is a serious, debilitating, and fatal disease that has mainly affected people in the prime of life, between the ages of 20 and 49 years. To be diagnosed as having AIDS, a person must have a clinical disease that indicates a cellular immunodeficiency and have no other reason to be cellularly immunodeficient except infection with the virus that causes AIDS and related disorders.

Pathophysiology/Etiology

The primary cause of AIDS is infection with a virus called the *human immunodeficiency virus* (HIV). This virus was previously known as HTLV-III, the human T cell lymphotrophic virus III, or LAV, the lymphadenopathy-associated virus. In 1986, the International Committee on the Taxonomy of Viruses recommended the use of HIV, human immunodeficiency virus, to name the virus that causes AIDS. HIV is a human retrovirus. Retroviruses, when infecting a cell, have the unique ability to integrate the viral genome (genetic make-up) into the genome of the cell. This alteration results in an abnormal cell, i.e., one that cannot perform its functions properly. At the same time, this cell, when activated and replicating, can produce more virus. HIV is transmitted

via sexual contact, via blood or blood products, and from mother to newborn child. Anyone who has sexual contact with an infected individual is at risk of acquiring the infection. HIV is not transmitted by casual contact in the home, school, or workplace. Although small amounts of virus have been isolated from saliva, kissing, sharing glasses, and other such activities in which saliva may be shared appear to be safe. In fact, there is some evidence that enzymes in saliva are capable of inactivating HIV.

The retrovirus HIV has a predilection for certain cells in the immune system, those with a T4 or CD4 marker (Fig. 27–1). The T4 lymphocyte is also called the helper-inducer cell. This cell plays a central role in human immunity because it is responsible for cell-mediated immunity and functions as a "conductor" of the immune orchestra by sending inducement signals to all other parts of the immune system (see Chap. 23). The person with AIDS has some infected T4 cells that do not function adequately, do not send normal inducement signals, and therefore contribute to overall malfunction of the whole immune system. The infected T4 cell is ultimately destroyed by HIV, so that over time the infected individual has fewer and fewer T4 cells. The results are (1) lymphocytopenia, with selective depletion of T4 cells; (2) an abnormal T cell function, as evidenced by the client's increased susceptibility to opportunistic infections (infection by organisms that take advantage of a defective immune system) and neoplasms, and an absent or diminished delayed cutaneous hypersensitivity response; (3) polyclonally activated B cells, as evi-

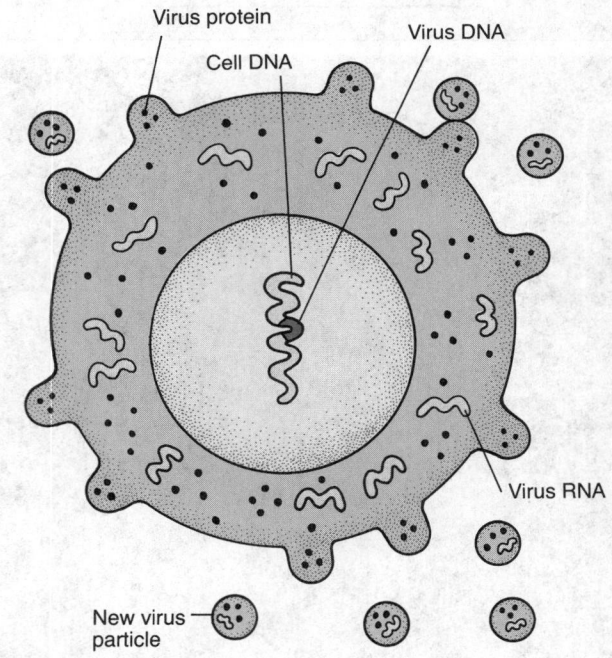

Figure 27–1

A T lymphocyte infected with HIV. The virus can be seen budding from the infected T cell.

KEY FEATURES OF DISEASE ■ Classification of the Centers for Disease Control of HIV Infection

I. Acute infection

II. Asymptomatic infection

III. Persistent generalized lymphadenopathy

IV. Other disease
   A. Constitutional disease
   B. Neurologic disease
   C. Secondary infectious diseases
      1. Secondary diseases specified in the CDC surveillance definition for AIDS
      2. Other specified secondary infectious diseases
   D. Secondary cancers
   E. Other conditions

---

denced by a hypergammaglobulinemia; and (4) abnormally functioning macrophages. It has also been shown that HIV can directly infect macrophages, including those in the central nervous system, which possibly leads to the complex of symptoms referred to as AIDS dementia complex.

AIDS is only one part of the spectrum of HIV infection (see the accompanying Key Features of Disease). Many individuals have HIV infection but no symptoms. Others are infected with HIV and have clinical problems like thrombocytopenia, lymphadenopathy (Centers for Disease Control [CDC] category III), or neurologic symptoms alone (CDC category IV, subgroup B). Still other HIV-infected individuals have a complex of constitutional symptoms such as persistent weight loss, fever, night sweats, diarrhea, fatigue, and the presence of some immune abnormalities by laboratory tests (CDC category IV, subgroup A). This group has previously been referred to as having AIDS-related complex or ARC.

Incidence

The incidence of AIDS has grown from only a handful of cases in 1979 and 1980 to approximately 100,000 cases in the United States by mid-1989, and the U.S. Public Health Service predicts that there will be approximately 365,000 cases by 1992. AIDS has become one of the leading causes of death for certain age groups in certain geographic areas. For example, in New York City, for men aged 30 to 39 years, AIDS is the leading cause of death; for women aged 30 to 34 years, it is the second leading cause of death. It is also clear that the number of known individuals who are HIV positive constitutes just the "tip of the iceberg." Although there have been approximately 100,000 (June 1989) persons diagnosed with AIDS in the United States, there are an estimated 1.0 to 1.5 million persons in the United States

who are infected with HIV but have no symptoms. The number of infected persons who will develop the full-blown disease AIDS is unknown, but current data have shown that it is approximately 35% within 5 to 6 years. Much remains to be learned about why one infected person remains symptom free and another develops AIDS.

Epidemiologic and demographic data have shown that of the individuals with AIDS in the United States, most have been homosexual and bisexual men, a smaller number have been intravenous drug abusers, and a much smaller number have been persons who had received contaminated blood or blood products, including factor VIII preparations (hemophiliacs). A relatively small but growing percentage of cases has occurred in heterosexual partners of infected persons. In the United States, more than 90% of cases have occurred in males, most of whom were between the ages of 20 and 49 years (U.S. Department of Health and Human Services [DHHS], 1987). Although most cases to date have occurred in New York, San Francisco, Los Angeles, and Miami, every state in the United States has reported a growing number of cases. AIDS has also been reported from most other countries in the world, and it has a particularly high incidence in central Africa, the Caribbean, and certain countries in Western Europe and South America.

In the United States as of mid-1989, there have been almost 2000 reported cases of AIDS in children. Most of these (79%) have occurred in children who were born to infected mothers, and some in children who had received blood or blood products, including hemophiliacs. Most of the children with AIDS are diagnosed between the ages of 3 and 24 months, and the distribution in males and females is equal.

In the United States, a disproportionate number of cases of AIDS have occurred in Black and Hispanic persons. Approximately 25% of AIDS cases have occurred in Black and 14% in Hispanic persons, who constitute approximately 12% and 6.5% of the population, respectively. The disproportion is even more dramatic in children and women.

AIDS is a disease with high mortality. The overall case fatality rate is about 55% (DHHS, 1987), meaning that just over half of all the people who have been diagnosed with AIDS are already dead. Two or 3 years from diagnosis, the case fatality rate is at least 80% (DHHS, 1987). To date there have been no reports of a cure or of a reversal of the immune defect.

PREVENTION

Most scientists, public policy experts, and the educated public believe that AIDS is a preventable disease. Adult cases of AIDS have been acquired through sexual contact, the sharing of contaminated needles, or receiving contaminated blood or blood products. As has happened with other communicable diseases, once the routes of transmission are understood, methods for reducing transmission can be instituted through education, public policy, behavioral changes, and laboratory testing. These have all begun to have an impact on the transmission of the disease in the United States.

Education about AIDS as a means of prevention must continue to be directed toward the general public, especially sexually active youth and adults; other high-risk individuals; clients, their families, and friends; and health care and public service personnel. In an effort to reduce transmission, the U.S. Public Health Service has published recommendations for persons who have had positive test results for antibody to HIV (see the accompanying Client/Family Education feature).

Since March of 1985, licensed commercial enzyme-linked immunosorbent assay (ELISA) tests have been available and are being used in all blood banks in the United States to screen blood for antibodies to HIV. Blood that reacts with antibody for HIV by ELISA is discarded. If the blood is reactive, the ELISA test is always repeated with a new sample from the same unit and/or is confirmed by another test called Western blot analysis before the individual is informed of the positive results. Red Cross data from the summer of 1985 indicate that less than 0.1% of random blood donors nationwide had positive test results for antibody to HIV. Although the antibody test was designed to test blood in blood banks, individuals who want to know their antibody status can be tested by their own physician, at a public health clinic, or at one of many alternative testing sites where confidentiality is ensured. Although most people agree that antibody testing should be widely available and used, much controversy exists about whether testing should be mandatory in certain circumstances. Testing is useful so that those who are infected will be able to protect themselves and others. There is also some evidence that treatment with azidothymidine (AZT) may prolong the onset of symptoms in asymptomatic infected individuals. On the other hand, information about antibody status can and is being used against people in discriminatory and damaging ways.

Research continues on the development of an effective vaccine to prevent AIDS and/or HIV infection. Phase I trials on candidate vaccines started in late 1987. Although the HIV genes have been isolated and cloned, the exact nature of the immune response that would protect an exposed person has yet to be elucidated.

COLLABORATIVE MANAGEMENT

 Assessment

Continuous, careful, and comprehensive assessment of the client who has AIDS or who is suspected of having AIDS is crucial in following the subtle changes that can occur in multiple systems, so that infections and other clinical problems can be found early and treated effectively.

History

A general history should include biographic data such as *age, sex, occupation,* and *residence.* The nurse elicits the client's perception of the reason for admission. The nurse thoroughly assesses the current complaint or current illness including its nature, when it started, severity of symptoms, associated problems, and any interventions to date. The nurse questions the client about when the diagnosis of AIDS was made and on what basis, and the nurse asks the client to give a chronology of infections and clinical problems since the diagnosis was made. The nurse assesses past medical history, including whether the client had ever received a blood transfusion. *Family medical history* is assessed for significant illnesses and causes of death. The client is questioned about *sexual practices* and history of *sexually transmitted diseases.* The nurse asks if the client takes any *medications* and if there is a history of allergy to any

---

CLIENT/FAMILY EDUCATION ■ U.S. Public Health Service Instructions for Persons with a Positive HIV Antibody Test Result

"Seek regular medical evaluation and follow-up."

"Either avoid sexual activity or inform your prospective partner of your antibody test results and protect him or her from contact with your body fluids during sex." ("Body fluids" includes blood, semen, urine, feces, saliva, and women's genital secretions.) "Use a condom and avoid practices that may injure body tissues (for example, anal intercourse). Avoid oral-genital contact and open mouthed, intimate kissing."

"Inform your present and previous sex partners, and any persons with whom needles may have been shared, of their potential exposure to HIV and encourage them to seek counseling and antibody testing from their physicians or at appropriate health clinics."

"Don't share toothbrushes, razors, or other items that could become contaminated with blood."

"If you use drugs, enroll in a drug treatment program. Needles and other drug equipment must never be shared."

"Don't donate blood, plasma, body organs, other body tissue, or sperm."

"Clean blood or other body fluid spills on household or other surfaces with freshly diluted household bleach — 1 part bleach to 10 parts water. (Do not use bleach on wounds.)"

"Inform your doctor, dentist, and eye doctor of your positive HIV status so that proper precautions can be taken to protect you and others."

"Women with a positive antibody test should avoid pregnancy until more is known about the risks of transmitting HIV from mother to infant."

environmental allergens, foods, or medications. The nurse assesses the client's level of knowledge regarding the diagnosis, symptom management, diagnostic tests, treatments, community resources, and modes of transmission of the virus. The client's familiarity with and use of safer sex practices is assessed, as well as the client's knowledge of the risks that are associated with reproduction.

Physical Assessment: Clinical Manifestations

Because the client with AIDS is susceptible to multiple infections and cancers, it is important for the nurse to look for many different signs and symptoms, including shortness of breath or cough, fevers, night sweats, fatigue, weight loss, lymphadenopathy, diarrhea, visual changes, headache, memory loss, confusion, seizures, personality changes, dry skin, rashes, skin lesions such as in KS or herpes, pain, and discomfort.

The most common malignancy that is associated with AIDS is *KS*, which occurs in approximately 11% of clients with AIDS. It presents as small, purplish-brown, palpable discrete lesions that are usually not painful or pruritic and can occur anywhere on the person's body. Most clients with KS present with cutaneous lesions, and many develop extracutaneous lesions, especially in the lymph nodes, gastrointestinal tract, or lungs. A small percentage of clients present with extracutaneous lesions but without cutaneous lesions. The nurse assesses the KS lesions for number, size, and location and monitors their progression over time. KS is diagnosed by biopsy and histologic examination of a possible KS lesion.

Opportunistic infections from a variety of organisms account for the majority of clinical manifestations seen in AIDS. The infections can be protozoal, viral, fungal, or bacterial (atypical types). Often, the nurse notes the presence of more than one infection in a client with AIDS.

P. carinii pneumonia, a protozoal infection, is the most common opportunistic infection in AIDS and occurs in more than 60% of clients. The client complains of tightness in the chest and shortness of breath, which gradually worsens. The nurse notes dyspnea, a persistent dry cough, and either low-grade or high fever. On auscultation of the lungs, the nurse notes rales. Another protozoal infection, encephalitis caused by *Toxoplasma gondii*, may cause subtle changes in personality, mild confusion, and headaches or may have an acute onset of seizures, lethargy, and confusion. The nurse does a comprehensive baseline mental status examination to detect subtle changes.

Cryptosporidium is a parasite that causes a gastroenteritis with diarrhea and abdominal discomfort. In AIDS this illness ranges from a mild diarrhea to a cholera-like syndrome with wasting and electrolyte imbalance. The nurse notes voluminous watery diarrhea, usually associated with weight loss.

Fungi that cause infections include *Candida albicans* and *Cryptococcus neoformans*. *Candida* stomatitis or esophagitis is a frequent finding in AIDS. A client with a *Candida* infection complains of food tasting "funny," mouth pain, and perhaps difficulty in swallowing and retrosternal pain. On examination of the mouth and the back of the throat, the nurse sees the characteristic cottage cheese–like white exudate and inflammation. Esophagitis is diagnosed by endoscopic biopsy and culture. *C. neoformans* causes severe debilitating meningitis and occasionally disseminated disease in AIDS. Clinical manifestations of meningitis include fever, headache, blurred vision, nausea and vomiting, stiff neck, mild confusion, and other mental status changes. The client sometimes presents with seizures and other focal neurologic abnormalities.

Bacterial infections are atypical in AIDS. The most common infection is with *Mycobacterium avium-intracellulare*, which is usually a disseminated infection, and positive cultures can often be obtained from lymph nodes, bone marrow, and sometimes blood. The clinical contribution of this bacterium is unclear because the associated symptoms are fairly nonspecific and could be caused by a number of other organisms that are also common in AIDS. Clinical manifestations include fever, debility, weight loss, malaise, and sometimes lymphadenopathy or organ disease. Other types of mycobacteria seen with some frequency in AIDS include *Mycobacterium tuberculosis* and *Mycobacterium kansasii*.

Viral infections, especially with cytomegalovirus (CMV), play a significant role in the morbidity and mortality that are associated with AIDS. CMV infection is responsible for many nonspecific constitutional symptoms such as fever, malaise, weight loss, fatigue, and lymphadenopathy. CMV can also cause a retinochoroiditis, with visual impairment ranging from slight to total bilateral blindness. On funduscopic examination, the skilled nurse sees evidence of inflammation and hemorrhage. Visual field cuts can be detected. CMV is also responsible for a colitis, which manifests as liquid diarrhea, abdominal bloating and discomfort, and weight loss. In addition, CMV can cause encephalitis, pneumonitis, adrenalitis, hepatitis, or disseminated infection. Herpes simplex virus infections in AIDS usually present as ulcerative lesions in the perirectal area, and less frequently in the oral or genital area. Symptoms include pain, bleeding, and rectal discharge.

Many clients have *neurologic symptoms* that are probably a result of direct infection of cells within the central nervous system with HIV. Headaches, personality changes (especially apathy and withdrawal), and dementia may occur. Peripheral neuropathies may also be noted, including paresthesias, pain, and gait changes.

Some clients have a severe *wasting syndrome* with no clear-cut infectious etiology or obvious mechanical problems. Weight loss is persistent and sometimes extreme, and the client may appear to be quite thin or emaciated. Many clients complain of dry, itchy, irritated skin, and sometimes diffuse rashes. The nurse may see evidence of eczema or psoriasis. The nurse or the client may note petechiae, blood in the urine or stool, or bleeding gums secondary to a low number of platelets.

Psychosocial Assessment

Psychosocial data collection for a client with AIDS is extremely important. The nurse asks about the client's family structure and significant others because often these clients have alternative support systems. The nurse assesses which family members and friends are aware of the client's diagnosis to help protect the client's confidentiality. Some clients, because of real or threatened discrimination, are quite selective about whom they tell about their diagnosis. Nurses respect the client's choices as much as possible without compromising care. Resources are offered to help with disclosure to sexual partners or family members. In many cases, the client is closest to a lover or a friend who is not legally recognized as next of kin. The nurse obtains the name and phone number of that person and finds out if a durable power of attorney document has been executed.

Information about the client's activities of daily living is elicited, as well as any changes that may have occurred since diagnosis. The nurse assesses the client's current employment status and occupation, social activities and hobbies, current living arrangements, and financial resources including health insurance. An assessment of the client's anxiety level, mood, and cognitive ability help in planning care and monitoring changes. The nurse asks the client about any experiences with discrimination and how they were handled. The nurse assesses the client's level of self-esteem, and together the nurse and client identify the client's strengths and coping strategies. The nurse gathers information about any suicidal ideation, depression, or other psychologic problems. Information about the client's involvement with support groups or other community resources is obtained.

Laboratory Findings

A lymphocyte count is generally done as part of a complete blood count with differential (see Chap. 66). The normal white blood cell count is between 4500 and 11,000 cells/mm³, with a differential of approximately 30% to 40% lymphocytes (an absolute number of 1500 to 4500). Clients with AIDS are often leukopenic, with white blood cell counts of less than 3500 cells/mm³, and are usually lymphopenic (less than 1500 cells/mm³).

Determinations of the percentage and number of T4 and T8 cells are often done as an important part of an immune profile. The number of T4 and T8 cells is currently determined most often by means of a *fluorescence-activated cell sorter*. This machine uses computerized laser beam technology and monoclonal antibodies to separate and count cells on the basis of cell surface markers. Persons with HIV infection usually have a lower than normal number of T4 cells; some clients with

AIDS have 100 cells/mm³ or fewer (the normal range is between 800 and 1200 cells/mm³). At the same time, the number of T8 cells is usually normal. The normal ratio of T4 to T8 cells is approximately 2:1. In AIDS, because of a low number of T4 cells, this ratio is low (<1).

HIV antibody can be measured by means of an *ELISA test*. Because of the sensitivity of the ELISA test, a person is considered to have a positive antibody test result only if the ELISA is repeatedly reactive or if it is confirmed by a positive Western blot analysis. The Western blot analysis is a more specific test that can detect antibody to specific parts of the virus. This test is not as widely available as ELISA and is complicated by subjective interpretation of results. If a person has a positive test result for antibody to HIV, it does not mean that he or she has AIDS, but that there has been infection with the virus. This person is considered to be infectious. A certain percentage of these infected individuals will later develop AIDS.

Technology is available with which to determine the presence of HIV itself. One method involves culturing the cells of an infected individual in a culture medium and over a 28-day period measuring the amount of reverse transcriptase activity and formation of syncytia. Reverse transcriptase is a viral enzyme that is necessary for replication of the virus within the cell. It is believed that the more reverse transcriptase that is present, the more actively the virus is replicating. A syncytium is in this case a characteristic clumping of infected and uninfected T4 cells resulting from HIV infection. The p24 antigen assay is a test that is used to quantify the amount of p24 (viral core protein) present in the patient's serum. Some studies have shown a correlation between high levels of p24 antigen and a declining clinical course. A newer technique, gene amplification, is accomplished by polymerase chain reaction. By this method, minute amounts of viral deoxyribonucleic acid (DNA) can be found in cells from a person who may have no other indication of infection with HIV.

Other laboratory tests are essential to (1) establish and monitor the overall condition of the client and (2) detect or diagnose any infections or secondary clinical processes. Standard tests that are done include SMAC, complete blood count with differential and platelets, prothrombin time and partial thromboplastin time, VDRL, hepatitis B surface antigen, and immunoglobulin levels. Tests that are sometimes done to further evaluate the immune profile of a client include skin testing for delayed hypersensitivity and bone marrow aspiration with biopsy and cultures. On the basis of the clinical symptoms with which the client presents, other *diagnostic tests* are chosen. Frequently included are tests of stool for ova and parasites; biopsies of skin, lymph nodes, lungs, liver, gastrointestinal tract, or brain; chest x-ray; gallium scans; bronchoscopy, endoscopy, or colonoscopy; liver and spleen scans; computed tomography scans; pulmonary function tests; and assays for arterial blood gases.

Analysis: Nursing Diagnosis

Usually, a person with AIDS is admitted to the hospital with the onset of symptoms that are consistent with one of the opportunistic infections. The typical client is a young, 20- to 40-year-old man, but men, women, and children of all ages can have AIDS. The client's health status ranges from seemingly fairly healthy to extremely debilitated or even terminally ill depending on the time since diagnosis, the number of infections or other clinical syndromes that have been experienced, and the presenting problem.

Common Diagnoses

The following nursing diagnoses are common in the client with AIDS:

1. Ineffective breathing pattern related to *Pneumocystis* pneumonia, CMV pneumonitis, pulmonary KS, and/or mycobacterial infection
2. Altered nutrition: less than body requirements related to infection, mechanical problems, or anorexia
3. Diarrhea related to infection or KS
4. Impaired skin integrity related to KS lesions or herpes simplex virus abscesses
5. Potential for infection related to cell-mediated immunodeficiency
6. Altered thought processes related to central nervous system lesions (toxoplasmosis, CMV, cryptococcosis, KS, lymphoma, HIV infection)
7. Self-esteem disturbance related to changes in body image or decreased self-esteem
8. Anticipatory grieving related to loss of control, health, independence, friends, social activities, job, home, life
9. Social isolation related to stigma, transmissibility of the virus, infection control practices, and/or fear

Additional Diagnoses

Many other diagnoses might be appropriate for some individuals with AIDS, such as

1. Activity intolerance related to fatigue, discomfort, central nervous system defect, weakness, or anemia
2. Potential for injury related to central nervous system deficit, mental status changes, depression, and/or thrombocytopenia
3. Pain related to KS, lymphadenopathy, high fevers, or infections
4. Sensory/perceptual alterations (visual) related to CMV retinitis and blindness
5. Sleep pattern disturbance related to physical discomfort, anxiety, depression, and/or night sweats
6. Ineffective individual coping related to the diagnosis of AIDS
7. Ineffective family coping related to the diagnosis of AIDS

 ## Planning and Implementation

The plan of care for clients with AIDS focuses on the most commonly seen nursing diagnoses (see the accompanying Client Care Plan). Certainly other diagnoses may be appropriate for individual cases.

Ineffective Breathing Pattern

The most common nursing diagnosis seen in AIDS is ineffective breathing pattern. Many clients are initially diagnosed with *P. carinii* pneumonia and with AIDS.

Planning: client goals. The major goals for this nursing diagnosis are that the client will (1) maintain adequate oxygenation and perfusion and (2) experience minimal dyspnea and discomfort.

Interventions: nonsurgical management. Appropriate drug therapy is initiated depending on identification of an infectious or neoplastic cause for respiratory difficulty. The treatment of choice for *P. carinii* pneumonia, the most common infection in AIDS, is trimethoprim-sulfamethoxazole (Bactrim). It can be given intravenously or orally depending on the severity of the infection. A high percentage of clients with AIDS have adverse reactions to this medication. The second drug of choice is pentamidine isothionate, usually given intravenously and sometimes intramuscularly. The nurse administers the drug appropriately and monitors the client carefully for adverse reactions by being alert to changes in the white blood cell count, rash, nausea or anorexia, and changes in liver or kidney function. It is recommended that prophylaxis for *Pneumocystis* infection be given with trimethoprim-sulfamethoxazole or aerosolized pentamidine to clients with fewer than 200 T4 cells.

In addition, the client needs appropriate nursing care to maintain respiratory function and to avoid complications. The nurse continuously assesses the client's respiratory status including vital signs; level of consciousness; rate, rhythm, and depth of respirations; and breath sounds. Arterial blood gas results are evaluated and monitored over time. The nurse provides the client with oxygen therapy as ordered, room humidification, mechanical ventilation, suctioning, and/or chest physical therapy as needed. The nurse is attentive to the client's fluid balance and helps the client to maintain an adequate fluid intake. The client's comfort is assessed by the nurse. Often a client will be more comfortable with the head of the bed elevated. The nurse monitors the client's temperature and administers antipyretics such as acetaminophen (Tylenol) or aspirin as indicated. The nurse helps the client to pace activities to minimize shortness of breath and exhaustion.

CLIENT CARE PLAN ■ The Client with AIDS*

Goal/Outcome Criteria	Interventions	Rationales
Nursing Diagnosis 1: Ineffective Breathing Pattern Related to Pneumocystis, CMV, KS, or MAI		
Client will experience minimal or no dyspnea or discomfort. ■ Has respiratory rate and depth within normal limits for activity level.	1. Use fluids, oxygen therapy, head of bed elevation. 2. Assess respiratory status: vital signs; level of consciousness; rate, depth, and rhythm of respirations; breath sounds.	1. These measures minimize dyspnea. 2. Changes should be monitored.
Client will experience adequate oxygenation or perfusion. ■ Has $PaO_2 > 80$ mmHg.	1. Monitor arterial blood gas levels. 2. Administer medication as ordered and watch for side effects.	1. These levels indicate oxygenation of blood. 2. Medication side effects are common.
Client will maintain patent airway. ■ Has no adventitious breath sounds on auscultation.	1. Ensure room humidification. 2. Use ventilation, suction, chest physical therapy as ordered.	1, 2. Most clients have a dry cough.
Client will be able to perform activities of daily living (ADL) and other activities.	1. Ensure activity moderation/pacing. 2. Assist with ADL. 3. Use antipyretics for fever. 4. Support client.	1, 2. Moderation and assistance minimize shortness of breath and exhaustion. 3. Reduction of fever lowers metabolic rate and conserves energy resources. 4. Providing supportive care as needed reduces the client's physical and emotional energy demands and conserves energy resources for other functions.
Nursing Diagnosis 2: Altered Nutrition: Less Than Body Requirements Related to Infection or Malignancy, with Weight Loss, Mechanical Problems, Pain, Anorexia, Nausea, Vomiting, or Diarrhea		
Client will maintain appropriate weight for height and body build. ■ Has no weight loss. ■ Shows weight increase in proportion to height and body build.	1. Monitor intake and output, calorie count. 2. Provide meals/snacks with high calorie and nutritional value. 3. Offer high-calorie supplements (e.g., Ensure, Sustacal). 4. Give enteral or parenteral feedings if needed.	1. These measures indicate fluid balance and adequacy of calorie intake. 2. Proper intake provides calories and improves nutrition. 3. Supplements provide many calories and nutrients in an easy-to-use can. 4. Clients who cannot get adequate calories orally need other types of feedings.
Client will maintain adequate nutrition and hydration. ■ Has fluid intake equal to amount of fluid lost plus 1000 mL. ■ Ingests a minimum of 2500 kcal/d. ■ Evidences no loss of weight from baseline.	1. Supplement with fluids and vitamins.	1. Supplements ensure adequate levels.
Client will identify foods tolerated. ■ Lists 25 preferred foods that do not cause discomfort.	1. Provide smaller meals, more often. 2. Use antiemetics, if needed. 3. Provide soft or bland diet. 4. Provide meticulous mouth care.	1. Smaller meals are usually better tolerated. 2. Antiemetics minimize nausea. 3. Foods that are easy to eat or digest will help if patient has mouth sores or abdominal pain. 4. Mouth care minimizes mouth soreness.
Nursing Diagnosis 3: Impaired Skin Integrity Related to KS, Herpes Simplex Virus Infection, Malnutrition, or Medication		
Client will not experience increased skin breakdown or secondary infection. ■ Develops no new skin lesions. ■ Evidences no redness or drainage from lesion sites.	1. Monitor progress of lesions. 2. Avoid pressure (use egg crates, air or water mattresses).	1. Monitoring allows institution of early treatment. 2. Pressure increases the possibility of skin breakdown.

CLIENT CARE PLAN ■ The Client with AIDS* *continued*

Goal/Outcome Criteria	Interventions	Rationales
Client will experience healing of existing lesions. ■ Has decreased lesion size and number from baseline. ■ Has re-epithelialization over all lesion sites.	1. Use careful hygienic measures.	1. Some clients have perirectal abscesses and massive diarrhea.
Client will remain comfortable. ■ Expresses comfort.	1. Provide skin care. 2. Give analgesics, if needed. 3. Use lotions, emollients for dry skin. 4. Use wound and skin precautions for herpes simplex virus.	1. Skin care allows maintenance of cleanliness and skin integrity. 2. Some skin lesions (e.g., herpes simplex virus lesions) are painful. 3. Dry skin is troublesome. 4. Virus is shed from the wound.

Nursing Diagnosis 4: Diarrhea Related to Cryptosporidiosis, CMV Colitis, Giardia or Amoeba Infection, Unknown Causes

Client will experience decreased diarrhea and stable fluid, electrolyte, and nutritional status.
■ Evidences no weight fluctuation > 1 lb/d.
■ Keeps serum sodium, potassium, calcium, and chloride values within normal ranges.
	1. Provide dietary counseling:
	  a. Less roughage, alcohol, spicy foods, sweets, fatty foods, lactate.
	  b. Smaller amounts of food more frequently.
	  c. Adequate amount of fluids, especially between meals.
	2. Offer antidiarrheals as needed.
		1. Dietary changes aid in decreasing diarrhea.
		
		2. Antidiarrheals such as diphenoxylate hydrochloride (Lomotil) or tincture of opium are often necessary.

Client will experience minimal or no incontinence. ■ Eliminates all wastes on bedpan or commode.	1. Provide commode or bedpan. 2. Support client and allow privacy.	1. Sometimes client cannot reach the bathroom. 2. Incontinence can be embarrassing.

Nursing Diagnosis 5: Altered Thought Processes Related to Toxoplasmosis, CMV Encephalitis, CNS Lymphoma, or HIV Infection

Client will maintain orientation and level of consciousness. ■ States correct date and location. ■ Correctly identifies known visitors and health care providers.	1. Assess mental status/neurovital signs. 2. Reorient the client and use clocks, calendars, windows, and so on.	1. Neurologic status should be followed. 2. Use of aids helps to reorient client.
Client and others will remain safe. ■ Incurs no injuries. ■ Experiences no seizure activity.	1. Provide a safe environment. 2. Use precautions for seizures. 3. Organize and pace activities. 4. Use anticonvulsants as necessary.	1. Environment can pose hazards. 2, 3. Use of standard seizure precautions and organized activities helps safety. 4. Some clients also need corticosteroids to reduce intracranial pressure.
Client will trust nurse. ■ Initiates open communication with nurse.	1. Structure and assist with ADL. 2. Offer emotional support to client and significant others.	1. These actions help to develop client's comfort and trust. 2. Neurologic problems are difficult to accept.

Nursing Diagnosis 6: Self-Esteem Disturbance Related to Body Image Changes, Decreased Self-Esteem, and Helplessness

Client will maintain normalcy and accept self. ■ Expresses positive feelings about self. ■ Verbalizes positive approaches to assist in adjustment process before and after discharge.	1. Provide a climate of acceptance. 2. Allow for privacy. 3. Offer a safe environment. 4. Encourage self-care, independence, control, decision-making. 5. Help formulate short-term goals that are attainable. 6. Be honest with feelings.	1. Client's self-acceptance is enhanced if others accept him or her. 2. Privacy respects the person. 3. A safe environment allows for expression of fears and anxiety. 4. These actions are normal. 5. Achieving goals enhances self-esteem. 6. Honesty from others shows respect for dignity of the person.

continued

CLIENT CARE PLAN ■ The Client with AIDS* continued		
Goal/Outcome Criteria	**Interventions**	**Rationales**
Nursing Diagnosis 7: Anticipatory Grieving Related to Loss of Control, Independence, Health, Energy, Job, Freedom, Friends, Love, or Life		
Client will experience healthy grieving ■ Verbalizes meaning of loss. ■ Identifies positive strategies to deal with feelings of grief, loss, and anger. ■ Identifies strategies to deal with decreased physical abilities.	1. Encourage sharing of grief with significant others. 2. Encourage verbalization. 3. Don't avoid difficult discussions. 4. Make appropriate referrals. 5. Help with future planning (e.g., insurance, wills, DPA). 6. Help with decisions about do not resuscitate orders, living wills, DPA, and so on. 7. Be there, act normal, touch, care.	1, 2. Verbalizing grief is healthy. 3. Client may need to discuss difficult losses with the nurse. 4. Nurse may need others (e.g., social worker, clergy or religious leader, lawyer) to help. 5, 6. Future planning, "putting things in order," reduces grief. 7. Some clients have said that this is the most important thing nurses can do.

*MAI, *Mycobacterium avium-intracellulare;* CNS, central nervous system; DPA, durable power of attorney.

Altered Nutrition: Less Than Body Requirements

Many clients with AIDS have difficulty maintaining their weight and nutritional status. This problem can be associated with anorexia, nausea, difficulty in eating, diarrhea, or a wasting syndrome. Sometimes, however, the problem is one of fatigue and thus inability to shop for or prepare food.

Planning: client goals. That the client will have a stable or increased weight via adequate nutrition and hydration is the major goal for this nursing diagnosis.

Interventions: nonsurgical management. Because there are multiple etiologies for alterations in nutrition in AIDS, the proper diagnostic procedures are undertaken to determine the etiology. Once the etiology is determined, appropriate therapy is initiated. For example, for the client with *Candida* esophagitis and difficulty in swallowing, therapy with ketoconazole (Nizorail) orally or with amphotericin B (Fungizone) intravenously is begun. For the client with giardiasis, metronidazole (Flagyl) is given. The client with KS of the small intestine may require chemotherapy.

Along with appropriate medical interventions, the nurse assesses and intervenes to maintain the client's weight and nutritional status at the optimal level. The nurse monitors the client's weight, intake and output, and, in some cases, calorie count. With the nurse's assistance, the client identifies foods that are appealing and available. The nurse instructs the client about foods that are high in caloric and nutritional value. In collabo-

ration with the dietitian, an appropriate diet is provided for the client that is high in calorie and vitamin content, and also soft or bland if the client has mouth sores or difficulty in swallowing. The use of supplemental vitamins and fluids is indicated in some cases. For the client who is unable to take a sufficient number of calories through food, the nurse provides high-calorie supplements such as Ensure or Sustacal. In more severe cases, tube feedings or total parenteral nutrition is needed.

For clients who are prone to oral ulceration or infection, the nurse provides meticulous mouth care. Rinses of sodium bicarbonate with normal saline every 2 hours or several times a day are helpful. The client is given a soft toothbrush and advised to drink plenty of fluids. For oral pain that interferes with the client's ability to eat, analgesics or viscous lidocaine may be necessary. Using antiemetics and providing smaller meals more often are helpful to the client who is nauseated.

Diarrhea

Clients with AIDS frequently suffer from diarrhea. Sometimes an infectious etiology (e.g., *Giardia* or *Amoeba*) can be determined and treated. Sometimes an infectious etiology is found, but no effective therapy is available, as in the case of cryptosporidiosis or CMV colitis. In some cases, clients with AIDS have diarrhea and no infectious etiology can be identified.

Planning: client goals. The major goals for this nursing diagnosis are that the client will (1) decrease diarrhea; (2) maintain fluid, electrolyte, and nutritional status; and (3) minimize incontinence.

Interventions: nonsurgical management. For most clients with AIDS and diarrhea, symptomatic management is all that is available. Antidiarrheals such as diphenoxylate hydrochloride (Lomotil) given on a chronic basis give the client some degree of relief. In collaboration with the dietitian, the nurse offers dietary counseling and helps to provide appropriate foods. Recommended dietary changes include less roughage and less fatty, spicy, or sweet food. Alcohol and caffeine are avoided. Some clients have symptomatic relief if they eliminate lactose from the diet. Clients are assisted to eat smaller amounts of food more often and to drink plenty of fluids, especially between meals.

The nurse provides the client with a bedside commode or a bedpan if needed. Some clients are unable to reach the bathroom in time because of inability or anal sphincter weakness, others only because of the urgency with which they have to move their bowels. The nurse provides privacy, support, and understanding for the client and helps to identify ways to make the diarrhea more manageable.

Altered Thought Processes

Neurologic changes and alterations in thought processes are major and important areas of concern for clients with AIDS. It is estimated that approximately 60% of all clients with AIDS have some degree of impairment or AIDS dementia related to HIV infection. In addition, several opportunistic infections and neoplasms can affect the central nervous system.

Planning: client goals. That the client will remain oriented and conscious is the major goal for this nursing diagnosis.

Interventions: nonsurgical management. Clients with AIDS suffer from enormous loss and psychologic stress, which complicates the assessment of any changes in behavior or affect. The nurse establishes a baseline neurologic status and mental status by using standard methods and tools. Examples of neurologic assessment tools are found in Chapter 32. All changes, subtle or not, can then be compared with this baseline. Subtle changes in memory, ability to concentrate, affect, and behavior are evaluated. Differential diagnosis is important to determine if the cause of the neurologic changes is treatable.

Drug therapy. If the client has *T. gondii* encephalitis, the treatment of choice is pyrimethamine (Daraprim) with sulfadiazine (Microsulfon). This is an effective regimen for toxoplasmosis, if tolerated. A high incidence of hypersensitivity and/or dose-limiting leukopenia is associated with the use of these drugs. For many clients, this combination of drugs is given long term because often when the drug is stopped the disease and symptoms recur. *C. neoformans* meningitis is treated with intravenous amphotericin B (Fungizone), sometimes with flucytosine. Amphotericin is quite toxic to the kidneys

and can also make a person nauseated and anorexic. Long-term treatment is also needed for *Cryptococcus*. The nurse administers these medications as ordered and monitors carefully for potential side effects.

Safety measures. Crucial to the well-being of the neurologically impaired client with AIDS is attention to safety. The client may not be aware of certain activities. Assistance may be needed with bathing, dressing, eating, ambulating, and other activities of daily living. The environment, whether it is the hospital room, long-term care facility, or home, is made safe and comfortable. Some clients are prone to seizures. Seizure precautions, including padded side rails and the availability of an airway, are instituted. Anticonvulsant medications may be added to the client's medications.

The nurse reorients the demented client to time, place, and person as needed. The nurse reminds the patient of who she or he is and explains what is to be done at any given time. Using calendars, clocks, and radios and putting the bed close to a window may all help to keep the person oriented. Activities should be paced, which allows independence, but assistance should be provided when needed to prevent undue frustration or problems. The nurse gives simple directions and uses short and uncomplicated sentences.

The nurse assesses the client with neurologic disease for signs and symptoms of increased intracranial pressure. Any changes in level of consciousness, vital signs, pupil size or reactivity, or limb strength are reported to the physician immediately for appropriate intervention. Some clients are given corticosteroids to reduce intracranial pressure.

The nurse works closely with the family and significant others of the neurologically impaired client. The trauma of seeing a loved one unable to provide self-care or behaving strangely or like a child is great. The nurse answers questions honestly and sensitively. The nurse encourages the family and significant others to help reorient the client and to continue to provide ongoing news of family happenings or current events.

Impaired Skin Integrity

The most common skin lesion seen in AIDS is KS. Frequently, no treatment is given to clients with KS. These lesions are often not problematic, but intervention may be necessary if they are open and weeping, painful, in an unusual location, or causing systemic symptoms. Another cause of impaired skin integrity is herpes simplex virus infection.

Planning: client goals. The major goals for this nursing diagnosis are that the client will (1) experience healing of any existing lesions and (2) avoid increased skin breakdown or secondary infection.

Interventions: nonsurgical management. KS can be treated with chemotherapy (single agent or combination). Chemotherapy is generally reserved for clients with rapidly progressive disease or with significant involvement of the gastrointestinal tract, lungs, or other organs. KS is also quite responsive locally to radiation therapy, but this treatment is only locally and transiently effective. Interferon-alpha has been approved for HIV-related KS and is quite effective, especially in clients with better immune function. Treatment of painful KS lesions may include radiation therapy or may be limited to the use of analgesics and comfort measures. KS lesions that are open and weeping must be kept clean and dressed to minimize the risk of secondary infection (see the accompanying Key Features of Disease).

Some clients with cutaneous KS are concerned about their appearance and the risk of being identified by others as having KS. The use of make-up, long-sleeved shirts, and hats may help.

For the client with a herpes simplex virus abscess, meticulous skin care is provided. The nurse cleans the abscess regularly with a diluted solution of povidone-iodine (Betadine) and leaves it open to the air or exposed to a heat lamp to help it dry. This infection can be painful and require the use of analgesics, assistance with position, and other comfort measures. In some clients with this type of abscess, Domeboro soaks have helped to promote healing. This viral infection is treated with acyclovir (Zovirax) given intravenously or by mouth, and in some cases topically depending on the severity of the infection. Acyclovir is potentially toxic to the kidney; therefore, the client must maintain adequate hydration. The nurse uses wound and skin precautions when caring for these clients.

Many clients with AIDS complain of dry or itchy skin. The nurse recommends the use of oils, lotions, and emollients to lessen the client's discomfort.

Potential for Infection

The major problem facing a client with AIDS is immunodeficiency secondary to HIV infection, which leaves him or her susceptible to opportunistic infections and cancers.

Planning: client goals. The client will (1) maintain immune function and (2) remain free from opportunistic diseases are the major goals for this nursing diagnosis.

Interventions: nonsurgical management. Several strategies can help the client to minimize the chances of acquiring an infection, but none at this time are foolproof. The accompanying Key Features of Disease gives treatments that are used for opportunistic infections and KS.

Intensive research is ongoing to find a drug that will inhibit the growth or infectivity of the virus in a client with HIV infection, without unacceptable side effects. Several medications have demonstrated antiretroviral effects in vitro and in animal studies; clinical trials of these compounds are being conducted at various centers. AZT or zidovudine (Retrovir) is an anti-HIV medication that was approved by the U.S. Food and Drug Administration in mid-1987 for use in persons with AIDS who have recently had *P. carinii* pneumonia or for those who have HIV infection and a T4 cell count lower than $200/mm^3$. In a multicenter phase II study, there were a significantly higher number of deaths (16) in the control group than there were in the group taking AZT (1). AZT can be given orally or intravenously; the usual dose is 200 mg every 4 hours orally. Side effects include a potentially severe macrocytic anemia often requiring regular transfusions; mild headache and nausea; and, less commonly, changes in white blood cell count or liver function tests. AZT and chemically similar compounds such as dideoxycytidine and dideoxyinosine are currently being tested in other persons with HIV infection.

Research is also being conducted to evaluate various modalities that may enhance or reconstitute the immune system of clients who are made immunodeficient by HIV infection. Some of these methods include bone marrow transplantation, lymphocyte transfusion, and the administration of lymphokines and other biologic response modifiers.

It has become evident that HIV can remain latent inside a cell for long periods and can cause an active infection when the cell is stimulated. What signals the cell to become activated, the so-called cofactors of HIV infection, are not known, but there are various possibilities. Other infections, especially viral and parasitic infections, activate T cells; several of these (e.g., CMV, Epstein-Barr virus, hepatitis B virus, and others) are considered to be potential cofactors. The nurse teaches the client to avoid exposure to infection as much as possible. The nurse also teaches the client about methods of safer sex, which are necessary not only for the prevention of transmission to others but also for the protection of the infected client. Guidelines for safer sex include avoidance of multiple partners and avoidance of sexual activity that results in exchanges of body fluids (including semen, urine, vaginal secretions, blood, and feces) with anyone who is infected with HIV or anyone whose infection status is not known. Avoidance of large crowds, travel to foreign places with poor sanitation, or exposure to infected individuals is important. The nurse teaches the client and supports him or her in efforts to remain healthy.

Self-Esteem Disturbance

The client with AIDS is susceptible to changes in self-esteem and self-concept. Contributing to this are real and often dramatic changes in appearance that alter the person's body image. In addition, many clients have significant changes in their relationships with others and in day-to-day activities, often including a job or other productive activity. All of these abrupt changes serve to disrupt one's self-concept. Self-esteem is also affected by the guilt or ambivalence that some clients feel about their choice of life style (e.g., homosexuality or intravenous drug use).

KEY FEATURES OF DISEASE ■ Treatment of Opportunistic Infections and Kaposi's Sarcoma

Problem	Treatment
Kaposi's Sarcoma	Local radiation therapy for palliation Single-agent chemotherapy (VP-16, vinblastine, others) Combination chemotherapy Interferon-alpha
Protozoal Infections	
P. carinii pneumonia	Trimethoprim-sulfamethoxazole (Bactrim), IV or PO for 14–21 d or longer Pentamidine isethionate by slow IV
T. gondii encephalitis	Pyrimethamine with sulfadiazine
Cryptosporidium gastroenteritis	Symptomatic treatment with antidiarrheals, fluids, and nutritional supplementation
Bacterial Infections	
M. avium-intracellulare	No known effective therapy Some use of antituberculosis medication Experimental treatment with ansamycin, clofazimine, and amikacin
M. tuberculosis	Isoniazid, rifampin, and ethambutol
Fungal Infections	
C. albicans stomatitis or esophagitis	Nystatin swish and swallow, clotrimazole troches, ketoconazole, amphotericin B
C. neoformans meningitis	Amphotericin B with or without flucytosine
Viral Infections	
Herpes simplex abscesses	Acyclovir
Cytomegalovirus retinochoroiditis, pneumonitis, colitis, encephalitis	Ganciclovir

Planning: client goals. The major goal for this nursing diagnosis is that the client will accept self and not withdraw or hide from others.

Interventions: nonsurgical management. The nurse and other members of the health care team provide a climate of acceptance for clients with AIDS. The nurse allows for the client's privacy but does not avoid or isolate the client. The nurse encourages the client's self-care, independence, control, and decision-making. The nurse helps the client to formulate short-term attainable goals and offers encouragement and praise when they are achieved. Many clients with AIDS become quite debilitated or have infections or lesions that alter their appearance considerably. The nurse accepts these changes, offers comfort and concern, but does not deny her or his own feelings.

Anticipatory Grieving

The client with AIDS grieves multiple losses from the day of diagnosis until the day of death. Clients lose control, independence, and health. Most feel frustrated by a loss of energy and ability to do things. Because of unfortunate misunderstandings, fear, and stigma, many clients have lost friends, jobs, and homes; even family members have turned away. Because HIV is a sexually transmitted disease and many clients abstain entirely from sex after learning of the diagnosis, they suffer from actual and perceived losses of affection and love. Ultimately, clients grieve for the loss of their own life, for they are only too aware of the fatal nature of this disease.

Planning: client goals. Major client goals for this nursing diagnosis are that the client will (1) grieve for the numerous losses being experienced in an appropriate manner and (2) verbalize the meaning of loss. In addition, family members and significant others will be involved in the grieving process, if possible.

Interventions: nonsurgical management. Nurses can assist the client and significant others with the grieving process. Nurses encourage the client to verbalize about the many losses and do not avoid difficult discussions about loss or death with the client. Nurses refer the client to the appropriate resources for help with future planning, e.g., writing a will, obtaining Social Security disability, and working out finances or living arrangements. Nurses encourage the client to share grief with significant others, which helps them to grieve and not feel isolated. Nurses are available to clients to show that they care and to discuss lighter topics (such as the latest movie, the weather, or recipes) as well as the meaning of loss and coping strategies. Nurses are available to help clients and significant others and to make appropriate referrals as decisions are required for the type and extent of care, durable power of attorney, resuscitation, and others.

Social Isolation

Many clients with AIDS experience discrimination, rejection, and isolation from others. Friends or health care workers sometimes exhibit avoidance behaviors or refuse to have anything to do with these clients. Misunderstanding and fear lead to misuse of proper infection control procedures so that clients are sometimes isolated in the hospital environment.

Planning: client goals. The major client goals for this nursing diagnosis are that the client will (1) verbalize an understanding of the infection control precautions and (2) maintain involvement with others and in activities.

Interventions: nonsurgical management. Nurses and health care workers consistently use universal infection control precautions (see Chap. 26) with all clients to minimize the risk of exposure to themselves. They explain these precautions and the rationale for their use to the client. Family, friends, and visitors, especially those who may assist with the client's care, are instructed about universal precautions. The use of precautions does not deter the nurse or other health care provider from entering the client's room and establishing a relationship with the client. No precautions need to be taken when entering the room to talk to the client, deliver medications, take vital signs, or perform other activities, except when the nurse will be handling blood or body fluids. Even if the nurse or health care worker is exposed

to contaminated blood or body fluids of an infected individual, the risk of acquiring an HIV infection is low. On the basis of several large prospective studies, the risk is estimated to be 0.5% after a needle stick or other percutaneous injury.

The nurse encourages the client to verbalize feelings about self, coping skills, and sense of ability to control the situation. The nurse helps the client to identify support systems, including those already in place for the client and those that need to be arranged.

The nurse does not isolate the client and establishes a therapeutic nurse-client relationship. The nurse shows understanding and concern while helping the client to find ways to minimize feelings of rejection and isolation.

■ Discharge Planning

The usual course of illness is one of intermittent acute infections interspersed with periods of relative wellness over a period of months or years, and ultimately a chronic progressive debilitation. Because of the fluctuating nature of this illness, the client often spends long periods at home between hospital admissions or clinic visits. In some instances, especially as the client's illness becomes more severe, referral may be needed to a long-term care facility, home health care agency, or hospice for care outside of the hospital.

When the client is discharged, the nurse, in collaboration with the social worker, dietitian, and other available resources, works with the client to plan what will be needed and how he or she will manage at home with self-care and activities of daily living. Appropriate referrals can help to prevent problems.

Home Care Preparation

If the client is discharged to home, a careful assessment of the client's status, ability to function, and actual or potential needs for care is undertaken. Some clients do not need care but need to maintain a link with the physician or primary care providers. Others need assistance or care in the home, which could range from assistance with activities of daily living for someone with weakness, debility, or limited function, to the need for round-the-clock supportive nursing care, medications, and nutritional support for someone who is more severely or terminally ill. The nurse assesses resources that are available to the client, including family members and significant others who are willing and able to function as caregivers, and helps to make arrangements for outside caregivers if needed. Clients may need referrals and/or help in planning housing, finances, insurance, legal services, funeral arrangements, and spiritual counseling.

Psychosocial Preparation

Clients with AIDS who are discharged to home or another care facility are often concerned about the possible social stigma and rejection that they may experience. The nurse is aware that this fear may be realistic and helps the client to identify ways to avoid problems as well as coping strategies for difficult situations. Family and significant others are supported in efforts to help the client and protect him or her from discrimination. The client is encouraged to continue as many usual activities as possible. Except when the client is too ill or too weak, clients can continue to work and to participate in most social activities. Because of the potential stigma and discrimination, clients are supported in their selection of friends and relatives with whom to discuss the diagnosis. Sexual partners and care providers should be informed; beyond that it is up to the client. Some clients experience severe depression or anxiety about the future. Almost all feel the burden of having a fatal disease that is widely considered to be unacceptable and thus feel compelled to maintain some secrecy about the illness. Referrals to community resources, mental health professionals, and support groups can help the client to verbalize fears and frustrations and to cope with the illness.

Client/Family Education

Education of the client and the client's family and significant others is a high priority, especially in preparation for discharge. The client should be carefully instructed about modes of transmission of the virus; about what behaviors will prevent transmission, including safer sex guidelines and not sharing toothbrushes, razors, and other blood-contaminated articles; and about notification of caregivers and sexual partners. The nurse teaches the client to identify signs and symptoms of potential infections and what to do if these appear. The nurse instructs the client about the importance of self-care strategies such as adequate nutrition, hygiene, balanced rest and exercise, skin care, mouth care, and safe administration of any ordered medications (including potential side effects). The nurse teaches the client about preventing infections by using safer sex guidelines; avoiding large crowds, especially in enclosed areas; maintaining a clean environment; and not traveling to countries with poor sanitation. Families and significant others need instruction and guidance about infection control precautions that they should observe while caring for the client in the home, to prevent their acquiring HIV and other infections; some nursing techniques for use in the home; and coping and support strategies.

Health Care Resources

In many cities in the United States, community organizations have been set up to assist the person with AIDS. These organizations are often composed of mainly volunteers, and they usually offer excellent services to the community. The types and number of services vary by agency and city, but many include HIV testing and counseling, clinic services, buddy systems,

support groups, respite care, education and outreach, referral services, and even residences. Examples of such community organizations include Gay Men's Health Crisis in New York, Los Angeles AIDS Project, Shanti Project in San Francisco, Health Education and Resource Organization in Baltimore, and Whitman-Walker Clinic in Washington, DC. Clients may also need referrals to other local resources such as home care agencies, companies that provide home intravenous therapy, community mental health agencies, Meals on Wheels, and others.

 Evaluation

On the basis of the identified nursing diagnoses, condition of the client, and clinical entities present, the nurse evaluates care for the client with AIDS. Expected outcomes for this client population include that the client

1. Maintains adequate respiratory function
2. Maintains weight and nutritional and fluid status
3. Remains adequately oriented and in a safe environment
4. Maintains skin integrity
5. Maintains immune function
6. Prevents, avoids, or minimizes opportunistic infections
7. Maintains self-worth and self-esteem
8. Grieves losses appropriately
9. Maintains support system and involvement with others
10. Complies with appropriate and available therapy

The overall goals for someone with AIDS are to maintain a high level of functioning for as long as possible, to minimize infections, and to maintain physiologic function and activity, quality of life, and dignity in the face of progressive illness. The nurse assists the client in meeting desired outcomes by providing assessment, care, teaching, and support as needed. Knowledgeable, sensitive, competent, nonjudgmental nursing care can make an enormous difference for this client population.

NUTRITION-RELATED DEFICIENCIES

Adequate and balanced nutrition is necessary for the proper functioning of the immune system. For example, lymphocytes are highly active metabolic cells that constantly shed surface components (such as immunoglobulin) and need appropriate nutrients for resynthesis of these components. Immunodeficiency that is related to nutrition is considered to be an acquired abnormality and results from multiple factors—biologic, political, economic, and cultural. Acquired immunodeficiencies from inadequate or inappropriate nutrition are potentially preventable and treatable. Malnutrition is a major cause of immunodeficiency in the world. It is seen with greatest frequency in developing countries, in the urban and rural poor of developed countries, and in the chronically ill. An important group at high risk for developing malnutrition are hospitalized adult medical-surgical clients. Four points should be kept in mind: (1) Anorexia that is associated with chronic disease, acute infection, and/or treatment often leads to reduced oral intake. (2) Absorption, assimilation, or utilization of nutrients is sometimes impaired because of gastrointestinal diseases or absorption problems. (3) Host defense mechanisms, which are called on in infection, result in increased demands for nutrients, and these demands are met at the expense of the body's stores. (4) Hospitalized clients are often placed on a semistarvation regimen with many hours of nothing by mouth because of procedures that will be performed, or with many hours of administration of intravenous fluids without essential nutrients. Malnutrition can impair any or all aspects of the immune system; the degree of impairment is related to the severity of the malnutrition. An excess of nutrients, especially fats and certain carbohydrates, can also have a detrimental effect on the immune system. Nutritional problems are almost never simple but are rather a complex of deficiency or excess of one or multiple nutrients.

PROTEIN-CALORIE MALNUTRITION

Protein-calorie malnutrition (PCM) affects all aspects of the immune system. The greatest impairment is noted in cell-mediated immunity, with a decreased number of T cells, reduced delayed hypersensitivity, and thymic changes. The result is anergy (no cutaneous delayed hypersensitivity response to common antigens) and an increased incidence of infection in the malnourished host. The incidence of PCM is unknown, but estimates range from 25% to 64% of children in developing countries, and from 25% to 50% of hospitalized adult medical-surgical clients (Marliss, 1985). PCM causes a deficiency in energy and protein synthesis, which necessitates the use of other body stores if available. The usual manifestations of PCM in adults include leanness and cachexia; decreased effort tolerance; lethargy; intolerance to cold; ankle edema; dry, flaking skin and various types of dermatitis; poor wound healing; and a higher than usual incidence of postoperative infections.

The management strategy is to treat the precipitating event and to supply protein and calories, sometimes with supplements of specific nutrients. In severe PCM, first any infections are treated and fluid and electrolyte imbalances are corrected. Then a gradual but steady repletion of protein and energy is undertaken. Often this refeeding begins parenterally because a severely malnourished gut undergoes atrophy of the mucosa and depletion of gastric enzymes, which result in an inability to tolerate food. Replenishment of protein and calories is accompanied by vitamin supplementation as appropriate, nutrition education, psychosocial stimulation, and a progressive increase in physical activity.

PCM is easier to prevent than it is to treat. The nurse is aware of hospitalized clients who are at risk of developing PCM. To prevent this risk, health care providers

1. Measure height and weight when the client is admitted to the hospital and weigh the client at least weekly

2. Monitor the client's ability to eat the ordered diet, and the amounts eaten

3. Obtain dietary consultations when needed

4. Evaluate whether the nutrients taken in are sufficient to meet basal and stress-related needs

5. Avoid prolonged use of intravenous fluids such as normal saline or dextrose and water; add protein, calories, and other nutrients after 3 to 5 days

6. Assess and monitor laboratory test values

7. Remember that hospital food, withholding of meals for tests, and anorexia caused by medications all contribute to potential malnutrition

IMMUNODEFICIENCIES RELATED TO OBESITY

The incidence and severity of infectious disease increase in obese individuals. Impaired cell-mediated immunity and decreased intracellular killing by neutrophils are associated with obesity, which make this population more susceptible to infection.

Excess dietary lipids are known to have a profound effect on immunity. Severe immunosuppression was noted in laboratory animals fed high-fat diets. Also, an increased incidence of cancer of the breast, prostate, and colon has been associated with the chronic intake of a high-fat diet. Although much more research is needed on the relationship between nutrition and immunity, nutrition is clearly a significant factor for maintaining or improving host defenses.

Congenital Immunodeficiencies

Congenital or primary immunodeficiencies are disorders in which the immunodeficient person is born with a defect in the development or function of one of the immune components. As a result, the immune response does not adequately protect the client from infection, and sometimes from malignancy or other disease. Fortunately, most congenital immunodeficiencies are rare. For example, the estimated incidence of agammaglobulinemia is 1 in 50,000 live births, and of severe combined immunodeficiency 1 in 100,000 to 1 in 500,000 live births (Buckley, 1983). The most common congenital immunodeficiency is selective immunoglobulin A (IgA) deficiency, with an estimated prevalence of 1 in 400 to 1 in 2500 live births (Waldmann et al., 1980).

KEY FEATURES OF DISEASE ■ Congenital
Immunodeficiencies

Humoral Immunodeficiencies

X-linked agammaglobulinemia (Bruton's)
Acquired hypogammaglobulinemia (common variable
    immunodeficiency)
Selective IgA deficiency

Cell-Mediated Immunodeficiencies

Congenital thymic aplasia (DiGeorge's syndrome)
Chronic mucocutaneous candidiasis

Combined Immunodeficiencies

Severe combined immunodeficiencies (SCID)
Wiskott-Aldrich syndrome
Immunodeficiency with ataxia-telangiectasia
Nezelof's syndrome

A great deal is known about the cellular abnormalities and functional impairment that are associated with primary immunodeficiencies, yet much remains to be learned about the fundamental biologic or genetic error. Some congenital immunodeficiencies are inherited as an X-linked trait (such as Bruton's disease or Wiskott-Aldrich syndrome), and some are autosomal recessive (such as immunodeficiency with ataxia-telangiectasia). For many congenital immunodeficiencies, however, the genetic defect and inheritance pattern have not been clearly identified. Examples of congenital immunodeficiencies are given in the accompanying Key Features of Disease. The pathophysiology and clinical manifestations of most primary immunodeficiencies can best be understood by classifying them according to the type of defect seen. A person with a congenital immunodeficiency usually has the first clinical signs and symptoms in early childhood. With appropriate treatment of infections, and with the use of new technologies that allow better care of the immunodeficient client, many of these people live into adulthood.

ANTIBODY-MEDIATED IMMUNODEFICIENCIES

B cell, or antibody-mediated, immunity normally protects the host from a variety of bacterial infections and some viral infections through the production of specific antibodies. Someone who lacks this protection generally has recurrent infections with encapsulated bacteria and/or a history of treatment failure. Laboratory evaluation reveals a hypogammaglobulinemia, i.e., low levels of circulating immunoglobulin, either a selective defi-

ciency (one class of immunoglobulin) or a panhypogammaglobulinemia (all classes of immunoglobulin).

A prototypic congenital antibody-mediated immunodeficiency is *Bruton's*, or *X-linked, agammaglobulinemia*. Boys born with this disease present at about 6 months of age with recurrent sinusitis, pneumonia, otitis, furunculosis, meningitis, and septicemia with extracellular pyogenic organisms like pneumococci, streptococci, and hemophilus. Except for clients who develop polio, chronic echovirus infection, or a lymphoreticular malignancy, the overall prognosis is fairly good if antibody replacement is begun early in life. Intravenous or intramuscular immune serum globulin is given to these clients on a regular basis, usually about 100 to 400 mg/kg every 3 to 4 weeks (see the Guidelines feature on p. 648 for immune serum globulin administration). The dosage and schedule should be individualized. Intermittent courses of antibiotics are used for specific infections, as well as long-term prophylactic antibiotic therapy in some cases. Despite therapy, some clients later develop severe sinopulmonary disease.

Common variable immunodeficiency, or *acquired hypogammaglobulinemia,* is a disease that is characterized by recurrent infections with pyogenic bacteria similar to those seen in clients with Bruton's disease, as well as low levels of circulating immunoglobulins of all classes (IgG, IgA, IgM). It differs from Bruton's disease in that it first appears later in life (usually in adolescents or young adults), occurs almost equally in males and females, and is associated with a less severe susceptibility to infection. Frequent complications include giardiasis (intestinal infection with the protozoa *Giardia lamblia*), bronchiectasis, gastric carcinoma, lymphoreticular malignancy, and cholelithiasis (gallbladder stones). Treatment for common variable hypogammaglobulinemia is similar to that for Bruton's disease, i.e., regular administration of intravenous or intramuscular immune serum globulin, and the use of antibiotics intermittently or chronically.

The individual with selective *IgA deficiency*, the most common congenital immunodeficiency, may be asymptomatic or may have chronic recurrent respiratory tract infections, atopic diseases, and/or collagen-vascular diseases. Because IgA is the major immunoglobulin in secretions, bacterial infections are seen primarily in the respiratory, gastrointestinal, and urogenital tracts. Some adults with IgA deficiency also have a malabsorption syndrome. Use of immune serum globulin is contraindicated in persons with IgA deficiency because of the presence of high levels of anti-IgA antibody. Therapy is limited to appropriate and vigorous treatment of infections. In some cases, nutritional supplementation (such as total parenteral nutrition) is necessary.

CELL-MEDIATED IMMUNODEFICIENCIES

T cells or cell-mediated immunity protects the host primarily against intracellular organisms and the accumulation of malignantly transformed cells or foreign cells.

GUIDELINES ■ Administration of Intravenous Immune Serum Globulin

Indications	Dosage	Interventions	Rationales
B cell or humoral immunodeficiencies Bruton's hypogammaglobulinemia Common variable immunodeficiency	Gamimune, 100–200 mg/kg or 2–4 mL/kg, IV once monthly or Sandoglobulin, 0.2–0.3 g/kg, IV once monthly	1. Observe client closely and monitor vital signs during infusion and for 30–60 min thereafter.	1. Monitoring detects signs of anaphylaxis and routine side effects. Side effects occur in 10% of clients and include skeletal pain, back pain, nausea, chills, headache, chest tightness, and abdominal cramps.
Combined immunodeficiencies Severe combined immunodeficiencies		2. Slow the rate of infusion or stop it temporarily if side effects occur.	2. Side effects appear to be related to the rate of infusion.
Others Pediatric AIDS			

Therefore, an individual who lacks cell-mediated immunity with a partial or absolute defect in T cell function clinically presents with recurrent infections with opportunistic fungi, viruses, and parasites. There is also a high incidence of malignancy. T cell–deficient individuals also frequently have growth retardation, wasting, and diarrhea. Because there is no effective therapy for many of the opportunistic infections seen in these clients and there is no effective way to replace cell-mediated immunity, the life span of these clients is short, with most not surviving beyond infancy or childhood. Treatment strategies for T cell deficiencies aim at reconstituting or enhancing T cell immunity. Methods that are being tried include bone marrow transplantation, fetal thymus transplantation, and enhancement with biologic response modifiers like thymosin and thymic factors. Some success has been seen with transplantation of bone marrow and fetal thymus.

COMBINED IMMUNODEFICIENCIES

A *combined immunodeficiency* is one in which both antibody-mediated and cell-mediated immunity are compromised or deficient. Clients with combined immunodeficiencies are characteristically extremely ill, have repeated and severe infections of various types and locations, and usually have a poor prognosis.

COLLABORATIVE MANAGEMENT

The nurse can be instrumental in helping the client with a congenital immunodeficiency to lead a relatively normal life. The nurse needs knowledge of the immune defect and the potential problems that the client faces because of it. Assessment and teaching skills, together with an awareness of and sensitivity to the client's situation, make a difference.

Assessment of the immunodeficient client is vitally important. The nurse should always look for signs and symptoms of infection, being aware that in some immunodeficient individuals the signs of infection may be less evident than in an immunocompetent host. Every complaint and even subtle objective changes should be explored further and followed up carefully. Any signs or symptoms of infection are responded to and treated as early and completely as possible. Congenitally immunodeficient individuals are at potential risk for developing different infections and clinical problems based on their specific defect, their history, and the sources of exposure.

The nurse is aware of potential hazards in the environment. Exposure to infected persons or contaminated articles poses a significantly greater risk to this client than to immunocompetent persons. Intravenous catheters, Foley's catheters, and invasive procedures provide a route of entry for microbes that the client may not be able to handle. Live, attenuated vaccines should not be given to people with combined immunodeficiencies or T cell deficiencies. Blood and blood products should be irradiated before administration.

Clients with congenital immunodeficiencies and their families need extensive education. As much as possible, the nurse teaches them about the immune defect, how it was inherited (if known), and what potential types of infection to watch for. The nurse informs them about signs and symptoms of infection, diagnostic procedures, treatments including medications, and general health and hygiene measures to reduce the possibility of infection.

Clients and families need support and encouragement to live as normal a life as possible. The client should be encouraged to play and interact with others so that growth and social and emotional development is less impaired. Genetic counseling should be provided.

Iatrogenic Immunodeficiencies

Specific immunodeficiencies may be secondary to other disease states that result in loss or destruction of immunoglobulins or T and B cells. For instance, there may be gastrointestinal loss of immunoglobulin as a result of protein-losing enteropathy or loss through the skin because of burns, eczema, or other skin diseases. Increased catabolism of immunoglobulin can occur in nephrotic syndrome or multiple myeloma, which also results in hypogammaglobulinemia. Many diseases cause a cell-mediated (or T cell) deficiency as well; an example is Hodgkin's lymphoma. The most common cause of secondary immunodeficiency is iatrogenesis.

An *iatrogenic* immunodeficiency is an immunodeficiency or immunosuppressive state that is induced in an individual by medical therapies or procedures performed on them. Many of the drugs and other treatment modalities that are used for various diseases can cause or result in immunosuppression. Sometimes this is a desired effect, as in the case of organ transplantation or the treatment of certain autoimmune disorders. At other times, immunosuppression is an undesirable and complicating side effect of therapy that is used for another intent, e.g., cancer chemotherapy, and may even necessitate an alteration in the therapeutic regimen. Different therapies cause different types and degrees of immunosuppression. The challenge is deriving maximal therapeutic effect without leaving the host overly immunosuppressed and therefore susceptible to potentially serious complications.

DRUG-INDUCED IMMUNODEFICIENCIES

Several classes of drugs have powerful and significant immunosuppressive effects. Some induce a general immunosuppression, whereas others are more specific and affect one part of the immune system more than another.

CYTOTOXIC DRUGS

Cytotoxic drugs are usually not selective but interfere with all rapidly proliferating cells. White blood cells, including immunocompetent lymphocytes and phagocytes, are rapidly proliferating and therefore susceptible to this type of destruction. The result is a decrease in the number of lymphocytes and phagocytic cells. Cytotoxic agents also interfere with the ability of lymphocytes to synthesize and release their products (i.e., lymphokines and antibodies), thereby causing a general immunosuppression. Most cytotoxic drugs are used in the treatment of malignancies. Chapter 25 provides more information concerning the actions of these agents.

CORTICOSTEROIDS

Corticosteroids are adrenocortical hormones that are used in the treatment of many immunologically mediated diseases, neoplasms, and several neurologic and endocrine disorders. Corticosteroids have both anti-inflammatory and immunosuppressive effects. They inhibit inflammation by stabilizing the vascular membrane, thereby blocking the migration and mobilization of neutrophils and monocytes. As immunosuppressants, it is believed that they sequester T cells in the bone marrow, which results in a lymphopenia and suppressed cell-mediated immunity. Corticosteroids are not cytotoxic; therefore, lymphocyte levels can return to normal within 24 hours after stopping the drug. Corticosteroids probably interfere with IgG synthesis and the binding of immunoglobulin to antigen. These drugs have many physiologic and immunologic effects, which can alter disease activity. There are also numerous side effects that are associated with corticosteroid therapy including

1. Central nervous system changes such as euphoria, insomnia, or psychosis
2. Cardiovascular changes such as hypertension and edema
3. Gastrointestinal tract effects such as gastric irritation, ulcers, and increased appetite (with weight gain)
4. Other changes such as cataracts, hyperglycemia and glucose intolerance, muscle weakness, osteoporosis, delayed wound healing, increased susceptibility to infection, redistribution of fat pads, and moon faces

The most commonly used oral corticosteroid is prednisone (Deltasone, Meticorten, others). The nurse instructs the client to take it early in the morning to minimize exogenous suppression of cortisol production and to take it with food or milk to minimize gastric irritation. The nurse teaches the client that corticosteroids must be tapered gradually, and never stopped abruptly. The nurse monitors the client's blood pressure, weight, blood glucose level, and fluid intake and output. Clients should also be instructed to eat a carefully balanced diet that has a low salt content and to watch for any signs or symptoms of infection.

CYCLOSPORINE

Cyclosporine (cyclosporin A) is a specific immunosuppressant that selectively suppresses the helper subset of T lymphocytes by blocking proliferation and development. Cyclosporine has been used primarily to prevent organ transplant rejection and has been approved by the U.S. Food and Drug Administration for use in kidney, liver, and heart transplantations. It is currently undergoing clinical trials for use in other disorders, such as uveitis, rheumatoid arthritis, and other autoimmune diseases.

Cyclosporine can be toxic to the liver and kidneys and may be associated with a higher than normal incidence of lymphoma. Studies show that its side effects are minimized by administering small doses and by a shorter duration of therapy.

RADIATION-INDUCED IMMUNODEFICIENCIES

X-rays are cytotoxic to proliferating and intermitotic cells. Most lymphocytes are sensitive to radiation, so exposure can induce a profound lymphopenia in lymphoid organs and in the circulation, thereby causing a general immunosuppression. Total nodal irradiation is used in certain diseases, such as Hodgkin's disease, to induce immunosuppression. This treatment results in a lymphopenia and a decreased T cell function and is being evaluated for use as a therapy for other diseases.

HYPERSENSITIVITIES

Hypersensitivity is a state of altered reactivity in which a previously sensitized immune system reacts in an exaggerated or inappropriate way with resultant tissue damage and pathology. It is clear that although the primary function of the immune system is protection of the host from harm, the same protective mechanisms sometimes have a deleterious effect and may produce damage or disease in the host.

Immune mechanisms that result in tissue damage to the host were classified in 1963 by Gell and Coombs into four basic types of hypersensitivity. These are type I or immediate hypersensitivity (anaphylactic) reactions,

KEY FEATURES OF DISEASE ■ Mechanisms and Examples of Types of Hypersensitivity

Type	Mechanism	Clinical Examples
Type I: immediate	Reaction of IgE antibody on mast cells with antigen, which results in release of mediators	Hay fever Allergic asthma Anaphylaxis
Type II: cytotoxic	Reaction of IgG with host cell membrane or antigen adsorbed by host cell membrane	Autoimmune hemolytic anemia Goodpasture's syndrome Myasthenia gravis
Type III: immune complex mediated	Formation of immune complex of antigen and antibody, which deposits in walls of blood vessels and results in complement release and inflammation	Serum sickness Vasculitis Systemic lupus erythematosus Rheumatoid arthritis
Type IV: delayed	Reaction of sensitized T cells with antigen and release of lymphokines, which activate macrophages and induce inflammation	Poison ivy Graft rejection Tuberculosis Sarcoidosis

type II or cytotoxic reactions, type III or immune complex–mediated reactions, and type IV or delayed hypersensitivity reactions (see the accompanying Key Features of Disease). Clinical manifestations of disease may be the consequence of one or any combination of these mechanisms of tissue injury.

Type I: Immediate Hypersensitivity Reactions

OVERVIEW

Type I, or *immediate, hypersensitivity* occurs when IgE responds to an otherwise harmless antigen such as pollen and causes the release of mast cell mediators, which results in an acute inflammatory reaction and symptoms such as bronchospasm, wheezing, and rhinorrhea (see the illustration on p. 653).

When first exposed to an *allergen* (an antigen that provokes allergic sensitization with IgE) the host responds by making specific IgE. IgE binds to certain cells in the body: the basophils in the circulation and the mast cells in connective tissue (especially skin, submucosa, peripheral nerves, and the reticuloendothelial system). Basophils and mast cells are similar in that both have large numbers of granules that contain powerful pharmacologically active mediators that can be released when stimulated (see Chap. 23). Basophils and mast cells also possess a receptor for IgE. IgE is referred to as the reaginic antibody. It is formed in response to exposure to a substance to which the individual is particularly sensitive. This sensitivity is most often genetically determined, as evidenced by the fact that atopic parents

have a 50% to 75% chance of having atopic children (*atopy* means a familial tendency to have certain allergic disorders).

Allergens can be categorized into those that are inhaled (e.g., plant pollens, fungal spores, animal dander, house dust, grass, and ragweed), ingested (e.g., foods, food additives, and drugs), injected (e.g., bee venom, drugs, or biologic substances such as contrast dyes and adrenocorticotropic hormone), and contacted (e.g., pollens and foods).

In a type I hypersensitivity reaction, the previously sensitized host is re-exposed to the provoking allergen. The allergen binds to two adjacent IgE molecules on the surface of a mast cell, bridges the IgE molecules, and causes distortion of the cell membrane. This distortion initiates a series of biochemical events, which causes the granules in the cell to swell, migrate, and fuse with the cell membrane. The granular contents are then expelled and released into the extravascular space; this process is called *degranulation*. The granular contents are pharmacologically active mediators that produce the pathologic manifestations of an allergic reaction. Functionally, there are three types of mediators: (1) chemotactic mediators, (2) vasoactive amines, and (3) tissue damage and repair substances.

The most important primary mediator is *histamine*, a short-acting vasoactive amine. Histamine causes increased capillary permeability, increased secretion of mucus (both nasal and bronchial), smooth muscle contractions (especially of bronchioles and small blood vessels), and an itching sensation or pruritus, sometimes accompanied by redness. These symptoms persist for approximately 10 minutes, with the maximum reaction occurring 1 to 2 minutes after the histamine is released. Other important mediators that contribute to physiologic changes and clinical symptoms include the leukotrienes like slow-reacting substance of anaphylaxis, which participates in contraction of bronchial small muscles, mucosal edema, and hypersecretion; chemotactic factors like eosinophil chemotactic factor, which attracts eosinophils to the site of activation; kinin-generating proteases, which result in the production of kinins (like bradykinin); and other substances, which cause vasodilation and increased vascular permeability.

Clinical examples of type I reactions include systemic anaphylaxis; allergic asthma; and atopic allergies such as hay fever, allergic rhinitis, and allergies to dust, animal dander, mold, grass, trees, drugs, foods, and other substances.

ANAPHYLAXIS

OVERVIEW

Anaphylaxis, the most dramatic example of a type I hypersensitivity reaction, is a rapid, systemic, simultaneous occurrence of these reactions in multiple organs. It generally occurs within seconds to minutes of exposure to a causative allergen. Anaphylaxis can be fatal.

Pathophysiology

On a second or subsequent exposure to a specific allergen, the sensitized host reacts to the histamine and other mediators that are released by the mast cells as a result of the allergen-IgE reaction (as described earlier). Pathophysiologically, three major systems are affected in anaphylaxis: respiratory, cardiovascular, and integumentary.

Etiology

Many substances can trigger anaphylaxis in a susceptible individual. The most common causative allergens are drugs, especially antimicrobials like penicillin, the cephalosporins, vancomycin, chloramphenicol, and amphotericin B; foreign proteins that are used as therapeutic agents, such as adrenocorticotropic hormone, insulin, vaccines, allergen extracts, and muscle relaxants; insect venom, especially from bees, wasps, hornets, and fire ants; and certain foods, such as shellfish, berries, chocolate, eggs, and nuts. There are many other potential triggers of anaphylaxis (see the Key Features of Disease, p. 654).

Substances such as aspirin, opiates, radiopaque dyes, and immune serum globulin can result in an anaphylaxis that is clinically similar to allergic anaphylaxis. However, the pathophysiologic mechanism is not an IgE-mediated immediate hypersensitivity event, but direct degranulation of mast cells.

Incidence

Anaphylaxis in humans is relatively uncommon, but it has always received a great deal of attention because of its rapid and unexpected nature and its potentially fatal outcome. Anaphylaxis from insect venom may be responsible for more than 50 deaths per year in the United States (Wallace, 1983).

PREVENTION

Because of the rapid onset of life-threatening symptoms and the potential for a fatal outcome, sometimes even with appropriate medical intervention, the prevention of anaphylaxis is of paramount importance. The nurse teaches the client with a history of allergic reactions to common allergens that can cause anaphylaxis to avoid these substances whenever possible, to wear a medical alert (Medic Alert) bracelet, and to alert health care personnel about their specific allergies. It is necessary for some clients to carry an emergency anaphylaxis kit, such as a bee sting kit with parenteral epinephrine, or an epinephrine injector such as EpiPen Auto-Injector (Center Laboratories), which is an easy-to-use, spring-loaded injector that delivers 0.3 mg of epinephrine per dose (in 2 mL).

The medical record of a client with a history of anaphylactic symptoms should prominently display the list of allergens to which that client is sensitive. A careful history is taken before the administration of *any* drug or therapeutic agent. Skin tests should be performed before the administration of substances with a high associated incidence of anaphylactic reactions, such as allergenic extracts or horse serums. Physicians and nurses should be aware of common cross-reacting agents. For example, a client with a history of sensitivity to penicillin is also likely to react to cephalosporins because they have a similar biochemical structure.

If an agent must be used despite a history of allergic reactions, precautionary measures should be taken. An intravenous solution should be started and intubation equipment and a tracheostomy set put at the bedside. The material should be given first intradermally, then subcutaneously, and then intramuscularly in increasing doses at 20- to 30-minute intervals so that the initial dose by the next route does not exceed the final dose by the previous route. When carefully done, this procedure is fairly safe.

COLLABORATIVE MANAGEMENT

 Assessment

History

A nursing history of someone who has had anaphylaxis or similar symptoms should focus on the symptoms, their cause, how quickly they appeared, and how

WHAT HAPPENS IN A TYPE I HYPERSENSITIVITY REACTION

On initial exposure to an allergen such as bee venom, B lymphocytes—aided by mature helper T lymphocytes—recognize the allergen as nonself and become sensitized to it. Each B lymphocyte then divides into two cells: an active plasma cell and a dormant memory cell (not shown). The plasma cells immediately start to manufacture the antibody IgE, which attaches to mast cells or to basophils. Some of these mast cells or basophils distort and release their granular contents in a process called degranulation. These granular contents are potent chemical mediators that cause the pathologic manifestations of an allergic reaction. At the first exposure to a particular allergen, however, relatively few cells degranulate, so clinical manifestations are usually mild if present at all.

On re-exposure to the same allergen, the previously sensitized plasma cells and the sensitized memory cells manufacture huge quantities of IgE. These IgE molecules immediately attach to mast cells or to basophils in clumps. Although only a limited number of these mast cells or basophils degranulated at the initial exposure to the allergen, now huge numbers of them release granular contents into the extracellular fluid. The process occurs with such speed and such magnitude that serious, even life-threatening, clinical manifestations develop, even while the bee is still stinging.

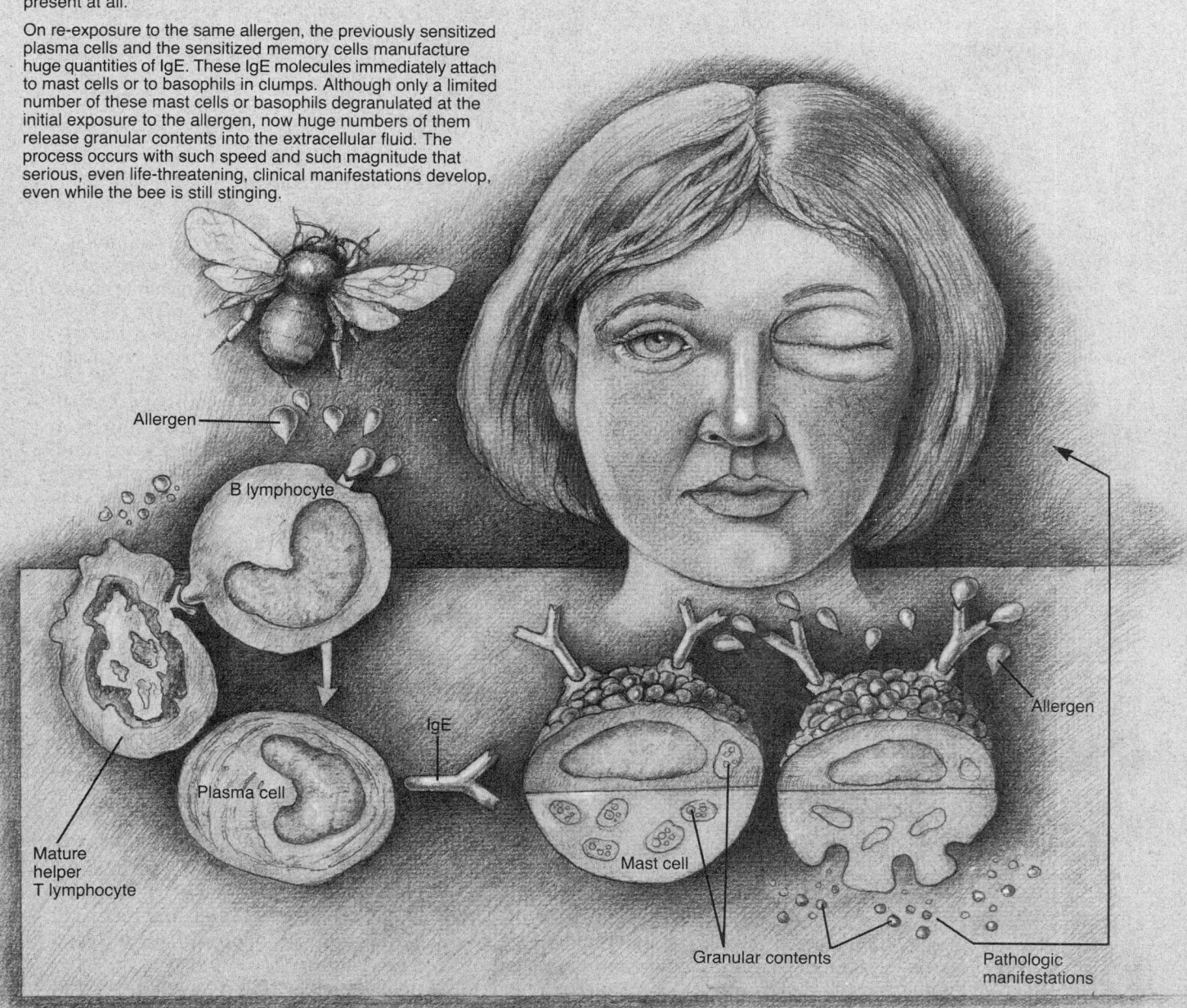

Allergen

B lymphocyte

Mature helper T lymphocyte

Plasma cell

IgE

Mast cell

Allergen

Granular contents

Pathologic manifestations

First exposure: limited IgE production, limited degranulation, limited manifestations
Re-exposure: copious IgE production, massive degranulation, serious to life-threatening manifestations

KEY FEATURES OF DISEASE ■ Agents that Cause Anaphylaxis

Drugs/Foreign Proteins

Antibiotics (penicillin, cephalosporins, tetracycline, sulfonamides, streptomycin, vancomycin, chloramphenicol, amphotericin B, others)

Adrenocorticotropic hormone, insulin, vasopressin, protamine*

Allergen extracts, muscle relaxants, hydrocortisone, vaccines, local anesthetics (lidocaine, procaine)*

Whole blood, cryoprecipitate, immune serum globulin*

Radiocontrast media*

Opiates*

Foods

Shellfish

Eggs

Legumes, nuts

Grains

Berries

Preservatives

Insects/Animals

Hymenoptera: bees, wasps, hornets

Fire ants

Snake venom

Other Agents

Pollens

Exercise

Heat/cold

Other

*Anaphylaxis that is caused by these substances is probably a result of direct mast cell degranulation, rather than an IgE-mediated hypersensitivity event.

rapidly they resolved, as well as a thorough history of other allergic symptoms or tendencies.

The nurse assesses specific *allergic symptoms* that the client has experienced and asks about manifestations such as urticaria (hives), angioedema (swelling), tingling around the mouth, swelling in the throat, vomiting, diarrhea, abdominal swelling, rhinorrhea (clear nasal discharge), wheezing, shortness of breath, and hypotension. The nurse asks the client to list allergens

that have caused symptoms, if they are known. The client's family history of allergies is also assessed. The nurse questions the client about current *medications* as well as any that were taken in the past to which there may have been a reaction, especially antibiotics, analgesics, and foreign proteins. Details are obtained about any medications that the client is taking for treatment of allergies. The nurse assesses the client's symptoms related to variations by time of day, month, or year, and also whether symptoms have changed since the first experienced episode. To do this, an account of the first episode is elicited, followed by a chronology of episodes and symptoms over time. The nurse asks the client about any prior skin testing for allergies and what the results were, and also about any previous desensitization therapy. Finally, the nurse assesses the client's level of knowledge about what allergens he or she is sensitive to, how to avoid or minimize contact with the allergen, and what to do if symptoms occur.

Physical Assessment: Clinical Manifestations

Typically, a client who is experiencing an anaphylactic reaction first complains of a feeling of *uneasiness, apprehension, weakness,* and a *feeling of impending doom.* The nurse notes that the client is *anxious* and *frightened.* These feelings are followed, often quickly, by a *generalized pruritus* and *urticaria.* The nurse sees *erythema (flushing)* and sometimes *angioedema of the eyes, lips, or tongue.* Frequently, *discrete cutaneous wheals* or *urticarial eruptions* appear that are intensely pruritic and that sometimes coalesce. Histamine, the leukotrienes, and prostaglandins cause bronchoconstriction and spasm as well as mucosal edema and hypersecretion of mucus. On respiratory assessment, the nurse notes *congestion, rhinorrhea, dyspnea,* and *increasing respiratory distress with audible wheezing.* On auscultation, *rales, wheezing,* and *diminished breath sounds* are detected. Laryngeal edema is usually experienced as a feeling of having a "lump in the throat," *hoarseness,* and *stridor* (a crowing sound). Distress increases as the tongue and larynx become more edematous and hypersecretion of mucus continues. The nurse may note increasing stridor and anxiety as the airway begins to occlude. Respiratory failure may follow quickly, secondary to laryngeal edema and suffocation or to lower airway bronchoconstriction causing hypoxemia (insufficient oxygenation of blood) and hypercapnia (increased carbon dioxide in blood).

In performing the cardiovascular assessment, the nurse usually finds *hypotension* and *a rapid, weak, possibly irregular pulse.* These findings are due to histamine and the kinins, which cause vasodilation and increased capillary permeability with resultant leakage of intravascular fluids. The client may be *syncopal* and *diaphoretic.* The nurse notes increasing anxiety, confusion, and eventually obtundation. *Arrhythmias, shock,* and *cardiac arrest* may occur within minutes as intravascular volume is lost. Less often, the client may complain of *abdominal cramping*, have *diarrhea,* or *vomit*. Death can be caused by respiratory failure (70% of deaths) and/or by shock and cardiac arrhythmias.

Psychosocial Assessment

The client with a history of anaphylaxis may feel anxious about the possibility of an episode's occurring unexpectedly and without appropriate intervention. The nurse assesses the client's level of anxiety and the degree to which this anxiety has affected his or her life and daily activities. The nurse assesses the client's willingness to take measures to avoid potentially offending allergens. The nurse also assesses the client's ability to remain calm and to take appropriate actions if symptoms occur, which in some cases means self-injecting with epinephrine and in all cases means seeking emergency help. The client's knowledge of emergency measures, phone numbers to call for help, and location of hospital emergency rooms is assessed. The nurse asks the client about the use of a Medic Alert bracelet or necklace that contains appropriate instructions. The nurse assesses the client's acknowledgment of and the ability to cope with the fact that anaphylaxis may be life-threatening.

 ## Analysis: Nursing Diagnosis

The client with anaphylaxis may be admitted to the hospital emergency room to begin treatment in the middle of an anaphylactic episode or to continue emergency treatment and recovery. The nurse may also encounter anaphylaxis in an inpatient unit of a hospital, a clinic, or a public place after the administration of a drug or the ingestion of an allergenic food.

Common Diagnoses

The following diagnoses are appropriate for most clients experiencing anaphylaxis:

1. Ineffective breathing pattern and ineffective airway clearance related to airway obstruction
2. Altered tissue perfusion: cardiopulmonary, cerebral, renal, or peripheral related to hypotension
3. Anxiety related to fear of death and a feeling of impending doom

Additional Diagnoses

In addition, the client may present with one or more of the following:

1. Impaired skin integrity related to pruritus or urticaria
2. Pain related to pruritus, urticaria, or abdominal pain
3. Diarrhea
4. Knowledge deficit related to avoidance of allergens

 ## Planning and Implementation

The following plan of care for a client undergoing anaphylaxis focuses on the common nursing diagnoses.

Ineffective Airway Clearance; Ineffective Breathing Pattern

Clients experiencing anaphylaxis almost invariably have difficulty breathing because of laryngeal edema and hypersecretion of mucus. Because respiratory failure is the major cause of death in anaphylaxis, this diagnosis is a priority one.

Planning: client goals. Major goals for this nursing diagnosis are that the client will (1) have a patent airway; (2) maintain an effective breathing pattern; (3) have adequate air exchange; and (4) remain free from atelectasis, infection, stasis of air or secretions, obstruction, and/or hypoxia.

Interventions: nonsurgical management. Emergency respiratory management is critical for the client having an anaphylactic reaction because the severity of the reaction and the gravity of the consequences increase with time. An airway must be established and/or stabilized immediately. The nurse may need to initiate cardiopulmonary resuscitation and to administer mouth-to-mouth resuscitation. Epinephrine (1:1000), 0.2 to 0.5 mL, should be given subcutaneously as soon as possible after an individual displays symptoms of systemic anaphylaxis. The same dose may be repeated every 15 to 20 minutes if needed.

H_1 antihistamines such as diphenhydramine (Benadryl), 25 to 100 mg, are usually given intravenously, intramuscularly, or orally to treat angioedema and urticaria. If the extent of upper airway narrowing requires it, a small endotracheal tube may need to be inserted or an emergency tracheostomy required.

If the client is able to breathe independently, supplemental oxygen should be given to minimize hypoxemia. Oxygen should be started via nasal cannula at 5 to 10 L or via face mask at 40% to 60% before arterial blood gas results are obtained. Arterial blood gas concentrations are monitored to determine the adequacy of the oxygenation with the PO_2 maintained between 80 and 100 mmHg. The nurse uses suction to remove excess secretions, if indicated, and closely assesses the client and records rate, rhythm, and depth of respirations as well as the presence of bronchospasm and adventitious breath sounds. The nurse elevates the client's bed to 45 degrees unless this maneuver is contraindicated because of hypotension. For severe bronchospasm, the client is given aminophylline, 6 mg/kg intravenously, over 20 to 30 minutes. If the person is taking aminophylline regularly, no more than 3 mg/kg should be given. Maintenance aminophylline (0.3 to 0.5 mg/kg per hour) is initiated. The client should be given an inhaled beta-adrenergic agonist such as metaproterenol (Alupent) or albuterol (Proventil) every 2 to 4 hours. For persistent symptoms (after 1 to 2 hours), corticosteroids are added to prevent the late recurrence of symptoms (Table 27–1).

Altered Tissue Perfusion

The client is at risk for developing decreased perfusion to the heart, brain, kidneys, and periphery because of severe hypotension experienced in anaphylactic shock.

Planning: client goals. The major goals for this nursing diagnosis are that the client will (1) maintain blood pressure and blood volume, (2) maximize tissue perfusion, (3) maintain function of vital organs, and (4) maintain cardiac output.

Interventions: nonsurgical management. As noted previously, as soon as anaphylactic symptoms are observed, the client is given epinephrine (1:1000), 0.2 to 0.5 mL subcutaneously, and this dose is repeated every 15 to 20 minutes if needed. The nurse monitors the client's vital signs every 15 minutes. Venous access should be obtained as quickly as possible with a large gauge (18 or 19) catheter. The client is placed in the recumbent position with legs elevated. Rapid infusion of normal saline is begun (sometimes as fast as 1 L in 20 to 30 minutes). After several liters of normal saline are given, many physicians add albumin or 5% plasma protein fraction as volume expanders. If the client has not responded to administration of volume fluids and subcutaneous epinephrine, intravenous epinephrine (1:1000) may be given. Some physicians use potent vasoconstrictors such as norepinephrine or dopamine instead of epinephrine. Clients receiving intravenous vasoconstrictors should have central venous pressure and/or pulmonary arterial and capillary wedge pressures monitored in a critical care setting. The nurse monitors the client's cardiac rate and rhythm because cardiac arrhythmias can occur secondary to anaphylaxis or to treatment. The nurse carefully monitors and records the client's intake and output because of the danger of fluid overload and assesses the client's mental status for changes, such as restlessness, confusion, changes in thought processes, and a diminished level of consciousness, which could occur because of cerebral hypoxia.

Anxiety

Anxiety is a common occurrence in anaphylaxis because most clients experience a sense of impending doom and an associated fear of death.

Planning: client goals. The major goal for this nursing diagnosis in the setting of anaphylaxis is that the client will experience a reduction in anxiety.

Interventions: nonsurgical management. The nurse stays with the client and provides reassurance that appropriate measures are being taken. It is important for nurses to speak slowly and calmly and not convey their own anxiety. The nurse uses short, simple sentences, gives concise directions, and uses touch to reduce anxiety. When anxiety is sufficiently diminished, the nurse assesses for unmet needs or expectations and helps the client to recall what he or she experienced immediately before the episode. Explanations and rationale are given to the client at this time.

■ Discharge Planning

The client with anaphylaxis can be discharged to home when the respiratory and cardiovascular systems have returned to baseline functioning.

Home Care Preparation

When discharged to home, the client must be aware of the danger of re-exposure to the inciting allergen. If possible, the allergen is removed from the environment. Clients who have had anaphylactic symptoms from certain foods should avoid those foods. Hypersensitivity reactions to drugs are reported and recorded. The nurse helps the client to obtain a Medic Alert bracelet and encourages the client to wear it at all times. Some clients need to carry with them an emergency anaphylaxis kit, which usually consists of an epinephrine automatic injector or syringes and epinephrine. The nurse teaches the client to use the injector if an injection is needed before going to a medical facility.

Psychosocial Preparation

Clients may fear having repeated episodes of anaphylaxis and/or being unable to get treatment in time. If the causative agent is unknown, this fear is increased. The nurse teaches the client and family what to do at the first suggestion of symptoms and offers them support. Appropriate referrals for counseling and support are made by the nurse.

Client/Family Education

The nurse teaches clients and their families about anaphylaxis—why it occurs, what to avoid to prevent it, and what to do if exposure to a known allergen occurs—and about drugs and treatments that are used for emergencies.

Health Care Resources

In the United States, several organizations provide information and referrals to the person with allergic disorders, including anaphylaxis. Examples are the American Academy of Allergy and Immunology and the Asthma and Allergy Foundation of America. The National Jewish Center for Immunology and Respira-

TABLE 27 – 1   Drugs Used in Treatment of Anaphylaxis

Drug	Mechanism	Side Effects
Sympathomimetics		
Epinephrine	Rapidly stimulates alpha- and beta-adrenergic receptors of autonomic nervous system (alpha: vasoconstriction; beta: bronchodilation)	Pallor, tachycardia and palpitations, nervousness, muscle twitching, sweating, anxiety, insomnia, hypertension, headache, hyperglycemia
Isoproterenol	Stimulated beta-adrenergic receptors, relaxing bronchial muscle and dilating vessels	Same as for epinephrine.
Ephedrine sulfate	Similar to isoproterenol, but with longer duration of action	Same as for epinephrine.
Antihistamines		
Diphenhydramine HCl	Competes with histamine for H_1 receptors on effector cells, thus blocking effects of histamine on bronchioles, gastrointestinal tract, and blood vessels	Drowsiness, confusion, insomnia, headache, vertigo, photosensitivity, diplopia, nausea, vomiting, dry mouth
Cimetidine	H_2 receptor antagonist; decreases secretion of gastric acid	Agranulocytosis, thrombocytopenia, increased blood urea nitrogen and creatinine levels, exfoliative dermatitis
Corticosteroids		
Prednisone (PO) Hydrocortisone sodium succinate (Solu-Cortef) (IV/IM) Methylprednisolone sodium succinate (Solu-Medrol) (IV/IM) Beclomethasone (inhalant)	Anti-inflammatory; inhibit mast cell degranulation	Fluid and sodium retention, hypertension, Cushingoid state, gastric distress, adrenal suppression, psychosis, osteoporosis, susceptibility to infection
Methylxanthines		
Aminophylline	Relaxes bronchial smooth muscle	Restlessness, dizziness, palpitations, tachycardia, nausea, vomiting, epigastric distress, headache, convulsions
Vasopressors		
Norepinephrine (Levophed)	Raises blood pressure and cardiac output in severely decompensated states	Headache, tachycardia, fibrillation, decreased urinary output, hypertension, metabolic acidosis
Dopamine		Arrhythmias, tachycardia, hypertension, dyspnea, nausea and vomiting, azotemia, headache

tory Medicine in Denver has an immunologic diseases hot line (1-800-222-LUNG), with nurses available to answer questions.

 Evaluation

The nurse evaluates care that is given to the client experiencing anaphylaxis on the basis of identified nursing diagnoses. Expected outcomes include that the client

1. Has blood pressure and blood volume restored to baseline and maintained
2. Has a patent airway and an uncompromised and effective breathing pattern
3. Has no or less urticaria, pruritus, and angioedema
4. Experiences reduced anxiety
5. Is aware of the offending allergen(s) (if known) and of symptoms to be noted
6. Is knowledgeable about the use of epinephrine automatic injector, if appropriate

The client who is prone to having anaphylactic reactions can live a relatively normal life with few or no episodes of anaphylaxis if she or he is aware of things to avoid, symptoms to respond to rapidly, and actions to take.

ATOPIC ALLERGY

OVERVIEW

Atopic reactions are allergic manifestations that occur in persons who are genetically predisposed to respond to a variety of environmental allergens by forming IgE. Once the person has sensitized IgE, allergic symptoms occur on re-exposure to the allergen via degranulation of mast cells (see earlier description of type I hypersensitivity). Conditions such as allergic asthma, allergic rhinitis, urticaria, and eczematous dermatitis are manifested alone or in combination. Allergic rhinitis is a symptom complex that includes hay fever and other seasonal allergies, as well as perennial allergic rhinitis (to dust, molds, animal dander, and other environmental stimuli not related to the seasons).

Pathophysiology

Allergic rhinitis is a type I hypersensitivity response to otherwise nontoxic substances such as pollens (trees, grasses, and weeds), dust, molds, and animal dander. Mast cells that are located primarily in the nasal mucosa and upper respiratory tract degranulate when presensitized IgE binds to an allergen. They then release histamine and other mediators, which cause the clinical symptoms of rhinorrhea (runny nose), sneezing, mucosal edema and congestion, pharyngeal and conjunctival itching, and lacrimation (tearing).

Etiology

The cause of allergic rhinitis is a genetic hypersensitivity to pollens such as tree pollens (oak, elm, maple, alder, birch, cottonwood), usually in the spring; grass pollens (Bermuda, timothy, sweet vernal, orchard, Johnson), in the summer; and weed pollens (ragweed), in the fall; or to other environmental substances (nonseasonal) including house dust, feathers, animal dander, and fungal spores.

Incidence

An estimated 8% to 10% of the U.S. population suffers from allergic rhinitis. There is a high familial correlation, with most clients coming from an atopic family, i.e., with a family history of allergies, rhinitis, eczema, asthma, or urticaria (Austen, 1983). The symptoms almost always appear before the fourth decade of life and gradually diminish with age. Hay fever, or ragweed allergy, and allergy to grass pollen are the most common seasonal allergies. Hay fever is a misnomer because no fever is involved and the allergy is not to hay.

PREVENTION

The primary means of preventing allergic rhinitis is avoidance of the offending allergen. Prevention is relatively straightforward for a client with a cat or a dog and an allergy to animal dander but is less so for clients who react to other allergens. The client with a seasonal allergy to pollen may have relief of symptoms if he or she moves to another geographic location with a different set of pollens. People with pollen sensitivities are advised to stay indoors on dry, windy days, to drive the car with windows closed, and to avoid working in the garden or being involved in other outdoor activities during the season in which they are most affected. Clients with known allergies to dust are advised to keep the home environment as free from dust as possible and, when feasible, to do minimal dusting and housecleaning and to wear a mask when cleaning. Minimizing dust-collecting furniture, carpets, and draperies and installing a high-efficiency air-filtering system are also helpful.

Clients who suffer from perennial allergic rhinitis for whom the allergen is unknown will be unable to benefit from avoidance, but they should always be alert to locations, environmental surroundings, and activities that improve or aggravate their symptoms.

COLLABORATIVE MANAGEMENT

 Assessment

History

An accurate history can be the best means of determining the allergens to which a client is sensitive. Reviewing the client's symptoms, their relation to the environment and their seasonal or situational variations, and the clinical course provides valuable information. The nurse asks the client about the *current complaint,* including substances to which he or she has been exposed, what symptoms are being experienced, and the extent of these symptoms. The client reports any *known allergies* and the results of any prior *skin testing.* The client is asked about substances that might *aggravate* symptoms such as alcohol, heat, cold, perfume, smoke, humidity, and chemicals. The nurse explores with the client *when* the symptoms occur; whether there are daily, weekly, monthly, or seasonal *variations;* when and under what circumstances the first episode occurred; and the most recent. Because many people are sensitized to substances in their environment, the nurse questions the client about the effect of *vacations* or *geographic changes;* about the effect of *school, work, or other specific environments;* and about the client's *home,* e.g., whether symptoms are worse in one room versus another, and what kind of mattress, pillows, and blankets the client uses. The nurse notes any *hyposensitization therapy* the client may have had, including when it was given, what antigens were used, how long therapy continued, and what reactions and response occurred. The nurse also notes a history of the use of any *allergic medications* (current or previous) such as antihistamines, bronchodilators, antibiotics, and steroids.

Physical Assessment: Clinical Manifestations

The nurse observes the client *sneezing* frequently and the presence of clear, watery *rhinorrhea.* The client will complain of *congestion* and *nasal pruritus.* The conjunctivae of the eyes appear *red, edematous,* and *pruritic,* and there is increased *lacrimation.* The ears may be itchy and feel full; the palate and pharynx also itch. The throat may feel sore, and there is often postnasal drip and increased secretion of mucus. Frontal headaches, irritability, anorexia, depression, and insomnia may occur. Especially with persistent symptoms, the nurse notes coughing, dyspnea, wheezing, increased sputum production, and sometimes chest pain. There may be urticaria of the skin as well.

Psychosocial Assessment

The client with atopic allergies may feel anxious about not being able to participate in activities or to go to places where symptoms are aggravated. The nurse assesses the client's level of anxiety. By gathering information about habits and activities, the nurse assesses the client's willingness and ability to avoid known allergens and to comply with drug therapy. By reviewing the stressors in the client's life, the association of these stressors or fatigue with aggravation of symptoms can be evaluated. The nurse also assesses the impact of allergy on the person's life style, environment, and relationships. In some cases, clients are struggling with how

to leave a job, move, or stop visiting a family member or friend. This measure may be made more difficult if there is resistance, reluctance, or lack of understanding on the part of significant others. Gathering this information helps the nurse to formulate a plan for intervention and to make appropriate referrals.

Diagnostic Tests

The most common and convenient test for the detection of IgE-mediated allergic reactions is the *skin test* (see the accompanying Guidelines feature). Solutions are made from extracts of common allergens and then applied either by a scratch test or intradermally. The intradermal method is more risky because of the potential of a systemic reaction (anaphylaxis). The *intradermal skin test* is done with a tuberculin syringe and a 26-gauge needle, usually with approximately 0.02 to 0.1 mL of test extract. The nurse injects the allergen extract intradermally in the forearm or in the subcutaneous fat of the upper arm. The nurse will see a small bleb rise while injecting. Wiping the site with alcohol after injection is avoided. Control tests are performed simultaneously with a diluent and either histamine or morphine (a mast cell degranulator), given intradermally. The diluent should produce a negative result, and the latter a wheal of approximately 1 cm or less. Nurses instruct clients who will be undergoing skin testing to stop taking all antihistamines at least 48 hours beforehand, the newer longer-acting antihistamines such as terfenadine (Seldane) 5 days beforehand, and hydroxyzine (Atarax, Vistaril) 1 week beforehand. Clients are told that they must remain under observation for at least 15 to 20 minutes after skin testing. Emergency drugs and equipment are kept readily available for the possibility of anaphylaxis. A positive skin test result is obvious about 15 minutes after the application, and the nurse will note the characteristic *wheal* (more than 0.5 cm larger than the diluent control) and *flare reaction.* The nurse measures and/or grades the reaction and records what was given, where it was given, and the reaction. Skin test results should always be correlated with the clinical history.

The *RAST (radioallergosorbent test)* may be performed in some cases. The RAST detects the presence of allergen-specific IgE. In this test, a known allergen is mixed with the client's serum in the laboratory. Any serum IgE that is specific for the allergen attaches to it. Radiolabeled anti-IgE antibody is then added, and the amount of allergen-specific IgE is measured.

Skin testing for food allergens is generally not reliable. (Food is rarely the cause of allergic rhinitis; it more likely causes urticaria or anaphylactic-type symptoms.) The most reliable and safe method of determining a food allergy is through the use of *elimination diets.* The client's diet is reduced to basic, relatively nonallergenic substances. Suspected foods and foods that are common allergens are added to the diet one at a time and are eaten regularly for 3 to 7 days or until symptoms recur. Aggravation or reappearance of symptoms after the ad-

GUIDELINES ■ Procedure for Skin Testing

Intradermal Allergy Skin Test

Purpose

To determine which allergens a client is sensitive to and to estimate the degree of sensitivity.

Equipment

Tuberculin syringes (one for each antigen to be injected).
26- or 27-gauge needles ½ or ¾ in long.
Alcohol pads.
Pen to mark site.
Ruler on skin test guide to measure reaction.

Procedure

1. Have emergency equipment and medications available.
2. Inform client of possible reactions.
3. Draw up ordered amount and concentration of allergen.
4. Label each allergen carefully if several are being used.
5. Eject all air from syringe and needle.
6. Select site and clean skin with alcohol.
7. Use thumb and forefingers to stretch skin.
8. Position bevel upward and place needle and syringe almost parallel to arm.
9. Insert needle until bevel is in the corium.
10. Advance plunger; observe the rise of a bleb of approximately 1 cm.
11. Remove needle and record what and where allergen was placed (do *not* wipe with alcohol after injection).
12. Repeat with other allergens as indicated (up to 20).

Results

1. Reaction is read approximately 15 to 30 min later. The nurse looks for erythema (flare) and wheal:
      − No reaction
     + 3- 4-mm wheal with erythema
    ++ 4- 8-mm wheal with erythema
   +++ Erythema and wheal without pseudopod
  ++++ Erythema and wheal with pseudopod form.
2. Results are documented in medical record.

Delayed Hypersensitivity Skin Testing

Purpose

To evaluate in vivo cell-mediated immunity.

Equipment

Same as for intradermal skin test.

Procedure

Same as for intradermal skin test except common antigens are used instead of allergens. Common antigens include purified protein derivative, mumps, trichophyton, streptokinase/streptodornase, candida, and tetanus toxoid.

Results

1. Results are read at 24 and/or 48 h.
2. Two diameters of induration are measured in millimeters.
3. Erythema is not measured.
4. A positive response requires an induration of at least 5 mm in diameter at 48 degrees. No response is referred to as *anergy*.
5. Results are documented in medical record.

dition of a specific food is evidence of allergy to it. The allergy should be verified by removing that food again for several days and restoring it while noting the effect on symptoms.

 Analysis: Nursing Diagnosis

A client with allergic rhinitis is rarely admitted to the hospital; this client is more often encountered in an outpatient clinic or in a physician's office. The following nursing diagnoses are applicable to these clients.

Common Diagnoses

The most frequently seen nursing diagnosis is potential for ineffective airway clearance related to chronic allergy.

Additional Diagnoses

In addition, there may be other diagnoses including

1. Pain related to conjunctival, nasal, palatine and pharyngeal pruritus, and swelling
2. Knowledge deficit related to avoiding allergens

 Planning and Implementation

Potential for Ineffective Airway Clearance

The following plan of care for a client with atopic allergic rhinitis focuses on potential for ineffective airway clearance.

Planning: client goals. The major goals for this nursing diagnosis are that the client will (1) maintain a patent airway, (2) maintain fluid secretions, and (3) participate in the preventive and treatment regimen.

Interventions: nonsurgical management. The major interventions for a client with allergic rhinitis include drug therapy for symptomatic relief, avoidance therapy, environmental control, and hyposensitization.

Drug therapy. The drugs most commonly used for symptomatic relief in allergic rhinitis are H_1 antihistamines. Chlorpheniramine maleate (Chlor-trimeton), 4 to 8 mg, and diphenhydramine hydrochloride, 25 to 50 mg every 4 to 6 hours, work well to block some of the uncomfortable effects of histamine release. Sympathomimetics are often used in combination with antihistamines for their decongestant properties. Examples are phenylpropanolamine, phenylephrine (Neo-Synephrine), or pseudoephedrine (Sudafed). Nasal decongestants are *not* recommended because their effect is short-lived, and there is often a rebound increase in nasal mucosal swelling. For nasal symptoms that are not adequately relieved by antihistamines, dexamethasone (Decadron) nasal spray is often used. Systemic corticosteroids are used rarely because in most cases the risks of use outweigh the benefits. Cromolyn sodium (Nasalcrom) may help to prevent the progression of symptoms because it acts as an inhibitor of mast cell degranulation.

Avoidance therapy. Avoidance of the offending allergen is the most effective way to relieve or prevent symptoms. It is not always the easiest, however, for it may necessitate that the client move, change jobs, give away a beloved pet, alter her or his eating habits, or make major changes in the environment.

Environmental control. Certain modifications in the client's environment may contribute to relieving symptoms, especially for the client with perennial allergic rhinitis. The nurse recommends the following measures to clients and explains their rationale: Clients should use nonallergenic materials for bedding (mattresses, pillows, blankets); enclose the mattress and box springs in airtight plastic covers; replace carpets with washable throw rugs and draperies with light, washable curtains; use pull shades rather than Venetian blinds; and launder bed linens frequently. If possible, clients should use a system of heating and cooling that both humidifies and filters the air (e.g., steam or hot-water heat). Avoiding rapid changes in temperature can be helpful. Avoiding smoking and smoke-filled areas also prevents aggravation of symptoms.

Hyposensitization. Hyposensitization, which is also referred to as desensitization or immunotherapy, is a process whereby the client is administered gradually increasing subcutaneous doses of allergen. Over time, the level of IgG to the specific allergen rises. IgG is thought to be a blocking antibody, i.e., it binds to the allergen and thus blocks binding by IgE. Exposure to the allergen in this way may also lead to tolerance, and in some clients the level of serum IgE declines. The recommended method for hyposensitization is weekly subcutaneous injections starting at 0.1 mL of a dilution in the range of 1 : 100,000 to 1 : 100,000,000. Doses are gradually increased until a maximal tolerated concentration is reached. After this, regular injections are given at a frequency ranging from every week to every month or even less often. The nurse observes the client for 30 minutes after each injection to watch for a possible systemic reaction. The nurse is prepared for the possibility of a systemic anaphylactic reaction to the injection by having the appropriate medications and equipment on hand (see under the heading Anaphylaxis). If these symptoms occur, the nurse applies a tourniquet above the injection site and gives 0.2 mL of epinephrine (1:1000) subcutaneously into the site and 0.3 mL into the other arm. Treatment for anaphylaxis is given if necessary. After all hyposensitization injections, the nurse measures the wheal and flare reaction and documents findings in the record. This reaction is a useful indication of the client's tolerance to the concentration given.

■ Discharge Planning

As mentioned earlier, most clients with atopic allergy are seen in a clinic or outpatient setting and live at home. The nurse working with the client can help to identify how the client can alter the home environment and can educate the client and family about how to minimize and manage symptoms.

Home Care Preparation

Home care preparation is crucial if the allergen is found in the home environment. For example, clients who are allergic to dust should keep the home as free from dust as possible by wet-dusting every day and by wearing a mask when dusting. Eliminating dust-collecting furniture, carpets, and draperies and using a high-efficiency air-filtering system also help (see under the heading Environmental Control). Clients who are allergic to animal dander should not have household pets. Clients with seasonal allergies should stay indoors during peak seasons, especially where the air quality index is poor. The nurse instructs clients to drive with car windows closed during the peak seasons and to avoid bicycle riding, jogging, hiking, gardening, and other outdoor activities during these seasons (see the accompanying Client/Family Education feature).

Client/Family Education

The teaching plan for a client with atopic allergies includes (1) avoidance of allergens, (2) management of symptoms, (3) drug therapy, and (4) desensitization (if appropriate). The nurse, along with other members of the health care team, helps the client to identify allergens to which he or she is sensitive and discusses realistic methods of avoiding them (see under the heading Avoidance Therapy).

The nurse teaches the client how to relieve or reduce symptoms. Once symptoms begin, the client can remove himself or herself from the environment to prevent symptoms from getting worse. Clients are taught about H_1 antihistamines like chlorpheniramine and diphenhydramine, which clients should carry with them and take to relieve symptoms. Clearly, the priority for the client is to maintain adequate respiratory function; therefore, the nurse instructs the client to go to a physician or an emergency room when respiratory status is compromised. The client is reminded that stress, fatigue, and anxiety all contribute to and aggravate allergic symptoms. Therefore, the nurse discusses stress and anxiety with the client and teaches relaxation and other stress management techniques.

The nurse teaches the client the correct dosage, side effects, and purpose of H_1 antihistamines and sympathomimetics. The correct procedure for administration of inhalant medication and/or nasal sprays (like dexamethasone) is taught. Clients are taught to avoid nasal decongestants because of their transient relief and aggravating rebound effect. The nurse carefully teaches

CLIENT/FAMILY EDUCATION ■ Instructions for Clients with Allergic Rhinitis During the Peak Season

Instructions	Rationales
1. "Keep your windows closed at night, and use an air conditioner if you have one."	1. Closed windows prevent pollen from entering the house, and air conditioners clean, cool, and dry the air.
2. "Minimize early morning activity."	2. Emission of pollen is greatest at 5 to 10 AM.
3. "Keep your car windows closed."	3–6. Exposure to pollen is minimized by avoidance measures.
4. "Stay indoors on windy days and days on which the humidity and pollen count are high."	
5. "Take vacations in more pollen-free places, such as beaches."	
6. "Do not mow the lawn, rake leaves, or work in the garden."	
7. "Take allergy medications as prescribed by your doctor."	7. Adherence to the prescribed regimen can minimize allergic episodes.
8. "Do not hang sheets and clothes outside to dry."	8. Damp fabrics gather airborne pollen.
9. "Do not keep many indoor plants if you are sensitive to molds."	9. Houseplants harbor molds, which may trigger allergic reactions in sensitive clients.

the client who is taking systemic corticosteroids about the many side effects and how to monitor for them, as well as about the importance of tapering the dosage and how it is done.

If the client is receiving desensitization injections, the nurse teaches the purpose and the method of injection, the characteristics of a reaction, and the meaning of a reaction. The client is alerted to the possibility of a systemic reaction to desensitization shots. Although the client is observed by the nurse for 30 minutes after each injection, the client should be aware of the possibility of a delayed reaction and should know to report to the physician when appropriate.

Psychosocial Preparation

Some clients are worried about their ability to avoid allergens and to manage symptoms. The nurse can be instrumental in allaying anxieties and helping clients to see that they can live a normal life as long as they take certain precautions. Families and significant others also need support for the changes they may have to make. For example, giving away the family dog or the rug that belonged to a favorite aunt has an impact on the whole family. Family members must be prepared to make small sacrifices to help the allergic individual be more comfortable. In some families, this expectation creates a great strain.

Health Care Resources

For more information, clients can contact the local chapter of the Asthma and Allergy Foundation of America (1-800-7-ASTHMA), the American Academy of Allergy and Immunology (1-800-822-ASMA), or the American Academy of Allergists (1-800-842-7777).

 Evaluation

On the basis of the identified nursing diagnoses and the interventions used, the nurse evaluates care given to the client with allergies. Expected outcomes include that the client

1. Has minimal symptoms of rhinitis and conjunctival, pharyngeal, and nasal itching by the appropriate use of antihistamines and decongestants
2. Is aware of offending allergen(s) and is taking appropriate measures to avoid exposure to them, including alterations in the environment, if indicated
3. If undergoing desensitization therapy, is compliant with and understands this therapy
4. Has a reduction in anxiety while demonstrating increasing control over allergic symptoms

The client with allergies, if aware of and attentive to substances that should be avoided, ways of manipulating the environment, and symptomatic relief with medications, can live with minimal disruption caused by allergies.

URTICARIA

Urticaria, also known as *hives*, is characterized by local wheals and erythema of the skin. Urticaria is an IgE-mediated event in which preformed IgE binds to aller-

gen, which causes mast cell degranulation and release of histamine. The histamine causes capillary dilation and increased permeability—the hive or urticarial lesion. Urticaria is essentially anaphylaxis that is limited to the skin. Urticaria can be due to exposure to drugs, insect stings, desensitization injections, and certain foods, especially eggs, shellfish, nuts, and berries. Urticaria can also be associated with a viral infection, such as hepatitis, infectious mononucleosis, or rubella, or with physical stimuli, such as cold, sunlight, heat, vibration, or exercise. In chronic urticaria, the inciting agent is often unknown.

The client experiencing urticaria initially reports pruritus, which is followed by the appearance of wheals. The nurse notes pink, raised, edematous, and pruritic areas that vary in size and shape; these areas are commonly called hives. Sometimes, larger wheals clear in the center and so appear as rings of erythema. The nurse observes that crops of hives appear, usually last a few hours, and then disappear as new ones appear in a different location. In some cases, the nurse sees urticaria associated with angioedema, particularly of the hands, eyelids, lips, and genitalia. Angioedema of the upper airway can obstruct breathing.

Most of the time, urticaria is self-limiting and will disappear within 7 to 10 days. Treatment during this time is symptomatic and usually includes an oral antihistamine such as diphenhydramine (Benadryl), 25 to 50 mg every 4 to 6 hours, cyproheptadine hydrochloride (Periactin), 4 to 8 mg three times a day, or hydroxyzine (Atarax, Vistaril), 25 to 50 mg three times a day. For a more severe reaction, especially urticaria with angioedema, corticosteroids may be used.

The nurse assists the client in identifying the allergen that caused the urticaria and strategies for avoiding exposure to that allergen. Nurses help clients suffering from chronic urticaria, for whom the allergen is often not known, to reduce stress in their lives and to avoid caffeine, tobacco, alcohol, and aspirin, all of which tend to aggravate symptoms. Chronic urticaria undergoes spontaneous remission within 2 years in approximately 50% of cases.

BRONCHIAL ASTHMA

Approximately 10% to 20% of the adult asthmatic population suffer from *extrinsic asthma*, i.e., asthma that is precipitated by allergenic exposure (e.g., to pollens, molds, dust, or animal dander). Extrinsic asthma is an IgE-mediated event in which mast cells in the respiratory tract release histamine and other mediators like the leukotrienes (slow-reacting substance of anaphylaxis), which cause bronchoconstriction, edema, and increased mucous production. Approximately 50% of adult asthmatics have *intrinsic asthma*, which is precipitated by nonallergenic factors, such as viral infection, exercise, cold, cigarette smoke, changes in temperature or humidity, gasoline fumes, and paint fumes. Emotional stress seems to aggravate an attack but may not have a primary etiologic role. In some adults, both allergenic and nonallergenic factors appear to play a significant role in triggering asthma attacks. Allergy is an important cause of asthma in infants and children.

Adult clients with asthma vary greatly in the frequency and severity of symptoms. Some have only occasional symptomatic episodes, which are relatively mild and brief. Others have a mild cough and wheeze most of the time, and on exposure to known allergens or other factors have a severe exacerbation of symptoms. The onset of symptoms may be acute or insidious. The client reports shortness of breath, cough, and a feeling of tightness or pressure in the chest. On assessment, the nurse notes dyspnea, tachypnea, nonproductive cough, audible wheezes, anxiety, and increasing respiratory distress. The client is usually sitting or even leaning forward, is using accessory muscles for breathing, is often hypertensive, and may be dehydrated. The client is unable to speak without stopping for air. Respirations will become increasingly rapid and shallow. The client then experiences fatigue and becomes cyanotic, confused, and lethargic as the PO_2 drops and PCO_2 rises. Pulmonary function test results are abnormal and arterial blood gas tests indicate hypoxemia and hypercapnia. Blood and sputum show eosinophilia.

Treatment of asthma centers on control of exacerbating factors, treatment of acute episodes, and maintenance drug therapy. An asthma attack is treated as an emergency, and the nurse intervenes promptly to interrupt symptoms. At the same time, the nurse acts calmly and confidently to reassure and support an anxious client. Medications that are used to treat an acute attack include beta-adrenergic agents (e.g., epinephrine, isoproterenol, ephedrine), which relax bronchial smooth muscle and inhibit mediator release; theophylline and derivatives, which act in a similar fashion; and, in some cases, corticosteroids. Oxygen is administered to maintain a PO_2 value higher than 60 mmHg. The nurse monitors fluid intake and output and electrolytes and administers intravenous fluids to replace loss. Asthmatic clients are usually given maintenance therapy with theophylline and bronchodilators or cromolyn sodium. For a more detailed discussion of bronchial asthma, see Chapter 62.

Type II: Cytotoxic Reactions

In a type II (cytotoxic) reaction, the host makes antibodies to self cells or tissues called *autoantibodies*. Autoantibodies react with the antigenic components of a self cell, or with a *hapten* (a substance of low molecular weight that becomes antigenic when attached to a carrier), which has been adsorbed by or coupled to a self cell. The autoantibody binds to the self cell and forms an antigen-antibody complex, or immune complex. The self cell, thus targeted, is then either destroyed by comple-

ment-mediated lysis (classic or alternative pathway) or destroyed via a cell with an Fc receptor and antibody-dependent cellular cytotoxicity (see Chap. 23). In either case, the cytotoxic reaction results in destruction of a self cell. Clinical examples of type II reactions include Coombs'-positive hemolytic anemias, thrombocytopenic purpura, pernicious anemia, hemolytic transfusion reactions, hemolytic disease of the newborn, Goodpasture's syndrome, and drug-induced hemolytic anemia.

An interesting variant of a type II reaction occurs when the autoantibody is made to a receptor. For example, in Graves's disease, the antibody known as LATS (long-acting thyroid stimulator) is made to the thyroid-stimulating hormone receptor on the thyroid gland. LATS binds with the receptor and stimulates it, which results in the production of abnormally high levels of thyroxine. Another clinical example involving an anti-receptor antibody is myasthenia gravis. In myasthenia gravis, an autoantibody is made to the acetylcholine receptor on muscle. The antibody binds to the receptor at the neuromuscular junction, which blocks acetylcholine and thus prevents transmission of the impulse that would stimulate the muscle. The result is profound muscular weakness. These disorders are discussed in more detail elsewhere in the text.

HEMOLYTIC BLOOD TRANSFUSION REACTION

A hemolytic transfusion reaction occurs when a recipient is given ABO-incompatible blood. Early in life, a person develops natural antibodies (agglutinins) to ABO antigens, which are found on erythrocyte membranes. If a client is transfused with incompatible blood, the agglutinins bind to the antigens on the donor's erythrocytes and coat them, and the cells agglutinate. Agglutination of cells results in blockage of small blood vessels and capillaries. The immune complex activates complement, which results in cytolysis (cell destruction) of erythrocytes. Through this destruction, hemoglobin is released, and ultimately the renal tubules are blocked and acute renal failure results.

The most common causes of hemolytic transfusion reaction are mistakes in labeling of blood and transfusion of blood to the wrong individual. Nurses can help prevent this type of reaction by ensuring that the client who is receiving blood has recently been typed and cross-matched and by double-checking the blood before use. Blood should always be administered slowly for the first 15 minutes, and the client is carefully monitored by the nurse (symptoms of transfusion reaction usually occur within the first 15 minutes). The client may complain of burning along the vein, facial flushing, headache, chest pain, and low back pain. The nurse monitors vital signs and detects fever, followed by chills and labored respirations. When the first symptom appears, the nurse stops the transfusion but continues intravenous administration of normal saline. The physician should be notified immediately. The nurse carefully monitors the client's vital signs and fluid output. If symptoms of shock develop, appropriate intervention is initiated with epinephrine, fluids, and oxygen. Samples of blood from the client are taken and sent to the blood bank, and urine is sent to the laboratory for determination of hemoglobin. The nurse remains calm and reassures the client that appropriate actions are being taken. If there is evidence of renal involvement, a potent diuretic such as mannitol (Osmitrol) is usually given (refer to Chap. 67).

DRUG-INDUCED HEMOLYTIC ANEMIA

Certain drugs precipitate a type II reaction to erythrocytes, and there are two main mechanisms by which this occurs. (1) Drugs such as penicillin and the sulfonamides act as haptens and form covalent bonds with the erythrocyte membrane. Antibodies are made, and the antigen-antibody reaction leads to agglutination and destruction of erythrocytes. (2) Methyldopa and some other drugs alter the erythrocyte surface chemically, thereby exposing an antigen that induces and reacts with an autoantibody and leads to agglutination and destruction of the cells.

Another mechanism that can occur, but that more often causes destruction of platelets rather than erythrocytes, is the "innocent bystander" phenomenon. In this case, antibodies are made to drugs like quinidine and form a soluble complex. The complex reacts with nearby platelets (the innocent bystander target cells) and causes lysis of the platelets, which results in thrombocytopenia.

Treatment of drug-induced hemolytic anemia starts with discontinuation of the offending drug. Otherwise, treatment is symptomatic. Complications such as hemolytic crisis and renal failure can be life-threatening.

Type III: Immune Complex Reactions

In a type III reaction, soluble immune complexes are formed, usually in the setting of antigen excess (see the illustration on p. 667). These circulating immune complexes are then deposited in the vessel wall, usually of small vessels, at the bifurcations of vessels, or where there is increased turbulence of blood flow. Common sites include the kidneys, skin, joints, and other small blood vessels. The deposited immune complex activates complement, which initiates a series of events including the migration of polymorphonuclear leukocytes and the release of their lysosomal proteolytic enzymes. Tissue or vessel damage results.

Examples of clinical conditions in which type III reactions play a role include serum sickness, systemic lupus erythematosus, polyarteritis nodosa, rheumatoid arthri-

tis, cryoglobulinemia, hypersensitivity pneumonitis, and the various vasculitides.

SERUM SICKNESS

Serum sickness is a complex of symptoms that occurs in an individual after the administration of foreign serum or certain drugs. It is caused by deposition of immune complexes in the walls of vessels in the skin, joints, and the glomeruli of the kidney. The most common causes of serum sickness today are penicillin and related drugs and some horse serum antitoxins. Serum sickness used to be quite common when vaccines were made with horse or rabbit serum, but now most are made with human serum or antigen fragments. Relatively new agents that can cause serum sickness are antilymphocyte globulin and antithymocyte globulin, both of which are used experimentally to suppress the immune response in transplantation of certain organs and are being tested in some other diseases.

The client experiencing serum sickness has symptoms of fever, arthralgia (achy joints), rash, lymphadenopathy, malaise, and possibly polyarthritis and nephritis, usually about 7 to 12 days after administration of the causative agent. The nurse alerts the client to the possibility of serum sickness and what symptoms to look for. When administering a foreign serum to a client, the nurse is also prepared for the possibility of a type I anaphylactic reaction and has emergency equipment and medications close at hand. Serum sickness is usually self-limiting, and symptoms subside after several days. Treatment is usually symptomatic, with antihistamines given for pruritus and aspirin for arthralgias. Prednisone is given if symptoms are severe. In some cases, the use of hydroxyzine or cyproheptadine decreases the incidence of symptoms.

IMMUNE COMPLEX DISORDERS

There are many immune complex disorders in which the type III reaction is the major mechanism of clinical manifestations. Many of these are known as collagen-vascular diseases or connective tissue disorders. For example, the clinical manifestations of rheumatoid arthritis are caused by immune complex deposition in the joint space followed by complement activation, recruitment of polymorphonuclear neutrophils, release of lysosomal enzymes, and destruction of tissue, and later scarring and fibrous changes. In rheumatoid arthritis, the antigen to which an autoantibody is made appears to be IgG. In a similar fashion, the clinical manifestations of systemic lupus erythematosus result from immune complex deposition in the vessels (vasculitis), the glomeruli (nephritis), the joints (arthralgia/arthritis), and other organs and tissues. In this disorder, the immune complex is composed of cellular DNA and anti-DNA antibodies. For a detailed discussion of these and other connective tissue disorders, please refer to Chapter 28.

Type IV: Delayed Hypersensitivity Reactions

In a type IV reaction, the important cell is the T lymphocyte. Antibodies and complement are not involved. Sensitized T lymphocytes (from a previous exposure) respond to an antigen by producing and releasing certain lymphokines. Important lymphokines released include macrophage chemotactic factor, macrophage migration inhibitory factor, and macrophage activation factor. These lymphokines act to recruit, retain, and activate macrophages that help to destroy the inciting antigen. Different from a type I hypersensitivity reaction, which takes place immediately, a type IV response typically occurs hours to days after exposure. A type IV reaction is characterized by an accumulation of lymphocytes and macrophages and the formulation of a granuloma. These events cause edema, ischemia, and tissue destruction at the site of response.

The type IV reaction is typified by a positive purified protein derivative test. In a client who had previously been exposed to tuberculosis, an intradermal injection of this agent causes sensitized T cells to accumulate at the injection site, release lymphokines, and recruit and activate macrophages. The nurse notes induration and sometimes tenderness and redness at the site of the injection approximately 24 to 48 hours later (see the Guidelines feature: Procedure for Skin Testing).

Clinical examples of type IV hypersensitivity reactions include contact dermatitis, allograft rejections, granulomas caused by intracellular organisms (such as *Mycobacterium tuberculosis* or *Mycobacterium leprae*), and granulomatous diseases in which the antigen is unknown (e.g., sarcoidosis, Wegener's granulomatosis).

TISSUE TRANSPLANT REJECTION

A *transplant* is simply the transfer of living cells from one individual to another. Surgical technology has made the transplant of almost any tissue feasible. However, transplantation of most organs is limited mainly because of the problem of immunologic rejection, which gradually or acutely destroys tissues after transplantation. In the 1980s, transplants of kidney, heart, liver, pancreas, bone marrow, cornea, and skin were all done with varying degrees of frequency and varying degrees of success. A better understanding of the immune mechanisms and methods for preventing rejection will allow more transplants, which may save the lives of people who would succumb to otherwise fatal diseases.

There are three types of transplant rejection, each involving a different immunologic mechanism. In *hy-*

peracute rejection, cytotoxic antibodies in the recipient's serum recognize the donor cells and quickly bind to and destroy them. This kind of rejection can occur before the surgical procedure is complete. Hyperacute rejection is usually avoided by the pretransplant cross-match of the recipient's serum with the donor's cells. If the serum contains reactive antibodies, another donor is sought.

Acute rejection is the most common type of rejection and is an example of the type IV hypersensitivity reaction. In an acute rejection, the recipient's mature T lymphocytes recognize the donor cells as foreign and respond by releasing lymphokines and recruiting macrophages and cytotoxic T cells in an effort to destroy the transplanted tissue. The infiltration of cells and resulting edema lead to thrombosis and tissue necrosis and sloughing. The vascularization to the new tissue is compromised, and the organ begins to fail. Acute rejection is usually seen within weeks to months after transplantation. Acute rejection is minimized by careful histocompatibility matching of donor and recipient before the transplant, which is done primarily via human leukocyte antigen (HLA) typing and the mixed lymphocyte culture. The ideal situation is to have a donor and a recipient with identical HLA types (A, B, C, and D), but this is extremely rare except in identical twins. A match at the D locus plus a match at as many other loci as possible creates an acceptable level of histocompatibility for some transplants. Because HLA genes are inherited from one's parents, siblings have a closer match than an unrelated person; therefore, siblings are often evaluated as possible donors. The *mixed lymphocyte culture* is also done to determine histocompatibility. In this test, the donor's lymphocytes and the recipient's lymphocytes are mixed in culture and the amount of resulting proliferation is measured. Rapid and significant proliferation of the recipient's cells indicates a high probability for rejection.

Acute rejection is also minimized by giving immunosuppressive medications to the recipient. Treatment usually begins before the transplant and continues after the transplant as chronic therapy. For example, in kidney transplantation, azathioprine (Imuran) or cyclosporine (cyclosporin A) is often given to the recipient before and after transplantation, usually in combination with corticosteroids. Kidney transplant recipients are maintained with chronic low-dose therapy with these medications. At the first indication of symptoms of rejection, the dose of these immunosuppressive medications is increased, which is often successful at aborting the episode of rejection.

Chronic rejection occurs over months to years and is characterized by gradual occlusion of the vascular supply to the transplanted organ. Chronic rejection is both a cell-mediated and a humoral event. Unlike acute rejection, an increase in immunosuppressive medications has little or no effect. Chronic rejection has a poor prognosis for the organ.

Graft-versus-host disease (GVHD) is an interesting, yet unfortunate, immune phenomenon that often occurs after bone marrow transplantation. GVHD can

WHAT HAPPENS IN A TYPE III (IMMUNE COMPLEX) REACTION

In a type III hypersensitivity reaction, antigen-antibody complexes accumulate in tissues of the kidney and other body organs. There they cause direct tissue damage and secondary damage related to obstructed fluid flow routes.

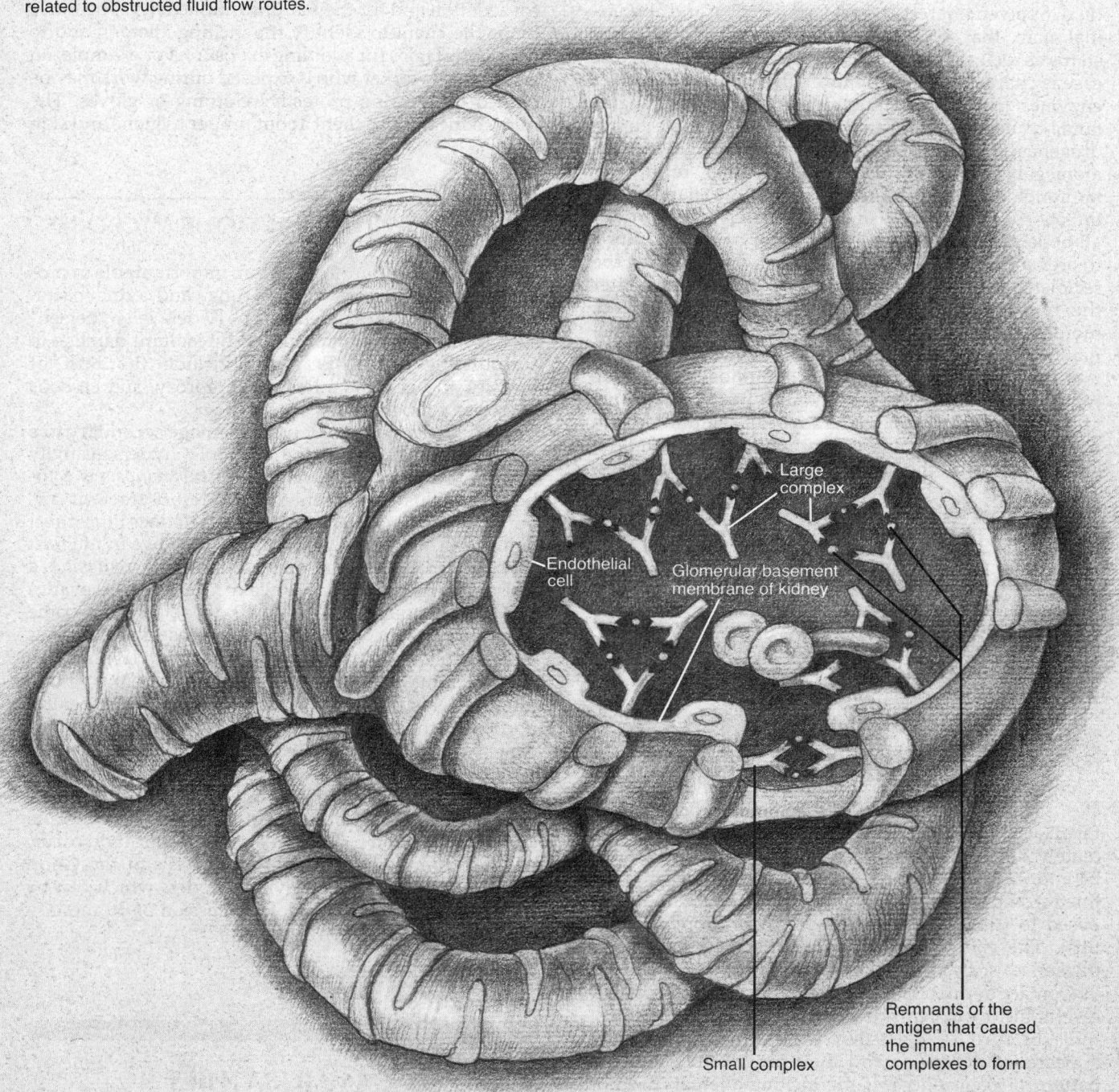

Large complex

Endothelial cell

Glomerular basement membrane of kidney

Remnants of the antigen that caused the immune complexes to form

Small complex

be thought of as rejection in reverse. In bone marrow transplantation, the tissue being transplanted contains mature T lymphocytes that are given to a recipient who is extremely immunosuppressed. The transplanted cells, therefore, immunologically reject the recipient's body. GVHD manifests primarily in the skin, gastrointestinal tract, and liver. A rash is usually a first sign. Gastrointestinal involvement results in severe diarrhea and abdominal pain that compromise the person's nutritional status as well as fluid and electrolyte balance. Liver disease is characterized by abnormally high levels of liver enzymes (aspartate aminotransferase, or serum glutamic-oxaloacetic transaminase [SGOT]; lactate dehydrogenase; bilirubin; alkaline phosphatase) and by hepatomegaly. GVHD also hinders the return of immunologic function, and many of these clients die of infection. GVHD occurs in approximately two-thirds of all bone marrow recipients and is not treatable. Efforts to prevent and/or minimize GVHD include treating the recipient with immunosuppressive medications after the transplant (most commonly methotrexate), and, more recently, treating the bone marrow before transplantation to eliminate mature T lymphocytes. Experimental methods to remove T lymphocytes include treating the bone marrow with anti–T cell monoclonal antibodies or treating it with a soybean agglutinin. Both methods are undergoing experimental trials, and both show promise for the future of bone marrow transplantation.

ALLERGIC CONTACT DERMATITIS

Contact dermatitis is an example of a type IV reaction of the skin in response to contact with a sensitizing agent. Allergens that are responsible for contact dermatitis include catechols from certain plants (poison ivy or poison oak), cosmetics, drugs, dyes, preservatives, metals (such as nickel and chromium), and certain dyes and chemicals used in agriculture and manufacturing. Clinical manifestations include erythema with papules and vesicles, scaling and pruritus, and sometimes large bullae filled with purulent fluid. Symptoms appear approximately 7 to 10 days after the first exposure and between 24 and 72 hours after re-exposure. Symptoms are confined to the region of contact with the allergen (as opposed to the widespread symptoms of atopic dermatitis). The client with chronic contact dermatitis has thickened, scaly, and lichenified lesions.

Contact dermatitis is diagnosed primarily through a careful history. Clients describe the onset of symptoms, the substance to which they were exposed, the initial appearance of lesions and their progression, and the pattern of recurrences. If the inciting allergen has not been identified, a *patch test* may be helpful. In a patch test, a low concentration of antigen is placed on the skin and covered with a dressing. The nurse observes the patch 48 hours later; the presence of an eczematous reaction indicates sensitivity to that allergen. Treatment of contact dermatitis consists of avoidance of the antigen and symptomatic therapy. Application of wet dressings and Burow's solution is helpful in relieving discomfort. Hydrocortisone (1%) cream is applied topically. In severe cases, systemic steroids in rapidly tapering doses are given. Antihistamines are sometimes used for sedation and for their antipruritic activity. The nurse helps the client to identify the inciting allergen and to devise strategies for avoiding exposure. For example, an agricultural worker who is exposed during work may be helped by wearing protective clothing or gloves. The nurse educates the client about proper hygiene and skin care.

REACTIONS TO INFECTIOUS MICROBES

Cell-mediated immunity plays an important role in protecting the host against viruses, fungi, and certain bacteria. In this process of defense, type IV delayed hypersensitivity reactions often occur, with resultant damage to surrounding tissue. Examples include the rash of measles and smallpox, lesions of leprosy, and caseous necrosis of tuberculosis.

The classic example of tissue damage secondary to a cell-mediated response and a type IV hypersensitivity reaction occurs in tuberculosis. *M. tuberculosis* is a tubercle bacillus that enters the respiratory tract via airborne transmission. The organism itself does little direct damage to lung tissue and actually may live in the host for a while before symptoms occur. *M. tuberculosis* is a resistant organism with a waxy coat, and it evades phagocytosis. Over time (7 to 12 days), T cells become sensitized to this organism and release lymphokines that recruit and activate macrophages. The macrophages clump together with epithelial cells and form a multinucleated giant cell or a granuloma. The central portion of the granuloma (called a Ghon tubercle) becomes necrotic and has a characteristic cheesy appearance called caseous necrosis. A cavity is formed by liquid's sloughing into the connecting bronchi, which allows airborne transmission of infectious particles. As the primary lesion heals, fibrosis and calcification occur. A Ghon complex is formed that consists of the Ghon tubercle and the regional lymph nodes, which can be seen on x-ray films. Complete discussion of pulmonary tuberculosis is found in Chapter 62.

GAMMOPATHIES

Gammopathies are disorders that involve abnormal proliferation of the lymphoid cells that produce immunoglobulins. More specifically, gammopathies are associated with abnormal proliferation of a single clone of immunoglobulin-secreting plasma cells, which are derived from B lymphocytes. Several terms other than gammopathies are used to describe this group of diseases: monoclonal gammopathies, plasma cell dyscrasias, paraproteinemias, dysproteinemias, and immunoglobulinopathies. Examples of diseases that are included in this group are multiple myeloma, Waldenström's macroglobulinemia, primary amyloidosis, and heavy-chain diseases.

To understand the gammopathies, an understanding of immunoglobulin structure, synthesis, and secretion is required. Immunoglobulins are synthesized by the plasma cell, which is the final stage in the differentiation of activated B lymphocytes. An immunoglobulin molecule is a protein that consists of four chains of amino acids, two heavy chains and two light chains, which are held together by disulfide bonds (see Chap. 23). A person usually has many diverse immunoglobulins that are the products of multiple different clones of plasma cells. In the gammopathies, one clone proliferates disproportionately, which results in production of homogeneous immunoglobulin, usually of the IgG class. A monoclonal gammopathy is often recognized by serum electrophoresis before symptoms of disease appear.

WALDENSTRÖM'S MACROGLOBULINEMIA

Waldenström's macroglobulinemia is a chronic lymphoproliferative disorder with a wide range of manifestations. It usually occurs in the middle-aged and elderly populations, and in males more often than in females. The diagnosis is made by the presence of a monoclonal IgM peak (spike) on protein electrophoresis, together with the typical symptoms and histologic evidence of plasma cell infiltrates that are identified by bone marrow aspiration or biopsy. The most common clinical features are a normochromic, normocytic anemia; lymphadenopathy; and the hyperviscosity syndrome. The client usually complains first of weakness, fatigue, and epistaxis. Recurrent infections, visual difficulties, weight loss, and neurologic symptoms are also common.

The hyperviscosity syndrome is a result of the increased serum concentration of IgM (the largest immunoglobulin molecule), which leads to slow blood flow or sludging. Resultant symptoms include neurologic signs such as confusion, peripheral neuropathy, paresis, headache, and dizziness; impaired vision with dilation and segmentation of retinal veins; and bleeding and oozing from mucous membranes.

The treatment of choice for a client with severe hyperviscosity syndrome and/or neurologic symptoms or bleeding is plasmapheresis. Plasmapheresis is effective because approximately 90% of the monoclonal protein

is intravascular. Because plasmapheresis only removes the tumor product and does not alter the underlying problem, clients are also treated with systemic chemotherapy. Chlorambucil (Leukeran) with or without prednisone (Meticorten, Deltasone) is given for 10 days and repeated approximately every 6 weeks. This regimen is effective in partially reducing the tumor volume in about 75% of clients (Alexanian, 1983).

MULTIPLE MYELOMA

Multiple myeloma is a malignant condition in which a clone of transformed plasma cells proliferates in bone marrow. The result is disruption of normal bone marrow function and eventual invasion and destruction of adjacent bone. The etiology of multiple myeloma is unknown, but genetic predisposition, oncogenic viruses, inflammatory stimuli, and chronic antigenic stimulation are all theoretical possibilities. Essentially, an excess number of abnormal plasma cells infiltrate the bone marrow and develop into tumors and ultimately destroy bone; they then invade lymph nodes, liver, spleen, and kidneys. These plasma cells produce an abnormal immunoglobulin, which is often referred to as a myeloma protein. Multiple myeloma occurs in middle-aged and elderly clients, and in males more often than in females.

The onset of multiple myeloma is generally slow and insidious, and most clients remain asymptomatic until the disease is somewhat advanced. Some clients are diagnosed without symptoms by the presence of Bence Jones proteinuria and an elevated total serum protein level. The major complaint is usually skeletal pain, especially in the pelvis, spine, and ribs. Clients also experience weakness, fatigue, and recurrent infection. Other clinical manifestations include osteoporosis and hypercalcemia related to destruction of bone. If the client has vertebral involvement and destruction, spinal cord compression and paraplegia are possible. Pathologic fractures are also common. Anemia is a major problem in this group. Anemia is due to infiltration of the bone marrow by plasma cells and, therefore, a failure of normal marrow function. Thrombocytopenia and granulocytopenia are also seen. Renal failure occurs in approximately 20% of clients and is due to calcium nephropathy, severe proteinuria, and hyperuricemia.

The diagnostic work-up shows pancytopenia, high total serum protein level, hyperuricemia, hypercalcemia, elevated serum creatinine level, and Bence Jones proteinuria. Radiograph and isotope scans show the extent of bony destruction. Treatment includes (1) systemic chemotherapy and (2) supportive care of complications. The chemotherapeutic agent that is most commonly used is melphalan (Alkeran), which is often given with corticosteroids and cyclophosphamide. Supportive care is important for control of symptoms and prevention of complications.

Clients need hydration (approximately 3 to 4 L/day)

to offset the potential problems of hypercalcemia and proteinuria. Intravenous sodium chloride and furosemide (Lasix) or other potent diuretics help to increase renal secretion of calcium. Clients are encouraged to ambulate to slow down bone resorption. Extremely high calcium levels must be treated as an emergency, often with corticosteroids and mithramycin (Mithracin).

The nurse is alert for focal back pain and the development of neurologic symptoms in the lower extremities. These symptoms may indicate impending spinal cord compression and should be diagnosed and treated (with surgery or radiation) as soon as possible to prevent paraplegia. The nurse teaches the client to recognize signs and symptoms of infection so that infections can be diagnosed and treated early and efficiently. Blood transfusions are often required for anemia. Pain control is essential. Analgesics, orthopedic supports, local radiation, and relaxation techniques are all helpful.

AUTOIMMUNITIES

Autoimmunity is a process whereby a host develops and expresses immunologic reactivity against self components. For unknown reasons, certain cells or tissues of the body are recognized as nonself or no longer tolerated as self, and immune reactions to them occur. The responses, both antibody and cell mediated, are similar to normal immune responses against nonself, although they are sometimes excessive and are usually inappropriate. Although the reasons for alterations in self-tolerance are not known, there are multiple theories.

Sequestered antigen theory. Some normal body antigens are sequestered within organs or away from circulatory and lymphoid immune cells (e.g., in the lens of the eye, testes, central nervous system, or thyroid). Tissue damage through trauma, infection, chemical exposure, or other means can release these antigens into the circulation, which provokes the production of autoantibodies. An example is Hashimoto's thyroiditis.

Alteration or mutation of tissues caused by viruses, tissue injury, or haptens. Certain viruses, trauma, necrosis, or drugs can alter the cell surfaces so that body tissues are no longer recognizable as self. An example is autoimmune hemolytic anemia.

Cross-reacting theory. Sometimes the structure of certain infectious agents is so similar to that of cellular components that antibodies made to the infectious agent mistakenly react with the tissue. This response is called a cross-reaction. An example is the anti–beta-hemolytic streptococcal antibodies that cross-react with myocardial cells in rheumatic heart disease.

Genetic instruction theory. For unknown reasons, the genetic instruction for antibody production is altered so that autoantibodies are made against certain self tissues. Many autoimmune diseases seem to occur in families, which lends support to this theory of genetic predisposition.

Immunoregulation theory. Again for unknown reasons, there may be an alteration in the normally sophisticated system of immunoregulation. In some diseases, B cell hyperreactivity is clearly demonstrated (e.g., systemic lupus erythematosus). This hyperreactivity may be due to a problem with the B cell itself or to faulty and inadequate T8 cell suppression or excessive T4 cell help signals.

Much research is ongoing in the area of autoimmunity, but there are still few confirmed, established data. Not only is the etiology of autoimmunity uncertain, but there is a lack of consensus as to which diseases are truly autoimmune. Diseases that are generally believed to be autoimmune include systemic lupus erythematosus, polyarteritis nodosa, rheumatoid arthritis, autoimmune hemolytic anemia, rheumatic fever, and Hashimoto's thyroiditis (see the accompanying Key Features of Disease).

Connective tissue disorders, also sometimes referred to as collagen disorders, are diseases that are characterized by changes in collagenous connective tissue. Many of these diseases are considered to be autoimmune diseases, and for most, autoantibodies have been detected. Connective tissue disorders include systemic lupus erythematosus, rheumatoid arthritis, scleroderma, and polyarteritis nodosa. Most of the connective tissue disorders are characterized as organ-nonspecific autoimmunities, which simply means that the autoantibodies and the tissue damage are not limited to a specific organ. These disorders can be differentiated from organ-specific autoimmunities in which tissue damage occurs in a specific organ (see Chap. 28).

Treatment of autoimmunities depends on the organ or organs affected. Common to most autoimmunities, however, is the use of anti-inflammatory drugs and immunosuppressive drugs.

SUMMARY

Although the immune system is highly integrated and efficient and seems to protect us against diseases on a 24-hour basis, sometimes it malfunctions. The malfunctions generally take the form of too little function (immunodeficiency), too much function (hypersensitivity), and inappropriate function (autoimmunity). All of these situations present clinical challenges to nurses and other health care providers. With a better understanding of

KEY FEATURES OF DISEASE ■ Characteristics of Probable Autoimmune Disorders*

Disorder	Autoantigen	Comments
Systemic or Organ-Nonspecific Disorders		
Systemic lupus erythematosus	DNA, DNA proteins	Autoantibodies to a number of entities; immune complex–mediated damage
Rheumatoid arthritis	IgG	Immune complex–mediated damage in joints (arthritis, fibrosis)
Progressive systemic sclerosis	DNA proteins	Autoantibodies against nuclear materials; sclerosis
Mixed connective tissue disease	DNA proteins	Autoantibodies to ribonucleoprotein
Organ-Specific Disorders		
Autoimmune hemolytic anemia	Erythrocytes	Killing of antibody-coated erythrocytes
Autoimmune thrombocytopenic purpura	Platelets	Killing of antibody-coated platelets or innocent bystander effect
Myasthenia gravis	Acetylcholine receptor	Blocking of impulse transmission by autoantibody to acetylcholine receptor on muscle
Graves' disease	Thyroid-stimulating hormone receptor	Stimulation by autoantibody to thyroid-stimulating hormone receptor
Rheumatic fever	Myocardial cells	Cross-reaction of antibody with myocardial cells
Idiopathic Addison's disease	Adrenal cell	Antibody- and cell-mediated adrenal cytotoxicity
Hashimoto's thyroiditis	Thyroid cell surface	Antibody- and cell-mediated thyroid cytotoxicity
Pernicious anemia	Intrinsic factor/parietal cell	Autoantibodies to intrinsic factor, intrinsic factor/B_{12} complexes, and parietal canalicula cells
Goodpasture's syndrome	Basement membrane	Anti–glomerular basement membrane antibodies, which also cross-react with pulmonary basement membrane
Glomerulonephritis	Glomerular basement membrane	Autoantibodies and/or immune complex–mediated damage
Uveitis	Uvea	? cell-mediated and humoral damage
Vasculitis	Unknown	Probably primarily immune complex–mediated damage

*Other inflammatory, granulomatous, degenerative, and atrophic disorders are thought to be autoimmune because there is no more reasonable alternative explanation.

the immune system and continued research into ways to prevent, diagnose, and treat immune system malfunctions, clients who suffer from immune system disorders will have quality care and a brighter future. The nurse has an essential role in the care, education, and support of this client population. Nurses who have the appropriate knowledge and preparation to meet this challenge can significantly affect the quality of life and clinical course of clients with immunodeficiencies, hypersensitivities, and autoimmunities.

IMPLICATIONS FOR RESEARCH

The science of immune disorders is relatively new. Much exciting research is being done in all areas of immunology, and the knowledge of immunology and immune disorders has increased manyfold over the past decade. Still, there are many unanswered questions.

A huge ongoing research effort has been to find a vaccine and a treatment for HIV infection, as well as to describe more accurately the natural progression and immunopathogenesis of HIV-related disease. More needs to be done in these areas to stem the tide of new cases and the associated morbidity and mortality.

In the area of other immunodeficiencies, continuous research into viable and safe methods of treatment is needed. Better and safer methods of preventing and treating infections and other secondary manifestations are also required. An extremely important area of research is development of more specific immunosuppressive medications and treatments so that iatrogenic immunosuppression is minimized.

Allergy research proceeds with several aims: to better understand the genetic control of IgE production, to develop newer ways of inhibiting mast cell degranulation, and to discover better antagonists for the various allergic mediators. More research on the mechanism underlying hives, food allergies, and identification of newer or previously unrecognized allergens is also important. Continued research on recognizing triggers of asthma, as well as diagnosis and treatment of clients with asthma, is necessary.

Research is needed to better describe and understand the mechanisms of autoimmunity. The search continues to identify autoantibodies or evidence of cell-mediated reactions against self so that disorders can be understood as autoimmune. Then, new and better ways to interrupt the immune system's attack on self, as well as to treat the symptoms that do occur, are indicated.

Nursing research is sorely needed in all of these areas. The human responses to immunodeficiency, hypersensitivity, and autoimmunity are only beginning to be studied. The relationship of psychologic stress to immune response is an important one. Nurses, through research, must define ways to help clients with immune disorders to cope better and manage their symptoms. For all of the disorders mentioned, client teaching is essential in the management of the disorder. The impact of an immune disorder on a client's life should be studied, and interventions to minimize the impact of the disorder should be devised and evaluated. Nurses are in a unique position from which to ask appropriate questions and try to find the answers through clinical research. Possible research questions include

1. What is the role of stress and fatigue in aggravating allergic symptoms, and what is the role of stress management and relaxation in relieving or minimizing symptoms?
2. What is healthy "immune" living; what should nurses teach clients about diet, exercise, and activity?
3. How effective is client teaching about infection in enhancing early detection and treatment of infection?
4. What nursing interventions are useful for minimizing the impact of AIDS, connective tissue disorders, multiple myeloma, and other disorders on a client's life?
5. How do nurses intervene effectively to support the client undergoing organ transplantation and his or her significant others? How do nurses effectively support a significant other who is the donor? What is the nurse's response if the organ fails?

REFERENCES AND READINGS

Armstrong, D., Gold, J., Dryjanski, J., Whimbey, E., Polsky, B., Hawkins, C., Brown, A., Bernard, E., & Kiehn, T. (1985). Treatment of infections in AIDS. *Annals of Internal Medicine, 103,* 738–743.

Austen, F. (1987). Diseases of immediate type hypersensitivity. In E. Braunwald, K. Isselbacker, R. Petersdorf, J. Wilson, J. Martin, & A. Fauci (Eds.), *Harrison's principles of internal medicine* (11th ed., pp. 1407–1414). New York: McGraw-Hill.

Barrick, B. (1988). Caring for A.I.D.S. patients: a challenge you can meet. *Nursing '88, 18*(11), 50–60.

Bennett, J. (1988). Helping people with AIDS live well at home. *Nursing Clinics of North America, 23,* 731–748.

Bowen, D. L., Lane, H. C., & Fauci, A. S. (1985). Immunopathogenesis of the acquired immunodeficiency syndrome. *Annals of Internal Medicine, 103,* 704–709.

Buckley, R. (1983). Immunodeficiency. *Journal of Allergy and Clinical Immunology, 72,* 627–635.

Buckley, R. H. (1988). Primary immunodeficiency diseases. In J. B. Wyngaarden & L. H. Smith, Jr. (Eds.), *Cecil textbook of medicine* (18th ed., pp. 1941–1948). Philadelphia: W. B. Saunders.

Carpenito, L. (1989). *Nursing diagnosis: Application to practice* (3rd ed.). Philadelphia: J. B. Lippincott.

Cochrane, C. G. (1988). Immune complex diseases. In J. B. Wyngaarden & L. H. Smith, Jr. (Eds.), *Cecil textbook of medicine* (18th ed., pp. 1960–1962). Philadelphia: W. B. Saunders.

Cooper, M., & Lawton, A. (1987). Immune deficiency diseases. In E. Braunwald, K. Isselbacker, R. Petersdorf, J. Wilson, J. Martin, & A. Fauci (Eds.), *Harrison's principles of internal medicine* (11th ed., pp. 1385–1391). New York: McGraw-Hill.

Corman, L. (1985). Effects of specific nutrients on the immune response. *Medical Clinics of North America, 69,* 759–774.

Doenges, M., & Moorhouse, M. (1985). *Nurse's pocket guide: Nursing diagnoses with interventions.* Philadelphia: F. A. Davis.

Donehower, M. (1987). Malignant complications of AIDS. *Oncology Nursing Forum, 14*(1), 57.

Durham, J., & Cohen, F. (Eds.). (1987). *The person with AIDS: Nursing perspectives.* New York: Springer.

Fauci, A. (1985). Acquired immunodeficiency syndrome. In J. B. Wyngaarden & L. H. Smith, Jr. (Eds.), *Cecil textbook of medicine* (17th ed., pp. 1861–1863). Philadelphia: W. B. Saunders.

Gallin, J., & Fauci, A. (Eds.). (1985). *Advances in host defense mechanisms: Vol. 5. Acquired immunodeficiency syndrome.* New York: Raven.

Grady, C. (1988). Host defense mechanisms: An overview. *Seminars in Oncology Nursing, 4*(2), 86–94.

Grady, C. (1988). HIV: Epidemiology, immunopathogenesis and clinical consequences. *Nursing Clinics of North America, 23,* 683–695.

Heller, B. (Ed.). (1984). Acquired immunodeficiency syndrome. *Topics in Clinical Nursing, 6*(2).

Kristal, A. R. (1986). The impact of the acquired immunodeficiency syndrome on patterns of premature death in New York City. *JAMA, 255,* 2306–2310.

Lawley, T., & Frank, M. (1987). Immune-complex diseases. In E. Braunwald, K. Isselbacker, R. Petersdorf, J. Wilson, J. Martin, & A. Fauci (Eds.), *Harrison's principles of internal medicine* (11th ed., pp. 261–262). New York: McGraw-Hill.

Lichtenstein, L. M. (1988). Anaphylaxis. In J. B. Wyngaarden & L. H. Smith, Jr. (Eds.), *Cecil textbook of medicine* (18th ed., pp. 1956–1958). Philadelphia: W. B. Saunders.

Lichtenstein, L., & Fauci, A. (1985). *Current therapy in allergy, immunology, and rheumatology.* St. Louis: C. V. Mosby.

Lockey, R. F., & Bukantz, S. C. (1987). *Principles of immunology and allergy.* Philadelphia: W. B. Saunders.

Longo, D., & Broder, S. (1987). Plasma cell disorders. In E. Braunwald, K. Isselbacker, R. Petersdorf, J. Wilson, J. Martin, & A. Fauci (Eds.), *Harrison's principles of internal medicine* (11th ed, pp. 1396–1402). New York: McGraw-Hill.

Marliss, E. (1985). Protein-calorie malnutrition. In J. B. Wyngaarden & L. H. Smith, Jr. (Eds.), *Cecil textbook of medicine* (17th ed., pp. 1183–1188). Philadelphia: W. B. Saunders.

McArthur, J., & Palenicek, J. (1988). Human immunodeficiency virus and the nervous system. *Nursing Clinics of North America, 23,* 823–829.

Meredith, T., & Acierno, L. J. (1988). Pulmonary complications of acquired immunodeficiency syndrome. *Heart and Lung, 17,* 173–178.

Pickersgill, F. (1987). Care of critically ill patients suffering from HIV infection. *Intensive Care Nursing, 3,* 106–109.

Quarterly report to the domestic policy council on the prevalence and rate of spread of HIV and AIDS—United States. (1988). *Mortality and Morbidity Weekly Report, 37,* 551–555.

Redgield, R., & Burke, D. (1988). HIV infection: The clinical picture. *Scientific American, 259*(4), 90–98.

Salmon, S. E. (1988). Plasma cell disorders. In J. B. Wyngaarden & L. H. Smith, Jr. (Eds.), *Cecil textbook of medicine* (18th ed., pp. 1026–1036). Philadelphia: W. B. Saunders.

Salvaggio, J. E. (1988). Allergic rhinitis. In J. B. Wyngaarden & L. H. Smith, Jr. (Eds.), *Cecil textbook of medicine* (18th ed., pp. 1951–1956). Philadelphia: W. B. Saunders.

Snyderman, R. (1988). Mechanisms of inflammation and tissue destruction in the rheumatic diseases. In J. B. Wyngaarden & L. H. Smith, Jr. (Eds.), *Cecil textbook of medicine* (18th ed., pp. 1984–1992). Philadelphia: W. B. Saunders.

Soter, N. A. (1988). Urticaria and angioedema. In J. B. Wyngaarden & L. H. Smith, Jr. (Eds.), *Cecil textbook of medicine* (18th ed., pp. 1948–1951). Philadelphia: W. B. Saunders.

Unanue, E., & Benacerraf, B. (Eds.). (1984). *Textbook of immunology* (2nd ed., pp. 299–307). Baltimore: Williams & Wilkins.

Update: Acquired immunodeficiency syndrome—United States 1989. (1990). *Morbidity and Mortality Weekly Report, 39,* 81–86.

U.S. Department of Health and Human Services. (1987). *Surgeon general's report on acquired immune deficiency syndrome.* Washington, DC: Author.

Volberding, P. (1985). Clinical spectrum of AIDS. *Annals of Internal Medicine, 103,* 729–733.

Waldmann, T. A., Strober, W., & Blaese, R. M. (1980). T and B cell immunodeficiency diseases. In C. W. Parker (Ed.), *Clinical immunology* (Vol. 1, pp. 314–375). Philadelphia: W. B. Saunders.

Wallace, J. (1987). Disorders caused by venoms, bites, and stings. In E. Braunwald, K. Isselbacker, R. Petersdorf, J. Wilson, J. Martin, & A. Fauci (Eds.), *Harrison's principles of internal medicine* (11th ed., pp. 831–838). New York: McGraw-Hill.

Yarchoan, R., Mitsuya, H., & Broder, S. (1988). AIDS therapies. *Scientific American, 259*(4), 110–119.

ADDITIONAL READINGS

Cohen, F. (1988, August). Acquired immunodeficiency syndrome research in critical care: A review and future directions. *Focus on Critical Care, 15*(4), 30–35.

This review is of research done with AIDS patients who were admitted to intensive care units. The research was related to outcome, survival, patterns of use of these units, economics, staff attitudes, and do not resuscitate decisions. The author also suggested future directions for nursing research in critical care.

Dickerson, M. (1988). Anaphylaxis and anaphylactic shock. *Critical Care Nursing Quarterly, 11*(1), 68–74.

This article presents a thorough review of the pathophysiology of the alterations in immune function that are responsible for anaphylactic shock and clearly stated management strategies. Nursing management techniques include detailed assessment criteria for the early detection of this rapid-onset health problem. Suggested interventions include appropriate drug therapy (with rationales) and specific nursing actions.

Larsen, E. (1988, January–February). Nursing research and AIDS. *Nursing Research, 37,* 60–62.

The author identifies several priority areas for nursing research in AIDS and HIV infection. She also describes the interest of the National Center for Nursing Research in HIV-related nursing research.

Lovejoy, N. (1988). The pathophysiology of AIDS. *Oncology Nursing Forum, 15*(5), 563–570.

The content of this article focuses on explanations of the molecular biology, mechanisms of cellular infection, modes of transmission, deficits of specific immune functions, pathologic effects on specific organs, and complications of AIDS. This information provides the nurse with a solid basis from which to assist clients and families to gain a better understanding of the AIDS disease process and its impact on health.

Moody, L., Wilson, M., Smyth, K., Schwartz, R., Tittle, M., & VanCott, M. (1988, November–December). Analysis of a decade of nursing practice research: 1977–1986. *Nursing Research, 37,* 374–379.

The authors conducted a study to analyze the research focus, theoretical bases, research designs, statistical methods, and research findings of 720 nursing practice research studies conducted between 1977 and 1986.

Pollock, S. (1987, September). Adaptation to chronic illness: Analysis of nursing research. *Nursing Clinics of North America, 22,* 631–644.

The author reviewed 54 nursing research studies conducted between 1980 and 1986 in the area of chronic illness. The author noted that interventions studied should be implemented by practitioners to promote adaptation to chronic illness and that more studies are needed in the area of prevention.

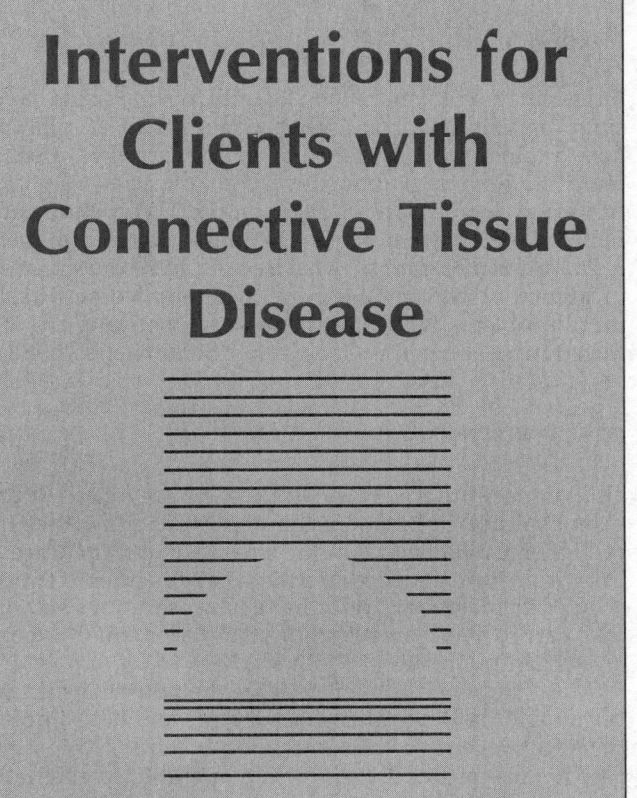

CHAPTER 28

Interventions for Clients with Connective Tissue Disease

Connective tissue disease (CTD) is the major component of *rheumatology*, the study of rheumatic disease. According to the American Rheumatism Association classification, any disease or condition involving the musculoskeletal system is categorized as a *rheumatic disease* (Schumacher, 1988). In this text, CTDs and other musculoskeletal conditions are discussed separately.

Much of the body is composed of connective tissue. The skin, joint structures, bone, nerve tissue, muscle, blood vessel walls, adipose tissue, and organ coverings are types of connective tissue. Primary functions of connective tissue include mechanical protection, metabolism, and provision of body structure, warmth, and elasticity needed for movement.

More than 37 million Americans, or 1 in 7, have one or more of over 100 CTDs. These illnesses result in annual health care costs of an estimated $30 billion or more (Schumacher, 1988). Most of these diseases have *arthritis*, or inflammation of joints, as a key feature. Consequently, the diseases are often incorrectly referred to as arthritis. Some CTDs have localized clinical manifestations, whereas others are systemic. Management of clients with CTDs requires a multidisciplinary approach, including nursing and physical and occupational therapy.

DEGENERATIVE JOINT DISEASE

OVERVIEW

Several terms are used to describe the most common CTD, *degenerative joint disease* (DJD). *Osteoarthritis* and *osteoarthrosis* are used interchangeably with DJD; however, this condition is not a primarily inflammatory disease, and thus osteoarthritis is not an accurate term.

Pathophysiology

DJD is characterized by the progressive deterioration and loss of articular cartilage in peripheral and axial joints. It is caused by prolonged or excessive use of these joints. Weight-bearing joints, the vertebral column, and hands are primarily affected because they are used most often and/or bear the stress of body weight. Because DJD is typically seen in the elderly population, it is also known as the wear and tear disease. Most clients have the *primary* form of the disease, but *secondary* DJD can result from other musculoskeletal conditions or from trauma.

In the joint, the normal bluish, translucent cartilage becomes soft, opaque, and yellow. Fissures and pitting develop, and the cartilage thins. As cartilage and subchondral bone beneath the cartilage begin to erode, the joint space narrows and osteophyte spur formation

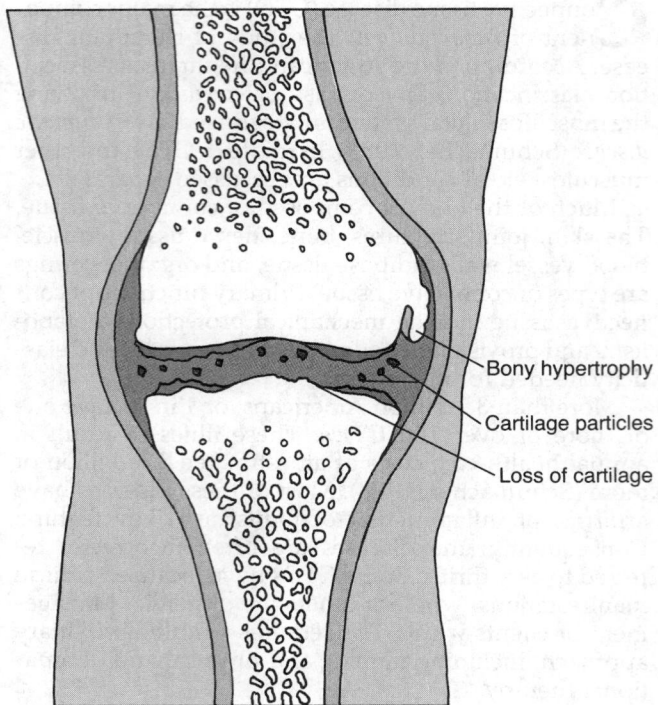

Figure 28-1

Joint changes in DJD.

Bony hypertrophy

Cartilage particles

Loss of cartilage

occurs, as seen in Figure 28-1. As a result of the alteration in cartilage metabolism, increased levels of destructive, inflammatory enzymes enhance tissue deterioration. The reparative process is unable to overcome the rapid process of degeneration. Bone cysts and secondary synovitis (synovial inflammation) are common in advanced disease. Eventually, subluxation and gross joint deformities cause marked immobility, pain, and muscle spasm.

Etiology

Although the causative mechanisms at the cellular level have not been well established, the risk factors for the disease have been identified. Aging causes degenerative changes in all tissues of the body; joints that are used most often are affected. Obesity also contributes to the likelihood of DJD, particularly in the hips and knees, the weight-bearing joints. Athletes stop participating in sports when overuse of certain joints causes chronic pain and degeneration. Joint hyperextensibility, as seen in gymnasts, predisposes the individual to DJD. The condition is also common in persons whose occupations involve mechanical stress to joints such as carpet layers, construction workers, jackhammer operators, and musicians. Congenital anomalies, trauma, and intra-articular sepsis can result in secondary DJD. Metabolic diseases, such as diabetes mellitus and Paget's disease, and hemophilia can also cause joint degeneration.

Some researchers support a genetic tendency for the disease, but this has not been proved. At present, the disease is not classified as autoimmune, but the possibility of involvement of the immune system in its development is being studied.

Incidence

It is estimated that more than 20 million Americans have symptomatic DJD, but probably more than 40 million have radiographic evidence of the disease. Prevalence increases with age; almost everyone over age 65 years has some degree of joint degeneration. Women are affected more often than men; the ratio of women to men is 2:1 after menopause. Men usually have the greatest incidence of hip involvement, whereas women have more problems with hands. Native Americans are affected twice as often as Caucasians (Schumacher, 1988).

PREVENTION

Unlike most other CTDs, DJD can be prevented to an extent. Although a person cannot prevent aging, weight reduction can alleviate undue stress on hips and knees. Proper posture can slow vertebral involvement. Those who participate in sports or have hazardous jobs should take care to avoid overexertion and placement of excessive strain on joints.

Many industries now recognize the potential risks of certain jobs to the health of employees and have implemented preventive measures. For example, to reduce the overuse of hand joints while operating machinery on an assembly line, employees rotate to different types of tasks every hour. Physical and emotional stressors are being addressed for U.S. workers in a variety of settings.

COLLABORATIVE MANAGEMENT

Assessment

History

The nurse collects the following information from the client at the initial interview that is specifically related to DJD. Because this disease is found more often in older women, *age* and *sex* are important factors for the nursing history. The nurse asks about the client's *occupation* and *nature of work,* history of *trauma,* and current or previous involvement in *sports.* Even if the client appears to be within the ideal range for body weight, the client is asked about a possible history of *obesity.* A *family history of "arthritis"* is also ascertained because many CTDs seem to have familial tendencies. Finally, the nurse determines if the client has a current or previous medical diagnosis that may cause joint manifestations. As with all musculoskeletal disorders, the nurse asks questions about the course of the disease, as described in Chapter 29.

Physical Assessment: Clinical Manifestations

The client's primary complaint is usually *joint pain,* which early in the course of the disease diminishes after rest and intensifies after activity. Later, the pain occurs with slight motion or even at rest. Because cartilage has no nerve supply, the pain is probably due to intra-articular and periarticular involvement and to muscle spasm. During examination of the joints, the nurse can often elicit pain or tenderness by palpation or by putting the joint through range of motion. *Crepitus,* a continuous grating sensation, may be felt or heard as the joint is put through range of motion. One or more joints are affected. The client may also complain of joint stiffness that lasts no more than 30 minutes.

On inspection, the joint is frequently enlarged because of *bony hypertrophy;* rarely does a joint appear to be hot and inflamed. Approximately one-half of clients with hand involvement display characteristic *Heberden's nodes* (at the distal interphalangeal joints) and *Bouchard's nodes* (at the proximal interphalangeal joints). Although DJD is not considered to be a bilateral, symmetric disease, these bony nodes appear in that pattern (Fig. 28–2). They may be painful and red, but some clients do not experience discomfort from their presence. These nodes have a familial tendency and are a cosmetic concern, particularly to women (the nodes occur in women 10 times more often than in men). Intra- and periarticular *effusions* (fluid accumulations) are common when knees are involved. The adjacent skeletal muscle is often atrophied from disuse, as shown in Figure 28–3. The vicious pain cycle discourages movement of painful joints, which then results in contractures, muscle atrophy, and further pain.

DJD of the spine usually affects the lumbar region, particularly L3-4, or the cervical area in C4-6. Compression of spinal nerve roots causes radiating pain, stiffness, and muscle spasms in one or both extremities. Spinal and vertebral arteries may also become compressed.

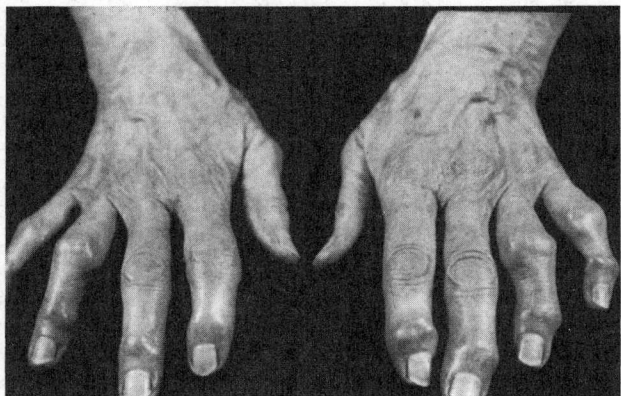

Figure 28–2

Bony nodules characteristic of DJD (Heberden and Bouchard nodes). (From the Arthritis Teaching Slide Collection, copyright 1980. Used by permission of the Arthritis Foundation.)

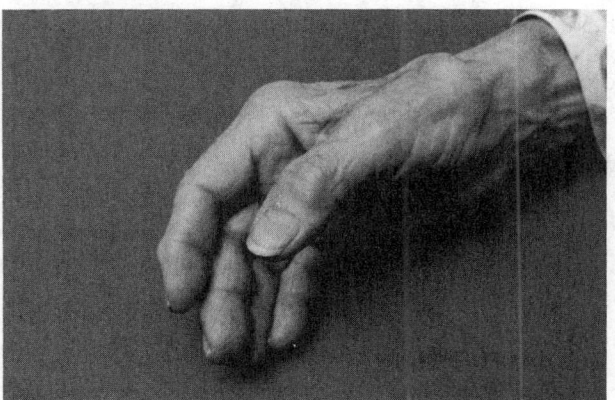

Figure 28–3

Thenar muscle atrophy from disuse and joint pain. (From the Arthritis Teaching Slide Collection, copyright 1980. Used by permission of the Arthritis Foundation.)

Physical assessment of the client with DJD includes determining the level of mobility and ability to perform activities of daily living (ADL). Severe pain and deformity interfere with ambulation and self-care. Chapter 21 describes ADL and mobility assessment in depth.

Psychosocial Assessment

DJD is a chronic condition that may cause permanent changes in the client's life style. The inability to care for one's self in advanced disease curtails socialization and results in role changes. Therefore, the client may exhibit a variety of behaviors indicative of the grieving process, such as anger and depression. Chapter 11 describes these behaviors in detail.

Deformities and bony nodules may cause an alteration in body image and self-esteem. The nurse observes the client's response to body changes: Does he or she ignore them or seem overly occupied with them? How does he or she refer to the changes—with anger, degradation, or humor? These clues help the nurse to assess the client's acceptance of body alterations. Further discussion of the assessment of body image is found in Chapter 9.

In severe DJD, the client may experience a role change in the family and/or workplace. The nurse assesses the roles of the client before disease development to ascertain changes that have been or need to be made. Adjustment and alternatives to change are determined, and problem areas are identified.

Laboratory Findings

There are no significant laboratory tests for this disease. The erythrocyte sedimentation rate (ESR) can be slightly elevated when secondary synovitis occurs (see Table 29-3 in Chap. 29).

Radiographic Findings

Routine x-ray films are useful in determining structural joint changes. Specialized views are taken when the disease cannot be visualized on standard x-ray films but is suspected. A computed tomography scan is used to determine vertebral involvement.

 Analysis: Nursing Diagnosis

After assessment of the client, the nurse summarizes the data and identifies relevant nursing diagnoses for the planning of care.

Common Diagnoses

Most clients with DJD present with the following common diagnoses:

1. Chronic pain related to cartilage disruption and joint deformity
2. Impaired physical mobility related to pain, deformity, and muscle atrophy

Additional Diagnoses

In addition to these diagnoses, the client may also have secondary problems caused by the pain and immobility common in DJD. These include

1. Activity intolerance related to pain, deformity, and decreased mobility
2. Altered nutrition: more than body requirements related to obesity
3. Total self-care deficit related to deformity, pain, and immobility
4. Self-esteem disturbance related to joint deformity and immobility
5. Knowledge deficit related to treatment regimen

 Planning and Implementation

Chronic Pain

Planning: client goals. The major concern of the client with DJD is pain relief. Therefore, the goal is that the client will experience a reduction in chronic pain.

Interventions. Pain relief may be accomplished by drug and nondrug measures. If these modalities become ineffective, surgery is performed to reduce pain.

Nonsurgical management. Management of chronic arthritic pain is difficult for both the client and the health care professional. A combination of modalities is often used. Chapter 7 elaborates on alternative methods of pain control.

Drug therapy. The purpose of drug therapy is to reduce pain, relieve muscle spasm, and reduce secondary inflammation if present. The drug class of choice is nonsteroidal anti-inflammatory drugs (NSAIDs) (Table 28–1). Salicylates in small doses may also be used. For temporary relief of pain in a single joint, the joint can be injected with a corticosteroid such as cortisone, but the number of injections is usually limited to three to four in a year. Muscle relaxants are sometimes given for severe muscle spasm. Potent analgesics are not appropriate for the client with DJD because of the chronic nature of the pain.

Rest. Several types of rest are used in the management of clients with DJD: local, systemic, and psychologic. *Local* rest is the immobilization of a joint with a splint or brace; cervical traction is used for severe cervical spine involvement. If a joint becomes acutely inflamed, the joint is rested until inflammation subsides. *Systemic* rest refers to the immobilization of the entire body, such as a nap. The client should sleep about 10 hours and nap for 1 to 2 hours each day. *Psychologic* rest is equally important because it allows relief from daily stresses that can enhance pain. Chapter 6 describes methods for relaxation and strategies for coping.

Positioning. Joints should be placed in their functional position, which may not be the position of comfort. When the client is in a supine position, a small pillow may be placed under the head or neck, but other pillows are avoided. A bed cradle or footboard keeps bed covers away from extremely painful joints. Flexion contractures quickly develop from use of large pillows under the knees or head. To reduce back discomfort, the client's legs may be elevated 8 to 12 in. Lying in a prone position twice a day is recommended. The nurse also reminds the client to use proper posture when standing and sitting to reduce undue strain on the vertebral column.

Heat. The client with DJD generally uses heat instead of cold to reduce pain. Cold application is usually reserved for acutely inflamed joints. The nurse can provide comfort to the client by using hot showers and baths, hot packs or compresses, and moist heating pads. Temperature of the client's room is also controlled so that the client does not chill. Special heat treatments such as paraffin dips, diathermy, and ultrasound are provided by a physical therapist. Usually a 15- to 20-minute heat application is sufficient to reduce pain, spasm, and stiffness. Regardless of modality, the nurse ensures that the hot pack is not too heavy or so hot as to cause burns. A temperature just above the body's temperature is adequate to promote comfort.

Diet therapy. There is no "arthritis diet," as has been proposed by the media and unknowledgeable authors. Foods high in protein and vitamin C are advocated to promote tissue healing. An obese client is encouraged to lose weight to lessen stress on weight-bearing joints. Less weight reduces pain and slows the disease process in affected joints.

Other pain relief measures. A variety of other modalities may be used for pain reduction. A transcutaneous electrical nerve stimulator (TENS) may be particularly helpful for vertebral involvement. Acupuncture, hypnosis, music therapy, and imagery are other methods that may be used by the client. The reader is referred to Chapters 6 and 7 for further explanation of these techniques.

TABLE 28-1   Drugs Used in the Treatment of Connective Tissue Disease*

Drug	Usual Daily Dosage	Interventions	Rationales
Salicylates, e.g., aspirin, buffered aspirin, Ecotrin, Ascriptin	12–18 tablets/d (4–6 g) are given in divided doses to achieve therapeutic effect.	1. Give with meals or snack. 2. Instruct client to observe for tinnitus, bleeding, or bruising (especially seen in *elderly* clients). Teach client to use soft-bristled toothbrush.	1. Aspirin products can cause gastrointestinal problems, including bleeding and ulcers, because of increased stomach acid production. Drugs can damage eighth cranial nerve and prevent platelet aggregation, which causes clotting. 2. Gums may bleed easily because of decreased clotting.
NSAIDs, e.g., naproxen (Naprosyn), sulindac (Clinoril), indomethacin (Indocin), ibuprofen (Motrin, Advil, Nuprin), mefenamic acid (Ponstel), phenylbutazone (Butazolidin), piroxicam (Feldene), diclofenac sodium (Voltaren), Ansaid (another NSAID)	Dose varies depending on which drug is used. Piroxicam and naproxen are given in fewer doses because of longer half-life. Indomethacin and phenylbutazone are not as commonly used because of tendencies to cause peptic ulcer and CNS changes.	1. Same as for salicylates above. 2. In addition, observe for fluid retention, increased blood pressure, and changes in renal function. 3. Monitor electrolyte and complete blood count values. 4. Observe for CNS changes, e.g., dizziness or confusion. 5. If a client is taking aspirin *and* an NSAID or is taking two NSAIDs, observe carefully for side effects or toxic effects.	1. Same as for salicylates above. 2. Most NSAIDs cause sodium retention, which can lead to edema formation, hypertension, renal damage, and/or congestive heart failure. Drugs should be used with caution in *elderly* population. 3. Most NSAIDs cause increased sodium levels and can cause bone marrow suppression. 4. Most NSAIDs can cause CNS effects, especially in the elderly. 5. Drugs are often used in combination, especially in clients with rheumatoid arthritis. Additive effects can cause serious complications.
Gold Auranofin (Ridaura)	Dose is 3 mg bid PO.	1. Observe for and instruct client to report gastrointestinal prob-lems, such as diarrhea, nausea/vomiting, abdominal cramping.	1. This side effect causes discomfort and can lead to electrolyte imbalance.
Gold sodium thiomalate (water-based gold) (Myochrysine)	After a 10-mg test dose, 25 mg and then 50 mg is given every week until monthly maintenance of 50 mg IM is reached.	1. Observe for rash or other skin change and for mouth ulceration (stomatitis).	1. Drug may be discontinued for a short period, then restarted.

Table continued on following page

TABLE 28–1 Drugs Used in the Treatment of Connective Tissue Disease* _Continued_

Drug	Usual Daily Dosage	Interventions	Rationales
Aurothioglucose (oil-based gold) (Solganal)	Same as for gold sodium thiomalate. If total of 1000 mg is used and no clinical change is seen, gold is discontinued.	1. Instruct client to expect metallic taste in mouth; teach importance of proper mouth care. 2. Monitor urine for protein and serum for CBC. If CBC is markedly decreased or if proteinuria is present, discontinue drug. 3. Give _deep_ IM, preferably by Z-track technique. 4. After IM administration, observe for nitroid crisis, a form of anaphylactic reaction.	1. Proper, frequent mouth care reduces risk of stomatitis and metallic taste. 2. These changes indicate serious toxic effects, and drug needs to be discontinued. 3. Drug is locally irritating to soft tissue. 4. Flushing, dyspnea, and anxiety may occur shortly after drug administration.
Hydroxychloroquine sulfate (Plaquenil)	200 mg PO each day is given.	1. Instruct client to have frequent (every 3–6 mo) ophthalmologic examination.	1. Drug can cause retinal damage.
Penicillamine (Cuprimine, Depen)	125–250 mg PO each day is used (may be given in two divided doses).	1. Same as for IM gold, except no nitroid crisis occurs.	1. Same as for IM gold.
Immunosuppressive agents, e.g., azathioprine (Imuran), cyclophosphamide (Cytoxan), methotrexate	Dose varies depending on disease activity and route of drug administration.	1. Observe for side effects and toxic effects, including, but not limited to, nausea/ vomiting, bone marrow suppression, and alopecia. 2. Teach client to avoid crowds and individuals with infections such as influenza.	1. Side effects and toxic effects of these drugs can be devastating. Drugs are reserved for severe forms of CTDs in which organ involvement is potentially life-threatening. 2. Bone marrow suppression or immune suppression increases risk of infection.
Prednisone (Deltasone)	Dose is 10–150 mg PO each day. For maintenance, attempt to give dose every _other_ day (to allow client's adrenal glands to function).	1. Observe for cushingoid changes, e.g., moon-face, buffalo hump, striae, acne, thin skin, bruising, fluid retention, and increased blood pressure. 2. Monitor electrolyte and glucose levels. 3. Observe for long-term effects of chronic steroid therapy, such as osteoporosis, cataracts, hypertension, or diabetes.	1. These changes are expected and tend to be dose related. Changes will diminish as dose decreases. 2. Chronic steroid therapy can cause sodium or fluid retention, potassium depletion, and elevated glucose level. 3. These complications may need to be treated with other drugs or modalities.

TABLE 28–1   Drugs Used in the Treatment of Connective Tissue Disease* *Continued*

Drug	Usual Daily Dosage	Interventions	Rationales
		4. Teach client to avoid crowds and individuals with infections such as influenza.	4. Drug suppresses immune system (lymphocytes) and increases risk of infection or decreased healing.

* NSAID, nonsteroidal anti-inflammatory drug; CNS, central nervous system; CBC, complete blood count; IM, intramuscularly; PO, orally.

Surgical management.   When all other measures are inadequate to provide pain relief, surgery is indicated. The two major surgeries performed for the client with DJD are *osteotomies* and *total joint replacements* (TJRs).

Osteotomy.   As the name implies, an osteotomy is a surgical procedure in which the bone is cut to promote realignment. In a client with DJD, joint deformity causes pain and abnormal stress on bone ends. In this procedure, a bone wedge may be removed or inserted, or the bone may be rotated to correct weight-bearing abnormalities. Hip and knee surgeries are most commonly performed.

The *preoperative nursing care* for a client undergoing this procedure is similar to that provided for the client who is having an open reduction, internal fixation, which is described in Chapter 31.

If the client has hip surgery, the *postoperative nursing care* is similar to that described in Chapter 31 for hip open reduction, internal fixation. A client with knee surgery generally has a tibial osteotomy to correct valgus (bowlegged) or varum (knock-kneed) deformities. The affected leg is wrapped with an elastic bandage from groin to heel, and one or two surgical drains remain in place until the bulky pressure dressing is removed. A knee immobilizer, as seen in Figure 31–20 in Chapter 31, prevents the knee from flexion; a hard or soft cast can be used instead of the bandage and immobilizer. Weight bearing and exercise are determined by the physician and physical therapist; crutches are used for ambulation.

Total joint replacement.   Any synovial joint of the body can be replaced with a prosthetic system consisting of at least two parts, one for each joint surface. A TJR is the major type of arthroplasty (surgical creation of a joint) that is performed. It is a procedure of last resort for pain and is used when all other methods of pain relief have been unsuccessful. Hips and knees are most commonly replaced, but replacements of hands, elbows, shoulders, and feet have gained popularity in the last 15 years. Although TJRs are performed most often for clients with DJD, other conditions cause joint damage requiring surgery. These disorders include rheumatoid arthritis, congenital anomalies, trauma, and avascular necrosis (bony necrosis secondary to lack of blood flow, usually from injury or chronic steroid therapy).

The primary contraindications for this procedure are infection anywhere in the body, advanced osteoporosis, and severe inflammation. An infection from a source in the body or from the joint being replaced can result in an infected TJR and subsequent prosthetic failure. If an individual has a urinary tract infection, for example, the infection is treated before consideration of surgery. Advanced osteoporosis could cause bone shattering during the procedure when the prosthetic device is inserted. A joint that is acutely inflamed is treated before surgery because the mechanical stress of the procedure could promote further inflammation and prosthetic failure.

As a group, TJRs are quite successful. Many clients who have lived with chronic, unbearable pain for years and have been unable to function independently in the home or workplace no longer experience pain and can once again be productive members of society after this procedure. The pain relief and psychologic lift outweigh the perioperative risks.

Total hip replacement.   The most commonly replaced joint is the hip. Clients of any age can have the surgery, but the procedure is done most often on elderly clients. The special needs and normal physiologic changes of elderly clients often complicate the perioperative period and may result in additional postoperative complications. The reader is referred to Unit 5 for further discussion of routine perioperative care and the special considerations needed for care of the elderly client.

As with any surgical procedure, *preoperative nursing care* begins with assessment of the client's level of understanding about the impending replacement. The physician explains the procedure and care expectations during the office visit, but this explanation may have occurred weeks or months before the surgery is scheduled. Elderly clients, in particular, may forget some of the information or may not know what questions to ask. Many orthopedic surgeons employ nurses in the office setting who can follow up and address any special concerns of the client. In addition, formal classes may be held in the hospital several weeks before surgery to answer questions and clarify information. The client is shown the prosthesis or a picture of the device as part of health teaching and is given written instructions or teaching booklets to reinforce the information.

In view of cost-containment efforts in the acute care setting, most clients are admitted on the morning of surgery and do not come to the orthopedic or medical-surgical unit until after surgery.

Because infection is a major complication of reconstructive surgery, the client may be required to have sputum and urine cultures to check for potential sources of infection. A dental examination is often advised to treat tooth decay or peridontal disease that could later lead to systemic infection. To reduce the flora that are normally present on the skin, the surgeon usually requests that the client clean the surgical site with povidone-iodine (Betadine) the night before and/or morning of surgery.

Before the start of the operative procedure, the operating room is specially cleaned and may be sealed to reduce the risk of infection. The surgery is usually scheduled early in the morning, and movement into and out of the room is kept to a minimum. Laminar airflow units are used in some operating rooms during surgery as an added precaution. The first dose of intravenous antibiotics, usually cephalosporins, is administered at least an hour before the initial surgical incision is made.

The client is placed under general, epidural, or spinal anesthesia for the procedure. Epidural or spinal induction reduces the risk of cardiopulmonary complications for which the elderly are at high risk. The approximately 10-in incision is usually longitudinal on the lateral or anterolateral thigh. A posterior incision may be used to preserve muscle, but postoperatively the client is more likely to experience hip dislocation if this type of incision is used. The hip is dislocated and the natural acetabulum is reamed to remove degenerated tissue. The area is prepared for the prosthetic acetabular cap, which is usually a metal cup with a plastic insert. If the prosthesis is cemented, *polymethyl methacrylate*, an acrylic fixating substance, is used.

The "old" femoral head is removed, and a tunnel is made within the femoral intramedullary canal in which the cement is placed. Some surgeons also remove the trochanters during prosthetic insertion, but union of bone may not occur after trochanter reattachment with wire. A number of trial prostheses are tried until the appropriate size is determined. After femoral implant insertion, the hip is relocated, and one or two surgical drains, such as a Hemovac, are inserted. A large, bulky dressing is applied to prevent hemorrhage.

If the implants are cemented, the procedure usually takes approximately 2 to 2½ hours. A recent advance in joint replacement surgery is the increased use of noncemented prostheses. Although polymethyl methacrylate is an excellent initial fixator, it has a finite life span and deteriorates over time, which causes loosening of the implant and pain. The average life span of a cemented hip is 10 years. When a prosthesis loosens, it is replaced; this procedure is sometimes called a *revision*. To prevent repeated replacements, a number of devices have been designed that do not require a fixating substance. Figure 28–4 illustrates a typical hip replacement system.

The most common mechanism that is used to avoid polymethyl methacrylate is a porous metal coating on the shaft of the femoral component and the back of the acetabular cap. By using a tight fit, known as a *press fit*, the implants are placed snugly against the bone tissue. Usually within 6 weeks, new bone tissue grows between the pores and "grafts" to the device. This bony ingrowth

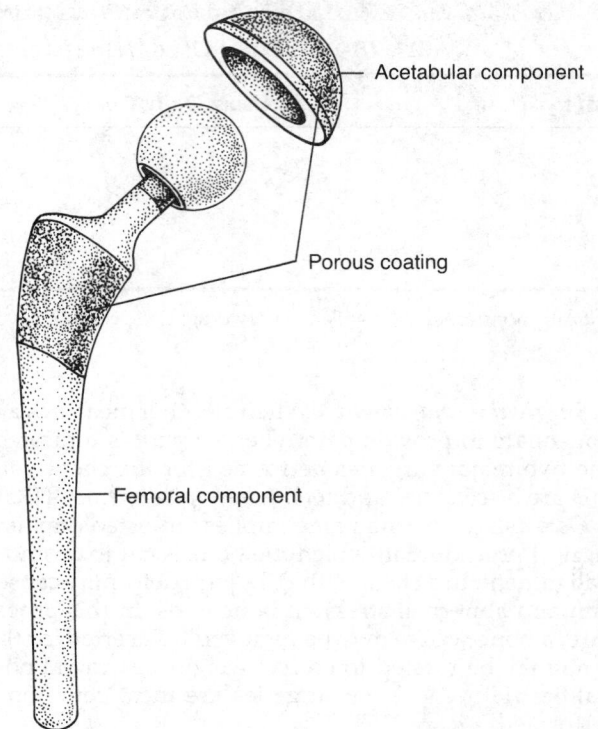

Figure 28–4

Noncemented, porous-coated hip replacement system.

serves as the fixating mechanism and ideally lasts a lifetime, although the follow-up periods have not yet been long enough to support this theory. Clients who are quite old and/or do not have sufficient bone mass are not candidates for the noncemented hip. The surgical time that is required to insert noncemented prostheses is usually less than that for traditional implants with cement, but this time depends on the type of noncemented prosthesis used.

Common complications of TJR surgery with nursing measures for prevention, assessment, and intervention are given in Table 28–2. The most common complication of total hip replacement is the possibility of *subluxation* or *dislocation*. Therefore, correct positioning must be maintained at all times. On return from the postanesthesia care unit, the client is placed in a supine position with the head slightly elevated. As shown in Figure 28–5, an abduction pillow, with or without straps, is usually placed between the client's legs to prevent adduction beyond the body's midline. Some hospitals no longer use this device because it is uncomfortable for the client; several regular bed pillows are used instead. The affected leg is placed and supported in neutral rotation by using a device such as the cradle boot (Fig. 28–6). The cradle boot not only prevents rotation but elevates the leg to the desired functional position and keeps the client's heel off the bed linen to prevent heel tissue breakdown. The client can usually be turned *toward* either side as long as the abduction or other pillow is in

TABLE 28–2   Nursing Measures to Prevent Complications of Total Joint Replacement Surgery

Complication	Prevention/Assessment Measure	Interventions
Dislocation	Position correctly. For hip, keep legs slightly abducted. For hip, prevent hip flexion beyond 90 degrees. Assess for pain, rotation, and/or extremity shortening.	Keep client in bed. Report immediately to physician.
Infection	Use aseptic technique for wound care and emptying of drains. Wash hands thoroughly when caring for client.	Culture drainage fluid. Monitor temperature. Report excessive inflammation and/or drainage to physician.
Deep vein thrombosis/ pulmonary embolism	Have client wear elastic stockings and/or sequential compression stockings. Teach leg exercises to client. Encourage fluid intake. Observe for signs of thrombosis (redness, swelling, or pain). Test for Homans' sign with client's legs flexed. Observe client for changes in mental status.	Keep client in bed. Do not massage legs. Do not use knee gatch on bed.
Hypotension, bleeding, or infection caused by use of polymethyl methacrylate	Take vital signs at least every 4 h. Observe client for bleeding.	Report excessively low blood pressure or bleeding to physician.

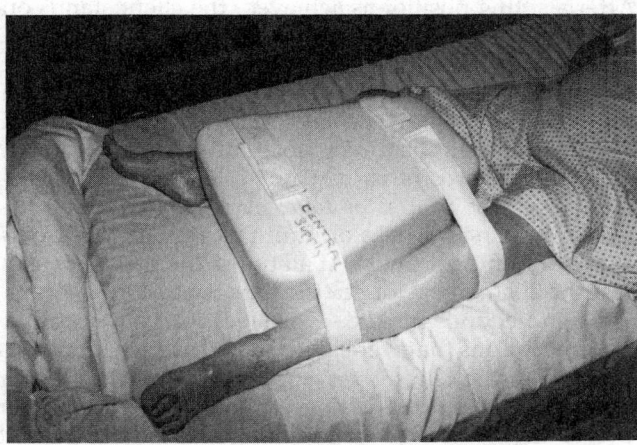

Figure 28–5

Typical abduction pillow used after a total hip replacement. (Photograph by Dave Bishop.)

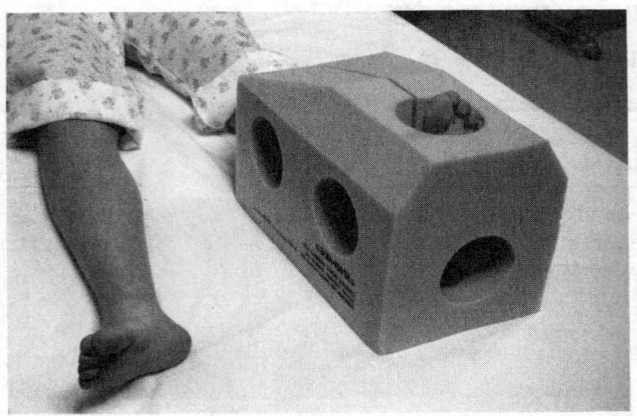

Figure 28–6

Cradle boot in place to prevent leg rotation and heel breakdown. (Courtesy of Span America Corporation.)

place. This policy varies depending on the surgeon's preference and policy of the hospital.

The nurse observes the client for possible signs of hip dislocation, which include increased hip pain, shortening of the affected leg, and leg rotation. If any of these clinical manifestations occur, the nurse keeps the client in bed and notifies the surgeon immediately. The treatment for repair of this problem is described in Chapter 31.

The second most common potential complication of hip replacement is *infection*, although this is the *most* common problem when considering all types of TJRs. The nurse monitors the surgical area and vital signs carefully — every 4 hours for the first several days — for signs of impending infection. Staples are often preferred to sutures because a lower infection rate is associated with their use. The surgical drains serve to remove exudate, which is an ideal medium for growth of pathogenic organisms. The nurse observes, measures, and empties the drainage fluid every shift. The total amount of drainage is usually less than 200 mL/8 hours. If the client has received a plasma expander such as dextran, this amount can increase to as much as 1000 mL/8 hours.

The drains and bulky pressure dressing are removed 48 to 72 hours postoperatively by the surgeon. For an elderly client, care must be taken to prevent tape burns when the surgical dressing is removed, especially when a heavy, elastic bandage (e.g., Elastoplast) is used. If the tape causes the skin to blister or open, the nurse uses the unit's standard of care for treating the skin lesion (e.g., Maalox application followed by exposure to a heat lamp).

Dry surgical dressings may be reapplied as needed by the nurse, but some physicians prefer an air-dry method for wound healing. For the latter method, no dressing is used, and the wound is cleaned with povidone-iodine solution or hydrogen peroxide several times a day.

As with other bone surgery, frequent neurovascular assessments, which are done along with vital signs, are necessary to monitor for possible compromise in circulation to the distal extremity. The technique for this nursing intervention is described in Chapter 31 in Table 31–2.

As soon as the client's bowel sounds return and the client is voiding in sufficient quantity, administration of continuous intravenous fluids is stopped, and the intravenous catheter is usually converted to a heparin lock for the continued administration of antibiotics for 48 to 72 hours. IV access is also needed if the client requires blood transfusions. Although most clients receive several units of blood during surgery, it is not unusual for the hematocrit to fall below the normal level so that additional blood is needed 2 or 3 days postoperatively. Autologous blood transfusions are common because TJRs are elective procedures (Brinkley, 1989). Intake and output are monitored for at least the first 24 hours.

Although it is sometimes difficult for the client to use a bedpan, the use of a Foley catheter is discouraged because it is a major source of infection. A fracture pan is used to minimize discomfort. Frequent linen changes and skin care are needed for the client who is incontinent. After the client is allowed to get out of bed, the incontinence often improves.

Although hip replacement is performed for relief of joint pain, the client experiences pain related to the surgical procedure. Many clients state that they have pain after surgery but that it is a different type and less excruciating than the pain before surgery. Pain control may be achieved by epidural analgesia, patient-controlled analgesia, TENS, intramuscular narcotic analgesia, or a combination of techniques. Chapter 7 discusses each of these modalities in detail, as well as the nursing care that is associated with each type. Regardless of the method used, most clients do not require parenteral analgesia after the first few days. Oral narcotics such as oxycodone plus acetaminophen (Percocet) are then commonly given until the client's pain can be controlled by NSAIDs.

Usually, the client with a total hip replacement is allowed to get out of bed the day after surgery. Activities that are allowed differ among surgeons and institutions, but prolonged bed rest can cause numerous complications. When getting the client out of bed, the nurse stands on the same side of the bed as the affected leg. After a sitting position is achieved, the client stands on the unaffected leg and pivots to the chair. Weight bearing on the affected leg is determined by the surgeon, type of prosthesis, and surgical approach. A client with a cemented implant is usually allowed partial weight bearing or weight bearing to tolerance immediately. An uncemented prosthesis can not tolerate weight until bony ingrowth occurs; *toe-touch only* is typically permitted for the first 6 weeks or until there is radiologic evidence of bony ingrowth. At all times, the nurse ensures that the client does not flex the hips beyond 90 degrees, as illustrated in Figure 28–7. Dislocation could result if the precautions that were just detailed are not followed.

Because the client does not resume full activity for several weeks, the risk of developing lower-extremity or pelvic thrombi is high. In addition, an elderly client is at

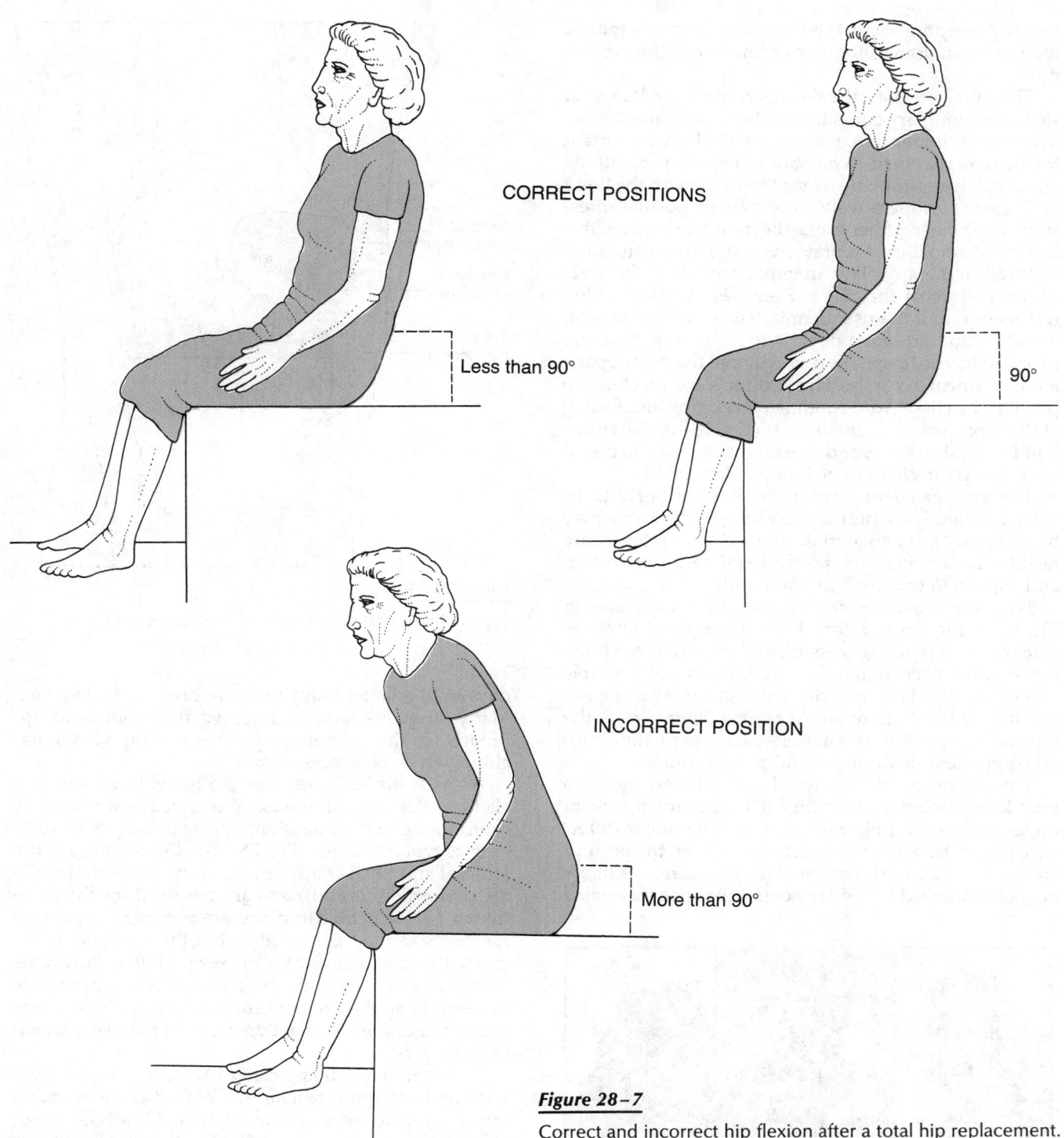

CORRECT POSITIONS

Less than 90°

90°

INCORRECT POSITION

More than 90°

Figure 28–7

Correct and incorrect hip flexion after a total hip replacement.

increased risk from age and probable compromised circulation before surgery. Clients who are obese or who have a history of deep vein thrombi are especially at risk for a recurrence of thrombi. Total hip replacement clients are predisposed to develop thrombi in the thigh, which more readily become emboli than calf or other thrombi. For this reason, thigh-high stockings, elastic bandages, and/or sequential compression devices are used during the hospital stay. Anticoagulants, such as

aspirin (Ecotrin or buffered aspirin), warfarin (Coumadin), or heparin, are given in maintenance doses. Leg exercises commence in the immediate postoperative period and include plantar flexion and dorsiflexion (heel pumping), circumduction of the feet, gluteal and quadriceps setting, and straight-leg raises. The client does gluteal exercises by pushing the heels into the bed; quadriceps setting is achieved by straightening the legs and pushing the back of the knees into the bed. In addition to preventing clots, these exercises improve muscle tone, which aids in restoration of function of the extremity.

The nurse assesses the client's respiratory status for signs of pulmonary emboli, atelectasis, and pneumonia. Vigorous pulmonary hygiene is particularly important for the elderly client, who should use deep breathing and incentive spirometry every 1 to 2 hours for the first 2 or 3 days postoperatively. Intermittent positive-pressure breathing treatments may be used for clients with a history of smoking or a previous respiratory condition.

Physical therapy plays an important role in the postoperative care of the client. Exercises, weight-bearing restrictions, and the use of ambulatory aids are taught. Assistive and adaptive devices to help with ADL are supplied by the hospital's occupational therapy department. Particularly important are tools for reaching to prevent the client from bending or stooping and flexing at the hips more than 90 degrees (Fig. 28–8). Extended handles on shoehorns and dressing sticks are also useful for helping the client to be independent in ADL.

The average client stays in the hospital for 7 to 10 days, but elderly clients may stay longer. Discharge may be to home, a rehabilitation unit, or a long-term care facility. Instructions for posthospital care are written and explained to the client and family.

Total knee replacement. The second most common TJR is for the knee. Before 1980, attempts at knee replacement were not successful, and most of these prostheses have been removed. The knee is not a simple hinged joint; it is a condylar joint and rotates slightly when flexed and extended. As seen in Figure 28–9, the typical knee prosthesis is a three-part system: the femoral component, tibial plate, and patellar button.

The preoperative care for the client undergoing a total knee replacement is similar to that for the client undergoing a total hip replacement. The major difference lies in the teaching, which depends on the postoperative protocol used. The client may come from surgery not being allowed to bend the operative knee for several

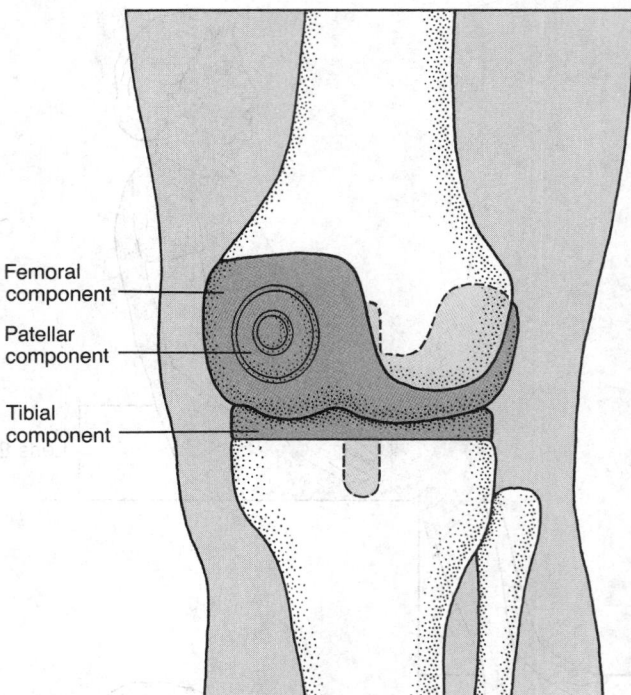

Figure 28–9

Typical three-part condylar knee replacement system.

days until a large, bulky pressure dressing is removed. Many surgeons have abandoned this traditional approach for the continuous passive motion (CPM) machine, which is discussed later.

As with the hip, the knee can be replaced with the client under general, epidural, or spinal anesthesia. A central longitudinal incision, approximately 8 to 10 in long, is typically made (Fig. 28–10). Osteotomies of the femoral and tibial condyles and of the posterior patella are performed; the surfaces are prepared for the prostheses. Noncemented implants are becoming as popular for knees as they are for hips, but they commonly increase the time required for the surgical procedure. One or two surgical drains are inserted, and a bulky pressure dressing is applied to prevent bleeding. If both knees need replacement, it is not uncommon to have bilateral knee surgery.

Postoperative nursing care of the client with a total knee replacement is similar to that for the client with a total hip replacement. The abduction pillow is not used; a CPM machine is often applied in the postanesthesia recovery area or in the orthopedic or medical-surgical area the next day (Fig. 28–11). The machine is preset by the surgeon, physical therapist, or technician for the appropriate range and cycles per minute. A typical beginning setting is 10 to 30 degrees range of motion at two cycles per minute, but this setting varies. The machine is used for 8 to 20 hours/day, and the range of motion is increased gradually. The current trend is intermittent use for several hours at a time. Although one

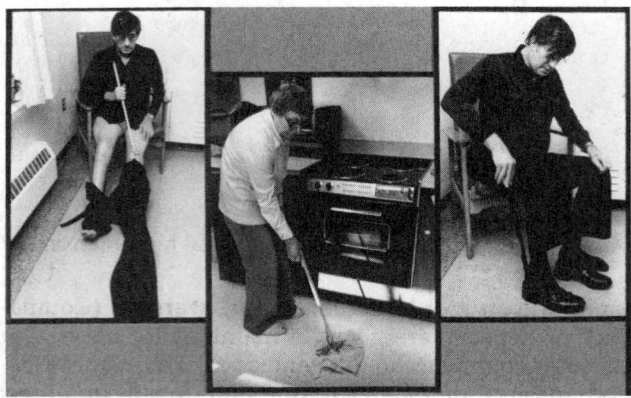

Figure 28–8

Long-handled devices to prevent bending at the waist. (From the Arthritis Teaching Slide Collection, copyright 1980. Used by permission of the Arthritis Foundation.)

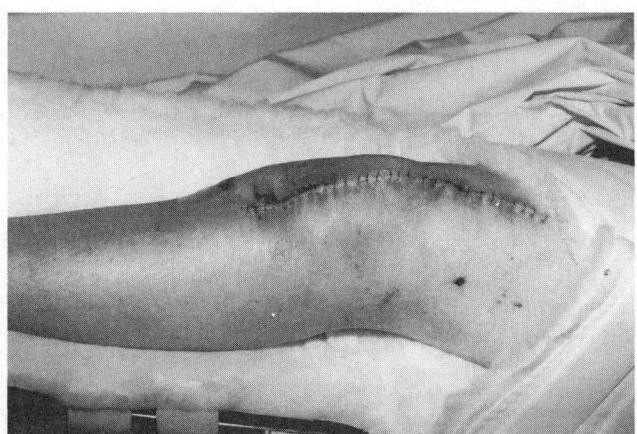

Figure 28–10

A central longitudinal incision for total knee replacement. (Photograph by Dave Bishop.)

might expect increased pain from use of the device compared with the traditional immobilization method, most clients tend to complain of less pain with the CPM machine. The use of this device prevents the development of scar tissue, which causes pain when the joint is put through range of motion. Another advantage is the achievement of the desired 90-degree flexion that is required before the client's discharge. With the traditional method, clients often returned to the operating room for manipulation of the knee to the desired flexion. One problem with the CPM machine, however, is the increase in bleeding. As a result, the device cannot be used for some clients until the first postoperative day. The client's response to the use of the device is noted daily. The accompanying Guidelines feature outlines the nurse's responsibility when caring for a client who is using the apparatus.

Dislocation is a rare problem for a client with a total knee replacement. Therefore, special positioning is not required. Other complications that were discussed earlier under postoperative care of total hip replacement clients may occur in these clients as well. After discharge from the hospital, the client should not hyperflex the knee or kneel for prolonged periods.

Total shoulder replacement. In the United States, replacement of the shoulder has not been as successful as other types of replacement. Because the joint is complex with many articulations, subluxation or dislocation is a major complication. The Neer prosthesis is most commonly used, with or without cement. Postoperatively, the client's affected arm is placed in a sling and swathed for 2 to 3 days until an exercise program begins to regain range of motion (Follman, 1988). An alternative to this protocol is the application of the CPM machine shortly after surgery (see Guidelines feature just cited). Frequent neurovascular assessments are important during the first few postoperative days.

Total elbow replacement. The elbow replacement is usually successful in increasing range of motion, but infection is common because of extensive tissue cutting during surgery. The Ewald prosthesis is commonly inserted, and the CPM device is often used postoperatively.

Finger and wrist replacements. Any joint of the hand can be replaced. The flexible, silicone prostheses are implanted without the use of polymethyl methacrylate. Postoperatively, a bulky dressing is used for 3 to 5 days, when it is replaced by a dynamic splint, brace, or cast (Fig. 28–12), or a CPM machine (Fig. 28–13). Edema formation is controlled by elevating the arm as much as possible. The rehabilitation program for finger arthroplasties lasts for months, until normal function and strength return.

Any bone of the wrist can be replaced, including the heads of the radius and ulna. The postoperative pressure dressing is removed in 3 to 5 days, and a splint or

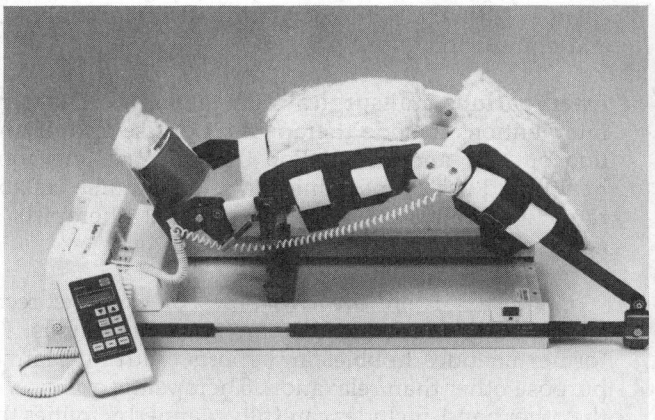

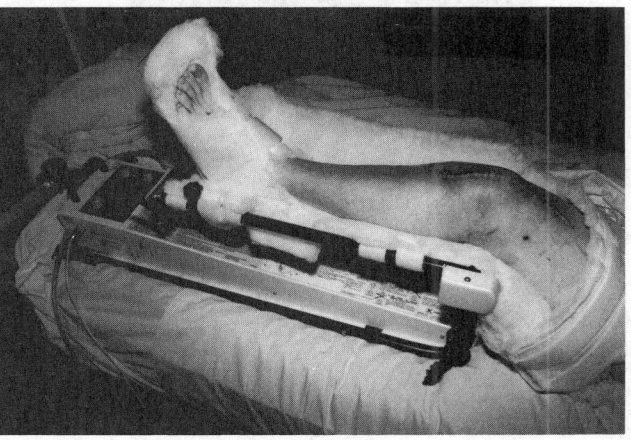

Figure 28–11

Two types of CPM machines, one shown in use after a total knee replacement. (Left photograph courtesy of Sutter Corporation.)

GUIDELINES ■ Care of the Client Who is Using a Continuous Passive Motion Machine

Interventions	Rationales
1. Ensure that the machine is well padded with sheepskin or other similar material.	1. The metal of the machine can damage skin and underlying tissues.
2. Check the cycle and range-of-motion settings at least once per shift (every 8 h).	2. The settings should be specified by the physician. The client or staff may change the settings unintentionally.
3. Ensure that the joint being moved is properly positioned on machine.	3. If the extremity is not properly positioned, nerve or soft-tissue damage can occur.
4. If the client is confused, place controls to the machine out of the client's reach.	4. A confused client may change the settings.
5. Assess the client's response to the CPM machine.	5. The machine may increase the client's pain or cause other concerns.
6. Turn off the machine while the client is having a meal in bed.	6. Motion and noise from the machine can prevent the client from eating.
7. When the machine is not in use, do not store it on the floor.	7. The machine may become soiled or damaged.

short arm cast is applied. The client usually regains full function within 6 to 12 weeks, but lifting may be restricted for a longer period. Usually, occupational therapists are involved with upper-extremity rehabilitation.

Total ankle and toe replacements. The ankles support approximately 25% of the body's weight; therefore, developing an implant that is both small and strong has been difficult. Usually when the ankle is replaced, an *arthrodesis*, or bone fusion, is performed for added stability. Replacing the ankle is not a common procedure.

The metatarsal implants are made of silicone and cannot bear excessive weight. Typically, the client has one or more osteotomies and fusions, which are immobilized by wires and a cast while healing occurs. Chapter 31 discusses this procedure and its associated nursing care.

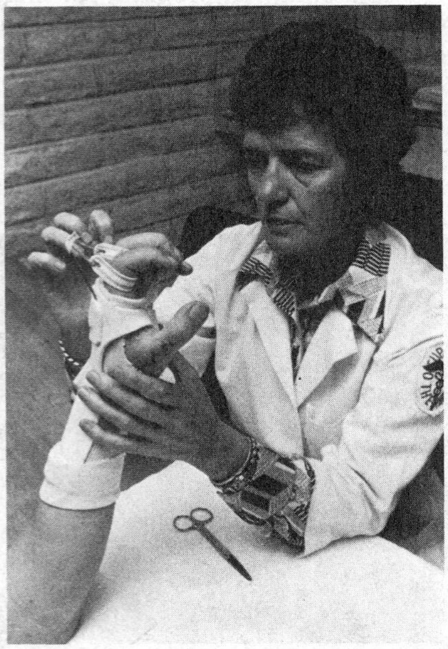

Impaired Physical Mobility

Planning: client goals. The primary goal is that the client will function independently in performing ADL and ambulation.

Interventions: nonsurgical management. The major interventions include therapeutic exercise and promotion of ADL and ambulation through teaching about health and use of mechanical aids. The nurse collaborates with physical and occupational therapists to achieve this goal.

Exercise. There are two types of exercise: recreational and therapeutic; they are not synonymous. The former includes hobbies and sports, with no planned purpose other than relaxation. Therapeutic exercise, on the other hand, includes carefully planned activities that are designed to improve muscle strength and tone and the range of motion of the joint. Certain recreational activities may be therapeutic, such as doing the breast

Figure 28–12

Dynamic splint used after finger implants. (From the Arthritis Teaching Slide Collection, copyright 1980. Used by permission of the Arthritis Foundation.)

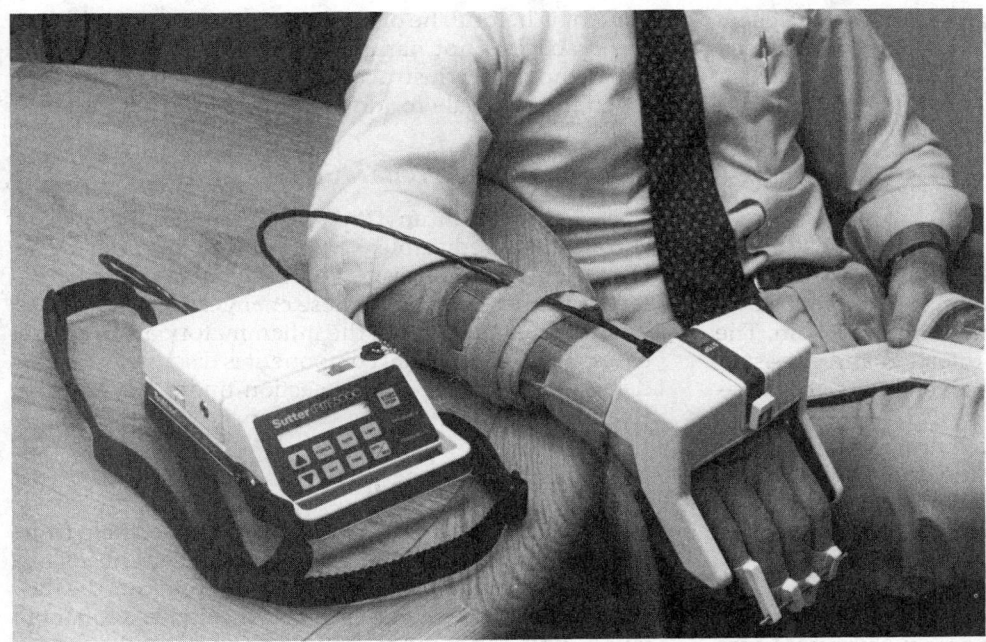

Figure 28–13
CPM machine used after finger implant surgery. (Courtesy of Sutter Corporation.)

stroke during swimming to enhance chest and arm muscles. Exercises are usually prescribed by the physical therapist, but the nurse reviews their techniques and principles. The ideal time for exercise is immediately after the application of heat. The instructions for exercise outlined in the accompanying Client/Family Education feature are followed rigorously so as not to cause further joint damage.

Use of assistive and adaptive devices. The client is evaluated by the physical therapist for the need for ambulatory aids such as canes, walkers, or platform crutches. Although many clients do not like to use these aids, they are important for prevention of further joint deterioration and pain. An occupational therapist evaluates the client's ability to perform ADL and can pro-

vide devices for assistance. Chapter 22 describes these assistive and adaptive devices and their uses.

■ Discharge Planning

Home Care Preparation

The client with DJD is not usually hospitalized for the disease except for evaluation or for surgery. If weight-bearing joints are markedly involved, the client may have difficulty going up or down stairs. Making arrangements to live on one floor with accessibility to all rooms is often the best solution. A community health nurse, social worker, or other health professional assesses the need for structural alterations to the home to

---

CLIENT/FAMILY EDUCATION ■ Exercise Instructions for the Client with Degenerative Joint Disease or Rheumatoid Arthritis

"Follow the exercise instructions that have been specifically prescribed for you." (There are no universal exercises; each client is treated on the basis of his or her own needs.)

"Do your exercises on both 'good' and 'bad' days. Consistency is important."

"Respect pain. If pain increases with exercise, discontinue the exercise and report this occurrence to your physician."

"Use active rather than active-assist or passive exercise whenever possible."

"Reduce the number of repetitions when the inflammation is severe (when you have more pain)."

"Do not substitute ADL or household tasks for the prescribed exercises."

"Avoid resistive exercises when your joints are severely inflamed."

accommodate ambulatory aids and to enable the client to perform ADL. For example, a kitchen counter may need to be lowered or a seat and handrails to be installed in the shower. If the client has a total hip replacement, a higher-level toilet seat is necessary to prevent excessive hip flexion.

Client/Family Education

The most important feature of client education is joint protection. Preventing further damage to joints slows the progression of the disease and minimizes pain. The nurse teaches general rules of protection and cites specific examples for illustration, as given in the accompanying Client/Family Education Feature.

As with other diseases in which drugs and diet therapy are used, the nurse teaches the drug protocol, side effects, and toxic effects to the client and family. The importance of reducing weight and eating the proper foods to enhance tissue healing is also emphasized.

Many clients with "arthritis" become frustrated and desperate about the course of the disease and treatment, and they look for a cure. Unfortunately, there is no cure for these diseases, even though tabloids, books (which are sometimes written by uninformed health care professionals), and the media frequently claim to have the curative remedy. Billions of dollars are spent each year on quackery, including liniments, special diets, and copper bracelets. More hazardous substances such as snake venom, industrial cleaners, and drugs that are available only outside the United States are also advertised as remedies. The nurse instructs the client to always check with The Arthritis Foundation about new "treatments" that propose to cure the disease. If the client believes that, for example, wearing a copper bracelet or eating more foods with a high vitamin C content is helpful, he or she is encouraged to continue if the practice is not harmful. If there is a potential for harm, the client is instructed to avoid the modality and is given the rationale for doing so.

Psychosocial Preparation

The client with any type of CTD must live with a chronic, unpredictable, and painful disorder. The client's roles, self-esteem, and body image may be affected by these diseases. These changes are often not as devastating in DJD as in the inflammatory arthritic diseases. The psychosocial component is discussed in more detail in the corresponding section under the heading Rheumatoid Arthritis.

Health Care Resources

The client who has surgery is likely to need help from community resources. After a TJR, the client needs extensive assistance with mobility. The client may be discharged to home, a long-term care facility, or a rehabilitation unit. The nurse collaborates with the social worker and physician to find the best placement for each client. If the client is discharged to home, home care nurses need to visit frequently for the first 6 to 12 weeks. A nursing assistant may come to the home to help with hygiene-related needs; a physical therapist works with the client on a daily basis. In addition, a client having a TJR is *never* discharged to be at home alone. A family member or significant other must be in the home at all times for at least the first 6 weeks, when the client needs the most assistance.

Regardless of whether the client goes home or to another inpatient facility, the nurse provides written instructions about the care that is required; communica-

---

CLIENT/FAMILY EDUCATION ■ Joint Protection Instructions

"Use large joints instead of small ones; e.g., place your purse strap over your shoulder instead of grasping the purse with your hand."

"Do not turn a doorknob clockwise. Turn it counterclockwise" (to prevent ulnar deviation).

"Use two hands instead of one to hold objects."

"Sit in a chair with a high, straight back."

"When getting out of bed, do not push off with your fingers; use the entire palm of both hands."

"Do not bend at the waist; bend your knees instead, while keeping your back straight."

"Use long-handled devices, such as a hairbrush with an extended handle."

"Use assistive and/or adaptive devices, such as Velcro closures and built-up utensil handles" (to facilitate independence and protect joints).

"Do not use pillows in bed, except a small one under your head" (to prevent flexion contractures).

"Avoid twisting or wringing your hands."

tion with the new care provider is ideal for continuity of care. Arrangements are made so that the client can return to the same acute care hospital if needed.

An important community resource for all clients with CTD is The Arthritis Foundation. This organization provides information to lay and health professionals and refers clients and their families to other resources as needed.

Evaluation

The nurse evaluates the care provided by determining whether the following desired outcomes for the client have been met, that the client

1. States that pain is reduced or alleviated
2. Ambulates without personal assistance (but a mechanical aid may be used)
3. Is ADL independent (may use assistive and adaptive devices)

In addition to these general outcomes, more specific criteria may be used. The American Nurses' Association together with nurses from the Arthritis Health Professions Nursing Task Force developed a set of standards

for rheumatology nursing in 1983. If surgery is performed, additional outcome criteria are established.

RHEUMATOID ARTHRITIS

OVERVIEW

Rheumatoid arthritis (RA) is the second most common CTD and is the most destructive. It is a chronic, progressive, systemic, inflammatory process that affects primarily synovial joints (see the accompanying Key Features of Disease).

Pathophysiology

The onset of the disease is characterized by *synovitis*, inflammation of the synovial tissue in joints. As shown in Figure 28–14, the synovium thickens and becomes hyperemic, fluid accumulates in the joint space, and a

KEY FEATURES OF DISEASE ■ Differential Features of Rheumatoid Arthritis and Degenerative Joint Disease

Characteristic	Rheumatoid Arthritis	Degenerative Joint Disease
Typical onset	At 35–45 yr	At > 60 yr
Sex affected	Female (3:1)	Female (2:1)
Risk factors or etiology	Probably autoimmune Emotional stress	Aging Obesity Trauma Occupation
Disease process	Inflammatory	Degenerative
Disease pattern	Bilateral, symmetric, multiple joints Usually affects upper extremities first Distal interphalangeal joints of hands spared Systemic	May be unilateral, single joint Affects weight-bearing joints and hands, spine Metacarpophalangeal joints spared Nonsystemic
Laboratory findings	Elevated rheumatoid factor, antinuclear antibody, ESR*	Normal or slightly elevated ESR
Drug therapy	Salicylates NSAIDs* Gold or penicillamine Corticosteroids Immunosuppressive agents Other analgesics	NSAIDs Acetaminophen (Tylenol) Other analgesics

* ESR, erythrocyte sedimentation rate; NSAIDs, nonsteroidal anti-inflammatory drugs.

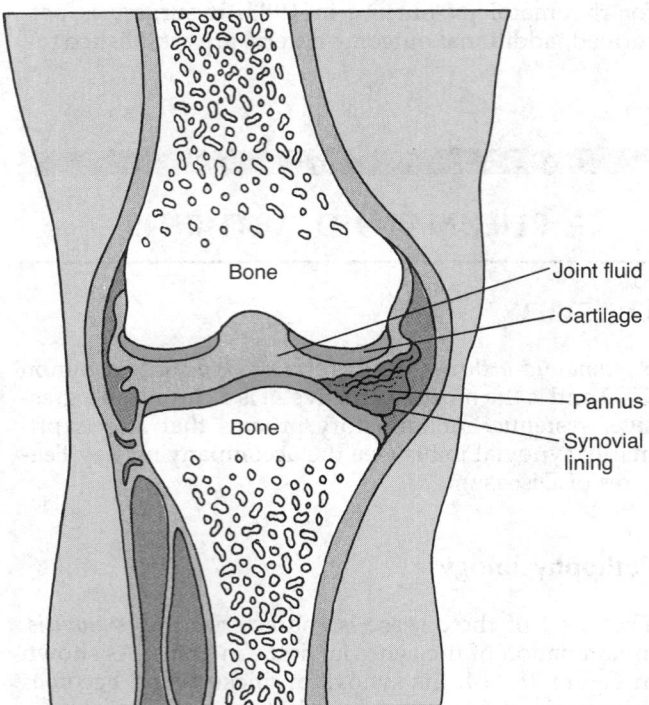

Figure 28–14

Joint changes in RA.

pannus forms. The *pannus* is vascular granulation tissue, composed of inflammatory cells, that erodes articular cartilage and eventually destroys bone. As a result, fibrous adhesions, bony ankylosis, and calcifications occur; bone loses density and secondary osteoporosis results.

If the client is diagnosed early in the course of the disease, permanent joint changes can often be avoided. Treatment can cause a remission of the disorder; about 25% of clients have a remission, which may last as long as 20 years. Spontaneous remissions and exacerbations can also occur without treatment.

RA is a systemic disease; i.e., areas of the body in addition to synovial joints can be affected. Inflammatory responses that are similar to those occurring in synovial tissue may be seen in any organ or body system in which connective tissue is prevalent. If blood vessel involvement, called *vasculitis*, occurs, the organ that is supplied by that vessel can be affected. The result is malfunction and eventual failure of an organ or system. These pathologic changes usually occur late in the disease process and cause life-threatening problems, as described under the later heading Physical Assessment: Clinical Manifestations.

Etiology

A number of theories have been postulated to explain the pathogenesis of RA. The most popular theory to date is the immune complex hypothesis. Unusual antibodies of the immunoglobulin (Ig) M and/or IgG type, termed *rheumatoid factor*, develop against IgG antigenic determinants to form complexes that lodge in synovium and other connective tissues. Local and systemic inflammatory responses result. RA has recently been found to be strongly associated with the human leukocyte antigen (HLA) DRw4. Other antigens have been identified but are found less frequently. Chapter 23, on cellular inflammation and the immune response, describes these processes in depth.

Although RA is considered to be a probable autoimmune disease, there is no clear explanation of the origin of rheumatoid factor. A genetic predisposition to developing the disease is most likely because the disease affects individuals with a family history of RA two or three times more often than the normal population.

Some researchers suspect that there is a hormonal influence on the development of the disease because RA affects women more often than men; others suspect that a virus (such as Epstein-Barr) could trigger the autoim-

NURSING RESEARCH

Increased Stress Translates into Increased *Dis*tress for Clients with Rheumatoid Arthritis.

Crosby, L. J. (1988). Stress factors, emotional stress and rheumatoid arthritis disease activity. *Journal of Advanced Nursing, 13,* 452–461.

Recent studies indicated a relationship between RA and emotional stress. The purpose of this study was to determine the relationship among stress-producing factors (as measured by the Daily Hassles Scale), emotional stress (as evidenced by a visual analogue scale and the State Trait Anxiety Inventory), and disease activity (as measured by the client's erythrocyte sedimentation rate and a compilation of clinical findings). One hundred one subjects were tested in a large rheumatology outpatient clinic. The researcher found positive correlations between emotional stress level and disease activity, and between the number or severity of stress factors and emotional stress.

Critique. The researcher used an adequate number of subjects in the study, although she stated that a larger group would have been preferred for the number of variables. Reliability and validity were established, and multiple measures of the variables were used when possible. The findings of this descriptive study lend themselves to further investigation with an experimental design to test interventions for stress reduction.

Possible nursing implications. Many of the stress-producing factors that were identified in this study, such as fatigue and anxiety, are amenable to nursing interventions. Teaching a client how to use stress management techniques may help to reduce emotional stress levels, which ultimately can decrease rheumatoid disease activity.

mune process. Studies have failed to support these theories. Physical stress and emotional stress have been linked to exacerbations of the disorder and are therefore probably contributing factors in its development (see the accompanying Nursing Research feature).

Incidence

RA affects women three times more often than men. Also, women who are taking or who have taken oral contraceptives are less likely to have RA. The onset of the disease is typically between ages 25 and 40 years, but it can occur at any age. The sex difference is not as great in the elderly population. There are no significant differences among geographic locations despite the common lay belief that warmer, drier climates cure the disease. Although joint pain may be less in these areas, the occurrence of the disease is as frequent. With the exception of Native Americans, there are no major differences among races or ethnic groups. Studies of several northern Native American tribes revealed RA prevalence rates that were three to seven times higher than those in Caucasians (Schumacher, 1988).

COLLABORATIVE MANAGEMENT

 Assessment

History

The nurse considers *age* and *sex* of the client because the disease begins most commonly in young women.

Other risk factors, such as *family history* and *previous viral infections,* are also determined. The nurse asks the woman whether oral contraceptives have been taken because clients who are taking this medication are less likely to have the disease. The client's ability to cope with *stress* is also ascertained because increased emotional stress is correlated with the onset of the disorder.

Physical Assessment: Clinical Manifestations

The manifestations of RA can be categorized as early and late disease and as articular (joint related) and extra-articular (see the accompanying Key Features of Disease). The onset of RA may be acute and severe or may be insidious with vague complaints lasting for several years before diagnosis.

The client typically complains of *fatigue, generalized weakness, anorexia,* and a *weight loss* of 2 or 3 lb (about 1 kg). Persistent low-grade *fever* may accompany the inflammatory process. In early disease, upper extremity joints are involved initially, usually the proximal interphalangeal and metacarpophalangeal joints of the hands. The joints may be slightly *reddened, warm, stiff, swollen,* and *tender* or *painful,* particularly on palpation. The typical pattern of joint involvement in RA is *bilateral* and *symmetric* (e.g., both wrists).

As the disease worsens, the joints become progressively inflamed, hot, and quite painful. The client complains of *morning stiffness* (also known as the gel phenomenon), which lasts between 30 minutes and several hours after awakening. On palpation, the joints feel soft because of synovitis and effusions (fluid accumulation).

KEY FEATURES OF DISEASE ■ **Early Versus Late Clinical Manifestations of Rheumatoid Arthritis**

Early Manifestations	Late Manifestations
Joint	
Inflammation	Deformities, e.g., swan neck or ulnar deviation
	Moderate to severe pain and morning stiffness
Systemic	
Low-grade fever	Osteoporosis
Fatigue	Severe fatigue
Weakness	Anemia
Anorexia	Weight loss
Paresthesias	Subcutaneous nodules
	Peripheral neuropathy
	Vasculitis
	Pericarditis
	Fibrotic lung disease
	Sjögren's syndrome
	Renal disease

The fingers often appear spindle-like. *Muscle atrophy* can result from disuse secondary to joint pain, and *range of motion decreases.*

Eventually, most or all synovial joints are affected. In severe disease, the temporomandibular and cricoarytenoid joints may be involved, but this involvement is not common. When the spinal cord is affected, the cervical joints are most likely to be affected. *Joint deformity* occurs as a late, articular manifestation, and secondary *osteoporosis* can cause bone fractures. Common deformities are illustrated in Figure 28–15. Extensive wrist involvement can result in *carpal tunnel syndrome* (see Chap. 31 for assessment and management). *Baker's cysts,* or enlargement of popliteal bursa, may occur and cause tissue compression and pain; *tendon rupture* is not uncommon.

Numerous extra-articular clinical manifestations are associated with advanced disease. Consequently, the nurse assesses other body systems to ascertain systemic involvement. Moderate to severe weight loss, fever, and extreme fatigue are common. Approximately 25% of clients have the characteristic round, movable, and nontender *subcutaneous nodules,* which are most often palpated on the ulnar surface of the arm. These nodules may disappear and reappear at any time and are associated with severe, destructive disease. They occasionally open and become infected, but otherwise they do not cause a problem.

Inflammation of the blood vessels results in *vasculi-tis,* particularly of small to medium-sized vessels. When arterial involvement *(rheumatoid arteritis)* occurs, major organs and body systems become ischemic and malfunction. Ischemic skin lesions appear in groups as small brownish spots, most commonly around the nail bed (periungual lesions). The nurse counts the lesions and notes their locations daily. Larger lesions on the lower extremities lead to ulcerations, which heal slowly.

About 10% of clients with RA have acute episodes of *pericarditis,* which is most common in males. Myocarditis and coronary arteritis are less common. *Respiratory complications* manifest as pleurisy, pneumonitis, diffuse interstitial fibrosis, and pulmonary hypertension. *Peripheral neuropathy* causing foot drop and paresthesias can occur, most often in the elderly. *Ocular involvement* is not unusual and manifests as iritis or scleritis.

Several syndromes are seen in clients with RA. The most common is *Sjögren's syndrome,* which includes a triad of dry eyes (keratoconjunctivitis sicca or the sicca syndrome), dry mouth (xerostomia), and dry vagina. Immune complexes and inflammatory cells are thought to obstruct secretory glands and ducts. This syndrome is usually found in persons with CTDs such as RA but may occur alone. Less commonly seen is *Felty's syndrome,* which is characterized by RA, hepatosplenomegaly (enlarged liver and/or spleen), and leukopenia. *Caplan's syndrome* is the presence of rheumatoid nodules in the lungs and pneumoconiosis, which is found primarily in coal miners and asbestos workers.

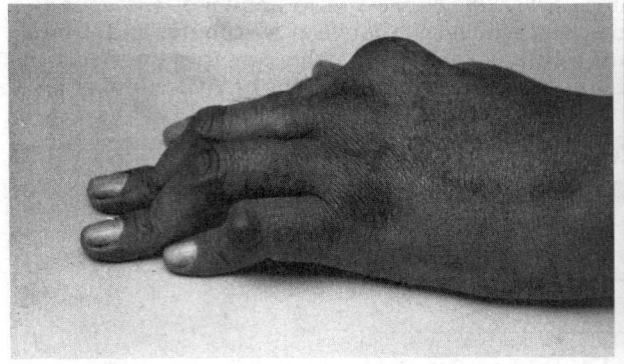

A

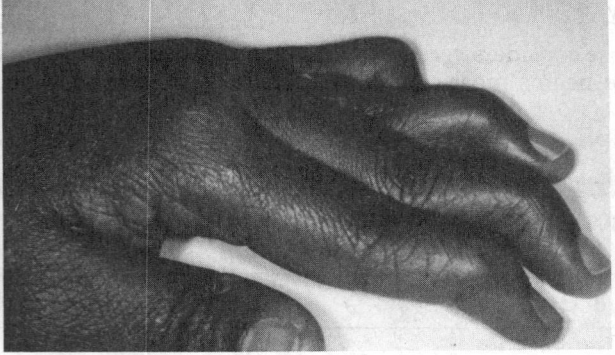

B

C

Figure 28–15

Common joint deformities seen in RA. *A,* Boutonniere, or buttonhole; *B,* swan neck; *C,* ulnar deviation (on left). (From the Arthritis Teaching Slide Collection, copyright 1980. Used by permission of the Arthritis Foundation.)

Psychosocial Assessment

RA *can* be a crippling disease. After 10 to 15 years of having the disease, less than one-half of clients are ADL independent. As many as 10% of clients are eventually confined to a wheelchair or a bed. These physical limitations result in role changes in the family and society. For example, the person may not be able to cook for the family or be an active sexual partner. Extreme fatigue often results in an early bedtime and a reluctance to socialize. The person with RA may not be able to work and support the family financially.

Changes of the body cause poor self-esteem and body image. Because U.S. society values a physically fit, attractive body, the client with RA is embarrassed to be seen in public places. The client grieves, and depression with suicide attempts is not uncommon. A feeling of helplessness may accompany loss of control over a disease that can "consume" the body. Living with a chronic disease and the pain that results is difficult for the client and family. The nurse assesses the client's emotional and mental status related to the disease and its problems. The client's support system and resources are also assessed. The reader is referred to Chapters 6, 11, and 21 on stress and coping, loss, and disabling and chronic diseases, respectively, for further information on psychosocial assessment for this type of client.

Laboratory Findings

Laboratory tests help to support a diagnosis of RA, but no single test or group of tests can confirm it. Table 28–3 summarizes the common laboratory tests that are used for diagnosis of CTD.

Rheumatoid factor. The test for rheumatoid factor measures the presence of unusual antibodies of the IgM and/or IgG type that develop in several CTDs. Two methods are used most commonly to ascertain the degree to which these antibodies are present in the body: Rose-Waaler and latex agglutination. Both procedures report values as titers. The Rose-Waaler test is more specific for a diagnosis of RA than the latex agglutination but is not sensitive. A client with a positive Rose-Waaler test result probably has RA and is *seropositive*; a client with a negative test result may or may not have the disease and is *seronegative*. About 80% of RA clients are seropositive and have a titer value higher than 1:80 by this test. The latex agglutination test, on the other hand, is sensitive but is not specific for RA. Its normal value is less than 1:120. The higher the titer, the more active the disease process.

Antinuclear antibody. The antinuclear antibody (ANA) test also measures the titer of unusual antibodies that destroy the nuclei of cells and cause tissue death. When the fluorescent method is used, the test is sometimes referred to as FANA. If this test result is positive (a value higher than 1:8), various subtypes of this antibody are identified and measured. As with the rheumatoid factor, the higher the titer, the more active the disease

process. The significance of these subtype values is described in Table 28–3.

Erythrocyte sedimentation rate. The "sed rate," as the ESR is sometimes called, is used to confirm inflammation or infection anywhere in the body. It is particularly useful in CTD because the value directly correlates with the degree of inflammation and later, with the severity of disease. Because several laboratory procedures are used to measure the ESR, normal values vary; women have higher normal values than men. As a general rule, a value of 20 to 40 mm/hour indicates mild inflammation; 40 to 70 mm/hour indicates moderate inflammation; and 70 to 150 mm/hour represents severe inflammation. This test is also used to monitor a client's response to anti-inflammatory drug therapy: the ESR should decrease if the drug dosage is effective.

Serum complement. In an attempt to destroy the immune complexes, complement (C') attaches to the complex. If a large amount of complement is used in the lytic process, the concentration of free-floating complement in the blood diminishes. Normal values vary considerably depending on the laboratory technique used. An abnormal finding is a decrease in serum complement and is seen primarily in clients with vasculitis.

Serum protein electrophoresis. The protein fractions of the plasma are measured by using electrical current to separate them. In acute inflammation, the level of alpha globulin is raised, but in chronic inflammatory conditions such as RA, the level of gamma globulin is increased because of the increase in immunoglobulins.

Immunoglobulins. The immunoglobulins can be separated into subtypes by using any one of various techniques. In chronic inflammation, IgG is needed to combine with the rheumatoid factor. Thus, in RA the IgG value is typically elevated.

Radiographic Findings

The standard x-ray film is used to visualize the joint changes and deformities that were described earlier. The computed tomography scan may help to determine the degree of cervical spine involvement.

Other Diagnostic Tests

Arthrocentesis is a common diagnostic procedure performed on clients with RA. It may be done at the bedside or in a physician's office. After use of local anesthesia, a large-gauge needle is inserted into a joint, usually the knee, to aspirate a sample of synovial fluid, which also relieves pressure. The fluid is analyzed by use of tests described in Table 28–3.

A bone or joint scan is frequently done to assess the extent of articular manifestations (this test is described under Other Diagnostic Tests in Chap. 29). Thermography detects the degree of inflammation by measuring the heat radiating from the skin's surface. It is not done as often as are other diagnostic procedures.

TABLE 28–3 Normal Values and Significance of Abnormal Findings in Common Laboratory Tests Used for Connective Tissue Disease*

Test	Normal Values	Significance of Abnormal Findings
Rheumatoid factor Rose-Waaler	< 1:80	*Elevations* of either titer (increase in number at right of colon) indicative of possible CTD *Increased* Rose's titer indicative of RA (seropositive); not a sensitive test
Latex agglutination	< 1:120	Latex titer not as specific to one disease, but quite sensitive test
ANA (total)	< 1:8 (if positive, types of ANA identified, e.g., anti-DNA, anti-DNP, anti-RNA, to indicate what part of cells involved)	*Elevations* common in SLE, PSS, RA, and other inflammatory CDTs (5% of healthy adults have positive ANA results)
Serum complement (C′ or CH$_{50}$)	Varies greatly among laboratories	*Decreased* value indicative of active autoimmune disease such as SLE
LE preparation	< 1:8	A type of ANA (anti-DNP); not reliable because negative result does *not* rule out SLE; can be used as screening test
SPEP		*Increased* levels of gamma globulins indicative of CTD (inflammatory type)
Albumin	52–68†	
Globulin	32–48	
Alpha$_1$ globulin	2.4–5.3	
Alpha$_2$ globulin	6.6–13.5	*Increased* level of alpha globulins possible in RA
Beta globulin	8.5–14.5	
Gamma globulin	10.7–21.0	
HLA testing (HLA-B27)	None	*Presence* of HLA-B27 indicative of Reiter's syndrome or ankylosing spondylitis
ESR	Described in Table 29-3 in Chapter 29	

* ANA, antinuclear antibody; DNP, dinitrophenol; SLE, systemic lupus erythematosus; PSS, progressive systemic sclerosis; LE, lupus erythematosus; SPEP, serum electrophoresis; ESR, erythrocyte sedimentation rate.
† SPEP values given as a percentage of total protein.

RA can affect multiple body systems, and therefore tests to diagnose specific systemic manifestations are performed as necessary. For example, electromyography helps to confirm peripheral neuropathy. Pulmonary function tests determine the presence of lung involvement.

 Analysis: Nursing Diagnosis

Several nursing diagnoses for the client with RA are the same as those for DJD. Joint pain and immobility are primary concerns in both diseases, although clients with RA have additional systemic manifestations.

Common Diagnoses

The client with RA typically presents with the following nursing diagnoses:

1. Chronic pain related to joint destruction and deformity

2. Impaired physical mobility related to pain, stiffness, and deformity

3. Total self-care deficit related to joint deformity, pain, and fatigue
4. Fatigue and activity intolerance related to chronic, systemic disease and probable decreased hemoglobin concentration and hematocrit
5. Body image disturbance, altered role performance, and self-esteem disturbance related to joint deformity, pain, and fatigue

Additional Diagnoses

In addition to the commonly seen nursing diagnoses, the client may present with any of the following diagnoses:

1. Ineffective individual coping related to chronic disease
2. Social isolation related to poor self-concept
3. Impaired gas exchange related to restrictive lung involvement
4. Impaired home maintenance management related to multiple physical and psychosocial problems associated with chronic illness
5. Altered oral mucous membrane related to dry mouth secondary to Sjögren's syndrome
6. Sexual dysfunction related to joint deformity, pain, and fatigue
7. Potential for infection related to Felty's syndrome
8. Sleep pattern disturbance related to pain
9. Altered nutrition: less than body requirements related to anorexia, fatigue, and anemia
10. Knowledge deficit related to drug regimen, joint protection, energy conservation, or exercise program

 Planning and Implementation

Chronic Pain

Planning: client goals. The primary goal is that the client will experience a reduction of joint pain. Total alleviation of pain is not realistic in this chronic disease.

Interventions. As in other types of arthritis, pain is managed by a combination of drug and nondrug measures. When these modalities are no longer effective, surgery is indicated.

Nonsurgical management. Although numerous pain relief modalities are available, the client with RA usually needs a variety of medications to relieve pain and/or slow the progression of the disease.

Drug therapy. Medications that are used for clients with RA have analgesic, antipyretic, and anti-inflammatory actions. The first drug type of choice is salicylates. As seen in Table 28–1, any one of several agents may be used. Aspirin is most commonly given unless gastrointestinal distress (nausea, vomiting, or ulcers)

occurs; buffered or enteric-coated forms are administered as alternatives. The initial dosage is 12 to 18 tablets each day in divided doses (usually four times a day) until a therapeutic serum salicylate level of 20 to 25 mg/100 mL is achieved, usually in 3 to 6 weeks. The dosage is regulated so that side effects are minimized and the serum level is less than 30 mg/100 mL. A level higher than this often results in signs of toxicity such as tinnitus. The nurse asks the client if he or she has experienced this symptom. If so, the daily dosage is reduced. Once the client's pain and other clinical manifestations are alleviated, the dosage can be adjusted to a maintenance level, which falls between 15 and 20 mg/100 mL.

If pain and inflammation are not decreased within 6 to 12 weeks, an NSAID is given in combination with aspirin. The choice of which drug to administer depends on the client's needs and the physician's preference. If after 6 weeks there is no clinical change, the NSAID is discontinued and another is tried instead. This process repeats until the appropriate drug is found for the individual client. Side effects and toxic effects of NSAIDs are the same as those of aspirin. In addition, many of these agents cause retention of sodium and fluids, which poses a risk when the drugs are given to clients, especially elderly clients, with hypertension or congestive heart failure.

When pain and inflammation are not reduced by aspirin and NSAIDs, gold therapy is usually added to the aspirin plus NSAID combination. Unlike the former drugs, gold can induce disease remission as well as reduce pain and inflammation. The most common parenteral preparation is gold sodium thiomalate (Myochrysine). After a small test dose of 10 mg intramuscularly to detect an allergy to the drug, weekly gold injections are given. The dosage increases from 25 to 50 mg/week until improvement is evident or until a cumulative total of 1000 mg is administered. If the client responds to the drug without showing toxic effects such as rash, blood dyscrasias, or renal involvement, the injections are slowly tapered to every 2 weeks, then to every 3 weeks, and then to once a month. Before each administration, the client's urine is tested for protein level, and a complete blood count is taken. If remission does not occur after a total of 1000 mg has been given, the drug is discontinued.

Because of painful administration of intramuscular gold preparations, auranofin (Ridaura), an oral gold product, may be used. This drug must be taken daily to achieve a therapeutic serum level. Its major side effect is gastrointestinal symptoms, especially diarrhea, nausea, and vomiting, which occur in 50% of clients who take the medication (Brassell, 1988).

Other remittive agents that can be used are hydroxychloroquine (Plaquenil) and penicillamine (Cuprimine, Depen). These drugs are not used as often as gold in RA because they have numerous common side and toxic effects and are often not as effective. Clients receiving hydroxychloroquine are monitored carefully for changes in vision because retinal toxicity is not uncommon. The side effects of penicillamine are similar to those of gold.

For clients who do not experience pain relief from the commonly administered medications, steroids, usually prednisone (Deltasone), are given for their anti-inflammatory and immunosuppressive ability. Unfortunately, chronic steroid therapy can result in devastating complications such as diabetes mellitus, infection, hypertension, osteoporosis, and glaucoma. As shown in Table 28–1, some drug effects are dose related, whereas others are not. Intra-articular steroid injections may be used for temporary relief in a single joint, but the number of injections is limited to three or four per year. The nurse observes the client for side effects of these medications and reports them to the physician.

Clients with life-threatening rheumatoid arteritis are given additional immunosuppressive drugs that are used for clients with cancer. The side effects and toxic effects of these agents range from alopecia to nausea and vomiting to blood dyscrasias. Chapter 25 describes these drugs in detail. Cyclophosphamide (Cytoxan), azathioprine (Imuran), and methotrexate are most commonly used. These medications may be given as a routine oral regimen or as *pulse* therapy, in which one or more doses are given intravenously in high concentrations. After remission of the condition is achieved, pulse therapy is discontinued until the next exacerbation, when the process is repeated.

Other analgesic drugs may be prescribed to supplement the anti-inflammatory medications that are specific for the disease, such as acetaminophen (Tylenol, Datril), propoxyphene (Darvon), and propoxyphene with acetaminophen (Darvocet-N 100). Although these agents are not narcotic, their use is monitored for side effects and possible overuse. The effects of NSAIDs and other drugs can be masked by administering such analgesics on a routine basis.

All of the drugs that are used for clients with RA are potent and can cause serious complications. The nurse teaches clients to look for potential side effects and toxic effects and to report them immediately to the health care provider. Nursing interventions for clients who are taking each drug type were summarized in Table 28–1.

Rest, positioning, and heat. Adequate rest, proper positioning, and heat application are important features of pain management and were discussed for DJD under the heading Chronic Pain. If there is acute inflammation, the nurse and client may decide that cold applications are better for pain relief until the acute inflammation improves. Ice packs are commonly used. Care is taken to prevent the packs from being too heavy and thus increasing discomfort. To relieve morning stiffness, a hot shower is usually better than a sponge bath or a tub bath. In addition, it is often difficult for the client with RA to get into and out of the bathtub.

Other pain relief measures. As in any client with arthritis, various other pain relief modalities are available. For example, some clients may achieve relief with TENS, hypnosis, acupuncture, imagery, or music therapy. Stress management is becoming more popular as a pain relief intervention. Chapters 6 and 7 describe these interventions in detail.

Surgical management. When nonsurgical pain management techniques are not effective in reducing pain, surgery is performed. In early disease, a synovectomy may be performed to remove excess synovial tissue, thus decreasing pressure on nerve endings in and around joints. In advanced disease, other surgical procedures (osteotomy and TJR) are used (see under the heading Surgical Management in the discussion of chronic pain in DJD for a description of these surgeries and their associated nursing care). Because of the common joint deformity and joint destruction that are caused by RA, clients having a joint replacement may not achieve increased mobility, but pain relief is usually gained.

Impaired Physical Mobility

The goals and interventions that apply to the client with RA who has impaired physical mobility are the same as those for the client with DJD who has this nursing diagnosis. Clients with RA are more likely to become restricted to a wheelchair or to bed than clients with DJD, but an aggressive mobilization program may prevent total dependence. Of special importance is the need for higher-level toilet seats, chairs, and wheelchairs to facilitate transfers.

Total Self-Care Deficit

Planning: client goals. The primary goal is that the client will independently perform ADL. The nurse collaborates with physical and occupational therapists to accomplish this goal.

Interventions: nonsurgical management. Although the physical appearance of a client with severe RA may lead the nurse to think that ADL independence is not possible, there are a number of alternative methods for performing these activities. It is not beneficial for the nurse to perform activities for the client; clients with RA do not want to be dependent. For example, hand deformities frequently prevent a client from opening packages of food such as crackers. The client may prefer to use his or her teeth to open the crackers rather than depend on someone else. In the hospital, a client may not eat because of the barriers of heavy plate covers, milk in cartons, small packages of condiments, and heavy cups. The client may be too embarrassed to ask the nurse to set up the tray. As an alternative, the nurse should discuss optional tray arrangements with the dietitian that would allow the client access to food and total eating independence.

When fine motor activities such as squeezing a tube of toothpaste become impossible, larger joints or body surfaces can substitute for smaller ones. In this case, the palm of the hand can press the paste onto the brush. Adaptive devices such as long-handled brushes can allow the client to brush his or her hair; dressing sticks can facilitate putting on pants. These examples illustrate the need for the nurse to assess the problem area, suggest alternative methods, and refer the client to an occupational therapist for special assistive and adaptive devices if necessary. Chapter 22 describes additional interventions for clients with self-care deficits.

Fatigue; Activity Intolerance

Planning: client goals.   Activity intolerance as a result of chronic fatigue is common in clients with RA. The client states that he or she is tired or exhausted and displays irritability and less capacity for work and other activities. The goals are that the client will experience (1) a decrease in fatigue and (2) an increased tolerance when performing daily activities.

Interventions: nonsurgical management.   Nursing interventions depend in part on determining contributing factors to fatigue. Anemia is a common cause of fatigue and is treated with iron (if an iron deficiency anemia is present), folic acid, and/or vitamin supplements. Chronic normochromic or chronic hypochromic anemia is frequently found in systemic disease. The nurse assesses for drug-related blood loss, such as that caused by salicylate therapy, by testing the stool for occult blood.

When fatigue results from muscle atrophy, an aggressive physical therapy program is instituted to strengthen muscles. When pain prevents adequate rest and sleep, fatigue is increased. Measures to facilitate sleep include promoting a quiet environment, giving warm beverages, and using hypnotics or relaxants if necessary; pain relief interventions have been discussed.

In addition to identifying and managing specific reasons for fatigue, the nurse assesses the client's daily activities and teaches principles of energy conservation. These principles include pacing activities, allowing rest periods, setting priorities, and obtaining assistance when possible. The accompanying Client/Family Education feature lists specific suggestions for conserving the client's energy and thus increasing activity tolerance.

Body Image Disturbance; Altered Role Performance; Self-Esteem Disturbance

Planning: client goals.   The specific goals for the client with a poor self-concept depend on the area affected, i.e., body image, self-esteem, or role performance. These areas are interrelated, however, such that an overall goal is that the client will verbalize an improvement in self-concept. An improvement in one area is usually followed by an improvement in another. For example, a better perception of one's body image usually increases self-esteem.

Interventions: nonsurgical management.   Not only may body image be affected by the disease process, it may be affected by drug therapy as well. Steroids, for instance, cause a moon-faced appearance, acne, striae, buffalo humps, and weight gain. The nurse determines the client's perception of these changes and the impact of family reactions to them. The most important intervention for the nurse is communicating acceptance of the client. When a trusting relationship is established, the nurse encourages the client to express his or her feelings.

Use of a hospital gown reinforces the sick role. The client is encouraged to wear his or her own nightclothes, brush his or her hair, and use make-up if desired. The nurse assists in making the client as presentable as possible. The use of colored bows for hair, nail polish, and perfume can improve the client's self-concept. Chapter 9 identifies additional strategies for care of a client with an altered body image.

The client may display behaviors indicative of loss and may attempt to use coping strategies ranging from denial or fear to anger or depression. In an attempt to regain control over the effects of the disease process, the client often appears to be manipulative and demanding and is sometimes referred to as having an "arthritis personality." This label, which has negative connotations, is a myth. Clients are trying to cope with the effects of their illness and should be treated with patience and understanding. The nurse continually assesses and accepts these behaviors but remains realistic in discussing goals to improve self-concept. The client's strengths are emphasized, and previously successful coping strategies

---

CLIENT/FAMILY EDUCATION ■ Energy Conservation Instructions for the Client with Arthritis

"Balance activity with rest, including one or two naps each day."

"Pace yourself; do not plan too much for one day."

"Set priorities. Determine which activities are most important, and do them first."

"Delegate responsibility and tasks to family members, significant others, and friends."

"Plan ahead to prevent last-minute rushing and stress."

"Learn your own activity tolerance and do not exceed it."

are identified. Further interventions for loss and coping are discussed in Chapters 6 and 11.

■ Discharge Planning

The client is usually managed at home but may be institutionalized in a long-term care setting if he or she becomes restricted to bed or a wheelchair. Some clients may be discharged to a rehabilitation facility for several weeks to aid in developing strategies, techniques, and skills for independent living at home.

Home Care Preparation

The amount of home care preparation depends on the severity of the disease. Structural changes may be necessary if there are deficits in ADL or mobility. Doors must be wide enough to accommodate a wheelchair or a walker if one is used. Ramps are needed to prevent the client from being homebound. If stairs cannot be negotiated, the client must have access to facilities for all ADL on one floor.

To promote continued homemaking functions, structural changes of counter tops and appliances may be needed. Handrails and higher-level chairs and toilet seats also help for transfers. Chapter 22 on rehabilitation discusses environmental adaptations in further detail.

Client/Family Education

Health teaching is the most important nursing intervention to promote the client's compliance with a treatment plan. Precautions regarding myths and quackery are important to protect the client from harm (see the corresponding discussion of quackery). Information about drug therapy, joint protection, energy conservation, rest, and exercise is reviewed with the client and family.

Psychosocial Preparation

The client with RA often complains of being on an "emotional roller coaster" from coping with a chronic illness every day of life. Control over one's life is an important human need. The client with an unpredictable chronic disease may lose this control, which adds to poor self-esteem. Health providers must allow the client to make decisions about care. Families and significant others must also include the client in decision-making. Although the client's behavior may be perceived as demanding or manipulative, the client's self-esteem cannot be improved without this important aspect of interpersonal relationships.

Increased dependency also affects the client's sense of control and self-esteem. Some clients ignore their health needs and portray a tough image for others by insisting that they need no assistance. The nurse emphasizes to the client and family that asking for help

may be the best decision at times to prevent further joint damage and disease progression.

Social and work roles are dramatically affected by this disease. The client may find new friends among others who have the same problem. Becoming active members of and volunteering for The Arthritis Foundation can help the client to meet social and work needs. Loss of income from being unable to be gainfully employed can be a major source of stress. The client may qualify for disability benefits through Social Security. If possible, the client can learn new, less stressful skills for a different career.

In addition to other interventions that were just described in the section on body image disturbance, altered role performance, and self-esteem disturbance, the nurse may need to refer the client to a counselor or to a religious or spiritual leader for emotional support and guidance during times of crisis. Other support systems within the family and community need to be identified and recommended for use when necessary.

Health Care Resources

The need for health care resources for the client with RA is the same as that for the client with DJD. A home care nurse or aide, physical therapist, and/or occupational therapist may be needed. These resources are identified and made available before the client is discharged from the hospital or other health care facility.

 Evaluation

The nurse, on the basis of the identified nursing diagnoses, evaluates the care provided for the client with RA. The desired outcomes include that the client

1. States that pain and stiffness are reduced
2. Ambulates without personal assistance
3. Is independent in ADL (may use assistive and adaptive devices)
4. States that fatigue is decreased
5. Increases tolerance to daily activities
6. States acceptance of altered body image and/or role performance

LUPUS ERYTHEMATOSUS

OVERVIEW

The name of this disorder comes from the Latin term for "wolf," *lupus*. In the mid-19th century, the facial rash that was seen in clients with the disease was thought to look like bites caused by a wolf. Also, the rash was usually red, and thus the term *erythematosus* was added to describe the disease.

Pathophysiology

There are two main classifications of lupus: *discoid lupus erythematosus* (DLE) and *systemic lupus erythematosus* (SLE). Less than 10% of clients with lupus have the DLE type, which affects only the skin. One in 20 clients with DLE, however, will develop systemic clinical manifestations. A unique feature of lupus is its variability: no two people have the same manifestations, and the disease progresses differently in each person.

The systemic disorder is a chronic, progressive, systemic, inflammatory CTD that can cause major body organs and systems to fail. It is characterized by spontaneous remissions and exacerbations, and it may have an acute or an insidious onset. The condition is potentially fatal, although the survival rate has dramatically improved over the past decade. Today, more than 95% of clients with SLE are alive 5 years after diagnosis is made. Improvements in determining its etiology, diagnosis, and treatment account for the prolonged survival of these clients.

Lupus is thought to be an autoimmune process: abnormal antibodies are produced that react with the client's tissues. These antinuclear antibodies primarily affect the deoxyribonucleic acid (DNA) within the cell nuclei. As a result, immune complexes form in the serum and organ tissues, which causes inflammation and damage. The complexes invade organs directly or cause vasculitis (vessel inflammation), which deprives the organs of arterial blood and oxygen.

Nearly all clients with SLE have some degree of kidney involvement—the leading cause of death. Renal biopsies show progressive changes within the glomeruli. In minimal lupus nephritis, the glomeruli are slightly irregular; immunoglobulins and complement are seen by electron microscopy. Focal, or mild, lupus nephritis is characterized by further glomerular changes, and immune complex deposits are common. In this type of lupus, the client begins to show clinical signs of renal impairment. In diffuse, severe proliferative nephritis, more than 50% of the glomeruli are affected, and the client is in renal failure.

The second major cause of death from SLE is cardiac involvement. Immune complexes lodge in the pericardium, myocardium, or coronary vessels and cause heart failure. Central nervous system involvement (central nervous system lupus) is the third cause of death, usually from a cerebral infarction.

Etiology

The theory of an autoimmune response has been strongly supported, but the origin of lupus antibodies has not yet been determined. The incidence of lupus increases in families with a history of the disease. Ge-

netic markers, such as HLA-DRw2 and HLA-DRw3, are associated with the disease. A bacterial or viral infection may initiate the immune response, but this origin has not been supported.

Certain factors have been identified that trigger the disease process and cause exacerbations. Sunlight and other forms of ultraviolet light, physical and emotional stress, and pregnancy are documented stressors. Drug-induced lupus occurs as an adverse reaction to several drugs, especially procainamide (Pronestyl) and hydralazine (Apresoline). Other medications, such as phenytoin (Dilantin) and phenobarbital, have been suspected of causing a lupus-like syndrome, but this suggestion has not been substantially validated. Discontinuation of the drug in question and short-term steroid therapy usually reverse the lupus or lupus-like syndrome.

Incidence

Lupus affects women between the ages of 15 and 40 years at a rate 8 to 10 times more often than men. The onset of the disease is most often during childbearing years, but it has been reported in children as young as 2 years and in adults as old as 97 years. About 1 in 700 women between the ages of 15 and 64 years have the disease; 1 in 250 Black women of this age group are affected. If one twin has SLE, there is a 60% to 70% chance that the other will develop the disease (Schumacher, 1988).

COLLABORATIVE MANAGEMENT

 Assessment

History

In view of the incidence and etiologic factors that are associated with lupus (SLE is primarily seen in young women), the nurse notes the *sex* and *age* of the client. The nurse asks about a family history of the disease or other related CTD and asks if the client is pregnant. The client's *reaction to ultraviolet light* is also important because many clients report that they burn or develop "splotches" after exposure to bright sunlight. A complete *medication history* is valuable because the client may be taking a drug that could cause drug-induced lupus.

Physical Assessment: Clinical Manifestations

It is impossible to describe a typical client with lupus because of the extreme variability of symptoms among individuals. The major and perhaps only manifestation of DLE is a dry, scaly, raised rash appearing on the face and/or upper body, which is sometimes referred to as *discoid (coin-like) lesions*. The nurse observes all skin changes and monitors changes daily.

Articular involvement is another common clinical manifestation occurring in 95% of clients with SLE. The initial joint changes are similar to those seen in RA, but deformities are not common. *Avascular necrosis* is seen in clients with SLE who have been treated for at least 5 years, usually with steroids. The hip is most commonly affected, and pain and decreased mobility result. *Muscle atrophy* can result from disuse or from skeletal muscle invasion by the immune complexes. *Myalgia*, or muscle pain, occurs in approximately 25% of SLE clients.

Because SLE is an inflammatory condition, *fever* is a common finding. The presence of fever is the cardinal sign of a flare, or exacerbation. Various degrees of generalized weakness, fatigue, anorexia, and weight loss occur, and these signs may be the only ones of impending disease, which makes diagnosis difficult.

Because lupus *nephritis* is the leading cause of death, the nurse carefully assesses the parameters indicative of renal involvement, e.g., changes in urinary output, proteinuria, hematuria, and fluid retention. About one-half of clients with SLE have some type of nephritis.

Pleural effusions are found in 40% of clients, but this complication is usually not life-threatening. Pulmonary restrictive or obstructive changes may not result in overt clinical signs, but progressive involvement can lead to dyspnea and arterial blood gas abnormalities, for which the nurse assesses. Acute lupus pneumonitis occurs in less than 5% of cases and is characterized by fever, nonproductive cough, and rales.

Pericarditis is the most common cardiovascular manifestation and causes tachycardia, chest pain, and myocardial ischemia. *Raynaud's phenomenon* is seen in 15% of clients with lupus: on exposure to cold, the client complains of the characteristic red, white, and blue color changes and pain in digits caused by arteriolar vasospasm.

Neurologic manifestations are varied. Central nervous system effects include psychoses, paresis, seizures, migraine headaches, and cranial nerve palsies. Peripheral neuropathies are also common. Assessment of the nervous system is detailed in Chapter 32.

Recurrent *abdominal pain* occurs frequently, but its cause may not be identified. Mesenteric arteritis, pancreatitis from arteritis of the pancreatic artery, and colonic ulcers can cause abdominal pain in the client with lupus. The nurse may note *liver enlargement* on assessment of the abdomen, but jaundice is rare. More than one-half of clients have *lymph enlargement*, and 10% have *splenomegaly*. A few clients have Sjögren's syndrome, as is seen in clients with RA.

Psychosocial Assessment

The psychosocial ramifications of lupus can be devastating. In either discoid or systemic disease, the rash can be disfiguring and embarrassing to the client. Adolescent girls who never had a blemish are confronted with a rash that cannot be completely covered with make-up. If steroid therapy is used, side effects such as acne, striae, fat pads, and weight gain intensify the problem of the already altered body image.

Chronic fatigue and generalized weakness prevent the client from being as active as in the past. The client may avoid social gatherings and withdraw from family activities. The unpredictability and chronicity of SLE can cause fear and anxiety. Fear may heighten if the client knows other individuals with the disease, particularly if the other person has more advanced, severe disease. The myth that lupus is a fatal condition remains prevalent.

The nurse assesses the client's feelings about the illness to identify areas that require intervention. Assessing an individual's usual coping mechanisms and support systems is vital before developing a plan of care. Additional information about psychosocial assessment of clients with chronic illness is found under the corresponding heading in Chapter 21 and in the section on RA in this chapter.

Laboratory Findings

DLE is not a systemic condition, and thus the only test that is significant is a skin biopsy. The examiner gently scrapes skin cells from the rash for microscopic evaluation. The characteristic lupus cell and a number of inflammatory cells confirm the diagnosis.

The immunologic-based laboratory tests that are used to diagnose SLE are the same as those performed for RA: rheumatoid factor, antinuclear antibody, ESR, serum protein electrophoresis, serum complement, and immunoglobulins. The lupus cell preparation may also be performed, but this assay is a poor indicator of disease; rather, the test is best used for screening. These tests are discussed under the corresponding heading for RA and are summarized in Table 28–3.

In addition to immunologic testing, a battery of tests is performed to evaluate possible involvement of major organs and body systems. A complete blood count commonly shows pancytopenia, or a decrease of all cell types, probably caused by direct attack of the blood cells by immune complexes. Serum electrolyte levels, renal function, cardiac and liver enzymes, and clotting factors are also routinely assessed.

Radiographic Findings

No x-ray studies are done specifically for lupus. If certain organs are suspected of being affected by the disease, the appropriate radiographic study is performed. For example, renal function can be determined by intravenous pyelography. A barium enema can determine the presence of colonic ulcerations. A computed tomography scan is commonly used when central nervous system lupus is suspected.

Other Diagnostic Tests

No other diagnostic study is specific for SLE, but ultrasonography, radioisotope scans, and magnetic resonance imaging may be ordered to confirm organ involvement.

Analysis: Nursing Diagnosis

Because it is difficult to typify a client with SLE, the nursing diagnoses vary greatly depending on the biologic and psychosocial problems of the client. The most common diagnoses are included here.

Common Diagnoses

The most likely diagnoses for a client with discoid and/or systemic lupus are

1. Impaired skin integrity related to rash, vasculitic lesions, and/or cushingoid effects of steroids (DLE and SLE)
2. Body image disturbance and self-esteem disturbance (DLE and SLE) related to altered role performance (SLE)
3. Chronic pain related to joint inflammation and/or avascular necrosis (SLE)
4. Fatigue and activity intolerance secondary to chronic disease, pain, weakness, and anemia (SLE)

Additional Diagnoses

There are numerous other nursing diagnoses depending on the individual client and the severity of the disease process. Unless otherwise specified, these diagnoses refer to the client with SLE and include

1. Impaired physical mobility related to joint pain or avascular necrosis
2. Self-care deficit related to fatigue, disease exacerbation, or joint deformity
3. Ineffective individual coping related to chronic, unpredictable, and potentially life-threatening disease
4. Ineffective family coping related to chronic, unpredictable, and potentially life-threatening disease
5. Impaired gas exchange related to pleural effusion or chronic lung disease
6. Decreased cardiac output related to pericarditis
7. Altered thought processes related to central nervous system involvement
8. Altered patterns of urinary elimination related to renal damage
9. Potential for injury (hemorrhage) related to thrombocytopenia
10. Altered nutrition: less than body requirements related to anorexia, weight loss, or anemia
11. Potential for infection related to leukopenia or chronic steroid therapy
12. Altered oral mucous membrane related to ulceration or Sjögren's syndrome
13. Altered tissue perfusion related to vasculitis
14. Sexual dysfunction related to chronic fatigue and pain
15. Fear related to uncertainty about disease process (DLE and SLE)
16. Knowledge deficit related to treatment regimen and resources

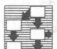 **Planning and Implementation**

Impaired Skin Integrity

Planning: client goals. The goal for this problem is that the client will have improved or healed skin lesions that are seen in both DLE and SLE. Many of the lesions do not disappear, but they fade when the disease is in remission.

Interventions: nonsurgical management. Potent drugs are used topically and systemically. In addition, precautions are taken to prevent further skin impairment.

Drug therapy. In DLE, the client's major concern is the rash or discoid lesions. Topical cortisone preparations help to reduce the inflammation and promote fading of the skin lesions. In addition, some clients are given hydroxychloroquine (Plaquenil) to decrease the inflammatory response, but other systemic medications are usually not used.

Skin protection. The client with lupus should avoid prolonged exposure to sunlight and other forms of ultraviolet lighting, including certain types of fluorescent light. The nurse instructs the client that long sleeves and hats with a large brim may need to be worn outdoors. The newer sun-blocking agents with an SPF (sun protection factor) of 25 or higher should be used on exposed skin surfaces.

In addition, the client cleans the skin with mild soap (such as Ivory) and avoids harsh, perfumed substances. The skin is rinsed and dried well, and lotion is applied. Excess powder and other drying substances are also avoided. Cosmetics are carefully selected and should include moisturizers and sun protectors. The nurse may refer the client to a medical cosmetologist who specializes in applying make-up for clients with skin lesions of all types.

The hair should receive special attention because alopecia is common. Mild protein shampoos are used, and harsh treatments such as permanents or frostings are avoided until the hair regrows during remission.

For clients with SLE, the aim of management is to treat the disease aggressively until remission, thereby resolving the common nursing diagnoses listed earlier. In addition to medications for skin lesions, chronic steroid therapy is given to treat the systemic disease process. In cases of renal or central nervous system lupus, the client is also administered immunosuppressive agents, as are sometimes used in RA. Although clinical manifestations improve during remission, maintenance doses of these drugs are continued to prevent further exacerbations of disease.

When drugs are not effective in improving the disease, newer, experimental techniques may be tried. Pulse therapy, in which high doses of steroids and/or immunosuppressives are administered intravenously, may be given with or without plasmapheresis. In the latter technique, the offending immune complexes are removed from the client's blood in an attempt to slow the progression of the disease.

Self-Esteem Disturbance; Chronic Pain; Activity Intolerance

The client goals and interventions for a client with lupus who has these problems are similar to those for clients with RA (see pages 697 to 699 for a discussion of these diagnoses).

■ Discharge Planning

Discharge planning for the client with lupus is not unlike that for clients with RA. The client is generally managed at home but has repeated hospitalizations during exacerbations of disease. Rehabilitation and long-term care facilities are usually not needed.

Many clients become frustrated that the disease is not well understood by their family or significant others or by the lay public. When lupus is in complete remission, the client appears to be healthy. However, an exacerbation can result in rapid admission to a critical care unit. This unpredictability disrupts the client's life.

Two major differences exist between SLE and RA in terms of education of the client and family. First, the client with SLE is taught how to protect the skin. The important points for teaching are summarized under the heading Impaired Skin Integrity. Second, body temperature is monitored carefully in SLE. Fever is the cardinal sign of an exacerbation during which the client can become seriously ill. Any other unusual or newly developed clinical manifestation is reported to the physician immediately.

Although The Arthritis Foundation is a general resource for all clients with CTD, the Lupus Foundation is a national organization, with chapters in every state, that provides information and assistance for clients with lupus. Support groups and services are offered without charge to the client.

 Evaluation

The nurse evaluates care for the client with lupus on the basis of goals for the common nursing diagnoses. The expected outcomes include that the client

1. Demonstrates an improvement in skin lesions as evidenced by a decreased number of lesions or less erythema
2. States that joint pain is reduced
3. States that fatigue has decreased
4. Increases tolerance of activities

5. States acceptance of disease and body changes, with an improving self-concept

The overall goal of medical management is a long-lasting remission of the disease, with no major body organ involvement.

PROGRESSIVE SYSTEMIC SCLEROSIS

OVERVIEW

Progressive systemic sclerosis (PSS) is one of a family of diseases and is often referred to as systemic scleroderma. *Scleroderma* means hardening of the skin, which is only one clinical manifestation of PSS. As the name implies, PSS is a systemic disease that is less common than lupus but has a greater associated mortality.

PSS is a chronic CTD that is characterized by inflammation, fibrosis, and sclerosis of the skin and vital organs. The inflammatory process of this disease is so similar to that of lupus that clients are often diagnosed as having SLE until the disease progresses. The inflamed tissue undergoes fibrotic and then sclerotic changes. The most obvious tissue affected is the skin, but renal involvement is the leading cause of death. Unfortunately, the disease does not respond well to steroids and immunosuppressants that are used for lupus, and the mortality rate is therefore higher.

The prognosis seems to be worst when the client presents with a group of manifestations that occur concurrently; the CREST syndrome: calcinosis (calcium deposits), Raynaud's phenomenon, esophageal dysmotility, sclerodactyly (scleroderma of the digits), and telangiectasia (spider-like hemangiomas). The disease tends to progress rapidly, but spontaneous remissions and exacerbations can occur.

Little is known about the cause of this disease, but autoimmunity is suspected. The occurrence of more than one case per family is extremely uncommon, although other CTDs may be noted in the family history.

PSS has been described in persons of all races and in all geographic areas. Women are affected three to four times more often than men. The onset of the disease is usually between the ages of 30 and 50 years; children rarely have PSS. Coal miners have a higher incidence of the disorder, which suggests that silicosis may be a predisposing or contributing factor.

COLLABORATIVE MANAGEMENT

Arthralgia (joint pain) and stiffness are common manifestations, which can be elicited by the nurse during the musculoskeletal examination. The acute inflammation that is seen in RA is not common, and deformities are rare.

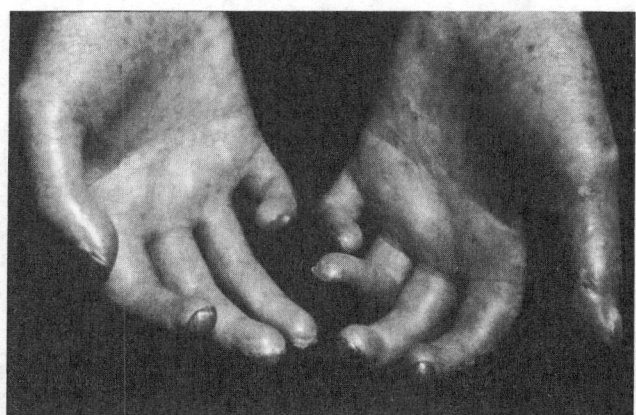

Figure 28–16

Skin changes seen in clients with PSS. (From the Arthritis Teaching Slide Collection, copyright 1980. Used by permission of the Arthritis Foundation.)

Findings on inspection of the skin depend on the stage of the scleroderma (Fig. 28–16). Typically, there is a painless, symmetric, pitting edema of the hands and fingers, which may progress to include the entire upper and/or lower extremities and face. In this *edematous* phase, the fingers are described as sausage-like. The skin is taut, shiny, and free from wrinkles. If diffuse scleroderma occurs, swelling is replaced by tightening, hardening, and thickening of skin tissue; this phase is sometimes called the *indurative* phase. The skin loses its elasticity, and range of motion is markedly decreased; ulcerations may occur. The client may develop joint contractures and may be unable to perform ADL independently. Figure 28–17 shows the facial appearance of a client.

The client with diffuse scleroderma is likely to develop major organ damage. Gastrointestinal tract involvement, particularly of the esophagus, is common. The esophagus loses its motility, and dysphagia and esophageal reflux result. A small, sliding hiatal hernia is often found. Reflux of gastric contents can cause esophagitis and subsequent ulceration, particularly in the lower two-thirds of the esophagus. Intestinal changes are similar to those of the esophagus. Peristalsis is diminished, which causes clinical manifestations similar to a partial bowel obstruction; malabsorption is a frequent complication.

In addition to assessing the digestive tract, the nurse observes for cardiovascular manifestations. Raynaud's phenomenon occurs in various degrees in as many as 98% of clients with PSS. On exposure to cold or emotional stress, the small arterioles in the digits of both hands and feet rapidly constrict, which causes decreased blood flow. In severe cases, the client experiences digit necrosis, excruciating pain, and autoamputation of distal digits (see Chap. 65 for a complete discussion of this disorder). Vasculitic lesions, often around the nail beds, can be found in many clients. Myocardial fibrosis, another common problem, is evidenced by electrocardiographic changes, cardiac arrhythmias, and chest pain.

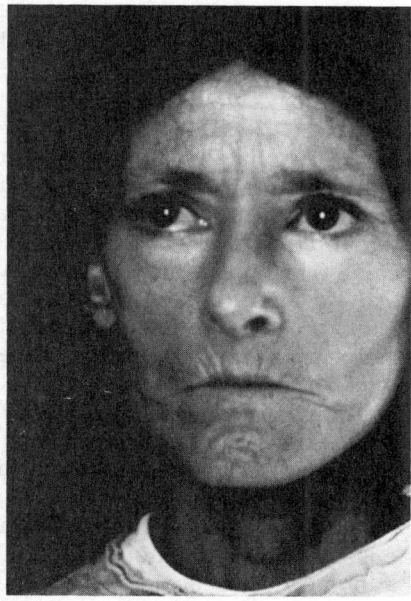

Figure 28–17

Typical "birdface" appearance of client with PSS. (From the Arthritis Teaching Slide Collection, copyright 1980. Used by permission of the Arthritis Foundation.)

Lung involvement may go undetected until autopsy. Fibrosis of the alveoli and interstitial tissues is present in almost all clients with PSS. Renal disease is an important aspect of the overall disease process and frequently causes malignant hypertension and death. The nurse assesses for signs of impending organ failure.

The laboratory findings in a client with PSS are not unlike those seen in a client with SLE. Clinical findings and the client's response to drug therapy help to differentiate the two diseases. Additional tests ordered for the client depend on which organs are suspected of being affected. Upper and lower gastrointestinal series are commonly performed because of the frequency of gastrointestinal clinical manifestations.

The aim of medical management is to force the disease into remission and thus slow disease progression. Drug therapy is used primarily for this purpose, but it is often unsuccessful. Systemic steroids and immunosuppressants are used in large doses and often in combination.

Local skin protective measures can help to maintain skin integrity. The nurse pays special attention to skin care by using mild soap, lotions, and gentle cleaning. The nurse inspects the skin daily for further changes or open lesions. Ulcers are treated according to their type and location (see Chap. 40 for ulcer care).

In addition to drug therapy to control the overall disease process, specific measures can be taken to provide comfort. The client with PSS not only experiences chronic joint pain, but also has severe, acute pain when episodes of Raynaud's phenomenon occur. A bed cradle and footboard keep bedcovers away from the skin in severe cases. The nurse adjusts the room temperature to prevent chilling, which can precipitate digit vasospasm.

If touching the affected areas is tolerated, the client can wear gloves and socks to increase warmth. Smoking and extreme emotional stress can also cause recurrence of symptoms and should be avoided or minimized as much as possible.

The client with esophageal involvement may need small, frequent feedings rather than the traditional three meals daily. The intake of foods and liquids that stimulate gastric secretion is minimized, e.g., spicy foods, caffeine, and alcohol. The nurse instructs the client to keep his or her head elevated for 1 to 2 hours after meals. Some clients may need to be in this position continuously. Histamine antagonists and antacids help to reduce and neutralize gastric acid.

Nursing care for the client with joint pain and decreased mobility is the same as that for the client with RA (see the earlier corresponding section in this chapter).

Discharge planning for the client with PSS is similar to that for the client with SLE or another CTD. The client is managed at home, and frequent hospitalizations are used if major organ involvement occurs during exacerbations.

GOUT

OVERVIEW

Unlike the previously discussed CTD, the cause and treatment of gout have been firmly established. The classic case of well-advanced disease is seldom seen today unless the client does not comply with the therapeutic regimen.

Pathophysiology

Gout, or gouty arthritis, is a systemic disease in which urate crystals deposit in joints and other body tissues. The two major types of gout are primary and secondary. *Primary* gout is the most common and results from one of several inborn errors of purine metabolism. An end product of purine metabolism is *uric acid,* which is usually excreted by the kidneys. In primary gout, uric acid production exceeds the kidneys' excretion capability, and sodium urate deposits in synovium and other tissues, which results in inflammation.

Secondary gout involves hyperuricemia, or excessive uric acid in the blood, that is caused by another disease. Renal insufficiency and diuretic therapy decrease the normal excretion of waste products, including uric acid. Disorders such as multiple myeloma and certain carcinomas increase uric acid production because of greater turnover of nucleic acids. Treatment of secondary gout involves management of the underlying disorder.

There are four phases of the disease process. The *asymptomatic hyperuricemic* phase is usually unknown to the client unless he or she has had a serum uric acid level determination. The client's serum level is elevated, but no overt signs of the disease are present. The first "attack" of gouty arthritis begins the *acute* phase, in which the client experiences excruciating pain and inflammation in one or more small joints, usually the metatarsophalangeal joint of the great toe. Seventy-five per cent of all clients with gout have inflammation of this joint (podagra) as the initial manifestation. Months or perhaps years can pass before additional attacks occur—this is the *intercritical,* or *intercurrent,* phase of the disease. The client is asymptomatic, and no abnormalities are found on examination of the joints. After repeated episodes of acute gout, the client develops deposits of urate crystals under the skin and within major organs, particularly of the renal system. The client is then classified as having *chronic tophaceous gout.* Urate kidney stone formation is more common than renal insufficiency in chronic gout.

Etiology

Primary gout is inherited as an X-linked trait; males are affected through female carriers. About one-fourth of clients have a family history of gout. The causes of secondary gout were just discussed under the heading Pathophysiology.

Incidence

Primary gout affects middle-aged and older men (85% to 90% of clients with gout) and postmenopausal women. The peak time of onset is the fourth and fifth decades of life. Secondary gout affects individuals of all ages. Gout is the leading inflammatory joint disease in men older than 40 years.

COLLABORATIVE MANAGEMENT

 Assessment

History

The historical data that the nurse collects include *age, sex,* and a *family history* of gout. This disorder affects men, particularly those who have relatives with gout. A *complete medical history* is needed to determine if gout could be caused by another problem. In women, especially, there is a tendency to overuse diuretics, which can lead to secondary gout.

Physical Assessment: Clinical Manifestations

Overt manifestations are present in the acute and chronic phases of gout. The nurse encounters a client with acute gout most often because chronic gout is not

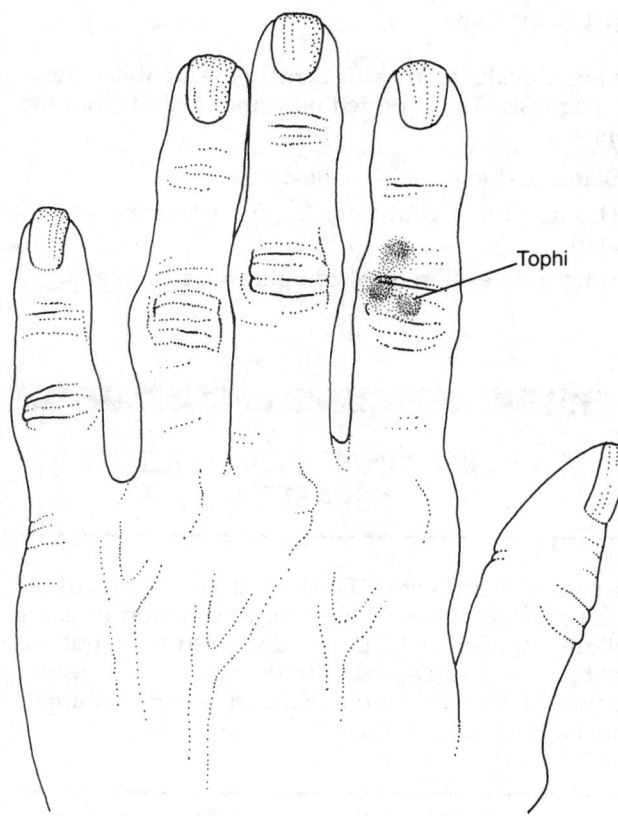

Tophi

Figure 28–18
Tophi on index finger, which are typical of chronic gout.

common today in the United States. *Joint inflammation* is the most frequent finding and is usually so painful that the client comes to the emergency room for treatment. The nurse uses inspection skills only; the inflamed area is too painful to be touched or moved.

In chronic gout, the skin is inspected for *tophi*, deposits of sodium urate crystals (Fig. 28–18). On palpation the tophi are hard, fairly large, and irregular in shape. When the skin is irritated, it may break open and a yellow, gritty substance is discharged. Infection may result.

Other manifestations include signs of *renal stones* or dysfunction. About 20% of clients with gout develop stones. In some cases, urate kidney stones occur before the arthritis. Chapters 57 and 58 describe the assessment and interventions for these complications.

Psychosocial Assessment

Gout is one of the easiest diseases to diagnose and treat in its early phases. If the client complies with drug therapy, the client will have no symptoms and no change in body image or life style. Fear of extremely painful episodes is alleviated by proper preventive actions.

Laboratory Findings

Serum uric acid levels are measured to ascertain hyperuricemia. Because the level can be altered by food intake, serial measurements are taken. A consistent level of more than 8 mg/100 mL is abnormal. Urinary uric acid levels are also determined; an overproduction of uric acid is confirmed by an excretion of more than 600 mg/24 hours after a 5-day restriction of purine intake. Renal function tests, such as blood urea nitrogen and serum creatinine level, are done to monitor possible kidney involvement.

Radiographic and Other Diagnostic Tests

Studies that are done routinely for clients with possible renal disorders are also performed for clients with gout. A definitive diagnostic test for the disease is synovial fluid aspiration (arthrocentesis) to detect the needle-like crystals that are characteristic of the disorder (refer to Other Diagnostic Tests in the section on RA).

 Analysis: Nursing Diagnosis

The client with gout presents with no nursing diagnoses in the asymptomatic and intercritical phases of the disease.

Common Diagnoses

These common diagnoses are for clients with acute gout because untreated chronic gout is rare:

1. Pain related to joint inflammation
2. Potential for altered patterns of urinary elimination related to renal stones or insufficiency

Additional Diagnoses

These diagnoses can apply to a client with chronic gout:

1. Impaired skin integrity related to tophi
2. Altered patterns of urinary elimination related to renal stones or insufficiency
3. Pain related to renal stones

 Planning and Implementation

Pain

Planning: client goals.   The primary goal is that the client will experience a reduction of both the pain and the inflammation causing the pain.

Interventions: nonsurgical management.   Drug therapy is the primary component of management. The inflammation subsides spontaneously within 3 to 5 days, but most clients cannot tolerate the pain for that long.

Drug therapy. The drugs used in acute gout are different from those used in chronic gout. A combination of colchicine and an NSAID is used in acute gout. These medications are given until the inflammation subsides, usually for 4 to 7 days, or until severe diarrhea occurs (a side effect of colchicine).

In chronic gout, drugs to promote uric acid excretion or to reduce its production are given on a continuous, maintenance basis. Allopurinol (Zyloprim) is the drug of choice. As a xanthine oxidase inhibitor, it prevents the conversion of xanthine to uric acid. Probenecid (Benemid) has also proved to be an effective uricosuric drug in gout (promotes excretion of excess uric acid). The nurse monitors serum uric acid levels to determine the effectiveness of these medications.

Diet therapy. Special dietary restrictions for a client with gout are controversial. Some clinicians advocate a strict low-purine diet, with avoidance of such foods as organ meats, shellfish, and oily fish with bones, such as sardines. Many physicians believe that limiting protein foods, especially red and organ meats, is sufficient. Still others do not believe that diet restrictions affect the treatment of the disease. It is well known, however, that excessive alcohol intake and fad "starvation" diets can cause a gouty attack. The nurse instructs the client to determine which foods precipitate an attack for him or her.

Avoidance of stressors. In addition to food and beverage restrictions, aspirin in any form and diuretics should be avoided because they can precipitate an attack. Likewise, excessive physical or emotional stress can exacerbate the disease. The nurse may need to teach stress management techniques, as described in Chapter 6.

Potential for Altered Patterns of Urinary Elimination

Planning: client goals. The goal is that the client will not develop uric acid renal stones.

Interventions: nonsurgical management. Forcing fluids is one of the best measures to prevent stone formation. Because uric acid is more soluble in urine that has a high pH, the urinary pH can be increased by intake of alkaline ash foods, such as citrus fruits and juices, and milk and certain dairy products. The value of adhering to a strict diet that is rich in these foods is questionable.

■ Discharge Planning

The client with a diagnosis of gout is seldom hospitalized unless renal complications develop. If the client follows the interventions described, he or she should not develop chronic tophaceous gout.

 Evaluation

The nurse evaluates nursing care for the identified nursing diagnosis. The expected outcomes include that the client

1. States that joint pain is alleviated
2. Has no further gouty attacks after treatment is initiated
3. Does not develop renal complications from gout

OTHER CONNECTIVE TISSUE DISEASES

The care of clients with CTDs is often similar regardless of the specific disease. Other fairly common diseases that are classified as CTDs are described here, but the nursing care is not specifically delineated. The reader should refer back to sections of the chapter for the applicable nursing interventions.

POLYMYOSITIS/DERMATOMYOSITIS

Polymyositis is a diffuse, inflammatory disease of striated muscle that causes symmetric weakness and atrophy. When a rash accompanies polymyositis, the disease is called *dermatomyositis.* Both diseases vary in their mode of onset and progression and are characterized by spontaneous remissions and exacerbations. Women are affected twice as often as men, and 30- to 60-year-old individuals are most prone to either disease.

In addition to proximal muscle and possible skin involvement, the client typically has polyarthritis, polyarthralgia, and Raynaud's phenomenon. Clients with dermatomyositis have the characteristic heliotrope (lilac) rash and periorbital edema. Malignant neoplasms occur more frequently in these clients than in the rest of the population, with as many as 30% of clients older than age 55 years having internal malignancies. Many clients have difficulty in swallowing and/or talking because of severe muscle weakness. Management includes the use of high-dose steroids, immunosuppressive agents, and supportive care, particularly attention to nutrition.

SYSTEMIC NECROTIZING VASCULITIS

Necrotizing vasculitis is a term that is used for a group of diseases whose primary manifestation is arteritis, or inflammation of arterial walls that causes ischemia in tissues that are usually supplied by the involved vessels.

Polyarteritis nodosa affects middle-aged men and involves every body system. Management is similar to that for SLE, but the prognosis is not as promising. Renal disorders and cardiac involvement are the most frequent causes of death.

Hypersensitivity vasculitis is the most common form of vasculitis and primarily causes skin lesions as an allergic response to drugs, infections, or tumors. *Takayasu's arteritis,* or the aortic arch syndrome, is commonly called the pulseless disease. Women in their 20s, particularly those of Japanese descent, are affected most often. Cerebral ischemia is manifested by visual changes, syncope, and vertigo. The drug of choice for most types of vasculitis is a steroid.

POLYMYALGIA RHEUMATICA

Polymyalgia rheumatica is a common clinical syndrome that is characterized by stiffness, weakness, and aching of the proximal musculature, i.e., the shoulder and pelvic girdles. Systemic manifestations such as fever, arthralgias, and weight loss occur in the majority of cases. The disease commonly occurs in women older than 50 years of age and typically responds to steroid therapy in 3 to 5 days. *Giant cell arteritis,* or temporal arteritis, is frequently associated with polymyalgia rheumatica. The branches of the aorta are vasculitic, which causes headaches and changes in vision. This disorder is easy to miss because most clients are elderly women who complain of declining vision (also an age-related change). Corticosteroids are highly effective in controlling giant cell arteritis.

ANKYLOSING SPONDYLITIS

Ankylosing spondylitis is also known as Marie-Strümpell disease and, more recently, as *rheumatoid spondylitis.* As shown in Figure 28–19, the disease affects the vertebral column and causes spinal deformities. Although this disorder is present in both sexes at any age in adulthood, young Caucasian males under age 40 years are most commonly affected. Other features include iritis, arthritis or arthralgia, and nonspecific systemic manifestations such as malaise and weight loss. Although the exact cause is unknown, the disease is associated with the HLA-B27 antigen. Compromised respiratory function because of a rigid chest wall is the major threat to health. Most clients function normally but live with chronic discomfort. Anti-inflammatory drugs and physical therapy are key components of management.

REITER'S SYNDROME

Like ankylosing spondylitis, *Reiter's syndrome* is associated with HLA-B27 antigen and most often affects

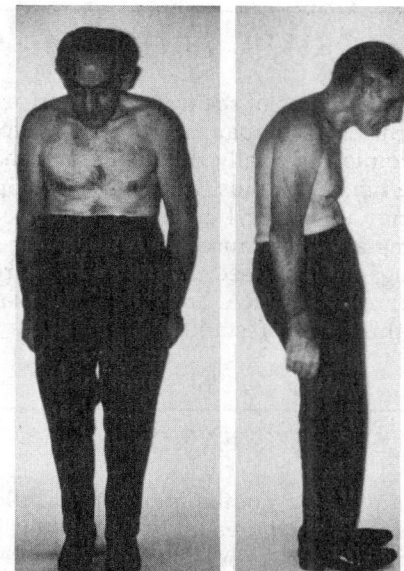

Figure 28–19
Spinal deformity and posture that are often seen in clients with advanced ankylosing spondylitis. (From the Arthritis Teaching Slide Collection, copyright 1980. Used by permission of the Arthritis Foundation.)

young Caucasian males. The complete syndrome is a triad of arthritis, conjunctivitis, and urethritis resulting from exposure to venereal disease or dysentery. Urethritis is therefore often the first clinical manifestation. Although the disease is characterized by this triad of manifestations, others such as circinate balanitis (ring-like inflammation of the glans penis) and skin lesions are equally significant for confirmation of the diagnosis. Management is symptomatic and may be complex if organ involvement occurs. Nonsteroidal anti-inflammatory drugs and physical therapy are generally used.

SJÖGREN'S SYNDROME

Sjögren's syndrome is a condition in which inflammatory cells and immune complexes obstruct secretory ducts and glands. As a result, the client has dry eyes (sicca syndrome), dry mouth (xerostomia), and dry vagina. In severe cases, swelling of the parotid and lacrimal areas and systemic manifestations such as fever and fatigue occur. Fifty per cent of clients with the syndrome have an associated CTD such as RA, as previously discussed. Local management includes meticulous mouth, eye, and perineal care, and use of artificial tears and saliva. Systemic steroids may also be administered. If the condition is not treated, the client can lose vision and develop oral ulcerations, dental caries, and difficulty in swallowing or talking.

PSORIATIC ARTHRITIS

Psoriatic arthritis is one of the most common arthritides in which arthritis accompanies another medical problem. Small joints, especially the distal interphalangeal joints of the hand, are most often affected. Spinal involvement may also occur, but effects in this area are not as devastating as those caused by ankylosing spondylitis. The drugs that are used for this disease are similar to those that are used for RA. Treating the psoriasis often helps the arthritic manifestations.

BEHÇET'S SYNDROME

Behçet's syndrome is a combination of oral ulceration, genital ulceration, and uveitis, which often leads to blindness. In addition, clients frequently develop skin lesions from vasculitis and synovitis. About 20% of clients acquire central nervous system complications, which can be fatal. The mean age of onset is 30 years, and women are affected twice as often as men. The use of systemic and topical corticosteroids and symptomatic care are the major modalities of management.

INFECTIOUS ARTHRITIS

Any infectious agent can invade the joint space and cause inflammation and tissue destruction. Certain pathogens such as *Staphylococcus aureus* destroy tissue rapidly, whereas others, especially viruses, do not cause irreversible damage. The hallmark of management is local and/or systemic antibiotic therapy.

LYME DISEASE

Lyme disease is a relatively newly named disorder that has been added to the list of CTDs. Unlike many CTDs, however, the cause has been identified: infected deer ticks (*Ixodes dammini*) transmit a bacterium (a spirochete) that causes a circular rash, malaise, fever, headache, and muscle or joint aches. If this disease is not diagnosed and treated, later complications such as arthritis, enlarged lymph tissue, and neurologic and cardiac problems can result. Prompt treatment with antibiotics, such as penicillin and tetracycline, is usually effective. The accompanying Health Promotion/Maintenance feature lists ways to prevent contracting this disease.

PSEUDOGOUT

Pseudogout is a disease that mimics the clinical manifestations of gout. The crystals that deposit in joints, however, are not sodium urate but are rather calcium pyrophosphate. These crystals migrate to cartilage most frequently, but they can also deposit in tendons, ligaments, and synovium. As in gout, men are affected more often than women. Anti-inflammatory drugs usually control the manifestations of the disease.

DISEASE-ASSOCIATED ARTHRITIS

A number of diseases can cause secondary arthritis. Tuberculosis, Crohn's disease, ulcerative colitis, hemophilia, and sickle cell anemia are typical examples. The management of joint involvement is the treatment of

---

HEALTH PROMOTION/MAINTENANCE ■ Methods of Prevention and Early Detection of Lyme Disease

Avoiding heavily wooded areas or those with thick underbrush

Using an insect repellent on skin and clothes when in an area where ticks are likely to be found

Wearing long-sleeved tops and long pants

Wearing closed shoes and a hat or cap

Bathing immediately after being in an infested area and inspecting for ticks (about the size of a pinhead), paying special attention to arms, legs, and hairline

Gently removing with tweezers or fingers any tick discovered and disposing of the tick by flushing it down the toilet (burning a tick could spread infection)

Waiting 4–6 wk after being bitten by a tick before being tested for Lyme disease (testing before this time is not reliable)

Reporting symptoms such as a rash or influenza-like manifestations to a physician

KEY FEATURES OF DISEASE ■ Disorders Associated
with Arthritis

Crohn's disease
Ulcerative colitis
Tuberculosis
Hemophilia
Whipple's disease
Intestinal bypass surgery
Hyperparathyroidism
Hyperthyroidism
Diabetes mellitus
Sickle cell anemia crisis
Psoriasis
Infection

the primary disease. For example, when a client with Crohn's disease has a remission, joint manifestations also subside. Conditions in which joint involvement can be seen are given in the accompanying Key Features of Disease.

MIXED CONNECTIVE TISSUE DISEASE

When a client presents with clinical manifestations that are not typical of any one CTD, a diagnosis of mixed CTD is made. Approximately 10% of clients with CTDs are classified as having mixed disease. Some of these are *overlap syndromes* in which two diseases occur concurrently. Examples are combinations of SLE plus PSS and RA plus SLE. Management depends on the clinical manifestations, but often the client is treated as having SLE.

FIBROSITIS

The term *fibrositis*, or *fibromyalgia*, is used to describe a syndrome that is characterized by trunk, extremity, and/or facial pain and tenderness without other objective findings. The primary manifestations are pain, stiffness, sensory changes, and exhaustion, which may be attributable to severe sleep disturbances. Tender areas, known as *trigger points*, can typically be palpated in a predictable, reproducible pattern. Physical therapy, nonsteroidal anti-inflammatory drugs, and muscle relaxants are commonly used to provide temporary relief. In most clients, the problem is the result of sleep deprivation, especially in stage 4. Hypnotics and other sleep-inducing methods may be needed to overcome this sleep disturbance. Secondary fibrosis syndromes can accompany any CTD, particularly lupus and RA, and may not be related to sleep patterns.

LOCAL INFLAMMATORY DISORDERS

Two of the most common inflammatory conditions are localized to specific connective tissues: *bursitis* and *tendinitis*. Both usually occur in the shoulder and are caused by aging and/or irritation. During middle age, the tendons become frayed, irregular, and calcified, which causes inflammation of tendons and adjacent bursae. This syndrome may be acute or chronic and occurs most often in women. The dominant arm is usually involved, but bilateral effects are found in 15% of cases. Intra-articular steroid injections and systemic anti-inflammatory drugs are administered.

SUMMARY

CTD is the major component of rheumatology. Although more than 100 types of CTD exist, most have arthritis as a common manifestation and a multitude of systemic complications. The nurse assesses every body system to identify problem areas and works with other members of the interdisciplinary team to resolve biopsychosocial nursing diagnoses. The goal of management is to force the disease into long-term remission, which slows the progression of the disease and improves the quality of life.

IMPLICATIONS FOR RESEARCH

Rheumatology is a relatively new branch of medicine, and research in the area has been limited. Only recently has federal funding for research increased. Management of CTD could improve if the etiologic factors were definitively established. It is known that many of the diseases have an autoimmune basis, but the triggering mechanisms are not clear. More definitive diagnostic testing and safer remission-inducing drugs are needed.

Because many of the diseases result in chronic pain and immobility, nursing needs to address the following research questions:

1. What are the most appropriate pain relief measures for chronic joint pain?
2. What methods can be used to accurately assess the client's level of mobility?
3. What is the relationship, if any, between mobility and dependence in the client with arthritis?

4. When are cold and heat applications most appropriate and beneficial?
5. How can the nurse best assess the client's degree of body image disturbance?

REFERENCES AND READINGS

Degenerative Joint Disease

Aglietti, P., Rinonapoli, E., Stringa, G., & Taviani, A. (1983). Tibial osteotomy for the varus osteoarthritic knee. *Clinical Orthopaedics and Related Research, 176*, 239–251.

American Nurses' Association and Arthritis Health Professionals Association Nursing Task Force. (1983). *Outcome standards for rheumatology nursing practice.* Kansas City: American Nurses' Association.

Arthritis Foundation. (1982). *Arthritis, diet, and nutrition: Facts to consider.* Atlanta: Author.

Blake, S. A. (1985). Noncemented femoral prosthesis: Intraoperative focus. *Orthopaedic Nursing, 4*(1), 40–42.

Boggs, J. (1982). *Arthritis, living and loving: Information about sex.* Atlanta: The Arthritis Foundation.

Bradley, L. A. (1985). Psychological aspects of arthritis. *Bulletin on the Rheumatic Diseases, 35*, 1–12.

Brinkley, L. B. (1989). Predeposit autologous blood for elective orthopaedic surgery. *Orthopaedic Nursing, 8*(1), 25–28.

Doheney, M. O. (1985). Porous coated prosthesis: Concepts and care considerations. *Orthopaedic Nursing, 4*(5), 43–45.

Dunajcik, L. M. (1989, April). The hip: When the joint must be replaced. *RN*, pp. 62–71.

Ehrlich, G. E. (1986). *Rehabilitation management of rheumatic conditions.* Baltimore: Williams & Wilkins.

Follman, D. A. (1988). Nursing care concerns in total shoulder replacement. *Orthopaedic Nursing, 7*(3), 29–31.

Greene, W. L. (1988). Thromboembolism prophylaxis with low-dose heparin. *Clinical Report on Aging, 2*, 1, 3.

Greenwald, R. A. (1986). Diet and arthritis: The myths and the facts. *Continuing Education for the Family Physician, 21*, 81–83.

Maly, B. J., Turk, M. A., & Kinney, C. L. (1988). Rehabilitation in joint and connective tissue diseases. *Archives of Physical Medicine and Rehabilitation, 69*(Suppl.), S71–S112.

Moskowitz, R. W. (1982). Management of osteoarthritis. *Bulletin on the Rheumatic Diseases, 31*, 31–34.

Panish, R. S., & Endo, L. P. (1986). Diet and unproven remedies. In W. Katz (Ed.), *The diagnosis and management of rheumatic diseases.* Philadelphia: J. B. Lippincott.

Pigg, J. S., Driscoll, P. W., & Caniff, R. (1985). *Rheumatology nursing: A problem-oriented approach.* New York: Wiley.

Salvati, E. A. (Ed.). (1988). Long term results of cemented joint replacement: Is cement obsolete? *Orthopedic Clinics of North America, 19*, 467–668.

Schumacher, H. R., Jr. (Ed.). (1988). *Primer on the rheumatic diseases.* Atlanta: The Arthritis Foundation.

Simpson, C. F. (1983). Heat, cold, or both. *American Journal of Nursing, 83*, 270–272.

Strand, C. V., & Clark, S. R. (1983). Adult arthritis: Drugs and remedies. *American Journal of Nursing, 83*, 266–270.

Sutton, J. D. (1984). The hospitalized patient with arthritis. *Nursing Clinics of North America, 19*, 617–625.

Walsh, C. R., & Wirth, C. R. (1985). Total knee arthroplasty: Biomechanical and nursing considerations. *Orthopaedic Nursing, 4*(2), 29–34.

Weiss, T., & Quinet, R. (1984). Clinical concepts of osteoarthritis: Part II. *Clinical Rheumatology in Practice, 2*, 4–16.

Zuckerman, J. D., & Sledge, C. B. (1985). Total joint replacement: Latest developments for the geriatric patient. *Geriatrics, 40*, 71–73, 77–78, 83–85, 88–90, 92.

Rheumatoid Arthritis

Benson, C. H. (1988). Arthritis and sexuality. *Journal of Urological Nursing, 7*, 370–372.

Brassell, M. P. (1988). Pharmacologic management of rheumatic diseases. *Orthopaedic Nursing, 7*(2), 43–51.

Calabro, J. J., & Londino, A. V. (1984). Drug therapy in rheumatoid arthritis: Based on an understanding of its natural history. *Clinical Rheumatology in Practice, 2*, 244–256.

Cella, J. H., & Watson, J. (1989). *Nurse's manual of laboratory tests.* Philadelphia: F. A. Davis.

Hess, E. V. (1988). Rheumatoid arthritis complicated by vasculitis. *Hospital Practice, 23*, 50–54, 57, 61–64+.

Hunder, G. G. (1982). Rheumatoid arthritis: Check for its systemic manifestations. *Consultant, 22*, 33–41.

Ignatavicius, D. D. (1987). Meeting the psychosocial needs of patients with rheumatoid arthritis. *Orthopaedic Nursing, 6*(3), 16–20.

Kaplan, H. (1985). Who should get gold and when? *Clinical Rheumatology in Practice, 3*, 53–57.

Koerner, M. E., & Dickinson, G. R. (1983). Adult arthritis: A look at some of its forms. *American Journal of Nursing, 83*, 255–262.

Malek, C. J., & Brower, S. A. (1984). Rheumatoid Arthritis: How does it influence sexuality? *Rehabilitation Nursing, 9*, 26–28.

Mooney, N. E. (1983). Coping with chronic pain in rheumatoid arthritis: Patient behaviors and nursing interventions. *Rehabilitation Nursing, 8*, 20–21, 24–25.

Navarro, A. H. (1983). Physical therapy in the management of rheumatoid arthritis. *Clinical Rheumatology in Practice, 1*, 125–130.

Nazaroff, K. S., Stanton, J. H., Magana, K. R., & Kaufman, R. L. (1988). Halo-body jacket immobilization in RA patients: Patients with cervical myelopathy. *Nursing Clinics of North America, 24*, 209–224.

Partridge, A. J. (1984). Determination of Social Security disability in rheumatic diseases. *Clinical Rheumatology in Practice, 2*, 275–280.

Riggs, G. K., & Gall, E. P. (Eds.). (1984). *Rheumatic diseases: Rehabilitation and management.* Boston: Butterworth.

Ziminski, C. M. (1985). Treating joint inflammation in the elderly: An update. *Geriatrics, 40,* 73–76, 79–81, 85, 88.

Systemic Lupus Erythematosus

Balow, J. E. (1988). Lupus as a renal disease. *Hospital Practice, 23,* 129–135, 139–140, 142–144.

Burlinghame, M. B., & Delafuente, J. C. (1988). Treatment of systemic lupus erythematosus. *Drug Intelligence and Clinical Pharmacology, 22,* 283–288.

Delany, P. (1983). Neurologic complications of systemic lupus erythematosus. *American Family Physician, 28,* 191–193.

Fessel, W. J. (1988). Epidemiology of systemic lupus erythematosus. *Rheumatic Disease Clinics of North America, 14,* 15–23.

Ginzler, E. M., & Schorn, K. (1988). Outcome and prognosis in systemic lupus erythematosus. *Rheumatic Disease Clinics of North America, 14,* 67–87.

Hooker, R. S. (1988). Systemic lupus erythematosus. *Physician Assistant, 12,* 71–72, 74–75, 79–80+.

Kirash, R. G. (1984). Psychologic responses of patients with systemic lupus and implications for rehabilitation. *Rehabilitation Nursing, 9*(3), 32–34.

Lewis, K. S. (1984). Systemic lupus erythematosus: The great masquerader. *Nurse Practitioner, 9,* 13–14, 16–22.

Lieberman, J. D., & Schatten, S. (1988). Treatment: Disease modifying therapies. *Rheumatic Disease Clinics of North America, 14,* 223–239.

Rothfield, N. F. (1989). The diagnostic pictures of systemic lupus erythematosus. *Hospital Practice, 24,* 37–46.

Steinberg, A. D. (1987). Systemic lupus erythematosus: Part I. *Hospital Medicine, 23,* 21, 25–26, 31+.

Steinberg, A. D., & Klinman, D. M. (1988). Pathogenesis of systemic lupus erythematosus. *Rheumatic Disease Clinics of North America, 14,* 25–41.

Townes, A. S. (1987). The "mask" of lupus. *Hospital Practice, 22,* 93–97, 101–103, 107–108.

Zeigler, G. C. (1984). Systemic lupus erythematosus and systemic sclerosis. *Nursing Clinics of North America, 19,* 673–695.

Other Connective Tissue Diseases

Calin, A., & Marks, S. (1982). Management of ankylosing spondylitis. *Bulletin on the Rheumatic Diseases, 31,* 35–38.

Chou, C-T., & Schumacher, H. R. (1983). Polymyalgia rheumatica. *Comprehensive Therapy, 9,* 33–37.

Diamond, H. S. (1983). The kidney in hyperuricemia and gout. *Clinical Rheumatology in Practice, 1,* 205–211.

Felts, W. R. (1982). Ankylosing spondylitis: The challenge of early diagnosis. *Postgraduate Medicine, 72,* 199–200.

Hawley, D. (Ed.). (1984). Symposium on arthritis and related rheumatic diseases. *Nursing Clinics of North America, 19,* 565–725.

Lee, B. C. (1989, April). Be ready for Lyme disease in your own back yard. *RN,* pp. 26–31.

Montanaro, A. (1988). Vasculitis in older patients: Presentations and significance. *Geriatrics, 43,* 75–96.

Norman, D. C., & Yoshikawa, T. T. (1983). Responding to septic arthritis. *Geriatrics, 38,* 83–91.

Schumacher, H. R., Jr. (Ed.). (1988). *Primer on the rheumatic diseases.* Atlanta: The Arthritis Foundation.

Smeltzer, K. J. (1987). Fibromyalgia: The frustration of diagnosis and treatment. *Orthopaedic Nursing, 6*(3), 28–31.

Wilske, K. R., & Healey, L. A. (1985). Polymyalgia rheumatica and giant cell arteritis. *Postgraduate Medicine, 77,* 243–248.

ADDITIONAL READINGS

Guccione, A. A. (1989). Understanding arthritis in the elderly. *Focus on Geriatric Care and Rehabilitation, 3*(5), 1–8.

This publication devoted an entire issue to the subject of arthritis in the elderly. The major types of arthritis seen in this population were described, and the management of each type was discussed. The author provided practical tips for helping the client manage the problems associated with arthritis.

Halfman, T. M., & Pigg, J. S. (1984). Nurses' perceptions of rheumatic disease problems as evidenced in nursing diagnoses, defining characteristics, etiologies, expected outcomes, and interventions. In M. J. Kim, G. K. McFarland, & A. M. McClane (Eds.), *Classification of nursing diagnosis: Proceedings of the fifth conference.* St. Louis: C. V. Mosby.

This study was an attempt to standardize the most common nursing diagnoses and nursing interventions that are used for clients with rheumatic disease. Client care plans were reviewed to identify those diagnoses and interventions. Alteration in comfort (pain), impaired physical mobility, and self-care deficit were three of the problems typically identified.

Miller, J. F. (1983). *Coping with chronic illness: Overcoming powerlessness.* Philadelphia: F. A. Davis.

Although this book has been available for nearly 10 years, it remains the most comprehensive, thorough publication on the topic. The author explained how to assess the client with chronic illness, such as arthritis, and then identified interventions to help the client cope with the illness.

Unit 8 Resources

Nursing Resources

Association of Nurses in AIDS Care (ANAC), 10141 Liberty Road, Randallstown, MD 21133. Telephone 301-922-1446; 215-750-1684.

Fosters professional development of nurses involved in all aspects of AIDS and promotes health, welfare, and rights of persons infected with HIV. Publishes the *Journal of the Association of Nurses in AIDS Care.*

Association for Practitioners in Infection Control, 505 East Hawley Street, Mundelein, IL 60060. Telephone 312-949-6052.

See Unit 7 Resources for more information.

Other Resources

American Academy of Allergy and Immunology, 611 East Wells Street, Milwaukee, WI 53202. Telephone 414-272-6071.

American College of Allergists, 800 East Northwest Highway, Suite 101, Mount Prospect, IL 60056. Telephone 800-842-7777.

Asthma and Allergy Foundation of America, 1717 Massachusetts Avenue NW, No. 305, Washington, DC 20036. Telephone 800-7ASTHMA.

Centers for Disease Control, Department of Health and Human Services, U.S. Public Health Service, GA 30333. Telephone 404-639-3534.

National Institute of Allergy and Infectious Diseases (NIAID), Building 10, Bethesda, MD 20892. Telephone 301-496-4000.

National Jewish Center for Immunology and Respiratory Medicine, 1400 Jackson Street, Denver, CO 80206. Immunologic diseases hot line 800-222-LUNG.

U.S. Public Health Service AIDS Hot Line 800-342-AIDS.

UNIT 9

PROBLEMS OF MOBILITY: MANAGEMENT OF CLIENTS WITH DISRUPTIONS OF THE MUSCULO-SKELETAL SYSTEM

CHAPTER 29

Assessment of the Musculoskeletal System

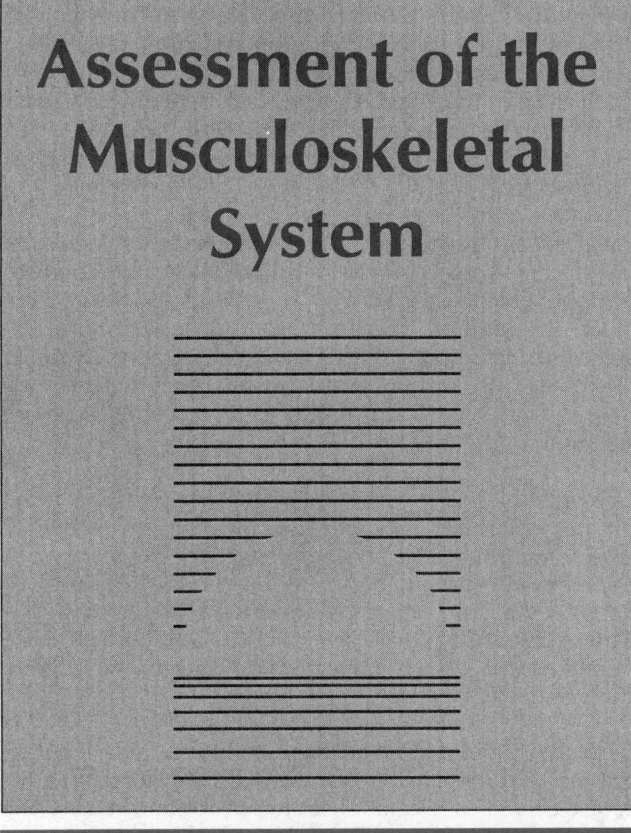

The musculoskeletal system includes bones, joints, and skeletal muscles and their supporting structures. Accounting for as much as 75% of the body's weight, the musculoskeletal system is one of the largest body systems. Disease and trauma frequently affect any part of the system, yet its assessment is often overlooked by the nurse. As the elderly population increases, the incidence of bone and muscle problems also increases. In the younger adult, an interest in sports and exercise often results in musculoskeletal injuries.

ANATOMY AND PHYSIOLOGY REVIEW

SKELETAL SYSTEM

The skeletal system consists of bones and joints. The growth and development of these structures occur during childhood and adolescence and are not discussed in this text.

BONES

Types

There are 206 bones of various types in the body. *Long bones,* such as the femora, are cylindric with rounded ends and often bear weight. By contrast, *short bones* are small and bear little or no weight, e.g., the phalanges. *Flat bones,* such as the sternum, protect vital organs and often contain blood-forming cells. Bones that have unique shapes are known as *irregular bones,* e.g., the carpal bones in the wrist. The *sesamoid* bone is the least common type and develops within a tendon; the patella is a typical example of this type.

Structure

As shown in the illustration on page 719, the outer layer of bone, or *cortex,* is composed of dense, *compact* bone tissue. The inner layer, in the *medulla,* contains spongy, *cancellous* tissue. Almost every bone has both tissue types, but in varying quantities. The long bone typically has a shaft, or *diaphysis,* and two knob-like ends, or *epiphyses.*

The structural unit of the cortical, compact bone is the *haversian system,* as seen in detail in the illustration on page 719. As a complex canal network, the haversian system contains microscopic blood vessels, which supply nutrients and oxygen to bone, and the *lacunae,* which are small cavities that house *osteocytes* (bone cells). As illustrated, the canals run longitudinally within the hard, cortical bone tissue.

The softer, cancellous tissue contains large spaces, or *trabeculae,* filled with red and yellow marrow. Hematopoiesis (production of blood cells) occurs in the red marrow. The yellow marrow contains fat cells, which can be dislodged and enter the blood stream, causing a life-threatening complication, fat embolism. *Volkmann's canals* connect bone marrow vessels with the haversian system and *periosteum,* the outermost covering of the bone. Osteogenic cells, which later differentiate into *osteoblasts* (bone-forming cells) and *osteoclasts* (bone-destroying cells), are found in the deepest layer of the periosteum.

In addition to cells, bone contains a *matrix,* also called osteoid, consisting chiefly of collagen, mucopolysaccharides, and lipids. Inorganic calcium salts (carbonate and phosphate) deposit in the matrix to provide the hardness of bone.

Bone is a vascular tissue, with an estimated total blood flow between 200 and 400 mL/min. Each bone has a principal nutrient artery, which enters near the middle of the shaft and branches into ascending and descending vessels; these vessels supply the cortex, the marrow, and the haversian system. Sympathetic and afferent (sensory) fibers constitute the sparse nerve supply to bone. Dilation of blood vessels is controlled by the sympathetic nerves, whereas the afferent fibers are responsible for pain experienced in primary lesions of the bone.

Growth and Metabolism

After puberty, bone reaches its maturity and maximal growth. Bone is a dynamic tissue, however, undergoing a continuous process of formation and resorption, or destruction, at equal rates until the age of 35 years. In later years, bone resorption accelerates, resulting in decreased bone mass and a predisposition to injury (see Chaps. 5 and 30 for a discussion of the effects of aging on bone metabolism).

Bone growth and metabolism are affected by numerous minerals and hormones: calcium, phosphorus, calcitonin, vitamin D, parathyroid hormone (PTH), growth hormone, glucocorticoids, and sex hormones. Each substance depends on the presence and action of others to promote a healthy skeleton.

Calcium and phosphorus. Bone accounts for approximately 99% of the calcium in the body and 90% of the phosphorus. The concentrations of calcium and phosphorus maintain an inverse relationship, e.g., when calcium levels rise, phosphorus levels decrease. When serum levels of these substances are altered, several hormones work to maintain equilibrium. If the calcium level of the blood is decreased, the bone (which stores calcium) releases calcium into the vascular system in response to stimulation by PTH.

Calcitonin. Calcitonin is produced by the thyroid gland and functions to decrease the serum calcium level if it is increased above its normal level. Calcitonin works by inhibiting bone resorption and increasing renal excretion of calcium and phosphorus as needed.

Vitamin D. Vitamin D and its metabolites are considered hormones. They are produced in the body and transported in the blood to promote the absorption of calcium and phosphorus from the small intestines. They also appear to enhance PTH activity in the release of calcium from the bone. A decrease in the body's vitamin D level can result in osteomalacia in the adult. A detailed explanation of vitamin D metabolism is provided in Chapter 30.

Parathyroid hormone. When serum calcium levels are lowered, PTH secretion increases and stimulates bone to promote osteoclastic activity and donate calcium to the blood. In addition, the hormone reduces the renal excretion of calcium and facilitates its absorption from the intestine. Conversely, when serum calcium levels increase, PTH secretion diminishes to preserve the bone calcium supply.

Growth hormone. Secreted by the anterior lobe of the pituitary gland, the growth hormone is responsible for increasing bone length and determining the amount of bone matrix formed before puberty. An increased or decreased secretion during childhood results in gigantism or dwarfism, respectively. In the adult, an increase causes *acromegaly,* characterized by bone and soft-tissue deformities (Chap. 49).

Glucocorticoids. The adrenal glucocorticoids regulate protein metabolism. When needed, the hormones increase or decrease catabolism to reduce or intensify the organic matrix of bone. They also aid in the regulation of intestinal calcium and phosphorus absorption.

Sex hormones. Estrogens stimulate osteoblastic activity and tend to inhibit the role of PTH. Androgens, such as testosterone, promote anabolism and increase bone mass. The reader is referred to Chapters 12 and 48 for discussions of the roles of the substances affecting bone growth and metabolism.

Function

The skeletal system serves several major functions. It

1. Provides a framework for the body
2. Supports the surrounding tissues (e.g., muscle and tendons)
3. Assists in movement through muscle attachment and joint formation
4. Protects vital organs, such as the heart and lungs
5. Manufactures blood cells in red bone marrow
6. Provides storage for mineral salts (e.g., calcium and phosphorus)

STRUCTURE OF A TYPICAL LONG BONE

The cortex, or outer layer, is composed of dense, compact tissue. The microscopic structure of this compact cortical tissue is the haversian system.

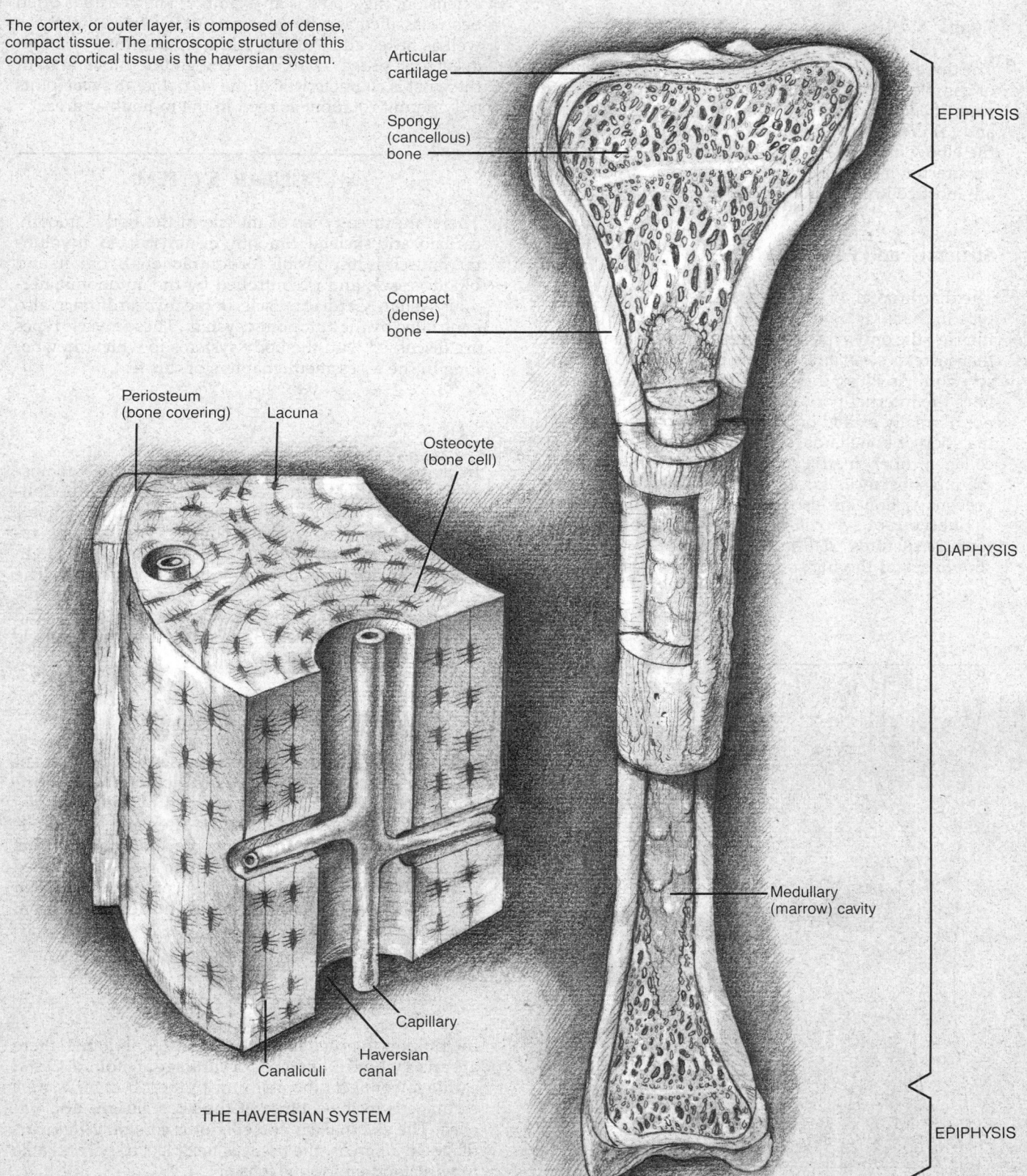

Articular cartilage

Spongy (cancellous) bone

Compact (dense) bone

EPIPHYSIS

DIAPHYSIS

Medullary (marrow) cavity

EPIPHYSIS

Periosteum (bone covering)

Lacuna

Osteocyte (bone cell)

Capillary

Canaliculi

Haversian canal

THE HAVERSIAN SYSTEM

JOINTS

Types

The three types of joints in the body are (1) *synarthrodial,* or completely immovable (e.g., in the cranium); (2) *amphiarthrodial,* or slightly movable (e.g., in the pelvis); and (3) *diarthrodial* (synovial), or freely movable (e.g., the elbow and knee). Although any of these joints can be affected by disease or injury, the diarthrodial joints are most commonly involved.

Structure and Function

The diarthrodial, or *synovial,* joint is the most common type in the body. Synovial joints are so named because they are the only type lined with *synovium,* a membrane that secretes *synovial fluid* for lubrication and shock absorption. As illustrated in Figure 29–1, the synovium lines the internal portion of the joint capsule, but does not normally extend onto the surface of the *cartilage* at the spongy bone ends. Articular cartilage consists of a collagen fiber matrix impregnated with a complex ground substance. *Bursae,* small sacs located at joints to prevent friction, are also lined with synovial membrane.

Subtypes of synovial joints are based on their anatomic structures. *Ball-and-socket* joints, such as the shoulder and the hip, permit movement in any direction. *Hinge* joints allow motion in one plane, flexion and extension; the elbow is an example. The knee has often been classified as a hinge joint, but it rotates slightly as well as flexes and extends. It is best described as a *condylar* type of synovial joint. The gliding movement of the wrist is characteristic of the *biaxial* joint. *Pivot* joints only permit rotation, as seen in the radioulnar area.

MUSCULAR SYSTEM

There are three types of muscle in the body: smooth, cardiac, and skeletal. Smooth, or nonstriated, involuntary muscle is responsible for contractions of organs and blood vessels and is controlled by the autonomic nervous system. Cardiac muscle, or the myocardium, is also controlled by the autonomic system. These muscle types are discussed with the body systems to which they belong in the assessment chapters of this text.

STRUCTURE

In contrast to smooth and cardiac muscle, skeletal muscle is voluntarily controlled by the central and peripheral nervous systems. The junction of a peripheral motor nerve and the muscle cells it supplies is sometimes referred to as a *motor end plate.* Muscle fibers are held in place by connective tissue in bundles, or *fasciculi.* The entire muscle is surrounded by dense, fibrous tissue, *fascia,* which contains the muscle's blood, lymph, and nerve supply (see Chap. 32 for a discussion of muscle innervation and physiology).

FUNCTION

The primary function of skeletal muscle is movement of the body and its parts. When bones, joints, and supporting structures are adversely affected by injury or disease, the adjacent muscle tissue is often involved, limiting mobility. During the aging process, muscle fibers decrease in size and number, even in well-conditioned individuals. This *senile atrophy* is compounded when muscles are not regularly exercised and deteriorate from disuse.

SUPPORTING STRUCTURES

In addition to articular cartilage located in joints, there are areas where other types of cartilage are found. *Costal* cartilage connects the sternum to the rib cage; *hyaline* cartilage is in the septum of the nose, larynx, and trachea. The external ear and epiglottis contain *yellow* cartilage. In all areas, the tissue is flexible, elastic, and able to withstand enormous tension.

Tendons are bands of tough, fibrous tissue that attach muscles to bones. Bones are attached to other bones by *ligaments* at joints.

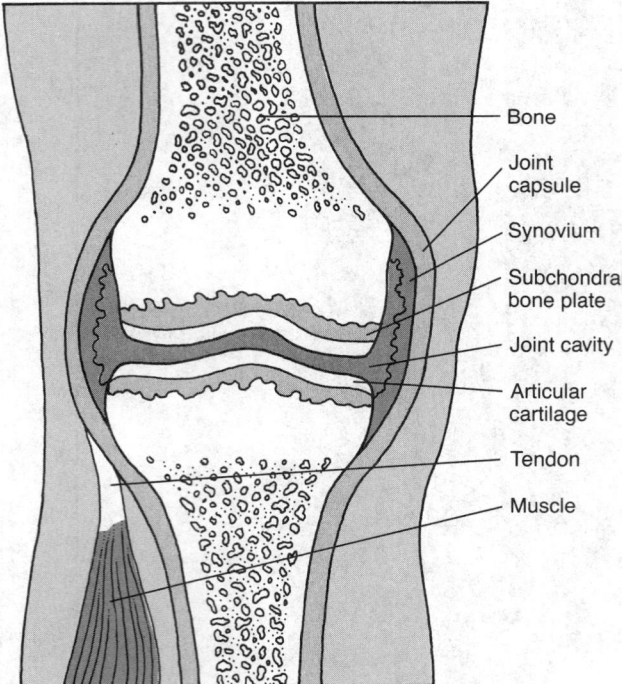

Bone
Joint capsule
Synovium
Subchondral bone plate
Joint cavity
Articular cartilage
Tendon
Muscle

Figure 29–1

Structure of a diarthrodial joint. Synovium lines the joint capsule, but does not extend into the articular cartilage.

FOCUS ON THE ELDERLY ■ Changes in the Musculoskeletal System Related to Aging

Structure	Change	Interventions	Rationales
Bone	Decreased density	Teach safety tips to prevent falls.	Porous bones are more likely to fracture.
	Prominent bony structure	Prevent pressure on bony prominences.	There is less soft tissue to prevent skin breakdown.
Vertebral column	Kyphotic posture; widened gait, shift in the center of gravity	Teach proper body mechanics; instruct the client to sit in supportive chairs with arms.	Correction of posture problems prevents further deformity; the client should have support for bony structures.
Synovial joint	Cartilage degeneration	Provide moist heat, such as shower.	Moist heat increases blood flow to the area.
	Decreased ROM	Assess the client's ability to perform ADL and mobility.	The client may need assistance with self-care skills.
Muscle	Atrophy, decreased strength	Teach exercises.	Exercises increase muscle strength.
	Slowed movement	Do not rush the individual; be patient.	The client may become frustrated if hurried.

MUSCULOSKELETAL CHANGES ASSOCIATED WITH AGING

As one ages, bone density decreases, causing postural changes and predisposing an individual to fracture. Synovial joint cartilage degenerates owing to repeated use of joints, especially weight-bearing joints, such as the hips and the knees. The result is often disabling degenerative arthritis. Muscle tissue atrophy occurs, but its rate may be slowed by increased activity and exercise. Collectively, these changes cause decreased coordination, gait changes, and predisposition to falls with injury. The accompanying Focus on the Elderly feature lists major physiologic changes and the associated nursing interventions.

HISTORY

When assessing a client with an actual or potential musculoskeletal problem, a detailed history aids in the identification of diagnoses and subsequent interventions.

DEMOGRAPHIC DATA

The *age* and *sex* of the client are important indicators in musculoskeletal disorders. For example, elderly women are most likely to have metabolic bone disease, whereas young men are at the greatest risk for trauma related to motor vehicle accidents.

PERSONAL AND FAMILY HISTORY

Previous illnesses and *accidents* may relate to a client's current problem. When taking a personal health history, the nurse asks questions about all traumatic incidents, regardless of date of occurrence. An injury to the lumbar spine 30 years previously may contribute to a client's current complaint of low-back pain. An automobile accident that results in no apparent personal injury can be the cause of musculoskeletal dysfunction years after the event. Previous or concurrent diseases may also affect musculoskeletal status. For example, a diabetic client treated for a foot ulcer is at high risk for acute or chronic osteomyelitis: in addition, diabetes slows the healing process. Certain disorders have a familial or genetic tendency. Osteoporosis, for instance, is often seen in several family generations; bone cancer also tends to be genetically linked. It is also important to determine a history of previous hospitalizations and illnesses or complications.

DIET HISTORY

An evaluation of the client's diet history is helpful in determining the cause of a musculoskeletal problem and anticipating complications resulting from an inadequate nutritional status. An *inadequate intake of calcium or protein foods* or *insufficient exposure to sunlight* predisposes the elderly individual to bone and muscle tone loss. Inadequate protein or insufficient vitamin C in the diet inhibits bone and tissue healing. *Obesity* places excess stress and strain on bones and joints, resulting in fractures and cartilage degeneration. In addition, obesity inhibits mobility in clients with musculoskeletal problems, which predisposes them to the hazards of immobility, such as respiratory and circulatory problems (Greipp, 1988).

SOCIOECONOMIC STATUS

When assessing a client with a possible musculoskeletal alteration, information regarding the life style is included. An individual's *occupation* could cause or contribute to an injury. For instance, fractures are not uncommon in clients with jobs requiring manual labor, such as carpenters and mechanics. Certain factory jobs may predispose an individual to carpal tunnel syndrome (entrapment of the median nerve in the wrist). Nurses and other health care professionals may experience back injury from prolonged standing and excessive lifting. Amateur and professional athletes frequently experience musculoskeletal injuries.

Socioeconomic status and *ethnic or cultural background* may be related to the client's occupation, and therefore affect an individual's likelihood of musculoskeletal alteration. Ethnic and cultural background may also be helpful in ascertaining a client's tolerance to pain. There may be differences in reactions to pain among cultural populations. The nurse uses this information to aid in pain assessment.

CURRENT HEALTH PROBLEM

The nurse gathers pertinent data regarding the client's presenting complaint, as follows:

1. Date and time of onset
2. Factors that cause or exacerbate the problem
3. Course of the problem (e.g., intermittent or continuous)
4. Clinical manifestations (as expressed by the client) and the pattern of their occurrence
5. Measures that improve clinical manifestations (e.g., heat)
6. Assessment of the type, duration, frequency, and nature of pain

PHYSICAL ASSESSMENT

Although bones, joints, and muscles are usually assessed simultaneously utilizing a head-to-toe approach, each subsystem is described separately for emphasis and understanding.

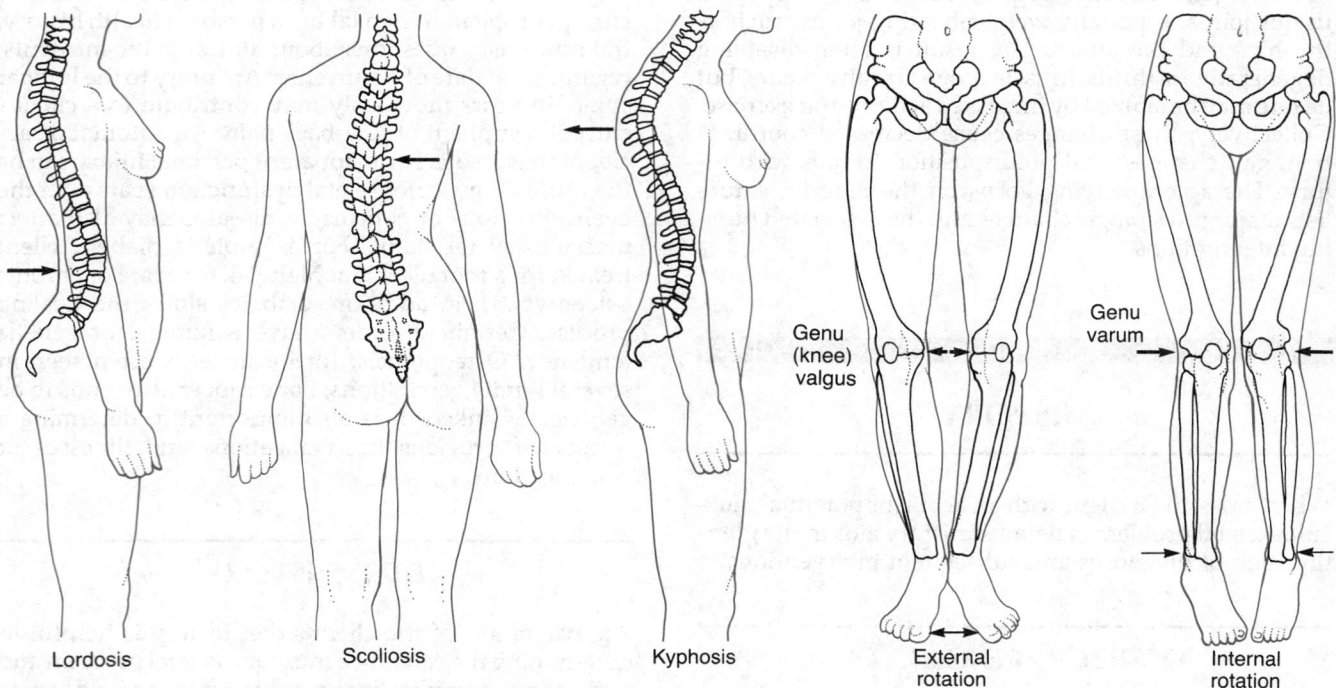

Lordosis   Scoliosis   Kyphosis   Genu (knee) valgus   External rotation   Genu varum   Internal rotation

Figure 29 – 2

Common musculoskeletal deformities.

ASSESSMENT OF THE SKELETAL SYSTEM

GENERAL INSPECTION

The nurse observes the client's posture, gait, and mobility for gross deformities and impairment. *Posture* includes the individual's body build and alignment when standing and walking. Curvature of the spine and the length, shape, and symmetry of extremities are inspected. Figure 29–2 shows common musculoskeletal deformities. *Muscle mass* is inspected for size and symmetry. The client's *gait* is evaluated for balance and steadiness, and ease and length of stride; a limp or other asymmetric leg movement or deformity is noted. The nurse observes the client's need for ambulatory devices during transfer from bed to chair and while walking and climbing stairs. *Mobility* is also assessed by asking the client to perform simple activities of daily living (ADL), such as donning shoes. Pain and deformity may limit physical mobility.

After a general evaluation is performed, the nurse assesses major bones, joints, and muscles by inspection, palpation, and determination of function. As shown in Figure 29–3, a *goniometer,* used commonly by physical therapists and clinical specialists, provides an exact measurement for joint range of motion (ROM), but the nurse can estimate the degree of joint mobility by putting each joint through its respective ROM. For each anatomic location, the nurse observes the skin for color, elasticity, and lesions that may relate to musculoskeletal dysfunction.

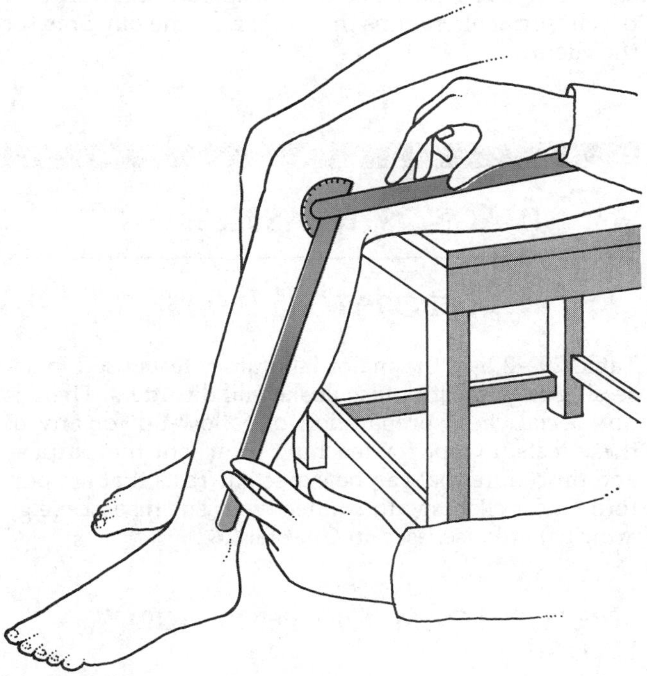

Figure 29–3
Goniometric measurement of the knee joint.

ASSESSMENT OF THE HEAD AND NECK

The nurse inspects and palpates the skull for *shape, symmetry, tenderness, and masses.* The temporomandibular joints (TMJs) are best evaluated by asking the client to open her/his mouth while the nurse palpates the TMJs. Common abnormal findings are tenderness or pain, crepitus (a grating sound), and a spongy swelling caused by excess synovium and fluid, which can be palpated.

Each vertebra of the spine in the neck is observed and palpated. Clinical findings may include malalignment, tenderness, and inability to flex, extend, and rotate the neck as expected.

ASSESSMENT OF THE VERTEBRAL SPINE

The thoracic spine, lumbar spine, and sacral spine are evaluated in the same manner as the neck. In addition, the nurse places both hands over the lumbosacral area and applies pressure with his/her thumbs to elicit tenderness. Clients often do not complain of discomfort until the area is palpated.

ASSESSMENT OF THE UPPER EXTREMITIES

The nurse assesses both extremities concurrently. For example, both shoulders are inspected and palpated for *size, swelling, deformity, malalignment, tenderness or pain,* and *mobility.* A shoulder injury may prevent the client from combing his/her hair with the affected arm, but severe arthritis may inhibit movement in both arms. Similarly, the elbows and wrists are assessed.

Assessment of hand function is perhaps the most critical part of the examination, as the hand has multiple joints in a single digit. The nurse inspects and palpates the metacarpophalangeal (MCP), proximal interphalangeal (PIP), and distal interphalangeal (DIP) joints, comparing the same digits on right and left hands (Fig. 29–4). ROM for each joint is also determined using active movement if possible.

ASSESSMENT OF THE LOWER EXTREMITIES

Evaluation of the hip joint relies primarily on determining its degree of *mobility,* as the joint is deep and thereby difficult to inspect or palpate. On the other hand, the knee is readily accessible for nursing assessment, particularly when the client is sitting and the knee is flexed. Fluid accumulation, or effusion, is easily detected in the knee joint, and limitations in movement with accompanying pain are common findings. The ankles and feet are often neglected in the physical examination, yet they contain multiple bones and joints that can be affected by disease and injury. Each joint should be observed, palpated, and tested for ROM.

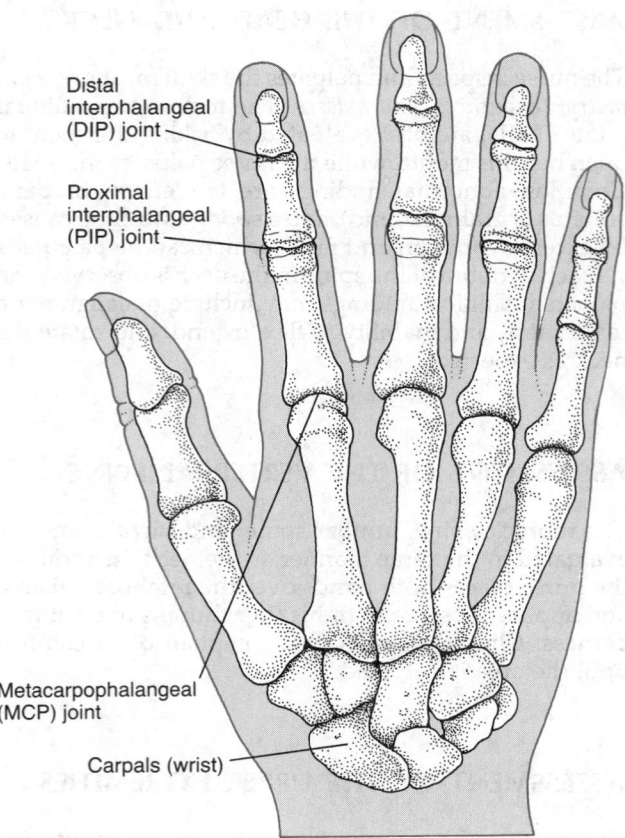

Figure 29–4

The small joints of the hand.

ASSESSMENT OF THE MUSCULAR SYSTEM

The nurse evaluates the *size, shape, tone,* and *strength* of major skeletal muscles. The circumference of each muscle is measured and compared symmetrically to estimate muscle mass. In addition to inspecting and palpating

TABLE 29–1	Lovett's Scale for Determining Muscle Strength
Rating	**Description**
5	*Normal:* ROM unimpaired against gravity with full resistance
4	*Good:* can complete ROM against gravity with some resistance
3	*Fair:* can complete ROM against gravity
2	*Poor:* can complete ROM with gravity eliminated
1	*Trace:* no joint motion and slight evidence of muscle contractility
0	*Zero:* no evidence of muscle contractility

the skeletal muscles, the nurse asks the client to demonstrate muscle strength. For instance, grip strength is often determined by asking the client to squeeze a sphygmomanometer bulb and recording the level of pressure achieved. This method provides a precise measurement that can be used to follow the improvement or deterioration of muscle ability. Another method is to apply resistance by holding the extremity and asking the client to move it. Although movement against resistance is not easily quantified, several scales are available for grading the client's strength; a commonly used scale is delineated in Table 29–1.

PSYCHOSOCIAL ASSESSMENT

The data from the history and physical examination provide clues for the nurse in anticipating psychosocial problems. For instance, the client with multiple fractures requiring extensive immobilization and therapy is at high risk for sensory deprivation (Chap. 8). Prolonged absence from employment or permanent disability may cause the client to lose his/her job or occupation. Further stress may be experienced if chronic pain ensues and the client cannot cope with numerous stressors simultaneously. Deformities resulting from musculoskeletal disease or injury can affect an individual's body image and self-concept (Chap. 9). Psychosocial ramifications of specific musculoskeletal problems are discussed in Chapters 30 and 31. The nurse continuously assesses for the presence or anticipated occurrence of psychosocial alterations that can affect the outcome for the client.

DIAGNOSTIC ASSESSMENT

LABORATORY TESTS

Table 29–2 lists the major laboratory tests used in assessing clients with musculoskeletal disorders. There is no special client preparation or follow-up for any of these tests, except for teaching the client the purpose and procedure that can be expected. Tests that are performed for clients with connective tissue diseases (e.g., arthritis) are discussed in Chapter 28.

SERUM CALCIUM AND PHOSPHORUS LEVELS

The concentrations of calcium and phosphorus, or phosphate (inorganic phosphorus), have an inverse re-

TABLE 29–2 Normal Findings and Significance of Abnormal Findings in Common Laboratory Tests in Musculoskeletal Assessment

Test	Normal Range for Adults	Significance of Abnormal Findings
Serum calcium level	8.0–10.5 mg/dL or 4.5–5.5 mEq/L	*Hypercalcemia* (increased calcium) Metastatic cancers of the bone Paget's disease Bone fractures in healing stage *Hypocalcemia* (decreased calcium) Osteoporosis Osteomalacia
Serum phosphorus level	2.5–4.0 mg/dL	*Hyperphosphatemia* (increased phosphorus) Bone fractures in healing stage Bone tumors Acromegaly *Hypophosphatemia* (decreased phosphorus) Osteomalacia
Alkaline phosphatase level	30–90 IU/L (slightly higher in elderly)	*Elevations* Metastatic cancers of the bone Paget's disease Osteomalacia
Erythrocyte sedimentation rate	*Westergren's method* Men 0–15 mm/h Women 0–20 mm/h *Wintrobe's method* Men 0–9 mm/h Women 0–15 mm/h	*Elevations* Infection Inflammation Carcinoma Cell or tissue destruction
Serum muscle enzyme level Creatine kinase (CK_3) (creatine phosphokinase)	15–150 IU/L	*Elevations* Muscle trauma Progressive muscular dystrophy Effects of electromyography
Lactate dehydrogenase (LDH_4 and LDH_5)	60–150 IU/L	*Elevations* Skeletal muscle necrosis Extensive cancer Progressive muscular dystrophy
Aspartate aminotransferase (AST, or SGOT)	10–50 mU/mL (slightly lower in women)	*Elevations* Skeletal muscle trauma Progressive muscular dystrophy
Aldolase A	1.3–8.2 U/dL	*Elevations* Polymyositis and dermatomyositis Muscular dystrophy

lationship. When calcium level decreases, phosphorus level increases, and vice versa. Bone and parathyroid gland disorders are often reflected in an alteration in serum calcium or phosphorus levels.

ALKALINE PHOSPHATASE LEVEL

Alkaline phosphatase (ALP) is an enzyme normally present in blood; its concentration increases when bone or liver damage occurs. In metabolic bone disease and bone cancer, the enzyme concentration rises in proportion to the osteoblastic activity, indicating bone forma-

tion. The level of ALP is normally slightly increased in the elderly (Garner, 1989).

ERYTHROCYTE SEDIMENTATION RATE

Although not a test specifically for musculoskeletal disorders, the erythrocyte sedimentation rate (ESR) is a sensitive indicator of inflammation and infection. For an unknown reason, in the presence of these conditions, red blood cells "settle" to the bottom of a test tube more rapidly than usual. The more severe the inflammation or infection, the higher the laboratory value is. A value between 20 and 40 mm/hour indicates a mild elevation, 40 to 70 mm/hour is a moderate level, and greater than 70 mm/hour denotes a severe problem. The normal value for women is usually slightly higher than that for men, and the normal value increases with age (Cella & Watson, 1989).

SERUM MUSCLE ENZYME LEVELS

The major muscle enzymes affected in skeletal muscle disease or injury are creatine kinase (CK), or creatine phosphokinase; aspartate aminotransferase (AST), formerly known as glutamic-oxaloacetic transaminase (SGOT); aldolase (ALD); and lactate dehydrogenase (LDH). As a result of damage, the muscle tissue releases additional amounts of these enzymes, resulting in increased serum levels. Serum CK level begins to rise in 2 to 4 hours after muscle injury and is elevated early in muscle disease, such as muscular dystrophy. The CK molecule has two subunits: M (muscle) and B (brain). Three isoenzymes have been identified. Skeletal muscle CK (CK-MM, CK_3) is the only isoenzyme that rises in concentration when damage occurs to skeletal muscle (Cella & Watson, 1989).

Moderate elevations of AST (three to five times normal) occur in certain muscle diseases, such as muscular dystrophy and dermatomyositis. The levels of the isoenzymes aldolase A (ALD A), LDH_4, and LDH_5 also increase in clients with these disorders (Cella & Watson, 1989).

RADIOGRAPHIC EXAMINATIONS

STANDARD RADIOGRAPHY

The skeleton and its supporting structures are readily visible using standard x-ray views. Radiographic testing begins with anteroposterior projections as a screening procedure. Other views, such as lateral or oblique approaches, are obtained, depending on the part of the skeleton to be evaluated. Observations of bone density, alignment, swelling, and intactness are made. The condition of joints, including the size of the joint space, the smoothness of articular cartilage, and synovial swelling, can be determined. Soft-tissue involvement is also evident. The nurse informs the client that the x-ray table is hard and cold and that the client should remain still during the filming process.

TOMOGRAPHY AND XERORADIOGRAPHY

Whereas standard radiographs superimpose one structure on another, tomography produces planes, or slices, for focus and blurs the images of other structures. This procedure is helpful in musculoskeletal assessment, as the many structures in proximity make visualization difficult. Xeroradiography highlights the contrast be-

tween structures, allowing margins and edges to be clearly seen (edge enhancement). Its disadvantages include the higher radiation dose to the client and the inability to determine tissue densities.

MYELOGRAPHY

Myelography requires the insertion of a contrast medium, or dye, into the subarachnoid space of the spine, usually via a lumbar puncture, to visualize the vertebral column, intervertebral disks, spinal nerve roots, and blood vessels. Although this test is commonly performed, it may become less popular as computed tomography (CT) and magnetic resonance imaging (MRI) replace such invasive diagnostic techniques.

Client Preparation. During the evening and morning before the study, the nurse provides increased amounts of oral or intravenous (IV) fluids to promote hydration. Most clients are allowed to have a clear or full liquid breakfast on the day of the test. Adequate hydration is essential to promote the manufacture of cerebrospinal fluid (CSF); prevent dehydration, which could result from posttest vomiting; and increase the rate at which the water-soluble contrast medium, if used, is excreted by the kidneys.

Phenothiazines and central nervous system (CNS) depressants and stimulants are not administered for 48 hours before the myelogram, as they decrease the seizure threshold and thus increase the risk of a seizure. The nurse asks if the client has a history of seizures, allergies to iodine or seafood, or renal or liver dysfunction. Most of the media are iodine based and may cause allergic reactions ranging from rashes to anaphylaxes. Metabolism and excretion of the water-soluble contrast medium depend on proper functioning of the liver and kidneys.

For the client having a myelogram, education regarding expectations during and after the procedure is crucial. The nurse needs to know what type of media will be used, as client care differs for each type.

Clients are frequently apprehensive about this procedure. They may fear discomfort or possible paralysis from having a needle inserted close to the spinal cord. The nurse assures the client that a local anesthetic helps to decrease discomfort, but that the client may experience a feeling of pressure at the needle site during insertion. Because the needle is placed below the level of the spinal cord, which ends between the first and second lumbar interspace, there is minimal risk of neurologic damage from needle insertion.

Procedure. Because of the nature and risks of myelography, the procedure is usually performed in a special procedures room in the radiology department or in the operating room. Emergency equipment is available, and clients are carefully monitored. The client is prepared as for surgery and therefore signs a consent form (see Chap. 18 for discussion of nurse's role in informed consent). Because CNS depressants are usually withheld, most clients do not receive heavy sedation before the test. Diazepam (Valium) is often administered intramuscularly for relaxation, anxiety reduction, and seizure prevention. To decrease swelling and the risk of allergy, methylprednisolone (Solu-Medrol), or other corticosteroid, or diphenhydramine (Benadryl) is given.

Three types of contrast media are available: air or oxygen, iophendylate (Pantopaque), and metrizamide (Amipaque). Air or oxygen is seldom used, except for individuals who are allergic to iodine-based media. Iophendylate is an oil-based iodine solution; metrizamide is a water-based iodine solution.

The spinal insertion site is typically in the lumbar region, although the cervical area is occasionally used. The client is placed in a prone position with a pillow under the abdomen, a sitting position flexed at the waist, or a side-lying, knee-chest position in preparation for the examination. After a local anesthetic is given, a large-gauge spinal needle is inserted into the third or fourth lumbar interspace. A larger needle is used for iophendylate, which is more viscous, than for the water-based medium. Approximately 6 to 15 mL of CSF is removed to allow room for the medium. An amount of contrast medium equal to the amount of CSF removed is slowly injected while observing for an immediate allergic reaction. The head of the examining table is tilted downward to allow the solution to ascend the spine for visualization of the cervical and thoracic regions via fluoroscopy. Serial radiographs are taken during this procedure. The client must not move so as not to dislodge the needle and must maintain neck hyperextension to prevent the solution from entering the cranium. If iophendylate is used, the solution is withdrawn after the films are obtained. As a water-soluble medium, metrizamide mixes with the CSF and cannot be removed.

Follow-up care. The client who was given iophendylate is placed flat in a supine position to prevent CSF leakage for at least 8 hours, depending on institutional policy. The client who received metrizamide is placed in a sitting position at a 15- to 45-degree angle for 8 to 16 hours to prevent ascension of the medium into the brain. This may be followed by an 8-hour period of remaining in a flat-lying position.

At the conclusion of the procedure, the nurse evaluates the client's neurologic status and monitors it carefully for the first 24 hours after myelography. The nurse assesses vital signs at frequent intervals, depending on institutional policy (usually every 4 hours); the client's ability to move the lower extremities; unusual sensation, such as tingling in the feet and legs; and complaints of radiating pain and discomfort in the lower back or extremities. The nurse immediately reports any change in motor or sensory status from pretest levels to the physician. (A description of neurologic assessment technique is found in Chap. 32.)

Although the client remains in bed for several hours, the nurse inspects the injection site by turning the client onto his/her side. Leakage of CSF (a clear fluid) or blood, or hematoma formation, is reported immediately. A large loss of fluid can result in a spinal headache, causing severe pain often not relieved by medication. If the headache lasts for a week or more, a "blood patch" may be performed in which 10 mL or more of the client's blood is inserted into the injection site for clotting and sealing the leak. This procedure is not commonly performed, as it is risky and must be performed by an anesthesiologist.

The client often complains of local discomfort at the injection site or muscle spasms triggered by manipulation during the test. Mild to moderate-strength analgesics are given, but potent narcotics (CNS depressants) are avoided for 24 hours to reduce the risk of a seizure. The elderly client may also experience discomfort caused by prolonged and uncomfortable positioning on a hard, cold table during the test. The nurse applies heat by heating pad or warm compresses to aching joints and muscles to promote comfort.

As a result of discomfort, temporary bed rest, and possible spinal nerve root damage, the client may not be able to void. The detrusor muscle of the bladder is innervated by the second through fourth sacral spinal nerves, which can be traumatized by the procedure. Male clients, in particular, have difficulty voiding in a supine position. If the client has received iophendylate, the physician often allows the client to stand at the bedside for voiding during the period of bed rest. The client who has been given metrizamide is usually allowed out of bed for bathroom privileges.

Headaches from CSF leakage occur most frequently in clients receiving the oil-based medium. Nausea, often accompanied by severe vomiting, is common in clients receiving metrizamide, particularly during the first 3 to 8 hours after the test. With either contrast medium, temporary or permanent neurologic deficits can occur. The accompanying Guidelines feature summarizes nursing interventions for the client who has undergone myelography. It is estimated that 20% to 25% of clients having a myelogram have at least one complication. The nurse carefully observes for signs of impending problems, which can then be treated and possibly reversed.

DISKOGRAPHY

Diskography is similar to myelography in that a contrast medium is injected for the purpose of visualizing intervertebral disks. The medium (1 mL or more) is injected directly into the disk targeted for examination, instead of into the subarachnoid space. Leakage of the solution often indicates a herniated disk. Because of the limitation of evaluating only one disk, the test is not as commonly employed as myelography or CT. The nursing care is similar to that discussed for myelography.

ARTHROGRAPHY

An arthrogram is an x-ray film of a joint after injection of a contrast medium (air or solution) to enhance its visualization. Double-contrast arthrography uses both air and

GUIDELINES ■ Care of the Client Who Has Undergone Myelography

Interventions	Rationales
1. Check the client's neurologic status immediately after the client returns to the room and every 1–2 h for the first 24 h (or according to institutional policy). If a change from pretest status is present, notify the physician immediately. a. Vital signs. b. Ability to move all extremities. c. Loss of sensation in extremities. d. Complaint of severe pain in back or extremities.	1. The contrast medium can temporarily or permanently injure the spinal cord, spinal nerves, or brain. The nurse compares pretest and posttest findings.
2. Check the needle puncture site for bleeding or other drainage when assessing neurologic status. If present, notify the physician immediately.	2. The spinal needle can cause local tissue trauma. If the site does not close, CSF can leak from the subarachnoid space, causing a CSF deficit and possibly severe headache.
3. Observe for adverse effects of contrast medium. a. Headache. b. Nausea or vomiting. c. Neurologic changes, such as disorientation or seizure.	3. These adverse effects can be uncomfortable or life-threatening and must be treated.
4. Maintain proper client positioning. a. The client remains flat in bed for 8–12 h after iophendylate administration (may turn from side to side). b. The client sits at 15- to 45-degree angle for 8–16 h, followed by 8 h flat in bed, after administration of metrizamide or other water-based medium.	4. Positioning depends on the type of dye used. a. Clients who received iophendylate have a CSF deficit of 6–15 mL from the procedure. If placed upright, the client can leak additional CSF, contributing to a severe headache. b. Clients who receive water-based media are at risk for its ascension into the brain tissue, causing neurologic damage.
5. Give prescribed pain medication as needed.	5. Clients often have mild to moderate discomfort at the needle site. They may also have a headache.
6. Check the client's ability to void. If the client has not voided within 8 h after the test, notify the physician.	6. The spinal needle can traumatize sacral nerves, which innervate the bladder.
7. Do not give CNS depressants or stimulants or phenothiazines for 24 h after the test. Observe for episodes of seizure.	7. These drugs lower a person's seizure threshold, increasing the risk of seizure activity.
8. Force oral fluids and maintain IV fluid administration if needed. Offer at least 8 oz/h.	8. Increasing fluid intake promotes CSF production, prevents dehydration from vomiting, and promotes excretion of water-based contrast media.
9. Explain interventions to the client.	9. Providing the client with information often promotes compliance and allays anxiety.

solution and is performed most commonly when a traumatic injury is suspected. The physician is often able to determine the presence of bone chips, torn ligaments, or other loose bodies within the joint.

Client preparation.   The most common joints studied are the knee and the shoulder. The nurse questions the client about allergy to seafood or iodine. The client is taken to the radiology department for the examination to be performed. The nurse informs the client that the test may be uncomfortable owing to pressure experienced at the needle insertion site. The client is also instructed that the joint will be swollen for several days after the test, and strenuous physical activity should be

avoided for 12 to 24 hours. After the test, the joint may be wrapped and ice may be applied at intervals for the first few hours to decrease swelling.

Procedure.   If the knee is examined, the client is placed in a sitting position to flex the joint. After administration of a local anesthetic, an iodine-based contrast medium is injected directly into the joint, using a medial or lateral approach. The client feels pressure, but should not experience pain. Radiographs are then taken of the joint, which may be put through ROM during the test.

Follow-up care.   Because the medium mixes with synovial fluid, it is not withdrawn after the procedure. As a result, the client's joint is enlarged and slightly uncomfortable. Some clients state that they feel the solution moving in the joint and hear "clicking" noises for several days until the solution is absorbed by the body. The client is instructed to resume usual activities, but to avoid strenuous exercise, such as participating in contact sports, for at least 12 hours after the test. An elastic bandage around the joint may be worn for several days; ice application may reduce some of the swelling.

COMPUTED TOMOGRAPHY

CT is gaining wide acceptance in the detection of musculoskeletal problems, particularly those of the vertebral column. It may be used with or without a contrast medium, which is given orally or intravenously. As a noninvasive procedure, it requires minimal nursing attention, except client education. During the procedure, the client must remain still on a hard table while encased in the machine. Complaints of claustrophobia and annoyance from the clicking sounds made by the scanner on rotation are common, but the nurse reassures the client that there is no danger from the machine.

OTHER DIAGNOSTIC TESTS

BONE BIOPSY

In a bone biopsy, a specimen of bone is extracted for microscopic examination, often confirming the presence of infection or neoplasm. Two techniques are used to retrieve the specimen: needle (closed) or incisional (open) biopsy.

Client preparation. The nurse teaches the client about the procedure and posttest care. The open technique is more invasive and requires the most care.

Procedure. The test may be performed in the client's room, a special procedures room in the radiology department, or the operating room under local or general anesthesia. After anesthesia is induced, a long needle is inserted into the bone cortex or a small incision is made to reveal the bone tissue. A sterile dressing is applied after extraction of the osseous tissue. If an incision is made, a pressure dressing is used.

Follow-up care. The nurse inspects the biopsy site for bleeding, swelling, and hematoma formation, the most common complications of bone biopsy. Because the pressure dressing inhibits observation, the nurse monitors the client's level of pain. If internal bleeding or marked swelling occurs, the client complains of severe pain, instead of the mild to moderate discomfort usually resulting from the procedure. To decrease the likelihood of bleeding, the affected extremity is immobilized for 12 to 24 hours. Vital signs, taken at least every 4 hours for the first 24 hours after the biopsy, not only help in ascertaining the presence of bleeding, but also indicate bone infection, the second most common complication of biopsy after hemorrhage. A mild analgesic often relieves the discomfort resulting from the procedure. The nurse reapplies sterile dressings daily over the incision site after an open biopsy, inspecting the wound for signs of inflammation or infection, such as redness, warmth, and tissue swelling.

MUSCLE BIOPSY

Muscle biopsies are done for the diagnosis of atrophy (as in muscular dystrophy) and inflammation (as in polymyositis). The procedure and care for clients having this procedure are the same as those for bone biopsy.

ELECTROMYOGRAPHY

Electromyography (EMG) is usually accompanied by nerve conduction studies to determine the electrical potential generated in an individual muscle. It is helpful in the diagnosis of neuromuscular, lower motor neuron, and peripheral nerve disorders.

Client preparation. The nurse informs the client that the test may cause temporary discomfort, especially when the client is subjected to episodes of electrical current. Some physicians order pretest baseline serum muscle enzyme determinations for comparison with posttest levels (7 to 10 days after EMG); the levels are sometimes increased as a result of the procedure. For selected clients, mild sedation is ordered. The physician may also order a temporary discontinuation of skeletal muscle relaxants several days before the procedure to prevent the effects of medication on test results.

Procedure. The test may be performed at the bedside or in an EMG laboratory. When both the EMG and nerve conduction studies are done, nerve conduction is usually tested first. Flat electrodes are placed along the nerve to be evaluated, and small doses of electrical current are passed via the electrodes to the nerve and muscle innervated. If nerve conduction is accomplished, the muscle contracts.

To test muscle potential, multiple needle electrodes, varying from 1.3 to 7.5 cm (½ to 3 in), are inserted. The client may be asked to perform activities to measure muscle potential during minimal and maximal contraction. The degree of nerve and muscle activity is recorded on an oscilloscope, providing a graphic readout for later interpretation.

Follow-up care. There are few medical complications of the procedure. The nurse provides comfort measures and inspects the needle sites for hematoma formation. The nurse can apply ice to prevent this complication. The client may complain of increased pain and anxiety after the test.

ARTHROSCOPY

An arthroscope is a tubular device inserted into a joint for direct visualization; the knee and shoulder are most commonly tested. In addition to a diagnosis, synovial biopsy and surgical procedures to repair traumatic injury can be accomplished with the arthroscope. A discussion of these uses of arthroscopy is in Chapter 31.

Client preparation. Because the knee is most commonly evaluated, the care described for the client undergoing this procedure relates to that joint. If the client is having a diagnostic procedure, it is performed on an ambulatory basis or as same-day surgery. Clients who cannot flex their knees at least 40 degrees or who have infected knees are not candidates for the test. The procedure requires knee flexion, and joint infection could worsen from the mechanical trauma of arthroscope insertion.

If possible, the client should have a physical therapy consultation before surgery to learn the leg exercises that are necessary after the test. Straight-leg raises (SLR) and quadriceps setting exercises (isometrics with the leg extended) are practiced in sets of 10 each. ROM exercises are also taught, but may not be allowed immediately after the test if arthroscopic surgery is performed. The nurse can teach these exercises or reinforce the information provided by the physical therapist. The nurse also explains the procedure and posttest care.

Procedure. The client is usually placed under light general, epidural, or spinal anesthesia. In some hospitals, a large tourniquet is used around the thigh to minimize bleeding during the procedure; medications promoting vasoconstriction to control bleeding may be used alone or in conjunction with the tourniquet. The knee is flexed to at least 40 degrees, and saline or Ringer's lactate is used to irrigate the knee. As shown in Figure 29–5, the arthroscope is inserted through a small incision less than 0.6 cm (1/4 in). Multiple incisions may be required to allow for inspection at a variety of angles. After the procedure, a bulky pressure dressing and elastic bandage may be applied, depending on the amount of manipulation used during the test or surgery.

Follow-up care. The nurse evaluates the neurovascular status of the client's affected leg frequently, in accordance with nursing standards of care. The typical protocol is every hour for the first 4 hours, decreasing to every 4 hours for the next 24 hours. The technique for this evaluation is described in Chapter 31. The client is encouraged to perform exercises as taught before the examination. For the mild discomfort experienced after the diagnostic arthroscopy, a mild analgesic, such as acetaminophen (Tylenol), is given. The client seldom has activity restrictions and often returns to normal daily activities immediately. When arthroscopic surgery is performed, a narcotic-analgesic combination, such as oxycodone and acetaminophen (Percocet), is usually prescribed.

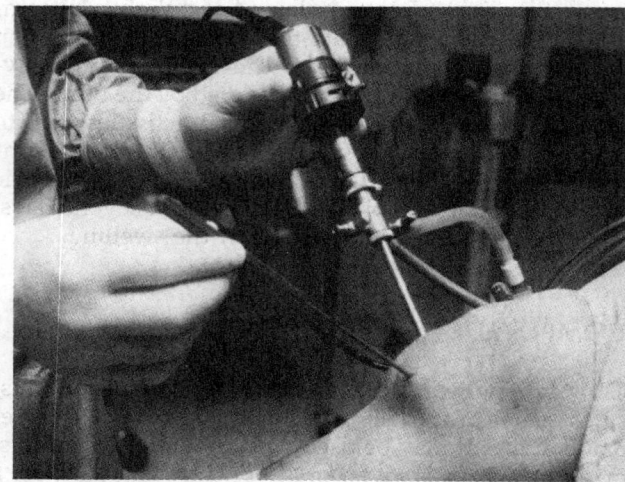

Figure 29–5

An arthroscope is used in the diagnosis of joint pathologic changes. (From Kelley, W. N., Harris, E. D., Jr., Ruddy, S., & Sledge, C. B. [1989]. *Textbook of rheumatology* [3rd ed., p. 11]. Philadelphia: W. B. Saunders.)

Although complications are not common, the nurse monitors and teaches the client to monitor for hypothermia (decreased body temperature) resulting from the use of the tourniquet during the procedure, increased joint pain attributable to mechanical injury, thrombophlebitis, and infection. Severe joint or leg pain after discharge from the hospital may be indicative of a possible complication and warrants that the client contact the physician immediately. The client is seen by the physician about 1 week after the test to check for complications.

BONE SCAN

The bone scan is a radionuclide test in which radioactive material is injected for visualization of the entire skeleton. It is used primarily for the detection of tumors, arthritis, osteomyelitis, osteoporosis, vertebral compression fractures, and unexplained bone pain.

Client preparation. The client is given the radioactive isotope technetium (^{99m}Tc) intravenously by a nuclear medicine physician or technician 2 to 3 hours before the scanning procedure. As a bone-seeking substance, the isotope migrates to bone. The nurse assures the client that the dose is minimal and that no complications will result from receipt of the material. The client is asked to void immediately before the scan to prevent an obliterated view of the pelvis.

Procedure. The client is taken to the nuclear medicine department and placed on the scanning table. The client must be able to lie still for 30 to 60 minutes while scanning occurs to provide an accurate image. Clients who are elderly, restless, or in pain may find this test uncomfortable and may need mild sedation. The examiner looks for areas of bone in which there is an increased uptake, or concentration, of the isotope. These hot lesions indicate abnormal bone metabolism, a sign of bone disease. Cold lesions, in which there is a decreased uptake, indicate poor blood flow to bone, as seen in severe arteriosclerosis.

Follow-up care.   The amount of radioactivity in the isotope is minimal and presents no hazard to the client or the nurse. The substance is excreted in urine and stool. Because there is rapid deterioration of the substance in the body, no special precautions are required when handling excreta. Repeated scans may be taken, but do not require additional injection of the radioisotope.

GALLIUM SCAN

The gallium scan is similar to the bone scan, but is more specific and sensitive in detecting bone problems. Gallium citrate (^{67}Ga) is the radioisotope used. This substance also migrates to brain, liver, and breast tissue and therefore is used to examine these structures when suspected of disease.

Client preparation.   Because bone takes up gallium more slowly than technetium, the material is administered by a nuclear medicine physician or technician 1 to 3 days before scanning. Tests that require contrast media or other isotopes cannot be given during this time. The nurse instructs the client that the radioactive material poses no threat to the client, as the material readily deteriorates in the body. Because gallium is excreted through the intestinal tract, it tends to collect in feces before the scanning procedure. Serial enemas may be given during the time between administration of the isotope and the scan to prevent a false test reading if the abdomen is scanned.

Procedure.   Depending on the tissue to be examined, the client is taken to the nuclear medicine department 1 to 3 days after injection. The procedure takes 30 to 60 minutes, during which time the client must lie still for accurate test results to be achieved. Mild sedation may be required to facilitate relaxation and cooperation during the procedure for confused elderly clients or those in severe pain.

Follow-up care.   There is no special care required after the test. The radioisotope is excreted via stool and urine, but no precautions are taken when handling the excreta. Follow-up scans may be taken to monitor excretion from the body.

INDIUM IMAGING

Indium imaging is used primarily in the detection of bone infection. The client's leukocytes are separated

from a blood sample, labeled (or tagged) with indium (^{111}In), and injected intravenously. In acute bone infection (osteomyelitis), the labeled leukocytes accumulate and can be seen on scanning. There is no special client preparation or follow-up care for this test.

MAGNETIC RESONANCE IMAGING

MRI can be used for diagnosis of musculoskeletal disorders. The image is produced through the interaction of magnetic fields, radiowaves, and atomic nuclei showing hydrogen density. For some tissues, the cross-sectional image is better than that produced by radiography or CT. The lack of hydrogen ions in cortical bone makes it easily distinguishable from soft tissues. The test is particularly useful in identifying problems with muscle, tendons, and ligaments.

The nurse ensures that the client removes all metal objects and checks for clothing zippers and metal fasteners. Although joint implants that are titanium or stainless steel based are safe, other devices such as pacemakers and surgical clips are not. A complete list of questions that the nurse must consider before the client has the test is provided in Table 29–3. Although MRI is a noninvasive procedure, the client may complain of discomfort and claustrophobia from lying still for 30 to 60 minutes while encased in a large machine (Zubay, 1988).

ULTRASONOGRAPHY

For soft-tissue disorders, such as masses and fluid accumulation, an ultrasound procedure in which sound waves produce an image of the tissue may be used. A jelly-like substance is applied to the skin over the site to

---

TABLE 29–3   Nursing Considerations for the Client Preparing for Magnetic Resonance Imaging

Is the client pregnant?

Does the client weigh more than 260 lb?

Does the client have magnetic metal fragments or implants, such as an aneurysm clip?

If the client has an IV catheter, can it be converted to a heparin lock temporarily?

Is the client claustrophobic?

Does the client have a pacemaker or electronic implant?

Can the client be without supplemental oxygen for an hour?

Can the client tolerate the supine position for 20–30 min?

Can the client lie still for 20–30 min?

Does the client need life-support equipment?

Can the client communicate clearly and understand verbal communication?

be examined to promote the movement of a metal probe. No special preparation or posttest care is necessary.

SUMMARY

Musculoskeletal assessment depends on a combination of accurate history taking, physical examination, and diagnostic studies. The nurse uses communication and physical assessment skills to identify nursing diagnoses for intervention. Clients having diagnostic tests are taught about the procedures and the follow-up care essential for the promotion of wellness.

REFERENCES AND READINGS

Bassett, L. W., Gold, R. H., & Webber, M. M. (1981). Radionuclide bone imaging. *Radiology Clinics of North America, 19*, 675–702.

Bates, B. (1987). *A guide to physical examination and history taking.* Philadelphia: J. B. Lippincott.

Bradley, W. G., & Sheldon, C. H. (1983). Nuclear magnetic resonance imaging. *American Journal of Surgery, 146*, 85–87.

Cella, J. H., & Watson, J. (1989). *Nurse's manual of laboratory tests.* Philadelphia: F. A. Davis.

Deutsch, S. D., & Gandsman, E. G. (1983). The use of bone scanning for the diagnosis and management of musculoskeletal trauma. *Surgical Clinics of North America, 63*, 567–585.

Farrell, J. (1986). *Illustrated guide to orthopedic nursing.* Philadelphia: J. B. Lippincott.

Garner, B. C. (1989). Guide to changing lab values in elders. *Geriatric Nursing, 10*, 144–145.

Genant, H. K. (1981). Computed tomography in diagnosis of bone and joint disorders. In D. Resnick & G. Niwayama (Eds.), *Diagnosis of bone and joint disorders.* Philadelphia: W. B. Saunders.

Greipp, M. E. (1988). Anthropometric considerations in the orthopaedic assessment. *Orthopaedic Nursing, 7(4)*, 36–40.

Kalbach, L. R. (1989). Spinal headache: Cause and care. *Orthopaedic Nursing, 8(2)*, 51–55.

Kirschner, P. T., & Simon, M. A. (1981). Radio-isotopic evaluation of skeletal disease. *Journal of Bone and Joint Surgery, 63A*, 673–681.

Magee, D. J. (1987). *Orthopaedic physical assessment.* Philadelphia: W. B. Saunders.

Malasanos, L., Barkauskas, V., Moss, M., & Stoltenberg-Allen, K. (1986). *Health assessment.* St. Louis: C. V. Mosby.

Moon, K. L., Genant, H. K., Helms, C. A., Chafetz, N. I., Crooks, L. E., & Kaufman, L. (1983). Musculoskeletal applications of nuclear magnetic resonance. *Radiology, 147*, 161–171.

Pellino, T. A., Mooney, N. E., Salmond, S. W., & Verdisco, L. A. (1986). *Core curriculum for orthopaedic nursing.* Pitman, NJ: Anthony J. Janetti.

Propst-Proctor, S. L., Dillingham, M. F., McDougall, I. R., & Goodwin, D. (1982). The white blood cell scan in orthopedics. *Clinical Orthopedics, 168*, 157–165.

Schneider, R. (1983). Percutaneous needle bone biopsy. *Orthopaedic Review, 12*, 119–125.

Sculco, T. P. (Ed.). (1985). *Orthopaedic care of the geriatric patient.* St. Louis: C. V. Mosby.

Stewart, J. R., & Thorne, R. P. (1985). Complications of metrizamide (Amipaque) myelography. *Orthopaedic Nursing, 4(4)*, 53–54.

Weissman, B. N., & Sledge, C. B. (1986). *Orthopedic radiology.* Philadelphia: W. B. Saunders.

Zubay, R. L. (1988). Understanding magnetic resonance imaging from a nursing perspective. *Orthopaedic Nursing, 7(6)*, 17–23.

ADDITIONAL READINGS

Huffer, J. M. (1988). The use of x-rays in caring for fracture, dislocation of the elbow. *Orthopaedic Nursing, 7*, 59–63.

This article discusses various types of radiographic examinations and their advantages in diagnosing fractures and dislocations. Tomography, CT, and MRI are especially sensitive in determining the presence or absence of fragments within a joint.

MacArthur, B. J. (1986). Arthroscopy of the shoulder. *Orthopedic Nursing, 5(4)*, 26–28.

This article emphasizes the usefulness of shoulder arthroscopy in the diagnosis and possible surgical treatment of shoulder trauma. The procedure is described, including the operating room set-up and equipment. Preoperative and postoperative nursing care is also discussed, with an emphasis on health teaching for discharge.

Schoen, D. C. (1986). Musculoskeletal assessment. In D. C. Schoen, *The nursing process in orthopaedics* (pp. 13–62). Norwalk, CT: Appleton-Century-Crofts.

This chapter describes musculoskeletal assessment, with emphasis on the physical examination. Specific instructions for the client are provided for the nurse to use when assessing ROM, and multiple illustrations demonstrate the movement of each joint.

Stearns, H. C., & Stearns, C. M. (1986). Orthopaedic radiology. *Orthopaedic Nursing, 5(2)*, 26–31.

The authors present concise, yet meaningful, descriptions of the radiologic studies utilized for musculoskeletal problems. They discuss the interpretation of common findings, focusing on deformity, joint congruity, bone density, and calcification. An etiologic classification of orthopaedic disorders is also presented.

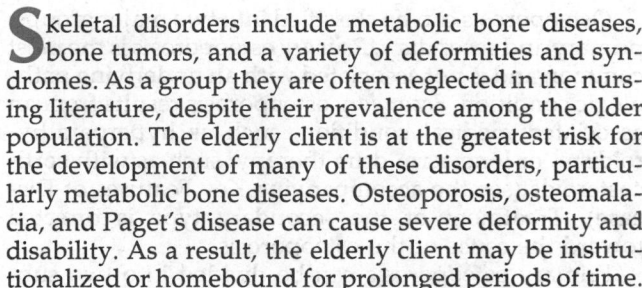

CHAPTER 30

Interventions for Clients with Musculoskeletal Disorders

Skeletal disorders include metabolic bone diseases, bone tumors, and a variety of deformities and syndromes. As a group they are often neglected in the nursing literature, despite their prevalence among the older population. The elderly client is at the greatest risk for the development of many of these disorders, particularly metabolic bone diseases. Osteoporosis, osteomalacia, and Paget's disease can cause severe deformity and disability. As a result, the elderly client may be institutionalized or homebound for prolonged periods of time.

The incidence of bone cancer is increasing in both the young and the elderly population. As technologic advances occur and clients survive longer with primary lesions, metastatic cancer becomes more prevalent. Care for clients with skeletal disorders is challenging and, at times, frustrating. Although cures are not always available, the nurse can help the client reach an optimal level of health through support and health teaching.

METABOLIC BONE DISEASES

OSTEOPOROSIS

OVERVIEW

Osteoporosis is an age-related metabolic disease in which bone demineralization results in decreased density and subsequent fractures. The wrist, the hip, and the vertebral column are most frequently affected. Osteoporosis is a major health problem in the United States, and the estimated cost for osteoporosis-related health care is more than $6 billion each year. Osteoporosis is the twelfth leading cause of death in the United States.

Pathophysiology

Bone is a dynamic tissue. Throughout the life span, new bone is formed by osteoblastic activity, while old bone is resorbed through osteoclastic activity. Bone mass, or density, peaks between 30 and 35 years of age. After the peak years, calcium stored in cancellous, or spongy, bone leaves the tissue, followed by a loss of calcium from the cortical, or compact, bone. As a result, more than 1.5 million fractures per year occur in persons older than 45 years (Consensus Conference, 1984).

Bone mass decreases rapidly in postmenopausal women as serum estrogen levels diminish. Approximately 40% to 45% of a woman's bone mass is lost during her life span. It is estimated that 50% of all women older than 65 years of age have symptomatic osteoporosis (Mundy, 1983).

Osteoporosis can be classified into two major groups: primary and secondary. *Primary* osteoporosis is the most common and is not associated with an underlying pathologic condition. *Secondary* osteoporosis results from an associated medical condition, such as hyperparathyroidism, or long-term drug therapy, such as with corticosteroids (see the accompanying Key Features of Disease). Treatment of the secondary type is directed toward the cause of the osteoporosis.

Primary osteoporosis can be divided into two subtypes. The *postmenopausal* type occurs in women between the ages of 55 and 65 years. Estrogen presumably prevents or decreases the rate of bone resorption in women and is therefore unavailable in sufficient quantities after menopause. Vertebral and wrist fractures are common in this group, as the predominant bone type in these areas is cancellous. *Senile* osteoporosis occurs in those older than 65 years of age, affecting women twice as often as men. Hip and vertebral fractures are frequently seen in persons with this type of disease.

The exact pathophysiology of osteoporosis remains a mystery. Two theories of disease development have been advocated. First, osteoporosis may result from decreased osteoblastic activity. The osteoblasts, or bone-forming cells, may have a shortened life span or be less efficient in the osteoporotic client. The second and more popular theory suggests an increase in osteoclastic, or bone resorption, activity. The latter theory has gained increased recognition over the past few years, and has directed treatment of the disease toward measures to prevent rapid bone resorption.

Etiology

The exact cause of osteoporosis is unknown; however, numerous risk factors have been identified as contributing to the likelihood that an individual will become osteoporotic. Osteoporosis most frequently occurs in women, in Caucasians, and after menopause. In addition, body build seems to predict the occurrence of the disease. Osteoporosis occurs more frequently in thin, lean-built individuals, particularly those who do not exercise regularly. Obese women can store estrogen in their tissues for use as necessary to maintain a normal level of serum calcium. Exercise decreases bone resorption and stimulates bone formation. Immobilization, such as prolonged bed rest, produces rapid bone loss.

The relationship of osteoporosis to dietary factors is not as well established. A diet deficient in calcium and vitamin D stimulates the parathyroid gland to produce parathyroid hormone (PTH), which triggers the release of calcium from the bony matrix. Malabsorption, caused by disease or drugs, also contributes to low serum calcium levels. Institutionalized or homebound persons who are not exposed to sunlight may be at risk, as they do not receive adequate vitamin D for the metabolism of calcium.

As aging occurs, the concentration of 1,25-dihydroxycholecalciferol, a vitamin D metabolite, decreases in the serum. In addition, osteoporosis is often accompanied by low levels of serum calcitonin, a hormone secreted by the thyroid gland that aids in maintaining a normal serum calcium level.

Protein deficiency may also contribute to the incidence of bone demineralization, although this theory is controversial. Because 50% of serum calcium is protein bound, protein is needed for calcium utilization. On the other hand, excessive protein intake may increase calcium loss in the urine.

Alcohol consumption and cigarette smoking have also been cited as possible risk factors. Although the exact mechanisms are not known, it is believed that these substances promote acidosis, which in turn increases bone loss. Excessive caffeine intake, for example, coffee and soft drinks, can increase calcium loss in the urine.

Hereditary factors may play a role, but this hypothesis has not been confirmed. Several of the suspected risk factors, such as body build, are determined in part by heredity; however, it is likely that heredity or a genetic influence alone does not predict osteoporosis. A recent study demonstrated that daughters of osteopo-

---

KEY FEATURES OF DISEASE ■ Causes of Secondary Osteoporosis

Diseases/Conditions

Diabetes mellitus
Hyperthyroidism
Hyperparathyroidism
Cushing's syndrome
Growth hormone deficiency
Metabolic acidosis
Female hypogonadism
Paget's disease
Osteogenesis imperfecta
Rheumatoid arthritis
Prolonged immobilization
Marfan's syndrome
Bone cancer
Cirrhosis
Chronic obstructive pulmonary disease

Drugs (Chronic Use)

Corticosteroids
Heparin
Anticonvulsants
Ethanol

rotic clients have lower bone mass than daughters of nonosteoporotic clients (Evans et al., 1988).

Incidence

More than 20 million Americans have osteoporosis. The incidence of the disease is greater in women than in men (at least 5:1), with Caucasian women being affected more often than Black. It is well documented that Black women have 10% more bone mass than Caucasian women. Postmenopausal women are at the highest risk, regardless of race.

In those older than 90 years of age, 32% of women and 17% of men experience at least one hip fracture as a result of osteoporosis (Consensus Conference, 1984). Women are at higher risk than men, as they have less bone mass. The mortality for elderly clients with hip fractures is more than 50%, and the debilitating effects can be devastating. (See Chap. 31 for discussion of hip fractures.)

PREVENTION

Osteoporosis is an irreversible osteopenia, or bone mass loss. Prevention is aimed toward minimizing risk factors and retarding the progress of the disorder. Aggressive preventive measures are reserved for women who are at the highest risk (i.e., Caucasian, thin, postmenopausal women). Preventive measures include drug therapy, diet therapy, and exercise.

Estrogen replacement is effective in preventing bone loss. Studies have shown a remarkable reduction of fractures in women undergoing estrogen therapy (Miller, 1985). It is recommended, however, that the drug be initiated within 3 to 5 years after menopause, as later induction may not be beneficial.

Low doses of conjugated estrogen, such as 0.625 mg of Premarin, are administered every day, as the side effects of the drug are potentially serious (Table 30–1). As a result of the side effects, some physicians do not utilize the drug for preventive purposes. Other physicians believe that the benefit of estrogen in preventing potentially debilitating and life-threatening fractures outweighs its risks. The woman who has a premature onset of menopause (for example, after surgical removal of the ovaries) is more likely to receive estrogen therapy than the woman who experiences a natural onset of menopause.

If an individual cannot ingest sufficient quantities of calcium in the diet, calcium supplements are used. Supplements are started as early as 40 years of age in the high-risk population, because bone resorption accelerates after age 35 years. Calcium carbonate, found in over-the-counter (OTC) drugs such as Tums, is probably the most efficacious. Forty per cent of calcium carbonate is elemental calcium that can be utilized by the body. For example, a 600-mg tablet contains about 240 mg of elemental calcium.

Calcium supplements should be taken under the supervision of a physician or nurse practitioner. As shown in Table 30–1, hypercalcemia, or excess serum calcium, can cause serious damage to the urinary system. The amount of calcium prescribed is affected by the addition of estrogen therapy and the presence of risk factors for the development of osteoporosis.

In the United States, the typical daily intake of dietary calcium is between 450 and 550 mg. The recommended daily allowance (RDA) of calcium is 800 mg (see the accompanying Nursing Research feature). Many clinicians and researchers believe that the RDA is insufficient to meet the calcium requirements of postmenopausal women. Studies indicate that the estrogen-

NURSING RESEARCH

Typical Calcium Intake of Young Women Is Below RDA — and Even RDA May Be Too Low.

Carter, L. W. (1987). Calcium intake in young adult women: Implications for osteoporosis risk assessment. *Journal of Obstetric, Gynecologic, and Neonatal Nursing, 16*, 301–308.

Insufficient dietary calcium intake is directly related to an increased incidence of osteoporosis and subsequent fractures. The RDA for calcium is 800 mg, but studies have demonstrated that this level should be increased to 1250 mg to decrease the risk of osteoporosis. This descriptive study surveyed a convenience sample of 41 healthy, Caucasian women, who were not pregnant or menopausal, to quantify their daily calcium intake. Their ages ranged from 25 to 35 years.

A written instrument was administered face-to-face to record a 3-day dietary recall. The research tool was tested for content validity, but reliability was not evaluated.

Eighteen of the 41 subjects consumed 0 to 800 mg (mean 484 mg), and 13 consumed 801 to 1250 mg daily (mean 968 mg). The primary source of calcium was milk products. Eleven women reported broken bones in either their mothers or grandmothers.

Critique. This study used a homogeneous convenience sample who relied on recall of the data needed to answer the research question. Although the tool was tested for content validity, no reliability was assessed. Generalizability of the findings is therefore limited.

Possible nursing implications. Nurses need to teach women about the importance of increasing their dietary calcium intake to prevent osteoporosis. The author suggested that teaching should begin as early as adolescence.

Nurses also need to place pressure on federal legislators regarding the need to raise the RDA from 800 to at least 1250 mg. In 1985, the National Research Council recommended this increase, but the group was disbanded by Congress before action could be taken.

TABLE 30–1 Drugs Used in the Prevention and Treatment of Osteoporosis

Drug	Usual Daily Dosage	Interventions	Rationales
Calcium, preferably calcium carbonate (e.g., Os-Cal, Tums, Caltrate-600, and Ca-Plus)	1.0.–1.5 g in divided doses PO	1. Give 1 h before meals.	1. Calcium may cause gastrointestinal irritation if taken when the stomach remains empty; free hydrochloric acid is needed for calcium absorption.
		2. Give a third of daily dose at bedtime. Push fluids.	2. Calcium is most readily utilized by the body when the client is fasting and immobile. Increased fluid intake aids in preventing the formation of calcium-based urinary stones.
		3. Assess for history of urinary stones.	3. Calcium supplements are not given to clients who are susceptible to urinary stone formation.
		4. Monitor serum calcium level.	4. Hypercalcemia, or calcium excess, is a side effect of calcium supplementation.
		5. Monitor urinary calcium level (no more than 4 mg/kg in 24 h).	5. The kidneys attempt to excrete excess calcium.
		6. Observe for signs of hypercalcemia.	6. Hypercalcemia can result in urinary stones, cardiac arrhythmias, and an increase or decrease in skeletal muscle tone.
Conjugated estrogen (e.g., Premarin, Estinyl, and Estrace) — may be given with progesterone on d 16–25	0.425–1.25 mg PO for 25 d/mo	1. Assess for history of tumors, hypertension, thromboembolytic disease, or liver or gallbladder disease.	1. Estrogen therapy is withheld from clients with susceptibility to an exacerbation of one or more of these problems.
		2. Teach the importance of gynecologic exams every 6 mo.	2. Endometrial and breast cancer can result from estrogen therapy.

treated woman needs at least 1000 mg/day, and that other postmenopausal women require as much as 1500 mg or more daily to prevent osteoporosis (Consensus Conference, 1984). An increased calcium intake may prevent bone loss in men as well. Foods rich in calcium include milk and dairy products and dark-green, leafy vegetables (see the Health Promotion/Maintenance feature on p. 738).

Vitamin D supplementation may be necessary for the institutionalized or homebound individual. An adequate level of vitamin D is needed for optimal calcium absorption in the intestines. The prescribed dosage is usually 400 to 800 IU/day. Higher doses can produce toxic effects, such as hypercalcemia and hyperphosphatemia.

Because consumption of alcohol and caffeine may

TABLE 30–1   Drugs Used in the Prevention and Treatment of Osteoporosis *Continued*

Drug	Usual Daily Dosage	Interventions	Rationales
		3. Teach breast self-examination.	3. Clients can detect potentially malignant lesions early so that treatment can begin immediately.
		4. Observe for vaginal bleeding.	4. Vaginal bleeding is a side effect of estrogen therapy and a sign of possible endometrial cancer.
		5. Monitor blood pressure.	5. Hypertension and other cardiovascular complications may result from combined estrogen-progesterone therapy.
		6. Observe for thrombus formation.	6. Thrombophlebitis is a complication of combined estrogen-progesterone therapy.
		7. Monitor serum liver enzyme and cholesterol levels.	7. An elevation of liver enzyme levels may be indicative of liver involvement resulting from estrogen. An elevated cholesterol level can result in hypertension and thrombus formation.
Vitamin D (e.g., ergocalciferol, calcitriol, and calcifediol)	7000–8000 IU PO	1. Observe for signs of hypercalcemia and hyperphosphatemia.	1. Calcium and phosphate excess can result from excessive vitamin D therapy.
		2. Monitor renal status.	2. Excessive serum calcium levels can result in urinary stone formation.
Sodium fluoride	40–90 mg in divided doses	1. Give 15 min before meals or with meals	1. Gastric irritation may result if sodium fluoride is given when the stomach is empty.
		2. Observe for synovitis or joint inflammation.	2. Synovitis is a side effect of sodium fluoride therapy.

contribute to the development of osteoporosis, these substances should be avoided. Smoking should also be discouraged.

Weight-bearing exercises are recommended to prevent bone resorption. A reasonable exercise program, including walking and swimming, may stimulate bone formation as well. Exercise should be performed up to the point at which bone pain occurs. Too much exercise can be as hazardous as too little. Trivial, or minimal, trauma caused by overexertion can lead to fractures and damage to other body systems.

Because most osteoporosis-related fractures occur in the elderly person, prevention of falls is also important. Drugs that cause incoordination and drowsiness should be used with caution in the elderly population. In addition, environmental hazards, such as a cluttered room

HEALTH PROMOTION/MAINTENANCE ■ Foods High in Calcium Content

Food	Serving Size	Calcium Content (mg)*
Milk (whole or skim)	8 oz	300
Cheese		
Swiss	1 oz	270
Cheddar	1 oz	205
American	1 oz	175
Cottage	1 c	130
Yogurt	8 oz	275–450†
Sardines with bones	3 oz	370
Green vegetables (cooked)‡		
Collard greens	1 c	360
Bok choy	1 c	250
Broccoli	1 c	135
Rhubarb (cooked)	1 c	210

* Approximate value.
† Depends on brand.
‡ Some green vegetables, e.g., spinach and beet greens, should be avoided as they contain oxalic acid, which binds calcium.

and scatter rugs, should be manipulated or eliminated to prevent falls.

COLLABORATIVE MANAGEMENT

 Assessment

History

When taking a history from a client with osteoporosis, the nurse keeps the risk factors for the disorder in mind. Data to collect from the client include *age, sex,* and *race,* as the disorder occurs most frequently in middle-aged and elderly, Caucasian, postmenopausal women. Because thin, petite women are more predisposed to rapid bone loss than heavier women, *body build, weight,* and *height* are important data to obtain. Other risk factors to look for are the client's usual *exposure to sunlight, cigarette and alcohol use,* and *caffeine consumption.* Each of these is thought to contribute to the development of osteoporosis.

The nurse takes a thorough *diet history* to determine daily calcium and vitamin D intake. The client is asked to recall a typical day's food and beverage intake at home. The nurse also asks whether the client *exercises* routinely and what type of exercise is performed. *Concurrent medical conditions* may contribute to the development of osteoporosis. If the client is unable to recall this information, previous medical records are obtained if possible. The nurse asks the client to list past and current *medications,* prescribed and OTC. It is important to know whether the client has been or is being treated for osteoporosis. In addition, a *family history* of the disorder is noted.

Because the client is often hospitalized for a fracture from osteoporosis, the client is asked to recall a past or current *history of falls or sudden movements.* The client usually complains of back pain or hip pain from a fall or jerky movement. The nurse asks whether the client has experienced a *previous fracture* and when it occurred.

In addition to information about the client, the nurse assesses the client's environment and daily routine. These data indicate the likelihood of a fall, which could result in life-threatening fractures. Of particular importance is information regarding the client's residence. For example, does the client need to use stairs? Is there adequate space to walk easily in each room? Are the floors waxed? carpeted? Are scatter rugs used?

Physical Assessment: Clinical Manifestations

Typically, osteoporosis is diagnosed after the client sustains a vertebral, wrist, or hip fracture. The client may be asymptomatic before admission with one or more bone fractures.

When performing a musculoskeletal assessment, the nurse inspects and palpates the vertebral column. The classic dowager's hump, or *kyphosis* of the dorsal spine, is usually present (Fig. 30–1). The client often states that height has been shortened, perhaps as much as 2 to 3 in within the previous 20 years. Accompanying the spinal

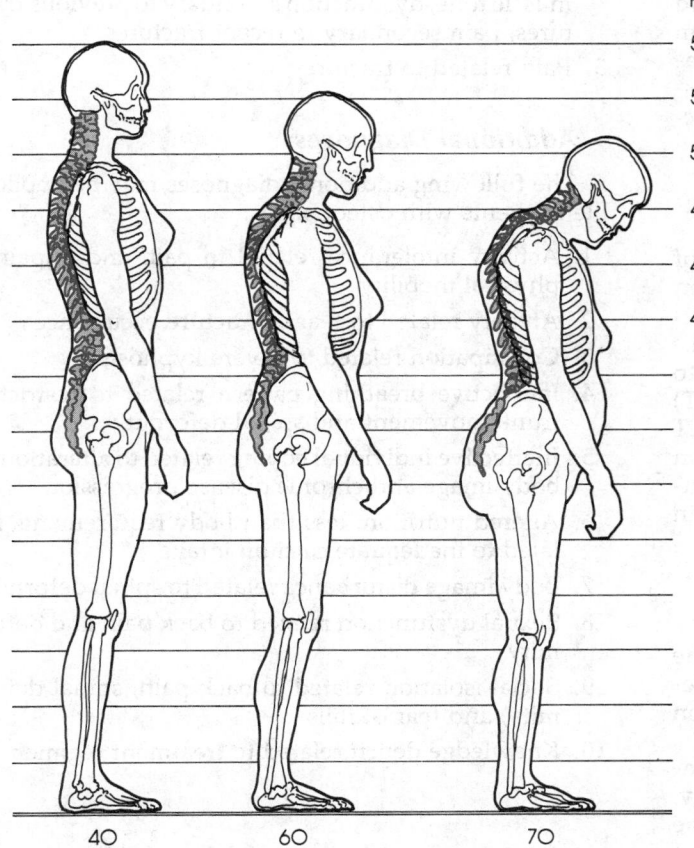

Figure 30–1

Normal spine at age 40 and osteoporotic changes at ages 60 and 70. These changes can cause a loss of as much as 6 to 9 in in height and can result in the so-called dowager's hump (far right) in the upper thoracic vertebrae.

deformity is the complaint of *back pain,* which frequently occurs after lifting, bending, or stooping. The pain may be sharp and acute in onset. Pain is worse with activity and is relieved by rest. Palpation of the vertebrae, particularly the lower thoracic and lumbar vertebrae, usually increases the client's discomfort. Therefore, palpation should be gentle.

Back pain accompanied by *tenderness* and *voluntary restriction of spinal movement* is indicative of one or more compression vertebral fractures, the most common type of osteoporotic fracture. Movement restriction and spinal deformity may result in constipation, abdominal distention, and respiratory compromise in severe cases. The most likely area for fracture occurrence is between T8 and L3.

Fractures are also common in the distal end of the radius and the upper third of the femur. Special attention is directed to these areas as part of the physical assessment. (See Chap. 31 for further discussion of wrist and hip fractures.)

Psychosocial Assessment

The typical clinical picture of the osteoporotic client is a postmenopausal woman with back pain who is predisposed to multiple bone fractures from trivial trauma. The nurse assesses the client's concept of body image, especially if the client is severely kyphotic. Finding clothes that fit properly may be a problem for the client.

The client may have curtailed social interactions because of a change in appearance or the physical limitations of being unable to sit in chairs in restaurants, movie theaters, and so forth. Alterations in sexuality may occur as a result of poor self-esteem or the discomfort imposed by positioning during intercourse.

The decrease in estrogen level as a result of menopause may also contribute to the client's psychologic status. The nurse assesses the client's response to the onset of menopause and her feelings about being a postmenopausal aging woman. Younger clients who are menopausal by surgical induction (by having their ovaries removed) may have more negative feelings toward menopause than clients who had a natural onset.

Because osteoporosis readily predisposes a client to fractures, the client must be extremely cautious about activities. As a result, the threat of fracture can create anxiety and fear. The nurse assesses for the presence of these feelings as they may affect the client's response to health care. For instance, the client may be anxious to the point that she/he will not exercise as prescribed for fear that a fracture will occur.

Laboratory Findings

There are no definitive laboratory tests that confirm a diagnosis of primary osteoporosis. A battery of tests is performed to rule out secondary osteoporosis or other metabolic bone diseases, such as osteomalacia and Paget's disease. These include determination of serum calcium, vitamin D, phosphorus, and alkaline phosphatase (ALP) levels. Urinary calcium levels are also assessed. Serum protein measurements and thyroid function tests are performed to exclude hyperthyroidism.

Radiographic Findings

Radiographs of the spine and long bones show loss of bone density and the presence of fractures. However, radiographic findings of bone density changes are evident only after a 25% to 40% bone loss has occurred.

In the search for a more sensitive diagnostic test to detect early bone changes, computed tomography (CT) has been used extensively, particularly for the spine. CT can visualize changes in the cancellous bone better than in the cortical bone. Because the vertebral column consists primarily of cancellous bone, the test is helpful in the early diagnosis of osteoporosis.

Other Diagnostic Tests

The only definitive diagnostic test to determine the cause of bone demineralization is the bone biopsy. Because this test is invasive, it is not practical to perform on everyone with suspected bone disease.

In the past few years, technologic advances have enabled the detection of early changes in bone density, some without the use of radiography. Some of the newer diagnostic tools are the single or dual photon absorptiometer (densitometer) and neutron activation analysis. *Photon absorptiometry*, used more commonly, is a screening test that measures bone mineral content at several sites on the client's nondominant arm; the client is exposed to minimal radiation for a short period of time. Bone loss of as little as 1% to 3% can be detected. There is no special client preparation or follow-up care required. These studies are complex, expensive, and not yet available in many parts of the country. Use of these techniques as standard procedures in the future will depend on their benefit versus financial cost to the client.

 Analysis: Nursing Diagnosis

Most often, the osteoporotic client is admitted to the hospital with a spinal fracture, although other types of fractures can result from the disorder. The typical client is a middle-aged or elderly, postmenopausal woman.

Common Diagnoses

Three nursing diagnoses are common to clients with osteoporosis:

1. Potential for injury (fracture) related to trivial accidents (striking an object) or falls
2. Impaired physical mobility related to decreased

muscle tone, dysfunction secondary to previous fractures, pain secondary to recent fractures
3. Pain related to fracture

Additional Diagnoses

The following additional diagnoses may be applicable to clients with osteoporosis:

1. Activity intolerance related to pain and impaired physical mobility
2. Anxiety related to fear of fracture occurrence
3. Constipation related to severe kyphosis
4. Ineffective breathing pattern related to restricted trunk movement and spinal deformity
5. Ineffective individual coping related to alteration in body image and chronic disease progression
6. Altered nutrition: less than body requirements related to inadequate calcium intake
7. Body image disturbance related to spinal deformity
8. Sexual dysfunction related to back pain and deformity
9. Social isolation related to back pain, spinal deformity, and fear of falls
10. Knowledge deficit related to treatment regimen

 Planning and Implementation

The following plan for care of osteoporotic clients focuses on the common nursing diagnoses (see the accompanying Client Care Plan).

Potential for Injury

Planning: client goals. The two major goals for this nursing diagnosis are that the client will (1) prevent falls and fractures resulting from falls and (2) avoid activities that could result in a fracture.

Interventions: nonsurgical management. Because the client is predisposed to fractures, drugs and diet therapy are used to retard bone resorption and form new bony tissue. These measures help to reduce the chance of fracture and subsequent complications.

Drug therapy. Estrogens, calcium supplements, and vitamin D, if necessary, are given for the treatment of osteoporosis, as well as for the prevention of the disease. Other agents have been given, but with limited success.

Sodium fluoride, in combination with estrogen and calcium, stimulates the formation of new bone and may inhibit bone loss. The side effects of the drug, however, must be considered in relationship to its benefits. Currently the drug is reserved for investigative settings or is used with extreme caution by the clinician. A recent study demonstrated that intermittent slow-release so-

Goal/Outcome Criteria	Interventions	Rationales
Nursing Diagnosis 1: Potential for Injury (Fracture) Related to Trivial Accidents or Falls		

Client will not experience falls and fracture resulting from falls.
■ Identifies and avoids potential environmental hazards.
	1. Create a hazard-free environment for the client while in hospital.
	  a. Get the client out of bed with bed height in lowest position.
	  b. Teach the client to wear nonskid slippers.
	  c. Inspect the floor for spills and the room for equipment that may cause tripping or stumbling.
	  d. Provide additional lighting for an elderly client.
	  e. Place necessary items close to bed within easy reach (e.g., water pitcher and call bell).
	  f. Keep side rails up, especially for elderly clients who are confused.
	  g. Teach the importance and the use of handrails in the bathroom.
		1. Creating a hazard-free environment reduces the risk of falls and subsequent fracture.

	2. Provide ambulatory support as needed.
	  a. Assess the need for a cane or a walker.
	  b. Consult with a physical therapist.
	  c. Teach the client to call for assistance.
	  d. Teach the client to take his/her time when getting out of bed and walking.
		2. Ambulatory aids provide additional support when walking and help prevent rushing, which contributes to falls. Elderly clients often hurry to the bathroom to prevent incontinence.

■ Avoids activities or drugs that could result in a fracture.	3. When helping with activities of daily living (ADL), prevent the client from accidentally hitting side rails, door frames, and so on.	3. Striking hard surfaces can cause bone fracture, as bones are porous from calcium loss.
	4. Teach the client to bend or stoop slowly; teach client not to lift or move heavy objects such as hospital furniture.	4. Quick body movements can easily lead to vertebral compression fractures in the osteoporotic client.
	5. Monitor drugs the client may be taking for concurrent medical conditions for side effects.	5. Drugs such as diuretics, phenothiazines, and tranquilizers can cause dizziness, drowsiness, and weakness, predisposing the client to falls.

■ Increases calcium intake in the diet.	6. Teach the importance of diet in preventing further osteoporosis.
	  a. Refer for dietary consultation.
	  b. Teach foods high in calcium content.
	  c. Teach the need to decrease caffeine and alcohol intake.
		6. Dietary calcium is needed to maintain serum level, thus preventing additional loss from bone. Caffeine excess can increase calcium loss in urine; alcohol excess can promote acidosis, which increases bone resorption.

	7. Teach the effect of cigarette smoking on bone remodeling (if client is a smoker).	7. Cigarette smoking can promote acidosis.

continued

CLIENT CARE PLAN ■ The Client with Osteoporosis *continued*

Goal/Outcome Criteria	Interventions	Rationales
Nursing Diagnosis 2: Impaired Physical Mobility Related to Decreased Muscle Tone, Dysfunction Secondary to Previous Fractures, or Pain Secondary to Recent Fractures		
Client will increase physical mobility to level of ADL independence. ■ Complies with daily exercise regimen.	1. Consult with physical therapist regarding an exercise program to include strengthening and weight-bearing exercises. a. Assist the client as necessary with exercises b. Teach the client that ADL do not replace prescribed exercises. c. Teach the importance of exercises.	1. Strengthening exercises increase joint movement, increase muscle tone, and stimulate blood circulation to bone and muscle tissue. Weight-bearing exercises decrease the rate of bone loss and increase bone formation.
	2. Assist with ADL as necessary, allowing the client to be as independent as possible.	2. Pain and poor muscle tone may limit the client's ability to be independent, especially after a fracture.
■ Uses assistive and adaptive devices as advised to independently perform ADL.	3. Assess the need for assistive and adaptive devices to perform ADL; consult with the occupational therapist to obtain appropriate equipment.	3. Devices may be needed for client to be ADL independent. Overuse and reliance, however, should be discouraged.
Nursing Diagnosis 3: Pain Related to Vertebral Fracture		
Client will experience alleviation or reduction of pain so that client can be independent in care.	1. Assess the need for pain medication: narcotic or nonnarcotic analgesics, muscle relaxants, or anti-inflammatory drugs.	1. Clients usually receive pain medication on a prn schedule. Elderly clients often do not request pain medication even if needed; therefore, the nurse must anticipate this need.
■ States that pain is reduced or alleviated.	2. Maintain orthotic devices for vertebral fracture. a. Check that the brace or corset fits properly. b. Inspect the skin where device causes pressure. c. Apply the device for use when the client gets out of bed.	2. Orthotic devices maintain spine alignment and provide spinal column support.
■ Utilizes pain relief measures independently as advised.	3. Apply moist heat to back (heat packs or hot compresses) as needed to reduce pain. (Physical therapist may do this.) (Also see Chap. 7.)	3. Heat increases blood circulation to affected areas, thus relieving muscle spasms, which cause pain.

dium fluoride given to osteoporotic women was successful and safe in forming new bone and reducing vertebral fractures (Pak et al., 1989).

Androgens have been used with some success in decreasing bone resorption. When given to postmenopausal women, however, the drug causes masculine traits and may lead to liver disease. Androgens may decrease bone resorption in men, particularly the elderly.

Calcitonin inhibits bone loss, but is expensive and administered by injection. These disadvantages prohibit its use in most settings over a long period of time. Another naturally occurring hormone, PTH, is being tested for its ability to strengthen bone by its bone formation capability.

Metabolites of vitamin D, such as 1,25-dihydroxy-vitamin D (calcitriol), are potentially helpful in inhibiting bone resorption, but remain experimental. At present there is little clinical evidence to support this hypothesis. Table 30–1 summarizes drug therapy in the osteoporotic client.

Diet therapy. The dietary considerations for the treatment of a client with a diagnosis of osteoporosis are the same as those for the prevention of the disease. Calcium and vitamin D intake is increased, and alcohol and caffeine consumption is discouraged. For the client who has sustained a fracture, protein, vitamin C, and iron are increased in the diet to promote bone healing.

Prevention of complications. The client must be careful to prevent falls and other activities that could cause a fracture. A hazard-free environment is necessary to meet this goal, and the nurse must teach the client about its importance.

While the client is in the hospital, the nurse employs safety measures and eliminates potential hazards. Accidents in the hospital occur most frequently between 6 and 9 PM and during peak activity times, such as mealtime. Because persons older than 60 years of age generally require twice as much lighting as a 20-year-old individual, extra lighting is important. The creation of glare is avoided, however, as glare can impede vision and lead to falls.

Drugs such as diuretics, phenothiazines, and tranquilizers can cause dizziness, drowsiness, and weakness. The nurse carefully monitors the client receiving these medications for side effects that could contribute to falls.

Impaired Physical Mobility

Planning: client goals. The primary goal for this diagnosis is that the client will increase physical mobility to the level of activities of daily living (ADL) independence. If this goal is not met, complications of impaired mobility may occur. (See Chap. 22 for a discussion of the complications of immobility and promotion of ADL independence.)

Interventions: nonsurgical management. Exercise is the major intervention employed. The nurse works with the physical therapist to plan and implement a structured exercise program geared to the individual client.

Strengthening exercises. Specific exercises are prescribed for strengthening the abdominal and back muscles to improve posture and provide an improved support for the spine. Abdominal isometrics, deep breathing, and pectoral stretching are stressed to increase pulmonary capacity. Exercises for the extremity muscles include isometric, resistive, and range-of-motion (ROM) exercises. The nurse encourages active ROM exercises, as they improve joint mobility and increase muscle tone. (Refer to Chap. 22 for discussion of ROM exercise techniques.)

Weight-bearing exercises. A general weight-bearing exercise program is implemented in addition to the muscle-strengthening component. Walking, both slow and fast, and bicycling are recommended daily activities. Recreational activities that could promote vertebral compression, such as bowling and horseback riding, are discouraged.

Pain

Planning: client goals. The major goal is that the client will experience the alleviation or reduction of pain associated with fracture. One of the most painful fractures is vertebral compression.

Interventions: nonsurgical management. The pain management program depends on the intensity and duration of the pain. Pain from spinal fractures often resolves in 6 to 8 weeks after injury with treatment, which usually includes drug therapy and orthotic devices.

Drug therapy. Analgesics, narcotic and nonnarcotic, are given during the acute phase of the pain, that is, from the time of injury through as long as several weeks. Muscle relaxants to ease the discomfort associated with muscle spasms are frequently used for spinal fractures. Anti-inflammatory medications are beneficial for pain relief and for decreasing spinal nerve root inflammation from crushed vertebrae. The nurse monitors the need for medication, as well as the side effects that could contribute to injury.

Orthotic devices. Back braces are useful in immobilizing the spine during the acute pain phase and providing spinal column support. Examples of braces include the Jewett hyperextension brace, the Knight-Taylor brace, a lumbosacral corset with metal stays, or a lightweight plastic molded orthosis (Fig. 30–2). Elderly clients usually tolerate these devices poorly, as they are uncomfortable and often somewhat cumbersome. The nurse works with the physical therapist to ensure proper placement of the brace on the client. The nurse inspects the skin for irritation, and the client's tolerance of the device is noted.

If medication and orthotic devices are ineffective in reducing or alleviating pain, surgery may be required to stabilize the spine. Chapter 31 describes surgery for spinal fractures.

■ Discharge Planning

The osteoporotic client with one or more fractures can be discharged to the home setting. In some instances, the client is discharged to a long-term care facility for rehabilitation or permanent residence when support systems are not available.

Home Care Preparation

If the client is discharged to a home setting, the environment must be assessed for potential hazards before discharge. The nurse uses the data base completed at time of admission to ascertain if alterations in the home environment are necessary. For example, if scatter rugs are used in the home, the client is advised to have these removed to prevent the chance of falling.

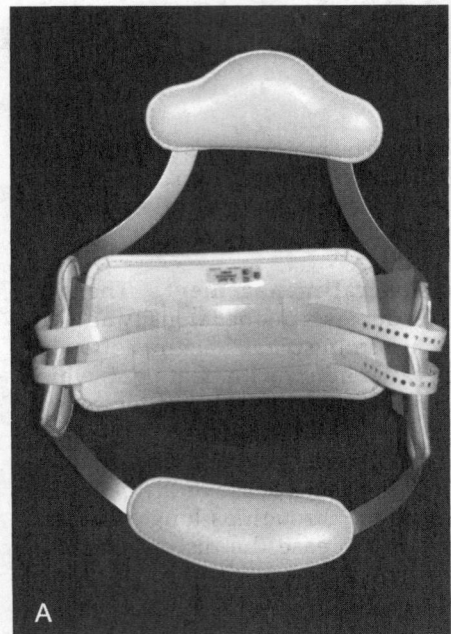
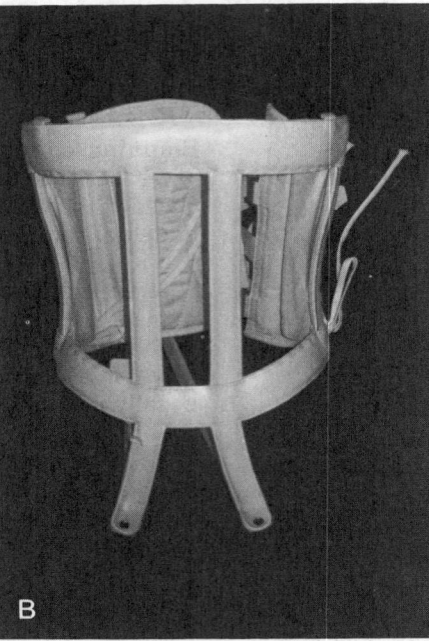

Figure 30–2

Typical back braces for lower vertebral compression fractures: *A*, Jewett's brace (worn anteriorly). *B*, Knight-Taylor brace (worn posteriorly). (Courtesy of Clarence Knight, orthotist, Baltimore, MD.)

A two-story house or apartment may be a problem if physical mobility is limited or if adequate support railing is not available to assist with stair climbing. The social worker, in conjunction with the nurse, helps the client identify adaptations that may have to be made to create as hazard free an environment as possible.

Assistive or adaptive devices for personal use may also be needed at home, if only for a short time. Devices to assist with ADL, such as a dressing stick to put on pants, are helpful in maintaining the client's independence. The occupational therapist works with the nurse to determine the need for assistive devices. Chapter 22 describes the promotion of ADL independence in detail.

The nurse and physical therapist assess the need for ambulatory aids in the home. A walker or cane may provide the additional support necessary to prevent falls.

Client/Family Education

The teaching plan for the client with osteoporosis includes (1) prevention of falls, (2) exercise, (3) diet therapy, and (4) drug therapy. The client must be extremely careful to prevent falls, especially in public places. Ambulatory aids should be used for additional support, although some clients refuse to be seen in public with a cane or walker. Similarly, clients may not wear back braces because of embarrassment or discomfort. A thorough explanation of the necessity and the proper method for using these devices is provided by the nurse and physical therapist.

A structured exercise program is prescribed by the physical therapist and reinforced by the nurse. Strengthening, ROM, and weight-bearing exercises are taught. Follow-up physical therapy visits ensure that the client has learned the exercises and is compliant.

A diet rich in calcium-containing foods is emphasized. A diet consultation before discharge can help the client select foods that are liked, yet high in the essential nutrients. If a fracture has occurred, foods rich in vitamin C, protein, and iron are encouraged. Clients are also instructed to decrease caffeine and alcohol consumption. Smoking should also be discouraged.

For a client who will be homebound or institutionalized, sunlight exposure should be promoted as an essential source of vitamin D. The importance of sunlight to this client should be stressed to the nursing home or long-term care facility where the client may be transferred.

Because most osteoporotic clients are elderly, compliance with the diet may not be achieved. Often the elderly client is used to eating less than the required daily nutrients. Consumption of milk and dairy products is usually minimal. As a result, calcium supplements are ordered for long-term maintenance. The nurse instructs the client to take only the prescribed amount, as too much can lead to hypercalcemia.

If placed on estrogen therapy, the client needs to have frequent gynecologic checkups to detect early signs of cervical cancer. The nurse teaches the client how to monitor for side effects. Follow-up visits to the internist or orthopedist are scheduled frequently to monitor calcium blood levels and determine further progression of the disease.

Psychosocial Preparation

Because clients are often afraid that they will sustain a fracture, it is extremely important to allay their fears to the extent possible. The degree of osteoporosis determines the likelihood of injury. The more severe the osteoporosis, the more limited the activities should be. For example, a severely osteoporotic woman may sustain vertebral compression fractures from stooping or bending. For most clients, an aggressive treatment plan will prevent fractures from trivial trauma.

Explaining the importance of orthotic and ambulatory aids in the prevention of injury increases compliance and decreases reluctance to use the devices. A supportive spouse, family member, or significant other can help to encourage the client to adhere to the treatment plan.

Health Care Resources

If the client cannot return home, a nursing home or long-term care facility placement may be needed, at least for a short time. The hospital nurse documents the client's needs on the transfer chart and communicates the special considerations required for this client.

If returning to a home environment, the client may need equipment for ADL and ambulation. Financial resources are assessed before equipment is obtained. If insurance or other third-party payer will not reimburse the client, other sources are explored. Religious and support organizations are possible resources for free materials. Items are often donated to these groups for use as needed in the community. Rental of equipment is also an option. The hospital or local medical supplier can provide estimates of renting versus purchasing the needed equipment. The equipment should be accessible before the client returns home.

A home care nurse may be needed for follow-up in the home environment. The nurse in this setting can be contacted to assist in the discharge planning for the client, to assess potential environmental hazards, and to obtain equipment and supplies. The need for physical or occupational therapy, social work, and homemaking personnel in the home is determined by the home care nurse.

In addition to home care resources, the Osteoporosis Foundation provides information to clients and health care professionals regarding the disease and its treatment. Large metropolitan hospitals often have osteoporosis specialty clinics and support groups for clients with the disease.

 Evaluation

On the basis of the identified nursing diagnoses, the nurse evaluates the care for the osteoporotic client. The expected outcomes for the client with osteoporosis include that the client

1. States that pain is reduced or alleviated
2. Identifies potential environmental hazards and avoids them
3. Uses assistive and adaptive devices as advised
4. Uses orthotic and ambulatory aids as prescribed
5. Complies with the daily exercise regimen
6. Increases calcium intake in the diet
7. Describes and complies with the drug regimen as ordered

By meeting the stated desired outcomes, the progression of osteoporosis should diminish and the likelihood of potential fractures should decrease. As a result, anxiety and fear will be alleviated and life style alterations will be minimal.

OSTEOMALACIA

OVERVIEW

Osteomalacia is a metabolic disease in which there is a defect in the mineralization of bone. Unlike the situation in osteoporotic tissue, in osteomalacia the amount and quality of bone matrix (osteoid) is normal, but mineralization is delayed or inadequate (see the accompanying Key Features of Disease).

KEY FEATURES OF DISEASE ■ **Differential Features of Osteoporosis and Osteomalacia**

Characteristic	Osteoporosis	Osteomalacia
Definition	Decreased bone mass	Demineralized bone
Pathophysiology	Lack of calcium	Lack of vitamin D
Radiographic findings	Osteopenia, fractures	Pseudofractures, Looser's zones, fractures
Calcium level	Normal	Low or normal
Phosphate level	Normal	Low or normal
PTH level	Normal	High or normal
ALP level	Normal	High

Pathophysiology

Osteomalacia is the adult equivalent of rickets, or vitamin D deficiency, in children. In its natural form, vitamin D is obtained from the ultraviolet radiation of the sun and certain foods. In combination with calcium and phosphorus, the vitamin is necessary for bone formation.

Vitamin D is actually a group of vitamins, including vitamins D_2 and D_3. The naturally occurring substance is D_2, or cholecalciferol, which is manufactured by photochemical activation in the skin when triggered by the sun's ultraviolet light. As illustrated in Figure 30–3, the D_2 from either the skin or food is carried to the liver bound to an alpha-globulin as transcalciferin. There, part of the substance is converted to 25-hydroxycholecalciferol, or calcidiol.

Calcidiol is then transported to the kidney for transformation into the major active vitamin D metabolite, 1,25-dihydroxycholecalciferol, or calcitriol. The amount of calcitriol produced is regulated by PTH and the blood level of phosphate, the inorganic form of phosphorus. An increase in calcitriol production occurs when there is an increase in PTH or a decrease in serum phosphate levels.

Calcitriol is needed for optimal intestinal absorption of calcium and works in combination with PTH for the release of calcium from bone to assist in serum calcium regulation. Consequently, calcitriol or vitamin D deficiency results in decreased calcium absorption from the gut, which in turn leads to PTH stimulation and a decrease in both serum phosphate and calcium levels.

In osteomalacia, a primary or secondary vitamin D deficiency causes insufficient bone mineralization. Nonmineralized or poorly mineralized osteoid accumulates over the surfaces of both cortical and cancellous bone.

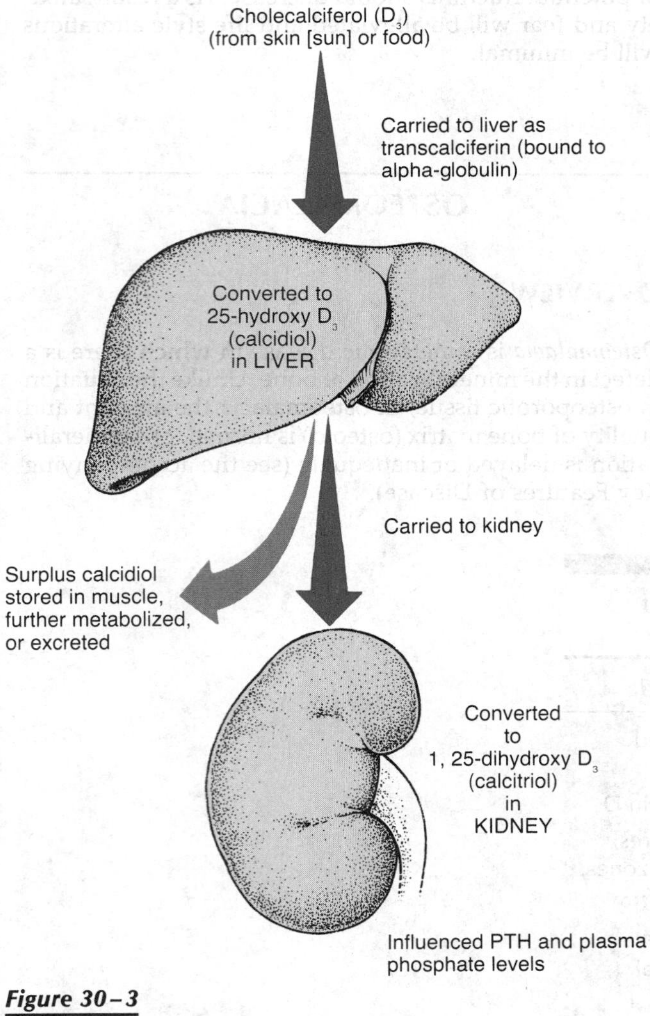

Etiology

In addition to primary vitamin D deficiency related to lack of sunlight exposure or dietary intake, vitamin D deficiency attributable to various pathologic conditions may result in osteomalacia (see the accompanying Key Features of Disease). Malabsorption of the vitamin from the small bowel is a common postsurgical complication

Cholecalciferol (D₃)
(from skin [sun] or food)

Carried to liver as transcalciferin (bound to alpha-globulin)

Converted to 25-hydroxy D₃ (calcidiol) in LIVER

Carried to kidney

Surplus calcidiol stored in muscle, further metabolized, or excreted

Converted to 1, 25-dihydroxy D₃ (calcitriol) in KIDNEY

Influenced PTH and plasma phosphate levels

Figure 30–3

Process of vitamin D metabolism in the body.

KEY FEATURES OF DISEASE ■ Causes of Osteomalacia

Vitamin D Disturbance

Inadequate production
  Lack of sunlight exposure
Dietary deficiency
Abnormal metabolism
  Drug therapy
    Phenytoin (Dilantin)
    Fluoride
    Barbiturates
  Liver disease
  Renal disese
Inadequate absorption
  Postgastrectomy
  Malabsorption syndrome
Inflammatory bowel disease

Kidney Disease

Chronic renal failure
Renal tubular disorders
  Acidosis
  Hypophosphatemia

Familial Metabolic Error

Hypophosphatemia

of partial or total gastrectomy and bypass or resection surgery of the small intestine. Small bowel disease, such as Crohn's disease, may cause decreased vitamin absorption.

Liver and pancreatic disorders interrupt vitamin D metabolism and decrease the production of usable substance. Renal failure or disease interferes with the synthesis of calcitriol, the most active vitamin metabolite.

Conditions that contribute to phosphate depletion, or hypophosphatemia, lead to osteomalacia. Osteomalacia is also a complication of the intake of certain drugs, particularly anticonvulsants, barbiturates, and fluoride. The exact mechanism for the drug effects is not known.

Incidence

Until recently, osteomalacia was considered nonexistent in the United States. Although the disease is not thought to be common, researchers and clinicians are beginning to explore its incidence in the elderly. In the geriatric population, there are significant numbers of people who are deprived of sun exposure, maintain poor diets, or both. Although there are no statistical data to indicate the incidence of osteomalacia in the United States, many health care professionals have studied its occurrence in nursing homes and other residences for the elderly (Barzel, 1983; Parfitt et al., 1982). As a result, osteomalacia is recognized as a health problem for the elderly population.

PREVENTION

Prevention of osteomalacia is determined by its possible causative factors. In the elderly, particularly those who are institutionalized or homebound, sun exposure is increased if possible. The elderly person should not be heavily clothed when exposed to sunlight.

The ingestion of foods rich in vitamin D is vital. The only foods that naturally contain vitamin D in significant amounts are eggs, swordfish, mackerel, sardines, and chicken liver. In the United States, milk and dairy products are fortified with the vitamin. The elderly individual usually does not consume large quantities of fortified foods and must therefore rely on other foods rich in vitamin D. These foods are relatively expensive for the limited budgets of the elderly, and oral supplementation becomes necessary.

The RDA of vitamin D is currently 10 μg, or 400 IU. Because the elderly are at risk for bone demineralization from aging, as well as osteomalacia, a safe and adequate daily requirement may be as high as 15 to 20 μg, or 600 to 800 IU (Parfitt et al., 1982).

In the increasingly health conscious society of the United States, meat consumption is declining in favor of other foods such as vegetables and fruits. Vegetarians are at risk of vitamin D deficiency, especially those with dark-pigmented skin in which vitamin metabolism is not as great as that for light-skinned individuals.

When a small bowel, liver, pancreatic, or kidney disorder occurs, the condition is treated and vitamin supplementation is given to prevent osteomalacia. Drugs that predispose an individual to osteomalacia are carefully monitored for the complication. If the disease is suspected, the drug dosage is decreased or the drug is discontinued.

COLLABORATIVE MANAGEMENT

 Assessment

History

The important data to obtain for a client with osteomalacia or suspected osteomalacia include *age, exposure to sunlight,* and *skin pigmentation.* The elderly individual who has been homebound or chronically institutionalized is at the greatest risk for the disease. Those individuals who have dark skin and consume minimal protein are more at risk than light-skinned persons with the same dietary habits. The nurse takes a thorough *diet history* also to determine the intake of vitamin D- and calcium-containing foods. If the client is taking *medications* known to contribute to the disease or has *other medical conditions* that can lead to osteomalacia, these are identified. The nurse asks the client if he/she has ever sustained a *fracture* and when the fracture occurred. The client's answer can provide information about the longevity of the disorder.

Physical Assessment: Clinical Manifestations

Osteomalacia is easily confused with osteoporosis. Not only are many of the clinical manifestations similar, but both disorders may occur at the same time.

In the early stages of osteomalacia, the manifestations are nonspecific. Muscle weakness and bone pain are often misdiagnosed as arthritis or rheumatism. In some cases, proximal muscle weakness in the shoulder and pelvic girdle areas is the only complaint.

Muscle weakness in the lower extremities may progress to a waddling and unsteady gait, which contributes to falls and subsequent fractures. Hypophosphatemia leads to an inadequate production of muscle cell adenosine triphosphate, thus resulting in a decrease in muscle cell energy. If hypocalcemia is present, muscle cramping may accompany the weakness.

The nurse assesses muscle strength and observes the client's gait. Complaints of muscle cramps and *bone pain* are recorded. The skeletal discomfort is often vague and generalized. The spine, the ribs, the pelvis, and the lower extremities are most often affected. The client usually describes the pain as aggravated by activity and worse at night.

In addition to the client's subjective complaint of pain, the nurse palpates the bones affected for tenderness. *Bone tenderness* can be elicited by pressure on the tibia or rib cage. The nurse observes skeletal malalignment as long bone bowing or spinal deformity, similar to that seen in osteoporosis. In extreme cases, the pelvis narrows such that vaginal childbirth is difficult.

If osteomalacia is untreated, vertebral, rib, and long-bone fractures may occur. The client may be misdiagnosed as having bone cancer or osteoporosis.

Psychosocial Assessment

Unlike osteoporosis, osteomalacia is a reversible condition. The fear of fracture and deformity may be present until the treatment of the disease becomes effective. If a client's diagnosis has not been confirmed, he/she may be apprehensive and fear bone cancer. The nurse identifies the client's level of anxiety regarding the suspected diagnosis or the possible occurrence of fracture or deformity.

Laboratory Findings

Alkaline phosphatase. In an attempt to form new bone, increased osteoblastic activity results in an increased level of serum ALP. The exact role of this enzyme in bone formation and mineralization is not known.

Serum phosphate. Hypophosphatemia frequently accompanies an increase in ALP level. This finding is probably the result of intestinal phosphate malabsorption, secondary hyperparathyroidism, lack of action of calcitriol on renal phosphate conservation, or a combination of these factors. Hypophosphatemia usually precedes hypocalcemia, or decreased levels of serum calcium.

Serum calcium. The blood level of calcium remains unchanged until osteomalacia becomes severe or is late in its course. Hypocalcemia results from intestinal malabsorption of calcium and the impaired action of PTH in maintaining bone calcium levels. Both contributing factors to a calcium decrease are due to a lack of active vitamin D metabolite.

Parathyroid hormone. The level of PTH may increase as a compensatory response to hypocalcemia. Changes in the PTH level are also seen in late, severe disease.

Vitamin D metabolites. The most sensitive index of vitamin D in the body is the plasma level of its metabolites. Most laboratory tests measuring metabolites cannot discriminate among types, for example, D_2 or D_3. The elderly individual often has a normally low level of vitamin D metabolites.

Radiographic Findings

Radiographs of bone tissue with osteomalacia show a decrease in the trabeculae of cancellous bone and lack of osteoid sharpness. The classic diagnostic finding specific to the disease, however, is the presence of radiolucent bands called Looser's lines or zones. Looser's zones

are pseudofractures; they represent stress fractures that have not mineralized. They often appear symmetrically in the inner femora, ribs, and inferior pubic rami and may progress to complete fractures with minimal trauma.

CT is used to detect vertebral compression fractures and confirm the changes in cancellous bone mineralization.

Other Diagnostic Tests

A bone biopsy is performed when the diagnosis of osteomalacia is suspected but not confirmed. Bone scans using radioactive isotopes may also be ordered to confirm the diagnosis.

 Analysis: Nursing Diagnosis

The nursing diagnoses for the client with osteomalacia are identical to those for the client with osteoporosis. The client is usually admitted to the hospital with muscle weakness and unexplained bone pain.

 Planning and Implementation

Because the nursing diagnoses for osteomalacia are the same as those for osteoporosis, the client goals are also similar. An increase in vitamin D through dietary intake, sun exposure, and drug supplementation is promoted for the treatment of the disease. The nurse teaches the client about foods high in vitamin D and the importance of frequent sun exposure for the manufacture of the vitamin. The dosage and side effects of vitamin D and calcium are emphasized as outlined in Table 30–1.

■ Discharge Planning

The client with osteomalacia usually recovers completely if the diagnosis is made before severe fractures and deformity occur. Therefore, the client is most often discharged to the home setting and assessed periodically to ensure compliance with therapy.

 Evaluation

The client outcomes are similar to those for the client with osteoporosis (see earlier).

PAGET'S DISEASE

OVERVIEW

Paget's disease, or osteitis deformans, is a metabolic disorder of bone remodeling, or turnover, in which increased resorption or loss results in bone deposits that are weak, enlarged, and disorganized. First described in 1876 by Sir James Paget, an English surgeon, the disease was thought to be an inflammatory process, infectious in origin. Until the 1960s, Paget's disease was considered a medical curiosity and given little attention. With a growing number of elderly in the United States, interest in the disease has increased and treatment has improved.

Pathophysiology

Three pathophysiologic phases of the disorder have been described. In the first phase, called the *active* phase, a prolific increase in osteoclasts causes massive bone destruction and deformity. The osteoclasts of pagetic bone are large and multinuclear, unlike those of normal bone tissue. In the *mixed* phase of the disease, the osteoblasts react in a compensatory manner to form new bone. The result is bone that is disorganized and chaotic in structure. The new trabecular bone has a mosaic pattern with a volume twice that of normal bone. When the osteoblastic activity exceeds the osteoclastic activity, the *inactive* phase occurs. The newly formed bone becomes sclerotic and ivory hard. The number of osteoclasts begins to return toward normal.

As a result of the metabolic bone process, the vascularity of the newly formed bone tissue is increased. The arterial capillaries of pagetic bone become hypertrophied, causing marrow sinus and venous system distention. Paget's disease occurs in one bone or in multiple sites. The most common areas of involvement are the vertebrae, the femur, the skull, the sternum, and the pelvis.

Etiology

The exact cause of Paget's disease is unknown, but it is thought to be the result of a latent viral infection contracted in young adulthood and manifesting as a disease 20 to 40 years later. Bone biopsy specimens have revealed an antigen from a respiratory virus and measles. Some researchers believe that a pneumovirus is responsible (Altman, 1984). A familial autosomal dominant pattern has been suggested, as the disorder is present in monozygotic twins. The disease has been found in up to 30% of persons with a positive family history for Paget's disease (Rebel, 1987).

Incidence

Paget's disease is primarily a disease of the older age group. It occurs in about 4% of the United States population less than 40 years of age, and about 10% of persons older than 80 years, or 3 million Americans. Because the disorder occurs more frequently in Europe and less often in Asia and Scandinavia, researchers are investigating a possible link between the disease and ethnic origin (Altman, 1984).

COLLABORATIVE MANAGEMENT

 Assessment

History

When collecting data from a client with suspected Paget's disease, the nurse focuses on his/her *age, sex,* and *family history of the disorder.* The most important data are elicited from the physical and psychosocial assessment.

Physical Assessment: Clinical Manifestations

Eighty per cent of clients with Paget's disease are asymptomatic. The diagnosis is often accidentally discovered during a routine laboratory or radiographic examination. In more severe disease, the manifestations are diverse and potentially fatal.

Bone pain causes the client to seek medical attention. The pain is aching, poorly described, deep, and aggravated by pressure and weight bearing. It is most noticeable at night or when the client is resting and is categorized as mild to moderate. Back pain and headache are common complaints.

The pain associated with the disorder may be from metabolic bone activity, secondary arthritis, impending fracture, or nerve impingement. Arthritis occurs at the joints of the affected bones, but its relationship to Paget's disease is unclear. Nerve impingement is particularly common in the lumbosacral area of the vertebral column, presenting as back pain that radiates along one or both lower extremities.

The nurse assesses the location and extent of the client's pain to determine the bone areas involved. The nurse also observes the client's posture, stance, and gait to identify gross *bony deformities* that exist in Paget's disease. Because of the enlargement of the vertebrae, loss of normal spinal curvature, and lower-extremity malalignment, the client is usually short (Fig. 30–4). Long-bone bowing in the arms and legs with subsequent varus deformity of the elbows and knees is often symmetric. Flexion contractures of the hips are commonly present.

When performing a musculoskeletal assessment, the nurse pays particular attention to the size and shape of the skull, which is soft, thick, and enlarged in Paget's disease. Involvement of the temporal bone may lead to deafness and vertigo, whereas basilar complications can compress any of the cranial nerves and result in neurologic compromise. Platybasia, or basilar invagination, causes brain stem manifestations that threaten life. In some cases, the bony enlargement of the skull blocks cerebrospinal fluid, resulting in hydrocephalus. Chapter 33 describes neurologic complications.

The nurse assesses the client's *skin* for its color and temperature. In Paget's disease, the skin is *flushed* and *warm* because of increased vascularity. In addition, the nurse assesses the energy level of the client. The client usually complains of *apathy, lethargy,* and *fatigue.*

Pathologic fractures may be the presenting clinical

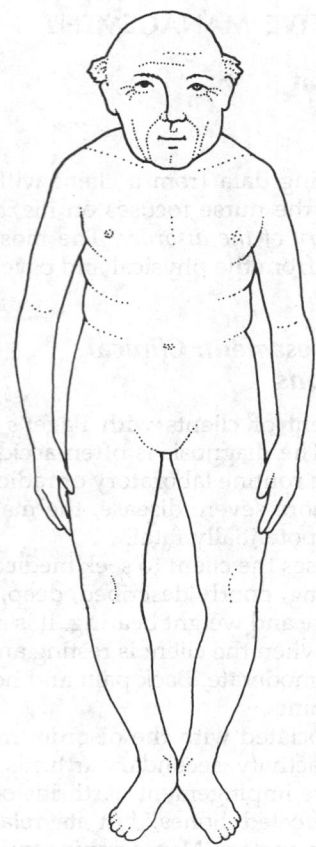

Figure 30–4

Client with Paget's disease of the bone.

manifestation of the disorder. As many as 30% of clients with Paget's disease sustain at least one incomplete or complete fracture. The femur and the tibia are most often affected, and fracture of these bones can result from minimal trauma. The fracture line is usually perpendicular to the long axis of the bone, and healing is unpredictable in view of abnormal metabolic activity within the bone.

The most dreaded complication of Paget's disease is *neoplasm*, most commonly osteogenic sarcoma (see later discussion of bone cancer). Sarcomas occur in about 1% of clients with pagetic bone. They appear primarily in the pelvis, the femur, and the humerus and carry a grave prognosis owing to early metastasis to the lung or extensive local invasion. Frequently, they are multifocal, and they occur more often in men. When severe bone pain is present in a client with Paget's disease, neoplasm is suspected.

Other less common manifestations of Paget's disease include *hyperparathyroidism* and *gout*. Secondary hyperparathyroidism leads to an increase in serum and urinary calcium levels. In severe cases, calcium excess results from prolonged immobilization. Calcium deposits occur in joint spaces or as stones in the urinary tract. Hyperuricemia, or serum uric acid excess, and gout occur, as the increased metabolic activity of bone creates an increase in nucleic acid catabolism.

In a few cases, increased vascularity causes an *increase in cardiac output, resulting in congestive heart failure.* Cardiac complications tend to occur only in cases in which more than 30% of the skeleton is involved.

Psychosocial Assessment

The psychosocial impact of the disease in a client who is not symptomatic is minimal when compared with the impact on the client with advanced disease. The more severe form of Paget's disease causes multisystem involvement and intense pain. Coping with pain and the fear of secondary bone cancer are important variables in the assessment.

The nurse assesses the effect of the chronic disorder on the client's ability to function as a family member and a productive member of society. The coping capacity of the client and the family or significant others is also evaluated. Specific techniques for assessing coping mechanisms are outlined in Chapter 6.

As in osteoporosis and osteomalacia, the client may fear fractures resulting from falls or trivial trauma. The nurse documents the fears and concerns regarding the course of the disease.

Laboratory Findings

Alkaline phosphatase. Increases in serum ALP and urinary hydroxyproline levels are the primary laboratory findings indicating the probability of Paget's disease. Overactive osteoblasts are responsible for the alteration in ALP level.

Hydroxyproline. An evaluation of the 24-hour urinary hydroxyproline level reflects an increase in bone collagen turnover and indicates the degree of the disease process. The higher the value of hydroxyproline, the greater the severity of Paget's disease is.

Serum and urinary calcium. The calcium levels in blood and urine are normal or elevated. The immobilized client is more likely to have an increase in calcium levels.

Serum uric acid. Paget's disease often causes an elevation of uric acid, as nucleic acid from overactive bone metabolism increases. This finding may be misinterpreted as primary gout.

Radiographic Findings

Bone radiographs of pagetic bone reveal radiolucent, or punched out, areas indicative of increased bone resorption (Fig. 30–5). Depending on the phase of the disease, the overall bone mass is enlarged and the cortices are thickened. Malalignment deformities, fractures, and secondary arthritic changes may be present.

The CT scan is useful in the detection of sarcomas, basilar invagination of the skull, and spinal cord or nerve compression.

Other Diagnostic Tests

Bone scans using radioactive isotopes are only slightly more sensitive than routine radiographs in delineating the bone changes of Paget's disease. When the diagnosis is difficult, a bone biopsy is performed.

 Analysis: Nursing Diagnosis

The data collected from the physical and psychosocial assessments are reviewed and analyzed to derive nursing diagnoses.

Common Diagnoses

If the client has symptomatic, advanced disease, the following diagnoses are appropriate:

1. Pain (bone) related to metabolic process, secondary arthritis, or impending fracture
2. Impaired physical mobility related to pain and deformity
3. Activity intolerance related to fatigue, pain, and deformity
4. Body image disturbance related to bone deformity
5. Potential for injury (fracture) related to trivial trauma or falls.

Additional Diagnoses

Because Paget's disease is a variable multisystem disease, numerous potential diagnoses may become actual for a specific client, including

1. Anxiety related to potentially fatal complications of the disease
2. Ineffective individual or family coping related to potential outcome, pain, and chronicity of disease
3. Fear related to potential for fractures and deformity
4. Anticipatory grieving related to potential disease outcome and chronicity of disease
5. Total self-care deficit related to bone deformity and fatigue
6. Sensory/perceptual alterations (visual, and auditory) related to cranial nerve damage
7. Sleep pattern disturbance related to severe pain
8. Social isolation related to self-care deficit and poor self-concept
9. Urinary retention related to presence of calcium-based urinary stone
10. Sexual dysfunction related to bone pain and deformity
11. Knowledge deficit related to treatment regimen

 Planning and Implementation

The plan of care for a client with Paget's disease may be complex, depending on the severity of the illness. A

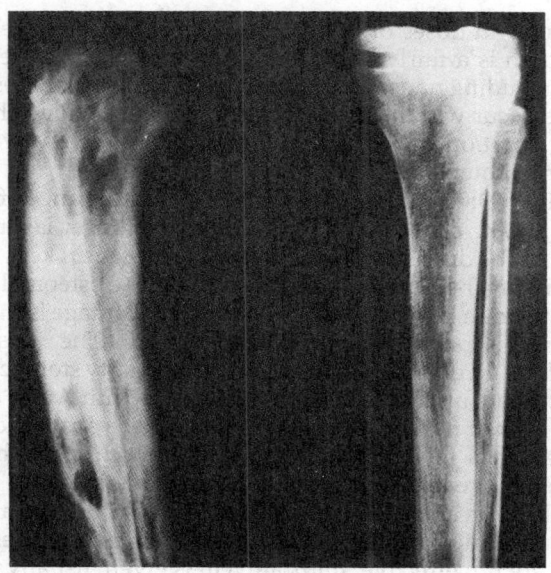

Figure 30–5

Radiographs of bowed tibia (left) and normal tibia in a client with Paget's disease. Note large punched-out area in lower left tibia. (From Siris, E. S., Jacobs, T. P., & Canfield, R. E. [1980]. Paget's disease of bone. *Bulletin of the New York Academy of Medicine, 56,* 285–304.)

basic plan founded on the nursing diagnoses seen in most clients is outlined.

Pain

Planning: client goals. The goal for bone pain is that the client will experience a reduction or alleviation of the discomfort.

Interventions. Nonsurgical or surgical management may be necessary to reduce the client's pain. Nonsurgical interventions are employed initially.

Nonsurgical management. Drug therapy is the primary intervention utilized for pain relief. Not only can drugs relieve pain, they may cause the disease to go into a remission for a period of time. Other pain relief measures are also employed.

Drug therapy. The purpose of drug therapy in Paget's disease is to relieve pain and to decrease bone resorption. Mild to moderate pain may be alleviated by aspirin or nonsteroidal anti-inflammatory drugs (NSAIDs), such as ibuprofen (Motrin) and indomethacin (Indocin). When the level is more than twice the normal value and multisystem disease is present, more potent drugs are given, such as calcitonin, etidronate disodium (EHDP), and mithramycin.

Calcitonin (calcitonin-salmon [Calcimar]) is a thyroid hormone that, when given to clients with Paget's disease, is 75% effective in initiating a remission of the disease, possibly by retarding bone resorption, and subsequent relief of pain. The drug often causes a dramatic decrease in the ALP level in a few weeks. Given subcutaneously in doses of 50 to 100 μg three times a week, calcitonin is a fairly safe medication, but with side effects including nausea, flushing, and rash. Most of these effects occur within 1 hour of drug administration. The usual duration of therapy is 6 months, followed by a 6-month course of EHDP.

EHDP (Didronel) is given orally in a dosage range of 5 to 20 mg/kg per day and tends to have a longer lasting effect on the disease than calcitonin. The dosage is kept to a minimum, because high dosages may cause osteomalacia or vitamin D deficiency. Its major disadvantage is that the drug is poorly absorbed from the gut. The nurse, therefore, gives EHDP to the client on an empty stomach, 1 to 2 hours after breakfast or at bedtime with water or juice. Milk or milk products inhibit the drug's absorption as well. In a few clients, diarrhea may occur, but this problem is treated with an antidiarrheal medication.

Calcitonin and EHDP are the first drugs given and are often used in combination. If repeated courses of these drugs are not effective, mithramycin is given, usually in concert with one of the initial medications.

Mithramycin (Mithracin) is a potent antineoplastic and antibiotic with many side effects. It is reserved for clients with marked hypercalcemia or severe disease with neurologic compromise. By suppressing both osteoblast and osteoclast activity, the drug can relieve bone pain in 4 to 5 days. The usual dosage range is 10 to 25 μg/kg per day intravenously, with 15 μg/kg the most commonly administered dosage. The nurse observes for signs of toxicity to the liver, gastrointestinal tract, and kidneys. Liver and kidney function test results and intake and output are monitored daily. Because mithramycin also suppresses platelets, daily platelet counts and bleeding precautions are taken (see under the heading Interventions in the section on venous disease of Chap. 65). When liver enzyme levels become extremely high, drug therapy is interrupted temporarily.

Other pain relief measures. In addition to administering medication, the nurse employs physical measures to reduce pain. These may include application of heat, massage, and institution of an exercise program and are performed in conjunction with a physical therapist. The client may be fitted for an orthotic device to immobilize and provide support for the vertebrae or long bones. Additional interventions for pain relief, such as relaxation techniques, are discussed in Chapter 7.

Surgical management. When a client with Paget's disease has secondary arthritis and pain relief is not achieved, the client may undergo a partial or total joint replacement. The care for a client having this surgery is discussed in Chapter 28.

Impaired Physical Mobility

Planning: client goals. The major goal is that the client will maintain or improve mobility so that the client can independently perform necessary transport and self-care activities. Prolonged immobilization of the client with Paget's disease promotes hypercalcemia and its sequelae.

Interventions. For most clients with Paget's disease, nonsurgical management is sufficient to maintain or improve mobility. Surgery is performed for clients with severe bone deformity.

Nonsurgical management. The nurse works with the physical therapist to plan and implement a structured exercise program. Strengthening and weight-bearing exercises are performed daily under careful supervision.

Surgical management. When bone deformity interferes with physical mobility, one or more osteotomies (bone resections) may be performed. The care for a client with an osteotomy is described in Chapter 28.

Activity Intolerance

Planning: client goals. The goals for this diagnosis are that the client will (1) have a decrease in fatiguability and (2) experience an improvement in tolerance for activity.

Interventions: nonsurgical management. The client with severe disease is easily prone to fatigue. The nurse plans care in an organized fashion to promote rest. Activities are distributed throughout the day so that care, diagnostic testing, and physical therapy are not all performed during the morning hours. In addition, the nurse allows the client time to nap during the afternoon and sleep uninterrupted for 8 to 10 hours at night.

Body Image Disturbance

Planning: client goals. The primary goal for a client with a body image alteration is that the client will have an improvement in self-concept. The deformities incurred by the disease do not improve or reverse, but further deformity can be prevented by disease remission.

Interventions: nonsurgical management. By meeting the goals of pain reduction, improved mobility, and activity tolerance, the client's self-concept will probably improve. Specific interventions for promoting a healthy self-concept in view of alterations in body image are described in Chapter 9.

Potential for Injury

The planning and implementation for the prevention of injury are the same as those for the client with osteoporosis and osteomalacia (see earlier). The client is at the greatest risk for fracture during the *active* phase of the disease.

■ Discharge Planning

The client with Paget's disease may be discharged to home or a long-term care facility. For clients with terminal osteogenic sarcoma, hospice care is an alternative.

Home Care Preparation

The client discharged to the home setting has many of the same needs as the client with osteoporosis (see earlier).

Client/Family Education

Teaching for the client with Paget's disease is determined by the extent of disease. In symptomatic illness, the client and the family or significant others are taught about pain relief with drugs and non–drug-related measures. The nurse teaches the actions, dosage, and side effects of each medication, as well as reinforcing other pain relief strategies that were effective in the hospital setting.

The importance of maintaining a prescribed exercise program and wearing orthotic devices, if warranted, is stressed. Follow-up care in the home by the home care nurse and physical therapist is initiated by the hospital nurse before discharge.

The physician follows the client to monitor the progress of the disease. Laboratory tests, especially for ALP and urinary hydroxyproline levels, are performed at least monthly. Radiographs are taken periodically to determine the phase of the disease process and its severity.

Psychosocial Preparation

If the client goes into remission, he/she may think that the disease is cured. The nurse emphasizes that a remission is not a cure and that exacerbations may cause the disease to progress. Drug therapy may be resumed if the exacerbation is severe.

The uncertainty of the disease course and its potential debilitating effects may alter the client's role in the family and society. Support systems are mobilized as quickly as possible to assist with role changes.

The client is also prepared to expect the possibility of life-threatening complications. Careful medical and nursing monitoring of the client may improve the prognosis when complications are treated early in their course.

Health Care Resources

In addition to the resources described for the client with osteoporosis, the client with Paget's disease can contact the Paget's Disease Foundation or the local chapter of The Arthritis Foundation.

 Evaluation

On the basis of the identified nursing diagnoses, the nurse evaluates the care for the client with Paget's disease. The expected outcomes include that the client

1. States that pain is reduced or alleviated
2. States that fatigue is less frequent than before nursing interventions

3. Complies with daily exercise program
4. Uses assistive and adaptive devices as needed for independent self-care
5. Uses orthotic and ambulatory aids as prescribed
6. States that self-concept regarding body image is improving
7. Describes and complies with the drug regimen as ordered

The goal for the client is to force the disease into a long-term remission, thus halting the progress of the disorder. Although some clients may have a 5-year remission, in others Paget's disease may progress to multiple and life-threatening complications.

BONE INFECTION

OSTEOMYELITIS

OVERVIEW

Osteomyelitis is the term used to describe any infection of the bone. Even with current antibiotic treatment options, osteomyelitis continues to be a common problem and a difficult challenge for the health care team.

Pathophysiology

Osteomyelitis is divided into two major types: acute and chronic. An infection lasting less than 4 weeks is classified as *acute;* an infection lasting longer than that time is *chronic* osteomyelitis.

Regardless of the type of osteomyelitis, the pathophysiologic process is the same. On invasion by one or more pathogenic microorganisms, the bone, and often the surrounding soft tissues, becomes inflamed. The resulting increased vascularity promotes edema formation. Within several days, vessel thromboses develop, causing ischemia, or decreased blood flow, to the involved bone, which consequently dies. The presence of necrotic bone, or *sequestrum,* retards bone healing and causes superimposed infection, often in the form of bone abscess. As shown in Figure 30–6, the cycle repeats itself as the superimposed infection leads to further inflammation, vessel thromboses, and necrosis. Increased attention has been given to the mechanisms by which pathogens invade bone tissue: hematogenous spread, direct inoculation, and contiguous spread.

Acute hematogenous osteomyelitis occurs more often in children, but is becoming increasingly common in adults, particularly the elderly. An infection occurring in another part of the body moves to and invades bone tissue, particularly the long bones, such as the femur, and the vertebra. Pathogenic microbes favor bone that has a rich vascular supply and a marrow cavity.

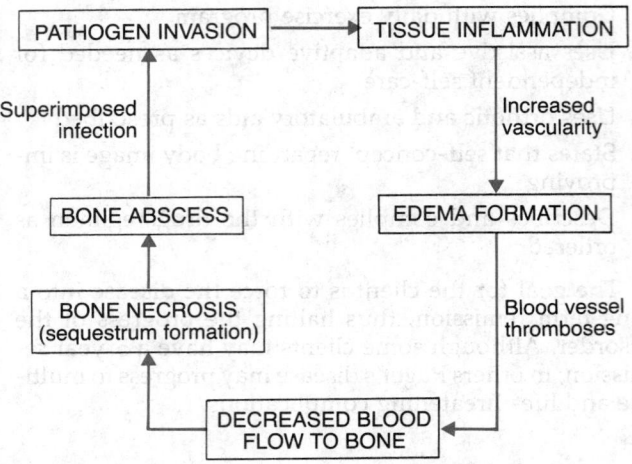

Figure 30–6

Infection cycle of osteomyelitis.

Osteomyelitis occurring from *direct inoculation* is seen frequently in adults. In this case, the client experiences penetrating trauma, which allows the offending organism direct access to bone tissue. The microbe may originate from the client's skin or from a penetrating object, such as a nail.

Contiguous spread of microorganisms occurs when surrounding soft tissue becomes infected. This mechanism is common in adults who have vascular compromise, as in diabetes or peripheral vascular disease. The client with vascular insufficiency is typically older than 50 years of age and has soft-tissue infections of the small bones in the feet or hands. Many different types of microbes invade the adjacent bone simultaneously.

Chronic osteomyelitis may result from any of the acute types. The adult with a compromised vascular supply is at the greatest risk for chronic infection. Advanced age and concurrent disease may prolong the course of the infection for as long as a year or more.

Etiology

Each type of bone infection has its own causative factors. Acute hematogenous spread results from bacteremia, underlying disease, or nonpenetrating trauma. Urinary tract infections, particularly in older men, tend to spread to the lower vertebrae. Long-term intravenous (IV) catheters, such as Hickman catheters, are primary sources of infection. Clients undergoing long-term hemodialysis and IV drug abusers are also at risk for osteomyelitis. Salmonella infections of the gastrointestinal tract may spread to bone. Clients with sickle cell anemia and other hemoglobinopathies frequently experience multiple episodes of salmonellosis, which can cause bone infection.

Minimal trauma of the nonpenetrating type can cause hemorrhages or small vessel occlusions, leading to

bone necrosis. Regardless of cause, many infections are caused by *Staphylococcus aureus.*

In contrast, penetrating trauma leads to acute osteomyelitis by direct inoculation. A concurrent soft-tissue infection may be present as well. Animal bites, puncture wounds, and bone surgery can result in bone infection. The most common offending organism is *Pseudomonas aeruginosa,* but other gram-negative bacteria may be found.

Contiguous spread occurs when adjacent soft tissues are infected. Poor dental hygiene and radiation therapy can predispose the mandible to infection. Malignant external otitis media involving the base of the skull and mastoid bones is seen in elderly diabetic clients. The most common case of contiguous spread is found in the client with diabetes or peripheral vascular disease who has a slow-healing foot ulcer. Multiple organisms are responsible for the subsequent osteomyelitis.

If bone infection is misdiagnosed or inadequately treated, chronic osteomyelitis occurs. Inadequate treatment results when the treatment period is too short or when the treatment is delayed or inappropriate. Gram-negative bacteria alone or mixed with gram-positive organisms account for nearly 50% of chronic bone infections (Gentry, 1987).

Incidence

Acute hematogenous osteomyelitis is decreasing in frequency, while contiguous infection associated with peripheral vascular disorders is increasing. The age distribution has shifted from children to the older population. In addition to *S. aureus,* gram-negative and mixed bacteria are becoming more common as the invasive organisms.

Chronic osteomyelitis remains a problem, occurring in as many as 25% of clients with acute hematogenous infection. Recurrence of infection years after its initial onset is common.

PREVENTION

Acute osteomyelitis is a preventable condition. Risk factors are identified and omitted or modified when possible. For example, strict aseptic technique is used for IV catheters. Foley's catheters are removed as quickly as possible to prevent urinary tract infection. Special precautions are used in the operating room when bone surgery is performed. The use of double masks, intraoperative antibiotics, and laminar airflow units are examples of measures taken to reduce the chance of bone infection.

High-risk clients—the elderly, diabetic persons, and those with peripheral vascular disease—are identified and monitored carefully. They are taught the preventive measures necessary to avoid osteomyelitis. If acute infection occurs, clients should seek medical attention and comply with long-term treatment to reduce the risk of chronic infection.

COLLABORATIVE MANAGEMENT

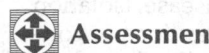 **Assessment**

History

When taking a history, the nurse records the presence of risk factors related to osteomyelitis. In addition to *age*, the nurse asks the client about a *history of drug abuse; previous infections anywhere in the body; concurrent medial conditions,* such as sickle cell anemia or diabetes mellitus; *nonpenetrating trauma; penetrating wounds; surgical procedures,* especially bone surgery; *use of tubes or catheters;* and *radiation therapy.* All of these factors are potential sources of infection.

In addition to the identification of risk factors, information about the client's overall health status is obtained. A malnourished client with a bone infection, for instance, is less likely to heal than a client who is adequately nourished.

Physical Assessment: Clinical Manifestations

The client with osteomyelitis manifests *fever*, usually above 101° F (38° C). The area around the infected bone *swells* and is tender when palpated. *Erythema,* or redness, and *heat* may also be present.

When vascular insufficiency is suspected, the nurse assesses circulation in the distal extremities. Neurovascular assessment technique is described in Chapter 31. *Draining ulcers* may be present on the feet or hands, indicating inadequate healing ability as a result of poor circulation.

Bone pain, with or without other manifestations, is a common complaint of clients with bone infection. The pain is described as a constant, localized, pulsating sensation that intensifies with movement. In severe vascular compromise, the client may not feel discomfort because of nerve damage from lack of blood supply.

Fever, swelling, and erythema are less common in chronic osteomyelitis. Ulceration resulting in sinus tract formation, localized pain, and drainage are more characteristic of chronic infection.

Psychosocial Assessment

The client with osteomyelitis often fears that the infection may not heal and that consequently disfiguring surgery, perhaps an amputation, may be needed. The nurse identifies and documents this concern.

Antibiotic therapy is intensive and given for 4 weeks or longer. If the treatment needs to be supervised in a hospital setting, the client can expect weeks and perhaps months of hospitalization. The nurse assesses the potential impact of this disruption in the client's life, particularly in relationship to family and occupation. If the client is to receive treatment in the home setting, the nurse assesses the available resources and support systems that can be utilized during the recovery phase of illness.

The client may be isolated from others, depending on the type of microorganisms found. The nurse elicits information regarding the client's feelings about being isolated, recognizing that a disturbance in self-concept may result.

Laboratory Findings

White blood cell count.   The client with osteomyelitis usually has an elevated leukocyte count, often double the normal value. In chronic infection, normal or slight elevations are not uncommon.

Erythrocyte sedimentation rate.   The erythrocyte sedimentation rate (ESR) may be normal early in the course of the disease, but rises as the condition progresses. It is not unusual for the rate to remain elevated for as long as 3 months after drug therapy is discontinued.

Blood culture.   If bacteremia is present, a blood culture identifies the offending organisms to determine which antibiotics should be used in treatment. Approximately 50% of clients with acute hematogenous infection have positive blood cultures (Lefrock et al., 1984).

Radiographic Findings

Radiographic findings are not usually helpful in the early course of the disease. Changes in bone tissue are not evident and are easily misinterpreted during the first few weeks.

Other Diagnostic Tests

Bone scans.   Although bone changes cannot be detected early with standard radiographic testing, changes in blood flow can be seen early in the course of the disease by radionuclide scanning. A bone scan, using technetium or gallium, is extremely helpful in the diagnosis of osteomyelitis and identifies about 90% of cases. Indium imaging has been used, but its results have not been adequately compared with technetium scanning findings.

Computed tomography and magnetic resonance imaging.   Some studies indicate that CT and magnetic resonance imaging are more sensitive in the diagnosis of osteomyelitis than traditional bone scanning. When cost and accessibility factors are considered, their usefulness may not outweigh the value of less costly techniques.

Bone biopsy.   The definitive diagnosis of osteomyelitis is made by bone biopsy. A culture of soft tissue or sinus tracts may not identify the offending microbes invading the bone. Often the organisms affecting soft tissue and bone are different, and each must be treated.

 Analysis: Nursing Diagnosis

If the client has had repeated episodes of chronic infection, his/her mental and emotional outlook may overshadow physical problems. The priority of nursing diagnoses drawn from the data depends, in part, on the severity of the disease.

Common Diagnoses

The typical nursing diagnoses for a client with osteomyelitis include the following:

1. Potential for injury related to bone infection
2. Pain related to infectious process
3. Impaired physical mobility related to pain and inflammation
4. Altered (peripheral) tissue perfusion related to inflammation and infection
5. Impaired skin integrity related to inflammation, wound, or ulceration

Additional Diagnoses

The following additional diagnoses may be applicable to the client with osteomyelitis:

1. Activity intolerance related to pain
2. Anxiety related to possible treatment failure and need for surgery
3. Fear related to possible disfiguring surgery
4. Anticipatory grieving related to possible amputation
5. Impaired home maintenance management related to lack of support systems
6. Altered nutrition: less than body requirements related to need for increased nutrients to promote healing
7. Body image disturbance related to isolation or surgery
8. Sleep pattern disturbance related to pain and round-the-clock antibiotic therapy
9. Altered (peripheral) tissue perfusion related to diabetes or other peripheral vascular disease
10. Knowledge deficit related to treatment regimen

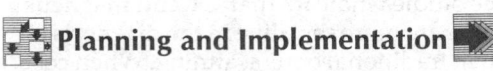

Planning and Implementation

Potential for Injury

Planning: client goals. The goals for resolving this problem are that the client will (1) not experience further infection, (2) not have any complications from the infectious process, and (3) have adequate bone and soft-tissue healing.

Interventions. The specific treatment protocol depends on the type and number of microbes present in the infected tissue. Surgical management may be needed when other measures fail to resolve the infectious process.

Nonsurgical management. Antibiotic therapy is initiated as soon as possible to reverse the disease. Isolation procedures (drainage and secretion precautions or contact isolation) prevent the spread of the offending organism to other clients and health personnel.

Drug therapy. IV antibiotic therapy is given for 4 to 6 weeks for acute osteomyelitis. Often more than one antibiotic is needed to combat the presence of multiple types of organisms. The nurse gives the drugs at specifically ordered times so that therapeutic serum levels are achieved. The nurse must become familiar with the drugs' actions, side and toxic effects, interactions, and precautions for administration. The nursing implications for major antibiotics are discussed in Chapter 26.

The optimal drug regimen for chronic osteomyelitis is not well established. Prolonged therapy for more than 3 months may be needed to eliminate the infection. Because of the cost of lengthy hospital stays, clients are being discharged to the home setting with IV catheters, such as the Hickman catheter, to self-administer their medications. After discontinuation of IV drugs, oral antibiotic therapy may be needed for weeks or months. A cost-saving alternative to IV drug therapy is the use of new oral quinolone antibiotics such as ciprofloxacin (Cipro). This drug is administered every 12 hours in doses of 250, 500, or 750 mg. The nurse cautions the client to avoid taking antacids because they decrease the absorption of the antibiotic (Martin, 1989).

In addition to drug administration, the wound may be irrigated, either continuously or intermittently, with one or more antibiotic solutions. The nurse is responsible for drug administration and uses sterile technique at all times. A technique in which beads are impregnated with an antibiotic and packed into the wound provides direct contact of the antibiotic with the offending organism.

Drainage precautions and contact isolation. If an open wound or ulcer is present, the client's treatment usually includes drainage precautions for limited infections in which the wound is covered. Contact isolation is reserved for more severe infections, particularly when the purulent material cannot be adequately contained by a dressing (see Chap. 26 for procedures). The open area is covered and strict aseptic technique is used when changing dressings to prevent further contamination. Wounds may be managed through the window of a cast, which must remain dry during dressing or irrigation procedures. Chapter 31 describes the nursing care for a client with a cast.

Surgical management. Antibiotic therapy alone may not be sufficient to meet the goals of treatment. New surgical techniques are being used to minimize the disfigurement that heretofore has been a devastating sequela. Most often surgery is reserved for clients with chronic osteomyelitis.

Sequestrectomy. Bone cannot heal in the presence of necrotic tissue. Therefore, a sequestrectomy is performed to débride the infected bone and allow revascularization of tissue.

Bone grafts. The excision of devitalized and infected bone often results in a sizable cavity, or bone defect. The use of cancellous bone grafts to obliterate bone defects began in the 1940s and is still used widely today. One of the most popular surgical techniques is referred to as the Papineau procedure, or open cancellous bone graft, and is used primarily with large bone and soft-tissue defects.

As a three-step procedure, the necrotic bone is excised, the bone is grafted, and the skin is covered, if necessary (Fig. 30–7). The donor bone is most often taken from the client's posterior ileum. Small chips of bone are packed tightly into the cavity and a pressure dressing is applied. In 4 or 5 days, the first postoperative dressing is done in the operating room under sterile conditions. Daily sterile dressings are applied until about 2 weeks later when the graft stabilizes. If needed, a skin graft, usually a simple split-thickness graft, is performed between 8 and 16 weeks after the bone graft. Chapter 40 describes the care for a client with a skin graft.

Bone segment transfers. When infected bone is extensively resected, reconstruction with microvascular bone transfers may be useful. In general, a bone transfer is reserved for skeletal defects longer than 6 cm (2.4 in); defects shorter than this receive cancellous bone grafting (Wood & Cooney, 1984).

The most common donor sites are the client's fibula and iliac crest. The bone graft may have an attached muscle or skin flap if necessary. The steps of the procedure are similar to those of cancellous grafting in that débridement precedes bone transfer.

Muscle flaps. If the bony defect is relatively small, a muscle flap may be the only surgery required. Local muscle flaps are used in the treatment of chronic osteomyelitis when soft tissue does not obliterate the dead space, or cavity, resulting from bone débridement. The flap provides wound coverage and enhances blood flow to promote healing. A split-thickness skin graft is often applied several days after the muscle flap.

Amputation. When the described surgical procedures are not appropriate or successful, the affected limb may be amputated. The physical and psychologic care for a client who has undergone an amputation is discussed in Chapter 31.

For all of the surgical procedures and their recovery phases, long-term antibiotic coverage is necessary. The postoperative nursing care is similar to that for repair of musculoskeletal trauma (Chap. 31).

Pain

Planning: client goals. The primary goal is that the client will experience reduction or alleviation of pain and discomfort.

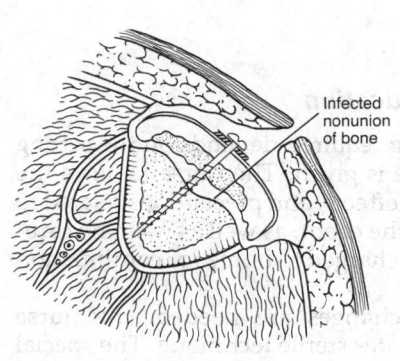
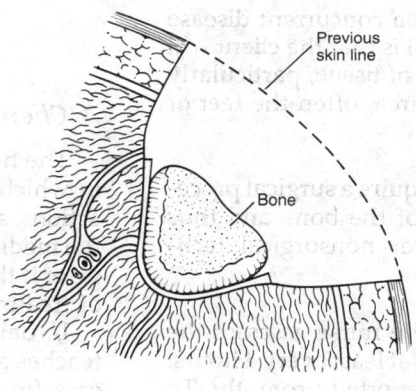

Figure 30–7

Three stages of the Papineau procedure: *A*, Stage I: excision and stabilization, allowing tissue to granulate. *B*, Stage II: open cancellous bone graft showing vascularization. *C*, Stage III: skin coverage if not spontaneous.

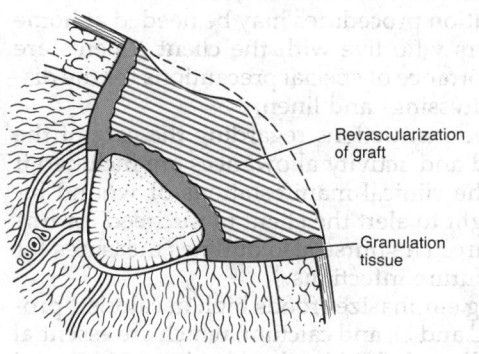
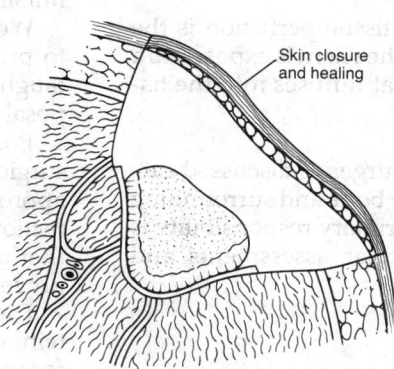

Interventions: nonsurgical management. The client with osteomyelitis frequently suffers chronic pain for many months or years. Potent analgesics and NSAIDs are given and alternated to prevent dependence. Pain management, both drug and non–drug related, is described in detail in Chapter 7.

Impaired Physical Mobility

Planning: client goals. The client may be able to provide self-care, but often has difficulty with ambulation because of the pain associated with the infection or the treatment required, for example, surgery. The goals, then, are that the client will (1) increase mobility and (2) not experience complications from prolonged impaired mobility.

Interventions: nonsurgical management. The nurse confers with the physical therapist to assess the need for ambulatory assistive devices, such as crutches. Instruction on ambulatory aids and transfer techniques is usually provided by the physical therapist and reinforced by the nurse. Strengthening and ROM exercises are important to increase mobility and prevent complications of immobility.

Altered (Peripheral) Tissue Perfusion

Planning: client goals. The client's alteration in tissue perfusion may be complicated by a concurrent disease such as diabetes mellitus. The goal is that the client will have an increase in the perfusion of tissue, particularly that distal to the bone infection area, often the feet or hands.

Interventions. The client may require a surgical procedure to increase the vascularity of the bone and thus promote healing, although newer nonsurgical techniques are being tested.

Nonsurgical management. The nurse assesses the extremity for neurovascular status at least every 4 hours. Any changes are recorded and reported promptly. To decrease edema formation, which may be impairing tissue perfusion, the nurse elevates the extremity on one or two pillows.

A new treatment to increase tissue perfusion is the use of the hyperbaric chamber. The client is exposed to a high concentration of oxygen that diffuses into the tissues to promote healing.

Surgical management. The surgeries discussed earlier increase the vascularity of the bone and surrounding soft tissues. Again, the nurse's primary responsibility is to perform frequent neurovascular assessments and record specific findings.

Impaired Skin Integrity

Planning: client goals. The client's skin integrity may be disrupted from an associated traumatic wound or ulceration or from surgery. In either case, the goal is that the client will have a restoration and maintenance of skin integrity.

Interventions: nonsurgical management. The nurse carefully observes the skin frequently for changes in color, temperature, size of lesion, and drainage. Open lesions require at least daily dressing changes using sterile technique. Nonpurulent drainage may be normal after grafting procedures.

To promote wound healing, the nurse increases the client's caloric and protein intake. Intake of vitamin C, calcium, and vitamin D is also encouraged.

■ Discharge Planning

The client with osteomyelitis may be treated in a hospital setting or receive treatment on an outpatient or home care basis.

Home Care Preparation

If the client is treated outside of the hospital, the nurse helps the client identify resources for assistance with care. The drug therapy and dressing change procedure may be so complex that the client needs help. Health teaching for the client and caregiver in the home is vital.

Client/Family Education

The health teaching required depends on the setting in which medical care is given. The nurse reviews the actions, side and toxic effects, and precautions related to the medications with the client, as well as with the caregiver if the client is discharged to home for continuation of treatment.

If daily dressing changes are needed, the nurse teaches and demonstrates sterile technique. The special care for long-term IV catheters is also demonstrated. The client should perform self-care, such as dressing changes and catheter care, several times under direct nursing supervision before discharge from the hospital.

Wound isolation procedures may be needed at home to protect others who live with the client. Clients are taught the importance of special precautions for the disposal of dirty dressings and linen.

Postoperative instructions regarding the care of the surgical wound and activity allowances are included if appropriate. The clinical manifestations of wound infection are taught to alert the client to the need for further medical care. The nurse also outlines measures for prevention of future infections.

Diet teaching emphasizes foods high in calories, protein, vitamins C and D, and calcium, which are essential for wound healing. A fluid intake of at least 3000 mL/day is encouraged to prevent renal complications from prolonged antibiotic use.

Psychosocial Preparation

The client with chronic osteomyelitis needs encouragement regarding response to treatment. The infection, especially in the presence of vascular compromise, may take months or years to cure. Clients fear repeated infections and consequent surgeries. The longevity of the course of illness may affect the client's role as a family member and cause financial burden if the client loses his/her job because of prolonged sick leave.

Health Care Resources

Treatment in the home requires supplies for medication administration, wound dressings, and IV catheter care. The nurse provides information to the client and the caregiver, perhaps a family member, as to where supplies can be obtained. The nurse also contacts the community health nurse for follow-up care, including wound monitoring and supervision in the home.

 Evaluation

On the basis of the identified nursing diagnoses, the nurse evaluates the care provided to the client with acute or chronic osteomyelitis. The expected outcomes include that the client

1. Complies with the prolonged treatment regimen
2. States that pain is reduced or alleviated
3. Restores and maintains skin integrity
4. Increases tissue perfusion to the affected area
5. Performs ambulation activities independently

The goal of medical treatment is to cure the infection and prevent its recurrence. The process is often long and frustrating.

BONE TUMORS

BENIGN BONE TUMORS

OVERVIEW

Benign bone tumors are often asymptomatic and may be discovered on routine radiographic examination or as the cause of pathologic fractures. Tumors may arise from several types of tissue. The major classifications include *chondrogenic* (from cartilage), *osteogenic* (from bone), and *fibrogenic* (from fibrous tissue; found in children) (see the accompanying Key Features of Disease). The cause of bone tumors, like other neoplasms, is unknown. Although many specific benign tumors have been identified, only the common ones are described here.

KEY FEATURES OF DISEASE ■ Classification of Bone Tumors	
Benign	**Malignant**
Chondrogenic	
Osteochondroma	Chondrosarcoma
Chondroma	
Osteogenic	
Osteoid osteoma	Osteosarcoma
Osteoblastoma	
Giant cell tumor	
	Fibrogenic
	Fibrosarcoma
	Unknown origin
	Ewing's sarcoma

Chondrogenic Tumors

Osteochondroma

Pathophysiology. The most common benign bone tumor is osteochondroma. Although its onset is usually in childhood, the tumor grows until skeletal maturity and may not be diagnosed until adulthood. The tumor may be a single growth or multiple growths and can occur in any bone. The femur and the tibia are most frequently involved.

On gross appearance, the tumor has a large cartilaginous cap with a bony stalk protruding away from the bone. As the cap grows, the tumor ossifies and may become malignant. About 10% of osteochondromas change into sarcomas.

Incidence. Osteochondromas account for about 40% of all benign bone tumors and typically affect males more often than females.

Chondroma

Pathophysiology. The chondroma, or endochondroma, is closely related to the osteochondroma in histologic presentation. Unlike the osteochondroma, however, the chondroma is a lesion of mature hyaline cartilage affecting primarily the hands and the feet. The ribs, the sternum, the spine, and the long bones may also be involved. Chondromas are slow growing and frequently cause pathologic fractures after trivial injury.

Incidence. Chondromas are found at any age, occur in both males and females, and can affect any bone.

Osteogenic Tumors

Osteoid Osteoma

Pathophysiology. The osteoid osteoma is distinguished by its pinkish, granular appearance, resulting from the proliferation of osteoblasts. Unlike other tumors, a single lesion is usually less than 1 cm in diameter. Any bone can be affected, but the femur and the tibia are most often involved. When the osteoid osteoma occurs in the spinal column and sacrum, the client has clinical manifestations resembling the lumbar disk syndrome. The client complains of unremitting bone pain, probably attributable to the increase in prostaglandin levels associated with the tumor.

Incidence. Approximately 10% of all benign bone tumors are osteoid osteomas. The lesion occurs in children and young adults, with a predominance among males.

Osteoblastoma

Pathophysiology. Often called the giant osteoid osteoma, the osteoblastoma affects the vertebrae and long bones. The tumor is larger than the osteoid osteoma and lies in cancellous bone. Its reddish, granular appearance facilitates diagnosis.

Incidence. The lesion accounts for less than 1% of primary bone tumors and affects male adolescents and young adults.

Giant Cell Tumor

Pathophysiology. The origin of the giant cell tumor remains uncertain. These lesions are aggressive and can be extensive. On gross examination, they are gray to reddish brown and may involve surrounding soft tissue. Although classified as benign, giant cell tumors can metastasize to the lung.

Incidence. Unlike most other benign bone tumors, giant cell tumors affect women older than 20 years of age, with the peak incidence in the third decade. Approximately 18% of all benign bone tumors are giant cell.

COLLABORATIVE MANAGEMENT

 Assessment

History

In addition to recording *age* and *sex*, the nurse collects data from the client that are linked with the occurrence of bone tumors. The nurse asks whether the client has experienced *trivial trauma*, *fractures*, or *neoplasms*. A *family history of neoplasms* is also elicited.

Benign bone tumors can recur, especially if all of the neoplastic tissue is not removed. Giant cell tumors have the highest recurrence rate.

Physical Assessment: Clinical Manifestations

If a client experiences clinical manifestations of a benign bone tumor, *pain* is the most frequent complaint. The pain can range from a mild to moderate level, as seen with chondromas, to the unremitting, intense pain typical with osteoid osteomas. Pain can be caused by direct tumor invasion into soft tissue, compressing peripheral nerves, or by a resulting pathologic fracture.

In addition to collecting information regarding the nature of the client's pain, the nurse observes and palpates the suspected involved area. When affecting the lower extremities or the small bones of the hands and feet, *local swelling* may be detected as the neoplasm enlarges. In some cases, *muscle atrophy* or *muscle spasm* may be present. The nurse palpates the bone and muscle to detect these changes and elicit tenderness.

Psychosocial Assessment

The client with a suspected or actual bone tumor is often fearful that the lesion is or may become malignant. Additionally, he/she may be anxious about the possibility or extent of surgery needed to remove the tumor. The nurse identifies the fears and concerns of the client so that appropriate interventions can be planned and implemented.

Laboratory Findings

Laboratory testing is not helpful in the diagnosis of benign tumors, but is useful in distinguishing benign from malignant lesions.

Radiographic Findings

Routine radiography and conventional tomography are extremely beneficial in localizing and visualizing neoplasms of the bone. Benign tumors are characterized by sharp margins, intact cortices, and smooth, uniform periosteal bone.

CT is less useful, except in complex anatomic areas, such as the spinal column and sacrum. The test is helpful in evaluating the extent of soft-tissue involvement.

Other Diagnostic Tests

Bone biopsy. When the diagnosis of a benign tumor is uncertain, an open or needle biopsy of the bone is performed. The open, surgical method is preferred to obtain a sufficient amount of tissue.

Bone scan. A bone scan is not specific in distinguishing a benign from a malignant tumor, but it visualizes the extent of the lesions better than most radiographic examinations.

Analysis: Nursing Diagnosis

After assessing the client, the nurse analyzes the data to identify the nursing diagnoses for a client with a benign bone tumor.

Common Diagnoses

The common nursing diagnoses for a client with a benign bone tumor are

1. Potential for injury related to pathologic fractures secondary to bone tissue changes
2. Pain related to direct tumor invasion or pathologic fracture

Additional Diagnoses

For extensive and invasive bone tumors, the following nursing diagnoses may be appropriate:

1. Activity intolerance related to pain
2. Anxiety related to possible surgical intervention
3. Fear related to possibility of sarcomatous tumor changes
4. Impaired physical mobility related to pain, muscle wasting, or surgical procedure
5. Impaired skin integrity related to surgical procedure
6. Sleep pattern disturbance related to pain secondary to osteoid osteoma
7. Knowledge deficit related to medical diagnosis and treatment regimen

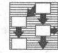 **Planning and Implementation**

Potential for Injury

Planning: client goals. The major goal for this diagnosis is that the client will not experience a fall or trivial trauma, which could result in a pathologic fracture. After the tumor is removed, the danger of fracture is minimized.

Interventions: nonsurgical management. The nursing interventions to prevent clients from experiencing a fracture are the same as those described for the client with osteoporosis (see earlier).

Pain

Planning: client goals. The goal for this diagnosis is that the client will experience alleviation or reduction of pain resulting from the bone tumor.

Interventions. Nonsurgical measures for relief of pain are usually combined with surgery to remove the tumor.

Nonsurgical management. Drug therapy and surgery are used in combination when possible. Nondrug pain relief measures are also employed.

Drug therapy. In addition to receiving analgesics to reduce pain, the client with osteoid osteoma is given one or more NSAIDs to inhibit prostaglandin synthesis and thus relieve pain. The nurse observes for drug actions and side effects, administering the drug after meals or with milk and crackers.

Other pain relief measures. Depending on the client's preference and tolerance, measures such as application of heat or cold may be helpful. In addition to physical interventions, the nurse can employ imagery and relaxation techniques (Chap. 7).

Surgical management. The most common surgical procedure used for clients with benign bone tumors is *curettage,* or simple excision of the tumor tissue. If the tumor is small, surgery may not be indicated. When the lesion is extremely extensive, as in giant cell tumor, the neoplasm is removed with care to restore or maintain the function of the adjacent joint, most often the knee. In some cases, the knee is replaced with a prosthetic device or is fused (arthrodesis). The nursing care for clients with these surgical procedures is discussed elsewhere in the text.

■ **Discharge Planning**

The client is discharged to home after stabilization postoperatively. The care and health teaching implemented by the nurse are the same as those for other general orthopedic surgery (Chap. 31).

 Evaluation

On the basis of the identified nursing diagnoses, the nurse evaluates the care provided to the client with a benign bone tumor. The expected outcomes may include that the client

1. States that pain is minimized after interventions
2. Avoids physical injury that could result in fracture
3. Returns to a functional life style

MALIGNANT BONE TUMORS

OVERVIEW

Malignant bone tumors may be *primary,* those that originate in bone, or *secondary,* those that originate in other tissues and metastasize to bone. Primary tumors occur most frequently in persons between 10 and 30 years of age and make up a small percentage of bone cancers. As for other forms of cancer, the exact cause of bone cancer is unknown. Metastatic lesions are found most often in the older age group and account for the majority of bone cancers.

Primary Tumors

Osteosarcoma

Pathophysiology. Osteosarcoma, or osteogenic sarcoma, is the most common type of primary malignant bone tumor. More than half occur in the distal femur, with the proximal tibia and humerus following in frequency of occurrence. Flat-bone and long-bone incidence is about equal in persons older than 25 years of age.

Osteosarcoma is a relatively large lesion, causing pain and swelling of short duration. The area involved is usually warm as the vascularity to the site increases. The central portion of the mass is sclerotic from increased osteoblastic activity, whereas the periphery is soft, extending through the bone cortex in the classic sunburst appearance associated with the neoplasm. An inward expansion into the medullary canal is also common.

Osteosarcoma may be categorized as osteoblastic, chondroblastic, or fibroblastic, depending on the tissue of origin. Regardless of source, the lesion typically metastasizes to the periphery of the lung within 2 years of treatment; metastasis usually results in death.

Incidence. Osteosarcoma occurs more often in males than in females (2:1) between ages 10 and 30 years and in older individuals with Paget's disease. Clients who have received radiation for other forms of cancer or who have benign lesions are at a high risk for the development of malignant tumor.

Ewing's Sarcoma

Pathophysiology. Although Ewing's sarcoma is not as common as other tumors, it is the most malignant. Like other primary tumors, it causes pain and swelling. In addition, systemic manifestations, particularly low-grade fever, leukocytosis, and anemia, characterize the lesions. The pelvis and the lower extremity are most often affected. Pelvic involvement is a poor prognostic sign.

Histologically, the tumor is similar to bone lymphoma. On x-ray film the characteristic mottled destructive pattern and onionskin appearance of the bone surface distinguish the neoplasm as Ewing's sarcoma. Like other malignant tumors, it is not encapsulated and often extends into soft tissue. Death results from metastasis to the lungs and other bones.

Incidence. Five per cent of all malignant bone tumors are Ewing's sarcoma. Although the tumor can be seen in clients of any age, it usually occurs in children and young adults in their 20s. Men are affected more often than women.

Chondrosarcoma

Pathophysiology. In contrast to the client with osteosarcoma, the client with chondrosarcoma experiences dull pain and swelling for a long period. The tumor typically affects the pelvis and proximal femur near the diaphysis. Arising from cartilaginous tissue, the lesion destroys bone and often calcifies. The client with this tumor has a better prognosis than one with osteogenic sarcoma.

Incidence. Chondrosarcoma occurs in middle- and older-aged individuals, with a slight predominance in men, and accounts for about 7% of all malignant bone tumors.

Fibrosarcoma

Pathophysiology. Arising from fibrous tissue, fibrosarcomas can be divided into subtypes. The most malignant subgroup is the malignant fibrous histiocytoma (MFH). Most often its clinical presentation is slow and insidious, without specific manifestations. Local tenderness, with or without a palpable mass, occurs in the long bones of the lower extremity. Like other bone cancers, the lesion can metastasize to the lungs.

Incidence. MFH affects persons of all ages, but typically occurs in middle-aged men. Fortunately, the lesion is not common.

Metastatic Bone Disease

Pathophysiology. Primary tumors of the prostate, the breast, the kidney, the thyroid, and the lung are called *bone-seeking* cancers, that is, they metastasize to the bone more often than other primary tumors. The vertebrae, the pelvis, the femur, and the ribs are the bone sites commonly affected. Simply stated, primary tumor cells or seeds are carried to bone through the blood stream. Almost all metastatic lesions are of epithelial origin and begin in the bone marrow.

Pathologic fractures, which occur in 10% to 15% of cases, are a major concern in management. The most commonly affected areas for fracture are the acetabulum and the proximal femur.

Incidence. Metastatic bone tumors greatly outnumber primary malignant neoplasms. Metastatic bone disease primarily affects persons older than 40 years of age. In a client with a history of cancer and local pain, metastasis is suspected. The incidence of bone metastasis ranges from 20% to 70%, depending on the statistical reporting source. It is suspected that the reported incidence is grossly underestimated.

COLLABORATIVE MANAGEMENT

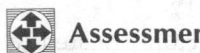 **Assessment**

History

The data collected for the client suspected of having a malignant tumor are similar to those required for the client with a benign growth. In addition, the nurse asks the client whether he/she has had *previous radiation therapy for cancer* and elicits information about the client's *general health state.*

Physical Assessment: Clinical Manifestations

The clinical manifestations seen in clients with malignant tumors or metastatic disease vary, depending on the specific type of lesion. Most often, the client has a group of nonspecific complaints including *pain, local swelling,* and a *tender, palpable mass.* Marked *disability* may be present in metastatic bone disease.

In a client with Ewing's sarcoma, a *low-grade fever* may occur because of the systemic features of the neoplasm. For this reason, Ewing's sarcoma is often confused with osteomyelitis. Fatigue and pallor resulting from anemia are also common.

In performing a musculoskeletal examination, the nurse inspects the involved area and palpates the mass for size characteristics and tenderness. The client's ability to perform mobility tasks and ADL is also determined. The nurse observes the client performing mobility skills and records results on an ADL or mobility assessment tool (Chap. 21). The degree of disability can then be determined for comparison with later measurements after medical and nursing intervention.

Psychosocial Assessment

Often the client with a malignant bone tumor is a young adult whose socially productive life is just beginning. Research has repeatedly demonstrated that the client needs support systems to help cope with the diagnosis and its treatment. Family, significant others, and health care professionals are major components of the needed support. The nurse assesses the systems available to the client.

Clients frequently experience a loss of control over their lives when a diagnosis of malignancy is made. As a result, they become anxious and fearful about the outcome of their illness. Coping with the diagnosis becomes a challenge. The client goes through the grieving process—initially, there is denial. The nurse identifies the anxiety level, and assesses the stage or stages of the grieving process experienced by the client. The nurse also identifies any maladaptive behavior, indicating ineffective coping mechanisms.

Chapter 25 further elaborates on the psychosocial assessment for the client with a malignancy.

Laboratory Findings

Alkaline phosphatase. The client with a malignant or metastatic bone tumor typically has an elevation of serum ALP levels, indicating the body's attempt to form new bone by increasing osteoblastic activity.

Complete blood cell count. The client with Ewing's sarcoma or metastatic bone lesions frequently has a normocytic anemia. In addition, leukocytosis is common with Ewing's sarcoma.

Serum calcium. In about 10% of clients with bone metastasis from the breast, the kidney, and the lung, the serum calcium level is elevated. Massive bone destruction stimulates release of the mineral into the blood stream.

Erythrocyte sedimentation rate. A client with Ewing's sarcoma and bone metastasis often has an elevated ESR, probably attributable to secondary tissue inflammation.

Other laboratory tests. In addition to the listed tests, a more thorough evaluation, including a platelet count and SMA-12 (12/60) analysis, is performed for clients with metastatic disease. The client's general health status is assessed to predict the treatment outcome.

Radiographic Findings

As for benign bone tumors, routine x-ray films and conventional tomography allow for adequate visualization of malignant lesions. Although each tumor type has its own characteristic radiographic pattern, certain findings are common to all. Malignant tumors typically show poor margination, bone destruction, irregular periosteal new bone, and cortical breakthrough (Fig. 30–8). Metastatic lesions may increase or decrease bone density, depending on the amount of osteoblastic and osteoclastic activity. CT is helpful in determining the extent of soft-tissue damage.

Other Diagnostic Tests

Bone biopsy. A bone biopsy is performed to diagnose tumor type. A needle biopsy is usually done when metastasis to the bone is suspected. An open method, through surgical incision, is preferred for primary lesions. The surgeon keeps the incision as small as possible. The biopsy scar is removed during bone cancer surgery to eliminate a possible source of tumor seeds.

After biopsy, the cancer is staged according to the grade of the tumor. One popular method is the *TNM* staging system, utilizing determinations of tumor size, nodal involvement, and evidence of metastasis. Another surgical staging method is to correlate the tumor grade (high or low), tumor site (intracompartmental or extracompartmental), and the presence of metastatic

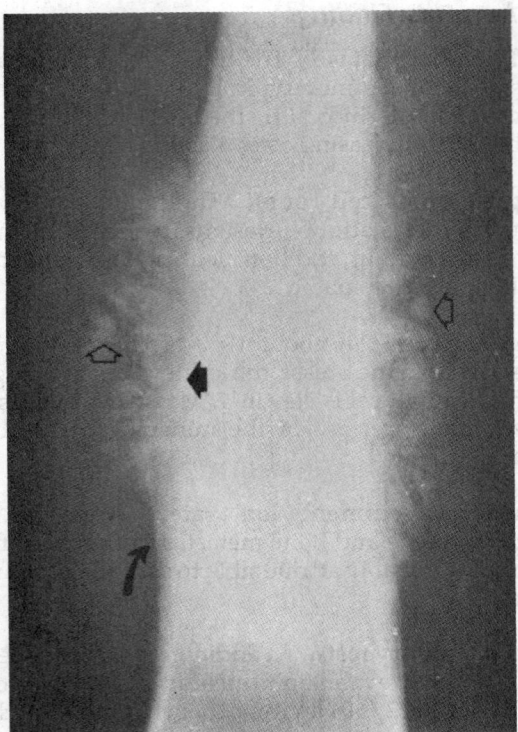

Figure 30-8

Radiograph of osteosarcoma. Cortical breakthrough (sunburst appearance) marked by black arrow. New bone formation shown by open arrows. (From Kricun, M. E. [1983]. Radiographic evaluation of solitary bone lesions. *Orthopedic Clinics of North America, 14,* 39–64.)

disease (positive or negative). Staging guides the health care team in their decision regarding treatment.

Bone scan. Although a bone scan is not helpful in determining the type of tumor, it serves to visualize the extent of the cancer. A scan is almost always ordered when bone metastasis is suspected.

 Analysis: Nursing Diagnosis

The client with a malignant or metastatic bone tumor presents a challenge to the health care team. The nurse gathers the initial data and formulates nursing diagnoses and goals in conjunction with the family and other team members.

Common Diagnoses

Before medical treatment is instituted, the following nursing diagnoses are common to clients with malignant bone lesions:

1. Pain related to direct tumor invasion into soft tissue
2. Anticipatory grieving related to change in body image or impending death

3. Body image disturbance related to possible chemotherapy, radiation therapy, or surgery
4. Potential for injury (pathologic fracture) related to bone demineralization secondary to bone tumor
5. Anxiety related to loss of control and need for support systems

Additional Diagnoses

In addition to the common diagnoses seen in most clients, one or more of the following diagnoses may be applicable on the basis of the assessment findings:

1. Fear related to medical diagnosis, possible disfiguring surgery, or impending death
2. Ineffective individual coping related to nonacceptance of medical diagnosis
3. Ineffective family coping: compromised related to nonacceptance of medical diagnosis
4. Dysfunctional grieving related to inability to cope with medical diagnosis
5. Impaired physical mobility related to size and extent of tumor
6. Altered nutrition: less than body requirements related to increased metabolic process secondary to cancer
7. Potential for injury (pathologic fracture) related to trivial trauma
8. Sleep pattern disturbance related to pain
9. Total self-care deficit related to impaired physical mobility
10. Altered role performance related to temporary or permanent inability to maintain role in family or community
11. Spiritual distress related to fear of death
12. Sexual dysfunction related to pain and immobility
13. Knowledge deficit related to treatment regimen

 Planning and Implementation

Pain

Planning: client goals. The goal is that the client will experience a reduction or alleviation of pain associated with the bone lesion. Because the pain is often due to direct tumor invasion, treatment is aimed at reducing the size of or removing the tumor.

Interventions. A combination of nonsurgical and surgical management is often employed to promote client comfort and eliminate the complications of bone cancer.

Nonsurgical management. In addition to analgesics for the relief of pain and other local pain relief measures, chemotherapeutic agents and radiation therapy are often administered in an attempt to cause tumor regression. In vertebral metastatic disease, bracing and immobilization with cervical traction reduce back pain.

Drug therapy. Chemotherapy may be given alone or in combination with radiotherapy or surgery. Certain proliferating tumors, such as Ewing's sarcoma, are sensitive to cytotoxic medications. Others, such as chondrosarcomas, are often totally drug resistant. Chemotherapy seems to work best for small, metastatic lesions and may be given before or after surgery.

For most tumors, the physician orders a combination of agents. The drugs selected are determined in part by the primary source of the cancer in metastatic disease. For example, when metastasis occurs from breast cancer, estrogens and progesterones are commonly used. Metastatic thyroid cancer is most sensitive to doxorubicin (Adriamycin). Table 30–2 lists drugs commonly given to clients with malignant and metastatic bone tumors.

Chapter 25 discusses the nursing care associated with the administration of cytotoxic agents. The nurse observes the client carefully for side and toxic effects and monitors laboratory tests diligently.

Radiation therapy. Radiation is employed for selected types of malignant tumors. Recent studies show that the treatment is as effective as disfiguring surgery in clients with Ewing's sarcoma. In early osteosarcoma, radiation may be the treatment of choice in reducing tumor size and thus reducing pain.

In metastatic disease, radiation is given primarily for palliation. The therapy is directed toward the painful sites in an attempt to provide a more comfortable life span for the client. One or more treatments are given, depending on the extent of disease. With precise planning, radiation therapy can be used with minimal complications. The nursing care for a client receiving radiation therapy is described in Chapter 25.

Surgical management. The treatment of primary bone tumors is surgery, often combined with radiation or chemotherapy. Wide or radical resection procedures are commonly performed for bone sarcomas. *Wide excision* is the removal of the lesion surrounded by an intact cuff of normal tissue and leads to cure of low-grade tumors only. A *radical resection* includes the removal of the lesion, the entire muscle, bone, and other tissues directly involved. It is the only procedure adequate for high-grade tumors of the bone.

In the past, limb amputation was commonly performed for bone tumors, with or without disarticulation, or joint removal. Today, advances in reconstructive surgery allow for the resection of the tumor and repair of the resulting bony defect to salvage the limb. Bone defects are corrected by total joint replacements with prosthetic implants, either whole or partial; custom metallic implants; or allografts from the iliac crest, the rib, or the fibula. In a few cases, arthrodesis, or joint fusion, may be the procedure of choice.

Total joint replacements are discussed in Chapter 28. As an alternative to total replacement, an allograft may be implanted with internal fixation for those clients who

do not have metastases. This is a common procedure for sarcomas of the proximal femur. Allografts for the knee are also performed, particularly on young adults. Preoperative chemotherapy is given to enhance the likelihood of success. Allografts with adjacent tendons and liga-

---

TABLE 30–2 Chemotherapeutic Agents Commonly Used for Malignant and Metastatic Bone Tumors

Alkylating agents

Mechlorethamine
Chlorambucil
Cyclophosphamide

Antibiotics

Doxorubicin
Bleomycin
Actinomycin D
Mithramycin
Mitomycin

Antimetabolites

Methotrexate
6-Mercaptopurine
5-Fluorouracil
Cytosine arabinoside

Plant alkaloids

Vincristine
Vinblastine
Etoposide (VP-16-213)

Enzymes

L-Asparaginase

Hormonal agents

Estrogens
Progesterones
Androgens
Antiestrogens
Corticosteroids

Synthetics

Cisplatin
Procarbazine
Hydroxyurea
Dacarbazine

Adapted from Bhardwaj, S., & Holland, J. F. (1982). Chemotherapy of metastatic cancer in bone. *Clinical Orthopaedics and Related Research, 169,* 30.

ments are harvested from cadavers and can be frozen or freeze-dried for a prolonged period. The graft is fixed with a series of bolts, screws, or plates. Twelve per cent of allografting procedures have one or more complications. The nurse observes for signs of hemorrhage, infection, and fracture (Racolin & Present, 1989).

In metastatic disease, intractable pain is surgically treated with percutaneous cordotomy, or cutting of the spinal nerve roots. Cryosurgery, or cold application, is performed to reduce pain and tumor size.

Preoperative care. Preoperatively, the client is thoroughly evaluated to assist the physician in the selection of the surgical procedure to be performed. In addition to the nature, progression, and extent of the tumor, the client's age and general health state are taken into consideration. Chemotherapy may be administered preoperatively.

As for any client preparing for cancer surgery, the client with bone cancer needs psychologic support from the nurse and other members of the health care team. The nurse assesses the level of understanding of the client and the family or significant others. As a client advocate, the nurse encourages the expression of concerns and questions and provides information regarding hospital routines and procedures. Spiritual support is important to some clients who prefer to contact their own clergyperson, rabbi, or spiritual leader or talk with the clergy affiliated with the hospital. The nurse helps to arrange for spiritual assistance if needed.

Postoperative needs are anticipated and planned for as much as possible before the client goes to surgery. The nurse informs the client what to expect postoperatively and how to help to ensure an adequate recovery.

Postoperative care. The surgical incision for a limb salvage procedure is often extensive. A pressure dressing with wound suction is maintained for 5 to 7 days.

The client who has undergone a limb salvage procedure has resulting impaired physical mobility and a self-care deficit. The nature and extent of the alterations depend on the location and extent of the surgery.

Usually, muscle strengthening and ROM exercises begin immediately postoperatively and continue for at least a year. For upper-extremity surgery, active-assistive exercises are possible by using the opposite hand to help achieve motions such as forward flexion and abduction of the shoulder. Continuous passive motion (CPM) using a CPM machine may be initiated as early as the first postoperative day for either upper- or lower-extremity procedures.

For lower-extremity surgery, the emphasis is on the strengthening of the quadriceps muscles by using passive and active motion when possible. Maintaining muscle tone is an important prerequisite to weight bearing, which progresses from toe touch or partial weight bearing to full weight bearing by 3 months postoperatively.

Surrounding tissues, including nerves and blood vessels, may be sacrificed during surgery. Vascular grafting is common; however, the lost nerve is usually not re-

placed. The nurse assesses the neurovascular status of the affected extremity and its digits thoroughly and frequently. Splinting or casting of the limb may also cause neurovascular compromise and needs to be checked for proper placement.

The client who has had a bone graft has a plaster cast that remains in place for several months. Weight bearing is prohibited until there is evidence that the graft is incorporated into the adjacent bone tissue. Chapter 31 discusses casting and ambulation aids.

During the recovery phase, the client needs assistance with ADL, particularly if the surgery involves the upper extremity. The nurse assists if needed, but at the same time, tries to encourage the client to do as much as possible unaided.

In addition to physical disabilities, the client often needs psychologic help coping with the surgery and its effects postoperatively. Having identified the available support systems preoperatively, the nurse helps to mobilize them for use after surgery.

The client experiences an alteration in body image as a result of most of the surgical procedures. The nurse can suggest ways to minimize cosmetic changes. For example, a shoulder droop can be covered by a custom-made pad worn under clothing. Lower-extremity defects can be covered by pants.

Pelvic lesions, although not commonly seen, are also excised. Reconstruction generally entails bone fusion with muscle and nerve preservation. A hip spica cast or brace may be necessary until graft incorporation has occurred. A cane may be needed for ambulation.

The major complications peculiar to reconstructive surgery for which the nurse should observe are superficial and deep wound infection, dislocation or loosening of the implants, and rapid neurovascular compromise. An increase in pain or temperature or a rapid deterioration in circulatory status should alert the nurse to notify the physician promptly.

Anticipatory Grieving

Planning: client goals. The goal is that the client will accept the medical diagnosis and its treatment. In some cases, the cure for cancer may be as devastating as the cancer itself, as when amputation is needed.

Interventions: nonsurgical management. Chapter 25 details the nursing care required to help the client meet the goal of acceptance. The most important role of the nurse is to allow the client and the family or significant others to verbalize their feelings and to be an attentive listener. Counselors and members of the clergy or spiritual leaders may provide additional assistance in promoting acceptance of the diagnosis, treatment, or, possibly, impending death.

The nurse acts as an advocate for the client and the family and often promotes the physician-client relationship. For instance, the client may not completely understand the medical or surgical treatment plan, but may be hesitant to question the physician. The nurse's intervention increases communication, which is essential in successful management of the client with cancer.

Body Image Disturbance

Planning: client goals. The client's perception of his/her own body image is closely associated with the ability to accept the illness. The goal is that the client will experience an improvement in his/her feelings about the alteration in body image and, it is hoped, accept the resulting physical changes. The client's perception may be complicated by the additional stress of prolonged immobilization.

Interventions: nonsurgical management. The nurse recognizes and accepts the client's view about the body image alteration. A trusting nurse-client relationship allows the client freedom to verbalize negative feelings. The client's strengths and remaining capabilities are emphasized. Realistic mutual goals regarding life style are established. Chapter 9 provides a comprehensive care plan for a client with an altered body image.

Potential for Injury

Planning: client goals. As with other bone diseases in which pathologic fracture is a possible complication (e.g., osteoporosis), the goal is that the client will prevent its occurrence by avoiding falls and minimizing trauma. In metastatic bone disease, fractures more readily occur and are not as preventable because of resulting destructive bone changes. A more realistic goal for this diagnosis, then, is that the client's pain will be minimized through treatment of the fracture.

Interventions. Radiation or surgery may be required to reinforce or replace the diseased bone to prevent fracture. In recent years, surgical techniques have also been improved for fracture fixation.

Nonsurgical management. Newer techniques in radiation therapy have improved the incidence of bone healing for actual and impending pathologic fractures. Chapter 25 describes the care for clients undergoing radiation therapy.

To improve muscle tone and consequently reduce the risk for fracture, strengthening exercises are performed. Physical therapy on an ambulatory basis is commonly prescribed.

Surgical management. The principles of surgery for metastatic fractures include replacing as much defective bone as possible, being thorough in technique to avoid a second procedure, and aiming to return the client to a functional state with a minimum of hospitalization and immobilization.

Fractures of the proximal femur are particularly common. Prosthetic replacement reinforced with poly-

methyl methacrylate is preferred over open reduction and internal fixation when feasible. Intramedullary devices and compression screws are used for more distal fractures. Prophylactic fixation may be done for microscopic fractures that cause chronic pain. Chapter 31 discusses the nursing management for clients with fractured hip repair.

Anxiety

Planning: client goals. The goal is that the client will experience a reduction in anxiety so that function is not impaired.

Interventions: nonsurgical management. The nurse assesses the level of anxiety and its causative factors. Loss of control over the situation can be reduced by allowing the client to be an active participant in the decision-making aspects of care.

Fear of the unknown also contributes to anxiety. The nurse explains procedures and aspects of care, including the rationale and importance of each aspect.

■ Discharge Planning

After medical treatment for a primary malignant tumor, the client is usually discharged to home with follow-up care. The client with metastatic disease may return home, or, when home support is not available, may go to a long-term facility for extended or hospice care.

Home Care Preparation

The nurse evaluates the client's home environment for structural barriers that may hinder mobility. The client may be discharged with a cast, crutches, or wheelchair.

Accessibility to eating and toileting facilities is essential to promote independence. Because the client with metastatic disease is prone to pathologic fractures, potential hazards that could contribute to falls or injury are removed.

Client/Family Education

The client receiving intermittent chemotherapy on an ambulatory basis is taught the importance of keeping appointments. The nurse reviews the side and toxic effects of the medications. The client is taught how to treat minor side effects and when to alert the physician. If the drugs are administered at home via long-term IV catheter, the nurse teaches the care involved with daily dressing changes and potential catheter complications. Chapter 25 describes the health teaching required for a client receiving chemotherapy at home.

Clients receiving radiation therapy are also taught the importance of keeping appointments and recognizing the complications of treatment. The nurse reviews interventions that can be employed at home for minor complications (see Chap. 25 for discussion of nursing interventions related to radiation therapy).

As a result of surgery, the client has a wound and limited mobility. The nurse teaches the client how to care for the wound and perform ADL and mobility activities independently. Physical and occupational therapists assist in ADL teaching and provide or recommend assistive and adaptive devices if necessary. The proper use of ambulatory aids, such as crutches, and exercises are also taught by the physical therapist and reinforced by the nurse.

Pain management can be a major problem, particularly in clients with metastatic bone disease. Nondrug pain relief measures are taught, including relaxation and music therapy. The nurse should review those techniques that worked during hospitalization.

Psychosocial Preparation

The client with bone cancer fears that the malignancy will return. The nurse acknowledges this possibility, but reinforces confidence in the health care team and medical treatment chosen.

Realistic goals regarding return to work, recreational activities, and so forth are mutually established. The client is encouraged to resume a functional life style, but may need to do so gradually. Certain activities, such as participating in sports, may be prohibited. A major facet of preparation is the identification and use of health care resources.

The client with advanced metastatic bone disease needs to prepare for death. The nurse and other support personnel assist the client through the stages of death and dying and identify resources that can help the client write a will, visit with distant family members, or do whatever he/she thinks is needed to die in peace.

Health Care Resources

In addition to family and significant others, cancer support groups available to anyone with cancer are helpful to the client with bone cancer. Organizations such as I Can Cope provide information and emotional support; others such as CanSurmount are geared more toward client and family education. A complete listing of resources can be found at the end of Unit 8.

The hospital nurse also ensures that follow-up care is available in the home, including nursing care and physical or occupational therapy. The client with terminal cancer may choose to become part of a hospice program (Chap. 11).

 Evaluation

On the basis of the identified nursing diagnoses, the nurse evaluates the care provided for the client with primary or metastatic bone cancer. The expected outcomes may include that the client

1. States that pain is reduced or alleviated

2. Performs ADL and ambulation activities independently

3. Seeks health care resources as needed, including cancer support groups

4. States that body image perception is improved

5. Returns to a functional life style (or accepts impending death in the case of advanced metastasis)

6. States that anxiety regarding medical diagnosis and treatment is decreased

The outlook for malignant primary bone tumors is improving, with current predictions of an 80% survival rate after treatment. The incidence of metastatic bone disease is increasing, however, as advanced technology enables clients with other types of cancer to survive longer.

DISORDERS OF THE HAND

CARPAL TUNNEL SYNDROME

OVERVIEW

Carpal tunnel syndrome (CTS) is a common condition in which the median nerve in the wrist becomes compressed, causing pain and numbness. It is also known as compression neuropathy of the median nerve in the carpal tunnel, tardy median palsy, median neuropathy, or thenar atrophy.

Pathophysiology

The carpal tunnel is a rigid canal lying between the carpal bones and a fibrous tissue sheet called the flexor retinaculum. As seen in Figure 30–9, a group of nine tendons enveloped by synovium share space with the median nerve in the carpal tunnel. When the synovium becomes swollen or thickened, the nerve is compressed.

The median nerve supplies the motor, sensory, and autonomic function for the first three digits of the hand and the palmar aspect of the fourth. Because of its proximity to other structures, wrist flexion causes nerve impingement against the flexor retinaculum; extension causes increased pressure in the distal portion of the carpal tunnel.

Etiology

CTS usually manifests as a chronic problem—acute cases are rare. Excessive hand exercise, edema or hemorrhage into the carpal tunnel, or thrombosis of the median artery can lead to acute CTS. Clients with a Colles

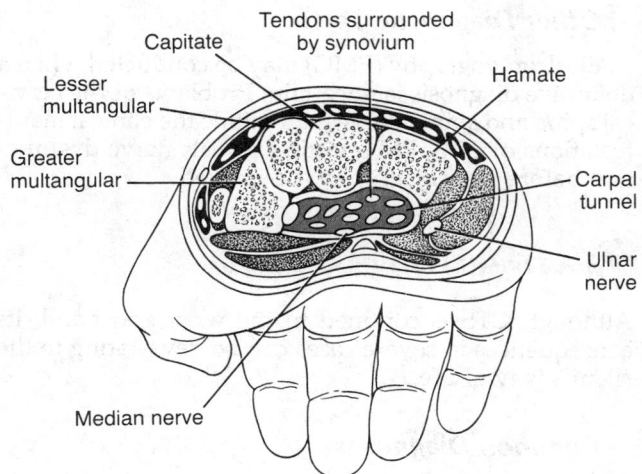

Figure 30-9

Carpal tunnel anatomy.

fracture or hand burns are particularly at risk for rapid CTS development.

In most cases, however, the causative factor or factors may not result in neurologic deficit for years. CTS is a common complication of certain metabolic and connective tissue diseases. For example, synovitis, or inflammation of the synovium, occurs in clients with rheumatoid arthritis. The hypertrophied synovium compresses the median nerve. In chronic disorders such as diabetes mellitus, inadequate blood supply can cause median nerve neuropathy, or dysfunction, resulting in CTS.

The problem is also a potential occupational hazard. Individuals with jobs that require repetitive hand activities involving pinch or grasp during wrist flexion, such as factory workers and jackhammer operators, are predisposed to CTS.

In a few cases, CTS may be a familial or congenital problem, manifesting itself in adulthood. Space-occupying lesions, such as ganglia, tophi, and lipomas, can also result in nerve compression.

Incidence

CTS occurs in adults of any age, but peaks between ages 30 and 60 years. Women are five times more likely to experience the problem than men. Most often the problem affects the dominant hand, but it can occur in both hands simultaneously.

PREVENTION

In some instances, CTS is a preventable condition. Proper medical treatment of metabolic and connective tissue diseases may prevent the occurrence of the syndrome. Rotation of factory jobs among workers reduces

the risk of CTS. Early control of the edema and hemorrhage can prevent acute nerve compression.

COLLABORATIVE MANAGEMENT

Assessment

History

When collecting data about the client with suspected CTS, the nurse includes *age, sex,* and *occupation,* which may contribute to the onset of CTS. The nurse asks if there is a *family history of the problem* and if the client has any *concurrent medical conditions,* such as rheumatoid arthritis, which can cause CTS. The nurse also asks whether the client has sustained a *recent wrist fracture or burn* and how the client *exercises.* Each of these risk factors is considered in evaluating a client with CTS.

Physical Assessment: Clinical Manifestations

On the basis of the client's history and complaint of *hand pain* and *numbness,* a medical diagnosis is often made without further assessment. The nurse questions the client regarding the nature, intensity, and location of the pain. Clients often state that the pain is worse at night as a result of flexion or direct pressure during sleep. The pain may radiate to the arm, the shoulder and neck, or the chest.

In addition to the complaint of numbness, *paresthesia,* or painful tingling, is also experienced by clients with CTS. Sensory changes usually precede motor manifestations by weeks or months.

Several tests can be performed by the nurse to elicit abnormal sensory findings. Phalen's wrist test produces paresthesia in the median nerve distribution within 60 seconds. The client is asked to relax the wrist into flexion or place the backs of the hands together and flex both wrists simultaneously (Fig. 30-10). Eighty per cent of clients with CTS have a positive Phalen's test finding.

The same sensation can be elicited by tapping lightly over the area of the median nerve in the wrist, called Tinel's sign. If the test is unsuccessful, a blood pressure cuff can be placed on the upper arm and inflated to the client's systolic pressure. The result is frequently pain and tingling.

Motor changes begin with a *weak pinch, clumsiness,* and *difficulty with fine movements,* then progress to *muscle weakness* and *wasting.* The nurse tests for pinching ability and asks the client to perform a fine-movement task such as threading a needle. Strenuous hand activity aggravates the subjective complaints.

In addition to inspecting for muscle atrophy and task performance, the nurse observes the wrist for *swelling* attributable to edema or lesions. The area is palpated, and characteristics are described.

Autonomic changes may be evidenced by skin discoloration; nail changes, such as brittleness; and increased or decreased palmar sweating.

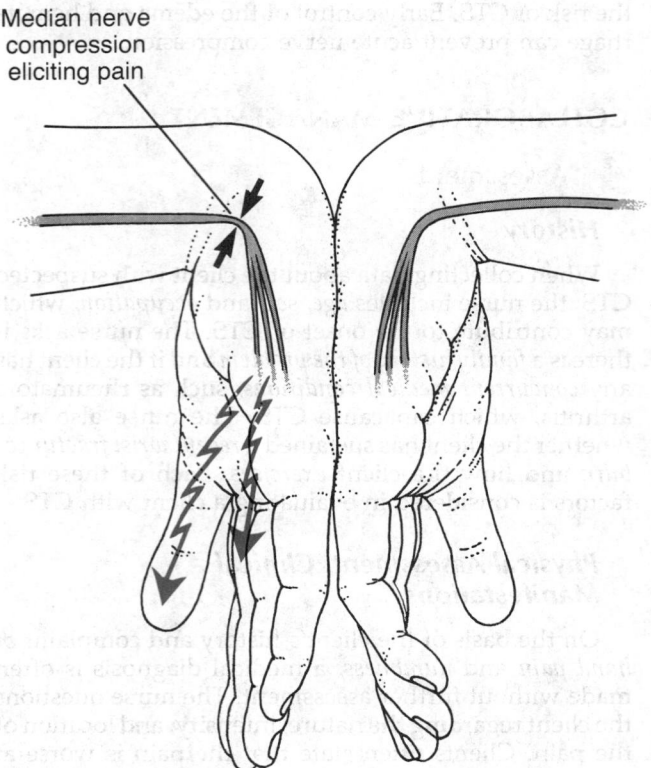

Median nerve compression eliciting pain

Figure 30-10

Phalen's wrist test for carpal tunnel syndrome.

Psychosocial Assessment

The client with CTS may fear that the manifestations are the result of a spinal problem. If the cause is job related, the client may have to decide whether to change his/her job or career or live with a worsening, chronic health problem. Many clients have repeated and lengthy medical treatment for CTS. On the other hand, clients with mild CTS sometimes have a spontaneous remission.

The nurse assesses the alterations in life style that the client has experienced. In addition to work-related activities, the client may have difficulty with the usual daily activities requiring fine movements or entailing lifting and carrying objects, such as grocery bags.

Laboratory Findings

There are no specific laboratory tests for CTS. If a client has a suspected or confirmed diagnosis of systemic disease that could cause the condition, laboratory tests that relate specifically to the disease are performed.

Radiographic Findings

Routine radiographs are ordered to visualize bone changes, space-occupying lesions, and synovitis. If these causative factors are not suspected, a client with CTS may not be radiographed.

Other Diagnostic Tests

Electromyography (EMG) may be conducted when a definitive diagnosis is uncertain. Problems of the cervical spine and spinal nerves can mimic the clinical manifestations of CTS. EMG testing reveals nerve dysfunction before muscle atrophy is observed.

 Analysis: Nursing Diagnosis

Although CTS is confined to the wrist and hand, its consequences in severe cases can be devastating to the client's way of life.

Common Diagnoses

The common diagnoses for a client with CTS include

1. Pain related to median nerve compression
2. Sensory/perceptual alterations (tactile) related to numbness from median nerve compression
3. Altered (peripheral) tissue perfusion related to median nerve compression

Additional Diagnoses

In severe cases of CTS, the following diagnoses may be applicable:

1. Activity intolerance related to inability to lift and carry objects secondary to muscle weakness and atrophy
2. Sleep pattern disturbance related to severe radiating pain
3. Ineffective individual coping related to need for job or career change
4. Ineffective family coping related to need for job or career change
5. Knowledge deficit related to treatment regimen

 Planning and Implementation

Pain

Planning: client goals. The primary goal is that the client will experience a reduction or alleviation of the pain associated with CTS.

Interventions. Conservative measures are tried before surgical intervention. With either type of treatment, however, the problem can recur.

Nonsurgical management. Drug therapy and immobilization of the wrist are the major components of nonsurgical management. The nurse teaches the importance of these modalities to the client in the hope of preventing surgical intervention.

Drug therapy. The most commonly used drugs for the relief of pain and inflammation, if present, are aspirin and NSAIDs. Diuretics may be given if edema is present.

Direct injection into the carpal tunnel with corticosteroids may also be helpful. If the client responds to the medication, several additional weekly or monthly injections are given.

When CTS is not related to systemic disease, pyridoxine hydrochloride (vitamin B_6) is sometimes effective. The usual dose is 100 to 200 mg/day orally for about 3 months. Vitamin B is essential for nerve tissue integrity and function.

As with any medication, the nurse's responsibility is to monitor the effects of the drug. Aspirin and NSAIDs are given with or after meals to reduce gastric irritation. Chapter 28 describes nursing implications for NSAIDs.

Immobilization. A splint may be used to immobilize the wrist during the day, night, or both. About 70% of clients experience temporary relief with splinting. The wrist is placed in the neutral position or slight extension. Even when a splint is not used, the client is instructed to minimize hand activities, at least temporarily.

Surgical management. Surgery is necessary in about 40% of clients with CTS. The purpose of surgery is to relieve the pressure on the median nerve, or nerve decompression. When CTS is a complication of rheumatoid arthritis, a *synovectomy*, or removal of excess synovium, may resolve the problem. Removal of a space-occupying lesion, if present, also decompresses the nerve.

Preoperative care. The nurse reinforces the teaching provided by the physician regarding the nature of the surgery. Postoperative care is reviewed so that the client knows what to expect.

Postoperative care. In addition to the routine care for any client having surgery, the client's pressure dressing is checked carefully for drainage and tightness. The client's hand and arm are elevated for 1 or 2 days to reduce swelling from surgery. The nurse checks the neurovascular status of the digits every hour during the first 12 hours postoperatively, encouraging the client to move all fingers of the affected hand frequently. (See Chap. 31 for neurovascular assessment technique.) Pain medication is offered every 3 to 4 hours.

Sensory/Perceptual Alterations

Planning: client goals. The goals are that the client will (1) prevent injury to the hand and (2) experience an improvement in tactile sensation in the hand and wrist.

Interventions. The most important nursing intervention is health teaching to prevent injury while the problem is causing a decrease in sensation.

Nonsurgical management. The client who experiences numbness in the affected hand may be unable to discern extreme temperatures; for example, the client should check bath water using the unaffected hand. If both hands are affected, the nurse checks the temperature for a safe range.

Picking up objects may be difficult, and the client may feel self-conscious about clumsiness if an object is dropped. The nurse emphasizes the need for the client to ask for help, rather than risk injury to self or others.

To improve circulation to the affected hand, exercises may be prescribed. Exercises that can exaggerate symptoms are avoided. Massage may also be beneficial, although this may increase pain in some clients. A physical therapy consultation can discriminate helpful from harmful modalities for increasing circulation.

Surgical management. The surgery described earlier resolves sensory deficits and the pain associated with CTS.

Altered (Peripheral) Tissue Perfusion

Planning: client goals. The goal is that the client will not experience further impairment in tissue perfusion in the affected hand and wrist.

Interventions. The nurse carefully assesses the circulation in the affected hand and wrist, regardless of whether the client has had surgery. Edema can severely impair the ability of the tissues to receive adequate oxygen.

Nonsurgical management. The nurse assesses the neurovascular status of the hand and wrist as a baseline, and notes changes that indicate worsening of the problem (Chap. 31). If edema is the causative factor, the arm is elevated and diuretic medications may be administered.

Surgical management. The surgical procedure for pain management is applicable.

■ Discharge Planning

Home Care Preparation

The client is not hospitalized for nonsurgical management. Surgery may require a 1- to 2-day stay in the hospital or may be performed on an ambulatory basis. Health teaching by the nurse is essential so that the client knows what to expect.

After surgery, the client is placed in a splint that allows thumb and finger movements. The splint is usually not applied until the sutures have been removed and is used for at least 2 weeks.

Client/Family Education

Hand movements, including lifting heavy objects, are restricted for 4 to 6 weeks. The client can expect weakness and discomfort for weeks or perhaps months. The nurse teaches the client how to assess for neurovascular status.

Psychosocial Preparation

The client must realize that the surgical procedure may not be a cure. For instance, synovitis may recur in clients with rheumatoid arthritis and recompress the median nerve. Multiple surgeries and other treatment modalities are not uncommon for CTS.

Health Care Resources

The client may need assistance with routine daily tasks or even self-care activities. The nurse ensures that assistance in the home is available, usually provided by the family or significant others.

 Evaluation

On the basis of the identified nursing diagnoses, the nurse evaluates the care provided for the client with CTS. Expected outcomes include that the client

1. States that pain is reduced or alleviated
2. States that numbness and paresthesia are reduced or alleviated
3. Avoids injury as a result of motor and sensory loss
4. Has an increase in tissue perfusion to the affected hand

DUPUYTREN'S CONTRACTURE

Dupuytren's contracture, or deformity, is a slowly progressive contracture of the palmar fascia resulting in flexion of the fourth or fifth fingers of the hand. The third digit is occasionally affected. Although it is a fairly common problem, its cause is unknown. It usually occurs in older men, tends to be familial, and can be bilateral.

When function becomes impaired, surgical release is required. A partial or selective *fasciectomy*, or removal of fascia, is performed. After removal of the dressing and drain, a splint is frequently used. The nursing care for the client is similar to that for the client with carpal tunnel repair.

GANGLION

A *ganglion* is a round, cyst-like lesion often overlying a wrist joint or tendon. The synovium surrounding the tendon degenerates, allowing the tendon sheath tissue to become weak and distended. Ganglia are painless on palpation, but can cause joint discomfort after prolonged joint use or minor trauma, such as a strain. The lesion can disappear, then recur. Persons aged 15 to 50 years are most likely to develop ganglia.

Although the fluid within the lesion can be aspirated, total excision is preferred. The postoperative care is the same as that for other hand surgeries.

DISORDERS OF THE FOOT

HALLUX VALGUS

The hallux valgus deformity, sometimes referred to as a *bunion,* is a common foot problem in which the great toe deviates laterally at the metatarsophalangeal (MTP) joint, as shown in Figure 30–11. Although the problem is frequently congenital, it can occur as a result of arthritis or poorly fitted shoes. As the deviation worsens, the bony prominence enlarges and causes pain, particularly when wearing shoes. Women are more frequently affected than men.

The surgical procedure, or simple *bunionectomy,* involves removing the bony overgrowth and bursa. When other toe deformities accompany the condition or if the bony overgrowth is large, several *osteotomies,* or bone resections, may be performed. In this case, clients usually have Kirschner's wires inserted vertically through the toes for about 3 weeks postoperatively until healing occurs (Fig. 30–12). If both feet are affected, one is treated at a time.

HAMMERTOE

Often, clients have hammertoes and hallux valgus deformities simultaneously. As shown in Figure 30–13, a *hammertoe* is the dorsiflexion of any MTP joint with plantar flexion of the adjacent PIP joint. The second toe

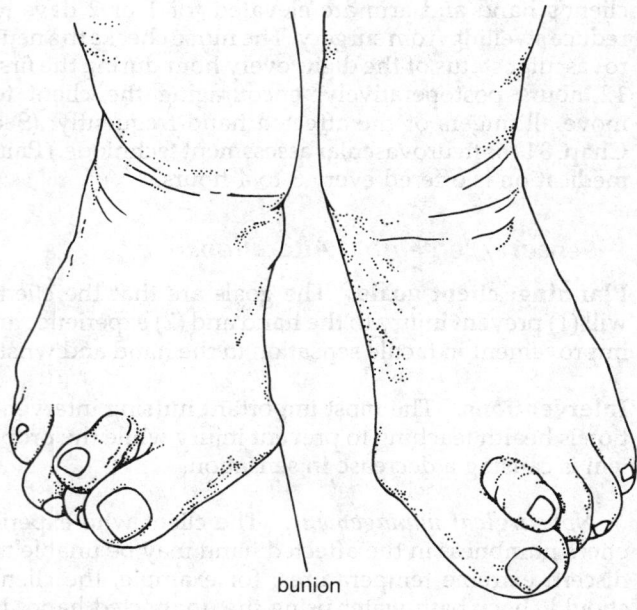

bunion

Figure 30–11

Hallux valgus with bunion.

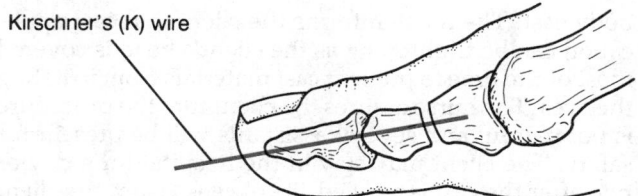

Figure 30-12

Use of Kirschner's wires to repair hallux valgus.

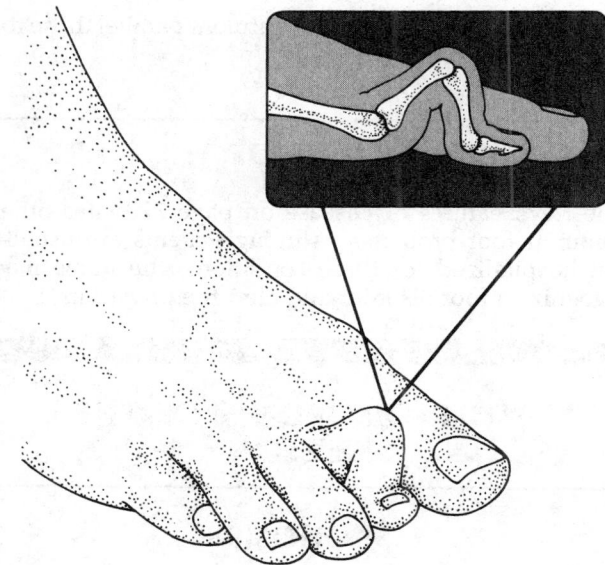

Figure 30-13

Hammertoe of second MTP joint.

is most often affected. As the deformity worsens, corns may develop on the dorsal side of the toe, whereas calluses may appear on the plantar surface. Clients are uncomfortable when wearing shoes and walking.

The treatment is the surgical correction of the deformity by osteotomies and the insertion of Kirschner's wires for fixation. The postoperative course is similar to that for hallux valgus repair. The client uses crutches until full weight bearing is allowed in 3 to 4 weeks postoperatively.

MORTON'S NEUROMA

The development of a small tumor in a digital nerve of the foot is called *Morton's neuroma,* or plantar digital neuritis. The pain is usually described as an acute, burning sensation in the web space and involves the entire surface of the third and fourth toes. Treatment is the surgical removal of the neuroma and pressure dressing application. Ambulation is usually permitted immediately after surgery.

TARSAL TUNNEL SYNDROME

Tarsal tunnel syndrome is the ankle version of the carpal tunnel syndrome. The posterior tibial nerve in the ankle becomes compressed, resulting in loss of sensation and pain in a portion of the foot. Typically, the median and lateral plantar branches, which supply the sole of the foot and the distal phalanges, are affected by the nerve

KEY FEATURES OF DISEASE ■ Treatment of Common Foot Problems

Problem	Description/Cause	Treatment
Corn	Induration and thickening of the skin caused by friction and pressure, painful conical mass	Surgical removal by podiatrist
Callus	Flat, poorly defined mass on the sole over a bony prominence caused by pressure	Padding and lanolin cremes, overall good skin hygiene
Ingrown nail	Nail sliver penetration of the skin, causing inflammation	Removal of sliver by podiatrist, warm soaks, antibiotic ointment
Hypertrophic ungual labium	Chronic hypertrophy of nail lip caused by improper nail trimming; results from untreated ingrown nail	Surgical removal of necrotic nail and skin, treatment of secondary infection

compression. Diagnosis and treatment parallel those for carpal tunnel syndrome.

OTHER PROBLEMS OF THE FOOT

The Key Features of Disease on page 773 cites other common foot problems. Although clients are usually not hospitalized for these conditions, the nurse may recognize a foot disorder and alert the physician.

OTHER DISORDERS OF THE SKELETON

SCOLIOSIS

OVERVIEW

Scoliosis is a C- or S-shaped lateral curvature of the vertebral spine (see Chap. 29, Fig. 29–4). Many individuals with this disorder are diagnosed and treated before adolescence. Information about caring for children with scoliosis is found in most pediatric nursing texts. In adult scoliosis, the impairment is usually cosmetic, although severe deviations of more than 50 degrees can compromise cardiopulmonary function. The abnormal curvature can cause lower-back pain for which treatment is initiated. Women are affected more frequently than men.

Methods of treating adult scoliosis are different from those used in the childhood condition. The adult spinal column is less flexible and therefore less likely to respond to exercises, weight reduction, bracing, and casting for correction of the deformity. In the adult, the disorder is progressive and can result in an additional 1 degree of deviation each year (Schoen, 1986).

COLLABORATIVE MANAGEMENT

Surgical intervention is the most common treatment for the adult and consists of surgical fusion and insertion of instrumentation. A *spinal fusion* is performed by packing cancellous bone chips, usually from the iliac crest, between the affected vertebrae for support and stabilization. The metal instrumentation straightens the spine and immobilizes the fused area during healing. One of four types of instrumentation can be used: Harrington, Dwyer, Luque, or Cotrel-Dubousset.

Harrington rod instrumentation uses a compression rod on the convex side of the spine and a distraction rod on the concave side. This system is used when a large portion of the vertebral column is fused. In preparation for the insertion of Harrington rods, many surgeons admit the client to the hospital 2 weeks preoperatively for the application of a Risser cast, a type of corrective

body cast. The nurse informs the client that cast application can be frightening as the client's head is covered most of the time to prevent cast materials from irritating the eyes. The nurse assures the client that the procedure is not painful and several assistants will be present for safety. The client may stay in the hospital for a day or two after the cast is applied. Two weeks later, the client is readmitted for surgery.

The client may or may not have a partial body cast after surgery. To keep the spine immobilized and aligned, the client may be placed on a Foster or Stryker frame (refer to Chap. 33 for discussion of these special beds). During the immobilization period, the client is predisposed to complications of immobility, such as pulmonary embolism. The nurse employs measures to prevent these complications, as described in Chapter 22.

Dwyer cable instrumentation requires an anterolateral surgical approach and involves entrance into the thoracic cavity with subsequent chest tube insertion. The bone graft for the spinal fusion is taken from a rib; screws are then placed laterally into the vertebrae. A cable is threaded through the heads of the screws. This procedure can also be used to correct *lordosis* (an increase in the concave curve of the spine), but this deformity is not as common as scoliosis.

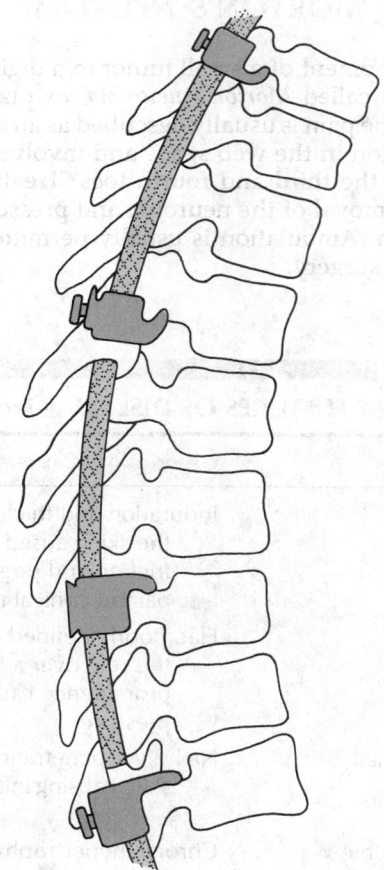

Figure 30-14

Corrected lateral spine contour with Cotrel-Dubousset instrumentation.

With the *Luque* rod system, the client does not need to wear a cast, but operative time and blood loss are greater for insertion. Loops of heavy stainless steel wire are placed under the affected laminae for insertion of the rods through each wire. The hospital stay for a client receiving this surgery is usually 6 to 7 days.

The newest addition to implantation techniques for scoliosis treatment is the *Cotrel-Dubousset* (C-D) system, a three-dimensional segmental instrumentation using noninvasive hooks to prevent neurologic complications (Fig. 30–14). Clients with this system are not immobilized by a brace or cast and can be discharged from the hospital in 5 to 6 days.

The nursing care of clients with corrective surgery for scoliosis is similar to that for the client undergoing a laminectomy (Chap. 31). The major difference is the length of postoperative immobilization, which can be several days in bed with Harrington or Dwyer procedures. Luque and C-D instrumentation allow the client to be out of bed the same evening or day after surgery. For Harrington rod insertion with casting, the nurse must incorporate cast care as part of postoperative management. Cast care is described in Chapter 31.

With the newer surgical techniques, the client may return to work in about 3 weeks and can resume activities such as swimming and bicycling. Recreational sports such as tennis are usually resumed in 6 weeks with C-D surgery, but other surgeries may prevent the client from performing these activities until 3 to 6 months postoperatively. Many clients are allowed to return to contact sports within a year or less.

OSTEOGENESIS IMPERFECTA

Although there are several types of osteogenesis imperfecta (OI), one type is more prevalent in adults (i.e., the milder tarda form with autosomal inheritance). In this rare, hereditary disease, a defect of connective tissue formation results in fragile and deformed bones. In addition to multiple fractures and poor skeletal development, the client may have blue sclera; soft, brownish teeth; and presenile deafness. The treatment is palliative, and the life span is frequently shortened.

MUSCULAR DISEASES

PROGRESSIVE MUSCULAR DYSTROPHIES

At least nine types of muscular dystrophy (MD) have been clinically identified; these can be broadly categorized as slowly progressive or rapidly progressive. The slowly progressive types are most commonly seen in the adult population.

There are five types of MD frequently seen in adults.

Each type has its own distinct characteristics and causes, but all are progressive (see the accompanying Key Features of Disease).

The exact pathophysiologic mechanisms are unknown, but three theories have been advocated. The *vascular* theory suggests that a lack of blood flow causes the typical degeneration of muscle tissue seen in muscular dystrophy. Microscopic necrotic areas in dystrophied muscle tissue support this hypothesis, although this finding does not explain the marked degree of degeneration frequently seen in the disease. The *neurogenic* theory proposes a disturbance in nerve-muscle interaction. Research has failed, however, to locate the nature of the disturbance. The most popular belief is the *membrane* theory, in which cell membranes are genetically altered, causing a compromise in cell integrity. An increase in the activity of muscle proteolytic enzymes may accompany the membrane alteration, leaving the muscle cell vulnerable to degeneration. Increased enzyme activity has been documented in clients with dystrophied muscles.

The cause of MD is unknown, but there is strong evidence to support a genetic influence for most of the major types. Some are transmitted as autosomal dominant or recessive traits, whereas others are sex linked. The most commonly occurring type of MD is the severe X-linked recessive variety initially described by Guillaume Duchenne in 1868. Each year 20 to 33 cases are reported per 100,000 live male births. In an X-linked recessive disorder, one-half of the male children of an unaffected mother, or carrier, manifest the disease. Becker's dystrophy is also inherited in an X-linked recessive manner, but is less common than Duchenne's dystrophy. The other types of MD seen in adults can occur in either sex.

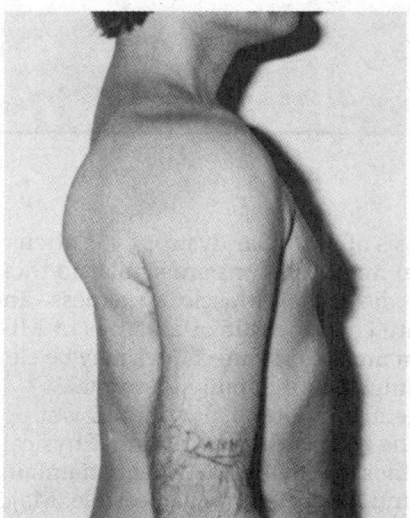

Figure 30–15

Muscle atrophy common in muscular dystrophy. (From Galdi, A. P. [1984]. *Diagnosis and management of muscle disease.* Great Neck, NY: P. M. A. Publishing.)

KEY FEATURES OF DISEASE ■ Differential Features of Common Muscular Dystrophies

Dystrophy	Onset	Genetics	Clinical Manifestations	Progression
Duchenne (severe X-linked)	Between 18 mo and 4 yr of age	Sex-linked recessive, expression in males	Symmetric pelvic and shoulder girdle muscle weakness, waddling gait, cardiac involvement common, mental retardation in one-third	Severely progressive, leading to inability to walk between 7 and 11 yr of age, death from cardiac or respiratory failure in second or third decade
Becker (benign X-linked)	5–25 yr of age	Sex-linked recessive, expression in males	Wasting of pelvic and shoulder muscles, normal cardiac and mental function	Gradual progression, inability to walk 25 yr after onset, usually normal life span
Limb-girdle	Usually second or third decade	Usually autosomal dominant, expression in either sex	Upper-extremity and neck muscles and lower-extremity and hip muscle weakness	Extremely variable, severe disability within 10–20 yr after onset, life span shortened by 10–20 yr
Facioscapulohumeral (Landouzy-Dejerine)	Usually in second decade	Autosomal dominant, expression in either sex	Facial and shoulder girdle muscle involvement	Usually benign, normal life span
Myotonic (Steinert)	Birth to fourth decade	Autosomal dominant, expression in either sex	Muscle atrophy with multiple organ involvement (e.g., heart, lungs, smooth muscle, and endocrine system)	Usually gradual if onset in adulthood

Diagnosis of muscular dystrophy is often difficult, as the clinical manifestations are similar to those of other muscular disorders. Muscle weakness and trophic changes are characteristic of all types of MD (Fig. 30–15). Serum muscle enzyme values may be elevated, and EMG findings are frequently abnormal.

Management of the client with MD is supportive and involves the entire health care team. Physical and occupational therapy helps the client maintain as much function and independence as possible. Major organ or body system involvement is medically managed, but the client's life span is often shortened from these manifestations of the disease. To date, no drug has been found to slow the progression of the disorder, although steroids and immunosuppressive agents have been tried. Nursing interventions focus on making the client as comfortable as possible and reinforcing techniques and exercises taught in the physical therapy program. The nurse's role in caring for a client with cardiac or other organ involvement is the same as for any client with dysfunction of these areas.

OTHER MUSCULAR DISORDERS

Most muscle diseases are classified as neuromuscular disorders, such as myasthenia gravis, or connective tissue diseases, such as polymyositis. Therefore, these disorders are discussed in Chapters 34 and 28, respectively.

SUMMARY

The major metabolic bone diseases include osteoporosis, osteomalacia, and Paget's disease. The older population is at the greatest risk for acquiring bone disease and certain forms of osteomyelitis and bone cancer. Technologic advances in the treatment of bone disorders have prolonged life, yet most of these diseases are chronic and treatments are costly.

Muscle involvement frequently accompanies other disorders of other body systems. MD, however, is a primary disease of skeletal muscle that can affect major organs and result in a decreased life span. Treatment is limited and management is supportive.

IMPLICATIONS FOR RESEARCH

Metabolic bone diseases are receiving increased attention in medical research. Questions regarding the amount of vitamin D and calcium needed to prevent these disorders are being investigated. Improved modalities for treatment are being tried in an attempt to retard disease progression for these disorders as well as for MD.

Nursing research needs to be conducted to answer the following questions related to the care of clients with musculoskeletal disorders:

1. What effect does health teaching have on the prevention of osteoporosis and osteomalacia?

2. What nondrug pain relief measures are effective in reducing or alleviating the chronic pain associated with bone disease?

3. How can the nurse best promote client independence in self-care and mobility?

4. What effect does health teaching have on the incidence of client falls and trivial trauma leading to pathologic fracture?

REFERENCES AND READINGS

Metabolic Bone Diseases

Altman, R. D. (1984). Paget's disease of bone (osteitis deformans). *Bulletin on the Rheumatic Diseases, 34,* 1–8.

Avioli, L. V. (1984). *The osteoporotic syndrome: Detection, prevention, and treatment.* New York: Grune & Stratton.

Barzel, U. S. (1983). Vitamin D deficiency: A risk factor for osteomalacia in the aged. *Journal of the American Geriatrics Society, 31,* 598–601.

Barzel, U. S. (1988). Estrogens in the prevention and treatment of premenopausal osteoporosis: A review. *American Journal of Medicine, 85,* 847–850.

Cawley, M. I. D. (1983). Complications of Paget's disease of bone. *Gerontology, 29,* 276–287.

Chase, J. A. (1985). Spine fractures associated with osteoporosis. *Orthopaedic Nursing, 4*(3), 31–34.

Chestnut, C. H., III. (1984). Treatment of postmenopausal osteoporosis. *Comprehensive Therapy, 10,* 41–47.

Consensus Conference. (1984). Osteoporosis. *JAMA, 252,* 799–802.

Doppelt, S. H. (1984). Vitamin D, rickets, and osteomalacia. *Orthopedic Clinics of North America, 15,* 671–685.

Evans, R. A., Marel, G. M., Lancaster, E. K., Kos, S., Evans, M., & Wong, S. Y. P. (1988). Bone mass is low in relatives of osteoporotic patients. *Annals of Internal Medicine, 109,* 870–873.

Heaney, R. P., Gallagher, J. C., Johnston, C. C., Neer, R., Parfitt, A. M., Chir, B., & Whedon, G. D. (1982). Calcium nutrition and bone health in the elderly. *American Journal of Clinical Nutrition, 36,* 986–1008.

Holm, K., & Hedricks, C. (1989). Immobilization and bone loss in the aging adult. *Critical Care Nursing Quarterly, 12,* 46–51.

Lane, J. M., & Vigorita, V. J. (1984). Osteoporosis. *Orthopedic Clinics of North America, 15,* 711–728.

Liddel, D. (1985). An in-depth look at osteoporosis. *Orthopaedic Nursing, 4*(4), 23–30.

Lindsay, R. (1989). Osteoporosis: An updated approach to prevention and management. *Geriatrics, 44,* 45–46, 51–52, 54.

Merkow, R. L., & Lane, J. M. (1984). Current concepts of Paget's disease of bone. *Orthopedic Clinics of North America, 15,* 747–763.

Miller, G. (1985). Osteoporosis. *Journal of Gerontological Nursing, 11,* 10–15.

Menczel, J., Robin, G. C., Makin, M., & Steinberg, R. (1982). *Osteoporosis.* Chichester: Wiley.

Mundy, G. R. (1983). The management of osteoporosis. *Comprehensive Therapy, 9,* 27–32.

Nugent, C. A., Gall E. P., & Pitt, M. J. (1984). Osteoporosis, osteomalacia, rickets, and Paget's disease. *Primary Care, 11,* 353–367.

Osteoporosis: Prevention and treatment. (1989). *Drug Therapy Bulletin, 27,* 1–4.

Pak, C. Y. C., Sakhaee, K., Zerwekh, J. E., Parcel, C., Peterson, R., & Johnson, K. (1989). Safe and effective treatment of osteoporosis with intermittent slow release sodium fluoride: Augmentation of vertebral bone mass and inhibition of fractures. *Journal of Clinical Endocrinology and Metabolism, 68,* 150–159.

Parfitt, A. M., Gallagher, J. C., Heaney, R. P., Johnston, C. C., Neer, R., & Whedon, G. D. (1982). Vitamin D and bone health in the elderly. *American Journal of Clinical Nutrition, 36,* 1014–1031.

Perry, G. R. (1988). Living with osteoporosis. *Geriatric Nursing, 9,* 174–176.

Rebel, A. (Ed.). (1987). Paget's disease. *Clinical Orthopaedics and Related Research, 199,* 4–170.

Ryan, W. G. (1983). Pathophysiology and modern management of Paget's disease. *Comprehensive Therapy, 9,* 64–69.

Siris, E. S. (1983). Diagnosis and treatment of Paget's disease of bone. *Comprehensive Therapy, 9,* 47–53.

Watts, N. B. (1988). Osteoporosis. *American Family Physician, 38,* 193–207.

Bone Infection

Cabanela, M. E. (1984). Open cancellous bone grafting of infected bone grafts. *Orthopedic Clinics of North America, 15,* 427–440.

Cierney, G., & Mader, J. T. (1984). Adult chronic osteomyelitis. *Orthopedics, 7,* 1557–1564.

Gentry, L. O. (1985). Role for newer beta-lactam antibiotics in treatment of osteomyelitis. *American Journal of Medicine, 78*(6A), 134–139.

Gentry, L. O. (1987). *Approach to the patient with chronic osteomyelitis: Current clinical topics in infectious diseases.* New York: McGraw-Hill.

Lefrock, J. L., Smith, B. R., & Molavi, A. (1984). Drug therapy for bacterial osteomyelitis. *American Family Physician, 30,* 213–216.

Martin, M. E. (1989). Oral antibiotics for treatment of patients with chronic osteomyelitis. *Orthopaedic Nursing, 8*(3), 35–38.

Merkel, K. D., (1984). Scintigraphic evaluation in musculoskeletal sepsis. *Orthopedic Clinics of North America, 15,* 401–416.

Ruttle, P. E., Kelly, P. J., Arnold, P. G., Irons, G. B., & Fitzgerald, R. H. (1984). Chronic osteomyelitis treated with a muscle flap. *Orthopedic Clinics of North America, 15,* 451–459.

Schmid, F. R. (1984). Infectious arthritis and osteomyelitis. *Primary Care, 11,* 295–306.

Sen, P., & Louria, D. B. (1983). Infectious complications in the elderly diabetic patient. *Geriatrics, 38,* 63–72.

Thompson, R. L., & Wright, A. J. (1984). Antimicrobial therapy in musculoskeletal surgery. *Orthopedic Clinics of North America, 15,* 547–563.

Wagner, D. K., Collier, B. D., & Rytel, M. W. (1985). Long-term intravenous antibiotic therapy in chronic osteomyelitis. *Archives of Internal Medicine, 145,* 1073–1078.

Wald, E. R. (1985). Risk factors for osteomyelitis. *American Journal of Medicine, 78*(6A), 206–211.

Wheat, J, (1985). Diagnostic strategies in osteomyelitis. *American Journal of Medicine, 78*(6A), 218–224.

Wood, M. B., & Cooney, W. P. (1984). Vascularized bone segment transfers for management of chronic osteomyelitis. *Orthopedic Clinics of North America, 15,* 461–471.

Worlock, P. (1988). The prevention of infection in open fractures: An experimental study of the effect of antibiotic therapy. *Journal of Bone and Joint Surgery, 70A,* 1341–1347.

Bone Tumors

Fedora, N. L. (1985). Fighting for my leg . . . and my life. *Orthopaedic Nursing, 4*(5), 39–42.

Gregorcic, N. J. R. (1985). Functional abilities following limb-salvage procedures. *Orthopaedic Nursing, 4*(5), 24–28.

Lamphier, P. C. (1985). Primary bone tumors. *Orthopaedic Nursing, 4*(5), 17–23.

Lewis, M. M. (Ed.). (1989). Bone tumors: Evaluation and treatment. *Orthopedic Clinics of North America, 20,* 273–512.

Malinin, T. I., & Gross, A. E. (Eds). (1985). Bone allografts in reconstructive surgery. *Clinical Orthopaedics and Related Research, 197,* 4–157.

Matzke, K. A., Gasner, D. M., Van Vugt, B. L., & Marquardt, R. A. (1985). Case study: Nursing care of a patient with osteogenic sarcoma. *Orthopaedic Nursing, 4*(5), 44–47, 69.

Piasecki, P. A., & Rodts, M. F. (1985). Bone banking: Its role in skeletal tumor reconstruction. *Orthopaedic Nursing, 4*(5), 56–60.

Racolin, A. A., & Present, D. A. (1989). Osteochondral allografts for limb salvage. *Orthopaedic Nursing, 8*(2), 35–39.

Spross, J. A., and Hope, A. (1985). Alterations in comfort: Pain related to cancer. *Orthopaedic Nursing, 4*(5), 48–52.

Other Disorders of the Skeleton

Allard, J. L., & Dibble, S. L. (1984). A look at Luque rods. *American Journal of Nursing, 84,* 609–614.

Bridwell, K. (1988). Cotrel-Dubousset instrumentation. *Orthopaedic Nursing, 7*(1), 11–16.

Conolly, W. B. (1984). *Treatment of carpal tunnel syndrome.* Oradell, NJ: Medical Economics Books.

Henning, J. H., Allard-Paliembo, J., Pellino, T. A., Wixson, N., & Rinsky, L. (1984). Preparation for the Luque procedure: Patient education booklet. *Orthopaedic Nursing, 3*(3), 50–51.

Karn, M. A., & Crawford, A. H. (1984). Postoperative nursing management of the patient following posterior spinal fusion. *Orthopaedic Nursing, 3*(3), 21–28.

Reeder, J. M. (1981). Adult scoliosis: A personal experience. *AORN Journal, 33,* 35–50.

Schoen, D. (1986). *The nursing process in orthopaedics.* Norwalk, CT: Appleton-Century-Crofts.

Smith, R., Francis, M. J. O., & Houghton, G. R. (1983). *The brittle bone syndrome: Osteogenesis imperfecta.* London: Butterworths.

Winter, R. B. (Ed.). (1988). Scoliosis. *Orthopedic Clinics of North America, 19,* 227–408.

Wynne-Davies, R., & Gormley, J, (1981). Clinical and genetic patterns in osteogenesis imperfecta. *Clinical Orthopaedics and Related Research, 159,* 26–35.

ADDITIONAL READINGS

National Institute of Arthritis and Musculoskeletal and Skin Diseases. (1986). *Osteoporosis: Cause, treatment, prevention.* Rockville, MD: National Institutes of Health.

This booklet presents the most current information regarding the etiology, prevention, and treatment of osteoporosis. It provides a comprehensive discussion of the disease for the lay person or health care professional.

Nirenberg, A. (1985). The adolescent with osteogenic sarcoma. *Orthopaedic Nursing, 4*(5), 11–16.

Special nursing interventions are discussed for the adolescent client who has bone cancer. The focus is on limb salvage procedures, which are particularly important for the psychologic well-being of a client in this developmental stage.

Pozzi, M., & Peck, N. (1986). An option for the patient with chronic osteomyelitis: Home intravenous antibiotic therapy. *Orthopaedic Nursing, 5*(5), 9–14.

With an increasing trend to shorten hospital stays, selected clients with chronic osteomyelitis are being discharged to home while still receiving IV antibiotic therapy. The nurse demonstrates the procedure for medication administration to the client and the caregiver and teaches side and toxic effects to be monitored. This article presents written instructions on changing the client's dressing and IV catheter cap and flushing the catheter with heparin solution (these are discussed and reviewed with the client and family before discharge).

Voznak, L. (1988). My life with scoliosis. *Orthopaedic Nursing, 1*(1), 22–26.

The author shares her experience with scoliosis. After multiple treatment modalities, she was able to have successful surgery. The psychosocial implications of this disorder are thoroughly discussed.

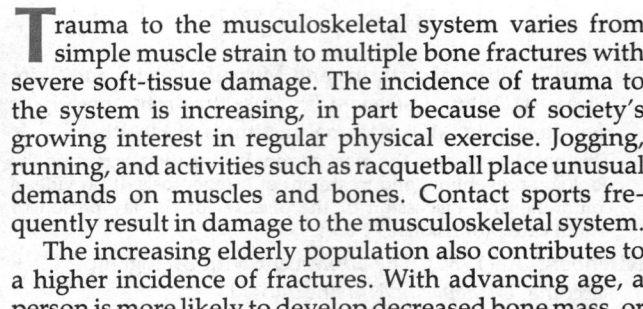

C H A P T E R 3 1

Interventions for Clients with Musculoskeletal Trauma

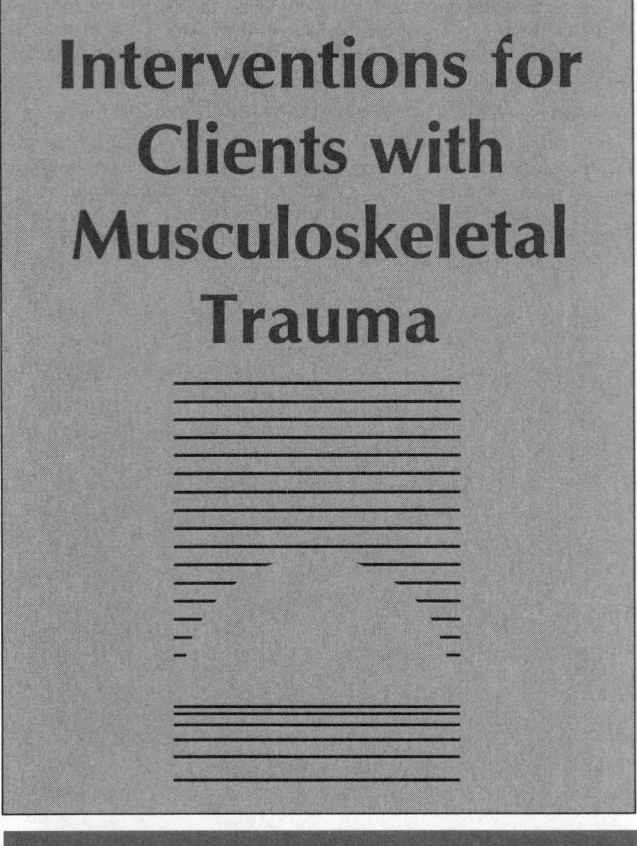

Trauma to the musculoskeletal system varies from simple muscle strain to multiple bone fractures with severe soft-tissue damage. The incidence of trauma to the system is increasing, in part because of society's growing interest in regular physical exercise. Jogging, running, and activities such as racquetball place unusual demands on muscles and bones. Contact sports frequently result in damage to the musculoskeletal system.

The increasing elderly population also contributes to a higher incidence of fractures. With advancing age, a person is more likely to develop decreased bone mass, or brittle bones, which break easily when the person falls. Hip, wrist, vertebral, and pelvic fractures are common in this age group. The resulting physical and psychosocial deficits are often devastating to the client and present a major challenge to nurses who provide care.

FRACTURES

OVERVIEW

A *fracture* is a break or disruption in the continuity of a bone. Fractures can occur anywhere in the body and at any age. The basic pathophysiology and nursing management are similar for all fractures regardless of their type or location.

Pathophysiology

Classification

A fracture is classified by type and extent of the break and its location. All fractures are either complete or incomplete. A *complete* fracture implies that the break is across the entire width of the bone such that the bone is divided into two distinct sections. In contrast, an *incomplete* fracture does not divide the bone into two portions as the break occurs through only part of the bone.

To describe the extent of associated soft-tissue damage, a fracture is described as open or closed. An *open*, or *compound*, fracture is one in which the skin surface over the broken bone is disrupted, which causes an external wound. These fractures are often graded to define the extent of tissue damage. Grade I indicates the least severe injury and involves minimal skin damage. In grade II, an open fracture is accompanied by skin and muscle contusions. The class of the most severe injury is grade III, in which there is damage to skin, muscle, nerve tissue, and blood vessels, and the wound is greater than 6 to 8 cm (2.4 to 3.2 in) in diameter (Pellino et al., 1986). A *closed*, or *simple*, fracture does not extend through the skin and therefore there is no visible wound. Figure 31–1 illustrates common classifications of fractures. The nurse needs to be familiar with the differences in

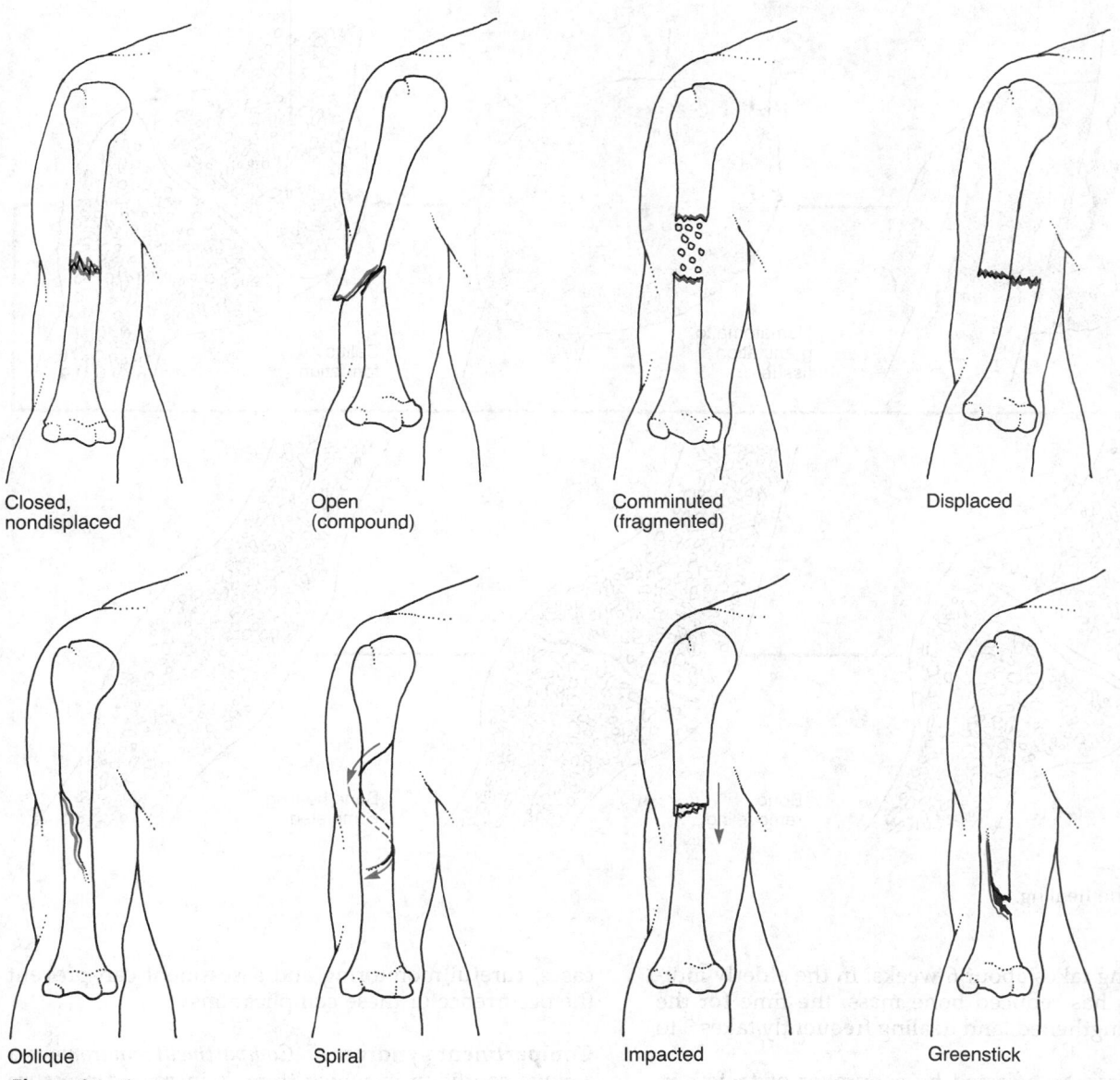

Closed, nondisplaced

Open (compound)

Comminuted (fragmented)

Displaced

Oblique

Spiral

Impacted

Greenstick

Figure 31–1

Common types of fractures.

these types because they often dictate the specific type of nursing care that is required for the client.

In addition to being identified by type, fractures are frequently characterized by their cause. A *pathologic* (spontaneous) fracture occurs after minimal trauma to a bone that has been weakened by disease. For example, it is quite common for a client with bone cancer to easily sustain a pathologic fracture. When a break results from excessive strain and stress on the bone, the injury is called a *fatigue* fracture.

Healing

When a bone is broken, the body immediately begins the healing process to repair the injury and restore the body's equilibrium. Within 48 to 72 hours of the injury, a hematoma forms at the site of the fracture because bone is extremely vascular. Blood supply to and within the bone usually diminishes, which causes an area of bone necrosis. Fibroblasts and osteoblasts migrate to the area to begin the granulation stage of healing. As a result of vascular and cellular proliferation, the fracture site is surrounded by new vascular tissue known as a *callus*. Callus formation is the beginning of a nonbony union. As healing continues, the callus is transformed from a loose, fibrous tissue into bone. Osteoclasts and phagocytes remove the debris, and necrotic bone is resorbed. This process of building and resorption of bone is often referred to as bone *remodeling*. Figure 31–2 summarizes the stages of bone healing. In the young, healthy adult

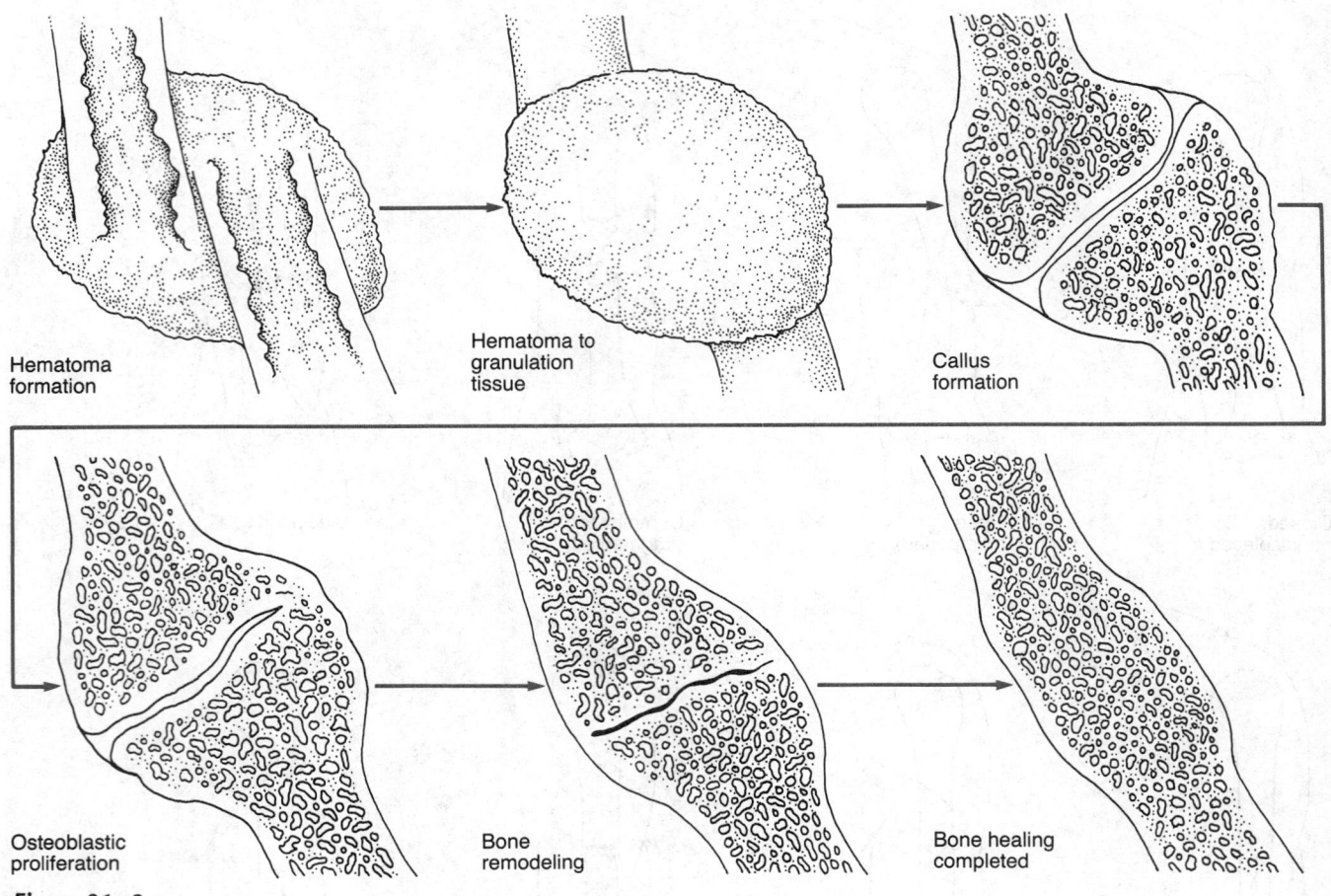

Hematoma formation

Hematoma to granulation tissue

Callus formation

Osteoblastic proliferation

Bone remodeling

Bone healing completed

Figure 31–2

Stages of bone healing.

bone, healing takes about 6 weeks. In the elderly individual who has reduced bone mass, the time for the process is lengthened, and healing frequently takes 3 to 6 months.

Healing can be affected by a number of factors in addition to the aging process. Bone formation and strength rely on adequate nutrition. Calcium, phosphorus, vitamin D, and protein are necessary for new bone production, as discussed in Chapter 30. A loss of estrogen, which occurs after menopause, is detrimental to the body's ability to form new bone tissue. The presence of concurrent diseases can also affect the rate at which bone heals. For instance, peripheral vascular diseases, such as arteriosclerosis, reduce arterial circulation to bone, and thus the bone receives less oxygen and nutrients that are needed for repair.

Complications

Regardless of the type or location of the fracture, several life-threatening complications can occur as a result of the injury. The nurse must be able to recognize the clinical manifestations of impending complications so that treatment can be started immediately. In some cases, careful monitoring and assessment can prevent the occurrence of these complications.

Compartment syndrome. *Compartment syndrome* is a serious condition in which there is increased pressure within one or more muscle compartments of the extremities, which causes massive compromise of circulation to the area. The distal portions of the upper and lower extremities contain more compartments than the proximal portions; therefore, the risk of developing complications is greater when a pathologic condition occurs in the lower leg or lower part of the arm. The pressure source can be external or internal. Tight, bulky dressings or casts are examples of external pressure sources; bleeding or fluid accumulation is a common internal source of pressure. This complication is not limited to clients with musculoskeletal problems. Clients with severe burns, insect bites, or massive infiltration of intravenous fluids are also susceptible to compartment syndrome, as edema increases pressure in compartments.

The primary physiologic changes that result from increased compartment pressure are sometimes referred to as the *ischemia-edema cycle.* Capillaries within the viable muscle dilate, which raises capillary pressure.

Capillaries become more permeable because of the release of histamine by the ischemic muscle tissue. As a result, plasma proteins leak into the interstitial fluid space, and edema occurs, which causes pressure on nerve endings and subsequent pain. Blood flow to the area is reduced, and further ischemia results. The color of the tissue pales, and pulses begin to weaken; the affected area is usually palpably tense. If the condition is not treated, cyanosis, tingling, numbness, paresis, and severe pain occur. The accompanying Key Features of Disease summarizes the pathophysiologic events that occur in a client with compartment syndrome.

Compartment syndrome is not common but creates an emergency situation when it does occur. There can be irreversible neuromuscular damage within 4 to 6 hours after the onset of compartment syndrome, and the limb can become useless in 24 to 48 hours (Pellino et al., 1986). Specific problems resulting from compartment syndrome include infection, persistent motor weakness

---

KEY FEATURES OF DISEASE ■ Physiologic Changes and Associated Clinical Findings in Compartment Syndrome

Physiologic Change	Clinical Findings
1. Increased compartment pressure	1. No change
2. Increased capillary permeability	2. Edema
3. Release of histamine	3. Increased edema
4. Increased blood flow to area	4. Pulses present; pink tissue
5. Pressure on nerve endings	5. Pain
6. Increased tissue pressure	6. Referred pain to compartment
7. Decreased tissue perfusion	7. Increased edema
8. Decreased oxygen to tissues	8. Pallor
9. Increased production of lactic acid	9. Unequal pulses; flexed posture
10. Anaerobic metabolism	10. Cyanosis
11. Vasodilation	11. Increased edema
12. Increased blood flow	12. Tense muscle swelling
13. Increased tissue pressure	13. Tingling; numbness
14. Increased edema	14. Paresthesia
15. Muscle ischemia	15. Severe pain
16. Tissue necrosis	16. Paresis

---

in the affected extremity, contracture, and myoglobinuric renal failure. *Infection* from the presence of necrotic tissue may become severe enough that amputation of the limb is warranted. *Motor weakness* from injured nerves is not reversible, and the client may require braces or other orthotic devices for assistance in movement. Reconstructive surgery can be performed on the affected muscles to improve function. *Volkmann's contractures* result from shortening of the ischemic muscle and nerve involvement. The most potentially fatal complication of compartment syndrome is *myoglobinuric renal failure.* Injured muscle tissues release myoglobulin (muscle protein) into the circulation, and the protein is then filtered by the kidneys. Although the exact pathophysiologic mechanisms are unknown, it is suspected that myoglobulin causes renal vasoconstriction or has a direct toxic effect on the kidney.

When multiple compartments are affected, a *crush syndrome* can occur, in which massive or prolonged muscle ischemia causes acidosis, as lactic acid production is increased; hyperkalemia (increased potassium level in serum), as the injured cells release potassium into the blood stream; shock, as a result of fluid imbalance; myoglobulinuria, as muscles release myoglobulin into circulation; and renal failure, as a result of shock and acidosis. These systemic effects result in death if the client is not treated immediately.

For clients in whom the risk of developing compartment syndrome is extremely high, the pressure within the compartments can be monitored with a wick or slit catheter, usually in a critical care setting. Clients with fractures seldom have a catheter inserted; clients with burns or other massive soft-tissue trauma are more likely candidates for the procedure. This apparatus alerts the nurse when slight increases in pressure occur.

Shock.   Bone is quite vascular, and therefore there is a risk of bleeding when an injury occurs. In addition, trauma can sever adjacent arteries and cause a hemorrhage. Consequently, hypovolemic shock can develop rapidly. The pathophysiology of hypovolemic shock is described in Chapter 17.

Fat embolism syndrome.   Fat embolism is a serious complication, usually resulting from a fracture, in which fat globules are released from the bone into the blood stream. The condition may also be seen, although less often, in pancreatitis, diabetic coma, osteomyelitis, and sickle cell anemia. Five to 10% of persons with fractures have the complication, and 8% of those individuals die as a result (Stevenson, 1985). Risk factors that increase an individual's susceptibility to having fat emboli include an elevated serum glucose or cholesterol level, increased capillary fragility, and an inability to cope with stress.

Fat emboli are most likely to occur if there are fractures of long bones or multiple fractures, although a break in any bone with sufficient bone marrow content can cause the complication. The problem can be seen at any age or in either sex, but young men between ages 20 and 40 years, and older persons between ages 70 and 80 years are at the greatest risk. The elderly client with a fractured hip is at the highest risk, but the condition is also common in clients with fractures of the pelvis.

Several theories have been offered to explain how fat is released from the bone marrow. The *metabolic* theory advocates that catecholamines, whose concentration is elevated as a result of trauma, cause the mobilization of free fatty acids, which leads to platelet aggregation and formation of fat globules. The *mechanical* theory suggests that the pressure within yellow bone marrow is greater than capillary pressure, and therefore fats are released directly from the bone. In either case, the globules deposit in small blood vessels that supply the major organs of the body, most commonly the lungs (Mims, 1989).

The client typically presents with respiratory distress, tachycardia, hypertension, tachypnea, fever, and *petechiae*, a macular, measles-like rash over the neck, upper arms, and/or chest and abdomen. The presence of petechiae is a unique characteristic of fat emboli, but the physiologic basis for their development is not known. Laboratory findings include an increased erythrocyte sedimentation rate, decreased serum albumin and calcium levels, decreased red blood cell and platelet counts, and increased serum lipase level. These changes in blood values are poorly understood, but they aid in diagnosis of the condition. Fat embolism usually occurs within 48 hours of the fracture and can result in respiratory failure or death, often from pulmonary edema. When the lungs are affected, the complication may be misdiagnosed as a blood clot embolism (see the accompanying Key Features of Disease).

Thromboembolic complications.   Deep venous thrombosis (DVT) is frequently seen in individuals who are immobile for prolonged periods because of trauma or disability. It is the most common complication of lower-extremity surgery or trauma and the most frequently fatal complication of orthopedic surgery. In persons older than 40 years of age, the incidence of DVT is as high as 40% to 60% if anticoagulant therapy is not used. Of the group who have DVT, 5% to 10% develop life-threatening pulmonary emboli (Aaron & Ciombor, 1983). A person who smokes, is obese, has heart disease, or has a history of thromboembolic complications is at an increased risk for developing this complication. The incidence of life-threatening embolic conditions is highest in elderly individuals, particularly during the first 2 to 3 days after musculoskeletal surgery. Fractures at certain sites cause more life-threatening thrombi than others. For example, clients with fractures of the lower extremities and pelvis are more likely to develop DVT that become pulmonary emboli than clients with fractures at other sites. Local venous stasis or trauma increases the chance of DVT in clients with musculoskeletal trauma. A further discussion of DVT is found in Chapter 65; pulmonary emboli are described in Chapter 62.

Infection.   Anytime there is trauma to tissues, the body's defense system is disrupted. Wound infections are the most common type of infection resulting from orthopedic trauma; they range from superficial skin infections to deep wound abscesses (Hoyt, 1986). Infection can also be caused by indwelling hardware, i.e., pins, plates, and rods, that is used to repair a fracture

---

KEY FEATURES OF DISEASE ■ Differential Features of Pulmonary Emboli: Fat Versus Blood

Characteristic	Fat Embolism	Blood Clot Embolism
Definition	Obstruction of pulmonary vascular bed by fat globules	Obstruction of pulmonary artery by blood clot(s)
Origin	95% from fractures of long bones; occurs usually within 48 h Altered mental status (earliest sign)	85% from deep vein thrombi in legs or pelvis; can occur anytime
Assessment findings	Increased respirations, pulse, temperature Dyspnea Decreased level of consciousness Petechiae (50%–60%) Retinal hemorrhage (not common) Mild thrombocytopenia	Same as for fat embolism, except no petechiae
Treatment	Bed rest Gentle handling Oxygen Hydration (intravenous fluids) Possibly steroid therapy	Preventive measures (e.g., leg exercises, antiembolism stockings) Bed rest Oxygen Possibly mechanical ventilation Heparin therapy Thrombolytics Possible surgery: ligation of vena cava, vena cava umbrella

surgically. Clostridial infections can result in gas gangrene or tetanus and can cause malunion. Bone infection, or *osteomyelitis,* is most commonly seen in open fractures in which skin integrity is lost, and after surgical repair of a fracture. A further discussion of osteomyelitis is found in Chapter 30. For clients experiencing trauma, there is an increased risk of hospital-acquired, or nosocomial, infections. Chapter 26 describes the infectious process in detail.

Avascular necrosis.   *Avascular necrosis* is sometimes referred to as *aseptic* or *ischemic* necrosis, or osteonecrosis. In certain types of fractures, the blood supply to bone is disrupted, which results in the death of bone tissue. This complication is most frequently seen in clients with hip fractures or any fracture in which there is displacement of bone. Surgical repair of fractures can also lead to avascular necrosis because the hardware used can interfere with circulation. Chapter 28 describes this problem as a complication of chronic steroid therapy.

Delayed union, nonunion, and malunion.   *Delayed union* is defined as a fracture that has not healed within 6 months from the time of injury. Some fractures never achieve union, i.e., they never completely heal; others heal incorrectly, which causes malunion. These problems occur most commonly in clients with tibial fractures, fractures for which a number of different treatment modalities have been used (e.g., cast, traction), and pathologic fractures. Union may also be delayed or not achieved in the elderly client. As a result of the lack of healing, the client experiences pain and immobility.

A relatively new procedure to the United States is sometimes used for malunion or nonunion fractures: the Ilizarov technique. Originating in the Soviet Union more than 30 years ago, this procedure uses a circular external fixation device that lengthens the bone by stimulating bone growth. It may also be used for congenital anomalies, joint contractures, and ischemia (Aronson et al., 1989). The care of the client with this device is similar to the care of the client with external fixation systems, which are discussed later in this chapter.

For selected clients, *electrical bone stimulation* may be successful for treating nonunion. This procedure was developed as a result of research showing that bone has inherent electrical properties that are used in healing. The exact mechanism of action of this method is unknown, but numerous reports of union after its use are found in the literature (Geier & Hesser, 1985). Table 31–1 provides important information about the types of stimulators that are currently available.

Another method of treating these complications is bone grafting. Chips of bone are taken from the client's iliac crest or other site and are packed or wired between the bone ends to facilitate union. Allografts from cadavers may also be used. These grafts are frozen or freeze-dried and stored under sterile conditions in a bone bank, usually within a hospital.

Reflex sympathetic dystrophy.   *Reflex sympathetic dystrophy* is a poorly understood complex syndrome of pain, trophic changes, and vasomotor instability caused by an abnormally hyperactive sympathetic nervous system. It is most often the result of traumatic injury. Treatment options include physical therapy, diuretics, pain management techniques, and edema control. Sympathetic anesthetic blockade or surgical sympathectomy may be performed if more conservative measures are unsuccessful (Seale, 1989).

Etiology

The primary cause of a fracture is trauma from a motor vehicle accident or fall. Sports, vigorous exercise, and malnutrition contribute to the incidence of fractures. The trauma experienced may be a direct blow to the bone or an indirect force from muscle contractions or pulling forces on the bone. In addition, bone diseases such as osteoporosis increase the risk of a fracture in the elderly (see Chap. 30 for a discussion of osteoporosis).

Incidence

The incidence of fractures depends on the location of the injury. Rib fractures are the most common type in the adult population; overall, however, the clavicle is most often fractured, with its highest incidence in children younger than 5 years of age (Pellino et al., 1986). Femoral shaft fractures occur most often in young and middle-aged adults, but the elderly population has the highest incidence of proximal femur (hip) fractures. Humeral fractures are common in adults; the older the person, the more proximal the fracture. Wrist (Colles) fractures are typically seen in the middle-aged and elderly population. It is estimated that more than 1 million fractures occur annually as a result of osteoporosis and that most fractures occur in the middle-aged and elderly groups.

PREVENTION

Most fractures are preventable. Using safety measures such as seat belts and obeying posted speed limits can reduce the number of motor vehicle accidents and the extent of injury when accidents occur. Caution when engaging in rigorous sports and physical exercise can also prevent fractures, particularly the fatigue type. A major goal in the management of bone disease is prevention of pathologic fractures by treating the disease and by implementing safety measures such as the use of padded side rails.

In the hospital setting, safety precautions are taken to prevent clients from falling. The elderly person, in particular, is prone to falling and needs assistance in creating a hazard-free environment by removing objects in the walking path, cleaning spills, and using ambulatory aids as necessary. The call bell for the nurse is placed

TABLE 31–1 Features of Electrical Bone Stimulation

Technique	Description	Duration of Treatment	Risk	Client Responsibilities
Noninvasive electromagnetic coils system	Uses external coils on skin or cast to induce weak electrical currents in bones called pulsing electromagnetic fields.	5–6 mo	None known because current is weak; system is not used on arms if client has pacemaker.	Use 10–12 h/d, preferably at night without interruption. Avoid weight bearing until consent given by physician. Notify physician if alarm signals, which indicates equipment malfunction.
Semi-invasive percutaneous stimulator	One or more electrodes placed at fracture site with one or more placed on skin (number depends on type, severity, and treatment of fracture).	3 mo	Local skin irritation from electrodes (anode or cathode); breakage of cathode pins.	Avoid weight bearing. Change anode pad every 48 h to avoid skin irritation.
Fully implantable, direct current stimulator	Entire system placed at fracture site under skin; no external apparatus.	5–6 mo	Usual risk of complications with bone surgery.	Follow physician's advice for weight bearing and activity; often, weight bearing can begin immediately after surgery.

within reach, and the client is taught to remain in bed until help arrives. Many elderly clients are afraid that they will be incontinent and climb out of bed by going over the side rails to get to the bathroom as quickly as possible. Research suggests that using side rails for some elderly persons can be more hazardous in causing falls and other injuries than not using them (Morris & Isaacs, 1980).

EMERGENCY CARE

A fracture may be accompanied by multiple injuries to vital organs. Therefore, the client is first assessed for respiratory distress, bleeding, and head injury. If any of these are present, the nurse provides lifesaving care before being concerned about the fracture.

The fracture injury is then assessed (see the accompanying Emergency Care feature). Clothing is cut away from the fracture site for best visualization. Bleeding from a suspected fracture is controlled by direct pressure on the area, accompanied by digital pressure over the proximal artery nearest the fracture. At the same time, the nurse treats the client prophylactically for shock by checking vital signs, placing the client in a supine posi-

tion, and keeping the client warm with coverings (see Chap. 17 for nursing interventions for hypovolemic shock).

The nurse also inspects the fracture site for intactness of skin, swelling, and deformity such as shortening and

EMERGENCY CARE ■ Extremity Fracture

1. Remove the client's clothing (cut if necessary) to inspect the affected area.
2. Apply direct pressure on the area if there is bleeding and pressure over the proximal artery nearest the fracture.
3. Keep the client warm and in a supine position.
4. Check the neurovascular status of the area distal to the extremity: temperature, color, sensation, movement, and capillary refill. Compare affected and unaffected limbs.
5. Immobilize the extremity by splinting; include joints above and below the fracture site.
6. Cover the affected area with clean cloth, e.g., handkerchief.

rotation. The area is *lightly* palpated to determine temperature (coolness), decreased sensation, and blanching. Distal pulses are assessed by comparing affected and unaffected extremities, if applicable. The nurse assesses for motor function by asking the client to move an area distal to the fracture. For example, if a femoral fracture is suspected, the client is asked to move the ankle and foot on the affected side. The upper portion of the leg remains immobilized.

The area of the fracture is immobilized by *splinting* to prevent further damage, reduce pain, and increase circulation. Any object or device that extends to the joints above and below the fracture can be used as a splint. If the nurse is at the scene of an accident, the nurse may need to improvise by using available materials such as a tree limb or board. If the skin is broken, a clean (preferably sterile) cloth is applied loosely to prevent further contamination of the wound.

COLLABORATIVE MANAGEMENT

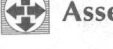 **Assessment**

History

The nurse elicits data to determine the causative factors of the fracture, which helps in developing an individualized plan of care for the client. *Age* and *sex* provide information about the possible type of injury and resultant extent of the fracture. The young male client most likely sustained an injury from a motor vehicle accident or a fall at work. The elderly female client probably fell as a result of osteoporosis, incoordination, and/or lack of balance.

The nurse asks the client to *recall the specific events* up to the time of the injury. Some type of force has led to most orthopedic injuries: incision, crush, acceleration or deceleration, shearing, and/or friction (Maher, 1986). As a result, several body systems are frequently affected. Incisional and crush injuries cause hemorrhage and a disruption of blood flow to major organs. Acceleration or deceleration injuries cause direct trauma to organs such as the spleen, brain, and kidney when they are moved from their fixed locations in the body. Shearing and friction trauma damage the skin and cause a high level of wound contamination.

By asking about the events leading to the injury, the nurse can determine which forces have been experienced and therefore which body systems or parts of the body to assess. For example, a forward fall often results in Colles fracture of the wrist because the individual tries to catch himself or herself with an outstretched hand.

A *medication history*, including substance abuse, is important regardless of age. For example, the young adult may have had an excessive amount of alcohol, which contributed to the motor vehicle accident or to the fall at the work site. Many elderly persons also consume alcohol and an assortment of prescribed and over-the-counter drugs, which can cause dizziness and loss of balance.

A *previous medical history* provides information about possible fracture causes and gives clues as to how long it will take for the bone to heal. Certain diseases such as bone cancer and Paget's disease cause pathologic fractures, which often do not achieve union.

The nurse asks about the client's *recreational* and *diversional activities.* Certain hobbies and activities are extremely hazardous, e.g., skydiving and parachute jumping. Contact sports such as football and ice hockey are likely to result in musculoskeletal injuries, including fractures. Other activities do not have such an obvious potential for hazard but can cause fractures nonetheless. For instance, daily jogging and frequent marching in a band can lead to fatigue fractures.

Because inadequate nutrition contributes to the occurrence of fractures and can inhibit bone healing, the nurse takes a complete *nutritional history*. The nurse asks the client to describe typical foods consumed for breakfast, lunch, and dinner. Also, it is not unusual for elderly clients to eat poorly because of losses of companionship and poor finances. They may be unable to prepare meals and thus rely on others for proper nutrition. A complete description of how a nurse takes a nutritional history is found in Chapter 41.

Physical Assessment: Clinical Manifestations

The client with a fracture often sustains trauma to other body systems. Consequently, the nurse assesses all major body systems for life-threatening complications, including head, thoracic, and abdominal injuries. The assessment of these areas is described in chapters on their respective body systems elsewhere in this text.

When inspecting the site of a possible fracture, the nurse observes for a *change in bone alignment.* The bone may appear to be deformed, or a limb may be internally or externally rotated. Accompanying these deviations may be an alteration in the length of the extremity, which is usually a *shortening*, and/or a *change in bone shape*, which is sometimes seen in fractures of the chest (ribs, clavicle, or sternum). The nurse asks the client if he or she can move the involved body part, and if pain is elicited, the movement is stopped immediately.

The nurse observes the skin for integrity. If the skin is intact, the area over the fracture may be *ecchymotic,* or bruised. *Subcutaneous emphysema,* the appearance of bubbles under the skin because of air trapping, is not uncommon but is seen later. *Swelling* at the fracture site occurs rapidly after injury and can result in marked neurovascular compromise. Therefore, the nurse performs a thorough *neurovascular assessment* and compares the injured area with its symmetric counterpart. Skin color and temperature, sensation, mobility, pain, and pulses are assessed distal to the fracture site. If the fracture involves an extremity, the nails are checked for capillary refill ability by applying pressure to the nail and observing for the speed of blood return to the area. If nails are

TABLE 31–2 Nursing Assessment of Neurovascular Status in Clients with Musculoskeletal Injury

Characteristic	Assessment Technique	Normal Findings
Skin color	Inspect area distal to injury.	There is no change in pigmentation when compared with other parts of body.
Skin temperature	Palpate area distal to injury (dorsum of hands is most sensitive to temperature.	Skin is warm.
Movement	Ask client to move affected area and/or area distal to injury (active motion). Move area distal to injury (passive motion).	Client can move without discomfort. There is no difference in comfort when compared with active movement.
Sensation	Ask client if numbness or tingling is present (paresthesia). Palpate with safety pin or paper clip (especially web space between first and second toes or web space between thumb and forefinger).	No numbness or tingling is present. There is no difference in sensation in affected and unaffected extremities. Loss of sensation in these areas indicates perineal nerve or median nerve damage.
Pulses	Palpate pulses distal to injury.	Pulses are strong and easily palpated; there is no difference in affected and unaffected extremities.
Capillary refill	Press nail beds distal to injury until blanching occurs (or skin near nail if nails are thick and brittle).	Blood returns (return to usual color) within 5 s.
Pain	Ask client about location, nature, and frequency of pain.	Pain is usually localized and is often described as stabbing or throbbing.

brittle or thick, the skin adjacent to the nail is assessed. Table 31–2 describes the procedure for a neurovascular assessment, which is sometimes called a circulation check ("circ. check") or CMS (circulation, movement, sensation) assessment.

For an open fracture, the nurse determines the degree of soft-tissue damage and the amount of *bleeding*. The area may be lightly palpated to determine if there is tenderness, but a sterile glove is worn if the skin is disrupted. Clients often complain of *moderate to severe pain* at the site of the fracture or in an adjacent or distal area. For example, clients with a fractured hip may have thigh pain or pain referred to the back of the knee. Pain is usually due to *muscle spasm* and edema, which result from fractures. In clients with one or more fractured ribs, severe pain occurs when deep breaths are taken. The nurse assesses the client's *respiratory status*, which may be severely compromised from a pneumothorax (lung collapse).

For fractures of the shoulder and upper arm, the assessment is best done with the client in a sitting or standing position if possible so that shoulder drooping or other abnormal positioning can be seen. The affected arm is supported and the elbow is flexed to promote comfort during the assessment. For more distal areas of the arm, the assessment is done with the client in a supine position so that the extremity can be elevated to reduce swelling.

The nurse places the client in a supine position for assessment of the pelvis and lower extremities. A client with an impacted hip fracture may be able to walk for a short time after injury, although this is not recommended. This client has pain and decreased range of motion in the hip. Like rib fractures, pelvic fractures can cause internal organ damage resulting in hemorrhage. The nurse assesses the client's vital signs, skin color, and level of consciousness for indications of possible hypovolemic shock. The urine is checked for blood, which indicates damage to the urinary system, often the bladder.

Psychosocial Assessment

The psychosocial status of a client with a fracture depends on the extent of the orthopedic injury and the presence of other complications. Hospitalization is not required for a single, uncomplicated fracture, and the client may return to usual daily activities within a few days. Healing usually is complete in a young adult in 4 to 6 weeks.

In contrast, a multiple trauma client can be hospitalized for weeks or months and may undergo many surgeries and other treatments. For these individuals, disruptions in life style can create a high level of stress. For example, if the client is the breadwinner of the family, income from employment may be eliminated if workers' compensation or disability pay is not available. In addition, the client may fear permanent disability that will prevent return to the previous job, sport, and/or recreational activities. The possibility of extended or repeated hospitalizations may cause financial concerns about health insurance coverage. Many health insurance plans do not pay 100% of the costs of in-hospital, rehabilitation, or home care.

The stresses that are created by musculoskeletal injuries that create a chronic condition affect relationships between the client and family members and/or significant others. The nurse assesses the client's feeling about himself or herself as a person and asks for information about the client's ability to cope with previously experienced stressful events. The client's body image and sexuality may be altered by deformity, treatment modalities that are used for fracture repair, and/or long-term immobilization. Chapters 5, 9, and 11 describe nursing assessment of these psychosocial concepts.

Laboratory Findings

No special laboratory tests are available for clients who have fractures. The client's hemoglobin level and hematocrit are often low because of bleeding caused by the injury. If extensive soft-tissue damage accompanies the fracture, the erythrocyte sedimentation rate may be elevated, which indicates the expected inflammatory response. During the healing stages, serum calcium and phosphorus levels are often increased as the bone releases these elements into the blood.

Radiographic Findings

Standard x-ray films confirm a diagnosis of fracture by revealing the bone disruption, malalignment, or deformity. In preparation for surgical repair, a venogram and/or arteriogram may be performed to assess vascular flow. Chapter 65 describes the nursing implications for these procedures.

The computed tomography (CT) scan is useful in detecting fractures of complex structures such as the hip and pelvis. It is also used in identifying compression fractures of the spine.

Other Diagnostic Tests

A bone scan can help in detecting certain types of fractures, particularly pathologic and fatigue fractures. It is impossible to visualize small bone or occult fractures by conventional x-ray films as early as by a bone scan. In addition, the bone scan can better determine fracture complications such as delayed bone healing, nonunion, infection, and avascular necrosis.

The magnetic resonance imaging scan is useful in determining the amount of soft-tissue damage that may have occurred with the fracture.

 Analysis: Nursing Diagnosis

The nursing diagnoses for a client with one or more fractures depend on the extent of the injuries and the

location of the fracture. If other body systems are affected or if medical complications arise as a result of the fracture, additional diagnoses are noted.

Common Diagnoses

Nursing diagnoses that are commonly seen in clients with fractures include

1. Pain related to bone fracture, muscle spasm, edema, and/or soft-tissue damage
2. Altered (peripheral) tissue perfusion related to compromised blood flow caused by injury
3. Potential for infection related to bone trauma and soft-tissue damage
4. Impaired physical mobility related to pain and treatment modalities for fracture
5. Altered nutrition: less than body requirements related to additional metabolic need for healing of bone and soft tissues
6. Anxiety related to pain, disability, and impaired mobility

Additional Diagnoses

In addition to the common diagnoses, a client with a fracture may present with one or more of the following diagnoses:

1. Activity intolerance related to pain and impaired mobility
2. Constipation related to prolonged immobility (particularly in the elderly)
3. Ineffective individual coping related to prolonged immobility, hospitalization, and/or life style changes
4. Ineffective family coping related to client's prolonged hospitalization and/or life style changes
5. Diversional activity deficit related to prolonged hospitalization
6. Anticipatory grieving related to altered life style
7. Self-care deficit related to pain and immobility
8. Body image disturbance related to deformity and/or treatment modality
9. Sexual dysfunction related to pain and immobility
10. Sleep pattern disturbance related to chronic pain and prolonged hospitalization
11. Fear related to possible nursing home placement and/or death (particularly in the elderly)
12. Impaired skin integrity and impaired tissue integrity related to open fracture
13. Knowledge deficit related to treatment regimen

These nursing diagnoses may occur in a client with an uncomplicated fracture and healing process. However, in an elderly client with a history of cardiopulmonary disease or other concurrent medical condition, the nurse identifies appropriate diagnoses related to the increased potential for problems in these areas. In addition, the nurse keeps in mind the normal physiologic changes of aging when identifying potential diagnoses. For example, because the client is aged, there is a greater likelihood of altered skin integrity (pressure ulcer) related to prolonged bed rest.

If a client develops one or more complications of fractures, e.g., pulmonary embolus or infection, the nurse identifies other diagnoses relevant to these problems or adds the problems as additional factors in an already established diagnosis. For instance, a client with a pulmonary embolus has a diagnosis of impaired gas exchange, and nursing care is planned accordingly.

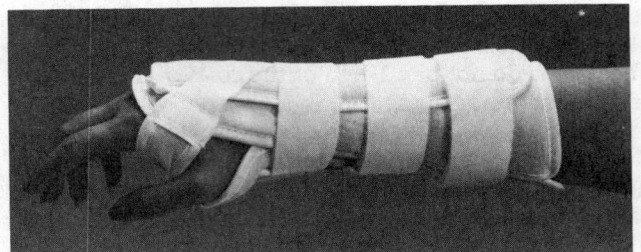

Figure 31-3

Universal wrist and forearm splint used for immobilization. (Photograph courtesy of Richards Medical Company.)

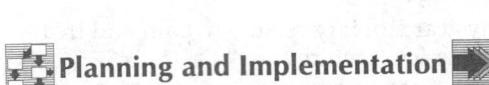 **Planning and Implementation**

Pain

Planning: client goals. The goal for this diagnosis is that the client will experience a reduction or alleviation of pain.

Interventions. Fracture management begins with the reduction and immobilization of the fracture to align the bone fragments for promote proper healing. *Reduction,* or realignment of bone ends, is accomplished by using a closed method (e.g., traction) or an open (surgical) procedure. *Immobilization* is achieved by the use of bandages, casts, traction, internal fixation, and/or external fixation. The physician decides on the method on the basis of the type, location, and extent of the fracture. These interventions reduce discomfort and prevent further injury, which would increase pain. The nurse is responsible for maintaining these modalities and for assessing for, preventing, and intervening for complications that can result from their use.

Nonsurgical management. Nonsurgical management typically involves closed reduction, which is often accompanied by immobilization with a bandage, splint, cast, or traction. Regardless of method chosen, the client usually requires drug and nondrug measures for the reduction of pain.

Closed reduction. Closed reduction is performed by the physician and involves manipulating the bone ends so that they realign, while applying a manual pull, or traction, on the bone. To ensure that the bone ends are approximated, a radiograph is taken before the bone is immobilized.

Bandages and splints. For certain areas of the body such as the scapula and clavicle, an elastic or muslin bandage may be used to immobilize the bone during healing. Because upper-extremity bones do not bear body weight, splints may be sufficient to keep bone fragments in place. A new, flexible material for splinting, Thermoplast, allows for custom-fitting to the client's body part. Figure 31–3 illustrates the use of a wrist splint for fracture immobilization. The nurse's pri-

mary responsibility is to assess the status of the area distal to the application of the bandage or splint for neurovascular compromise to determine if the device is too tight. The client usually complains of increased discomfort that is not relieved by analgesics if the splint or bandage is not properly fitted. The nurse teaches the client how to assess for circulatory changes and reminds the client to keep the device as dry and clean as possible to prevent skin breakdown and infection.

Casts. For more extensive fractures or fractures of the lower extremity, a cast is applied to hold bone fragments in place after reduction. The use of a cast also allows early mobility, corrects and prevents deformity, and reduces pain. A cast is a rigid device that immobilizes the affected body part while allowing other body parts to move. Although its most common use is for fractures, a cast is also used for correction of deformities such as a rotated ankle or for prevention of deformities such as those that may be seen in clients with rheumatoid arthritis.

Several types of materials are used to make the cast, which is applied by the physician or orthopedic technician or assistant. The traditional *plaster of Paris* (anhydrous calcium sulfate) cast requires application of a well-fitted stockinet. If the stockinet is too tight, it may cause circulation impairment; if it is too loose, wrinkles can lead to the development of pressure ulcers and subsequent skin breakdown. Web padding is applied over the stockinet, followed by wet plaster rolls wrapped around the extremity or other body part. The cast feels hot because an immediate chemical reaction occurs, but it soon becomes damp and cool. This type of cast takes from 24 to 72 hours to dry depending on the size and location of the cast. A wet cast feels cold, smells musty, and is grayish. The cast is dry when it feels hard and firm, is odorless, and has a shiny, white appearance.

In addition to being heavy and cumbersome, the plaster cast has rough edges that often crumble, which causes skin irritation. To resolve this problem, the cast should be *petaled* if the underlying stockinet does not cover the edges of the cast. Small strips of tape, or petals, are placed over the rough edges to protect the skin. If the skin under the cast was disrupted, a *window* is cut into the cast so that the wound can be observed and cared for. A window is also used as access for taking pulses, removing wound drains, or relieving abdominal distention when the client is in a body or spica cast.

If the cast is too tight, it may be cut with a special cutter to relieve pressure or to allow for tissue swelling. The physician may choose to *bivalve* the cast, or cut it lengthwise into two equal pieces, if complete bone healing has almost occurred. The nurse can remove either half of the cast for inspection or for provision of care. The two pieces are reunited by an elastic bandage wrap.

Several new types of synthetic materials are also used for casts, including *fiber glass* and *polyester-cotton knit* (Fig. 31–4). These materials are lighter weight and require minimal drying time compared with traditional materials. Fiber glass casts are dry within 10 to 15 minutes and can bear weight 30 minutes after application. Polyester-cotton casts take 7 minutes to dry and can withstand weight bearing in approximately 20 minutes (Schoen, 1986). Some physicians use plaster of Paris casts for lower extremities and synthetic casts for upper extremities because the former can bear more weight for a longer time.

Casts can be divided into four main groups: upper extremity, lower extremity, cast brace, and body or spica cast. Table 31–3 describes specific casts that are used for various parts of the body. When a client is in bed with an *arm* cast, the nurse uses a sling to elevate the arm above the client's head to reduce swelling. Ice may be applied for the first 24 to 48 hours. When the client is out of bed, the arm is supported by a sling that is placed around the neck to alleviate fatigue of the arm caused by the weight of the cast. The sling should distribute the weight over a large area of the client's body, not just the neck.

A *leg cast* permits mobility and requires the client to use ambulatory aids such as crutches. A cast shoe or boot that attaches to the foot or a rubber walking pad

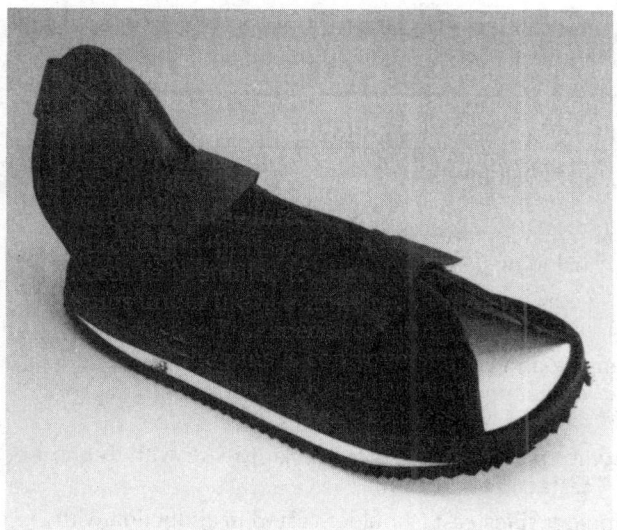

Figure 31–5

Cast shoe used to facilitate walking with leg cast. (Photograph courtesy of Richards Medical Company.)

attached to the sole of the cast assists the client in ambulation and helps to prevent falls or damage to the cast (Fig. 31–5). The nurse elevates the affected leg on several pillows to reduce swelling and applies ice for the first few days if needed.

To enable the client to bend unaffected joints while the fracture is healing, a *cast brace* may be used. The fracture must show signs of healing and minimal tissue edema before application of this cast. Two cylindrical casts are made and connected by a hinge to allow joint movement. As healing occurs, the casts may be removed and replaced with a soft brace (Fig. 31–6).

A *body cast* encircles the trunk of the body; a *spica cast* encases a portion of the trunk and one or two extremities. A client with either of these types of casts presents a special challenge for nursing care. Potential complications related to severe impairment in mobility include skin breakdown; respiratory dysfunction, such as pneumonia and atelectasis; constipation; and joint contractures. In addition to these physical limitations, the client may experience a *cast syndrome*, which is similar to a claustrophobic reaction. The client exhibits behaviors of acute anxiety such as hyperventilation, diaphoresis, hypertension, and increased heart rate. Other physiologic manifestations are due to decreased gastrointestinal motility, which results in nausea, vomiting, and abdominal distention from a paralytic ileus (cessation of peristalsis). Paralytic ileus is thought to be related to traction on the superior mesenteric artery, which reduces blood flow to the bowel (Pellino et al., 1986). The management of an ileus is the same for this client as for any client with the complication (see Chap. 20 for care of client with a paralytic ileus).

Before the client has a cast applied, the nurse explains

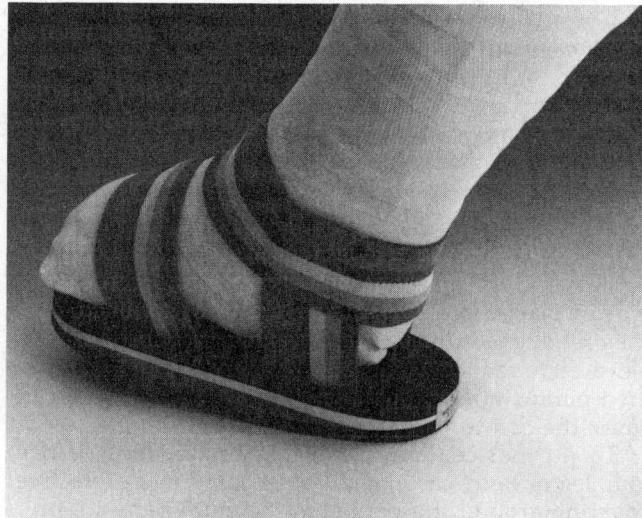

Figure 31–4

Fiber glass synthetic cast with cast sandal. (Photograph courtesy of Richards Medical Company.)

TABLE 31-3 **Types of Casts Used for Musculoskeletal Trauma**

Type and Characteristics of Cast	Use
Upper-Extremity Casts	
Short-arm cast (SAC) (extends from below elbow to and including part of hand)	Stable fractures of wrist (metacarpals, carpals, or distal radius)
Long-arm cast (LAC) (includes upper arm to and including part of hand)	Unstable fractures of wrist, distal humerus, radius, and/or ulna
Hanging-arm cast (same as LAC, but heavier, with added loop at mid-forearm)	Humerus fractures that cannot be aligned by LAC; light traction possible while client is in bed or by attached strap that extends around neck
Thumb spica (gauntlet) cast (similar to SAC with thumb casted in abduction)	Fractures of thumb
Shoulder spica cast (shoulder casted in abduction with elbow flexed)	Unstable fractures of shoulder girdle or humerus; dislocations of shoulder
Lower-Extremity Casts	
Short-leg cast (SLC) (from below knee to base of toes)	Fractures of ankle, metatarsals, and/or foot
Long-leg cast (LLC) (from mid-upper thigh to base of toes)	Unstable fractures of tibia, fibula, and/or ankle
Walking cast (walking device on bottom of SLC or LLC)	Same as for SLC or LLC
Leg cylinder (similar to SLC, but ankle and foot not casted)	Stable fractures of tibia, fibula, and knee
Long-leg cylinder (similar to LLC, but ankle and foot not casted)	Stable distal femur, proximal tibia, and knee fractures
Cast Braces (or Brace Casts)	
Patellar weight-bearing cast (similar to SLC or leg cylinder)	Midshaft or distal shaft fractures of femur
External polycentric knee hinge cast (hinge connects lower and upper leg and allows 90 degrees knee flexion)	Same as for patellar weight-bearing cast
Body Casts	
Hip spica (extends from below nipple line down affected leg [single], down leg and half of unaffected leg [1½], or down both legs [double])	Dislocation of hip; pelvic and hip injuries
Risser's cast (body jacket extends from shoulders to beyond iliac crests and hips, with large opening over anterior chest)	Scoliosis; thoracic spinal fractures
Halo cast (body jacket contains halo brace)	Fractures of cervical spine

the purpose and procedure of cast application. For a *plaster* cast, it is particularly important to warn the client about the heat that will be felt immediately after the cast is applied. The new cast, sometimes called a *green* cast, is not covered to facilitate air drying. When a client with a wet plaster cast is moved and turned, the cast is handled with the palms of the hands to prevent indentations and resulting areas of pressure on the skin. The client is turned every 1 to 2 hours to allow air to circulate and dry all parts of the cast. A sign should be placed at the head of the client's bed to remind health care personnel that the cast is wet and requires special handling. The client

may be placed on a firm mattress or fracture bed to keep the cast aligned during the drying period. If the cast is elevated to reduce swelling, the nurse uses a cloth-covered pillow, not one that is encased in plastic that can cause the cast to retain heat and prevent drying.

To prevent contamination by urine or feces, a dry long leg or body cast should be encased in a protective covering around the perineum. Fracture pans are preferred to traditional bedpans because they are smaller and more comfortable for the client. The nurse is careful to prevent spillage onto the cast.

The nurse checks to ensure that the cast is not too

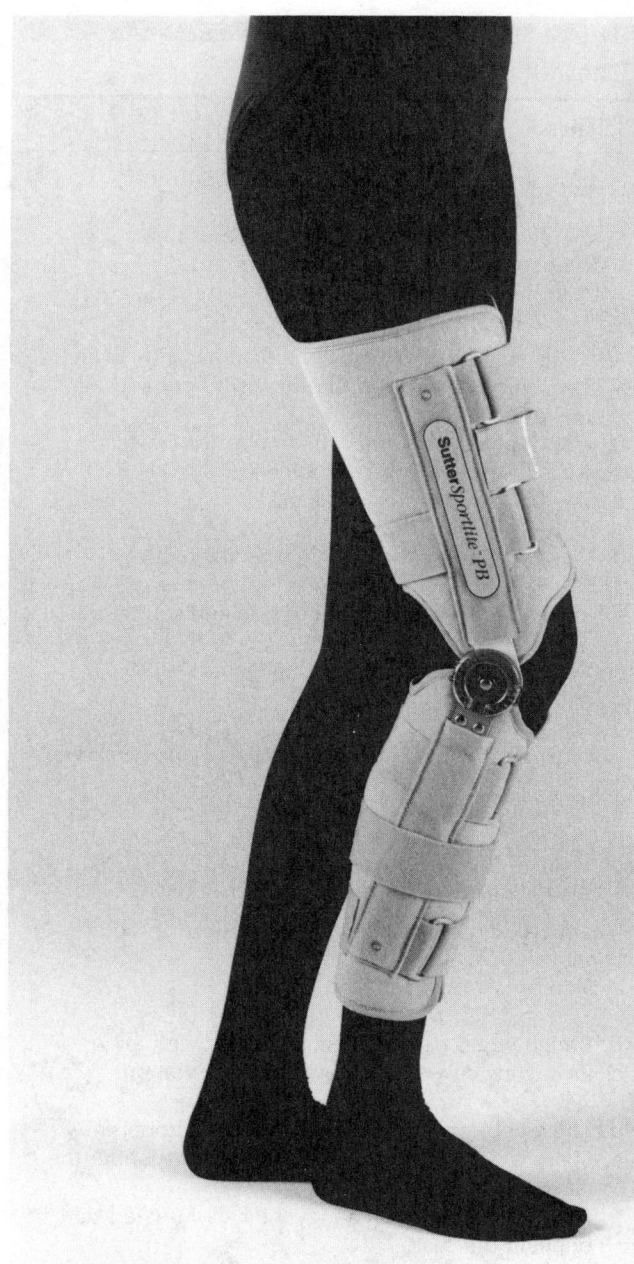

Figure 31–6

Sportlite PB postoperative knee brace. (Photograph courtesy of Sutter Corporation.)

tight and frequently monitors the client's neurovascular status, usually every hour for the first 24 hours after application (see Table 31–2 for a description of the procedure and normal findings). The nurse should be able to insert a finger between the cast and skin.

Once the cast is dry, the nurse inspects the cast at least once daily for drainage, cracking, crumbling, alignment, and fit. Areas of drainage on the cast are circled, dated, and monitored for change. It is not unusual, however,

for bloody drainage to seep through the cast from an open fracture site. The nurse reports sudden increases in the amount of drainage or a change in the integrity of the cast to the physician immediately. After swelling decreases, it is not uncommon for the cast to become too loose and need replacement.

Other complications resulting from casting can be serious and life-threatening, such as infection, circulation impairment, and peripheral nerve damage. *Infection* most often results from breakdown of skin underneath the cast. The client typically complains of a "hot spot" under the cast, and the cast may feel warmer in the affected area. The nurse smells the suspected infected area for a mustiness or unpleasant odor that would indicate infected material. If the infection progresses, the client may develop a fever.

Circulation impairment, peripheral nerve damage, and *pressure necrosis* can result from constriction of the cast. The nurse performs frequent neurovascular assessments, as described in Table 31–2. A client with a new cast may require hourly assessments; a client with a cast that is 3 or 4 days old usually requires assessments every 8 hours. Because of prolonged immobilization, a joint may become *contracted,* usually in a fixed state of flexion, or may develop *degenerative arthritis* from lack of weight bearing that is necessary for cartilage viability. *Muscle atrophy* can also occur from lack of exercise during prolonged immobilization of the affected body part, usually an extremity.

The client with a cast may be immobilized for a prolonged period depending on the extent of the fracture and type of cast. The nurse assesses for complications of immobility such as skin breakdown, thromboembolism, and constipation. Nursing assessment, preventive measures, and interventions for these problems are discussed elsewhere in this chapter. Before the cast is removed, the nurse informs the client that the cast cutter will not injure the skin, but that the client may feel heat during the procedure. Specific nursing interventions that are required for a client with a cast are delineated in the accompanying Guidelines feature.

Traction. Traction is the application of a pulling force to a part of the body to provide reduction, alignment, and rest. It can also decrease muscle spasm, thus relieving pain, and prevent or correct deformity. A client in traction is usually hospitalized longer than one who has a cast, but can generally move and exercise more readily without the weight and limitations of a cast.

Mechanical traction can be continuous, as in fracture treatment, or intermittent, as for relief of muscle spasm in other types of musculoskeletal trauma such as low-back pain (LBP). Traction may also be classified as running traction or balanced suspension. In *running traction,* the pulling force is in one direction and the client's body acts as countertraction. Moving the body or bed position can alter the countertraction force. *Balanced suspension* provides the countertraction such that the pulling force of the traction is not altered (Fig. 31–7).

Traction is classified as one of four types: skin, skeletal, plaster, or brace. *Skin* traction involves the use of

GUIDELINES ■ Care of a Client with a Cast

Interventions	Rationales

1. Monitor neurovascular status of casted extremity every 1–2 h for the first 24 h and every 4 h thereafter.
  a. Perform circulation check as described in Table 31–2
  b. Ask client if cast feels too tight.
  c. Have cast cutter available.
	1. Neurovascular status indicates tissue perfusion.
	  a, b. Adequate tissue perfusion prevents tissue necrosis and compartment syndrome.
	  c. If the cast restricts circulation, it must be cut to relieve pressure.

2. Maintain integrity of cast.
  a. Turn client every 1–2 h.
 	
  b. Use palms of hands when handling wet cast.
 	
  c. Do not turn client by holding on to abductor bar, e.g., hip spica.
  d. Do not cover a wet cast or place it on a plastic-coated pillow.
  e. Protect other parts from irritation from the rough surface of cast made from synthetics.
  f. Keep set plaster cast dry during bathing by covering it completely with plastic (also, tuck plastic into ends to prevent water seepage under the cast).
  g. Immerse synthetic cast in water during bathing, if permitted.
  h. Clean soiled plaster cast with mild detergent and damp cloth as necessary.
  i. Inspect cast when performing circulation checks for crumbling and cracking.
	2. A disrupted cast can cause complications in healing.
	  a. Repositioning allows a plaster cast to dry and prevents skin breakdown.
	  b. Use of palms prevents indentations of the cast, which can cause pressure ulcers.
	  c. The bar can bend or break.
	
	  d. Coverings and plastic prevent drying of a cast.
	
	  e. The rough surface can injure skin and soft tissue.
	
	  f. Wetting a plaster cast can change its shape.
	
	  g. Most synthetic casts do not change shape when wet.
	
	  h. Extreme soiling can cause skin infection.
	
	  i. A disruption in cast integrity can reduce its effectiveness in immobilization.

3. Maintain skin integrity.
 	
  a. Examine skin around cast edges for redness and irritation.
  b. Trim edges of cast to prevent roughness
  c. Petal edge with 1- to 2-in adhesive strips if stockinet edging is not used.
  d. Do not use lotions or powder on skin around cast.
  e. Teach client not to place foreign objects beneath cast (e.g., wire hanger to scratch under cast).
  f. Smell cast for foul odor and palpate for hot areas every shift.
  g. Inspect cast for increase in drainage every shift.
	3. Healthy skin prevents infection, irritation, and other complications.
	  a. Skin breakdown can lead to infection.
	
	  b. Rough edges can cause skin breakdown.
	  c. Protecting cast edges prevents skin irritation.
	
	  d. These substances provide media for bacterial growth.
	  e. Sharp objects can cause skin breakdown under the cast.
	  f. Foul odor and hot area may indicate infected skin beneath the cast.
	  g. Increased drainage may indicate bleeding or purulent exudate from infected area under cast.

traction tape (which is rarely used because of skin damage), Velcro (hook and loop) boot (Buck's traction) (Fig. 31–8), belt, or halter, which is attached to the skin and soft tissues. The purpose of this type of traction is to decrease painful muscle spasms that accompany fractures. The weight that is used as a pulling force is limited (5 to 10 lb), to prevent injury to the skin.

In *skeletal* traction, pins (e.g., Steinmann's), wires (e.g., Kirschner's), tongs (e.g., Crutchfield's), or screws are surgically inserted directly into bone and therefore allow the use of a longer traction time and heavier weights, usually from 15 to 30 lb. Skeletal traction aids in bone realignment. *Plaster* traction involves a combi-nation of skeletal traction and a plaster cast. A *brace* traction device exerts a pull to correct alignment deformities. *Circumferential* traction uses a belt around the body, such as pelvic traction for low-back problems. Table 31–4 describes commonly used types of traction for various parts of the body.

The nurse may set up or assist in the set-up of traction. Once traction is applied, the nurse is responsible for maintaining the correct balance between traction pull and countertraction force. Weights are not removed without a physician's order; they are not manually lifted or allowed to sit on the floor. Weights must be freely hanging at all times. The nurse teaches this important

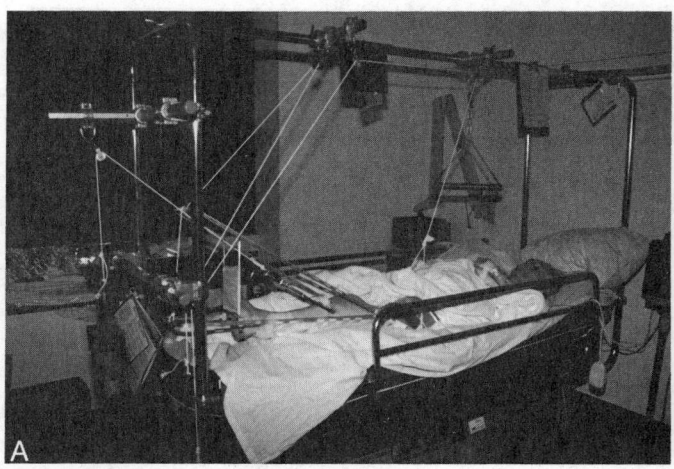
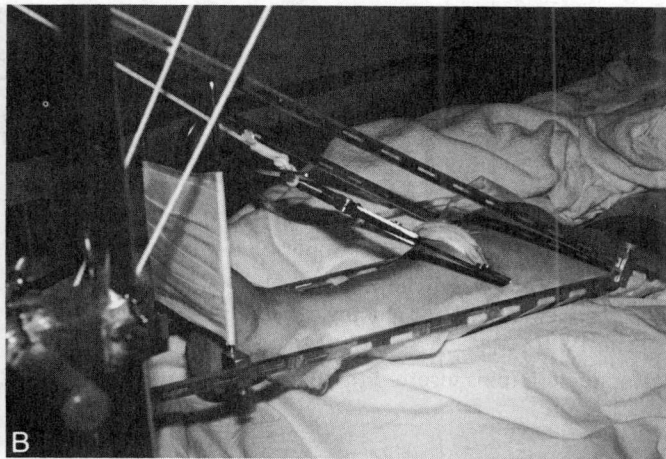

Figure 31–7

A, Balanced suspension with Thomas' splint and Pearson's attachment. *B,* Pin placement in tibia to provide skeletal traction. (Photographs by Dave Bishop, Easton, MD.)

point to other staff members on the unit and to personnel in departments such as radiology.

The skin is inspected every 8 hours for signs of irritation and inflammation. When possible, the belt or boot that is used for skin traction is removed for inspection under the device. Elderly clients often have peripheral vascular disease, connective tissue disease, and/or diabetes, so they are at high risk for developing problems caused by skin or skeletal traction because of inadequate circulation. Traction of any type is not the ideal treatment for the elderly client because it necessitates a prolonged period of immobilization, which can result in serious complications like pneumonia and pulmonary emboli.

The nurse pays particular attention to the points of entry of pins, wires, or screws at the skin for signs of inflammation and/or infection when skeletal traction is used. Some hospitals and physicians prefer that sterile pin care be provided by the nurse once or twice a day (see the accompanying Nursing Research feature). The pins and areas surrounding the pins are typically cleaned with hydrogen peroxide and/or saline. Some

NURSING RESEARCH

Is Pin Care a Waste of the Nurse's Time?

Jones-Walton, P. (1988). Effects of pin care on pin reactions in adults with extremity fracture treated with skeletal traction and external fixation. *Orthopaedic Nursing, 7*(4), 29–33.

This qualitative study examined the effectiveness of pin care provided by nurses for clients with a single upper- or lower-extremity fracture who had skeletal traction or external fixation for at least 3 weeks. A retrospective study of medical records was done for 12 subjects; 9 received some type of pin care, all with hydrogen peroxide alone or in combination with another agent. Five subjects developed reactions during the hospital stay. Pin care had no effect on the outcome regarding pin reaction.

Critique. Although the study sample was small, the investigator conducted an in-depth evaluation of the benefit of a routine nursing task that is performed for most clients with skeletal pins. There is no standard protocol for pin care in orthopedic nursing. This study should stimulate further investigation because it raises questions about nursing practice and the standard of care.

Possible nursing implications. If pin care is not effective in helping to prevent pin reactions, nurses may want to consider omitting it as a daily, time-consuming task. Nurses often perform tasks routinely without evaluating their value during this time of sophisticated technology and increased demands on professional nursing time.

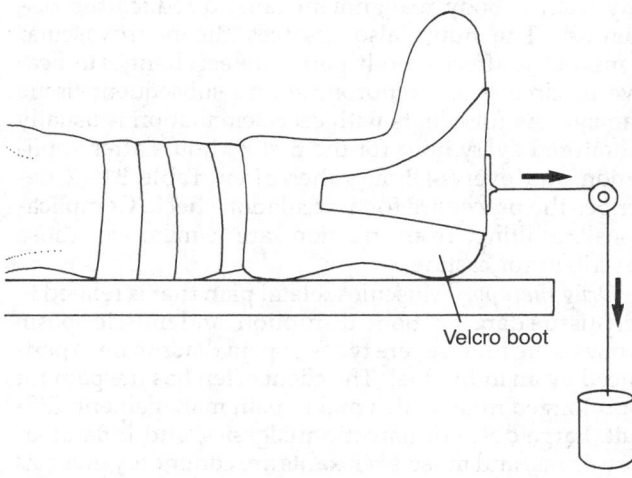

Velcro boot

Figure 31–8

Buck's traction with Velcro boot, commonly used for fractured hip.

TABLE 31–4 Types of Traction Used for Musculoskeletal Trauma

Type and Characteristics of Traction	Use
Upper-Extremity Traction	
Sidearm skin or skeletal traction (forearm is flexed and extended 90 degrees from upper part of body)	Fractures of humerus with or without shoulder and clavicle involvement
Overhead, or 90–90 traction, skin or skeletal (elbow is flexed and arm is at right angle to body over upper chest)	Same as above (depends on physician's preference)
Plaster traction (pins inserted through bone are fixed in cast)	Fractures of wrist
Lower-Extremity Traction	
Buck's extension traction (skin) (affected leg in extension)	Fractures of hip or femur preoperatively; prevention of hip flexion contractures; reduction of low back muscle spasms (bilateral Buck's); hip dislocation
Russell's traction (similar to Buck's but sling under knee to suspend leg)	Fractures of end of tibia
Balanced skin or skeletal traction (usually limb elevated in a Thomas splint with Pearson's attachment, or Böhler-Braun splint used)	Fractures of femur and/or pelvis
Spinal Column and Pelvic Traction	
Cervical halter (strap under chin)	Cervical muscle spasms, strain/sprain, or arthritis
Cervical skeletal, e.g., halo brace, Crutchfield's tongs	Cervical fractures of spine; muscle spasms
Pelvic belt (strap around hips at iliac crests attached to weights at foot of bed)	Pain, strain, sprain, or muscle spasms in lower back
Pelvic sling (wide strap around hips attached to overhead bar to keep pelvis off bed)	Pelvic fractures and other pelvic injuries

physicians and nurse specialists believe that cleaning disrupts the skin's natural barrier to infection and advise against this care. In any case, the pin sites are observed at least daily for drainage, color, odor, and severe redness, which indicate inflammation and possible infection. Infection of the pin tract can easily result in osteomyelitis.

The nurse is responsible for checking traction equipment to ensure its proper functioning. All ropes, knots, and pulleys are inspected at least every 8 hours for loosening, fraying, and positioning. The nurse checks the weight for consistency with the physician's order. At times, the physician or qualified technician changes the weight without notifying the nurse or modifying the written order; the nurse contacts the person responsible for a new order for confirmation of the change. Sometimes one of the weights is accidentally displaced by a staff member or visitor who bumps into them. The nurse replaces the weights if they are not correct and notifies the physician.

If the client complains of severe pain from muscle spasm, the weights may be too heavy or the client may need realignment. The nurse reports the pain to the physician if body realignment fails to reduce the discomfort. The nurse also assesses the neurovascular status of the affected body part to detect changes indicative of circulation compromise and subsequent tissue damage. As for clients with casts, circulation is usually monitored every hour for the first 24 hours after application and every 4 hours thereafter. Table 31–2 describes the procedure for a circulation check. Complications resulting from traction are similar to those described for casting.

Drug therapy. Musculoskeletal pain that is related to soft-tissue damage, bone disruption, and muscle spasm is one of the most severe types of pain that can be experienced by an individual. The client often has the pain for a prolonged time, which makes pain management difficult. Large doses of narcotic analgesics, anti-inflammatory drugs, and muscle relaxants are commonly given as needed. Mild tranquilizers such as diazepam (Valium) may also be used to promote a calming effect, to minimize muscle spasm, and to reduce anxiety, which can heighten the intensity of pain. For clients with chronic, severe pain, narcotic and nonnarcotic drugs are alternated or are given together to prevent drug dependence. The nurse and client mutually decide on the best times to administer the strong pain relievers, e.g., before a complex dressing change and at bedtime. The nurse observes the client carefully for the effectiveness of the medication and its side effects. An early sign of compartment syndrome is often the sudden inability of pain medication to relieve pain. Chapter 7 discusses the various methods of pain management, including epidural analgesia and patient-controlled analgesia.

Nondrug measures.   With chronic, severe pain, the client cannot depend solely on drugs for relief. The nurse uses temporary pain relief measures such as ice or heat, depending on the cause of the pain. If swelling causes pressure on the affected area, ice and elevation of the affected body part may be appropriate. Muscle spasms are best relieved by application of heat and massage. Other physical measures include a warm, soothing bath and back rub, and the use of therapeutic touch.

If these measures are not effective in reducing pain, the nurse uses distraction, imagery, or music therapy as alternatives. The nurse teaches the client relaxation techniques, such as deep breathing, for use during periods of severe pain. Chapter 7 discusses these techniques in detail.

Surgical management.   For some types of fractures, casts and traction are not appropriate or sufficient treatment modalities. Open reduction with internal fixation (ORIF) remains a common method of reducing and immobilizing a fracture. When this method is not feasible, external fixation with closed reduction is used. Although the nurse does not make the decision about which surgical technique is used, it is important to understand the procedures to enhance client teaching and care.

Open reduction, internal fixation.   Open reduction allows the surgeon direct visualization of the fracture site and permits early client mobilization. Consequently, it is often the preferred surgical method for an elderly client who is prone to complications of immobility. Internal fixation involves the use of pins, screws, rods, plates, and/or prostheses to immobilize the fracture during healing. The surgeon implants the device by making an incision to gain access to the broken bone. After the bone achieves union, the hardware may be removed depending on the location and type of fracture. Specific types of internal fixation devices are discussed under the later heading Fractures of Specific Sites.

External fixation.   An alternative modality for initial management of fractures is use of an external fixation apparatus, as shown in Figure 31–9. After fracture reduction, small percutaneous incisions are made so that pins may be implanted into the bone. Several small holes are drilled into the bone, and a series of metal pins are inserted through or into the bone. The pins are held in place by a large, external metal frame to prevent bone movement.

External fixation has several advantages over other immobilization techniques. First, there is minimal blood

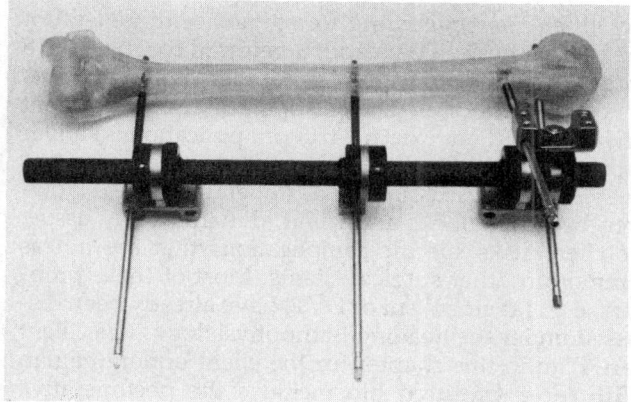

Figure 31–9

Hex-Fix external fixation system for tibial fracture. (Photograph courtesy of Richards Medical Company.)

loss when compared with internal fixation. The device allows for early ambulation and exercise of the affected body part while relieving pain. In open fractures, in which skin and tissue trauma accompanies the fracture, the device permits easy access to the wound and promotes healing. This method is often preferred to the use of a window in a cast for wound care.

A major disadvantage of external fixation is the risk of pin tract infection, which is seen in about 10% of all clients with an external fixator. Pin tract infections can lead to osteomyelitis, which is a serious and difficult to treat infection (see Chap. 30 for discussion of osteomyelitis). To prevent these infections, some agencies have a pin care procedure that is performed once or twice a day. The procedure is similar to that described for skeletal traction pins under the heading Traction. As with skeletal traction, the need for special cleaning of the pins and the area around the pins is controversial. Regardless of whether or not pin care is done, the nurse inspects the pin sites at least daily for severe redness, swelling, and drainage.

As with any fracture treatment, the nurse assesses the neurovascular status of the extremity or part distal to the fracture. External fixators may be used for an extremity or for fractures of the pelvis. External fixation is not long-term treatment for fractures. After a fixator is removed, the client is typically placed in a cast until healing is complete.

The client with an external fixator may experience a body image disturbance. The frame is large and bulky, and the affected area may have massive tissue damage with dressings. The nurse is sensitive to this possibility for planning care.

Preoperative care.   Before an ORIF surgery, the client may be placed in traction for several days to stabilize the fracture. This procedure is typical of the management of a fractured hip, in which Buck's traction (5 to 7 lb) is often used (see Fig. 31–8). The nurse teaches the client, family, and/or significant others what to expect during and after the surgery. The preoperative care for a client undergoing musculoskeletal surgery is similar to that for any other client preparing for surgery with general or spinal anesthesia. The reader is referred to Chapter 18 for a thorough discussion of preoperative nursing care.

Postoperative care. The postoperative care for a client having an ORIF or external fixator application is similar to that provided for any client undergoing surgery (see Chap. 20 for discussion of postoperative care). However, because bone is a vascular, dynamic body tissue, the client risks specific complications that are not as common in other surgical clients. Most of these problems, e.g., fat embolism or DVT, have already been discussed under the heading Pathophysiology. The Client Care Plan in this chapter for the client undergoing an ORIF for a fractured hip includes the postoperative nursing care for a client having musculoskeletal surgery.

Altered (Peripheral) Tissue Perfusion

Planning: client goals. For this diagnosis, the primary goal is that the client will maintain a sufficient blood flow to provide adequate oxygen and nutrients to tissues, particularly distal to the fracture.

Interventions. The nurse uses the assessment techniques that were described in Table 31–2 to monitor local tissue perfusion. If a severe impairment occurs, surgery may be performed to relieve the compression of nerves and blood vessels and to restore circulation. Tissue perfusion may also be reduced as a result of a lower hemoglobin level and hematocrit. Bone bleeds easily, and blood loss that results from the injury can lead to anemia and possibly hypovolemic shock.

Nonsurgical management. The nurse assesses the client's circulation after a fracture at least every hour for the first 24 hours after the injury, every 2 hours for the next 12 to 24 hours, and every 4 hours for the next few days. Unit nursing standards and the individual's needs may necessitate a deviation from this schedule. If assessment of the client reveals findings that are different from the expected normal findings, the nurse monitors circulation more frequently, perhaps every half hour, to evaluate perfusion ability, and the physician is notified immediately.

The nurse also monitors the client's complete blood count for indications of anemia resulting from blood loss. The area of injury is assessed for the amount of bleeding that has occurred or is occurring. The client with a fracture may receive several units of packed red blood cells or whole blood. If the client is elderly, malnourished, or alcoholic, vitamin and iron supplements are given to help restore the essential nutrients that are needed for manufacture of red blood cells.

Surgical management. As described under the heading Pathophysiology, compartment syndrome can result from a fracture and can cause permanent tissue damage (necrosis). If this complication occurs, the source of pressure is identified and removed if possible.

For example, if a cast is too tight, the cast is cut. If the pressure is caused by edema and bleeding within the tissues, a *fasciotomy* is performed by the surgeon to relieve the pressure on blood vessels, muscles, and nerve tissue. The surgeon makes an incision through the compartments into the fascia, which is left open. The nurse applies wet-to-dry dressings for 5 to 7 days after the procedure to débride the wound. The wound is then usually grafted and closed.

Potential for Infection

Planning: client goals. The goal for this nursing diagnosis is that the client will not experience a wound or bone infection.

Interventions: nonsurgical management. When caring for a client with a fracture, particularly an open fracture, the nurse uses strict aseptic technique for dressing changes, wound irrigations, and pin care. Signs of local inflammation with purulent drainage are reported immediately to the physician. The nurse monitors the client's vital signs for increases in temperature and pulse, which often indicate systemic infection. Chapter 26 describes prevention of infection, and Chapter 30 discusses osteomyelitis.

Most clients with an open fracture are given a broad-spectrum antibiotic prophylactically. This treatment is especially important in clients with fractures requiring surgical repair.

Impaired Physical Mobility

Planning: client goals. The goals are that the client will (1) not experience complications of impaired mobility and (2) be independent in ambulation and/or mobility, such as transferring from bed to chair.

Interventions: nonsurgical management. The interventions necessary for this diagnosis can be grouped into two types: those that help to prevent complications of impaired mobility and those that help to increase mobility of the client.

Prevention of complications. The nurse plays a vital role in preventing and assessing complications that can occur in immobilized clients with fractures. Additional information about the nursing care that is required to prevent these problems is found in Chapter 22. The risk of each complication is dramatically increased if surgery is performed. The elderly client is at the greatest risk of having these complications as sequelae of aging, and prolonged immobility and surgery add to this predisposition.

Thromboembolic disease. When prolonged bed rest is anticipated, as in clients with skeletal traction, measures are taken to prevent DVT, especially in the lower extremities. The nurse applies knee-high or thigh-high antiembolism stockings, like TEDS, which are removed once each day during bathing. Thigh-high stockings are commonly used because thigh thrombi more readily become emboli than calf thrombi. The stockings apply pressure on the venous walls, which promote venous blood return to the heart and thus prevents venous stasis, which could lead to DVT.

Newer antiembolism devices such as Venodyne and sequential compression devices are gaining popularity. These devices are attached to pumps that apply pressure to the legs alternately or sequentially. They may be used alone or over TED stockings.

The nurse obtains a physical therapy consultation to teach the client appropriate isometric and isotonic exercises to be performed in bed. The technique and frequency (usually every hour in sets of 10) of quadriceps and gluteal setting and of ankle pumping (by alternating dorsiflexion and plantar flexion) are taught to clients who are limited to the bed or those with limited time out of bed. The nurse reinforces the way to perform the exercises. Quadriceps setting is done by having the client straighten the legs, push his or her knees against the bed, and tense the quadriceps muscle. Gluteal setting is accomplished by instructing the client to push the heels into the bed. The client is allowed to get out of bed as soon as possible, which is particularly important for the elderly individual.

Most orthopedic surgeons prescribe anticoagulant therapy to prevent clot formation. Low doses of some form of aspirin (Ascriptin, Bufferin, Ecotrin) or warfarin (Coumadin) are given once or twice a day. Dipyridamole (Persantine) may be used as an alternative or as a supplement to these other drugs. Some physicians prescribe heparin sodium, which is a more potent drug acting directly in the blood stream and which cannot be given orally. Five thousand units is given subcutaneously every 8 to 12 hours. The nurse carefully monitors coagulation studies, such as prothrombin and partial thromboplastin times, and observes the client for signs of excessive bleeding, e.g., blood in the stool or the urine. Because the maintenance drug doses are relatively small, the danger of hemorrhage is minimal, but it should not be negated. An alternative or adjunct to anticoagulant medication is the use of plasma volume expanders such as dextran.

The nurse assesses the client at least once daily for the presence of DVT, with special attention to the lower extremities. The calves and thighs are compared with each other for size, color, temperature, and pain. The circumference of each leg is measured and recorded daily if DVT is suspected (swelling is a common indication of clot formation). The nurse tries to elicit the Homans sign by briskly dorsiflexing the ankle while the knee is flexed. A positive sign is the client's complaint of calf pain during the procedure and signifies possible DVT, although a client may have DVT without a positive Homans sign. The nurse reports a positive Homans finding to the physician immediately.

Respiratory complications.   For clients whose fracture(s) and treatment require prolonged immobility or use of a body cast, the risk of hypostatic pneumonia and atelectasis, or lung collapse, is high, especially in the elderly. The nurse teaches and reinforces the need and technique for deep breathing and coughing every 2 hours, as described in Chapter 18. In addition, the nurse initiates the use of an incentive spirometer, such as Triflows, to expand the lungs and thus prevent respiratory complications. For the heavy smoker or the client with chronic obstructive pulmonary disease, more aggressive pulmonary hygiene measures, such as intermittent positive-pressure breathing, may be used. The nurse assesses the client's need for these interventions and consults with a respiratory therapist if available. The nurse assesses the client's breath sounds daily for indications of pneumonia or atelectasis; this procedure is described in Chapter 60. To mobilize pulmonary secretions, the client is turned at least every 2 hours, if feasible, and is assisted out of bed as soon as possible.

Contractures or muscle atrophy.   While on bed rest, the client must exercise to prevent these complications of immobility. The nurse consults with the physical therapist for initiation of isometric and range-of-motion exercises. For the lower extremity, quadriceps setting is performed by the client every hour. Gluteal setting for the buttocks and biceps and triceps setting are also performed. Active range-of-motion exercises are preferred to passive, but if the client is unable to perform these exercises alone, the nurse assists the client in active-assist exercise.

Skin impairment.   The elderly client is at extremely high risk for developing pressure ulcers as a result of impaired mobility. The nurse inspects all bony prominences and pays special attention to the sacrum and heels, where the problem typically begins. In addition to turning and massage, the nurse uses special materials or devices for the bed such as heel and elbow protectors, an eggcrate mattress, and/or an alternating pressure mattress. Numerous products are available for prevention of skin breakdown.

Alterations in elimination.   The elderly client is extremely vulnerable to developing constipation and urinary retention leading to infection and stone formation. Normal physiologic changes of aging include decreased muscle tone in the intestines and the bladder (detrusor muscle). The nurse carefully observes and records the client's patterns of elimination and increases the fluid intake to between 2500 and 3000 mL/day if this amount is not otherwise medically contraindicated. A diet high in fiber, including raw fruits and vegetables, bran, and/or prunes, often promotes fecal elimination. Stool softeners and bulk laxatives are usually given on a regular basis. An indwelling urinary catheter is not routinely inserted because it is frequently responsible for urinary tract infections.

Cerebral dysfunction.   One of the most important challenges to nursing care of an elderly client who has impaired mobility is altered thought processes. A client who had been alert, oriented, and independent in self-care can become confused, disoriented, and dependent after admission to a health care facility. The nurse's primary goal is to help the client become oriented to the environment. A large clock and calendar placed close to the client's bed may help this orientation. Having the client's family bring familiar personal items from home can reduce anxiety, which may contribute to altered thought processes. The elderly client is likely to climb out of bed at night in response to "sundowning," a phenomenon in which the client becomes confused when darkness occurs. A protective vest and side rails help to ensure the client's safety. The nurse needs to be creative in this situation.

For any client who is immobilized for a prolonged period because of the use of traction or complex casting, the nurse assesses and intervenes for sensory deprivation. The client is isolated in the hospital setting and needs stimulation to prevent this problem. The reader is referred to Chapter 8 for assessment and prevention of sensory deprivation.

Promotion of mobility. To increase mobility and assist in ambulation, the client uses crutches or a walker but may progress to use of a cane. *Crutches* are the most commonly used ambulatory aid for many types of musculoskeletal trauma, e.g., fractures, sprains, and amputations. In most hospitals, the physical therapist fits the client for crutches and teaches the client how to ambulate with them on flat surfaces and stairs. The nurse's role is to reinforce the instructions provided and evaluate whether the client is using the crutches correctly.

Walking with crutches requires strong upper extremities, balance, and coordination. For these reasons, crutches are not used as often for the elderly client. To prepare for using crutches, the client practices upper-extremity strengthening exercises. The unaffected extremity and gluteal muscles are also strengthened because they carry the weight that is usually supported by the affected extremity.

The tips and axillary bars of the crutches are padded to prevent the tips from slipping and the bars from damaging the axillae. To prevent pressure on the axillary nerve, there should be two to three finger widths between the axilla and the top of the crutch when the crutch tip is at least 15 cm (6 in) diagonally in front of the foot. The crutch is adjusted so that the elbow is flexed no

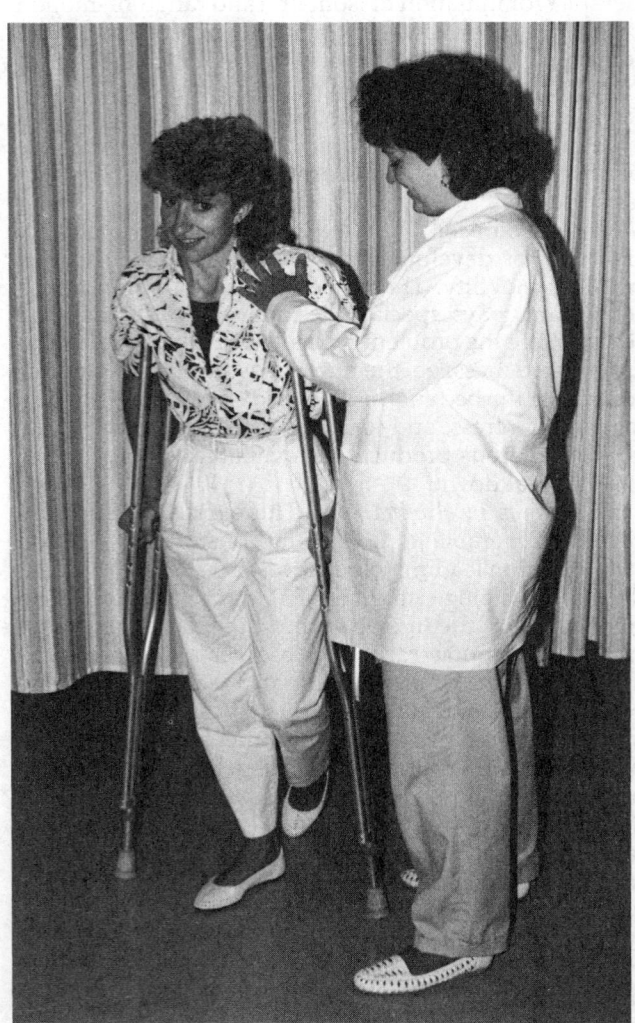

Figure 31–10

Assisting client with walking with crutches. Note guarding by therapist, with client's elbows at no more than 30 degrees of flexion.

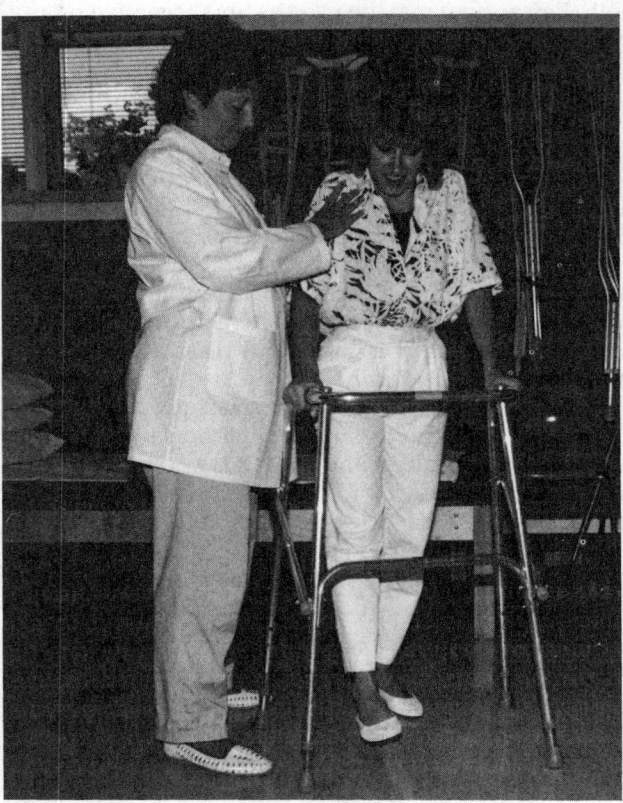

Figure 31–11

Teaching client how to use walker.

more than 30 degrees when the palm is on the handle (Fig. 31–10).

Although there are several types of gaits for walking with crutches, the most common one for musculoskeletal injury is the three-point gait. The client advances both crutches and affected leg at the same time, while the body's weight is supported by the crutches and unaffected leg. The client then swings the involved extremity to the crutches. The client is initially taught the use of crutches by the physical therapist, but the nurse reviews this information and observes the client for correct use of these aids.

A *walker* is most often used by the elderly client who needs additional support for balance. Upper-extremity and unaffected leg strength are assessed and improved with exercise as needed. As seen in Figure 31–11, the client advances the walker and steps forward. A *cane* is sometimes used if the client needs only minimal support for an affected leg. It is placed on the *unaffected* side and should create no greater than 30 degrees flexion of the elbow. The top of the cane should be parallel to the greater trochanter of the femur, as shown in Figure 31–12.

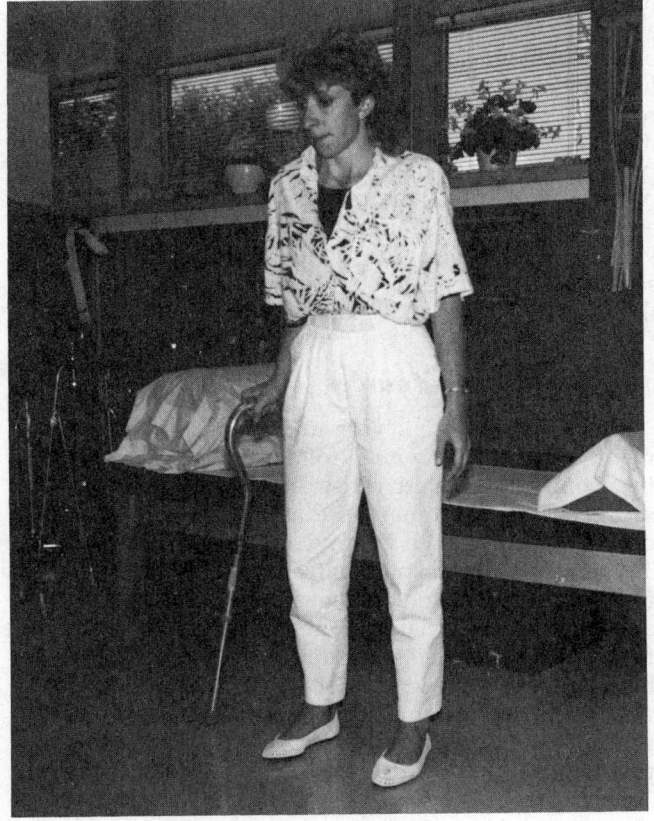

Figure 31–12

Using cane to ambulate. Note that top of cane is parallel to greater trochanter of femur.

Altered Nutrition: Less Than Body Requirements

Planning: client goals.   The primary nutritional goal is that the client will maintain an adequate dietary intake to promote healing and to prevent complications.

Interventions: nonsurgical management.   Nursing interventions focus on meeting the client's nutritional needs. The nurse assesses the client's food likes and dislikes and works with the dietitian to plan meals that are both appealing and nutritional. To promote bone and tissue healing, the client needs a high-protein, high-calorie diet. Supplements of vitamins B and C are also required for tissue nutrition. Many clients with fractures are immobilized for extended periods, and thus they are predisposed to hypocalcemia, which results in loss of calcium from bone and in subsequent bone fragility. The nurse teaches the client to increase intake of foods high in calcium, particularly milk and milk products.

In 7 to 10 days after injury, an immobilized client can develop a negative nitrogen balance because of an increase in catabolism without compensatory protein intake. The nurse offers frequent small feedings and supplements of high-protein liquids such as Ensure. Milk shakes are also an excellent protein and calorie supplement, as well as a source of calcium.

Because of less weight bearing, the immobilized client with a fracture frequently becomes anemic. In addition, blood loss from the injury or reparative surgery contributes to the anemic state. Intake of foods high in iron content is encouraged, and an oral iron supplement may be prescribed. It is not uncommon for the client to receive a daily multivitamin with iron preparation.

Anxiety

Planning: client goals.   The goal is that the client will state that anxiety about the consequences of the injury is reduced.

Interventions: nonsurgical management.   The client who is hospitalized for a prolonged period because of extensive bone and tissue damage is more likely to become extremely anxious than one who is casted and sent home to recuperate. The immobilized client experiences a number of emotions during the hospital stay, any or all of which can increase anxiety. For example, the client may be concerned about family functioning during the hospitalization. If the client is the breadwinner, there is often worry that there will be insufficient funds to meet the family's needs. An elderly client who cares for his or her spouse at home will worry about the possibility that the spouse may not be cared for properly. Many clients often experience "hospitalitis," a state of boredom and frustration from being in the hospital for a long time. They may become depressed or agitated and use the nursing staff as a scapegoat for their frustrations. The nurse cannot help the client deal with anxiety until feelings about the injury and its ramifications are identified.

After assessing the causes of anxiety, the nurse focuses on ways to reduce it. Severe anxiety can impede a person's recovery and can increase pain. The most therapeutic action for the nurse to implement is to encourage the client to ventilate feelings, sometimes by asking a direct question, such as "What are you feeling now?" The nurse helps the client to solve personal problems but recognizes that unsolicited advice is not warranted. The nurse discusses the client's potential need for professional counseling with the physician, and consultation with a counselor, psychologist, or other health care professional may be arranged.

■ Discharge Planning

Home Care Preparation

The client with an uncomplicated fracture is usually discharged to home. Elderly clients with hip or other fractures or clients with multiple trauma are often transferred to a rehabilitation setting, or to a long-term care facility for rehabilitation or permanent residence if there is total incapacitation. The discharge nurse or the discharge planner in the hospital, or both communicate the client's plan of care to the facility receiving the client to ensure continuity of care.

Clients should not be discharged to home alone because they usually need assistance with care during the healing phase. The nurse assesses the home environment for structural barriers to mobility, e.g., stairs. A cast is bulky and requires room for maneuvering and ambulating. Scatter rugs and other items that could contribute to falls are removed to create a hazard-free environment. The rooms should not be cluttered with furniture to allow the client to maneuver with crutches, a walker, or a cane. An elevated toilet seat may be required to promote independence in toileting.

Client/Family Education

The client with a fracture may be discharged from the hospital with a bandage, splint, cast, or external fixator. The nurse provides verbal and written instructions for the client on the care of these devices. The accompanying Client/Family Education feature describes the care required for the affected extremity after removal of the cast.

The client may also need to continue wound care while at home. The nurse instructs the client and caregiver how to assess and dress the wound to promote healing and to prevent infection. Wound care at home is discussed in Chapter 40. The client is taught how to recognize complications (discussed earlier in this chapter) and when and where to contact professional health care should complications occur.

Additional educational needs depend on the type of

> **CLIENT/FAMILY EDUCATION** ■ Care of the Extremity After Cast Removal
>
> "Remove scaly, dead skin carefully by soaking—do not scrub."
> "Move the extremity carefully, expect discomfort, weakness, and decreased range of motion."
> "Support the extremity with pillows or your orthotic device until strength and movement return."
> "Exercise slowly as instructed by your physical therapist."
> "Wear support stockings or elastic bandages to prevent swelling" (for lower extremity).'

fracture and fracture repair. Care of external fixators and casts was discussed earlier in this chapter.

Psychosocial Preparation

The nurse identifies potential or actual problems in the hospital and arranges for follow-up care at home. For example, professional counseling may need to continue for depression after the client's discharge from the hospital. A social worker may need to help the client apply for funds to pay medical bills. If there is severe bone and tissue damage, the nurse must be realistic and help the client understand the long-term nature of the recovery period, particularly if the client experiences a major complication, such as infection, while in the hospital. Multiple treatment modalities and surgeries may be required for these complications and can be mentally and emotionally draining for the client and family. A vocational counselor may be needed to help the client seek a different type of job, depending on the nature of the fracture.

Health Care Resources

The client with a severe injury and multiple treatment modalities may need follow-up care in the home by a community health nurse. In addition, an elderly or incapacitated client may need assistance with activities of daily living, which is provided by home care aides. The nurse in the hospital anticipates the client's needs for these services and arranges them, usually with the assistance of the social worker. It is extremely important for the hospital nurse to communicate the client's needs to the nurse or aide who will care for the client at home. A physical therapist may come to the home, or the client may go to a clinic, hospital, or private office for follow-up physical therapy after discharge from the hospital. An occupational therapist may be needed in the home to assess the environment, to assist with retraining for activities of daily living, and to make adaptations in the home to enable the client to be independent.

Evaluation

The nurse evaluates the care provided to the client with a fracture on the basis of the identified nursing diagnoses. Expected outcomes include that the client

1. States that pain is reduced or alleviated
2. Maintains adequate tissue perfusion, as evidenced by bone healing
3. Does not acquire an infection of the bone or soft tissues
4. Independently ambulates with or without ambulatory aids and provides self-care
5. Does not experience complications of immobility
6. Maintains an adequate nutritional intake, as evidenced by healing
7. States that anxiety is reduced
8. Verbalizes knowledge of treatment regimen

FRACTURES OF SPECIFIC SITES

Upper Extremity

Clavicle

Fractures of the clavicle typically occur as a result of a fall on an outstretched hand, fall on the shoulder, or direct injury. Most clavicular fractures are self-healing; a splint or bandage is used for immobilization. Complicated fractures, although uncommon, may require ORIF with pins, wires, or screws.

Scapula

Scapular fractures are not common and are usually caused by direct impact to the area. The shoulder is immobilized with a sling until healing occurs, which is generally uneventful.

Humerus

Fractures of the proximal humerus, particularly impacted or displaced fractures, are quite common in the elderly population. An impacted injury is usually treated conservatively, with a sling for immobilization. A displaced fracture often requires ORIF with pins or a prosthetic device.

Humeral shaft fractures are generally corrected by closed reduction and the application of a hanging arm cast or splint. If necessary, the fracture is surgically repaired with an intramedullary rod or metal plate and screws, or with external fixation. Nonunion of the bone and radial nerve palsy are frequent complications of this type of fracture, each occurring in about 12% of clients with humeral fractures (Schoen, 1986). Bone grafting is performed to facilitate union; prolonged splinting is necessary while the radial nerve regenerates.

A direct blow to the condyles of the distal humerus can cause either or both condyles to fracture, usually in a T- or Y-shaped configuration. The most serious complication in this fracture is damage to the brachial or median nerves. Fracture treatment is usually ORIF with a series of screws, although skeletal traction and casting can be used.

Olecranon

Fractures of the olecranon are relatively common in adults and typically result from a fall on the elbow. Many are successfully treated by closed reduction and the application of a cast, although the healing process usually takes more than 2 months. Several additional months may be needed before full use of the elbow is achieved. For displaced fractures, ORIF is performed, and a splint is worn during the healing phase.

Radius and Ulna

Forearm fractures of the ulna without accompanying injury to the radius are rare. As with other fractures of long bones, closed reduction with casting may be the appropriate treatment. If the fracture is displaced, ORIF with intramedullary rods or plates and screws is required.

A Colles fracture, or distal radius fracture, is common in the elderly population (particularly women) because it results most often from a fall on an open hand. The distal radius has a large percentage of cancellous bone, the type that is initially affected by osteoporosis. Chapter 30 describes osteoporosis, or loss of bone mass, in detail. The options for reduction and immobilization include splinting, casting, plaster-and-pin fixation, or external fixation with a frame.

Wrist and Hand

A fracture of one or more of the bones in the wrist and hand can occur, but the most common involves the carpal scaphoid and occurs in young adult men. It is also one of the most misdiagnosed fractures because it is poorly visualized on an x-ray film. Closed reduction and casting for 6 to 12 weeks is the treatment of choice. If healing does not occur, open reduction and bone grafting are performed.

Fractures of the metacarpals and phalanges are usually not displaced, which makes their treatment and healing less difficult than for other fractures. Metacarpal fractures are immobilized for 3 to 4 weeks; phalangeal fractures are immobilized in finger splints for 10 to 14 days.

Lower Extremity

Hip

Hip fractures include those involving the upper third of the femur and are classified as *intracapsular* or *extra-*

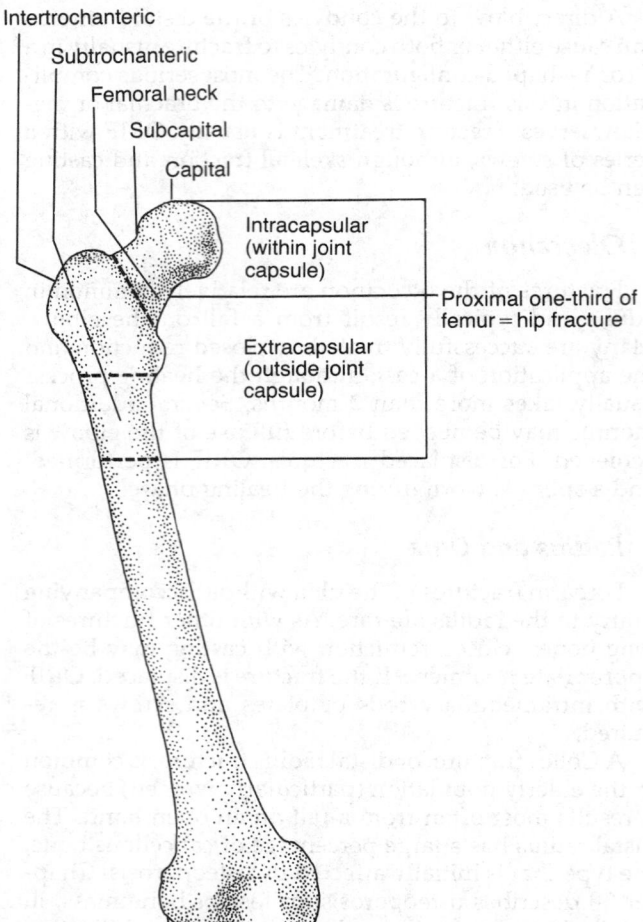

Figure 31-13

Types of hip fractures.

TABLE 31-5   Internal Fixation Devices for Fractured Hips

Location of Fracture	Type of Surgical Hardware
Subtrochanteric	Intramedullary devices (rods), e.g., Ender rod, Zickel rod
	Sliding nail plates, usually compression screw (e.g., Richards)
	Fixed blade plate, similar to osteotomy plate (not commonly used)
Intertrochanteric	Compression screw, e.g., Richards
	Pins, e.g., Ender, Knowles Harris or Ambi nail
Femoral neck or head	Compression screw, e.g., Richards
	Prosthesis, e.g., Austin Moore, bipolar

used. If the femoral neck or head is fractured, a prosthetic device is implanted. Table 31-5 identifies the types of hardware used for their respective locations. Figures 31-14 and 31-15 illustrate examples of these devices. Nonsurgical options are skin traction, usually Buck's, and skeletal traction followed by use of a cast brace.

Because hip fractures are common, with more than 250,000 per year in the United States, nurses in all health care settings need to know how to care for the special needs of the elderly client with this type of frac-

capsular, within or outside the joint capsule, respectively. These classifications are further divided according to fracture location (Fig. 31-13). Hip fractures occur most frequently in elderly persons, particularly among women who have osteoporosis. It is estimated that nearly one-half of elderly clients who sustain a hip fracture die within 1 year after injury from medical complications caused by the fracture or by immobility that occurs after the fracture.

Falls cause most hip fractures, often resulting in impaction or displacement, especially of the femoral neck. If the degree of osteoporosis is so severe that it prevents surgical intervention, the client may be incapacitated for the remainder of his or her life. The treatment of choice is surgical repair when possible to allow the elderly client to get out of bed. Depending on the exact location of the fracture, ORIF may include an intramedullary rod, pins, prosthesis, or fixed sliding plate such as a compression screw. The client with a compression screw can usually ambulate a few days after surgery and has a decreased chance of infection and nonunion when compared with clients for whom other procedures are

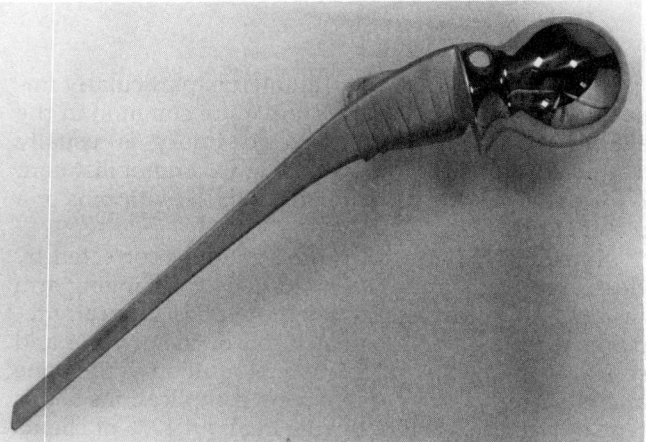

Figure 31-14

Moore's prosthesis used for hip fractures. (Photograph courtesy of Richards Medical Company.)

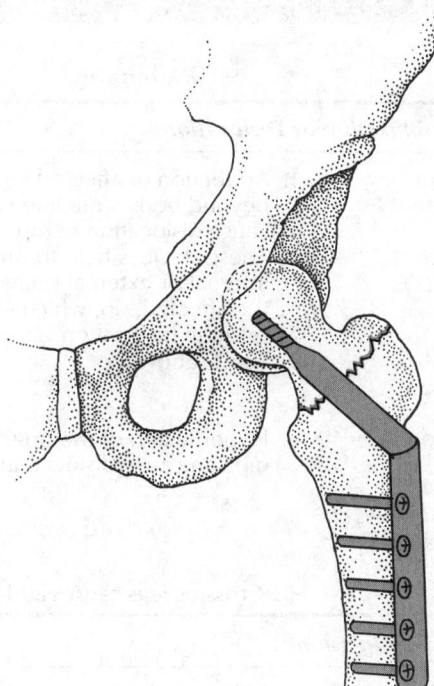

Figure 31–15

Compression hip screw used for ORIF of hip.

ture. The accompanying Client Care Plan describes common nursing diagnoses and care required for this client.

Femur

Fractures of the lower two-thirds of the femur are usually the result of trauma, often a motor vehicle accident. A femoral fracture is seldom immobilized by casting because the powerful muscles of the thigh become spastic, which causes displacement of bone ends. Skeletal traction followed by a cast brace or hip spica cast is the typical nonsurgical treatment. Surgery is an ORIF with nails, rods, or compression screw. In a few cases, external fixation may be employed.

Patella

Like most other fractures, patellar fractures result from direct impact. Fracture repair is done by closed reduction and casting or internal fixation with screws.

Tibia and Fibula

Trauma to the lower leg most often results in fractures of both the tibia and the fibula, particularly the lower third. The three basic modalities of treatment are closed reduction with casting, internal fixation, and external fixation. If closed reduction is used, the client wears a cast for at least 8 to 10 weeks. It is not unusual for delayed union to occur with this type of fracture.

Internal fixation with nails or a plate and screws followed by a long-leg cast for 4 to 6 weeks is another option. When the fractures cause extensive skin and soft-tissue damage, the initial treatment may be external fixation, often for 6 to 10 weeks.

Ankle and Foot

Ankle fractures are described by their anatomic place of injury. For example, a bimalleolar (Pott's) fracture involves the medial malleolus of the tibia and the lateral malleolus of the fibula. Because of the instability of the ankle joint, the fracture can result from supination and eversion, pronation and abduction, or pronation and eversion. These forces generally create spiral, transverse, or oblique breaks, which are often difficult to treat and present problems in healing. A combination of closed and open techniques may be used depending on the severity and extent of the fracture. An arthrodesis (fusion) may be needed if the bone does not heal.

Fractures of the foot or phalanges are treated similarly to other fractures, with either closed or open reduction. Phalangeal fractures are more painful but not as serious as most types of fractures.

Ribs and Sternum

Chest trauma may cause fractures of the ribs or sternum; the most commonly fractured ribs are numbers four through eight. The chest may be immobilized by an elastic bandage or chest strap, although these devices are being used less commonly because they can restrict lung expansion and breathing. The major concern with rib and sternal fractures is the potential for puncture of the lungs, heart, or arteries by bone fragments or ends. Fractures of the lower ribs may damage underlying organs such as the liver, spleen, or kidneys.

Pelvis

Because of the proximity of the pelvis to major organs and arteries, the chief concern in fracture management is assessing and treating associated internal damage. Pelvic fractures are the second most common cause of death from trauma, after head injuries. These fractures typically result from motor vehicle accidents or falls from buildings in young adults and from falls in the elderly population. Internal abdominal trauma is assessed by checking for the presence of blood in the urine and stool and by watching the abdomen for the development of rigidity or swelling. The trauma team may use peritoneal lavage for assessment of hemorrhage, as described in Chapter 45.

Fractures of the pelvis are divided into two broad categories: non–weight bearing and weight bearing. When a non–weight-bearing part of the pelvis is fractured, treatment can be as minimal as bed rest on a firm

CLIENT CARE PLAN ■ The Client with a Fractured Hip Who Has Had Open Reduction, Internal Fixation

Goal/Outcome Criteria	Interventions	Rationales
Nursing Diagnosis 1: Potential for Injury Related to Subluxation or Dislocation		

Client will not experience subluxation or dislocation of operative hip during hospital stay.
■ Does not adduct affected leg beyond body's midline.
■ Does not flex hip beyond 90 degress
■ Does not sustain dislocation of hip (as evidenced by pain, leg rotation, and leg shortening).
	1. Place abduction pillow or splint between client's legs while in bed.
	
	2. Use leg cradle or similar device to align affected leg.
	
	3. Turn client carefully toward either side to prevent adduction (check physician's order).
	4. Do not flex operative hip beyond 90 degrees.
	  a. Use elevated toilet seat
	  b. Have client sit in supporting chair with straight back and seat.
	5. Teach client not to cross legs.
		1. Adduction of affected leg beyond body's midline can cause dislocation of hip.
		2. These devices help to prevent internal or external rotation of the affected hip, which could result in dislocation.
		3. See 1, above.
		
		4. Hyperflexion of the operative hip can cause dislocation.
		
		5. Crossing legs causes adduction.

Nursing Diagnosis 2: Pain Related to Surgical Incision		
Client will experience alleviation or reduction of surgical pain. ■ States that pain is alleviated or reduced. ■ Participates in physical therapy program without severe pain.	1. Give pain medication as needed; anticipate client's need if client is unable to verbalize (may use epidural or patient-controlled analgesia). 2. Give pain medication after physical therapy session or other periods of increased activity. 3. Use fracture pan instead of traditional bedpan. 4. Assess appropriateness of using transcutaneous electrical nerve stimulation unit (consult with physician). 5. Use nondrug pain relief measures such as distraction, music, and relaxation exercises as needed.	1, 2. Relieving the client's pain helps the client to participate more fully in plan of care. 3. Fracture pan does not require as much lifting by the client, which increases pain. 4, 5. Nondrug pain relief measures may reduce use of narcotic analgesia.
Nursing Diagnosis 3: Potential for Infection Related to Impaired Skin Integrity		
Client will not experience surgical wound infection. ■ Manifests signs and symptoms of wound infection. ■ Experiences healing without complication.	1. Inspect surgical dressing for drainage and document type and amount. 2. Monitor and measure drainage collected in surgical drain, such as Hemovac (keep suction device compressed to prevent hematoma formation, which increases risk of infection). 3. After removal of surgical dressing, inspect incision for redness, swelling, and warmth. 4. If dressing is used, change dressing by using sterile technique. 5. Monitor vital signs every 4 h for 1–3 d.	1. Purulent drainage indicates wound infection. 2. Drains allow removal of exudate, which can be a medium for bacterial growth. 3. Signs of inflammation may indicate an infectious process. 4. Sterile conditions reduce chance of infection. 5. Elevated pulse and temperature may indicate wound infection.

continued

CLIENT CARE PLAN ■ The Client with a Fractured Hip Who Has Had Open Reduction, Internal Fixation *continued*

Goal/Outcome Criteria	Interventions	Rationales
Nursing Diagnosis 4: Impaired Physical Mobility Related to Hip Precautions and Surgical Pain		

Client will experience increased physical mobility.
■ Ambulates and makes transfers independently with or without ambulatory devices.
■ Independently performs activities of daily living (ADL) using assistive-adaptive devices.
	1. Reinforce transfer and ambulation techniques (walker or crutches) as taught by physical therapist.
	  a. Have trapeze and overhead frame on bed before surgery and teach client to use this device.
	  b. Teach client to bear weight to tolerance (or to bear weight partially for at least 6 wk postoperatively).
	2. Assess client's need for assistive-adaptive devices to perform ADL independently; consult with occupational therapist.
	3. Assess for and prevent complications of prolonged immobility, e.g., DVT, skin breakdown, or hypostatic pneumonia. (See Chap. 22 and earlier sections of this chapter for nursing assessment and prevention of complications.)
		1, 2. Increasing mobility promotes client's independence and return to society as functional member.
		
		3. Complications of immobility cause client discomfort and prolonged hospitalization.

mattress or bed board. This type of fracture can be quite painful, and the client may need stool softeners to facilitate defecation. A weight-bearing fracture may require the use of a pelvic sling, skeletal traction, double hip spica cast, or external fixator.

Other Fracture Sites

Because the skull and vertebral columns protect the brain and spinal cord, the discussion of these fractures is found in Chapter 33. The nurse must be aware of the special care required for these clients because of possible neurologic damage resulting from these fractures. Fractures of the jaw, nose, and other facial trauma are discussed elsewhere in the text.

AMPUTATIONS

OVERVIEW

An *amputation* is the surgical removal of a part of the body. The nurse recognizes that the psychosocial rami-

fications of the procedure are often more devastating than the physical impairment that results. The loss experienced by the client is complete and permanent and causes a change in body image and often in self-esteem. As in other types of loss, the client can be expected to progress through phases of the grieving process.

Pathophysiology

Amputations range from removal of part of a digit to removal of nearly half the entire body. An amputation is performed by one of two methods: open, or guillotine, and closed, or flap. The *open* method is used for clients who have or are likely to develop an infection. The wound remains open with drains to allow drainage to escape from the site until the infection clears. The skin flaps may be sutured over the wound at a later time. In the *closed* technique, skin flaps are pulled over the bone end and are sutured in place as part of the amputation procedure. In either method, the surgeon attempts to preserve as much of the part as possible and to keep major joints intact for maximal postoperative mobility.

Not all amputations are surgically planned; some, classified as traumatic amputations, occur when a body part is severed unexpectedly, e.g., by a saw. Because the amputated part in these clients is usually healthy, attempts to replant it may be made.

Levels of Amputation

Lower extremity. Loss of any or all of the small toes presents a minor disability, but loss of the great toe is significant because it affects balance, gait, and "push off" ability during walking. Midfoot amputations and the Syme procedure are commonly performed for peripheral vascular disease. In the Syme amputation, most of the foot is removed but the ankle remains. The advantage of this surgery over traditional amputations below the knee is that weight bearing can be accomplished without use of a prosthesis and without pain.

There is intense effort today to preserve knee joints by performing a below-knee amputation (BKA) rather than above-knee amputation (AKA). When the cause for the amputation extends beyond this level, however, above-knee or higher amputations are performed. Hip disarticulation, or removal of the hip joint, and hemipelvectomy procedures are more common in the younger client than in the elderly client, who cannot easily handle the cumbersome prostheses that are required for ambulation. The higher the level of amputation, the more energy is required for ambulation. These higher-level procedures are typically done for cancer of the bone.

Upper extremity. An amputation of any part of the upper extremity is generally more incapacitating than one of the leg. The arms and hands are necessary for activities of daily living such as feeding, bathing, dressing, and driving a car. Typically, as much length as possible is saved to maintain function. Early replacement with a prosthetic device is vital for the client with this type of amputation. Amputations of the upper extremity are not as common as those of the lower extremity.

Complications of Amputations

As with any surgical procedure, *infection* can occur in the wound or the bone. The elderly client who is debilitated and confused is at the greatest risk because excreta may soil the wound and because the client may remove the dressing and pick at the incision.

Phantom limb pain is a frequently occurring complication of amputation. The client complains of pain in the removed body part, most often immediately after surgery. The pain is described as severe, burning, crushing, or cramping. In addition, some clients state that they feel as if the removed part is in a distorted, uncomfortable position, and they experience numbness and tingling as well as pain. Some clients report that the most distal area of the removed part feels as if it is retracted into the stump end. For most clients, the pain is triggered by touching the stump, concurrent illness, fatigue, and emotional stress. If the pain is long-standing, any stimulus can cause the pain, including touching any part of the body. The nurse recognizes that the pain is real to the client and must be treated to avoid increasing the client's anxiety and to ensure the client's compliance with the therapeutic regimen.

Because the client experiences reduced mobility as a result of surgery, complications such as atelectasis, pneumonia, thromboembolism, and skin breakdown can readily occur. Each of these problems is discussed in detail under the heading Pathophysiology in the section on fractures earlier in this chapter.

Formation of a *neuroma*, which is a sensitive tumor consisting of nerve cells found at severed nerve endings, occurs most often in amputations of the upper extremity but can occur anywhere. *Flexion contractures* of the hip or knee are seen in clients with amputations of the lower extremity. This complication must be avoided to enable the client to ambulate with a prosthesis.

Etiology

The primary indication for surgical amputation is *ischemia* from peripheral vascular disease in the elderly client (see Chap. 65 for discussion of this disease). The client may have arteriosclerosis or diabetes mellitus, both of which contribute to poor blood supply and thus reduced tissue perfusion.

Most knowledge about amputations was obtained during World War II when *trauma* frequently necessitated a loss of one or more body parts. Today, with the advent of highly sophisticated microsurgery for revascularization of tissues to save limbs, amputations related to trauma are less likely to be needed. Amputations are also performed less often for *thermal injuries*, such as frostbite and burns; *tumors*; *infections*; *metabolic disorders*, such as Paget's disease; and *congenital anomalies*. Limb salvage procedures such as those described in Chapter 30 (under the heading Interventions in the section on bone cancer) have reduced the need for amputation.

Traumatic amputations most often result from accidents. An individual may be cleaning lawn mower blades or a snow blower without disconnecting the machine. A motor vehicle or industrial machine accident may also cause an amputation.

Incidence

Surgical amputations are not as common as they were 20 years ago. The typical client undergoing the procedure is a middle-aged or elderly diabetic man with a lengthy history of smoking. The client most likely has failed to care for his feet properly, which has resulted in a nonhealing, infected foot ulcer and possibly gangrene, or tissue necrosis. The second largest group having amputations consists of young men who experience motorcycle or other vehicular accidents or who are injured at work by machines used in industry. These individuals either may experience a traumatic amputation or may have a surgical amputation because of a severe crushing injury and massive soft-tissue damage.

PREVENTION

Many amputations can be prevented by teaching clients about proper health practices. The client with poor circulation that is caused by diabetes or other illness must pay special attention to the feet, which are the part of the body farthest from the heart and subsequently are the slowest to heal when injured. Foot care is described thoroughly in Chapter 51.

Safe driving habits and proper use of industrial and recreational machinery prevent traumatic injury, which can result in amputation. Although young men in particular like to take certain risks, the dangers that are associated with these machines cannot be underestimated.

COLLABORATIVE MANAGEMENT

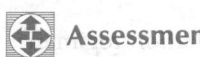 Assessment

History

The nurse collects information about *historical events* that led to tissue destruction so that teaching about health care can be individualized for the client. For example, if the diabetic client has not practiced proper foot care, the nurse assesses a need for teaching about foot care.

The client's *age* and *sex* are also important because there is a greater incidence of peripheral vascular disease in elderly persons, especially men. The nurse asks the client about *concurrent illnesses* such as heart disease, which can contribute to poor circulation, and about *smoking.* Smoking constricts blood vessels and thus impedes blood flow.

The nurse asks the client if he or she has experienced coolness of distal extremities (e.g., the feet) and if the distal area is painful (because of ischemia). A history of skin changes, such as cyanosis, or swelling is elicited from the client or family. Often an amputation of a limb precedes an amputation of another limb for the same reason.

Physical Assessment: Clinical Manifestations

Preoperatively, the nurse's primary concern is to assess circulation in other parts of the body when the client has peripheral vascular disease. The nurse assesses *skin color, temperature, sensation,* and *pulses* in both affected and unaffected extremities. *Capillary refill ability* is evaluated by applying pressure to the nail bed and waiting for the return of a normal color. In the elderly client, however, this test may be difficult to do because the nails may be thick and opaque. In this situation, the skin near the nail bed can be assessed.

Psychosocial Assessment

People react differently to the loss of a body part. The nurse needs to be aware that an amputation of a portion of one finger can be traumatic to the client, and therefore the loss must not be underestimated. The client undergoing an amputation faces a complete, permanent loss. The nurse assesses the client's psychologic prepa-

ration for a planned amputation and expects the client to experience the grieving process. Adjustment to a traumatic, unexpected amputation is often more difficult than accepting a planned one. The young client is frequently bitter, hostile, and uncooperative. In addition to loss of a body part, the client may lose a job, the ability to participate in favorite recreational activities, and/or a social relationship if the other person cannot accept the body change. Chapter 11 discusses the nursing assessment for a client experiencing loss.

The client is faced with an altered self-concept. The physical alteration that results from an amputation affects one's body image and self-esteem. For example, a client may think that an intimate relationship with a mate is no longer possible. An elderly client may feel a loss of independence. The nurse assesses the client's feelings about himself or herself to identify areas in which the client needs emotional support. The reader is referred to Chapter 9 on body image for a complete discussion and assessment tools.

The nurse tries to determine the client's willingness and motivation to withstand a prolonged rehabilitation after the amputation. Asking questions about how the client has dealt with previous life crises can provide clues. The client's willingness to change careers or other activities is also determined. Adjustment to the amputation is less difficult if the client is willing to make the changes that may be necessary.

In addition to assessing the client's psychosocial status, the nurse assesses the family's reaction to the surgery. The family's response usually correlates directly with the client's progress during recovery and rehabilitation. The family can be expected to grieve for the loss and must be allowed to adjust to the change in the client.

The nurse also assesses the client's coping abilities and helps the client identify personal strengths and weaknesses. The nurse ascertains the client's religious or spiritual beliefs because certain groups require that the amputated body part be stored for burial with the body later. Chapter 6 describes coping mechanisms that can be used by the client having an amputation.

Laboratory Findings

There are no special tests for a client having an amputation. The routine preoperative tests as described in Chapter 18 are performed.

Radiographic Findings

Routine preoperative x-rays, such as a chest x-ray, are done as for any client having surgery. The surgeon determines which tests are done to assess for viability of the limb. Angiography is not as common today as it was 10 or 15 years ago because it has been replaced with newer technology for determining blood flow.

Other Diagnostic Tests

Surgeons need to assess the viability of limb tissues, especially the skin, to ensure wound healing. A large number of noninvasive techniques are available to assist in this evaluation; for complete accuracy, no single test is relied on. One of the most common procedures is measurement of segmental blood pressure in the limb. If the segmental pressure is 35% to 40% of the brachial systolic pressure, an amputation at that level is appropriate (Burgess, 1983).

Blood flow in an extremity can also be assessed by use of isotope scans and a Doppler flowmeter, a local ultrasound device that emits signals indicating sufficient blood flow. Blood flow to the skin can be evaluated by thermography. The adequately perfused areas emit more heat than those that are not well perfused. A thorough discussion of vascular testing is found in Chapter 65.

 ### Analysis: Nursing Diagnosis

Common Diagnoses

The nurse identifies common diagnoses for the client with an amputation. These diagnoses include

1. Impaired physical mobility related to loss of body part
2. Body image disturbance related to change in physical appearance and possible changes in life style
3. Anticipatory grieving related to permanent loss
4. Pain related to trauma and phantom limb sensation
5. Impaired skin integrity related to wound
6. Potential for altered (peripheral) tissue perfusion related to decreased circulation

Additional Diagnoses

In addition to the common diagnoses, one or more of the following diagnoses may be noted for certain clients:

1. Potential for infection related to impaired skin integrity

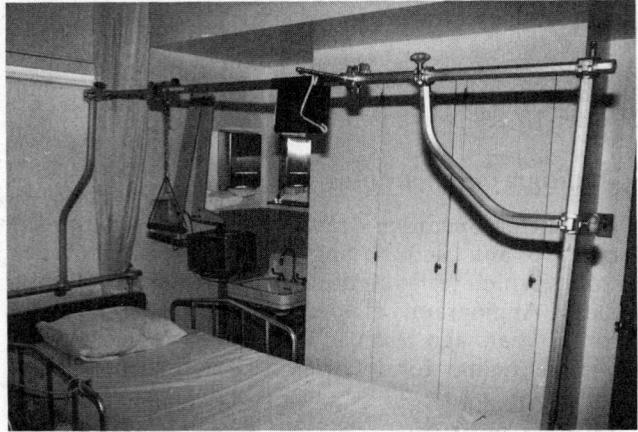

Figure 31–16

Placement of overhead frame and trapeze on bed.

2. Sleep pattern disturbance related to stump pain and phantom limb pain
3. Constipation related to immobility
4. Ineffective individual coping related to change in physical appearance and possible changes in life style
5. Ineffective family coping related to client's physical appearance and possible changes in life style
6. Dysfunctional grieving related to permanent loss
7. Impaired home maintenance management related to structural barriers to mobility
8. Self-care deficit related to loss of part or all of upper extremity
9. Knowledge deficit related to rehabilitation regimen

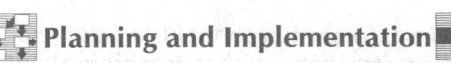 ### Planning and Implementation

Impaired Physical Mobility

Planning: client goals.   The primary goals for this diagnosis are that the client will (1) independently ambulate, with ambulatory aids if necessary, and (2) not experience complications of immobility.

Interventions: nonsurgical management.   Most clients undergoing amputation today are not confined to a wheelchair. Advancements in the design of and knowledge about prosthetics have enabled clients to become independent in ambulation. Therefore, complications from extended bed rest are not common, even for the elderly client.

Promotion of ambulation.   The nurse or physician consults with a physical therapist to initiate exercises as soon as possible after surgery. If the amputation is a planned one, the therapist often works with the client before surgery to start muscle-strengthening exercises and to evaluate the need for aids such as crutches. If the client can be instructed preoperatively in the use of these devices, learning how to ambulate after surgery is facilitated.

The client is also taught how to perform range-of-motion exercises to prevent flexion contractures, particularly of the hip and knee. A trapeze and overhead frame, as shown in Figure 31–16, aid in strengthening the upper extremities and allow the client to move independently while in bed.

A firm mattress is essential for the client with a lower-extremity amputation to prevent a contracture. The nurse assists the client into a prone position every 3 to 4 hours for 20- to 30-minute periods. This position may be uncomfortable for the client initially but is necessary to prevent hip flexion contractures. The nurse instructs the prone client to pull the stump close to the other leg and contract the gluteal muscles of the buttocks. For below-knee amputations, the nurse also teaches the client to push the residual limb down toward the bed while supporting it on a pillow. After the sutures are removed, the physical therapist may begin resistive exercises with a "sling and spring" apparatus, which can also be used at home.

Elevating a lower-leg stump on a pillow while the client is in a supine position is controversial. Some practitioners advocate avoiding this procedure at all times because it promotes hip or knee flexion contracture. Others allow elevation for the first 24 hours to reduce swelling and subsequent discomfort. The nurse inspects the residual limb daily to ensure that it lies flat on the bed surface.

For an elective amputation, the nurse arranges for the client to see a prosthetist to begin planning for the client's postoperative needs. It is especially important to arrange for replacement of an upper extremity so that the client can provide self-care. Clients are sometimes fitted with a temporary prosthesis at the time of surgery. Other clients, particularly the elderly client with vascular disease, are fitted later, after the stump has healed.

Prevention of complications of immobility. For the elderly client who is confused and debilitated, there is a risk of developing medical complications associated with bed rest or reduced mobility. The nursing interventions for preventing these problems are described under the heading Impaired Physical Mobility in the section on fractures.

Body Image Disturbance

Planning: client goals. The primary goals for this diagnosis are that the client will (1) state that he or she has an improved body image and self-esteem and (2) participate actively in rehabilitation and self-care.

Interventions: nonsurgical management. The client often experiences feelings of inadequacy as a result of losing a body part, especially the elderly person who was in poor health before surgery. If possible, the nurse arranges for the client to meet with a rehabilitated amputee. If the client is elderly, an elderly amputee is the ideal person with whom the client should interact.

Using the word *stump* when referring to the remaining portion of the limb is controversial. Clients have reported feeling as if they were part of a tree when the term was used. However, rehabilitation specialists who routinely work with amputees believe that the term is appropriate because it forces the client to realize what has happened and it enhances adjustment to the amputation (Farrell, 1986).

The nurse assesses the client's verbal and nonverbal references to the affected area. Some clients behave euphorically and seem to have accepted the loss. The nurse should not jump to the conclusion that acceptance has occurred. The nurse asks the client to describe his or her feelings about changes in body image and self-esteem. The client may verbalize acceptance but refuses to look at the area during a dressing change. This inconsistent behavior is not unusual and should be noted by the nurse. The reader is referred to Chapter 9 for further

nursing interventions for the client with an altered body image.

The client may believe that it will be impossible to return to a previous life style, including intimate relationships, job, and recreational activities. With advancements in prostheses, many clients can return to their jobs and other activities. Professional athletes who use prostheses are quite successful in sports. Clients with amputations ski, hike, bowl, and participate in other activities that are physically demanding. If a job or career change is necessary, the nurse consults with a vocational counselor for evaluation of the client's other skills that can be used in another capacity. A supportive family or significant other is important for the client's adjusting to this change. The client may also think that an intimate relationship is no longer possible because of physical changes. The nurse works with the sexual partner to help in the client's adjustment to the amputation. Professional assistance from a sexual counselor or psychologist may be needed.

For any client with an amputation, the nurse helps the client to set realistic goals, to take one day at a time. The nurse helps the client recognize personal strengths, which are emphasized and taken into account when setting goals. If the client is not realistic, frustration and disappointment may dampen the client's motivation during rehabilitation. Basic principles of rehabilitation are discussed in Chapter 22.

Anticipatory Grieving

Planning: client goals. The goal is that the client will state acceptance of the body change after a period of grieving.

Interventions: nonsurgical management. Clients grieve for various amounts of time; acceptance is usually not achieved until after discharge from the hospital. As part of preoperative teaching, the nurse describes the care that is necessary and the sensations that may be experienced by the client after surgery.

In addition to interventions that were described in the previous section on body image, the nurse may seek spiritual assistance for the client. The nurse asks the client to identify the person with whom he or she prefers to talk. If the client has no special spiritual leader or clergy, the nurse contacts the ministerial department in the hospital for consultation. For further information on nursing interventions for a client experiencing loss, the reader is referred to Chapter 11.

Pain

Planning: client goals. The goal for this diagnosis is that the client will experience a reduction in pain.

Interventions: nonsurgical management. Pain management for the client with an amputation is not unlike that for any client in pain (see Chap. 7). If the client complains of phantom limb pain, the nurse recognizes that the pain is real. It is not therapeutic for the nurse to remind the client that the limb cannot be hurting because it is missing. Pain medication is given as requested for phantom limb pain or for stump pain. The nurse handles the stump carefully when assessing the site or changing the dressing.

Impaired Skin Integrity

Planning: client goals.   The primary goal is that the client will have complete wound healing without complications such as infection.

Interventions: nonsurgical management.   The initial pressure dressing and drains are removed 48 to 72 hours after surgery. The nurse inspects the wound site for signs of inflammation, e.g., redness and swelling, and monitors the healing process. The characteristics of drainage are recorded. The dressing is changed every day until the sutures are removed. The nurse or physician wraps the stump with an elastic bandage to hold the dressing in place and to shape the stump in a functional manner. Figure 31–17 illustrates a typical method of

stump wrapping. A stump shrinker, a heavy stockinet sock, is sometimes used in place of the bandage for the client who has difficulty keeping an elastic bandage in place.

Potential for Altered (Peripheral) Tissue Perfusion

Planning: client goals.   The goal is that the client will have adequate tissue perfusion to promote healing and to prevent complications such as tissue necrosis and infection.

Interventions: nonsurgical management.   The nurse's primary focus is to monitor for signs indicating that there is sufficient tissue perfusion. The skin flap at the end of the stump should be pink in a light-skinned individual and not discolored (lighter or darker than other skin pigmentation) in a dark-skinned client. The area should be warm but not hot. The nurse assesses the closest proximal pulse for strength and compares it with that for the other extremity. If the client has bilateral

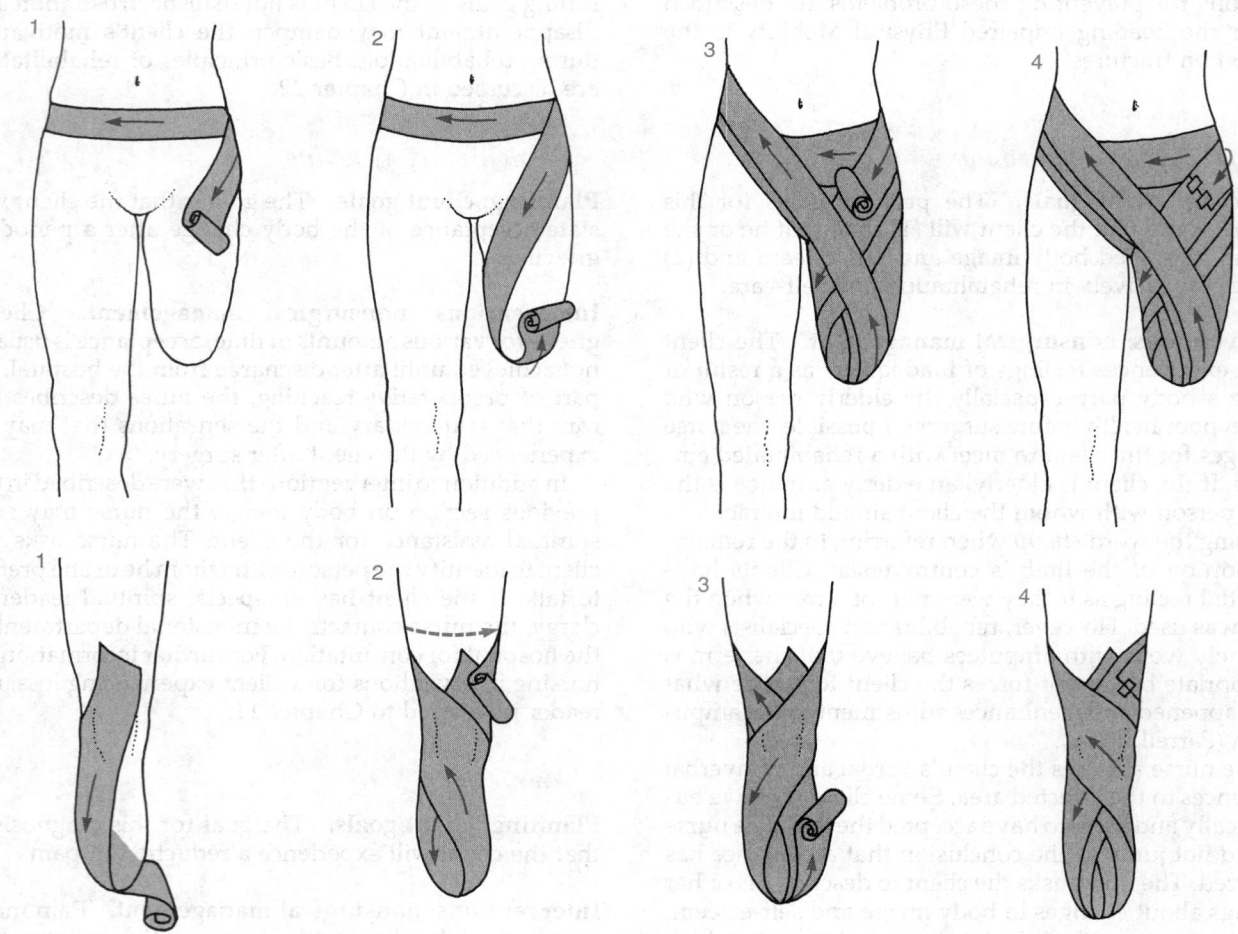

Figure 31–17
Common method used to wrap stump.

vascular disease, however, comparing limbs is not an accurate way to measure blood flow.

■ Discharge Planning

Home Care Preparation

The client is discharged directly to home or to a rehabilitation facility, depending on the extent of the amputation. In the few cases when rehabilitation is not feasible (e.g., in a debilitated, confused elderly client), the client may be discharged to a long-term care facility.

The client with amputation of a lower extremity needs to have enough room at home to maneuver a wheelchair if the leg prosthesis is not yet available. The client must be able to use toileting facilities and have access to areas necessary for self-care such as the kitchen. Structural changes may be required before the client goes home. Chapter 22 describes home modifications in detail.

Client/Family Education

The nurse teaches the client how to care for the stump and prosthesis if available. The stump should be rebandaged with clean bandages every day by the client or family member and should be inspected for signs of inflammation or skin breakdown. After the stump is healed, it is cleaned each day with the rest of the body during bathing with soap and water, and it is inspected for signs of inflammation or skin breakdown. Prostheses require special care to ensure their reliability and proper function. The accompanying Client/Family Education feature summarizes discharge teaching for the amputee with a prosthesis.

Psychosocial Preparation

A client who seemed to adjust to the amputation during hospitalization may realize that it is difficult to cope with the loss after discharge from the hospital. The nurse in the hospital setting should tell the client that this can happen. During the hospital stay, the nurse helps the client to identify strong support systems on which the client can rely after discharge.

Health Care Resources

For the elderly client or for one who has an extensive amputation such as a hemipelvectomy, the hospital nurse arranges for follow-up care in the home by a community health nurse. Physical therapy may continue in the home or on an outpatient basis. Arrangements are made for vocational and/or family counseling as needed. Some clients are discharged to a rehabilitation facility for 4 to 6 weeks for these services. Chapter 22 describes the rehabilitation phase of health care in detail.

Evaluation

The nurse evaluates nursing care on the basis of the nursing diagnoses identified for the client with an amputation. Expected outcomes include that the client

1. Ambulates independently with or without ambulatory aids or a wheelchair
2. States that body image has improved
3. Accepts the amputation as evidenced by actively engaging in activities such as work
4. States that pain is reduced or alleviated
5. Maintains skin integrity as evidenced by wound healing
6. Maintains adequate tissue perfusion as evidenced by wound healing
7. Verbalizes knowledge of treatment regimen

BACK PAIN

OVERVIEW

Back pain is second only to headache as the most common complaint of individuals in the United States. It is estimated that 80% of the population will have at least one episode of back pain in a lifetime (Schoen, 1986). The areas of the back that are most commonly affected are the cervical and lumbosacral vertebrae.

Pathophysiology

Cervical Back Pain

Cervical involvement usually results from a herniation of the nucleus pulposus in an intervertebral disk. As

---

CLIENT/FAMILY EDUCATION ■ **Care of a Prosthesis**

"Have a wooden prosthesis refinished at least once every 6 months."

"Clean the prosthesis socket with mild soap and water and dry it completely."

"Replace worn inserts and liners when they become too soiled to clean adequately."

"Check all mechanical parts, such as bolts, periodically for unusual sounds or movements."

"Grease the mechanical parts as instructed by your prosthetist."

"Use garters to keep socks or stockings in place."

"Replace your shoes, when they wear out, with new ones of the same height and type."

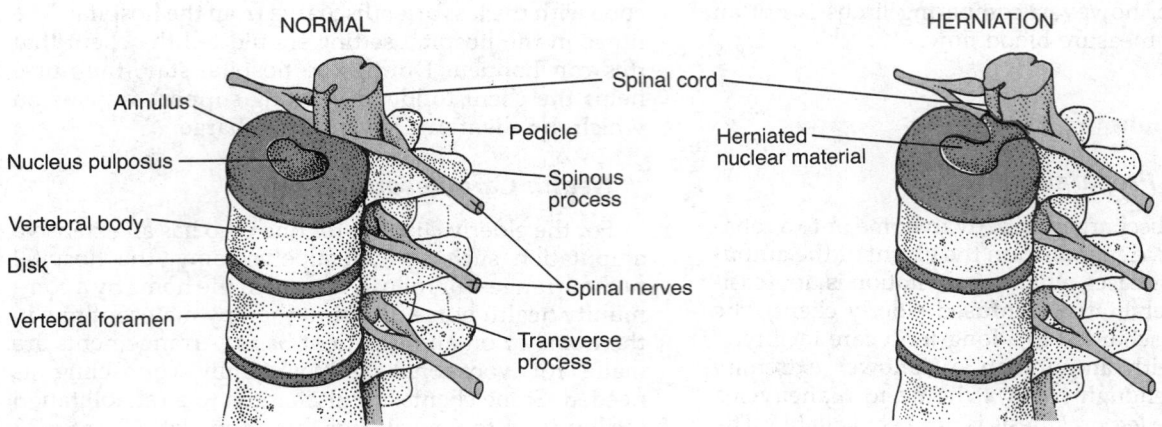

NORMAL

Annulus
Nucleus pulposus
Vertebral body
Disk
Vertebral foramen

Spinal cord
Pedicle
Spinous process
Spinal nerves
Transverse process

HERNIATION

Herniated nuclear material
Spinal cord

Figure 31–18

Herniation of nucleus pulposus.

seen in Figure 31–18, the herniation occurs laterally where the *annulus fibrosus* is weakest and the posterior longitudinal ligament is thinnest. The result is spinal nerve root compression, with subsequent motor and sensory manifestations. The disk between the fifth and sixth cervical vertebrae (C5-6) is affected most often. In cases in which the disk does not rupture, nerve compression may be caused by osteophyte formation from degenerative joint disease. The osteophyte presses on the intervertebral foramen, which results in narrowing of the disk. The client with this type of problem often has continuous or intermittent chronic pain.

Cervical pain—acute or chronic—may also occur from muscle strain or ligament sprain.

Lumbosacral Back Pain

Low-back pain (LBP) is more common than cervical pain. Acute pain is caused by a herniated nucleus pulposus, ligament sprain, disk injury from hyperflexion, or muscle strain and/or spasm. If the pain continues for 3 months or if repeated episodes of pain occur, the client is diagnosed as having chronic back pain. Herniated disks occur most often between the fourth and fifth lumbar vertebrae (L4-5) or fifth lumbar and first sacral vertebrae (L5-S1). The sciatic spinal nerve root is frequently compressed, which causes motor and sensory deficits. The pain is usually aggravated by sneezing, coughing, or straining.

Etiology

Back pain usually results from trauma. The client typically hyperflexes or twists the back during a vehicular accident or when lifting a heavy object. Obesity places increased stress on back muscles and can contribute to the occurrence or the severity of back pain. Congenital spinal conditions and scoliosis can also lead to back discomfort. For elderly clients, the cause is usually de-

generative joint disease, a type of arthritis that is seen with aging (see Chap. 28 for description of this disease).

Chronic back pain in women may result from poor posture or from wearing high-heeled shoes. Excessively high heels cause the body to compensate to maintain balance: the lower back becomes more lordotic, which strains back muscles.

Incidence

Elderly individuals, especially women, are more predisposed to cervical pain from joint disease. LBP occurs most frequently in men between 30 and 50 years of age. Seventy per cent of clients with LBP have ligament sprain from twisting the lower back. Also, women who wear high heels on a regular basis are predisposed to LBP.

PREVENTION

Many back injuries can be prevented. For example, people should be taught about proper body mechanics, including maintaining correct posture and keeping the back straight while using large leg muscles when lifting an object. Before moving or lifting an object or person, the individual should determine whether assistance is needed. The back should not be twisted or hyperflexed. Pushing an object is better than pulling it. In addition, women should wear low-heeled shoes for prolonged standing or walking.

COLLABORATIVE MANAGEMENT

 Assessment

History

The most important information for the nurse to collect from the client is a history of the *precipitating event*

HEALTH PROMOTION/MAINTENANCE ■ Use of Proper Body Mechanics to Prevent Back Injury

Size up the load to determine the number of persons needed to perform task.

When lifting an object, keep your back straight, do not bend at the waist, lift with the large thigh muscles.

Push objects rather than pull them.

Do not twist your back.

Avoid prolonged sitting or standing.

Sit in chairs with good support; sleep on a firm or semifirm mattress.

Avoid shoulder stooping — use proper posture.

Do not walk or stand in high heels for prolonged period (for women).

---

or injury. What did the client do before the onset of back pain? The activity may not be done immediately before the pain occurs; the pain may not begin until the next day or later.

The nurse notes the client's *age* and *sex* because young to middle-aged males have the highest incidence of lower-back problems. The client's *occupation* is a clue that the pain could be the result of a work-related injury. A client history or family history of *arthritis* is important because the disease can affect the cervical spine.

For clients with chronic pain, the client's *medical history* as it relates to previous back pain episodes is essential. The nurse asks the client about what treatments were used in the past, including spinal surgeries. A *weight history* is obtained to determine if there is a correlation between weight changes and the onset of back pain. Increased body weight can place extra stress on the back.

Physical Assessment: Clinical Manifestations

The nurse assesses the client's *posture* and *gait*. Some clients have so much pain that they walk in a stiff, flexed state, or they may be unable to bend at all. For LBP, the nurse may note a limp, which may indicate sciatic nerve impairment. Walking on heels or toes often causes the client severe pain in the affected leg and/or back.

The nurse inspects the back for vertebral alignment and swelling caused by muscle spasm. Local *muscle spasms* are common in clients with back pain, and muscle spasms in the affected extremity are not uncommon. It is thought that a compressed nerve becomes inflamed and irritates adjacent muscle tissue. Clients complain of a knife-like, continuous pain in the muscle close to the affected disk. *Pain* radiates down one arm in the case of cervical injury, and down the posterior leg in lumbosacral involvement. The pain usually does not extend the entire length of the limb, e.g., the client with LBP complains of sharp, burning posterior thigh or calf pain.

The client may also complain of the same type of pain in the middle of one buttock.

The nurse palpates the back and involved extremity for *tenderness*, which is frequently present. The nurse assesses for *sensory changes* by asking the client if there is paresthesia or numbness present in the involved limb. Both extremities should be tested for sensation by using a pin or paper clip and cotton ball for comparison assessment of light and deep touch. The client may be able to feel sensations in both limbs but may have stronger sensation in the unaffected side.

If the sciatic nerve is compressed, the client complains of severe pain when raising a straight leg. To complete the neurologic assessment, the nurse evaluates *muscle tone* and *strength*. In severe, chronic conditions, muscles in the extremity or in the back atrophy. The client has difficulty with movement, and certain movements elicit more pain than others. The client with cervical pain may lose hand grip strength and be unable to carry as much weight as before the injury.

Psychosocial Assessment

The client with a first-time acute episode of back pain is usually not incapacitated for a prolonged period. If the injury is work related, workers' compensation often pays for medical care costs. However, chronic pain can result in repeated hospitalizations, treatments, and surgeries for the client. Changes in life style, particularly employment and recreational activities, may be necessary.

The nurse assesses the client's feelings about the problem and recognizes the frustration and depression that typically accompany chronic back pain. The family's reaction is also determined.

Laboratory Findings

There are no special laboratory tests for back pain, but if the client has surgery, routine preoperative testing is performed (see Chap. 18 for discussion of these tests).

Radiographic Findings

The client's radiographic evaluation begins with flat plate x-ray films with anterior, posterior, and lateral views. A CT scan, done with or without contrast media enhancement, is frequently performed to visualize the herniated disk. Many clients have a myelogram, which is an invasive procedure that may or may not detect the problem. Chapter 29 describes the nursing implications of these tests in detail.

Other Diagnostic Tests

Herniations of intervertebral disks can usually be visualized by magnetic resonance imaging. This procedure takes longer to complete than the CT scan but is becoming more widely available. Chapter 29 discusses the procedure and nursing implications of this method.

Analysis: Nursing Diagnosis

Common Diagnoses

After analyzing the subjective and objective data obtained for a client, the nurse formulates the following common diagnoses:

1. Pain (acute or chronic) related to nerve compression and/or muscle spasm
2. Impaired physical mobility related to severe pain and/or treatment, e.g., pelvic traction
3. Sensory/perceptual alterations (tactile) related to sensory deficit from nerve compression

Additional Diagnoses

In addition to the above-mentioned diagnoses, the client with severe involvement or chronic pain may have the following diagnoses:

1. Urinary retention related to prolonged sacral nerve compression
2. Ineffective individual coping related to unremitting chronic pain, repeated hospitalizations, or treatment modalities
3. Sleep pattern disturbance related to severe pain
4. Self-care deficit related to severe pain
5. Sexual dysfunction related to acute or chronic pain
6. Knowledge deficit related to treatment regimen

 Planning and Implementation

Pain

Planning: client goals.   The primary goal is that the client will experience a reduction or alleviation of pain.

Interventions.   Treatment for the client with back pain varies with the severity and chronicity of the problem. Both the client and nurse can become frustrated when pain relief measures are ineffective. Conservative measures are initially implemented, but if these are unsuccessful, surgery is indicated.

Nonsurgical management.   Nonsurgical management for back pain includes drug therapy, back exercises, heat, bracing, diet therapy, traction, positioning, and nondrug measures such as transcutaneous electrical nerve stimulation. Because exercise also increases physical mobility, it is discussed under the next diagnosis of Impaired Physical Mobility.

Drug therapy.   The client is medicated with muscle relaxants, such as cyclobenzaprine hydrochloride (Flexeril), and nonsteroidal anti-inflammatory drugs, such as aspirin or ibuprofen (Motrin). The physician may also prescribe an analgesic to be given as necessary. The nurse monitors the effects of the medications in relieving pain as well as the side effects, which may indicate the need for a reduction in dosage. In some cases, the physician may give an epidural steroid injection. Chapter 7 describes nursing interventions for a client with chronic pain.

Heat.   Many clients experience temporary relief from application of heat, which increases blood flow to the area and promotes healing of injured nerves. Moist heat in the form of heat packs and hot showers or baths is beneficial. Deep heat therapy such as ultrasound treatments and diathermy is administered by a physical therapist. The nurse monitors the effects of heat treatment by assessing the client's skin condition.

Bracing.   For some types of LBP, immobilization by the use of a lumbosacral brace or corset may reduce pain. A custom-fitted, light-weight orthosis is preferred to ensure support and proper fit.

Diet therapy.   Weight control frequently helps to reduce back pain. If the client's weight exceeds the ideal by more than 10%, caloric restriction is necessary. The nurse reinforces the need for the client to lose weight to prevent or lessen chronic back pain.

Traction.   The purpose of traction in clients with back pain is to separate the vertebrae and thus relieve pressure on the impinged nerve. In clients with cervical injuries, a head halter or skeletal traction, e.g., halo traction, is used with bed rest (see Chap. 33). After discharge from the hospital, the client may wear a soft collar to immobilize the neck.

Three types of traction are available for clients with LBP: pelvic traction (Fig. 31–19), bilateral Buck's traction, and hanging traction. In pelvic traction, the client has the option of independently removing the weights at intervals. A typical regimen is to apply traction for 4 hours and then to remove the weights for 30 minutes, with this cycle being repeated continuously while the client is awake. The Williams position is more comfortable and therapeutic for the client with LBP. The client is placed in the semi-Fowler position, and the knees are flexed to relax the muscles of the lower back and to relieve pressure on the spinal nerve root. Bilateral Buck's traction and hanging traction are used less commonly.

Positioning.   Some clients benefit from a bed board placed under the mattress to provide back support. A flat position is particularly helpful for clients with a muscle injury. For a client with a herniated disk causing spinal nerve root compression, a flat position may aggravate the pain. The client usually has pain relief from flexing the knees while in a reclining position, which alleviates the pressure placed on the nerve by the affected disk (Williams' position). The benefit of special beds such as water beds is controversial.

Nondrug pain relief measures.   Transcutaneous electrical nerve stimulation (TENS) is used for chronic, unremitting pain. Two electrodes attached to a small generator are secured to the skin over the painful areas of the back. The device emits a small electrical current, which produces a tingling sensation that masks the pain. The physician or physical therapist works with the client to identify the best location for the electrodes and the strength of the electrical impulse.

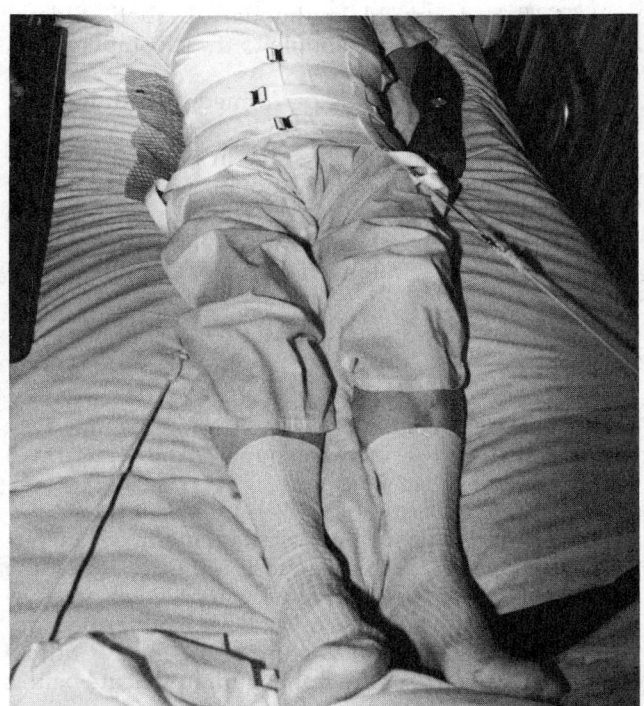

Figure 31–19

Use of pelvic traction for LBP (weights are attached to ropes present but are not shown). (Photograph by Dave Bishop, Easton, MD.)

Other measures to reduce pain include distraction, imagery, and music therapy. Chapter 7 describes nondrug measures for chronic pain relief in detail.

Surgical management. When conservative measures fail to relieve pain and neurologic deficits progress, the client usually has a *laminectomy.* A laminectomy is removal of one or more vertebral laminae, plus osteophytes and the herniated nucleus pulposus, through a 3-in longitudinal incision. The standard hospital stay is 2 to 3 days. When repeated laminectomies are performed or the spine is unstable, a spinal *fusion* is done to stabilize the affected area. Chips of bone are removed, typically from the client's iliac crest, and are placed between the vertebrae for support and grafting to strengthen the back. The hospital stay is a few days longer with this procedure.

Three alternatives to a laminectomy that are gaining popularity are chemonucleolysis, percutaneous lateral diskectomy, and microdiskectomy. The primary advantage of these surgical procedures is a shortened hospital stay or the possibility of having the procedure done on an outpatient basis. In *chemonucleolysis,* the client's affected disk is injected with an enzymatic substance, chymopapain (Chymodiactin), under local anesthesia and fluoroscopy, a type of x-ray visualization. This procedure is not used for serious neurologic deficits or for persons who had previous back surgeries. Eighty per

cent of properly selected clients obtain relief from this method, which can be performed as same-day surgery. The major complication is an immediate, severe anaphylactic reaction, which can result in death. The fluoroallergosorbent test (FAST) is used before the procedure is done to determine whether a client is sensitive to chymopapain. Women, particularly Black women, are more likely to experience this anaphylactic reaction. After chemonucleolysis, the client follows special exercises and precautions for 2 to 3 months before resuming full activity. Some clients complain that the procedure causes an exacerbation of their symptoms for at least 6 weeks, but then they obtain relief.

Because of the problems associated with chemonucleolysis, *percutaneous lateral diskectomy* may be performed. Local anesthesia is used for insertion of a metal cannula adjacent to the affected disk under fluoroscopy. A special cutting tool is threaded through the cannula for removal of pieces of the disk that are compressing the nerve root. The primary risks of this surgery are infection and nerve root injury. The client is discharged in 48 to 72 hours and follows precautions similar to those for clients who receive chymopapain injection.

A *microdiskectomy* involves microscopic surgery through a 1-in incision, which increases operating time over the previously described procedure. The complications of this procedure include infection, dural tears, and missed disk fragments.

Preoperative care.   Because the lumbar laminectomy is performed most often for a herniated nucleus pulposus, preoperative care and postoperative care for this procedure are mentioned here. Preoperative care of the client preparing for a laminectomy is similar to that for any client undergoing surgery and is described in Chapter 18. The nurse teaches the client what to expect postoperatively and how to move in bed. The client should be warned that various sensations may be experienced in the affected leg or both legs because of manipulation of nerves and muscles during surgery.

Postoperative care.   As for any surgical client, the nurse measures vital signs at least every 4 hours during the first 24 hours to assess for fever and for hypotension, which indicates bleeding. The surgical dressing is inspected for blood or any other type of drainage. Clear drainage may mean cerebrospinal fluid leakage and must be reported to the surgeon immediately. A complete neurologic assessment is performed with vital signs. Of particular importance is the client's ability to feel sensation in and move extremities. The nurse carefully checks the client's ability to void. Pain and remaining in a flat position in bed make voiding difficult, especially for men. Inability to void may indicate damage to the sacral spinal nerves, which control the detrusor muscle in the bladder. The client usually gets out of bed with assistance on the evening of surgery, which may facilitate voiding for men.

Turning the client in bed is especially important. The client is logrolled by at least two people every 2 hours from side to back and vice versa. The client is turned as one unit while the back is kept straight. For large clients, a turning sheet may be used. Two nurses are needed for either turning method. When the nurse assists the client in getting out of bed, the client's back is kept straight and the client is placed in a straight-backed chair, with feet resting comfortably on the floor.

As for any postoperative client, the client is instructed to deep breathe and cough every 2 hours to prevent atelectasis (lung collapse) and pneumonia. Until independent ambulation is accomplished, the client wears antiembolism stockings and/or another antiembolism device such as a sequential compression device to prevent DVT and possible pulmonary emboli. Elderly clients are especially susceptible to these complications of immobility.

When a spinal fusion is performed in addition to a laminectomy, more care is taken with mobility and positioning. The client usually stays in bed for 24 to 48 hours and is logrolled every 2 hours. A brace or other type of thoracolumbar support, which must be worn when the client is out of bed, is fitted for the client by the physical therapist. Prolonged sitting or standing is discouraged.

Impaired Physical Mobility

Planning: client goals. The goals for this diagnosis are that the client will (1) increase mobility and (2) return to a previous life style.

Interventions: nonsurgical management. The primary intervention for this diagnosis is the use of exercise to strengthen the back and to relieve pressure on compressed nerves. The type of exercises prescribed depends on the location and nature of the injury and the type of pain. Exercises are not begun until acute pain is reduced by other modalities. Several exercises are given in the accompanying Client/Family Education feature.

Sensory/Perceptual Alterations (Tactile)

Planning: client goals. The goals are that the client will (1) regain sensation and (2) prevent injury to the affected extremity.

Interventions: nonsurgical management. The nurse teaches the client to be careful when exposing an affected arm or leg to hot water because decreased sensation can result in a burn. For clients with sensory compromise in the feet, the client must make sure when walking that the foot is placed firmly on the ground with each step. Otherwise, the client can easily miss a step and sustain a fall. Surgical intervention may allow the client to regain sensation if the nerve is decompressed.

■ Discharge Planning

Home Care Preparation

The client should have a firm mattress to provide support for the entire vertebral column. If the client's mattress is worn and soft and the client cannot afford to purchase a new one, a bed board or large piece of plywood placed under the mattress may suffice. After back surgery, the client is not allowed to climb stairs for several weeks. It is essential that facilities to meet personal needs are on one level in the home. The client can usually return to work in 2 to 4 weeks, depending on the nature of the job. Weight that may be lifted is initially limited to 5 lb, and the amount gradually increased as healing occurs.

CLIENT/FAMILY EDUCATION ■ Typical Exercises for Chronic or Postoperative Low-Back Pain

Exercise	Instructions
Extension Exercises	
Stomach lying	"Lie face down with a pillow under your chest."
Upper trunk extension	"Lie face down with your arms at your sides and lift your head and neck."
Prone pushups	"Lie face down on a mat and, keeping your body stiff, push up to extend your arms."
Flexion Exercises	
Pelvic tilt	"Lying on your back with your knees bent, tighten your abdominal muscles to push your lower back against the mat."
Semi-sit-ups	"Lying on your back with your knees bent, raise your upper body at a 45-degree angle and hold this position for 5–10 seconds."
Knee to chest	"Lying on your back with your knees bent, tighten your abdominal muscles to push your lower back against the mat. Now bring one or both knees to your chest and hold this position for 5–10 seconds."

Client/Family Education

The nurse teaches the client to continue with a weight reduction diet, if needed; the use of moist heat; and strengthening exercises as initiated in the hospital setting. Principles of body mechanics are reviewed and demonstrated by the nurse. The client is then asked to demonstrate these principles for the nurse. The client may also continue to take medications such as anti-inflammatory drugs and muscle relaxants. The nurse reminds the client and family about side effects of drugs and what to do about them if they occur. If the client has a spinal fusion, he or she must wear a brace or thoracolumbar support for 3 to 6 months while the fusion heals completely. The client may not be able to return to full functioning for 6 to 12 months after a spinal fusion.

Psychosocial Preparation

The client with an acute episode of back pain typically returns to usual activities but may fear a recurrence. The nurse reminds the client that if caution is exercised, the client may never have another episode. For the client with chronic pain, however, the continuous or repeated pain can be frustrating and tiring. Surgery is performed if pain is unremitting. The nurse teaches the client and family to set short-term goals and to take steps toward recovery slowly.

In a few clients, back surgery is not successful. Repeated diskectomies, laminectomies, and fusions often discourage this individual, who must continue nonsurgical management of pain after these operations.

The nurse identifies support systems for the client, e.g., family and clubs. For example, a spouse may help the client with exercises or may perform the exercises with the client.

Health Care Resources

The client with back pain often continues physical therapy on an outpatient basis after discharge from the hospital. For unresolved pain, clients may be referred to pain clinics, which are usually found in large metropolitan hospitals.

 Evaluation

The nurse evaluates the client's care on the basis of the nursing diagnoses. Expected outcomes include that the client

1. States that pain is alleviated or reduced
2. Maintains increased mobility to function independently in society
3. Regains sensation and movement in an affected extremity
4. Complies with treatment regimen

SPORTS-RELATED INJURIES

In addition to the bone- and muscle-related problems already discussed, trauma can affect other tissues of the body such as cartilage, ligaments, and tendons. Many musculoskeletal injuries are the result of participation in sports or other strenuous physical activities. These injuries have become so common that large metropolitan hospitals frequently have clinics and physicians for the specialty of sports medicine. Although numerous specific types of injuries can occur, this chapter includes only the most common ones seen by the nurse in a hospital setting. The principles of injury to one part of the body are analogous to those of similar injuries in other parts. For example, a tendon rupture in a knee is cared for in the same manner as a tendon rupture in the wrist. Because the knee is most frequently injured, it is discussed as typical of other areas of the body. The accompanying Emergency Care feature lists general emergency measures for these traumas.

KNEE INJURIES

Trauma to the knee results in *internal derangement*, a broadly used term for disturbances of an injured knee joint. When surgery is required to resolve the problem, most surgeons prefer to perform the procedure through an arthroscope when possible. A general description of arthroscopy is found under the heading Diagnostic Assessment in Chapter 29.

Menisci Injuries

There are two semilunar cartilages, or *menisci*, in the knee joint: medial and lateral. These pads act as shock absorbers, but they can tear, usually as a result of twisting the leg when the knee is flexed and the foot is placed firmly on the ground. The medial meniscus is nine times

---

EMERGENCY CARE ■ Sports-Related Injuries

1. Do not move victim until spinal cord injury is ascertained (see Chap. 33 for assessment of spinal cord injury).
2. Immobilize injured part; immobilize joint above and below injury by applying splint.
3. Apply ice intermittently for first 24–48 h (heat may be used thereafter).
4. Elevate affected limb to decrease swelling.
5. Always assume that the area is fractured until x-rays are taken.
6. Assess neurovascular status in area distal to injury.

more likely to tear than the lateral meniscus because it is less mobile (Schoen, 1986). Internal rotation causes an injury to the medial meniscus; external rotation causes a tear in the lateral meniscus.

Tears can be anterior or posterior, longitudinal or transverse. In the medial meniscus, a longitudinal tear, or "bucket handle" injury, often causes the knee to lock, i.e., the torn cartilage jams between the femur and tibia and prevents extension of the knee. Surgery is frequently required for this type of injury. In transverse tears, the knee does not lock, and surgery may not be required for treatment.

The client with a torn meniscus has pain, swelling, and tenderness in the knee. A clicking or snapping sound when moving the knee can often be heard. A common diagnostic technique is the McMurray test in which the examiner flexes and rotates the knee and then presses on the medial aspect while slowly extending the leg. A test is positive if a clicking sound is palpated or heard. A negative finding, however, does not rule out a tear.

For a locked knee, the treatment is usually manipulation followed by casting for 3 to 6 weeks. If the problem recurs, a partial or total *meniscectomy* is performed. An *open* meniscectomy requires a surgical incision to remove all or part of the meniscus. Most surgeons prefer to remove only the affected portion, which can be accomplished via an arthroscope, during a *closed* meniscectomy. As described in Chapter 29, an arthroscope is a metal tubular instrument that is used for diagnosis or surgery of joints. One or more small incisions (less than 0.6 cm [¼ in] long) are made in the knee for insertion of the arthroscope. A cutting device is threaded through the arthroscope for removal of the torn cartilage while the knee is irrigated with saline or Ringer's lactate solution. A bulky pressure dressing is applied after the procedure, and the affected leg is wrapped from groin to ankle in elastic bandages.

As in any postoperative client, the nurse checks the surgical dressing for bleeding and monitors the client's vital signs after the client is readmitted to the unit. Circulation checks, as outlined in Table 31–2, are performed every hour for the first 12 to 24 hours or as dictated by the unit standards. The client begins leg exercises immediately after surgery to strengthen the leg, prevent thrombophlebitis, and reduce swelling. Quadriceps setting, in which the client straightens the leg while pushing the knee against the bed, is done in sets of 10 or more. Straight-leg raises are also performed as soon as the client awakens from anesthesia. Range-of-motion exercises are usually not started for several days. To prevent the client from bending the affected knee, a knee immobilizer such as the one shown in Figure 31–20 is frequently used. The nurse elevates the leg on one or two pillows and applies ice to reduce postoperative swelling. Full weight bearing is restricted for several weeks, depending on the amount of cartilage removed. The client is usually discharged with crutches in 1 or 2 days.

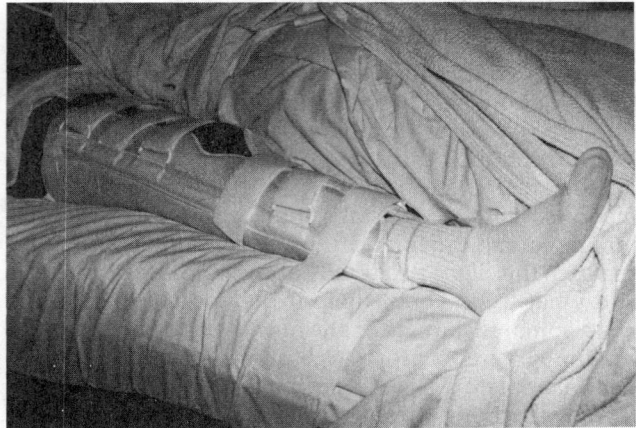

Figure 31–20

Use of knee immobilizer to prevent knee flexion. (Photograph by Dave Bishop, Easton, MD.)

Ligament Injuries

The collateral and cruciate ligaments in the knee are predisposed to injury, often from sports or vehicular accidents. Ligament damage is referred to as a *sprain*. Sprains are classified according to severity. A first-degree, or mild, sprain involves tearing of a few fibers of a ligament; function of the joint is not impaired. In a second-degree injury, or moderate sprain, more fibers are torn but stability of the joint remains intact. Severe sprains are third-degree injuries and cause marked instability of the joint. Pain and swelling characterize ligament injuries.

The treatment for mild sprains is minimal and includes rest and the use of ice and a compression bandage, which is applied for a few days to reduce swelling and to provide joint support. Second-degree sprains require casting for 4 to 6 weeks while the tear heals. In severe ligament damage, surgery is the treatment of choice. The surgeon repairs the tears by reattaching the torn portions of the ligaments, and the client is placed in a cast. If the ligament cannot be repaired, reconstructive surgery by grafting is performed. In the past several years, the U.S. Food and Drug Administration has approved several artificial knee ligaments. The Gore-Tex ligament is a permanent implant; the ligament augmentation device is used temporarily while an autograft heals. Both of these materials can be implanted through an arthroscope (Peters & Fox, 1988). *Complete* healing of knee ligaments after surgery can take 6 to 9 months or longer. Nursing management is similar to care of any client in a cast, which is described earlier in this chapter.

Tendon Rupture

Rupture of the patellar tendon is common in young adults who participate in strenuous sports. In the elderly client, quadriceps tendon rupture occurs from a fall down several steps. As for severe ligament damage, the tendon is surgically repaired and the leg is immobilized in a cast for 6 to 8 weeks. If the tendon is beyond repair, a tendon transplant, also known as tendon reconstruction, is performed. A tendon is removed from one part of the body and transplanted to the affected area. The nursing care for these clients is similar to that discussed earlier for a client with a cast.

DISLOCATIONS AND SUBLUXATIONS

Dislocation of a joint occurs when the articulating surfaces are no longer in proximity. If dislocation is not complete, the joint is partially dislocated, or *subluxed.* Dislocation can occur in any diarthrodial (synovial) joint but is commonly seen in the shoulder, hip, knee, and fingers. This injury is most often the result of trauma but can be congenital or pathologic, resulting from joint disease such as arthritis.

The typical manifestations are pain, immobility, alteration in contour of the joint, deviation in length of the extremity, and rotation of the extremity. The physician performs a closed manipulation, or reduction, of the joint and forces it back into its original position while the client is anesthetized. The joint is immobilized by a cast or bandage until healing occurs. Recurrent dislocations are common in the knee and shoulder. For this problem, the joint is fixed with wires to prevent further displacement, and a cast, splint, or traction is applied for 3 to 6 weeks.

STRAINS AND SPRAINS

A *strain* is an excessive stretching of a muscle and/or tendon when it is weak or unstable. Falls, lifting heavy items, and exercise are often responsible for this injury. As described earlier for knee injuries, a *sprain* is an injury to a ligament as a result of forcing a joint beyond its usual range of motion. Twisting motions from a fall or sports activity typically precipitate the injury. Both sprains and strains are graded by severity of injury; treatment is implemented accordingly.

SUMMARY

Musculoskeletal trauma results in a number of physical impairments. Some injuries, like mild sprains, are minor, whereas others, such as multiple fractures, are devastating to the client both physically and emotionally. Trauma can be treated on an outpatient basis or by a prolonged hospitalization. Young adults are most fre-

quently predisposed to trauma from strenuous physical activities and vehicular accidents. Elderly individuals are more likely to have falls cause a traumatic injury. The nurse considers the age and overall health of the client when planning and implementing care. For conditions requiring periods of prolonged immobility, the nurse pays particular attention to preventing life-threatening complications that can result.

Musculoskeletal trauma often causes changes in the client's life style, body image, and self-concept. The nurse helps the client adjust to these changes and accepts the client's behavioral response.

IMPLICATIONS FOR RESEARCH

Technologic advances in medical treatment of trauma have resulted in the proliferation of hardware for internal fixation and the use of electrical bone stimulation to promote bone growth. Research needs to continue to perfect these devices and to make them readily available.

Because there is a high incidence of thromboembolic complications associated with musculoskeletal surgery, more research needs to be conducted on preventive measures, particularly drug therapy. A variety of anticoagulants are used, but there is little evidence to show which drugs are most effective and what is the best protocol for therapy.

For nursing research, the following questions need to be investigated:

1. Is pin care for skeletal traction and external fixators necessary? If so, what is the best protocol to prevent pin tract infection?
2. What are the most appropriate nursing interventions for the client who is frustrated and depressed from prolonged immobility and hospitalization?
3. What is the best method of immobilizing a fractured hip in a disoriented, elderly client?
4. How can the nurse effectively help a client with an amputation improve body image and self-esteem?
5. How effective are leg exercises in the prevention of deep venous thrombi?

REFERENCES AND READINGS

Fractures

Aaron, R. K., & Ciombor, D. (1983). Venous thromboembolism in the orthopedic patient. *Surgical Clinics of North America, 63,* 529–537.

Aronson, J., Johnson, E., & Harp, J. H. (1989). Local bone transportation for treatment of intercalary defects by the

Ilizarov technique. *Clinical Orthopaedics and Related Research, 243,* 71–79.

Crocker, C. G. (1986). Acute postoperative pain: Cause and control. *Orthopaedic Nursing, 5*(2), 11–18.

Dickinson, S., & Bury, G. M. (1989). Pulmonary embolism—anatomy of a crisis. *Nursing '89, 19*(4), 34–41.

Dunwoody, C. J. (1987). Patient-controlled analgesia: Rationale and essential factors. *Orthopaedic Nursing, 6*(5), 31–36.

Eaton, J. A. (1988). Continuous meperidine infusion for postoperative pain. *Orthopaedic Nursing, 7*(6), 29–34.

Farrell, J. (1984). Orthopedic pain: What does it mean? *American Journal of Nursing, 84,* 466–469.

Farrell, J. (1986). *Illustrated guide to orthopaedic nursing.* Philadelphia: J. B. Lippincott.

Farrell, N. (1985). Cast syndrome. *Orthopaedic Nursing, 4*(3), 61–64.

Fitzgerald, J., Fagan, L., Tierney, W., & Dittus, R. (1987). Changing patterns of hip fracture before and after implementation of the prospective payment system. *JAMA, 258,* 218–221.

Frese, S. M. (1985). Coping with trauma. *Orthopaedic Nursing, 4*(2), 58–60.

Geier, K. A., & Hesser, K. (1985). Electrical bone stimulation for treatment of nonunion. *Orthopaedic Nursing, 4*(2), 41–51.

Genge, M. L. (1986). Orthopaedic trauma: Pelvic fractures. *Orthopaedic Nursing, 5*(1), 11–18.

Genge, M. L. (1988). Epidural analgesia in the orthopaedic patient. *Orthopaedic Nursing, 7*(4), 11–19.

Groth, F. (1988). Effects of wheat bran in the diet of postsurgical orthopaedic patients to prevent constipation. *Orthopaedic Nursing, 7*(3), 41–46.

Hansell, M. J. (1988). Fractures and the healing process. *Orthopaedic Nursing, 7*(6), 43–50.

Harper, A. (1985). Initial assessment and management of femoral neck fractures in the elderly. *Orthopaedic Nursing, 4*(3), 55–58.

Hendrickson, R., & Ogden, J. A. (1984). Geriatric hip fractures. *Geriatrics, 39,* 75–84.

Hoyt, N. J. (1986). Infections following orthopaedic injury. *Orthopaedic Nursing, 5*(4), 15–24.

Johnson, J. (1986). Respiratory complications of orthopaedic injuries. *Orthopaedic Nursing, 5*(1), 24–29.

Kidd, P. A. (1989). Action stat! Ruptured bladder. *Nursing '89, 19*(1), 33.

Kostopoulos, M. R. (1985). Reducing patient falls. *Orthopaedic Nursing, 4*(6), 14–15.

Krug, B. M. (1989, April). The hip: Nursing fracture patients to full recovery. *RN,* pp. 56–61.

Kustaborder, M. J., & Rigney, M. (1983). Interventions for safety. *Journal of Gerontological Nursing, 9,* 159–162.

Lavin, R. J. (1989, February). The high pressure demands of compartment syndrome. *RN,* pp. 22–25.

Maher, A. B. (1985). After the emergency is over: Delayed and occult injuries in the trauma patient. *Orthopaedic Nursing, 4*(3), 25–28.

Maher, A. B. (1986). Early assessment and management of musculoskeletal injuries. *Nursing Clinics of North America, 21,* 717–727.

Mims, B. C. (1989). Fat embolism syndrome: A variant of ARDS. *Orthopaedic Nursing, 8*(3), 22–25.

Morris, E. V., & Isaacs, B. (1980). The prevention of falls in a geriatric hospital. *Age and Ageing, 9,* 181–185.

Morris, L., Kraft, S., Tessem, S., & Reinisch, S. (1988, February). Special care for skeletal traction. *RN,* pp. 24–29.

Mubarak, S. J., & Hargens, A. R. (1983). Acute compartmental syndromes. *Surgical Clinics of North America, 63,* 539–565.

Newschwander, G. E., & Dunst, R. M. (1989). Limb lengthening with the Ilizarov external fixator. *Orthopaedic Nursing, 8*(3), 15–21.

Omer, G. E. (1985). Assessment of hand trauma. *Orthopaedic Nursing, 4*(2), 29–33.

Osborne, L. J. (1987). Traction: A review with nursing diagnoses and interventions. *Orthopaedic Nursing, 6*(3), 13–19.

Pellino, T., Mooney, N., Salmond, S., & Verdisco, L. (1986). *Core curriculum for orthopaedic nursing.* Pitman, NJ: Anthony Jannetti.

Pradka, L. (1985). Use of the wick catheter for diagnosing and monitoring compartment syndrome. *Orthopaedic Nursing, 4*(3), 17–18.

Redheffer, G. (1989). Treating wounds on the scene, part 2. *Nursing '89, 19*(8), 47–49.

Redheffer, G. M., & Bailey, M. (1989). Assessing and splinting fractures. *Nursing '89, 19*(6), 51–59.

Reinhard, S. C. (1988). Case managing community services for hip fractured elders. *Orthopaedic Nursing, 7*(5), 42–49, 71.

Robinson, J. E., & Marx, L. O. (1985). Nail-safe method. *American Journal of Nursing, 85,* 158–161.

Schoen, D. (1986). *The nursing process in orthopaedics.* Norwalk, CT: Appleton-Century-Crofts.

Seale, K. S. (1989). Reflex sympathetic dystrophy of the lower extremity. *Clinical Orthopaedics and Related Research, 243,* 80–85.

Southwick, J. R., & Callahan, D. J. (1985). A study of blood-drainage patterns on synthetic cast materials. *Orthopaedic Nursing, 4*(1), 72–76.

Sproles, K. (1985). Nursing care of skeletal pins: A closer look. *Orthopaedic Nursing, 4*(1), 11–19.

Stevenson, R. C. K. (1985). Take no chances with fat embolism. *Nursing '85, 15,* 58–63.

Wittert, D., & Barden, R. M. (1985). Deep vein thrombosis,

pulmonary embolism, and prophylaxis in the orthopaedic patient. *Orthopaedic Nursing, 4*(3), 27–32.

Amputations

Bates, M., Kneer, K., & Logan, C. (1989). Medicinal leech therapy. *Orthopaedic Nursing, 8*(2), 12–17.

Burgess, E. M. (1983). Amputations. *Surgical Clinics of North America, 63,* 749–770.

Cushing, M. (1989). Who's responsible for too-early discharge? *American Journal of Nursing, 89,* 471–472.

Farrell, J. (1982). Helping the new amputee. *Orthopaedic Nursing, 1,* 18–21.

Farrell, J. (1986). *Illustrated guide to orthopedic nursing.* Philadelphia: J. B. Lippincott.

Gandy, E. D., & Veigh, G. (1984). Help the amputee stand on his own again. *Nursing '84, 14,* 46–49.

Karcher, W. C. (1983). Anxiety reduction in lower limb amputees. *Rehabilitation Nursing, 8,* 15–19.

McAndrew, M. P. (Ed.). (1989). The severely traumatized lower limb: Reconstruction versus amputation. *Clinical Orthopaedics and Related Research, 243,* 3–99.

O'Hara, M. M. (1988). Leeching: A modern use for an ancient remedy. *American Journal of Nursing, 88,* 1656–1658.

Robinson, K. A. (1987). Modified stump shrinker sock. *Clinical Management in Physical Therapy, 7,* 37.

Walters, J. (1981). Coping with a leg amputation. *American Journal of Nursing, 81,* 1349–1352.

Back Pain

Anderson, L. (1989). Educational approaches to management of low back pain. *Orthopaedic Nursing, 8*(1), 43–46.

Hausman, D., Gates, S. J., & Peters, R. G. (1984). Percutaneous lateral discectomy: Another approach for the treatment of a herniated nucleus pulposus. *Orthopaedic Nursing, 3*(2), 9–17.

Jacobson, S. (1988). Lumbar percutaneous diskectomy. *Bulletin of the Hospital for Joint Diseases, 48,* 67–73.

Lawles, G. F., & McCoy, C. E. (1983). Psychological evaluation: Patients with chronic pain. *Orthopedic Clinics of North America, 14,* 527–538.

Liang, M. H. (1988). Acute low back pain: Diagnosis and management of mechanical back pain. *Primary Care, 15,* 827–847.

Lucas, P. R. (1983). Low back pain. *Surgical Clinics of North America, 63,* 515–528.

Mooney, V. (1983). The syndromes of low back disease. *Orthopedic Clinics of North America, 14,* 505–516.

Musolf, J. (1983). Chemonucleolysis: A new approach to herniated intervertebral disks. *American Journal of Nursing, 83,* 882–886.

O'Brien, J. P. (1983). The role of fusion for chronic low back pain. *Orthopedic Clinics of North America, 14,* 639–648.

Wiltse, L. L. (1983). Chemonucleolysis in the treatment of lumbar disc diseases. *Orthopedic Clinics of North America, 14,* 605–622.

Sports-Related Injuries

Connelly, J. F. (1983). Shoulder subluxations and dislocations. *Emergency Medicine, 15,* 69–84.

Folcik, M. A. (1988). Winter sports injuries: An overview. *Orthopaedic Nursing, 7*(6), 25–28.

Hoshowsky, V. M. (1988). Chronic lateral ligament instability of the ankle. *Orthopaedic Nursing, 7*(3), 33–40.

Hubbard, L. F., & Herndon, J. H. (1983). Microsurgery in orthopedics. *Surgical Clinics of North America, 63,* 737–748.

Lowe, E. B. (1983). Diagnostic and operative arthroscopy. *Surgical Clinics of North America, 63,* 599–605.

MacArthur, B. J. (1986). Arthroscopy of the shoulder. *Orthopaedic Nursing, 5*(4), 26–28.

Peters, V. J., & Fox, J. M. (1988, July). Knee surgery clears a hurdle. *RN,* pp. 20–25.

Schoen, D. (1986). *The nursing process in orthopaedics.* Norwalk, CT: Appleton-Century-Crofts.

Stover, C. N., & Debald, M. (1986). Guide to lateral ankle sprain management. *Orthopaedic Nursing, 5*(3), 34–39.

Wittert, D. D. (1986). Rotator cuff tears. *Orthopaedic Nursing, 5*(4), 17–24.

ADDITIONAL READINGS

Clay, K. L., & Stirn, M. L. (1986). Documentation of discharge teaching of patients who had hip surgery. *Orthopaedic Nursing, 5*(6), 22–24, 28.

With clients being discharged quickly from hospitals to contain health care costs, nurses need to thoroughly teach clients and their families the care that will be necessary in the home environment. This article stressed the need to document discharge teaching and related how one hospital designed its discharge documentation system. The development and revision of teaching criteria for clients discharged after hip surgery were discussed in detail.

Lisanti, P. A. (1989). Perceived body space and self-esteem in adult males with and without chronic low back pain. *Orthopaedic Nursing, 8*(3), 49–56.

This study examined body space and self-esteem in two matched groups of young males, one with chronic back pain and the other healthy and without pain. There was no difference in either perceived body space or self-esteem between the two groups.

Lukens, L. (1986). Six months after hip fracture. *Geriatric Nursing, 7,* 202–206.

This study investigated elderly clients' mobility and activity levels 6 months after hip surgery. The author found that 17 of 20 individuals in the sample were less active after the surgery than before, but that the levels varied among the subjects. Activity levels were directly related to age, i.e., the older the person, the less active both before and after surgery.

Wells, D. L., & Saltmarche, A. (1986). Voiding dysfunction in geriatric patients with hip fracture: Prevalence rate and tentative nursing interventions. *Orthopaedic Nursing, 5*(6), 25–28.

This article described a study of elderly clients who had hip fractures with associated voiding problems, i.e., incontinence or retention. Of the 142 clients in the sample, 47% presented with one or more of these problems. The authors provided nursing interventions for these clients to minimize voiding dysfunction, including intermittent catheterization, intake and output recording, and fluid intake increase.

UNIT 9 RESOURCES

Nursing Resources

American Radiological Nurses Association (ARNA), 2462 Stantonsburg Road, Suite 162, Greenville, NC 27834. See Unit 7 Resources for more information.

National Association of Orthopaedic Nurses (NAON), North Woodbury Road, PO Box 56, Pitman, NJ 08071. Telephone 609-582-0111.

Promotes high standards in orthopedic nursing practice, educates practitioners, and fosters research. Publishes *Orthopaedic Nursing (bimonthly journal) and other materials.*

Orthopaedic Nurses Certification Board, North Woodbury Road, PO Box 56, Pitman, NJ 08071. Telephone 609-582-0111.

Certifies nurses specializing in orthopedics.

Other Resources

Arthritis Foundation, 1314 Spring Street NW, Atlanta, GA 30309. Telephone 404-872-7100.

National Institute of Arthritis and Musculoskeletal and Skin Diseases, National Institutes of Health, Bethesda, MD 20892. Telephone 301-496-4000.

Osteoporosis Foundation, 612 North Michigan Avenue, Suite 510, Chicago, IL 60611.

Paget's Disease Foundation, PO Box 2772, Brooklyn, NY 11202. Telephone 718-596-1043.

Scoliosis Association, PO Box 51353, Raleigh, NC 27609. Telephone 919-846-2639.

UNIT 10

Problems of Mobility and Coordination: Management of Clients with Disruptions of the Nervous System

CHAPTER 32

Assessment of the Nervous System

This is an exciting time to study neurologic function and dysfunction. Advances in the development of laboratory equipment, computers, and technical procedures have enabled increased understanding of the function of specific tissues of the nervous system. The living nervous system is no longer hidden from view as it was for the early anatomists. Most of the early study was done on cadavers. This was satisfactory for exploring anatomy, but did not help physiologic or functional understanding. As even more physiologic knowledge is gained, neurologic problems will not seem so difficult or mysterious.

Scientists are now describing and naming various nervous system elements for their functional roles. In the past, many parts of the nervous system were named for the discoverer of the tissue or for what the tissue resembled (colliculus = small hill; hippocampus = sea horse), simply because early anatomists were unable to determine function. Some older names and new names still coexist.

ANATOMY AND PHYSIOLOGY REVIEW

The nervous system is responsible for the maintenance and control of itself, as well as the control of the rest of the body. The peripheral nerves, the spinal cord, and the lower portion of the brain stem are capable of sustaining vegetative life without control or direction from cerebral structures. Cerebral structures are capable of more complex function and exert control over the lower structures. The cerebral structures are those that make humans different from animals. The major divisions of the nervous system are the *central nervous system* (CNS) and the *peripheral nervous system* (PNS). The nervous system contains two types of cells, *neurons* and *glial cells.*

NERVOUS SYSTEM CELLS

NEURONS

Structure

Each neuron has a cell body, or *soma; dendrites* and an *axon* extend from the nerve cell (Fig. 32–1). Dendrites may have many branches or few. Each dendrite synapses with another cell body, axon, or dendrite, and brings information to the cell body from other neuronal cells. The dendritic process can also be described as an *afferent pathway* (Latin *ad* meaning "to" + *ferre* meaning "to carry"). There is only one axon extending from each neuron, but it may have few or many branchings. The

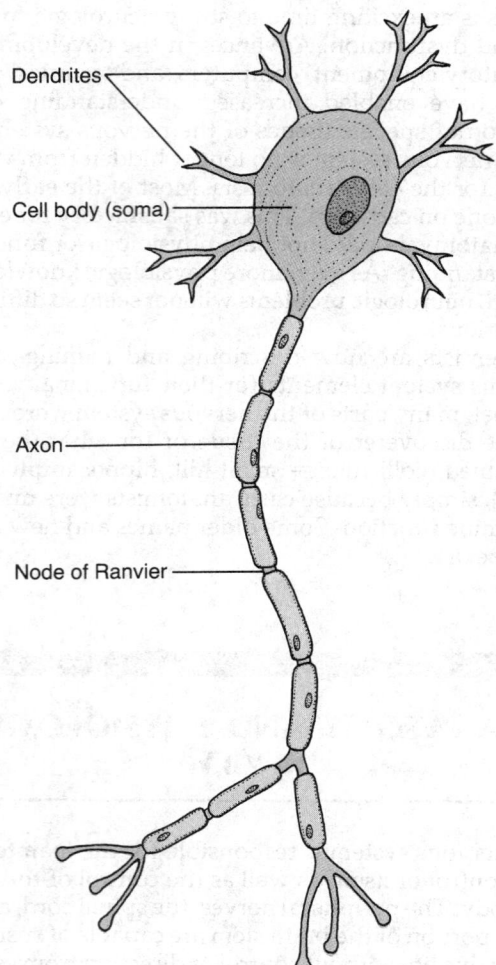

Figure 32–1

Typical neuron structure.

axonal process is called the *efferent pathway* (Latin *effere*, "to carry away"). An axon transmits impulses from its cell body to other neurons and may be myelinated or unmyelinated. *Myelinization* is a process whereby lipid cells derived from oligodendrocytes (type of glial cell) form a coating. The myelinated axons appear whitish and are therefore also referred to as *white matter*. The nonmyelinated axons have a grayish cast and are called *gray matter* (these axons actually do have a thin layer of myelin sheath, although this cannot be visualized without sophisticated equipment). Myelinated axons have gaps in the myelin called *nodes of Ranvier*, which play a major role in impulse conduction, as shown in Figure 32–1. The distal end of each axon is enlarged and is called the *synaptic*, or *terminal*, *knob*. Within the synaptic knobs are the mechanisms for manufacturing, storing, and releasing a transmitter substance. Each neuron produces a specific transmitter substance, such as acetylcholine or serotonin, that is capable of either enhancing or inhibiting the impulse, but not both (see discussion of impulse transmission later).

Types

Neurons range from large to small. The larger cells are also called *principal* cells because their axons carry the impulse from the cell to other cells of the nervous system. The smaller cells are called *interneurons*, internuncial cells, intercalary cells, or intercalated cells (referred to as interneurons in this text). Interneurons are located between other neurons in the brain and the spinal cord to form complex circuits. Neurons are also referred to as *unipolar*, *bipolar*, and *multipolar*, depending on the number of processes (axon and dendrites) for each cell (see Fig. 32–1).

Function

The function of the neuron is *impulse conduction*. At present, it is thought that each neuron transmits a specific type of impulse. For example, some neurons are sensory, some are motor, some are responsible for processing information, and some are responsible for retention of information.

Mechanism for Nerve Impulse Conduction

The electrical potential for each cell of the body occurs in almost the same manner for all cells of the body, regardless of task. Therefore, neuron cellular action is briefly reviewed. At the nerve cell membrane, the action potential occurs, as for other cells of the body. A stimulus causes the membrane to become permeable to sodium, and the process of depolarization begins. Studies have shown that there are specific routes for the movement of sodium and potassium. Certain proteins within the membrane function as gates, or channels, which open for either sodium or potassium, but not both. With depolarization, sodium diffuses through the membrane first (calcium plays a part in controlling the amount of sodium that diffuses by probably controlling the gates). After sodium has entered the cell, potassium begins to leave the cell. Sodium is actively pumped out of the cell, and repolarization occurs. In nerve membrane, as an action potential or impulse occurs at one point on the membrane, it excites adjacent cells so that the impulse is conducted all along the nerve fiber membrane. If the impulse is not of sufficient strength, there will be no action potential (the all-or-nothing principle).

The rate of speed with which the entire membrane is excited depends on whether the nerve axon is myelinated or unmyelinated and on the size of the fiber. The action potential in myelinated fibers "jumps" from node to node of Ranvier through the extracellular fluid (ECF) surrounding the axon. The ECF facilitates transmission. Action potentials in unmyelinated fibers travel the length of the fiber, which requires more time. Additionally, fiber diameter affects the speed with which an action potential is transmitted—the larger the fiber, the greater the conduction rate is. A large myelinated fiber conducts impulses faster than a small myelinated fiber, and a myelinated fiber of any size conducts impulses faster than an unmyelinated fiber of comparable size.

Because nerve membrane is excitable, it responds to varied stimuli. *Electrical* stimuli are used in laboratory testing and for pain control or diagnostic testing; *chemical* stimuli include any of the transmitters or other chemicals, such as acids or bases; and *mechanical* stimuli include crushing, pinching, or even slight pressure in some areas.

Synapses

Impulses are transmitted to their eventual destination through synapses. There are two distinct types of synapses: *neuron to neuron* and *neuron to muscle* (or gland). Between the terminal knob and the next cell is a small space called the *synaptic cleft*. The knob, the cleft, and the portion of the cell to which the impulse is being transmitted constitute the *synapse.*

Neuron to neuron. Neuron-to-neuron transmission occurs when an impulse goes from the axon of one neuron to the dendrites, the soma, or the axon of another neuron. A synapse may be either excitatory or inhibitory, but not both. An *excitatory* potential occurs when sodium enters the cell, causing depolarization. An action potential is then initiated, and the impulse is carried by the axon to its destination — a synapse with the dendrites of another neuron.

An *inhibitory* postsynaptic potential occurs when the postsynaptic membrane becomes permeable to potassium and chloride, but not to sodium. Potassium then diffuses out and the inside of the cell becomes more negatively charged than usual. That cell needs a stronger-than-normal stimulus to fire an impulse. This is the inhibitory sequence that occurs in the higher centers (cerebrum and cerebellum), according to present knowledge. Inhibition lower in the nervous system occurs when an inhibitory knob synapses with an excitatory axon. This action results in the release of a smaller amount of transmitter substance and is called *presynaptic* inhibition.

After the transmitter substance has completed transfer of the impulse, it is released from the receptor cells and deactivated. Deactivation occurs by either enzyme degradation or reabsorption into the presynaptic knob.

Neuron to muscle. Neuron-to-muscle synapses are somewhat different than neuron-to-neuron. One important difference is that the junction with the muscle is in the middle of the muscle. This allows an impulse to travel in both directions to facilitate contraction (nerve-to-nerve impulses occur in only one direction). The synapse between nerve and muscle membrane is called the neuromuscular end plate, or *neuromuscular junction,* as shown in the illustration on page 831. The junction can be with either skeletal or smooth muscle.

Skeletal muscle innervation. One nerve with all the muscle fibers it innervates is called a *motor unit.* Approx-

imately 200,000 motor units originate in the spinal cord. A nerve fiber stimulates between 3 and 2000 muscle fibers, depending on the degree of muscle function complexity. For example, each nerve fiber innervating the eye is responsible for far fewer muscle fibers than a nerve innervating thigh muscle fibers.

The peripheral axon has two additional sheaths over the myelin — a neurilemmal sheath and a delicate outer endoneural sheath. The latter sheath extends beyond the terminal ending of the axon to join with the sheath of the muscle, resulting in a "roof" over the junction. The subsynaptic membrane directly across from the presynaptic plate lies in folds, which greatly increases the area of exposure to the transmitter substance. Normally, only the subsynaptic membrane portion of the muscle is receptive to the transmitter substance. However, studies have shown that if the axon is removed, causing motor end plate degeneration, the rest of the muscle membrane becomes responsive to the transmitter (*acetylcholine* for skeletal muscle). If the nerve is reattached, this situation reverses and again only the subsynaptic membrane responds to acetylcholine.

When the nerve impulse reaches the axon terminal, the presynaptic membrane becomes permeable to calcium and calcium ions enter from the ECF. Vesicles within the terminal knob release packages (quanta) of acetylcholine. As shown in the illustration on page 831, acetylcholine diffuses across the cleft to the receptor site (specific proteins) on the motor end plate. As acetylcholine molecules reach the receptor sites, some molecules diffuse out of the cleft and some are degraded by acetylcholinesterase present in the folds of the synaptic cleft. These molecules are broken down into choline and acetic acid and are immediately reabsorbed into the terminal for synthesis of more acetylcholine. Those molecules reaching the postsynaptic receptor membrane are also degraded by acetylcholinesterase within 1 to 2 milliseconds.

Smooth muscle innervation. There are two types of smooth muscle. *Multiunit* muscle fibers, such as those of the ciliary eye muscles, the iris, or hair follicle (piloerector) muscles, have precise, discrete functions. These fibers are often innervated by a single nerve ending and operate independently of adjacent fibers. The fibers are protected from stimulation by neighboring nerves by a glycoprotein substance on their surface. The other type of fiber is *unitary.* These are present in the visceral smooth muscles found in most organs. The fibers are in such close contact that their cell membranes fuse or almost fuse. When one fiber is stimulated, the stimulus is transmitted to neighboring fibers. The synapse between nerve and smooth muscle may be one of two types — contact or diffuse.

The two transmitter substances for smooth muscle innervation are *acetylcholine* and *norepinephrine*. It is thought that the receptor sites contain a substance determining which of the two will excite the muscle fiber, as smooth muscle tissue can be either excited or inhibited by acetylcholine or norepinephrine. Usually, one substance excites and the other inhibits a given muscle fiber, although this is not always the case. The degradation of the transmitter substance involves the same process as that for skeletal muscle.

Factors Affecting Transmission

Several factors affect the transmission of an impulse. *Distance* is one of the established factors. Synapses that are on or near the body of the cell have greater influence than those farther along the dendrite. The impulse loses strength as it travels from the dendrite to the body of the cell. The strength of the stimulus can also be influenced by a variety of other mechanisms: *inhibition* by another neuron, *inadequate supply* of transmitter substance, or *ECF changes.* ECF deficits of calcium or sodium or an increase in ECF magnesium content decreases vesicle release and thus the amount of transmitter substance. Changes in extracellular *pH* affect neuron transmission. For example, acidosis depresses nerve cell activity. Lack of oxygen or the use of hypnotics and anesthetics can quickly depress nerve cell activity. Alkalosis, on the other hand, excites nerve cells. Increased nerve cell activity occurs with some *drugs,* such as caffeine (in coffee), theophylline (in tea and asthma drugs), theobromine (in cocoa), and strychnine. *Repetition* also affects transmission. If a nerve cell is stimulated repeatedly and then allowed to rest, the next response to a stimulus is likely to be more easily elicited (posttetanic facilitation). This may represent a part of the learning process.

Research involving impulse transmission and transmitters is an exciting area of study. Studies have shown that, during mental stress, calcium absorption tends to decrease, whereas calcium excretion tends to increase. This could then affect the vesicle release of transmitter substance. Some transmitters may be affected by dietary or plasma levels of protein *precursors,* with implications for certain diseases. It appears that the amines are in this category—serotonin, the *catecholamines* (epinephrine and norepinephrine), and *acetylcholine.* The manufacture of serotonin depends on plasma tryptophan; of the catecholamines, on tyrosine; and of acetylcholine, on choline (dietary lecithin). Tryptophan and tyrosine cannot be manufactured in the body. Choline can be manufactured in the body, but diet is still the main source. Therefore, dietary amines are necessary for the production of these transmitters.

Transmitters

Some transmitters, such as acetylcholine, act directly to open ionic gates of the postsynaptic membrane, thus creating the membrane potential or impulse. Others, such as the catecholamines, act through an enzyme process and use adenosine 3',5'-cyclic phosphate (cAMP) to open the postsynaptic ionic gates (cAMP is known as the second messenger).

Some substances have been definitely identified as *transmitters.* These include acetylcholine, serotonin, dopamine, norepinephrine, gamma-aminobutyric acid (GABA), substance P, and the endorphins and enkepha-

lins. Other substances, although not specifically identified as transmitters, are considered *putative* (probably) transmitters or are believed to have influence on the sensitivity of a neuron so that it responds to another transmitter. The latter are called *neuromodulators.* As research continues, the identification of the transmitters, probable transmitters, and neuromodulators changes. Although opinions among researchers concerning the actual status of some of these chemicals vary, Table 32–1 summarizes what is currently known about them.

GLIAL CELLS

There is much less information about glial cells than about neurons.

Structure

The glial cells vary in size and shape. Some cells have only a few processes extending from the cell body, whereas others have many. Glial cells are thought to have evolved from the ectoderm layer of the nervous system.

Type

There are four main types of glial cells. *Astroglia* (star shaped) are found around capillaries and larger vessels and in the gray and white matter. *Oligodendrocytes* are found wherever there are myelinated axons in the CNS. *Microglia* are found in gray and white matter; *ependymal* cells are found in the ventricles.

Function

Astroglia provide the physical support for the neurons, regulate the chemical environment, and nourish the neurons. Oligodendrocytes form the myelin sheath around the axons in the CNS (Schwann's cells perform this function in the PNS). Some microglia appear to be phagocytic, as they are found at the site of disease, but the function of other microglia is not known. The ependymal cells form the lining of the ventricles and the central canal of the spinal cord. They are also part of the *blood-brain barrier* (discussed later). Because of the close proximity of each ependymal cell to the next, passive movement of plasma proteins into the cerebrospinal fluid (CSF) is prohibited. Ependymal cells also help regulate the composition of CSF.

NERVOUS SYSTEM DIVISIONS

The two divisions of the nervous system are the CNS and the PNS. Because of the hierarchy of nervous sys-

HOW A NERVE IMPULSE CAUSES SKELETAL MUSCLE TO CONTRACT

When the brain commands a skeletal muscle to contract, a complex series of biochemical events occurs. An electrical impulse makes its way from the brain, through the nervous system, and to the synaptic (terminal) knob of an axon. There, nerve and muscle meet at a junction called the neuromuscular end plate (neuromuscular junction). When the electrical nerve impulse reaches the synaptic knob, the impulse causes the presynaptic membrane to become permeable to calcium in the extracellular fluid. Calcium ions enter the neuromuscular end plate and alter its delicate chemical balance. This change in chemical balance causes the acetylcholine vesicles to release acetylcholine across the synaptic cleft to acetylcholine receptors on the postsynaptic membrane. A wave of muscular contraction is generated and spreads to both ends of the skeletal muscle.

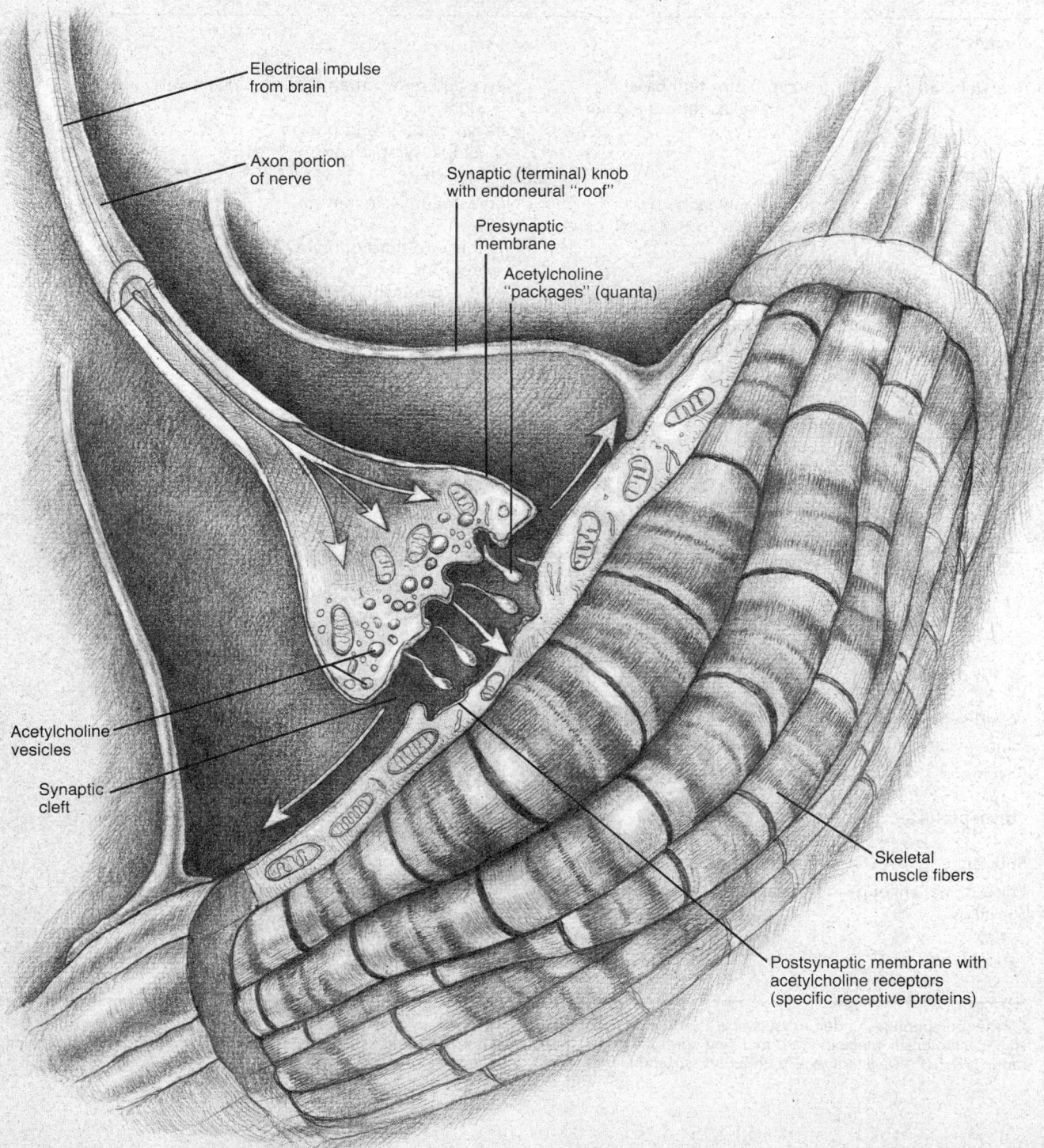

Electrical impulse from brain

Axon portion of nerve

Synaptic (terminal) knob with endoneural "roof"

Presynaptic membrane

Acetylcholine "packages" (quanta)

Acetylcholine vesicles

Synaptic cleft

Skeletal muscle fibers

Postsynaptic membrane with acetylcholine receptors (specific receptive proteins)

TABLE 32–1   Sites, Functions, and Actions of Transmitters, Probable Transmitters, and Neuromodulators

Transmitter Substance*	Site	Function/Comments	Action
Amines			
Acetylcholine	Brain, brain stem basal ganglia, autonomic nervous system	Nerve and muscle transmission Parasympathetic and preganglionic sympathetic system	Excitatory, but some inhibitory
GABA	Brain, brain stem, basal ganglia, spinal cord, cerebellum	Nerve and muscle transmission Possibly one-third of brain neurons GABA as a transmitter	Inhibitory
Histamine	Brain, spinal cord, PNS	Not many data	Questionable
Serotonin	Medial brain stem, hypothalamus, dorsal horn of spinal cord	Possible onset of sleep, mood control; pain pathway inhibitor in spinal cord	Inhibitory
Catecholamines			
Dopamine	Substantia nigra to basal ganglia	Complex movements, emotional response regulation, attention	Usually inhibitory
Norepinephrine (epinephrine parallels)	Hypothalamus, brain stem reticular formation, cerebellum, sympathetic nervous system	Maintenance of arousal, reward system, dreaming sleep, mood regulation	Mainly excitatory
Amino Acids			
Aspartic acid	Brain, spinal cord interneurons	Sensation	Excitatory
Glutamic acid	Sensory pathways	Sensation	Excitatory
Glycine	Spinal cord interneurons	Muscle control	Inhibitory
Polypeptides*			
Substance P	Brain, neurons in spinal cord	Pain transmission	Excitatory
Endorphins, enkephalins	Thalamus, hypothalamus, spinal cord, pituitary	Pleasure sensation, reward system, analgesia (inhibits release of substance P), released with ACTH during stress	Probably excitatory

* Other polypeptides under investigation as probable transmitters are vasopressin (ADH), gastrin, cholecystokinin, glucagon, insulin, somatostatin, angiotensin, melanocyte-stimulating hormone (MSH), luteinizing hormone-releasing hormone (LH-RH), and thyrotropin-releasing hormone (TRH). Prostaglandins, also under investigation, are thought to be modulators.

tem tissue, survival is possible with only portions of the nervous system intact (see earlier).

PERIPHERAL NERVOUS SYSTEM

The PNS is composed of the *peripheral sensory nerves* transmitting information to the spinal cord, the *lower motor neurons* leaving the spinal cord, and the *autonomic nervous system*. The autonomic nervous system is reviewed with the cranial nerves.

Spinal Nerves

There are 31 pairs of spinal nerves (8 cervical, 12 thoracic, 5 lumbar, 5 sacral, and 1 coccygeal) exiting from the spinal cord. Each of the nerves has a posterior and an anterior branch (Fig. 32 – 2). The posterior branch carries sensory information to the cord (afferent pathway), and the anterior branch transmits motor impulses to the muscles of the body (efferent pathway).

The posterior nerve impulses are transmitted through the sensory spinal ganglion (a group of neurons) located just outside the spinal cord, but inside the vertebra. The spinal ganglion is the origin of the cell bodies of the sensory nerves. The pathway continues into the spinal cord through the *intervertebral foramen*. The anterior motor axons exit through the intervertebral foramen to form an anterior root (where branches come together), which then joins the posterior root just outside the vertebral column to form a *spinal nerve*. Parasympathetic and sympathetic fibers are added to the spinal nerve through other pathways.

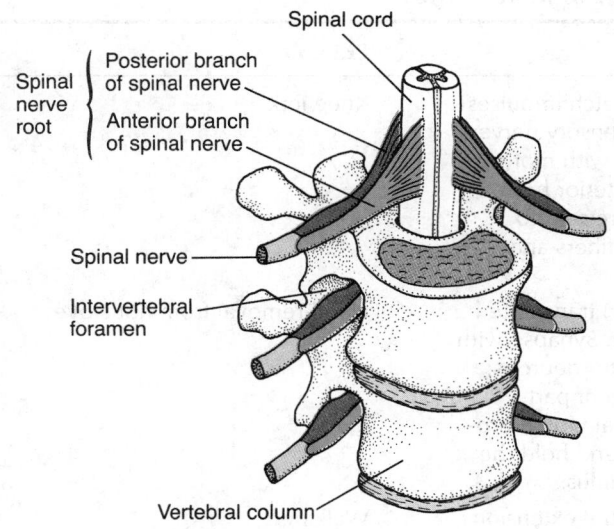

Spinal cord

Posterior branch of spinal nerve

Spinal nerve root

Anterior branch of spinal nerve

Spinal nerve

Intervertebral foramen

Vertebral column

Figure 32 – 2

Spinal nerve branches exiting from the spinal cord through the intervertebral foramen of a vertebra.

Each spinal nerve is responsible for the muscle innervation and sensory reception of a given area. The cervical and thoracic spinal nerves are relatively close to their areas of responsibility, whereas the lumbar and sacral spinal nerves are some distance from theirs. The spinal cord ends between L-1 and L-2, so the axons of the lumbar and sacral cord extend downward before exiting the appropriate intervertebral foramen. The area controlled by each spinal nerve is roughly reflected in the dermatomes (see Chap. 33, Fig. 33 – 15).

Sensory Receptors

Sensory receptors throughout the body monitor and transmit impulses of pain and temperature, touch, vibration, pressure, visceral sensation, and equilibrium, as well as those sensations of the special senses — vision, taste, smell, and hearing. At the present time, it is thought that each of these sensations (except pain and temperature) has specific receptors and corresponding pathways.

Lower Motor Neurons and Plexus

The cell bodies of the anterior spinal nerves are located in the anterior gray matter (anterior horn) of each level in the spinal cord. As each nerve axon leaves the spinal cord, it joins other spinal nerves to form *plexuses*. Plexuses continue as trunks, divisions, and cords, and finally branch into individual peripheral nerves. The major plexuses are the cervical, brachial, lumbar, and sacral (the latter two are also referred to as lumbosacral). An awareness of the location of plexuses is helpful, because there is a major concentration of nerves present. Additionally, the nerves of each plexus pass through or are surrounded by bone. Injury to the area or entrapment of a nerve by bone can cause multiple problems.

Reflexes

Much of human body movement and function occurs at an unconscious and automatic level. If this were not true, one would be exhausted just trying to breathe. This automatic movement occurs at the spinal cord level and is called a *reflex*. Reflexes consist of sensory input from the muscles, tendons, skin, organs, and special senses; small cells in the spinal cord lying between the posterior and anterior gray matter (interneurons); and the anterior motor neurons, along with the muscles they innervate (Fig. 32 – 3). Sensory data from a specific peripheral location account for a change in the motor impulses going to that location. This is a closed circuit and is called the *reflex arc*.

Muscle tone is achieved by special fibers in the middle of the muscle. The ends of these special fibers (muscle spindle or intrafusal fibers) are attached to the surrounding muscle, and they are able to contract only at

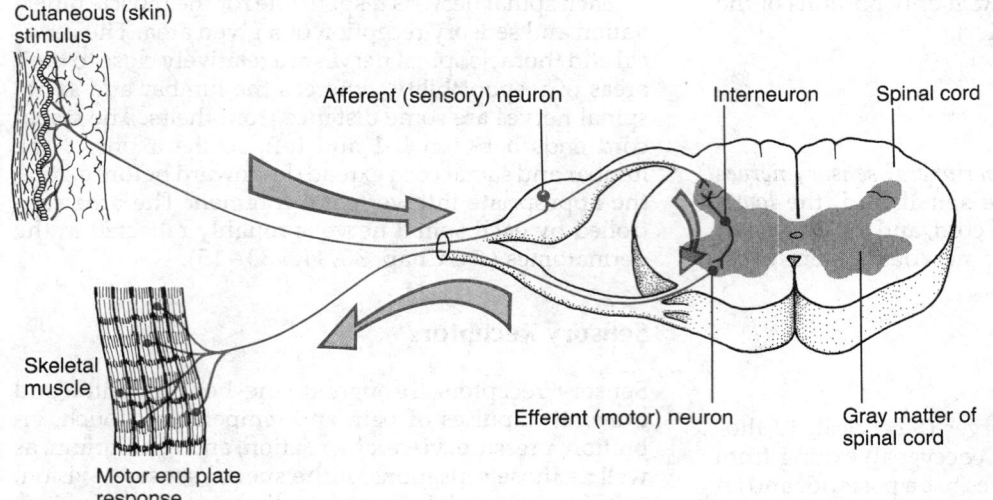

Cutaneous (skin) stimulus

Afferent (sensory) neuron

Interneuron

Spinal cord

Skeletal muscle

Motor end plate response (contraction)

Efferent (motor) neuron

Gray matter of spinal cord

Figure 32–3

Example of reflex activity: stimulation of skin results in involuntary muscle contraction (reflex arc).

their ends. The contractible ends are innervated by special motor fibers from the anterior horn. The middle portion of the intrafusal fibers contains special receptors that measure the *degree* of stretch of the muscle. These receptors are responsible for identifying a change in length of the muscle, as well as measuring the *rate* of change in length. There are two types of intrafusal fibers. Both are innervated by sensory fibers that transmit impulses quickly only while the muscle is in the process of stretching. Another type of sensory fiber transmits at a slower rate, but continues as long as the

muscle is stretched. The types of reflexes and their mechanisms are listed in Table 32–2.

CENTRAL NERVOUS SYSTEM

The CNS is composed of the *spinal cord* and *brain*. The cord initiates reflex activity and transmits impulses to and from the brain. The brain directs the regulation and function of the nervous system, as well as all other systems of the body.

TABLE 32–2 Mechanisms of Reflex Types

Reflex Types	Mechanism	Example
Stretch (one synapse)	Degree and rate of stretch impulses to cord through sensory nerves. Impulse synapses with motor neurons in the anterior horn. Motor impulses are sent to change intrafusal fibers and muscle itself.	Knee jerk
Withdrawal or flexor (multiple synapses)	Pain sensation (usually) transmitted to the spinal cord. Synapse with interneurons. Motor neurons: initiate withdrawal of part, inhibit muscles that would prohibit withdrawal, and hold the part from the stimulus.	Hand removal from hot stove
Crossed extensor (multiple synapses)	The flexor reflex plus the extension of the opposite limb.	Walking
Gamma reflex loop (multiple synapses)	Descending motor impulses impose tension control over the reflex arc.	Maintaining a position because it is necessary, even though uncomfortable

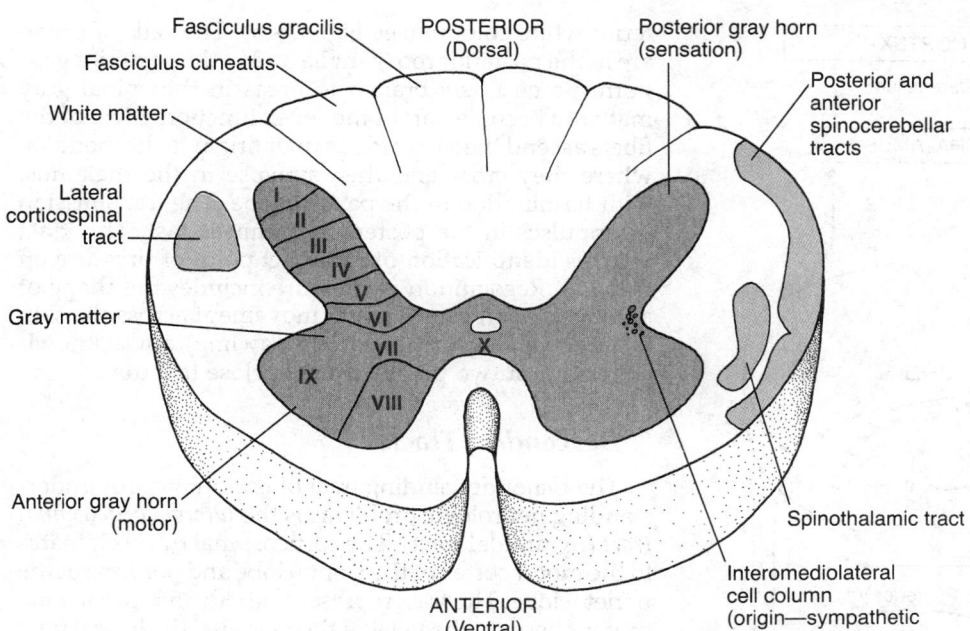

Figure 32-4

Cross-section of the spinal cord with common tracts.

Spinal Cord

The spinal cord contains gray matter (neuron cell bodies) and white matter (myelinated axons). The white matter is divided into posterior, lateral, and anterior columns. Groups of cells in the white matter (ascending and descending tracts) have been fairly well identified (Fig. 32-4). The gray matter divisions are posterior, intermediolateral, and anterior. Certain areas of the gray matter have been only recently identified by cell type and function (laminae of Rexed [I to X]). Generally, the posterior gray cells are sensory receivers from the periphery and the origin of the ascending sensory tracts. The lateral or intermediolateral gray cells (T-1 to L2-3) are the origin of sympathetic fibers, visceral sensory receptors, and visceral motor fibers. The anterior gray cells are the origin of the lower motor neurons.

As impulses enter the cord, some terminate immediately on the anterior gray cells (stretch reflex); some travel up or down several segments through segmental cells to meet with other impulses on interneurons; and others ascend the cord for interpretation at higher levels. Impulses that must be interpreted at a higher level are transmitted by specific ascending tracts. Motor impulses are also transmitted down the cord by specific descending tracts.

Ascending Tracts

Three ascending tracts are important for understanding the client with neurologic problems: spinothalamic, spinocerebellar, and fasciculi gracilis and cuneatus.

Spinothalamic tracts.* The spinothalamic tracts carry sensations of pain, temperature, light (or simple) touch, and pressure. The impulses enter the posterior gray matter, travel up one to four segments, and synapse in specific laminae of the posterior horn. Most touch and pressure sensations terminate in laminae III and IV, whereas those of pain and temperature terminate in laminae I, II (old name was substantia gelatinosa), and V. Even though sharp and dull pain sensations are transmitted by different types of fibers, their terminal is the same (some impulses go directly to motor cells for immediate action). It is probable that pain impulses are changed or modified in some way by other impulses in lamina II before further transmission. The cell origin of the spinothalamic axons is in the posterior gray matter. The axon fibers from the cells decussate (cross) the anterior white and gray commissures to the opposite side and become the contralateral (situated on the opposite side) spinothalamic tract. These fibers continue up to the thalamus, with some branches terminating in the *reticular formation* of the medulla and pons. A pain or temperature impulse then enters the posterior horn on the same side that the pain occurs, transmits to other cells in several laminae, is further propelled to the opposite spinothalamic tract, laminae, and continues up to its ultimate destinations—the thalamus and the parietal lobe (Fig. 32-5).

Posterior and anterior spinocerebellar tracts. The *posterior* spinocerebellar tract transmits impulses of pro-

---

* Most texts separate the spinothalamic tract into the lateral and anterior spinothalamic tracts. Current investigation indicates there is no division (Barr & Keirnan, 1988).

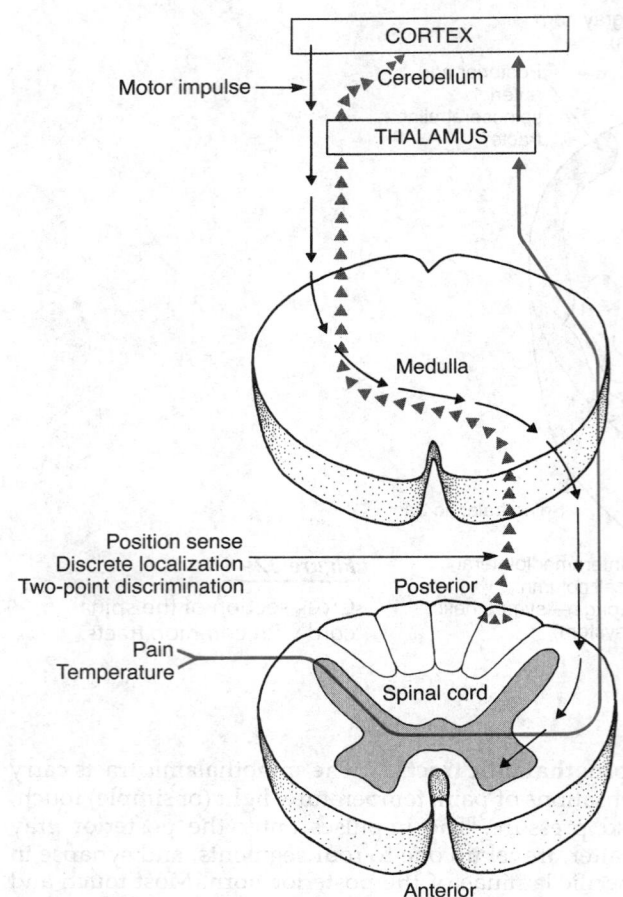

Figure 32–5

Examples of common spinal tract pathways.

prioception (awareness of position and movements of body parts), or kinesthesia, from the extremities (mostly lower). The impulses enter the posterior gray horn and synapse with tract cells in lamina VII. Spinocerebellar axons then form the tract on the *same* side. This tract begins at the second lumbar level and ascends to the medulla and then to the cerebellum.

The *anterior* spinocerebellar tract begins lower in the lumbar spine than the posterior tract. These fibers cross immediately and ascend as a contralateral tract, transmitting proprioceptive impulses from the lower extremities. The fibers cross again in the midbrain on their way to the cerebellum. Because these fibers have crossed the midline twice, the sensations terminate on the side where they originated. The *right* cerebellum receives information about the *right* side of the body, and the *left* cerebellum receives data about the *left* side.

Fasciculus gracilis and fasciculus cuneatus (posterior white column). Sensation of proprioception from muscles, joints, and tendons plus vibratory sense, light touch from the skin, discrete localization, and two-point discrimination is transmitted to the thalamus by the pos-

terior white column (see Fig. 32–5). The cells of origin are in the posterior root ganglia and in the posterior gray horn. Some fibers branch to areas in the spinal gray matter to become part of the reflex function. Most of the fibers ascend the *same* side as their origin to the medulla, where they cross and then synapse in the thalamus, with termination in the parietal lobe. The transmission of impulses in the posterior column is fast. This tract enables identification of the exact point of pressure on the skin. Recognition of pressure includes the shape of an object (with eyes closed), movement across the skin (a number being written or a fly crawling), and acknowledgement of two points of touch close together.

Descending Tracts

The major descending tract of importance for understanding neurologic problems is the *lateral corticospinal tract* (pyramidal tract). The corticospinal tract originates in the motor cortex of the frontal lobe and portions of the parietal lobe. The tract represents about 85% of the total motor fibers. At the level of the medulla, the lateral tract fibers cross to the opposite side (pyramid of the medulla). After crossing, the fibers descend to a predetermined level and synapse with interneurons of the gray matter. A few fibers connect directly with lower motor neurons. The cervical area has a high concentration of fibers synapsing with interneurons, possibly reflecting the complexity of hand and finger movements.*

Spinal Cord Circulation

The blood supply for the cord comes from three main arteries. The *anterior spinal artery* originates from a branch of the vertebral arteries, whereas the two *posterior spinal arteries* originate from either the vertebral or posterior inferior cerebellar artery. Additional circulation is supplied by branches of the descending aorta.

Brain

Brain Stem and Diencephalon

The spinal cord continues upward beyond the cervical cord to the brain stem, which includes the medulla, the pons, and the mesencephalon (midbrain) (Fig. 32–6). Although the diencephalon developmentally is considered part of the cerebrum, it is continuous anatomically. The diencephalon includes the thalamus, the hypothalamus, the subthalamus, and the epithalamus. Throughout the brain stem are special cells that constitute *reticular formation* tissue.

---

* The motor neurons of the other descending tracts and the basal ganglia were formerly referred to as an extrapyramidal system. It was thought that pyramidal neurons initiated voluntary muscle activity and the extrapyramidal neurons initiated automatic or nonvoluntary muscle action. The descending tracts and the basal ganglia are necessary for the smooth function of *all* motor activity. Clinically, the term extrapyramidal is still often used to connote the origin of abnormal spontaneous movement.

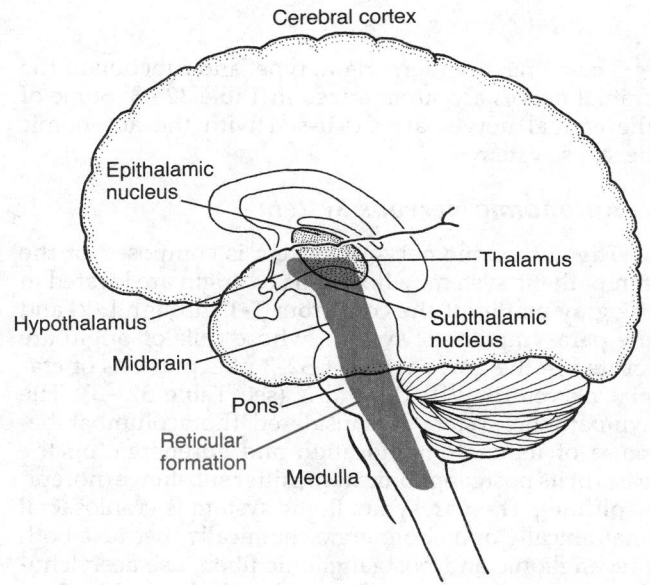

Figure 32-6

Structures of the brain stem and the diencephalon.

Most reticular formation tissue is responsible for controlling awareness or alertness. For example, this tissue awakens one from sleep when an arm or leg has become ischemic ("gone to sleep"), when there is abdominal pain, or because it is time to rise. Many sensory fibers branch and terminate here, and the reticular formation area has abundant connections with the brain, the rest of the brain stem, and the cerebellum. This is referred to as the *reticular activating system* (RAS). Within the reticular formation tissue are groups of specific neurons that have been found to have functions other than controlling alertness. These neurons are referred to as *brain stem nuclei.*

Medulla. The medulla is the lowest section of the brain stem. Motor tracts pass downward through the anterior medulla (pyramid); ascending sensory tracts continue upward through the medulla. Reticular formation tissue is present throughout the medulla, and within the reticular tissue is a cardiac-slowing center and a respiratory center (Fig. 32-7). The latter cannot initiate rhythmic respirations. The medulla has many reciprocal connections with the rest of the brain stem, the cortex, and the cerebellum that transmit continuous data to higher centers of control and initiate physiologic changes as necessary for homeostasis. Cranial nerves IX (glossopharyngeal), X (vagus), XI (spinal accessory), and XII (hypoglossal) emerge from the medulla, as do portions of cranial nerves VII (facial) and VIII (acoustic).

Pons. The pons contains three tracts (peduncles) to and from the cerebellum. The reticular formation tissue of the pons contains cardiac acceleration and vasoconstriction centers. The pneumotaxic center of the superior pons helps control respiratory pattern and rate. Four cranial nerves originate from the pons: VI (abducens), VII, VIII, and V (trigeminal).

Mesencephalon (midbrain). The mesencephalon is the small section between the pons and diencephalon containing motor and sensory pathways, as well as the inferior and superior colliculi—centers for auditory and visual reflexes. It contains a small canal between the third and fourth ventricles called the cerebral aqueduct (aqueduct of Sylvius). Just surrounding the canal is tissue called the *periaqueductal gray*. Stimulation of this area abolishes pain and is the focus of pain control research. Cranial nerves located here are III (oculomotor) and IV (trochlear). Cranial nerve I originates in olfactory epithelium (olfactory bulb). Cranial nerve II (optic) originates in the retinal cells.

Figure 32-7

Autonomic control centers of the brain stem and the diencephalon.

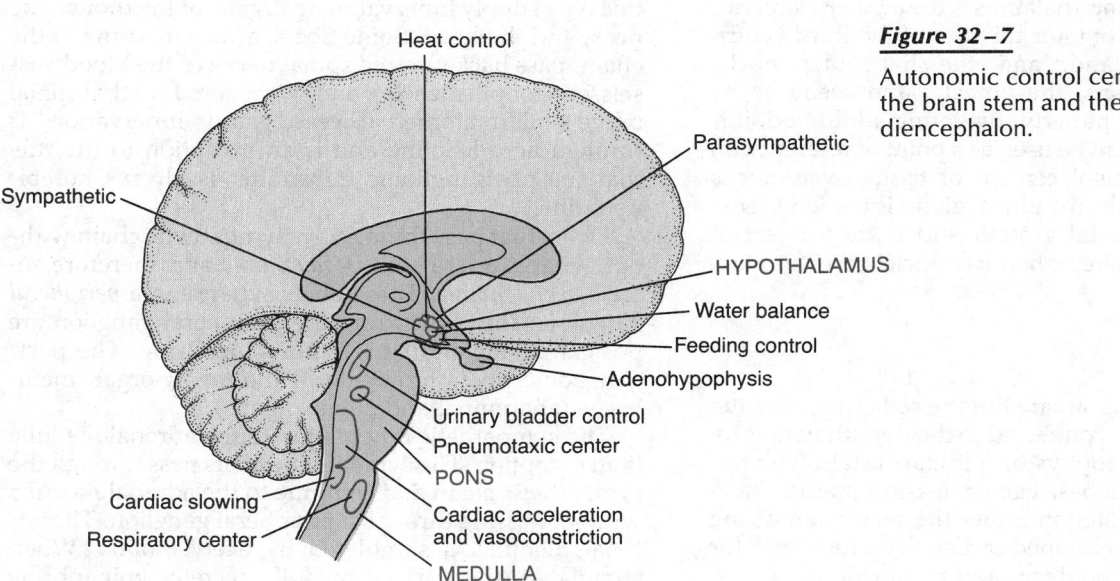

Thalamus. The thalamus is divided into two lobes by the third ventricle and is the major relay station, or central switchboard, for the CNS. Almost every area of the cortex is represented in the thalamus, and there are communicating tracts for each area. *Smell* is the only sensation that does not synapse in the thalamus before reaching its final destination. Without cerebral interpretation, sensation perceived at the thalamic level is crude and cannot be localized or quantified.

Some neurons and tracts within the thalamus have the specific function of transmitting only certain stimuli, such as auditory stimuli to the temporal lobe, optic impulses to the occipital lobe, or general body sensations to the parietal sensory area. Other neurons have connections with the association or interpretive areas of the cortex, but have no input from ascending tracts. These latter neurons are involved with basic emotional drives concerned with self-preservation and as such are considered part of the *limbic system* (discussed later).

Hypothalamus. The hypothalamus is an integral part of the autonomic nervous system and plays an essential role in intellectual function. It is located just above the pituitary gland between the third ventricle and the subthalamus. The hypothalamus regulates the internal environment, such as temperature, through the sympathetic and parasympathetic nervous systems. Hormonal activity is governed by the hypothalamus as well. Posterior pituitary (neurohypophysis) hormones are synthesized in the hypothalamus, and anterior pituitary (adenohypophysis) hormone excretion is controlled by the hypothalamus. The emotional components of the hypothalamus are related to those emotions and drives basic to self-preservation.

Subthalamus. The subthalamus contains sensory tracts and reticular formation tissue. There are connections to the basal ganglia, which are reciprocal.

Epithalamus. The epithalamus is the area just superior to the thalamus. It contains the roof of the third ventricle, the pineal gland, and the habenular nuclei (neurons). In humans, the pineal gland seems to be nonfunctional after puberty. By young adulthood, it is often calcified and can be used as a point of reference on x-ray films when displacement of tissue by tumor is suspected. In animals, the pineal gland is related to sexual and developmental growth and is the subject of ongoing research. The habenular nuclei receive olfactory impulses.

Hypophysis

The hypophysis is situated in the sella turcica of the ethmoid bone and is connected to the hypothalamus by tissue called the hypophyseal (pituitary) stalk. The hypophysis has two lobes, each releasing specific hormones into the circulation under the regulation of the hypothalamus, as mentioned earlier. See Chapter 48 for discussion of the hypophysis and its functions.

Cranial Nerves

The name, number, origin, type, and function of the cranial nerves are summarized in Table 32-3. Some of the cranial nerves are discussed with the autonomic nervous system.

Autonomic Nervous System

The autonomic nervous system is composed of the sympathetic system, whose cells of origin are located in the gray matter of the cord from T-1 through L-2, and the parasympathetic system, whose cells of origin are located in the gray matter of S2-3 plus portions of cranial nerves III, VII, IX, and X (see Table 32-3). The sympathetic system is considered thoracolumbar because of its anatomic location and adrenergic on the basis of its postganglionic transmitter substance (norepinephrine). The parasympathetic system is craniosacral anatomically and cholinergic chemically, because both preganglionic and postganglionic fibers use acetylcholine as a transmitter. (These chemical classifications have been used as the basis for names of drugs acting on the autonomic nervous system.)

Sympathetic division. The sympathetic nervous system, although participating in normal functioning of the body, has the ability to increase its activity when necessary for any type of need. For example, the stress of an examination, going into battle, injury, illness, fear, or anxiety can increase sympathetic outflow. The stressor can be external or internal.

Lying beside the spinal cord on either side is a chain of ganglia extending the length of the cord; this is called the *sympathetic chain*. Sympathetic axons leave the spinal nerve immediately and enter the sympathetic chain. Some fibers synapse within the sympathetic chain, and others do not.

The axons leaving the chain *after* synapsing secrete *norepinephrine* and are called *postganglionic*. Fibers of this type supply innervation to organs of the thorax, the neck, and the head. Some fibers, after synapsing in the chain, pass back into the spinal nerve to the blood vessels, erector pili muscles, and sweat glands of that spinal nerve's dermatome. (Sweat gland innervation is through acetylcholine and is an exception to the rule that the postganglionic transmitter is always norepinephrine.)

Fibers that pass through the sympathetic chain without synapsing are still *preganglionic* and therefore secrete *acetylcholine*. These fibers synapse in a *peripheral* ganglion. The axons from the peripheral ganglion are postganglionic and secrete norepinephrine. The postganglionic fibers terminate in the target organ membrane (abdominal and pelvic organs).

The sympathetic innervation to the adrenal medulla is an exception. The sympathetic fibers pass through the sympathetic chain and continue to the adrenal medulla without passing through a peripheral ganglion. The adrenal medulla is stimulated by acetylcholine. When stimulated, the adrenal medulla secretes epinephrine

TABLE 32-3   Origins, Types, and Functions of the Cranial Nerves

Cranial Nerve	Origin	Type	Function
I: Olfactory	Olfactory bulb	Sensory	Smell
II: Optic	Midbrain	Sensory	Vision
III: Oculomotor	Midbrain	Motor to eye muscles	Eye movement via medial and lateral rectus and inferior oblique and superior rectus muscles; lid elevation via the levator muscle
		Parasympathetic-motor	Pupil constriction; ciliary muscles
IV: Trochlear	Lower midbrain	Motor	Eye movement via superior oblique muscles
V: Trigeminal	Pons	Sensory	Sensation from the skin of the face and scalp and the mucous membranes of the mouth and nose
		Motor	Muscles of mastication (chewing)
VI: Abducens	Inferior pons	Motor	Eye movement via lateral rectus muscles
VII: Facial	Inferior pons	Sensory	Pain and temperature from ear area; deep sensations from the face; taste from anterior two-thirds of the tongue
		Motor	Muscles of the face and scalp
		Parasympathetic-motor	Lacrimal, submandibular, and sublingual salivary glands
VIII: Vestibulocochlear	Pons-medulla junction	Sensory	Hearing Equilibrium
IX: Glossopharyngeal	Medulla	Sensory	Pain and temperature from the ear; taste and sensations from the posterior one-third of the tongue and the pharynx
		Motor	Skeletal muscles of the throat
		Parasympathetic-motor	Parotid glands
X: Vagus	Medulla	Sensory	Pain and temperature from the ear; sensations from the pharynx, the larynx, and thoracic and abdominal viscera
		Motor	Muscles of the soft palate, larynx, and pharynx
		Parasympathetic-motor	Thoracic and abdominal viscera; cells of secretory glands; cardiac and smooth muscle innervation to the level of the splenic flexure
XI: Spinal accessory	Medulla (anterior gray horn of the cervical spine)	Motor	Skeletal muscles of the pharynx and larynx and sternocleidomastoid and trapezius muscles
XII: Hypoglossal	Medulla	Motor	Skeletal muscles of the tongue

and norepinephrine into the circulatory system, which enhances and potentiates the effect of the sympathetic system.

Sympathetic nerve endings terminate on one of two known types of receptor cells, alpha-receptor and beta-receptor. These receptor cells determine the effect of the neurotransmitter. As for the parasympathetic system, knowledge of the action of the two types of receptor cells has aided in producing drugs that can stimulate, inhibit, block, or mimic a specific type of receptor, transmitter, or enzyme.

If almost any portion of the sympathetic system is stimulated, the whole system responds (the flight-or-fight response). During periods of excessive sympathetic stimulation, skeletal muscle vessels dilate, the heart pumps faster, the liver releases extra glucose, the thyroid is stimulated, sweat glands are overactive, kidney vessels are constricted, and peristalsis is decreased. During true emergencies this is a useful mechanism, but with false emergencies (such as being unduly anxious), this mechanism wastes resources. The sympathetic system functions without control from the hypothalamus, the limbic system, or the cortex in the event of injury to the upper spinal cord (descending impulses are blocked). Table 32–4 compares the action of sympathetic and parasympathetic systems on the body.

Parasympathetic division. The parasympathetic system conserves the body's resources. Parasympathetic axons synapse with ganglia in or near their target organs. The transmitter substance of both *preganglionic* and *postganglionic* axons is *acetylcholine*. The postganglionic axon is short (located in or close to its target membrane), and, because acetylcholine is destroyed quickly, the parasympathetic system is described as having discrete function. For example, stimulation of the salivary glands does not stimulate cardiac muscle. As for the sympathetic system, there are two types of receptor cells (muscarinic and nicotinic) in the target membrane that determine the effect of the transmitter on the organ.

Parasympathetic fibers to the viscera also have some sensory ability in addition to motor function. Sensations of irritation, stretching of an organ, or a decrease in tissue oxygen are transmitted to the thalamus through pathways not yet fully understood. Because pain from internal organs is often felt below the body wall served by the spinal nerve, it is presumed there are connections between the viscera and body structure that relay pain sensations. The following are some important autonomic reflexes that illustrate the precise nature of the parasympathetic system.

Control of arterial pressure. Increased arterial pressure causes stretching of parasympathetic fibers located in the aortic arch and common carotid artery bifurcation. This initiates the sending of impulses to the cardiac center in the reticular formation of the medulla. From there, the impulses are transmitted to the vagus nerve to slow the heart *rate* and the reticulospinal tract to inhibit the sympathetic cells of the spinal cord. Inhibition of the sympathetic system permits *vasodilation* of the vessels. The slowed heart rate and vasodilation decrease arterial pressure. The dilation results from impulses transmitted through a central tract in the spinal cord, which occurs only if the cord is intact.

Control of respiration. Respiratory centers are located in the reticular formation of the medulla and the pons. The two medullary centers are for inspiration and expiration. The *pontine* (pneumotaxic) center regulates the rhythm of respirations. Carbon dioxide in the circulation stimulates the inspiratory center, which then transmits impulses to the diaphragm and intercostal muscles. Inspiration is also stimulated through nerve cells in the carotid and aortic bodies (acting as *chemoreceptors*) if a decrease in oxygen concentration occurs. A decrease in circulating oxygen causes impulses to be transmitted to the pontine and medullary centers to increase the rate and depth of inspiration. Expiration occurs when nerve endings in the bronchial branches are stretched by lung expansion. Impulses to the expiratory center result in inhibition of the action of the diaphragm and the intercostal muscles.

Gastrointestinal reflexes. Smell and taste of food are stimuli that cause the facial, vagal, and glossopharyngeal parasympathetic fibers to initiate secretion for digestion in the mouth, the stomach, and the intestine. At the distal end of the gastrointestinal tract, another reflex is involved in the elimination of waste products. When the rectum becomes distended, this sensation is relayed to the sacral parasympathetic fibers of the cord. A parasympathetic motor response is initiated, and movement of feces begins. Emptying of the rectum is under voluntary control.

Bladder control. Bladder emptying is also controlled through the sacral parasympathetic system. With bladder wall distention, motor parasympathetic impulses contract the bladder wall (detrusor) muscle and relax the sphincter (trigone). This reflex is under voluntary control after early childhood.

Sexual reflex. Erection is a sacral parasympathetic reflex that can be elicited by psychic stimulus, genital stimulus, or both, and is under voluntary control in the normal adult. Erection after psychogenic stimulation originates in the cerebrum. The impulses are transmitted through the limbic system, the hypothalamus, and the spinal cord to a thoracolumbar erection center and then to the sacral cord. External stimulation of the genitalia produces a *reflex* erection via parasympathetic outflow from the sacral cord. The reflex arc encompasses stimuli from the genitalia to the sacral cord and the motor response back to the penis or clitoris. Spinal cord injury above the sacral level leaves the parasympathetic system intact, as cranial nerves III, V, VII, IX, and X (which carry parasympathetic fibers) have exited the CNS above the cervical cord level. If the sacral portion of the cord has not been injured, the client with a spinal cord injury has the potential for reflex erection, but has no voluntary control.

Control of the autonomic nervous system. The autonomic nervous system is under the higher control of the hypothalamus, the limbic system, and some parts of the frontal lobe. Although most vegetative functions are governed by the hypothalamus, the regulation of body water also requires the posterior pituitary, which releases vasopressin (antidiuretic hormone [ADH]). Research has identified the limbic system as an integral part of autonomic function.

Cerebellum

The cerebellum is a complex structure consisting of several types of neurons and many interconnections between the various cerebellar cells, the brain stem, and the cortex. The cerebellum receives instantaneous and

TABLE 32–4   Effects of the Autonomic Nervous System on Various Organs of the Body

Organ	Effect of Sympathetic Stimulation	Effect of Parasympathetic Stimulation
Eye		
Pupil	Dilated	Constricted
Ciliary muscle	Slight relaxation	Constricted
Glands		
Nasal	Vasoconstriction and slight secretion	Stimulation of copious (except pancreas) secretion (containing many enzymes for enzyme-secreting glands)
Lacrimal		
Parotid		
Submandibular		
Gastric		
Pancreatic		
Sweat glands	Copious sweating (cholinergic)	None
Apocrine glands	Thick, odoriferous secretion	None
Heart		
Muscle	Increased rate	Slowed rate
	Increased force of contraction	Decreased force of contraction (especially of atrium)
Coronary arteries	Dilated (beta$_2$); constricted (alpha)	Dilated
Lungs		
Bronchi	Dilated	Constricted
Blood vessels	Mildly constricted	? Dilated
Gut		
Lumen	Decreased peristalsis and tone	Increased peristalsis and tone
Sphincter	Increased tone (most times)	Relaxed (most times)
Liver	Glucose released	Slight glycogen synthesis
Gallbladder and bile ducts	Relaxed	Contracted
Kidney	Decreased output and renin secretion	None
Bladder		
Detrusor	Relaxed (slight)	Excited
Trigone	Excited	Relaxed
Penis	Ejaculation	Erection
Systemic arterioles		
Abdominal	Constricted	None
Muscle	Constricted (alpha-adrenergic)	None
	Dilated (beta$_2$-adrenergic)	
	Dilated (cholinergic)	
Skin	Constricted	None
Blood		
Coagulation	Increased	None
Glucose	Increased	None
Basal metabolism	Increased up to 100%	None
Adrenal medullary secretion	Increased	None
Mental activity	Increased	None
Piloerector muscles	Excited	None
Skeletal muscle	Increased glycogenolysis	None
	Increased strength	

From Guyton, A. C. (1986). *Textbook of medical physiology* (7th ed.). Philadelphia: W. B. Saunders.

continuous information about the condition of muscles, joints, and tendons. When a directive is received by the cerebellum from the motor cortex, it reviews the order, comparing it with data received from the periphery (the state of the involved peripheral muscles, joints, and tendons), and then alters or corrects the original directive as necessary. Cerebellar function enables one to keep a moving part from overshooting the intended destination, move from one skilled movement to another in an orderly sequence, predict distance or gauge the speed with which one is approaching an object, control voluntary movement, and maintain equilibrium.

Cerebellar control of the body is *ipsilateral* (situated on the same side). The right side of the cerebellum controls the right side of the body, and the left cerebellum controls the left side of the body.

Cerebrum

The cerebral cortex forming the outermost portion of the cerebrum has three to six layers of cells. It is the six-layer portion (neocortex) that is highly developed in humans, allowing a greater level of function than in any other species. The dominant hemisphere in most humans is the *left* hemisphere (even for many left-

handed people). The cerebral hemispheres are divided into lobes by sulci (fissures) and are named the same as the overlying bone, with the exception of the limbic lobe. Within the cerebral cortex, there are many interconnections and circuits between cells, layers of cells, rows of cells, the lobes, and the two hemispheres. The hemispheres are in communication with each other through the corpus callosum (the connecting path between the two). The right and left lateral ventricles are situated in the inner, lower aspect of the cerebral hemispheres. Since the early 1900s, there have been attempts to classify neurons by their cellular structure and then relate that to function. Brodmann's map represents one such attempt and is used most frequently (Fig. 32–8).

Limbic lobe. The limbic lobe consists of the tissue immediately surrounding the upper part of the brain stem —the medial aspect of the cerebral hemispheres. It consists of the cingulate gyrus, the hippocampus, and the parahippocampal gyrus. This portion of the cortex appeared early in cerebral development. The limbic *system* includes those structures plus the amygdaloid body, the hypothalamus, the thalamus, and the habenular nuclei of the epithalamus. Limbic lobe or system function is related to emotional and visceral patterns connected

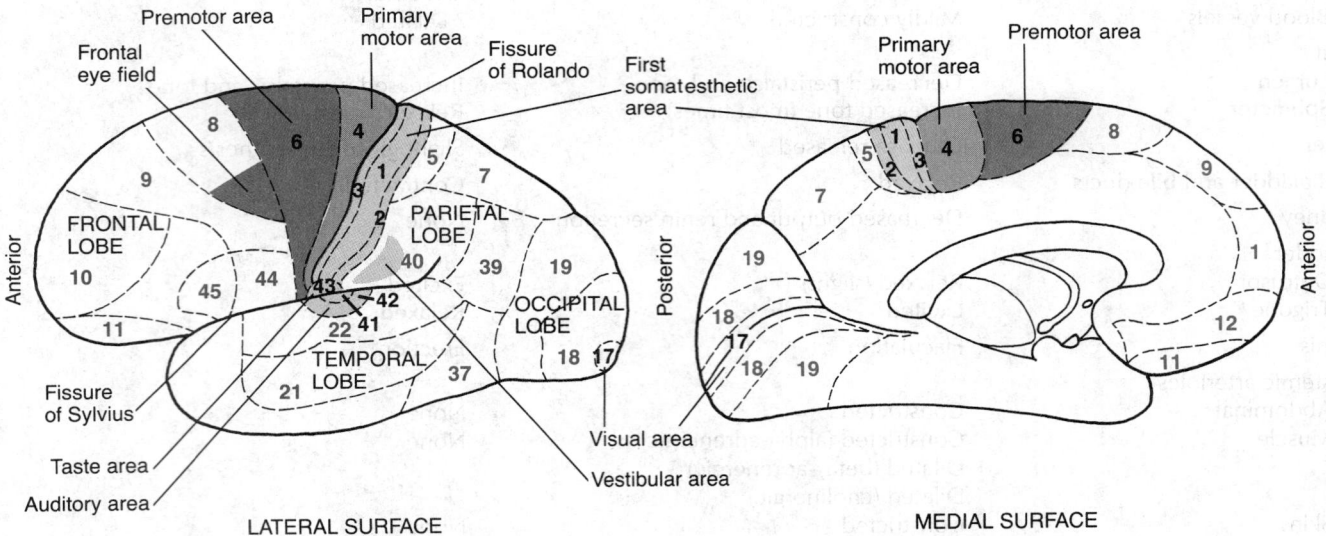

Figure 32–8

Functions of the brain according to Brodmann's map. Key: 1, 2, and 3: primary somatic sensory area (overlap with 4); 4: primary motor area; 5: somatesthetic association cortex; 6: premotor area; 7: somatesthetic association cortex; 8: frontal eye field; 9 through 14: prefrontal or orbitofrontal association cortex (judgment, foresight, behavior), autonomic centers (respiratory, circulatory, renal, gastrointestinal) (11 and 12: no clearly assigned function); 17: visual area; 18 and 19: visual association cortex; 21 and 22: ideation, sensory, language, also 37 (posterior part: auditory association cortex [Wernicke's area]) 37: see 21 and 22; 39 and 40: ideation, sensory, language, angular gyrus; 41: auditory area; 42: may also function as auditory area; 43: taste area; 44 and 45: dominant hemisphere (motor speech centers and related functions), lips and tongue (Broca's center); 47: no clearly assigned function. (Modified from Barr, M. L., & Kiernan, J. A. [1988]. *The human nervous system: An anatomical viewpoint* [5th ed]. Philadelphia: J. B. Lippincott.)

with survival. Research indicates that the hippocampus plays a major role in learning and memory.

Frontal lobe. The frontal lobe is below the frontal bone and extends anteriorly from the central sulcus (fissure of Rolando) and upward from the lateral fissure (fissure of Sylvius). It contains the primary motor area (also known as the motor "strip"), a premotor area, Broca's speech center on the dominant side, and an eyefield (Brodmann's areas 4, 6, 44 and 45, and 8, respectively).

The *primary motor area* contributes about 30% of the fibers of the corticospinal (pyramidal) tract for the contralateral side of the body. Cells in this area are responsible for voluntary muscle contraction of specific muscle groups. The *premotor area* also contributes about 30% of the fibers of corticospinal tract; this area is just anterior to the motor strip. In addition to supplying the fibers of the corticospinal tract, the premotor area contributes fibers to other descending tracts and directly affects the primary area. The premotor area directs the movement for skilled voluntary action, either for a new movement or when a previously learned one is changed. *Broca's area* is composed of neurons responsible for the formation of words. This requires respiratory activation of the vocal cords, which must occur at the same time as tongue and mouth movements. The neuronal cells of the *eyefield* permit voluntary movement of the eyes and control eyelid movement.

The rest of the frontal lobe (Brodmann's areas 9, 10, 11, and 12) is called the prefrontal cortex and has many connections with the parietal, occipital, and temporal lobes. These connections provide access to current sensory data and to past information or experience. There are also connections to thalamic nuclei that guide the affective response to a situation. The prefrontal cortex regulates behavior that is based on judgment and foresight. All of the various interconnections in the frontal lobe help the individual guide behavior, make judgments, prevent distraction, develop long-term goals, weigh the pros and cons of a situation or action, and elaborate thought. These factors contribute to one's personality.

Parietal lobe. The parietal lobe extends posteriorly from the central sulcus to the parieto-occipital fissure and down to the *angular gyrus* (the junction of the temporal, occipital, and parietal lobes). The rest of the corticospinal tract fibers (about 35%) originate in the parietal lobe. The primary and secondary somatesthetic (body consciousness) sensory areas are located here (Brodmann's areas 1, 2, and 3), as well as a large number of sensory association cells (Brodmann's areas 5, 7, 39, and 40). The *primary* areas interpret simple sensations, whereas the *association* areas are responsible for more complex interpretation. The parietal lobe enables one to understand texture, size, shape, and spatial relationships. Comparisons are made with previous experiences. The right parietal lobe seems to be involved with three-dimensional (spatial) perception and is important for singing, playing musical instruments, and process-

ing nonverbal visual experiences. Interpreting the spatial relationship of body parts to the whole is a function of the parietal lobe. Taste impulses also terminate in the parietal lobe for interpretation. Taste sensations terminate in the lower parietal area, where it folds deep into the lateral (sylvian) fissure (Brodmann's area 43). This area lies close to or even on the tongue portion of somatic area I.

Temporal lobe. The temporal lobe extends from the lateral fissure down and posterior to the area of the angular gyrus. It contains auditory centers (Brodmann's areas 41 and 42), where impulses are received (simple sounds are interpreted), and association areas, where interpretation of complex sounds occurs. This latter area (Wernicke's area) plays a significant role in higher-level brain function. It enables processing of words heard into coherent thought and recognizing the idea behind written or printed words. It is also believed that this area is responsible for complicated memory patterns. It is unknown whether those patterns are stored here or elsewhere. Wernicke's area is larger in the left lobe than in the right lobe in the majority of people, even at birth. Sensations of smell are transmitted to anterior medial parts of the brain and brain stem. However, the primary olfactory cortex is located in the dorsomedial portion of the anterior temporal cortex. Impulses arriving here have not been relayed to the thalamus first. All the areas concerned with smell have interconnecting fibers, lending emotional and visceral components to actual smell interpretation.

Occipital lobe. The occipital lobe is the most posterior part of the cortex and is just above the cerebellum. Within the occipital lobe is a primary visual center (Brodmann's area 17) receiving stimuli from the retinas. Adjacent to the primary centers are the visual association areas (Brodmann's areas 18 and 19) where interpretation of more complex sights occurs. Fibers from the occipital lobe extend forward to the angular gyrus.

General interpretative area. Association fibers from the parietal, temporal (Wernicke's), and occipital lobes all synapse in the posterior part of the superior temporal lobe and the anterior angular gyrus. This area enables one to process complex thoughts, remember the notes of music, recite a speech heard or read long ago, recall childhood experiences, and so forth. Damage to this area on the dominant side after the age of 5 years is catastrophic.

Cerebral Circulation and the Blood-Brain Barrier

The cerebral circulation originates from the carotid and vertebral arteries (Fig. 32–9). The *internal carotid* arteries branch into the *anterior* and *middle cerebral* arteries. The two *posterior vertebral* arteries become the *basilar* artery, which then divides into two *posterior cerebral* arteries. The anterior, middle, and posterior cerebral

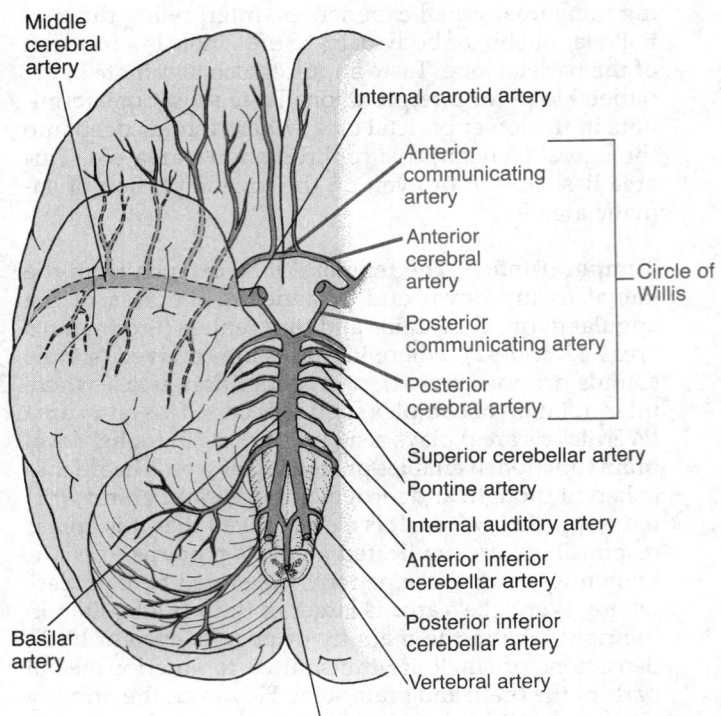

Figure 32–9

Cerebral circulation and the circle of Willis at the base of the brain.

arteries are joined together by small communicating arteries to form a ring, the *circle of Willis.* The circle of Willis is about the level of the pons or the level of the upper nose or lower border of the eye. The middle cerebral artery supplies the lateral surface of the cerebrum from about the mid-temporal lobe upward, i.e., the area for hearing and upper body motor and sensory neurons. The anterior cerebral artery supplies the midline, or medial, aspect of the same area—lower body motor and sensory neurons. The posterior cerebral arteries supply the area from the mid-temporal region down and posteriorly (occipital lobe), as well as much of the brain stem. Table 32–5 identifies the origin of blood supply to the brain.

Venous drainage occurs through the cerebral veins into the *dural sinuses*—large venous reservoirs between the inner and outer dura mater. From the dural sinuses, the blood drains into the jugular vein and then into the superior vena cava. Cerebral veins have no values, and therefore intracranial pressure can be affected by central venous pressure. Two sinuses are of particular importance. The *superior sagittal sinus* receives CSF after it circulates through the ventricular system. The *cavernous sinus* is located near the eye and receives venous blood from the eye. In addition, the carotid artery passes through the cavernous sinus (the only place in the body that an artery passes through a vein); thus, there is the potential for development of a fistula between an artery and a vein (usually from trauma).

The *blood-brain barrier* seems to exist because the endothelial cells of the cerebral capillaries, along with ependymal cells, are tightly joined together. This keeps some substances in the plasma out of the cerebrospinal circulation and out of brain tissue. Substances that can pass through are oxygen, carbon dioxide, alcohol, anesthetics, and water.

Cerebrospinal Fluid Circulation

CSF is the fluid that surrounds and cushions the brain and spinal cord. CSF is secreted primarily by the *choroid plexuses* (clusters of blood vessels covered by ependymal cells), which are located in the floor of the lateral ventricles and the roof of the third and fourth ventricles. Additional fluid is secreted by the surfaces of the ventricles. Between 500 and 800 mL of CSF is formed every day, but only 125 to 140 mL is normally present at one time (Cella & Watson, 1989). The properties of CSF are different from those of plasma (CSF has more chloride, less potassium, and less glucose), indicating that it is not simply a filtrate of plasma. The circulation of the CSF is as follows: lateral ventricles through the interventricular foramen (Monro's) to the third ventricle, through the cerebral aqueduct (sylvian aqueduct) to the fourth ventricle, where it passes out into the subarachnoid space through three foramina, a middle one called Magendie's and two lateral foramina called Luschka's (Fig. 32–10). While circulating through the subarachnoid space, the

---

TABLE 32–5   Blood Distribution to the Brain

Artery	Distribution
Internal Carotid Artery Branches	
Hypophyseal	Posterior pituitary
Ophthalmic	Eye, frontal scalp, frontal and ethmoid sinuses
Anterior choroidal	Choroid plexus (lateral), optic tract, uncus, amygdaloid body, hippocampus, globus pallidus, lateral geniculate nucleus, internal capsule
Middle cerebral	Insula; lateral frontal, parietal, occipital, and temporal lobes (involves major motor and sensory areas)
Lenticulostriate branches	Putamen, caudate nucleus, globus pallidus, internal capsule, corona radiata
Other branches	Choroid plexus (lateral ventricles), hippocampus, globus pallidus
Anterior cerebral	Medial surface of frontal and parietal lobes, corpus callosum, superior or lateral strip of frontal and parietal lobes
Vertebral Artery Branches	Medulla
Posterior cerebellar	Posterior cerebellum, inferior vermis, cerebellar nuclei, choroid plexus (fourth ventricle), posterolateral medulla
Basilar Artery Branches	
Anterior inferior cerebellar	Cortex and inferior surface cerebellum, cerebellar nuclei, upper medulla, lower pons
Internal auditory	Inner ear
Pontine	Pons
Superior cerebellar	Cortex, white matter and nuclei of cerebellum, pons, superior cerebellar peduncle, inferior peduncle, inferior colliculus
Posterior Cerebral Artery Branches	Medial, inferior temporal, and occipital lobes
Calcarine branch	Visual cortex
Other branches	Posterior and lateral thalamus, subthalamus, pituitary, mamillary bodies, and midbrain; choroid plexus of lateral and third ventricle, dorsal thalamus
Circle of Willis Branches	Hypothalamus, caudate nucleus, putamen, globus pallidus, internal capsule, external capsule, thalamus, subthalamus, cerebral peduncles

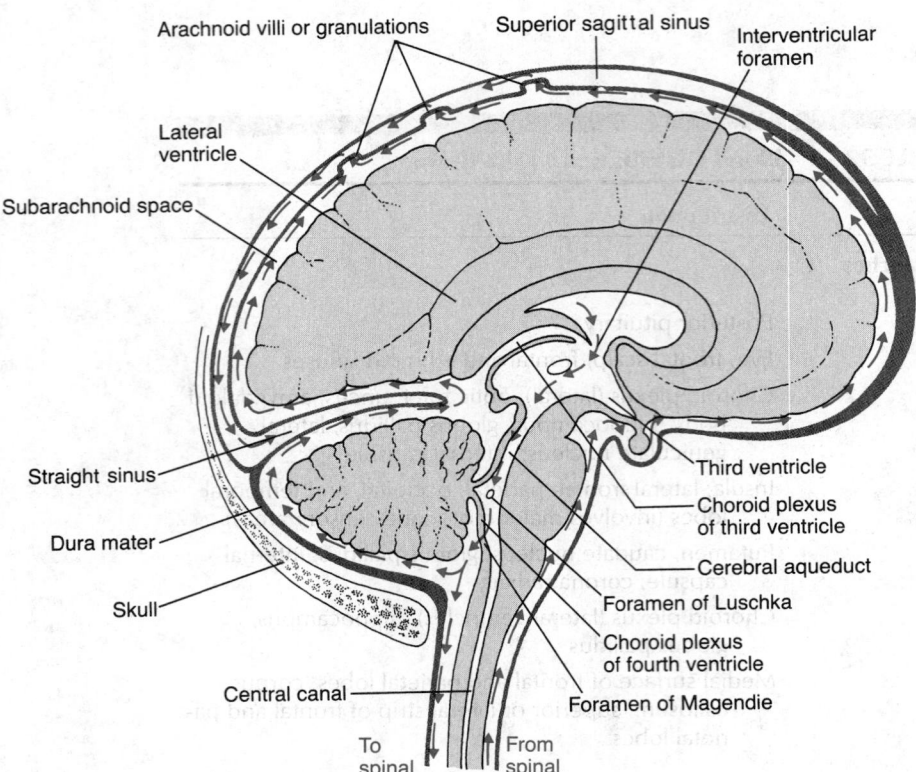

Figure 32–10

Circulation of cerebrospinal fluid. Note that the fluid also extends down into the spinal column.

fluid is continuously reabsorbed by the *arachnoid villi* and then channeled into the superior sagittal sinus. Expanded areas of subarachnoid space, where there are large amounts of CSF, are called *cisterns*. The largest cistern is the lumbar cistern — the site of lumbar puncture (L2-S2).

Central Nervous System Protection

Meninges

The meninges form the immediate protective covering of the brain and the spinal cord. The covering adhering to the brain and the spinal cord is the *pia mater*, a thin, delicate, and vascular membrane. The next layer is the *arachnoid*. It is thin and delicate, but also fibrous, with the CSF filling the web-like tissue. The outer layer, the *dura mater,* is heavy, fibrous, and nonelastic. There are actually two layers of dura; the outer is adhered to the cranium and becomes the periosteum, whereas the inner layer covers the brain. Between the two layers of dura are the venous sinuses. The inner layer of dura dips down between the two hemispheres and is called the *falx.* The dura also goes between the cortex and the cerebellum and is called the *tentorium.* The purpose of the falx and the tentorium is to decrease or prevent the transmission of force from one hemisphere to another and to protect the lower brain stem, respectively. Clinical references may be made to something (e.g., a tumor) as being *supratentorial* or, if in the cerebellum, *infratentorial.*

Bone

The brain and spinal cord are encased in the cranium and the vertebral column and, for the most part, are well protected. However, there are some areas of vulnerability, such as the nasal sinuses, the palate of the throat, the ears, and the cervical spine. The upright position of humans creates additional strain on the vertebrae and musculature. The cranial bones are named the same as the cerebral lobes they cover. There are 7 cervical, 12 thoracic, 5 lumbar, 5 sacral (fused), and 4 coccygeal (fused) vertebrae. Although there are some differences in structure, the purposes of the vertebrae remain the same, that is, to protect the spinal cord and give structure to the body (Fig. 32–11).

NEUROLOGIC CHANGES ASSOCIATED WITH AGING

Motor changes in the elderly are interrelated with sensory function and musculoskeletal status (see the accompanying Focus on the Elderly feature). Any problems affecting nerves, bones, muscles, or joints affect motor ability. The elderly individual may have tremors

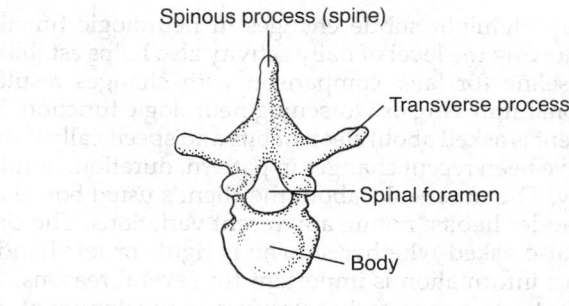

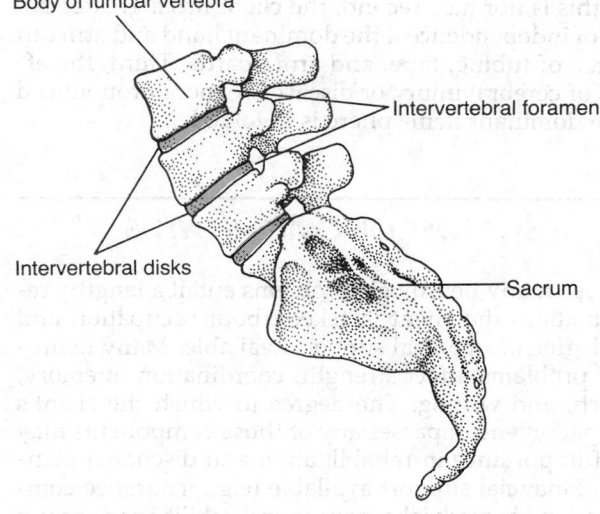

Spinous process (spine)

Transverse process

Spinal foramen

Body

Body of lumbar vertebra

Intervertebral foramen

Intervertebral disks

Sacrum

Figure 32–11
Major structural components of the vertebrae.

without rigidity, and deep tendon reflexes may be hypoactive. Balance and coordination may be impaired as a result.

Sensory changes in the elderly can affect their daily activities. Pain sensation tends to decrease, so that what might be an acute pain in a younger person may be perceived as a dull ache in the older client. Pupils decrease in size, restricting the amount of light entering the eye. The pupils also adapt more slowly. Touch sensation decreases, which may precipitate falls, as the elderly may not feel pebbles or small objects underfoot. Vibration sense may be lost in the ankles and feet. Hearing also decreases.

Intellect does not decline solely as a result of aging. However, a decrease in intellectual level may be caused by insufficient oxygen supply to the CNS. The elderly may lose some complex skills, such as problem-solving and completing analogies and number series. It is thought that loss of these skills may be from disuse, rather than from neurologic impairment. The elderly individual may need more time than a younger person to process questions.

Memory changes are typical for many elderly persons. Distant memory seems better than recent memory. The elderly may need more time to retrieve information. Learning that also requires *unlearning* is the most difficult for the elderly. These changes may be partly due to the loss of CNS neurons, which is associated with the aging process.

Mental status studies have shown that there is a substantial incidence of insomnia, anxiety, and depression among the elderly, which was not previously recognized. Circadian rhythm disorders lead to wakefulness until later at night with extended sleeping in the morning (the opposite of most health care facility routines). Alcohol and medication side effects or inappropriate dosages also cause insomnia, anxiety, and depression.

FOCUS ON THE ELDERLY ■ Neurologic Changes Related to Aging

Change	Interventions
Recent memory loss	Reinforce teaching by repetition and written teaching aids.
Decreased touch sensation	Remind client to look where his/her feet are placed when walking.
	Instruct the client to wear shoes that provide good support when ambulating.
	If the client is unable, change client's position frequently (every hour) while in bed or chair.
Change in perception of pain	Ask the client to describe the nature and specific characteristics of pain.
	Monitor additional assessment variables to detect possible health problems.
Change in sleep patterns	Ascertain individual sleep patterns and preferences.
	Adjust the client's daily schedule to sleep pattern and preference as much as possible, e.g., evening versus morning bath.
Altered balance or coordination	Instruct the client to move slowly when changing positions.
	If needed, advise the client to hold on to handrails when ambulating.
	Assess the need for an ambulatory aid, such as a cane.

HISTORY

The nursing history and assessment of the client with a neurologic problem proceed as for any client, with the nurse providing privacy and making the person as comfortable as possible. If the client appears confused or has trouble speaking or hearing, the nurse asks a family member or significant other to stay with the client during the history taking to help secure accurate information.

DEMOGRAPHIC DATA

The *age* and *sex* of the client may be indicators of certain neurologic problems. For example, younger people have a higher incidence of arteriovenous malformations than the elderly, and certain types of tumors are more likely to be found in the elderly rather than in younger people.

PERSONAL AND FAMILY HISTORY

Questions about the *client's past medical history,* as well as the *family history,* are necessary for any bearing they might have on the present problem. Prior injuries or congenital problems could be related to the present problem. Chronic diseases, such as hypertension, diabetes mellitus, and lung disease, have a direct effect on the nervous system. The nurse asks the client about any previous neurologic problem such as headaches, seizures, head or spine trauma, or eye problems. These questions are important because the current problem could be related to a pre-existing health problem. The client might not consider previous problems worth mentioning if he/she is not asked. The client is questioned about any food, drug, or environmental *allergies,* as well as the *medications* (prescribed, illicit, and over the counter) in use, as these can affect the nervous system. The nurse asks the client about *pain tolerance,* the usual medications taken, and the behaviors used to ease the pain (for example, go to bed, ignore it, or use an icebag). The client is asked about usual *recreational activities,* including physical activity and hobbies. The nurse questions the client about alcohol consumption and use of recreational drugs (including the frequency and last incidence of use). Alcohol and other chemicals directly affect the nervous system, and the type of physical recreational activity or hobbies the client engages in may have relevancy for rehabilitation or discharge planning. *Ethnic and cultural background* may be an influence, depending on the degree of socialization to the health care system. As more is learned about the effects of dietary intake on the nervous system, diet history may become an important aspect of the history.

Questions about the client's *level of daily activity* may highlight subtle changes in neurologic function. Knowing the level of daily activity also helps establish a baseline for later comparison with changes resulting from improving or worsening neurologic function. The client is asked about sleep habits and specifically if there have been recent changes in pattern, duration, or intensity. The nurse asks about the client's usual bowel and bladder habits, noting any recent variations. The client is also asked whether she/he is right- or left-handed. This information is important for several reasons. The client may be somewhat stronger on the dominant side, and this is normal. Second, the client has a greater degree of independence if the dominant hand and arm can be free of tubing, tape, and arm boards. Third, the effects of cerebral injury or disease are more pronounced if the dominant hemisphere is involved.

SOCIOECONOMIC STATUS

Because many neurologic problems entail a lengthy rehabilitation, the client is asked about occupation and the degree of financial support available. Many neurologic problems affect strength, coordination, memory, speech, and writing. The degree to which the client's occupation encompasses any of those components may be of importance in rehabilitation and discharge planning. Financial support available (e.g., insurance compensation for medical expenses or disability or a second wage earner in the home) is important because of the length of time that may be needed for recovery.

CURRENT HEALTH PROBLEM

The nurse asks the client specific questions related to the current problem. The following information is obtained:

1. Date of onset and the initial signs and symptoms
2. Factors predisposing to or precipitating the condition and the progression since its onset
3. Measures used to relieve the problem (e.g., medications and behaviors)
4. Effect on livelihood, emotions, body image, family life, and activities of daily living
5. Level of understanding the client has about the problem (e.g., the reason for admission, the plan of treatment, and expected outcomes)

PHYSICAL ASSESSMENT

The nurse may not perform the initial physical examination, but must be aware of and knowledgeable about those components that are within the scope of nursing practice. There are times when the nurse is the first person to see the client and, as such, performs a neurologic examination as a part of the complete physical examination. Establishment of baseline data for the client is most important. Nurses must constantly make comparisons with each assessment (e.g., to findings 5 minutes or an hour earlier, to the client's normal, between the right and left sides, and to the expected progression for the client). Much of the neurologic examination can be done with the client sitting or lying down. If the client is experiencing increased headache pain during the assessment, the nurse suspects increasing intracranial pressure, which should be reported to the physician immediately.

ASSESSMENT OF MENTAL STATUS

While collecting the history data, the nurse makes observations especially about the client's mental status, speech, and behavior. Are the answers appropriate? Is the client's behavior appropriate? Is the speech pattern of normal tone, rate, rhythm, and volume? Are the answers complete? Is his/her appearance neat or untidy? Is the client cooperative, hostile, or anxious? Although the mental status examination is often left until last, it may be better to complete it as part of the initial physical assessment, especially if neurologic problems have been noted. Although normal mental status in the elderly varies considerably, there are some general considerations to be aware of during the mental status assessment. Elderly persons often take longer to process and answer questions, particularly if they do not see the relevancy. Their attention span may be short, and they may be guided by internal rather than external motivation. Depending on age, previous occupation, and retirement activities, some of the cognitive tests may be difficult or impossible to perform. The questions should then be changed to focus on their immediate life. If the client's behavior seems appropriate, the mental status assessment can be shortened considerably. Of primary importance for mental status is assessing *level of consciousness* (LOC) and *memory.*

LEVEL OF CONSCIOUSNESS

LOC is determined by asking the client questions that indicate orientation to *person, place,* and *time.* During the history taking, the client's ability to relate the onset of symptoms, the name of her/his physician, the year or month, the client's address, and the name of the referring physician or institution all indicate orientation to person, place, and time. Factors such as advanced age, time of day, medications, and need for sleep affect a client's responses. Assessment of the client who is less than alert because of trauma, surgery, and so forth is discussed in Chapter 33. In the past, clients who were less than alert were labeled as lethargic (sleepy but

arousable), stuporous (arousable with difficulty), and comatose (not arousable). To better identify the client's exact state of consciousness, these categories should be augmented by descriptions of the client's behavior in response to stimulation.

MEMORY

Memory is one of the most important criteria in assessing the client with a neurologic condition. If the client cannot remember, most of the verbal assessment tests will be either not feasible or at best unreliable. Loss of memory, especially recent memory, tends to be an *early* sign of neurologic problems. There are three facets of memory to test—*remote, recent,* and *new.* The elderly client may not be as capable with recent or new memory, and this may be acceptable for that person.

Remote, or long-term, memory is tested by asking the client about his/her birthdate, schools attended, the city of birth, or anything from the past. The nurse must be able to verify the answers. One question often asked is the maiden name of the mother, as this is sometimes listed on the admission form and can be checked. *Recent* memory can be tested fairly well during the history taking by assessing the accuracy of the medical history, dates of clinic appointments, the time of admission, physicians seen within the past few days, or mode of transportation to the hospital or clinic. *New* memory is tested by giving the client two or three unrelated words, such as "apple," "street," "chair," and asking her/him to repeat them to make sure the words were heard. After about 5 minutes, while continuing with the examination, the client is asked to repeat the words. Normally, a person should be able to do this correctly.

ATTENTION

The nurse asks the client to repeat three numbers, such as 4, 7, 3, and increases the series by one number with each successful repetition until seven or eight digits are achieved. If the client has difficulty at any level (cannot repeat the series), the nurse repeats the numbers again. If the client cannot repeat, the nurse stops the procedure. Next, the nurse asks the client to repeat the numbers backward, starting again with three digits and increasing by one each time. Normally, a person should be able to repeat *five to eight digits forward* and *four to six backward.* Education, occupation, interest, culture, anxiety, and depression all affect mental status, and what is considered normal may not be so for a particular client. The *serial seven* test can also be used to test attention. The client is asked to count backward from 100 by 7 (the examiner stops when the client reaches 63 successfully). Depending on education and other factors, it may be much better to ask the person to subtract by three or to add forward by five. The nurse must use judgment in deciding which of these tests to use.

LANGUAGE AND COPYING

Most of language and copying can be tested during the initial interview. Language comprehension is demonstrated by the client's ability to follow the nurse's directions regarding admission (e.g., getting undressed and providing a urine specimen). Was there any hesitancy in speech, indicating that the client groped for words? If so, the nurse asks him/her to name items to which the examiner points, such as a drinking glass, the door, or the bed. Reading comprehension is tested by writing a simple command and giving it to the client (e.g., "close your eyes"). Writing can be tested by asking the client to write a sentence. Copying ability is usually tested by having the client copy something the examiner has drawn. The figures used most frequently are a cross, a circle, a diamond, and square. Those drawn by the client should look similar to those of the nurse.

COGNITION

Higher *intellectual* function is assessed by asking information about favorite hobbies, current events, the names of the last few presidents, or the meaning of a statement. *Abstract reasoning* is usually tested by asking the meaning of proverbs (e.g., "A stitch in time saves nine" or "A rolling stone gathers no moss"). *Judgment* can also be assessed, at least partially, during the interview. Did the client make rational decisions in dealing with his/her symptoms? Judgment can be evaluated by asking questions such as "What would you do if stopped for speeding?" and "What would you do if there was a fire in the wastepaper basket?"

ASSESSMENT OF CRANIAL NERVES

CRANIAL NERVE I: OLFACTORY

With the client's eyes closed, one nostril at a time is tested (the client occludes the other with a finger). The nurse has the client identify familiar *odors*, such as coffee, tobacco, mint, or soap. Alcohol sponges and ammonia are not used, as these stimulate the trigeminal nerve, not the olfactory. Lack of or decreased smell sensation may not be significant, as loss or decrease occurs with age, smoking, colds, and allergies. The client's report that smell was suddenly lost without a predisposing factor or that odors are distorted is more significant.

CRANIAL NERVE II: OPTIC

Each eye is tested alone with the other eye covered but open. *Central* vision is tested by the Snellen chart, asking the client to read out loud from a pocket reader card, a magazine, or a newspaper. The test should be done with glasses if the client uses glasses for far or near vision.

Peripheral vision can be tested by asking the client to focus his/her eye on the examiner's nose. The nurse wiggles one finger of each hand in the superior visual field, asking the client to indicate where the movement is. He/she should see movement on both sides. The nurse then repeats in the inferior visual field. To begin testing the second eye, the nurse wiggles the finger of only one hand to prevent the client from repeating the previous answers. The nurse then tests the superior and inferior fields using a finger of each hand. If the client cannot see the fingers in one or more of the fields, further testing is required. The *fundus*, or internal eye, is inspected with the ophthalmoscope to check for vascular problems, retinal disease, papilledema, or optic atrophy. Special training is required for the nurse to operate the ophthalmoscope.

CRANIAL NERVE III: OCULOMOTOR

Eye movement (medial, superior and medial, superior and lateral, and inferior and lateral) is tested with the assessment of cranial nerve VI. *Pupil constriction* is tested with the room darkened, if possible. The nurse brings the penlight in from the side or from above or below and shines the light in the client's eye. The pupil should constrict and stay constricted. The nurse repeats with the other eye and watches for *consensual* (involuntary) constriction in the eye not being tested (consensual response will be less than direct response). Pupils should be equal in size, round, regular, and react to light and accommodation (PERRLA). The pupils should react to light with the *same rate* of speed and to the *same degree*. Glaucoma, cataract surgery, and iridectomy may influence the shape and size of the pupil, as well as its reaction to light. A pupil may dilate slightly after constricting with the light stimulus still present (Gunn's pupil sign); this reaction may be normal. However, if the dilation is marked, it may represent optic nerve or retinal pathologic changes. A few people have one pupil larger than the other (Adie's pupil); this may also be normal, if there are no other eye symptoms. The client is usually aware of the size difference. Adie's pupil is slow to react to light and constricts only a little. *Accommodation* is tested by bringing an object from far to near the client's eyes. The pupils should constrict and the eyes converge (turn in to focus on the object). Accommodation need not be tested if constriction to light is normal. Some medications may affect constriction and dilation. To assess for *lid elevation*, the upper eyelid should rest approximately at the top or slightly below the top of the pupil. Strength and closure of the lid are a function of cranial nerve VII, but can be tested with the eye examination.

CRANIAL NERVE IV: TROCHLEAR

Eye movement (inferior and medial) is tested with assessment of cranial nerve VI.

CRANIAL NERVE V: TRIGEMINAL

The client's eyes are closed for the *sensory* portion of the testing. The nurse asks the client to indicate when touched by saying "now." By stroking a piece of cotton over the client's skin (*light touch*), the nurse tests all three branches of the trigeminal nerve (ophthalmic—forehead, maxillary—cheek, mandibular—jaw), alternating sides for comparison. Next, the nurse asks the client to indicate whether the sensation is sharp or dull while using an object that has sharp and dull components (e.g., a safety pin) and then repeats the process. The *motor* aspect can be done with the client's eyes open. The nurse palpates the temporal and masseter (jaw) muscles (with one hand on each side) for strength and equality while the client clenches her/his teeth. The *corneal reflex* has traditionally been tested by using a wisp of cotton and touching the edge of the cornea, which normally causes blinking. However, that procedure can cause abrasion to the cornea. In a routine examination, blinking will be seen by the examiner and the corneal reflex need not be tested. If there is concern that the corneal reflex is absent, there are two safer ways to test. One is to bring a fist quickly toward the client's face in a threatening motion. If the client has vision, this will cause blinking. Alternatively, the nurse can use a syringe full of air and expel it toward the eyes. Blinking will result if the reflex is intact.

CRANIAL NERVE VI: ABDUCENS

Eye movement, a function of cranial nerves of III, IV, and VI, is tested by checking the *six cardinal positions of gaze*. The nurse asks the client to follow the examiner's finger or a held object while keeping his/her head still. The nurse starts at 1 o'clock position and moves clockwise through the six positions shown in Figure 32–12. The nurse pauses in the horizontal and vertical positions to check for *nystagmus* (involuntary oscillation of the eyes) or deviation. Some nystagmus in the extreme lateral position is normal. Severe lateral nystagmus or nystagmus in any other position is abnormal. If there is weakness or paralysis of a particular muscle, the eye will not turn in that direction.

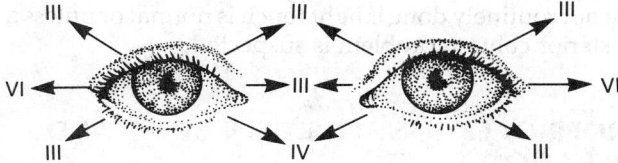

Figure 32–12

Checking extraocular movements in the six cardinal positions indicates the functioning of cranial nerves III, IV, and VI.

CRANIAL NERVE VII: FACIAL

Only the *motor* aspect is tested. Testing of taste on the anterior portion of the tongue is done with cranial nerve IX testing. The nurse asks the client to *frown, smile, wrinkle the forehead*, and *puff out the cheeks*, while looking for symmetry of both sides. *Eyelid closure and strength* are tested by asking the client to close the eyes tightly and keep them closed while the examiner tries to pry them open.

CRANIAL NERVE VIII: VESTIBULOCOCHLEAR (ACOUSTIC)

Hearing is tested initially with the client's eyes closed. The nurse rubs a thumb and finger together next to the client's ear and asks where sound is heard and then repeats this maneuver for the other ear. A watch can also be used, or the examiner can whisper close to each ear. The Weber and Rinne tests (with the client's eyes open) are done to check for conductive or sensorineural hearing loss. *Conductive* hearing loss occurs because of external-ear and middle-ear problems (e.g., excessive cerumen, presence of pus, ossicle fusion, or a damaged eardrum. *Sensorineural* loss occurs because of cochlear or nerve damage. In the *Weber* test, in which a vibrating tuning fork is placed on top of the head or the forehead, the client should hear sound equally in both ears. (Touching the fork tines will stop the vibration; therefore, the fork must be held by the handle only.) With conductive loss, the sound is heard louder in the ear with the deficit because the sound bypasses the obstruction. The sound will be louder in the better ear in sensorineural loss. The *Rinne* test, in which a vibrating tuning fork is placed on the mastoid bone until sound is no longer heard and then moved near the external ear canal, measures the difference between bone and air conduction. Normal, or *positive*, results occur when the client hears the sound about twice as long by air conduction as by bone. In conductive hearing loss, the client hears the sound longer through bone (*negative* Rinne's test). The sound is heard longer by air than by bone (positive) in sensorineural loss (see also p. 1083). *Equilibrium*, although controlled by cranial nerve VIII, is generally tested with cerebellar testing at the end of the examination to avoid having the client stand and sit excessively.

CRANIAL NERVE IX: GLOSSOPHARYNGEAL

The *motor* portion is tested with cranial nerve X assessment. *Taste* (posterior one-third of tongue) is often not tested unless the client reports loss of taste. When testing taste, it is important to remember the tongue must be rinsed in between the sweet, sour, bitter, and salt samples. Taste only occurs when the substance is in solution, so the tongue must be moist for a true test result.

CRANIAL NERVE X: VAGUS

The *motor* portion is tested by asking the client to say "Ah" when the examiner looks into the throat. The uvula and palate should rise bilaterally and equally. Stimulating the gag reflex with a tongue blade reflects sensitivity to a stimulus. Ability to *swallow* and *normal phonation* also imply intact nerves IX and X.

CRANIAL NERVE XI: SPINAL ACCESSORY

The *strength* of the sternocleidomastoid and trapezius muscles is tested by having the client turn his/her head against the resistance (provided by the examiner's hand on the side of the face toward the turn) and then repeat in the other direction. The second test requires the client to shrug his/her shoulders upward against the resistance of the examiner's hands placed on the client's shoulders.

CRANIAL NERVE XII: HYPOGLOSSAL

Motor innervation to the tongue is tested by asking the client to stick out her/his tongue. The nurse checks for deviation to one side or the other. The tongue deviates toward the same side where the lesion has occurred in the brain. *Strength* may be tested by asking the client to push against a tongue blade held at one side of the tongue and then repeat on the other side.

ASSESSMENT OF SENSORY FUNCTION

Sensory examination of the client is done in as expedient a manner as possible, as the entire procedure soon causes fatigue and makes test results questionable. A few tests can be done to give an accurate assessment for the client who has not complained of any sensory loss. Sensory testing of the face is completed when testing the trigeminal nerve.

PAIN AND TEMPERATURE

Pain and *temperature* sensations are transmitted by the same nerve endings. Therefore, if one sensation is tested and found to be intact, it can be safely assumed the other is intact. The testing of temperature sensation is usually not accurate because it is difficult to keep vials of water at the appropriate temperatures (hot and cold) during testing. Pain sensation is relatively easy to test and is more reliable. Pain can be tested with any objects that are perceived as being sharp or dull. A safety pin has a sharp and a dull end. A needle is sharp and the hub end is dull (the needle cap can be used for the dull component). The nurse instructs the client to keep her/his eyes closed and to indicate whether the touch is sharp or dull.

It may be necessary to first demonstrate with the client's eyes open what will be done. The sharp and dull stimuli should be interchanged at random so the client does not anticipate the type of the next stimulus. Not all dermatomes need to be tested. Testing at one site on the upper arm, the lower arm, the hand, the thigh, the lower leg, and the foot suffices. If testing is begun on the hands and feet, there is no need to test the more proximal parts of the extremities, as the tracts transmitting pain and temperature sensations are intact. The nurse compares reactions on each side. A sensation reported as dull when the stimulus was actually sharp necessitates more finite testing. A client with sensory loss is generally aware of the loss and points it out to the examiner.

LIGHT TOUCH

Light touch is tested by taking a piece of cotton or a cotton swab and lightly stroking the client's skin over some of the dermatomes. While the client's eyes are closed, the nurse asks the client to say "now" when touched. Testing once on each hand or wrist and each ankle or foot should be sufficient. It is unlikely that light touch discrimination is abnormal if pain and temperature sensations are intact.

TOUCH DISCRIMINATION AND TWO-POINT DISCRIMINATION

With the client's eyes closed, the nurse touches the client with a finger and asks that he/she point to the area touched. This procedure is repeated at various points on each extremity, by randomly picking points rather than in sequence. Next, the nurse touches the client on each side of the body on corresponding sites at the same time. The client should be able to point to both sites. Inability to sense touch on one side is called the *extinction phenomenon* (a subtle test for sensory loss). Then, with two objects such as cotton-tipped applicators, the nurse touches the client in two places on the same extremity. Normally a person can identify two points fairly close together, depending on where the stimuli are. The more nerve innervation an area has, the closer is *two-point discrimination*. For instance, two points around the mouth, on the fingers and the feet, or around the eyes can be identified at closer range than can two points the same distance apart on the leg or the back. These tests are not routinely done if light touch is normal or unless a posterior column problem is suspected.

PROPRIOCEPTION: POSITION SENSE AND VIBRATION SENSE

Position sense is tested with the client's eyes closed. The nurse grasps the great toe on either side between thumb and index finger and moves the toe *up* or *down*, asking the client to indicate the direction of movement. It is important not to grasp the toe by the anterior and posterior aspects because the pressure of the fingers will indicate the direction of movement. The same test is done on the thumbs if upper-extremity problems are apparent.

Vibration sense is tested with the use of the tuning fork. After the client closes his/her eyes, the nurse places a vibrating tuning fork on the bony part of the ankle or the wrist. The client indicates the *onset* and *cessation* of vibration. The length of time the client feels the vibration can be compared with a normal response by using the nurse as a control. This posterior column function decreases with age, and in the elderly there may be a normally decreased duration of vibration sensation.

GRAPHESTHESIA AND STEREOGNOSIS

Graphesthesia is tested by using an object, such as a capped pen, to write a number or a letter on the palm of the client's hand. Normally, the letters or numbers are identified correctly. *Stereognosis* is the recognition by *feel* alone of an object placed in the hand. A key, a coin, and a pen are ordinary objects that should be recognized. Both tests are performed with the client's eyes closed.

ABNORMAL SENSORY FINDINGS

Abnormal sensory findings may have a PNS or a CNS cause. Those attributable to a PNS cause include the neuropathies of diabetes, malnutrition, or vascular problems, and generally involve the whole extremity or both extremities. Damage to a specific spinal nerve may not show significant sensory loss because the spinal nerves overlap. Injury to several adjacent spinal nerves is manifested as decreased or absent sensation in the dermatomes of those nerves. CNS problems can occur within the spinal cord, the brain stem, the cerebellum, and the cortex. Sensory deficits attributable to spinal cord damage vary with the location of the damage. Involvement of only the posterior column leads to lost proprioception below the level of the damage on the same side or on both sides (if both right and left posterior columns are involved). A lesion involving only the *right spinothalamic tract* results in loss of pain and temperature sensation below the lesion on the *left* side. Problems in the brain stem, the thalamus, and the cortex generally result in loss of sensation on the *contralateral* side of the body. Cerebellar lesions affect sensation on the same side of the body as the lesion.

ASSESSMENT OF MOTOR FUNCTION

Throughout the examination, the client can be observed for involuntary tremors or movements. The characteristics of these movements, if present, need to be described as accurately as possible, for example, "pill rolling with the thumbs and fingers at rest" or "intention tremors of both hands" (tremors occurring when the person tries to do something).

Motor function is best tested by putting each joint and extremity through range of motion with and without resistance. The head and neck muscles are tested during the examination of the cranial nerves. *Hand strength* is measured by asking the client to grasp and squeeze two fingers of each of the examiner's hands. The nurse then compares the grasps for equality of strength. After comparison, the nurse tries to withdraw the fingers from the grasp and compares the ease or difficulty as another means of evaluating strength. The client should release the grasps on command, which is another assessment of consciousness.

Cerebral or *brain stem integrity* is assessed in the following procedure: The nurse asks the client to close his/her eyes and hold the arms perpendicular to the body with palms up for 15 to 30 seconds. If there is a cerebral or brain stem reason for muscle weakness, the arm on the weak side will start to fall, or "drift," with the palm pronating (turning inward). The same can be done for the lower extremities with the client lying on his/her stomach with the legs bent upward at the knees. However, it is easier for most clients to sit on the side of the bed and extend the legs outward.

Testing for strength *against resistance* is usually done by asking the client to resist the examiner's bending or straightening the client's arm, hand, leg, or foot, whichever is being tested at the time. A rating scale is commonly used (see Chap. 29, Table 29–1). The results of testing are sometimes recorded as 5/5, 3/5, and so forth, indicating the criteria that were used and the status of the client at that testing. It is important to evaluate and compare strength on each side. Later testing is compared with these and other previous results to indicate progress or regression.

Peripheral motor problems occur because of injury, neuropathies, vascular problems, or a localized lesion in the opposite motor cortex. Tremors, unintentional movements (clonus), and changes in gait or posture represent problems in the *basal ganglia* or specialized nuclei of the *brain stem*. Motor cortex lesions, such as cerebrovascular accidents (stroke), cause weakness or paralysis on the contralateral side of the body.

ASSESSMENT OF CEREBELLAR FUNCTION

Most of the assessment of cerebellar function can be done with the client sitting on the side of the bed or examining table. Fine coordination of muscle activity is tested. With the client's eyes closed, the nurse asks the client to perform the following: run the heel of one foot down the shin of the other leg and repeat with the other leg (the client should be able to do this smoothly and keep the heel on the shin); place the hands palm up and then palm down on each thigh, repeating as fast as possible (normally, this can be done rapidly); with arms out at the side, touch finger to nose, two or three times with eyes open and then with eyes closed (this can be done with alternating arms or with each arm individually). *Gait* and *equilibrium* can be tested at the end of the examination (see later).

If the client is unable to perform any of the above-mentioned activities smoothly, the problem is manifested on the same side as the cerebellar lesion. If both lobes of the cerebellum are involved, the incoordination is bilateral.

ASSESSMENT OF REFLEX ACTIVITY

Deep tendon reflexes assessed in a routine neurologic examination are the tendons of the biceps, triceps, brachioradialis, quadriceps, and Achilles' reflexes. The *cutaneous* (superficial) reflexes usually tested are the plantar reflexes and sometimes the abdominal reflexes (Table 32–6). The striking of the tendon with the hammer should cause contraction of the muscle (Fig. 32–13). The appropriate muscle contraction is indicative of an intact reflex arc. The nurse taps each tendon quickly, but not with too much force. The biceps reflex is tested by tapping the examiner's thumb placed over the tendon rather than tapping the tendon directly, as for the other reflexes. It sometimes helps to relax the client if the examiner supports the part being tested.

The *plantar reflex* is tested by using a pointed, but not sharp, object such as the handle end of the hammer or the rounded end of bandage scissors. The sole of the foot is stroked from the heel up the lateral side and then across the ball of the foot to the medial side. The normal response is plantar flexion of all toes. Dorsiflexion of the great toe and fanning of the other toes (*Babinski's sign*) is abnormal in anyone older than 2 years of age and represents the presence of *upper motor neuron* (CNS) disease. (Clinically, the terms positive Babinski's sign, meaning an abnormal response, and negative Babinski's sign, meaning a normal response, are used, but this is not exactly correct. Babinski's sign is present if the reaction is abnormal.) Babinski's sign can occur with drug and alcohol intoxication or after a seizure. It is a normal occurrence in infants and children younger than 2 years of age. The *abdominal reflex* is tested by stroking the abdomen in all four quadrants diagonally toward the umbilicus. The umbilicus should deviate toward the stimulus, but obesity may mask the reflex. It can be absent in both upper and lower (PNS) motor neuron disease.

Hyperactive reflexes are indicative of possible upper motor neuron disease, tetanus, or hypocalcemia. *Hypoactive* reflexes may result from lower motor neuron disease (damage to the spinal cord), disease of the neuromuscular junction, muscle disease, or metabolic diseases (diabetes mellitus, hypothyroidism, or hypokale-

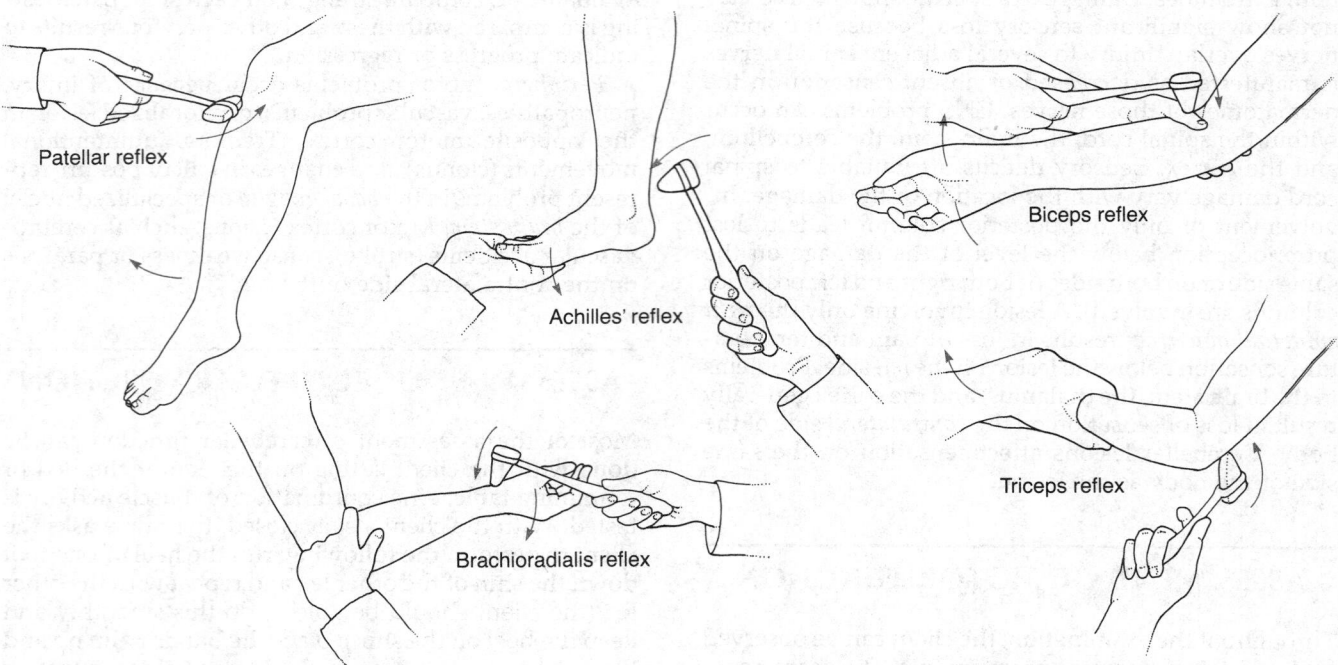

Figure 32–13

Procedures for testing deep tendon reflexes.

TABLE 32–6 Deep Tendon and Superficial Reflexes

Deep Tendon Reflexes

Jaw closure

Biceps

Triceps

Brachioradialis

Patellar

Achilles'

Superficial Reflexes

Corneal

Palatal

Pharyngeal

Abdominal (upper and lower)

Cremasteric

Gluteal

Plantar

mia). Although individuals can display hyperactive, hypoactive, or even absent reflexes, *asymmetry* is an important finding, as it likely indicates a disease process. The usual way to record the results of reflex testing is to use a stick figure and a 0 to 4 scale (Fig. 32–14). A score of 2 (++) is considered normal, although scores of 1 or 3

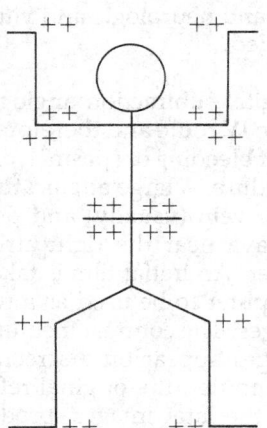

0	Absent, no response
1 (+)	Weaker than normal, hypoactive
2 (++)	Normal
3 (+++)	Stronger or more brisk than normal
4 (++++)	Hyperactive
	(Note: 1 and 3 may be normal for some individuals)

Figure 32–14

Stick figure and scale for recording reflex activity.

(hypoactive and hyperactive, respectively) may also be normal for a particular client.

REMAINING CEREBELLAR ASSESSMENT

The last part of the examination requires that the client stand to test *gait* and *equilibrium*. First, the nurse asks the client to walk across the room and return and observes the client for inequality in steps, difficulty maneuvering, and so forth. The nurse then asks the client to stand on one foot and then the other to evaluate balance. Tiptoe walking and heel-to-toe walking also can demonstrate cerebellar problems. Knee bends and one-leg squats are used as part of the testing, but these may be normally impossible for the elderly or nonathletic persons.

Equilibrium is tested by asking the client to stand with arms at his/her side, with feet and knees close together, and eyes open. The nurse checks for swaying and then asks the client to close his/her eyes and maintain position. The examiner should be close enough to the client to prevent falling should the client not have the ability to stay erect. If the client sways with the eyes closed, but not when open, it is probably a *proprioceptive* problem, which is referred to as a positive Romberg sign. If the client sways with eyes open and closed, the neurologic disturbance is probably *cerebellar* in origin.

DIAGNOSTIC ASSESSMENT

LABORATORY TESTS

For clients with a neurologic problem resulting from or concomitant with systemic infection, *blood cultures* are necessary to ascertain the causative agent of the infection. Although any client must have the cause of infection determined, this is especially true for clients with CNS disease. The blood-brain barrier is often not intact in neurologic disease, and the client is more susceptible to infection of the nervous system (meningitis).

RADIOGRAPHIC EXAMINATIONS

FLAT PLATE AND DECUBITUS

Plain x-ray films of the skull and spine are used to determine body fractures, curvatures, bone erosion, bone dislocation, and possible calcification of soft tissue, which can damage the nervous system. Several views are taken—anteroposterior, lateral, oblique, and, when necessary, special views of the facial bones. In head trauma and multiple injuries, cervical fracture must be ruled out by radiography as one of the first priorities.

The nurse explains that the procedure for obtaining x-ray films is similar to that for a chest x-ray, that the client will have to remain still during the procedure, and that the exposure to radiation is minimal. If the client is in traction, the nurse may need to accompany the client to assist with positioning if a portable x-ray unit is not available. Any client who cannot walk from a wheelchair to the x-ray table should go to the radiology department on a stretcher. The client is positioned for each of the views desired and is asked not to move just before the taking of each picture. Follow-up care is not required.

CEREBRAL ANGIOGRAPHY

Cerebral angiography (arteriography) illuminates cerebral circulation by injecting contrast medium into an artery (usually the femoral) and taking x-ray films sequentially as the contrast medium flows with the blood to visualize carotid, vertebral, and cerebral circulation. The purpose is to diagnose vascular aneurysms, malformations, displacements, and occluded or leaking vessels.

Contrast Media Method

Client preparation. The nurse ascertains that there are no allergies to contrast agents or iodine. The procedure is explained to the client initially by the person obtaining the written consent. The nurse can clarify the explanation by answering questions and reinforcing the following: the necessity for not moving during the procedure, the necessity for immobilization of the head, and the expectation of heat sensation from the contrast medium as it is injected. The client is allowed nothing by mouth for 6 to 8 hours before the test. Most health care institutions require that a preoperative check list be completed. The following interventions are performed: hairpins, jewelry, hearing aids, and dentures are removed; signed consent is obtained before preangiography sedation; neurologic and vital signs are recorded; and the client should be asked to empty his/her bladder. The nurse then administers the preangiography hypnotic, sedative, or analgesic as ordered.

Procedure. The client is placed on an examining table and secured with straps, and his/her head is placed within a headrest device or immobilized with tape. The artery to be used is located either by cutdown or palpation, and a catheter is threaded into the artery. Although the carotid or vertebral artery can be used, the femoral or brachial artery is preferred because the incidence of complications is decreased. Patency of the catheter is maintained with intravenous (IV) fluid. Contrast medium is injected (usually 40 to 50 mL), and a series of x-rays films are taken automatically as the contrast material moves through the circulation. The major risks are allergic response to the contrast medium and vaso-

spasm, either of which may result in discontinuation of the test. The vasospasm may be severe enough to cause occlusion and subsequent clotting. The resulting tissue ischemia can cause hemiparesis, paralysis, or speech difficulties, depending on the artery in spasm. This risk is about 0.5% to 1%. After the catheter is removed, pressure is maintained over the puncture site for 5 minutes or more to prevent arterial bleeding.

Follow-up care. The client is restricted to bed rest for 6 to 24 hours, with the extremity kept straight and immobilized for approximately the length of the bed rest. The nurse checks the extremity for adequate circulation, demonstrated by skin color and temperature, pulses distal to the injection site, and capillary refill. The injection site is checked frequently for evidence of bleeding. A pressure dressing, sandbag, icebag, or a combination of the three may be maintained over the site for 6 to 12 hours to prevent bleeding, swelling, or hematoma formation. The nurse checks neurologic and vital signs frequently for the first hour or two and compares them with the preangiography signs. Oral or IV fluid intake is increased, if not contraindicated, to help the client excrete the contrast material (for approximately 24 hours).

Digital Subtraction Method

Client preparation. The nurse determines if the client has allergies to contrast agents or iodine. Food intake is restricted for 2 hours before the test, but fluids are not. Instructions for remaining still (as for the contrast method) are given to the client by the nurse. Individual health care institutions may require a signed consent. A preprocedural check list may or may not be necessary, depending on the institution, but the client must empty her/his bladder and neurologic and vital signs must be taken and recorded.

Procedure. Digital subtraction angiography (DSA) is done through the IV route and therefore has the advantage of less risk of bleeding or spasm. It can be done as an outpatient procedure. A large angiocatheter is threaded into the brachial vein (usually) and positioned in the superior vena cava near the right atrium. IV fluid is given via catheter. An initial film is taken; the image is placed in a computer to be used as a reference for the subsequent images. The contrast medium is injected. As subsequent images appear on a screen and are transferred to the computer, the original reference image is *subtracted* from the later images, producing a heightened image. Although not quite as satisfactory as the contrast method, DSA is the best choice for some clients.

Follow-up care. The nurse checks the extremity for adequate circulation, as outlined for the contrast media method, and checks the IV injection site for any drainage (because of the large size of the catheter). The nurse encourages the client to increase fluid intake for 24 hours after the procedure to help contrast medium excretion, unless increased fluid intake is contraindicated. There are no bed rest restrictions.

MYELOGRAPHY

Myelography involves the injection of a liquid or air contrast substance into the lumbar subarachnoid space to visualize the spinal structures. The reader is referred to Chapter 29 for further description of the procedure, client preparation, and follow-up care.

COMPUTED TOMOGRAPHY

Computed tomography (CT) has been a significant tool in advancing neurologic diagnoses. With the aid of a computer, pictures are taken at many horizontal levels, or slices, of the brain or spinal cord. The resulting pictures distinguish bone and soft tissue, such as the brain, the vascular system, and the ventricular system.

Client preparation. The nurse explains the procedure and ascertains whether the client has allergies to iodine. The client is instructed to remove hairpins, hair pieces, or wigs from the head. Food may or may not be withheld for 4 to 6 hours before the test if contrast medium is used. Fluids are generally not withheld. The nurse alerts the physician if the client seems unduly anxious, fearful, or unable to cooperate. Preprocedure sedation may be ordered, although it is not usually necessary.

Procedure. The client is placed on a movable table with his/her head positioned in a holding device, which is then secured. The angles for the desired pictures are determined. The client must be completely still during the test, which may be difficult for some individuals. The table is then positioned within the machine (a large cylinder-type structure). Some clients are fearful of the machine or being confined in a small space. A noncontrast series of pictures is taken first. Contrast media enhance the visualization of the vascular system and are frequently used. Other than the injection of contrast media, the procedure is noninvasive. The entire procedure takes 10 minutes or less with the newer machines, and 40 minutes with older machines or the use of contrast media.

Follow-up care. The nurse checks for delayed allergic response to contrast medium, if it was used. If contrast medium was used, the resulting diuresis may require the administration of replacement fluids.

OTHER DIAGNOSTIC STUDIES

LUMBAR PUNCTURE

Lumbar puncture (spinal tap) is the insertion of a spinal needle into the subarachnoid space between the third and fourth lumbar vertebrae (sometimes the fourth and fifth lumbar vertebrae). Lumbar puncture is used to

1. Obtain pressure readings with a manometer
2. Obtain CSF for analysis
3. Check for spinal blockage attributable to a spinal cord lesion
4. Inject contrast medium or air for diagnostic study (Chap. 29)
5. Inject anesthetic (spinal anesthesia) (Chap. 7)
6. Inject certain medications
7. Reduce mild to moderate increased intracranial pressure in certain conditions

The procedure is contraindicated in clients with symptoms suggestive of increased intracranial pressure, except under extreme conditions (the procedure is then different from the one described here) because of the danger of sudden release of CSF pressure. The sudden release causes a sudden shift of cranial tissue known as uncal herniation, which results in more damage. The procedure is also contraindicated in clients with skin infections at or near the puncture site because of the danger of introducing infective organisms into the CSF.

Client preparation. The nurse asks the client if he/she has had the procedure before. The procedure is similar to the myelogram described in Chapter 29. If the answer is yes, the nurse determines what the client remembers about the procedure, such as any discomfort or difficulty. The client who has not had the test needs an explanation. A specific signed consent may or may not be necessary, depending on the policy of the health care institution. The nurse asks the client to empty his/her bladder as a comfort measure and then positions the client on whichever side he/she is most comfortable, with the back close to the edge of the bed or examining table. When the physician is ready, the nurse asks the client to bring the knees up as close as possible to the trunk and to assume a "fetal" position (using his/her arms to hold the knees in place) with head bent forward. Some clients need help in achieving and maintaining this position. The nurse grasps the client behind the knees and the back of the lower neck to help maintain the position. A pillow under the head and between the knees aids body alignment.

Procedure. The skin site is thoroughly cleaned. The injection site is determined, and a local anesthetic is injected. A few minutes after the anesthetic is injected, the physician inserts a spinal needle with stylet between the third and fourth vertebrae. After proper placement in the subarachnoid space is determined by removing the stylet and seeing CSF, the client is instructed to relax a little so the pressure reading will be more accurate. Opening and closing pressure readings are taken and recorded. Usually three to five test tubes of CSF are collected and numbered sequentially. After the specimens are collected, the needle is withdrawn; slight pres-

TABLE 32–7 Significance of Cerebrospinal Fluid Findings

Findings	Significance
Pressure	
70–180 mmH$_2$O (5–13 mmHg)	Normal range.
65–195 mmH$_2$O (4–15 mmHg)	Upper limits of normal.
Color/Appearance	
Clear, colorless	Normal.
Pink-red to orange	Red blood cells present.
Yellow	Bilirubin present owing to hemolysis of red blood cells. Possible causes include subarachnoid hemorrhage, jaundice, increased CSF protein, hypercarotenemia, or hemoglobinemia.
Brown	Methemoglobin present, indicating prior meningeal hemorrhage.
Unclear or hazy	Cell count greater than 200/mL.
Cells	
0–5 small lymphocytes/mm³	Normal range.
More than 5 lymphocytes/mm³	Reaction to infection, tumor, chemical substance, or blood.
Proteins	
Total	
15–45 mg/100 mL (or less than 1% of serum levels)	Normal range.
45–100 mg/100 mL	Paraventricular tumor.
50–200 mg/100 mL	Viral infection.
More than 500 mg/100 mL	Bacterial infection, Guillain-Barré syndrome.
Less than 15 mg/100 mL	Meningismus, pseudotumor cerebri, hyperthyroidism, normal finding after lumbar puncture.
Immune Gamma Globulin (IgG, the most important protein)	
3%–12% of *total* protein	Normal range.
More than 3%–12% of total protein	Multiple sclerosis, neurosyphilis, or viral infection.
Albumin/Globulin Ratio	
8:1	Normal range.

sure is applied; and an adhesive bandage strip is placed over the insertion site. The nurse may or may not be able to help with the collection and numbering of the specimens, depending on the client's ability or inability to remain quiet. If the client is restless or unable to cooperate, the procedure may need two people assisting in-stead of one. The nurse considers this possibility before beginning the procedure.

Examination of CSF has been a useful diagnostic tool for some time, and recent technical advances are increasing the number of analyses that can be done on CSF. The normal characteristics of CSF and some of the

TABLE 32–7   Significance of Cerebrospinal Fluid Findings *Continued*

Findings	Significance
Glucose	
45–80 mg/100 mL	Normal range.
Less than 45 mg/100 mL (usually accompanied by the presence of pathologic organisms)	Bacterial, fungal, or viral meningitis; CNS leukemia; or cancer.
Electrolytes and Minerals	
Sodium	
144–154 mEq/L	Normal range (abnormal values are not disease specific).
Potassium	
2.4–3.1 mEq/L	Normal range (abnormal values are not disease specific).
Chloride	
118–132 mEq/L	Normal range (abnormal values are not disease specific).
Calcium	
2.1–2.7 mEq/L	Normal range (abnormal values are not disease specific).
Other Characteristics	
Lactic Acid	
10–20 mg/dL	Normal range.
More than 10–20 mg/dL	Systemic acidosis or increased CSF glucose metabolism.
Urea	
10–15 mg/dL	Normal range.
More than 10–15 mg/dL	Uremia, meningitis, or urea administration.
Glutamine	
Less than 20 mg/dL	Normal range.
More than 20 mg/dL	Hepatic coma or cirrhosis of liver.
Lactate Dehydrogenase	
10% of serum level	Normal value.
More than 10% of serum level	Bacterial meningitis, inflammatory diseases of CNS.

more common abnormalities are given in Table 32–7. Gram's stain smears are done to test for particular types of meningitis, such as tubercular meningitis. CSF can be cultured, and sensitivity studies are performed to determine the best choice of antibiotic if an infection is diagnosed. A specific test for neurosyphilis is the fluorescent treponemal antibody absorption (FTA-ABS) test. Cytologic studies can be performed on CSF to identify tumor cells.

Follow-up care.   The client is restricted to bed rest in a flat position for 4 to 12 hours, as prescribed by the physician or determined by institutional policy to prevent CSF leakage from the puncture site. The nurse encourages the client to increase fluid intake (to 3000 mL) for 24 to 48 hours to facilitate CSF production. A decrease in CSF may cause the client to experience a severe, throbbing headache. Analgesics can be given for headache if it occurs. If the lumbar puncture was done to reduce intracranial pressure, the assessment of neurologic signs, especially level of consciousness, should be performed more frequently until stability is ensured. Complications of lumbar puncture are not common, but include infection, CSF leakage, and hematoma formation.

ELECTROENCEPHALOGRAPHY

Electroencephalography (EEG) is the recording of the electrical activity of the cerebral hemispheres. Each graphic recording represents the changes in voltage in various areas of the brain (determined by recording the difference between two electrodes). The test is done to

1. Determine the general activity of the cerebral hemispheres
2. Determine the origin of seizure activity (epilepsy)
3. Determine cerebral function in pathologic conditions other than epilepsy (tumors, abscesses, cerebrovascular disease, hematomas, injury, metabolic diseases, degenerative brain disease, and drug intoxication)
4. Differentiate between organic and hysterical or feigned blindness or deafness
5. Monitor cerebral activity during surgical anesthesia
6. Diagnose sleep disorders (all-night EEG)
7. Determine brain death

Client preparation. The nurse explains the test. If the EEG is ordered with the client "sleep deprived," the client should be kept awake from about 2 to 3 AM through the night. CNS depressants and stimulants are usually not administered for 24 hours before the test. The physician indicates whether anticonvulsants are to be withheld; if withheld, the nurse monitors the client for signs of seizure activity. The nurse withholds coffee, tea, and other stimulants, but food and other fluids *are* given because *hypoglycemia* affects brain activity. The nurse checks to make sure the hair is clean and free from hairpins, sprays, or oils.

Procedure. The client is placed on a reclining chair or bed. Usually, 16 to 24 electrodes are attached to the scalp with a jelly-like substance, according to an internationally accepted procedure, and connected to the machine. A glue is placed over the electrodes to prevent slippage. The client must lie still with the eyes closed during the initial recording. The rest of the test involves the client in certain activities (activating procedures). These include hyperventilation, photic stimulation, and sleep.

Hyperventilation produces cerebral vasoconstriction and alkalosis, which increases the likelihood of seizure activity; the client is asked to breathe deeply 20 to 30 times for 3 minutes.

In *photic stimulation,* a strobe light (a bright light) is placed in front of the client; frequencies of 1 to 20 flashes per second are used with the client's eyes open and then closed. The EEG shows waves corresponding to each flash of light or waves indicating seizure activity if the client's seizures are photosensitive in origin.

Sleep is either natural or induced by an oral or IV sedative. Waves indicative of temporal lobe epilepsy can be best demonstrated during sleep.

Throughout the test, which takes 40 to 60 minutes, the examiner watches the client closely and records any movement. These movements alter the record and must be labeled as artefacts. Examples of artefacts are tongue movement, eyeblinking, muscle tenseness, and nervousness.

Follow-up care. The nurse removes the jelly-like substance and glue from the scalp and hair, if this is not done in the EEG laboratory, with acetone and then shampoo. Any medications that were withheld are reinstituted, and provision for a nap made if client was deprived of sleep before the test.

MAGNETIC RESONANCE IMAGING

Magnetic resonance imaging is one of the newest diagnostic tools used to detect neurologic problems. Through the use of a large magnetic field and the introduction of a specific radio frequency, protons of the body absorb and emit energy, which is then converted to a picture or an image on a screen or magnetic tape. The resulting images are clear for all densities of tissue. It surpasses the CT in clarity for many types of tissue and lesions, does not involve exposure to radiation, and is noninvasive. This diagnostic procedure is also discussed in Chapter 29.

POSITRON EMISSION TOMOGRAPHY

Positron emission tomography is another new diagnostic tool available only in larger medical centers at present. The client is injected with the radioisotope oxyglucose. The isotope emits activity in the form of positrons, which are scanned and converted into an image by computer. The image is displayed in color. The more active a given part of the brain is, the greater the glucose uptake is. This test is being used extensively in the diagnosis of and research on Alzheimer's disease. The level of radiation is equivalent to that experienced when five or six x-ray films are obtained, but much less than the exposure during CT. One problem at present is that the radioisotopes have such a short life that there must be a cyclotron on the premises to prepare them, which limits the number of medical centers able to offer the test.

Client preparation.   The nurse explains the test and withholds caffeine, alcohol, and tobacco for 24 hours before the test. The client should eat a meal 3 to 4 hours before the procedure (with insulin, if the client is diabetic; no insulin is given before the test). The nurse withholds any other drugs that alter glucose metabolism.

Procedure and follow-up care.   The client sits on a reclining chair in front of the scanner. An IV line is started in each hand or arm — one to inject the isotope and the other to obtain blood samples. The arm used for blood samples is warmed to get arterial (shunted) and venous blood. The client may be blindfolded and have earplugs inserted for all or part of the test and must be still for an hour to an hour and a half. The client is asked to perform certain mental functions, which then activate different areas of the brain. The radioisotope is eliminated in the urine, which requires no special precautions. Follow-up care is not required.

ELECTROMYOGRAPHY

Electromyography records the electrical activity of peripheral nerves by testing muscle activity (see Chap. 29 for description of client preparation, procedure, and follow-up care).

CALORIC TEST OR ELECTRONYSTAGMOGRAPHY

Testing of vestibular function is accomplished by caloric stimulation or electronystagmography (ENG). *Caloric testing* involves the instillation of cold and then warm water into the ear canals to elicit nystagmus. The *ENG test* is done by placing electrodes near the eyes; these transmit eye movements, which are recorded on graph paper. The two tests can be done separately or in conjunction.

Client preparation.   The nurse explains the test and withholds food and fluids for 6 to 8 hours before the caloric test to lessen the incidence of vomiting. (There are no restrictions for the ENG test.) The client is asked to empty the bladder as a comfort measure. For the caloric test, the tympanic membranes must be intact (with no perforations), which is checked by the *person ordering the test* or the *person performing the test*. For the ENG test, the nurse asks the client to remove any makeup around the eyes.

Procedure.   The client is positioned on a chair (usually in a diagnostic laboratory) with the head tilted forward 30 degrees. The client is instructed to maintain eye con-

tact with a certain object, which enables the examiner to observe eye movement during the test. One ear is irrigated with cold water (7° C below body temperature) for 30 seconds. The normal result is *slow* movement of the eyes *toward* the side of irrigation followed by *fast* movement to the *opposite* side. After a wait of 5 minutes, the ear is irrigated with warm water (7° C above body temperature). The normal result is nystagmus to the irrigated side. The other ear is then tested in the same way. The instillation of fluid usually produces nausea, vertigo, and occasionally vomiting. The client may be placed in another position or asked to perform some cerebellar assessments (finger-to-nose touch or Romberg's test). Abnormal findings of no nystagmus or nystagmus in directions other than normal are found in Meniere's disease, coma, certain brain tumors, and brain stem pathologic states.

For ENG, the client is recumbent and electrodes are secured to the skin near the eyes and then attached to a machine that records the eye movements graphically. The client must keep his/her eyes closed during the entire test and may be asked to change positions at various intervals. A small amount of cold or warm water (0.2 mL) may be instilled into the ear canal as a stimulus.

Follow-up care.   For the caloric test, the client is restricted to bed rest until abatement of any nausea, vomiting, or vertigo. The ENG requires no follow-up care unless a caloric stimulus was used.

OCULOPLETHYSMOGRAPHY

Oculoplethysmography is a study of carotid artery blood flow by monitoring one of its branches, the ophthalmic artery. The systolic pressure of each ophthalmic artery is measured by raising the *intraocular* pressure above *systolic* ophthalmic arterial pressure. This is accomplished by instilling anesthetic eyedrops, placing suction cups that resemble contact lenses on the cornea, and applying pressure. The pressure is then released and the reappearance of pulsation is measured as the systolic pressure of the ophthalmic artery. The eyes are compared for circulatory assessment. Other than explaining the test and checking for corneal abrasion after the procedure, there is no client preparation or follow-up care.

CEREBRAL BLOOD FLOW DETERMINATION

Cerebral blood flow can be determined for many areas of the brain. A radioactive substance is injected intravenously, or the client inhales a radioactive gas. Sensors placed over the scalp follow the isotope flow through the brain circulation. Local blood flow increases can be seen with any neuronal activity, such as reading, hand movement, seizures, and temperature elevation (up to 42° C). Local blood flow decreases with degenerative disease, comas of metabolic origin, increased intracranial pressure, and subarachnoid hemorrhage.

Client preparation. The nurse explains the test and withholds CNS depressants and stimulants if drugs have previously been ordered, for 24 hours before the test. The nurse checks to make sure the client's hair is clean and hairpins are removed.

Procedure and follow-up care. The client must be able to relax mentally and physically. Sensors or probes connected to a computer are attached to the scalp. The radioactive isotope (usually xenon) is injected intravenously or the client inhales the radioactive gas (xenon) through a mouthpiece (with the nostrils occluded) or a mask for 1 minute. The client receives various stimuli during the test. The results are studied in light of the client's suspected neurologic problem. Follow-up care is not required.

EVOKED POTENTIALS

Evoked potentials are recordings of electrical potentials of the brain's response to external stimuli. The cortical activity of the sensory organs (eyes or ears) and peripheral nerves is processed by computer to identify conduction problems along a given pathway. Visual evoked potentials (VEP) can identify retrobulbar problems in clients with no overt signs of visual impairment.

Auditory pathways can be tested via auditory evoked potentials. This test is also referred to as brain stem auditory evoked potentials. Peripheral nerve pathways and the cortical somatosensory area are tested in a like manner. The median, peroneal, and tibial nerves are used for those tests. The somatosensory tests are somatosensory evoked potentials (SEP) or short-latency SEP. Problems in conduction can be identified in the spinal roots, the posterior column, the brain stem, and the parietal cortex. Monitoring SEP on a continuous basis as an assessment tool is currently being tried in some critical care units.

Client preparation. The nurse explains the test and checks to be sure the client's hair is clean and hairpins are removed.

Procedure and follow-up care. The procedure may be done in the EEG laboratory or other diagnostic laboratory and can take up to 45 minutes to complete. The electrodes are secured with a paste substance to the scalp. VEP requires electrode placement near the eyes, the parietal lobe, and the occipital lobe. The client is shown a changing checkerboard pattern (or a flashing light), one eye at a time, as a stimulus (use of the checkerboard requires a cooperative client). The activity is recorded graphically. The electrodes for auditory testing are placed on the ear lobe and over the top of the head (vertex). The client is exposed to a clicking noise in each ear. Peripheral testing is done by applying electrical stimuli (which is painless) over the ulnar, median, peroneal, or tibial nerve. Electrodes are placed over the lumbar and cervical spine, the clavicle, and the opposite parietal lobe, depending on which extremity is being tested. A delay in conduction between any of the sites — peripheral and lumbar, lumbar and upper spine, or upper spine and parietal lobe — locates the conduction defect. Cleaning hair of glues as necessary is all that is required for follow-up care by the nurse.

BRAIN SCAN

The *brain scan* is a radionuclide imaging study using a radioactive substance to detect certain pathologic conditions. The test is especially useful in evaluating vascular abnormalities, such as aneurysms, and locating tumors, hematomas, and abscesses. As technologic advances in diagnostic testing continue, this test may be performed less frequently.

Client preparation. The nurse explains the test and asks the client to empty her/his bladder as a comfort measure. A signed consent may be necessary.

Procedure and follow-up care. The client is injected with a radioactive isotope, usually 99^mTc. There is a delay in the test of up to 2 hours while waiting for absorption of the isotope by the brain. The client is placed on a table and must remain still with the hands at his/her side for the duration of the test. The test takes 1 to 2 hours, depending on the number of scannings used. For follow-up care, the nurse provides fluid to promote isotope elimination (urine does not need special handling).

CAROTID PHONOANGIOGRAPHY AND CAROTID DOPPLER FLOW ANALYSIS

These tests are performed to determine carotid artery narrowing or occlusion. The lumen size of the carotid arteries can be measured through the use of amplified sound, which is then converted to a graphic picture. An electronic microphone is placed over the client's carotid arteries for the phonoangiography; a directional Doppler probe is used in the flow analysis. Other than explaining these tests, there is no client preparation or follow-up care.

SUMMARY

Knowledge of the anatomy and physiology of the nervous system guides the nurse in the assessment and management of the client with a neurologic problem.

Careful and accurate observations by the nurse assist the entire health care team in identifying diagnoses and interventions for a particular client. Increasingly advanced technology has made, and continues to make, neurologic tests more accurate, safer, and more tolerable for the client.

REFERENCES AND READINGS

Adams, R. D., & Victor, M. (1985). *Principles of neurology* (3rd ed.). New York: McGraw-Hill.

Barr, M. L., & Kiernan, J. A. (1989). *The human nervous system: An anatomical viewpoint.* (5th ed.).

Bates, B. (1987). *A guide to physical examination* (4th ed.). Philadelphia: J. B. Lippincott.

Carlson, N. R. (1986). *Physiology of behavior* (3rd ed.). Boston: Allyn & Bacon.

Cella, J. H., & Watson, J. (1989). *Nurse's manual of laboratory tests.* Philadelphia: F. A. Davis.

Giubilato, R. T., & Metcalf, J. (1984). Evoked potentials: Nursing perspectives. *Journal of Neurosurgical Nursing, 16,* 241–247.

Goldberg, S. (1984). *The four-minute neurological exam.* Miami: MedMaster.

Guyton, A. C. (1986). *Textbook of medical physiology* (7th ed.). Philadelphia: W. B. Saunders.

Hickey, J. (1986). *The clinical practice of neurological and neurosurgical nursing.* Philadelphia: J. B. Lippincott.

Hummelgard, A. B., Martin, E. M., & Singer, J. (1984). Prognostic value of brainstem auditory evoked potentials in head trauma. *Journal Neurosurgical Nursing, 16,* 181–187.

Lord-Ferolie, K., & Maguire-McGinty, M. (1985). Toward a more objective approach to pupil assessment. *Journal of Neurosurgical Nursing, 17,* 309–312.

Maida, M. J. (1982). Regional cerebral blood flow: Patient correlations. *Journal of Neurosurgical Nursing, 14,* 309–314.

Malasanos, L., Barkaukas, V., Moss, M., & Stoltenberg-Allen, K. (1986). *Health assessment* (3rd ed.). St. Louis: C. V. Mosby.

Marchette, L., & Holloman, F. (1985). A first hand report on the new body scanners. *RN, 48*(11), 28–31.

Mitchell, P. H., Cammermeyer, M., Ozuna, J., & Woods, N. F. (1984). *Neurological assessment for nursing practice.* Reston, VA: Reston Publishing.

Price, M. B., & DeVroom, H. L. (1985). A quick and easy guide to neurological assessment. *Journal of Neurosurgical Nursing, 17,* 313–320.

Rogers, A. E., & Dykstra, F. (1989). EEG's: A closer look at a familiar test. *Journal of Neuroscience Nursing, 21,* 227–233.

Rudy, E. B. (1984). *Advanced neurological and neurosurgical nursing.* St. Louis: C. V. Mosby.

Rudy, E. B. (1985). Magnetic resonance imaging: New horizons in diagnostic techniques. *Journal of Neurosurgical Nursing, 17,* 331–337.

Sherburne, E. (1985). Continuous somatosensory evoked potential monitoring in the NICU. *Journal of Neurosurgical Nursing, 17,* 247–252.

Smith, K. A., Cobb, C. A., & French, B. N. (1983). CAT scans: What do they tell us? *Journal of Neurosurgical Nursing, 15,* 222–227.

Snyder, M. (Ed.). (1983). *A guide to neurologic and neurosurgical nursing.* New York: Wiley.

Vogt, G., Miller, M., & Esluer, M. (1985). *Mosby's manual of neurological care.* St. Louis: C. V. Mosby.

ADDITIONAL READINGS

Cohen, S. N. (1987). The neurologic examination: Practical points, part 1. *Hospital Medicine, 23*(9), 21–42.

Cohen, S. N. (1987). The neurologic examination: Practical points, part 2. *Hospital Medicine, 23*(10), 27–42.
These articles discuss the fundamentals of the neurologic examination. Although written for the family practice physician, the material is presented in a clear, concise manner that will help nurses learn how to perform a complete neurologic physical assessment.

Stevens, S. A. (1988). A simple, step-by-step approach to neurologic assessment, part 1. *Nursing '88, 18*(9), 53–61.

Stevens, S. A. (1988). A simple step-by-step approach to neurologic assessment, part 2. *Nursing '88, 18*(10), 51–58.
These articles present a comprehensive, simplified system for performing a neurologic nursing assessment. The text is enhanced by illustrations that help the nurse understand the techniques used in the examination.

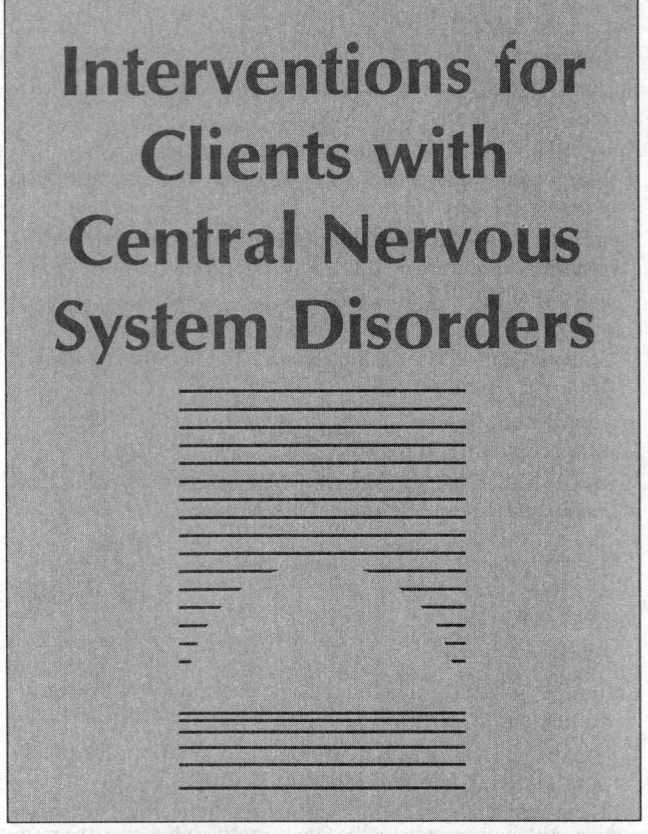

CHAPTER 33

Interventions for Clients with Central Nervous System Disorders

Dysfunction of the central nervous system (CNS) may be a mild disorder that a person can learn to live with, a devastating one that drastically affects the client and the family, or a degree between the two extremes. With better diagnostic tools and improved treatment methods, the rate and the quality of recovery and rehabilitation are improving steadily. Neurologic impairment tends to involve many aspects of the person's life—the neurologic problem itself, family life alteration or disruption, occupational changes, body image and self-worth conflicts, and, frequently, the realization of a continuous need for external resources to survive.

HEADACHES

There are probably few persons who have not experienced a headache. Headache is one of the most common problems for which individuals seek medical attention and is also one of the most commonly self-treated problems. Headaches occur when pain-sensitive areas of the head have been stimulated, although much of the brain is not pain sensitive (Table 33–1).

MIGRAINE HEADACHE

OVERVIEW

Migraine headaches tend to have the same clinical manifestations each time they occur in an individual and may result in absence from regular activities for several days if the headache cannot be abated in the early stage. Although the clinical picture and treatment have been documented for some time, the cause and mechanism of migraines are only beginning to be understood.

Pathophysiology

Before the actual onset of the headache, or during the *prodromal* phase, cerebral arterial constriction occurs, with a rise in plasma serotonin level. After this vasoconstriction phase, dilation, stretching, and swelling of intracranial and extracranial vessels occur, causing the headache and a fall in the serotonin level. Although the headaches tend to occur during periods of premenstrual tension and fluid retention, the estrogen and progesterone levels throughout the menstrual cycle of women with migraines do not differ from those of women who do not have migraines. The onset of the migraine in the premenstrual period is related to the estrogen rather

TABLE 33-1 Pain-Sensitive and Non-Pain-Sensitive Areas of the Head

Pain-Sensitive Areas

Skin, subcutaneous tissue, muscles, and periosteum of the skull

Extracranial and intracranial vessels

Eye, ear, nasal cavity, and sinuses

Dura mater at the base of the brain

Cranial nerves V, IX, and X

First three cervical nerves

Non-Pain-Sensitive Areas

Skull bone

Most of pia, arachnoid, and dura mater

Brain parenchyma

Ependyma and choroid plexus

---

than the progesterone level. Other chemicals thought to be implicated in migraine headache are being investigated, with inconsistent results to date. Reserpine (Serpasil) can precipitate a migraine in a susceptible person but not in the nonmigrainous person. Some persons with migraines excrete increased amounts of epinephrine and nonrepinephrine end products, in addition to serotonin end products. Bradykinin, histamine, and the prostaglandins are also under investigation.

Etiology

Migraine headache is a familial disorder, as it appears that there is an inherited vascular response to certain chemicals. The vascular changes possibly follow or are a result of electrical or metabolic disturbances in the brain. Several studies have focused on an important area of the brain called the *locus coeruleus,* which contains, among other functions, sympathetic (adrenergic) control of cerebral blood flow and vascular permeability (refer to Chap. 32 for review of autonomic function). This same area is also closely associated with maintenance of the sleep-wake cycle, which could explain the frequent occurrence of the early morning onset of many migraine headaches. Some migraines occur during a period of rest after a period of stress; therefore, stress is also considered a precipitating factor by some researchers. The stress factor has not been a consistent finding. A relationship between migraine and neurosis was an early hypothesis that has not been demonstrated, nor has it been established that there is an association with a specific personality type. The reference to personality types can still be seen in current literature, however. No one theory to date explains all the findings.

Incidence

Migraine headaches occur in 3% to 5% of the population and 15% of women in their reproductive years. They are twice as common in women as in men and tend to occur before menses. The attacks begin in early childhood or near puberty and continue periodically, with diminishing severity, until middle age. Menopause may cause an exacerbation. Migraine headaches can continue into old age, although this is not typical. Classic migraine episodes tend to increase in frequency during pregnancy, whereas the common migraine incidence decreases in about 80% of pregnant women. Contraceptive hormones increase the frequency and severity of migraine and can also be a precipitating factor.

PREVENTION

Migraine headaches are not preventable in the sense of eliminating all attacks, but the incidence and severity can be lessened in most instances. General health measures, such as adequate sleep, diet, and recreation, are important factors. The amount of sleep required by a given client should be determined and then adhered to as much as possible on a daily basis. Diet is of particular importance, as some clients can identify foods and beverages that cause an attack. The most common of these are animal fats, eggs, chocolate, raw fruit (especially apples, oranges, tomatoes, and onions), mushrooms, cheese, beef products, and alcohol. After migraine headaches have been diagnosed, alcohol consumption in any form should be discontinued. Alcohol intake, menses, and increased stress constitute the three most common triggers for a migraine (Whitney & Daroff, 1988). Regular periods of recreation provide exercise and release of tension. Contraceptive pills may precipitate an attack and should be discontinued when this happens. Eyestrain attributable to a refractive problem can precipitate an attack; therefore, refractory errors should be corrected.

Because stress may be a precipitating factor, new ways to cope with stress must be identified. Increasingly, behavior therapy is considered an adjunct to medication treatment. Such behavior therapy, including relaxation tapes, exercise classes, and biofeedback, helps prevent attacks. Researchers are finding that younger people tend to have positive results with behavior therapy.

COLLABORATIVE MANAGEMENT

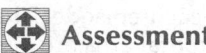 **Assessment**

History

Data to be collected specifically from the client with migraine headaches include *sex, age, onset of menses* if female, *use of contraceptive hormones,* and the *age at onset of the first headache.* The nurse carefully helps the client identify the *sequence of events* for the headache. Included in the sequence are any *precipitating factors,* including foods. Is there an *aura* (a consistent subjective sensation that precedes each attack)? The *time between the aura and the onset of the headache* should also be noted. If *nausea* or *vomiting* occurs during the attack, the nurse helps the client identify when this occurs and for how long. Last, the *length* of the entire attack is ascertained.

The client's treatment regimen is important. The nurse needs to identify what the client does at home to ease the attack. This includes *prescribed* and *nonprescribed drugs.* A nonprescribed drug can be an over-the-counter (OTC) medication, or it could be a drug given to the client by a friend. Another aspect of self-treatment is the *behaviors* utilized by the client for relief, such as lying down in a darkened room and using ice bags or earplugs. The nurse also asks the client about *foods* that are either avoided or eliminated from the diet because they precipitate an attack. *Alcohol* intake must also be determined during the history taking. Because migraine headaches may involve stress, the nurse asks the client about his or her *job* and to *recall a typical week's activities.* Notation is made of any other *family members* with migraine headaches, because migraines are familial.

Physical Assessment: Clinical Manifestations

There are two main types of migraine headaches, with variations from person to person within each category. The *classic,* or typical, migraine begins with a neurologic manifestation much like an aura before seizure activity. For 25% of those having an early warning, it is a visual disturbance within homonymous (same side) half-fields, for example, the left field of each eye. The visual disturbance is most often a shimmering or zigzag light that may have a colored outline. This may be followed or accompanied by other neurologic signs, such as numbness or tingling of the lips or tongue, slowness or slight confusion of thought, aphasia (difficulty speaking), vertigo, or drowsiness. The headache, nausea, and vomiting begin as the other disturbances lessen. The pain begins in one area (usually the temple) and spreads over the entire affected side. It gradually increases in intensity and becomes throbbing within an hour. The headache, nausea, and vomiting may last a few hours or up to several days if untreated. Classic migraine seems to be precipitated by strong sensory stimuli, such as light, smells, and noises. The same manifestations tend to be repeated with each episode. The superficial vessels over the frontotemporal area are distended and pulsating on the affected side. There may be congestion of the nasal mucosa and conjunctiva. The client's discomfort caused by the pain of the headache is obvious to the nurse.

The *common,* or atypical, migraine begins without a prodromal sign before the onset of the headache, or, if present, the prodrome may be unrecognized as such. The early warning, if present, is usually a mood change, such as euphoria, irritability, or depression. The headache is the same, beginning in one area and spreading over the entire side. It may spread to both hemispheres and may or may not be accompanied by nausea and vomiting. The onset of the common migraine often occurs in the early morning hours or during a period of rest after a period of increased stress.

Psychosocial Assessment

An important part of the psychosocial assessment is to investigate the client's work ethic, perceived ability to function under stress, coping mechanisms, and means of relaxation. The common migraine headache is thought by some to occur more often after periods of stress and during the subsequent period of relaxation. Recall of a typical week's events before an attack may lead to some insight as to the degree of stress experienced by the client. The degree to which the attacks are incapacitating is also important. Is time lost from work? Is time lost caring for children or others? Is activity with spouse or significant others curtailed? In the past there has been some social stigma placed on the client with migraine because it occurs in women more often and is associated with the menses. The nurse explores self-image with the client by asking about her/his perception of the migraine headaches and the views held by significant others.

Laboratory Findings

There are few tests for migraine headache that are conclusive. Plasma serotonin level is elevated during the prodromal phase and is decreased during the headache phase. If an isotopic blood flow study is done in the early phase, a decrease in cerebral blood flow can be identified.

 Analysis: Nursing Diagnosis

The client with migraine headache may be managed as an outpatient for the most part. Hospital admissions are most likely to be the result of complications of drug therapy. For instance, ergotamine intoxication makes the headache constant and more severe.

Common Diagnoses

The following nursing diagnoses are typically seen in the client with migraine headache:

1. Pain related to the vasodilation phase of the migraine attack (increased blood flow)
2. Fear related to the pain and the inability to control the pain

Additional Diagnoses

The client may additionally have one or more of the following nursing diagnoses:

1. Knowledge deficit (self-care management techniques) related to unfamiliarity with information resources
2. Ineffective individual coping related to absence of problem-solving and information-seeking skills or failure to incorporate into future planning
3. Sleep pattern disturbance related to physical discomfort of headache
4. Anxiety related to concern about possible loss of job or inability to perform activities of daily living (ADL)

 ## Planning and Implementation

The plan of care encompasses the two common diagnoses (see the accompanying Client Care Plan).

Pain

Pain can be severely disruptive for the client with migraine headaches. ADL are interrupted, and often an absence from work is necessary. Families or significant others may be affected as well.

Planning client goals.   The main goals for this nursing diagnosis are that the client will (1) have reduced pain and (2) experience no future pain.

Interventions: nonsurgical management.   The interventions include drug therapy and measures initiated by the nurse, which are directed toward abatement of the attack. The nursing measures are an important factor in migraine therapy.

Drug therapy.   The client may be started on a beta-blocker, such as propranolol (Inderal), or an ergot derivative, such as methysergide (Sansert), to prevent attacks. Antidepressants may also be used. These drugs are not without risk, and the client must be under close supervision while taking them, as well as understand the dosage, side effects, contraindications, and indications for notifying the physician.

The drug aimed at alleviating pain after the headache has started is primarily ergotamine tartrate (Ergomar, Gynergen), although other drugs, such as indomethacin (Indocin) or naproxen (Naprosyn), have been used with

---

CLIENT CARE PLAN ■ The Client with Migraine Headache

Goal/Outcome Criteria	Interventions	Rationales
Nursing Diagnosis 1: Pain Related to the Vasodilation Phase of the Migraine Attack		
Client will experience reduced pain. ■ States the attack was less painful than previous attacks. ■ States the attack was of shorter duration than prior attacks. ■ Has no nausea or vomiting. ■ Temporal vessels on the affected side are visibly no larger or more prominent than vessels on the unaffected side.	1. Give medication at the client's first awareness of an impending attack. 2. Completely close blinds or pull privacy curtains (in a multiple-bed room). 3. Avoid turning on strong lights unless necessary. 4. Provide cover for the client's eyes if desired. 5. Provide an emesis basin. 6. If the client is able to sleep, allow him/her to sleep undisturbed until awakening.	1. Headache can be lessened in severity or eliminated entirely. 2–4. Clients are often photosensitive. Strong light sometimes acts as a stimulus. 5. Client can stay in bed. 6. Sleep can shorten the attack.
Client will not experience pain in the future. ■ Has no attacks or experiences an increase in the interval between attacks.	1. Give maintenance medication on time. 2. Provide dietary referral for elimination of suggested foods. 3. Adjust the blinds to deflect the light toward the ceiling or pull the shades halfway. 4. Suggest that sunglasses be worn if the client's eyes are sensitive. 5. Provide for uninterrupted sleep.	1. Properly spaced medication maintains plasma level. 2. Even if client is unaware of a food trigger, it should be given a trial. 3, 4. See 2–4 above. 5. Regular amounts of sleep help to decrease the frequency and degree of attacks.

continued

CLIENT CARE PLAN ■ The Client with Migraine Headache *continued*

Goal/Outcome Criteria	Interventions	Rationales
Nursing Diagnosis 2: Fear Related to the Pain and Inability to Control the Pain		

Client will be educated regarding her/his therapy regimen.
 ■ Surrenders drugs for safekeeping if has them.
 ■ Has hours of sleep verified by observation and client confirmation.
 ■ Is able to name those foods that are to be avoided.
 ■ Is able to name the drugs being taken, their purpose or action, dosage and timing of administration, side effects, contraindications, and special instructions.
	1. Determine whether the client brought medications to the hospital.
	 2. Ask the client to identify optimal hours of sleep and provide for that amount while hospitalized.
	 3. List those foods that are implicated in triggering attacks and discuss with the client.
	 4. Teach the client about the drugs.
	   a. Name.
	   b. Purpose or action.
	   c. Dosage and timing of administration.
	   d. Side effects.
	   e. Contraindications.
	   f. Special instructions.
		1. If being given a rest from a drug (such as ergotamine), the client may be reluctant to be without that security.
		 2. Each person requires an individualized amount of sleep.
		 3. Foods are considered factors until disproved. *Newly* prescribed drugs during this admission may require avoidance of foods with tyramine.
		 4. Knowledge aids in control of pain and helps prevent overdosage or underdosage. Client is better able to comply with therapy and is less likely to self-prescribe during future attacks.

■ Indicates a plan for including regular exercise in daily activities.	5. Discuss with the client the types of exercises that can be enjoyed and explore ways to include exercise on a regular basis.	5. Regular exercise aids relaxation and decreases tension caused by stress, which is thought to be a precipitating factor in some clients.
■ Is able to identify undue stress (or lack of it).	6. Ask the client to recall the past week's activities and indicate possible stress points.	6. Evaluation may indicate whether stress is a factor for this client.

Client will take advantage of resources for alternative methods or adjunctive methods of controlling pain.
 ■ Asks for more information and help with referral.
	1. Explain the types of resources available.
	   a. Biofeedback (Biofeedback Society of America maintains list of certified practitioners).
	   b. Progressive relaxation.
	   c. Exercise classes.
	   d. Guided imagery.
		1. Alternative methods can help in pain control.
		   a. Biofeedback works well in physiologic dysfunction, such as headache and stress.
		   b. Relaxation can be helpful.
		   c. Exercise promotes relaxation and decreases tension.
		   d. Imagery works well for clients with chronic pain, helps relaxation, and decreases nausea.

	2. Help the client obtain referral to appropriate centers or resource personnel.	2. Clients may be willing to try, but lack the initiative to seek the resource on their own.

some success. Antimetics are used to help control nausea and vomiting. Table 33-2 summarizes the drug therapy utilized for migraine headaches.

Other pain relief measures. At the beginning of the attack, the client can often alleviate pain if allowed to go to bed and have the room darkened. The nurse pulls the blinds or privacy curtains. The client may want his/her eyes covered as well and should be allowed to sleep undisturbed until awakening. If the client's migraine

signs and symptoms include nausea or vomiting, the nurse places an emesis basin within reach of the client.

Fear

There are helpful adjuncts to control the pain of migraines. The client must be aware of these aids and incorporate them into his/her life style to lessen the effects of migraine headaches. The ability to be in con-

Text continued on page 873

TABLE 33–2   Drugs Used in the Prevention and Treatment of Migraine Headaches

Drug	Usual Daily Dosage	Interventions	Rationales*
Agents That Decrease Platelet Aggregation			
Acetylsalicylic acid (aspirin)	600 mg daily PO	1. Assess for prior salicylate intolerance.	1. Drug can cause hearing impairment, tinnitus, gastric bleeding or irritation, and depressed plasma ascorbic acid level.
		2. Check for petechiae.	2. Drug prolongs bleeding time.
Dipyridamole (Persantine)	50 mg tid PO	1. Give with a glassful of water.	1. Water aids absorption and decreases gastric distress.
		2. Observe for signs of gastric distress.	2. Drug may need to be taken with meals.
Agents Used for Prevention of Attacks			
Propranolol (Inderal)	60 mg in divided doses initially and increased gradually to 240 mg in divided doses orally	1. Administer the last dose of the day at bedtime.	1. Bedtime administration prevents early morning vasodilation.
		2. Check for petechiae.	2. Drug decreases platelet aggregation.
		3. Teach the client to take pulse.	3. Drug causes bradycardia. Notify the physician if pulse is slower than baseline or irregular. Pulse may not rise in response to stress, such as fever and exercise.
		4. Teach slow position changes.	4. Drug lowers blood pressure, and the client may become hypotensive, especially when changing position.
		5. Assess other drug use.	5. Propranolol is contraindicated if the client is taking MAO inhibitors.
		6. Assess overall health status.	6. Propranolol is contraindicated if the client has asthma or acute congestive heart failure.
		7. Ensure gradual withdrawal.	7. Gradual withdrawal prevents severe symptoms.
Methysergide (Sansert)	2–6 mg in divided doses PO	1. Administer with meals	1. Food helps prevent GI disturbances.
		2. Assess for fibrotic, cardiovascular, and CNS complications.	2. There is a high incidence of side effects: fibrotic—retroperitoneal fibrosis (oliguria, dysuria, urinary obstruction, and in-

Table continued on following page

TABLE 33–2 Drugs Used in the Prevention and Treatment of Migraine Headaches *Continued*

Drug	Usual Daily Dosage	Interventions	Rationales*
Methysergide (Sansert)			creased BUN) and pleuropulmonary fibrosis (dyspnea, chest pain, pleural friction rubs, and effusion) (*drug should be stopped every 3 months for at least 2 weeks to prevent fibrosis*); cardiovascular — peripheral edema, phlebitis, claudication, postural hypotension, and heart murmurs; and CNS — insomnia, vertigo, confusion, euphoria, feelings of depersonalization, distortion of body image, anxiety, depression, hallucinations, nightmares, ataxia, and paresthesia.
		3. Teach slow position changes.	3. Drug can cause orthostatic hypotension.
		4. Withdraw gradually.	4. Gradual withdrawal prevents rebound headache.
Cyproheptadine (Periactin)	2 mg tid PO	1. Give with food or milk.	1. Food or milk prevents gastric distress.
		2. Assess other drug use.	2. Drug may increase and prolong effects of alcohol, barbiturates, narcotic analgesics, tranquilizers, and other CNS depressants. Contraindicated if the client is taking MAO inhibitors.
		3. Assess overall health status.	3. Drug is contraindicated if the client has asthma or glaucoma.
Phenelzine (Nardil) or tricyclic antidepressant, such as imipramine hydrochloride (Tofranil)	30–60 mg daily in divided doses	1. Teach avoidance of foods and liquids containing tryamine.	1. MAO inhibitor increases norepinephrine in tissues. Tyramine forms *pressor* amines in body.
		2. Teach slow position changes.	2. Drugs have some paradoxic hypotensive effects.
		3. Assess for appearance of GI, mental, renal, muscular, or neural symptoms.	3. Side effects can be often eliminated by adjusting the dosage.

TABLE 33–2   Drugs Used in the Prevention and Treatment of Migraine Headaches *Continued*

Drug	Usual Daily Dosage	Interventions	Rationales*
Phenelzine (Nardil) or tricyclic anti-depressant, such as imipramine hydro-chloride (Tofranil)		4. Assess for headache or palpitation.	4. Drugs are discontinued if prodromal signs of hypertensive crisis occur.
		5. Slow withdrawal.	5. Gradual withdrawal prevents rebound headache.
Ergotamine	0.3 mg	1. Frequent oral hygiene.	1. Mouth dryness may be a problem.
Phenobarbital	20 mg	1. Assess overall health status.	1. Drug is contraindicated in peripheral vascular and coronary disease, renal or hepatic disease, and glaucoma.
Belladonna, phenobarbital, and ergotamine tartrate (Bellergal-S)	0.1 mg AM, noon, and h.s. PO	1. None specified.	

Agents Used for Early Alleviation of Attacks

Drug	Usual Daily Dosage	Interventions	Rationales*
Ergotamine tartrate (Gynergen)	1–2 mg sublingually, no more than 4–6 mg/wk	1. Give immediately at onset.	1. Relief of pain is directly proportional to early treatment. Sublingual administration provides rapid effect and lower effective dose. Drug is poorly absorbed from GI tract.
		2. Monitor peripheral vasculature.	2. Vasoconstrictive drug leads to muscle pain, claudication, weakness, and cold or numb digits.
		3. Teach avoidance of overuse.	3. Drug is accumulated in the body and eliminated slowly, contributing to ergotamine poisoning. Poisoning is enhanced by sepsis, renal and vascular disease, heavy smoking, malnutrition, pregnancy, contraceptive hormones, and fever.
Caffeine–ergotamine tartrate combination (Cafergot)	100 mg, caffeine, 1.0 mg ergotamine: 2 tablets at start of attack, then 1 tablet every 30 min PO	1. Watch timing of administration	1. Dose late in the day may prevent sleep.
		2. Assess overall health status.	2. Drug is contraindicated in peripheral vascular and coronary artery disease, hypertension, and renal or hepatic disease. Dosage should not exceed 6 tablets per attack.

Table continued on following page

TABLE 33-2 Drugs Used in the Prevention and Treatment of Migraine Headaches *Continued*

Drug	Usual Daily Dosage	Interventions	Rationales*
Indomethacin (Indocin) or Isometheptene, dichloralphenazone, and acetaminophen (Midrin)	150–200 mg in divided doses PO 2 capsules, can repeat once	1. Give with meals or milk. 2. Last dose at bedtime.	1. Food or milk decreases gastric irritation. 2. Bedtime administration reduces the incidence of frontal morning headache. If frontal headache persists, the dosage may be reduced or the drug stopped.
Naproxen sodium (Anaprox) Naproxen (Naprosyn)	275-mg tablets — 3 tablets, then 2 more in 1 h if no result 250-mg tablets — 3 tablets, then 1 more in 1 h if no results	3. Assess overall health status. 4. Monitor weight. 5. Assess for possible infections.	3. Contraindicated if the client is sensitive to aspirin or has renal or hepatic disease. 4. In cardiovascular disease, water and sodium retention occur. 5. Drug may mask signs and symptoms of latent infections.
Agents Used for Control of Nausea or Vomiting			
Metoclopramide (Reglan)	10–20 mg PO	1. Give at onset of attack and 30 min before other migraine drugs. 2. Assess overall health status. 3. Assess for CNS symptoms (extrapyramidal).	1. Drug helps regain peristalsis and aids absorption of other drugs. 2. Drug is contraindicated for those with epilepsy or history of breast cancer. 3. These are most likely to occur in younger adults — restlessness, involuntary movements, facial grimacing, rigidity, and tremors.
Promethazine hydrochloride (Phenergan)	50 mg PO once (or IM)	1. Give with food, milk, or glassful of water. 2. Teach slow position changes. 3. Assess overall health status. 4. Encourage frequent oral hygiene. 5. Assess other medications being taken.	1. Food, milk, or water minimizes GI distress. 2. Drug has a hypotensive effect. 3. Drug is contraindicated in angle-closure glaucoma, epilepsy, and urinary retention. 4. Mouth dryness may be a problem. 5. OTC medications should not be taken without physician approval, nor should CNS depressants, including alcohol.

TABLE 33–2   Drugs Used in the Prevention and Treatment of Migraine Headaches *Continued*

Drug	Usual Daily Dosage	Interventions	Rationales*
Promethazine hydrochloride (Phenergan)		6. IM injection is given deeply in large muscle. 7. Teach avoidance of sunlamps and prolonged exposure to the sun.	6. Subcutaneous injections can cause irritation and necrosis. 7. Photosensitivity may occur with promethazine.

* MAO, monoamine oxidase; BUN, blood urea nitrogen.

trol of the therapy regimen or to have input has a positive effect on the degree of pain for most clients.

Planning: client goals.   The goals for this diagnosis are that the client will (1) demonstrate understanding of the therapy regimen and (2) identify the available resources for controlling pain by means other than drugs.

Interventions: nonsurgical management.   The nurse structures education sessions with the client to cover the following aspects: diet; sleep needs; recreational activity; purpose, action, dosage, and side effects of all drugs; and stress identification in daily living. An educated client has the power to control some aspects of the pain and therefore reduces fear.

The possibility or feasibility of using behavior therapy in conjunction with drug therapy is explored by the nurse. This includes biofeedback, exercise classes, and relaxation techniques, which are generally offered in a center such as a headache clinic. Often, a combination of these alternative methods is recommended for best results. These resources are becoming more available and provide clients with active participation in their program of pain control. An additional positive factor is that these programs usually allow the client to interact with others with the same or similar problems. Knowledge that one is not alone helps relieve fear and allows the client an opportunity to exchange ideas with others. Chapters 6 and 7 discuss stress reduction and pain relief methods.

■ Discharge Planning

Planning for discharge of the client with migraine headaches, as for any other client, begins on admission. Successful planning likely prevents readmission for the same problem in the near future. The nurse reviews each of the following categories to assess the individual needs of a particular client.

Home Care Preparation

The client with migraine headache is discharged to home or his/her prior setting. There is little home care preparation unless the client has identified that a bed-

room needs to be modified for a quiet environment. The lighting and blinds or shades need to provide control of the degree of light, depending on whether the client is photosensitive.

Client/Family Education

It is beneficial to have some member of the family with the client during the teaching process, if possible. This provides further support to the client regarding the importance of regular rest, recreational activities to reduce stress, and avoidance of specific foods if those are factors. A family member or responsible person needs to be included for all education sessions for a young teenager or a mentally disabled client.

Psychosocial Preparation

The psychosocial adjustment should be minimal if the client is educated to manage his/her own therapy with the continued support of the health care team and significant others. If stress has been identified as a factor, the client needs access to the various forms of stress reduction techniques with the opportunity to try several to identify the ones that are most successful. The nurse helps the client identify those activities that induce stress and encourages alternative activities that would be less stressful.

Health Care Resources

The client may be referred to a behavior therapy clinic or a headache clinic. The nurse completes whatever documents are necessary for the referral and helps with appointments as necessary. If contraceptive hormones were the precipitating factor, the client may desire referral for another form of birth control.

Evaluation

Evaluation of the care of the client with migraine headache is based on the determined nursing diagnoses. The expected outcomes are that the client

1. States that the attack was less painful than previous attacks

2. States that the attack was of shorter duration than prior attacks

3. Has no or less nausea and vomiting

4. States that there have been no further attacks or the interval between attacks has increased

5. Has identified those aspects of his or her life that may need to be modified

6. Indicates a reasonable plan for including regular exercise in daily activities

7. Is able to name the drugs that have been prescribed, as well as their purpose or action, dosage and administration times, side effects, contraindications, and special instructions

8. States that he/she is no longer afraid of not being able to control the pain

CLUSTER HEADACHE

OVERVIEW

Cluster headaches have been identified for more than 100 years and have been called by a variety of names, including *angioparalytic hemicrania, migrainous neuralgia, ciliary neuralgia, greater superficial petrosal neuralgia,* and *histamine cephalalgia.* The headaches have been known as *cluster headaches* since the early 1950s. Whether cluster headaches are a type of migraine headache is still unresolved.

Pathophysiology

The pain of these unilateral, oculotemporal or oculofrontal headaches is described as excruciating, boring, and nonthrobbing. They occur every 8 to 12 up to 24 hours daily at the same time for about 6 to 8 weeks (hence the term cluster), followed by a period of remission for 9 months to a year. This episodic form is the most common, although there is a chronic form in which there has not been a remission for more than a year. The average duration of each headache is 10 to 45 minutes. The headache is accompanied by ipsilateral (same side) lacrimation (tearing of the eye), rhinorrhea (excess nasal secretion) or congestion, ptosis (drooping of the eyelid), and miosis (abnormal contraction of the pupil). There may be bradycardia (slow heartbeat), flushing or pallor of the face, increased intraocular pressure, and increased skin temperature. The pain may radiate to the forehead, the temple, or the cheek. The temporal artery may be prominent and tender. Physical activity during the attack consists of pacing, walking, or sitting and rocking. This is the only headache type in which this behavior occurs. During periods of remission, alcohol does not induce a headache (as it does during the headache period). The onset of the headaches is associated with relaxation, napping, or rapid eye movement (REM) sleep.

Etiology

The cause of cluster headaches is unknown. There is no genetic or family link, diet has no effect, and the disorder is unrelated to personality types. Some studies have shown decreased blood flow in selected superficial vessels, with increase in cerebral blood flow during the headache. Other studies showed an increased serum and urine histamine level during the headache compared with preheadache levels, but later studies did not confirm those findings. Because of bradycardia in some persons, the autonomic nervous system is thought to be implicated. Precipitating factors include nitroglycerin and histamine (in experimental situations), altitude, and alcohol.

Incidence

The actual incidence of cluster headaches is unknown, but they occur preponderantly in young men. Studies have shown a male/female ratio from 4 : 1 to as great as 7 : 1, with the average age at onset being 27 to 30 years. Data from headache clinics seem to indicate a higher incidence in Black persons than in the Caucasian population.

PREVENTION

Preventive measures focus on the precipitation aspect of cluster headaches. Afternoon naps should be avoided. Alcohol, including beer and wine, should not be consumed, as alcohol precipitates a headache while the person is in the cluster period (alcohol does not cause a headache when the person is in remission). Owing to poor toleration of light and glare during the active phase, sunglasses should be worn and the person should sit with his/her back to the outdoor light. Behaviors to be avoided are bursts of anger, prolonged anticipation, excitement, and excessive physical activity, as the headaches are likely to occur *after* those behaviors during a period of relaxation. If the client is in remission, these behaviors may begin the onset of cluster headaches. Another activity to be avoided is alteration in sleep-wake patterns, such as occur with vacations and new occupations. This is thought to be one of the most important factors. Drugs used to prevent attacks are methysergide (Sansert), prednisone (Deltasone, Lisacort), lithium citrate (Cibalith-S), and ergotamine (Gynergen).

COLLABORATIVE MANAGEMENT

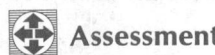 **Assessment**

History

Data to be collected specifically from the client with cluster headaches include *sex, age, race,* and the *age at onset of the headaches.* The nurse helps the client identify the *sequence of events* for the headaches. This includes the *precipitating factors, duration, frequency in 24 hours,* and *number of weeks before remission.* The *characteristics* of the headache need to be determined. Characteristics include the origin of the headache, spread, tenderness of arteries, presence of lacrimation, rhinorrhea or congestion, facial flushing or pallor, presence of bradycardia (client may not be aware of this), and behavior during the headache, such as pacing, walking, or sitting and rocking.

The nurse asks the client about *prescribed drugs* for both prevention and alleviation and *nonprescribed drugs* (anything the client may be taking). *Alcohol intake* must also be determined. If alcohol is used, the type, amount, and frequency of consumption are ascertained. The client is asked to recall a typical week's *activities* and to specifically identify bedtimes and arisal times, which helps the nurse assess extremes in activity or lack of continuity in the sleep-wake cycle.

Physical Assessment: Clinical Manifestations

There are no observable findings unless the client is having a headache at the time of the assessment. During a headache, the facial skin may be pale or flushed, and the temperature of the skin may be elevated on the side of the headache. There may be lacrimation, rhinorrhea, or congestion. The temporal artery may be distended and tender on the affected side. Ptosis and miosis may also occur on the side of the headache. Most noticeable is the client's inability to sit still or lie down. Pacing, walking, and rocking while sitting are considered characteristic of cluster headaches. The nurse assesses heart rate, as bradycardia may be present.

Psychosocial Assessment

The nurse assesses the client's ability to cope with the irritations of daily living by specifically asking about the type of job the client performs, relationships with co-workers and superiors, and daily pressures of work. Living relationships are also assessed. The nurse can ask the client directly how excitement, anger, and prolonged anticipation are handled. Reaction to irritations, prolonged anticipation, and excitement may need to be verified with a significant other.

Laboratory Findings

No consistent laboratory findings have been identified. Cerebral blood flow is increased during a headache, while flow in superficial vessels seems to be decreased. Serum and urine histamine level studies have not been conclusive.

 Analysis: Nursing Diagnosis

As is the case with migraine headache, it is likely that the client with cluster headaches is seen in clinic facilities

rather than the hospital setting, unless the client has been hospitalized for another reason.

Common Diagnoses

There is one nursing diagnosis common to clients with cluster headaches: pain related to increased blood flow to the brain.

Additional Diagnoses

The client may additionally have one or more of the following nursing diagnoses:

1. Ineffective individual coping related to disruption in life style
2. Knowledge deficit (self-care management techniques) related to unfamiliarity with information resources

 Planning and Implementation

Pain

Pain is not as disruptive for the client with cluster headaches as it is for the client with migraines. Because the headaches are cyclic and therefore predictable, much can be done to prevent or abort the attack. The length of the attack is also shorter than that of migraine headache.

Planning: client goals. The main goals for this nursing diagnosis are that the client will (1) block the pain at onset and (2) prevent the pain of future attacks.

Interventions: nonsurgical management. The interventions for pain relief and prevention include drug therapy and other measures initiated by the nurse. The client's understanding of the preventive measures is important in the management of cluster headaches.

Drug therapy. Ergotamine (Gynergen), 2 mg, administered 2 hours before the onset of the expected attack or immediately at the onset usually stops the headache. The client knows when an attack will occur. Prophylactically, the client is started on a regimen of methysergide (Sansert), 6 to 8 mg/day; prednisone (Deltasone), 40 mg/day for 3 weeks and then tapered; or lithium citrate (Cibalith-S), 600 to 1200 mg/day. Table 33–2 outlines the nursing implications for clients taking methysergide and ergotamine. Serious side effects of prednisone include ulcers, hypertension, diabetes, and masking of infection. Serious side effects of lithium are avoided by keeping the blood level below 1.2 mg/dL. Because an informed person is better able to comply with the therapeutic plan, the client must be educated in all aspects of the drugs being taken. Those aspects include the name, the purpose and action, the dosage and timing of administration, side effects, and any special instructions.

Other pain relief measures. During the periods of attack, the nurse instructs the client to wear sunglasses and sit facing away from the window, which helps to decrease exposure to light and glare. If oxygen administration is ordered, the nurse gives 100% oxygen via mask at 7 L/minute with the client in a sitting position. The oxygen is administered for no longer than 15 minutes, but is discontinued when the headache is relieved. Oxygen reduces cerebral blood flow and inhibits activity of the carotid bodies. To prevent future attacks brought on by precipitating factors, the nurse discusses the relationship between precipitating factors (bursts of anger, prolonged anticipation, excessive physical activity, and excitement) and the postactivity period and the onset of cluster headaches. The nurse also explains the necessity and importance of a consistent sleep-wake cycle.

■ Discharge Planning

Home Care Preparation

The client with cluster headaches is discharged to home or his/her prior setting. There is no special home preparation required. The client and the family may have to make some alteration to allow the client to sleep alone if necessary to provide the opportunity for a consistent sleep-wake cycle.

Client/Family Education

It is beneficial to have some member of the family with the client during the teaching process, if possible. This provides further support to the client regarding the need for regular patterns of sleep, as well as the necessity for a stable emotional environment.

Psychosocial Preparation

The adjustment should be minimal if the client understands the medication regimen. If behaviors need to be modified, the nurse helps the client understand that this will take patience and time and may not occur quickly. Keeping a record or diary of the occurrence of undesired behaviors may help the client to focus on implementing change or decreasing the frequency of those behaviors.

Health Care Resources

If the client has decided that additional direction is needed to control anger, avoid undue excitement, or focus on short-range anticipation, there are many facilities and teams able to provide these services. The nurse assists the client in locating the resource best suited to the particular needs of the client.

▼ Evaluation

Evaluation of the care of the client with cluster headaches is determined on the basis of the identified nursing diagnosis. The expected outcomes are that the client

1. Has no attacks of cluster headache
2. Can describe the name, the purpose and action, the dosage and timing of administration, the side effects, and any special instructions regarding the drugs being taken
3. Indicates those behaviors that need to be modified and begins change

OTHER TYPES OF HEADACHE

Headaches occur from a variety of other causes (see the accompanying Key Features of Disease). Discussion of headaches caused by common nonneurologic problems is presented elsewhere in the text.

CEREBROVASCULAR ACCIDENT

OVERVIEW

A *cerebrovascular accident* (CVA), commonly referred to as a *stroke*, is a disruption in the normal blood supply to the brain. It often occurs suddenly and produces focal neurologic deficits. Although the number of stroke deaths has decreased during the past several years, CVA remains the third most common cause of death in the United States. Of the estimated 400,000 new strokes that occur annually in the United States, more than half are associated with or caused by hypertension (Bronstein et al., 1986).

Pathophysiology

Blood to the brain is supplied by the right and left common carotid arteries, which branch to form the internal and external carotid arteries. Within the cranial vault, the *internal carotid arteries* branch to form the ophthalmic, posterior communicating, anterior choroidal, and anterior and middle cerebral arteries. These arteries and their numerous branches supply blood to most of the cerebral hemispheres. The *external carotid arteries* together with their branches supply blood to the face, the orbits, and the dura mater. An important function of the external carotid arteries is their ability to supply blood to the brain in the event of occlusion or blockage of the internal carotid arteries.

The two vertebral arteries arise from the subclavian artery and join at the base of the brain to form the basilar artery. Anatomically, the basilar artery is located over the pons, the middle structure of the brain stem. Branches of the basilar artery provide blood to the brain stem. The two posterior cerebral arteries, which branch

KEY FEATURES OF DISEASE ■ Differential Features of Common Headache Types

Type	Pathophysiology, Signs, and Symptoms	Treatment Approaches	Comments
Ophthalmoplegic migraine	Headache with paralysis of cranial nerve III (usually) persists for days or weeks. Ptosis occurs. Pupil is usually not affected.	Carotid aneurysm and tumors must be ruled out.	Paralysis may become permanent.
Basilar artery migraine	Brain stem symptoms of giddiness (vertigo), ataxia, dysarthria, and loss of consciousness are present. More commonly occurs in young girls and women. Lasts 10–30 min and is followed by occipital headache.	Tumors must be ruled out.	
Tension headache	Pathophysiology is unknown. Usually bilateral in occipital-nuchal, temporal, or frontal region. May be diffuse over top of the head. Pain is dull and aching. Descriptions include feeling of fullness, tightness, or vise or band around head. Gradual onset, but lasts days, weeks, months, or years. More common in women than in men, and occurrence almost as great as that for migraine. Most likely to begin in middle age or when anxiety and depression are present.	Massage, relaxation. Antianxiety drugs include diazepam (Valium), meprobamate (Equanil), phenobarbital (Luminal), and chlordiazepoxide (Librium). One of the above plus amitriptyline (Elavil) in presence of depression.	Aspirin does not help. Psychotherapy does not help.
Traumatic headache from head injury	Often occurs from subdural hematoma. Pain is deep seated and steady. Unilateral or generalized and accompanied by drowsiness, confusion, stupor, coma, or hemiparesis.	Identification and correction of possible focus. Settlement of litigation (if present) as soon as possible.	See text.
Meningeal irritation headache from infection or hemorrhage	Dilation and congestion of inflamed vessels. Irritation of nerve endings in meninges from serotonin, plasma kinins, or possibly increased ICP. Acute	Rest, time, and antibiotics if infection is cause.	See text.

Continued

Type	Pathophysiology, Signs, and Symptoms	Treatment Approaches	Comments
	onset of pain, which is severe, generalized, deep seated, and constant with nuchal rigidity.		
Post–lumbar puncture headache	No satisfactory pathophysiologic explanation at present. Possible reasons—leakage of CSF through needle tract or low CSF pressure causes brain to exert painful traction on vessels or dural attachments. Pain is occipital, frontal, and nuchal. Steady pain is evident after LP on arising.	Time, fluids to aid CSF production.	If severe neck and head pain continues, bacteria introduced by needle must be considered. See Chapter 32.
Headaches from disease of ligaments, joints, or muscles of upper spine from arthritis or whiplash	Pain referred to occiput and nape of neck. Steady ache and often more painful after immobility.	Massage, heat.	See Chapter 28.
Ocular—hypermetropia (hyperopia) or astigmatism	Sustained contraction of frontotemporal muscles during prolonged close use. Steady ache.	Correction of visual defect.	See Chapter 36.
Cranial arteritis			See Chapter 28.
Sinus headache from infection or blockage	Pressure and irritation of sinus walls.		See Chapter 63.
Headaches occurring during sexual activity	Pathophysiology unknown. Resembles pain of ruptured aneurysm, except there are no other symptoms. Severe, throbbing, explosive type at time of orgasm. Persists for several minutes to hours.	None.	Hypertensive hemorrhage, rupture of aneurysm or AVM does occur during sexual activity.
Headaches related to medical problems: Hypertension Fever Carbon monoxide exposure Chronic pulmonary disease with hypercapnia Hypothyroidism Cushing's disease Corticosteroid withdrawal Chronic ergotamine ingestion			

KEY FEATURES OF DISEASE ■ Differential Features of Common Headache Types *Continued*

Type	Pathophysiology, Signs, and Symptoms	Treatment Approaches	Comments
Chronic exposure to nitrites			
Adrenal insufficiency			
Aldosterone-producing adrenal tumors			
Pheochromocytoma			
Acute anemia with hemoglobin below 10 g/dL			
Constipation			
Birth control hormones			

from the basilar artery, provide blood to the temporal and occipital lobes of the brain.

An important area at the base of the brain is the circle of Willis (see Chap. 32, Fig. 32–9), a network of blood vessels composed of the two anterior cerebral, one anterior communicating, two posterior cerebral, and two posterior communicating arteries. The circle of Willis functions as a type of collateral circulation between the blood vessels of the two cerebral hemispheres and between the carotid and vertebrobasilar circulation. Branches of the basilar artery supply the diencephalon and the basal ganglia.

If blood flow through the cerebral vessels is interrupted, the brain is often able to receive an adequate blood supply through collateral circulation or the shunting of blood via other pathways. Although this is helpful, it does not entirely eliminate the problems of inadequate cerebral tissue perfusion.

The brain must receive a constant flow of blood for normal function, as it is unable to store oxygen or glucose. In addition, blood flow is important for the removal of metabolic waste, carbon dioxide, and lactic acid. If deprived of its blood flow, the brain can be damaged irreparably within a few minutes.

Through the processes of cerebral autoregulation, blood flow is maintained at a fairly constant rate of 750 mL/minute. In response to blood pressure changes, or changes in carbon dioxide tension, the cerebral arteries dilate or constrict.

In the event of a CVA, ischemia (decreased or altered blood supply) occurs in the brain tissue supplied by the involved vessel, and brain dysfunction occurs. Ischemia leads to hypoxia (decreased oxygen supply) or anoxia (absent oxygen supply) and hypoglycemia. These processes then cause infarction or death of the neurons, glia, and vasculature of the involved area. In addition, brain metabolism after stroke is affected in the involved area, as well as in the contralateral (opposite side) hemisphere through a phenomenon known as diaschisis.

Small lacunar infarcts may occur. Lacunae are small, deep cavities within the brain that result from occlusion

of a small vessel, leading to infarct and necrosis of the area of the brain supplied by the affected vessel. Lacunar infarcts occur almost exclusively in the internal capsule, the basal ganglia, and the pons and rarely in the thalamus. Lacunar infarcts produce either a pure motor or a pure sensory deficit.

CVAs are classified as ischemic or hemorrhagic. *Ischemic stroke* is caused by occlusion of a cerebral artery by either a thrombus or an embolus (Fig. 33–1). A stroke that is caused by a thrombus is referred to as a thrombotic stroke, whereas a stroke caused by an embolus is referred to as an embolic stroke. Hemorrhage into the brain tissue generally results from a ruptured saccular aneurysm, rupture of an arteriovenous malformation (AVM), or, more commonly, hypertension.

A *thrombotic stroke* is commonly associated with the development of atherosclerosis of the blood vessel wall (see Fig. 33–1). Arteriosclerosis is a noninflammatory degenerative disease affecting almost any cerebral blood vessel. As a result of plaques or atheromatous deposits that gradually build up on the interior of the vessel wall, the vessel loses its elasticity and becomes hardened. The thrombus extends along the interior of the artery, gradually occluding the lumen of the artery. This process may occur over many years, and often collateral circulation to the involved area develops. As the artery becomes completely occluded, blood flow to the area is markedly diminished; this causes transient ischemia, which progresses to complete ischemia and infarction of the brain tissue. Within 72 hours, the area is edematous and necrotic, and cavities develop. Large vessels, such as the internal carotid, proximal middle cerebral, and anterior cerebral arteries, are most often involved. Because of the gradual occlusion of the arteries, thrombotic strokes tend to have a slow onset.

An *embolic stroke* is caused by an embolus or a group of emboli that break off from one area of the body and travel to the cerebral arteries via the carotid artery (see Fig. 33–1). The usual source of the emboli is as follows: mural thrombosis in the left atrium or ventricle, septic

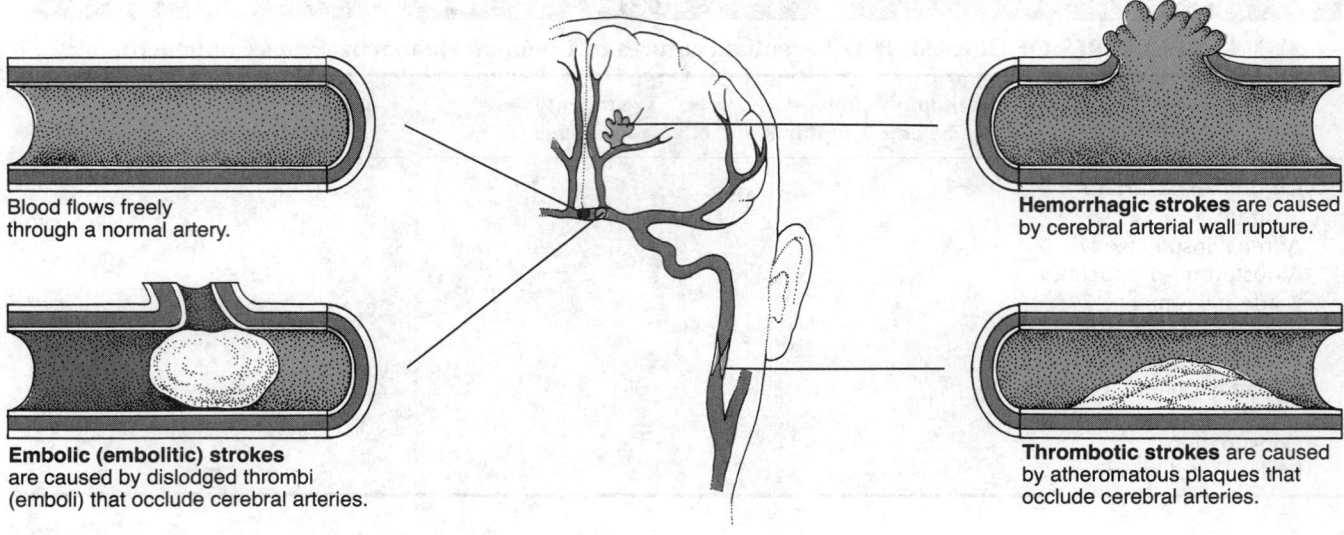

Blood flows freely
through a normal artery.

Embolic (embolitic) strokes
are caused by dislodged thrombi
(emboli) that occlude cerebral arteries.

Hemorrhagic strokes are caused
by cerebral arterial wall rupture.

Thrombotic strokes are caused
by atheromatous plaques that
occlude cerebral arteries.

Figure 33–1

The types of stroke.

emboli from bacterial endocarditis, or atrial fibrillation. Another source of emboli may be plaque that breaks off from the carotid sinus or the internal carotid artery. Emboli tend to become lodged in the smaller cerebral blood vessels at their point of bifurcation or where the lumen narrows. The middle cerebral artery is most frequently involved. As the emboli occlude the vessel, ischemia develops, and the client experiences signs and symptoms of the stroke. However, as often occurs, the occlusion is temporary, and the embolus breaks into smaller fragments, enters smaller vessels, and is absorbed. For these reasons, embolic strokes are characterized by the sudden development and rapid occurrence of focal neurologic deficits, followed by clearing of the symptoms over several hours or a few days. It must be remembered, however, that a cerebral hemorrhage may occur if significant damage to the wall of the involved vessel has occurred.

Ischemic strokes are frequently preceded by *warning* signs, such as a transient ischemic attack (TIA) or reversible ischemic neurologic deficit (RIND) (see the accompanying Key Features of Disease). Both cause transient focal neurologic dysfunction attributable to a brief interruption in cerebral blood flow, possibly owing to cerebral vasospasm or transient systemic arterial hypertension. The difference between a TIA and an RIND is the length of time the client is symptomatic. A TIA lasts a few minutes to less than 24 hours, whereas symptoms of an RIND last longer than 24 hours but less than a week. It should be noted that both TIAs and RINDs cause damage to the brain tissue, which is evidenced by magnetic resonance imaging (MRI) or computed tomography (CT).

The second major classification of stroke is *hemorrhagic* (see Fig. 33–1). In this type of stroke, the integrity of the vessel is interrupted and bleeding occurs into the brain tissue or subarachnoid space. The most common cause of a hemorrhagic stroke is hypertension. Although the exact mechanisms involved are unknown, it is hypothesized that elevated systolic and diastolic pressures cause changes within the arterial wall that leave it prone to rupture. An intracerebral hemorrhage occurs when the vessel ruptures. Over time, the bleeding seeps into the subarachnoid space and ventricles.

A ruptured cerebral *aneurysm* is another cause of

KEY FEATURES OF DISEASE ■ Clinical Manifestations of Transient Ischemic Attack

Visual Deficits

Blurred vision
Diplopia (double vision)
Blindness in one eye
Tunnel vision

Motor Deficits

Transient weakness (arm, hand, or leg)
Gait disturbance (ataxic)

Sensory Deficits

Transient numbness (face, arm, or hand)
Vertigo

Speech Deficits

Aphasia
Dysarthria (slurred speech)

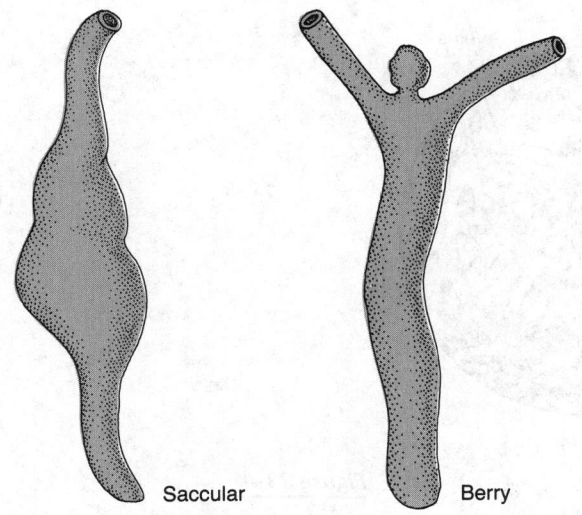

Figure 33-2

Two common types of cerebral aneurysms.

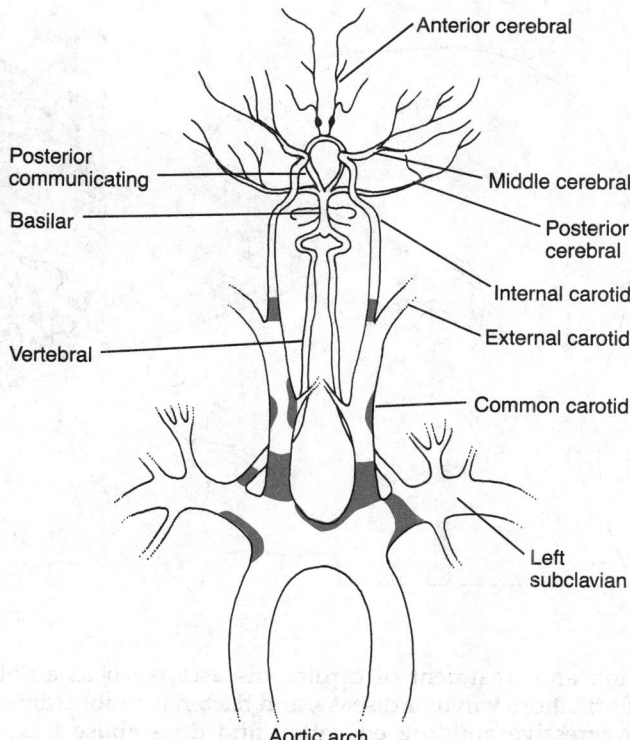

Figure 33-3

Common locations for cerebral aneurysms.

hemorrhagic stroke. An aneurysm is an abnormal ballooning or blister on the involved artery (Fig. 33-2). It is a developmental defect in the media and elastica of the vessel wall. Continued force on the weakened vessel wall from the elevated blood pressure causes it to become stretched and quite thinned. Although rupture may occur at any time, it usually occurs during activity. Aneurysms are often found at branchings of major cerebral arteries (Fig. 33-3). Rupture of the aneurysm causes bleeding into the subarachnoid space or directly into the ventricles and the development of an intracerebral hematoma. Vasospasm often occurs after a cerebral hemorrhage, leading to cerebral ischemia and infarction and further neurologic dysfunction.

An AVM is a developmental abnormality that occurs during embryonic development. It is a tangled or spaghetti-like mass of malformed, thin-walled, dilated vessels (Fig. 33-4). These vessels form an abnormal communication, or fistula, between the arterial and the venous systems. The vessels may eventually rupture, causing bleeding into the subarachnoid space or into the intracerebral tissue.

Etiology

Strokes are caused by an occlusion in an artery attributable to a thrombus or an embolus, hemorrhage resulting from hypertension, or a ruptured aneurysm or AVM. Certain risk factors have been identified that increase the likelihood of cerebrovascular disease. The three major risk factors are hypertension, diabetes, and cardiac disease. Other risk factors include smoking, substance abuse (particularly cocaine), obesity, sedentary life style, high stress levels, and elevated serum cholesterol, lipoprotein, and triglyceride levels.

Incidence

CVAs occur 10% to 15% more frequently in males than in females. Blacks are affected more frequently than other races, possibly owing to the high frequency of hypertension in this group. Stroke may occur at any age; however, it occurs more often in those older than 45 years of age, with an increased frequency in those older than 65 years. The number of strokes occurring in the younger population is increasing as a result of drug abuse; these clients are at risk for septic emboli and arteritis.

It is estimated that 2 million Americans are currently disabled because of stroke. In the United States, approximately 400,000 strokes occur each year, with almost half the affected individuals dying. Strokes tend to occur more often in the southern states, which is probably related to the geographic distribution of the older population.

PREVENTION

Prevention and control of hypertension are the single most important factors in the prevention of CVAs. Additional preventive measures include avoiding smoking, maintaining an appropriate weight, and avoiding foods that are high in fat and cholesterol. Many embolic strokes could be prevented through the prompt recogni-

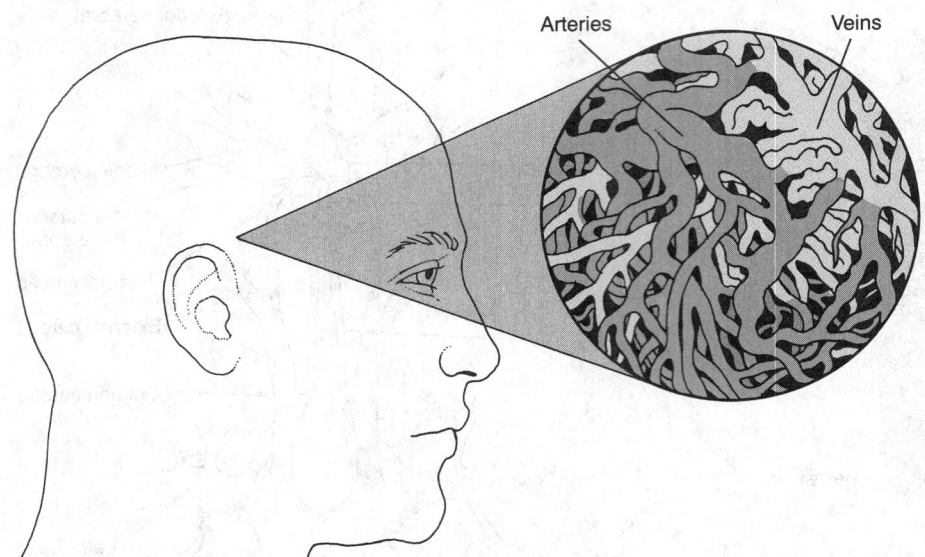

Figure 33–4

Arteriovenous malformation. Note dilated, entangled blood vessels.

tion and treatment of cardiac diseases, such as atrial fibrillation, valvular disease, and bacterial endocarditis. Aggressive antidrug education and drug abuse treatment programs may reduce the incidence of strokes from arteritis or endocarditis in clients who use illegal intravenous (IV) drugs.

COLLABORATIVE MANAGEMENT

 Assessment

History

An accurate history is important in the diagnosis of a stroke. The information obtained assists in the identification of the area of the brain involved, as well as the cause of the stroke (see the Key Features of Disease on p. 883). The nurse obtains a history concerning the client's *activity* when the stroke began. Ischemic strokes frequently occur during sleep, whereas hemorrhagic strokes tend to occur during activity. Next, the nurse asks the client or a family member how the *symptoms progressed* and elicits a history of the onset of the stroke. Symptoms of an embolic or hemorrhagic stroke tend to occur abruptly, whereas thrombotic strokes tend to have a more stepwise progression. The nurse must also determine the *severity* of the symptoms, for example, whether they got worse after the initial onset (hemorrhagic) or began to improve (embolic). It is important to determine whether the symptoms come and go, possibly indicating a TIA or RIND.

Throughout the interview process, the nurse observes the client's *level of consciousness* and assesses for indications of *intellectual or memory impairments* or difficulties with *speech* or *hearing*. The nurse questions the client or a family member regarding the presence of any *sensory or motor changes, visual problems,* problems with

balance or gait, and a change in *reading or writing* abilities.

In addition, the nurse elicits information concerning *past medical history,* with specific attention directed toward a history of head trauma, diabetes, hypertension, cardiac disease, anemia, obesity, and headache. The nurse obtains a list of any *medications* the client currently takes, including prescribed, OTC, and recreational drugs. Medications that the nurse should be alert for include anticoagulants, aspirin, vasodilators, and illegal drugs, as this information may provide clues as to the cause of the stroke or affect treatment options. To complete the history taking, the nurse obtains data regarding the client's social history, including education, employment, travel, leisure activities, and personal habits (e.g., smoking, diet, exercise pattern, and alcohol use).

Physical Assessment: Clinical Manifestations

The typical client with a CVA is a man older than 60 years of age with a history of hypertension and often diabetes. The client has sensorimotor dysfunction; language problems, if the dominant hemisphere is involved; and often intellectual or memory impairments.

The nurse performs a complete neurologic examination of the client as outlined in Chapter 32. Specific neurologic and other signs and symptoms exhibited by the client depend on the extent and location of the insult (see the Key Features of Disease: Signs and Symptoms of Stroke Syndromes on p. 884).

In addition to changes in *level of consciousness,* the client may exhibit a variety of *cognitive problems.* The nurse assesses the client for indications of denial of illness; neglect syndrome (see later in this section) or hemiparesis; spatial and proprioceptive (awareness of

KEY FEATURES OF DISEASE ■ Differential Features of the Types of Stroke

Feature	Thrombotic	Embolic	Hemorrhagic
Evolution	Intermittent or stepwise improvement between episodes of worsening Completed stroke	Abrupt development of completed stroke Steady progression	Usually abrupt onset
Onset	Daytime (10 AM–12 PM) Gradual (min to h)	Daytime Sudden	Daytime Sudden, may be gradual if caused by hypertension
Level of consciousness	Preserved (client is awake)	Preserved (client is awake)	Deepening stupor or coma
Contributing associated factors	Hypertension Atherosclerosis	Cardiac disease	Hypertension Vessel disorders
Prodromal symptoms	TIA	Home	Home
Neurologic deficits	Deficits over first few weeks Slight headache Speech deficits Visual problems Confusion	Maximal deficit at onset Paralysis Expressive aphasia	Focal deficits Severe frequent
CSF	Normal, possibly presence of protein	Normal	Bloody
Seizures	No	No	Usually
Duration	Improvements over weeks to months Possibly permanent deficits	Rapid improvements	Variable, possibly permanent neurologic deficits

body position in space) dysfunction; impairment of memory, judgment, or problem-solving and decision-making abilities; and decreased ability to concentrate and attend to tasks. The client's dysfunction in one or more of these areas may be more pronounced, depending on the hemisphere involved (see the Key Features of Disease: Differential Features of Left and Right Hemisphere Cerebrovascular Accidents on p. 884). The right cerebral hemisphere is more involved with visual and spatial awareness and proprioception. A person with a stroke involving the right cerebral hemisphere often is unaware of any deficits and may be disoriented to time and place. The left cerebral hemisphere, the dominant hemisphere in all but about 15% to 20% of the population, is the center for language, mathematical skills, and analytic thinking. A left hemisphere CVA results in aphasia, alexia (reading problems), and agraphia (difficulty writing).

The *motor examination* provides information concerning which cerebral hemisphere is involved. A right hemiplegia or hemiparesis indicates a stroke involving the left cerebral hemisphere. Conversely, a left hemiplegia or weakness indicates a right hemisphere CVA. In addition to assessing motor strength, the nurse gauges the client's muscle tone. The client with hypotonia or flaccidity is unable to overcome the forces of gravity, and the extremities tend to fall to the side; the extremities feel heavy and muscle tone is inadequate for right-

ing, equilibrium, or protective mechanisms. Hypertonia tends to cause fixed positions or contractures of the involved extremities. Range of motion (ROM) of the joints is restricted, and shoulder subluxation may easily occur. Other motor areas to be assessed by the nurse include proprioception, head and trunk control, balance, coordination, and gait. Muscle weakness and cognitive dysfunction usually lead to a spastic, uninhibited bladder and bowel function, resulting in incontinence.

The *sensory examination* conducted by the nurse evaluates the client's response to touch and painful stimuli. In addition, the nurse determines the client's ability to distinguish between two tactile stimuli presented simultaneously. Finally, the nurse assesses the client's ability to respond to stimuli that require proprioceptive and tactile processing together with cortical integration. The client who has had a stroke may be unable to write, comprehend reading material, use an object correctly (agnosia), or carry out a purposeful motor activity (apraxia).

The nurse also evaluates the client for indications of *neglect syndrome*, which is particularly evident with right hemisphere strokes. In this syndrome, the client is unaware of the existence of his/her left or paralyzed side. The typical picture is that of the client sitting in a wheelchair leaning to the left with the arm caught in the wheelchair wheel. When questioned, the client often

KEY FEATURES OF DISEASE ■ Signs and Symptoms of Stroke Syndromes

Middle Cerebral Artery

Contralateral hemiparesis: arm > leg
Contralateral sensory deficit
Homonymous hemianopia
Unilateral neglect or inattention
Aphasia, anosmia, alexia, agraphia, and acalculia
Impaired vertical sensation
Spatial deficit
Perceptual deficit
Visual field deficit
Altered level of consciousness: drowsy to comatose

Posterior Cerebral Artery

Perseveration
Aphasia, amnesia, alexia, agraphia, visual agnosia, and ataxia
Loss of deep sensation
Decreased touch sensation
Possible choreoathetoid movements
Stupor; coma

Internal Carotid Artery

Contralateral hemiparesis
Sensory deficit
Hemianopia, blurred vision, blindness
Aphasia (dominant side)

Internal Carotid Artery

Headache
Bruit

Anterior Cerebral Artery

Contralateral hemiparesis: leg > arm
Bladder incontinence
Personality and behavior changes
Aphasia, gait apraxia, and amnesia
Positive grasp and sucking reflex
Perseveration
Sensory deficit (lower extremity)
Memory impairment
Apraxic gait

Vertebrobasilar Artery

Headache and vertigo
Coma
Memory loss and confusion
Flaccid paralysis
Areflexia, ataxia, and vertigo
Cranial nerve dysfunction
Dysconjugate gaze
Visual deficits (uniorbital) and homonymous hemianopia
Sensory loss: numbness

KEY FEATURES OF DISEASE ■ Differential Features of Left and Right Hemisphere Cerebrovascular Accidents

Feature	Left Hemisphere*	Right Hemisphere
Language	Aphasia Agraphia Alexia	Impaired sense of humor
Memory	No deficit	Disoriented to time, place, and person Cannot recognize faces
Vision	Unable to discriminate words and letters Reading problems Deficits in right visual field	Visual spatial deficits Neglect of left visual field Loss of depth perception
Behavior	Slow Cautious Anxious when attempting a new task Depression or catastrophic response to illness Sense of guilt Feeling of worthlessness Worries over future Quick anger and frustration	Impulsive Unaware of neurologic deficits Confabulates Euphoric Constantly smiles Denies illness Poor judgment Overestimates abilities (risk for injury)
Hearing	No deficit	Loses ability to hear tonal variations

* Location for speech in all but 15% to 20% of people.

states that everything is fine and believes that he/she is sitting up straight in the chair.

Another important examination focuses on the client's *visual* system. Infarction or ischemia involving the carotid artery may cause pupillary abnormalities, ptosis, visual field deficits, or pallor and petechiae of the conjunctiva. *Amaurosis fugax,* a brief episode of monocular blindness, results from retinal ischemia caused by ophthalmic or carotid artery insufficiency. *Hemianopia,* or blindness in half of the visual field, results when there is damage to the optic tract or the occipital lobe. Most often this deficit occurs as *homonymous hemianopia,* in which there is blindness in the same side of both eyes. The client with this condition must turn his/her head to scan the complete range of vision. Otherwise, the client does not see half of the visual field; for example, the client eats only half of a meal because that is the only portion seen.

The nurse conducts a review of each *cranial nerve,* with particular attention to abnormalities of cranial nerves V, VII, IX, X, and XII. Damage to these cranial nerves may cause difficulties with chewing (V), facial paralysis or paresis (VII), dysphagia (inability to swallow) (IX and X), an absent gag reflex (IX), or impaired tongue movement (XII). The client may have a great deal of difficulty chewing or swallowing foods and liquids correctly and is at risk for aspiration pneumonia. In addition, the client may become constipated from inadequate fluid intake.

At the completion of the neurologic examination, the nurse performs a complete physical examination. Of particular importance is the assessment of the client's *cardiac system.* Clients with embolic strokes often have heart murmur, arrhythmias, or hypertension. It is not unusual for the client to be admitted to the hospital with a blood pressure value greater than 180–200/110–120. Although a somewhat higher blood pressure (150/100) is needed to maintain cerebral perfusion after a stroke, pressures above this limit may lead to another stroke.

Psychosocial Assessment

The typical client with a stroke is older than age 60 years, is hypertensive, and has varying degrees of motor weakness. Language and cognitive deficits may also occur, and the client may experience behavior and memory problems.

The nurse determines the client's reaction to illness, especially in relation to changes in body image, self-concept, and ability to perform ADL. In collaboration with the client's family and friends, the nurse identifies any difficulties in coping mechanisms or personality changes.

The nurse assesses the client's financial status and occupation, as these aspects of the client's life may be altered by the residual neurologic deficits from the CVA. Clients who do not have disability insurance may worry about how their family will cope financially with the disruption in their life.

The nurse also assesses the client for emotional lability, especially if the frontal lobe of the brain has been affected. In such cases, the client will laugh and then cry unexpectedly for no apparent reason. It is important that the nurse explain these uncontrollable emotions to the family or significant others so that they do not feel responsible for the client's reactions.

Laboratory Findings

There are no definitive laboratory tests to confirm the diagnosis of a stroke. Elevated hematocrit and hemoglobin levels are associated with a more severe stroke. An elevated white blood cell count may indicate the presence of an infection, possibly subacute bacterial endocarditis or a response to physiologic stress. Generally, a prothrombin time (PT) and partial thromboplastin time (PTT) are obtained to establish baseline coagulation information in the event that anticoagulation therapy is initiated. These diagnostic tests may also provide supportive evidence that a hemorrhagic stroke has occurred. If there is no indication of increased intracranial pressure (ICP), a lumbar puncture is performed to obtain cerebrospinal fluid (CSF) for analysis. Blood in the spinal fluid or a high CSF red blood cell count is indicative of a subarachnoid hemorrhage.

Radiographic Findings

CT assists in the differential diagnosis of a stroke. The primary purpose of the initial scan is to identify the presence of hemorrhage or a cerebral aneurysm. This diagnostic test shows the presence of ischemia and is invaluable in establishing baseline information for future comparison, should the client's condition deteriorate. In addition, the scans enable the physician to identify pathologic changes that may mimic a stroke, such as a brain tumor or a hematoma, both of which are unrelated to cerebrovascular disease. As the stroke progresses, later CT scans may show the presence of edema and tissue necrosis not evident on the initial scan. Information about the status of the cerebral vessels is obtained by angiography, digital subtraction angiography, or digital IV angiography. These studies reveal abnormal vessel structures or identify the area of vessel wall rupture. Skull radiography is generally not performed, although it may detect the presence of abnormal calcification of a vessel or a pineal shift, both of which may indicate the presence of cerebral hemorrhage.

Other Diagnostic Studies

MRI also assists in the differential diagnosis of a stroke. Ultrasound or Doppler studies provide additional information about the cerebral vasculature. These noninvasive procedures are particularly useful for the diagnosis of blocked arteries. An electroencephalogram (EEG) shows focal slowing in the presence of a stroke, as well as other neurologic diseases. To assist in the determination of a cardiac cause of a stroke, electrocardiography, Holter's monitor test, and echocardiography are performed. As with other neurologic diseases, it is not unusual to find the following changes on the electrocardiogram (ECG): inverted T wave, ST depression, and QT elevation and prolongation.

 Analysis: Nursing Diagnosis

The client with cerebrovascular disease is admitted to the hospital with hemiplegia, varying degrees of sensory/perceptual loss, and a variety of cognitive dysfunctions.

Common Diagnoses

The following nursing diagnoses are commonly noted in clients with a stroke:

1. Altered (cerebral) tissue perfusion related to impaired cerebral blood flow, increased ICP, and hypoxia
2. Sensory/perceptual alterations related to decreased sensation, neglect, or visual impairment
3. Impaired physical mobility and self-care deficit related to hemiparesis or hemiplegia, decreased level of consciousness, or cognitive dysfunction
4. Total (urinary) incontinence and bowel incontinence related to decreased sensation, cognitive dysfunction, immobility, or expressive aphasia
5. Impaired verbal communication related to aphasia (left hemisphere lesion) or cognitive deficits
6. Impaired swallowing related to weakness of muscles required for swallowing and decreased gag reflex

Additional Diagnoses

In addition to the common diagnoses, the client may have one or more of the following diagnoses:

1. Ineffective airway clearance, impaired gas exchange, and ineffective breathing pattern related to pooling of secretions, diminished ability to cough or clear secretions, decreased level of consciousness, and/or immobility
2. Body image disturbance and altered role performance related to physical or cognitive disability
3. Potential impaired skin integrity related to immobility
4. Potential for injury related to denial of deficits, impulsiveness, or visual problems
5. Anxiety and fear related to hospitalization, limited understanding of the disease process, and apprehension about the outcome
6. Altered sexuality patterns or sexual dysfunction related to disability

 Planning and Implementation

The following care plan for clients with a diagnosis of stroke focuses on the common nursing diagnoses.

Altered (Cerebral) Tissue Perfusion

Planning: client goals. The major goals for this nursing diagnosis are that the client will (1) maintain or improve level of consciousness and (2) not experience additional neurologic problems.

Interventions. The client is at risk for continued progression of the stroke or increased ICP. A comprehensive neurologic assessment is performed when the client is admitted to the hospital and at the beginning of each nursing shift. Neurologic checks using the Glasgow Coma Scale (Table 33–3) are performed by the nurse at least every 4 hours or more often as indicated by the client's condition. The client is at most risk for increased ICP resulting from edema during the first 72 hours after admission. The nurse must be alert for symptoms of increased ICP (see the discussion of head injury later) and report any deterioration in the client's neurologic status to the physician.

Nonsurgical management. The head of the client's bed should be elevated 30 to 45 degrees, and the client's head should be maintained in a midline, neutral position to facilitate venous drainage from the brain. The nurse plans the client's care to avoid activities and procedures that may increase ICP, particularly if the client has focal neurologic deficits and indications of cerebral

---

TABLE 33–3 Glasgow Coma Scale*

Eye Opening	
Spontaneous	4
To sound	3
To pain	2
Never	1
Motor Response	
Obeys commands	6
Localizes pain	5
Normal flexion (withdrawal)	4
Abnormal flexion	3
Extension	2
Nil	1
Verbal Response	
Oriented	5
Confused conversation	4
Inappropriate words	3
Incomprehensible sounds	2
None	1

* Highest possible score is 15.

edema. These measures include positioning the client to avoid extreme hip and neck flexion. Extreme hip flexion may increase the intrathoracic pressure, whereas extreme neck flexion prohibits venous drainage from the brain. Additional management measures include avoiding the clustering of nursing procedures (such as giving a bath followed immediately by changing the bed linen) and hyperoxygenating the client before suctioning is performed. A quiet environment is particularly important for the client experiencing a headache, which frequently occurs in the presence of an aneurysm or increased ICP attributable to blood in the subarachnoid space or pressure within the cranial vault.

The client's vital signs are monitored closely, at least every 4 hours. The nurse asks the physician for acceptable limits for the client's blood pressure. Generally, the physician allows the client to be slightly hypertensive (blood pressure of 150/100) to facilitate adequate cerebral tissue perfusion. A higher blood pressure could lead to hypertensive stroke or rebleeding of an aneurysm (if present). Clients admitted to a critical care unit are connected to a cardiac monitor and observed for indications of arrhythmias. A cardiac assessment is performed, with particular attention directed toward auscultation of heart sounds to identify the presence of cardiac murmurs.

Drug therapy. An occlusive (thrombotic) stroke is often treated with anticoagulant therapy. Sodium heparin is given subcutaneously or via a continuous IV infusion. Baseline PT and PTT values are obtained *before* the initiation of heparin therapy, 6 to 8 hours after the start of the infusion, and every morning while the client is receiving heparin therapy. The therapeutic goal is to achieve one and a half times the client's normal baseline PT and PTT. (The PT is used to monitor oral anticoagulation therapy, whereas the PTT is used to monitor heparin therapy.) Heparin and other anticoagulants, such as warfarin sodium (Coumadin), may cause bleeding. The nurse observes for signs of blood in the urine or stool of the client and for signs of easy bruising. Anticoagulation therapy is contraindicated in clients with ulcers, uremia, and hepatic failure.

Enteric-coated or other forms of aspirin or dipyridamole (Persantine) have proved useful to forestall thrombotic and embolic strokes by preventing clotting of the blood through reducing platelet adhesiveness. Anticoagulants and antiplatelet medications are contraindicated in the presence of hemorrhagic stroke, as they may cause further bleeding.

Anticonvulsants, such as phenytoin (Dilantin), may be given to prevent seizures. Epsilon-aminocaproic acid (Amicar) is an antifibrinolytic agent used to stabilize a clot over the site of a ruptured aneurysm. It works by preventing the production of plasmin, which is responsible for the breakdown of the clot. It is important for the clot to remain intact until the aneurysm is surgically treated, as this prevents the vessel from further rebleeding into the brain tissue.

Calcium channel blockers (e.g., nimodipine) are used to treat cerebral vasospasm or chronic spasm of the vessel, which inhibits blood flow to the area and worsening ischemia. These drugs work by relaxing the smooth muscles of the vessel wall. It is believed that this could prevent arterial narrowing that occurs when a vessel is in spasm, as well as possibly dilate collateral vessels to ischemic areas of the brain. Cerebral vasospasm is responsible for almost 40% of the deaths that occur after rupture of a cerebral aneurysm.

Aneurysm precautions. Aneurysm precautions are implemented for all clients with a ruptured aneurysm or AVM. Although the restrictions vary from hospital to hospital, they generally consist of the following: complete bed rest with the head of the bed elevated 30 to 40 degrees; a quiet, dark room, with television, radio, and reading material restricted; no hot or cold beverages and no caffeine products; limited visitors; and no straining or vigorous coughing. Sedation may be used to help the client rest and comply with these restrictions. Chapter 65 discusses aneurysms and their treatment.

Surgical management. The two most widely used surgical procedures to treat occlusive strokes are a carotid endarterectomy and a superior temporal artery–middle cerebral artery (STA-MCA) anastomosis. Both procedures are not without risk, including the possibility of another more serious stroke, hemorrhage, or edema. These procedures have come under increasing scrutiny, as some long-term studies indicate that medical management is as effective as surgical intervention, except in selected cases. An *endarterectomy* is done to remove atherosclerotic plaque from the inner lining of the artery, usually the carotid artery. It is hoped that this will open the artery enough to re-establish blood flow. The STA-MCA anastomosis consists of bypassing the blocked artery by making a graft or bypass from the superior temporal artery to the middle cerebral artery. The procedure establishes blood flow around the blocked artery and re-establishes blood flow to the involved areas. The procedure is used only in selected clients in whom it is believed that more conservative therapy would not be beneficial.

A craniotomy is also indicated in the treatment of AVMs or cerebral aneurysms. The usual treatment of an AVM involves the injection of small silicone (Silastic) beads into the carotid artery (Fig. 33–5). The beads travel through the cerebral circulation to the involved vessels, where they become lodged and cause the vessels to thrombose. Whenever possible, total surgical removal of the involved vessels is done. The vessels are ligated, and the defect is removed. Morbidity and mortality rates have been significantly reduced by improved microsurgical techniques, and this procedure is becoming the treatment of choice in many medical centers.

Cerebral aneurysms are repaired as soon as the client's condition is stabilized. Surgery may be postponed for clients with a grade IV or V aneurysm (see the accompanying Key Features of Disease), as their condition makes them high-risk surgical candidates. The aneurysm is clipped, or a clamp is placed at the base, or neck, of the aneurysm, which prevents blood from entering the area. If the aneurysm does not have a neck, it may be wrapped with muscle, muslin, or a plastic

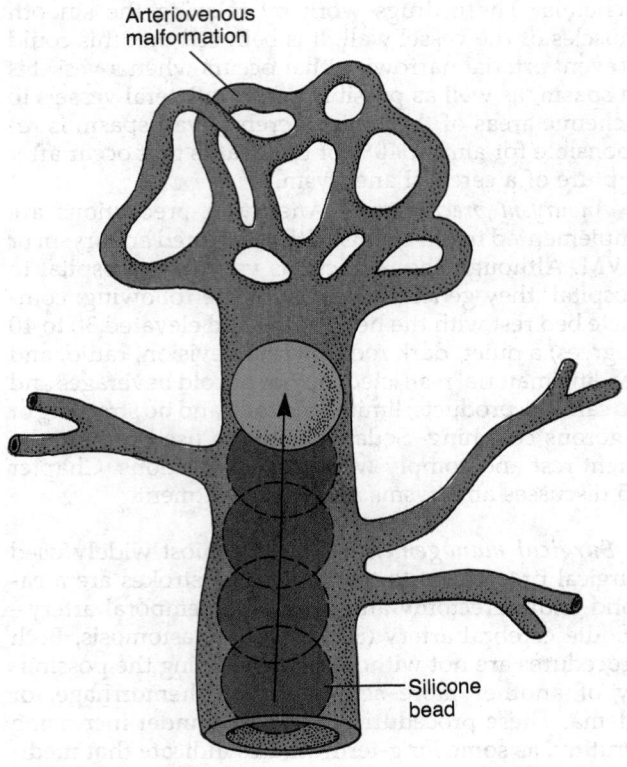

Figure 33–5

Embolization procedure to treat an AVM. Silicone (Silastic) beads travel to the area to cause vessel thrombosis.

(methyl methacrylate) coating to reinforce the wall to prevent rebleeding. Chapter 65 describes these procedures.

Sensory/Perceptual Alterations

Planning: client goals. The two major goals for clients with this diagnosis are that the client will (1) adapt to visual or spatial problems and (2) be free of injury.

Interventions: nonsurgical management. Clients with right hemisphere brain damage have difficulty with visual-perceptual or spatial-perceptual tasks. They have problems with depth and distance perception and with discriminating right from left or up from down. Because of these problems, they have difficulty performing routine ADL. The nurse can help the client adapt to these disabilities by using frequent verbal and tactile cues and by breaking tasks down into small steps. The client should be approached from the nonaffected side. The client who has experienced a stroke may have difficulties ambulating and may lack depth perception and proprioception. The nurse teaches the client with visual field deficits to turn his/her head from side to side and scan with the eyes to compensate for the disability. Objects should be placed within the client's field of vision; a mirror may be helpful to assist the client to visualize more of the environment. If the client has diplopia, a patch may be placed over the affected eye. The nurse ensures a safe environment by removing clutter from the room.

The client with a left hemisphere lesion generally experiences memory deficits and may show significant changes in ability to carry out simple tasks. To assist the client with memory problems, the nurse should reorient the client to the month, year, day of the week, and circumstances surrounding admission to the hospital. The nurse establishes a routine or schedule for the client that is structured, repetitious, and consistent. Information should be presented in a simple, concise manner. A step-by-step approach is often most effective because the client can master one step before moving to the next.

KEY FEATURES OF DISEASE ■ Classification of Cerebral Aneurysms		
Grade	Amount of Bleeding	Neurologic Findings
I	Minimal	Neurologically intact Slight headache
II	Mild	Minimal neurologic deficit, alert Severe headache Stiff neck
III	Moderate	Facial deficits Drowsy, sleepy Headache, stiff neck
IV	Moderate to severe	Hemiparesis Increasing neurologic deficits Stuporous, obtunded
V	Severe	Comatose Decorticate or decerebrate posturing

When possible, the family should bring in pictures and other objects that are familiar to the client.

The client may be unable to plan and execute tasks in an organized manner. Typically, the client exhibits a slow, cautious, and hesitant behavior style. Neglect syndrome (discussed earlier) places the client at additional risk for injury owing to an inability to recognize her/his physical impairment or to a lack of proprioception.

Impaired Physical Mobility; Self-Care Deficit

Planning: client goals.   The major goals for this nursing diagnosis are that the client will (1) increase tolerance and endurance for therapies, (2) not exhibit complications of immobility, and (3) become independent in ADL.

Interventions: nonsurgical management.   Clients who have experienced a stroke may exhibit hypotonia (flaccidity) or spasticity. The nurse performs passive ROM exercises at least once during each nursing shift for involved extremities and teaches the client to do active ROM exercise for unaffected areas. Careful positioning is necessary to maintain proper alignment of the body and to decrease spasticity or increase muscle tone in flaccid extremities. The affected hand or lower leg may need splinting to prevent contractures. The nurse collaborates with therapists (physical or occupational) to determine the most appropriate positions for lying, sitting, and transferring from bed to chair. Chapter 22 discusses interventions for assisting clients to increase mobility and promote ADL independence.

A major complication of immobility is the development of deep venous thrombosis. The nurse provides care to prevent this complication by the correct application of antiembolism stockings, frequent positioning changes, and mobilization of the client. The nurse should report any indications of deep venous thrombosis to the physician and document the finding in the client's chart. Immobile clients should have weekly measurements of their thighs and calves; an abnormal increase in the size of the leg or a positive Homan's sign may indicate venous stasis.

Total (Urinary) Incontinence; Bowel Incontinence

Planning: client goals.   The major goal for this nursing diagnosis is that the client will become continent of urine and stool.

Interventions: nonsurgical management.   The client may be incontinent of urine and stool owing to an altered level of consciousness, cognitive deficits, muscle weakness, or an inability to communicate the need to urinate or defecate. Before beginning a training program to correct these problems, the nurse must first establish the cause or causes. Most often, both bowel and bladder control can be relearned by the client with a CVA. The client with bladder dysfunction attributable to an upper motor neuron (UMN) lesion may initially require an intermittent catheterization program. To begin a *bladder training* program, the nurse places the client on the bedpan or commode, or offers the urinal, every 2 hours. Unless contraindicated, the nurse encourages the client to have a total fluid intake of 2000 mL or more per day.

Before establishing a *bowel training* program, the nurse determines the client's normal time for bowel elimination and any routine that helps to ensure an acceptable evacuation. If possible, this routine is followed, and the client is placed on the bedpan or commode at the same time as at home. A diet high in bulk and fiber is provided. The nurse encourages the client to drink apple or prune juice to help promote bowel elimination. A complete discussion of bowel and bladder training is found in Chapter 22.

Impaired Verbal Communication

Planning: client goals.   The major goal for this nursing diagnosis is that the client will develop strategies for alternative methods of communication.

Interventions: nonsurgical management.   Language or speech problems are usually the result of a stroke involving the dominant hemisphere. In all but 15% to 20% of the population, the left cerebral hemisphere is the speech center. Language problems may be the result of *aphasia*, an inability to use or comprehend language, or *dysarthria*, problems with the rate or rhythm of speech or with articulation. Although aphasia is caused by hemisphere damage, dysarthria is due to loss of motor function to the tongue or muscles of speech.

Aphasia is classified as expressive, receptive, or global (mixed). An *expressive* (Broca's or motor) aphasia is due to damage in Broca's area of the frontal lobe. It is a motor *speech* problem—the client generally understands what is said but is unable to verbally communicate. A *receptive* (Wernicke's or sensory) aphasia is due to injury involving Wernicke's area in the temporoparietal area. The client is unable to understand the spoken and often the written word. More often, the client exhibits *language* dysfunction in both the areas of expression and reception; this is known as a *global*, or mixed, aphasia.

The aphasic client requires repetitive directions to understand or complete a task. Each task should be broken down into component parts and given to the client one step at a time. The nurse faces the client and speaks slowly and clearly. The client should be given sufficient time to understand and process the information and to respond. The nurse encourages the client to communicate and positively reinforces this behavior. Family members or the nurse repeats the names of objects used on a routine basis; for example, the nurse states, "This is the toothbrush," when assisting the client to brush his/her teeth. If necessary, a picture board or communication board should be developed for the client who has Broca's aphasia. It consists of a picture of an activity (e.g., someone eating) and the printed description below. The client can point to the activity or object desired.

It is difficult to understand the client who is dysarthric. The same techniques used by the nurse for the client with aphasia can be used for the individual with dysarthria. Facial muscle exercises may be performed to strengthen the muscles used for speech. Many clients who are dysarthric are also aphasic. The client with communication impairments is usually referred to a speech and language pathologist.

Impaired Swallowing

Planning: client goals. The major goals for this nursing diagnosis are that the client will (1) eat each meal without aspiration and (2) maintain or attain ideal body weight.

Interventions: nonsurgical management. Positioning the client to facilitate the swallowing process is important. The client should eat all meals sitting in a chair or sitting straight up in bed. The client's head and neck are positioned slightly forward and flexed. Generally, clients with swallowing problems are able to tolerate or swallow soft or semisoft foods and fluids (mechanically soft or dental diet, junior baby foods) better than thin liquids (water, juice, or broth) or a regular meal. The nurse instructs the client to place food in the back of the mouth on the unaffected side to prevent trapping food in the affected cheek.

Some clients are able to swallow without difficulty, but, because they are easily distracted and impulsive, they are at risk for aspiration. These clients require a distraction-free environment with minimal disruption from television, visitors, or other environmental noise. The nurse observes the client for indications of fatigue, as this can significantly interfere with the desire and ability to eat.

■ Discharge Planning

The client with a CVA may be discharged to home, a rehabilitation center, or long-term care facility, depending on the extent of the disability. Many clients experience no significant neurologic dysfunction as a result of their stroke and are able to return home and live independently or with minimal support. Other clients are able to return home, but require ongoing assistance with ADL, as well as supervision to prevent accidents or injury. Speech, physical, or occupational therapy is conducted in the home or on an outpatient (ambulatory) basis. Clients admitted to a rehabilitation or long-term care facility require continued or more complex nursing care, as well as extensive physical, occupational, recreational, and speech or cognitive therapy. The goal of rehabilitation is to maximize the client's abilities in all aspects of life.

Home Care Preparation

If the client is discharged to the home setting, needs for adaptive or safety equipment must be identified. The extent of this assessment is dependent on the disabilities experienced by the client. The home of the client with hemiparesis should be free of scatter rugs or other obstacles in the walking pathways. The bathtub and toilet should be equipped with grab bars. Antiskid patches or strips should be placed in the bathtub to prevent the client from slipping. The physical or occupational therapist works with the client and the family to obtain all needed assistive devices *before* discharge from the hospital. Appointments for outpatient speech, physical, and occupational therapy must also be arranged before discharge.

Client/Family Education

The teaching plan for the client with a stroke includes the medication schedule, mobility transfer skills, and self-care skills. The client must take the prescribed medication to prevent another stroke and to keep hypertension under control. The nurse teaches the client and the family the name of the drug, the dosage, the timing of administration and how to take it, and possible side effects. In collaboration with the physical and occupational therapists, the nurse teaches the client how to safely climb stairs, transfer from bed to chair, and get into and out of the car, as well as how to use any aids to mobility. Finally, the client and family members are taught how to use any adaptive equipment recommended to increase independence in self-care skills. The most important information the nurse provides the client concerns what to do in an emergency and whom to call for nonemergency questions.

Psychosocial Preparation

It is not unusual for clients to become depressed within 6 months after discharge from the hospital. Generally, this is self-limiting, although the client may require antidepressants, such as amitriptyline (Elavil), for a short period of time.

Families may feel overwhelmed by the continuing demands placed on them by the client. Depending on the location of the lesion, the client may be anxious, slow, cautious, and hesitant and lack initiative (left hemisphere), or impulsive and seemingly unaware of any deficit. The family members need to spend time away from the client on a routine basis to continue to provide full-time care without sacrificing their own physical and emotional health.

Health Care Resources

Resources available to the client include a variety of publications from the American Heart Association, including *Stroke: A Guide for Families* or *Stroke: Why Do They Behave That Way?* There is a National Stroke Foundation, and many local health care institutions sponsor stroke support groups or clubs.

Evaluation

On the basis of the identified nursing diagnoses, the nurse evaluates the care for the client with CVA. The expected outcomes include that the client

1. Maintains adequate cerebral tissue perfusion
2. Improves his/her level of consciousness
3. Adapts to sensory/perceptual alterations in vision, proprioception, and sensation
4. Improves endurance in mobility
5. Uses adaptive devices as needed
6. Obtains and maintains bowel and bladder control
7. Communicates in an understandable manner or uses gestures or phrases to make needs known
8. Eats an appropriate diet without choking or aspiration

By meeting the desired outcomes, the client should be able to function well in the home and the community.

EPILEPSY

OVERVIEW

A *seizure* is an abnormal, sudden excessive discharge of electrical activity within the brain. Seizures generally signal underlying central nervous system (CNS) dysfunction, such as a brain tumor or meningitis. Seizures may also be caused by metabolic disorders, acute alcohol withdrawal, or electrolyte disturbances. *Epilepsy* is a chronic disorder characterized by recurrent seizure activity and is a symptom of brain or CNS irritation. In spite of intense public education programs, social barriers and discriminatory practices continue to exist.

Pathophysiology

The neuron consists of the cell body, a single axon, and multiple dendrites. Surrounding the cell body is the semipermeable cell wall. Within the cell body are numerous positively charged particles, potassium ions. Outside the cell membrane in the interstitial space are sodium and chloride ions, both of which are also positively charged. In the presence of an intense stimulus, an action potential is created and sodium and potassium ions cross the cell membrane of the axon, causing depolarization of the neuron and transmission of the impulse along the unmyelinated nerve. This entire process takes a few milliseconds before repolarization occurs and the cell membrane returns to its resting potential. Nerve conduction along a myelinated nerve occurs as a result

of ion (sodium and potassium) exchange at the nodes of Ranvier. The impulse "jumps" from one node of Ranvier to another, resulting in faster transmission of the impulse than in nonmyelinated fibers. Impulse transmission from one neuron to another takes place at the synapse through the coordinated efforts of the presynaptic terminals, synaptic cleft, and postsynaptic membrane.

The exact mechanisms responsible for the development of seizure activity is not fully understood. What is known is that a triggering mechanism causes a sudden, abnormal burst of activity, which disrupts the brain's usual system for nerve conduction. If the disruption is widespread, a generalized seizure occurs; if it is more localized, a partial seizure occurs.

The International Classification of Epileptic Seizures (Santilli & Sierzant, 1987) recognizes three types of seizure disorders, namely, generalized, partial, and unclassified (see the accompanying Key Features of Disease). Four types of *generalized* seizures may occur. The first is a generalized *tonic-clonic* seizure, which used to be called a grand mal seizure. This seizure begins with a tonic phase characterized by stiffening or rigidity of the muscles, particularly of the arms and legs, and immediate loss of consciousness. It is followed by clonic or rhythmic jerking of all extremities. Occasionally, only tonic or clonic movement may occur. *Absence* seizures, previously referred to as petit mal seizures, are more common in children and consist of brief (often just seconds) periods of loss of consciousness, as though the person is daydreaming. The third type of a generalized seizure is a *myoclonic* seizure, which is a brief generalized jerking or stiffening of the extremities, which may occur singly or in groups. *Atonic* (akinetic) seizures (formerly referred to as drop attacks) are characterized by sudden loss of muscle tone, which in most cases causes the client to fall.

Partial seizures, frequently referred to as focal sei-

KEY FEATURES OF DISEASE ■ Classification of Seizure Disorders

Generalized Seizures

Generalized absence (petit mal)

Generalized tonic-clonic (grand mal)

Myoclonic

Atonic

Partial Seizures (Focal Seizures)

Simple partial

Complex partial

Unclassified Seizures*

* Incomplete data.

zures, are further subdivided into two main classes. Complex partial seizures cause the client to lose consciousness, or black out, for a few seconds. Characteristic behavior known as automatism (because the client is not aware of the behavior) may occur, such as lip smacking, patting, picking at clothes, and so forth. The area of the brain most often involved in this type of epilepsy is the temporal lobe, and for this reason complex partial seizures are often called psychomotor seizures or temporal lobe seizures.

Clients with a simple partial seizure remain conscious throughout the episode. The client often reports an aura before the seizure takes place. This may consist of a déjà vu phenomenon, perception of an offensive smell, or sudden onset of pain.

Idiopathic, or unclassified, seizures account for about half of all seizure activity. They occur for no known reason and do not fit into the generalized and partial classifications.

Etiology

Seizures are often symptoms of underlying brain pathologic conditions, such as scar tissue from a head injury, vascular disease, brain tumors, aneurysm, or meningitis. They may also occur in the presence of metabolic and electrolyte disorders, drug withdrawal, acute alcohol intoxication, or kidney and liver failure.

Heredity may play a part in the development of absence, akinetic, or myoclonic seizures. Studies are inconclusive about the role of heredity in the development of partial seizures.

Incidence

Many clients attempt to hide their seizure disorder because of the fears and social stigma associated with this disorder. This makes it difficult to determine the actual incidence of epilepsy. In the United States, estimates vary from as low as 1 million to as high as 2.5 million people currently affected, with 100,000 new cases diagnosed annually (DeVroom & Considine, 1987; Santilli & Sierzant, 1987).

COLLABORATIVE MANAGEMENT

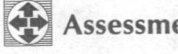 Assessment

History

A complete description of the *type of seizure activity* that occurs and events surrounding the seizure assists in determining the best treatment plan. Information to be obtained from the client and the family about the seizure includes how often they occur, a description of the seizure (e.g., tonic-clonic and staring spells), if more than one type occurs, the sequence of seizure progres-

sion, how long it lasts, when the last seizure took place, whether it is preceded by an aura (warning sign) or whether anything seems to precipitate the seizure, if the client knows a seizure has taken place, what the client does after the seizure, how long it takes for the client to return to preseizure status, and whether the client becomes incontinent of bowel or bladder during the seizure.

Some clients are able to predict when a seizure will occur through the presence of an *aura.* An aura is a peculiar sensation that warns the client of an impending seizure. The sensation may include dizziness, numbness, or visual or auditory disturbances. The nurse elicits specific information about the nature of the client's aura if it has been experienced in the past.

The nurse obtains detailed information concerning the client's current *medication* schedule. This includes the name of the medication, the dosage, the frequency of administration, and when the medications were last taken. The client should be asked if he/she takes the medicine on time in the dosage prescribed and if he/she ever routinely skips or misses the medication. If the client does not take the medication as prescribed, the nurse should attempt to find out why the client is unable to comply with the medication schedule.

Physical Assessment: Clinical Manifestations

The nurse performs a complete neurologic assessment and routine physical assessment to determine the presence of any deficits that may signal underlying pathologic changes. In the event of a seizure, the nurse observes the *type and progression of seizure activity* that occurs and attempts to identify any factors that may have precipitated the seizure. It is important to note all physical signs exhibited by the client throughout the seizure, such as eye fluttering, head and eye deviation to one side or another, changes in pupil size, movement and progression of motor activity, lip smacking or other automatisms, and level of consciousness alterations. Other physical manifestations of a generalized tonic-clonic seizure include apnea, cyanosis, copious salivation, incontinence of urine or stool, and tongue or lip biting. When the seizure is complete, the nurse records how long the seizure lasted and the client's *postictal behavior.* Postictally, the client may resume normal behavior and be completely unaware that a seizure has taken place, or may be drowsy, be difficult to arouse, and sleep for several hours.

Psychosocial Assessment

The client with newly diagnosed epilepsy may have difficulty adjusting to the diagnosis. Many clients fear that they will have a seizure at work or in social situations. They are concerned about the possibility of losing their jobs or friends and the effects of the diagnosis on their family. Often they strive to hide the diagnosis from anyone except close family members and friends. Denial of the problem is not unusual. Therefore, the nurse assesses the client's ability to utilize coping mechanisms that helped in the past to handle other difficult situations. The nurse should also assess close family members and friends for their reaction to the client's diagnosis and assist them to cope with their feelings or make an appropriate referral to other health care professionals.

Laboratory Findings

A variety of laboratory tests may be done to determine an underlying cause for the seizure activity. These may include a complete blood count (CBC), serum electrolyte determinations, liver function tests, and urinalysis.

Radiographic Findings

CT may be done to determine the presence of underlying CNS pathologic changes, which may be the cause of the seizures.

Other Diagnostic Tests

Electroencephalography is the most definitive test used to diagnose epilepsy. An EEG measures the electrical activity of the brain and records it as alpha, beta, delta, and theta brain waves. Clients with epilepsy exhibit a distinctive pattern on the EEG, which identifies the specific type of seizure disorder. For example, a generalized tonic-clonic seizure is characterized by high-voltage fast spike waves in all leads. In addition, the EEG is often able to pinpoint the focus or source of the seizure. Special techniques may be employed to further identify the type of seizure. These procedures include having the client hyperventilate, flashing lights in the client's eyes, providing auditory stimulation, or recording the EEG while the client is asleep.

MRI may also be done to determine the presence of pathologic CNS changes.

 ### Analysis: Nursing Diagnosis

The client with epilepsy is generally managed on an outpatient basis. Hospitalization may occur for more comprehensive testing and treatment or occasionally for medication adjustment. The client is at risk for injury during a seizure and may have difficulty adjusting to the diagnosis and complying with the treatment plan.

Common Diagnoses

The following diagnoses are common in clients with a diagnosis of epilepsy:

1. Potential for injury related to seizure activity
2. Ineffective individual coping and ineffective family coping related to perceived social stigma, potential

changes in employment or leisure activity, and chronicity of the disease

Additional Diagnoses

In addition to the common diagnoses, the client may have one or more of the following diagnoses:

1. Ineffective airway clearance related to seizure activity and postictal status
2. Self-esteem disturbance related to diagnosis of epilepsy
3. Social isolation related to self-esteem disturbance and change in body image
4. Noncompliance (failure to follow prescribed treatment plan) related to lack of understanding concerning consequences of failing to take medication; lack of money to buy medications; and failure to understand need to continue medication when seizure activity does not occur

 ## Planning and Implementation

The following plan of care for the client with epilepsy focuses on the common nursing diagnoses.

Potential for Injury

Planning: client goals.   The major goal for this nursing diagnosis is that the client will not be injured if a seizure occurs.

Interventions.   Approximately 80% of all seizures can be completely or almost completely controlled through the administration of anticonvulsants for specific types of seizures.

Nonsurgical management.   Drug therapy is the hallmark of management (Table 33–4). Generally, one drug at a time is introduced to achieve seizure control. If the chosen drug is not effective, the dosage may be increased or another drug introduced. At times seizure control is achieved only through a combination of medications. The dosage of medications is adjusted to achieve therapeutic blood levels without causing major side effects. The nurse administers the medications on time to maintain therapeutic blood levels and maximal effectiveness. In addition to giving the medication on time, the nurse must be cognizant of factors that could interfere with the absorption or metabolism of the anticonvulsant.

If clients are at risk for seizure activity, *seizure precautions* should be implemented, according to institutional policies. Generally, however, all facilities recommend that oxygen and suctioning equipment be readily available. It may be appropriate to insert a heparin lock in clients who are at significant risk for generalized tonic-clonic seizures (e.g., clients who have been weaned from

TABLE 33–4 Drugs Used in the Treatment of Epilepsy

Drug	Therapeutic Blood Level (μg/mL)	Remarks and Interventions
Carbamazepine (Tegretol)	8–12	Give with meals. Monitor for side effects; diplopia or blurred vision, ataxia, vertigo, vomiting, and leukopenia (check CBC monthly or every 3–6 mo). Contraindicated if glaucoma or cardiac, renal, or hepatic disease is present.
Clonazepam (Clonopin)	—	Monitor CBC. Contraindicated in glaucoma. Monitor for side effects: lethargy, ataxia, vertigo, hypotonia, anorexia, and thrombocytopenia.
Diazepam (Valium)	—	Monitor closely for respiratory distress if given intravenously. Given to stop the motor activity associated with status epilepticus.
Ethosuximide (Zarontin)	30–100	Monitor CBC and liver function test every 4–6 mo. Contraindicated in renal or liver disease. Monitor for side effects: nausea, vomiting, anorexia, lethargy, and blood dyscrasias.
Phenobarbital (Luminal)	10–30	Monitor for side effects: lethargy and nystagmus. Observe for respiratory distress if given intravenously. Drug potentiates phenothiazines; is potentiated by valproic acid; decreases warfarin absorption; and increases digoxin metabolism.
Phenytoin (Dilantin)	10–20	Check CBC and calcium levels. Monitor for side effects: gingival hyperplasia, gastric distress, hirsutism, anemia, ataxia, and nystagmus. For IV administration, flush IV line before and after with normal saline only. Give slowly, no more than 50 mg/min. Metabolism is inhibited by warfarin, chloramphenicol, isoniazid, and phenothiazines; decreased therapeutic blood levels occur when given with carbamazepine, clonazepam, prednisone, and digoxin.
Primidone (Myidone)	5–12	Monitor for side effects: vertigo and lethargy (same as for phenobarbital); potentiated by isoniazid; drug interactions same as for phenobarbital.
Valproic acid (Depakene)	50–100	Monitor CBC and AST. Monitor for side effects: nausea, vomiting, lethargy, impaired PT and PTT, hair loss, leukopenia, and liver toxicity. Increases serum phenobarbital levels and alters serum phenytoin levels.

their medication or those under extreme stress), as this provides ready access if IV medication must be given to stop the seizure. It is usually inappropriate to pad the side rails of the client's bed, as they are rarely the source of significant injury. More importantly, padded side rails may cause significant embarrassment to the client and the family. Padded tongue blades do not belong at the bedside and should *never* be inserted into the client's mouth after a seizure begins. The jaw clenches down as soon as the seizure begins; forcing a tongue blade into the mouth is more likely to chip the client's teeth and

increase the risk of aspiration of tooth fragments than to prevent the client from biting the tongue.

When a seizure occurs, the nurse takes precautions to prevent the client from injury. The actions taken by the nurse should be appropriate for the type of seizure experienced by the client. For example, all that may be necessary for a simple partial seizure is to observe, document, and time the length of the seizure. Clients engaged in activities that may cause harm should be directed away from the activity. The client who loses consciousness during a seizure, usually during a generalized tonic-clonic or complex partial seizure, should be turned on his/her side if possible, or the client's head should be turned to the side to prevent aspiration and allow secretions to drain. Any objects that could injure the client should be moved out of the way. It is not unusual for the client to become cyanotic during a generalized tonic-clonic seizure, and precautions must be taken to maintain an open airway. This is generally self-limiting and requires no treatment, although some physicians prefer to give high-risk clients (e.g., elderly, critically ill, or debilitated individuals) oxygen by nasal cannula or face mask throughout the seizure and during the postictal period. The client should never be restrained unless he/she is in grave danger of causing severe injury. Restraining the client may cause injury and often aggravates the situation, causing more seizure activity. Clients with atonic seizures may benefit from a protective device when sitting in a chair to keep them from falling. Again, the decision to restrain must be weighed carefully against the possibility that a seizure will take place.

The nurse carefully observes the seizure and documents the time the seizure began; the part or parts of the body affected; the progression of the seizure and the type or character of movements; eye deviation, nystagmus (involuntary rhythmic oscillation of eyes), or changes in pupil size; the client's condition throughout the seizure; and postictal status.

Status epilepticus (seizure that lasts longer than 4 minutes or seizures that occur in rapid succession) is a potential complication of all types of seizures. It is a neurologic emergency in clients with generalized tonic-clonic seizures and must be treated promptly to prevent irreversible brain damage and possibly death from anoxia, cardiac arrhythmias, or lactic acidosis. The physician is notified immediately. An adequate airway must be established promptly (intubation may be necessary), and oxygen should be given as indicated by the client's condition. The usual causes of status epilepticus include sudden withdrawal from anticonvulsant medication, infections, acute alcohol withdrawal, head trauma, cerebral edema, and metabolic disturbances. Medications used to treat this problem include IV diazepam (Valium) to stop motor movement, phenytoin (Dilantin), phenobarbital, or a combination of all three. The client's respiratory status may be further compromised when diazepam and phenobarbital are given intravenously. Phenytoin should never be given faster than 50 mg/minute, as this may lead to cardiac arrhythmias. Other medications used to control status epilepticus include paraldehyde and thiopental sodium. General anesthesia may be used as a treatment of last resort to stop the seizure activity. Additional nursing care for the client in status epilepticus includes inserting a nasogastric tube to prevent aspiration and vomiting, monitoring cardiac status and blood pressure, preventing hyperthermia, and observing the client for side effects or signs of toxicity from the medications used to stop the seizures. Serum blood levels should be closely monitored for the first 3 days after the start of the anticonvulsant medication and thereafter as indicated.

Surgical management. As noted earlier, 20% of clients with epilepsy cannot be fully controlled with medications. When all other treatment options are exhausted, surgery may be indicated to improve the quality of the client's life. The more traditional approach is a *corpus callosotomy,* which is used to treat tonic-clonic or atonic seizures. In this procedure, the corpus callosum is severed, preventing neuronal discharges from passing between the two hemispheres of the brain. It usually reduces the number and severity of the seizures, making them more amenable to more conventional drug therapy.

The second procedure involves identifying the seizure focus through elaborate procedures involving continuous recording of the client's EEG, close observation, and, in many institutions, video monitoring of the client at all times, except during personal care activities. After the focus is identified, electrodes are surgically implanted into the brain tissue to identify the extent of the focal area. This is followed by additional continuous EEG and, when possible, video monitoring of the client at all times and close observation by the nursing staff. The area is excised if it can be safely removed without affecting vital areas of brain function. Preoperative and postoperative nursing care is similar to that described for craniotomy (see later).

Ineffective Individual Coping; Ineffective Family Coping

Planning: client goals. The major goal for these nursing diagnoses is that the client and the family will begin to develop strategies to adjust to the diagnosis.

Interventions: nonsurgical management. The nurse helps the client and the family to identify strategies that they have successfully used to cope with difficult situations in the past. Often the client's and the family's difficulties in coping with the diagnosis stem from a lack of understanding about epilepsy and misconceptions about changes that will take place in their lives as a result of the diagnosis. Many of their fears and anxieties can be relieved with a thorough education program.

■ Discharge Planning

Home Care Preparation

The diagnostic work-up of clients with epilepsy is performed on an outpatient basis. Approximately 20% of clients with epilepsy are unable to be managed with anticonvulsant medications alone, and surgery may be helpful for some. The majority of clients can easily be treated on an outpatient basis; hospitalization for epilepsy alone is rare. Home care preparation is minimal. If the client's seizures are not readily controlled, additional precautions must be taken to prevent injury during activities such as bathing and toileting. These may include grab bars in the bathtub or shower area, a signal device the client can use if help is needed, and a mechanism to easily enter a locked bathroom door from the outside.

Client/Family Education

An educational program for the client with epilepsy includes discussion of what it is and what it is not; anticonvulsant therapy; precautions to be taken when ill, under stress, or fatigued or when workload or social activities increase; diet and effects of alcohol; and driving or operating any type of motorized vehicles (see the accompanying Client/Family Education feature).

Information about epilepsy should be presented to the client and the family in a manner that can be easily understood. The nurse ascertains what the client and the family understand about the disorder. Any misinformation should be corrected, and new information is presented as they are able to assimilate and comprehend it.

Information given to the client about the medications includes the name of the drug, the dosage, and the side effects and symptoms of toxicity and what should be done if any of these occur. The nurse should stress the need to keep all health care appointments and the importance of maintaining serum levels of the drugs by administration at prescribed intervals. The nurse collaborates with the client to develop an appropriate medication schedule. Many clients are reluctant to take their medications at work or school, and this is a major reason for noncompliance. The medication schedule should be adjusted to meet the following: the ease and convenience of administration, the half-life of the drug, and the avoidance of factors that may interfere with absorption and metabolism. The nurse must stress to the client that the medication must *not* be stopped because the seizures have stopped, as this could lead to the recurrence of seizures or the life-threatening complication of status epilepticus. Some clients may stop taking the medication simply because they do not have the money to purchase their drugs. Clients with limited incomes should be referred to the social services department for financial assistance. The client should ask the physician what action to take in the event that a medication dose is missed or vomited. If only one dosage is missed, this generally does not present a problem. If more than one dosage is missed, the client should notify the appropriate health care worker (physician, clinic nurse, or nurse practitioner).

Most clients with a seizure disorder should avoid alcohol consumption altogether or drink little. Fatigue, stress, and excessive excitement may trigger a seizure. The client should be instructed to keep a log to identify factors that cause seizures to occur. After a pattern is identified, steps can be taken to prevent or minimize the risk of a seizure. The client should learn to recognize warning signs of a seizure so that precautions can be taken to avoid injury.

Although most clients are reluctant to do so, they should be encouraged to wear a medical alert (Medic Alert) bracelet or necklace. In any event, the client should have this information on personal identification cards.

Although state laws differ, most people with epilepsy are unable to drive or operate motorized vehicles (cars, trucks, tractors, airplanes, and so forth) until they have been seizure free (with or without medications) for a period of time, usually 1 to 2 years. All states prohibit discrimination against people who have epilepsy. Clients who work in occupations in which a seizure could cause serious harm to themselves or others (e.g., construction worker, dangerous equipment operator, pilot, and railroad engineer) may need to find alternative employment. Strenuous or potentially dangerous

---

CLIENT/FAMILY EDUCATION ■ Instructions for the Client with Epilepsy

Instructions	Rationales
1. "Take medication as prescribed; do not miss any dose."	1. Therapeutic levels of the drugs are maintained.
2. "Avoid alcohol consumption and excessive fatigue."	2. These predispose the individual to seizure.
3. "Do not take any medication, including OTC drugs, without asking the physician."	3. Other drugs may interact with the seizure medication or lower the client's seizure threshold.
4. "Wear a medical alert (Medic Alert) bracelet or necklace."	4. In case of emergency, anyone can recognize the client's condition.
5. "Contact the Epilepsy Foundation of America or other organized epilepsy group."	5. Support for the client and information are available.
6. "Check with state laws regarding driving and operating machinery as an epileptic."	6. Laws vary among states.

physical activity may need to be curtailed or modified to prevent harm to the client. Restriction of recreational activities should be discussed with the physician.

Psychosocial Preparation

The client and the family must be prepared for some rejection or social and work setting discrimination by those who are misinformed about the diagnosis of epilepsy. Friends may be afraid of the client and fear that a seizure may occur and they will not know what to do. If the client has a positive attitude and resumes or maintains a usual life style, friends will be more comfortable and supportive. Employers may fear that the client will utilize more sick time or be involved in more workers' compensation injuries, even though most studies dispute this point. The client may find it difficult to obtain life and health insurance.

Health Care Resources

The client with epilepsy should be referred to the Epilepsy Foundation of America, National Epilepsy League, Inc., or National Association to Control Epilepsy.

 Evaluation

On the basis of the identified nursing diagnoses, the nurse evaluates the care for the client with epilepsy. The expected outcomes include that the client

1. Is free of injury
2. Takes anticonvulsant medication as prescribed
3. Implements appropriate precautions when at increased risk for seizures to occur (e.g., during times of stress or fatigue)
4. Asks appropriate questions about the diagnosis and maintains social contacts (family or significant others as well)

INFECTIONS

MENINGITIS

OVERVIEW

Meningitis is an inflammation of the arachnoid and pia mater (leptomeninges) of the brain and the spinal cord. Bacterial and viral agents are most often responsible for meningitis, although fungal agents may also be involved. Bacterial meningitis occurs most frequently; early detection and treatment are associated with a more favorable outcome. Viral meningitis is usually self-limiting, and the client has a complete recovery.

Pathophysiology

The brain and spinal cord are covered by the three-layered meninges—dura mater, arachnoid, and pia mater. CSF produced within the choroid plexus of the ventricles travels via the subarachnoid space within the ventricular system and around the brain and spinal cord. It is reabsorbed via the arachnoid villi, which are finger-like structures in the arachnoid layer of the meninges.

The organisms responsible for meningitis enter the CNS via the blood stream at the blood-brain barrier. Direct routes of entry occur as a result of penetrating trauma, surgical procedures, or a ruptured cerebral abscess. Otorrhea (ear discharge) or rhinorrhea, which may be caused by a basilar skull fracture, may lead to meningitis owing to the direct communication of CSF with the environment. The invading organisms are able to migrate throughout the CNS via the subarachnoid space. The presence of the pathologic organism in the subarachnoid space produces an inflammatory response in the pia, the arachnoid, the CSF, and the ventricles. The exudate formed may spread to both cranial and spinal nerves, causing further neurologic deterioration. In addition, the exudate may block the normal flow of CSF and lead to the development of hydrocephalus.

Etiology

Meningitis is caused by a wide variety of organisms (see the accompanying Key Features of Disease). Most often, the client has a predisposing condition, such as a fractured skull, infection, or brain or spinal surgery, that increases the likelihood of meningitis.

Bacterial Meningitis

The most frequently involved organisms responsible for bacterial meningitis include *Haemophilus influenzae*, *Streptococcus preumoniae*, *Neisseria meningitidis*, and *Staphylococcus aureus*. The body recognizes the protein

---

KEY FEATURES OF DISEASE ■ **Bacteria Responsible for Meningitis**

Haemophilus influenzae

Neisseria meningitidis (meningococcal)

Diplococcus pneumoniae (pneumococcal)

Streptococci, group A

Staphylococcus aureus

Escherichia coli

Klebsiella

Proteus

Pseudomonas

within the bacteria as a foreign substance and sets up an inflammatory response. Neutrophils, monocytes, lymphocytes, and other inflammatory cells respond. An exudate consisting of bacteria, fibrin, and leukocytes is formed in the subarachnoid space. It accumulates within the CSF and may cause the normally thin, watery CSF to become thickened. This may interfere with the normal flow of CSF around the brain and spinal cord, as well as interfere with its absorption at the arachnoid granulation and lead to hydrocephalus. In addition, the presence of the exudate within the subarachnoid space can cause a further inflammatory response and increased ICP. The exudate is deposited over the brain, cranial nerves, and spinal nerve roots. The meningeal cells become edematous, as the cell membrane is no longer able to regulate the flow of fluid into or out of the cell. Rapid vasodilation of the cerebral vessels occurs, which may lead to engorgement, rupture, or thrombosis of the vessel walls. The brain tissue may become infarcted, leading to a further increase in ICP. These processes may result in a secondary infection of the brain if the bacteria are able to extend into the brain tissue, causing encephalitis and further neurologic impairment.

Viral Meningitis

This type of meningitis is often referred to as *aseptic meningitis*. It often occurs as a sequela to a variety of viral illnesses, including measles, mumps, herpes simplex, and herpes zoster. The formation of exudate that is common in bacterial meningitis does not occur, and no organisms are cultured from the CSF. Inflammation occurs over the cerebral cortex, the white matter, and the meninges. The susceptibility of the brain tissue to the virus varies, depending on which type of cell is involved. The herpes simplex virus alters cellular metabolism, which quickly results in necrosis of the cells. Other viruses cause an alteration in the production of enzymes or neurotransmitters, which cause dysfunction of the cells and possible neurologic defects.

Incidence

There are no known statistics on the overall incidence of meningitis. Pneumococcal meningitis occurs most often in adults older than 40 years of age. Bacterial meningitis is seen most often in the fall and winter seasons when upper respiratory tract infections commonly occur.

PREVENTION

Meningitis can be prevented by prompt recognition and treatment of predisposing conditions, such as otitis media and upper respiratory tract infection. Health care personnel must continue to emphasize the need to complete the course of all prescribed medications, even though the symptoms of the infection have completely

disappeared. The client who is immunosuppressed, receiving chemotherapy or radiation therapy, or receiving long-term steroids must be educated about the risk for and indications of meningitis.

After the presence of meningitis is recognized, prompt action must be taken to identify the causative organism and to begin organism-specific treatment to prevent serious complications.

COLLABORATIVE MANAGEMENT

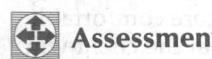 **Assessment**

History

The diagnosis of meningitis is based on the findings of a complete history and physical examination of the client. This information identifies the probable cause, as well as the types of organisms responsible for the development of meningitis. The nurse asks the client to *describe the symptoms* currently being experienced; when they began; whether they stayed the same, improved, or became worse; and what, if anything, aggravates or relieves the symptoms. Next, the nurse questions the client about his/her past *medical history* to include information about any viral or respiratory tract diseases; head trauma or skull fracture; ear, nose, or sinus infections; heart disease, diabetes mellitus, or cancer; and current immunosuppressive therapies (e.g., steroids), chemotherapy, and previous surgical procedures, especially neurologic surgery or procedures involving the ear and nose.

The nurse elicits information concerning exposure to communicable disease, the presence of a rash, and animal or insect bites. The nurse asks about travel outside of the United States, what countries were visited, and where the client stayed (e.g., urban or rural area, in hotel, or with local family or camping).

Physical Assessment: Clinical Manifestations

The nurse begins the examination by assessing the client's level of consciousness, orientation to person, place, and year, pupil reaction and eye movements, and motor response. In the early stages of the disease, the client may exhibit mild *lethargy, memory changes,* a short attention span, bewilderment, and personality and *behavior changes.* As the disease progresses, the client becomes increasingly stuporous. Clients with a mild case of meningitis, and particularly with viral meningitis, may exhibit few symptoms, including severe headache and generalized muscle aches and pains.

Although the pupils are generally reactive to light, the client may complain of *photophobia* when light is shined directly into the eyes. While checking the pupils, the nurse observes for *nystagmus*, as well as any other abnormal eye movements. Owing to the formation of exudate, inflammation, and vascular engorgement, dysfunction of cranial nerves III, IV, and VI may be seen.

If cranial nerves VII and VIII are involved, the client shows signs of facial paresis and has difficulty hearing. The client may also experience dizziness owing to the involvement of cranial nerve VIII.

Findings from the client's motor examination are usually within normal limits in the early stages of the disease. Later, hemiparesis, hemiplegia, and decreased muscle tone may occur.

Other indicators of meningeal irritation include nuchal rigidity and a positive Kernig's or Brudzinski's sign. *Nuchal rigidity* is manifested by a stiff neck and soreness, particularly when the client's neck is flexed. The nurse may elect to test both Kernig's and Brudzinski's signs. A positive response occurs in the presence of bacterial meningitis and is absent in viral meningitis. Both tests are performed with the client lying supine in bed. The nurse flexes the client's leg at the hip, brings the knee to a 90-degree angle (Fig. 33–6), and then attempts to straighten the knee. *Kernig's sign* is pain in the client with meningeal irritation and spinal nerve root inflammation (from exudate around the roots). To test the *Brudzinski reflex*, the nurse gently flexes the client's head and neck onto the chest. A positive response is indicated by flexion of the hips and knees.

Other signs of meningitis include *headache, nausea, vomiting, fever, chills,* and *tachycardia.* These early symptoms are often mistaken for an influenza-like illness. A distinguishing characteristic is that the headache experienced by those with meningitis is severe and unrelenting, whereas the headache with influenza is less severe and tends to resolve within 24 hours. The client may develop a red macular rash, especially in the presence of meningococcal meningitis. Viral meningitis may be characterized by the additional symptoms of abdominal and chest pain.

The nurse also assesses the client for complications that may occur, including *increased ICP* resulting from the presence of exudate, which can lead to hydrocephalus and cerebral edema. Left untreated, increased ICP can lead to herniation of the brain and death (see later for more information on increased ICP).

Seizure activity may be caused by irritation of the cerebral cortex or from hyponatremia. Owing to abnormal stimulation of the hypothalamic area, excessive amounts of antidiuretic hormone (ADH) (vasopressin) are produced. This results in water retention and dilution of serum sodium attributable to increased excretion of sodium by the kidneys. This syndrome of inappropriate antidiuretic hormone (SIADH) production may lead to increased ICP (see later).

The assessment of the client's vascular status includes observation of the color and temperature of the extremities, determination of the presence of peripheral pulses, and identification of any indicators of abnormal bleeding. Septic emboli in the blood may block circulation in the small vessels of the hands and feet, leading to gangrene. Excessive fibrinolysis that occurs in bacteremia and infections from viruses, fungi, or protozoa may lead to disseminated intravascular coagulation. Vascular involvement of the cerebral arteries, veins, and venous sinuses may lead to seizures and hemiparesis. (Refer to Chap. 65 for a complete discussion of these cardiovascular problems.)

Psychosocial Assessment

The client with meningitis often has complaints of fever, severe headache, nausea, vomiting, and sleepiness. The family typically reports subtle to overt changes in mental status, behavior, or personality. Owing to the clinical course of the disease, the client may feel frightened and anxious. The nurse assesses these behaviors to assist in planning appropriate care.

Laboratory Findings

The most significant laboratory test to diagnose meningitis is the analysis of the client's CSF. A lumbar puncture should *not* be done in the presence of increased ICP, as this may cause downward herniation of the brain tissue onto the medulla and subsequent cardiopulmonary arrest. The CSF is analyzed for cell count and protein and glucose concentrations, and a culture and sensitivity test are performed. Counterimmunoelec-

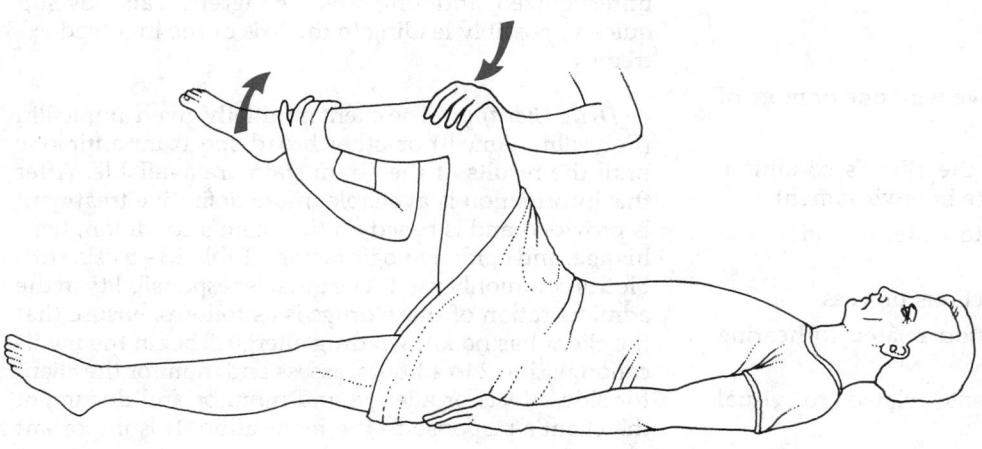

Figure 33–6

Kernig's sign to test for meningitis. Flexion of the hip and knee causes pain.

trophoresis (CIE) may be performed to determine the presence of viruses or protozoa in the CSF. CIE is also indicated if the client has received antibiotics before the CSF was obtained. To identify a possible bacterial source of infection, cultures of the blood, the urine, the throat, and the nose are also performed.

A CBC is performed, with attention to the white blood cell count, which is generally elevated well above the normal value. Serum electrolyte and glucose values are studied to identify the presence of electrolyte abnormalities, especially hyponatremia. The serum glucose result is compared with the CSF glucose level. Normally, the CSF glucose level is two-thirds that of the serum glucose. In the presence of meningitis (except viral meningitis), the CSF glucose level is normal to slightly decreased.

Radiographic Findings

CT may be performed to determine the presence of cerebral edema or other neurologic disease. Results are usually normal, unless the disease has markedly progressed. Skull films to identify the presence of infected sinuses may be obtained if clinically indicated.

 Analysis: Nursing Diagnosis

The client with meningitis is admitted to the hospital with fever and changes in normal neurologic functioning.

Common Diagnoses

Four nursing diagnoses are commonly noted in clients with meningitis, as follows:

1. Altered (cerebral) tissue perfusion related to increased ICP or cerebral edema
2. Altered (peripheral) tissue perfusion related to decreased blood supply to the hands and feet
3. Pain related to headache, meningeal irritation, or photophobia
4. Potential for injury related to seizures, changes in mental status, and altered level of consciousness

Additional Diagnoses

In addition, the client may have with one or more of the following:

1. Anxiety and fear related to the client's condition, knowledge deficit, and change in environment
2. Fluid volume excess related to water retention and SIADH
3. Hyperthermia related to infectious process
4. Impaired verbal communication related to hearing loss
5. Sensory/perceptual alterations related to visual changes

6. Ineffective family coping related to client's overall condition

 Planning and Implementation

The following plan of care for the client with meningitis focuses on the common nursing diagnoses.

Altered (Cerebral) Tissue Perfusion; Altered (Peripheral) Tissue Perfusion

The primary concern in the client with meningitis is to prevent complications resulting from the alterations in cerebral and peripheral tissue perfusion.

Planning: client goals. The goals for these nursing diagnoses are that the client will (1) return to his/her preillness neurologic status and (2) be free of vascular complications.

Interventions: nonsurgical management. The client's vital signs and neurologic status are assessed every 4 hours or more often if clinically indicated. The nurse assesses for complications, including cerebral edema, hydrocephalus, and increased ICP. All interventions for increased ICP (discussed later) are initiated. Of particular importance for the client with meningitis is to avoid flexion of the neck, as this can cause severe pain.

Owing to the potential involvement of the cranial nerves, the nurse includes complete cranial nerve testing as part of the routine neurologic assessment. Particular attention is given to cranial nerves I, III, IV, VI, and VIII, as discussed earlier. A sixth cranial nerve defect (inability to move the eyes laterally) may indicate the development of hydrocephalus. Other indicators of hydrocephalus include the usual signs of increased ICP and the presence of urinary incontinence in the previously continent client.

A complete vascular assessment is performed during each nursing shift or more often, if indicated, to prevent and detect early vascular compromise from septic emboli. This severe complication is most frequently seen in circulation to the hand. If vascular compromise is left unrecognized and untreated, gangrene can develop quickly, possibly leading to the loss of the involved extremity.

Drug therapy. The client is initially given ampicillin (Polycillin, Amcill) or other broad-spectrum antibiotic until the results of the Gram stain are available. After this information is available, more definitive treatment is provided and is based on the client's condition, her/his age, and epidemiologic factors. Table 33–5 lists antibiotics commonly used. The nurse's responsibility in the administration of these drugs is as follows: ensure that the client has no known drug allergies, begin the medication within 2 to 4 hours, assess and monitor the client for side effects or allergy, and monitor and document the client's response to the medication. It is important

TABLE 33-5 Antibiotics Specific to Organisms Causing Meningitis

Antibiotic	Organisms
Pencillin G	Pneumococci
	Meningococci
	Streptococci
Gentamicin	*Klebsiella*
	Pseudomonas
	Proteus
Chloramphenicol	*Haemophilus influenzae*

for medications to be given on time to maintain therapeutic effectiveness.

Isolation. Isolation precautions should be followed for the first 24 hours after the start of antimicrobial therapy for clients with bacterial meningitis. Clients with viral meningitis require precautions for urine and stool only. More specific guidelines on isolation can be obtained from the Centers for Disease Control or the hospital's infection control manual (see Chap. 26).

Pain

The inflammatory and infectious process involving the meninges can cause severe headache, which increases the client's anxiety level as well.

Planning: client goal. The major goal for this nursing diagnosis is that the client will state that pain is reduced or alleviated.

Interventions: nonsurgical management. The client with meningitis usually has a severe headache and photophobia. The environment is kept as quiet as possible, and the lights are dimmed. Muscle aches and pain related to fever can be relieved by frequent positioning changes, moist heat, or back rubs. Analgesics, such as acetaminophen (Tylenol) or codeine, may be given to relieve more severe pain. The nurse plans activities and treatments to allow the client to have uninterrupted periods of rest. This may include restriction of visitors to immediate family.

Potential for Injury

The client with meningitis is predisposed to seizure activity and must be protected from injury.

Planning: client goals. The major goal for this nursing diagnosis is that the client will remain injury free.

Interventions: nonsurgical management. The client is at risk for seizure activity and loss of consciousness. Routine seizure precautions are implemented by the nurse to include keeping the side rails up at all times and the bed in low position. Suction apparatus and oxygen are placed at the bedside. In the event of a seizure, the nurse records a description of the event, the length of seizure, whether eye deviation occurred, and any interventions (e.g., medications and oxygen) used to treat the seizure. To further protect the client from injury, all harmful objects are removed from the immediate environment. The client should be visually checked each hour to ensure safety.

■ Discharge Planning

The client with meningitis is discharged to the home setting. In cases in which the client has residual neurologic deficits, discharge to a rehabilitation facility may be warranted.

Home Care Preparation

Most clients with meningitis are discharged with few or no neurologic problems. If neurologic problems persist, routine assessment of the home for potential hazards and accessibility should be done. This includes ensuring that the client can enter the house, that scatter rugs and unnecessary clutter are removed, and that there is accessibility to the bathroom, kitchen, and sleeping quarters.

Client/Family Education

The client may need to continue antimicrobial therapy at home. The client should be instructed on the name and purpose of the medication, as well as the time to take it and any side effects. The nurse stresses the importance of taking all medications until completely depleted. Some clients may think it acceptable to stop the medication as soon as they feel better. The client should be encouraged to call the physician, the clinic, or the nurse practitioner if any questions arise after discharge from the hospital.

Families and other close contacts of the clients with meningococcal or *H. influenzae* meningitis may be required to take rifampin (rifamycin) as a preventive measure. Side effects of rifampin include headache, orange-colored urine, permanent orange discoloration of contact lenses, and interference with the effectiveness of birth control pills. The client should be instructed about the causes of meningitis and what measures to take to prevent recurrence.

Psychosocial Preparation

Many clients are concerned that they will develop a recurrence of meningitis at a later date. This is especially true when the disease has occurred after a seemingly simple ear or sinus infection. To alleviate their fears, the nurse should instruct clients on appropriate preventive techniques. The importance of keeping the follow-up medical appointment and complying with all therapeutic modalities should be stressed.

Health Care Resources

If the client requires adaptive equipment at home, it should be ordered and delivered before discharge from the hospital. The physical or occupational therapist can help the client learn to use it safely.

 Evaluation

On the basis of the identified nursing diagnoses, the nurse evaluates the care for the client with meningitis. The expected outcomes include that the client

1. Remains afebrile
2. States that pain is alleviated
3. Describes and complies with the medication program as ordered

By meeting the desired outcomes, the client should experience minimal discomfort and complications from meningitis.

ENCEPHALITIS

OVERVIEW

Encephalitis is an inflammation of the brain parenchyma (brain tissue) and often the meninges. It affects the cerebrum, the brain stem, or the cerebellum. It is most often caused by a viral agent, although an ameba may also be involved. Viral encephalitis is almost always preceded by a viral infection.

Viruses are composed of both deoxyribonucleic acid (DNA) and ribonucleic acid (RNA) and depend on living tissue for reproduction. Because of this, the virus-invaded tissues redirect their normal activities to concentrate on reproduction of the virus. Certain viruses show a propensity for certain areas of the brain; for example, the herpesvirus is most often found in the temporal lobe.

The virus gains access to the CNS via the blood stream, or along peripheral or cranial nerves, or is already present in the meninges (in meningitis). After the virus invades the brain tissue, it begins to reproduce, causing an inflammatory response. Unlike the case with meningitis, this does not cause exudate formation. Inflammation extends over the cerebral cortex, the white matter, and the meninges, with concomitant degeneration of the neurons of the cortex. Owing to the destruction of the white matter, demyelination of axons occurs in the involved area. This leads to hemorrhage, edema, necrosis, and the development of small lacunae within the cerebral hemispheres. Widespread edema can cause compression of blood vessels, leading to further increase in ICP. Death may occur from herniation and increased ICP.

The viruses most often responsible for the development of encephalitis are the arboviruses, enteroviruses, and herpes simplex type 1 virus. Arboviruses can be transmitted to humans through the bite of an infected mosquito or tick. The most common types of encephalitis seen are eastern and western equine, St. Louis, and California. Echovirus, coxsackievirus, poliovirus, and viruses that cause mumps and chicken pox are the common enteroviruses associated with encephalitis. Herpes simplex type 1 causes the third type of viral encephalitis, the most frequently occurring nonepidemic encephalitis in North America.

Amebic meningoencephalitis is caused by the amebae *Naegleria* and *Acanthamoeba*. Both are found in warm freshwater and can enter the nasal mucosa of people swimming in ponds or lakes. The amebae may also be found in soil and decaying vegetation. Although this has not been seen frequently in the past, its incidence in North America is increasing.

Few statistics are available regarding the overall incidence of encephalitis. Each year, the Centers for Disease Control receives reports of several thousand new cases. Mortality rates for herpes simplex type 1 encephalitis can be as high as 40% to 50%, whereas mortality for the other types is much lower. The morbidity rates with encephalitis, particularly those caused by the arboviruses and herpes simplex virus, remain high.

Encephalitis associated with tick bites tends to occur more frequently in the spring, whereas that associated with mosquitoes occurs in middle to late summer. The incubation period for both is 5 to 15 days. Summer is also the peak time for encephalitis caused by the enteroviruses, with the exception of the mumps virus, which is more prevalent in early winter. The incubation period varies depending on the virus involved.

Prevention of encephalitis caused by the arboviruses is directed toward eliminating breeding sources for mosquitoes and effective mosquito control. During the summer and spring months, people who have been outdoors, particularly in wooded areas, should check for the presence of ticks everywhere on their bodies.

Prevention of encephalitis related to the enteroviruses can be accomplished to some degree through immunization against measles, mumps, and poliomyelitis. Other measures include the prompt and aggressive treatment of all viral illness and careful attention to the signs and symptoms of encephalitis. Early detection and treatment are associated with a more favorable outcome.

COLLABORATIVE MANAGEMENT

The diagnosis of encephalitis is complicated because the presenting signs and symptoms are similar to those of a variety of other neurologic diseases, including subarachnoid hemorrhage, brain abscess, meningitis, and septic emboli. Therefore, the history is important to help differentiate encephalitis from these other problems.

To verify the diagnosis of herpes simplex encephalitis, the nurse elicits information about the presence of cold sores or lesions or ulcerations of the oral cavity. This should include both recent or past history and the frequency of cold sores.

The nurse queries the client about a recent history of mosquito or tick bites and the client's response to them. For example, did a bite cause a large reddened area or become infected? Often, the client is unaware of tick bites, so the nurse questions the client about outdoor activities. Additional information should be obtained concerning swimming in freshwater lakes and ponds, particularly in countries outside of North America.

Enteroviruses are associated with echovirus and coxsackievirus infections and mumps, and the nurse inquires about exposure to any infectious diseases, as well as travel to areas in which these diseases are prevalent.

The typical client with encephalitis has changes in level of consciousness and mental status, meningeal irritation, motor dysfunction, focal neurologic deficits, and, often, symptoms of increased ICP.

The nurse assesses the level of consciousness using the Glasgow Coma Scale. The client may be lethargic, stuporous, or comatose. Mental status changes include confusion, disorientation, irritability, and personality and behavior changes (especially noted in the presence of herpes simplex). The nurse examines the client for signs of meningeal irritation by assessing for the presence of nuchal rigidity and Kernig's or Brudzinski's sign (described earlier). Motor changes exhibited by the client may vary from a mild weakness to hemiplegia. The client may have muscle tremors, spasticity, an ataxic gait, myoclonic jerks, and increased deep tendon reflexes. Seizure activity is not uncommon. The client often complains of fever, nausea, vomiting, headache, and vertigo.

Cranial nerve involvement is exhibited by ocular palsies, facial weakness, and nystagmus. The herpes zoster lesion affects cranial and spinal nerve root ganglia, which is clinically manifested by a rash, severe pain, itching, burning, or tingling in the areas innervated by these nerves.

In severe cases of encephalitis, the client may exhibit increased ICP resulting from cerebral edema, hemorrhage, and necrosis of brain tissue. The client's vital signs are observed for indications of a widened pulse pressure, bradycardia, and irregular respirations. The client's pupils become increasingly dilated and less responsive to light. Left untreated, increased ICP leads to herniation of the brain tissue and possibly death.

There are few specific tests to diagnose encephalitis. A lumbar puncture is performed, unless contraindicated, and the CSF is analyzed for cell count and protein and glucose levels. Culture and sensitivity testing, Gram's stain, and CIE may be done to determine the involved organism. However, the findings are often normal, and the virus is not identified, particularly with the arbovirus or herpesvirus. The serum white blood cell count may be elevated, indicating that an infection is present.

CT is done to rule out other causes of disease, such as a brain abscess or a subarachnoid hemorrhage, and to determine the presence of cerebral edema.

The interventions for this disorder are similar to those for meningitis, with the exception of drug therapy. Supportive nursing care and the prompt recognition and treatment of increased ICP are essential components of treatment. The nurse also maintains a patent airway to prevent the development of atelectasis or pneumonia, which could lead to further brain hypoxia from inadequate amounts of oxygen in the circulating blood. The client is encouraged to turn, cough, and deep breathe at least every 2 hours. Deep tracheal suctioning may be performed, even in the presence of increased ICP if the findings of the respiratory assessment indicate that the client's respiratory status is compromised, possibly causing cerebral hypoxia.

The client's vital signs and neurologic signs are checked every 2 hours or more frequently if clinically indicated. The head of the bed is elevated 30 to 45 degrees, unless contraindicated (e.g., after lumbar puncture or with severe hypotension). The client is positioned to avoid aggravating or increasing ICP.

Vidarabine (Vira-A; adenine arabinoside, Ara-A) is used to treat herpes encephalitis. Therapy is most effective if used early, before the client becomes stuporous or comatose, which usually occurs within 4 to 6 days after the appearance of the initial neurologic symptoms. No specific drug therapy is available for infection by arboviruses or enteroviruses. Acyclovir has recently been approved for the treatment of herpes simplex type 1 and is associated with a significantly lower mortality rate than vidarabine, although the morbidity rate remains essentially the same.

Because of permanent neurologic disabilities, the client with encephalitis is usually discharged to a rehabilitation setting or a long-term care facility. Clients with minimal neurologic problems are discharged to home.

BRAIN ABSCESS

OVERVIEW

A *brain abscess* is a purulent infection of the brain in which pus forms in the extradural, subdural, or intracerebral area of the brain. The causative organisms are most often bacteria, which invade the brain directly or indirectly.

Organisms from the ear, sinus, or mastoid area generally enter the brain by traveling along the wall of the cerebral veins and therefore may spread to any area of the brain. At times, the organisms (especially those from the ear) erode the bone, form a tract, and directly enter the brain. Septic emboli from the heart, the lungs, or a dental or peritonsillar abscess may break off and enter the systemic circulation. These organisms may become lodged in a cerebral vessel and produce a localized infection. Penetrating trauma, open head injuries, and neurosurgical procedures provide a potential means for the direct entry of an organism into the brain.

The organisms cause a local infection, with acute inflammation surrounding the involved area. Within a few days, necrosis of the tissue takes place and pus formation and liquefaction of the tissue occur. This is followed by the development of cerebral edema owing to localized vascular congestion in response to inflammation. Over the subsequent 2 weeks, the area becomes encapsulated, first by fibrous granulation tissue and later by collagenous connective tissue. The abscess usually occurs deep within the cerebral hemisphere and involves the white matter of the brain. Occasionally, the abscess does not become encapsulated; instead, it spreads through the brain tissue to the subarachnoid space and ventricular system.

An *epidural* or extradural abscess usually results from a skull fracture or osteomyelitis. The overwhelming majority of *subdural* abscesses, more correctly referred to as a subdural empyema, are caused by a sinus or ear infection. *Intracerebral* abscesses usually are due to ear infections.

The organisms most often involved in the formation of brain abscesses are bacteria, such as *Streptococcus, Staphylococcus,* or *Streptococcus pneumoniae.* Fungi and parasites are rarely involved in cerebral abscess formation, unless the client is immunosuppressed or has acquired immunodeficiency syndrome (AIDS).

According to recent statistics, 80% of all brain abscesses occur in the cerebral hemispheres, with the remaining 20% occurring in the cerebellum (Thompson et al., 1986). It is estimated that 5% to 20% of affected clients have more than one abscess. Mortality rates vary from 40% to 60%; those caused by the *Streptococcus* organism are associated with higher mortality.

COLLABORATIVE MANAGEMENT

The nurse questions the client about a history of previous sinus, ear, mastoid, or tonsillar infections; pneumonia, endocarditis, or diverticulitis; head injury, including any that may have occurred several years earlier; and prior invasive neurosurgical procedures. Additional data to collect from the client include information concerning chronic infections or a history of immunosuppressive therapy.

The client with a brain abscess is usually admitted to the hospital with symptoms of a mass lesion and mildly increased ICP. The nurse begins the examination by performing a complete neurologic assessment. The client is usually mildly lethargic and somewhat confused. The pupillary response to light is normal in the early stages; as increased ICP progresses, the pupils dilate and become nonresponsive. Examination of the client's visual fields often reveals a temporal field blindness (decrease in peripheral vision). If the abscess affects the cerebellar hemisphere, nystagmus and a dysconjugate gaze may be noted. Motor examination reveals a generalized weakness. More significant motor problems, such as a hemiplegia, may be apparent in the presence of a frontal lobe abscess. An ataxic gait is seen with cerebellar abscess. Sensory impairment varies, although the client often exhibits no sensory deficits. The client may have varying degrees of aphasia in the presence of a frontal or temporal lobe abscess. Seizure activity may occur owing to irritation of the cortical tissue. Late in the disease process, more severe symptoms of increased ICP occur, including severe headache, coma, a widened pulse pressure, bradycardia, and irregular respirations.

A CBC and erythrocyte sedimentation rate (ESR) are done. The white blood cell count and ESR are usually elevated, indicating the presence of infection. If the abscess is encapsulated, the white blood cell count may be normal. Aerobic and anaerobic (when possible) cultures of the blood, ear, nose, and throat are done to determine the primary source of infection.

CT is done to determine the presence of cerebritis or an encapsulated abscess. A brain scan is useful in the diagnosis of multiple abscesses and is more sensitive than a CT scan in identifying an abscess in the early stages of formation. An EEG can localize the lesion in most cases and shows high-voltage slow-wave activity; electrical silence may be noted in the area of the abscess. Radiography of the sinuses and the mastoid is often indicated.

The client is assessed by the nurse using the Glasgow Coma Scale at least every 2 hours or more often if clinically indicated (Table 33–3). Included in this assessment are the client's vital signs. The client is at risk for increased ICP, which may be initially manifested by a change in the level of consciousness. Late signs of increased ICP include seizures, pupillary changes, and a widened pulse pressure and bradycardia. The head of the client's bed is elevated 30 to 45 degrees to promote venous drainage from the head. Other interventions for increased ICP are discussed earlier.

IV antibiotics, such as penicillin G (Bicillin), chloramphenicol (Chloromycetin), or nafcillin (Nafcil, Unipen), are given to treat the specific organism involved. Metronidazole (Flagyl) may be used if an anaerobic organism is the causative agent. These agents are particularly useful in the early stages (cerebritis) of abscess formation. A combination of antibiotics is used, particularly if the abscess resulted from septic emboli. Anticonvulsants, such as phenytoin (Dilantin), may be used prophylactically to prevent seizures. Strict adherence to the medication schedule is important to maintain therapeutic blood levels. Analgesics are used to treat the client's headache.

Although surgical drainage of an encapsulated abscess is considered somewhat controversial, it is sometimes done to reduce the mass effect of the lesion. The decision to perform surgery is based on the client's general condition, the stage of abscess development, and the site of the abscess. The nurse provides routine preoperative and postoperative care for the client with a craniotomy (see later).

The client with a brain abscess is discharged to home if few or no neurologic deficits are present. Those with severe dysfunction are usually transferred to a long-term care or rehabilitation facility.

POLIOMYELITIS

Poliomyelitis (polio) is an acute viral disease characterized by destruction of the motor cells of the anterior horn of the spinal cord, the brain stem, and the motor strip in the frontal lobe. This communicable disease may be relatively asymptomatic or may lead to paralysis or death. The incubation period is 7 to 10 days.

The virus is transmitted either through droplet infection or via the fecal or oral route and the gastrointestinal (GI) tract. After the virus gains entrance to the body, it settles in the lymph nodes of the throat and ileum and multiplies. The virus then invades the CNS, causing inflammation, scarring, and shrinking of the cell body of the involved motor cell. If the disease progresses, necrosis of the neuron occurs and results in permanent neurologic dysfunction.

Poliomyelitis, although rare in North America today, is seen most often in the summer and fall months. It affects males more often than females; males are more at risk for paralysis. The disease can be prevented by immunization with Salk's or Sabin's vaccine.

The signs and symptoms of poliomyelitis include fever; chills; excessive perspiration; severe muscle aches and weakness, especially of the legs, the neck, and the back; and drowsiness, irritability, increased deep tendon reflexes, abdominal tenderness, nausea, vomiting, dysphagia, and headache. Diagnosis is based on clinical presentation and positive throat or stool cultures for the poliovirus.

Treatment is symptomatic. Analgesics are given to relieve pain. Antibiotics may be indicated to prevent secondary infections. Nursing interventions are directed at providing supportive care and preventing complications of immobility. The client's respiratory status is carefully monitored to prevent respiratory arrest resulting from paralysis of the muscles of respiration.

POSTPOLIO SYNDROME

Recently, a syndrome known as *postpolio syndrome,* or *postpolio sequelae* (PPS), has been discovered in individuals who have recovered from poliomyelitis. It refers to the new onset of weakness, pain, and fatigue in persons who had poliomyelitis 30 or more years previously. The exact cause is not known, but physical and emotional stressors have been named as contributing factors. Temporary or permanent disability can result from PPS.

The client suspected of having or being predisposed to PPS should have a complete physical examination and diagnostic tests for muscular, neurologic, and pulmonary function. If the results of these tests are abnormal, the interdisciplinary health care team teaches the client how to make life style modifications to preserve energy and physiologic function. Swimming in warm water is widely recommended to promote comfort and flexibility. Adaptive and orthotic devices may be needed to prevent high energy consumption and maintain muscle function.

Having PPS is a frightening experience. The client who survived the initial disease has to face the chronic, potentially debilitating sequelae. Support groups are becoming readily available around the country and information is available through the Polio Network News (Smith, 1989).

BOTULISM

Botulism is a neurotoxic disorder caused by the bacterium *Clostridium botulinum.* The most common cause of botulism is eating improperly canned foods. Less often, the bacterium can enter the body through a wound and produces the toxin in the traumatized area. A third type of botulism is seen exclusively in infants.

The bacterium impairs the release of acetylcholine (ACh) at the motor nerve synapse. This causes a motor paralysis that affects both voluntary and involuntary motor activity.

The disease is manifested by extraocular and facial muscle paralysis, bulbar palsies, blurred vision, diplopia, dysarthria, flaccid paralysis, dysphagia, nausea, and vomiting. Paralysis of the respiratory muscles is not uncommon. Diagnosis is based on history, clinical presentation, and isolation of the *C. botulinum* organism in the stool. Anaerobic blood cultures may also isolate the organism.

Treatment consists of the rapid administration of trivalent botulism antitoxin. Secondary bacterial infections are treated with antibiotics. Other care is supportive to prevent respiratory complications and other complications of immobility and to provide nutritional support.

TETANUS

Tetanus, also known as lockjaw, is caused by *Clostridium tetani* and is easily prevented through immunization. It is frequently transmitted through a wound contaminated with the bacterium, which is commonly found in soil. On entering the wound, it multiplies rapidly and produces the toxin *tetanospasmin.* The toxin enters the CNS and spinal motor ganglia though the blood stream. The toxin interferes with the normal activity of the inhibitory postsynaptic potentials. This causes the anterior horn cells to become overstimulated and transmit excessive stimuli to the muscles, causing opisthotonos (spasm causing head and feet flexion), tonic rigidity, cramps, and muscle spasms and stiffness. Diagnosis is made on the basis of history and clinical findings almost exclusively, and there are no definitive tests for tetanus.

Treatment includes the prompt intramuscular (IM) administration of the antitoxin, human tetanus immune globulin, or hyperimmune equine or bovine serum. Sedatives, antianxiety agents, and muscle relaxants are given to decrease muscle spasms and increase the client's comfort. If necessary, propranolol (Inderal) is given to treat cardiac irregularities. Aggressive respiratory support and intervention are provided. Other interventions are directed toward preventing the complications of immobility. The mortality rate for untreated tetanus is high.

CREUTZFELDT-JAKOB DISEASE

Creutzfeldt-Jakob disease is a rare, progressive, fatal disease caused by a slow virus. The incubation period is unknown, and the disease is transmitted via contact with infected blood, CSF, and brain tissue. Onset of the disease occurs in middle life (approximately age 55 years); both sexes are affected equally. In the absence of other neurologic disease, the presence of myoclonus, personality changes, and dementia is highly suggestive of the diagnosis of Creutzfeldt-Jakob disease. Other symptoms include extrapyramidal signs, fasciculations, cerebellar ataxia, and possibly seizure activity. Coma and death generally occur within 2 years of the onset of symptoms.

There is no known cure for the disease; treatment is symptomatic and supportive. Although isolation is not required, special precautions should be taken in addition to proper hand washing techniques. Gloves should be worn when in contact with the client's urine, stool, blood, CSF, or body tissue. Any needles (e.g., spinal, injection, and EEG electrodes) that come in contact with the client are disposed in a separate, marked container. In addition to these measures, the nurse provides support and guidance for the client and the family.

MULTIPLE SCLEROSIS

OVERVIEW

Multiple sclerosis (MS) is a progressive degenerative disease that affects the myelin sheath and conduction pathway of the CNS. It is one of the leading causes of neurologic disability in persons 20 to 40 years of age. This chronic disease is characterized by periods of remission and exacerbation. As the severity and duration of the disease progress, the periods of exacerbation become more frequent.

Pathophysiology

A neuron is composed of a cell body, an axon, and dendrites. Nerve impulses are transmitted from one nerve cell to another along unmyelinated fibers or via the nodes of Ranvier in myelinated axon fibers. In the presence of MS, *plaque* forms along the myelin, causing an inflammatory response; perivascular edema; gliosis, or scarring; and destruction of the myelin. The white fiber tracts that connect the neurons in the brain and spinal cord are involved. Especially affected areas include optic nerves, pyramidal tracts, posterior columns, brain stem nuclei, and the periventricular region. Although the myelin surrounding the axon is involved, the axon itself is relatively spared until late in the disease process when scarring occurs. Initially, however, recovery of the myelin occurs with remission of symptoms. Eventually, with repeated exacerbations of the disease, damage becomes permanent.

Three types of MS are seen. The *classic* picture of exacerbation followed by remission occurs most often. The course of the disease may be benign, mild, or moderate, depending on the degree of disability. *Progressive* MS is characterized by the absence of periods of remission. Progressive deterioration occurs over several years. The third type, *combined*, begins with the classic presentation of MS and at some point converts to a progressive course.

Etiology

The exact cause of MS remains unknown. Research continues on viral, immunologic, and genetic etiologic factors. The viral theory of MS suggests that it is caused by a slow virus that has been dormant for many years. Specific antibodies found to be elevated in clients with MS include those to herpes simplex type 1, measles, mumps, and influenza viruses.

The immune theory suggests that an unidentified factor (probably a virus) triggers the immune response. This theory is supported by research data that immunoglobin G (IgG) and oligoclonal bands in the CSF of clients with MS are elevated. In addition, some studies have noted that IgG can be found at the site of demyelination surrounding areas of plaque formation.

Although no genetic pattern of transmission has been found, immediate relatives of clients with MS have a 15 times greater risk of developing the disease than the general population. The risk is 300 times greater if an identical twin has MS.

Incidence

MS usually occurs between the ages of 20 and 40 years, although cases may occur in those younger than 15 and older than 50 years. Approximately 500,000 people in the United States are currently affected. Women are affected slightly more often than men (3 : 2), and there is a greater prevalence in the Caucasian population.

MS is seen more often in the colder climates of the northeastern, Great Lakes, and Pacific northwestern states. Studies have indicated that, if one relocates after the age of 15 years from an area of high incidence to one of a lower incidence, the risk factor of the higher area is carried. For those less than 15 years of age, the risk factor is not carried. These studies suggest that the risk factor for developing MS occurs about the age of 15 years. Life expectancy for those with MS is about 85% of that of the general population, or about 35 years after onset of symptoms.

COLLABORATIVE MANAGEMENT

 Assessment

History

MS often mimics other neurologic diseases. Therefore, obtaining a thorough history is essential for accurate diagnosis. The nurse begins by asking the client for a *history of changes* in vision, motor skills, and sensations, all *early indicators of MS*. The symptoms are often vague and nonspecific in the early stages of the disease. Of significance is the client's report that symptoms were first noticed several years ago, but, because they disappeared, medical attention was not sought. The nurse questions the client about the progression of symptoms, with particular attention toward delineating whether the symptoms are intermittent or if they are becoming progressively worse. It is important to ascertain the date (month and year) when the client first noticed the clinical manifestations.

Next, the nurse questions the client about *factors that aggravate* the symptoms. These factors may include fatigue, stress, overexertion, temperature extremes, or a hot shower or bath. The client and the family are questioned about any *personality or behavior changes* that have occurred (e.g., euphoria, poor judgment, and inattentiveness). In addition, they are questioned about family history of MS.

Physical Assessment: Clinical Manifestations

The nurse performs a *complete neurologic assessment.* Typical clinical findings from assessment of the client's visual acuity, visual fields, and pupils include blurred vision, diplopia, and decreased acuity; scotoma, or changes in peripheral vision; and nystagmus.

Next, the nurse assesses the client's motor status. The client often complains of increased fatigue and stiffness of the extremities, particularly of the legs. Flexor spasms at night may awaken the client from sleep. Further examination of the client reveals increased, or hyperac-

tive, deep tendon reflexes; clonus; positive Babinski's reflex; and absent abdominal reflexes. The client's gait may be unsteady owing to weakness of the legs and spasticity.

Significant cerebellar findings exhibited include intention tremor (tremor when performing an activity), dysmetria (inability to direct or limit movement), and dysdiadochokinesia (inability to arrest one motor impulse and substitute another). Motor movements are often clumsy; the client may lose her/his balance easily and exhibit signs of incoordination.

During examination of the cranial nerves and brain stem function, the client may complain of tinnitus, vertigo, and hearing loss. The client may show indications of facial weakness and have difficulty swallowing. Speech problems exhibited by the client with MS include dysarthria, ataxia, and slow, scanning speech.

The sensory examination findings include hypalgesia, paresthesia, and facial pain. The client may complain of numbness, tingling, burning, or crawling sensations.

If demyelination of the spinal cord has occurred, the client may experience bowel and bladder problems, as well as alterations in sexuality. The client may have an areflexic bladder or experience frequency, urgency, or nocturia. Bowel problems include altered rectal tone or constipation, as well as incontinence. Problems with sexuality include impotence, difficulty sustaining an erection, frigidity, and decreased vaginal secretion. Finally, the nurse examines the client for mental status changes. Cognitive changes are usually seen late in the course of the disease and include memory loss, decreased ability to perform calculations, inattentiveness, and impaired judgment.

Psychosocial Assessment

After the initial diagnosis of MS, the client is often quite anxious. Apathy, emotional lability, and depression are not uncommon. The client may be euphoric or giddy, either as a result of the disease itself or because of the medications used to treat the disease. The nurse assesses the client's previously used coping and stress management skills in preparing the client for a chronic, usually debilitating disease.

Laboratory Findings

No one specific procedure can definitively diagnose MS. However, the collective results of a variety of tests are usually conclusive. During an acute attack, changes are evident. Abnormal CSF findings include an elevated cell count and protein level and a slight increase in the white blood cell count. CSF electrophoresis reveals an increase in the myelin basic protein and the presence of oligoclonal bands (IgG). IgG bands are seen in more than 90% of those with MS.

Radiographic Findings

CT is usually performed and may show an increased density in the white matter and MS plaques.

Other Diagnostic Tests

The EEG may demonstrate slow-wave activity during the acute stage and no changes while the client is in remission. It is not unusual for the EEG to be normal throughout the course of the disease. Results of visual, auditory, and brain stem evoked potential studies are often abnormal. In cases of advanced disease, the electromyogram (EMG) findings may be grossly abnormal. MRI is usually done and may show similar findings to CT.

Analysis: Nursing Diagnosis

Most often the client is admitted to the hospital or seen in the neurologist's office with complaints of weakness, incoordination, dizziness, and loss of balance. Visual changes are not infrequent.

Common Diagnoses

The following diagnoses are commonly found in clients with MS:

1. Sensory/perceptual alterations related to visual, motor, and sensory changes
2. Impaired physical mobility and total self-care deficit related to muscle weakness, awkward movements, and incoordination
3. Body image disturbance and altered role performance related to changes caused by the disease process
4. Knowledge deficit related to the effect of the disease process and how to manage the disease, especially medications

Additional Diagnoses

In addition to the common diagnoses, the client may have one or more of the following diagnoses:

1. Sleep pattern disturbance related to flexor spasms
2. Altered nutrition less than body requirements related to dysphagia
3. Pain related to sensory changes and flexor spasm
4. Activity intolerance related to fatigue
5. Impaired adjustment related to disability
6. Constipation related to decreased mobility, changes in dietary habits, or the disease process
7. Altered patterns of urinary elimination related to urgency, frequency, and the disease process itself
8. Ineffective family coping related to changes in role performance
9. Altered thought processes related to changes in memory, judgment, and cognitive skills

10. Sexual dysfunction related to motor and sensory alterations

  ## Planning and Implementation

The plan of care for the client with MS focuses on the common nursing diagnoses.

Sensory/Perceptual Alterations

Planning: client goals. The major goals for this nursing diagnosis are that the client will (1) learn strategies to maximize vision and (2) remain free of injury attributable to motor and sensory impairment.

Interventions: nonsurgical management. On the basis of the result of the visual assessment, the nurse assists the client in developing compensatory strategies. An eyepatch that is alternated from eye to eye every few hours usually relieves diplopia. If the client has peripheral vision deficits, the nurse provides instruction in scanning techniques. Changes in visual acuity may be assisted by corrective lenses. The nurse orients the client to the environment and keeps it free of clutter. The environment should be as standardized as possible to enable the client to memorize or anticipate the placement of objects.

Because of changes in sensation, the client must be protected from injury and treated for any discomfort. The client should avoid overexposure to heat, cold, or pressure. The nurse instructs the client to use a thermometer to test the temperature of water for bathing or washing dishes. The client should wear shoes at all times to avoid foot injuries. Carbamazepine (Tegretal) or acetaminophen (Tylenol) may be used to treat pain and paresthesias.

Impaired Physical Mobility; Total Self-Care Deficit

Planning: client goals. The two major goals for this nursing diagnosis are that the client will (1) maintain maximal mobility for the stage of the disease and (2) experience no complications of immobility.

Interventions: nonsurgical management. The client with MS is weak and easily fatigued. She/he is instructed by the nurse on the importance of planning activities and allowing sufficient time to complete activities. For example, the client should check that all items needed for work are gathered before leaving the house. Items used on a daily basis should be easily accessible.

In collaboration with physical and occupational therapists, the nurse develops an exercise program to include ROM, stretching, and strengthening exercises. The client is encouraged to ambulate as tolerated, using assistive ambulation devices as needed, including canes, walker, wheelchair, or electric cart (Amigo). Additional assistive-adaptive devices may be needed to enable the client with tremor, spasticity, and weakness to remain independent in ADL. Chapter 22 describes additional interventions to increase physical mobility and promote ADL independence.

The nurse instructs the client on the importance of avoiding activities that cause an increase in body temperature. This may lead to increased fatigue, as well as decreased motor ability and visual acuity resulting from changes in the conduction abilities of the injured axons.

Body Image Disturbance; Altered Role Performance

Planning: client goals. The major goals for these nursing diagnoses are that the client will (1) adjust to changes in body image, role performance, and self-esteem and (2) state that he/she has developed a positive self-image.

Interventions: nonsurgical management. The nurse encourages the client to maintain independence in all activities as the condition allows. The client is encouraged to ventilate her/his feelings of frustration or anger. The family, the nurse, and the client should stress the abilities the client *has* and work together to develop strategies to minimize the impact of disabilities. The client is encouraged to continue usual activities as much as possible, including social activities with family and friends and work. Vocational counseling may be needed if the client's condition does not allow return to her/his former employment. Most importantly, the client must be given usable information and be assisted to identify realistic short- and long-term goals. A referral to a support group, psychologist, or psychiatrist may be necessary.

Knowledge Deficit

Planning: client goals. The major goals for this nursing diagnosis are that the client will (1) identify the actions and side effects of medications and other treatment modalities and (2) experience no or few adverse effects of prescribed treatment.

Interventions: nonsurgical management. A wide variety of medications are used to treat and control the disease. Adrenocorticotropic hormone (ACTH) and corticosteroids (prednisone, dexamethasone [Hexadrol]) are used to reduce edema and the inflammatory response. These medications often decrease the length of time the client's symptoms are exacerbated and often improve the degree of recovery. Adverse effects of ACTH and other steroids include hyponatremia or hypernatremia, hypokalemia, fluid retention and pedal edema, congestive heart failure and hypertension, gastric ulceration, hyperglycemia, increased risk of infection, and personality changes. Common nursing interventions while the client is receiving these medications include careful monitoring of fluid and electrolyte levels; testing the client's serum glucose concentration;

providing dietary or supplemental potassium; observing for indications of GI bleeding, such as gastric pain or blood in the stool; documenting any changes in personality (e.g., euphoria and insomnia); and minimizing the client's exposure to communicable or infectious diseases.

Immunosuppressive therapy with a combination of cyclophosphamide (Cytoxan) and ACTH is used for treatment of progressive MS to stabilize the disease process. Clients receiving cyclophosphamide usually develop alopecia 4 to 5 weeks after the institution of treatment; hair growth returns within 2 to 3 months. Before commencing this treatment regimen, the nurse advises the client to purchase a wig, hair piece, or other appropriate cover if desired. In addition to alopecia, the client generally experiences nausea, vomiting, and anorexia, which can be controlled with antiemetics.

Another possible side effect of cyclophosphamide is hemorrhagic cystitis. The nurse tests the urine daily for microscopic hematuria. In addition, at least 3 L of oral or IV fluid should be given daily, unless contraindicated. This increased fluid intake may complicate the bladder problems that most clients with MS develop. Interventions to treat these problems, such as intermittent catheterization for retention, should be developed before the start of treatment. The clients should be placed on strict intake and output measurements and weighed daily.

Gonadal suppression may occur. Cyclophosphamide is excreted in breast milk; breastfeeding *must* be discontinued before the initiation of therapy. In addition, congenital anomalies have been reported when the drug was administered during pregnancy.

■ Discharge Planning

The client with MS is usually followed closely in the outpatient setting. Hospitalization occurs for the administration of medication during periods of exacerbation or for treatment of complications.

Home Care Preparation

The client's home is assessed for any hazards before discharge from the hospital. Any items that could interfere with mobility, such as scatter rugs, are removed. In addition, care must be taken to prevent injury resulting from visual problems. The home environment should remain as structured and free of clutter as possible. Later, as the disease progresses, the home may need to be adapted for wheelchair accessibility. Any assistive-adaptive device needed by the client should be available before discharge from the hospital.

Client/Family Education

The client receives instruction about all discharge medications, including the time and route of administration, dosage, purpose, and side effects. The client is taught how to differentiate expected side effects from adverse or allergic reactions and is given the name of a resource person to call if the client has questions.

An exercise program is developed in collaboration with physical, occupational, or speech therapists. The program should be appropriate for the client's tolerance level. The client is instructed concerning techniques for self-care, daily living skills, and the use of required adaptive equipment. It is important to include information on the following programs: bowel and bladder management, skin care, nutrition, and positioning techniques.

The results of a 35-year long-term study suggest that a low-fat diet may help clients with MS live longer and with fewer neurologic complications (Swank & Grimsgaard, 1988). The regimen restricted saturated fat intake to 20 g/day and limited intake of animal fats, coconut and palm oils, margarine, and peanut butter.

Psychosocial Preparation

The client is encouraged to obtain adequate rest and to avoid undue stress. It is equally important for the client to engage in regular social diversional activities. Often, the client is anxious about discharge from the hospital and worries about how long the remission will last or when the disease will progress further. Personality changes are not unusual, and the family is instructed regarding strategies that will enable them to cope with these changes. For example, the family may develop a nonverbal signal to alert the client of potentially inappropriate behavior (e.g., a talkative person may be reminded to be quiet if a family member displays prearranged signal). This action avoids client embarrassment.

Health Care Resources

The client with MS is able to live independently throughout the early stages of the disease. As the client's condition deteriorates, the assistance of a home care nurse or a family member may be required. Another alternative may be placement in a long-term care facility.

The client and the family should be referred to the local and national MS society. Other community resources available include meal delivery services (e.g., Meals on Wheels), transportation services for the disabled, and homemaker services.

Evaluation

On the basis of the identified nursing diagnoses, the nurse evaluates the care of the client with MS. The expected outcomes include that the client

1. Develops strategies to minimize the effects of visual disturbances
2. Demonstrates adjustment to changes in body image and self-concept

3. Demonstrates few or no complications of immobility
4. Maintains maximal activity and mobility for level of disability
5. Complies with the medication regimen and states the name, dose, time of administration, use, and side effects of all medications

By meeting the desired outcomes, the client with MS should be able to function independently as long as possible.

PARKINSON'S DISEASE

OVERVIEW

Parkinson's disease, also referred to as paralysis agitans, is a movement disorder involving the basal ganglia and substantia nigra. It is characterized by resting tremors, decreased postural reflexes, rigidity, and bradykinesia.

Pathophysiology

Motor activity requires the integrated action of the cerebral cortex, the basal ganglia, and the cerebellum. Through its influence on the pyramidal and extrapyramidal pathways, the cerebral cortex influences the activity of the lower motor neurons. The major influence of the basal ganglia and the cerebellum on motor activity is through their connections to the motor cortex.

The basal ganglia are located deep within the cerebral hemisphere at the base of the brain, near the lateral ventricles and internal capsule. They are composed of the following structures: caudate nucleus, putamen, globus pallidus, and amygdaloid. The largest component of the basal nuclei is the corpus striatum, which is primarily concerned with voluntary motor movement. Two distinctive parts of the conus striatum are the caudate nucleus and the putamen (neostriatum). The substantia nigra, although not a part of the basal nuclei, has close connection with the corpus striatum.

In addition to the above structures, two neurotransmitters are involved in motor activity, namely, dopamine and ACh. Dopamine is produced in the substantia nigra, as well as in the adrenal glands, and has an inhibitory function on the basal ganglia and consequently integrates voluntary motor activity. ACh is produced in the nerve endings, as well as being found in high concentrations within the striatum. It is inhibitory to the function of dopamine or blocks the release of dopamine. Normally, the two neurotransmitters work to form balanced antagonist systems to produce coordinated motor movements, or a balance between inhibition and excitation of the neuron groups.

In the presence of Parkinson's disease, degenerative changes within the substantia nigra occur, leading to a decrease in the amount of dopamine in the corpus striatum and substantia nigra. Dopamine produced in the adrenal glands is not available, as it is quickly metabolized in the periphery. The imbalance between dopamine and ACh results in excessive unbridled excitation of selected neuron groups that are no longer inhibited by dopamine. Therefore, owing to dopamine deficiency, the client is unable to initiate movement.

Six major categories of Parkinson's disease are used to classify the disease according to the processes that affect the substantia nigra and corpus striatum.

Primary (idiopathic) parkinsonism occurs most often. A few clients have *postencephalitic parkinsonism* as a sequela of encephalitis. Antipsychotic phenothiazine drugs may lead to *iatrogenic parkinsonism.* Although Parkinson's disease primarily occurs in those older than 50 years of age, a *juvenile parkinsonism* may occur in those less than 40 years of age and is associated with Wilson's disease, progressive lenticular degeneration, Hallervorden-Spatz disease, or Huntington's chorea. The fifth classification is *secondary parkinsonism,* which results from damage to the substantia nigra as a consequence of trauma or ischemia. Finally, *pseudoparkinsonism* encompasses a wide variety of disorders (benign essential familial tremor, hypothyroidism, and severe psychomotor retardation) that have several characteristics of Parkinson's disease; however, further investigation rules out *true* Parkinson's disease.

In addition to the six classifications described above, Parkinson's disease is separated into stages, depending on the symptoms and degree of disability (see the accompanying Key Features of Disease). *Stage 1* is mild disease with unilateral limb involvement. Bilateral limb involvement occurs in *stage 2,* whereas in *stage 3* the client exhibits significant gait disturbances and moderate generalized disability. *Stage 4* is characterized by severe disability, akinesia, and rigidity. The client with *stage 5* disease is completely dependent in all ADL.

Etiology

The cause of Parkinson's disease remains unknown. There may be a hereditary connection, although this remains unproved. In some cases, Parkinson's disease is related to the use of phenothiazine drugs or exposure to carbon monoxide. Viral and vascular causes may also be possible.

Incidence

Parkinson's disease occurs preponderantly after the age of 50 years, with a median age of 55 years. It affects men and women equally. The incidence in the United States is estimated to be almost 1 million, with 50,000 new cases reported annually (Lannon et al., 1986).

COLLABORATIVE MANAGEMENT

 Assessment

History

The nurse collects data related to the *time and progression of symptoms* noticed by the client or the family. The nurse questions the client about *gait problems,* such as difficulty with ambulation, and *changes in posture,* such as a stooped posture when standing or walking. The client may experience *bradykinesia* (slow movements) and have problems performing two activities at once, such as walking while talking. The nurse obtains a history of tremor and should note if it occurs only at rest, under stress, during sleep, or when performing voluntary motor activities. Data are obtained from the client about problems with speech, swallowing, and bladder and bowel continence. Owing to possible *involvement of the autonomic nervous system,* the nurse elicits information suggestive of orthostatic hypotension, excessive perspiration, blepharospasm (spasm of the orbital muscles of the eye), oily skin, and seborrhea. Finally, the nurse questions the client about changes in handwriting, which typically becomes small and can be accomplished only slowly.

KEY FEATURES OF DISEASE ■ Stages of Parkinson's Disease

Stage 1: Initial Stage

  Unilateral limb involvement
  Minimal weakness
  Hand and arm trembling

Stage 2: Mild Stage

  Bilateral limb involvement
  Mask-like facies
  Slow, shuffling gait

Stage 3: Moderate Disease

  Gait disturbances increase

Stage 4: Severe Disability

  Akinesia
  Rigidity

Stage 5: Complete Dependence

Physical Assessment: Clinical Manifestations

The nurse begins the assessment of the client by checking for evidence of rigidity. The *rigidity* is defined as cogwheel, plastic, or lead pipe and is evaluated as the nurse performs passive ROM of the extremities. Cogwheel rigidity is manifested by a rhythmic interruption of the muscle movement. Plastic rigidity is defined as mildly restrictive movement, whereas lead-pipe rigidity is total resistance to movement. This symptom is present early in the disease process and progresses over time. The nurse further observes the client's ability to relax a muscle or move a selected muscle group.

Changes in facial expression or a *mask-like facies* (Fig. 33–7) with wide-open, fixed, staring eyes is caused by rigidity of the facial muscles. This can lead to difficulties in chewing and swallowing, particularly if the pharyngeal muscles are involved. Uncontrolled drooling may occur.

Next, the nurse assesses the client's respiratory status. Rigidity of the intercostal muscles required for respiration may be manifested by restricted chest wall expansion, decreased breath sounds, and labored respiration. The client's speech is assessed by the nurse. The client typically has a soft, low-pitched voice and is *dysarthric* owing to rigidity of the vocal cords. Other speech problems exhibited by the client include echolalia (automatic repetition of what another person says) and repetition of sentences.

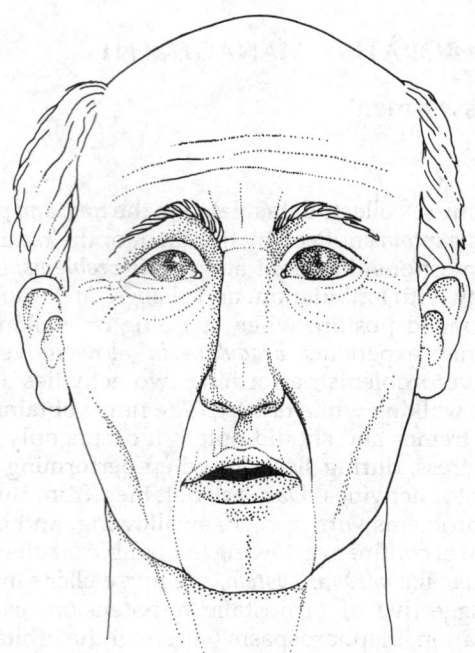

Figure 33–7

Mask-like facial expression typical of clients with Parkinson's disease.

The nurse assesses the client for changes in posture and gait. Typically, the client has a *stooped posture* with a flexed trunk. Because of the truncal rigidity, the client tends to move his/her body as a unit. Rolling over in bed and changing from a sitting to standing position are difficult. When the client is standing, fingers are abducted and flexed at the metacarpophalangeal joint; the wrist is slightly dorsiflexed. When walking, the client's arms tend not to move and often characteristic mannerisms, such as "talking with the hands," are absent. The client's gait is slow and shuffling, with short, hesitant steps. The client may have a propulsive gait, one that is slow to initiate but accelerates almost to a trot. In addition, the client may have difficulty stopping quickly. In a few cases the client may demonstrate reverse propulsion or retropulsion, walking backward when intending to walk forward.

Bradykinesia may progress to the point at which the client is unable to move. The nurse assesses the client for the ability to perform rapid alternating movement by asking the client to rapidly pronate and supinate the palms of her/his hands. In addition, the nurse observes for indication of "freezing" (akinesia) when the client is asked to perform two activities at the same time, such as walking while talking. The client is often unable to perform either.

A distressing symptom to the client is the presence of *tremors*. The tremors occur *at rest* and are absent during sleep. Emotional stress and fatigue increase frequency of the tremors. The fingers are most often involved, with the classic "pill rolling" movement in which the thumb moves along the distal second and third digits of the hand.

In addition to the previously mentioned behaviors, the nurse assesses the client for orthostatic hypotension, excessive perspiration, oily skin, and seborrhea. Other indicators of autonomic dysfunction include flushing, changes in skin texture, and GI dysfunction, such as severe constipation.

Psychosocial Assessment

The typical client with Parkinson's disease is emotionally labile, and the nurse observes for signs of depression and paranoia. The client may become easily upset and have rapid mood swings. Commonly, the client may have cognitive impairments and demonstrate a delayed reaction time. For example, the client may be slow to respond to questions or to complete a task. The client should be observed for signs of dementia, which may be associated with the disease or may be a result of medications.

Laboratory Findings

Diagnosis of Parkinson's disease is based on the clinical findings. There are no specific diagnostic tests. Analysis of CSF may show a decrease in dopamine level, although the results of other studies are usually normal.

Analysis: Nursing Diagnosis

The client with Parkinson's disease is generally not admitted to the hospital, but is followed on an outpatient basis. The client has alterations in movements, rigidity, and often tremors. Early symptoms are usually vague and may be confused with those of other conditions. The disease may vary from mild and slowly progressive course to a rapid progression to complete disability.

Common Diagnoses

The following diagnoses are commonly noted in clients with Parkinson's disease:

1. Total self-care deficit (the level depends on the stage of disease) related to rigidity and tremors
2. Impaired physical mobility related to alterations in movement.
3. Impaired verbal communication related to tremors, dysarthria, or low voice
4. Altered nutrition: less than body requirements related to dysphagia
5. Self-esteem disturbance and body image disturbance related to tremors, gait changes, or drooling

Additional Diagnoses

In addition to the common diagnoses, the client may have one or more of the following diagnoses:

1. Ineffective airway clearance and ineffective breathing pattern related to rigidity of the intercostal muscles and immobility
2. Sleep pattern disturbance related to rigidity and immobility
3. Pain related to rigidity and tremors
4. Constipation related to immobility and altered nutrition or hydration
5. Potential for injury related to gait changes, tremors, and rigidity
6. Social isolation related to changes in body image
7. Ineffective individual coping and ineffective family coping related to changes in life style, role performance, and self-concept

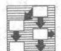 **Planning and Implementation**

The plan of care for clients with Parkinson's disease focuses on the common nursing diagnoses.

Total Self-Care Deficit

Planning: client goals. The major goal for this nursing diagnosis is that the client will be as independent as possible in the performance of ADL.

Interventions: nonsurgical management. The nurse encourages the client to participate as much as possible in the performance of self-care skills. Sufficient time must be allowed for these activities to be completed. The nurse should schedule client appointments and activities late in the morning or during the early afternoon to prevent the need to rush through bathing and dressing activities. The environment should be conducive to independence in activity and as stress free as possible. Consultations with occupational and physical therapists should be obtained for ADL training and the use of adaptive devices if needed. Chapter 22 discusses additional interventions for clients with self-care deficits.

Impaired Physical Mobility

Planning: client goals. The two goals for this nursing diagnosis are that the client will (1) ambulate independently or with assistance for as long as possible and (2) be free of contractures and impairment of skin integrity.

Interventions. The client with Parkinson's disease slowly loses the ability to care for himself/herself owing to decreased physical mobility. Drug therapy, physical or occupational therapy, and, as a last resort, palliative surgery may be performed to assist the client in remaining mobile for as long as possible.

Nonsurgical management. In collaboration with the physical therapist, the nurse plans and implements an active and passive ROM and muscle-stretching program. The exercise program includes exercises for the muscles of the face and tongue to facilitate swallowing and speech. The client is encouraged to ambulate as tolerated, to avoid sitting for long periods, and to reposition the body frequently. A cane or a walker may be needed for ambulation and to prevent falls. Because of the potential for respiratory problems, the client is taught how to perform breathing exercises. The client with orthostatic hypotension is instructed to change positions slowly, especially when moving from a sitting to a standing position, to allow for adequate cerebral blood flow.

A variety of medications are used to control tremor and rigidity. Medication administration must be closely monitored, and the dosage should be adjusted or the medication changed as the client's condition warrants. The drugs of choice to treat rigidity are the dopaminergics. These include levodopa (L-dopa) and carbidopa-levodopa combination (Sinemet). The drug amantadine hydrochloride (Symmetrel), an antiviral agent, is being used more often as the drug of choice for conservative medical management. It acts by increasing the release of dopamine. Carbidopa-levodopa combination potentiates the effects of levodopa in the basal ganglia and has fewer side effects than levodopa.

Anticholinergic drugs, such as biperiden (Akineton), trihexyphenidyl (Artane), and benztropine mesylate

(Cogentin), decrease the excitatory effects of ACh. They are given to augment levodopa therapy and are particularly beneficial for the client whose primary symptom is tremor. The antihistamine diphenhydramine hydrochloride (Benadryl) is given in conjunction with anticholinergics to inhibit dopamine uptake or synapses.

A dopamine agonist, bromocriptine mesylate (Parlodel), crosses the blood-brain barrier and stimulates dopaminergic receptors. It is especially useful in those clients who have experienced such side effects as dyskinesias or orthostatic hypotension while receiving levodopa.

Clients on long-term drug therapy regimens often develop drug tolerance or drug toxicity. Drug toxicity is evidenced by confusion, decreased effectiveness of the drug, or hallucinations. When drug tolerance is reached, the client finds that the medication's effects do not last as long as previously. This "on-off" phenomenon may occur as a complication of long-term therapy and is manifested by periods of absence or significant reduction of symptoms, alternated with periods of immobility or akinetic spells. Treatment of drug toxicity or tolerance includes a reduction of medication dosage, a change of medications or frequency of administration, or a drug holiday (particularly with levodopa therapy). During a drug holiday, which typically lasts up to 10 days, the client receives no medications. The client must be carefully monitored during this time.

Surgical management.   In the past, a thalamotomy was performed to surgically treat Parkinson's disease. It consisted of destroying areas of the globus pallidus or ventrolateral nucleus of the thalamus to control tremor and rigidity. This procedure is infrequently done today, because a wider variety of medications are available to treat these symptoms.

An experimental surgical procedure currently being conducted at several medical centers throughout the country consists of transplanting small pieces of the client's own adrenal gland into the caudate nucleus of the brain. A right adrenalectomy is performed, followed by a right frontal craniotomy. A collection reservoir is implanted during the procedure to enable the surgeon to easily obtain CSF for postoperative analysis of dopamine content. This surgical procedure is considered palliative rather than curative at present.

Impaired Verbal Communication

Planning: client goals.   The major goal for this nursing diagnosis is that the client will be able to communicate verbally or with a communication board as appropriate.

Interventions: nonsurgical management.   The client should be encouraged to speak slowly and clearly and to pause and take deep breaths at appropriate intervals during each sentence. Unnecessary environmental noise should be eliminated to maximize the listener's ability to hear and understand the client. The nurse and the family ask the client to repeat words they do not understand and watch the client's lips and nonverbal expressions for cues as to the meaning of conversation. The client is instructed to organize thoughts before speaking and is encouraged to use facial expression and gestures (if possible) to augment communication. In addition, the client should exaggerate words to increase the listener's ability to understand.

If the client is unable to verbally communicate, alternative methods of communication must be used, such as a communication board, mechanical voice synthesizer, computer, or electric typewriter.

Altered Nutrition: Less Than Body Requirements

Planning: client goals.   The major goals for this nursing diagnosis are that the client will (1) maintain an adequate caloric intake and (2) maintain ideal body weight.

Interventions: nonsurgical management.   The nurse should carefully monitor the client's swallowing and chewing abilities. Usually, a soft diet or thick cold fluids are more easily tolerated. Several small meals several times each day may assist the client who has difficulty swallowing. The client should be positioned properly with his/her head elevated to facilitate swallowing.

When possible, medications are scheduled so that peak action occurs during mealtime to assist in independence in feeding. The client is weighed weekly, and his/her caloric intake is measured daily. Supplemental feedings with high-protein, high-calorie liquids or puddings may be given several times a day to maintain weight.

Self-Esteem Disturbance; Body Image Disturbance

Planning: client goals.   The primary goal for these diagnoses is that the client will state that she/he is able to maintain positive self-esteem and body image.

Interventions: nonsurgical management.   The client with Parkinson's disease often has no cognitive dysfunction, yet appears demented. The client experiences changes in gait and tremors that are uncontrollable. In the late stages of the disease, the client is unable to move without assistance, has difficulty with articulation, has minimal facial expression, and may drool. Clients with this disorder often state that they are embarrassed and tend to avoid social events or groups of people. Clients should not be forced into situations in which they feel ashamed of their appearance. Activities that do not require small muscle dexterity may be undertaken, such as light, modified aerobic exercises.

The nurse emphasizes the client's abilities or strengths and provides positive reinforcement when the client has met daily goals. The client, the family, and the nurse mutually set realistic goals that can be achieved. Assisting the client with grooming and hygiene is also important in maintaining a positive body image. Chapter 9 offers many suggestions for improving or maintaining body image.

■ Discharge Planning

As mentioned earlier, the client with Parkinson's disease does not require hospitalization for diagnostic evaluation. Hospitalization occurs when the client requires a drug holiday or experiences complications related to immobility or respiratory distress. In stage 4 or 5 of the disease, the client often requires placement in a long-term care facility.

Home Care Preparation

In the early stages of the disease process, the home is assessed for potential hazards. In particular, any item that could impede the client's gait is removed (e.g., scatter rugs or small tables). Possible physical adjustments that might be necessary include making the entryway more accessible, installing a chair lift to get to the second floor, or providing adaptations to the bathroom, such as grab bars in the bathtub or elevation of the commode seat.

Client/Family Education

The teaching plan for the client with Parkinson's disease includes medications, exercise program, and self-care skills. The client is instructed about the name, use, dosage and timing of drug administration, and side effects of all medications. The client is also given information about what action to take if a dose is missed or side effects develop.

The exercise program is particularly important for the client to maintain mobility and functional motor skills for as long as possible. The program includes ROM and stretching exercises, as well as exercises for the muscles of the face and speech. In collaboration with the physical and occupational therapists, the nurse teaches the client how to use adaptive devices properly.

Psychosocial Preparation

The client may exhibit signs of irritability, anger, and depression. The nurse explores coping strategies with the client and the family and assists them to develop new strategies as appropriate. The client is encouraged to maintain his/her usual life style as long as possible, including work and leisure activities. The client or the family should report any unusual behavior or psychologic problems (hallucinations, paranoia, and delirium) to the physician, as these behaviors may be caused by side effects of the medications.

Health Care Resources

The client should be referred to the local and national support groups for persons and families with Parkinson's disease. These include the American Parkinson's Disease Association Inc., Parkinson Disease Foundation, and National Parkinson's Foundation.

A home care nurse may be needed as the disease progresses to provide physical care of the client, monitor the effects of the medication, and provide support to the client and the family. The physician, the clinic nurse, and the home care nurse should communicate frequently to optimize continuity of care.

 Evaluation

On the basis of the identified nursing diagnosis, the nurse evaluates the care for the client with Parkinson's disease. The expected outcomes include that the client

1. Demonstrates maximal independence in self-care activities as his/her condition permits
2. Demonstrates maximal mobility for the stage of the disease
3. Demonstrates no contractures and no areas of impaired skin integrity
4. Describes and complies with the drug regimen as ordered
5. Complies with the daily exercise regimen
6. Demonstrates compensatory strategies to communicate
7. Maintains appropriate fluid and caloric intake and appropriate body weight
8. States plans for follow-up care

By meeting the desired outcomes, the client should be able to maintain a functional life style for as long as his/her condition permits.

ALZHEIMER'S DISEASE

OVERVIEW

Alzheimer's disease (also known as senile dementia, Alzheimer's type [SDAT]) is a chronic, progressive, degenerative disease that accounts for almost half of the dementias occurring in persons older than 65 years of age. It is also seen in people in their 40s and 50s, which is referred to as *presenile dementia*, Alzheimer's type. Alzheimer's disease is characterized by loss of recent memory for events, persons, and places. Over time, those affected become increasingly confused and disoriented;

severe physical deterioration takes place and death occurs.

Pathophysiology

The brain of the older adult weighs less and occupies less space in the cranial vault than that of a younger person. Other changes in the brain that occur with aging include widening of the cerebral sulci, narrowing of the gyri, and enlargement of the ventricles. In the presence of Alzheimer's disease, these normal changes are greatly accelerated. Brain weight is reduced further, and there is marked cerebral atrophy. The cerebral sulci and fissures, as well as the ventricles, are enlarged more than those of persons of the same age without Alzheimer's disease. Areas of the brain particularly affected include the precentral gyrus of the frontal lobe, the superior temporal gyrus, the hippocampus, and the substantia nigra.

Microscopic changes of the brain found in those with Alzheimer's disease include neurofibrillary tangles, senile or neuritic plaques, and granulovascular degeneration. *Neurofibrillary tangles* are a classic finding at autopsy in the brains of clients with Alzheimer's disease. They consist of tangled masses of fibrous elements throughout the neuron. The same tangles are found in clients with Down's syndrome, and it is reported that all those with Down's syndrome who live long enough eventually develop Alzheimer's disease (Gray-Vickrey, 1988). *Senile plaques* are composed of degenerating nerve terminals and are found particularly in the hippocampus. Although granulovascular degeneration occurs in the normally aging brain, its presence is significantly increased in Alzheimer's disease and accounts for loss of the ability of nerve cells to function properly. This pathologic change contributes to the mortality of this disorder.

In addition to the structural changes in the brain associated with Alzheimer's disease, abnormalities in the neurotransmitters ACh, norepinephrine, and dopamine occur. ACh in the nucleus olivaris of Meynert is reduced as much as 75% and leads to a reduction in the amount of acetyltransferase in the hippocampus. This loss is significant because the decrease in acetyltransferase interferes with cholinergic innervation to the cerebral cortex, resulting in dysfunction of cognition, recent memory, and the ability to acquire new memories. The exact role that the reduction of norepinephrine and dopamine plays in the development of Alzheimer's disease is not well understood.

Recent research is focusing on the role that changes in the cerebral blood flow, blood-brain barrier, and brain metabolic activity of clients with Alzheimer's disease have in the development of the disease process.

Etiology

The exact cause of Alzheimer's disease is unknown. It is believed that there may be two forms of the disease, familial and sporadic. Research has focused on the following areas: heredity and familial incidence, a cholinergic defect, the role of ACh and other neurotransmitters, environmental agents, and immunologic changes. Recent studies indicate that there is a hereditary predisposition to the development of the disease, possibly related to a defect in chromosome 21. Viral agents and aluminum toxicity have been suggested as environmental causes, although recent research has generally eliminated both factors as causes of this disease. More research is being conducted on the roles of other elements, such as calcium and magnesium. A study conducted by the University of California suggests that clients who have experienced a head injury may be more at risk for Alzheimer's disease and at an earlier age than others. Research concerning immunologic causes of Alzheimer's disease has been inconclusive, and further studies continue (Burns & Buckwalter, 1988).

Incidence

Alzheimer's disease may affect anyone older than 40 years of age, although it occurs more often in those older than 65 years. Currently, more than 3 million people in the United States older than age 65 years have Alzheimer's disease, and 350,000 new cases are reported annually (Gray-Vickrey, 1988). Of those affected, more than 80,000 are in their 40s and 50s. Each year, some 120,000 victims of Alzheimer's disease die, making this the fourth leading cause of death, after heart attacks, cancer, and strokes. The cost to care for those with the disease is estimated at over $40 billion annually.

COLLABORATIVE MANAGEMENT

 Assessment

History

A thorough history is necessary to differentiate Alzheimer's disease from other dementias and neurologic disorders. Information is obtained from the client, as well as the family, as the client may be unaware of the problems, denying their existence or covering them up. The nurse queries the client and the family about *changes in memory* or *increasing forgetfulness*. Further information obtained includes current employment status, work history, and ability to fulfill household responsibilities, including grocery shopping, preparing meals, and cleaning. The nurse elicits a history concerning changes in driving ability, ability to handle routine financial transactions, and language and communication skills. In addition, any changes in *personality* and *behavior* are recorded.

The history taking concludes with a review of the client's past medical history. A history of head trauma, viral illness, and exposure to metal or toxic waste and a family history of Alzheimer's disease are explored further by the nurse.

Physical Assessment: Clinical Manifestations

The clinical manifestations associated with Alzheimer's disease have been grouped into four broad stages on the basis of the progress of the disease (see the accompanying Key Features of Disease). The client does not necessarily progress from one stage to the next in an orderly fashion. A stage may be bypassed, or the client may exhibit symptoms of one or several stages. Stage I, or early Alzheimer's, is characterized by forgetfulness. Confusion is seen in stage II, and the classic symptoms of dementia occur in stage III. Stage IV of the disease is considered terminal, and clients usually die within 1 year of reaching this stage from complications of immobility.

The primary focus of the neurologic examination of clients with Alzheimer's disease is to identify abnormalities in cognition, including language, personality, and behavior. Focal neurologic dysfunction (seizures or ataxia) tends to occur late in the disease process.

Cognition refers to the ability of the brain to process, store, retrieve, and manipulate information. Therefore, the nurse assesses the client for deficits in attention and concentration, judgment and perception, learning and memory, communication and language, and speed of information processing. Typical symptoms experienced by the client include memory impairment, including new memories, and defects in information retrieval resulting from dysfunction in the hippocampal, frontal, or parietal regions. Alterations in communication abilities, such as apraxia, aphasia, dysarthria, and agnosia, are due to dysfunction of the temporal and parietal lobes. Visuoconstructive problems come late with lesions in the parietal lobe. Frontal lobe impairment produces difficulties with judgment, inability to make decisions, decreased attention span, and diminished ability to concentrate. As the disease progresses, the client loses all cognitive abilities, is totally unable to communicate, and becomes less aware of the environment.

Changes in self-care skills observed by the family or the nurse include decreased interest in personal appearance, selection of clothing that is inappropriate for the weather or event, loss of bowel and bladder control, and nutritional deficits related to dysphagia. As the disease progresses, the client may wander and become lost. Over time, the client becomes less mobile, muscle contractures develop, and the client becomes totally immobile.

Other neurologic changes observed by the nurse include the presence of *tremors, myoclonus,* and *seizure activity.* In the terminal stage, the nurse is easily able to elicit a positive grasp and sucking reflex, which is abnormal in the adult client.

KEY FEATURES OF DISEASE ■ Stages of Alzheimer's Disease

Stage I
(2–3 yr or longer)

Forgetfulness

Mild memory lapse

Short attention span

Decreased interest in personal affairs

Subtle changes in personality and behavior

Stage II
(1–2 yr)

Confusion, problems with judgment

Obvious memory loss, especially short-term memory

Long-term memory generally intact

Hesitant speech

Misplaces item, may claim items stolen

Ritualistic, repetitive behavior

Stage III
(1–2 yr)*

Dementia

Disoriented to time, place, and person

Increasing motor deficits

Wanders, becomes lost

Aphasia, incontinence, and decreased muscle coordination

Stage IV
(mo to 1 yr)*

Terminal stage

Severe physical deterioration

Mental status significantly deteriorated

Does not recognize family members or significant others

Completely dependent on others for all ADL

* Some texts combine stages III and IV.

Psychosocial Assessment

The cognitive changes, as well as biochemical and structural dysfunctions, affect personality and behavior. The nurse assesses the client's reactions to changes in routine or environment. It is not unusual for the client to exhibit a catastrophic response or overreact to change. Apathy, social isolation, disinterest in hobbies, loss of interest in current events, irritability, and anxiety are often reported by the family as behaviors exhibited by the client. As brain function deteriorates (resulting from limbic system dysfunction), the client may become suspicious, paranoid, and verbally and physically abusive. Hallucinations and delusions late in the disease process are not uncommon.

Laboratory Findings

There are no laboratory tests to confirm the diagnosis of Alzheimer's disease; it is diagnosed by examination of the brain tissue, which confirms the presence of neuro-fibrillary tangles and neuritic plaques. A brain biopsy is rarely done to obtain a definitive diagnosis owing to the seriousness of the procedure and the potential complications. The diagnosis is often confirmed by a postmortem brain biopsy.

A variety of laboratory tests are done to rule out other treatable causes of dementia. These tests include a CBC; determination of serum electrolyte, vitamin B_{12}, and folate levels; thyroid and liver function tests; a serologic test for syphilis; and drug toxicity screening tests.

Radiographic Findings

CT or positron emission tomography (PET) may be performed to rule out other causes of neurologic diseases. The scans typically show cerebral atropy and ventricular enlargement. The PET scan, which measures glucose in living cells, shows a significant decrease in metabolic activity in the brains of persons with Alzheimer's disease. Chest radiography is performed to rule out cardiac disease, which may cause symptoms similar to those of Alzheimer's disease.

Other Diagnostic Tests

MRI may also be done to rule out other neurologic disease causes, and the ECG, to rule out cardiac disease.

The EEG shows slow-wave delta activity indicative of dementia.

In an effort to clearly identify the nature and extent of the client's cognitive dysfunction, several neuropsychologic tests are employed. These include the Wechsler's Adult Intelligence Scale test, the Folstein Mini-Mental State Examination (MMSE) (Fig. 33–8), and the Alzheimer's Disease Assessment Scale.

 Analysis: Nursing Diagnosis

The client with Alzheimer's disease is usually maintained in the home environment for as long as possible. As dementia and behavior problems develop and the client becomes increasingly dependent in all aspects of daily living, nursing home or long-term care placement becomes inevitable.

Common Diagnoses

The following nursing diagnoses are commonly noted in clients with Alzheimer's disease:

1. Altered thought processes related to decreased awareness of the environment, memory deficits, and the disease process

---

Maximum Score	Score	
		Client _____ Examiner _____ Date _____
		Orientation
5	( )	What is the (year) (season) (date) (day) (month)?
5	( )	Where are we (state) (country) (town) (hospital) (floor)?
		Registration
3	( )	Name 3 objects: 1 second to say each. Then ask the client all 3 after you have said them. Give 1 point for each correct answer. Then repeat them until he/she learns all 3. Count trials and record.
		Trials _____
		Attention and Calculation
5	( )	Serial 7's. 1 point for each correct answer. Stop after 5 answers. Alternatively spell "world" backward.
		Recall
3	( )	Ask for the 3 objects repeated above. Give 1 point for each correct answer.
		Language
2	( )	Name a pencil and watch. (2 points)
1	( )	Repeat the following "No ifs, ands, or buts." (1 point)
3	( )	Follow a 3-stage command: "Take a paper in your hand, fold it in half, and put it on the floor." (3 points)
1	( )	Read and obey the following: CLOSE YOUR EYES. (1 point)
1	( )	Write a sentence. (1 point)
1	( )	Copy design. (1 point)
_____		Total Score

Figure 33–8

The mini–mental state examination. (Reprinted with permission from *Journal of Psychiatric Research, 12,* Folstein, M. E., & Folstein, S. E., Mini-mental state: A practical method for grading the cognitive state of patients for the clinician, Copyright 1975, Pergamon Press plc.)

2. Potential for injury related to memory loss, wandering, behavior changes, and seizure activity

3. Ineffective family coping: compromised and altered family processes related to the client's deteriorating condition and constant care demands

4. Sleep pattern disturbance related to the disease process

Additional Diagnoses

In addition to the common diagnoses, the client may exhibit one or more of the following diagnoses:

1. Impaired verbal communication related to aphasia, agnosia, and apraxia

2. Altered nutrition: less than body requirements related to self-care deficit and dysphagia

3. Total (urinary) incontinence and bowel incontinence related to cognitive and self-care deficits

4. Social isolation related to personality and behavior changes

5. Impaired physical mobility related to contractures or myoclonus

6. Potential impaired skin integrity related to immobility or impaired nutritional status

7. Self-care deficit related to cognitive deficit

8. Potential for violence related to behavior changes

 Planning and Implementation

The plan of care for the client with Alzheimer's disease focuses on the common nursing diagnoses.

Altered Thought Processes

Planning: client goals. The major goals for this nursing diagnosis are that the client will (1) recognize self and family, (2) remain at home for as long as possible, and (3) remain as independent as possible in ADL.

Interventions: nonsurgical management. The client with memory problems benefits from a structured and consistent environment. Objects should be kept in the same place (e.g., furniture, hairbrush, and glasses). A daily routine is established, posted in view of the client, and followed as much as possible. Changes in routine are explained before the occurrence and again immediately before they take place. Clocks and single-date calendars help the client maintain day-to-day orientation to the environment. The presence of an activity calendar and familiar objects is useful for the client with dementia. Family members and health care professionals should frequently reorient the client to his/her environment.

Every effort should be made to allow the client to maintain independence in daily living skills as long as possible. For example, complete clothing outfits (e.g., shirt, slacks, underwear, and socks) can be placed on a single hanger, and the client selects from these group-

ings. When possible, the client should participate in meal preparation, grocery shopping, and other household routines. Adaptive devices, such as grab bars in the bathtub or shower area, elevated commode, and adapted silverware, are obtained to enable the client to maintain independence in grooming, toileting, and feeding for as long as possible. The client can remain continent of bowel and bladder for long periods of time if taken to the bathroom every 2 hours during the day and less frequently at night. It is helpful to limit the client's fluid intake in the evening to decrease the number of times the client may need to be taken to the bathroom at night.

As the disease progresses, the client may develop *prosopagnosia* (inability to recognize self and other familiar faces). The nurse encourages the family to provide the client with pictures of family members and close friends that are labeled with the person's name on the picture. Additionally, the family should be encouraged to reminisce with the client about pleasant experiences from the past. It is not unusual for the client to talk to his/her image in the mirror, and this behavior should be allowed as long as it is not harmful.

The nurse can assist the client with communication problems and nonlistening behaviors by attracting the client's attention before conversing. The environment should be free of distractions. The nurse should speak directly to the client in a slow and distinct manner. Sentences should be clear and short. The client should be asked to perform one task at a time, and sufficient time must be allowed for completion.

A variety of drugs are used or under investigation to improve the client's cognitive abilities. Ergoloid mesylates (Hydergine, Niloric) may be used in the early stages of the disease. Although cognitive abilities usually improve for a short period of time, side effects, such as orthostatic hypotension and dizziness, frequently occur. A variety of cholinergic drugs are under investigation in the hope that they will improve the client's memory. To date no improvement has been seen in clients who are given ACh precursors. Physostigmine (Antilirium) and tacrine (tetrahydroaminoacridine [THA]) are ACh esterase inhibitors that have improved cognitive function for short periods of time. Both drugs remain under investigation; their use may be limited because of side effects, especially from THA, which causes liver damage when given for long periods of time.

Many clients with Alzheimer's disease develop depression and may be treated with amitriptyline (Elavil), doxepin (Sinequan), or imipramine (Tofranil). Other antidepressants that may be used include desipramine (Norpramin), maprotiline (Ludiomil), and trazodone (Desyrel). The nurse observes for the effects of these medications and reports untoward effects to the physician.

Potential for Injury

Planning: client goals. The major goals for this nursing diagnosis are that the client will (1) remain free from physical harm and (2) not injure anyone else.

Interventions: nonsurgical management. The client with Alzheimer's disease tends to wander and may easily become lost. The client should always wear an identification badge or bracelet. The nurse checks the client frequently and places the client in a room that can be monitored easily, ideally close to the nurse's station and away from exits and stairs. Restlessness may be decreased if the client is taken for frequent walks. Restraints should be used only when absolutely necessary, as they may increase the client's restlessness and agitation. The client may become injured because he/she is unable to recognize objects or situations as harmful. All dangerous objects (e.g., knives, needles, and cleaning solutions) are removed or secured. The client is often unaware that his/her driving ability is impaired and usually wants to continue this activity. Automobile keys must be secured and the client appropriately counseled. In the event of agitated behavior, the nurse talks calmly and softly and attempts to redirect the client to a more positive behavior or activity. If the client remains agitated, the nurse ensures the client's safety and leaves the room after explaining that he/she will return later. Frequent visual checks must be done during this time.

Late in the disease process, the client may develop seizure activity. Seizure precautions should be instituted and appropriate action taken during a seizure episode (see earlier discussion of the care of clients experiencing seizures).

Seizures occur in 10% to 20% of clients with Alzheimer's disease and are usually treated with phenytoin (Dilantin). Agitation, assaultiveness, or hyperactivity may be treated with hypnotics or neuroleptics. Hypnotics used include diphenhydramine (Benadryl), triazolam (Halcion), and chloral hydrate. For more severe behavior problems, the neuroleptics, such as haloperidol (Haldol), thioridazine (Mellaril), and loxapine (Loxitane), have been found to be somewhat effective. The nurse observes for drug side effects, including increased confusion and extrapyramidal symptoms (e.g., tremors) and promptly reports these to the physician.

Ineffective Family Coping: Compromised; Altered Family Processes

Planning: family goals. The major goal for these nursing diagnoses is that the family will obtain appropriate support services to enable them to adjust and cope with the client's physical and mental problems.

Interventions: nonsurgical management. The client with Alzheimer's disease requires continual supervision. Severe cognitive changes leave the client unable to manage finances, property, and personal care. The nurse advises the family to seek legal counsel regarding the client's competency and the need to obtain guardianship or durable power of attorney. The family is referred to the local Alzheimer's support group and is provided with literature concerning the disease. The nurse establishes a supportive environment for family members and encourages them to express their feelings

to other family members. Family members are encouraged to maintain their own social network and obtain respite from care of the client. The nurse assists the family in developing strategies to cope with the long-term consequences of the disease process. Health teaching and referral to activity, physical, and occupational therapists are done as needed.

Sleep Pattern Disturbance

Planning: client goals. The major goal for this nursing diagnosis is that the client will sleep through the night.

Interventions: nonsurgical management. The client with Alzheimer's disease often has difficulty sleeping at night. To facilitate sleep, a pre-bedtime ritual should be established. The routine consists of personal hygiene activities (bathing, toileting, and brushing teeth) and environmental control measures to reduce noise and eliminate distractions. A back rub or small snack may help the client prepare for sleep.

The client's treatment and medication schedule are adjusted to provide for uninterrupted sleep. If more conventional measures fail to induce sleep, medications that may be used include chloral hydrate, triazolam, and flurazepam (Dalmane).

Another important factor to facilitate sleep at night is to keep the client active during the day. A daily routine that consists of a balance between passive activities and those requiring more strenuous exercise, such as walking or stretching activities, usually facilitates sleep at night. The client may want to take a nap in the late afternoon, but this should be discouraged.

■ Discharge Planning

The client with Alzheimer's disease is usually maintained at home for as long as possible. Usually, in stage III or IV of the disease process, the client is placed in a long-term care facility.

Home Care Preparation

Special precautions are taken to safely maintain the client at home. The environment must be uncluttered, consistent, and structured. All hazardous items (e.g., cleaning fluids, power tools, and insect spray) are removed or secured. All electrical sockets not in use should be covered with safety plugs. Handrails and grab bars should be installed in the bathroom; handrails should be along all stairways and a guardrail placed around porches or open stairwells. Because of the client's tendency to wander, especially at night, the family may want to install alarms to all outside doors, basement, and the client's bedroom. All outside and basement doors should have deadbolt locks to prevent the client from going outside unsupervised. The temperature of the water heater should be adjusted to prevent accidental burns. Night-lights should be used in the client's bedroom, hallway, and bathroom.

Client/Family Education

Usually the client with Alzheimer's disease is cared for in the home until late in the disease process. The care is typically provided by family members, as health insurance and family finances are usually insufficient to cover the services of a private duty nurse or home care aide. The client care plan developed by the nurse in conjunction with the family must be reasonable and realistic for the family to implement.

The family is taught how to assist the client with bathing, dressing, toileting, and other self-care activities. The nurse and the occupational therapist collaborate to teach the family and the client how to use assistive-adaptive equipment, such as a brace, a sling, a cane, or adapted eating utensils. The client may have difficulty chewing, swallowing, or tasting foods and may not be able to eat without assistance. The nurse, the family, and the dietitian should develop a diet plan to maximize the client's nutritional intake.

The nurse teaches the family what to do in the event of a seizure and how to prevent the client from injury. The family should be instructed to notify the physician if the seizure is prolonged or if the client's seizure pattern changes.

The name, time of administration, the dosage, the route of administration, and the side effects of all medications should be explained to the family. The family should be instructed to check with the client's physician before using any OTC medications.

It is important for the client to have an established exercise program to maintain mobility as long as possible, as well as to prevent complications of immobility. The nurse collaborates with the family and the physical therapist to develop an individualized exercise program.

Psychosocial Preparation

The client may begin to withdraw from friends and social events as memory impairments and personality and behavior changes become more apparent. This increases the family's responsibilities to minimize the impact of social isolation and decreased activity. The family may begin to decrease their own social activities as the demands of the client's care take more of their time. It is important for the nurse to emphasize to the family the importance of maintaining their own social contacts and leisure activities. It is now possible in many areas of the country for the family to arrange respite care. The client may be placed in a respite facility for the weekend or for several weeks to give the family a break from the constant care demands of the client. It may also be possible to obtain respite care in the home through a home care agency. The nurse stresses that respite care is for a short period of time; it is not a permanent placement. Many long-term care facilities have opened day care centers or specialty units for clients with Alzheimer's disease. In the day care center, the client spends all or part of the day at the facility and participates in activities as his/her condition permits. These centers are usually open only on weekdays.

The family should be trained in defensive techniques to use when the client becomes restless, agitated, or combative. In addition, they should be advised in strategies to use to orient the client to everyday activities.

Health Care Resources

When the client can no longer be cared for at home, referral to a nursing home or a long-term care facility may be needed. The nurse should advise the family early in the course of the disease that placement may be needed in the late stages of the disease. This allows the family to begin the search process for an appropriate facility before a crisis develops and immediate placement is needed.

All families should be referred to the Alzheimer's Disease and Related Disorders Association. This organization provides information and support services to clients and their families.

 Evaluation

On the basis of the identified nursing diagnoses, the nurse evaluates the care of the client with Alzheimer's disease. The expected outcomes include that the client

1. Remains at home for as long as possible
2. Maintains independence in ADL and self-care skills as long as possible
3. Remains free of injury from falls, seizure activity, or environmental hazards
4. Demonstrates positive coping skills
5. Obtains appropriate support services
6. Sleeps throughout the night or for at least 6 hours
7. Complies with the drug regimen as ordered

By meeting the desired outcomes, the client should be able to stay in the home environment until physical and psychosocial problems render home care impossible.

HUNTINGTON'S CHOREA

Huntington's chorea is a hereditary disorder transmitted as an autosomal dominant trait at the time of conception. The offspring of a parent with the disease has a 50% chance of eventually manifesting the disease. In the United States, 10,000 to 25,000 people have the disease, with another 20,000 to 50,000 thought to carry the gene (Jackson, 1987). Men and women are equally affected, and symptoms begin between 35 and 45 years of age.

The two main symptoms of the disease are progressive mental status changes, leading to dementia, and choreiform movements. Dementia is related to the destruction of neurons within the cerebral cortex; it may also be associated with excessive amounts of dopamine found within the cerebral cortex and limbic systems of those affected.

Two structures within the basal ganglia are involved in the development of Huntington's chorea, namely, the caudate nucleus and the putamen. Both structures have close connections to the cerebral cortex and are closely associated with neurotransmitters. Neurotransmitters are secreted at the synapse, or junction, of one neuron with another, and through their specific excitation or inhibition of neurons, fine, controlled, integrated motor activity occurs.

In the presence of Huntington's disease, there is a decrease in the amount of gamma-aminobutyric acid (GABA), an inhibitory neurotransmitter. This creates an imbalance between dopamine, an excitatory neurotransmitter, and GABA at the synapse and causes uninhibited motor activity. The result is brisk, jerky, purposeless movements, particularly of the hands, the face, the tongue, and the legs, which the client is unable to stop.

There is no known cure or treatment of the disease. The only way to prevent transmission of the gene is for those affected to refrain from having children. Genetic counseling is important for children of clients with the disease. It is now possible to test individuals at risk for the disease to determine if they have the gene present on chromosome 4. However, the test is still under investigation, and large-scale studies have not been completed. Therefore, the results of testing may be subject to error, although this risk has been greatly reduced recently. Before the testing procedure is undertaken, counseling must be done to ensure that the client has voluntarily decided in favor of testing and is not being pressured by family or friends. In addition, counseling helps to determine if the benefits of knowing the results outweigh the risks of a positive result (e.g., depression or suicide).

The diagnosis of Huntington's disease is based on a family history of the disease, clinical assessment, and laboratory findings. Clinical manifestations of the disease include choreiform movements, poor balance, hesitant or explosive speech, dysphagia, impaired respiration, and bowel and bladder incontinence. Mental status changes include decreased attention span, poor judgment, memory loss, personality changes, and, later in the disease process, dementia.

Management is symptomatic. Nursing interventions are directed toward treating the following nursing problems: impaired physical mobility; altered nutrition: less than body requirements; total incontinence; bowel incontinence; total self-care deficit; body image disturbance and altered role performance; potential for injury; and ineffective airway clearance, ineffective breathing pattern, and impaired gas exchange. As the symptoms progress, the client's status deteriorates, and death occurs from complications of immobility, such as pneumonia or sepsis.

AMYOTROPHIC LATERAL SCLEROSIS

Amyotrophic lateral sclerosis (ALS), also known as Lou Gehrig's disease, is a progressive degenerative disease involving the motor system. Unlike many other degenerative diseases, the sensory and autonomic nervous systems are not involved. Mental status changes do not occur as a result of the disease.

ALS may occur at any age; however, it is commonly seen in the fourth and fifth decades of life. The exact cause is unknown, although genetic, autoimmune, and metabolic factors are currently under investigation. The incidence is estimated at 3 in 100,000 persons, with men significantly more frequently affected than women, and Caucasians affected more often than Blacks (Thompson et al., 1986). Death occurs within 3 to 5 years after the onset of symptoms and is attributable to respiratory failure.

Degeneration and destruction of the neurons occur within the precentral gyrus of the cerebral cortex, along the corticospinal tract, and within the anterior horn cells of the spinal cord. The brain stem nuclei of cranial nerves V, VII, X, and XII, as well as the pyramidal tract, may be involved.

The clinical manifestations of ALS include fatigue, muscle atrophy, and weakness. Early symptoms include fatigue while talking, tongue atrophy, dysphagia, weakness of the hands and arms, fasciculations of the face, nasal quality of speech, and dysarthria. As the disease progresses, muscle atrophy, particularly of the trapezius and sternocleidomastoid muscles, develops. Muscle weakness and atrophy extends until the client develops a flaccid quadriplegia. Eventually, the respiratory muscles become involved, leading to respiratory compromise, pneumonia, and death.

Diagnosis of ALS is based on clinical and diagnostic test findings. The EMG reveals a normal conduction time; however, a decreased number of motor units may be found. A muscle biopsy specimen typically demonstrates small, angulated, atrophic fibers. Other diagnostic studies reveal motor strength deficits in serial muscle testing; abnormal pulmonary function test results, such as a decreased vital capacity (less than 2 L); and dysphagia. CT, MRI, and myelography findings are often normal.

There is no known cure for the disease, and treatment is symptomatic. Nursing interventions are directed toward treating the following nursing diagnoses: impaired physical mobility; total self-care deficit; altered nutrition: less than body requirements; impaired verbal communication; ineffective breathing pattern, ineffective airway clearance, and impaired gas exchange; and total (urinary) incontinence and bowel incontinence. In addition to the above problems, the nurse provides ongoing support and counseling to the client and the family as they begin to cope with the impact of this terminal disease.

SYRINGOMYELIA

Syringomyelia is a disease involving the formation of a cavity in or the dilation of the central canal of the spinal cord resulting from a direct or indirect communication with the fourth ventricle. Over time, the cavity enlarges and may extend upward to the medulla or downward to the lower cervical or high thoracic region. The disease occurs almost exclusively within the cervical spinal cord. If the cavity is filled with blood instead of spinal fluid, the disorder is referred to as *hematomyelia*.

Initial symptoms of syringomyelia include loss of deep tendon reflexes in the arms (biceps and triceps reflexes) and decreased or absent sensation below the level of the lesion. As the lesion expands, damage to the corticospinal tracts, the motor neurons of anterior horn cells, and the spinothalamic tract occurs, causing significant motor loss and additional sensory findings. Paresthesias, weakness, muscle atrophy, and fasciculations occur. The signs are bilateral, but not symmetric. Of significance with this disease is the loss of pain and temperature sensation in the hands and inner areas of the forearms. This leaves the client at risk for injuries, such as burns or osteomyelitis.

Diagnosis of this dysfunction is based on clinical findings, as well as radiographic studies of the cervical vertebral column. Myelography, CT, and MRI show an enlarged vertebral column and spinal cord.

Management is directed toward surgically correcting the defect that allows flow of CSF between the fourth ventricle and the central canal. A ventriculocisternal shunt may be inserted or, if the foramen of Magendie is obstructed, it may be dissected until open. In addition, a cervical laminectomy is performed to relieve pressure on the spinal cord. Although some function may return, the client has residual neurologic dysfunction.

Nursing interventions are directed toward treating the following nursing diagnoses: sensory/perceptual alterations; impaired physical mobility; total incontinence; bowel incontinence; total self-care deficit; and self-esteem disturbance. With appropriate rehabilitation, the client is able to maintain a productive quality of life. See Chapter 22 for rehabilitation nursing interventions.

HEAD INJURY

OVERVIEW

Craniocerebral trauma, commonly referred to as head trauma, is a traumatic insult to the brain caused by an external physical force that may produce a diminished or altered state of consciousness. It may result in impairment of cognitive abilities or physical functioning, as well as disturbance of behavior or emotional functioning. These impairments may be either temporary or permanent and cause partial or total functional disability or psychosocial maladjustment. In the United States, head injury has taken more lives of people 18 to 34 years of age than all other diseases combined for that age group. Total expenses for brain injury cost American families $4 billion annually, which does not include lost productivity and potential wages.

Pathophysiology

Various terms are used to describe brain injuries that are produced when a mechanical force is applied either directly or indirectly to the brain. A force produced by a blow to the head is a *direct* injury, whereas a force applied to another body part with a rebound effect to the brain is an *indirect* injury. The brain responds to these forces by forward movement within the rigid cranial vault. The brain may also rebound or rotate on the brain stem, causing diffuse axonal injury (shearing injuries). This moving brain may be contused or lacerated as it moves over the inner surfaces of the cranium, which is irregularly shaped and sharp. Damage most frequently occurs to the frontal and temporal lobes of the brain.

Primary Brain Injury

Primary brain damage results from the physical stress (force) within the brain tissue caused by open or closed trauma. An open head injury occurs when there is a fracture of the skull or the skull is pierced by a penetrating object. The integrity of the brain and dura is violated, and there is exposure to outside, or environmental, contaminants. Damage may occur to the underlying vessels, the dural sinus, the brain, and the cranial nerves. A closed head injury is the result of blunt trauma; the integrity of the skull is not violated. It is the more serious of the two types of injury, and the damage to the brain tissue is dependent on the degree and mechanisms of injury.

Open head injury. The types of fractures associated with an open head injury are linear, depressed, and open. A *linear* fracture is a simple, clean break in which the impacted area of bone bends inward, whereas the area around it bends outward; linear fractures account for about 80% of all skull fractures. In a *depressed* fracture, the bone is pressed inward into the brain tissue to at least the thickness of the skull. In an *open* fracture, the scalp is lacerated, creating a direct opening to the brain tissue. A unique fracture that may occur is a *basilar* skull fracture. It occurs at the base of the skull, usually along the paranasal sinus, and results in CSF leakage from the nose or ears. Of significance with this fracture is the potential development of hemorrhage caused by damage to the internal carotid artery; damage to cranial nerves I, II, VII, and VIII; and infection.

The majority of penetrating injuries to the skull are

caused by gunshot wounds and knife injuries. The degree of injury to the brain tissue is dependent on the velocity, mass, shape, and direction of impact. High-velocity injuries produce the greatest damage to brain tissue. As with any open head injury, the client with a penetrating injury is at high risk for infection from the object that pierces the skull, as well as from other environmental contaminants.

Closed head injury. Closed head injuries, caused by blunt trauma, lead to concussions, contusion, and lacerations of the brain. The damage to the brain may be mild, as occurs in a concussive injury, or it may be more severe, causing diffuse axonal injury or widespread injury to the white matter of the brain. A *concussion* is characterized by a brief loss of consciousness; damage occurs to the gray matter of the cerebral cortex or possibly to the diencephalon or the brain stem. The damage to the axons is functional, not structural (some authorities believe that both are involved), which is why permanent neurologic dysfunction is generally not seen. A *contusion* is a bruising of the brain tissue and is most frequently found at the site of impact (coup) or in a line opposite the site of impact (contrecoup) (Fig. 33–9). The base of the frontal and temporal lobes is most often involved. A *laceration* causes actual tearing of the cortical surface vessels, which may lead to secondary hemorrhage, and is therefore more serious than a contusion.

Types of force. Other factors that must be considered in the discussion of the dynamics of head injury are the type of force and mechanisms of injury involved (Fig. 33–10). An *acceleration injury* is caused by the head in motion. A *deceleration injury* occurs when the head is suddenly stopped or hits a stationary object. These forces may be sufficient to cause the cerebrum to rotate about the brain stem, resulting in shearing, straining, and distortion of the brain tissue, particularly of the axons in the brain stem and cerebellum. Small areas of hemorrhage may develop around the blood vessels that sustain the impact of these forces (stress), with destruction of adjacent brain tissue. Particularly affected are the basal nuclei and the hypothalamus.

Secondary Responses/Insult

Secondary responses to brain injury include any neurologic damage that occurs after the initial injury. Secondary injuries or responses increase the morbidity and mortality after head trauma. The most frequently occurring response is the development of increased ICP attributable to edema, hemorrhage, impaired cerebral

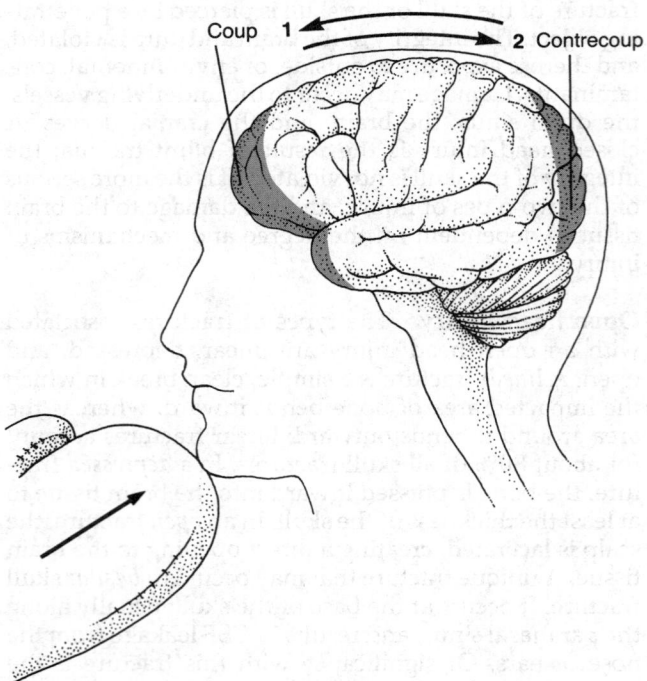

Figure 33–9

Coup (site of impact) injury to frontal area of brain and contrecoup injury to frontal and temporal areas of the brain.

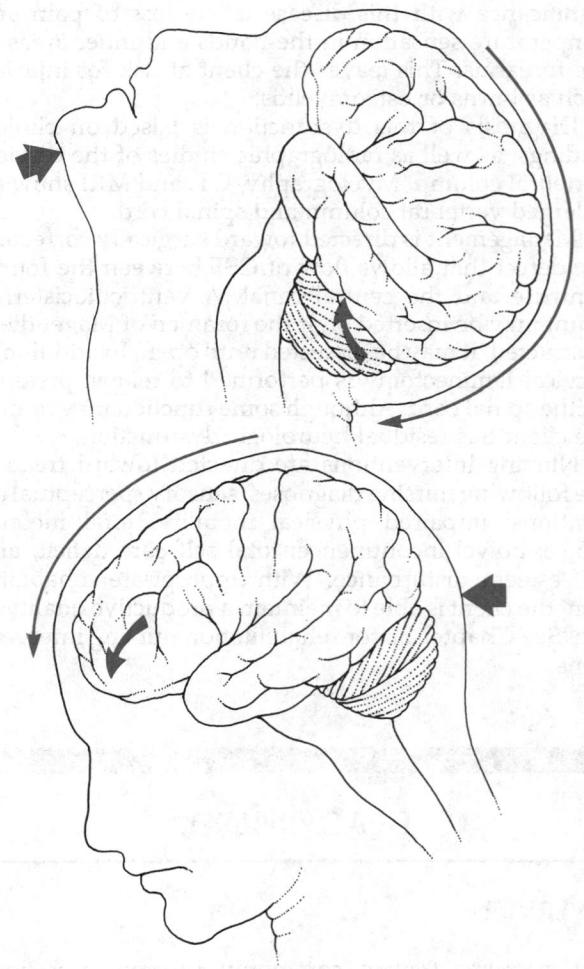

Figure 33–10

Movement of the head during acceleration-deceleration injury typically seen in motor vehicle accidents.

autoregulation, and hydrocephalus. Hypoxemia, hypercapnia, and systemic hypotension may precipitate increased ICP. Damage to the brain tissue occurs primarily because the delivery of oxygen and glucose to the brain is interrupted.

Increased intracranial pressure. The brain, composed of brain tissue, blood, and CSF, is encased in the relatively rigid skull. Within this space, there is little room for any of the components to expand or increase in volume. Through the processes of accommodation and compliance, the ICP is maintained at its normal pressure of 10 to 15 mmHg, despite transient increases in pressure that occur with straining during defecation, coughing, or sneezing. According to the Monroe-Kellie hypothesis, any increase in the volume of one component must be compensated for by a decrease in the volume of one of the other components. As a first response to an increase in volume of any of these components, the CSF is shunted or displaced from the cranial compartment to the spinal subarachnoid space, or the rate of CSF absorption is increased. An additional response, if needed, is a decrease in cerebral blood volume by the displacement of cerebral venous blood into the sinuses. As long as the brain is able to compensate for the increase in volume and to remain compliant, there are minimal increases in ICP.

Increased ICP is the leading cause of death from head trauma in clients who reach the hospital alive. It occurs when compliance no longer takes place and the brain cannot accommodate further volume changes. As the ICP increases, cerebral blood flow decreases, leading to tissue hypoxia, a decrease in serum pH, and an increase in carbon dioxide level. This process causes cerebral vasodilation, edema, and a further increase in the ICP, and the cycle begins anew. If this condition is untreated, the brain herniates downward toward the brain stem, causing irreversible brain damage and possibly death.

Two types of edema may cause increased ICP. A third type occurs in the presence of acute brain swelling. *Vasogenic edema* is seen most often as a cause of increased ICP in the adult. It is characterized by an increase in brain tissue volume caused by an abnormal permeability of the walls of the cerebral vessels, which allow protein-rich plasma infiltrate to leak into the extracellular space of the brain. The fluid collects primarily in the white matter. In addition to vasogenic edema, *cytotoxic or cellular edema* may occur as a result of a hypoxic insult, which causes a disturbance in cellular metabolism, the sodium pump, and active ion transport. The brain is quickly depleted of available oxygen, glucose, and glycogen and converts to anaerobic metabolism. The sodium pump fails, and sodium enters the cells and pulls water from the extracellular space. A concomitant decrease in serum sodium level to less than 120 mEq/L occurs. As a result, there is an abnormal accumulation of fluid in the brain cells and a decrease in the extracellular fluid space. Cytotoxic edema may lead to vasogenic edema and further increase in ICP. *Interstitial edema* occurs in the presence of acute brain swelling and is associated with elevated blood pressure or CSF pressure. Edema develops rapidly in the perivascular and periventricular white space and can be controlled through measures to reduce the client's blood pressure or decrease the CSF pressures.

Hemorrhage. Hemorrhages are caused by vascular damage from the shearing force of the trauma. An *epidural hematoma* (Fig. 33–11), arterial bleeding into the space between the dura and the inner table of the skull, is frequently caused by a fracture of the temporal bone, which houses the middle meningeal artery. A *subdural hematoma* (see Fig. 33–11), venous bleeding into the space beneath the dura and above the arachnoid, occurs most frequently as a result of tearing of the bridging veins within the cerebral hemispheres or from laceration of the brain tissue. An *intracranial hemorrhage* (see Fig. 33–11) is the accumulation of blood within the brain tissue caused by the tearing of small arteries and veins in the subcortical white matter. Brain stem hemorrhage occurs as a result of direct trauma, fractures, or torsion injuries to the brain stem. All hematomas are potentially life-threatening, as they act as space-occupying lesions and are surrounded by edema.

Loss of autoregulation. Through the process of cerebral autoregulation, the blood flow to the brain remains relatively constant, despite variations in systemic blood pressure. Loss of autoregulation causes the cerebral blood flow to fluctuate passively with the systemic blood pressure. Systemic hypertension may cause an increase in ICP (from an increase in cerebral blood flow) and potential development of vasogenic edema. Hypoxemia and hypercapnia cause marked cerebral vasodilation and therefore an increase in cerebral blood flow, which contributes to increased ICP.

Hydrocephalus. An abnormal increase in the CSF volume is caused by dilation of the cerebral ventricles, resulting either from the impairment of CSF absorption in the arachnoid villi or from obstruction of the CSF circulation pathway. This increase in the CSF volume may lead to the development of increased ICP.

Herniation. In the presence of increased ICP, the brain tissue may shift and herniate downward. Of the several types of herniation syndromes that may occur (Fig. 33–12), *uncal*, or transtentorial, herniation is the most clinically significant. It is caused by a shift of one or both areas of the temporal lobe, known as the uncus. This shift creates pressure on the third cranial nerve and results in dilated and nonreactive pupils, ptosis, and a rapidly deteriorating level of consciousness. *Central* herniation is caused by a downward shift of the brain stem and the diencephalon from a supratentorial lesion. It is clinically manifested by Cheyne-Stokes respirations and pinpoint nonreactive pupils. A shift of the cingulate gyrus below the falx cerebri is known as *cingulate* herniation. A type of infratentorial herniation, *cerebellar tonsillar* herniation, occurs when the cerebellar tonsils shift and compress the medulla. This may lead to respiratory and cardiovascular compromise or arrest. All

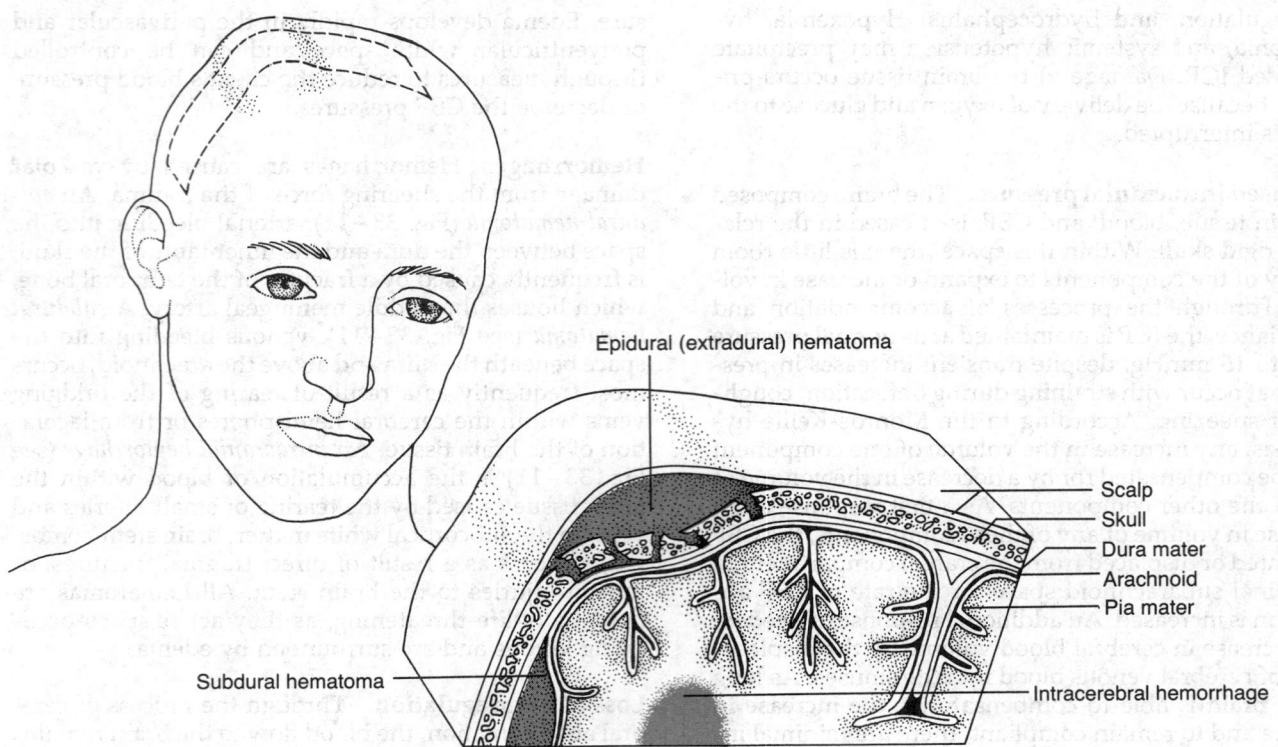

Figure 33–11

Epidural hematoma (outside the dura mater of the brain), subdural hematoma (under the dura mater of the brain), and intracranial hemorrhage (within the brain tissue).

herniation syndromes are potentially life-threatening, and the physician must be notified immediately when they are suspected.

Etiology

The most common cause of head injury in the United States is accidents involving motor vehicles, which include both automobiles and motorcycles. Falls are the second most frequent cause of head injury. In a National Institutes of Health survey, the majority of falls occurred in those younger than 15 years of age; however, a University of Virginia study showed that elderly individuals, particularly those older than 70 years, were affected more often (Rimel & Jane, 1983). Penetrating injuries to the brain are most frequently caused by gunshot or knife wounds.

Incidence

Approximately 10 million head injuries occur in the United States each year. Of these individuals, 500,000 are hospitalized, 100,000 die, and some 70,000 are left with permanent neurologic dysfunction. Head injuries occur two to three times more often in males than in females. More than 70% occur in clients between the ages of 10 and 39 years, with a peak incidence between 15 and 24 years of age. Although the overall incidence of head injury in those older than 70 years of age is less than 3%, the number of injuries within that age group is statistically significant at 30 per 10,000 population. Studies indicate that the summer and spring months and weekends are associated with a high number of injuries. Five million days of hospitalization and 30 million lost workdays occur annually as a direct result of head trauma (Jennett, 1983; Walleck, 1989).

PREVENTION

Many head injuries could be entirely prevented or their seriousness reduced through the proper use of automobile seat belts. The use of seat belts can reduce the number of fatalities from head trauma, as well as protect against chest and spinal cord injuries. Protective headgear has been shown to reduce the severity of injury from motorcycle and bicycle accidents. Programs need to be developed to educate the public on the effects of excessive speed, drugs, and alcohol on driving. Physical education programs need to stress safety in sports and leisure activities. Many injuries at work could be avoided through following the standards set by the Oc-

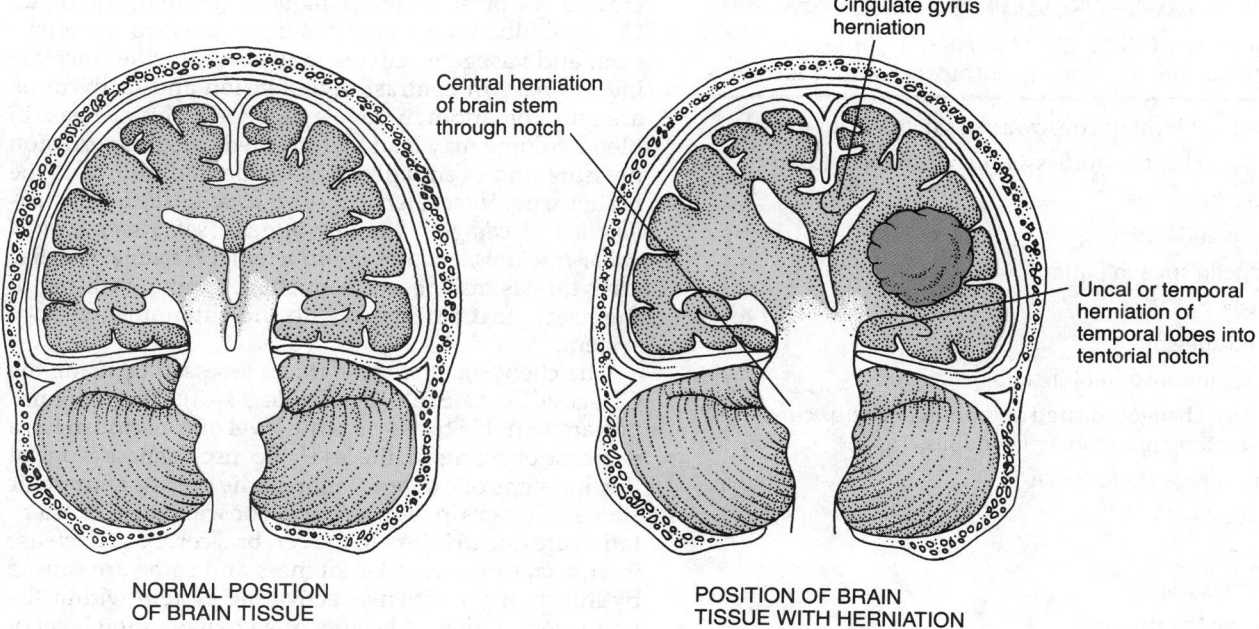

NORMAL POSITION
OF BRAIN TISSUE

POSITION OF BRAIN
TISSUE WITH HERNIATION

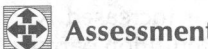

Figure 33–12

Herniation syndromes.

cupational Safety and Health Administration (OSHA). Programs for senior citizens should be developed to emphasize home safety, particularly the prevention of falls.

COLLABORATIVE MANAGEMENT

Assessment

History

Obtaining an accurate history from a client with craniocerebral trauma may be difficult because of either the seriousness of the injury or the presence of amnesia. It is not unusual for the client to experience retrograde or anterograde amnesia—loss of memory for the events before or after the injury, respectively. The client with a serious head injury is admitted to the hospital unconscious or in a confused and combative state. If the client is unable to provide information, the history can be obtained from rescue workers or witnesses to the injury. Important information to obtain is when, where, and how the injury occurred. Did the client lose consciousness? If so, for how long was the client unconscious, and has there been a change in the level of consciousness?

The nurse obtains information concerning the events immediately after the injury. Clients with a severe injury may have several different reactions. The client may be completely unresponsive after the injury or may initially be responsive and within a few minutes to several hours may deteriorate rapidly. In another typical presentation, the client is initially unconscious for a few

minutes as a result of the primary brain injury, returns to a normal level of consciousness, and then rapidly deteriorates as a result of the consequences of secondary insult to the brain. The nurse determines whether the client experienced any *seizure activity* before or after the injury or if there is a history of a seizure disorder. It is important to obtain precise information concerning the circumstances of falls, particularly in the older client, to differentiate a head injury attributable to a fall from a head injury caused by a stroke, an aneurysm, or a heart attack. Other pertinent information includes hand dominance, any diseases of or injuries to the eyes, and any allergies to medications or food, particularly seafood. People allergic to seafood are often allergic to contrast media used in diagnostic tests. The nurse obtains a history regarding alcohol or drug use and abuse, as drugs or alcohol may mask the symptoms of increased ICP. In addition, routine questions concerning the client's medical history should be asked in accordance with the hospital's policies.

Physical Assessment: Clinical Manifestations

No two injuries are alike—the client with a head injury may have a variety of signs and symptoms depending on the severity of injury and the resulting increase in ICP (see the accompanying Key Features of Disease). The goals of the nursing assessment are the establishment of baseline data and the early detection of and prevention of increased ICP, systemic hypotension, hypoxia, and hypercapnia. Through the early detection

KEY FEATURES OF DISEASE ■ Clinical Manifestations of Increased Intracranial Pressure

Decreased level of consciousness (lethargy to coma)

Behavior changes: restless, irritable, and confused

Headache

Nausea and vomiting

Change in speech pattern

Aphasia

Slurred speech

Change in sensorimotor status

Pupillary changes: dilated and nonreactive or constricted and nonreactive pupils

Cranial nerve dysfunction

Ataxia

Seizures

Cushing's triad

Abnormal posturing
  Decerebrate } latest stage
  Decorticate

of subtle changes in the client's neurologic status, the health care team is able to prevent or treat potentially life-threatening complications.

It is estimated that 5% to 20% of clients with head trauma have associated cervical spinal cord injuries. All those with craniocerebral trauma must be treated as though they have spinal cord injury until radiographic studies prove otherwise. It is important that adequate visualization of the cervical vertebrae take place. Other indicators of spinal cord injury are loss of motor and sensory function, tenderness along the spine, and abnormal head tilt. The client may experience respiratory problems and diaphragmatic breathing, and her/his reflexes may be diminished or absent.

The *first* priority is the assessment of the client's *airway and breathing pattern*. Hypoxia and hypercapnia are best detected through arterial blood gas analysis. Injuries to the brain stem may cause a change in the client's breathing pattern, such as Cheyne-Stokes respirations, central neurogenic hyperventilation, or apneustic, cluster, or ataxic breathing. The accompanying Key Features of Disease describes common respiratory patterns of comatose clients.

The mechanisms of *autoregulation* are frequently impaired as the result of craniocerebral trauma. The more serious the injury, the more severe is the impact on autoregulation. The client's blood pressure and pulse are taken and recorded to alert the nurse to possible changes in cerebral blood flow caused by impaired autoregulation as a result of hypotension or hypertension. The Cushing reflex, a classic yet late sign of increased ICP, is manifested by severe hypertension with a widened pulse pressure and bradycardia. As the ICP increases, the pulse becomes thready, irregular, and rapid. Cerebral blood flow increases in response to hypertension, and vasogenic edema may occur, further increasing the ICP. In contrast, hypotension and tachycardia are symptomatic of hypovolemic shock. This decrease in blood volume may lead to decreased cerebral perfusion pressure and eventually to ischemia and infarct of the brain tissue. *Hypovolemic shock is usually due to intra-abdominal bleeding or bleeding into the soft tissue around major fractures, and not to intracranial bleeding.* Cardiac arrhythmias may result from chest trauma, bruising of the heart, or interference with the autonomic nervous system.

The client's *neurologic status* is assessed by using the Glasgow Coma Scale (see Table 33–3). The most important variable to assess is the level of consciousness; a decrease or change in the level of consciousness is one of the first signs of a deterioration in the client's neurologic status. Changes in the content of consciousness or orientation are due to injury to the cerebral cortex. A decrease in arousal or increased sleepiness and coma are caused by injury in the reticular activating system within the brain stem. Other indicators of a change in the level of consciousness include behavior changes, such as restlessness or irritability.

The client's *pupils* are checked for size and reaction to light. Bilaterally dilated and nonreactive pupils are indicative of central dysfunction or a defect in the area of the diencephalon; a unilateral nonreactive pupil signifies peripheral dysfunction of cranial nerves II and III. Pinpoint and nonresponsive pupils are indicative of brain stem dysfunction at the level of the pons. Of particular importance is the ovoid pupil, which is regarded as the midstage between a normal-sized and a dilated pupil and heralds the development of increased ICP. Gross vision is checked, if the client's condition permits, by having the client read any printed material, such as the nurse's name tag, or count the number of fingers held within his/her visual field. Loss of vision is usually caused by injury to the occipital lobe, which produces temporary cortical blindness. If the client is able to cooperate, cranial nerves III, IV, and VI are tested. Extraocular movements may be diminished owing to the presence of increased ICP and hydrocephalus. Damage to the optic chiasm, optic tract, or optic radii may cause visual field deficits or diplopia. In the unconscious client, the oculocephalic and oculovestibular tests are performed to test the integrity of the brain stem and the integrity of cranial nerves III, VI, and VII.

Bilateral motor responses are assessed to avoid missing lateralizing signs. The client's motor loss or dysfunction usually appears contralateral to the site of the lesion. For example, a left-sided hemiparesis is indicative of an injury to the right cerebral hemisphere. A deterioration in motor function or the development of posturing or flaccidity is another indicator of increased ICP attributable to dysfunction within the pyramidal system or cerebral peduncles. Brain stem or cerebellar injury may cause ataxia, decreased or increased muscle tone, and weakness.

KEY FEATURES OF DISEASE ■ Respiratory Patterns in Comatose Clients

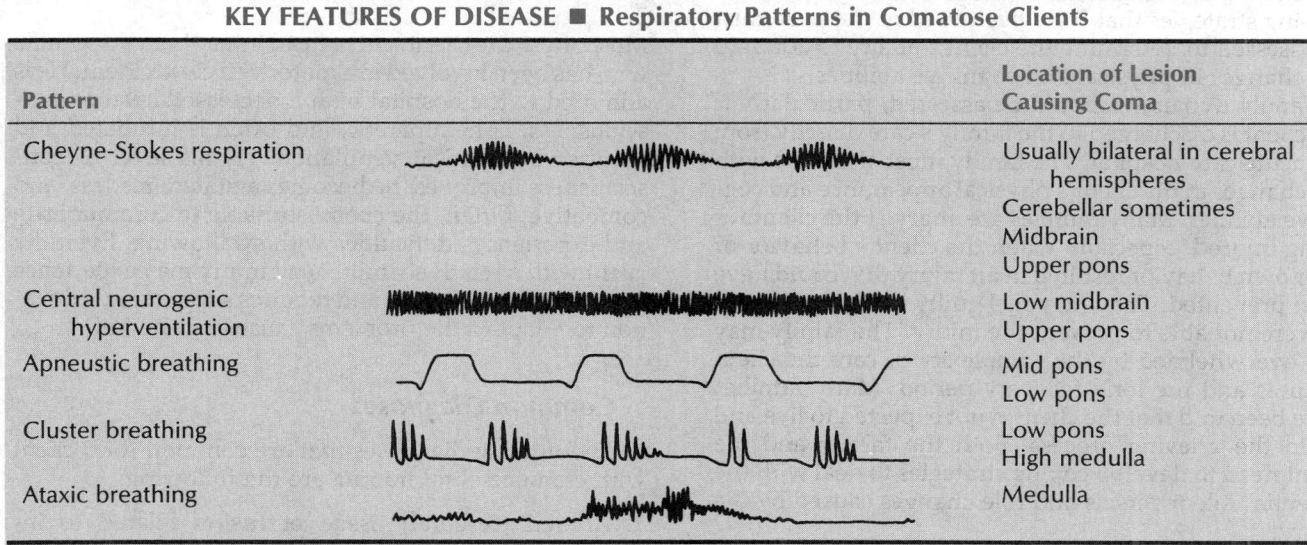

Pattern		Location of Lesion Causing Coma
Cheyne-Stokes respiration		Usually bilateral in cerebral hemispheres
		Cerebellar sometimes
		Midbrain
		Upper pons
Central neurogenic hyperventilation		Low midbrain
		Upper pons
Apneustic breathing		Mid pons
		Low pons
Cluster breathing		Low pons
		High medulla
Ataxic breathing		Medulla

If the client is able to cooperate, a full neurologic assessment is completed as outlined in Chapter 32. Particular attention is paid to cranial nerves I, V, VII, IX, and X. The first cranial nerve is frequently damaged where the frontal lobe passes over the irregularly shaped bones of the anterior and middle fossa; this results in the loss of smell. Cranial nerves V, VII, IX, and X are important for chewing and swallowing abilities and phonation. The client's ability to speak must be assessed, with particular attention directed toward differentiating aphasias (caused by injury to the cerebral cortex) from communication impairments (caused by damage to the cranial nerves and cerebellum). Damage to the cranial nerves occurs from disruption of the nerve trunk, either intracranially or along its extracranial course in the skull or face, as a result of direct trauma or from compression associated with pressure or hemorrhage.

Other signs of *increased ICP* include severe headache, nausea, vomiting, seizures, and papilledema. Papilledema is always a sign of increased ICP. Headache and seizures are a response to the injury and may or may not be associated with increased ICP. Abdominal injuries, such as a lacerated bowel, may cause nausea and vomiting. In general, a single neurologic finding is not indicative of increased ICP. The nurse must keep in mind, however, that the client can have a marked increase in ICP, yet be relatively asymptomatic.

The client's ears and nose are examined for any signs of *CSF leaks* that result from a basal skull fracture. CSF placed on a white absorbent background can be distinguished from other fluids by the "halo" sign, a yellowish stain surrounded by bloody drainage. In addition, CSF will test positively for glucose when a strip testing method (Dipstix) is used. In the presence of a CSF leak, the client should be assessed for any signs of nuchal rigidity, which would indicate infection or blood in the CSF. Nuchal rigidity is not checked until a spinal cord injury has been ruled out.

The client's head is palpated to detect the presence of fractures or subgaleal hematomas. The nurse looks for areas of ecchymosis, tender areas of the scalp, and lacerations.

Clients with a minor head injury must be assessed for signs and symptoms of posttraumatic sequelae. The symptoms include a wide array of physical and cognitive problems, ranging from persistent headache, weakness, and dizziness, to personality and behavior changes, loss of memory, and problems with perception, reasoning abilities, and concept formation. The symptoms may persist for a few days or weeks to several months after injury. For some, severe physical and cognitive problems remain, despite a relatively benign initial clinical presentation and normal CT or MRI findings.

Psychosocial Assessment

The person who has had a head injury is never quite the same as before the injury. Most often, the client with a major head injury has personality changes manifested by temper outbursts, depression, risk-taking behavior, and denial of disability. The client may become talkative and develop a gregarious outgoing persona. Memory, especially recent or short-term memory, is affected, which should not be confused with problems of aphasia. The client's ability to learn new information and concentration may be affected. Finally, the client may exhibit problems with insight and planning. All of these problems may lead to difficulties within the family structure and with social and work-related interactions. Coping strategies that have been used in the past must be assessed to determine the client's ability to adapt to the changes in physical and cognitive abilities.

Family dynamics should be assessed, particularly if the client is discharged to the family's care directly from the acute care hospital. The family must also cope with the changes in the client's physical appearance and cognitive abilities. Many families are angry at the client for being injured, especially when the client's behavior or their own behavior resulted in an injury that could have been prevented. They may feel guilty that they did not or were not able to prevent the injury. The family may feel overwhelmed by the complexity of care the client requires and the long recovery period. Many families have been told that the client is not expected to live and begin the grieving process. Both the family and the client need to develop coping strategies to deal with the potential role reversals and role changes caused by the injury.

Laboratory Findings

There are no laboratory tests to diagnose primary brain injury; however, several laboratory tests are used to diagnose or indicate measures to prevent secondary brain insult. Arterial blood gases are analyzed, with particular attention to oxygen and carbon dioxide levels. A CBC and determination of serum electrolyte levels and osmolarity are routinely performed to monitor the client's hemodynamic status or identify electrolyte imbalance or the presence of infection.

Radiographic Findings

CT is done to identify the extent and scope of injury to the brain. MRI is particularly useful in the diagnosis of diffuse axonal injury. Most importantly, either of these diagnostic tests can identify the presence of a lesion that requires surgical intervention, such as an epidural or subdural hematoma. Radiography of the cervical spine and the skull is done to rule out fractures and dislocations. A chest x-ray film is taken to identify fractured ribs or other chest injuries. A flat plate of the abdomen may be obtained to assist in the diagnosis of abdominal bleeding or bowel laceration.

Other Diagnostic Tests

As the client's condition stabilizes, other diagnostic tests may be performed to identify the extent of the injury to the brain. The integrity of the cerebral vessels is measured through the use of Doppler flow studies or an arteriogram; cerebral perfusion is measured by cerebral blood flow studies. An EEG is obtained to determine the presence of seizure activity, which frequently occurs after a severe head injury. A brain stem evoked potential is done to assess the integrity of the brain stem and its ability to transmit information for hearing and vision.

 ## Analysis: Nursing Diagnosis

Most often, the client with a head injury is a young male who has been involved in a motor vehicle accident. He is admitted to the hospital with a decreased level of consciousness, is hemiparetic, and often is intubated and requires mechanical ventilation. As his level of consciousness improves, he becomes agitated, restless, and combative. Often, the client is unable to communicate and experiences difficulties with swallowing. Even the client with a relatively mild head injury may experience posttraumatic sequelae and requires support and education to adapt to the problems caused by the injury.

Common Diagnoses

The nursing diagnoses that are common for a client with craniocerebral trauma are the following:

1. Altered (cerebral) tissue perfusion related to increased ICP, hypoxia, or impaired autoregulation
2. Sensory/perceptual alterations related to decreased level of consciousness, damage to the parietal lobe, or injury to the olfactory nerve
3. Impaired physical mobility related to hemiplegia, hemiparesis, spasticity, or fatigue
4. Potential for injury related to seizures, agitation, restlessness, and confusion
5. Impaired gas exchange related to pooling of secretions, poor cough reflex, and altered breathing pattern
6. Body image disturbance and altered role performance related to cognitive dysfunction and physical disabilities
7. Altered nutrition: less than body requirements related to inability to chew or swallow

Additional Diagnoses

In addition, the client may have one or more of the following diagnoses:

1. Total self-care deficit (depends on the degree of injury) related to cognitive impairment and impaired physical mobility
2. Impaired verbal communication related to aphasia
3. Powerlessness related to physical disabilities and cognitive impairments
4. Ineffective family coping: compromised related to changes in the client's role and physical and cognitive disabilities
5. Posttrauma response related to sudden and unexpected injury
6. Impaired skin integrity related to impaired physical mobility
7. Pain related to traumatic injuries or headache

Planning and Implementation

The plan of care for a client with craniocerebral trauma focuses on the common nursing diagnoses.

Altered (Cerebral) Tissue Perfusion

Planning: client goals.   The major goals for this nursing diagnosis are that the client will (1) maintain a normal ICP, (2) maintain appropriate vital signs and arterial blood gas values, and (3) achieve improvement in level of consciousness.

Interventions.   The client with a severe head injury is admitted to the critical care unit or trauma center. Clients with mild head injuries are admitted to the general nursing unit, where they are closely observed for at least 24 hours. Nursing interventions for all clients with a head injury are directed toward preventing or detecting increased ICP, promoting fluid and electrolyte balance, and monitoring the effects of treatments and medications. If these measures fail, surgery may be indicated to remove necrotic brain tissue, tips of the temporal lobe, or part of the frontal lobe. These procedures are used only if more conservative measures to treat increased ICP or cerebral edema fail.

Nonsurgical management.   The client's vital signs are taken and recorded every 1 to 2 hours. Medications may be required to prevent severe hypertension or hypotension. The client in the critical care unit is connected to a cardiac monitor to detect any cardiac dysrhythmias. Nonspecific ST segment or T wave changes may occur, possibly in response to stimulation of the autonomic nervous system or an increase in the level of circulating catecholamines. Cardiac irregularities should be documented and reported to the physician.

Positioning.   The nurse positions the client to avoid extreme flexion or extension of the neck and to maintain the head in the midline, neutral position. The client is logrolled when turned to avoid extreme hip flexion. The head of the bed is elevated 30 to 45 degrees. All of these measures are used to enhance venous drainage, which helps prevent increased ICP.

Hyperventilation.   The client who requires mechanical ventilation is hyperventilated to maintain an arterial carbon dioxide pressure (PCO_2) of 25 to 30 mmHg, as hyperventilation causes vasoconstriction and leads to a decrease in cerebral blood volume. The arterial PCO_2 must not be allowed to fall to less than 20 mmHg, which may result in hypoxia caused by *severe* vasoconstriction. Arterial oxygen levels (PO_2) are maintained between 80 and 100 mmHg to prevent cerebral vasodilation resulting from hypoxemia. Arterial blood gas values are monitored at least twice per day and after each change in the ventilator setting.

Recent studies suggest that hyperventilation may worsen ischemia because of the variability of cerebral hemodynamic response to routine hyperventilation (Walleck, 1989). Additional studies continue to further identify the response of the injured brain to hyperventilation.

Barbiturate coma.   The client with a severe head injury may be placed in a barbiturate coma using pentobarbital or thiopental to decrease elevated ICP by decreasing the metabolic demands of the brain and cerebral blood flow. The dosage is adjusted to maintain complete unresponsiveness. As a consequence, it is difficult to recognize subtle or not-so-subtle neurologic changes. The client requires mechanical ventilation, sophisticated hemodynamic monitoring, and ICP monitoring. Complications of barbiturate coma include cardiac arrhythmias, hypotension, and fluid and electrolyte disturbances. As an alternative to barbiturate coma, some institutions are using narcotic sedation to control the ICP and cerebral metabolic rate, as well as the agitation often seen in clients with head injuries. Narcotics can increase ICP, but this effect can be minimized through the use of controlled mechanical ventilation with hyperventilation. The advantage of this therapy is that it can more easily be reversed using naloxone (Narcan).

Drug therapy.   Glucocorticoids (dexamethasone or methylprednisolone) may be used to reduce cerebral edema, although their effectiveness is being questioned. The nurse monitors serum glucose concentrations, as steroids may cause hyperglycemia, which generally does not require insulin administration. Osmotic diuretics, such as mannitol (Osmitrol) and urea, are used to treat cerebral edema by pulling water out of normal (not edematous) brain tissue. They may also increase cerebral blood flow by decreasing ICP. Mannitol should be given through a filter in the IV tubing or, if given by IV push, drawn up through a filtered needle to eliminate microscopic crystals. Increasingly, emphasis has been placed on using loop (high-ceiling) diuretics, such as furosemide (Lasix), to treat increased ICP. Loop ceiling diuretics are associated with less fluid and electrolyte imbalance and osmolality dysfunction, but are less reliable in controlling ICP. The client receiving either osmotic or loop ceiling diuretics is strictly monitored for intake and output and is observed for severe dehydration and indications of acute renal failure. Foley's catheter must be inserted to maintain strict measurement of output.

Paralytic agents, such as pancuronium (Pavulon), are used if the client is mechanically ventilated to control restlessness and agitation in those clients who are at high risk for developing increased ICP. Anticonvulsants, such as phenytoin (Dilantin), are given to prevent seizures. Acetaminophen (Tylenol) and aspirin are given to clients who are febrile (temperature >39° C [101° F]) to reduce fever.

Fluid and electrolyte monitoring.   The client with craniocerebral trauma is at risk for diabetes insipidus, SIADH, and hyperglycemia. Therefore, serum and urine electrolyte levels and osmolarity are monitored frequently. Serum sodium level may fall to as low as 120 mEq/L or less. Hyperglycemia occurs after the administration of steroids. Urine specific gravity is measured every hour. The client's fluid intake is usually restricted, and the client may become markedly dehydrated, leading to renal failure. Fluid overload can occur in the client with multiple trauma from the rapid administration of IV fluids, plasma expanders, or corticosteroids.

Surgical management. The physician may elect to insert an ICP monitoring device to evaluate the client's pressure more closely. All devices are inserted through a bur hole that is placed in the skull using a twist drill. Each device is connected to a transducer that is connected to a monitor; the monitor is able to record the pressure waves and provide a digital readout of the pressure.

Intracranial pressure monitoring. Three types of devices may be used (Fig. 33–13). An *intraventricular catheter* is a small tube that is inserted into the anterior horn of the lateral ventricle of the nondominant cerebral hemisphere. The advantage of this system is that CSF can be drained and specimens obtained for laboratory analysis. The *subarachnoid screw* or *bolt* is a hollow device that is placed into the subarachnoid space for direct pressure measurement. A disadvantage of the system is that CSF cannot be drained to treat increased ICP. An *epidural monitor* is a transducer that is placed between the skull and the dura, leaving the dura intact. Its major advantage is the decreased risk of infection from an open dural space. The nurse follows facility protocols for the management of these devices. The waveform should be observed for signs of damping, which indicates that the device is not functioning and the pressure that is displayed may not be accurate. If this occurs, the nurse checks that the transducer is at the level of the ventricle. The transducer is recalibrated and rebalanced, and the tubing is checked for air bubbles. If the waveform remains damped, the nurse should notify the physician.

Craniotomy. If the client's ICP cannot be controlled, the physician may elect to perform a craniotomy to remove ischemic tissue or the tips of the temporal lobes.

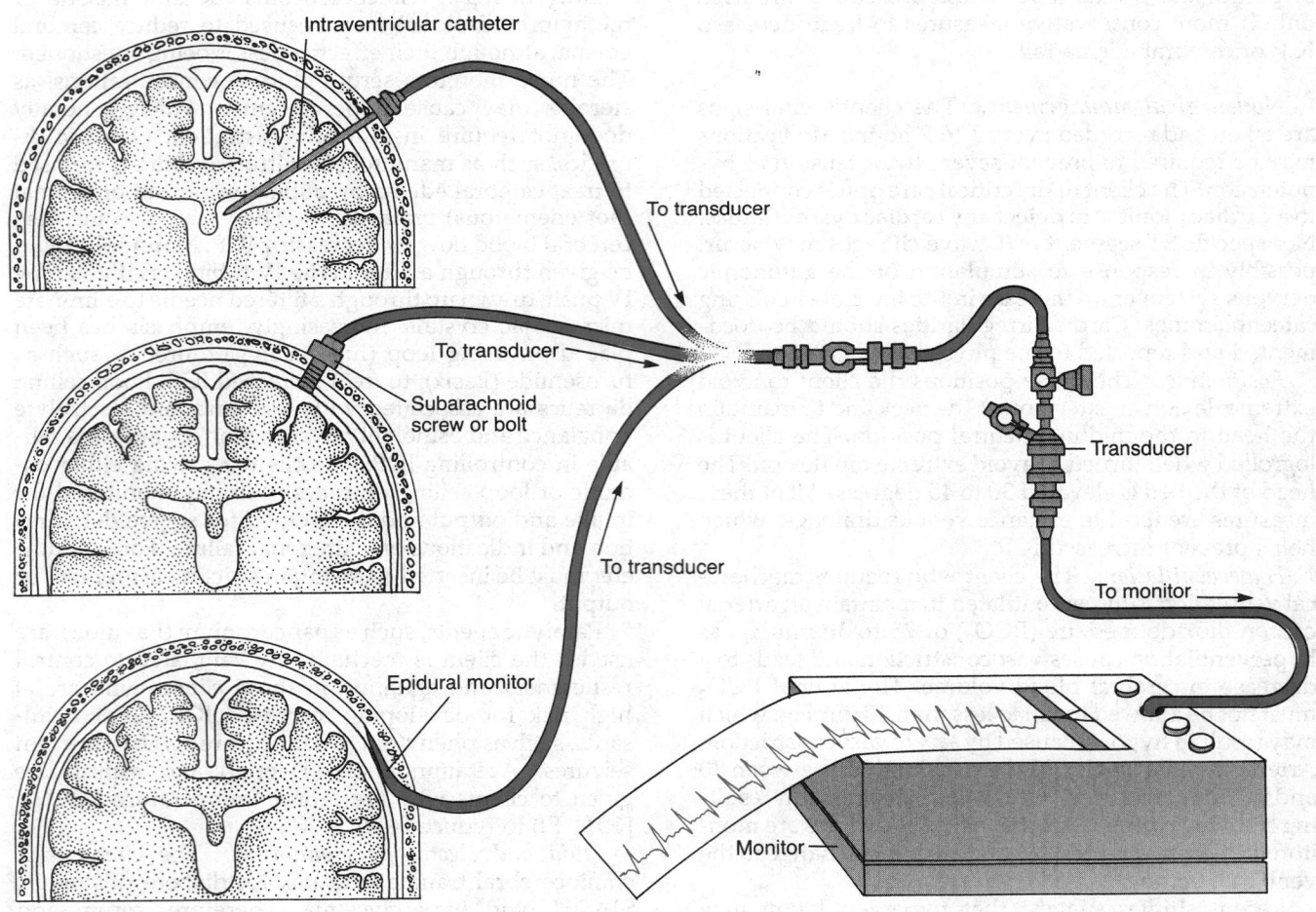

Figure 33–13

Common types of ICP monitoring devices: ventricular catheter, subarachnoid screw or bolt, and epidural monitor.

The removal of nonvital brain tissue allows for expansion of brain tissue without further compromise of the ICP. A craniotomy may also be performed to remove epidural or subdural hematomas. The nursing care for clients undergoing craniotomy is discussed later.

Sensory/Perceptual Alterations

Planning: client goals. The major goal for this nursing diagnosis is that the client will develop strategies to adapt to the residual neurologic dysfunction.

Interventions: nonsurgical management. The client with this diagnosis may exhibit changes in the following areas: sense of smell; ability to taste, swallow, or feel the presence of food within the oral cavity; and changes in vision, pain, and temperature sensation. As a result, he/she is at risk for nutritional deficits, which may interfere with the healing process. The client may be injured from falling over objects outside the field of vision, or burn injuries could occur because of the inability to perceive variations in water temperatures.

Mealtime should be a pleasant experience. The tray should be presented in an attractive manner, and every effort should be made to serve the food and beverages that the client enjoys. The nurse positions the client to maximize swallowing ability, and strategies are taught to prevent food from accumulating in the cheek of the affected side. Attention is directed to the environment: extraneous noise is reduced and bedpans and urinal are removed from the client's line of vision.

In the presence of a large lesion of the parietal lobe, the client may experience loss of sensation for pain, temperature, touch, and proprioception. This may prevent the client from responding appropriately to environmental stimuli. A hazard-free environment is necessary to prevent injury that could occur, for example, from burns if the client's coffee is too hot or falls if the side rails on the bed are not kept up. A sensory stimulation program should be integrated into the comatose or stuporous client's routine care activities. Sensory stimulation is done to facilitate a meaningful response to the environment by the client. Visual, auditory, or tactile stimuli are presented one at a time. The purpose and the type of stimuli presented are explained to the client. For example, the nurse shows a picture of the client's mother and says to the client, "This is a picture of your mother." The picture is shown to the client several times and the same words used to describe the picture. If auditory tapes are used, they should not be longer than 10 to 15 minutes. If the stimulus is presented for a longer period, it simply becomes white noise, or meaningless background noise (see the accompanying Nursing Research feature).

The client may be disoriented and experience a short-term memory loss. The nurse always introduces himself/herself to the client before any interaction. Explanations of procedures and activities are short and simple and are done immediately before and throughout the procedure. A sleep-wake cycle must be maintained,

NURSING RESEARCH

Does What Nurses Say at the Bedside Change a Comatose Client's Intracranial Pressure?

Johnson, S. M., Omery, A., & Nikas, D. (1989). Effects of conversation on intracranial pressure in comatose patients. *Heart and Lung, 18,* 56–63.

A number of studies have begun to examine the effects of nursing interventions on the ICP of comatose clients, but many questions remain unanswered. The purpose of this research was to measure the effect of two types of conversations on ICP—the first type was a report of the client's condition and the second was dialogue unrelated to the client.

There was no significant difference between baseline ICP and ICP during the conversations at the bedside. In addition, there was no difference in ICP measurements relative to the type of conversation presented. Although these findings were unexpected, the researchers did note that ICP for all 8 subjects was decreased during the second type, or non–client-related conversation. The conclusion was that response is individual and perhaps related more to the individual's level of consciousness or other variables.

Critique. The small convenience sample was drawn from two hospitals according to guidelines attempting to make the study group as homogeneous as possible. Interrater observer reliability was determined at 100%, and the equipment was carefully calibrated to improve its reliability. This study needs to be replicated using a larger sample.

Possible nursing implications. Although the research hypotheses were rejected, the study found that ICP decreased during conversation not related to the client's condition. Nurses should not discuss the client's condition at the client's bedside, even if the client is comatose. Talking to the client about other topics may decrease anxiety and lower ICP in the comatose client.

with scheduled rest periods. The nurse orients the client to day, month, year, and place and explains the reason for the client's hospitalization. The client is reassured by the nurse that his/her family knows where he/she is and that he/she is safe. The nurse should ask the family to bring in familiar objects, such as pictures. Orientation cues within the environment, such as a large clock with numbers or a single-date calendar, should be provided.

Impaired Physical Mobility

Planning: client goals. The major goal for this nursing diagnosis is that the client will not experience complications of immobility.

Interventions: nonsurgical management. For a complete discussion of the complications of immobility, refer to Chapter 22.

Pulmonary care. It is especially important to prevent pulmonary complications, as they may further compromise the client's neurologic status. The client is turned at least every 2 hours. Chest physiotherapy can be done if attention is directed toward preventing increased ICP. It may be necessary to sedate the client before the procedure or to avoid placing the client in Trendelenburg's position. The client should wear thigh-high antiembolism stockings until fully mobile to prevent venous stasis that could lead to either a pulmonary embolus or deep venous thrombosis.

Exercise and splints. The nurse provides passive or active-assistive ROM exercises at least once per nursing shift, with particular attention given to the joints of the fingers and the wrist. Splints for the affected limbs should be fashioned by physical or occupational therapists. High-topped tennis shoes to prevent foot drop are used for feet that are flaccid. They may be used in the client who is spastic only after consultation with the occupational or physical therapist. Splints and supportive shoes must be removed and the skin inspected for signs of irritation several times each day.

Potential for Injury

Planning: client goals. The major goal for the client with this nursing diagnosis is that the client will not experience injuries that may occur as a result of seizure activity, restlessness, agitation, or confusion. The client is at risk for seizure activity, and actions are taken as outlined in the discussion of epilepsy (see earlier).

Interventions: nonsurgical management. The nurse keeps the bed in a low position with the side rails up. A chest restraint may be necessary to keep the client in the bed or a chair. If the client pulls out the IV line or nasogastric tube, the nurse may use hand mittens. Restraint of extremities should be employed only if absolutely necessary and should begin with single-limb restraint or opposite restraints. Restraining all four extremities increases the client's agitation and fear. The nurse always obtains a physician's order for the use of restraints of any kind.

The nurse should orient the client to his/her surroundings and provide a quiet environment. The nurse should closely monitor the client's response to television programs or the radio; often, the client is unable to differentiate these situations or programs from what is happening within his/her own environment.

Impaired Gas Exchange

Planning: client goals. The goals for a client with this nursing diagnosis are that the client will (1) be free of respiratory infection and atelectasis and (2) have adequate arterial blood gas values.

Interventions: nonsurgical management. Pulmonary secretions tend to pool as a result of a decreased level of consciousness, ineffective cough, or an altered breathing pattern. The secretions may be thick because of the fluid intake restriction used to prevent cerebral edema. Chest physiotherapy, frequent turning, and suctioning are done as indicated by the results of the respiratory assessment. Chapter 62 describes these techniques in detail.

Body Image Disturbance; Altered Role Performance

Planning: client goals. The major goals for the client with these nursing diagnoses is that the client will develop confidence in her/his abilities and begin to adapt to changes in physical appearance and abilities.

Interventions: nonsurgical management. To assist the client in developing a positive self-concept, the nurse must first establish a trusting relationship with the client. This is accomplished by employing a nonjudgmental attitude and providing open and honest communication. The nurse encourages the client to ask questions about his/her care and to participate as much as

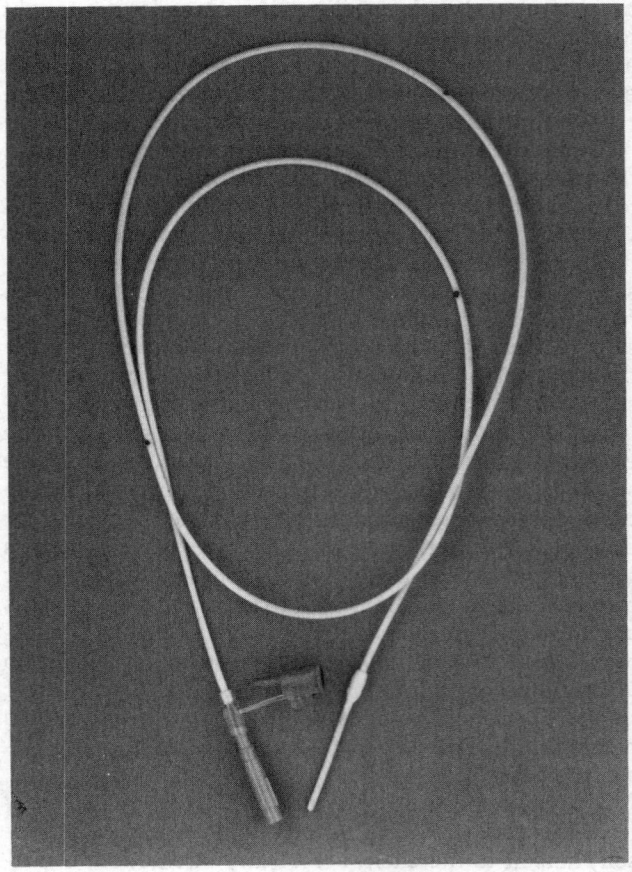

Figure 33–14

Typical small-lumen nasogastric feeding tube.

possible in all decision-making regarding treatment. The client is encouraged to verbalize her/his thoughts, fears, and anxieties. The nurse emphasizes the client's abilities while assisting him/her to adapt to disabilities. The nurse should answer any questions honestly and correct any misinformation. The nurse allows the client privacy; however, the client should be encouraged to balance a need for privacy with appropriate social interaction.

Altered Nutrition: Less Than Body Requirements

Planning: client goals. The primary goals for this diagnosis are that the client will (1) maintain body weight within 10% of ideal body weight and (2) maintain adequate hydration.

Interventions. The client who is moderately to severely injured usually has a decreased level of consciousness, at least temporarily. As a result, the client is unable to chew or swallow and must receive nutrition and fluids by an alternate method.

Nonsurgical management. The client initially receives IV fluids until stabilized. If there is no improvement in level of consciousness long-term nutritional support via enteral feeding is usually instituted. A small-lumen nasogastric or nasoduodenal tube is used for continuous feeding (Fig. 33–14). The tube is made of a flexible, low-pressure, silicone material that prevents nasal and esophageal irritation or erosion. Insertion of the tube follows the procedure described in Chapter 44. Care of the client with continuous enteral feeding is summarized in the accompanying Guidelines feature.

Surgical management. Although the design of nasogastric feeding tubes has improved, life-threatening aspiration can occur with this type of nutritional support. For this reason, a gastrostomy tube may be inserted directly into the stomach. The surgeon makes a small opening in the skin and stomach for the insertion of the tube; a single suture holds the tube in place to prevent dislodging. The procedure may be done in the operating room or at the client's bedside. With the use of either type of tube, the nurse weighs the client daily to determine if caloric needs are being met and monitors serum

---

GUIDELINES ■ Care of the Client Receiving Nasogastric Tube Feeding

Interventions	Rationales
1. Check tube for placement in stomach every 8–12 h by injecting 30 mL of air into the tube while listening over the stomach area with stethoscope (should hear a "swooshing" sound).	1. Prevents feeding from entering lungs.
2. Flush tube every 4 h with 30–50 mL of water (may not be necessary if a continuous feed is used). Flush well when medications are given.	2. Maintains patency of the tube.
3. Secure the tube to the nose with tape so that the tube does not cause pressure on the nares; change the tape every 1–2 d.	3. Prevents tube dislodgement; prevents pressure necrosis of the nares.
4. Provide feeding at hourly rate prescribed by the physician or dietitian.	4. Provides adequate calories and other nutrients to meet the client's daily requirements. (Water is given as a bolus to maintain adequate fluid and electrolyte balance.)
5. Keep the head of bed elevated.	5. Helps to prevent aspiration of the feeding solution into the lungs.
6. Check for residual in the stomach every 4 h or according to hospital policy or physician's orders.	6. Prevents overdistention of the stomach, which can cause nausea and vomiting.
7. Monitor the client's weight and serum albumin and serum electrolyte values.	7. Determines if the client's daily nutritional needs are being met.

albumin level to ensure adequate protein intake. The client is assessed daily for signs of dehydration, such as dry mucous membranes and poor skin turgor. Chapter 13 describes nursing assessment and interventions for the client with dehydration, as well as a discussion of the various types of commercial supplemental feedings available for tube feeding.

■ **Discharge Planning**

The client with a mild head injury is usually discharged to home. Clients with more severe injuries are discharged to facilities that specialize in head injury rehabilitation. Chapter 22 discusses the care of the client in a rehabilitation setting.

Home Care Preparation

Little home care preparation is needed for the client with a concussion unless she/he is experiencing symptoms of posttraumatic sequelae. The client's home should be assessed for potential hazards before discharge from the hospital. This includes functioning smoke and fire alarms, as the client with a head injury often loses the sense of smell. This information can be obtained from the admission data or by a home visit. Home adaptations and referrals to outside agencies should be completed before the client is discharged from the hospital.

Information concerning the selection of a head injury rehabilitation facility can be obtained from the National Head Injury Foundation (NHIF). Other preparation includes the development of a detailed client care plan to be given to the rehabilitation facility. This will enable the provision of consistent care and decrease the initial anxiety related to the change that the client may experience. The nursing discharge summary should include the following information: medications, including dosage, reactions, and special preparation; the current client care plan; techniques used to motivate or calm the client; and strategies to assist the family to adapt to the situation.

Client/Family Education

The teaching plan for the client with craniocerebral trauma includes strategies to adapt to sensory dysfunction and to cope with the personality or behavior problems that may arise.

The same strategies used in the hospital to treat sensory/perceptual alterations are taught to the family and the client. In addition, the nurse instructs the family on the importance of not moving furniture or other objects in the home to a different place, as this could lead to an injury in the client with visual problems or confuse the client with cognitive impairments.

Clients with personality and behavior problems respond best to an environment that is structured and consistent. The nurse instructs the family to develop a home routine that provides for structure, repetition, and consistency. The family must be instructed on the importance of reinforcing positive behavior and not reinforcing negative behaviors.

The nurse teaches the client who has sustained a minor head injury, for example, a concussion, that *posttrauma syndrome* may occur. This syndrome is a group of clinical manifestations including, but not limited to, personality changes, irritability, headaches, dizziness, restlessness, nervousness, and insomnia. Although many clients with head injuries experience some of these manifestations during recovery, some individuals have these problems for weeks, months, or even years to the extent that they interfere with daily activities, such as employment. The prolonged pattern is classified as posttrauma syndrome. The exact cause of the phenomenon is not known, but physiologic and psychologic theories have been espoused. Support groups and professional counseling are the most effective interventions.

Psychosocial Preparation

Most clients who had moderate to severe craniocerebral trauma are discharged with physical as well as cognitive disabilities. Changes in personality and behavior are not unusual. The family must learn to cope with the client's increased fatigue, irritability, temper outbursts, depression, and memory problems. Frequently, these clients require constant supervision at home, and eventually the families feel socially isolated. The nurse instructs the family to plan for regular respite care, either in a structured day care respite program or through relief provided by a friend or a neighbor. The family members, particularly the primary caretaker, may become depressed, with feelings of loneliness, and experience isolation, increased responsibilities, and role reversals. In addition, they may feel angry at the client because of the additional responsibilities (financial or emotional) that his/her care has placed on them. To help the family cope with these problems, the nurse suggests that they join and actively participate in the local head injury support group.

The client needs assistance in identifying realistic expectations for discharge. Owing to the cognitive deficits, it may not be possible for the client to return to previous employment or educational pursuits. The client may experience a sense of isolation and loneliness, as his/her personality and behavior changes make it difficult to resume or maintain preinjury social contacts.

Health Care Resources

Families and clients should be referred to the NHIF, as well as to the local or state group, for information and support. The NHIF and its state chapters maintain lists of rehabilitation facilities for clients with head injuries. The NHIF will send family members and other interested persons guidelines for selecting a rehabilitation facility. Families should inquire about the facility's experience in caring for the person with a head injury, how many admissions the facility had in the previous 2 to 3 years, and the results or outcome statistics on those clients (e.g., how many went home and at what functional recovery level — poor, fair, or good).

Other helpful groups include the National Easter Seal Society and National Institute of Handicapped Research.

Evaluation

On the basis of the identified nursing diagnoses, the nurse evaluates the care of the client with craniocerebral trauma. The expected outcomes include that the client

1. Maintains an adequate cerebral tissue perfusion and the level of consciousness stays the same or improves
2. Experiences no seizure activity
3. Remains free of injury
4. Demonstrates strategies to begin adaptation to sensory/perceptual changes
5. Demonstrates improved level of mobility (spasticity of affected limbs is minimal)
6. Demonstrates an adequate airway
7. Maintains adequate nutrition and hydration

By meeting the expected outcomes, the client should be able to fully participate in a rehabilitation program and experience minimal medical complications.

SPINAL CORD INJURY

OVERVIEW

Loss of motor function, sensation, reflex activity, and bowel and bladder control may occur as a result of a spinal cord injury. In addition, the client may experience significant behavior and emotional problems as a result of changes in body image, role performance, and self-concept.

Pathophysiology

The spinal vertebral column consists of seven cervical, twelve thoracic, five lumbar, five fused sacral, and five fused coccygeal vertebrae. Support for the spine is provided by a series of ligaments, intervertebral disks, and the muscles of the neck and trunk. The physical structure of the vertebral column allows for the motions of flexion, extension, and rotation. The cervical spine and thoracolumbar junction are highly mobile areas and therefore are more prone to injury. The thoracic area is less flexible and more stable owing to the attachment of the ribs and their anatomic structure.

The spinal cord is enclosed within the spinal or vertebral canal. In the adult, it extends from the base of the brain, or the medulla, to the second lumbar vertebra, where it tapers to form the conus medullaris. Thirty-one pairs of spinal nerves originate from the spinal cord and exit from the spinal column through the intervertebral foramina. Each spinal nerve is composed of both a sensory or posterior (dorsal) root and a motor or anterior (ventral) root. The area of skin innervated by a single nerve root is called a dermatome (Fig. 33–15). Sensory and motor nerve roots join at the dorsal root ganglion to form a mixed sensory and motor nerve (see Chap. 32, Fig. 32–3).

Within the CNS are groups of neurons called upper motor neurons (UMNs) and lower motor neurons (LMNs). UMNs originate within the cerebral cortex and brain stem and form tracts (corticospinal, reticulospinal, vestibulospinal, and rubrospinal) that terminate or synapse in all levels of the anterior horn cells of the spinal cord. These UMNs control or mediate motor function, particularly fine motor and postural reflexes. Damage or injury to these neurons causes a *spastic* paralysis and hyperreflexia because the spinal reflex remains intact below the level of the lesion.

LMNs are located in the anterior horn cells of the spinal cord and brain stem motor nuclei; they terminate in skeletal muscle. The function of LMNs is to maintain muscle tone and transmit impulses for reflex activity, as well as voluntary muscle action. If damage occurs to an LMN, the muscle served by that neuron no longer receives stimuli and therefore is unable to contract, causing a *flaccid* paralysis and hyporeflexia.

Within the spinal cord are the preganglionic and postganglionic fibers of the autonomic nervous system. Sympathetic fibers are located within the gray matter of all the thoracic and first two lumbar spinal cord segments. Sympathetic fibers innervate the abdominal and thoracic viscera and organs. Parasympathetic fibers arise from several of the cranial nerves, as well as from the sacral segments of the spinal cord. These fibers innervate the smooth muscles of the bowel, the bladder, and the reproductive tract.

Specific syndromes seen after spinal cord injury and damage to the autonomic nervous system are spinal shock and autonomic dysreflexia. *Spinal shock* occurs immediately after the injury as a result of disruption in the communication pathways between UMNs and LMNs. It is also known as neurogenic shock and is characterized by flaccid paralysis, loss of reflex activity below the level of the lesion, bradycardia, paralytic ileus (sometimes), and hypotension. It may last for a few days to several months.

Autonomic dysreflexia, or hyperreflexia, is usually seen only in injuries above the level of the sixth thoracic vertebra. It usually occurs after the period of spinal shock is completed. This syndrome results from uninhibited sympathetic discharge; that is, the sympathetic nervous system is no longer controlled by higher centers

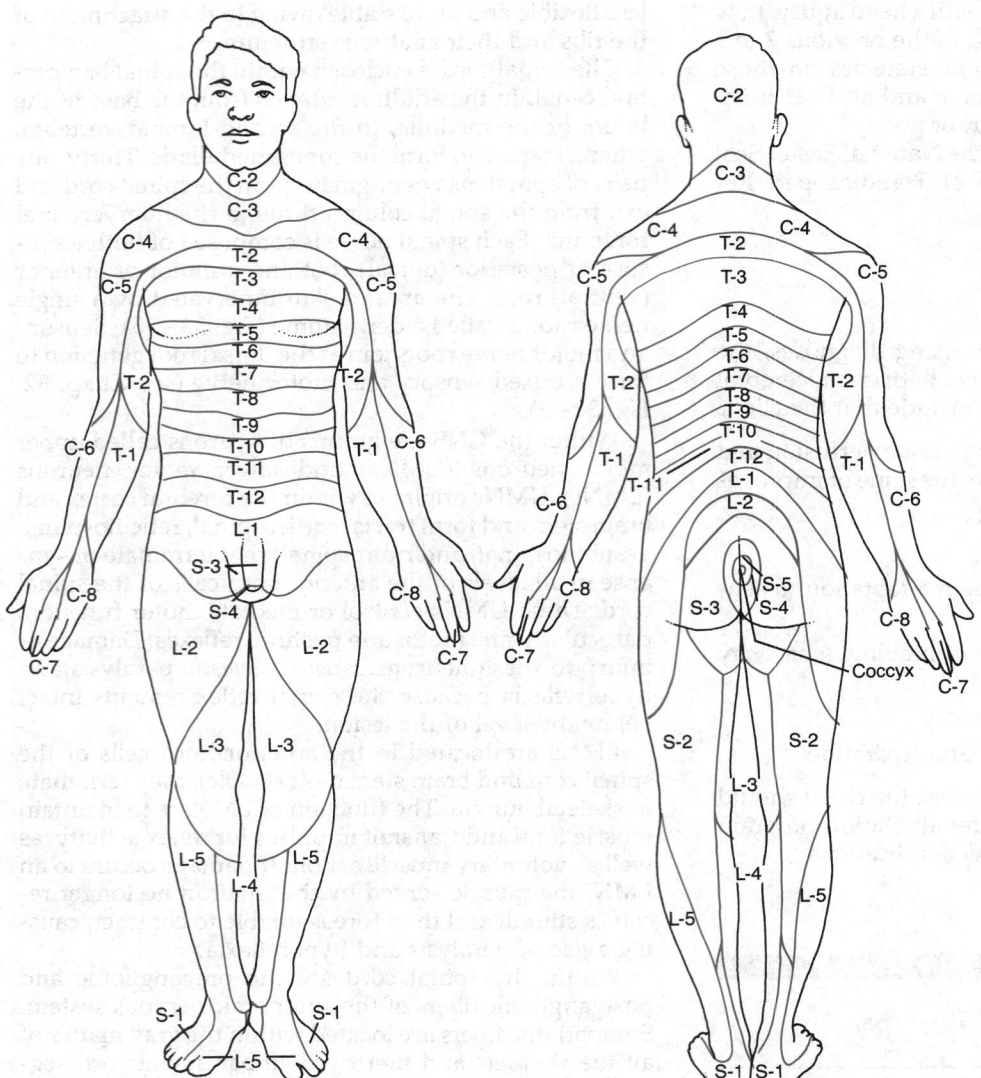

Figure 33-15

Dermatomes (cutaneous innervation of spinal nerves).

in the cerebral cortex owing to disruption in impulse transmission. The accompanying Emergency Care feature summarizes nursing assessment and interventions for this life-threatening complication.

Mechanisms of injury. When sufficient *force* is applied to the spinal cord, damage results in neurologic deficits. Sources of force include injury to the vertebral column (fracture, dislocation, and subluxation) or penetrating trauma (gunshot or knife wounds). Although in some cases the cord itself may remain intact, at other times the cord undergoes a destructive process caused by a contusion, compression, or concussion.

Four mechanisms that may result in spinal cord injury are hyperflexion; hyperextension; axial loading, or vertical compression; and penetrating wounds. A *flexion injury* (Fig. 33-16) occurs when the head is suddenly and forcefully accelerated forward, causing extreme flexion of the neck. Flexion injury to the lower thoracic

and lumbar spine may occur when the trunk is suddenly flexed on itself, as occurs in a fall on the buttocks. The posterior ligaments can be stretched or torn, or the vertebrae may fracture or dislocate. Either process may disrupt the integrity of the spinal cord, causing hemorrhage, edema, and necrosis.

Hyperextension injuries (Fig. 33-17) occur most often in automobile accidents in which the client's vehicle is struck from behind or falls where the chin is struck. The head is suddenly accelerated and then decelerated. This stretches or tears the anterior longitudinal ligament, fractures or subluxates the vertebrae, and perhaps ruptures an intervertebral disk. As with flexion injuries, the spinal cord may easily be damaged.

Diving accidents cause most of the injuries attributable to *axial loading (vertical compression)* (Fig. 33-18). The blow to the top of the head causes the vertebrae to shatter. Pieces of bone enter the spinal canal and damage the cord.

Penetrating injuries to the spinal cord are classified by

EMERGENCY CARE ■ Autonomic Dysreflexia

Clinical Manifestations

Severe headache

Markedly *increased* blood pressure; severe hypertension

Tachycardia—may lead to arrhythmias, diaphoresis above the level of lesion

Flushed skin above the level of lesion; pallor below the level of lesion

Nasal congestion

Visual disturbances

Goose flesh

Piloerection

Interventions

1. Place the head of the bed in high Fowler's position.
2. Check Foley's catheter for patency; if kinked, release.
3. Check the rectum for stool impaction; if present, remove.
4. Check the room for cool drafts; cover the client with light spread or blanket.
5. Call the physician immediately; prepare for administration of fast-acting antihypertensive medication, such as IV or IM hydralazine hydrochloride (Apresoline).

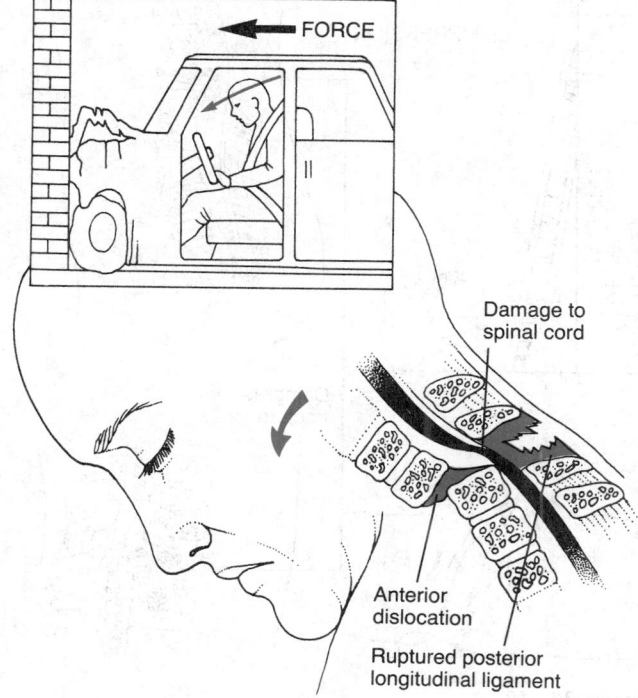

Figure 33–16

Flexion injury of the cervical spine.

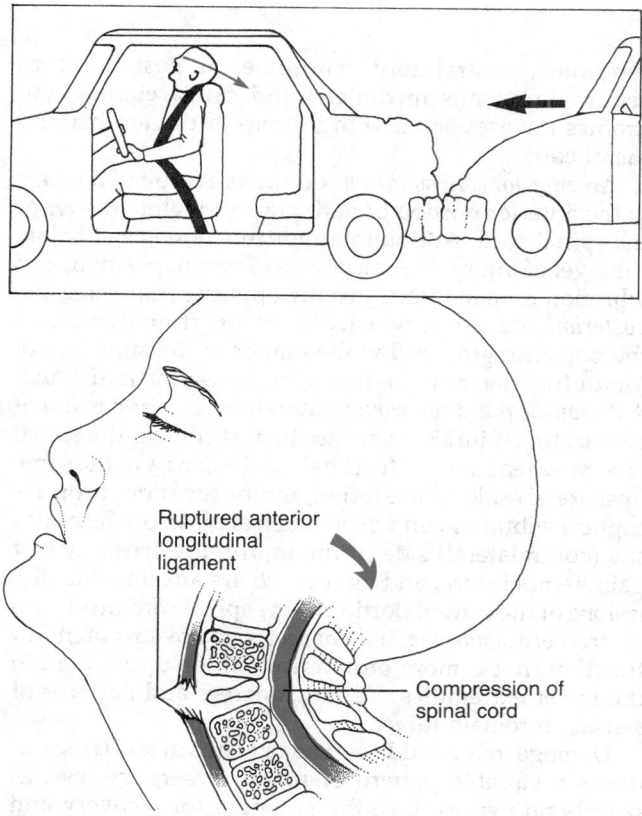

Figure 33–17

Hyperextension injury of the cervical spine.

the velocity of the vehicle (e.g., knife or bullet) causing the injury. Low-velocity, or impact, injuries cause damage directly at the site or localized damage to the spinal cord or spinal nerves.

In contrast, high-velocity injuries that occur from gunshot wounds cause both direct and indirect damage. As mentioned earlier, the spinal cord may be contused, lacerated, or compressed as a result of the injury. Petechial hemorrhage into the central gray matter, and later into white matter, can be caused by contusion and laceration of the spinal cord. Together with compression of the cord from hemorrhage of a lacerated blood vessel or bony fragments, spinal cord edema develops. Necrosis of the spinal cord occurs from compromised capillary circulation and venous return.

Extent of injury. Injury to the spinal cord is classified as either complete or incomplete. A *complete lesion* is characterized by total loss of motor, sensory, and reflex activity below the level of the lesion. A complete lesion means that the cord is completely transected; it is an infrequent occurrence.

What occurs more typically is an *incomplete lesion* with preservation of a mixed pattern of motor, sensory, and reflex function. Specific syndromes occur as a result of incomplete lesions (Fig. 33–19). Cervical injuries may result in anterior cord syndrome, Brown-Séquard

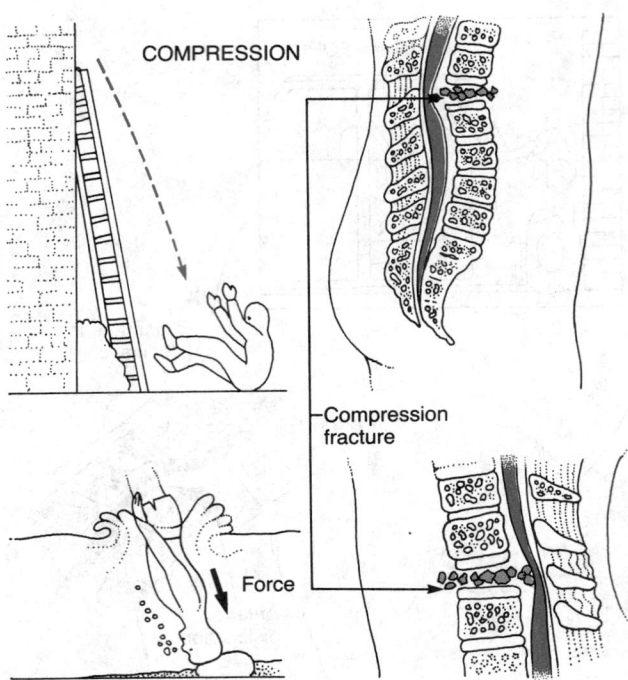

Figure 33 – 18

Axial loading (vertical compression) injury of the cervical spine and the lumbar spine.

syndrome, central cord syndrome, or posterior cord syndrome. Conus medullaris and cauda equina syndromes are associated with injuries to the lumbar and sacral cord.

An *anterior cord syndrome* occurs as a result of damage to the anterior portion of both gray and white matter of the spinal cord. Although motor function is lost below the level of injury, the sensations of touch, position, and vibration remain intact. Just the opposite transpires in a *posterior cord lesion*, which also occurs from damage to the posterior gray and white matter of the spinal cord. Motor function remains intact, but sensation is affected. A *Brown-Séquard syndrome* generally occurs as a result of penetrating injuries that cause hemisection of the spinal cord or when injury affects half of the cord. On the same (ipsilateral) side of the lesion, motor function, proprioception, vibration, and deep touch are lost; on the opposite (contralateral) side of the injury, the sensations of pain, temperature, and light touch are affected. Finally, lesions of the central portion of the spinal cord produce a *central cord syndrome*. It is characterized by loss of motor function that is more pronounced in the upper than in the lower extremities. Varying degrees and patterns of sensation remain intact.

Damage to the cauda equina or conus medullaris produces a variable pattern of motor or sensory loss, as peripheral nerves have the potential for recovery and regrowth. In addition, this usually results in neurogenic bowel and bladder.

Etiology

Trauma is the leading cause of spinal cord injuries, with almost half occurring as a result of motor vehicle accidents. The second leading cause is falls, followed by acts of violence. Diving, football, and skiing are other activities that commonly contribute to the incidence of spinal cord injuries.

Although not as common as brain tumors, tumors of the spinal cord also cause spinal neurologic deficits. Unlike trauma, these deficits occur insidiously and progress slowly. Spinal cord tumors are classified as *intramedullary* (within the spinal cord tissue) or *extramedullary* (outside the spinal cord tissue). Benign tumors, such as meningiomas, are the most common, but malignant tumors do occur. Chapter 25 describes radiation therapy that may be used if surgery is not successful in removing the malignant spinal cord tumor.

Incidence

It is estimated that there are over 200,000 persons in the United States with spinal cord injuries, and 10,000 new injuries occur each year (Zejdlik, 1983). The typical client with a spinal cord injury is an unmarried male between the ages of 15 and 30 years, with 19 years of age being the most common age. The client is hospitalized for 6 months or longer, including acute care and rehabilitation. Peak months of incidence for injury are in the summer or warmer months. Spinal tumors are most common in young and middle-aged adults.

PREVENTION

Most spinal cord injuries can be prevented through the use of proper safety precautions. Lower speed limits, use of seat belts and helmets (motorcycle and bicycle), and safe driving practices can reduce the number and severity of injuries from motor vehicle accidents. The slogan of "feet first" must be universally emphasized to help decrease diving and other water-related accidents. Injuries from sports can be decreased through proper coaching, emphasis on safety while learning and participating in sports, and proper use of protective sports equipment. Public education should be directed toward prevention of falls in the home and community.

After a spinal cord injury has occurred, great care must be taken to prevent extension of the injury. This is accomplished through extensive training of rescue personnel, as well as education of the public. It is important to know when to move or, more critically, when not to move the client with a potential spinal cord injury. Proper spinal immobilization is critical to the eventual outcome of a spinal cord injury. Immobilization techniques consist of the application of a rigid cervical collar, the placement of sandbags around the client's head to further restrict movement, and transport on a spinal board.

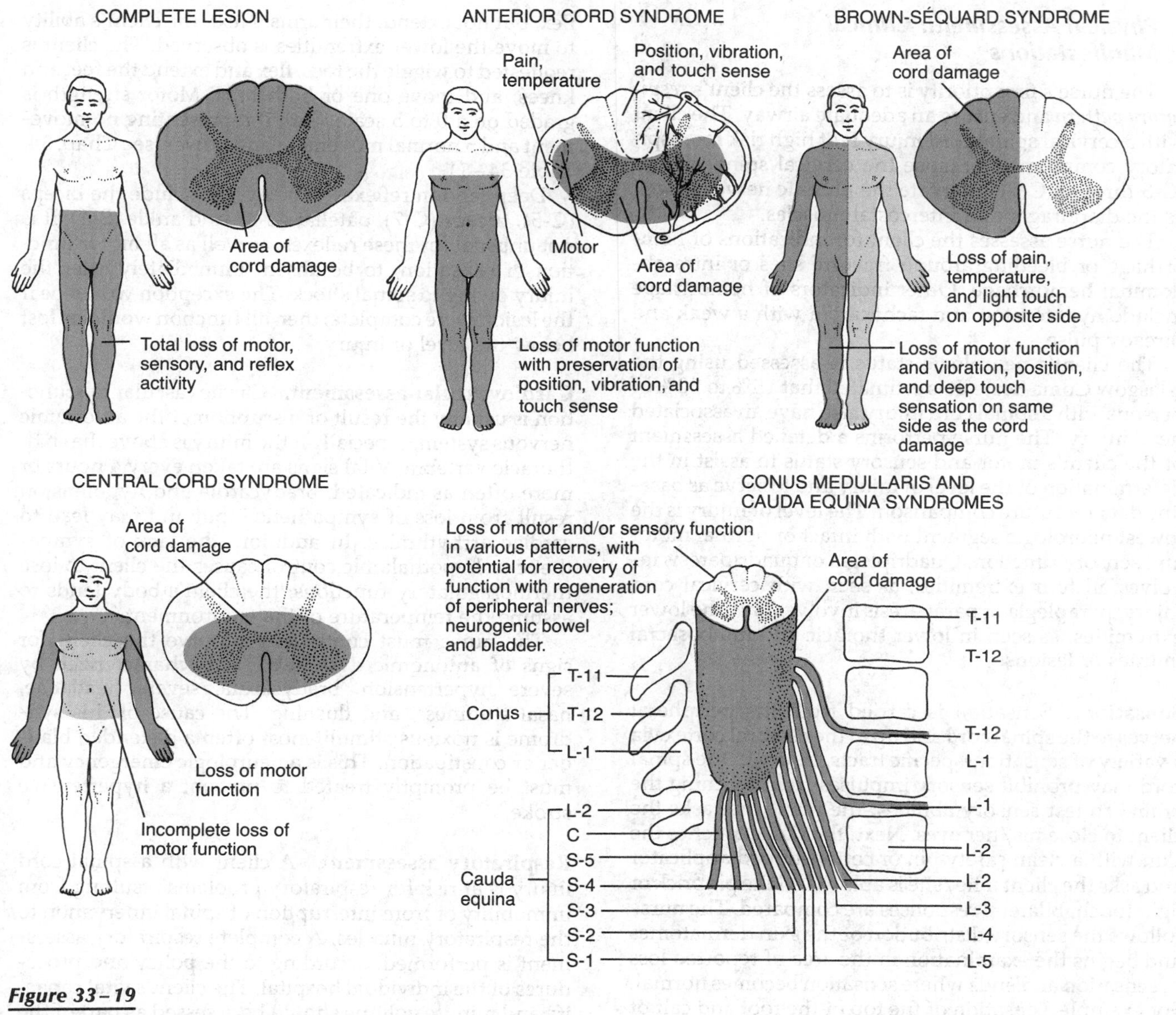

COMPLETE LESION

Area of cord damage

Total loss of motor, sensory, and reflex activity

ANTERIOR CORD SYNDROME

Pain, temperature

Position, vibration, and touch sense

Motor

Area of cord damage

Loss of motor function with preservation of position, vibration, and touch sense

BROWN-SÉQUARD SYNDROME

Area of cord damage

Loss of pain, temperature, and light touch on opposite side

Loss of motor function and vibration, position, and deep touch sensation on same side as the cord damage

CENTRAL CORD SYNDROME

Area of cord damage

Loss of motor function

Incomplete loss of motor function

CONUS MEDULLARIS AND CAUDA EQUINA SYNDROMES

Loss of motor and/or sensory function in various patterns, with potential for recovery of function with regeneration of peripheral nerves; neurogenic bowel and bladder.

Area of cord damage

Conus — T-11, T-12, L-1

Cauda equina — L-2, C, S-5, S-4, S-3, S-2, S-1

T-11
T-12
T-12
L-1
L-1
L-2
L-2
L-3
L-4
L-5

Figure 33–19

Common spinal cord syndromes.

COLLABORATIVE MANAGEMENT

 Assessment

History

When obtaining a history from a client with a spinal cord injury, it is useful to obtain as much data as possible concerning *how the accident occurred* and the *probable mechanism of injury*. Specific information to be obtained by the nurse includes the position of client immediately after the injury, what symptoms occurred after the injury, and what changes have occurred since the initial appearance of signs and symptoms. In addition, the nurse questions rescue personnel about the type of im-

mobilization devices used and whether any problems occurred during extrication and transport of the client. The nurse also obtains information about the medical treatment given at the scene of injury or in the emergency room (e.g., medications and IV fluids).

The client's *past medical history* must be determined. Information specific to obtain for the person with spinal cord injury is a history of arthritis of the spine, congenital deformities, osteoporosis or osteomyelitis, cancer, and previous injury or surgery on the neck or back. These health problems may cause or contribute to the development of a spinal cord insult. If the client has experienced a cervical spinal cord injury, a detailed history of any respiratory problems should be documented by the nurse.

Physical Assessment: Clinical Manifestations

The nurse's first priority is to assess the client's *respiratory pattern* and ensure an adequate airway. The client with a cervical spinal cord injury is at high risk for respiratory compromise because the cervical spinal nerves (C-3 through C-5) innervate the phrenic nerve, as well as the diaphragm and intercostal muscles.

The nurse assesses the client for indications of hemorrhage or bleeding around fracture sites or intra-abdominal hemorrhage. Other indicators of hemorrhage include hypotension and tachycardia with a weak and thready pulse.

The client's neurologic status is assessed using the Glasgow Coma Scale. It is estimated that 15% to 20% of persons with a spinal cord injury also have an associated head injury. The nurse performs a detailed assessment of the client's motor and sensory status to assist in the determination of the level of injury and to serve as baseline data for future comparison. The level of injury is the lowest neurologic segment with intact or normal motor and sensory function. Quadriplegia or quadriparesis involves all four extremities, as seen with cervical cord injury; paraplegia or paraparesis involves only the lower extremities, as seen in lower thoracic and lumbosacral injuries or lesions.

Sensation. Sensation is carried from the peripheral nerves to the spinal cord and up to the cerebral cortex via a variety of sensation-specific tracts. Injury to the spinal cord may prohibit sensory impulses from reaching the brain. To test sensory abilities, the nurse first asks the client to close his/her eyes. Next, the nurse touches the skin with a clean safety pin or cotton-tipped applicator and asks the client if he/she is able to feel the pinprick or light touch. Bilateral responses are compared. The nurse follows the sensory distribution of the skin dermatomes and begins the examination in the area of reported loss of sensation and ends where sensation becomes normal. For example, sensation of the top of the foot and calf of the leg is spinal skin segment (dermatome) level L-3, L-4, and L-5. The area at the level of the umbilicus is T-10, the clavicle is C-3 or C-4, and finger sensation is C-7 and C-8. The client may report a complete sensory loss, hypoesthesia (decreased sensation), or hyperesthesia (increased sensation).

The nurse may elect to determine the client's proprioceptive function. The client is again asked to close his/her eyes. Next, one of the client's fingers or toes is moved up or down. The client is asked to identify the position of the digits.

Motor ability. In addition to performing a routine motor evaluation of the client, the nurse evaluates selected muscles in a more systematic fashion. The client is asked to shrug the shoulders, flex and extend the elbows, elevate both arms off the bed, and flex and extend the wrists and fingers. Clients with spine injuries at the fifth or sixth cervical vertebra are often able to flex, but not extend, their arms. Next, the client's ability to move the lower extremities is observed. The client is requested to wiggle the toes, flex and extend the feet and knees, and move one or both hips. Motor strength is graded on a 0 to 5 scale, with 0 representing no movement and 5 normal movement and power (see Chap. 34, Table 34–1).

Deep tendon reflexes to be tested include the biceps (C-5), triceps (C-7), patellar (L-3), and ankle (S-1). It is not unusual for these reflexes, as well as all motor function or sensation, to be absent immediately after the injury owing to spinal shock. The exception would be if the lesion were complete; then all function would be lost below the level of injury.

Cardiovascular assessment. Cardiovascular dysfunction is usually the result of disruption of the autonomic nervous system, especially if the injury is above the sixth thoracic vertebra. Vital signs are taken every 4 hours or more often as indicated. Bradycardia and hypotension result from loss of sympathetic input and may lead to cardiac arrhythmias. In addition, the lack of sympathetic or hypothalamic control causes the client to lose thermoregulatory functions; the client's body tends to assume the temperature of the environment.

The nurse must continually observe the client for signs of autonomic dysreflexia. It is characterized by severe hypertension, bradycardia, severe headache, nasal stuffiness, and flushing. The cause of this syndrome is noxious stimuli, most often a distended bladder or constipation. This is a neurologic emergency and must be promptly treated to prevent a hypertensive stroke.

Respiratory assessment. A client with a spinal cord injury is at risk for respiratory problems resulting from immobility or from interruption of spinal innervation to the respiratory muscles. A complete respiratory assessment is performed, according to the policy and procedures of the individual hospital. The client's vital capacity and minute volume should be assessed as part of the examination. Periodic repetition of these tests should be done as the client's clinical status indicates. Respiratory complications that must be observed for include impaired gas exchange, pneumonia, pulmonary emboli, and atelectasis.

Gastrointestinal and genitourinary assessment. The nurse assesses the client's abdomen for indications of hemorrhage or distention. Hemorrhage may result from the trauma or may occur later owing to the development of a stress ulcer or the administration of steroids. The client may develop a paralytic ileus within 72 hours of admission. During the period of spinal shock, peristalsis decreases, leading to a loss of bowel sounds and gastric distention. This lack of or interference with autonomic innervation may lead to a reflux or hypotonic bowel.

Autonomic dysfunction initially causes an areflexic bladder, which later leads to urinary retention and a neurogenic bladder. The client is at risk for urinary tract infection from an indwelling urinary catheter or from bladder distention, stasis, and overflow.

Musculoskeletal assessment. The nurse assesses the client's muscle tone and size. Muscle wasting occurs as a result of a flaccid paralysis. Incomplete lesions may cause spasticity, which can lead to contractures. The nurse assesses the condition of the client's skin, especially over pressure points, at least twice daily. Another complication of immobility is heterotrophic ossification (bony overgrowth, often into muscle). It is evidenced by swelling, redness, warmth, and decreased ROM of the involved extremity. Changes in the bony structure are not evidenced until several weeks after the initial symptoms appear.

Psychosocial Assessment

The nurse assesses the client's preinjury psychosocial status by obtaining information about the client's usual methods of coping with illness, difficult situations, and disappointments. It is also important to elicit information about the client's level of independence or dependence and his/her comfort level in discussing feelings and emotions with family or close friends. Clients who are emotionally secure, with a positive self-image, a supportive family, and financial and job security, often are better able to adapt to their injury. Information about the client's religious or cultural beliefs also assists the nurse in developing the care plan. The client with a spinal cord injury has to cope with changes in body image, self-esteem, independence, role relationships, and sexuality.

In addition, the family members are assessed by the nurse to determine how well they are coping with the client's injury and changes in their roles. Many of the clients are young and without adequate health insurance; the families are particularly concerned about financial matters.

Laboratory Findings

Routine laboratory studies are performed on the client with a spinal cord injury to establish baseline data or in preparation for surgery. A urinalysis checks for the presence of blood in the urine after trauma. Arterial blood gas analysis is used to follow the respiratory status of a client at risk for respiratory insufficiency. The findings should be within normal limits, unless the client has a history of heavy smoking, preinjury lung disease, or developing respiratory failure as indicated by decreased oxygen and increased carbon dioxide levels and respiratory acidosis.

Radiographic Findings

A complete spine radiographic series is taken to identify vertebral fractures, subluxation, or dislocation. CT may be performed to determine the degree and extent of damage to the spinal cord and to detect the presence of blood and bone within the spinal column.

Other Diagnostic Tests

An EMG, evoked potentials, and somatosensory evoked potentials may be obtained to identify which level of the spinal cord is intact. These studies measure the electrical conduction within the muscle. MRI may also be done to detect spinal cord damage.

 Analysis: Nursing Diagnosis

The client with a spinal cord injury is admitted to the hospital with varying degrees of sensory and motor dysfunction, as well as possible involvement of the autonomic nervous system. The client may have loss of voluntary bowel and bladder function. In addition, the client usually exhibits problems with adjusting to potential disability and accompanying changes in body image, self-esteem, and sexuality.

Common Diagnoses

The nursing diagnoses that are commonly found in clients with a spinal cord injury include the following:

1. Altered (spinal cord) tissue perfusion related to compression, contusion, or edema
2. Ineffective airway clearance, ineffective breathing pattern, and impaired gas exchange related to loss of innervation to muscles of respiration or immobility
3. Impaired physical mobility and/or total self-care deficit related to quadriplegia or quadriparesis or paraplegia or paraparesis
4. Altered patterns of urinary elimination and bowel incontinence related to neurogenic bowel and bladder
5. Impaired adjustment related to depression, change in body image, or role performance

Additional Diagnoses

In addition to the common diagnoses, the client may have one or more of the following:

1. Potential impaired skin integrity related to immobility
2. Altered sexuality patterns and sexual dysfunction related to loss of or decreased innervation to reproductive organs
3. Pain related to trauma, spasticity, or immobility
4. Anxiety and fear related to threat to self-concept, change in biologic integrity, change in environment, and potential change in job or school activities
5. Ineffective thermoregulation related to autonomic nervous system dysfunction
6. Potential for injury related to immobility and decreased sensation
7. Altered health maintenance related to immobility and self-care deficits

Planning and Implementation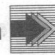

The care plan for the client with a spinal cord injury focuses on the common nursing diagnoses.

Altered (Spinal Cord) Tissue Perfusion

Planning: client goals. The major goal for this nursing diagnosis is that the client will exhibit no further deterioration in neurologic status.

Interventions. If the client has experienced fractured vertebrae, the primary concern is to reduce and immobilize the fracture as for any fracture. Nonsurgical techniques using traction or external fixation are typically employed, but surgery may be necessary to stabilize the spine and prevent further spinal cord damage.

Nonsurgical management. The client with a cervical spine injury is usually placed in a traction or immobilization device to realign the vertebrae and to prevent further damage.

Immobilization. The most commonly used devices are cervical (Gardner-Wells or Crutchfield-Vinke) tongs and the halo fixation device (Fig. 33–20). Cervical tongs are inserted by the physician into the outer aspect of the client's skull. Traction is added, and the physician prescribes the amount of weights to be used to reduce the fracture. The weights should hang free at all times. Releasing the traction could cause further neurologic damage. The nurse maintains the client in alignment and ensures that the ropes for the traction remain within the pulley. Postprocedure nursing care includes monitoring the client for any changes in neurologic status. The insertion site of the tongs is monitored for signs of infection; the nurse follows hospital policy for sterile pin site care, which may specify solutions such as saline or ointments such as bacitracin. With a halo fixation device, four pins are inserted into the client's skull. The fixation device and halo jacket or cast are then applied. The client's neurologic status is monitored for changes in movement or decreased strength every hour for 4 hours, then every 2 hours for 6 hours after the halo device is applied. If the client remains stable, routine neurologic assessments are done according to hospital policy. The client should never be moved or turned by holding or pulling on the halo device. The client's skin is checked frequently to ensure that the jacket or cast is not causing pressure. The nurse should be able to insert one finger easily under the jacket or cast. The pin sites of both the cervical tongs and the halo device should be checked to ensure a tight and secure fit. Chapter 31 describes nursing care for clients in traction.

Drug therapy. Corticosteroids, such as dexamethasone (Decadron), are used for their anti-inflammatory effects, although some physicians believe that cortico-

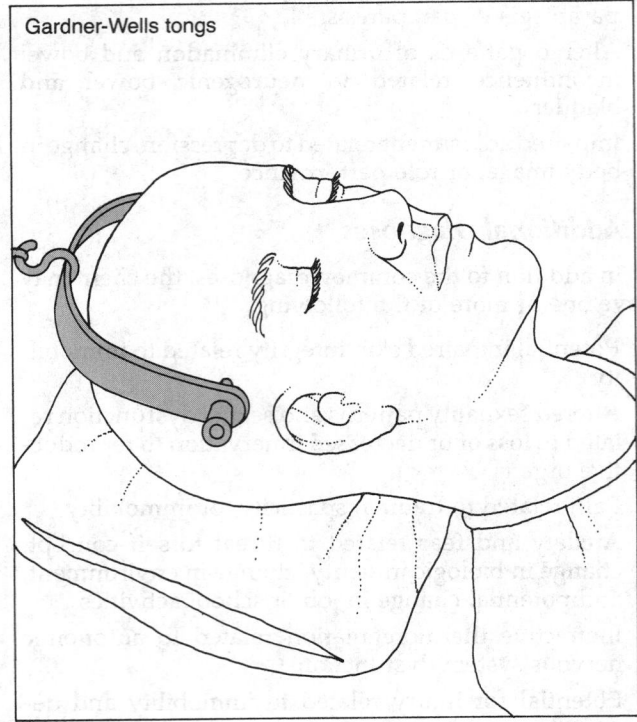

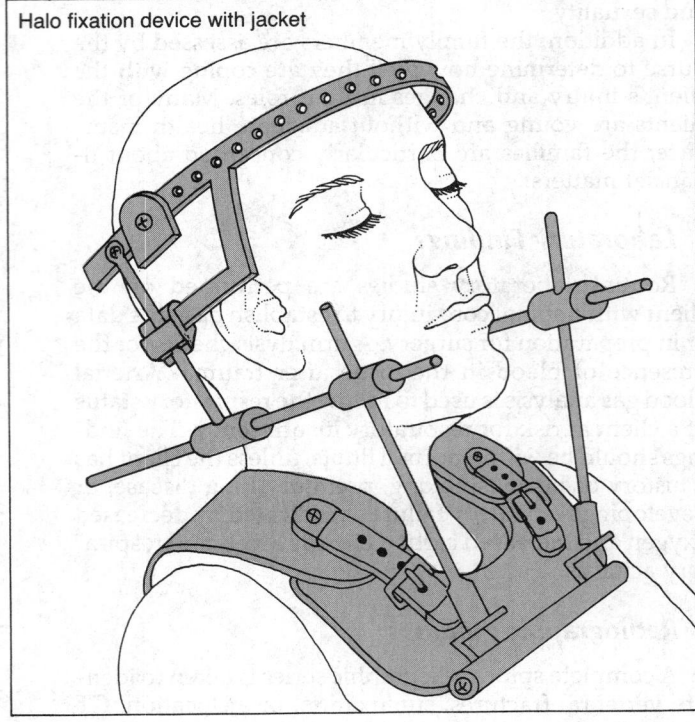

Figure 33–20

Types of cervical spine traction.

steroids interfere with healing. Dextran, a plasma expander, may be used to increase capillary blood flow within the spinal cord and to prevent or treat hypotension. Atropine sulfate is used to treat bradycardia if the pulse rate falls below 50 to 60 beats per minute. Hypotension, if severe, is treated with a dopamine (Intropin) drip, which is generally used only in a critical care unit. Medications to treat spasticity include dantrolene (Dantrium) and baclofen (Lioresal).

A controversial technique used to treat spinal cord injuries is hyperbaric oxygenation. The client is placed in a hyperbaric chamber, and the atmospheric pressure is increased as the client breathes pure oxygen. The blood is able to absorb more oxygen because of the pressure changes. It is believed that improving diffusion into the injured cord lessens potential damage from ischemia. This procedure should begin within 12 to 24 hours after injury.

Surgical management.   Emergency surgery may be indicated if there is evidence of spinal cord compression. The procedure is usually necessary to remove bone fragments from a vertebral fracture, evacuate a hematoma, or remove penetrating objects, such as a bullet. A *decompressive laminectomy* is performed to allow for cord expansion from edema if other more conventional measures fail to prevent neurologic deterioration.

Surgical procedures to stabilize and support the spine may be performed at the discretion of the physician, depending on the client's condition and the extent of the injury. Typical procedures include a spinal fusion and the insertion of metal or steel rods, such as Harrington's rods, to stabilize *thoracic* injuries. Postoperatively, the client usually wears a brace, corset, or lumbosacral support to keep the operative area immobilized during recovery. Although not a widely accepted form of treatment, cooling, or hypothermia, of the spinal cord within a short time after injury (4 to 6 hours) is done at selected medical centers. The procedure involves cooling the cord to 6° C (43° F) for 3 to 4 hours to reduce edema and improve circulation.

Postoperative care specific for the client with a spinal cord injury is as follows: the client's motor status and vital signs are taken at least every hour for the first 4 to 6 hours after surgery, and then, if the client is stable, every 4 hours. Complications of surgery, such as the development of a hematoma or edema, are manifested by a deterioration in neurologic status. Owing to loss of sympathetic innervation, the client is at risk for cardiovascular instability. The client should be logrolled when being moved to maintain skeletal alignment. A complete discussion of postoperative nursing care for the client with spinal surgery is found in Chapter 31.

Ineffective Airway Clearance; Ineffective Breathing Pattern; Impaired Gas Exchange

Planning: client goals.   The goals for these nursing diagnoses include that the client will (1) maintain a respiratory rate of between 16 and 24 respirations per minute and (2) not develop respiratory complications, such as pneumonia or atelectasis.

Interventions: nonsurgical management.   Clients with injury at and above the sixth thoracic vertebra are at risk for respiratory complications owing to impaired functioning of the respiratory muscles; the client is turned at least every 2 hours and instructed to breathe deeply. To facilitate independence in deep breathing, the nurse instruct the client to take a few deep breaths during commercial breaks on the television or radio or after receiving medications or visitors. The nurse can assist the quadriplegic client to cough by placing his/her hands on either side of the rib cage or upper abdomen below the diaphragm. As the client inhales, the nurse gently pushes upward to help the client expand the lungs. The nurse encourages the client to use blow bottles, an incentive spirometer, or Thompson's respirator (compressed air to expand the lungs) every 4 hours. The nurse performs a respiratory assessment during each nursing shift to determine the effectiveness of these strategies. It may be necessary to perform oral or nasal suctioning if the client is unable to effectively clear the airway of secretions.

Impaired Physical Mobility

Planning: client goals.   The major goal for this nursing diagnosis is that the client will not develop complications of immobility.

Interventions: nonsurgical management.   The client is especially at risk for deep venous thrombosis, pulmonary emboli, and pressure sores. The client is turned at least every 2 hours while in bed. When sitting in a chair, he/she is repositioned every 30 minutes. Pressure relief maneuvers are discussed more completely in Chapter 22. The client's skin is inspected frequently to determine tolerance for sitting as well as to detect the presence of reddened areas. The nurse attempts to blanch the reddened areas over the ischial tuberosities. If unable to blanch, the area is prone to breakdown. ROM exercises are performed at least once per nursing shift. The nurse collaborates with physical and occupational therapists to determine the most appropriate positioning and exercise techniques, to assess the need for hand splints, and to develop a plan to prevent foot drop (usually clients wear high-topped tennis shoes for prevention).

The client's lower extremities are assessed for indications of deep venous thrombosis. The calf and thigh circumferences are measured each day. Thigh-high antiembolism stockings are used. They are removed during every nursing shift for 1 hour, and the client's skin is checked for any signs of redness or impairment. Sodium heparin, 5000 units every 12 hours subcutaneously, or warfarin sodium (Coumadin) in therapeutic dosages may be ordered to prevent deep venous thrombosis or embolus formation. Further discussion of measures to prevent complications is found in Chapters 22 and 31.

Altered Patterns of Urinary Elimination; Bowel Incontinence

Planning: client goals.   The major goal for these nursing diagnoses is that the client will achieve continence of stool and urine. A more complete discussion of bowel and bladder programs is presented in Chapter 22.

Interventions: nonsurgical management.   Clients with spinal cord injuries have reflex or neurogenic loss of bowel and bladder control. Many of these clients can become continent if they rigorously adhere to an established program. The type of program depends on the client's usual elimination pattern and whether the injury involved UMNs or LMNs.

Bowel program.   The essential elements of this program are a consistent time for bowel elimination, a high fluid intake (2000 mL/day) unless fluid intake is restricted, high-fiber diet, suppository program, and, if needed, stool-softener medications such as docusate sodium (Colace) or docusate sodium and casanthranol (Peri-Colace). If the client sustained a LMN injury, the resulting flaccid large bowel may require the client to perform or have manual disimpaction. Additional stimuli used to facilitate a bowel movement include scheduling toileting 30 minutes to 1 hour after meals to optimize the gastrocolic reflex and teaching the client to perform Valsalva's maneuver or massaging the abdomen from right to left along the outline of the large intestine.

Bladder program.   As soon as the client is medically stable, the indwelling Foley's catheter is removed. Initially, an intermittent catheterization program is instituted. The client is catheterized every 4 hours and more frequently if the urinary output is greater than 500 mL. Over time, the intervals between catheterizations are increased and adjusted to the client's fluid intake and sleep times. After the acute care phase has passed, the client may be able to initiate voiding by using specific techniques. Clients with UMN bladder problems (injury above the sacrum) may be able to stimulate voiding by stroking the inner thigh, pulling on pubic hair or hair of the upper thigh, pouring warm water over the perineum, or tapping the bladder area to stimulate the detrusor muscle. Clients with injuries to the sacrum (LMN) may achieve emptying of the bladder by performing Valsalva's maneuver or tightening the abdominal muscles. To ascertain the effectiveness of these maneuvers, the client should be catheterized for residual urine after voiding. Some clients rely on catheterization twice or three times daily to empty their bladders. As with the bowel program, the client is encouraged to drink 2000 to 2500 mL of fluid each day. Clients with LMN injury often decrease fluid intake after 6 or 7 PM each evening.

Impaired Adjustment

Planning: client goals.   The major goals for this nursing diagnosis are that the client will (1) begin to cope with the changes caused by the injury and (2) verbalize his/her feelings about the situation.

Interventions: nonsurgical management.   The nurse uses the information obtained from the psychosocial assessment to identify strategies to help the client adjust to the disability. The client is invited to ask questions, which should be answered openly and honestly. Questions regarding prognosis and potential for complete recovery should be referred to the physician because the timing and extent of recovery vary for each individual. The nurse encourages the client to discuss his/her perceptions of the situation and what coping strategies can be utilized. The client should feel free to express personal feelings and emotions in an acceptable manner. Often, the client behaves in a socially unacceptable manner (excessive anger, verbal abuse, and use of illegal drugs), and the nurse attempts to redirect this behavior. In addition, the nurse begins a client education program to clarify misconceptions, as well as to provide health teaching. Referrals to clergy, rabbi, or spiritual leaders or to a psychologist or a psychiatric liaison nurse may be needed to help clients adjust to their unexpected life change.

■ Discharge Planning

The client with a spinal cord injury is often discharged to a rehabilitation facility before returning home. However, a client with minimal neurologic dysfunction can be directly discharged to home from the hospital and receive physical or occupational therapy on an outpatient basis.

Home Care Preparation

If the client is discharged to home or returns to home for a weekend visit from the hospital, the environment must be assessed to ensure that it is free from hazards and will accommodate the client's special needs (e.g., wheelchair). It is particularly important that ease of accessibility is offered to the entrance of the home, as well as the bathroom, kitchen, and bedroom. The height of the client's bed may need to be adjusted to facilitate smooth transfer into or out of the bed.

All adaptive devices the client will use at home should be ordered and delivered to the hospital. This enables the nurse and other therapists to ensure that the item fits correctly and that the client knows how to use it correctly.

Client/Family Education

The teaching plan for the client with a spinal cord injury includes physical mobility and activity skills, ADL skills, bowel and bladder program, skin care, medication regimen, and sexuality. Mobility skills are important to learn to enable the client to negotiate movement on sidewalks, carpeting, and other flooring surfaces. The client must also be able to negotiate sidewalk curbs while walking independently with crutches or a cane or while in a wheelchair.

ADL training includes a structured exercise program to promote strength and endurance. The client is instructed in the correct use of all adaptive equipment. Family members or the caregiver must be instructed in transfer skills, feeding, bathing, dressing, positioning, and skin care as appropriate. Included within this program is nutritional training to maintain an ideal body weight and to promote bowel and bladder elimination. The individualized bowel and bladder program is reinforced. The client is instructed in the procedures to follow should problems such as diarrhea or infection develop.

The client is instructed on the name, the purpose, the dosage and timing of administration, and side effects of all medications. It is important for the client to understand the possible interaction of prescribed medication with OTC medication or illegal drugs and alcohol.

The goal of sexuality education in the acute care setting is to answer the client's questions and correct any misinformation. Unless the nurse has specific training or experience in sexuality counseling of people with spinal cord injuries, more detailed questions should be directed to a sexuality counselor. The reader is referred to Chapters 10 and 22 for specific nursing interventions for these clients.

Psychosocial Preparation

Psychosocial adaptation is one of the critical factors in determining rehabilitation success. The acute care nurse can help the client prepare for discharge or transfer to a rehabilitation hospital by assisting the client to verbalize feelings and fears regarding body image, self-concept, role performance, and self-esteem. The nurse should prepare the client for the reactions of those outside the hospital. In the acute care setting, this can be accomplished by having the nurse, family members, or friends take the client to the hospital lobby or, if permitted, to the cafeteria or outside on the hospital grounds. The nurse should tactfully and nonjudgmentally let the client know when behavior is unacceptable for the time and place where it occurred as well as encourage more positive behaviors. The use of role playing or anticipating responses to potential problems is helpful. For example, the client can practice answering questions from children about why he/she is in a wheelchair or cannot move.

Health Care Resources

The client and his/her family should be referred to the local, state, and national organizations for those with spinal cord injuries. These include the National Spinal Cord Injury Association and the Spinal Cord Injury Hotline. A variety of consumer-oriented books, journals, and films are also available.

If the quadriplegic client returns home, a full-time caretaker is usually required. The caretaker may be a family member or nursing assistant employed to provide care and companionship.

 Evaluation

On the basis of the identified nursing diagnoses, the nurse evaluates the care of the client with a spinal cord injury. The expected outcomes include that the client

1. Demonstrates adequate spinal cord tissue perfusion as evidenced by stable neurologic and vital signs
2. Maintains an adequate airway, breathing pattern, and gas exchange
3. Demonstrates no or minimal complications of immobility
4. Uses adaptive devices correctly
5. Maintains bowel and bladder continence or controlled incontinence
6. Consumes an adequate fluid intake and appropriate diet to maintain hydration and weight
7. Complies with exercise programs and medication schedule
8. Begins to adjust or adapt to the disabilities

BRAIN TUMORS

OVERVIEW

Brain tumors can arise anywhere within the brain structures and are named according to the cell or tissue from which they originate. Primary tumors originate within the CNS and rarely metastasize outside this area. Secondary brain tumors occur as a result of metastasis from other areas of the body, such as the lungs, the breast, the kidney, or GI tract.

Pathophysiology

Primary brain tumors occur as a rapid proliferation or abnormal growth of cells normally found within the CNS. Secondary brain tumors occur as malignant cells from tumors outside the CNS metastasize to the brain. Regardless of the origin, the tumor expands in an irregular fashion and invades, infiltrates, or compresses normal brain tissue. This leads to cerebral edema, increased ICP, focal neurologic deficits, obstruction of the flow of CSF, and pituitary dysfunction.

Complications

Cerebral edema, or more specifically *vasogenic edema*, occurs as a result of changes in capillary endothelial tissue permeability, which allow plasma to seep into the extracellular spaces. This leads to increased ICP, and herniation of the brain tissue may occur. A variety of focal neurologic deficits result from edema, infiltration, and compression of surrounding brain tissue. The cerebral blood vessels may become compressed because of edema and increased ICP, and this compression leads to ischemia of the area supplied by the vessel. In addition, the tumor may infiltrate the walls of the vessel, causing it to rupture and hemorrhage into the tumor bed or adjacent brain tissue. Approximately one-third of clients with brain tumors experience seizure activity attributable to interference with the brain's normal conduction pathways.

Increased ICP may also occur as a result of obstruction of the flow of CSF or displacement of the lateral ventricles by the expanding lesion. Typically, a tumor obstructs the aqueduct of Sylvius or one of the ventricles or encroaches on the subarachnoid space. Posterior fossa tumors may obstruct the flow of CSF from the fourth ventricle to the foramen of Luschka or Magendie. In any event, the obstruction of normal CSF flow causes hydrocephalus and eventually leads to increased ICP.

Classification

Brain tumors are generally classified as *malignant* or *benign*, as shown in the accompanying Key Features of Disease. Although benign tumors are generally associated with a more favorable outcome, this is often not the case. If the tumor cannot be completely removed or treated, it continues to grow. As it invades other brain tissue, cerebral edema, focal neurologic deficits, and increased ICP occur. Herniation of the brain tissue eventually leads to death. Further, within 3 to 5 years, benign tumors often undergo histologic changes and become malignant.

KEY FEATURES OF DISEASE ■ Classification of Brain Tumors

Benign

Acoustic neuroma

Meningioma

Pituitary adenoma

Astrocytoma
   Grade 1 (may undergo changes and become malignant)

Malignant

Astrocytoma
   Grade 2
   Grade 3
   Grade 4 (also known as glioblastoma multiforme)

Oligodendroglioma

Ependymoma

A second classification system is based on *location.* Supratentorial tumors, which occur most often in the adult, are located in the area above the tentorium, the tent-like fold of dura that surrounds the cerebellar hemisphere and supports the occipital lobe. In other words, *supratentorial* tumors are located within the cerebral hemispheres. Located beneath the tentorium is the *infratentorial* area, the area of the brain stem structures and cerebellum.

A third classification system is according to the *cellular, anatomic,* or *histologic* origin of the tumor. The nervous system is composed of two types of cells: neurons, which are responsible for nerve impulse conduction, and neuroglial cells, which provide support, nourishment, and protection for neurons. Four specific types of cells make up neuroglial cells: (1) astrocytes, (2) oligodendroglia, (3) ependymal cells, and (4) microglia.

A fourth classification system has been developed by several pathologists to address some of the shortcomings in the grading system discussed. This system categorizes the tumors on the basis of their *histologic features.* The three categories are well-differentiated astrocytoma, astrocytoma with atypical or anaplastic foci, and glioblastoma multiforme.

Gliomas are malignant tumors; they account for 45% to 60% of all adult brain tumors and arise from the neuroglial cells of the brain and the brain stem. They infiltrate and invade surrounding brain tissue. The most common type of glioma is the *astrocytoma,* which may be found anywhere within the cerebral hemispheres. It is usually treated by surgery, followed by radiation and chemotherapy. *Oligodendrogliomas,* another type of glioma, are generally located within the temporal lobes of the brain. These are slow-growing tumors and usually are calcified. Surgical removal is possible, and the long-term prognosis for the client is good. A *glioblastoma* is a highly malignant, rapidly growing, invasive astrocytoma. Although improved surgical techniques and advanced treatment have improved the outlook and quality of life for a client with this type of tumor, the prognosis remains poor for long-term survival. *Ependymomas* arise from the lining of the ventricles and are difficult to treat surgically because of their location. Radiation and shunting procedures to control hydrocephalus caused by the tumor's blocking normal CSF flow are the treatment of choice. Chemotherapy may also be used for these tumors.

Gliomas are graded according to their cellular differentiation or how closely the tumor cells resemble normal cells. Grade I tumors are well differentiated; grade II are moderately so; grade III are poorly differentiated and may rapidly change to grade IV tumors, which are poorly differentiated. A grade III or IV astrocytoma is referred to as *glioblastoma multiforme* and is associated with a poor outcome. Like benign tumors, grade I and II tumors frequently undergo cellular changes and become grade III or IV.

Meningiomas arise from the coverings of the brain (the meninges). They account for 15% of brain tumors in adults and occur more frequently in women than in men. This tumor is benign, is highly vascular, and causes compression and displacement of surrounding brain tissue. Although complete removal of the tumor is possible, it tends to recur.

Pituitary tumors that occur in the anterior lobe account for 7% to 12% of brain tumors and may cause endocrine dysfunction. The majority of pituitary tumors are *chromophobic adenomas* and produce hypopituitary signs (loss of body hair, diabetes insipidus, sterility, visual field defects, and headaches). *Basophilic adenomas* produce Cushing's syndrome signs, including moon facies, thin arms and legs, muscle weakness, obesity, fatigue, and hypertension. An *eosinophilic adenoma* produces gigantism before puberty and acromegaly after puberty. These tumors are benign and frequently occur in young and middle-aged adults.

An *acoustic neuroma* arises from the sheath of Schwann's cells in the peripheral portion of cranial nerve VIII. It is also referred to as a cerebellar pontine angle tumor to describe its anatomic location. This benign tumor compresses brain tissue and tends to surround adjacent cranial nerves (VII, V, IX, and X), making surgical removal difficult without causing permanent cranial nerve dysfunction.

The remainder of adult brain tumors are of miscellaneous origin, such as those involving blood vessels (hemangioblastoma), or are metastatic. Metastatic tumor cells from the lungs, the breast, the colon, the pancreas, and the kidney travel to the brain via the blood and lymphatic system.

Etiology

The exact cause of brain tumors is unknown. Several types of tumors seen in children are thought to be of congenital or hereditary origin. Genetic factors may also account for acoustic neuromas seen in young adults.

Several factors have been identified that were thought to place the client at increased risk for a brain tumor. However, recent studies have found no relationship between head trauma and family predisposition and brain tumors (Bauman & Zumwalt, 1989). Exposure to chemical carcinogens, selected viruses, and certain immunosuppressive agents remains under investigation. A relationship between exposure to high-dose radiation and tumors and between breast cancer and meningioma has been established.

Incidence

Brain tumors account for 2% of all cancer deaths. Each year in the United States, 36,000 new cases of brain tumors are diagnosed (Bauman & Zumwalt, 1989). Brain tumors in the adult population are seen primarily in clients between 35 and 50 years of age, with an incidence of 4.5 per 100,000 population. Overall, males and females are equally affected, with two exceptions. Meningiomas are seen more frequently in middle-aged women, whereas gliomas are seen slightly more often in men.

COLLABORATIVE MANAGEMENT

 ### Assessment

History

When possible, the nurse obtains a history from the client, as well as the family. General information is obtained to identify *risk factors*, such as exposure to radiation or chemical agents.

Next, information concerning *current signs and symptoms* is obtained. The majority of clients with a brain tumor complain of a generalized headache, which is more severe in the morning or on awakening. The client may report vomiting shortly after awakening that is not accompanied by nausea. The client may eat a full breakfast without further episodes of emesis. Papilledema (edema of the optic disk) may cause the client to experience decreased visual acuity, double vision, or a visual field deficit.

Family members may report that the client has exhibited personality or *behavior changes* or appears depressed. In addition, they may report that the client is forgetful and that responses are slow or delayed.

The nurse elicits the following information concerning each symptom reported by the family or client. First, when did the symptom originally occur? Has it changed in any way since that time, for example, increased or decreased in severity? Is there a time or place pattern (e.g., time of day or location)? Is there a particular activity or event that triggers the symptom, or does the presence of the symptom vary with activity? The last question concerns the actions taken to relieve the symptoms. Of particular importance is information concerning any medication or treatment utilized by the client to relieve the symptoms and the effectiveness of these measures.

Physical Assessment: Clinical Manifestations

The nurse performs a complete neurologic assessment of the client to establish baseline data and to determine the nature and extent of neurologic deficits. The manifestations exhibited by the client depend on the areas of the brain affected by the tumor.

The most frequent complaint of the client with a brain tumor is *headache*. The client reports that it is of moderate intensity, always present, and more severe on awakening. *Vomiting* often occurs shortly after awakening and is related to increased ICP or pressure on the medulla. Nausea generally does not occur, nor is vomiting related to eating.

Papilledema, or edema of the optic disk, is easily visualized as a swollen, reddish disk during ophthalmoscopic examination and occurs in the majority of clients with a brain tumor. It is also evidenced by changes in visual acuity, visual field deficits, and diplopia. The client may also have difficulty moving the eye to the side or outward, which indicates pressure on cranial nerve VI.

The nurse may observe a *hemiparesis* or *hemiplegia* if

the tumor involves the motor strip or precentral gyrus. Hypokinesia (decreased movement) or akinesia may also be noted. Jacksonian or generalized *seizure* activity may occur.

The client may experience significant changes in *sensation*, particularly in the presence of a large parietal lobe tumor. Hyperesthesia, paresthesia, and loss of tactile discrimination may occur. Other sensory findings include astereognosis (inability to recognize objects by feeling shape), agnosia (inability to recognize familiar objects), apraxia (inability to use objects appropriately), and agraphia (inability to write). The client may lose body-half awareness or awareness of body parts contralateral to the lesion. For example, men may shave only half of their face or women apply make-up to only one side of their face. Body image changes and lack of attention to personal grooming may occur.

If the lesion is present in the client's dominant hemisphere, aphasia may occur. An expressive, or Broca's, aphasia occurs in the presence of a frontal lobe tumor, whereas receptive, or Wernicke's, aphasia occurs in temporal lobe tumors. Aphasia is discussed earlier.

Tumors involving the brain stem frequently cause *cranial nerve dysfunction*. An acoustic neuroma, for example, involves cranial nerve VIII, and loss of hearing occurs. In addition, this tumor frequently involves cranial nerves V, VII, IX, and X. When these nerves are involved, the client experiences facial pain and weakness, dysphagia, decreased appreciation of taste, loss of gag reflex, nystagmus, and hoarseness. Cerebellar tumors or involvement of the cerebellar hemisphere produces ataxia and dysarthria.

The client with a pituitary tumor exhibits symptoms of endocrine dysfunction. Often, these symptoms cause the client to see a physician, and a pituitary tumor is discovered during the routine endocrine evaluation. Additional information about specific tumors is found elsewhere in the text.

Psychosocial Assessment

Personality and behavior changes are often reported by the family of a client with a frontal lobe tumor. The nurse may observe inappropriate behavior, particularly in social situations, as well as wide mood swings. The client may have difficulty making a decision or act impulsively. Often the client is depressed and has a flat affect.

During the assessment of the client, the nurse must be alert for indications of anxiety and fear. The typical client is anxious about the hospitalization, diagnostic tests, and pending surgery. The client may fear that surgery will cause significant disability and disfigurement. Some clients fear that surgery will result in death. In addition, the client may be concerned about the potential loss of employment income in the event of a prolonged illness. Both the family and the client are usually anxious over the changes in their roles and relationships that occur as a result of the diagnosis and treatment of a brain tumor. Additional information

to help the nurse assess the client is found in Chapter 11.

Laboratory Findings

A lumbar puncture may be performed if there is no indication of clinically significant increased ICP. In the presence of a brain tumor, the CSF pressure is elevated, the protein count is high, and cytologic studies may find the presence of cancerous cells.

Radiographic Findings

CT is performed to identify the size, location, and extent of the tumor. CT also identifies the presence of edema, midline cranial shift, and hydrocephalus. A cerebral angiogram often is not indicated to diagnose a brain tumor. However, it may be performed to provide additional information about the vascular supply to the tumor. A brain scan or echoencephalogram may be indicated to provide further information about the tumor site and location. If the lesion is a secondary tumor, x-ray films of the chest, the kidneys, and other organs can identify the source of the metastatic tumor.

Skull films often reveal the presence of a calcified pineal gland, erosion of the clinoid process or sella turcica, or the presence of intracranial calcifications.

Other Diagnostic Tests

An EEG may be obtained to determine the presence of seizure activity, as well as to assist in the localization of the lesion. MRI may be done for reasons similar to those for doing CT. Visual field studies are performed to provide more precise information on the extent of any visual field deficits. If a pituitary tumor is suspected, a variety of laboratory tests are performed to identify the extent of pituitary or endocrine dysfunction.

 ### Analysis: Nursing Diagnosis

The client with a brain tumor is usually first diagnosed between 35 and 55 years of age. Typical symptoms experienced by the client include headache, vomiting, visual field or visual acuity changes, possibly seizure activity, and/or motor weakness. Personality and behavior changes may also occur.

Common Diagnoses

The following diagnoses are common in clients with a brain tumor:

1. Altered (cerebral) tissue perfusion related to increased ICP
2. Pain related to increased ICP
3. Potential for injury related to seizures, change in level of consciousness, or visual problems
4. Anxiety and fear related to diagnosis and surgery

Additional Diagnoses

In addition to the common diagnoses, the client may have one or more of the following diagnoses:

1. Total self-care deficit related to hemiparesis or change in level of consciousness
2. Impaired verbal communication related to aphasia
3. Impaired physical mobility related to hemiparesis
4. Ineffective airway clearance and impaired gas exchange related to immobility
5. Altered nutrition: less than body requirements related to decreased level of consciousness or dysphagia
6. Body image disturbance and altered role performance related to physical disabilities
7. Hopelessness related to diagnosis

 Planning and Implementation

The plan of care for a client with a brain tumor focuses on the common nursing diagnoses.

Altered (Cerebral) Tissue Perfusion

Planning: client goals. The primary goals for this diagnosis are that the client will (1) maintain normal ICP and (2) demonstrate an improvement in neurologic status.

Interventions. The client with a brain tumor may be treated by nonsurgical techniques, such as drugs and radiation, or may require surgery for tumor removal. The management selected by the physician depends on the size, the location, and the nature of the tumor tissue.

Nonsurgical management. The client's vital signs and neurologic status are assessed at least every 4 hours. A deterioration in the client's neurologic status should be reported to the physician immediately. Routine measurement of intake and output is instituted; strict measurement should be done if the client is vomiting or nauseated, as usually occurs during radiation or chemotherapy. To enhance venous drainage of CSF and minimize the risk of increased ICP, the head of the bed is elevated 30 to 45 degrees and the client's head is maintained in a midline, neutral position.

Drug therapy. A variety of medications are used to treat the client's symptoms and to prevent complications. Analgesics, such as codeine or acetaminophen (Tylenol), are given for headache. Dexamethasone (Decadron) is usually given to control cerebral edema. Phenytoin (Dilantin) or phenobarbital is used to prevent seizure activity. Clients receiving steroids or under stress are given antacids, such as magnesium hydroxide (Mylanta, Maalox), to reduce gastric irritation. Cimetidine (Tagamet) or ranitidine (Zantac) is given to reduce gastric secretion and prevent the development of stress ulcers. Prochlorperazine (Compazine) and other antiemetics are used to treat nausea and vomiting.

Radiation therapy. Radiation therapy may be used alone, after surgery, or in combination with chemotherapy to treat a brain tumor. The purpose of radiation therapy is to destroy rapidly dividing cancer cells by altering the cell membrane. Because radiation also destroys normal tissue, care must be taken to radiate only the area of the tumor. This is accomplished by accurately measuring the location of the tumor and using a "cross fire" technique. Radiation is delivered by either a linear accelerator or a cobalt machine, which rotates (cross fire) around the head to radiate the tumor from different angles; this increases the ability of the radiation to penetrate the tumor more deeply and destroy more tumor cells. The total dose of radiation is usually 50 to 80 Gy given in increments, or fractions, over a 6- to 8-week period. The radiation dose is based on tumor type and location and the client's response to or tolerance of the treatment.

Radiation therapy causes the skin to become reddened and irritated. Alopecia always occurs; hair growth recurs after treatment is completed. As the treatment continues, the skin becomes dry and flaky—similar to a severe sunburn. Alcohol, powder, oils, or creams are *never* used without the written permission of the physician, as these products can cause a severe burn during the next treatment. It is acceptable to wash the skin with non–oil-based soap and water. If the skin has been marked to outline the area of radiation, care must be taken to avoid washing the marks off.

A second group of side effects from radiation therapy include nausea, vomiting, anorexia, and dry mouth. The nurse encourages the client to maintain excellent oral hygiene. Hard candy may relieve dryness of the mouth. Small frequent meals often minimize the effects of nausea. The client is instructed to drink at least 1500 to 2000 mL of fluids each day. Citrus juices or other fluids with a high acid content are avoided if the client's oral cavity is irritated.

The treatments may cause a mild, temporary increase in ICP from cerebral edema, which can be treated with low-dose corticosteroids, such as dexamethasone. The client may experience an increase in fatigue during this time and is instructed to rest frequently. Any significant deterioration in the client's neurologic status needs to be reported to the physician.

Chemotherapy. Chemotherapy is used primarily as an adjunct to surgery. It may be given alone or in combination with radiation therapy or surgery. Although chemotherapeutic agents may be given intravenously, this method is not as effective and causes severe side effects that may outweigh the benefits. Usually, the medications are injected intrathecally or intraventricularly. The intrathecal injection of chemotherapeutic drugs is accomplished by withdrawing an equal amount of CSF as drug (usually 10 to 15 mL) to be given from the fourth or fifth lumbar space and injecting the chemotherapeutic agent into the subarachnoid space. A disadvantage of this method is that it results in an uneven distribution of the medication within the CSF and, consequently, a reduction in its effectiveness. An Ommaya reservoir is inserted to give intraventricular medication. The reservoir consists of a small-diameter catheter, which is placed in the anterior horn of the lateral ventricle, attached to a small mushroom-shaped reservoir (Fig. 33–21). To inject the medication, the physician or nurse aspirates a small amount of CSF (up to 5 mL) and then slowly injects the medication. After this step, the aspirated CSF is used to flush the reservoir and ensure that all medication enters the ventricle. This direct approach enhances the concentration of the chemotherapeutic agent in the brain.

Chemotherapeutic agents act by interfering with the reproductive cycle of the cells. They attack both cancer and normal cells. Because all cells are not in the process of reproduction at any given time, chemotherapy is best given in divided doses. It is also more effective when given in high doses. Brain tumors usually contain more than one type of cell, necessitating the use of a combination of drugs rather than one particular drug.

Side effects of chemotherapy include severe nausea, vomiting, diarrhea, and anorexia. Alopecia generally, but not always, occurs. Irritation of the oral mucosa is not uncommon. The client should be encouraged to maintain meticulous oral hygiene. Hard candy may relieve some of the discomfort caused by stomatitis. Antiemetics should be given before the chemotherapy and as often as needed at the completion of the treatment. If severe nausea and vomiting occur, the client may need IV fluid administration to maintain an adequate fluid intake.

Chemotherapy may cause bone marrow suppression. Consequently, the client's CBC must be monitored. In addition, the white blood cell count may be so low as to necessitate special precautions (protective isolation) to minimize the client's exposure to infections (see Chap. 25).

The factors that most influence the success or failure of chemotherapy include the client's age and neurologic status and the stage of the disease at diagnosis. Clients who are younger with few neurologic deficits and are diagnosed early in the course of the disease tend to have a better outcome. Another significant factor related to outcome is the type of tumor. Clients with gliomas, for example, have a less favorable outcome.

Surgical management. Surgical treatment of a brain tumor involves performing a *craniotomy*. In this procedure, a skin incision is made and muscle is stripped away from the skull. Next, four or five bur holes are drilled into the skull. The bone between the bur holes is cut, using a bone saw called a craniotome. The bone flap is turned down or completely removed. If the bone is removed the procedure is more correctly referred to as a craniectomy. After the bone flap is secured, the dura is incised and the brain exposed.

Conventional dissection, laser, or a stereotaxic approach may be used, depending on tumor type, size, and location. A conventional dissection involves cutting through the brain and blood vessels to expose the tumor. The tumor is excised, using suction and conventional surgical instruments. Often, the surgeon elects to use a laser to remove the tumor after it has been exposed. The laser acts by emitting carbon dioxide, a low-wave element, which is absorbed by water within the tissue and converted to heat. Water within the intracellular and extracellular tissues reaches a flash boiling point and the tissue is vaporized. The advantage of the laser is that minimal damage occurs to normal tissue, and less edema occurs. In addition, blood loss is minimized, as small vessels are coagulated during the application of the laser beam to the tumor. A stereotaxic procedure is used to treat deeply embedded small tumors or tumors close to vital centers that are not amenable to more conventional approaches. The procedure involves the placement of a stereotaxic ring, CT scan, and surgery. The ring is secured to the client's skull by four stainless steel pins. Next, a CT scan of the head is done. Using a specialized computer program, the exact location of the tumor is determined. The stereotaxic ring is adjusted to enable the surgeon to later place a probe through the frame directly into the tumor. The client is taken to the operating room after the ring is fixed to the skull and placement is verified by CT scan. A craniotomy or bur hole is performed, and the dura is incised. The probe and cutting devices are inserted through the

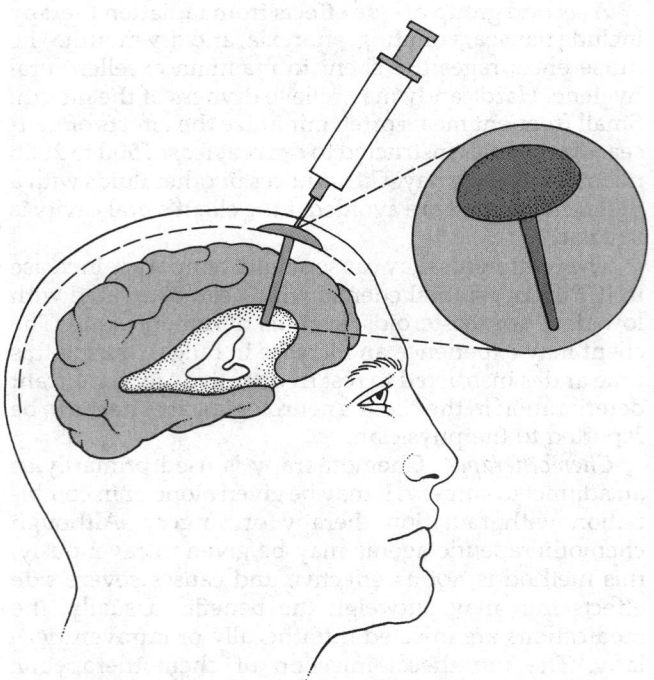

Figure 33–21

Ommaya reservoir used to inject chemotherapeutic agents directly into the CNS.

ring and into the brain tissue; the tumor is excised or tissue biopsies are taken. The procedure may also be used for implantation of interstitial radiation to treat malignant gliomas.

Preoperative care.   The nurse should be present when the physician explains the procedure to the client to ensure that consistent information is provided during the preoperative teaching sessions conducted by the nurse. The nurse encourages the client to ask questions and reassures the client that questions and fears are normal. Information presented to the client includes who will perform the surgery; where, when, and what will be done; where the client will go after surgery (e.g., recovery room or critical care unit); what the client's role is, and when the family will be permitted to visit. The client's head will be shaved, and plans for an appropriate head covering should be made before surgery if appropriate. The family should be told exactly where they should wait during surgery. Most clients are admitted to the critical care unit after surgery. When possible, the family and the client should tour the unit or meet the nurses who will provide postoperative care. The family should be informed that they will not be able to see the client immediately after admission to the unit; it usually takes 1 hour or more for the critical care nurse to complete the admission assessment and stabilize the client.

Postoperative care.   The focus of postoperative nursing interventions is to stabilize the client, detect changes in status, and prevent or minimize complications. The client's neurologic and vital signs are assessed every 30 minutes for the first 4 to 6 hours after surgery and then every hour. If the client is stable for 24 hours, the frequency of these checks may be decreased to every 2 to 4 hours. Potential neurologic deficits include decreased level of consciousness, motor weakness or paralysis, aphasia, visual changes, and personality changes. Periorbital edema and ecchymosis of one or both eyes is not unusual and is treated with cold compresses. The nurse irrigates the affected eyes with warm saline solution or artificial tears to improve the client's comfort.

The client in the critical care unit is routinely connected to the cardiac monitor and observed for arrhythmias. Arrhythmias may occur after posterior fossa surgery or be due to fluid and electrolyte imbalance. Other nursing interventions include strict recording of the client's intake and output and a fluid intake restriction to 1500 mL/day. ROM exercises to all extremities are performed at least once per nursing shift. The client is assisted to turn, cough, and deep breathe every 2 hours. Antiembolism stockings are worn until the client is ambulatory to prevent the development of deep venous thrombosis.

The client should not be positioned on the operative site, especially if the bone flap has been removed, as the brain has no bony covering on the affected site. The head of the bed is elevated 30 to 45 degrees to promote venous drainage from the client's head. The nurse positions the client to avoid extreme hip or neck flexion and maintains the head in a midline, neutral position.

The head dressing is checked frequently for signs of drainage. The area of drainage is marked once during each nursing shift for baseline comparison. A small or moderate amount of drainage is to be expected. Many clients have a Hemovac or Jackson-Pratt surgical drain in place for 24 hours after surgery. This drainage is measured during each nursing shift and the amount and color recorded; a typical amount of drainage is 30 to 50 mL/shift. Manufacturer and physician instructions should be followed to maintain the suction within the Hemovac or other type of drain. Excessive amounts of drainage (saturated head dressing or greater than 50 mL/shift) should be reported immediately to the physician.

Laboratory studies that are followed postoperatively include CBC, serum electrolyte levels and osmolarity, PT and PTT, and arterial blood gas measurements. The client's hematocrit and hemoglobin concentration may be abnormally low from blood loss during surgery or perhaps elevated if the blood loss was replaced. Hyponatremia may occur as a result of fluid volume overload, SIADH, or steroid administration. Hypokalemia may cause cardiac irritability. Weakness, change in level of consciousness, and confusion are symptoms of hyponatremia and hypokalemia. Hypernatremia may be caused by meningitis, dehydration, or diabetes insipidus. It is manifested by muscle weakness, restlessness, extreme thirst, and dry mouth. If untreated, hypernatremia may lead to seizure activity. Arterial blood gas values are monitored to ensure adequate cerebral oxygenation.

Often, the client is electively mechanically ventilated and hyperventilated for the first 24 to 48 hours after surgery to prevent increased ICP. The goal of hyperventilation is to maintain the client's arterial carbon dioxide level at 25 mmHg, with normal arterial oxygen levels. If the client is awake or attempting to breathe at a rate other than that set on the ventilator, medications such as fentanyl (Sublimaze) are given. The client who is intubated is suctioned if indicated by the findings of frequent respiratory assessments. The nurse remembers to hyperoxygenate the client before suctioning.

Medications.   Medications routinely given postoperatively include anticonvulsants, antacids or histamine receptors, and corticosteroids. Analgesics such as codeine are given for pain and acetaminophen is given for fever or mild pain. Some physicians may elect to administer prophylactic antibiotics to prevent infection.

Prevention of complications.   The major postoperative complication is *increased ICP* from cerebral edema, hemorrhage, or obstruction of the normal flow of CSF. Symptoms of increased ICP include severe headache, deteriorating level of consciousness, restlessness, irritability, and dilated or pinpoint pupils that are slow to react or nonreactive to light. Other symptoms include increased motor weakness, seizure activity, and, late in the postoperative recovery process, bradycardia and hypertension. Without prompt recognition and treatment, herniation syndromes develop and the client could expire.

Treatment of increased ICP includes placing the client supine with the head of the bed elevated 30 to 45 degrees, unless contraindicated. The client's head should be maintained in a midline, neutral position to facilitate venous drainage from the brain. Osmotic diuretics such as mannitol (Osmitrol), glucocorticoids, or loop diuretics may be given to decrease cerebral edema. After CT or other diagnostic tests to determine the exact cause of increased ICP, the client may be connected to a respirator and hyperventilated. An ICP monitoring device may be inserted to more accurately measure ICP. Surgery may be needed to correct the problem (e.g., hematoma) or to relieve pressure. Treatment of increased ICP is discussed more fully earlier.

Cerebral edema is frequently present before surgery and may be further increased by tissue manipulation during the surgical procedure. Edema usually reaches a peak within 72 hours after surgery and, if no further complications occur, gradually subsides over the next few weeks. Cerebral edema is manifested by a change in the level of consciousness and other symptoms of increased ICP.

Subdural and epidural hematomas and intracranial hemorrhage are manifested by severe headache, change in level of consciousness, progressive neurologic deficits, and herniation syndromes. Bleeding into the posterior fossa may lead to sudden cardiovascular and respiratory arrest. Treatment of a hematoma requires surgical removal, whereas an intracranial hemorrhage is treated with aggressive medical management (e.g., osmotic diuretics and ICP monitoring).

Hypovolemic shock is caused by loss of blood during or after surgery, inadequate replacement of fluid loss, or dehydration from fluid restriction or osmotic diuretics. The client in shock has a rapid, thready pulse; hypotension; pallor; and cold, clammy skin. Treatment consists of replacing the lost fluid volume.

Hydrocephalus is caused by obstruction of the normal CSF pathway from edema, an expanding lesion such as a hematoma, or blood in the subarachnoid space. Rapidly progressive hydrocephalus produces the classic symptoms of increased ICP. Slowly progressive hydrocephalus is manifested by headache, decreased level of consciousness, irritability, blurred vision, and urinary incontinence. Often, this is self-limiting and resolves without any treatment or with daily lumbar punctures to remove CSF. If treatment is required, a surgical shunt is inserted to drain CSF to another area of the body. Usually, a ventriculoperitoneal, or, less often, a ventriculoatrial or lumbar peritoneal shunt procedure is performed. A major complication of a shunting procedure is a subdural hematoma from tearing of bridging veins. Additional information about shunts may be found in the literature about critical care.

Respiratory complications include atelectasis, pneumonia, and neurogenic pulmonary edema. Atelectasis and pneumonia can be prevented by providing appro-

priate pulmonary hygiene, frequent turning, and encouraging the client to take several deep breaths to expand the lungs each hour. Humidified air and incentive spirometry are useful techniques to treat these complications. Other treatment modalities include endotracheal or oral tracheal suctioning and chest physiotherapy. Although these measures may cause an increase in the client's ICP, their benefit may outweigh the potential risk involved.

Neurogenic pulmonary edema is a life-threatening complication of neurosurgical procedures that infrequently occurs. Its symptoms are the same as those of acute pulmonary edema; however, there are no associated cardiac problems. In spite of aggressive treatment, most clients with neurogenic pulmonary edema do not survive the insult.

Wound infections occur more often in older and debilitated clients and those with a history of diabetes, long-term steroid use, obesity, and previous infections. The client may contribute to the problem by rubbing or scratching the wound. If infection is present, the wound appears reddened and puffy. It may begin to separate, is sensitive to touch, and feels warm. The client may or may not be febrile. Treatment is based on the degree and extent of the infection. A localized infection may be treated by simply cleaning with alcohol or applying local antibiotics. For more severe infection, systemic antibiotics may be required. If the underlying bone is involved, it may need to be removed.

Meningitis is an inflammation of the meninges and may occur as a result of wound infection, a CSF leak, or contamination during surgery. The reader is referred to the discussion of meningitis earlier for a more complete explanation of this complication.

Complications related to fluid and electrolyte imbalance include diabetes insipidus and SIADH. Diabetes insipidus is seen most often after surgery on the pituitary gland or in the area of the hypothalamus or third ventricle. Failure of the posterior pituitary gland to secrete ADH leads to failure of the renal tubules to reabsorb water. The client's urinary output increases dramatically (may be up to 10 L/day) and the urine specific gravity drops to below 1.005. Urine osmolarity decreases, whereas serum osmolarity increases. The client may become dehydrated and if this condition is left untreated, hypovolemic shock develops. If fluid replacement fails to correct the problem, synthetic ADH may be given. Vasopressin (Pitressin) tannate in oil is effective for up to 24 to 36 hours. Aqueous vasopressin is short-acting, lasting only 6 to 8 hours. For long-term replacement therapy, desmopressin acetate (DDAVP) or lypressin (Diapid) may be used. The client receiving a synthetic ADH preparation must be closely monitored for water intoxication, as manifested by muscle cramps, restlessness, seizure activity, and coma.

SIADH occurs when the posterior pituitary gland secretes too much ADH, causing water retention. The client becomes anuric, with a urinary output of less than 20 mL/hour. Sodium concentration in the urine is normal or elevated, whereas serum sodium level falls. Other indications of SIADH are loss of thirst, irritability, muscle weakness, and decreased level of consciousness.

Clients with complications related to fluid and electrolyte imbalance have strict measurement of their intake and output. Daily weight measurement is an essential aspect of treatment. The client must be assessed carefully for indications of fluid overload or dehydration throughout the treatment process. Serum electrolyte levels and osmolarity are measured daily or more often if clinically indicated.

Other treatment modalities. Experimental treatment modalities are currently under investigation in several medical centers around the country. Hyperthermia is used to treat malignant gliomas as an adjunct to conventional therapy. This treatment involves implanting catheters into the tumor bed and applying heat. The tumor bed is "heated" for 3 of every 4 hours, for a total treatment time of 72 hours.

Interstitial radiation treatment involves implanting radium isotopes directly into the tumor, most often a malignant glioma. This treatment modality requires the nurse to implement special techniques to prevent overexposure to radiation (see Chap. 25).

Pain

Planning: client goals. The major goal for this diagnosis is that the client will be free of pain.

Interventions: nonsurgical management. Before the administration of analgesics, the severity, location, and extent of the headache should be assessed. Analgesics, such as codeine phosphate and acetaminophen, are usually sufficient to relieve the discomfort from surgery. Brain tissue has no pain receptors; therefore, stronger analgesics are usually not necessary. The client with a severe headache accompanied by nausea or vomiting should be assessed for other indicators of increased ICP.

Potential for Injury

Planning: client goals. The major goal for this diagnosis is that the client will be free of injury from seizures.

Interventions: nonsurgical management. The postoperative craniotomy client is at risk for seizure activity. Anticonvulsants, such as phenytoin, are given prophylactically. Routine seizure precautions are instituted, including keeping the bed in the lowest position with side rails up and placing suction equipment and an airway at the bedside. In the event of a seizure, the client should be turned on either side and protected from injury. A padded tongue blade or other object should never be forced into the client's mouth during a seizure. The nurse documents the seizure according to the guidelines discussed earlier.

The client with an altered level of consciousness or visual problems must be protected from injury. Nursing interventions include placing the call light within easy reach; frequent visual checking of the client; using a seat belt when the client is sitting in a chair, or keeping the side rails up while the client is in bed; and placing objects within the client's reach. The client with an alteration in level of consciousness usually benefits from a quiet, nonstimulating environment. The nurse frequently orients the client to time, place, and event throughout the day. When possible a normal day-night cycle should be maintained. For example, the television or radio should be off at night and the lights turned down.

Anxiety; Fear

Planning: client goals. The major goals for the diagnoses are that the client will (1) communicate his/her thoughts and feelings regarding the diagnosis and treatment and (2) state that anxiety and fear have lessened.

Interventions: nonsurgical management. The nurse encourages the client and the family to discuss their concerns regarding the diagnosis and treatment and reassures them that these feelings are normal. Preoperative and postoperative teaching are essential to provide the client and the family with the information they need to fully participate in the treatment plan. In addition, this knowledge often reduces the anxiety and fear associated with the unknowns (e.g., "Will my hair be removed?" "Will I be given pain medicine?"). Questions out of the scope of nursing practice should be referred to the physician. To ensure that the client and the family have the information they need, the nurse assists them to develop a list of questions to ask the physician. The nurse should advise the physician of the client's concerns to enable the surgeon to plan sufficient time to answer these questions at the next visit. The client with unresolved anxieties and fears may require the services of a psychologist, a clinical specialist in mental health nursing, or a clinical social worker.

■ Discharge Planning

The client with a brain tumor is usually discharged to home. Clients with residual neurologic deficits may be discharged to a rehabilitation facility, usually on a short-term basis. If the tumor was malignant, radiation or chemotherapy may be given on an outpatient basis.

Home Care Preparation

Unless the client has a permanent disability, no special home care preparation is needed. Clients with hemiparesis need assistance to ensure that their home is accessible, depending on their method of mobility (e.g., cane, walker, or wheelchair). The environment should be made safe to prevent falls. For example, scatter rugs should be removed and grab bars placed in the bathroom.

Information concerning the selection of a rehabilitation facility can be obtained from the social worker. The facility selected should have experience providing care for the neurologically impaired client. It is also important that a psychologist formally trained in the administration of neuropsychologic testing be available to provide input into the interdisciplinary treatment team evaluation regarding the cognitive disabilities often exhibited by the client.

Client/Family Education

It is important that the client and the family fully understand the importance of any recommended follow-up health care appointments. The date, time, and place should be written on a card and given to the client. The nursing discharge summary should state the name of the person who was given follow-up information.

The client should receive instructions on all medications to be taken after discharge from the hospital. Information given to the client includes the name of the medication, the dosage, the timing of administration and number of days to take the medication, and any side effects. In addition, the client is instructed on what to do or who to call if any adverse reactions occur. The client is taught to refrain from taking any OTC medication unless authorized by the physician.

The client is instructed to maintain a program of regular physical exercise within the limits of any disabilities. Referral to the dietitian may be necessary to ensure adequate caloric intake for the client receiving radiation or chemotherapy.

Seizures are a potential complication that can occur at any time for as long as 1 year or more postoperatively. The nurse provides the client and the family with information about seizure precautions and what to do should a seizure occur.

Psychosocial Preparation

Recent literature reports that many clients who have undergone a craniotomy experience subtle cognitive or emotional changes (Hannegan, 1989). These changes, if any, should be identified before discharge to enable the family or caretaker to develop strategies to manage these problems.

Health Care Resources

The client and the family should be referred to the Association for Brain Tumor Research and the local chapter of the NHIF. Home care agencies are available to provide both physical and rehabilitative care the client may need.

 Evaluation

On the basis of the identified nursing diagnoses, the nurse evaluates the care of the client with a brain tumor. The expected outcomes include that the client

1. Maintains an adequate cerebral perfusion
2. Experiences an improvement in level of consciousness and neurologic status
3. Experiences no seizures
4. Remains free of injury
5. States that pain is relieved
6. Maintains compliance with follow-up treatments and appointments
7. Maintains compliance with medications
8. Verbalizes feelings of anxiety and fear and implements strategies to reduce or eliminate them

By meeting the expected outcomes the client should be able to fully participate in community living within the limits of any neurologic deficits that may be present.

SUMMARY

The nervous system is the basis for all human function. It is the center of thinking, memory, judgment, sensation, movement, cognition, communication, behavior, and personality. In addition to its direct control over many processes, the nervous system innervates many other body systems and thus indirectly influences their functions. For example, damage to the spinal nerves that innervate the diaphragm may result in respiratory arrest. Clients with neurologic dysfunction may be encountered throughout the health care system in various settings, including the acute care hospital, the ambulatory care center, the rehabilitation facility, and the home. Disorders of the nervous system can range from acute life-threatening emergencies to chronic, long-term conditions resulting in significant impairments, disability, or handicap. Therefore, the nurse employs numerous skills when caring for clients with these conditions.

IMPLICATIONS FOR RESEARCH

Research in the area of CNS dysfunction is expanding with the development of sophisticated technology that allows measurement of neuronal function in the body. Studies that examine the physiology of increasing ICP have recently been undertaken by nurse physiologists, but broader research to validate nursing diagnoses and nursing interventions for clients with CNS problems is needed.

Possible questions for future nursing research include the following:

1. What is the best method for communicating with a client with a CVA?

2. What effects do routine nursing tasks have on ICP?

3. What are the most effective nondrug pain management modalities for the client experiencing a migraine headache?

4. How can the nurse best assist the client with Parkinson's disease to maintain positive self-esteem and body image?

REFERENCES AND READINGS

Headaches

Amery, W. K., & Vandenbergh, V. (1987). What can precipitating factors teach us about the pathogenesis of migraine? *Headache, 27,* 146–150.

Derman, H. (1988). Migraine headache: Old, newer, and new treatments. *Consultant, 28,* 31–38.

Diamond, S. (1988). Headaches that herald intracranial emergencies. *Emergency Medicine, 20,* 20–32.

Diamond, S., & Shapiro, D. B. (1983). Cluster headaches. *Neurology and Neurosurgery Update Series, 4,* 1–8.

Eating to prevent migraine. (1988). *Patient Care, 22,* 147–148.

Kirn, T. (1987). Discussion, ideas abound in migraine research, consensus remains elusive. *Journal of the American Medical Association, 257,* 9–12.

Smith, L. S. (1988). Evaluation and management of the muscle contraction headache. *Nurse Practitioner, 13,* 20–27.

Whitney, C. M., & Daroff, R. B. (1988). An approach to migraine. *Journal of Neuroscience Nursing, 20,* 284–289.

Cerebrovascular Accident

Bronstein, K., Murray, P., Licata-Gehr, E., Banko, M., Kelly-Hayes, M., Fast, S., & Kunitz, S. (1986). Stroke Data Bank project: Implications for nursing research. *Journal of Neuroscience Nursing, 18,* 132–134.

Doolittle, N. D. (1988). Stroke recovery: Review of the literature and suggestions for future research. *Journal of Neuroscience Nursing, 20,* 169–173.

Hickey, J. (1985). *The clinical practice of neurological and neurosurgical nursing.* Philadelphia: J. B. Lippincott.

Hufler, D. R. (1987). Helping your dysphasic patient eat. *RN, 50*(9), 36–38.

Hummel, S. K. (1989). Cerebral vasospasm: Current concepts of pathogenesis and treatment. *Journal of Neuroscience Nursing, 21,* 216–224.

Lundgren, J. (1986). *Acute neuroscience nursing concepts and care.* Boston: Jones & Barlett.

Epilepsy

DeVroom, H., & Considine, E. P. (1987). Advances in localization of epileptic foci for surgical resection. *Journal of Neuroscience Nursing, 19,* 77–82.

Graham, O. (1989). A model for ambulatory care of patients with epilepsy and other neurological disorders. *Journal of Neuroscience Nursing, 21,* 108–112.

Hartshorn, J. (1986). Nursing interventions for anticonvulsant drug interactions. *Journal of Neuroscience Nursing, 18,* 250–256.

Santilli, N., & Sierzant, T. L. (1987). Advances in the treatment of epilepsy. *Journal of Neuroscience Nursing, 19,* 141–155.

Infections

Coderre, C. B. (1989). Meningitis: Dangers when the diagnosis is viral. *RN, 52*(8), 50–54.

Ellner, J. J. (1985). Central nervous system infection in the intensive care unit. In R. J. Henning & D. L. Jackson (Eds.), *Critical care neurology and neurosurgery.* (pp. 186–208). New York: Praeger.

Neatherlin, J. S. (1988). Creutzfeldt-Jacob disease. *Journal of Neuroscience Nursing, 20,* 309–313.

Prendergast, V. (1987). Bacterial meningitis update. *Journal of Neuroscience Nursing, 19,* 95–99.

Smith, D. W. (1989). Polio and postpolio sequelae: The lived experience. *Orthopaedic Nursing, 8,* 24–28.

Thompson, J. K., McFarland, G. K., Hirsch, J. E., Tucker, S. M., & Bowers, A. C. (1986). *Clinical nursing.* St. Louis: C. V. Mosby.

Multiple Sclerosis; Parkinson's Disease; Alzheimer's Disease; Huntington's Chorea; Amyotrophic Lateral Sclerosis

Berry, P., & Ward-Smith, P. (1988). Adrenal medullary transplant as a treatment for Parkinson's disease: Perioperative considerations. *Journal of Neuroscience Nursing, 20,* 356–361.

Burns, E. M., & Buckwalter, K. C. (1988). Pathophysiology and etiology of Alzheimer's disease. *Nursing Clinics of North America, 23,* 11–27.

Delgado, J., & Billo, J. M. (1988). Care of the patient with Parkinson's disease: Surgical and nursing interventions. *Journal of Neuroscience Nursing, 20,* 141–150.

Ferguson, J. M. (1987). Helping an MS patient live a better life. *RN, 50*(12), 22–27.

Gray-Vickrey, V. P. (1988). Evaluating Alzheimer's patients—the importance of being thorough. *Nursing '88, 18*(12), 34–41.

Holland, N., Francabandera, F., & Wiesel-Levinson, P. (1986). International scale for assessment of disability in multiple sclerosis. *Journal of Neuroscience Nursing, 18,* 39–44.

Hurwitz, A. (1988). The benefits of a home exercise regimen for ambulatory Parkinson's disease patients. *Journal of Neuroscience Nursing, 20,* 180–184.

Jackson, L. (1987). A predictive test for Huntington's disease: Recombinant DNA technology and implications for nursing. *Journal of Neuroscience Nursing, 19,* 244–250.

Kassier, M. R. (1987). Pain in multiple sclerosis. *American Journal of Nursing, 87,* 968–969.

Kelly, B. (1988). Nursing care of the patient with multiple sclerosis. *Rehabilitation Nursing, 13,* 238–243.

Lannon, M. C., Thomas, C. A., Bratton, M., Jost, M. G., & Lockhart-Pretti, P. (1986). Comprehensive care of the patient with Parkinson's disease. *Journal of Neuroscience Nursing, 18,* 121–131.

Samonds, R., & Cammermeyer, M. (1989). Perceptions of body image in subjects with multiple sclerosis: A pilot study. *Journal of Neuroscience Nursing, 20,* 190–194.

Swank, R., & Grimsgaard, A. (1988). MS: The lipid relationship. *American Journal of Clinical Nutrition, 48,* 1387.

Head Injury

Alves, W. M., Colohan, A. R. T., O'Leary, T., Rimel, R. W., & Jane, J. A. (1986). Understanding post traumatic symptoms after head injury. *Journal of Head Trauma Rehabilitation, 1,* 1–12.

Baggerly, J. (1986). Rehabilitation of the adult with a head trauma. *Nursing Clinics of North America, 21,* 577–587.

Bourdon, S. E. (1986). Psychological impact of neurotrauma in the acute care setting. *Nursing Clinics of North America, 21,* 629–640.

Burtkowski, H. M., & Lovely, M. P. (1986). Prognosis in coma and the persistent vegetative state. *Journal of Head Trauma Rehabilitation, 1,* 1–5.

Gardner, D. (1986). Acute management of the head injured adult. *Nursing Clinics of North America, 21,* 555–562.

Gennarelli, T. A. (1986). Mechanisms and pathology of cerebral concussion. *Journal of Head Trauma Rehabilitation, 1,* 23–29.

Germon, K. (1988). Interpretation of ICP waves to determine intracerebral compliance. *Journal of Neuroscience Nursing, 20,* 344–349.

Hegeman, K. M. (1988). A care plan for the family of a brain trauma client. *Rehabilitation Nursing, 13,* 254–258.

Hinkle, J. (1988). Nursing care of patients with minor head injury. *Journal of Neuroscience Nursing, 20,* 8–14.

Jennett, B. (1983). Scale and scope of the problem. In M. Rosenthal, E. Griffith, M. Bond, & J. D. Miller (Eds.), *Rehabilitation of the head injured adult.* Philadelphia: F. A. Davis.

Jennett, B., & Teasdale, G. (1984). *Management of head injuries.* Philadelphia: F. A. Davis.

Nikas, D. (1987). Critical aspects of head trauma. *Critical Care Nursing Quarterly, 10,* 19–44.

Palmer, M., & Wyness, M. A. (1988). Positioning and handling: Important considerations in care of the severely head injured patient. *Journal of Neuroscience Nursing, 20,* 39–42.

Pollack-Latham, C. L. (1988). Intracranial pressure monitor-ing: Part I, physiologic principles. *Critical Care Nurse, 7,* 40–52.

Pollack-Latham, C. L. Intracranial pressure monitoring: Part II, patient care. *Critical Care Nurse, 7,* 53–72.

Rimel, R. W., & Jane, J. A. (1983). Characteristics of the head injured patient. In M. Rosenthal, E. Griffith, M. Bond, & J. D. Miller (Eds.), *Rehabilitation of the head injured adult* (pp. 9–22). Philadelphia: F. A. Davis.

Walleck, C. W. (1989). Controversies in the management of the head injured patient. *Critical Care Nursing Clinics of North America, 1,* 67–74.

Willis, D., & Drake-Harbit, M. (1989). A fatal attraction: Cocaine related subarachnoid hemorrhage. *Journal of Neuroscience Nursing, 20,* 171–174.

Spinal Cord Injury

Barker, E., & Higgins, R. (1989). Managing a suspected spinal cord injury. *Nursing '89, 19*(4), 52–59.

Browner, C. M., Hadley, M., Sonntag, V. K. H., & Mattingly, L. G. (1987). Halo immobilization brace care: An innovative approach. *Journal of Neuroscience Nursing, 19,* 24–30.

Lyons, M. (1987). Immune function in spinal cord injured males. *Journal of Neuroscience Nursing, 19,* 18–23.

Mathews, P. J., & Carlson, C. E. (1987). *Spinal cord injury: A guide to rehabilitation nursing.* Rockville, MD: Aspen Publishers.

Meyer, P. R., & Gireesan, G. T. (1987). Management of acute spinal cord injured patients by the Midwest regional spinal cord injury care system. *Topics of Acute Care and Trauma Rehabilitation, 1,* 1–31.

Zejdlik, C. M. (1983). *Management of spinal cord injury.* Monterey, CA: Wadsworth Health Sciences.

Brain Tumors

Bauman, C. K., & Zumwalt, C. B. (1989). Intracranial neoplasms: An overview. *AORN Journal, 50,* 240–256.

Cammermeyer, M., & Evans, J. E. (1988). A brief of neurobehavioral exam useful for detection of postoperative complications in neurosurgical patients. *Journal of Neuroscience Nursing, 20,* 314–323.

Hannegan, L. (1989). Transient cognitive changes after craniotomy. *Journal of Neuroscience Nursing, 21,* 165–169.

Harper, J. (1988). Use of steroids in cerebral edema: Therapeutic implications. *Heart and Lung, 17,* 70–73.

Hodges, K. (1988). Meningioma, astrocytoma, germinoma: Case presentations of 3 intracranial tumors. *Journal of Neuroscience Nursing, 21,* 113–121.

Markin, D. A. (1986). Preoperative concerns of the patient undergoing craniotomy. *Journal of Neuroscience Nursing, 18,* 275–278.

Mitchen, H. L. (1984). A CT guided stereotactic apparatus: A new approach to biopsy and removal of brain tumors. *Journal of Neuroscience Nursing, 16,* 231–236.

Welsh, D. M., & Zumwalt, C. B. (1988). Volumetric interstitial hyperthermia: Nursing implications for brain tumor treatment. *Journal of Neuroscience Nursing, 20,* 229–235.

Zumwalt, C. B., & Bauman, C. K. (1989). Malignant glioma: A case study. *AORN Journal, 50,* 240–256.

ADDITIONAL READINGS

Franges, E. Z., & Beideman, M. E. (1988). Infections related to intracranial pressure monitoring. *Journal of Neuroscience Nursing, 20,* 94–103.

This article described one of the complications of ICP monitoring —infection. Placing a foreign object into the ventricles of the brain allows invasion of bacteria or other organisms into the body. Encephalitis and meningitis are two of the infections discussed.

Lanuza, D., Robinson, C. R., Marotta, S. F., & Patel, M. K. (1989). Body temperature and heart rate rhythms in acutely head-injured patients. *Applied Nursing Research,* 2(3), 135–139.

This descriptive nursing research examined the circadian rhythms of heart rate and temperature in clients with head injuries and investigated if there was any relationship between these variables. Using a convenience sample of 10 clients, the researchers did not find rhythm disruptions in these clients, but noted a low correlation between the study variables.

Reimer, M. (1989). Head injured patients: How to detect early signs of trouble. *Nursing '89,* 19(3), 34–41.

This article described some of the subtle changes that the nurse must assess for in a client with a suspected head injury. In addition, complications of untreated head injury were discussed with practical nursing interventions.

Spica, M. M. (1989). Sexual counseling standards for the spinal cord injured. *Journal of Neuroscience Nursing, 21,* 56–59.

Counseling the client with a spinal cord injury is often difficult. Most of the injuries occur in young men unexpectedly from trauma, usually a motor vehicle or diving accident. This article provided practical, accurate information to guide the nurse or other health care professional when counseling these clients.

CHAPTER 34

Interventions for Clients with Peripheral Nervous System Disorders

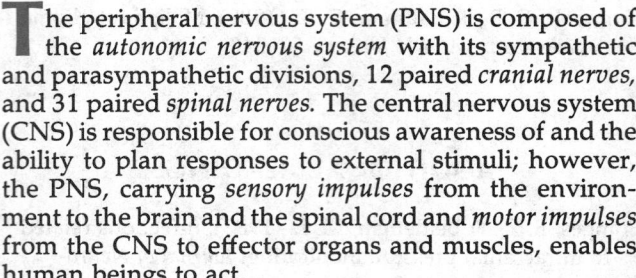

The peripheral nervous system (PNS) is composed of the *autonomic nervous system* with its sympathetic and parasympathetic divisions, 12 paired *cranial nerves,* and 31 paired *spinal nerves.* The central nervous system (CNS) is responsible for conscious awareness of and the ability to plan responses to external stimuli; however, the PNS, carrying *sensory impulses* from the environment to the brain and the spinal cord and *motor impulses* from the CNS to effector organs and muscles, enables human beings to act.

PNS disorders range in severity from life-threatening conditions, such as *Guillain-Barré syndrome* and *myasthenia gravis* (which may require intensive nursing care), to relatively benign conditions, such as *polyneuritis, peripheral nerve trauma,* and *cranial nerve disorders,* (e.g., *trigeminal neuralgia* and *Bell's palsy*). Although hospitalization is rarely required for these less serious dysfunctions, the nurse may encounter them as secondary disorders in hospitalized individuals, as well as in clients in outpatient (ambulatory) or community settings. These conditions may be extremely painful, and disfigurement may result. Often, these less serious PNS conditions are so irritating and annoying that help is desperately sought by those affected.

GUILLAIN-BARRÉ SYNDROME

OVERVIEW

Guillain-Barré syndrome is also called acute idiopathic polyneuritis, infectious polyneuritis, acute immune-mediated polyneuritis, Landry-Guillain-Barré-Stohl syndrome, Landry's paralysis, polyradiculoneuropathy, acute polyradiculitis, acute polyneuropathy, and acute inflammatory demyelinating polyradiculoneuropathy. It is a condition in which the client's life and ultimate potential for rehabilitation depend almost entirely on the effectiveness of nursing care. The nurse's expertise in providing individualized care, monitoring for and preventing complications, and offering emotional support for the client and significant others is essential, for with skilled care, the mortality rate can be as low as 1.5% (Miller, 1985).

Pathophysiology

Segmental demyelination, the destruction of myelin between the nodes of Ranvier (see Chap. 32, Fig. 32–1), is the major pathologic finding in Guillain-Barré syndrome. *Saltatory conduction,* the leaping of impulses from node to node of Ranvier, is thus affected, leading to dispersion of impulses, slow conduction velocities, or conduction block in the late stages of the disease. Because the more heavily myelinated cranial and motor nerves are affected more frequently than the thinly myelinated pain, touch, and temperature nerve fibers, sensory functions may be spared. Microscopically, aggregates of lymphocytes are seen at the points of myelin breakdown, yet the axons usually remain intact. In some instances, there may be secondary damage to the cell body, the neurolemma, or the axon, resulting in delayed recovery or permanent deficits.

Three stages have been identified in the *acute course* of Guillain-Barré syndrome: (1) the *initial period,* which begins with the onset of the first definitive symptom and ends when no further deterioration is noted, is usually 1 to 3 weeks; (2) a *plateau period* lasts from several days to 2 weeks; and (3) the *recovery phase,* which is thought to coincide with remyelination and axonal regeneration, lasts 4 to 6 months. Clients who have sustained axonal injury require more extensive rehabilitation. In this case, rehabilitation may last up to 2 years, and complete recovery may not occur.

Etiology

The cause of Guillain-Barré syndrome remains obscure, although most of the evidence implicates a cell-mediated immunologic reaction. Research suggests that the humoral immune system is involved as well. Defects of T lymphocytes (T cells) and B lymphocytes (B cells) of the lymphatic system are thought to be the basis of the syndrome. T cells are responsible for cell-mediated immunity and the phagocytosis of bacteria. B lymphocytes produce and secrete immunoglobulins, which form the humoral arm of the immune system. Normally, these antibodies combine with antigens, such as viruses, and prevent the organisms from having a harmful effect. This antigen-antibody combination also induces an inflammatory reaction by attracting T cells.

Frequently, the client with Guillain-Barré syndrome relates a history of acute illness, trauma, surgery, or immunization 1 to 4 weeks before the onset of neurologic signs and symptoms. Other risk factors that have emerged from epidemiologic studies include an upper respiratory tract infection or gastrointestinal (GI) illness in 50% of cases and positive antibodies to cytomegalovirus or Epstein-Barr virus. Vaccinations have been implicated in 15% of cases, with a significant number of cases occurring after inoculation for swine influenza (Koski et al., 1986). It is believed that the prodromal event causes a limited malfunction of the immune system, sensitizing the T cells to the client's myelin. Apparently, in response to several antigens, some clients form a demyelinating antibody that has a direct toxic effect on nerves or attracts a cellular immune response, which ultimately destroys myelin (Griswold et al., 1984).

Incidence

The annual incidence of Guillain-Barré syndrome ranges from 0.6 to 1.9 cases per 100,000 population in the United States (Koski et al., 1986). It has worldwide distribution, is not seasonal, and affects persons of all races and ages. Higher rates, however, have been noted among persons 45 years of age or older, among Caucasians as opposed to Blacks (50% to 60% higher among Caucasians), and among men as opposed to women (Koski et al., 1986). Guillain-Barré syndrome is the most common cause of acute weakness in clients younger than 40 years of age.

In 3% to 10% of cases, clients develop a chronic or recurrent Guillain-Barré syndrome, which has been linked to the use of immunosuppressive agents, such as corticosteroids (e.g., prednisone) or cyclophosphamide (Cytoxan), for the treatment of this disorder.

COLLABORATIVE MANAGEMENT

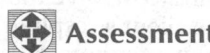 **Assessment**

History

In addition to biographical data, such as *age, sex,* and *race,* the nurse collects a complete medical and surgical history. The occurrence of any *antecedent illness* (infection or other illness) 3 to 4 weeks before the onset of Guillain-Barré syndrome is explored. A *description of the symptoms,* in the client's own words (if possible) and in chronologic order, is elicited.

Physical Assessment: Clinical Manifestations

Although many variations may be encountered, most individuals relate an *abrupt onset of symptoms, paresthesias* (numbness or tingling), *pain* resembling that of a charley horse or a deep strain, *facial weakness, difficulty walking, motor weakness,* and less often, problems controlling *bladder or bowel function.* In addition, the sensory and motor disturbances are most often described as having characteristic clinical patterns — usually ascending, distal to proximal. Neurologic symptoms may be summarized as muscle weakness or flaccid paralysis without muscle atrophy, paresthesias or other sensory changes, and, in some cases, *autonomic dysfunction,* evidenced by *orthostatic hypotension* or *tachycardia.* The syndrome is fairly, although not precisely, symmetric and includes *decreased or absent deep tendon reflexes* and *cranial nerve involvement* evidenced by *facial weakness, dysphagia* (difficulty swallowing), and *diplopia* (double vision). *Respiratory compromise or failure* is a common complication if the respiratory musculature is affected, and the nurse assesses the client at frequent, regular intervals for dyspnea, decreased breath sounds on auscultation, and decreasing tidal volume and vital capacity. Guillain-Barré syndrome does not affect the client's level of consciousness, cerebral function, or pupillary signs.

Several clinical variations, which reflect the areas of earliest or most severe involvement, have been identified. *Ascending* Guillain-Barré syndrome is the most common clinical pattern, with weakness and paresthesias beginning in the lower extremities and progressing upward to include the trunk and arms or affect the cranial nerves. The nurse may observe an ascending flaccidity, or weakness, evolving over a period of hours to several days (1 to 10 days), with the extent of motor deficit ranging from mild paresis to total quadriplegia. In about 50% of these cases, the nurse observes some degree of respiratory compromise. Although diminished during the initial examination, deep tendon reflexes are absent in limbs that become paralyzed. *Pure motor* Guillain-Barré syndrome is identical to the ascending variant, except sensory signs and symptoms are absent.

In clients with *descending* Guillain-Barré syndrome, the nurse initially observes weakness of the face or bulbar muscles of the jaw, the sternocleidomastoid muscles (head rotators), and the muscles of the tongue, pharynx, and larynx, which progresses downward to involve the limbs. This type may quickly affect the client's respiratory function, and the nurse carefully monitors the client for breathlessness during speech, shallow respirations, dyspnea, and decreased tidal volume. In addition, this variation often includes *ophthalmoplegia* (paralysis of the eye muscles), causing diplopia, or, if the pupillary response to light is affected, functional blindness may result. Thus, the nurse assesses visual function, while providing information, explanation, and support to the client experiencing visual disturbances. In this variation, numbness is more common in the hands than in the feet. Decreased or absent deep tendon reflexes occur.

The *Miller-Fisher variant* consists of a triad of *ophthalmoplegia, areflexia,* and *severe ataxia.* The nurse usually observes normal motor strength and intact sensory function. Occasionally, the nurse notes that the pupillary response to light is affected by the ophthalmoplegia, resulting in *functional blindness.* Although respiratory complications are rare in clients with this variant, *respiratory function* is monitored frequently.

With any of the variants, *cranial nerve* involvement most often affects the facial nerve (cranial nerve VII), resulting in the inability to smile, frown, whistle, or drink from a straw. In addition to monitoring these functions of cranial nerve VII, the nurse assesses for dysphagia and paralysis of the larynx. Less frequently affected cranial nerves include the glossopharyngeal (IX), vagus (X), spinal accessory (XI), and hypoglossal (XII). The client's inability to cough, gag, or swallow results from involvement of cranial nerves IX and X. In addition, the nurse closely monitors the client for varying blood pressures (hypertensive and hypotensive episodes or postural hypotension) and tachycardia, symptoms characteristic of *autonomic dysfunction,* which is linked to vagal nerve (X) deficit. The nurse assesses cranial nerve XI (spinal accessory) by asking the client to perform shoulder shrugs. Hypoglossal nerve (XII) deficit is evidenced by deviation or paralysis of the tongue.

Psychosocial Assessment

In addition to determining the client's usual roles and responsibilities, occupation, motivation, and available support systems, the nurse assesses the client's ability to cope with this devastating illness and the accompanying fear and anxiety. Research has identified psychologic accompaniments to the three phases of the syndrome discussed earlier. Severe anxiety, fear, and panic were found in the initial period when symptoms were progressing. During the plateau phase, anger and depression were observed. When improvement began, severe depression occurred as clients contemplated the long, slow recovery or permanent neurologic deficit. The nurse assesses the client during each of these phases by remaining alert to the speed and tone of voice, posture, and other body language, as well as physical symptoms, physical appearance, cognitive ability, and the client's verbalizations.

Laboratory Findings

Although there is no single clinical or laboratory finding that confirms the diagnosis of Guillain-Barré syndrome, lumbar puncture is performed for the evaluation of cerebrospinal fluid (CSF). Albuminocytologic dissociation, an increase in CSF protein level without an increase (or only a slight to moderate increase) in the cell count, is a distinguishing feature of Guillain-Barré syndrome; however, high protein levels may not be noted until after 1 to 2 weeks of illness, reaching a peak in 4 to 6 weeks. The CSF lymphocyte count is normal.

Peripheral blood tests may initially show a moderate leukocytosis early in the illness, which rapidly returns to normal levels in the absence of complications or concurrent illness. The erythrocyte sedimentation rate is typically within normal limits.

Other Diagnostic Tests

Electrophysiologic studies demonstrate demyelinating neuropathy, although the degree of abnormality found on testing does not always correlate with the clinical severity. Soon after paralysis develops, nerve conduction velocities are slowed, with denervated potentials (fibrillations) developing in some cases later in the illness. Electromyographic (EMG) findings, reflecting peripheral nerve function, are normal early in the illness; electrophysiologic changes appear only after denervation of muscle has been present for 4 weeks or longer.

Because respiratory function is frequently compromised in clients with Guillain-Barré syndrome, there may be decreased vital capacity and abnormal arterial blood gas values (decreased PO_2, increased PCO_2, or increased pH).

 Analysis: Nursing Diagnosis

Nursing diagnoses for clients with Guillain-Barré syndrome vary, depending on the severity of the illness and the phase of its clinical course.

Common Diagnoses

The following nursing diagnoses are seen in clients with Guillain-Barré syndrome:

1. Ineffective breathing pattern related to respiratory muscle weakness or paralysis

2. Ineffective airway clearance related to inability to cough and deep breathe

3. Impaired gas exchange related to respiratory muscular weakness or paralysis, immobility, or pulmonary congestion

4. Impaired physical mobility related to weakness, paralysis, and ataxia

5. Impaired skin integrity and potential impaired skin integrity related to altered sensation, altered nutrition, or immobility

6. Powerlessness related to the inability to perform activities of daily living (ADL) and usual role responsibilities

7. Anxiety related to powerlessness, uncertain prognosis, and fear of the unknown

8. Anticipatory grieving related to loss of function and inability to perform usual roles and responsibilities

9. Total self-care deficit related to inability to perform ADL unassisted

Additional Diagnoses

Many clients with Guillain-Barré syndrome may also have one or more of the following nursing diagnoses:

1. Knowledge deficit related to disease process, treatment, and outcome

2. Sensory/perceptual alterations (tactile, kinesthetic, and visual) related to paresthesias and diplopia

3. Impaired verbal communication related to cranial nerve paralysis

4. Body image disturbance and self-esteem disturbance related to loss of body function, physical changes, and dependency

5. Altered nutrition: less than body requirements related to difficulty chewing, dysphagia, paralysis of extremities, anxiety, or depression

6. Fluid volume deficit and potential fluid volume deficit related to cranial nerve paralysis, dysphagia, paralysis of the extremities

7. Constipation, diarrhea, and bowel incontinence related to inadequate oral intake, immobility, and impaired communication

8. Pain related to paresthesias or immobility

9. Decreased cardiac output related to autonomic dysfunction

 Planning and Implementation

Ineffective Breathing Pattern; Ineffective Airway Clearance; Impaired Gas Exchange

Although not all clients with Guillain-Barré syndrome experience respiratory compromise, assessment and maintenance of respiratory function are essential, especially during the initial phase when symptoms may be progressing rapidly.

Planning: client goals. The primary goal for these diagnoses is that the client will demonstrate effective air exchange as evidenced by clear lung sounds on auscultation, vital capacity within acceptable limits, and arterial blood gas levels within normal limits.

Interventions: nonsurgical management. In the acute (initial) phase, the nurse monitors the client closely, generally in a critical care unit, for signs of respiratory distress, such as dyspnea, air hunger, confusion (resulting from hypoxia), or subjective complaints of shortness of breath. In addition, the nurse monitors respiratory rate, rhythm, and depth every 1 to 4 hours; checks the client's temperature every 4 hours; and auscultates the lungs at 4-hour intervals. Arterial blood gas values are monitored for acid-base abnormalities and decreasing oxygen saturation. Generally, vital capacity is measured every 2 to 4 hours. Deterioration of vital capacity to less than 15 to 20 mL/kg and the inability to clear secretions may be indications for elective intubation. (See Chap. 62 for the care of a ventilator-dependent client.) Equipment for performing a tracheostomy and a ventilator are kept available in case of respiratory emergency.

The nurse maintains (or assists the client to maintain) a patent airway by correct positioning, suctioning, and adjusting endotracheal or nasotracheal airways. When suctioning, sterile technique is maintained to prevent infection, and the color, consistency, and amount of secretions are assessed and documented. Chest physiotherapy and frequent position changes are combined with breathing exercises (coughing and deep breathing) to prevent pneumonia and atelectasis. Administration of oxygen by nasal cannula may be prescribed at a flow rate determined by the physician.

Because pulmonary emboli are frequent complications of immobility, subcutaneous heparin injections may be prescribed every 12 hours. Antiembolism stockings may be used and may be removed every 8 hours by the nurse for 15 to 30 minutes to assess skin condition and circulation. Range-of-motion (ROM) exercises are performed every 2 to 4 hours, and the client is assisted in transfers from bed to chair as tolerated. A tilt table may be used to decrease severity of orthostatic hypotension.

Impaired Physical Mobility

Planning: client goals. The goals for this diagnosis are that the client will (1) participate, actively or passively, in mobilization and (2) not develop complications related to immobility.

Interventions: nonsurgical management. During the initial period, when symptoms may be developing rapidly, the nurse assesses motor function every 2 to 4 hours using a reproducible method that is readily understood by all members of the health care team. The Medical Research Council (MRC) Scale (Table 34–1) may be used to evaluate the specific muscle groups (Table 34–2). Nursing interventions to provide for mobility and prevent complications depend on the degree

---

TABLE 34 – 1 Medical Research Council Scale for Power Grading

---

0 No contraction

1 Flicker or trace of contraction

2 Active movement with gravity eliminated

3 Active movement against gravity

4 Active movement against gravity and resistance

5 Normal power

From Griswold, K., Guanci, M. M., & Ropper, A. H. (1984). An approach to the care of patients with Guillain-Barré syndrome. *Heart and Lung, 13*, 66–72.

of motor deficit. To ensure the client's safety, the nurse assists with ambulation, transfers from bed to chair, position changes, and maintenance of proper body alignment, always encouraging maximal independence. Gentle ROM exercises are performed actively or passively every 2 to 4 hours, and the nurse instructs family members in these techniques. Collaboration of the nurse with physical and occupational therapists enables continuity of care. (Chap. 22 discusses interventions for prevention of complications related to immobility.)

Drug therapy. Treatment of Guillain-Barré syndrome depends on ventilatory assistance and supportive nursing care, for, in the majority of cases, the disease is self-limiting and recovery is complete. Table 34–3 lists drugs used in the treatment of Guillain-Barré syndrome. Although a therapeutic trial of prednisone (Deltasone), 45 to 60 mg/day, may be utilized by some physicians, this treatment is controversial. Recent research suggests that administration of corticosteroids during

---

TABLE 34 – 2 Muscles Routinely Tested with the Medical Research Council Scale

---

Sternocleidomastoid: rotates head to opposite side

Deltoid: abducts arm

Triceps: extends forearm

Biceps: flexes and supinates forearm

Wrist dorsiflexors

Grasp ability

Iliopsoas: flexes hip

Hamstrings: flexes knee

Quadriceps: extends knee

Anterior tibialis: dorsiflexes and inverts foot

Gastrocnemius: plantar flexes foot

Extensor hallucis longus: extends great toe

From Griswold, K., Guanci, M. M., & Ropper, A. H. (1984). An approach to the care of patients with Guillain-Barré syndrome. *Heart and Lung, 13*, 66–72.

the acute phase of the syndrome may predispose the client to chronic Guillain-Barré syndrome and may counteract the effectiveness of plasmapheresis. Adrenocorticotropic hormone (ACTH), 25 to 40 units three times a day intramuscularly or subcutaneously, has been noted to shorten the syndrome's duration, although further investigation is needed to determine its therapeutic usefulness. Other immunosuppressive agents, such as cyclophosphamide (Cytoxan) and azathioprine (Imuran), have met with variable success.

Plasmapheresis. In plasmapheresis, plasma is selectively separated from whole blood, and its abnormal constituents are removed or the plasma is exchanged with normal plasma or a colloidal substitute. The use of this measure has led to reductions in the length of hospitalization, in the period of ventilatory dependency, and in the amount of time required for the client to resume walking. If instituted 3 weeks or longer after the onset of illness, however, the procedure seems to be of little value. In clients with chronic, recurrent Guillain-Barré syndrome, beneficial responses, although temporary, can be maintained with repeated plasmapheresis or with the addition of immunosuppressive therapy. Research suggests that an exchange of 200 to 250 mL/kg during 7 to 14 days (Koski et al., 1986), with a total of five exchanges of 3 L each during 8 to 10 days, is adequate for the normal-sized adult. Nursing care for the client undergoing plasmapheresis includes providing information and emotional support and monitoring the client for signs of complications (see the Guidelines feature on p. 967).

Impaired Skin Integrity; Potential Impaired Skin Integrity

Paresthesias and paralysis, with resulting inability to sense pressure and pain or to move independently, place the client at risk for skin breakdown. In addition, the client may be nutritionally compromised or incontinent of urine or feces, thus compounding the problem.

Planning: client goals. The goal for these nursing diagnoses is that the client will maintain skin integrity as evidenced by dry, intact skin surfaces.

Interventions: nonsurgical management. The client's motor and sensory function and skin condition (integrity, color, temperature, and turgor) are assessed by the nurse every 4 hours and as necessary. While monitoring for incontinence, the nurse assists the client to change position at intervals of 2 hours or less, massaging the skin and bony prominences with lotion to promote circulation. The skin is kept clean and dry, using a commercial skin wash and protective ointment after episodes of incontinence. The nurse keeps bed linens taut and free from wrinkles or ridges, minimizing excessive pressure on the client's bony prominences. Pressure prevention devices, such as cushions, flotation devices, eggcrate or alternating pressure mattresses, air-fluidized

TABLE 34-3 Drugs Used in the Treatment of Guillain-Barré Syndrome

Drug	Usual Daily Dosage	Interventions*	Rationales
ACTH (corticotropin, Acthar)	25–40 units tid IM or SC	1. ACTH treatment should be preceded by verification of adrenal function and tests for hypersensitivity. 2. Observe for and report exaggerated euphoria, insomnia, nervousness, and depression. 3. Provide low-sodium, high-potassium diet. Provide potassium supplements as prescribed. 4. Evaluate for concurrent disease or infection.	1. Drug cannot elicit a hormonal response from a nonfunctioning adrenal gland. 2. These are indications for dosage reduction or stopping the drug. Sedatives may be prescribed. 3. These measures minimize drug-induced edema and hypokalemia. 4. ACTH may mask the signs of chronic disease and decrease the client's resistance to and ability to localize infection.
Azathioprine (Imuran)	3–5 mg/kg daily initially PO; maintain at 1–2 mg/kg per d; varies according to client's response	1. Decrease the dosage to ¼ or ⅓ of normal dosage if client is also taking allopurinol. 2. Watch for clay-colored stools, dark urine, jaundice, and increased alkaline phosphatase, bilirubin, SGOT (AST), and ALT levels. 3. Monitor hemoglobin level, WBC, and platelet count weekly. 4. Advise client to avoid conception for at least 4 months after drug therapy. 5. Warn client that some alopecia may occur. 6. Avoid IM injections in clients with decreased platelet levels.	1. Allopurinol impairs the inactivation of azathioprine. 2. These indicate hepatotoxicity. 3. Drug may cause bone marrow suppression, leukopenia, anemia, and pancytopenia. 4. This agent is potentially teratogenic. 5. Nurse can allay anxiety over this side effect. 6. Bleeding may occur with IM injection.
Cyclophosphamide (Cytoxan, Procytox)	2–4 mg/kg per d for 10 d initially, then maintenance 1.5–3.0 mg/kg per d	1. Monitor client for leukopenia, thrombocytopenia, and hepatic or renal disease. 2. Give an antiemetic before drug administration. 3. Push fluids to 3 L/d. 4. Do not give the drug at bedtime. 5. Instruct the client to void frequently at night. 6. Monitor for hematuria, and instruct the client to continue this practice for several months after drug therapy. 7. Warn the client that alopecia may occur. 8. Administer anticoagulants cautiously. Watch for signs of bleeding. 9. Avoid IM injections if platelet count is low.	1. These are side effects of the drug. 2. Nausea is associated with the drug. 3, 4. Hemorrhagic cystitis is associated with the drug. 5. Frequent voiding prevents cystitis. 6. Cystitis can occur months after therapy has been stopped. 7. Nurse can allay anxiety over this side effect. 8. Thrombocytopenia is associated with the drug. 9. Bleeding may occur with IM injection.

Table continued on following page

TABLE 34-3 Drugs Used in the Treatment of Guillain-Barré Syndrome *Continued*

Drug	Usual Daily Dosage	Interventions*	Rationales
Prednisone (Deltasone, Meticorten, Orasone, Paracort)	45-60 mg/d, in 2-4 divided doses PO	1. Give with food, milk, or antacid, unless contraindicated. 2. Tell client not to discontinue drug abruptly. Gradually reduce dosage on physician's order after long-term therapy. 3. Titrate drug to lowest effective dosage on physician's order. 4. Monitor blood pressure, sleep patterns, and blood glucose and serum potassium levels. 5. Weigh client daily. Report sudden weight gain. 6. Give salt-restricted diet rich in potassium and administer potassium supplements on physician's order.	1. Drug causes peptic ulcer and GI irritation. 2. Sudden withdrawal may result in increased weakness, lethargy, depression, dyspnea, and fainting. 3. Side effects include GI irritation, euphoria, insomnia, edema, hypertension, hyperglycemia, and hypokalemia, which are dose dependent. 4. Side effects may require dosage adjustments. Diabetic clients may require increased insulin administration. 5. Drug causes edema and weight gain. 6. Salt increases fluid retention and potassium levels should be restored.

* SGOT, serum glutamic-oxaloacetic transaminase; ALT, alanine aminotransferase; AST, aspartate aminotransferase; WBC, white blood cell count.

mattresses (such as Clinitron), or low air-loss beds (such as Rotorest or Mediscus), may be utilized (see Chap. 22). The client's nutritional intake is monitored by the nurse in consultation with the dietitian. If necessary, assistance is provided to ensure adequate intake of foods and fluids. Enteral feedings may be initiated if inadequate intake cannot be maintained orally.

Powerlessness

Planning: client goals. Goals for this nursing diagnosis include that the client will (1) increase the ability to identify factors that are under independent control; (2) make decisions regarding care, treatment options, and the future, when possible; and (3) participate in care within the limitations of the illness.

Interventions: nonsurgical management. The nurse assesses feelings of powerlessness by encouraging the client to verbalize feelings concerning the illness and its effects. Previous decision-making patterns, roles, and individual responsibilities are examined. By asking the client and the family to describe their usual life styles and situations during which they coped both effectively and ineffectively, the nurse may identify factors that influence coping ability. The nurse is then better able to identify interventions that facilitate a greater sense of control for the client and the family.

The nurse provides information regarding the patho-physiology and natural progression of the syndrome, as well as tests, procedures, and routines, as increased knowledge enhances the client's sense of control. The client is encouraged to make choices and to participate in care as much as possible, while positive feedback is given for doing so.

The client's own cosmetics, personal hygiene items, and clothing are utilized, when feasible, to provide a sense of the familiar. In addition, the nurse ensures environmental control by keeping the call light, television control, telephone, and other necessary items within the client's reach. Alternate communication methods, such as chalk and blackboard, may be needed if the client cannot verbally express his/her needs.

Anxiety; Anticipatory Grieving

These nursing diagnoses affect both the client and the family system and have similar interventions.

Planning: client goals. The primary goal is that the client and the family will cope effectively, adapting to the changes in roles and responsibilities associated with the disease process and verbalizing feelings related to anxiety, fear, and grief.

Interventions: nonsurgical management. The nurse assesses the client and family members for verbal and nonverbal behaviors indicative of anxiety, fear, and

GUIDELINES ■ Interventions for Complications of Plasmapheresis

Complication	Interventions
Trauma or infection at site of vascular access	Keep the site clean and dry. Monitor the site for redness, swelling, drainage, or other signs of infection.
Hypovolemia with resulting hypotension, tachycardia, dizziness, and diaphoresis	Monitor fluid and electrolyte status and vital signs. Administer fluids as prescribed. Provide an explanation of side effects and reassure the client.
Hypokalemia and hypocalcemia	Monitor fluid and electrolyte balance. Administer replacement electrolytes. Observe for cardiac arrhythmias.
Temporary circumoral and distal extremity paresthesias, muscle twitching, and nausea and vomiting related to administration of citrated plasma	Add calcium gluconate or calcium chloride to exchange fluids, as prescribed. Provide explanations, comfort measures, and reassurance.

grieving. Sadness, depression, anger, guilt, crying or the inability to cry, denial, and withdrawal may be noted. The nurse helps to establish a trusting, therapeutic nurse-client relationship, and the client and the family are encouraged to discuss fears and concerns. Usual coping strategies and remaining strengths are identified and capitalized on. The family is encouraged to spend time with the client and to assist with care, providing ROM exercises, massages, and other comfort measures. The nurse provides as much information as needed and initiates referrals to social services department, the hospital chaplain or appropriate religious leader, and local support groups, if indicated.

Total Self-Care Deficit

The inability to perform ADL may be total or partial, depending on the severity or stage of the client's illness.

Planning: client goals.   During the acute phase, the client may be totally dependent on others for performing even the most basic ADL. The goal for this phase is that the client will accept dependency, coping with the deficits through acceptance of realistic long-term goals and planning for optimal daily living skills.

In less severe cases, or as the client's condition improves, goals shift toward rehabilitation through physical and occupational therapy, use of assistive devices, and the ability to direct others in providing assistance with care.

Interventions: nonsurgical management.   The nurse assesses the client's ability to perform ADL while monitoring her/his emotional and mental status to determine the client's level of acceptance of the disability. Necessary assistance is provided; however, the client is encouraged to perform activities independently, if possible. The response to or tolerance of activity is monitored, and adequate rest periods are provided between activities and therapy sessions. Activities are coordinated with interventions of other health care team members (occupational, speech, and physical therapists.). Assistive devices and instructions for their use are provided for the client. Positive feedback is given liberally by the nurse for any gains noted in the client's self-care activities. The family is encouraged to become involved in all aspects of the rehabilitation process.

■ Discharge Planning

The severity and course of this illness are extremely variable, making it difficult to predict prognosis for a particular individual. Neurologic deterioration may continue for several days or several weeks; however, many clients never develop total quadriparesis or respiratory paralysis necessitating tracheostomy and assisted ventilation. The course of the rehabilitation phase is even more variable and may require from 2 weeks to 2 years.

Planning for discharge of the client who has Guillain-Barré syndrome begins on admission. Successful planning provides a smooth transition from the hospital or rehabilitation setting to the home. The nurse reviews each of the following areas, assessing individual and family needs particular to each situation.

Home Care Preparation

The client with Guillain-Barré syndrome may be discharged to home or, in more severe cases, to a rehabilitation setting for further therapy before returning home.

In most cases, little preparation of the home setting is needed. If the client is discharged while still dependent on assistive devices, the nurse, in consultation with occupational and physical therapists, makes certain that the necessary equipment has been delivered. In the case of items such as grab bars for bathtub and toilet transfers, the nurse checks to see that they are properly installed. In addition, any modifications to the arrangement of the home need to be completed before the client's arrival. Throw rugs should be removed if they pose a hazard; ramps should be installed, doorways widened, and commodes provided if the client remains wheelchair dependent.

Client/Family Education

The nurse carefully assesses the client's and the family's knowledge and understanding of the disease, their learning needs, and their readiness and ability to learn. Among the many factors affecting ability or readiness to learn are pain, anxiety, denial, disbelief, levels of development and motivation, education, language, ethnic background, and health care beliefs and practices. Offering encouragement and reassurance, the nurse provides oral and written information, reinforces the teaching provided by other health care disciplines, and makes appropriate referrals to local or community agencies for assistance in the home setting after discharge from the hospital.

If feasible, a family member or significant other is included in education processes throughout the client's hospitalization. By the time the client is discharged to home, major problems, such as respiratory paralysis, have been resolved. The most likely residual effects seen at discharge are related to mobility, self-care, and perhaps sensory alteration and disturbed self-concept.

The client and the family are given both oral and written instructions in techniques to facilitate mobility and prevent skin breakdown. If mobility remains markedly impaired, the need for ROM exercises, positioning and frequent turning techniques, and the use of massage are emphasized. The nurse makes certain that the client and the family understand how to use assistive devices safely and properly, providing written instructions and diagrams, as necessary. If paresthesias persist, the nurse instructs the client and the family to visually examine the affected limbs several times daily. After discharge from the hospital, the client must be monitored for recurrent disease.

Psychosocial Preparation

The psychosocial adjustment needed may be minimal to dramatic, depending on the client's residual deficit, age, sex, usual roles and responsibilities, usual coping strategies, available support systems, and occupation. As the client begins to function in familiar surroundings, it is likely that an improved self-concept will result. Rarely, residual deficits require permanent changes in life styles or roles. The nurse encourages the client and the family to discuss their feelings with one another, which provides necessary support.

Health Care Resources

Self-help groups for clients with chronic illness abound. The nurse consults with the client and the physician and seeks referrals to these groups if indicated. The Guillain-Barré Foundation provides information about local resources and information for clients and their families.

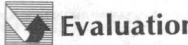 **Evaluation**

Evaluation of the nursing care plan for the client with Guillain-Barré syndrome is based on the identified nursing diagnoses. The expected outcomes are that the client

1. Demonstrates an effective respiratory rate, coughs effectively, and has adequate gas exchange in the lungs

2. Participates in mobilization to the greatest extent possible, demonstrates use of adaptive devices, and does not develop complications related to immobility

3. Maintains skin integrity and participates in the prevention of pressure sores; and describes causative and preventive factors in skin breakdown and the rationale for interventions

4. Identifies factors that are under independent control and makes decisions concerning care, treatment, and the future, when possible

5. Verbalizes feelings relative to emotional status and coping abilities, utilizing family members, the nurse, and other sources for support (with the family)

6. Develops appropriate coping strategies on the basis of personal strengths and previous experiences (with the family)

7. Demonstrates increasing ability to accomplish self-care and ADL through improved motor function, the ability to make use of adaptive devices, and the ability to direct others who are providing or assisting the client with those activities

8. Describes the disease process, proper use of prescribed medications, and other therapeutic interventions, as well as realistic plans for care after discharge (with the family)

MYASTHENIA GRAVIS

OVERVIEW

Myasthenia gravis (MG) means "grave muscle weakness." It is characterized by remissions and exacerbations. MG is a chronic, neuromuscular, autoimmune disease, which involves a decrease in the number and effectiveness of acetylcholine (ACh) receptors at the neuromuscular junction. Nursing care of the myasthenic client involves providing anticholinesterase drugs and related client teaching, assisting with self-care activities and energy conservation measures, and helping the client and the family cope with the effects of chronic illness through emotional support and education.

Pathophysiology

Normally, the neurotransmitter *ACh* is released at the neural side of the neuromuscular junction, diffuses across the synaptic gap, and unites with *ACh receptor sites* in the postsynaptic membrane of the muscle fiber (see the figure on p. 831). This changes the membrane's permeability to sodium and potassium, leading to depolarization. When the threshold is reached, an *action potential* is generated, which propagates along the sarcolemma, resulting in contraction of the muscle fiber. ACh is destroyed by the enzyme *acetylcholinesterase* after transmission across the neuromuscular junction has occurred.

The major pathologic defect in MG is that nerve impulses are not transmitted to the skeletal muscle at the neuromuscular junction. The defect appears to result from a deficiency of ACh released from the presynaptic membrane terminals or a reduced number of normal ACh receptors, possibly as a result of autoimmune injury. Antibodies to ACh receptor protein have been found in 60% to 90% of persons with MG and in infants with neonatal myasthenia (Adams & Victor, 1985). It is speculated that these antibodies bind to ACh receptor sites on the postsynaptic membrane, making them unavailable to bind with ACh.

There is no evidence of central or peripheral nervous system disease in MG. The muscle appears normal macroscopically, usually without evidence of atrophy. Microscopically, lymphocytic infiltrates may be seen within muscles and other organs, yet these findings have been inconsistent.

The *thymus gland* is often abnormal. *Thymoma* (encapsulated thymus gland tumor) occurs in approximately 15% of cases, and 80% of the remaining cases show hyperplasia of the thymus (Adams & Victor, 1985). The precise role of the thymus remains unclear, but it is suspected that some antigenic stimulus in the gland perpetuates the production of anti–ACh receptor antibody. There is also a very strong association between MG and hyperthyroidism.

Etiology

Although the precipitating event remains unclear, research strongly suggests that myasthenic weakness results from circulating antibodies to ACh receptor. It has been hypothesized that myoid cells (cells in the thymus that resemble skeletal muscle cells) are the site of origin of the disease. A virus might be responsible for the injury to these cells, which results in the antibody formation. Other researchers have shown that thymic lymphocytes from persons with myasthenia gravis can synthesize this ACh receptor antibody (AChRab) in vitro and in vivo, suggesting a different mode of thymic involvement.

Although the disease is not hereditary, approximately 15% of infants born to myasthenic mothers exhibit transient symptoms of the disease, such as muscular weakness, a weak cry, ptosis (drooping of the eyelid), difficulty sucking, and respiratory insufficiency. These symptoms disappear when the antibodies in the infant's blood disappear, 7 to 14 days after birth, supporting the theory that antibodies are responsible for the symptoms of the disease.

Incidence

Although it may begin at any age, onset of MG during the first decade or after the seventh decade of life is rare. The peak age at onset is between 20 and 30 years. Before age 40 years, females are affected two to three times more often than males, whereas in later life the incidence in the sexes is about equal. Males predominate among myasthenic persons with thymoma, and these male clients tend to be 50 to 60 years of age (Adams & Victor, 1985).

The incidence of MG is estimated to be from 1 in 10,000 to 1 in 50,000 of the U.S. population (Adams & Victor, 1985). Family occurrence is rare, but infants of myasthenic mothers may show symptoms at birth, which diminish within a few days or weeks.

COLLABORATIVE MANAGEMENT

 Assessment

History

In addition to the standard biographical data and medical-surgical history, the nurse assesses the client for the rapid onset of *fatigue* and for subjective complaints of *muscular weakness* that increases on exertion or as the day wears on and improves with rest. The nurse elicits a description of symptoms in the client's own words, if possible, specifically noting the affected muscle groups and any limitation or inability of the client to perform ADL. Additional areas of inquiry include any history of *ptosis* or *diplopia,* difficulty *chewing* or *swallowing,* and the type of diet best tolerated. Complaints of *respiratory difficulty, choking,* or *weakness of the voice* are elicited by the nurse, as well as whether the client experiences difficulty holding up the head, brushing the teeth, combing the hair, or shaving. The nurse also inquires about the presence of *paresthesias* or *aching* in weakened muscles. Last, any history of *thymus gland tumor* is elicited.

Although the onset of MG is usually insidious, some instances of fairly rapid development, occasionally preceded by *infection, emotional upset, pregnancy,* or *anesthesia,* have been reported. Thus, the nurse inquires about any history of these events. In addition, temporary increase in weakness may be noted after vaccination, menstruation, and exposure to extremes in environmental temperature.

Physical Assessment: Clinical Manifestations

Assuming that the client can cooperate fully, the diagnosis of MG may be established by the demonstration of *progressive paresis* of affected muscle groups that is resolved by rest, at least in part. The most common symptoms (exhibited by more than 90% of clients) are related to involvement of the levator palpebrae or extraocular muscles. The nurse assesses the client for the presence of *ocular palsies, ptosis, diplopia,* and *weak or incomplete eye closure.* These symptoms may last only a few days at the onset, then resolve only to return weeks or months later. Normal pupillary responses to light and accommodation are present.

In 80% of affected clients, the muscles of *facial expression, chewing,* and *speech* are affected. The nurse notes the client's smile, which may be transformed into a snarl, and the jaw, which may hang so that the client must prop it up with the hand. Difficulty in chewing and swallowing may lead to considerable weight loss, and the nurse inquires about the client's nutritional status and any recent loss of weight. It may be more difficult for the client to eat after talking, and after extended conversations the voice may become weaker or may exhibit a nasal twang. In some clients, the tongue may exhibit one central and two lateral longitudinal fissures.

Less often involved are the muscles of the shoulders, the flexors of the neck, and the hip flexors. *Limb weakness* is more often *proximal,* so that the client may have difficulty climbing stairs, lifting heavy objects, or raising the arms overhead. Neck weakness may be mild or severe enough to cause difficulty holding the head erect. Among the trunk muscles, the erector spinae are most frequently affected, resulting in difficulty sustaining a sitting or walking posture. The nurse carefully assesses the client for deficits in these areas.

All muscles are weakened in the most advanced cases, including those associated with *respiratory function* and the control of *bladder and bowel function.* Thus, in severe cases, the nurse inquires about bowel and bladder function. Respiratory function is assessed regularly.

Although rarely marked in degree, *atrophy* of myasthenic muscles occurs in approximately 10% of affected females and 20% of males with MG. Tendon reflexes, although seldom altered even after repeated tapping of the tendon, are examined by the nurse. In addition, the nurse assesses for pain, which is seldom a major complaint; however, many clients report some *aching* of the weakened muscles. *Paresthesias* affecting the muscles of the face, the hands, and the thighs have been reported, but are not associated with any loss of sensation. Lost or *decreased sensations* of *smell* and *taste* have been reported. There is no alteration of consciousness.

In *Eaton-Lambert syndrome,* a special form of myasthenia often observed in combination with small cell carcinoma of the lung, the muscles of the trunk and the pelvic and shoulder girdles are most frequently affected. Although increasing weakness after exertion is exhibited in this syndrome, there may be a temporary increase in muscle strength during the first few contractions, followed by rapid decrements.

Osserman (1958) introduced a clinical staging classification for MG, which has been adopted by many medical centers (see the accompanying Key Features of Disease: Osserman's Clinical Staging of Myasthenia Gravis). Precipitants of myasthenic crisis or worsening of symptoms are given in the Key Features of Disease on page 971.

Psychosocial Assessment

The nurse notes the client's age, sex, occupation, usual roles and responsibilities (including developmental level), usual coping methods, motivation, acceptance of the condition, financial status, and available support systems. The myasthenic client or the family faces a future of uncertainty, exacerbations and remissions of disease, altered body image, and family system disruption, which lead to feelings of loss, fear, helplessness, and grief. Thus, the nurse remains alert for signs of ineffective coping and provides needed support.

KEY FEATURES OF DISEASE ■ Osserman's Clinical Staging of Myasthenia Gravis

Class I	Ocular myasthenia Ptosis and diplopia Mild; no mortality
Class II	A. Mild Generalized Myasthenia with Slow Progression No crises Drug responsive Low mortality B. Moderate Generalized Myasthenia Severe skeletal and bulbar involvement No crises Drug response less than satisfactory Low mortality
Class III	Acute fulminating myasthenia Rapid progression with respiratory crises Poor drug response High incidence of thymoma High mortality
Class IV	Late severe myasthenia Progression during 2 years from class I to class II Poor response to medication High mortality

Adapted with permission from Adams, R. D., & Victor, M. (1985). *Principles of neurology* (3rd ed.). New York: McGraw-Hill.

KEY FEATURES OF DISEASE ■ Factors Precipitating or Worsening Myasthenia Gravis

Medications
  Anticholinesterase drugs
  Potassium-depleting diuretics or laxatives, or enemas
  Tranquilizers or sedatives
  Antibiotics
    Aminoglycosides
    Tetracyclines
    Polymyxins
  Antiarrhythmics
    Procainamide
    Quinine or quinidine
  Narcotic analgesics
  Diphenhydramine
Alcohol, mixers containing quinine
Hormonal changes
Stress
Infection
Seasonal or temperature changes
Heat
Surgery

Laboratory Findings

In virtually all cases, the diagnosis of MG is obvious from the history and physical examination findings and may be immediately confirmed by the client's response to cholinergic drugs. A standard series of laboratory studies is usually performed for clients with known or suspected MG. In addition, thyroid function should be tested and serum protein electrophoresis used to evaluate the client for immunologic disorders. Thyrotoxicosis is present in approximately 5% of myasthenic clients, and rheumatoid arthritis, systemic lupus erythematosus, and polymyositis are associated with the disease as well.

Testing for AChRab has become an important diagnostic criterion: 85% to 95% of persons with MG have AChRab, and there are virtually no false-positive results. Thus, a positive antibody test result confirms the diagnosis, but a negative finding does not exclude the disease, as up to 15% of those affected have no demonstrable antibodies.

Other Diagnostic Tests

Because 10% to 15% of persons with MG have a thymoma, the client is assessed for the possible presence of this condition. The thymus, an H-shaped gland located in the upper mediastinum beneath the sternum, is one organ in which AChRabs are formed. Although thymoma can often be seen on the routine frontal and lateral chest x-ray films, special studies of any suspicious area in the anterior mediastinum should be done. The nurse prepares the client for these tests, computed tomography and magnetic resonance imaging, by explaining the equipment and what the client may expect during the tests.

Although electrical testing of the normal neuromuscular junction produces no change in the amplitude of muscle contraction, slow (2403 Hz), supramaximal, repetitive stimulation of a defective junction does not always result in depolarization of the postsynaptic membrane. Thus, the amplitude of the muscle response diminishes with progressive stimulation. A decrease in amplitude of more than 10% between the first and fifth responses generally indicates defective neuromuscular transmission characteristic of, although not unique to, MG. To increase the likelihood of detecting an abnormality, several muscles may be tested, and testing may be performed after exercise or the exposure of the muscle to curare or to ischemia.

Single-fiber EMG represents an even more sensitive method of detecting defects in neuromuscular transmission. This test compares the stability of the firing of one muscle fiber with that of another fiber that is innervated by the same motor neuron. Normally, the time interval between the two firings shows a minor degree of variability, called jitter. Defective transmission results in increased jitter or in the actual blocking of successive discharges.

These electrical tests are performed by inserting needle electrodes into the muscle to be examined. The nurse prepares the client for these procedures by explaining that momentary discomfort may accompany insertion of the electrode needles and that the client will be asked to contract and relax particular muscles during the tests. In addition, the nurse answers any questions the client has and provides necessary emotional support.

Pharmacologic tests using the cholinesterase inhibitors edrophonium chloride (Tensilon) or neostigmine bromide (Prostigmin) have been used since the 1950s. Edrophonium is used more often because of its rapid onset and brief duration of action. This drug inhibits the breakdown of ACh at the postsynaptic membrane, thereby increasing its availability for excitation of postsynaptic receptors. To perform the test, the physician first estimates the strength of certain cranial muscles. Initially, 2 mg (0.2 mL) is injected intravenously; if this is tolerated, an additional 8 mg (0.8 mL) is injected after 30 seconds. Within 30 to 60 seconds of the first dose, most myasthenic clients demonstrate a marked improvement in muscle tone, lasting 4 to 5 minutes. False-positive test results may be due to increased muscular effort by the client, whereas false-negative findings may be seen if the tested muscle is extremely weak or refractory to the drug.

This test may also be utilized to help determine whether increasing weakness in the previously diagnosed myasthenic client is due to *cholinergic crisis* (overmedication with anticholinesterase drugs) or to *myasthenic crisis* (undermedication with cholinesterase inhibitors). In cholinergic crisis, there is no improvement after the administration of edrophonium; instead, weakness may actually increase, and fasciculations (muscle twitching) may be noted around the eyes and face. The edrophonium test poses a danger of ventricular fibrillation and cardiac arrest, although these complications are rare. Atropine sulfate is the antidote for edrophonium and must be available in case these emergencies occur.

The neostigmine test is much less frequently used for the diagnosis of MG. In this test, 1 to 2 mg of neostigmine is injected intramuscularly, with improvement of muscle tone seen in the myasthenic client within 30 minutes and lasting 2 to 3 hours. Atropine sulfate (0.6 mg) should be available to counteract side effects, such as nausea, vomiting, sweating, or salivation. Neostigmine may be given intravenously in a dose of 0.5 mg, but it should be preceded by atropine administration to decrease the danger of ventricular fibrillation and cardiac arrest. Oral neostigmine may also be given as a test dose, with both the onset and duration of action being increased.

The curare test is used only when the diagnosis remains uncertain after both the edrophonium and neostigmine tests. Respiratory support, similar to that used during anesthesia induction, must be available whenever this test is performed. Two per cent of the normal curarizing dose of 3 mg of *d*-tubocurarine per 18 kg (40 lb) body weight is given to the client with findings suggestive of MG. If no respiratory difficulty develops within 5 minutes, a total of 5% of the dose is injected. Increased weakness at this low dose indicates MG or Eaton-Lambert syndrome.

Although all of these tests are performed by the physician, the nurse may be required to provide assistance with preparation or administration of the drugs, monitoring of the client for effects and side effects, and documentation of test results and the client's tolerance. In addition, the nurse provides emotional support for the client and the family while assessing their understanding of the procedures and providing information, as necessary.

Analysis: Nursing Diagnosis

Nursing diagnoses for the client with MG vary, depending on the severity of the illness and the client's response to drug treatment.

Common Diagnoses

The following nursing diagnoses are seen among clients with MG:

1. Ineffective airway clearance and ineffective breathing pattern related to muscle weakness
2. Impaired gas exchange related to muscle weakness and possible aspiration
3. Impaired physical mobility and activity intolerance related to muscle weakness and fatigue
4. Total self-care deficit related to muscle weakness
5. Potential for injury related to muscle weakness, visual disturbances, and incomplete eyelid closure (potential for corneal damage)
6. Sensory/perceptual alterations (visual) related to weakness of the eye muscles with resulting ptosis, ocular palsy, and diplopia
7. Impaired verbal communication related to muscle weakness
8. Altered nutrition: less than body requirements related to muscle weakness, fatigue, GI dysfunction, and dysphagia
9. Body image disturbance and self-esteem disturbance related to muscle weakness, self-care deficit, loss of independence, and inability to perform usual roles
10. Anticipatory grieving related to actual or perceived loss of function and loss of independence

Additional Diagnoses

Many clients with MG may exhibit one or more of the following nursing diagnoses:

1. Impaired skin integrity related to altered nutrition and immobility
2. Ineffective individual coping and ineffective family coping related to the episodic nature of the disease, loss of independence, changes in role function, and loss of well-being
3. Fear related to uncertainty about the future
4. Sleep pattern disturbance related to immobility, loss of well-being, and fear
5. Potential for infection (pulmonary) related to respiratory muscle weakness
6. Knowledge deficit related to disease, treatment, and prognosis or outcome

Planning and Implementation

Ineffective Airway Clearance; Ineffective Breathing Pattern; Impaired Gas Exchange

Although not all clients with MG exhibit respiratory compromise, ongoing assessment and maintenance of respiratory function by the nurse are essential, because both myasthenic crisis (undermedication) and cholinergic crisis (overmedication) increase muscle weakness and the client's risk for respiratory compromise. The diaphragm and the respiratory and intercostal muscles may be affected, resulting in inhibition of the client's ability to maintain adequate ventilation, breathe deeply, or cough effectively. In addition, dysphagia may result in the aspiration of foods, fluids, or saliva, compounding the respiratory problems. Owing to their respiratory muscle involvement, many of these clients have an increased risk of pulmonary infections.

Planning: client goals. The primary goal for these nursing diagnoses is that the client will demonstrate effective gas exchange as evidenced by bilateral lung ventilation without adventitious breath sounds, tidal volume and vital capacity within acceptable limits, and absence of symptoms of respiratory distress.

Interventions: nonsurgical management. In the acute care setting, the nurse monitors the client closely for signs of respiratory distress, such as dyspnea, or subjective complaints of shortness of breath, air hunger, labored breathing, or increasing confusion (from hypoxia). The nurse monitors respiratory rate, rhythm, and depth and encourages the client to turn, cough, and deep breathe every 2 hours. In addition, the nurse auscultates the client's lungs and measures vital signs, tidal volume, and vital capacity every 2 to 4 hours; monitors the arterial blood gas values for acid-base abnormalities or decreasing oxygen saturation; and notifies the physician promptly of any significant changes.

The nurse assists the client to maintain a patent airway by providing gentle suctioning using aseptic technique if the client is unable to cough effectively. The nurse may need to teach assisted cough technique similar to that used by quadriplegics (see Chap. 33). Chest physiotherapy consisting of postural drainage, percussion, and vibration mobilizes secretions and helps prevent pneumonia and atelectasis. An Ambu bag, equipment for oxygen administration, and endotracheal intubation equipment are kept at the bedside in case of respiratory distress. Because breathing difficulty or the inability to breathe easily is frightening, it is important for the nurse to remain cognizant of the client's mental and emotional status during periods of respiratory compromise and to provide information and support to the client and significant others. Finally, the nurse administers the medications prescribed for muscle weakness, bronchodilation, and pulmonary congestion, while monitoring and documenting the client's response.

Impaired Physical Mobility; Activity Intolerance

Planning: client goals. The primary goals for these nursing diagnoses are that the client will (1) participate, actively or passively, in mobilization; (2) remain free of complications associated with immobility; and (3) be able to participate in activities without excess fatigue.

Interventions. The hallmark of MG is muscular weakness that increases when the client is fatigued and limits the client's mobility and ability to participate in activities. Treatment efforts for this disease fall into two categories: those that affect its symptoms without influencing the actual course of the disease (anticholinesterases or cholinergic drugs) and those efforts aimed at inducing remission, such as the administration of immunosuppressive drugs or corticosteroids, plasmapheresis, and thymectomy (removal of the thymus gland).

Nonsurgical management. The nurse assesses and monitors the client's motor strength before and after

periods of activity, providing assistance with mobilization as necessary to avoid undue fatigue. The nurse teaches the client to participate in activities early in the day or during the energy peaks that follow the administration of medications; the nurse also helps the client to plan the periods of rest necessary to avoid excess fatigue.

During periods of maximal weakness, it may be necessary for the nurse to provide assistance with ambulation, transfers from bed to chair or toilet or commode, position changes, and the maintenance of body alignment. In addition, the nurse performs active or passive ROM exercises every 2 to 4 hours and assesses skin integrity; the nurse also instructs family members in these techniques. The client is repositioned and bony prominences are massaged every 2 hours to prevent skin breakdown and contractures. The nurse also uses heel and elbow protectors, eggcrate or alternating pressure mattresses, and other pressure ulcer prevention devices. The physical and occupational therapy departments may be consulted by the nurse for assistance with mobility, self-care, and energy conservation techniques.

Drug therapy. Three groups of drugs—anticholinesterases, immunosuppressants, and corticosteroids—are prescribed for the treatment of MG (Table 34–4). The nurse's responsibility in the administration of these medications includes providing them *on time* to maintain blood levels and thus facilitate increased muscle strength. The nurse is also responsible for monitoring and documenting the client's responses and providing instructions for the client and the family concerning the indications, effectiveness, and side effects of drugs used in the treatment of MG.

Anticholinesterase drugs increase the response of muscles to nerve impulses, thus improving strength. Neostigmine, 7.5 to 45.0 mg every 2 to 6 hours orally; pyridostigmine (Mestinon), 60 to 180 mg two to four times daily; and ambenonium (Mytelase), 5 to 25 mg every 3 to 4 hours, are the anticholinesterase drugs of choice. The dosages are highly individualized, and the nurse may expect day-to-day variations in dosage, depending on the client's fluctuating symptoms. Small doses of atropine may be given to manage the side effects of these drugs. It is important for the nurse to administer these medications on time to maintain consistent blood levels. In addition, the nurse administers the medications with a small amount of food to help alleviate GI side effects and instructs the client to eat meals 45 minutes to 1 hour after taking these medications. Drugs containing magnesium, morphine or its derivatives, curare, quinine, quinidine, procainamide, and hypnotics or sedatives should be avoided, as these substances may increase the client's weakness. Antibiotics such as neomycin, kanamycin, streptomycin, polymyxin B, and certain tetracyclines have been shown to impair transmitter release and increase myasthenic symptoms as well (Adams & Victor, 1985).

Sudden increases in weakness and the inability to clear secretions, swallow, or breathe adequately indicate that the client is experiencing crisis. There are two types

TABLE 34–4 Drugs Used in the Treatment of Myasthenia Gravis

Drug	Usual Daily Dosage	Interventions	Rationales
Anticholinesterases			
Neostigmine (Prostigmin) bromide Neostigmine (Prostigmin) methylsulfate	7.5–45 mg PO q 2–6 h Exacerbations: 0.5–2 mg q 1–3 h IM or IV	1. Monitor response and tolerance to side effects. 2. Observe for nausea, vomiting, cramps, diarrhea, increased weakness, facial muscle twitching, and dyspnea. 3. Administer regularly and on time, and instruct the client to do so at home. 4. Administer before activities, such as eating, ADL, work or sports, and instruct client to do so at home. 5. Avoid morphine and its derivatives, curare, quinine, quinidine, procainamide, mycin-type antibiotics, and drugs containing magnesium, and instruct client to do so at home. 6. Administer with a small amount of food. 7. Instruct the client and the family about crises (see text). a. Myasthenic. b. Cholinergic.	1. Goal is optimal response with minimal side effects; dosage is highly individualized. 2. These may indicate toxicity or impending cholinergic crisis. 3. Fluctuating blood levels may increase weakness. 4. Drug lessens dysphagia and fatigue and increases muscle strength. 5. These drugs may reverse cholinergic effects on muscle, which would increase weakness. 6. This measure decreases GI side effects. 7. These are medical emergencies requiring treatment. a. Because of undermedication with anticholinesterases. b. Because of overmedication with anticholinesterases.
Pyridostigmine bromide* (Mestinon, Regonol)	60–180 mg bid or qid PO (usual dose 600 mg/d, but may be up to 1500 mg/d)	1. Same as for neostigmine. 2. If extended-release tablets are prescribed, explain how they work. Administer at same time each day, at least 6 h apart.	1. Same as for neostigmine. 2. Extended-release tablets work for 6 h. Instruct the client to avoid overdose.
Ambenonium chloride†	5–25 mg q 3–4 h PO; may range from 5–75 mg per dose	1. Same as for neostigmine.	1. Same as for neostigmine.
Corticosteroids			
Prednisone (Deltasone, Meticorton, Orasone, Paracort)	20–25 mg and gradually increase; optimal dose 40–45 mg/d; up to 100 mg/d administered on alternate days	1. Administer in a hospital setting. 2. Start drug in low dosages, with respiratory support readily available. 3. Administer on alternate days on physician's order after optimal dosage is attained. 4. Titrate to lowest effective dosage on physician's order after improvement occurs.	1. Worsening of symptoms during first 7–10 d may be expected. 2. Low initial dosages minimize worsening of symptoms. 3. Side effects of long-term therapy are reduced. 4. GI upset, electrolyte imbalance, weight gain, edema, and hyperglycemia are dose dependent.

TABLE 34–4   Drugs Used in the Treatment of Myasthenia Gravis *Continued*

Drug	Usual Daily Dosage	Interventions	Rationales
		5. Administer anticholinesterase drugs concurrently on physician's order.	5. Concurrent administration increases effectiveness of medications.
		6. Give drug with food, milk, or antacid, unless contraindicated.	6. Drug causes peptic ulcer and GI irritation.
		7. Tell the client not to discontinue the drug abruptly. Gradually reduce the dosage on physician's order after long-term therapy.	7. Sudden withdrawal may result in increased weakness, lethargy, depression, dyspnea, fainting, or death.
		8. Monitor blood pressure, sleep pattern, and blood glucose and serum potassium levels.	8. Side effects may require dosage adjustment. Diabetic clients may require increased insulin.
		9. Weigh client daily. Report sudden weight gain.	9. Drug causes edema and weight gain.
		10. Give salt-restricted diet rich in potassium, and administer potassium supplements on physician's order.	10. Salt increases fluid retention and potassium levels should be restored.
Immunosuppressants			
Azathioprine (Imuran)	3–5 mg/kg daily PO initially; maintain at 1–2 mg/kg per d; varies according to client's response	1. Decrease dosage to ¼ or ⅓ of normal dosage if client is also taking allopurinol.	1. Allopurinol impairs the inactivation of azathioprine.
		2. Watch for clay-colored stools, dark urine, jaundice, and increased alkaline phosphatase, bilirubin, AST, and ALT levels.	2. These are signs of hepatotoxicity.
		3. Monitor hemoglobin level, WBC, and platelet count weekly.	3. Drug may cause bone marrow suppression, leukopenia, anemia, and pancytopenia.
		4. Advise client to avoid conception for at least 4 months after drug therapy.	4. This agent is potentially teratogenic.
		5. Warn client that some alopecia may occur.	5. Nurse can minimize anxiety over this side effect.
		6. Avoid IM injections in clients with decreased platelet count.	6. Bleeding may occur with IM injections.
Cyclophosphamide (Cytoxan, Procytox)	2–4 mg/kg per d for 10 d initially, then maintenance 1.5–3.0 mg/kg per d	1. Monitor client for leukopenia, thrombocytopenia, and hepatic or renal disease.	1. These are side effects of the drug.
		2. Give an antiemetic before drug administration.	2. Nausea is associated with the drug.
		3. Push fluids to 3 L/d.	3, 4. Hemorrhagic cystitis is associated with the drug.
		4. Do not give the drug at bedtime.	
		5. Instruct the client to void frequently at night.	5. Frequent voiding prevents cystitis.
		6. Monitor for hematuria, and instruct the client to continue this practice for several months after drug therapy.	6. Cystitis can occur months after therapy has been stopped.

Table continued on following page

TABLE 34–4 Drugs Used in the Treatment of Myasthenia Gravis *Continued*

Drug	Usual Daily Dosage	Interventions	Rationales
		7. Warn client that alopecia may occur.	7. Nurse can allay anxiety over this side effect.
		8. Administer anticoagulants cautiously. Watch for signs of bleeding.	8. Thrombocytopenia is associated with the drug.
		9. Avoid IM injections if platelet count is low.	9. Bleeding may occur with IM injections.

*Available in extended-release tablets that have the longest duration of any cholinergic used for MG.
†Used for clients who cannot take neostigmine bromide or pyridostigmine bromide.

of crises: myasthenic crisis, an exacerbation of the myasthenic symptoms caused by undermedication with anticholinesterase drugs, and cholinergic crisis, an acute exacerbation of muscle weakness caused by overmedication with cholinergic (anticholinesterase) drugs. In either crisis, an adequate airway and artificial respiration must be maintained. Because myasthenic and cholinergic crises have many common characteristics, it is necessary to identify the type of crisis the client is experiencing to provide effective treatment (see the accompanying Key Features of Disease). In many clients, increasing myasthenic symptoms lead to overdose of anticholinesterase drugs. As a result, the client may experience a mixed crisis. Use of the edrophonium test (described earlier), although not always conclusive, is an important procedure for differentiation. Edrophonium produces a temporary improvement in myasthenic crisis, but no improvement or worsening of symptoms in cholinergic crisis.

Nursing management of the client in crisis is directed at early detection of the type of crisis and maintenance of adequate respiratory function. The acutely ill client may need intensive nursing care to monitor and maintain body functions. If in myasthenic crisis, the client may be maintained on a respirator. Anticholinesterase drugs are withheld because they increase respiratory secretions and may cause the development of cholinergic crisis. Administration of medications is reinstituted gradually and at lower dosages. In cholinergic crisis, anticholinergic drugs are withheld while the client is maintained on a ventilator. Atropine (1 mg intravenously) may be given and atropine administration repeated, if necessary. When atropine is given, the nurse must observe the client carefully, as secretions are thickened by the drug, causing more difficulty with airway clearance and possibly development of mucous plugs. Unless complications, such as pneumonia or aspiration, develop, the client in crisis improves rapidly after the appropriate drugs have been given. The nurse continues to provide assistance as necessary because the client continues to tire easily after minimal exertion.

Corticosteroids, such as prednisone (Deltasone), may be used with anticholinesterase drugs in the treatment of MG. Worsening of symptoms during the first 7 to 10 days of prednisone therapy should be expected, and the client is thus hospitalized and observed carefully by the nurse for respiratory difficulty. The drug is given in low dosages of 20 to 25 mg/day; the dosage is gradually

KEY FEATURES OF DISEASE ■ Characteristics of Myasthenic and Cholinergic Crises

Myasthenic Crisis	Cholinergic Crisis	Mixed Crisis
Increased pulse and respiration	Nausea	Apprehension
Rise in blood pressure	Vomiting	Restlessness
Anoxia	Diarrhea	Dyspnea
Cyanosis	Abdominal cramps	Dysphagia
Bowel and bladder incontinence	Blurred vision	Dysarthria
Decreased urinary output	Pallor	Increased lacrimation
Absence of cough and swallow reflex	Facial muscle twitching	Increased salivation
	Pupillary miosis	Diaphoresis
	Hypotension	Generalized weakness

increased to minimize the initial period of increased weakness. After optimal doses have been obtained (usually 40 to 45 mg daily, but up to 100 mg daily), many neurologists change to alternate-day drug administration, giving the same daily total dosage, to reduce the incidence of side effects related to long-term steroid therapy. Improvement occurs in the subsequent few weeks, and prednisone is then reduced to the lowest effective dosage. In addition to administering the prednisone, the nurse observes for untoward side effects, such as electrolyte imbalance, weight gain, acne, glucosuria, GI upset, and blood in the stools. The nurse may also administer potassium supplements and antacids as needed to counteract these side effects. Anticholinesterase drugs are usually given simultaneously, and, as the client's condition improves, the dosage of these drugs may be reduced as well.

Immunosuppression with drugs such as azathioprine (Imuran), methotrexate (Mexate), and cyclophosphamide (Cytoxan) has been utilized, resulting in some clinical improvement and reduction in AChRab levels. Occasionally, paralyzing doses of curare (*d*-tubocurarine) may be administered for several weeks while the client's respiration is maintained mechanically and anticholinesterase drugs are discontinued to restore the client's sensitivity to anticholinesterase drugs. Gradually, the medication is restarted and the dosage is adjusted until the client attains maximal strength.

Plasmapheresis.   Plasmapheresis is a method by which autoantibodies are removed from the plasma. Immunosuppressive drugs are administered concurrently to decrease the formation of additional antibodies. An antecubital vein or shunt is utilized for the procedure, which takes 2 to 5 hours to complete. Nursing responsibilities for the client undergoing plasmapheresis include providing information and reassurance to the client, teaching the client to eat well before the procedure, weighing the client before and after the procedure, and administering proper care to the shunt, especially maintaining shunt patency, checking for bruits every 2 to 4 hours, keeping double bulldog clamps at the bedside, and observing the puncture site for bleeding or ecchymosis. In addition, the nurse monitors the client for side effects of anticholinesterase drugs, as dosage of these medications may need to be decreased. Complications and nursing management of the client undergoing plasmapheresis are presented in earlier discussion of Guillain-Barré syndrome.

Surgical management.   For clients with myasthenia gravis, thymectomy is an alternative method of treatment. The procedure is not always immediately effective, and it may take several years for remission to occur, if at all. Clients who have the surgery within 2 years of the onset of myasthenic symptoms show the most marked improvement. One of two surgical approaches may be used: the transcervical incision or the sternal split. Advocates of the transcervical approach claim a lower morbidity rate and more rapid recovery with less

postoperative discomfort, with the client often requiring only a small dressing and an intravenous (IV) line. The sternal split, however, allows the surgeon to directly visualize the mediastinum, thus ensuring more precise and complete removal of all thymic tissue, and may be the approach of choice (Mulder et al., 1986). When thymoma is present, all contiguous involved structures, such as the pericardium, the innominate vein, a portion of the superior vena cava, and a portion of the lung, are removed (Mulder et al., 1986). A single chest tube is placed in the anterior mediastinum, and the client may be admitted to the critical care unit postoperatively.

Preoperative care.   The nurse teaches the client coughing and deep breathing exercises and the use of incentive spirometry and demonstrates airway suctioning. In addition, wound care, IV infusions, and the critical care unit environment (if indicated) should be discussed. Because there is no way to predict if and when remission or improvement will occur, it is important to avoid making promises, although optimism is warranted.

Immediately before surgery, the nurse may administer pyridostigmine (Mestinon) with a small amount of water to keep the client stable during and after surgery. If steroids have been used, they are also given before surgery and are tapered during the postoperative period. The nurse also administers antibiotics immediately before and for several days after surgery. Plasmapheresis may be used preoperatively and postoperatively to decrease circulative antibodies more quickly.

Postoperative care.   Although clients with adequate respiratory function may be extubated immediately after the procedure, most clients require a gradual weaning from the ventilator (see Chap. 62 for care of ventilator-dependent clients). Prolonged ventilatory assistance, however, is rare. After the client is extubated, conscientious attention is given by the nurse to pulmonary toilet. The nurse provides suctioning as necessary and encourages the client to turn, cough, and breathe deeply and to use incentive spirometry every 2 hours. In addition to observing respiratory function and providing bronchial hygiene, the nurse observes for signs of pneumothorax or hemothorax, such as chest pain, sudden shortness of breath, diminished or delayed chest wall expansion, diminished or absent breath sounds, and restlessness or a change in vital signs (decreasing blood pressure or weak, rapid pulse), while providing routine chest tube and wound care. The nurse also remains alert for signs of infection, such as increasing or purulent drainage; redness, warmth, or swelling around the wound; or elevated temperature. Finally, the nurse provides appropriate client and family teaching to prepare the client for discharge from the hospital. See Chapter 20 for additional postoperative nursing care.

Total Self-Care Deficit

Generalized weakness and fatigue have an impact on the myasthenic client's ability to participate in ADL. In addition, impaired fine-motor control and shoulder weakness, resulting in difficulty raising the arms, often compound the problem. Self-care deficits may be complete or partial, depending on the severity of the illness, the client's response to drugs, and the client's ability to tolerate activity without excessive fatigue.

Planning: client goals. Goals for this nursing diagnosis depend on the degree of impairment. For the severely impaired client, appropriate goals may be that the client will cope effectively with the deficits and accept dependency on others, whereas other clients may realistically expect to regain total independence.

Interventions: nonsurgical management. The nurse assesses the client's ability to perform ADL to establish abilities and limitations. Although encouraging the client to perform activities as independently as possible, the nurse provides whatever assistance is necessary to avoid undue frustration and fatigue. Activities are planned to follow the administration of medication to maximize independence and successful attempts at self-care. The nurse monitors and documents the client's response or tolerance to activity, providing alternating periods of activity and rest. Rest is critical because increased fatigue can precipitate a crisis. In addition, the nurse may consult occupational and physical therapists for assistive-adaptive devices as necessary and for assistance in teaching the client and the family energy conservation techniques and ideas for making work and self-care easier after discharge from the hospital.

Potential for Injury; Sensory/Perceptual Alterations (Visual)

The ptosis, ocular palsy, and diplopia that result from weakness of the ocular muscles often limit the myasthenic client's vision. In addition, the client's inability to completely close the eyes may lead to corneal abrasions, further compromising both vision and comfort.

Planning: client goals. The major goals for these nursing diagnoses are that the client will (1) be able to interpret incoming visual stimuli, (2) remain free from injury, and (3) keep the eyes moist and free from corneal abrasion.

Interventions: nonsurgical management. The nurse assesses cranial nerve function (III, IV, VI, and VII) to determine deficits and abilities (see Chap. 32). The nurse allays fears and limits potential injury in the visually compromised client by providing orientation to the surroundings and explaining the need for assistance with ADL and mobility. In addition to providing needed assistance, the nurse encourages the client to verbalize feelings of frustration or helplessness by listening and offering emotional support.

During the day, the nurse applies artificial tears to the client's eyes to keep the corneas moist and free from abrasion. A lubricant gel and shield may be applied to the eye at bedtime to provide more extensive coverage. To relieve diplopia, the nurse alternately patches each eye for 2 to 3 hours.

Impaired Verbal Communication

Weakness of speech and facial muscles often results in dysarthric and nasal speech. Thus, it may be difficult for myasthenic clients to make their speech understood by others.

Planning: client goals. The major goal for this nursing diagnosis is that the client will establish an effective means of communication, which results in minimal frustration for the client and the listener.

Interventions: nonsurgical management. The nurse assesses the functions of cranial nerves V, VII, IX, X, and XII (see Chap. 32) to determine the client's ability to communicate. The client is instructed to speak slowly while the nurse attempts to lip read, repeating the information to verify that it is correct. Questions that can be answered with "yes" or "no" responses or gestures may be used along with alternative communication systems, such as eye blinking, flash cards, magic slates, notebook and pencil, or picture, letter, or word boards. The nurse may also contact the speech therapist for suggestions and support. In addition, it is important for the nurse to provide empathy for the client experiencing communication problems.

Altered Nutrition: Less Than Body Requirements

The client may have difficulty maintaining an adequate intake of food and fluid, as the muscles needed for chewing and swallowing become weakened and tire easily. In addition, loss of fine-motor control and weakness in the arms limit the client's ability to eat independently. Finally, many of the medications used to treat MG have side effects, such as nausea, diarrhea, constipation, and cramping, that may affect the client's desire to eat and drink.

Planning: client goals. The primary goals for this nursing diagnosis is that the client will (1) maintain an optimal nutritional status with minimal or no weight loss and no aspiration of food or fluid and (2) maintain an optimal fluid intake to avoid dehydration and constipation.

Interventions: nonsurgical management. The nurse assesses the client's gag reflex and ability to chew and swallow without undue fatigue or aspiration. Frequent oral hygiene is encouraged to maximize the client's appetite and comfort. Food preferences and dislikes are discussed, and preferred foods are provided to help motivate adequate intake. The nurse provides small, frequent meals and high-calorie snacks, which help to provide nutrients with minimal abdominal discomfort. The nurse consults speech and occupational therapists, as well as the dietitian, for recommendations and coordinates their suggestions into a workable nutrition program. In addition, the nurse monitors the effectiveness of the nutrition program by recording calorie counts, intake and output, and daily weights.

The nurse administers anticholinesterase medications 45 minutes to 1 hour before meals to maximize the client's muscular strength and prevent aspiration. A mechanically soft diet may be required, and the nurse encourages the client to eat slowly and take small bites, providing whatever assistance is necessary. Boluses of food with pudding or mashed potato consistency are preferred; liquids readily cause choking. During meals, the nurse observes the client for choking, nasal regurgitation, and aspiration, providing suctioning if indicated. The physician should be informed of any problems with eating. The nurse may initiate tube feeding and IV feeding on the physician's order if the client is unable to maintain sufficient nutrition and hydration by mouth. If nausea and vomiting are a problem, the nurse administers antiemetics as prescribed, keeping the call light and emesis basin within the client's reach.

Bowel evacuation is assessed for diarrhea or constipation, bowel sounds are auscultated every 8 hours, and the client's intake of fiber or diarrhea-producing foods is monitored by the nurse. To maintain optimal bowel function, the nurse establishes a bowel program in collaboration with the client. If diarrhea is present, the call light and bedpan are kept within reach of the client. Antidiarrheal medications may be prescribed, but diphenoxylate (Lomotil) should be avoided because of its atropine-like effects. For constipation, the nurse provides a high-fiber diet, gives prune juice, and administers stool softeners or suppositories as prescribed. Strong cathartics, especially those containing magnesium, enemas, and hot liquids are avoided as they may increase weakness. In addition, the nurse assists the client with mobilization and encourages increased activity to promote peristalsis. After meals, the nurse provides necessary assistance with toileting to facilitate more complete bowel evacuation.

Body Image Disturbance; Self-Esteem Disturbance; Anticipatory Grieving

The muscle weakness, as well as the treatment, may cause body-image changes related to the inability to communicate verbally, the inability to smile, a lack of mobility, the actual or potential inability to work, and so forth. In addition, the client and family face an uncertain future, which will be influenced by exacerbations and remissions of the disease; this further interferes with role performance and self-esteem.

Planning: client goals. The goal for these nursing diagnoses is that the client and the family will demonstrate adaptation to changes in body image and life style by verbalizing their feelings and using significant others for support.

Interventions: nonsurgical management. The nurse must first establish a trusting and therapeutic relationship with the client and the family by listening, providing emotional support, and just being there for them. In addition, the nurse reinforces the client's capabilities by focusing on abilities rather than on disabilities, keeps the client and the family informed of progress, and encourages their participation in care. The nurse also encourages the client and the family to talk about the future and provides information about local self-help groups for myasthenics and others with chronic illness.

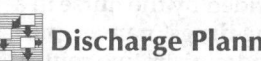 Discharge Planning

Clients with MG are usually managed at home, with hospitalization restricted to the diagnostic and evaluation processes, myasthenic or cholinergic crisis resulting in respiratory failure, or periods of exacerbation when respiratory function is threatened, regardless of the cause. Discharge planning begins on admission, as the nurse reviews each of the following areas, considering individual and family needs particular to each situation.

Home Care Preparation

Unless the client requires assistive devices, little preparation of the home setting is required. In consultation with physical and occupational therapists, the nurse makes certain that needed equipment has been delivered and properly installed. In addition, the nurse makes sure that the client and family members are able to use the equipment safely. If the client is wheelchair dependent, the nurse ensures that any necessary modifications to the home, such as the installation of ramps or widening of doorways, have been completed before the client's discharge from the hospital.

Client/Family Education

The more that the client and the family know about the disease and the drugs used for treatment, the less likely it is that complications will develop. Thus, the essence of discharge planning is client and family teaching. The nurse carefully assesses the client's and the family's knowledge and understanding of the disease, their learning needs, and their ability and readiness to learn. The nurse considers such factors as anxiety, denial, education levels, motivation, and prior health care practices and beliefs that may have an impact on learning ability and readiness. The nurse provides oral and written information and instructions throughout the client's hospitalization. Information about the disease process, life style changes, medications, myasthenic and cholinergic crises, and community resources is provided, and the client and the family are encouraged to ask questions.

Specific points concerning the disease process that are covered by the nurse include its episodic nature (exacerbations and remissions) and factors that predispose the client to exacerbation, such as infection, stress, surgery, hard physical exercise, sedatives, and enemas or strong cathartics (see Key Features of Disease: Factors Precipitating or Worsening Myasthenia Gravis). In addition, the nurse stresses the importance of making such life style adaptations as avoiding heat (e.g., sauna, hot tubs, and sunbathing), crowds, overeating, erratic changes in sleep habits, or emotional extremes. Signs of exacerbation, such as increased weakness, increased diplopia, ptosis, and problems with chewing or swallowing, are discussed, and the client is told when to contact the physician or nurse practitioner.

The medication regimen is provided by the nurse in a written format, which includes the drugs' names, purposes, dosages, times scheduled, administrative routes, and side effects. The nurse explains that the drugs are normally taken before such activities as eating, participating in sports, or engaging in work and informs the client of the importance of maintaining therapeutic blood levels by taking the medications on time as prescribed and not missing or postponing doses. In addition, the nurse informs the client of the side effects of anticholinesterase drugs, including lacrimation, salivation, increased bronchial secretions, diaphoresis, abdominal cramps, nausea, vomiting, diarrhea, frequency of urination, and facial muscle twitches. Finally, the nurse advises the client to avoid such medications as morphine, curare, quinine, quinidine, procainamide, mycin-type antibiotics, and drugs containing magnesium as these agents markedly increase muscle weakness.

In preparing the client for discharge, the nurse also explains the signs and symptoms of both myasthenic and cholinergic crises and the need to contact the physician or other health care professional whenever either type of crisis is suspected. Because respiratory compromise often occurs in myasthenic clients, family members are encouraged to gain skills in resuscitation procedures. An Ambu bag, suctioning equipment, and oxygen should be available in the home for clients prone to crisis, and family members should be instructed in their proper use.

Psychosocial Preparation

The episodic nature of this disease, the potential or actual loss of independence, and the body image changes that result (e.g., the inability to smile) have an impact on the client's adjustment. In addition, such factors as age, sex, usual roles and responsibilities, available support systems, occupation, and financial status are considered during discharge planning. Because the client's and the family's need for psychosocial adjustment may range from minimal to dramatic, the nurse remains sensitive to their needs and provides information and support while encouraging family members to discuss their feelings with one another.

Health Care Resources

In consultation with the physician and the client and the family, the nurse may initiate referrals to home care agencies and to local self-help groups for persons who have chronic illnesses and their families. The Myasthenia Gravis Foundation has education and research programs and provides assistance with financial aid and community resources. Finally, the client is encouraged to obtain and wear a medical alert (Medic Alert) bracelet or necklace and to carry identification at all times.

Evaluation

Evaluation of the nursing care plan of the client with MG is based on the identified nursing diagnoses. The expected outcomes are that the client

1. Demonstrates an effective respiratory rate and airway clearance with normal tidal volume, normal vital capacity, and adequate air exchange in the lungs
2. Is mobile, participates in activities without undue fatigue, and does not develop complications related to immobility
3. Performs self-care activities with maximal independence, using adaptive devices, if necessary, or directs others in providing assistance with these activities
4. Maintains orientation to surroundings, interprets incoming visual stimuli, and remains free from corneal abrasion or other injury related to visual deficits
5. Demonstrates an effective means of communication, verbal or nonverbal, which results in minimal frustration for the client and the listener
6. Maintains body weight within 10% of weight on admission, swallows without aspiration or tolerates tube feeding, and has regular soft-formed bowel movements
7. Verbalizes feelings concerning his/her emotional status, coping abilities, and plans for the future (with the family)
8. Describes the disease process and life style changes necessary for adaptation
9. Lists medications and their schedule of administration, dosages, and side effects
10. Distinguishes between myasthenic and cholinergic crises and verbalizes appropriate treatment

POLYNEURITIS AND POLYNEUROPATHY

OVERVIEW

Systemic diseases, infections, trauma, vascular or metabolic disturbances, and exogenous substances such as alcohol, medications, industrial agents, or heavy metals may damage cranial and peripheral nerves. Although the term *polyneuritis* implies an inflammatory process, it may be used to denote noninflammatory lesions as well. Thus, the terms *polyneuritis, polyneuropathy,* and *peripheral neuropathy* may be used to describe syndromes whose clinical hallmarks are muscle weakness with or without atrophy, pains and paresthesias or loss of sensation, impaired reflexes, and autonomic manifestations, or combinations of these symptoms.

The most common type is a symmetric polyneuropathy in which the client experiences decreased sensation, along with feeling that an extremity is asleep, and tingling, burning, tightness, or aching sensations, usually starting in the feet and progressing to the level of the knee before being noted in the hands (glove and stocking neuropathy). Other clients may complain of unsteadiness, clumsiness, the inability to recognize objects by feel, and injury without pain. Diabetic neuropathy is a common example, as are the neuropathies resulting from renal or hepatic failure, alcoholism, acquired immunodeficiency syndrome (AIDS), and drug or toxic exposures. Common factors associated with polyneuropathy are presented in the accompanying Key Features of Disease.

COLLABORATIVE MANAGEMENT

Although peripheral neuropathy is rarely the primary problem necessitating hospitalization, the nurse is likely to encounter clients with this condition in a variety of settings, particularly among the elderly or in clients with a related illness. Nursing assessment includes a detailed medical history and examination of the client's sensory and motor abilities. Often, the client can best outline a specific area of sensory deficit. Because the client may be unaware of decreased sensation, the nurse assesses the distal extremities for light touch and pain using cotton balls or cotton-tipped applicators and a safety pin. Position sense, or kinesthetic sensation, is assessed by gently grasping the involved digit or extremity on its sides. With the client's eyes closed, the nurse changes the position of the digit or extremity. The client is asked to describe how the position was changed. The client should be able to acknowledge even slight movements. A tuning fork may be placed on bony prominences to test for sensitivity to vibration. The examination is started at distal sites and more proximal areas are tested only if the client fails to perceive the duration of the vibration at the distal site. The nurse examines the extremities for any signs of injury of which the client may be unaware. Last, the nurse assesses the client for orthostatic hypotension; abnormal sweating; miosis (abnormal constriction of the pupil); sphincter disturbances, such as loss of bowel and bladder control; and other autonomic dysfunctions that may accompany the neuropathy. All abnormal findings are documented and brought to the physician's attention.

Treatment of clients with peripheral neuropathy consists of removal or treatment of the underlying cause

KEY FEATURES OF DISEASE ■ Factors Associated with Polyneuropathy	
Diseases	**Drug Use**
Amyloidosis	Nitrofurantoin
Alcoholism	Vincristine
Carcinomas	Isoniazid
Diabetes mellitus	Phenytoin
Diphtheria	Amitriptyline
Hepatic failure	Hydralazine
Malabsorption or malnutrition	
Porphyria	**Environmental**
Renal failure (uremia)	**Exposures**
Trauma	
Vascular disease	Heavy metals
	Industrial solvents
Vitamin Deficiencies	
Vitamin B_1 (thiamine)	
Vitamin B_6 (pyridoxine)	
Vitamin B_2 (riboflavin)	
Vitamin B_c (folic acid)	
Vitamin B_{12}	
Niacin	

and symptomatic therapy, including supportive care and physiotherapy. The diet is generally supplemented with vitamins, especially if vitamin deficiency is an underlying cause. However, there is no evidence that vitamins in excess of those contained in a well-balanced diet have any effect on forms of polyneuropathy unrelated to vitamin deficiency. With removal of the toxic agent or correction of the metabolic defects, recovery may be rapid, if the continuity of the nerves has not been interrupted. If there has been axonal destruction, recovery may require several months. After severe degeneration, there may be permanent weakness, atrophy, decreased reflexes, and sensory deficits.

The nurse is responsible for extensive client teaching. For clients with decreased sensation in feet and legs, the nurse explains the importance of proper foot care, instructing the client to wash, apply lanolin ointment or other appropriate lubricant, and visually inspect the feet and legs daily. The nurse instructs the client to wear white or color-fast stockings and to change them daily. The client is instructed to purchase high-quality, well-fitting shoes and avoid going barefoot. In addition, the nurse assists the client with decreased sensation to recognize potential hazards, such as exposure to extremes of environmental temperature (e.g., frostbite), bathwater or dishwater that may be too hot, contact of the feet with heat sources (such as heating pads or radiators) while sleeping, and burns associated with cooking. Smoking is discouraged by the nurse, as the resulting vasoconstriction may worsen the neuropathy. The importance of maintaining adequate nutrition is emphasized. Clients with postural hypotension are taught to arise slowly and wear support or elastic stockings to minimize blood pooling in the legs.

Many clients, especially those with the acute forms of polyneuropathy associated with drugs or exposure to toxic substances, experience anxiety, ineffective coping, and changes in such family processes as role responsibilities and sexual functioning. Thus, it is vital for the nurse to establish a trusting nurse-client relationship and to provide psychosocial support. In consultation with the physician, social worker, chaplain or religious leader, and physical and occupational therapists, the nurse focuses on the client's abilities and strengths and helps to identify new ways of coping, meeting needs, and restructuring activities.

PERIPHERAL NERVE TRAUMA

OVERVIEW

The peripheral nerves are subject to injuries associated with military conflict, mechanical or vehicular acci-
dents, certain sports, injection of particular drugs (or improper injection technique), and acts of violence such as knife or gunshot wounds. Specific mechanisms of injury include partial or complete severance of a nerve or nerves; contusion, stretching, constriction, or compression of a nerve or nerves; ischemia; and electrical, thermal, or radiation injury. Most commonly affected are the median, ulnar, and radial nerves of the upper extremities and the peroneal, femoral, and sciatic nerves of the legs (Fig. 34–1).

After transection of a nerve, degeneration and retraction of the nerve distal to the injury occur within 24 hours. Motor and sensory dysfunction distal to the lesion coincides with the loss of electrical excitability as the nerve fibers degenerate. Recovery occurs as Schwann's cells of the neurolemma proliferate from both the proximal and distal stumps. Dividing mitotically, these cells form neurolemmal cords, which act as guidelines for the regenerating axon. Tiny unmyelinated sprouts are generated at the proximal axon and grow 1 to 4 mm each day. Some are able to cross the transected gap through guidance by the neurolemma to find their way to the distal stump (see the illustration on p. 983). The more well aligned the union, the more normal the functional return is.

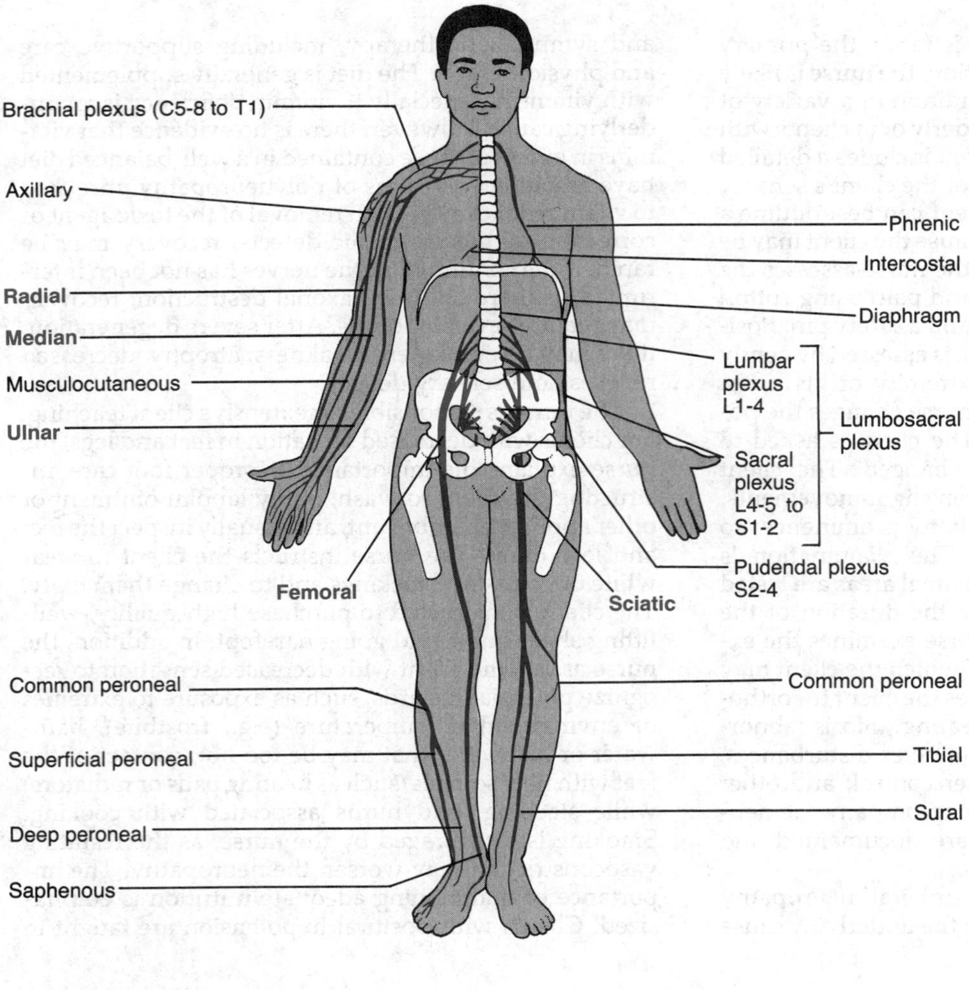

Figure 34–1

Distribution of selected peripheral nerves in the body.

Brachial plexus (C5-8 to T1)
Axillary
Radial
Median
Musculocutaneous
Ulnar
Femoral
Common peroneal
Superficial peroneal
Deep peroneal
Saphenous

Phrenic
Intercostal
Diaphragm
Lumbar plexus L1-4
Sacral plexus L4-5 to S1-2
Pudendal plexus S2-4
Lumbosacral plexus
Sciatic
Common peroneal
Tibial
Sural

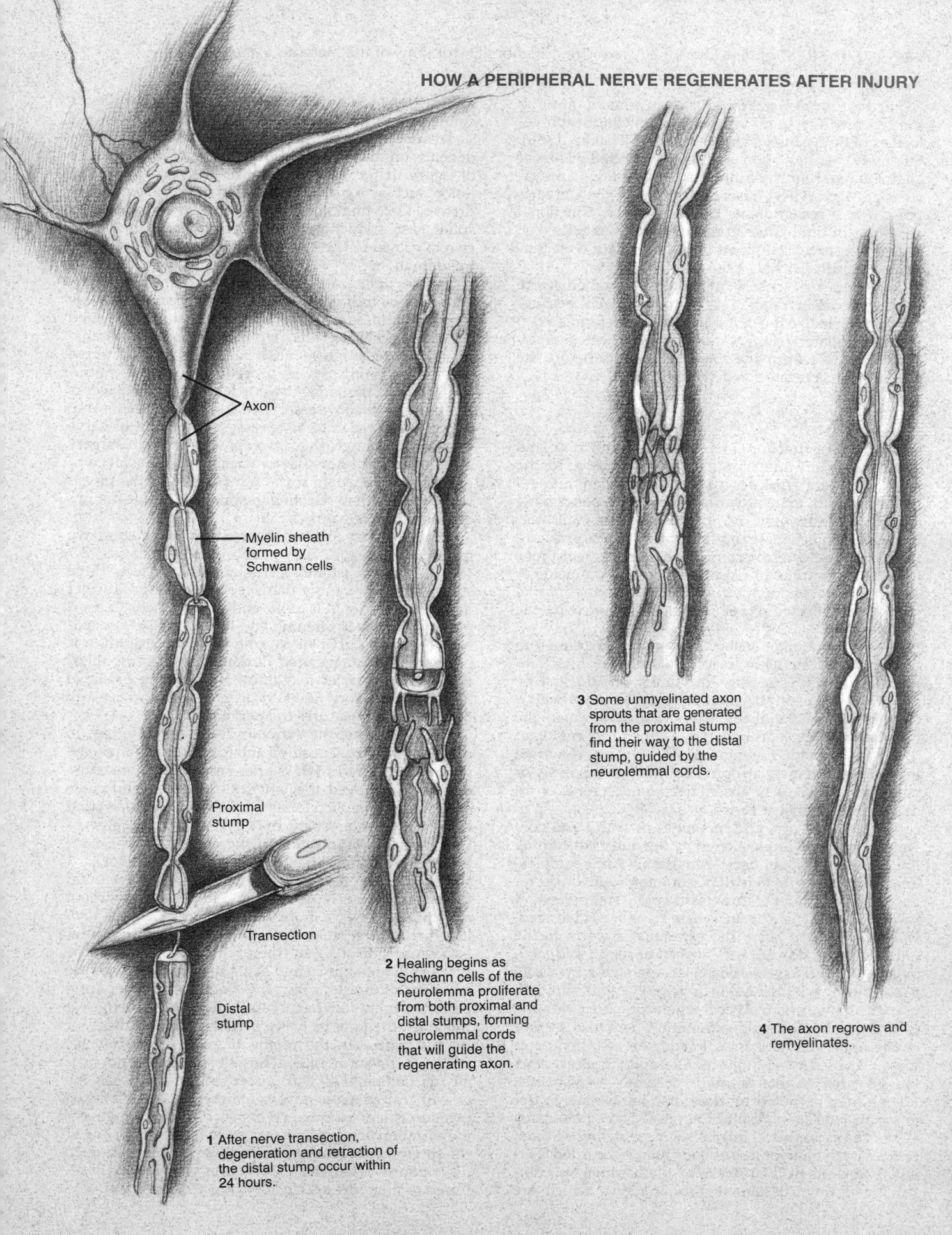

Axon

Myelin sheath formed by Schwann cells

Proximal stump

Transection

Distal stump

1 After nerve transection, degeneration and retraction of the distal stump occur within 24 hours.

2 Healing begins as Schwann cells of the neurolemma proliferate from both proximal and distal stumps, forming neurolemmal cords that will guide the regenerating axon.

3 Some unmyelinated axon sprouts that are generated from the proximal stump find their way to the distal stump, guided by the neurolemmal cords.

4 The axon regrows and remyelinates.

Successfully realigned nerves remyelinate, grow to their former size, and eventually claim conduction velocities of 80% of their former capacity (Hickey, 1986). Successful reinnervation is adversely affected by loss of anatomic continuity of the nerve, infection, and increasing age. Where disorganization of the nerve is present or if realignments are mismatched, functional weakness or unintentional muscle movements, as well as poor sensory discrimination and localization of stimuli, may result (Hickey, 1986).

Some return of sensory function may be noted before the regeneration process can occur. This is because nerves proximal to the injured neurons are stimulated to produce collateral innervation to the affected areas. These collaterals provide some innervation before the axon itself has regenerated sufficiently.

COLLABORATIVE MANAGEMENT

Assessment of function, maintenance of function, and rehabilitation are primary nursing considerations for the client with peripheral nerve trauma. The client may relate a history of extremity or pelvic trauma, penetrating injury, recent surgery, use of crutches, or pain after medication injections. In addition to weakness or flaccid paralysis, the client may complain of burning sensations distal to the trauma or pain that increases on tactile or environmental stimulation. A history of skin and nail changes of affected extremities may be noted by the client as well.

Physical examination by the nurse is performed to determine which neurologic functions are intact. In acute traumatic situations, the injury should first be evaluated by the physician to determine if movement is contraindicated. If movement is not contraindicated, the nurse assesses motor function by asking the client to put the limb through the normal ROM. Any abnormal movements, tremor, atrophy, contractions, paresis or paralysis, and weak or absent deep tendon reflexes are documented. Sensory function is tested using a wisp of cotton, a safety pin, and test tubes of warm and cold water. The client is questioned by the nurse concerning the occurrence of abnormal sensations. After complete denervation, the extent of vasomotor function is reflected in skin temperature, skin color, and edema. A "warm" phase and a "cold" phase have been identified. During the *warm phase* the extremity is warm to the touch, and the skin appears flushed or rosy. Gradually, over 2 to 3 weeks, this phase is superseded by a *cold phase,* during which the skin appears cyanotic, mottled, or reddish blue and feels cool when compared with the contralateral, unaffected extremity. The dorsal surface of the nurse's hand is used to compare skin temperatures because the abundance of temperature receptors in this area facilitates more accurate assessments. Edema may be noted by the nurse immediately after injury or later, as a result of surgical procedures. Any evidence of trophic changes, such as scaling of skin, brittleness of nails, or loss of body hair, is recorded. This initial assessment then serves as the baseline for comparison during subsequent examinations, which are done every 2 to 4 hours or less frequently as the client's condition indicates.

Treatment of the client with peripheral nerve trauma depends on the location, as well as the type and degree of injury. If the nerve trauma results from a primary lesion such as a tumor, the underlying problem is addressed first. Immobilization of the involved area by splint, cast, or traction may be prescribed by the physician to provide the rest needed to limit and resolve any inflammation.

In cases of laceration or transection of the nerve, surgery may be indicated. Restorative procedures include resection and suturing to reapproximate the severed nerve ends, nerve grafts, and nerve and tendon transplants. Since surgeons first began to repair injured nerves, the timing of these procedures has been controversial. In the past, repairs were delayed for 3 to 8 weeks after injury to allow associated injuries to heal and to permit the surgeon to better assess the extent of nerve damage. Although the development of microsurgery and the use of lasers have increased the incidence of primary nerve repair at the time of injury, the physician's judgment in selecting the optimal time and surgical procedure remains crucial.

After an injury, the two severed nerve segments have contracted and each may have formed scar tissue. Before surgical anastomosis, the surgeon dissects these stumps to remove any damaged nerve tissue, further decreasing the lengths of the ends to be joined. To compensate for this shortening and to avoid excessive tension on the sutured nerve, the involved extremity is positioned in exaggerated flexion. The surgeon aligns the segments under magnification, bringing proximal motor and sensory fibers to distal motor and sensory fibers, and then sutures the nerve tissue.

After suturing, the extremity is placed in a cast to maintain the flexed position and to avoid tension on the suture line. Ten to 14 days after nerve repair, the entire dressing is removed, the joint flexion is eased, and a new splint may be applied for an additional 2 weeks. At that time, a removable splint may be applied and physiotherapy begun. Protection of the nerve sutures is continued for a minimum of 6 weeks (Wilkins, 1986).

If a large segment of nerve has been damaged and direct anastomosis would be impossible without stretching the nerve more than 10% to 15% of its total length, the surgeon may interpose a nerve graft. Motor and sensory axons may then regenerate through the graft, joining proximal and distal segments through the two sites of anastomosis. The amount of sensory and motor regeneration that occurs depends on the length of the graft, the kind of nerve involved, the condition of the end plates, and the number of axons able to traverse the graft and suture sites. Thus, the results are not usually as favorable as with direct reanastomosis. In the case of grafted nerve repairs, maintenance of the flexed position is less essential (Wilkins, 1986), although immobilization using splints or casts to facilitate healing of the surgical sites remains imperative. For more detailed descriptions of surgical procedures, the reader is referred to literature specific to surgery of the hand.

Splints are usually held in place with elastic (Ace) wrapping or hook and loop (Velcro) closures, which can become too tight if edema develops. The skin around splints and casts is checked frequently (hourly, initially) by the nurse for tightness, warmth, and color. If the client complains of discomfort, tingling, or coolness or if the color is blanched, the cast or splint may be too tight and the nurse promptly informs the physician. Any indication of drainage under a splint or cast is immediately reported by the nurse.

Skin care is essential, as atrophy of the epidermis and underlying tissue causes the skin to become more fragile and more susceptible to injury and breakdown. The decreased skin nutrition and vascularity associated with denervation causes delayed healing, further compounding the problem. The nurse thoroughly examines the skin for evidence of irritation or injury and assists or instructs the client to wash and dry the involved areas carefully. If the skin is dry, lanolin or cocoa butter may be used as a lubricant. In addition, because sensation may be absent or inhibited, the nurse instructs the client to protect involved areas from extremes in temperature or other sources of potential additional trauma.

Depending on the extent and type of injury, as well as the selected mode of treatment, the rehabilitation process may be limited or quite extensive. While fostering a positive, trusting relationship, the nurse helps the client set realistic goals by providing information and support. Extensive teaching may be needed for the client to regain the greatest possible level of independence. Physiotherapy is the major approach used for rehabilitation after surgical repair. Because this may be a slow and painful process, the nurse reinforces and helps the client perform exercises learned in these sessions. Because the regeneration of nerves and subsequent return of sensory and motor function may be extremely slow, the client may become discouraged and depressed. If the disability is permanent, the client needs encouragement and assistance to cope with the changes in body image, self-esteem, and life style. Many clients experience feelings of frustration, hostility, anger, loss, grief, and bereavement, resulting from their loss of power, lack of control over the situation, and changes in role function. Therefore, it is important for the nurse to provide psychosocial support and initiate necessary referrals to other members of the health care or rehabilitation team. Often, these clients continue treatment on an outpatient basis with physical and occupational therapists in cooperation with the physician and the community health nurse.

DISEASES OF THE CRANIAL NERVES

The nurse may encounter clients with cranial nerve disease in various practice settings, such as clinics, physician's offices, home care agencies, or hospitals. Al-

though the cranial nerves may be affected in association with other disorders of the nervous system or as a result of trauma, only the most common disorders, those affecting cranial nerves V (trigeminal) and VII (facial), are discussed.

TRIGEMINAL NEURALGIA

OVERVIEW

Trigeminal neuralgia, or *tic douloureux,* appears usually in persons older than 50 years of age, affecting the elderly at a frequency of 155 cases per million with a female/male ratio of 3:2 (Adams & Victor, 1985). This disorder entails a specific type of facial pain, which occurs in abrupt, intense paroxysms; is usually provoked by minimal stimulation of a trigger zone; and is unilateral and confined to the area innervated by the trigeminal nerve, most often the second and third branches (Fig. 34–2). Terms used by clients when describing the pain include sharp, shooting, piercing, burning, and jabbing. Between bursts of pain, which last from seconds to minutes, there is usually no pain. The nurse usually finds no sensory or motor deficits on examination, although the condition can be agonizing for the client. The fear of precipitating attacks often causes clients to avoid talking, smiling, eating, or attending to hygienic needs, such as shaving, washing the face, and brushing the teeth.

Although the cause of trigmeninal neuralgia has not been firmly established, both intrinsic lesions within the nerve and extrinsic pressure against the nerve have been implicated. In addition, trauma and infection of the teeth, jaw, or ear may be contributing factors.

The course of trigeminal neuralgia is characterized by bouts of pain for several weeks or months, followed by spontaneous remissions. The length of these remissions

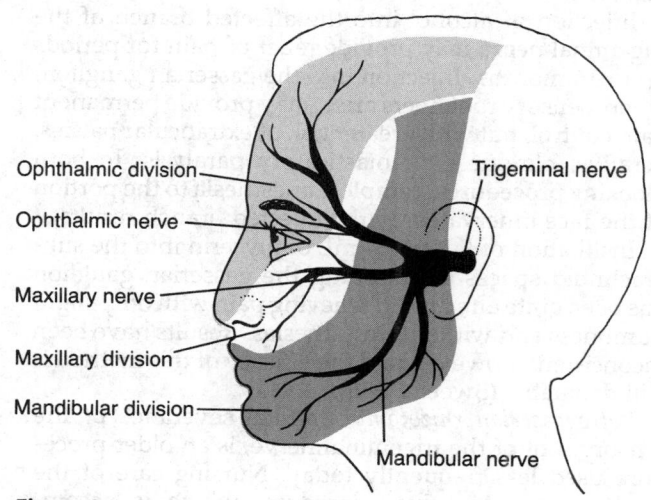

Figure 34–2

Distribution of the trigeminal nerve and its three divisions: ophthalmic, maxillary, and mandibular.

may vary from days to years, but there is a tendency for attack-free periods to become shorter as the client grows older. Permanent disappearance of symptoms is rare.

COLLABORATIVE MANAGEMENT

Medical management is accomplished with the use of drugs, such as carbamazepine (Tegretol), phenytoin (Dilantin), baclofen (Lioresal), and occasionally amitriptyline (Elavil) or diazepam (Valium). In addition, local nerve blocking by injection of alcohol or glycerol may provide temporary relief. Initial therapy should always be nonsurgical, and drugs may be utilized singly or in combination. Surgical management may be considered if the client and the physician agree that the pain or the toxic effects of drug therapy are worse than the risk of surgery.

Approximately 70% of clients respond to carbamazepine, 20 to 1200 mg daily, alone or in combination with phenytoin, in average daily dosages of 200 to 400 mg. Phenytoin may also be given intravenously to abort an acute attack. Both of these drugs are anticonvulsants, and it is believed that their action decreases the paroxysmal afferent impulses in much the same way as when these drugs are used in the treatment of seizure disorders. The nurse monitors the client for medication side effects, such as headache, nausea and vomiting, rash, vertigo, ataxia, drowsiness, and blood dyscrasias (e.g., aplastic anemia and leukopenia). Regular (weekly in the beginning) complete blood count (CBC) and close monitoring by the physician and the nurse are required for both drugs. The nurse teaches the client the early indications of potential problems, including fever, sore throat, easy bruising, ulcers in the mouth, and petechial hemorrhage or purpura. The nurse instructs the client to contact the physician at once if any of these symptoms appear. It is important to detect any changes in CBC early because aplastic anemia may be reversed in some persons.

Injection of alcohol into the affected branch of the trigeminal nerve may provide relief of pain for periods up to 16 months. Injection into the gasserian ganglion, where sensory root fibers arise, may provide permanent pain control, but with greater risk of extraocular palsies, keratitis, blindness, or masticatory paralysis. In both blocking procedures, complete anesthesia to the portion of the face innervated by the injected branch results.

Instillation of 0.2 to 0.4 mL of glycerin into the subarachnoid spaces surrounding the gasserian ganglion has been quite effective in relieving pain with only slight numbness and without dysesthesias. Results have been inconsistent, however, and the efficacy of this method is still debatable (Sweet, 1986).

Retrogasserian rhizotomy, or total severance of the sensory root of the trigeminal nerve, is an older procedure used less frequently today. Nursing care of the client undergoing this procedure, which is accomplished by craniotomy, follows the principles of care for craniotomy outlined in Chapter 33. This procedure produces permanent anesthesia of the innervated area, yet the client may experience paresthesias—a burning, itching, or scratching sensation in the anesthetized area (anesthesia dolorosa). Facial paralysis, corneal ulceration, and extraocular palsies are other possible complications.

In addition to routine postcraniotomy care, the nurse evaluates the client's corneal reflex, extraocular muscles, and facial nerve during each examination. The corneal reflex may be tested by touching the cornea lightly with sterile cotton or by making a threatening motion with the fist close to the eye. The client will blink if the reflex is intact. Extraocular muscles are assessed by asking the client to follow a finger through the six cardinal positions (see Chap. 32) while the nurse observes for conjugate eye movements. The facial nerve is tested by asking the client to wrinkle the forehead, frown, wink, squeeze the eyes closed, whistle, and blow air out of the cheeks. Last, the nurse evaluates the client for abnormal sensations and pain, as well as assessing the client's ability to chew. Any abnormal findings are documented by the nurse and reported to the physician.

In some clients, a small artery compresses the trigeminal nerve as it enters the pons. This artery may be relocated surgically to relieve the pain of trigeminal neuralgia without compromising facial sensation. The *Jannetta procedure* accomplishes this through a posterior fossa craniotomy. Under microscopic vision, the loop of artery is carefully lifted off the nerve and a small silicone (Silastic) sponge is placed between the vessel and the nerve. Complications associated with this procedure include headache, facial pain, and those complications seen with posterior fossa surgery. Postoperatively, the nurse provides routine care; as soon as the client is alert, an assessment of the trigeminal neuralgia pain is conducted by the nurse and compared with the client's preoperative assessment.

Electrocoagulation or *percutaneous radio frequency rhizotomy* may provide lasting relief of pain without compromising touch or motor function. During this procedure the client is sedated with small doses of diazepam (Valium) or fentanyl (Sublimaze), but is alert and able to respond verbally to questions. A needle electrode is then inserted and advanced under radiographic control to the appropriate area where a heat lesion is then made. After each needle insertion, the corneal and ciliary reflexes, as well as sensation in the face, are checked. The advantages of this procedure include long-term pain relief, relatively short hospital stays, tolerance by the elderly, absence of facial paralysis, and preservation of the sensation of touch. The possibility of puncturing the internal carotid artery and the occurrence of anesthesia dolorosa are disadvantages (Hickey, 1986). The affected side is permanently insensitive to pain.

Postoperatively the nurse applies an ice pack to the operative site on the jaw for 4 hours. A soft diet is prescribed, and the client is discouraged from chewing on the affected side until the paresthesia is abated. Client teaching includes instructing the client to avoid rubbing the eye on the affected side, as the protective mechanism of pain will no longer warn of injury (see the accompanying Client/Family Education feature). In addi-

---

CLIENT/FAMILY EDUCATION ■ Instructions After a Trigeminal Nerve Rhizotomy

Instructions	Rationales
1. "Avoid rubbing your eye on the affected side."	1. The eye's protective pain mechanism is removed, and eye injury may occur if the eye is rubbed.
2. "Inspect your eye daily for redness and irritation."	2. Without pain as a warning sign, inflammation or injury to the eye may go undetected.
3. "See your dentist regularly for examinations."	3. Dental pain from tooth caries or gum disease will not be present.
4. "When possible, chew your food on the unaffected side."	4. Food particles may become lodged in the cheek of the affected side owing to loss of sensation. In addition, the client may unknowingly bite the inside of the cheek and cause injury.

tion, the client is instructed to inspect the eye daily for redness or irritation and to report this or the occurrence of blurred vision to the physician. The nurse also encourages the client to schedule regular dental examinations because the absence of pain may not warn the client of potential problems.

Psychosocial considerations for the client with trigeminal neuralgia include disappointment with ineffective drug protocols or surgical procedures, as well as fear that the pain may recur with any activity. The client may fail to move the face in an attempt to prevent pain. This behavior may be misinterpreted by others as withdrawal, antisociability, or depression. The nurse's goal is to help the client cope with the condition and to develop strategies to deal with identified problems.

FACIAL PARALYSIS

OVERVIEW

Facial paralysis, or *Bell's palsy,* acute paralysis of cranial nerve VII, was first described by Sir Charles Bell of England in 1821. The incidence of this condition is 23 per 100,000, with men and women equally affected. Although the incidence may be slightly higher among diabetics, the condition occurs among all ages and at all times of the year (Adams & Victor, 1985).

The onset is acute, with maximal paralysis attained within 48 hours in about half of the clients and within 5 days in almost all clients. Pain behind the ear or on the face may precede paralysis by a few hours or days. The disorder is characterized by a drawing sensation and paralysis of all facial muscles on the affected side. The client is unable to close the eye, wrinkle the forehead, smile, whistle, or grimace. The face appears mask-like and sags. Taste is usually impaired to some degree, but this seldom persists beyond the second week of paralysis. Although the cause of Bell's palsy remains obscure, it is believed to be due to an inflammatory process. Although these clients are rarely hospitalized for the Bell's palsy, the nurse may encounter them in outpatient settings, such as clinics or physician's offices.

COLLABORATIVE MANAGEMENT

Medical management consists of prednisone (Deltasone), 30 to 60 mg daily during the first week after the onset of symptoms. Analgesics may be helpful in relieving the pain. Nursing care is directed toward managing the major neurologic deficits and providing psychosocial support. Because the eye does not close, the cornea must be protected from drying and subsequent ulceration or abrasion. The nurse instructs the client to manually close the eyelid at intervals and to instill artificial tears four times daily. The eye may be patched or taped closed at bedtime.

The client may be unable to chew, sip fluids through a straw, or control drooling on the affected side. Thus, mealtime may become a problem for the client. The nurse may be needed to provide emotional support and suggestions for coping and adapting. Frequent, small meals may be better tolerated, and clients may require a soft diet.

The nurse teaches the client simple techniques of massage; application of warm, moist heat; and facial exercises. A facial sling may be provided to prevent drooping of the affected side. As muscle tone improves, the nurse instructs the client to grimace, wrinkle the brow, force the eyes closed, whistle, and blow air out of the cheeks three or four times daily for 5 minutes in front of a mirror.

Although 80% of clients recover fully within a few weeks or months, approximately 15% to 20% show some residual weakness and 2% to 4% have permanent neurologic deficits. Thus, these clients require a great deal of support, as body image and self-esteem are drastically affected. The nurse is a valuable source of both information and psychosocial support.

SUMMARY

PNS dysfunctions have a variety of clinical manifestations, ranging from life-threatening conditions, such as respiratory distress, to severe facial pain, as seen in trigeminal neuralgia. Nurses may therefore see these clients in all types of practice settings and often work with other health care professionals, including physical and occupational therapists, to meet client goals.

IMPLICATIONS FOR RESEARCH

Research on PNS disorders has concentrated on determining the exact causes of these diseases. Nursing research related to PNS disorders has been limited. Possible questions for nursing research include the following:

1. How can adequate nutrition be ensured for the client with painful trigeminal neuralgia?

2. What nondrug measures can the nurse use to help relieve the pain associated with disorders of the cranial nerves?

3. How can the nurse assist the client in developing coping strategies for disorders that often cause major life style changes?

4. How can the nurse collaborate more effectively with other health care professionals in the delivery of quality care for clients with PNS disorders?

REFERENCES AND READINGS

Adams, R. D., & Victor, M. (1985). *Principles of neurology* (3rd ed.). New York: McGraw-Hill.

Blanco, K., & Cuomo, N. (1983). From the other side of the bedrail: A personal experience with Guillain-Barré syndrome. *Journal of Neurological Nursing, 15,* 355–359.

Bowes, D. (1984). The doctor as patient: An encounter with Guillain-Barré syndrome. *Canadian Medical Association Journal, 131,* 1343–1348.

Caine, R. M., & Bufalino, P. M. (1987). *Nursing care planning guides for adults.* Baltimore: Williams & Wilkins.

Fisher, M. A. (1981). Peripheral neuropathy. In W. J. Weiner and C. G. Goetz (Eds.), *Neurology for the non-neurologist.* Philadelphia: Harper & Row.

George, M. R. (1988). Neuromuscular respiratory failure: What the nurse knows may make the difference. *Journal of Neuroscience Nursing, 20,* 110–117.

Griswold, K., Guanci, M. M., & Ropper, A. H. (1984). An approach to the care of patients with Guillain-Barré syndrome. *Heart and Lung, 13,* 66–72.

Hickey, J. V. (1986). *The clinical practice of neurological and neurosurgical nursing* (2nd ed.). Philadelphia: J. B. Lippincott.

Jefferson, D. (1985). Peripheral nerve disease. In R. W. Russell & C. M. Wiles (Eds.), *Integrated clinical science: Neurology.* Chicago: Year Book Medical.

Koski, C. L., Khurana, R., & Mayer, R. F. (1986). Guillain-Barré syndrome. *American Family Practice, 34* (3), 198–210.

Loh, L. (1986). Neurological and neuromuscular disease. *British Journal of Anaesthesia, 58,* 190–200.

Miller, R. G. (1985). Guillain-Barré syndrome: Current methods of diagnosis and treatment. *Postgraduate Medicine, 77*(7), 57–64.

Mulder, D. G., White, K., & Herrmann, C. (1986). Thymectomy: Surgical procedure for myasthenia gravis. *AORN Journal, 43,* 640–646.

Oosterhuis, H. J. G. H. (1984). *Myasthenia gravis.* New York: Churchill Livingstone.

Osserman, K. E. (1958). *Myasthenia gravis.* New York: Grune & Stratton.

Parker, B. C. (1988). Rehabilitative aspects of nerve injuries of the hand. *Orthopaedic Nursing, 7*(1), 29–34.

Provenzale, J. M. (1987). Treatment modalities in Guillain-Barré syndrome. *Hospital Practice, 15,* 93–102.

Ravits, J. (1988). Myasthenia gravis: A well understood neuromuscular disorder. *Postgraduate Medicine, 83*(1), 219–223.

Rhynsburger, J. (1989). How to fight MG fatigue. *American Journal of Nursing, 89,* 337–340.

Ropper, A. H. (1986). Severe acute Guillain-Barré syndrome. *Neurology, 36,* 429–432.

Rowland, L. P. (1984). Cranial and peripheral nerves. In L. P. Rowland (Ed.), *Merritt's textbook of neurology* (7th ed.). Philadelphia: Lea & Febiger.

Sellman, M. S., & Mayer, R. F. (1985). Treatment of myasthenic crisis in late life. *Southern Medical Journal, 78,* 1208–1210.

Seybold, M. E. (1983). Myasthenia gravis: A clinical and basic science review. *JAMA, 250,* 2516–2522.

Shearn, M. A., & Shearn, L. (1986). A personal experience with Guillain-Barré syndrome: Are the psychologic needs of patient and family being met? *Southern Medical Journal, 79,* 800–803.

Shumak, K. H., & Rock, G. A. (1984). Therapeutic plasma exchange. *New England Journal of Medicine, 310,* 762–771.

Sweet, W. H. (1986). Medical intelligence current concepts, the treatment of trigeminal neuralgia (tic douloureux). *New England Journal of Medicine, 315,* 174–177.

Therapeutic Plasmapheresis — Consensus Conference. (1986). The utility of therapeutic plasmapheresis for neurological disorders. *JAMA, 256,* 1333–1337.

Thompson, J. M., McFarland, G. K., Hirsch, J. E., Tucker, S. M., & Bowers, A. C. (1986). *Clinical nursing.* St. Louis: C. V. Mosby.

Verbanets, J. A. (1988). Cranial nerves: An often overlooked area of the peripheral nervous system. *Topics in Acute Care and Trauma Rehabilitation, 3,* 75–90.

Vogt, G., Miller, M., & Esluer, M. (1985). *Manual of neurological care.* St. Louis: C. V. Mosby.

Wilkins, R. H. (1986). Peripheral nerve injuries. In D. C. Sabiston, Jr. (Ed.), *Textbook of surgery.* Philadelphia: W. B. Saunders.

UNIT 10 RESOURCES

Nursing Resources

American Association of Neuroscience Nurses (AANN), 218 North Jefferson Street, Suite 204, Chicago, IL 60606. Telephone 312-993-0043.

Promotes the health, welfare, and education of the general public through education, research, and high standards of practice in neuroscience nursing. Publishes the *Journal of Neuroscience Nursing* (bimonthly), *Synapse* (bimonthly newsletter), the *Core Curriculum for Neuroscience Nursing,* and other print and audiovisual materials.

American Association of Spinal Cord Injury Nurses (AASCIN), 75–20 Astoria Boulevard, Jackson Heights, NY 11370. Telephone 718-803-3782.

Promotes education, research, and professional development as a means of achieving excellence in providing care for clients with spinal cord injuries. Publishes *SCI Nursing* (quarterly), *Educational Guidelines for Professional Nursing Practice,* and the *SCI Patient/ Family Education Manual for Nurses.*

American Board of Neuroscience Nursing (ABNN), c/o Professional Examination Service, 475 Riverside Drive, New York, NY 10115. Telephone 212-733-3971.

Certifies registered nurses in neuroscience nursing on the basis of demonstration of requisite knowledge and endorsement by colleagues.

American Society for Parenteral and Enteral Nutrition (ASPEN), 8630 Fenton Street, Suite 412, Silver Spring, MD 20910. Telephone 301-587-6315.

Promotes optimal nutrition care.

National Board of Nutrition Support Certification (NBNSC), 8630 Fenton Street, Suite 412, Silver Spring, MD 20910.

Certifies registered nurses with experience in nutrition support.

Other Resources

Alzheimer's Disease and Related Disorders Association, 70 East Lake St., Chicago, IL 60601. Telephone 800-621-0379.

American Parkinson's Disease Association Inc., 116 John Street, New York, NY 10038. Telephone 212-732-9550.

Association for Brain Tumor Research, 6232 North Pulaski Road, Suite 200, Chicago, IL 60646. Telephone 312-286-5571.

Epilepsy Foundation of America, 815 15th Street NW, Suite 528, Washington, DC 20005. Telephone 202-638-5229.

Guillain-Barré Foundation, 129 North Carolina Avenue SE, Washington, DC 20003. Telephone 202-387-2216.

Myasthenia Gravis Foundation, 61 Gramercy Park North, New York, NY 10010. Telephone 212-533-7005.

National Association to Control Epilepsy, 22 East 67th Street, New York, NY 10021.

National Easter Seal Society, 2023 West Ogden Avenue, Chicago, IL 60612. Telephone 312-243-8400.

National Head Injury Foundation, 333 Turnpike Road, Southborough, MA 01722. Telephone 508-485-9950.

National Multiple Sclerosis Society, 205 East 42nd Street, New York, NY 10010. Telephone 212-532-3060.

National Parkinson's Foundation, 1501 NW 9th Avenue, Miami, FL 33136. Telephone 305-547-6666.

National Spinal Cord Injury Association, 600 West Cumming Park 3200, Woburn, MA 01801. Telephone 800-962-9629.

Parkinson Disease Foundation, Medical Center, William Black Medical Research Building, 640 West 168th Street, New York, NY 10032. Telephone 212-923-4700.

UNIT 11

Problems of Sensation: Management of Clients with Disruptions of the Sensory System

Assessment of the Eye

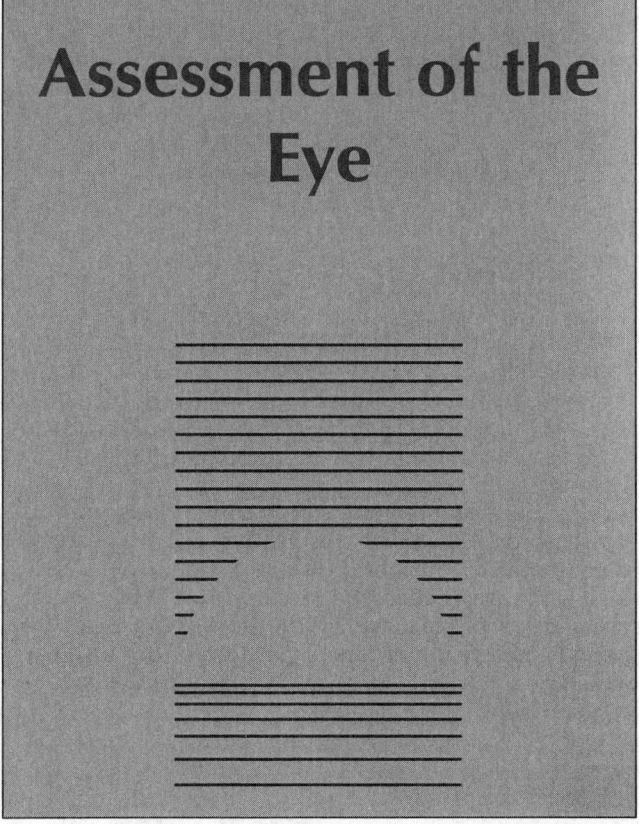

The eye is an invaluable sensory organ that is responsible for gathering visual stimuli to assist individuals in communicating with the world around them. Nurses need an understanding of the structure and function of the eye and related organs, as well as the relationship of the eye to the body, when caring for clients with ophthalmic disorders.

Visual screening is an essential component of the physical assessment process. Nurses in settings such as schools, emergency rooms, clinics, industries, and public health systems are instrumental in conducting these assessments. After an assessment and evaluation of the eye and visual processes, the nurse refers clients to an ophthalmologist or optometrist for further diagnosis if necessary.

An *ophthalmologist* is a physician (MD or DO) specializing in medical and surgical treatment of eye diseases and disorders. Ophthalmologists perform eye examinations as well as diagnose and treat orbital injuries and diseases. Ophthalmologists prescribe corrective lenses and medications and also perform ocular and laser surgery. An *optometrist* is a doctor of optometry (OD) who is trained to perform a complete eye examination, prescribe corrective lenses, and detect eye diseases. Optometrists may prescribe exercises for muscle imbalance, and in some states they are permitted to treat certain eye diseases and prescribe ophthalmic medications. An *optician* is licensed to fit, adjust, and dispense glasses and contact lenses, which have been ordered by a licensed ophthalmologist or optometrist. The *ocularist* prepares and fits ocular prostheses.

ANATOMY AND PHYSIOLOGY REVIEW

STRUCTURE

The eyeball is a spherical organ, about 1 in (2.5 cm) in diameter, which is located in the anterior portion of the orbit. The *orbit* is the bony structure of the skull that surrounds the eye and offers protection to the eye as well as to the associated muscles, nerves, vessels, and most of the lacrimal (tear) apparatus.

LAYERS OF THE EYEBALL

The eye has three layers, or coats, as shown in Figure 35–1. The external layer, the *fibrous* coat, supports the eye and consists of the *sclera,* which is an opaque white tissue that comprises the posterior five-sixths of the eye, and the *cornea,* which is a dense, transparent layer that completes the remaining anterior one-sixth.

The *middle layer,* or *uvea,* the second layer of the eyeball, is vascular and heavily pigmented. This layer

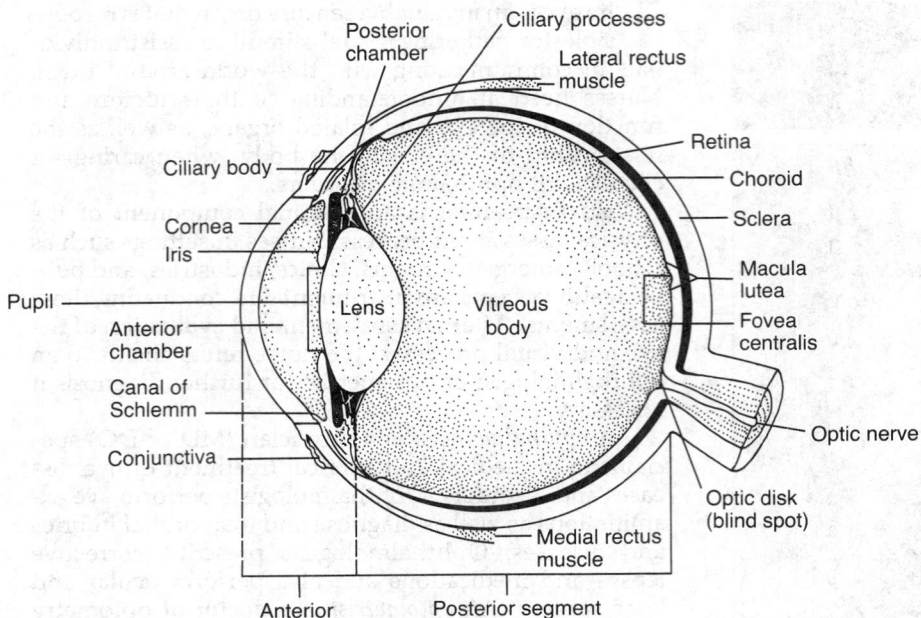

Figure 35–1

Anatomic features of the eye.

consists of the choroid, the ciliary body, and the iris. The *choroid*, a dark brown membrane located between the sclera and the retina, forms the largest part of the middle layer. It lines most of the sclera. The choroid is firmly attached to the retina, but it can be easily detached from the sclera. Located in the choroid are many blood vessels that are responsible for supplying nutrients to the adjacent retina.

The *ciliary body* connects the choroid with the circumference of the iris. Ciliary processes are folds on the internal surface of the ciliary body that secrete aqueous humor, one of the two fluid-like substances that help give the eye its shape. The *iris* is the colored portion of the eye and appears characteristically blue, green, hazel, gray, or brown. It is situated in front of the lens and has a central circular opening called the *pupil*. During waking hours, the size of the pupil varies as the amount of light entering the eye is regulated.

The most internal layer is the *retina*—a thin, delicate structure through which the fibers of the optic nerve are distributed. It is bordered externally by the choroid and sclera and internally by the vitreous. The vitreous is a gel-like substance that maintains the eye's spherical shape. The retina contains blood vessels, which supply nourishment to the retinal fibers, and two classes of photoreceptors, called *rods* and *cones*. The rods function at reduced levels of illumination and are responsible for peripheral vision. The cones function at bright levels of illumination and are responsible for color vision and for central vision. There are usually about 110 to 125 million rods and about 6.5 million cones in a single retina (Friedman, 1981).

At the posterior pole of the eye (posterior to the ciliary processes) is the *optic fundus*. Within this area is the *optic disk*, which is a creamy pink to white depressed area in the retina. The *optic nerve* enters and exits the eyeball at this point. The optic disk is sometimes referred to as the

blind spot because it contains only nerve fibers and no photoreceptor cells and is insensitive to light. Lateral and temporal to the optic disk is a small, oval, yellowish-pink area called the *macula lutea*. The central depressed part of the macula is the *fovea centralis,* where the most acute vision occurs. If portions of the fovea or macula are damaged, visual acuity is reduced, and central vision blindness may result.

REFRACTIVE MEDIA

Light waves pass through the following structures of varying densities on the way to the retina: the cornea, aqueous humor, lens, and vitreous humor. Each of these structures causes the light waves to bend, or *refract*, to some degree. These structures constitute the *refracting media* of the eye.

The cornea, as previously described, is the transparent layer that forms the external coat of the anterior portion of the eye. The *aqueous humor* is a clear, watery fluid that fills the anterior and posterior chambers of the eye (see Fig. 35–1). The *anterior chamber* of the eye lies between the cornea and iris. The *posterior chamber* lies between the iris and lens. Aqueous humor is produced by the ciliary processes and passes from the posterior chamber through the pupil and into the anterior chamber. This fluid drains through spaces at the *iridocorneal angle* (filtration angle), which opens into a circular venous canal called the *canal of Schlemm*. This canal permits the aqueous fluid to drain out of the eye into the systemic circulation so that a fairly constant intraocular pressure (pressure within the eye) is maintained.

The *lens* is a circular, biconvex structure that lies behind the iris and in front of the vitreous body. It is normally transparent. The lens bends rays of light entering through the pupil so that they fall on the retina.

The curvature of the surfaces of the lens varies, which enables a person to focus on objects near or distant. The curvature of the lens is adjusted by contraction and relaxation of fibers, called *zonules,* that hold the lens in place.

The *vitreous body* consists of a gelatinous substance that occupies the vitreous chamber, the space between the lens and the retina. This gelatinous body transmits light and gives shape to the posterior eye. *Vitreous humor* is composed of about 99% water and constitutes about four-fifths of the volume of the eyeball. Unlike the aqueous humor, the vitreous humor is not continuously replaced.

EXTERNAL STRUCTURES

The *eyelids* are thin, delicate, movable folds of skin that when closed protect the eyes from entry of a foreign body, shut out light during sleep, and aid in the propulsion of tears to keep the cornea moist. The upper eyelid is larger than the lower one and when open partly covers the iris. The place at which the two eyelids meet is called the *canthus,* or corner of the eye.

The *conjunctivae* are thin, transparent mucous membranes. The *palpebral conjunctiva* lines the posterior surface of each eyelid. Located over the sclera is the *bulbar conjunctiva.* The area where the conjunctivae meet is called the *fornix. Cul-de-sac* is the term for the lower

fornix. The *eyelashes,* or *cilia,* are tiny hairs that are arranged in two or three irregular rows in the margins of the eyelids. The lashes are quite sensitive to touch and serve to protect the eyeball from dust or small particles. The *eyebrows* are the small hairs that form an arch on the upper part of the orbit of the eye and protect the eyeball from perspiration.

Tears are produced by a small *lacrimal gland,* which is located in the upper temporal part of each orbit. The tears flow and are propelled across the eye toward the nose and into the *lacrimal lake* at the inner lower canthus. They are drained out through the *punctum,* which is found at each of the innermost lid margins, into the *lacrimal duct* and *sac,* and then into the nose through the nasolacrimal duct. The structure of the tear apparatus is seen in Figure 35–2. The lacrimal fluid moistens the corneal surface. When the cornea becomes dry, the eye blinks and the eyelids carry a film of lacrimal fluid over the eye. In this way, foreign materials such as dust particles are removed from the cornea and are carried to the medial canthus of the eye. When an individual cries, or if excess tears are produced, the lacrimal lake overflows, and tears roll down onto the cheeks.

MUSCLES

There are seven voluntary muscles of the orbit, six of which can rotate the eyeball in any direction and coordinate eye movements (Fig. 35–3). Four of these extraocular muscles are *rectus* (straight): the superior, inferior, lateral, and medial rectus muscles. Two extraocular muscles are *oblique:* the superior and inferior oblique muscles. Coordinated eye movements and adequate visual acuity are needed to enable the fovea centralis of the macula of each eye to receive an image at the same time. The focused image from the fovea of each eye is transmitted to the optic area of the cerebral cortex,

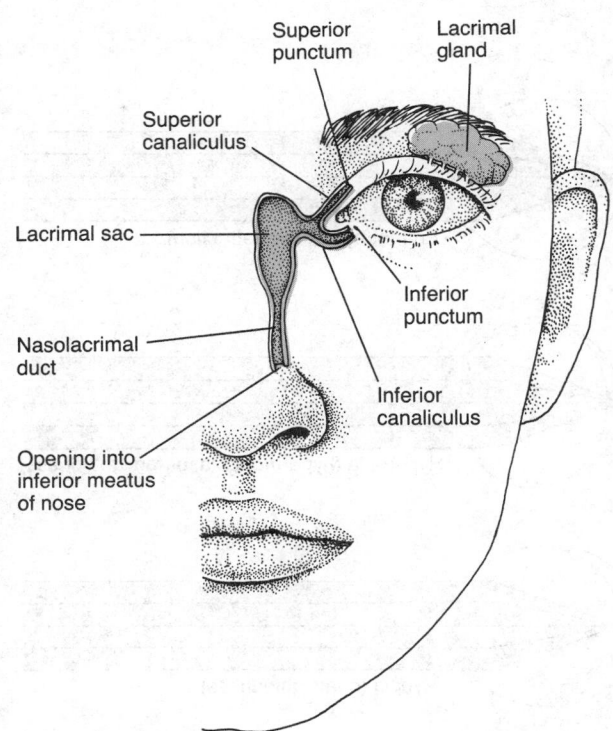

Figure 35–2

Anterior view of the eye and adjacent structures.

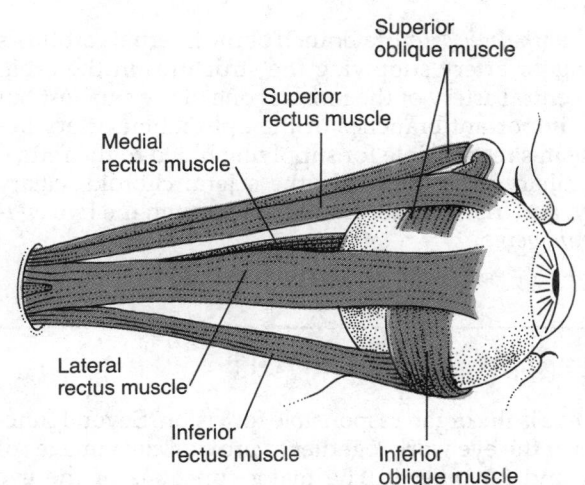

Figure 35–3

The extraocular muscles.

where the brain interprets the two images as a single one.

When an extraocular muscle contracts, it rotates the eye in the direction of the pull. Rectus muscles exert their pull when the eye is turned temporally (toward the temple). Oblique muscles have the greatest action when the eye is turned nasally (toward the nose) (Boyd-Monk & Steinmetz, 1987). The lateral rectus muscle abducts the eye. The superior rectus muscle and inferior oblique muscle control upward movement of the eye. Adduction of the eye is controlled by the medial and inferior rectus muscles. The superior oblique muscle controls downward movement of the eye. These muscles do not work independently, but rather in conjunction with the muscle that produces the opposite movement. Smooth eye movements are achieved by contraction and relaxation of these muscles in concert with each other.

The seventh orbit muscle, the levator palpebrae, acts to elevate the upper eyelid. This muscle does not insert into the eyeball and therefore cannot move it.

NERVES

The extraocular muscles are innervated by the following cranial nerves: oculomotor (cranial nerve III), trochlear (cranial nerve IV), and abducens (cranial nerve VI). The *optic nerve* (cranial nerve II) is the nerve of sight. It connects the optic disk to the brain. The ophthalmic division of the trigeminal nerve (cranial nerve V) innervates the sensory portion of the blink reflex, which is stimulated when the cornea is touched. The facial nerve (cranial nerve VII) innervates the lacrimal glands and musculature involved in lid closure. These nerves are discussed in Chapter 32.

BLOOD VESSELS

The *ophthalmic artery* (a branch of the internal carotid) is the major artery supplying the structures in the orbit. The central artery of the retina is one of the smallest but most important branches of the ophthalmic artery because it is responsible for supplying blood to the retina. The ciliary arteries supply the sclera, choroid, ciliary body, and iris. Venous drainage is through the two *ophthalmic veins*.

FUNCTION

The eye is the organ responsible for vision. Several functions of the eye work together to provide clear images of near and far objects. The major functions of the eye include refraction, pupillary constriction, and accommodation.

REFRACTION

Refraction is the process of bending light rays so as to focus an image on the retina. The eye manifests its refracting power in the form of several curved surfaces, each separated by media with different indices of refraction. The most important surfaces are in the anterior and posterior cornea and lens. *Emmetropia* is the term used to describe ideal refraction of the eye. In this state, with the lens at rest (unaccommodated), parallel light rays from a distant source (6 m or more) are focused into a sharp image on the fovea. Figure 35–4 shows the normal refraction of light that occurs within the eye.

Several common conditions occur in which there is an error of refraction. *Hyperopia*, which is also called hypermetropia or farsightedness, is a refractive error in which the eye possesses insufficient refracting power. The cause of this error is invariably a short anteroposterior diameter of the eye. In the case of a hyperopic eye, objects converge to a point behind the retina (see Fig. 35–4). Vision beyond 20 ft is normal, but near vision is poor. The appropriate correction is done by use of a convex lens.

Myopia (nearsightedness) is a type of refractive error in which the refracting power of the eye is too great for the anteroposterior diameter. This condition may be due to an enlargement of the anteroposterior diameter of the eye or to an excess of corneal refracting power. Parallel rays coming from an object are focused in front of the retina, at a point in the vitreous (see Fig. 35–4). Near

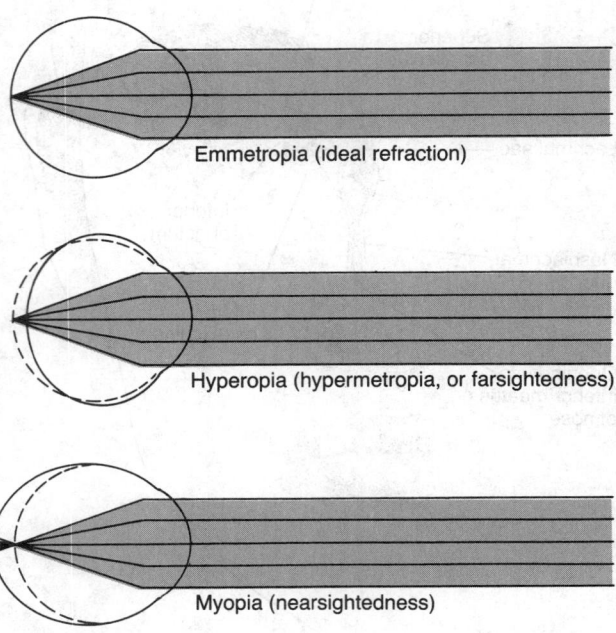

Figure 35–4

Refraction in emmetropia, hyperopia, and myopia.

vision is normal, but distant vision is defective. To correct this condition, a biconcave lens is used.

Astigmatism is a refractive error resulting from an alteration in the curvature or spherical refracting surface that causes visual distortion. Optical distortion most often results from irregular corneal curvature. Astigmatism may be hyperopic or myopic, depending on where the point of focus falls.

PUPILLARY CONSTRICTION

The pupils modulate the amount of light that enters the eye and eventually reaches the retina. If the level of illumination of one or both eyes is increased, both pupils constrict. The amount of constriction depends on the strength of the light stimulus, the state of adaptation of the retina, and other factors such as the individual's emotional state and alertness. Darkness produces dilation of the pupil.

ACCOMMODATION

In the healthy state, the eye possesses the ability to focus sharp images on the retina. The process by which a clear visual image is maintained as the gaze is shifted from a distant to a near point is known as *accommodation.* The ability of the eye to change its focusing power is mediated through a change in the curvature of the lens, which results from contraction and relaxation of the zonules, the fibers that hold the lens in place.

EYE CHANGES ASSOCIATED WITH AGING

Visual acuity is less than 20/40 in the majority of the population older than age 65 years (Cotran et al., 1989) (see the accompanying Focus on the Elderly feature). Along with physiologic changes that occur within the eye and nervous system, structures supporting the eye undergo degenerative changes that affect visual function.

In the elderly, eyes appear to be sunken because of a loss of subcutaneous fat, decreased elastic tissue under the skin, and decreased muscle tone. As the levator muscle grows weaker, the elderly individual is less able to maintain an upward gaze and has more difficulty in sustaining convergence. *Arcus senilis,* an opaque ring formed within the circumference of the cornea, is a result of deposition of fatty globules. Although this problem is not a universal effect of aging, the nurse frequently sees this ring when assessing the eyes of an elderly client.

The transparency of the cornea decreases with age. However, the most important corneal change is its over-

FOCUS ON THE ELDERLY ■ Eye Changes Related to Aging

Structure/Function	Change
Appearance	Eyes appear to be sunken. Arcus senilis forms. Sclera yellows.
Cornea	Cornea flattens, which causes astigmatism and blurring of vision.
Ocular muscles	Muscle strength is reduced, resulting in a diminished capacity to maintain an upward gaze and to sustain convergence.
Lens	Elasticity is lost, which increases the near point of vision. Lens hardens and becomes compact. Cataracts form.
Iris	Decrease in ability to dilate results in small pupil size and poor adaptation to darkness.
Pupil	Aperture size takes longer to change, which reduces ability to see in dim light.
Color vision	Discrimination of short-wavelength colors (green, blue, violet) decreases.
Tears	Tear production is diminished, resulting in dry eyes.

all change in shape. After age 65 years, the cornea flattens and has an irregular curvature of its surface. This change produces an astigmatism or a change in a previous astigmatism. As a result, refraction of light occurs at varying angles, and a distorted and blurred visual image is produced.

Changes are also noted in other structures. Degenerative changes occur in the sclera: fatty deposits cause the sclera to develop a yellowish tinge. As the sclera thins, a bluish color may be noted. The color change is due to the increased visibility of the underlying choroid. With increasing age, the iris has less ability to dilate. This change is particularly problematic during adaptation to a darkened environment. The average pupil size at night in a 20-year-old individual is 3.3 mm compared with 0.2 mm in an 80-year-old individual (Sullivan, 1983). Adjustments in pupillary aperture size are slower to occur. This change can be particularly troublesome when the eye adjusts to dim light. During the aging process, the lens undergoes changes that affect the ability of the eye to transmit and focus light. Changes in the lens occur in most people after 40 years of age. The lens continues to grow throughout the life span, as layers of epithelial tissue are added. As new cells are added, the lens hardens, loses water, and becomes compact. This layering effect plays a role in the development of cataracts.

As the lens loses elasticity, the ciliary muscle has less effect on the zonules attached to the lens. The ability of the eye to accommodate is gradually lost with age. As the accommodation power is lost, the *near point*, the closest distance at which the eye can see an object clearly, increases, and near objects (especially reading material) must be placed farther from the eye to be clearly seen. This age-related change is termed *presbyopia*. The *far point*, or the farthest point at which an object can be distinguished, decreases. Therefore, the elderly person has a narrower visual field. Reading glasses to supplement the eye's accommodative capacity help to alleviate this problem.

Current research shows that older clients undergo changes in visual threshold and color perception, in addition to decreased visual acuity. More light is needed to stimulate the visual receptors. Color sensitivity across the entire light spectrum is lost, as is discrimination among colors of short wavelengths such as green, blue, and violet. The fact that the lens yellows with age and absorbs light of short wavelengths is one possible cause of the loss of color discrimination.

HISTORY

In assessing a client's vision, the nurse first completes a thorough history. Many factors can affect the visual process, and knowledge of the following information is helpful as the nurse begins to collect data, generate nursing diagnoses, and plan appropriate nursing interventions and referrals.

DEMOGRAPHIC DATA

The *age* of the client is an important factor in assessing the visual processes and the structure of the eye. During aging, the incidence of conditions such as glaucoma and the formation of cataracts increases. The severity of myopia tends to increase in individuals younger than 30 years. Presbyopia begins to occur in the 4th decade.

Information about the client's *ethnic background* is important because some conditions are more prevalent in certain groups. For example, Jewish individuals are more susceptible to Tay-Sachs disease, which has ocular manifestations.

The *sex* of the client may also be significant. For example, retinal detachments are more common in males.

The client's address and telephone number are requested. The nurse also notes whether the client lives locally or whether travel for follow-up care could be a potential problem. The name and address of a person to call in an emergency are also solicited. If no friends or family members live nearby, transportation may be a problem.

PERSONAL AND FAMILY HISTORY

The nurse asks the client if there is a *family history* of eye problems because some conditions show a familial tendency.

The client is questioned about past *accidents, injuries, surgeries,* or *blows to the head* that may have led to the present findings. Nurses may need to inquire specifically about previous laser surgeries or procedures because clients frequently do not classify laser treatment as surgery. It is essential to know the types of *sports* in which the client participates because some injuries are more common to participation in specific sports.

The nurse asks the client about the presence of any *systemic medical conditions*, such as diabetes, hypertension, lupus erythematosus, sarcoidosis, sexually transmitted disease, sickle cell anemia, acquired immunodeficiency syndrome, or multiple sclerosis, which could have ocular involvement. In addition, prescribed ocular medications may adversely affect some pre-existing medical conditions.

The client is also questioned about the type of *medications* currently being used. Particularly important drugs to note include decongestants and antihistamines, for their ocular effects and complaints of dry eyes are well documented. Many clients do not consider over-the-counter eyedrops to be a medication. The name, strength, dosage, and schedule of administration are noted for all ophthalmic medications. This information is critical because measurements of intraocular pressure can be affected by these factors. Many drugs given systemically can have ocular effects, which cause disturbances of various degrees. Clinical manifestations resulting from drugs include pruritus (itching), foreign body sensation, redness, tearing, photophobia (sensitivity to light), and the development of acquired disorders such as cataract and glaucoma.

The nurse questions the client about known *allergies* to specific medications and differentiates between allergic reactions and expected side effects. Cross-allergies between drugs, such as between penicillin and cephalosporins, are kept in mind. A list of substances to which the client is allergic is reviewed and updated each time the client visits the health care facility.

DIET HISTORY

The nurse asks questions about *foods* that the client eats because some ocular problems are associated with various vitamin deficiencies. Deficient intake of vitamins usually occurs because of malnutrition. Clients who have inadequate dietary intake are questioned about their use of multivitamin supplements.

SOCIOECONOMIC STATUS

Visual acuity and a full field of vision are required in some occupations in which the individual must read gauges, operate equipment, or prepare written materials. The nurse asks the client about the nature of the client's work and the extent to which the eyes are used. In occupations such as computer programming, constant use of the eye for reading monitor screens may lead to eyestrain and the need for eyeglasses. Many types of jobs such as machine operators are hazardous to the eyes because of the high velocities at which particles can be thrown at the eye. The nurse questions clients who work in industrial settings about the use of protective eyewear, such as goggles. Individuals who are exposed to chemical fumes may complain of eye irritation unless there is sufficient exhaust ventilation. If the intensity of infrared or ultraviolet lights is greater than normal, workers can develop photophobia and/or cataract.

CURRENT HEALTH PROBLEM

The nurse gathers information about the client's present complaint. The client is questioned about the onset of visual changes. Has the change occurred rapidly or slowly? Any client with a sudden or persistent loss of vision occurring within the past 48 hours should be seen immediately by an ophthalmologist, as should clients experiencing trauma, a foreign body in the eye, or sudden pain in the eye.

The following questions are asked if an ocular injury or eye trauma is involved: How long ago was the injury? What was the client doing when it happened? If a foreign body might be involved, what was its source? Was any first aid administered at the scene? If so, what actions were taken?

It is important to determine if any precipitating factors, such as recent administration of medication, may have caused the distress. For example, clients with hypertension who have their blood pressure lowered rapidly may complain of ocular effects. The nurse asks the client to estimate the duration of the problem and to describe the clinical manifestations and pattern of their occurrence. Are the symptoms present in one or both eyes? Are both eyes affected equally, or is one affected more than the other? The client is also asked what measures, such as cool compresses, rest, or discontinuing use of contact lenses, have been used with or without success to relieve or improve the clinical manifestations.

PHYSICAL ASSESSMENT

In doing a physical assessment of the client's eyes and visual system, the nurse uses observational skills and performs various examinations of the visual system. Nurses who have received instructions in the use of the direct ophthalmoscope, an instrument for assessing the external eye and retina, may also include the use of instrumentation in completing a physical assessment of the eye.

INSPECTION

The nurse first observes the client's *appearance* and *posture*. The nurse looks for any unusual clothing combinations, which may indicate a color vision defect, as well as head tilting or noticeable postural characteristics that could offer clues about compensatory stances to attain clear vision. For example, the client who has double vision may cock his or her head to the side in an attempt to focus images into one image.

The nurse observes for *symmetry* in the appearance of the left and right eyes. The client's facial symmetry is assessed for placement of the eyes; the nurse looks to see that they are placed an equal distance from each other. The eyes are also assessed for their placement in the orbits. The nurse checks for one eye that is larger, more prominent, or bulging forward by examining the resting position of the upper eyelid. No sclera should be visible between the lower edge of the eyelid and the edge of the iris. *Exophthalmos*, or *proptosis*, is a condition in which the eyeball(s) protrude or are pushed forward. *Enophthalmos* describes eyeballs that are sunken. An *exophthalmometer* is used to measure from the outer edge of each eye's lateral margin to the cornea in each eye.

The *eyebrows* and *eyelashes* are assessed for distribution of hair growth. Direction of the eyelashes is carefully determined. Eyelashes should extend outward and away from the insertion of the eyelashes into the eyelid. The nurse asks the client to raise or elevate the eyebrows to determine any differences between the left and right sides. The nurse also looks at the eyelid to determine the presence of *ptosis* (drooping), redness, tenderness, lesions, or swelling. The lids should normally close completely, with the upper and lower lid margins approximating. When the eyes are open, the upper lid covers a small portion of the iris and overlying cornea. The margin of the lower lid lies below the junction line of the cornea and sclera. No sclera should be visible between the eyelid and the iris.

If the nurse thinks that there might be a *stye* (hordeolum) or *chalazion* present, the upper and lower eyelids must be everted, as shown in Figure 35–5. Refer to Chapter 36 for more information on these two external ocular problems. The lower lid is everted by drawing the margin downward against the cheek while having the client look upward. To evert the upper lid, the nurse asks the client to look down. The nurse gently grasps the eyelid near the base of the eyelashes and gently pulls downward. A cotton-tipped applicator is placed on the skin side of the upper lid. While pushing down on the skin side of the lid, the nurse flips the eyelid over the applicator. Gentle pressure keeps the upper lashes against the superior part of the lid and maintains eversion as the client continues to look down. While the eyelid is everted, the nurse looks for any redness, swelling, or presence of foreign bodies. The conjunctiva is normally pale pink and glistening.

The nurse can observe part of the *lacrimal gland* by retracting the upper lid and asking the individual to look down. The lacrimal gland is examined for swelling. The nurse can press on the lacrimal sac, inside the lower inner orbital rim, to check for obstruction of the nasolacrimal duct. The puncta can also be observed by gently pulling the lower eyelid down against the cheek.

The *sclera* is examined for color; it is usually white. A yellowish color may indicate jaundice or systemic problems. However, in dark-skinned persons, the normal sclera may also appear yellow, and small, dark, pigmented dots may be visible.

The *cornea* is best observed by directing a light at it obliquely from several angles. The cornea should be transparent, smooth, shiny, and bright; any cloudy areas or specks may be the result of accidents or injuries.

The nurse may check the *corneal reflex*. If the client is conscious and the blink reflex is present, or if the client is wearing contact lenses, this reflex is not tested. To perform this assessment, the nurse brings a fist quickly toward the client's face in a threatening motion. If the client has vision, this movement will cause blinking. Alternatively, the nurse can use a syringe full of air and expel it toward the eyes. Blinking results if the reflex is intact.

The *pupils* are usually round and of equal size. Approximately 5% of individuals may normally have a slight but noticeable difference in the size of the pupils (Malasanos et al., 1986). This variance is termed *anisocoria*. The size of pupils varies in individuals who are exposed to the same amount of light. Pupils are smaller in older adults. Individuals with myopia (nearsightedness) have larger pupils, whereas hyperopic (farsighted) persons have smaller pupils. The normal pupil diameter is between 2 and 6 mm. Pupils smaller than 2 mm are considered to be *constricted*, whereas pupils larger than 6 mm are termed *dilated*.

Pupils are assessed for response to light. The pupillary response to light is more readily observed when the test is performed in a darkened room. However, in individuals with dark brown eyes, it is more difficult for the nurse to detect changes. Constriction of both pupils is the normal response to direct light. Increasing illumination causes pupillary constriction, whereas decreasing illumination causes dilation. Pupils also constrict in response to accommodation (the change in focus as the gaze is shifted from a distant to a near object). The nurse assesses pupillary reaction to light by asking the client to look straight ahead while quickly bringing the beam of a flashlight in from the side and directing it at the right (oculus dexter or O.D.) pupil (see Chap. 32). The con-

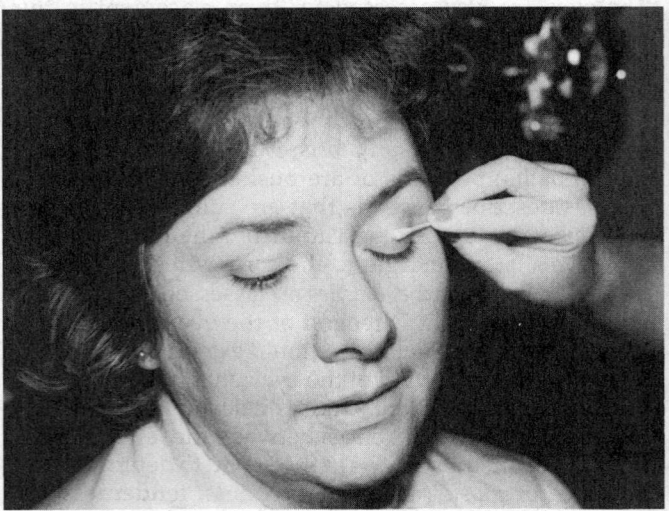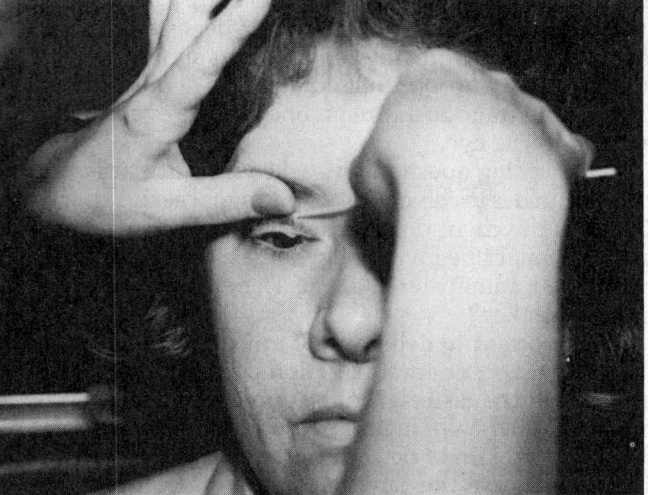

Figure 35–5

Left, Placement of cotton-tipped applicator for eyelid eversion. *Right*, Eversion of eyelid.

striction of the O.D. pupil is a *direct* response to the shining of the flashlight into *that* eye. Constriction of the left (oculus sinister or O.S.) pupil while shining the light at the O.D. pupil is known as a *consensual* response. Direct and consensual responses should be evaluated for each eye.

The pupils also are individually evaluated for speed of reaction. Immediate constriction should occur when a light is directed at the pupil. This rapid response is termed *brisk*. If the pupil constricts but the constriction occurs over a slightly longer period, such as over more than a second, the response is termed *sluggish*. Pupils that fail to react are referred to as *nonreactive* or *fixed*. Reactivity speed of O.D. and O.S. pupils should be compared, and any discrepancy noted.

In assessing for *accommodation*, the nurse holds the index finger about 12 to 18 cm from the client's nose and moves it toward the client's nose. The client's eyes should converge while the finger is watched, and the pupils should constrict equally. When accommodation stops, the pupils begin to enlarge and return to their normal size.

Although the rapidity of the pupillary responses to light and accommodation varies in healthy persons, the nurse must note the presence of the responses and whether the responses in both eyes are equal. The notation *PERRLA* stands for pupils equal, round, react to light, and accommodation.

ASSESSMENT OF VISION

ASSESSMENT OF ACUITY

Testing visual acuity is the most important measure of ocular function and should be a part of the routine eye examination. Visual acuity tests measure client's distant and near vision. Failure to see the letters on an eye chart may be a traumatic experience for some clients, and they try to deny this finding. The nurse may assist the client by maintaining an empathic attitude and by recognizing that performance on an acuity test may be affected by variables such as fatigue or anxiety. The *Snellen chart* is one of the more simple tools that the nurse can use to record distance vision. For adults, the chart is available with letters, numbers, pictures, or a single letter presented in various positions (Fig. 35–6). The letter *E* or *C* is most frequently used in single-letter charts. The client stands 20 ft from the chart, covers the left eye, and uses the right eye to read the line that appears most clearly. If the client is able to do this accurately, the nurse asks him or her to read the next lower line. This sequence is repeated until the client is unable to correctly identify more than half of the characters on the line. The procedure is repeated for the other eye. Findings are recorded as a comparison between what the client can read at 20 ft and the number of feet normally required by an individual to read the same line. For example, 20/50 means that the client is able to read at 20 ft from the

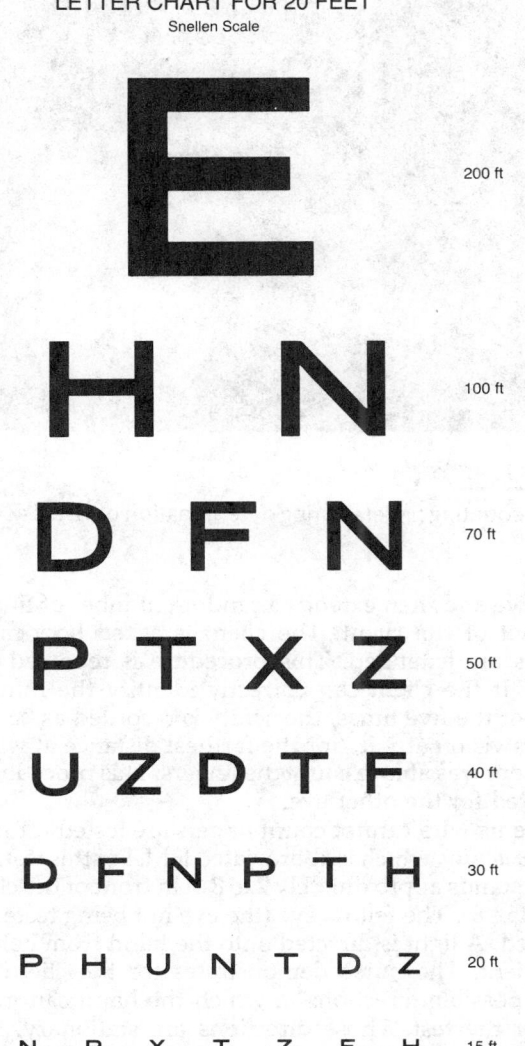

LETTER CHART FOR 20 FEET
Snellen Scale

Figure 35–6

A typical Snellen chart. (Courtesy of the National Society to Prevent Blindness.)

chart what a "healthy eye" can read at 50 ft. If an exact measurement of visual acuity is needed, the acuity can be further specified by noting the number of characters that the client failed to identify on the line, such as 20/25 (−2).

Clients who wear corrective lenses other than for reading should have their vision tested with the lenses in place. The notation of the acuity should reflect whether the client was wearing corrective lenses: s̄c indicates the absence of corrective lenses during testing and c̄c indicates with correction.

For clients who are in a confined space or who are unable to see the 20/400 character, the nurse can determine visual acuity by holding fingers in front of the client's eyes and asking the client to *count the number of fingers* (Fig. 35–7). The nurse asks the client to cover the

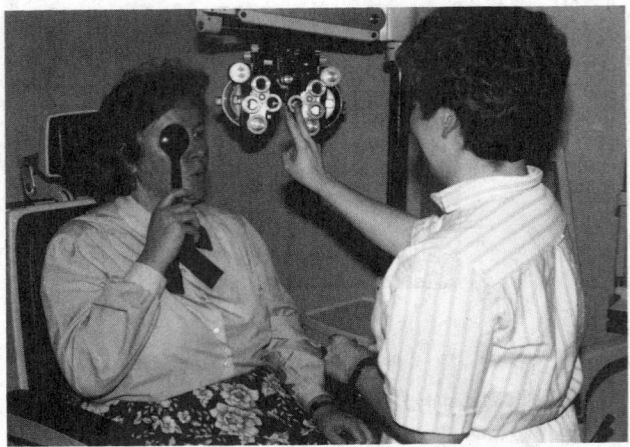

Figure 35–7

Client counting fingers during determination of visual acuity.

O.S. eye and then extends a random number of fingers in front of the client. The client is asked how many fingers are extended. This procedure is repeated five times. If the client can correctly identify the number three of the five times, the acuity is recorded as "count fingers vision at 5 ft," or the farthest distance at which the client was able to count the fingers. This procedure is repeated for the other eye.

Clients who cannot count fingers are tested for *hand motion acuity,* which is abbreviated HM. For this test, the nurse stands approximately 2 to 3 ft in front of the client (Fig. 35–8). The fellow eye (the eye not being tested) is covered. A light is directed onto the hand from behind the client. The nurse demonstrates for the client the three possible directions in which the hand can move during the test. Those directions are stationary, left-right, or up-down. The nurse moves the hand slowly (1

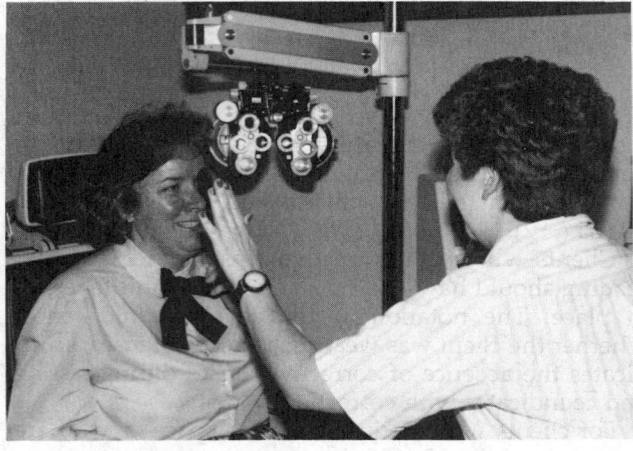

Figure 35–8

Client indicating hand motions during determination of visual acuity.

second per motion) and asks the client, "What is my hand doing now?" This procedure is repeated at least five times. If the client correctly identifies the direction three of five times, the visual acuity is recorded as "hand motion at the farthest the client correctly identifies the majority of directional movement." The other eye is then tested.

If the client cannot detect hand movement, acuity is tested by measuring *light perception,* which is abbreviated LP. The nurse first asks the client to cover the O.S. eye. In a darkened room, from a distance of about 2 to 3 ft, the nurse directs the beam of an indirect ophthalmoscope or penlight at the O.D. eye for 1 to 2 seconds. Clients should be instructed to say "on" when the beam of light is perceived and "off" when it is no longer detected. This procedure is repeated five times. If the client correctly identifies the presence or absence of light three times or more, the acuity is recorded as light perception. Clients who are unable to detect the stimuli correctly have an acuity that is termed *no light perception* (NLP).

The measurement of contrast sensitivity is being explored as an alternative to the use of the Snellen eye chart for acuity testing. Low-contrast letters appear on a white background. The contrast of the letters is progressively reduced. Notation of where the client is unable to distinguish the letters from the background is made.

Near vision testing. A gross assessment of near vision is performed for the client who complains of difficulty in reading and in persons older than 40 years. The nurse can use a newspaper clipping with various sizes of print or a small, hand-held Snellen chart (called a *Jaeger card*) (Fig. 35–9) to check near vision. The card has different-sized printed letters, numbers, and/or shapes. It is held by the client 14 in away from the eyes. The client is instructed to read the letters from the card. Eyes are tested separately and then together. The nurse notes the Jaeger value that is assigned to the lowest line in which the client can identify more than half of the characters. For example, the acuity might read "J2 at 14 inches."

Visual acuity is tested in each eye separately (monocular) and then in both eyes together (binocular). The nurse needs to be aware of clients who squint or who attempt to memorize the letters. Such a client can be directed to read the line backwards or to use a different chart.

Testing for blindness. *Legal blindness* is defined as a best lens-corrected visual acuity, with the better-seeing eye, of 20/200 or less, or a widest diameter of the visual field of no greater than 20 degrees.

ASSESSMENT OF VISUAL FIELDS

A *confrontational* test is used to examine the client's *visual fields,* or *peripheral vision.* During the test, the nurse and the client sit facing each other (Fig. 35–10). The client is asked to continue looking directly into the nurse's eyes throughout the test. The nurse covers his or

ROSENBAUM POCKET VISION SCREENER

		Point	Jaeger	distance equivalent
95				$\frac{20}{800}$
874				$\frac{20}{400}$
2843		26	16	$\frac{20}{200}$
638 EШƎ XOO		14	10	$\frac{20}{100}$
8745 ƎMШ OXO		10	7	$\frac{20}{70}$
63925 MEƎ XOX		8	5	$\frac{20}{50}$
428365 ШEM OXO		6	3	$\frac{20}{40}$
374258 ƎШƎ X X O		5	2	$\frac{20}{30}$
937826 ШmE x o o		4	1	$\frac{20}{25}$
428739 EШm o o x		3	1+	$\frac{20}{20}$

Card is held in good light 14 inches from eye. Record vision for each eye separately with and without glasses. Presbyopic patients should read thru bifocal segment. Check myopes with glasses only.

DESIGN COURTESY J. G. ROSENBAUM, M.D., CLEVELAND, OHIO

PUPIL GAUGE (mm.)

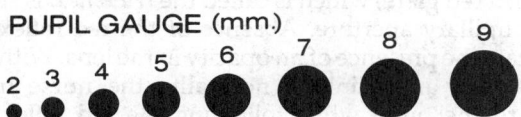

2 3 4 5 6 7 8 9

Figure 35–9

A typical Jaeger card. (Courtesy of SMP Division, Cooper Laboratories [P.R.], Inc., San German, P.R.)

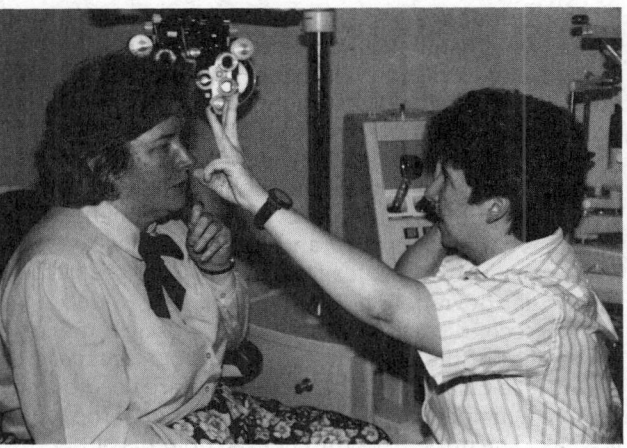

Figure 35–10

Confrontational assessment of visual fields.

her right eye (O.D.) while the client covers the left eye (O.S.), so that both individuals have approximately the same visual field. The nurse moves a finger or an object from a nonvisible area into the client's line of vision. Both the nurse and the client should see the finger at approximately the same time. When the client sees the nurse's fingers coming into the line of vision, the client informs the nurse. The nurse and client cover the opposite eye and repeat the procedure. This test assumes the nurse or examiner has normal peripheral vision. When testing visual fields, the nurse should note that the client is alert, is not medicated, can follow directions, and can focus as directed. Sedation can interfere with the client's

ability to respond and with the speed of response. Interference in either area can result in inaccurate measures of the visual fields.

Findings from this test are recorded as "confrontational fields full with or without correction." If visual perception is decreased, the nurse records which quadrant is affected, e.g., "confrontational field full with decrease in superior, inferior, temporal, or nasal quadrant." Visual field findings are usually greater temporally (90 degrees) than nasally (60 degrees). Upward fields are 50 degrees, whereas downward fields are 70 degrees.

This test provides only a crude estimate of the individual's visual fields and is used to detect large field defects such as hemianopia, quadrantanopia, or large scotomas. *Hemianopia* is blindness for one-half of the field of vision in one or both eyes. *Quadrantanopia* is blindness in one-fourth of the field of vision in one or both eyes. A *scotoma* is a blind spot in the visual field. Clinical use of this test is limited to gross screening. A client with a possible finding of reduced peripheral vision is referred to an ophthalmologist for more quantitative measurements.

Other methods are used to determine visual fields. The stimulus is presented to the eye by an examiner or a computer. Clients are asked to respond to their seeing the stimulus by pressing a button. Areas of response and of lack of response are noted and graphed.

ASSESSMENT OF EXTRAOCULAR MUSCLE FUNCTION

Assessment of extraocular muscle function includes three components: the corneal light reflex, the six cardinal positions of gaze, and the cover-uncover test. A basic element in each of these is the nurse's observation of the parallelism of the eyes and smoothness of ocular movements.

The *corneal light reflex* is used to determine the parallelism, or alignment of the two eyes. After asking the client to stare straight ahead, the nurse shines a penlight at both corneas from a distance of 12 to 15 in. The bright dot of light that is reflected from the shiny surface of the cornea should be located in a symmetric position, e.g., at the 1 o'clock position in the right eye and at the 11 o'clock position in the left eye. An asymmetric reflex indicates a deviating eye and probable muscle imbalance. A weak extraocular muscle is usually the cause of this ocular deviation.

The second means of assessing muscle function is movement of the eyes through the *six cardinal positions of gaze* (see Chap. 32). These positions are used because the eye will not turn to a particular position if the muscle is weak. The nurse asks the client to hold his or her head still and to move the eyes to follow a small object, such as a pen or a bottle of eyedrops, which is moved to the following positions: (1) to the client's right (lateral), (2) upward and right (temporal), (3) down and right, (4) to the client's left (lateral), (5) upward and left (temporal), and (6) down and left. While the client moves the eyes to these positions, the nurse observes for (1) conjugate (parallel) movements of the eye or (2) any deviation of movement of the eye, such as *nystagmus*, which is an involuntary rhythmic, rapid twitching of the eyeball. It is a normal finding for the far lateral gaze; it may be caused by abnormal innervation or prolonged reduced vision. Movements may be vertical, horizontal, rotary, or a combination of two movements (mixed). The nurse records the direction of nystagmus (direction of the quicker movements).

A different method of assessing muscle function is the *cover-uncover test.* Eyes are usually maintained in a parallel position, which makes binocular vision possible. A muscle imbalance can be observed when one eye is covered. The nurse asks the client to use both eyes and look at a specific fixed point, such as the nurse's nose. One of the client's eyes is covered with an opaque card. The nurse observes the uncovered eye to see if it moves to fix on the object. If the eye moves, it was not straight before the other eye was covered. The nurse then removes the cover and observes for any movement in the eye just uncovered. Usually, when an eye is covered, the image of an object on the retina is suppressed, and the eye remains in its former position. If there is a muscle weakness in the eye that is covered, it relaxes and drifts to a different resting position. When the eye is uncovered, the eye jerks back into position so that the visual image again appears on the retina.

The nurse records any deviations of eye movement (*strabismus*) and the direction of the muscle deviation. *Exodeviation* describes a turned-out eye; *esodeviation* refers to a turned-in eye.

ASSESSMENT OF COLOR VISION

Normal color vision is essential for certain occupations. About 8% of men and 0.5% of women have a congenital color vision defect (Boyd-Monk & Steinmetz, 1987). The defect is usually the inability to perceive red/green or blue. There are several methods available to test color vision. The most frequently used tool is the *Ishihara chart,* which consists of numbers that are composed of colored dots, located within a circle of colored dots. Testing each eye separately, the nurse or examiner asks the client what numbers are seen on the chart. The ability to read the numbers depends on the normal functioning of the client's color vision. This test is sensitive for diagnosis of red/green blindness but is not effective for detection of defective discrimination of blue.

OPHTHALMOSCOPY

An instrument that is used to view the external structures and the interior of the eye is the *direct ophthalmoscope.* It is easiest to examine the fundus when the room is dark because the pupil will dilate. When performing direct ophthalmoscopy, the nurse holds the instrument with the right hand when examining the O.D. eye, and with the left hand when examining the O.S. eye. The nurse stands on the same side as the client's eye that is being examined. The client is instructed to look straight ahead at an object located on the wall behind the nurse. A thumb is placed on the client's eyebrow to assist the examiner in knowing the distance from the ophthalmoscope to the client (Bates, 1984). The ophthalmoscope is held firmly against the nurse's face and is aligned so that the examiner's eye sees through the sight hole (Fig. 35–11).

When using the ophthalmoscope, the nurse approaches the client's eye from about 12 to 15 in away and approximately 15 degrees lateral to the client's line of vision. As the ophthalmoscope is directed at the pupil, a red glare, which is called the *red reflex,* is seen in the pupillary aperture. Absence of the red reflex may indicate the presence of an opacity in the lens. With both eyes open and blinking normally, the nurse moves toward the pupil while following the red reflex. The retina should be visible through the ophthalmoscope. It is suggested that the following sequence be used during examination of the optic fundus: (1) optic disk, (2) optic vessels, (3) fundus, and (4) macula. The nurse begins by looking for the *optic disk.* If it is not immediately visible, a blood vessel can be followed toward the center until the disk is seen. To bring the disk into focus, the examiner adjusts the lens of the ophthalmoscope. Color, margins, cup size, and rings should be assessed. *Color* is usually creamy yellow to white. *Margins* should be clear and distinct, although the nasal margin may be somewhat blurred. If a cup-like depression is noted in the center of the disk, *cup size* should be no less than one-half the diameter of the disk. The presence of any unusual *rings* or *crescents* around the disk should be noted.

After viewing the disk, the nurse follows each of the four main blood vessels away from the disk toward the periphery of the retina. The nurse observes the *size, color,* and *light reflection* of the vessels. *Arterioles* are

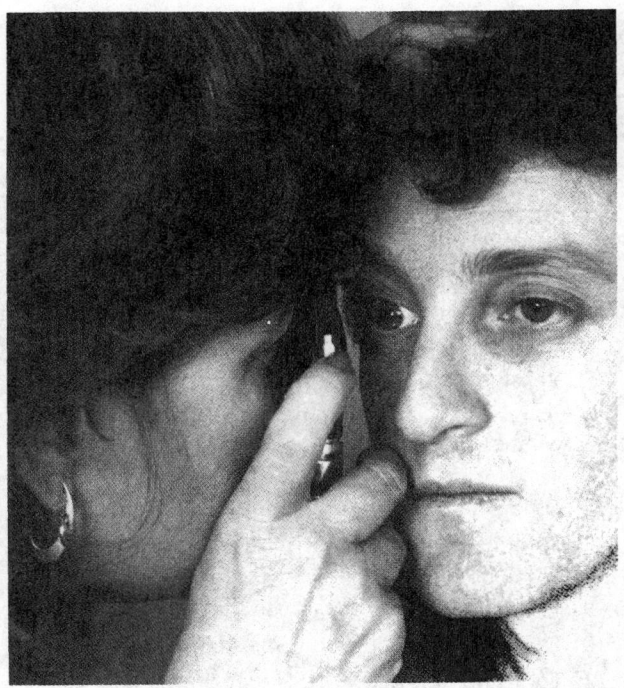

Figure 35–11

Nurse using proper technique for direct ophthalmoscopic visualization of the retina. (From Swartz, M. H. [1989]. *Textbook of physical diagnosis: History and examination.* Philadelphia: W. B. Saunders.)

smaller, lighter red, and brighter in reflectivity than veins. Areas of arteriole-venule crossings are observed for nicking or narrowing.

The *retinal background,* or *fundus,* should be examined systematically for color and regularity of appearance. It is usually creamy pink. Any hemorrhage, lesion, hole, or tear is noted.

The *macular area* is examined last because of the discomfort that is caused by shining a bright light at the center of acute vision. The ophthalmoscope is directed temporally while the client is asked to gaze into the light. A bright foveal reflection enables the nurse to see the relative absence of blood vessels in the area.

PSYCHOSOCIAL ASSESSMENT

Vision is an important sense because it provides a means for contact with the environment. Anyone undergoing changes in visual perception may express anxiety and fear related to a loss of vision. Clients with severe visual defects may be unable to perform normal activities of daily living. The feelings of dependency resulting from diminished vision affect the individual's self-esteem.

The nurse needs to ask questions about the client's feelings regarding the visual disturbances and to assess the effectiveness of the client's coping techniques. The nurse also discusses the client's concerns with family members or significant others to determine the availability of support for the client. Current knowledge and use of available services for the visually impaired by the client should be determined and referrals to social services agencies made as necessary.

DIAGNOSTIC TESTS

LABORATORY TESTS

Cultures and *smears* made from corneal or conjunctival swabs and scrapings are used to aid in the diagnosis of infections. Suspicious exudate should be cultured and stained with Gram's stain before antibiotics or topical anesthetics are instilled. Swabs should be taken from the conjunctivae and ulcerated or inflamed areas. Refer to Chapter 26 for a description of the procedure used to obtain cultures.

RADIOGRAPHIC EXAMINATIONS

FLUORESCEIN ANGIOGRAPHY

Fluorescein angiography is a test that provides a detailed imaging and permanent record of the ocular circulation by means of a series of photographs that are taken in rapid succession after the administration of dye. This test is particularly useful for diagnosis of conditions affecting the circulation of the retina, such as diabetic retinopathy and hypertensive retinopathy, or for the differential diagnosis of intraocular tumors. Pregnancy or a history of allergic response to fluorescein dye is a contraindication to the test. It is performed with caution in clients who have experienced allergic reactions to other contrast media.

Client preparation. The nurse explains the procedure to the client, asks about allergies and previous reactions to dyes, and instills mydriatic (a drug causing pupil dilation) eyedrops about an hour before the test. The accompanying Guidelines feature gives the steps for correct instillation of eyedrops. An informed consent to the procedure must be obtained from the client or responsible party. At this time, the nurse warns the client that the dye may cause the skin to appear yellow for several hours after the test. The stain is gradually eliminated through the urine.

Procedure. Venous access must be obtained. After validating the presence of the catheter in the antecubital

---

GUIDELINES ■ Procedure for Instillation of Ophthalmic Drops

Interventions	Rationales
1. Wash your hands.	1. To remove surface microorganisms.
2. Don gloves if secretions are present.	2. To protect from exposure to secretions.
3. Explain the procedure to the client.	3. To reduce the client's anxiety.
4. Check the name, strength, and expiration date of the medication.	4. To ensure correct medication (old medications may have altered chemical properties).
5. Instruct the client to tilt the head backward, open the eyes, and look up.	5. To position the head for easiest access to ocular structures.
6. Pull the lower lid downward against the cheekbone or grasp the skin of the lower lid with the thumb and index finger and pull forward.	6. To create a pocket into which drops of medication will be placed.
7. Hold the bottle like a pencil, with the tip downward.	7. To facilitate control of the bottle.
8. Rest the wrist of the hand that is holding the bottle on the client's cheek.	8. To bring the bottle close to the eyeball without touching it or the eyelashes.
9. Squeeze the bottle gently.	9. To allow *one* drop to fall into the sac.
10. Gently release the lower eyelid.	10. To keep medication from splashing out.
11. Instruct the client to *close* the eyes *gently, not squeeze them.*	11. To distribute medication (squeezing causes medication to be forced into the nasolacrimal system, which decreases absorption).
12. Wait 5 min before instilling another drop.	12. To promote maximal absorption of the drug.

---

vein, 5 mL of a 10% solution of fluorescein is injected into the vein in the client's arm. The dye undergoes excitation by the light emitted from the camera. The fluorescent dye is photographed by means of successive exposures as it passes through the vessels of the retina and choroid. The procedure takes only minutes because the vessels fill quickly.

Complications. Clients may experience mild side effects during the procedure such as nausea, vomiting, sneezing, paresthesia of the tongue, pain at the injection site, and dizziness. Hives may also develop during the procedure. If hives appear, an oral or intramuscular antihistamine such as diphenhydramine (Benadryl) can be given. If the dye leaks subcutaneously, the client may complain of intense tissue burning.

Serious side effects, such as laryngeal edema, syncope, bronchospasm, and respiratory arrest, are also possible. Emergency resuscitation equipment must be immediately available. All caregivers must know their role in delivering emergency care to the ophthalmic client.

Follow-up care. After the test, the client may feel weak and nauseated. After the nausea resolves, clients are encouraged to drink fluids, to remove the dye from their system. The nurse encourages the client to rest and reminds the client that any yellow staining of the skin will disappear in a few hours. After the test, urine is bright green until the dye is excreted. Avoiding direct sunlight for a few hours after the test is also communicated.

Photophobia will continue until pupil dilation returns to normal.

COMPUTED TOMOGRAPHY

Computed tomography is a radiographic diagnostic method in which a cross-sectional image is formed by use of computers. Data are obtained by scanning the skull and orbits with a beam of x-rays. This diagnostic technique has replaced some of the previously used tests and is particularly valuable in visualizing the globes, extraocular muscles, and optic nerves. It is a sensitive method for detecting tumors that are restricted to the orbital space. Contrast material is not usually administered because it does not significantly help visualization of the normal intraorbital structures. Therefore, no special client preparation or follow-up care is required. The nurse informs the client that there is no pain involved with this test. However, the client is required to be positioned in a confined space and to keep the head still during the procedure.

OTHER DIAGNOSTIC STUDIES

EXAMINATION BY SLIT LAMP

The *slit lamp*, as shown in Figure 35–12, is an instrument that permits examination of anterior ocular struc-

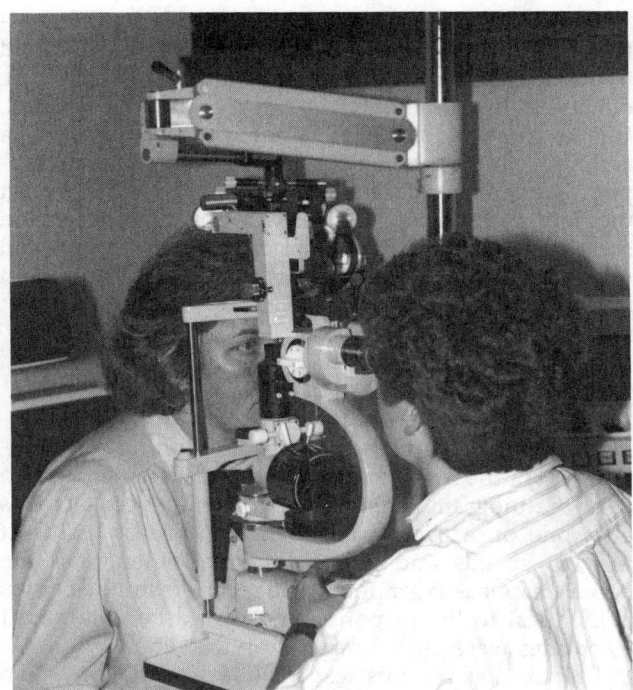

Figure 35–12

Slit-lamp ocular examination.

tures under microscopic magnification. The client leans on a chin rest to stabilize the head while a narrowed beam (slit) of light is aimed so that it brightly illuminates only a narrow segment of the eye. This technique allows the examiner to accurately localize the positon of any abnormality in the cornea, lens, or anterior vitreous humor. The slit beam is also helpful in determining the presence of cells in the aqueous humor. Clients are advised about the brightness of the light and the need to look forward at a point over the examiner's ear. There is no special client preparation or follow-up care for this test.

CORNEAL STAINING

Corneal staining consists of the instillation of fluorescein or other topical dye into the conjunctival sac (cul-de-sac) to outline irregularities of the corneal surface that are not easily visible. The use of corneal staining is indicated in cases of known or suspected corneal trauma; pathologic conditions caused by contact lens; the presence of foreign bodies; corneal abrasions or ulcers; or other corneal disorders. This test is valuable for evaluating suspected corneal injury in emergency rooms, physicians' offices, or industrial settings in which a slit lamp is not available.

Client preparation. Before staining the eye, the nurse asks the client to remove contact lens(es) if present. The nurse explains the procedure and informs the client that

the test is brief and painless. It should be reinforced that the test involves only the application of a solution in contact with the eye because many clients think that the dye will be injected into the eye and are fearful.

Procedure. Several topical dyes are used to aid in the evaluation of superficial corneal defects. The most commonly used dye is fluorescein. Because the corneal epithelium may be interrupted, the risk of infection is great. The nurse begins by washing his or her hands. Fluorescein dye is available in eyedrop form or in filter strips. Either must be applied carefully to the cul-de-sac to maintain sterility. The client is instructed to blink after the dye has been applied. This action will distribute the fluorescein evenly across the cornea. When the eye is viewed through a blue filter, a bright green color indicates areas of nonintact corneal epithelium.

Follow-up care. After the procedure, the nurse cleans the client's cheeks with a moistened cotton ball to remove any dye. If an ophthalmic topical anesthetic was used to moisten the fluorescein strip, the client is advised not to rub the eye until the anesthetic has worn off. Contact lenses should not be reinserted until the examiner informs the client that there is no corneal abnormality.

TONOMETRY

A tonometer is an instrument that is used to measure intraocular pressure. A normal intraocular pressure reading is 10 to 21 mmHg. Tonometer readings should be taken for all clients older than age 40 years. Clients with a family history of glaucoma should have their intraocular pressure measured on a regular basis (one or two times a year) during their adult years.

Several methods are available to measure intraocular pressure, e.g., use of the *noncontact tonometer* (NCT). The NCT directs a puff of air against the cornea, which causes *indentation.* No instrument actually touches the cornea. The client may become startled when the air puff comes in contact with the eye. Advantages of the NCT include the fact that no anesthetic is needed to anesthetize the cornea and the rapidity with which the test can be performed. Thus, the NCT is the ideal instrument to use for screening. A client with any intraocular pressure reading that falls outside the normal range should be referred to an ophthalmologist for evaluation with more sensitive and accurate equipment.

Applanation tonometry is one of the most popular and accurate methods to measure intraocular pressure. In this method, the quantity of force that is required to *flatten* the cornea is determined.

Client preparation. The nurse explains the test to the client and emphasizes that the procedure is safe, of short duration, and painless. The client sits upright at the slit lamp in the examination chair (Fig. 35–13). Each eye is anesthetized by instilling an anesthetic agent into the conjunctival sacs. After the eyedrops are instilled, the

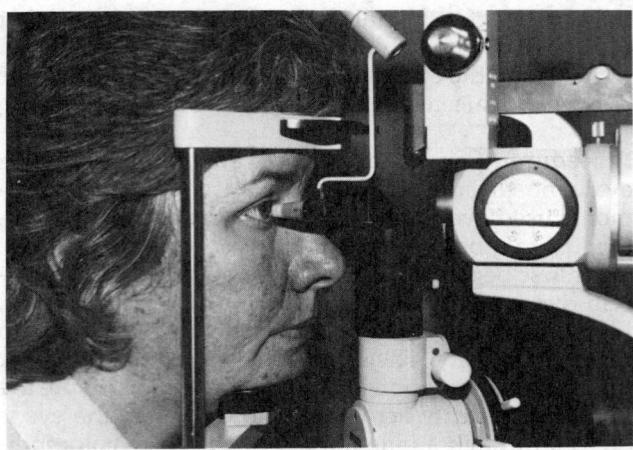

Figure 35–13
Measurement of intraocular pressure by applanation tonometry.

nurse instructs the client not to rub the eyes. The anesthesia has a desensitizing effect, and rubbing the eyes could cause corneal abrasions.

Procedure. After the eye is anesthetized, the client is asked to stare forward at a point above the nurse's ear. A flattened cone is brought into contact with the anesthetized cornea. The amount of pressure that is needed to flatten the cornea is measured by the tonometer. Several measurements are taken for each eye. The procedure is then repeated for the fellow eye.

Follow-up care. After taking the readings for each eye, the nurse reminds the client that the cornea has been anesthetized by eyedrops before the procedure. Therefore, the client must avoid rubbing the eye because it is possible to scratch the cornea.

ULTRASONOGRAPHY

Ultrasonography is the examination of the orbit and eye by using sound waves. This noninvasive test aids in the diagnosis of trauma, intraorbital tumors, proptosis, and choroidal and/or retinal detachments. It has become extremely helpful in calculating the axial length of the eye to determine the strength of a lens implant and in determining gross outline changes in the eye and the orbit of clients who have cloudy corneas or lenses that prevent examination of the fundus.

Two forms of ultrasonography exist. In *contact ultrasonography,* sound waves are transmitted through a transducer by using a gel conductor to make contact with the closed eyelid. In *immersion ultrasonography,* a saline water bath is used to transmit the sound waves through the eye. This latter method is used in cases of trauma in which pressure from the transducer might cause extrusion of the ocular contents.

Client preparation includes the instillation of anesthetic drops into the cul-de-sac. The client is cautioned to avoid rubbing the eye because of the desensitizing effects of the anesthetic. Next, the client is positioned. Clients are seated upright for contact ultrasonography; a reclining position is used for immersion ultrasonography. The probe is placed on the closed lid for the contact method and in the saline bath for the immersion method. Sound waves are bounced through the eye and return to the instrument, which creates a permanent image.

ELECTRORETINOGRAPHY

Electroretinography is the process of graphing the measurement of the retina's response to light stimulation. An electroretinogram is obtained by placing a contact lens electrode on a client's anesthetized cornea. Lights at varying speeds and intensities are flashed, and the neural response is graphed. The record from the cornea is identical to the response that would be obtained if electrodes were placed directly on the retina.

Preparation for this test includes instillation of an anesthetic into the eye. Afterwards, the client is reminded to avoid rubbing the eye until the effects of the anesthetic have disappeared.

This procedure is especially helpful in detecting and evaluating vascular changes, such as diabetic or hypertensive retinopathy; traumatic alterations to the retinal blood supply, such as those occurring with a retinal detachment; toxic changes resulting from the use of drugs, such as hydroxychloroquine sulfate (Plaquenil) (*Physician's Desk Reference,* 1989); and systemic disorders, such as vitamin A deficiency (Boyd-Monk & Steinmetz, 1987).

RADIOISOTOPIC SCANNING

Radioisotopes are used to locate tumors and lesions in various body organs. ^{32}P studies are used to differentiate the diagnosis of intraocular tumor and hemorrhage, especially in the choroid layer.

Client preparation. The client receives a tracer dose of the isotope either orally or by injection. Before the scanning procedure is performed, the client waits until the radioisotope is assimilated by the eye.

Procedure. The individual is asked to lie still and breathe normally while the scanner measures the radioactive atoms that are concentrated in the area being studied to determine the presence of a tumor. Clients who are restless, anxious, or agitated may require sedation.

Follow-up care. The nurse assures the client that the amount of radioisotope that is used as a tracer is extremely small and that the body absorbs a minimal amount of radiation. It is often necessary to reinforce the fact that the client is not radioactive.

SUMMARY

Ocular functions are of extreme importance in assisting clients with daily activities and in maintaining sensory contact with the world. Assessment and early detection of visual disorders can result in prompt treatment and achievement of optimal vision. Nurses play important roles in assessing the function of the eye and associated structures and in referring the client for additional help.

REFERENCES AND READINGS

Barnhart, E. (1989). *Physicians' desk reference* (43rd ed.). Oradell, NJ: Medical Economics.

Bates, B. (1984). *A guide to physical examination* (3rd ed.). Philadelphia: J. B. Lippincott.

Blocker, G. (1981). Glaucoma screening. *Occupational Health Nursing, 29*(6), 25–27.

Boyd-Monk, H. (1981). Practical methods of how to examine the external eye. *Occupational Health Nursing, 29*(6), 10–14.

Boyd-Monk, H., & Steinmetz, C. (1987). *Nursing care of the eye.* Norwalk, CT: Appleton & Lange.

Bryant, W. (1981). Common toxic effects of systemic drugs on the eye. *Occupational Health Nursing, 29*(6), 15–17.

Caird, F., & Williamson, J. (Eds.). (1986). *The eye and its disorders in the elderly.* Bristol, England: John Wright and Sons.

Coakes, R., & Holmes, P. (1985). *An outline of ophthalmology.* Bristol, England: John Wright and Sons.

Cotran, R. S., Kumar, V., & Robbins, S. L., (1989). *Robbins pathologic basis of disease* (4th ed.). Philadelphia: W. B. Saunders.

Crafts, R. (1979). *A textbook of human anatomy* (3rd ed.). New York: Wiley.

Faye, E. (1984). *Clinical low vision* (2nd ed.). Boston: Little, Brown.

Friedman, A. (1981). *Vision: the optyl atlas of the human eye.* Morristown, NJ: Compton.

Galloway, N. (1985). *Common eye diseases and their management.* New York: Springer-Verlag.

Gillin, S. (1981). Simple nursing procedures for the occupational health nurse. *Occupational Health Nursing, 29*(6), 18–20.

Gittinger, J. (1984). *Ophthalmology.* Boston: Little, Brown.

Glasspool, M. (1982). *Problems in ophthalmology.* Philadelphia: F. A. Davis.

Guyton, A. C. (1986). *Textbook of medical physiology* (7th ed.). Philadelphia: W. B. Saunders.

Hammerschlag, S., Hesselink, J., & Weber, A. (1983). *Computerized tomography of the eye and orbit.* Norwalk, CT: Appleton-Century-Crofts.

Hollinshead, W., & Cornelius, R. (1985). *Textbook of anatomy* (4th ed.). Philadelphia: Harper & Row.

Kwitko, M., & Weinstock, F. (Eds.). (1985). *Geriatric ophthalmology.* Orlando, FL: Grune & Stratton.

Malasanos, L., Barkauskas, V., Moss, M., & Stoltenberg-Allen, K. (1986). *Health assessment* (3rd ed.). St. Louis: C. V. Mosby.

Moore, K. (1980). *Clinically oriented anatomy.* Baltimore: Williams & Wilkins.

Paron-Langston, D. (Ed.). (1984). *Manual of ocular diagnosis and therapy.* Boston: Little, Brown.

Rooke, F., Rothwell, P., & Woodhouse, D. (1980). *Ophthalmic nursing.* New York: Churchill Livingstone.

Rubin, M. (Ed.). (1984). *Dictionary of eye terminology.* Gainesville, FL: Triad Publishing.

Sloane, A., & Garcia, G. (Eds.). (1979). *Manual of refraction* (3rd ed.). Boston: Little, Brown.

Smith, J., & Nachazel, D., Jr. (1980). *Ophthalmologic nursing.* Boston: Little, Brown.

Steinmetz, C. (1981). Practical anatomy and physiology of the eye and orbit. *Occupational Health Nursing, 29*(b), 7–9.

Sullivan, N. (1983). Vision in the elderly. *Journal of Gerontological Nursing, 9,* 228–235.

Wilensky, J., & Read, J. (Eds.). (1984). *Primary ophthalmology.* Orlando, FL: Grune & Stratton.

CHAPTER 36

Interventions for Clients with Eye and Visual Disorders

Vision is the sense that is used with greatest frequency during our waking hours. It enables us to recognize the faces of loved ones as well as hazards to our safety in the environment. Vision is the medium by which 83% of learning occurs (*Strategies for Improving Visual Learning*, 1978).

The eyes hold unique and special meanings for each person. It is important to note the historical attitudes of society toward vision, for they may be evidenced in the attitude and behaviors of the ophthalmic client. People also refer to eyesight frequently in idiomatic phrases. A few examples are, "There is more than meets the eye," "Out of sight, out of mind," "If looks could kill," and "Beauty is in the eye of the beholder." Vision is also used in warnings of danger, such as, "Look before you leap," "See here," and "Look out."

Acute or chronic conditions can affect a person's ability to process sensory information. These conditions can evolve over a lifetime, such as cataract, or they can happen in a moment, such as a corneal laceration from a BB gun. Visual changes affect each client in a unique manner, and a holistic approach must be used to guide the client's care.

BLINDNESS

OVERVIEW

Blindness is a term that evokes the image of total darkness, a world of nonsight. However, varied forms of blindness exist. In color vision blindness, the client is unable to distinguish certain colors. These clients are unable to see certain primary colors, which they perceive as gray. Color perception can also be altered by abnormal physiologic states.

The legal definition of blindness is used most frequently to describe impaired sight. Clients are classified as *legally blind* if their best visual acuity, with corrective lenses, in the better eye is 20/200 or less, or if the widest diameter of the visual field in that eye is no greater than 20 degrees.

Central vision is used to recognize faces, read a book, watch television, or drive a car. It can be impaired by diseases involving the macula, such as macular edema or macular degeneration.

Loss of peripheral vision is associated with glaucoma. The loss of side vision affects the client's ability to drive or to be aware of hazards in the periphery.

Blindness can occur in one or both eyes. When one eye is affected, the horizontal field of vision is narrowed and depth perception is impaired.

COLLABORATIVE MANAGEMENT

Many negative attitudes exist about blindness and nonsighted people. Many sighted people treat the blind as inadequate or inferior. The blind may be thought of as unattractive and of lower socioeconomic status. Nurses must be aware of these perceptions because the client may have had negative experiences either within or outside of the health care system. Clients who are newly blind are advised of the possibility of encountering these attitudes in the community.

To enable the client to better use existing vision, the nurse can offer the following helpful hints. Moving the head slightly up and down can enhance a three-dimensional effect. When shaking hands or pouring water, line up the object and move toward it. Choose a position that favors the good eye. For example, people with vision in the right eye should position people and items on their right.

When providing care to a client experiencing a temporary or permanent partial or total visual impairment, the nurse must balance the client's need for independence with the necessity to provide a safe environment. Nursing interventions for the client with reduced sight may be classed into four areas: orientation, ambulation, self-care, and support.

Orientation

Most clients seen in health care settings have various degrees of sight. Most clients who are referred to as "blind" had had sight at some time and thus have a background knowledge of size and shape on which the nurse can rely when providing information. When conversing with an individual who has limited sight or is blind, the nurse uses a normal tone of voice. Clients are first oriented to the immediate environment. The approximate size of the room is communicated. One object in the room, such as an examination chair or hospital bed, serves as the focal point during the nurse's explanation of the environment (Smith & Nachazel, 1980). The nurse guides the client to the focal point and provides further orientation to the environment from that location. For example, the nurse might say, "To the left of the bed is a chair." All other objects are described to the client in relation to the focal point. The nurse accompanies the client to other important areas, such as the bathroom, so that their locations may be known. The nurse highlights the location of the toilet, sink, and toilet paper holder. The client may wish to touch the objects in the room because the tactile stimuli assist in determining their size. Knowing the location of objects in the room decreases anxiety and increases independence. An individual with limited sight should never be left in the center of an unfamiliar room.

Clients with limited sight prefer to establish the location of personal objects such as the nurse's call bell, water pitcher, and clock. Once the location of these objects has been settled, they should not be moved without the client's consent.

At mealtime, assistance with setting up the tray may be needed. The *clock placement* of foods on the tray can be used to orient the client. For example, "There is sliced ham at 6 o'clock; peas are located at 3 o'clock; to the right of the plate is coffee; salt and pepper are next to the coffee." Help with liquids is usually appreciated. For example, the nurse helps the client to avoid spillage by tearing lids only halfway off the cup of juice. Pouring liquids may be especially difficult when one eye is covered by a patch because depth perception is lost.

Ambulation

When assisting an individual with limited sight to ambulate, the nurse allows the client to grasp his or her arm at the elbow. The arm is kept close to the nurse's body so that the client can detect the direction of movement. It is usually comfortable for the client to remain one step behind the nurse. If a narrow doorway or obstacles are noted in the path ahead, the nurse must alert the client. Because the client is unable to see furniture placement, the location of movable items, e.g., chairs, stools, and wastebaskets, is not disturbed without consultation with the client.

Clients may use a cane to help in detecting obstacles such as furniture, walls, or curbs. This cane is differentiated clearly from other canes by its straight white shape and red tip. Because it is used for safety and guidance, not mobility, the cane is held in the dominant hand several inches off the floor. The cane sweeps the ground where the client's foot will be placed next. If the left foot is forward, the cane sweeps in front of the right foot to determine the presence of obstacles.

Self-Care

The ability to control the environment is important to the client with a sight defect. Health care providers should knock on the door before entering the client's environment, whether it is an examination room, hospital room, or living area. The knock alerts the client to someone's approach and demonstrates respect. The caregiver's name and reason for visiting should be stated when the room is entered.

The passage of time seems slow for clients with impaired sight. To assist in passing time, as well as to facilitate reorientation, a radio can be played, tuned to a station of the client's choice. Clocks that give the time orally and Braille watches are also available from local agencies that assist the blind.

Many items are available at low-vision clinics to help clients care for themselves. Reading materials with large print are available on a variety of topics and include cookbooks, *Reader's Digest,* and popular newspapers. Special lighting and magnifiers are available to maximize favorable conditions for reading. If these devices do not provide adequate assistance, "talking books" are available.

Support

Reaction to the loss of sight is similar to that when there is the loss of a body part. Newly blind clients may experience a brief period of physical or psychologic immobility. A period of grieving is needed for the "dead" (nonseeing) eye. Hopelessness and denial are frequently experienced. Anger usually gives way to acceptance. The ability to cope may begin within days or weeks, but some clients may need months to mourn. Suicidal feelings and sleep disturbances have been observed. Clients benefit by the honest, empathic support that nurses can provide. They need to hear that it is acceptable to mourn, to cry, and to feel the loss. Having the nurse validate these feelings of grief as normal reassures the client. However, the client must be encouraged to move beyond the grief to greater functioning. The achievement of mastering self-care activities is frequently the turning point in the client's adaptation to the loss. Nurses can help clients move toward acceptance by encouraging the mastery of one task at a time and by providing positive reinforcement for each small success.

EXTERNAL EYE DISORDERS

Eyelid Disorders

The eyelid comprises small muscles and thin skin. The eyelid is responsible for protection of the external ocular surface as well as the maintenance and distribution of tears. Disorders can be related to changes in the structure, function, or position of the eyelid. Lid structure may also be altered by age. Aging causes a loss of skin elasticity and wrinkling. Dropping of the eyelids may result.

ENTROPION

OVERVIEW

An *entropion* is an inversion of the eyelid margin, which results in eyelashes' rubbing against the eyeball. It may be a congenital condition or may develop at a certain point in an individual's lifetime, usually after age 40 years. This condition can be caused by spasms of the retractor muscle of the eyelid, the orbicularis oculi, as well as by scarring and deformity of the tarsal plate from trauma, chemical or thermal burns, atonia, or inflammation. Elderly clients are prone to developing an entropion because of the loss of tissue support.

The client usually presents with the complaint of a foreign body sensation—"feeling something in the eye." Pain and tearing may also be present. On inspection, the eyelid is deviated inward and the conjunctiva may look inflamed. A corneal abrasion may be present because of irritation from the eyelashes.

COLLABORATIVE MANAGEMENT

Surgery may correct the position of the eyelid either by tightening the orbicular muscle and causing eversion of the eyelid to a normal position or by directly preventing inward rotation of the eyelid margin. After surgery, the eye is usually covered with a patch, and the client is discharged a few hours later. The patch is removed the next day.

Nursing interventions for the time before the procedure include assessing the eye for symptoms of dryness or infection. The nurse also demonstrates the instillation of eyedrops and evaluates the client's ability to perform this function. Figure 36–1 shows a client correctly instilling eyedrops. All of the client's questions should be answered. The nurse instructs the client to leave the patch in place until the client is seen by the ophthalmologist the next day. The client is encouraged to inform the ophthalmologist of any drainage under the patch or of complaints of severe pain. If the client is to care for sutures, the nurse demonstrates how to clean the suture line with a cotton swab and the prescribed solution. A small amount of antibiotic ointment may be applied (Fig. 36–2). The Guidelines feature on page 1014 describes the correct technique for application of ophthalmic ointment. Table 36–1 summarizes important information on ophthalmic drugs.

ECTROPION

OVERVIEW

An *ectropion* is the outward sagging and eversion of the eyelid. It may also be a congenital condition but is more frequently associated with aging. Types of ectropion include *atonic*, which is caused by the relaxation of the orbicular muscle that is associated with aging; *paralytic*, which is caused by injury or paralysis of the seventh cranial nerve; and *cicatricial*, which results from the scarring produced from trauma, burns, or ulcers.

This abnormal lid position does not permit tears to wash adequately over the anterior surface of the eye. Tears wash onto the cheek, and an enzyme that is present in tears, lysozyme, may cause skin excoriation. Corneal drying and ulceration also may result from the inability to keep the cornea moist. Clients frequently complain of constant tearing. Outward deviation of the eyelid is noted on close observation.

COLLABORATIVE MANAGEMENT

Surgery is required to restore proper lid alignment. After surgery, the eye is covered with a patch and the client is

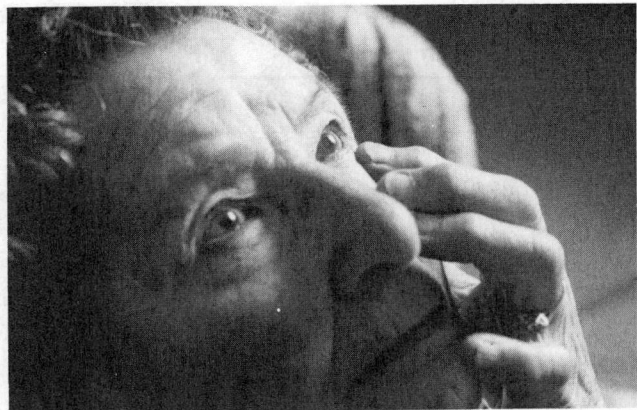

1. The client tilts her head back, opens her eyes, and looks up.

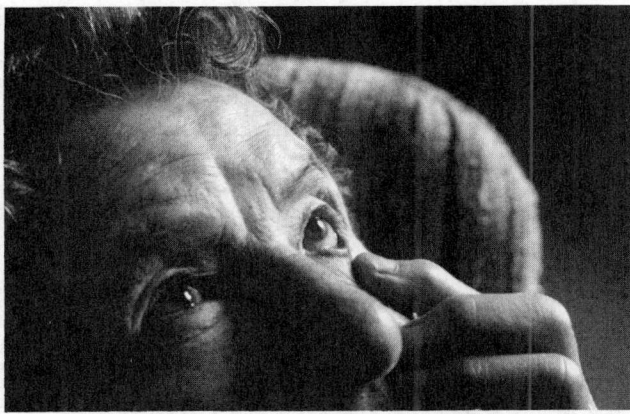

2. The client pulls the lower eyelid downward, against her cheekbone.

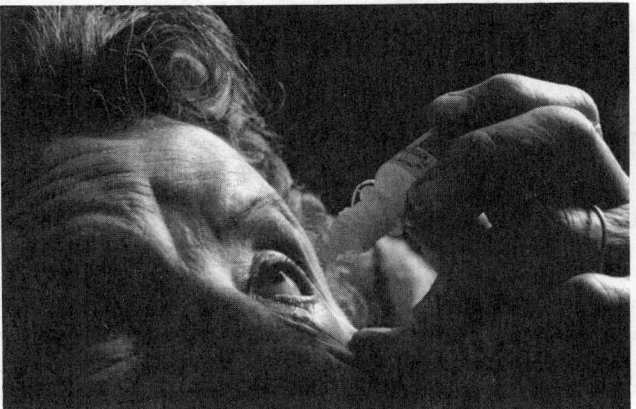

3. The client holds the bottle like a pencil, with the tip downward, and squeezes the bottle gently, allowing one drop to fall into the sac.

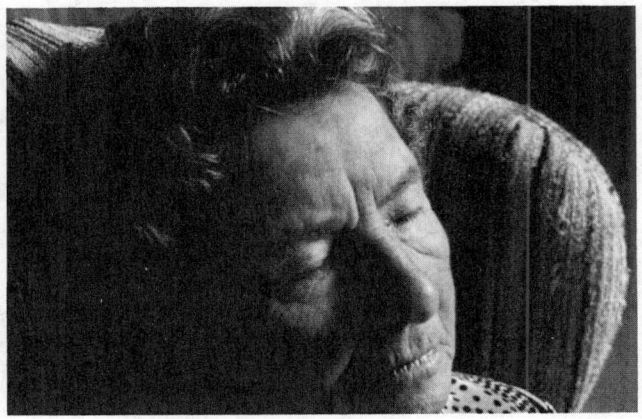

4. The client gently *closes* her eyes.

Figure 36–1

Client demonstrates proper technique for instillation of eyedrops.

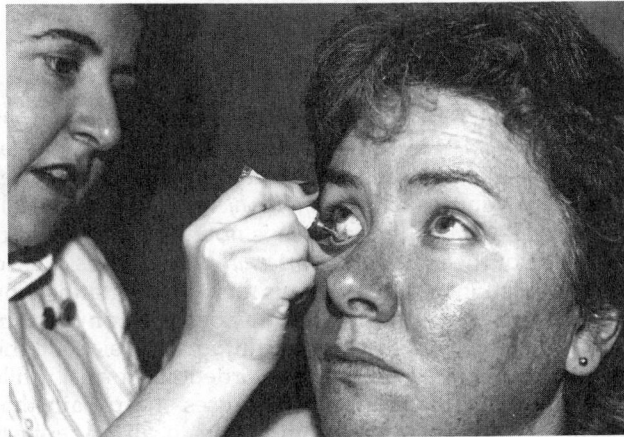

Figure 36–2

Application of ophthalmic ointment.

discharged from the facility. Nursing interventions are the same as those for the client with an entropion.

PTOSIS

OVERVIEW

Ptosis is the drooping of, or the inability to use, the upper eyelid. This disorder can be genetically transmitted or can have other causes. *Acquired* ptosis can be neurogenic, myogenic, mechanical, or traumatic. *Neurogenic* ptosis results from interference with the third cranial nerve, which controls the levator muscles. *Myogenic* ptosis is related to altered myoneural impulse function. *Mechanical* ptosis is caused by abnormal weight of the eyelids from edema, inflammation, or a tumor that can prevent the lid from elevating fully. *Traumatic* ptosis is

---

GUIDELINES ■ How to Instill Ophthalmic Ointment

Interventions	Rationales
1. Wash your hands.	1. To remove surface microorganisms.
2. Don gloves if secretions are present.	2. To protect from exposure to secretions.
3. Explain the procedure to the client.	3. To reduce anxiety.
4. Check the name, strength, and expiration date of the medication.	4. To ensure correct medication (medications with expired dates may have altered chemical properties).
5. Instruct the client to tilt the head backward, open eyes, and look up.	5. To position the head properly.
6. Pull the lower lid *gently* downward against cheekbone or gently grasp the skin of the lower lid with the thumb and index finger and pull forward.	6. To create a pocket into which ointment will be placed.
7. Hold the ointment tube near BUT NOT TOUCHING the eye or eyelashes.	7. To prevent touching the eye or eyelashes, which could cause ocular injury, and to prevent contamination of the ointment.
8. Squeeze a *thin* ribbon of ointment along the lining of the sac from the inner to the outer canthus.	8. To apply from a clean area to a dirty area.
9. Gently release the lower eyelid.	9. To prevent ointment from being pushed out of the pocket.
10. Instruct the client to close the eyes gently.	10. To distribute ointment.
11. Instruct the client that vision may be blurred by the ointment.	11. To allay anxiety and prevent injury.

---

caused by any injury to the third cranial nerve or the levator muscle that reduces the eyelid's ability to elevate.

COLLABORATIVE MANAGEMENT

The nurse asks the client when the ptosis began and if any change in vision has resulted. Because ptosis may be associated with myasthenia gravis, a thorough medical evaluation should also be conducted.

If the ptosis is slight and does not alter appearance or visual function, no intervention is needed. Surgery can be performed to improve elevation of the eyelid if visual acuity or appearance is adversely affected. The goal is to have the eyelids rest at the superior and inferior limbus, where the cornea and sclera meet. Eyelid surgery is performed almost exclusively on an outpatient basis.

The nurse determines the client's knowledge of the procedure to be performed and reviews the information that the client received before arriving at the health care facility. The nurse assesses the eye and eyelid for redness or purulent drainage. Any evidence of infection should be communicated to the ophthalmologist. The eye usually does not receive a patch after the procedure. Cool compresses are applied to decrease edema formation. A shield may be used to protect the eye. A mild analgesic, such as acetaminophen (Tylenol) or Tylenol with Codeine, is usually prescribed for control of pain.

Nursing interventions include instilling an ophthalmic antibiotic or an antibiotic-steroid combination ointment, such as neomycin sulfate, polymyxin B sulfate, plus dexamethasone (Maxitrol), to prevent corneal dryness, and teaching the client how to do this procedure. The client is instructed to keep the eye as clean as possible and to avoid rubbing the eyelid. It is possible to overcorrect the ptosis and cause part of the sclera to remain exposed when the lids are closed. The client is instructed to notify the ophthalmologist if dry, burning eyes or redness develops.

HORDEOLUM

OVERVIEW

A hordeolum is frequently referred to as a *stye*. An *external hordeolum* is an infection of the glands of Moll or Zeis. This infection occurs near the exit of the eyelashes from the eyelid, called the *eyelid-eyelash margin*. A localized, red, swollen, tender area is noted on the skin surface side of the margin. An *internal hordeolum* is caused by an infection of the sebaceous meibomian glands. The small, beady, edematous area may be noted on the skin side of the eyelid or on the conjunctival side of the eyelid-eyelash margin. As the hordeolum forms, it fills with purulent material, which causes sharp pain that becomes dull. The hordeolum and its localized redness usually affect only one eyelid at a time. Vision is not affected. *Text continued on page 1024*

Drug	Usual Daily Dosage (D) and Use (U)	Action	Side Effects	Contraindications (C) and Interactions (I)	Interventions	Rationales
Topical Anesthetics						
Proparacaine HCl (Alcaine, Ophthetic, Ophthaine), 0.50% solution	D: 1–2 gtt; can repeat q 5–10 min prn during procedure (up to 5–7 doses) U: tonometry, removal of foreign body, suture removal.	Produces anesthesia by preventing initiation and transmission of impulses at nerve cell membrane Onset: 20 s Duration: up to 15 min	Conjunctival redness Possible delayed wound healing Stinging Burning	C: should be used cautiously in client with cardiac disorder	1. Remind client not to rub or touch eye while it is anesthetized. 2. Protect eye with patch if client leaves facility before anesthetic wears off. 3. Do not let client leave facility with bottle of anesthetic. 4. Do not use discolored solution. 5. Store bottle tightly closed.	1. Touching may injure eye. 2. Patch prevents injury such as corneal abrasion. 3. Client may use other drops for comfort; these agents retard wound healing. 4. Discoloration may be a sign of drug's altered composition. 5. Air may cause contamination and oxidation of drug.
Tetracaine HCl (Pontocaine), 0.5% solution	D: same as for proparacaine U: minor surgical procedures and same as for proparacaine	Same as for proparacaine Onset: within 1 min Duration: 15–20 min	Transient stinging, epithelial damage with long-term use Sensitization on repeated use	I: sulfonamides (interferes with antibacterial action	1. Wait ½ h after anesthesia before instilling sulfonamide. 2. Same as 2–5 for proparacaine.	1. Waiting avoids additive effects of successive doses. 2. Same as 2–5 for proparacaine.
Cocaine HCl 1%–4%	D: same as for proparacaine U: same as for proparacaine, and removal of corneal epithelium	Same as for proparacaine Onset: within 20 s Duration: 30 min	Pupillary dilation may affect intraocular pressure; epithelial damage; central nervous system excitation with absorption		1. Follow narcotic control procedures. 2. Use nasal punctal occlusion. 3. Same as 1–5 for proparacaine.	1. Appropriate documentation and recording are required. 2. Technique decreases systemic absorption and side effects. 3. Same as 1–5 for proparacaine.

Table continued on following page

TABLE 36-1   Drugs Used in the Diagnosis and Treatment of Ophthalmic Disorders *Continued*

Drug	Usual Daily Dosage (D) and Use (U)	Action	Side Effects	Contraindications (C) and Interactions (I)	Interventions	Rationales
Anti-infective Agents						
Gentamicin (Gentacidin, Genoptic), 3.0 mg/mL solution, 3.0 mg/g ointment	D: 1–2 gtt q 4 h (may be increased to q 1 h; ointment ½ in bid or tid U: effective against pseudomonas, gram-negative bacilli, staphylococcus	Bactericidal (inhibits protein synthesis resulting from misreading of RNA) Onset: 1 h	Ototoxicity, nephrotoxicity, stinging	I: possibly synergistic with carbenecillin and ampicillin. Incompatible with erythromycin C: not effective against pneumococcus or streptococcus Hypersensitivity Increase in nonsusceptible organisms possible with prolonged use	1. Be sure culture is taken before use. 2. Monitor blood levels of gentamicin if systemic administration is used. 3. Reinforce importance of strict adherence to administration schedule. 4. Warn client not to share washcloths. 5. Clean exudate from eyes before administering drops. 6. Teach symptoms that signal a hypersensitivity reaction, e.g., eyelid itching or burning. 7. Apply pressure over the lacrimal sac for 1 min after instillation.	1. Use of antibiotic before culture has been obtained may alter culture results. 2. Drugs can be nephrotoxic and ototoxic if blood levels are too high. 3. Compliance is critical to maintain a therapeutic level of medication. 4. Sharing personal items increases the potential for disease transmission. 5. Cleaning decreases the chance of contaminating the eyedrop bottle. 6. Such knowledge facilitates rapid detection of side effects. 7. Pressure decreases systemic absorption and promotes local absorption.
Tobramycin (Tobrex), 3.0 mg/mL solution, 3.0 mg/g ointment	D: same as for gentamicin U: effective against gram-positive and gram-negative pathogens but more effective against pseudomonas	Same as for gentamicin	Lid itching, swelling conjunctival erythema Same as for gentamicin. Signs of overdose: keratitis, erythema, increased tearing, eyelid edema	I: hypersensitivity	1. Monitor signs and symptoms of overdose. 2. Same as 2 for gentamicin.	1. Monitoring promotes rapid detection of problems. 2. Same as 2 for gentamicin.

Drug	Action	Dosage (D) / Use (U)	Side Effects	Contraindications	Nursing Implications	Rationale
Erythromycin (Ilotycin), 0.5%–1.0% ointment	Bactericidal (inhibits bacterial protein synthesis) Onset: 4 h Effective against gram-positive organisms including *Neisseria*	D: ½ in qd to bid U: trachoma caused by chlamydia; ophthalmia neonatorum	Slows corneal wound healing Overgrowth of nonsusceptible organisms	C: known hypersensitivity	1. Apply within 1 h of birth. 2. Warn client that drug may cause blurred vision. 3. Same as 3–5 for gentamicin.	1. Timing is critical to rapid treatment of infection. 2. Blurred vision is a safety hazard. 3. Same as 3–5 for gentamicin.
Combination antibiotics: neomycin sulfate, polymyxin B sulfate, and dexamethasone (Maxitrol), suspension/ointment	Bactericidal (similar to gentamicin) Anti-inflammatory: decreased cellular exudation and collagen-forming activity Decreases excessive capillary permeability	D: 1–2 gtt 4–6 times per day U: allergic conjunctivitis, uveitis, keratitis	Prolonged wound healing Posterior subcapsular cataract	C: possible increased intraocular pressure with long-term use Hypersensitivity Fungal disease or herpes simplex keratitis Untreated purulent infection	1. Taper dosage. 2. *Shake bottle well before use to achieve appropriate drop composition.* 3. Same as 3–5, 7 for gentamicin.	1. Tapering decreases chance of recurrence of infection. 2. Medication must be evenly distributed in suspension. 3. Same as 3–5, 7 for gentamicin.

Topical Antiviral Agents

Drug	Action	Dosage (D) / Use (U)	Side Effects	Contraindications	Nursing Implications	Rationale
Idoxuridine (IDU) (Stoxil, Herplex), 0.1% solution, 0.5 % ointment	Substitutes for thymidine in DNA synthesis, resulting in production of faulty DNA and destroying destructive capacity of virus	D: 1 gtt q 1 h during day and 1 gtt q 2 h at night ½-in strip of ointment q 4 h U: herpes simplex keratitis	Ocular irritation, pain, itching, edema of lids, photophobia, corneal clouding	C: hypersensitivity Long-term use: If no improvement in 5–7 d, change to vidarabine Deep ulcers	1. Refrigerate. 2. Protect from light. 3. Warn client not to share washcloths. 4. Clean exudate from eyes before using medication. 5. Wear gloves if secretions are present. 6. Taper dosage at end of treatment. 7. Be sure client knows how to apply medication.	1, 2. Refrigeration ensures stability of medication. 3. Sharing personal items increases the potential for transmission of microorganisms. 4. Cleaning decreases the chance of contaminating medication and increases the surface area of absorption. 5. Wearing gloves decreases the potential for transmission of microorganisms. 6. Tapering decreases chance for recurrence of ulcer. 7. Knowledge facilitates compliance with regimen.

Table continued on following page

Drug	Usual Daily Dosage (D) and Use (U)	Action	Side Effects	Contraindications (C) and Interactions (I)	Interventions	Rationales
Vidarabine (Vira-A), 3% ointment	D: ½ in 5 times/d U: herpes simplex keratitis and acute keratoconjunctivitis, continued until corneal epithelium is healed	Appears to interfere with early DNA synthesis	Lacrimation, foreign body sensation, conjunctival redness, photophobia	C: hypersensitivity Deep ulcers	1. Same as 1 for idoxuridine. 2. Monitor for signs of sensitivity (itching lids and burning). 3. Advise client to report these signs to physician. 4. Stress importance of compliance with frequent use of eyedrops.	1. Same as 1 for idoxuridine. 2, 3. Sensitivity to drug is common, and monitoring promotes rapid detection and treatment of symptoms. 4. Compliance is critical to maintain a therapeutic level of medication.
Trifluridine (Viroptic), 1% solution	D: 1-2 gtt q 2 h; maximum 9 doses/d until re-epithelialization occurs, then q 4 h for 1 wk U: herpes simplex virus types 1 and 2	Interferes with DNA synthesis	Fewer than for other viral agents Mild corneal and conjunctival irritation on instillation	C: long term use: can be too toxic after 21 d; if no improvement after 7 d, discontinue	Same as above	
Topical Steroids						
Prednisolone acetate (Pred Mild, Econopred, 0.125%-Pred Forte, 1.0% suspension	D: 1-2 gtt up to every h U: allergic conjunctivitis, uveitis, scleritis, interstitial keratitis, postsurgical inflammation Must be tapered before stopping Use lowest concentration possible to treat problem	Decreases fibrinous exudation and tissue infiltration; inhibits fibroblast activity; reduces excessive permeability of inflamed capillaries Has 3-5 times inflammatory potency of hydrocortisone	Prolonged wound healing, susceptibility to common infections, cataract	C: hypersensitivity Fungal disease, active viral disease, untreated purulent infection, diseases causing corneal thinning; also, use with caution in clients with glaucoma	1. Check label carefully; several strengths are available. 2. Advise client to report decreased vision and/or pain *immediately* to ophthalmologist. 3. Reinforce necessity of *vigorous shaking* of bottle before use. 4. Monitor client for signs of corneal ulceration.	1. Correct medication must be administered. 2. Signs of infection require discontinuing use of medication. 3. Medication is in suspension. Shaking is required to evenly distribute medication in solution. 4. Steroid use predisposes client to infection.

Drug	Action	Dosage and Use	Side Effects	Contraindications and Interactions	Nursing Considerations (Rationale)
					5. Instruct client not to store remaining medication for future eye problems. (5. Medication could become contaminated or client could change potency.)
Prednisolone phosphate (Inflamase Mild), 0.125% Inflamase Forte, 1.0% solution		D: 1–2 gtt up to every hour; decrease to q 4 h as soon as response noted. U: use lowest possible effective concentration. Taper dosage before stopping use	Same as for prednisolone acetate. Secondary ocular infections, stinging, and burning	Same as for prednisolone	1. Advise client not to use leftover medication for new problems. (1. Same as 5 for prednisolone acetate.) 2. Advise client not to share eyedrops with family members. (2. Disease transmission is possible with sharing.) 3. Remind client to frequently have eye pressure checked if receiving long-term steroid therapy. (3. Steroids can be associated with increased intraocular pressure.)
Dexamethasone (Maxidex), 0.1% suspension, 0.5% ointment		D: same as for prednisolone acetate. U: inflammatory conditions of conjunctival cornea and anterior segment. Dosage must be tapered before stopping drug	Same as for prednisolone acetate	C: herpes dendritic keratitis, viral disease, after foreign body removal, varicella	1. Shake vigorously before use. (1. Medication is in suspension. Shaking is required to evenly distribute medication in solution.) 2. Same as 2 for prednisolone acetate. (2. Same as 2 for prednisolone acetate.)
Miotics					
Pilocarpine HCl (Pilocar, Isopto-Carpine), 0.25%–10% solution, 4% gel	Decreases formation and increases outflow of aqueous humor. Onset: 60 min	D: 1 gt 4–6 times/d Gel: ½ in at h.s. U: open- and closed-angle glaucoma. Also, break adhesions when used with atropine. Counteracts mydriatics and cycloplegics after eye examination	Systemic: sweating, nausea, vomiting, diarrhea, pulmonary edema, salivation, lacrimation, bronchospasm. Transient myopia and brow pain common when treatment initiated	I: Carbachol (additive) Phenylephrine HCl (inhibits dilation) C: Acute iritis, or anterior segment inflammation, or corneal abrasion	1. Warn client that vision may be blurred temporarily. 2. Instruct client that gel can blur vision and to avoid fine work or driving after use of gel. 3. Note that pupillary variation can cause a change in visual field. (1, 2. Blurred vision can predispose to injury. 3. Treatment decisions are frequently made based on visual field results.)

Table continued on following page

TABLE 36–1 Drugs Used in the Diagnosis and Treatment of Ophthalmic Disorders *Continued*

Drug	Usual Daily Dosage (D) and Use (U)	Action	Side Effects	Contraindications (C) and Interactions (I)	Interventions	Rationales
						4. This form requires less frequent administration.
Carbachol (Isopto-Carbachol), 0.75%–3.0% solution	D: 1 gt 3–4 times/d U: narrow- and open-angle glaucoma	Mimics effects of parasympathetic system in inhibiting the effects of cholinesterase Onset: slow	Accommodative spasms, headache, conjunctival vasodilation, headache, brow pain, diarrhea, sweating, flushing	C: iritis, corneal abrasion Use cautiously in clients with Parkinson's disease, heart failure, urinary tract obstruction	1. Stress importance of compliance with treatment regimen. 2. Tell client to contact ophthalmologist if side effects are noted. 3. Use nasal punctal occlusion.	1. Compliance is critical to maintaining therapeutic control of intraocular pressure. 2. Rapid notification of physician results in rapid treatment of side effects. 3. Occlusion decreases systemic absorption and side effects.
Adrenergics (Sympathomimetics)						
Dipivefrin HCl (Propine), 0.1% solution	D: 1 gt q 12 h U: open-angle glaucoma	Prodrug form of epinephrine, converted to epinephrine in the eye, after which it decreases aqueous humor production and enhances outflow	Prodrugs produce fewer side effects: transient burning and stinging, deposits on conjunctiva and cornea, macular edema, tachycardia, arrhythmias, hypertension	C: narrow-angle glaucoma, unstable cardiovascular disease Use with caution in clients with hypertension, heart disease, or aphakia	1. Monitor vital signs in hypertensive and cardiovascular clients. 2. Instruct client to perform punctal occlusion.	1. Adrenergic drugs can increase heart rate and blood pressure. 2. Procedure reduces systemic absorption and side effects of drug.

Beta Blockers

Drug	Dosage/Use	Action	Contraindications/Interactions	Side Effects	Nursing Interventions	Rationale
Timolol maleate (Timoptic), 0.25%–0.5% solution	D: 1 gt q 12 h; begin with 0.25%, increase to 0.5% if ineffective. U: chronic open-angle glaucoma, secondary glaucoma	Reduces aqueous humor formation; may increase aqueous outflow. Nonspecific beta blocker, affecting both $beta_1$- and $beta_2$-receptors in eye, heart, and lung	C: asthma, heart failure, severe cardiac disease, severe chronic obstructive pulmonary disease. I: e.g., beta-blocking drugs, propanolol HCl (Inderal). Increased ocular and systemic effects	Headache, depression, fatigue, slight decrease in resting heart rate, anorexia, hypotension, bradycardia, syncope, exacerbation of asthma and congestive heart failure with systemic absorption; reduced corneal sensitivity with long-term use; hypotension during anesthesia; may mask symptoms of hypoglycemia	1. Instruct client in nasal punctal occlusion. 2. Monitor vital signs. 3. Advise diabetics of potential masking of hypoglycemic symptoms. 4. Reinforce importance of reporting side effects to ophthalmologist immediately. 5. Remind client that he/she may need to change position and begin activity gradually.	1. Procedure decreases systemic absorption and side effects of drug. 2. Medications have potential to alter vital signs. 3. Delayed recognition can delay initiation of treatment and can be life-threatening. 4. Such reporting promotes rapid detection and treatment of side effects. 5. Medications may cause orthostatic hypotension.
Betaxolol HCl (Betoptic), 0.5% solution	D: 1 gt q 12 h. U: chronic open-angle glaucoma, ocular hypertension	Specific beta blocker; does not affect $beta_2$-receptors in lungs	C: sinus bradycardia, cardiogenic shock. Use with caution in clients with history of cardiac failure, diabetes, or heart disease	Insomnia, masked symptoms of hypoglycemia	1. Stress importance of compliance. 2. Same as 2, 3 for timolol maleate.	1. Compliance is critical to maintain therapeutic control of intraocular pressure. 2. Same as 2, 3 for timolol maleate.

Mydriatics and Cycloplegics

Drug	Dosage/Use	Action	Contraindications/Interactions	Side Effects	Nursing Interventions	Rationale
Sympathomimetic Phenylephrine HCl (Neo-Synephrine), 2.5%–10% solution	D: 1–2 gtt before examination; 1 drop q 10–15 min 3 times before surgery	Potentiates action of epinephrine, causing activation of dilator muscle of iris. Duration: 3 h	C: narrow-angle glaucoma, Shallow anterior chambers. I: monoamine oxidase inhibitors, tryclic antidepressants	Iris floaters	1. Instruct client to wear sunglasses until effects of drug wear off. 2. Advise client of burning sensation when drops are instilled. 3. Refrigerate drops if burning is uncomfortable. 4. Advise client to avoid hazardous activity during treatment.	1. Glasses promote comfort while decreasing effects of photophobia. 2. Knowledge decreases anxiety. 3. Coolness promotes comfort. 4, 5. Blurred vision can be a safety hazard.

Table continued on following page

Drug	Usual Daily Dosage (D) and Use (U)	Action	Side Effects	Contraindications (C) and Interactions (I)	Interventions	Rationales
					5. Warn client not to drive or operate heavy machinery while vision is blurred.	
					6. Dim lights as needed for comfort.	6. Photophobia is common
					7. Teach client nasal punctal occlusion.	7. Procedure decreases systemic absorption of drug.
Parasympatholytic Tropicamide (Mydriacyl), 0.5%–1.0% solution	D: 1–2 gtt q 5 min × 3 U: diagnostic purposes	Shortest-acting cycloplegic Duration: 4–6 h	Flushing, blurring of vision, dry mouth, confusion, burning on instillation of drops	C: narrow-angle glaucoma Shallow anterior chamber	1. Same as 1–6 for phenylephrine.	1. Same as 1–6 for phenylephrine
Cyclopentolate (Cyclogyl), 0.5%–2.0% solution	D:1–2 gtt before examination U: cycloplegia for eye examination	Duration: up to 24 h	Burning on instillation of drug, psychosis, ataxia, restlessness, speech changes, disorientation, increased blood pressure	C: narrow-angle glaucoma	1. Same as 1–6 for phenylephrine.	1. Same as 1–6 for phenylephrine
Atropine (Atropisol), 0.5%–3% solution	D: 1 gt bid U: acute iritis, uveitis, amblyopia	Most potent mydriatic Duration: up to 14 d	Flushing, dryness of mouth, tachycardia, increased blood pressure, conjunctivitis, blurred vision, abdominal distention, confusion, irritability, drowsiness, restlessness	C: angle-closure glaucoma Hypersensitivity Use with caution in the elderly, children, or clients with cardiovascular disease	1. Same as 1–6 for phenylephrine	1. Same as 1–6 for phenylephrine
Flurbiprofen (Ocufen), 0.5% solution	D: 1 gt q 1/2 h beginning 2 h before surgery (total of 4 doses) U: inhibition of intraoperative miosis	Inhibits miosis by constricting iris sphincter Nonsteroidal anti-inflammatory action	Burning and stinging on drug instillation, ocular irritation, may prolong wound healing	C: epithelial herpes simplex Use with caution if a history of bleeding tendencies I: Use with caution with aspirin and anticoagulants	1. Have client instill drops preoperatively while nurse observes technique. 2. Advise client to report symptoms of infection immediately.	1. Demonstration enables nurse to observe client's technique. 2. Use of medication can slow wound healing.

Carbonic Anhydrase Inhibitors

Agent	Dosage (D) / Uses (U)	Action / Onset	Side Effects	Contraindications	Nursing Implications	Rationale
Acetazolamide (Diamox), 125- to 250-mg tablets, 500-mg capsules, 500-mg vials	D: 250 mg qid PO or 500 mg bid PO; 500 mg IV. U: (IV) angle-closure glaucoma or for rapid reduction in intraocular pressure; (PO) adjunct treatment of open-angle glaucoma	Reduces aqueous secretion by inhibiting ciliary body carbonic anhydrase. Onset (PO): 2 h. Onset (IV): 5 min	Potassium depletion gastrointestinal upset, nausea, vomiting, diarrhea, renal calculi, depression, numbness and tingling of extremities, anorexia, transient myopia, blood dyscrasias	C: sulfonamide derivative, allergies, Addison's disease and adrenal insufficiency	1. Instruct client in signs and symptoms of hypokalemia. 2. Monitor K+ levels. 3. Encourage intake of K+-rich foods. 4. Be aware that side effects can be uncomfortable and discouraging for client. 5. Reinforce importance of notifying ophthalmologist when side effects develop. 6. Monitor electrocardiograms during drug use.	1. Rapid detection of symptoms is important. 2. Monitoring promotes rapid detection before symptoms are present. 3. Increased intake will help to maintain normal K+ levels. 4. Awareness enables nurse to provide support to client. 5. Rapid detection of side effects is critical 6. Hypokalemia causes potentially life-threatening arrhythmias.
Methazolamide (Neptazane), 50-mg tablets	D: 1-2 tablets tid. U: adjunct treatment of open-angle glaucoma	Similar to acetazolamide. Onset: 2 h. Duration: 10-12 h	Drowsiness, fatigue, malaise, minimal gastrointestinal upset		1. Same as 1-5 for acetazolamide.	1. Same as 1-5 for acetazolamide.

Osmotic Agents

Agent	Dosage (D) / Uses (U)	Action / Onset	Side Effects	Contraindications	Nursing Implications	Rationale
Mannitol (Osmitrol), 20% solution	D: 1.5 g/1 kg body weight, given over 45 min. U: acute angle-closure glaucoma; rapid reduction of intraocular pressure before surgery	Acts as diuretic. (Increased osmotic pressure of plasma in relationship to aqueous humor lowers intraocular pressure) Onset: within 30 min	Increased cardiovascular workload, diuresis, headache, confusion, tachycardia, blurred vision, rhinitis, nausea, urinary retention	C: severe congestive heart failure, impaired renal function, pulmonary edema, anuria	1. Monitor vital signs and output during administration. 2. Give IV through filter. 3. Check solution frequently for precipitates.	1. Volume depletion can cause hypotension. 2. Use of filter prevents precipitates from entering blood vessel. 3. Rapid detection of precipitates is critical.
Isosorbide solution (Ismotic) 100 mg/220 mL	D: 1.5 g/kg body weight. U: same as for mannitol	Same as for mannitol	Nausea, vomiting, headache, confusion, disorientation	Same as for mannitol	1. Give over chipped ice or with lemonade. 2. Keep emesis basin handy.	1. Ice or lemonade improves taste. 2. Medication can cause nausea.

COLLABORATIVE MANAGEMENT

Treatment includes use of warm compresses four times a day. An antibacterial ointment, such as sulfacetamide sodium (Sodium Sulamyd), may be prescribed. When the lesion opens, either spontaneously or after use of warm compresses, the purulent material drains and pain subsides.

Nursing interventions include applying a clean washcloth compress and instructing the client in this application. The accompanying Guidelines feature describes the proper technique for application of ocular compresses. Thorough hand washing is necessary before and after applying the compresses. The washcloth is folded once lengthwise and once widthwise and is then moistened with warm water from the sink. The water should be quite warm, but not an uncomfortable temperature to the wrist. Once the compress is applied to the closed eye, a second washcloth should be placed under the water to warm. Compresses are held in place over the closed eye until they become cool (usually 2 to 5 minutes). The washcloth can be reapplied by using a fresh side each time it is placed over the eye. The nurse also instructs the client to separate these washcloths from the washcloths of other members of the household. After the compresses have been applied for the prescribed time, the antibiotic ointment is instilled. The nurse also advises the client that the use of ointments may cause the vision to be blurred and that care must be exercised when ambulating. Ointment should be removed from the eye before driving or operating machinery. To remove the ointment, the eye is closed and the closed eyelid is wiped gently from the inner canthus outward. Vigorous wiping is avoided because of the potential of applying pressure on the eye. Clients are advised to refrain from wearing make-up because it may be a source of irritation.

CHALAZION

OVERVIEW

A *chalazion* is a sterile, granulomatous inflammation of the meibomian gland (Vaughan & Asbury, 1986). It begins with inflammation and tenderness, similar to the hordeolum, and is characterized by a gradual painless swelling at the gland. In its fully developed state, no inflammatory signs are present. Most chalazia point on the conjunctival side of the eyelid. Left untreated, the chalazion can press on the cornea or globe and cause astigmatism. The client may also complain of eye fatigue and sensitivity to light. *Epiphora*, excessive tearing, may also be present.

COLLABORATIVE MANAGEMENT

Treatment includes the use of warm compresses for 15 minutes four times a day followed by instillation of ophthalmic ointment. The chalazion is excised if it is large enough to affect vision, is cosmetically unsatisfactory to the client, or recurs frequently. After excision, antibiotic ointment is instilled and the eye is covered with a patch. Steps for proper application of a nonpressure eyepatch are described in the Guidelines feature on page 1025.

The nurse makes sure that the eye is closed before applying the patch. Clients are instructed to leave the eyepatch intact for 4 to 6 hours and then to remove the patch and to begin applying warm, moist compresses. Antibiotic eyedrops, such as gentamicin (Genoptic) or sulfacetamide sodium (Bleph 10), are instilled after the use of the compresses. The nurse reviews the use of warm compresses and eyedrop instillation with the client. The client is instructed to report any evidence of

---

GUIDELINES ■ How to Apply Ocular Compresses

Interventions	Rationales
1. Wash your hands.	1. To reduce the numbers of microorganisms and debris on skin.
2. Explain the procedure to the client.	2. To reduce anxiety.
3. Fold a clean washcloth into fourths.	3. To facilitate molding the cloth to ocular contours (four applications are used).
4. Moisten the cloth with water until it is warm to the touch on your inner wrist.*	4. To prevent use of excessively warm water; wrist sensitivity roughly approximates that of globe.
5. Position the cloth against the client's *closed* eyelid.	5. To prevent corneal irritation.
6. Hold the compress in place until the warmth fades (approximately 2–5 min).	6. To judge when to repeat process; when warmth fades, additional application is necessary.
7. Repeat steps 4–6 for three additional applications.	7. To rewarm the cloth, maintaining warmth against the eyelid.
8. Use a separate fold of the cloth against the eye each time.	8. To keep a clean surface against the eye, which reduces the spread of microorganisms.

* If cool compresses are desired, change water temperature and follow same procedure.

GUIDELINES ■ How to Apply an Eyepatch

Interventions	Rationales

Nonpressure Eyepatch

1. Assemble equipment:
   a. Eyepatch.
   b. Skin preparation.
   c. Nonallergenic paper tape.
2. Explain the procedure to the client.
3. Wash your hands.

4. Apply a skin preparation to the client's forehead and cheek.
5. Instruct the client to gently close both eyes.
6. Place a patch over the closed eyelid (Fig. A).
7. Apply tape from the cheek to the middle of the forehead in a diagonal line. Pull the tape snugly enough that the cheek is pulled slightly upward (Fig. B).
8. Cover the patch with overlapping pieces of tape (Fig. C).

Pressure Eyepatch

1. Assemble equipment:
   a. Two eyepatches for each eye requiring treatment.
   b. Skin preparation pad.
   c. Nonallergenic paper tape.
2–5. Follow corresponding steps under Nonpressure Eyepatch.
6. Fold one eyepatch in half, place over the closed eyelid, and apply a second eyepatch (unfolded) over the folded one (Fig. D).
7, 8. Follow corresponding steps under Nonpressure Eyepatch.

Rationales column:

1. To ensure availability of equipment.

2. To decrease anxiety.

3. To decrease the potential for cross-contamination between clients.

4. To provide a surface for tape adherence and decrease the potential for skin irritation.
5. To facilitate complete eyelid relaxation.
6. To exert slight pressure against the eyelid.
7. To hold the patch against the closed eyelid.

8. To ensure even pressure against the eyelid.

1. To ensure availability of equipment.

6. To exert pressure against the closed eyelid and to maintain the patch against it.

A

B

C

D

infection, increasing redness, purulent drainage, or reduced vision to the ophthalmologist immediately. Women are instructed to refrain from the use of makeup because it is a common allergen and a good medium for growth of microorganisms.

Lacrimal Apparatus Disorders

The lacrimal system is responsible for making tears, bathing the external eye with tears to moisten the cornea, and removing tears from the external surface of the eye. Problems can arise from insufficient tear production as well as from infection or inflammation in any part of the lacrimal system.

KERATOCONJUNCTIVITIS SICCA

OVERVIEW

Keratoconjunctivitis sicca is also referred to as *dry eye syndrome*. It results from a deficiency in the composition of tears, from lacrimal gland malfunction, or from factors that alter the distribution of tears. Tears have three components: *aqueous, mucin,* and *lipids.* An enzyme, *lysozyme,* is also present in tears to inhibit the growth of many microorganisms. If the goblet cells of the eyelid fail to produce sufficient mucin, the tears will not spread evenly across the external eye. Tears will break up, leaving areas of the cornea exposed and resulting in patchy dryness. A deficiency of mucin production is associated with rheumatoid arthritis, vitamin A deficiency, and chronic conjunctivitis. Decreased tear production can also occur during the use of antihistamines, beta-adrenergic blocking agents, and drugs containing atropine. Diseases that are associated with decreased tear production include rheumatoid arthritis, leukemia, sarcoidosis, and lymphoma (Newell, 1986).

Lacrimal gland function may be affected by congenital or acquired disorders. In the former, the nasolacrimal duct may fail to develop fully or to open. Acquired lacrimal gland dysfunction occurs as a result of systemic disease, trauma, or infection. Systemic diseases that are associated with altered lacrimal gland function include mumps and multiple sclerosis. Trauma from irradiation or chemical burns can also decrease lacrimal system function. Injury to the facial nerve (cranial nerve VII) can also inhibit tearing.

Tear distribution can be affected by mechanical factors, including the misuse of contact lenses, altered structure or function of the eyelid, and the forward protrusion of the eyeball, which is called proptosis or exophthalmos. The client complains of a foreign body sensation, burning and itching eyes, and photophobia. The corneal light reflex may be dulled or distorted. Tear film of the client may contain strands of mucus.

COLLABORATIVE MANAGEMENT

Tests to evaluate dry eye syndrome and tear disorders include Schirmer's test and rose bengal staining. Treatment depends on the severity of the symptoms. Artificial tears (Hypotears, Refresh) are prescribed for daytime use to reduce dryness. These liquids can be used as often as necessary. At night, a lubricating ointment (Lacri-Lube S.O.P., Refresh PM). is used. If the dry eye syndrome is caused by an abnormal eyelid position or function, surgery may be required.

Nursing interventions include explaining the diagnostic tests to the client and assessing the eyes for symptoms of dryness. Suggestions for increasing moisture in the environment, such as a humidifier, are discussed with the client. The ability of the client to instill eyedrops and ointments is assessed. The nurse stresses the importance of avoiding dry, irritating environments and noxious odors or fumes.

Conjunctival Disorders

The *conjunctiva* is a thin mucous membrane composed of two portions that act as a protective coating for the eye. The anatomic features of the conjunctivae are described in Chapter 35. Because of its location, the conjunctiva is subject to direct environmental injury from trauma or exposure to noxious gases. It is susceptible to infection because of its proximity to the eyelids and eyelashes. Also, because it is close to the cornea, it can be an avenue for the spread of disease.

Subconjunctival Hemorrhage

OVERVIEW

Subconjunctival blood vessels are somewhat fragile and can break after localized increased pressure that results from vigorous sneezing or coughing or from vomiting. In certain instances, these hemorrhages may be associated with hypertension or blood dyscrasias.

The small well-defined area of hemorrhage appears bright red under the shimmering conjunctiva. The client is usually quite concerned about its development and appearance. However, no pain or visual impairment accompanies the hemorrhage, and it resolves gradually over a 10- to 14-day period, with no treatment required.

COLLABORATIVE MANAGEMENT

Nursing interventions include eliciting a detailed history. The development of a subconjunctival hemorrhage may be linked to hypertension, so the nurse assesses and documents the client's blood pressure. Baseline visual acuity is also noted.

Conjunctivitis

Conjunctivitis is an inflammation or infection of the conjunctiva. *Inflammatory* conjunctivitis can result from exposure to allergens or irritants and is not contagious. *Infectious* conjunctivitis occurs frequently as a result of bacterial or viral infection and is readily transmitted from person to person.

ALLERGIC CONJUNCTIVITIS

OVERVIEW

Allergic conjunctivitis is one of the most frequently occurring external eye diseases (Boyd-Monk & Steinmetz, 1987). This form of conjunctivitis may be seasonal and is associated with a sensitivity to pollens, animal protein, feathers, dust, certain foods or materials, insect bites, or drugs (including atropine and antibiotics of the mycin family such as neomycin). Allergic conjunctivitis may also occur after exposure to noxious chemicals, such as hair spray, make-up, smog, or tobacco smoke. Asthma, hay fever, and eczema are also associated with allergic conjunctivitis.

Symptoms include minimal to severe edema of the conjunctiva, a sensation of burning, and vascular injection (engorgement of blood vessels). Excessive tearing sometimes occurs. Itching is most severe in this form of conjunctivitis (Vaughan & Asbury, 1986).

COLLABORATIVE MANAGEMENT

Treatment includes the instillation of vasoconstrictors. Corticosteroid eyedrops such as prednisolone acetate (Poly-Pred) may be prescribed for short-term use in severe cases, but long-term use of steroid eyedrops is not encouraged because of possible cataract formation and the development of glaucoma.

Nursing interventions include obtaining a baseline measure of visual acuity and assisting the client to identify possible sources of allergens. Women are instructed to refrain from using make-up until all symptoms of conjunctivitis subside. If the cause of the allergic conjunctivitis has not been determined at that point, make-up can be reintroduced gradually. The nurse also suggests ways of reducing exposure to allergens, such as wearing sunglasses or avoiding irritating environments. The nurse also assesses the client's ability to instill eyedrops and provides assistance as necessary.

BACTERIAL CONJUNCTIVITIS

OVERVIEW

Bacterial conjunctivitis is also referred to as *pink eye.* This form of easily transmitted conjunctivitis is usually caused by *Staphylococcus aureus.* It may also occur after exposure to *Haemophilus influenzae* or *Neisseria gonorrhoea* (Vaughan & Asbury, 1986).

Symptoms include marked blood vessel dilation, mild conjunctival edema, and tearing. Discharge is watery at first from the increased tearing but it gradually becomes thicker, with shreds of mucus, and progresses to a purulent state that causes the eyelids to adhere together in a closed position. Exudation is most profuse in this type of conjunctivitis (Vaughan & Asbury, 1986). Small breaks in the corneal epithelium may be noted (Boyd-Monk & Steinmetz, 1987).

COLLABORATIVE MANAGEMENT

The causative microorganism is identified by culturing the discharge. A smear of the discharge may also be made. Treatment is aimed at controlling the infection with topical antibiotics. A broad-spectrum topical antibiotic is administered initially until specific sensitivities of the microorganisms are determined.

Nursing interventions are focused on preventing the spread of the disease. Bacterial conjunctivitis usually occurs unilaterally; however, cross-contamination may cause involvement of the other eye. The nurse obtains a detailed history of the present problem and notes any recent eye injuries or exposure to nonhygienic environments. All cases of gonococcal conjunctivitis must be reported to the local health department. The amount, color, and type of drainage are noted. Hygienic principles are reviewed with the client. Hands are a major source of cross-infection. Thus, hands must be washed before and after wiping the eye and instilling eyedrops. Clients are warned not to touch the unaffected eye without first washing their hands. The client is also cautioned against rubbing the eye or carelessly disposing of tissues. Family members are advised to avoid sharing washcloths and towels with the client to prevent cross-contamination. The nurse is also responsible for appropriate cleaning of equipment after the client's examination.

VIRAL CONJUNCTIVITIS

OVERVIEW

Viral conjunctivitis usually results from infection with the human adenovirus or from the systemic viral diseases mumps and mononucleosis. The most frequently occurring adenoviral inflammation is *epidemic kerato-conjunctivitis.*

Symptoms of this type of keratoconjunctivitis include enlargement of the preauricular lymph nodes, photophobia, and sensation of a foreign body in the eye. Profuse tearing is a predominant symptom (Vaughan & Asbury, 1986), and periorbital pain may be present. In approximately 50% of cases, the cornea is involved and corneal opacities are noted (Boyd-Monk & Steinmetz, 1987). The conjunctiva is noticeably reddened. Minimal exudates are noted.

COLLABORATIVE MANAGEMENT

Treatment consists of rest and a mild analgesic, such as acetaminophen or acetaminophen with codeine, which is prescribed for pain. An antibiotic is sometimes prescribed to prevent a secondary infection.

Nursing interventions for this disorder are the same as those for bacterial conjunctivitis.

TRACHOMA

OVERVIEW

Trachoma is a chronic, bilateral scarring form of conjunctivitis. Caused by *Chlamydia trachomatis,* it is *the chief cause of blindness in the world* (Newell, 1986). The prevalence and severity of the disease depend on the standards of living, personal hygiene, and climate. A higher incidence of trachoma is noted in warm, moist climates where hygienic practices are substandard. In the United States, trachoma is rare except among Native Americans of the Southwest (Vaughan & Asbury, 1986). Contamination also occurs through vectors such as flies and gnats.

The incubation period is between 5 and 14 days. Initially, trachoma resembles bacterial conjunctivitis. Early symptoms include tearing, photophobia, edema of the eyelids, and conjunctival edema. Follicles form on the palpebral conjunctiva near the superior tarsus and at the corneal limbus. A profuse drainage is noted (Vaughan & Asbury, 1986). As the disease progresses, the eyelid scars and turns inward, which causes the eyelashes to abrade the cornea. This irritation stimulates *pannus,* the growth of new blood vessels in from the corneal-scleral margin.

COLLABORATIVE MANAGEMENT

Cultures and smears are taken of areas in question to ascertain the causative organism. Trachoma is treated with a 3- to 4-week course of oral tetracycline (Achromycin) or erythromycin (E-Mycin, E.E.S.). Topical use of these same drugs may be added or used in place of systemic agents if the systemic drugs are unavailable or are not tolerated by the client.

Conjunctival scarring frequently results from trachoma. The scarring can close access to the lacrimal system, which alters the tear film. Corneal ulcerations and infections may result.

The critical focus for nursing interventions is the establishment or restoration of sanitary conditions. Control of the fly population should be encouraged. Water for cleaning faces and eyes should be heated before use. When discharge from the eye is present, hands must be washed before and after touching the eyes. If crusty drainage is a problem, the use of warm, moist compresses can be suggested. Families are advised to keep the washcloths of the client away from unaffected household members and to launder them separately. The client is advised to avoid entering crowded public areas.

Extraocular Muscle Disorders

As described in Chapter 35, eye movements are coordinated by six extraocular muscles. Coordinated eye movements enable the eyes to receive an image simultaneously, which results in the visualization of a single image. Problems with extraocular muscle function result in specific visual disturbances, such as strabismus (upward, downward, inward, or outward deviation of the eyes). In adults, the treatment of choice is surgical adjustment of specific extraocular muscles.

Corneal Disorders

OVERVIEW

The cornea is referred to as our "window to the world" because all visual stimuli must pass through its transparent avascular structure to be focused on the retina. As the first refracting surface of the eye, production of a sharp image on the retinal receptors requires the cornea to be transparent and intact. Covering the anterior one-sixth of the eye, it is in a particularly vulnerable location for injury or infection, and corneal disease is one of the leading causes of visual impairment in the United States.

Corneal tissue is complex, with each layer having its own properties, responsibilities, and characteristic pathologic conditions. The cornea is composed of five layers (Fig. 36–3). The *epithelium,* the most anterior layer of regenerating tissue, is continuous with the conjunctival epithelium. The eye can heal an epithelial injury without a scar. Approximately 70 nerve endings from the trigeminal nerve (fifth cranial nerve) innervate the epithelium (Boyd-Monk & Steinmetz, 1987). Any irritant or injury is rapidly noted by the nerve ends, and an im-

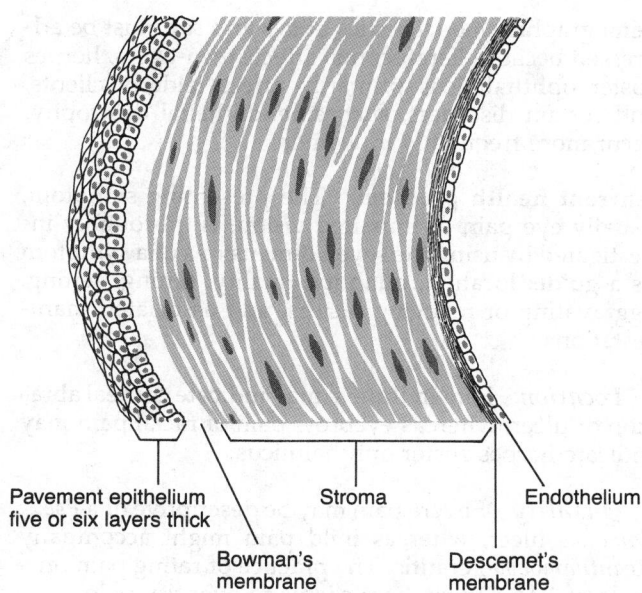

Figure 36 – 3

Anatomy of the cornea.

pulse is immediately forwarded to the brain, and a response is elicited such as eyelid closure or tearing. *Bowman's membrane* is composed of tightly packed, nonregenerating connective tissue fibers. It forms a protective barrier against trauma and microorganisms. Injury here results in scar development. The *stroma* is composed of many collagen fiber bundles. It accounts for 90% of corneal thickness. Injury here results in scarring. The appearance of the stroma is similar to that of ground glass. *Descemet's membrane* is a thin elastic membrane that is located on the inner surface of the stroma. It is normally not seen unless it is pathologically changed, resulting in folds or tears. The *endothelium* is a single layer of hexagon-shaped cells that keeps the cornea dehydrated through its pumping action. These cells are unable to regenerate. Any injury to or compromise of the intactness of this layer, such as from surgery or inflammation, causes a reduction in cell number. Reduced membrane efficiency is noted because the healthy cells must stretch out to cover the endothelium. This reduced efficiency limits the effectiveness of the pump, and water is allowed to enter the cornea.

Corneal transparency is due to the uniform anatomic structure of the layers, the absence of blood vessels, and the dehydrated state of the cornea. If water is allowed to enter the cornea, edema results and transparency is diminished.

Pathophysiology and Etiology

A variety of diseases and conditions change the structure and function of the cornea. The pathophysiology and etiology are addressed separately for each condition.

Keratoconus

Keratoconus is a degenerative disease that causes generalized thinning and forward protrusion of the cornea, which results in a cone-shaped appearance (Fig. 36 – 4). Linear scars occur at the base of the cone. Although the exact etiology is unknown, this disorder appears to be inherited as an autosomal recessive trait and is associated with the following diseases: Down's syndrome, aniridia, Marfan's syndrome, asthma, atopic dermatitis, and retinitis pigmentosa (Vaughan & Asbury, 1986).

Blurred vision is the only symptom and is related to the unstable progressive astigmatism that is caused by the altered corneal shape. This altered shape is evidenced by a distorted corneal light reflex. The onset of symptoms usually occurs in the teenage years, with progression noted as the person approaches age 30 years.

Dystrophies

Dystrophies are characterized by the abnormal deposition of substances, which cause changes in the corneal structure. These disorders usually affect both eyes. Dystrophies are classified as epithelial, stromal, or endothelial, depending on the anatomic location of the abnormal deposits.

The degree of visual impairment depends on the number and location of endothelial infiltrates, the degree and location of stromal opacities, and the presence or absence of bullae.

Keratitis

Keratitis is inflammation of the cornea. The inflammation may be caused by irritation or infection.

Exposure keratitis. This inflammation results from inadequate coverage of the cornea by the upper eyelid and is the most common form of irritation keratitis. It occurs most frequently in clients with exophthalmos (forward protrusion of the eye) and in clients who are unable to close the eyelid after a stroke or while comatose.

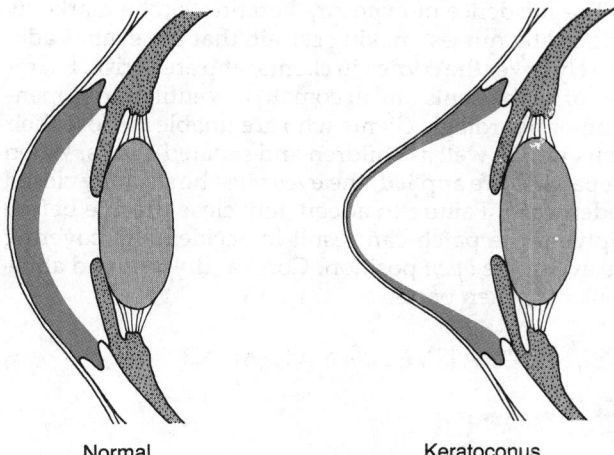

Normal   Keratoconus

Figure 36 – 4

Profiles of the normal eyeball and one with keratoconus.

Acanthamoeba **keratitis.** This inflammation is caused by ameba living in water, soil, and air. These organisms feed on bacteria and can be found in contaminated distilled water. This form of keratitis is seen with increasing frequency in clients who prepare their own saline solution from distilled water and salt tablets for use in cleaning, disinfecting, and storing contact lenses. It is unclear if the contamination occurs after the solution is prepared or if it is due to pre-existing contamination of the distilled water ("New Warning," 1988).

Corneal Ulcers

Any break in the normally intact corneal epithelium can provide an entrance for bacteria, viruses, and fungi. The integrity of the corneal epithelium can be destroyed by inflammation, corneal drying, and chemical or mechanical injury. An ulcer may involve the epithelium, stroma, or endothelium. If the lesion extends into the stroma or beyond, the healing process is slow and accompanied by scar formation. Common symptoms associated with corneal ulcers of any type include increased tearing, photophobia, and ocular irritation. Treatment varies according to the causative organism.

PREVENTION

Several corneal disorders are preventable. Prevention is achieved by reducing exposure to causative factors and by slowing the clinical course of the disorders. Several types of corneal ulcers can be reduced in severity or prevented. Clients are instructed to use protective eyewear when mowing the grass, doing yard work, or when cross-country skiing. A pair of glasses, sunglasses, or safety glasses can significantly reduce the exposed and vulnerable corneal surface area.

The use of corticosteroids should be limited to cases in which it is absolutely necessary. When corticosteroids are used, the client should be instructed to report signs and symptoms of infection to the physician immediately.

The incidence of exposure keratitis can be markedly reduced by nurses' making certain that the eyelids adequately cover the cornea in clients who are at risk. Examples of such clients are all comatose, ventilation-dependent, or neurologic clients who are unable to close their own eyes, as well as children and sedated adults. When eyepatches are applied, the eyes *must* be securely closed underneath. Failure to adequately close the eye before applying the patch can result in accidentally covering the eye in the *open* position. Corneal dryness and abrasions may then occur.

COLLABORATIVE MANAGEMENT

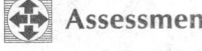 Assessment

History

Demographic data. When taking a history from a client with known or suspected corneal disease, the demographic characteristics of *age* and *sex* must be addressed because keratoconus affects teen-agers, herpes zoster ophthalmicus primarily affects elderly clients, and certain disorders, such as endothelial dystrophy, occur more frequently in women.

Current health problem. The presenting symptom, usually eye pain or impaired vision, is thoroughly investigated by using the seven dimensions of a symptom as a guide: location, quantity, quality, timing, setting, aggravating or relieving factors, and associated manifestations.

Location. Pain in the eye may indicate corneal abrasion or ulcer, whereas eyebrow pain or facial pain may indicate herpes zoster ophthalmicus.

Quantity. Severe pain may be descriptive of a *Pseudomonas* ulcer, whereas mild pain might accompany *Acanthamoeba* keratitis. The practice of rating pain on a scale of 1 to 10 may help clients to quantify pain.

Quality. The pain of herpes zoster ophthalmicus may be described as burning, whereas corneal ulcer pain may be described as a foreign body sensation.

Timing. The length of time from the onset of visual impairment to the present complaint may vary. *Pseudomonas* ulcers can cause impaired vision over several hours, whereas keratoconus may take much longer.

Setting. The location of the client when the symptom began is important. If the pain began on arising, a recurrent corneal erosion may be suspected. Special note should be made of recent travel to tropical environments or areas with poor sanitation.

Aggravating or relieving factors. If vision improves after contact lenses are removed for a few days, the lens care routine should be examined because the chemicals used for care may be causing corneal irritation.

Associated manifestations. Mucopurulent drainage accompanied by a foreign body sensation may be indications of a corneal ulcer.

Vision history. The nurse takes a thorough vision history. Any recent or remote eye surgery or injury is explored in detail. Recent or frequent changes in the client's prescription eyewear are noted. The client's visual environment, both work and home, is assessed for dryness and for the presence of irritants and chemicals.

Concurrent medical conditions. Concurrent medical conditions or their treatment may contribute to the development of or be associated with corneal dystrophies, keratoconus, or corneal ulcers.

Medication history. The nurse also requests the client to list current and past medications, including over-the-counter drugs. Information on the use of either prescription or over-the-counter eyedrops is specifically requested because the client may not consider eyedrops to be medication.

Physical Assessment: Clinical Manifestations

The client is usually diagnosed with a corneal disorder after presenting with complaints of *pain* or *reduced vision*. Visual acuity is frequently less than the client's normal level as measured with the Snellen chart. The nurse asks clients to describe their vision behaviorally by saying, "Tell me what your vision is like." Common descriptions include "It is as if I am looking through a dirty windshield" or "seeing the world through a foggy watch crystal." In all situations in which visual acuity is assessed, the nurse must keep in mind the client's normal acuity. For example, a visual acuity of 20/50 is not significantly deficient. However, an acuity of 20/50 is markedly reduced for a client whose baseline acuity is 20/20.

The nurse may observe the *photophobic* client's use of sunglasses and lack of comfort in a well-lighted room. The client may also be observed keeping both eyes closed. Closing the eyes decreases lid movement across the cornea and keeps light from reaching the cornea. For these clients, the examination should be completed under subdued lighting conditions.

Secretions from the eye are common. Cloudy fluid evidencing an infection may be present. Purulent discharge may be noted on the eyelids or eyelashes. A hypopyon may be evident in the anterior chamber.

The *cornea* may look hazy or cloudy. An altered corneal light reflex may be noted. The cornea may no longer be intact: patchy areas or scattered dot-like areas may be visible on examination. When fluorescein is used, these areas appear green.

Psychosocial Assessment

Clients with corneal disorders range in age from the adolescent with keratoconus to the older adult with corneal dystrophy. The nurse should therefore consider the client's level of maturational development during the psychosocial assessment. Although the altered corneal shape of keratoconus is not readily observable, the adolescent is quite concerned about his or her appearance, and the concept of body image may be significantly affected.

The client who is diagnosed with corneal disease usually has experienced a reduction in vision and grieves for this loss. If the vision loss is permanent, the grief may be more noticeable. If the vision loss is temporary, such as that occurring in epithelial dystrophies or from a superficial ulcer, anxiety about the possibility of not regaining perfect vision may be noted.

Corneal disorders and the associated reduction in vision may alter the client's ability to enter or practice the chosen vocation, and the client's self-esteem may be affected. Loss of role identity may also occur. The nurse

should assess how the reduced vision has affected the client's life style.

If vision is significantly reduced, the client may choose to limit activities in unfamiliar environments, such as a restaurant or theater, for fear of injury or of having others see a need for assistance. Clients often choose to remain in familiar environments where they are able to exercise a greater degree of independence. The nurse must carefully assess the client's feelings of preferred isolation because they may have a negative impact on the client's willingness to seek health care.

Laboratory Findings

There are no definitive tests to confirm the presence of corneal disease. However, several tests are done to determine which organism is causing a corneal ulcer, including tissue culture and corneal scrapings. For tissue culture, swabs from the ulcer and its margins are obtained and sent to the laboratory where the anaerobic and aerobic microorganisms will be identified. For corneal scrapings, the cornea is anesthetized with a topical agent such as tetracaine hydrochloride (Tetracaine, Pontocaine). A sterile spatula is used to remove samples from the center and edge of the ulcer. The specimen is sent to the laboratory for staining. Each microorganism has distinctive characteristics that are evident after staining.

Other Diagnostic Tests

Endothelial cell counts may be obtained. A picture is taken of the corneal endothelium. The ophthalmologist can then determine the number and size of endothelial cells. Endothelial cells are usually polygonal and number approximately 500,000. With disease, the number of cells may decrease, which causes the size of each cell to increase so that the spaces caused by cell loss are filled.

 Analysis: Nursing Diagnosis

Clients with corneal disorders are usually treated on an ambulatory basis. The most common disorders include corneal dystrophies and corneal ulcers. The adolescent to the geriatric client may be affected. The degree of visual impairment can fall anywhere on a continuum from not significant to reducing the client's self-care abilities. The following nursing diagnoses are possible.

Common Diagnoses

Several nursing diagnoses are common in clients with a corneal disorder. These include

1. Sensory/perceptual alterations (visual) related to reduced corneal transparency
2. Potential for injury related to difficulty in processing sensory information and in seeing environmental hazards
3. Pain related to irritation of corneal nerve endings

Additional Diagnoses

The following diagnoses may be appropriate for the client with a corneal disorder:

1. Anxiety related to potential of further visual impairment and possible failure to regain useful vision
2. Anticipatory grieving related to actual or potential loss of vision
3. Body image disturbance related to altered appearance of cornea
4. Ineffective individual coping related to temporary or permanent difficulty in maintaining familial and community roles
5. Social isolation related to fear of injury, reluctance to leave familiar environment, or fear of embarrassment
6. Knowledge deficit related to lack of previous information about treatment regimen
7. Powerlessness related to impact of vision loss on life style
8. Sleep pattern disturbance related to inability to rest because of the need for frequent use of eyedrops
9. Self-care deficit related to poor vision

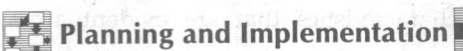

Planning and Implementation

The following care plan for the client with a corneal disorder focuses on the specific nursing diagnosis.

Sensory/Perceptual Alterations (Visual)

Planning: client goals. The two goals for this nursing diagnosis are that the client will (1) experience improved vision and (2) demonstrate maximal ability to use existing vision.

Interventions: nonsurgical management. The treatment regimen for the client with a corneal disorder is aimed at reducing symptoms, restoring corneal clarity, and enhancing the client's ability to use the remaining vision.

Drug therapy. The specific ocular pharmacologic agents used to treat corneal disorders have been previously described under the heading Pathophysiology. Antibiotics, antifungal agents, and antiviral drugs are prescribed to prevent replication of the microorganisms. Steroids may be used in selected cases of herpes zoster ophthalmicus to reduce the inflammatory response in the eye (Boyd-Monk & Steinmetz, 1987). The side effects of using a steroid, including the potential for fungal overgrowth, must be weighed against the benefits. Drugs can be administered topically as eyedrops, injected subconjunctivally, or administered intravenously. Intravenous administration of medications is reserved for severe corneal disorders. The nurse plays a pivotal role in the pharmacologic treatment plan. The following principles are used in eyedrop administration.

Because drugs are administered at frequent intervals,

timing of administration is critical. The corneal ulcer client is often given several broad-spectrum antibiotics. If each drug is administered every hour, separate dosage schedules should be created. For example, antibiotic A is given at 7:00, 8:00, 9:00, and 10:00. Then, antibiotic B is given at 7:30, 8:30, 9:30, and 10:30.

If two medications must be administered *at the same time, 5 minutes should separate their instillation.* For example, a client with glaucoma and a bacterial ulcer should receive timolol (Timoptic) at 7:00 and tobramycin (Tobrex) at 7:05.

If the same medication is required for both eyes and one is infected, *separate bottles of medication* are used and clearly labeled OS and OD.

Gloves are worn when ocular drainage is present.

Hand washing before and after administering eyedrops is necessary.

The client's compliance with a drug therapy plan is critical to its success at saving sight. The nurse explains the reason that each medication has been ordered and its name, dosage, and frequency of administration. A schedule of administration is established that best integrates the client's life style into the regimen. This consideration is especially critical if the client is managed on an outpatient basis.

Vision enhancement. The second role of the nurse is to assist clients in using their functional vision. If glare creates difficulties for clients, sunglasses and indirect lighting can be suggested. If clients are unable to continue to work in their current job, assistance should be obtained through the state bureau of vocational rehabilitation. Clients may find assistive devices such as magnifiers and special light fixtures helpful. These devices can be obtained through local offices of services for the visually impaired.

Interventions: surgical management. *Keratoplasty,* or corneal transplant, is the surgical removal of the client's diseased corneal tissue and replacement with tissue from a human donor cornea. It is performed to restore vision by removing corneal opacities or scars created by injury or infection, or to correct a corneal dystrophy. There are two approaches to performing a keratoplasty. In *lamellar keratoplasty,* or partial-thickness keratoplasty, the superficial cornea is removed and replaced with donor tissue. *Penetrating keratoplasty* involves removing the full thickness of the client's cornea and replacing it with donor tissue. Penetrating keratoplasty is the most frequently used procedure because it produces optimal visual clarity. The surgery (Fig. 36–5) consists of removing the center 7 to 8 mm of the client's diseased cornea with a round-edged knife called a *trephine.* Trephines work in the same manner as a cookie cutter. The same trephine is used to cut a button of tissue from the donor cornea. The donor corneal button, also called the *graft,* is positioned on the eye and sutured into place by using a running suture. The suture material is finer than a human hair. A single knot is located at the superior limbus where it is covered by the conjunctiva to make a water-tight closure. Figure 36–6 shows the actual ap-

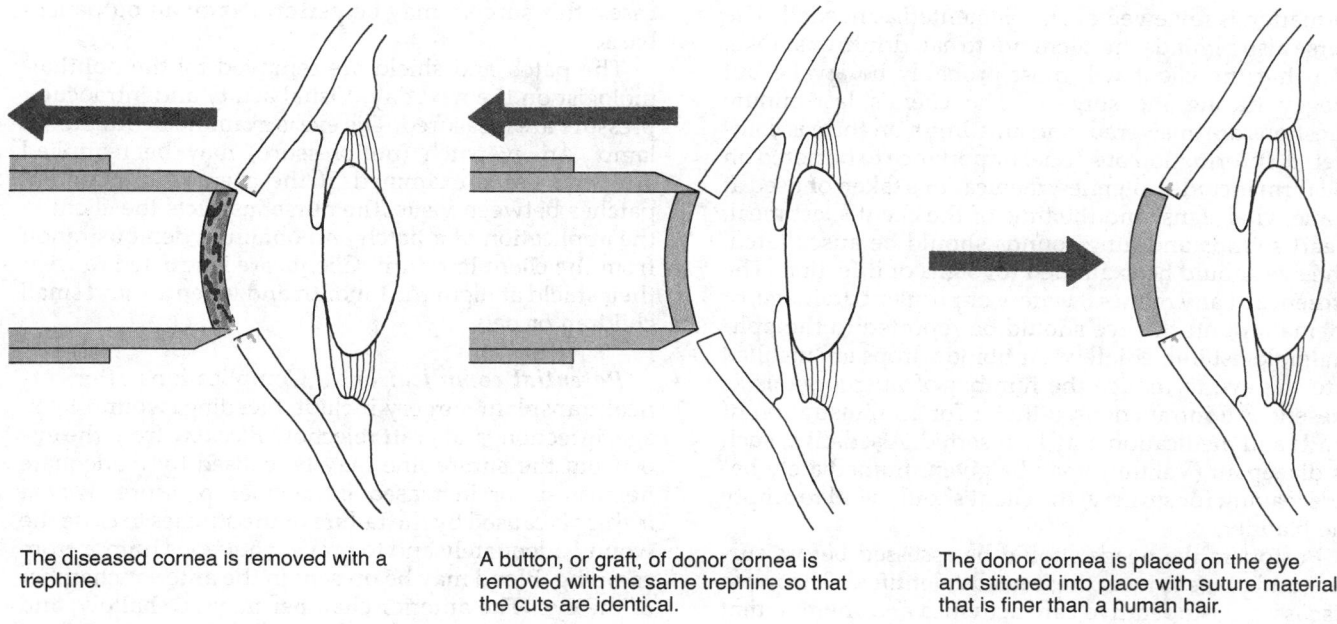

The diseased cornea is removed with a trephine.

A button, or graft, of donor cornea is removed with the same trephine so that the cuts are identical.

The donor cornea is placed on the eye and stitched into place with suture material that is finer than a human hair.

Figure 36-5

Steps involved in corneal transplantation (penetrating keratoplasty).

pearance of the eye with sutures in place after a corneal transplant.

Tissue for a keratoplasty is obtained from a local eye or tissue bank. An eye bank obtains its supply of corneal tissue from volunteer donors. These volunteer donors must be free from infectious disease at the time of their death and must meet the requirements set forth by the local chapter of the Eye Bank Association of America. Many states have implemented "required request" legislation that mandates health care professionals to ask the families of deceased hospitalized clients about their wishes regarding organ and tissue donation. All donors are checked for the presence of human immunodefi-

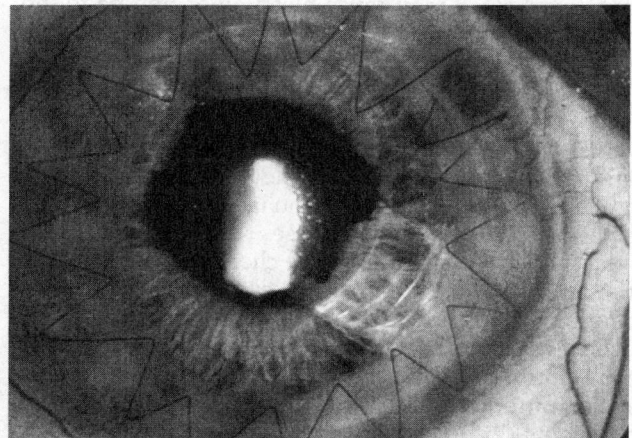

Figure 36-6

Appearance of eye with sutures in place after corneal transplant. (Courtesy of John A. Costin, MD.)

ciency virus. If the nurse believes a deceased client to be a potential eye donor, the following actions are implemented: Raise the head of the bed 30 degrees. Instill antibiotic eyedrops such as neosporin or tobramycin. Close the eyes and apply a small ice pack to the closed eyes. The eyes should be removed within 4 to 5 hours of death.

Keratoplasty is usually performed with the client under facial and retrobulbar anesthesia. The nerves around and behind the eye are numbed so that the client cannot move or see out of the eye. Because the client is awake, the importance of lying still must be reinforced. If the client will be unable to lie still for the procedure, general anesthesia can be used.

Penetrating keratoplasty can be performed together with other eye surgeries. During a *combined procedure,* a cataract extraction is done at the time of the corneal transplant. A *triple procedure* combines a cataract extraction with an intraocular lens implant and a corneal transplant.

Preoperative care. Currently, corneal transplants are not operations that can be scheduled in advance because the surgery must be performed when donor tissue becomes available. The recipient is told of the tissue availability several hours to 1 day before the surgery. On arrival at the health care facility, the client can be quite anxious. These feelings of anxiety can occur in response to the upcoming surgery, as well as in response to the rush to reach the facility. The nurse's calm approach in settling the client into the room is appreciated. After orienting the client to the surroundings, the nurse assesses the client's knowledge of the surgery to be performed, as well as pre- and postoperative routines. Information is reviewed or supplemented as needed. The nurse also reminds the client not to eat, drink, or smoke, and that the client will most probably be awake but groggy during the surgery. The client's last-minute questions are answered, and an admission form is completed. Information of special importance to be noted on the form includes allergies, medications taken or used at home, vital signs, and the time of the client's last meal. Heart sounds and lung sounds should be auscultated. The eye should be examined for signs of infection. The presence of any redness, watery or purulent drainage, or edema around the eye should be reported to the ophthalmologist immediately. Antibiotic drops are instilled into the eye to reduce the number of microorganisms present. An intravenous catheter for administration of fluids and medication may be inserted. A sedative, such as diazepam (Valium), may be given. Immediately before leaving for surgery, the client should void to empty the bladder.

Postoperative needs should be assessed before surgery and plans to meet these needs identified. The nurse discusses postoperative care activities and the role that the client will play in this care.

Postoperative care. After the corneal transplant is completed, a subconjunctival injection of an antibiotic is given and an antibiotic ointment is instilled. The eye is covered with a pressure patch (see Guidelines: How to Apply an Eyepatch) and a protective shield made of metal or plastic. This initial dressing is left in place until the next day. It is not removed or changed by the nurse without a specific order from the ophthalmologist. The pressure patch dressing is left intact to prevent the eye from opening under the patch, which would irritate the suture line. Preventing eyelid movement against the cornea also promotes healing of the epithelium.

On the client's return to the room, the nurse assesses *vital signs, level of consciousness,* and *dressing* immediately. The ophthalmologist should be notified of any significant changes in vital signs or of drainage on the dressing. Vital signs are taken every ½ hour for 2 hours.

The nursing diagnosis of sensory/perception alterations (visual) remains appropriate for the corneal transplant client during the immediate postoperative period. In this period, the client cannot see out of the affected eye because of the presence of the eyepatch and shield. Reorientation of the client to the environment remains important. Equipment, such as the telephone and call bell for the nurse, is placed within the client's sight and reach. Other sources of stimulation, such as quiet music and conversation, may give enjoyment and comfort to the client. Visitors are instructed to sit near the client's unaffected side because the client cannot see out of the affected eye and is discouraged from lying on the operative side. If vision in the fellow eye is poor, nurses and other persons should announce their entrance to and exit from the room, as well as their names and purpose of the visit.

Overnight is the usual length of stay in the hospital for the client having corneal transplant surgery. In some cases, this surgery may be performed on an outpatient basis.

The patch and shield are removed by the ophthalmologist on the next day. Visual acuity and intraocular pressure are measured. The eye is examined with the slit lamp. An eyepatch (nonpressure) may be reapplied after the eye is examined. If the client is to maintain patches between visits, the nurse instructs the client in the application of a patch and obtains a demonstration from the client in return. Clients are instructed to wear their shield at night for 1 month and when around small children or pets.

Potential complications. Complications after corneal transplant surgery include bleeding, wound leakage, infection, and graft rejection. *Bleeding* from the eye or from the suture line may be caused by inadequate hemostasis or increased intraocular pressure. *Wound leakage* is caused by the failure of the stitches to close the wound adequately and to prevent aqueous humor from escaping. Blood may be present in the anterior chamber of the eye. The anterior chamber may be shallow, and aqueous humor may also cause blanching of the conjunctival blood vessels nearby. As with any surgery, an entrance for microorganisms is created, and *infection* may result. The eye may become reddened, clear drainage may become purulent, and pain may increase. Although the cornea has no blood supply, *graft rejection* is still possible. The inflammatory process starts in the donor cornea near the graft margin and moves centrally (Newell, 1986). Vision is reduced significantly. The cornea becomes slightly cloudy. Treatment consists of the frequent topical use of corticosteroids (Newell, 1986). If the rejection process continues, the cornea becomes opaque and blood vessels may begin to branch into the opaque tissue.

Potential for Injury

Planning: client goals. The goal is that the client will not experience an injury while in the health care facility. Any injury or fall may cause bleeding or trauma to the eye and may negatively affect the outcome of the surgery.

Interventions: nonsurgical management. Postoperatively, the eye on which surgery has been performed is covered with a patch and shield, which renders the client sightless in that eye. Vision in the fellow eye may also be limited. The nurse assesses the functional status of the fellow eye and assists the client accordingly. Reorientation of the client to the environment remains important. Placing needed objects, including the nurse's call bell, within sight and reach is also important. Assistance is provided at mealtime, and orientation to the location of foods and utensils on the tray is provided so that clients do not poke themselves in the eye with a straw or a fork or burn themselves with hot liquids.

The nurse assesses the environment for any hazards. Beds are left in the low position. Any low pieces of furniture or footstools are removed. Wastebaskets are removed from areas through which the client is likely to walk.

Depth perception is altered postoperatively while the eyepatch is in place, which may affect the client's judgment of distance. The nurse advises the client to call for assistance before moving around the room. Protection must always be worn in front of an eye that has had a corneal transplant to prevent injury. During the day, glasses or sunglasses are an acceptable alternative to the shield. The shield must be applied and taped securely over the eye at night for approximately 1 month. This shield protects the eye from rubbing by the client during sleep and from the irritating edge of the bedclothes.

Pain

Planning: client goals.   The goal is that the client will report reduction or absence of pain ½ hour after the selected nursing intervention.

Interventions: nonsurgical management.   Preoperatively, comfort may be altered because of irritation of corneal nerves by the disease. After surgery, the presence of the incision may irritate the nerve endings. Because retrobulbar and topical anesthesia is used, the client may not perceive any pain for several hours. As the anesthesia wears off, the nerve endings in the tissue are stimulated, which causes perception of pain. The nurse carefully examines the client's complaints of pain. After eye surgery, pain is usually dull and achy and is relieved by oral analgesics such as acetaminophen with codeine. Severe pain or pain accompanied by nausea is an indicator of increased intraocular pressure and must be reported immediately to the ophthalmologist. The nurse elevates the head of the bed at least 30 degrees to reduce edema formation. A quiet, restful environment is encouraged, especially during complaints of pain. If the level of light bothers the client, shades are lowered and lighting is subdued.

■ Discharge Planning

Home Care Preparation

Preparing the home for the client's return after corneal transplant surgery may be difficult because of the short time frame between the client's notification that the procedure has been scheduled and entrance into the health care facility. If possible, the client should make the necessary environmental modifications when her or his name is placed on the waiting list for corneal tissue. Because the client is not permitted to bend over from the waist (this position increases intracranial pressure and intraocular pressure), objects in low cupboards should be moved to counter height. Feeding animals may pose a problem because the client is unable to bend over and fill the dish. To avoid this problem, these dishes are placed on a low chair, and the client reaches the dish by sitting down on a chair and reaching forward. Depth perception may be altered, so a piece of brightly colored tape can be placed at the edge of each step. Other important spots, such as the "off" position of electrical devices and stove burners, should be clearly marked.

Safety hazards in the home environment should also be examined. Loose throw rugs should be removed from the floors. Areas with poor lighting should have better light. Bathtub rails should be firmly attached.

The location of telephones in the home should be noted. At least one telephone should be at desk level so that if the client falls, the desk phone can be reached from the floor to summon help. A list of emergency numbers, including a friend or family member nearby, should be placed next to each phone.

If there will be no one at home to assist the client, a few meals should be prepared in advance and frozen. A supply of foods that are easy to prepare, such as canned soup or boxed dinners, may make the first few days at home more manageable. A program such as Meals on Wheels may be an alternative to cooking for the first few days after the client returns to the home environment.

Client/Family Education

The teaching plan for the client after corneal transplant surgery should address activities, administration of medications, detection of complications, and plans for follow-up care.

Activities.   Activities that are permitted after corneal transplant surgery include riding in a car, watching television or reading, light housekeeping such as doing dishes and meal preparation, walking, and climbing stairs. Care should be taken to avoid bending from the waist; rubbing, bumping, or scratching the eye; lifting more than 15 to 20 lb; yard work; or driving. The ophthalmologist discusses when these activities can be resumed. The nurse also reminds clients about the following self-care activities.

Shield application.   For the first month after surgery, the shield should be securely taped in place at bedtime or when clients are in the same area as small children or pets.

Eyelid care.   For the first few weeks after surgery, a thick, yellow-white, crusty drainage may be noted on the eyelids and eyelashes. This drainage, called *mattering,* is easily removed. Instruct clients to moisten a cotton ball with ophthalmic irrigation solution (Dacriose or Blinx), close the eyes, and then gently wipe across the eyelashes from the medial canthus to the lateral canthus. A new cotton ball is used for each wipe across the closed eyelid.

Vision check.   One of the early signs of graft rejection is a decrease in vision. Clients are instructed to check their vision daily, with the same object as a focal point. If vision is reduced or if previously clear objects appear to be out of focus, the ophthalmologist is notified immediately.

Administration of medications. Clients are usually told to use ophthalmic medications beginning on the first postoperative day, after removal of the eyepatch and shield by the ophthalmologist. Clients are usually placed on a medication regimen that includes an antibiotic such as gentamicin or tobramycin and a corticosteroid such as prednisolone acetate (Pred-Forte). Aseptic instillation of these drops is essential. Clients are taught the reasons for the use of these medications and their schedule of administration. Before clients leave the health care facility, their eyedrop instillation technique should be observed. Steps for instilling eyedrops should be reviewed as needed (see Guidelines: Procedure for Instillation of Ophthalmic Drops, in Chap. 35).

Detection of complications. The specific complications of corneal transplant surgery have already been addressed. Clients must be able to state signs and symptoms of these problems and the importance of immediately notifying the ophthalmologist should they occur.

Plans for follow-up care. The schedule of postoperative visits for the corneal transplant client is individualized. Clients are usually seen 1, 3, and 7 days after discharge from the health care facility. Further visits are planned on the basis of the client's condition at that time.

Psychosocial Preparation

Clients with corneal disease may experience frustration and depression associated with reduced vision. They may place a tremendous amount of hope in the surgery to restore their vision. The nurse helps clients to realize that clear sight may not be achieved immediately. The healing process after corneal transplantation may take up to a year. The client may compare this lengthy time for restored vision to the immediate return of sight that is associated with cataract surgery. Frequent reassurance as healing progresses is helpful.

Health Care Resources

If the client is reluctant or unable to return home immediately, alternative arrangements should be considered. A few days of staying with a friend or family member may be all the assistance that is needed.

A referral to a home care agency should be completed if the nurse questions the safety of the home environment or the client's ability to comply with the treatment regimen. The nurse communicates special needs of the client to this agency via the transfer form.

Financial concerns may be present. If the client indicates limited financial resources, a referral to the billing counselor should be made. Community agencies or civic organizations, such as the Lion's Club, may be of assistance.

The Ambassadors of Corneal Transplantation is a volunteer program of individuals who have had corneal transplant surgery. It is conducted through the Eye Bank Association of America. These volunteers speak to clients awaiting corneal transplant surgery who have questions or who desire to speak with someone who has also had the procedure.

Evaluation

The nurse evaluates the plan of care for the client with a corneal disorder on the basis of the nursing diagnoses. Progress toward the mutually identified goal is noted. The expected outcomes for the client with a corneal disorder include that the client

1. Demonstrates improved visual function
2. States that pain is reduced or alleviated
3. Removes environmental hazards and remains free from injury
4. Verbalizes fear regarding vision loss
5. Describes and complies with treatment regimen
6. Adapts life style to adjust to visual abilities

Scleral Disorders

The *sclera* is the white fibrous outer coat of the eye that is attached anteriorly to the cornea and posteriorly to the dural sheath of the optic nerve. It is approximately 1 mm thick, except at the insertion of the rectus muscles where it is 0.3 mm thick (Vaughan & Asbury, 1986). The sclera is covered by a thin layer of vascular elastic tissue called the *episclera*.

EPISCLERITIS

OVERVIEW

Episcleritis is a localized inflammation of the episclera, usually close to the corneal margin. The cause is not known, but hypersensitivity reactions may be a factor. It is a common finding in clients with rheumatoid arthritis, syphilis, herpes zoster, or tuberculosis. Episcleritis is unilateral in most cases and affects men and women equally.

Symptoms include ocular redness, pain, lacrimation, and photophobia. The eyeball appears pink or purple, with edema of the episclera and hyperemia of the episcleral vessels. Diagnosis is based on the clinical symptoms and ocular examination.

COLLABORATIVE MANAGEMENT

Episcleritis is usually self-limiting and disappears in 1 to 2 weeks. Topical corticosteroids, such as dexamethasone (Maxidex), may be used to reduce the inflammation (Vaughan & Asbury, 1986). When corticosteroids are used, the clinical course of episcleritis is shortened to 3 to 4 days. Recurrences of episcleritis are common. Episcleritis usually does not progress to scleritis.

If topical corticosteroid drops will be used, the client's ability to aseptically instill the drops into the conjunctival sac should be assessed by the nurse. Because corticosteroids may predispose the client to the development of a corneal ulcer, instructions must be given to report any ocular injury or abrasion to the ophthalmologist. Signs and symptoms of an infection, including increasing redness, photophobia, reduced visual acuity, foreign body sensation, and watery or pus-like drainage, must also be explained.

INTRAOCULAR DISORDERS

Lens Disorders

CATARACT

OVERVIEW

The crystalline lens is a biconvex, avascular, transparent, refractive elastic structure that is suspended behind the iris by zonule fibers that attach it to the ciliary body.

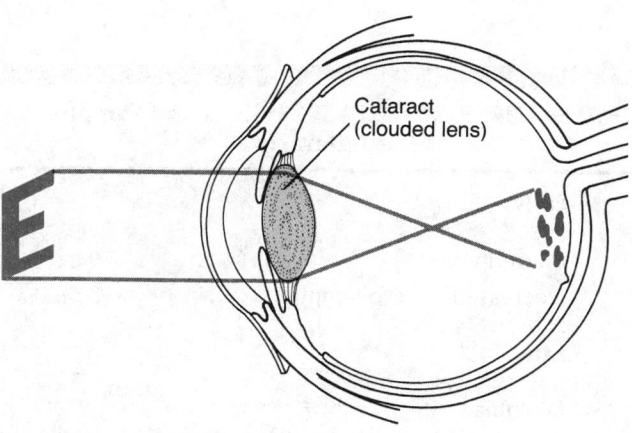

Figure 36–7

Visual impairment produced by the presence of a cataract.

The lens is transparent because its cells do not have nuclei, and its components have similar abilities to transmit light. A *cataract* is an opacity of the lens that distorts the image projected onto the retina (Fig. 36–7). Aging accounts for 95% of all cataracts, with the remaining 5% caused by congenital disorders, trauma, toxicity, or systemic disease (McCoy, 1981). The degree of disability that is created by the cataract is affected by the location and density of the opacification as well as the age, occupation, leisure pursuits, and living arrangements of the individual. Intervention is indicated when the visual acuity has been reduced to a level that the client finds to be unacceptable or adversely affecting life style. A visual acuity of 20/50 may be unacceptable to an architect or an anesthesiologist, yet not inconvenience a 75-year-old hospital volunteer.

Pathophysiology

The lens consists of 65% water, 35% protein, and a trace of minerals. With aging, the lens gradually loses water and increases in size and density. This increased density results from the central compression of older lens fibers. As new lens fibers are produced in the cortex, the older fibers are compressed toward the center. The lens comprises three separate areas. A *capsule*, or transparent envelope, surrounds the *cortex*, which is composed of putty-like material, and the centrally located *nucleus*. Opacities may develop in any part of the lens or its capsule. A cataract is formed as oxygen uptake is reduced (Vaughan & Asbury, 1986), water content is decreased, calcium content is increased, and soluble protein becomes insoluble (Newell, 1986). The compacting of lens fibers over time causes a progressive loss of transparency that is painless and frequently bilateral; however, the rate of progression in each eye is seldom similar.

Etiology

Cataracts are classified by nature or by timing of onset. They may be present at birth or develop at any time during the life cycle. Cataracts may be age related or may form as a result of trauma or exposure to toxic substances. In addition, the formation of cataracts is associated with specific diseases and other ocular disorders.

Age-Related Cataract

The most common cataract is the age-related cataract. The Framingham Eye Study noted that cataracts were present in 18% of persons ages 65 to 74 years and in 45.9% of persons 75 to 84 years of age (Kahn et al., 1977). Some degree of cataract formation is expected in anyone over age 70 years.

Traumatic Cataract

Any event that destroys the integrity of the lens capsule can cause a traumatic cataract to develop. Such trauma includes blunt or penetrating blows; the presence of intraocular foreign bodies; or overexposure to excessive heat, x-rays, or radioactive material. The time for development of traumatic cataracts can vary from hours to years.

Toxic Cataract

After ingestion of or exposure to certain chemicals or substances, toxic cataracts may develop. Extended use of corticosteroids, chlorpromazine (Thorazine), or miotic agents for the treatment of glaucoma has been implicated in formation of this type of cataract.

Associated Cataract

Systemic diseases such as diabetes mellitus, hypoparathyroidism, Down's syndrome, and atopic dermatitis can predispose an individual to developing a cataract. In diabetes, the excess glucose within the lens is chemically reduced to its alcohol, called L-sorbitol. The lens capsule is impermeable to the sugar alcohol and prevents it from leaving. In an effort to restore normal osmolarity, the lens takes in water (Newell, 1986).

Complicated Cataract

Cataracts may also develop as a result of ocular disorders. Intraocular diseases that are associated with the development of cataracts include retinitis pigmentosa, glaucoma, and retinal detachment. These cataracts are usually unilateral.

Incidence

It is estimated that 5 to 10 million individuals become visually impaired by cataracts every year (Newell, 1986). In the United States alone, 300,000 to 400,000 cataract extractions are performed annually. The highest incidence of cataract formation occurs in the elderly population.

PREVENTION

Because lens opacities often develop as a sequela of aging, there is no known effective prevention for the most frequently occurring form of cataracts. Use of safety precautions in the workplace may reduce the incidence of traumatic cataracts caused by radiation, heat, or x-ray exposure. The use of protective eyewear while mowing grass, clipping weeds and hedges, working with metal, or participating in sports can significantly decrease the incidence of traumatic cataracts by preventing the injury. Careful regulation of diabetes, hypo-

parathyroidism, and atopic dermatitis may reduce the incidence of cataracts associated with these systemic diseases.

COLLABORATIVE MANAGEMENT

 Assessment

History

When taking a history from a client with known or suspected cataracts, *age* is an important factor to note because this ocular disease is most common in elderly clients. The nurse also asks questions about the presence of other predisposing factors, which include *trauma* to the eye, both recent and in the past; *exposure* to radioactive materials or x-rays; the presence of *systemic disease* such as diabetes mellitus, hypoparathyroidism, Down's syndrome, or atopic dermatitis; *use of medications* such as corticosteroids, chlorpromazine, or miotic drugs; or the presence of *intraocular disease* such as recurrent uveitis.

The nurse asks clients to describe their vision in behavioral terms with open-ended questions. For example, the nurse might ask the client, "Tell me what you can see well and what you have difficulty seeing." Use of this technique helps the nurse know the impact of the visual deficit on the client.

Physical Assessment: Clinical Manifestations

Early symptoms of cataract development include slightly blurred vision and a decrease in color perception (see the accompanying Key Features of Disease). As the lens nucleus begins to yellow, it filters out the shorter-wavelength colors of blue, green, and purple. These colors are perceived as varying shades of gray. As lens opacification continues, clients complain of a decrease

---

KEY FEATURES OF DISEASE ■ Signs and Symptoms of Cataracts

Early

Blurred vision
Decreased color perception

Late

Diplopia
Reduced visual acuity progressing to blindness
Absence of red reflex
Presence of white pupil

in vision that adversely affects their performance of daily activities. Central lens opacities may divide the visual axis, which creates the optical defect of seeing two blurred images. When the lens nucleus is involved, the refractive ability of the eye (the ability to focus images on the retina) is improved. This ability, which is called *second sight*, may enable the client to read without glasses. The visual deterioration can progress to blindness if no surgical intervention is performed. *No pain or eye redness is associated with age-related cataract formation.* Hypermature cataracts can leak lens protein into the eyeball, which causes increased intraocular pressure and ocular redness.

Visual acuity can be tested by the use of *Snellen's chart* and *brightness acuity testing* (Chap. 35). It is important to evaluate acuity by using various lighting conditions because the different conditions will assist in determining the exact location of the cataract in the lens and the degree of visual disability that the client is experiencing. Visual acuity among clients with cataracts is significantly reduced.

The nurse can examine the lens with the direct ophthalmoscope. The diopter of the hand-held ophthalmoscope is turned to at least +15. Any observed densities are described by size, shape, and location. Cataracts are most easily observed after they reach the mature stage. As the cataract matures, the opacification makes visualization of the retina increasingly difficult. Eventually, fundus reflection is absent, as evidenced by the inability to elicit a red reflex. When this occurs, the pupil is white (Fig. 36–8). A white pupil is the most easily detected symptom of a cataract.

Psychosocial Assessment

The loss of eyesight is usually gradual, and the client may deny that the change has occurred until the loss significantly affects activities such as reading, meal preparation, walking, or driving. Fear of losing eyesight

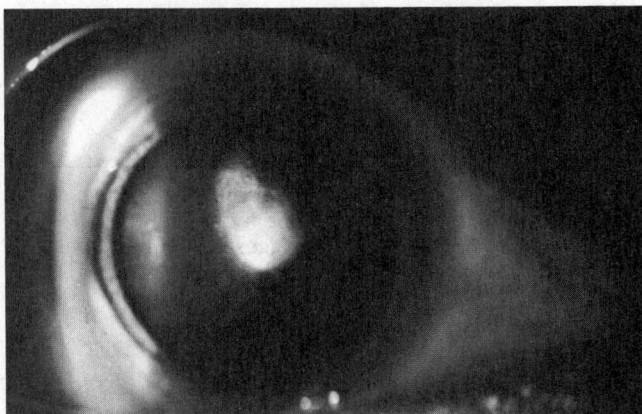

Figure 36–8

Appearance of the eye with a mature cataract. (Courtesy of John A. Costin, MD.)

can be frightening. There is often great anxiety when the client seeks an ocular evaluation. The nurse uses a calm approach and demonstrates an understanding of the fears that the client is experiencing when questioning a client about eyesight. All of the nurse's perceptions must be validated by the client.

 Analysis: Nursing Diagnosis

The client with cataracts is usually an elderly individual whose vision has deteriorated to the point that it adversely affects the client's normal activities of daily living and life style. The following nursing diagnoses are derived from the data that are compiled by the nurse.

Common Diagnoses

The most common diagnosis applicable to the client with a cataract is sensory/perceptual alterations (visual) related to ocular lens opacity.

Additional Diagnoses

In addition to the common diagnosis, the client may present with one or more of the following diagnoses:

1. Fear related to loss of eyesight, scheduled surgery, or inability to regain eyesight
2. Potential for injury related to decreased vision, age, or presence in an unfamiliar environment
3. Social isolation related to reduced visual acuity, fear of injury, decreased ability to navigate in the community, or fear of embarrassment
4. Self-care deficit related to visual impairment
5. Knowledge deficit (cataract pathophysiology and treatment) related to lack of information or misinterpretation of previously acquired information
6. Impaired home maintenance management related to age, limited vision, or activity restrictions imposed by surgery

 Planning and Implementation

Sensory/Perceptual Alterations (Visual)

The care for the client with a cataract focuses on the actual nursing diagnosis, as shown in the accompanying Client Care Plan.

Planning: client goals. The goal for this nursing diagnosis is that the client will possess improved ability to process visual stimuli.

Interventions: surgical management. Surgery and a variety of nursing interventions are necessary to facilitate the client's recovery of vision. The cataractous lens is removed by extracapsular extraction or intracapsular

CLIENT CARE PLAN ■ The Client with a Cataract

Goal/Outcome Criteria	Interventions	Rationales
Nursing Diagnosis 1: Sensory/Perceptual Alterations (Visual) Related to Ocular Lens Opacity		

Client will demonstrate improved ability to process visual stimuli and communicate visual limitations.
 	
■ Identifies factors that affect ocular function.
	1. Assess and document baseline visual acuity.
	2. Elicit functional description of what client can and cannot see.
	3. Adapt environment to client's visual needs.
	  a. Orient client to environment.
	  b. Place frequently used articles within client's view (call light, television control, water pitcher, tissues).
	  c. Provide amount of lighting that client finds most helpful.
	
	  d. Avoid glare.
	
	  e. Place articles in consistent locations.
	
	  f. Use materials with large print and high contrast (black print on off-white paper).
	  g. Avoid use of the colors blue, green, and purple in printed materials.
	
	  h. Use the "clock hour" system to orient client to the location of foods on the plate.
		1. To determine how well client sees.
		2. To provide baseline data on how accurate vision is and how it affects care.
		3. To enhance client's self-care, which decreases reliance on nurse.
		  a. To facilitate independent safe movement
		  b. To enhance independent action and promote safety.
		
		  c. To improve vision. Location of cataract will influence whether dim or bright light is better.
		  d. To prevent distress. Cataracts split light beams, which causes distress.
		  e. To reinforce use of memory as a replacement for seeing objects.
		  f. To facilitate reading.
		
		  g. To facilitate reading. Yellowing of the lens filters out these colors and causes them to appear as shades of gray.
		  h. To assist client in eating.

■ Identifies alternative sources of stimuli.	4. Assess amount and type of stimuli that are preferred by client. 5. Advise client of alternative forms of stimuli (radio, television, and conversation). 6. Provide source of stimuli as requested. 7. Refer client to services that provide aids such as talking books.	4–7. To promote stimulation. As vision becomes limited, some clients substitute other stimuli such as radio and television for reading.
Nursing Diagnosis 2: Potential for Injury (Fall) Related to Difficulty in Processing Visual Images and Altered Depth Perception		

Client will not experience injury or visual compromise resulting from fall.
■ Identifies reasons for increased potential for falls.
 	
■ Identifies and removes potential hazards from the environment.
■ Reports no falls.
	1. Advise client that covering an eye with a patch and/or shield causes monocular vision, which changes depth perception and narrows the visual field.
	2. Eliminate potential hazards from the client's environment.
	  a. Lock wheel of cart or bed.
	  b. Provide adequate lighting.
	  c. Get client out of bed with bed in the low position, and on client's unaffected side.
	  d. Keep side rails up.
	  e. Remove small or loose objects such as wastebaskets, tissues, or low stools from ambulation path.
		1. To promote compliance. The client may be more likely to integrate suggested interventions if the rationale is given.
		
		2. To prevent injury.

CLIENT CARE PLAN ■ The Client with a Cataract *continued*

Goal/Outcome Criteria	Interventions	Rationales
Nursing Diagnosis 2: Potential for Injury (Fall) Related to Difficulty in Processing Visual Images and Altered Depth Perception		
	f. Place articles such as call bell, tissues, phone, or television control within easy reach on client's nonaffected side. g. Encourage client to use bathroom rails if available. h. Monitor floor for spills and loose objects such as tissues and pencils.	
■ Avoids activities associated with increased potential for injury.	3. Teach client to change position slowly.	3. To prevent dizziness.
	4. Teach client to avoid reaching for objects for stability when ambulating.	4. To prevent falls related to altered depth perception. Objects may not be located where they are perceived. Excessive reaching alters the center of gravity, which can precipitate a fall.
	5. Encourage client to use adaptive equipment (cane, walker) for ambulation as needed.	5. To provide a source of stability.
	6. Advise client to go up and down steps one at a time.	6. To enhance the sense of balance.
■ Uses measures to reduce potential for injury.	7. Reinforce the importance of wearing an ocular shield when participating in high-risk activities such as ambulating at night and playing with small children or pets.	7. To prevent injury.
Nursing Diagnosis 3: Impaired Home Maintenance Management Related to Age, Limited Vision, or Activity Restrictions Imposed by Surgery		
Client will return home able to care safely for self in chosen environment.	1. Discuss client's desired location for postoperative recovery.	1. To promote recovery. Clients know best where they wish to recover.
	2. Discuss current ability of client to meet self-care needs and activities of daily living.	2. To determine needs for assistance, which will in part be based on current functional level.
	3. Evaluate how client's current functional ability will be affected by activity restrictions and postoperative care needs.	3. To determine client's awareness of limitations. Clients may not realize care requirements and how normal activities may need to be altered.
	4. Help client to decide on a realistic site for postoperative recovery.	4. To facilitate acceptance of plan. Clients should be involved in decision-making.
■ Develops a plan for self-care in the desired living arrangement.	5. Teach client required self-care activities: a. Personal care. b. Shield application. c. Eyedrop instillation. d. Activities permitted. e. Activity restrictions. f. Medications. g. Monitoring for complications.	5. To promote compliance. Clients must possess knowledge before they can implement a care regimen at home.
	6. Assist client to determine what activities will require assistance: a. Personal care. b. Meal preparation. c. Eyedrop instillation. d. Shopping.	6. To determine need for assistance. Clients have the best knowledge of what assistance they need.

continued

CLIENT CARE PLAN ■ The Client with a Cataract *continued*

Goal/Outcome Criteria	Interventions	Rationales
Nursing Diagnosis 3: Impaired Home Maintenance Management Related to Age, Limited Vision, or Activity Restrictions Imposed by Surgery		
	7. Evaluate sources of assistance: a. Friends/family. b. Home health care (skilled nursing care, home care aide).	7. To determine availability of assistance. Clients may need a variety of assistance—from shopping (because they are unable to drive) to assistance with use of eyedrops. Many clients require the aid of nonskilled personnel for housework and shopping. Skilled nursing time is usually spent teaching a neighbor how to administer eyedrops.
	8. Critique safety of home: a. Location of phone. b. Emergency plan. c. Presence of loose rugs or carpets.	8. To ensure that the client has a plan to deal with emergencies. Falls in this client population are common. Desk phones can be reached from the floor. Discussion of emergency plan may assist client to adjust to stressful environment.
	9. Adapt the home environment to facilitate adherence to activity restrictions: a. Place needed articles at counter height. b. Prepare meals in advance. c. Remove loose objects from floor.	9. To promote compliance. Nonadherence to activity restrictions can increase intraocular pressure and threaten visual acuity.

extraction. Figure 36–9 depicts surgical removal of the cataractous lens.

The procedure most commonly used is the *extracapsular cataract extraction.* During this extraction, performed with the use of a microscope in the operating room, the anterior portion of the capsule is ruptured and removed. The lens cortex and nucleus are then expressed or removed. Any remaining lens material is carefully removed from the eye. The posterior lens capsule is left inside the eye. The posterior capsule is left in place to prevent forward movement by the vitreous, to protect the retina from ultraviolet light, and to provide support for the intraocular lens implant.

In *intracapsular cataract extraction,* the lens is removed completely within the capsule. The advantage of this extraction is the ease with which the procedure is performed. Its major disadvantage is the removal of the protective posterior capsule, which places the eye at greater risk for retinal detachment and removes a supportive structure for the intraocular lens implant.

Preoperative care. Providing clients with accurate information that is needed so that they can make informed decisions about treatment is an important responsibility of the nurse.

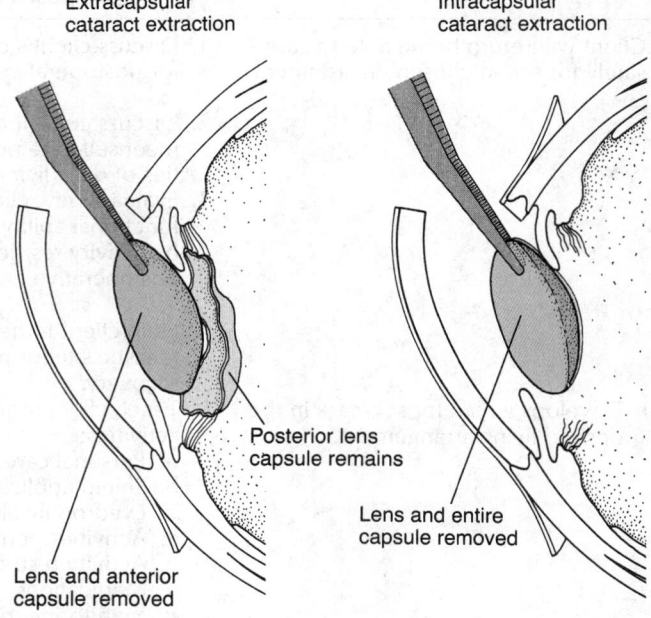

Figure 36–9

Surgical approaches to lens removal for cataracts.

A number of myths exist about the exact nature of cataracts and their formation. Common misconceptions include: a cataract is a film over the eye that must be stripped away; cataracts must be "ripe" before they can be removed; cataracts are a form of cancer; the eye is removed during surgery, then reinserted; and cataracts can be removed by the use of a laser. The nurse must know about these inaccurate pieces of data because the client may have heard them from friends or read them in nonscientific journals or magazines. The nurse presents factual information to the client and dispels myths.

The nurse teaches the client about the nature of cataracts, their progression, and their treatment. As with any instructional session, the nurse must assess what information the client seeks and the client's readiness to learn. Special attention is directed to how the information is communicated on the basis of the age of the client. Because auditory function frequently is reduced with aging and responses are slower, the nurse speaks in a normal tone, but slower, and sits facing the client. As short-term memory deficits occur with aging, the nurse provides written information for the client to read after leaving the health care facility. The nurse conducts the educational session in a quiet place, free from interruptions and background noise, because these can affect the elderly client's ability to process information. Once the environment is set for the education session, and the client has decided to undergo surgical intervention, the nurse may begin discussing the surgical experience that is planned for the client.

Preoperatively, the client may be filled with anxieties related to the possible loss of eyesight or the possible failure to regain eyesight after the surgery. The nurse needs to listen to the client and provide support while these concerns are expressed. While the client is in the health care facility, it is important for the nurse to assess how well the client's vision allows participation in daily living skills such as dressing, eating, and ambulating. For the client with reduced vision, the nurse provides orientation to the environment, explains the location of objects in the room, demonstrates the use of call systems, and discusses necessary safety precautions.

Once the client is settled in the room, the nurse discusses the events that will occur before surgery. Cataract surgery is usually performed by using local and retrobulbar anesthesia. An anesthesiologist is usually present to monitor the client's vital signs and administer any necessary medication. An intravenous infusion may be started in the client's room or in the operating room. Diazepam (Valium), given by mouth, is the usual preoperative sedative. Oral acetazolamide (Diamox) or methazolamide (Neptazane) may be given on the morning of surgery to reduce intraocular pressure. A series of sympathomimetic drugs, such as phenylephrine (Neo-Synephrine), are instilled preoperatively to achieve mydriasis and vasoconstriction. Parasympatholytic drops, such as tropicamide (Mydriacyl) or cyclopentolate hydrochloride (Cyclogyl), are also administered to induce paralysis and render the ciliary muscles unable to move the lens.

After drops have been administered and the client has voided, he or she is transported to the surgical area. Surgery is performed with the client under local anesthesia, which paralyzes the nerves around and behind the eye. The client may receive an intravenous injection of methohexital sodium (Brevital) to create a few minutes of light anesthesia during the administration of local anesthesia.

Rehabilitation options. The nurse discusses options for visual rehabilitation after cataract surgery with the client. This discussion must occur before surgery because most lens implantations occur at the time of the cataract extraction.

After removal of the lens by surgery, the eye is *aphakic* (without a lens). The eye has no accommodative power and has lost a great share of its refractive ability. A replacement lens is required to focus light rays in the retina. Aphakia must be corrected by use of eyeglasses, contact lenses, or an intraocular lens implant to attain clear, functional vision.

Eyeglasses. Called *aphakic spectacles,* this appliance for visual rehabilitation must be worn during waking hours for the rest of the client's life if this option is selected. This method of visual rehabilitation is the least expensive and safest one. Adjustment to cataract glasses can be difficult and frustrating and may take a period of several weeks. A disadvantage is that the thick, heavy "Coke bottle" glasses distort images by 25% to 33%, which causes vertical lines such as doorways and lampposts to look curved. Peripheral vision is lost because images must be viewed through the center of the lens to appear clear and in focus. This distortion can be particularly dangerous for unsteady clients because they may lose their balance, misjudge distances, and lose confidence in their ability to navigate. If only one eye has been operated on, the two eyes cannot be made to function together because the difference in the size of the image reaching the retina is great. The two images cannot be fused together into one by the brain, and diplopia, or double vision, results.

Contact lenses. The use of contact lenses is an alternative corrective method for aphakia. Lenses are available in hard, semisoft, and soft plastic materials. The chief advantage of contact lenses over eyeglasses is that image size with a contact lens is only 7% larger than normal so that images from both eyes can be fused into one image. The visual field is neither distorted nor constricted with a contact lens. Unfortunately, the manual dexterity required to insert and remove contact lenses does limit the type of client who can manage them without assistance. The development of extended wear contact lenses has greatly increased the availability and benefits of this option to the older adult. One disadvantage of this option is that it requires an adequate amount of tears be present, and tearing is reduced with age. Other disadvantages include the potential for corneal abrasions and infection of the eye, as well as expenses related to lens care products, insurance for lenses, and replacement lenses if lenses are lost.

Intraocular lens implants. At the time of surgery or at a later date, a small, clear, high-density plastic lens composed of polymethyl methacrylate can be implanted. The major advantages of an intraocular lens implant include the minimal (1% to 3%) distortion of the image produced, immediate return to binocular vision, and the perceived satisfaction of the client with the achieved visual acuity. Disadvantages include a 3% higher rate of complications than a cataract extraction without such an implant, as well as the possibility of rejection of the lens and the higher cost. McCoy (1981) identified the following indications for lens implantation:

1. Persons who are unable to manage removal, cleaning, and reinsertion of contact lenses
2. Presence of ocular conditions that contraindicate the wearing of contact lenses, such as dry eyes
3. Workplace, such as a dry or dusty environment, which makes wearing contact lenses impossible.

Postoperative care. Immediately after the surgery is completed, an antibiotic such as (gentamicin) is administered subconjunctivally, and an antibiotic plus steroid ointment (neomycin sulfate, polymyxin B sulfate, and dexamethasone [Maxitrol]) is instilled. The closed operated eye is covered with a patch and a protective shield. Clients are positioned on their backs in semi-Fowler's position or on the unoperated side. The nurse observes the dressing for any evidence of drainage. Any drainage visible on the eye pad must be reported to the surgeon immediately. Vital signs are taken and recorded per hospital policy. The ophthalmologist usually performs the first dressing change and examines the eye with a slit-lamp microscope the next day. In certain cases, ophthalmologists may request that the client be advised to remove the eyepatch and shield 6 to 8 hours after surgery and to begin using eyedrops. Steroid-antibiotic eyedrops (neomycin sulfate, polymyxin B sulfate, and dexamethasone) are instilled. As an alternative, separate antibiotic and steroid eyedrops may be ordered. Mild itching is normal and is caused by the small stitches that are used to close the incision. Cool compresses are usually of benefit.

Discomfort at the site is usually controlled by use of a mild analgesic such as acetaminophen (Tylenol). Aspirin is avoided for several days because of its effects on blood coagulation. The presence of pain may indicate a serious complication such as increased intraocular pressure or hemorrhage. If pain occurs, especially associated with nausea and vomiting, the client needs to be advised to contact the ophthalmologist.

After the dressing is removed, eye protection must be worn at all times. During the day, glasses or sunglasses may be worn instead of the protective shield. At night, the protective shield must be worn to guard against injury from the client's rubbing the eye or irritation from bed linens.

Prevention of complications. One of the major postoperative complications is an *increased, intraocular pressure.* To minimize intraocular pressure, the nurse needs to enforce some activity restrictions during the postoperative period and to teach these to the client and family. Activities that can cause a sudden rise in intraocular pressure include coughing, bending at the waist, vomiting, sneezing, lifting more than 15 lb, squeezing the eyelids, straining with bowel movements, and sleeping or lying on the operative side. Constipation, severe nausea, and cold symptoms should be treated with appropriate medications to avoid jeopardizing the healing process.

The second major complication is *infection.* The nurse observes the client for increasing redness of the eye, change in visual acuity, tearing, or photophobia. The presence of creamy white, dry, crusty drainage on the eyelids and lashes is normal. If the nurse observes yellow or green drainage, however, the opthalmologist is contacted.

Bleeding into the anterior chamber of the eye may also occur, usually several days after surgery. Blood may come from the incision, iris, or ciliary body. Causes of intraocular hemorrhage include defective wound healing, inadequate suturing, trauma (such as rubbing or bumping the eye), and increased intraocular pressure. Any change in vision should be reported to the ophthalmologist by the client.

After cataract surgery, the *posterior capsule may become cloudy.* Lens fibers adhere to the posterior capsule, light is prevented from reaching the retina, and vision is once again dim. This *secondary membrane,* or *secondary cataract,* must be altered for light to again reach the retina. A neodymium:yttrium-aluminum-garnet (Nd:YAG) laser is aimed at the cloudy membrane of the capsule, and a hole is burned in it. This "cold" laser treatment is successful in treating 90% of secondary cataracts. Surgical removal is an option for the rare failures.

Retinal detachments can also occur after cataract surgery (Jaffe, 1981). The incidence of this problem is higher for intracapsular cataract extraction, in which the posterior capsule is removed. With sharp, sudden movements by the client, the vitreous can move forward, pulling the retina away from its supportive structure. Symptoms include seeing dark spots, having an increase in the number of floaters, seeing bright flashes of light, or losing all or part of the visual field. Clients are instructed to report any of these symptoms to the ophthalmologist immediately.

■ Discharge Planning

The client undergoing cataract surgery is often discharged on the day of operation. Because of an early discharge, the nurse is essential in helping the client and family with plans for the return home. Discharge planning should begin at the time of the decision to proceed with surgery. Meals can be prepared ahead and frozen and groceries purchased in sufficient amounts so that the client will not need to make frequent trips to the store. Articles in low kitchen cupboards can be moved to the counter tops. If the client has difficulty in inserting eyedrops, a supportive neighbor, friend, or family member can be taught the procedure. Adaptive equipment that positions the bottle of eyedrops directly over the eye can also be purchased. When this system is used, the client merely opens the eye and squeezes the bottle. If the client has difficulty in holding the eyelids open, using the adaptive equipment may be problematic.

Home Care Preparation

Safety is a primary concern on the client's return to home. An eyeshield is worn at night on the operative eye for several weeks after surgery. If the client has a cataract in the opposite eye, vision may be severely reduced. The client needs to be well oriented to the home environment. Placement of furniture needs to be reviewed with the client, and pathways should be maintained free from clutter, throw rugs, or obstacles.

Client/Family Education

Signs and symptoms of complications after cataract surgery should be reviewed again with the client and family before the client's discharge. These signs include sharp, sudden pain; bleeding or increased discharge; lid swelling; decreased vision; and seeing flashes of light or floaters. The nurse instructs the client to wear a shield over the operative eye at night to prevent accidental injury to the eye during sleep. The procedure for instilling eyedrops is reviewed with the client or the person who will be performing this task after discharge. If the client is concerned that the drop may not reach the correct place, the nurse may instruct the client to refrigerate the eyedrops. Then, when the eyedrop falls into the conjunctival sac, a cool feeling is detected by the client. The nurse also checks with the pharmacist to make sure that the drops may be refrigerated.

The nurse also tells the client to avoid activities that might increase intraocular pressure, such as straining for a bowel movement; bending at the waist; and lifting heavy objects, pets, or grandchildren. If an intraocular lens implant was not performed, the nurse instructs the client about the proper use of cataract eyeglasses. The eyeglasses should first be used while the client is seated, until the client adjusts to the distortion that they cause. The client is instructed to look through the center of the corrective lenses and to turn the head, rather than only the eyes, when looking to the side. Clear vision is possible only through the center of the lens. Peripheral vision is poor because of distortions caused by the strong lenses. Family members can be taught to help the client practice eye-hand coordination. Walking and climbing steps should be practiced with assistance. Coordinated movements such as drinking from a cup or pouring liquids must be relearned because spatial perceptions are altered. Contact lenses are usually fitted 4 to 6 weeks after the eye has healed.

Hair washing may begin several days after surgery, if this can be performed with the head tilted back, such as in a beauty salon or barber shop. For the immediate postoperative period, the client should be advised to stand in the shower with the face held away from the shower head. Washing hair or standing in the shower in the usual manner would permit soap and water too near the eye. Allowing soap and water near the eye might cause irritation and predispose the client to infection. Cooking and light housekeeping are permitted, but vacuuming should be avoided for several weeks because of the forward flexion involved and the rapid, jerky movements required. Clients are advised to refrain from driving, operating machinery, and participating in certain sports such as golfing until given specific permission for these activities from the ophthalmologist.

Psychosocial Preparation

After cataract removal, the individual may experience anxieties during the adjustment to visual changes. Clients with intraocular implants regain vision immediately after surgery and adjust quite readily. However, individuals who are fitted with cataract eyeglasses experience great frustrations because altered spatial perception affects the performance of tasks of daily living. These individuals may refuse to go outside of the home because of difficulties in walking, crossing the street, or climbing stairs. As a result, social isolation and depression may occur.

Support by the nurse and assistance by family members in the adjustment after surgery are essential. Positive reinforcement and encouragement to be as independent as possible help the client to assume a more positive outlook about capabilities.

Health Care Resources

If the client lives alone and has no family or significant others, arrangements should be made for a home care nurse to assess the client and home situation. If the client is uncomfortable with being alone in the immediate postoperative period, arrangements can be made with a local nursing agency to place an aide or sitter in the home. In certain areas of the country, professional nursing care may be available in the home through a visiting nurse or home care agency. When possible, arrangements for postoperative home care should be made *before* the operation.

Instillation of eyedrops is necessary, and the client may be unable to perform this task independently. A friend, neighbor, or family member can be taught this technique. If assistance is required in the areas of personal care, a home care aide may be of benefit to the client.

 Evaluation

The nurse evaluates the care for the client with cataracts on the basis of the nursing diagnoses identified. The expected outcomes include that the client

1. Demonstrates improved vision
2. Recognizes signs and symptoms of complications after cataract removal

3. Instills eyedrops correctly
4. States activities to avoid that could increase intraocular pressure
5. Remains free from injury after cataract removal
6. Uses cataract eyeglasses as prescribed

Glaucoma

OVERVIEW

Glaucoma is a group of ocular diseases that are characterized by increased intraocular pressure. When the intraocular pressure is greater than the tissues can tolerate, damage occurs to the ganglion cells of the retina; optic nerve atrophy can also occur. If the condition is untreated, blindness may result. Glaucoma is the second most common cause of blindness in the United States (Epstein & Pavan-Langston, 1980). It is often referred to as a "thief in the night" because in its most common form, vision is lost gradually and painlessly, without the individual's awareness.

Pathophysiology

Glaucoma is basically a problem of increased intraocular pressure, which is a measure of fluid (aqueous humor) pressure. Chapter 35 describes the structures and mechanisms that are involved in the production, circulation, and reabsorption of aqueous humor. Normal intraocular pressure (10 to 21 mmHg) is maintained as long as there is a balance between production and outflow of aqueous humor. Intraocular pressure can be raised by an abnormally high resistance to outflow of aqueous fluid through the anterior chamber. It can also be increased by the excess production of aqueous humor. In glaucoma, aqueous humor builds up inside the eye, and the increased pressure compromises blood flow to the optic nerve and retina. The sensitive nerve tissue becomes ischemic and dies. Tissue damage usually starts in the periphery and moves in toward the fovea centralis. Left untreated, glaucoma results in blindness. The lost vision is evidenced as blind spots in the visual field. The degree of increased intraocular pressure that is capable of causing organic damage varies. Some individuals tolerate pressures that might rapidly blind another.

There are several causes and types of glaucoma. Glaucoma is classified as primary, secondary, or congenital.

Primary glaucoma is the most frequently occurring form of glaucoma, in which the structures that are involved in circulation and/or reabsorption of the aqueous humor undergo direct pathologic change. This type of glaucoma includes *open-angle glaucoma* and *angle-closure glaucoma*, which are differentiated according to the position of the iris with regard to the iridocorneal angle. Open-angle glaucoma is the most common form of primary glaucoma. It is usually bilateral and produces no symptoms in the early stages. This form of glaucoma occurs in people who have normal open chamber angles (the angle between the iris and cornea). There is a resistance to the outflow of aqueous humor through the chamber angle. The resistance may be in the trabecular meshwork, Schlemm's canal, or the aqueous veins. Because aqueous humor cannot leave the eye at the same rate as it is produced, the intraocular pressure gradually builds.

Angle-closure glaucoma, a much less common form, has a sudden onset and must be treated as an emergency. Other terms used to describe this form of glaucoma include *closed-angle glaucoma, narrow-angle glaucoma,* and *acute glaucoma*. The basic mechanisms that are involved in the pathophysiology of acute angle-closure glaucoma are a narrowed angle and an anteriorly displaced iris. Anterior displacement of the iris against the cornea narrows or closes the chamber angle, which obstructs the outflow of aqueous humor.

Secondary glaucoma results from ocular diseases that cause a narrowed angle or an increased volume of fluid within the eye. These diseases or conditions indirectly disrupt the activity of the structures involved in circulation and/or reabsorption of aqueous humor.

Congenital glaucoma results from the failure of mesodermal tissue to create a functioning trabecular meshwork. This condition is caused by inheritance of an autosomal recessive trait and is usually bilateral (Boyd-Monk & Steinmetz, 1987).

Etiology

Aging and heredity seem to be principal causes of adult open-angle glaucoma. Individuals older than age 40 years are at higher risk of developing glaucoma. Glaucoma is more common in individuals with family members who have been diagnosed as having glaucoma, as well as in clients with diabetes, hypertension, severe nearsightedness, retinal detachment, and central retinal vein occlusion (Boyd-Monk & Steinmetz, 1987). Degenerative changes occurring with aging have been found to reduce the rate of aqueous production. However, greater limitations on the effectiveness of the outflow channels are noted. Uveitis, iritis, neovascular disorders, trauma, tumors, degenerative diseases, and postsurgical procedures performed on the eye can cause secondary glaucoma.

Incidence

One to 2% of the U.S. population older than age 40 years, or more than 1 million people, have been diagnosed with increased intraocular pressure (Shields, 1987). As a result of glaucoma, 500,000 persons have visual impairment and 56,000 are legally blind (Vaughan & Asbury, 1986). Non-Caucasians have a higher incidence of glaucoma than Caucasians.

PREVENTION

Although many of the factors causing glaucoma cannot be prevented, early detection of glaucoma through routine tonometry is the best means of preventing permanent damage and vision loss. Several warning signs of glaucoma should be taught to all individuals older than age 40 years, especially those with a hereditary predisposition to development of the condition. These warning signs include occasional brow aching and seeing halos or colored rings around lights.

COLLABORATIVE MANAGEMENT

 Assessment

History

When taking a history from a client with known or suspected glaucoma, the nurse first considers the demographic data of *age* and *race*. Glaucoma occurs most frequently in clients older than age 40 years and in non-Caucasians. The nurse questions the individual about the presence of glaucoma, severe nearsightedness, or hypertension in other family members.

Although secondary glaucoma is less common, the nurse asks questions about previous or existing eye-related problems such as recent surgical procedures, trauma to the eye, or the presence of uveitis, tumors, or degenerative disease. Questions related to the use of antihistamines are also asked because these drugs dilate the pupils and may precipitate an attack of angle-closure glaucoma.

The nurse also asks questions about the presence of any visual disturbances, how long the visual disturbance has been present, when the last eye examination

occurred, and whether the client has had tonometry tests to measure intraocular pressure.

Primary open-angle glaucoma develops slowly and usually without symptoms. The gradual losses of visual field that are associated with this disease remain undetected because central vision remains unaffected. At times, foggy vision and diminished accommodation occur. The client may note a mild aching in the eyes or headaches and may require frequent changes in eyeglass prescriptions.

Late symptoms of glaucoma that occur after irreversible damage to optic nerve function include visual field losses, decreased visual acuity not correctable with glasses, and the appearance of halos around lights (see the accompanying Key Features of Disease).

Physical Assessment: Clinical Manifestations

Examination with an ophthalmoscope reveals *cupping and atrophy of the optic disk.* The disk becomes wider and deeper and takes on a white or gray color. If the nurse holds a finger over the covered eyeball, a crude estimation of increased intraocular pressure can be detected. The increased pressure creates a firmer globe, which is noted on palpation.

To determine the extent of *peripheral field losses,* visual fields are measured. A visual field examination maps the areas seen by the eye while it fixates on a central point. The test searches for *scotomas,* or blind spots. In chronic open-angle glaucoma, the visual fields initially show a small crescent-shaped defect that gradually progresses to a nasal and superior field defect. In acute angle-closure glaucoma, the visual fields can quickly become significantly decreased.

The *clinical manifestations* of acute angle-closure glaucoma are quite different from those of open-angle glaucoma. In the former, the onset of symptoms is acute, and the client complains of sudden, excruciating pain around the eyes that radiates over the sensory distribution of the fifth cranial nerve. A headache or brow ache may also be present. Nausea, vomiting, and abdominal discomfort are associated with the pain. Other symptoms may include seeing colored halos around lights and sudden blurred vision with decreased light perception. On examining the eyeball, the nurse may note that the sclera appears reddened and the cornea steamy. An ophthalmoscopic examination reveals a shallow anterior chamber, turbid aqueous humor, and a moderately dilated nonreactive pupil. Sclera of the affected eye is injected or reddened, with blood vessels radiating outward from the iris.

In the beginning, the individual may experience transitory attacks, usually after being in a darkened environment. These attacks may last only a few hours and recur at intervals of weeks or years before a full-blown prolonged attack of acute glaucoma occurs. Each acute attack reduces vision and the peripheral visual field. A typical attack is unilateral.

KEY FEATURES OF DISEASE ■ Signs and Symptoms of Glaucoma

Early

Increased intraocular pressure
Diminished accommodation

Late

Diminished visual fields (loss of peripheral vision)
Decreased visual acuity not correctable with glasses
Halos around lights
Headache or eye pain (acute closed-angle glaucoma)

In secondary glaucoma, the client frequently complains of increasing pain and other specific symptoms depending on the causative ocular disease. Symptoms of congenital glaucoma include photophobia, blepharospasm, and epiphora (excessive tearing). Other signs include large eyes and a large, cloudy cornea.

Psychosocial Assessment

Clients who perceive a threat to their vision or who experience loss of sight may be anxious. Some anxiety about vision loss is normal, and it may motivate clients to comply with treatment regimens. The nurse must be alert to the degree of anxiety demonstrated by the client. Severe anxiety may limit the client's ability to focus on necessary information. Clients who are quite anxious may experience a reduction in their ability to concentrate. When assessing client anxiety, the nurse observes the client's posture, gestures, and speech patterns. Anxious clients may speak rapidly, change topics frequently, and use repetitive gestures. They may experience difficulty in concentrating on a subject and frequently ask to have information repeated. The anxious client may misinterpret statements about the size, location, and presence of blind spots as indicating that total blindness will result. Careful and sensitive correction of misperceptions is necessary. When verbal or nonverbal symptoms of anxiety are observed, the nurse validates the observations with the client and discusses the anxieties and concerns.

Clients grieve for the vision that they have lost or believe that they may lose. Their process of coping may follow the stages of grieving for any loss and thus may include denial, anger, bargaining, depression, and acceptance (see Chap. 11). The nurse assesses the stage at which the client is currently functioning, as the client may move from one stage to another.

When assisting a client with glaucoma to deal with the disease, its symptoms, its treatment, and its complications, the nurse identifies what the client believes may happen, as well as how stressed or anxious the client is in response to the disease. It is helpful to discuss how the client has dealt with similar stressful events in the past, i.e., what coping strategies have been used and how effective these coping strategies have been.

Diagnostic Tests

Tonometry. Intraocular pressure, as measured by tonometry, is elevated in glaucoma. If an elevated reading is found, several readings are taken over a period of time and at various times of the day to determine a pattern. A discussion of the instruments that are commonly used to measure intraocular pressure is presented in Chapter 35. In open-angle glaucoma, the tonometry reading will be between 22 and 32 mmHg (a normal intraocular pressure reading is 10 to 21 mmHg). In angle-closure glaucoma, the tonometry reading may be 30 mmHg or higher.

Tonography. Another method that is used to diagnose glaucoma is tonography, which combines use of an electronic indentation tonometer with a recording device. The facility of outflow of aqueous humor from the eye is measured while a weight rests on the globe. The slope of the graph is significant. A flat tracing indicates interference with the rate of outflow, as in glaucoma. A steep downhill tracing indicates that drainage is adequate.

Gonioscopy. A special lens that eliminates the corneal curve is used in this technique to facilitate the examiner's view of the drainage angle in the anterior chamber of the eye. A direct view of the trabecular structure can be attained via this lens, along with a slit lamp. The entire 360-degree circumference of the iridocorneal angle is examined to provide vital information for diagnosis. The presence of adhesions, aberrant blood vessels, sites of previously undiagnosed trauma, and other data are noted as possible causes of secondary glaucoma.

 Analysis: Nursing Diagnosis

Common Diagnoses

The most frequently demonstrated common diagnosis for clients with glaucoma is sensory/perceptual alterations (visual) related to destruction of nerve fibers by increased intraocular pressure.

Additional Diagnosis

The following diagnoses may also be applicable to the glaucoma client:

1. Pain related to increased intraocular pressure
2. Noncompliance (with treatment regimen) related to side effects of medication, lack of motivation, difficulty in remembering treatment regimen, or financial implications
3. Knowledge deficit (about disease process, current clinical status, or treatment plan) related to lack of information and/or misperception of information previously acquired
4. Anxiety and fear related to actual or potential loss of eyesight or to perceived impact of chronic illness on life style
5. Potential for injury related to reduced peripheral vision
6. Self-care deficit related to visual deficits
7. Social isolation related to reduced peripheral vision, fear of injury, or negative response of society to visual handicap
8. Anticipatory grieving related to actual or anticipated loss of vision

Planning and Implementation

Sensory/Perceptual Alterations (Visual)

Planning: client goals.   The major goal for this nursing diagnosis is that the client will maintain existing vision.

Interventions: nonsurgical management.   Blindness from glaucoma can frequently be prevented by early detection, lifelong treatment, and a commitment to close monitoring and follow-up care. Glaucoma can be controlled, but no cure is available.

Drug therapy.   Drug therapy for glaucoma focuses on reducing intraocular pressure. Two mechanisms for reducing this pressure include (1) physically constricting the pupil so that the ciliary muscle is contracted, which allows better circulation of the aqueous humor to the site of absorption, and (2) inhibiting the production of aqueous humor.

Agents that enhance pupillary constriction.   Miotics, which constrict the pupil and contract the ciliary muscle, are the most commonly used drugs to treat glaucoma. Pilocarpine hydrochloride (Pilocar, Isopto-Carpine) is a frequently used miotic. In acute angle-closure glaucoma, the constriction of pupil size is also a desired effect as it stretches the iridocorneal angle and enhances aqueous outflow. Carbachol (Isopto Carbachol) may be used in addition to or may be substituted for pilocarpine. Echothiophate iodide (Phospholine Iodide) enhances the effect of acetylcholine on the iris and ciliary muscle, thus producing miosis and increasing outflow. It is occasionally used in combination with other agents for glaucoma, although potential side effects of this drug include retinal detachment and cataract formation. The nurse must remind the client that miotics may cause blurred vision for 1 to 2 hours after use and that adaptation to dark environments is difficult because of the pupillary constriction. Miotic eyedrops are frequently instilled three or four times a day. Recently, a gel form of pilocarpine hydrochloride (Pilocarpine HS Gel) has become available and is administered once a day, usually at night. Pilocarpine is also available as a thin, flexible, controlled-release wafer (Ocusert), which is placed on the palpebral conjunctiva of the lower eyelid. This form of medication delivers pilocarpine to the eye at a constant rate of 20 or 40 mg/day for a week. The timed-release forms of pilocarpine are of benefit to clients who do not have the dexterity to insert eyedrops.

Agents that inhibit formation of aqueous humor.   Timolol (Timoptic) is a nonspecific beta-adrenergic blocking agent. When used as eyedrops, it is thought to reduce aqueous humor production without pupil constriction. Advantages of using timolol over pilocarpine include the small amount needed to maintain normal intraocular pressure without fluctuations, a reduction in the undesirable effects of miosis, and an easier administration schedule because timolol is administered twice a day rather than three or four times a day. Other beta-block-

ing agents that are specific for beta-receptors are betaxotol (Betoptic) and levobunolol (Betagan).

Carbonic anhydrase inhibitors, such as acetazolamide (Diamox) and methazolamide (Neptazane), reduce production of aqueous humor to help maintain a lowered intraocular pressure. Side effects of numbness, tingling of the hands and feet, and nausea or malaise are common. Epinephrine, 0.5% to 2%, and dipivefrin hydrochloride (Propine) also lower aqueous humor production. Dipivefrin is a prodrug form of epinephrine. It is not active in its stored state, and it must be transformed in the eye before therapeutic activity can occur. This prodrug form is more easily absorbed, which makes it a more effective delivery system. However, these epinephrine-containing agents are not used in angle-closure glaucoma because of pupillary dilation caused by sympathomimetic action.

Osmotic agents may be administered systemically to the client with angle-closure glaucoma as part of the emergency treatment to reduce intraocular pressure. Oral glycerin (Osmoglyn) should be administered in lemon or lime juice, or over ice. The high osmolarity of these agents is used to draw fluid into the intravascular space, which lowers the intraocular pressure.

Nursing interventions during drug therapy. Interventions are directed at assisting the client to understand the need for, and comply with, a lifelong treatment plan because studies have shown the relationship between knowledge and compliance (Parkin et al., 1976). Information is provided to the client regarding the disease itself, suggested treatments, and possible complications of disease and/or treatment. Clients are told that vision loss is permanent but that further vision loss may be preventable if intraocular pressure is controlled. Because the administration of eyedrops is the major treatment strategy, the nurse must validate that the client knows how to properly administer eyedrops.

A second area that requires the nurse's attention is facilitating the client's compliance with the treatment plan. The drug treatment plan for glaucoma can be complex and involve unpleasant side effects. During the initial discussion and at each subsequent interaction, the nurse discusses the client's perception of the need for compliance. To facilitate compliance, the nurse teaches the client the reason for each medication, its name, dosage schedule, and side effects. The nurse should assist the client in integrating the treatment plan and medication schedule into the life style.

Glaucoma clients require frequent remotivation to adhere to the treatment plan. If vision loss has occurred, the client may wonder why the plan must continue. The nurse emphasizes the fact that the medications are a sight-saving mechanism, even though lost sight cannot be restored.

The nurse should also be alert to indications of noncompliance, such as the client's inability to state the name of the drugs, schedule of medications, or last administered dose, or a measure of an intraocular pressure greater than the client's normal value. On noting these indications, the nurse validates the suspected noncompliance with the client and discusses the factors contributing to noncompliance with the client, such as financial concerns, memory error or impairment, or side effects of medication. The nurse can assist the client to develop strategies for improving compliance, such as memory aids (e.g., calendars, notes, or calls from friends), a set schedule, and written instructions. If the cause of noncompliance is related to side effects of medications, the nurse can collaborate with the ophthalmologist to change the medication, if possible, or to minimize the side effects by administering the medication at times when the impact on the client's vision can be reduced, such as at bedtime.

Laser therapy. When a medical regimen for the open-angle glaucoma client has been ineffective at controlling intraocular pressure, laser therapy is indicated. A *laser trabeculoplasty* is performed with the client under local anesthesia to produce scars in the trabecular meshwork, which causes the meshwork fibers to tighten. This tightening of the fibers allows increased outflow of aqueous humor and thus a reduction in intraocular pressure. With this procedure, up to 85% of the clients have a significant decrease in intraocular pressure (Vaughan & Asbury, 1986). The effects of laser trabeculoplasty may fade over time, and pharmacologic treatment may need to be resumed.

Laser therapy is also indicated for the client with angle-closure glaucoma. The laser is used to create a hole in the periphery of the iris, which allows aqueous humor to flow from the posterior chamber to the anterior chamber and then into the trabecular meshwork.

Nursing interventions for this treatment plan include informing the client about the laser procedure, the expected sights and sounds that are commonly heard during use of the laser, and expected outcomes. The nurse reinforces information given to the client during the informed consent process. Clients are asked to arrange for someone to drive them home. Because laser procedures can sometimes cause an increase in intraocular pressure, clients must wait at the facility for at least 1 hour after the procedure to have the intraocular pressure re-evaluated. The client may be prescribed an ocular steroid such as prednisolone acetate (Polypred). Before going home, the client is instructed to report symptoms of headache that are unrelieved by acetaminophen or that are accompanied by nausea, brow pain, or a change in visual acuity. An appointment for follow-up care, usually in 1 to 3 days, is made.

Interventions: surgical management. When pharmacologic and laser therapy fails in open-angle glaucoma, or in selected cases of angle-closure glaucoma, surgical intervention is required. Most surgical procedures for glaucoma involve creation of a new route for aqueous humor to drain into an area where reabsorption into systemic circulation is possible. Such procedures include filtering procedure, fistulizing sclerectomy, peripheral iridectomy, and cyclodialysis.

If these procedures are not effective, cyclocryotherapy is performed. A cryoprobe is touched to the sclera overlying the ciliary body. Parts of the ciliary body are destroyed by the freezing effect of the probe. After parts of the ciliary body are destroyed, aqueous humor production is decreased.

Preoperative care. Before surgery, the nurse discusses the planned intervention thoroughly with the client. The client may be filled with great apprehension and fears about the upcoming eye surgery or about the sudden onset of symptoms (as in angle-closure glaucoma). Other areas of concern include possible complications such as postoperative infection, cataract formation, loss of vision, loss of the eye, and an unsuccessful outcome of surgery, which may not be able to lower intraocular pressure and prevent further vision loss. The nurse corrects any misinformation, such as "intraocular pressure is like blood pressure," "the eye is removed during surgery," or "the client will be able to see instruments approaching the eye during surgery." Listening in a supportive manner and providing accurate information may assist clients in controlling their anxiety.

After the client's anxiety or fear has been reduced to a level that allows the client to function, education regarding the surgical experience can begin. The nurse assesses how much information the client has about the surgery and reviews it as necessary. Glaucoma surgery is performed either in a hospital or on an outpatient basis. The average length of stay is several hours to several days. Medications to lower intraocular pressure will be administered topically (as eyedrops) or intravenously. Antibiotic eyedrops will also be instilled. Preoperative sedation with diazepam (Valium) is frequently ordered. Because glaucoma surgery can be performed with the client under local or general anesthesia, the client may or may not have to avoid food and fluids. One effect of the medication that is to lower intraocular pressure is diuresis, so the client should void immediately before going to the operating room.

Postoperative care. At the conclusion of the procedure, an antibiotic is administered subconjunctivally by the ophthalmologist. The eye is covered with a patch after an antibiotic-steroid ointment (neomycin sulfate, polymyxin B sulfate, and dexamethasone [Maxitrol]) is inserted. A protective shield is applied over the dressing.

On return to the room, the client can have the head of the bed raised to any height and can eat and ambulate after the effects of the preoperative sedation have worn off. Clients are instructed not to lie on the operative side.

The nurse assesses the condition of the dressing while taking care not to remove the shield. Any drainage on the dressing is reported to the physician at once. The original dressing should not be removed without a specific order. The nurse instructs the client to report symptoms of brow pain, severe eye pain, or nausea because these may indicate a change in intraocular pressure.

Discomfort in the eye is usually controlled by use of a

mild analgesic such as acetaminophen. Aspirin is avoided because of its effect on platelet function.

Prevention of complications. A major postoperative complication is a change in intraocular pressure. *Hypotony,* or low intraocular pressure, may occur if the bleb the end point of the newly created drainage channel is functioning too well, or if a leak exists in the wound closure. The anterior chamber may become shallow. The most serious complication of hypotony after glaucoma surgery is choroidal hemorrhage. If intraocular pressure is too low to maintain normal pressure relationships, fluid may enter the suprachoroid located between the choroid and the sclera. This movement may result in a choroidal detachment (Newell, 1986). The accumulation of fluid in this space may strain the many blood vessels that are located there (Gressel et al. 1984). Symptoms of choroidal hemorrhage include pain deep in the eye, with a definite onset (Hutchison, 1986), diaphoresis, or change in vital signs. Should any or all of these symptoms be demonstrated, the ophthalmologist is notified immediately.

If the surgical pathway becomes blocked and/or the angle become closed, *intraocular pressure may rise.* Symptoms of increased intraocular pressure include ocular pain, pain above the eyebrow, and nausea. To prevent an elevated intraocular pressure, the client should avoid bending from the waist, lifting heavy objects, straining while having a bowel movement, coughing, and vomiting.

Infection may also occur after glaucoma surgery. The nurse monitors the client's vital signs and instructs the client about the symptoms of infection. Infection must be prevented because it can ultimately cause the client to lose vision or to lose the eye itself.

Scar tissue may form over time and reduce the effectiveness of the new pathway. Topical steroids, such as prednisolone acetate (Poly-Pred) or prednisolone sodium phosphate (Inflamase), may be used because a side effect of steroid use is prolonged wound healing.

■ Discharge Planning

Discharge planning should occur at every visit to the ophthalmologist and should begin most intensely when the decision to operate is made.

Home Care Preparation

Because the client returns to the home rapidly after laser treatment or surgery, the nurse is essential in assisting the family and client develop a plan for home care. With adequate notice, the home environment can be made ready, with meals cooked ahead and objects placed in easily accessed areas. Should assistance with personal care or housekeeping be needed, appropriate referrals could be made before surgery.

The nurse assists the client who has had a laser procedure or surgery performed to develop a plan to deal with an emergency should one arise. Clients should be able to state who they would notify if they needed urgent assistance and how they would notify the person.

Client/Family Education

Signs and symptoms of complications should be reviewed with the client and family before the client leaves the health care facility. The client should be reminded to wear the ocular shield over the operated eye at night, and to wear protective eyewear during the day to prevent accidental injury.

The nurse should review all medications, including eyedrops, that the client will use at home. A demonstration of eyedrop instillation technique should be performed for the client and/or family as needed. In return, the client should demonstrate the technique before leaving the health care facility.

Plans for follow-up care should also be reviewed. The client should know the date and time of the follow-up appointment before leaving for home.

Psychosocial Preparation

Anxiety may continue to be experienced by the client. To many people, glaucoma is associated with blindness. Concerns may be expressed about how well the treatment regimen is maintaining the intraocular pressure at an acceptable level. Other concerns include grieving over lost sight or anticipating future vision loss. The nurse listens supportively and suggests ways in which clients can control their anxieties, such as speaking with a supportive person and complying with the treatment regimen.

Health Care Resources

Referrals to governmental and community agencies may reduce the client's anxiety by providing another source of information and may enable the client to interact with others experiencing similar problems. Such agencies include the Glaucoma Research Foundation, local sight centers, Centers for the Visually Handicapped, and other support groups.

If the diagnosis of noncompliance related to financial difficulties is identified, the nurse refers the client to local social services agencies or civic organizations. There are organizations that target the needs of the visually impaired as their service projects, such as the Lions Club.

Should the diagnoses of self-care deficit related to limited vision or sensory/perceptual alterations (visual) related to peripheral vision loss be identified, the client should be referred to the state bureau of visual rehabilitation and sight center for vocational counseling and low-vision assistive devices such as magnifiers.

 ## Evaluation

The nurse evaluates the plan of care for the glaucoma client on the basis of the identified nursing diagnoses.

The expected outcomes for this population include that the client

1. Maintains existing vision and does not experience further loss of vision
2. Realizes that vision loss from glaucoma is permanent
3. Complies with a mutually established therapeutic regimen
4. Instills eyedrops correctly and aseptically
5. Describes the importance of maintaining intraocular pressure at a safe level
6. Identifies activities that can raise intraocular pressure
7. Remains free from infection after glaucoma surgery

Ocular Chamber Disorders

The vitreous is the avascular gelatinous body that makes up the posterior two-thirds of the eye. Located between the lens and the retina, it provides the eye's shape. Any condition or disease that damages the transparency of the vitreous results in some degree of visual impairment.

VITREOUS HEMORRHAGE

OVERVIEW

Vitreous hemorrhage is defined as bleeding into the vitreous cavity. Vitreous hemorrhage may result from aging, concomitant diseases, or trauma. It may also occur spontaneously. As the client ages, the vitreous may spontaneously detach from the retina. If blood vessels are torn, bleeding into the vitreous may result. Diseases that alter the integrity of the retinal blood vessels, such as hypertensive retinopathy and proliferative diabetic retinopathy, may cause the blood vessels to leak into the vitreous. In diabetic retinopathy, fragile blood vessels rupture easily, which causes blood to be released into the vitreous. Trauma to adjacent vascularized structures by penetration, rupture, or contusion can cause bleeding into the vitreous. Spontaneous bleeding into the vitreous may also occur.

Symptoms of vitreous hemorrhage include a reduction in visual acuity, with the degree of reduction varying with the severity of the hemorrhage. A mild hemorrhage may cause the client to see a series of vitreous floaters. Moderate hemorrhage may be graphically described by the client as seeing "black streaks" or "tiny black dots." Severe hemorrhage may cause the client's visual acuity to be reduced to hand motion only (Vaughan & Asbury, 1986). Examination of the eye shows a noticeably reduced red reflex because light rays have difficulty in reaching the retina. The fundus is difficult to visualize with the indirect ophthalmoscope.

Ultrasonography may be used to determine the location and extent of the hemorrhage.

COLLABORATIVE MANAGEMENT

A vitreous hemorrhage may absorb slowly with no treatment. If the hemorrhage is still present several months later, a *vitrectomy*, surgical removal of the vitreous, is performed.

A thorough history, including occurrence of trauma, presence of disease, and time of onset of symptoms, should be elicited from the client. Baseline visual acuity should be assessed. The client will be noticeably concerned about the reduction in visual acuity. A supportive approach by the nurse can reduce the client's anxiety. Resolution of the hemorrhage may take time, and the client may become frustrated with the apparent lack of progress. Validating the client's frustration and noting the progress made are important functions of the nurse. Because vitreous hemorrhage may occur with systemic diseases of diabetes and hypertension, the client's blood pressure and blood glucose level should be reviewed.

Uveal Tract Disorders

The uveal tract is composed of three separate but interrelated parts, the iris, the ciliary body, and the choroid. All of these structures contribute to the ability of the eye to focus an image in the proper area of the retina. Chapter 35 discusses the functions of these various structures. Problems with any or all of these structures result in some degree of visual impairment. The most common problem associated with these structures is inflammation. Inflammatory diseases of the uveal tract are characterized by location and extent. They can be acute or chronic.

UVEITIS

OVERVIEW

Uveitis is a general term for inflammatory diseases of the uveal tract. One or more segments of the eye may be involved at any given time because a common blood supply nourishes these areas.

Anterior uveitis includes iritis, which is inflammation of the iris; iridocyclitis, which is inflammation of both the iris and the ciliary body; and cyclitis. The etiology of anterior uveitis is unknown but may be related to exposure to allergens, fungi, bacteria, viruses, or chemicals; anterior uveitis can also follow surgical or accidental trauma. Systemic diseases such as rheumatoid arthritis, ankylosing spondylitis, herpes simplex, and herpes zoster may predispose an individual to development of anterior uveitis.

Symptoms of anterior uveitis include moderate periorbital aching, tearing, blurred vision, and photophobia, which is due to the pain that accompanies contraction of the inflamed iris in bright lights. A small, irregular, nonreactive pupil is caused by the adhesions that form between the iris and the lens during inflammation. Engorgement of the episcleral vessels near the corneal-scleral limbus creates a purplish discoloration called *ciliary flush* (Boyd-Monk & Steinmetz, 1987). Fibrinous material or a hypopyon, which is an accumulation of purulent matter in the anterior chamber, may be noted in severe cases.

Posterior uveitis is the common term for retinitis, which is inflammation of the retina, and chorioretinitis, which is inflammation of both the choroid and the retina. Posterior uveitis is usually associated with infectious processes such as tuberculosis, syphilis, and toxoplasmosis. The onset of symptoms is slow and insidious. Visual impairment in the affected eye is the primary symptom. It results from the exudation of protein-rich fluid, fibrin, and cells into the vitreous cavity (Newell, 1986). The location and extent of visual impairment depend on the size and site of inflammation. The vision loss appears to be more severe than the amount of choroid or retina involved.

On examination, the pupil is seen to be small, nonreactive, and irregularly shaped because of the adhesions that bind the iris to the lens. Vitreous opacities composed of fibrin and inflammatory cells are seen as black dots against the red background of the fundus. Chorioretinal lesions are seen as grayish-yellow, defined patches on the retinal surface.

COLLABORATIVE MANAGEMENT

Treatment of anterior and posterior uveitis is largely symptomatic because the etiology is difficult to determine. The treatment plan includes putting the ciliary body to rest with a cycloplegic agent such as atropine. The pupil is dilated to prevent adhesions between the iris and the lens. Steroid drops, e.g., prednisolone acetate (Pred-Forte), are administered every hour to decrease the inflammatory response of the eye and to prevent adhesions of the iris to the cornea and lens. Ointments such as dexamethasone phosphate (Maxidex) are also used. Subconjunctival injections of steroids may be used in posterior uveitis or when topical steroids have been ineffective. If inflammation causes intraocular pressure to increase, the use of timolol (Timoptic) may be initiated. Treatment is also aimed at controlling the causative systemic disease. If the iritis is due to tuberculosis, appropriate drug therapy for the infection is instituted. Early syphilitic lesions respond well to antibiotics. Analgesics such as acetaminophen (Tylenol or Tylenol with Codeine) are ordered for pain. Antibiotics may be initiated for the client with posterior uveitis (Boyd-Monk & Steinmetz, 1987).

Any client who complains of reduced or blurred vision should be thoroughly questioned, and a baseline visual acuity should be measured before further evaluation of the eye. The client presenting with blurred vision or visual impairment may be anxious about the actual change and may fear that they may not regain useful vision. Careful and sensitive listening by the nurse to these concerns can allay much anxiety. Warm compresses may be used for complaints of ocular pain. Darkening the room and encouraging the client to wear sunglasses reduce the complaints of photophobia. Because vision will be blurred from the use of cycloplegic drops, the client should be advised not to drive or to operate machinery. Signs and symptoms of bacterial and fungal ulcers, for which steroid eyedrops have been prescribed, must be reviewed with the client. Eyedrop instillation by the client should be observed by the nurse before the client leaves the health care facility. Indications of increased intraocular pressure should be reviewed with the client.

The client may become irritable and restless because of sleep deprivation associated with frequent eyedrop administration. The nurse should facilitate the client's resting whenever possible.

Retinal Disorders

HYPERTENSIVE RETINOPATHY

OVERVIEW

More than 22 million Americans have hypertension, 50% of whom may be unaware that they have the disease. It affects Black persons with a greater frequency than it affects Caucasians and occurs in approximately 5% of the general population. In hypertensive disease, vascular changes occur in the eyes, kidney, brain, and heart.

Hypertensive retinopathy is classified by grades. With each increasing grade, progressive changes are noted in the retina. A direct relationship exists between arteriole narrowing and elevation of the diastolic blood pressure. In *grade I*, minimal narrowing of the arterioles occurs, and mild hypertension is noted. *Grade II* changes include localized and generalized arteriole narrowing. The arterioles take on a characteristic "copper wire" appearance. *Nicking*, or narrowing, of the vessel at arteriovenous crossings can be found. Blood pressure is higher and remains elevated. In *grade III*, areas of localized ischemia that are known as *soft exudates* or *cotton wool spots* develop, caused by occlusion of the arteriole. Hard yellow-white exudates are found around the macula and produce a macular scar. Small "dot and blot" and "flame-shaped" hemorrhages may be noted. The client may also complain of headaches and vertigo. With successful therapy, cotton wool spots and arteriole changes can be resolved (Vaughan & Asbury, 1986).

Grade IV changes include edema of the optic disk. In addition to the symptoms of the previous grades, headaches and visual disturbances can be described by the client. Left untreated, hypertensive retinopathy can produce serous retinal detachments.

COLLABORATIVE MANAGEMENT

Nursing interventions include monitoring the blood pressure of all clients. As a case finder, the nurse can alert clients to elevated blood pressure and can refer them for a thorough medical evaluation. The impact of weight, exercise, and sodium intake on blood pressure and, as a result, on hypertensive retinopathy cannot be stressed too frequently. Clients may require assistance from the nurse in modifying their life style to accommodate self-care activities of weight reduction, more exercise, and reduced sodium intake. The importance of adhering to any prescribed antihypertensive medication regimen and of reporting side effects should be discussed.

DIABETIC RETINOPATHY

OVERVIEW

Diabetic retinopathy refers to the vascular complications of diabetes that develop in the retina. It is a major cause of blindness and disability in the United States and is responsible for 10% of new cases of blindness per year (Boyd-Monk & Steinmetz, 1987). Diabetic retinopathy is the leading cause of vision loss in young adults (Boyd-Monk & Steinmetz, 1987). The longer the individual has diabetes, the greater the incidence and severity of retinopathy. Approximately 80% of individuals have some degree of diabetic retinopathy after a 15-year history of diabetes. A second factor influencing the severity of retinopathy is control of the blood glucose level. Good control of the blood glucose level in the years after diagnosis is believed to lessen the severity of the disease.

There are two classifications of diabetic retinopathy: background and proliferative. In *background diabetic retinopathy,* the supporting cells of retinal vessels die. The capillary walls of the retina thicken and allow fluid to leak through. As this fluid is absorbed, thick yellow-white deposits, called *hard exudates,* are formed. Outpouches in the walls of capillaries, called *microaneurysms,* are formed. These fragile capillaries bleed easily and cause intraretinal dot and blot and flame-shaped hemorrhages in the nerve fiber layer of the retina. Small soft infarcts (cotton wool spots) also occur in the nerve fiber layer. Macular edema results from fluid accumulating under the macula. Visual acuity is affected by reduction of the capillary blood supply to the retina or by macular edema.

Proliferative diabetic retinopathy is differentiated from background diabetic retinopathy by the development of a network of fragile new blood vessels that leak blood and protein into the surrounding tissue. These blood vessels are stimulated to develop by the hypoxic state of the retina that results from poor capillary perfusion of retinal tissues. Poor capillary perfusion causes retinal pallor. Hard and soft exudates continue to form. New blood vessels grow in the retina, encroach onto the iris, and grow into the posterior face of the vitreous. These vessels become fibrous over time. The vitreous contracts and pulls away from the retina, taking the new blood vessels along. The pulling force on the fragile vessels causes them to break and bleed into the vitreous. A retinal detachment can result.

COLLABORATIVE MANAGEMENT

Treatment of diabetic retinopathy depends on the degree of retinal involvement. The goal of background retinopathy treatment is to control the level of blood glucose early in the course of the disease. Reducing the retina's need for oxygen is the goal of proliferative retinopathy treatment. *Laser photocoagulation,* or *panretinal photocoagulation,* uses a laser beam of intense light focused on the retina, where it is absorbed by pigmented epithelial cells. The laser light is converted to heat, which coagulates retinal tissue. Oxygen requirements are decreased when laser burns are scattered across the peripheral retina. The decreased oxygen demand causes neovascularization to regress. Peripheral vision is decreased slightly by the photocoagulation, but central vision is not affected because great care is taken to avoid the macula.

A *vitrectomy* is performed if frequent bleeding occurs into the vitreous and the body is unable to reabsorb it, or if fibrin bands threaten to detach the retina. Fibrin bands within the vitreous are severed with a cutter and then flushed away. As blood and fibrin bands in the vitreous humor are removed, the volume is replaced continually with a balanced salt solution. Silicone oil or a gas such as sulfahexafluoride (SF6) can be used to hold the retina in place (Boyd-Monk & Steinmetz, 1987). Postoperatively, a pressure patch and an ocular shield are applied over the eye, and the care of the client is similar to that required after retinal detachment surgery. If silicone oil or a gas was used during the procedure, specific orders for positioning and activity will be noted. The goal of positioning is to promote the placement of the gas or oil in the desired location.

Nursing interventions include detection of diabetes and education and support of the client. The nurse may be performing a general physical examination and may identify background changes in the retina. The client should be referred for a medical work-up.

Also, the client needs to learn what diabetes is and how hyperglycemia can affect vision. Every effort should be made to develop a treatment plan, together with the client's internist, with which the client is able to comply.

The third area of nursing intervention is support for the client experiencing decreased vision. Macular edema creates an alteration in central vision that makes reading, writing, recognizing faces, and close work more difficult. As retinopathy progresses and rebleeding occurs, vision may become more compromised. The client may feel frustrated and may be forced to change occupations and/or give up important activities such as driving. The nurse's gentle, attentive listening approach will facilitate expression of a client's concerns. Changes in roles may develop, as the client may need to rely on others for help. The client may need assistance in dealing with these new stressors. A referral to the state bureau of vocational rehabilitation for job assistance and to the local services for the visually impaired for assistive devices such as magnifiers and high-intensity lighting is warranted.

MACULAR DEGENERATION

OVERVIEW

Macular degeneration involves deterioration of the macular portion of the retina. This degeneration can be atrophic (age related; also referred to as *dry degeneration*) or exudative (referred to as *wet*). Atrophic degeneration is characterized by sclerosing of retinal capillaries, which causes macular cells to become ischemic and necrotic. Central vision steadily declines with this type of degeneration, and clients describe the vision changes as "mild blurring and distortion." Exudative degeneration is characterized by a sudden decrease in vision in response to a serous detachment of pigment epithelium in the macular area. Blood vessels invade this injured area and cause fluid and blood to accumulate under the macula, which results in progressive distortion of vision.

COLLABORATIVE MANAGEMENT

Management of clients with exudative macular degeneration is geared toward halting the initiating process and identifying further changes in visual perception. Fluid and blood may resorb in a small percentage of clients with exudative degeneration. In addition, laser sealing of leaking blood vessels in or near the macula may also limit the extent of the disorder in some clients. Visual perception is monitored with an Amsler grid, a special sheet of graph paper with a dot in the center. Clients are asked to describe their perceptions of the straight lines on the grid while they stare at the dot in the center. New or increased distortions in the lines indicate continued degeneration.

The treatment of atrophic macular degeneration is geared toward assisting the client to maximize the use of the remaining vision. The associated loss of central vision may interfere with the client's ability to read, write, and drive a motor vehicle. The nurse assists the client

with suggestions of alternative strategies (such as use of books with large print and public transportation) and referrals to community organizations that provide a wide range of adaptive equipment.

RETINAL HOLES, TEARS, AND DETACHMENTS

OVERVIEW

The retina is responsible for receiving visual stimuli and converting the stimuli into a form that the brain can interpret. It covers the inner aspect of the posterior two-thirds of the eye. The retina is composed of many layers of neural tissue attached to a single layer of pigmented epithelial cells, which closely approximate Bruch's membrane. The neural layer, composed of photoreceptors, converts images into nerve impulses that are transmitted to the visual cortex of the brain. The retinal pigmented epithelium provides the background pink-orange color of the fundus. The retina itself is transparent.

Blood is supplied to the retina from two sources. The choriocapillaries supply the outer one-third of the retina, which includes photoreceptors, the fovea centralis, and the pigmented epithelium. Providing blood to the inner two-thirds of the retina is the central retinal artery.

Pathophysiology

A *retinal hole* is a break in the integrity of the peripheral sensory retina that is frequently associated with trauma or that occurs with aging. A *retinal tear* is a more jagged and irregularly shaped break in the retina that occurs as a result of traction on the retina. A *retinal detachment* is the separation of the sensory retina from the pigmented epithelium. The two layers are usually lightly held together (Boyd-Monk & Steinmetz, 1987). Separation of the layers creates a subretinal space. Fluid can accumulate in this "third space" and is referred to as subretinal fluid. Retinal detachments are classified by the nature of their development. *Rhegmatogenous detachments* occur after the development of a hole or tear in the retina that creates an opening for the vitreous to filter into the subretinal space. When sufficient fluid collects in this space, the retina detaches. *Traction detachments* are created when the retina is pulled away from the epithelium by bands of fibrous tissue in the vitreous. *Exudative detachments* are caused by fluid accumulation in the subretinal space as a result of an inflammatory process (such as uveitis), in association with a systemic disease (such as toxemia), or by ocular tumors (Boyd-Monk & Steinmetz, 1987). An exudative detachment is not characterized by a break in the retina. If the underlying problem can be resolved, the subretinal fluid is absorbed without intervention. However, if the fluid continues to accumulate, the sensory retina is separated from the pigmented epithelium.

Etiology

Rhegmatogenous detachments result from atrophic holes in the retina or from tears caused by a mechanical force. Traction detachments follow the contraction of vitreous fiber bands that pull the sensory retina away from the pigment epithelium. Exudative detachments occur as the result of fluid that has accumulated in the subretinal space that causes detachment of the retina from the pigmented epithelium.

Incidence

Rhegmatogenous detachments rarely occur in younger clients unless trauma is involved. The incidence of retinal detachment increases during the fourth decade of life and peaks during the fifth and sixth decades. Three factors are known to increase the potential for retinal detachments: aphakia, degeneration of the retina or vitreous, and myopia. Removal of the human lens (resulting in aphakia) can permit forward movement of the vitreous. In severe myopia, the anteroposterior length of the eye is enlarged. As the size of the posterior chamber increases, so does the force that can be exerted on the retina. Severe myopia is present in two-thirds of the clients who are diagnosed with a retinal detachment (Boyd-Monk & Steinmetz, 1987).

PREVENTION

Retinal detachments cannot be directly prevented. Efforts at decreasing their occurrence must be focused toward the particular etiology. Rhegmatogenous detachments that result from the mechanical force of trauma may be prevented by wearing protective eyewear during high-risk activities, such as participating in sports involving high-speed objects (e.g., tennis and racquetball) or working with high-speed equipment (e.g., saws, sanders, lawn mowers, and weed removers). The early treatment of retinal holes and tears can potentially prevent a retinal detachment. Traction detachments from proliferative retinopathy might be reduced by controlling the blood glucose level.

Symptoms of retinal detachments should be taught to all clients who are at high risk of developing this disorder. They should be instructed to inform the ophthalmologist immediately should symptoms occur. This notification may facilitate rapid detection and treatment and thus prevent an extension of the detachment.

COLLABORATIVE MANAGEMENT

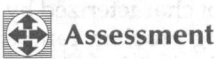 Assessment

History

The *risk factors* that are associated with retinal detachment—aphakia, increased age, vitreoretinal de-

generation, and myopia—should be kept in mind by the nurse during the assessment. Any client who complains of a sudden decrease in vision should be evaluated immediately. A description of the situation in which the client first noted the decreased vision is obtained. The client is requested to describe previous *ocular and medical history*. Any history of ocular surgery or injury is recorded. The nurse attempts to facilitate the client's description of symptoms by asking if the visual changes are noted in one or both eyes, the length of time since the onset of symptoms, the severity of symptoms, and if anything improves or worsens symptoms.

The onset of a retinal detachment is usually sudden and painless because no pain fibers are located in the retina (Smith & Nachazel, 1980). Clients frequently complain of suddenly seeing bright flashes of light or floating dark spots in front of the affected eye. These dark spots are caused by the breaking of capillaries, which releases red blood cells into the vitreous. These blood cells cast shadows on the retina, which are perceived as black spots. The flashes of light are related to the vitreous' pulling on the retina. During the initial phase of the detachment or if the detachment is partial, the client may describe the sensation of a curtain's being pulled over part of the visual field. The visual field loss corresponds to the area of detachment. The temporal retina is affected by detachments more frequently, so clients complain of defects in the nasal area of vision. Central vision defects are noted by the client if the macular area is involved.

Physical Assessment: Clinical Manifestations

To assess the entire retina adequately, the *pupil must be widely dilated.* Phenylephrine (Neo-Synephrine) and tropicamide (Mydriacyl) are used. The indirect ophthalmoscope, consisting of a hand-held magnifying lens and a head-mounted light source, is used to evaluate, diagram, and describe the presence of retinal holes, tears, and detachments. The fellow eye is also examined for these disorders. Detachments are seen as gray bulges or folds in the retina that quiver with movement. This appearance is in marked contrast to the flat pink-orange color of the choroid as it shows through the transparent retina. Depending on the cause of the detachment, a hole or tear may be seen at the edge of the detachment. A tear is usually shaped like an arrowhead or a horseshoe.

Psychosocial Assessment

The client who perceives a threat to vision, such as a sudden loss of sight, may be anxious. The nurse must be alert to the degree of anxiety of the client. Severe anxiety impairs the client's ability to process new information. Posture, gestures, and speech patterns of the client are noted. The anxious client may appear distracted, may change topics frequently, and may ask for information to be repeated. Anxious clients can also misinterpret information. They may hear only a portion of what is said and fill in the gaps later themselves. Careful and sensitive correction of misperceived information is necessary. Frustration may be noted in clients who previously have experienced traction detachment related to diabetic retinopathy or who have experienced a previous detachment of the retina. Diabetic clients may see this development as a further complication of the disease that greatly affects their life style.

Whenever the nurse assists the client through a stressful event, information must be obtained about how the client has previously dealt with similar experiences, including the client's coping strategies and the effectiveness of these strategies.

Diagnostic Tests

Indirect ophthalmoscopy involves a thorough evaluation of the retina, via a widely dilated pupil, that must be performed to detect, document, and diagram all holes, tears, and detachments of the retina. An indirect ophthalmoscope is composed of a hand-held magnifying lens and used in conjunction with a head-mounted light source. A scleral depressor is also used to facilitate examination of the retina. It flattens the retina and makes it easier for the ophthalmologist to review difficult and hidden places.

 Analysis: Nursing Diagnosis

Common Diagnoses

The most frequent nursing diagnoses for the client with a retinal hole, tear, or detachment are

1. Sensory/perceptual alterations (visual) related to impaired ability to process visual stimuli
2. Self-care deficit related to impaired mobility and activity restrictions

Additional Diagnoses

Other diagnoses that may be applicable to this client population include

1. Anxiety related to sudden loss of vision and potential failure to regain vision
2. Pain related to surgical manipulation of tissue
3. Knowledge deficit (pre- and postoperative self-care activities and routine) related to lack of information or misinterpretation of previously acquired information
4. Potential for infection related to surgical interruption of body surface integrity
5. Impaired physical mobility related to poor vision and presence in nonfamiliar environment
6. Potential for injury related to limited vision and altered depth perception

 Planning and Implementation

Sensory/Perceptual Alterations (Visual)

Planning: client goals. The goal is that the client will experience an increased ability to receive visual stimuli resulting in improved vision

Interventions: surgical management

Repair of retinal tears and holes. If a retinal hole or tear is discovered before it causes a detachment, the ophthalmologist may elect to seal the break. Closure prevents the accumulation of fluid under the retina, which reduces the likelihood of a detachment. The goal of treatment is to create an inflammatory response that will bind the retina and choroid together around the break. This inflammatory response can be created through cryotherapy, photocoagulation, or diathermy. In *cryotherapy*, a supercooled metal probe is placed on the conjunctiva over the area that corresponds to the retinal break. The freezing selectively destroys cells but leaves ocular structures intact. *Photocoagulation* involves focusing a laser light on the pigmented epithelium. The epithelium absorbs the light and converts it to heat. This method is used to seal holes and tears in the posterior portion of the eyeball. *Diathermy* involves the use of a high-frequency current. When applied to the sclera directly over the site of the break, the current causes a burn that creates a local inflammatory response, which results in the sealing of the retinal break (Vaughan & Asbury, 1986).

Repair of retinal detachments. Spontaneous reattachment of the retina is rare. Surgical repair is thus required to place the retina in contact with the underlying structures. One such repair procedure is the *scleral buckling procedure*. During a scleral buckling procedure, the ophthalmologist repairs wrinkles or folds in the retina so that the retina can again assume its normal smooth position. The sclera is flattened against the retina. To promote reattachment, a small piece of silicone is placed against the sclera and held in place by an encircling band. These devices keep the retina in contact with the choroid and sclera. Any subretinal fluid is drained.

To further encourage retinal reattachment, gases such as sulfahexafluoride (SF6) or silicone oil can be used. These agents have a specific gravity of less than that of the vitreous or air and can float up against the retina (Charles, 1987).

At the conclusion of the procedure, a subconjunctival injection of an antibiotic such as gentamicin is administered. An antibiotic-steroid ointment, neomycin, sulfate, polymyxin B sulfate and dexamethasone (Maxitrol), is instilled. As an alternative, separate antibiotic and steroid eyedrops can be used. A patch and metal shield are then applied to cover the eye.

Approximately 90% of retinal detachments can be successfully repaired with one operation. Should the retina fail to reattach, additional surgery may be required.

Preoperative care. Clients requiring retinal surgery are noticeably anxious. They have experienced a sudden and unexpected loss of vision. Fears of failure to regain useful vision may be voiced. Providing accurate information and the calm reassurance of the nurse will assist in allaying fears.

Activity restrictions may be involved and depend on the location and size of the retinal break. Unless the macula is threatened, bathroom privileges will be permitted. The client is positioned as ordered by the ophthalmologist. These restrictions are discussed later.

The nurse must assess the client's understanding of the planned surgery and needed preoperative activities. It is important to discern what the client knows and what information the client wishes to know. Certain clients may find information beneficial, whereas others may find the same information overwhelming.

An eyepatch may be placed over the affected eye to reduce eye movement. Topical medications are used to inhibit accommodation and constriction of the pupil. The pupil must be widely dilated to facilitate viewing of the retina during surgery. Commonly used agents include phenylephrine hydrochloride, tropicamide, and cyclopentolate hydrochloride (Cyclogyl).

Because the procedure is performed with the client under general anesthesia, food and fluid are withheld for a specified interval before the surgery. A mild sedative, diazepam (Valium), may be ordered preoperatively. Immediately before leaving for surgery, clients are asked if they have any last-minute questions and are assisted to the bathroom to void.

Postoperative care. After a scleral buckling procedure, the client's vital signs should be monitored in accordance with established hospital policy, usually every 15 to 30 minutes until they are stable. The eyepatch and shield should be evaluated for the presence of drainage. Any drainage noted on the dressing should be reported to the ophthalmologist immediately. The initial eyepatch and shield are not removed without a specific order. Activity status will vary. If gas was used to assist in promoting retinal reattachment, the client is positioned to allow the gas to float against the retina. These same activity restrictions may be ordered when silicone oil is used. Positioning the patient on the abdomen with the head turned to the operative eye is frequently ordered. The head is turned to the operative side, so the client lies with the unaffected eye down. This facedown position is maintained for several days, until the gas has been absorbed. As an alternative to this position, the client can sit on the side of the bed and place the head on a bedside stand. Bathroom privileges are allowed once the client is fully awake. Care should be taken to avoid placing the client in a position in which gas or oil can come into contact with the lens of the eye because cataracts can develop if this occurs (Hosein, 1988).

Nausea is a frequently occurring problem after retinal surgery. Food and fluids should be avoided until the client is fully awake without complaints of stomach upset. Antiemetics such as prochlorperazine (Compazine) should be administered as soon as the client complains of nausea because vomiting increases intraocular pressure.

The client may experience pain postoperatively. Analgesics such as meperidine (Demerol) or acetaminophen and codeine (Tylenol with Codeine) are usually administered. Nonpharmacologic interventions such as distraction and guided imagery may be of benefit. Any complaint of a sudden increase in pain or pain accompanied by nausea should be reported to the ophthalmologist because these may indicate the development of complications.

Activities that are known to increase intraocular pressure (e.g., sneezing, vomiting, bending over from the waist, and straining to move bowels) should be avoided. A laxative should be administered if necessary.

The eyepatch and shield are removed the day after surgery by the ophthalmologist to assess the status of the retinal breaks and the amount of subretinal fluid. Redness of the eye is common because of manipulation of the eye during surgery. Antibiotic-steroid eyedrops, such as neomycin sulfate, polymyxin B sulfate, and dexamethasone, are ordered to prevent infection and reduce irritation. Cycloplegic agents such as atropine are used to dilate the pupil and to rest the muscles that are used for accommodation. The client should be advised that vision will be blurred while these eyedrops are in use.

Activity restrictions in the first week after retinal detachment surgery include the avoidance of reading, writing, and performing close work such as needlepoint. These activities should be avoided because they cause rapid eye movements.

Complications

Increased intraocular pressure can result after retinal detachment surgery. The canal of Schlemm and the trabecular meshwork can become obstructed by cells and tissue particles that are a by-product of the inflammatory process. The use of silicone oil or gas can also affect intraocular pressure and cause it to rise. Symptoms of increased intraocular pressure—brow pain, eye pain, and nausea—should be reported immediately.

Failure of retinal reattachment or repeat detachment may follow retinal surgery. Symptoms include seeing bright flashes of light, dark spots in front of the eye, or a "curtain" in the visual field. The client should be able to detect these symptoms after the eyepatch and shield are removed and should be instructed to notify the nurse if they occur.

Infection can also occur because the integrity of the eye has been altered by surgery. The nurse should monitor the eye for the presence of increasing water or purulent drainage, or for a reduction in visual acuity. The client's temperature is also evaluated, and any elevation is reported.

Self-Care Deficit

Planning: client goals.   The goal is that the client will participate in self-care activities to the maximal degree permitted by visual and activity restrictions.

Interventions: nonsurgical management.   The degree of activity restriction depends on the size and location of the retinal hole, tear, or detachment. Clients with small holes or tears in the periphery of the retina that will be treated with the laser demonstrate no self-care deficit. In cases of retinal detachment, especially if the macula is threatened, severe restrictions on activity and eye movement will be imposed, which creates a potential for self-care deficit. Preoperatively, a patch is placed over the eye to reduce eye movement. In rare cases, bilateral eye patches are applied to further restrict eye movement.

When significant activity restrictions are necessary, a deficit in self-care ability can result. The client for whom gas is used to enhance retinal reattachment must maintain a face-down position for several days until the gas bubble is absorbed. Lying prone in bed is one way to achieve the face-down position. The nurse must creatively identify how to assist clients to care for themselves.

As long as the face must be held in the down position, the client can sit on the side of the bed, and the client's head can be positioned on an overbed table supported by pillows. Care must be taken because these tables do not lock. It is possible for the client to misjudge distances and fall over, causing injury. At mealtime, plates can be placed on the client's lap. Activities of daily living can be difficult to perform from these positions. It is helpful to encourage the client to order foods eaten with fingers such as fried chicken and sandwiches. If visual acuity is poor in the fellow eye, the client may need assistance in setting up the tray for eating. It is helpful to describe the type of food and to use the hours of a clock to describe the location of the food on the plate. To wash, the client can lie on the edge of the bed and a basin of water be placed on a chair nearby.

When one eye is covered with a patch, binocular vision and depth perception are altered. Clients must be advised to exercise caution when using sharp or pointed objects such as knives or drinking straws. It is easy to injure the eye with a drinking straw because with altered depth vision objects can be closer than they appear to be.

■ Discharge Planning

Discharge planning should begin at the time that the client is informed of the need for surgery. The short time from diagnosis to surgery does not permit a great deal of advance preparation for discharge. Retinal detachment surgery and the scleral buckling procedure are usually performed on a semiurgent basis to prevent further detachment. If the macula is threatened, surgery is performed as soon as possible.

Home Care Preparation

Clients having the scleral buckling procedure have an average length of stay in the hospital of between 2 and 4 days. While the client is hospitalized, the home environment can be made ready by family or neighbors, with meals prepared ahead and objects placed in easily accessed areas. The home environment should be examined for potential hazards to safety, such as loose throw rugs, long electrical cords, and small, quietly moving pets. These hazards should be removed because a fall could potentially cause another retinal detachment. If the client will require assistance with personal care or housekeeping, a referral to a home care agency can be made.

As the time approaches for the client's discharge, the nurse should provide assistance in developing a plan for dealing with emergencies. The client should be able to state the names of several people to contact in the event of an emergency or if assistance is needed on an urgent basis, as well as how to contact these individuals. The likelihood of needing to activate this plan is small; however, the client must be prepared.

Client/Family Education

Signs and symptoms of complications should be explained to the client and family before the client leaves the health care facility, as well as whom to notify should any of these complications be noted. Self-care activities should be reviewed. The client should be reminded to wear the shield over the eye at night and to use protective eyewear during the day to prevent accidental injury.

The nurse should review the discharge medication regimen with the client and family. The name, purpose, dose, and frequency of administration for each medication should be explained. Written sets of instructions should be provided to the client and family members. It is helpful to provide the family with a copy because many clients turn to the family for answers to questions.

Plans for follow-up care should also be reviewed. The first follow-up appointment should be made for the client before discharge from the health care facility.

Psychosocial Preparation

The return of complete vision after retinal detachment surgery is not immediate. Return of vision is related to the length of time between detachment of the retina and reattachment surgery. If the nerve fiber layer remains detached from its blood supply, it degenerates. Vision improves over days to weeks after the surgery. Clients sometimes expect to have 100% improvement when the patch and shield are removed the day after surgery. They need to be reassured that vision will continue to improve as the subretinal fluid is absorbed.

Health Care Resources

Referrals to outside agencies can facilitate a smooth transition to the home for the client. If assistance is needed in the client's home, a home care agency should be contacted and a referral initiated. If a client refuses assistance in the home and the nurse is concerned about the client's safety, Adult Protective Services should be contacted.

 Evaluation

The nurse evaluates the plan of care for the client receiving treatment for a retinal hole, tear, or detachment on the basis of the identified nursing diagnoses. The expected outcomes for this population include that the client

1. Experiences no further vision loss and recovers lost visual function
2. Cares for self to the extent permitted by visual limitations
3. Ambulates safely without falls or injury
4. Discusses feelings of anxiety
5. Possesses adequate information to make informed decisions about, and participate in, own care
6. States that an acceptable level of comfort is present
7. Demonstrates no sign of infection

REFRACTIVE ERRORS

OVERVIEW

The optical ability of the eye is similar to the workings of a camera. Just as the camera lens focuses images on the film, the lens system of the eye focuses light rays onto the retina. Camera film is similar to the retina because images are projected onto each.

The ability of the eye to focus images on the retina depends on the anteroposterior diameter of the eye and the refractive power of the lens system. *Refraction* is defined as the bending of light rays. Problems in either of these areas can result in refractive errors.

Myopia

Myopia is also referred to as *nearsightedness*. The refractive ability of the eye is too strong for the anteroposterior length. Images are bent in such a way that they fall in front of and not on the retina.

Hyperopia

Hyperopia is also called *hypermetropia* or *farsightedness*. The refractive ability of the eye is too weak, causing images to be focused behind the retina. A shorter anteroposterior diameter of the eye may contribute to the development of hyperopia.

Presbyopia

As individuals age, the crystalline lens loses its elasticity and is less able to alter its shape to focus the eye for close work. As a result, images fall behind the retina. This loss of close work ability is usually noticed in the fourth decade of life.

Astigmatism

Astigmatism occurs when the curvature of the cornea is greater in one place than another. Light rays are not refracted equally in all directions, so a focus point on the retina cannot be achieved.

Aphakia

Aphakia is defined as the absence of the crystalline lens. It exists after removal of a cataractous or a dislocated lens. Without the focusing ability of the lens, images fall behind the retina.

COLLABORATIVE MANAGEMENT

Diagnosis. Refractive errors are diagnosed through a process known as *refraction*. The client is asked to view an eye chart while lenses of different strengths are systematically placed in front of the eye. The client is asked if the lenses sharpen or worsen vision. These lenses either are placed in a trial frame or are located in a machine called a Phoropter. The Phoropter is an instrument containing a series of lenses that can be dialed into the client's view while he or she looks through the openings at an eye chart. The power or strength of the lens necessary to permit focusing of the image on the retina is expressed in measurements called *diopters*. Cyclopentolate hydrochloride eyedrops may be administered to paralyze the focusing ability of the eye. Examining the eye with the muscles at rest permits a more definitive measurement of refractive error.

Interventions: nonsurgical management. Errors of refraction must be corrected to permit light rays to be focused on the retina. This correction is achieved through the use of a lens. In myopia, vision is corrected to bring the image forward onto the retina with a concave lens. Hyperopic vision is corrected with convex lenses to move the focused image back to the retina. Hyperopic correction is also used to treat presbyopia and is usually "added" to the client's distance vision lenses. If the client does not require distance correction, half glasses or "readers" that contain the presbyopia correction can be worn.

Eyeglasses are used frequently to hold the lenses necessary to correct errors of refraction. Advantages of eyeglasses include ease of use, durability, availability, and low cost when compared with other strategies for refractive error correction. Disadvantages include an alteration in physical appearance, weight of the frame on the nose, and reduced peripheral vision because vision is corrected only when the client looks through the center of the lens.

Contact lenses are a second form of medical treatment for refractive errors. These round plastic disks are designed to rest against the cornea and fit under the eyelid. Contact lenses are fitted by measuring the size and shape of the cornea and the refractive power needed. Care must be taken to provide sufficient oxygen to the cornea. Tear fluid is forced under the contact lens to moisten the cornea and to remove debris during each blink.

Hard contact lenses have been used to treat refractive errors for many years. With recent developments in contact lens technology, some forms of astigmatism may now be treated with contact lenses. Contact lenses are able to correct refractive errors by changing the shape of the cornea, which increases its refracting ability, and by placing the specific refractive power and shape needed in front of the eye so that light rays can be correctly focused onto the retina. Contraindications to wearing contact lenses include insufficient tear film quality because of abnormal eyelid position or function; life styles or occupations involving an environment containing dust, dryness, or fumes; lack of motivation to maintain lens care and sterilization protocols; inadequate manual dexterity to insert and remove lenses; and impaired corneal sensation.

Contact lenses can be inserted by the client or the nurse. The Guidelines features on pages 1061 and 1062 describe the techniques of insertion and removal of hard contact lenses, as well as their cleaning.

Complications of contact lens wearing include corneal edema that occurs when contact lenses are worn for an extended period. Corneal abrasions can result from the overwearing of contact lenses, which dries the epithelium and causes minute breaks, or from the irritating surface of the contact lens against the cornea. An additional complication, giant papillary cell conjunctivitis, which is an inflammation of the palpebral conjunctiva, usually on the upper eyelid, may occur. It is usually due to a sensitivity reaction and occurs in long-term contact lens wearers. Symptoms include conjunctival redness and tearing, and the conjunctiva takes on a characteristic elevated cobblestone appearance.

Soft contact lenses are larger but are better tolerated than hard contact lenses. They can be worn for longer periods because the hydrophilic character of the material allows greater access of moisture and oxygen to the cornea. Disadvantages of soft contact lenses include easy damage to lenses (tears or holes), increased tend-

---

GUIDELINES ■ How to Clean Hard Contact Lenses

Interventions	Rationales
1. Wash your hands thoroughly.	1. To remove microorganisms present on the skin.
2. Explain the procedure to the client.	2. To decrease anxiety.
3. Place a towel or a cloth on a smooth surface away from an open drain.	3. To prevent loss of the lens.
4. Place the lens in the palm of a dry hand, concave side up.	4. To avoid damaging the lens and to place the cleaning solution.
5. Fill the lens completely with cleaning solution.	5. To provide a sufficient amount of solution to clean the lens.
6. Distribute the solution evenly over both sides of the lens using your finger pad—not your fingertip.	6. To clean all sides of the lens without damaging it. The finger pad is less likely to damage the lens than is the fingertip, which is close to the nail.
7. Rinse the lens with soaking solution while holding the lens by its edges.	7. To maximize the surface area reached by the rinsing solution.
8. Hold the lens up to a light.	8. To check for cleanliness and nicks.
9. Place one drop of wetting solution on each side of the lens.	9. To prepare the lens for insertion.

GUIDELINES ■ How to Insert and Remove Hard Contact Lenses

Interventions	Rationales
Insertion	
1. Wash your hands.	1. To reduce microorganisms and debris.
2. Explain the procedure to the client.	2. To reduce anxiety.
3. Moisten the index finger of your dominant hand with wetting solution.	3. To provide a platform for the lens.
4. Moisten both surfaces of the lens.	4. To promote easier insertion.
5. Place the lens concave side up near the fingertip of the index finger of your dominant hand.	5. To place concave edge next to cornea.
6. Instruct the client to flex the chin slightly and to look straight ahead.	6. To position the eye to receive the lens.
7. Hold the client's lower lid near the eyelash margin against the orbital rim using the index finger of your nondominant hand.	7, 8. To provide maximum exposure of the cornea.
8. Hold the client's upper lid near the eyelash margin up against the bony margin of the brow using the middle finger of your nondominant hand.	

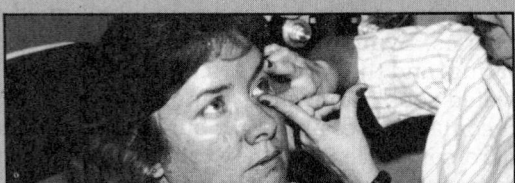

9. Raise the finger holding the lens until it touches the sclera.	9. To bring the contact lens in contact with the external eye.
10. Remove the finger holding the lens.	10. To leave the lens in position.
11. Slowly release the lower, then the upper eyelid, allowing the lids to close. The lens will center itself on the cornea.	11. To prevent the lens from being dislodged from the eye.
12. Stand still until you are sure that the lens is on the cornea.	12. To prevent loss of a lens that has become dislodged.
Removal	
1. Wash your hands.	1. To decrease microorganisms and debris.
2. Explain the procedure to the client.	2. To reduce anxiety.
3. Fill lens case with storage solution.	3. To keep lenses moist between wearing.
4. Instruct the client to flex the chin down and look forward into your hand.	4. To position the client for lens removal.
5. Place a towel on a surface below the client's head.	5. To prevent loss of a dropped lens.
6. Instruct the client to open the eyes wide.	6. To uncover the edge of the lens.
7. To remove the right lens, place your right hand against the client's right cheek. To remove the left lens, place your left hand against the client's left cheek.	7. To provide a surface onto which the lens will fall.
8. Pull the eyelid up and outward toward the ear with your middle finger.	8. To position the eye for easy lens removal.
9. Instruct the client to blink.	9. To force the lens away from the cornea and into your hand.
10. Place the lens in its storage case.	10. To protect lenses between wearing.

GUIDELINES ■ How to Insert and Remove Soft Contact Lenses

Interventions	Rationales
Insertion	
1. Wash your hands thoroughly.	1. To remove surface microorganisms and debris.
2. Explain the procedure to the client.	2. To reduce anxiety.
3. Retrieve the lens from its dome or the cup of its storage case. Use your finger pad, not your fingertip.	3, 4. To prevent lens damage by the fingernail.
4. Place the lens on the pad of the index finger of your dominant hand.	
5. Instruct the client to flex the chin slightly.	5. To position the head for insertion.
6. Pull the client's lower lid down against the cheek from the eyelash margin with the middle finger of your nondominant hand.	6, 7. To provide exposure for lens insertion without exerting pressure against the globe.
7. Pull the client's upper lid up against the eyebrow from the eyelash margin.	
8. Instruct the client to look slightly upward.	8. To expose the area where the lens is applied.
9. Bring your index finger carrying the lens up toward the eye and place the lens on the sclera below the cornea, or against the cornea.	9. To position the lens.
10. Bring your index finger away from the client's eye.	10. To leave the lens in position.
11. Slowly release the client's eyelids.	11. To prevent dislodging the lens.
12. Instruct the client to close the eyes.	12. To center the lens.
Removal	
1. Wash your hands.	1. To remove microorganisms and debris.
2. Fill the lens case with the desired solution.	2. To prevent damage. Soft lenses will dehydrate quickly if they are not kept moist, which causes damage.
3. Instruct the client to look up.	3. To provide exposure of the area from which the lens will be removed.
4. Pull the client's lower lid down against the cheekbone with the pad of the finger of your dominant hand.	4. To increase exposure.
5. Slide the lens off the cornea and onto the sclera.	5. To prevent discomfort. The sclera is less sensitive than the cornea.
6. Capture the lens between the thumb and index finger of your dominant hand.	6. To secure attachment to lens.
7. Remove the lens from the sclera.	7. To complete the procedure.
8. Place the lens on the dome or cup of its storage case.	8. To prevent damage.

ency of lenses to absorb chemicals and medications, and a reduced ability to correct astigmatism. Two types of soft contact lenses exist: daily wear lenses, which are worn during waking hours, and extended wear contact lenses, which can be worn continuously for several days to several weeks depending on the client's environment, activities, and tolerance of the lenses. Extended wear lenses are thinner than daily wear lenses to permit increased oxygenation and have a higher water content to bathe the corneal surface. Insertion, removal, and

cleaning of soft contact lenses are explained in the Guidelines features on pages 1063 and 1064.

The nurse helps the client to select a method of visual correction for the refractive error. Advantages and disadvantages of contact lenses should be reviewed with the client so that an informed decision can be made. If the client selects eyeglasses, support must be provided during the adaptation phase.

If the client selects contact lenses, the safe, aseptic cleaning, storage, insertion, and removal of the lens

---

GUIDELINES ■ How to Clean Soft Contact Lenses

Interventions	Rationales
1. Wash your hands.	1. To remove microorganisms from the surface.
2. Explain the procedure to the client.	2. To reduce anxiety.
3. Fill the lens storage case with normal saline.	3. To prepare the case for storage.
4. Place the lens in the palm of your hand.	4. To provide a safe surface area on which to clean the lens.
5. Apply several drops of cleaning solution to the lens.	5. To remove particles from the lens.
6. Distribute the cleaning solution evenly over both sides of lens with the pad of your finger.	6. To protect the lens from the damage by the fingernail.
7. Rinse the lens with normal saline.	7. To remove cleaning solution, which is irritating to the eye.
8. Hold lens up to a light.	8. To inspect for cleanliness and damage.
9. Place the lens on its dome or in its case.	9. To prevent damage. The case provides protection. If a dome is present, it provides a surface on which the lens rests.
10. If case has a dome and covering arm, position the arm in place over the lens. Press until a click is heard.	10. To lock the lens in place.

---

must be discussed and demonstrated. Before the client leaves the health care facility with the contact lenses, the client must provide a return demonstration of these skills. Symptoms of problems should be reviewed with the client, who should be instructed to remove the lenses and report the symptoms to the contact lens professional immediately.

Interventions: surgical management. Surgery is becoming an alternative to the previously described interventions for refractive errors. *Radial keratotomy* is an outpatient surgical procedure for the treatment of mild to moderate myopia. Eight to 16 diagonal incisions are made through 90% of the peripheral cornea. The central cornea is not incised, so vision is not affected. These incisions flatten the cornea, which decreases the anteroposterior length of the eye and allows the image to be focused closer to the retina.

Candidates for radial keratotomy are clients who are intolerant of contact lenses or whose work, interests, or life style requires good visual acuity and clear peripheral vision. Slight over- or undercorrection of the refractive error is possible, which requires the client to still wear some form of visual correction after the surgery. Other complications of this surgery include corneal scars, if the incisions are made too deep, and failure to achieve adequate correction, if the incisions are made too shallow.

Another surgical procedure to correct refractive errors is *epikeratophakia*, the surgical grafting of donor corneal tissue onto the client's own cornea to alter its refractive ability. Although the donor tissue used for this procedure is unacceptable for a full-thickness corneal transplant, it is usable for grafting by being frozen and reshaped to the specific strength and size needed by the client.

TRAUMATIC DISORDERS

The eye is well protected by the bony prominence of the forehead and the ocular orbit. Retrobulbar fat also acts as a cushion to minimize the effect of force applied to the eye. Despite these safeguards that are built into the anatomic structure and function of the eye, injuries occur. Trauma to the eye or periorbital area can result from naturally occurring objects such as tree branches or wood chips, as well as from manufactured articles and devices such as BB guns, slingshots, lawn darts, drills, lawn mowers, electric weed removers, and fireworks. It is estimated that 1.3 million eye injuries occur annually in the United States, permanent visual impairment occurs in 40,000 of these injuries (Parke & Hamill, 1988).

Blunt Trauma

HYPHEMA

OVERVIEW

A *hyphema* is defined as the presence of blood in the anterior chamber. It is produced when a force is sufficient to alter the integrity of the blood vessels located in the eye. This force can be applied to the eye directly, such as a penetrating injury from a BB pellet, or indirectly, such as from striking the forehead on a steering wheel during an accident. The blood may fill all or part of the anterior chamber. Because blood is thicker and heavier than aqueous humor, it settles to the lower part of the anterior chamber. If the hyphema is sufficiently large, it may obstruct the pupil and reduce visual acuity. Other symptoms include pain and photophobia. Hemolysis of the blood occurs, and it is filtered out of the eye through the trabecular meshwork. If the hemolyzed blood obstructs the trabecular meshwork, an increased intraocular pressure will be noted.

COLLABORATIVE MANAGEMENT

Diagnosis of the hyphema follows examination of the eye at the slit lamp.

The client with a hyphema is treated by bed rest in semi-Fowler's position to assist gravity in keeping the hyphema away from the optical center of the cornea. Minimal or no sudden eye movements are permitted for 3 to 5 days to decrease the likelihood of rebleeding. Bleeding recurs in approximately 10% to 30% of these clients. Cycloplegic eyedrops, such as atropine, may be ordered to place the eye at rest. The eye is protected by a shield and may be covered with a patch. The use of television and reading may be restricted. The hyphema usually resolves in 5 to 7 days.

Nursing interventions include monitoring visual acuity, monitoring adherence to the activity restrictions, and providing alternative forms of sensory stimulation such as music or conversation. A sudden increase in eye pain should be reported immediately to the ophthalmologist, as it may indicate rebleeding.

CONTUSION

OVERVIEW

A contusion of the eyeball and surrounding tissue is produced by traumatic contact with a blunt object. The forces of the contact push the eye back in the orbit. The globe is compressed, which decreases its length. As a compensatory mechanism, the width increases (Parke & Hamill, 1988). Stretching of the ocular soft tissues (retina, choroid, and iris) occurs, which can produce damage. Results of the injury may not be immediately seen. These results include edema of the eyelids, a subconjunctival hemorrhage, corneal edema, or a hyphema. Periorbital ecchymosis, which is also known as a black eye, may be present.

A common contusion injury, the black eye is usually caused by blunt trauma to the area from a fist, baseball, or racquetball. Bleeding into the soft tissue occurs, which creates the characteristic purple ecchymosis. The purple color fades to green and then yellow; discoloration disappears in approximately 10 days. Visual acuity is usually not affected. Other symptoms are orbital pain, photophobia, and eyelid edema. Diplopia may occur in some cases.

COLLABORATIVE MANAGEMENT

Treatment begins at the time of injury. Ice should be applied immediately. The client should receive a thorough eye examination to rule out the presence of other eye injuries.

Nursing interventions include preventing contusion injuries by educating the public and athletes to the importance of protective eyewear. The nurse should act as a role model by wearing protective eyewear for sporting events. As a care provider, the nurse may apply ice at the scene of the injury and encourage the injured client to sit upright.

Foreign Bodies

OVERVIEW

Eyelashes, dust, fingernails, dirt, and airborne particles can come in contact with the conjunctiva or cornea and produce a mechanical *irritation* or *abrasion*. If nothing is seen on the cornea or conjunctiva, the eyelids are everted to examine the palpebral and bulbar conjunctivae.

The client complains of a foreign body sensation ("feeling something in my eye") or of blurry vision. Pain is a common symptom if the corneal epithelium is injured because the cornea contains many sensory nerves, which are located beneath the epithelium. Tearing and photophobia may be noted.

COLLABORATIVE MANAGEMENT

Treatment is preceded by evaluating vision. Any client with a suspected or known corneal abrasion should have the eye examined with fluorescein followed by ocular irrigation with normal saline (0.9%) to facilitate gentle removal of the particles. The procedure for an ophthalmologic irrigation is described in the accompanying Guidelines feature. Care must be taken to direct the flow of the solution across the cornea to the lateral canthus, where a collection device, such as an emesis basin, has been placed. This position will also prevent contaminating the fellow eye.

Nursing interventions include obtaining a thorough history from the client, including the setting of the injury and a description of symptoms. Visual acuity is assessed and documented before any treatment occurs, for medical baseline and legal reasons. The client's comfort is assessed frequently during the irrigation, and additional anesthetic drugs are instilled as needed. After the foreign body is removed and the eyepatch is applied, the client is instructed about the length of time that the

GUIDELINES ■ How to Perform Extensive Ocular Irrigation

Interventions	Rationales

1. Assemble the following equipment:
  a. Normal saline IV (1000-mL bag).
  b. Macrodrip IV tubing.
  c. IV pole.
  d. Topical anesthetic (proparacaine hydrochloride [Alcaine]).
  e. Eyelid speculum or irrigating contact lens.
  f. Gloves (nonsterile).
  g. Collection receptacle.
  h. Towels.
  i. pH paper.
	1. To ensure availability of equipment.

2. Quickly obtain a history from the client while flushing the tubing or irrigating the contact lens with normal saline.
  a. Nature and timing of injury.
  b. Irritant or chemical (if known).
  c. First aid given at scene.
  d. Allergy to drugs of "caine" family.
	2. To obtain only essential information. Time is of the essence.
	
	a–c. To plan care.
	
	  d. To avoid precipitating an allergic reaction.

3. *Briefly* explain the procedure.	3. To enhance client's cooperation.
4. Evaluate the client's visual acuity as soon as possible, and *before* treatment is initiated.	4. To plan care and document status before nurse rendered care.
5. Don gloves.	5. To protect the nurse's skin from chemicals or irritants.
6. Place a strip of pH paper in the cul-de-sac of the client's affected eye.	6. To identify the chemical to be removed.
7. Instill proparacaine hydrochloride (ophthetic) as ordered, or per protocol. Repeat as needed for the client's comfort.	7. To anesthetize the external surface, which promotes the client's comfort.
8. Place the client in a supine position, with the head turned slightly toward the affected side.	8. To facilitate drainage away from the unaffected eye.
9. Position the eyelid speculum or irrigating contact lens. Do not use an irrigating contact lens if the potential irritant was particulate matter.	9. To facilitate irrigation without injury. The speculum holds eyelids apart. An irrigating contact lens could embed particulate material in cornea. The protective reaction is to close the eyelids.
10. Direct the flow of irrigating solution across the globe toward the lateral canthus and into the receptacle.	10. To prevent recontamination of the eye.
11. Assess the client's comfort throughout the procedure.	11. To enhance cooperation.
12. Provide reassurance and support throughout the procedure.	12. To decrease anxiety.
13. If both eyes are affected, irrigate them simultaneously, but using separate equipment and personnel.	13. To minimize the time during which a chemical irritant is in contact with the eye.

patch must be left in place. In most instances, it is left in place overnight. The nurse advises the client to prevent further injuries by wearing glasses, safety glasses, or goggles when cutting hedges, mowing grass, or using a weed remover. The client is reminded to seek follow-up care to have the patch removed and the eye examined because rust rings may develop after the injury. Signs and symptoms of ocular infection are also reviewed with the client.

Lacerations

OVERVIEW

Lacerations are caused by sharp objects such as scissors, knives, sticks, fishhooks, and projectiles such as fireworks or BB pellets. Lacerations can occur to any part of the eye. The most common areas involved are the eyelids and the cornea. Eyelid lacerations bleed heavily and look more severe than they actually are.

COLLABORATIVE MANAGEMENT

Initially, the eye is closed and a small ice pack is applied to decrease bleeding. One or two ice cubes that have been crushed and placed in a self-sealing bag that is covered with a washcloth will suffice. The client should be transported to receive medical attention as soon as possible. If tissue is missing, the nurse attempts to locate it at the scene of the accident and sends it with the client packed in a self-sealing bag that is placed in a second self-sealing bag filled with ice and water.

Treatment includes checking visual acuity, if the client is able to open the eye, and cleaning the eyelids. Minor lacerations of the eyelid can be sutured in an emergency department, an urgent care center, or an ophthalmology office. Lacerations involving the eyelid margin or lacrimal system, those involving a large area, or those with jagged edges require use of a microscope located in the operating room. If the client is quite uncomfortable or is a young child, the repair may be performed with the client under general anesthesia. Care must be taken to ensure the smooth approximation of wound edges, or a notch will be created as the eyelid heals.

Corneal lacerations are more serious than eyelid lacerations because ocular contents may prolapse through the laceration. These lacerations are treated as an ocular emergency. Symptoms include severe eye pain, photophobia, tearing, and decreased visual acuity. As a protective mechanism, the client may be unable or unwilling to open the eyelid. If the laceration is the result of a penetrating injury, the object may be noted protruding from the eye. *This object must NEVER be removed except by the ophthalmologist because it may be holding ocular structures in place.*

Antibiotics are initiated to reduce the likelihood of an infection. Repair of the laceration by use of the operating room microscope is necessary. A general anesthetic is the method of choice, providing the client has not eaten recently. Depending on the depth of the laceration, scarring may develop. If the scar alters vision, a corneal transplant may be needed later. If the ocular contents have prolapsed through the laceration or if the injury is severe, an enucleation may need to be performed.

Nursing interventions include supporting the client, who is usually extremely anxious and fearful. Acknowledging these fears and the presence of pain, combined with a quiet, gentle approach, facilitates the examination. If an object is noted protruding from the eye, it is stabilized before transporting the client, but it is not removed. If no object is noted protruding from the eye, a temporary shield should be made at the scene of the injury from a paper cup, glass, or plastic top of a spray can. Care must be taken to avoid putting any pressure on the eye when the temporary shield is applied and taped in place. The shield should be removed by a phy-

sician, and a visual acuity measure obtained, if possible, for medical documentation and legal protection. The nurse elicits a thorough history and asks the client to describe how the accident occurred. The nurse also determines the date of the client's last tetanus shot and the time of the last meal and fluids.

Penetrating Injuries

OVERVIEW

Penetrating ocular injuries have the poorest visual prognosis (Parke & Hamill, 1988). Glass, high-speed metallic or wood particles, BB pellets, and bullets are common causes of penetrating injuries. The particles can enter the eye through the eyelid, sclera, or cornea. They may lodge in or behind the eyeball.

The client usually complains of some eye pain and relates a history of "suddenly feeling hit in the eye." An entrance wound may be visible. Depending on the location of the entrance and the resting place of the projectile, vision may be affected. X-ray films and computed tomography scans of the orbit are taken. These studies assist in determining the nature and location of the projectile. Ultrasonography of the globe and orbit may also be performed. This procedure is helpful when the ocular fundus cannot be observed because of a hemorrhage or a cataract.

COLLABORATIVE MANAGEMENT

Surgery usually is performed to remove the foreign object. Metallic foreign bodies are removed by using an intraocular magnet. Removal of some foreign bodies requires a vitrectomy to be performed. Intravenous antibiotics are started before surgery to reduce the chance of an infection. A tetanus booster is administered if necessary.

The nurse obtains a detailed description of the setting and the events related to the complaint of having an object in the eye. It is imperative that visual acuity be assessed and documented. A standard eye chart is not necessary. The nurse can use whatever is available, such as a newspaper, a poster, or a label on a carton. If the client is unable to see print, it is critical to note if he or she is able to count fingers or see directional movement of the nurse's hand. If the client cannot see movement, the ability to see light must be assessed. The date of the client's last tetanus shot is noted, as is the time of the client's last meal. The nurse attempts to discern the probable size, speed, and composition of the suspected projectile. Preoperative teaching is the same for any client who is undergoing intraocular surgery. The client may be quite anxious. An opportunity to discuss his or her fears may be of benefit to the client.

Postoperative care includes administering antibiotics and monitoring the eye for signs and symptoms of infection. Adherence by the client to activity restrictions should be facilitated. Because a patch and shield are applied to the eye after surgery, the nurse places objects in the client's field of vision.

Chemical Burns

OVERVIEW

Chemicals can be splashed onto the eyelids or into the eye from a variety of sources. Acids and alkaline compounds are the two most common sources of injury-causing chemicals. Any chemical coming in contact with the eye should be treated as a severe injury and an ocular emergency. When acids such as battery acid come in contact with ocular tissue, coagulation occurs in the cornea, causing a haze, but it protects the rest of the eye. Alkaline products such as magnesium hydroxide (such as in fireworks) or sodium hydroxide (lye) penetrate the corneal epithelium and cause the release of proteases and collagenases. Liquefactive necrosis of the cornea and sclera may occur. If the cornea is involved, melting and severe intraocular inflammation and vascularization and perforation of the cornea may eventually result. Corneal transplants after alkaline burns have not been especially successful.

COLLABORATIVE MANAGEMENT

Treatment must begin immediately. Emergency care is described in the accompanying Emergency Care feature. Eyelids should be copiously irrigated at the site of the injury with water or nonirritating liquid such as commercially available irrigating solution (Blinx, Dacriose) for at least 15 minutes, even before seeking treatment. Any chemical in contact with the eye should be flushed out for a minimum of 20 minutes. If the client is unable to hold the eye open because of pain, assistance should be obtained. After the client reaches the health care facility, the eye should be anesthetized with a drop of proparacaine hydrochloride (ophthetic), and a piece of litmus paper should be dabbed onto the conjunctiva to determine the acid or alkali nature of the irritant. Visual acuity is assessed. The nurse can quickly determine if the client can count the number of fingers held up by the nurse. The presence or absence of the ability to perceive light is important to note for medical and legal reasons. No attempt is made to neutralize the chemical because this generates heat and causes further damage to the cornea. The eye is irrigated copiously with a gentle solution such as normal saline or ophthalmic irrigating solution. The irrigant solution is directed across the cornea and toward the lateral canthus. The stream should also be directed into the superior and inferior fornices to remove any particles or debris (Parke & Hamill, 1988). The client's comfort should be assessed throughout the procedure and additional topical anesthetics instilled as needed. After the irrigation is complete, a measure of visual acuity is again obtained for medical and legal reasons. An antibiotic-steroid ointment, such as neomycin sulfate, polymyxin B sulfate, and dexamethasone (Maxitrol), is applied. The eye is covered with a pressure patch.

Nursing interventions include preventing chemical burns through public education about the importance of using chemicals safely and of wearing safety glasses or goggles when performing high-risk activities. The nurse elicits a history from the client after the eye has been

---

EMERGENCY CARE ■ CHEMICAL BURNS OF THE EYE

Interventions	Rationales
1. Irrigate eye(s) immediately with a large amount of clean liquid such as water or irrigating solution for minimum of 10 min.	1. To reduce contact of the chemical with ocular tissue.
2. Restrain the client's hands as necessary.	2. To maximize eye access. The client's natural reaction is to cover the eyes with the hands as if for protection. However, this action limits access to the eye.
3. Hold the client's eyelids open during irrigation.	3. To increase the surface area exposed to irrigation.
4. Assess the client's visual acuity.	4. To provide baseline information for medical and legal reasons.
5. Obtain a sample of chemical involved.	5. To assist the physician in determining the source of the irritation.
6. Transport the client to the hospital.	6. To complete assessment and treatment which require equipment available at a hospital.
7. Have someone telephone the hospital to alert emergency personnel of your arrival.	7. To allow hospital personnel to prepare the necessary equipment before the client's arrival.

anesthetized and during the irrigation. If both eyes are involved, simultaneous irrigations should be performed, preferably by two nurses. Gloves should be worn by the nurse to prevent contact dermatitis.

OCULAR TUMORS

Extraocular Tumors

Tumors can occur outside or inside the eye and can be benign or malignant. Many can be detected because they are readily visible or alter the structure or function of the eye.

BASAL CELL CARCINOMA

OVERVIEW

Basal cell carcinoma is the most common of all malignant epithelial tumors (Newell, 1986). It occurs most frequently in the lower eyelid, but occurrences on the upper lid have been noted. The growth of basal cell carcinoma is slow and painless. The cancerous lesion begins as a tiny wart-like growth with a raised nodular border. Surrounding tissue may be eroded by the tumor that begins to bleed and scab over. These tumors do not metastasize. Multifacial lesions may be present. Vision is altered only when the tumor size, location, or weight affects ocular functioning. Left untreated, the tumor can continue growing and fill the entire orbit.

COLLABORATIVE MANAGEMENT

The only way to diagnose basal cell carcinoma definitively is through biopsy of the lesion.

Treatment for basal cell carcinoma is surgical excision of the lesion. A frozen section should be taken to determine if the excision is complete. This excision can be performed in the ophthalmologist's office or as an outpatient procedure in the hospital.

Nursing interventions for the client with basal cell carcinoma include assessing the client's knowledge about the diagnosis. When the diagnosis of cancer is first mentioned to a client, he or she may become visibly anxious. The client may think of friends, relatives, and colleagues who have died from cancer. The client needs to be assisted in working through these feelings. The client should also be advised to maintain a regular schedule of follow-up visits to facilitate rapid detection of a recurrence.

Intraocular Tumors

MELANOMA

OVERVIEW

Melanoma is believed to occur in between 2 and 6 per 10,000 of the total eye client population in the United States (Vaughan & Asbury, 1986). This unilateral tumor most frequently occurs in the fourth and fifth decades of life. The uveal tract is the most frequent site of origin. Eighty-five per cent of tumors are noted in the choroid, 9% in the ciliary body, and 6% in the iris (Vaughan & Asbury, 1986).

A malignant melanoma lesion can spread easily because of its rich blood supply and vascular channels. Common pathways for metastatic spread include directly through the sclera or indirectly through invasion of other intraocular structures.

Symptoms of malignant melanoma may not be readily apparent; the lesion may be found during a routine examination. Blurring of vision may be evident if the macular area is invaded. Visual acuity is reduced if the tumor grows inward toward the center of the eye from the choroid, thus altering the visual pathway. Increased intraocular pressure can result if the tumor invades the canal of Schlemm, which obstructs outflow of aqueous humor. A change in iris color may occur if the tumor infiltrates the iris. Sudden loss of a portion of the visual field may result from the tumor's invading the subretinal space, which produces detachment of the overlying retina. The lesion is visible when the eye is examined with the indirect ophthalmoscope and looks mushroom shaped. Subretinal fluid may also be noted.

COLLABORATIVE MANAGEMENT

Diagnostic tests for a malignant melanoma lesion depend on the size and rate of growth of the lesion. Ultrasonography is performed to determine the location and size of the lesion. Melanomas are measured in diameter and height.

Treatment depends on the size and growth rate of the lesion and the condition of the other eye. Small lesions of the iris not affecting the iris root are not excised but are monitored until growth is observed. Lesions of the choroid can be treated by surgical enucleation of the eye or by radiation therapy with radioactive cobalt plaque.

Enucleation

Enucleation is the surgical removal of the entire eyeball. The procedure is usually performed with the client under general anesthesia, but it can be performed with local anesthesia if the client's medical condition precludes use of a general anesthetic. After the eye is removed, a ball implant is inserted to provide a firm base

GUIDELINES ■ How to Insert and Remove an Ocular Prosthesis

Interventions	Rationales
Insertion	

1. Assemble equipment:
   a. Prosthesis.
   b. Gloves.
   c. Towel.
	1. To ensure availability of equipment.

2. Explain the procedure to the client.	2. To decrease anxiety.
3. Wash your hands.	3. To remove surface microorganisms and debris.
4. Cover the work area with a cloth or towel.	4. To protect the prosthesis should it be dropped.
5. Don gloves.	5. To prevent exposure to the client's secretions.
6. Remove the prosthesis from its container and rinse it with tepid water.	6. To remove any soaking solution.
7. Lift the client's upper lid using your nondominant hand.	7. To expose the socket fully.

8. Place the prosthesis between the thumb and forefinger of your dominant hand. The notched end of the prosthesis should be closest to the client's nose.	8. To maximize dexterity. The notched end most closely parallels orbital socket.

9. Insert the prosthesis with the top edge slipping under the upper lid. Continue until most of the iris is covered by the upper lid.	9. To position the upper edge of the prosthesis in the socket.

GUIDELINES ■ How to Insert and Remove an Ocular Prosthesis *Continued*

Interventions	Rationales
10. Gently release the upper eyelid.	10. To end upper eyelid traction.
11. Retract the lower lid slightly until the bottom edge of the prosthesis slips behind it.	11. To permit the bottom edge of the prosthesis to position itself.
12. Release hands slowly.	12. To prevent dislodging the prosthesis.

Removal

Interventions	Rationales
1. Assemble equipment: a. Normal saline–filled labeled container. b. Gloves.	1. To ensure availability of equipment.
2. Explain the procedure to the client.	2. To decrease anxiety.
3. Wash your hands.	3. To reduce surface microorganisms.
4. Don gloves.	4. To prevent exposure to secretions.
5. Instruct the client to sit up and tilt the head slightly downward.	5. To position the prosthesis for easy removal.
6. Place your hand against the client's cheek, palm side up.	6. To create a platform on which the prosthesis can rest on when removed.
7. Pull the lower lid slightly down and laterally.	7. To increase surface area, promoting easy removal of the prosthesis.
8. Allow the prosthesis to slide out onto your hand, or pull gently if necessary.	8. To prevent injury.
9. Place the prosthesis in normal saline–filled container labeled with the client's name and cover the container.	9. To protect the prosthesis.

for the socket prosthesis and to facilitate the best cosmetic result. It is covered with surrounding tissue, muscles, and conjunctiva. A plastic conformer is placed over the conjunctiva to maintain the shape of the eyelids until a prosthesis can be fitted, in approximately 1 month. After the dressing is removed, a pressure patch is placed over the eye for 24 hours.

Postoperatively, the nurse monitors vital signs every 15 to 20 minutes until they are stable. The orbit is a highly vascularized area, so the potential for hemorrhage exists. Any change in vital signs or the presence of bright red drainage on the dressing should be promptly brought to the ophthalmologist's attention. The client's level of comfort is evaluated.

Whenever a body part is removed, a loss results. The client may mourn the loss of the eye, as well as the life style changes that the surgery imposes. No longer will the client have binocular vision. A scanning type of vision (head turning side to side) must be used. The client must relearn to judge distances because depth perception is changed. The nurse must support the client's early attempts at judging distances and assist in maintaining a safe environment. Initially, side rails of the bed should be up, and the client should be instructed to call for assistance before getting out of bed. Assistance with meal trays should be offered if vision in the remaining eye is poor.

As the time of discharge approaches, information about how to care for the eye socket should be reviewed with the client. The socket is rinsed with an irrigating solution daily. Until the prosthesis is fitted, usually 1 month after surgery, an antibiotic-steroid ointment such as neomycin sulfate, polymyxin B sulfate, and dexamethasone may be inserted into the cul-de-sac once a day.

Steps for the insertion and removal of the prosthesis are given in the accompanying Guidelines feature and are reviewed with the client by the ocularist. The prosthesis, usually made of porcelain, is custom-made for the client and matches the fellow eye in color. It should be washed only with warm water or normal saline, as explained in the Guidelines feature on page 1072.

GUIDELINES ■ How to Clean an Ocular Prosthesis

Interventions	Rationales

1. Assemble equipment:
   a. Clean container with lid.
   b. Mild soap.
   c. Normal saline–filled container.
	1. To ensure availability of equipment.

2. Explain the procedure to the client.	2. To decrease anxiety.
3. Wash your hands.	3. To remove surface microorganisms.
4. Cover the work area with a cloth or towel.	4. To protect the prosthesis should it be dropped.
5. Close the drain of the sink.	5. To prevent loss of the prosthesis.
6. Don nonsterile gloves.	6. To protect the nurse from contact with secretions.
7. Rinse the prosthesis with tepid water from the tap.	7. To remove surface secretions.
8. Place the prosthesis in the palm of your nondominant hand.	8. To provide a platform on which prosthesis can rest for cleaning.
9. Apply a small amount of mild soap to the prosthesis and distribute it with the finger pad of your dominant hand.	9. To reduce surface tension, allowing for easy removal of secretions. The finger pad will not scratch the prosthesis as a brush or cloth might.
10. Rinse the prosthesis with tepid water.	10. To remove soap without damaging the prosthesis. Extreme temperatures can damage the prosthesis. Rinsing removes soap residue, which can be irritating to ocular tissue.
11. Examine the prosthesis.	11. To detect surface deposits caused by tears and scratches, which can irritate the eyelid.
12. Place the prosthesis into a container filled with normal saline and labeled with the client's name.	12. To protect the prosthesis.

The nurse also reviews the importance of maintaining the safety of the remaining eye. The client should be advised to wear eye protection when performing any activity that might be hazardous. Goggles or safety glasses should be worn during yard work or when drilling on metal, plastic, and wood. Many practitioners advocate fitting the client with a pair of eyeglasses to protect the fellow eye, even if no correction is needed.

Radiation Therapy

Cobalt plaque therapy can be used to reduce the size and thickness of malignant melanomas for small tumors, as well as for medium to large tumors when a good visual prognosis is expected, and for large tumors when the client's only seeing eye is affected. The *plaque*, a round, flat disk about the size of a dime, is sutured to the sclera overlying the tumor site. The plaque contains a radioactive material such as cobalt-60 or iodine-125 in a sealed source. The length of time the plaque remains sutured to the sclera depends on the size of the tumor and the dose of radiation to be delivered.

Complications of radiation therapy include radiation tumor vasculopathy, radiation retinopathy, and cataract formation. Vitreous hemorrhage may develop as the tumor gets smaller.

Nursing interventions include supporting the client through the diagnostic and treatment processes. An empathetic, supportive response by the nurse encourages the client to express his or her feelings. The advantages and limitations of plaque therapy should be discussed. While the plaque is in place, the client may or may not have the eye covered with a patch. Cycloplegic eyedrops, such as cyclopentolate hydrochloride (Cyclogyl), and an antibiotic-steroid combination, such as neomycin sulfate, polymyxin B sulfate, and dexamethasone, will be ordered. Because of the proximity of the plaque to the cul-de-sac, the client should be taught how to instill eyedrops. The nurse must follow appropriate precautions to limit exposure to radiation. These precautions are discussed in Chapter 25.

OCULAR MANIFESTATIONS OF ACQUIRED IMMUNODEFICIENCY SYNDROME

Acquired immunodeficiency syndrome (AIDS) affects many ocular structures and can significantly impair visual function. The ocular effects of this disease are seen in three of four clients who are diagnosed with AIDS (Mines & Kaplan, 1986; Newsome et al., 1984). Chapter 27 discusses the general care for clients with AIDS.

Ocular manifestations of AIDS can be divided into two categories. These categories are based on location of the pathology and are referred to as External Manifestations and Internal Manifestations.

External Manifestations

OVERVIEW

Kaposi's sarcoma (KS) is the most common lesion noted in the anterior segment of the eye of AIDS clients. It is present in approximately 30% of clients diagnosed with AIDS (Centers for Disease Control, cited in Rao & Biswas, 1988). The most common sign of KS is the presence of a nontender reddish-purple discoloration or nodule in the lower fornix (Freeman & Gross, 1988) or on the eyelid. It may also appear on the palpebral or bulbar conjunctiva, or as a bright red subconjunctival mass (Rao & Biswas, 1988). Other signs include edema of the eyelid, chronic blepharitis, and recurrent subconjunctival hemorrhages. If the lesion impairs closure of the eyelid, signs of exposure keratitis may be noted. Pain is the most common symptom of KS, although KS lesions elsewhere on the body are usually painless. If the lesion occupies space so as to press against ocular structures or disturb function, discomfort may result.

COLLABORATIVE MANAGEMENT

Treatment goals for ocular KS are to remove the sarcoma with the smallest degree of structural alteration possible and to preserve visual function. Treatment is geared toward palliation of symptoms because many AIDS clients die of other causes (Freeman & Gross, 1988).

Conjunctival lesions of KS are usually well encapsulated and poorly adherent to the surrounding tissue, which facilitates their excision. These factors are important because incomplete removal tends to cause a local recurrence (Herman & Palestine, 1988). Careful excision is critical because of the vascular nature of the sarcoma. The preoperative and postoperative care of the client undergoing biopsy and/or removal of a KS lesion is similar that for the client undergoing an entropion or ectropion repair, described earlier in this chapter.

Radiation therapy may be the treatment of choice for large lesions for which excision would create defects in eyelid structure or function (Herman & Palestine, 1988). Parts of the eye that are not being irradiated should be protected.

Infection is primarily responsible for other external manifestations of AIDS. The deficient immune system causes increased susceptibility of clients to opportunistic organisms. Such organisms include herpes zoster, which can cause herpes zoster ophthalmicus, as well as fungi that cause serious corneal ulcers (Parrish et al., 1987). These pathologic conditions were discussed earlier in this chapter.

Internal Manifestations

RETINAL INVOLVEMENT

OVERVIEW

The retina is the internal ocular structure that is most frequently affected by HIV. The vasculopathy that is associated with AIDS presents itself most commonly as *cotton wool spots, retinal hemorrhages,* or *retinitis.* Cotton wool spots are fluffy white opacities that indicate focal retinal ischemia. The retinal ischemia involves the nerve fiber layer and is caused by the occlusion of retinal arterioles and capillaries (Pomerantz et al., 1987). Areas of retinal capillary nonperfusion were noted in 100% of a small number of clients (13) with cotton wool spots by Newsome et al. (1984).

Retinal hemorrhages are seen in both the superficial and the deep layers of the retina. Hemorrhages have been noted in the following shapes: dots and blots, and flames when the ocular fundi of AIDS clients are examined. Roth's spots, areas of hemorrhage with a white central area, have also been observed.

COLLABORATIVE MANAGEMENT

No treatment is indicated for cotton wool spots. They are monitored as indicators of microvascular perfusion. Treatment of retinal hemorrhage and retinitis for the client with AIDS is the same as that for other clients with these retinal disorders.

CYTOMEGALOVIRUS RETINITIS

OVERVIEW

The most common opportunistic infection in people with AIDS is cytomegalovirus (CMV) retinitis (Fay et al., 1988). CMV is a member of the herpes family. Direct invasion of retinal cells by the virus occurs, which causes damage and necrosis.

CMV retinitis presents with granular white dots on the retina that somewhat resemble cotton wool spots. However, these dots are deep and represent an increased density. These lesions tend to occur in proximity to blood vessels and coalesce to form patches of opacification (Shields et al., 1988). Left untreated, these patches expand and affect large portions of the retina. Blood vessel occlusion occurs in the involved retinal areas. Changes in the optic nerve such as atrophy and papilledema can also occur (Rao & Biswas, 1988). Hemorrhages shaped as dots, blots, and flames are also present. Left untreated, CMV retinitis can progress to acute retinal necrosis.

COLLABORATIVE MANAGEMENT

The diagnosis of CMV retinitis is based on ocular findings. These findings result in a characteristic clinical appearance. Atrophic areas of white retinal tissue peel off and flake into the vitreous. Other indications of this sight-threatening disorder include ocular pain, marked vision loss, and retinal edema.

Treatment of CMV retinitis involves use of the drug dihydroxypropoxymethylguanine (ganciclovir) (Fay et al., 1988). This relatively new antiviral drug is similar to acyclovir. It has been shown to slow the prolific nature of the disease (Henderly et al., 1987). Dosage is established by body weight. Once the CMV retinitis has been controlled, maintenance doses of ganciclovir are needed to reduce inflammation and edema. Although the antiviral agent halts DNA replication and controls the CMV infection, it may have retinal side effects. Freeman et al. (1987) reported a 29% incidence of retinal detachments in 17 clients receiving this drug.

SUMMARY

The major causes of vision loss include cataracts, glaucoma, and corneal disease. The older client is also at risk for developing macular degeneration.

Technologic advances including the development of lasers, microsurgical instruments, and suture materials have promoted a more ambulatory focus to the care of the ophthalmic client. These developments have also reduced the incidence of complications after eye surgery.

Ophthalmic clients are presented with the unique challenge of coping with a temporary or permanent visual deficit. A calm, supportive approach by the nurse can assist the ophthalmic client in dealing with anxiety and can facilitate the client's coping abilities.

IMPLICATIONS FOR RESEARCH

The need to investigate the impact of visual alterations is becoming increasingly important. Clients are living longer, which predisposes them to the chronic visual diseases of glaucoma, cataracts, and macular degeneration. The number of clients who are affected by trauma continues to grow.

Nursing research needs to be conducted to answer the following questions related to the care of the ophthalmic client:

1. What is the effect of activity restriction on the final visual outcome after retinal surgery?

2. Can factors be identified that predict compliance with a glaucoma treatment regimen?

3. What interventions can the nurse use to facilitate self-care, mobility, and independence in the visually impaired client?

4. How can nurses best assist clients to deal with a sudden vision loss?

5. Do clients with sudden vision loss and those with chronic vision loss use similar or different coping mechanisms?

REFERENCES AND READINGS

Boyd-Monk, H., & Steinmetz, C. (1987). *Nursing care of the eye.* Norwalk, CT: Appleton & Lange.

Chan, P. (1989, July). *Ocular pharmacology review.* Paper presented at a meeting of the American Society of Ophthalmic Registered Nurses, Philadelphia, PA.

Charles, S. (1987). *Vitreous microsurgery,* (2nd ed). Baltimore: Williams & Wilkins.

Easterlin, M. (1986). Cobalt plaque therapy: A conservative approach to posterior uveal melanoma. *Journal of Ophthalmic Nursing and Technology, 5,* 140–142.

Epstein, D. L. (Ed.) (1986). *Chandler's and Grant's glaucoma* (3rd ed.). Philadelphia: Lea & Febiger.

Epstein D. L., Pavan-Langston, D. (1980). Glaucoma. In D. Pavan-Langston (Ed.), *Manual of ocular diagnosis and therapy.* Boston: Little, Brown.

Fay, M., Freeman, W., Wiley, C., Hardy, D., & Bozette, S. (1988). Atypical retinitis in patients with acquired immunodeficiency syndrome. *American Journal of Ophthalmolgy, 105,* 483–490.

Freeman, W., & Gross, J. (1988). Management of ocular disease in AIDS patients. *Ophthalmology Clinics of North America, 1,* 91–100.

Freeman, W., Henderly, D., Wan, W., Causey, D., Trousdale, M., Green, R., & Rao, N. (1987). Prevalence, pathophysiology, and treatment of rhegmatogenous retinal detachments in treated cytomegalovirus retinitis. *American Journal of Ophthalmology, 103,* 527–536.

Freeman, W., Lerner, C., Mines, J., Lash, R., Nadel, A., Starr, M., & Tapper, M. (1984). Prospective study of the ophthalmic findings in the acquired immune deficiency syndrome. *American Journal of Ophthalmology, 97,* 133–142.

Gressel, M., Parrish, R., Heuer, D. (1984). Delayed nonexpulsive suprachoroidal hemorrhage. *Archives of Ophthalmology, 102,* 1757–1759.

Henderly, D.E., Freeman W. R., Smith R. E., Causey, D., & Rao, N. A. (1987). Cytomegalovirus retinitis as the initial manifestation of the acquired immune deficiency syndrome. *American Journal of Ophthalmology, 103,* 316–320.

Henkind, P., Walsh, J., & Berger, A. (1985). *Physician's desk reference for ophthalmology.* Oradell, NJ: Medical Economics.

Herman, D., & Palestine, A. (1988). Ocular manifestations of Kaposi's sarcoma. *Ophthalmology Clinics of North America, 1,* 73–80.

Hosein, A. (1988). The use of silicone oil in vitreoretinal surgery. *Journal of Ophthalmic Nursing and Technology, 7,* 126–129.

Hutchison, B. T. (1986). Post-operative choroidal hemorrhage. In D. Epstein (Ed.)., *Chandler and Grant's glaucoma* (3rd ed.). Philadelphia: Lea & Febiger.

Jaffe, N. (1981). *Cararact surgery and its complications.* St. Louis: C. V. Mosby.

Kahn, H., Leibowitz, H., Ganley, J., Kini, M., Colton, T., Nickerson, R. E., Dawger, T. (1977). The Framingham Eye Study; I, Outline and major prevalence findings. *American Journal of Epidemiology, 106,* 17–32.

McCoy, K. (1981). Cataracts and intraocular lenses: Cloudy to clear. *Nursing Clinics of North America, 16,* 405–414.

Mines, J., & Kaplan, H. (1986). Acquired immunodeficiency syndrome (AIDS). *International Ophthalmology Clinics, 26,* 73–78.

Newell, F. (1986). *Ophthalmology principles and concepts.* St. Louis: C. V. Mosby.

Newsome, D., Green, W., Miller, E., Kiessling, L., Morgan, B., Jabs, D., & Polk, B. (1984). Microvascular aspects of acquired immune deficiency syndrome retinopathy. *American Journal of Ophthalmology, 95,* 590–601.

New warning for contact lens tablets. (1988). *FDA Drug Bulletin, 18,* 6.

Parke, D., & Hamill, M. (1988). Injury to the eye. In K. Mattox, E. Moore, & D. Feliciano (Eds.), *Trauma.* Norwalk, CT: Appleton & Lange.

Parkin, D. M., Henney, C. R., Quirk, J., & Crooks, J. (1976). Deviation from prescribed drug treatment after discharge from hospital. *British Medical Journal, 2,* 686–688.

Parrish, C., O'Day, D., & Hoge, T. (1987). Spontaneous fungal ulcer as an ocular manifestation of AIDS. *American Journal of Ophthalmology, 104,* 302–307.

Pederson, K., & Nulty, G. (1987). Nursing grand rounds: Herpes zoster ophthalmicus. *Journal of Ophthalmic Nursing and Technology, 6,* 151–155.

Pomerantz, R., Kuritzkes, D., De La Monte, S., Rota, T., Baker, A., Albert, D., Bor, D., Feldman, E., Schooley, R., & Hirsch, M. (1987). Infection of the retina by human immunodeficiency virus type I. *New England Journal of Medicine, 317,* 1643–1647.

Rao, N., & Biswas, J. (1988). Ocular pathology in AIDS. *Ophthalmology Clinics of North America, 1,* 63–72.

Shields, M. B. (1987). *Textbook of glaucoma* (2nd ed.). Baltimore: Williams & Wilkins.

Shields, W., Ai, E., & Fujikawa, L. (1988). Cytomegaloviral retinitis. *Ophthalmic Clinics of North America, 1,* 81–90.

Smith, J. F., & Nachazel, D. P. (1980). *Ophthalmologic Nursing.* Boston: Little, Brown.

Stinson, E. (1986). Acanthamoeba keratitis in soft contact lens wearers. *Journal of Ophthalmic Nursing and Technology, 5,* 132–134. *Stratgies for improving visual learning (1978).* State College, PA: Learning Services.

Vaughan D., & Asbury, T. (1986). *General ophthalmology* (11th ed.). Norwalk, CT: Appleton & Lange.

CHAPTER 37

Assessment of the Ear

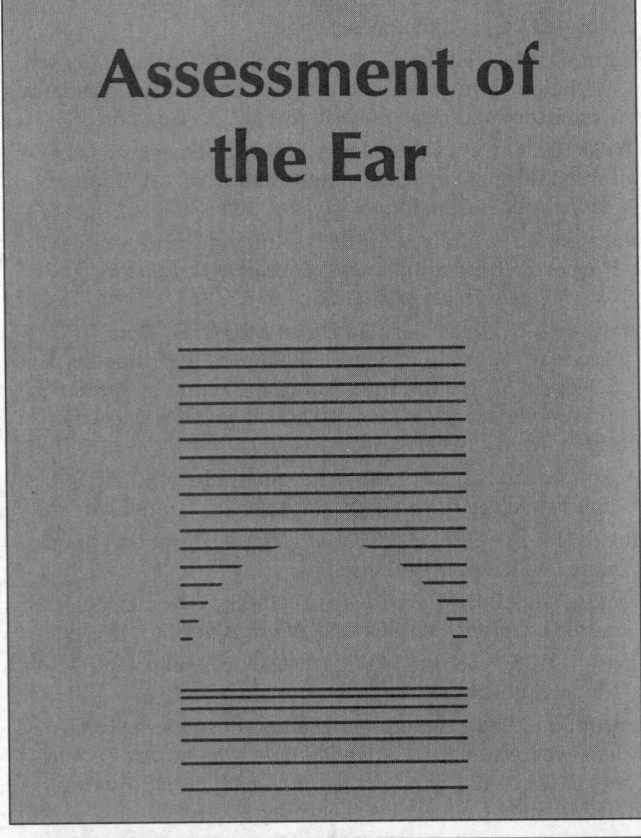

The ear is a sensory organ whose function includes both hearing and the sense of balance. Nurses who work with clients who have ear disorders need a thorough understanding of the normal anatomy and physiology of the external ear, middle ear, and inner ear, as well as the process and nature of hearing. Auditory screening is conducted from the neonatal period throughout life. If problems with the ear or with hearing are suspected, the nurse refers clients to a physician and/or audiologist for specialized diagnostic assessments. An audiologist is a health care professional who is educated in the science of hearing, including the treatment and rehabilitation of persons with impaired hearing.

ANATOMY AND PHYSIOLOGY REVIEW

STRUCTURE

The ear consists of three structural parts: external, middle, and inner. Each of these structures and their functions are significant and integral parts of the process of hearing.

EXTERNAL EAR

The external ear is developed in embryonic life at the same time that the kidneys and urinary tract are developed. Hence, defects of the external ear may be present in conjunction with congenital renal anomalies.

The external ear is embedded in the temporal bone bilaterally at the level of the eyes, at approximately a

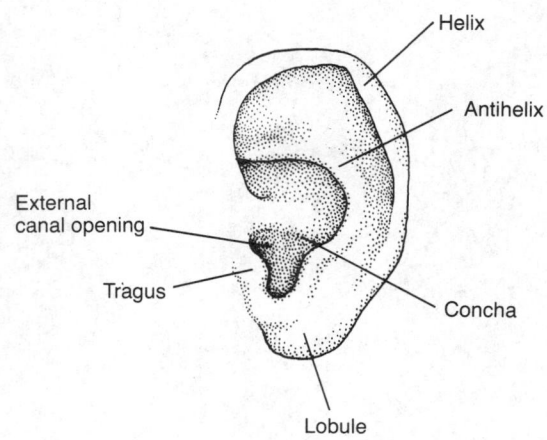

Figure 37–1

Anatomic features of the external ear.

10-degree angle with the head. Cartilage and skin attach the external ear to the head. The external ear extends from the visible auricle, or pinna, through the external canal to the lateral side of the tympanic membrane, or eardrum. The *pinna* is composed of the helix, antihelix, tragus, concha, external canal opening, and lobule (Fig. 37–1). The external ear canal is slightly S shaped and is lined with cerumen (wax)-producing glands, sebaceous glands, and hair follicles. The hair follicles and cerumen serve to protect the tympanic membrane and the middle ear. The length of the external canal varies with age. In the adult, the distance from the opening of the external canal to the tympanic membrane is approximately 2.5 to 3.75 cm (1 to 1½ in). In addition, the external ear includes the *mastoid process,* the bony ridge located over the temporal bone behind the pinna, which covers the mastoid air cells.

MIDDLE EAR

The middle ear consists of the medial side of the tympanic membrane and a compartment called the *epitympanum,* or attic, which contains the three bony *ossicles:* malleus, incus, and stapes (Fig. 37–2). In addition, the proximal end of the eustachian tube opens in the middle ear. The *tympanic membrane* is a thick, transparent sheet of tissue, 9 mm (0.35 in) in diameter, that provides a barrier between the external ear and the middle ear. The entire tympanic membrane is embedded in the temporal bone surrounded by the mastoid air cells. The landmarks on the tympanic membrane include the annulus, pars flaccida, and pars tensa (Fig. 37–3). The *annulus* is the site where the tympanic membrane attaches itself to

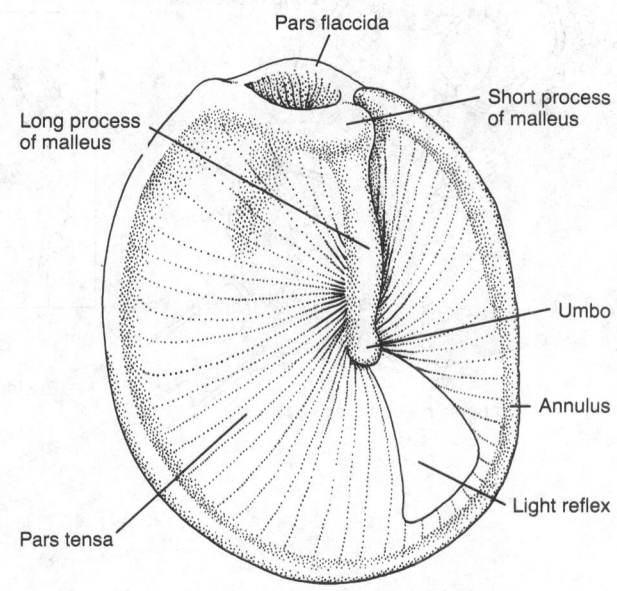

RIGHT TYMPANIC MEMBRANE

Figure 37–3

Landmarks on the tympanic membrane.

the external canal; it cannot be visualized directly as it is embedded in the temporal bone. The *pars flaccida* is that portion of the tympanic membrane above the short process of the malleus, which is usually less transparent and less mobile than the pars tensa portion of the tympanic membrane. The *pars tensa* is that portion of the tym-

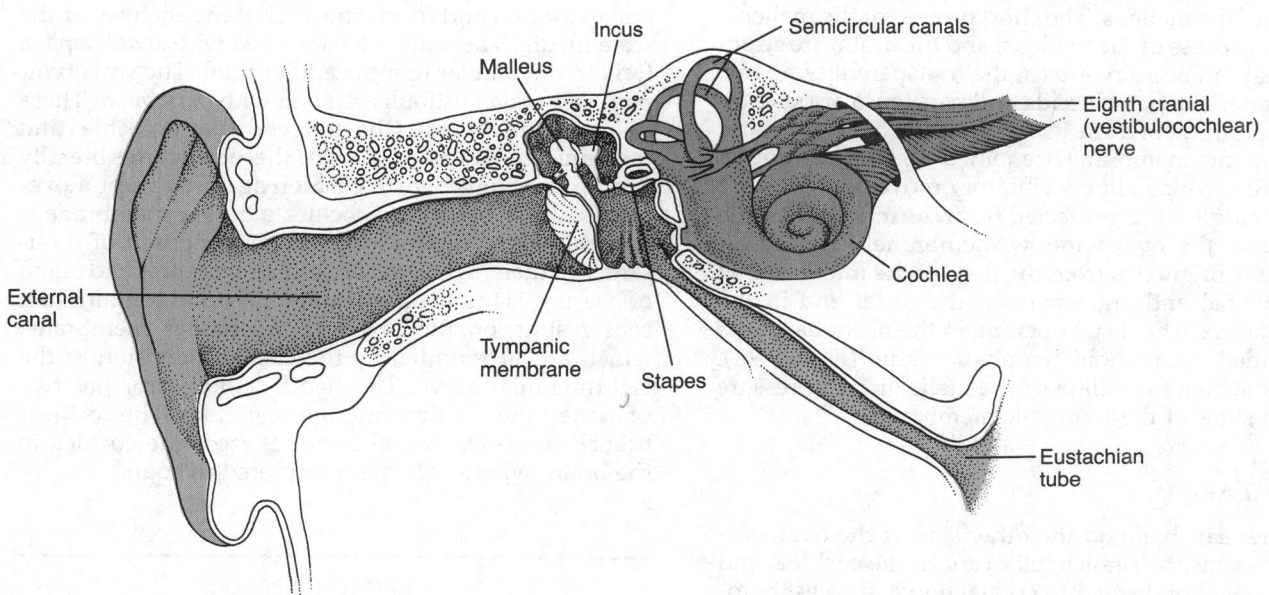

Figure 37–2

Anatomic features of the internal ear.

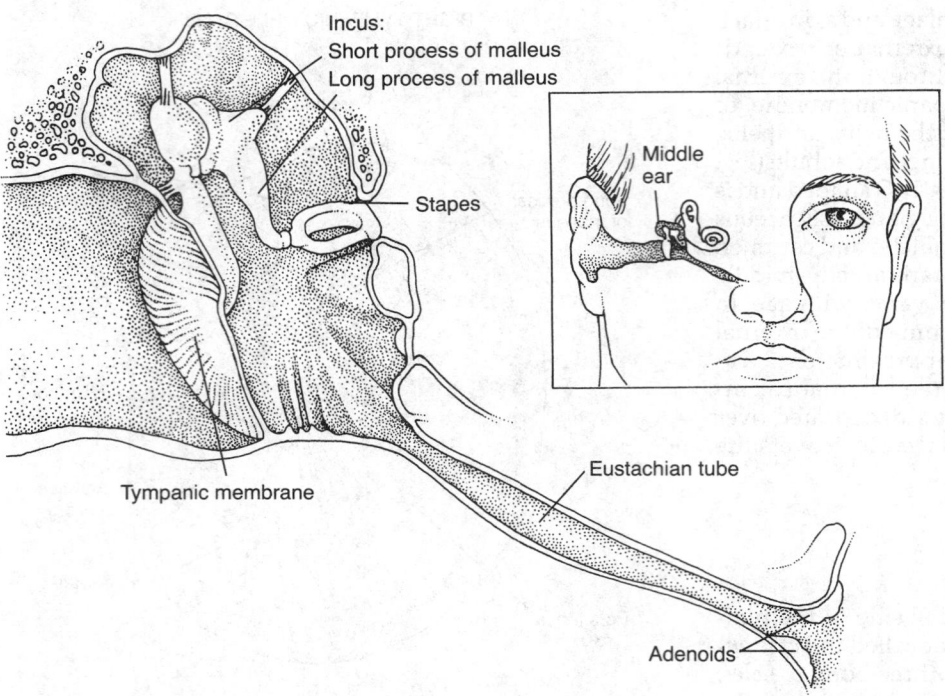

Figure 37–4

Anatomic features and attached structures of the middle ear.

panic membrane surrounding the long process of the malleus. It is usually referred to as transparent, opaque, or pearly gray and is mobile when air is injected into the external canal. The tympanic membrane is attached to the first bony ossicle, the *malleus*, at a site designated the *umbo* (see Fig. 37–3). The umbo is seen through the tympanic membrane as a white dot at the end of the long process of the malleus. The short process of the malleus, the long process of the malleus, and the umbo are structures that can be seen *through* the transparent tympanic membrane. The pars flaccida and pars tensa are sites on the tympanic membrane itself. The bony ossicles behind the tympanic membrane are joined together, although not rigidly, which allows vibratory movement.

The middle ear is protected from the inner ear by the round and the oval window membranes. The eustachian tube originates from the floor of the middle ear at the proximal end and opens at the distal end in the nasopharynx. The distal opening in the nasopharynx is surrounded by adenoid lymphatic tissue (Fig. 37–4). The eustachian tube allows for equalization of pressure on both sides of the tympanic membrane.

INNER EAR

The inner ear, lying on the other side of the oval window, contains the semicircular canals, the cochlea, and the distal end of the eighth cranial nerve, the vestibulo-cochlear nerve (see Fig. 37–2). The *semicircular canals* are structures containing fluid and hair cells, which are connected to the sensory nerve fibers of the vestibular portion of the eighth cranial nerve. They help to main-

tain a person's sense of balance, or equilibrium. Separating the semicircular canals from the cochlea are the utricle and saccule, which are vestibular receptors that respond to the position of the head.

The *cochlea* is the spiral-shaped organ of hearing that is divided into two parts, the scala tympani and the scala vestibuli. Reissner's membrane stretches across the scala vestibuli and forms the duct of the cochlea, or the scala media. The scala media is filled with *endolymph*, a fluid that is similar to intracellular fluid. The scala tympani and scala vestibuli are filled with *perilymph*. These fluids are important in the protection of the cochlea and the semicircular canals because these structures literally float in the fluids, which cushion against abrupt movements of the head. The cochlea's basilar membrane is approximately 30 mm long and is composed of thousands of fibers. The *organ of Corti*, the receptor end organ of hearing, is found on this membrane and contains hair cells resting on the fibers of the basilar membrane, which are surrounded by the cochlear division of the eighth cranial nerve. The *eighth cranial nerve* has two branches: the cochlear and the vestibular. The cochlear branch transmits neural impulses from the cochlea to the brain, where they are interpreted as sound.

FUNCTION

The main physiologic functions of the ear are hearing and the maintenance of balance. Hearing is accomplished when sound is delivered through the air to the external ear canal and the temporal bone covering the mastoid air cells. The sound waves strike the mastoid and the movable tympanic membrane, which is connected to the first bony ossicle, the malleus. The sound wave vibrations are transferred from the tympanic membrane to the malleus, the incus, and the stapes. From the stapes, the vibrations are transmitted to the cochlea. Receptors there transduce the vibrations into action potentials, which are conducted to the brain as neural impulses by the cochlear portion of the eighth cranial nerve. Thus, sound is processed and interpreted by the brain.

The semicircular canals are part of the vestibular apparatus. They are filled with fluid and composed of hair cells that are connected to the sensory nerve fibers of the vestibular portion of the eighth cranial nerve. When the client's head position changes, the hair cells are bent by the flow of fluid in the semicircular canals, which apprises the central nervous system of the client's relative position.

FOCUS ON THE ELDERLY ■ Ear and Hearing Changes Related to Aging

Structure/Function	Change	Interventions	Rationales
Pinna	The pinna becomes elongated because of normal loss of subcutaneous tissue and decreased tissue elasticity.		
Hair	Hair becomes coarser and longer, especially in men.		
Cerumen-producing glands	Glands decrease in number and function. However, cerumen tends to be drier in older clients; it becomes impacted, which causes hearing loss.	1. Irrigate ear canal weekly. 2. Place 1–2 drops of oil into ear canal 8 h before irrigation.	1. To remove excess cerumen, thus preventing impaction and enhancing transmission of sound waves. 2. To soften impacted cerumen, thus facilitating its removal.
Tympanic membrane	The membrane loses elasticity; it may normally appear dull and retracted.		
Bony ossicles	Ossicles have decreased movement.		
Cochlea	The cochlea undergoes degenerative changes.		
Vestibular function	Disturbed vestibular function results in occasional dizziness, vertigo, and sensations of unsteadiness in 50%–60% of older clients.	1. Assist client with standing and initial ambulation.	1. To provide a stable point of reference and to decrease the risk of falling as a result of vestibular disorientation.
Hearing acuity	Acuity diminishes with advancing age. The ability to hear high-frequency sounds is nearly gone by age 60 years, which affects speech reception and increases auditory reaction time greatly. Clients have particular difficulty with the f, s, sh, and pa sounds. Some older clients hear a persistent noise (tinnitus). Presbycusis (a sensorineural type of hearing loss) is common in the aged.	1. Establish that a hearing deficiency exists. 2. When speaking to an older client with a hearing deficiency, use the following measures. a. Provide a quiet environment. b. Face the client. c. Speak slowly in a deeper voice.	1. To determine whether interventions 2a–c are needed. Not all elderly clients have diminished hearing acuity. 2. To make it easier for client to hear and communicate. a. To reduce extraneous noise that may interfere with client's auditory perception. b. To allow client to see lip movement. c. To use frequencies that client may be able to discern more easily.

EAR AND HEARING CHANGES ASSOCIATED WITH AGING

Ear and hearing changes that are related to aging are summarized in the Focus on the Elderly feature on page 1079. Some of these changes are harmless; others pose serious threats to older clients and call for nursing interventions.

HISTORY

A thorough history is obtained from the client. Informal hearing assessment begins during the history taking as the client listens to and answers the nurse's interview questions. The nurse notes the client's posture and appropriateness of responses during the history taking to provide additional information about the client's hearing acuity.

During the interview, the nurse sits in good light facing the client, which allows the client to see the nurse speaking. The nurse is careful to use terminology that is understandable to the client and collects demographic data and information about personal and family history, use of medication, socioeconomic status, and current health problems.

DEMOGRAPHIC DATA

Establishment of *sex* is important in assessing hearing because some auditory disorders (e.g., otosclerosis) are more common in females, whereas others (e.g., Meniere's disease) are more common in males. Increasing *age* is a significant factor in hearing loss. The older client with hearing loss may rely on viewing the nurse's lip movement during conversation to understand speech sounds that they cannot hear. Most hearing loss beyond age 50 years is caused by either presbycusis or otosclerosis. *Race* is also determined because cerumen is generally moist and tan or brown in Caucasian and Black individuals but is dry and light brown to gray in Asians and Native Americans.

PERSONAL AND FAMILY HISTORY

Personal history includes information on past or current signs and symptoms of ear pain; ear discharge; vertigo; tinnitus; hearing change, including decreased hearing or difficulty in understanding people talk; and hearing noises. The nurse asks the client about any history of ear trauma, ear surgery, past infections, excessive cerumen,

ear itch, any invasive instruments that are routinely used to clean the ear, the type and pattern of ear hygiene, exposure to loud noise or music, air travel (especially in unpressurized aircraft), swimming habits, and the use of protective ear devices for swimming or noisy environments. The client is questioned about the use of a hearing aid and how well it works; and the date of the last hearing test, the type of test (audiometry or tympanometry [see under the later heading Other Diagnostic Studies]) given, and its results. Information on allergies; upper respiratory tract infection; hypothyroidism; arteriosclerosis; head trauma; and recent head, facial, or dental surgery is obtained because all of these conditions may contribute to hearing or equilibrium pathologic conditions. In addition, the nurse asks questions about occupation and hobbies that involve exposure to excessive environmental noise or music. The nurse investigates the client's use of protective ear devices and/or the use of any devices inserted into the ear such as telephone operator headsets or stethoscopes. Information about the incidence and type of hearing loss among family members is important to obtain because some types of hearing loss are hereditary or have a genetic component.

TABLE 37–1 Impact of Ototoxic Substances on Auditory and Vestibular Function

Drug	Auditory Problems*	Vestibular Problems*
Antibiotics		
Amikacin (Amikin)	+ to ++	+
Chloramphenicol (Chloromycetin)	+ to ++	+
Erythromycin (E-Mycin)	+ to ++	+
Gentamicin (Garamycin)	+ to ++	+
Streptomycin	+ to ++	+
Tobramycin (Nebcin)	+ to ++	+
Vancomycin (Vancocin)	++	+
Diuretics		
Acetazolamide (Diamox)	++	+
Furosemide (Lasix)	++	+
Ethacrynic acid (Edecrin)	++	+
Other Drugs		
Cisplatin (Platinol)	+	+
Nitrogen mustard	+	+
Quinine (Quinamm)	+	++
Quinidine (Quinaglute)	+	++
Alcohol	+	++

*Symbols: +, slight; ++, significant.

MEDICATION HISTORY

A thorough medication history is crucial because many drugs are ototoxic to the cochlea and vestibule and others cause dizziness (Table 37–1). Drugs that should provoke concern are alkylating agents, aminoglycosides, antimalarials, aspirin, quinine, and diuretics (ethacrynic acid, furosemide). Drugs that cause dizziness are antihypertensives, barbiturates, estrogens, oral contraceptives, and phenothiazines. These drugs cause dizziness not by damaging the inner ear, but by altering the function of the central nervous system.

SOCIOECONOMIC STATUS

The nurse needs to assess the socioeconomic status of the client and family to determine the availability of health care. Frequently, clients of lower socioeconomic status do not seek health care for ear-related problems until the damage to the hearing is extensive and difficult to treat or rehabilitate. However, clients at any position on the socioeconomic spectrum might hesitate to have their hearing loss diagnosed because they do not enjoy the thought of wearing a hearing amplification device.

CURRENT HEALTH PROBLEM

Current health problems related to the ear should be elicited by the nurse. The nurse asks if the client has noticed any "trouble with" his or her ears or has ear pain or ear discharge, including any problems with ear wax. The nurse asks the client if he or she has noticed any changes in hearing or any associated problems like ringing in the ears. If there are changes, the nurse asks whether one or both ears are involved and whether the changes occurred suddenly or gradually. The nurse also asks the client if there are any problems with balance or if there is a sense of dizziness.

The existence of current medical conditions that are not strictly associated with the ear and their treatments should be determined. Such conditions as allergies, upper respiratory tract infections, diabetes mellitus, hypothyroidism, hypertension, arteriosclerosis, head trauma, and recent head, facial, or dental surgery, as well as the medications used to treat them, may cause hearing and/or equilibrium problems.

PHYSICAL ASSESSMENT

Inspection and *palpation* are the only examination techniques that are used for assessment of the ear. The ears are not auscultated or percussed. The examination begins by placing the client in either a sitting or a supine position. Uncooperative clients are carefully restrained to prevent injury to the external canal. If the client wears a hearing aid, the client should remove it and carefully place it on a safe surface during the examination. The nurse inspects the hearing aid for cracks and debris and for a proper fit after the otoscopic examination.

Assessment of the ears is divided into (1) examination of the external ear and mastoid, (2) the otoscopic examination, and (3) tests of auditory and vestibular function.

EXTERNAL-EAR AND MASTOID ASSESSMENT

The *mastoid process* is inspected for redness and swelling indicative of inflammation. The nurse gently taps with one finger over the mastoid process. Pressure or a tapping over the mastoid process normally does not elicit pain. The nurse compresses the tragus with one finger to assess for tenderness. Tragus compression is also normally painless. For an adult, the nurse manipulates the external pinna forward and back. If there is any tenderness caused by pressure over the mastoid, manipulation of the pinna, or compression of the tragus, an inflammatory process in either the external canal or the mastoid is suspected.

The entire *external ear*, or pinna, is bilaterally inspected for configuration, location or attachment to the head, and condition of the visible external canal. The normal pinna is uniformly shaped without evidence of additional skin tags or deformity. The pinna should be attached vertically to the side of the head with no greater than a 10-degree posterior angle, and it should fall within or touch the eye-occiput line. The eye-occiput line is an imaginary line drawn from the greatest protuberance on the occiput to the lateral canthus of the eye. If the top of the pinna falls below the level of the eye-occiput line, the angle of attachment varies, and/or the pinna configuration reveals deformity, the client should be examined for congenital renal anomalies or chromosomal aberrations. The normal pinna has no lesions. Abnormalities include nodules and lesions. In chronic gout, accumulations of sodium urate crystals result in hard, irregular, painless nodules called tophi that are seen on the helix and antihelix portions of the pinna. Other painless nodules on the pinna might be due to basal cell carcinoma or rheumatoid arthritis. A small, crusted, ulcerated or indurated lesion on the pinna that fails to heal promptly could be a squamous cell carcinoma.

The normal external canal is free from lesions and is dry, clean, and not reddened. The nurse assesses for abnormalities including furuncles (circumscribed inflammation of a single hair follicle), large accumulations of cerumen resulting from poor hygiene, scaliness, redness, and swelling or drainage from the ear that could be associated with the presence of a foreign object, trauma, or infection. Drainage can be blood, cerebrospinal fluid, pus, or serous fluid.

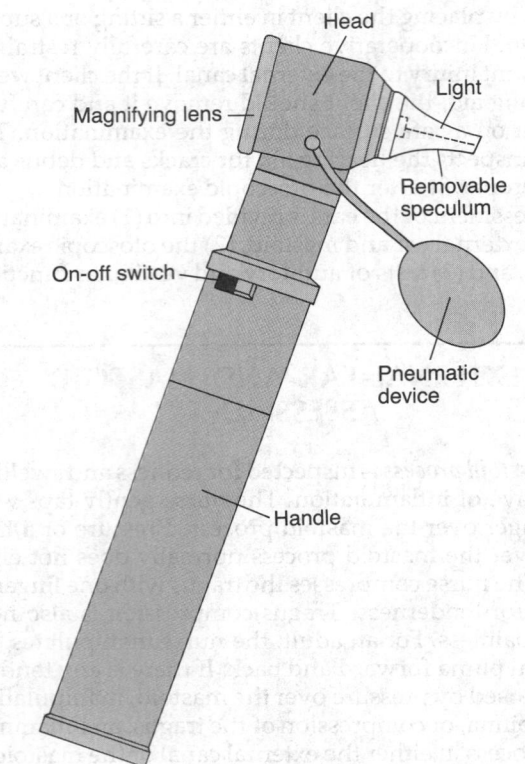

Head

Light

Magnifying lens

Removable speculum

On-off switch

Pneumatic device

Handle

Figure 37–5

Functional components of an otoscope.

OTOSCOPIC ASSESSMENT

A special instrument called an *otoscope* is used to examine the ear. Many types are available, but they all consist of the following parts: light, handle, magnifying lens, and pneumatic device attachment for injecting air into the external canal to test mobility of the tympanic membrane (Fig. 37–5).

Otoscopes have specula of various sizes that are attached to the head of the otoscope. The specula vary in the size of the diameter opening. The largest diameter that most comfortably fits the client's external canal is selected for the examination. Because the length of the external canal to the tympanic membrane varies with age, the speculum is never blindly introduced into the external canal because of the risk of perforating the tympanic membrane. The light of the otoscope should be bright and white. If the light appears to be yellowish or dim, the power source for the otoscope handle needs to be checked. Otoscope handles are powered by either alkaline or rechargeable batteries.

If any pain is elicited during examination of the external ear, a cautious otoscopic examination is attempted because the speculum causes extreme pain if it comes in contact with inflamed tissue in the external canal. It is especially important that the nurse become familiar with and memorize all the structures of the

tympanic membrane and middle ear before attempting to visualize these structures with an otoscope.

When performing an otoscopic examination, the nurse tilts the client's head slightly away and holds the otoscope upside down as if it were a large pen, as shown in Figure 37–6. This position permits the nurse's hand to lie against the client's head for support. If the client were to move, both the nurse's hand and otoscope would move with the client's head, thus preventing damage to the highly sensitive and friable external canal. The nurse holds the otoscope in the dominant hand and displaces the pinna with the nondominant hand. The nurse pulls the pinna up and back to straighten the external canal to accept the otoscope speculum. The nurse visualizes the external canal while slowly inserting the speculum. The nurse uses caution and avoids jamming the speculum into the walls of the external canal, which causes pain.

After the pinna is correctly displaced and the otoscope is comfortably introduced in the external canal, the following observations are noted: color, intactness, presence of lesions, and amount and consistency of cerumen and hair. The normal external canal is pink, intact, without lesions, and with various amounts of soft, tan, brown, or gray cerumen and fine little hairs.

Next, the nurse bilaterally assesses the *tympanic membranes* for intactness, the normal structures seen through the tympanic membrane (the long process of the malleus, the short process of the malleus, and the umbo), sites on the tympanic membrane itself (light reflex [see later], pars flaccida, and pars tensa), and color, shape, lesions, and mobility. The normal tympanic membrane is always intact, not perforated. Careful visualization of the entire tympanic membrane, including the complete border of the annulus, pars tensa, and pars flaccida, is conducted. The long process of the malleus is seen through the tympanic membrane as a whitish streak extending from the short process of the malleus to the umbo. A normal variation that is seen in some persons with allergies is evidence of vascularity over the long process, although this vascularity might be an early indication of otitis media.

The short process of the malleus is seen through the tympanic membrane as a white structure, which seems more three-dimensional than the other structures on the tympanic membrane. It also seems to project out toward the otoscope. The umbo is the site where the malleus is connected to the tympanic membrane, and it appears as a round, white dot.

The long process of the malleus, the short process of the malleus, and the umbo are always easily identified in the normal ear. Abnormal variations of these structures are caused by serous otitis media and otitis media, among other disorders.

The otoscope light reflecting off the tympanic membrane reveals what is called the *light reflex*. In the normal ear, there should be a clearly demarcated triangle of light, with the base of the triangle on the annulus and the point of the triangle on the umbo. The base of the light reflex is to the right in the right ear and to the left in

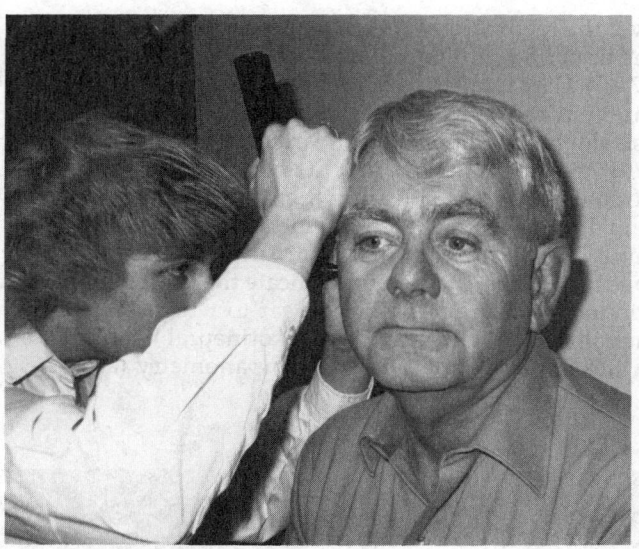

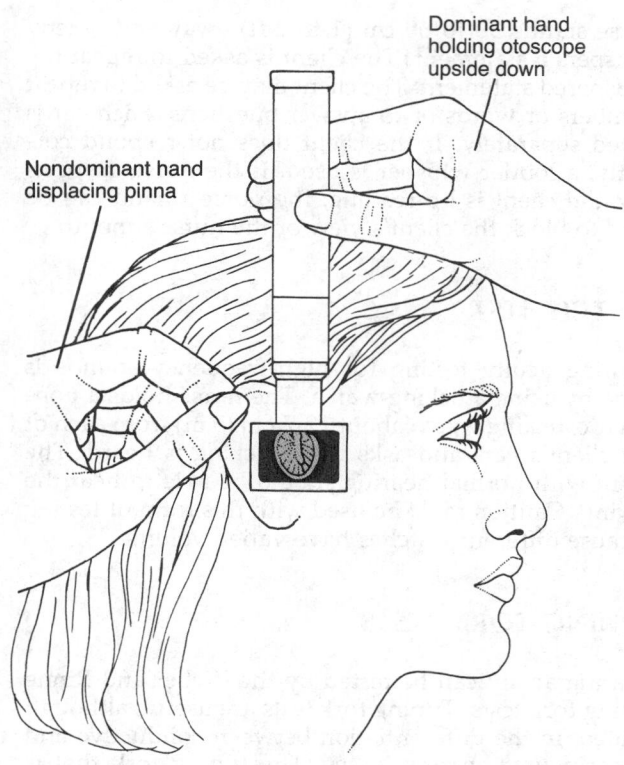

Dominant hand
holding otoscope
upside down

Nondominant hand
displacing pinna

Figure 37–6

Proper technique for an otoscopic examination.

the left ear. When the light reflex is spotty or multiple as a result of a changed shape of the tympanic membrane from either retraction or bulging, the light reflex is referred to as diffuse.

The color of the tympanic membrane is normally described as transparent, opaque, or pearly gray. Abnormal variations include red (often called injected), as seen in otitis media, and dull or retracted, as often seen in serous otitis.

The normal shape of the tympanic membrane is slightly concave. The shape of the tympanic membrane allows the pars tensa portion of the membrane to move gently when tested with a puff of air from the pneumatic device on the otoscope. Variations in the shape of the tympanic membrane result from obstruction of the eustachian tube or from excessive fluid in the middle ear. These variations and changes in consistency limit the mobility of the tympanic membrane.

The normal tympanic membrane is free from lesions. The most common lesion is scarring caused by previous ear infection and perforation. A scar thickens the tympanic membrane and makes it difficult or impossible to see through the membrane at the point of the scar. A scar can also reduce the mobility of the tympanic membrane.

Mobility of both tympanic membranes is tested by injecting a small puff of air via the pneumatic device on the otoscope into the external canal and watching for the pars tensa portion of the tympanic membrane for movement. The normal tympanic membrane moves gently with this procedure. Decreased or absent mobil-

ity of the tympanic membrane results from scarring, retraction, or bulging.

AUDITORY ASSESSMENT

After completing bilateral external-ear and otoscopic examinations, the nurse assesses the client's hearing acuity. Sound is transmitted by two routes, *air conduction* and *bone conduction*. Air conduction normally takes two to three times longer than bone conduction. If hearing acuity is decreased, the hearing loss is categorized into three types: conductive, sensorineural, and mixed conductive and sensorineural.

A *conductive hearing loss* is due to any physical obstruction to the transmission of sound waves, such as a foreign body in the external canal, a retracted or bulging tympanic membrane, or fused bony ossicles. A *sensorineural hearing loss* is due to a defect in the organ of hearing (cochlea), in the eighth cranial nerve (auditory nerve), or in the brain itself. A *mixed conductive-sensorineural hearing loss* results in a profound hearing loss. Each of the auditory function tests is devised to determine presence of hearing loss, as well as to differentiate the type of loss.

VOICE TEST

A simple hearing acuity test can be accomplished by asking the client to block one external canal while the nurse stands 30 to 60 cm (1 to 2 ft) away and quietly whispers a statement. The client is asked to repeat the whispered statement. The client may be asked to repeat numbers or words or to answer questions. Each ear is tested separately. If the client does not respond correctly, a louder whisper is used. If the nurse suspects that the client is lip-reading, the nurse's hand can be used to block the client's view of the nurse's mouth.

WATCH TEST

Hearing acuity testing for high-frequency sounds is done by using a ticking watch. The nurse holds a non-electric, ticking watch about 12.7 cm (5 in) from each of the client's ears and asks if the ticking is heard. The client with normal hearing should be able to hear the ticking. Caution must be used with this form of testing because different watches have varied volume.

TUNING FORK TESTS

Hearing acuity can be tested by the Weber and Rinne tuning fork tests. Tuning fork tests are useful, although limited, in the differentiation between conductive and sensorineural hearing losses. The tuning fork that is used for these tests is one that corresponds to the frequency range of normal speech, i.e., 512 or 1024 cycles per second (cps), or hertz. Hertz (Hz) is an international term that is equivalent to cycles per second, or the measurement of the number of vibrations per second. The client sits for the assessment while the nurse stands in front of the client.

The *Weber tuning fork test* is performed by placing the vibrating tuning fork in the middle of the client's head, at the midline of the forehead, or above the upper lip

over the teeth. Many clients object to the vibration over the upper lip, so the preferred site is midline skull (Fig. 37–7). Care is taken to hold the vibrating tuning fork by the stem only, not by the vibrating forks. The client is asked whether the sound is heard equally in both ears or whether the sound is louder in one ear or the other. The normal test result is hearing the sound equally in both ears. If the client hears the sound louder in one ear, the term *lateralization* is applied to the side hearing the loudest. Such a finding may indicate that the client has a conductive hearing loss in the ear to which the sound lateralized, or that there is a sensorineural hearing loss in the opposite ear. Without tympanometry (a test of

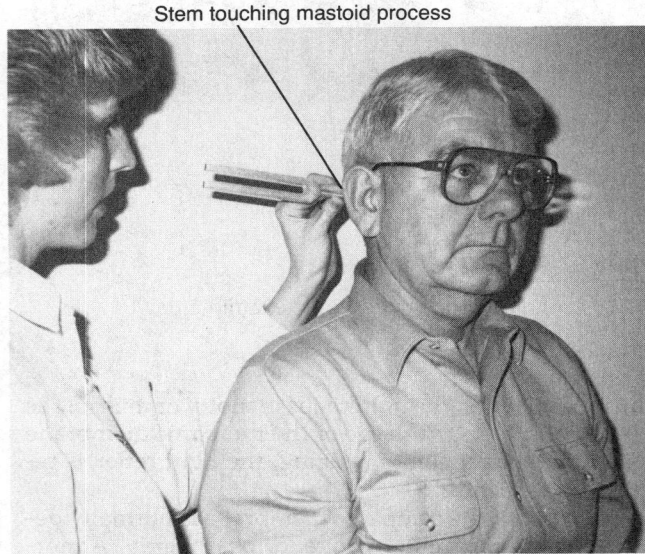

Stem touching mastoid process

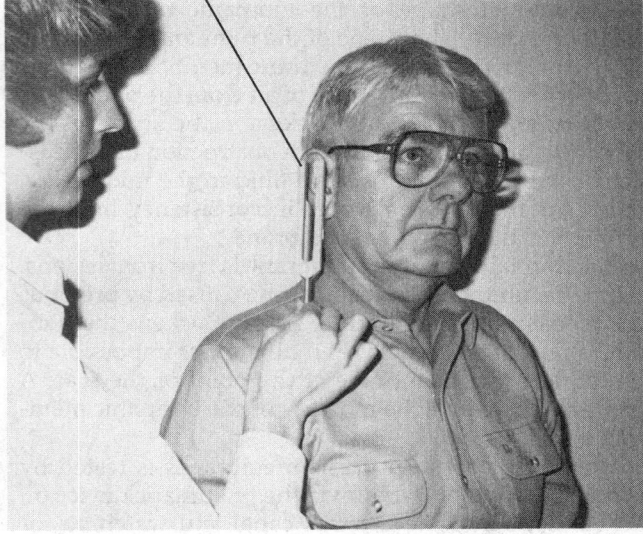

Tuning fork held in front of, but not touching, client's ear

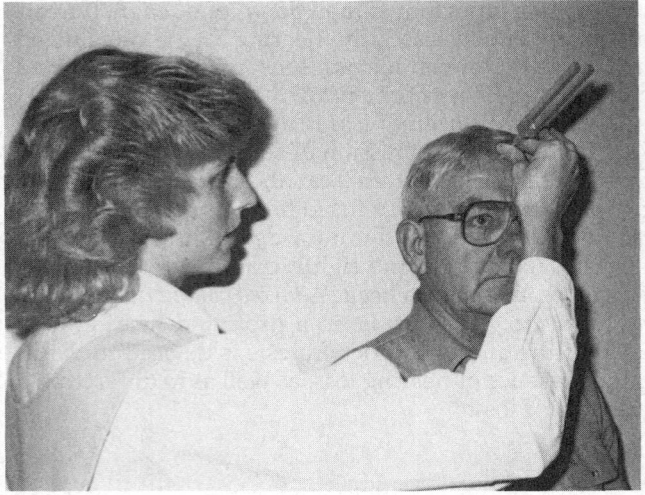

Figure 37–7
Correct placement of the tuning fork for the Weber test.

Figure 37–8
Correct placement of tuning forks for the Rinne test.

tympanic membrane mobility), the nurse is not able to distinguish the type of hearing loss.

The *Rinne tuning fork test* compares the client's hearing by air conduction and bone conduction. Normally, air conduction is two to three times greater than bone conduction. The Rinne tuning fork test is performed by placing the vibrating tuning fork stem on the client's mastoid process and asking the client to indicate when he or she no longer hears the sound. As the client indicates this moment, the nurse quickly brings the tuning fork in front of the pinna without touching the client and asks the client to indicate if he or she still hears the sound (Fig. 37–8). The nurse records the duration of both phases, bone conduction followed by air conduction, and compares the times. The client normally continues to hear the sound two times longer in front of the pinna after not hearing it with the tuning fork touching the mastoid process. Such results are a *positive* Rinne test. If the client is unable to hear the sound through the air in front of the pinna, the client may have a conductive hearing loss on the side tested because bone conduction is greater than air conduction. These results are a *negative* Rinne test. Because air conduction is normally greater than bone conduction with a sensorineural hearing loss, the Rinne tuning fork test is of no value in determining sensorineural hearing loss.

VESTIBULAR ASSESSMENT

The vestibular function of the ear can be evaluated by the test for falling (Romberg's test), the test for past pointing, assay of gaze nystagmus, or the Hallpike maneuver (see also under the later heading Vestibular Tests in the section on other diagnostic studies). To conduct the *test for falling,* the nurse asks the client to stand with feet together, arms hanging loosely at the sides, and eyes closed. The client is assured that the nurse is nearby to prevent a fall if there is a loss of balance. The client normally remains erect with only slight swaying. A significant sway or a fall is a positive Romberg sign, and referral to a physician is needed.

The *test for past pointing* is conducted with the client sitting in front of the nurse. The nurse instructs the client to close the eyes and extend the arms in front, pointing both index fingers at the nurse. The nurse holds and touches his or her own extended index fingers under the extended index fingers of the client to give the client a point of reference. The nurse instructs the client to raise both arms and then lower them, attempting to return to the nurse's extended index fingers. The normal test result is for the client to easily return to the point of reference. Clients with vestibular function problems lack a normal sense of position and are unable to return their extended fingers to the point of reference. Instead, they deviate to either the right or the left of the reference point.

Gaze nystagmus evaluation is done by examining the client's eyes as they look straight ahead, 30 degrees to each side, upward and downward. Any spontaneous nystagmus (a constant, involuntary, cyclic movement of the eyeball in any direction) represents problems with the vestibular system.

The *Hallpike maneuver* assesses for benign paroxysmal positional vertigo or induced dizziness. In this test, the client assumes a supine position. The head is rotated to one side for 1 minute. A positive test results in nystagmus (eye movements) after 5 to 10 seconds, and a follow-up referral is needed.

PSYCHOSOCIAL ASSESSMENT

Clients may behave in an irritable manner if they are frustrated by an inability to hear and to respond appropriately. Depression may also result from the sensory isolation that hearing loss sometimes involves. The nurse needs to be sensitive to the client and conduct the interview at a pace that is appropriate for the client.

The inability to hear results in frustrating experiences and often isolates clients from the world in which they live and work. The nurse investigates the client's social and work relationships in an attempt to see if the client experiences isolation as a result of hearing problems. In addition, the nurse encourages the client to express feelings related to the sensory loss and to discuss what changes in daily living activities have been tried to cope with the loss. It may be valuable to obtain information from family members as well, especially if the client denies problems with hearing. Throughout the assessment, the nurse remains patient and empathic.

DIAGNOSTIC ASSESSMENT

LABORATORY TESTS

Infections of the external canal can be assessed if discharge from the auditory canal exists. The etiologic agent is determined via microbiologic culture and sensitivity assays. However, the presence of certain organisms in the external ear usually reflects normal microbial flora. These organisms include a fungus, non–*albicans Candida* species, and the following bacteria: *Bacillus* species, diphtheroids, *Gaffkya tetragena, Lactobacillus* species, *Klebsiella* species, *Propionibacterium acnes, Staphylococcus* species, *Streptococcus mitis,* and *Streptococcus pneumoniae.* The middle ear and inner ear are normally sterile. Bacteria are the most common pathogens invading the middle and inner ear.

Collection of ear discharge is conducted with aseptic

technique in which a sterile cotton-tipped swab and sterile collection container are used. The external ear is first cleaned before the culture procedure to remove contaminating bacteria on the surface. The external ear is cleaned with a 1:1000 aqueous solution of benzalkonium chloride, a detergent. The nurse swabs any discharge firmly, without rubbing the culture site, and transports the specimen to the laboratory as soon as possible.

A complete blood cell count with differential may be useful in detecting systemic inflammation with its origin in the ear. In this case, there is an increased white blood cell count (leukocytosis) with a left shift differential of neutrophils. In addition, any clear fluid drainage from the ear or from a surgical ear incision is tested for the presence of cerebrospinal fluid. This test is done by determining the presence of glucose (a normal component of cerebrospinal fluid) in the drainage with a Dextrostix.

RADIOGRAPHIC EXAMINATIONS

TOMOGRAPHY

Tomography is an x-ray method that allows examination of a single layer or plane of tissue by blurring the tissues above and below the level being examined. This method provides exacting detail and can be used to assess the mastoid, middle-ear structures, and inner-ear structures for the presence of pathologic conditions. This highly sophisticated test aids in the diagnosis of both conductive and sensorineural hearing losses.

Client preparation. Careful explanation of the procedure and the purpose of tomography should be given the client before the procedure. The nurse informs the client that tomography requires approximately 45 minutes to complete. The nurse asks women clients if they are pregnant because clients in the first trimester of pregnancy should delay tomography. All jewelry is removed before the procedure.

Procedure. Women in the latter phases of pregnancy are protected with a lead apron over the abdomen and pelvic areas. All clients are shielded with lead eyeshields covering the cornea to diminish the radiation dose to the eyes. Clients must remain quite still in a supine position during the procedure.

Follow-up care. No special follow-up care is needed.

PLANE FILM X-RAY STUDIES

Routine x-ray films of the temporal bone are not of significant value except for diagnosis of glomus tumors of the ear because of the blurring effect of plane x-rays.

POLYTOME X-RAY STUDIES

Polytome x-ray films, with or without contrast, are especially helpful in the diagnosis of any lesion of the temporal bone. Several polytome cuts of 1 mm are made, which allow extreme clarity of all structures within the temporal bone.

COMPUTED TOMOGRAPHY

Computed tomography (CT), with or without contrast, in which multiple x-ray films of the head are made and a computer averages the responses, can reveal the structures of the ear in great detail. CT is especially helpful in the diagnosis of acoustic tumors.

ARTERIOGRAPHY AND VENOGRAPHY

When the polytome x-ray films are positive and a tumor is suspected, arteriography may be done. This technique involves inserting a catheter in the carotid artery to determine the vascularity and origin of blood supply for the tumor by roentgenography. Venography is usually done if the polytome x-ray films do not clearly show involvement of the jugular bulb of the carotid canal. This procedure involves roentgenography after threading a catheter into the jugular vein or the femoral vein.

OTHER DIAGNOSTIC STUDIES

MAGNETIC RESONANCE IMAGING

Magnetic resonance imaging (MRI) is a noninvasive, nonradioactive diagnostic tool that generates images via a computer. There are few known biologic hazards with MRI, which has numerous advantages over plane roentgenography and CT in the evaluation of the eighth cranial nerve. It is quite sensitive to soft-tissue changes, and, because of its superior contrast resolution so that no bony artifacts can obscure tissue, it can detect subtle alterations in tissue. Clients with internal metal vascular clips cannot have MRI.

AUDIOMETRY

Audiometry is the measurement of hearing acuity. To understand audiometry, the nurse must first understand certain terms that are used in audiometric testing.

Frequency refers to the highness or lowness of tones, expressed in hertz, or the number of vibrations per second. The greater the number of vibrations per second, the higher the frequency (pitch) of the sound. The fewer the number of vibrations per second, the lower the frequency of the sound.

Persons with loss of hearing primarily high-frequency sound (e.g., persons who have been exposed to high levels of noise or those with presbycusis, or hearing loss in older age) usually demonstrate difficulty in understanding the speech of others. This situation exists because approximately one-third of the sounds of American English are of high frequency.

The *intensity* of sound is expressed in decibels (dB). The lowest intensity at which a young normal ear can just detect the presence of sound about 50% of the time is 0 dB. Sound at 110 dB is so intense (loud) that it would be painful for most persons who have normal hearing. Conversational speech is generally around 60 dB. A soft whisper is usually around 20 dB (Table 37 – 2). A hearing loss of 45 to 50 dB would render the person unable to hear speech without the use of a hearing aid. A person with a hearing loss of 90 dB may not be able to hear speech even with the use of a hearing aid.

Threshold is the lowest level of intensity at which pure tones and speech are heard by a particular client about 50% of the time.

Pure tones are sounds generated by an *audiometer* (Fig. 37 – 9) for the purpose of determining the acuity of hearing. Pure tone audiometers have been used as devices for determining thresholds of hearing for almost 100 years.

There are two types of audiometry: pure tone audiometry and speech audiometry.

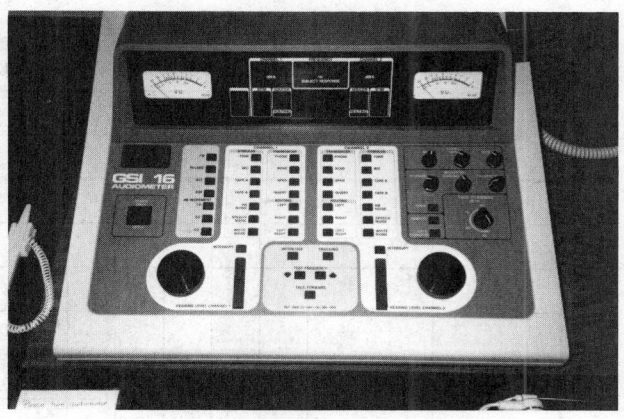

Figure 37 – 9

A pure tone audiometer.

In *pure tone audiometry*, tones generated by an audiometer are presented to the client at various frequencies that are important for hearing speech, music, and other sounds of the environment. Pure tone audiometry is performed by air conduction testing or bone conduction testing. *Pure tone air conduction testing* is used to determine whether a client's hearing is within normal limits or whether there is a hearing loss. *Pure tone bone conduction testing* is used to determine whether the loss detected by air conduction testing is due to conductive or sensorineural factors, or to a combination of the two. It is used only when the results of air conduction testing are abnormal. The results of pure tone audiometry are plotted on an *audiogram* (Fig. 37 – 10).

They are designed to test air conduction hearing sensitivity (through earphones) at frequencies of 125, 250, 500, 750, 1000, 1500, 2000, 3000, 4000, 6000, and 8000 Hz, but thresholds are usually confined to the frequencies of 250, 500, 1000, 2000, 4000, and 8000 Hz. The intensities for administering the pure tone testing generally range from −10 to 110 dB.

For testing by bone conduction, there are restrictions on both frequency and intensity of the sound produced by the device. The frequencies are usually restricted to those between 250 and 4000 Hz. Maximal outputs for bone conduction are also lower, mainly because the power required to drive a bone conduction oscillator enough to cause the skull to vibrate is great.

In addition to air conduction and bone conduction capabilities, a *masking* control is often provided to allow for introduction of a noise to the ear not being tested as needed during audiometric testing. The use of masking is important if the hearing loss in one ear is severe. In this case, the tester will want to be assured that the non – test ear is not participating in the test. If masking is not used in the non – test ear, the intensity of the tone being presented to the test ear can stimulate the non – test ear, and the client being tested begins responding to

TABLE 37 – 2 Decibel Intensity and Safe Exposure Time for Common Sounds

Sound	Decibel Intensity (dB)	Safe Exposure Time*
Threshold of hearing	0	
Whispering	20	
Average residence or office	40	
Conversational speech	60	
Car traffic	70	> 8 h
Motorcycle	90	8 h
Chain saw	100	2 h
Rock concert, front row	120	3 min
Jet engine	140	Immediate danger
Rocket launching pad	180	Immediate danger

*For every 5-dB increase in intensity, the safe exposure time is cut in half.

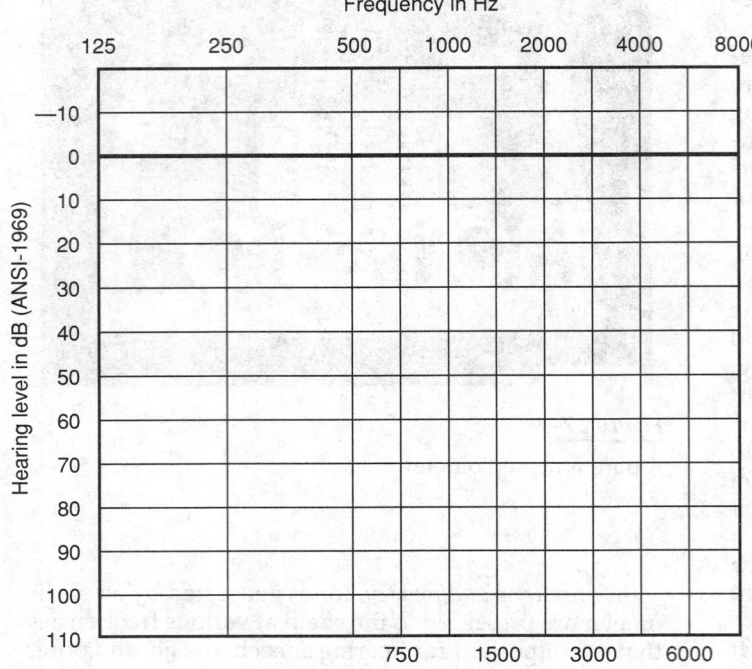

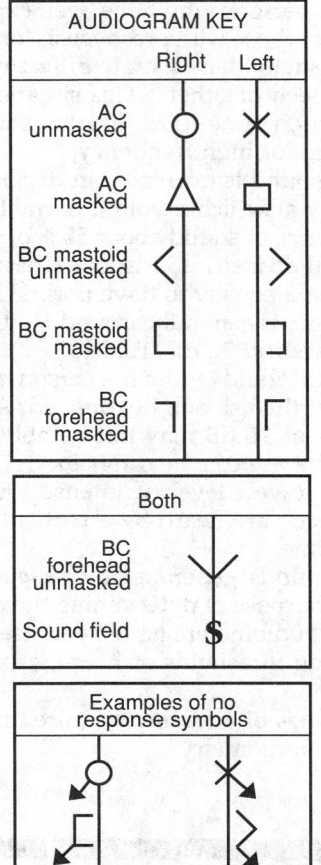

Figure 37–10

A typical audiogram. (Hayes A. Newby/Gerald R. Popelka, AUDIOL-OGY, 5e, © 1985, pp. 146, 151, 152, 155. Adapted by permission of Prentice-Hall, Inc., Englewood Cliffs, New Jersey.)

what is heard by the non–test ear instead of the ear that is being tested.

In *speech audiometry*, the client's ability to hear spoken words is measured through a microphone connected to an audiometer (see under later heading Speech Audiometry). The two components of speech audiometry are the speech reception threshold and speech discrimination. The speech reception threshold is the level of intensity at which a client can repeat simple words. Speech discrimination testing establishes the client's ability to discriminate among similar sounds or among words that contain similar sounds.

Pure Tone Audiometry

Air Conduction Testing

Client preparation. The client is placed in a sound-isolated room in which the ambient noise level does not exceed standards established by the American National Standards Institute. The room need not be commercially

prefabricated, but it should be carefully designed and constructed to meet these standards.

The nurse sits facing the client because the client's facial expressions are frequently helpful in evaluating responses. Hearing-impaired clients may benefit from being able to lip-read the nurse's instructions. The nurse instructs the client as follows.

"I am going to test your hearing. The object of the test is to find the point at which you can just barely hear the tones that I will present. The tones will sound like those of soft bells or tuning forks. Every time you hear one, no matter how soft it is, signal by raising your hand (or pushing the button) on the side on which you hear the tone. [If the client is unable to raise a hand or push a button because of physical or motor disabilities, it is appropriate to use a "yes-no" verbal response.] When you no longer hear the tone, lower your hand (or release the button). These are your signals to let me know when you hear the tone and when the tone goes away.

"Do you hear better in one ear than in the other? If so, we will test the ear with better hearing first. If not, we will begin with your right ear. Remember, no matter how soft the tone becomes, raise your hand on the side on which you hear it. Now, we will begin."

Procedure. Before beginning the actual test, the nurse checks the audiometric equipment, as follows:

1. Set the frequency control at 1000 Hz and the hearing level control at 40 dB.
2. Put on the earphones and listen to the tone as you switch from one ear to the other.
3. In each earphone, listen to the tone as you gradually turn the hearing level control toward the 0-dB hearing level. If you have normal hearing, you should still be able to hear the tone at the near 0-dB level.
4. If you plan to have the client use the signal cord and light during the procedure, test them to make sure that they are working.

The nurse follows the steps given in the accompanying Guidelines feature to obtain a profile of a client's hearing for pure tones across the frequencies tested, from low to high frequencies. The frequencies usually tested are 250 (middle C on the piano), 500, 1000, 2000, 4000, and 8000 Hz.

Follow-up care. No special follow-up care is needed.

Bone Conduction Testing

Client preparation. The nurse explains that hearing sensitivity for bone conduction is now going to be checked and that the sounds and type of response to them will be the same as those used for air conduction testing.

Procedure. Theoretically, the ear with greater acuity should be tested first, as in air conduction testing. However, it is difficult to tell which ear possesses better hearing for bone conduction without further testing. It is desirable to perform the Weber test, as described earlier, to determine the better-hearing ear by bone conduction. If neither ear is "better," it makes no difference which ear is tested first.

The bone conduction vibrator is placed behind the pinna, firmly on the mastoid process. If masking is not used during the bone conduction testing, the opposite ear must not be covered with an air conduction earphone. To do so creates a moderate degree of air conduction loss in the opposite ear. The tone may cross over to that ear, and the testee may then actually be responding to sound in the wrong ear.

The nurse then follows steps 4 through 9 of the Procedure for Pure Tone Air Conduction Audiometry, as given in the Guidelines feature just cited. However, *it is important to remember the restrictions that are placed on both the intensity and the frequency used in bone conduction testing.* They are usually described on the face of the audiometer.

Follow-up care. No special follow-up care is needed.

GUIDELINES ■ Procedure for Pure Tone Air Conduction Audiometry

1. After explaining the procedure to the client as outlined under the text heading Client Preparation, the nurse places the earphones on the client, making sure that the side marked *left* is on the left ear and the side marked *right* is on the right ear. The earphones must cover the ears.
2. Test the ear with better hearing first if the client reports a probable difference between the two ears.
3. Begin the testing at 1000 Hz because this frequency is near the middle of the ear's sensitivity spectrum. Also, it has been demonstrated to have good test-retest reliability.
4. Adjust the audiometer so that the tone is inaudible unless the interrupter switch is depressed. Start with the hearing level control at its minimal reading, either 0 or −10 dB. Depress the interrupter switch and gradually increase the intensity of the tone until the client signals that the tone is heard. Increase the intensity of the tone beyond this point by about 20 dB to give the client an opportunity to hear it well.
5. Now, reduce the intensity of the tone in 5-dB steps until the client indicates that the tone is no longer heard. Note the last intensity level, in the 5-dB decrement steps, at which the client signaled that the tone was still heard. The last point at which the client indicated that the tone was still heard should be his
   or her threshold for hearing for that frequency. The threshold can be tested for reliability by increasing the tone by 20 dB once again and then descending in 5-dB steps until once again the lowest point in intensity at which the client last responded is reached.
6. If you have succeeded in obtaining a consistent threshold picture at 1000 Hz, change the frequency control to 500 Hz and start again. The preferred method is to test the lower frequencies first (500 and 250 Hz) and then to move to those higher than 1000 Hz, usually 2000, 4000, and 8000 Hz. At each frequency, the procedure is the same as that suggested for 1000 Hz.
7. After completing the threshold measurements on the first ear, switch the output selector to the opposite earphone and proceed in the same manner to obtain thresholds for the other ear, also beginning at 1000 Hz.
8. If the thresholds of the second ear appear to differ by 40 dB or more from those of the first ear, masking of the better-hearing ear is indicated to rule out its participation in the test.
9. Make sure that in operating the interrupter switch, you do not fall into rhythmic patterns that the client can follow. The pattern of tonal presentations should be irregular so that the client cannot predict when the tone will be presented.

Interpretation of Results

Audiometric evaluation is conducted to determine whether the client being tested possesses hearing that is within normal limits, or, in the instance of a hearing impairment, whether the hearing loss is conductive, sensorineural, or mixed. The type can be determined by observing the configuration of the audiogram on completion of pure tone air and bone conduction audiometry.

In the hands of an experienced clinician, the audiometer is a useful tool for obtaining measures of the extent and type of hearing loss. When evaluating results of a hearing test, the individual who performed the test and the reliability of the responses of the client must be considered. Unfortunately, some physicians and educators tend to accept audiograms at face value, without regard for the conditions under which the tests were administered, or by whom, or on whom. The audiogram is the best *estimate* by the diagnostician of the state of the client's hearing, based on the observations of the client's auditory behavior in the testing situation.

Normal hearing. Figure 37–11 is an audiogram showing normal results of air conduction and bone conduction tests. Hearing is generally considered to be normal when the pure tone thresholds are at 10 dB or better. The 0-dB line on the audiogram represents the hearing thresholds of a young person who possesses an optimally functioning hearing mechanism.

Conductive hearing loss. Figure 37–12 shows the audiometric configuration of a conductive loss. A *pure* conductive loss is a result of a middle-ear pathologic condition or of a blockage of sound from passing along the external auditory meatus. The inner ear (cochlea) may be perfectly functional, but sound is blocked from stimulating it. The audiometric results reveal normal to near-normal hearing by bone conduction and a hearing loss by air conduction. Even though the majority of conductive hearing losses are shown in a relatively flat audiometric configuration, this configuration cannot be used alone when diagnosing a conductive hearing loss. Sensorineural hearing losses can also show a flat audio-

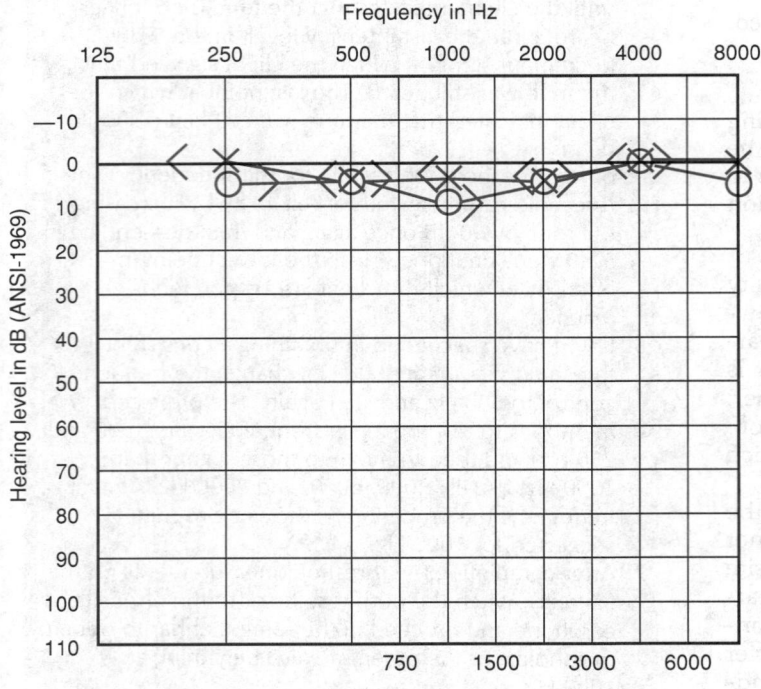

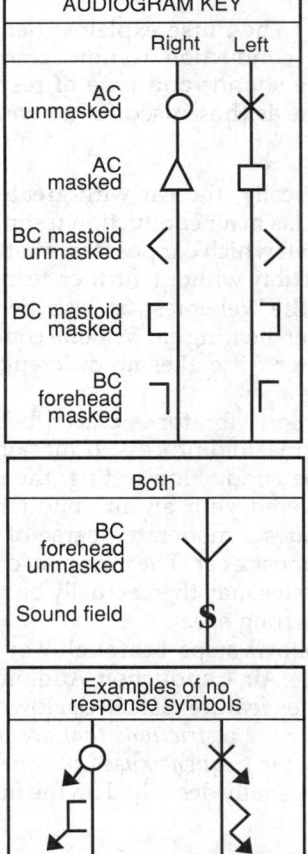

Figure 37–11

Audiogram pattern depicting normal hearing. (Hayes A. Newby/Gerald R. Popelka, AUDIOLOGY, 5e, © 1985, pp. 146, 151, 152, 155. Adapted by permission of Prentice-Hall, Inc., Englewood Cliffs, New Jersey.)

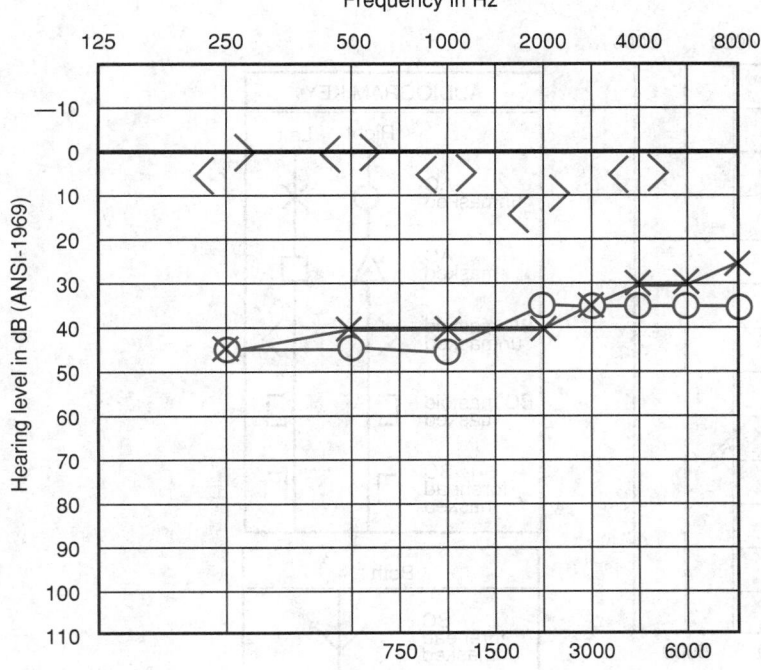

Frequency in Hz

AUDIOGRAM KEY

Figure 37–12

Audiogram pattern depicting conductive hearing loss. (Hayes A. Newby/Gerald R. Popelka, AUDIOLOGY, 5e, © 1985, pp. 146, 151, 152, 155. Adapted by permission of Prentice-Hall, Inc., Englewood Cliffs, New Jersey.)

metric configuration. Both air and bone conduction scores must be included in the evaluation.

Sensorineural hearing loss.   Figure 37–13 is an audiogram that reveals a sensorineural hearing loss. Typically, but not always, the audiometric configuration shows a greater loss of hearing in the higher frequencies than in the lower frequencies. However, sensorineural losses can also be relatively equal in the extent of loss, and a flat configuration across the audiogram can be seen. In all cases, air and bone conduction scores are essentially equal. That is, the scores by bone conduction match the audiometric hearing thresholds by air conduction. It is not unusual to find individuals who possess better hearing in one ear than the other.

The etiology of sensorineural hearing impairments cannot be determined by the audiometric results.

Mixed hearing loss.   Figure 37–14 is an audiogram that reveals a mixed type of hearing loss. The configuration is that of a loss of hearing sensitivity for both bone

conduction and air conduction. For example, the individual may possess middle-ear pathologic features caused by infection and may also have previously sustained a sensorineural loss caused by excessive noise exposure. This situation would be revealed audiometrically as a conductive hearing loss in the low frequencies and a sensorineural hearing loss in the high frequencies.

Speech Audiometry

Speech Reception Threshold

In testing the threshold for the reception of speech, the nurse tries to determine how intense a simple speech stimulus must be before the client can hear it well enough to repeat it correctly. The purpose is to find the intensity level at which the client can repeat simple words. This level is referred to as the client's *speech reception threshold.* In one common test, lists of two-syllable words are used. These words are referred to as *spondee,* i.e., words in which there is generally equal

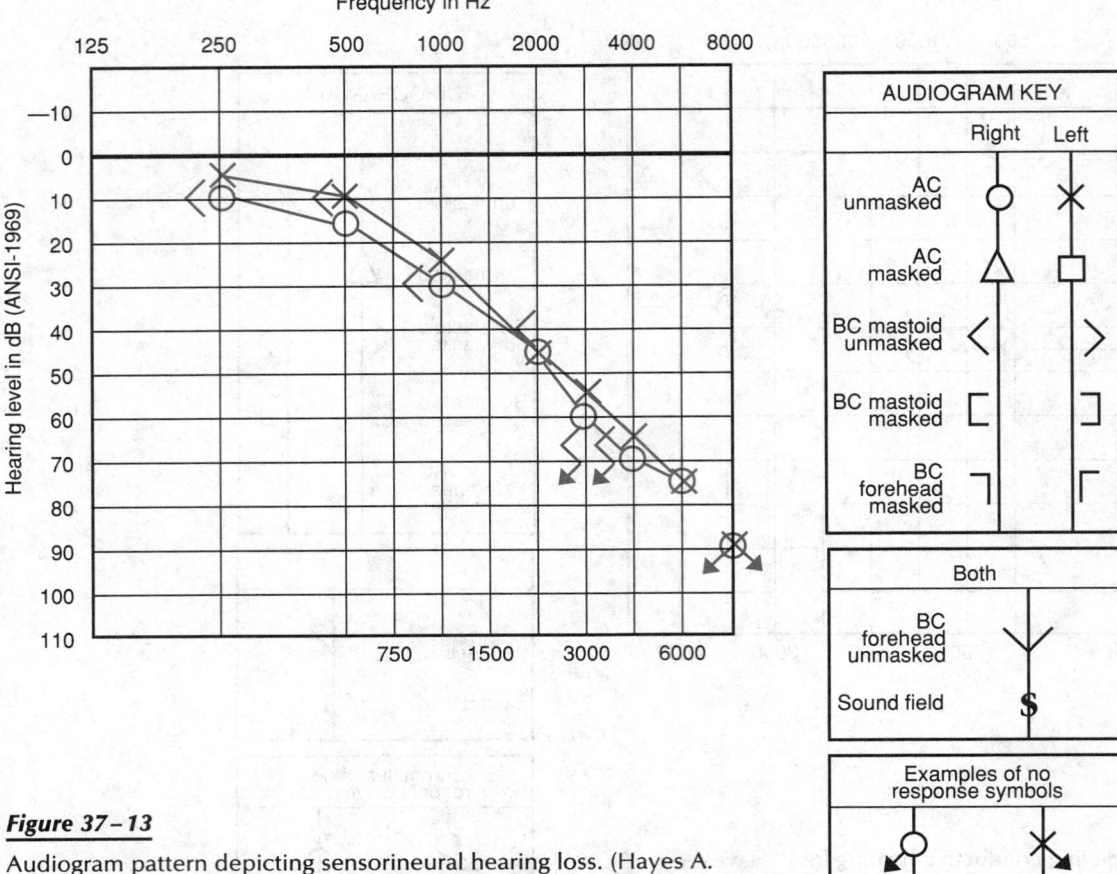

Figure 37–13

Audiogram pattern depicting sensorineural hearing loss. (Hayes A. Newby/Gerald R. Popelka, AUDIOLOGY, 5e, © 1985, pp. 146, 151, 152, 155. Adapted by permission of Prentice-Hall, Inc., Englewood Cliffs, New Jersey.)

stress on each syllable, such as airplane, railroad, hot dog, and cowboy.

The speech reception threshold is defined as the hearing level, obtained through the use of the audiometer, at which the client can repeat simple words correctly 50% of the time. The test is administered in essentially the same way as the pure tone tests, but with the microphone activated through the audiometer. The intensity dial on the audiometer is used to regulate the level of intensity of the words.

Speech Discrimination

The ability to understand speech must be considered the most important measurable aspect of human auditory function. Assessment of speech discrimination ability provides an indication of the client's understanding of speech. The handicap of a hearing loss may consist not only of decreased sensitivity to sound, but also of impaired understanding of what is being said. A test for speech discrimination is one that examines a client's ability to discriminate among similar sounds or among words that contain similar sounds.

A standard format for this assessment consists of the presentation of 50- or 25-word lists of monosyllabic words (one-syllable words such as carve, day, toe, and ran) that are phonemically balanced (designed to include the phonemes of American English in the proper proportion) and that are balanced for word difficulty between lists. The lists are presented to the client via earphones at a comfortable loudness level, generally around 30 to 40 dB above the speech reception threshold, or depending on the client's most comfortable listening level. A percentage score is derived from the number of words that are repeated correctly. For example, if four words were repeated incorrectly out of a 50-word list in the right ear, the score would be 92%. Each ear is tested individually, unless the test is conducted through loudspeakers that are housed in the sound suite.

TYMPANOMETRY

Tympanometry is an objective procedure that assesses tympanic membrane mobility or the compliance of the structures of the middle ear as a function of systematically varied air pressure in the external auditory canal.

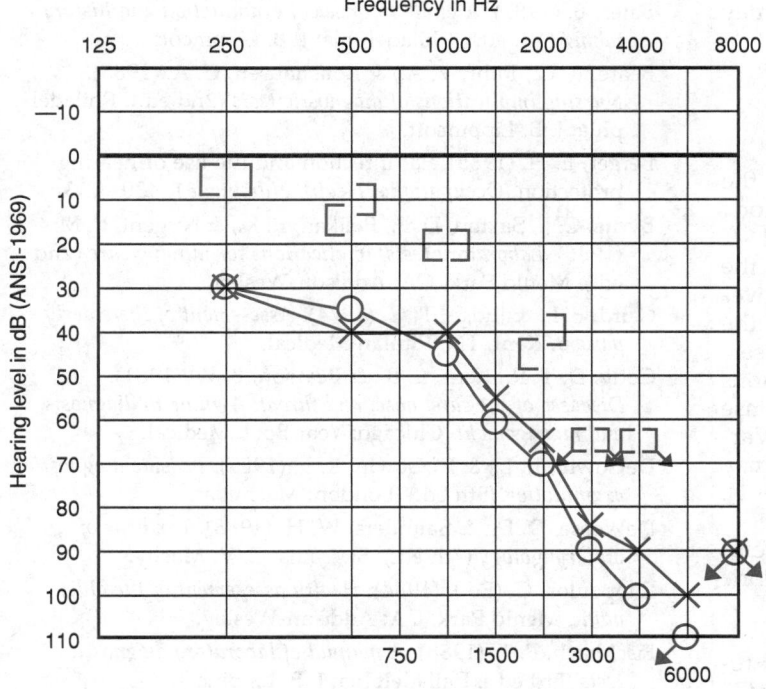

Frequency in Hz

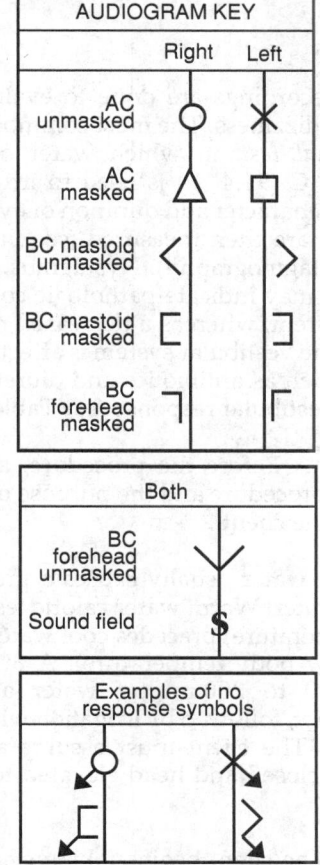

AUDIOGRAM KEY

Figure 37–14

Audiogram pattern depicting mixed conductive and sensorineural hearing loss. (Hayes A. Newby/Gerald R. Popelka, AUDIOLOGY, 5/e, © 1985, pp. 146, 151, 152, 155. Adapted by permission of Prentice-Hall, Inc., Englewood Cliffs, New Jersey.)

The progression and/or resolution of otitis media can be accurately monitored. This test is helpful in distinguishing middle-ear pathologic conditions such as otosclerosis, ossicular disarticulation, otitis media, and perforation of the tympanic membrane. It is also valuable for assessing eustachian tube patency and for following postsurgical recovery of middle-ear function.

VESTIBULAR TESTS

Electronystagmography

Electronystagmography is a specialized diagnostic procedure to evaluate both spontaneous and induced eye movements known as nystagmus. *Nystagmus* is the constant, involuntary, cyclic movement of the eyeball in any direction. The purpose of electronystagmography is to distinguish between normal nystagmus and either drug-induced nystagmus or nystagmus caused by a lesion in the central or peripheral vestibular pathway. Electronystagmography records the changing electrical

field with movement of the eye as monitored by electrodes placed on the skin around the eyes.

Client preparation. Before the procedure, careful explanation of the procedure and the purpose of electronystagmography should be given to the client. The client receives nothing by mouth 3 hours before the testing; any unnecessary medications are also omitted for 24 hours before the testing. The client should bring any prescribed eyeglasses to the examination.

Procedure. During the procedure, the client sits and is instructed to gaze at lights, focus on a moving pattern, focus on a moving point, and sit with eyes closed. While sitting in a specially designed chair, the client is rotated clockwise and turned upside down. In addition, the client's ears are irrigated with both cool and warm water (see under the heading Caloric Tests), which might result in nausea and vomiting. The client requires much support during the long and tiring procedure.

Follow-up care. The client begins taking clear fluids slowly and cautiously after the test in the event of nausea and vomiting. In addition, assisted ambulation may be necessary in the event of any ataxia.

Caloric Tests

Caloric response recordings are done to evaluate the client experiencing dizziness. The most common caloric test is the *bithermal test*, in which water of 44° C (111.2° F) and 33° C (91.4° F) is used to irrigate the external canal. The character and duration of eye movements (nystagmus) are then measured (see under the heading Electronystagmography). Nystagmus, nausea, vomiting, or ataxia may indicate pathologic conditions of the labyrinth system, whereas a decreased response may indicate that the vestibular system is affected. Various medications such as antibiotics and diuretics may interfere with the vestibular response (see Table 37–1).

Client preparation. Before the procedure, a careful explanation of the procedure and the purpose of caloric testing is given to the client.

Procedure. Warm water usually causes a greater response than cold water. Warm water caloric testing (7° C above body temperature) precedes cool water caloric testing (7° C below body temperature). A 30-second irrigation with 180 to 200 mL of water at 44° C (111.2° F) is used first, followed by irrigation with water at 33° C (91.4° F). The client must assume a supine position with eyes closed and head elevated to 30 degrees.

Follow-up care. The client begins taking clear fluids slowly and cautiously after the test in case of nausea and vomiting. In addition, the nurse assists the client in ambulation in case of any ataxia.

SUMMARY

The auditory system is complex and requires technical assessment with specialized equipment and procedures. These assessments should not be overlooked because of the devastating effect on communication that hearing loss presents. Early detection of ear and hearing problems often aids in the treatment and rehabilitation of the client.

REFERENCES AND READINGS

Anderson, R. G., Simpson, K., & Roeser, R. (1983). Auditory dysfunction and rehabilitation. *Geriatrics, 38*(9), 101–112.

Bates, B. (1987). *A guide to physical examination and history taking* (4th ed.). Philadelphia: J. B. Lippincott.

Beare, P. G., Rahr, V. A., & Ronshausen, C. A. (1985). *Nursing implications of diagnostic tests* (2nd ed.). Philadelphia: J. B. Lippincott.

Berger, E. H. (1985). Ear infection and the use of hearing protection. *Occupational Health Nursing, 31*, 430–433.

Byrne, C. J., Saxton, D. F., Pelikan, P. K., & Nugent, P. M. (1986). *Laboratory tests, implications for nursing care* (2nd ed.). Menlo Park, CA: Addison-Wesley.

Caird, F. I., & Judge, T. G. (1974). *Assessment of the elderly patient.* Kent, TN: Pitman Medical.

Cody, D. T. R., Kern, E. B., & Pearson, B. W. (1981). *Diseases of the ears, nose, and throat: A guide to diagnosis and management.* Chicago: Year Book Medical.

DeGowin, E. L., & DeGowin, R. L. (1987). *Bedside diagnostic examination* (5th ed.). London: Macmillan.

DeWeese, D. D., & Saunders, W. H. (1988). *Textbook of otolaryngology* (7th ed.). St. Louis: C. V. Mosby.

Eliopoulos, C. (Ed.). (1984). *Health assessment of the older adult.* Menlo Park, CA: Addison-Wesley.

Fischbach, F. T. (1988). *A manual of laboratory diagnostic tests* (3rd ed.). Philadelphia: J. B. Lippincott.

Giolas, T., & Randolph, K. (1977). *Basic audiometry, including impedance measurement.* Lincoln, NE: Cliffs Speech and Hearing Series.

Guyton, A. C. (1986). *Textbook of medical physiology* (7th ed.). Philadelphia: W. B. Saunders.

House, J. W., & O'Connor, A. F. (1987). *Handbook of neurotological diagnosis.* New York: Marcel Dekker.

Hughes, G. B. (1985). *Textbook of clinical otolaryngology.* New York: Thieme-Stratton.

Jahn, A., & Santos-Sacchi, J. (Eds.) (1988). *Physiology of the ear.* New York: Raven.

Jerger, J., & Northern, J. L. (Eds.) (1980). *Handbook of clinical impedance audiometry* (2nd ed.). New York: Thieme Medical.

Kenney, R. A. (1982). *Physiology of aging: A synopsis.* Chicago: Year Book Medical.

Malasanos, L., Barkauskas, V., Moss, M., & Stoltenberg-Allen, K. (1986). *Health assessment* (3rd ed.). St. Louis: C. V. Mosby.

Malkiewicz, J. A. (1982). How to assess the ears and test hearing acuity. *RN, 45*(3), 56–63.

Martin, F. N. (1986). *Introduction to audiology* (3rd ed.). Englewood Cliffs, NJ: Prentice-Hall.

Newby, H. A., & Popelka, G. R. (1985). *Audiology* (5th ed.). Englewood Cliffs, NJ: Prentice-Hall.

Penrod, J. (1986). Speech discrimination testing. In J. Katz (Ed.), *Handbook of clinical audiology* (3rd ed.). Baltimore: Williams & Wilkins.

Petrakis, N. L. (1969). Dry cerumen—a prevalent genetic trait among American Indians. *Nature, 222*, 1080–1081.

Petrakis, N. L., Pringle, U., Petrakis, S. J., & Petrakis, S. L. (1971). Evidence for a genetic cline in earwax types in the Middle East and Southeast Asia. *American Journal of Physiological Anthropology, 35*(1), 141–144.

Potter, D. O. (Ed.). (1982). *The nurse's reference library: Assessment.* Springhouse, PA: Intermed Communications.

Price, S. A., & Wilson, L. M. (1986). *Pathophysiology: Clinical concepts of disease processes* (3rd ed.). New York: McGraw-Hill.

Roberts, A. (1985). Setting up the systems: Development of the ear; part 31. *Nursing Times, 81*(46), 47.

Schill, H. (1986). Thresholds for speech. In J. Katz (Ed.), *Handbook of clinical audiology* (3rd ed.). Baltimore: Williams & Wilkins.

Seidel, H. M., Ball, J. W., Dains, J. E., & Benedict, G. W. (1987). *Mosby's guide to physical examination.* St. Louis: C. V. Mosby.

Sherman, J. L., & Fields, S. K. (1988). *Guide to patient evaluation* (5th ed.). Garden City, NJ: Medical Examination Publishing.

Voke, J. (1984). Aspects of hearing/one: Physiology of the ear. *Nursing Times, 80*(33), 28–30.

Wilber, L. (1986). Calibration: Puretone, speech and noise signals. In J. Katz (Ed.), *Handbook of clinical audiology* (3rd ed.). Baltimore: Williams & Wilkins.

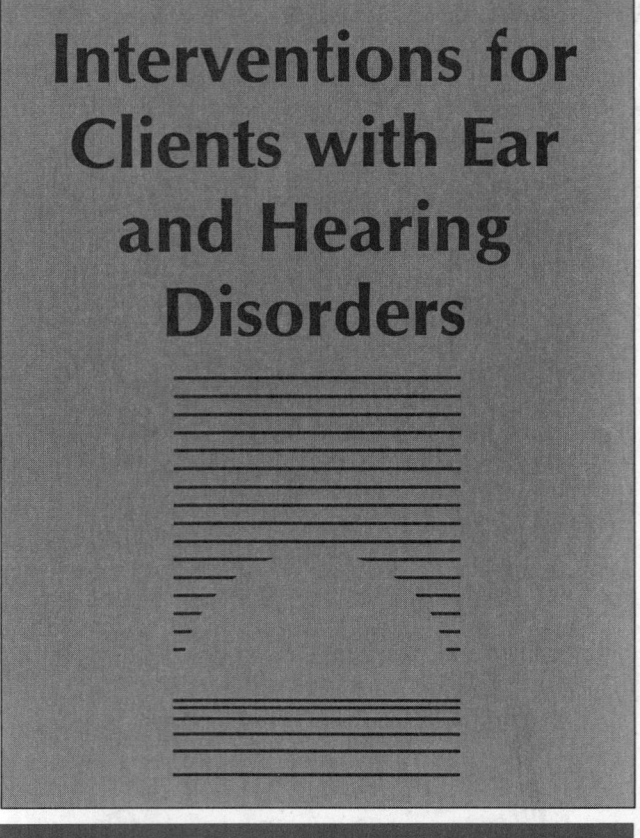

CHAPTER 38

Interventions for Clients with Ear and Hearing Disorders

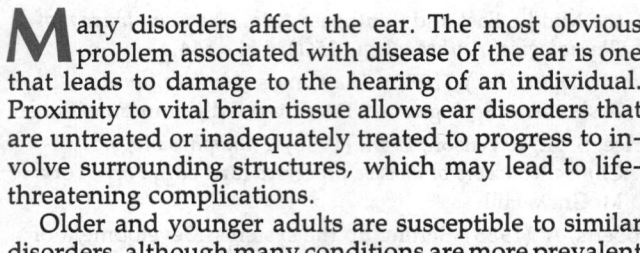

Many disorders affect the ear. The most obvious problem associated with disease of the ear is one that leads to damage to the hearing of an individual. Proximity to vital brain tissue allows ear disorders that are untreated or inadequately treated to progress to involve surrounding structures, which may lead to life-threatening complications.

Older and younger adults are susceptible to similar disorders, although many conditions are more prevalent in particular age groups. It is important for the nurse to understand the different ear disorders, especially with respect to location, so that complications can be recognized early and appropriate interventions initiated.

HEARING LOSS

OVERVIEW

Hearing loss is one of the most common physical handicaps in the United States. A definitive diagnosis of hearing loss is done through an audiologic examination. Approximately 16 million people in the United States are diagnosed as having a hearing loss, with many more having some degree of undiagnosed hearing impairment (Campbell, 1984). Not only is communication affected by decreased hearing, but many other pleasures of life, such as music, television, and the sound of birds singing, are diminished. In addition, safety needs of the hearing-impaired person become a special concern. When hearing is impaired, the individual is unable to heed auditory warnings, such as an ambulance siren, a child's cry for help, or a shout alerting of immediate danger.

Hearing loss is generally thought of as conductive, sensorineural, or a combination of the two (Fig. 38–1). When sound waves are blocked from coming to inner-ear nerve fibers because of external-ear or middle-ear disorders, the term *conductive* hearing loss is used. If there is a pathologic process of the inner ear or of the sensory fibers that lead to the cerebral cortex, the hearing loss is termed *sensorineural*. The combination hearing loss is known as *mixed conductive-sensorineural*.

Differential features of conductive and sensorineural forms of hearing loss are summarized in the Key Features of Disease on page 1098. Infection, trauma, and obstruction can each cause hearing loss of both varieties. The etiology determines the degree to which the hearing loss can be corrected and the amount of normal hearing that will return after appropriate treatment.

Disorders that lead to a conductive hearing loss can often be corrected with no damage to hearing or minimal permanent hearing loss. Sensorineural hearing loss is often permanent, and measures must be taken to reduce further damage or to attempt to amplify sounds as a means of improving hearing to some degree.

Any inflammatory process or obstruction of the external or middle ear leads to a conductive hearing loss. An otoscopic examination reveals or rules out many etiologic factors. Direct observation allows the nurse to detect a collapse in the external canal. Cerumen or a foreign object can be seen by direct inspection or by use of the otoscope. Changes in the tympanic membrane such as bulges, retractions, or perforations may indicate damage to middle-ear structures, which leads to conductive hearing loss. Tumors, otosclerosis, and the build-up of scar tissue on the ossicles from previous middle-ear surgery all lead to forms of conductive hearing loss that are not obvious to the nurse on inspection. Tuning fork tests are used to assist with diagnosis. In the Weber test, the client tends to be able to hear sounds well in the ear suspected of having a conductive hearing loss because of the preserved bone conduction. In the Rinne test, the client reports that sound transmitted by bone conduction is louder and more sustained than that transmitted by air conduction.

When the inner-ear structures or the auditory nerve (cranial nerve VIII) has been damaged, a sensorineural hearing loss develops. Damage can result from a variety of factors. Prolonged exposure to loud noise can damage the hair cells of the cochlea. Many drugs are toxic to the inner-ear structures. A variety of mechanisms, including toxic levels of drugs in the perilymph fluid, may damage the hair cells in the organ of Corti. Another cause of damage from drugs is through enzymatic changes in the inner ear. Effects on hearing loss from ototoxic drugs can be transient or permanent, unilateral or bilateral, and dose related or non–dose related. In addition to auditory function tests, it is essential that renal function be monitored in clients who are being treated with ototoxic drugs so that the clinician is assured of adequate clearance of drugs and drug by-products. Older clients are especially prone to developing ototoxicity because of a decline in renal function.

Presbycusis is a common cause of sensorineural hearing loss that is associated with aging. Hearing loss is bilateral, with a gradual yet progressive nature. Clients often state that they have no problem with hearing but that they cannot understand what the words are. The client might think that the speaker is mumbling. Hearing loss is caused by changes in several areas of the ear structure. These changes appear to be related to degeneration or atrophy of the ganglion cells in the cochlea, loss of elasticity of the basilar membrane, and compromise of the vascular supply to the inner ear. It is generally believed that the catabolic process of aging is the greatest cause of presbycusis.

Other causes of sensorineural hearing loss include

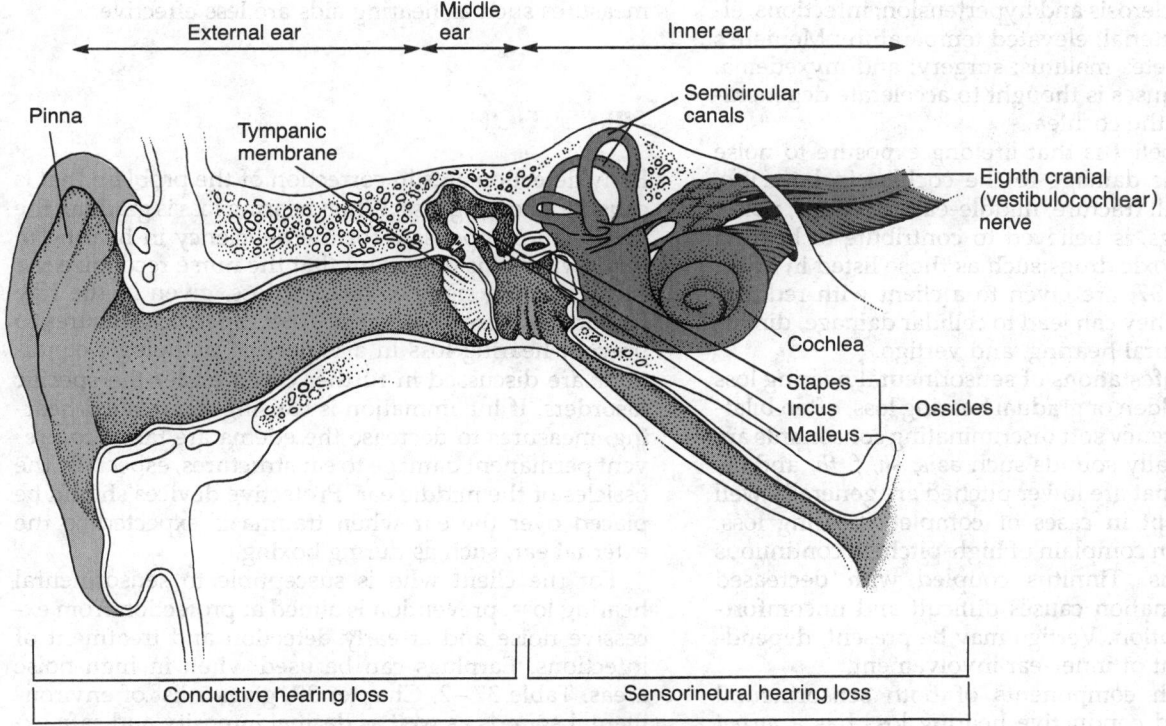

Figure 38–1

Anatomy of hearing loss. Hearing loss can be divided into three types: conductive (difficulty in the external or the middle ear), sensorineural (difficulty in the inner ear or the acoustic nerve), and mixed conductive-sensorineural (a combination of the two other types of hearing loss).

KEY FEATURES OF DISEASE ■ Differential Features of Conductive and Sensorineural Hearing Loss

Feature	Conductive Hearing Loss	Sensorineural Hearing Loss
Causes	Cerumen Foreign body Perforation of the tympanic membrane Edema Infection of the external or middle ear Tumors Otosclerosis	Prolonged exposure to noise Presbycusis Ototoxic substances Meniere's syndrome Acoustic neuroma Diabetes mellitus Labyrinthitis Infection Myxedema
Assessment findings	Evidence of obstruction with otoscope Abnormality in tympanic membrane Speaking softly Hearing best in a noisy environment Rinne's test: air conduction greater than bone conduction Weber's test: lateralization to affected ear	Normal appearance of external canal and tympanic membrane Tinnitus common Occasional dizziness Speaking loudly Hearing poorly in loud environment Rinne's test: air conduction less than bone conduction Weber's test: lateralization to unaffected ear

inherited disorders; metabolic and circulatory disorders, such as arteriosclerosis and hypertension; infections, either viral or bacterial; elevated temperature; Meniere's syndrome; diabetes mellitus; surgery; and myxedema. Each of these causes is thought to accelerate degenerative changes of the cochlea.

A common belief is that lifelong exposure to noise causes traumatic damage to the cochlea in later life. Trauma, via skull fracture, middle-ear infections, noise, or ototoxic drugs, is believed to contribute to hearing loss. When ototoxic drugs such as those listed in Table 37–1, Chapter 37, are given to a client with reduced renal function, they can lead to cellular damage, diminished sensorineural hearing, and vertigo.

Clinical manifestations of sensorineural hearing loss may include sudden or gradual hearing loss, often bilateral. High-frequency soft discriminating consonants are lost first, especially sounds such as s, sh, f, th, and ch. Vowel sounds that are lower pitched are generally well preserved, except in cases of complete hearing loss. Clients also often complain of high-pitched, continuous bilateral tinnitus. Tinnitus coupled with decreased speech discrimination causes difficult and uncomfortable communication. Vertigo may be present, depending on the extent of inner-ear involvement.

A client with components of both sensorineural hearing loss and conductive hearing loss has a *mixed conductive-sensorineural hearing loss.* For example, a client with presbycusis who also has a build-up of cerumen in the external canal would have a mixed hearing loss. The consequences of this type of hearing loss are that hearing is generally worse than with just sensori-

neural or conductive hearing loss and that corrective measures such as hearing aids are less effective.

PREVENTION

Early detection aids in correction of the problem that is causing a hearing loss. When hearing loss is gradual, the client can compensate for the deficiency in hearing in other ways. It is important that the nurse recognize the early warning signs of hearing loss, given in the Key Features of Disease on page 1099. Specific measures to prevent hearing loss in a variety of pathologic conditions are discussed in further detail under the specific disorders. If inflammation is causing diminished hearing, measures to decrease the edema are taken to prevent permanent damage to ear structures, especially the ossicles of the middle ear. Protective devices should be placed over the ear when trauma is expected to the external ear, such as during boxing.

For the client who is susceptible to sensorineural hearing loss, prevention is aimed at protection from excessive noise and at early detection and treatment of infections. Earplugs can be used when in high-noise areas. Table 37–2, Chapter 37, gives a list of environmental sounds as well as decibel intensity and safe exposure times. Prevention of sustained and widespread infections at an early age may limit the severity of presbycusis as the client ages. For clients with other systemic diseases that tend to increase hearing loss, a balance between exercise and rest, a well-balanced diet, and

KEY FEATURES OF DISEASE ■ Early Warning Signs of Hearing Loss

Frequently asking people to repeat statements

Better understanding in small groups

Withdrawing from social interactions

Straining to hear

Turning head to favor one ear or leaning forward

Shouting in conversation

Ringing in the ears

Failing to respond when not looking in the direction of the sound

Irritability

Answering questions incorrectly

Raising the volume of television or radio

Avoiding large groups

control of the disease are important factors that may help to prevent degenerative changes. Medications are reviewed for possible contributory ototoxicity, which makes hearing loss worse. Renal status must be monitored closely to ensure adequate excretion of ototoxic substances.

COLLABORATIVE MANAGEMENT

Facilitating Communication

The most obvious means of communicating with a client with a hearing problem is by the written word if the client is able to see, read, and write. Pictures of familiar phrases and objects can also be used. Some television programming is now closed-captioned for the hearing impaired. Subtitles that communicate in writing what is being said in the program are flashed on the screen.

Talking in a room without distracting noises can assist anyone to communicate better. The client can thus concentrate on the person's voice without distractions. If the client has a high-frequency hearing loss, the nurse talks in lower tones. Shouting to the client who cannot hear is of little benefit because the sound may be projected at a higher frequency and the client is less able to understand. Moving closer to the client and speaking slowly and clearly do much to improve oral communication.

Many devices are useful for clients with permanent progressive hearing loss. Telephone amplifiers increase the volume of the sound that is carried by the telephone, which allows the caller speaking in a normal voice to be heard. Flashing lights that are activated by the ringing

telephone or doorbell alert the client visually rather than by auditory means. In some cases, the client may be referred for use of a specially trained dog that helps the client to be aware of sounds in the same manner that a Seeing Eye dog assists the blind. The dog alerts the client to telephones, doorbells, cries of other people, and potential dangers.

Cochlear implantation is a new and experimental means of assisting a client with a sensorineural hearing loss. A small computer converts sound waves into electronic impulses. Electrodes are placed by the internal ear, with the computer device attached to the external ear. The electronic impulses then directly stimulate nerve fibers. Some clients have a 50% return of their hearing with this method.

People can be educated to use two tools that enhance communication: lip reading and sign language. In a formal lip-reading class, clients are taught the special cues to look for when lip reading, as well as how to understand body language. It is important to point out that the very best lip reader still misses more than 50% of what is being said. Because hearing is assisted by even minimal lip reading, clients are encouraged to wear their glasses when talking with someone to improve vision so that subtle movements of the lips can be seen. The nurse faces the client to facilitate lip reading.

For clients with a more severe hearing loss, a special language has been developed, the American Sign Language. This language combines speech with hand movements that signify letters, words, or phrases. The language takes time and effort to learn. Many people are unable to use this language, just as many people cannot speak different verbal languages. As the hearing-impaired person is less able to function, he or she may become motivated to learn this different form of communication.

Additional steps can be taken by the nurse to ensure continued communication. The nurse instructs the client and the family about different techniques that can be used. The accompanying Guidelines feature lists steps that should be taken when communicating with the hearing-impaired client.

Using Hearing Aids

A common means of improving communication is the use of a hearing aid. A hearing aid is a miniature electronic amplifier. Hearing aids are usually used for clients with a conductive hearing loss. The hearing aid can help the client who has a sensorineural loss, although not as effectively. The amplifier can be worn in one or both ears. With bilateral hearing loss, the use of binaural hearing aids enhances hearing more than the use of monaural amplification by providing a stereo effect, which aids in speech discrimination.

Health care personnel use educational instruction and psychologic support when introducing hearing aids

---

GUIDELINES ■ How to Communicate with a Hearing-Impaired Client

Position yourself directly in front of the client.

Make sure that there is plenty of light in the room.

Get the attention of the client before you begin to speak.

Do not shout; this only raises the frequency of the sound of the voice and often makes understanding more difficult.

Keep hands and other objects away from your mouth when talking to the client.

Attempt to have conversations in a quiet room with minimal distractions.

Validate with the client the understanding of statements made by asking the client to repeat what was said. If the client is asked whether he or she understands, the reply is often yes even when the client does not understand.

Rephrase sentences and repeat information to aid in understanding.

Move closer to the better-hearing ear.

Use appropriate hand movements.

Write messages on paper if the client is able to read.

---

to hearing-impaired clients. Clients must learn to use the hearing aid for maximal benefit. Special aural rehabilitation classes are offered by local agencies for the hearing impaired, which assist the new hearing aid wearer in getting the most benefit from this device.

Some special tips that help the client adjust to the new type of hearing are necessary. It is important to remember that hearing with a hearing aid can be much different from natural hearing. The client is encouraged to start using the hearing aid slowly to develop an appreciation for the device, initially wearing the hearing aid only at home and only during part of the day. Listening to television and radio and reading aloud are practice tools that help get the client used to new sounds. The tone or volume of the hearing aid can be adjusted to fit the situation. The most important and yet difficult aspect associated with the use of a hearing aid is the amplification of background noise as well as voices. Clients must learn to concentrate on the sounds that are to be heard and to filter out amplified background noises. When fatigued, the client should remove the hearing aid so that continued efforts to ignore background noise can be avoided.

The client must also learn how to care for the hearing aid, as described in the accompanying Client/Family Education feature. Hearing aids are delicate electronic devices that can assist the client greatly and should be handled only by people who know how to care for them properly. The cost of the aids varies greatly, but in all

cases an investment is required. Proper care ensures a long life for the device.

Managing Psychosocial Concerns

Communication for the person with a hearing loss can become a struggle. People often isolate themselves because it is too much of an effort to talk and to listen to others. Social isolation can lead to depression, fear, and despair. The nurse must be aware of changes in emotional state and behavior that may be related to reduced hearing and a decline in conversational skills.

To prevent social isolation, the client must use remaining resources to make social contact satisfying. The most obvious way to decrease social isolation is by improving communication as previously described. The client must be made aware that changes in communication patterns or styles are necessary with increasing physical limitation.

Clients often become irritated easily when the nurse asks many questions in an effort to obtain a thorough history. When possible, the nurse asks household members about the client's understanding of hearing loss and comprehension of general conversations, and about changes in behavior, such as withdrawal. If the client lives alone, the nurse asks about past or present diversional activities. This information helps the nurse assess the most satisfying activities and social interactions and determine the amount of effort necessary for the client to continue to engage in these activities. A plan can be made with the client to alter certain activities to maximize the client's satisfaction. Someone who is used to going to large gatherings of people might choose to be with a smaller number of people instead. A quiet evening meal at home with friends might substitute for dinner in a noisy restaurant.

Information and support for the client can come from different organizations such as the American Speech-Language-Hearing Association. This organization publishes papers that are helpful resources to clients and discusses ways to reduce hearing loss. Many public and private institutions offer hearing evaluations. The National Association of Hearing and Speech Agencies and Self-Help for Hard-of-Hearing People (Shhh) both have programs for clients with hearing disorders. These agencies supply information and counseling for many clients.

CONDITIONS AFFECTING THE EXTERNAL EAR

Many conditions affect the structures of the external ear and cause problems. Congenital malformation, trauma,

CLIENT/FAMILY EDUCATION ■ How to Care for a Hearing Aid

Instructions	Rationales
1. "Clean the earmold with mild soap and water while avoiding excessive wetting. Keep the hearing aid dry."	1. Dirt in the earmold inhibits the effectiveness of the device and increases the risk of external otitis.
2. "Clean debris from the ear cannula, the hole in the middle of the part that goes in the ear, with a toothpick or pipe cleaner."	2. Blockage of the hole decreases the effectiveness of sounds transmitted through the hole.
3. "Turn off the hearing aid and remove the battery when not in use."	3. Disconnecting the battery prolongs its effective life.
4. "Check and replace the battery correctly and frequently. Keep extra batteries on hand."	4. The device operates most effectively when batteries are fresh and fully charged. Old batteries may leak corrosive substances, which damage the device.
5. "Keep the hearing aid in a safe place; avoid dropping and extremes of heat and cold."	5. Device is a delicate electronic instrument with numerous internal connections. Dropping may cause disconnections. Temperature extremes cause wires and other connections to become brittle and to crumble more easily.
6. "Adjust the volume to the minimal hearing level to prevent feedback squeaking."	6. Feedback squeaking increases background noise and decreases the client's reception and perception of more critical sounds.
7. "Avoid use of hair spray, oils, or other hair and face products that might come into contact with the receiver."	7. These products may clog the opening in the device and increase the rate of decomposition of the plastic housing.
8. "If the hearing aid does not work, change the battery, check the connection between the earmold and receiver, check the on/off switch, clean the cannula, adjust the volume, or take the hearing aid to a service center authorized to repair that brand and model."	8. The device cannot assist the client to hear better unless it is fully functional.

and infectious or noninfectious lesions of the pinna, auricle, or auditory canal may exist. Congenital anomalies range from a crumpling or falling forward of the pinna to the absence, or atresia, of the auditory canal. Congenital disorders of the external ear do not necessarily mean that there will be problems with middle-ear and inner-ear structures because each develops differently in the embryo. The auricle and external canal can also be damaged or destroyed through trauma. Surgical reconstruction, done in phases, is performed to re-form the pinna by using skin grafts and plastic prostheses.

Trauma to the auricle that results in a hematoma leads to the hardening of the hematoma and results in what is called a *cauliflower ear*. For any hematoma formation in the external ear, blood is removed via needle aspiration to prevent calcification and hardening.

Benign cysts or polyps of the auricle or external canal need to be surgically removed if they grow large enough to block the canal and affect the hearing of the client. Malignant cells can also be found on the pinna. The most common type is basal cell carcinoma. In general, simple excision of the tumor is the treatment. As the lesion becomes larger, the closeness to the skull and facial nerve makes treatment more difficult.

EXTERNAL OTITIS

OVERVIEW

External otitis is an infective, inflammatory, or allergic response involving structures of the external auditory canal or the auricle. It may present as an acute, recurrent, or chronic condition. The lesion is usually localized to the external ear.

Pathophysiology

An irritating or infective agent comes into contact with the epithelial layer of the external ear, which leads to either an allergic response or signs and symptoms of an infection. The skin becomes red, swollen, and tender to touch or movement. Extensive swelling of the canal can lead to a conductive hearing loss because of obstruction of the canal.

Necrotizing external otitis is the most virulent form of external otitis and can have a 60% to 80% mortality. In necrotizing, or malignant, external otitis, the organism spreads beyond the external auditory canal into the adjacent structures of the ear and skull. Hearing loss, which may or may not be present, is caused by swelling of the auditory canal. The high mortality that is seen with malignant external otitis is related to the wide variety of complicating disorders. With the extension of infective materials into the brain, one or more of the following disorders might develop: meningitis, brain abscess, or destruction of certain cranial nerves, especially the facial nerve (cranial nerve VII).

Etiology

Irritating agents vary from individual to individual depending on the person's particular sensitivities. Common causes of allergic external otitis are cosmetics, hair sprays, earphones, earrings, and at times even hearing aids. Viral infections of the external ear are rare; infecting agents are more often bacterial or fungal. The most common organisms are *Pseudomonas aeruginosa, Streptococcus, Staphylococcus,* and *Aspergillus.* The accompanying Key Features of Disease compares external otitis and otitis media.

External otitis occurs more often in hot, humid environments, especially in the summer months. It has been termed *swimmer's ear* because of the increased incidence after submersion of the head in water such as during swimming. The increased incidence in swimmers has a twofold etiology. Swimming or diving tends to clear cerumen (wax) out of the ear at a greater rate than normal. Because one of the primary functions of cerumen is to gather bacteria and debris for removal, the rapid removal of cerumen eliminates this protective mechanism. Loss of cerumen coupled with the introduction of a pathogenic agent from lake or pool water leads to an infection. Individuals who have traumatized the external auditory canal with sharp objects such as hairpins and cotton-tipped applicators resulting in an open lesion are more prone to developing external otitis.

Incidence

External otitis is more common in children and younger adults. The necrotizing form is seen most often in older clients with diabetes, but it can also be found in other immunosuppressed or chronically debilitated individuals such as the elderly adult, clients diagnosed with a neoplasm, or clients who are being treated with chemotherapeutic or corticosteroid agents.

KEY FEATURES OF DISEASE ■ Differential Features of External Otitis and Otitis Media

Problem	Etiology	Clinical Manifestations	Treatment	Interventions	Rationales
External otitis	Allergic reaction Bacterial or viral infection Swimming Local trauma	Pain Itching Hearing loss Plugged feeling in ear Redness and edema Exudate	Topical antibiotics Corticosteroids Oral analgesics Local heat	1. Institute nonpharmacologic pain relief measures. 2. Educate client about medications and means of prevention.	1. To enhance comfort. 2. To enhance compliance and prevent recurrence of infection.
Otitis media	Bacterial or viral infection Sterile accumulation of fluid	Pain Pressure in ear Hearing loss Tinnitus Fever Malaise Nausea/vomiting Bulging tympanic membrane Fluid behind tympanic membrane	Systemic antibiotics Analgesics Local heat Antipyretics Antihistamines Decongestants Myringotomy	1. Institute nonpharmacologic pain relief measures. 2. Follow special communication techniques. 3. Educate client about medications. 4. Monitor progress of infection.	1. To enhance comfort. 2. To aid in client's education and to relieve anxiety. 3. To enhance client's compliance. 4. To detect worsening.

PREVENTION

Elimination of irritating or infecting agents is always the best means of prevention. The ear should be kept clean and dry. Although cerumen has a protective component, it can swell when wet, and thus excessive amounts can occlude the canal. Cleaning old wax and debris from the canal through irrigation is important for initial healing and for prevention of a new occurrence of external otitis. The proper way to irrigate an ear for removal of excess cerumen and debris is given in the accompanying Guidelines feature and in Figure 38–2.

The use of earplugs is recommended for clients who have recurrent episodes of otitis after swimming. After the inflammatory process has subsided, alcohol may be dropped into the ear to keep it clean and dry. Cotton-tipped applicators should not be used to dry ears because their use could lead to trauma to the canal, either directly or by packing cerumen into the canal, and could thus increase the client's susceptibility to infection or inflammation.

If earphones or hair products are suspected of being the irritating agents, their use should be discontinued until the irritation is healed. Alternative materials might be tried, although close observation for recurrence is important.

COLLABORATIVE MANAGEMENT

 Assessment

History

Data collection includes a *review of the present illness, its course, and its severity* and a *discussion of possible etiologies.* The client is questioned about swimming and bathing habits, use of earphones, recent changes in hair or other cosmetic products, or changes in soap or laundry detergents. *Similar complaints in other family members* are also noted to identify multiple irritating or infective sources. When taking a history, the nurse must be aware of small changes in the client's activities of daily living and use of toiletries to assess the cause of the disease adequately.

GUIDELINES ■ How to Irrigate an Ear

Interventions	Rationales
1. Gather proper equipment: basin, appropriate syringe, otoscope, and towel.	1. To avoid delaying procedure.
2. Warm tap water to body temperature.	2, 3. To decrease vestibular stimulation.
3. Fill syringe with warm water.	
4. Place a basin under the ear to be irrigated as well as a towel around the client's neck to avoid getting the client wet.	4. To enhance the client's comfort.
5. Use otoscope to check the location of the impacted cerumen.	5, 6. To enable nurse to aim above or below to help create back-pressure and free cerumen.
6. Place the tip of the syringe at an angle so that the fluid pushes at one side of the impaction and not directly on the impaction. This helps to loosen the cerumen and avoids pushing it further back in the canal.	
7. Watch fluid return for signs of cerumen plug removal.	7. To be aware of when irrigation can be stopped.
8. Continue to irrigate the ear with approximately 70 mL of fluid. If the cerumen does not drain out, wait about 10 min and repeat the procedure.	8. To soften the cerumen, which absorbs water, and loosen it from the external canal. By waiting, the soft cerumen will drain out easier with the next irrigation. Excessive irrigation can cause trauma and discomfort for the client.
9. Monitor the client for signs of nausea during the procedure. If the client becomes nauseated, stop the procedure.	9. To detect and correct excessive vestibular stimulation, which causes nausea and dizziness.
10. If the cerumen cannot be removed by irrigation, the client may drop mineral oil into the ear three times a day for 2 days, after which irrigation may be repeated.	10. To loosen cerumen, which makes irrigation easier.

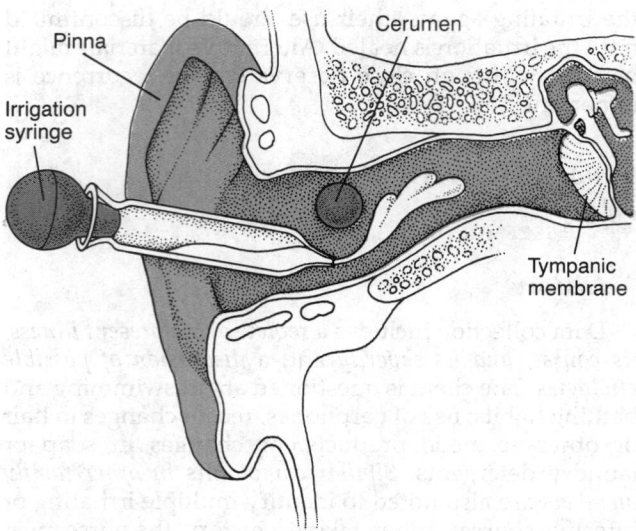

Figure 38-2

Irrigation of the external canal. Cerumen and debris can be removed from the ear by irrigation with warm water. The stream of water is aimed above or below the impaction to allow back-pressure to push it out rather than further down the canal.

Clients are also questioned about *recent trauma or injury* to the ear or external canal. This trauma might be caused by a variety of items, such as a cotton-tipped applicator, other sharp objects used to clean the ear, or any foreign object that might have been lodged and removed, causing direct trauma to the canal.

As with many other disorders, the nurse should document the *age* and *general physical condition* of the client. Age is an important factor to consider because external otitis is more common in younger persons. For the older client, the nurse asks about the presence of *past or present medical problems,* such as diabetes, because possible complications of external otitis are more likely to occur in clients with this diagnosis.

Physical Assessment: Clinical Manifestations

Clinical manifestations of external otitis may include a variety of different complaints ranging from *mild itching* to *pain* with movement of the pinna or tragus. Clients typically have pain with physical manipulation of the pinna and tragus or when upward pressure is applied to the external canal. Clients complain that they feel as if the ear is plugged and their hearing is changed. Hearing loss is caused by swelling of the auditory canal.

Redness and *swelling* of the external structures are seen either by direct observation or by use of an otoscope. In severe cases, the edema can be so extensive that it is impossible to examine the ear with the otoscope. Extreme caution is used with the otoscope not to exert pressure on the walls of the external canal, which would cause excessive pain. Drainage from the ear,

when present, is often greenish white. The nurse is careful to dispose of the otoscope tip and to wash hands thoroughly between examining alternate ears to prevent cross-contamination.

In severe cases, clients might complain of a large amount of *drainage* from the ear. This drainage is the result of a ruptured furuncle or localized external otitis (see under the later heading Furnucle for further description). Hearing loss can be severe on the affected side when the inflammatory process causes obstruction of the tympanic membrane. Occasionally, preauricular or postauricular lymph nodes might be tender and palpable.

The onset and duration of external otitis vary with the type of infecting or irritating agent. Clinical manifestations of bacterial infections generally appear 12 to 24 hours after introduction of the agent. Fungal infections usually take 2 to 3 days to show clinical manifestations.

The redness and irritation are usually localized to the ear without signs and symptoms of systemic infection such as elevated temperature, malaise, anorexia, and fatigue.

Psychosocial Assessment

Localized external otitis occurs most commonly in children and young adults. The need to eliminate etiologic factors like swimming or use of earphones may be problematic, and it is hard to gain compliance of the client. Swimming is sometimes allowed with consistent use of occlusive earplugs after the infection is cleared. Care is taken to ensure the client's understanding of the need to change habits to avoid the recurrence of the problem.

Occasionally, hearing aids are the irritating agents, and the client needs to discontinue their use during treatment and healing. If the client uses a hearing aid, the nurse makes arrangements for different forms of communication. For most clients, this can be a disturbing situation. The nurse allows the client time to discuss concerns and indicates that the situation is temporary while acknowledging the client's expressed fears.

For clients with malignant external otitis, the high mortality rate must be considered. The nurse supports the client and the family during this difficult time. Fear of death is real, and the nurse must be able to listen and to give comfort without expressing false hopes.

Laboratory Findings

Laboratory tests have limited use in the diagnosis and treatment of external otitis because treatment is generally based on signs and symptoms. Routine cultures are rarely performed unless excessive drainage is present. Cultures to determine the exact etiology are obtained only if initial therapy is ineffective in relieving signs and symptoms. Complete blood counts with differential are indicated only if systemic involvement from the external otitis is suspected. White blood cell counts may be elevated.

Radiographic Findings

In the typical form of external otitis, no radiographic studies are necessary. If the client is an older diabetic with suspected malignant external otitis, radiographic studies help to determine the extent of involvement beyond the external canal. Skull x-ray films are used to evaluate bony involvement, and computed tomography of the head aids in determining soft-tissue involvement.

 Analysis: Nursing Diagnosis

Clients present with pain in the ear or changes in sensory perception related to the feeling of fullness in the ear. Diagnoses are determined from subjective and objective data. The following nursing diagnoses are derived from these data.

Common Diagnoses

Two nursing diagnoses are common in clients with external otitis:

1. Pain related to inflammatory process and edema
2. Sensory/perceptual alterations (auditory) related to obstruction of the external auditory canal

Additional Diagnoses

In addition to the actual diagnoses, the client may present with one or more potential diagnoses. These include

1. Potential for injury related to altered auditory perception
2. Activity intolerance related to pain
3. Anxiety related to inability to communicate
4. Body image disturbance related to alterations in appearance
5. Social isolation related to inability to communicate
6. Knowledge deficit related to treatment plan and etiologic factors

 Planning and Implementation

The following plan of care for clients with external otitis focuses on the two common diagnoses.

Pain

Planning: client goals.   The main goal for this nursing diagnosis is that the client will experience a reduction of pain after a decrease in edema and inflammation.

Interventions: nonsurgical management.   Treatment of pain focuses on measures that reduce local inflam-mation and edema. These measures alleviate the factors causing pain and prevent further discomfort.

Local relief.   Heat may be applied locally for 20 minutes three times a day. Towels may be warmed with water and then wrapped in a plastic bag to apply heat. Heating pads placed on a very low setting may also be used. Bed rest is often helpful because head movements are limited, which thereby reduces pain.

Drug therapy.   Topical antibiotic therapy and steroid therapy are the most effective means of decreasing the causes of pain. If edema has caused an obstruction of the external canal, an earwick is inserted past the blockage, with medicated drops applied to the outside end (Fig. 38–3). A long piece of gauze dressing serves as an earwick and is inserted by the physician using forceps to carefully push through the blocked external auditory canal to the tympanic membrane. The earwick may be removed when medication can flow freely into the canal. Care is taken for proper disposal of the earwick because it contains highly contaminated material. Thorough hand washing is strictly enforced. The nurse must be aware that any antibiotic placed in the ear might cause a contact dermatitis, which will increase the pain if the treatment continues. Systemic oral or intravenous antibiotics are used in severe cases, especially when a cellulitis is present or auricular lymph nodes are enlarged. Examples of antibiotics that are used include penicillin (Pen-Vee-K), ampicillin (Polycillin), and cephalosporins such as cephalothin (Keflin).

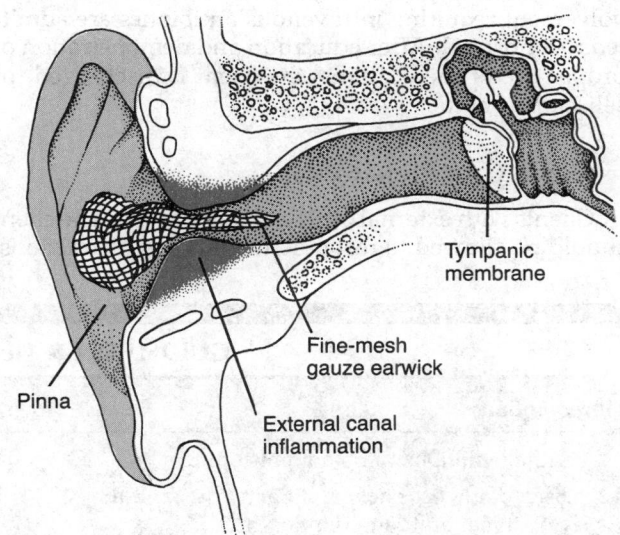

Figure 38–3

Earwick for instillation of antibiotics into the external canal. When edema occludes the external auditory canal, it is difficult for antibiotic solutions to enter the canal adequately. An earwick is placed through the meatus. Solutions placed on the external portion of the earwick are absorbed through the canal.

Analgesics are required during the initial days of therapy. The pain may be so severe that narcotics may be required for relief of pain. Acetylsalicylic acid (aspirin) or acetaminophen (Tylenol) can be given to relieve less severe pain. However, their antipyretic effect must be considered when the nurse is following the client for elevations in temperature as an indication of systemic infection.

Sensory/Perceptual Alterations (Auditory)

Planning: client goals. The main goal for this nursing diagnosis is that the client will have a decrease in the obstruction of the external auditory canal that is causing the hearing loss.

Interventions: nonsurgical management. Treatment of sensory/perceptual alterations focuses on measures that reduce local inflammation and allow the transmission of sounds through the external canal. Both local relief and drug therapy aid in the reduction of inflammation and therefore improve hearing. During the acute phase of the disease, the client's hearing is diminished or distorted. Measures should be taken to maintain a quiet environment, free from excessive noises, so that the client is able to rest. Communication is maintained through use of the unaffected ear. The nurse moves to the side of the unaffected ear and speaks in a normal voice.

■ Discharge Planning

Only clients with extensive bone and soft-tissue involvement requiring intravenous antibiotics are admitted to a hospital. After education and demonstration of proper use of medications, the client is discharged for self-care at home.

Home Care Preparation

Clients with external otitis experience pain. The client should be allowed to rest quietly with few distractions. Proper medications, analgesics and antibiotics, as well as a heating pad, for local relief of pain, need to be placed so that the client has easy access to them.

Client/Family Education

Pain and inflammation should be reduced by prescribed medications and local treatment. The client or a responsible party must know the proper route, administration times, and duration of the medication therapy. The nurse reassures the client that when the inflammation subsides, the pain and itching will be reduced. The client must be prevented from scratching or further traumatizing the affected area. In older adults, this can be achieved by placing a dressing over the ear.

Because topical antibiotics and steroids are often used, the nurse reviews with the client the proper way to self-instill eardrops or ointment, as shown in the accompanying Guidelines feature. The client should then be observed to make sure that proper technique is used. The head should be tilted in the opposite direction of the affected ear, thus making sure that all surfaces are covered with the medication. If heat is applied, care must be taken to prevent burns. Extremely low heat settings on a heating pad should be used for only short periods.

If the external otitis is caused by an irritating substance rather than an infective agent, care must be taken to identify the causative agent and to avoid its use. The nurse systematically helps the client to identify the irritating substance by asking questions about personal hygiene, use of cosmetics, and activities such as swimming, which might cause problems.

Psychosocial Preparation

In most cases, the clinical manifestations of external otitis are resolved with proper therapy. Clients who must make life style changes such as wearing earplugs while swimming, changing toiletry brands, discontinuing the use of earphones, or not wearing a hearing aid

---

GUIDELINES ■ How to Administer Eardrops

Interventions	Rationales
1. Gather solutions to be administered.	1. To avoid delaying client.
2. Discard any ear packing. Irrigate the ear if the tympanic membrane is intact.	2. To allow the solution to touch all surfaces thoroughly.
3. Place the solution in a bowl of warm water.	3. To decrease vestibular stimulation.
4. Tilt the client's head in the opposite direction of the affected ear and place the drops in the ear.	4–6. To keep medication in the canal and to cover all affected areas.
5. With the head so tilted, move the head back and forth.	
6. Insert a cotton ball into the ear canal to act as packing.	

need help with the best ways to institute these changes. The nurse is careful not to make these life style changes seem small and insignificant. Most clients are willing to make changes to prevent the irritation or infection, but any alteration in normal activities has some type of consequence. The nurse explores with the client the meaning of all changes to self-esteem and health.

Health Care Resources

For the client with repeated infections and inflammation, a home care nurse may be brought into the home to evaluate that environment. The client can then demonstrate methods of medication administration and routine irrigation. The nurse evaluates anything that is placed over or near the ear.

 Evaluation

The nurse evaluates the care given on the basis of the identified client diagnosis. Expected outcomes for a client with external otitis include that the client

1. States the pain is reduced or alleviated
2. Returns to the preinfection hearing level
3. Describes proper ways to provide ear care
4. Identifies potential hazards to the external ear and avoids them
5. Demonstrates proper techniques when using eardrops or ointment

By meeting the desired outcomes, the signs and symptoms of external otitis should be alleviated quickly and the potential complications avoided. After the acute phase is over, the major goal becomes prevention. If the desired outcomes are met, the likelihood of chronic recurrence is diminished.

FURUNCLE

Often called localized external otitis, a *furuncle* is caused by bacterial infection of a hair follicle. A furuncle is located on the outer half of the external canal. The infecting organism is usually *Staphylococcus*. Clinical manifestations of a furuncle include intense local pain to light touch. The area is swollen and pink, with tight skin covering the area. There may or may not be evidence of a purulent head. No drainage is noted unless the furuncle has ruptured, spilling its contents. Hearing is impaired if the lesion is large enough to occlude the canal.

Treatment is consistent with other types of external otitis: local and systemic antibiotics and localized heat. An earwick may be used with 10 drops of one-half strength Burow's solution to relieve pain. The furuncle itself might need to have an incision and drainage if it does not resolve with the use of systemic antibiotics.

CERUMEN OR FOREIGN BODIES

Many objects can enter or be placed in the external auditory canal. *Cerumen*, or wax, is the most common cause of an impacted canal, but the list of possible foreign objects is almost endless. Vegetables, beads, pencil erasers, and insects are all common items that may enter the canal, either with or without the help of the client. Although uncomfortable, this condition is rarely a true emergency, and care must be taken when removing cerumen or foreign bodies.

Clients generally complain of a sensation of fullness in the ear, with or without associated hearing loss. There may also be complaints of pain, itching, or bleeding from the ear.

If the occluding material is cerumen, the nurse may be instructed to irrigate the canal with a mixture of water and hydrogen peroxide at body temperature (see Fig. 38–2). Guidelines for proper irrigation should be followed (see Guidelines: How to Irrigate an Ear). Removal of wax by irrigation is a slow process, and the nurse cannot always expect to remove all material at one sitting. Between 50 and 70 mL of solution is about the maximal amount that the client can tolerate at one sitting. Irrigation is contraindicated in clients with a history of tympanic membrane perforation.

If the cerumen is thick and dry or unable to be removed easily, the physician may prescribe the use of a cerumenolytic product such as Cerumenex to soften the wax before an attempt is made to remove it. Another way to soften cerumen is to add three drops of glycerine to the ear at bedtime and three drops of hydrogen peroxide twice a day. After several days of this treatment, the cerumen is more easily removed through irrigation. In some cases, a small curette or cerumen spoon may be used to scoop out the wax. Only persons with special knowledge and skill should use this method because damage to the canal or tympanic membrane is likely with improper technique.

When the foreign object is vegetable matter, irrigation is used with care because this material expands with hydration. A better treatment is to use a bent curette or small forceps for removal of the object. Special care is taken to avoid pushing the object further into the canal and damaging the tympanic membrane. In some cases, surgical removal with general anesthesia is necessary. As attempts are made to remove the object, the canal becomes more edematous and painful. Surgical removal of the object is through a transcanal route by using a wire that is bent at a 90-degree angle and that can thus be passed around the object and used to pull the object out. The painful nature of this procedure makes general anesthesia necessary.

Insects should be killed before removal unless they can be coaxed out by a flashlight or a humming noise. Mineral oil or alcohol is instilled into the ear to suffocate the insect, which is then removed by using ear forceps. If there has been local irritation, an antibiotic or steroid ointment may be applied to prevent infection and to reduce local irritation. Hearing acuity is tested if hearing loss is not resolved by removal of the object.

CONDITIONS AFFECTING THE MIDDLE EAR

OTITIS MEDIA

OVERVIEW

The three most common forms of otitis media are acute and chronic otitis media and serous otitis media. Each affects the middle-ear structures but has a slightly different pathology, etiology, and incidence. Different forms range from simple accumulation of sterile fluid in the middle ear to extensive infection of the middle-ear structures, which leads to perforation of the tympanic membrane. If the condition progresses or remains untreated, permanent conductive hearing loss may occur.

Pathophysiology

Acute otitis media and *chronic otitis media,* which are also known as suppurant or purulent otitis media, are similar in their pathophysiology. An infecting agent introduced into the middle ear causes an inflammatory process within the mucosa, which leads to swelling and irritation of the bones, or ossicles, within the middle ear. This process is followed by formation of purulent inflammatory exudate. Onset is sudden, with the acute disease being of relatively short duration, 3 weeks or less. Chronic otitis media usually follows repeated acute episodes, has a longer duration, and can be associated with greater morbidity or injury to the middle-ear structures. There is usually bilateral ear involvement.

In either acute or chronic cases, signs and symptoms of the disease are caused by pressure of the fluid in the middle-ear cavity. The eustachian tube and mastoid, connected to the middle ear by a continuation of cells, are also affected by the infective process. Destruction of the bones of the middle ear develops as a result of an infection that is untreated or resistant to treatment. If the tympanic membrane perforates and infective materials spill into the external ear, the disease and treatment may be complicated by external otitis. Etiologic factors are usually such that there is bilateral ear involvement.

Serous otitis media, or catarrhal otitis media, is characterized by an accumulation of sterile fluid behind the tympanic membrane. Serous otitis media can precede or can be a long-term complication of acute otitis media. The effusion or fluid may remain in the middle ear for up to several months.

When the fluid remains longer and begins to thicken, a complication called *adhesive otitis media* results. Untreated serous or chronic otitis media causes thickening and scarring in the middle-ear structures and bones. Necrosis of the ossicles leads to destruction of the middle-ear structures. Surgical reconstruction of the ossicles is necessary to correct the resulting hearing loss.

Etiology

The middle ear is a sterile cavity connected to the nasopharynx by the eustachian tube. Migration of organisms causing an upper respiratory tract infection through the eustachian tube to the middle ear is the primary route of transmission of the infection in otitis media. A major etiologic factor in some individuals is the angle at which the eustachian tube is positioned. With a straight angle of the eustachian tube, bacteria and viruses migrate more easily to the middle ear. Common infecting agents include *Streptococcus, Staphylococcus,* and *Haemophilus influenzae.*

In rare cases, a traumatic perforation of the tympanic membrane allows an organism to enter the middle ear from the outside and to cause otitis media. External otitis rarely progresses to otitis media unless there is a previous perforation of the eardrum.

Incidence

Adults may have a diagnosis of acute otitis media, but more commonly they have the chronic form of the disease. Adults who are at higher risk for otitis media include Eskimos and Native Americans and persons with Down's syndrome. In these individuals, the eustachian tube is at a straighter angle than that of the general adult population. Otitis media has a greater incidence in Caucasian than Black persons and in males than females. The rate of infection is greater in persons who have frequent viral upper respiratory tract infections and in persons who have allergies that affect the upper respiratory tract. This situation can be attributed to the increased fluid within the eustachian tube, which makes for easier migration of infective agents to the middle ear.

PREVENTION

Prevention and early treatment of upper respiratory tract infections are the best precaution against adult otitis media. To prevent upper respiratory tract infections, the client needs to avoid individuals who are infected. To prevent transfer of infections within the family, members of the family need to use care when discarding tissues, to thoroughly wash their hands before touching articles used by other family members, and to wash dishes thoroughly to prevent cross-contamination.

If an individual already has an upper respiratory tract infection, use of decongestants and antibiotics is sometimes helpful. Decongestants help clear the eustachian tube and prevent migration of infecting organisms to the middle ear. Antibiotic therapy, when warranted for the upper respiratory tract infection, often helps to control the growth of bacteria before they can infect the middle ear.

COLLABORATIVE MANAGEMENT

 Assessment

History

One of the first questions that must be answered when taking a history of a client who complains of ear pain is, "Has there been a *recent upper respiratory tract infection?*" Along with this question, the nurse asks the client if *allergies affecting the upper respiratory system* are present. Examples of such allergies include irritation resulting from contact with flowers, grasses, dust, molds, and air pollutants.

Because there is usually a high degree of recurrence, the client is asked about any *past diagnosis of acute otitis media*. If the client has had a recent episode of otitis media, the nurse asks about the treatment used and exactly how well the client followed the directions (see the accompanying Nursing Research feature). It is not uncommon for clients to stop following prescribed treatment when they are feeling well but before the treatment is fully effective.

Age is an important factor to note with documentation because the acute form is more common in children and younger adults. Chronic otitis media is diagnosed more often in the older adult.

Physical Assessment: Clinical Manifestations

The chief complaint of the client with *acute or chronic otitis media* is ear *pain* with or without manipulation of the external-ear structures. Pain experienced with chronic otitis media is much less severe than that associated with the acute form of the disease. As the pressure in the middle ear increases, there is a greater sensation of fullness in the ear, and hearing is diminished and distorted. The client may complain of a sticking or cracking sound in the ear with yawning or swallowing. When it is present, *tinnitus*, or ringing in the ear, develops as a low hum or a low-pitched sound. *Hearing loss* that develops is a conductive hearing loss or some physical obstruction to the transmission of sound waves. *Headaches* are not uncommon. Signs and symptoms of systemic involvement can occur such as malaise, fever, nausea, and vomiting. As the pressure on the middle ear impinges on the inner ear, the client may begin to complain of slight *dizziness* or *vertigo*.

Physical findings from examination of the ear vary

NURSING RESEARCH

Nursing Interventions Increase Clients' Compliance with Follow-up After Treatment for Otitis Media.

Jones, S., Jones, P., & Katz, J. (1989). A nursing intervention to increase compliance in otitis media patients. *Applied Nursing Research*, 2(2), 68–73.

Some people are prone to having repeated episodes of otitis media. The number of these episodes decreases when clients return for a follow-up visit after antibiotic therapy to determine if fluid remains and if further treatment is needed. However, once otitis media symptoms have been relieved, many clients do not return for this follow-up visit.

This study attempted to increase client compliance for follow-up after treatment for otitis media by implementing a health belief model that relied on clinical intervention and/or telephone intervention. The number of clients who scheduled and kept a follow-up appointment after either or both of the two interventions was significantly greater than the number of clients who scheduled and kept follow-up appointments in the control group. The telephone intervention was determined to be more cost-effective than the clinical intervention in accomplishing the stated goal.

Critique. The results of this well-organized study support the hypothesis that clients may increase health-seeking behaviors if they perceive these behaviors to be beneficial. Nursing interventions can help clients to perceive the benefits of specific health-seeking behaviors.

Possible nursing implications. The interventions used in this study can be applied to other clinical situations in which follow-up care is critically important in preventing recurrence of a specific health problem. Because nurses are the primary health care providers who engage in client education activities, the nurse may be the most influential factor in successful health-promoting practices.

depending on the stage of the disease. The *tympanic membrane* is initially retracted, which allows clear visualization of the ear landmarks. At this early stage, the client has only vague complaints of ear discomfort. As the disease progresses, the tympanic membrane has dilation of the blood vessels and begins to appear red. The client begins to have otalgia, or ear pain, without any hearing loss. In the third stage, if the examiner has had an opportunity to see each stage, the tympanic membrane becomes red, thickened, and bulging, with a loss of landmarks. There is also a loss of mobility of the membrane when it is inspected with a pneumatic otoscope. With close observation, the nurse may be able to see an exudate behind the membrane.

Should the disease progress, the tympanic membrane spontaneously perforates, and pus or blood drains from the ear. This discharge may be pulsating when viewed through the otoscope. When the membrane ruptures, the client notices a marked decrease in pain. The perforation relieves the pressure on middle-ear structures, and pain is relieved. *Chronic otitis media* is almost always associated with a *perforation*. The perforation is usually central (Fig. 38–4). Perforations may heal if the infection is controlled; the membrane covering will always appear thinner over the healed perforation location. If the infection continues, the client may notice mucoid *otorrhea*, or ear drainage, during episodes of upper respiratory tract infection. A simple central perforation itself does not interfere with hearing unless the ossicles of the middle ear are damaged or the perforation is large.

The client with *serous otitis media* complains of the sensation of fullness and change in sounds within the ear. There is an absence of pain, fever, and systemic symptoms such as malaise and nausea. When visualized, the tympanic membrane often has a characteristic *ground glass* amber discoloration. A clear fluid level or bubbles are often detected, and the mobility of the membrane is impaired. Fluid within the middle ear limits the movement of the bony structures and leads to a conductive hearing loss.

During an examination, the nurse inspects both ears to determine if signs and symptoms of the infection or inflammation exist bilaterally. In view of the etiology, it is uncommon for the client to have absolute unilateral involvement. At times, the client may complain of more pain in one ear even though the physical examination shows bilateral changes. If symptoms persist with continued therapy, cancer of the ear or nasopharynx must be ruled out.

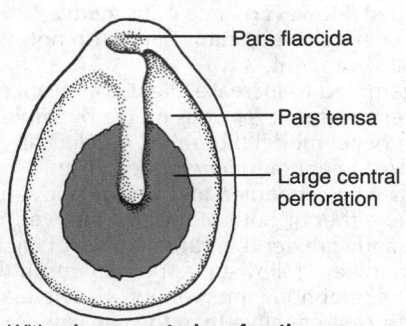

With a **large central perforation,**
clients complain of significant hearing loss.

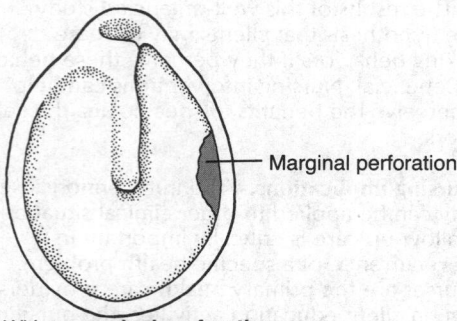

With a **marginal perforation,**
clients might complain of significant hearing loss.

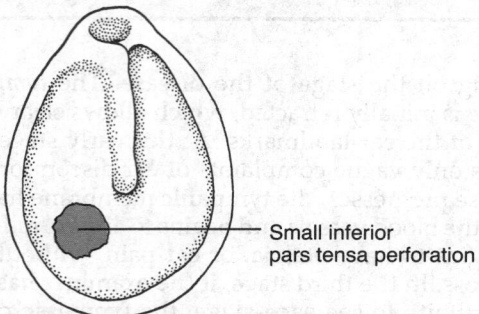

With a **small inferior pars tensa perforation,**
clients do not complain of much interference with hearing.

Figure 38–4

Perforations of the tympanic membrane. Central perforations heal more quickly than do marginal perforations. Marginal perforations that do not heal allow cholesteatoma formation.

Psychosocial Assessment

Pain, changes in auditory perception, and systemic symptoms interfere with the client's ability to interact with others. Systemic symptoms limit the client's desire to be active. For some clients, loss of time at work can have serious financial effects. The nurse assures the client that loss of work time will be limited and that return to work is possible as soon as the body temperature is normal.

Hearing loss and distortions in sounds are usually quite disturbing for the client. The nurse speaks slowly and in a soft voice while reassuring the client that the hearing loss will resolve with treatment of the infection. Clients can become quite frightened when they are told that a perforation has occurred or that a myringotomy, or surgical perforation of the tympanic membrane, is necessary (see under later heading Surgical Management). The nurse assures the client that this procedure does not permanently impair hearing unless bony structures have already been damaged.

Laboratory Findings

White blood cell counts are elevated in the client with acute or chronic otitis media. In the client with serous otitis media, blood values are normal because there is no infective process.

Cultures of the drainage after a perforation from uncontrolled otitis media may reveal the infecting agent. Cultures are usually not taken unless previous treatment has been ineffective. In cases in which the tympanic membrane is not perforated, a needle aspiration or myringotomy is used to obtain fluid for culture.

Analysis: Nursing Diagnosis

As with external otitis, clients present with pain and changes in sensory perception of hearing, and diagnoses are determined from subjective and objective data. The following nursing diagnoses are derived from these data.

Common Diagnoses

Three nursing diagnoses are common in clients with otitis media:

1. Pain related to inflammatory process and fluid in middle ear
2. Potential for injury related to the inflammatory process
3. Sensory/perceptual alterations (auditory) related to obstruction and/or damage in the middle ear

Additional Diagnoses

In addition to the actual diagnoses, the client may present with one or more potential diagnoses. These include

1. Knowledge deficit related to treatment and preventive measures
2. Activity intolerance related to pain
3. Anxiety related to inability to communicate
4. Social isolation related to pain and decreased hearing
5. Potential for injury related to altered auditory perception

 Planning and Implementation

The following plan of care for clients with otitis media focuses on the above-mentioned common diagnoses, although additional diagnoses must be considered for comprehensive care.

Pain

Planning: client goals. The main goals for this nursing diagnosis are that the client will (1) experience a reduction in pain after a reduction of fluid retention in the middle ear and (2) experience a decrease in inflammation.

Interventions. The management of pain involves nonsurgical treatment in the form of drugs. If nonsurgical methods do not relieve pain, surgical intervention is necessary.

Nonsurgical management. Pain relief is focused on measures that decrease the amount of fluid in the middle ear and of local inflammation. Treatment can be as simple as leaving the client in a quiet environment without distractions. Bed rest limits head movements and prevents movements that intensify the pain. Localized heat may be applied by using a heating pad adjusted to a low setting to hasten resolution of the infection and to relieve pain. Application of cold may occasionally relieve pain.

Systemic antibiotic therapy plays an important role in decreasing pain by reducing inflammation. Specific drug therapy can be found under the later nursing diagnosis heading Potential for Injury.

Analgesics are also required to aid in pain relief. Acetylsalicylic acid (aspirin) or acetaminophen (Tylenol) is frequently used. The antipyretic effect of these agents aids in helping the client feel better by relieving an elevated temperature. When the client complains of severe pain, narcotic analgesics such as codeine and meperidine (Demerol) may be necessary.

Oral and nasal antihistamines and decongestants are prescribed to decrease mucus production in the nasopharynx and to decrease levels of fluid in the middle ear. The body can thus reabsorb the fluid, and pressure from the fluid and pain in the ear are reduced.

Surgical management. If the pain persists after initial antibiotic therapy and the tympanic membrane continues to bulge, a *myringotomy* is performed. A myringotomy is a surgically performed perforation of the pars tensa of the tympanic membrane. Myringotomies result in drainage of middle-ear fluids and thus in almost immediate relief of pain. The small surgical incision can be performed in the doctor's office and heals rapidly. An alternative to the myringotomy is to remove fluid from the middle ear via needle aspiration. For relief of pressure caused by serous otitis media, a small grommet may be surgically placed through the tympanic membrane to allow continuous drainage of the middle-ear fluids (Fig. 38–5).

Preoperative care. Clients should be reassured that the myringotomy will relieve pain. This procedure is usually performed without anesthesia. Many people are apprehensive about a perforation and its effect on hearing. To help relieve some of the anxiety, the nurse discusses reasons for the procedure with the client: pain relief, relief of pressure from the middle-ear structures to prevent damage leading to hearing loss, and increased effectiveness of localized antibiotic therapy. Relaxation techniques such as deep breathing before and during the procedure help to calm the client and relieve anxiety.

Systemic antibiotic therapy continues before and after this procedure. The external canal is cleaned with a bacteriostatic solution such as povidone-iodine (Betadine) before the myringotomy is performed.

Postoperative care. Eardrops can be used to treat otitis media after the myringotomy. With a direct access to the middle-ear structures, the nurse places antibiotic drops such as neomycin sulfate (Myciguent) or bacitracin (Baciguent) in the canal for localized treatment of the

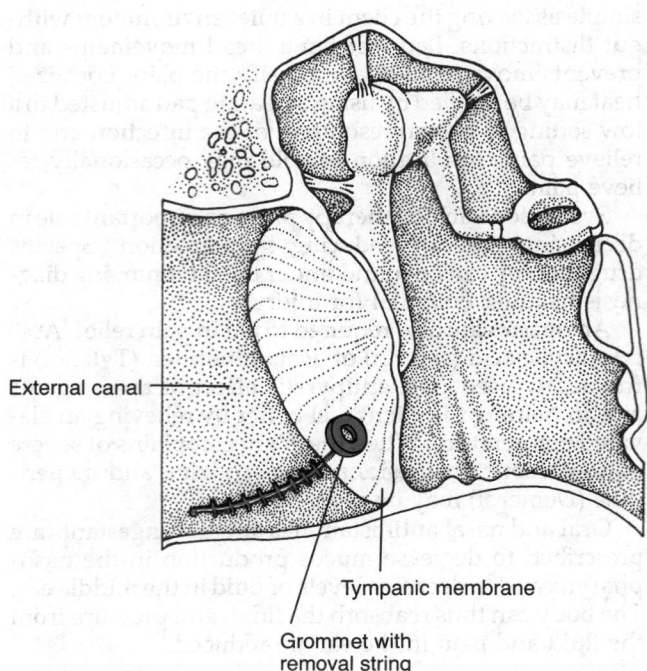

External canal

Tympanic membrane

Grommet with
removal string

Figure 38-5

Grommet through the tympanic membrane. A small grommet is placed through the tympanic membrane away from the margins, which allows prolonged drainage of fluids from the middle ear. The grommet can be removed later and the tympanic membrane allowed to heal naturally or patched with a small piece of homogeneous tissue.

infection. A cotton plug is placed in the external canal to help keep the medication in the ear. Care must be taken to keep the external ear and canal free from other substances while the incision is healing. The client needs to keep his or her head dry by avoiding washing hair or showering for several days. Instructions for clients to follow during the postoperative period are given in the accompanying Client/Family Education feature.

Potential for Injury

Planning: client goals. The major goal for this diagnosis is that the client will remain free from complications of prolonged or extended inflammation.

Interventions. Prevention of injury involves nonsurgical treatment in the form of drugs, diet, and rest. If nonsurgical methods do not relieve the inflammation, surgical intervention is necessary to prevent injury.

Nonsurgical management. In all except the severely immunosuppressed clients, the body attempts to control infections and to prevent their spread. To aid clients to use their own body defenses, it is important that the nurse is aware of the factors that complicate or enhance this process.

Diet therapy. A balanced diet with increased fluid intake is necessary. The client may not feel hungry but needs a balanced diet to supply the proper nutrients for tissue repair and production of antibodies to fight the infection. With an elevated temperature, the need for an increased amount of fluids is essential. These oral fluids replace those lost through perspiration. The fluids also help to cool the body and to reduce temperature to normal levels.

Therapeutic activity. Adequate rest is essential so that the body is able to repair damaged tissue without expending the energy on other activities; complete bed rest is not necessary. Some mild activities, such as walking and routine nonstrenuous activities, are necessary to prevent muscle wasting, which might make the client more prone to further infections.

Drug therapy. Systemic antibiotics are usually required to eliminate the infection completely from the middle ear. Examples of commonly used antibiotics include penicillin V potassium (Pen · Vee K), erythromycin (E-Mycin), cephalexin monhydrate (Keflex), and amoxicillin (Larotid). The nurse emphasizes the importance of taking the medication for the full prescribed course, which is usually 10 to 14 days depending on the antibiotic used.

In mild cases and in the chronic form of otitis media, antibiotic eardrops or powders such as polymyxin B sulfate (Aerosporin) or neomycin (Myciguent) may be of help. Ear irrigation helps with removal of debris in the external canal so that the antibiotic can reach infected tissue. A solution of 2% acetic acid is commonly used for irrigation of the ear.

Prevention of complications. If the tympanic membrane is perforated, it is important to protect the middle ear from invasion by external pathogenic organisms. Clients are instructed to keep water from entering the ear. A cotton ball that is coated with petroleum jelly provides an effective barrier against water.

In cases of severe otorrhea, the client must protect the neck from coming into contact with infective drainage. A cotton ball that is coated with petroleum jelly also helps to protect the spread of infection to external structures. When the cotton is removed, care must be used to discard it in a place where no one comes in contact with it. The client is also instructed to perform thorough hand washing after touching contaminated materials.

Surgical management. A myringotomy is performed to reduce the pain caused by otitis media, but it is also used when fever persists, hearing loss worsens, or the client complains of vertigo. Increased hearing loss indicates that the fluid levels and infection are not being treated adequately by the systemic antibiotics, and the fluid and purulent materials need to be drained for effective treatment. When clients with otitis media complain of vertigo, infection and pressure have spread to the inner ear. Prompt relief of pressure is necessary to prevent a sensorineural hearing loss. Pre- and postoper-

CLIENT/FAMILY EDUCATION ■ Instructions for the Client Recovering from Ear Surgery

Instructions	Rationales
1. "Avoid straining when you have a bowel movement, when you drink through a straw, and when you travel by air, and avoid excessive coughing for 2–3 weeks."	1. To avoid increased middle-ear pressure.
2. "Avoid people with colds."	2. To prevent recurrent infection.
3. "If you need to blow your nose, blow one side at a time with your mouth open for the first 2–3 weeks."	3. To avoid increased middle-ear pressure.
4. "Avoid washing your hair, showering, and getting your head wet for 1 week."	4, 5. To keep contaminated material out of the middle ear.
5. "Keep your ear dry for 6 weeks by keeping a ball of cotton coated with petroleum jelly, such as Vaseline, in your ear."	
6. "Avoid rapid head movements, bouncing, and bending over for 3 weeks."	6. To avoid increased middle-ear pressure and dislodging the graft.
7. "Change your ear dressing every 24 hours as directed."	7. To prevent secondary infection.
8. "Report excessive drainage immediately to your physician."	8. To detect and treat infection quickly.

ative care for a myringotomy is discussed earlier under the heading Surgical Management.

Sensory/Perceptual Alterations (Auditory)

Planning: client goals. The major goal for this diagnosis is that the client who is experiencing a hearing loss will experience a return of hearing to a functional level.

Interventions. The management of alterations in hearing involves nonsurgical treatment in the form of special communication needs. If the hearing loss persists, surgical intervention is necessary to correct the damage causing the hearing loss.

Nonsurgical management. The client's understanding of the treatment plan may be limited because of decreased hearing or the distortion of sounds. A low-pitched hum in the ear makes communication and understanding difficult. When giving instructions to the client, the nurse ensures that the environment is quiet and does not have additional distractions. Information is given slowly in a soft voice. Loud voices simply cause reverberation of fluids within the middle ear and distort the sounds to a greater degree. Written instructions aid the client with diminished hearing if he or she is able to read.

Surgical management. In some cases of chronic otitis media, surgical treatment is necessary to restore hearing. *Tympanoplasty,* or reconstruction of the middle ear, may be attempted to improve the conductive hearing loss. The surgical procedures for this operation can vary from simple reconstruction of the tympanic membrane, or *myringoplasty,* to replacement of the ossicles within the middle ear. The term type I tympanoplasty has been given to the myringoplasty. As the amount of damage and need for reconstruction increase, the nurse sees higher grades of tympanoplasties such as type II through type V (Fig. 38–6).

The tympanic membrane can be repaired with numerous materials including temporal muscle fascia, a split-thickness skin graft, or venous tissue. If the ossicles are damaged, more extensive measures must be taken to repair or replace these tiny bones. The ossicles are reached in one of three ways: a transcanal approach, an endaural incision, and via the postauricular route by performing a mastoidectomy (Fig. 38–7). Diseased tissue is removed, and the middle-ear cavity is cleaned. The ossicles can then be more closely assessed for damage or for the extent to which repair or replacement is necessary. Materials that are used to repair or replace the ossicles include autogenous cartilage or bone, cadaver ossicles, stainless steel wire, or Teflon components.

Surgical treatment is initiated only if the middle ear is free from infection at the time of surgery and the condition of the eustachian tube does not promote continued infection. If an infection is present, the graft is more likely to become infected and not heal properly.

Preoperative care. Specific care that is given to clients who are scheduled for a tympanoplasty is directed at clearing the ear of debris. Antibiotic drops are used to eliminate any remaining infecting organism. Before surgery, a solution of equal parts of vinegar and sterile water is used to irrigate the ear to restore its normal pH. The client follows measures aimed at decreasing chances of infection preoperatively. Clients are advised

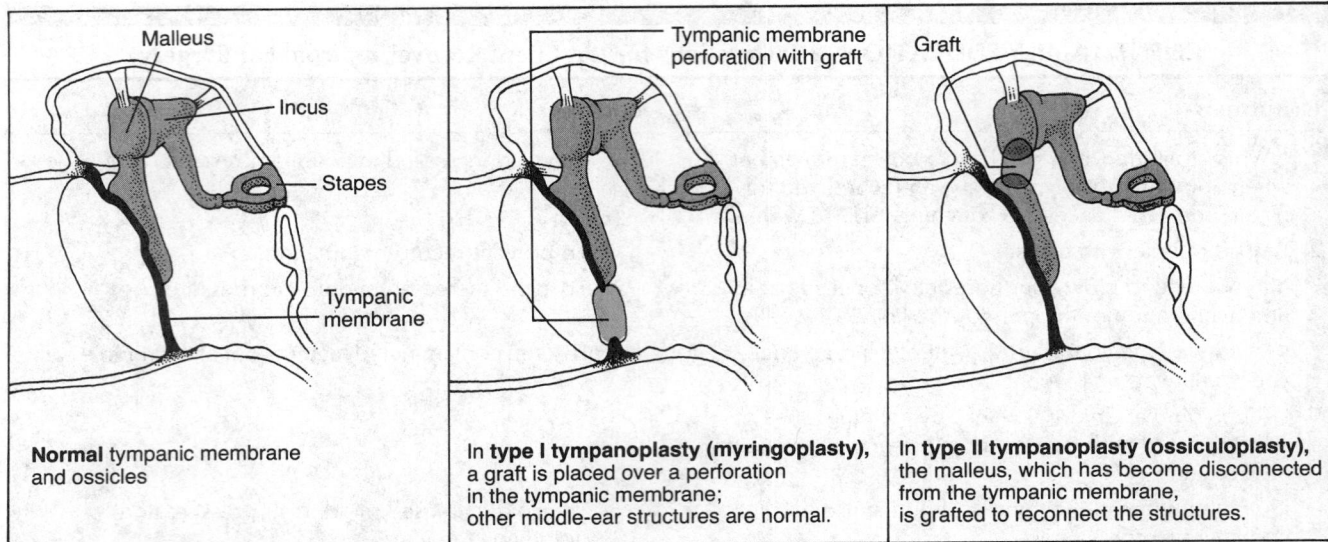

| | Tympanic membrane perforation with graft | Graft |

Figure 38–6

A normal tympanic membrane and two types of tympanoplasties.

to avoid persons with upper respiratory tract infections, to get adequate rest, and to eat a balanced diet, and to maintain an adequate fluid intake.

Surgery of the tympanic membrane and ossicles requires use of a microscope and is considered to be a delicate procedure. Local anesthesia can be used, although general anesthesia is often chosen to prevent the client from moving. The nurse explains the procedure to be used and what the client can expect postoperatively. The client is instructed about the importance of deep breathing postoperatively. Coughing is also used, but forceful coughing, which increases pressure in the middle ear, is avoided.

The nurse assures the client that the procedure is being performed to improve hearing. Initially, hearing is diminished because of the packing in the canal. The client is told this preoperatively to allay anxiety.

Postoperative care. The type of dressing used depends on the type of procedure. Either a direct incision through the external canal and tympanic membrane or a postauricular incision, behind the ear, is performed. In either case, an antiseptic-soaked gauze, such as iodoform gauze (Nugauze), is packed in the auditory canal. If the postauricular or endaural incision is used, an external dressing is placed over the operative site. Dressings should be kept clean and dry, and the nurse uses sterile technique when changing dressings. The client is kept flat with the operative ear up for at least 12 hours postoperatively. Prophylactic antibiotic therapy is often used to prevent subclinical infections from recurring. Hearing improvement is generally reported after the canal packing is removed. Until that time, the nurse uses techniques for communication with the hearing impaired and directs conversation to the unaffected ear. Teaching guidelines for clients who have had ear surgery should be followed and given to the client (see the feature Client/Family Education: Instructions for the Client Recovering from Ear Surgery).

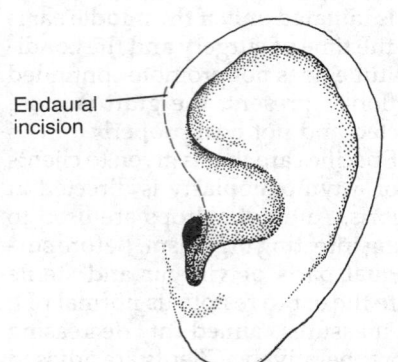

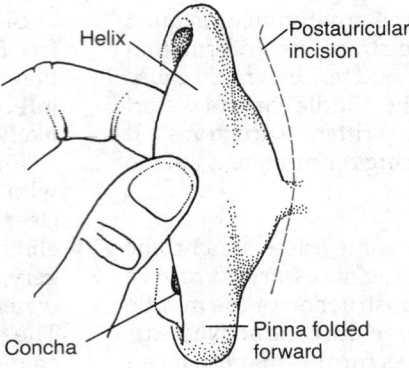

Figure 38–7

Surgical approaches for the ear. The endaural approach is used when the external canal is too small to use for a transcanal approach (not shown because no external incision is used). The postauricular approach is used for more extensive repair of the middle-ear and inner-ear structures.

■ Discharge Planning

Hospitalization is rare unless parenteral antibiotic therapy is necessary after oral and nonsurgical means of therapy have failed. If surgical repair is necessary and the procedure is completed without complications, the duration of hospitalization is only 2 to 3 days.

Home Care Preparation

Clients are allowed to go home for treatment but probably will not feel well enough to return to usual daily activities. As for any client with an infectious process, adequate rest and fluid intake and a balanced diet are necessary for proper wound healing. The client may return to work when the temperature is normal and the client feels well enough—about 3 weeks postoperatively.

Client/Family Education

Clients are given written instructions about how to take medications and when to come back for follow-up care. If the client is unable to read, the nurse gives these instructions to a family member who may assist with care. The nurse follows client teaching guidelines for instillation of eardrops (see Guidelines: How to Administer Eardrops), and for ear irrigation (see Guidelines: How to Irrigate an Ear), to demonstrate these techniques; a return demonstration by the client ensures use of the proper technique.

Submersion of the head in water, as well as trauma to the canal and tympanic membrane, is avoided during active otitis media. Trauma can be caused internally by forceful blowing of the nose. Air travel and drinking from a straw cause increased pressure on the tympanic membrane, and these activities need to be avoided by any client who has an upper respiratory tract infection and a history of otitis media.

Psychosocial Preparation

Persistent conductive hearing loss is a complication of all forms of otitis media. The degree of hearing loss that develops varies from client to client. In the days before antibiotic therapy, hearing loss was an almost certain outcome of chronic otitis media. The nurse needs to assure the client that not all people with hearing loss during the acute phase continue with that deficit. Surgical repair of the middle ear and tympanic membrane is not always totally successful in returning hearing to its preinjury functioning level. The nurse is aware of this and not unrealistic when discussing possible outcomes. However, the nurse allows the client to remain hopeful. Treatment for hearing loss is discussed earlier under the heading Collaborative Management in the section on hearing loss, along with special psychosocial considerations for these clients.

Health Care Resources

In rare cases, home care nurses are assigned to visit clients with otitis media. The nurse evaluates the client's use of oral and topical medications. For the client with a tympanoplasty, the surgical site is monitored for healing and any signs of infection.

Follow-up hearing tests are scheduled for the client when the lesion is well healed, in about 6 to 8 weeks. Pretreatment and posttreatment audiograms are compared. At this time, evaluation begins regarding the need for further surgical treatment or prescribing a hearing aid to improve conductive hearing.

 Evaluation

On the basis of the identified diagnosis, the nurse evaluates the care given to the client. Expected outcomes for a client with otitis media include that the client

1. States that the pain is reduced or alleviated
2. Describes proper use of antibiotic therapy
3. Demonstrates proper techniques when using eardrops, ointments, powders, or irrigation liquids
4. Identifies and avoids potential causes of otitis media
5. States that the hearing loss has been at least partially relieved
6. States the importance of having follow-up hearing assessments

By meeting the desired outcomes, the infection is resolved in almost all cases. Complications occasionally occur that require further treatment and education for the client. The nurse is always alert to the early signs of possible complications.

MASTOIDITIS

OVERVIEW

The epithelial lining of the middle ear is continuous with the epithelial lining of the mastoid air cells, which are embedded in the temporal bone. Mastoiditis is a secondary disorder resulting from an untreated or inadequately treated chronic or acute otitis media. Mastoiditis itself can be either acute or chronic. The term *chronic mastoiditis* is used when an acute infection is superimposed over a chronic infection that has invaded the mastoid cells, often secondary to cholesteatoma production. In the days before antibiotic therapy, mastoiditis was a leading cause of death in children and of hearing loss in adults. Today, antibiotic therapy is aimed at treating the middle-ear infection before it progresses to mastoiditis.

Clinical manifestations of mastoiditis include swelling behind the ear and pain with minimal movement of the tragus, pinna, or head. Pain is not relieved by myringotomy, or perforation of the tympanic membrane. A cellulitis develops on the skin or external scalp over the mastoid process. Otoscopic examination reveals a reddened, dull, thick, immobile tympanic membrane, with or without perforation. Postauricular lymph nodes are tender and enlarged. Clients with mastoiditis also complain of generalized systemic illness: low-grade fever, malaise, and anorexia.

COLLABORATIVE MANAGEMENT

General nursing care as described in the section on otitis media applies for clients with mastoiditis. In addition, surgical removal of infective material is necessary. Antibiotic therapy is aimed at preventing the continued spread of infection from the otitis media or mastoiditis, but it has limited use in the actual treatment of mastoiditis because of the difficulty of achieving effective antibiotic levels within the bony structure of the mastoid. Cultures are done to determine sensitivities of infecting organisms to specific antibiotics, culture material being obtained from the ear drainage or by myringotomy, so that the most effective antibiotic is chosen for treatment.

Surgical removal of the infected tissue is necessary if the client does not respond to nonsurgical treatment within a few days. A simple or modified radical mastoidectomy with tympanoplasty is the most common treatment. Only tissue that is infected is removed, and a tympanoplasty is performed to reconstruct the ossicles and tympanic membrane in an attempt to restore maximal hearing. It is essential that all infected tissue is removed so that the infection does not spread to other structures.

Complications arise when complete removal of the infective material has not been achieved or when there is contamination to other structures outside the mastoid and middle ear. Complications of mastoiditis include damage to the abducens and facial cranial nerves (nerves VI and VII, respectively). This damage is exhibited by an inability to look laterally (cranial nerve VI) and a drooping of the mouth on the affected side (cranial nerve VII). Other complications include meningitis, brain abscess, chronic purulent otitis media, and wound infection. The client may experience vertigo if the infection spreads into the labyrinth.

The nurse observes the client for dizziness, stiff neck, and vomiting. The wound dressing may be changed in 24 hours. The surgical incision is observed for edema, drainage, and redness. Dressings are reapplied.

Immediately after surgery, the client lies flat with the operative side up. If reconstruction of the ossicles has taken place, precautions are taken, as with any tympanoplasty, to prevent dislodging of the graft (see the feature Client/Family Education: Instructions for the Client Recovering from Ear Surgery). Clients are restricted to the bed with bedside commode privileges for 24 hours and are instructed to ask for assistance in getting out of bed to prevent falling and injury should dizziness persist as a problem.

TRAUMA

OVERVIEW

Trauma, and therefore damage, may occur to the tympanic membrane and ossicles by infection, by direct damage to the structures, or through rapid changes in the middle-ear cavity pressure. Foreign objects placed in the external canal may exert pressure on the tympanic membrane and cause perforation. If the objects continue through the canal, the bony structure of the stapes, incus, and malleus may be damaged. Blunt injury to the basal skull and ears can damage middle-ear structures through fractures extending to the middle ear. Rapid slapping of the external ear increases the pressure in the external auditory canal, which when great enough tears the eardrum in the same fashion as overinflating a balloon. The tympanic membrane has a limited stretching ability and gives way under high pressure. Excessive nose blowing and rapid changes of pressure that occur with nonpressurized air flight (barotrauma) can cause an increase in the pressure within the middle ear. High pressure damages the ossicles and can cause outward perforation of the eardrum.

COLLABORATIVE MANAGEMENT

Tympanic membrane perforations usually heal within 24 hours. Repeated perforations, especially from chronic otitis media, are slower to heal, and tympanic scarring increases. Depending on the amount of damage to the ossicles, hearing loss may or may not return. Hearing aids can improve hearing. Surgical reconstruction of the ossicles and tympanic membrane through a tympanoplasty or myringoplasty may also be performed to improve hearing (refer to the earlier discussion of nursing care after a tympanoplasty).

Preventive measures should be taken to avoid trauma. Clients are instructed to avoid inserting objects into the external canal. Ear protectors can be used when blunt trauma is likely to be experienced, especially in sports such as boxing. Most airplanes are pressurized to prevent barotrauma by rapid altitude changes.

OTOSCLEROSIS

OVERVIEW

Otosclerosis is a disease of the labyrinthine capsule of the middle ear that results in a bony overgrowth of the tissue surrounding the ossicles. Diagnosis is primarily made through evaluation of clinical manifestations, family history, and the absence of other disorders that might cause similar complaints.

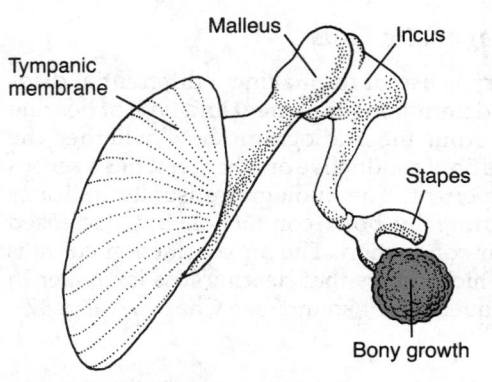

Otosclerosis at the anterior footplate

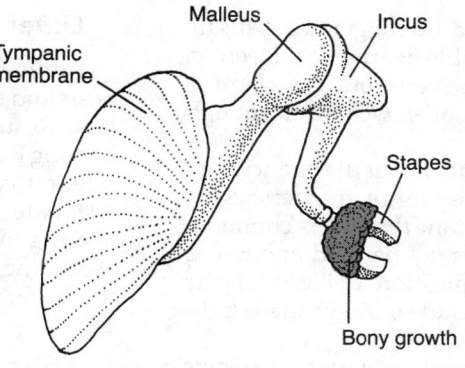

Otosclerosis at the junction
of the incus and stapes

Figure 38-8
Common sites of otosclerosis. Otosclerosis can cause fixation of the stapes by spongy growth of bone around the anterior footplate or at the junction of the incus and stapes.

Pathophysiology

Otosclerosis is characterized by development of irregular areas of new bone formation. As the otosclerotic bone grows, it usually involves the footplate of the stapes and causes the fixation of the footplate within the oval window (Fig. 38-8). One or more sites of bone growth can be present in the capsule. Occasionally, the lesion increases in size and involves structures of the inner ear such as the vestibule or cochlea. Stapes fixation leads to a conductive hearing loss. If the disease involves the inner ear, sensorineural hearing loss is present. It is not uncommon to have bilateral involvement, although hearing loss may be worse in one ear.

Etiology

The etiology of otosclerosis is unknown, but it is thought to have a familial tendency. A positive family history can be obtained in more than half of the cases. Clinical manifestations of otosclerosis begin or worsen during or soon after pregnancy, although it is unclear how pregnancy exacerbates the progress of the disease.

Incidence

The onset of symptoms is usually restricted to adults between the second and fifth decades of life. Otosclerosis occurs more frequently in Caucasian than in Black persons. The incidence of the disease in women is twice that in men, and otosclerosis is frequently associated with hormonal changes seen with pregnancy (Hall & Colman, 1987).

PREVENTION

There are no known measures that prevent the development of otosclerosis because its exact etiology is unknown. Women with a strong family history of the disorder may consider the possibility of limiting the number of pregnancies as a means of prevention.

COLLABORATIVE MANAGEMENT

Assessment

History

The major clinical manifestation of otosclerosis is *hearing loss.* When taking a history, the nurse should document, if possible, the *time of onset of any hearing deficit.* Symptoms typically progress slowly, and it is difficult for the client to determine the exact time when a deficit began. Onset and progress of hearing loss are important in making the differential diagnosis of otosclerosis versus other disorders that also lead to diminished hearing.

Heredity, race, sex, and *age* are important factors to assess for a diagnosis of otosclerosis. If there is a positive family history of otosclerosis, the nurse is more likely to suspect the client of having an otosclerotic lesion. If the client is a woman of childbearing age, the nurse questions her about changes and clinical manifestations during pregnancy.

The nurse reviews the client's *history of ear infections* or other complaints. Clients may attribute hearing loss to chronic infections of the middle ear. A high incidence of middle-ear infections has little correlation with the occurrence of otosclerosis.

Physical Assessment: Clinical Manifestations

The most common complaint of clients with otosclerosis is a *slowly progressing conductive hearing loss.* Hearing loss is *bilateral,* although the progression of the disease is different in each ear, which gives the effect of having one "good" ear and one "bad" ear. Otosclerosis and the associated hearing deficit most commonly begin to develop in early adulthood but are often ignored until middle age when the client can no longer compensate for the increasing loss. Measurable hearing loss (seen on an audiogram) may be quite severe, but the client is often able to discriminate the spoken word well enough for daily conversation.

Initial hearing loss is of the lower frequencies of sound; the loss then progresses to all frequencies. A ringing or roaring type of constant *tinnitus* is common, and this sound within the ear may be loud enough to disturb the rest and communication abilities of the client. Chewing also causes a loud sound in these individuals.

A physical examination reveals a *normal tympanic membrane.* Occasionally, the eardrum has a pinkish discoloration (*Schwartze's sign*) and indicates vascular changes within the middle ear. The two tuning fork tests, Rinne's and Weber's, both used to test for conductive hearing loss, are useful when assessing clients suspected of having otosclerosis. The Rinne test result is negative, i.e., bone conduction is greater than or equal to air conduction. In the Weber test, clients with otosclerosis have *lateralization* of the sound to the ear with the most conductive hearing loss.

Psychosocial Assessment

During the initial phase of the disease, little or no psychosocial support related to otosclerosis is necessary. As the disease progresses and before a diagnosis is made, clients may begin to feel uncomfortable with their surroundings because of diminished hearing. With the insidious progress of the disability and the difficulty of making a diagnosis before hearing loss is severe, a client may go many years feeling that something is wrong but unable to identify the cause. Clients and their families need to express their feelings and to discover ways to support each other.

As the client notices continued hearing loss, uneasy feelings are substituted by fear of permanent deafness. It is important that the nurse work with the client to find ways of coping with the disability and to review ways of managing the hearing loss. The client needs to understand that the hearing loss will continue to progress and that there is no treatment to prevent the progression. There are treatments, such as surgery or wearing a hearing aid, to improve hearing in most clients, but these treatments do not guarantee the return of normal hearing.

Radiographic Findings

Diagnosis of otosclerosis is usually made by noting clinical presentation and the absence of other causative factors. Recently, the use of tomography has allowed examiners to identify the otosclerotic lesion. This technique is especially useful before surgical treatment so that the exact location and extent of the lesion may be seen. Tomography is also useful in cases in which the clinical manifestations could be a mixture of otosclerosis and another disease.

Other Diagnostic Tests

Audiometry is useful for making a differential diagnosis and for determining the extent and type of hearing loss. Results from the audiogram show whether the hearing loss is only conductive or whether it has a sensorineural component. The audiogram usually indicates adequate hearing by bone conduction but decreased hearing by air conduction. The air conduction curve is ascending, which shows that hearing loss is greater in the lower frequencies of sound (see Chap. 37, Fig. 37–12).

 ### Analysis: Nursing Diagnosis

Clients present with progressive hearing loss over a prolonged time. Diagnoses are determined from subjective and objective data. The nursing diagnoses are derived from these data.

Common Diagnoses

The nursing diagnosis that is common in clients with otosclerosis is sensory/perceptual alterations (auditory) related to changes in the bony structures of the middle ear.

Additional Diagnoses

Other nursing diagnosis that may be present include

1. Fear related to possible permanent hearing loss
2. Social isolation related to inability to communicate
3. Ineffective individual coping related to prolonged period of perceptual changes without a diagnosis
4. Self-esteem disturbance related to loss of body function
5. Impaired verbal communication related to reduced hearing
6. Knowledge deficit related to treatment modalities

 ### Planning and Implementation

The following plan of care for clients with otosclerosis focuses on the most common diagnosis.

Sensory/Perceptual Alterations (Auditory)

Planning: client goals. The major goal for this nursing diagnosis is that the client will regain maximal hearing abilities with minimal complications associated with treatment plans.

Interventions. Treatment for otosclerosis includes nonsurgical interventions that promote improvement in hearing through amplification. The client may also decide to have surgical intervention to remove the bony growth causing the hearing loss.

Nonsurgical management. Nursing measures are aimed at assisting the client to maintain optimal communication ability. Usually, clients with otosclerosis are able to understand daily conversations. After the client is assessed for the extent of hearing loss, the nurse initiates interventions to promote better hearing. Communication needs to take place in an area with minimal distractions. Low-frequency hearing loss means that deep, low sounds are missed more often than high-frequency sounds. After a period of long-term hearing loss, clients often begin to agree with people most of the time, even when they do not fully comprehend what is being said. The nurse needs to validate the client's understanding of instructions by asking for return demonstrations or a repeat of the instructions.

In cases of severe otosclerosis with bilateral involvement and complete hearing loss, alternative methods of communication are necessary. Writing paper, magic slates, or computerized communication devices help the client who is able to read. For those clients who cannot read or understand the language used by the nurse, a basic form of communication is necessary. Flash cards with pictures of frequently used ideas are available in many health care facilities through the speech and language pathology department, school supply stores, or toy stores.

Hearing aids can be quite useful for many clients. If there is only a conductive hearing loss, the hearing aid amplifies sounds enough to make hearing easier. Clients must learn certain techniques for proper use of the hearing aid for optimal effectiveness. Education of the client on the use of a hearing aid is discussed under the heading Using Hearing Aids in the section on hearing loss.

Surgical management. The most effective intervention that is used to correct hearing loss is a *partial stapedectomy* or *complete stapedectomy* with prosthesis. A stapedectomy involves removal of the head, neck, or crura of the stapes, and less often removal of the footplate. After removal of the immobile bone, a small hole is drilled in the footplate, and a metal or plastic prosthesis in the shape of a piston is connected between the incus and the footplate (Fig. 38-9). This procedure is called *fenestration.* Sounds cause the prothesis to vibrate in the same manner as did the stapes. Both stapedectomy and fenestration have high success rates, with up to 90% of clients experiencing restoration of practical hearing.

Preoperative care. A stapedectomy is usually performed with the client under local anesthesia and is a transcanal procedure, through the external auditory canal. Local anesthetics are used along with medications to relax the client during the procedure to reduce positional discomfort.

To prevent introduction of infective material to the middle-ear structures, it is essential that no signs or symptoms of external otitis are present at the time of surgery. Clients are instructed to follow measures that prevent occurrence of middle-ear or external-ear infections: avoidance of excessive nose blowing, no placement of objects in the canal for cleaning, and removal of

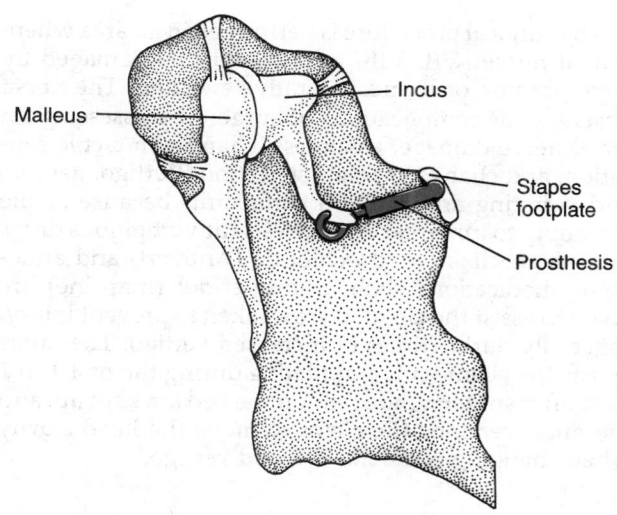

Figure 38-9
Prosthesis used with stapedectomy. The stapes is removed, leaving the footplate. After a hole is drilled in the footplate, a metal or plastic prosthesis is connected to the incus and inserted through the hole to act as a vibration device, much as the stapes worked before the development of otosclerosis.

a hearing aid 2 weeks before surgery to ensure the integrity of local tissue.

Hearing is initially worse after the surgical procedure to correct otosclerosis. The success rate of this procedure is high, but, as with all procedures, it carries a risk of failure that might lead to total deafness on the affected side or damage to the cranial nerves. The client is informed of this risk preoperatively and may continue to be concerned about the potential outcome even after the procedure is completed.

Clients must be informed of expected outcomes (amount and progression of hearing restoration) and possible complications, including complete hearing loss, prolonged vertigo, infection, and facial nerve damage. A decision to proceed with surgery should be made with full knowledge and understanding of these complications.

Postoperative care. Clients need to be told that noticeable improvement in hearing may take as long as 6 weeks after surgery. Initially, the Gelfoam ear packing interferes with hearing. Gelfoam is an absorbable gelatin sponge that serves to decrease bleeding. Postoperative swelling in the ear continues to affect hearing until the edema has resolved. Medications for pain assist the client in maintaining comfort and cooperation. Antibiotics such as neomycin (Miciguent) are given prophylactically to lessen the chance of infection at the surgical site. The client is told to use the postoperative instructions given earlier (see the feature Client/Family Education: Instructions for the Client Recovering from Ear Surgery). Changes in middle-ear pressure could dislodge the graft or prosthesis.

The surgical procedure is performed in an area where cranial nerves VII, VIII, and X might be damaged by direct trauma or by postoperative swelling. The nurse observes for complications of surgery by assessing for facial nerve damage, weakness, changes in tactile sensation, and changes in taste sensation. Vertigo, nausea, and vomiting are common complaints because of the proximity to inner-ear structures. Antivertiginous drugs such as meclizine hydrochloride (Antivert) and antiemetic medications such as droperidol (Inapsine) are given to assist the client. Care is taken to prevent injury, especially during times of increased vertigo. The nurse assists the client with ambulating during the first 1 to 2 days after surgery. Side rails on the bed are kept up, and the nurse reminds the client to move the head slowly when changing positions to avoid vertigo.

■ Discharge Planning

Home Care Preparation

With persistent vertigo, the client remains in danger of falling. The home environment needs to be assessed for potential hazards. In addition, the nurse assesses the client's home situation to determine if family members or significant others are available to assist the client in the home with meal preparation and activities of daily living. Home care nurses and nonprofessionals contacted earlier can help greatly.

Client/Family Education

To prevent late postoperative infections, clients are instructed to avoid persons with upper respiratory tract infections, to avoid showering and getting the head and wound wet, and to refrain from using small objects such as cotton-tipped applicators to clean the external canal. Rapid, extreme changes in air pressure caused by quick head movements, sneezing, nose blowing, straining during a bowel movement, and changes in altitude should also be avoided. For more information, see the feature Client/Family Education: Instructions for the Client Recovering from Ear Surgery.

If a hearing aid is used by the client, he or she is taught how to use it most effectively. Learning to use a hearing aid and care of the device are described earlier under the heading Using Hearing Aids and in the feature Client/Family Education: How to Care for a Hearing Aid.

Psychosocial Preparation

Clients are informed of the success rate with surgical correction of otosclerosis. A complication of an unsuccessful surgery is continued disability or complete loss of hearing in the affected ear. Surgery is performed on the ear with the greatest hearing loss. If the surgery does not improve the hearing, the client must decide either to attempt surgical correction of the other ear or to con-

tinue to use an amplification device. The progressive nature of the disease makes this decision a difficult one for the client. The nurse supports the client by listening to her or his concerns and giving additional information when needed.

Health Care Resources

If the client does not have family or friends to help during the postoperative period, a referral to a home care agency is necessary. Assistance with meal preparation, cleaning, and personal hygiene can be contracted with the hospital discharge planners before discharge.

Evaluation

On the basis of the identified diagnoses, the nurse evaluates the care given. Expected outcomes for a client with external otitis include that the client

1. States that hearing loss has been at least partially relieved
2. Demonstrates proper technique for using a hearing aid when applicable
3. Participates in communication appropriately
4. Avoids nose blowing and sneezing
5. Identifies potential hazards postoperatively
6. Seeks assistance with activities of daily living until vertigo and dizziness have subsided

By meeting the desired outcomes, hearing will be improved and communication will be easier for the client. Postoperative complications are avoided that might lead to the return or worsening of hearing loss.

CHOLESTEATOMA

OVERVIEW

Cholesteatoma is a benign growth of squamous cell epithelium. Formation of a cholesteatoma can occur in several ways. It is most common in clients who have chronic otitis media with a perforation of the tympanic membrane that fails to heal on its own. A perforation of the tympanic membrane, especially a marginal perforation, leaves an open access for tissue from the external canal to grow into the middle ear (Fig. 38–10). Another way in which a cholesteatoma is formed is by a retraction of the tympanic membrane into the middle ear. In either case, debris is deposited into the sac, and the epithelial tissue begins to grow and to invade the ossicles of the middle ear, mastoid, labyrinth, facial nerve, or other intracranial structures.

The general appearance of a cholesteatoma is a grayish-white, shiny mass behind or involving the tympanic membrane; the mass is often described as having a

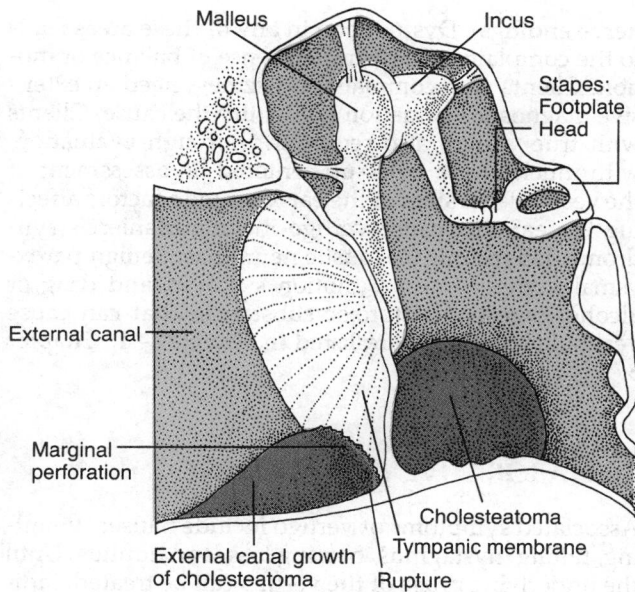

Figure 38-10

The cholesteatoma shown here resulted from growth of squamous cell tissue of the external canal through a marginal perforation of the tympanic membrane into the middle-ear cavity.

cauliflower-like appearance. If there is no perforation of the tympanic membrane, it becomes difficult to diagnose the presence of a cholesteatoma. Destruction of one or more structures by the cholesteatoma determines which clinical manifestations are seen. If the growth is limited to the middle ear and is associated with chronic otitis media, complaints are similar to those for otitis media without cholesteatoma. Hearing might be diminished to a greater extent than usual because of the obstruction or invasion and destruction of the ossicles by the cholesteatomatous mass.

If the labyrinth becomes involved, the client complains of vertigo and experiences a sensorineural hearing loss. Facial paralysis is produced by erosion of cranial nerve VII.

COLLABORATIVE MANAGEMENT

If there is an infectious process, antibiotic therapy is initiated after a culture is obtained and sensitivity of the organism is determined. Antibiotics are given orally, parenterally, or topically through the external canal. Care is taken to clean debris from the canal so that the medication can reach the infections. Usually, surgical removal of the cholesteatoma is necessary; the exact location determines the surgical approach. If the growth is limited to the middle ear, removal takes place through the external canal. The procedure called a *myringoplasty* is used to repair the tympanic membrane. A *tympanoplasty* is performed to repair or replace the ossicles to

improve conductive hearing. For more extensive growths, a *mastoidectomy* might be necessary, or an incision behind the tragus is made for access to the growth. More information about these procedures is presented under the heading Surgical Management for the diagnosis Sensory/Perceptual Alterations (Auditory) in the section on otitis media. While the nurse describes the need to remove the cholesteatoma to prevent further damage to other structures, especially the cranial nerves or inner ear, the nurse also discusses the possibility of permanent hearing loss with the client.

NEOPLASMS

OVERVIEW

Tumors of the middle ear are rare. The most common type of tumor is the *glomus jugulare,* which is a highly vascular benign lesion arising from the jugular vein. When this type of lesion is limited to the middle ear, the name *tympanicum* is used. Growth of any lesion within the middle-ear fossa leads to disruption of conductive hearing, erosion of the ossicles, and potential for involvement of the inner ear and adjacent cranial nerves. Clients complain most often of progressive hearing loss and tinnitus. Infection, drainage, and pain are rarely associated with glomus jugulare tumors. A physical examination reveals bulging of the tympanic membrane or even a mass extending to the external auditory canal. The highly vascular nature of the glomus jugulare tumor gives it a reddish color and a visible pulsation when seen through the eardrum.

COLLABORATIVE MANAGEMENT

Diagnosis is made by physical examination, tomography, and angiography. Extremely rare malignant tumors include primary adenocarcinoma, adenoid cystic carcinoma, and mucoepidermoid carcinoma. At times, cholesteatomas and infectious lesions may be mistakenly diagnosed as neoplasms.

Neoplasms are removed by surgery, which generally sacrifices hearing in the affected ear. If all the margins of the tumor can be seen clearly through the tympanic membrane, a transcanal approach is used to remove the lesion. When the tumor margins extend past the tympanic membrane, further diagnostic tests are necessary to determine the extent of growth and vascular involvement. Radiation therapy is used to decrease the vascularity of the glomus jugulare tumor but is not the preferred method of treatment for these or other middle-ear tumors. Benign lesions are removed because with continued growth, cranial structures other than the middle ear can be affected, with further damage of the facial nerve (cranial nerve VII) or the trigeminal nerve (cranial nerve V). When possible, reconstructive surgery of the middle-ear structures is performed at a later date in an attempt to restore conductive hearing.

CONDITIONS AFFECTING THE INNER EAR

TINNITUS

OVERVIEW

Tinnitus is one of the most common complaints of clients with otologic disorders, especially disorders involving the inner ear. Symptoms of tinnitus range from mild ringing in the ear, which can go unnoticed during the day, to a loud roaring in the ear, which can interfere with the individual's thinking process. When clients complain of tinnitus, the nurse is alert to the wide variety of pathologic disorders and other factors that cause tinnitus: presbycusis, otosclerosis, Meniere's syndrome, certain drugs, exposure to loud noise, and other abnormalities of the inner ear.

COLLABORATIVE MANAGEMENT

The exact pathophysiology of tinnitus varies with the underlying cause. Clients and nursing staff are frustrated in efforts to treat tinnitus unless the accompanying disorder is resolved. When no underlying cause can be found or the disorder is untreatable, therapy focuses on ways to mask the tinnitus. Background sound, noise-makers, and music help to mask the sound during the sleeping hours. Earmold hearing aids can be used to amplify sounds to drown out the tinnitus. Many clients learn to adjust their lives so that the ear noise is less disturbing. The American Tinnitus Association is a helpful resource for clients to assist them in coping with tinnitus when medical therapy has been unsuccessful.

VERTIGO AND DIZZINESS

OVERVIEW

Vertigo and dizziness, like tinnitus, are common clinical manifestations of many ear disorders. *Dizziness* is described as a disturbed sense of the proper relationship to space. Different clients vary greatly in what sensations they call dizziness. The term *vertigo* is often used interchangeably with dizziness, but the definition, as well as the etiology, is somewhat different. True vertigo is a sense of whirling or turning in space. Clients might say that they are turning or that the room is spinning. With vertigo, there is a real sense of motion, in contrast to dizziness, which is usually defined as a disturbed sense of uneasiness with spatial relations.

Three systems combine to give input to the cerebellum regarding the balance of the individual: the visual system, the vestibular system (cochlea, semicircular canals), and the proprioceptive system (muscles and nerve endings). Dysfunction in any of these areas leads to the complaint of a disturbed sense of balance or motion. Clients who complain of dizziness need an extensive diagnostic evaluation to identify the cause. Clients with true vertigo also require a thorough evaluation, with much of the work-up centered on assessment of the vestibular system of the ear. Common factors affecting the ear that cause vertigo include Meniere's syndrome, labyrinthitis, acoustic neuromas, benign paroxysmal vertigo, trauma, motion sickness, and drug or alcohol ingestion. Ototoxic substances that can cause vestibular problems are listed in Table 37–1, Chapter 37.

COLLABORATIVE MANAGEMENT

Associated symptoms of vertigo include nausea, vomiting, falling, nystagmus, hearing loss, and tinnitus. Until the underlying cause of the vertigo can be treated, individual clinical manifestations are treated. Clients are advised to restrict head motions or to move more slowly; to maintain adequate hydration, especially when vomiting has occurred; and to take medications that have antivertiginous effects such as dimenhydrinate (Dramamine), diazepam (Valium), and scopolamine (Transderm Scōp, Triptone). Many clients are dissatisfied with treatment because side effects of the medications, especially drowsiness, can be worse than the vertigo. The nurse cautions clients to maintain a safe, uncluttered environment to prevent accidents during periods of vertigo. Use of a cane or a walker helps in maintaining balance. The nurse instructs the client not to drive or to operate machinery when taking drugs that cause vertigo.

LABYRINTHITIS

OVERVIEW

Labyrinthitis is an infection of the labyrinth, which occasionally occurs as a complication of acute or chronic otitis media. Infection results from an erosion of the bony capsule that allows infective materials to invade the structure. Labyrinthitis often results from growth of a cholesteatoma from the middle ear into the lateral semicircular canal. Other etiologies of labyrinthitis include infections introduced by surgery to the semicircular canal or to the stapes footplate and meningitis. When the infecting organism is viral, the labyrinthitis may be part of a systemic viral infection such as an upper respiratory tract infection or infectious mononucleosis. Infection is usually unilateral.

Clinical manifestations include hearing loss, tinnitus, and spontaneous nystagmus to the affected side. The client also complains of vertigo with associated nausea and vomiting. Meningitis may be the source of infection of the labyrinth. Even if meningitis is not the source of infection, it is the most common complication.

COLLABORATIVE MANAGEMENT

The nurse observes the client for signs and symptoms of meningitis such as headache, stiff neck, and lethargy. A lumbar puncture is performed for analysis of cerebrospinal fluid and detection of white blood cells when the client is suspected of having meningitis.

Treatment includes use of systemic antibiotics such as ampicillin (Omnipen). Clients are advised to stay in bed, especially in a darkened room, until the clinical manifestations have diminished. Antiemetics such as chlorpromazine (Thorazine) and antivertiginous medications such as dimenhydrinate are useful for relief of symptoms.

The client needs a great deal of psychosocial support. Hearing loss may be permanent on the affected side. The client is reassured that the vertigo will subside as the inflammation resolves. Balance problems that persist can be improved with gait training through physical therapy.

MENIERE'S SYNDROME

OVERVIEW

Meniere's syndrome is characterized by a triad of symptoms: *tinnitus, unilateral sensioneural hearing loss,* and *vertigo.* These symptoms occur in attacks that are self-limiting but at times last for several days. Clients are almost totally incapacitated during an attack, and several days are needed to fully recover. The initial hearing loss is reversible, but as the frequency of attacks continues, hearing loss becomes permanent.

Pathophysiology

Another name given to Meniere's syndrome is *endolymphatic hydrops,* which refers to dilation of the endolymphatic system, either by overproduction or decreased reabsorption of endolymphatic fluid. The increase in fluid causes a distortion of the entire system of the inner canal, thereby causing decreased hearing from dilation of the cochlear duct, vertigo because of damage to the vestibular system, and tinnitus with an unknown etiology. The fluctuating nature of the attacks and clinical manifestations is thought to be due to leaking endolymph into surrounding tissues, which worsens the symptoms. As the fluid is slowly reabsorbed, a type of remission occurs. Repeated damage to the cochlea, caused by increased fluid pressure, leads to permanent hearing loss. Endolymphatic hydrops is usually unilateral.

Etiology

The etiology of Meniere's syndrome is unknown, but several theories have been considered (Wilmot, 1984).

Any factor that increases endolymphatic secretion in the labyrinth could lead to the symptoms associated with Meniere's syndrome. Factors that increase fluid include viral or bacterial infections, allergic reactions, and biochemical disturbances. A vascular disturbance producing changes in the microcirculation of the labyrinth is another possible etiologic factor. Psychologic factors cannot be ignored. Relatively mild long-term stress seems to be associated with the development of Meniere's syndrome. In cases in which stress appears to be a factor, there has usually been no outlet for expressing the emotions for a long time. Family history is often positive for Meniere's syndrome, which might indicate a genetic component or a familial tendency to deal with stress in a certain fashion.

Incidence

The onset of symptoms of Meniere's syndrome usually occurs in the third to fifth decades of life. The prevalence is greater in males. In females, Meniere's syndrome appears to be linked to the sexual cycle, which makes symptoms worse in the later stages of pregnancy and during the premenstrual period. Meniere's syndrome is more common in Caucasians than non-Caucasians.

PREVENTION

Because the exact etiology of Meniere's syndrome is unknown, measures to prevent the disease have not been described. If prolonged stress is an etiologic factor, stress reduction techniques may help to prevent symptoms. After the client has experienced an attack of vertigo, hearing loss, and tinnitus, it becomes increasingly difficult to lessen anxiety while the client awaits another episode. Identification of allergies and infections with early treatment might also help to prevent the development of Meniere's syndrome.

COLLABORATIVE MANAGEMENT

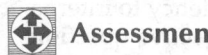 Assessment

History

The history is an important component in obtaining a differential diagnosis. Many disorders can cause tinnitus, vertigo, and hearing loss and therefore mimic Meniere's syndrome. The nurse documents the *duration of the episodes,* their *intensity,* and the *time between episodes.*

In an effort to review possible etiologic factors, the nurse discusses the client's history of *viral and bacterial infections; allergies,* especially to environmental antigens; and *any exposure to drugs or chemicals.* In clients who have been exposed to these factors, it remains unclear what length of time and how much exposure are required before symptoms occur.

Physical Assessment: Clinical Manifestations

The nurse documents the type of clinical manifestations that the client experiences. The classic symptoms of Meniere's syndrome include *tinnitus, vertigo,* and *hearing loss.* Times of severe, debilitating attacks alternate with periods that are almost free of symptoms. A *feeling of fullness in the ear* precedes the more severe trilogy. Clinical manifestations are unilateral in 60% to 70% of the cases.

Clients describe the tinnitus as a continuous, low-pitched roar or a humming sound, which is present much of the time but worsens just before and during a severe attack. Hearing loss is initially of the low-frequency tones but worsens to include all levels after repeated episodes. The loss of hearing is worse during an attack. In the early stages of the disease, periods of remission are marked by normal or nearly normal hearing. A permanent hearing disability develops as the number of attacks increases.

When questioned, the client describes the vertigo as periods of whirling, which might even cause him or her to fall to the ground. The vertigo is so intense that even while lying down, clients hold the bed or ground in an attempt to prevent the whirling. The severe vertigo usually lasts 3 to 4 hours, but the client continues to complain of a sense of dizziness long after the attack. *Nausea* and *vomiting* are common. Other clinical manifestations include *nystagmus, rapid eye movements,* and *severe headaches.*

Psychosocial Assessment

The strong evidence of a stress component with Meniere's syndrome leads the nurse to make a thorough assessment of the client's stressors and review his or her coping style (see Chap. 6). The nurse questions the client about the amount of stress perceived in the client's life, both at home and at work. The client is then asked how he or she copes with that stress. As for other disorders with a psychosomatic component, clients often do not feel overly stressed because of the tendency to internalize many feelings. The nurse asks objective questions about daily routines and personal coping such as, "Do you take time in the day to relax?" "How do you react to very unpleasant or upsetting news?" Life style changes will be imposed on the client because of the debilitating nature of the disorder. During an attack, the client will not be able to work or care for himself or herself. Forced dependency makes the client feel powerless.

Laboratory Findings

There are no specific laboratory tests for diagnosis of Meniere's syndrome. A test to rule out syphilis is done because syphilis can cause hydrops, which leads to symptoms similar to those of Meniere's syndrome.

Radiographic Findings

Radiographic tests are performed to rule out other disorders. X-ray films are taken to diagnose an acoustic neuroma, which might lead to tinnitus, vertigo, and hearing loss on the affected side.

Diagnostic Tests

Pure tone audiometry shows a loss of low-tone hearing with low-tone tinnitus in the affected ear during the early stages of the disease. There is also evidence of *recruitment,* or an abnormal sensation of loudness with a minimal increase in the intensity of the test sound. Speech discrimination is well preserved until later in the disease. *Diplacusis,* a pure tone heard differently in each ear, is another common finding.

 Analysis: Nursing Diagnosis

Clients with Meniere's syndrome complain of many problems related to vertigo, hearing loss, and tinnitus. Diagnoses are determined from subjective and objective data. The following nursing diagnoses are derived from these data.

Common Diagnoses

Two nursing diagnoses are common to clients with Meniere's syndrome:

1. Potential for injury related to changes in space perception caused by vertigo
2. Sensory/perceptual alterations (auditory) related to progression of the disease process

Additional Diagnoses

The following additional diagnoses may be found in some clients with Meniere's syndrome:

1. Sleep pattern disturbance related to tinnitus, anxiety, and/or vertigo
2. Potential fluid volume deficit related to nausea and vomiting
3. Social isolation related to altered state of wellness
4. Anxiety related to the threat to health
5. Ineffective individual coping related to situational crises

 Planning and Implementation

The following plan of care for clients with Meniere's syndrome focuses on the common diagnoses.

Potential for Injury

Planning: client goals. The main goal for this diagnosis is that the client will remain free from injury.

Interventions. The nurse assesses the client's status and the client's environment to prevent injury and to provide the client with a safe environment. Factors potentially causing injury are controlled.

Nonsurgical management. Clients often have certain clinical manifestations before an attack of vertigo, such as headaches, increasing tinnitus, and a feeling of fullness in the affected ear. It becomes important for the nurse to instruct the client in ways of preventing injury during an acute attack of vertigo. Clients must avoid driving when an attack is imminent. It is helpful for the client to lie down in a quiet environment, free from the responsibilities of daily living. A calm, stressor-free environment may help the client to avoid an attack of vertigo or may lessen the effects. Clients need help with walking to the bathroom or should use a bedpan when the vertigo is severe to prevent falling and injury. Clients are instructed to make slow head movements to prevent worsening of the vertigo.

Dietary changes that reduce the amount of endolymphatic fluid have been proposed. Salt and fluid restriction may help. Clients are advised to stop smoking because of its vasoconstrictive effects.

The main aims of drug therapy are to control the vertigo and vomiting and to restore normal balance. By controlling these factors, the client is less likely to be in a position where injury is possible. Nicotinic acid has been found to be useful because of its vasodilatory effect. Antihistamines like diphenhydramine (Benadryl) and dimenhydrinate (Dramamine) have been helpful in reducing the severity of or in stopping an acute attack by reducing the production of histamine and the inflammation that it causes. Antiemetics such as chlorpromazine (Thorazine), droperidol (Inapsine), and trimethobenzamide (Tigan) assist in the prevention of possible aspiration of vomitus if the client is in the supine position. Diazepam (Valium) not only calms the anxious client but also has an effect on controlling vertigo, nausea, and vomiting and allows the client to rest quietly during an attack.

The great variety of drugs used indicates a wide range of treatment modalities for Meniere's syndrome. There are so many etiologic factors that various drugs are used. Many clients are not helped by any of the above-mentioned treatments, and the physician uses different medications in an attempt to find those that are most beneficial for a particular client.

Surgical management. Surgical treatment for Meniere's syndrome remains controversial because the remaining hearing in the affected ear is sacrificed. When medical therapy is ineffective and the functional level of the client has decreased significantly, surgery is performed. The most radical procedure involves resection of the vestibular nerve or total removal of the labyrinth, or *labyrinthectomy.* The labyrinthectomy is done via the transcanal route. The footplate of the stapes is moved aside, and the labyrinth is removed through the oval window with fine forceps. These steps are taken so that the client may remain physically functional, especially when severe hearing impairment is already present. Often, attacks of vertigo cease after complete hearing loss from the disease.

Another procedure that is performed early in the course of the disease is an *endolymphatic drainage and shunt.* This procedure is performed by going through the mastoid process. The endolymphatic sac is drained, and a small tube is inserted to assist with drainage of excess fluid. Some clients report relief of vertigo while hearing remains preserved.

Preoperative care. Teaching and reassurance of the client are the most important aspects of preoperative care. The client may already have an impairment in hearing. The nurse assesses the understanding of the client before surgery and answers questions frankly and correctly. Most clients who elect to have surgery have had many years of problems with vertigo and increasing hearing loss, and they decide to undergo surgical treatment for control of the vertigo. The nurse reassures the client that each of these surgical options is designed to relieve the vertigo. General anesthesia is used for surgery on the endolymphatic sac. The client is instructed about the need to turn, cough, and deep breathe after surgery (see Chap. 18).

Postoperative care. Specific nursing care varies according to the type of surgical route used. If a transcanal approach has been used for the labyrinthectomy, the nurse expects to find packing and a dressing directly on the ear. The nurse takes care to speak to the side of the unaffected ear. Nerve resection requires a cranial approach. Neurologic assessments, such as level of consciousness, pupil size, and facial and eye movements, are necessary to monitor for the potential effects of edema on adjacent structures.

If an endolymphatic decompression has been performed, the nurse expects to find a dressing in the mastoid region. Manipulation of the vestibular structures of the inner ear causes postoperative vertigo. The client is informed of this possibility but is reassured that the vertigo is due to the surgical procedure rather than the disease process and that it is temporary. Side rails of the bed remain in the elevated position. Clients are supplied with a bedside commode and are instructed to call the nurse for assistance in getting out of bed. Antivertiginous and antiemetic drugs are helpful in treating postoperative vertigo and nausea and vomiting.

Sensory/Perceptual Alterations (Auditory)

Planning: client goals. The major goals of this diagnosis are that the client will (1) not have increased hearing impairment and (2) be able to cope with the present hearing disability.

Interventions. Actions that prevent the occurrence of acute attacks of Meniere's syndrome will decrease hearing loss. Interventions are the same as those performed to reduce vertigo and prevent injury because the cause of the vertigo is the same as the cause of hearing loss.

Nonsurgical management. If the amount of endolymphatic fluid is decreased or vasoconstriction eliminated, attacks can be avoided. Salt and fluid restriction as well as cessation of smoking helps to decrease damage caused by dilation of the endolymphatic system.

Surgical management. An endolymphatic drainage is performed to prevent further loss of hearing. A thorough description of this procedure, including pre- and postoperative care, is discussed earlier.

■ Discharge Planning

Clients are seldom admitted to the hospital setting unless parenteral medications are needed to control or to stop an acute attack or unless surgery is required. At times, hospitalization occurs before a diagnosis of Meniere's syndrome has been made. However, if the client has had an episode of severe vertigo of unknown etiology, admission to a hospital for a differential diagnosis is usually done. Much of the testing, especially audiometry, is performed on an outpatient basis.

Home Care Preparation

Methods to prevent injury, such as keeping the environment uncluttered, should be discussed with the client and family. Walkers and canes may be of assistance when the vertigo is less severe. The client should have easy access to the bathroom. Most clients prefer a quiet, dark environment, especially during times of vertigo. Home care personnel or nonnursing personnel can assist the client who has little support from family or friends with cleaning and meal preparation.

Client/Family Education

Clients need to be educated about recurrences and the progressive nature of the disease. With the vast array of possible medications that may be prescribed, it is essential that the client be knowledgeable about the indications for use of drugs and about their side effects. Overmedication is possible during acute attacks, while the client attempts to treat the severe vertigo and nausea.

Psychosocial Preparation

The recurrent nature of the disease makes psychosocial measures to control anxiety and fear necessary throughout the course of the disease. Clients who have been diagnosed with Meniere's syndrome should be assured that they do not have a brain tumor or another life-threatening disease that might cause similar severe clinical manifestations. Stress reduction techniques,

such as meditation, deep breathing, or directed muscle relaxation, used daily during symptom-free times may help to reduce the severity of the attack and assist the client in maintaining a quiet and calm emotional state during an acute attack.

In addition, long-term psychotherapy can help. Clients must live with a disease that is debilitating at times. Hearing loss is evident after several attacks, so the fear of deafness is well founded. Psychotherapy is used to aid the client in exploring feelings and to give the client ways of expressing rather than internalizing emotions.

Health Care Resources

Many communities have support groups for clients with this disease. These groups allow clients to discuss personal needs and potential treatment regimens. There is no curative treatment for Meniere's syndrome, but many forms of supportive care are necessary.

 Evaluation

On the basis of the identified client diagnoses, the nurse evaluates the care given. Expected outcomes for a client with Meniere's syndrome include that the client

1. Describes methods of preventing injury secondary to vertigo
2. Demonstrates knowledge of proper medications to use in the treatment of the various symptoms
3. Uses a variety of methods to mask tinnitus and is able to sleep at night
4. Expresses fears and anxiety about the disease and identifies ways of coping
5. Develops alternative forms of communication when bilateral involvement is present
6. Learns to cope with the disease

By meeting the desired outcomes, the client is able to learn methods for coping with Meniere's syndrome. This disorder is not usually curable, except possibly through surgical means. Therefore, the client must evaluate the many treatment methods available and seek out those that are the most beneficial. Continued fear and anxiety must be evaluated from the perspective of the client.

ACOUSTIC NEUROMA

OVERVIEW

An *acoustic neuroma* is a benign tumor of the vestibular, or acoustic, nerve. Although the tumor is benign, its location makes it a destructive lesion. Depending on the size and exact location of the tumor, damage can be done to hearing and to facial movements and sensation;

other neurologic pathologic disorders associated with a lesion that occupies intracranial space may also result. Tumor formation is unilateral.

Clinical manifestations begin with tinnitus and progress to gradual sensorineural hearing loss. More than 90% of clients complain of hearing loss. Later, clients complain of constant mild vertigo. As the tumor enlarges, damage to adjacent cranial nerves can be expected.

COLLABORATIVE MANAGEMENT

Diagnosis of an acoustic neuroma is made by use of tomography and computed tomography scanning. Either method gives the exact location and size of the tumor. Another diagnostic technique is electronystagmography, which reveals rapid nystagmus, or oscillating movement of the eye, toward the side of the lesion. Audiograms are used to diagnose a sensorineural hearing loss. Cerebrospinal fluid assays show increased pressure and positive results for protein.

Surgical removal via a craniotomy is necessary, and the remaining hearing is sacrificed. Extreme care is taken to preserve the function of the facial nerve (cranial nerve VII). Clients are taken to a critical care unit immediately after the operation. Routine postcraniotomy care is discussed in Chapter 33. Acoustic neuromas rarely recur after surgical removal.

SUMMARY

Disorders of the ear can be classified to reflect which part of the ear is affected most: the external, middle, or inner ear. Problems associated with the ear are categorized into a variety of groups including infection, trauma, mass, obstruction, chemical or enzymic changes, and degeneration of the structures. Medical treatment for ear disorders has been greatly assisted by availability of antibiotic treatment and microsurgical techniques. Common clinical manifestations include pain; hearing loss, either sensorineural or conductive; tinnitus; and vertigo. The specific clinical manifestations that occur are determined by the structures involved and the type of disease process.

Psychosocial needs focus on alterations in perception, which influence the client's social interaction and coping skills. Fear of permanent, irreversible hearing loss is real. The client must learn to cope with the loss and to use reserves such as friends, family, and support groups to maintain functional ability.

Loss of hearing and total deafness are the most devastating consequences of ear problems. Many clients can be aided with communication skills by aural reha-bilitation methods. Clients should make adjustments so that the quality of life does not suffer.

IMPLICATIONS FOR RESEARCH

Little nursing research has been performed with regard to ear disorders and hearing loss, although medical researchers have continued to do many physiologic studies on the effect of disease and drug therapy on hearing. Questions of concern to the nurse focus on physiologic needs of clients with infections, obstructions, or hearing loss. Psychosocial needs of the client with ear or hearing problems are also important parts of nursing research.

Typical research questions include

1. What are the consequences of hearing impairment for the client and his or her family?
2. What is the effect of hearing loss on the physical and psychosocial needs of the elderly?
3. What nursing measures best decrease the recurrence of otitis media in young adults?
4. Which psychosocial support measures lead to reduced stress in clients with Meniere's syndrome?

REFERENCES AND READINGS

Alberti, P. (1987). Tinnitus in occupational hearing loss: Nosological aspects. *Journal of Otolaryngology, 16*(1), 34–35.

Anderson, R. G., Simpson, D., & Roeser, R. (1983). Auditory dysfunction and rehabilitation. *Geriatrics, 38*(9), 101.

Ballenger, J. (1985). *Diseases of the nose, throat, ear, head and neck.* Philadelphia: Lea & Febiger.

Baloh, R. (1984). *Dizziness, hearing loss, and tinnitus: The essentials of neurotology.* Philadelphia: F. A. Davis.

Barnes, L., & Peel, R. L. (1985). Diseases of the external auditory canal, middle ear, and temporal bone. In L. Barnes (Ed.), *Surgical pathology of the head and neck* (Vol. 1, pp. 467–486). New York: Marcel Dekker.

Becker, W., Buckingham, R. A., Holinger, P. H., Steiner, W., & Jaumann, M. P. (1984). *Atlas of ear, nose and throat diseases, including bronchoesophagology* (2nd ed.). Philadelphia: W. B. Saunders.

Bentley, M. (1984). Left stapedectomy. *Nursing Times, 80*(14), 40–44.

Berger, E. H. (1985). Ear infection and the use of hearing protection. *Occupational Health Nursing, 33*(9), 430–433.

Bonikowski, F. P. (1983). Differential diagnosis of dizziness in the elderly. *Geriatrics, 38*(2), 89–92, 97, 101ff.

Bordley, J. E., Brookhouser, P. E., & Tucker, C. F. (1986). *Ear, nose and throat disorders of children.* New York: Raven.

Callaway, T., & Tucker, C. M. (1986). Rehabilitation of deaf black individuals: Problems and intervention strategies. *Journal of Rehabilitation, 52*(4), 53–56.

Calvani, D. (1985). How well do your clients cope with hearing loss? *Journal of Gerontological Nursing, 11*(7), 16–20.

Campbell, S. L. (1984). Some sound advice for managing a hearing-impaired patient. *Nursing '84, 14*(12), 46.

Carruth, J. A., & Simpson, G. T. (1988). *Lasers in otolaryngology.* Chicago: Year Book Medical.

Caruso, V. G. (1980). When the patient has otitis externa. *Geriatrics, 35*(5), 35–42.

Chovaz, C. (1989). Nursing the hearing impaired patient. *Canadian Nurse, 85*(3), 34–36.

Clarcq, J. R. (1983). Technology: A tool to facilitate the career development and employment of hearing impaired individuals. *Journal of Rehabilitation, 49*(3), 31–34.

DeWeese, D. D., Saunders, W. H., Schuller, D., & Schleunign, A. (1988). *Otolaryngology—head and neck surgery* (7th ed.). St. Louis: C. V. Mosby.

Eichenwald, H. (1985). Developments in diagnosing and treating otitis media. *American Family Physician, 31*(3), 155–164.

Eliopoulos, C. (Ed.). (1984). *Health assessment of the older adult.* Menlo Park, CA: Addison-Wesley.

Farmer, H. S. (1980). A guide for the treatment of external otitis. *American Family Physician, 21*(6), 96–101.

Feigin, R. D. (1982). Otitis media: Closing the information gap. *New England Journal of Medicine, 306,* 1417.

Fitzgerald, K. C. (1985). The aging ear. *American Family Physician, 31*(27), 225–232.

Graber, R. F. (1986). Removing impacted cerumen. *Patient Care, 20*(1), 151–153.

Hall, I. S., & Colman, B. (1987). *Diseases of the nose, throat, and ear.* Edinburgh: Churchill Livingstone.

Hanson, C., & Roffo, F. (1985). Comprehensive care of patients undergoing stapedectomy for otosclerosis. *Perioperative Nursing Quarterly, 1*(2), 21–28.

Hughes, B. G. (1985). *Textbook of clinical otology.* New York: Thieme-Stratton.

Innes, A. J., & Gates, N. (1985). *ENT surgery and disorders.* London: Faber and Faber.

Jahn, A., & Santos-Sacchi, J. (1988). *Physiology of the ear.* New York: Raven.

Jerger, J. (Ed.). (1984). *Hearing disorders in adults.* San Diego, CA: College-Hill.

Johnson, C. A. (1988). Hearing loss following the application of topical neomycin. *Journal of Burn Care Rehabilitation, 9*(2), 162–164.

Karmady, C. S. (1983). *Textbook of otolaryngology.* Philadelphia: Lea & Febiger.

Katz, A. E. (1986). *Manual of otolaryngology: Head and neck therapeutics.* Philadelphia: Lea & Febiger.

King, J. (1988). Interacting with the deaf. *Nursing Homes, 37*(1), 20–21.

Krump, M. A., Schroeder, S. A., & Tierney, L. M. (1987).

Current medical diagnosis and treatment. Norwalk, CT: Appleton & Lange.

Lamb, C. (1983a). Otitis media: Pinpointing the diagnosis. *Patient Care, 17*(15), 94–107.

Lamb, C. (1983b). Otitis media: Selecting the therapy. *Patient Care, 17*(15), 108–129.

Lim, D. L., Bluestone, C. D., Klein, J. O., & Nelson, J. D. (1984). *Recent advances in otitis media with effusion.* Philadelphia: B. C. Decker.

Lyon, M., & Lyon, D. (1986). Early detection of hearing loss: A follow-up study. *Canadian Journal of Public Health, 77,* 221–224.

Mader, J. T., & Love, J. T. (1982). Malignant external otitis. *Archives of Otolaryngology, 108,* 38.

Magilvy, J. K. (1985). Quality of life of hearing-impaired older women. *Nursing Research, 34,* 140–144.

Marshall, K. G., & Attia, E. L. (1983). *Disorders of the ear: Diagnosis and management.* Boston: John Wright PSG.

Nathan M. (1981). Protecting the elderly against drug-induced hearing loss. *Geriatrics, 36*(6), 95.

Nomura, Y. (Ed.). (1985). *Hearing loss and dizziness.* Tokyo: Igaku-Shoin.

Oosterveld, W. J. (1984). *Otoneurology.* Chichester: Wiley.

Paparella, M. M., & Goycoolea, M. V. (Eds.). (1982). *Clinical problems in otitis media and innovations in surgical otology.* Baltimore: Williams & Wilkins.

Rambur, B. (1989). Sudden hearing loss. *Nurse Practitioner, 14*(1), 8, 11, 14.

Ruenes, R., & De La Cruz, A. (1986). *Otologic radiology with clinical correlations.* New York: Macmillan.

Salomon, G., Vesterager, V., & Jagd, M. (1988). Age-related hearing difficulties. I: Hearing impairment, disability and handicap. *Audiology, 27*(3), 164–178.

Scura, K. (1988). Audiological assessment program. *Journal of Gerontological Nursing, 14*(10), 19–25.

Shimotakahara, S., Ruby, R., & Lampe, H. (1989). Otitis media with effusion in the adult. *Journal of Otolaryngology, 18*(3), 85–89.

Soliman, S. (1987). Low-frequency sensorineural hearing loss: A syndrome. *Audiology, 26*(6), 332–338.

Stair, T. O. (1986). *Practical management of eye, ear, nose, mouth, and throat emergencies.* Rockville, MD: Aspen Publications.

Surjan, L., & Godo, G. (1982). *Borderline problems in otorhinolaryngology.* Amsterdam: Excerpta Medica.

Turner, J. S. (1982). Treatment of hearing loss, ear pain, and tinnitus in older patients. *Geriatrics, 37*(8), 108–113.

Upchurch, D. T. (1982). Removing foreign bodies from ears, nose and throat. *Consultant, 22,* 283.

Vesterager, V., Salmon, G., & Jagd, M. (1988). Age-related hearing difficulties. II: Psychological and sociological consequences of hearing problems. *Audiology, 27*(3), 179–192.

Watking, S., Moore, T. H., & Phillips, J. (1984). Clearing impacted ears. *American Journal of Nursing, 84,* 1107.

Wilmot, T. (1984). *Meniere's and its management.* Springfield, IL: Charles C Thomas.

ADDITIONAL READINGS

Kopac, C. A. (1983). Sensory loss in the aged: The role of the nurse and the family. *Nursing Clinics of North America, 18,* 373–383.

This article is useful for any student or nurse who works with clients who have some type of sensory loss. An overview of the effect of hospital environments on sensory loss is presented. The article is divided among vision, hearing, touch, taste, and smell. Helpful tips regarding common concerns, assessment, and nursing interventions are included.

Lees, R. E., Roberts, H., & Wald, Z. (1985). Noise induced hearing loss and leisure activities of young people. *Canadian Journal of Public Health, 76*(3), 171–173.

This article describes the amount of hearing loss in people between 16 and 25 years of age. Forty per cent of the subjects had evidence of a hearing loss. A high correlation was found between noise exposure and hearing loss.

Magilvy, J. K. (1985). Experiencing hearing loss in later life: A comparison of deaf and hearing-impaired older women. *Research in Nursing and Health, 8,* 347–353.

This descriptive research study discusses the degree and type of handicap experienced by older women who are deaf or hearing impaired. Women with recent-onset hearing loss were compared with women with long-standing hearing loss. Hearing loss is described as a problem for each group, although the two groups expressed the problem differently. Emotional and situational problems were emphasized in the late-onset deaf and hearing-impaired women, whereas women with early-onset deafness expressed mostly communication difficulties.

UNIT 11 RESOURCES

Nursing Resources

American Society of Ophthalmic Registered Nurses (ASORN), 655 Beach Street, PO Box 3030, San Francisco, CA 94119. Telephone 415-561-8513.

Promotes the role of registered nurses specializing in ophthalmic care to enhance the quality of care of clients with ophthalmic problems. Certifies registered nurses in ophthalmic nursing through the National Certifying Board for Ophthalmic Registered Nurses. Publishes *Insight* (bimonthly).

National Certifying Board for Ophthalmic Registered Nurses, 655 Beach Street, PO Box 3030, San Francisco, CA 94119. Telephone 415-561-8500.

Certifies registered nurses in ophthalmic nursing.

Society of Otorhinolaryngology and Head/Neck Nurses, 439 North Causeway, New Smyrna Beach, FL 32069. Telephone 904-428-1695.

Other Resources

American Academy of Ophthalmology, PO Box 7424, San Francisco, CA 94119. Telephone 415-561-8500.

American Foundation for the Blind, 15 West 16th Street, New York, NY 10011. Telephone 212-620-2000.

American Speech-Language-Hearing Association, 10801 Rockville Pike, Department AP, Rockville, MD 20852. Telephone 301-897-5700.

American Tinnitus Association, PO Box 5, Portland, OR 97207. Telephone 503-248-9985.

Eye Bank Associations of America, 1725 Eye Street NW, Suite 308, Washington, DC 23006. Telephone 202-775-4799.

National Association of Hearing and Speech Agencies, 919 18th Street NW, Washington, DC 20006.

National Society to Prevent Blindness, 500 East Remington Road, Chaumburg, IL 60173. Telephone 312-843-2020.

Self-Help for Hard-of-Hearing People (Shhh), 4848 Battery Lane, Department E, Bethesda, MD 20814. Telephone 301-657-2248.

UNIT 12

Problems of Protection: Management of Clients with Disruptions of the Integumentary System

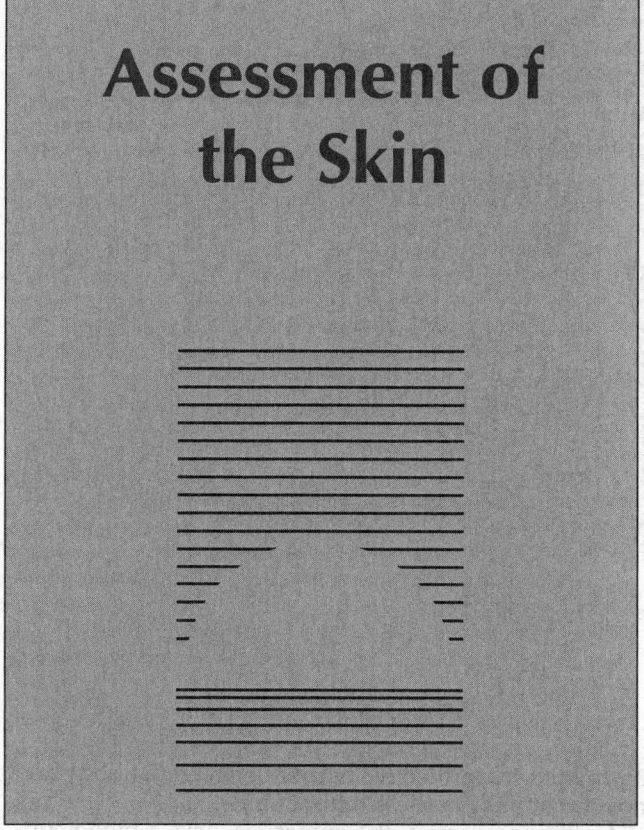

CHAPTER 39

Assessment of the Skin

As the largest organ of the body, the skin may be thought of as a multilayered suit of armor continuously shielding the fragile inner organs from the external environment. In its protective capacity, it not only regulates many important physiologic functions, such as body temperature and fluid and electrolyte balance, but also acts as a physical barrier to invasion by harmful microorganisms. Throughout a person's life span, the skin's appearance and functioning may be altered by a number of factors, including the aging process, emotional stress, injury, and disease.

For the nurse, one of the most important characteristics of the skin is its ability to communicate information. Skin appearance and texture, as well as subjective reports of pain, itching, heat, cold, and pressure, can provide important clues about a client's well-being. Likewise, the sensory function of the skin allows the nurse to use touch as a therapeutic intervention—to comfort, relieve pain, and communicate caring.

ANATOMY AND PHYSIOLOGY REVIEW

SKIN STRUCTURE

As shown in Figure 39–1, skin has three distinct anatomic layers, each with unique characteristics that contribute to the skin's ability to maintain its complex functions.

SUBCUTANEOUS FAT (ADIPOSE TISSUE)

The innermost layer of skin overlying muscle and bone is the major site for fat formation and storage. Fat cells act as a thermal insulator for the body, while providing the necessary padding over internal structures to absorb shock and protect against mechanical injury. The distribution of fat is highly variable, differing not only with anatomic area and age, but also between the sexes. Numerous blood vessels of varying sizes perforate the fatty layer, extending into the dermal layer of the skin to form complex capillary networks, which supply nutrients and aid in the removal of waste products.

DERMIS (CORIUM)

Above the subcutaneous fat lies a layer of essentially noncellular connective tissue composed of interwoven collagen and elastic fibers that give the skin both flexibility and mechanical strength. The principal fibrous component of dermal tissue, *collagen,* is a protein found in the lining of bone, as well as in tendons and ligaments. The fibrous collagen bundles are continually

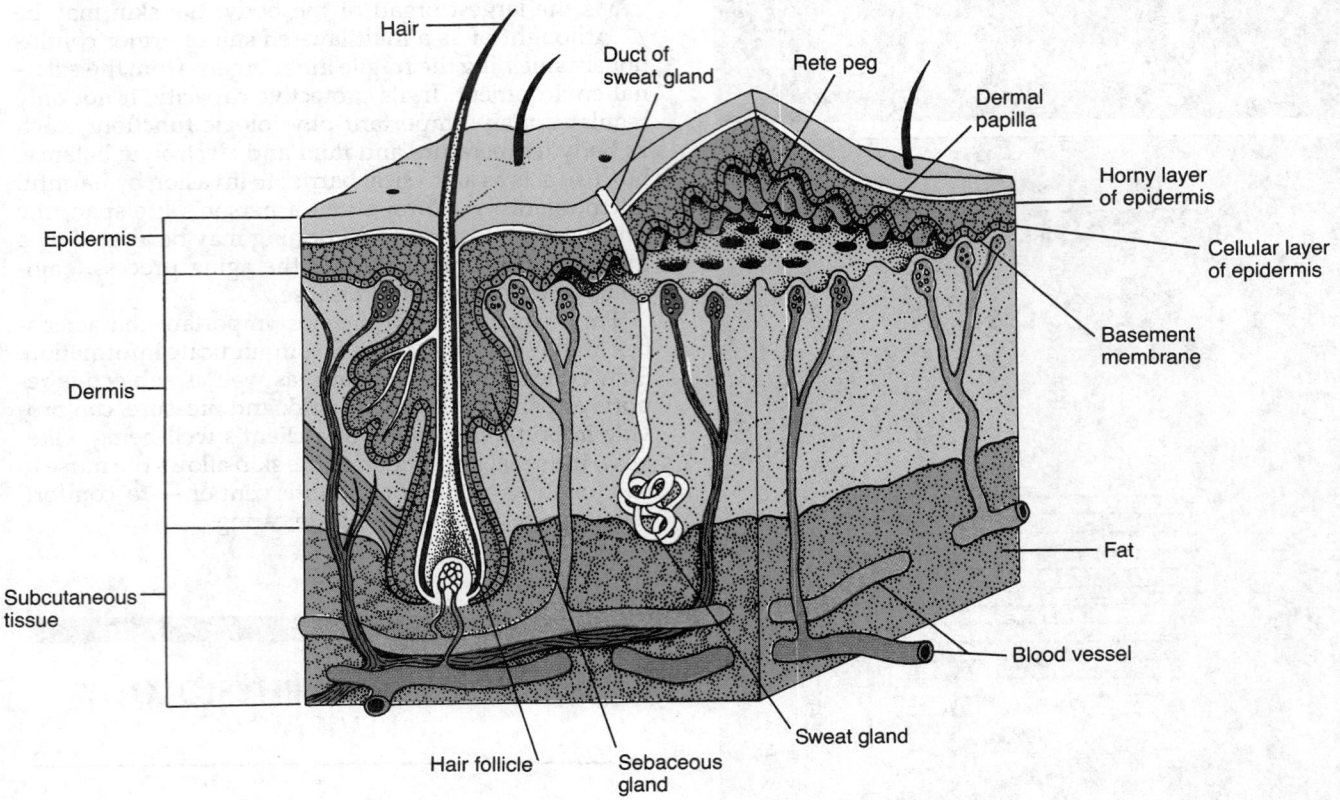

Figure 39–1

Anatomy of the skin.

being broken down and resynthesized by dermal cells called fibroblasts. *Fibroblasts* are migrating cells; they play an important role in wound healing. In addition to producing collagen, fibroblasts are responsible for the production of ground substance, a lubricating mucopolysaccharide material that surrounds the dermal cells and fibers and is thought to contribute to the skin's normal suppleness and turgor. The elasticity of the skin depends on both the quantity and the quality of the elastic fibers, which are interspersed among the collagen fibers. The major component of the elastic fiber is *elastin*, a protein found in relatively small concentrations in the skin when compared with its concentration in other connective tissues of the body. In addition to housing a network of capillaries and lymph vessels where the exchange of oxygen and heat takes place, the dermis is also rich in myelinated and nonmyelinated sensory nerves responsible for transmitting the sensations of touch, pressure, temperature, pain, and itch.

EPIDERMIS

Anchored to the dermis by finger-like projections of dermal tissue called *dermal papillae* is the outermost layer of skin, the *epidermis*. The corresponding interlocking fingers of epidermal tissue are termed *rete pegs*. The epidermis is less than 1 mm in thickness; however,

it provides the protective barrier between the body and noxious stimuli in the environment.

Unlike the dermis, the epidermis lacks a blood supply. It receives its nutrients from the highly vascular dermal layer through a porous membrane at the dermal-epidermal junction called the *basement membrane*. Attached to the basement membrane is a single layer of functional cell units called the *keratinocytes*. Keratinocytes account for 95% of the cells of the epidermis. Through the process of mitosis, the basal cells continuously divide to form new cells, pushing older keratinocytes upward to compose the characteristic stratified layers of the epithelium (also referred to as the malpighian layers). As keratinocytes move toward the surface, they flatten and eventually die, forming the outermost skin layer composed of dead cells, which is called the *stratum corneum* (horny layer). *Keratin*, the chemical protein produced within the cells of the malpighian layers, contributes to the highly waterproof properties of the horny layer. It takes approximately 28 to 45 days for a keratinocyte to complete its journey from the basement membrane to the skin surface, where it is shed or exfoliated.

Also occurring primarily within the stratified epidermal layer is the synthesis of vitamin D, a process activated by ultraviolet (UV) light. Although this endocrine function of the epithelial cell is of little importance during childhood and young adulthood, Vitamin D deficiency is thought to be related to an increased incidence of bone fractures in the elderly population.

Melanocytes are found at the level of the basement membrane at a frequency of about 1 melanocyte for every 10 keratinocytes. These pigment-producing cells give color to the skin and therefore are responsible for the racial differences in skin tone. Interestingly, the darker skin tones are *not* attributable to increased numbers of melanocytes, but rather to the size of the pigment granules *(melanin)* contained in each cell. Melanin production is stimulated by UV light and therefore helps protect against the harmful effects of sun exposure. In addition, increased melanin production may occur in localized areas in response to endocrine changes or inflammation.

The *Langerhans' cell* is found midway in the stratified epithelium. Although there is considerable controversy regarding the actual purpose of this cell, it is thought to be a type of macrophage responsible for detecting harmful antigens that may adhere to the outer skin surface. Subsequently, these cells transmit useful information to the immune system when a cutaneous inflammatory reaction is indicated.

SKIN APPENDAGES

HAIR

Human *hair*, an evolutionary remnant of the thick protective pelt worn by most mammals, serves primarily as an adornment to modern humans. Hair growth varies with race and sex, and individual hairs can differ in both structure and rate of growth, depending on body location. Even though hair follicles are located primarily in the dermal layer of the skin (see Fig. 39–3), these hair follicles are actually extensions of the epidermal layer. Within each hair follicle, a cylindric column of keratin is produced to form the substance of a mature hair shaft. The increased sulfur content of hair keratin, as opposed to that of the keratin found in the cells of the stratum corneum, contributes to the toughness of the hair shaft as it is formed. As with skin, hair color is genetically determined by the individual's quantity of melanin production.

Hair growth occurs in cycles—a growth, or anagen, phase followed by a resting, or telogen, phase. Local and systemic stressors can alter the growth cycle significantly, resulting in a temporary hair loss that can have a significant impact on an individual's perceived body image. On the other hand, permanent baldness, such as common male baldness, is usually of genetic origin and is seldom attributable to either internal or external stimuli.

NAILS

Well-groomed *fingernails* and *toenails* have cosmetic value; in addition, the nails serve as useful tools with

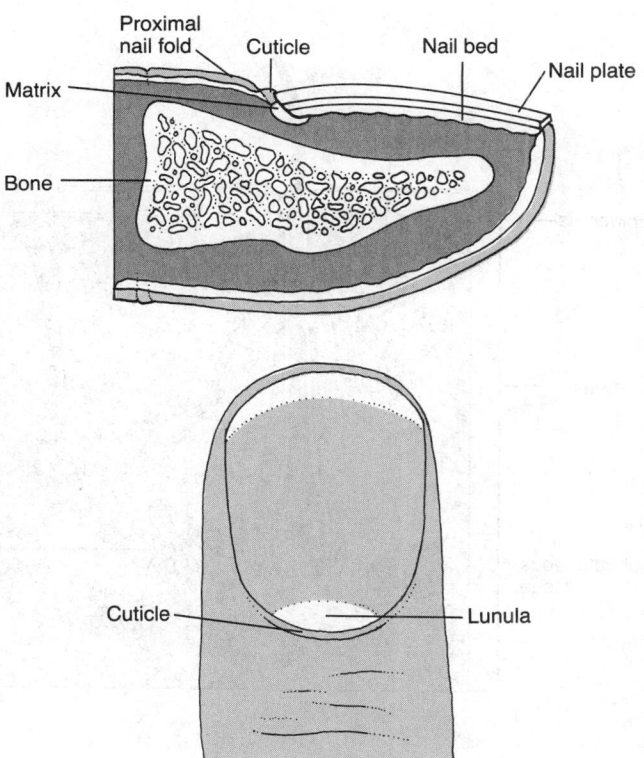

Figure 39–2
Anatomy of the nail.

which to scrape and grasp. Like hair follicles, the nail appendages are extensions of the keratin-producing epidermal layers of the skin. Unlike hair growth, which is cyclic, the production of nail keratin is a continuous process, occurring at a rate of about 0.1 mm/day. As illustrated in Figure 39–2, the white crescent-shaped portion of the nail visible at the proximal end of the nail plate (called the *lunula*) is a reflection of the underlying nail matrix, where nail keratin is formed. The *cuticle*, a layer of keratin produced by the epithelial cells of the proximal nail fold, attaches the nail plate to the soft tissue of the nail fold. The nail body is largely translucent with a pinkish hue reflective of a rich capillary blood supply beneath the nail surface. Nail growth and appearance are frequently altered during systemic disease or serious illness.

GLANDS

Sebaceous glands are distributed over the entire skin surface, with the exception of the palms and the soles. A majority of these glands are structurally connected to the hair follicles, as shown in Figure 39–3. Those of the eyelids, nipple areolae, and genitalia are freestanding. Sebaceous glands continuously produce *sebum*, a mildly bacteriostatic lipid-containing substance, which lubricates the skin and minimizes evaporative water loss

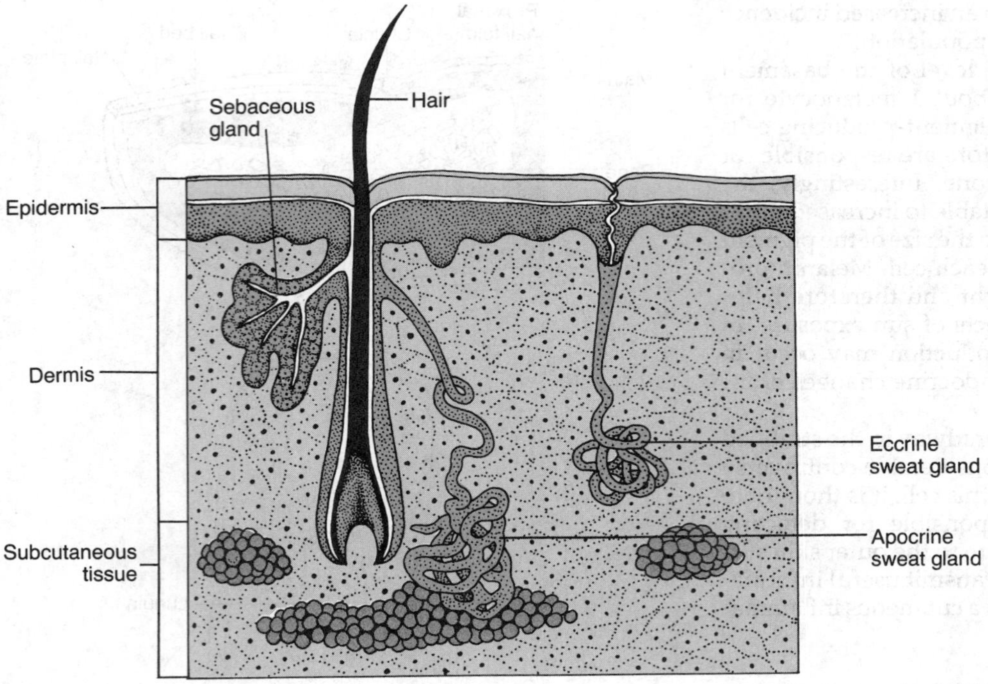

Figure 39–3

Anatomy of the hair follicle and sebaceous and sweat glands.

from the skin surface. The overproduction of sebum during puberty contributes to the problem of acne in some individuals.

The sweat glands of the skin are of two types— eccrine and apocrine. *Eccrine* sweat glands originate from epithelial cells and are found over the entire skin surface as distinct structures, unassociated with the hair follicle. The odorless, colorless, isotonic secretions of the eccrine glands are the single most important factor in the regulation of body temperature. As sweating is stimulated by either physiologic or psychologic mechanisms, sweat is delivered from the glands through tightly coiled ducts to the skin surface, where it evaporates and cools both the skin and the blood flowing through it. Stimulation of the eccrine sweat glands and the resulting evaporative water loss enables the body to lose as much as 10 to 12 L of fluid in a single day.

Unlike eccrine glands, *apocrine* sweat glands communicate directly with the hair follicle and are found primarily in the areas of the axillae, the perineum, the nipple areolae, and the periumbilicus. Interaction of skin bacteria with the secretions of the apocrine glands is responsible for the characteristic body odor.

SKIN FUNCTIONS

The skin is a complex body organ responsible for the regulation of many important body functions throughout the life span (Table 39–1). Although the skin has mainly protective and regulatory functions, the dynamic interrelationship between the skin and the outside world makes it an important vehicle for communication of a client's state of health.

SKIN CHANGES ASSOCIATED WITH AGING

The process of aging begins at birth. As changes in physiologic processes progress with aging, so does the skin undergo age-related alterations in both structure and function (see the Focus on the Elderly feature on pp. 1138 and 1139). An awareness of these changes is essential for the assessment of elderly clients with both potential and actual impairments in skin integrity.

There are individual differences in how quickly and to what degree the skin ages. Although such factors as genetic background, hormonal changes, and presence of systemic disease may greatly contribute to changes in the appearance of the skin over time, chronic sun exposure is the single most important factor leading to degeneration of the various skin components.

HISTORY

Before examining the skin, the nurse obtains an accurate history from the client so that actual and potential skin problems can be readily identified (Table 39–2). The nurse begins by gathering information about integumentary changes, including current skin care practices, from the client. The degree to which the interviewer elicits information about the skin depends on whether the client has a specific skin-related complaint.

TABLE 39–1 Functions of the Skin

Epidermis	Dermis	Subcutaneous Tissue
Protection		
Keratin provides protection from injury by corrosive materials	Provides fibroblasts for wound healing	Mechanical shock absorber
Inhibits proliferation of microorganisms because of dry external surface	Provides mechanical strength Collagen fibers Elastic fibers Ground substance	
Mechanical strength through intracellular bonds	Lymphatic and vascular tissues respond to inflammation, injury, and infection	
Homeostasis (water balance)		
Low permeability to water and electrolytes prevents systemic dehydration and electrolyte loss		
Temperature Regulation		
The eccrine sweat glands allow dissipation of heat through evaporation of sweat secreted onto the skin surface	Cutaneous vasculature, through dilation or constriction, promotes or inhibits heat conduction from the skin surface	Fat cells act as insulators and assist in retention of body heat
Sensory Organ		
Transmits a variety of sensations through neuroreceptor system	Encloses extensive network of free and encapsulated nerve endings for relaying sensations to the brain	Contains large pressure receptors
Vitamin Synthesis		
7-Dehydrocholesterol present in large concentrations in malpighian cells; photoconversion to vitamin D takes place		
Psychosocial		
Body image alterations result with many epidermal diseases, such as generalized psoriasis	Body image alterations seen with many dermal diseases, such as scleroderma	Body image alterations may result from increases, decreases, and redistribution of body fat stores

From Rosen, T., Lanning, M. B., & Hill, M. J. (1983). *The nurse's atlas of dermatology* (p. 176). Boston: Little, Brown. Copyright 1983.

FOCUS ON THE ELDERLY ■ Skin Changes Related to Aging

Physical Changes	Clinical Findings	Changes in Functional Ability
Epidermis		
Decreased thickness in epidermal layer	Increased skin transparency and fragility	Decreased cell replacement
Decreased epidermal mitotic activity	Delayed wound healing	
Decreased epidermal mitotic home-ostasis	Skin hyperplasias, such as hyperker-atoses and skin cancers (especially in sun-exposed areas)	
Increased epidermal permeability	Increased susceptibility to irritant reactions	Decreased barrier function
Decreased number of Langerhans' cells	Decreased cutaneous inflammatory response	Decreased injury response
Decreased number of active melanocytes	Increased sensitivity to sun exposure	
Hyperplasia of melanocytes at the dermal-epidermal junction (especially in sun-exposed areas)	Mottled hyperpigmentation and hypopigmentation (e.g., liver spots and age spots)	
Decreased vitamin D production	Increased susceptibility to osteoma-lacia	Decreased vitamin D production
Flattening of the dermal-epidermal junction	Increased susceptibility to shearing forces, resulting in blisters, purpura, skin tears, and pressure-related skin problems	
Dermis		
Decreased dermal blood flow	Increased susceptibility to dry skin (xerosis)	Decreased chemical clearance
Decreased vasomotor responsive-ness	Increased thermoregulatory alter-ations (predisposition to heat stroke and hypothermia)	Decreased vascular responsiveness
Decreased dermal thickness	Paper-thin, transparent skin with an increased susceptibility to trauma	Decreased injury response
Degeneration of elastic fibers	Decreased tone and elasticity (wrinkles)	Body image alterations
Benign proliferation of capillaries	Cherry hemangiomas	
Abnormal nerve endings	Alterations in sensory perception	Decreased sensory perception
Subcutaneous Layer		
Redistribution of adipose tissue	"Bags," cellulite, double chin, abdominal apron	Body image alterations
Thinning of subcutaneous fat layer	Increased susceptibility to hypother-mia	Decreased thermoregulation
	Decreased resistance to mechanical injury (especially pressure necrosis)	Decreased injury response
Hair		
Decreased number of hair follicles and rate of growth	Increased hair thinning	Decreased cell replacement
Decreased number of active melanocytes in follicle	Gradual loss of hair color (graying)	Body image alterations

FOCUS ON THE ELDERLY ■ Skin Changes Related to Aging *Continued*

Physical Changes	Clinical Findings	Changes in Functional Ability
Nails		
Decreased rate of growth	Increased susceptibility to fungal infections	Decreased cell replacement
Decreased blood flow beneath nail bed	Longitudinal nail ridges	
Glands		
Decreased sebum production, despite sebaceous gland hyperplasia	Increased size of pores (especially on nose); large comedones in malar region	Decreased sebum production
Decreased eccrine and apocrine gland activity	Increased susceptibility to dry skin	Decreased sweat production
	Decreased perspiration, leading to decreased cooling effect	Decreased thermoregulation
	Decreased need for antiperspirants	

DEMOGRAPHIC DATA

The nurse obtains demographic data from clients with actual or potential skin disorders. *Age* is an important factor because many alterations in the integumentary system are normal manifestations of the aging process. *Race* and *nationality* can also be important; some irregularities in skin appearance are normal cutaneous manifestations among clients of specific races and nationalities and abnormal for clients of other races or nationalities. Information regarding the client's *occupa-*

TABLE 39–2 Important Points in the Nursing History of Clients with Skin Problems

Medical-Surgical History

Does the client have any current or prior medical problems?
Has the client had any recent or prior surgeries?

Family History

Is there any family tendency toward chronic skin problems?
Do any members of the immediate family have recent skin complaints?

Medication History

Is the client allergic to any systemic or topical medication? If so, have the client describe the reaction.
What prescription drugs has the client taken recently? When was the drug administration started? What is the dosage or frequency of administration? When was the last dose taken?
What OTC drugs has the client taken recently? When was the drug administration started? What is the dosage or frequency of administration? When was the last dose taken?

Social History

What is the client's occupation?
What recreational activities does the client enjoy?
Has the client traveled recently?
What is the client's nutritional status?

Current Health Problem

When did the client first notice the skin problem?
Where on the body did the problem begin?
Has the problem gotten better or worse?
Has a similar skin condition ever occurred before? If so, have the client describe the typical course and how it was treated.
Is the problem associated with any of the following: itching, burning, stinging, numbness, pain, fever, nausea and vomiting, diarrhea, sore throat, cold, stiff neck, exposure to new foods, new soaps or cosmetics, new clothing or bed linens, or stressful situations?
Does anything seem to make the problem worse (e.g., sun exposure, medications, heat or cold, and menses)?
Does anything seem to make the problem better?

tion and *hobbies* can provide clues to chronic skin exposure to chemicals, abrasive substances, and other environmental factors that may contribute to the development of a skin problem.

PERSONAL AND FAMILY HISTORY

The nurse obtains information about the client's medical history, including prior or current medical illnesses and surgeries to determine if skin changes are a manifestation of an underlying systemic disorder. Because the predisposition to many skin diseases is genetically determined, the nurse also explores any family tendency toward chronic skin problems. In addition, an examination of the immediate family's current health status is helpful when considering the possibility of a communicable disease that has been transferred between family members.

MEDICATION HISTORY

Because cutaneous reactions to systemic medications are common, the nurse seeks information about recent exposure to both prescription and over-the-counter (OTC) preparations (e.g., laxatives, antacids, and cold remedies). Obtaining accurate information often requires persistence on the part of the nurse, as many clients may overlook the importance of nonprescription drugs in causing skin rashes. The nurse asks when the administration of each medication was started, the dosage and frequency, and the time the last dose was taken. The potential for cross-reactions between medications of similar chemical composition makes it important to investigate the details of any rash that the client is aware of having experienced as a result of receiving a medication. A medication history is also helpful in identifying skin changes that can be attributed to the treatment of other medical problems, such as the changes that occur with chronic steroid or anticoagulant therapy.

DIET HISTORY

The nurse notes the client's weight, height, and body build and explores food preferences. Inadequate nutrition in the form of protein deficiencies, vitamin deficiencies, and obesity can predispose a client to skin lesions, as well as delay wound healing. Fat-free diets and chronic alcoholism can lead to fatty acid deficiencies and associated skin changes. In addition, some skin diseases, such as chronic urticaria and acne, are exacerbated by certain foods or food additives.

SOCIOECONOMIC STATUS

The nurse seeks information about a client's social and economic background as a means of identifying environmental factors that could contribute to skin disease. Recent travel is noted as a potential source of skin infections or unusual lesions. If the client is well-tanned, the nurse inquires about the amount of time spent in the sun and tanning booths and asks if there have been any skin problems in the past associated with sun exposure. Because skin problems related to poor hygiene are common, clients from low socioeconomic environments are questioned about living conditions and the availability of running water.

CURRENT HEALTH PROBLEM

If a skin problem is identified, diagnosis can often be facilitated by obtaining additional information about the specific complaints. When did the client first notice the rash? Where on the body did the rash begin? Has the problem gotten better or worse? If a similar problem has occurred before, the nurse asks the client to describe the typical course of the skin lesion and how it was treated. Association of the problem with specific symptoms, such as itching, burning, numbness, pain, fever, nausea and vomiting, sore throat, or stiff neck, is sought. Finally, the nurse asks if the client can identify anything that seems to make the problem better or worse.

PHYSICAL ASSESSMENT

SKIN INSPECTION

Skin changes not only are related to specific skin diseases, but are also frequently a reflection of underlying systemic disorders. In addition, some skin problems become manifest only during periods of severe psychologic stress. By developing skin assessment skills, the nurse is in a unique position to identify both obvious and subtle clues about a client's state of wellness.

A thorough assessment of the skin is best accomplished with the client partially or completely disrobed. As skills are developed, the nurse may find it easier to maintain privacy by incorporating visual inspection and systematic uncovering of specific body surfaces with the physical examination of each organ system. For example, the skin of the anterior and posterior neck and chest can be observed while auscultating breath sounds. Monitoring for actual and potential impairments in skin integrity should become a routine part of daily care during bathing of the client or while assisting the client with other personal hygiene measures.

Actual inspection of the skin surfaces is performed in a well-lighted room, preferably with natural or bright fluorescent lighting to enhance visualization of subtle skin changes. Although no special equipment is needed, a penlight is often helpful for close inspection of lesions and for illumination of the oral cavity. During the physical examination, the nurse systematically inspects each skin surface, including the scalp, the hair, the nails, and mucous membranes. Particular attention is given to the skin fold areas, where a moist, warm environment can often harbor opportunistic microorganisms, such as yeast and bacteria. The nurse notes obvious changes in color and vascularity, as well as the presence or absence of moisture, edema, and skin lesions. In addition, the cleanliness of the various body areas may indicate a need for further evaluation of self-care activities.

COLOR

Skin color is affected by a number of factors, including blood flow, oxygenation, body temperature, and pigment production. In addition to these factors, the wide variability in natural skin tones often makes color assessment difficult for the beginning nurse.

In general, changes in skin color are described by their appearance (Table 39–3). The nurse documents not only the observable alterations in color, but also whether the distribution is generalized or localized. Inspection of the areas of least pigmentation, such as the buccal mucosa, the sclera, nail beds, and palms and soles, where color changes are accentuated, may often help confirm more subtle color alterations of the general body areas. Although transient changes in color (such as the flush that accompanies high fever) usually reflect a systemic reaction to illness, chronic color changes are more often associated with localized alterations in pigmentation from increased or decreased melanin production.

LESIONS

Skin disease is clinically described in terms of primary and secondary lesions (see the illustration on pp. 1144–1145). *Primary* lesions represent the initial reaction to an underlying problem that results in an alteration in one of the structural components of the skin. *Secondary* lesions are changes in the appearance of the primary lesions that occur with normal progression of the underlying disease or in response to therapeutic intervention in the form of topical or systemic treatments. For example, an acute dermatitis frequently occurs as primary vesicles with an associated pruritus. Secondary lesions in the form of crusts become evident as the vesicles are disrupted and the serous exudate dries. In chronic dermatitis, the skin often becomes *lichenified*, or thickened, owing to continuous rubbing of the epidermis by the client to relieve the pruritus.

In addition to describing the lesions observed and whether they are primary or secondary, the nurse notes their color and location and whether the lesions occur as isolated changes or are grouped to form a distinct pattern. Table 39–4 defines terms commonly used to describe lesion configurations.

In describing the location of lesions, the nurse identifies whether the lesions are generalized or localized and, if localized, what specific body regions are involved. Involvement of only the sun-exposed areas of the body is important information when considering possible cause. Rashes limited to the skin fold areas, such as on the axillae, beneath the breasts, and in the groin, should alert the nurse to problems associated with friction, heat, and excessive moisture. The importance of clear communication in describing skin changes cannot be overemphasized. Because certain patterns of skin lesions are so closely linked to specific disease entities, an explicit description of clinical observations is the key to timely and therapeutic intervention for the client.

EDEMA

Edema, or swelling of the tissues, is caused by leakage of water and low-molecular-weight proteins from the vasculature into the surrounding tissue. The fluid tension within edematous tissue often causes the skin to appear shiny, taut, and paler in color than uninvolved skin. During skin inspection, the nurse notes the location, distribution, and color of any areas of edema.

Skin *elasticity* is also affected by the presence of edema. The nurse presses the tip of the index finger against edematous tissue with moderate pressure to determine the degree of indentation, or pitting (see Chaps. 13, 59, and 64 for more information on edema).

MOISTURE

The nurse examines the skin carefully for moisture content. Normally, increased moisture in the form of perspiration can be expected with increased activity or elevated environmental temperatures. In addition, dampness of the skin fold areas is common because of decreased air circulation where the skin surfaces touch. However, in bedridden and debilitated clients, excess moisture can contribute to maceration and eventual skin breakdown. Areas of macerated (water-logged) skin over the buttocks and perineum should alert the nurse to potential impairments in skin integrity related to fecal or urinary incontinence.

Overly dry skin can be caused by a number of factors, including a dry environment, improper skin lubrication, inadequate fluid intake, and the normal processes of aging. Dry skin is characterized by scaling of the stratum corneum and may be especially marked in areas of limited circulation, such as the distal lower extremities. In general, dry skin becomes a problem for most adults during the winter months, when the air contains less

TABLE 39–3   Causes, Locations, and Significance of Common Alterations in Skin Color

Alteration	Underlying Cause	Location	Significance
White (pallor)	Decreased hemoglobin level	Conjunctivae	Anemia
	Decreased blood flow to the skin (vasoconstriction)	Mucous membranes	Shock or blood loss
		Nail beds	Chronic vascular compromise
		Palms and soles	Sudden emotional upset
		Lips	Edema
	Genetically determined defect of the melanocyte (decreased pigmentation)	Generalized	Albinism
	Acquired patchy loss of pigmentation	Localized	Vitiligo; tinea versicolor
Yellow-orange	Increased total serum bilirubin level (jaundice)	Generalized	Increased hemolysis of red blood cells
		Mucous membranes	Liver disorders
		Sclera	
	Increased serum carotene level (carotenemia)	Perioral	Increased ingestion of carotene-containing foods (carrots)
		Palms and soles	
		Absent in sclera and mucous membranes	Pregnancy
			Thyroid deficiency
			Diabetes
	Increased urochrome level	Generalized	Chronic renal failure (uremia)
		Absent in sclera and mucous membranes	
Red (erythema)	Increased blood flow to the skin (vasodilation)	Generalized	Generalized inflammation (e.g., erythroderma)
		Localized (to area of involvement)	Localized inflammation (e.g., sunburn, cellulitis, trauma, and rashes)
		Face, cheeks, nose, and upper chest	Fever; increased alcohol intake
		Area of exposure	Exposure to cold
Blue	Increase in deoxygenated blood (cyanosis)	Nail beds	Cardiopulmonary disease
		Mucous membranes	Methemoglobinemia
		Generalized	
	Bleeding from vessels into tissue:		
	Petechiae (1–3 mm)	Localized	Thrombocytopenia
	Ecchymosis (>3 mm)		Increased blood vessel fragility
Reddish-blue	Increased overall amount of hemoglobin	Generalized	Polycythemia vera
	Decreased peripheral circulation		
Brown	Increased melanin production	Localized (to area of involvement)	Chronic inflammation
		Pressure points, areolae, palmar creases, and genitalia	Exposure to sunlight
			Addison's disease
		Face, areolae, vulva, and linea nigra	Pregnancy; oral contraceptives (melasma)
	Café au lait spots (tan-brown patches)		
	<6 spots	Localized	Nonpathogenic
	>6 spots	Generalized	Neurofibromatosis
	Melanin and hemosiderin deposits (bronze or grayish-tan color)	Distal lower extremities	Chronic venous stasis
		Exposed areas or generalized	Hemochromatosis

**TABLE 39–4   Terms Commonly Used to Describe
Skin Lesion Configurations**

Annular: Ring-like with raised borders around flat clear
centers of normal skin

Circinate: Circular

Circumscribed: Well-defined with sharp borders

Clustered: Several lesions grouped together

Coalesced: Lesions that merge with one another and
appear confluent

Diffuse: Widespread, involving most of the body with
intervening areas of normal skin; generalized

Linear: Occurring in a straight line

Serpiginous: With wavy borders, resembling a snake

Universal: All areas of the body involved, with no areas of
normal-appearing skin

---

moisture, and in the hospital environment, where humidity is often poorly controlled. Excessive scaling is frequently associated with dehydration and is seen in conjunction with dry mucous membranes, a loss of skin turgor, and parched or cracked lips.

VASCULAR MARKINGS

Vascular changes are classified as either normal or abnormal, depending on the cause. Bleeding from the vasculature into the tissue results in purpuric lesions: petechiae and ecchymosis. *Petechiae* are small, non-blanchable vascular lesions measuring less than 0.5 mm in diameter and are frequently indicative of increased capillary fragility. *Ecchymoses,* or bruises, are larger areas of hemorrhage that vary in size from several millimeters to many centimeters. Petechiae and ecchymoses may be round or have irregular borders and may be flat or raised, depending on the amount of associated edema. In the elderly population, bruising is common after minor trauma to the skin, especially in sun-exposed areas of the body. Another common finding is petechiae of the lower extremities associated with stasis dermatitis, a condition frequently seen in clients who have a history of chronic venous insufficiency. Abnormal cutaneous bleeding unrelated to the altered vascular support that occurs with aging is seen in thrombocytopenic disorders, including the leukemias, systemic lupus erythematosus, and some drug reactions (see Chaps. 28 and 67).

Normal vascular markings include birthmarks, cherry angiomas, spider angiomas, and venous stars (Table 39–5).

INTACTNESS

The nurse examines more thoroughly those areas where an actual breakdown in skin integrity has occurred. For example, owing to a flattening of the dermal-epidermal junction with aging, skin tears are a common finding in the elderly. The thin, fragile skin is easily disrupted by the application of friction or shearing forces, especially if areas of ecchymosis are already present. The nurse looks for skin tears in areas where constricting clothing rubs against the skin surface, on the upper extremities where one often grasps the skin when assisting a client to ambulate, and in areas where adhesive tapes or dressings have been applied and removed. Furthermore, the nurse remains alert to the presence of multiple abrasions or early pressure-related skin changes that may signal previously unrecognized impairments in physical mobility or alterations in sensory perception.

Actual breaks in the intactness of the skin are described in terms of location, size, color, distribution, and the presence or absence of signs of infection. If needle marks are evident, the nurse documents the approximate number and their distributions to support additional assessments of possible substance abuse. Evaluation of partial- and full-thickness wounds, including a discussion of objective criteria that describe progress toward healing, is found in Chapter 40.

CLEANLINESS

An evaluation of the cleanliness of the skin gives the nurse important information about health maintenance needs. The hair, the nails, and the skin are inspected closely for excessive soiling and offensive odor. Depending on a client's degree of self-care deficit, hard-to-reach areas, such as the perirectal and inguinal skin folds, the axillae, and the feet, may be less clean than other skin surface areas.

SKIN PALPATION

Palpation is used concurrently with skin inspection to gather additional information about skin lesions, moisture content, temperature, turgor, and texture (Table 39–6). Inspection alone can often be misleading. Palpation is helpful in confirming the lesions' size and whether the lesions are flat or slightly raised. The consistency of larger lesions can vary from soft and pliable to firm and solid. If the nurse closes his/her eyes, the more subtle changes, such as the difference between a fine macular (flat) and papular (raised) rash, can be detected. Tenderness on palpation is not a common finding with most skin lesions. If tenderness is present, a chronic skin problem with secondary bacterial infection is suspected.

The nurse touches areas of excess moisture to determine the thickness of *secretions* and whether the secretions are watery or oily in consistency. In areas of excess dryness, the nurse rubs a finger against the skin surface to better observe the degree of flaking or scaling.

Both generalized and localized changes in skin *temperature* are detected by placing the back of a hand on the skin surface. Before assessing for changes in skin

HOW SKIN LESIONS ARE DESCRIBED

PRIMARY LESIONS

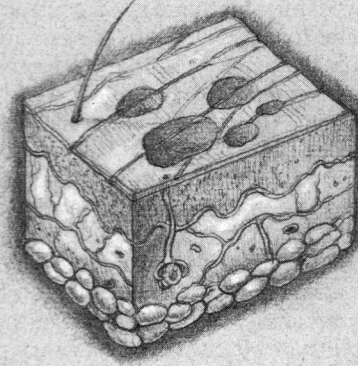

Macules (such as *freckles, flat moles,* or *rubella*) are flat lesions of less than 1 cm in diameter. Their color is different from that of the surrounding skin—most often white, red, or brown.

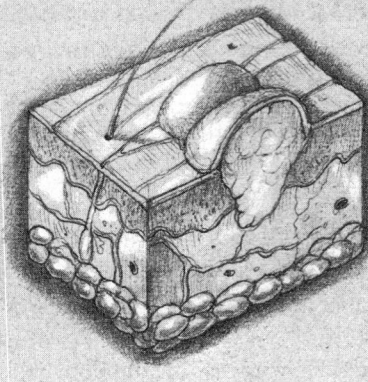

Nodules (such as *lipomas*) are elevated, marble-like lesions more than 1 cm wide and deep.

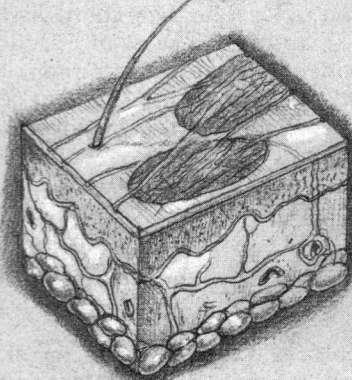

Patches (such as *vitiligo* or *café au lait spots*) are macules that are larger than 1 cm in diameter. They may or may not have some surface changes—either slight scale or fine wrinkles.

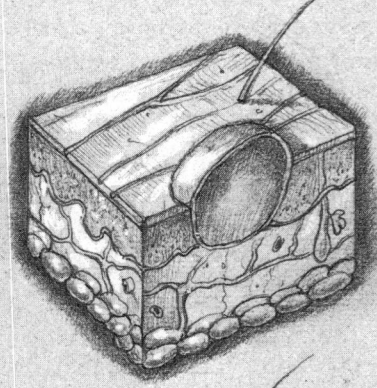

Cysts (such as *sebaceous cysts*) are nodules filled with either liquid or semisolid material that can be expressed.

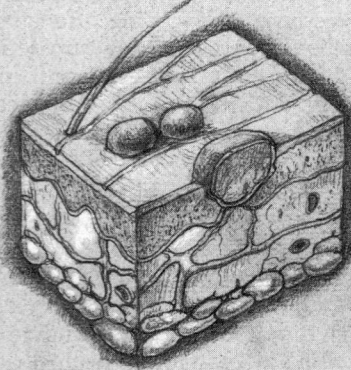

Papules (such as *warts* or *elevated moles*) are small, firm, elevated lesions less than 1 cm in diameter.

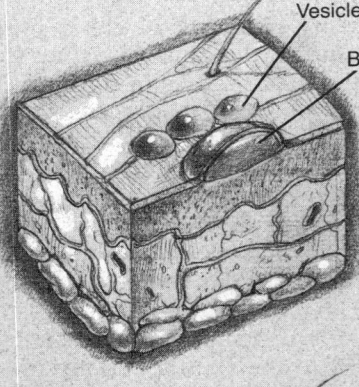

Vesicle

Bulla

Vesicles (such as in *acute dermatitis*) and **bullae** (such as *second-degree burns*) are blisters filled with clear fluid. Vesicles are less than 1 cm in diameter, and bullae are more than 1 cm in diameter.

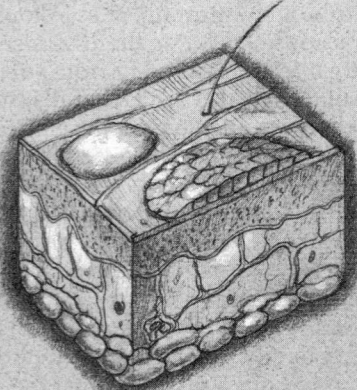

Plaques (such as in *psoriasis* or *seborrheic keratosis*) are elevated, plateau-like patches more than 1 cm in diameter that do not extend into the lower skin layers.

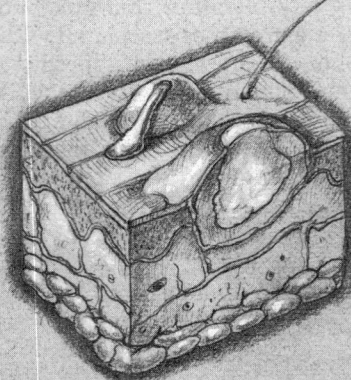

Pustules (such as in *acne* and *acute impetigo*) are vesicles filled with cloudy or purulent fluid.

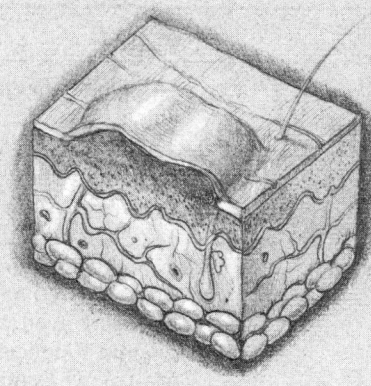

Wheals (such as *urticaria* and *insect bites*) are elevated, irregularly shaped, transient areas of dermal edema.

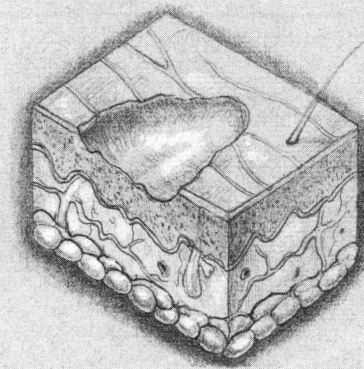

Erosions (such as in *varicella*) are wider than fissures but involve only the epidermis. They are often associated with vesicles, bullae, or pustules.

SECONDARY LESIONS

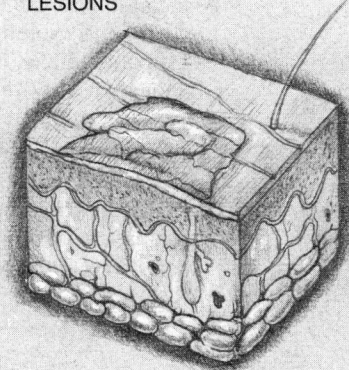

Scales (such as in *exfoliative dermatitis* and *psoriasis*) are visibly thickened stratum corneum. They appear dry and are usually whitish. They are seen most often with papules and plaques.

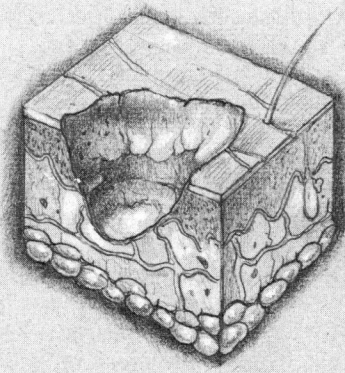

Ulcers (such as *stage 3 pressure sores*) are deep erosions that extend beneath the epidermis and involve the dermis and sometimes the subcutaneous fat.

Crust   Oozing

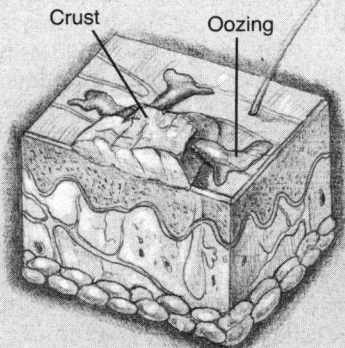

Crusts and **oozing** (such as in *eczema* and *late-stage impetigo*) are composed of dried serum or pus on the surface of the skin, beneath which liquid debris may accumulate. Crusts frequently result from broken vesicles, bullae, or pustules.

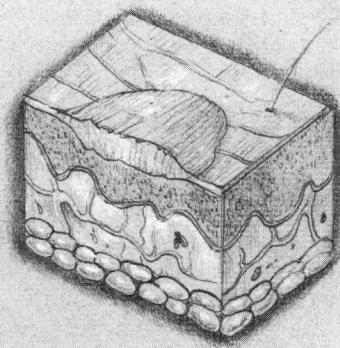

Lichenifications (such as in *chronic dermatitis*) are palpably thickened areas of epidermis with accentuated skin markings. They are caused by chronic rubbing and scratching.

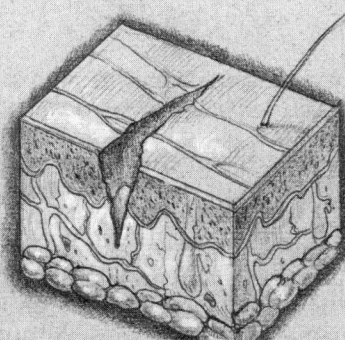

Fissures (such as in *athlete's foot*) are linear cracks in the epidermis, which often extend into the dermis.

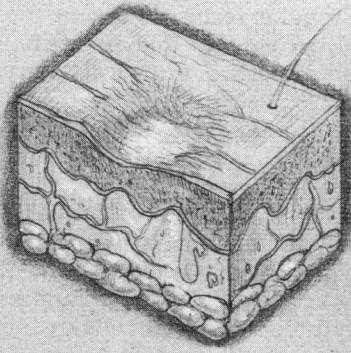

Atrophy (such as *striae* [stretch marks] and *aged skin*) is characterized by thinning of the skin surface with loss of skin markings. The skin is translucent and paper-like. Atrophy involving the dermal layer results in skin depression.

TABLE 39-5   Clinical Findings, Location, and Significance of Common Vascular Skin Lesions

Lesion	Clinical Findings	Location	Significance
Cherry angioma (senile angioma)	Bright to dusky red, dome-shaped papule 2-5 mm in diameter. Adjacent lesions may vary in size and color. Partial blanching on palpation.	Chest and back	Normal skin change with aging.
Spider angioma	Bright red, star-like lesion varying in size from small to 2 cm. Center of "star" is sometimes raised and may pulsate when palpated.	Face, neck, and upper trunk	Associated with liver disease, pregnancy (change in estrogen level), and vitamin B deficiency. May occur as normal finding.
Telangiectasia	Reddish-blue linear or star-like lesion caused by enlargement of the superficial blood vessels.	Face and trunk	Associated with sun exposure and prolonged alcohol intake. May also be seen in systemic scleroderma and after continued use of potent topical steroids.
Venous star	Spider-like, blue marking varying in size from small to several inches. May have a "cascading" appearance. Does not blanch with pressure.	Legs (near veins) and anterior chest	Associated with increased pressure in superficial veins (varicose veins).
Port-wine stain	Large dark red to purple area of discoloration. Does not blanch with pressure.	Face, scalp, and groin	Congenital abnormality. If on the face, may be associated with neurologic disorders and ocular abnormalities.

temperature, the nurse makes certain to have warm hands. Cold hands interfere with accurate assessment and cause unnecessary discomfort for the client.

The skin surfaces are palpated to assess *texture*, which differs according to body region and exposure to environmental irritants. For example, areas of chronic sun exposure have a rougher texture than protected skin surfaces. Clients with occupations that require repeated skin exposure to harsh soaps or chemicals may show changes related to the exposure. Increased thickness of the skin attributable to scarring, lichenification, or edema usually results in decreased elasticity; mobility may be affected if a joint is involved.

The *turgor* of the skin is an indication of the amount of skin elasticity and can be altered by a number of factors, including water content and age. The skin is pinched gently between a thumb and forefinger and then released. If skin turgor is normal, the skin immediately returns to its original state when released. Poor skin turgor is evidenced by "tenting" of the skin, with gradual return to the original state. Normal loss of elas-

ticity with aging makes assessment of skin turgor difficult in elderly clients. If the client is in a supine position, using the forehead or abdominal tissue to test turgor gives the best indication of skin hydration.

HAIR

During the skin assessment, hair growth is inspected and palpated for *cleanliness, distribution, quantity,* and *quality.* Normally, hair is found in an even distribution over most of the body surfaces, with hair on the scalp, in the pubic region, and in the axillary folds being thicker and coarser than body hair found on the trunk and extremities. Although wide variations in color and growth patterns occur, sudden or marked changes in hair characteristics may be reflective of an underlying disease process. As with skin changes, the nurse investigates any abnormal findings further by obtaining an in-depth history of the circumstances surrounding any change.

TABLE 39–6 Common Clinical Findings in Skin Palpation

Clinical Finding	Cause	Location	Examples of Predisposing Conditions
Edema			
Localized	Inflammatory response	Area of injury or involvement	Trauma
Dependent or pitting	Fluid and electrolyte imbalance	Ambulatory: dorsum of foot and medial ankle	Congestive heart failure Renal disease
	Venous and cardiac insufficiency	Bedridden: buttocks, sacrum, and lower back	Hepatic cirrhosis Venous thrombosis or stasis
Nonpitting	Endocrine imbalance	Generalized, but more easily seen over the tibia	Hypothyroidism (myxedema)
Moisture			
Increased	Autonomic nervous system stimulation	Face, axillae, skin folds, palms, and soles	Fever, anxiety, activity Hyperthyroidism
Decreased	Dehydration Endocrine imbalance	Buccal mucous membranes with progressive involvement of other skin surfaces	Fluid loss Postmenopause Hypothyroidism Normal aging
Temperature			
Increased	Increased blood flow to the skin	Generalized Localized	Fever, hypermetabolic states Inflammation
Decreased	Decreased blood flow to the skin	Generalized	Impending shock, sepsis, anxiety Hypothyroidism
		Localized	Interference with vascular flow
Turgor			
Decreased	Decreased elasticity of dermis (tenting when pinched)	Abdomen, forehead, or radial aspect of the wrist	Severe dehydration Sudden severe weight loss Normal aging
Texture or Thickness			
Roughness or thickness	Irritation, friction	Pressure points (e.g., soles, palms, and elbows)	Calluses Chronic eczema Atopic skin diseases
	Sun damage	Areas of sun exposure	Normal aging
	Excessive collagen production	Localized or generalized	Scleroderma Keloids
Softness or smoothness	Endocrine disturbances	Generalized	Hyperthyroidism

How well the hair is groomed, including the cleanliness of areas of thicker hair growth, can often confirm information that has already been gathered about a client's social history and health care needs. Although parasite infestation can occur even with meticulous grooming, it is most often associated with less-than-adequate living conditions and poor hygiene practices. Pruritus is a common symptom of louse infestation. If the client complains of intense itching or scratches continuously, the nurse examines the scalp and pubis carefully for the presence of lice and nits (lice eggs). Excoriations from repeated scratching can result in secondary bacterial infections, with crusting, matting of the hair, and foul odor. The nurse also inspects the scalp for excessive scaling, redness, or tenderness, symptoms associated with fungal infections, such as ringworm (*tinea capitis*).

Dandruff is a common occurrence; an accumulation of patchy or diffuse white or gray scales is found on the surface of the scalp. Although dandruff is mainly a cosmetic problem, inflammatory changes can occur if the scalp is excessively oily, resulting in erythema and pruritus. Severe inflammatory dandruff can extend to involve the eyebrows, as well as the skin of the face and neck. If severe dandruff is not treated, hair loss can occur.

Although gradual hair loss is often associated with aging, the sudden occurrence of areas of asymmetric or patchy hair loss at any age is of concern. *Alopecia areata* occurs as round, smooth, and patchy areas of baldness without obvious skin changes. This condition can occur anywhere on the body, but is most noticeable on the scalp. A single cause of alopecia is not known; however, its occurrence has been associated with genetic predisposition, autoimmune disorders, and emotional stress. Fungal infections, repeated hair treatments (coloring and permanent waves), chemotherapy, and hyperthyroidism can also contribute to abnormal hair loss.

Increased hair growth across the face and anterior chest in the female client is a sign of *hirsutism*. If hirsutism is apparent, the nurse looks for associated changes in fat distribution and capillary fragility, which can occur in Cushing's disease, or for clitoral enlargement and deepening of the voice, indicating a possible ovarian tumor.

NAILS

Because dystrophic (abnormal) nails are often a reflection of serious systemic illness or a sign of local skin disease involving the epidermal keratinocytes, the nurse evaluates the fingernails and toenails for *color, shape, thickness, texture,* and the presence of *lesions.* Many individual variations in color, texture, and grooming of the nails are influenced by factors unrelated to disease, e.g., occupation. When assessing the elderly client, the nurse notes minor variations associated with the aging process, such as gradual thickening of the nail plate, the appearance of longitudinal ridges, and a yellowish-gray discoloration.

The color of the nail plate is dependent on many factors, including the thickness and transparency of the nail, blood composition, the adequacy of arterial blood flow, and the presence of pigment deposits (Table 39–7). In addition, changes in color can be attributed to external factors, such as the chemical damage from dyes and detergents encountered in some occupations and the chronic use of nail polish.

During examination, the fingers and toes should be free of any surface pressure that might interfere with local blood flow and alter the appearance of the digits. To differentiate between color changes attributable to the underlying vascular supply and those resulting from pigment deposition, the nail bed is blanched to see if a significant color change occurs with pressure. The nurse gently squeezes the end of the finger or toe, exerting downward pressure on the nail bed, and then releases the pressure. Color caused by vascular alterations changes as pressure is applied and returns to the original state when pressure is released. Color caused by pigment deposition remains unchanged.

In addition to color, an evaluation of nail shape may indicate early or late changes consistent with systemic disease. For example, fingernail clubbing is a valuable diagnostic indicator of impaired gas exchange, even though the exact mechanism by which physical changes in the nail occur is not fully understood. To evaluate nail shape, the curvature of the nail plate and surrounding soft tissue is systematically observed from all angles. The nurse palpates the fingertips to define areas of sponginess, tenderness, or marked edematous infiltration. Table 39–8 summarizes important information on common variations in nail shape.

Increased thickening of the nail plate can occur as a result of trauma, chronic dermatologic disease, or decreased arterial blood flow. If the client is elderly, the nurse looks for a "heaped-up" appearance of the toenails, which is commonly associated with fungal infection (*onychomycosis*). The great toe is more prone to such involvement, and destruction of the nail plate can occur if the infection is untreated. The elderly frequently ignore this condition because of an absence of discomfort and difficulty seeing the nail changes. Onychomycosis is aggravated by pressure from poorly fitting shoes.

Differences in nail consistency are described as hard, soft, or brittle. Nail plates may become hard, with increased thickening, requiring warm water soaks or lubrication with petroleum jelly to soften the nail plates before they can be trimmed. Soft nail plates, which are thin and bend easily with pressure, have been associated with malnutrition, chronic arthritis, myxedema, and peripheral neuritis. Brittle or friable nails are prone to splitting, as is seen in onychomycosis or advanced psoriasis. Splitting of the nail plate has also been attributed to repeated exposure to water and detergents, which causes damage to the plate over time.

Separation of the nail plate from the nail bed (*onycholysis*) creates an air pocket beneath the nail plate that is initially seen as a grayish-white area of opacity. As dirt and keratin collect in the pocket, the color may change and the area becomes malodorous. Onycholysis of the great toenail is common with fungal infections and after trauma. Separation of the nail plate may also be seen in psoriasis or as a result of prolonged contact with chemical irritants.

The nurse inspects the soft-tissue folds around the nail plate for localized redness, heat, swelling, and tenderness. Inflammation of the skin around the nail (*acute paronychia*) is usually associated with a torn cuticle or an

TABLE 39–7   Clinical Findings and Significance of Common Alterations in Nail Color

Alteration	Clinical Findings	Significance
White	Horizontal white banding or areas of opacity	Chronic hepatic or renal disease (hypoalbuminemia)
	Generalized pallor of nail beds	Shock Anemia Early arteriosclerotic changes (toenails) Myocardial infarction
Yellow-brown	Diffuse yellow to brown discoloration	Jaundice Peripheral lymph-edema Bacterial or fungal infections of the nail Psoriasis Diabetes Cardiac failure Staining from tobacco, nail polish, or dyes Chronic tetracycline therapy Normal aging (yellow-gray color)
	Vertical brown banding extending from the proximal nail fold distally	Normal finding in Black clients Nevus or melanoma of nail matrix in Caucasian clients
Red	Thin, dark red vertical lines 1–3 mm in length (splinter hemorrhages)	Bacterial endocarditis Trichinosis Trauma to nail bed Normal finding in some clients
	Red discoloration of lunula	Cardiac insufficiency
	Dark red nail beds	Polycythemia vera
Blue	Diffuse blue discoloration that blanches with pressure	Respiratory failure Methemoglobinuria Venous stasis disease (toenails)

ingrown toenail. If acute paronychia occurs in an immunocompromised host, an opportunistic infection with *Staphylococcus* is suspected. Chronic paronychia is a more common occurrence and is characterized by inflammation that persists for months. Persons thought to be at high risk for chronic paronychia are men and women with frequent intermittent exposure to water, such as homemakers, bartenders, and laundry workers. Both gram-negative and gram-positive bacteria have been implicated as causative agents, and secondary colonization with *Candida albicans* may contribute to the chronicity of the problem.

SPECIAL CONSIDERATIONS FOR ASSESSMENT OF DARK SKIN

The recognition of pallor, erythema, cyanosis, and other color changes reflective of a client's physical state is

TABLE 39–8 Clinical Findings and Significance of Common Variations in Nail Shape

Nail Shape	Clinical Findings		Significance
Normal	Angle of 160 degrees between nail plate and proximal nail fold. Nail surface slightly convex. Nail base firm when palpated.		Normal finding
Clubbing Early clubbing	Straightening of angle between nail plate and proximal nail fold to 180 degrees. Nail base spongy when palpated.		Hypoxia Lung cancer
Late clubbing	Angle between nail plate and proximal nail fold exceeds 180 degrees. Nail base visibly edematous and spongy when palpated. Enlargement of the soft tissue of fingertips, giving "drumstick" appearance when viewed from above.		Prolonged hypoxia Advanced lung cancer

Spoon nails
  (koilonychia)
  Early koilonychia
	Flattening of the nail plate with an increased smoothness of the nail surface.		Iron deficiency (with or without anemia)
			Poorly controlled diabetes of >15 yr duration

Late koilonychia	Concave curvature of the nail plate.		Local injury Psoriasis Chemical irritants Developmental abnormality
Beau's grooves	1-mm-wide horizontal depressions in nail plates caused by growth arrest (involves all nails).		Acute, severe illness Prolonged febrile state Isolated periods of severe malnutrition
Pitting	Small, multiple pits in the nail plate. May be associated with plate thickening and onycholysis. Most often involves the fingernails, several or all.		Psoriasis Alopecia areata

more difficult in people who have naturally dark skin tones. Although physiologic processes are the same for both light-skinned and dark-skinned clients, the amount of skin pigmentation greatly alters how the skin appears in response to physiologic alterations. Consequently, one must develop assessment skills to detect the more subtle color changes that can occur. The nurse

should become familiar with the normal appearance of a dark-skinned client's mucous membranes, nail beds, and skin tone so that variations from normal can be identified.

To detect generalized pallor, the nurse inspects the mucous membranes for an ashen-gray color. If the lips and the nail beds are not heavily pigmented, they appear paler than normal for that client. The skin is examined under appropriate lighting for the absence of the underlying red tones that normally give heavily pigmented skin a healthy glow. With generalized decreased blood flow to the skin, brown skin appears yellow-brown and very dark brown skin is ashen gray.

Cyanosis is even more difficult to detect than pallor. If impaired gas exchange is anticipated, the nurse examines the lips, tongue, nail beds, conjunctivae, and palms and soles at regular intervals for subtle color changes. With cyanosis, the lips and tongue are gray and the palms, soles, conjunctivae, and nail beds have a bluish tinge. To support these observations, the nurse assesses for the more obvious signs accompanying hypoxia, such as changes in respiratory rate and rhythm, decreased breath sounds, changes in level of consciousness, and increased amount and viscosity of secretions.

If areas of acute inflammation are suspected, the back of the hand is used to palpate for the increased warmth that occurs when blood flow to the skin increases. With the fingertips, the nurse palpates to further assess for hardened areas deep in the tissue which may give the skin a "woody" feeling on palpation. Inflamed skin is tender and edematous. If edema is extensive, the skin is taut and shiny.

Areas of the body where inflammation, such as an inflammatory rash or cellulitis, has recently resolved appear darker than the normal skin tone. This is due to stimulation of the melanocytes during the inflammatory process and to increased pigment production, which continues after inflammation subsides. On the other hand, more extensive injury to the skin, resulting in destruction of melanocytes (such as a deep ulcer or a full-thickness burn) may produce healing with color changes that are lighter than the normal skin tone. Unlike acute changes, chronic inflammatory changes seldom produce tenderness on palpation. If scar tissue is present, the skin may feel less supple, especially over joints. If chronic inflammatory changes are suspected, the client is questioned about a history of skin problems in that area of the body.

Jaundice is best seen by inspecting the oral mucosa, especially the hard palate, for yellow discoloration. Inspection of the conjunctivae and adjacent sclera may be misleading owing to normal deposits of subconjunctival fat that produce a yellowish hue when seen in contrast to the dark periorbital skin. Therefore, the nurse examines the sclera closest to the cornea for a more accurate determination of jaundice. Similarly, the palms and soles of dark-skinned clients may appear yellow if calloused, which should not be mistaken for jaundice.

Purpuric lesions may be difficult to detect, depending on the degree of skin pigmentation. In general, areas of ecchymosis appear darker than normal skin and may be tender and easily palpable, depending on whether hematoma is present. In most cases, the client relates a history of trauma to the area to confirm the assessment. Petechiae are rarely visible in dark skin and may be evidenced only in the oral mucosa and conjunctival areas.

PSYCHOSOCIAL ASSESSMENT

Actual impairments in skin integrity are commonly associated with altered perceptions in body image, especially if the more visible skin surfaces, such as the face, the hair, or the hands are involved. The nurse assesses the client's body language for clues indicating a disturbance in self-concept. For example, avoidance of eye contact or the use of garments to cover the affected areas communicates concern about physical appearance. In chronic skin diseases, the client often relates a history of social isolation, attributable to fear of rejection by others or a belief that the skin problem is contagious.

Skin changes associated with poor hygiene are common in clients from low socioeconomic backgrounds. The nurse assesses the client's overall appearance for excessive soiling, matted hair, body odor, and similar self-care deficits. Unsanitary living conditions are confirmed by obtaining a social history. Often, the client relates similar skin problems among family members, friends, and sexual contacts. If skin problems related to poor hygiene are identified in an elderly client, the nurse also evaluates any physical limitations that could be contributing to poor health maintenance. For example, problems with vision or limited mobility can result in difficulty seeing or reaching skin surfaces to clean them.

DIAGNOSTIC ASSESSMENT

CULTURES

Fungal, bacterial, or viral pathogens may be suspected as the cause of certain skin changes; confirmation by microscopic examination is necessary. For example, when superficial fungal (dermatophyte) infections are suspected, scales are gently scraped from the skin lesions into a Petri dish or a similar clean container and transported to the diagnostic laboratory for implantation into a suitable culture medium. Fingernail clippings and hair are collected in a similar manner.

Deeper fungal infections require a piece of tissue for culture, which the physician usually obtains by punch biopsy. The biopsy specimen may be sent for histopathologic analysis and special fungal stains, necessitating the tissue specimen to be bisected or two separate biopsy specimens to be obtained.

Bacterial cultures are obtained from intact primary lesions (bullae, vesicles, or pustules), if possible. Material is expressed from the lesion, collected with a cotton-tipped applicator, and placed in a bacterial culture medium. Intact lesions may require unroofing with a sterile small-gauge needle before material can be easily expressed. If secondary lesions in the form of crusts are present, the nurse removes the crusts and swabs the underlying exudate. As with deep fungal infections, deep bacterial infections may require a biopsy to isolate the organism for culture. If bacterial cellulitis is suspected, nonbacteriostatic saline can be injected deep into the tissue and aspirated, and the aspirant sent for culture.

Viral cultures are indicated if lesions resulting from herpes virus are suspected. By using a cotton-tipped applicator, vesicle fluid is obtained from intact lesions as described earlier. Unlike bacterial and fungal specimens that can remain at room temperature until transport to the laboratory, viral culture tubes should be placed in a cup of ice immediately after the culture is obtained.

SKIN BIOPSY

To establish an accurate diagnosis or assess the effectiveness of a therapeutic intervention, it is often necessary for the physician to obtain a small piece of skin tissue for histopathologic study. Skin biopsies may be performed by punch excision, shave excision, or scalpel excision, depending on the size, depth, and location of the skin changes. Before preparing the client, the nurse checks with the physician to determine the number, location, and type of skin biopsies to be performed.

The *punch biopsy* is the most basic technique used and is performed with a small, circular cutting instrument, or punch, ranging in size from 2 to 6 mm in diameter. A cylindric plug of tissue is cut to the depth of the subcutaneous fat and removed with forceps and scissors; the biopsy site is closed with one or two sutures. Some physicians may elect to allow the biopsy site to heal without suturing.

A *shave biopsy* removes only that portion of the skin elevated above the plane of the surrounding tissue by injection of the local anesthetic. A scalpel or razor blade is moved parallel to the skin surface to remove the tissue specimen. Shave biopsies are usually indicated for superficial or raised lesions and do not require suturing.

In rare instances, larger or deeper specimens are obtained via excision of tissue with a scalpel. An *excisional biopsy* is performed using deep elliptic incisions that are sutured after the specimen is removed. Unlike the punch or shave biopsy, excisional biopsies usually involve more discomfort for the client while the site is healing.

Client preparation. As with any invasive procedure, the client is prepared for a biopsy procedure with a brief explanation of what to expect. Because many clients express anxiety, the nurse emphasizes that a biopsy is a minor procedure with few, if any, complications. If a punch or shave biopsy is planned, the client is reassured that scarring is minimal owing to the small size of the piece of tissue removed. If an excisional biopsy is planned, the nurse tells the client to expect a cosmetic

result similar to that which occurs when a surgical incision heals.

Procedure. The nurse prepares for the biopsy procedure by establishing a sterile field and assembling biopsy instruments, gauze pads, cotton-tipped applicators, forceps, scissors, and a needle holder with suture if indicated. A syringe with the physician's choice of local anesthetic should also be available. A small-gauge needle (No. 25) is attached to the syringe to minimize discomfort during injection. Biopsy site preparation differs according to the physician's preference. Usually, the nurse shaves any hair from the area and cleans the skin gently with an antibacterial soap or solution.

The most uncomfortable time for the client is during the injection of local anesthetic, which usually produces a burning or stinging sensation. The client is reassured that the discomfort will subside as the anesthetic takes effect. Talking the client through the procedure with a quiet voice, combined with gentle touch, has a calming effect. During the procedure, the physician may request that the nurse don sterile gloves and assist by blotting away blood or holding pressure on the biopsy site until sutures can be placed.

After removal, tissue specimens for routine histopathologic study are placed directly in 10% formalin for fixation. Specimens for culture are placed in sterile saline solution. Bleeding of the biopsy site is sometimes controlled with a topical hemostatic agent, such as Monsel's solution or absorbable gelatin sponge (Gelfoam).

Follow-up care. After bleeding is under control and any sutures have been placed, the site is covered with an adhesive bandage (Band-Aid) or a dry gauze dressing. The nurse instructs the client to keep the dressing dry and in place for a minimum of 8 hours. After dressing removal, the site is cleaned three times a day with a cotton-tipped applicator saturated with hydrogen peroxide. The physician may also prescribe application of an antibiotic ointment to minimize local bacterial colonization. The healing biopsy site may be left open, unless a covering is preferred for cosmetic reasons or because of location (an area frequently soiled). The nurse instructs the client to report any erythema or excessive drainage at the site. Suture removal is usually performed 7 to 10 days after biopsy.

WOOD'S LIGHT EXAMINATION

A hand-held, long-wavelength ultraviolet (black) light or Wood's light is sometimes used during physical examination; areas of blue-green or red fluorescence are associated with certain skin infections. In addition, hypopigmented skin becomes more prominent when viewed under black light, greatly facilitating examination of pigmentary changes in fair-skinned individuals. Examination of the skin under a Wood's light is always carried out in a darkened room.

DIASCOPY

Diascopy is a technique used to eliminate erythema caused by increased blood flow to the skin and thereby facilitate the inspection of skin lesions associated with the erythema. A glass slide or lens is pressed down over the area to be examined, blanching the skin and revealing the shape and configuration of the underlying lesions.

SKIN TESTING

Patch Testing

If a client's rash is thought to be an allergic contact dermatitis, *patch testing* may prove a valuable diagnostic tool in identifying the responsible allergen. Contact with a substance to which the client is allergic results in a delayed hypersensitivity reaction, which takes from 48 to 96 hours to develop.

Test chemicals are applied to uninvolved skin under occlusive tape patches. After the patches are removed, the areas of chemical contact with the skin are examined closely for localized erythema, swelling, and vesicular eruption indicative of a cutaneous allergic response. For a positive patch test result to have clinical relevance, a history of exposure to substances containing the chemical is also required.

Client preparation.   To prevent suppression of the inflammatory response to an allergen, the administration of systemic corticosteroids is discontinued for at least 48 hours before the test application. Topical steroid therapy may be continued. If testing is performed in the outpatient (ambulatory) setting, it is also helpful to give the client advance warning that testing will involve three separate visits to the dermatologist: one to apply the test patches, the second for an initial reading, and the third for detection of any delayed hypersensitivity reactions. Finally, many clients assume that patch testing involves pricking the skin with needles. The nurse explains the difference between patch testing and intradermal skin testing to allay any unnecessary anxiety.

Procedure.   The preferred location for application of test patches is the upper back, where increased vascularity and flat skin surfaces ensure better contact with the chemicals and optimal results. After the client has disrobed, the back is inspected for evidence of rash and the presence of hair. If rash is present, alternative sites for test applications are the flanks, the lower back, and the upper arms. Any hair is shaved to prevent poor contact and subsequent false-negative results. In addition, defatting of the skin with alcohol to remove skin oils is helpful in promoting adhesiveness of the patches.

Small quantities of chemicals and solutions in standardized concentrations are placed in separate metal chambers backed with hypoallergenic adhesive tape. The tape is then carefully applied to the skin so that each chemical is held in contact with the skin surface. The individual chambers are marked for later identification. As many as 60 or more chemicals may be tested simultaneously. The nurse instructs the client to keep the test sites dry at all times. If the client is used to taking showers, baths are substituted until testing is complete. The nurse emphasizes caution when washing the hair to avoid getting the patches wet and discourages excessive physical activity that will result in perspiration. Reapplication by the client of patches that come loose can interfere with an accurate interpretation of true allergic reactions. The nurse reinforces the necessity of removing loose or nonadherent test patches for reapplication by the physician or nurse at a later date.

The initial reading is performed 2 days after application. The tape containing the chemical-filled chambers is peeled away from the skin, and each area of contact is marked with indelible ink for future reading. Any initial allergic or irritant reactions are noted in the client's medical record. Final reading of the test results is performed 2 to 5 days later, depending on the physician's preference.

Follow-up care.   If a potential allergen is identified, the client is given a list of items containing that chemical to avoid. Follow-up visits to the dermatologist are necessary to monitor the progress of the rash. Removal of the offending agent does not always result in cure. Episodes of allergic contact dermatitis can often be exacerbated by other irritants, causing a perpetuation of symptoms.

Scratch Testing

A *scratch,* or *prick test,* differs from a patch test in that it evokes an *immediate* hypersensitivity reaction to an allergen. Scratch tests are used for routine allergy testing to determine the possible cause of urticaria (hives). Allergens introduced to the skin through a superficial scratch or prick cause a localized reaction (wheal) when the test is positive. The inadvertent intradermal injection of solutions used for scratch testing may induce an anaphylactic reaction. Consequently, resuscitation equipment should be readily available when scratch tests are performed.

SUMMARY

Skin disorders have important implications for the physical and psychologic well-being of clients, and early recognition of skin changes presents a unique challenge to the nurse. Skin findings alert the nurse to potential problems that can complicate the course of treatment or herald the onset of serious systemic illness. The physical discomfort and emotional distress frequently associated with skin disorders require continual nursing assessment so that interventions remain timely and therapeutic.

REFERENCES AND READINGS

Bryant, R. (1988). Saving the skin from tape injuries. *American Journal of Nursing, 88,* 189–191.

Caughman, S., Mayer, R., & Russo, G. (1989). Cutaneous signs of internal cancer. *Patient Care, 22*(2), 28–41.

Chapel, T., Riley, H., Russo, G., & Septimus, E. (1988). Cutaneous signs of infection. *Patient Care, 22*(13), 185–197.

Fenske, N., Grayson, L., & Newcomer, V. (1989). Common problems of aging skin. *Patient Care, 23*(7), 225–234.

Fenske, N. A., & Lober, C. W. (1986). Structural and functional changes of normal aging skin. *Journal of the American Academy of Dermatology, 15*(4, Pt. 1), 571–585.

Gilchrest, B. A. (1984). *Skin and aging processes.* Boca Raton, FL: CRC Press.

Jaubovic, H. R., & Ackerman, A. B. (1985). Structure and function of skin. In S. L. Moschella & H. J. Hurley (Eds.), *Dermatology* (2nd ed., Vol. 1, pp. 1–74). Philadelphia: W. B. Saunders.

Klein, L. (1988). Maintenance of healthy skin. *Journal of Enterostomal Therapy, 15*(6), 227–231.

Kreisberg, S., Ledger, W., Schulze, R., & Speroff, L. (1989). Skin signs in endocrine disease. *Patient Care, 23*(6), 73–86.

Lookingbill, D. B., & Marks, J. G., Jr. (1986). *Principles of dermatology.* Philadelphia: W. B. Saunders.

Millington, P. F., & Wilkinson, R. (1983). *Skin.* Cambridge: Cambridge University Press.

Nasemann, T., Sauerbrey, W., & Burgdorf, W. H. C. (1983). *Fundamentals of dermatology.* New York: Springer-Verlag.

Orentreich, D. S., & Orentreich, N. (1985). Alterations in the skin. In R. Andes, E. L. Bierman, & W. R. Hazzard (Eds.), *Principles of geriatric medicine* (pp. 354–386). New York: McGraw-Hill.

Pritchard, V. (1988). Geriatric infections: Skin and soft tissue. *RN, 51*(6), 60–63.

Roach, L. B. (1977). Color changes in dark skins. *Nursing '77, 7,* 48–51.

Robinson, J. K. (1986). *Fundamentals of skin biopsy.* Chicago: Year Book Medical.

Rosen, T. R., Lanning, M. D., & Hill, M. J. (1983). *The nurse's atlas of dermatology.* Boston: Little, Brown.

Sauer, G. C. (1985). *Manual of skin diseases* (5th ed.). Philadelphia: J. B. Lippincott.

Sherman, J. L., Jr., & Fields, S. K. (1982). *Guide to patient evaluation.* New York: Medical Examination Publishing.

Silvers, D. M. (1982). The skin: Basic pathophysiology. In A. N. Domonkos, H. L. Arnold, Jr., & R. B. Odom (Eds.), *Andrews' diseases of the skin* (7th ed., pp. 1–14). Philadelphia: W. B. Saunders.

ADDITIONAL READINGS

Dangel, R. B., (1986). Pruritus and cancer. *Oncology Nursing Forum, 13*(1), 17–21.

Pruritus is a rare but distressing symptom experienced by clients with cancer. Dangel presents a review of the literature describing the relationship of pruritus to specific diagnostic categories of cancer. A discussion of nursing assessment variables, goals, and interventions is also applicable to non–cancer-related pruritus.

Gaskin, F. C., (1986). Detection of cyanosis in the person with dark skin. *Journal of the National Black Nurses Association, 1*(1), 52–60.

Assessment of subtle changes in skin color reflective of life-threatening physiologic alterations is much more difficult in dark-skinned clients. This article discusses the techniques for detecting cyanosis in the client with dark skin.

Huether, S. E., & Jacobs, M. K. (1986). Determination of normal variation in skin blood flow velocity in healthy adults. *Nursing Research, 35,* 162–165.

Cutaneous blood flow is altered with aging and the coexistence of circulatory pathophysiology. Decreased circulation to the skin predisposes clients to impairments in skin integrity, such as arterial and venous ulcers or poor healing of surgical wounds. This study investigated the use of a laser Doppler velocimeter for noninvasive assessment of cutaneous blood flow. Indications for the use of such an instrument include the assessment of the relative degrees of pathophysiology, as well as objective documentation of the effectiveness of nursing interventions.

CHAPTER 40

Interventions for Clients with Skin Disorders

SKIN DISORDERS

Rarely is a client admitted to the hospital with an isolated medical or surgical problem. More than likely there is evidence of multisystem involvement, which is often accompanied by a variety of skin disorders, ranging from minor irritation to major skin disease. Immunosuppression, as a result of either the underlying disease process or anti-inflammatory medications, predisposes a client to opportunistic skin infections with bacterial, fungal, and viral organisms. Many oral and intravenous (IV) drugs can trigger a cutaneous drug reaction. Surgical intervention can also result in wound infection and delayed healing.

The elderly client is of particular concern, not only because age-related skin changes increase the chance of hospital-acquired skin lesions, but also because the elderly are often admitted with previously undiagnosed skin disease. For example, the nurse may be the first to recognize a suspicious lesion later found to be a skin cancer. Furthermore, skin irritations are common among the elderly and, when bed rest and immobility are contributing factors, can progress to serious complications that prolong hospitalization and contribute to increased morbidity and mortality. Both early assessment and timely intervention are essential for the elderly client.

MINOR IRRITATIONS

DRYNESS

Dry skin is a common problem, especially in elderly clients. Although there are currently few data to support the actual cause of the dry, rough quality of old skin, changes in the functioning of the sebaceous glands, with a loss of natural lubrication and increased evaporative water loss, are thought to play a role. Dry skin is seen as a fine flaking of the stratum corneum (outermost skin layer), which may appear more pronounced over the distal lower extremities in clients with vascular insufficiency. In addition to visible skin changes, severe dehydration of the stratum corneum (*xerosis*) is often accompanied by complaints of a generalized pruritus. In chronic conditions, unrelieved pruritus may result in secondary skin lesions, excoriations, and lichenification (thickening), as the client scratches and rubs the skin in an attempt to relieve the intense itching.

Xerosis is exacerbated in dry climates. Central heating and air conditioning reduce the available humidity in the air and help advance the dryness of the skin. Wind, cold, and sunlight also contribute to the problem. Frequent bathing with harsh soap and hot water further robs the skin of natural lubrication, often resulting in an annoying skin eruption that is common in elderly clients known as winter itch. To re-establish skin integrity, the nurse plans interventions to maintain adequate skin lubrication and minimize the loss of moisture from the outer skin layers.

Immediate nursing intervention is aimed at rehydration of the skin and relief of any associated pruritus. A 20-minute soak in a tepid bath, followed by application of an emollient cream or lotion, is often sufficient to rehydrate the stratum corneum and promote comfort. If the client is bedridden or if tub baths are contraindicated, the trunk and extremities can be wrapped in warm moist towels covered by plastic sheeting and additional blankets to prevent chilling. The nurse always applies skin creams or lotions to slightly damp skin after the above procedures or within 2 to 3 minutes after routine bathing. Contrary to popular belief, the cream or lotion is *not* what makes the skin soft and supple. Water softens the outer skin layers and the lubricant seals in the moisture, promoting suppleness and preventing flaking. Some skin lotions are hydrophilic and actually draw moisture from the skin and contribute to the dryness if not applied directly to damp skin.

Further intervention involves educating the client or significant other in measures to maintain healthy skin. For example, in the home, room humidifiers are often helpful in combating dry air, especially during the winter months. Although soap and water are useful in cleaning oily skin, soap can often contribute to irritation and pruritus if winter itch is a problem. Total body bathing with soap every other day is usually sufficient for most people if the face, the axillae, and the perineum are bathed daily. A mild, nonalkaline soap should be used and should be rinsed thoroughly from the skin before drying. The nurse instructs the client to avoid very warm or hot water, as it promotes lipid loss from the skin. If the client is accustomed to using bath oil, the nurse explains that adding bath oil to the water at the *end* of the bath will allow the skin time to become hydrated before sealing the surface with the oil. Finally, the nurse explores with the client ways to maintain adequate fluid intake so that systemic dehydration and subsequent skin cell dehydration can be avoided. A daily fluid intake of 3000 mL is suggested for maintaining hydration, if not contraindicated for other medical reasons.

PRURITUS

Pruritus, or itching, is an often-distressing cutaneous symptom that may or may not be associated with skin disease. Although pruritus was previously thought to result from low-threshold stimulation of pain receptors in the skin, studies indicate that pruritus is caused by stimulation of itch-specific nerve fibers at the dermal-epidermal junction. Physical or chemical agents either act directly on these nerve fibers or activate chemical mediators, such as histamine, which, in turn, act on itch receptors.

As a subjective sensation similar to pain, pruritus varies from client to client in distribution and severity.

Regardless of the underlying cause, pruritus is usually reported to be worse at night, probably owing to an increased awareness of discomfort with removal of daytime distractions. In addition, poor skin hydration, increased skin temperature, perspiration, and emotional stress may aggravate the symptom.

Relief from pruritus is usually sought by scratching or rubbing the skin, a protective reflex that further stimulates the itch receptors and initiates a pattern referred to as the itch-scratch-itch cycle. When the pruritus is associated with skin lesions, effective relief can usually be obtained by treatment of the underlying dermatologic disorder with appropriate topical and systemic medications. Certain systemic diseases, such as hepatic and venous disorders, can also result in pruritus, without the presence of skin lesions. In these instances, treatment is often complicated because the underlying biochemical mechanisms causing the itching are poorly understood.

The nurse plans care to promote comfort and prevent alterations in the skin's protective mechanism that can result from vigorous scratching. Dry skin is often a contributing factor, requiring that the nurse emphasize proper bathing and skin lubrication techniques (see nursing interventions for dry skin). The nurse encourages the client to keep fingernails trimmed short, with rough edges filed, to minimize excoriation. Mittens or splints can be worn at night to prevent inadvertent scratching during sleep. Finally, a cool sleeping environment combined with the administration of a larger dose of antihistamine at bedtime (when the associated drowsiness is welcome) may be sufficient to provide an uninterrupted night's sleep. Therapeutic baths (balneotherapy) containing colloidal oatmeal preparations or tar extracts may prove helpful in providing temporary relief (Table 40–1).

If antihistamines are ordered, the nurse administers them promptly and closely monitors the client's response to therapy so that the dosage can be adjusted accordingly. In addition, the anti-inflammatory properties of any topical steroid preparations that may be ordered can be maximized if the nurse applies the ointment or cream to slightly damp skin. Additional nursing measures that promote comfort include tepid or cool baths and cool compresses to increase vasoconstriction and the use of distraction or relaxation techniques to allay anxiety, which can often worsen pruritic episodes.

PRICKLY HEAT

Miliaria rubra, or prickly heat, occurs as small vesicles or papules on an erythematous base. This often pruritic skin eruption is commonly found on the posterior trunk or in the large skin fold areas where moisture accumulates and obstructs the sweat glands. Contributing factors include high fevers with diaphoresis, an overly warm environment, or activity resulting in excessive perspiration.

The nurse minimizes any stimulus to sweating by promoting a cool, dry environment. Although an air-

TABLE 40–1   Uses of Therapeutic Baths

Agents	Disease	Purpose
Antibacterial Baths		
Potassium permanganate (1:32,000; 1:64,000)	Infected eczema	Lower skin bacterial load
Acetic acid	Dirty ulcerations	Prevent pemphigus
Hexachlorophene	Furunculosis	
Povidone-iodine		
Colloidal Baths		
Starch and baking soda (1 c each/tub)	Any red, irritated, oozing condition	Relieve itching
Aveeno Colloidal Oatmeal (1 c/tub)	(e.g., atopic eczema)	Soothe
Aveeno Oilated Colloidal Oatmeal		
Emollient Baths*		
Bath oils; Alpha Keri, Lubath	Any dry skin condition	Clean and hydrate the skin
Mineral oil		
Tar Baths*		
Bath oils with tar: Balnetar, Zetar, Polytar	Scaly dermatoses (e.g., psoriasis)	Loosen scale
Coal tar concentrate (Liquor carbonis detergens)		Relieve itching
		Potentiate UVA or UVB light therapy

* For emollient and tar baths, add 3 to 6 capfuls of therapeutic agent per standard bathtub.

From Theodore Rosen, Marilyn B. Lanning, & Marcia J. Hill, *The nurse's atlas of dermatology*, p. 176. Copyright © 1983 by Theodore Rosen and Marilyn B. Lanning. Reprinted by permission of Little, Brown and Company.

conditioned room is ideal, the use of a small fan also helps to circulate the air. If the client is bedridden, the nurse places a folded cotton bath blanket or mattress pad on the bed to absorb excess moisture and keep the skin dry. The use of waterproof pads directly next to the skin should be avoided when possible, as they contribute to maceration of the skin and pruritus. The client is positioned to promote optimal air circulation to the involved areas. For example, a side-lying position is encouraged if the posterior trunk is involved. In addition, loose-fitting cotton clothing and the use of a bed cradle to tent the sheets allow for more effective air circulation and cooling of the skin. Although absorbent powders, such as talc, can sometimes prove effective in maintaining a dry skin surface, cornstarch should be avoided as a drying agent because it supports the growth of fungal organisms. Finally, to prevent further blockage of the eccrine glands, the nurse uses water-soluble creams or lotions to lubricate the skin in place of the more greasy emollient preparations.

SUNBURN

Sunburn is an example of a first-degree burn and one of the most common skin injuries. Excessive exposure to ultraviolet (UV) light results in injury to the superficial dermis, with subsequent dilation of the capillaries, erythema, tenderness, edema, and occasionally vesicle and bulla formation. Involvement of large areas of the body may also produce systemic symptoms, such as headache, nausea, and fever.

As for most injuries, the best treatment for sunburn is prevention. Fair-skinned clients are at greater risk owing to decreased production of melanin by the melanocytes at the basement membrane of the dermis. In addition, certain drugs and other chemical agents can *photosensitize* the skin, making clients more susceptible to sunburn, regardless of their skin tone.

Education of the client is guided by individual skin color, past experiences with sun exposure, and the amount of exposure anticipated. The nurse encourages the liberal use of commercial sunscreens during outdoor activities and warns against exposure between 11 AM and 3 PM when UV radiation is strongest. The ability of a sunscreen preparation to reflect or absorb UV light is expressed as a sunburn protection factor (SPF). The higher the SPF, the more efficient a product is in preventing sunburn. For a sunscreen to remain effective, it must be applied frequently and in adequate amounts. Both perspiration and swimming can contribute to dilution of the screening agent and loss of protection. Shade offers only partial protection from UV radiation. Complete protection can be afforded by covering the skin with opaque clothing.

After sunburn has occurred, erythema and discomfort begin within a few hours after exposure and gradually increase in intensity for 1 to 2 days before subsiding. Treatment is directed toward symptomatic relief of discomfort using cool baths and soothing lotions, such as calamine or refrigerated moisturizing lotions. Antibiotic ointments are indicated only if blistering of the skin results in secondary infection. The use of topical corticosteroids may decrease the inflammation temporarily if discomfort is severe; however, systemic corticosteroids and nonsteroidal anti-inflammatory agents have been reported to be of little use in treatment of established sunburn.

URTICARIA

Urticaria, or hives, is characterized by white or red edematous papules or plaques of varying sizes, shapes, and distribution. The individual lesions are transient, resolving and reappearing over short periods of time. Urticaria may be associated with severe pruritus; however, owing to the transient nature of the disorder, excoriations are uncommon. Hives are also sometimes accompanied by deep subcutaneous swelling called *angioedema,* which frequently involves the lips and the eyes.

In general, urticaria results from exposure to a specific noxious stimulus, which causes the release of histamine in the dermal tissue, vasodilation, and subsequent leakage of plasma protein to form the characteristic lesions, or wheals. Unfortunately, a definitive cause of urticaria is identified in only a small number of cases. Factors that have been implicated include drugs, food products, infections, autoimmune diseases, malignancies, and psychogenic and physical factors.

Treatment is aimed at removal of the potentially harmful stimulus and relief of any associated symptoms. Because the cutaneous reaction is associated with histamine release, antihistamines are the drugs of choice. In addition, the nurse instructs the client to avoid situations that may contribute to vasodilation and subsequent exacerbation of symptoms, such as overexertion, alcohol consumption, and warm environments. Reassurance that urticaria is a relatively common occurrence is often welcomed by the client, especially if a specific cause cannot be identified.

TRAUMA

OVERVIEW

Skin trauma can vary from a neat, aseptic surgical incision performed in a controlled environment to a grossly infected, draining pressure ulcer with significant tissue destruction. In each of these examples, injury to the skin results in a predictable series of events aimed at repairing the defect and thus re-establishing the continuity of the body's protective barrier. Normally, wound healing occurs in phases: (1) the inflammatory, or "lag," phase; (2) the fibroblastic, or connective tissue repair, phase; and (3) the maturation, or remodeling, phase. The length of each phase depends largely on the circumstances surrounding the injury and whether the wound is allowed to heal by first, second, or third intention (see the illustration on page 479). For example, a wound without tissue loss, such as a clean laceration or a surgi-

NURSING RESEARCH

Proper Technique Reduces the Incidence of Skin Damage Associated with Subcutaneous Medications.

Woolridge, J., & Jackson, J. (1988). Evaluation of bruises and areas of induration after two techniques of subcutaneous heparin injection. *Heart and Lung, 17,* 476–482.

Two different subcutaneous injection techniques were used on the same clients to determine if any differences in skin trauma resulted. Fewer incidences of skin trauma, as measured by the formation of bruises and induration, were noted by the subcutaneous injection method that included changing the needle between drawing up medication and administering it, sealing the medication in the tissues with an air bubble, and using a dry sponge over the needle during withdrawal.

Critique. This study controlled for client variables, as well as drug administration variables, by using two different injection techniques for each client. This method increases the likelihood that the observed differences in skin damage are attributable to the actual differences in injection technique.

Possible nursing implications. For some types of treatment-induced skin and tissue trauma, changes in nursing care techniques can make a significant difference. Identification of possible areas where changes in nursing care can reduce client discomfort or the incidence of treatment-induced problems should be a major focus of clinical nursing research.

cal incision, can be closed primarily with sutures or staples. The wound edges are immediately brought together, with the skin layers approximated and held in place until healing is complete. Because the defect can be easily corrected and dead space eliminated, healing by *first intention* shortens the phases of tissue repair considerably. Inflammation resolves quickly and connective tissue repair is minimal, resulting in a thin scar. On the other hand, a wound with tissue loss, such as a chronic pressure ulcer or venous stasis ulcer, results in a cavity-like defect that requires gradual filling in of the dead space with connective tissue. Consequently, healing by *second intention* prolongs the repair process. Wounds with a high potential for infection, such as surgical incisions that enter a nonsterile body cavity or traumatic wounds that occur under unclean conditions, may be intentionally left open for several days. After debris and exudate have been removed and inflammation has subsided, the wound is closed by first intention. Healing by delayed primary closure, or *third intention*, results in a scar similar to that found in wounds that heal by first intention. As can be seen in the accompanying Key Features of Disease, healing can be impaired by a number of stressors, including alterations in the client's immune response, lack of sufficient wound oxygen attributable

COLOR PLATES

ASSESSMENT FINDINGS COMMON IN ELDERLY CLIENTS
NORMAL FINDINGS

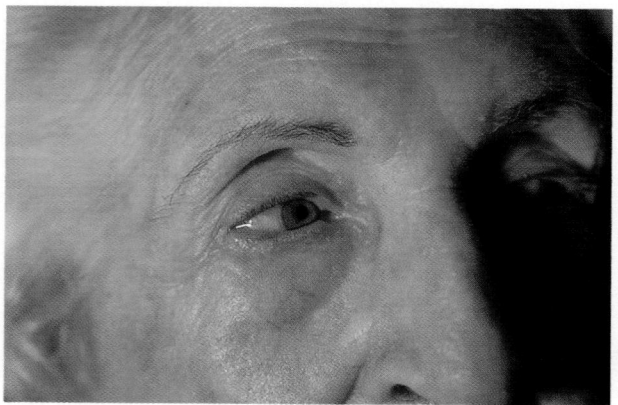

Plate 1

Eyelid eversion. Changes in the elasticity of the skin cause loosening around the eyelids, particularly the lower lids, which results in exposure of the conjunctiva. (Chaps. 35, 39)

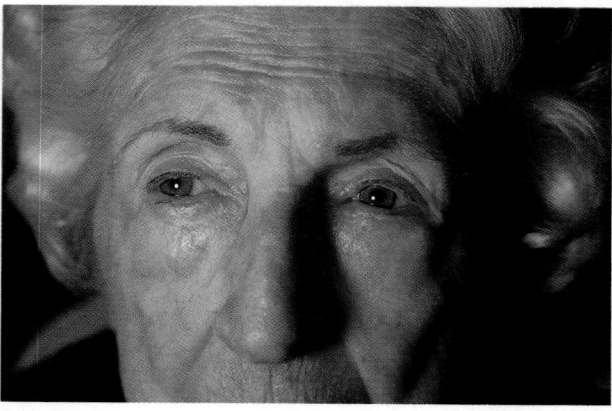

Plate 2

Deepening of the orbital cavity. Loss of orbital tissue causes the eyes to sink deeper into the orbit. (Chap. 35)

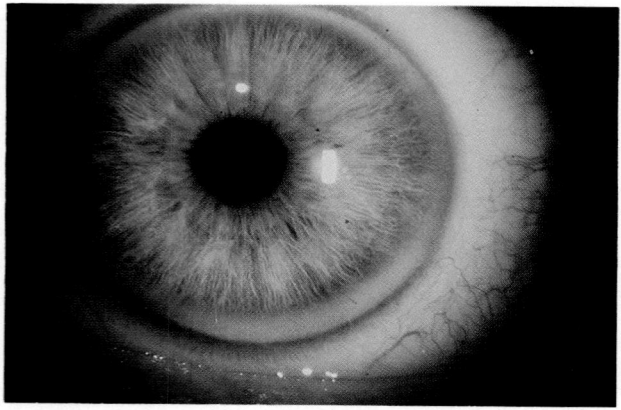

Plate 3

Arcus senilis of the iris. (Chap. 35)

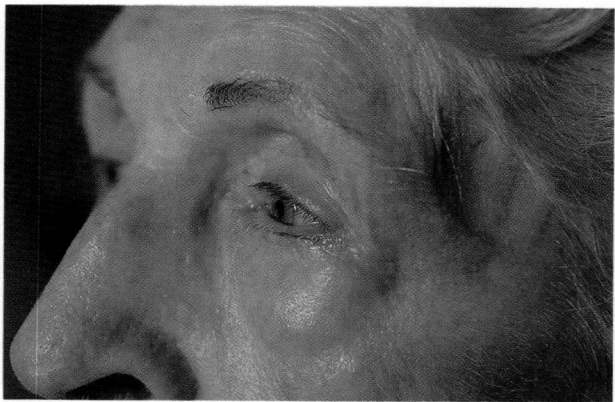

Plate 4

Changes in body contour. Redistribution of adipose tissue, combined with changes in skin elasticity, results in obvious changes in body contour, such as a double chin and "bags" under the eyes. (Chaps. 35, 39)

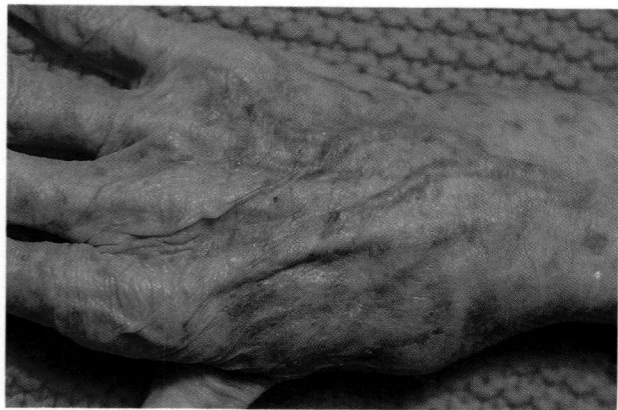

Plate 5

Paper-thin, transparent skin. The fragile, translucent appearance of the skin of elderly clients is caused by thinning of the dermis. (Chap. 39)

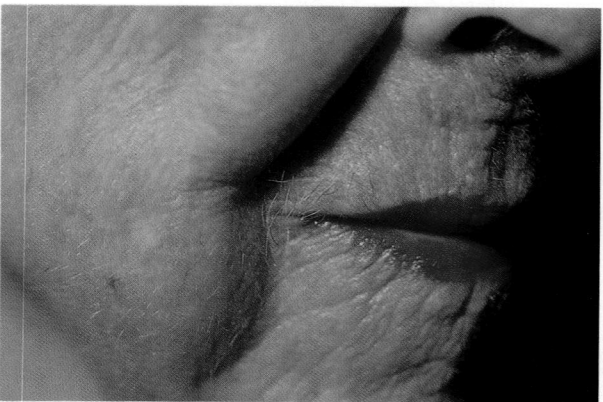

Plate 6

Wrinkles. Gradual degeneration of elastic fibers and thinning of the dermis contribute to loss of skin tone and the characteristic wrinkles of old age. (Chap. 39)

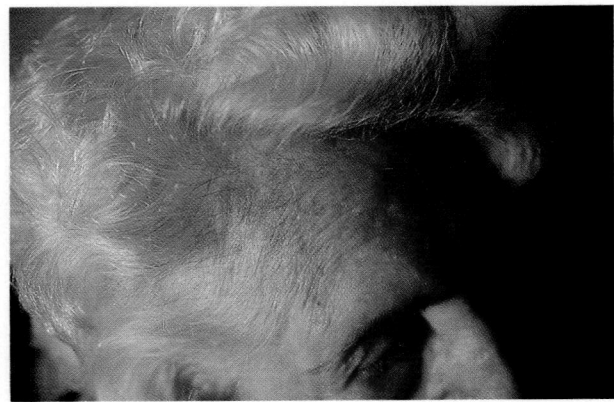

Plate 7

Hair thinning. Progressive loss of functional melanocytes in the hair bulb and a gradual decrease in the number of active hair follicles cause the scalp hair to turn gray and to thin. (Chap. 39)

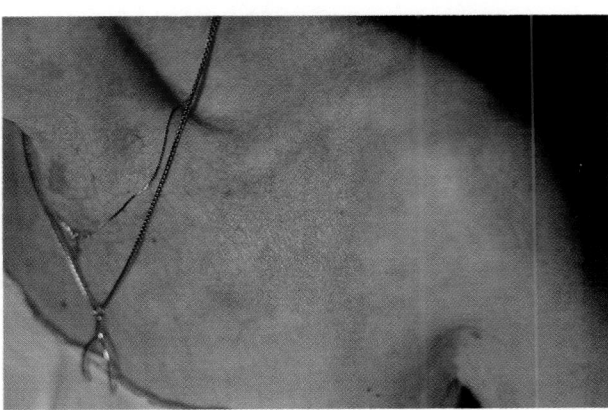

Plate 8

Xerosis (dry skin). The dry, rough quality of aging skin can be attributed in part to decreased dermal blood flow. Although the distribution may be generalized, xerosis is usually more prominent on the lower extremities. The condition tends to worsen during the winter months, and the associated intense pruritus often leads to breaks in the skin from scratching. Note the reddened skin on the client's shoulder, which is caused by scratching. (Chap. 39)

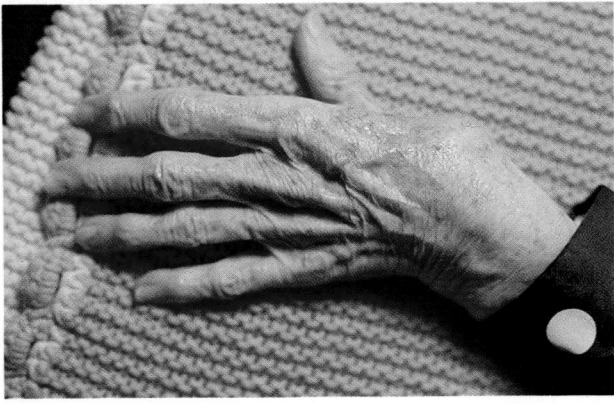

Plate 9

Actinic purpura. Increased fragility of blood vessels from exposure to sun and from aging may lead to ecchymotic macules on the dorsum of the hands and lower arms as a result of minor trauma. (Chap. 39)

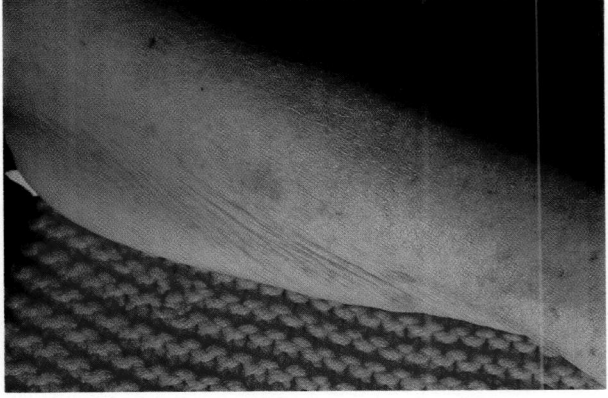

Plate 10

Actinic lentigo (liver spots). Hyperpigmented macules resembling large freckles are a common finding on sun-exposed areas of the head, neck, arms, and shoulders in the elderly. Cumulative damage from ultraviolet radiation causes some melanocytes to produce more pigment. In contrast to the name, these lesions are not associated with abnormal liver function. (Chap. 39)

Plate 11

Senile (cherry) hemangioma. These dusky red, dome-shaped papules are most often found on the upper trunk. Caused by a benign increase in proliferation of capillaries with aging, these lesions may vary considerably in size and color on the same client. (Chap. 39)

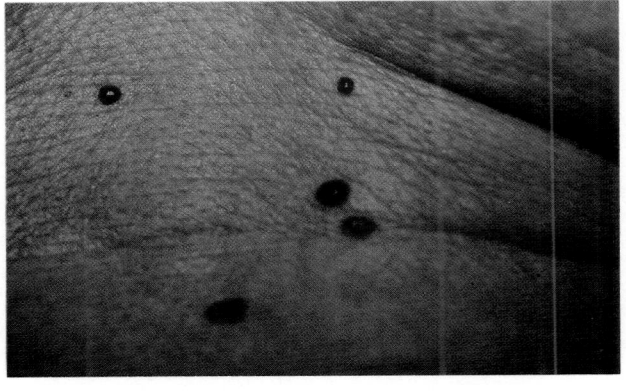

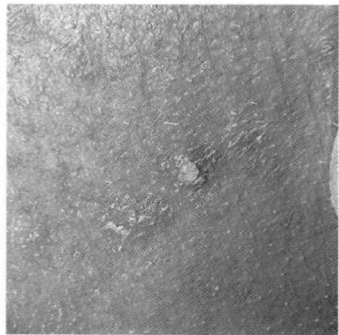

Plate 12

Actinic (solar) keratosis. These premalignant lesions are commonly found in elderly clients with sun-damaged skin that has a yellowish color, wrinkles, and freckled pigmentation. (Chap. 39)

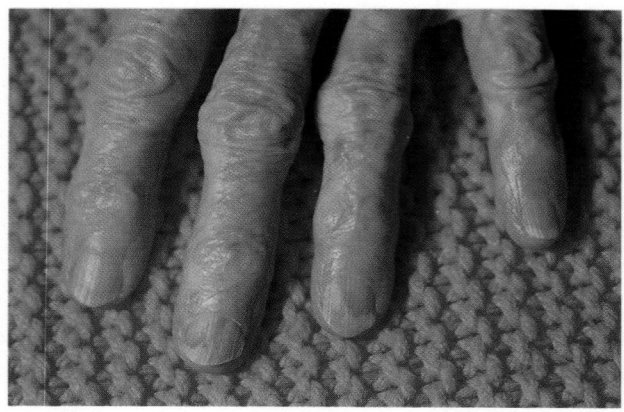

Plate 13

Nail changes. Fingernails and toenails develop longitudinal ridges (onychorrhexis) with aging. Toenails may thicken considerably as a result of poor circulation or frequent trauma. (Chap. 39)

PATHOLOGIC FINDINGS

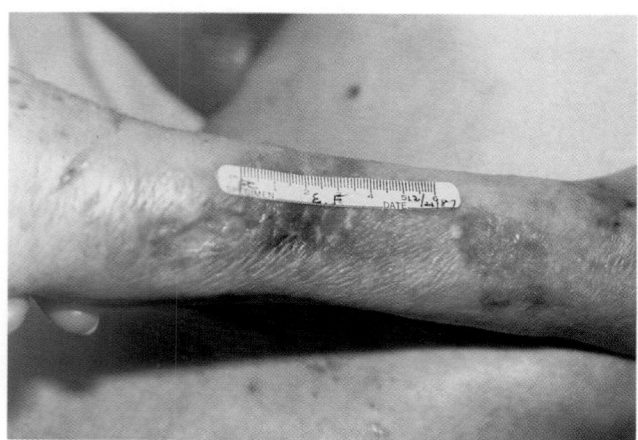

Plate 14

Skin tears. With aging, a flattening of the attachment between the epidermis and dermis makes the skin more susceptible to shearing forces. Skin tears are not uncommon. Often associated with purpura, these traumatic lesions are frequently seen on the forearms, a place that is often grabbed when a family member or staff person assists with positioning or ambulation. (Chap. 40)

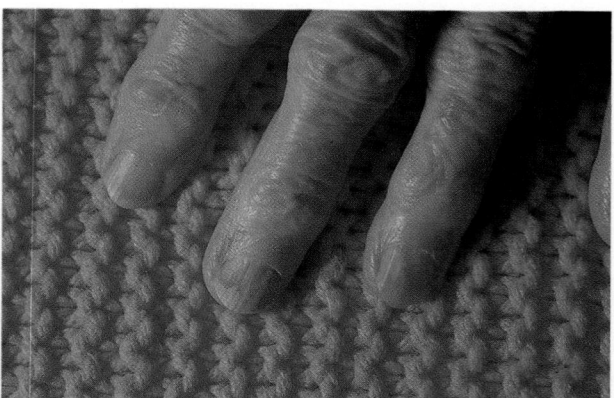

Plate 15

Fungal infection of the nails, visible on the middle finger of this elderly client. (Chaps. 26, 40)

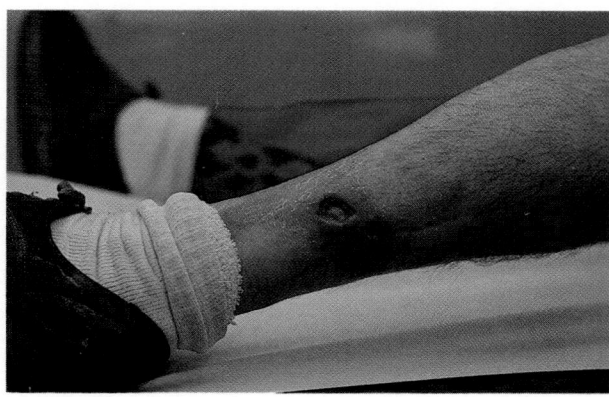

Plate 16
Venous stasis ulcer. (Chaps. 40, 65)

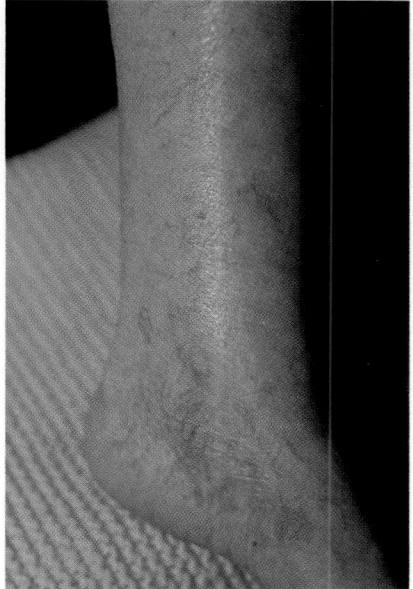

Plate 17
Nonpitting edema. (Chaps. 13, 40, 64)

ASSESSMENT FINDINGS COMMON IN DARK-SKINNED CLIENTS
NORMAL FINDINGS

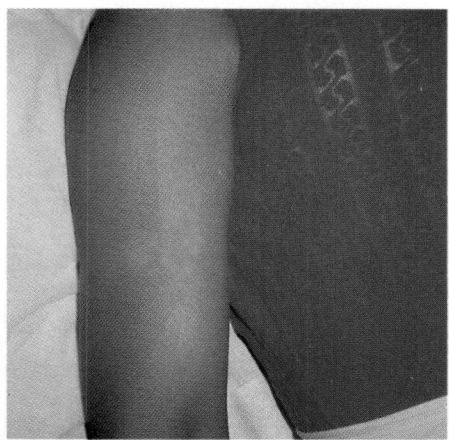

Plate 18
Futcher's or Voight's line. A sharp line of demarcation between dark and light skin, usually on the upper arms, is a common finding in Black persons. The mark is usually bilateral and symmetric. Futcher's line also occurs in about 4% of the Japanese population. (Chap. 39)

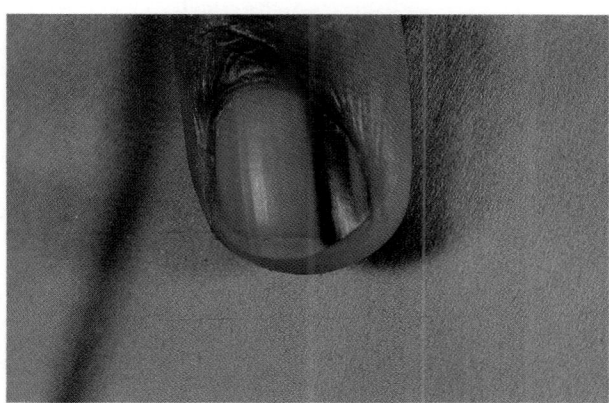

Plate 19
Linear nail pigmentation. Longitudinal, linear stripes of pigment ranging in width from 1 mm to several millimeters may be found in the nail plates of Black individuals. Both the darkness or prominence of these dark stripes and the number of nails involved tend to increase with age. The nurse carefully assesses the client to distinguish this normal variant from pathologic conditions of pigment deposition such as subungual melanoma or nevus. (Chap. 39)

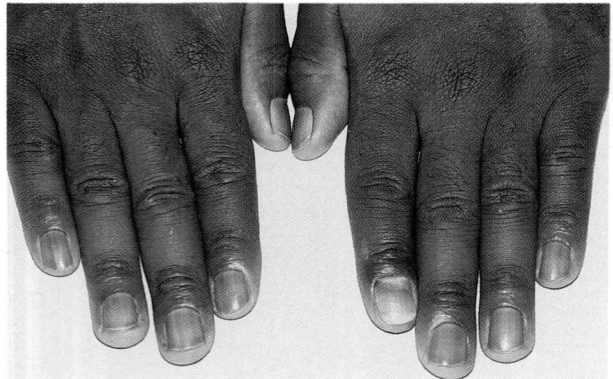

Plate 20

Diffuse nail pigmentation. Diffuse nail pigmentation of the entire nail plate is a normal skin variant and may involve one or more nail plates. (Chap. 39)

PATHOLOGIC FINDINGS

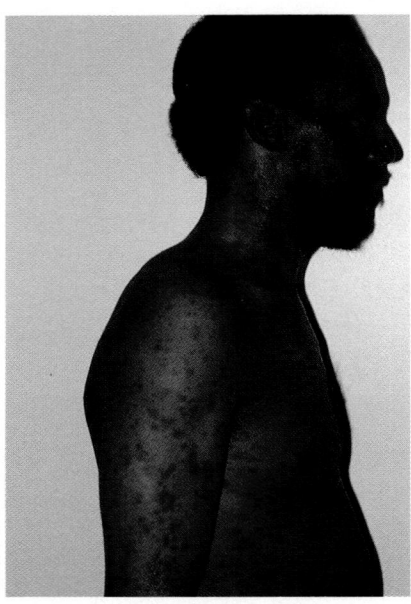

Plate 21

Postinflammatory hyperpigmentation. Areas of persistent skin darkening may occur in Black clients when melanocytes are stimulated by inflammation. Hyperpigmentation can occur after any traumatic injury, skin infection, or inflammatory skin disease. (Chap. 40)

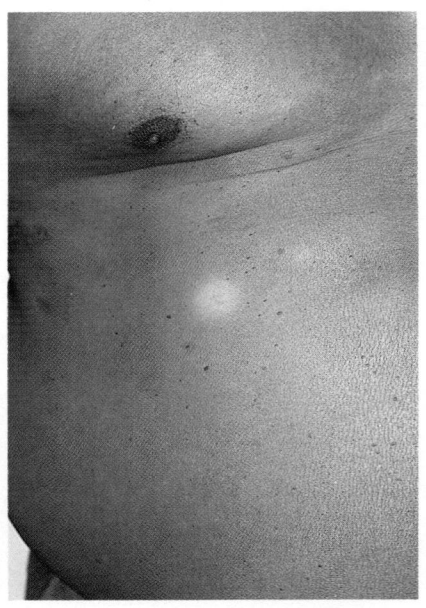

A

B

Plate 22

Postinflammatory hypopigmentation. *A*, Some disease processes cause patchy areas of depigmentation that are more noticeable in dark skin because of the color contrast. *B*, Permanent pigment loss occurs when the melanocytes in the skin have been totally destroyed, such as in this full-thickness burn that has healed by secondary intention. (Chaps. 16, 40)

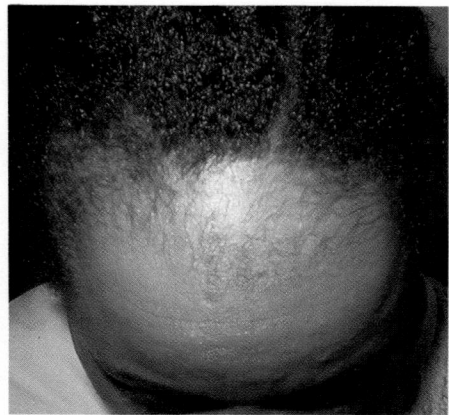

Plate 23

Hair loss caused by tension on the scalp. Patchy hair loss can result from prolonged tension on scalp hair. The Black custom of tightly plaiting the hair leads to gradual damage to the hair follicles, hair thinning, and hair loss. (Chap. 40)

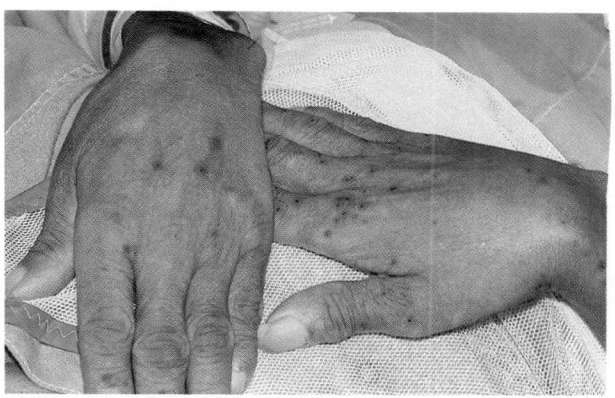

Plate 24

Petechiae. Intradermal or submucosal bleeding causes pinpoint purplish-red lesions. They are usually observable only on the oral mucosa or conjunctivae of a dark-skinned client, but in this client they are visible on the dorsal aspects of the hands. (Chaps. 40, 67)

Plate 25

Some lesions, such as this scarlatiniform rash, may show no changes in pigmentation in dark-skinned clients. (Chap. 40)

EYE ASSESSMENT

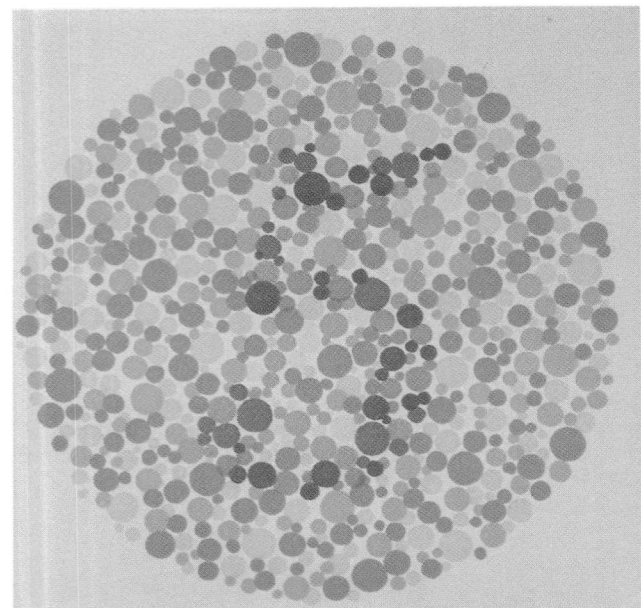

Plate 26

A typical pseudoisochromatic plate for testing color vision. (Chap. 35)

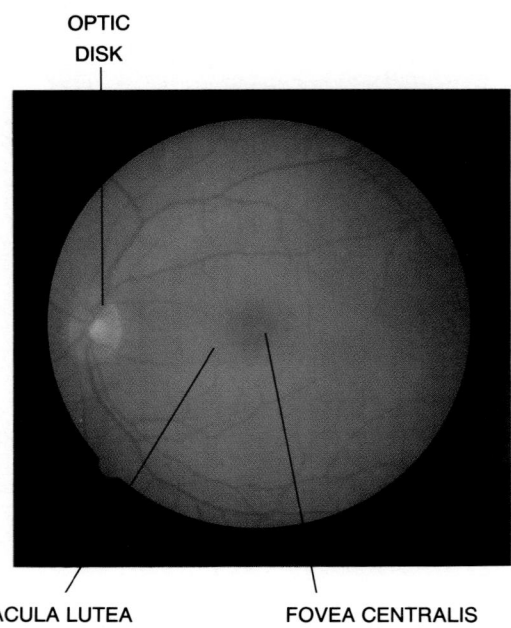

OPTIC DISK

MACULA LUTEA

FOVEA CENTRALIS

Plate 27

A normal optic fundus. (Chap. 35)

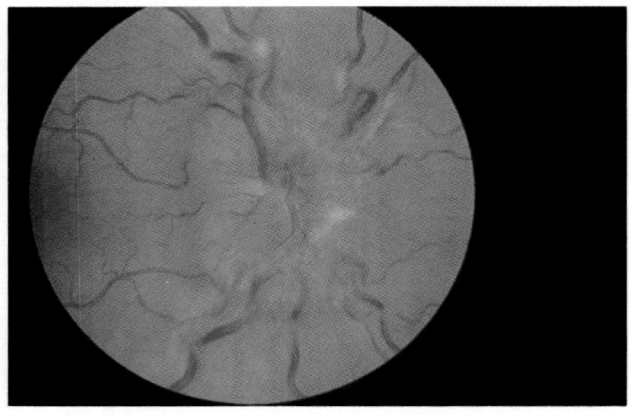

Plate 28

Optic fundus of a client with increased intracranial pressure (causing papilledema). (Chaps. 33, 36)

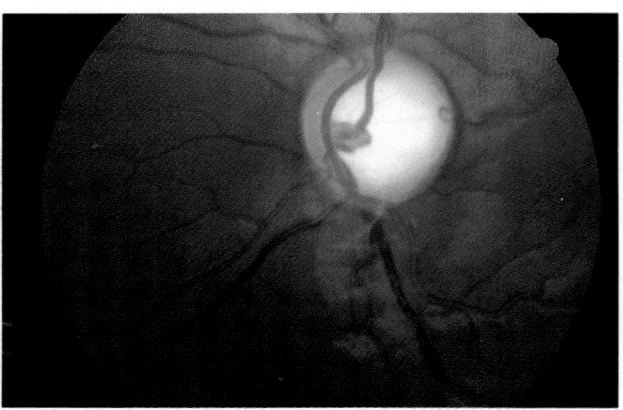

Plate 29

Optic fundus of a client with glaucoma. (Chap. 36)

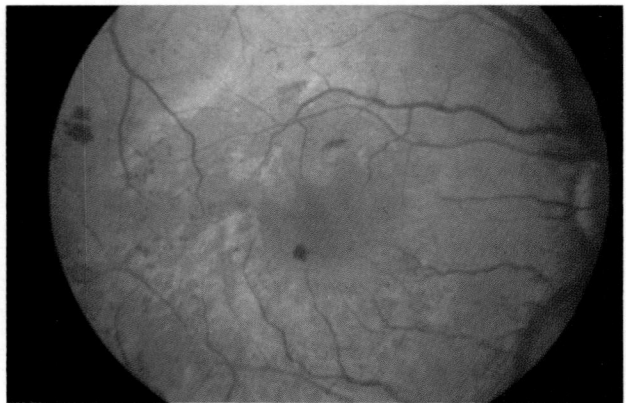

Plate 30

Optic fundus of a client with diabetes. (Chaps. 36, 51)

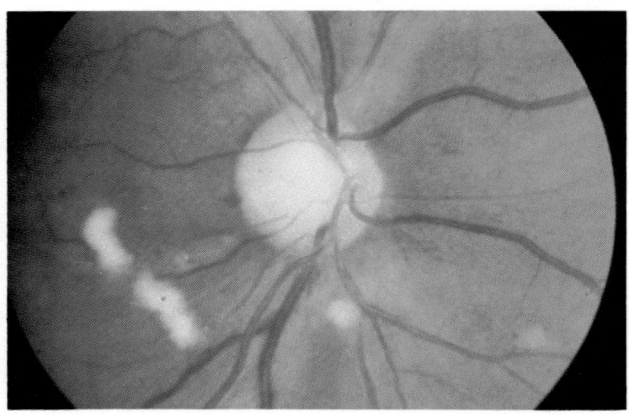

Plate 31

Optic fundus of a client with hypertension. (Chaps. 36, 65)

EAR ASSESSMENT

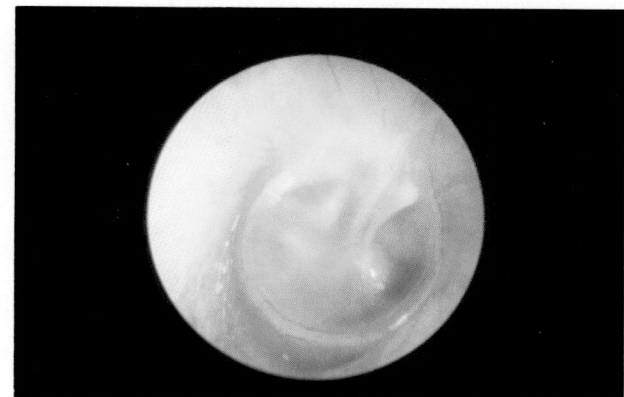

Plate 32
A normal tympanic membrane. (Chap. 37)

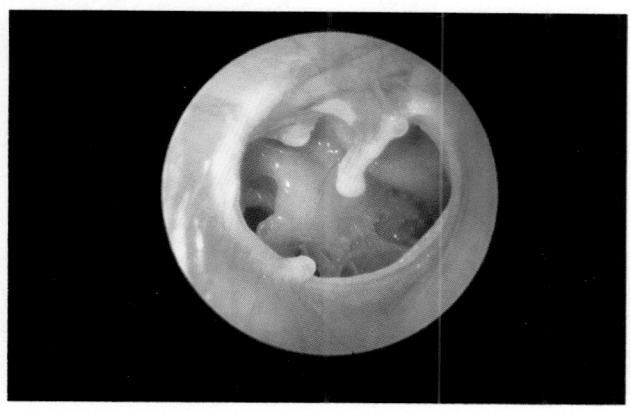

Plate 33
A perforated tympanic membrane. (Chap. 38)

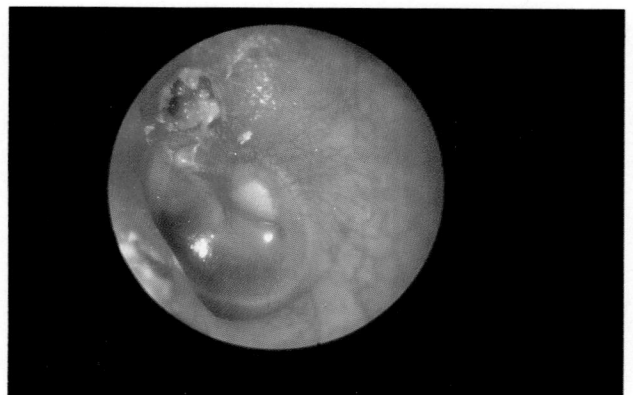

Plate 34
Cholesteatoma. (Chap. 38)

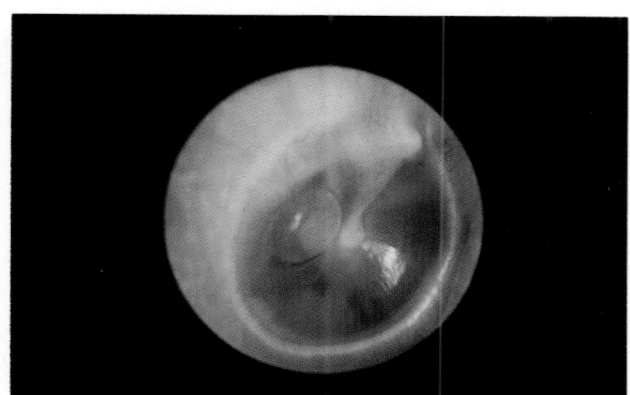

Plate 35
Otitis media. (Chap. 38)

ASSESSMENT OF THE ORAL CAVITY

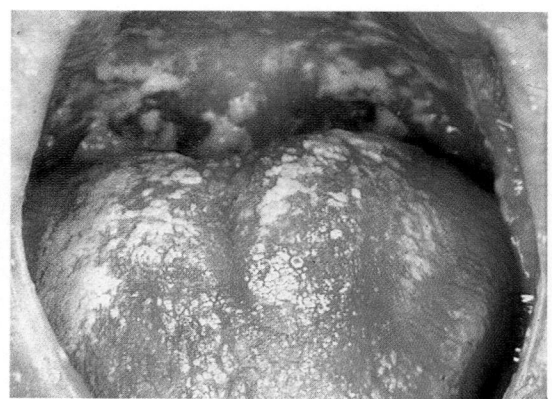

Plate 36
Oral candidiasis. (Chaps. 26, 42)

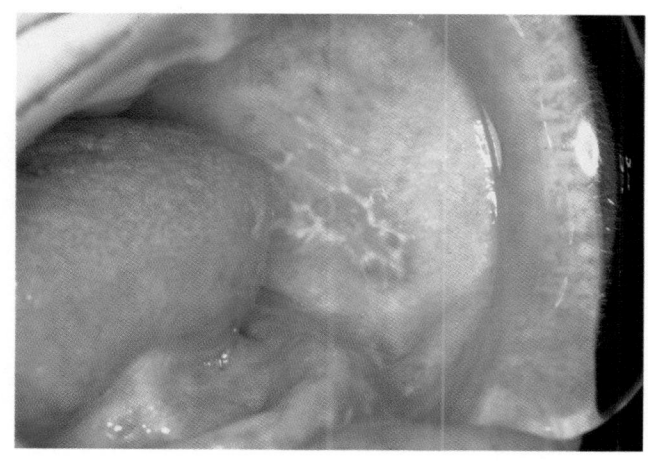

Plate 37
Oral lichen planus. (Chaps. 26, 42)

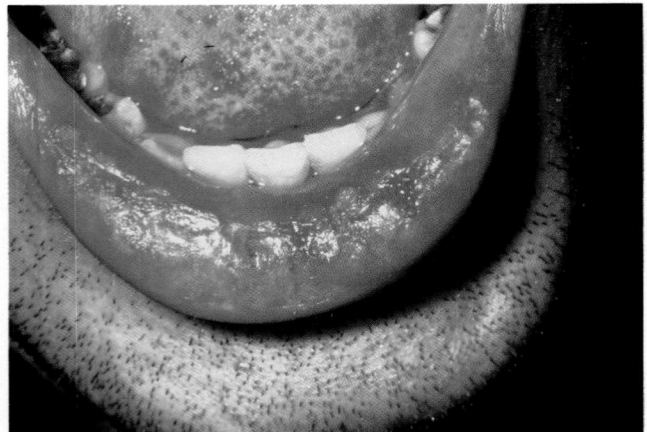

Plate 38
Recurrent herpetic stomatitis. (Chaps. 26, 42, 56)

SKIN ASSESSMENT

Plate 39
Miliaria rubra. (Chap. 40)

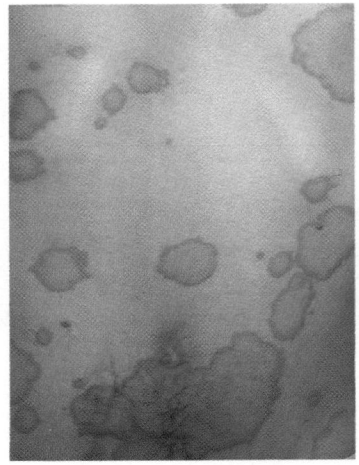

Plate 40
Urticaria. (Chaps. 27, 40)

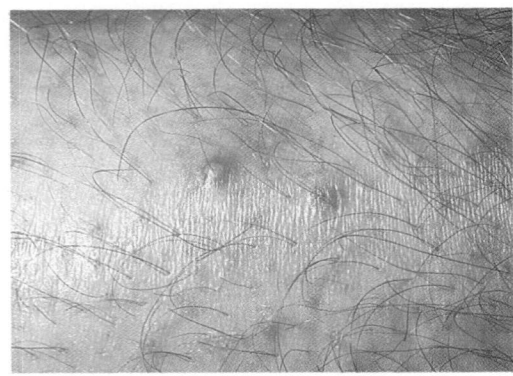

Plate 41
Folliculitis. (Chap. 40)

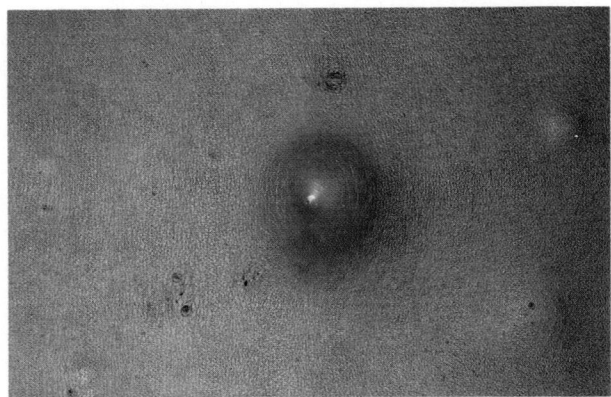

Plate 42
Furuncle. (Chap. 40)

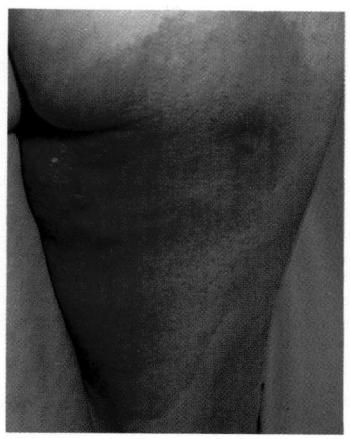

Plate 43
Cellulitis. (Chap. 40)

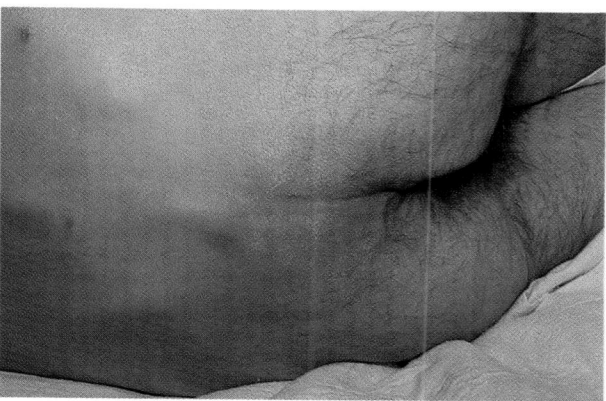

Plate 44
Stage I pressure ulcer. (Chap. 40)

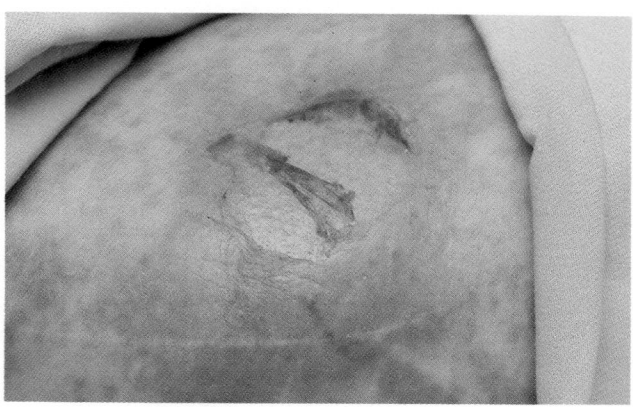

Plate 45
Stage II pressure ulcer. (Chap. 40)

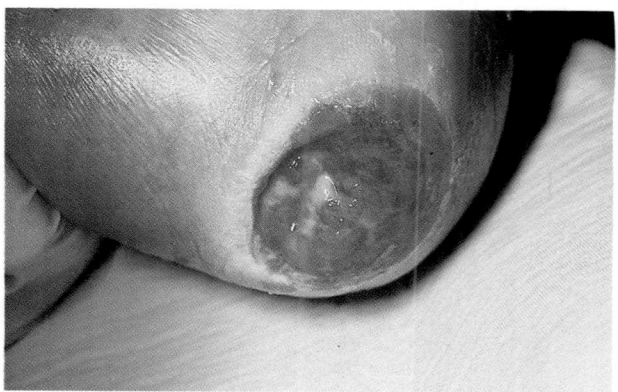

Plate 46
Stage III pressure ulcer. (Chap. 40)

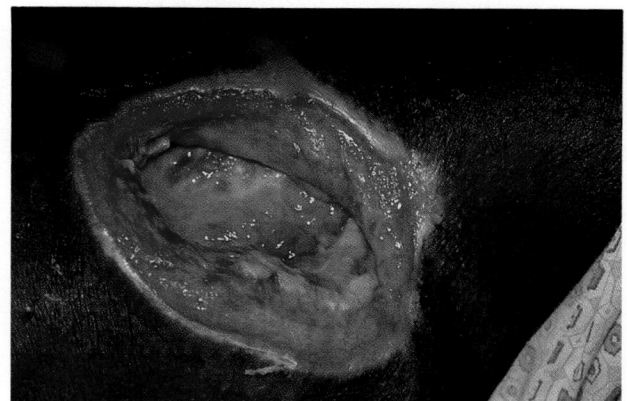

Plate 47
Stage IV pressure ulcer. (Chap. 40)

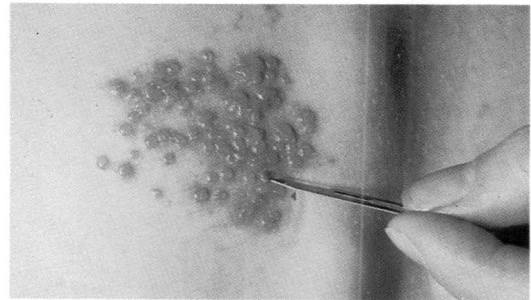

Plate 48
Herpes simplex. (Chaps. 26, 40, 56)

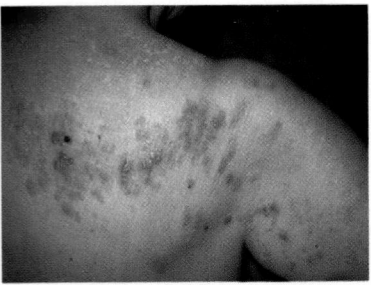

Plate 49

Herpes zoster. (Chaps. 26, 34, 40)

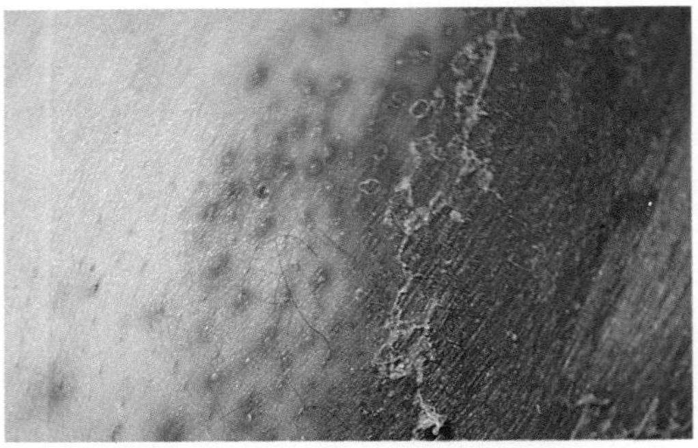

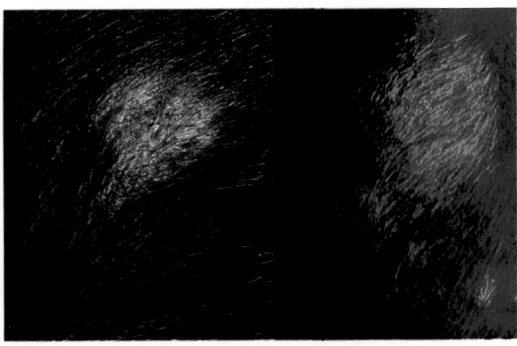

Plate 50

Candidiasis of the skin. (Chaps. 26, 40)

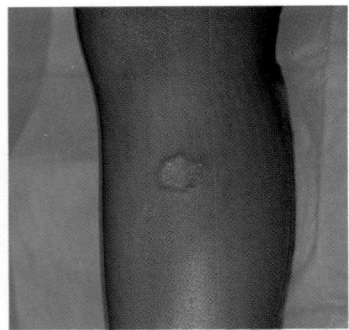

Plate 51

Tinea corporis. (Chaps. 26, 40)

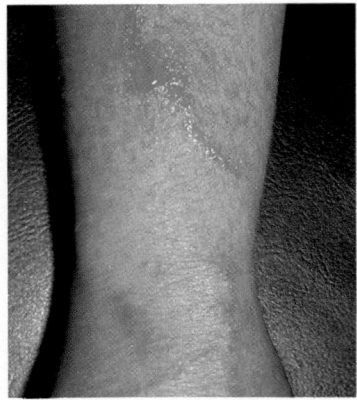

Plate 52

Tinea capitis. *Left,* Clinical appearance; *right,* appearance under Wood's lamp. (Chaps. 26, 40)

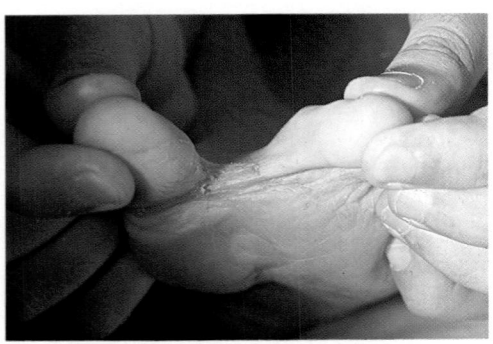

Plate 53

Tinea pedis. (Chaps. 26, 40)

Plate 54

Contact dermatitis. (Chaps. 27, 40)

Plate 55

Atopic dermatitis. (Chaps. 27, 40)

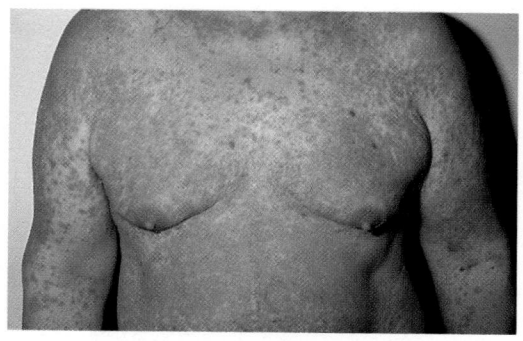

Plate 56

Drug-caused eruption. (Chap. 40)

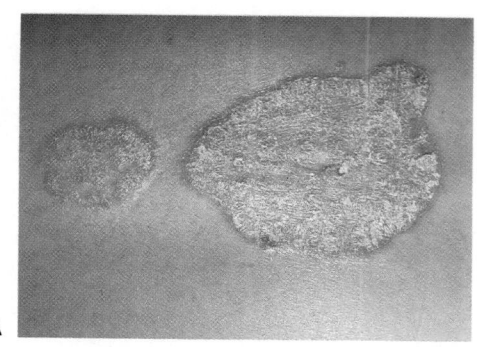

A

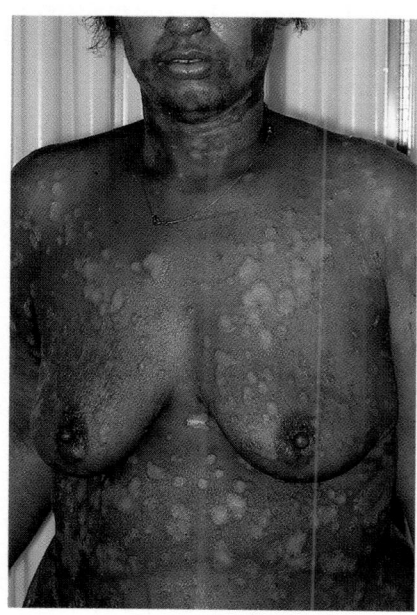

B

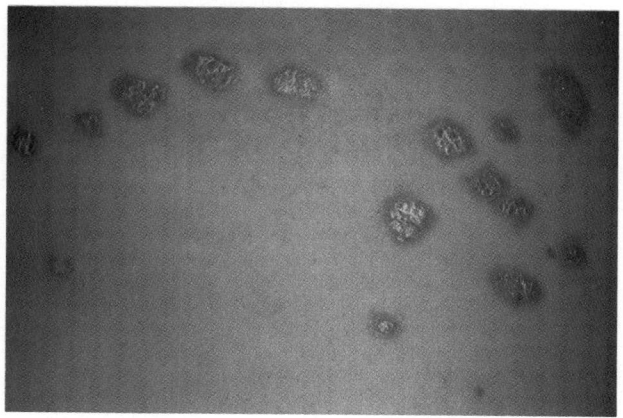

Plate 58

Guttate psoriasis. (Chap. 40)

Plate 57

Psoriasis vulgaris. *A,* In a Caucasian client. *B,* In a Black client. An uncommon disease in the Black population, psoriasis vulgaris may be difficult to detect in a Black client. The typical bright red color is not present. The plaques assume a blue or violaceous hue because of stimulation of melanocytes. The silvery scale is often absent. (Chap. 40)

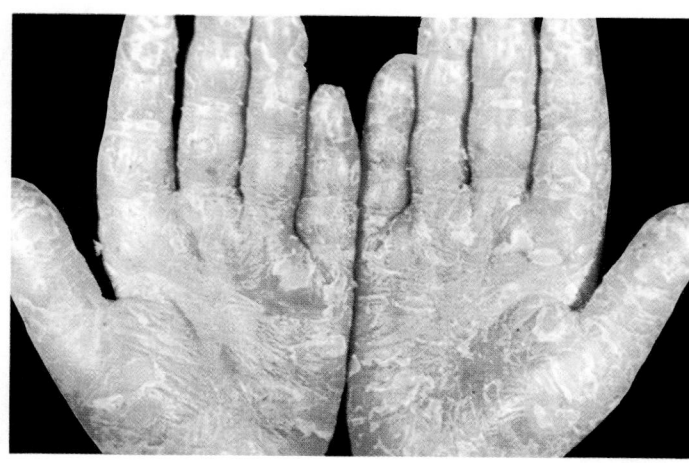

Plate 59

Exfoliative psoriasis. (Chap. 40)

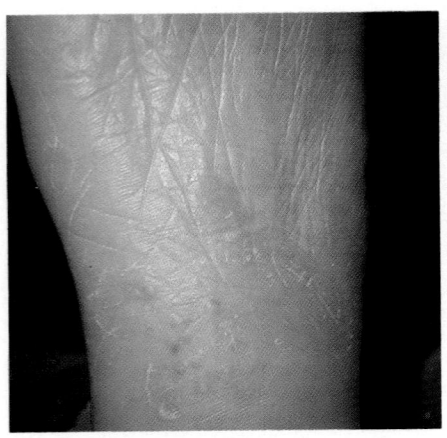

Plate 60
Pustular psoriasis. (Chap. 40)

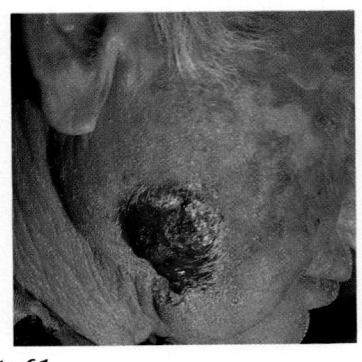

Plate 61
Squamous cell carcinoma. (Chaps. 25, 40)

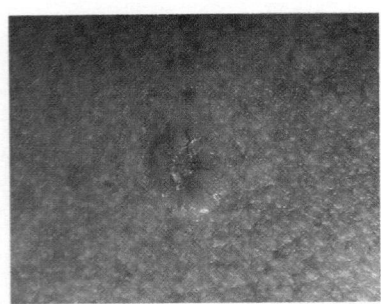

Plate 62
Basal cell carcinoma. (Chaps. 25, 40)

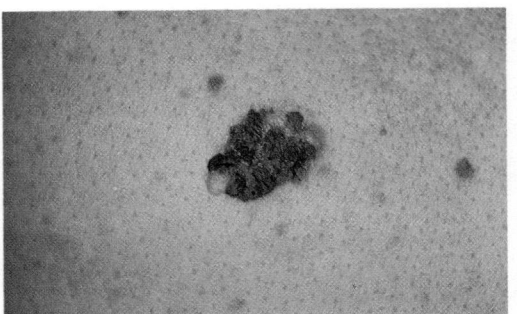

Plate 63
Melanoma. (Chaps. 25, 40)

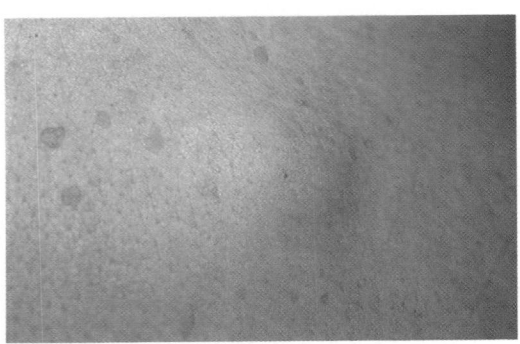

Plate 64
Epidermal inclusion cyst. (Chap. 40)

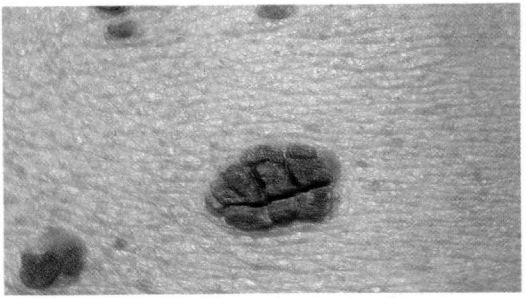

Plate 65
Seborrheic keratosis. (Chap. 40)

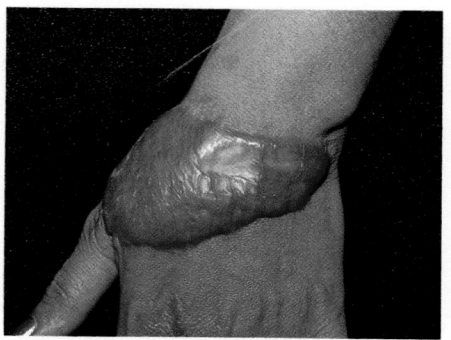

Plate 66

Keloid. (Chap. 40)

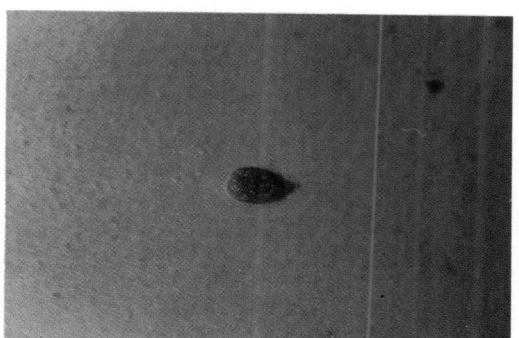

Plate 67

Compound nevus. (Chap. 40)

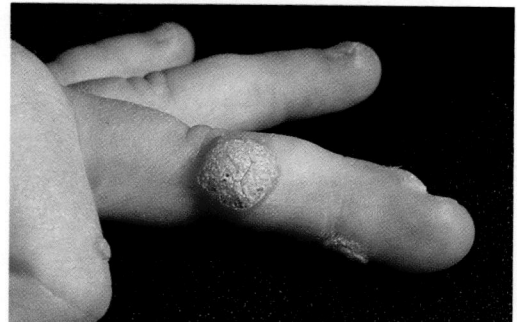

Plate 68

Common wart. (Chaps. 26, 40)

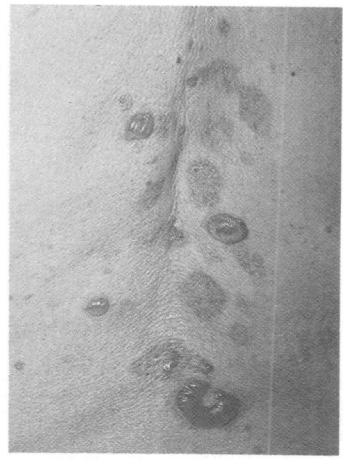

Plate 69

Pemphigus vulgaris. (Chap. 40)

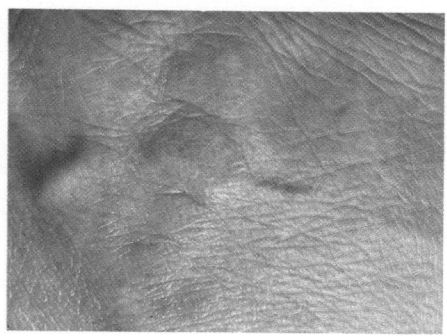

Plate 70

Lichen planus of the skin. (Chaps. 26, 40)

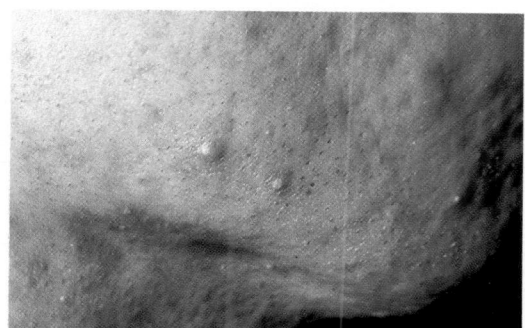

Plate 71

Acne. (Chap. 40)

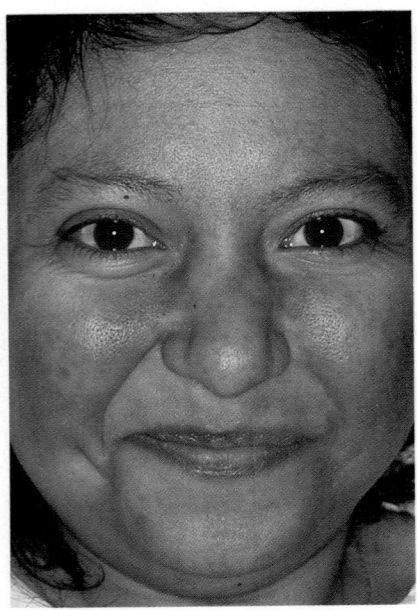

Plate 72

Butterfly rash of systemic lupus erythematosus. (Chap. 28)

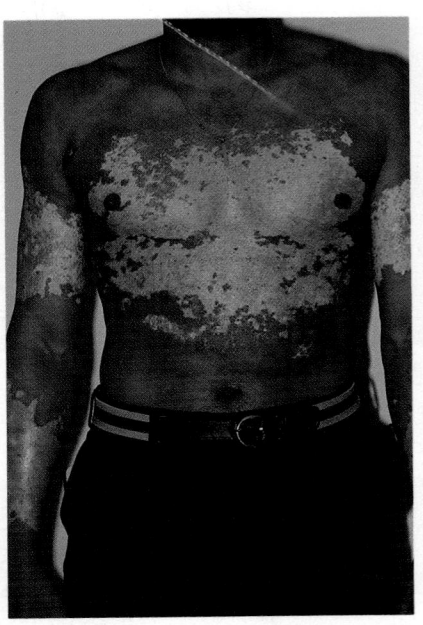

Plate 73

Discoid lesions of systemic lupus erythematosus. (Chap. 28)

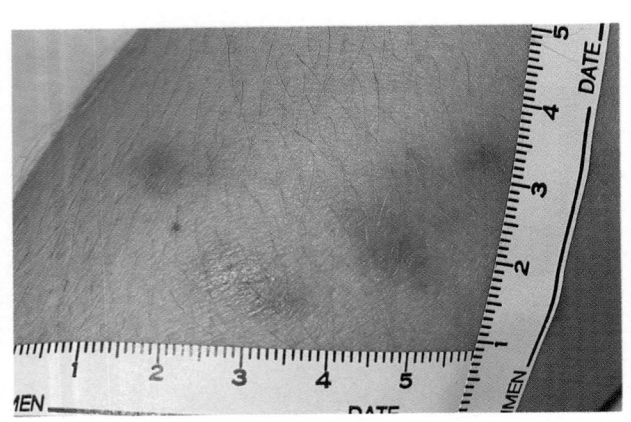

Plate 74

Kaposi's sarcoma. (Chaps. 25–27, 40, 56)

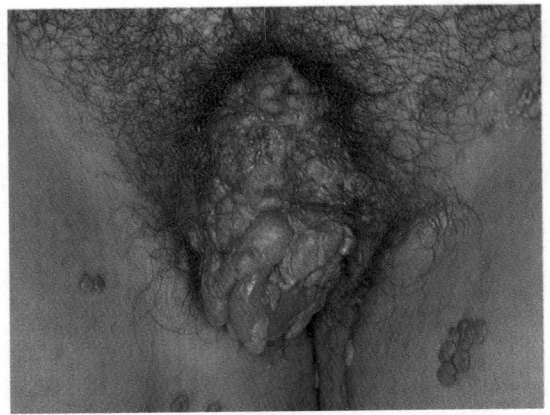

Plate 75

Genital warts. (Chaps. 26, 54–56)

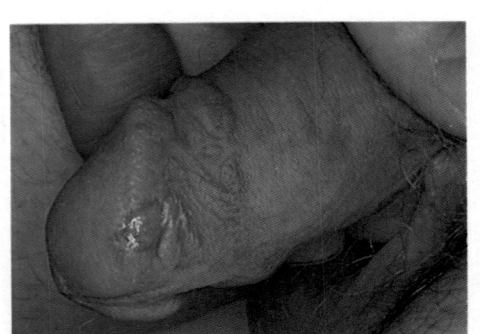

Plate 76

Primary syphilis. (Chaps. 26, 54–56)

KEY FEATURES OF DISEASE ■ Causes of Impaired Wound Healing

Cause	Mechanism
Altered Inflammatory Response	
Local	Altered local tissue circulation, resulting in ischemia, impaired leukocytic response to wounding, and increased probability of wound infection
Arteriosclerosis	
Diabetes	
Vasculitis	
Thrombosis	
Venous insufficiency	
Lymphedema	
Pharmacologic vasoconstriction	
Irradiated tissue	
Crush injuries	
Primary closure under tension	
Systemic	Systemic inhibition of leukocytic response, resulting in impaired host resistance to infection
Leukemia	
Prolonged administration of high-dose anti-inflammatory drugs	
Corticosteroids	
Aspirin	
Impaired Cellular Proliferation	
Local	Prolonged inflammatory response, which can result in low tissue oxygen tension and further tissue destruction
Wound infection	
Foreign body	
Necrotic tissue	
Repeated injury or irritation	
Movement of wound (e.g., across a joint)	
Wound desiccation or maceration	
Systemic	Impaired cellular proliferation and collagen synthesis. Decreased wound contraction
Aging	
Chronic stress	
Nutritional deficiencies	
Calories	
Protein	
Vitamins	
Minerals	
Water	
Impaired oxygenation	
Pulmonary insufficiency	
Heart failure	
Hypovolemia	
Cirrhosis	
Uremia	
Prolonged hypothermia	
Coagulation disorders	
Cytotoxic drugs	

to poor local blood supply, nutritional deficiencies, and specific therapeutic interventions, such as steroid or radiation therapy.

The *inflammatory phase* of repair begins at the time of injury or cell death. An immediate response of vasoconstriction and clot formation at the site of injury is followed within about 5 to 10 minutes by vasodilation of the same vessels. As the capillaries dilate, the permeability of the vessel wall increases, allowing plasma containing fibrinogen and white blood cells (polymorphonuclear neutrophils) to leak into the surrounding tissue. The white blood cells gradually increase in number, and phagocytic macrophages begin actively engulfing bacteria and dead tissue in an attempt to clean up the wound. As these cells continue to remove unwanted materials from the injury site, they gradually disintegrate and release intracellular enzymes and debris in the form of wound exudate. Simultaneously, the lymph channels become blocked with fibrin plugs, preventing reabsorption of extravascular tissue fluid. Localized accumulation of fluid compresses sensory nerves within the wounded tissue. These events result in the classic signs of inflammation: localized swelling, erythema, heat, and pain. Inflammation is the body's normal response to injury and must occur for wound healing to progress (Chap. 23). In clean wounds with minimal tissue destruction, the acute inflammatory response subsides within 3 to 5 days as capillary permeability returns to normal, lymphatic vessels open to allow drainage of tissue fluid, and healing progresses. A prolonged inflammatory phase with delayed healing, or sudden recurrence of the signs and symptoms of inflammation, is usually associated with a wound infection.

The *fibroblastic phase* of repair begins about the fourth day after injury and continues for the subsequent 2 to 4 weeks, depending on the size and depth of the wound. Using strands of fibrin contained within the inflammatory exudate as a framework, fibroblasts migrate into the wound and proliferate, laying down large amounts of collagen and ground substance to replace the damaged tissue. The amount of collagen deposited in a wound is controlled by simultaneous collagen breakdown and reabsorption. During active wound healing, the disorderly fashion in which collagen bundles are deposited gives the wound structural stability, a factor that also results in the inflexibility of scar tissue when compared with uninjured tissue. If nutritional deficiencies are present and the rate of collagen breakdown exceeds the rate of collagen synthesis, the wound loses strength, and opening of a closed wound may occur. Soon after the migration of fibroblasts, new vascular tissue moves into the area. This revascularization occurs as undamaged, dilated capillaries adjacent to the injury begin budding and growing toward the wound space. The budding of capillaries, combined with collagen synthesis, creates the red, thick, pebble-like appearance of granulation tissue. As might be expected, wounds closed by first intention with good approximation of the tissue planes have minimal collagen deposits when compared with open wounds allowed to heal by second intention.

During the *maturation phase,* through continued collagen degradation and synthesis, the scar tissue within the wound is remodeled to have increased strength and less bulk. This process begins as early as 3 weeks after wounding and can continue for a year or more. A mature scar is one that no longer blanches with pressure and, although slightly firm and inelastic when palpated, is not raised above the skin surface.

The body restores skin integrity through two major processes: epithelialization and contraction. The degree to which these processes are used to obtain wound closure depends on the depth of injury and the extent of tissue loss. For example, sutured wounds require minimal resurfacing of the stratum corneum to re-establish the skin's protective barrier. On the other hand, open wounds take significantly longer to heal. Understanding the mechanisms of epithelialization and contraction can be simplified if two categories of injuury are considered: partial thickness and full thickness.

Pathophysiology

Partial-thickness or superficial wounds heal by *epithelialization,* the reproduction of new skin cells by epithelial cell remnants in the dermal layer of the skin and at the base of the epidermal appendages (Fig. 40–1). On

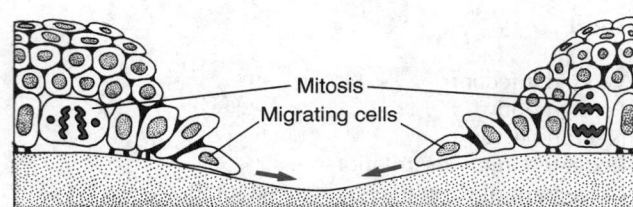

Skin cells at the edge of the wound begin multiplying and migrate toward the center of the wound.

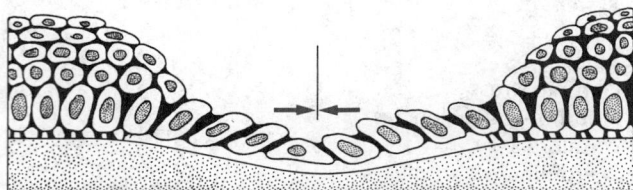

Once advancing epidermal cells from the opposite sides of the wound meet, migration halts.

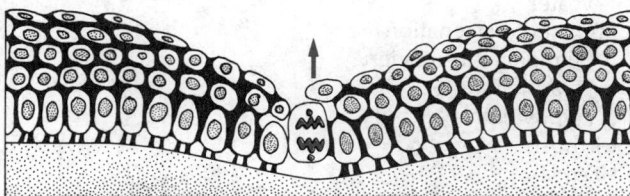

Epithelial cells continue to divide until the thickness of the new skin layer approaches normal.

Figure 40–1

Epithelialization. (Modified from Swaim, S. F. [1980]. *Surgery of traumatized skin.* Philadelphia: W. B. Saunders.)

injury, a fibrin clot forms. Undamaged epithelial cells at the level of the basement membrane and at the base of the hair follicles and glands undergo a burst of mitotic activity. Movement of the new skin cells is directed into "cell-free" spaces on the wound surface, where the fibrin clot acts as a scaffold. Resurfacing, initially only one cell layer thick, proceeds with thickening or restratification of the new epidermis and, eventually, rete peg formation and keratin production. In a healthy client, healing of a partial-thickness wound by epithelialization takes approximately 5 to 7 days. Granulation tissue formation is not required for epidermal migration; however, migration is facilitated by tissue that is well hydrated, is well oxygenated, and has few micro-organisms.

In deeper or *full-thickness* wounds, most if not all of the epithelial remnants have been destroyed, with the exception of those remaining at the wound margins. Healing of full-thickness wounds requires active removal of the nonviable tissue so that gradual filling in of the defect with granulation tissue can progress. Occurring concomitantly with collagen synthesis and wound revascularization is the drawing together of the wound edges, a mechanism of healing known as *contraction* (Fig. 40–2). Unlike epithelialization, in which new tissue is formed, wound contraction is a cell-mediated phenomenon that acts to decrease the surface area of a full-thickness wound by stretching and thinning the existing tissue surrounding the wound. Contractile fibroblasts in the wound bed exert a mechanical force on the wound edges, causing the wound to decrease in size at a uniform rate of about 0.6 to 0.75 mm/day. As might be expected, complete closure of a wound by contraction depends on the dermal mobility of the surrounding skin as tension is applied to it.

If tension in the surrounding skin meets or exceeds the force of contraction, wound closure ceases and the wound remains open until epithelial cells at the wound edges eventually bridge the remaining defect. Unlike epithelialization in partial-thickness wounds in which the skin integrity soon returns to normal, the migration of epithelial cells from wound margins over fibrous connective tissue results in an unstable epithelial surface that is poorly attached to the underlying tissue and

thus prone to reinjury. A venous stasis leg ulcer is an example of a skin defect in an area where effective movement of the surrounding skin is usually not sufficient to allow wound healing by contraction. As a result, the thin epithelial covering is unable to withstand environmental hazards and abrades easily.

It soon becomes evident that wound contraction can prove detrimental as well as beneficial. Contraction over joints, where the skin is particularly mobile, can result in loss of function (contracture). Likewise, contraction of large wounds in areas of limited dermal mobility results in poor quality of repair.

The mechanisms of epithelialization and contraction do not continue indefinitely. The presence of infection, pressure, or mechanical obstacles, such as a poorly applied dressing, can slow or even halt natural healing processes. In the case of chronic wounds, cessation of healing can occur spontaneously and without a clearly defined cause. An understanding of the mechanisms of wound healing is important to set realistic goals and plan nursing interventions that result in an optimal environment for healing.

Etiology

Partial-thickness wounds can occur as a result of a number of factors, including thermal or chemical injury, mechanical trauma, and tissue anoxia. Examples of partial-thickness wounds attributable to trauma include second-degree burns, superficial abrasions, and split-thickness skin graft donor sites. In incontinent clients, prolonged skin contact with urine or feces can result in chemical irritation and superficial skin loss. Elderly clients are at particular risk for skin trauma owing to the presence of age-related skin changes. Progressive flattening of the dermal-epidermal junction predisposes the elderly client to skin tears from mechanical shearing forces, such as the removal of adhesive tape and friction from tightly applied restraints. In addition, friction over bony prominences can lead to partial-thickness skin destruction and early pressure ulcer formation. If pressure is unrelieved, tissue destruction progresses to full-thickness injury.

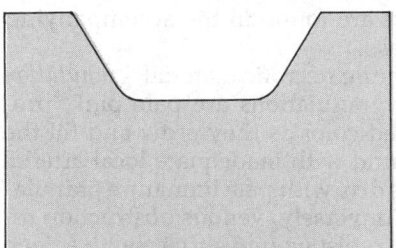

Full-thickness skin loss resulting in a cavity-like defect.

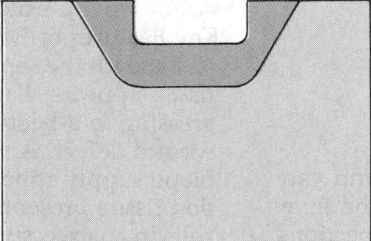

As the wound space gradually fills with granulation tissue, the wound margins begin to pull together. The force of the pull stretches the skin and subcutaneous tissue around the wound.

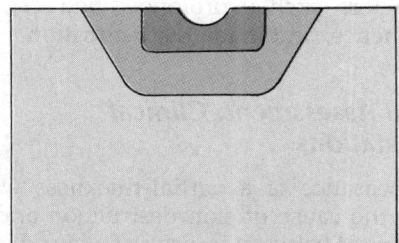

The wound continues to contract until tissues around it can stretch no further.

Figure 40–2

Wound contraction.

Full-thickness wounds occur as a result of acute trauma, such as third-degree burns, or if the skin has gradually lost the ability to maintain its integrity owing to bacterial invasion, prolonged tissue anoxia, or normal wear and tear. Examples of this latter category include deep pressure necrosis, radiation ulcers, venous and arterial leg ulcers, and dehiscence of surgical wounds.

Incidence

Because of the many variables that contribute to tissue injury, the overall incidence of partial- and full-thickness wounds would be impossible to calculate. However, the incidence of some of the more commonly encountered wounds can be estimated by reviewing specific wound categories. For example, pressure sores have been found to occur in about 3% to 4.5% of hospitalized clients, with 70% of the total occurring in those 70 years of age or older (Cooney & Reuler, 1984).

COLLABORATIVE MANAGEMENT

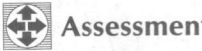 Assessment

History

When taking a history from a client with a partial- or full-thickness wound, the nurse attempts to identify the *underlying cause of skin loss*, as well as *factors that may be associated with impaired healing*. In addition, the nurse investigates the specific *circumstances surrounding the skin loss*. In general, clients with chronic skin ulcerations are able to relate a history of delayed healing or recurrence of the ulcer after healing has occurred. Subjective descriptions of any associated pain may prove helpful in confirming the cause. Skin ulcerations resulting from a compromised arterial blood supply are associated with more severe pain than ulcerations produced by venous insufficiency. Likewise, clients with diabetes may have full-thickness foot ulcers of which they are unaware owing to an associated neuropathy. Finally, because pressure-related skin loss is a common problem among the severely debilitated, the nurse remains alert to contributing factors, such as prolonged bed rest, immobility, incontinence, and inadequate nutrition.

Physical Assessment: Clinical Manifestations

The appearance of a partial-thickness wound can differ with the cause of skin destruction and the time that has elapsed between injury and wound inspection. If injury to the epidermal tissue is uniformly distributed, such as when friction is applied over a bony prominence, the damaged epidermis separates from the underlying dermis as fluid seeps from the dilated capillaries into the wound space. The result is a fluid-filled *bulla* or blister with a nonviable epidermal roof. Contin-

ued pressure or friction causes the bulla to break, revealing a shallow wound with a slightly moist and pink base. If the wound remains exposed to air over a period of time, blood and plasma on the wound surface clot and dry, forming a crust or scab, which, if left undisturbed, serves as a dressing until healing is complete. Traumatic removal of epidermis can occur without bulla formation. Sudden application of mechanical forces to already impaired skin can result in tears or progressive removal of epidermal cells, such as that which occurs with repeated stripping of the skin with adhesive tape. Although wound infection is a more common complication of deeper tissue injury, secondary bacterial infections of partial-thickness wounds with *Staphylococcus* or *Streptococcus* can sometimes lead to invasive infection, especially if the client is immunosuppressed. The nurse inspects the wound margins for *cellulitis*, inflammation of the skin cells extending well beyond the area of injury and usually accompanied by fever. Excessive amount of wound exudate or progressive tissue destruction, as reflected by an increase in the size or depth of the wound, usually indicates impairment in the client's ability to resist infection.

Full-thickness wounds have characteristic colors and textures that reflect the stage of healing and, therefore, direct intervention. The nurse inspects the wound for the presence or absence of *necrotic tissue.* Owing to the depth of tissue destruction, a full-thickness wound is initially covered by a layer of black or brown, nonviable, denatured collagen called a wound *eschar.* In the early stages of wound healing, the eschar is dry and leathery with firm attachment to the wound surface. As the inflammatory phase of wound healing begins and removal of wound debris progresses, the eschar starts to lift up and separate from the tissue beneath. When disrupted, this nonviable eschar serves as an excellent culture media for bacteria normally found on the skin surface, as well as those inadvertently introduced by other means. As bacteria increase in number, they release proteolytic enzymes, which further hasten the liquefaction of necrotic tissue. This tissue becomes softer in consistency and more yellow. In the presence of bacterial colonization, wound exudate increases substantially; the color and odor of wound exudate indicate the predominant microorganism present. The characteristics of wound exudate are found in the accompanying Key Features of Disease.

Beneath the separating necrotic material, *granulation tissue* appears. Early granulations are pale pink, progressing to a beefy-red color as they grow and fill the wound defect. A wound with inadequate local arterial blood supply appears dry, with pale immature granulation tissue present. Conversely, venous obstruction results in an excessively moist wound surface with a deep red color reflective of the deoxygenated blood beneath the wound surface. Severe nutritional deficiency promotes collagen catabolism and impairs granulation formation. The nurse palpates the wound to determine the texture of the mature granulations. Healthy granulations have a slightly spongy texture. On occasion, the

KEY FEATURES OF DISEASE ■ Characteristics and Significance of Types of Wound Exudate

Type	Characteristics	Significance
Serosanguineous	Blood-tinged amber fluid consisting of serum and red blood cells	Normal for first 48 h after injury Sudden increase in amount precedes wound dehiscence in primarily closed wounds
Purulent	Creamy yellow pus	Colonization with *Staphylococcus*
	Greenish-blue pus, causing staining of dressings and accompanied by a "fruity" odor	Colonization with *Pseudomonas*
	Beige pus with a "fishy" odor	Colonization with *Proteus*
	Brownish pus with a "fecal" odor	Colonization with aerobic colliform and *Bacteroides* (usually occurs after intestinal surgery)

tissue rapidly fills the wound space, becoming boggy in consistency and protruding above the surface of the surrounding skin. These so-called *hypertrophic* granulations present a physical impediment to wound healing via contraction and epithelialization and require removal before wound closure can occur by natural forces.

Deep, chronic wounds, such as pressure ulcers, may have more extensive tissue destruction than is first evident on inspection. If pressure-related skin changes are suspected, the nurse palpates the bony prominences for deep hardening of the surrounding soft tissue, which is often suggestive of early tissue ischemia well beneath the surface of the skin. After ischemia has occurred, continued pressure over the area of injury results in progress of tissue destruction from the deep tissue layers toward the surface. This "hidden" wound may first be observed as a small opening in the skin through which purulent drainage exudes. If such an opening is found, the nurse uses a cotton-tipped applicator to gently probe for a much larger pocket of necrotic tissue beneath. Similar hidden wounds with draining sinus tracts can be associated with osteomyelitis and rectal abscesses.

Psychosocial Assessment

Wounds are commonly associated with perceived alterations in body image. Depending on the cause of the wound, ineffective coping patterns may emerge as the client strives to comply with significant changes in life style necessary to facilitate healing. In addition, chronic slow-healing ulcers are often painful and costly to treat. The nurse assesses the client's knowledge of the goals of treatment at each stage of the healing process, as well as compliance with the prescribed treatment regimen. The nurse further assesses individual skills in wound cleaning and dressing application. Noncompliance with wound care procedures may reflect an inability to accept the diagnosis or cope with the pain, the cost, or the potential scarring associated with prolonged healing. Depending on the location of the wound, the client may need the assistance of a family member or visiting nurse to adequately care for the wound in the home environment. Finally, the nurse explores with the client specific changes in activities of daily living (ADL) that are required to promote healing of the wound. For example, chronic ulcerations resulting from prolonged venous hypertension require frequent bed rest with elevation of the legs for healing to occur; these interventions could make it difficult for a homemaker or a secretary to perform usual job expectations.

Laboratory Findings

Bacterial cultures and sensitivity studies are done to identify the causative microorganism in suspected wound infection. The difference between bacterial colonization of a wound and true wound infection is an important concept to understand when interpreting culture results. All wounds allowed to heal by second intention become colonized by bacterial flora on the skin and in the environment. In most cases local tissue defenses are adequate to keep the numbers of bacteria at a minimum. However, if wounds are extensive, if clients are severely immunocompromised, or if local blood supply to the wound is impaired, bacterial growth may exceed the body's ability to defend against invasion into deeper tissue layers. The result is deep wound infection and, eventually, bacteremia and sepsis (systemic infection). Swab cultures are helpful only in identifying the types of bacteria present on the wound surface and are not reflective of the relative concentration of bacteria in the underlying tissues. Tests such as quantitative wound biopsies are available and allow the numbers of bacteria to be analyzed. Unfortunately, these tests are time-consuming, costly, and rarely indicated, except in large extensive wounds. Therefore, the clinical indicators of infection, such as cellulitis, progressive increase in wound size or depth, changes in the quantity and quality of wound exudate, and systemic signs of bacteremia, are important criteria in the diagnosis and subsequent treatment of an established wound infection.

Other Diagnostic Tests

Any additional laboratory studies are based on the suspected cause of the wound. For most chronic ulcers to show progress toward healing, the underlying problem must be diagnosed and treated. For example, noninvasive and invasive arterial blood flow studies are indicated if an ischemic ulcer is suspected. Similarly, blood tests to establish specific nutritional deficiencies are helpful in treating the debilitated, malnourished client with a wound.

 ### Analysis: Nursing Diagnosis

The client with partial- or full-thickness skin trauma is usually admitted to the hospital for treatment of another more life-threatening condition that is either the underlying cause of a chronic ulcer or is significantly contributing to delayed healing. Severely debilitated and elderly clients are at considerable risk for skin wounds in the hospital owing to their generally poor skin integrity and the many factors that can contribute to skin breakdown in the hospital environment. Treatments requiring surgical intervention, such as tracheotomy and chest tube placement, result in chronic wounds and are common occurrences in the acute care setting. After skin loss occurs, the added risk of nosocomial wound infection becomes a primary concern.

Common Diagnoses

The nursing diagnoses most commonly found in clients with skin trauma are

1. Impaired skin integrity related to vascular, hematologic, and infectious diseases; neoplasms; and iatrogenic and traumatic circumstances
2. Potential for infection related to disruption of the skin's protective barrier, impaired local blood supply, and immunosuppression

Additional Diagnoses

The client may have one or more additional diagnoses, depending on the cause of the skin loss. These diagnoses include

1. Pain related to skin trauma, wound infection, and wound treatment
2. Body image disturbance related to loss of skin
3. Ineffective individual coping related to the chronicity of the wound, alteration in body image, and changes in life style required to promote healing
4. Altered nutrition: less than body requirements related to inadequate intake of calories, protein, vitamins, and minerals
5. Altered (peripheral) tissue perfusion related to vascular disease and prolonged alterations in fluid volume

6. Bowel incontinence related to underlying disease process or side effect of medical treatment
7. Altered patterns of urinary elimination related to inability to control bladder function (or emptying)
8. Knowledge deficit related to lack of information about or unclear explanation of the treatment regimen

 ### Planning and Implementation

The following plan of care for clients with established skin trauma focuses on the common nursing diagnoses.

Impaired Skin Integrity

Planning: client goals. The goals for a client with an open wound are that the client will (1) protect the viable cells on the wound surface until healing is completed and (2) experience complete wound healing.

Interventions: nonsurgical management. Wound care techniques vary according to the individual client's needs and the physician's preference. Although aggressive removal of necrotic tissue by surgical excision may be indicated in a severely immunosuppressed client who is likely to develop a life-threatening wound infection, a nonsurgical approach to wound débridement is preferred for an elderly client who has adequate host defenses but is too ill or debilitated to undergo surgery. Nonsurgical management of open wounds is often left to the discretion of the nurse who must select a method of wound dressing on the basis of the identified goal of wound management (Table 40–2).

Dressings. A properly designed dressing can expedite healing by removing unwanted debris from the wound surface, protecting exposed viable tissues, and re-establishing a temporary barrier between the body and the environment until wound closure is complete. A draining, necrotic wound requires a dressing designed to remove excessive wound exudate and loose debris without damaging migrating epithelial cells or newly formed granulation tissue. If necrosis is extensive and the eschar is thick, surgical removal of the nonviable tissue is necessary before further débridement with dressings proves effective. Depending on the dressing material used, dressings contribute to removal of debris either through mechanical entrapment and detachment of dead tissue or by creating an environment that promotes self-digestion of necrotic material by the bacterial enzymes' *autolysis.*

After all of the nonviable tissue has been removed, protection of any exposed vital structures, such as tendon, bone, and newly formed collagen, becomes a primary objective of wound care. The ideal physiologic environment for healing by epithelialization and contraction is a clean, *slightly* moist wound surface with minimal bacterial colonization. Excessive moisture from

TABLE 40-2 Mechanism of Action of Common Dressing Techniques Used for Wound Débridement

Technique	Mechanism of Action
Wet-to-dry saline-moistened gauze	Dry, necrotic debris is softened by the saline, allowing it to become more effectively entrapped in the interstices as the gauze dries and shrinks. Dressing may also entrap healing tissue.
Wet-to-damp saline-moistened gauze	As with the wet-to-dry technique, necrotic debris is mechanically removed, but with less trauma to healing tissue.
Continuous wet gauze	The wound surface is continually bathed with a wetting agent of choice, promoting dilution of viscous exudate and softening of dry eschar.
Topical enzyme preparations	Proteolytic action on thick, adherent eschar causes breakdown of denatured protein and more rapid separation of necrotic tissue.
Hydrophilic beads	Exudative wounds are dried by capillary action, and surface bacteria are removed.
Synthetic dressings	Spontaneous separation of necrotic tissue is promoted by autolysis.

an excessively secreting wound or a too-wet dressing can interfere with healing by promoting the growth of microorganisms and causing maceration of healthy tissue. Likewise, if a clean wound surface is exposed to air, or if highly absorbent dressing materials are used for prolonged periods, the subsequent drying effect can lead to dehydration of viable surface cells, scab formation, and conversion to a deeper injury.

The nurse assesses the wound for the presence or absence of nonviable tissue and the quantity of wound exudate. A dressing material with properties that promote an optimal environment for healing is selected (Table 40-3). For example, a material that is nonadherent to the wound surface and does not remove fragile epithelial cells when changed is the dressing of choice for protecting new tissue. Depending on the amount of drainage, either a hydrophobic or hydrophilic material can be used. The nurse selects a *hydrophobic* (nonabsorbent, waterproof) material when the wound is relatively free of drainage and the objective is to protect the wound from external contamination, for instance, urine or feces. A *hydrophilic* (absorbent) material draws excessive drainage away from the wound surface, preventing maceration. A variety of synthetic materials with hydrophilic and hydrophobic properties are available, which, unlike cotton gauze dressings, may be left intact for extended periods. In addition, biologic skin substitutes, such as homograft (human cadaver skin), heterograft (pigskin), and amniotic membrane, prevent tissue dehydration and provide an environment conducive to healing (see Chap. 16).

In general, the frequency of dressing changes depends on the amount of necrotic material or exudate present. Dry gauze dressings should be changed when "strike through" occurs, or the outer layer of the dressing first becomes saturated with exudate. Gauze dressings used for débridement such as those placed on a wound wet, allowed to dry, and then removed should be changed frequently enough to actively take off any loose debris or exudate. Synthetic dressings should be

changed when accumulation of exudate causes the adhesive seal to break and leakage occurs. Before reapplying any dressing, the nurse gently cleans the wound surface with saline or a dilute antibacterial soap as prescribed. If soap is used, the nurse rinses and dries the surface thoroughly before applying the dressing.

Physical therapy. As an adjunct to the use of dressings for wound débridement, mechanical removal of dead tissue can be facilitated by daily whirlpool treatments. The wound is immersed in warm tap water to which an antibacterial cleaning agent has been added. Continuous agitation of the water serves to mechanically loosen the debris and wash away exudate and particulate matter. During the treatment, gentle cleaning of the wound surface with a gauze pad is accomplished. After the treatment, the therapist often uses instruments to trim away any obvious bits of dead tissue that are still loosely attached to the wound surface.

Drug therapy. Clean, healthy granulation tissue is highly vascular and capable of providing white blood cells and antibodies to the wound surface to combat infection. However, if extensive necrosis is present or when local tissue defenses are impaired, topical antibacterial agents are often indicated to control bacterial growth. Chapter 16 provides a complete description of the advantages and uses of topical antimicrobial agents. In the absence of established wound infection, the use of prophylactic antibiotics is usually avoided because of the danger of the development of resistant strains of bacteria.

Diet therapy. Successful wound healing depends on adequate nutritional stores of calories, protein, vitamins, minerals, and water. Nutritional deficiencies are common among the elderly and chronically ill clients, contributing to increased risk of skin breakdown, as well as delayed healing of established wounds. Severe protein deficiency inhibits all stages of the healing process

TABLE 40-3 Properties of Commonly Used Dressing Materials

	Polyurethane Films	Hydrocolloidal Wafers	Hydrogel Dressings	Biologic Dressings	Cotton Gauze Dressings
Examples	Op Site Tegaderm Bioclusive	DuoDerm Comfeel Ulcus J & J Ulcer Dressing	Vigilon Geliperm sheets	Porcine heterograft Cadaver homograft Amnion Cultured epithe-lium	Continuous dry Continuous wet Wet to damp Wet to dry
Indications	Débridement* Protection (partial-thick-ness lesions)	Débridement* Absorption Protection	Débridement* Absorption Protection	Débridement after eschar removal* Protection Test before skin grafts (pigskin and cadaver skin)	*Continuous dry:* Absorption Protection (non-adherent contact layer) *Continuous wet:* Delivery of topical agent Débridement (autolysis) Protection *Wet to damp:* Atraumatic me-chanical débridement *Wet to dry:* Aggressive mechanical débridement
Advantages	Wound visualiza-tion Good adhesion Waterproof Reduces pain Cost effective Easy to store	Absorbent Excludes bacteria Waterproof Reduces pain Easy application Easy to store	Absorbent Nonadhesive Reduces pain Conducive to use with topical agents Conforms to uneven wound sur-faces Cost effective if rehydrated Easy to store	Most "natural" wound covering Reduces pain Conforms to un-even wound surfaces Available in a vari-ety of sizes and types (pigskin)	Readily available Good mechanical débridement *if used properly* Effective delivery of topical agents (continuous wet)
Disadvantages	Difficult to apply properly Nonabsorbent Adhesive to normal and healing tissue Limited to superficial lesions	Nontransparent Softening and loss of shape with pressure, heat, and fric-tion Odor with dressing removal Expensive Requires use of granules for deep, draining lesions	Poor barrier function Only partial wound visual-ization Requires addi-tional dressing to secure Can promote the growth of *Pseudomonas* and other organisms	Requires addi-tional dressing to secure Time consuming to apply Potential allergen Requires special storage Expensive	Delayed healing if used improp-erly Pain on removal Requires frequent dressing changes
Dressing changes	Necrotic base: every 24 h Clean base: on leakage of ex-udate	Necrotic base: every 24 h Clean base: on leakage of ex-udate	Necrotic base: every 6-8 h Clean base: every 24 h	Every 24 h until adherent, then every 5-7 d as needed	Necrotic base: every 4-6 h Clean base: every 12-24 h

* Use with caution in patients with leukopenia or macrovascular or microvascular disease.

and impairs local host defenses against bacterial invasion. To promote healing, the nurse encourages the intake of a well-balanced diet, with emphasis on foods containing nutrients vital to epidermal proliferation and the synthesis of collagen (see the accompanying Health Promotion/Maintenance feature). If sufficient amounts of food cannot be taken orally, nasogastric feedings and hyperalimentation via central venous catheter may become necessary to reverse negative nitrogen balance (see Chap. 13).

HEALTH PROMOTION/MAINTENANCE ■ Foods That Promote Wound Healing

Food	Function	Food	Function
Protein Sources		**Zinc Sources**	
Meat	Maintenance and	Usually same as protein	Tissue repair (zinc-defi-
Fish	healing of body	sources, especially:	cient diet causes
Poultry	tissues	Beef	poor wound
Milk	Antibody production	Organ meats	healing, decreased
Cheese	Energy	Shellfish	ability to taste, and
Eggs		Salmon	poor appetite)
Soybeans		Meats	Protein synthesis
Legumes		Poultry	
Nuts		Cheese	
Nutritional supplements		Whole grains	
		Dried beans	
Carbohydrate Sources			
		Iron Sources*	
Whole grains (preferable	Energy		
to enriched because	Spare protein (if diet	Liver	Cellular respiration
of higher nutritional	does not contain	Meat	Hemoglobin
and fiber content)	sufficient nonpro-	Baked beans	
Enriched grain and	tein calories, protein	Dried fruits	
cereal products	from body tissues	Legumes	
Fruit	will be broken down	Eggs	
Juices	to supply energy)	Dark green leafy	
Vegetables (especially	Wound healing	vegetables	
starchy ones: corn,		Blackstrap molasses	
peas, and potatoes)		Whole grain breads and	
Milk		cereals	
Desserts and sweets			
		Sources of Vitamin B₁₂	
Sources of Vitamin C			
		Liver	Protein synthesis
Berries	Collagen synthesis	Organ meats	
Broccoli	Immunity	Muscle meats	
Brussels sprouts		Fish	
Cabbage		Eggs	
Citrus fruits and juices		Shellfish	
Green peppers		Milk	
Kale		Yogurt	
Melons		Cheese	
Spinach and dark green			
vegetables		**Sources of Vitamin B₆**	
Tomatoes			
Vitamin C–enriched		Meats	Amino acid metabolism
juices		Liver	

Continued

HEALTH PROMOTION/MAINTENANCE ■ **Foods That Promote Wound Healing** *Continued*

Food	Function	Food	Function
Sources of Vitamin B₆		**Folate Sources**	
Some vegetables		Fresh oranges	
(including potatoes)		Whole-wheat products	
Wheat germ			
Wheat bran		**Water Sources**	
Whole-grain cereals		Water	Maintain condition of the skin
(enriched breads do not		Milk	(dehydration can lead to
contain B₆)		Juices	tissue breakdown, poor ap-
Fish		Gelatin	petite, and constipation)
Brewer's yeast		Tomatoes	
Dried beans		Citrus fruits	
		Melons	
Folate Sources		Berries	
Liver	Protein synthesis	Vegetables	
Yeast		Broths	
Leafy vegetables		Soups	
Dried beans		Tea	
Green vegetables		Coffee	
Nuts		Carbonated beverages	

* Iron cooking utensils add iron to the diet.

From Ross, R., & Noe, J. M. (1983). *Chronic problem wounds* (p. 60). Boston: Little, Brown.

Prevention of complications. Complications associated with wound healing are avoided by diligent monitoring of wound progress. Sudden deterioration of the wound, as evidenced by an increase in the size or depth of the lesion, changes in the color or texture of the granulation tissue, or changes in the quantity, color, or odor of wound exudate, is reported to the physician. The nurse also remains alert for the classic signs of wound infection: increased erythema, edema, purulent and malodorous drainage, and tenderness of the wound margins, which may or may not be accompanied by clinical signs of bacteremia, such as fever and positive blood cultures.

Interventions: surgical management. Surgical management of an open wound includes sharp débridement of nonviable tissue, as well as skin grafting to re-establish skin integrity in wounds that cannot heal by the processes of epithelialization and contraction.

Débridement. Sharp excision of thick, adherent wound eschar using a scalpel or scissors is sometimes undertaken to hasten the removal of the devitalized tissue, which is a potential source of infection. Surgical débridement is particularly indicated in severely immunosuppressed clients or those with extensive areas of necrosis, such as burns or large full-thickness ulcers, in whom the time required for spontaneous separation of eschar places the client at risk for systemic sepsis or prolonged hospitalization. Depending on the size and depth of the wound and projected blood loss, excision can be performed at the bedside, in the treatment room, or in an operating room.

Grafting. Full-thickness wounds unable to close by second intention owing to the extent of the injury or forces inhibiting contraction, as well as wounds in which natural healing results in loss of joint function or unacceptable cosmetic results, require autografting to achieve satisfactory wound closure. Successful grafting of skin requires a clean granulating or freshly excised wound bed. Partial-thickness (split-thickness) or full-thickness strips of skin are removed from a donor area as seen in Figure 40–3, transferred to the wound, and sutured or stapled in place. Full-thickness *free grafts* and flaps are used to cover deep, massive wounds or wounds in which vital structures, such as bone or tendon, are exposed. Unlike free grafts, a *pedicle flap* is a full-thickness flap of skin that is raised and rotated to cover the defect, with one edge of the flap still attached to the site of origin to provide a blood supply (Fig. 40–4). Because all skin layers are removed, full-thickness donor sites are closed primarily or covered with additional split-thickness skin grafts. Partial-thickness donor sites heal by epithelialization if secondary infection is avoided.

Preoperative care. Preoperative care is focused on preparing the wound to accept a skin graft. The nurse

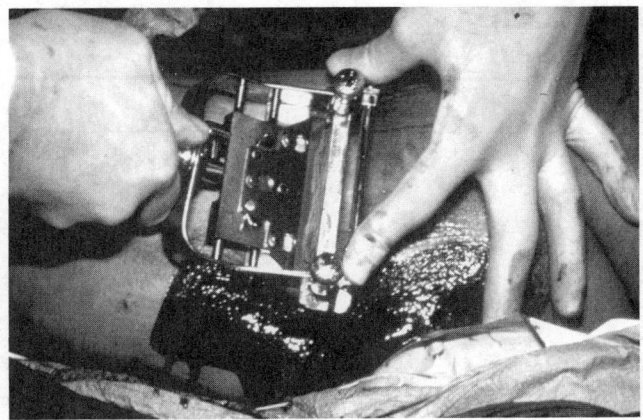

Figure 40–3

Removal of a partial-thickness (split-thickness) skin graft.

carefully monitors potential donor sites, taking care to maintain the integrity of the donor skin and avoid minor injuries that could result in infection and graft loss.

Postoperative care. Postoperative graft sites are immobilized with bulky cotton pressure dressings for 3 to 5 days to allow vascularization, or "take," of the newly grafted skin. The nurse does not disturb the dressing and encourages elevation and complete rest of the grafted area, including prohibition of any activity that could cause movement of the dressing against the body and separation of the graft from the wound. After dressings are removed, the nurse monitors the graft for signs of failure to vascularize: nonadherence to the wound or graft necrosis. If a pedicle flap has been used to cover the wound, the nurse inspects the edges of the flap frequently for changes in color. A pale flap with delayed capillary filling when blanched may have inadequate arterial perfusion. A dusky color or sharp line of color demarcation suggests inadequate venous or lymphatic drainage.

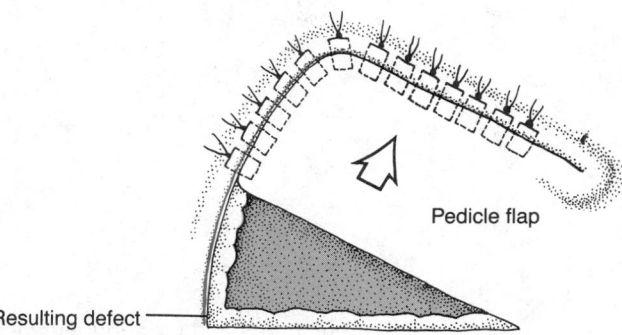

Figure 40–4

A full-thickness pedicle flap of skin is separated and rotated to cover the wound. Blood vessels are left intact. The resulting defect is either primarily closed or covered with skin grafts. The flap is held in place with staples or sutures.

Postoperative care of donor sites is aimed at protecting the area from injury and infection until healing can occur and promoting client comfort. Some surgeons elect to cover donor sites with synthetic dressings, such as Op Site or Duoderm, to promote moist wound healing. Others prefer to use dry fine-mesh gauze or an ointment-impregnated dressing, while encouraging dry exposure. Whichever method is chosen, the client usually returns from surgery with a pressure dressing in place over the donor area to promote hemostasis. After 24 to 48 hours, this outer dressing is removed.

If the donor site is treated with dry exposure, the nurse promotes air circulation to the wound by positioning the client to avoid pressure on the site and using an overbed cradle to tent the sheets. When the use of heat lamps is ordered, the nurse places the bulb (60 to 100 watt) at least 2 feet from the wound to prevent thermal injury to the skin. After a scab has formed, the wound is left undisturbed until healing is evident (10 to 14 days). As the donor site heals, the gauze and scab lift away from the new epithelium beneath. Trimming the separating gauze close to the skin surface minimizes the chance of the client's catching the loose end of the dressing on an object and removing the still adherent gauze before healing is complete. Because exposed donor sites are initially more painful than graft sites, the nurse administers pain medication as ordered and provides other comfort measures as needed. Repositioning the client during the immediate postoperative period to promote comfort is acceptable only if movement of the graft site can be avoided. Back rubs are offered to help relieve muscle spasms that occur with bed rest and immobility.

Graft and donor sites involving the posterior body surfaces present a particular problem. For the graft or flap to become fully vascularized or donor sites to dry, the client must be immobilized in a side-lying or prone position for 7 to 10 days. An alternative to difficult positioning is the use of special low-pressure beds referred to as low air-loss systems. These beds minimize ischemia of the graft or flap while the client is in a supine position by keeping the skin-mattress interface pressures lower than skin capillary filling pressure with inflatable pillows. Also available is the air-fluidized system consisting of microscopic silicone beads through which warm air is circulated. The beads are covered by a polyester filter sheet, and the result is a fluid-like surface that relieves pressure and promotes drying of donor sites via air circulation. A major limitation to the use of these special beds is cost.

Potential for Infection

Planning: client goals. The major goal for this nursing diagnosis is that the client will not experience a wound infection and subsequent systemic sepsis. These complications are more common in clients who are elderly, are severely immunosuppressed, or have wounds with a poor microvascular or macrovascular blood supply.

TABLE 40–4 Objective Criteria for Monitoring Wound Infection

Objective Criteria	Frequency of Assessment	Rationales
Wounds Without Tissue Loss		
Examples		
Surgical incisions and clean lacerations closed primarily by sutures or staples		
Observations		

Check for the presence or absence of
  Localized tenderness.
  Swelling of the incision line.
  Erythema of the incision line
  >1 cm on each side of wound.
  Localized heat.
	At least every 24 h until sutures or staples are removed	To detect cellulitis (bacterial infections originating in tissue)*

Check for the presence or absence of
  Purulent drainage from any portion of the incision site.
  Localized fluctuance (from fluid accumulation) and tenderness beneath a *portion* of the wound when palpated.
	At least every 24 h until sutures or staples are removed	To detect abscess formation related to presence of foreign body (suture material) or deeper wound infection*

Check for the presence or absence of approximation (sealing) of wound edges with or without serosanguineous drainage.	At least every 24 h until sutures or staples are removed	To detect potential for wound dehiscence
Wounds with Tissue Loss		
Examples		
Partial- or full-thickness skin loss caused by pressure necrosis, vascular disease, trauma, and so forth, and allowed to heal by second intention		
Observations		
WOUND SIZE		
Measure wound size at greatest length and width using a metric ruler or, for asymmetric ulcers, by tracing the wound onto a piece of plastic film or sheeting (plastic template). Compare all subsequent measurements against the initial measurement.	At least every week	To detect progress toward wound closure
ULCER BASE		

Check for the presence or absence of
  Necrotic tissue (loose or adherent).
  Presence or absence of foul odor from wound when dressing is changed.
Note the frequency of dressing changes or dressing reinforcements owing to drainage.
	At least every 24 h	To detect the need for débridement or the response to treatment (necrotic tissue) and to detect local wound infection (frequent dressing changes and foul odor)

TABLE 40–4   Objective Criteria for Monitoring Wound Infection *Continued*

Objective Criteria	Frequency of Assessment	Rationales
Observations		
WOUND MARGINS		
Check for the presence or absence of Erythema and swelling extending outward >1 cm from wound margins. Increased tenderness at wound margins.	At least every 24 h or at each dressing change	To detect wound infection*
SYSTEMIC RESPONSE		
Check for the presence or absence of elevated body temperature.	At least every 12 h	To detect bacteremia

* The wounds of clients who are severely immunosuppressed or those wounds with compromised blood supply may not exhibit a typical inflammatory response to local wound infection.

Interventions: nonsurgical management. Because of the many intrinsic factors that can affect a client's resistance to infection, emphasis is placed on close monitoring of wound progress so that timely treatment with topical and systemic antibiotics can be initiated if wound deterioration occurs. Steps are taken to minimize introduction of pathogenic organisms to the wound through direct contact.

Monitoring wound progress. Frequent monitoring of wound appearance using objective criteria allows the nurse to recognize early signs of impending infection and evaluate response to treatment. Table 40–4 outlines objective indicators of local infection for wounds with and without tissue loss. Clients who are at highest risk for infection—those who have white blood cell disorders, are receiving steroid therapy, or have wounds with a compromised blood supply—may exhibit a subdued inflammatory response to infection.

Precautionary measures. Because of the great variety of microorganisms in the hospital environment, keeping a wound totally free of bacteria is impossible. Therefore, optimal wound management is based on maintaining acceptably low levels of microorganisms through meticulous local wound care and minimizing contamination with pathogenic organisms. The nurse takes necessary precautions to prevent direct contact with wound secretions and cross-contamination between clients. Thorough hand washing is performed before and after dressing changes, and soiled dressings and linens are disposed of properly.

■ **Discharge Planning**

In most instances, clients with chronic slow-healing wounds are discharged from the hospital before complete wound closure is obtained. Discharge may be to the home setting or to a long-term care facility, depending on the degree of debilitation.

Home Care Preparation

Care of the wound in the home environment is not unlike care in the hospital setting. Most dressing supplies can be easily obtained at the local pharmacy or medical supply store. If mechanical débridement of the wound is still needed, a hand-held shower device or forceful irrigation of the wound with a 20-mL syringe can be substituted for whirlpool therapy.

Client/Family Education

The client or family member who will be performing the wound care should demonstrate facility in dressing removal, wound cleaning, and dressing application before the client is discharged. When choosing a dressing to be used in the home environment, the nurse considers the client's or family member's ability to apply the dressing properly, as well as the cost of the dressing material if finances are limited. Some dressings may be easier to apply and less expensive than other materials. Additional teaching includes knowledge of the signs and symptoms of wound infection.

A balanced diet, with frequent high-protein snacks,

should be encouraged. The nurse discusses diet preferences with the client and suggests foods that promote wound healing (see Table 40–4). Vitamin and mineral supplements may also be ordered if dietary deficiencies are present.

Psychosocial Preparation

Clients with chronic wounds are often depressed about their debilitated state, which may affect compliance with wound care measures. Many clients are unable to change their own dressing because of distress over altered body image or the pain experienced with dressing removal. Others are totally dependent on family members or support personnel owing to limited physical mobility or inability to reach the wound.

For some clients, drastic changes in daily activities will be necessary to promote healing. For example, clients with leg ulcers may need frequent rest periods with leg elevation. Immobile clients with pressure sores require round-the-clock repositioning as often as every 3 to 4 hours to prevent further breakdown, which takes its toll on family members or caregivers. The nurse explains the rationale for activity changes and explores with the client and the family alternative ways of coping with these changes.

Health Care Resources

A home care nurse may be needed to follow wound progress after the client is discharged from the hospital. Detailed communication of wound size and appearance and any special wound care needs by the hospital nurse is important so that the nurse in the home can accurately judge changes in wound appearance. The same is true if the client is discharged to a nursing home or long-term care facility.

Proper use of dressing materials is emphasized to minimize waste and help decrease the overall cost of treatment. Nonsterile supplies are acceptable for treatment of chronic wounds and are less costly than sterile products. Nonsterile dressing materials can often be purchased in bulk from a local medical supply store at reduced cost.

Routine outpatient visits to the primary physician are needed to monitor the progress of wound healing and evaluate response to treatment.

 Evaluation

On the basis of the identified nursing diagnoses, the expected outcomes for the client with skin trauma include that the client

1. Describes the cause of the wound
2. Demonstrates skills necessary to care for the wound in the home environment
3. Incorporates modifications of life style related to promotion of healing in ADL

4. Lists the signs and symptoms of wound infection
5. Makes the necessary changes in dietary intake to correct any nutritional deficiencies

---

COMMON INFECTIONS

BACTERIAL INFECTIONS

The majority of cutaneous bacterial infections are caused by gram-positive organisms: *Staphylococcus* or *Streptococcus*. Because of the prevalence of these organisms in the hospital environment, nosocomial cutaneous bacterial infections are not uncommon.

Pathophysiology

Typical primary bacterial lesions involve the hair follicle, where bacteria can easily accumulate and flourish in the warm, moist environment. *Folliculitis* is a relatively superficial staphylococcal infection involving only the upper portion of the follicle and is associated with mild discomfort. Streptococcal folliculitis is rare. *Furuncles* (boils) are also caused by *Staphylococcus*, but the infection is much deeper in the follicle. *Cellulitis* is a generalized nonfollicular infection with either *Staphylococcus* or *Streptococcus*, which involves the deeper connective tissue. Secondary staphylococcal infection of already established breaks in skin integrity is not uncommon.

Etiology

Minor skin trauma usually precedes the appearance of folliculitis and furuncles and may or may not be associated with the development of cellulitis. It is not unusual for folliculitis to continue to spread as new areas of the body are inoculated by the fingernails. Furuncles are more likely to develop in the presence of heat and moisture, such as in the hair-bearing skin fold areas. Recurrent superficial bacterial infections are sometimes associated with the overuse of hair oils or bath oils.

Cellulitis can occur as a result of secondary bacterial infection of an open wound or be unrelated to skin trauma. Clients with chronic lymphedema are particularly susceptible to this infection, which may be recurrent. Immunocompromised clients remain at risk for progression of the infection and sepsis if it remains untreated.

Incidence

The incidence of bacterial infections is greater in environments in which the concentration of gram-positive microorganisms is high, such as in the hospital setting. The recurrence rate of folliculitis and furunculosis is also higher in clients who are nose and throat carriers of *Staphylococcus.*

VIRAL INFECTIONS

Recurrent viral infections are a common occurrence and may result in multiple complications if the client is severely immunosuppressed. Early recognition and treatment of these infections is vital in this population owing to the potential for systemic dissemination of the virus.

Pathophysiology

Herpes simplex virus (HSV) infections are of two types. Type 1 virus (HSV$_1$) infections are responsible for the classic cold sore, with the initial infection commonly occurring in childhood and recurrent infections appearing throughout adulthood. Genital herpes caused by the type 2 virus (HSV$_2$) is also recurrent. After a primary infection by direct exposure to another infected individual, the virus resides in a dormant state in the dorsal root ganglia, during which time the client is asymptomatic. Reactivation of the infection stimulates the virus to travel the pathway of sensory nerves to the skin, where lesions reappear. In general, recurrent disease is less severe than the primary infection and differs in clinical presentation. The time span between episodes and the severity of individual attacks vary. Outbreaks of oral herpes simplex usually last 3 to 10 days, and active shedding of the virus and contagion are possible for the first 3 to 5 days. The client may experience tingling or burning of the lip before any lesion is evidenced. Recurrent genital herpes may persist for 7 to 18 days or longer, with contagion most likely during the first 3 to 4 days. Some clients remain contagious even when they are asymptomatic. Generally, genital herpes is more painful than oral disease, as evidenced by prodromal symptoms of burning, tingling, buttock pain, and back pain in about 50% of cases. The most typical clinical presentation of both type 1 and type 2 herpes simplex virus infection is isolated or grouped vesicles on an erythematous base.

Analogous to the pathophysiology of herpes simplex, *herpes zoster* (shingles) is caused by reactivation of the latent varicella-zoster virus in clients who have previously had chickenpox. Dorsal root ganglia of the sensory cranial and spinal nerves are involved. The individual lesions of herpes zoster infections are similar to those of herpes simplex, but with a different distribution pattern. Multiple lesions occur in a dermatomal (segmental) distribution in the skin area innervated by the infected nerve. Herpes zoster eruptions are preceded by several days of pain, which may vary from minor irritation and itching to severe, deep pain. The course of eruption usually lasts several weeks. Postherpetic neuralgia, pain persisting after the lesions have resolved, is a common complication in elderly clients and may persist to the point of becoming disabling.

Etiology

In relatively healthy individuals, recurrence of herpes simplex virus infection is triggered by physical or psychologic stress: sunburn, trauma, fever, menses, or fatigue. Furthermore, the virus can be spread by direct contact between an actively infected individual and a susceptible host. Autoinoculation, transfer of either viral type from one part of the body to another, is also possible. Although primary infections do occur in the hospitalized client as a result of direct exposure or cross-contamination, recurrent infection is more common. *Herpetic whitlow* is a form of herpes simplex infection occurring on the fingertips of medical personnel who have come in contact with viral secretions and is a potential source of client inoculation. Immunosuppressed clients are at a particular risk for severe and persistent eruptions that can lead to life-threatening complications.

Herpes zoster is essentially a disease of immunosuppression, occurring with increased frequency and severity in the elderly population owing to age-related alterations in host resistance. As with herpes simplex infections, herpes zoster presents a considerable risk to the hospitalized client who is severely immunocompromised. Dissemination of the virus can be accompanied by fever and malaise, often progressing to visceral involvement. Herpes zoster is contagious to those individuals who have not been previously exposed to chickenpox. Complications can include ophthalmic infection and scarring if the virus is introduced into the eye, Bell's palsy, and full-thickness skin necrosis.

Incidence

Recurrent oral-facial HSV infection is a common problem and affects 25% to 40% of people in the United States (Crumpacker, 1987). Genital HSV infection is most common in sexually active adults, as evidenced by the occurrence of an estimated 95% of cases after sexual exposure. The incidence of genital infection has increased markedly over the past two decades, and genital HSV infection is the most common sexually transmitted disease among the well-educated, middle-class population (see Chap. 56). In the hospital environment, approximately 70% of all clients with HSV infections experience recurrence when undergoing cancer chemotherapy or organ transplantation (Zaia, 1986).

Herpes zoster is an age-related disease, with more than two-thirds of reported cases occurring in individuals older than 50 years of age. The incidence of herpes zoster in clinically immunocompromised clients is increased 20- to 100-fold.

FUNGAL INFECTIONS

Superficial fungal *(dermatophyte)* infections can differ in lesion appearance, anatomic location, and species of the

KEY FEATURES OF DISEASE ■ Locations of Various Tinea Infections

Infection	Location
Tinea pedis	Feet (athlete's foot)
Tinea manus	Hands
Tinea cruris	Groin (jock itch)
Tinea corporis	Smooth skin surfaces (ringworm)
Tinea capitis	Scalp
Tinea barbae	Beard

infecting organism. The term *tinea* is used to describe dermatophytoses. The accompanying Key Features of Disease gives the corresponding anatomic locations of the various categories of infection. A somewhat deeper fungal infection, candidiasis, is classified separately.

Pathophysiology

Depending on the species, dermatophytes reside predominantly in the soil, on animals, and on humans. Superficial infection can be initiated only if suitable conditions exist for inoculation and maintenance of the organism in the outer layers of the skin. Predisposing factors for dermatophytosis include impairment of the barrier function of the stratum corneum in warm, humid environments followed by minor skin trauma. After inoculation, the fungi digest and subsist on keratin.

Candidiasis of the skin and mucous membrane is largely an opportunistic infection, which occurs when host defenses are minimal. The *Candida* organism is a yeast that commonly colonizes the mucous membrane and skin surfaces of warm-blooded animals. Certain factors have been associated with increased incidence of cutaneous infection by these organisms, including nutritional deficiencies, certain systemic illnesses, and specific medications. In addition to the skin lesions, *Candida* can produce lesions in the mouth, vagina, gastrointestinal tract, and lungs. Infection may progress to septicemia in the immunocompromised client.

Etiology

Dermatophyte infections occur when the infecting organism comes in contact with an impaired skin surface in a susceptible host. Most infections are spread by direct contact with infected humans or animals. Certain types of dermatophytoses, such as tinea capitis and tinea corporis, can be transmitted by means of inanimate objects. For example, tinea capitis is associated with poor personal hygiene and the subsequent sharing of contami-nated combs, brushes, hats, pillowcases, and similar objects.

Although predisposing factors play an important role in host susceptibility to candidiasis, the most important factor that encourages cutaneous spread of the organism is moisture. Skin fold areas where perspiration collects, skin areas covered with moist dressings or occlusive garments, and skin around ostomy sites are often involved. Among the more common precursors to cutaneous candidiases in the hospitalized client are broad-spectrum antibiotic therapy and diabetes. Administration of broad-spectrum antibiotics changes the body's normal flora of microorganisms, allowing yeast organisms to predominate. Host defenses are altered in uncontrolled diabetes, predisposing the client to opportunistic infections.

Incidence

Dermatophyte infections occur more frequently in warm, humid climates. Incidence of infection by specific species of fungi has been shown to vary according to sex, age, race, geographic location, and genetic predisposition. For example, tinea cruris is almost exclusively a problem of the male population, with sexual transmission between husband and wife being rare.

The incidence of *Candida* infection is not affected by sex. Hospitalized clients are at greater risk owing to the number of predisposing factors in the hospital environment. Extremes of age, antibiotic or corticosteroid therapy, pregnancy, endocrine disease, immunodeficiency, and iron deficiency are commonly associated with increased incidence.

COLLABORATIVE MANAGEMENT

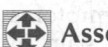 Assessment

History

The clinical manifestations of the cutaneous infection provide direction for collection of data to confirm a suspected diagnosis. To differentiate among the possible causes of the lesions, the nurse concentrates on those risk factors associated with each type of infection. If the location and appearance of lesions are highly suggestive of a bacterial infection, the nurse explores any *recent history of skin trauma*, as well as *past or current staphylococcal or streptococcal infections*. Associated symptoms of fever and malaise are also noted.

Lesions appearing on the lips, in the oral cavity, or in the genital region alert the nurse to a possible viral infection. The nurse seeks information about a *past history of similar lesions* in the same location; prodromal signs of burning, tingling, or pain; and recent stress factors that could have precipitated the outbreak. Acknowledgement by the client of the recurrent nature of lesions is often important in helping to differentiate between viral and bacterial lesions, especially those occurring in the perianal region. In addition, if herpes zoster is suspected, the nurse confirms *previous exposure to chickenpox* and inquires if the client has a history of shingles.

The data sought from a client with probable dermatophyte infection depend on the anatomic location of the lesions. Tinea corporis and tinea capitis require further assessment of social and environmental factors that may have contributed to inoculation, such as direct contact with an infected individual, poor personal hygiene practices, or frequent contact with animals. If tinea cruris and tinea pedis are suspected, the nurse asks about the type and frequency of athletic activities. Confirmation of *factors that contribute to decreased host resistance* is indicated if the client has signs of *Candida*

infection. Is the client presently receiving immunosuppressive drugs or antibiotics? Do past or present medical problems include diabetes or cancer? Does the client have nutritional problems? nutritional deficiencies? obesity?

Physical Assessment: Clinical Manifestations

Because most skin infections are contagious, the nurse takes necessary precautions to prevent the spread of infection when performing a physical assessment. The accompanying Key Features of Disease summarizes the clinical manifestations of common skin infections.

KEY FEATURES OF DISEASE ■ Clinical Manifestations of Common Skin Infections

Infection	Clinical Manifestations	Distribution
Bacterial		
Folliculitis	Isolated erythematous pustules occurring singly or in groups; hairs growing from centers of many of the lesions. Occasional papules. Little or no associated discomfort. No residual scarring.	Areas of hair-bearing skin, especially buttocks, thighs, beard area, and scalp.
Furuncle	Small, tender erythematous nodules become pus filled and more tender over time. Lesions may be single or multiple and also recurrent. Regional lymphadenopathy is sometimes present; fever is rare. Occasional scarring.	Areas of hair-bearing skin, especially buttocks, thighs, abdomen, posterior neck regions, and axillae.
Cellulitis	Localized area of inflammation may enlarge rapidly if not treated. Redness, warmth, edema, tenderness, and pain are present. On rare occasions, blisters are present. Often accompanied by lymphadenopathy and fever.	Lower legs, areas of persistent lymphedema, and areas of skin trauma (leg ulcer, puncture wound, and so forth).
Viral		
Herpes simplex	Grouped vesicles on an erythematous base. Vesicles evolve to pustules, which rupture, weep, and crust. Older lesions may appear as punched out shallow erosions with well-defined borders. Lesions are associated with itching, stinging, or pain. Secondary bacterial infection with necrosis is possible in immunocompromised clients.	Type 1 classically on the face and type 2 on the genitalia, but either may develop in any area where inoculation has occurred. Recurrent infections occur repeatedly in the same skin area.

Continued

KEY FEATURES OF DISEASE ■ **Clinical Manifestations of Common Skin Infections** *Continued*

Infection	Clinical Manifestations	Distribution
Viral		
Herpes zoster	Lesions are similar in appearance to herpes simplex and also progress with weeping and crusting.	Anterior or posterior trunk following involved dermatome; face, sometimes involving trigeminal nerve and eye.
	Grouped lesions present unilaterally along a segment of skin following the pathway of a spinal or cranial nerve (dermatomal distribution).	
	Eruption preceded by deep pain and itching.	
	Postherpetic neuralgia is common in the elderly.	
	Secondary infection with necrosis is possible in immunocompromised clients.	
Fungal		
Dermatophytosis	Annular or serpiginous patches with elevated borders, scaling, and central clearing.	Anywhere on the body.
	Pruritus is common.	
	Lesions may be single or multiple.	
Candidiasis	Erythematous macular eruption with isolated pustules or papules at the border (satellite lesions).	Skin fold areas: perineal and perianal region, axillae, beneath breasts, and between the fingers; under wet or occlusive dressings.
	Associated with burning and itching.	
	Oral lesions (thrush) appear as creamy-white plaques on an inflamed mucous membrane.	
	Cracks or fissures at the corners of the mouth may be present.	Lesions may also be present on the oral or vaginal mucous membranes.

Psychosocial Assessment

In general, psychosocial assessment focuses on family and social interactions that may have resulted in inoculation. Depending on how contagious the skin infection is, intimate contact (skin to skin and/or sexual) may have to be avoided until the infection has subsided. Recurrent genital herpes can prove quite distressing to a sexually active adult. It is sometimes helpful to explain that recurrent attacks often become less frequent and may cease entirely as time progresses. The pain associated with postherpetic neuralgia can also be distressing and may persist in spite of analgesic therapy.

As with any skin condition, perceived alterations in body image need to be addressed. Usually, concern over appearance only occurs with facial involvement. However, because a skin infection is contagious, a client may feel "dirty" and actively withdraw from social interactions.

Laboratory Findings

In bacterial infections in which pustules are present, the infecting organism is confirmed by swab culture of the purulent material. In immunocompromised clients,

anaerobic cultures may also be indicated. The responsible organism in cellulitis is not easily recovered. Blood cultures may prove helpful, especially if the client is showing clinical signs of bacteremia. Occasionally, nonbacteriostatic saline is injected into the cellulitic area and aspirated, and the aspirant is sent for Gram's stain and culture; however, this procedure is only 50% effective in isolating a pathogen.

Viral infections are confirmed by *Tzanck's smear* and viral culture. Tzanck's smear is a cytologic examination that involves examination of cells from the base of a lesion under a microscope. The presence of multinucleated giant cells confirms a herpetic infection. Tzanck's smear is less likely to be positive in lesions that have crusted, with viral cultures usually being more reliable. In chronic herpetic erosions, failure to isolate the virus is common.

Fungal infections are confirmed by a potassium hydroxide (KOH) test. Scrapings of scales from the lesions are obtained and, after preparation, examined under a microscope. The presence of fungal hyphae confirms the diagnosis. In addition to a KOH test, a fungal culture is sometimes indicated. Occasionally, a skin biopsy is performed, but only in rare instances.

Analysis: Nursing Diagnosis

The client with a skin infection may first be seen in the outpatient (ambulatory) setting or in the hospital. In the hospital setting, a majority of the clients are elderly and debilitated. The degree to which the client's immune system is compromised determines both the severity and the persistence of the infection. Because many superficial infections are asymptomatic, the problem may go undetected in healthy individuals.

Common Diagnoses

The nursing diagnosis most commonly noted in clients with skin infections is impaired skin integrity related to bacterial, viral, or fungal infection.

Additional Diagnoses

The client may have one or more additional diagnoses, depending on the cause of the infection.

1. Pain related to herpes simplex, herpes zoster, or cellulitis
2. Chronic pain related to postherpetic neuralgia
3. Ineffective individual coping related to recurrent skin infections
4. Sexual dysfunction related to contagious skin infections
5. Altered oral mucous membrane related to herpes simplex or oral candidiases
6. Body image disturbance related to skin lesions
7. Social isolation related to potential for spread of infection or altered body image
8. Knowledge deficit related to lack of information about or unclear explanation of the treatment regimen

 Planning and Implementation

The plan of care for clients with skin infection focuses on the common nursing diagnosis of impaired skin integrity.

Impaired Skin Integrity

Planning: client goals. The major goal for this nursing diagnosis is that the client will participate in a treatment regimen designed to restore skin integrity.

Interventions: nonsurgical management. Emphasis is placed on meticulous skin care to the involved areas to facilitate resolution of lesions and adherence to general isolation precautions. In some instances, drug therapy is also warranted.

Skin care. For bacterial infections, daily bathing with an antibacterial soap is indicated. The nurse instructs the client to gently débride any pustules or crusts so that topical medications are more easily absorbed.

Application of warm compresses twice a day to furuncles or areas of cellulitis often promotes comfort by increasing blood flow to the area and decreasing edema.

Application of astringent compresses, such as Burow's solution, to viral lesions for 20 minutes three times a day promotes crust formation and healing. Compresses are also useful in helping to relieve the irritation and pain associated with herpetic infection. The client should avoid constricting garments that might rub the lesions and increase irritation.

Most superficial skin infections resolve more quickly if the involved skin is allowed to dry between treatments with moist compresses. Excessive moisture, especially under occlusion, promotes growth of microorganisms. Interventions are similar to those for miliaria rubra (see earlier). If the client is bedridden, the nurse positions the client for optimal air circulation to the area and avoids occlusive dressings or garments. Drying of the infected areas is particularly important in cutaneous candidiases. *Candida* infections of the groin require that the client assume a frog-leg position when supine. A pillow between the knees is helpful when the client assumes a side-lying position. Finally, if the skin fold of the breasts is involved, the nurse places a rolled washcloth beneath the breasts to separate the skin surfaces and promote air circulation.

Isolation precautions. Precautions should be taken to minimize the spread of pathogenic organisms to other individuals. For most superficial bacterial infections, attention to proper hand washing is sufficient to prevent cross-contamination. However, hospitalized clients can become colonized with *Staphylococcus* that is resistant to antibiotic therapy, requiring strict adherence to isolation procedures to prevent spread to other clients.

The nurse instructs clients with recurrent herpes infections to avoid sexual contact as long as lesions are present. Some physicians believe that the use of condoms is helpful in minimizing transmission between outbreaks, when asymptomatic shedding of virus can occur. Yearly Papanicolaou's smears are important for infected women, with repeated cultures being performed during late pregnancy to determine whether cesarean section is needed to prevent transmission of the virus to the fetus during passage through the birth canal. In the case of herpes zoster, susceptible children exposed to the herpes zoster lesions can contract chickenpox.

Of the dermatophyte infections, tinea capitis, tinea corporis, and tinea pedis have the highest incidence of cross-transmission. The nurse instructs clients to avoid sharing potentially contaminated personal items, such as hairbrushes, articles of clothing, or footwear. Infection rates for tinea pedis are increased for those who use communal baths or swimming pools. Repeated infections transmitted by dogs or cats may necessitate getting rid of a family pet for the infections to be controlled.

Drug therapy. Commonly used topical medications for the treatment of bacterial, viral, and fungal skin infections are listed in Table 40–5.

TABLE 40-5 Topical Drugs Used in the Treatment of Skin Disorders

Drug	Usual Daily Dosage	Interventions	Rationales
Antibacterial Drugs			
Ointments			

Neomycin sulfate
  Combination antibiotics
  (Neosporin, Bacitra-
  cin, Polysporin,
  Mycitracin)
Gentamicin (Garamycin)
Chloramphenicol (Chloro-
  mycetin)
Povidone-iodine (Beta-
  dine)
	Apply a thin layer to the affected area tid. Dressing is optional.	1. Gently clean affected areas with saline, half-strength peroxide, or tap water before applying ointments.
		
		2. Avoid rubbing oint-ment into skin. Apply with downward strokes in direction of hair growth.
		3. Assess for worsening of problem in spite of topical therapy. Discontinue use if rash appears.
			1. Atraumatic cleaning promotes healing by preventing further injury to skin cells. Cleaning helps to re-move exudate, crusts, and residual medication and to increase the effec-tiveness of therapy.
			2. Ointments can irritate hair follicles and lead to folliculitis.
			
			3. Client may become allergic to active ingredients, the oint-ment base, or added preservatives.

Creams			
Silver sulfadiazine (Silvadene, SSD)	Apply in layer approxi-mately 1/16-in thick to affected areas tid and prn. Dressing is optional.	1. Assess for allergy to sulfa drugs. 2. Gently clean affected areas with saline, half-strength hydrogen peroxide, or tap water before reapplying. 3. If affected areas are left open without dress-ings, reapply cream prn between cleanings to maintain a layer of cream at all times. 4. Monitor white blood cell count for drop to <5000/mm³.	1. Use should be avoided in clients with a suspected or known sulfa allergy. 2. Cleaning removes crusts, exudate, and caked-on medication while promoting percutaneous absorption of drug. 3. Cream base melts with increase in body or room temperature and is easily rubbed off with movement if left uncovered. 4. Use of silver sulfadiazine over large skin surface areas has been associated with a transient leukopenia (cause unknown).

TABLE 40–5   Topical Drugs Used in the Treatment of Skin Disorders *Continued*

Drug	Usual Daily Dosage	Interventions	Rationales
Antifungal Drugs			
Ointments and Creams			
Clotrimazole (Lotrimin, Mycelex) Nystatin (Mycolog, Mycostatin, Nilstat) Ciclopirox olamine (Loprox) Miconazole nitrate (Monistat-Derm 2%) Econazole (Spectazole) Tolnaftate (Tinactin) Haloprogin (Halotex) Undecylenic acid (Desenex)	Apply a thin layer to the affected area tid.	1. Teach the importance of thoroughly drying the skin before applying medication. 2. Position bedridden clients for maximal air circulation to involved areas. 3. Emphasize wearing of nonconstricting cotton garments to absorb perspiration.	1. Moist environment promotes the growth of fungal organisms. 2. Increasing air circulation to the affected areas promotes drying. 3. Cream base is easily removed with perspiration, decreasing the effectiveness of therapy.
Powders			
Nystatin (Mycostatin) Tolnaftate (Zeosorb-AF 1%)	Apply a thin dusting of powder to the affected area tid.	1. Teach the client to thoroughly dry skin before applying powder.	1. In addition to discouraging the growth of fungal organisms, a dry skin surface minimizes caking of powder in skin fold areas.
Oral Preparations			
Nystatin (Mycostatin oral suspension, Nilstat oral suspension)	Rinse mouth qid with 4–6 mL (400,000–600,000 units) and swallow	1. Teach the client to coat the entire oral cavity with medication and hold the suspension in mouth for several minutes before swallowing.	1, 2. Effectiveness of medication is dependent on good contact of medication with mucous membrane surfaces.
Clotrimazole (Mycelex troche)	1 troche five times daily.	2. Teach the client to let troche dissolve slowly in the mouth.	

Table continued on following page

TABLE 40-5 Topical Drugs Used in the Treatment of Skin Disorders *Continued*

Drug	Usual Daily Dosage	Interventions	Rationales
Anti-inflammatory Drugs			
Steroid Preparations			
POTENT FLUORINATED Clobetasol propionate (Temovate 0.05%) Triamcinolone acetonide (Aristocort 0.5%, Kenalog 0.5%) Amcinonide (Cyclocort 0.1%) Betamethasone dipropionate (Diprosone 0.05%) Diflorasone diacetate (Maxiflor 0.05%, Florone 0.05%) Halcinonide (Halog 0.025%) Fluocinonide (Lidex 0.05%, Topsyn gel 0.05%) Fluocinolone acetonide (Synalar-HP 0.2%) Desoximetasone (Topicort 0.25%) Betamethasone benzoate (Uticort 0.025%)	Apply a small amount to affected areas no more than four times in 24 h.	1. Teach the client to use the least amount of medication possible to cover the treatment site and to use the medication *only* under the direction of a physician. 2. Never apply highly potent steroid preparations to the face, genital area, or skin fold areas.	1. Overuse of topical steroid preparations can cause serious side effects, including skin thinning (atrophy), superficial dilated blood vessels (telangiectasia), acne-like eruptions, and adrenal suppression. The incidence of side effects increases proportionately with the potency of the steroid and is most common with prolonged widespread use of the high-potency preparations. 2. Absorption of topical steroids is much higher in these areas, and the associated side effects are more severe.
Medium-Potency Fluorinated Triamcinolone acetonide (Kenalog 0.025%, 0.1%; Aristocort 0.025%, 0.1%) Flurandrenolide (Cordran 0.05%, 0.025%) Fluocinolone acetonide (Fluonid 0.025%, Synalar 0.025%) Desoximetasone (Topicort LP 0.05%) Betamethasone valerate (Valisone 0.1%)			

TABLE 40-5   Topical Drugs Used in the Treatment of Skin Disorders *Continued*

Drug	Usual Daily Dosage	Interventions	Rationales
Anti-inflammatory Drugs			
Low-Potency		1. Teach the client to hydrate the skin before applying a topical steroid.	1. Skin hydration increases percutaneous absorption and maximizes the effectiveness of topical treatment.
Nonfluorinated			
Hydrocortisone 0.5%, 1.0%, 2.5% Desonide (Tridesilon) Hydrocortisone valerate (Westcort)			
Antiviral Drugs			
Ointments Acyclovir (Zovirax)	Apply to affected areas six times a day.	1. Teach the client to use topical acyclovir only under the direction of a physician for primary infections.	1. Topical acyclovir has no proven clinical benefit in the prevention or treatment of recurrent infections.
		2. Emphasize precautionary measures to prevent transmission of infection while the lesion is present.	2. There is no evidence that topical treatment prevents transmission of infection.

Mild bacterial infections of the skin usually resolve with topical antibacterial treatment. Extensive infections, including those with associated fever or lymphadenopathy, require oral or parenteral antibiotic therapy.

Acyclovir is the drug of choice for the treatment of viral infections. Topical acyclovir ointment decreases the numbers of active virus on the skin surface and reduces pain in primary herpetic infections and localized lesions in immunocompromised clients. Topical treatment is of little benefit in recurrent infection. Oral antiviral drugs are effective against both primary and recurrent genital infections. IV administration is limited to severe primary infections and immunosuppressed clients with symptoms of systemic involvement.

Topical antifungal agents are indicated for dermatophyte and yeast infections. An imidazole cream is applied to the infected skin twice a day until the lesions have cleared. The therapy is usually continued for 1 to 2 weeks after clearing to discourage recurrence. In some instances antifungal powders may also prove useful in suppressing fungal growth. For widespread or resistant fungal infections, systemic antifungal agents are administered.

Prevention of complications. Complications are rare, except in immunosuppressed clients. Emphasis is placed on early recognition and treatment of skin infections in the immunosuppressed population.

Interventions: surgical management. Surgical intervention is uncommon in superficial skin infections, with the exception of incision and drainage of furuncles. Occasionally, in severely immunocompromised clients, superficial lesions progress to extensive full-thickness wounds requiring surgical excision.

■ Discharge Planning

The hospitalized client is frequently discharged before a skin infection has completely resolved. Continuation of treatment in the home environment with appropriate follow-up care is indicated.

Home Care Preparation

Elderly clients may require assistance in carrying out daily skin care needs. If family members are unavailable, the nurse arranges for a neighbor or home care nurse to assist with treatments and monitor progress of the infection.

Client/Family Education

The nurse assesses the client's understanding of the treatment of the skin infection and any precautions that need to be taken to prevent the spread of infection in the home environment. For example, the nurse encourages the client to use separate towels and washcloths and to change bed linen frequently. It is often helpful to have family members or sexual partners present when discussing precautions so that individual questions can be addressed and any misunderstandings corrected. Follow-up appointments with the physician are usually indicated until the infection has resolved.

Psychosocial Preparation

Clients requiring the most psychologic support are those with genital herpes. Feelings of embarrassment and disbelief eventually give way to frustration. Because there is no cure, the client often feels controlled by the infection and may express anxiety about the possibility of infecting sexual partners. Anticipation of recurrent outbreaks increases the client's stress and may actually potentiate recurrences. Providing information in a matter-of-fact way is important in enabling these clients to communicate their fears and anxieties and in minimizing feelings of social isolation (see Chap. 56).

Health Care Resources

Because of the increasing incidence of sexually transmitted herpes, many self-help groups have formed to provide information and support, as well as encourage social interaction among people with a common problem. Often, the client is unaware that such support mechanisms exist. In addition, written materials for lay people are available through several national health care organizations.

 Evaluation

On the basis of the identified nursing diagnoses, the nurse evaluates care of the client with a skin infection. Expected outcomes include that the client

1. Demonstrates knowledge and skills necessary to continue local skin care in the home environment
2. States the effect of diagnosis on personal habits, coping behaviors, sexuality, and perceived body image
3. Describes precautions necessary to prevent the spread of infection in the home environment
4. Describes and complies with drug therapy as ordered
5. Describes resources available in the community (if applicable)

By meeting the stated desired outcomes, the client should show rapid resolution of the skin infection, and the frequency of transmission and recurrence should be minimized.

COMMON INFLAMMATIONS

OVERVIEW

The inflammatory skin conditions have a variety of nonspecific epidermal manifestations, including marked pruritus, lesions with indistinct borders, and different distribution patterns. The eruption may have an identifiable cause, or its cause may remain a mystery. As with many of the skin diseases, inflammatory rashes can evolve from acute to chronic conditions.

Pathophysiology

The pathogenesis of cutaneous inflammatory rashes is related to the immune response. Impairments in the barrier function of the stratum corneum result in exposure of the internal environment to toxins, irritants, and potentially infectious agents. The result is tissue destruction or epidermal alteration induced by humoral or cellular mediators of the immune system. A more detailed description of these immune mechanisms can be found in Chapter 23.

Etiology

The inciting agent of inflammatory rashes is not always identified. When this is the case, the catchall diagnosis of nonspecific eczematous dermatitis, or *eczema,* is often used. To add to the confusion, the terms eczema and dermatitis are used interchangeably to describe the appearance of the lesions common to these skin changes.

Contact dermatitis is an acute or chronic eczematous rash caused either by direct contact with an irritant substance, resulting in toxic injury to the skin, or by contact with an allergen, resulting in a cell-mediated immune reaction. Irritant dermatitis is most often due to contact with strong acids, alkalis, solvents, and detergents. Some of the more common sensitizers in allergic dermatitis are nickel, rubber, plants, and topical medications. Genetic predisposition to contact allergies does not occur.

Atopic dermatitis is a chronic rash that is associated with genetic predisposition to respiratory allergies and atopic skin disease. Although the exact mechanism is unknown, atopic dermatitis is exacerbated by a number of factors, including dry or irritated skin, food allergies, chemicals, and stress.

Inflammatory skin changes can also occur when clients are allergic to systemic medications. The list of medications associated with *drug eruptions* is exhaustive; however, the more common causative drugs include the antibiotics (particularly sulfonamides) and antineoplastic agents. Progression of drug eruptions can sometimes result in the shedding of large sheets of epidermis similar in appearance to that occurring with a partial-thickness burn. When large surface areas are involved, hypothermia and dehydration are potential complications.

Incidence

The incidence of inflammatory rashes depends on the cause of the disease. As might be expected, nonspecific eczema accounts for a majority of rashes seen in both inpatient and outpatient settings. Often, this diagnosis is used until further investigation points to a more specific cause.

Surprisingly, contact dermatitis accounts for more than 60% of occupational injury, excluding accidents. One in 1000 workers is affected, at a cost of millions of dollars a year in the United States (Lookingbill & Marks, 1986). Atopic dermatitis, on the other hand, is predominantly a disease of childhood and usually resolves before puberty. Recurrent episodes of the disease in adulthood are not common.

Finally, drug eruptions can account for as many as 7% of dermatologic consultations in the inpatient setting (Lookingbill & Marks, 1986). The high incidence of drug-related allergy occurs because most hospitalized clients receive an average of nine oral or IV medications.

COLLABORATIVE MANAGEMENT

 Assessment

History

Because all of the inflammatory skin eruptions have similar clinical presentations, data collected from the client are often the determining factor in identifying the cause. When taking a history from the client with an inflammatory rash, the nurse inquires about *present or past history of allergies to any substances,* including medications, foods, topical preparations, and jewelry. *Past or recent exposure to potential irritants or allergens* is also explored by having the client describe his/her occupation, hobbies, and hygiene practices. Identifying specific *situations that make the rash better or worse* helps limit the number of possible offending agents. If atopic dermatitis is suspected, the nurse asks about any *past personal or family history of cutaneous inflammation, asthma, or allergic rhinitis.* To rule out drug reactions as a possible cause of the rash, a *recent medication history,* including over-the-counter as well as prescription drugs, is taken. The *presence of associated symptoms,* such as severe pruritus or fever, alerts the nurse to the possibility of a secondary bacterial infection.

Physical Assessment: Clinical Manifestations

Although the clinical appearance of eczematous dermatitis lesions is similar, the chronicity of the disease, the distribution of lesions, and associated symptoms may vary (see the accompanying Key Features of Disease).

Psychosocial Assessment

Psychosocial assessment focuses on problems related to self-concept, as well as complaints of pruritus. Many of the eczematous rashes involve body areas that are not hidden by clothing. Clients have concerns about appearance, as well as fear that the rash may be contagious. Pruritus is often the chief complaint. Itching can be constant or episodic, and the intensity often interrupts sleep or interferes with ADL. Increased stress levels have been associated with flares of dermatitis in some individuals, especially those with atopy.

Laboratory Findings

Diagnosis is usually based on historical and clinical data. Although skin biopsies are sometimes performed, the information obtained from these tests is diagnostic for only the general findings of eczematous skin changes. In atopic dermatitis, serum immunoglobulin E levels are frequently elevated. If crusted or oozing lesions are present, swab cultures are diagnostic for secondary infection with bacteria or yeast.

Other Diagnostic Tests

If allergic contact dermatitis is suspected, *patch tests* may be performed in an attempt to identify the causative chemical. Commercially available solutions and ointments containing common chemical sensitizers are applied topically to the skin under occlusion to see if a local allergic reaction occurs. Although patch testing is a rather simple procedure, proper application of the test patches and interpretation of results are essential to an accurate diagnosis. In addition, results of patch testing are considered meaningful only if the client's history of exposure is consistent with test findings. For more information on patch testing, see Chapter 39.

 Analysis: Nursing Diagnosis

Whether a client with inflammatory skin disease is in the inpatient or outpatient setting, successful management depends on a thorough history and physical assessment to identify the probable cause, followed by intervention aimed at removing the offending agents. If a cause is not identified, symptomatic treatment of the rash is indicated. Often, a complaint of pruritus is the first sign of an impending inflammatory rash.

Common Diagnoses

The nursing diagnoses that are most commonly found in clients with inflammatory skin disease are

1. Impaired skin integrity related to inflammatory rash
2. Pain related to intense pruritus

Additional Diagnoses

The client may have one or more additional diagnoses.

KEY FEATURES OF DISEASE ■ Clinical Manifestations of Common Inflammatory Skin Conditions

Condition	Clinical Manifestations	Distribution
Nonspecific eczematous dermatitis	Evolution of lesions from vesicles to weeping papules and plaques. Lichenification occurs in chronic disease. Oozing, crusting, fissuring, excoriation, or scaling may be present. Pruritus is common.	Anywhere on the body. Localized eczema commonly involves the hands or feet.
Contact dermatitis	Localized eczematous eruption with well-defined, geometric margins that is consistent with contact by an irritant or allergen. Usually seen in the acute form, but may become chronic if exposure is repeated. Allergy to plants (e.g., poison ivy or oak) classically occurs as linear streaks of vesicles or papules.	Cosmetic/perfume allergy: head and neck. Hair product allergy: scalp. Shoe/rubber allergy: dorsum of feet. Nickle allergy: ear lobes. Mouthwash/toothpaste allergy: perioral region. Airborne contact allergy (e.g., paint and ragweed): generalized.
Atopic dermatitis	Hallmark in adults is lichenification with scaling and excoriation. Extremely pruritic. Face involvement is seen as dry skin with mild to moderate erythema, perioral pallor, and skin folds beneath the eyes (Dennie-Morgan lines). Associated with linear markings on the palms.	Face, neck, upper chest, and antecubital and popliteal fossae.
Drug eruption	Bright red erythematous macules and papules are found. Skin blisters in extreme cases. Lesions tend to be confluent in large areas. Moderately pruritic. Fever is rare. Dehydration and hypothermia can occur with extensive involvement. Condition clears only after offending medication has been discontinued.	Generalized. Involvement begins on trunk and proceeds distally (legs are the last to be involved).

1. Body image disturbance related to skin disease
2. Ineffective individual coping related to altered body image, chronicity of disease, or unrelieved pruritus
3. Sleep pattern disturbance related to pruritus
4. Social isolation related to altered body image and ineffective individual coping
5. Potential for infection related to impaired skin integrity
6. Knowledge deficit related to lack of information about or unclear explanation of the treatment regimen

 Planning and Implementation

Impaired Skin Integrity

Planning: client goals.   The goals for the client with an inflammatory rash are that the client will (1) prevent or minimize contact with any offending agents and (2) experience increased comfort through the treatment of associated symptoms.

Interventions: nonsurgical management.   If the cause of the rash is identified, avoidance therapy is used in an attempt to reverse the reaction and clear the rash. Even when the cause is unclear, certain irritants in the environment may cause progression of the rash and increase discomfort. Additional interventions are aimed at promoting comfort through suppression of the inflammatory response.

Avoidance therapy.   In the case of contact dermatitis, complete avoidance of a sensitizing agent is not always possible. Protective clothing is sometimes helpful in providing an additional barrier for the skin, and, in certain situations, a less toxic substance can be substituted for the offending material. Many occupation-related allergies result in time away from the job for extended periods. If contact with a proven allergen cannot be avoided, the client's only option is to change jobs.

In suspected drug reactions, every effort is made to identify the medications responsible for the problem and discontinue its administration. Usually the onset of symptoms occurs 3 to 7 days after the introduction of a new medication. If the culprit cannot be readily identified, the number of medications administered is reduced to the absolute minimum or substitutions are made.

When a food allergy is thought to contribute to recurrent atopic dermatitis, controlled food challenges and elimination diets can be used to confirm the allergen. Clients with this skin disease have a particular problem with overly dry skin and should avoid those factors that promote drying, especially during the winter months. Furthermore, wool clothes often need to be avoided because of skin irritation from the wool lanolins.

Drug therapy.   Topical, intralesional, or systemic steroids are used to suppress inflammation. In general, the vehicle used to deliver a topical steroid depends on the body area involved. The nurse does not apply ointments and pastes in the sweaty skin fold areas because increased maceration and blocking of pores may result in folliculitis. Instead, creams, which are more water soluble, are the vehicle of choice for these areas. Lotions and gels prevent matting of the hair and are more appropriate for hairy areas, such as the scalp. Finally, stiff pastes are used to apply therapy to localized areas, because this vehicle clings to the skin where it is applied and resists spreading to uninvolved skin. Cream preparations are indicated in acute dermatitis when oozing and weeping are present. Chronic dermatitis responds more favorably to ointments that seal in moisture and help combat dryness and scaling.

Antihistamines provide some relief of pruritus, but may fail to keep the client totally symptom free. The nurse can minimize sedative effects of these drugs by having the client take most of the daily dose near bedtime.

Therapeutic baths and dressings.   Cool moist compresses and tepid baths with bath additives may be ordered. These measures have a soothing effect, decrease inflammation, and help débride crusts and scale. Colloidal oatmeal preparations, tar extracts, oils, or cornstarch is often added to baths to promote relief of pruritus (see

Table 40–1). The nurse can moisten dressings with warm tap water to place over topical steroid preparations for short periods of time to facilitate absorption.

Pain

Measures for relieving pruritus and preventing secondary excoriation are discussed earlier under the heading Pruritus.

■ Discharge Planning

Client/Family Education

Because inflammatory skin diseases are often chronic, continued treatment in the home setting is likely. Often, these rashes get better, only to flare when irritant substances are introduced or seasons change. The nurse assists the client in identifying substances that need to be avoided in the home and work environments and suggests ways of preventing contact. A rule of thumb is "If something makes the rash worse, stay away from it." When medication allergy is the problem, the nurse stresses the importance of communicating the allergy to future health care providers.

Regardless of the cause of the rash, the nurse emphasizes the need for good skin care, particularly prevention of dry skin (see earlier). Dry skin serves to exacerbate pruritus and frequently promotes excoriation and secondary infection.

The nurse discusses topical and systemic drug therapy with the client and the family. Proper application of topical steroids to slightly damp skin to increase the effectiveness of topical therapy is stressed. A common side effect of prolonged use of topical steroids is thinning of the skin, telangiectasia (dilated superficial blood vessels), and striae formation (stretch marks). The stronger the steroid preparation, the greater the chance of adverse reactions is. The nurse instructs the client to apply the medication in a *thin* layer and no more often than recommended by the physician. Highly potent steroid preparations should never be applied to the skin fold areas or the face because these areas are more prone to atrophy. In addition, acne-like eruptions may occur on the face if the steroid used is too potent.

Prednisone is the most commonly prescribed systemic steroid preparation for inflammatory skin disease, with use usually limited to severe cases of contact dermatitis or extensive drug eruptions. A side effect of oral corticosteroid administration is adrenal suppression. Prolonged administration in chronic conditions may result in Addison's disease–like symptoms, delayed wound healing, gastric ulceration, and increased susceptibility to infections. If the client has been receiving long-term therapy, the nurse warns against abrupt discontinuation of the drug without consulting the physician. Tapering of dosages is indicated to allow adrenal gland function to return to normal before the drug administration is stopped. An important point to remember is that *corticosteroids never cure.* During active disease, they are used to keep the disease from manifesting itself and to relieve associated discomfort. When the dosage is tapered or drug administration stopped, it is not unusual for a rebound effect to occur, with a return of symptoms that may be worse than the original condition.

The nurse instructs clients receiving antihistamines to avoid driving or operating machinery owing to lengthened reaction times from the sedative effect of these drugs. As mentioned earlier, sedation can be minimized by nighttime administration. Anticholinergic side effects include dry mouth, blurred vision, and impaired micturition.

Psychosocial Preparation

Psychosocial preparation is focused on placing clients in control of treatment of their rash. Because of the chronicity of the problem, frustration and anger often arise when a specific cause cannot be identified and recurrent flares occur. The nurse stresses the need for clients to put aside personal time, uninterrupted by family, to take care of their skin needs. For chronic conditions, it may also be helpful for some clients to keep a log of activities and how those activities correlate with skin improvement. Often, writing experiences down, gives the client insight into potential offending agents and the relationship of psychologic stress to flares.

Follow-up visits to the dermatologist are scheduled as needed. Usually, the frequency of follow-up visits depends on the severity of symptoms and the response to treatment.

 Evaluation

On the basis of the identified nursing diagnoses, the nurse evaluates care of the client with inflammatory skin disease. The expected outcomes include that the client

1. Identifies potential environmental agents that cause exacerbation of the disease and avoids them
2. States that pruritus is reduced or alleviated
3. Describes and complies with the drug regimen as ordered

By meeting the stated desired outcomes, progression from acute to chronic disease may be prevented and associated complications minimized.

PSORIASIS

OVERVIEW

The term "heartbreak of psoriasis" is not without justification. *Psoriasis* is a lifelong disorder characterized by exacerbations and remissions. Lesions may occur any-

where on the body and may be limited to one or two localized plaques or involve large areas of the epidermis, including the scalp and the fingernails. Psoriasis is also associated with a rare form of arthritis, which can be crippling. Even though this disease cannot be cured, control of symptoms can usually be achieved with proper treatment.

Pathophysiology

Psoriasis is a scaling disorder with underlying dermal inflammation. Pathogenesis involves an abnormality in the proliferation of epidermal cells in the outer skin layers. Normally, cells at the basement membrane of the epidermis take about 27 days to reach the outermost stratum corneum, where they are shed. In psoriasis, the rate of cell multiplication is speeded up so that cells are shed every 4 to 5 days. This abnormality in reproduction of cellular tissue may be related to a disturbance of amino acid synthesis.

Etiology

The cause of psoriasis is not known. A genetic predisposition has been recognized in some cases; however, often, there is no family history of the disease. Many different environmental factors have been found to precipitate outbreaks and influence the severity of clinical symptoms, but these vary significantly from individual to individual. Triggering factors may be local or systemic. Often a psoriatic lesion appears after skin trauma (Koebner's phenomenon). The phenomenon occurs in about 50% of clients with psoriasis after surgery, sunburn, excoriation, or similar compromise in skin integrity. The influence of climate is controversial. Generally, the disease seems to improve in warmer climates, where there is more exposure to sunlight. Systemic factors that can aggravate the disease are well documented. These include infection (severe streptococcal throat infection, *Candida* infection, and upper respiratory tract infection), hormonal changes (during puberty and menopause), psychologic stress, certain drugs (lithium, beta-blocking agents, indomethacin, and antimalarials), and general health factors (obesity and disease).

Incidence

The initial outbreak of psoriasis may occur at any age, with the average age at onset being about 27 years. The earlier the disease starts, the worse the prognosis is. Overall prevalence of the disease in the general population is estimated at about 0.9%, with a lower incidence in the darker-skinned races. A positive family history for psoriasis is found in about one of three clients with psoriasis. Incidence is equally distributed among males and females.

COLLABORATIVE MANAGEMENT

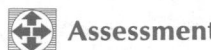 **Assessment**

History

When taking a history from a client with psoriasis, the nurse collects information that helps establish the individual pattern of presentation, including potential precipitating factors. In addition to routine epidemiologic data, information to collect from the client includes any *family history* of psoriasis. *Age at onset* of the disease and a *description of disease progression*, with emphasis on the *pattern of recurrences*, is obtained. The nurse has the client describe the *current flare* of psoriasis including, whether the onset was gradual or sudden, where the lesions first appeared, any observed changes in severity over time, and the presence of associated symptoms (e.g., fever and pruritus). *Possible precipitating factors* are explored, including recent skin trauma, upper respiratory tract infection, recent surgeries, menopause status (if female), past and current use of medication, and recent stress-provoking occurrences. Finally, the nurse investigates *previous treatment modalities* and the effectiveness of each in initiating and maintaining remission of the disease.

Physical Assessment: Clinical Manifestations

The appearance of psoriasis and the course it takes vary from client to client. Typically, during flares of the disease, lesions thicken and extend to involve new areas of the body. As psoriasis responds to treatment, individual lesions become thinner with less scaling. The color of psoriatic plaques is the last thing to change, progressing from red to brown before fading completely. The lower extremities are usually the last body area to clear.

Psoriasis vulgaris, the most common presentation of psoriasis, is characterized by thick erythematous papules or plaques surmounted by silvery-white scales. Borders between the lesions and normal skin are sharply defined. Patches may appear less red and more moist in skin fold areas owing to maceration from perspiration. Lesions are usually distributed symmetrically, with the more common sites being the scalp, the elbows, the trunk, the knees, the sacrum, and extensor surfaces of the limbs. Involvement of the facial skin is rare. The client may have only a few isolated lesions, or the entire skin surface may be affected. As associated nail involvement is present in about 50% of clients with psoriasis. Small lesions resembling ice pick depressions in the nail plate are visible, and onycholysis (separation of the nail plate from the nail bed) can also occur if a plaque of psoriasis forms in the distal nail bed.

Less common presentations include guttate psoriasis, exfoliative psoriasis, and pustular psoriasis. *Guttate psoriasis* occurs as isolated droplet-shaped papules, primarily scattered over the trunk and sparing the palms and the soles.

Exfoliative psoriasis (erythrodermic psoriasis) is an explosively eruptive form of the disease characterized by generalized erythema and scaling without obvious lesions. A similar presentation may be seen in severe drug reactions and other situations, requiring that diagnosis be supported by history, nail involvement, and histologic examination. The nurse inspects and palpates for signs of dehydration and hypothermia or hyperthermia related to this severe inflammatory reaction. The vasodilation and increased blood flow to the skin that occur with inflammation can cause alterations in fluid volume resulting from increased evaporative water loss from the skin surface. Alterations in body temperature result from interference in the thermoregulatory function of the skin.

Generalized *pustular psoriasis* is a rare manifestation that is often fatal. On inspection, the skin appearance is similar to that of exfoliative psoriasis with the added feature of pustules. Initially, the pustules are sterile; however, secondary infection can occur. The nurse palpates the skin for severe tenderness and elevated skin temperature that often accompanies the disease. More common is a localized form of pustular psoriasis occurring as typical plaques studded with pustules, but without the severe systemic complications associated with generalized disease.

Psychosocial Assessment

Because of the subjective nature of emotional factors, the relationship between psoriasis and stress remains controversial. Although many authors do not support a causal relationship, there is general agreement that stress can precede the onset or relapse of disease. A study by Seville (1983) showed a high correlation between self-knowledge or insight and prognosis. Those clients who were willing to acknowledge the impact of emotional disturbances and stress on recurrence of disease had a better prognosis than those who were without insight. In addition to acknowledged emotional stresses, the impact of an altered body image as an additional stressor needs to be considered.

The nurse questions the client about stressful situations that occurred within the month preceding the onset or exacerbation of symptoms. Attention to body language and voice tone is important in providing clues to factors that need further investigation. The nurse phrases questions in such a way that the client is encouraged to be reflective. For example, asking a client what seems to make his/her psoriasis better or worse may help identify a common stress factor preceding past episodes.

Observation of body language between the client and family members or friends also alerts the nurse to problems with self-concept. Many individuals who are not knowledgeable about psoriasis assume that it is contagious and may project these feelings to the client, causing further stress. In addition, observation of family interactions can provide an important clue to unacknowledged tensions.

Laboratory Findings

Diagnosis is usually based on history and clinical presentation. Occasionally, skin biopsy is warranted to confirm the diagnosis in unusual presentations. Additional blood studies or cultures are indicated to rule out systemic precipitating factors.

 Analysis: Nursing Diagnosis

Psoriasis can vary from a mild to a severe and disabling chronic disease. Clients may be seen in the outpatient setting or, if the disease is extensive, require hospitalization for more intensive therapy. Even those clients with less severe symptoms remain at risk for rapid spread of the lesions if a precipitating factor occurs.

Common Diagnoses

The nursing diagnoses most commonly noted in clients with psoriasis are

1. Impaired skin integrity related to psoriatic lesions or generalized erythema
2. Pain related to pruritus
3. Ineffective individual coping related to primary stress factors
4. Body image disturbance related to skin disease

Additional Diagnoses

The client may have one or more additional diagnoses.

1. Social isolation related to altered body image and ineffective individual coping
2. Chronic pain related to psoriatic arthritis
3. Fluid volume deficit and potential fluid volume deficit related to generalized exfoliative or pustular psoriasis
4. Hypothermia related to exfoliative psoriasis or generalized pustular psoriasis
5. Potential for infection related to psoriatic lesions, excoriation, or complications of topical therapy
6. Knowledge deficit related to lack of information about or unclear explanation of the treatment regimen
7. Noncompliance (with treatment regimen) related to denial, unacceptable changes in daily activities, or apathy related to chronicity of disease

 Planning and Implementation

The plan for care of psoriatic clients focuses on the nursing diagnoses (see the accompanying Client Care Plan). With the exception of the tar preparations and systemic chemotherapy, most of the assessments and interventions for psoriasis are also applicable to the care of clients with other skin disorders.

Impaired Skin Integrity

Planning: client goals. The major goal for this nursing diagnosis is that the client will restore skin integrity by complying with the medical treatment regimen. In the hospital setting, emphasis is placed on teaching the client proper skin care practices, with progression toward total independence in care before discharge from the hospital. If this goal is not met, the chance of readmission for recurrence of symptoms is increased.

Interventions: nonsurgical management. A number of different approaches to therapy can be used and are based on the physician's preference and how resistant the psoriasis is to treatment. In general, medical therapy is aimed at decreasing epidermal proliferation and underlying inflammation through the use of topical agents alone or in combination with ultraviolet (UV) light treatments. Occasional use of a systemic agent is warranted in widespread disease that does not respond to topical therapy.

Topical therapy. The pharmacologic and physical topical agents employed in the treatment of psoriasis are (1) topical steroids, (2) topical tar and anthralin preparations, and (3) UV light. Topical medications are further described in Table 40–5.

Topical steroids. The corticosteroids have anti-inflammatory properties; in addition, their application to psoriatic lesions suppresses mitotic activity and increases the transit time of keratinocytes from the basement membrane to the skin surface. The effectiveness of a topical steroid depends on its potency and ability to be absorbed into the skin. In general, the more potent preparations are used in the treatment of psoriasis, and the vehicle (e.g., cream, ointment, and lotion) is chosen on the basis of the criteria for selection in inflammatory skin conditions.

A popular procedure for enhancing the percutaneous penetration of these agents is for the nurse to apply the steroid to the skin followed by warm, moist dressings and an occlusive outer wrap of plastic film, plastic gloves, booties, or similar garments. When large surface areas are involved, occlusive therapy is usually limited to 12 hours per day owing to the increased risk of local and systemic side effects. In addition, plastic occlusion is uncomfortable and can precipitate outbreaks of miliaria and bacterial and yeast infections.

Tar preparations. Although their exact mechanism of action is unknown, tar preparations suppress mitotic activity and produce an anti-inflammatory effect when applied to the skin. Preparations containing crude coal tar and derivations of crude coal tar are available as solutions, ointments, lotions, gels, and shampoos. The use of crude coal tar ointments is usually limited to inpatient care because they are messy, cause staining, and

Text continued on page 1194

CLIENT CARE PLAN ■ The Client with Psoriasis Vulgaris

Goal/Outcome Criteria	Interventions	Rationales
Nursing Diagnosis 1: Impaired Skin Integrity Related to Psoriatic Lesions		

Client will experience progressive clearing of psoriatic lesions.

Goal/Outcome Criteria	Interventions	Rationales

■ Identifies factors that could exacerbate the flare and avoids them.	1. Teach factors that could exacerbate the flare and assist the client in avoiding them.
	  a. Assess for indications of emotional stress and encourage the client to identify possible causes of stress.
	  b. Assess factors that increase anxiety in the hospital environment (lack of privacy, difficulty sleeping, and so forth) and correct them as needed.
	  c. Instruct the client to request antihistamines as needed.
	
	  d. Instruct the client to keep the skin well lubricated at all times.
	  e. Instruct the client to report any sensations of burning or tenderness after UV light treatments.
	  f. Instruct the client in the use of sunscreens or how to shield sunburned areas as ordered by the physician.
		1. To minimize the possibility of flares, giving the client control over the disease.
		  a. To help the client manage stress, which precipitates a flare and also contributes to slow clearing of lesions.
		  b. To decrease anxiety, which contributes to emotional stress.
		
		  c. To prevent uncontrolled pruritus, which can lead to excoriation and result in the Koebner phenomenon.
		  d. To reduce pruritus.
		  e. To prevent and detect overexposure to UVB light, which can percipitate the Koebner phenomenon.
		  f. To prevent further skin damage, which can lead to spread of lesions.

■ States the rationale and potential side effects of treatment.	2. Depending on the individualized treatment protocol, teach the rationale behind each step in the medical regimen, including how to minimize side effects.
	  a. Therapeutic baths.
	    ■ Instruct the client in the purpose of the bath.
	
	    ■ Demonstrate how to *gently* rub the lesions with a washcloth using a circular motion.
	    ■ Instruct the client to use only warm water.
	
	    ■ Instruct the client to dry the skin using a patting motion.
		2. To allow the client to apply general principles of skin treatment in the home environment.
		
		  a. To promote clearing of lesions.
		    ■ To enhance compliance. Therapeutic baths or showers serve to remove topical medications, hydrate the skin, facilitate débridement of loose scales, and deliver therapeutic agents.
		    ■ To remove any loose scale. Rough washing can precipitate the Koebner phenomenon.
		    ■ To prevent increased erythema and itching caused by use of hot water.
		    ■ To prevent brisk rubbing of the skin, which can precipitate the Koebner phenomenon.

continued

CLIENT CARE PLAN ∎ The Client with Psoriasis Vulgaris *continued*

Goal/Outcome Criteria	Interventions	Rationales
	Nursing Diagnosis 1: Impaired Skin Integrity Related to Psoriatic Lesions	
	b. Steroid creams, ointments, and lotions.	b. To promote clearing of lesions.
	■ Explain the purpose of topical steroid preparations.	■ To enhance compliance. Steroids are anti-inflammatory and also inhibit skin cell growth, thereby promoting flattening of lesions.
	■ Explain the purpose of placing steroid preparations under occlusion if ordered.	■ To enhance compliance. Occlusion increases percutaneous absorption of steroid preparations and intensifies the treatment.
	■ Teach the client why certain vehicles are used only in specific body areas.	■ To prevent injury. Application of ointments to skin fold areas can promote maceration and folliculitis.
	■ Stress the importance of using topical steroids only under the direction of the physician.	■ To minimize side effects, which are associated with long-term use of potent topical steroids. Close monitoring is required. Potent steroids should never be used on the face or in skin fold areas.
	■ Demonstrate proper application of steroid lotions or gels to the scalp.	■ To enhance compliance. Application is facilitated by having the client part the hair in segments and apply the lotion to the parts. Scalp treatments are best applied to a freshly washed scalp.
	c. Tar preparations.	c. To promote clearing of lesions.
	■ Explain the purpose of the use of tar in conjunction with UVB light.	■ To enhance compliance. UVB light inhibits skin cell growth and tends to result in longer remission times.
	■ Demonstrate how to apply tar ointment in a thin layer in the direction of hair growth.	■ To minimize plugging and irritation of the hair follicle, which can result in tar folliculitis.
	■ Reinforce the need to reapply tar frequently during the day to maintain an adequate amount of medication on the lesions.	■ To promote healing. Tar tends to rub off onto pajamas and bed linen with movement.
	d. Anthralin.	d. To promote clearing of chronic lesions.
	■ Explain the purpose of anthralin therapy.	■ To enhance compliance. Anthralin ia a potent irritant that inhibits skin cell growth and helps flatten chronic lesions.
	■ Demonstrate proper application of anthralin to chronic lesions only, avoiding normal skin and not exceeding the recommended treatment time.	■ To prevent chemical burns of normal skin and lesions resulting in Koebner's phenomenon. It should never be applied to acute lesions.

CLIENT CARE PLAN ■ The Client with Psoriasis Vulgaris *continued*

Goal/Outcome Criteria	Interventions	Rationales

Nursing Diagnosis 1: Impaired Skin Integrity Related to Psoriatic Lesions

Goal/Outcome Criteria	Interventions	Rationales
	■ Teach client to avoid unnecessary activity, protect clothing and furniture, and avoid touching lesions during therapy.	■ To prevent permanent staining. A "no touch" approach is best to avoid spreading the agent to uninvolved areas or inadvertently introducing it into the eyes.
	e. UVB treatments.	e. To enhance treatment with topical preparations.
	■ Explain the purpose of UVB treatments.	■ To enhance compliance. UVB treatment inhibits skin cell growth and promotes flattening of the lesions.
	■ Instruct the client to notify a nurse or physician if burning or tenderness occurs in association with light treatments.	■ To minimize erythema and prevent cellular damage.
	■ Teach safety precautions associated with UVB treatments.	■ To prevent injury. Safety goggles must be worn during treatment to prevent eye injury. The client must avoid direct contact with the bulbs to prevent burns.
	f. PUVA treatments.	f. To enhance treatment with topical preparations.
	■ Explain why psoralen needs to be ingested 2 h before the UVA treatment.	■ To enhance compliance. Psoralen is a photosensitizing agent that, when taken by mouth, travels to the skin and increases the effects of the UVA light.
	■ Instruct the client to notify a nurse or physician if swelling, redness, or tenderness of the skin occurs after treatment.	■ To detect and prevent recurrence of overexposure to UVA light, which can result in severe burns.
	■ Teach safety precautions associated with PUVA treatments.	■ To prevent injury. Safety glasses must be worn during treatment and dark glasses worn for the entire day after taking psoralen because of photosensitivity and the possibility of corneal damage.
	g. Methotrexate.	g. To promote clearing of recalcitrant lesions.
	■ Explain the purpose of methotrexate.	■ To enhance compliance. Methotrexate is a chemotherapeutic drug used in low-dose form to treat psoriasis that does not respond to other forms of therapy or that is particularly disabling.

continued

Goal/Outcome Criteria	Interventions	Rationales
	Nursing Diagnosis 1: Impaired Skin Integrity Related to Psoriatic Lesions	
	■ Teach precautions to take during methotrexate therapy: avoid excessive alcohol intake, avoid taking aspirin and aspirin-like drugs, and practice contraception while receiving therapy.	■ To prevent injury. Salicylates interact with methotrexate, and excessive alcohol intake can promote the toxic effects of the drug. A mutagenic risk is associated with therapy.
	■ Teach signs and symptoms that need to be brought to the attention of a physician, specifically jaundice or increased bleeding tendency.	■ To detect liver toxicity.
■ Demonstrates skills necessary to perform skin care independently or with a minimum of assistance.	3. Have the client perform return demonstration of skin care practices and exhibit progress toward independence in following the skin care regimen.	3. To ensure that the client will assume responsibility for care and gain confidence in self-care activities.
■ Actively participates in planning and self-care activities during hospitalization.	a. Prepare a schedule of the treatment regimen, review the schedule with the client, and leave it at the bedside for easy reference.	a. To minimize confusion.
	b. Assess the client's level of compliance with the scheduled treatments daily.	b. To detect problems with acceptance of the diagnosis or lack of understanding of expectations.
	c. Assist the client in applying topical medications to difficult-to-reach lesions as needed.	c. To promote healing. Depending on distribution of lesions, the client may need assistance. A family member can also be taught how to assist.
	d. Before discharge from the hospital, have the client describe plans for treatment in the home environment.	d. To evaluate readiness for discharge. Outpatient treatment usually involves a less complex skin care regimen, but requires planning of treatment and ADL.
■ Describes the expected appearance of the lesions as they clear.	4. Teach the client how to monitor response to treatment.	4. To detect progress toward clearing of lesions.
	a. Have the client assess the distribution, color, and thickness of plaques on admission and daily thereafter.	a. To detect gradual flattening of the plaques with central cleaning and less scaling, which indicate healing. Color should progress from red to brown to normal color. Lower extremities clear last.
	b. Have the client assess skin areas daily for erythema associated with burning or tenderness, folliculitis, or spread of psoriatic lesions.	b. To detect complications associated with treatment.
	c. Reinforce that response to treatment is usually rapid at first, then may slow.	c. To minimize frustration if progress slows. Clients need to know that this is a normal response.

Goal/Outcome Criteria	Interventions	Rationales
Nursing Diagnosis 2: Pain Related to Pruritus		

Client will experience relief of discomfort associated with pruritus.
■ States that pruritus is relieved or controlled.
	1. Assess factors that can contribute to pruritus:
	  a. Overly dry environment.
	  b. Bathing in water that is too hot.
	  c. Use of harsh soaps.
	  d. Time between treatments when skin is not being lubricated by a topical agent.
	2. Teach the client methods to avoid contributing factors:
	  a. Using room humidifier when available.
	  b. Using tepid to warm water when bathing.
	  c. Avoiding the use of harsh soaps.
	  d. Keeping the skin lubricated with petrolatum when the skin is not covered with another agent (e.g., after bath, during light treatment).
	3. Medicate the client as needed.
	  a. Administer antihistamines as ordered.
	  b. Instruct the client to contact a nurse if pruritus persists.
	  c. Assess the need for bath additives and notify the physician as indicated.
	4. Assess for complications associated with pruritus and its treatment.
	  a. Examine the skin daily for evidence of excoriation.
	  b. Observe the client for signs of lethargy associated with antihistamine use, and, if present, have the physician consider adjusting the dose accordingly.
		1. To minimize causative factors, which will minimize pruritus.
		
		2. To control pruritus.
		
		3. To control pruritus by maintaining adequate blood levels of antihistamines and to provide additional relief with bath additives.
		
		4. To prevent excoriation and initiation of the Koebner phenomenon. Overmedication with antihistamines can result in lethargy and diminished reaction time. A larger dose given at bedtime helps to maintain adequate blood levels when drowsiness is welcome.

Nursing Diagnosis 3: Ineffective Individual Coping Related to Primary Stress Factors		

Client will gain insight into emotional factors that may have precipitated the flare.
■ Discusses possible emotional problems that could have precipitated the psoriatic flare.
■ Identifies ways to minimize identified stressors.
	1. Assess verbal and nonverbal cues that indicate a possible precipitating stress factor.
	  a. Observe the client's reaction to visitors or significant others.
	  b. Explore situations that the client perceives as contributing to a worsening of symptoms.
	  c. Observe for reluctance to discuss a subject or a tendency to change the subject during conversation.
	2. Considering the client's degree of insight, explore with the client alternative ways to minimize stress (e.g., physical exercise, relaxation techniques, and professional counseling).
		1. To detect the presence of a stress factor. Not all clients are able to relate a stressful occurrence to their flare. Many clients may be unwilling to discuss stress factors or unconsciously suppress them.
		
		2. To promote coping with stress. Client must be willing to acknowledge stress before intervention can be therapeutic.

continued

CLIENT CARE PLAN ■ The Client with Psoriasis Vulgaris *continued*

Goal/Outcome Criteria	Interventions	Rationales
Nursing Diagnosis 4: Body Image Disturbance Related to Skin Disease		

Client will experience enhanced self-esteem.
■ Interacts with staff, visitors, and other psoriatic clients.
	1. Encourage interaction with other clients who have psoriasis.
	  a. Introduce the psoriatic client to other clients with the same or similar skin problems.
	  b. Hold group discussions including family members to address common problems and concerns.
	  c. Reinforce that psoriasis is *not* contagious.
	2. Communicate acceptance of the client and the skin problem.
	  a. Use touch frequently, avoiding gloves when possible.
	  b. Encourage the client to verbalize feelings regarding altered body image.
	  c. Reinforce that, with time and treatment, the skin returns to normal appearance without scarring.
		1. To promote self-acceptance. Psoriasis is a temporarily disfiguring skin disease that involves body areas not always covered by clothes. In-hospital treatment promotes withdrawal from socialization owing to the unpleasant appearance and odor of tar and fear of contagion.
		2. To promote self-esteem by initiating interaction with the client.

have an unpleasant odor. Although the response to treatment is usually delayed when tar ointments are used, remission time after clearing is reported to be longer than with steroid preparations. This is probably due in part to the rebound effect associated with discontinuation of steroid therapy. Tar preparations are sometimes combined with salicylic acid or a similar keratolytic (keratin-dissolving) agent that helps hasten the removal of scales.

Topical therapy with anthralin (dithranol), a hydrocarbon with similar action to that of tar, is also effective for chronic psoriasis. It is used in a variety of potencies alone and in combination with coal tar baths and UV light *(Ingram's technique)*. The stronger concentrations of anthralin cause staining and skin irritation.

High-potency anthralin, suspended in a stiff paste, is applied to individual lesions by the nurse for short periods of time, not exceeding 2 hours. Short-contact therapy is gaining popularity as a practical way to treat chronic psoriasis at home or in day care facilities. Progress of treatment is monitored by the degree of anthralin staining to psoriatic lesions. Because anthralin is a strong irritant and can cause chemical burns, the nurse observes for local tissue reaction and prevents inadvertent contact with uninvolved skin. Anthralin is not indicated for the treatment of acute, spreading psoriasis because of the probability of inducing the Koebner phenomenon.

Ultraviolet light therapy. UV radiation is a physical agent commonly employed as a topical treatment in many skin conditions, including psoriasis. Of the broad spectrum of electromagnetic radiation that reaches the earth's surface from the sun, the UV spectrum includes those wavelengths between x-ray and visible light. Ultraviolet B (UVB) light, which has a comparatively shorter wavelength and therefore produces more energy, is responsible for the obvious biologic effects of the sun, such as burning. Ultraviolet A (UVA) light, on the other hand, emits a lower level of energy, requiring longer exposure time before cellular destruction occurs. Although the sun is the least expensive source of UV radiation, control of both availability and intensity in skin treatment is best obtained with artificial light sources. These sources include high-intensity mercury vapor lamps or specially constructed cabinets containing vertical UV fluorescent tubes.

The therapeutic action of UVB light is attributed to its action in decreasing epidermal growth rate, resulting from biochemical inhibition of deoxyribonucleic acid (DNA) synthesis. Artificial UVB light exposure is often used in the inpatient setting in conjunction with tar, a photosensitizing agent, for treatment of extensive psoriasis *(Goeckerman's treatment)*.

In general, UV therapy is governed by the potency and distance of the source from the skin, as well as the exposure time. In UVB therapy, potency and distance remain constant and the time of exposure is gradually increased to achieve a minimal erythema, or mild sunburn effect, without burning or tenderness. Skin type, ranging from fair to darkly pigmented, reflects the client's susceptibility to burning and is the basis for determining initial and subsequent exposure times. Because of the extremely high intensity of most artificial UVB light sources, daily treatments are measured in seconds of exposure; eye protection during treatment is required. Onset of the erythema response is seen 6 to 8 hours after treatment.

The nurse carefully inspects the skin daily for signs of overexposure, especially to body areas that are usually covered with clothing. Complaints of tenderness on palpation, combined with clinical signs of severe erythema or vesicle and bullae formation, require prompt notification of the physician before therapy is resumed. In less severe overexposure, the physician orders local application of sunscreens or requests that the areas be draped with towels during treatments until symptoms resolve. A burn can result in Koebner's phenomenon in some clients, causing a flare of disease and prolonging hospitalization.

Psoralen and UVA *(PUVA)* treatments are more commonly employed on an outpatient basis (Fig. 40–5). PUVA requires the ingestion of a photosensitizing agent, psoralen, 2 hours before exposure to UVA light. The psoralen interacts with various cellular components in the skin, causing absorption of the longer-wavelength energy and photochemical reactions that inhibit epidermal growth. Because UVA produces less energy than UVB light, the onset of erythema and pigmentation may be delayed as long as 96 hours after exposure. Therefore, to monitor for possible side effects, treatments are limited to two to three times a week and are not given on consecutive days. Exposure is measured in energy units called joules and is gradually increased until tanning occurs. As with UVB exposure, dosage corrections are adjusted according to the erythema reaction of normal skin, as well as the response of psoriatic lesions. The nurse observes for generalized erythema with edema and tenderness, which requires interrup-

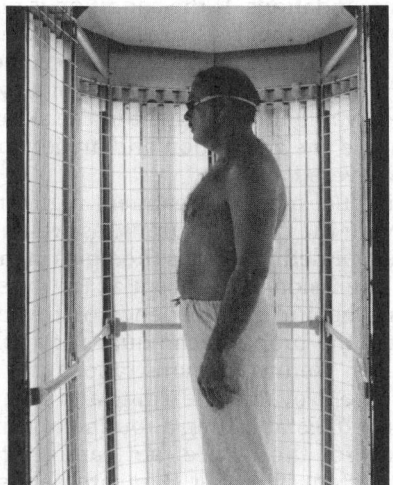

Figure 40–5

Client receiving PUVA treatment. (Courtesy of the Department of Dermatology, Baylor College of Medicine, Houston, TX.)

tion in treatment until symptoms subside. The strong photosensitizing properties of psoralen necessitate the wearing of dark glasses during treatment and for the remainder of the day. Long-term side effects of both UVB therapy and PUVA include premature aging of the skin, actinic keratosis, and increased incidence of cutaneous malignancies.

Systemic therapy. In rare situations, clients have severe and disabling psoriasis that is resistant to topical therapy. In these instances, systemic treatment with a cytostatic (slows cell growth) agent is warranted. Methotrexate is a folic acid antagonist with antipsoriatic action directed toward interruption of the epidermal cell growth cycle. Because of the hepatotoxic side effects of methotrexate, a liver biopsy is indicated before the initiation of therapy and yearly thereafter. Relatively small doses are required to obtain clearing of lesions. This last-resort treatment is contraindicated in the presence of liver damage, bone marrow depression, impaired renal function, or a poor nutritional status.

Pain

Planning: client goals. The primary goal for this diagnosis is that the client will experience relief of pruritic discomfort associated with skin inflammation. If this goal is not met, excoriation can initiate the Koebner phenomenon and result in spread of the lesions to previously uninvolved areas.

Interventions: nonsurgical management. In addition to the scaling associated with psoriasis, an added drying effect on the skin is caused by light treatments and frequent bathing. Interventions to minimize drying include those discussed earlier, with emphasis on providing antihistamine therapy and maintaining adequate skin lubrication between treatments.

Ineffective Individual Coping

Planning: client goals. The primary goal for this diagnosis is that the client will gain insight into emotional factors that may have precipitated the flare. The gaining of insight will not occur during a single hospitalization; it is a gradual process that requires an acceptance of the stressor and a willingness on the part of the client to readjust.

Interventions: nonsurgical management. If a possible precipitating stress factor is identified, the nurse encourages the client to talk about it. It is important to remember that not all clients are able to relate a stressful occurrence as a factor in the flare. Furthermore, many clients suppress the problem or are unwilling to discuss it. The nurse observes the client during unguarded moments and notes reactions to visitors, expressions of joy, or irritability. If the client is suppressing a problem, periods of silence can occur if a subject is particularly bothersome. Skin symptoms also give a clue to the problem. One client reported an increased tingling in his skin accompanied by pruritus on particularly busy days at work. Further investigation revealed that he was not taking needed breaks on those days, but continuing to work while eating at his desk.

After a client is willing to acknowledge that stress may play a role in the disease, nursing intervention is aimed at assisting the client to find ways of dealing with the stress. Relaxation techniques and physical exercise are helpful for some clients. If the problem is severe enough, professional counseling may be indicated before successful control of the psoriasis can be accomplished (see Chap. 6).

Body Image Disturbance

Planning: client goals. The primary goal for this diagnosis is that the client will increase self-esteem. If this goal is not met, behaviors consistent with withdrawal from social interactions are observed.

Interventions: nonsurgical management. Often, problems of self-esteem arise not only from the presence of skin lesions, but also from the unpleasantness associated with some of the treatment modalities. Tar not only looks dirty, it has an extremely objectionable odor! Bed linen and pajamas become stained, further discouraging social interaction. The nurse promotes contact with other clients who have similar problems. Group discussions involving family members are often helpful in increasing the socialization process. In addition, the use of touch with these clients takes on an added significance. For example, the nurse shakes the client's hand during introduction or places a hand on the client's shoulder when explaining a procedure. Gloves are not worn during these social interactions. Touch, more than any other gesture, communicates acceptance of the person and the skin problem.

■ Discharge Planning

Many clients can be taught to care for their psoriasis effectively in the home environment, thereby avoiding repeated hospitalizations. Also gaining in popularity are psoriasis day care centers where treatment times can be individualized to the client's needs and work schedules.

Home Care Preparation

Often, the client is encouraged to purchase a home light box, so that UVB treatments can continue in the privacy of the home. Portable units are available commercially or a clothes closet can be easily converted to a light cabinet. The advantages of home light therapy are many. After the psoriasis has cleared, controlled UVB exposure once or twice a week can help maintain remission. If psoriasis recurs in spite of intermittent exposure, a modified form of the hospital tar treatment can be initiated promptly before the flares get out of hand. An

added advantage is that scheduling of light treatments in the home environment is more flexible, allowing the clients freedom to return to work, as well as plan other activities around skin care.

As might be expected, the decision by the physician to recommend the purchase of a home unit depends on the severity of skin disease, the pattern of recurrences, and the individual client's compliance with skin care recommendations. During hospitalization, the nurse assesses each client's knowledge and skills in relation to the medical regimen. If the purchase of a home light unit is recommended, the nurse further assesses the client's financial resources. Although this one-time purchase can prevent future hospitalizations, most insurance companies require a letter of medical justification and provide only partial reimbursement for this equipment.

Client/Family Education

The teaching plan for a client with psoriasis includes knowledge of factors that precipitate flares, rationale of the treatment regimen, and proper application and side effects of topical therapeutic agents. Knowledge of the disease and skill in managing the skin care regimen depends on when the disease was first diagnosed and past experiences with flare. Clients with newly diagnosed psoriasis need extensive education with frequent reinforcement throughout their hospitalization to gain confidence in managing their condition. On the other hand, clients who have experienced repeated hospitalizations for psoriasis are usually quite adept at discussing their skin care needs and demonstrating proper skin care techniques.

When discussing etiology, the nurse emphasizes that, although no cure is currently available, control of psoriasis is possible through identification of precipitating factors and personal motivation to comply with treatment recommendations. If the condition is newly diagnosed, the nurse further reassures the client that the skin will return to its normal appearance when the psoriasis clears. Warning the client that periods of slow progress with no observable improvement in the skin is normal may help avoid the frustration and anxiety often associated with severe flares.

The individual medical treatment regimen depends on how severe the current flare is, as well as how the client has responded to various therapies in the past. On the client's admission to the hospital, the nurse explains the rationale behind the sequence of treatments and demonstrates the proper techniques for application of topical agents. Return demonstrations by the client allow the nurse to evaluate learning and give reinforcement as needed. Establishing a routine of skin care can be confusing for the novice, but careful attention to detail is important if proper skin care habits are to be formed and optimal results obtained. To minimize confusion, the nurse sits down with the client and writes out a step-by-step schedule with the specific time when each medication or treatment is due. This schedule is left at the bedside and serves as a reminder to the client until the routine becomes familiar. Although the complexity of hospital treatment regimens usually exceeds the daily care required to continue treatment at home, an understanding of the principles of skin care is important if the client is going to maintain control over this chronic skin disease.

Psychosocial Preparation

The nurse works with the client to obtain total independence in care before discharge from the hospital. The client's ability to participate in planning and assume accountability for the daily skin care regimen reflects the degree to which the client is coping with the diagnosis. Failure to comply with self-care activities alerts the nurse to the need for further psychologic assessment.

Problems related to poor self-concept are usually on the way to being resolved by the time discharge nears. When compared with skin appearance on admission to the hospital, the gradual flattening of the thick, unsightly lesions with the added visual enhancement of a total body tan is welcomed by the client. The nurse offers reassurance that any remaining lesions or areas of altered pigmentation eventually return to normal with continued care after discharge. The client needs to consider how skin care requirements can best be accomplished at home while meeting job and household responsibilities. For example, if a home light unit is purchased, the client may decide to wake up earlier in the morning so that a skin treatment can be done before working hours. On the other hand, clients expected to visit the dermatologist's office several times a week for light exposure need to make specific arrangements with their employer.

Health Care Resources

Except in the case of elderly or severely debilitated clients, home treatment of psoriasis rarely requires the assistance of a visiting nurse. Monitoring of progress is usually accomplished by frequent visits to the dermatologist. Less severe flares can be easily managed on an outpatient basis or by having the client visit a local psoriasis day care center.

Additional information about psoriasis and its treatment can be obtained by having the client contact the National Psoriasis Foundation. This foundation publishes a quarterly newsletter and annual report, which provides updates on research and treatment. In addition, information is available on how clients can correspond with other psoriatics or obtain discount medications through a mail-order pharmacy service.

 Evaluation

On the basis of the identified nursing diagnoses, the nurse evaluates the care of the client with psoriasis. After inpatient teaching, the expected outcomes include that the psoriatic client

1. Discusses the rationale and potential side effects of the medical treatment regimen
2. Actively participates in planning and self-care activities during hospitalization
3. Demonstrates skills necessary to perform skin care after discharge
4. States that pruritus is relieved or controlled
5. Identifies factors that could exacerbate a flare and avoids them
6. Discusses possible emotional factors that could have precipitated the psoriatic flare
7. Explores with the nurse ways to minimize identified stressors
8. Interacts with staff members, visitors, and other psoriatic clients
9. Describes the expected appearance of the lesions as they clear

CANCER

OVERVIEW

Although there are a number of factors associated with the development of skin cancers, overexposure to sunlight is the major cause of cutaneous malignancy. Because sun damage is an age-related skin finding, screening for suspicious lesions is an integral part of routine physical assessment of the elderly. Although prevention remains the treatment of choice, early diagnosis is the key to timely intervention and cure.

The most common skin cancers include actinic or solar keratosis, squamous cell carcinoma, basal cell carcinoma, and malignant melanoma. The neoplasms originate in different cell types of the epidermis and vary in their potential to metastasize to adjacent tissues.

Pathophysiology

Actinic keratoses are actually premalignant lesions involving the keratinocytes of the epidermis. These lesions are quite common in individuals with chronically sun-damaged skin and, in spite of treatment, may continue to appear spontaneously throughout the latter years of life. Progression to squamous cell carcinoma is possible if the lesions are untreated.

Squamous cell carcinomas are malignant neoplasms of the epidermis characterized by local invasion and potential for metastasis. Lesions on the ear, the lip, and the external genitalia are more inclined to early invasion with metastasis via the lymphatics than those found elsewhere on the body. In addition to sun exposure, chronic epithelial damage resulting from repeated injury or irritation predisposes to this malignancy.

Basal cell carcinomas arise in the basal cell layer of the epidermis. Early malignant lesions often go unnoticed, and, although metastasis is rare, underlying tissue destruction can progress to include vital structures, such as bone, blood vessels, and cartilage. Genetic predisposition and chronic irritation are risk factors in the development of lesions; however, UV radiation remains the primary carcinogen.

Melanomas are pigmented malignant lesions originating in the melanin-producing cells of the epidermis. Risk factors include genetic predisposition and the presence of one or more precursor lesions that resemble unusual moles. This skin cancer is highly metastatic, and survival is dependent on early diagnosis and treatment.

Etiology

As mentioned earlier, skin cancers are largely age-related diseases, resulting from the cumulative effects of sunlight throughout the life span. Fair-skinned individuals with blond or red hair have less protective pigmentation to prevent penetration of the skin by UV radiation. The result is an increased susceptibility to burning and a greater risk of injury and cellular alteration. Although the most common form of UV radiation is natural sunlight, repeated exposure to artificial sources of radiation, such as with radiotherapy treatments or the use of tanning salons, can also cause skin cancer.

In addition to UV radiation, occupational hazards present an added risk to some clients. Most chemical carcinogens are carefully controlled; however, repeated skin exposure to arsenic, pesticides, and similar carcinogenic agents can result in epidermal skin cell mutation. The occupations at highest risk include farmers, miners, and metal workers.

Finally, scar tissue formed in chronic, slow-healing wounds, such as a burn wound, is susceptible to the growth of an uncommon type of squamous cell carcinoma called *Marjolin's ulcer*. Although the exact mechanism of cell mutation is not known, alteration in local immune response is thought to play a role.

Incidence

The incidence of skin cancer is highest among the light-skinned races and men older than 60 years, with almost 50% of the population having experienced a skin cancer by the age of 65 years (Kopf, 1988). Geographic prevalence favors the Sunbelt, where sun-bathing is a common recreational activity. The incidence is higher among individuals who work outdoors and have an added risk of occupational exposure to arsenic or other chemical carcinogens. Clients who have sustained burns or those with chronic leg ulcers are also at greater risk for developing Marjolin's ulcer. The incidence of malignant melanoma has rapidly increased during the past 30 years; melanoma accounts for 2% of all cancers and 1% of all cancer deaths (Lookingbill & Marks, 1986). A concomitant rise in the incidence of diagnosed skin cancers in low-risk individuals is attributed to grad-

ual destruction of the earth's ozone layer, which filters cancer-causing rays.

PREVENTION

Unlike many malignancies, skin cancer is a preventable disease that seldom receives any attention until treatment is warranted. Evidence suggests that skin habits taught in childhood could have a major influence on the development of skin cancer in an adult.

In addition to the daily use of sunscreens and avoidance of overexposure to the sun, preventive measures are directed toward early detection of potentially dangerous lesions. Monthly self-examination of the skin surfaces in susceptible individuals greatly reduces the associated risks and minimizes the potentially disfiguring effects of surgery. Many clients avoid routine self-assessment owing to fear of what might be discovered.

A large number of changes in skin appearance that occur with aging are unrelated to cancer. Knowing what is normal and understanding the significance of early detection can often prevent unnecessary anxiety. After monthly inspection of warts, moles, birthmarks, and scars, warning signs that need to be brought to the attention of a physician include the following:

1. A change in the color of a lesion, especially if it darkens or shows evidence of spreading
2. A change in the size of a lesion, especially rapid growth
3. A change in the shape of a lesion, such as a sharp border becoming irregular or a flat lesion becoming raised
4. Redness or swelling of the skin around a lesion
5. A change in sensation, especially itching or increased tenderness of a lesion
6. A change in the character of a lesion, such as oozing, crusting, bleeding, or scaling

COLLABORATIVE MANAGEMENT

 Assessment

History

When taking a history from a client with suspected skin cancer, the nurse elicits information to confirm the presence of any risk factors. In addition to age and race, data to collect from the client include any *family history of skin cancer* and any *past surgeries for removal of skin growths. Recent changes in the size, color, or sensation of any mole, birthmark, wart, or scar* are also significant. The nurse verifies the role of repeated sun exposure by inquiring about the *geographic regions where the client has lived and is currently residing* and *occupational and recreational activities* in relation to sun exposure. Finally, an occupational history of *exposure to chemical carcinogens* (e.g., arsenic, coal tar, pitch, radioactive waste, and radium) is explored.

In addition to assessing for high-risk factors, the nurse inquires about any skin growths that are subject to repeated irritation by the rubbing of clothes against them. Although the role of chronic inflammation and injury in the development of skin malignancy is not well understood, most physicians prefer to remove irritated warts or moles as a preventive measure.

Physical Assessment: Clinical Manifestations

The skin cancers vary in their appearance and distribution. In general, the majority of cancerous lesions are found in sun-exposed areas of the body; however, skin inspection should include the *entire* skin surface. The nurse systematically examines the skin for any *unusual lesions*, paying particular attention to the appearance of moles, warts, birthmarks, and scars. Hair-bearing areas of the body, such as the scalp and genitalia, are also examined. Palpation is used to determine the surface texture of lesions. As any normal or suspicious growth is noted, the nurse documents the location, size, color, and surface characteristics, as well as any subjective reports of associated tenderness or itching. The accompanying Key Features of Disease summarizes important features of common skin cancers.

Psychosocial Assessment

Many clients with skin cancer are unaware of the lesion or choose to ignore it, either because of fear of cancer or failure to recognize the significance of the skin change. In addition, elderly clients often have poor vision and are unable to see the lesions. The nurse assesses the client's understanding of the diagnosis and associated risk factors. Reactions to a diagnosis of skin cancer may vary from extreme anxiety to hopelessness, even when such reactions are unwarranted. If the diag-

KEY FEATURES OF DISEASE ■ Important Features of Common Skin Cancers

Skin Cancer	Clinical Manifestations	Distribution	Course
Actinic keratosis (premalignant)	Small (1–10 mm) macule or papule with dry, rough, adherent yellow or brown scale Base may be erythematous Associated with yellow, wrinkled weather-beaten skin Thick indurated keratoses more likely to be malignant	Cheeks, temples, forehead, ears, neck, backs of hands, and forearms	May disappear spontaneously or reappear after treatment. Slow progression to squamous cell carcinoma is possible.
Squamous cell carcinoma	Firm, nodular lesion topped with a crust or with a central area of ulceration Indurated margins Fixation to underlying tissue with deep invasion	Sun-exposed areas, especially head, neck, and lower lip Sites of chronic irritation or injury (e.g., scars, irradiated skin, burns, and leg ulcers)	Rapid invasion with metastasis via the lymphatics occurs in 10% of cases. Larger tumors are more prone to metastasis.
Basal cell carcinoma	Pearly papule with a central crater and rolled, waxy borders Telangiectasias and pigment flecks visible on close inspection	Sun-exposed areas, especially head, neck, and central portion of face	Metastasis is rare. May cause local tissue destruction. 50% recurrence rate related to inadequate treatment.
Melanoma	Irregularly shaped, pigmented papule or plaque Variegated colors, with red, white, and blue tones	Can occur anywhere on the body, especially where nevi (moles) or birthmarks are evident Commonly found on upper back and lower legs Soles of feet and palms in Asians and Blacks	Horizontal growth phase followed by vertical growth phase. Rapid invasion and metastasis with high morbidity and mortality.

nosis of invasive or metastatic skin cancer is confirmed, the nurse remains sensitive to the client's fear of disfigurement.

Laboratory Findings

Punch, shave, or excisional biopsy of suspicious lesions is necessary to confirm the diagnosis of a malignancy. In the case of actinic keratosis, diagnosis is usually based on clinical findings, with biopsy indicated only for thick, indurated lesions.

 ### Analysis: Nursing Diagnosis

The typical client with skin cancer is elderly and is admitted to the hospital for treatment of other medical problems. The lesion is often first detected by the nurse who is performing an assessment or assisting with personal hygiene.

Common Diagnoses

The nursing diagnoses commonly found in clients with skin cancer include

1. Impaired skin integrity related to premalignant or malignant skin lesions
2. Anxiety related to fear of death or disfigurement

Additional Diagnoses

In addition to the common diagnoses, the client may have one or more of the following diagnoses:

1. Potential for infection related to surgical intervention
2. Body image disturbance related to surgical excision of malignant lesions
3. Ineffective individual coping related to invasive or metastatic skin cancer
4. Hopelessness related to the diagnosis of invasive malignant melanoma
5. Knowledge deficit related to lack of information about or unclear explanation of the treatment regimen

 ### Planning and Implementation

The plan of care for the client with skin cancer focuses on the common nursing diagnoses. Additional diagnoses are considered, depending on the size and severity of the malignancy and the extent of surgical intervention.

Impaired Skin Integrity

Planning: client goals. The major goals for this diagnosis are that the client will (1) maintain skin integrity by

prompt medical intervention and (2) minimize complications related to treatment modalities.

Interventions: nonsurgical management. Nonsurgical treatment modalities for skin cancers include drug therapy and radiation therapy. The decision to choose any one modality is based on the type and severity of the skin cancer, the location of the lesion, the age of the client, and general health considerations.

Drug therapy. Topical chemotherapy with 5-fluorouracil cream is reserved for treatment of multiple actinic keratoses or, in rare instances, widespread superficial basal cell carcinoma that would require several surgical procedures to eradicate. The medication is applied sparingly twice a day to the obvious areas of sundamaged skin, resulting in a therapeutic inflammation of the actinic lesions. Therapy is continued for several weeks, during which time the treated areas become increasingly tender and inflamed as the lesions crust, ooze, and erode. The nurse prepares the client for an unsightly appearance during therapy and offers frequent reassurance that the cosmetic result of topical treatment is positive. After discontinuation of treatment, cool compresses and topical corticosteroid preparations help to decrease inflammation and promote comfort.

Systemic chemotherapeutic agents are rarely indicated in the treatment of cutaneous malignancy. Occasional use of these agents is seen in disease with poor prognosis, such as advanced metastatic melanoma. The response rate to chemotherapy alone is only about 20% in metastatic melanoma, with less than 5% showing complete disappearance of the disease (Sober et al., 1986).

Radiation therapy. Radiation therapy of malignant skin lesions is limited to elderly clients with large, deeply invasive basal cell tumors and those who are poor risks for surgery. In addition, the gradual skin changes associated with radiation therapy and the increased chance of initiating a new cancer with repeated exposure have fewer implications in the elderly than in younger clients. Primary malignant melanoma is resistant to radiation therapy; however, radiation therapy has proved of some value in treatment of metastatic disease when used in combination with systemic corticosteroids.

Interventions: surgical management. Surgical intervention ranges from local treatment of individual lesions, with minimal discomfort and positive cosmetic results, to massive excision of large areas of the skin.

Cryosurgery. This technique involves the local application of liquid nitrogen ($-200°$ C) to isolated lesions, causing cell death and tissue destruction. Local anesthesia is seldom needed, as only minor discomfort is experienced during the procedure. However, the nurse prepares the client for swelling and increased tenderness of the treated area when the skin thaws. Tissue freezing is followed in 1 or 2 days by hemorrhagic blister formation. Most physicians prefer that the blisters remain intact, as they will progressively flatten and peel away when healing is complete in 2 to 3 weeks. The nurse instructs the client to clean the treatment sites with hydrogen peroxide to prevent secondary infection. A topical antibiotic preparation may also be ordered.

Curettage and electrodesiccation. In small lesions with well-defined clinical borders, curettage and electrodesiccation are used to destroy the cancerous cells while minimizing damage to the surrounding uninvolved tissue. After a local anesthetic is administered, a dermal curette with a curved, semisharp blade is used to scrape away the cancerous tissue. The difference in consistency between the softness of the tumor and the hard, normal collagen beneath allows the physician to define the tumor margins by feel with a relatively high degree of accuracy.

After curettage is complete, electrodesiccation of the resulting wound is performed. An electric probe is placed on the wound surface and malignant remnants of the tumor are destroyed by thermal and mechanical energy. Electrodesiccation also provides hemostasis, and many physicians elect to reverse the above procedure, cauterizing the tumor before removing it with the curette.

Wounds treated by curettage and electrodesiccation are allowed to heal by second intention. Scarring is usually minimal owing to the superficial nature of well-differentiated, noninvasive tumors. The nurse instructs the client in the care of the wound, including cleaning, the use of any antibacterial medications, and the application of dressings as dictated by the physician. Potential complications of treatment include secondary infection of the wound and possible recurrence of the cancer if all of the malignant tissue is not destroyed.

Excision. Large or poorly defined skin cancers, recurrent tumors, and deeply invasive cancers require wide scalpel excision to remove the malignancy. If the size and location of the lesion permit, surgical excision with primary closure is the preferred therapy. If the tumor has already been removed several times or the surrounding skin has been damaged by radiation therapy, healing by second intention is indicated, so that the wound can be carefully monitored for recurrence of the cancer. Skin grafts and flaps are used to repair large defects with deep tissue destruction. Whatever the method of wound closure, the nurse selects interventions to promote an optimal environment for healing (see earlier).

A specialized form of excision used in the treatment of basal and squamous cell carcinomas is *Mohs' surgery.* This technique involves horizontal sectioning of the cancerous tissue in layers, with histologic examination of each layer to determine the exact location of residual tumor cells. Although the procedure is long and tedious, high cure rates and less sacrifice of healthy tissue is reported when compared with less meticulous excision.

Anxiety

Planning: client goals. The major goal for this diagnosis is that the client will experience minimal anxiety associated with fear of death or disfigurement.

Interventions: nonsurgical management. The nurse assesses the client's understanding of the diagnosis and associated risk factors. Many individuals automatically associate cancer with death, and fears may be out of proportion to the severity of the diagnosis. The nurse allays any unnecessary anxiety by encouraging the client to verbalize fears and by answering questions openly and honestly.

Clients who must undergo large excisions are often understandably anxious about the potential cosmetic outcome. Unrealistic expectations are not uncommon. The nurse assists the client to place concerns in the proper perspective. Surgical excision to remove invasive skin cancer is a lifesaving intervention. The method of surgical repair, as well as the possible need for reconstructive surgery in the future, must be guided by the severity of the cancer if a cure is to be obtained.

■ Discharge Planning

Client/Family Education

Client and family education is focused on wound care to minimize the potential for infection after destruction or removal of a cancerous skin growth. The type of care needed at home depends on the extent of surgical intervention and whether the resulting wound is closed by first or second intention. The nurse teaches the procedure for wound cleaning and applying dressings and observes return demonstrations as needed. Clinical manifestations of wound infection are reviewed in the discussion of trauma earlier.

Psychosocial Preparation

The client who has had a precancerous or cancerous lesion removed is often fearful that the cancer will return. The nurse directs this fear in a positive manner by emphasizing the high rate of cure with early detection and treatment. Preventive measures are emphasized, with family members included in the discussion when possible. The nurse reviews risk factors and suggests alternatives for avoiding overexposure to sunlight. Monthly skin inspection is encouraged, and warning signs are reviewed as needed. Compliance with regular skin self-inspection may be poor owing to the client's fear of discovering another lesion. Female clients may find it easiest to include skin inspection as part of their monthly breast self-examination. Spouses or sexual partners are encouraged to assist with the monitoring of areas not easily visualized by the client.

Health Care Resources

The need for follow-up in the home environment by a home care nurse depends on the extent of surgical intervention and the ability of the client to follow through with wound care recommendations. Often, family members are able to assist, especially if the client is elderly or has problems with vision. Frequent visits to the physician are indicated until healing is complete. Periodic re-examination is necessary to monitor for recurrence or to evaluate the need for cosmetic reconstruction.

Information for the general public about skin cancer, sun protection, and sunscreens is available through the Skin Cancer Foundation, a national nonprofit organization concerned solely with prevention and treatment.

 Evaluation

On the basis of the identified nursing diagnoses, the nurse evaluates the care of the client with skin cancer. The expected outcomes include that the client

1. States the risk factors associated with the development of skin cancer
2. Verbalizes fears associated with the diagnosis or planned interventions
3. Demonstrates skills needed to care for the wound in the home environment and complies with recommended treatments
4. Describes measures to prevent or minimize the risk of recurrence

By meeting the stated desired outcomes, risks associated with surgical intervention are minimized and the potential for recurrence of disease is diminished. In addition, any anxiety associated with fear of the unknown is alleviated.

PLASTIC AND RECONSTRUCTIVE SURGERY

OVERVIEW

The main purpose of plastic or reconstructive surgery is to correct functional defects and alter physical appearance, processes that directly influence a person's concept of self. Unlike a medical illness that is unexpected, plastic surgery is usually an elective procedure. Surgical intervention is sought by clients who are unable to perform ADL owing to an anatomic malformation or by those unsatisfied with their body image. Although a number of anatomic alterations can change a person's appearance, facial changes are the most visible and

therefore tend to have a greater impact on the client's sense of self.

Pathophysiology

In American society, the decision to have plastic surgery is frequently a response to established social and cultural norms. The client becomes self-conscious about unsightly scars, obvious facial lesions, disproportionate anatomic features, or changes in physical features associated with aging. In some instances, severe trauma or extensive surgical excision of soft tissue leads to acquired functional defects that warrant surgical correction. For example, breast reconstruction is commonly performed after radical mastectomy. This type of plastic surgery not only serves an aesthetic purpose for some clients, but also replaces lost anatomy and negates the need for a prosthesis.

Both skin trauma and the natural progression of some skin disorders can result in healing with obvious scar formation. For example, acne can cause facial scars ranging from ice pick–type pitting of the skin to extensive and deep defects. Burn scars are particularly disfiguring, often resulting in severe mutilation of facial features that require repeated surgeries to correct. In another example, poor healing of a surgical incision may result in an unsightly closure, requiring scar revision to obtain acceptable cosmetic results. In general, the degree of scar formation after tissue destruction depends on several factors, including the extent of tissue damage and the timing and method of wound closure. Extensive tissue trauma with infection and chronic inflammation is more likely to produce an unsightly scar than a carefully sutured clean laceration.

Benign facial lesions can contribute to an altered body image. Telangiectasias, pigmented nevi, birthmarks, keloids, or skin tumors may result in an uneven appearance of features or distract from the overall image. The extent to which any of these lesions can be considered unsightly or distracting depends on the number of lesions and their location.

It is not uncommon for clients to request plastic surgery as a remedy for the normal changes in skin appearance that occur with aging. Loss of skin elasticity and redistribution of adipose tissue is progressive and especially noticeable around the eyes, near the cheeks, and on the neck. Fine facial wrinkles of the periorbital and perioral skin are one of the first signs of aging, followed by gradual stretching and downward displacement of the soft tissue of the lower two-thirds of the face. Similar changes in skin texture contribute to wrinkling and flaccidity of skin on the upper extremities, the chest, the abdomen, buttocks, and thighs, a problem also seen after dramatic weight loss. In addition, balding and the gradual appearance of skin lesions associated with chronic sun exposure may cause the aging client concern.

Disproportionate anatomy is either developmental or acquired. For example, slight degrees of breast asymmetry are quite common. Significant discrepancies in breast size can occur if breast tissue fails to form at puberty or if congenital chest wall or skeletal deformities are present. Acquired breast asymmetries can result from trauma, inflammation, or neoplasm.

In rare cases, plastic surgery is used as a last resort to remove excess adipose tissue and striae-marked skin from clients who are obese. Diet control is the preferred treatment for obesity and is usually attempted before tissue excision is considered.

Etiology

The causes of the more common conditions associated with plastic surgery are presented in the sections dealing with aging, skin trauma, and specific skin disorders. In most cases, gradual changes in skin appearance occur throughout the life span, with more sudden alterations, such as severe nasal deformity or facial laceration, related to traumatic events. Congenital deformity can also occur. The degree of disfigurement with each condition is based entirely on subjective data—the client's perception of ideal body image.

Incidence

A distinctive feature of plastic surgery is that 85% to 90% of clients are female, whereas a majority of plastic surgeons are male. Because insurance plans rarely cover these procedures unless there is an associated functional defect, one would expect to find a majority of clients among the financially secure upper middle class.

COLLABORATIVE MANAGEMENT

 Assessment

History

When taking a history from a client who elects to have plastic surgery, the nurse is careful not to assume the reason for surgery on the basis of physical appearance. Often, what might appear to be unsightly to the nurse is of little concern to the client, who wishes to change something else. Besides actively listening and encouraging the client to verbalize, the nurse also observes for any nonverbal communication that might establish the emotional state of the individual or reveal frequently associated feelings of embarrassment or guilt. The nurse encourages the client to *describe the problem* in his/her own words, including *why the problem is bothersome* and *what the client expects as a result of the change.* An exploration of *past surgeries* and the *client's emotional reactions* to those surgeries may reveal a personality disorder that requires professional intervention before plastic surgery is considered. A *past and current history of medical problems,* including obesity and

trauma, is also important to better predict the amount of surgery needed to correct the defect and potential complications.

Physical Assessment: Clinical Manifestations

Clients seeking plastic surgery may have alterations in appearance ranging from minor to significant deformity. In general, physical alteration needs to be significant enough to warrant the risk of a surgical procedure. Depending on the location of the deformity, the client may need to disrobe before the examination. Many of these clients are embarrassed by their problem, and the nurse takes necessary steps to ensure privacy as needed.

The nurse begins the physical assessment by closely examining the area of involvement to determine the extent of the deformity. Having the client assume different postures, for example, normal sitting and standing postures, may provide better visualization of nonfacial defects. Depending on the presenting problem, the nurse notes any asymmetry of anatomic features, wrinkling or skin redundancy, scars or disfiguring skin marks, and obvious skin lesions.

Psychosocial Assessment

Of particular importance in the psychosocial assessment of the client is information related to the client's expectations of surgery. Often, those seeking reconstructive operations have unrealistic expectations or are uncertain about what they really want. For example, clients with minor deformities who are seeking perfection are sure to be disappointed. Those who are having an operation mainly because their spouse is requesting that they have it done are also poor candidates. A positive psychologic outlook before surgery is important if results are to be therapeutic.

Laboratory Findings

There are no specific laboratory findings associated with plastic surgery. Preoperative testing includes only those designated as standard by the hospital unless the client has a specific health problem.

 Analysis: Nursing Diagnosis

The typical client seeking consultation with a plastic surgeon is usually a young woman concerned about facial scarring or disproportionate anatomic features or an older woman who wishes to recapture youth. Similar diagnoses apply to clients undergoing plastic surgery for severe disfigurement or functional defects.

Common Diagnoses

The nursing diagnoses commonly found in clients undergoing cosmetic surgery are

1. Impaired skin integrity related to cosmetic surgery
2. Pain related to surgical incision and edema
3. Body image disturbance related to perceived or actual physical deformity

Additional Diagnoses

Depending on the degree of deformity and the client's perceived changes in body image, one or more of the following diagnoses may also apply:

1. Social isolation related to perceived or actual deformity
2. Sexual dysfunction related to poor body image
3. Ineffective individual coping related to severe disfigurement
4. Potential for infection related to impaired skin integrity
5. Knowledge deficit related to lack of information about or unclear explanation of the treatment regimen
6. Anxiety (mild) related to surgical procedure and expected results

 Planning and Implementation

Impaired Skin Integrity

Planning: client goals. Ironically, plastic surgery requires the inflicting of a potentially disfiguring wound to correct existing skin deformities. Although the final result is largely dependent on surgical technique, the goal is that the client will restore skin integrity and minimize complications associated with surgical intervention so that optimal healing and correction of the deformity can occur.

Interventions: surgical management. Depending on the planned intervention, either surgery is performed in the outpatient setting under local anesthesia or the client is hospitalized. The majority of clients scheduled for plastic surgery will have had several office consultations with their physician to discuss the planned intervention, possible complications, and postoperative expectations. The indications and complications of common cosmetic procedures are summarized in Table 40–6.

Many plastic surgeons use photography both as a visual aid when discussing the client's problems and as a means of documentation before and after surgical intervention. Photographs taken at the time of initial consultation allow the surgeon to point to specific areas of concern while explaining the operative plans, a process that helps the client visualize the outcome of the proposed surgery. Furthermore, sharing postoperative photographs of individuals who have had similar surgery may identify discrepancies between the client's expectations and those of the surgeon. Pictures taken of clients are confidential. Showing clients pictures of

other clients is done only after proper consent is obtained.

Preoperative care. Because of the large amount of blood loss associated with skin, and particularly facial, surgery, the client may be instructed by the surgeon to avoid ingestion of salicylates or to discontinue anticoagulation medications for several weeks before and after the procedure. Immediate preoperative care is focused on collection of any routine laboratory test data required before general anesthesia and preparation of the operative site. In most cases, the procedure for shaving and washing the skin is dictated by physician's preference (see Chap. 18). Clients undergoing facial surgery, specifically *rhytidectomy* (face lift), are frequently asked to wash their hair several times with antibacterial soap to decrease bacterial flora near the incision site. The nurse also instructs these clients to remove any make-up and avoid use of face creams before surgery. If a *rhinoplasty* (cosmetic reconstruction of the nose) is scheduled, the nurse prepares the client for the early postoperative period by explaining the need for nasal packing to control bleeding and reviewing mouth-breathing techniques.

Postoperative care. Postoperative care is focused on monitoring for complications associated with surgical intervention (see Chap. 20). Pressure dressings may be applied at the time of surgery and left in place for several days to control both hemorrhage and edema formation. The nurse checks dressings and any nasal packing for bright red bleeding, along with monitoring changes in vital signs and level of consciousness indicative of active hemorrhage. Repeated swallowing followed by belching after rhinoplasty is a sign of postnasal bleeding and is immediately reported to the surgeon. Clients who have had breast surgery may have drains in place postoperatively, and the nurse monitors the amount and color of drainage. If a rhytidectomy, blepharoplasty (removal of "bags" around the eyes), or rhinoplasty has been performed, the nurse places the client in semi-Fowler's position to minimize edema and promote comfort. Additional comfort measures, such as the application of ice packs or cold compresses, are instituted as ordered. Special support garments are often indicated after breast surgery to minimize edema and tension on the suture line from the weight of the breast tissue.

The nurse monitors for signs and symptoms of wound infection and progress toward healing. Of particular concern are any areas of skin necrosis or eschar formation near the operative site, a complication related to excessive tension on the suture line from edema and subsequent obstruction of microcirculation. For a description of criteria used to monitor wound infection, refer to Table 40–4.

Pain

Planning: client goals. The goal of care is that the client will experience an alleviation of the pain associated with the surgical incision or wound and accompa-

TABLE 40-6 Indications for and Complications of Common Plastic Surgical Procedures

Procedure	Description	Indications	Complications
Blepharoplasty	Excision of bulging fat and redundant skin of the periorbital area with primary closure	Bags under the eyes	Hematoma Ectropion Corneal injury Visual loss (rare) Wound infection (rare)
Breast augmentation (augmentation mammaplasty)	Insertion of synthetic breast-shaped implants through a skin incision	Inadequate breast volume or contour	Hematoma or hemorrhage Wound infection (with gram-positive organisms) Phlebitis
Breast reduction (reduction mammaplasty)	Excision of excessive breast tissue and skin with primary closure	Hypertrophy of breast tissue caused by elevated hormone levels, endocrine abnormalities, or obesity	Hematoma or hemorrhage Nipple, areola, and skin flap necrosis Wound infection Fat necrosis Wound dehiscence
Dermabrasion	Abrasive removal of the facial epidermis and a portion of the dermis followed by healing by second intention	Moderate to severe acne scars Deep wrinkling Multiple actinic keratoses Hyperpigmentation (postinflammatory or after the use of estrogens)	Hypertrophic scarring Altered skin pigmentation Acne flare Wound infection (rare)
Rhinoplasty	Removal of excessive cartilage and tissue from the nose with correction of septal defects if indicated	Disproportionate nasal anatomy Posttraumatic nasal deformity Congenital or acquired deviated septum	Hematoma or hemorrhage Ecchymosis and edema (temporary) Wound infection (with gram-positive organisms) Septal perforation Minor skin irritation
Rhytidectomy (face lift)	Removal of excess skin and tissue from the face at the level of the hairline followed by primary closure	Excessive wrinkling or sagging of facial skin	Hematoma or hemorrhage Facial nerve damage (temporary or permanent) Wound infection Ecchymosis and edema (temporary) Skin necrosis Hair loss

nying edema. The degree of discomfort is usually directly related to the amount of tissue manipulation required during correction of the deformity.

Interventions: nonsurgical management. The discomfort experienced by a client after plastic surgery varies with the anatomic area involved and the amount of tissue swelling. For example, rhinoplasty is particularly uncomfortable, owing to prolonged nasal obstruction, sinus congestion, headaches, and altered senses of taste and smell. Surgery in the vicinity of the eyes can also cause edema of the periorbital skin, significantly impairing vision and requiring that the client be assisted with ADL until it subsides. Temporary numbness of the lower lip and cheeks is not uncommon after rhytidectomy and can prove bothersome to the client, as can heaviness of the breast tissue after breast surgery. Finally, the wound inflicted by dermabrasion is similar to a partial-thickness burn and can cause increasing discomfort until healing occurs. The nurse offers reassurance that these symptoms are normal and administers pain medication as ordered. Additional comfort measures may be instituted on the basis of the type of surgery performed. For example, frequent oral hygiene is offered to the client who is mouth breathing after rhinoplasty.

Occasionally, a client's complaint of pain may signal a problem requiring medical intervention. For example, unilateral facial pain after rhytidectomy is sometimes indicative of hematoma formation. The pain may or may not be associated with edema and facial pallor. Eye pain after blepharoplasty is uncommon and should be reported to the physician.

Body Image Disturbance

Planning: client goals. The major goal for this diagnosis is that the client will have decreased anxiety related to postoperative expectations. Clients who have sought surgical intervention to improve their self-image are understandably preoccupied with the outcome and will be anxiously looking forward to their new image after surgery.

Interventions: nonsurgical management. Regardless of the planned procedure, the nurse prepares the client preoperatively for edema and discoloration of the operative site. Swelling and ecchymosis can significantly alter the facial features and may not resolve completely for several weeks after surgery. The nurse reinforces postoperatively that the true results of surgery will not be visible until healing is complete, usually 6 months to a year or longer postoperatively.

■ Discharge Planning

If cosmetic surgery is performed in the outpatient setting, the client proceeds with immediate postoperative care in the home environment. Clients admitted to the hospital for general anesthesia may be discharged shortly after surgery while dressings are still in place. A family member should be available to drive the client home.

Client/Family Education

When teaching the client and the family after cosmetic surgery, the nurse focuses on wound care. Many surgeons prefer to have the client return to the clinic for dressing changes, especially the initial removal of any pressure dressings. If wound cleaning or application of topical antibiotics is indicated, the nurse reviews the procedure with the client. Written instructions are helpful, as they provide an easy reference for clients who are often anxious. The nurse also emphasizes observations that require professional intervention, including excessive bleeding at the operative site and signs of wound infection. Heavy lifting or straining is discouraged, as it can renew bleeding and potentially contribute to wound dehiscence. In particular, clients who have had a rhinoplasty are told to avoid blowing the nose. Finally, on the basis of the physician's preference, the client is instructed when it is safe to resume bathing, shampooing, and applying make-up.

Clients who have undergone facial surgery may require assistance in the home environment if vision is temporarily impaired owing to edema. The family is taught to use pillows to elevate the head. Liquids and soft foods that require minimal chewing are preferred for the first 1 to 2 days postoperatively.

Psychosocial Preparation

As might be expected, the client is often hesitant to be seen by anyone except family members until her/his appearance has returned to near-normal. In addition, feelings of guilt and embarrassment are not unusual because of the assumption that others may think the surgery unnecessary and a result of excessive vanity. Because concerns over body image are heightened immediately after surgery, social isolation is warranted at this time. The client may prefer to take an extended vacation or sick leave until healing is complete. However, reluctance to socialize after the results of surgery are evident usually indicates continuing problems with self-concept related to body image.

Health Care Resources

Frequent follow-up by the surgeon is indicated until healing is complete or for as long as the client feels it is necessary. Even with visible improvement in appearance, some clients may have difficulty accepting small incision scars or are genuinely disappointed in the outcome of surgery. In these cases, physician referral to a cosmetic counselor is helpful. The client can be taught the creative use of make-up and hair pieces to effectively camouflage residual flaws. Professional counseling may be indicated for clients with severe disturbances in self-concept.

 Evaluation

On the basis of the identified nursing diagnoses, the nurse evaluates care of the client undergoing plastic surgery. The expected outcomes include that the client

1. Describes and institutes measures to minimize complications after surgery
2. Demonstrates skills necessary to care for the wound in the home environment

3. States that postoperative discomfort is reduced or alleviated

4. Describes postoperative problems requiring professional intervention

5. Describes the usual appearance of the operative site after surgery

6. States that anxiety related to the expected cosmetic result is reduced or alleviated

By meeting the stated outcomes, corrections of the client's deformity will be maximized and anxiety related to unrealistic expectations allayed.

BENIGN TUMORS

CYSTS

Cysts are firm, flesh-colored nodules that contain liquid or semisolid material. Unlike malignant growths, which are hard and firmly attached to underlying structures, a cyst is characterized by fluctuance and mobility on palpation. Often, there is a central pore through which material can be expressed if the lesion is squeezed.

The most common cyst is an *epidermal inclusion cyst.* These benign growths often occur spontaneously and are asymptomatic. They can be located anywhere on the body, but are found most frequently on the head and trunk. The content of epidermal inclusion cysts is macerated keratin, which has a cheesy consistency and a foul odor. The most common cyst found on the scalp is the sebaceous, or *pilar, cyst.* The growth arises from the sebaceous structure within the epidermis and, on physical examination, is often indistinguishable from an epidermal inclusion cyst.

Therapy to remove cysts is rarely indicated. If the client prefers that the cyst be removed, surgical excision with primary closure is performed under local anesthesia. It is important that the entire cyst wall be removed during excision to prevent recurrence.

A *pilonidal cyst* is a lesion found in the sacral area that is often associated with a sinus track extending into deeper tissue structures. Proximity of this lesion to the perineum may result in secondary infection, requiring surgical incision and drainage.

SEBORRHEIC KERATOSES

Seborrheic keratoses are a common malady of the elderly population. These benign epidermal neoplasms are gradually acquired after middle age and are often mistaken for actinic keratoses or pigmented skin cancers. On inspection, they appear as multiple "pasted-on" papules or plaques ranging in color from flesh tones to brown or black. The surface of the lesion has a rough, greasy, wart-like texture on palpation. These growths may occur anywhere on the body, but are more commonly found on the face, the neck, the upper trunk, and the arms.

Removal of seborrheic keratoses is indicated only for cosmetic reasons or if a lesion becomes irritated owing to friction or excoriation. Removal is performed using cryosurgery or curettage with or without local anesthetic.

KELOIDS

A *keloid* is essentially overgrowth of a scar resulting from an excessive accumulation of collagen and ground substance after skin trauma. On physical examination, it appears as an elevated, protuberant nodule or tumor that extends well beyond the boundaries of the original injury. These growths are common in Black persons and often arise at sites of surgical incisions, burns, and ear piercing.

Treatment of these cosmetically disfiguring lesions is difficult and not always successful. Surgical excision alone can result in a larger, more protuberant scar. Consequently, surgery is usually combined with another form of therapy, such as intralesional steroid injections or low-dose radiotherapy. Pressure dressings or elastic garments worn over the skin for 1 year after excision or steroid injection may also prove beneficial in keeping the lesion flat.

NEVI

A *nevus,* or *mole,* is a normal skin finding representing a benign neoplasm of the pigment-forming cells. Nevi may be either congenital or acquired, with the majority being acquired between the ages of 1 year and 35 years. These lesions are classified according to the location of the neoplasm within the layers of the skin. For example, a *junctional nevus* is confined to the epidermis and occurs as a light to dark brown macular lesion, whereas a *compound nevus* is papular and involves both the dermis and the epidermis.

Normal nevi have regular, well-defined borders and are uniform in color, ranging from light colors to dark brown. The lesion's surface may be rough or smooth. Because about one-half of malignant melanomas arise from moles, nevi with irregular or spreading borders and those with variegated colors should be considered highly suspicious. Other abnormal findings include sudden changes in size and complaints of itching or bleeding.

Unsightly nevi or those subject to repeated irritation or trauma can be excised. Biopsy of any suspicious lesions should be performed to rule out malignancy.

WARTS

Warts, or *verrucae,* are small tumors caused by infection of the keratinocytes with the papillomavirus. They may occur singly or in groups and are classified according to their anatomic location. *Common warts* are raised, flesh-colored papules with a rough, hyperkeratotic surface.

Although they may grow anywhere on the skin surface, they are frequently found on the hands and fingers. *Flat warts* range in size from 2 to 4 mm and appear as slightly elevated reddish-brown or flesh-colored papules with flat tops and minimal scale. These warts often multiply and affect the hands and the face. Another often painful wart occurring on the bottom of the foot is the *plantar wart*. Plantar warts are usually covered with thick callus that when removed reveals tiny black dots (thrombosed capillaries). *Venereal warts*, or condyloma acuminata, are sexually transmitted neoplasms that can involve the external genitalia, the rectum, the urethra, the vagina, and the cervix. They are often referred to as moist warts because of their soft, cauliflower-like appearance. The association of venereal warts with the development of squamous cell genital carcinomas necessitates biopsy of persistent or suspicious condylomata. In addition, routine Papanicolaou's smears are recommended for all female clients with genital lesions (see Chap. 54).

The treatment of warts is aimed at destroying the keratinocytes containing the virus, a process that can be destructive and painful. Surgical excision, electrodesiccation and curettage, and cryosurgery are acceptable treatment modalities; however, cryosurgery is usually preferred, because local anesthetic is not required and scarring is less likely. Topical caustic agents, including salicylic acid and lactic acid, are also employed. These agents are painted onto the surface of the lesion and result in destruction of the cells and peeling of the infected skin area.

Venereal warts can be particularly problematic, especially if they are extensive. Limited areas of involvement are usually treated topically with caustic or antimetabolic agents. Electrodesiccation and cryosurgery are also used, particularly if warts are resistant to topical therapy. Treatment of extensive involvement with carbon dioxide (CO_2) laser therapy is especially promising. The CO_2 laser generates an intense strong beam of light that, when directed at a lesion, causes thermal vaporization of the tissue. The advantages of this therapy over electrodesiccation and cryosurgery include more efficient and effective treatment of large areas of abnormal tissue with control of hemorrhage.

HEMANGIOMAS

Hemangiomas, or angiomas, are vascular neoplasms and represent one of the most common of the benign tumors. Clinical presentation varies from lesions that appear shortly after birth and gradually regress to lesions that are present at birth and gradually expand in size with growth.

Nevus flammeus is a congenital vascular neoplasm involving the mature capillaries. These lesions favor the face and the upper body and occur as well-demarcated macular patches ranging in color from pink to bluish purple. Although nevus flammeus may gradually fade during the first years of life, a form of this neoplasm called the port-wine stain grows proportionately with

the child and remains unchanged in adult life. Port-wine stains usually occur as solitary lesions, but may vary in size. With aging, the surface of the lesion often becomes papular in texture, representing an overgrowth of angiomatous tissue.

The significance of nevus flammeus is largely cosmetic. Depending on the size of the lesion, surgical excision with or without skin grafting may be indicated. Treatment with laser therapy appears to be an acceptable alternative to surgery and is currently under evaluation. Noninvasive treatment consists of masking the lesion by covering it with an opaque make-up.

A common hemangioma found in elderly clients is the *cherry hemangioma*. These lesions are small, dome-shaped papules ranging in color from red to purple. Treatment is not usually indicated. However, lesions can be removed by excision or electrodesiccation if the client requests removal because of cosmetic reasons.

A less common proliferating capillary neoplasm is the *pyogenic granuloma*. This lesion often arises at the site of trauma as a small erythematous papule, which rapidly enlarges to a lobulated lesion with overhanging edges. Solitary lesions not exceeding 1 cm in size are most common. Secondary infection results in crusting with purulent exudate. Lesions may be excised or destroyed by electrodesiccation; however, incomplete removal of the neoplasm results in recurrence.

Arterial spiders, or *spider angiomas*, are not true tumors, but result from dilation of superficial arteries. These lesions are common in pregnancy, and multiple lesions may also be associated with liver disease. Arterial spiders favor the neck, the upper chest, and the face and occur as small, bright red erythematous papules with radiating legs resembling a spider. Lesions associated with increased estrogen levels usually disappear spontaneously. Permanent lesions may be treated with electrodesiccation.

PARASITIC DISORDERS

The parasitic skin disorders are most commonly associated with poor hygiene and less-than-adequate living conditions. Clients who show obvious signs of self-care deficit should be thoroughly examined for these contagious parasitic infections.

PEDICULOSIS

The term *pediculosis* refers to infestation by human lice: pediculosis capitis (head lice), pediculosis corporis (body lice), and pediculosis pubis (pubic or crab lice). Human lice are oval in shape and measure approximately 2 to 4 mm in length. The female louse lays hundreds of eggs called *nits*, which are deposited at the base of the hair shaft in hair-bearing areas. The most prominent symptom of pediculosis is pruritus, which may or may not be accompanied by excoriation. In addition to the discomfort caused by human lice, these parasites can also be vectors of systemic disease, such as typhus and recurrent fever.

Pediculosis capitis is more commonly found in women, especially on the sides and back of the scalp. Pruritus, caused by biting of the scalp by the parasites, is usually intense; the development of a secondary staphylococcal infection from scratching is possible with severe infestation. Because the louse is difficult to see on inspection, the nurse examines the scalp for visible white flecks, which are the nits of the female louse. Matting and crusting of the scalp accompanied by a foul odor alert the nurse to the probability of secondary infection.

Pediculosis corporis is caused by lice that live and lay eggs usually in the seams of clothing. The parasites also cause itching and the only visible sign of infestation may be excoriations on the trunk, the abdomen, or the extremities.

Pruritus of the vulvar or perirectal region alerts the nurse to the possibility of *pediculosis pubis*. Pubic lice, which are more compact and crab-like in appearance than body lice, can be contracted from infested bed linen or during sexual intercourse. Although the louse is usually confined to the genital region, infestation of the axilla, the eyelashes, and the chest can also occur.

The treatment for pediculosis is chemical killing of the parasites with agents such as lindane (Kwell) or topical malathion. In the case of pediculosis capitis, areas where the client's head has rested should also be treated. Clothing and bed linens require thorough washing in hot water or dry cleaning. The removal of nits from an infested scalp can be facilitated by the use of a fine-toothed comb. In all cases of louse infestation, social contacts are treated when possible. In the hospital setting, care is taken to isolate a client with pediculosis until treatment can be initiated. All clothing and personal belongings are considered potential vectors of infection and are disinfected accordingly.

SCABIES

Scabies is a contagious skin disease characterized by epidermal curved or linear ridges and follicular papules. The pruritus associated with this mite infestation is more intense than that of pediculosis, and the client frequently reports that the itching becomes unbearable at night. The visible white epidermal ridges are formed by burrowing of the mite into the outer skin layers. The nurse closely examines the skin between the fingers and on the palms and volar aspects of the wrists, where these ridges are most common. A hypersensitivity reaction to the mite results in excoriated erythematous papules, pustules, and crusted lesions found primarily on the elbows, the nipples, the lower abdomen, the buttocks, and the thighs and in the axillary folds. Male clients can also have excoriated papules on the penis.

Scabies infections are transmitted by close and prolonged contact with an infested companion or bedding.

Although infestation is a common problem among clients of lower socioeconomic status, the scabies mite is also carried by pets and occurs endemically among schoolchildren and institutionalized elderly clients; thus, one should never preclude the possibility of infection on the basis of the client's social status. Suspected infestation is confirmed by taking a scraping of a lesion and examining it under the microscope for mites and eggs. Close contacts are also monitored for the possibility of infestation.

Treatment consists of chemical disinfection with scabicides, such as lindane (Kwell) or topical sulfur preparations, applied daily for one or two applications. Clothes and personal items are laundered, but do not require disinfection. Residual pruritus, which may last for 1 to 2 weeks after treatment, requires topical antipruritic preparations, such as calamine lotion, to control discomfort.

OTHER DISORDERS

INSECT BITES

Reactions to insect bites or stings can vary from local inflammatory reactions to systemic hypersensitivity. Local skin reactions are either acute, with urticaria-like lesions, or chronic, as evidenced by an erythematous papular eruption. Insect bites are common and rarely require medical attention unless the reaction is severe.

Although most stinging insects, such as wasps, bees, and fire ants, are encountered outdoors, biting insects are usually found indoors. The bites of fleas, spiders, and occasionally bedbugs are more often characterized by a delayed reaction, with itching being the first sign that a bite has occurred.

Insect bites resolve spontaneously and require only symptomatic treatment. In highly allergic individuals, stings can lead to serious anaphylactic reactions requiring *prompt* therapy. If honeybee stings occur, stingers should be removed to prevent continuing release of venom into the circulation. Topical steroid preparations and antihistamines are indicated for more subacute and chronic bites (see Chap. 27 for further discussion of allergic reactions).

RABIES

Rabies is a severe and often fatal neurologic disease caused by a virus that is transmitted via a bite by a rabid mammal. In most cases, the skin must be broken for the virus to be transmitted. However, contamination of scratches or similar breaks in skin integrity with the saliva of a rabid animal can also result in infection.

Regardless of the suspected risk of rabies infection, all animal and human bites or potentially contaminated cuts should be thoroughly cleaned with detergent and running water for a minimum of 5 minutes, followed by application of a topical antiseptic. Antiseptics that are most effective against viruses are 70% alcohol and povidone-iodine. Deep wounds may require exploration to remove foreign objects or allow débridement of nonviable tissue. Bite wounds are rarely closed by first intention because of the danger of inoculating the rabies virus into deeper tissue and the increased chances of abscess formation. Occlusive dressings are also avoided, as a moist wound surface can promote the growth of viral organisms. Instead, the rabies virus is killed by exposure and drying.

PEMPHIGUS VULGARIS

Pemphigus vulgaris is a rare and chronic blistering disease associated with high morbidity and mortality. It is caused by an autoimmune disorder that occurs predominantly during middle and old age. The acute lesions occur on nonerythematous, normal-appearing skin or mucous membrane surfaces as fragile, flaccid bullae. Disruption of the bullae leaves partial-thickness wounds that bleed, weep, and eventually form crusts. Distribution is generalized; the initial lesions usually occur on the oral mucosa, with subsequent bullae formation on the trunk. Spread of the disease is characterized by the appearance of new lesions, particularly on the face and in skin fold areas, while older lesions are in the process of healing. Oral involvement is a common symptom of pemphigus and can interfere with chewing and swallowing, potentially contributing to malnutrition in untreated clients. Secondary infection of broken bullae is also a concern in severely debilitated clients.

Treatment of pemphigus is aimed at suppressing the immune response that causes the blister formation. Systemic steroids and cytotoxic agents are used to obtain remission. Although these agents have been successful in decreasing the morbidity and mortality of the disease, long-term use of these drugs is associated with a high incidence of drug toxicity. Topical antibiotic creams or ointments are used to minimize bacterial colonization of the unhealed lesions.

TOXIC EPIDERMAL NECROLYSIS

Toxic epidermal necrolysis (TEN) is a rare and acute epidermal drug reaction characterized by diffuse erythema and bullae formation. Mucous membranes are often involved, and marked systemic toxicity is evident. The drugs most frequently implicated in triggering this disease are the sulfonamides, pyrazolones, barbiturates, and antibiotics. Removal of the offending agent is usually followed by gradual healing in 2 to 3 weeks, with widespread peeling of the epidermis.

Administration of the drug thought to be causing the reaction is stopped, and therapy is aimed at systemic support and prevention of secondary infection. These clients are often admitted to burn units where fluid and electrolyte balance, caloric intake, and potential prob-

lems with hypothermia can be closely monitored. Topical antibacterial agents are used to suppress bacterial growth until re-epithelialization can occur. Systemic steroids have not been found to be of benefit in the treatment of TEN and, because of the potential for bacterial infection, are avoided. Long-term prognosis depends on successful management of systemic sequelae. Scarring and keloid formation are possible. The mortality associated with TEN is approximately 20% (Wintroub et al., 1987).

LICHEN PLANUS

Lichen planus is a fairly common skin disorder characterized by purple, flat-topped papules that are pruritic. Lesions are usually distributed over the wrists and the inner surfaces of the forearms, but may also be present on the lower legs, the genitalia, and other body areas. Oral lesions of lichen planus may occur alone or in combination with skin changes. Unlike the skin lesions, mucosal lesions have a characteristic white lace-like appearance, which predominantly involves the buccal mucosa and is often confused with thrush.

Although viral infections and emotional stress have been suggested as possible causes of lichen planus, it remains an idiopathic disorder. The course of the disease can be chronic, or spontaneous resolution can occur. Treatment is symptomatic, with topical steroids used to decrease inflammation and antihistamines to control pruritus. Occasionally, systemic steroids are warranted for widespread involvement, but long-term use is avoided because of the associated toxicity.

FROSTBITE

Cold injury of the skin depends on several factors, including the temperature, the duration of exposure, and the relative hypoxia of the tissues at the time of exposure. Cell death occurs as a result of microvascular vasoconstriction and subsequent interference with blood flow and stasis. With continued exposure, vascular necrosis and gangrene is imminent. Cold injuries are becoming more common owing to the popularity of winter sports and the increasing numbers of homeless in the population. Factors that place an individual at increased risk for cold injury include age, immobility, alcohol use, vascular disease, and psychiatric disorders.

Acute frostbite is ideally treated in the hospital setting, with rapid and continuous rewarming of the tissue in a water bath (32° to 42° C) for 15 to 20 minutes or until flushing of the skin occurs (Purdue & Hunt, 1986). Slow thawing or interrupted periods of warmth are avoided, as they can contribute to increased cellular damage. Thawing can cause considerable pain, and the nurse administers analgesics as ordered. After thawing, the extremity is left exposed so that local tissue changes can be monitored. At this stage, nursing intervention is aimed at preventing further trauma and secondary infection. Blisters are usually left intact. With time, the degree of actual tissue destruction becomes evident as an eschar forms. After an eschar is evident, local care of the wound is similar to that discussed earlier for skin trauma. Although low-molecular-weight dextran and heparin have been suggested as treatments to prevent progressive thrombosis and minimize tissue destruction, the use of these agents remains controversial. Long-term complications of cold injury include amputation, scarring, depigmentation, and thickened nail plates.

LEPROSY

Leprosy, or Hansen's disease, is a chronic, highly contagious systemic mycobacterial infection of the peripheral nervous system complicated by secondary skin involvement. The clinical course of the disease is either progressive or self-limiting, depending on the immunologic status of the host. Although often thought of as an extinct problem, the disease is regularly introduced into the United States by legal and illegal aliens. The areas of the country where a majority of the new cases are reported include Florida, Louisiana, Texas, New York, California, and Hawaii.

The exact mechanism for transmission of the disease to a susceptible host remains unknown. Clinical investigations have supported transmission via the airborne route, by insects, and through direct contact with skin lesions. The armadillo, chimpanzee, and certain species of monkey have been found to be animal reservoirs of the infection. Protective immunity against leprosy varies, although a majority of individuals are resistant to the disease.

Clinical manifestations of leprosy, including any skin changes, are directly related to the degree of individual resistance to the mycobacteria. Localized, or high-immunity, leprosy is characterized by one or two isolated, erythematous, anesthetic plaques that are hairless and sometimes scaly in texture. On the other hand, generalized, or low-immunity, leprosy involves widespread faintly erythematous macules, papules, nodules, and plaques. Varying degrees of diminished skin sensation of the lesions are attributed to the concomitant peripheral nerve damage.

Treatment is best approached on an outpatient basis owing to the potentially infectious nature of the disease. Management is aimed at controlling bacterial proliferation and minimizing associated physical deformities. The drug of choice in treatment of leprosy is dapsone, a sulfone with relatively few side effects that must be taken for life. In the case of sulfone-resistant disease, other antibacterial drugs are indicated.

ACNE

Acne is an erythematous pustular eruption affecting the sebaceous glands of the epidermis. Lesions occur as a result of increased sebum production stimulated by ele-

vated androgenic hormones and gradual obstruction of the sebaceous canal outlet. Accumulation of debris leads to proliferation of anaerobic bacteria and eventual rupture of the gland into the surrounding dermis with inflammation. This progressive disorder results in the clinical appearance of several types of lesions, including noninflammatory comedones (blackheads and whiteheads), inflammatory papules, pustules, and cysts. Distribution of lesions is usually limited to the face and upper trunk.

Acne is a common disease that, despite popular belief, is not confined to the adolescent population. Treatment is usually sought because of concerns about body image. Control of the disorder is possible, with spontaneous remission occurring in time. However, severe disease can lead to extensive scarring, which further perpetuates disturbances in self-concept.

For superficial lesions and comedones, topical agents, such as retinoic acid, benzoyl peroxide, and antibiotic solutions, are employed. Systemic antibiotics, tetracycline being the drug of choice, are indicated in inflammatory disease. Clients with severe disease have shown dramatic improvement with oral retinoic acid (Accutane) administration. The side effects of this drug include elevated liver function test results and dry, chapped skin. However the most important concern is the teratogenic effect of systemic retinoic acid. A pregnancy test is required before therapy, and strict birth control measures are used during therapy.

NAIL DISORDERS

INGROWN TOENAIL

Although seemingly a minor problem, an ingrown toenail *(unguis incarnatus)* can be troublesome. Pain and local infection, common complications of both the disorder and the treatment, result when the edge of the nail plate grows into the soft pulp of the toe. Conservative management is aimed at controlling local infection while encouraging the nail edges to grow beyond the level of the pulp where the nail plate can be trimmed transversely. This is accomplished by having the client soak the foot in warm water (to which an antiseptic has been added) for 20 to 30 minutes, then gently lifting the softened nail plate and inserting a small piece of gauze between the nail and the flesh on each side. This procedure is repeated twice daily until the nail has grown beyond the flesh so that it can be cut. More aggressive treatment consists of surgical wedge excision of the nail plate. However, the pain of surgical removal can be severe, and recurrence is possible if the nail bed is not completely destroyed. The problem of ingrown toenails takes on an added significance in the diabetic client who is much more prone to infection. Diabetics with peripheral neuropathy and similar symptoms of progressive disease should always be followed by a podiatrist as a prophylactic measure.

HYPERTROPHY

Thickening of the nail place (*onychauxis*) is associated with a number of disorders, including fungal infections, psoriasis, lichen planus, and chronic dermatitis. Unfortunately, treatment of specific causes is not always successful. Topical preparations, such as antifungal agents, are unable to penetrate the thickened nail plate. For this reason, oral antifungal agents are the treatment of choice if fungus is a problem. Local PUVA treatments and oral vitamin A have been reported helpful in treating hypertrophy caused by psoriasis; however, response to any treatment (regardless of the underlying cause) is slow.

SUMMARY

Planning care of the client with an impairment in skin integrity presents a special challenge to the nurse. The emphasis, placed on wound care and evaluation, ultimately affects progress toward healing. For clients with extensive inflammatory skin disease, the attention given to detail in planning the skin care regimen directly influences both the immediate response to treatment and the long-term results. Repeated client observation allows the nurse to detect early changes in skin integrity and initiate timely intervention, which has been shown to have significant impact on the morbidity and mortality of elderly and immunosuppressed clients.

IMPLICATIONS FOR RESEARCH

Nurses are in a unique position to make a difference in client outcome when an actual or potential impairment in skin integrity is identified. Close client contact and easy accessibility to the skin when giving care offer the nurse an added advantage over most health care professionals. Although a number of investigators have looked at the significance of touch in nursing practice, few have addressed the impact of nursing intervention on actual skin problems.

Skin trauma, and more specifically chronic wound management, is an area of care that is falling more and more within the realm of nursing practice. Of the few nursing studies dealing with wound healing, most address the relative effects of environmental factors, such as various dressing materials, on the healing process. However, because of the many endogenous and exogenous variables that affect wound healing, well-controlled studies in the clinical setting are difficult to design. Considerably more effort has been directed toward prevention of skin breakdown. Several nursing investigators have identified risk factors that predispose the elderly client to pressure necrosis. Most of these studies have concentrated on the nursing home population. Few researchers have attempted to validate specific risk factors related to skin breakdown in the acute care setting or to question the relationship between prolonged surgical procedures and altered skin integrity.

A unique problem and one that holds important implications for nursing intervention is the observed relationship between emotional stress and flares of skin disease. This observation has not only been made with psoriasis, but also with pruritus, skin infections, and some of the inflammatory skin diseases. Surprisingly, few studies have been done to support this observation in the clinical setting.

Finally, although disturbances in self-concept are an accepted problem of altered body image, no nursing studies have addressed the client's perception of self in relation to nonfacial skin diseases. On the basis of a review of the literature and identified needs for study that will directly affect the practice of nursing, the following research questions are raised:

1. What risk factors in the acute care setting predispose a client to skin breakdown?
2. What is the relationship between the length of a surgical procedure under general anesthesia and the incidence of skin breakdown?
3. What is the relationship between perceived emotional stress and subjective reports of pruritus?
4. What is the relationship between perceived emotional stress and the course of a skin disease?
5. What effect does nonfacial skin diseases have on perceived body image?

REFERENCES AND READINGS

Trauma

Alper, J. C., Welch, E. A., Ginsberg, M., Bogaars, H., & Maguire, P. (1983). Moist wound healing under a vapor permeable membrane. *Journal of the American Academy of Dermatology, 8,* 347–353.

Alper, J. D., Welch, E. A., & Maguire, P. (1984). Use of the vapor permeable membrane for cutaneous ulcers: Details of application and side effects. *Journal of the American Academy of Dermatology, 11,* 858–866.

Carrico, T. J., Mehrhof, A. I., & Cohen, I. K. (1984). Biology of wound healing. *Surgical Clinics of North America, 64,* 721–733.

Clark, R. A. F. (1985). Cutaneous tissue repair: Basic biologic considerations. I. *Journal of the American Academy of Dermatology, 13,* 701–725.

Cooney, T. G., & Reuler, J. B. (1984). Pressure sores. *Western Journal of Medicine, 140,* 622–624.

Eaglestein, W. H. (1985). Experiences with biosynthetic dressings. *Journal of the American Academy of Dermatology, 12,* 434–439.

Katz, S., McGinley, K., & Leyden, J. J. (1986). Semipermeable occlusive dressings: Effects on growth of pathogenic bacteria and reepithelialization of superficial wounds. *Archives of Dermatology, 122,* 58–62.

Lewis, C. M. (1986). *Nutrition and nutritional therapy in nursing.* Norwalk, CT: Appleton-Century-Crofts.

May, S. R. (1984). Physiology, immunology, and clinical efficacy of an adherent polyurethane wound dressing: OpSite. In D. L. Wise (Ed.), *Burn wound coverings* (Vol. 2). Boca Raton, FL: CRC Press.

Mertz, P. M., Marshall, D. A., & Eaglestein, W. H. (1985). Occlusive wound dressings to prevent bacterial invasion and wound infection. *Journal of the American Academy of Dermatology, 12,* 662–668.

Peacock, E. E., Jr. (1984). *Wound repair* (3rd ed.). Philadelphia: W. B. Saunders.

Pruit, B. A., & Levine, N. S. (1984). Characteristics and uses of biologic dressings and skin substitutes. *Archives of Surgery, 119,* 312–322.

Reed, B. R., & Clark, R. A. F. (1985). Cutaneous tissue repair: Practical implications of current knowledge. II. *Journal of the American Academy of Dermatology, 13,* 919–944.

Roe, D. A. (Ed.). (1986). *Nutrition and the skin.* New York: Alan R. Liss.

Rudolph, R., & Noe, J. M. (1983). *Chronic problem wounds.* Boston: Little, Brown.

Zitelli, J. A. (1984). Delayed wound healing with adhesive wound dressings. *Dermatological Surgery and Oncology, 10,* 709–710.

Infections

Crumpacker, C. S. (1987). Herpes simplex. In T. B. Fitzpatrick, A. Z. Eisen, K. Wolff, I. M. Freedberg, & K. F. Austen (Eds.), *Dermatology in general medicine* (3rd ed., pp. 2193–2248). New York: McGraw-Hill.

Oxman, M. N. (1987). Varicella and herpes zoster. In T. B. Fitzpatrick, A. Z. Eisen, K. Wolff, I. M. Freedberg, & K. F. Austen (Eds.), *Dermatology in general medicine* (3rd ed., pp. 2314–2340). New York: McGraw-Hill.

Roberts, R. B. (1986). *Infectious diseases: Pathogens, diagnosis, and therapy.* Chicago: Year Book Medical.

Swartz, M. N., & Weinberg, A. N. (1987). Infections due to gram-positive bacteria. In T. B. Fitzpatrick, A. Z. Eisen, K. Wolff, I. M. Freedberg, & K. F. Austen (Eds.), *Dermatology in general medicine* (3rd ed., pp. 2100–2121). New York: McGraw-Hill.

Weinberg, A. N., & Swartz, M. N. (1987). General considerations of bacterial diseases. In T. B. Fitzpatrick, A. Z. Eisen, K. Wolff, I. M. Freedberg, and K. F. Austen (Eds.), *Dermatology in general medicine* (3rd ed., pp. 2089–2100). New York: McGraw-Hill.

Zaia, J. (1986). When to anticipate herpes viruses in immunocompromised patients. In *The immunocompromised host* [Highlights of a special teleconference sponsored by Burroughs Wellcome Co.]. New York: World Health Communications.

Inflammations

Fisher, A. A. (1986). *Contact dermatitis* (3rd ed.). Philadelphia: Lea & Febiger.

Rothstein, M. S. (1983). Guidelines for the use of topical medications. *Journal of Enterostomal Therapy, 10*(6), 203–206.

Soter, N. A., & Fitzpatrick, T. B. (1987). Cutaneous changes in disorders of altered reactivity: Eczematous dermatitis. In T. B. Fitzpatrick, A. Z. Eisen, K. Wolff, I. M. Freedberg, and K. F. Austen (Eds.), *Dermatology in general medicine* (3rd ed., pp. 1367–1383). New York: McGraw-Hill.

Wintroub, B. U., Stern, R. S., & Arndt, K. A. (1987). Cutaneous reactions to drugs. In T. B. Fitzpatrick, A. Z. Eisen, K. Wolff, I. M. Freedberg, & K. F. Austen (Eds.), *Dermatology in general medicine* (3rd ed., pp. 1353–1366). New York: McGraw-Hill.

Psoriasis

Dunn, M. D., Cockerline, E. B., & Rice, M. R. (1988). Treatment options for psoriasis. *American Journal of Nursing, 88,* 1082–1087.

Lowe, N. J. (1986). *Practical psoriasis therapy.* Chicago: Year Book Medical.

Meir, P. D., & van der Kerhof, P. C. M. (Eds.). (1986). *Textbook of psoriasis.* Edinburgh: Churchill Livingstone.

Roenigk, H. H., Jr., & Maibach, H. I. (Eds.). (1985). *Psoriasis.* New York: Marcel Dekker.

Seville, R. H. (1983). Psoriasis: Stress, insight and prognosis. *Seminars in Dermatology, 2,* 213–216.

Cancer

Fewkes, J., & Mohs, F. E. (1987). Dermatologic surgery: Microscopically controlled surgical excision (the Mohs technique). In T. B. Fitzpatrick, A. Z. Eisen, K. Wolff, I. M. Freedberg, & K. F. Austen (Eds.), *Dermatology in general medicine* (3rd ed., pp. 2557–2563). New York: McGraw-Hill.

Gilchrest, B. A. (1986). When to refer: Geriatric skin problems. *Hospital Practice, 21,* 59–60.

Kopf, A. (1988). Prevention and early detection of skin cancer/melanoma. *Cancer, 62*(Suppl. 8), 1791–1795.

Longman, A. J., & Graham, K. Y. (1986). Living with melanoma: Content analysis of interviews. *Oncology Nursing Forum, 13*(4), 58–64.

Miaskowski, C. (1983). Potential and actual impairments in skin integrity related to cancer and cancer treatment. *Topics in Clinical Nursing, 5*(2), 64–71.

Schultz, S., & Mastrangelo, M. (1989). The pathophysiology and staging of cutaneous malignant melanoma. *Seminars in Oncology, 16*(Suppl. 1), 27–33.

Sober, A. J., Rhodes, A. R., Mihm, M. C., Jr., & Fitzpatrick, T. B. (1986). Neoplasms: Malignant melanoma. In A. Rook, D. S. Wilkinson, F. J. B. Ebling, R. H. Champion, & J. L. Burton (Eds.), *Textbook of dermatology* (4th ed., Vol. 3, pp. 947–966). Oxford: Blackwell Scientific.

Stewart, D. (1987). Indoor tanning: The nurse's role in preventing skin damage. *Cancer Nursing, 10*(2), 93–99.

Plastic and Reconstructive Surgery

Beeson, W. H., & McCollough, E. G. (Eds.). (1986). *Aesthetic surgery of the aging face.* St. Louis: C. V. Mosby.

Regnault, P., & Daniel, R. K. (Eds.). (1984). *Aesthetic plastic surgery: Principles and techniques.* Boston: Little, Brown.

Stal, S., & Spira, M. (1986). Dermabrasion and chemical peel. In R. Rudolph (Ed.), *Problems in aesthetic surgery: Biological causes and clinical solutions* (pp. 339–372). St. Louis: C. V. Mosby.

Stegman, S. J., & Tromovitch, T. A. (1984). *Cosmetic dermatologic surgery.* Chicago: Year Book Medical.

Miscellaneous Disorders

Adams, F., Cruz, L., Deachman, M., & Zamora, E. (1989). Plaques may complicate subcutaneous opioid infusions. *American Journal of Nursing, 89,* 109–110.

Beaven, D. W., & Brooks, S. E. (1984). *Color atlas of the nail in clinical diagnosis.* Chicago: Year Book Medical.

Browne, S. G. (1987). Mycobacterial diseases: Leprosy. In T. B. Fitzpatrick, A. Z. Eisen, K. Wolff, I. M. Freedberg, & K. F. Austen (Eds.), *Dermatology in general medicine* (3rd ed., pp. 2180–2193). New York: McGraw-Hill.

DeWitt, S. (1988). Skin conditions common to the urology patient. *Journal of Urologic Nursing, 7,* 476–482.

Hagermark, O. (1985). Pruritus. In L. Fry (Ed.), *Skin problems in the elderly* (pp. 267–291). Edinburgh: Churchill Livingstone.

Jopling, W. H. (1984). *Handbook of leprosy.* London: William Hienemann Medical.

Kaplan, C., Turner, G. S., & Warrell, D. A. (1986). *Rabies: The facts* (2nd ed.). Oxford: Oxford University Press.

Kelly, A. (1988). Keloids. *Dermatologic Clinics, 6,* 413–424.

Lookingbill, D. B., & Marks, J. G., Jr. (1986). *Principles of dermatology.* Philadelphia: W. B. Saunders.

Lowy, D. R., & Androphy, E. J. (1987). Wart. In T. B. Fitzpatrick, A. Z. Eisen, K. Wolff, I. M. Freedberg, & K. F. Austen (Eds.), *Dermatology in general medicine* (3rd ed., pp. 2355–2364). New York: McGraw-Hill.

Marks, R. (1987). *Skin disease in old age.* Philadelphia: J. B. Lippincott.

Moschella, S. L., & Hurley, H. J. (Eds.). (1985). *Dermatology* (2nd ed.). Philadelphia: W. B. Saunders.

Nardacci, A. W. (1986). Urticaria: Evaluation and treatment. *Comprehensive Therapy, 12,* 58–63.

Parrish, J. A., & Tian Tan, O. (1987). Laser photomedicine. In T. B. Fitzpatrick, A. Z. Eisen, K. Wolff, I. M. Freedberg, & K. F. Austen (Eds.), *Dermatology in general*

medicine (3rd ed., pp. 1558–1566). New York: McGraw-Hill.

Purdue, G. F., & Hunt, J. L. (1986). Cold injury: A collective review. *Journal of Burn Care and Rehabilitation, 7,* 331–342.

Rook, A., Wilkinson, D. S., Ebling, F. J. B., Champion, R. H., & Burton, J. L. (Eds.). (1986). *Textbook of dermatology* (4th ed.). Oxford: Blackwell Scientific Publications.

Rosen, T. R., Lanning, M. B., & Hill, M. J. (1983). *The nurse's atlas of dermatology.* Boston: Little, Brown.

Sauer, G. C. (1985). *Manual of skin diseases* (5th ed.). Philadelphia: J. B. Lippincott.

Seville, R. H., & Martin, E. (1981). *Dermatological nursing and therapy.* Oxford: Blackwell Scientific.

Stoddard, C. J., & Smith, J. A. R. (1985). *Complications of minor surgery.* London: Bailliere Tindall.

Wheeland, R. G. (1988). *Lasers in skin disease.* New York: Thieme Medical.

ADDITIONAL READINGS

Cuzzell, J. Z. (1985). Wound care forum: Artful solutions to chronic problems. *American Journal of Nursing, 85,* 162–166.

This article reviewed the various treatment modalities for clients with chronic "problem" wounds. Emphasis was placed on planning nursing intervention on the basis of a specific goal of wound management as it relates to the stage of the healing process. Techniques for wound débridement, dressing application, and dressing removal were discussed.

Cuzzell, J. Z. (1988). Wound care forum: The new RYB color code. *American Journal of Nursing, 88,* 1342–1346.

Wound assessment in the clinical setting is an important aspect of nursing practice. However, none of the traditional wound classification systems provide adequate information on which to base therapy. This article introduced a new concept for assessing wound healing by second intention. Based on predictable color changes of the tissue as the wound progresses through the phases of tissue repair, the RYB classification system provides the nurse with a simple tool to guide intervention.

Frantz, R. A., & Kinney, C. K. (1986). Variables associated with skin dryness in the elderly. *Nursing Research, 35,* 98–100.

The authors investigated the role of sebum and other external variables as contributing to dry skin problems in the elderly. Findings supported the frequent occurrence of dry skin in this population, but failed to validate reduced sebaceous activity or loss of skin moisture as isolated causes.

Shell, J. A., Stanutz, F., & Grimm, J. (1986). A comparison of moisture vapor permeable (MVP) dressings to conventional dressings for management of radiation skin. *Oncology Nursing Forum, 13*(1), 11–26.

Impairments in skin integrity related to radiation treatment for cancer continue to present a challenge to nursing. This study compared the management of radiodermatitis with MVP polyurethane film dressings and lanolin-impregnated gauze. Findings supported an increased healing time, less discomfort, and reduced nursing time required for dressing changes with the MVP dressing.

UNIT 12 RESOURCES

Nursing Resources

American Society of Plastic and Reconstructive Surgical Nurses (ASPRSN), North Woodbury Road, PO Box 56, Pitman, NJ 08071. Telephone 609-589-6247.

Promotes quality nursing care of clients undergoing plastic and reconstructive surgery. Supports the collaborative relationship among nurses engaged in clinical practice, education, administration, and research. Publishes *Plastic Surgical Nursing* (quarterly) and *ASPRSNews* (bimonthly newsletter).

Dermatology Nurses Association (DNA), North Woodbury Road, PO Box 56, Pitman, NJ 08071. Telephone 609-582-1915.

An association of more than 1000 nurses caring for dermatology clients. Publishes *Dermatology Nursing* (bimonthly).

Enterostomal Therapy Nursing Certification Board (ENTCB), 2081 Business Center Drive, Suite 290, Irvine, CA 92715. Telephone 714-476-0268.

See Unit 13 Resources for more information.

International Association for Enterostomal Therapy (IAET), 2081 Business Center Drive, Suite 290, Irvine, CA 92715. Telephone 714-476-0268.

See Unit 13 Resources for more information.

Plastic Surgical Nursing Certification Board, North Woodbury Road, PO Box 56, Pitman, NJ 08071. Telephone 609-589-6247.

Certifies nurses in plastic surgical nursing.

Other Resources

HELP (Herpes Resource Center), PO Box 100, Palo Alto, CA 94302. Telephone 919-361-2120.

National Psoriasis Foundation, 6443 Southwest Beaverton Highway, Suite 210, Portland, OR 97221. Telephone 503-297-1545.

Psoriasis Research Institute, PO Box V, Stanford, CA 94305. Telephone 415-326-1848.

Skin Cancer Foundation, 475 Park Avenue South, New York, NY 10016. Telephone 212-725-5176.

Provides informative pamphlets and brochures, a quarterly newsletter, education programs, and screening clinics.

UNIT 13

Problems of Digestion, Nutrition, and Elimination: Management of Clients with Disruptions of the Gastrointestinal System

CHAPTER 41

Assessment of the Digestive System

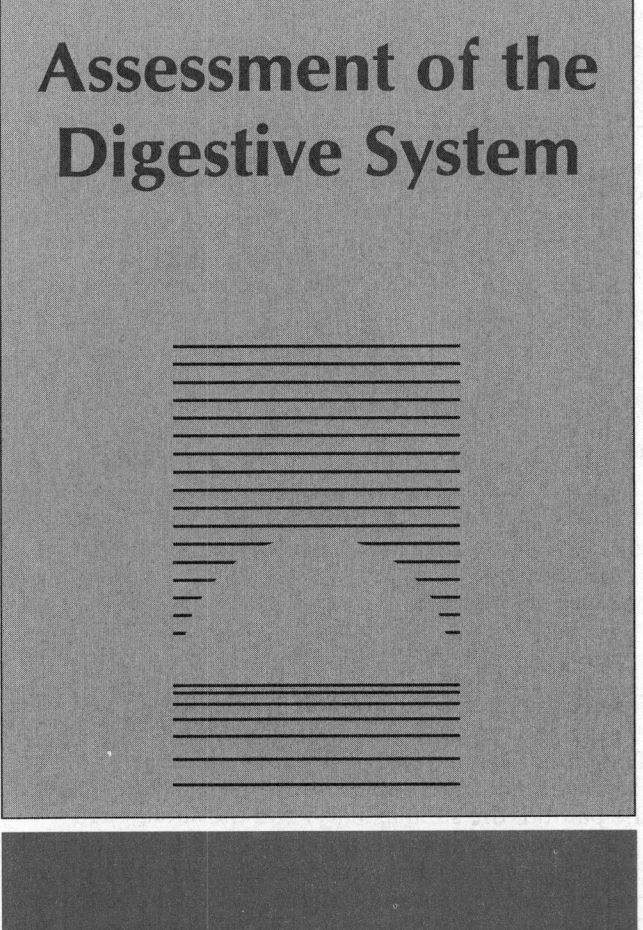

OVERVIEW OF THE GASTROINTESTINAL TRACT

STRUCTURE

The gastrointestinal (GI) tract is a tube that extends from the mouth to the anus (see the illustration on p. 1221). It has generally the same structure throughout its 25-ft length. The hollow part of the tube, or the *lumen,* is surrounded by a layer of surface and epithelial cells called the *mucosa.* The mucosa also includes a thin layer of smooth muscle and some exocrine gland cells, which secrete digestive and protective juices. This layer is surrounded by the *submucosa,* which is made up of connective tissue and additional exocrine gland cells. The outermost layer is made up of both circular and longitudinal smooth muscles, which work to keep contents moving through the tract.

FUNCTION

The GI tract has three major functions: transport, digestion, and absorption. *Transport* of water and food through the GI tract is the first function. After food is ingested, it is swallowed, propelled along the lumen, and eliminated as waste products of digestion.

Digestion, the second function of the GI tract, is a mechanical and chemical process whereby complex foodstuffs are broken down into simpler forms that can be used by the body. During digestion, the GI tract secretes many hormones and enzymes that aid in food breakdown. After the digestive process is complete, the tract functions to absorb the nutrients. This third function, *absorption,* is carried out as nutrients pass through the intestinal walls into the body's circulatory system for uptake by individual cells (Fig. 41-1).

NERVE SUPPLY

Innervation of the GI tract occurs in two ways, as shown in the illustration just cited. Local contractile stimulation is provided by two internal nerve plexuses: the *myenteric plexus,* an outer plexus found in the longitudinal and circular smooth muscle; and the *submucosal plexus,* an inner nerve plexus found in the submucosa. These nerve plexuses connect with each other along the entire length of the GI tract to maintain the tone of the smooth muscle and to stimulate movements. The second type of innervation is provided by the autonomic nervous system, which connects with nerve fibers from the intrinsic nerve plexuses. *Parasympathetic stimulation* is provided

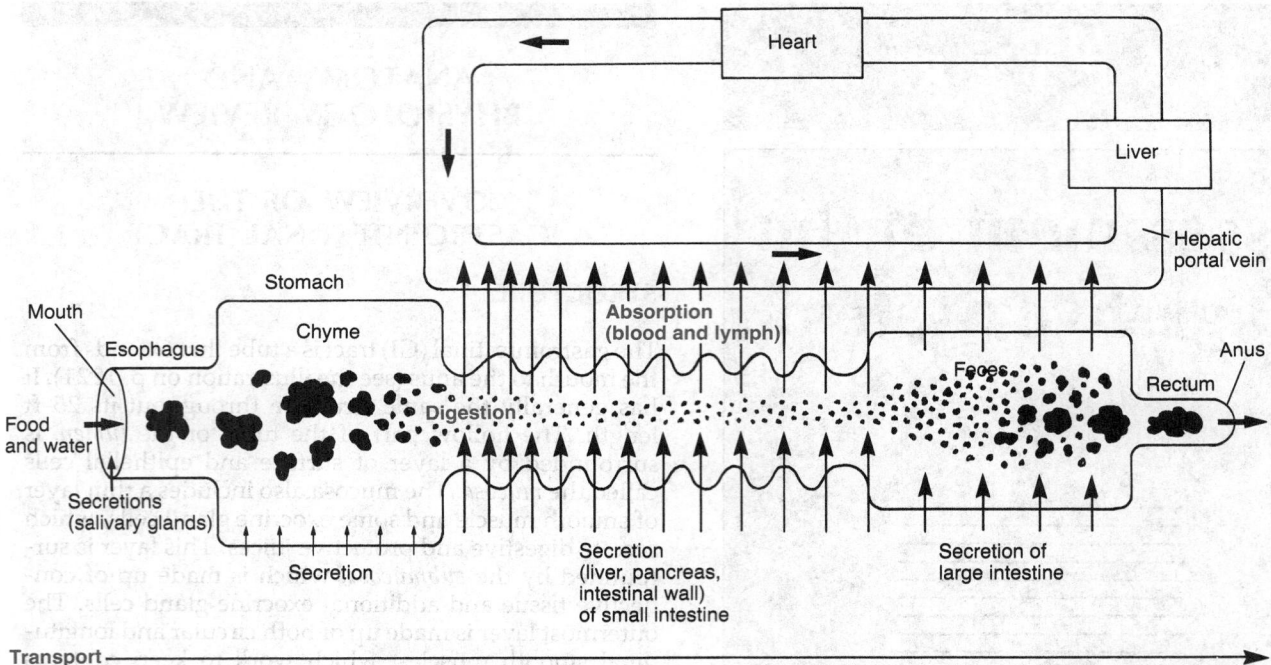

Figure 41–1

Conceptual view of the gastrointestinal system. (From Vander, A. J., Sherman, J. H., & Luciano, D. S. *Human physiology* [3rd ed.]. Copyright © 1980 by McGraw-Hill, Inc. Used by permission of McGraw-Hill Book Company.)

mainly by the vagus nerve, which innervates the esophagus, stomach, and, to a lesser extent, the small intestines, gallbladder, and part of the large intestine. This stimulation causes increased motor and secretory activity and relaxation of sphincters. *Sympathetic stimulation* via the thoracic and lumbar splanchnic nerves is provided to all parts of the GI tract and functions to slow movement, inhibit secretions, and contract sphincters.

BLOOD SUPPLY

The blood supply to the GI tract originates from the aorta and branches to the many arteries throughout the length of the tract: celiac, gastric, splenic, common hepatic, internal and external iliac, and superior and inferior mesenteric. The blood flow accounts for approximately 20% of the cardiac output. The venous system that carries absorbed nutrients away from the lumen of the GI tract includes the gastric vein, the splenic vein, and others that drain into the portal vein of the liver. This blood circulates through the liver to the hepatic vein and returns to the heart via the inferior vena cava.

MOUTH AND PHARNYX

STRUCTURE

The mouth and pharynx are the beginning pathway of digestion (Fig. 41–2). The *mouth*, or *buccal cavity*, is

formed by the hard and soft palates (the roof); the cheeks, or sidewalls; the tongue (the floor); and the lips. The mouth is lined with mucous membranes and contains the teeth, gums, and three pairs of salivary glands: the parotid, the submaxillary, and the sublingual.

The *pharynx*, which is also called the *throat*, extends from the soft palate to the esophagus. It is lined with mucous membranes and contains three pairs of organs: the adenoids, the lingual tonsils (at the base of the tongue), and the palatine tonsils.

FUNCTION

The act of *swallowing*, or *deglutition*, begins after food is taken into the mouth and chewed by the teeth. Saliva is secreted in response to the presence of food in the mouth and begins to soften the food. Saliva contains mucin and an enzyme, *amylase*, which begins the breakdown of carbohydrates. As the food softens, the tongue forces the bolus of food to the rear of the mouth toward the pharynx. This process is the first phase of swallowing, or the *voluntary* phase. The second, or *pharyngeal*, phase is under reflex control and is thus no longer a voluntary act. As the bolus is forced into the pharynx, the soft palate elevates, which seals the nasal cavity. At this time, the swallowing reflex also inhibits respirations and allows for the opening of the esophagus so that the food can enter. The *esophageal* phase begins as a peristaltic wave and passes the food down the esophagus to the stomach, which takes about 9 sec-

THE GASTROINTESTINAL SYSTEM

The gastrointestinal system (GI tract) can be thought of as a tube (with accessory structures) extending from the mouth to the anus for a 25-foot length. The structure of this tube (shown enlarged) is basically the same throughout its length.

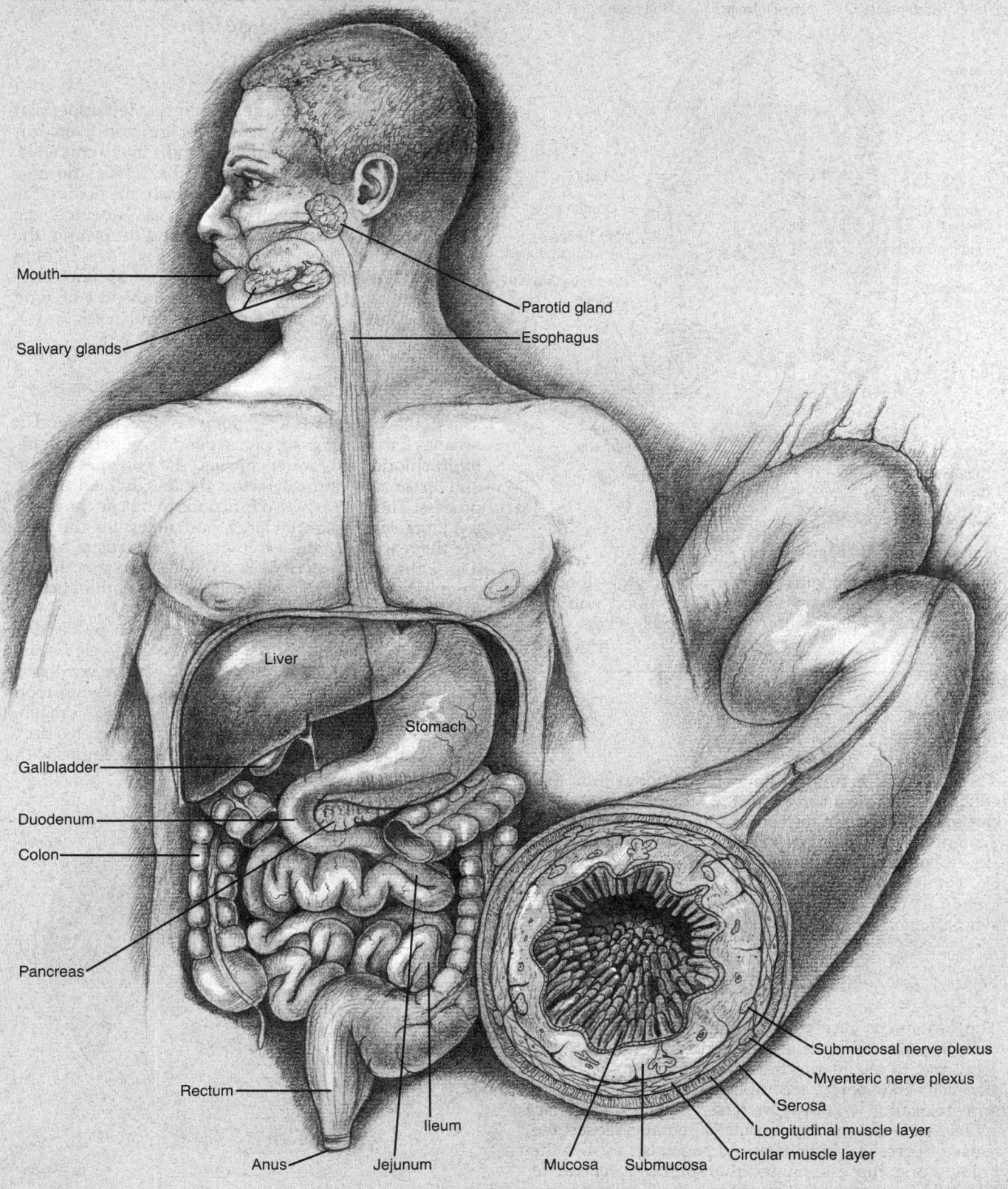

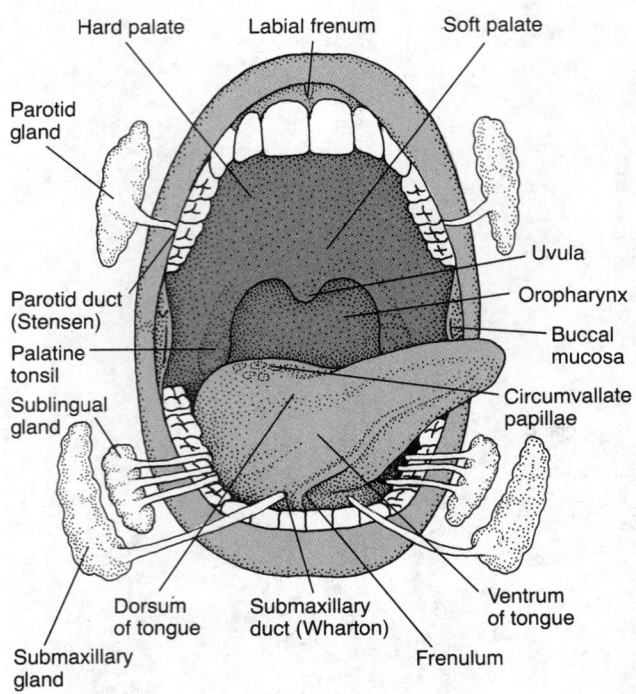

Figure 41–2
Anatomy of the oral cavity.

onds. The bolus may take longer to reach the stomach depending on the consistency of the food and the amount of fluid present in the esophagus.

ESOPHAGUS

STRUCTURE

The *esophagus* is a 10-in-long (25-cm-long) tube that extends from the pharynx to the stomach and passes through the hiatus in the center of the diaphragm. It lies posterior to the trachea. The esophagus is lined with skeletal muscle in the upper one-third and smooth muscle in the lower two-thirds, and it contains mucus-secreting glands. The esophagus is innervated by both sympathetic and parasympathetic fibers.

FUNCTION

The esophagus receives the bolus of food from the pharynx, and its walls secrete mucus to lubricate the food and to aid in the transport of the bolus to the stomach. Transport is accomplished through peristalsis and relaxation of the *gastroesophageal*, or *cardiac*, *sphincter*. This sphincter normally remains closed because of pressure differences. As peristalsis pushes the bolus along the esophagus, the sphincter relaxes to allow the bolus to enter the stomach. This protective mechanism also prevents the highly acid contents of the stomach from refluxing into the esophagus.

STOMACH

STRUCTURE

The *stomach* is located in the midline and left upper part of the abdomen, below the diaphragm and liver. It is approximately 10 in (25 cm) long and 4 in (10 cm) wide. The stomach has four divisions: the *cardia*, the area where the esophagus joins the stomach; the *fundus*, the enlarged left area above the esophageal opening; the *body*, the main area of the stomach; and the *pylorus*, the lower area that meets the duodenum (Fig. 41–3). Both ends of the stomach are guarded by sphincters—cardiac and pyloric—which aid in transport of food through the GI tract and which prevent backflow.

FUNCTION

The stomach serves as a temporary reservoir for food. It secretes 2 to 3 L of gastric juice per day, which contains hydrochloric acid, water, mucus, the enzymes pepsin and lipase, and intrinsic factors that begin the digestive process. The stomach also functions to mix or churn the food, breaking apart the large food molecules and mixing them with gastric secretions to form *chyme*, which has a thick consistency. It regulates the amount of chyme that enters the small intestine for continuation of digestion and absorption of nutrients.

The mechanism of gastric secretion can be divided into three phases. The first, or *cephalic*, phase occurs before the food reaches the stomach. Gastric secretions begin as a result of smelling, tasting, or chewing food and are regulated by the vagus nerve to the stomach. Hydrochloric acid, pepsin, and mucus are secreted during this phase. The second, or *gastric*, phase begins with

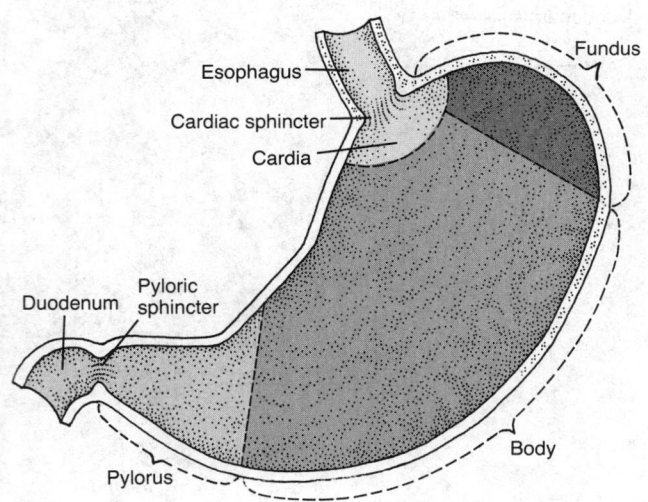

Figure 41–3
Anatomy of the stomach.

the presence of food in the stomach. *Gastrin,* a hormone that is released by the cells in the wall of the stomach in response to the presence of food and its chemical composition, regulates the continued secretion of hydrochloric acid until a pH of 1.5 is reached. The last, or *intestinal,* phase begins as the chyme passes from the stomach into the duodenum. The intestine secretes a hormone, *secretin,* that inhibits further acid production and decreases gastric motility.

PANCREAS

STRUCTURE

The *pancreas* is a smooth-surfaced, carrot-shaped organ that has sharp borders and distinct lobules. Its broad right extremity is called the *head,* which is connected to the main part, or *body,* by a slightly constricted area called the *neck.* The left narrow portion is called the *tail.* It is 4 to 8 in (10 to 20 cm) long and 1 to 2 in (3 to 5 cm) wide. It lies retroperitoneally in the upper abdominal cavity behind the stomach and extends horizontally

from the duodenal C loop to the spleen. It has a rich blood supply from the splenic and superior mesenteric arteries.

The pancreas has two major ducts (Fig. 41–4). The first one, the *duct of Wirsung,* which is also called the *pancreatic duct,* runs through the pancreas from left to right, with other ducts emptying into it at right angles. It comes quite close to the common bile duct, with both ducts passing into the wall of the duodenum to form the *ampulla of Vater.* The second duct, the *accessory duct of Santorini,* drains the lower part of the head of the pancreas and enters the duodenum about 0.79 in (2 cm) above the duct of Wirsung, through the sphincter of Oddi.

The pancreas receives its nerve supply from the vagus and splanchnic nerves. The vagus controls pancreatic secretion during the cephalic and gastric phases of digestion. The splanchnic nerve controls the sensation of pain.

FUNCTION

Two major cellular bodies within the pancreas serve separate functions: exocrine and endocrine. The *exo-*

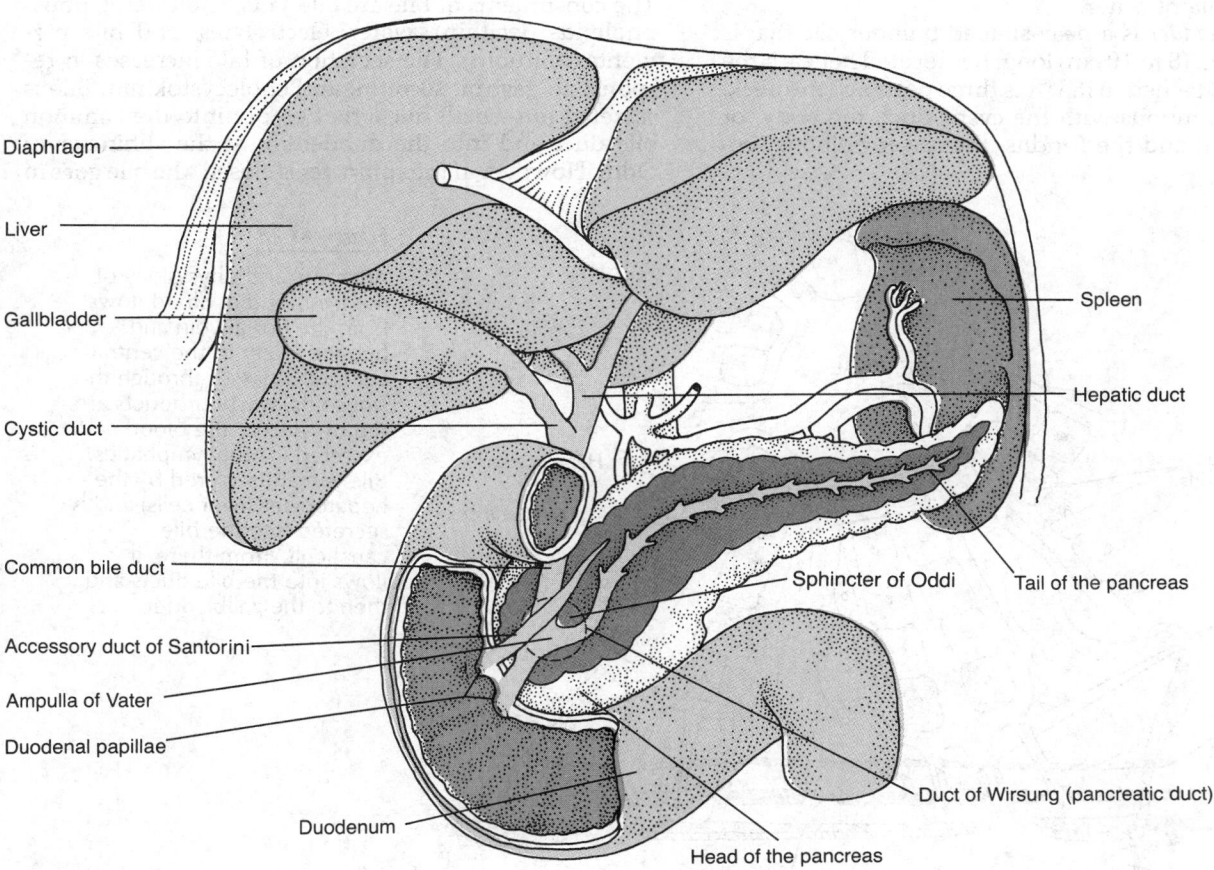

Figure 41–4

Anatomy of the pancreas, liver, and gallbladder.

crine pancreas consists of acinar cells, which secrete the enzymes that are necessary for digestion of carbohydrates, fats, and proteins: *trypsinogen, chymotrypsinogen, amylase,* and *lipase.* The *endocrine pancreas* is made up of the islets of Langerhans, with alpha cells producing glucagon and beta cells producing insulin.

LIVER AND GALLBLADDER

STRUCTURE

The *liver* is the largest organ in the body and is located in the right upper quadrant. It has two major lobes, a larger right lobe and a smaller left lobe, that are divided by the falciform ligament, which attaches the liver to the diaphragm. The liver is made up of functioning units called *lobules* (Fig. 41–5) and has a connective tissue covering, called the *Glisson's capsule,* which provides protection to the organ. *Hepatocytes,* or liver cells, are arranged into cellular plates, which radiate from a central vein. Small bile channels fit between the plates and empty into terminal bile ducts. These merge into a single hepatic duct, which joins the cystic duct of the gallbladder to form the *common bile duct.* This duct empties into the duodenum at the ampulla of Vater.

The *gallbladder* is a pear-shaped bulbous sac that is about 3 to 4 in (8 to 10 cm) long. It is located beneath the liver and is attached to it. It has three portions: the neck, which is continuous with the cystic duct; the body, or main portion; and the fundus, the lower bulbous section.

FUNCTION

The liver performs more than 400 functions in three major categories: storage, protection, and metabolism. The liver serves a *storage* function for several minerals and vitamins: copper, iron, magnesium, vitamin B_{12}, folic acid, vitamin B_6, niacin, and the fat-soluble vitamins A, D, E, and K. The *protective* function of the liver involves phagocytic Kupffer's cells, which are part of the body's reticuloendothelial system. They function to engulf harmful bacteria and worn-out red blood cells. The liver also detoxifies potentially harmful compounds such as some hormones, drugs, chemicals, and alcohol that are ingested. The liver functions in *metabolism* of proteins that are vital for human survival. It functions to break down amino acids to remove ammonia (NH_3), which is then converted to urea and is excreted via the kidneys. In addition, the liver synthesizes several plasma proteins, such as albumin, prothrombin, and fibrinogen. The liver's role in carbohydrate metabolism involves storing and releasing glycogen as the body's energy requirements change. The liver synthesizes, breaks down, and temporarily stores fatty acids and triglycerides.

The liver forms and continually secretes *bile,* which is essential for the digestion of fat in the small intestine. The constituents of bile are bile salts, cholesterol, phospholipids (lecithin), water, electrolytes, and bile pigments (bilirubin). The secretion of bile increases in response to gastrin, secretin, and cholecystokinin. Bile is secreted into small ducts that empty into the common bile duct and into the duodenum at the sphincter of Oddi. However, if the sphincter is closed, the bile goes to

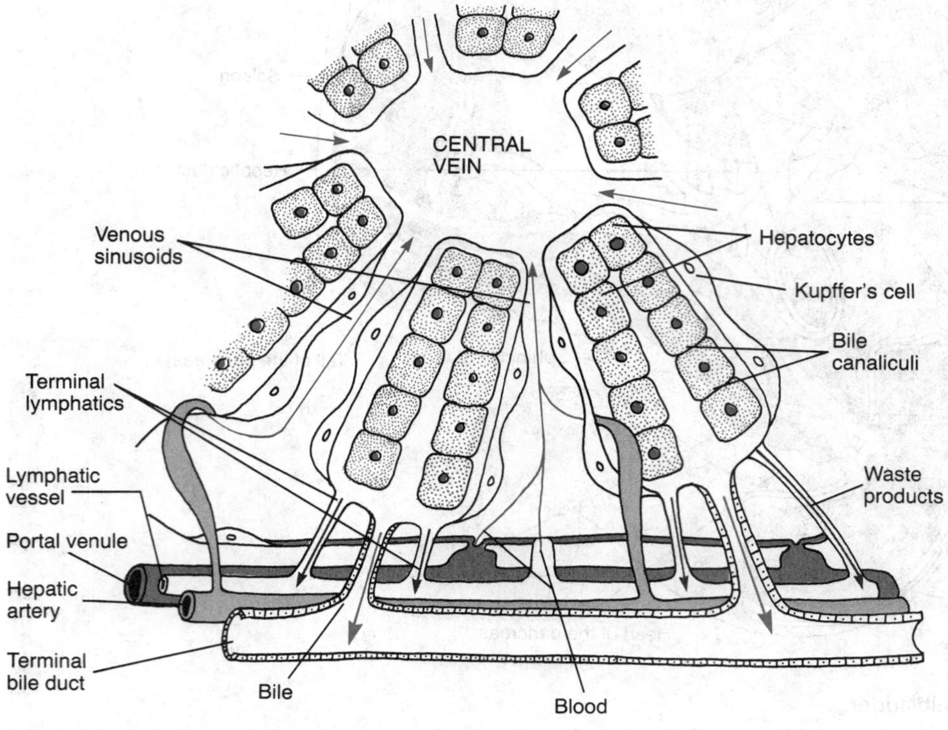

Figure 41–5

Anatomy and physiology of the liver lobule. Blood flows from the portal vein and hepatic artery to the central vein. As it passes through the sinusoids, waste products are removed from the blood and excreted via the lymphatics. Bile is manufactured by the hepatocytes (liver cells) and is secreted into the bile canaliculi. From there, it flows into the bile ducts and then to the gallbladder.

the gallbladder. The gallbladder functions to concentrate and store the bile that has come from the liver. It releases the bile into the duodenum via the common bile duct when fat is present and being digested in the small intestine.

SMALL INTESTINE

STRUCTURE

The small intestine is a 1-in-round tube that is 10 to 13 ft long and consists of three divisions: the duodenum, the jejunum, and the ileum. The *duodenum* is the first 10 in (25 cm) of the small intestine and is attached to the distal end of the pylorus. It is C shaped, curving left around the head of the pancreas and bending behind the transverse portion of the large intestine. After bending forward and downward, the small intestine is termed the *jejunum* for the next 4 ft. For the last 8 ft, it is called the *ileum.*

The inner surface of the small intestine has circular folds of mucosa and submucosa called *plicae circulares,* which project into the lumen to increase the surface area for digestion and absorption. *Villi,* which are microscopic finger-like projections, cover the plicae circulares to further increase the absorptive surface of the small intestine.

FUNCTION

The small intestine has three main functions: movement (mixing and peristalsis), digestion, and absorption. The small intestine mixes and transports the chyme by movements called *segmental contractions.* The contents are moved back and forth over short distances, thereby allowing the chyme to mix with many digestive enzymes. It takes an average of 3 to 10 hours for the contents to be propelled by peristalsis through the small intestine. The ileocecal valve, between the small and large intestines, opens only to allow the passage of chyme. It is usually closed to provide increased absorp-

tion time and to prevent bacteria in the large intestine from invading the small intestine.

The small intestine finishes the digestion of the chyme. Many digestive hormones (Table 41–1) and enzymes (Table 41–2) aid in this process, each having a specific function. Carbohydrates, fats, proteins, vitamins, water, and electrolytes are *absorbed* by both diffusion and active transport, which are described in Chapter 12.

LARGE INTESTINE

STRUCTURE

The large intestine is a tube, 2.5 in (6 cm) in diameter, that is the last 5 to 6 ft of the GI tract. It begins at the *cecum,* a pouch that extends below the junction with the ileum. The *appendix* is an outgrowth of the cecum. The *colon* consists of four divisions: the ascending, transverse, descending, and sigmoid colons. The sigmoid colon empties into the *rectum.* The large intestine is made up of smooth muscle and secretes only mucus to protect the bowel wall against the fecal contents. Its surface area is much smaller than that of the small intestine because it has no villi and no plicae circulares.

FUNCTION

The large intestine's functions are movement, elimination, and absorption. *Movement* in the large intestine consists of mainly segmental contractions, like those in the small intestine, to allow enough time for absorption of water. These contractions are called *haustral contractions,* or *haustrations.* In addition, three or four strong peristaltic contractions per day are triggered by colonic distention in the proximal large intestine to propel the contents toward the rectum. Here, the material is stored until the urge to defecate occurs, which is usually 12 to 24 hours after a meal is ingested. *Absorption* of water and some electrolytes occurs in the large intestine to

TABLE 41–1   Sources and Effects of Gastrointestinal Hormones

Hormone	Source	Effect
Gastrin	Secreted by gastric mucosa in presence of peptides	Stimulates gastric motility and secretion of hydrochloric acid
Secretin	Secreted by duodenum in presence of hydrochloric acid	Stimulates secretion of pancreatic juice and bile from liver
Pancreozymin	Secreted by duodenum in presence of hydrochloric acid and peptides	Stimulates secretion of pancreatic juice
Cholecystokinin	Secreted by duodenum in presence of amino acids and fatty acids	Stimulates secretion of pancreatic enzymes and bile from the gallbladder

TABLE 41–2   Sources, Substrates, and End Products of Major Digestive Enzymes and Bile

Name of Substance	Source	Substrate	End Product
Salivary amylase (ptyalin)	Salivary glands	Starch	Dextrins, maltose
Gastric pepsin (protease)	Stomach	Proteins	Polypeptides
Gastric lipase	Stomach	Emulsified fats	Fatty acids* and glycerol*
Bile (contains no enzymes)	Liver; stored and released from gallbladder	Unemulsified fats	Emulsified fats
Trypsin	Pancreas	Proteins and polypeptides	Polypeptides and amino acids*
Chymotrypsin	Pancreas	Proteins and polypeptides	Polypeptides and amino acids*
Carboxypeptidase	Pancreas	Polypeptides	Smaller polypeptides
Amylase	Pancreas	Starch	Maltose, lactose, and sucrose
Lipase	Pancreas	Bile and emulsified fats	Glycerol* and fatty acids*
Enterokinase	Duodenal mucosa	Trypsinogen	Trypsin
Peptidases	Intestine	Peptides	Amino acids*
Lactase	Intestine	Lactose (milk sugar)	Glucose* and galactose*
Maltase	Intestine	Maltose (malt sugar)	Glucose*
Sucrase	Intestine	Sucrose (cane sugar)	Glucose* and fructose*

* End product ready for digestion.

reduce the fluid volume of the chyme, which creates a more solid material, the feces, for *elimination.*

DIGESTIVE CHANGES ASSOCIATED WITH AGING

Physiologic changes of the digestive system are known to occur with aging. They are summarized in the accompanying Focus on the Elderly feature.

HISTORY

DEMOGRAPHIC DATA

Demographic data about the client, such as *age, sex, race, religion,* and *occupation,* are helpful for GI tract assessment. This information can provide hints to the nurse about predispositions to particular GI tract disorders. For example, many cancers of the GI tract are familial and are seen more frequently in males than in females. Many GI tract cancers are also correlated with age, the elderly being at high risk. In addition, the incidence of

hiatal hernia increases with each decade of life. Diverticulosis and gallstones are also seen increasingly in persons over 40 years of age. Ulcerative colitis occurs more frequently in young and middle-aged adults and is more prevalent among Jewish individuals. Gastrointestinal ulcers correlate with certain demographic data. They are seen more frequently in persons with high-stress occupations and in males more than in females. Duodenal ulcers are seen more frequently in young adults, whereas gastric ulcers are more common in middle-aged adults.

PERSONAL AND FAMILY HISTORY

A review of the client's *overall health status* is an important part of every history. The nurse questions the client about previous *GI tract disorders* or *abdominal surgery.* The nurse assesses whether the client currently has or previously had diabetes mellitus, liver disease, pancreatic disease, heart disease, cancer, jaundice, hemorrhoids, bleeding disorders, hernia, ulcers, colitis, gallbladder disease, abdominal aneurysm, or alcoholism.

The nurse also asks the client about his or her *family's health status,* and whether any family members have had diabetes mellitus, liver disease, pancreatic disease, heart disease, bleeding disorders, cancer, alcoholism, ulcers, or colitis. Many of these disorders have a high incidence within families. If close family members are

FOCUS ON THE ELDERLY ■ Digestive Changes Related to Aging

Structure	Changes	Disorders Related to Changes	Interventions	Rationales
Stomach	Atrophy of gastric mucosa is characterized by a decrease in the ratio of gastrin-secreting cells to somatostatin-secreting cells. This change leads to decreased hydrochloric acid (hypochlorhydria).	Decreased hydrochloric acid leads to decreased absorption of iron and vitamin B_{12} and to proliferation of bacteria. Atrophic gastritis occurs secondary to bacterial overgrowth.	1. Encourage frequent feedings of bland foods high in vitamins and iron. 2. Assess for epigastric pain.	1. To prevent gastritis and to ensure adequate intake of vitamins and iron. 2. To detect gastritis.
Large intestine	Peristalsis decreases and nervial impulses are dulled.	Decreased sensation to defacate can result in postponement of bowel movement, which leads to constipation and impaction.	1. Encourage high-fiber diet and 1500 mL of fluids daily (if not contraindicated). 2. Encourage as much activity as tolerated.	1, 2. To increase sensation to defacate.
Pancreas	Distention and dilation of pancreatic ducts change. Calcification of pancreatic vessels occurs with a decrease in lipase production.	Decreased lipase results in decreased fat absorption and digestion. Steatorrhea, or excess fat in the feces, occurs because of decreased fat digestion.	1. Encourage small, frequent feedings. 2. Assess for diarrhea.	1. To prevent steatorrhea. 2. To detect steatorrhea.
Liver	A decrease in the number and size of hepatic cells leads to decreased liver weight and mass. This change and an increase in fibrous tissue lead to decreased protein synthesis and changes in liver enzymes. Enzyme activity and cholesterol synthesis are diminished.	Decreased enzyme activity depresses drug metabolism, which leads to accumulation of drugs, possibly to toxic levels.	1. Assess all clients for adverse effects of all drugs, even those administered in normal doses.	1. To detect toxicity.

deceased, the nurse asks the client to relate the age and cause of death.

The nurse asks the client what *medications* are being taken, how much, when, and why they have been prescribed. The practice of taking over-the-counter medications, which the client may buy and use independently, is also explored. Many clients do not consider drugs that they can buy on their own to be important. In particular, the nurse asks whether aspirin, vitamin supplements, laxatives, antacids, or enemas are taken. Large amounts of aspirin can predispose the client to GI ulcer disease. Similarly, long-term use of laxatives or enemas can cause dependence on such stimulation.

A final area for investigation includes the client's *travel history.* The nurse asks the client if he or she has traveled out of the country recently. This information may give some clue about a possible cause of a GI tract symptom such as diarrhea.

DIET HISTORY

A *diet history* is important when assessing GI tract function. The nurse determines if the client is eating a special diet. The client is asked to describe the usual foods that are eaten daily and the times of the meals. The nurse thus gains information about the client's knowledge of the four basic food groups and the importance of a balanced diet.

The nurse explores with the client any changes that have occurred in *eating habits* as a result of illness. The nurses assesses the diet and the usual and current *appetite* and notes any changes. The occurrence of nausea, vomiting, heartburn, and/or reflux is also assessed, along with a description of each symptom in terms of frequency, duration, and association with meals. *Taste* is assessed, and any alterations are noted. Difficulty or pain in *swallowing* (dysphagia) is also assessed. The nurse asks the client if any foods are avoided and why they are avoided. Particular attention is paid to *alcohol and caffeine consumption* because both substances contribute to many GI tract disorders.

Cultural and religious patterns are important to a GI tract history. Many cultures use spices or hot pepper in cooking, which can aggravate or precipitate GI tract complaints such as heartburn or indigestion. Religious patterns of fasting or abstinence are also important to note.

SOCIOECONOMIC STATUS

Knowledge of the client's socioeconomic status can give the nurse valuable clues for determining the client's ability to obtain food, medications, and medical care. Individuals who have limited budgets, such as the elderly, may not be able to obtain a balanced diet. They may also substitute less expensive over-the-counter medications for prescription medications, which may not have the same effects or protective coatings.

CURRENT HEALTH PROBLEM

GI tract signs and symptoms are often vague and difficult for the client to describe. The nurse explores each complaint in detail, assessing the location of the problem, what precipitates or alleviates it, when it is worst, and how long it lasts. The following examples are topics to explore with clients about specific GI tract symptoms.

A *change in bowel habits* is a significant complaint. The nurse explores with the client: how often bowel movements occur; color and consistency of the feces; occurrence of diarrhea or constipation; effective action taken to relieve diarrhea or constipation; the meaning of diarrhea and constipation to the client; and the presence of abdominal distention or gas.

An unexplained *weight gain* or *weight loss* is often an early warning sign to the client that something is wrong. The nurse assesses the client for his or her normal weight; weight gain or weight loss; period of time for weight change; and change in appetite or oral intake.

Smoking predisposes the client to developing several oral cancers. The nurse asks if the client has ever smoked. If the client smokes, the nurse obtains a *smoking history* from the client, including the number of packs of cigarettes smoked per day for how many years. If the client has stopped smoking, the nurse asks when and why this was done.

Pain is a common complaint with GI tract disorders. The nurse questions the client about the presence of pain; the location of the pain; radiation to another site; what makes the pain worse; what makes the pain better; and the time of day when the pain is worst.

Changes in the skin can result from several GI tract disorders such as liver and biliary system obstruction. The nurse asks the client about skin discolorations or rashes; itching; jaundice; increased susceptibility to bruising; and increased tendency to bleed.

PHYSICAL ASSESSMENT

Physical assessment of the GI system involves a comprehensive examination of the client's nutritional status, the mouth and pharynx, the abdomen, and the extremities.

NUTRITIONAL ASSESSMENT

HEIGHT AND WEIGHT

The nurse determines the client's height in inches or centimeters with a measuring stick on a weight scale. The client is usually weighed while wearing hospital garments. The amount of clothing that the client is wearing is noted so that subsequent measurements can be done in a like manner. For daily or sequential weights, the nurse notes the time and obtains the weight at the same time each day. See Table 41–3 for height and weight norms for women and men.

ANTHROPOMETRIC ARM MEASUREMENTS

The *triceps skin fold thickness* measurement gives some indication about the client's subcutaneous fat stores and can be most helpful in assessing obesity.

To measure triceps skin fold thickness (Fig. 41–6), the nurse (or dietitian) locates and marks the midpoint on the client's upper arm by using a tape measure. The nurse then grasps the client's arm skin about 1 cm above the midpoint and places the calipers at the midpoint. The nurse applies the calipers and records the measurement. The standard measurement for adult men is 12.5 mm; that for adult women is 16.5 mm.

To measure the *midarm circumference* (Fig. 41–7), the nurse returns to the midpoint on the client's upper arm

TABLE 41–3 Height and Weight Norms for Women and Men

Height		Weight (lb)		
Feet	Inches	Small Frame	Medium Frame	Large Frame
Women				
4	10	102–111	109–121	118–131
4	11	103–113	111–123	120–134
5	0	104–115	113–126	122–137
5	1	106–118	115–129	125–140
5	2	106–121	118–132	128–143
5	3	111–124	121–135	131–147
5	4	114–127	124–138	134–151
5	5	117–130	127–141	137–155
5	6	120–133	130–144	140–159
5	7	123–136	133–147	143–163
5	8	126–139	136–150	146–167
5	9	129–142	139–153	149–170
5	10	132–145	142–156	152–173
5	11	135–148	145–159	155–176
6	0	138–151	148–162	158–179
Men				
5	2	128–134	131–141	138–150
5	3	130–136	133–143	140–153
5	4	132–138	135–145	142–156
5	5	134–140	137–148	144–160
5	6	136–142	139–151	146–164
5	7	138–145	142–154	149–168
5	8	140–148	145–157	152–172
5	9	142–151	148–160	155–176
5	10	144–154	151–163	158–180
5	11	146–157	154–166	161–184
6	0	149–160	157–170	164–188
6	1	152–164	160–174	168–192
6	2	155–168	164–178	172–197
6	3	158–172	167–182	176–202

Courtesy Metropolitan Life Insurance Company.

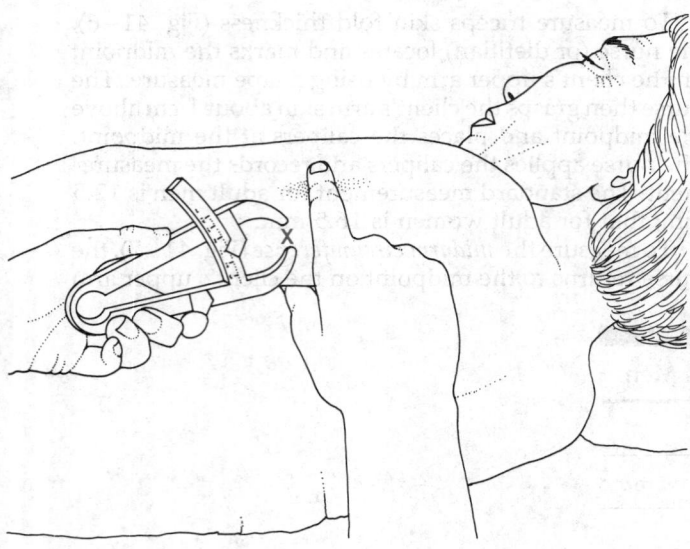

Figure 41–6
Technique for measurement of triceps skin fold thickness.

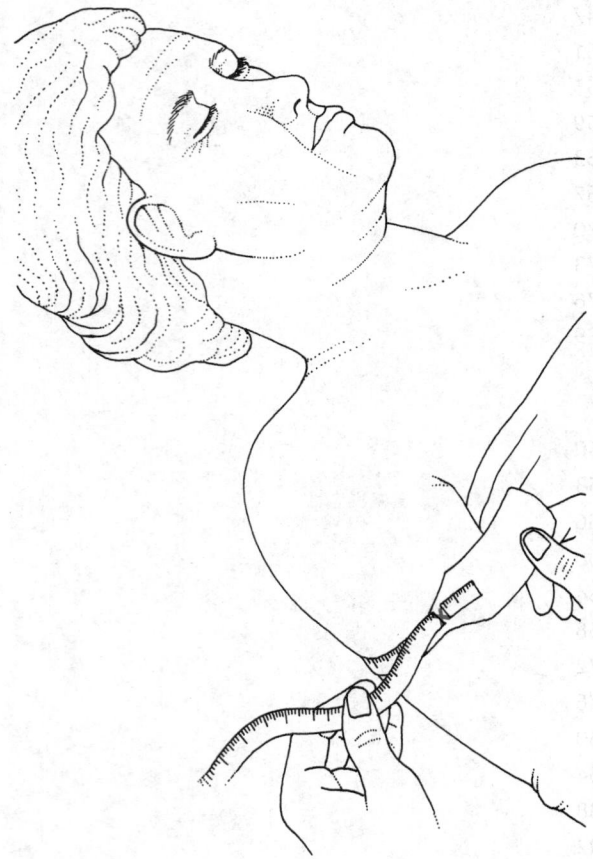

Figure 41–7
Technique for measurement of midarm circumference.

and measures the circumference. The standard measurement for adult men is 29.3 cm; that for adult women is 28.5 cm.

The *midarm muscle circumference* indicates the client's protein or muscle mass reserve. To determine this measurement, the nurse multiplies the triceps skin fold thickness (in centimeters) by 3.1413 and then subtracts the figure obtained from the midarm circumference. The standard measurement for adult men is 25.3 cm; that for adult women is 23.2 cm.

All three of these measurements for the client are compared with the standard measurements and are recorded as percentages. A finding of higher than 90% of the standard indicates adequate energy reserves; a finding of lower than 90% of the standard indicates inadequate protein and calorie reserves.

MOUTH AND PHARYNX

Assessment of the mouth involves *inspection* and *palpation.* To begin the examination of the mouth, the nurse puts on gloves, faces the client, and inspects the lips for color, symmetry, and any abnormalities, such as ulcers. The nurse asks the client to open and close the mouth and notes the ability to perform this movement and its symmetry. To continue, the nurse needs a penlight and a tongue depressor. The nurse inspects the inner surfaces of the lips and the oral mucosa, starting on the client's left side and moving in a clockwise fashion, and notes the color and condition of the membranes. The nurse asks the client to stick the tongue out of the mouth for a better view. The tongue is inspected for color, coating, ulcers, and variations in size and shape. The nurse inspects the teeth and gums for gross evidence of dental caries, absence of teeth, and inflammation or signs of bleeding. If the client wears dentures, they are removed. A recommendation can be made to the client to seek follow-up dental care if the nurse detects any notable problems. Throughout this examination, the nurse is alert to any significant mouth odors that suggest disease.

For further examination of the oral cavity, the nurse asks the client to open his or her mouth wide to inspect the pharynx. The nurse observes color and any signs of inflammation. The presence of the tonsils and exudate, ulcerations, or swellings are noted. The nurse asks the client to say "ah" and observes the normal retraction of the uvula with an intact vagus nerve (cranial nerve X).

ABDOMEN

During the abdominal examination, the nurse usually begins at the client's right side and proceeds in a systematic fashion: right upper quadrant, left upper quadrant, left lower quadrant, and right lower quadrant (Fig. 41–8).

The nurse determines from the history whether there is pain or tenderness and examines the area of pain last.

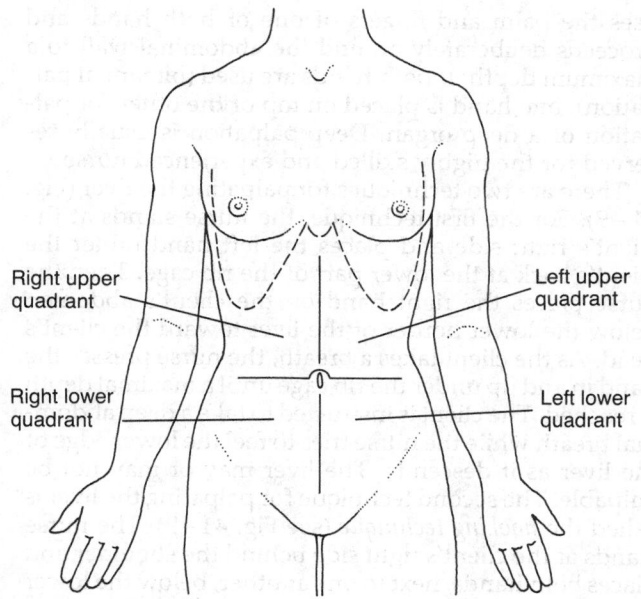

Right upper quadrant

Left upper quadrant

Right lower quadrant

Left lower quadrant

Figure 41–8
Topographic division of the abdomen.

This sequence should prevent the client from tensing abdominal muscles because of the pain, which would make the examination difficult. The nurse examines any area of tenderness cautiously and instructs the client to state if it is too painful. The client's face is observed for signs of distress or pain.

The nurse assesses the client's abdomen by using the four techniques of examination but in a different sequence: *inspection, auscultation, percussion,* and *palpation.* This sequence is preferred so that palpation and percussion do not increase intestinal activity and hence increase bowel sounds. The nurse instructs the client to empty his or her bladder, to lie in a supine position with the knees bent, and to keep the arms at the side to prevent inadvertent tensing of abdominal muscles.

INSPECTION

The nurse inspects the *skin* and notes overall color of the abdomen; hair distribution; and the presence of discolorations, such as rashes, lesions, striae, petechiae, scars, distended superficial veins, jaundice, and any other pigmentation changes. The nurse also checks for edema and/or ascites by noting the presence of marked abdominal distention, bulging flanks, and taut, glistening skin.

The nurse assesses the *architecture* of the client's abdomen by observing its contour and symmetry. The contour of the abdomen is the client's abdominal profile and is either rounded, flat, concave, or distended. The nurse notes whether the contour is symmetric or asymmetric. An asymmetric abdomen could be the result of a hernia, tumor, or previous abdominal surgery. The

nurse inspects the shape and position of the umbilicus for any deviations.

Finally, the nurse inspects the client's *abdominal movements,* including the normal rising and falling of inspiration and expiration, and notes any distress during movement. Occasionally, pulsations may be visible, particularly in the area of the abdominal aorta. Peristaltic movements are rarely seen on inspection. If such movements are observed, the nurse notes the quadrant of origin and the direction of peristaltic flow. This finding is reported to the physician because it could indicate an intestinal obstruction.

AUSCULTATION

Auscultation of the abdomen is performed with the diaphragm of the stethoscope. The nurse places the stethoscope lightly on the abdominal wall and listens for bowel sounds in all four quadrants. Bowel sounds are created as air and fluid move through the GI tract. They are normally heard as soft clicks and gurgles every 5 to 15 seconds, with a normal frequency range of 5 to 34 per minute. The nurse listens for the character and frequency of the sounds. Bowel sounds may be irregular, and the nurse needs to listen for at least 5 minutes in each quadrant to confirm the absence of bowel sounds. Bowel sounds are diminished or absent after abdominal surgery or in the client with peritonitis or paralytic ileus (see Chap. 45). Increased bowel sounds, especially loud gurgling sounds, are a result of hypermotility of the bowel. These sounds are usually heard in the client with diarrhea or gastroenteritis.

The nurse can also auscultate the abdomen for circulatory sounds, especially bruits. A *bruit* is heard with the bell of the stethoscope placed lightly on the abdomen and usually indicates a constriction of a vessel. The sound is similar to the blowing or swooshing sound of a systolic murmur. The nurse can listen over the aorta, the renal arteries, and the iliac arteries. A bruit heard over the aorta usually indicates the presence of an aneurysm. If this sound is heard, the nurse discontinues the examination and notifies the physician immediately.

There are two other abnormal circulatory sounds for which the nurse can auscultate. A *friction rub,* which sounds like two pieces of leather rubbing together, can be heard over the spleen or liver and indicates the presence of a splenic infarct or a hepatic tumor. A continuous *venous hum* is heard in the periumbilical region in the presence of engorged liver circulation, as in hepatic cirrhosis.

PERCUSSION

Percussion is used when assessing the abdomen to determine the size of solid organs and to detect the presence of masses, fluid, and air. Percussion notes are elicited by placing the middle finger of one hand over the area to be percussed. The nurse strikes the abdomen lightly once or twice and systematically assesses each quadrant by comparing sounds over different areas. The percussion notes heard in the abdomen are termed *tympany* (the high-pitched, loud, musical sound of an air-filled intestine) or *dull* (the medium-pitched, softer, thud-like sound over a solid organ such as the liver).

To percuss the size of the liver span, the nurse begins from below the right nipple in the midclavicular line and is careful to percuss between ribs. The percussion note should change from resonance of the lung tissue to dullness of the liver when the upper liver border is reached. The area where percussion tones change is noted. Then the nurse percusses up from the iliac crest in the midclavicular line until the percussion note changes from tympany of the bowel to dullness of the liver at the lower border. Again the nurse marks this area. The distance between the two marks is the approximate liver span, which is normally 2 to 4 in (6 to 12 cm).

Percussion is used to determine the size and position of the spleen at the tenth intercostal space in the left midaxillary line. Percussion can also be used to detect a distended bladder. Again, the percussion notes that are elicited are dull because these are solid organs.

PALPATION

The technique of *light palpation* is used to detect large masses and areas of tenderness and to help the client achieve muscular relaxation. The nurse places the palm and fingers of the hand lightly on the abdomen and proceeds smoothly and systematically from quadrant to quadrant; the nurse depresses to a 1- to 2-cm depth. Any areas of tenderness or guarding are noted. These areas should be examined last and cautiously during deep palpation. While performing light palpation, the nurse is alert to signs of rigidity or muscle spasticity. If the nurse thinks that the client is relaxed, which is best determined while palpating abdominal muscles on expiration, rigidity is probably involuntary. This rigidity could indicate the presence of peritoneal inflammation.

Deep palpation is used to further determine the size and shape of abdominal organs and masses. The nurse uses the palm and fingers of one or both hands and proceeds deliberately around the abdominal wall to a maximum depth. If both hands are used (bimanual palpation), one hand is placed on top of the other for palpation of a deep organ. Deep palpation is usually reserved for the highly skilled and experienced nurse.

There are two techniques for palpating the liver (Fig. 41–9). For the first technique, the nurse stands at the client's right side and places the left hand under the client's back at the lower part of the rib cage. Then the nurse places the right hand on the client's abdomen below the lower border of the liver toward the client's head. As the client takes a breath, the nurse presses the hand in and up under the rib cage until a maximal depth is reached. The client is instructed to take a deep abdominal breath while the nurse tries to feel the lower edge of the liver as it descends. The liver may or may not be palpable. The second technique for palpating the liver is called the *hooking technique* (see Fig. 41–9). The nurse stands at the client's right side behind the shoulder and places both hands, next to one another, below the lower border of the liver. The client is instructed to take a deep breath while the nurse presses in with the fingers of both hands at the costal margin. The nurse attempts to feel the lower border of the liver as it descends.

Palpation is also used to detect an enlarged spleen; however, the spleen must be three times its original size before it is palpable. The same two techniques for palpating the liver are used for the spleen, but on the left side. The pancreas, gallbladder, and kidneys are usually not palpable in most adults.

EXTREMITY FINDINGS

The nurse inspects the skin of the neck, shoulders, and chest for the presence of *spider telangiectases*, which are red, vascular lesions indicative of liver cirrhosis. The nurse also assesses the lower extremities for thigh and leg edema, and if it is present, checks circulation to the tissue by evaluating the dorsalis pedis and posterior tibial pulses.

A clinical finding known as *asterixis*, which is also

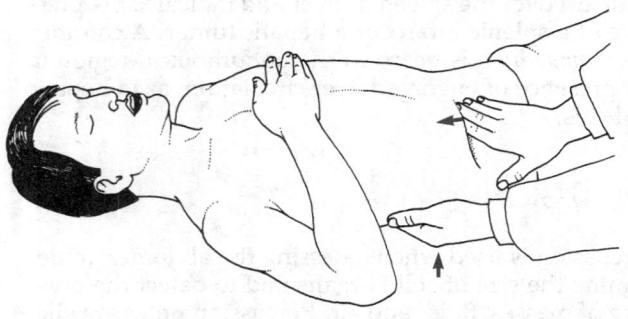
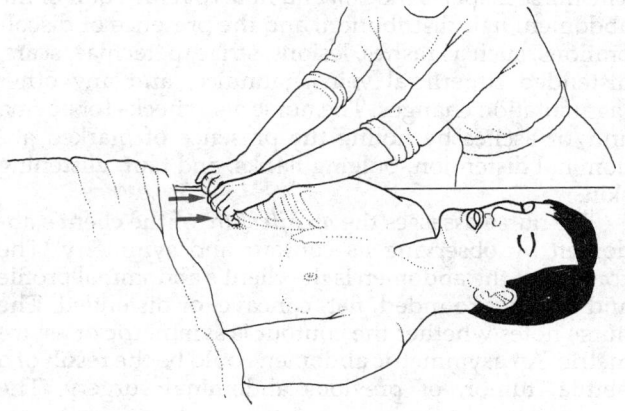

Figure 41–9
Techniques for palpation of the liver.

called liver flap, can be assessed by asking the client to put both arms on a flat surface and extend the hands upward. The nurse notes whether the client's fingers flap while in this position, which indicates hepatic encephalopathy. Axterixis can also be assessed initially by changes in the client's handwriting.

PSYCHOSOCIAL ASSESSMENT

Psychosocial assessment focuses on how the current complaint affects the client's life style. The nurse asks the client if there has been any interruption of or disturbance to usual activities, including employment. For example, has the client been able to work or has he or she had to stay away from work because of illness? The nurse questions the client about the stress level of the job or any other recent emotional stresses experienced. Stress in one's life can lead to the development GI tract disorders.

Another important area for psychosocial assessment includes asking about the client's current financial status. Financial problems can be a source of stress and may precipitate GI tract disorders. In addition, poor finances, especially in the elderly, may prevent the client from obtaining appropriate medical care or a proper diet.

DIAGNOSTIC ASSESSMENT

LABORATORY TESTS

To make an accurate assessment of the many possible causes of GI tract abnormalities, blood, urine, and stool specimen tests can be performed (Tables 41–4 and 41–5).

A complete blood count is a test that evaluates the blood's formed elements, such as the red blood cells, hemoglobin concentration, hematocrit, and white blood cells. It is used to aid in the diagnosis of anemia and to detect changes in the blood's formed elements. Another blood test, the prothrombin time, measures coagulation factors produced in the liver. This test is useful in evaluating these clotting factors, whose levels are abnormally increased in diseases of the liver. Serum protein electrophoresis is also useful for evaluation of GI tract disorders. It is a test to measure the serum protein fractions in the blood, which are important for maintenance of oncotic and capillary pressures.

Calcium and potassium are two electrolytes whose levels are altered in GI tract dysfunctions. Calcium is necessary for the regulation of blood coagulation, for development of bones and teeth, and for many enzyme actions. Calcium is absorbed in the GI tract. It is measured to detect blood clotting deficiencies, GI tract malabsorption, and renal and endocrine disorders. Potassium is necessary for muscle activity and for enzyme reactions. A measure of potassium is useful in the evaluation of renal and endocrine disorders.

Many blood studies are important in the evaluation of liver function. SGOT (serum glutamic-oxaloacetic transaminase), most recently referred to as aspartate aminotransferase (AST), and SGPT (serum glutamic-pyruvic transaminase), most recently called alanine aminotransferase (ALT), are two enzymes found in the liver and other organs. These enzymes are released into circulation when the liver is damaged. LDH (lactate dehydrogenase) is an enzyme that is necessary for the conversion of lactic acid to pyruvic acid. One form of LDH is found in the liver. Serum levels of alkaline phosphatase, which is an enzyme that is found in the liver and intestines, are elevated in clients with biliary obstruction on liver disease. Bilirubin is the primary pigment in bile, which is normally conjugated and excreted by the liver and biliary system. Bilirubin is measured as total serum bilirubin, conjugated (direct) bilirubin, and unconjugated (indirect) bilirubin. These measurements are important in the evaluation of jaundice and of liver and biliary tract functioning.

In addition, a measure of urine urobilinogen, a form of bilirubin that is converted by the intestinal flora, is useful in the evaluation of hepatic and biliary obstruction.

The serum level of ammonia is also measured to evaluate hepatic function. Ammonia is normally used to rebuild amino acids or is converted to urea for excretion. Elevated ammonia levels are seen in cirrhosis of the liver.

Several laboratory tests are useful in measuring pancreatic function. Serum glucose checks the absence or deficiency in the secretion of insulin, which maintains glucose levels within normal limits. It is useful in the evaluation of diabetes mellitus. Serum amylase and serum lipase are evaluated for acute pancreatic dysfunction. Amylase is an enzyme that is formed by the pancreas for digestion of starches, and lipase is necessary for the digestion of fats. The level of amylase in urine is also measured for the evaluation of acute or chronic pancreatitis. After an attack of acute pancreatitis, levels of amylase remain high in the urine after serum levels have returned to normal.

Cholesterol, which is metabolized in the liver and secreted in the bile, is also measured to evaluate fat metabolism in the body.

D-Xylose absorption measures the body's absorption of D-xylose, a sugar that is absorbed in the small intestine. It is useful in the evaluation of malabsorption.

Several stool examinations are used in the evaluation of GI tract dysfunction. Stool for occult blood measures the presence of blood in the stool from GI bleeding and

TABLE 41–4 Normal Findings and Significance of Abnormal Findings in Common Laboratory Tests Used in Gastrointestinal Assessment

Test	Normal Range	Major Significance of Abnormal Findings
Complete blood count		*Decreased values indicate possible:*
Red blood cell count	3.6–5.0 million/mm³ (women)	Anemia
	4.2–5.5 million/mm³ (men)	
Hemoglobin	12–15 g/dL (women)	Recent hemorrhage
	14–16.5 g/dL (men)	
Hematocrit	37%–45% (women)	*Increased values indicate possible:*
	42%–50% (men)	Hemoconcentration caused by dehydration
		Blood loss
Prothrombin time	11.0–12.6 s	*Increased values indicate possible:*
		Deficiency in prothrombin, fibrinogen, or extrinsic factors
		Liver disease
		Vitamin K deficiency
Calcium	8.0–10.5 mg/dL	*Decreased values indicate possible:*
		Malabsorption
		Renal failure
		Acute pancreatitis
Potassium	3.5–5.0 mg/L	*Decreased values indicate possible:*
		Vomiting
		Gastric suctioning
		Diarrhea
		Drainage from intestinal fistulas
Serum protein electrophoresis	Total protein 6.5–8.0 g/dL	*Decreased values indicate possible:*
Albumin	3.5–5.0 g/dL	Hepatic disease
Alpha₁-globulin	0.1–0.4 g/dL	GI disorders
Alpha₂-globulin	0.5–1 g/dL	Peptic ulcer
Beta-globulin	0.7–1.2 g/dL	Acute cholecystitis
Gamma-globulin	0.5–1.6 g/dL	Malabsorption
AST or SGOT*	10–50 mU/mL	*Increased values indicate possible:*
		Viral hepatitis
		Cirrhosis
		Acute pancreatitis
		Other liver damage
ALT or SGPT*	5–35 mU/mL	*Increased values indicate possible:*
		Liver disease
		Hepatitis
		Cirrhosis
LDH (lactate dehydrogenase)	60–150 IU/L	*Increased values indicate possible:*
		Damaged liver caused by hepatitis and other hepatocellular disorders
Alkaline phosphatase	30–90 IU/L	*Increased values indicate possible:*
		Hepatic disease
		Biliary obstruction
Bilirubin		
Total serum	0.2–1.0 mg/dL	*Increased values indicate possible:*
		Hemolysis, biliary obstruction, or hepatic damage.
Conjugated (direct)	0.1–0.3 mg/dL	*Increased values indicate possible:*
		Biliary obstruction
Unconjugated (indirect)	0.2–0.8 mg/dL	*Increased values indicate possible:*
		Hemolysis or hepatic damage

TABLE 41–4   Normal Findings and Significance of Abnormal Findings in Common Laboratory Tests Used in Gastrointestinal Assessment *Continued*

Test	Normal Range	Major Significance of Abnormal Findings
Ammonia	Less than 50 mg/100 mL	*Increased values indicate possible:* Hepatic disease such as cirrhosis
D-Xylose absorption	25–40 mg/dL in 2 h 3.5 g in 5 h 5.0 g in 24 h	*Decreased values in blood and urine indicate possible:* Malabsorption in small intestine
Serum amylase	60–160 Somogyi units/dL	*Increased values indicate possible:* Acute pancreatitis
Serum lipase	20–60 mm/mL	*Increased values indicate possible:* Acute pancreatitis
Glucose (fasting)	60–100 mg/dL	*Increased values indicate possible:* Diabetes mellitus Chronic hepatic disease
Cholesterol	140–200 mg/dL	*Increased values indicate possible:* Pancreatitis Biliary obstruction *Decreased values indicate possible:* Liver cell damage

* AST, aspartate aminotransferase; SGOT, serum glutamic-oxaloacetic transaminase; ALT, alanine aminotransferase; SGPT, serum glutamic-pyruvic transaminase.

TABLE 41–5   Normal Findings and Significance of Abnormal Findings in Common Urine and Stool Tests Used in Gastrointestinal Assessment

Test	Normal Range	Significance of Abnormal Findings
Urine bilirubin	Negative	*Increased values indicate possible:* Biliary obstruction Cirrhosis Hepatitis
Urobilinogen	Urine: 0.1–1 Ehrlich unit/mL	*Increased values indicate possible:* Hepatitis Cirrhosis *Absence indicates possible:* Obstructive jaundice
Urine amylase	Various levels depending on unit of measure	*Increased values indicate possible:* Acute pancreatitis Pancreatic obstruction
Stool for occult blood	Negative	*Presence indicates possible:* Carcinoma Peptic ulcer Ulcerative colitis
Ova and parasites	Negative	*Presence is diagnostic of infection*
Fecal fat	2–5 g/24 h with normal diet	*Increased values indicate possible:* Crohn's disease Malabsorption syndrome Pancreatic disease

other GI tract disorders. Stool samples for ova and parasites are collected to aid in the diagnosis of intestinal infection caused by parasites and their ova. Stool samples tested for fecal fats are evaluated for steatorrhea and malabsorption. Fat is normally absorbed in the small intestine in the presence of biliary and pancreatic secretions. In malabsorption, fat is abnormally excreted in the stool.

RADIOGRAPHIC EXAMINATIONS

FLAT PLATE OF ABDOMEN

A *flat-plate x-ray film* is done to visualize organs in the abdomen. This simple film has the ability to reveal abnormalities such as masses, tumors, and obstructions or strictures to normal movement. This x-ray investigation is generally the first one done when diagnosing a GI tract problem. There is no required client preparation, except that the client should wear a hospital gown and remove any jewelry or belts, which may interfere with the film.

BARIUM SWALLOW

A *barium swallow* is a test of the pharynx and esophagus done to detect tumors, strictures, ulcers, or other motility disorders. It is often performed for a client with a complaint of heartburn or dysphagia.

Client preparation. The client is permitted nothing by mouth (NPO) after midnight the evening before the test. The nurse instructs the client about the barium preparation and its consistency.

Procedure. This test is performed with the client in an upright position. During the test, the client must swallow a barium sulfate mixture, and fluoroscopy is used to follow the passage of the barium down the esophagus. The client may be placed in other positions, lying flat or moved from side to side. This test should be done *after* a barium enema or gallbladder series to prevent the mixture used in the barium swallow from interfering with the other examinations.

Follow-up care. The nurse assesses the abdomen for distention and bowel sounds. A laxative should be ordered. The nurse evaluates the client's stools to ensure that all barium is expelled and that stools return to a brown color. Abdominal distention and/or decreased or absent bowel sounds associated with constipation or obstipation may indicate barium impaction.

UPPER GI SERIES AND SMALL BOWEL SERIES

An *upper GI series* is an x-ray visualization of the lower esophagus, stomach, and duodenum. The *small bowel series* continues the tracing of the barium through the small intestines up to and including the ileocecal junction. These tests are performed for a client with complaints of heartburn, abdominal pain, nausea, vomiting, and/or weight loss.

Client preparation. The client is NPO after midnight the evening before the test. The nurse instructs the client about the barium preparation and its consistency and that he or she will have to drink about 16 oz of the barium. The nurse also tells the client about the rotating x-ray table and the many positions that are required for this test.

Procedure. The client drinks a mixture of barium sulfate, and fluoroscopy is used to trace the barium through the esophagus and stomach, which takes about 30 minutes. If a small bowel series is included, the client drinks more barium, and more x-ray films are taken at 30-minute intervals. This series can take from 2 to 6 hours, depending on how long it takes the barium to reach the cecum.

Follow-up care. Follow-up care for either of these series includes giving an ordered laxative, usually 30 mL of milk of magnesia, to allow for natural elimination. The client should be instructed that stools may be white for 24 to 72 hours as barium is excreted. As with the barium swallow, the nurse assesses that the client passes all barium and resumes passing brown stools. If the client is at home, the nurse instructs him or her to report abdominal fullness, pain, or delay in return to brown stools.

BARIUM ENEMA OR LOWER GI SERIES

A *barium enema* or *lower GI series* is an x-ray visualization of the large intestine. This test is usually ordered for a client with a complaint of blood or mucus in the stool or a change in bowel pattern (e.g., diarrhea or constipation).

Client preparation. Client preparation for a barium enema is quite important. Whenever possible, the client is placed on a low-residue diet 2 days before the test. The client must have clear liquids (no milk products) the evening before the examination and is NPO after midnight until the test is completed. In addition, the client is usually ordered a potent laxative and an oral liquid preparation for cleaning the bowel the evening before the examination.

Procedure. During the test, a rectal catheter is inserted, the barium mixture is instilled by gravity slowly, and the client is instructed to hold the barium while films are being taken. The client may have abdominal cramps and the urge to defecate as the barium enema is given. This procedure can be extremely uncomfortable, especially for the elderly. The client is instructed to take slow, deep breaths and to hold the anal sphincter as tightly closed as possible. The test takes about 45 minutes.

Follow-up care.   Follow-up care should include a mild laxative or cleaning enema, as ordered, after the examination is completed. The nurse informs the client that the stools will be white for 24 to 72 hours. The nurse encourages the client to drink plenty of liquids, unless contraindicated, to ensure adequate hydration and prevent fecal impaction.

PERCUTANEOUS TRANSHEPATIC CHOLANGIOGRAPHY

Percutaneous transhepatic cholangiography is x-ray visualization of the biliary duct system with an iodine dye. This test is usually performed for a client who has jaundice and/or persistent upper abdominal pain even after cholecystectomy.

Client preparation.   There is no formal preparation, but the client is asked about allergies to iodine or seafood.

Procedure.   During the test, clients are instructed to hold their breath, and a needle is inserted into the liver under x-ray visualization. The dye is injected as the needle is removed. X-ray films are taken as the dye reaches the biliary duct system. The test usually takes 30 minutes.

Follow-up care.   The client should be confined to the bed for 8 hours, and the nurse inspects the injection site for bleeding or swelling. The nurse checks vital signs frequently, as ordered, and observed the client for abdominal distention or tenderness.

ORAL CHOLECYSTOGRAPHY OR GALLBLADDER SERIES

Oral cholecystography is x-ray visualization of the gallbladder made possible through oral ingestion of radiopaque dye. This test is commonly used to detect gallbladder disease. In the presence of disease, there is poor visualization of the gallbladder because biliary obstruction prevents the passage of the dye into the gallbladder. Oral cholecystography should precede any barium studies.

Client preparation.   The nurse checks with the client about any allergies to iodine or seafood. Client preparation involves eating a fat-free dinner on the evening before the test. The client takes six radiopaque iodine tablets by mouth at approximately 8:00 PM the evening before the test. The client is NPO until after the test is completed in the morning.

Procedure.   The client is in the x-ray department for 30 to 60 minutes. If the gallbladder is visualized, the client

may be given a fatty meal, and subsequent films are taken to check for gallbladder contraction.

There is no follow-up care for this test.

INTRAVENOUS CHOLANGIOGRAPHY

Intravenous (IV) *cholangiography* is x-ray visualization of the gallbladder and biliary ducts. This test is performed if the gallbladder is not visualized by oral cholecystography or if biliary symptoms occur in a client who has had a cholecystectomy.

Client preparation.   The nurse checks with the client about any allergies to iodine or seafood.

Procedure.   The client is in the x-ray department for 2 to 4 hours. The client is given an IV injection of a contrast material, and films are taken at 20-minute intervals for 1 hour or until the biliary ducts are visualized. The gallbladder should be visualized in 1 to 2 hours.

No follow-up care is needed for this test.

COMPUTED TOMOGRAPHY

Computed tomography (CT) is a cross-sectional x-ray visualization that is used to detect tissue densities and abnormalities in the liver, pancreas, spleen, and biliary tract.

Client preparation.   Client preparation involves education about the procedure. CT equipment is quite threatening to the client because it is large and may be noisy. The client *may* be NPO after midnight before the test.

Procedure.   The nurse instructs the client to lie still and to hold the breath when asked. The nurse reassures the client that the scan is painless. The client is placed on the x-ray table, and a series of x-ray films are taken. *Contrast media* may be ordered to be given by IV injection for a second set of x-ray films to enhance the pictures.

No follow-up care is needed for this test.

OTHER DIAGNOSTIC STUDIES

ENDOSCOPY

Endoscopy is direct visualization of the GI tract by using a flexible fiberoptic endoscope. Endoscopes of different sizes are used for different areas of the GI tract. Visualization of the esophagus, the stomach, the biliary system, and the bowel is possible. Endoscopy is usually ordered to evaluate bleeding, ulceration, inflammation, masses, tumors, and cancerous lesions. Biopsy and cytologic studies are possible through the endoscope if cancer is suspected. There are several types of endoscopic examinations, each of which is discussed.

Upper GI Endoscopy

Upper GI endoscopy is a visual examination of the esophagus, stomach, and duodenum.

Client preparation. The client is usually NPO after midnight the evening before the test. The nurse explains to the client that during the test, a flexible tube is passed down the esophagus. Medication such as benzodiazepine (Valium) may be administered to relax the client. Atropine may be administered to dry secretions. In addition, a local anesthetic is sprayed into the client's throat to allow passage of the tube. The nurse explains to the client that this anesthetic will calm the gag reflex and that swallowing will be difficult. If the client has dentures, they should be removed.

Procedure. After the medications are administered, the client is asked to swallow and the tube is passed through the mouth and into the esophagus (Fig. 41–10). The client is positioned with the neck hyperextended throughout the examination.

Follow-up care. The nurse checks the client's vital signs frequently, as ordered. The client remains NPO for 2 to 4 hours until the gag reflex returns. The nurse observes the client for signs of perforation, such as pain, bleeding, or fever.

Endoscopic Retrograde Cholangiopancreatography

Endoscopic retrograde cholangiopancreatography includes visual and radiographic examination of the liver, gallbladder, and pancreas.

Client preparation. The client is prepared in the same manner as for upper GI endoscopy, including being NPO after midnight.

Procedure. The endoscopic portion of this procedure is similar to upper GI endoscopy, except that the endoscope is advanced farther, to the duodenum and into the biliary tract. Contrast medium is injected, and x-ray films are taken to evaluate the biliary tract.

Follow-up care. The nurse assesses vital signs every 15 minutes for 1 hour, every 30 minutes for 2 hours, and then hourly for 4 hours. The client remains NPO for 2 to 4 hours until the gag reflex returns. The nurse assesses the client for signs of cholangitis or perforation, which include fever, chills, hypotension, tachycardia, or abdominal pain, especially in the right upper quadrant.

Colonoscopy

Colonoscopy is visual examination of the entire large bowel.

Client preparation. The client should have a liquid diet for 24 hours before the examination and is NPO after midnight the evening before the procedure. An oral liquid preparation for cleaning the bowel such as GoLYTELY is given to the client the evening before the examination. This solution produces a mild diarrhea and usually clears the bowel in 4 to 5 hours.

Procedure. The client is usually given medication to aid in relaxation. The client is placed on the left side with knees drawn up while the endoscope is passed through the bowel.

Follow-up care. The nurse checks the client's vital signs frequently, as ordered. The nurse observes the client for signs of perforation, such as abdominal pain, bleeding, and fever.

Sigmoidoscopy and Proctoscopy

Sigmoidoscopy is visual examination of the sigmoid colon, and *proctoscopy* is visual examination of the lower rectum and anal mucosa.

Client preparation. The client should have a liquid diet for at least 24 hours before the examination and

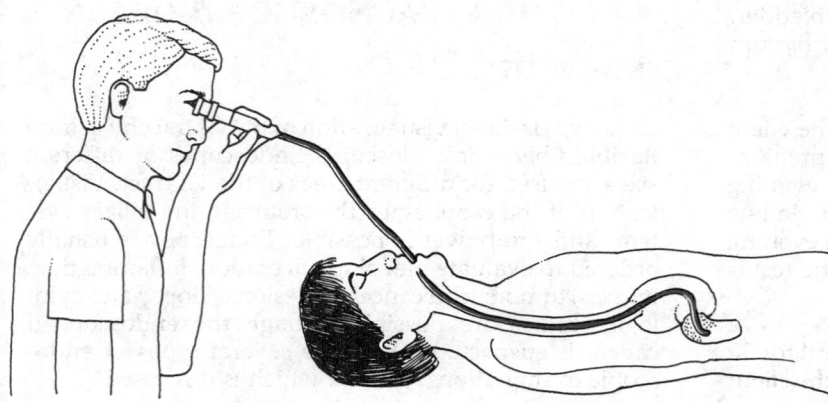

Figure 41–10

Upper GI endoscopy allows visualization of the esophagus, stomach, and duodenum. If the esophagus is the focus of the examination, the procedure is called esophagoscopy. If the stomach is the focus, the term gastroscopy is used.

usually receives a cleaning enema or sodium biphosphate (Fleet) enema the morning of the procedure. A laxative may be ordered.

Procedure.   The client is placed on the left side in the knee-chest position, or on a special table in the proctoscopic position. The sigmoidoscope is passed first. The nurse instructs the client to bear down as the instrument is inserted. The proctoscope is inserted next. This insertion is less uncomfortable for the client than the first one. The examination lasts 30 to 60 minutes.

Follow-up care.   The client is observed for signs of perforation, such as pain, bleeding, and fever. Sitz baths may be ordered to relieve discomfort.

GASTRIC ANALYSIS

Gastric analysis is used to measure the stomach's secretion of hydrochloric acid and pepsin, for evaluation of stomach and duodenal disorders. There are two tests in gastric analysis: *basal gastric secretion* and *gastric acid stimulation.*

Basal gastric secretion is used to measure the secretion of hydrochloric acid between meals.

Client preparation.   The client is NPO for at least 12 hours before the test. A nasogastric (NG) tube is inserted, and the residual contents of the stomach are removed and discarded.

Procedure.   The NG tube is attached to suctioning equipment, and the contents are collected at 15-minute intervals for 1 hour. The nurse collects each sample and labels the time and volume of each specimen.

Gastric acid stimulation is a follow-up test to basal gastric secretion if only small amounts of secretion are collected. The NG tube is left in place, and a drug that stimulates gastric acid secretion (e.g., pentagastrin, histalog) is given to the client. Fifteen minutes after the injection of the drug, specimens are again collected at 15-minute intervals for 1 hour. The nurse collects, labels, and measures the specimens.

Depressed levels of gastric secretion suggest the presence of gastric carcinoma. Increased levels of gastric secretions indicate Zollinger-Ellison syndrome and gastric and duodenal ulcers.

ULTRASONOGRAPHY

Ultrasonography is a technique in which very high frequency, inaudible vibratory sound waves are passed through the body. Echoes of the sound waves that are created vary with tissue density changes. It is commonly used to image soft tissues, such as the liver, spleen, pancreas, gallbladder, and biliary system.

Client preparation.   The client is usually ordered to be NPO for 8 to 12 hours before ultrasonography of the abdomen. The nurse informs the client that it will be necessary to lie still during the study.

Procedure.   The client is placed in a prone or a supine position. Insulating gel is applied to the end of the transducer and on the area of the abdomen under investigation. This gel allows for airtight contact of the transducer to the client's skin. The transducer is moved back and forth over the skin until desired visualizations are obtained. The study takes about 15 to 30 minutes.

No follow-up care is necessary.

LIVER SCAN

A *liver scan* is a nuclear medicine technique. It is more correctly called a liver-spleen scan because an IV injection of a radioactive colloid is given that is taken up primarily by the liver and secondarily by the spleen. It is used to evaluate the liver and spleen for tumors or abscesses.

Client preparation.   The nurse instructs the client to lie still once the examination begins and to hold his or her breath at brief intervals. The client is assured that the colloid injection has only extremely small amounts of radioactivity and is not dangerous.

Procedure.   The injection is given through an IV line, and a wait of about 15 minutes is required for uptake. The client is placed in many different positions while the scanning takes place.

No follow-up care is necessary.

SUMMARY

GI tract assessment can be quite difficult and often produces signs and symptoms that are vague and nonspecific. Knowledge of GI anatomy and physiology is important in distinguishing signs and symptoms of disorders and relating them to the structures involved. Physical assessment of the GI system includes evaluation of nutrition, the mouth, the abdomen, and the extremities. Many laboratory and diagnostic tests can be done to aid in the diagnosis of a GI tract disorder.

REFERENCES AND READINGS

Elias, E., & Hawkins, C. (1985). *Lecture notes on gastroenterology.* Boston: Blackwell Scientific.

Evans, W. (1983). *Anatomy and physiology* (3rd ed.). Englewood Cliffs, NJ: Prentice-Hall.

Fischbach, F. (1988). *A manual of laboratory diagnostic tests* (3rd ed.). Philadelphia: J. B. Lippincott.

Given, B., & Simmons, S. (1984). *Gastroenterology in clinical nursing.* St. Louis: C. V. Mosby.

Groth, K. (1988). Age-related changes in the gastrointestinal tract. *Geriatric Nursing, 9*(5), 278–280.

Guyton, A. C. (1987). *Human physiology and mechanisms of disease* (4th ed.). Philadelphia: W. B. Saunders.

Hamilton, H., & Rose, M. B. (Eds.). (1985). *Gastrointestinal disorders.* Springhouse, PA: Springhouse Corp.

Helleman, J., & Vantrappen, G. (1984). *Gastrointestinal tract disorders in the elderly.* New York: Churchill Livingstone.

Jensen, D. (1980). *The principles of physiology* (2nd ed.). Norwalk, CT: Appleton-Century-Crofts.

Langley, L. L., Telford, I. R., & Christensen, J. B. (1980). *Dynamic anatomy and physiology* (5th ed.) New York: McGraw-Hill.

Malasanos, L., Barkauskas, V., Moss, M., & Stoltenberg-Allen, K. (1985). *Health assessment* (3rd ed.). St. Louis: C. V. Mosby.

Matteson, M. A. (1988). Age-related changes in the gastrointestinal system. In M. A. Matteson & E. S. McConnell (Eds.), *Gerontological nursing: Concepts and practice* (pp. 265–278). Philadelphia: W. B. Saunders.

Potter, D. O. (Ed.). (1982). *Assessment.* Springhouse, PA: Intermed Communications.

Selkurt, E. E. (1982). *Basic physiology for the health sciences* (2nd ed.). Boston: Little, Brown.

Vierling, J. M. (1982). Physiology and diseases of the digestive system in the aged. In R. W. Schrier (Ed.), *Clinical internal medicine in the aged.* Philadelphia: W. B. Saunders.

Weinreb, E. L. (1984). *Anatomy and physiology.* Reading, MA: Addison-Wesley.

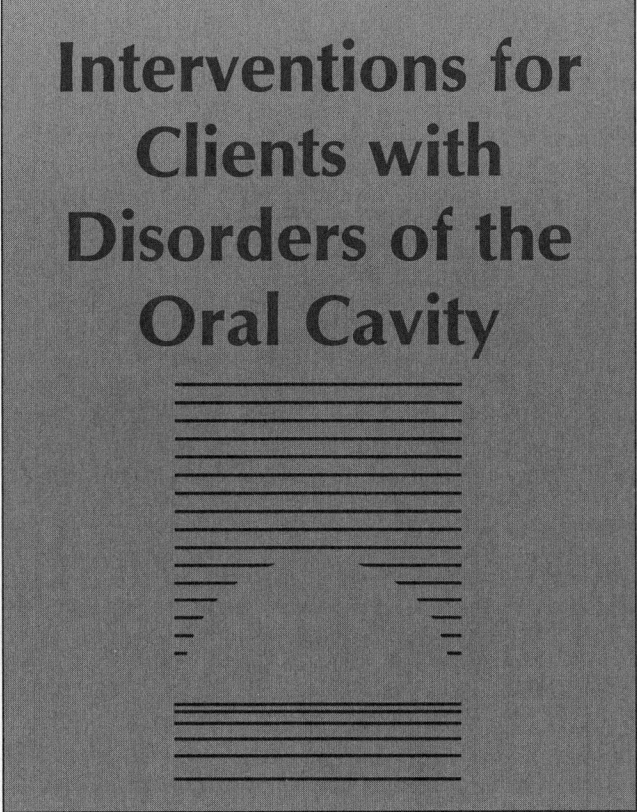

CHAPTER 42

Interventions for Clients with Disorders of the Oral Cavity

Problems of the oral cavity, although seemingly limited to a small anatomic area, pose numerous actual and potential difficulties for clients. Basic functions of eating, breathing, and speaking can be severely impaired by disease of or trauma to the oral cavity. Psychologically, the body image and self-concept of the client are strongly linked to the functioning and appearance of the oral cavity. Nurses must be aware of the impact that disorders of the oral cavity can have on clients' health, life styles, and psychologic well-being. Client education that is focused on prevention and self-care measures can minimize the disability accompanying problems of the oral cavity.

INFLAMMATIONS AND INFECTIONS

DENTAL DISEASE

OVERVIEW

Plaque, a compound consisting of saliva, food debris, bacteria, and organic acids, is the primary factor in loss of permanent dentition. When accumulated over time, plaque erodes the enamel of the teeth, producing dental caries (tooth decay), and inflames gingival tissues.

Pathophysiology

Dental Caries

Plaque and calculus can cause progressive demineralization and destruction of the outer enamel of the tooth. Eventually, over months or years, damage to the pulp occurs (Fig. 42–1). Plaque tends to collect along and under the gingival margins, between the teeth, in deep fissures of the teeth, on malaligned teeth, and along orthodontic appliances. These areas are not well exposed to the regular cleaning actions of saliva, abrasive foods, or physical contact with the tongue or the cheeks.

Periodontal Disease

Periodontal disease can be viewed as existing on a continuum, with gingivitis (inflammation of the gingiva) as an early phase and pyorrhea (periodontitis) as a late phase. Periodontal disease is often characterized by waxing and waning in its severity. Manifestations can progress from early symptoms of swelling of the gums, bleeding when traumatized, pain, and occasional alteration in color of the gingiva to inflamed gingiva with craters or pockets. As the disease progresses, saliva pools in the pockets, creating an environment for bacteria to flourish. Eventually, if periodontal disease is un-

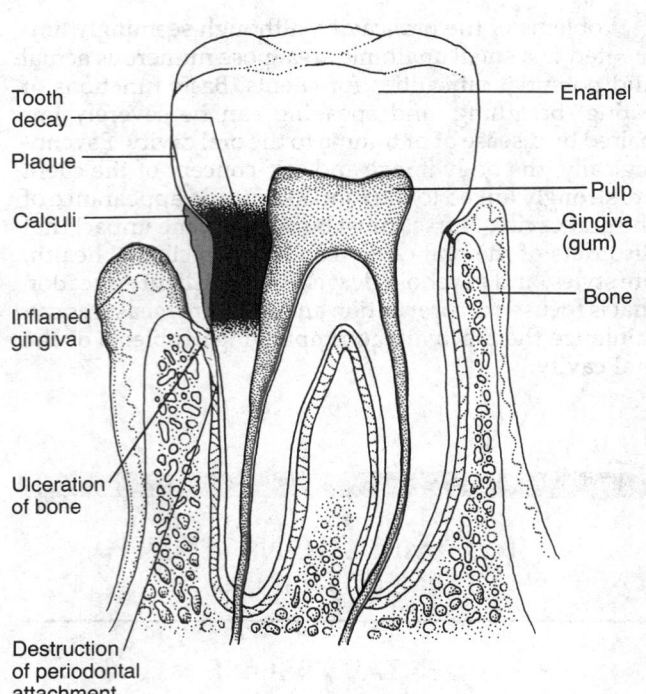

Figure 42-1

Pathophysiology of tooth decay and periodontal disease.

controlled, underlying tissues, including alveolar bone (bone of the maxilla or the mandible underlying gingival tissues), can be destroyed.

Etiology

Accumulation of plaque is the major cause of dental caries and periodontal disease. When allowed to build up, plaque contributes to the formation of *calculus*, a cement-like compound, which can be removed only by skilled professional instrumentation.

The degree of resistance of tooth enamel and the type of dietary intake are also factors in the formation of dental caries. Dental enamel that is softened or has decreased resistance (owing to genetic factors or inadequate dietary intake) has increased susceptibility to destruction by plaque. Dietary sugar intake, particularly sticky carbohydrates (such as caramel), has been shown to increase bacterial metabolism, which in turn increases plaque formation. Between-meal snacking, even of non–sugar-containing foods, changes the composition and quality of normal saliva and thereby retards the remineralizing effect of normal saliva on softened dental enamel.

Incidence

Dental caries and periodontal disease are common health complaints of the United States population. It has been estimated that 90% to 99% of the population have experienced a dental disorder (Chasteen, 1984). Males and females seem to experience dental disorders in equal proportions.

PREVENTION

Prevention of plaque accumulation is the best defense against the development of dental caries and periodontal disease. The nurse instructs the client in the techniques of brushing, auxiliary plaque control efforts, and other oral hygiene measures that concentrate on strengthening tooth resistance to decay. The addition of fluoride to the water in many communities in the concentration of one part fluoride per million parts water reduces the incidence of dental caries in those communities by 40% to 60% (Chasteen, 1984). The action of fluoride compounds makes tooth enamel more resistant to erosion by bacterial acids. Fluoridated water is available to only 45% of the United States population; however, fluoride compounds are available in drops and tablets for systemic use or in gels for topical application.

COLLABORATIVE MANAGEMENT

 Assessment

History

While obtaining the history from the client with actual or potential dental disease, the nurse assesses for and obtains information concerning *previous difficulty with dentition*, specifically a *history of dental caries, periodontal disease,* and *difficulty with occlusion.* Recurrent or chronic dental caries or periodontal disease may be symptomatic of a need for more vigorous dental hygiene. Difficulty with occlusion may result in discomfort or altered chewing ability. Information concerning the prior dental history can also indicate the client's willingness to seek dental help and the client's response to dental therapy. The nurse assesses the client for the *presence of discomfort,* as oral pain often dictates changes in oral hygiene, eating habits, and life style. The nurse questions the client about the *presence of dentures or orthodontic appliances.* Special dental hygiene practices are often needed with dental prostheses. The nurse also assesses the client with dental appliances for specific complaints related to the equipment, such as difficulty with eating, discomfort, and body image discrepancy. The nurse determines the client's *current pattern of dental hygiene,* including the *availability of fluoride in the water* and the *frequency of dental visits,* to determine the effectiveness of the current regimen, the need for alteration in the current regimen, and the client's feelings concerning professional dental care. A history of any *medications* the client is currently taking is obtained by the nurse, as many medications (such as phenytoin [Dilantin]) can affect the gums or the resistance of the tooth enamel to decay. The nurse questions the client about *nutritional status, eating habits* (including snacking), and *ability to chew* to determine the need for any changes to prevent dental disease, as well as for any education for the client to alter poor nutritional habits.

Physical Assessment: Clinical Manifestations

During any examination of the oral cavity, the nurse wears nonsterile gloves for protection against obvious or subclinical infection. Adequate lighting and a tongue blade facilitate the examination of the oral cavity.

Nursing assessment of the teeth and the gingiva is limited to observation and palpation. The nurse asks the client to remove any dentures and then assesses the teeth and the gingiva. The normal mucosa of the gingiva is shiny, is smooth, and has an uneven pale red color, called *stippling.* Brownish coloration of the gums is frequently seen in dark-skinned clients. The nurse assesses the gingival area for increased redness or swelling, which could indicate gingivitis or ill-fitting dentures. Edema or hypertrophy of the gums is occasionally seen as a normal accompaniment to pregnancy. Hypertrophy of the gums is a common side effect of phenytoin (Dilantin) therapy (Fig. 42–2). Stippling often disappears or is decreased with gingivitis, and the gums may also bleed easily. Periodontitis is often seen as enlarged debris-filled pockets between the gum and the teeth. The gingiva may appear to have receded, exposing the roots of the teeth. The nurse palpates the gums for edema and tenderness.

The nurse examines the teeth for decay, broken teeth, poor alignment, and malocclusion. The teeth are tapped with the tongue blade to elicit tenderness and are palpated for looseness. The nurse looks for chalky-white spots on the tooth enamel, the first sign of caries. In later stages of decay, this area becomes discolored and stained, and begins to soften and decay the tooth. The

nurse notes attrition of the teeth, which occurs in elderly clients owing to long use—the enamel appears worn away, exposing the brownish-yellow dentin layer. The nurse assesses for gum or mucosal inflammation from denture irritation or broken teeth.

Psychosocial Assessment

The nurse determines the client's educational level, need and desire for dental education, and motivation for improvement of dental health; the priority the client places on dental hygiene; and any ethnic or cultural barriers to education or dental hygiene. The appearance of the teeth and gums is often a clue to how the client feels about body image and appearance. The nurse assesses the client's feelings about self-concept and the importance of the status of the oral cavity in particular. If the client has a dental prosthesis, the nurse assesses the psychosocial adjustment to the appliance.

It is also important for the nurse to assess the client's willingness to seek professional dental care. Fear of the dentist and the associated feelings of loss of control and pain are probably the most common reasons for not seeking early dental intervention for dental problems.

 Analysis: Nursing Diagnosis

Common Diagnoses

A common nursing diagnosis for the client with dental disease is potential for infection related to dental disease.

Additional Diagnoses

In addition, the client may exhibit one or more of the following nursing diagnoses:

1. Altered oral mucous membrane related to dental disease
2. Pain related to altered oral mucous membrane
3. Altered nutrition: less than body requirements related to pain
4. Noncompliance (dental hygiene regimen) related to knowledge deficit of causes of dental disease
5. Potential for injury related to broken dentition
6. Knowledge deficit related to dental hygiene, prophylaxis, and nutrition
7. Body image disturbance related to change in oral or dental structure
8. Anxiety and fear related to dental procedures

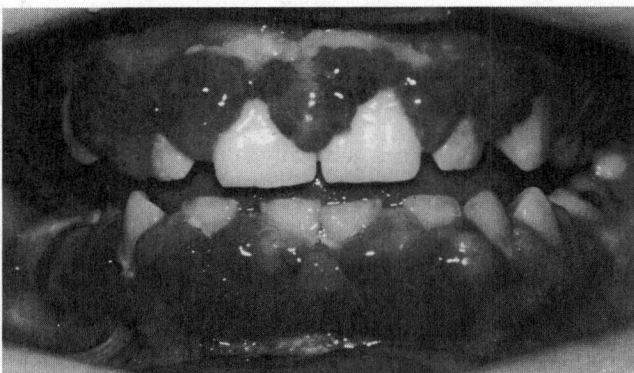

Figure 42–2

Gingival hyperplasia from phenytoin therapy. (From Adams, G. L., Boies, L. R., Jr., & Hilger, P. A. [1989]. *Boies fundamentals of otolaryngology: A textbook of ear, nose, and throat diseases* [6th ed.]. Philadelphia: W. B. Saunders.)

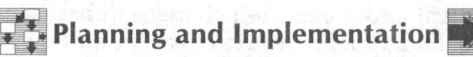 **Planning and Implementation**

The plan of care for the client with dental caries or periodontal disease focuses on the common nursing diagnosis.

Potential for Infection

Planning: client goals. The major goals for clients with potential for infection related to dental disease are that the client will (1) prevent infection by establishing a regular course of dental hygiene and maintaining a balanced diet, and (2) identify early clinical manifestations of infection.

Interventions: nonsurgical management. Prevention of oral infection and its sequelae is the aim of client education concentrated on establishing a regular course of dental hygiene and a properly balanced diet.

Dental hygiene. The nurse assesses the client's current course of dental hygiene and modifies it to include appropriate brushing, flossing, and rinsing. Modifying the current practices of the elderly client is often more easily facilitated and more readily accepted by the client than attempting to change lifelong habits. The nurse instructs the client in toothbrushing for the secondary purpose of stimulating oral tissues to assist in maintaining optimal condition. The nurse instructs the client to brush five to eight strokes over each dental area or for a total of 2 to 3 minutes after each meal and snack. This process removes most accumulated plaque in areas easily accessible to the brush and allows the surfaces of the teeth to be acted on by the remineralizing effects of saliva and fluoridated water.

The nurse demonstrates the use of dental floss to allow cleaning and massaging of the interproximal area (the area between adjacent teeth), where plaque tends to accumulate and access by the brush is difficult. The nurse instructs the client in oral rinsing as an adjunct to brushing to further remove debris loosened by brushing. Oral rinsing is advised when brushing is not possible. The client's need for specialized dental equipment, such as a floss holder or waterpick (Water Pik), is assessed. Electric toothbrushes are available, with a variety of actions and rotations. The large handles on these brushes often make them easier to use for clients with arthritis or those with hand or arm disabilities. Dental appliances, dentures, and professional assistance with dental needs can be costly. The nurse assesses the client's need for financial assistance, as many elderly clients are on fixed incomes without dental insurance.

Nutrition. The nurse instructs the client and the family as to the essential elements of a balanced nutritious diet, with special emphasis on the elimination of sugar and foods with hidden sugars (see the accompanying Health Promotion/Maintenance feature). The nurse addresses the special educational needs of the client who wears dentures for the first time. The nurse cautions the client about expected changes in oral sensation of foods. Full upper dentures cover the surface of the hard palate and thereby alter the client's ability to perceive the texture and the temperature of foods. The nurse instructs the client that increased time and care in chewing are needed, as the decreased sensation of foods in the oral cavity can make the client with dentures more prone to choke on large particles of food.

Fluoride. If the client has access to a fluoridated water supply, the nurse encourages the client to drink 6 to 10 glasses of water a day, barring any medical restrictions. In addition to being the accepted amount of fluid for general body requirements, this amount of water provides the client the benefit of ingested fluoride to strengthen tooth enamel and prevent infection. The nurse encourages the client to buy concentrated juices and beverage mixers that require water for reconstitution rather than purchasing ready-to-drink fluids. If the client has no access to fluoridated water, the nurse refers the client for professional dental evaluation of the need for supplementary topical or systemic fluoride treatments.

Early detection of infection or inflammation. The client and the family are given written as well as oral instructions regarding the clinical manifestations of infection. Clients are particularly advised to be alert for oral swelling, soreness, redness, pain on chewing, and pain referred to the ear. The client is instructed regarding who and when to call concerning suspicion of infection.

Interventions: surgical management. Surgical management of the client with dental disease is directed at either removing the entire tooth (extraction) or preserving the tooth by pulpectomy (root canal surgery).

Tooth extraction. Extraction of diseased dentition can be limited to the removal of a single tooth or a few teeth or can involve extraction of all teeth in preparation for prosthetic dentures. If only one or a few teeth are to be removed, the procedure is usually performed with local anesthesia. General anesthesia or heavy sedation is an option for the client having several extractions or a full-mouth extraction.

Pulpectomy. In pulpectomy, the entire pulp of the tooth is removed, and then the cavity aseptically filled and sealed to eliminate further infection. Although without living pulp, the tooth usually remains well rooted in the gingiva and can be of use to the client. The pulpectomy procedure generally takes from 1 to 2 hours to complete and is usually performed with local anesthesia.

Preoperative care. The nurse instructs the client preoperatively regarding the type of anesthesia to expect, whether or not sutures will be present, and postoperative care.

Postoperative care. Postoperatively, the care of the client is centered on the goals of (1) preventing postoperative dislodgement of the clot, which can result in excessive bleeding; (2) preventing infection; and (3) providing comfort measures to the client.

Inpatients and outpatients are instructed to keep pressure on the extraction site by biting on moist gauze

HEALTH PROMOTION/MAINTENANCE ■ Examples of Hidden Sugars in Food

Food Item	Size of Portion	Approximate Sugar Content (tsp)	Food Item	Size of Portion	Approximate Sugar Content (tsp)
Beverages					
Coca-Cola	12 fl oz	3	Canned fruit juice	12 fl oz	1–2
Dr. Pepper	12 fl oz	2½	Canned fruit cocktail	1 c	9–12
Fanta root beer	12 fl oz	4½	Canned peaches	2 halves and 1 tbsp of syrup	3½
Grape Tang	12 fl oz	7¼			
Hawaiian Punch	12 fl oz	5			
Kool-Aid Punch	12 fl oz	6	**Dairy Products**		
Pepsi Cola	12 fl oz	1¾			
7-Up	12 fl oz	3	Chocolate milk	1 c	3
Sprite	12 fl oz	6½	Cocoa	1 c	3–4
			Ice cream (vanilla)	⅓ pt (3½ oz)	2
Cakes, Cookies, and Doughnuts					
			Jams and Jellies		
Angel food cake	4-oz piece	5–7			
Applesauce cake	4-oz piece	4–5	Apple butter	1 tbsp	1
Banana cake	2-oz piece	2	Jelly	1 tbsp	4–6
Cheesecake (plain)	4-oz piece	2	Strawberry jam	1 tbsp	4
Chocolate cake (plain)	4-oz piece	5–6	**Desserts**		
Pound cake	4-oz piece	5			
Brownies	¾ oz	2	Apple pie	1 slice (average)	7
Gingersnaps	1	2	Berry pie	1 slice	10
Macaroons	1	4	Mincemeat pie	1 slice	4
Oatmeal cookies	1	2	Pumpkin pie	1 slice	5
Doughnut (plain)	1	3	Banana pudding	½ c	2
Doughnut (glazed)	1	4–5	Chocolate pudding	½ c	4
			Tapioca pudding	½ c	3
Candies					
			Breads		
Baby Ruth	2-oz bar	3			
Chunky	1-oz bar	2½	Hamburger bun	1 bun	⅛
Fudge	1-oz square	4	White bread	1 slice	⅛
Hershey's (plain)	1½-oz bar	2¼			
Marathon	1¼-oz bar	2¾	**Cereals (with ½ cup of ½% milk)**		
Milky Way	1½-oz bar	4			
Munch	1³⁄₁₆-oz bar	1¼	40% Bran flakes	1 oz	3½
Nestle's Crunch	1¹⁄₁₆-oz bar	3	Corn flakes	¾ oz	3
Peanut brittle	1-oz piece	3½	Frosted Flakes	1 oz	5¼
Snickers	1½-oz bar	2½	Fruit Loops	¾ oz	4¾
Three Musketeers	1¾-oz bar	2½	Product 19	1 oz	2¾
Tootsie Roll	1⅛-oz bar	1¾	Raisin Bran	1¼ oz	3¼
			Rice Krispies	⅝ oz	3
Canned Fruits and Juices			Special K	⅝ oz	2¾
Canned apricots	4 halves and 1 tbsp of syrup	3½			

Reproduced by permission from Chasteen, J. E., *Essentials of clinical dental assisting* (3rd ed.). St. Louis, 1984, The C. V. Mosby Co.

for 30 minutes. Some oozing from the extraction site is expected for 15 to 30 minutes; however, the physician is notified if bleeding continues after 1 hour. If bleeding does occur, the nurse instructs the client to expectorate the blood rather than swallow it so that the exact amount of bleeding can be determined and nausea and vomiting can be prevented. Local application of ice over the extraction site for half-hour periods for several hours and elevation of the head of the bed to 30 to 45 degrees decrease edema.

If the client is in an inpatient facility, the nurse assesses and documents the status of the oral cavity at regular intervals and monitors vital signs. The nurse assesses the client's need for analgesics and documents the effectiveness of medications administered. The client is allowed to eat soft foods but should avoid hot or cold foods for several days. The use of a straw is contraindicated, as the suction needed could dislodge the clot. Frequent oral hygiene measures with normal saline rinses often soothe the extraction site, but rinsing of the mouth or brushing of the remaining teeth should be deferred until the subsequent day.

After pulpectomy, there are no sutures or extraction sites, so postoperative nursing care is limited to instruction of the client and the family about comfort measures. These include administration of analgesics, elevation of the head of the bed to at least 30 degrees to decrease edema, local applications of ice over the operative site for half-hour periods over several hours, and ingestion of a soft diet with avoidance of extremely cold or hot foods for 1 or 2 days postoperatively.

■ Discharge Planning

Home Care Preparation

Minimal home care preparation is required for the client with dental disease. The nurse questions the client as to the availability of fluoride in the water and the need for special orthodontic appliances or equipment. If fluoridated water is not available, the client should be referred to a dental program for evaluation of the need for fluoride supplements.

Client/Family Education

Client education for home care includes supplying oral and written instructions regarding a balanced diet, routine oral hygiene, and early symptoms of infection (see earlier). The nurse addresses the special educational needs of the client who is given dentures to wear for the first time. The nurse also instructs the client in the care of the new dentures. Client demonstration of all skills involved increases retention of the information and documents the client's understanding of the processes and treatments involved.

Psychosocial Preparation

Body image adjustment of the client to an edentulous (without teeth) state, new dentures, or orthodontic ap-

pliance is assessed to mobilize home support systems for the client and to identify reluctance to adhere to the treatment regimen. The client is encouraged to express concerns about the diagnosis and treatment of dental disease.

Health Care Resources

Appropriate referrals to social workers, health care workers, and public health nurses can provide the client with resources for self-care. Social workers can assist the client and the family to obtain necessary equipment and supplies. Referral to local food stamp or welfare services can increase the quality of nutritional intake or help the client obtain necessary prescriptions. Community services can be sought for the client to ease the financial burden.

 Evaluation

Expected outcomes for a client with dental caries or periodontal disease include that the client

1. Adheres to a regular regimen of dental hygiene
2. Seeks professional prophylaxis and assessment on a regular basis
3. Maintains nutritional status by eating a balanced diet
4. Recognizes early signs and symptoms of infection and reports such to appropriate health care providers

STOMATITIS AND PHARYNGITIS

OVERVIEW

Inflammations and infections of the oral cavity other than dental disease can be generalized as stomatitis or pharyngitis, although the two can occur simultaneously. *Stomatitis* is considered inflammation of the oral cavity or mouth. The boundaries of the oral cavity are from the lips to the first tonsillar arch (see Chap. 41, Fig. 41–2).

Pharyngitis, or inflammation of the pharynx, occurs within the pharyngeal boundaries of the first tonsillar arch (including the arch, the tonsils, and the soft palate) to the posterior pharyngeal wall. Technically, the pharynx is divided into the nasopharynx, the oropharynx, and the hypopharynx.

Stomatitis

Stomatitis is classified on the basis of the cause of the inflammation as primary or secondary. Primary stomatitis includes aphthous stomatitis, herpes simplex stomatitis, Vincent's stomatitis, and traumatic ulcers. Secondary stomatitis is generally the result of infection by opportunistic viral or bacterial agents when the host resistance is lowered by a local or systemic disorder. The oral mucosa is often the first site to evidence a systemic disease. Implicated as etiologic factors in stomatitis are bone marrow disorders, allergy, systemic diseases, drugs, nutritional disorders, and emotional disturbance.

Primary Stomatitis

Aphthous stomatitis

Pathophysiology. *Aphthous stomatitis, aphthous ulcers,* or *canker sores* are recurrent small ulcerated lesions of questionable etiology. The lesions begin as small, erythematous, circular areas, which quickly undergo central necrosis. The resulting lesion is circular, white, and extremely painful and is surrounded by a red, often indurated, well-defined margin (Fig. 42–3). The lesions measure approximately 2 to 5 mm in diameter, remain for 5 to 7 days, and then heal within 2 weeks, leaving no scarring. The lesions are localized to the oral cavity, but can occur anywhere within the oral cavity. No systemic involvement has been noted.

Various causes have been explored, including autoimmune responses and psychosomatic causes, as these lesions are similar to gastrointestinal ulcerations with psychosomatic causes. The lesions often appear after periods of stress.

Incidence. Aphthous stomatitis is the most common form of ulcerative stomatitis (Jackler & Kaplan, 1988). Females are more prone to the lesions than are males. Young adults are most frequently affected, although the ulcers can occur in all age groups.

Herpes simplex

Pathophysiology. Stomatitis caused by the *herpes simplex virus* (HSV) occurs as a primary or secondary (or recurrent) infection, with secondary infections being

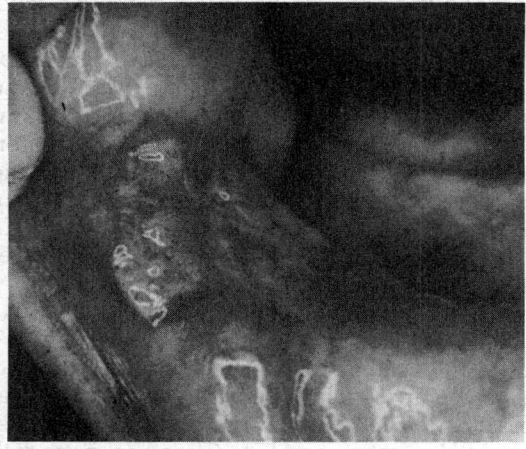

Figure 42–3

Aphthous stomatitis. (From Shafer, W. G., Hine, M. K., & Levy, B. M. [1983]. *A textbook of oral pathology* [4th ed.]. Philadelphia: W. B. Saunders.)

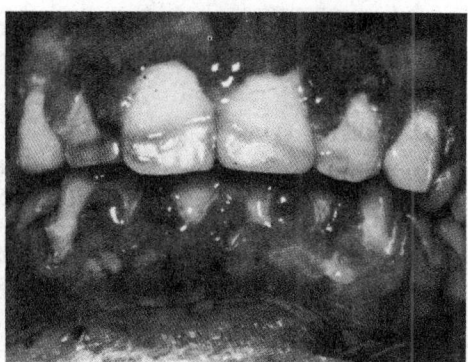

Figure 42–4

Acute herpetic stomatitis. (From Adams, G. L., Boies, L. R., Jr., & Hilger, P. A. [1989]. *Boies fundamentals of otolaryngology: A textbook of ear, nose, and throat diseases* [6th ed.]. Philadelphia: W. B. Saunders.)

more common. Two types of HSV have been identified: HSV type 2, causing genital lesions, and HSV type 1, responsible for nongenital lesions.

Primary HSV infections result from the initial exposure to the virus. The lesions appear in the oral cavity as uniformly sized vesicles, which occur most frequently on the tongue, the palate, and the buccal and labial mucosae. The vesicles rupture soon after appearing, leaving painful ulcerated areas surrounded by erythematous margins (Fig. 42–4). The lesions at this stage appear similar to aphthous ulcers. The ulcerated areas heal within 10 to 14 days.

The mucosal vesicles are generally accompanied by acute inflammation of the gingiva, occasionally with herpetic lesions on the gingiva. The tongue has a characteristic white coating, and the client complains of a foul odor to the breath. Primary HSV infections are accompanied by symptoms of generalized infection, including malaise and fever.

A secondary herpes simplex lesion occurs as a typical cold sore or fever blister. This is caused by a recurrent HSV infection. The current theory postulates that the virus lies dormant after a primary exposure (which is often subclinical, not resulting in generalized symptoms or stomatitis) and is reactivated by an upper respiratory tract infection, a febrile episode, exposure to actinic radiation (sunlight), trauma, or emotional stress. The lesions consist of a group of vesicles surrounded by erythema. These usually occur on the lip at the edge of the labial mucosa; the lesions can also occur in other regions. There may be a single vesicular lesion or several. The vesicles erupt soon after appearing, crust over, and heal within 7 to 10 days.

Incidence. Primary herpetic stomatitis is usually a disease of young children because the clinical manifestations are the result of the initial exposure to HSV. It can be seen in adulthood, however. Secondary herpes simplex is often seen in immunosuppressed clients, such as those receiving chemotherapy for cancer and those with human immunodeficiency virus (HIV) infection or acquired immunodeficiency syndrome (AIDS).

Vincent's stomatitis

Pathophysiology. *Vincent's stomatitis,* or necrotizing stomatitis, is an acute bacterial infection of the gingiva. The disease has a sudden onset and is related to the decreased resistance of tissues to normal oral bacterial flora. Systemic etiologic factors that decrease tissue resistance include poor nutrition, leukemia, and severe infections, such as pyelonephritis. Poor oral hygiene and extreme emotional stress have also been suggested as possible contributing factors. The disease is characterized by erythema, ulceration, and necrosis of the gingival margins, leaving a slough of skin that is easily scraped off. The gingival papillae that are normally between the teeth appear worn away and raw (Fig. 42–5). Clients complain of severe pain, foul breath, thick ropy secretions, and increased salivation. The gingivae often bleed spontaneously or from mild irritation, such as chewing. Systemic clinical manifestations can include malaise, poor appetite, and occasionally enlargement of cervical (neck) lymph nodes.

Incidence. Necrotizing gingivitis occurs frequently in adults, with the incidence appearing to increase with aging, probably owing to increased susceptibility to infections with advancing age.

Traumatic ulcers

Pathophysiology. *Traumatic ulcers* can be differentiated from aphthous ulcers on the basis of history and clinical manifestations. The client is usually able to recall injury as the etiologic factor. Similar in appearance to aphthous ulcers, traumatic oral lesions are less sharply defined and are generally not as exquisitely painful as aphthous ulcers.

Incidence. Traumatic ulcers are commonly found in clients with malocclusion, ill-fitting dentures, or broken teeth and in those who chew their oral mucosa.

Secondary Stomatitis

Lichen planus

Pathophysiology. *Lichen planus* is a chronic dermatosis involving both skin and oral mucous membrane. Oral lesions are present in many cases of lichen planus and are often the first manifestations of the disease. Symmetric, white oral lesions of various patterns (linear, interlacing lines, spots, or plaques) appear most commonly in the pharynx, but also are found on the tongue and the buccal or labial mucosa. The lesions tend to be domed and shiny, although those on the tongue are often flat and dull in appearance. The floor of the mouth is infrequently involved. These oral lesions rarely

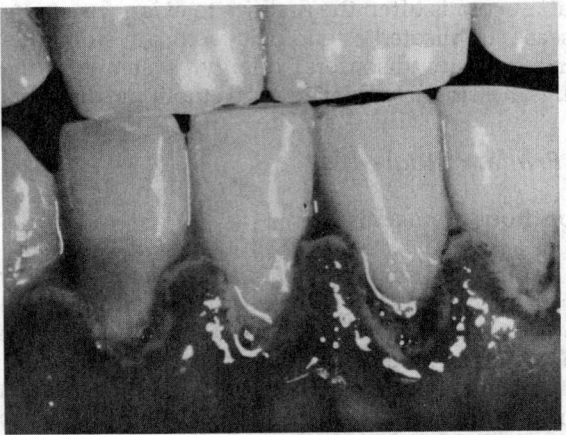

Figure 42–5

Vincent's stomatitis. (From Adams, G. L., Boies, L. R., Jr., & Hilger, P. A. [1989]. *Boies fundamentals of otolaryngology: A textbook of ear, nose, and throat diseases* [6th ed.]. Philadelphia: W. B. Saunders.)

ulcerate and are generally asymptomatic. Clients occasionally complain of a burning feeling, especially from lesions on the tongue. The disease process can last from months to years.

Etiologic factors proposed are psychosomatic, genetic, allergic, and infectious processes. Prognosis for cure is poor, and preventive methods are best aimed at exploring with the client the possible causes in hopes of bringing about a remission. Spontaneous flares and remissions are hallmarks of the disease.

Incidence. Lichen planus occurs with equal frequency in males and females and is usually a disease of middle-aged Caucasians.

Candidiasis (moniliasis)

Pathophysiology. *Candida albicans,* the causative organism of *candidiasis* (or thrush), is part of the normal flora of the oral cavity. With recurrences of candidiasis, as with all secondary stomatitis, a causative systemic disorder should be sought. Candidiasis appears as white patches, often described as milk curds, on the tongue, the palate, and the buccal mucosa (see Illustration in color insert). The lesions are anchored rather firmly and are difficult to strip away from the mucosa. Clients rarely complain of actual pain, but describe the lesions as dry or hot.

Incidence. Candidiasis of the oral cavity is commonly seen in clients who are undergoing immunosuppressive therapy (chemotherapy, radiation to head, or steroids), and in clients with immunodeficiency disease, such as HIV infection or AIDS. Clients who are diabetic, pregnant, malnourished, under stress, or taking antibiotics also have a high incidence.

Cheilitis (angular stomatitis)

Pathophysiology. *Cheilitis* describes stomatitis limited specifically to one or both corners of the lips. Rather than manifesting as discrete lesions, cheilitis is first seen as pallor of the area, which later develops fissuring (Fig. 42–6). Clients with cheilitis often complain of pain, especially on opening the mouth widely. Underlying disorders that can be responsible for cheilitis include nutritional deficiencies (specifically riboflavin deficiency), a recent febrile episode, neurotic habits such as chewing or licking the corners of the mouth, drooling, and candidiasis.

Constant maceration of the angles of the lips because of the presence of saliva can lead to cracking of the mucous membrane in these areas and the development of cheilitis. Loss of the normal tooth structures is responsible for excessive folding of the mucosa at the junction of the lips, which can also cause maceration of these tissues.

Incidence. Cheilitis is seen in clients with nutritional deficiencies. Clients with weakness or paralysis of the tongue or the lips after a cerebrovascular accident or surgery may experience oral incontinence, which can lead to cheilitis. Angular stomatitis is also seen in elderly clients with tooth attrition and tooth loss.

Pharyngitis

Acute Pharyngitis

Pathophysiology. Acute pharyngitis can be of viral or bacterial origin. The most common form of viral pharyngitis is caused by the coxsackievirus A—the pharyngitis might precede or follow an upper respiratory tract infection with symptoms of mild sore throat, low-grade fever, and mild dysphagia. Viral pharyngitis usually runs its course in 4 to 6 days and is generally responsive to symptomatic treatment.

Bacterial pharyngitis is most commonly caused by group A hemolytic streptococci. With streptococcal pharyngitis, the client notes abrupt onset of the disease accompanied by fever, chills, headache, and muscle aches. The client complains of severe sore throat and difficulty with swallowing. Obtaining a definitive diagnosis of streptococcal pharyngitis is important, as rheumatic fever is a possible sequela of severe streptococcal pharyngitis.

Incidence. Acute pharyngitis is common; viral pharyngitis occurs more frequently.

Vincent's Angina

Pathophysiology. The same organism responsible for Vincent's stomatitis also causes *Vincent's angina,* an extremely painful infection that affects the oropharynx rather than the gingiva alone. The client complains of a foul taste in the oral cavity and a feeling of choking, and the clinician objectively notes foul breath, fever, and enlarged lymph nodes.

Vincent's angina is generally secondary to systemic disease affecting normal oral tissue resistance. The disease is rarely seen after the tonsils have been removed.

Incidence. Although Vincent's stomatitis is common in adults, Vincent's angina of the oropharynx is rare.

Tonsillitis

Pathophysiology. Differentiating between acute tonsillitis and pharyngitis is often difficult. Clients with tonsils usually have inflammation of the tonsils when pharyngitis is present. Tonsillitis is often caused by beta-hemolytic streptococci. The client complains of abrupt onset of clinical manifestations, with fever, malaise, chills, and severe sore throat and difficulty with swallowing. When treated with systemic antibiotics, acute tonsillitis usually runs a course of 4 to 6 days.

Chronic tonsillitis is characterized by myalgias, occasional fever, and recurrent sore throat. The pharyngeal pain is usually not as acute as with pharyngitis and acute tonsillitis. Between episodes of acute tonsillitis, the client complains of mild sore throat.

Incidence. Acute tonsillitis is usually a disease of children and adolescents. Chronic tonsillitis is a disease of adults.

Peritonsillar Abscess (Quinsy)

Pathophysiology. *Peritonsillar abscess* is caused by *Streptococcus pyogenes* or *Staphylococcus aureus,* which spreads into the tissue between the tonsil and the un-

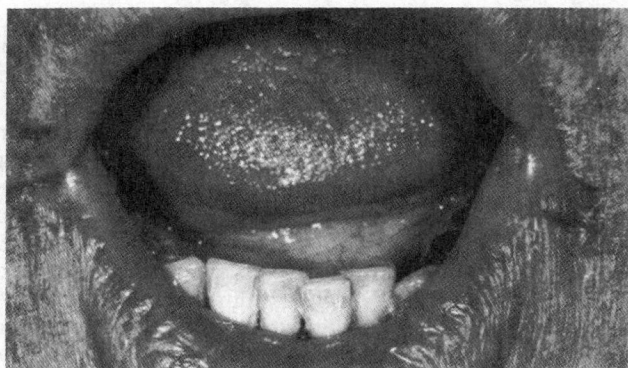

Figure 42–6

Cheilitis. (From Regezi, J. A., & Sciubba, J. J. [1989]. *Oral pathology: Clinical-pathologic correlations.* Philadelphia: W. B. Saunders.)

derlying muscle fascia and creates an abscess. If untreated, the infection can spread deeper into the neck, with the potential for eroding a large vessel. Another complication of untreated peritonsillar abscess is aspiration of purulent drainage if the abscess ruptures when the client is asleep.

The client with a peritonsillar abscess gives a history of sore throat for several days, with progression of clinical manifestations, including malaise and fever. The client complains of increasing unilateral pain and difficulty in swallowing thickened oral secretions. Occasionally, the dysphagia is so severe that the client drools rather than swallowing the saliva. Pain is often referred to the ear on the same side. Because of pain and swelling in the area, the client often speaks with a "hot potato voice"—a speech pattern adopted to decrease the pain caused by opening the mouth. Peritonsillar abscesses tend to recur; therefore, the client is advised to undergo tonsillectomy after recovery from peritonsillar abscess.

Incidence. Peritonsillar abscess is an uncommon but serious complication of acute bacterial pharyngitis.

COLLABORATIVE MANAGEMENT

 Assessment

History

When beginning to assess the client with stomatitis and pharyngitis, the nurse obtains a history of the current problem, which includes information concerning the *onset of the disease process* (sudden or insidious) and the *location and duration of the symptoms.* Rapidity of onset often signals whether the disease is a primary infection, a recurrence, or a symptom of an underlying disease. *Previous history of a similar problem* is discussed with the client to determine the presence of a chronic or recurring process. The nurse assesses the *presence of pain,* the *location* of the pain, and the effect that oral discomfort has on the client's daily routine. The *presence of systemic symptoms,* such as fever, malaise, nausea, and vomiting, is assessed, as well as *disability resulting from the condition.*

The nurse asks the client about his/her *routine oral hygiene regimen,* the presence of *dentures or orthodontic appliances,* and *the effectiveness of the current regimen* to determine changes needed in the oral hygiene routine. The client's *nutritional habits, ability to chew and swallow,* and *nutritional status* are assessed to determine any alterations in nutritional habits and status dictated by the current oral problem.

Physical Assessment: Clinical Manifestations

The nurse assesses the oral cavity of the client with stomatitis for *lesions, coating, cracking,* and *fissures.*

NURSING RESEARCH

An Oral Assessment Guide Assists in Communicating Changes in the Oral Cavity.

Eilers, J., Berger, A. M., & Peterson, M. C. (1988). Development, testing, and application of the oral assessment guide. *Oncology Nursing Forum, 15,* 325–330.

Oral cavity changes are a major problem for clients undergoing treatment for cancer. Despite this, a clear, concise, clinically useful tool for assessing stomatitis resulting from chemotherapy or radiation has been lacking. This pilot study was undertaken to assess the clinical usefulness of a newly developed oral assessment guide.

A clinical trial of the tool was conducted by studying the oral complications of 20 clients undergoing bone marrow transplantation. Nurses caring for these clients completed oral assessments before and during the transplant course. Scores increased as the condition of the mouth worsened, and decreased as the oral condition improved. The nurses using the tool showed a high level of compliance in their use of the tool.

Interrater reliability was established by this group of registered nurses using Pearson's correlation with $r = .912$.

Critique. This pilot study supported the interrater reliability of the oral guide. It also supported the guide's usefulness as a tool in quantifying changes in the oral cavity when used by nurses knowledgeable about its use.

Possible nursing implications.. Nurses may quantify their assessments of the oral cavity, which would result in better communication, more accurate record keeping, and improved care for clients with oral changes. The availability of a reliable and valid research tool would allow the opportunity to evaluate treatment for stomatitis. More studies involving larger client populations with variable disorders need to be done with this tool.

Characteristics of the lesions are described in terms of their location, size, shape, color, and drainage. Odors are also described.

Assessment of the oropharynx is limited to observation; a tongue blade is used to avoid stimulating the gag reflex. The client with bacterial pharyngitis has an erythematous and edematous pharynx with yellow exudate, often on the tonsils, if present. Viral pharyngitis is characterized by an erythematous pharynx without exudate. A client with Vincent's angina manifests an erythematous oropharynx, with yellow pustules somewhat detached from the underlying mucosa at the edges. The nurse assesses a client with tonsillitis as having enlarged, often erythematous tonsils with crypts filled with purulent exudate. Tender anterior lymphadenopathy is often present. Examination of a peritonsillar abscess reveals a red, edematous area above the tonsil

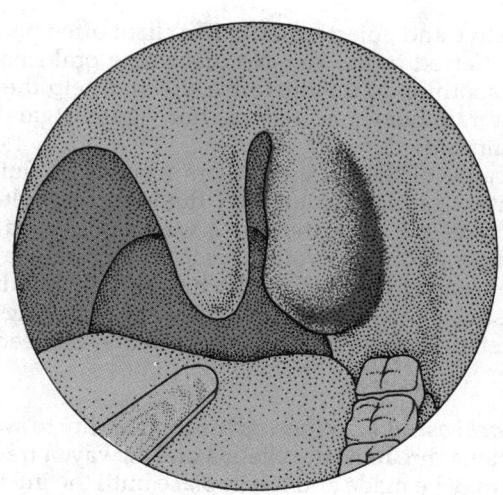

Figure 42–7
Peritonsillar abscess (quinsy).

between the soft palate and the tonsil, often displacing the uvula (Fig. 42–7). Edema of the area may threaten the patency of the airway.

Laboratory Findings

White blood cell count.   Clients with bacterial pharyngitis, Vincent's angina, tonsillitis, and peritonsillar abscess often have an elevated white blood cell (WBC) count. Clients with secondary stomatitis, such as herpes simplex or candidiasis, often have a diminished WBC count.

Culture.   Viral cultures may be performed on fluid from herpetic vesicles in herpes simplex stomatitis. Bacterial cultures are performed on exudate of pharyngeal mucosa to validate Vincent's stomatitis, bacterial pharyngitis, tonsillitis, and peritonsillar abscess.

Smears.   Gram's stains or smears of scrapings from white candidiasis lesions reveal hyphae.

Psychosocial Assessment

A large number of oral lesions suggest emotional stress; therefore, psychosocial assessment of the client by the nurse includes an in-depth evaluation of the client's perceptions of current stressors. The nurse inquires about changes in current life style, emotional trauma, or crises that have recently occurred or are anticipated. The nurse explores feelings of fear of malignancy; perceived pressures of life style, job, or school; and adjustment and coping patterns. As the functioning and appearance of the oral cavity are strongly linked with body image and sexuality, the nurse assesses the impact of the oral lesions on the self-concept of the client.

 Analysis: Nursing Diagnosis

Common Diagnoses

Common nursing diagnoses for the client with stomatitis or pharyngitis are

1. Potential for infection related to altered oral mucous membrane
2. Pain related to altered oral mucous membrane
3. Altered nutrition: less than body requirements related to oral discomfort or underlying systemic disease

Additional Diagnoses

In addition, the client may have one or more of the following nursing diagnoses:

1. Knowledge deficit related to treatment protocol, hygiene measures, and balanced nutrition
2. Altered oral mucous membrane related to pharyngitis or stomatitis
3. Body image disturbance related to altered oral mucous membrane
4. Anxiety and fear related to increased oral discomfort, treatment regimen, and suffocation
5. Ineffective breathing pattern related to edema and secretions

 Planning and Implementation

The plan of care for the client with stomatitis or pharyngitis is based on the common nursing diagnoses.

Potential for Infection

Planning: client goals.   The major goal for the client with stomatitis or pharyngitis is that the client will prevent infection or the spread of infection to other oral structures.

Interventions: nonsurgical management

Oral hygiene.   The nurse assesses the client's current regimen of oral hygiene and suggests modifications that might be needed owing to oral discomfort. Use of gauze sponges might replace brushing during painful episodes of stomatitis, or the nurse suggests oral rinses with normal saline as a helpful adjunct to brushing and flossing. Rinses can help debride oral structures, as well as provide a soothing effect. Clients who experience difficulty in swallowing increased or tenacious secretions can use oral suction equipped with a dental tip or a tonsil tip to evacuate saliva.

Drug therapy.   Systemic antibiotics are administered to clients with bacterial pharyngitis, tonsillitis, peritonsillar abscess, Vincent's stomatitis, and Vincent's angina. When inflammation and edema threaten the airway, the client is hospitalized for observation and treated with systemic steroids, as well as intravenous (IV) antibiotics.

Antibiotics are of little value, however, in viral or fungal stomatitis and pharyngitis unless there is evidence of superinfection. Systemic antibiotics are also ineffective and generally not recommended for clients with lichen planus.

Clients who are immunocompromised and contract herpes simplex stomatitis are started on a regimen of IV acyclovir (Zovirax) at the first sign of the infection. Acyclovir is administered to clients with normal renal function at a dosage of 5 mg/kg, infused at a constant rate over 1 hour, every 8 hours for 7 days. Clients with competent immune systems may be given acyclovir in oral or topical form.

Clients with *Candida* in the oral cavity are given an antifungal agent, such as nystatin (Mycostatin) oral suspension 600,000 units four times daily for 7 to 10 days. Systemic steroids can be of benefit in long-standing lichen planus.

Interventions: surgical management. The surgical management of pharyngitis includes tonsillectomy and tracheostomy.

Tonsillectomy. Indications for tonsillectomy include three to five documented episodes of streptococcal tonsillitis in 1 year, an episode of peritonsillar abscess, and exceedingly large tonsils.

Preoperative care. Before tonsillectomy, the nurse assesses the client's knowledge of the procedure and postoperative routines and supplements information as needed. The nurse discusses the continued need for routine oral hygiene preoperatively to prevent infection, the type of anesthesia, any preoperative medications, and the postoperative procedures and limitations, including IV therapy, pain and pain-relieving medications, diet, and activity.

Postoperative care. Early in the posttonsillectomy period, the client is placed in a side-lying position to prevent aspiration. The nurse instructs the client to avoid excessive harsh coughing, which could dislodge the eschar (scab) at the operative site. A small amount of bloody oozing is normal for the first 1 to 2 hours postoperatively; however, the nurse observes the client carefully for bleeding and encourages the client to expectorate saliva rather than swallow it so that the amount of bleeding can be determined and nausea and vomiting can be prevented.

The nurse keeps the head of the bed raised to 30 degrees at all times after the client is awake to assist in decreasing edema. An ice collar placed over the anterior neck, in addition to prescribed narcotics, often provides pain relief.

The nurse assesses the client's need for analgesics and the effectiveness of medications given, relying on subjective and objective data. The client often perceives pain referred to the ear. Normal saline oral rinses are often soothing to the operative site and help the client expectorate bloody secretions, but vigorous gargling is contraindicated.

Because of the pain, the client receives IV fluids for hydration until adequate oral fluids can be tolerated. Soft foods are suggested for 2 weeks postoperatively, and citrus juices are avoided, as they may cause a burning sensation. The client is discharged to home the day after surgery with written instructions regarding activity, diet limitations, and what to do in case of bleeding at home.

Tracheostomy. When edema or inability to swallow secretions threatens the client's oral airway, a tracheostomy may be made and left in place until the inflammation of the oral cavity responds to treatment and the oral airway is again secure. The client is hospitalized postoperatively, but generally is decannulated (has the tracheostomy tube removed) before discharge to home. (Refer to Chap. 61 for nursing care of the client with a tracheostomy.)

Pain

Planning: client goals. The major goal for clients with pain caused by stomatitis or pharyngitis is that the client will experience relief of pain, allowing proper nutritional intake and participation in activities of daily living (ADL).

Interventions: nonsurgical management. Nonsurgical management of discomfort from stomatitis or pharyngitis includes the administration of analgesics (both systemic and topical) and corticosteroids, cautery, dietary changes, and oral rinses.

Drug therapy. Analgesics, narcotic and nonnarcotic, are often required for the client with stomatitis and pharyngitis, as the conditions can manifest with extreme oral pain. The nurse assesses the need for analgesics and the effect of the chosen regimen on the basis of subjective and objective symptoms of pain and pain relief.

Topically applied agents often provide temporary relief of severe oral pain. Coating agents, such as kaolin and milk of magnesia, relieve severe oral pain associated with aphthous ulcers. The coating agents provide a soothing feeling, as well as protect the lesions from further irritation. Gentian violet, 0.5% to 1% aqueous solution, can also be painted on *Candida* lesions every other day for 1 week to decrease local irritation. Topical swishes are available, such as 50:50 diphenhydramine hydrochloride (Benadryl) and kaolin with pectin, lidocaine (Xylocaine) viscous, and dyclonine hydrochloride (Dyclone); these provide topical analgesia as well as local anti-inflammatory effects. Topical swishes are often prescribed for HSV and lichen planus. These suspensions can be offered to the client in frozen form, which provides longer-lasting analgesia owing to the numbing effects of the cold. Topical corticosteroids are indicated for aphthous ulcers and primary HSV lesions. Triamcinolone cream, applied with the finger or a cotton-tipped applicator, is frequently used with these lesions, or the corticosteroid can be injected directly into the lesion.

The use of cautery for painful lesions, especially aphthous ulcers, can decrease pain by destroying nerve endings. Phenol and silver nitrate are the agents most commonly used to cauterize ulcerative lesions.

Diet therapy. A change in the client's diet to liquids only or to soft, puréed foods can ease the discomfort of maintaining nutritional intake with painful oral lesions. A change in food consistency often eliminates irritation. Avoiding citrus juices and spicy or hot foods also prevents oral irritation. Cold, icy drinks are usually well accepted. The nurse assesses the client's nutritional status and ability to maintain adequate hydration and nutrition by mouth. In severe cases of pharyngitis and stomatitis, nutrition may have to be supplemented by IV fluids or nasogastric feedings.

Oral care. Gentle mouth care using lukewarm, soothing solutions is generally welcomed by the client with lesions of the oral cavity. Commercial mouthwashes are contraindicated, as they have a high alcohol content, which causes a burning sensation when in contact with irritated or ulcerated oral mucosa. Mouth rinses with normal saline, baking soda (1 tsp in 8 oz of water), or half-strength hydrogen peroxide are tolerated better than commercial products and soothe inflamed tissues. Frequent gentle mouth care enhances gentle débridement of ulcerated lesions and can prevent superinfections. Frequent oral care also tends to promote general feelings of well-being.

Altered Nutrition: Less Than Body Requirements

Planning: client goals. The major goal for the client with altered nutrition related to inflammation or infection of the oral cavity is that the client will maintain an adequate nutritional status to be independent in ADL and to have resistance to infection.

Interventions: nonsurgical management. In addition to promoting the changes in diet recommended earlier for decreasing oral discomfort while eating, the nurse assesses the client's general level of nutrition to determine the need for further intervention. Poor nutrition in general can decrease tissue resistance to pathogenic organisms. Chronic vitamin deficiencies can be primarily responsible for the development of oral lesions. The nurse requests assistance from a registered dietitian as appropriate because many clients with inflammations of the oral tissues experience dysphagia, taste changes,

and anorexia. Foods that are well tolerated may need to be substituted for others in the diet.

Severe cases of inflammation or infections of the oral cavity can prevent the client from taking adequate oral nutrition because of pain, edema, dysphagia, malaise, or nausea. If a decrease in oral nutrition is anticipated to last more than a day or two, nasogastric feedings, the administration of IV fluids, or IV hyperalimentation might become necessary (Chap. 13). Severe lesions of the pharynx often contraindicate nasogastric tube placement.

■ Discharge Planning

Home Care Preparation

Home care preparation for the client with stomatitis or pharyngitis involves assessing the specialized needs of the client who requires nutrition by alternative routes or oral suction. Clients with severe stomatitis who are receiving nasogastric feedings often benefit from referral to home care companies, which can provide nursing care personnel as well as nutritional supplies.

Client/Family Education

The nurse supplies written as well as verbal instructions regarding medications, diet, early symptoms of infection or recurrence, and measures to prevent the spread of infection. Client and family demonstration of all skills involved will increase retention of the information, as well as document understanding of the treatments involved. The nurse instructs the client and the family in how to assess the quantity and quality of nutritional intake and provides guidelines concerning when and who to notify about decreased intake. Reinforcement of instructions can be accomplished by the primary nurse by telephone conversations or follow-up visits or by the community health nurse during home visits.

Psychosocial Preparation

If the nurse anticipates that the client might experience disturbance in self-concept, the topic is introduced to the client and the family to encourage verbalization of concerns. Disturbance of sexuality is often a problem for clients with long-standing stomatitis (such as lichen planus) or with recurrent HSV lesions. These clients may benefit from referral for counseling (Chap. 10).

Another source of anxiety for the client with stomatitis and pharyngitis is airway clearance. Edema or increased secretions with these diseases can threaten the oral airway. Difficulty with breathing is one of the most terrifying experiences for the client. Although the possibility of airway obstruction may be remote, the nurse addresses the client's fears should the client display concern on this topic. Often, merely supplying the client with resources to call on at home allays much of the fear.

Health Care Resources

Two major health care resources for the client with stomatitis or pharyngitis are the social worker and the community health nurse. Consultation with a social worker is often sought for clients who require specialized equipment or nutritional resources at home. The social worker assists in assessing the financial needs of the client and makes referrals to government, community, lay, and church organizations as needed to augment the client's financial position and need for supplies. Referral to community resources for meal provision (e.g., Meals on Wheels or church groups) can provide increased stimulation during mealtime and a variety of foods as well. The community health nurse is consulted to assess the home situation, to determine the ability of the client and the family to perform the needed treatments at home, and to provide ongoing evaluation or information concerning home care, nutritional status, pain control, and the need for additional health care workers.

 Evaluation

Considering the actual nursing diagnoses, the nurse evaluates the care of the client with stomatitis or pharyngitis. Expected outcomes include that the client

1. Adheres to a regimen of oral hygiene
2. Maintains nutritional status by eating a balanced diet
3. Recognizes early signs and symptoms of infection or recurrence
4. Understands the cause of recurrent lesions and takes measures to avoid situations provoking recurrences
5. States that pain is alleviated or controlled

TUMORS

OVERVIEW

Tumors of the oral cavity, whether benign or malignant, have the potential for affecting many aspects of the client's daily routine. Swallowing or chewing may be altered, speech may be affected, or tumors may be immediately obvious to others. Pain may affect the client's ability to perform ADL. Tumors of the oral cavity often have a profound impact on the client's body image as well. The nurse must be aware of the many implications of tumors of the oral cavity as he/she assists the client to

decide on a treatment regimen and maintain independence and control while undergoing treatment.

The oral cavity includes the oral structures from the lips to and including the tonsils and the tonsillar pillars (see Chap. 41, Fig. 41–2). Tumors of the oral cavity can be classified as *premalignant, malignant,* or *benign.* Most benign lesions in the oral cavity are of salivary gland origin, arising from the many minor salivary glands located in the oral mucous membrane (see later discussion of salivary gland neoplasms).

Premalignant Lesions

Leukoplakia

Pathophysiology. Leukoplakia is described as a white spot or patch on the oral mucous membrane that is not due to other processes, such as lichen planus or candidiasis. The lesion can occur in any area of the mucous membrane, but is most commonly seen on the buccal mucosa. The lesion is usually asymptomatic, but clients may complain of slight burning or itching in the area of the lesion.

The presence of leukoplakia is important in that the lesions are considered potentially premalignant. In approximately 2% to 6% of cases, leukoplakia represents early squamous cell carcinoma (Jackler & Kaplan, 1988).

The major etiologic factors implicated in the development of oral leukoplakia are mechanical factors, such as poorly fitting dentures, broken or poorly repaired teeth, neurotic habits of cheek nibbling, and problems with occlusion that result in long-term irritation of the oral mucous membrane. The dryness, heat, and tobacco products associated with smoking, as well as excessive heat from food and beverages, are also implicated. The client may also have inherited a trait rendering him/her at risk for these lesions. Poor nutrition can enhance susceptibility to leukoplakia by lowering the resistance of the mucous membrane.

Incidence. Leukoplakia of the oral mucous membrane is a relatively commonplace disorder, usually seen in the fifth decade of life. Males are twice as likely to have leukoplakia as females; however, the incidence of leukoplakia in females is rising.

Erythroplakia

Pathophysiology. Erythroplakia is a red, velvety-appearing patch on the oral mucosa that is believed to be an early manifestation of oral carcinoma. Erythroplakic lesions are generally asymptomatic, are not raised or indurated, and are often discovered on routine oral examinations. About 90% of erythroplakia is early squamous cell carcinoma (Jackler & Kaplan, 1988).

Incidence. Erythroplakia occurs most often in people 60 to 70 years of age, with equal distribution between the sexes (U.S. Department of Health and Human Services [DHHS], 1988).

Malignant Tumors

Squamous Cell Carcinoma

Pathophysiology. Squamous cell carcinomas arise from tiny flat cells that line various parts of the oral cavity, most often the lips, the buccal mucosa, the gingivae, the floor of the mouth, the tongue, and the tonsils. Because these tumors usually grow slowly, the lesion may be quite large before the onset of symptoms, unless ulceration is present. Symptoms of a tumor include the presence of a sore or lesion in the oral cavity or in the neck (cervical metastasis), trouble with wearing dentures, mild irritation of the tongue, sore throat, loose teeth, or pain in the tongue or ear.

The American Joint Committee on Cancer has devised classification systems for tumors of the lip and oral cavity and for tumors of the pharynx. Each lesion is accorded a T (size or degree of penetration of tumor), N (the presence, size, number, and location of involved cervical lymph nodes), and M (presence of distant metastasis) rating (see the accompanying Key Features of Disease on pp. 1255 and 1256).

Overuse of tobacco and alcohol, in combination, is the primary causative factor of oral carcinomas. Excessive tobacco use alone is implicated, as is a history of a large alcohol intake, but the two factors combined appear to be especially destructive to the oral mucosa. Smokeless tobacco and snuff, which is tucked between the lip and the gum and held in place for long periods, are also implicated in the development of neoplasms of the lip, alveolar ridge, and floor of the mouth. As with leukoplakia, poor nutritional status appears to accom-

---

KEY FEATURES OF DISEASE ■ TNM Classification for Tumors of the Lip and Oral Cavity

Primary Tumor (T)

TX   Primary tumor cannot be assessed
T0   No evidence of primary tumor
Tis   Carcinoma in situ
T1   Tumor 2 cm or less in greatest dimension
T2   Tumor more than 2 cm but not more than 4 cm in greatest dimension
T3   Tumor more than 4 cm in greatest dimension
T4   (lip) Tumor invades adjacent structures, e.g., through cortical bone, tongue, and skin of neck
T4   (oral cavity) Tumor invades adjacent structures, e.g., through cortical bone, into deep (extrinsic) muscle of tongue, maxillary sinus, and skin

Lymph Node (N)

NX   Regional lymph nodes cannot be assessed
N0   No regional lymph node metastasis
N1   Metastasis in a single ipsilateral lymph node, 3 cm or less in greatest dimension
N2   Metastasis in a single ipsilateral lymph node, more than 3 cm but not more than 6 cm in greatest dimension, or multiple ipsilateral lymph nodes, none more than 6 cm in greatest dimension, or bilateral or contralateral lymph nodes, none more than 6 cm in greatest dimension
   N2a   Metastasis in a single ipsilateral lymph node more than 3 cm but not more than 6 cm in greatest dimension
   N2b   Metastasis in multiple ipsilateral lymph nodes, none more than 6 cm in greatest dimension

Lymph Node (N)

   N2c   Metastasis in bilateral or contralateral lymph nodes, none more than 6 cm in greatest dimension
N3   Metastasis in a lymph node more than 6 cm in greatest dimension

Distant Metastasis (M)

MX   Presence of distant metastasis cannot be assessed
M0   No distant metastasis
M1   Distant metastasis

Stage Grouping

0	Tis	N0	M0
I	T1	N0	M0
II	T2	N0	M0
III	T3	M0	M0
	T1	N1	M0
	T2	N1	M0
	T3	N1	M0
IV	T4	N0	M0
	T4	N1	M0
	Any T	N2	M0
	Any T	N3	M0
	Any T	Any N	M1

From American Joint Committee on Cancer. (1988). Beahrs, O. H., Henson, D. E., Hatter, R. V., & Myers, M. H. (Eds.). *Manual for staging of cancer* (3rd ed.). Philadelphia: J. B. Lippincott.

KEY FEATURES OF DISEASE ■ TNM Classification for Tumors of the Pharynx (Including the Base of the Tongue, Soft Palate, and Uvula)

Primary Tumor (T)

TX   Primary tumor cannot be assessed
T0   No evidence of primary tumor
Tis Carcinoma in situ

Oropharynx

T1   Tumor 2 cm or less in greatest dimension
T2   Tumor more than 2 cm but not more than 4 cm in greatest dimension
T3   Tumor more than 4 cm in greatest dimension
T4   Tumor invades adjacent structures, e.g., through cortical bone, soft tissues of neck, and deep (extrinsic) muscle of tongue

Nasopharynx

T1   Tumor limited to one subsite of nasopharynx
T2   Tumor invades more than one subsite of nasopharynx
T3   Tumor invades nasal cavity and/or oropharynx
T4   Tumor invades skull and/or cranial nerve(s)

Hypopharynx

T1   Tumor limited to one subsite of hypopharynx
T2   Tumor invades more than one subsite of hypopharynx or an adjacent site, without fixation of hemilarynx
T3   Tumor invades more than one subsite of hypopharynx or an adjacent site, with fixation of hemilarynx
T4   Tumor invades adjacent structures, e.g., cartilage of soft tissues of neck

Lymph Node (N)

NX   Regional lymph nodes cannot be assessed
N0   No regional lymph node metastasis
N1   Metastasis in a single ipsilateral lymph node, 3 cm or less in greatest dimension

Lymph Node (N)

N2   Metastasis in a single ipsilateral lymph node, more than 3 cm but not more than 6 cm in greatest dimension, or multiple ipsilateral lymph nodes, none more than 6 cm in greatest dimension, or bilateral or contralateral lymph nodes, none more than 6 cm in greatest dimension
  N2a Metastasis in a single ipsilateral lymph node more than 3 cm but not more than 6 cm in greatest dimension
  N2b Metastasis in multiple ipsilateral lymph nodes, none more than 6 cm in greatest dimension
  N2c Metastasis in bilateral or contralateral lymph nodes, none more than 6 cm in greatest dimension
N3   Metastasis in a lymph node more than 6 cm in greatest dimension

Distant Metastasis (M)

MX   Presence of distant metastasis cannot be assessed
M0   No distant metastasis
M1   Distant metastasis

Stage Grouping

0	Tis	N0	M0
I	T1	N0	M0
II	T2	N0	M0
III	T3	M0	M0
	T1	N1	M0
	T2	N1	M0
	T3	N1	M0
IV	T4	N0	M0
	T4	N1	M0
	Any T	N2	M0
	Any T	N3	M0
	Any T	Any N	M1

From American Joint Committee on Cancer. (1988). Beahrs, O. H., Hanson, D. E., Hatter, R. V., & Myers, M. H. (Eds.). *Manual for staging of cancer* (3rd ed.). Philadelphia: J. B. Lippincott.

---

pany many cases of oral cancer. Family history often reveals a trend in familial cancer incidence, which might indicate an inherited trait. Poor oral hygiene is associated with oral cancer. Deficient oral hygiene might be a factor in rendering the mucous membrane less resistant to infection and trauma.

Incidence. Oral cancers represent 3% of all cancers in the United States, with squamous cell carcinomas accounting for the vast majority. More than 90% of oral cancers occur in individuals older than 45 years of age, with a higher frequency in Blacks than in Caucasians (DHHS, 1988).

Basal Cell Carcinoma

Pathophysiology. Basal cell carcinoma of the oral cavity occurs primarily on the lips. The lesion is asymptomatic and resembles a raised scab. With time, the lesion evolves into a characteristic ulcer with a heaped-up pearly border. Basal cell carcinomas do not metastasize, but can be aggressive in involving the skin of the face. The major etiologic factor in basal cell carcinoma is exposure to sunlight.

Incidence.   Basal cell carcinoma is the second most common type of oral cancer, but occurs much less frequently than squamous cell carcinoma. Clients with outdoor employment are more likely to have basal cell carcinomas, especially Caucasians with fair skin, which poorly tolerates sun exposure.

PREVENTION

Prevention of leukoplakia and malignant tumors of the oral cavity can primarily be aimed at abstaining from or decreasing the use of both tobacco products and alcohol. Discontinuing or reducing smoking can often make the leukoplakic lesion fade away. Routine oral hygiene, which increases the resistance of the oral mucous membrane, and attention to early intervention for dental problems can decrease mechanical irritation, which is implicated in the etiology of leukoplakia.

The nurse counsels clients to avoid overexposure to the sun. If the client has an outdoor occupation, wearing a sunscreen and protective clothing is advised. Improvement of nutritional status is encouraged to strengthen the quality of the oral mucosa. The client with a strong family history of cancer, history of leukoplakia, history of heavy tobacco or alcohol use, or a combination of these is counseled to have frequent physical examinations, including thorough oral examinations.

COLLABORATIVE MANAGEMENT

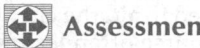 Assessment

History

When beginning to assess the client with a tumor of the oral cavity, the nurse obtains a history of the current problem, which includes information concerning *occupation* and *exposure to known oral carcinogens or irritants.* These include sunlight, mechanical irritation, exposure to heat (from foods or tobacco products), and the use of alcohol and tobacco. In discovering causes of possible insult to the oral tissues, the nurse identifies areas of client education needed to alter behaviors that are potentially harmful to the mucosa. The nurse obtains a *family history of cancer and a history of previous oral cancer,* factors that alert health care workers to be especially vigilant for appearance of neoplastic disease.

The nurse assesses the client's *routine oral hygiene regimen* and *the presence of dentures or oral appliances,* which might add to discomfort or mechanically irritate the mucosa. The nurse questions the client in regard to a history of *hemoptysis,* which might indicate an ulcerative lesion. Modifications to the client's oral hygiene regimen may be necessary owing to the inadequacy of

the current routine or discomfort experienced when performing oral care.

The nurse determines the status of the client's past and current *appetite* and *nutritional state,* including difficulty with chewing or swallowing. A continuing trend of weight loss may be related to metastasis, heavy alcohol intake, disability in eating or chewing, or an underlying disorder.

Physical Assessment: Clinical Manifestations

The nurse performs a thorough assessment of the oral cavity, looking closely for any *lesions,* evidence of *pain,* or *restriction of movement.* The nurse notes any *alteration in speech* attributable to tongue restriction.

Owing to the relatively high incidence of cervical metastasis with lesions of the buccal mucosa and the tongue, the nurse completes the physical assessment of the client with a lesion of the oral cavity by assessing the *cervical lymph nodes.* The nurse palpates for enlarged nodes in the cervical area (Fig. 42–8) using enough pressure to palpate structures underlying the skin, rather than rubbing the fingers over the tissues.

Psychosocial Assessment

Fear of cancer is probably the most important factor in the client's failure to seek professional assessment when oral lesions are noted. The nurse explores the client's fears and anxieties, providing information as

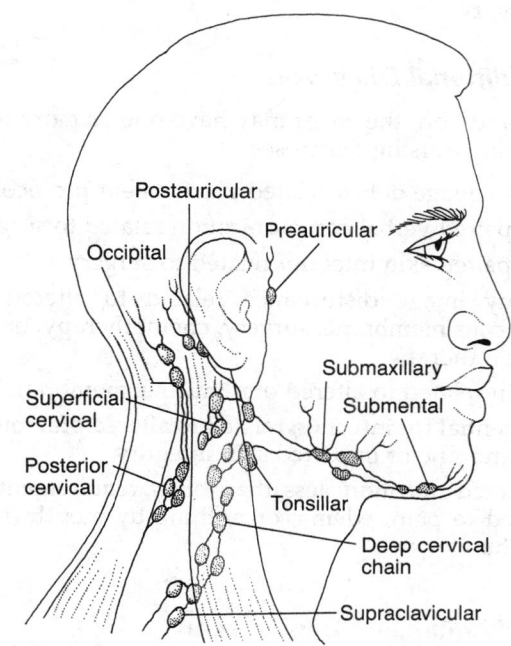

Figure 42–8

Lymph nodes of the cervical region.

needed concerning the diagnosis and treatment of oral lesions. The meaning of cancer to the client is assessed, as this often varies; some fear death, others fear pain or loss of family roles. The nurse assesses the client's support system and past mechanisms of coping. This facilitates the identification of available supports during the current crisis of diagnosis of oral cancer.

As the functioning and the appearance of the oral cavity are strongly linked with body image and sexuality, the nurse assesses the impact of oral lesions on the client's self-concept. In addition, the nurse assesses the client for any educational or cultural limitations to instruction or therapy.

Diagnostic Tests

A biopsy of the oral tissue is obtained to assess for malignancy or premalignancy. Biopsies can be performed with local anesthesia or with the client under general anesthesia, in which case they are usually combined with endoscopy (bronchoscopy, esophagoscopy, laryngoscopy, or a combination of these).

 ## Analysis: Nursing Diagnosis

Common Diagnoses

Common nursing diagnoses for the client with an oral tumor are

1. Ineffective breathing pattern related to tumor, edema, or secretions
2. Altered oral mucous membrane related to tumor or surgery

Additional Diagnoses

In addition, the client may have one or more of the following nursing diagnoses:

1. Knowledge deficit related to treatment protocol
2. Impaired verbal communication related to surgery
3. Impaired skin integrity related to surgery
4. Body image disturbance related to altered oral mucous membrane, surgery, chemotherapy, or radiation therapy
5. Pain related to altered oral mucous membrane
6. Potential for infection related to altered oral mucous membrane or impaired skin integrity
7. Altered nutrition: less than body requirements related to pain, edema, or nothing by mouth (NPO) status

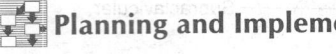 ## Planning and Implementation

The plan of care for the client with an oral tumor is based on the common nursing diagnoses. A complete client

care plan for the client undergoing excision or resection of a tumor of the oral cavity is found later under the heading Altered Oral Mucous Membrane.

Ineffective Breathing Pattern

Planning: client goals. The major goal for the client with ineffective breathing pattern caused by tumor of the oral cavity is that the client will maintain a patent airway. This is accomplished by removing oral secretions and decreasing oral edema.

Interventions: nonsurgical management. Maintaining airway patency is the goal of nursing measures centered on decreasing the tenacity of oral secretions, enabling the client to expectorate oral secretions, and decreasing edema in the head and neck area.

Measures to decrease oral secretions. The nurse assesses the client's current regimen of oral hygiene and suggests modifications that might be needed because of oral discomfort, bleeding, or edema. The nurse suggests the use of gauze sponges, vigorous rinsing, and the use of a waterpick as possible alternatives to brushing. Clients with ulcerative or bleeding lesions may be unable to use chemical mouth rinses. Many commercial mouth rinses have a high alcohol content, which can cause a burning sensation in the area of the lesion. The nurse modifies the rinse solution according to whether the secretions need to be vigorously evacuated or merely thinned and rinsed out. A solution of ½ tsp of baking soda in 8 oz of water is soothing and well tolerated by many clients. The nurse may elect to use a solution of half hydrogen peroxide and half normal saline to rinse the oral cavity. If the oral cavity appears to require more vigorous cleaning action, the nurse uses oral suction with a dental tip or a tonsil tip as needed to aid the client in expectorating oral secretions. The nurse often leaves the suction equipment for the client to use as needed.

The nurse also assesses the fluid balance and hydration state of the client with ineffective breathing pattern attributable to tenacious secretions. Increasing and improving general hydration have the effect of thinning the oral secretions, thereby facilitating removal.

Measures to decrease edema. Clients at risk for ineffective breathing pattern caused by edema are often receiving steroids to reduce inflammation. Antibiotics are given in case an infectious process in the lesion adds to the inflammation and edema.

The nurse elevates the head of the bed to at least 30 degrees to aid in decreasing edema by gravity drainage and assesses the need for supplying a cool mist via face tent to aid in oxygen transport and control of edema.

Interventions: surgical management. Occasionally, the client with an oral lesion is unable to sustain a normal breathing pattern preoperatively owing to the presence of tumor, secretions, edema, or a combination of these. A *tracheotomy* re-establishes a patent airway and can be performed under local or general anesthesia. The tracheostomy tube is usually left in place until the edema resolves and the oral airway is again patent. If the tumor is the major cause of the oral airway blockage, however, the tracheostomy may be maintained through the perioperative period until the tumor has been excised and oral healing begins. After postoperative edema is resolved, the client is decannulated (the tracheostomy tube is removed). (Refer to Chap. 61 for nursing care of the client with a tracheostomy.)

Altered Oral Mucous Membrane

Planning: client goals. The major goal for the client with altered oral mucous membrane caused by oral cancer is that the client will maintain or re-establish oral mucosal integrity by cooperating with medical and nursing care protocols during therapy.

Interventions: nonsurgical management. The two standard nonsurgical therapies for clients with cancer of the oral cavity are radiation therapy and chemotherapy. The two modalities can be given separately, but are often combined for an additive effect.

Radiation therapy. Radiation therapy for oral cancers can be given by external beam, in which the radiation passes through the skin or mucous membrane to the tumor site, or by implantation of radioactive substances directly into the tumor area (interstitial radiation therapy). The choice of radiation therapy is based on the tumor site and staging.

Interstitial radiation is used for smaller lesions that do not infiltrate surrounding tissues. The radioactive materials can be supplied via seeds, which are permanently implanted into the tissue; needles or wires, which are extracted at the end of therapy; radiation catheters or holders, which are later loaded with radioactive materials; or a "mold" of radioactive material placed directly over the lesion for specific time periods. Interstitial therapy delivers the radiation close to the tumor area and rarely involves adjacent tissues. The dosage administered, however, is often difficult to calculate, and the client must remain hospitalized and radiation isolation precautions must be instituted while the materials are active or in place. A tracheostomy may be required when interstitial implants are present owing to edema and increased oral secretions. (See Chap. 25 for nursing care of clients undergoing radiation therapy.)

Chemotherapy. The response of oral carcinomas to numerous chemotherapeutic agents is being evaluated (Table 42–1). The advantages of chemotherapy instead of surgery or radiation for cancer of the oral cavity remain to be determined. The nurse instructs the client undergoing chemotherapy regarding anticipated side effects of the medication, which vary with each agent. The nurse provides the client with antiemetic medications as prescribed and provides other comfort measures as needed (Chap. 25).

TABLE 42–1   Some Chemotherapeutic Drugs Commonly Used in Clients with Squamous Cell Carcinoma of the Head and Neck
Methotrexate
Bleomycin
Cisplatin (*cis*-platinum)
Cyclophosphamide
Doxorubicin (Adriamycin)
Vincristine
5-Fluorouracil
Hydroxyurea

Interventions: surgical management. Small, noninvasive lesions of the oral cavity can often be excised in an outpatient (ambulatory) setting with local anesthesia. The surgical defect is usually small enough to be closed by sutures. These smaller lesions are also responsive to *laser therapy*, which can be performed as an outpatient procedure, but which requires general anesthesia (Chap. 19). Small oral cancers are equally as responsive to radiation therapy as to surgery. However, excision is often more appealing to the client because outpatient surgery or at most a 1- to 2-day hospital stay is preferred to commuting daily for weeks to undergo external beam radiation.

More invasive, extensive lesions require more extensive surgical excision, usually in combination with radiation therapy. Not all lesions are able to be excised by the peroral (through the mouth) approach (Fig. 42–9). An external approach is often necessary—the surgeon may approach the oral cavity from underneath the

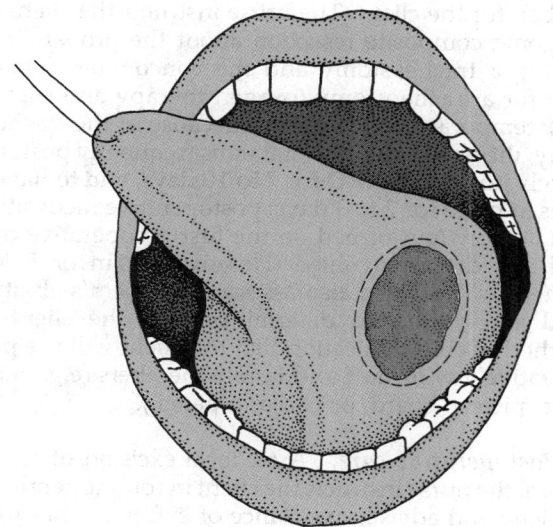

Figure 42–9

Peroral incision for surgery of the oral cavity.

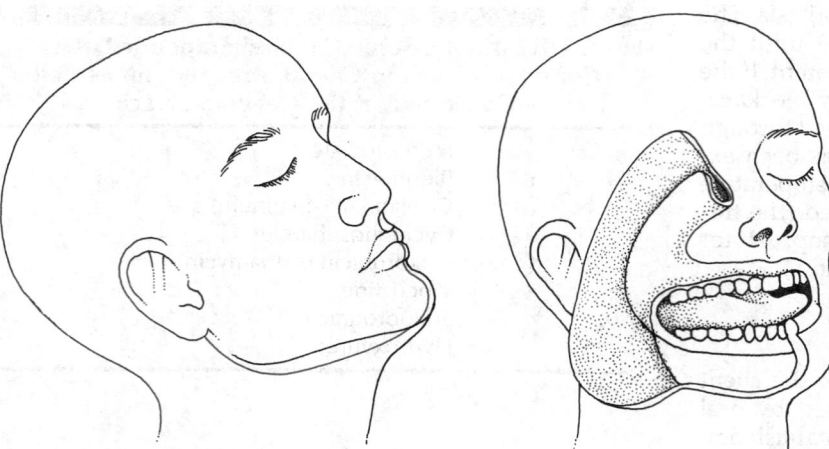

Figure 42 – 10

External approach for surgery of the oral cavity. (From Thawley, S. E., & Panje, W. R. [1987]. *Comprehensive management of head and neck tumors.* Philadelphia: W. B. Saunders.)

mandible or may split the lower lip and retract the lips and cheek for exposure (Fig. 42 – 10). Occasionally, the mandible is split as well and pushed aside for oral access; it is rewired at the end of the operation. The most extensive oral operation is the *composite resection* or *commando* (co-mandible) *procedure,* in which a segment of the mandible is excised with the oral lesion, usually in conjunction with a radical neck dissection (Chap. 61).

Preoperative care.   Before excision of a lesion of the oral cavity, the nurse assesses and documents the client's level of understanding of the disease process, the rationale for the surgery, and the planned intervention. Information is supplied as needed. Family and support persons are identified by the nurse and included in all teaching. The nurse discusses the type of anesthesia, any preoperative medications, and any postoperative limitations. For small local excisions, postoperative instructions by the nurse include informing the client of the routines of liquid diet for a day, then soft foods; no activity limitations; and analgesics that will be prescribed for the client. The nurse instructs the client undergoing composite resection about the probability of having a tracheostomy and the concomitant nursing care for a tracheostomy (oxygen therapy and suctioning); temporary loss of speech because of the tracheostomy; the need to obtain vital signs frequently postoperatively, to remain NPO for 7 to 10 days, and to have IV lines in place for 2 to 3 days; postoperative medications and activity (out of bed on the first preoperative day); and any drains involved (Hemovac drain or Foley's catheter). The nurse also assesses the client's ability to read and write and determines with the client the method of communication that the client will use postoperatively with staff and family members (e.g., magic slate, picture board, or pad and pencil).

Postoperative care.   After local excision of an oral lesion, the nurse instructs the client in routine gentle oral hygiene and advises avoidance of extremely hot foods and beverages, spicy foods, hard or crisp foods, and alcohol until the area is fully healed.

After extensive excision or composite resection, the nurse focuses on the clinical problems of ineffective airway clearance, impaired verbal communication, potential for infection, and altered nutrition: less than body requirements (see the accompanying Client Care Plan). The client may not recall on awakening from anesthesia that a tracheostomy tube is in place. Initially, the client may panic because of the inability to speak. The nurse reminds the client on awakening of the reason why he/she cannot speak and reassures the client that the vocal cords are intact. The nurse provides the client with the mutually predetermined method of communication. After oral edema has decreased and the tracheostomy tube has been changed to a noncuffed type, the nurse determines with the physician the appropriateness of instructing the client in how to speak by plugging the stoma with the finger. Clients who have undergone extensive resection may have slurred speech or difficulty in phonating. The nurse assesses the need for consultation with a speech therapist.

The nurse protects the oral suture line from trauma by prohibiting any oral hygiene, oral suctioning, and oral temperature checks until cleared by the physician. After healing has begun, the nurse provides the client with gentle mouth care to help clean away tenacious secretions, as well as to stimulate continued salivary flow. The nurse elevates the head of the bed to at least 30 degrees to assist in decreasing edema by gravity and encourages the client to be out of bed after the first postoperative day. If skin grafting was done, the nurse inspects the donor site (generally on the anterior thigh) during every nursing shift for bleeding or clinical manifestations of infection. (For specific nursing care for the client with a radical neck dissection, refer to Chap. 61.)

The nurse assesses the client's need for analgesics and the effectiveness of the medications given, relying on subjective and objective data. The client who has undergone a split-thickness skin graft often perceives the greatest amount of pain at the donor site. Comfort measures related to a painful donor site include providing a mechanism for keeping bed linens off of the site and consulting with the physician about using a heat lamp three times a day.

Clients who have undergone extensive resections of

CLIENT CARE PLAN ■ The Client Undergoing Excision of a Tumor of the Oral Cavity

Goal/Outcome Criteria	Interventions	Rationales
Nursing Diagnosis 1: Ineffective Airway Clearance Related to Edema		
Client will maintain a patent airway.	1. Provide nursing care for the client with a tracheostomy (see Chap. 61). 2. Utilize methods to decrease edema as instructed. a. Keep the head of the bed elevated to at least 30 degrees. b. Monitor and record intake and output, including output from drains, during each nursing shift. c. Ensure patency of Hemovac drains. Document and report any significant change in the color or character of drainage and any obstructing clots. d. Notify the physician if leaks or whistling is noted from the Hemovac drain. Apply bacitracin ointment over the leak to attempt to seal the site. e. Avoid pressure on flaps. If the client has a tracheostomy, check to see that ties are not constricting the flap. Prevent kinking of the flap by head position.	1. See Chap. 61. 2. Edema can obstruct the upper airway. a. Elevation of the head of the bed decreases edema by gravity drainage. b. Monitoring can indicate fluid overload or retention and the patency of drains. c. Hemovac drains are a major means of removing serous drainage and blood after surgery. Continuous suction provided by Hemovac drains is necessary for the viability of flaps after surgery. d. Leaks or whistling can indicate malfunction of the Hemovac system. e. Pressure on the flap impedes gravity drainage of edema. Pressure also impedes blood flow to the flap and can compromise flap viability.
Nursing Diagnosis 2: Impaired Verbal Communication Related to Tracheostomy		
Client will demonstrate the ability to communicate with family and staff members postoperatively.	1. Use methods to provide client with means of communication. a. Assess and document the ability to hear and understand the spoken voice preoperatively. b. Assess and document the literacy level preoperatively. Have the client demonstrate the ability to write. c. Discuss and agree on an alternative system of communication, such as pad and pen, magic slate, or picture board. Document the system agreed on. d. Consult with a speech therapist postoperatively as appropriate. e. Postoperatively, remind the client of the temporary nature of lack of speech as appropriate (for example, because of tracheostomy or edema).	1. Communication assistance provides a means for the client to express feelings and needs to health care professionals and family. a. A baseline of communication abilities is established. b. Assessment provides a baseline for determining choices of nonverbal communication. c. Documentation of a prearranged system of communication will inform other health care workers and provide continuity of communication between the client and the family. d. Speech therapists can assist the client in determining alternative communication methods and provide the client with input and a sense of control over his/her environment. e. Speech loss or difficulties due to surgery for oral tumors are often temporary and can be restored by plugging the tracheostomy to speak or waiting until edema has decreased. *continued*

Goal/Outcome Criteria	Interventions	Rationales
Nursing Diagnosis 3: Potential for Infection Related to Altered Mucous Membranes		

Client will have no signs or symptoms of infection or trauma at the surgical site.	1. Prevent trauma to the surgical site.
	  a. Do not reposition or replace the nasogastric tube in a client with pharyngeal anastomoses.
	  b. Do not start oral care until cleared by the physician.
	  c. Do not suction the oral cavity without a physician's order.
	  d. Avoid pressure on the donor site if skin grafting was done (site is usually on the thigh; prevent bed linens, etc., from rubbing the site).
	  e. Do not obtain oral temperatures for the client undergoing oral surgery.
	2. Monitor the surgical site for early detection of infection or complications.
	
	  a. Assess the cutaneous suture line for redness, drainage, and other signs of infection.
	  b. Clean sutures during each nursing shift with half-strength hydrogen peroxide; dry the area and apply a small amount of antibacterial ointment.
	  c. Assess the donor site during each nursing shift. Document and report signs of bleeding or infection.
	  d. Apply the heat lamp to the donor site per physician's order three times a day for 10 min.
	
	  e. After drains are removed, clean Hemovac drain sites with half-strength hydrogen peroxide; dry the area and apply a small amount of antibacterial ointment. Assess drain sites while performing care for early signs of infection.
	  f. Monitor vital signs as per physician's orders. Document and report any significant changes.
	
	  g. Assess potentially compromised skin flaps (see Chap. 61).
		1. Trauma could puncture or irritate the intraoral incision, the donor site, or cutaneous sutures; trauma could open a potential route of infection.
		
		2. Monitoring can detect complications and early signs of infection as soon as possible.
		  a. Redness, drainage, and tenderness can be early signs of infection.
		  b. Crusts and secretions could be ideal media for bacterial growth.
		
		  c. Frequent assessments can lead to early detection of complications.
		
		  d. Heat lamp promotes drying of the donor area if a skin graft was done; prevents bacterial infection by preventing the formation of a warm, wet medium; and is soothing to the client.
		  e. Crusts and secretions provide good media for bacterial growth.
		
		  f. Increased pulse and temperature can be early indications of infection. Discrete bleeding can be indicated by increased pulse and decreased blood pressure.
		  g. Continual assessment and documentation monitor flap progress.

Nursing Diagnosis 4: Altered Nutrition: Less Than Body Requirements Related to NPO Status		

Client will maintain adequate nutritional intake by nasogastric tube until oral feedings are begun.	1. Use methods to provide nutritional support while client is NPO.
	  a. Remind the client of NPO status when the client is alert.
		1. Nutrients are provided and tissue growth is promoted while client is NPO.
		  a. Elderly clients may demonstrate memory deficit; clients are often NPO until the intraoral incision has healed.

Goal/Outcome Criteria	Interventions	Rationales
	Nursing Diagnosis 4: Altered Nutrition: Less Than Body Requirements Related to NPO Status	
	b. Monitor IV hydration while the client is NPO and before tube feedings are begun; monitor and record intake and output during every nursing shift.	b. Evaluation of hydration status can alert the nurse to fluid overload or retention; the elderly are often susceptible to overload of fluids.
	c. Assess and document bowel sounds during every nursing shift until tube feedings are well tolerated.	c. A baseline for bowel sounds is established; the return of bowel sounds postoperatively is often an indication to begin tube feedings.
	d. Measure and record weight daily.	d. Weight changes indicate fluid status.
	e. Maintain proper functioning of the nasogastric tube: While the client is attached to suction, measure and record drainage during every nursing shift. When tube feedings are begun, flush the tube carefully with water after each feeding or medication administration.	e. Patency of the tube is noted by continued drainage and by flushing of the tube.
■ Demonstrate ability to assist with tube feedings.	2. Provide the client with written and oral instructions regarding tube feedings.	2. Written instructions provide the client with resources when the nurse is not available. Elderly clients often benefit from being able to review procedures several times owing to memory deficits.
	a. Include the family in all teaching.	a. Including the family ensures support for the client to perform the procedures.
	b. Have client perform return demonstration of procedure.	b. Return demonstration aids in retention of the learned procedure, as well as providing a means of evaluation for the nurse.
■ Maintain adequate oral nutritional intake with minimal dysphagia or aspiration.	3. When oral fluids are begun, assess and document difficulty in swallowing, aspiration, or leakage.	3. Clients occasionally have difficulty with oral feeding after oral excisions; assessment provides documentation of real or perceived difficulty.
	a. If the client is experiencing difficulty in swallowing, check with the physician about a consultation with speech therapist for assessment of or assistance with swallowing.	a. Speech therapists are often expert at evaluating swallowing disorders; providing the client with techniques of head positioning and breath holding or oral exercises can help overcome minor swallowing difficulties.
	b. Offer encouragement to continue to practice eating. Assure the client that this impairment is often temporary.	b. Clients often become discouraged at the inability to perform a previously reflexive maneuver. Providing the client with encouragement and hope often increases motivation and dedication to practice.
	c. Consult with the dietitian as appropriate.	c. Often a change in food consistency eases swallowing difficulties. Liquids are often poorly tolerated at first; semisolids are tolerated best.
	d. When oral feedings are begun, check with the physician about starting oral care measures.	d. Providing the client with oral hygiene can aid in cleaning the oral cavity of tenacious secretions, which often hinder swallowing efforts, and also provides the client with a sense of oral normalcy and well-being.

the oral cavity are often NPO for 7 to 10 days to allow for healing in the oral cavity before food products contact the incision. Nasogastric feeding or total parenteral nutrition is needed during this time. The tubes are usually inserted in the operating room.

When oral fluid intake is begun, the nurse assesses for and documents difficulty in swallowing, aspiration, or leakage of saliva or fluids from the suture line. A speech therapist is often consulted to assist the client with swallowing techniques. A swallowing impairment may be a problem, but it is usually temporary. The client is usually encouraged to practice swallowing.

■ Discharge Planning

Home Care Preparation

Minimal home care preparation is required for the client undergoing biopsy or minor excision of a lesion of the oral cavity. Home care needs for the client who has undergone extensive excision depend on the condition of the client at the time of discharge. Often, the client who has been decannulated is taking a soft diet by mouth before discharge. Occasionally, however, clients are discharged from the hospital while still requiring tracheostomy suction, oral suction, and nasogastric feedings. Suction equipment, nutritional supplies, and nursing care can often be provided by home care companies. (Refer to Chap. 13 for home care preparation for the client receiving home hyperalimentation, and to Chap. 61 for home care preparation for the client with a tracheostomy.)

Client/Family Education

The nurse supplies the client and the family with instructions regarding medications, diet or feedings, any treatments (such as tracheostomy care, suture line care, and dressing changes), and early symptoms of infection. The nurse consults a dietitian as needed to discuss food preparation and eating schedule with the client and the family food preparer. The client and the family demonstrate all skills involved to increase retention of the information, as well as to document understanding of the treatments. The nurse instructs the client and the family in how to assess the quantity and quality of nutritional intake of the client who is just beginning to eat and provides the client with guidelines concerning who and when to notify about decreased nutritional intake.

Psychosocial Preparation

The nurse assesses the readiness of the client and the family for self-care at home and consults with a social worker for counseling and referral for financial assistance as needed. Community health nurses can evaluate anticipated home care problems.

Clients who undergo composite resection often experience depression related to change in body image. Excision of a portion of the mandible can leave the client with a facial defect that may be difficult to hide. Speech is often affected as well. The nurse accepts the feelings the client displays and encourages him/her to verbalize fears and concerns. The nurse consults the social worker or other health care professionals for assistance with client and family counseling as needed (Chap. 9).

Health Care Resources

Social workers and community health nurses are two major health care resources for the client returning home after extensive excision for carcinoma of the oral cavity. Social worker consultation is sought by the nurse for assistance for the client who requires special equipment or nutritional resources at home. The social worker assists in assessing the financial needs of the client and makes referral to government, community, lay, and religious organizations as needed to assist the client financially. The community health nurse assesses the home situation and the ability of the client and family to perform treatments at home, provides emotional support, and performs ongoing evaluation of home care, nutritional status, pain control, and the need for other health care workers.

 Evaluation

Considering the common nursing diagnoses, the nurse evaluates the care of the client with a tumor of the oral cavity. The expected outcomes include that the client

1. Maintains a patent oral airway by handling oral secretions
2. Maintains nutritional status by eating a balanced diet
3. Communicates thoughts and feelings to family members, friends, and health care personnel
4. Maintains the integrity of the oral mucous membrane

DISORDERS OF THE SALIVARY GLANDS

ACUTE SIALADENITIS

Acute sialadenitis, the inflammation of a salivary gland, can be of bacterial, viral, or allergic origin. The most common causative organisms include *S. aureus*, *S. pyogenes*, *Streptococcus pneumoniae*, and *Escherichia coli*. This disorder most commonly affects the parotid or submandibular gland in adults. The precipitating event for the development of acute sialadenitis is usually a decrease in salivary production, as is often seen in dehydrated or debilitated clients or in clients who are NPO postoperatively for an extended time. The bacteria or viruses enter the gland through the ductal opening in the oral cavity.

Systemic medications, such as phenothiazines, chloramphenicol, and oxytetracycline, can also precipitate an episode of acute sialadenitis. Untreated infections of the salivary glands can evolve into abscesses with the potential for rupturing and spreading infection into the tissues of the neck and the mediastinum.

Assessment findings include pain and swelling of the face over the affected gland, which increases with meals. Fever and general malaise also occur, and purulent drainage can often be massaged from the affected duct in the oral cavity. Treatment includes the administration of IV antibiotics and measures to increase salivary flow, such as hydration, application of warm compresses, massage of the gland, and use of sialagogues (substances that stimulate salivary flow). Sialagogues include lemon slices and fruit- or citrus-flavored candy. Massage is accomplished by milking the edematous gland with fingertips moving toward the ductal opening. Elevation of the head of the bed also promotes gravity drainage of the edematous gland.

Prevention of acute sialadenitis is best accomplished by adherence to practices of routine oral hygiene to prohibit infections from ascending to the salivary glands from the oral cavity.

POSTIRRADIATION SIALADENITIS

The salivary glands are sensitive to ionizing radiation from radiation therapy or radioactive iodine used for the treatment of thyroid cancers. Exposure of the glands to such radiation produces *xerostomia* (severe reduction in salivary flow) within 24 hours. Radiation to the salivary glands can also produce pain and edema of the glands, which generally abates after several days.

Xerostomia resulting from radiation may be temporary or permanent, depending on the dosage of radiation and the percentage of total salivary gland tissue irradiated. There is little that can be done to relieve the client's dry mouth during the course of radiation therapy. Frequent sips of water and frequent mouth care, especially before meals, are the most effective interventions. After the course of radiation therapy has been completed, saliva substitutes may provide moisture for 2 to 4 hours at a time. Over-the-counter solutions are available, or solutions may be mixed using methylcellulose (Cologel), glycerin, and saline.

CALCULI

Salivary calculi, or stones, can occur within the gland itself or in the gland's ductal system. In general, calculi within the gland produce few symptoms unless an infectious process is present. Salivary calculi within the ducts, however, unless naturally expelled, often cause obstruction of salivary flow.

Symptoms of obstruction by salivary calculi include sudden pain and swelling of the affected gland, occurring most commonly when the client is eating. Treatment includes attempts to pass the calculus spontaneously by dilating the duct and the duct opening with increasingly larger sizes of bougies (dilators) and milking the gland. If dilation and massage fail to remove an obstructing calculus, surgical removal may be necessary.

NEOPLASMS

Tumors of the salivary glands are relatively rare, constituting only 3% of all tumors. The parotid gland is the salivary gland most affected by neoplastic disease. The most common benign tumor of the salivary gland is the *mixed tumor*. A mixed tumor usually occurs as a small, slow-growing mass. The client is usually asymptomatic.

Malignant tumors of the salivary glands are most commonly classified as mucoepidermoid, epidermoid, and adenoid cystic carcinomas. Malignant neoplasms are characterized by more rapid growth than benign tumors and are generally associated with pain. Facial nerve involvement is more common with malignancies, resulting in facial weakness or paralysis (partial or total) on the affected side.

Biopsy of suspected salivary gland malignancy is contraindicated as a precaution against rupturing the capsule (tumor covering) of the mass and thereby potentially spreading tumor cells into unaffected tissues.

The treatment of choice for both benign and malignant tumors of the salivary glands is surgical excision; however, radiation therapy is frequently employed for salivary gland cancers that are large, have recurred, show evidence of residual disease after excision, or are highly malignant.

Clients who have undergone parotidectomy or submandibular gland surgery are at risk for weakness or loss of function of the facial nerve, as the nerve courses directly through the gland. The nurse assesses the client's ability to wrinkle the brow, raise the eyebrows, squeeze the eyes shut, wrinkle the nose, pucker the lips, puff out the cheeks, and grimace or smile.

MALOCCLUSION

OVERVIEW

Pathophysiology

Malocclusion (abnormal occlusion of the teeth) is primarily related to altered position of the teeth or altered position of the mandible or maxilla to which the teeth are attached. Specifically, fractures of the teeth or mandible are most often responsible for the acute onset of malocclusion (as opposed to chronic malocclusion attributable to congenital facial deformity or uncorrected malposed teeth).

Fractures of the mandible create malocclusion when the fractured bone fragment is displaced. Fractures of the mandible are rarely fatal, but require treatment to prevent further malocclusion or deformity resulting from improper healing.

Fractures of the teeth cause malocclusion by changing the pattern of the fit of the maxillary teeth against the mandibular teeth. Malocclusion caused by tooth fractures also requires professional treatment to prevent infection of the pulp of the tooth, as well as to correct the malocclusion.

Etiology

Tooth fractures and mandibular fractures result from trauma. Many occur from motor vehicle accidents, work accidents, sports, and assault. The facial bones absorb the impact of the trauma and protect the spinal cord and the brain from injury. Fractures of the mandible are also caused by falls in the elderly, who are more prone to osteoporosis. Mandibular fractures are common owing to the prominence and rigidity of the mandible.

Tooth fractures occur from trauma similar to that causing mandibular fractures. Teeth can also be fractured by biting down on hard objects (e.g., bone or foreign objects) in foods. Teeth can become more prone to fracture as a result of decay or poor nutrition, which can soften teeth.

Incidence

Incidence figures for tooth fractures vary, but fractures are fairly common, especially in the elderly and those with devitalized teeth. Fractures of the mandible occur more often than other facial fractures (with the exception of nasal fractures), in part because of the mandible's prominent position.

PREVENTION

Strong tooth and bone growth from proper diet, the prevention of osteoporosis, the prevention of falls in the elderly, a decrease in automobile accident injury from seat belt use, and the use of correct sports equipment are all means of preventing mandibular fractures. Dental fractures can be prevented by careful chewing habits, proper dental routine, regular professional dental care, and proper nutrition.

COLLABORATIVE MANAGEMENT

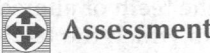 Assessment

History

While obtaining the history from the client with malocclusion from tooth or mandibular fracture, the nurse inquires about the *onset of malocclusion*, when the malocclusion was first noted, to determine whether the problem is chronic or is a result of a recent incident. The nurse obtains a complete *dental history*, as poor hygiene, improper nutrition, or lack of professional attention to dental problems can increase the possibility of tooth fractures. The nurse questions the client as to *recent trauma* to the head and neck, including biting down on hard objects in food. The client's *nutritional status* is assessed, including past nutritional habits, which affect tooth and bone formation, as well as the current nutritional status. The nurse obtains from the client information about recent changes or difficulties in eating caused by perceived malocclusion or pain.

Physical Assessment: Clinical Manifestations

The nurse observes the client while obtaining the history for deformity of facial structure. It is helpful to carefully observe the client when the facial muscles are at rest, as well as in motion, such as during talking or eating. As the client opens and closes the jaw, the nurse gently palpates over the area of the teeth and mandible, assessing for *pain*, abnormality or restriction of *movement*, *crepitance* (grinding sensation and sound caused by bone fragments), or *change in sensation*. The interior of the oral cavity is inspected; the nurse notes the presence of *broken teeth*, the status of the *dentition*, and the *intactness of the oral mucous membrane*. Teeth can be tapped with a tongue blade to elicit tenderness. The mandibular rim in the oral cavity can be palpated using techniques similar to those for the external examination, assessing for abnormal movement, pain, and crepitance.

Edentulous clients who do not wear dentures may be unaware of a mandibular fracture because of a lack of symptoms of malocclusion. Symptoms of mandibular fracture include pain on motion, lack of sensation from damage to cranial nerve V, drooling (pain often overstimulates the salivary glands), disfigurement, and disability in opening the mouth.

Psychosocial Assessment

The nurse assesses the client's psychosocial reaction to fractures within the oral cavity. As the functions and the appearance of the oral cavity and face are strongly linked with body image and sexuality, the nurse inquires about the impact of the fracture on the client's self-concept. If the disorder is due to trauma, the nurse assesses the client's reaction to and recovery from the event. If the fracture is the result of an altercation, the nurse evaluates the need for counseling or intervention by a social worker to evaluate the client's interpersonal relationships. Elderly clients who sustain fractures because of osteoporosis or falls are assessed for the need for assistance at home. The nurse explores with the client the meaning and consequence of any disability or life style change (such as inability to eat or pain) attributable to the fracture. In addition, the nurse assesses the client's education level, determines the need and desire for information, and identifies any ethnic or cultural barriers to education or instruction.

Radiographic Findings

If tooth fracture is present, dental x-rays are often required to determine the status of the tooth pulp. Other facial x-rays might be ordered, including panoramic radiography (Panorex), which produces a picture of the entire mandible as opposed to only one section.

 ## Analysis: Nursing Diagnosis

Common Diagnoses

A common nursing diagnosis for the client with malocclusion resulting from tooth or mandibular fracture is potential for infection related to impaired tissue integrity.

Additional Diagnoses

In addition, the client may exhibit one or more of the following nursing diagnoses:

1. Pain related to fracture
2. Ineffective airway clearance related to pooling of secretions and oral edema
3. Body image disturbance related to injury to the facial area
4. Altered oral mucous membrane related to injury
5. Knowledge deficit related to treatment protocol
6. Anxiety and fear related to diagnostic procedures and treatment
7. Altered nutrition: less than body requirements related to oral pain or malocclusion

 ## Planning and Implementation

Potential for Infection

Planning: client goals. The major goals for the client with potential for infection related to tooth or mandibular fracture are that the client will (1) adhere to a regimen of oral hygiene, (2) maintain reduction until healing is complete, and (3) maintain balanced nutritional intake while in intermaxillary fixation (IMF).

Interventions: nonsurgical management

Medications. Clients who have experienced trauma to the oral cavity often receive prophylactic antibiotics because of the possibility of wound contamination from foreign objects or normal oral flora. Narcotic and nonnarcotic analgesics are often required, as fractures of the teeth or mandible can be painful, especially when eat-

ing. Efficient use of analgesics can enhance client compliance with the treatments required for the fracture.

Alternative comfort measures. Much of the discomfort of tooth or mandibular fracture is related to pressure from edema. The nurse instructs the client to keep the head of the bed elevated or to sleep on several pillows to encourage gravity drainage of edema. The nurse also cautions the client to avoid sleeping on the injured side to prevent further discomfort. The nurse recommends the application of ice packs to the affected area to decrease swelling during the first 24 hours after the fracture; the ice often provides an analgesic effect as well.

Oral hygiene. Oral hygiene measures often need to be altered when malocclusive fractures occur, as vigorous brushing or commercial rinse agents may increase discomfort. The nurse advises the client to maintain adequate oral hygiene by using lukewarm saline or sodium bicarbonate rinses and brushing with a soft brush when and where appropriate. The use of a waterpick set on a gentle setting can be effective. By instructing the client to maintain oral hygiene, the nurse assists the client to prevent infection, as well as to promote feelings of oral well-being. The nurse assesses and evaluates the method of oral hygiene used and alters the regimen as needed to increase compliance by eliminating uncomfortable elements.

Diet therapy. The nurse counsels the client and the family food preparer concerning recommended diet changes to lessen discomfort. Soft foods that require little or no chewing or puréed liquids are often recommended if the client has pain caused by pressure from chewing. Hot and cold foods and beverages are also avoided, as thermal extremes can stimulate exposed tooth pulp or nerves. The nurse provides the client and the family with guidelines to ensure that a proper balance of nutritional elements is maintained while the client requires an alteration in food consistency.

Interventions: surgical management. Surgical management of malocclusion resulting from tooth fracture or mandibular fracture involves tooth extraction, pulpectomy, repair of the tooth with a crown, or reduction of the mandibular fracture. Crown repair entails restoring the contours of the tooth with gold, porcelain, or a blend of these materials by a dentist. The client may or may not require a pulpectomy before crown placement. (The reader is referred to earlier discussion of the nursing care of the client undergoing tooth extraction and pulpectomy.)

Reduction of mandibular fracture involves placing the mandible in proper alignment and maintaining reduction until the fracture is healed, usually for a period of 6 weeks. Clients with nondisplaced fractures are often placed in IMF (the mandibular teeth are occluded to the maxillary teeth and wired or banded without requiring further reduction) (Fig. 42–11). Displaced frac-

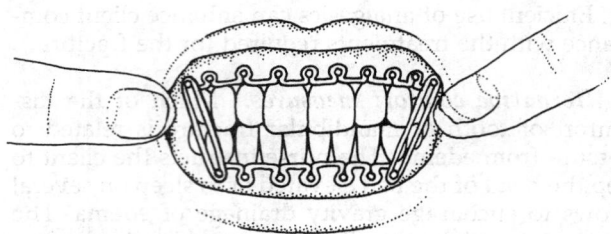

Figure 42–11

Teeth wired in intermaxillary fixation.

tures often require open reduction, a surgical incision to expose the mandible and reduce the fracture during surgery. Postoperatively, the client is placed in IMF.

Preoperative care. Clients who do not require open reduction of mandibular fractures are often treated with topical anesthetics while the wires are placed. The nurse discusses with these clients the need for a liquid diet while in IMF, continued oral hygiene while in occlusion, and the presence of pain and analgesics available.

The nurse instructs clients undergoing open reduction to expect the following postoperatively: IV fluids for 24 hours or until able to take a liquid diet without nausea, nasogastric suction for 24 hours (if the teeth are placed in occlusion during the surgery), the presence of pain and analgesics available, the ability to get out of bed the first postoperative day, and the application of dressings over the incision if the reduction is not done through an intraoral incision.

Postoperative care. The nurse monitors the client's airway closely as the client wakes from general anesthesia in IMF. Vomitus or oral secretions are extremely difficult to clear from the airway when the teeth are wired or banded in occlusion. The nurse takes care to visualize the positioning of the bands or wires that will require cutting should the client experience airway difficulty. Prevention of vomiting is a major nursing goal. Often, the client is not banded or wired until fully awake from anesthesia to circumvent the problem of vomiting after general anesthesia. If the client is placed in IMF in the operating room, the client may have a nasogastric tube to suction and empty the stomach of gastric contents until fully awake. After the client in IMF is fully alert and begins to take a liquid diet, the nurse instructs the client and the family to notify the nursing staff for symptoms of nausea. Antiemetics can be administered to overcome nausea. If the client begins to vomit, the nurse will have to cut the wires with wire cutters kept at the bedside or cut the bands with scissors to clear the client's oral airway. Suction equipment is often kept at the bedside for emergencies to help in clearing the oral airway in these circumstances. Bands or wires will also be cut for other respiratory emergencies, such as respiratory arrest and the need for cardiopulmonary resuscitation.

The nurse inspects the incision for signs of infection or bleeding. Cutaneous suture lines are cleaned two to four times a day with half-strength hydrogen peroxide (half hydrogen peroxide, half normal saline), and a small amount of antibacterial ointment is applied to prevent infection, prevent crusting, and decrease scarring.

The nurse instructs the client in oral care to maintain dental health, as well as to prevent infection if there is an intraoral incision. With the teeth wired in occlusion, brushing of the lingual aspects of the teeth is impossible. The nurse checks with the physician about the advisability of using a soft brush to clean the outer aspects of the teeth as appropriate. Oral rinses are the most effective methods of oral cleaning to date for the client in IMF. Rinse agents applied under pressure, such as with a waterpick or bulb syringe, provide débridement. The nurse also supplies the client with a lip emollient to prevent cracked lips, as clients in IMF also are unable to lick their lips.

For comfort measures, the nurse raises the head of the client's bed to at least 30 degrees after the client is fully awake from general anesthesia to assist in decreasing edema. The nurse assesses the client's subjective and objective symptoms of discomfort to determine the need for analgesics and the effectiveness of the analgesic regimen. The nurse carefully assesses the level of analgesia achieved to prevent oversedation and decrease in important reflexes, especially the gag reflex. Wires used to place the client in IMF often press against the gingivae and lips and can be painful for the client, especially if oral edema is placing the wires in direct contact with oral structures. The nurse assesses the need for topical anesthetics. Bone wax, beeswax, or dental wax can be rubbed over protruding wires to soften sharp edges and prevent further trauma. Assisting the client to be more comfortable in IMF often increases client compliance with measures needed during IMF and encourages the client not to tamper with bands and wires.

Clients in IMF are unable to chew and must take all nutrition in liquid or puréed liquid form. The nurse consults with a dietitian to instruct the client and the family food preparer in the preparation of the diet and in maintenance of nutritional balance while the client is ingesting a liquid diet. Often, the food preparer must be creative to provide enough variation in a potentially monotonous diet. Clients in IMF often lose 10 to 20 lb in 6 weeks. Special care must be taken to assess the client's nutritional status and prevent excessive weight loss.

■ **Discharge Planning**

Home Care Preparation

Little home care preparation is needed for the client who has undergone repair or extraction of a fractured tooth. For clients who have had repair of a fractured mandible, the nurse assesses the client's need for a blender for diet preparation and a waterpick for oral care.

Client/Family Education

The nurse instructs the family and the client regarding treatments (such as suture line care and dressing changes), oral care, medications, diet, and early detection of infection.

The nurse counsels the client in IMF about safety precautions while the teeth are wired in occlusion. The nurse cautions the client to have scissors or wire cutters with him/her at all times and instructs the client in which wires to cut in an emergency. Swimming and water activities are contraindicated, as the water entering the oral cavity is difficult to clear quickly while in IMF. The nurse instructs the client to avoid carbonated beverages because the fizzing in the oral cavity can often cause sensations of choking. Alcoholic beverages are contraindicated while the client is maintained in IMF, not only because of the potential for vomiting after excessive alcohol intake, but also because of the effect of alcohol on decreasing the gag reflex. The client is advised to avoid contact sports or any activities that could result in re-injury to the fracture area.

The nurse also advises the client to seek professional dental assistance after the wires are removed, as the minimal hygiene measures during the 6-week period of IMF often result in numerous caries, which require attention.

Psychosocial Preparation

As for clients with other disorders of the oral cavity, clients who have undergone tooth repair or extraction because of fracture or who are in IMF for mandibular fracture often experience a disturbance in self-concept. The appearance of oral disorders is often difficult to hide. In addition, the client in IMF experiences changes in speech pattern and eating. If the nurse anticipates that the client may experience a disturbance in self-concept, the topic is introduced to the client and the family before discharge from the hospital to encourage verbalization of these feelings and to assure the client that such feelings are common and to be expected.

Health Care Resources

The social worker is often sought to assist the client with financial needs, procure equipment, supply special dietary needs at home, or assist in counseling the client who is experiencing difficulty returning to social roles. Community health nurses assess the home situation, ascertain the ability of the client and the family to perform the treatment or supply the diet at home, provide ongoing evaluation of the client at home (for example, assess nutritional status and pain control), provide emotional support to the client and the family, and determine the need for other health care workers at home.

 ## Evaluation

On the basis of the common nursing diagnoses, the nurse evaluates the care of the client with malocclusion resulting from a tooth or mandibular fracture according to the expected client outcomes. The expected outcomes include that the client

1. Adheres to a regimen of oral hygiene
2. States that pain is alleviated or controlled
3. Recognizes early clinical manifestations of infection
4. Maintains balanced nutrition while in IMF

SUMMARY

Problems and potential problems of the oral cavity are numerous and often have varied clinical manifestations. However, the effects of these disorders on the client and the client's life style are often similar. Oral discomfort can affect the ability to speak, eat, or manage oral secretions. Edema or lesions are often obvious to others. Physical changes in the head and neck area are difficult to hide. Owing to the effect of oral disease on the client's ADL, diseases of the oral cavity often have a profound effect on the client's self-concept and body image. Even clients with benign oral lesions often require counseling and emotional support to resume normal activities and social roles.

Awareness by the nurse of the clinical manifestations of oral diseases and the profound effect these diseases can have on the client can aid in instituting nursing interventions early. These interventions are aimed at decreasing or avoiding the physical and psychologic difficulties associated with lesions of the oral cavity.

IMPLICATIONS FOR RESEARCH

Little information is available in the literature about the role of the nurse in multimodal research of problems of the oral cavity. Nurses are well prepared to assess and evaluate the client and the client's understanding of oral lesions and their treatment, as well as to assess the client's response to illness. The area most often researched by nurses is the assessment and evaluation of oral care and oral hygiene measures, particularly oncology nursing of stomatitis (see earlier Nursing Research feature).

Potential research questions for nurses regarding oral lesions include

1. What topical methods provide the most effective relief of pain from aphthous stomatitis?
2. What oral care measures provide the best débridement of the oral cavity for clients in IMF?
3. What factors motivate clients to adhere to a regimen of dental and oral hygiene?
4. Is there a role for stress management in the treatment of stomatitis?

REFERENCES AND READINGS

Auld, E. M. (1988). Oral health. *Geriatric Nursing, 9,* 340–341.

Chasteen, J. E. (1984). *Essentials of clinical dental assisting* (3rd ed.). St. Louis: C. V. Mosby.

Cummings, C. W., & Schuller, D. (Eds.). (1986). *Otolaryngology–head and neck surgery* (Vol. 1). St. Louis: C. V. Mosby.

DeWeese, D. F., & Saunders, W. H. (Eds.). (1982). *Textbook of otolaryngology* (6th ed.). St. Louis: C. V. Mosby.

Harris, N. O., & Christen, A. (1982). *Primary preventive dentistry.* Reston, VA: Reston Publishing.

Hilderley, L. J. (1987). Radiotherapy. In S. L. Groenwald (Ed.), *Cancer nursing: Principles and practice* (pp. 320–344). Boston: Jones & Bartlett.

Isselbacher, K. J., Adams, R. D., Braunwald, E., Pettersdorf, R. G., & Wilson, J. D. (Eds.). (1980). *Harrison's principles of internal medicine* (9th ed.). New York: McGraw-Hill.

Jackler, R. K., & Kaplan, M. J. (1988). Ear, nose and throat. In S. A. Schroeder, M. A. Krupp, & L. M. Tierney (Eds.), *Current medical diagnosis and treatment* (pp. 110–131). Norwalk, CT: Appleton & Lange.

Knauer, C. M., & Silverman, S. (1988). Alimentary tract and liver. In S. A. Schroeder, M. A. Krupp, & L. M. Tierney (Eds.). *Current medical diagnosis and treatment* (pp. 342–428). Norwalk, CT: Appleton & Lange.

Lynch, M. A. (Ed.). (1984). *Burket's oral medicine* (8th ed.). Philadelphia: J. B. Lippincott.

Mason, D. K., & Chisholm, D. M. (1975). *Salivary glands in health and disease.* Philadelphia: W. B. Saunders.

McCarthy, P., & Shklar, G. (1980). *Diseases of the oral mucosa* (2nd ed.). Philadelphia: Lea & Febiger.

Paparella, M. M., & Shumrick, D. A. (Eds.). (1980). *Otolaryngology* (2nd ed., Vol. 3). Philadelphia: W. B. Saunders.

Peterson, D. E. (1986). Oral complications associated with hematologic neoplasms and their treatment. In D. E. Peterson, et al. (Eds.), *Head and neck management of the cancer patient* (pp. 351–361). New York: Martinus Nijhoff.

Suen, J. Y., & Myers, E. N. (Eds.). (1981). *Cancer of the head and neck.* New York: Churchill Livingstone.

U.S. Department of Health and Human Services. (1988). *Oral cancers* (NIH Publication No. 88–2876). Bethesda, MD: National Cancer Institute.

Yuska, C. (Ed.). (1989). Head and neck cancer. *Seminars in Oncology Nursing, 5*(3).

Zinner, S. H., Belcher, A. E., & Murphy, C. (1988). *Assessing the risk of herpes in immunocompromised patients* (Monograph No. 729). Research Triangle Park, NC: Burroughs Wellcome Co.

ADDITIONAL READINGS

Blaney, G. M. (1986). Mouth care—basic and essential. *Geriatric Nursing, 7,* 242–243.

This article delineates medical conditions, medications, and other stressors that affect the health of oral cavity tissues. Various nursing measures and oral hygiene techniques are discussed.

Kahn, R. (1986). Renewing the commitment to oral hygiene. *Geriatric Nursing, 7,* 244–247.

This article outlines a teaching program for clients and nurses to promote self-care of the teeth, gums, and tongue.

Ofstenhage, J. C., & Magilvy, K. (1986). Oral health and aging. *Geriatric Nursing, 7,* 238–241.

This article provides a discussion of age-related changes in oral cavity structure and function, including teeth, salivary glands, mucosa, taste perception, and motor function.

O'Laughlin, J. (1986). A dental program for nursing home residents. *Geriatric Nursing, 7,* 248–250.

Description of a care plan is provided in this article, which was written by a dentist. The purpose of this work was to teach nursing staff in long-term care facilities proper oral care for clients.

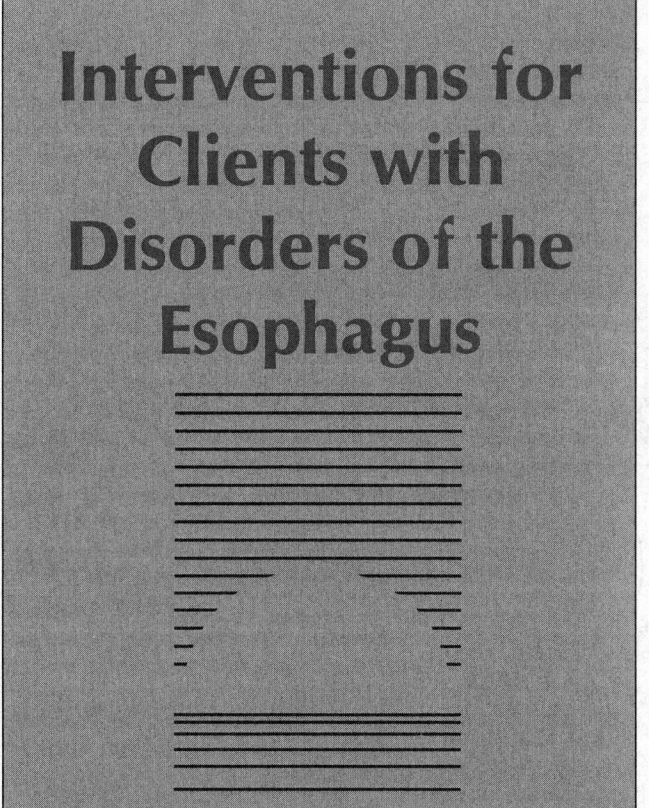

CHAPTER 43

Interventions for Clients with Disorders of the Esophagus

The esophagus is a hollow tube, located behind the trachea, that passes through the diaphragm at the esophageal hiatus (Fig. 43–1). The esophagus serves primarily as a food conduit, transporting the bolus of food from the mouth to the stomach while preventing the backward flow of gastrointestinal (GI) contents. The upper one-third of the esophagus is composed of skeletal muscle and the remaining two-thirds, smooth muscle. Despite its basic simplicity, the esophagus is vulnerable to a variety of inflammatory, structural, motor, and neoplastic health problems. These disorders range in severity from mild and annoying to life-threatening. The nurse plays a significant role in successful disease management because many of the treatment strategies involve diet and life style modifications rather than definitive medical or surgical therapy. Appropriate client teaching, family counseling, and support can influence the client's overall adaptation and self-care ability in a positive way.

GASTROESOPHAGEAL REFLUX DISEASE

OVERVIEW

Esophageal reflux, which involves the backward flow of GI contents into the esophagus, is estimated to account for up to 90% of all esophageal disease (Henderson, 1986). *Gastroesophageal reflux disease* (GERD) is a term that is used to describe a heterogeneous syndrome that can result from esophageal reflux. Reflux produces its characteristic symptoms by exposing the esophageal mucosa to the irritating effects of gastric and/or duodenal contents, which gradually break down the mucous barrier of the esophagus. An individual with acute symptoms of inflammation is often described as having *reflux esophagitis,* but this term is not as descriptive or inclusive as GERD.

Pathophysiology

The reflux of gastric contents into the esophagus is normally prevented by the presence of two esophageal sphincters, which remain closed except during the act of swallowing. These sphincters are not really distinct anatomic structures but are zones of high pressure at the upper and lower ends of the esophagus that are under muscular, hormonal, and neural control. The function of the lower esophageal sphincter (LES) is supported by its anatomic placement in the abdomen, where the surrounding pressure is significantly higher than in the low-pressure thorax. Sphincter function is also augmented by the acute angle (angle of His) that is formed as the normal esophagus enters the stomach.

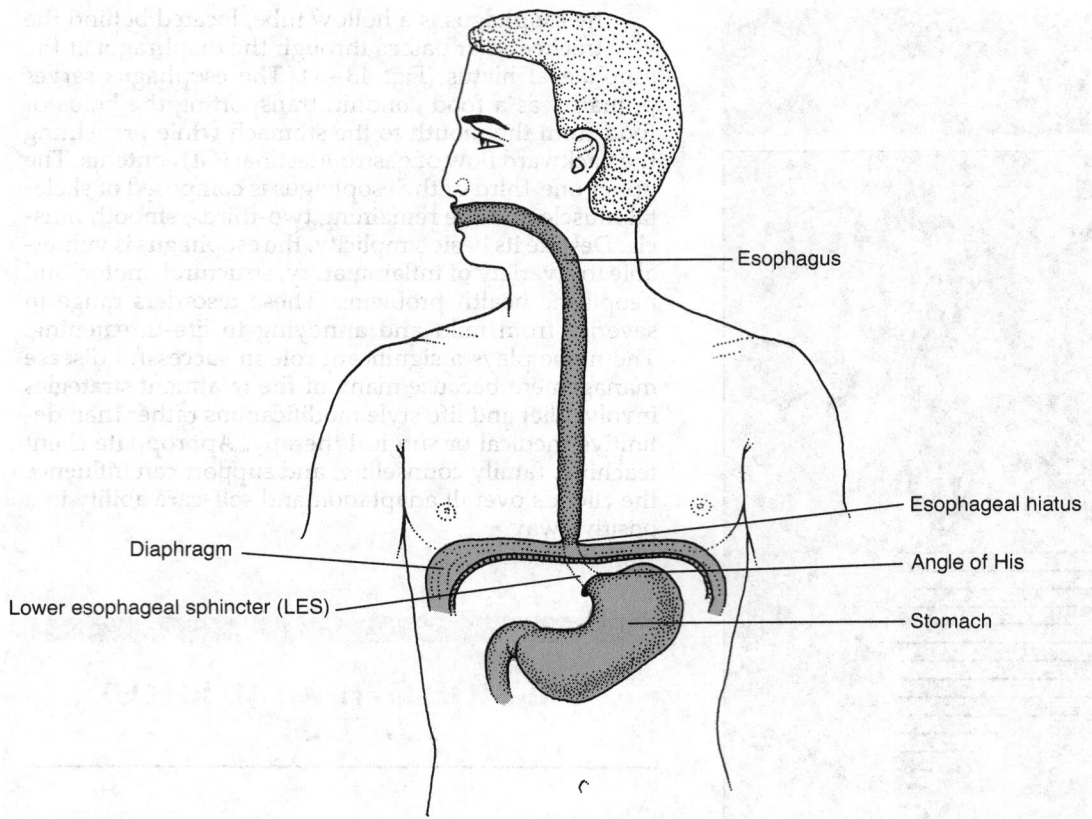

Figure 43–1

Esophagus and related structures.

Esophageal reflux can occur when gastric volume or intra-abdominal pressure is elevated, or when the sphincter tone of the LES is decreased. It can also occur when the LES undergoes inappropriate relaxation. Virtually everyone occasionally experiences reflux. Clients may even experience frequent episodes of reflux and be unaware of their occurrence because the episodes are asymptomatic. However, the esophagus has only a limited resistance to the damaging effects of acidic GI contents. GERD develops when the esophageal mucosal barrier breaks down and an inflammatory response is initiated. The degree of esophageal inflammation appears to be related to the acid concentration of the refluxed material, the number of reflux episodes, and the length of time during which the esophagus is exposed to the irritating material. Refluxed material is returned to the stomach by a combination of peristalsis and gravity. An inflamed esophagus is not able to eliminate the refluxed material as quickly or efficiently as normal, and the duration of exposure is therefore increased with each reflux episode. The duration of exposure is thought to be more important than the actual frequency of reflux episodes in determining the degree of damage.

Hyperemia and erosion occur in the esophagus in response to the chronic inflammation. Pepsin and gastric acid cause most of the injury. Minor capillary bleeding frequently accompanies the erosion, although frank hemorrhage is relatively rare. During the process of healing, the body may substitute a columnar epithelium called Barrett's epithelium for the normal squamous cell epithelium of the lower esophagus. This new tissue is more resistant to acid and therefore supports esophageal healing, but it has been found to be premalignant tissue that is associated with an increased risk of adenocarcinoma. The fibrosis and scarring that also accompany the healing process can produce esophageal stricture, which results in a progressive difficulty in swallowing. Uncontrolled esophageal reflux not only produces significant symptoms but also creates the risk of other serious complications such as esophageal ulceration, hemorrhage, and aspiration.

Etiology

The inappropriate relaxation of the LES in response to an unknown stimulus is believed to be the primary cause of GERD. Many clients experiencing symptoms are found to have resting LES pressures that are within normal limits or only slightly low. Nighttime reflux is considered to be important. The nighttime swallowing rate decreases by two-thirds, and the recumbent position of sleep significantly interferes with the ability of the esophagus to clear the refluxed material. Therefore, the duration of exposure to this material is significantly increased.

For many years, it was assumed that the presence of a sliding hiatal hernia, which displaced the LES into the thorax, was the primary etiologic feature in GERD. An extremely high incidence of hiatal hernia is found in individuals with GERD, but the two conditions are now considered to be separate. Hiatal hernia has been found to be much more common in the general population than was previously estimated, and although most clients with hiatal hernias experience reflux, not all clients who experience reflux have hiatal hernias. The symptoms of GERD appear to correlate better with incompetency of the LES than they do with the presence of a hernia. Any condition that delays gastric emptying and thereby maintains a high gastric volume and pressure can also contribute to reflux.

A number of environmental and physical factors have also been identified that appear to influence the tone and contractility of the LES. LES pressure is lowered by fatty meals, the nicotine in cigarette smoke, the xanthine-containing drinks (tea, cola, coffee), ganglionic stimulants, beta-adrenergic agents, and high levels of estrogen and progesterone. LES tone can be increased by gastrin release, protein ingestion, and cholinergic and alpha-adrenergic agents.

Other conditions besides GERD can produce esophagitis, although GERD is by far the most common cause. Herpes and monilial infections of the esophagus can produce acute inflammation. Ingestion of corrosive substances produces severe esophagitis and can cause irreversible esophageal damage. Radiation to the lung, esophagus, or mediastinum frequently produces an acute esophagitis that is directly dose related.

Incidence

GERD can occur in any age group, and its actual incidence is probably significantly underestimated because many individuals with mild disease simply accept it as a normal condition and relate it to episodes of stress or dietary indiscretion. It is estimated to produce daily symptoms in as much as 10% of the population and at least monthly symptoms in approximately one-third (Castell, 1986).

COLLABORATIVE MANAGEMENT

 Assessment

History

Obtaining a careful and complete history is an essential part of the assessment of GERD because many clients with the disorder can be diagnosed through the history of clinical manifestations alone. A full diagnostic work-up is not indicated for every client.

The nurse identifies what *symptoms* the client has been experiencing, when they started, whether they have increased in frequency or severity, and what environmental factors the client associates with their occurrence. A complete history needs to include the possibility of ingestion of corrosive substances, radiation treatment to the head and neck region, and the occurrence of frequent infections involving structures of the mouth. The nurse performs a careful assessment of *diet pattern* and assists the client to identify situations in which symptoms typically occur. The nurse also assesses the methods that the client has used to deal with the symptoms at home, particularly the use of any *over-the-counter medications.* The client's *work* and *leisure time activities* are also assessed.

Physical Assessment: Clinical Manifestations

The nurse assesses the client's general *physical appearance* and *nutritional status* and assists the client to locate the pain anatomically. The nurse also observes the client's *swallowing* and assesses the smoothness of laryngeal movement.

Although clients can be asymptomatic with reflux, they usually exhibit characteristic clinical manifestations that may vary substantially in severity. The nurse carefully assesses the client's pain pattern because *heartburn (pyrosis)* is the primary symptom of GERD. This pain is commonly described as a *burning sensation* that moves up and down the chest like a wave. Pyrosis is the result of increased mucosal sensitivity and typically occurs in the epigastric region. If severe, the pain may radiate to the neck or jaw or may be referred to the back. The pain is typically aggravated by bending over, straining, or being in a recumbent position. With severe GERD, the pain occurs after each meal and persists for 20 minutes to 2 hours. Clients usually experience prompt relief with the ingestion of fluids or antacids. Some clients experience *atypical pain,* which closely mimics angina and needs to be carefully differentiated from cardiac disease.

Regurgitation, which is not associated with either belching or nausea, is another common symptom. The client reports the occurrence of warm fluid traveling up the throat. If the fluid reaches the level of the pharynx, the client notes a sour or bitter taste in the mouth. This effortless regurgitation frequently occurs with the client in the upright position. When it occurs with the client in a recumbent position, the danger of aspiration is quite high. If the client experiences regurgitation, the nurse carefully auscultates the chest for any evidence of *aspiration.* The nurse assesses for the occurrence of any recent episodes of respiratory infections or distress, which may be related to recumbent regurgitation.

Water brash is another common symptom. It involves a reflex salivary hypersecretion that occurs in response to reflux and must be carefully distinguished from regurgitation. The client reports a sensation of fluid in the throat but because the fluid is saliva, it does not have a sour or bitter taste.

Progressive GERD often involves *dysphagia,* or difficulty in swallowing. This symptom is usually fairly mild and not progressive and occurs with the first swallow of each meal. It does not interfere with oral nutrition or produce weight loss. If a client reports progressive or persistent dysphagia, careful assessment is required because it usually indicates the presence of a stricture or a tumor. The nurse assesses the degree of dysphagia; whether it occurs with ingestion of solids, liquids, or both; and whether it is intermittent or occurs with each swallowing effort.

Odynophagia, or painful swallowing, is another possible symptom, although it is relatively rare in uncomplicated reflux disease. Severe and long-lasting *chest pain* may be present if spasms occur in the esophagus that cause the muscle to contract with excess force. The pain that is experienced by the client can be agonizing and can last for hours.

Belching and a feeling of *flatulence* or bloating after eating are other common complaints. *Nausea* and *vomiting* occur infrequently, and *unplanned weight loss* is quite rare.

Psychosocial Assessment

A disorder that involves chronic episodes of pain that are associated with eating can produce serious disruptions in a client's daily life style. The nurse assesses the client's response to the disease and its symptoms and how the disease has affected the client's usual activities of daily living. The nurse assesses the client's knowledge about the disorder and what coping mechanisms the client uses to deal with stress. The client's living situation is also assessed, and the nurse identifies resources and supports available to assist the client in dealing with the disease and the treatment regimen.

Laboratory Findings

Standard laboratory tests are of limited value in the diagnosis of GERD. Esophageal erosion may produce a chronic low-grade bleeding, which is evidenced as an iron deficiency anemia.

Radiographic Findings

The barium swallow with fluoroscopy is the most widely used test of esophageal function. It outlines both the structure of the esophagus and its pattern of peristalsis. Client positioning maneuvers are performed to attempt to produce the spontaneous reflux of barium. It is neither a sensitive nor a specific measure of GERD, and the esophagus is usually evaluated as being normal unless gross disease is present.

Other Diagnostic Tests

Esophageal manometry. These tests, which are also called *motility tests,* are performed when the diagnosis is unclear. Water-filled catheters are inserted via the nose or mouth and are connected to transducers that record pressures from various sites in the esophagus as the catheters are withdrawn. Manometry quantifies the resting pressure of the LES and helps to evaluate sphincter competence.

Bernstein's test. This test involves infusion of an acid solution via a tube into the distal esophagus. Clients with normal esophageal mucosa experience no symptoms when acid is infused, whereas clients with esophagitis experience immediate heartburn.

Standard acid reflux test. This test involves the placement of pH probes 5 cm above the LES. Acid is then placed into the stomach, and the client is moved through a series of positions in an attempt to document reflux. This pH testing is the most sensitive and accurate measure of reflux.

Gastroesophageal scintigraphy. This technique involves preloading the stomach via mouth or tube with a liquid radioisotope. Scintillation counts are then taken over the lower esophagus and compared with counts obtained over the stomach. If a client is experiencing frequent reflux, the radioisotope will be refluxed back into the esophagus, which significantly elevates the scintillation counts over the lower esophageal region.

Esophagoscopy. This method is usually used to determine the severity of the disease, to identify the extent of esophageal injury, to take tissue scrapings for biopsy, and to identify structural complications.

 ### Analysis: Nursing Diagnosis

Common Diagnoses

The most common nursing diagnosis associated with GERD is pain related to the irritation caused by acid reflux in the esophagus.

Additional Diagnoses

In addition, one or more of the following nursing diagnoses may be appropriate:

1. Knowledge deficit related to diet and life style modifications to control reflux
2. Potential for ineffective individual coping related to chronic pain or to the restrictions of a medical regimen
3. Potential for impaired gas exchange related to regurgitation and aspiration
4. Potential for altered nutrition: less than body requirements related to dysphagia and/or odynophagia

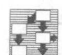 **Planning and Implementation** ➡

Pain

Planning: client goals. The major goal for the client with a diagnosis of pain is that the client will experience a reduction or elimination of the pain by decreasing gastric acidity and by preventing or reducing the incidence of reflux.

Interventions: nonsurgical management. Interventions begin with thorough teaching about GERD as a chronic disease that requires ongoing management. This knowledge base is essential for the client's understanding of and compliance with the prescribed regimen of drugs, diet therapy, and life style modifications.

Diet therapy. In relatively mild cases of GERD, diet therapy alone may be sufficient to significantly relieve the client's symptoms. The nurse explores the client's basic meal patterns, likes, and dislikes and then works with both the client and the family to discover modifications that may decrease reflux symptoms. It is essential that the family members who do the shopping and cooking be included in this discussion if compliance at home is to be successful. Fatty foods, coffee, tea, cola, chocolate, and alcohol have all been shown to decrease LES pressure, so the nurse counsels the client to limit or eliminate these foods in the daily diet. Spicy foods and acidic foods such as orange juice should also be restricted until esophageal healing can occur because they typically produce heartburn.

The nurse encourages the client to eat four to six small meals each day rather than three large ones because large meals both increase the pressure in the stomach and delay gastric emptying. Because reflux episodes are most damaging at night, the nurse teaches the client to avoid evening snacking and to eat no food for at least 3 hours before going to bed. This restriction may be the most difficult one for the client. Eating slowly and chewing thoroughly facilitate digestion and prevent eructation (belching).

The nurse encourages the client to investigate which particular diet modifications reduce the incidence and severity of the symptoms. One of the most sensitive areas involves teaching the client about the importance of not smoking. Smoking causes an almost immediate and significant drop in LES pressure and should be eliminated from the client's life style if at all possible.

Positioning. Teaching the client to elevate the head of the bed by 6 to 8 or even 12 in for sleep is the single most important aspect of client teaching for GERD. Nighttime reflux is extremely common, and infrequent swallowing in combination with a recumbent position significantly impairs esophageal clearance. The client must have a good understanding of the disease process to comprehend the crucial nature of this intervention. Elevation of the bed may be initially unacceptable to the client or the client's spouse or partner. Sleeping on multiple pillows or foam wedges is not an adequate substitute because the client typically rolls off the pillows during sleep. The nurse emphasizes the importance of this intervention and investigates all possible approaches to compliance.

If the client is obese, the nurse examines approaches to weight reduction. Decreasing intra-abdominal pressure reduces reflux symptoms in many clients. Other life style factors also cause increased abdominal pressure, and the nurse explores these with the client. Constrictive clothing, lifting heavy objects or straining, and working in a bent over or stooped position should all be avoided. The nurse emphasizes that these general life style adaptations are extremely effective and should be permanently incorporated into the client's daily routines.

Drug therapy. Drug therapy for GERD begins with antacid therapy, and in uncomplicated cases this prescription may be sufficient to control the heartburn. Antacids are used for their acid-neutralizing effect and usually produce prompt relief. Either aluminum or magnesium salts may be used. Because aluminum salts typically cause constipation and magnesium salts often cause diarrhea, clients frequently tolerate combination products such as Maalox or Mylanta best. The nurse instructs the client to take 30 mL of the antacid 1 hour before and 2 to 3 hours after each meal. When the stomach is empty, antacids are quickly removed from both the esophagus and the stomach, which limits their effectiveness for nighttime use.

Gaviscon, a combination of alginic acid and antacid, is occasionally prescribed. It forms a viscous foam that floats on top of the gastric contents and theoretically decreases the incidence of reflux. If reflux occurs, the foam enters the esophagus first and buffers the acid in the refluxed material. The effectiveness of Gaviscon appears to be similar to that of antacids.

Clients with moderate to severe disease whose reflux symptoms cannot be controlled with antacids alone may be prescribed a histamine receptor antagonist such as cimetidine (Tagamet) or the longer-acting ranitidine (Zantac). Although these drugs have no direct effect on the occurrence of reflux, they reduce gastric acid secretion and provide symptomatic improvement as well as support healing of the inflamed esophageal tissue. Cimetidine may be administered at intervals throughout the day or in a single large dose at bedtime to significantly reduce the effects of nighttime reflux. If cimetidine is prescribed for use four times a day, the nurse instructs the client to take the drug with meals during the day. The nurse also informs the client of frequently occurring drug side effects, including headache, fatigue, diarrhea, male impotence, and mild gynecomastia (breast enlargement in the male). Ranitidine is a longer-acting drug that requires less frequent routine administration and appears to produce fewer side effects.

Bethanecol (Urecholine) or metoclopramide (Reglan)

TABLE 43-1   Drugs Used in the Treatment of GERD

Drug	Usual Daily Dosage	Interventions	Rationales
Antacids, either aluminum or magnesium salts	30 mL PO PRN throughout the day and at bedtime	Give 1 h before meals, 2–3 h after meals, and at bedtime. Give prn as instructed by physician. Observe the client for constipation or diarrhea. Suggest alternating use of aluminum and magnesium products.	Antacids are used to neutralize the acid and usually produce prompt relief. Common side effects can be reduced by alternating the preparations.
Gaviscon, antacid plus alginic acid	1 tablet or 10–20 mL PO throughout the day and at bedtime	Give after meals and at bedtime.	Alginic acid forms a viscous foam that floats on top of the gastric contents, impeding reflux or buffering its effects when it occurs.
Histamine receptor antagonists: Cimetidine (Tagamet)	300 mg qid PO or 900–1200 mg PO at bedtime	Instruct the client to take the drug with meals. Observe the client for side effects; fatigue, headache, and diarrhea are common.	These drugs reduce acid secretion. Ranitidine appears to cause fewer and less severe side effects.
Ranitidine (Zantac)	150 mg bid PO		
Bethanecol (Urecholine)	25 mg qid PO	Instruct the client to take the drug 30–60 min before meals. Continue with antacids and histamine receptor antagonists as ordered. Observe the client for typical side effects: abdominal cramping, diarrhea, urinary urgency, and increased salivation. Counsel the client about their control.	This drug increases LES pressure and increases the rate of esophageal clearance. Bethanecol has cholinergic effects and increases the secretion of gastric acid. Typical associated cholinergic effects occur with the use of bethanecol.
Metoclopramide (Reglan)	10 mg tid or qid PO	Instruct the client to take the drug before meals. Teach the client to report the occurrence of neurologic or psychotropic side effects such as restlessness, anxiety, ataxia, or hallucinations.	This drug increases the rate of gastric emptying. Long-term drug use produces untoward side effects in up to one-third of clients.

may be added to the drug regimen for clients who experience severe and ongoing symptoms of reflux. Bethanecol has been shown to increase LES pressure and to significantly increase the rate of esophageal clearance.

Because bethanecol is a cholinergic drug, it increases the secretion of gastric acid and usually requires the simultaneous administration of a histamine receptor antagonist as well as antacids. It is typically prescribed in

25-mg doses four times a day. The nurse teaches the client to take bethanecol 30 to 60 minutes before meals and warns the client about typical side effects, which include abdominal cramping and diarrhea, increased salivation, and urinary urgency.

The primary action of metoclopramide is to increase the rate of gastric emptying. It does not cause a concurrent increase in gastric secretions, and it does not appear to assist directly in the healing of existing esophageal lesions. Metoclopramide is typically administered orally four times a day in 10-mg doses. The nurse instructs the client to take the drug before meals and warns the client about the high incidence of side effects associated with metoclopramide. Up to one-third of clients using the drug on a long-term basis experience neurologic or psychotropic side effects such as fatigue, restlessness, acute anxiety, cerebellar ataxia, and hallucinations.

The nurse also questions the client about other drugs that are used routinely or intermittently. Anticholinergics, calcium channel blockers, theophylline, and diazepam all appear to decrease LES pressure or to delay gastric emptying and should be avoided if at all possible. Table 43–1 summarizes the data about drugs used commonly in the treatment of GERD.

Interventions: surgical management. Antireflux surgery is generally used with otherwise healthy clients who have not responded positively to aggressive medical management. Several different surgical procedures may be used. The three major surgeries include the Nissen fundoplication, Belsey's repair, and Hill's repair. The Nissen procedure (shown in Fig. 43–4) is used most frequently. Each of these procedures involves wrapping and suturing the gastric fundus around the esophagus, which anchors the LES area below the diaphragm and reinforces the high-pressure area. The accompanying Client Care Plan outlines nursing care of clients undergoing all types of esophageal surgery. Clients who undergo surgery are encouraged to continue to follow the basic antireflux regimen because the rate of recurrence is still fairly significant.

The placement of the synthetic Angelchik prosthesis may also be used for clients with severe reflux. This relatively minor surgical procedure is an alternative for clients who are unable or unwilling to face the major surgery required for the other procedures. In this surgery, a laparotomy is performed and a C-shaped silicone prosthesis filled with gel is tied around the distal esophagus (Fig. 43–2). The prosthesis both anchors the LES in the abdomen and reinforces sphincter pressure.

Preoperative care. Preoperative nursing care concerning the Angelchik prosthesis focuses on client teaching. The nurse teaches the client exercises for deep breathing and reinforces the importance of these exercises in the postoperative period, especially for clients who smoke. Other preoperative care is routine and includes doing laboratory studies, taking chest x-ray films, and ensuring that the client takes nothing by mouth (NPO) before surgery (see Chap. 18 for routine preoperative care).

Postoperative care. Postoperative care closely parallels that used for any laparotomy surgery (see Chap. 20). The nurse pays special attention to respiratory care because the surgery is performed near the diaphragm. The nurse provides adequate analgesia so that the client can cough effectively and clear the airway. The client has a nasogastric (NG) tube for the first postoperative day but is promptly given clear liquids and is progressively advanced to a diet as tolerated over approximately 2 weeks. The nurse teaches the client that initial mild dysphagia is quite common but resolves in time. The client is cautioned to eat smaller meals to avoid overdistending the stomach. After the initial adjustment period, most clients adapt to the prosthesis extremely well and experience minimal problems.

■ Discharge Planning

Clients with GERD are only rarely hospitalized for diagnostic work-up, treatment of complications, or surgery. The emphasis of nursing intervention is on successful home management of reflux symptoms.

Home Care Preparation

Minimal home care preparation is needed. The major home adaptation required is elevation of the head of the bed on blocks. Concerns about appearance, furniture damage, and safety are carefully explored because these barriers could prevent implementation of this essential intervention.

Client/Family Education

Education of the client is the key to successful management of uncomplicated GERD. The nurse provides the client with written instructions concerning diet modifications, side effects of medications, and life style modifications to reinforce oral teaching. The nurse includes the spouse and family when possible in all teaching about diet modifications because any changes in meal size, composition, and frequency have an impact on the entire family. Meal pattern routines are deeply ingrained in a family's daily life pattern, and changes are not easy to accomplish.

Psychosocial Preparation

GERD frequently occurs in otherwise healthy clients who must be knowledgeable and committed to long-term self-care for a chronic and sometimes progressive disorder. Major life style adaptations are not usually necessary, but the nurse explores with the client the demands of a job, hobbies, or interests for which heavy lifting or working in a stooped position is required. These activities are contraindicated and will need to be modified if possible. The necessity to alter daily activity patterns may be devastating to the client who may re-

CLIENT CARE PLAN ■ The Client Undergoing Surgery of the Esophagus

Goal/Outcome Criteria	Interventions	Rationales
Nursing Diagnosis 1: Potential for Infection Related to Surgical Incision		
Client will manifest no signs or symptoms of infection.	1. Do not reposition or replace nasogastric tube. Do not perform endotracheal suctioning on a client with esophageal anastomosis or repair.	1. Moving the tube can cause trauma, which could puncture or irritate incision; trauma to the area could open a potential route of infection.
	2. Encourage client to suction or expectorate oral secretions rather than swallow them.	2. Clients are kept NPO* to avoid active peristalsis.
	3. Assess cutaneous suture line for redness, drainage, and other signs of infection. Observe dressing for bleeding; document and report any findings to the physician.	3. Monitor client to detect complications and early signs of infection as soon as possible.
	4. Clean sutures once each shift with half strength peroxide; dry the area and apply a small amount of antibacterial ointment.	4. Cleaning removes crusts and secretions, which could be ideal media for bacterial growth.
	5. Monitor vital signs as per the physician's orders. Document and report any significant changes to the physician.	5. Monitoring provides early detection of and intervention for hemorrhage or infection.
Nursing Diagnosis 2: Potential for Altered Nutrition: Less Than Body Requirements Related to NPO Status and Surgical Disruption of the Esophagus		
Client will maintain adequate nutritional intake by nasogastric tube until oral feedings are begun.	1. Remind client of NPO status when client is alert.	1. Elderly clients may demonstrate memory deficit; clients are often NPO until an intraoral incision is healed.
	2. Monitor IV* hydration while client is NPO and before tube feedings are begun; monitor and record intake and output every shift.	2. Monitor hydration status for overload or retention; elderly clients are often susceptible to overload of fluids.
	3. Assess and document bowel sounds every shift until tube feedings are well tolerated.	3. Establish a baseline for bowel sounds; return of bowel sounds postoperatively is often an indication to begin tube feedings.
	4. Measure and record weight daily.	4. Weight gives information on fluid status.
	5. Maintain proper functioning of nasogastric tube; while it is attached to suction, measure and record drainage every shift. When tube feedings are begun, flush the tube carefully with water after each feeding or medication administration.	5. Monitor and maintain patency to permit drainage and to allow route for administration of medications and nutrition.
	6. Elevate head of bed 30 degrees at rest and 90 degrees for feeding and for ½ h after feeding.	6. Raising the head helps prevent reflux; the incidence of reflux is greatest during and ½ h after tube feedings.

CLIENT CARE PLAN ■ The Client Undergoing Surgery of the Esophagus *continued*

Goal/Outcome Criteria	Interventions	Rationales
Nursing Diagnosis 2: Potential for Altered Nutrition: Less Than Body Requirements Related to NPO Status and Surgical Disruption of the Esophagus		
Client will demonstrate ability to assist with tube feedings.	1. Provide client with written and oral instructions regarding tube feedings. 2. Include family in all teaching. 3. Have client give a return demonstration of procedure.	1. Written instructions as well as oral provide the client with resources when the nurse is not available. 2. Including the family ensures support for the client to perform the procedures. 3. A return demonstration aids in retention of the learned procedure as well as provides a means of evaluation for the nurse.
Client will maintain adequate oral nutritional intake with minimal dysphagia or reflux.	1. When oral fluids are begun, assess and document difficulty in swallowing, aspiration, or leakage, including signs of increased pulse rate, increased temperature, increased respiratory rate, subcutaneous emphysema, or change in chest tube drainage indicating contamination from GI tract. 2. If the client is experiencing difficulty in swallowing, check with physician about consulting speech therapist for assessment or assistance in swallowing. 3. Consult with dietitian as appropriate. 4. Observe client for any epigastric burning, retrosternal or back pain, or pain radiating to the chin or shoulder indicative of esophageal reflux; document any findings.	1. Clients occasionally have difficulty in swallowing after esophageal surgery; assessment provides documentation of real or perceived difficulty. The nurse observes carefully for signs of leakage from the esophageal anastomosis site or from a perforation. 2. Speech therapists are often expert at evaluating swallowing disorders; providing the client with techniques of head positioning, breath holding, or oral exercises can help overcome minor swallowing difficulties. 3. Often a change in food consistency eases swallowing difficulties. 4. Esophageal reflux, once documented, can be treated by client positioning or dietary changes; analgesics may be required before mealtimes.
Nursing Diagnosis 3: Pain Related to Incision or Reflux		
Client will verbalize control of pain, facilitating adequate nutritional intake and participation in ADL*.	1. Assess and document the level of pain, relying on subjective and objective symptoms of pain and pain relief. Assess and document relief obtained from analgesic regimen. 2. Assess client for pain related to esophageal reflux or perforation: epigastric burning; pain radiating to shoulder, chin, or back; change in vital signs; change in character of chest tube drainage (if present); subcutaneous emphysema. Document and report all findings to the physician.	1. Clients are often unwilling to demonstrate evidence of pain and are often unwilling to use analgesics, particularly narcotics, as often as prescribed. 2. Early detection of esophageal perforation is imperative to begin effective treatment; documentation of reflux communicates need to prevent reflux aspiration to other health care workers.

continued

CLIENT CARE PLAN ■ The Client Undergoing Surgery of the Esophagus *continued*

Goal/Outcome Criteria	Interventions	Rationales
	Nursing Diagnosis 3: Pain Related to Incision or Reflux	
	3. Instruct client to keep head of bed raised 30 degrees at all times and 90 degrees at meals and for ½ h after meals.	3. Raising the head of the bed not only reduces edema by facilitating gravity drainage, but also facilitates food passage and prevents esophageal reflux.
	4. Explore dietary modifications with client to alleviate discomfort related to reflux.	4. Smaller, more frequent meals with change in food consistency can reduce discomfort associated with reflux.
	5. Explore various changes in client positioning to facilitate food passage and alleviate symptoms of reflux.	5. Varying positions assumed while eating and after eating can reduce discomfort associated with reflux or dysphagia.
	6. Instruct client to use analgesic medication ½ h before meals, chest physiotherapy, and other treatments as needed.	6. Assuring a peak analgesic effect during activities that the client reports as being most uncomfortable can increase compliance with those activities and can increase efforts to obtain adequate nutritional intake.
	7. Instruct client and family about medications prescribed: timing, side effects, and restrictions; provide written as well as oral instructions.	7. Written and oral instructions are given because the client may have memory loss.
	8. Instruct client to monitor his or her own comfort.	8. Client gains a feeling of control concerning discomfort.

*NPO, nothing by mouth; IV, intravenous; ADL, activities of daily living.

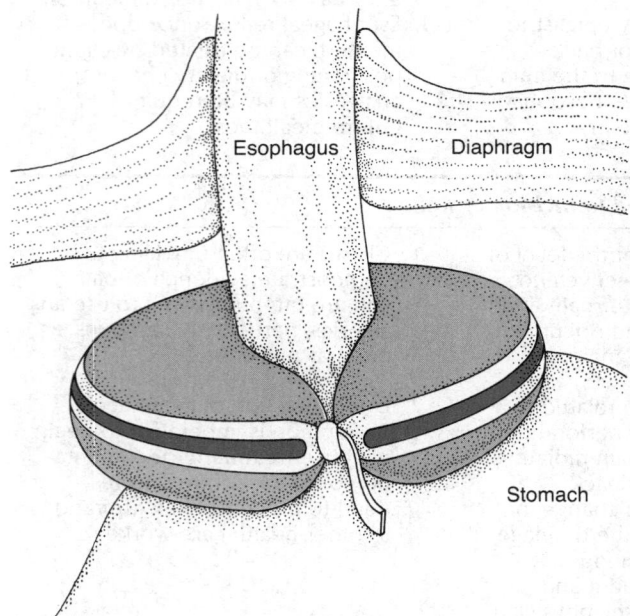

Figure 43–2
Placement of the Angelchik antireflux prosthesis.

quire significant support. Clients only rarely need support or assistance from other community health care resources.

Health Care Resources

Most GERD clients manage their symptoms at home with only transient support from their physician and nurse. The family therefore becomes the major resource for client support. In addition, the nurse refers the client as appropriate to community support groups to assist with weight loss and cessation of smoking.

 Evaluation

Evaluation is based on the specific diagnoses and the stated client goals. Expected outcomes include that the client

1. States that reflux pain is absent or significantly reduced

2. Maintains an optimal nutritional status and appropriate body weight

---

HIATAL HERNIA

OVERVIEW

The *esophageal hiatus* is the opening in the diaphragm through which the esophagus passes from the thorax to the abdomen. *Esophageal hiatal hernias*, which are also called diaphragmatic hernias, occur when the lower portion of the esophagus, or a portion of the stomach, or both move into the thorax through the hiatus. Clients with hiatal hernias may be completely asymptomatic or may experience daily symptoms that are usually similar to the symptoms of GERD. Either medical or surgical management may be used for hiatal hernias. The decision to use a specific type of management is based on the severity of the client's symptoms and the risk of serious complications.

Pathophysiology

There are two major types of hiatal hernias: sliding hernias and paraesophageal, or rolling, hernias. *Sliding hernias* are by far the most common and account for 90% of the total number of hernias (Payne & Ellis, 1984). In sliding hernias, the esophagogastric junction and a portion of the fundus of the stomach are displaced upward through the hiatus into the thorax (Fig. 43–3). The hernia generally moves freely and slides into and out of the thorax when there are changes in position or intra-abdominal pressure. Although the classic hernia-related risks of volvulus (twisting) or obstruction do exist, they rarely occur. The major concern with sliding hernias is the development of esophageal reflux and its complications. The development of reflux appears to be related to the chronic exposure of the LES to the low pressure of the thorax, which significantly reduces the effectiveness of the LES. The actual hernia itself appears to cause few, if any, problems.

With *paraesophageal*, or *rolling, hernias,* the gastroesophageal junction stays below the diaphragm, but the fundus and possibly portions of the stomach's greater curvature roll into the thorax beside the esophagus (see Fig. 43–3). The herniated portion of the stomach may be small or quite large. In rare cases the stomach completely inverts into the thorax. Reflux is rarely a concern

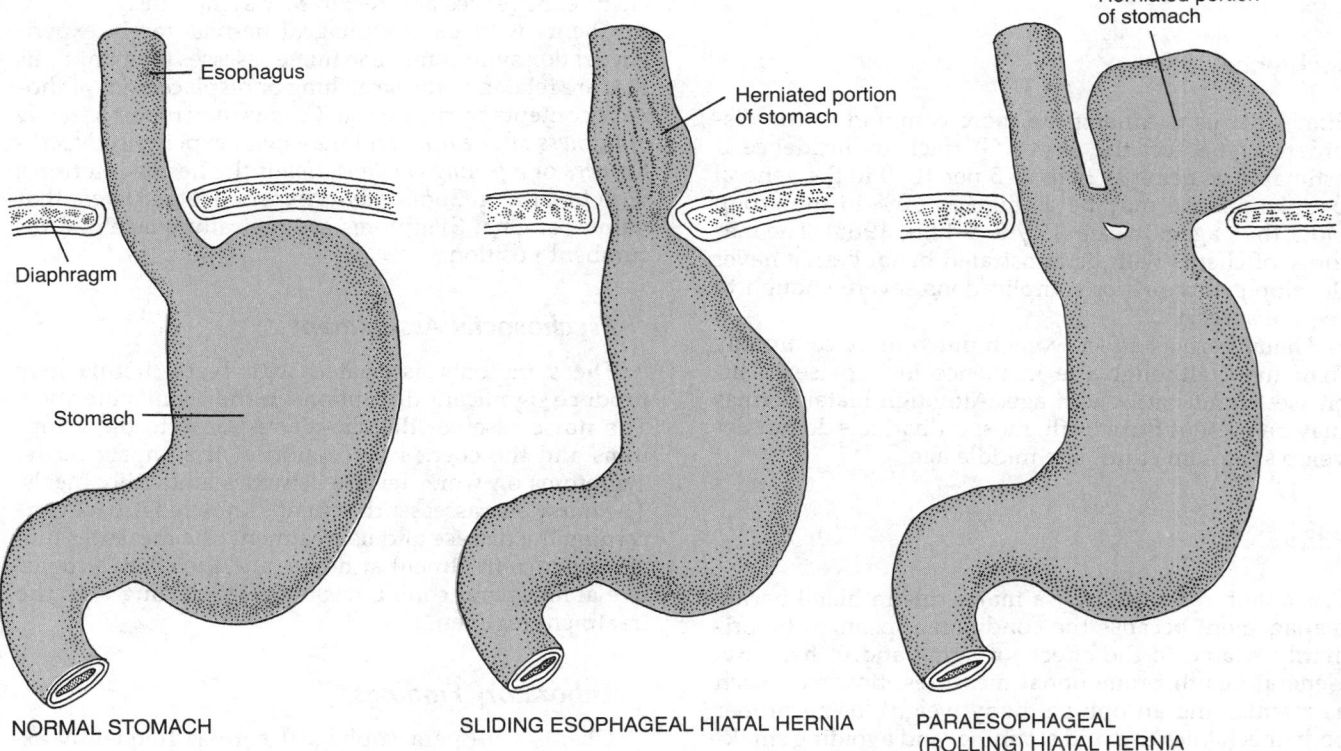

NORMAL STOMACH — Esophagus, Diaphragm, Stomach

SLIDING ESOPHAGEAL HIATAL HERNIA — Herniated portion of stomach

PARAESOPHAGEAL (ROLLING) HIATAL HERNIA — Herniated portion of stomach

Figure 43–3

Comparison of the normal stomach and sliding esophageal and paraesophageal (rolling) hiatal hernias.

with paraesophageal hernias because the LES remains anchored below the diaphragm, but the risks of developing volvulus, obstruction, and strangulation are quite high. Clients also typically develop iron deficiency anemia from chronic blood loss that is caused by either local pressure from the hiatus or stasis erosion in the herniated sac of the stomach. Clients rarely develop mixed hernias that exhibit features of both major types of hiatal hernia.

Etiology

Sliding hiatal hernias are believed to develop from muscle weakening in the esophageal hiatus, which loosens the esophageal supports and permits the lower portion of the esophagus to rise into the thorax. It is a straight-forward type of muscle weakness that appears to be consistent with the aging process, although congenital weaknesses, trauma, or surgery may play a significant role. The actual development of the hernia is the result of the combined effects of weakened support structures and prolonged increases in abdominal pressure.

Muscle weakening does not appear to play a major role in the development of paraesophageal hernias. Instead, it is theorized that the stomach was not properly anchored below the diaphragm and that the hernia thus results from an anatomic defect rather than a structural weakness.

Incidence

Hiatal hernia is among the more common of the disorders that affect the upper GI tract. Its incidence is estimated as being as high as 5 per 1000 in the general population and may be as high as 60% in the group older than age 60 years (Payne & Ellis, 1984). The majority of clients with demonstrated hiatal hernia never develop symptoms or complications severe enough to require surgery.

Hiatal hernias affect women much more commonly than men, although the incidence in both sexes increases significantly with age. Although hiatal hernias may be present from birth, most individuals do not develop symptoms until late middle age.

PREVENTION

Prevention does not play a major role in hiatal hernia management because the condition appears to be primarily related to the effects of aging and to heredity. General health promotional measures, however, such as maintaining an optimal body weight, using proper body mechanics to avoid straining, and avoiding smoking, all decrease the effects of elevated intra-abdominal pressure and may prevent or delay the development of symptoms.

COLLABORATIVE MANAGEMENT

 Assessment

History

Most clients are asymptomatic until LES pressure is decreased and they begin to experience persistent reflux. There appears to be little correlation between the size of the hernia and the severity of symptoms experienced by the client.

The nurse assesses the client's *age, sex, weight,* and *body build* because these factors are often important correlates of hiatal hernia. The nurse assesses the client's daily *work and leisure activities,* as well as the usual *diet pattern,* and assists the client to recognize relations between the occurrence of symptoms and specific foods or activities.

Physical Assessment: Clinical Manifestations

The nurse assesses the client's general physical appearance and nutritional status and assists the client to identify the location of any pain. Because the primary symptoms of sliding hiatal hernias are those associated with reflux, the nurse carefully assesses for *heartburn, regurgitation, pain, dysphagia,* and *belching.* The nurse also auscultates the thorax and lungs, particularly if the client experiences any respiratory symptoms.

Clients with paraesophageal hernias rarely experience reflux symptoms. The nurse assesses for symptoms that are related to the stretching or displacement of thoracic contents by the hernia. Clients may report a *feeling of fullness after eating* and may even experience *breathlessness* or a *feeling of suffocation* if the hernia interferes with breathing. Some clients experience *chest pain* that mimics angina. Symptoms are typically worse in a recumbent position.

Psychosocial Assessment

The symptoms associated with hiatal hernia may produce significant disruptions in the client's life style. The nurse assesses the client's response to the symptoms and the client's perception of the impact of the symptoms on work, leisure activities, and daily meals. The nurse also assesses the client's knowledge base concerning the disease and its treatment, the measures that are used for treatment at home, and the client's cognitive abilities and coping resources for dealing with the treatment regimen.

Laboratory Findings

Clients with paraesophageal hernias frequently experience chronic low-grade bleeding in the herniated portion of the stomach. These clients may present with low hemoglobin and hematocrit values.

Radiographic Findings

The barium swallow with fluoroscopy is the diagnostic test that is most specific to the identification of hiatal hernia. Paraesophageal hernias are usually clearly visible, and sliding hernias can often be demonstrated as the client is moved through a series of positions that increase intra-abdominal pressure.

Other Diagnostic Tests

Clients with sliding hernias usually experience the symptoms of reflux. Therefore, any or all of the diagnostic tests that are used with GERD may be used to fully evaluate the extent of reflux and the degree of esophageal damage (see earlier under the heading Other Diagnostic Tests for a more complete description of these tests).

 Analysis: Nursing Diagnosis

Common Diagnoses

Most clients with hiatal hernias are treated conservatively with medical management that duplicates the interventions for GERD. The most common nursing diagnosis is pain related to the irritation of acid reflux in the esophagus.

Additional Diagnoses

In addition, the client may experience one or more of the following nursing diagnoses:

1. Potential for impaired gas exchange related to aspiration or to pressure of the herniated stomach in the thorax
2. Potential for ineffective individual coping related to the symptoms of chronic reflux

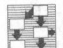 Planning and Implementation

Pain

Planning: client goals.   When clients are treated conservatively with medical management, the goal is that the client will experience a reduction in or alleviation of discomfort.

Interventions: nonsurgical management.   Basic interventions for the client with hiatal hernia closely follow the regimen that was outlined for GERD, including drug therapy, diet therapy, and life style modifications. The nurse carefully instructs the client about the underlying condition to increase understanding of the disorder and compliance with the treatment regimen.

Drug therapy.   Antacids, histamine receptor antagonists, and cholinergic drugs are prescribed in an attempt

to control reflux and its symptoms, as outlined in Table 43–1.

Diet therapy.   Diet therapy is an integral part of the conservative management of hiatal hernia and follows the guidelines discussed earlier for GERD. It is particularly important that the client not snack at night to ensure that the stomach is empty before going to bed. The nurse also works with the client to modify the diet to reduce body weight if appropriate because obesity increases intra-abdominal pressure and worsens both the hernia and the symptoms of reflux.

Positioning.   Teaching about positioning as outlined earlier for GERD is also extremely important for clients with hiatal hernia. It is essential that clients sleep at night with the head of the bed elevated 6 to 12 in, avoid lying down for several hours after eating, avoid straining or excessive vigorous exercise, and not wear clothing that is tight or constrictive around the abdomen.

Interventions: surgical management.   Surgery is usually scheduled when the risk of complications becomes high or the damage from chronic reflux becomes severe. Clients with paraesophageal hernias are usually scheduled for surgery even when they do not have serious symptoms because the risk of major complications is constantly present.

The repair of paraesophageal hernias is similar to other hernia procedures in that straightforward anatomic repair is the primary focus. There is no need to alter or modify LES function. Simple repair of the defect in the diaphragm, however, does not successfully control the reflux problems associated with sliding hiatal hernias. All of the current surgical approaches for sliding hernias also involve reinforcement of the LES to restore sphincter competence and prevent reflux. Eventual recurrence can be a problem with both types of hernias.

Although several different hiatal hernia repair procedures are in current use, each involves LES reinforcement through some degree of fundoplication. This procedure involves wrapping a portion of the stomach fundus around the distal esophagus to anchor it and reinforce the LES. The *Nissen repair,* shown in Figure 43–4, is one of the most commonly used and effective techniques. An abdominal approach is usually used, and the fundus is wrapped a full 360 degrees around the lower esophagus. The sphincter reinforcement is quite tight and usually extremely effective in controlling reflux. The *Hill repair* also uses an abdominal approach but the fundoplication is 180 degrees around the esophagus. It also restructures the angle of His to accentuate the angle at which the esophagus enters the stomach. The *Belsey repair* usually involves a 280-degree esophageal wrap and a thoracic approach. There is no agreement about which surgical repair is either most appropriate or most effective because each surgery has unique advantages and disadvantages.

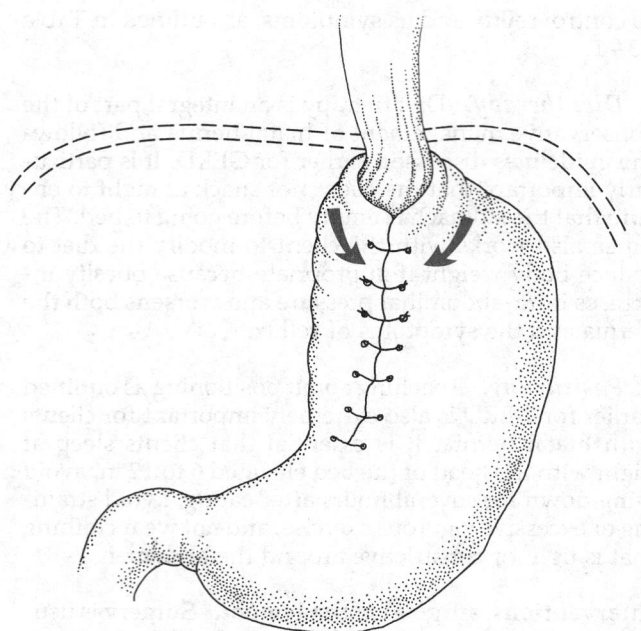

Figure 43–4

Nissen fundoplication for hiatal hernia repair.

Preoperative care. The nurse must know which surgical approach is planned because a thoracic incision necessitates teaching the client about chest tubes. Clients who are overweight are encouraged to lose weight before surgery. It is essential that clients attempt to quit or significantly reduce smoking. The nurse also informs the client that an NG tube will be inserted during surgery and will remain in place for several days, although oral intake is gradually restarted with clear liquids after peristalsis is re-established.

The nurse carefully instructs the client in techniques for effective coughing and deep breathing. Because the surgery involves the diaphragm, these exercises are essential to prevent postoperative respiratory complications. The high incision also makes these exercises extremely painful for the client. Teaching and reassurance about adequate postoperative analgesia are important routes to client cooperation and compliance.

Postoperative care. Postoperative care after hiatal hernia repair closely follows that required after any abdominal surgery, as discussed in Chapter 20. Prevention of respiratory complications is the primary focus. The head of the bed is elevated 30 degrees to lower the diaphragm and facilitate lung expansion. The nurse assists the client to get out of bed and walk as soon as possible. The incision line must be supported during coughing to reduce pain and to prevent excessive strain on the suture line, especially with obese clients. Incentive spirometers and chest physiotherapy are routinely used to aid in keeping the airway open. Adequate analgesia is essential for client compliance and should be

routinely offered 30 minutes before each session of chest physical therapy. Clients with a smoking history or chronic obstructive pulmonary disease require even more aggressive respiratory management.

The surgeon inserts a large-diameter NG tube during surgery to prevent making the fundoplication wrap too tight around the esophagus, and the tube must be carefully monitored postoperatively. The drainage is initially dark brown with old blood but should become normal yellowish-green gastric secretions within the first 8 hours. The nurse ensures that the NG tube is properly anchored and cannot be displaced because it cannot be safely reinserted without risking perforation of the incisional area. Patency of the NG tube is regularly evaluated because it is essential to keep the stomach decompressed to avoid retching or vomiting, which could strain or rupture the stomach sutures. Accurate measures of intake and output are recorded, and the nurse assesses the client's hydration status regularly. Adequate fluid replacement is important to help keep respiratory secretions thin. Frequent oral hygiene is an important comfort measure because the tube is quite irritating.

Oral intake with clear fluids is begun after active peristalsis is re-established, and the client progresses to a near-normal diet over and during the first 6 weeks. The nurse carefully supervises the first oral feedings because *temporary dysphagia* is a common problem. If dysphagia persists, it usually indicates that the fundoplication is too tight, and dilation may be required (see p. 1287). Few foods are either restricted or eliminated from the diet. The food storage area of the stomach is reduced by the surgery, however, and meals need to be both smaller and more frequent.

Another common complication of fundoplication surgery is the *gas bloat syndrome* in which clients are unable to voluntarily eructate (belch). It is usually temporary but may persist. The nurse teaches the client to avoid drinking carbonated beverages, eating gas-producing foods, and drinking with a straw. Many clients have also developed the habit of *aerophagia*, or air swallowing, from attempting to reverse or clear acid reflux. The nurse teaches these clients to consciously relax before and after meals and to eat and drink slowly, chewing all food thoroughly. Air in the stomach that cannot be removed by belching can be extremely uncomfortable for the client. Frequent position changes and ambulation are effective interventions to assist peristalsis to clear air from the GI tract. Lying supine should be avoided.

■ Discharge Planning

Home Care Preparation

Minimal home care preparation is required after hiatal hernia repair. Climbing stairs is restricted, and the home situation may need modification during the first days of limited activity. The nurse ensures that the client has adequate help to perform safe self-care activities without straining the incision through physical exertion.

Client/Family Education

Activity is restricted during the standard 6-week postsurgical recovery period, and the nurse carefully instructs the client to avoid straining during this time. Preventing constipation is an important part of the instruction. For long-term management, the nurse teaches the client about appropriate diet modifications, but the use of stool softeners or bulk laxatives is recommended for the first postoperative weeks until healing is complete. Lifting is also contraindicated.

The nurse instructs the client to inspect the healing incision daily and to report any incidence of swelling, redness, tenderness, discharge, or fever to the physician or other health care provider. The nurse advises the client to avoid individuals with respiratory infections and to contact the physician if symptoms of a cold or influenza develop. Persistent coughing could cause the incision or the fundoplication to dehisce. If at all possible, the client should stop smoking.

The nurse works with the entire family for diet education. Full support of the family is essential for the client to successfully modify the size and timing of meals. Relatively few ongoing diet restrictions are needed, but eating too much or eating the wrong kinds of foods can produce serious discomfort if the client cannot belch. The client is the best judge of what foods produce discomfort, and the nurse encourages cautious experimentation with new foods. The nurse instructs the client to report the recurrence of reflux symptoms to the physician.

Psychosocial Preparation

Most clients experience a sense of relief when the chronic symptoms of reflux are surgically relieved. But unrealistic expectations can be a problem for some clients. Although severe surgical complications are relatively rare, conditions such as gas bloat syndrome and dysphagia are common and may persist. The nurse assists the client to prepare for these problems, as well as for the potential that reflux may not be completely controlled or may occur again in the future. Although surgery controls the condition, a cure is rare, and life style modifications may need to be ongoing.

Health Care Resources

Most clients recover from surgery without sequelae and require only routine support. The family unit provides for most needs. The nurse refers the client to community resources for weight loss and smoking cessation programs as appropriate. These factors could significantly increase the client's risk of relapse of reflux symptoms.

 Evaluation

Evaluation is based on the nursing diagnoses and the stated client goals. Expected outcomes include that the client

1. States that the symptoms of reflux are minimal or absent
2. Achieves and maintains an optimal body weight
3. Recovers from surgery without respiratory or wound complications

ACHALASIA

OVERVIEW

Achalasia is a condition of progressively worsening dysphagia that is evidenced by chronic and sometimes vague complaints of difficulty in swallowing and of a feeling of food "sticking in the throat." Clients occasionally complain of postprandial substernal pain, but for many clients the condition is painless. Many clients with achalasia experience regurgitation of ingested foods into the back of the throat when lying down.

Pathophysiology

The pathophysiology of achalasia is still being explored. Current theories favor a lack of peristalsis related to neuromuscular factors coupled with inadequate relaxation (or spasm) of the LES. Over time, the esophagus can become extremely dilated, which further slows the passage of food.

Etiology

Achalasia is considered to be idiopathic and is a chronic disease, with dysphagia progressing over years. Occasionally, the onset of achalasia can be related to an acute episode of difficulty in swallowing. The clinical manifestations of achalasia are often exacerbated by emotional stress, overeating, or gulping of foods and liquids. Some documented cases of achalasia indicate a possible familial factor.

Incidence

Considered to be a fairly uncommon disorder, achalasia affects both sexes equally. The condition appears most often in middle-aged persons.

COLLABORATIVE MANAGEMENT

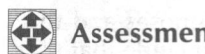 **Assessment**

History

In obtaining a history from the client with achalasia, the nurse notes the *symptoms* the client is experiencing, such as dysphagia, pain, or regurgitation. The nurse explores with the client the *onset* and/or *duration of symptoms.* Achalasia is often a chronic condition; however, many times the symptoms worsen over time, which makes the client more aware of the problems. The nurse questions the client about *factors that aggravate the symptoms,* such as position or diet changes, as well as *medications* or *home treatments that relieve the symptoms.* The nurse obtains from the client a history of *previous esophageal surgery or trauma,* which could add to the progressive dysphagia. *Respiratory history* and *current respiratory difficulties* are assessed because respiratory complications are possible in the presence of reflux or regurgitation. The nurse obtains from the client a *nutritional history* including diet habits, food tolerances, nutritional status, and any weight loss to determine the effect of the esophageal symptoms.

Physical Assessment: Clinical Manifestations

There is little for the nurse to assess in terms of physical manifestations of achalasia because the esophagus is not easily evaluated by physical assessment.

The nurse notes the presence of *halitosis* (foul mouth odor), which could be due to regurgitation of previously ingested food. The nurse assesses the client's *weight* and compares it with the client's report of past weight.

Psychosocial Assessment

The nurse assesses the client's psychosocial reaction or adjustment to the disease process, including the client's feelings of self-concept related to the eating disorder, chronic pain, life style changes, regurgitation, and halitosis. Fear of malignancy is prevalent in clients with achalasia. The nurse encourages the client to verbalize fears, concerns, or anxieties about the diagnosis. The nurse also assesses the client's history of coping and coping mechanisms and identifies psychosocial supports for the client facing this potentially chronic disorder.

Radiographic Findings

A barium swallow may demonstrate the presence of an air-fluid level in a dilated esophagus. Cinematic radiographic studies may demonstrate a lack of esophageal peristalsis in segments of the esophagus.

Other Diagnostic Tests

Endoscopy often corroborates radiographic findings of esophageal dilation.

 Analysis: Nursing Diagnosis

Common Diagnoses

The most common nursing diagnosis for clients with achalasia is potential for altered nutrition: less than body requirements related to dysphagia and/or odynophagia.

Additional Diagnoses

In addition, the client may present with one or more of the following nursing diagnoses:

1. Pain related to stasis of food in the esophagus
2. Knowledge deficit related to diet and other therapy
3. Potential for ineffective individual coping related to chronic disease
4. Potential for impaired gas exchange related to nocturnal regurgitation

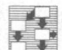 **Planning and Implementation**

The following plan of care for the client with achalasia is based on the most common nursing diagnosis of altered nutrition.

Potential for Altered Nutrition: Less Than Body Requirements

Planning: client goals. The major goal for the client with altered nutrition related to achalasia is that the client will maintain an adequate nutritional status to be independent in activities of daily living and to have increased resistance to infection.

Interventions: nonsurgical management. Nonsurgical management of decreased nutrition related to achalasia is achieved by the use of medications aimed at relaxing the LES or at increasing innervation of the esophagus: analgesics to decrease discomfort associated with meals; changes in diet; and positioning.

Drug therapy. Various categories of medications have been investigated to lower esophageal pressures and/or to relax the LES. Anticholinergic drugs, nitrates, GI hormones, and calcium channel blockers have all been used with varying effects. Narcotic and nonnarcotic analgesics may be administered, and the effectiveness of pain control is documented. The nurse assesses any effect of analgesic medications on the clinical manifestations of achalasia, such as increasing feelings of nausea or further impairing esophageal motility, as evidenced by increased pressure or regurgitation.

Diet therapy. The nurse advises the client to experiment with changes in diet because they can often ease the pressure and reflux associated with achalasia. The nurse discusses with the client any food habits that he or she has noted that aggravate or relieve the symptoms.

Semisoft foods are often better tolerated, as are warm foods and liquids. Eating several smaller meals during the day facilitates the passage of food compared with eating three larger meals. The nurse seeks consultation from a registered dietitian for additional suggestions about diet changes and nutritional balance.

Positioning.   Nocturnal reflux of foods and liquids from the dilated esophagus into the hypopharynx and oral cavity can often be prevented by having the client sleep with the head of the bed raised on blocks or by having the client sleep in a semisitting position. The nurse also advises the client to experiment with various changes in position while eating because these changes can also reduce pressure sensations during meals. Some clients benefit from arching the back while swallowing. The nurse also cautions the client to avoid wearing restrictive clothing, which can increase esophageal pressure and regurgitation.

Interventions: surgical management.   Surgical procedures for achalasia are aimed at facilitating the passage of food by dilating the unrelaxing esophageal sphincter (esophageal dilation) and enlarging the sphincter, or myotomy. For long-term refractory achalasia, excision of the affected portion of the esophagus may be attempted, with or without replacement by a segment of colon or jejunum (refer to the later heading Interventions: Surgical Management in the section on potential for infection for trauma for nursing care of the client undergoing blunt esophagectomy).

In general, dilation of the esophagus for achalasia requires considerably more force than that provided by passing progressively larges sizes of esophageal *bougies* (dilators). Sphincter dilation for achalasia is done with local anesthesia in the radiology suite by using a bougie with a pneumatized dilator, which is a pressurized bag filled with air or water (Fig. 43–5). A hydrostatic dilator (water-filled bag) is most frequently used. A bougie and then the pneumatized dilator are passed into the esophagus. Correct positioning is determined by fluoroscopy, after which the pneumatized bag is inflated to a predetermined level. After 30 to 60 seconds, the bag is deflated, and then it is reinflated for 30 to 60 seconds. The bag is rarely inflated more than twice.

Myotomy is a more complex surgical treatment for achalasia than dilation in that general anesthesia is required and the client is hospitalized for several days. A thoracotomy approach is used to expose the esophagus; muscle fibers around the LES are cut to open the sphincter and thereby provide less obstruction to food passage.

Preoperative care.   The nurse instructs clients undergoing any esophageal procedure about the necessity of remaining NPO after midnight before the surgery. The nurse informs the client of any preoperative medications that he or she will receive, such as an intramuscular narcotic analgesic.

Clients undergoing dilation are told that they will be awake throughout the procedure, but that a local anes-

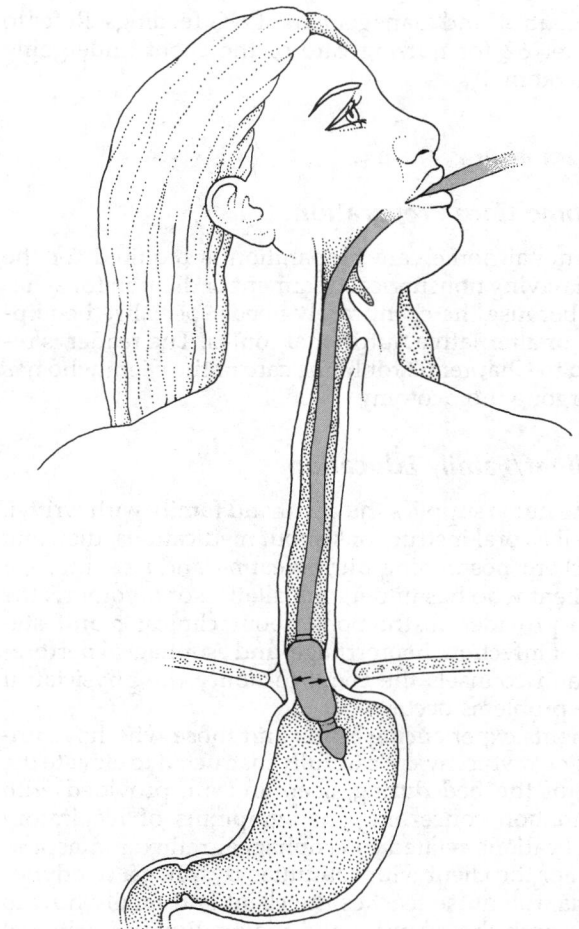

Figure 43–5

Balloon dilation of the lower esophagus.

thetic such as benzocaine (Cetacaine) is sprayed on the oropharynx.

The client is reminded that the procedure does not interfere with the ability to breathe, and the nurse instructs the client to continue to breathe in long, slow breaths during the passage of the bougies. The nurse advises the client of a brief feeling of discomfort as the bag is inflated.

Postoperative care.   After dilation, the nurse assesses the client for hemoptysis and teaches the client to expectorate rather than swallow secretions that accumulate in the oral cavity to evaluate for and quantify any bleeding. The nurse observes the client for symptoms of esophageal perforation including elevated temperature, chest pain, shoulder pain, subcutaneous emphysema in the chest and neck, and change in discomfort. The client is kept NPO for 1 hour after the procedure and is allowed only liquid food for 24 hours.

Clients undergoing myotomy or esophagectomy are observed postoperatively for management of chest tubes and drains, healing of the thoracotomy incision, pain control, and management of NG feedings. Refer to Chapter 62 for nursing care of the client undergoing thoracotomy.

■ Discharge Planning

Home Care Preparation

Minimal home care preparation is required for the client having nonsurgical treatment or dilation for achalasia because the client rarely needs specialized equipment or alternative nutritional routes. The reader is referred to Chapter 62 for home care of the client who has undergone thoracotomy.

Client/Family Education

The nurse supplies the client and family with written as well as oral instructions about medications, diet, and any client positioning during eating and sleeping. For the client who has undergone dilation or myotomy, the nurse provides instructions about clinical manifestations of infection, hemorrhage, and esophageal perforation and counsels the client to notify the physician if these problems occur.

Clients experiencing reflux and those who have undergone myotomy are carefully instructed to elevate the head of the bed during sleep and are provided with information concerning the symptoms of respiratory complications related to esophageal reflux and aspiration. For the client with continued dysphagia or odynophagia, the nurse teaches the client and family how to assess both the quantity and the quality of nutritional intake.

Psychosocial Preparation

The nurse assesses the client's readiness for self-care at home. If the nurse anticipates that the client might experience a disturbance in self-concept from a change in nutrition, he or she introduces the topic to the client and family to encourage verbalization of concerns.

Health Care Resources

Consultation with a social worker is often sought for clients who require financial assistance, specialized equipment, nutritional resources, or counseling for coping with a chronic disorder. The community health nurse is consulted to assess the home situation; to assess the ability of the client and family to perform any necessary treatments at home; and to provide ongoing evaluation and information concerning home care, nutritional status, pain control, and the need for other health care workers.

▼ Evaluation

On the basis of the most common nursing diagnosis, the nurse evaluates the care of the client with achalasia

according to expected client outcomes. Expected outcomes include that the client

1. Maintains nutritional status by eating a balanced diet of appropriate consistency
2. States that pain is alleviated or controlled

TUMORS

OVERVIEW

Both benign and malignant tumors may occur in the esophagus. Benign tumors, usually in the form of *leiomyomas*, are extremely uncommon and are usually asymptomatic. They require no specific treatment unless they produce symptoms and then are generally excised locally. Malignant tumors, however, produce widespread disabling effects in clients and at present cannot be successfully controlled by medical management. Cancer of the esophagus is almost always fatal, although there is no evidence that it is any more lethal than any other type of cancer. The tumor is, however, almost never diagnosed early enough to allow for effective intervention.

Pathophysiology

Cancer may develop at any point within the esophagus. The vast majority of esophageal cancers are squamous epidermoid tumors, which usually develop in the middle third or less frequently in the upper third of the esophagus. The remainder of the tumors are adenocarcinomas, which develop in the lower third of the esophagus and are believed to often evolve from Barrett's epithelium, which may be created by the presence of chronic reflux. Current research indicates that esophageal tumors of all types evolve as part of a slow process that begins with initially benign tissue changes.

Esophageal tumors exhibit rapid local growth because there is no serosal layer to limit their extension. Because the esophageal mucosa is richly supplied with lymphatics, early spread of tumors to lymph nodes is common. The tumors themselves are typically intraluminal ulcerating lesions with a tendency to encircle the wall of the esophagus as well as to extend up and down its length. Cancer of the esophagus is a progressive disease, and complications are an unfortunate but expected occurrence. Most clients experience pulmonary complications related to fistula formation and aspiration, and these are a frequent cause of death. The close anatomic relationships of the various structures in the neck and chest also contribute to the early development of symptoms associated with obstruction and compression within other structures. Total esophageal obstruction is an inevitable outcome if therapy is not successful. Invasion of the tumor into major vessels can produce life-threatening hemorrhage.

Because early diagnosis is rare, tumors less than 10 cm in size are considered to be small. Metastasis is frequently present at the time of diagnosis. Tumor complications are related to nutritional compromise; fistula formation in the trachea, lungs, or bronchi; and widespread invasion with the potential for bleeding. In addition, clients who are treated surgically are vulnerable to a wide variety of potentially life-threatening complications.

Etiology

Geographic and environmental factors appear to play a significant role in the development of esophageal cancer, and the disease exhibits an erratic worldwide incidence pattern. Chronic trauma and the long-term effects of other esophageal problems such as achalasia (failure of relaxation of the LES, producing dysphagia), stricture, and hiatal hernia also influence the incidence statistics, but in only a minor way. Research indicates that in the Western world, the long-term heavy consumption of alcohol and use of tobacco contribute significantly to the eventual development of esophageal cancer. In other parts of the world where esophageal cancer is extremely common, however, the incidence appears to be linked to high levels of nitrosamines and other contaminants in the soil and foodstuffs. Diets that are chronically deficient in fresh fruits and vegetables, vitamins, and proteins also appear to contribute to the development of this cancer.

Incidence

Cancer of the esophagus accounts for approximately 1.5% of all cancers and 7% of all tumors involving the GI tract in the United States (Livstone & Skinner, 1985). There have been statistically significant annual increases in the incidence of cancer of the esophagus in the U.S. over the last several decades, particularly in the Black population. Esophageal cancer mortality rates for this population group are now second only to cancer of the lung. Cancer of the esophagus is extremely virulent, and the 5-year survival statistics do not exceed 5% to 10% despite aggressive treatment (Knauer & Silverman, 1988).

These relatively low incidence statistics are unique to the United States and the Western world, however. In areas of northwest China, around the Caspian Sea in the Soviet Union and Iran, and in the Transkei region of southern Africa, the incidence of cancer of the esophagus is extremely high. Residents of some provinces in China have a 30% to 40% probability of dying of esophageal cancer (Tollefson, 1985). The causes of these extreme variations are being extensively researched but have not yet been satisfactorily explained.

In the United States, cancer of the esophagus typically affects men between the ages of 50 and 80 years. Men are affected four times as often as women, and Black persons are affected four times as often as Caucasian. Asian males also develop the disease more frequently.

PREVENTION

The incidence of the disease in the United States is related to heavy and long-term use of alcohol and tobacco, either smoked or chewed. The use of both products definitely potentiates the client's risk of developing cancer. To a lesser extent, the presence of stricture, achalasia, reflux, or chronic poor oral hygiene also increases the risk. Prevention strategies focus on the moderation or elimination of tobacco and alcohol in a client's life style and on prompt and effective treatment of associated esophageal disorders. The Black male population is specifically targeted for all prevention efforts.

COLLABORATIVE MANAGEMENT

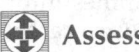 **Assessment**

History

The nurse assesses the client's *race, age,* and *sex,* as well as any pertinent history of *alcohol consumption* or *tobacco use.* The nurse also assesses for any history of other esophageal problems such as *stricture* or *reflux.*

Cancer of the esophagus is a silent tumor in its early stages, with few if any signs to identify on assessment. By the time the tumor causes symptoms, it has usually spread rather extensively. A *weight loss* of up to 40 to 50 lb over a 2- to 3-month period is common. The weight loss is a nonspecific assessment feature, which may be related to *anorexia,* dysphagia, or the discomfort produced by the tumor's presence. The nurse carefully assesses the client's *diet pattern* and any modifications that have been made in response to the symptoms.

Physical Assessment: Clinical Manifestations

The nurse assesses the client's general physical appearance and nutritional status and obtains data about recent weight loss.

The most important diagnostic feature is *dysphagia,* which is present in virtually every client. The nurse carefully assesses its severity and extent. Clients usually report a sensation that food is sticking in the throat or the substernal area. Tumor-induced dysphagia is both persistent and progressive. It is initially associated with swallowing solids, particularly meat, and then progresses rather rapidly over a period of weeks or months to difficulty in swallowing soft foods and liquids. Late in the disease, even saliva can induce choking. Careful assessment of the dysphagia is an important part of the diagnosis because the dysphagia that is associated with other esophageal disorders typically is not continuous. Dysphagia does not usually appear until at least 60% of the esophageal diameter is narrowed by the tumor (Mayer, 1988).

Odynophagia, or painful swallowing, is present in most clients and is reported as a steady, dull, substernal pain that may radiate. The presence of *pain* that is severe or persistent often indicates tumor invasion of mediastinal structures. The nurse also assesses for the occurrence of *regurgitation,* or *vomiting; foul breath;* and chronic *hiccups,* which often accompany advanced disease. The majority of clients also develop pulmonary complications at some point, and the nurse assesses for the presence of *chronic cough, increased secretions,* and a history of recent infections. Tumors in the upper esophagus may involve the larynx and thus cause *hoarseness.*

Psychosocial Assessment

The symptoms and diagnosis of esophageal cancer can affect a client in profound ways. The disease produces significant daily symptoms, requires major modifications in basic eating patterns, and is terminal. The fear of choking can transform normal mealtimes into frightening experiences to be avoided. The nurse carefully assesses the client's response to the diagnosis and prognosis and explores the client's coping strengths and resources. The nurse thoroughly assesses the impact of the disease on the client's usual pattern of activities. The client's home situation is assessed, including family members and friends who can provide support or direct assistance with care. The nurse also assesses the potential financial impact of the disease and its treatment.

Laboratory Findings

Slow occult bleeding from the tumor may produce a drop in hemoglobin and hematocrit values, but laboratory tests are not definitive for esophageal cancer.

Radiographic Findings

The barium swallow with fluoroscopy is the first test used to diagnose esophageal cancer. The tumor margins of large masses can often be outlined in this way. A negative test does not rule out cancer, however, and further work-up is usually carried out.

Other Diagnostic Tests

Esophagoscopy is performed to inspect the esophagus visually and to obtain specimens for cytologic studies and biopsy. Multiple samples are frequently required when the suspected tumor is in the distal esophagus because clear tissue samples are difficult to obtain.

If surgery is planned, the physician may also use computed tomography, gallium scans, and bronchoscopy to help determine the extent of the disease.

 Analysis: Nursing Diagnosis

Common Diagnoses

The most common nursing diagnosis that is associated with cancer of the esophagus is altered nutrition: less than body requirements related to impaired swallowing secondary to tumor obstruction of the esophagus.

Additional Diagnoses

In addition, one or more of the following nursing diagnoses may be appropriate:

1. Pain related to the pressure of the tumor mass in the esophagus or mediastinum
2. Potential for impaired gas exchange related to regurgitation, fistula, and aspiration
3. Impaired swallowing related to obstruction by tumor or effects of radiation
4. Potential for ineffective individual coping or for ineffective family coping related to disease effects and terminal prognosis
5. Anticipatory grieving related to declining physical status and terminal prognosis
6. Spiritual distress related to impending death

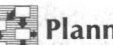 **Planning and Implementation**

Altered Nutrition: Less Than Body Requirements

Planning: client goals. Appropriate goals are determined by the individual client's situation and response to the disease, treatment regimen, and prognosis. The primary goal for this nursing diagnosis is that the client will ingest sufficient balanced nutrients to meet the body's needs and to maintain a stable weight.

Interventions. Treatment options for cancer of the esophagus include radiation therapy, dilation of strictures, prosthesis insertion, chemotherapy, nutritional support, and radical surgery. None of the available approaches have significantly improved either the 5-year survival rates or the terminal prognosis. There is, therefore, little agreement about how aggressively individual clients should be treated. Clients with cancer of the esophagus almost always suffer greatly, and relieving symptoms becomes an essential consideration.

Nonsurgical management. Treatment decisions are based on the location and size of the tumor, the presence of metastasis, and the client's concurrent health status and ability to withstand radical surgery. Nonsurgical interventions are usually directed at the palliation of symptoms and are selected when a client is either unable or unwilling to undergo extensive surgery.

Radiation therapy.   Radiation therapy is the treatment of choice for palliation. Radiation reduces the tumor's size and offers clients consistent short-term relief. High doses of radiation can, however, result in esophageal stricture or stenosis that may require dilation. Normal esophageal tissue is quite sensitive to the effects of radiation, and the treatment is typically administered during a 6- to 8-week period in an attempt to minimize these negative effects. Radiation therapy, therefore, is a successful palliative measure that improves the client's quality of life, but it also consumes a significant portion of the client's remaining time.

In the first weeks of treatment, radiation produces edema and epithelial desquamation, which create acute esophagitis and odynophagia. These symptoms may be quite severe. It also produces profound anorexia and may cause nausea and vomiting. Symptoms persist until treatment is completed. The nurse assesses the client frequently and determines the incidence and severity of symptoms. Systemic analgesics are often required to control discomfort, and the nurse administers oral lidocaine (Xylocaine Viscous) before each attempt at oral feeding. The nurse works with the client to modify the diet to meet nutritional needs and maintain comfort. Small, frequent soft or semiliquid feedings are offered. Sweet light foods are often tolerated best, and protein powder may be used to supplement the nutritional content of the diet. The nurse maintains accurate calorie counts, intake and output records, and daily weights and assesses skin turgor and mucous membranes regularly. Frequent gentle mouth care is important. Clients are at risk for developing monilial esophagitis, and the nurse must be alert to any abrupt worsening of the client's symptoms. Chapter 25 describes additional nursing interventions for the client undergoing radiation therapy.

Esophageal dilation.   Esophageal dilation may be performed as necessary throughout the course of the disease to achieve temporary symptomatic relief of dysphagia. Dilation is used to reduce the tumor obstruction and to treat the strictures that frequently follow radiation therapy. In the hands of a skilled physician, malignant tumors may be dilated safely, and the treatment should be repeated as often as needed to preserve the client's ability to swallow (see under earlier heading Interventions: Surgical Management in the section on achalasia).

Prosthesis insertion.   A semirigid prosthesis may be inserted to bypass disabling dysphagia and to prevent aspiration in clients with advanced disease or in those who develop tracheoesophageal or esophagobronchial fistulas. Prosthesis insertion successfully maintains an open esophagus and preserves the client's ability to take oral nourishment, but the procedure is not without risk. The prosthesis can become dislodged or can migrate and can perforate the esophagus as tumor bulk increases.

The nurse's primary emphasis is the prevention of aspiration because the tube interrupts the function of the LES and permits free reflux of gastric contents. The nurse supervises the client closely, offers small oral feedings, and ensures that the client does not lie flat in bed.

Drug therapy.   In recent years, chemotherapy combining several antineoplastic drugs has been used more frequently as part of the primary treatment, along with surgery and radiation. Other drugs used to treat clients with esophageal cancer include antacids and analgesics to relieve the symptoms of pyrosis (heartburn) and odynophagia.

Diet therapy.   Maintaining adequate nutrition is an essential ongoing goal for clients with esophageal cancer. Interventions often take different forms as the disease process progresses. The emphasis is on diet modification while dysphagia develops. The nurse teaches the client to select soft or semiliquid foods and to enrich these meals with skim milk powder or commercial protein supplements. Small frequent feedings are usually better tolerated. Attempts are made to prepare and serve meals as attractively as possible, and the client's personal likes and dislikes should be carefully considered.

Ongoing efforts are made to preserve the client's ability to swallow, but feeding tubes may be needed on a temporary basis when dysphagia is severe. In cases of complete obstruction or life-threatening fistula formation, it may be necessary to create a feeding gastrostomy or jejunostomy. Because these measures radically disrupt normal eating and do not enable clients to swallow even saliva, they are considered to be the least desirable option. When tube feedings are used, puréed regular foods with liberal additional water are preferable to commercial products because they are less likely to induce diarrhea. Short-term hyperalimentation is also used to improve a client's nutritional status quickly, particularly before surgery (see Chap. 13 for a discussion of nursing responsibilities associated with tube feeding and hyperalimentation). Daily weights, calorie counts, and intake and output are all monitored carefully to evaluate the client's response to the interventions.

Positioning.   Careful positioning is essential for clients who are experiencing frequent regurgitation or have prosthetic tubes inserted to keep the esophagus patent. The nurse teaches the client to remain upright for several hours after meals and to completely avoid lying flat. The head of the bed should always be kept elevated 30 degrees or more to prevent reflux.

Surgical management.   Radical surgery represents the only definitive treatment for esophageal cancer and is the preferred treatment for otherwise healthy clients. The surgeries are extensive, however, and have a high mortality rate, especially for elderly clients with concurrent health problems.

Subtotal or *total esophagectomy* is usually required be-

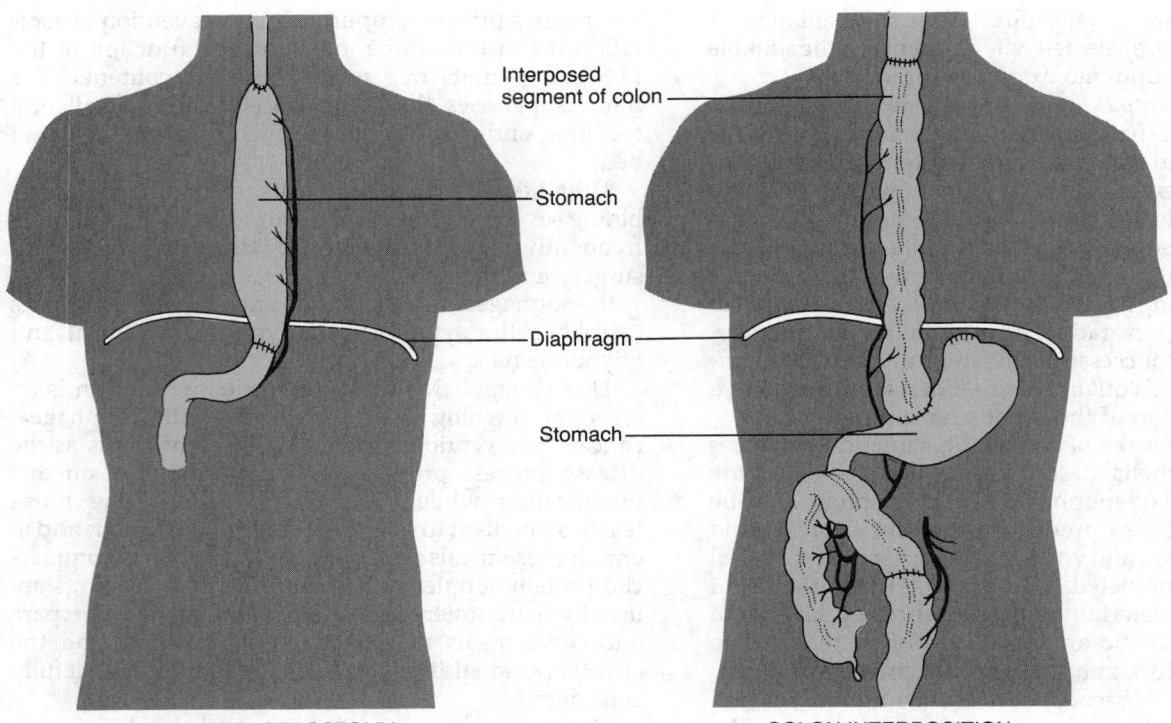

ESOPHAGOGASTROSTOMY   COLON INTERPOSITION

Figure 43–6

Surgical approaches to the treatment of esophageal cancer.

cause tumors are frequently quite large and involve distant lymph nodes. Several procedures are used, but the preferred surgery, an *esophagogastrostomy*, involves removing the diseased portion of the esophagus and anastomosing the cervical portion to the stomach, which is brought up into the thorax through the esophageal hiatus (Fig. 43–6). This procedure is the simplest, yet it involves both laparotomy and thoracotomy incisions. Tumors in the upper esophagus may also require radical neck dissection and laryngectomy because of spread of the disease to the larynx. When the tumor involves the stomach or the stomach is otherwise unsuitable for anastomosis, the surgeon may instead perform a colon interposition by removing a section of right or left colon and bringing it up into the thorax to substitute for the esophagus (see Fig. 43–6).

In addition to the usual surgical risks of shock, hemorrhage, and infection, these radical surgeries create a serious risk of leakage at the anastomosis site. This situation is especially true with colon interpositions because several anastomosis sites are vulnerable to the effects of tension, poor blood supply, and delayed healing. If the client successfully recovers from surgery, he or she is still at serious risk for aspiration from regurgitation because the sphincter effect of the lower esophagus has been eliminated.

Preoperative care. To adequately prepare a client for surgery may require anywhere from 5 days to 2 to 3 weeks of nutritional support. Ideally, this supplementation is given orally, but in fact clients usually require tube feeding or hyperalimentation. The client's weight, intake and output, and fluid and electrolyte balance are carefully monitored. Meticulous oral care is performed four times daily to decrease the risk of postoperative infection. Clients may also receive radiation therapy before surgery.

The remainder of preoperative nursing care focuses on teaching and psychologic support. The client may have ambivalent feelings about signing permission for this radical surgery. The nurse ensures that the client is knowledgeable about the surgery and its outcomes. The physician's instructions are clarified and reinforced as needed. The nurse teaches the client about the number and sites of all incisions, wound drainage tubes, chest tubes, NG tube, and intravenous lines. The critical care unit is visited if possible, and contacts are initiated with staff.

The client receives instructions about routines for turning, coughing, and deep breathing, as well as about chest physical therapy. The client demonstrates the learning as appropriate. The crucial nature of postoperative respiratory care is emphasized. The probable need for ventilator support should also be addressed because respiratory management is a major focus of postoperative care. If colon interposition is planned, the client will also undergo a complete bowel preparation with laxatives and enemas.

The client faces extensive surgery with a high surgical mortality rate. It is natural for the client to be extremely anxious and ambivalent. The nurse encourages the client to talk about personal feelings and fears and involves the family in all preoperative teaching and discussions. A primary nurse to provide continuity of care and support to the entire family is extremely helpful.

Postoperative care. The client requires meticulous postoperative care and is at risk for developing multiple serious complications. See Chapters 20 and 62 for a general discussion of care needs after abdominal and thoracic surgery.

Respiratory care is the highest priority, and the client may be temporarily placed on a respirator in a critical care unit. The nurse assesses the client's respiratory status every 1 to 2 hours and implements turning and coughing routines. Chest physiotherapy is used as ordered. Incisional support and adequate analgesia are essential to effective coughing and should be routinely administered if the client's vital signs remain stable. The client is maintained in semi-Fowler's or high Fowler's position to support ventilation and to prevent reflux. Prophylactic antibiotics and supplemental oxygen are given routinely, and blood gases are monitored regularly. Chest tubes are in place, and the nurse ensures the patency of the water seal drainage system.

Wound management is another significant postoperative concern because the client has multiple incisions and drains. Incisional support during turning and coughing is essential to prevent dehiscence. Anastomosis leakage is a dreaded complication, which may appear about 5 to 7 days after surgery. The nurse carefully assesses for fever, fluid accumulation, general signs of inflammation, and symptoms of early shock such as tachycardia and tachypnea. Prompt identification of signs of leakage is essential.

The NG tube is monitored for patency and is carefully secured to prevent dislodgement, which could disrupt the sutures at the anastomosis. The nurse *does not* irrigate or reposition the NG tube in clients who have had esophageal surgery. Unless another time interval is specified, the client is NPO for 4 to 5 days until GI motility is well established. The client receives intravenous fluids or hyperalimentation but is kept slightly dehydrated to avoid circulatory overload. The initial NG drainage is bloody but should change to a greenish-yellow color by the end of the first postoperative day. The continued presence of blood could indicate bleeding at the suture line. The nurse provides oral hygiene every 2 to 4 hours while the tube is in place. After initial stabilization, the client is given 3 to 5 mL of water every 15 to 30 minutes. If this fluid is satisfactorily tolerated, the quantity is increased to an ounce at a time. The nurse supervises the client during all initial swallowing efforts and ensures that the client is in an upright position. The NG tube is left in place while feedings are initiated to keep the area decompressed. The nurse continues to assess for signs of leakage.

If leaks do not appear, the client slowly progresses to puréed and semisolid foods. The nurse works with the client to establish what quantity of food can be safely and comfortably swallowed and to provide or review teaching about the importance of eating small meals and maintaining an upright position. The food storage area of the stomach has been radically decreased, and gravity is the client's only real defense against reflux.

■ Discharge Planning

Home Care Preparation

Most clients require a significant amount of assistance at home after discharge, particularly if the client lives alone or with an elderly spouse. Treatment of esophageal cancer is radical, and, even if major postoperative complications do not occur, the client is likely to be discharged with ongoing concerns about respiratory care, incisional healing, and nutritional support. The nurse gathers accurate and detailed data concerning the client's social situation and assists the physician to make decisions related to home care needs.

Client/Family Education

The care given in the hospital is continued to at least some degree after discharge, and it is essential that both the client and family are well informed about the care needed. Ongoing respiratory care is a priority, and family members are instructed to assist with ambulation, splinting incisions, or providing chest physiotherapy. The nurse teaches the family to protect the client from infection and to contact the physician immediately if signs of respiratory infection develop. The client is encouraged to be as active as possible and to avoid excessive bed rest and its complications at all costs.

Wound healing is also an ongoing concern. The nurse teaches the client and family to inspect the incisions daily for redness, tenderness, swelling, and discharge. The nurse prepares written instructions about the signs of anastomosis leakage and the importance of reporting them to the physician or other health care provider immediately.

Nutritional support also remains a concern. The client is encouraged to continue to increase oral feedings as tolerated and to emphasize a high-calorie, high-protein diet that contains soft and easily swallowed foods. Meals should be small and frequent, and nutritionally empty foods should be avoided. Eggnogs and milk shakes may be easily prepared and enriched to supplement the feedings. The family may be taught to manage tube feedings or hyperalimentation at home if necessary. The nurse emphasizes the importance of keeping the client upright after meals and elevating the head of the bed on blocks. Families are counseled that dysphagia or odynophagia may recur because of stricture or tumor regrowth. These symptoms should be promptly reported to the physician.

Psychosocial Preparation

Despite radical surgery, the client with cancer of the esophagus still has a terminal illness and a relatively short life expectancy. Emphasis is placed on the improved quality of life that surgery provides. Realistic planning is important as the client's condition eventually worsens, and the client and family should be assisted to plan together for the future. The nurse assists the family members to explore a variety of sources for support and encourages them to accept formal and informal sources of support.

Health Care Resources

The nurse initiates referrals to appropriate community or home care organizations to assist the family in providing the care required at home. In addition, the nurse provides the family with information about the services and supports that are available through the American Cancer Society. The nurse may also acquaint the family with area hospice services for future planning.

 Evaluation

Evaluation is based on the individual client's specific nursing diagnoses and the stated goals. It also reflects the understanding that the client's disease is ultimately fatal. Desired outcomes include that the client

1. Takes in sufficient balanced nutrients to meet the body's needs
2. Maintains a stable weight
3. Can swallow without discomfort
4. Maintains a patent airway and is free from respiratory infection
5. Adapts to the stresses of the diagnosis and receives meaningful support from family or significant others

DIVERTICULA

OVERVIEW

Diverticula in the esophagus are outpouchings that result in a blind pouch in which ingested foods and liquids are trapped, later often to be regurgitated. Clients complain of symptoms similar to those of achalasia (discussed earlier), such as regurgitation, nocturnal cough, halitosis, sour taste in the mouth, dysphagia, and feelings of pressure or fullness.

Pathophysiology

Diverticula are often subdivided into two categories: traction and pulsion. *Traction* diverticula occur when the esophageal mucosa is pulled outward from the wall of the esophagus. *Pulsion* diverticula are created when the esophageal mucosa pushes outward through a defect in the muscles covering the esophagus. Traction diverticula are most commonly located in the middle esophagus, whereas pulsion diverticula are most frequently found in the upper esophagus. The most common esophageal diverticulum is *Zenker's diverticulum,* commonly located near the hypopharynx. Clients with esophageal diverticula can be at risk for development of esophageal perforation because the esophageal mucosa is without protection of the normal esophageal muscle layer. Perforations can occur during surgical procedures, from accidental esophageal intubation, during routine esophagoscopy, or from the presence of a sharp foreign body in the esophagus, such as a bone.

Etiology

The etiology of pulsion diverticula is unclear. A congenital defect causing weakness in the esophageal wall could be responsible for the evagination of the esophageal mucosa through the wall. Prior esophageal trauma is another possible etiologic factor in esophageal wall weakness.

Traction diverticula, in which the esophageal mucosa is pulled as opposed to being pushed through the esophageal wall, are caused by the traction of scar tissue or by inflammation in the area.

Incidence

Esophageal diverticula are generally considered to be rare. Zenker's diverticula are more commonly seen in males than in females.

COLLABORATIVE MANAGEMENT

 Assessment

History

In obtaining a history from clients with esophageal diverticula, the nurse ascertains the *symptoms* the client has been experiencing, such as dysphagia, regurgitation, feeling of fullness, halitosis, or altered taste. Pain is a rare clinical manifestation of diverticula. The nurse explores with the client the *onset* and/or *duration of symptoms,* whether they occur only at mealtimes or whether they are exacerbated at night. The nurse questions the client about *factors that aggravate the symptoms,* including positioning and diet, as well as home *treatments that relieve the symptoms.* A history of *previous esophageal surgery or trauma* is also assessed. *Respiratory history* and *current respiratory difficulties,* including nocturnal cough, are assessed because respiratory complications are possible from regurgitation. The nurse also obtains a *nutritional history,* including diet habits, food tolerances, nutritional status, and recent weight loss.

Physical Assessment: Clinical Manifestations

There is little for the nurse to assess in terms of physical manifestations of an esophageal diverticulum because the esophagus is not easily evaluated by physical assessment.

The nurse assesses the client's chest and lungs because aspiration pneumonia, nocturnal cough, and other respiratory complications resulting from regurgitation often accompany esophageal diverticula. The nurse auscultates over the neck to detect any *gurgling sounds* suggestive of diverticula. *Halitosis* is noted and is due to regurgitation of food particles from the diverticulum.

Psychosocial Assessment

The nurse assesses the client's psychosocial reaction or adjustment to the disease process, including feelings about self-concept related to an eating disorder, life style changes, and symptoms of regurgitation and halitosis. The nurse assesses the client's history of coping and coping mechanisms and identifies psychosocial supports for the client who faces life style changes and/or surgery.

Radiographic/Other Diagnostic Findings

The barium swallow is routinely performed to look for filling of diverticula. The diagnosis can be made based on this finding. Endoscopy is rarely used because of the risk of perforation of the diverticulum with the esophagoscope.

 ## Analysis: Nursing Diagnosis

Common Diagnoses

The most common nursing diagnosis for clients with diverticula is pain related to dysphagia and substernal pressure.

Additional Diagnoses

In addition, the client may present with one or more of the following nursing diagnoses:

1. Potential for altered nutrition: less than body requirements related to dysphagia
2. Knowledge deficit related to diet and other therapy
3. Potential for impaired gas exchange related to regurgitation and aspiration

 ## Planning and Implementation

The following plan of care for the client with diverticula is based on the most common nursing diagnosis of pain. A complete Client Care Plan for the client undergoing surgery of the esophagus was given earlier.

Pain

Planning: client goals.   The major goal for the client with pain related to diverticula is that the symptoms causing discomfort will be alleviated or reduced so that the client can continue with normal activities and daily routines and can maintain a nutritionally balanced diet.

Interventions: nonsurgical management.   Nonsurgical management of discomfort related to regurgitation from a diverticulum is achieved through dietary changes and client positioning.

Diet therapy.   The nurse advises the client to experiment with changes in diet because variation in food consistency and in frequency and size of meals can often ease the pressure and reflux associated with diverticula. The nurse discusses with the client any food habits he or she has noted that exacerbate or relieve the clinical manifestations. Semisoft foods are often better tolerated. Eating several smaller meals instead of three large meals also facilitates the passage of food through the esophagus. The nurse also analyzes information obtained in the history to determine whether education is needed about maintaining balanced nutrition. The nurse seeks consultation from a registered dietitian for additional suggestions regarding dietary changes and nutritional balance for the client.

Positioning.   Nocturnal reflux, which is manifested by nocturnal coughing, can often be prevented by having the client sleep with the head of the bed raised on blocks or by having the client sleep in a semisitting position. Postprandial (after meal) reflux caused by diverticula can be controlled by having the head raised for at least 2 hours after meals. The nurse cautions the client against vigorously exercising or lying down immediately after meals. The nurse encourages the client to experiment with various positions while eating to evaluate changes perceived in the amount of regurgitation occurring. The nurse also cautions the client to avoid wearing restrictive garments, which cause pressure on the abdomen or esophagus.

Interventions: surgical management.   Surgical management of diverticula is aimed at excision of the diverticulum and reapproximating the esophageal mucosa. The esophageal mucosa is violated during this surgery, and the client must be maintained NPO for several days to allow mucosal healing. The most commonly excised diverticulum is Zenker's diverticulum, excision of which requires a cervical (neck) incision as opposed to a thoracotomy approach.

Preoperative care.   The nurse discusses the routines accompanying general anesthesia, as described in Chapter 18. The client is also told that he or she will be NPO postoperatively, will have an NG tube in place, and will have a neck dressing and a drain.

Postoperative care.   After excision of an esophageal diverticulum, nursing care measures are aimed at prevention and/or early detection of hemorrhage or esophageal perforation, at relief of discomfort, and at management of fluid and nutritional requirements. The nurse provides routine postoperative care after general anesthesia, as described in Chapter 20. The nurse also maintains NG suction immediately after the operation, measures and records drainage each shift, and observes for bloody drainage or external bleeding. The nurse *does not* irrigate or reposition the NG tube after esophageal surgery until ordered to do so by the surgeon. The nurse observes the client for symptoms of esophageal perforation, including elevated temperature, chest pain, and subcutaneous emphysema.

For comfort measures, the nurse raises the head of the bed at least 30 degrees at all times after the client is fully awake to assist in decreasing edema. The nurse assesses the client's subjective and objective clinical manifestations of discomfort to determine the need for analgesics and to assess the effectiveness of the analgesic regimen. Frequent oral hygiene is offered to increase comfort and feelings of well-being. The client's comfort is also enhanced by careful explanation of procedures and equipment.

While the client's NG tube is connected to suction, the client receives intravenous fluids for hydration until fluid feedings are begun by tube. The client is reminded to take care when ambulating or changing position to avoid possible dislodgement of the NG tube. When fluids and nutritional supplements are begun by tube, the nurse assesses and documents the client's response, and the nutritional plan is altered as necessary. The client is encouraged to participate in care as appropriate. The client is carefully evaluated for complications related to the nutritional route, such as infection, dehydration or fluid overload, constipation or diarrhea, or disturbance in self-concept (see Chap. 13 for nursing care of the client receiving supplemental feedings). When the NG tube is removed, the nurse assesses the client's ability to swallow.

■ Discharge Planning

Home Care Preparation

Clients are occasionally discharged with an NG tube in place for home tube feedings to allow for additional time for healing. The ability of the client or family to obtain supplies or equipment needed to prepare special foods at home is assessed.

Client/Family Education

The nurse supplies the client and family with written and oral instructions about medications, diet, and any positioning needed during mealtimes and at night. For the client who has undergone resection of a diverticulum, the nurse provides instructions about identification of symptoms of infection, hemorrhage, and esophageal perforation and advises the client to notify the physician if these symptoms occur. Clients experiencing reflux are instructed to elevate the head of the bed while sleeping

and are informed of the clinical manifestations of respiratory complications related to esophageal reflux and aspiration.

Psychosocial Preparation

The nurse assesses the client's readiness for self-care at home. If the nurse anticipates that the client might experience a disturbance in self-concept, he or she introduces the topic to the client and family to encourage verbalization of concerns.

Health Care Resources

The major health care resources for the client with an esophageal diverticulum are the same as those needed for the client with achalasia (see earlier section on achalasia).

 Evaluation

On the basis of the most common nursing diagnosis, the nurse evaluates the care of the client with esophageal diverticulum according to the expected client outcomes. Expected outcomes include that the client

1. States that discomfort related to regurgitation is alleviated or controlled
2. Maintains nutritional status by eating a balanced diet of appropriate consistency

TRAUMA

OVERVIEW

Trauma to the esophagus occurs from extrinsic or intrinsic causes. Esophageal rupture or perforation can occur from blunt injuries to the chest, such as in automobile accidents; as a complication of surgery; as a consequence of an esophageal burn; or as a result of spontaneous vomiting. Trauma to the esophagus places the client at risk for complications involving related or nearby organ systems, such as pulmonary or mediastinal complications, and necessitates nursing assessment of the client's ability to swallow and to maintain nutrition.

Pathophysiology

Esophageal Rupture or Perforation

When excessive pressure is exerted on the esophageal mucosa, whether from extrinsic sources such as instruments or from intrinsic sources of increased pressure, the mucosa can be perforated and can rupture, or it can weaken and rupture later from additional stress. Esophageal perforation or rupture allows caustic esophageal secretions and contents to enter the mediastinal cavity.

Cervical and thoracic esophageal perforations are serious, and certain types of tears have a mortality rate close to 90%. Esophageal and gastric secretions have the potential for beginning digestive processes on nearby tissues. The mortality figures for untreated esophageal perforations are high because of ensuing shock, respiratory difficulty, and infection from mediastinal contamination.

Chemical Injury

When strong alkaline or acidic substances come in contact with the esophageal mucosa, damage to the layers of the mucosa can quickly result. Alkaline materials tend to cause more severe tissue damage because of deep penetration of the esophageal wall, whereas acid burns are generally more superficial. Acid substances produce a coagulum layer on the surface of the mucosa, which often acts as a barrier to deeper penetration of the acid into the mucosa.

As the mechanism for injury for chemical burns of the esophagus is most commonly oral ingestion of the acid or alkali, damage to the mucosa of the oral cavity often accompanies esophageal chemical injury. The corrosive substance begins mucosal damage almost immediately on ingestion. Perforation of the esophagus can occur with very strong alkalis in less than 1 minute after ingestion.

Complications from caustic burns of the esophagus include pneumonia from aspirating the caustic substance or vomitus (if choking or retching occurred during the incident), hemorrhage from mucosal injury, and esophageal perforation. A late complication of burn injury to the esophagus is esophageal stricture from the formation of scar tissue.

Etiology

Esophageal Rupture or Perforation

Esophageal rupture can occur spontaneously or after blunt trauma. Spontaneous rupture most often accompanies severe episodes of vomiting, as can result from chemotherapy, hyperemesis gravidarum (nausea and vomiting during pregnancy that are severe and long-lasting), and excessive alcohol and/or food intake. Blunt trauma that can cause esophageal rupture includes crush injuries to the chest. Surgical perforations occur during endoscopy or other neck and mediastinal procedures, as well as during placement of NG tubes (see the accompanying Key Features of Disease).

Chemical Injury

Chemical injury of the esophagus is generally due to accidental or intentional swallowing of caustic sub-

> **KEY FEATURES OF DISEASE** ■ Causes of Esophageal Perforation
>
> Straining
> Convulsions
> Trauma
> Foreign objects
> Instruments or tubes
> Chemical injury
> Complications of esophageal surgery
> Ulcers

stances. The amount of chemical injury depends on the nature and concentration of the corrosive agent. Alkaline substances most commonly cause corrosive injury to the esophagus because they are found more frequently than acid substances in the home setting. Table 43–2 provides names and active ingredients of some caustic materials frequently found in the home.

Incidence

Esophageal Rupture or Perforation

Esophageal rupture is considered to be a rare occurrence, primarily because of the elasticity of the esophagus, which makes the esophagus tolerate rapid changes in pressure fairly well. The incidence of esophageal perforations as complications of surgical procedures is also relatively low.

Chemical Injury

The incidence of corrosive burn injuries of the esophagus is relatively uncommon in adults. When they occur, the injuries are most frequently due to accidental ingestion of corrosive substances, but they can also result from deliberate trauma from a suicide attempt. Storage of corrosive substances in containers other than original packaging (such as storing the substances in soda bottles) contributes to the incidence of accidental poisoning and esophageal burns.

COLLABORATIVE MANAGEMENT

 Assessment

History

The client after trauma to the esophagus is usually first seen in an emergency situation; therefore, initial history taking by the nurse is confined to pinpointing the *process* and the *time of the injury* and to determine any *respiratory difficulty* related to the injury. While the client is being stabilized, the nurse consults the family regarding the remainder of the history of the current

TABLE 43-2 Common Household Corrosives and Their Active Ingredients

Type	Corrosive	Active Ingredient
Acids		
Liquid	Mister Plumber	Sulfuric acid 8.5%
	Lysol Toilet Bowl Cleaner	Hydrochloric acid
	Sno-Bol Toilet Bowl Cleaner	Hydrochloric acid 15%
Granular	ZUD Rust and Stain Remover	Oxalic acid
	Sani-Flush Toilet Bowl Cleaner	Sodium bisulfite 75%
	Vanish Toilet Bowl Cleaner	Sodium acid sulfate 62%
	Rooto	Sulfuric acid
Alkalis	Liquid Drano	Sodium hydroxide 9.5%
	Crystal Drano	Sodium hydroxide 80%
	Liquid Plumr	Sodium hypochlorite and hydroxide 8%
	Easy-Off Liquid Oven Cleaner	Sodium hydroxide
	Mr. Muscle Oven Cleaner	Sodium hydroxide
	Industrial/Professional Drano	Sodium hydroxide 32%
	Ammonia	Ammonium hydroxide
Bleaches	Clorox	
	Peroxide	
Thermal agents	Dry Ice	
	Hot water	
	Clinitest Tablets*	
Detergents	Oxydol (laundry)	Sodium tripolyphosphate
	Cascade (dish)	Sodium tripolyphosphate
	Amway (dish)	Sodium tripolyphosphate

*Also have direct corrosive effects.
From Range, D., Hirokawa, R., & Bryarly, R. (1983). Caustic ingestion. *Ear, Nose, and Throat Journal, 62*, 47.

problem. If the client has only a minor caustic injury or a minor perforation, the nurse obtains the history directly from the client.

The nurse obtains a history of *previous esophageal surgery, dysphagia,* or *odynophagia.* If the client has suffered a spontaneous rupture, the nurse questions the family about *recent vomiting.* The nurse assesses the client's *nutritional status* and *ability to swallow* by asking the client about a recent change in food habits, the types and consistency of foods he or she can swallow, whether choking accompanies swallowing, and any recent weight loss.

Physical Assessment: Clinical Manifestations

The esophagus is not easily evaluated by physical assessment. The oral cavity is assessed for any redness or irritation from contact with corrosive materials.

Psychosocial Assessment

In nonemergency situations, the nurse assesses the client's psychosocial reaction to the injury, in particular, the client's feelings of self-concept. The nurse encour-

ages the client to verbalize fears, concerns, or anxieties about the diagnosis. The nurse also assesses the client's history of coping and coping mechanisms and identifies psychosocial supports for the client with an esophageal injury. In cases of chemical injury, the client is assessed for suicidal ideation.

Radiographic Findings

Esophagography. X-ray film may be used to assess for a patent esophagus or perforation. A finding of air in the mediastinum could indicate an esophageal tear or rupture.

Barium swallow. This test may be done in cases of corrosive burns, but it would probably be avoided if perforation were suspected.

Other Diagnostic Tests

Esophageal endoscopy is performed if a ruptured esophagus is suspected. If corrosive burns of the esophagus are suspected, this procedure may be avoided because of the risk of perforating damaged tissues.

Analysis: Nursing Diagnosis

Common Diagnoses

The most common nursing diagnosis for clients with esophageal trauma is potential for infection (mediastinal) related to esophageal perforation.

Additional Diagnoses

In addition, the client may present with one or more of the following nursing diagnoses:

1. Pain related to esophageal injury
2. Altered nutrition: less than body requirements related to esophageal injury
3. Altered oral mucous membrane related to esophageal injury
4. Potential for impaired gas exchange related to esophageal injury

 Planning and Implementation

The following plan of care for the client with esophageal trauma is based on the most common nursing diagnosis.

Potential for Infection

Planning: client goals.   The major goal for this diagnosis is that the client will prevent infection by adhering to dietary restrictions (NPO) until healing is complete and by adhering to the medication regimen.

Interventions: nonsurgical management.   Nonsurgical management is achieved by the restriction of oral intake to prevent esophageal contents from contaminating mediastinal structures and by the administration of medications to reduce inflammation and prevent infection.

Diet therapy.   Clients with esophageal perforation, rupture, or potential for perforation (such as those with severe esophageal burns and/or tissue injury) are usually maintained NPO with an NG or gastrostomy tube attached to suction. Prevention of oral intake and removal of gastric contents prevent esophageal secretions and foods from passing through the perforation into the mediastinum and affecting adjacent organs and tissues. Occasionally, the client with a pinpoint perforation is allowed an oral diet, but the nurse observes the client closely for clinical manifestations of leakage.

Healing of damaged esophageal tissues begins approximately 10 days after injury, at which time gastric suction is discontinued and the client receives nutritional supplements by NG tube.

Drug therapy.   In addition to medications administered to the client with esophageal trauma to counteract the effects of shock and blood loss, the nurse administers corticosteroids and broad-spectrum antibiotics. Adults with corrosive chemical injury to the esophagus often receive high dosages of steroids in an attempt to prevent later formation of esophageal strictures. Broad-spectrum antibiotics are administered to prevent infection of local and adjacent tissues if esophageal perforation is present or anticipated.

Analgesics, narcotic and nonnarcotic, are often required for the client who has experienced esophageal trauma. Clients with burns often have damage to the oral mucous membranes, with accompanying oral pain. Topically applied agents often provide temporary relief of severe oral pain. The coating agents provide a soothing feeling as well as protect the lesions from further irritation. Topical swishes are available, such as 50:50 diphenhydramine hydrochloride (Benadryl) and kaolin with pectin (Kaopectate), and topical lidocaine (Xylocaine Viscous), which provide topical analgesia as well as local anti-inflammatory effects. Care must be taken if the client is NPO that oral preparations and swishes are not swallowed.

Interventions: surgical management.   Surgical management of esophageal trauma is aimed at exploring the area of injury to determine the extent of injury, at providing drainage to prevent mediastinal complications, and at re-establishing esophageal function. Cervical or thoracic incisions are made to assess damage to the esophagus, to search for perforation, to provide repair if possible at that time, and to provide drainage to prevent mediastinal contamination from esophageal secretions. Severe injuries or strictures may require resection of a segment of esophagus (*blunt esophagectomy*) with or without replacement by a segment of bowel or by gastric repositioning. Blunt esophagectomy requires a thoracic or a midsternal incision. The damaged portion of esophagus is excised, and the two remaining segments of the esophagus can be reapproximated and anastomosed. For excisions involving larger segments of the esophagus, the esophagus can be repaired with a segment of colon or jejunum (*colon interposition*), or the stomach can be brought up to anastomose with the esophagus or pharynx (*gastric pull-up*), as for esophageal cancer (see Fig. 43–6).

Preoperative care.   If a thoracic incision is anticipated or the client is undergoing blunt esophagectomy, the nurse discusses chest tubes, dressings, incisional pain management, and oxygen therapy with the client. The client undergoing blunt esophagectomy often requires cardiac monitoring and arterial lines and often spends 24 to 48 hours in a critical care unit or step-down unit immediately after the operation. The nurse discusses with the client and family the monitoring routines and the expected progression from operating room to special care units.

Postoperative care.   After cervical or thoracic exploration of esophageal trauma, nursing care measures are directed at maintenance of the airway and gas exchange, prevention and/or early detection of hemorrhage and esophageal perforation, relief of discomfort, and management of fluid and nutritional requirements. The client undergoing blunt esophagectomy is usually in a critical care setting for several days postoperatively. Nursing care is also directed at early detection of cardiac arrhythmias during this time. The client who is alert is positioned with the head of the bed elevated 30 degrees to aid in diaphragm excursion, and clients are turned every 2 hours to promote bilateral lung expansion. Oxygen therapy and chest tube suction are maintained as appropriate. Chest tube drainage is noted and recorded every 4 to 8 hours (see Chap. 62 for care of the client with a chest tube). Routine postoperative interventions are discussed in Chapter 20.

The nurse assesses the client for symptoms of esophageal perforation, which include fever, chest pain, and subcutaneous emphysema in the area of the perforation. The nurse maintains gastric suction and measures and records gastric drainage, being alert for signs of bleeding.

The client is reminded to take care not to dislodge the NG tube when turning in bed or ambulating, and the nurse does not reposition or irrigate the tube until instructed to do so by the surgeon. When fluids and nutritional supplements are begun by tube, the nurse documents the client's tolerance of nutritional treatments and alters the nutritional plan as needed.

For comfort measures, the nurse raises the head of the bed after the client is alert to assist in decreasing edema. Use of pillows to aid in positioning can reduce discomfort associated with thoracic incision. See the earlier Client Care Plan for other specifics of caring for the client after surgery of the esophagus.

■ Discharge Planning

Home Care Preparation

When the client is discharged with a feeding tube, nutritional supplies will need to be purchased. Home preparation of nutritional supplements can be facilitated if the family is able to obtain a blender. Clients who have undergone surgery may require assistance with activities of daily living and incisional care.

Client/Family Education

The nurse provides family education concerning the causes of esophageal trauma and preventive measures. If excessive alcohol intake or binge-eating is the suspected cause of the esophageal rupture or perforation, the nurse teaches the client about moderation and facilitates mental health counseling if the client and family indicate such a need. Ingestion of caustic substances can be prevented by leaving them in their original containers.

Before discharge of the client from the hospital, the nurse instructs the family and client in all treatments

(e.g., suture line care, dressing changes, and tube feedings), medications, diet, and early detection of infection. The client and family are asked to demonstrate the skills involved to document understanding as well as to help retention of the information. For the client who has undergone esophageal exploration or blunt esophagectomy, the nurse provides instructions about early identification of signs of perforation or hemorrhage and instructs the client to notify his or her physician or nurse if these symptoms occur.

Clients who had a blunt esophagectomy are provided with dietary instructions, including drinking large amounts of fluids during meals if colon interposition has been performed. The liquid intake facilitates food passage through the colon segment. Because reflux is a potential problem for these clients, the nurse instructs the client to eat smaller, more frequent meals and to avoid lying down for several hours after meals. The nurse consults with a registered dietitian and/or speech therapist as needed to assist in discharge instructions regarding diet and swallowing difficulties. Instructions to the client are reinforced by phone conversations with the client and family or by community health nurses on home visits.

Psychosocial Preparation

Because mealtimes are often social occasions, trauma to the esophagus can affect the client's manner of eating and therefore can alter social interactions. If the nurse anticipates that the client might experience a disturbance in self-concept related to change in nutritional route or habits, the topic is introduced to the client and family before the client's discharge to encourage verbalization of concerns. Social workers or other health care professionals can assist the client and family in coping with potential changes in body image and social roles.

If the esophageal injury resulted from an accident, the client or family might express feelings of guilt about not having foreseen the accident and/or prevented it. The nurse assesses the client's and family's need for counseling and facilitates referral to an appropriate agency.

The nurse also assesses the client's readiness to participate in self-care at home. Community health nurse referral can be made to evaluate anticipated home care problems.

Health Care Resources

The major health care resources for the client with esophageal trauma are the community health nurse and the social worker. The community health nurse is consulted to assess the home situation and the ability of the family and client to provide the necessary care measures at home. This nurse also provides ongoing evaluation of home care, including nutritional status, pain control, re-entry into former social roles, and the need for other health care workers. The social worker is often sought to assist the client with financial needs, to procure equipment or nutritional supplements, and to provide counseling for the client and family.

 Evaluation

On the basis of the most common nursing diagnosis, the nurse evaluates the care of the client with esophageal trauma according to the expected client outcomes. Expected outcomes include that the client

1. States that pain is alleviated or controlled
2. Maintains a balanced nutritional intake
3. Maintains adequate respiratory status
4. Adheres to dietary and medication regimen

SUMMARY

Diseases of the esophagus range from mild to life-threatening disorders. Many diseases, such as hiatal hernia or reflux esophagitis, are common to a large percentage of the population. Many manifest as a chronic disease or develop chronic sequelae, such as strictures from esophageal trauma. Nurses play a major role in providing instructions about diet, activity, positioning, medications, and physical care changes related to esophageal surgery. Because of these many life style changes, nurses are also involved in psychosocial support and counseling for clients to assist them to resume daily activities and independence despite having a chronic disorder. Psychosocial support by nurses is also extended to families with a family member who has acute esophageal trauma or the poor prognosis of esophageal carcinoma.

Awareness by the nurse of the clinical manifestations and the impact on life style of disorders of the esophagus can facilitate early nursing interventions aimed at supporting the client in resuming normal activities and social roles.

IMPLICATIONS FOR RESEARCH

Nurses play a large role in caring for clients with disorders of the esophagus. Most esophageal disorders represent a chronic process in which nurses are instrumental in teaching the client and family various life style modifications related to, for example, diet, activities, and positioning.

Potential research questions for nurses regarding esophageal disorders include

1. What is the relationship between meal size and the frequency and severity of esophageal reflux?
2. What diet manipulations provide the most effective reduction of numbers of reflux episodes?
3. Can relaxation strategies positively influence perceived dysphagia in clients with cancer of the esophagus?
4. What dietary plans best support maintenance of appropriate body weight in clients with cancer of the esophagus?

REFERENCES AND READINGS

Bachrach, W., Boyce, H. W., & Jackson, D. (1981). Problems in swallowing and esophageal carcinoma. *Heart and Lung, 10,* 525–531.

Castell, D. O. (1986). Medical therapy for reflux esophagitis: 1986 and beyond. *Annals of Internal Medicine, 104,* 112–114.

Castell, D. O., & Johnson, L. F. (Eds.). (1983). *Esophageal function in health and disease.* New York: Elsevier Biomedical.

Cohen, D. J., & Starling, J. R. (1986). Surgery for reflux esophagitis. *AORN Journal, 43,* 858–864.

Cohen, S., & Soloway, R. D. (Eds.). (1982). *Contemporary issues in gastroenterology: Vol. I. Diseases of the esophagus.* New York: Churchill Livingstone.

Dabaghi, R. E., & Scott, L. D. (1986). Evaluation of esophageal diseases. *American Family Physician, 33,* 119–129.

Enterline, H., & Thompson, J. (1984). *Pathology of the esophagus.* New York: Springer-Verlag.

Frank-Stromberg, M. (1989). The epidemiology and primary prevention of gastric and esophageal cancer. *Cancer Nursing, 12,* 53–64.

Given, B. A., & Simmons, S. J. (1984). Esophageal disorders. In *Gastroenterology in clinical nursing* (3rd ed., pp. 220–243). St. Louis: C. V. Mosby.

Henderson, R. D. (1986). Gastroesophageal reflux. In C. W. Cummings (Ed.), *Otolaryngology—head and neck surgery* (Vol. 3, pp. 2377–2400). St. Louis: C. V. Mosby.

Knauer, C. M., & Silverman, S. (1988). Alimentary tract and liver. In S. A. Schroeder, M. A. Krupp, & L. M. Tierney (Eds.), *Current medical diagnosis and treatment* (pp. 342–428). Norwalk, CT: Appleton & Lange.

Livstone, E. M. & Skinner, D. B. (1985). Tumors of the esophagus. In J. E. Berk, W. S. Haubrich, M. H. Kalser, J. L. A. Roth, & F. Schaffner (Eds.), *Bockus gastroenterology* (Vol. 2, 4th ed., pp. 818–850). Philadelphia: W. B. Saunders.

Mayer, R. (1988). Gastrointestinal cancer. In E. Rubenstein & D. Federman (Eds.), *Scientific American medicine* (pp. 1–17). New York: Scientific American.

McNamara, J. P. (1982). Esophageal cancer. *Nursing '82, 12*(3), 64.

Morton, J. M., Poulter, C. A., & Pandya, K. J. (1983). Alimentary tract cancer. In P. Rubin (Ed.), *Clinical oncol-*

ogy for medical students and physicians: A multidisciplinary approach (6th ed, pp. 154–176). Rochester, NY: American Cancer Society.

O'Connor, K. W. (1985). Diagnosis and treatment of gastroesophageal reflux, or reflux revisited. *Comprehensive Therapy, 11*(12), 6–13.

Payne, W. S., & Ellis, F. H., Jr. (1984). Esophagus and diaphragmatic hernias. In S. I. Schwartz, G. T. Shires, F. C. Spencer, & E. H. Storer (Eds.), *Principles of surgery* (4th ed., pp. 1063–1112). New York: McGraw-Hill.

Pope, C. E., II. (1988). Diseases of the esophagus. In J. B. Wyngaarden & L. H. Smith, Jr. (Eds.), *Cecil textbook of medicine* (18th ed., pp. 679–689). Philadelphia: W. B. Saunders.

Quinn, R., Gregg, J., & Wood, C. D. (1982). *Benign diseases of the esophagus.* Garden City, NY: Medical Examination Publishing.

Ropka, M. E. (1982). Hiatal hernia. *Nursing '82, 12*(4), 126–131.

Rosenberg, J. C., Lichter, A. S., Roth, J. A., & Kelsen, D. P. (1985). Cancer of the esophagus. In V. T. DeVita, Jr., S. Hellman, & S. A. Rosenberg (Eds.), *Cancer: Principles and practice of oncology* (2nd ed., pp. 621–657). Philadelphia: J. B. Lippincott.

Shaw, L. M. (1982). Treating GI reflux with a prosthesis. *AORN Journal, 35,* 1303–1306.

Skinner, D. B. (1985). Pathophysiology of gastroesophageal reflux. *Annals of Surgery, 202,* 546–556.

Symbas, P. N., Hatcher, C. R., & Harlaftis, N. (1978). Spontaneous rupture of the esophagus. *Annals of Surgery, 187,* 634–640.

Thompson, J. J. (1982). Esophageal cancer and the premalignant changes of esophageal diseases. In S. Cohen & R. D. Soloway (Eds.), *Contemporary issues in gastroenterology* (Vol. 1, pp. 239–276). New York: Churchill Livingstone.

Tollefson, L. (1985). The use of epidemiology, scientific data, and regulatory authority to determine risk factors in cancer of some organs of the digestive system. 2. Esophageal cancer. *Regulatory Toxicology and Pharmacology, 5,* 255–275.

Vantrappen, G., & Janssens, J. (1985). Medical management of reflux esophagitis. *Digestion, 32*(Suppl. 1), 51–58.

Willis, B. L., Thompson, L. F., & Howard, J. C. (1988). Esophageal perforation: A nursing diagnosis approach. *Critical Care Nurse, 8*(5), 20–30.

ADDITIONAL READINGS

Kadas, N. (1983). The dysphagic patient: Everyday care really counts. *RN, 46*(11), 38–41.

A practical overview of an important problem. This article discusses the process of swallowing and characteristics of clients who are at risk for dysphagia. Detailed swallowing assessment criteria were provided and specific guidelines offered for facilitating safe swallowing efforts.

Range, D. R., Hirokawa, R. H., & Bryarly, R. C. (1983). Caustic ingestion. *Ear, Nose and Throat Journal, 62,* 46–63.

A comprehensive discussion of injury to the esophagus from caustic substances, including mechanisms of injury, clinical evaluation, treatment factors, and early and late therapy.

Simmons, S., & Given, B. (1981). Nissen fundoplication for hiatus hernia repair. *AORN Journal, 34,* 35–46.

A comprehensive overview of hiatal hernia—incidence, pathophysiology, and symptoms. This article discusses the Nissen fundoplication procedure thoroughly from a nursing perspective including preoperative care, intraoperative concerns, and postoperative course and complications.

Sweet, K. (1983). Hiatal hernia. *Nursing '83, 13*(12), 38–45.

A case study presentation of a complex hiatal hernia client situation. The described client experienced multiple serious complications, which are thoroughly discussed from a nursing perspective and compared throughout with routine care.

CHAPTER 44

Interventions for Clients with Disorders of the Stomach

Three stomach problems are commonly seen in nursing practice: gastritis, peptic ulcer disease, and gastric cancer. The nurse has a vital role in caring for clients with these problems. For hospitalized clients, nursing care is important in preventing complications, promoting comfort, and teaching and guiding clients and families. As clients prepare for discharge from the hospital, education and guidance assume an even more important role; clients must acquire the knowledge and skills needed to comply with the therapeutic regimen and to cope with their stomach problems.

GASTRITIS

OVERVIEW

The term *gastritis* implies inflammation of the gastric mucosa and refers to any diffuse lesion in the gastric mucosa that is histologically identified as inflammation. Gastritis may be classified as acute or chronic. The categories refer to the pattern of inflammation rather than a specific time course.

Pathophysiology

The stomach's mucosal barrier normally protects this muscular sac from digesting itself, a process termed *acid autodigestion.* Prostaglandins provide this protection. When this mucosal barrier fails, gastritis results. After the barrier is broken, mucosal injury occurs and is worsened by histamine release and cholinergic nerve stimulation. Hydrochloric acid can then diffuse back into the mucosa and cause injury to small vessels, which results in edema, hemorrhage, and erosion of the gastric lining. Alcohol, aspirin, and reflux of duodenal contents are known to alter the diffusion barrier.

Pathologic changes that occur with gastritis include vascular congestion, edema, acute inflammatory cell infiltration, and degenerative changes in the superficial epithelium. The early pathologic manifestation of gastritis is a thickened, reddened mucous membrane with prominent rugae, or folds. As the disease progresses, the walls and lining of the stomach thin and atrophy. Progressive gastric atrophy from chronic mucosal injury results in deteriorating function of the chief and parietal cells. When function of the acid-secreting cells deteriorates, the source of the intrinsic factor is lost. Vitamin B_{12} can no longer be formed, and body stores of vitamin B_{12} are eventually depleted, which results in pernicious anemia. Degeneration may be found in the chief and parietal cells. Stomach secretions gradually decrease in amount and concentration of acid until they consist of only mucus and water. The risk of developing gastric cancer is said to be increased after 10 years of chronic gastritis. Hemorrhage may occur after an episode of acute gastritis or with ulceration caused by chronic gastritis.

Acute Gastritis

Inflammation of the gastric mucosa or submucosa after exposure to local irritants is called gastritis. There are various degrees of mucosal necrosis and inflammatory reaction in *acute gastritis*. The diagnosis of acute gastritis cannot be based solely on clinical symptoms without histologic confirmation. Complete regeneration and healing usually occur within a few days, and complete recovery usually ensues with no residual evidence of gastric inflammatory reaction, if the muscularis is not involved.

Chronic Gastritis

The diffuse chronic inflammatory process involving the mucosal lining of the stomach is defined as *chronic gastritis*. Inflammation of the gastric mucosa may be divided into three categories: superficial gastritis, atrophic gastritis, and gastric atrophy. Intestinal metaplasia is one of the important features of chronic gastritis. Chronic gastritis usually heals without scarring, but it can progress to hemorrhage and the formation of an ulcer.

The main changes in *superficial gastritis* consist of infiltration of the lamina propria by lymphocytes and plasma cells and occasional eosinophils. This inflammatory band is localized in the outer area of the mucosa, and it does not occupy the space between the fundal glands, which look normal. Superficial gastritis causes an inflamed, edematous mucosa with hemorrhages and small erosions. *Atrophic gastritis* occurs in all layers of the stomach, with a decreased number of fundal, parietal, and chief cells, and is seen in association with gastric ulcer and gastric cancer. The muscularis is thickened and inflammation is present. Complete recovery usually ensues in 1 to 2 days unless extensive damage is sustained to the gastric mucosa. The symptoms are due to visceral afferent nerve stimulation and are not related to the actual extent of the inflammation. *Gastric atrophy* refers to total loss of fundal glands, minimal inflammation, and thinning of the gastric mucosa.

Etiology

Gastritis is thought to be an autoimmune response to a stressor. *Acute gastritis* is caused by local gastric irritation from agents such as drugs, including alcohol, analgesics (especially anti-inflammatory agents) in large dosages, cytotoxic agents, caffeine, corticosteroids, antimetabolites, indomethacin (Indocin), and phenylbutazone (Butazolidin). Bacterial endotoxins from staphylococci, *Escherichia coli*, or salmonella may cause acute gastritis. Accidental or intentional ingestion of corrosive substances including acids or alkalis, such as Lysol, Mis-

ter Plumber, Drano, or Clinitest, may also result in acute gastritis. In the noneating client, such as the burn client, the trauma client, or the postoperative client, gastritis may also occur because of lack of stimulation of normal secretions (see the accompanying Key Features of Disease). The temperature of foods and the use of spices have not been documented to cause or result in acute gastritis.

Chronic gastritis is associated with atrophy of the gastric glands and may be due to any condition that results in reflux of bile and bile acids from the duodenum into the stomach. Peptic ulcer disease (PUD) or gastrojejunostomy may result in chronic gastritis. Chronic local irritation by alcohol, drugs, smoking, radiation, and environmental agents may result in chronic gastritis. Endogenous factors such as age, genetic factors (e.g., pernicious anemia), and illness (e.g., diabetes and renal disease) may also result in chronic gastritis. Drugs, including nonsteroidal anti-inflammatory drugs, aspirin,

---

KEY FEATURES OF DISEASE ■ **Etiologic Factors in Acute and Chronic Gastritis**

Acute

Local Irritants

Drugs
Acids or alkalis (corrosive agents such as lye, Drano, or Mister Plumber)
Reserpine
Anti-inflammatory agents, aspirin, or indomethacin
Cytotoxic agents
Corticosteroids

Bacterial Endotoxins

Staphylococci or salmonella

Life Style

Heavy cigarette smoking
Use of alcohol

Chronic

Endogenous Causes

Reflux of bile and bile acid
Pancreatic enzymes
Radiation
Peptic ulcer disease
Renal disease

Chronic Irritants

Alcohol
Other drugs such as salicylates and digitalis

and steroids, may contribute to chronic gastritis. Age is related to the atrophic gastritis that occurs after age 60 years.

Atrophic gastritis is seen most frequently in the elderly; occurs after exposure to toxic substances in the workplace (e.g., benzole, lead, and nickel); is associated with infection, disease, and sepsis; is associated with brain lesions; and is seen in clients with renal failure. Cigarette smokers may be vulnerable to gastritis as a result of the reduced bicarbonate content of pancreatic secretion and a decreased pyloric sphincter pressure, which allows reflux.

Incidence

The incidence of gastritis is higher in men than in women, is highest in the fifth and sixth decades of life, and is greater in heavy smokers and in alcoholics. There are no exact incidence numbers given in the literature. Acute gastritis, however, is responsible for 10% to 30% of upper gastrointestinal (GI) tract bleeding (Berk, 1985).

PREVENTION

Prevention of gastritis includes precaution in the ingestion of drugs and other gastric irritants. After an episode of gastritis, the client should avoid irritating substances, including drugs. Enteric-coated aspirin, such as Ecotrin or Easprin, is used to prevent gastric irritation. Histamine$_2$ (H$_2$) antagonists may prevent drug-induced lesions. Alcohol should be used in moderation and its use discontinued if symptoms of gastric irritation occur. The mixture of alcohol and salicylates should be avoided.

Signs and symptoms of gastric irritation related to gastritis are associated with numerous conditions including shock, hepatic cirrhosis, portal hypertension, uremia, and central nervous system lesions. Medical treatment such as chemotherapy and radiation may also result in gastritis. Early detection, diagnosis, and treatment of these primary conditions will help to prevent the secondary problems of potential hemorrhage and ulceration.

COLLABORATIVE MANAGEMENT

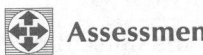 **Assessment**

History

The history focuses on risk factors for gastritis. The nurse assesses the client's *age, sex, health practices,* and perceived *stress.* The client's *diet,* with attention to the use of alcohol and caffeine, patterns of eating, and overall life style, including the use of *cigarettes,* are also assessed.

The nurse questions the client about the use of prescription and over-the-counter *drugs,* particularly corti-

costeroids and anti-inflammatory agents, and about any history of exposure to therapeutic *radiation.* Duodenal, gastrointestinal, and autoimmune diseases are the focus of the nurse's assessment of *concurrent medical conditions.*

Physical Assessment: Clinical Manifestations

The nurse assesses the general appearance of the client with gastritis. Signs and symptoms of gastric distress and location of pain are determined. Assessment determines the client's subjective report of epigastric discomfort, abdominal tenderness, cramps, indigestion, nausea, or vomiting. The assessment includes *onset, duration, location, and frequency of symptoms,* as well as aggravating or alleviating factors. The degree of disability in activities of daily living is assessed.

Objective data collected by the nurse include a description of the client's *general appearance,* which may show signs of distress, such as facial grimacing, restlessness, or moaning. Tense body posture and a *change in vital signs* may be present. The abdominal examination may reveal tenderness over epigastric area, guarding, distention, or increased bowel sounds or peristaltic waves. The physical examination does not yield significant data in uncomplicated gastritis.

Nutritional status is also assessed, including *weight, skin color and turgor,* and *adipose tissue distribution.* Nutritional deficits would indicate chronic disease or potential gastric cancer.

After exposure to an etiologic agent, there is a rapid onset of epigastric discomfort, anorexia, cramping, nausea, vomiting, and gastric hemorrhage. The symptomatic state is limited to a few hours or days and varies with the cause. Aspirin-related gastritis may result in dyspepsia or heartburn. Gastritis from alcohol abuse may lead to vomiting and hematemesis. Gastritis that is caused by endotoxins such as staphylococcal endotoxin is abrupt and violent, often occurring within 5 hours of ingestion of the contaminated food.

Chronic gastritis often produces vague complaints or may cause epigastric pain simulating ulcer-like distress with periodicity and relief on ingestion of food, but the pain is most often less radiating. Some clients develop anorexia and pain exacerbated by eating and vomiting. Intolerance of spicy or fatty foods may occur. Weight loss that occurs may mimic the situation with gastric cancer, but bleeding is uncommon. Pernicious anemia may occur over the long term because of depletion of vitamin B$_{12}$ stores. The discomfort from atrophic gastritis is not relieved by antacid therapy, nor do clients experience pain at night. Fifty per cent of gastric ulcer clients have associated chronic gastritis. Approximately 7% to 10% of persons with atrophic gastritis develop gastric carcinoma (Berk, 1985; Siler, 1985).

Psychosocial Assessment

The nurse assesses the client with gastritis for life style patterns that may predispose to the development of gastritis. Clients with personal habits including heavy alcohol, coffee, tobacco, and drug abuse may be at high risk for gastric irritation.

The nurse may also find an anxious, nervous individual because of an acute or chronic crisis or stress situation. The psychologic stress or crisis may lead to alcohol or drug abuse. The gastric irritation and resulting discomfort from these substances and the stress can cause disruption of the client's pattern of sleep and rest.

In assessing the family unit, the nurse may see other family members with similar risk factors. Including family members in the teaching program may enhance client compliance and adherence to treatment objectives. Compliance should also reduce the client's risk for the development of gastric problems and complications.

Laboratory Findings

Laboratory findings are not definitive for clients with gastritis. Hemoglobin and hematocrit values may be used to determine anemia that may occur from bleeding. Stools may be tested for the presence of occult blood. Serum gastrin levels may be low or normal. Serum vitamin B_{12} levels may be measured to assess for vitamin B_{12} deficiency.

Radiographic Findings

A barium swallow may be completed to rule out other gastric diseases.

Other Diagnostic Tests

Gastroscopy is the most effective tool for diagnosing gastritis. Superficial mucosal changes of gastritis may not be visualized. Visual interpretations of gastritis do not often correlate well with histologic findings. Biopsy is the procedure needed to establish a definitive diagnosis of the type of gastritis or the presence of gastric cancer. A cytologic examination is used to rule out the presence of gastric cancer.

 Analysis: Nursing Diagnosis

Individuals with gastritis are not often seen in the acute care setting unless they have an exacerbation of acute or chronic gastritis resulting in fluid and electrolyte imbalance or bleeding. Management is directed toward supportive care to relieve the symptoms. The following nursing diagnoses may be noted in clients with gastritis.

Common Diagnoses

1. Pain related to gastric irritation or atrophy of gastric glands
2. Altered nutrition: less than body requirements related to decreased appetite, food intolerance, nausea and/or vomiting, and pain

Additional Diagnoses

1. Noncompliance (preventive or treatment measures) related to anxiety, negative side effects of prescribed treatment, life style alterations necessary, expense of therapy, and/or nonsupportive family
2. Sleep pattern disturbance related to pain, nausea, or anxiety
3. Fluid volume deficit related to decreased fluid and electrolyte intake, vomiting, or bleeding
4. Ineffective individual coping related to persistent stress, inadequate psychologic resources, and/or significant life style alterations
5. Knowledge deficit related to causative factors of gastritis and therapeutic regimen

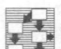 **Planning and Implementation**

The following plan of care focuses on the common nursing diagnoses.

Pain

Planning: client goals. The major goals for this nursing diagnosis are that the client will (1) experience relief of pain and discomfort and (2) not experience an exacerbation of gastritis by removing the irritating stimuli.

Interventions. Treatment is directed toward the removal of the cause of the discomfort. Acute gastritis is treated symptomatically and supportively because the healing process is spontaneous, usually within a few days. If the cause is removed, pain and discomfort usually subside. If hemorrhage occurs and is severe, a transfusion may be necessary; fluid replacement is indicated in clients with severe fluid loss. Gastrectomy, pyloroplasty, and vagotomy may be indicated for clients with major bleeding or ulceration.

Nonsurgical management. Because the client frequently experiences gastritis from noxious agents, the pain can often be relieved by identifying and eliminating causative factors. Assisting the client to identify and select strategies to avoid the stimuli are important, as discussed earlier under the heading Prevention. Drugs and diet therapy are used for clients with gastritis. In the acute phase, when discomfort is present, physical rest is recommended.

Drug therapy. In the acute phase, the nurse directs actions toward pain and discomfort relief. Blocking and buffering gastric acid secretions with medications may relieve pain. H_2 antagonists are used to block gastric secretions. These agents include cimetidine (Tagamet), ranitidine (Zantac), famotidine (Pepcid), and nizatidine. Antacids used as buffering agents commonly include aluminum hydroxide with magnesium hydroxide (Maalox), aluminum hydroxide with simethicone and magnesium hydroxide (Mylanta), or magaldrate (Riopan). Pain medications may be necessary. The therapeutic effectiveness and side effects of these medications are determined. If effectiveness is not achieved, the physician should be notified.

Topical anesthetics, such as oxethazaine, 10 mg with 1 tsp of aluminum hydroxide three or four times per day, may be useful. Vitamin B$_{12}$ may be necessary in clients with chronic gastritis to prevent and/or treat pernicious anemia.

Clients should be instructed about the side effects of certain medications that are associated with gastric irritation. These medications include chemotherapeutic agents, aspirin, corticosteroids, and nonsteroidal anti-inflammatory agents. Other drugs causing irritation include reserpine, chlortetracycline hydrochloride (Aureomycin), phenylbutazone, ferrous salts, indomethacin, and histamine. Medications may be altered if symptoms of gastric irritation appear that are related to medication ingestion. Clients are taught to examine the labels of over-the-counter medications for the presence of aspirin.

Diet therapy.   The client with gastric disease should be instructed by the nurse to have moderate intake of foods and spices if they cause distress, although these substances do not cause gastritis. Tea, coffee, cola and chocolate (caffeine), mustard, paprika, cloves, pepper, and Tabasco sauce (hot spices) may increase the client's discomfort.

After an acute episode of gastritis, the nurse helps the client to identify foods that aggravate discomfort. New foods should be introduced one at a time. Avoidance of substances that cause symptoms is important. Clients seem to progress better with a soft, bland diet and are instructed to avoid large, heavy meals.

Stress reduction.   The nurse assesses factors that decrease pain or discomfort tolerance (e.g., lack of knowledge, anxiety, and fatigue). The effects of fatigue and anxiety on discomfort should be explained. The client may be assisted with various techniques to reduce discomfort, such as progressive relaxation, cutaneous stimulation, guided imagery, and distraction. Chapter 6 discusses these stress reduction techniques.

Surgical management.   Partial gastrectomy, pyloroplasty, vagotomy, or even total gastrectomy may be indicated for clients with major bleeding from severe erosive gastritis. Such surgery is necessary only if other, more conservative measures have not controlled the bleeding. These measures, as well as surgical interventions, are discussed later under the heading Interventions: Surgical Management in the section on peptic ulcer.

Altered Nutrition: Less Than Body Requirements

Planning: client goals.   The major goals for this nursing diagnosis are that the client will (1) experience improved nutritional intake by eating a balanced diet and (2) achieve or maintain ideal weight.

Interventions: nonsurgical management.   It is important to meet the metabolic requirements and to correct any nutritional deficits. Promotion of comfort helps to achieve this goal.

Drug therapy.   If nausea, pain, or other discomfort is interfering with the client's desire or ability to eat, anti-emetic or pain medication should be given 1 hour before mealtimes. Buffering agents (e.g., antacids) and histamine antagonists such as cimetidine are used. Parenteral vitamin B$_{12}$ may be needed to correct a deficit.

Diet therapy.   A diet history should be taken before any diet management plan is formulated. Foods and beverages that can be consumed without causing gastric upset should be identified, and those contributing to distress should be eliminated. Clients are encouraged to have nothing by mouth (NPO) until discomfort or nausea and vomiting abate. Assessment for fluid and electrolyte deficits is conducted by the nurse (see Chap. 13). Consultation with or referral to a dietitian may be needed. If special foods can be brought from home that would appeal to the client, the family should be encouraged to bring them. If needed, numerous liquid supplements are available that could be offered between meals to supply needed nutrients. If severe nutritional deficit occurs, consideration of cultural or ethnic eating habits and usual food preferences may help long-term management.

■ Discharge Planning

Home Care Preparation

The client with gastritis is usually managed in the home. The client and family should have a plan to prevent recurrences and exacerbations by the avoidance of the causative agents of gastritis. They also need to be instructed about signs and symptoms that require immediate medical attention, i.e., hematemesis; blood in stools or dark, tarry stools; fatigue; faintness; shortness of breath; or abdominal pain.

Client/Family Education

Teaching about personal habits and strategies to bring about life style changes should be initiated. Regular medical follow-up is necessary because the incidence of gastric cancer is higher with clients with gastritis.

Avoidance of foods that have an extremely high roughage (fiber) content (such as corn and nuts) or of extreme temperatures may be necessary for some clients. Although there is not a clear association of these foods with the disease, they may cause symptoms in some clients. The nurse can assist the client and family to determine actions to take to solve problems, to deal with cooking, and to modify eating habits. Further, clients should use precautions in preventing food spoilage, thus avoiding ingestion of foods potentially contaminated with bacteria (e.g., staphylococci, *Clostridium botulinum, Clostridium perfringens*).

The nurse stresses the need for cessation of smoking, reduction of caffeine ingestion, and avoidance of foods and drugs that may be causative agents and works with the client to determine and implement a plan for life style modification. The client and family must be aware that these life style changes are not temporary measures but that they are lifelong changes that must be followed to prevent recurrences.

Family members need to be aware of these changes and the support that they can provide. Client compliance is more likely to be enhanced when the family is supportive and involved in necessary habit and life style changes.

Psychosocial Preparation

Some clients may not perceive that they have the ability to maintain the life style changes. They need to feel confident in their own strength and ability to carry out the needed therapeutic plan. These life style changes should include effective measures for coping with stress and anxiety, which may necessitate family counseling sessions to educate the entire family unit about potential sources of stress and to teach effective coping skills. In addition, support from a spouse, family, significant others, and various community support groups or social agencies may also enhance compliance.

Health Care Resources

Resources (family, community, medical, or nursing) should be used to assist with problems. Alcoholics Anonymous (AA) is a primary resource for the client who has an alcohol abuse problem. Attendance at AA meetings for the client and Al-Anon for Family Members is encouraged.

There are usually stress management programs available in the community that may be offered through local hospitals or community colleges. The client's health care provider is consulted about a high-quality program to attend.

If the client has any concerns about diet therapy, a dietitian based at a local hospital or home care agency is consulted. A pharmacist or the health care provider is consulted before any over-the-counter medications are taken.

 ### Evaluation

On the basis of the identified nursing diagnoses, the nurse evaluates the response of the client with gastritis. The expected outcomes include that the client

1. States that no pain exists and that comfort has been achieved

2. Prevents exacerbations by identification and avoidance of noxious stimuli or situations

3. Reports strategies used to manage treatment.

4. Maintains weight at ideal level or achieves the ideal by following proper diet without exacerbation of gastritis signs and symptoms

5. Avoids complications of GI tract hemorrhage by prompt reporting of early symptoms of gastric irritation to health care professional

6. Describes and complies with prescribed therapeutic regimen

7. Reports specifically how she or he follows the therapeutic diet

PEPTIC ULCER DISEASE

OVERVIEW

Ulcers of the stomach and duodenum are common and represent a major health problem, in terms of both individual suffering and cost to society. Approximately 4 to 8 million Americans have symptoms related to active ulcer disease, and the cost to society is in excess of $1 billion per year (Thompson, 1986). Peptic ulcers occur in the stomach, proximal duodenum, and rarely in the lower esophagus.

Peptic ulcer disease (PUD) is defined as a break in the continuity of the mucosa and may occur in any part of the GI tract that comes in contact with hydrochloric acid and pepsin. The term *peptic* is not adequate to discuss the disorder because there are anatomic differences in physiology and cause of the various types of ulcers. In this chapter, PUD, a chronic disorder, refers to gastric and duodenal ulcers.

Pathophysiology

Types of Ulcers

A *gastric ulcer* is a break in the gastric mucosa that extends into the muscularis mucosae. Gastric ulcers are usually found at the junction of the fundus and the pylorus, but smaller ulcers may also occur in the antrum. Gastritis often surrounds the gastric ulceration. Gastric ulcers are probably caused by a break in the mucosal barrier. This barrier overlies the gastric epithelium and differs from the glycoprotein mucus that covers the epithelium. When there is a break, the hydrochloric acid injures the epithelium. Gastric ulcers may then occur as a result of *back-diffusion* of acid or *pyloric sphincter dysfunction* (Fig. 44–1). The integrity of the mucosal barrier is enhanced by the rich blood supply of the mucosa of

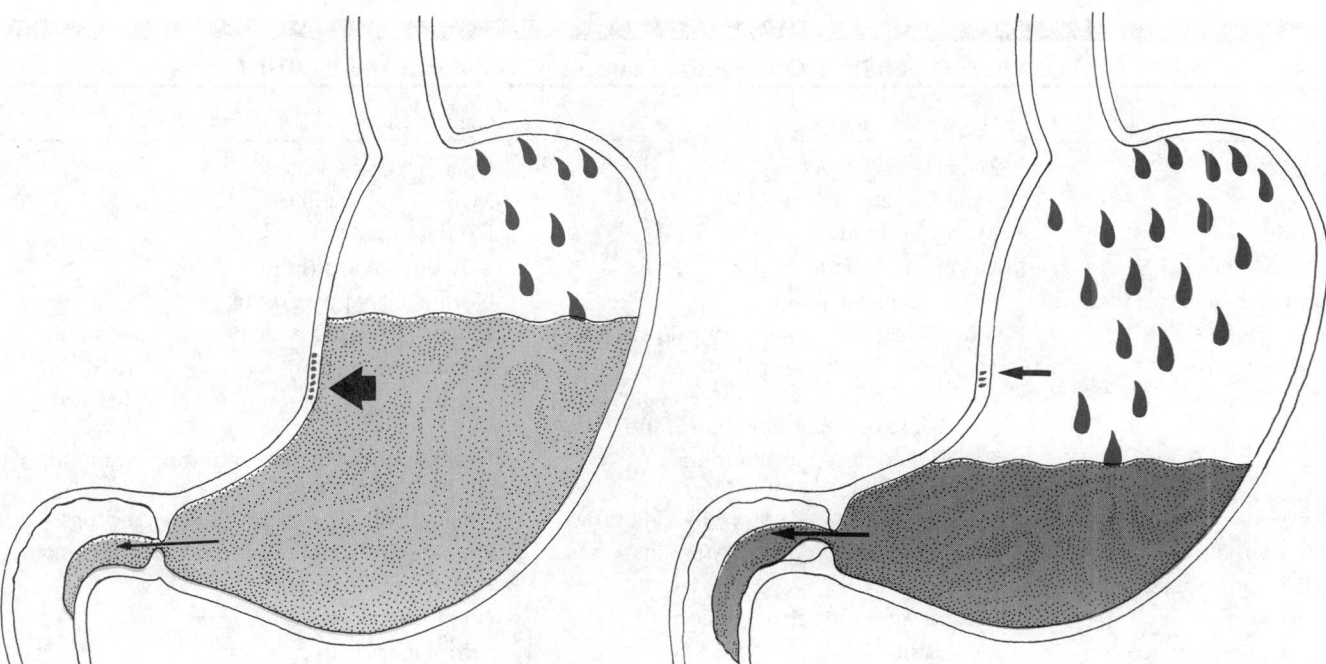

Conditions favoring the development of **gastric ulcers** are normal gastric acid secretion and normal stomach emptying with *increased diffusion of gastric acid back into the stomach tissues.*

Conditions favoring the development of **duodenal ulcers** are normal diffusion of acid back into stomach tissues with *increased secretion of gastric acid* and *increased stomach emptying.*

Figure 44 – 1

Pathophysiology of peptic ulcer.

the stomach and duodenum. In gastric ulcers, the pyloric sphincter may not function normally or may not respond to secretin or cholecystokinin, which increases the pressure and prevents reflux. Without normal functioning and competence of the pyloric sphincter, bile refluxes into the stomach. This reflux of bile acids may break the integrity of the mucosal barrier and produce hydrogen ion back-diffusion, which leads to mucosal inflammation. Toxic agents and bile may destroy the lipid plasma membrane of the gastric mucosa. Antral motility near the ulcer is often decreased with gastric ulcers. A decreased blood flow to the gastric mucosa may also alter the defense barrier, thereby allowing ulceration to occur.

Agents that break the mucosal barrier, such as acetylsalicylic acid (aspirin), alcohol, and indomethacin (Indocin), disrupt the mucosal protection, and hydrochloric acid flows back into the mucosa. Histamine is released, which results in greater acid production, vasodilation, and increased capillary permeability.

The great majority of gastric ulcers occur on the lesser curvature of the stomach near the pylorus (Fig. 44 – 2).

In contrast to a gastric ulcer, a *duodenal ulcer* is a chronic break in the duodenal mucosa extending through the muscularis mucosa that leaves a scar with healing (see the accompanying Key Features of Disease). Duodenal ulcers are the most common type of peptic ulcer. The duodenal ulcer is usually 0.5 in (1 cm) in diameter and is located ¼ to 1 in (0.5 to 2.0 cm) from the pylorus.

Duodenal ulcers are associated with increased acid secretion, which is due to greater parietal cell mass or vagal activity, which increases the response to produce acid, or to the decreased inhibition of gastric secretion.

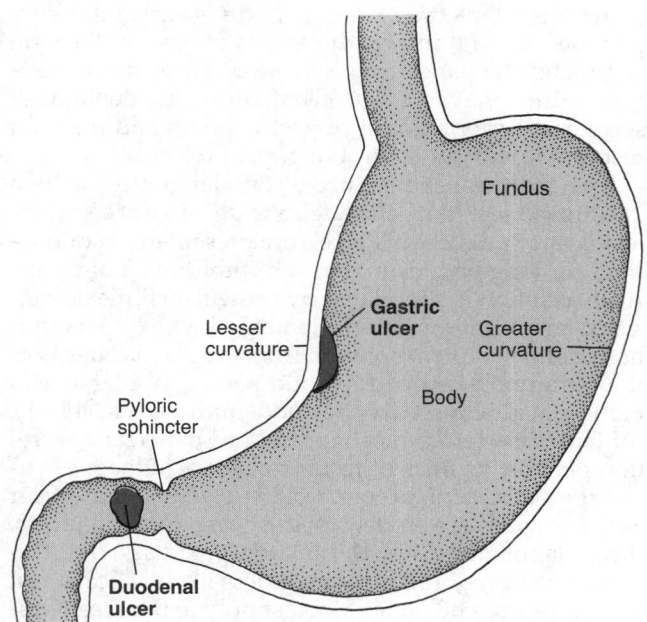

Figure 44 – 2

Most common sites for peptic ulcers.

KEY FEATURES OF DISEASE ■ Differential Features of Duodenal and Gastric Ulcers

Feature	Duodenal Ulcer	Gastric Ulcer
Age	Usually 40–50 yr	Usually 50 yr and older
Sex	Male/female ratio of 4 : 1	Male/female ratio of 2 : 1
Blood group	Most frequently O	No differentiation
General nourishment	Usually well nourished	May be malnourished
Stomach acid production	Hypersecretion	Normal or hyposecretion
Occurrence	Mucosa exposed to acid-pepsin secretion	Mucosa exposed to acid-pepsin secretion
Clinical course	Healing and recurrence	Healing and recurrence
Pain	Occurs 2–3 h after a meal; at night: often awakens client between 1 and 2 AM	Occurs ½–1 h after a meal; at night: rarely
	Relieved by ingestion of food	Not helped by ingestion of food, sometimes even increased
Response to treatment	Healing with H_2 receptor blocking drugs	Healing with H_2 receptor blocking drugs
Hemorrhage	Melena more common than hematemesis	Hematemesis more common than melena
Malignancy possibility	Rare	Perhaps in less than 10%
Recurrence	Occurs after modest resection	Less likely after surgery
Surrounding mucosa	No gastritis	Atrophic gastritis

With vagal stimulation, the parietal cells and G cells are stimulated to release gastrin. Production of pepsin and hydrochloric acid is also stimulated.

Gastric activity affects the regulation of secretions. Gastrin is stimulated by the presence of protein or distention of the antrum. Individuals with a duodenal ulcer are sensitive to gastrin and have increased secretion of gastric hydrochloric acid. A pH of 2.5 to 3.0 inhibits the secretion of gastrin and limits the amount of acid secreted. Acid chyme from the stomach inhibits gastric secretions. Cholecystokinin, secretin, gastric inhibitory peptides, and fat inhibit the effects of gastrin. Secretin stimulates the pancreas to secrete bicarbonates to neutralize duodenal acid. The client with a duodenal ulcer secretes a larger amount of gastric juices and may not respond to normal control of gastrin release.

The characteristic feature of duodenal ulcer is high gastric acid secretion, although a wide range of secretory levels is found. Low pH levels are present in the duodenum for long periods in persons with duodenal ulcers. Acid secretion is stimulated by protein-rich meals, calcium, and vagal excitation. Combined with hypersecretion, a rapid emptying of food from the stomach reduces the buffering effect of food and results in a large acid bolus that is delivered to the duodenum (see Fig. 44–1). Inhibitory secretory mechanisms and pancreatic secretion may be insufficient to control the acid load.

When ulceration occurs rapidly, bleeding may occur as vessel walls are eroded. With slower-forming ulcers, the inflammatory and thrombotic processes result in ulcer symptoms, and bleeding is less likely. Ulcers heal slowly because of a poor blood supply to the area. Gastric ulcers tend to heal less quickly and more complications tend to occur in older individuals.

A *stress ulcer* is the term given to an ulcer that occurs after an acute medical crisis or trauma such as head injury, burn, respiratory failure, shock, or septic state. Bleeding is the principal manifestation of acute stress ulcers, and it is due to gastric erosions. Lesions are multiple and occur in the proximal portion of the stomach. They begin as focal areas of ischemia and evolve into erosions and sometimes ulcerations that may progress to massive hemorrhage. Little is known about the etiology of stress ulcers, but probably ischemia is a contributing factor. In the presence of elevated hydrochloric acid, ischemia can progress to erosive gastritis and subsequent ulcerations. Increased hydrogen ion back-diffusion and mucosal ischemia may result.

Complications of Ulcers

Intractable disease. One-third of all clients with ulcers have a single episode with no recurrence. Intractability may develop from other complications of ulcers, stressors in the client's life, and the inability to make the necessary life style changes. Primarily in intractable disease, the client no longer responds to conservative management, or recurrences of symptoms interfere with activities of daily living. In general, the client continues to have recurrent pain and discomfort.

Hemorrhage. Bleeding from ulcers varies from minimal, which is manifested by occult blood in the tarry stool (melena), to massive, in which the client vomits bright red or coffee-ground blood (hematemesis) (see the accompanying illustration). Bleeding is the most serious complication of peptic ulcer; it accounts for 40% of deaths and occurs in 15% to 20% of all persons with

COMMON CAUSES OF UPPER GI BLEEDING

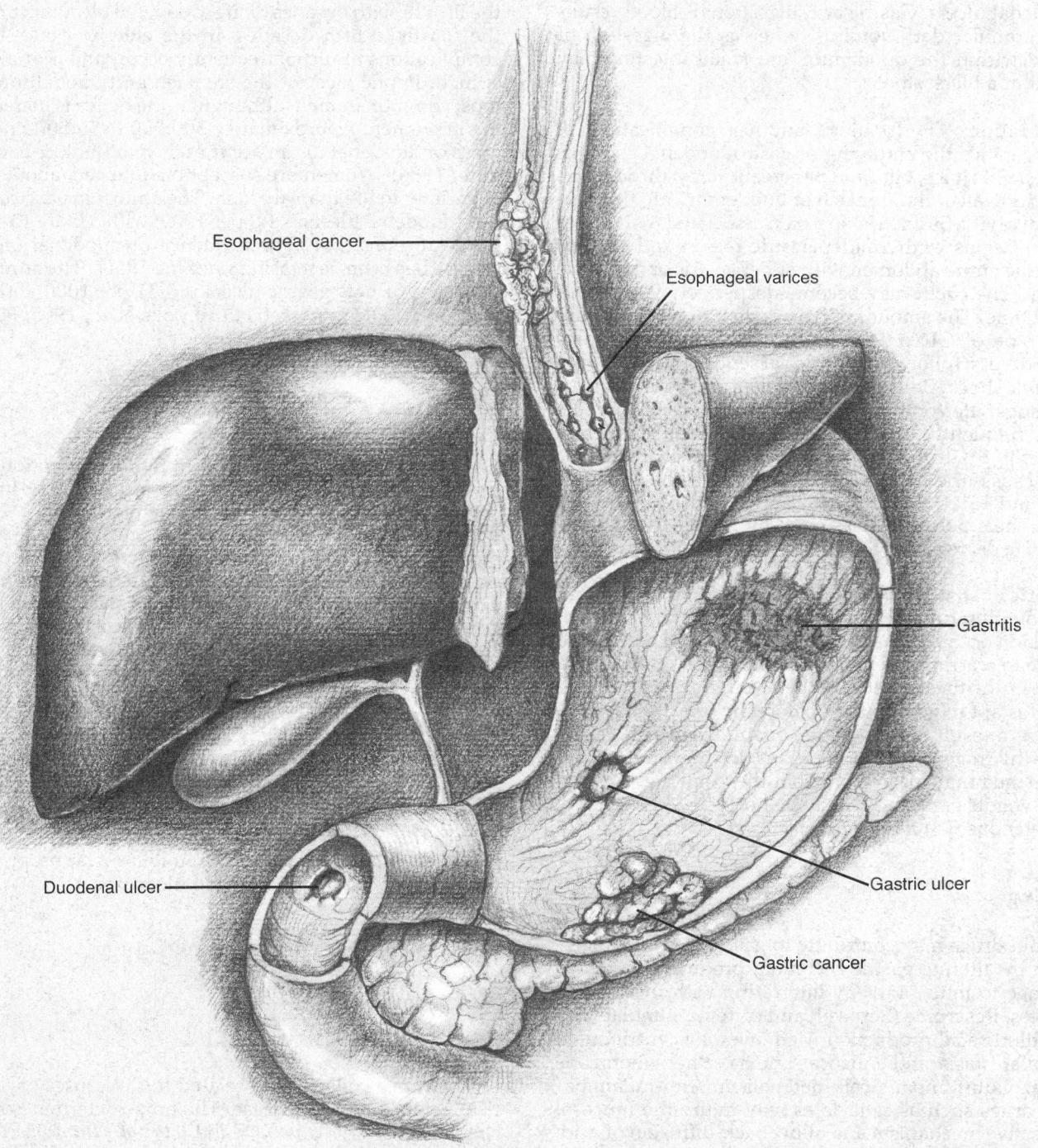

Esophageal cancer

Esophageal varices

Gastritis

Duodenal ulcer

Gastric ulcer

Gastric cancer

ulcer disease (Brooks et al., 1985). Hemorrhage tends to occur more often in clients with gastric ulcers and in the elderly. Hematemesis usually indicates bleeding at the duodenojejunal junction. Melena may occur in clients with gastric ulcers but is more common in those with duodenal ulcers. Gastric acid digestion of blood results in a granular dark vomitus, whereas the digestion of blood within the duodenum and small intestine may result in a black stool.

Perforation. Perforation, another complication of PUD, entails the emptying of gastroduodenal contents (acid peptic juice, bile, and pancreatic juice) through the anterior wall of the stomach or duodenum into the peritoneal cavity. Sudden, sharp pain associated with perforation begins in the midepigastric region and spreads over the entire abdomen with either gastric or duodenal ulcers. The client may become desperately ill within a short time. The amount of pain depends on the amount and type of GI contents spilled. Chemical peritonitis soon occurs, followed by bacterial septicemia and hypovolemic shock. Peristalsis diminishes and paralytic ileus develops. Perforation, a surgical emergency, occurs most frequently in clients with duodenal ulcers and occurs in 5% to 10% of ulcer clients. The characteristic pain causes the client to be apprehensive; the abdomen is found to be tender, rigid, and board-like; and the knee-chest position is assumed by the client in an attempt to decrease the tension on the abdominal muscles.

Pyloric obstruction. Pyloric obstruction is manifested by vomiting caused by stasis and gastric dilation. Obstruction occurs at the pylorus, at the gastric outlet, and is due to scarring, edema, or inflammation, or to a combination of these factors. When vomiting persists, the client is apt to go into hypochloremic (metabolic) alkalosis as a result of losing large quantities of acid gastric juice (hydrogen and chloride ions) in the vomitus. Hypokalemia may also result from the vomiting. A client who vomits persistently may be hospitalized to receive intravenous (IV) fluids and electrolytes.

Etiology

Certain drugs may contribute to gastroduodenal ulceration by altering gastric secretion, producing localized damage to mucosa, or by interfering with the healing process. Reserpine (Serpasil) and caffeine stimulate hydrochloric acid production. Caffeine may contribute to vascular stasis and mucosal anoxia. Phenylbutazone (Butazolidin) impairs cell metabolism. Anti-inflammatory drugs such as salicylates may injure the mucosal protective mechanism and allow back-diffusion of acid. The relationship between smoking and gastric ulcers has been described. The use of corticosteroids results in an increased incidence of peptic ulceration. Peptic ulceration is also associated with pancreatitis, Crohn's disease, hepatic disease, and Zollinger-Ellison syndrome because of the altered effect of these diseases on the inhibition and stimulation of gastric secretion.

Incidence

It is estimated that about 10% of the population in the United States will suffer from ulcer disease during their lifetime. The peak incidence of gastric ulcers is found in the fifth to sixth decades of life; duodenal ulcers occur in the fourth to fifth decades. In the elderly group, the complications of ulcers frequently occur, and mortality is high. Peptic ulcer of the stomach and duodenum is most common in men, although its incidence is increasing in women. Approximately 300,000 to 500,000 new cases of duodenal ulcers occur each year (Fink & Longmire, 1986). Women are susceptible to ulcers about 10 years later in life than are men. The annual incidence of new duodenal ulcers is 1.3 per 1000, with a male-to-female ratio of 2.2 : 1. The incidence of duodenal ulcer disease has been decreasing since the 1950s. The annual incidence of new gastric ulcers is 0.31 per 1000 with a male-to-female ratio of 1.1 : 1 (Brooks et al., 1985; Fink & Longmire, 1986).

PREVENTION

Cessation of smoking is important in the prevention of initial PUD as well as of recurrent disease. Low-fiber diets should be encouraged to prevent recurrence. Reduced intake of foods or substances such as protein-rich meals and calcium is encouraged to decrease acid secretion and thus the acid load delivered to the duodenum. The client is instructed to avoid drugs such as anti-inflammatory agents, salicylates, and corticosteroids in an attempt to prevent recurrence or initial disease. Alcohol, cola, and caffeine should be consumed in small amounts, if at all.

Stress experienced over a prolonged time has aggravated symptoms of ulceration of the GI tract. However, the role of stress in the cause and exacerbation of PUD remains controversial (Brooks et al., 1985). Although the ideal situation is avoidance of stress-producing situations, this is not always possible. Developing stress management and relaxation techniques is appropriate for clients at risk for developing ulceration.

COLLABORATIVE MANAGEMENT

 Assessment

History

The nurse collects data related to the causes of and risk factors for ulcer disease. The nurse determines the client's *age, sex, occupation,* and *level of education.* The client's overall *life style* is evaluated, with a focus on actual and perceived daily stressors. The nurse questions the client about *diet factors* such as caffeine and alcohol intake, intake of irritants, and overall eating patterns. The nurse determines the client's *use of cigarettes.*

A history of current or past *medical conditions* focuses

on GI tract problems and autoimmune disease. The nurse determines whether the client has taken or is taking any prescription or over-the-counter *drugs*, such as corticosteroids, salicylates, indomethacin, and phenylbutazone and whether the client has ever undergone *radiation treatments*.

The history of the present complaint includes the frequency, onset, and duration of signs and symptoms such as *pain* and *GI upset*. The nurse assesses for similar features of any previous attacks and their response to therapy. The nurse assesses any patterns of pain.

It is often necessary for the nurse to use several synonyms — "discomfort," "ache," "pressure," or even "hunger pain" — to elicit the client's complete description of the nature of pain. The occurrence of and pattern of pain of PUD and when it occurs in relation to the intake of food may give some information about the possible location of the ulceration and may help to distinguish the pain of PUD from that of other disorders. The pain is often exacerbated by certain foods, such as tomatoes, hot spices, fried food, and onions, or alcohol. Clients may exacerbate their discomfort by taking antacids that contain aspirin, e.g., Alka-Seltzer.

Physical Assessment: Clinical Manifestations

The principal clinical manifestation that the nurse assesses in taking the health history is the presence of aching, burning, cramp-like, or gnawing *pain*. The classic symptoms have a definite relationship to eating: discomfort is relieved by eating food or taking antacids. The pain of ulcer occurs after meals. Pain may radiate around the costal border or to the back. Early satiety, anorexia, and nausea are common and are often experienced by individuals in the early phase of development of the ulcer.

Discomfort and pain, the chief symptoms, are usually described as circumscribed in an area about 1 to 5 in (2 to 10 cm) in diameter, located between the xiphoid cartilage and umbilicus in the epigastrium or just to the right of the midline. Gastric ulcer pain often occurs in the upper epigastrium, with localization to the left of the midline; duodenal ulcer pain is in the right epigastrium. Steady pain near the midline of the back between the sixth and tenth thoracic vertebrae may indicate a perforated posterior wall caused by the duodenal ulcer. The nurse then assesses for the presence of a feeling of fullness or hunger. Distention of the duodenal bulb produces epigastric pain, which may radiate to the back and thorax.

The typical client with gastric or duodenal ulcer is diagnosed after an episode of GI upset. Ulcer pain is characterized as having periodicity. The overall clinical course of PUD is characterized by long periods of remission and periods of exacerbation that may last from days to months. Individuals with gastric ulcers may report exacerbation after eating, especially after drinking warm liquids. The most important differential characteristic of the pain is that pain related to a duodenal ulcer often wakens the individual from sleep. After relieving the pain with food or antacid, the individual returns to sleep and awakens in the morning without pain.

Heartburn (dyspepsia, or indigestion), a burning substernal discomfort, is common in clients with duodenal ulcer because of regurgitation of acid into the esophagus. Even during an exacerbation, the pain usually lasts for only a few hours at a time. A change in the pattern of pain to that of continuous pain that is no longer relieved by antacid usually signifies penetration of the ulcer through the posterior wall of the stomach. Pain is less frequently the initial complaint in the elderly; melena is a more frequent presenting sign of ulcer disease in this group.

Vomiting is a symptom that may occur with ulcer disease, most commonly with pyloric sphincter dysfunction. Vomiting results from gastric stasis associated with pyloric obstruction. *Appetite* is generally maintained in clients with peptic ulcer unless pyloric obstruction is present.

Psychosocial Assessment

The nurse assesses the impact of ulcer disease on an individual's life style, occupation, family, and social and leisure activities. Contrary to popular perception, ulcers do not occur more often in individuals with high pressure such as executives but in the unskilled and assembly line workers. The ability and willingness to alter the work environment and daily schedules to reduce occupational stressors or to integrate and accommodate therapeutic plans are important to assess. Family and individual stressors should be assessed, and usual patterns of coping and problem-solving should be ascertained.

Low income and low levels of education are associated with higher rates of ulcer disease for reasons that remain unclear. The nurse assesses the impact of life style changes that the chronic disease will have on the client. Questions about life style, occupation, and leisure can yield important information. This assessment is important to determine the client's abilities to comply with the prescribed treatment regimen and to obtain the needed social support to alter life style. Early signs and symptoms of recurrence or complications should be taught to the client and family.

Laboratory Findings

A complete blood count of hemoglobin and hematocrit values may be low, indicating the presence of bleeding. The stool specimen may be positive for occult blood if bleeding is present.

Radiographic Findings

An upper GI series (barium swallow) may show evidence of PUD. This series is often the initial test for a client who does not have severe symptoms.

Other Diagnostic Tests

The major diagnostic test for PUD is fiberoptic endoscopy, which is often done when there is active bleeding to find the cause immediately. Visualization of the ulcer crater by endoscopy (gastroscopy) also provides the opportunity for biopsy and cytologic studies that are necessary to rule out gastric cancer. Endoscopy may be repeated at 4- to 6-week intervals to evaluate the progress of healing in response to therapy.

 ### Analysis: Nursing Diagnosis

Common Diagnoses

The common nursing diagnoses for clients with ulcers include

1. Pain related to gastric and duodenal injury
2. Potential for injury related to complications (e.g., intractability, hemorrhage, perforation, or obstruction)

Additional Diagnoses

In addition to common diagnoses, the client may present with one or more additional diagnoses, including

1. Ineffective individual coping related to intractable progressive disease requiring significant life style alterations
2. Altered nutrition: less than body requirements related to anorexia, nausea, or diet constraints
3. Altered health maintenance related to diet constraints and self-control of anxiety
4. Sleep pattern disturbance related to discomfort
5. Knowledge deficit related to therapeutic regimen and strategies needed for coping

 ### Planning and Implementation

The following plan of care for the client with ulcer disease focuses on the common nursing diagnoses.

Pain

Planning: client goals. The major goal for this diagnosis is that the client will verbalize the absence of pain after the therapeutic regimen.

Interventions: nonsurgical management. Diet and medications are used to promote comfort of clients with PUD. The nurse assists the client to understand the meaning of discomfort and the importance of following the treatment regimen to relieve the signs and symptoms by decreasing stimulation. Clients with dyspepsia should be treated symptomatically for 6 to 8 weeks. If their symptoms do not disappear after this period, if they have no relief within 10 days, or if complications occur, further diagnostic evaluation should take place. Repeated upper GI x-ray films should be taken to document healing. If healing has not occurred, gastroscopy

and biopsy should be repeated. Ulcer disease is a chronic disease, and treatment programs are not curative but are used to heal the ulcer.

Drug therapy. The primary objective of the treatment of peptic ulcers is to provide rest for the stomach. The rationale for using drugs in the treatment of peptic ulcers involves different mechanisms: the reduction of secretions (hyposecretory drugs), the neutralization of buffering of acid (antacids), and the protection of the mucous barrier (mucosal barrier fortifiers) by decreasing the activity of pepsin and hydrochloric acid. Hyposecretory drugs, which cause a reduction in acid secretions, include histamine antagonists, anticholinergics, and prostaglandin analogues. See Table 44–1 for drugs commonly used in PUD.

H_2 antagonists. Drugs that block histamine-stimulated gastric secretions are effective in management of ulcer disease. H_2 receptor antagonists block the action of the H_2 receptors of the parietal cells. The most common drugs are cimetidine (Tagamet) and ranitidine (Zantac). Ranitidine is at least twice as effective as cimetidine against acid secretion. Famotidine (Pepcid) and nizatidine are newer H_2 antagonists. These drugs inhibit gastric acid secretion in response to all stimuli.

Antacids. The ideal antacid is one that decreases acidity; is effective for a prolonged period; is pleasant to take orally; is not constipating or cathartic in effect; and is not absorbed to cause systemic side effects. Antacids buffer gastric acid and prevent the formation of pepsin. Clients need to understand that antacids do not influence healing or prevent recurrence but that they do appear to decrease pain and discomfort. The client is instructed that for therapeutic effect, sufficient antacid is used to neutralize the hourly production of acid. For optimal effect, the nurse gives the antacids about 2 hours after meals to reduce the hydrogen ion load in the duodenum. Antacids may be effective from 30 minutes or up to 3 hours after ingestion. Antacids taken with an empty stomach are quickly evacuated, thus reducing the neutralizing effects.

Calcium carbonate is a potent antacid but may cause constipation, and it triggers gastrin release, which causes a rebound acid secretion. Magnesium carbonate and magnesium oxide are also potent antacids but are laxatives; they are sometimes prescribed to counteract the constipating effects of calcium carbonate. The nurse instructs the client to take these drugs alternately or balances dosages of each to produce a stool of the desired consistency. Aluminum hydroxide, aluminum phosphate, and aluminum carbonate are less effective because they only partially neutralize the acid. The combined magnesium and aluminum preparations are more palatable to the client. Sodium bicarbonate is a potent antacid, but its effects are brief and it is absorbed systemically. The nurse needs to ensure that the client understands the negative effects of sodium bicarbonate.

Antacids can also interact with certain drugs and interfere with their effectiveness. The nurse assesses the client to determine what other drugs are being used

TABLE 44 – 1   Drugs Commonly Used in the Treatment of Peptic Ulcer Disease

Drug	Usual Daily Dosage	Interventions	Rationales
Antacids			
Magnesium hydroxide with aluminum hydroxide (Maalox, Mylanta)	Maalox, 30 mL qid or 2–4 tablets qid Mylanta, 5–10 mL or 1–2 tablets qid	1. Give 1 h after meals and at bedtime. 2. Use liquid rather than tablets if palatable. 3. Do not give other drugs within 1–2 h of antacids. 4. Assess client for history of renal disease. 5. Assess client for history of congestive heart failure. 6. Observe client for side effect of diarrhea.	1. Hydrogen ion load is high after ingestion of food. 2. Suspensions are more effective than chewable tablets. 3. Antacids interfere with absorption of other drugs. 4. Hypermagnesemia may result. 5. These antacids have high sodium content. 6. Magnesium often causes diarrhea.
Aluminum hydroxide (Amphojel)	5–10 mL or tablets of 300–600 mg	1. Give 1 h after meals and at bedtime. 2. Use liquid rather than tablets if palatable. 3. Do not give other drugs within 1–2 h of antacids. 4. Observe client for side effect of constipation. 5. If constipation occurs, consider alternating with magnesium antacid. 6. Use for clients with renal failure.	1. Hydrogen ion load is high after ingestion of food. 2. Suspensions are more effective than chewable tablets. 3. Antacids interfere with absorption of other drugs. 4. Aluminum causes constipation. 5. Magnesium has a laxative effect. 6. Aluminum binds with phosphates in GI tract.
H_2 Antagonists			
Cimetidine (Tagamet)	200–300 mg qid or 900–1200 mg PO at bedtime. 200–300 mg every 6–8 h IV	1. Give clients age 60 yr and older reduced dose. 2. Give single dose at bedtime. 3. IV administration requires slow infusion. 4. Give 1 h before or after antacids. 5. Watch clients with impaired renal or hepatic function closely for side effects.	1. Side effect of confusion occurs most often in elders. 2. Bedtime administration suppresses nocturnal acid production. 3. Bradycardia or cardiac arrest may occur with rapid administration. 4. Antacids interfere with absorption. 5. Metabolism by liver and elimination by kidney will increase drug level.

Table continued on following page

TABLE 44–1   Drugs Commonly Used in the Treatment of Peptic Ulcer Disease *Continued*

Drug	Usual Daily Dosage	Interventions	Rationales
H₂ Antagonists			
Ranitidine (Zantac)	150 mg bid PO; 50 mg every 8 h IV	1. Give single dose at bedtime.	1. Bedtime administration suppresses nocturnal acid production.
Famotidine (Pepcid)	40 mg once a day or in 2 divided doses	1. Give single dose at bedtime.	1. Bedtime administration suppresses nocturnal acid production. Compliance may improve with less frequent administration.
Mucosal Barrier Fortifiers			
Sucralfate (Carafate)	1 g qid	1. Give 1 h before meals and at bedtime.	1. Food may interfere with drug's adherence to mucosa.
		2. Do not give within 30 min of giving antacids or other drugs.	2. Antacids may interfere with effect.

before a specific antacid is recommended. Medications are administered 1 to 2 hours before or after administration of an antacid. Clients are told that flavored antacids, especially wintergreen, are avoided because the flavoring increases the emptying time of the stomach, thus negating the desired effect of the antacid.

Clients with congestive heart failure should be instructed to avoid antacids with a high sodium content, such as some aluminum hydroxide, magnesium hydroxide, and simethicone combination products (Gelusil and Mylanta). Magaldrate (Riopan) has the lowest sodium concentration. Aluminum hydroxide (Alternagel) and some combination products (Maalox Plus Tablets, Mylanta-II Tablets, and Gelusil tablets) have a high sugar content. The aluminum and magnesium hydroxide combination products (Maalox and Mylanta-II) neutralize well at small doses. Combination therapy of H₂ antagonists plus antacids is common and appears to be effective.

Mucosal barrier fortifiers. Sucralfate (Carafate) is sulfonated disaccharide that forms complexes with proteins at the base of a peptic ulcer, thus making a protective coat that prevents further digestive action of both acid and pepsin. Sucralfate does not inhibit acid secretion and has minimal acid-neutralizing ability, but it has been shown to be effective in the treatment of ulcers. It may be used in conjunction with H₂ antagonists and antacids but should not be administered within 1 hour of the antacid. It is given on an empty stomach 1 hour before each meal and at bedtime. Constipation is its main side effect.

Carbenoxolone (Biogastrone), an extract of licorice, is effective in promoting gastric ulcer healing. The precise mode of action is unknown, but probably mucosal resistance such as mucous secretion is enhanced. In addition to ulcer healing, this drug affords symptomatic relief from pain. The nurse cautions the client to observe for potential adverse effects, including signs of sodium and fluid retention and of potassium loss. Clients are instructed to observe for sudden weight gain and swelling of hands or feet. Elderly clients should avoid the use of this drug because it is contraindicated in clients with hypertension, congestive heart failure, and renal impairment.

Anticholinergics. Anticholinergics decrease vagal stimulation by blocking the action of acetylcholine on smooth muscles, thus reducing gastric motility and inhibiting gastric secretion. This effect is largely limited to the relief of pain that does not respond to other medications. Because they commonly cause side effects such as blurred vision, constipation, urinary retention, and tachycardia, they are not used frequently.

Clients are instructed to stop taking anticholinergics if bleeding begins because the stomach may become distended and gastric dilation may result.

Antimuscarinics. Pirenzepine is a tricyclic pyridobenzodiazepine compound that acts much like an anticholinergic by inhibiting gastric acid secretion, principally by decreasing the secreted volume without the typical anticholinergic side effects just mentioned. It is taken ½ hour before meals and is an alternative to H₂ receptor antagonists.

Prostaglandin analogues. Prostaglandins are naturally abundant in the GI tract. They are thought to inhibit acid secretion and contribute to the gastric mucosal barrier. Misoprostol (Cytotec) is a new drug in this category. A significant adverse effect of this drug is that it can cause miscarriage; thus, it is contraindicated for pregnant women.

Diet therapy. The value of diet in the management of ulcer disease is a highly controversial issue. There is no evidence that restriction of diet promotes or accelerates healing. If diet treatment is used, it may be directed toward neutralization of acid and reduction of hypermotility, which may alleviate symptoms.

Food itself acts as an antacid by producing neutralization for 30 to 60 minutes after eating. An increased rate of secretion, called *rebound,* may follow. Clients are instructed to avoid substances that increase acid secretion, including caffeine-containing beverages such as coffee, tea, and cola. Decaffeinated coffee may be allowed if tolerated, but both caffeinated and decaffeinated coffees contain peptides that stimulate gastrin release. The nurse instructs the client that any foods that cause discomfort should also be excluded. Often during the acute symptomatic phase, the diet is bland and nonirritating and contains little fiber. For some clients, six daily feedings may help, but this regimen is no longer a regular part of therapy. Milk may be taken in small amounts but is a poor neutralizer. Alcohol and tobacco should be avoided because of their stimulatory effects.

Rest and decreased activity. Clients should avoid intense physical activity as a means to reduce motor activity that stimulates gastric secretions. Physical and mental rest should be achieved. The number and intensity of environmental stimuli are decreased to prevent increased gastric acid stimulation. When ulcer symptoms occur, the nurse assists the client to realize the importance of altering a stressful work routine. The nurse should help the client to implement a plan that enables physical rest periods. Coping and relaxation techniques should be taught. Strategies should be identified that are specific to the type of stressor identified. (See the later Client Care Plan.)

Potential for Injury

Planning: client goals. The major goal for this nursing diagnosis is that the client will not experience complications of ulcer disease such as hemorrhage, perforation, or obstruction.

Interventions: nonsurgical management. Monitoring and early recognition of potential complication are critical to the successful management of PUD. The nonsurgical approach to treatment depends on the type of complication.

Management of hemorrhage. The nurse observes the symptoms to determine the severity of the hemorrhage. Insertion of a nasogastric tube (Fig. 44–3) is carried out to ascertain the presence or absence of blood in the stomach, to assess the rate of bleeding, to prevent gastric dilation, and to administer saline lavage (see the accompanying Nursing Research and Guidelines features). In mild bleeding (less than 500 mL), only slight weakness and perspiration may be present. Blood loss of more than 1 L/24 hours may cause signs and symptoms of shock, such as hypotension; weak, thready pulse; chills; palpitations; and diaphoresis. In severe bleeding, the nurse keeps an accurate and up-to-date record of the client's hemoglobin and hematocrit values, which may

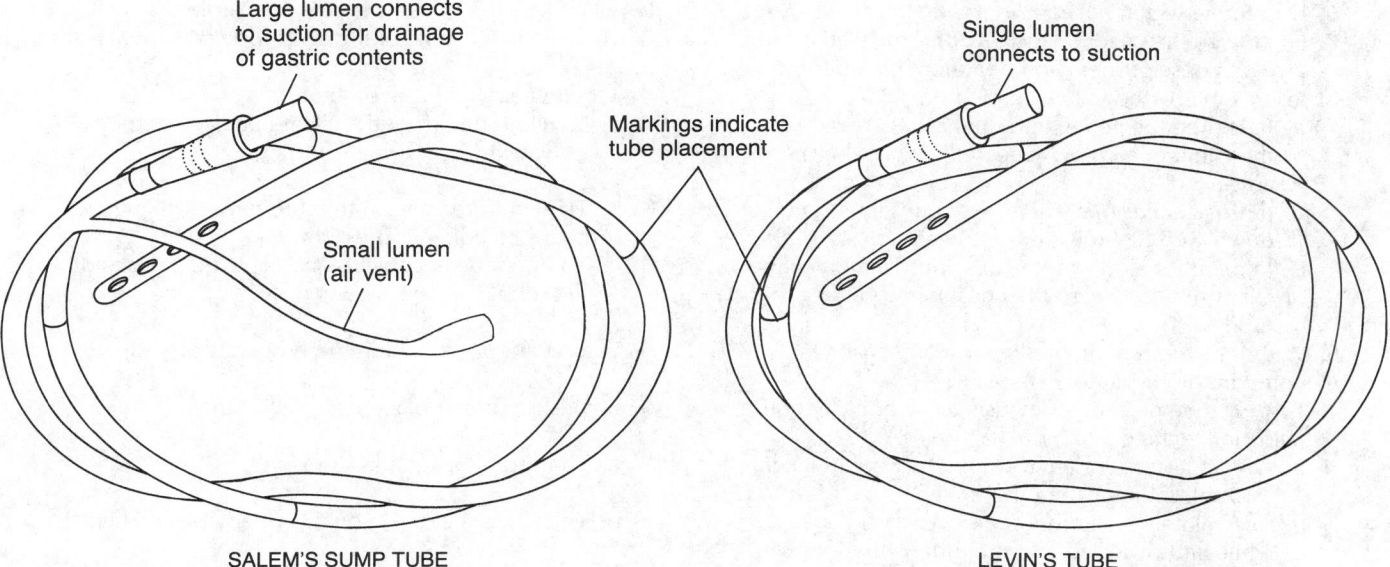

Large lumen connects to suction for drainage of gastric contents

Small lumen (air vent)

Single lumen connects to suction

Markings indicate tube placement

SALEM'S SUMP TUBE

LEVIN'S TUBE

Figure 44–3

Nasogastric tubes.

GUIDELINES ■ How to Insert a Nasogastric Tube and Care for Clients with a Tube in Place

Interventions	Rationales
1. Inform the client about the procedure and potential discomfort.	1. To alleviate apprehension and foster cooperation.
2. Position client sitting with pillows behind shoulders.	2. To facilitate passage of the nasogastric (NG) tube into the cardia of stomach and to decrease the gag reflex, make swallowing easier, and facilitate passage of the tube past the epiglottis into stomach.
3. Place the NG tube on ice or in a refrigerator.	3. To stiffen the tube for easier insertion, especially if the client is intubated.
4. Lubricate the tube with water-soluble lubricant.	4. To lessen irritation of the mucosa; water-soluble lubricant will be broken down if aspirated into lungs or if the NG tube is inadvertently passed into lungs.

5. Measure the length of the tube to be passed.
  a. Measure from the bridge of the nose to the earlobe to the xiphoid process.
  b. Indicate this length with a piece of tape on the tube.
	5. To approximate the length of the tube needed to reach the stomach.

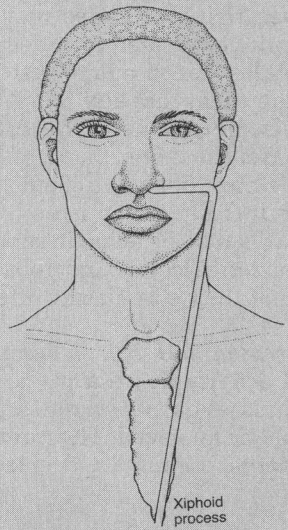

Xiphoid process

Interventions	Rationales
6. Determine which nostril is more patent.	6. To choose the nostril with the best airflow.
7. Encourage the client to swallow or drink water if the level of consciousness and treatment plan permit.	7. To facilitate passage of the NG tube and suppress the gag reflex.

8. Insert tube by the following method.
  a. Pass the tube gently into the nasopharynx. Ask the client to swallow repeatedly while the tube is advanced.
  b. If resistance is met, rotate the tube slowly, aiming downward and toward the closer ear.
  c. In the intubated or semiconscious client, flex the client's head toward the chest while passing the tube.
	8. To allow easy passage of the tube.
	  a. To avoid trauma and facilitate passage of tube downward.
	
	  b. To avoid pressure on the turbinates, which may cause bleeding or pressure.
	  c. To open the esophagus and facilitate passage of the tube.

9. Withdraw the tube immediately if any change is noted in the respiratory status.	9. To prevent placement in the bronchus or lung.

10. Test for tube placement by using one or more of the following techniques.
  a. Obtain gastric contents sample by aspirating with a 50-mL catheter-tipped syringe.
  b. Auscultate with stethoscope over gastric area while air is inserted into the tube with a syringe.
  c. Obtain an order for an x-ray film to confirm placement.
	10. To ensure proper placement.
	
	  a. To ensure location in stomach.
	
	  b. To ensure that the tube is properly placed (a rush of air should be heard).
	  c. Absence of bubbling or auscultation of air does not confirm proper location within the stomach.

Interventions	Rationales
11. Connect the tube to suction at low pressure.	11. To decrease the chance of trauma to the mucosa and facilitate drainage of GI contents.
a. Levine's tube is connected to intermittent low suction.	
b. Salem's sump or Anderson's tube is connected to continuous low suction.	
12. Secure the tube to the client's nose with adhesive tape and to the client's gown.	12. To prevent tugging on the tube when the client moves and to enable movement.
a. Tie a slipknot around the tube with a rubber band.	
b. Pin a rubber band to the client's gown.	
13. Check the client's intake and output every 4 h or more often as indicated.	13. To allow for evaluation of patency of the tube and proper location of the tube within the stomach.
14. Observe the client for nausea and vomiting and for abdominal fullness or distention.	14. To determine proper positioning or to determine whether tube is nonpatent.
15. If irrigation indicated, use only a normal saline solution.	15. To maintain electrolyte balance.
16. Observe the amount and color of drainage.	16. To provide information related to hemorrhage and fluid status.
17. Observe the client for fluid and electrolyte balance.	17. To prevent excessive NG drainage, which may predispose the client to fluid volume deficit, hypokalemia, hyponatremia, hypochloremia, and metabolic alkalosis.
18. If indicated, instruct the client about movement that will not dislodge the NG tube or cause nasal irritation.	18. To allow for more client independence.
19. Remove adhesive tape that secures the tube to the nose daily and prn to clean skin and reapply tape.	19. To prevent skin breakdown from pressure of the NG tube and tape against nares.

indicate significant blood loss. Any client who is suspected of having active bleeding is cared for in the critical care unit.

Traditionally, saline lavage has been accomplished by inserting a large-bore nasogastric tube and manually instilling iced saline in volumes of 50 to 200 mL, followed by repeated withdrawal of the saline and blood until returns are clear or light pink, without clots. To protect against exposure to blood, practitioners may use a closed system for irrigation and suction (Fig. 44–4). A Y connector is attached to the nasogastric tube, with a bag of normal saline and tubing attached to one end of the Y connector, and tubing to wall suction attached to the other end of the connector. After the stomach is initially drained via suctioning, the tubing attached to suction is clamped off, and up to 200 mL of normal saline is allowed to drain into the client via the nasogastric tube. After the saline is instilled, the tube connecting the saline to the nasogastric tube is clamped off, and the clamp to suction is released. Clients should lie on the left side during this procedure to limit the flow of saline out of the stomach and to help prevent aspiration.

There is considerable controversy about the value of using iced saline for lavage. Iced saline has been used to control bleeding through its vasoconstrictive effect. The concern about using iced saline is that it might cause a decrease in perfusion to the gastric mucosa, thus leading to more mucosal damage. It can also stimulate a vagal response, which decreases systemic perfusion. Because of these effects, some practitioners advocate the use of

NURSING RESEARCH

What's the Best Way to Test Placement of Nasogastric and Nasointestinal Tubes?

Metheny, N. (1988). Measures to test placement of nasogastric and nasointestinal feeding tubes: A review. *Nursing Research*, 37, 324–326.

A literature review regarding recommended measures to test nasogastric and nasointestinal tubes is presented. Discussion includes aspiration of gastrointestinal contents, auscultation of insufflated air, measurement of pH of gastrointestinal secretions, and observation for coughing and choking. Fallibilities of these methods are described.

Critique. This review provides valuable information on techniques to avoid complications associated with the use of feeding tubes. Nursing research comparing various techniques of intubation and measures to test placement is needed.

Possible Nursing Implications. Metheny suggests that flexing the head toward the chest closes off the glottis as an attempt to prevent entry to the trachea. Radiography may be needed to confirm proper placement. pH measurement of aspirated gastric sections is recommended. Administration of antacids and gastric acid inhibitors may interfere with the accuracy of these pH readings.

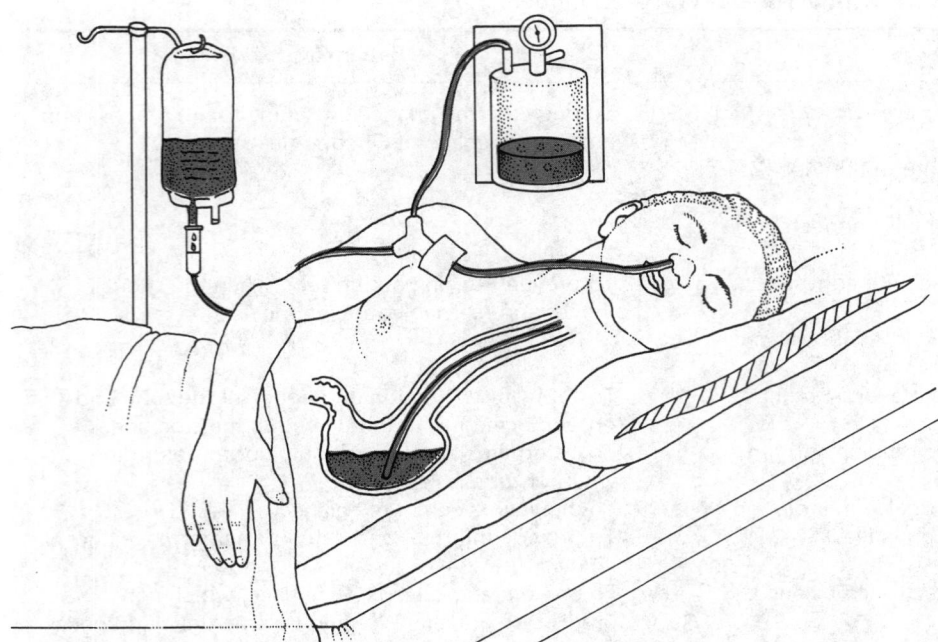

Figure 44–4

Saline lavage can be accomplished through a closed three-way system by using a Y connector and clamps.

saline at room temperature, which is cooler than body temperature yet not as cold as an iced solution.

Arterial administration of *vasopressin* (via infusion pump) has been successfully used to control acute hemorrhage. The preferred route of vasopressin administration is IV (peripheral). Complications from the pharmacologic effect of vasopressin that the nurse should be alert for include pain at the injection site or local necrosis, gangrene, chest pain (angina; pain related to myocardial infarction), difficulty in urinating, nausea and vomiting, abdominal or stomach cramps, belching, diarrhea, and water intoxication (evidenced by drowsiness, listlessness, headache, confusion, and weight gain). This procedure is contraindicated for cardiac patients.

Another approach to the control of bleeding is selective *arterial embolization*. The emboli may consist of autologous blood clots with or without absorbable gelatin sponge (Gelfoam). A modified clot may be made with a mixture of the client's own blood, aminocaproic acid (Amicar), and platelets. Laser photocoagulation, electrocoagulation, and norepinephrine injection combined with aethoxyscleral are other newer approaches being used to control hemorrhage. These latter approaches require much further testing before they will be applicable for general use.

The nurse provides a careful description and documentation of bleeding, including the occurrence of hematemesis and melena; the color, amount, and consistency of blood; and frequency of bleeding. Bright red blood signifies new bleeding, whereas dark red blood indicates old bleeding. Immediate notification of the physician is imperative in major episodes of hemorrhage.

Therapy for massive bleeding is aimed at treating hypovolemic shock, preventing dehydration and elec-

trolyte imbalance, stopping the bleeding, and providing rest. Early endoscopy is used to determine the necessity of surgery to control the bleeding. Clients are confined to bed, are kept on NPO status, and are given IV fluids until the bleeding has subsided. The nurse ensures by irrigation that the nasogastric tube remains patent and does not become obstructed with clotted blood.

Absolute bed rest to keep the blood pressure down and to decrease intestinal motility is essential for several days after bleeding has subsided. When bleeding stops, bathroom privileges are permitted. Narcotics, if used, are administered with caution. Morphine sulfate can cause nausea and vomiting, but it may be used for the client who is extremely restless or apprehensive.

During the first few days after hemorrhaging, gastric pH should be increased to between 5.5 and 7.0 and maintained at that level to control secretory activity. To accomplish this, the administration of cimetidine every 4 hours for a few days may be recommended. The use of antacids complements the effectiveness of cimetidine to maintain the pH level of gastric secretions. Anticholinergics are not recommended for clients with gastric hemorrhage because gastric motility is decreased. Cimetidine or ranitidine may be required every 30 minutes after the intake of food or fluids has begun. The recommended dosage of antacid is 3 mEq (30 mL) hourly during the day for 1 week.

Management of perforation. Treatment of perforation includes immediate replacement of fluid, blood, and electrolytes and administration of antibiotics to prevent peritonitis from the GI contents that have entered the peritoneum as a result of the perforation. Nasogastric suction is instituted to drain gastric secretions and, thus, to prevent further peritoneal spillage. The client is kept on NPO status, and intake and output are monitored carefully. The nurse checks the client's vital signs at least at hourly intervals and monitors the client for signs and symptoms of toxic shock such as fever, pain, tachycardia, lethargy, anxiety, and prostration (see Chap. 45 for surgical management and care of clients with peritonitis).

Management of pyloric obstruction. Pyloric obstruction is caused by edema, spasm, or scar tissue.

KEY FEATURES OF DISEASE ■ Surgical Management of Peptic Ulcer Disease

Surgery	Description	Possible Adverse Effects
Vagotomy		
Truncal (total abdominal vagotomy)	Cuts vagus nerve at the esophageal level. Severs both anterior and posterior trunks. Destroys vagal and abdominal innervation. Destroys gastrointestinal motility.	Gastric emptying is inhibited; pyloroplasty or antrectomy must be performed to prevent gastric stasis. Some clients experience problems of a feeling of fullness after eating (33%), dumping syndrome (10%), or diarrhea (10%).
Selective	Cuts vagus nerve to stomach, but other abdominal innervation remains. Acid production stops.	Gastric emptying is inhibited; pyloroplasty or antrectomy must be performed to prevent gastric stasis.
Proximal, or parietal cell (can be done without pyloroplasty or antrectomy)	Cuts parietal branches of vagus nerve. Alters innervation to acid-producing cells but does not alter gastric motility.	Few negative consequences because innervation of the antrum and the pyloric sphincter remains.
Vagotomy with antrectomy	Cuts the vagus nerve and removes the antrum (lower half) of stomach. Removes source of gastrin secretion.	Some clients may have a feeling of fullness after eating, dumping syndrome, diarrhea, anemia, or malabsorption.
Pyloroplasty	Enlarges pylorus by surgically enlarging the pyloric sphincter.	Stomach may empty too rapidly.
Vagotomy and pyloroplasty	Cuts the right and left branches of the vagus nerve. Widens the existing pyloric sphincter to prevent stasis and to enhance emptying of the stomach.	Stomach may empty too quickly.
Subtotal gastrectomy		
Billroth I (gastroduodenostomy after resection) hemigastrectomy	Removes the distal one-third to one-half of the stomach and anastomoses with the duodenum. Removes antral portion of the stomach and the pylorus.	Dumping syndrome, anemia, malabsorption, weight loss, or bile reflux may occur.
Billroth II (gastrojejunostomy after resection)	Removes distal segment of stomach and antrum and anastomoses with the jejunum. Retains duodenum; secretions of the liver and pancreas mix with the duodenal contents. Preferred procedure.	Infection in the duodenum, malabsorption-related weight loss, or vitamin B_{12} deficiency may occur.
Total gastrectomy (esophagojejunostomy)	Removes stomach from level of lower esophageal sphincter to duodenum and anastomoses the duodenum to the esophagus.	Gastric function is destroyed, and food remains undigested. Dumping syndrome and anemia may occur.

Symptoms of obstruction related to difficulty in emptying the stomach include feelings of fullness, distention, or nausea after eating, or vomiting of copious amounts of undigested food. Treatment of obstruction is directed toward restoring fluid and electrolyte balance and decompressing the dilated stomach; if necessary, surgical intervention is used. Obstruction related to edema and spasm generally responds to medical therapy. First, the stomach must be decompressed with nasogastric suction; then, metabolic alkalosis and dehydration are treated. After about 72 hours, the client's nasogastric tube is clamped and the client is checked for retention of gastric contents. If the amount retained is not more than 350 mL in 30 minutes, oral fluids may be initiated.

Interventions: surgical management. Surgery of the stomach is used to (1) reduce the acid-secreting ability of the stomach, (2) treat a surgical emergency that develops as a complication of PUD, or (3) treat clients who do not respond to medical therapy or who develop complications. Most chronic, recurring ulcers are eventually treated surgically. When an ulcer does not respond to intensive medical therapy or when a definitive diagnosis cannot be made by roentgenography and gastroscopy, surgery is performed. About 20% of duodenal ulcer clients require surgery for complications such as hemorrhage, perforation, obstruction, or intractability (Berk, 1985; Brooks et al., 1985).

If a *perforation* occurs, surgery entails closure of the perforation after the escaped gastric contents have been evacuated. If the perforation is small and closes immediately by adhering to the adjacent tissues, the loss of gastric contents is small. In this instance, the client may recover without surgery. Vagotomy and hemigastrectomy or vagotomy and pyloroplasty can provide definitive control of both the ulcer and the complication. Surgical treatment is usually limited to closure of the perforation by patching it with omentum. The peritoneal cavity is flushed out with an antibiotic or normal saline solution. Antibiotics are administered to prevent peritonitis.

Acute obstruction, perforation, and hemorrhage that is unresponsive to medical treatment are usually treated as emergencies by surgical intervention. Common surgeries used in PUD and their possible adverse effects are noted in the Key Features of Disease on page 1321.

The *vagotomy* is done to eliminate the acid-secreting stimulus to gastric cells and to decrease responsiveness of parietal cells. Three types of vagotomy can be done: truncal, selective, and proximal. In a vagotomy, each branch of the vagus nerve may be completely cut *(truncal)*; partially cut so as to preserve the hepatic and celiac branches *(selective)*; or partially cut so as to denervate only the parietal cell mass, thus preserving innervation of both the antrum and the pyloric sphincter *(superselective)*. Cutting the vagal nerve fibers selectively avoids the problems of impaired emptying and diarrhea that follow the truncal vagotomy. Vagotomy also eliminates the necessity for a drainage anastomosis to offset the gastric stasis, yet it reduces acid secretion and preserves the function of the antrum. In the *proximal* (parietal cell)

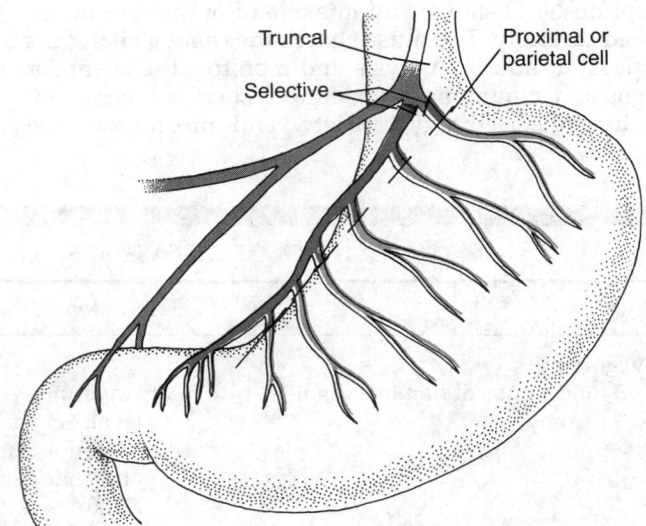

Figure 44–5

Types of vagotomies.

vagotomy, only the gastric portion of vagal nerves that innervate the upper two-thirds of the stomach is severed (Fig. 44–5).

Vagotomy and *pyloroplasty* involve cutting the right and left vagus nerves and widening the exit of the pylorus, respectively. The most commonly used procedure is the Heineke-Mikulicz pyloroplasty (Fig. 44–6). This procedure is done to prevent stasis and the resultant feeling of fullness, belching, and weight loss and to enhance emptying of the stomach.

A *simple gastroenterostomy* permits neutralization of gastric acid by regurgitation into the stomach of alkaline duodenal contents. This benefit may be offset by interference with acid inhibition of gastrin release, which results in a net increase in acid secretion. If the gastroen-

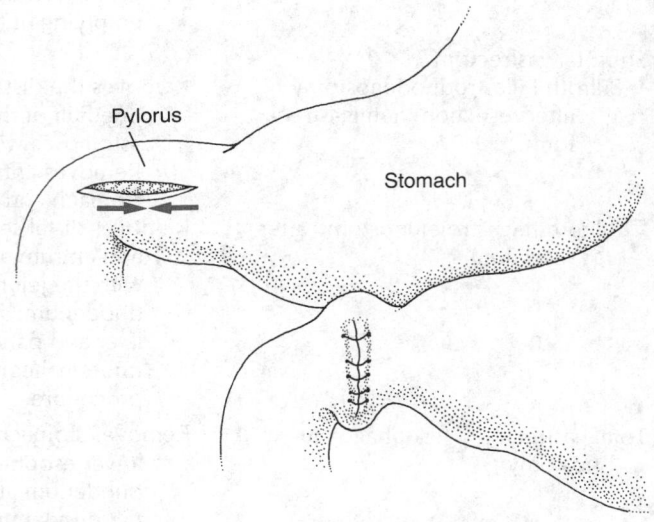

Figure 44–6

The Heineke-Mikulicz pyloroplasty.

terostomy drains the stomach, it reduces motor activity in the pyloroduodenal area. Drainage of the gastric contents diverts acid away from the ulcerated area to facilitate healing. However, the secretory capacity of the parietal cell mass of the stomach has not been reduced, and the gastrin mechanism continues to function. A vagotomy is usually combined with gastroenterostomy for reduction in the vagal influences (Fig. 44–7).

Antrectomy is the removal of the antrum of the stomach, with the remaining portion of the stomach anastomosed to the duodenum. This procedure is done to reduce the acid-secreting portions of the stomach.

A *subtotal gastrectomy* may be formed by means of either a Billroth I or a Billroth II procedure. In the *Billroth I procedure,* a part of the distal portion of the stomach is removed, including the antrum, with an anastomosis of the remainder to the duodenum; this procedure is more properly called a *gastroduodenostomy* (Fig. 44–8). This procedure removes the gastrin source in the antrum of some of the acid pepsin–secreting parietal cells and decreases the incidence of the dumping syndrome that often occurs after the surgery.

In a Billroth I procedure, the proximal end of the distal stomach is anastomosed to the duodenum. A *Billroth II resection,* or *gastrojejunostomy,* involves anastomosis of the proximal remnant of the stomach and the proximal jejunum and is most often the procedure that is used for gastric ulcer. The Billroth II technique is preferred for the treatment of duodenal ulcer because recurrent ulceration develops less frequently. The duodenal stump is preserved to permit bile flow to the jejunum, as shown in Figure 44–9.

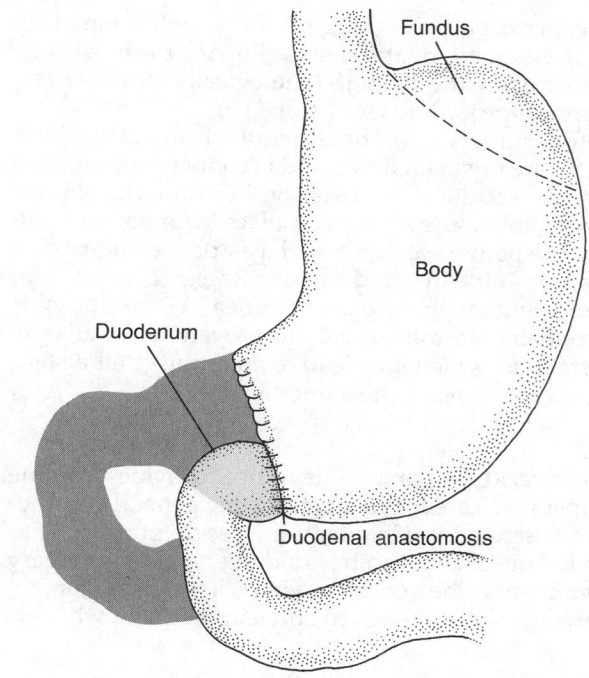

Figure 44–8

The Billroth I procedure (gastroduodenostomy). The distal portion of the stomach is removed and the remainder anastomosed to the duodenum. The shading shows the portion removed.

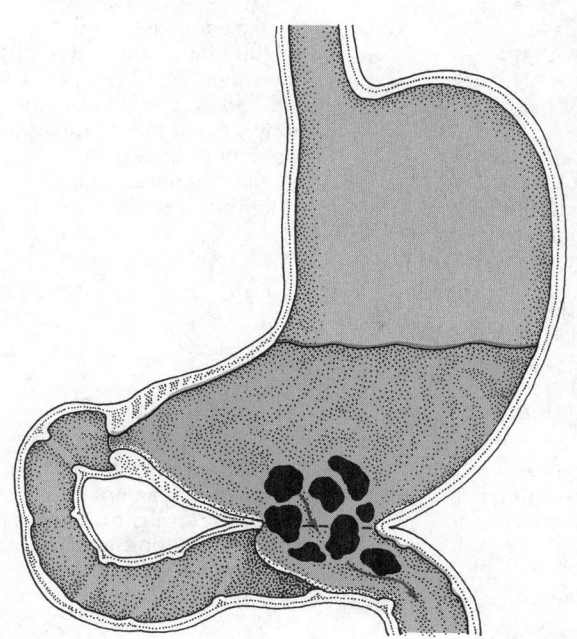

Figure 44–7

Gastroenterostomy, which is creation of a passage between the body of the stomach and the jejunum.

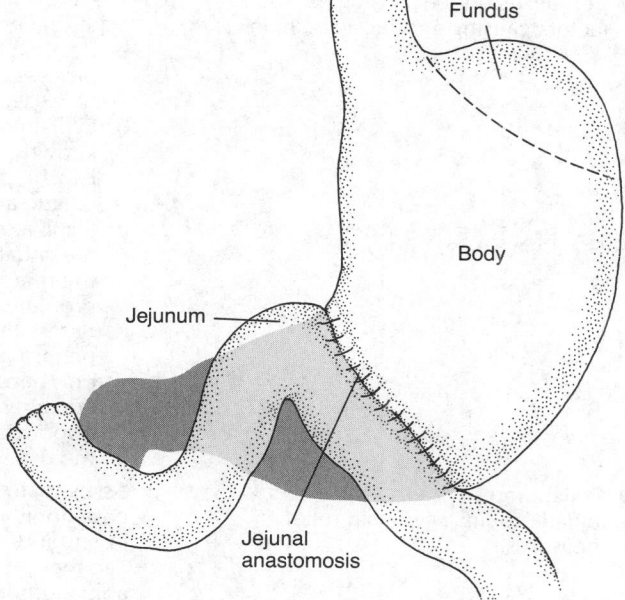

Figure 44–9

The Billroth II procedure (gastrojejunostomy). The lower portion of the stomach is removed, and the remainder is anastomosed to the jejunum. The shading shows the portion removed. A remaining duodenal stump is closed.

Preoperative care. Surgery for complications may be of an emergency nature, thus allowing the nurse little time to prepare the client psychologically for the stressful surgical procedure (see Chap. 18).

Before surgery, a nasogastric tube is inserted, if this has not already been done, and is connected to suction to remove secretions and empty the stomach. This removal enables surgery to take place without contaminating the peritoneal cavity with gastric secretions. (See the earlier Guidelines and Nursing Research features for care of clients with nasogastric tubes.) The nasogastric tube remains postoperatively to prevent accumulation of secretions, which may lead to vomiting or GI distention and pressure on the suture line.

Postoperative care. The nurse provides routine postoperative care for clients receiving general anesthesia, as described in Chapter 20. Specific nursing measures for the client who has undergone gastric surgery are outlined in the accompanying Client Care Plan.

Patency of the nasogastric tube in the client who has had gastric surgery is critical to prevent the retention of gastric secretions. The nurse assesses that no more than a scant amount of blood drains from the tube and that the client does not develop abdominal distention. If these problems occur, the nurse reports them immediately. The nurse never irrigates or repositions the nasogastric tube after gastric surgery.

Gastrojejunocolic fistula is a postoperative complication that is associated with recurrent PUD. The fistula arises from perforation of a recurrent ulceration at the gastrojejunal anastomosis site. The symptoms are caused by bacterial overgrowth in the small intestine. The nurse assesses for symptoms including fecal vomiting, diarrhea, weight loss, and anorexia. Belching of fecal-smelling gas may occur. Surgery may be necessary to correct the fistula.

Afferent loop syndrome may occur when the duodenal loop is partially obstructed after a Billroth II resection. Pancreatic and biliary secretions fill the intestinal loop, which becomes distended. Painful contractions occur in an effort to propel these secretions from the loop. When secretions finally enter the jejunum, the excessive pres-

CLIENT CARE PLAN ■ The Client Recovering from Gastric Surgery

Goal/Outcome Criteria	Interventions	Rationales
Nursing Diagnosis 1: Pain Related to Nausea, Vomiting, and Indigestion Caused by Ulcer and Surgery		

Client will experience reduced pain.
■ Verbalizes understanding of factors causing and reducing pain.
	1. Teach client about pain experiences.
	  a. Relate a typical disease process or course with realistic expectations.
	  b. Explain the cause of pain, if known.
	  c. Explain possible effects of fatigue and anxiety.
	  d. Instill a sense of control of the situation in relation to the temporary nature of the problem.
	  e. Assess the client's sleep pattern and influence of pain on sleep.
	  f. Encourage rest and provide opportunity for rest during the day.
		1. To reduce the client's anxiety level and fatigue. Increased anxiety and fatigue ultimately lead to an intensification of the pain experience by reducing the body's or mind's adaptive capacity to deal with uncomfortable stimuli or situations.

■ Collaborates with the nurse to initiate noninvasive pain relief measures.	2. Assess pain relief measures commonly used by the family or support people and encourage the use of mutually acceptable methods.
	3. Teach techniques commonly used.
	  a. Relaxation.
	  b. Cutaneous stimulation.
	  c. Massage.
		2–5. To enable the client and family to manage pain and discomfort, thus promoting a sense of control and avoiding use of invasive methods.

CLIENT CARE PLAN ■ **The Client Recovering from Gastric Surgery** *continued*

Goal/Outcome Criteria	Interventions	Rationales
Nursing Diagnosis 1: Pain Related to Nausea, Vomiting, and Indigestion Caused by Ulcer and Surgery		
■ Identifies factors that initiate pain.	4. Teach positioning to improve chest expansion, i.e., semi-Fowler's position or reclining or R side. 5. Teach client to splint incision during coughing. 6. Assist client in assessing for factors leading to exacerbations of pain or discomfort. 7. Avoid, or use with caution, drugs that decrease mucosal resistance (acetylsalicylic acid, nonsteroidal anti-inflammatory agents, adrenocorticotropic hormone, steroids) or drugs that alter gastric acid production (reserpine, catecholamines). 8. Discontinue and avoid use of stimulants (e.g., caffeine and nicotine) or spices (e.g., mustard, paprika, pepper, and Tabasco sauce), which are known to cause pain or discomfort. 9. Eliminate use of alcohol. Avoid concurrent use of alcohol and aspirin. 10. Encourage adequate diet to meet nutritional needs. Emphasize inclusion of nonirritating foods.	6–10. To eliminate individualized pain triggers. Some are known gastric irritants, yet not all factors affect each client.

■ Describes pain relief with use of prescribed medications.	11. Administer medications as ordered to
	  a. Block histamine-stimulated gastric secretions (H$_2$ receptor antagonists [e.g., cimetidine]).
	  b. Neutralize or buffer gastric acids (antacids).
	  c. Protect the mucous barrier (mucosal barrier fortifiers [e.g., carbenoxolone]).
	12. Assess the response of the medication.
	  a. Return in ½ h to determine effect.
	  b. Rate severity of pain and amount of relief.
	  c. Identify when the pain begins to increase.
	13. Consult primary care provider if dosage or interval change is required.
	14. Reduce or eliminate common medication side effects.
		11–14. To reduce pain through the use of medications that provide the stomach an opportunity to rest. This rest leads to decreased gastric acid secretion and promotes tissue healing and an ultimate reduction in pain and discomfort.

continued

CLIENT CARE PLAN ■ The Client Recovering from Gastric Surgery *continued*

Goal/Outcome Criteria	Interventions	Rationales
Nursing Diagnosis 1: Pain Related to Nausea, Vomiting, and Indigestion Caused by Ulcer and Surgery		
■ Verbalizes no discomfort from intake of foods and fluids.	15. Gradually increase food until client is able to eat three to six meals per day. 16. If discomfort recurs, decrease the size of meals and the amount of fluids. 17. Instruct client to report signs of complications, a feeling of fullness, weakness, and hematemesis.	15–17. To evaluate return of function of the stomach and intestines.
Nursing Diagnosis 2: Potential Fluid Volume Deficit Related to Nausea, Vomiting, and Possible Hemorrhage or Perforation		
Client will maintain vascular, cellular, and intracellular perfusion. ■ Demonstrates intact mental status. ■ Has stable blood pressure. ■ Has warm, dry skin. ■ Has urinary output of at least 30 mL/h.	1. Assess for nausea, vomiting, black or bloody stools, occult blood in stools, thirst, diaphoresis, pain, increased pulse, and decreased blood pressure; also assess urinary output and hemoglobin and hematocrit values.	1. To detect fluid volume deficit and evaluate its severity. If fluid volume deficit occurs, these same interventions allow for assessment of effectiveness of treatment.

sure forces them back into the stomach and vomiting occurs. The nurse observes and reports these symptoms if they occur. Treatment usually consists of nasogastric suction until operative edema subsides.

In the immediate postoperative period, *acute gastric dilation* produces epigastric pain, tachycardia, and hypotension. The client complains of a feeling of fullness, hiccups, or gagging. This situation rapidly improves after insertion of a nasogastric tube or the clearing of a plugged tube. Intake and output monitoring and fluid replacement are important nursing activities.

Several *problems of nutrition* develop from removal of the stomach, including a deficiency of vitamin B_{12}, folic acid, and iron; impaired calcium metabolism; and reduced absorption of calcium and vitamin D. These problems are caused by a shortage of the intrinsic factor that results from the resection and by inadequate absorption owing to rapid entry of food into the bowel. In the absence of intrinsic factor, symptoms of pernicious anemia occur. These symptoms are corrected by administration of vitamin B_{12}. Folic acid or iron preparations may also be given.

The *dumping syndrome*, which occurs after gastric resection in which the pylorus is bypassed, is a postprandial problem that is secondary to the rapid entry of ingested food into the jejunum without proper mixing and without the normal digestive processes of the duodenum having been accomplished. Observation for early manifestations of this syndrome should occur 5 to 30 minutes after eating. Symptoms include the vasomotor

disturbances of vertigo, tachycardia, syncope, sweating, pallor, palpitation, and the desire to lie down. The client's blood pressure is monitored by the nurse; the pulse may either rise or fall. The nurse observes for intestinal manifestations that include epigastric fullness, distention, diarrhea, abdominal cramping, nausea with only occasional vomiting, and borborygmi. Some clients experience a strong desire to defecate. Pain is not a part of this syndrome. The early manifestations are thought to be due to the rapid movement of extracellular fluids into the bowel to convert the hypertonic bolus that entered so rapidly into an isotonic mixture. This rapid fluid shift decreases the circulating blood volume, which causes the symptoms. The late manifestations, which are expected to occur 2 to 3 hours after eating, are caused by a release of an excessive amount of insulin, which follows a rapid rise in the blood glucose level resulting from the rapid entry of high-carbohydrate food into the jejunum. Having the jejunum distended with food and fluid increases intestinal peristalsis and motility, which causes the intestinal manifestations.

The dumping syndrome is treated by decreasing the amount of food taken at one time and giving a high-protein, high-fat, low-carbohydrate diet, as shown in the accompanying Health Promotion/Maintenance feature. Pectin administered in the form of a dry powder may prevent the syndrome. Gastric emptying can be delayed by not taking fluids with meals, by eating in a recumbent or semirecumbent position, or by lying down after meals. Sedatives and antispasmodics are given to

HEALTH PROMOTION/MAINTENANCE ■ Diet for Dumping Syndrome

Food Group	Foods Allowed or Encouraged	Foods to Use with Caution	Foods That Must Be Excluded
Soups		Fluids 30–45 min after meals	Spicy soups
Meat and meat substitutes	5 oz or more per day: fish, poultry, beef, pork, veal, lamb, eggs, cheese, and peanut butter		Spicy meats or meat substitutes
Potato and substitutes	Potato, rice, and pasta	Foods made with milk	Highly spiced potatoes or substitutes
Bread and cereal	White breads, rolls, muffins, crackers, and refined cereals	Whole-grain breads, rolls, crackers, and cereals	Breads with frosting, jelly, sweet rolls, and coffee cake
Vegetables	Two or more cooked vegetables	Gas-producing vegetables such as cabbage, onions, broccoli, or raw vegetables	
Fruits	Limit three per day: unsweetened canned fruits	Unsweetened juice or fruit drinks 30–45 min after meals; fresh fruit	Sweetened fruit or juice
Beverages	Dietetic drinks	Limit to 30–45 min after meals; 2 c of milk if tolerated; caffeine-containing beverages such as coffee, tea, and cola; if tolerated, diet carbonated beverages	Milk shakes, malts, and other sweet drinks; regular carbonated beverages and alcohol
Fats	Margarine, oils, shortening, butter, bacon, and salad dressings	Mayonnaise	Any fats with milk products
Desserts	Fruit (see under Fruits above)	Sugar-free gelatin, pudding, and custard	All sweets, cakes, pies, cookies, candy, ice cream, and sherbet
Seasonings and miscellaneous	Milk, spices, diet jelly, diet syrups, sugar substitutes	Excessive amounts of salt	Excessive amounts of spices, sugar, jelly, honey, syrup, or molasses

delay gastric emptying. This syndrome, which is most likely to occur after a Billroth II procedure, occurs soon after surgery and subsides in 6 months to 1 year.

Alkaline reflux gastritis is recognized as a sequela of gastric surgery in which the pylorus is bypassed or removed, such as pyloroplasty, gastric resection with gastroduodenostomy (Billroth I procedure), and gastrojejunostomy (Billroth II procedure). The reflux of duodenal contents with bile acids results in reflux gastritis. Injury to the gastric mucosal barrier by the bile acids may allow back-diffusion of hydrogen ions. Symptoms include a persistent pain and nausea and vomiting that are accentuated after meals. Epigastric burning is only partially relieved by vomiting.

Delayed gastric emptying is often present after gastric surgery and usually resolves within 1 week. The mechanical causes may be secondary to edema at the anastomosis or adhesions obstructing the distal loop. Metabolic causes such as hypokalemia, hypoproteinemia, or hyponatremia should be considered. The edema is resolved with nasogastric suction and maintenance of fluid and electrolyte balance and proper nutrition.

■ Discharge Planning

Home Care Preparation

Clients are discharged to home to continue recuperation. Clients who have undergone surgery or have had complications such as hemorrhage may require assistance with activities of daily living. Teaching individual risk factors to prevent recurrence of the ulcer is the focus of home care preparation.

Client/Family Education

Clients and families are given instructions about associated factors that are related to the development of an ulcer. Individual risk assessments are done to assist clients in identifying irritants and life style stressors. Strategies to make life style changes are mutually developed with the client. The nurse teaches and has the client describe symptoms that should be brought to the attention of the health care provider after discharge from the hospital, such as abdominal pain; nausea and vomiting; black, tarry stools; and weakness or dizziness. Clients are also taught diet patterns to be used to avoid postprandial distention or the dumping syndrome (see earlier).

After the individual is discharged, former patterns of living may require significant alteration. Strategies can be mutually identified by clients, families, and nurses to influence those required changes in a positive way.

For postsurgical clients, especially those with partial stomach removal, a smaller meal size may be required. Clients are instructed to have small, more frequent meals and to avoid drinking liquids with meals. Clients should be advised not to skip meals or go a long time without eating. In some cases, hot, spicy foods may cause symptoms and should be avoided. Clients are instructed to eliminate caffeine and alcohol consumption and to stop smoking. They are taught to avoid any product containing aspirin or ibuprofen. Regular follow-up visits to health care professionals should be scheduled.

Psychosocial Preparation

The client should be assisted in identifying how stress affects his or her life, in identifying situations that are stressful, in describing feelings during stressful situations, and in developing an awareness of patterns of coping with stressors. The nurse encourages the client to learn and use relaxation techniques such as exercise, yoga, biofeedback, humor, and imagery (see Chap. 6). Psychotherapy may be indicated to help some clients cope with stress.

The recurrence rate in gastric ulcer clients is lower than that in individuals with duodenal ulcers. It is essential for the client and family to understand how mod-

ified living, working, and eating habits are important in ulcer therapy to prevent recurrence.

Health Care Resources

No special equipment is needed. On occasion, clients may require dressings after surgical intervention. Referral to home care agencies may be indicated if clients or family members require instruction on any dimension of follow-up care such as dressing changes, IV therapy, monitoring of potential complications, or continued nutritional problems. Family members may need help, especially with follow-up after surgery, to modify eating habits and patterns.

▶ Evaluation

On the basis of the identified nursing diagnosis, the nurse evaluates the care for the client with ulcer disease. The expected outcomes include that the client

1. States that pain is reduced or alleviated and that comfort is achieved
2. States that nausea and vomiting are alleviated and that comfort is achieved
3. Identifies potential causes and risks for recurrence
4. Follows a nutritious diet that includes essential nutrients
5. Knows and reports early symptoms of recurrence or complications
6. Adheres to a plan for follow-up care and returns to the prior level of function in 6 to 8 weeks

ZOLLINGER-ELLISON SYNDROME

The *Zollinger-Ellison syndrome* is a hormonally induced peptic ulcer that is associated with autonomous secretion of gastrin by a rare islet cell tumor in the pancreas. The characteristic features are hypersecretion of acid with a high ratio of basal to maximal acid output and hypergastrinemia.

In addition to the peptic ulcers that are associated with gastrinomas, diarrhea may occur as a manifestation of this disorder. The diarrhea may be secondary to fat maldigestion from a low level of duodenal-inactivating pancreatic lipase or to malabsorption related to acid-induced injury of the villi.

The clinical manifestations of the Zollinger-Ellison syndrome are largely related to gastric acid hypersecretion. In part, this situation is due to hyperplasia of the gastric mucosa that is induced by the trophic effect of gastrin. The aim of therapy is to suppress acid secretion. Control of the hypersecretion controls the client's symptoms. In most clients, large doses of cimetidine or ranitidine are required. Anticholinergic drugs supplement the use of cimetidine. Two-hour gastric aspirations or 24-hour pH monitoring is used to evaluate control. Endoscopy is also indicated to evaluate clinical responses. If medical therapy fails, vagotomy and pyloroplasty may supplement the use of H₂ receptor blocking agents to control hypersecretion. A total gastrectomy becomes the surgical approach of choice for this disorder if vagotomy, pyloroplasty, and medical therapy are inadequate.

CARCINOMA

OVERVIEW

Gastric carcinoma refers to malignant neoplasms and tumors found in the stomach. Adenocarcinomas are the most common type of cancer, with malignant lymphoma the second most common.

Although the incidence of gastric cancer is decreasing in the United States, it is the sixth most common cause of cancer-related death. The onset is insidious, and the disease is often far advanced when detected.

Pathophysiology

Gastric adenocarcinoma develops from the mucous membrane within the stomach. Early gastric cancer is defined in pathologic terms (disease involving only the mucosa or submucosa) but is seldom symptomatic. Microscopically, the cells resemble intestinal metaplasia. The majority of gastric cancers develop in the pyloric and antral regions.

Gastric cancers have several methods of extension, including spread within the gastric wall and into regional lymphatics, as well as direct invasion of adjacent organs (e.g., liver, pancreas, transverse colon, and mesocolon). Hematogenous spread via the portal vein to the liver and via the systemic circulation to the lungs and bones are the most common modes of metastasis. Peritoneal seeding into the involved gastric serosa to the omentum, peritoneum, ovary, and pelvic cul-de-sac also occurs. Peritoneal seeding may produce a firm metastatic mass, which is referred to as a rectal shelf or Blumer's shelf and which is an indicator of advanced carcinomatosis.

The intramural lymphatics readily allow horizontal spread within the gastric wall. Extramural lymphatics carry tumor deposits to lymph nodes in more than 50%

of operable cases; nodes adjacent to the tumor are most often invaded, but up to 25% of cancers initially spread to lymph nodes that are distant from the tumor (Preece et al., 1986).

In advanced gastric cancer, there is invasion of the muscularis or beyond. These lesions are not amenable to curative resection, and overall there has not been significant improvement in results of treatment during the past 40 years. (See Chap. 24 for more specific information on the pathophysiology of carcinoma.)

Five-year survival rates are approximately 90% for stage I disease, 50% for stage II disease, and 10% for stage III disease; 5-year survival is exceedingly rare for individuals with stage IV disease. Unfortunately, most clients in the United States have stage III or IV disease when diagnosed (American Cancer Society, 1987). Lesions at the cardia or fundus have a poor prognosis because they are usually advanced when detected. The prognosis and treatment depend on the stage of disease and the general health status of the client. The American Joint Committee on Cancer classification system for gastric carcinoma is given in the accompanying Key Features of Disease.

Etiology

No etiologic factor has conclusively been proved to result in the development of gastric cancer. Pernicious anemia, gastric polyps, chronic atrophic gastritis, and achlorhydria appear to be factors that are associated with an increased risk for gastric cancer. Because of changes in the gastric mucosa, there may be more absorption of carcinogens when gastritis has been present. Gastric cancer appears to be positively correlated with ingestion of starch, pickled foods, salted fish, meat, and nitrates from processed foods and with a high salt consumption. It is *negatively correlated* with ingestion of whole milk, fresh vegetables, and vitamin C. Cigarette smoking is associated with gastric carcinoma, and genetic factors may play a role because there is an increased incidence in direct relatives.

There appears to be evidence that gastric surgery, especially a Billroth II procedure for benign conditions, increases the risk for gastric cancer, probably because of the development of atrophic gastritis. Bile reflux may also result in mucosal changes. Most cancers occur 20 years after the original surgical procedure (Berk, 1985; Preece et al., 1986).

Incidence

In the United States, the incidence of gastric carcinoma has decreased fivefold, from 25 to 5 per 100,000, during the past 50 years (American Cancer Society, 1987). The decline in the death rate is believed to be due primarily to the decreasing incidence of the disease rather than to improvements in treatment. Gastric cancer occurs more

KEY FEATURES OF DISEASE ■ TNM Classification for Gastric Carcinoma

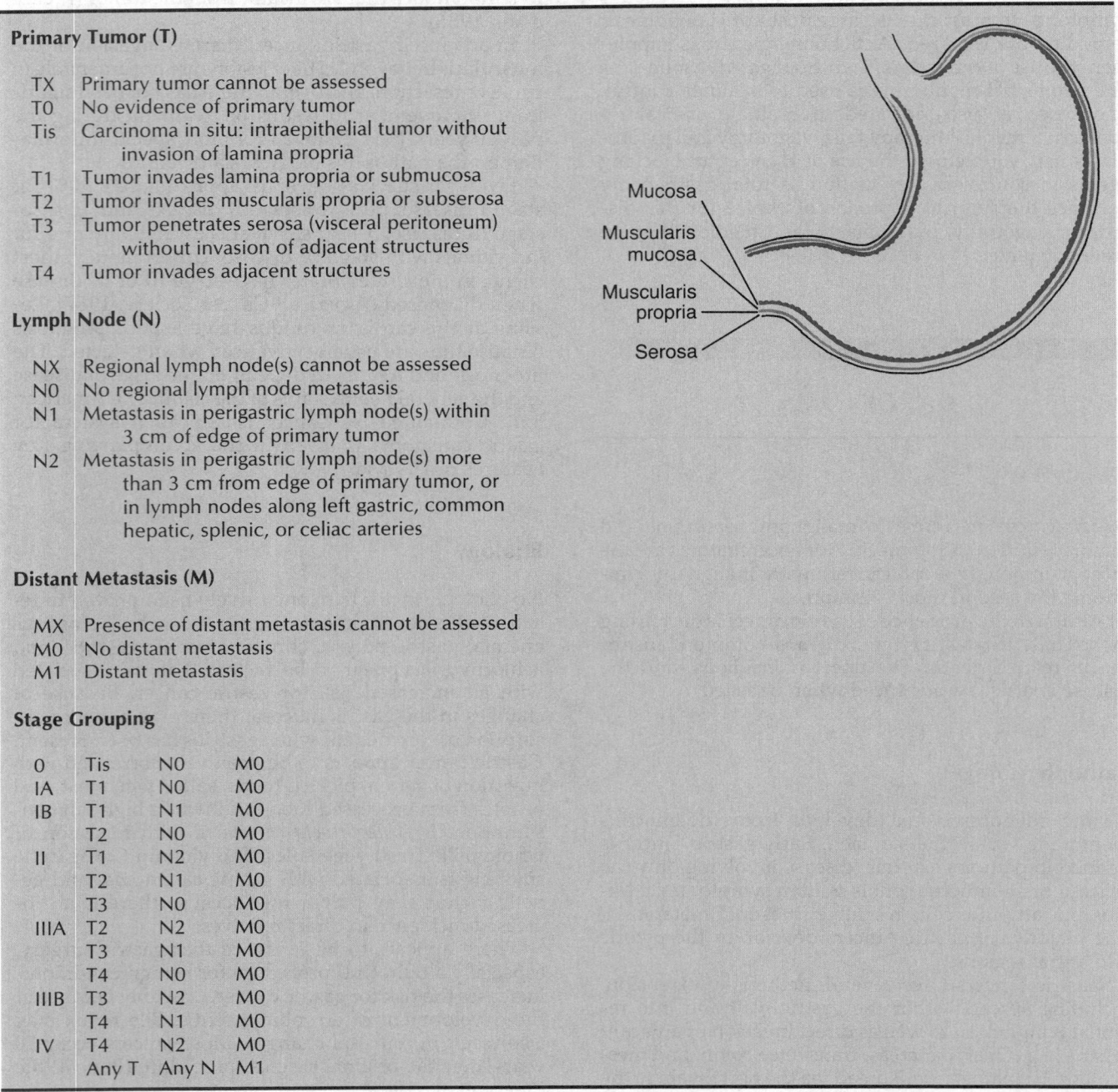

Primary Tumor (T)

TX	Primary tumor cannot be assessed
T0	No evidence of primary tumor
Tis	Carcinoma in situ: intraepithelial tumor without invasion of lamina propria
T1	Tumor invades lamina propria or submucosa
T2	Tumor invades muscularis propria or subserosa
T3	Tumor penetrates serosa (visceral peritoneum) without invasion of adjacent structures
T4	Tumor invades adjacent structures

Lymph Node (N)

NX	Regional lymph node(s) cannot be assessed
N0	No regional lymph node metastasis
N1	Metastasis in perigastric lymph node(s) within 3 cm of edge of primary tumor
N2	Metastasis in perigastric lymph node(s) more than 3 cm from edge of primary tumor, or in lymph nodes along left gastric, common hepatic, splenic, or celiac arteries

Distant Metastasis (M)

MX	Presence of distant metastasis cannot be assessed
M0	No distant metastasis
M1	Distant metastasis

Stage Grouping

0	Tis	N0	M0
IA	T1	N0	M0
IB	T1	N1	M0
	T2	N0	M0
II	T1	N2	M0
	T2	N1	M0
	T3	N0	M0
IIIA	T2	N2	M0
	T3	N1	M0
	T4	N0	M0
IIIB	T3	N2	M0
	T4	N1	M0
IV	T4	N2	M0
	Any T	Any N	M1

From American Joint Committee on Cancer. (1988). Beahrs, O. H., Henson, D. E., Hutter, R. V. P., & Myers, M. H. (Eds.). *Manual for staging of cancer* (3rd ed., p. 73). Philadelphia: J. B. Lippincott.

frequently in males than in females, with the incidence and mortality rates increasing with age, in Black persons, and in lower socioeconomic groups. The highest incidence of gastric cancer is in males older than 70 years of age. The disease remains common in Japan, Chile, Columbia, and Iceland, yet in the United States more than 25,000 new cases are diagnosed per year and there are more than 14,500 deaths (American Cancer Society,

1987). The incidence of gastric cancer is higher in the north central and northeast regions of the United States.

PREVENTION

After multiple bouts of gastritis that are unresponsive to treatment or recurrent symptoms after gastric surgery, clients need to have medical follow-up. A long lag time often occurs between the onset of symptoms and a diagnosis because of the vague and ill-defined nature of the complaints. Intractable symptoms need to be reported and medical assistance sought. Early detection, diagnosis, and treatment in the early stages of cancer will enable resection of lesions and a better prognosis. The public should be provided with information via the media regarding the need to seek medical evaluation for signs and symptoms such as recurrent heartburn, stomach upset, or pain. Self-medication for recurrent symptoms should be discouraged.

COLLABORATIVE MANAGEMENT

 Assessment

History

The nurse notes predisposing and risk factors to the development of gastric carcinoma when obtaining a client's history. Risk factors include a history of *gastric polyps, benign tumors, chronic gastritis, pernicious anemia, gastric surgery, male sex,* and *age more than 50 years.* The nurse takes a thorough *diet history* to determine whether the client frequently ingests large amounts of nitrates, salty foods, salted meats, pickled foods, or starch. Change in appetite and eating habits with or without a weight loss is also assessed, along with a *smoking history.* The presence of *pain* is assessed, including onset, duration, frequency, location, aggravating factors, alleviating factors, and resulting disability. A thorough *history of the present symptoms* is important because the early symptoms of gastric cancer are similar to those of ulcer disease.

Physical Assessment: Clinical Manifestations

There are no physical findings specifically associated with early gastric cancer. Any physical findings suggest advanced disease.

Five per cent to 10% of clients have complaints similar to those with ulcer disease (Preece et al., 1986). Symptoms or physical findings are rarely associated with "early" carcinoma of the stomach. When symptoms do occur, they are quite vague and ill defined. Symptoms are generally not produced until the tumor is advanced and of sufficient size to interfere with the motor activity of the stomach or to block the gastric luminal passage. Vomiting is a sign that usually occurs with pronounced dilation, thickening of the stomach wall, or pyloric obstruction. Obstructive symptoms appear earlier with tumors located near the pylorus than with fundic lesions.

In advanced gastric carcinoma, physical examination findings may be negative or an epigastric mass may be palpable, suggesting hepatomegaly from metastatic disease, or ascites. The presence of hard, enlarged lymph nodes in the left supraclavicular chain, left axilla, or umbilicus may be the result of metastasis from a gastric cancer. Except for cancer of the antrum, cancer of the

stomach, if palpable, is left of the midline. Masses on the right suggest metastasis in the perigastric lymph nodes or liver. Signs of distant metastasis include Virchow's (or sentinel) node (an enlarged supraclavicular lymph node, especially on the left), Blumer's shelf (resulting from peritoneal seeding), infiltration of the umbilicus, and Krukenberg's tumor (Berk, 1985; Preece et al., 1986). The most common physical findings are pallor and cachexia.

Acanthosis nigricans, a dermatosis with roughness and pigmentation, indicates cancer of the stomach. Recurrent episodes of phlebitis (Trosier's sign) that are unexplained by local findings in the extremities should warn the nurse of the possibility of an intra-abdominal (especially gastric and pancreatic) cancer.

Psychosocial Assessment

There do not appear to be particular psychologic characteristics of clients with gastric carcinoma. However, because of the poor prognosis associated with the diagnosis, the client may be anxious, depressed, and fearful. The client's coping mechanisms, strengths, and support systems are included in the assessment. The nurse assesses the family for the reaction to the diagnosis and the level of coping with the diagnosis of gastric cancer. Both the client and family require ongoing psychosocial counseling and support to deal with the adjustment and new information to deal with the diagnosis and radical treatments. Expressions by the client during the diagnostic phase such as denial, depression, withdrawal, and anger are to be expected. The nurse assists the client and family in dealing with these feelings.

Laboratory Findings

In clients with advanced disease, laboratory evidence of anemia as evidenced by a low hematocrit may develop. Clients may have macrocytic or microcytic anemia secondary to decreased iron or vitamin B_{12} absorption. The stool may be positive for occult blood. Hypoalbuminemia and abnormal liver tests (such as bilirubin and alkaline phosphatase occur with advanced disease and with hepatic metastasis. The level of carcinoembryonic antigen is elevated in advanced cancer of the stomach.

Radiographic Findings

An upper GI series is usually the first diagnostic test done. A polypoid mass, ulcer crater, or thickened fibrotic gastric wall may be evidence of gastric cancer.

Other Diagnostic Tests

Gastroscopy is also used for definitive diagnosis of gastric cancer because the lesion can be viewed directly, and benign and malignant lesions can be delineated. Cytologic brushing or gavage and biopsy may be used to determine the presence of cancer cells.

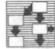 **Analysis: Nursing Diagnosis**

Common Diagnoses

The common diagnoses for clients with carcinoma of the stomach include

1. Potential for injury related to possible metastasis
2. Pain related to cancer
3. Altered nutrition: less than body requirements related to decreased appetite, nausea, vomiting, and pain

Additional Diagnoses

In addition, the client with advanced cancer may experience

1. Ineffective individual coping related to diagnosis and poor prognosis
2. Anticipatory grieving related to loss of former health status
3. Anxiety related to surgery, hospitalization, diagnosis, and role and life style changes
4. Fear related to life-threatening illness and treatment
5. Activity intolerance related to impaired physical mobility and malnourishment
6. Fluid volume deficit related to vomiting
7. Sleep pattern disturbance related to pain, hospitalization, and anxiety
8. Knowledge deficit related to treatment regimen for cancer
9. Impaired physical mobility related to pain and activity intolerance

 Planning and Implementation

Potential for Injury

Planning: client goals. The major goal for this diagnosis is that the client will not have metastasis or recurrence of gastric cancer.

Interventions. Individuals and families need to be taught how to adjust to metastatic disease should it occur. If there is no metastasis, family members and clients are taught to be aware of early signs of recurrence and are encouraged not to delay in seeking health care if symptoms occur.

Nonsurgical management. Nonsurgical management is used together with surgery and includes chemotherapy and, less frequently, radiation.

Drug therapy. Chemotherapy may be used with advanced disease (stage III or IV), but the results are poor. Combination-drug therapies are more effective than single agents, but the median survival time in responders is only approximately 1 year with both approaches.

At present, the procedure of choice appears to be the use of chemotherapy as an adjunct to surgical treatment.

The combination of fluorouracil, doxorubicin (Adriamycin), and mitomycin C (part of the FAM regimen of fluorouracil, doxorubicin, and mitomycin) or methyl CCNU (semustine) seems particularly efficacious. Removal of as much tumor as possible to reduce the tumor burden may enhance the response to chemotherapy. This fact supports the practice of resection of the gastric tumor. The combination of radiotherapy with chemotherapy after resection has also been recommended.

Radiation therapy. Radiation therapy is not the treatment of choice. However, high doses of radiation may be used, and radiation may be done in conjunction with surgery.

Surgical management. In early gastric cancer, surgery is usually curative. Distal subtotal resection, combined with adequate lymph node dissection, is the therapy of choice. Curative resection can be offered to only 40% to 60% of clients, however, because the remainder have advanced disease. Most of the latter clients are candidates for palliative surgical treatment (Berk, 1985). Demonstration of metastatic involvement by Virchow's nodes, in inguinal lymph nodes, in the liver, in the umbilicus, or by Blumer's shelf indicates that the opportunity for cure by resection is lost.

The type of gastric surgery performed depends on the location of the tumor in the stomach and the extent of the disease. The procedures involve wide excision of the cancer site, possibly including adjacent tissues. The excision may be a subtotal or a total gastrectomy and may include resection of a portion of the esophagus for cancer of the proximal stomach and a portion of the duodenum for cancer of the distal stomach.

Definitive radical surgical resection should be limited to lesions confined to the stomach and neighboring lymph nodes. When the lesion is in the distal two-thirds of the stomach, surgery involves a *subtotal gastrectomy,* with omentum and the relevant nodes en bloc; the spleen and its nodes are included in the resection. Alimentary continuity after subtotal resection is restored by a gastroduodenostomy (a Billroth I procedure), if the ends of the stomach and duodenum can be approximated without tension, or by a gastrojejunostomy (a Billroth II procedure) (see earlier).

Palliative resection may significantly improve the quality of life for a client suffering from obstruction, hemorrhage, or pain. Palliative treatment is all that can be offered to the 40% to 60% of clients with gastric cancer. Appropriate gastroenterostomy or intubation may achieve palliation for lesions at the gastric outlet (see earlier). The prognosis for clients who do not have a curative surgical resection is poor.

A growth in the upper one-third of the stomach requires a *total gastrectomy,* with en bloc removal of the spleen and omentum (Fig. 44–10). Total gastrectomy should not be performed as a palliative procedure and is not used on a routine basis unless lesions are near the esophagogastric junction. With a total gastrectomy, ei-

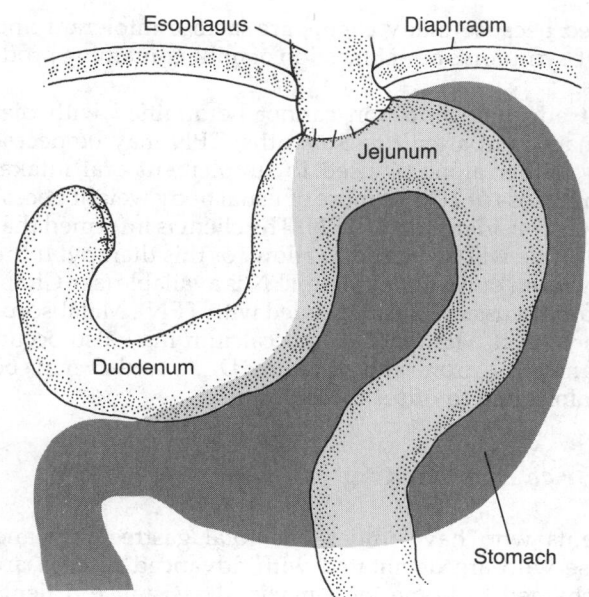

Figure 44-10

Total gastrectomy with anastomosis of the esophagus to the jejunum (esophagojejunostomy) is the principal medical intervention for extensive gastric cancer.

ther the esophagus is sutured to the duodenum or the jejunum is positioned between the esophagus and the remaining small bowel to reconstruct the continuity of the GI tract. After total gastrectomy, the resulting disability is a fair exchange when there is a hope of cure but not in the presence of incurable disease. For clients with cardioesophageal cancer, esophagogastrostomy may be used.

Preoperative care. The client is given an explanation of the disease and the treatment options available (potentially curative or palliative). The nurse reinforces and clarifies the information given. This knowledge aids the client in making decisions about care.

Some of the most common concerns of cancer clients and families are fear of alienation from family, friends, or health care providers; mutilation, particularly if radical surgery is the treatment of choice; and vulnerability, dependence, or lack of control. To assist clients and families in coping with these concerns, the nurse provides hope while avoiding false optimism by using a gentle, unhurried manner in expressing concern and by focusing on clients' strengths rather than weaknesses.

Opportunity is provided for clients and families to discuss their feelings and concerns about the diagnosis, treatment, and expected treatment outcome. Their expectations about the outcome of surgery are assessed in terms that are realistic to the situation. Specific information must be provided about preparatory procedures for surgery (e.g., laboratory tests, NPO status, and IV catheters); informed consent for surgery (including information on type and length of surgery); and expected recov-

ery course (including the client's condition after surgery, altered level of functioning, anticipated problems, and potential complications).

Postoperative care. Clients receive routine postoperative care that is given to clients who receive general anesthesia (see Chap. 20).

Complications that may follow gastric surgery include duodenal stump leakage, hemorrhage, obstruction, gastric dilation resulting in reflux gastritis, delayed gastric emptying, anemia, nutritional deficiency, and dumping syndrome. These complications are described earlier under the heading Peptic Ulcer Disease.

Pain

Planning: client goals. The major goal for this nursing diagnosis is that the client will experience a reduction or alleviation of pain.

Interventions: nonsurgical management. Many clients with pain do not obtain the relief that they need or desire from pain. Improperly treated discomfort results in interference with eating, sleeping, and socializing. Untreated pain results in weight loss, decreased strength, and overall deterioration in physical and mental status. It is imperative that pain be managed. Chapter 7 discusses pain management in detail.

The pain that is associated with gastric cancer because of tumor growth and metastasis may develop late in the course of the disease. Clients report epigastric distress, tenderness, pain, or nausea.

Assisting the client to identify and develop strategies that provide optimal pain relief is the focus of nonsurgical intervention.

Drug therapy. Pain may require medication for control in the advanced stages of the disease. Nonnarcotic (e.g., acetaminophen) or narcotic (e.g., codeine, meperidine [Demerol], and morphine sulfate) analgesics are provided as ordered. Clients may control the pain with use of pumps for IV analgesics. The nurse assesses the therapeutic effects of medications, possible side effects, and the need for titration of medication related to worsening pain or level of somnolence.

Stress reduction. Fear and anxiety with resultant fatigue often exacerbate the pain experience and result in an ever-increasing cycle of pain. Noninvasive measures to increase comfort by reducing stress include relaxation techniques, cutaneous stimulation, and visual imagery. Clients are counseled about possible methods for relieving stress (see Chap. 6).

Altered Nutrition: Less Than Body Requirements

Planning: client goals. The goal for this nursing diagnosis is that the client will increase nutritional intake to meet metabolic requirements and to maintain normal body weight.

Interventions: nonsurgical management. Alterations in nutrition related to decreased appetite, nausea and vomiting, and pain may be present before surgery. This altered nutritional state is then exacerbated in the postoperative client. The presence of malnutrition may lead to decreased blood volume, hemoconcentration, alterations in fluid and electrolyte balance, and decreased resistance to infection.

Nutritional therapy is an important aspect of preoperative and postoperative management of the client with gastric cancer. Severe tissue wasting is of major clinical significance to clients with advanced disease. Early satiety, abdominal distention, and pain may contribute to inadequate intake of nutrients. Weight loss up to 10% may occur. Steatorrhea related to malabsorption may contribute to this problem if a total gastrectomy has been performed.

Pain medication may relieve discomfort and allow the client to eat or drink more comfortably. Medications for relief of nausea, such as prochlorperazine (Compazine) and thiethylperazine (Torecan), may also improve the client's appetite.

To correct malnutrition before surgery, supplements to the diet and total parenteral nutrition (TPN) may be used. Vitamins with minerals, iron, and protein supplements are essential to correct nutritional deficits. To improve caloric intake, the nurse works with the client and family to determine food preferences, cultural norms, and the usual eating habits of the client. Clients tend to do better with frequent small meals and avoidance of spicy foods. The nurse guides the client and family to provide the most nutrients and calories for the client. Counseling about methods and types of food to increase caloric and protein intake is essential. Intake, output, and calorie counts are kept on a daily basis. Weights are recorded on at least a weekly basis.

Postoperative diet management may include the use of TPN to provide necessary nutrients and to prevent further deficiencies until oral intake is adequate. Oral intake should begin with fluids and should progress to solids as tolerated by the client. For clients who had esophageal or stomach surgery, regurgitation may result from eating too much or too fast. After oral feedings have been reinstituted, clients should be observed for signs and symptoms of the dumping syndrome. Clients should be taught the manifestations of the syndrome and how to avert it by frequent feedings and intake of high-protein, high-fat, low-carbohydrate foods. This diet is intended for clients who have recovered sufficiently from gastric surgery to eat regular foods but who are experiencing, or are likely to experience, the dumping, or jejunal, syndrome, which is caused by the formation of a concentrated hyperosmolar solution. The basic principles of the diet are the same as those for the postgastrectomy diet, with the exception that regular foods are used in place of bland foods. The diet is high in protein and fat and low in carbohydrate; food is given in six small daily feedings. Liquids should not be taken with meals. Milk and dairy products are usually eliminated because many clients are lactose intolerant and have symptoms after ingestion of milk-containing products.

If adequate nutrition cannot be attained with diet management after 2 to 3 months, TPN may be necessary, either alone or used to supplement oral intake. Weight loss of 10% or more of usual body weight necessitates consideration of TPN. The client is informed that an IV line will be placed to allow for this therapy. If the client is an outpatient, home TPN is available (see Chap. 13 for discussion of care needed with TPN). Malabsorption of iron, vitamin B_{12}, and calcium may also occur. Vitamin B_{12}, iron, and vitamins D, A, and B may be administered to offset these deficits.

■ Discharge Planning

Clients who have undergone total gastrectomy and those who are debilitated with advanced disease are discharged to home with maximal assistance. Clients who have undergone a subtotal gastrectomy without debilitation may be discharged to home with partial assistance for activities of daily living. Many clients have recurrence of the cancer and need regular follow-up examinations and radiographic assessments.

Home Care Preparation

The client and family need a list of medications to be taken and when they should be given. The nurse demonstrates home treatments such as dressing changes, and the client and family members responsible for care demonstrate these procedures in return.

The home of the client is assessed for the actual physical set-up and the ease of reaching the bathroom, bedroom, and kitchen facilities to enable the client to have mobility and care. It is important to know who will help care for the client at home and who will provide relief and/or assistance for the family caregiver.

Client/Family Education

The nurse gives instructions about recommended nutritional therapy, pain management, and medications. If clients are discharged with dressings, the nurse teaches the family about clean dressing changes and the signs and symptoms of incisional infection for which to watch and report, such as fever, redness, and drainage. Clients who will be receiving radiation therapy or chemotherapy require instructions related to the side effects of these treatments. See Chapter 25 for education for clients receiving chemotherapy or radiation therapy.

Psychosocial Preparation

Clients may have fears postoperatively about returning home related to their inability to care for themselves adequately and to control or minimize pain. Enlisting family and health care resources for the client may ease some of the anxiety about returning home. The family needs to have adequate information and support systems available to make the transition to home care easier for the client. If family members are still trying to cope with the diagnosis and poor prognosis of the client, their coping abilities will be impaired. If prognosis is poor, the client and the family need continued professional support to cope with death and dying. Chapter 25 discusses the psychosocial aspects of cancer, and Chapter 11 describes nursing interventions for the dying client.

Clients and families need to have continued support and an empathic approach from the nurse. It is essential that clients for whom cure is not possible, those for whom relapse has occurred, and those who do not respond to treatment do not feel abandoned. Clients and families must be included in making all decisions about further care. In many clients with gastric cancer, a trade-off of quality of life must be made against a possible survival. The psychosocial dimensions of care are as important a consideration as are the diagnostic and therapeutic dimensions.

It may be important to facilitate a support group contact. Clients can better communicate the feelings experienced in response to cancer with each other.

Health Care Resources

A home care nursing referral provides ongoing assessment, assistance, and encouragement to the client and family at home. A home care nurse can help the client and family with physical care procedures and can provide valuable psychologic support as well. This combination of resources helps to minimize anxieties of the individual and family.

Other referrals that might be necessary are to a dietitian, professional counselor, clergy or religious or spiritual leader, and hospice team. The coordinator of the client's care should be the person to arrange the referrals to ensure comprehensive care for the client and family. Appropriate support groups such as I Can Cope, provided by the American Cancer Society, can be a major resource (see Chap. 25).

 Evaluation

On the basis of the identified nursing diagnoses, the nurse evaluates the care of the individual with gastric cancer. The expected outcomes include that the client

1. Verbalizes feelings related to emotional state, identifies coping patterns and personal strengths, and receives support from family, friends, and health care professionals
2. Manages the pain and states that increased comfort has been achieved
3. Experiences adequate nutrition through oral intake, TPN, or a combination of therapies

SUMMARY

The success and ongoing effectiveness of care of the client with gastric disorders depend on the prevention of recurrence and complications, compliance with the therapeutic regimen, and client and family teaching and follow-up. Often the occurrence and course of the illness can be influenced by the client's behavior, e.g., an early response to symptoms. The nurse has an important role in assisting clients to achieve a high level of self-care and control. In general, little change has occurred in the management of these conditions during the past few years.

IMPLICATIONS FOR RESEARCH

Little research specific to gastric disorders is found in the nursing literature. A review of pertinent journals spanning 10 years revealed *no references related to gastric cancer, gastritis, or PUD.* Clearly, nursing research is needed to document common procedures and practices, and important work is needed to understand compliance behaviors for long-term therapy for PUD, strategies for the prevention of gastritis, and early detection and symptom control for the client with stomach cancer. The mechanisms related to management of symptoms of PUD need to be described.

Some specific research questions include

1. What is the quality of life after various surgical procedures for clients with gastric disease, e.g., Billroth II, total gastrectomy, and Billroth I?
2. What are the requirements of home care needs for clients with gastric cancer, for those with total gastrectomy, and for those with or without chemotherapy?
3. How long before diagnosis of gastric cancer do clients have vague and ill-defined symptoms of distress?
4. What is the compliance of PUD clients for following a specified diet, for taking antacids, or for making other life style alterations? How does the compliance relate to disease control?
5. What are barriers to seeking early health care for clients with gastric symptoms? What nursing strategies are effective in reducing those barriers?

REFERENCES AND READINGS

General

Alexander-Williams, J. (1984). Evaluation and management of postgastric operative system. In J. S. Najarian & J. P. Delaney (Eds.), *Advances in gastrointestinal surgery* (5th ed., pp. 205–212). Chicago: Year Book Medical.

Bates, B. (1985). *A guide to physical examination* (3rd ed.). Philadelphia: J. B. Lippincott.

Berk, J. E. (Ed.). (1985). *Bockus gastroenterology* (4th ed., Vols. 2 & 7). Philadelphia: W. B. Saunders.

Carpenito, L. J. (1983). *Nursing diagnosis: Application to clinical practice.* Philadelphia: J. B. Lippincott.

Clemente, C. (1985). *Gray's anatomy* (13th ed.). Philadelphia: Lea & Febiger.

Dworken, H. (1981). *Gastroenterology: Pathophysiology and clinical applications.* Stoneham, MA: Butterworth's.

Given, B. A., & Simmons, S. J. (1984). *Gastroenterology in clinical nursing* (4th ed.). St. Louis: C. V. Mosby.

Grabinar, J. (1987). Upper GI pain: Causes, clues and action. *Geriatric Medicine, 47*(8), 67–70.

Hamilton, H., & Rose, M. B. (1985). *Gastrointestinal disorders.* Springhouse, PA: Springhouse Corp.

Knauer, C. M., & Silverman, S. (1988). Alimentary tract and liver. In S. A. Schroeder, M. A. Krupp, & L. M. Tierney (Eds.), *Current medical diagnosis and treatment* (pp. 342–428). Norwalk, CT: Appleton & Lange.

Moore, K. (1985). *Clinically oriented anatomy* (2nd ed.). Baltimore: Williams & Wilkins.

Skinner, S. M. (1985, December). Gastric lavage. *Nursing '85,* 56M–56O.

Spiro, H. M. (1983). *Clinical gastroenterology* (3rd ed.). New York: Macmillan.

Stewart, J. (1986). *Clinical anatomy and physiology for the frustrated health professional.* Miami: MedMaster.

Thompson, J. M., McFarland, G. K., Hirsch, J. E., Tucker, S. M., & Bowers, A. C. (1986). *Clinical nursing.* St. Louis: C. V. Mosby.

Vander, A. (1985). *Human physiology: The mechanism of body function.* New York: McGraw-Hill.

Walt, A. J. (1986). Erosive gastritis. In D. C. Sabiston, Jr. (Ed.), *Textbook of surgery: The biological basis of modern surgical practice* (13th ed., pp. 862–868). Philadelphia: W. B. Saunders.

Gastritis

Cheli, R., Perasso, A., & Giacosa, A. (1987). *Gastritis: A critical review.* New York: Springer-Verlag.

Martin, L. F., Larson, G. M., & Fry, D. E. (1985). Bleeding from stress gastritis. Has prophylactic pH control made a difference? *American Surgeon, 51,* 189–193.

Siler, W. (1985). Pathogenic factors in erosive gastritis. *American Journal of Medicine, 29,* 45–48.

Strickland, R. G. (1983). Acute and chronic gastritis. *Hospital Medicine, 19,* 148, 153–154.

Peptic Ulcer Disease

Achkar, E. (1985). Peptic ulcer disease: Current management in the elderly. *Geriatrics, 40*(9), 77–83.

Bardhan, K. D. (1986). Gastric ulcer: Sparing patients from surgery. *Geriatric Medicine, 40*(5), 41–44.

Brooks, F. P., Cohen, S., & Soloway, R. D. (1985). *Peptic ulcer disease: Contemporary issues in gastroenterology* (Vol. 3). New York: Churchill Livingstone.

Connor, P. (1988). Management of upper gastrointestinal tract hemorrhage. *Update in medical-surgical nursing.* Proceedings of the meeting at Lahey Clinic Medical Center, Burlington, MA.

Farinati, F., Cardin, F., Di Mario, F., Battaglia, G., Cannizzaro, R., Penon, G., and Naccarato, R. (1988). Gastric ulcer and stomach aging: Pathophysiology and clinical implications. *Gerontology, 34,* 297–303.

Fink, A. S., & Longmire, W. P., Jr. (1986). Carcinoma of the stomach. In D. C. Sabiston, Jr. (Ed.)., *Textbook of surgery: The biological basis of modern surgical practice* (13th ed., pp. 881–896). Philadelphia: W. B. Saunders.

Isenberg, J. I., Peterson, W. L., Elashorf, J. D., Sandersfeld, M. A., Reedy, T. J., Ippoliti, A. F., Van Deventer, G. M., Frankl, L. H., Longstreth, G. F., & Anderson, D. S. (1983). Healing of benign gastric ulcer with low-dose antacid or cimetidine. A double-blind, randomized, placebo-controlled trial. *New England Journal of Medicine, 308,* 1319–1324.

Jaup, B. H., Stockbrugger, R., & Dotevall, G. (1982). Pirenzepine: A new antisecretory compound for the therapy of peptic ulcer disease. In C. J. Pfeiffer (Ed.), *Drugs and peptic ulcer: Therapeutic agents for peptic ulcer disease* (Vol. I). Boca Raton, FL: CRC Press.

Jensen, R. T., Collen, M. J., Pandol, S. J., Allende, H. D., Raufman, J. P., Bissonnette, B. M., Duncan, W. C., Durgin, P. L., Gillin, J. C., & Gardner, J. D. (1983). Cimetidine-induced impotence and breast changes in patients with gastric hypersecretory states. *New England Journal of Medicine, 308,* 883–887.

Nelis, G. F., Boeve, J., & Misiewicz, J. J. (1985). *Peptic ulcer disease: Basic and clinical aspects.* Boston: Martinus Nijhoff.

Thompson, J. C. (1986). The stomach and duodenum. In D. C. Sabiston, Jr. (Ed.), *Textbook of surgery: The biological basis of modern surgical practice* (13th ed., pp. 810–853). Philadelphia: W. B. Saunders.

Cancer

American Cancer Society. (1986). Gastric cancer. *CA: A Cancer Journal for Clinicians, 36.*

American Cancer Society. (1987). *Cancer facts and figures.* New York: Author.

American Joint Committee on Cancer. (1988). Beahrs, O. H., Henson, D. E., Hutter, R. V. P., & Myers, M. H. (Eds.). *Manual for staging of cancer* (3rd ed.). Philadelphia: J. B. Lippincott.

Craven, J. L., & Cuschieri, A. (1984). Treatment of gastric cancer. *Clinics in Oncology, 3,* 309–325.

Cushman, K. E. (1986). Symptom management: A comprehensive approach to increasing nutritional status in the cancer patient. *Seminars in Oncology Nursing: Nutrition and Cancer, 2*(1), 30–35.

Douglass, H. O. (1986). Current management of gastric cancer: Analysis of recent advances. *Current Concepts in Oncology, 8*(3), 3–8.

Groenwald, S. L. (1987). *Cancer nursing: Principles and practice.* Boston: Jones & Bartlett.

Koga, S., Takebayaski, M., Kaibara, N., & Nishido, H. (1987). Pathological characteristics of gastric cancer that develop hematogenous recurrence, with special reference to the site of recurrence. *Journal of Surgical Oncology, 36,* 239–242.

Lindsey, A. M. (1986). Cancer cachexia: Effects of the disease and its treatment. *Seminars in Oncology Nursing: Nutrition and Cancer, 2*(1), 19–29.

Mayer, R. (1988). Gastrointestinal cancer. In E. Rubenstein & D. Federman (Eds.), *Scientific American medicine* (pp. 1–17). New York: Scientific American.

Preece, P. E., Cuschieri, A., & Weelwood, J. M. (1986). *Cancer of the stomach.* New York: Grune & Stratton.

Schafer, L. W., Larson, D. E., Melton, L. J., Higgins, J. A., & Ilstrup, D. M. (1983). The risk of gastric carcinoma after surgical treatment for benign ulcer disease. *New England Journal of Medicine, 309,* 1210–1213.

Viste, A., Haugstvedt, T., Eide, G. E., & Sreide, O. (1988). Postoperative complications and mortality after surgery for gastric cancer. *Annals of Surgery, 207,* 7–13.

ADDITIONAL READINGS

Frank-Stromberg, M. (1989). The epidemiology and primary prevention of gastric and esophageal cancer. *Cancer Nursing, 12*(2), 53–64.

This article discusses the epidemiology and primary prevention of gastric and esophageal cancer throughout the world. The author, a nurse, identifies risk factors, early signs and symptoms, and early detection procedures for both types of cancer.

Konopad, E., & Noseworthy, T. (1988). Stress ulceration: A serious complication in critically ill patients. *Heart and Lung, 17,* 339–348.

This article discusses the pathophysiology of stress ulceration in critically ill clients. Although the pathophysiology of stress ulceration is not completely understood, a number of factors have been identified. The authors state that primary prevention is the cornerstone of management, with the goal being the maintenance of gastric pH greater than 3.5. Management of stress ulceration includes the administration of antacids, histamine receptor antagonists, sucralfate, and/or prostaglandins, all of which are discussed.

Patras, A, Paice, J., & Lanigan, K. (1984). Managing GI bleeding: It takes a two-track mind. *Nursing '84, 14*(7), 26–33.

This article discusses causes and sites of GI bleeding, key questions to be used for obtaining a history from clients with GI bleeding, and diagnostic tests. Medication therapy and surgical procedures for treatment of GI hemorrhage are briefly outlined.

U.S. Department of Health and Human Services. (1988). *Cancer of the stomach* (NIH Publication No. 88-2978). Bethesda: National Cancer Institute.

This research report describes the different types of stomach cancer, as well as their incidence, associated factors in development, and methods of detection, diagnosis, staging, and treatment. Information on clinical trials and on how to obtain other cancer resources available through the National Cancer Institute (NCI) is provided in this pamphlet. To obtain this and other NCI publications, call the Cancer Information Service at 1-800-4-CANCER.

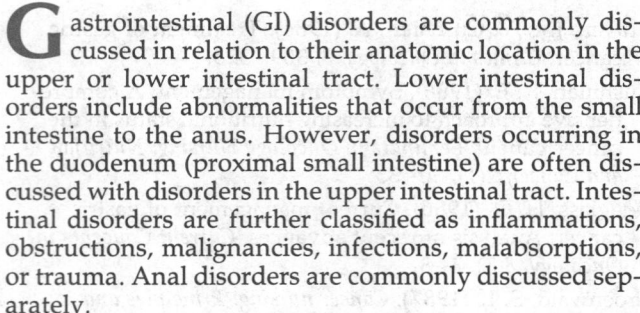

CHAPTER 45

Interventions for Clients with Intestinal Disorders

Gastrointestinal (GI) disorders are commonly discussed in relation to their anatomic location in the upper or lower intestinal tract. Lower intestinal disorders include abnormalities that occur from the small intestine to the anus. However, disorders occurring in the duodenum (proximal small intestine) are often discussed with disorders in the upper intestinal tract. Intestinal disorders are further classified as inflammations, obstructions, malignancies, infections, malabsorptions, or trauma. Anal disorders are commonly discussed separately.

Clinical manifestations of many intestinal disorders commonly include changes in stool pattern, abdominal pain, and rectal bleeding (see the accompanying illustration). These symptoms can be vague and insidious or can occur abruptly with significant insult to the client. Identification of the specific disorder is often difficult owing to common symptoms among intestinal diseases. The nurse's involvement in assessing and managing intestinal disorders is essential to early diagnosis and successful treatment.

GASTROENTERITIS

OVERVIEW

Gastroenteritis is an inflammation of the mucous membranes of the stomach and the intestinal tract. It primarily affects the small bowel and can be either viral or bacterial in origin. Both viral and bacterial forms of gastroenteritis have similar manifestations and are generally considered self-limiting in their course, unless complications occur. All organisms that are implicated in gastroenteritis cause diarrhea; however, these organisms have distinguishing characteristics.

Authors vary with regard to classifying the infectious diseases described as gastroenteritis. Some investigators include shigellosis when discussing gastroenteritis; others discuss shigellosis separately as a dysentery. Dysenteries affect the large bowel, and gastroenteritis is defined as affecting the small bowel. Other authors classify infectious disease of the intestine as bacterial, viral, and parasitic, without using the term gastroenteritis. Food poisoning is sometimes described in conjunction with gastroenteritis, specifically referring to the organism responsible for the food poisoning. Gastroenteritis, however, differs from food poisoning with regard to transmission in the body, incubation time, and effect on immunity. The discussion of gastroenteritis in this text includes epidemic viral gastroenteritis, rotavirus gastroenteritis, *Campylobacter* enteritis, *Eschericia coli* gastroenteritis, and shigellosis. (Organisms associated with food poisoning and parasitic infections are discussed later.)

COMMON CAUSES OF LOWER GI BLEEDING

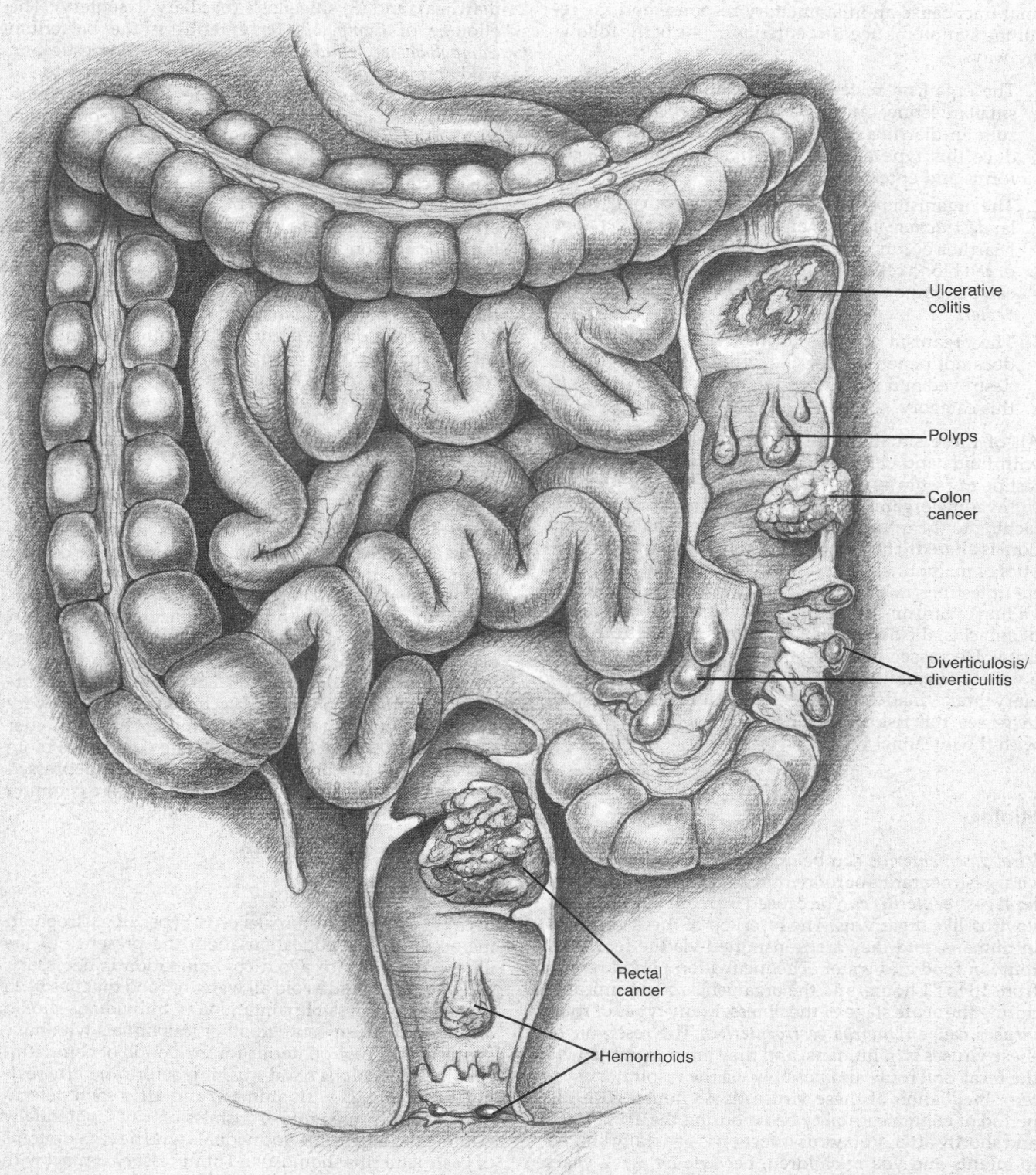

Ulcerative colitis

Polyps

Colon cancer

Diverticulosis/ diverticulitis

Rectal cancer

Hemorrhoids

Pathophysiology

Both viral and bacterial organisms entering the intestinal tract cause an inflammatory response and the resulting symptoms of gastroenteritis in one of the following ways:

1. The organism releases enterotoxin that acts on the small intestine, causing *local inflammation,* which results in diarrhea. Examples of organisms that produce this type of gastroenteritis are some *Shigella* forms and enterotoxigenic *E. coli.*

2. The organism *penetrates* the intestine, causing cellular *destruction, necrosis,* and a potential for *ulceration.* Diarrhea occurs, often with white blood cells (WBCs) or red blood cells (RBCs). Examples of organisms that can penetrate the intestine are *Shigella* and *Campylobacter.*

3. The organism attaches to mucosal epithelium, but does not penetrate it. Cells of the intestinal villi are destroyed and malabsorption results. Rotavirus is in this category.

All of these situations result in *increased* GI motility, with fluids and electrolytes being secreted into the intestine at fast rates.

Invading organisms have increased capabilities of attaching to the intestinal mucosa if the normal intestinal flora is altered. This can occur in clients receiving antibiotics or malnourished and debilitated clients. The pH of the intestines normally defends the intestine from invading organisms. If the pH is elevated, as with the use of antacids, the defense mechanism is not as effective as usual. Decreased intestinal motility, which can occur in a variety of conditions (e.g., immobility, inadequate dietary intake, inadequate fiber intake, and drug therapy), increases the risk of pathogens' establishing contact with the intestinal wall.

Etiology

Viral gastroenteritis can be classified as either epidemic viral gastroenteritis or rotavirus gastroenteritis. *Epidemic viral gastroenteritis* can be caused by many types of parvovirus-like organisms. The reservoir of these viruses is in humans, and they are transmitted via the fecal-oral route in food and water. The incubation period ranges from 10 to 51 hours, and the organism is communicable during the acute stage of the illness. Many types of rotaviruses cause *rotavirus gastroenteritis.* The reservoir of these viruses is in humans, and they are transmitted via the fecal-oral route and possibly via the respiratory system. Incubation of these viruses is 48 hours, with the period of communicability being during the acute stage and shortly after. Rotavirus infection is generally limited to infants and young children, because by age 2 years most individuals have acquired antibodies against most types of these viruses.

Bacterial gastroenteritis can be divided into three general types: (1) *Campylobacter* enteritis (traveler's diarrhea), (2) *E. coli* diarrhea (also referred to as traveler's diarrhea), and (3) shigellosis (bacillary dysentery). The etiology of *Campylobacter* enteritis is the bacterium *Campylobacter jejuni.* Its reservoirs are domestic and wild animals and birds. It is transmitted by ingestion of water or food contaminated with feces, by contact with infected animals or infants, and via the fecal-oral route. Incubation ranges from 1 to 10 days, and it is communicable for several days to weeks throughout the course of the infection (usually 2 to 7 weeks). Carriers of the bacteria are rare. The reservoirs of *E. coli* are humans, who are often asymptomatic. Transmission of the organism is via fecally contaminated food, water, or fomites.

Shigellosis is caused by different groups of *Shigella* bacteria, which have many strains. The reservoirs of these bacteria are humans, and direct or indirect fecal-oral transmission can occur from an infected person or carrier. Incubation is 1 to 7 days. The illness can be communicated during the acute phase to 4 weeks after. A person may be a carrier of this illness for months after the acute illness.

Incidence

Epidemic viral gastroenteritis occurs throughout the world and is common. As its name suggests, this disease often occurs in epidemic outbreaks among groups of people. *Campylobacter* enteritis occurs worldwide, commonly in epidemic outbreaks. Its incidence is highest during warm months. Diarrhea caused by *E. coli* also occurs worldwide, commonly in epidemics, with its highest incidence being in areas of poor sanitation during warm months. *Shigellosis* occurs worldwide in every age group, but is most frequent among children under the age of 10 years. Children and the elderly are more susceptible to this organism because of their depressed immune systems. Outbreaks of shigellosis are common in areas with crowded living conditions.

PREVENTION

Because epidemic outbreaks of all types of gastroenteritis occur, public education about the presence of the illness and ways to avoid contamination is necessary. Individuals should avoid all water or food that has been identified as a possible contaminant. Individuals should also limit their exposure to other individuals who have symptoms of gastroenteritis for the period of communicability. Meticulous hand washing before and after eating, after contact with animals, and after each defecation would prevent transmission of potentially pathogenic organisms. Individuals who have symptoms of gastroenteritis should avoid unnecessary contact with others during the acute stage and possibly up to several months after the illness, depending on the type of gastroenteritis (e.g., one can be a carrier of shigellosis for months).

Nurses and others who care for clients with gastroenteritis should consistently use blood and body fluid precautions (Chap. 26).

COLLABORATIVE MANAGEMENT

 Assessment

History

Most clients with gastroenteritis describe an acute onset of diarrhea. Data the nurse collects include the *age* and *sex* of the client, a description of the *first symptoms of diarrhea,* whether nausea and vomiting were present, and the date that symptoms first began. The nurse asks the client about the health of those in the client's household and contacts outside the home. The client is also asked about recent and past *travel* and specific locations visited. Ingestion of contaminated food or water and common symptoms with others who ingested the same food or water could indicate gastroenteritis or food poisoning.

It is particularly important to identify the *sequence in which symptoms occurred.* Abdominal pain that occurs *before* the onset of nausea, vomiting, and diarrhea is more characteristic of appendicitis.

Physical Assessment: Clinical Manifestations

All clients with gastroenteritis classically have *diarrhea.* The consistency and amount varies with the causative organism. *Shigellosis* causes stools with blood and mucus, which can continue for up to 5 days. *Campylobacter* enteritis causes foul-smelling stools with blood, which can number 20 to 30 per day up to 7 days. *E. coli* gastroenteritis may or may not cause blood or mucus in the stool, and diarrhea can last for up to 10 days. *Rotavirus* gastroenteritis causes watery diarrhea, lasting up to 8 days; rectal bleeding can occur. Diarrhea associated with *epidemic viral gastroenteritis* is typically limited to 24 to 48 hours. *Nausea* and *vomiting* can occur with all types, but are usually limited to the first 1 or 2 days of the illness.

The client usually appears ill. Temperature can be normal or elevated from 101° to 103° F (38.2° to 39.2° C). With *Campylobacter* enteritis or shigellosis, the client's temperature may be as high as 105° F (40° C). *Abdominal pain* typically occurs with *Campylobacter* enteritis and shigellosis. *Myalgia, headache,* and *malaise* are often reported with epidemic viral gastroenteritis. The abdominal examination may reveal slight distention. Auscultation reveals hyperactive bowel sounds, and there is diffuse tenderness on palpation. However, there should be *no* rebound tenderness, which would indicate peritonitis. Depending on the amount of fluids lost

through diarrhea and vomiting, the client may have varying degrees of *dehydration* manifested by poor skin turgor, dry mucous membranes, orthostatic blood pressure changes, hypotension, and oliguria. Dehydration may be severe, with shock occurring if diarrhea is prolonged.

Psychosocial Assessment

The client with gastroenteritis may be fearful and embarrassed about the clinical manifestations of this illness. Society views one's elimination habits as personal, and the client may be reluctant to provide the health care provider with information about his/her bowel habits.

The client may fear that he/she may lose control of his/her bowel. Fears about harboring an infectious organism and concerns about being viewed as contagious are also assessed by the nurse.

Laboratory Findings

Gram's stain of stool is done before culture. Many WBCs on Gram's stain are indicative of shigellosis. The presence of WBCs and RBCs in stool indicates *Campylobacter* gastroenteritis.

Stool culture positive for enterotoxigenic *E. coli* is diagnostic of *E. coli* diarrhea. Culture of stool that is positive for *Shigella* when there are pus cells or WBCs present on examination of stool is diagnostic of shigellosis.

Sophisticated electron microscopy or immunoassay procedures are available to identify epidemic viral gastroenteritis or rotavirus gastroenteritis, but such examinations are rarely done because these tests are tedious to perform and expensive.

 Analysis: Nursing Diagnosis

Common Diagnoses

Because the predominant clinical manifestation of all types of gastroenteritis is diarrhea, and vomiting is a concomitant condition in many cases, the following are common nursing diagnoses that apply:

1. Fluid volume deficit related to loss of GI fluids and decreased oral intake
2. Diarrhea related to intestinal hypermotility

Additional Diagnoses

In addition, clients may have the following diagnoses:

1. Pain related to diarrhea, vomiting, malaise, and myalgia
2. Altered nutrition: less than body requirements related to nausea, vomiting, and diarrhea

3. Activity intolerance related to fluid and electrolyte losses
4. Impaired skin integrity related to increased contact of GI contents with the anal area
5. Knowledge deficit related to the cause and the communicability of illness and the treatment plan

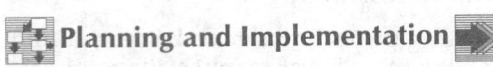 **Planning and Implementation**

Fluid Volume Deficit

Planning: client goals. The primary goal is that the client will have restoration of fluid volume loss and maintenance of a balanced fluid volume.

Interventions: nonsurgical management. Treatment is supportive for most types of gastroenteritis. It focuses on fluid replacement, with the amount and route of fluid administration determined by the individual client's fluid status. If the client has severe fluid volume depletion, he/she is admitted to the hospital for administration of intravenous (IV) fluids. The nurse obtains weight, orthostatic blood pressure readings, and other vital signs at the time of admission. Hypotonic IV fluids, such as half-strength normal saline (0.45% sodium chloride), are infused. Vital signs are checked every 4 hours or more often as indicated by the client's status. Weights are obtained using the same scale at the same time daily and recorded on a graph. A rapid gain or loss of 1 kg (2.2 lb) of body weight is equivalent to the gain or loss of 1 L of fluid. The nurse measures and records the intake and output of all fluids. Blood and body fluid precautions (or enteric precautions) are consistently used when handling all vomitus and stool, *regardless of whether a communicable disease has been documented.*

A potassium supplement is ordered to be added to IV fluids if warranted by the client's serum potassium level. The nurse verifies that the client is voiding before and during potassium replacement to help assess renal function and prevent hyperkalemia.

The client is advised to rest in bed, especially during periods of nausea or vomiting. The nurse advises the client to avoid quick movements, which could make nausea more severe.

Depending on the type of gastroenteritis, the local health department may need to be notified. It is mandatory that every case of shigellosis be reported. *Campylobacter* enteritis needs to be reported on a case-by-case basis in some endemic areas. Other types of gastroenteritis have to be reported only if they occur in epidemic proportion and not on a case-by-case basis.

Diet therapy. Diet therapy is the same for the client who remains at home and the client who is admitted to the hospital. If the client is not actively vomiting, he/she is advised to take small volumes of clear liquids with electrolytes (such as ginger ale) for 24 hours. The frequency and amount of oral intake can be increased if

nausea and vomiting are *not* present. If nausea and vomiting continue, the nurse withholds food and fluids until these symptoms subside. The nurse advises the client *not* to drink water because it does not contain any electrolytes to replace those lost. All clients have diets advanced after 24 hours of clear liquids, to include saltine crackers, toast, and jelly. When this is well tolerated, bland foods, such as nonfatty soup, custard, yogurt, cottage cheese, mashed or baked potatoes, and cooked vegetables, may be added. The client may progress to a regular diet as tolerated.

Diarrhea

Planning: client goals. The primary goal is that the client will have resolution of diarrhea.

Interventions: nonsurgical management. The nurse examines all stools for blood and mucus. A stool count chart is used as part of intake and output records. The most accurate way to evaluate output is to collect all stool in calibrated receptacles and measure it.

Diet therapy. As for fluid volume deficit, clear liquids with electrolytes are initially taken in small amounts, and then increased as tolerated for the first 24 hours. The diet then progresses as described earlier. The client should avoid milk and milk products for a week or more after the diarrhea resolves.

Drug therapy. Drugs that suppress intestinal motility, such as anticholinergics and antiemetics, are *not* given for bacterial or viral gastroenteritis. Use of these drugs could be dangerous because the infecting organisms need to be eliminated from the body, and these agents might interfere with the evacuation of the organisms.

If the gastroenteritis is due to shigellosis, anti-infective agents such as sulfamethoxazole with trimethoprim (Septra, Bactrim) are administered.

For relatively short-term diarrhea (i.e., 24 to 48 hours), the diagnosis is primarily based on history and clinical manifestations, without validation by examination of stool. When diarrhea is severe or persists for long periods of time, the stool is examined in an effort to determine the causative organism and begin specific treatment. It should be determined if diarrhea is caused by *Salmonella* or parasites, because these organisms respond to specific medications (see later discussion of parasites and *Salmonella*). Any diarrhea that continues longer than 10 days requires a thorough investigation for its etiology because it is probably *not* due to gastroenteritis.

Frequent stools that are rich in electrolytes and enzymes and frequent wiping and washing of the anal region can cause irritation to the skin. After the area is cleaned, application of a repellent cream (e.g., zinc oxide, petroleum jelly [Vaseline], Desitin ointment,

Sween cream) can protect the skin from further irritation. The application of witch hazel compresses or sitz baths may also be implemented in an attempt to relieve irritated skin.

■ Discharge Planning

The client who requires hospitalization for gastroenteritis is discharged after fluid volume has been replenished and diarrhea has resolved. Most clients with gastroenteritis, however, are treated on an outpatient (ambulatory) basis.

Home Care Preparation

The nurse assesses the client's ability to obtain and prepare food and to obtain adequate rest. If limitations in activities of daily living (ADL) exist, the nurse assesses the client's need for support to meet these needs.

The elderly or debilitated client who is seen in the acute stage of gastroenteritis and treated on an outpatient basis requires assessment of the ability to obtain fluids, food, and rest. The nurse determines whether these clients are able to ambulate, swallow, and use their hands and arms to eat and drink and perform skin care.

Client/Family Education

When the client is being treated on an outpatient basis, the nurse needs to educate the client and the family about the illness itself, how to minimize transmission of the infecting organism, diet therapy, and symptoms that need to be watched for and reported.

The nurse informs the client and the family that gastroenteritis can be caused by a virus or bacteria and that it is usually self-limiting. No medication cures this illness, except in the case of shigellosis. The client with shigellosis needs instruction on taking the anti-infective medication prescribed. Instruction includes oral and written information about the dosage, the schedule of administration, and side effects of the drug. The nurse stresses the need to finish *all* the medication in the prescription, regardless of how well the client might feel.

The nurse also teaches the client and the family about the importance of minimizing the risk of transmission of gastroenteritis. The client is advised to wash hands meticulously, especially after bowel movements; restrict the use of glasses, dishes, and eating utensils to the client only; maintain clean bathroom facilities to avoid exposure to stool; and maintain good personal hygiene. These precautions should be adhered to for up to 7 weeks after the illness, or up to several months if shigellosis was the offending organism.

The nurse advises clients to restrict their diets as described earlier. Clients who are normally on restricted diets need to be educated about the need to temporarily modify their diets. For example, the client who is usually on a sodium-restricted diet may not want to take carbonated beverages and saltine crackers, thinking that these will cause harm. The nurse explains that fluid and electrolyte requirements are different with the loss of large amounts of GI contents, and the diet should be changed temporarily to meet these needs.

The client and the family are informed orally and in writing about symptoms they should watch for and report. These include any increase or change in abdominal pain, persistent vomiting, blood in stools, diarrhea that continues for longer than 7 to 10 days, and fainting or weakness.

For the client who has been hospitalized, the nurse gives information on diet, which is based on what foods the client has tolerated by the time of discharge. The client is also informed about precautions that need to be taken to minimize the risk of transmission (described earlier).

Psychosocial Preparation

The client who is being treated on an outpatient basis may have concerns about the communicability and frequent elimination patterns inherent to this illness. The nurse assesses how much contact the client has with others and the availability of bathroom facilities. Information about time frames for and modes of transmission is provided by the nurse, in an effort to give the client some control in preventing this illness in others. The nurse emphasizes that the precautions outlined should help prevent transmission of the illness. The nurse also informs the client that, with time, the frequency and amount of stool diminish.

Health Care Resources

Clients are informed that each local health department has information about epidemics of gastroenteritis and individual cases of shigellosis. Clients may want to investigate the possibility of epidemics in areas they intend to travel to, so they might take precautions to avoid contracting the illness.

 Evaluation

The expected outcomes for the client with gastroenteritis include that the client

1. Gains and maintains stable weight
2. Has moist mucous membranes and good skin turgor
3. Has resolution of diarrhea
   a. Within 48 hours (viral gastroenteritis)
   b. Within 4 days (*Campylobacter*)
   c. Within 5 days (shigellosis)
   d. Within 8 days (rotavirus)
   e. Within 10 days (*E. coli*)

APPENDICITIS

OVERVIEW

Appendicitis is the inflammation of the vermiform appendix, the small, finger-like pouch attached to the cecum of the colon. It is about the thickness of a pencil and from 2 to 6 in long. The usual location of the appendix is the right iliac region, just below the ileocecal valve. However, it can be positioned in another area of the abdomen. Acute appendicitis is the most common cause of acute inflammation in the right lower quadrant. Consequently, it is one of the most common indications for emergency abdominal surgery.

Pathophysiology

The appendix has no known function. As part of the cecum, it fills with food and empties on a regular basis. Inflammation of the appendix can occur when there is ulceration of the mucosa or when the lumen of the appendix is obstructed. Inflammation leads to infection, as bacteria invade the wall of the appendix.

When the lumen is obstructed, the mucosa continues to secrete fluid, until the pressure within the lumen exceeds venous pressure. Blood flow to the appendix is restricted, and infection causes more swelling, which further impedes blood flow. Gangrene from hypoxia or perforation (rupture) can occur in 24 to 36 hours. If this process occurs slowly, adjacent organs may wall off the appendiceal area, and a localized abscess develops. However, rapid progression of the infectious process can cause peritonitis. All complications of peritonitis are serious (see later discussion of peritonitis). It is thought that chronic infection of the appendix can occur, but that it is not usually the cause of abdominal pain that lasts for weeks or months. Recurrent acute appendicitis does occur, often with complete remission of inflammation between acute attacks.

Etiology

Ulceration of the appendiceal mucosa is the initial event in the majority of acute appendicitis cases. The link between ulceration and subsequent appendicitis is not well understood. It is possible that the inflammation that results from the ulceration might transiently cause obstruction of the appendiceal lumen. Obstruction can also be caused by contents within the colon (such as a fecalith [a stone-like mass of feces]), kinking of the appendix, enlarged lymphoid follicles associated with viral infections, trapped barium, worms (e.g., pinworms), or tumors.

Incidence

Although appendicitis may occur at any age, the peak incidence is between the ages of 20 and 30 years. Males and females are affected with equal frequency, except between the ages of puberty and 25 years, when males predominate in a 3:2 ratio (Silen, 1987).

Appendicitis is relatively rare at extremes in age; however, perforation is relatively more common in infants and the elderly, with higher mortality occurring in these age groups. The diagnosis of appendicitis is difficult to establish for people in these age groups, which may account for the higher rates of perforation and mortality. Infants and young children are not able to describe the symptoms. Elderly people have a decreased response to normal pain signals and therefore often have vague or mild symptoms with appendicitis. Delay in diagnosis and treatment occurs because the symptoms in these client populations are nonspecific.

PREVENTION

Action to prevent the occurrence of appendicitis is aimed at reducing the risks of obstruction or inflammation of the appendiceal lumen. Bowel elimination patterns of all clients are assessed for regularity. Because fecalith obstruction has been associated with inadequate amounts of dietary fiber, high-fiber diets assist in preventing the occurrence of appendicitis. Treatment of intestinal worms also diminishes the risk. Prompt recognition of the signs and symptoms of appendicitis minimizes the chance of gangrene, perforation, and peritonitis.

COLLABORATIVE MANAGEMENT

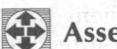 Assessment

History

Data that the nurse collects from the client with possible appendicitis include the client's *age* and *sex*, a history of *abdominal surgery* (specifically appendectomy), a history of *other medical conditions*, recent *barium intake* either by mouth or rectally, and a *diet history* with emphasis on fiber intake.

Physical Assessment: Clinical Manifestations

The nurse obtains information about the client's symptoms, with specific attention to the location and sequence of pain in relation to other symptoms. With classic appendicitis, *abdominal pain* is the *initial* symptom and it begins in the epigastric or periumbilical area. *Nausea* and *vomiting* begin *after* the initial symptom of pain, and vomiting is rarely profuse. The pain shifts to the right lower quadrant within a few hours after the initial onset. Pain may not be localized, however, and can actually exist anywhere in the abdomen or flanks. Pain is often described as sudden in onset. *Anorexia* and the *urge to defecate* or *pass flatus*, neither of which relieve the distress, are often present. Abdominal pain that increases with cough or movement and is relieved by flexion of the right hip or knees is indicative of a perforated appendix with peritonitis.

Physical findings vary, depending on the time of symptom onset, the location of the appendix, and the occurrence of perforation or peritonitis. The nurse gently palpates the abdomen to assess for tenderness. *Tenderness* is sometimes absent in the early stages of inflammation, or there may be diffuse tenderness in the umbilical or epigastric areas. In later stages of inflammation, tenderness becomes more localized and is noted with palpation of the right lower quadrant. This area is referred to as *McBurney's point*; it is located midway between the anterior iliac crest and the umbilicus in the right lower quadrant (Fig. 45–1). The nurse may feel tenseness of the muscles over the tender area, which is called *muscle rigidity*. Rigidity over the whole abdomen with tense positioning and guarding is indicative of a perforated appendix with peritonitis. *Rebound tenderness* describes a sensation of pain that occurs after deep pressure is applied and released. Performing this maneuver is controversial because it can elicit a painful response. If it is performed, the examiner should press his/her finger into the abdomen at a point away from the site where the client reports pain.

The client's temperature is usually normal or slightly elevated at 99° to 100.5° F (37.2° to 38° C), and a temperature of 101° F (38.2° C) suggests the presence of peritonitis. Tachycardia is present if fever exists.

The symptoms of many other medical conditions are similar to those of acute appendicitis, and it is often difficult to diagnose. It is important for the nurse to determine the sequence of symptoms. For example, nausea and vomiting that precede abdominal pain are often indicative of gastroenteritis.

Delay of surgical treatment for appendicitis may result in perforation of the appendix and subsequent peritonitis. However, peritonitis often occurs because the diagnosis is difficult to make and clients often delay in seeking medical treatment.

Symptoms that do not follow the classic pattern can also occur. Atypical symptoms are often due to variations in the anatomic location of the appendix. The appendix can be located deep in the pelvis, in the right upper quadrant, or even in the left lower quadrant. These variations are seen in 40% to 50% of cases (Silen, 1987).

Psychosocial Assessment

The client with appendicitis is faced with an abrupt illness. The nurse assesses the client's concerns related to separation from significant others and scheduled commitments. The nurse also evaluates concern about the physical discomfort of the disorder and hospital procedures. Because the onset of appendicitis is usually abrupt and prompt surgical treatment is necessary to prevent perforation, clients often receive little preoperative teaching. This lack of information can increase the psychologic stress, causing fear and anxiety.

Laboratory Findings

Laboratory findings do not establish the diagnosis, but there is often a moderate elevation of the WBC count (leukocytosis) to 10,000 to 18,000/mm³ with a "shift to the left" (an increased number of immature WBCs). WBC count elevation to greater than 20,000/mm³ may indicate perforation.

Radiographic Findings

X-ray films are rarely of value. However, some clients show a fecalith in the right lower quadrant on abdominal x-ray films. Occasionally, a localized ileus may also be present.

 ### Analysis: Nursing Diagnosis

Common Diagnoses

The most common diagnosis for a client with appendicitis is altered (gastrointestinal) tissue perfusion related to the inflamed appendix.

Additional Diagnoses

In addition, the client may have one or more of the following nursing diagnoses:

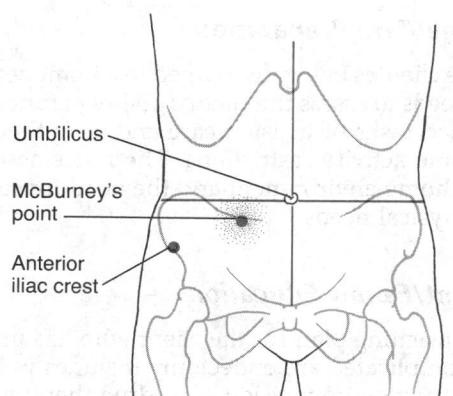

Figure 45–1
McBurney's point is located midway between the anterior iliac crest and the umbilicus in the right lower quadrant. This is the classic area for localized tenderness during later stages of appendicitis.

1. Pain related to the inflamed appendix and the surgical incision
2. Fluid volume deficit related to anorexia, vomiting, and nothing by mouth (NPO) status preoperatively and postoperatively
3. Ineffective breathing pattern related to abdominal and incision pain, anesthesia, and immobility
4. Altered nutrition: less than body requirements related to anorexia, vomiting, and NPO status preoperatively and postoperatively
5. Knowledge deficit related to treatment regimen during hospitalization and after discharge
6. Fear related to pain, abruptness of hospitalization, treatment, and separation from significant others

Planning and Implementation

Altered (Gastrointestinal) Tissue Perfusion

Planning: client goals. The primary goal is that the client will not experience complications of appendicitis from altered tissue perfusion (e.g., perforation, abscess, or peritonitis).

Interventions. All clients with suspected or diagnosed appendicitis are hospitalized. If the diagnosis is questionable, clients are observed before surgical exploration. The nurse monitors the client's pattern of *pain* to assist in establishing a medical diagnosis and definitive treatment plan.

Nonsurgical management. The client admitted to the hospital with suspected or known appendicitis is kept NPO to prepare for the possibility of emergency surgery and to avoid aggravating the inflammatory process. IV fluids are administered by the nurse to prevent fluid and electrolyte imbalance and replenish fluid volume. Analgesics are usually *not* given to clients until a definitive diagnosis of appendicitis is made, to prevent masking of symptoms. The nurse explains the rationale for withholding pain medication to the client and the family, emphasizing that the assessment of the pattern of pain is essential to making a definite diagnosis. The nurse minimizes movement of the client to avoid undue pain. After the diagnosis of appendicitis is established, surgical intervention is implemented. Narcotics may be administered by the nurse as the client is being prepared for surgery. The client with suspected appendicitis should not receive laxatives or enemas, as these could cause perforation of the appendix. No heat should ever be applied to the abdomen, because this could increase circulation to the appendix and lead to perforation.

Surgical management. Treatment of appendicitis requires surgical removal of the appendix (appendectomy) as soon as possible. If the diagnosis is not defini-

tive, but the client is at high risk for complications from suspected appendicitis, the client might undergo exploratory laparotomy to rule out appenditis. Even if the appendix is not found to be inflamed, it is usually removed at this time to avoid future risk of appendicitis.

Preoperative teaching is often limited, because the client is in pain or because the client is transferred to the operating room for emergent surgery.

Preoperative care. The nurse prepares the client for general anesthesia and surgery as described in Chapter 18.

Postoperative care. Postoperative care of the client who has undergone an appendectomy includes the care required for any client who has received general anesthesia (Chap. 20). The incision is located over McBurney's point if the appendix was in the typical location. It may extend the length of the abdomen, depending on what area needed to be explored in surgery and depending on the location of the appendix. Drains may protrude from the incision site if an abscess was present or if the appendix perforated. The drains are left in place for 3 to 5 days. If peritonitis occurred, the client will have a nasogastric tube in place to prevent GI distention. If an abscess or peritonitis occurred, the nurse administers antibiotics as ordered by the physician. Narcotic analgesics are administered for pain as needed. The client is often out of bed on the evening after surgery or the first postoperative day as ordered by the physician.

■ Discharge Planning

The client who has had appendicitis and undergone uncomplicated appendectomy should recover rapidly. He/she is usually discharged to home on the third postoperative day and should return to normal activity in 2 to 4 weeks. If surgery was complicated by perforation or peritonitis, the client is discharged in 1 to 2 weeks.

Home Care Preparation

If the client is being discharged to a home setting, the nurse needs to assess the client's ability to function with the added tasks of incision care and drug therapy and with some activity restrictions. The nurse assesses the client's home environment and the need for support to meet physical needs.

Client/Family Education

The teaching plan for the client who has undergone an uncomplicated appendectomy includes written and oral instruction on incision care, drug therapy, and activity limitations. The nurse teaches the client or the appropriate family member to observe the incision daily. Swelling, redness, bleeding, drainage, or warmth at the site should be reported to the health care provider. The client is also instructed on proper hand washing technique. If there is a surgical dressing, the client is instructed in proper dressing change technique. The nurse informs the client when he/she can shower or bathe, according to the physician's instructions. The nurse tells the client to watch for and report temperature of 101° F (38.2° C) or greater, or abdominal pain. A prescription for a narcotic analgesic is given to the client with instructions on how often it should be taken and possible side effects.

Because it may take up to 6 weeks for complete healing of abdominal tissues and muscles, the nurse instructs the client to refrain from lifting any heavy objects, such as a filled laundry basket, for 6 weeks. The client should follow the physician's recommendations with regard to driving and return to work. The type of work often dictates when the client can resume employment.

Psychosocial Preparation

Even though clients generally recover well from an uncomplicated appendectomy, the nurse needs to be aware of the client's perception of hospitalization and surgery.

The nurse teaches the client that the appendix has no known function and that there are no long-term physiologic deficits after it is removed. The nurse elicits concerns that the client has regarding discharge from the hospital. Common concerns include incision care, drug therapy, activity restrictions, and information on the amount of time necessary for full recovery.

Health Care Resources

If a client has a pre-existing illness or restriction in ADL and does not have a support system to assist with incision care and drug therapy, or if necessary activities are affected by the postoperative activity restrictions, the assistance of a home care nurse or home care aide may be necessary. The home care nurse can be contacted to arrange times to visit and assess wound healing and the proper administration of medications.

 Evaluation

On the basis of the identified nursing diagnoses, the nurse evaluates the care of the client with appendicitis. The expected outcomes include that the client

1. States that pain similar to that on admission to the hospital has resolved and that incision pain is reduced or alleviated
2. States the signs and symptoms that he/she should watch for and report to the appropriate health care provider, i.e., swelling, warmth, redness, and bleeding or drainage at the incision site; temperature of 101° F (38.2° C) or greater; or abdominal pain.

PERITONITIS

OVERVIEW

Peritonitis is an inflammation of the peritoneum (the lining of the abdominal cavity). It can be primary or secondary, localized or generalized. Peritonitis is a life-threatening illness, which is often associated with various abdominal disorders, and is routinely assessed for in all clients with abdominal complaints or symptoms.

Pathophysiology

When the peritoneal cavity is contaminated, the body initially produces an inflammatory reaction that walls off a localized area to fight the infection. This local reaction involves vascular dilation and increased capillary permeability, allowing for transport of leukocytes and subsequent phagocytosis of the offending organisms. This walling-off process can result in abscess formation or fibrous adhesions, which may or may not cause further pathologic change. If the peritonitis is contained, generalized peritonitis need not occur. However, if the offending stimulus is too massive to be contained, diffuse peritonitis occurs, leading to serious systemic insult.

Vascular dilation continues along with hyperemia and a fluid shift. The body responds to the infectious process by shunting extra blood to the area of inflammation. Fluid is shifted from the extracellular fluid (ECF) compartment into the peritoneal cavity, connective tissues, and the GI tract. This shift of fluid out of the vascular space can result in a significant decrease in circulatory volume. The rate of decreasing circulatory volume is proportional to the degree of peritoneal involvement. Decreased circulatory volume can result in insufficient perfusion of kidneys, leading to renal failure with electrolyte imbalance.

Peristalsis slows or stops in response to severe peritoneal infection, and the lumen of the bowel becomes distended with gas and fluid. Fluid that normally flows to the small bowel and the colon for reabsorption accumulates in the intestine in volumes of 7 to 8 L daily.

The toxins or bacteria responsible for the peritonitis can also enter the blood stream from the peritoneal area, leading to bacteremia and septicemia.

Respiratory problems can occur owing to increased abdominal pressure against the diaphragm from intestinal distention and fluid shifts to the peritoneal cavity. Pain can interfere with ventilatory efforts at a time when the client has increased oxygen demand because of the infectious process.

Etiology

The etiology of peritonitis is contamination of the peritoneal cavity by bacteria or chemicals. Peritonitis can be primary or secondary. *Primary* peritonitis is an acute bacterial infection that is *not* associated with a perforated viscus. Bacterial infection is the usual cause and is thought to be associated with an infection by the same organism somewhere else in the body, which reaches the peritoneum via the vascular system. Tuberculous peritonitis, which originates from tuberculosis elsewhere in the body, is a type of primary peritonitis. Clients with alcoholic cirrhosis and ascites, in the absence of a perforated organ, often manifest peritonitis, which may be due to leakage of bacteria through the wall of the intestine.

Secondary peritonitis is most often caused by bacterial invasion as a result of *perforation* or *rupture* of an abdominal viscus. However, it can also result from severe chemical reactions to pancreatic enzymes, digestive juices, or bile released into the peritoneal cavity.

The most common causes of bacterial invasion of the peritoneal cavity are *perforation* associated with appendicitis, peptic ulcer, diverticulitis, gangrenous gallbladder, gangrenous obstruction of the small bowel, incarcerated hernia, volvulus, spleen or liver conditions, and an ectopic pregnancy. Other stimuli include perforating tumors, ulcerative colitis, or foreign bodies (from blunt trauma). Leakage or contamination during a surgical procedure or contamination from a trochar or catheter used for peritoneal dialysis or the administration of intraperitoneal chemotherapy could also cause peritonitis. Bacterial invasion can also occur from an ascending infection through the reproductive tract, as in salpingitis or septic abortion.

Bacteria responsible for peritonitis include *E. coli,* streptococci, staphylococci, pneumococci, and gonococci.

Incidence

Primary peritonitis accounts for approximately 1% of the cases of peritonitis (Broadwell & McGarity, 1981). The incidence of secondary peritonitis is difficult to determine because data usually relate to the underlying cause, such as appendicitis or peptic ulcer. Data on the incidence of secondary peritonitis are lacking.

PREVENTION

Prevention of peritonitis focuses on prompt recognition and treatment of conditions that could lead to perforation of abdominal viscera or any conditions that foster the release of bacteria or chemicals into the peritoneal cavity. The ingestion of high-fiber diets and the administration of laxatives or enemas after barium ingestion help prevent appendicitis or diverticulitis. However, if acute appendicitis or diverticulitis is present, high-fiber diets and laxatives or enemas need to be avoided to prevent peritonitis. Clients with peptic ulcers and ulcerative colitis need to have treatment plans conducive to keeping their disease processes under control. All clients with vaginal, cervical, or pelvic infections need to be treated with appropriate antibiotics and instructed on the importance of taking all antibiotics as prescribed. Aseptic technique when handling trochars and catheters for peritoneal dialysis or chemotherapy can prevent organisms from contacting and invading the peritoneum.

COLLABORATIVE MANAGEMENT

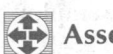 **Assessment**

History

The nurse collects data specifically relating to peritonitis for all clients who exhibit clinical manifestations of conditions known to be associated with peritonitis (see earlier discussion of etiology). For the client with known peritonitis, data should be sufficient to detect the many possible life-threatening complications. Data include a history of *abdominal pain,* which in the early stages is diffuse and vague, but then becomes localized at the area of inflammation. In the later stages, abdominal pain increases to moderately severe levels but remains localized if the peritonitis is limited, or walled off. Pain is severe but *widespread* if generalized peritonitis exists. The nurse elicits a history of abdominal pain that is aggravated by movement, including respiratory effort. The client might also report keeping the knees flexed to help reduce the abdominal pain. There may be a history of abdominal distention, anorexia, nausea, vomiting, elevated temperature with chills, and an inability to pass feces or flatus. The nurse obtains a history of recent *surgeries* and current and past *medical conditions.* For female clients, the date of the last menstrual period, along with information regarding a possible pregnancy, is also obtained to rule out a ruptured ectopic pregnancy.

Physical Assessment: Clinical Manifestations

Physical findings of peritonitis depend on whether it is early or late in the disease course and whether the body has been able to localize the process or it has progressed to generalized peritonitis.

The client appears acutely *ill,* lying still, possibly with knees flexed. Movement is guarded, and there are verbalization and manifestations of pain (e.g., facial grimacing) with cough or movement of *any* type. *Pain* may be sharp and localized in the abdomen, poorly localized in the abdomen, or referred to either the shoulder or the thoracic area. The abdomen may be *rigid, distended,* or both. The nurse may auscultate bowel sounds, but these usually disappear with progression of the inflammation. In the case of localized peritonitis, the nurse notes that the abdomen is *tender* on palpation in a well-defined area of the abdomen, with *rebound tenderness* in this area. With generalized peritonitis, tenderness is generalized. A *high fever* is often present because of the infectious process, with tachycardia occurring in response to the fever. The nurse assesses whether the client has *dry mucous membranes* with poor tissue turgor and a *low urinary output.* Low urinary output occurs because fluid accumulates in the peritoneal cavity, the GI tract, and connective tissues, resulting in a fluid deficit in the vascular space. Hiccups may occur owing to diaphragmatic irritation. Depending on the severity of peritonitis, the nurse may find that the client has a compromised respiratory status.

Psychosocial Assessment

The client with peritonitis is faced with a life-threatening illness that often occurs abruptly. The nurse assesses client's fears and concerns about the illness itself and the treatment, which is essential and often overwhelming. Clients with peritonitis are often so ill that clinical manifestations may intensify their fears and concerns, leading to interference with coping mechanisms. The nurse assesses the family's understanding of the causes, the planned interventions, and the client's responses to the illness and its treatment. The needs of the family of the client who responds quickly to treatment are different from those of the family of the client who develops complications from the illness, such as renal failure, respiratory failure, and sepsis.

Laboratory Findings

WBC counts are commonly elevated to 20,000/mm³ (see earlier), with a high neutrophil count. Blood cultures are done to determine whether bacterial invasion of the blood (bacteremia) has occurred and to identify the causative organism to enable appropriate therapy.

In addition to obtaining blood studies used specifically to identify peritonitis, laboratory testing is done to assess fluid and electrolyte balance and renal status (electrolyte, blood urea nitrogen [BUN], creatinine, and hemoglobin levels and hematocrit).

Arterial blood gas values may also be obtained to assess respiratory function and acid-base balance.

Radiographic Findings

Abdominal x-ray films are evaluated, specifically looking for free air or fluid in the abdominal cavity, which is indicative of perforation. Abdominal x-ray films may also show dilation, edema, and inflammation of the small and large intestines.

Other Diagnostic Tests

Peritoneal aspiration may be performed. The bacteria in peritoneal fluid are cultured to help determine the

cause of the peritonitis, as well as proper antibiotic therapy. The peritoneal fluid shows a WBC count greater than 300/mm³ with more than 25% neutrophils in most clients with spontaneous bacterial peritonitis. Cloudy or turbid fluid from a peritoneal tap may also be indicative of peritonitis. Bile-stained green fluid may indicate a ruptured gallbladder or perforated intestine, which could lead to chemical peritonitis.

 Analysis: Nursing Diagnosis

Nursing diagnoses for each client with peritonitis vary, depending on how severe the peritonitis is and to what degree other systems of the body are involved. The nurse considers the pathophysiology of peritonitis to include nursing diagnoses that might not have obvious clinical manifestations in the early stages of the disease.

Common Diagnoses

These diagnoses are commonly noted in clients with peritonitis.

1. Altered (gastrointestinal) tissue perfusion related to peritoneal inflammation
2. Fluid volume deficit related to abdominal third spacing

Additional Diagnoses

The client may also have the following nursing diagnoses:

1. Pain related to inflamed peritoneum
2. Altered nutrition: less than body requirements related to NPO status or restriction to a clear-liquid diet
3. Ineffective breathing pattern related to pain and abdominal distention
4. Decreased cardiac output related to vascular volume deficit
5. Activity intolerance related to pain, nutritional deficits, fluid volume deficits, electrolyte imbalance, and altered cardiac output and respiratory function
6. Fear related to pain and uncertainty about treatment
7. Knowledge deficit related to the illness and the treatment regimen

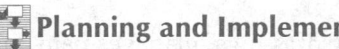 **Planning and Implementation**

Altered (Gastrointestinal) Tissue Perfusion

Planning: client goals. The primary goal is that the client will *not* experience complications of peritonitis, such as shock, renal failure, respiratory failure, or sepsis.

Interventions. All clients with peritonitis are hospitalized because of the critical nature of the illness. If the complications are extensive, the client may be in a critical care unit. The most important nursing intervention is thorough assessment of all body systems to identify complications early.

Nonsurgical management. IV fluids and broad-spectrum antibiotics are administered immediately after the diagnosis of peritonitis. A nasogastric tube is inserted to decompress the stomach and the intestine, and the client is maintained on NPO status. Oxygen is administered, the amount and mode of administration being based on the client's respiratory status.

Surgical management. Abdominal surgery is the optimal treatment to identify and repair the cause of the peritonitis. However, if the client is critically ill so that surgery is life-threatening, it may be delayed. The surgical approach focuses on controlling the contamination, removing foreign material from the peritoneal cavity, and draining collected fluid. The specific surgical procedure depends on the cause of the peritonitis. Examples of procedures to control contamination are an appendectomy for removal of an inflamed appendix and a colon resection and colostomy for a perforated colon.

The peritoneum is irrigated with antibiotic solutions during the surgical procedure, and two to four catheters may be inserted to drain the cavity and occasionally to provide irrigation.

Preoperative care. After surgery is planned, the nurse administers narcotic analgesics, sedatives, and anticholinergics as ordered by the surgeon and the anesthesiologist. The purpose of these medications is to alleviate pain and anxiety, minimize secretions, and prepare the client for anesthetic induction. The nurse instructs the client about the importance of coughing, deep breathing, moving, and exercising the legs postoperatively, as described in Chapter 18. Practice of these techniques may not be appropriate preoperatively because of abdominal pain. The nurse assures the client that pain medication will be available postoperatively as needed.

Postoperative care. The nurse monitors the client's pain, vital signs, level of consciousness, respiratory status (breath sounds and respiratory rate), abdominal signs (distention, bowel sounds, and nasogastric tube patency and output), IV infusion, and urinary output, *at least hourly.* The client is maintained in semi-Fowler's position, so that peritoneal contents drain to the inferior region of the abdominal cavity. This position also facilitates adequate respiratory excursion, in that the diaphragm and abdominal contents are not impinging on respiratory muscles.

The nurse checks any dressings, manages pain, and facilitates mobility and repositioning as for clients undergoing surgery with general anesthesia (Chap. 20). If peritoneal irrigation is ordered, the nurse determines that the client is *not* retaining irrigant by evaluating the client for the absence of abdominal distention and pain and by measuring the amount of irrigant with strict intake and output measurements. The client is likely to

have multiple incisions. This occurs when there is too much contamination for the surgeon to close the wound at the time of surgery. These wounds do not heal with the edges well approximated (by first intention), but by second or third intention. They require meticulous care, involving manual irrigation or packing as ordered by the physician.

Often, these clients have been so ill from systemic complications, such as sepsis, fluid and electrolyte imbalance, respiratory failure, or renal failure, that their activity tolerance is significantly limited. When activity is allowed, the nurse assists the client with dangling, assessing for orthostatic blood pressure changes and symptoms of dizziness. When dangling is well tolerated, the activity level is gradually increased.

Fluid Volume Deficit

Planning: client goals. The goal is that the client will retain and maintain a balanced systemic fluid volume.

Interventions: nonsurgical management. IV fluid replacement and maintenance are indicated for all clients with peritonitis because of the loss of fluids from the extracellular space to the GI space and peritoneal cavity. Fluid volume losses also result from nasogastric suctioning and the NPO status of the client. Normal saline or a balanced salt intravenous infusion with potassium is administered according to electrolyte, BUN, and serum creatinine values. The nurse monitors the client's vital signs, urinary output, skin turgor, integrity of mucous membranes, and weight to assess fluid volume. The nurse also assesses for edema from third spacing.

The client with peritonitis is characteristically thirsty owing to fluid losses. The nurse provides frequent mouth care to help maintain moist mucous membranes. The use of lemon-glycerin swabs should be avoided, because they can increase dryness.

■ Discharge Planning

The client with peritonitis is hospitalized for *at least* 1 to 2 weeks. The actual length of hospitalization depends on how localized the infectious process is and how severe the systemic reaction is. Clients who have a localized abscess drained and *respond* to antibiotics and IV fluids, without respiratory, renal, or cardiac complications, are discharged in 1 to 2 weeks. Clients who experience complications of peritonitis, along with sepsis or shock, may require mechanical ventilation or hemodialysis, with hospital stays lasting for weeks to months. Discharge planning varies with the degree of involvement of all body systems.

Home Care Preparation

If the client is being discharged to a home setting, the nurse assesses the client's ability to function at home with the added task of incision care and a diminished activity tolerance.

Client/Family Education

The nurse provides written and oral instructions about reporting any drainage, swelling, bleeding, redness, warmth, or odor from the wound; temperature greater than 101° F (38.2° C); or abdominal pain. Proper hand washing and dressing change techniques are also taught; the client is directed to dress wounds separately to avoid cross-contamination.

The client receives a prescription for a narcotic analgesic and possibly an antibiotic. The nurse reviews the type of drug, the dosage, the recommended schedule of administration, side effects, and the rationale for each prescription with the client. Diet and activity limitations are also reviewed. Diet depends on the type of surgery performed and the client's specific food tolerances at the time of discharge from the hospital. All clients are told to refrain from any lifting for *at least* 6 weeks. Other activity limitations are made on an individual basis with the physician's recommendation.

Psychosocial Preparation

Peritonitis is a life-threatening and consequently frightening illness. Incision care can be demanding, and activity intolerance can be overwhelming. If complications have resolved, the nurse reassures the client that the resumption of the previous life style is a realistic expectation. Convalescence is often longer than that required for other types of surgery, however, because of the multisystemic involvement.

Health Care Resources

Clients with incisions healing by second or third intention may require dressings, solution, and catheter-tipped syringes to irrigate the wound. The nurse may arrange for a home care nurse to assess, irrigate, or pack a wound and change a dressing as needed. If a client needs assistance with ADL, a home care aide or temporary placement in an extended care facility may be indicated.

 Evaluation

The nurse evaluates the client with peritonitis according to identified nursing diagnoses specific to each client's degree of illness. The expected outcomes for the client with peritonitis include that the client

1. States that pain similar to that on admission to hospital is alleviated and that incision pain is reduced or alleviated
2. Has adequate hydration
3. Has incision healing by first, second, or third intention without evidence of infection
4. Approaches a level of activity similar to that before the illness

ULCERATIVE COLITIS

OVERVIEW

Ulcerative colitis is a chronic inflammatory process of the bowel that results in poor absorption of vital nutrients. Over time, the client experiences episodes of physical discomfort and disruption of life style. The disease can range from minor periodic health problems, requiring only ambulatory care, to malnutrition, and physical debilitation, requiring multiple hospitalizations.

The clinical presentation is similar to that of Crohn's disease (see the accompanying Key Features of Disease). This makes diagnosis and treatment difficult.

KEY FEATURES OF DISEASE ■ Differential Features of Ulcerative Colitis and Crohn's Disease

	Ulcerative Colitis	Crohn's Disease
Location	Begins in the rectum and proceeds in a continuous manner toward the cecum	Most often in the terminal ileum, with patchy involvement through all layers of the bowel
Etiology	Unknown	Unknown
Peak incidence at age	15–35 yr	15–30 yr
Stools	10–20 liquid, bloody stools per day	5–6 soft, loose stools per day, rarely bloody
Complications	Hemorrhage Perforation Fistulas Nutritional deficiencies	Fistulas Nutritional deficiencies

Pathophysiology

Ulcerative colitis is classified as an inflammatory bowel disease. It is characterized by diffuse inflammation of the intestinal mucosa, resulting in a loss of surface epithelium with ulceration and possibly abscess formation. Generally, the disease begins in the rectum and proceeds in a uniform, continuous manner proximally toward the cecum.

With acute ulcerative colitis, there is vascular congestion, hemorrhage, edema, and ulceration of the bowel mucosa. As the disease course progresses, however, chronic changes are noted: muscle hypertrophy occurs, deposits of fat and fibrous tissue are evident, and the bowel becomes thicker, narrower, and shorter. The disease is characterized by periods of remission and exacerbation.

Other complications can include abscess formation, stenosis of the bowel, and bowel perforation, with resultant peritonitis, fissures, and fistula formation. All individuals who have had ulcerative colitis for 10 years or longer have a 10% to 20% risk for development of cancer of the bowel (Wyngaarden & Smith, 1988). Complications of ulcerative colitis can affect many body systems. Anemias can develop from the chronic loss of iron, and coagulation defects can occur if vitamin K is poorly absorbed.

Etiology

The cause of ulcerative colitis is unknown. Many theories have been formulated regarding possible causes, including infectious agents (bacterial, fungal, or viral) or allergy. There appears to be a genetic predisposition, as indicated by familial clustering of the disease. Immunologic theories, including autoimmune dysfunction, have been explored owing to the extraintestinal manifestations of the disease. Psychologic factors, such as stress and hostile feelings, have also been implicated as possible causes. However, it is believed that these factors only contribute to the severity of the attack, rather than being direct causes.

Incidence

Ulcerative colitis has demonstrated a familial tendency and is commonly found more often in females than in males. The annual incidence of ulcerative colitis is approximately 2 to 7 new cases per 100,000 persons, with a prevalence of 40 to 100 cases per 100,000 Americans. There is one peak incidence between the ages of 15 and 20 years, and another peak between ages 55 to 60 years. (Wyngaarden & Smith, 1988).

PREVENTION

Because the cause of the disease is unknown, there currently are no suggested methods of prevention. Mainte-

nance drug therapy has been helpful in reducing the amount of disease activity, but does not necessarily prevent exacerbations. Psychologic intervention, such as counseling, has assisted in reducing disease activity for some clients, but again does not prevent exacerbations. Occasionally, diet therapy (lactose-free diet) also may contribute to lessened disease activity. Astute assessment is necessary for early awareness of complications of the disease and aids in minimizing their effects on the individual and the family. Education regarding the familial tendency of the disease is important, and a referral for genetic counseling may be helpful.

COLLABORATIVE MANAGEMENT

 Assessment

History

The nurse collects data on *family history* of inflammatory bowel disease, and *previous and current therapy* for illness, including dates and types of surgery. *Diet history* is essential and should include the client's usual dietary patterns and the relationship of elimination patterns to intolerance of milk and milk products and greasy, fried, spicy, or hot foods. The nurse obtains information on the symptoms of acute ulcerative colitis, which often include 10 to 20 liquid, bloody stools per day, anorexia, and fatigue.

Physical Assessment: Clinical Manifestations

The client with ulcerative colitis may have symptoms varying with the acuteness of onset and with complications of the disease process. The nurse assesses for the presence or absence of bowel sounds.

Palpation may reveal areas of increased or localized *tenderness. Rebound tenderness* may be indicative of peritonitis. Localized areas of *abdominal pain* or *cramping* may be noted over areas of diseased bowel.

The nurse also assesses the *bowel elimination pattern,* noting the color, consistency, and character of stool and the presence or absence of blood in all stools. The relationship between the occurrence of diarrhea and the timing of meals, pain, emotional distress, and activity is also assessed. The client may be *febrile* and *tachycardiac,* indicating possible complications such as peritonitis, dehydration, or bowel perforation.

Psychosocial Assessment

The nurse evaluates the client's understanding of his/her illness and its impact on the life style. The client is encouraged and supported while exploring the relationship of life events to disease exacerbations, job-related stress factors that produce symptoms, effects of smoking and alcohol on the frequency of stool and the occurrence of crampy pain, the effect of pain and diarrhea on sleep habits, and family and social support systems.

Many clients are extremely apprehensive regarding the frequency of stools and the presence of blood. The uncontrollability of the disease symptoms, particularly diarrhea, can be disruptive and stress producing.

More severe illness can limit the client's activities outside the home. The individual may become dependent on the proximity of a bathroom owing to excessive diarrhea. Food and eating may be associated with pain and cramping, as well as an increased frequency of stools. Mealtimes may become unpleasant experiences for clients.

Laboratory Findings

The hematocrit and hemoglobin level may be low owing to chronic blood loss. An increased WBC count and elevated erythrocyte sedimentation rate are consistent with inflammatory disease. Sodium, potassium, and chloride concentrations may be depleted by the frequent diarrheal stools and the malabsorption that results from the diseased bowel.

Viral and bacterial dysenteries can cause symptoms similar to those of ulcerative colitis. Before an invasive diagnostic work-up, examination of stools for occult blood, as well as ova and parasites, and cultures are performed. It is essential that other problems are ruled out before making a definitive diagnosis of ulcerative colitis.

Radiographic Findings

Barium enemas with air contrast demonstrate differences between Crohn's disease and ulcerative colitis, as well as identifying complications, mucosal patterns, and the distribution and depth of involvement.

Other Diagnostic Tests

The sigmoidoscopic examination is probably the most definitive diagnostic procedure for ulcerative colitis. It allows direct visualization of the sigmoid and the transverse colon. In ulcerative colitis, edematous, friable bowel mucosa with a loss of vascular pattern and frequently ulcerations are noted.

 Analysis: Nursing Diagnosis

Common Diagnoses

The following diagnoses are frequently identified by nurses caring for clients with ulcerative colitis:

1. Diarrhea related to inflamed bowel mucosa
2. Pain related to cramping

Additional Diagnoses

On the basis of the diversity of manifestations of ulcerative colitis, the nurse may need to formulate additional diagnoses, including the following:

1. Altered nutrition: less than body requirements related to diarrhea and malabsorption
2. Fluid volume deficit related to diarrhea
3. Body image disturbance related to change in body function
4. Potential impaired skin integrity related to fissures, fistula, and skin irritation
5. Activity intolerance related to generalized weakness
6. Knowledge deficit related to the disease process
7. Ineffective individual coping related to physical illness and hospitalization

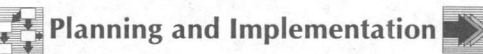 **Planning and Implementation**

Diarrhea

Planning: client goals. The goal is that the client will experience decreased diarrhea through control of the inflammation of the intestinal lining.

Interventions. Measures are used to relieve symptoms and reduce intestinal motility, decrease inflammation, and promote intestinal healing.

Nonsurgical management. Medical management of inflammatory bowel disease is the preferred and initial treatment option.

Diet therapy. The severity of the disease determines the type of diet. Clients with severe symptoms are kept NPO to ensure bowel rest. These clients are usually given total parenteral nutrition (TPN) (see Chapter 13). Clients with slightly less severe symptoms may be given elemental formulas, such as Vivonex or Ensure. These formulas are absorbed in the upper bowel, thus minimizing bowel stimulation. Clients with significant but less severe symptoms may be restricted to a low-residue diet. The low-residue diet provides all four food groups and essential nutrients, limiting high-roughage foods. Foods such as whole-wheat grains, nuts, and raw fruits or vegetables are avoided in low-residue diets (see the accompanying Health Promotion/Maintenance feature). Smoking, caffeinated beverages, pepper, and alcohol are GI stimulants and should be avoided. The client may begin with one form of diet therapy and progress to a more advanced diet as symptoms minimize, with the goal of preventing hyperactive bowel activity.

The nurse needs to provide detailed explanation of prescribed diet therapy and carefully monitor dietary intake (including calorie count) and intake and output. If eating has produced uncomfortable or unpleasant symptoms, anxiety can develop at mealtimes. The nurse encourages the client to verbalize concerns and, if possible, spends time with clients before and during mealtime.

Drug therapy. To provide symptomatic management of diarrhea, antidiarrheal agents are commonly used. The nurse's role is to administer these medications as

HEALTH PROMOTION/MAINTENANCE ■ Low-Residue Diet

Foods Allowed	Foods Not Allowed
Beverages	
Only 2 glasses of milk, if allowed, boiled or evaporated; strained fruit juices, coffee, tea, and carbonated beverages	Alcohol
Eggs	
Prepared in any manner, except fried	Fried
Cheese	
Cottage, cream, milk, American, and Tillamook (use in small amounts)	Highly flavored
Meats or Poultry	
Roasted, baked, or broiled tender beef, ham, lamb, liver, veal, fish, chicken, or turkey	Tough meats, pork; fried or highly spiced meats
Soups	
Bouillon, broth, and strained cream soups from foods allowed	Any others
Fats	
Butter, margarine, oils 30 mL (1 oz) of cream daily	None
Vegetables	
Canned or cooked vegetables, such as asparagus, beets, carrots, peas, pumpkin, squash, spinach, and young string beans; tomato juice	Raw or whole cooked vegetables
Fruits	
Strained fruit juices; cooked or canned apples, apricots, Royal Ann cherries, peaches, pears, dried fruit purée, and ripe banana and avocado; all of the above *without skins or seeds*	All other raw or cooked fruits
Bread and Crackers	
Refined bread, toast, rolls, and crackers	Pancakes, waffles, and whole-grain bread or rolls
Cereals	
Cooked cereal, such as Cream of Wheat, Malt-O Meal, strained oatmeal, cornmeal, cornflakes, puffed rice, Rice Krispies, and puffed wheat	Whole-grain cereals; other prepared cereals
Potatoes	
Potatoes, white rice, macaroni, noodles, and spaghetti	Fried potato, potato chips, and brown rice
Desserts	
Gelatin desserts, tapioca, angel food or sponge cake, plain custards, water ice or ice cream without fruit or nuts, and rennet or simple puddings	Rich pastries, pies, and anything with nuts or dried fruit

HEALTH PROMOTION/MAINTENANCE ■ Low-Residue Diet *Continued*

Foods Allowed	Foods Not Allowed
Sweets	
Sugar, jelly, honey, syrups, gumdrops, hard candy, plain creams, milk chocolate	Other candy; jam, marmalade
Miscellaneous Foods	
Cream sauce and plain gravy	Nuts, olives, popcorn, rich gravies, pepper, spices, and vinegar

From Williams, Sue Rodwell: *Nutrition and diet therapy*, ed. 6, St. Louis, 1989, Times Mirror/Mosby College Publishing.

ordered, assess and document their effectiveness in controlling symptoms, and observe for possible side effects, including constipation. Common antidiarrheal products include diphenoxylate hydrochloride and atropine sulfate (Lomotil), loperamide (Imodium), and camphorated tincture of opium (paregoric) (Table 45–1). Codeine sulfate and morphine sulfate can also be effective. These drugs decrease the frequency of stools, usually by reducing the volume of liquid in the stools.

Antimicrobial agents often are used to help prevent secondary infections. Treatment with Sulfasalazine (Azulfidine) has been useful in decreasing the frequency of remissions. Sulfasalazine is a sulfonamide that acts by blocking folic acid synthesis, thus making bacteria susceptible to destruction by this drug. The dosage ranges from 3 to 4 g/day orally in divided doses. These drugs can cause photosensitivity, agranulocytosis (a serious and acute disease attributable to extreme drop in WBC count), aplastic anemia, nausea, vomiting, and diarrhea. It is important that clients with ulcerative colitis consistently take their medication, even when they are feeling well and are less symptomatic.

Corticosteroid therapy is often used orally or intravenously during exacerbations. Prednisone, 30 to 60 mg

TABLE 45–1   Drugs Used in the Treatment of Diarrhea

Drug	Usual Daily Dosage	Interventions	Rationales
Diphenoxylate hydrochloride and atropine sulfate (Lomotil)	1 tablet 6 times per day; no more than 6 in 24 h	1. Assess for abdominal distention, pain, and fever.	1. These symptoms may indicate a bacterial organism in the GI tract. Diarrhea should not be suppressed in the presence of GI infection.
		2. Assess for sedation, dry mouth, urinary retention, and rash.	2. These are common side effects.
Loperamide (Imodium)	2 mg after each loose stool; maximum of 16 mg daily	1. Assess for abdominal distention, pain, and fever.	1. These symptoms may indicate a bacterial organism in the GI tract. Diarrhea should not be suppressed if GI infection is present.
		2. Assess for drowsiness, fatigue, and dry mouth.	2. These are common side effects.
Camphorated tincture of opium (paregoric)	0.6 mL qid PO; no more than 6 mL daily	1. Assess for abdominal distention, pain, and fever.	1. These symptoms may represent a bacterial infection.
		2. Assess for nausea and vomiting.	2. These are side effects.

daily, can be given orally, whereas adrenocorticotropic hormone (ACTH) is given intravenously. For rectal symptoms, topical steroids in the form of small retention enemas are given. There are also many other forms of topical steroids, such as foams and steroid suppositories.

Immunosuppressive drugs alone have not been effective, but, when combined with corticosteroids, they have produced a more rapid remission and allowed earlier decrease of steroid therapy after remission is achieved. The drug most commonly used is azathioprine (Imuran). The nurse observes for side effects, such as diarrhea, secondary infections, dermatitis, alopecia, and bone marrow depression.

Altered activity level. The client's activity is generally restricted at the onset of treatment. This aids in reducing intestinal activity, promotes comfort, and assists the client in receiving required rest to promote healing. The client should have easy access to a bedpan, commode, or bathroom in case of urgency or tenesmus (persistent spasm of the anal area).

Surgical management. On the basis of the response to medical management, the type and severity of symptoms, and the length of time the client has experienced symptoms, a decision for surgical management may be reached by the client and the physician. Three possible surgical interventions can be undertaken and result in great reduction in symptoms. The three procedures are total proctocolectomy with permanent ileostomy, Kock's ileostomy, and ileoanal reservoir. *Total proctocolectomy with permanent ileostomy* includes removal of the colon, the rectum, and the anus with closure of the anus. The end of the terminal ileum is brought out through the abdominal wall and forms a *stoma,* or *ostomy.* The stoma is usually placed in the right lower quadrant of the abdomen, below the belt line (Fig. 45–2).

Initially after surgery, ileostomy output is loose, dark green liquid and may contain some blood. Over time, a process called ileostomy adaptation occurs by which the small intestine begins to absorb increased amounts of sodium and water, a function of the large intestine that was removed by surgery. Stool volume decreases and becomes more thickened (paste-like), and the color becomes yellow green or yellow brown. The effluent (fluid material) usually has little odor or a sweet odor. Any foul or unpleasant odor may be a symptom of some underlying problem (e.g., blockage and infection).

Owing to the frequency and irritation of stool drainage, a pouch system must be worn at all times. Reusable pouch systems were frequently seen in ileostomy care in the past. However, disposable systems are most often used at present.

Prevention of skin problems (irritation, excoriation, and ulceration) is critical for the client with an ileostomy. Output from the small intestine is high in proteolytic enzymes and bile salts, which can quickly irritate and cause injury to the skin. A pouch system that has some type of skin barrier (gelatin or pectin) provides sufficient prevention for most clients. Other products are also available.

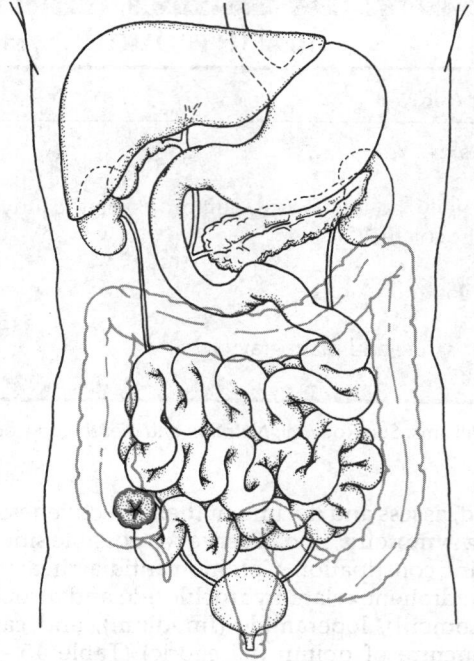

Figure 45–2

Total proctocolectomy with permanent ileostomy. This involves removal of the colon, the rectum, and the anus with closure of the anus. Note missing colon, rectum, and anus with resultant stoma in the right lower quadrant.

In the late 1960s, the Swedish surgeon Kock developed a procedure whereby an intra-abdominal pouch or reservoir was constructed from the terminal ileum (Fig. 45–3), and stool could be stored in the pouch until drained by the client. This procedure, called *Kock's ileostomy,* involves the connection of the pouch to the stoma, which is constructed with a nipple-like valve made from an intussuscepted portion of the ileum. The stoma is flush with the skin (see Fig. 45–3).

The advantages of this procedure are that an external pouch does not need to be worn for collection of stool, minimal skin problems are encountered, and there is no leakage of flatus or stool. Because the client controls evacuation, this type of ostomy is called a continent ostomy. Over time, the pouch capacity reaches 500 to 700 mL, and the client needs to drain the pouch several times per day. The client feels a sensation of fullness when the pouch needs to be emptied. The client then drains the pouch by inserting a urinary catheter. The client needs to wear a small dressing over the stoma to keep it moist and to protect clothing from the moist stoma.

In the late 1970s a procedure was developed to preserve the rectal sphincter muscles and prevent the need for an ostomy. This procedure, called the *ileoanal reservoir,* occurs in two steps (Fig. 45–4). The first stage consists of excision of the rectal mucosa, abdominal colectomy, construction of the reservoir or pouch to the anal canal, and a temporary loop ileostomy. The client

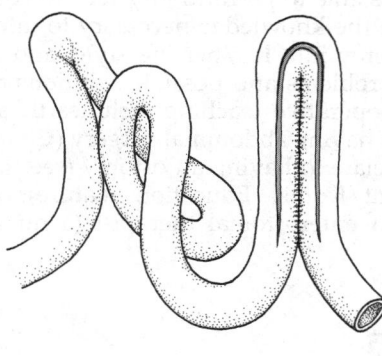
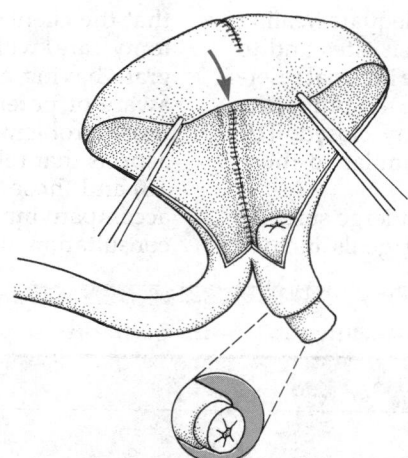
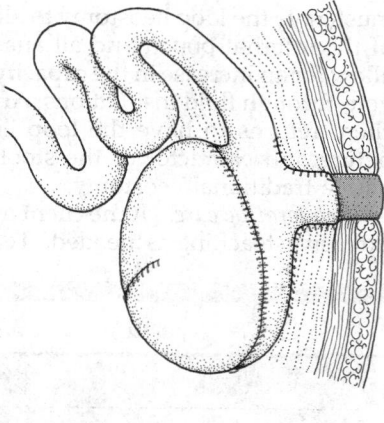

1. A reservoir, in which the client will retain stool until draining it, is constructed from a loop of ileum that is folded and sutured together and then cut.

2. A portion of the ileum is intussuscepted to form a nipple valve, and the upper part of the stitched and cut ileum is pulled down and sutured to form a pouch.

3. The nipple valve, which shuts tight against pressure from a filled pouch, is pulled through the stoma and is sutured flush with the abdomen.

Figure 45–3

Creation of Kock's, or continent, ileostomy.

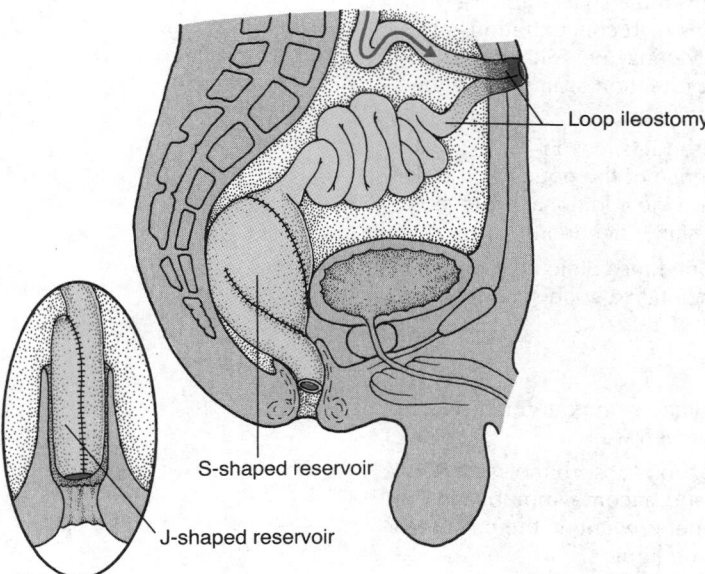
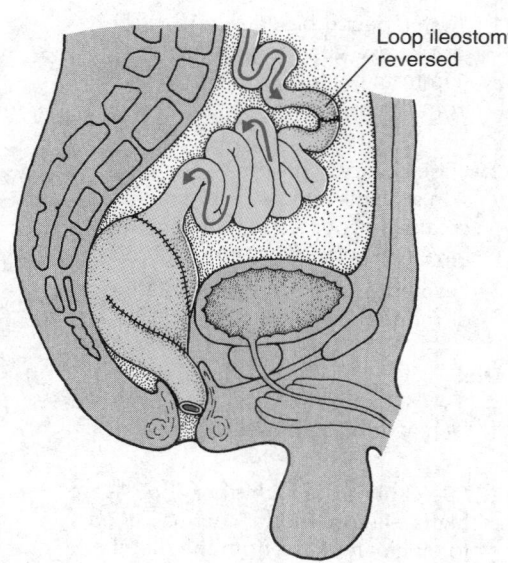

Stage 1.
After removal of the colon, a temporary loop ileostomy is created and an ileoanal reservoir is formed. The reservoir is created in an S-shaped reservoir (using three loops of ileum) or a J-shaped reservoir (suturing a portion of ileum to the rectal cuff, with an upward loop).

Stage 2.
After the reservoir has had time to heal—usually several months—the temporary loop ileostomy is reversed, and stool is allowed to drain into the reservoir.

Figure 45–4

Creation of an ileoanal reservoir.

must have the loop ileostomy to allow adequate healing of the internal pouch and all anastomosis sites and to allow for an increase in the capacity of the internal reservoir, through fluid instillations. After 3 to 4 months, the client returns to have the loop ileostomy closed. The nature and character of the stool are similar to those with a traditional ileostomy.

Preoperative care. If the client must undergo surgery, extensive teaching is needed. Teaching goals include

that the client will be able to perform his/her own ostomy care, will have the knowledge necessary to integrate having an ostomy into his/her life style, and is aware of potential problems and possible solutions to those problems. Preoperative teaching includes those aspects that relate to having abdominal surgery (Chap. 18) and those that relate to having an ostomy (see the accompanying Client/Family Education feature). A consultation with an enterostomal therapist (a nurse

---

CLIENT/FAMILY EDUCATION ■ How to Care for an Ileostomy

Instructions	Rationales
Pouch Care	
1. "Empty your pouch when it is ⅓ to ½ full."	1. Weight of a full pouch will undermine the seal at the base of the stoma.
2. "Change the pouch during inactive times, such as before meals, before retiring at night, on waking in the morning, and 2–4 hr after eating."	2. There will be less chance of stomal functioning during the changing procedure and increased ease with the pouch change.
3. "Change the entire pouch system every 3–7 d."	3. Individual wearing time is dependent on the style of the pouch, the stoma shape, and the condition of peritoneal skin surface.
Skin Protection	
1. "Use a pectin-based skin barrier (not karaya gum) to protect your skin from contact with contents from the ostomy."	1. Fluid from the small intestine contains high concentrations of digestive enzymes. Skin needs good protection against these enzymes.
2. "Use skin care products, such as skin sealants and ostomy skin creams, if your skin continues to have contact with ostomy contents."	2. Skin products may increase adherence of the pouch to the skin and provide additional protection of the skin if needed.
3. "Watch your skin for any irritation or redness."	3. It is sometimes difficult to obtain and maintain a good seal.
Diet	
1. "Chew food thoroughly."	1. Foods may come out undigested if not chewed well.
2. "Be cautious of high-fiber and high-cellulose foods. You may need to eliminate these from the diet if they cause severe problems (diarrhea, constipation, or blockage). Examples of these foods are popcorn, peanuts, coconut, Chinese vegetables, string beans, tough fiber meats, shrimp and lobster, rice, bran, and skinned vegetables (tomatoes, corn, and peas)."	2. These foods absorb moisture. They swell and become immobile in the intestine, preventing the passage of food and liquid.

trained and certified in ostomy care) is indicated preoperatively for recommendations on the location of the ostomy. A visit from an ostomate (a client with an ostomy) may be appropriate preoperatively, if the client agrees to this.

Postoperative care. The nurse provides routine postoperative interventions as for clients who have undergone abdominal surgery (Chap. 20). All clients requiring surgical intervention for ulcerative colitis have an ab-

dominal incision. Depending on the specific procedure performed, some clients have an ostomy, and some have a perineal wound (with removal of the rectum and anus). Initially, most clients are maintained on NPO status, and a nasogastric tube is used for suction.

Clients who undergo Kock's ileostomy have a gastrostomy tube that is inserted through the abdominal wall directly into the stomach. This tube, which is connected to suction, has been shown to be more effective

---

CLIENT/FAMILY EDUCATION ■ How to Care for an Ileostomy *Continued*

Instructions	Rationales
Medications	
1. "Avoid taking enteric-coated and capsule medications."	1, 2. Owing to the possibility of a shortened bowel from surgery, there may not be adequate digestion and absorption of heavily coated medications.
2. "Inform any physician who is prescribing medications for you that you have an ostomy. Inform your pharmacist that you have an ostomy, before having prescriptions filled."	
3. "Do not take any laxatives or enemas. You should usually have loose stool and should contact a physician if no stool has passed in 6–12 h."	
Symptoms to Watch For	
1. "Report any drastic increase or decrease in drainage to your physician."	1. Ileostomy normally drains about a pint of yellow-brown-green paste-like contents in 1 d. Some change in consistency normally occurs when different foods are ingested.
2. "If stomal swelling, crampy abdominal pain, or distention occurs or ileostomy contents stop draining, do the following: a. Remove the pouch with faceplate. b. Lie down, assuming a knee-chest position. c. Begin abdominal massage. d. Apply moist towels to the abdomen. e. Drink hot tea. If none of these maneuvers are effective in resuming ileostomy flow, or if abdominal pain is severe, call your physician right away."	2. These signs may indicate blockage, and the suggested maneuvers promote peristalsis. If these maneuvers are not successful, a blockage needs medical attention.

than a nasogastric tube in preventing discomfort and complications. These clients also have an indwelling Foley's catheter within the pouch, which is connected to low intermittent suction and irrigated as ordered.

When peristalsis returns, nasogastric and gastrostomy tubes are discontinued as ordered, and a clear-liquid diet is begun slowly. The diet is gradually increased to low-residue and then regular diet as tolerated.

Most clients undergoing surgical intervention for ulcerative colitis have lived with chronic illness for some time. Often, surgery is welcomed, for it provides a sense of relief from the multiple problems that occurred before surgery. However, initially, life with an ileostomy may not be perceived as a positive alternative. The client must have the opportunity to discuss any feelings regarding the effect of the illness and the perceived effect that surgical interventions will have.

Surgery results in a loss of a body organ and the partial or total loss of a body function. There is also a change in the physical appearance of the body. Client goals include the ability to provide self-care, adaptation of the life style to include care of an ostomy, and resumption of presurgery activities. If the client had a limited life style owing to illness before surgery, the goal is a more positive and productive life style after surgery.

Pain

Planning: client goals. The primary goal is that the client will experience relief from painful abdominal cramping that occurs with the disease.

Interventions: nonsurgical management. Disease symptoms can cause physical discomfort for the client, which also can contribute to emotional discomfort. The use of a variety of symptom-reducing interventions and supportive measures can provide increased comfort.

Pain monitoring. The nurse assesses for pain, and particular attention is given to any changes in the client's complaints of and responses to pain. Changes in the pain experience may be indicative of disease complications, such as increased inflammation, obstruction, hemorrhage, or peritonitis. Pain assessment includes the character, pattern of occurrence (e.g., before or after meals, during the night, and before or after bowel movements), and duration.

Drug therapy. Antidiarrheal medications are used to control the diarrhea and thereby reduce the resulting discomfort (see Table 45–1). Anticholinergics, such as propantheline bromide (Pro-Banthine), may be given before meals to provide relief from the pain and cramping that may occur with diarrhea. Narcotics are used sparingly and cautiously. These drugs can mask symptoms of life-threatening complications.

Diet therapy. The use of dietary measures in controlling the disease is discussed under Diarrhea earlier. These measures assist in controlling the disease symptoms and thereby promote relief from discomfort. The nurse's responsibility includes ongoing evaluation of the effect of dietary measures implemented in controlling symptoms and providing increased comfort.

Perineal skin care. The perineal skin can be irritated by the frequent contact of the diarrheal stool and frequent cleaning. This can be a major contributor to the client's discomfort. Cleaning with mild soap and warm water after each bowel movement keeps the skin free of any stool. Frequent sitz baths may be helpful, particularly after a bowel movement. Application of a thin coat of mineral oil, petroleum jelly, vitamin A and D ointment, or medicated foam applications may provide relief. Use of medicated wipes with witch hazel (e.g., Tucks) provides soothing relief to the client whose rectal area may be tender and sensitive from the use of toilet tissue.

Various ostomy manufacturing companies (e.g., Hollister and Bard) produce a three-product system for skin care that may be helpful in preventing and healing perineal skin irritation, thus relieving discomfort. Such systems include a skin cleaning solution that is gentle and soothing to the skin, a moisturizing and healing cream, and a petroleum jelly–like ointment that prevents contact of moisture and stool with the skin.

Other measures. The nurse assists the client in altering the pain experience by using measures such as changes in position, reduction of physical pressure on the site of pain, application of heat, diversional activities, adequate rest and activity, involvement of the client in plans of care, provision of information and explanation, and the allowance of opportunities for the client to voice feelings and concerns. Such measures contribute to a therapeutic environment and assist the client in acquiring the ability to deal with pain.

■ Discharge Planning

Home Care Preparation

The client is assessed for the ability to procure medications, to obtain rest, and to follow dietary restrictions after discharge. Clients who have undergone surgery are also assessed for their ability to provide incision and possibly ostomy, or Kock's pouch, care.

Client/Family Education

The client is educated about the nature of the disease with regard to its acute episodes and remissions and symptom management. It is essential that the client understand that, even though the cause is unknown, relapses can be resolved with proper health care.

If the client has undergone a surgical diversion to manage colon effluent, the client is given an explanation and demonstration of the required care as shown in Client/Family Education: How to Care for an Ileostomy. The client is encouraged to demonstrate self-care of the ileostomy.

Clients with ileostomies are also taught to include adequate amounts of salt and water in their diets, because the ileostomy promotes the loss of these elements. Clients are taught to be cautious in situations that promote profuse sweating or fluid loss, such as during strenuous physical activities, when environmental heat is excessive, and during episodes of diarrhea and vomiting.

Psychosocial Preparation

Leaving the relative safety and security of the hospital may initiate concerns about relapses and coping with responsibilities at home or in other settings, such as at work. Clients should have ample time to prepare for discharge from the hospital and to utilize problem-solving strategies for any anticipated concerns (see the accompanying Nursing Research feature). Opportunities to verbalize concerns and worries promote problem-solving skills. If a client has an ileostomy, there may be multiple concerns regarding management at home and sexual and social adjustments. Considering possible sexual issues assists the client to identify and discuss these concerns with the sexual partner. Social situations may precipitate some anxieties. Assisting the client to explore possible concerns is essential in the process of addressing and resolving these potentially stressful events.

Health Care Resources

If a client requires assistance with ADL, services of a home care aide may be arranged.

If the client is discharged from the hospital with an ileostomy, a referral is made to a home care agency. A visiting nurse can provide guidance in integrating ostomy care into the client's life style and possibly provide wound care, including the monitoring of wound healing. The client needs to know where to purchase ostomy supplies, along with the name, size, and manufacturer's order number to purchase the correct supplies. Local and regional supply houses should be contacted regarding price and availability. The local stoma support group can be identified by contacting the United Ostomy Association. A local support group and the National Foundation of Ileitis and Colitis may be of assistance in obtaining supplies. The client and the family are also informed of available ostomy outpatient clinics and enterostomal therapists. If the client agrees, a visit from an ostomate can be initiated or continued on an outpatient basis.

 Evaluation

On the basis of the identified nursing diagnoses, the nurse evaluates the care of the client with ulcerative colitis. The expected outcomes include that the client

---

NURSING RESEARCH

Most Ostomates Adjust Well to Having an Ostomy — with the Assistance of an Enterostomal Therapist.

Kelman, G., & Minkler, P. (1989). An investigation of quality of life and self-esteem among individuals with ostomies. *Journal of Enterostomal Therapy, 16,* 4–11.

The creation of an ostomy is a traumatic event with psychosocial and physiologic effects. Adaptation to this event requires internal and external resources. Adapting to a chronic illness has been shown to affect individuals' ability to care for themselves and their quality of life and self-esteem. This descriptive study surveyed a convenience sample of 346 individuals with ostomies. Eighty-one questionnaires were returned, and 50 were completed and used in the study. Thirty-eight percent of the subjects had a sigmoid colostomy; 42%, a standard ileostomy; 10%, a transverse colostomy; 8%, an ileal conduit; 2%, a continent ileostomy; and 2% had another type of colostomy.

A questionnaire and two instruments were mailed and returned by mail by the participants. The instruments included Geraldine Padilla and Marcia Grant's Quality of Life Index for colostomy patients and Morris Rosenberg's self-esteem scale. The Quality of Life Index has previously been shown to be reliable and valid, and the self-esteem scale has been shown to be highly reliable.

The study indicated that there is a relationship between quality of life and self-esteem among individuals with ostomies. The overall population had positive perceptions of their ostomy and management routine.

Critique. A limitation of the study was that questionnaires were not completely answered, thus contributing to the small sample size. Information regarding who was most responsible for the ostomate's learning to manage the ostomy was significant, with 46% reporting that source to be an enterostomal therapy nurse.

Possible Nursing Implications. Enterostomal therapists have been influential in ostomates' adaptation to an ostomy. Nurses need to continue to utilize this resource to assist clients after ostomy surgery. Because hospital stays are shorter, nurses need to ensure that ostomates receive adequate support to aid in adaptation to their ostomy.

---

1. Is free of diarrhea, rectal bleeding, or cramping
2. Maintains adequate hydration
3. Has an awareness of factors that influence active disease and uses this knowledge to adapt his/her life style for better control of exacerbations
4. Maintains ideal body weight
5. Is aware of and adheres to the prescribed drug regimen

Additionally, the client with an ileostomy

6. Is able to perform his/her own pouch care
7. Maintains peristomal skin integrity
8. Is able to verbalize diet restrictions
9. Demonstrates behaviors that integrate the ostomy into his/her life style
10. Verbalizes signs and symptoms of stomal complications

CROHN'S DISEASE

OVERVIEW

Crohn's disease, also known as regional enteritis, can affect any part of the GI tract, as well as all layers of the intestinal wall. An inflammatory bowel disease, Crohn's disease is similar to ulcerative colitis in that the cause is unknown. It is a chronic illness that is accompanied by a variety of serious complications.

Pathophysiology

Crohn's disease can occur anywhere in the GI tract, though the terminal ileum is most frequently involved. The lesions are patchy and often extend through all bowel layers, at which point bowel fistulas can develop.

Chronic changes include thickening of the bowel wall and thus narrowing of the bowel lumen. This inflammatory bowel disease is also characterized by remissions and exacerbations. In advanced disease, the bowel mucosa demonstrates nodular swellings intermingled with deep ulcerations. Fistulas form, probably beginning as ulcerations. Those that extend through the serosa and into nearby loops of bowel are called enter-

oenteric fistulas. Fistulous tracts may form from diseased segments of the bowel to the skin, umbilicus, and perineum. These are called enterocutaneous fistulas (Fig. 45 – 5). Fistulas can also extend from the bowel to other organs and body cavities, such as the bladder or the vagina. A fistula between two portions of intestine is termed enteroenteric.

Other complications include malnutrition, anemia, dehydration, and electrolyte imbalances. These complications occur when inflammatory changes within the bowel mucosa alter the absorption of nutrients and fluids. Mechanical intestinal obstruction may also occur owing to narrowing of the intestinal lumen.

Etiology

As for ulcerative colitis, the cause of Crohn's disease is unknown. Research suggests that the cause may be related to infectious, immune or psychologic factors.

Incidence

In the United States, there are 50,000 to 100,000 known cases of Crohn's disease, with 5000 to 10,000 new cases being diagnosed each year (Wyngaarden, 1988). In most surveys, women and men are affected with equal frequency. This disorder has its highest incidence in the teen years to age 30 years. A later peak incidence may occur between the ages of 55 and 60 years (Wyngaarden, 1988). A positive family history can be identified in 20% to 50% of cases.

PREVENTION

As the causes of Crohn's disease are unknown, it is difficult to institute preventive measures. Critical to the process of caring for clients with Crohn's disease is the early detection of illness and the prevention of complications. Emotional factors have not been shown to cause

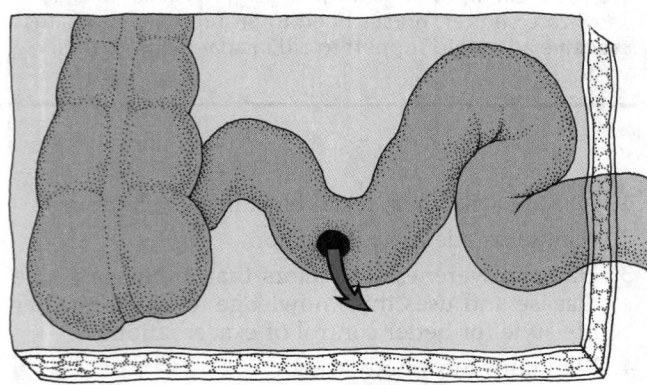
External enterocutaneous

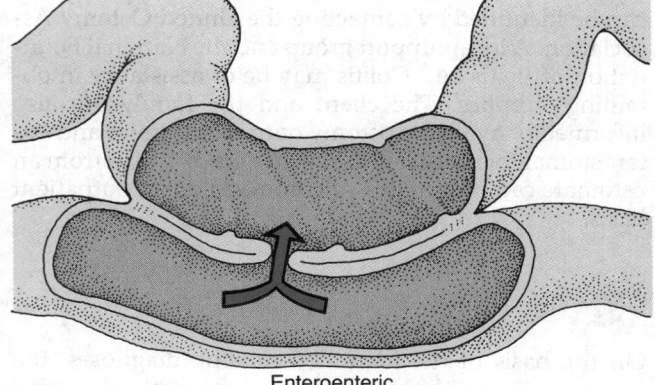
Enteroenteric

Figure 45 – 5

Types of fistulas that are complications of Crohn's disease.

Crohn's disease; however, psychologic and sociologic factors may play an important role in the individual's ability to cope with the stress of a chronic illness.

COLLABORATIVE MANAGEMENT

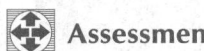 **Assessment**

History

When caring for a client with Crohn's disease, the nurse obtains an assessment in a format similar to that for a client with ulcerative colitis (see earlier). In addition, the nurse collects data regarding current or past *history of fistulas,* as these are frequent complications of this illness.

Physical Assessment: Clinical Manifestations

The clinical presentation of Crohn's disease can vary greatly from client to client. Initially, the client frequently complains of *right lower quadrant pain, diarrhea,* and *low-grade fever.* The physical examination findings are often consistent with those in acute appendicitis (tenderness, guarded movement, and palpable mass in the right lower quadrant).

Depending on the parts of the bowel involved, the nurse can identify a variety of symptoms. Most clients report diarrhea, abdominal pain, and fever. If the disease occurs only in the ileum, diarrhea occurs five to six times per day, often with a soft, loose stool. Stool may contain blood, but this is a rare finding.

Abdominal pain results from the inflammatory process and usually is constant and is located in the right lower quadrant. Clients also experience *periumbilical pain* before and after bowel movements, and, if the lower colon is diseased, pain is often experienced in both lower abdominal quadrants. *Steatorrhea* is a common occurrence. *Fever* is commonly present with complications such as fistulas.

Weight loss may indicate serious *nutritional deficiencies.* Nutritional problems occur frequently, as clients often experience anorexia, self-imposed dietary restrictions, the decreased absorption of multiple nutrients, and fluid and electrolyte loss. The marked inflammatory changes of the bowel decrease the small bowel's ability to absorb nutrients. These problems may be worsened by surgery and fistulas.

The nurse is acutely aware of how important it is to detect clinical manifestations of peritonitis, bowel obstruction, and nutritional and fluid imbalances. The early detection of a change in the client's status helps to minimize complications.

Psychosocial Assessment

The individual experiencing Crohn's disease needs a complete psychosocial assessment, as for the client with ulcerative colitis (see earlier). The chronicity of the problem and the troublesome complications often have great impact on clients and their families. The assessment should be ongoing and continuously reflect the client's status as well as the family's.

Laboratory Findings

A number of laboratory studies are performed for clients with Crohn's disease; however, no disease-specific tests are available to confirm the diagnosis. The process of diagnosis occurs by ruling out disorders with similar signs and symptoms. Findings noted in Crohn's disease include negative stool cultures, occult blood in stool, and low serum albumin level resulting from protein loss due to poor absorption. Liver function test values may or may not be elevated. Serum levels of folic acid and cobalamin (vitamin B_{12} group) are generally low because of malabsorption. A decreased hemoglobin level and hematocrit are generally noted, as a result of slow blood loss. WBCs in the urine may indicate infection, which may be caused by ureteral obstruction or enterovesical (bowel to bladder) fistula.

Radiographic Findings

The findings of the contrast barium enema often provide specific diagnostic information. The radiologic findings show narrowing, ulcerations, strictures, and fistulas consistent with Crohn's disease. In the acute illness, the barium enema is often deferred until the risk of perforation lessens.

Other Diagnostic Tests

Depending on the specific areas of the bowel that are diseased, the sigmoidoscopy examination may not be diagnostic. However, if the rectosigmoid is involved, the examiner may see ulcerations and inflamed mucosa. In addition, the examiner may visualize areas of fissure, fistula, and abscess formation of the perianal and perirectal areas.

Colonoscopy is used in the diagnostic process only when other tests, especially the barium enema, have not led to a specific diagnosis.

 Analysis: Nursing Diagnosis

The care of the client with Crohn's disease is similar to that for the client with ulcerative colitis. Similar nursing diagnoses are identified (see earlier), as well as impaired skin integrity related to fistula formation.

 Planning and Implementation

Impaired Skin Integrity

The plan of care for the client with Crohn's disease is consistent with that for the client with ulcerative colitis (see earlier).

Planning: client goals. The major goal for the client with a fistula is that the client will experience healing of the fistula.

Interventions. Dealing with a GI fistula often leaves clients frustrated and embarrassed as they deal with pain and medical problems. In Crohn's disease, fistulas may form as a result of surgery or the illness itself. Clients with fistulas are often experiencing complications such as systemic infections, skin problems, malnutrition, and fluid and electrolyte imbalances. The degree of associated problems depends on the site of the fistula, the client's general health status, and the character and amount of discharge from the fistula.

Nonsurgical management. Treatment is multidimensional and includes nutrition and electrolyte therapy, skin care, and prevention of infection.
Nutrition and electrolyte therapy. Establishing adequate nutrition and fluid and electrolyte balances must take priority in the care of the client with a fistula. GI secretions are high in volume, electrolytes, and enzymes.

Fluids and electrolytes are replaced by oral liquids and nutrients, as well as IV fluids. Frequently, an antidiarrheal agent, such as diphenoxylate hydrochloride and atropine sulfate (Lomotil), is used to decrease volume. Usually, when a fistula begins to develop, the nutritional status is compromised. After the fistula has developed, the nutritional status worsens. The client requires at least 3000 kcal/day to promote healing of the fistula. If the client is unable to take adequate oral fluids and nutrients, TPN may be indicated. The nurse carefully monitors the client's tolerance to diet; assists the client in making high-calorie, high-protein meal selections; offers supplements; and works with the dietitian to conduct calorie counts.
Prevention of infection. Clients with fistulas are at extremely high risk for intra-abdominal abscesses and sepsis. The treatment for intra-abdominal fistulas includes careful nursing observations, wound drainage, and antibiotic therapy. The nurse observes for subtle signs of infection or sepsis, such as fever, abdominal pain, or change in mental status.
Skin therapy. The presence of proteolytic enzymes or bile contributes to the problem of skin denudation. Skin irritation needs to be prevented; this is usually is accomplished through the use of skin barriers, application of pouches, and insertion of drains (Fig. 45–6). By applying a pouch to the draining fistula, the nurse prevents skin irritation and is also able to measure the effluent (drainage).

An approach to drainage management is to cover the area surrounding the fistula with barriers, such as Stomahesive, or DuoDerm, and then to apply a wound drainage system over the fistula, securing it to the protective dressing. The skin adjacent to the fistula is cleaned with normal saline solution and gently patted dry. Gaps may be filled in the skin barrier (e.g., Stomahesive) with karaya gum.

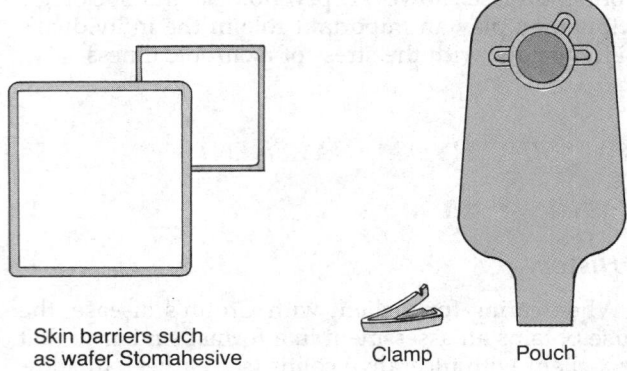

Skin barriers such as wafer Stomahesive | Clamp | Pouch

Figure 45–6

Skin barriers, such as wafers, are cut to fit ⅛ in around the fistula. A drainable pouch is applied over the wafer. Effluent should drain into the bag and not contact the skin.

An enterostomal therapist is an excellent resource in providing wound management. It is imperative that wound drainage *never* be allowed in direct contact with skin without prompt cleaning because intestinal fluid enzymes are caustic.

Surgical managment. Surgery to remove diseased portions of intestine is controversial because of considerable risk of disease recurrence. Recently, however, clients who have symptoms after long-term medical treatment more often undergo surgical treatment, commonly small bowel resection and anastomosis with or without colon resection. Preoperative and postoperative care is similar to care for clients undergoing other types of abdominal surgery (Chaps. 18 and 20).

■ Discharge Planning

The discharge care plan for the client with Crohn's disease is similar to that for the client with ulcerative colitis (as described earlier). If the client has a draining fistula, the nurse needs to help the client plan for care of the fistula at home.

Home Care Preparation

The client's home should be arranged so the client has easy access to the bathroom, as well as opportunities for privacy to perform fistula care and to rest. To ensure adequate nutrition, the client should have easy access to a well-supplied kitchen of readily prepared foods.

Client/Family Education

Before discharge from the hospital, the client is given an explanation and demonstration of fistula care. The client also needs to have opportunities to practice that care in the hospital. Ideally, the client should be independent in fistula care before leaving the hospital. However, many times (because of perirectal or vaginal location of the fistula or obese abdomen), the client needs assistance in this care. If this is the case, a family member or a caregiver must learn and practice the care, or the nurse can arrange for home health care services.

The teaching plan for the client with Crohn's disease is similar to that for the client with ulcerative colitis (see earlier). Clients who have undergone bowel resection are given instructions similar to those given to clients who have undergone abdominal surgery (Chap. 20).

Psychosocial Preparation

Like the client with ulcerative colitis, the client with Crohn's disease must identify stressors and methods to eliminate or reduce the impact of stressors. The nurse provides an atmosphere of trust and caring and encourages verbalization of the client's concerns. Interventions should build self-esteem and promote independence.

Health Care Resources

The client with Crohn's disease benefits from the same health care resources as the client with ulcerative colitis. If the client needs equipment for fistula care, such as skin barriers (e.g., Stomahesive) and wound drainage bags, medical supply houses are contacted to ascertain their availability and price. The nurse assesses the client's and the family's capability of carefully monitoring the progress of fistula healing and watching for signs and symptoms of infection and sepsis. The assistance of a home care nurse may be considered for monitoring fistula care and status. A home care aide might be considered for clients who are unable to meet their nutritional needs, for assistance with meal preparation and procurement of groceries.

 Evaluation

On the basis of the identified nursing diagnoses, the nurse evaluates the care of the client with Crohn's disease. The expected outcomes are that the client

1. Has a decrease in frequency of diarrhea
2. Has an awareness of factors that influence active disease and uses this knowledge to make life style changes for better control of exacerbations
3. Does not manifest complications of Crohn's disease

IRRITABLE BOWEL SYNDROME

OVERVIEW

Irritable bowel syndrome (IBS), also called spastic bowel and mucous colitis, is probably the most common digestive disorder affecting Americans today. It is not a true

colitis in that there is no inflammation present. It primarily entails a change in bowel habits, with abdominal pain and no actual organic disease.

Pathophysiology

The diagnosis of IBS is made through the exclusion of any other disease processes that mimic its symptoms. Diagnostic studies strongly suggest that IBS is a disorder of GI motility. This change in motility may be the result of anxiety, depression, fear, food, drugs, toxins, or colonic distention. As a result of motility changes, the bowel elimination pattern changes to one of diarrhea, constipation, or alternating diarrhea and constipation. Individuals may report an onset of IBS in adolescence or even later in life. Individuals experience a progressive change in bowel function and eventually form a characteristic bowel pattern, most commonly alternating diarrhea and constipation. The course of the illness is generally individual specific and most clients can identify factors, such as stress, diet, or anxiety, that precipitate exacerbations. There are no changes in the bowel mucosa and therefore no serious health consequences. However, the irregular bowel patterns and associated cramps often play havoc with the individual's life style.

Etiology

The exact etiology of IBS is unknown, and IBS is considered a functional disorder. Physical factors, such as diverticular disease, ingestion of coffee or other gastric stimulants, or lactose intolerance, may contribute to IBS.

Incidence

IBS is the most common disorder of the gastrointestinal tract in western societies (Wyngaarden, 1985), but reliable data regarding its incidence are not available. More than two-thirds of those affected are women. There is a higher incidence among Caucasians and Jews than in other groups. Most individuals report symptoms before the age of 35 to 40 years, and, for most clients, IBS follows a chronic pattern with periods of remission and periods of exacerbation characterized by constipation, diarrhea, pain, abdominal distention, belching, and passage of flatus.

PREVENTION

The individual can take many steps to prevent the symptoms of IBS. Most clients find it extremely helpful to avoid rich foods, such as ice cream and butter, and fatty foods, such as bacon and sausage. If certain foods, such as fruits, or medications, such as antibiotics, cause diarrhea, they should be avoided. The elimination of gas-producing foods, such as carbonated beverages, beans, and cauliflower, helps to control bloating. Eating a well-balanced diet, planning regular mealtimes, and maintaining adequate fluid intake are often helpful in preventing uncomfortable symptoms. Keeping a diet history helps the client identify foods that cause symptoms. Chewing foods slowly helps reduce the amount of swallowed air. Alcohol consumption and cigarette smoking should be eliminated, as they are both gastric stimulants.

Achieving balance in all aspects of the client's life is important. The client needs to reduce and manage stressors, and counseling may be indicated. A regular exercise program is vital for many purposes. Even a 20- to 30-minute walk each day may relieve tension and frustration, as well as promote regular bowel patterns. Consistency in obtaining adequate rest and sleep is also helpful, promoting stress reduction and the ability to cope with everyday life.

COLLABORATIVE MANAGEMENT

 Assessment

History

When taking a history from the client with IBS, the nurse considers contributing factors. Data to collect include the *sex, age,* and *race* of the client. Knowledge of the individual's occupation may help identify potential sources of stress. Information about habits such as cigarette, alcohol, and caffeine use are obtained, including the frequency of use. Assessment of current and ongoing *stressors,* usual *dietary patterns,* and report of *bowel patterns,* including the character, color, and consistency of stools, as well as associated factors, is also included. The client's current and past *medical history,* including a history of stress-related illness, is obtained. The client is also asked about any *recent weight loss,* as this may point to problems other than IBS.

Physical Assessment: Clinical Manifestations

The typical client with IBS is diagnosed after many bouts of *diarrhea* or *constipation.* Usually, a flare consisting of *worsening cramps, abdominal pain,* or diarrhea or constipation brings the client to the health care provider. The most common symptom of IBS is *pain* in the left lower quadrant of the abdomen. The client reports increased pain after eating and relief after a bowel movement. *Nausea* associated with mealtime and defecation may also be reported. The crampy abdominal patterns are accompanied by constipation or diarrhea. The constipated stools are small and hard, generally followed by several softer stools. The diarrheal stools are soft and watery, and mucus is frequently seen in the stools.

Clients with IBS frequently complain of other symptoms, including belching, gas, anorexia, and bloating. Some clients may also experience fatigue, anxiety, headaches, and difficulty in concentrating.

In performing the abdominal examination, the nurse inspects and auscultates the abdomen. Bowel sounds are generally within normal range and may be somewhat quiet if constipation is present.

When percussing the abdomen, the nurse may find that there are tympanic sounds over loops of filled bowel. On palpation, there may be diffuse tenderness, which is generally worse if the sigmoid colon is palpable. The rectal examination may show hard or soft stool.

The client generally looks well, but perhaps fatigued. Weight is stable, and nutritional and fluid status are within normal ranges.

Psychosocial Assessment

Clients with IBS often appear tense and anxious. They may have undergone a recent period of stress or emotional tension. Many times, the client is unaware of any correlation between stressors and changes in bowel patterns. Assisting the client to correlate pertinent events to bowel patterns (e.g., via a life event time line) is often helpful.

Laboratory Findings

There are no specific laboratory tests that confirm the diagnosis of IBS. A battery of tests are performed to rule out more serious problems, such as ulcerative colitis or Crohn's disease.

Radiographic Findings

A barium enema is routinely performed. Colonic spasm is often noted during the procedure; however, this finding is not diagnostic. In the absence of other diagnostic findings, the presence of colonic spasm supports the diagnosis (Fig. 45 – 7).

Other Diagnostic Tests

The evaluation of IBS is not complete without sigmoidoscopy. This examination often demonstrates intense spastic contractions, which frequently stimulate painful sensations. Otherwise, the bowel mucosa appears continuous, smooth, and pink.

 Analysis: Nursing Diagnosis

Most often, the client with IBS is cared for on an outpatient basis. Frequently, the client is a woman in her 20s or 30s.

Common Diagnoses

The typical diagnoses associated with IBS include

1. Diarrhea and constipation related to changes in motility
2. Ineffective individual coping related to feelings of limited control over the illness

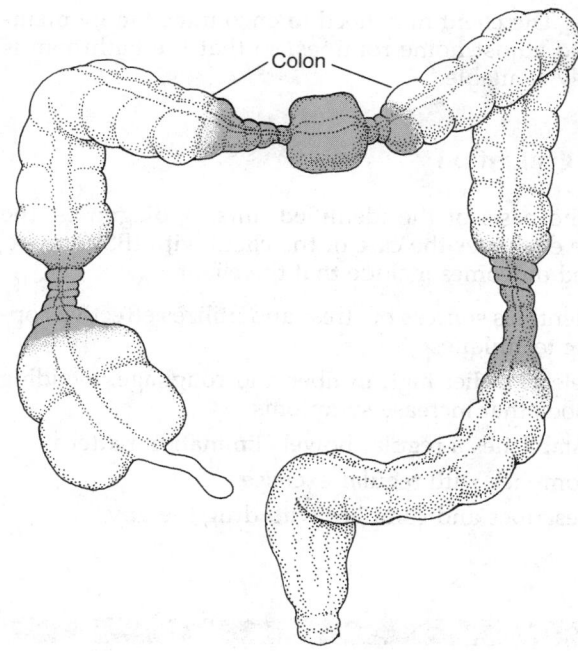

Figure 45–7

Spastic contractions of the colon, as they occur with IBS.

Additional Diagnoses

In addition, the client may also exhibit diagnoses such as

1. Altered nutrition: less than body requirements related to diarrhea, fatigue, abdominal pain, or dietary self-restriction
2. Chronic pain related to changes in GI motility
3. Knowledge deficit related to control or treatment of IBS

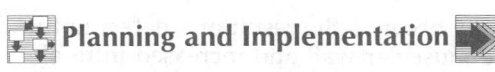

Planning and Implementation

Diarrhea; Constipation

Planning: client goals. The major goal is that the client will have a regular bowel pattern.

Interventions: nonsurgical management. In treating the client with IBS, a number of treatment modes are used, including drug therapy, diet management, exercise, and modification of routines.

Drug therapy. Bulk-forming laxatives, antidiarrheal agents, and cholinergic products are used in the treatment of IBS. The use of one or a combination of products can often be helpful in managing unpleasant symptoms.

The bulk-forming laxatives such as psyllium hydrophilic mucilloid (Metamucil) or calcium polycarbophil (Mitrolan) are generally taken at mealtimes with a glassful of water. The hydrophilic properties of these medications help prevent dry, hard, or liquid stools.

Antidiarrheal agents, such as diphenoxylate hydrochloride with atropine sulfate (Lomotil), loperamide (Imodium), or camphorated tincture of opium (paregoric), are used to help decrease cramping and frequent stools (see Table 45–1). These drugs carry a certain risk of dependency, and long-term therapy is generally not recommended because they all have a narcotic base.

Cholinergic receptor blocking agents, such as dicyclomine hydrochloride (Bentyl) and propantheline bromide (Pro-Banthine), help relieve abdominal cramping and intestinal spasm. If clients experience postprandial discomfort, the nurse gives these medications 30 to 45 minutes before mealtime.

Diet therapy. Adding fiber and bulk helps produce bulky, soft stools and establishes regular bowel habits. The client should ingest approximately 30 to 40 g of fiber per day. Eating regular meals, drinking 8 to 10 c of liquid each day, and chewing food slowly help promote normal bowel function.

Exercise and modification of routines. Regular exercise is important in stress management and the promotion of regular bowel elimination. The client needs to be alert to the urge to defecate and evacuate promptly to avoid straining. The client should plan to allow time and privacy in the bathroom. The nurse assists the client in maintaining a stool count and determining the consistency, color, and character of the stools in relationship to ADL.

Ineffective Individual Coping

Planning: client goals. The major goal is that the client will verbalize an increasing ability to cope with IBS and ongoing stressors.

Interventions: nonsurgical management. After completing a detailed psychosocial assessment, the nurse and the client set goals and plan appropriate interventions for *stress management.* Having clients learn and use relaxation techniques can help them feel that they have some skills in managing their illness. Assisting clients in understanding the illness empowers them to take certain actions (e.g., diet modification and exercise) that can have a significant impact on the course of illness.

If clients are in a stressful work or family situation, personal counseling may be helpful. The nurse assists the client in making appointments or makes appropriate referrals. The opportunity to discuss problems and attempt creative problem-solving is often helpful. Chapter 6 describes additional nursing interventions to assist clients and increase their coping skills.

■ Discharge Planning

Home Care Preparation

The client with IBS most usually is seen in the outpatient setting. The nurse helps the client modify work and home schedules to ensure adequate time and facilities for toileting, exercise routines, and a high-fiber diet.

Client/Family Education

The client is taught to make every effort to establish regular bowel patterns that most carefully coincide with his/her life style. The nurse explains the importance of responding to the messages of the bowel and of defecating regularly to avoid constipation.

The client is taught that regular exercise reduces stress, promotes a feeling of well-being, and promotes regular bowel activity. The exercise program should be a type of activity enjoyed by the client, which provides physical activity with minimal inconvenience.

The nurse encourages a high-fiber diet with adequate fluids (see Health Promotion/Maintenance: Fiber Content of Some Common Foods). The client identifies and eliminates offending or upsetting foods. Regular mealtimes are emphasized, as well as avoidance of alcohol, excess caffeine, and other gastric irritants. Milk and milk products should be avoided if the individual has a documented lactose intolerance or if the client can specify milk as an aggravating factor.

Stress identification and management is critical. Clients often benefit from the opportunity to discuss stressors. The nurse aids in establishing a regular plan for stress management that best prepares the client for successful management of stressors.

Drug therapy, usually with psyllium hydrophilic mucilloid and an antispasmodic and antidiarrheal agent, needs to be fully explained to the client, and a schedule for medication administration is established. When initiating therapy with a bulk-forming laxative, it make take a full week for the client to notice a change in bowel habits. The nurse explains side effects to the client for monitoring purposes.

Psychosocial Preparation

By the time a client has a definitive diagnosis of IBS, he/she may have experienced the changes in bowel patterns and abdominal cramping for months or years. The client may have severely curtailed activities both at work and at home and severely limited the diet in an attempt to handle symptoms.

Knowing the diagnosis and the treatment provides some answers, but the client faces many adjustments and changes. The client needs support in adapting to a new diet, medications, and activities. Re-establishing social and work activities may provide new challenges and stressors. The client requires nursing support while confronting past and present stressors.

Health Care Resources

Most clients with IBS are caring for their illness in the home situation. The office or home care nurse should be aware of special considerations for this client. The client needs easy access to a bathroom, both at work and at home. The client may need to encourage family members to adjust home routines, so that the bathroom is readily available.

Evaluation

On the basis of the identified nursing diagnoses, the nurse evaluates the care of the client with IBS. The expected outcomes include that the client

1. Identifies sources of stress and utilizes effective coping techniques
2. Selects a diet high in fiber and roughage, avoiding foods that increase symptoms
3. Establishes a regular bowel elimination pattern
4. Complies with regular exercise
5. Describes and complies with drug therapy

HERNIATION

OVERVIEW

A *hernia* is a weakness in the abdominal muscle wall through which a segment of the bowel or other abdominal structure protrudes. Hernias can also penetrate through any other defect in the abdominal wall, through the diaphragm, or through other structures in the abdominal cavity.

Pathophysiology

Hernias generally occur as the result of a defect in the integrity of the muscular wall and increased intra-abdominal pressure. Defects in the muscular wall result from weakened collagen or widened spaces at the inguinal ligament. These muscle weaknesses can be inherited or acquired as part of the aging process. Increased intra-abdominal pressure results from pregnancy and obesity. Similar increases in intra-abdominal pressure can occur from heavy lifting and coughing.

The most common types of hernias are indirect, direct, femoral, umbilical, and incisional (Fig. 45–8). *Indirect* inguinal hernias occur through the inguinal ring and follow the spermatic cord through the inguinal canal. These hernias frequently become large and often descend into the scrotum. *Direct* inguinal hernias, in contrast, pass through the abdominal wall in an area of muscular weakness.

Femoral hernias occur through the femoral ring. They occur as a plug of fat in the femoral canal, which enlarges and eventually pulls the peritoneum and often the urinary bladder into the sac.

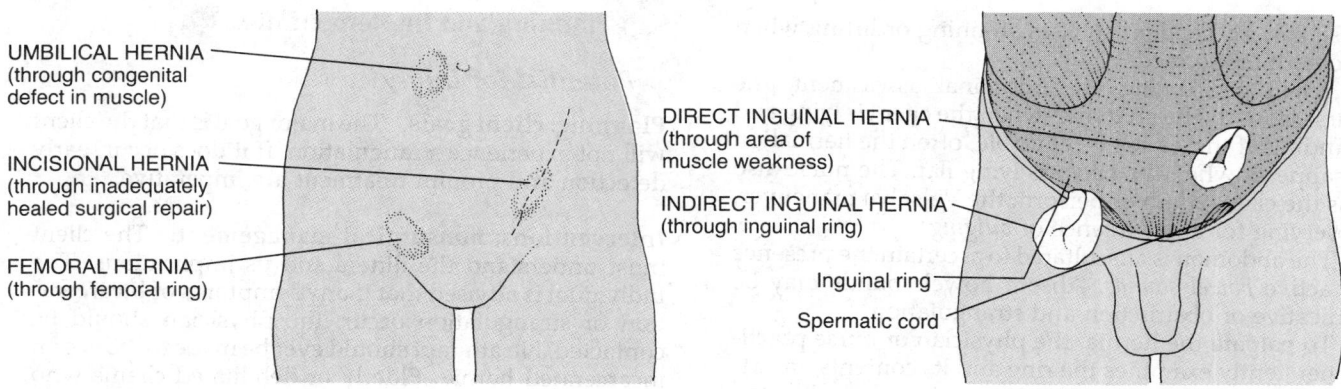

UMBILICAL HERNIA
(through congenital
defect in muscle)

INCISIONAL HERNIA
(through inadequately
healed surgical repair)

FEMORAL HERNIA
(through femoral ring)

DIRECT INGUINAL HERNIA
(through area of
muscle weakness)

INDIRECT INGUINAL HERNIA
(through inguinal ring)

Inguinal ring

Spermatic cord

Figure 45–8

Types of abdominal hernia.

Umbilical hernias are congenital or acquired. Congenital umbilical hernias occur in infancy. Acquired umbilical hernias occur as a direct result of increased intra-abdominal pressure. They are most frequently seen with obese individuals.

Incisional, or *ventral,* hernias occur at the site of a previous surgical incision. These hernias frequently occur as the result of inadequate healing of the incision, most often caused by postoperative wound infections, inadequate nutrition, and obesity.

Hernias may be reducible, irreducible, incarcerated, or strangulated. A *reducible* hernia occurs when the contents of the hernial sac can be replaced into the abdominal cavity by gentle pressure. *Irreducible,* or *incarcerated,* hernias cannot be reduced or placed back into the abdominal cavity. *Strangulated* hernias occur when the blood supply to the herniated segment of the bowel is cut off by pressure from the hernial ring (the band of muscle around the hernia). If a hernia is strangulated, there is ischemia and obstruction of the bowel loop. This can lead to necrosis of the bowel and possibly bowel perforation. Abdominal distention, nausea, vomiting, pain, fever, and tachycardia are signs of strangulation. Any of these symptoms require immediate medical and eventually surgical intervention. Any hernia that is not reducible requires immediate and careful surgical evaluation.

Etiology

The most important elements in the development of a hernia include the congenital or acquired muscle weakness and the increased intra-abdominal pressure. The most significant factors contributing to increased intra-abdominal pressure are obesity, pregnancy, and lifting of heavy objects.

Incidence

Hernias can occur at any age. Indirect inguinal hernias are the most common type and occur most frequently in men. Direct hernias occur more often in the elderly, whereas femoral and adult umbilical hernias are most common in obese or pregnant women. Incisional hernias occur most frequently in individuals who have undergone surgery.

PREVENTION

Congenital muscle weakness cannot be prevented; however, muscle strengthening exercises may possibly be helpful. Maintaining normal body weight, being physically fit, and using proper lifting techniques may prevent herniation. Early recognition and diagnosis of herniation are helpful in the prevention of strangulation. After the herniation occurs, the individual should seek medical attention and avoid lifting and straining, which contribute to strangulation.

COLLABORATIVE MANAGEMENT

 Assessment

History

When taking a history from a client with possible herniation, the nurse keeps risk factors for this disorder in mind. Data to collect from the client include *sex, age, body build, weight* and *height,* a history or presence of concurrent *medical conditions,* past and current use of prescribed and over-the-counter (OTC) *medications, exercise routine, occupation* (any lifting?), a history of *previous herniation,* and any *associated symptoms* (e.g., pain or change in bowel habits).

Physical Assessment: Clinical Manifestations

The typical client with a hernia comes to the physician's office or the emergency room with a complaint of a "bunch" noted on the abdomen. The client frequently describes an incident such as straining or lifting when "something popped."

When performing an abdominal assessment, the nurse inspects the abdomen when the client is lying and standing. If the hernia is reducible, often the herniation disappears when the client is lying flat. The nurse also has the client strain or perform the Valsalva maneuver, observing for any evidence of *bulging*.

The abdomen is auscultated to ascertain the presence of active *bowel sounds*. Absent bowel sounds may be indicative of obstruction and strangulation.

To palpate the hernia, the physician or nurse practitioner gently examines the ring and its contents, inserting a finger in the ring and noting any changes when the client coughs. The nurse never forces the hernia to reduce, as this maneuver can cause the rupture of a strangulated gut.

If the male client suspects a hernia in the groin, the nurse has the client stand and, using the right hand for the client's right side and the left hand for the client's left side, invaginates the loose scrotal skin with the index finger, following the spermatic cord upward to the external inguinal cord. At this point, the client is asked to cough, and the nurse notes any palpable herniation.

Psychosocial Assessment

The nurse completes a psychosocial assessment on all clients with hernias. Surgery is generally indicated, and the effects of hospitalization and surgery may be complex. The nurse assesses the family, work, and home responsibilities. If the individual's occupation involves heavy lifting, certain work modifications may be required. If the herniation results in strangulation, hospitalization occurs on an emergency basis. The client may need assistance in making family arrangements (e.g., for child care).

 Analysis: Nursing Diagnosis

Most clients with herniation are candidates for elective surgery.

Common Diagnoses

Pending surgery, the common nursing diagnosis for a client with herniation is potential for injury related to possible strangulation of the hernia.

Additional Diagnoses

In addition, the client with a hernia may exhibit the following diagnoses:

1. Altered (gastrointestinal) tissue perfusion related to hernial ring
2. Potential impaired skin integrity related to the use of a truss

 Planning and Implementation

Potential for Injury

Planning: client goals. The major goal is that the client will not experience strangulation. If it does occur, early detection and prompt treatment are imperative.

Interventions: nonsurgical management. The client must understand the illness and its implications. The individual is advised that if any symptoms of incarceration or strangulation occur, the physician should be contacted. No attempt should ever be made to reduce an incarcerated hernia. Elderly or debilitated clients who are poor surgical risks may use a truss to help keep the abdominal contents from protruding into the hernial sac. A truss is a pad made with firm material that is held in place over the hernia with a belt. If a truss is used, it should be applied only after the hernia has been reduced. The appliance is usually applied before arising. The skin should be assessed daily and protected with powder.

Interventions: surgical management. Herniorrhaphy is the treatment of choice for hernias. This procedure involves replacing the contents of the hernial sac into the abdominal cavity and closing the opening. A less frequently performed procedure is a hernioplasty. In this procedure, the weakened muscular wall is reinforced with mesh, fascia, or wire.

Preoperative care. The nurse prepares the individual for surgery as one would prepare the client for general surgery (Chap. 18). If the procedure is performed on an outpatient basis, the nurse assists the client to make appropriate arrangements for travel home and home care.

Postoperative care. Postoperative care of the client is the same as that described in Chapter 20, except that clients who undergo surgery for hernias are told to avoid coughing. Deep breathing and frequent turning are encouraged to promote lung expansion. If the client has had an indirect inguinal hernia repair, a scrotal support and ice bags applied to the scrotum help reduce swelling, which often contributes to pain. Elevation of the scrotum with a soft pillow and bed rest will help control swelling. If not contraindicated by scrotal swelling or pre-existing conditions, early ambulation is encouraged and often helps promote comfort and the feeling of well-being.

The client may experience difficulty with voiding. Having the male client stand allows gravity to facilitate voiding and bladder emptying. Techniques to stimulate voiding, such as allowing water to run, may be used. Careful monitoring of intake and output alerts the nurse to voiding problems early. The nurse carefully palpates the abdomen for distention. The intake of at least 1500 to 2400 mL of fluids per day prevents dehydration and maintains urinary function. Most surgeons order catheterization of the client every 6 to 8 hours if the client is unable to void. The interval between catheterizations should not be prolonged, as a distended bladder can stress the incision and increase discomfort.

■ Discharge Planning

Home Care Preparation

Clients undergoing herniorrhaphy or hernioplasty are able to return to their previous living situation with a minimal recovery period. A great number of hernia surgeries are performed on an outpatient basis, with clients returning to full activities within 2 weeks.

Client/Family Education

The nurse teaches the client to resume his/her usual diet, whether regular or special. He/she may need to be encouraged to include all four food groups and roughage in the usual amounts.

Generally, surgeons allow clients to return to their usual activities, avoiding straining and lifting for 2 weeks after surgery. Depending on the site and the extent of repair and the client's general physical condition, this period may be extended to 6 weeks.

The client is instructed orally and given a written list of symptoms to report. This list includes fever, chills, wound drainage, redness or separation of incision, and increasing incision pain.

The client is instructed to keep the wound dry and clean and replace the sterile dressing daily if indicated. If the physician allows, showering is permitted.

If the client is receiving any medication at home, the nurse instructs him/her about the purpose, the dosage, the frequency and timing of administration, and potential side effects. Many agents for pain relief may cause constipation and thus increase straining. The client should be instructed by the nurse about steps to take if these effects occur. The nurse suggests increased fluid and fiber intake; the physician may order small amounts of laxatives.

Psychosocial Preparation

The client going home after hernia surgery faces some temporary adjustments. The individual may require support as adaptation to postoperative recovery takes place. Some individuals fear a recurrence of the herniation. All clients need a thorough explanation of the healing process and instructions regarding proper body mechanics and lifting.

Health Care Resources

If returning home, the client needs dressing supplies for 3 to 5 days. If the client is unable to perform incision care independently, visits by a home care nurse can be arranged for follow-up at home.

Evaluation

On the basis of the identified nursing diagnoses, the nurse evaluates the care of the client undergoing surgical repair of a hernia. The expected outcomes include that the client

1. States that pain is controlled
2. Verbalizes the understanding of discharge instructions (e.g., medications, diet, follow-up care, signs and symptoms to report, and any activity restrictions)
3. Voids without difficulty
4. Has wound healing by first intention

DIVERTICULAR DISEASE

OVERVIEW

The term *diverticular disease* is used to describe the illnesses that traditionally have been identified as diverticulosis and diverticulitis. *Diverticulosis* is the presence of several abnormal outpouchings or herniations in the wall of the intestine. These herniations are called *diverticula*. *Diverticulitis* is the inflammation of one or more of these diverticula.

Pathophysiology

Diverticula can be present in any part of the small or large intestines, but occur most frequently in the sigmoid colon (Fig. 45–9). This is because high pressures are generated in the sigmoid colon to push stool into the rectum. In themselves, diverticula cause few problems. Clients most often do not even have symptoms associated with diverticula and are unaware of them until discovered incidentally during an x-ray examination. However, inflammation or hemorrhage of diverticula can occur. If undigested food or bacteria become trapped in a diverticulum, blood supply to that area diminishes and bacteria invade the diverticulum. Diverticulitis results when the diverticulum perforates and a local abscess forms. The perforated diverticulum can also progress to an intra-abdominal perforation with generalized peritonitis. Obstruction can occur when diverticula have trapped fecal contents recurrently, and the content leaks out. This leakage causes inflammatory changes and thickening and scarring of the colonic wall, which can lead to bowel obstruction. Extension of the

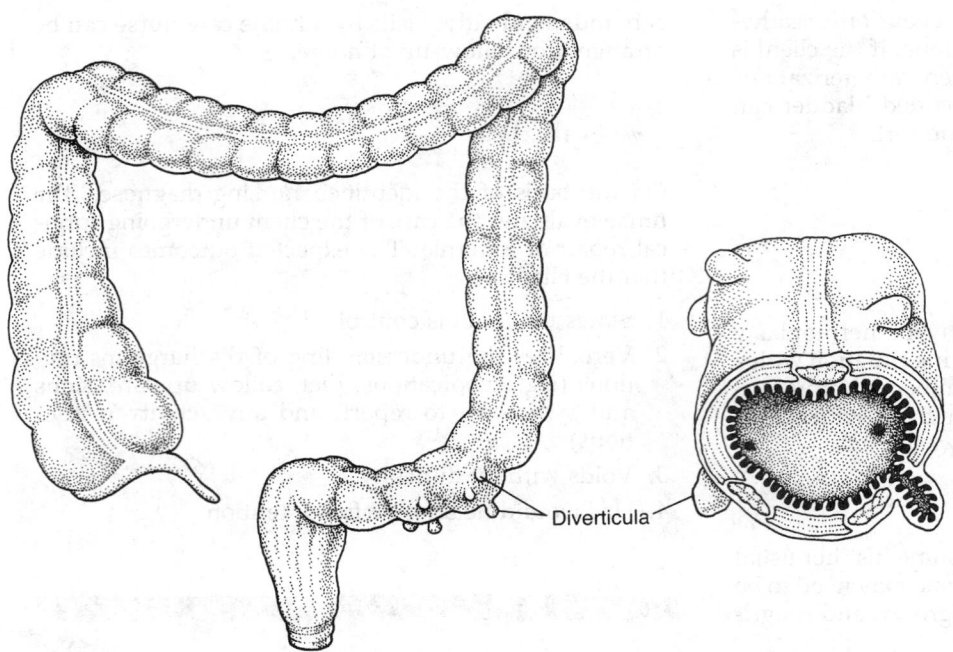

Figure 45-9

Several abnormal outpouchings, or herniations, in the wall of the intestine, which are diverticula. These can occur anywhere in the small or large intestine, but are found most often in the sigmoid as shown in this figure. Diverticulitis is inflammation of a diverticulum that occurs when undigested food or bacteria become trapped in a diverticulum.

Diverticula

inflammation can also result in fistulas to other organs, such as the bladder and the vagina. Bleeding from diverticula can occur, ranging from minor localized bleeding to massive hemorrhage. Minor bleeding is often due to localized inflammation in areas of vascular granulation tissue at the base of the diverticulum. Hemorrhage can occur when a blood vessel is eroded within a diverticulum. This erosion occurs when a mass, such as undigested food, becomes trapped in the diverticulum and irritates the vessel that traverses that diverticulum. Recurrent diverticulitis can lead to narrowing of the bowel lumen, which may result in obstruction.

Etiology

A diverticulum is caused when significantly high pressure in the lumen of the intestines pushes the intestine out, creating a herniation. It is thought that diverticula tend to occur at points of weakness in the intestinal wall, often at areas where blood vessels interrupt muscular continuity. The muscle weakness that in part accounts for the formation of diverticula develops as part of the aging process.

Diets with small amounts of fiber have been implicated in the development of diverticula, in that they cause less-bulky stool and possibly constipation. Both of these conditions require an increase in intraluminal pressure and muscle contractions to move fecal material through the colon.

The etiology of diverticulitis is thought to be retained undigested food in diverticula, which compromises the blood supply to that area and facilitates bacterial invasion of the sac.

Incidence

Diverticular disease is more common in Western countries. Australia, the United States, the United Kingdom, and France have high rates of diverticular disease. African, Asian, and Third World countries have low rates. However, epidemiologists have reported that when Black individuals from Africa started eating a characteristically Western diet, they developed diverticular disease (Shearman & Finlayson, 1982). Approximately one-third of the population older than 60 years of age have diverticular disease. Less that 5% of individuals with this illness are younger than 40 years of age (Shearman & Finlayson, 1982). Approximately 20% of individuals with diverticula develop diverticulitis (Spivak & Barres, 1983).

PREVENTION

Prevention of diverticular disease can be achieved with proper diet. Cellulose and hemicellulose are specific types of fiber that have been shown to be effective against constipation, which is associated with the development of diverticula. These fiber types are found in wheat bran and whole-grain breads and cereals.

Recommended amounts of cellulose and hemicellulose in a daily diet can be obtained with 15 g of bran (e.g., four slices of 100% whole-wheat bread and a 3-oz serving of all-bran cereal). There are many types of fiber, each with a different effect on the digestive system. Fruits and vegetables with high fiber content, such as seedless grapes, carrots, fresh peaches, and lettuce, add bulk to stools, thus promoting good elimination patterns and preventing constipation. However, clients with known diverticulosis should avoid high-fiber foods that contain indigestible roughage or seeds, such as nuts, corn, popcorn, cucumbers, celery, fresh tomatoes, figs, strawberries, or caraway seeds, because these foods may block the neck of a diverticulum and cause diverticulitis.

If clients cannot tolerate bran, bulk agents such as psyllium hydrophilic mucilloid (Metamucil) can be used. These OTC products can be purchased without a prescription.

COLLABORATIVE MANAGEMENT

 Assessment

History

The diagnosis of *diverticulosis* is usually made incidentally when a client has radiography of the GI tract to rule out other illnesses. Occasionally, diverticulosis causes symptoms. For clients with uncomplicated diverticulosis, the nurse obtains the client's *age* and *sex*, a history of intermittent *pain* in left lower quadrant, and a history of *constipation*.

When collecting data from the client with *diverticulitis*, the nurse collects information about changes in *bowel function*, including constipation or diarrhea and the presence of blood in stool. The nurse asks the client about the presence of diverticula and their location. Some individuals may be aware that they have diverticula because of previous episodes of diverticulitis or radiography of the GI tract. The nurse also collects information about *diet*, specifically the amount of bran, wheat bread, fruits, and vegetables in the diet. Recent intake of indigestible roughage or seeds, as in popcorn, nuts, corn, cucumbers, celery, fresh tomatoes, figs, strawberries, or caraway seeds, is also obtained because these foods can block the neck of the diverticulum and result in diverticulitis.

Physical Assessment: Clinical Manifestations

When assessing the client with *diverticulosis*, the nurse may find no clinical manifestations specific to this disorder. Occasionally, the nurse may elicit tenderness on abdominal palpation.

The client with *diverticulitis* has *abdominal pain*, which is often abrupt in onset, localized to the left lower quadrant, episodic, dull, or steady, which increases with coughing, straining, or lifting. There is occasionally right lower quadrant pain in female clients because drainage from perforated diverticula is shifted to the right pelvic area by the uterus. Abdominal pain is generalized if peritonitis occurs. The client has *temperature elevation* ranging from a low-grade fever to 101° F (38.2° C) with chills. Tachycardia is due to fever. A high temperature

may be absent in the elderly client because body temperature in the elderly client is generally lower owing to less subcutaneous fat and less heat production. *Nausea* and *vomiting* frequently occur.

On examination of the abdomen, the nurse may observe *distention*, and *tenderness* on palpation may be elicited over the area involved (usually the left lower quadrant). The colon may be palpable. If localized peritoneal irritation is present, localized muscle spasm, guarded movement, and rebound tenderness is present. If generalized peritonitis is present, abdominal muscle spasm, guarding, and rebound tenderness are more diffuse (see earlier discussion of peritonitis).

On examination of the rectum, the nurse may palpate a *tender mass* if the perforated diverticulum is close to the rectum. *Blood* may be present in the stool usually in microscopic amounts (a positive result is noted in testing with guaiac), but it can be present in larger amounts and is manifested by mahogany or bright red blood in stool. Small amounts of blood are thought to be due to inflammation with vascular granulation tissue at the base of the diverticulum. A large amount of bleeding occurs when the diverticulum is inflamed and large blood vessels over the dome of the sacs are affected. Blood pressure checks may show orthostatic changes. If bleeding is massive (rare with diverticulitis), the client could have hypotension and dehydration that result in shock. If generalized peritonitis has occurred, sepsis can ensue, along with the manifestations of hypotension and shock.

Psychosocial Assessment

Because diverticulosis is often asymptomatic and is discovered incidentally, the client may have concerns about its origin and significance. The client with diverticulitis often has concerns about the abrupt onset of symptoms and the outcome of treatment. Most clients are treated medically, but, depending on the client's response to treatment and the occurrence of complications, surgery is sometimes necessary.

The nurse assesses for client anxiety and fear related to the uncertainty about what treatments will be necessary. Consideration of treatment options can be particularly frightening and anxiety provoking for the client, because surgery might include the formation of a colostomy.

Laboratory Findings

Laboratory studies are not indicated for the client with uncomplicated diverticulosis. The client with *diverticulitis* has an elevated WBC count, with a shift to the left. Stools are tested for reaction to guaiac or occult blood, and positive results are found in 20% of clients (Knauer & Silverman, 1988).

Urinalysis may show a few RBCs if the left ureter is in proximity to a perforated diverticulum.

Radiographic Findings

X-ray films of the intestinal tract with barium contrast show diverticula. An upper gastrointestinal radiography series shows diverticula of the small intestine, and barium enema shows diverticula of the large intestine. Radiography is usually not indicated in cases of uncomplicated diverticulosis, because clients are usually asymptomatic or only minimally symptomatic.

The client with *diverticulitis* does *not* undergo invasive x-ray studies (e.g., barium enema) in the acute phase of the illness because of the risk of perforating a local abscess. The diagnosis of diverticulitis is usually based on history, clinical manifestations, and an elevated WBC count. A barium enema may be done after the client has been treated with antibiotics and the inflammation has resolved. A flat plate of the abdomen may reveal a mass. The finding of free air on abdominal x-ray films indicates perforation.

Other Diagnostic Tests

Sigmoidoscopy or colonoscopy may be performed *after the acute phase* of the illness, usually to rule out the presence of a tumor in the large intestine, particularly if the client has rectal bleeding. There is, however, a high risk for perforation of a diverticulum if the sigmoidoscope or colonoscope enters a diverticulum. Bleeding from diverticula usually stops spontaneously. If bleeding continues, angiography may be done to identify the location of the bleeding. Some clients with diverticulitis may have ultrasonography of the abdomen because it is noninvasive and thus safe.

 Analysis: Nursing Diagnosis

The client with uncomplicated diverticulosis can potentially have the same nursing diagnoses as the client with diverticulitis. However, the client with diverticulitis is more likely to exhibit several diagnoses.

Common Diagnoses

The diagnosis found in all clients with *diverticulitis* is altered (gastrointestinal) tissue perfusion related to perforated diverticulum. Clients with *diverticulosis* are at risk for experiencing this diagnosis if their diverticula become blocked and inflamed.

Additional Diagnoses

In addition, the following are frequently associated with diverticulitis:

1. Pain related to perforated diverticulum
2. Fluid volume deficit related to perforated diverticulum, bleeding, and NPO status
3. Altered nutrition: less than body requirements related to NPO status
4. Fear related to uncertainty about treatment regimens and the possibility of a colostomy

 Planning and Implementation

The following is a care plan for the client with diverticular disease, specifically diverticulitis.

Altered (Gastrointestinal) Tissue Perfusion

Planning: client goals. The primary goal is that the client will have increased tissue perfusion.

Interventions. When the client's symptoms are mild, temperature is less than 101° F (38.2° C), and the WBC count ranges from 13,000 to 15,000/mm³, the client may be treated as an outpatient.

Nonsurgical management. The preferred treatment is medical management of the inflammatory process.

Rest. The client should remain in bed during the acute phase. The client should also refrain from lifting, straining, coughing, or bending to avoid an increase in intra-abdominal pressures, which could lead to perforation of the diverticulum.

Diet therapy. Diet is restricted to clear liquids during the acute phase of the illness. Clients who have more severe symptoms are admitted to the hospital and are kept on NPO status. A nasogastric tube is inserted if nausea, vomiting, or abdominal distention is severe. IV fluids are administered as needed for hydration. Regular diet is resumed, or dietary intake is increased slowly as symptoms subside. When inflammation has resolved and bowel function returns to normal, a fiber-containing diet is introduced gradually. However, if active diverticulitis recurs, fiber intake is stopped for the acute phase of the illness.

Drug therapy. Clients with mild diverticulitis who are being treated on an outpatient basis receive prescriptions for broad-spectrum antibiotics, such as oral ampicillin (Omnipen) or tetracycline hydrochloride (Sumysin). Clients who are admitted to the hospital with mild diverticulitis may receive IV ampicillin or cephalexin (Keflex). In cases of severe diverticulitis, clients might receive gentamicin (Garamycin), clindamycin (Cleocin), tobramycin sulfate (Nebcin), or cefoxitin (Mefoxin). For clients with mild diverticulitis who are being treated on an outpatient basis, mild nonopiate analgesics such as propoxyphene napsylate (Darvon-N) are sometimes prescribed for pain. Anticholinergics, such as propantheline bromide (Pro-Banthine), may also be ordered to reduce the hypermotility of the intestine.

If the diverticulitis is severe, the client is hospitalized and a narcotic analgesic, such as meperidine hydrochloride (Demerol), is ordered to help alleviate pain.

Prevention of complications. The client who is being treated on an outpatient basis should be monitored for any prolongation or increase in fever, abdominal pain, leukocytosis, or blood in stool. A temperature greater than 101° F (38.2° C), persistent abdominal pain for more than 3 days, or an increase in pain requires hospitalization for more intense treatment, such as IV fluid and antibiotic administration and possibly nasogastric suctioning.

The nurse monitors the hospitalized client with diverticulitis for all of the above clinical manifestations. Laxatives are avoided because they increase intestinal motility. Enemas are avoided, as they increase intraluminal pressure. The nurse assesses the client for clinical manifestations of fluid and electrolyte imbalance on an ongoing basis.

Surgical management.   The client with diverticulitis may need to undergo surgery if one of the following occurs: peritonitis, pelvic abscess, bowel obstruction, fistula, presence of a mass and suspected tumor, persistent fever or pain after 4 days of medical treatment, or uncontrolled bleeding. Emergency surgery is performed if peritonitis, bowel obstruction, or pelvic abscess is present.

All clients undergo an exploratory laparotomy. The specific procedure performed depends on what the surgeon finds when the abdominal cavity is explored. The surgical approach recommended for the client with diverticulitis is a resection of the involved section of the colon, with a primary anastomosis. However, at the time of surgery, the inflammation and infectious process might not make it feasible to perform a primary anastomosis. If this is the case, a diverting colostomy is made with a mucous fistula or closure of the distal bowel into the pelvis (Hartmann's procedure). Often, this colostomy is done as a temporary measure and is considered part of a staged treatment for the intestinal inflammation. The surgeon may often allow the bowel to rest for 3 to 6 months, then bring the client back to surgery for closure of the colostomy with re-establishment of intestinal continuity. However, a permanent colostomy may be necessary, depending on the condition of the bowel.

Preoperative care.   Preparation of the client for surgery depends on the individual circumstances. The surgery may be done on an emergency basis, with a few days' notice (after unsuccessful medical treatment), or with a few weeks' notice (as when resection is being done for recurrent diverticulitis). The surgeon informs the client if there is a chance that a temporary or permanent colostomy might be required.

If the client is *not* in the acute stage of diverticulitis, a thorough bowel preparation *may* be given, consisting of enemas and laxatives daily for 2 to 3 days before surgery. However, because of the risk of perforation, the surgeon may elect to forego an aggressive bowel preparation. If a client has an acutely inflamed diverticulum or if the client has persistent fever and abdominal pain, the bowel preparation is most likely *withheld.*

The client who has been hospitalized for treatment of diverticulitis and requires surgery is already receiving IV antibiotics. For clients without active inflammation who are undergoing surgery, anti-inflammatory agents or antibiotics may be given orally or rectally before surgery.

The client who is to undergo emergency surgery or who has not responded to medical intervention is maintained on NPO status with a nasogastric tube in place.

These clients receive IV fluids with appropriate electrolyte replacements.

For clients without acute inflammation, a well-structured preoperative diet is given as part of the bowel preparation. The client has a low-residue diet for 4 to 5 days, followed by a full-liquid diet for 2 days, then a clear-liquid diet the evening before surgery.

Other preoperative interventions are similar to those described in Chapter 18 for clients undergoing abdominal surgery with general anesthesia. Preoperative teaching about colostomies depends on the surgeon's plan and how certain the need for colostomy is. The nurse need not discuss colostomy care in detail unless the client wants this information. The nurse should, however, describe the function and purpose of a colostomy when used in this situation (i.e., to allow the bowel to rest).

Postoperative care.   The immediate physical care for clients undergoing colon resection for diverticulitis is the same as described for clients undergoing abdominal surgery in Chapter 20. There is usually a drain in place at the incision site for 2 to 3 days. If a colostomy is performed, it may be covered with a dressing because it does not drain for approximately 2 days, or a colostomy bag may be placed over the stoma. If the stoma is visible, the nurse monitors its color and integrity. The stoma should be cherry red without retraction or prolapse into the abdomen.

If the client has had a colostomy, the nurse gives the client an opportunity to express feelings regarding the ostomy. The nurse needs to discuss these feelings with the client, acknowledging that anger and depression are normal responses. When the client is physically able, the nurse encourages him/her to look at the stoma and touch the apparatus (see later discussion of colostomy care).

The client is kept on NPO status after colon resection, with or without a colostomy, with a nasogastric tube in place for 2 to 4 days, until peristalsis returns. When peristalsis returns, the nasogastric tube is removed by the nurse, per physician's order, and clear liquids are introduced *slowly.*

The client's diet is advanced to solids gradually, depending on the return of peristalsis and bowel function.

If the client has a colostomy, it should start functioning in 2 to 4 days. Most clients who undergo surgery and colostomy formation for diverticulitis have a sigmoid colostomy, as the sigmoid colon is the most common site of diverticulitis. Drainage from a sigmoid colostomy is initially loose stool, but eventually it becomes formed. A tight seal around the stoma is essential to avoid contact of feces with the skin.

▪ Discharge Planning

The length of hospitalization for diverticulitis ranges from 1 to 2 weeks, depending on the client's response to medical treatment and the need for surgery. Discharge plans vary, depending on the treatment.

Home Care Preparation

For the client with diverticulitis who has responded to medical treatment, home care focuses on proper diet. The nurse assesses the client's ability to obtain and prepare the recommended high-fiber foods.

The client who has required surgical intervention has the added responsibilities of incision care and possibly colostomy care, with some temporary limitations placed on activities.

Client/Family Education

All clients with diverticular disease need instructions on proper diet and the rationale for this diet. The client with *diverticulosis* is encouraged to eat a diet high in cellulose and hemicellulose types of fiber (see the accompanying Health Promotion/Maintenance feature). These substances can be found in wheat bran, whole-grain breads, and cereals. At least 15 g of bran should be ingested daily. This could be derived from 4 slices of 100% whole-wheat bread and a 3-oz serving of all-bran cereal. The nurse also tells the client to eat fruits and vegetables with a high-fiber content to add bulk to stools. Recommended fruits and vegetables are seedless grapes, fresh peaches, carrots, and lettuce. The client should *avoid* foods that contain indigestible roughage or seeds that may block the neck of a diverticulum, such as nuts, corn, popcorn, cucumbers, celery, fresh tomatoes, figs, strawberries, or caraway seeds. Clients should also *avoid any fiber* when they have symptoms of diverticulitis, because these foods are irritating. The client who is

not accustomed to eating high-fiber foods should add them to the diet gradually to avoid flatulence and abdominal cramping. If the client cannot tolerate the recommended fiber, a bulk-forming laxative, such as psyllium hydrophilic mucilloid (Metamucil), should be taken to increase fecal size and consistency.

The nurse also informs the client that hot or cold foods and liquids cause gas, and these should be avoided. Alcohol should also be avoided, because it irritates the bowel.

The client who is overweight is advised to begin weight reduction because excessive weight aggravates the symptoms of diverticular disease. A variety of techniques to assist the client to lose weight are suggested. Such techniques include establishment of goals for weight loss, 24-hour recall of diet to identify problem areas, calorie counting, the use of sample diets and menus, consistent follow-up, and support groups.

The nurse provides the same information to the client with active diverticulitis, emphasizing that the recommended fiber should *not* be taken until fever and abdominal pain have totally resolved. The client who has undergone surgery is taking solid food by the time of discharge from the hospital.

Clients who have had abdominal surgery need oral and written instructions on incision care and the signs and symptoms to watch for and report; these are similar to the instructions given to clients after other types of abdominal surgery (Chap. 20). Clients who have had a colostomy should receive instruction on colostomy care (see the accompanying Client/Family Education feature).

Clients *with any type of diverticular disease* are instructed orally and in writing with regard to signs and symptoms of acute diverticulitis, including fever, abdominal pain, and bloody, mahogany, or tarry stools. *All clients* are advised to avoid the use of laxatives (other than bulk-forming laxatives) and enemas. *All clients* can also benefit from avoiding the activities that increase intra-abdominal pressure, such as straining at stool, bending, or lifting heavy objects.

Psychosocial Preparation

The nurse encourages the client with *diverticulosis* that this disorder need not cause problems if proper diet is followed.

The nurse informs the client with *diverticulitis* that this illness does not commonly recur and that, with proper diet and elimination patterns, the client can help prevent its recurrence and potential complications.

The client with a colostomy has special needs with regard to the alteration in body image and loss of body function. The nurse also encourages the client to verbalize concerns about body image (see Chapter 9).

Health Care Resources

Clients who have undergone surgery may need assistance with incision and colostomy care. The nurse arranges for a home care nurse to assess wound healing

---

HEALTH PROMOTION/MAINTENANCE ■ Diet for Clients with Diverticular Disease *Without* Symptoms of Diverticulitis

Recommended Foods

Wheat bran
Whole-grain breads and cereals
Whole-wheat bread
Seedless grapes
Fresh peaches
Fresh carrots
Fresh lettuce

Foods to Avoid

Nuts
Corn
Popcorn
Cucumbers
Celery
Fresh tomatoes
Figs
Strawberries
Caraway seeds

CLIENT/FAMILY EDUCATION ■ How to Care for a Colostomy

Instructions	Rationales
Pouch Care	
1. "Empty the pouch when it is ⅓ to ½ full."	1. Excessive drainage causes increased weight in pouch and may pull down on the seal, causing leakage around the seal.
2. "If using a two-piece system, remove and empty drainage into the toilet. You may sit on the toilet or on a chair in front of the toilet to empty the pouch."	2. Sitting makes the client more comfortable and facilitates management of colostomy equipment.
3. "To clean the pouch, use a small squeeze bottle with lukewarm water."	3. Water aimed onto the skin facilitates removal of drainage.
4. "Change the total pouch system every 4–7 d for a permanent or two-piece system, and every 1–3 d for a one-piece system."	4. Pouch system should be changed before leakage occurs. Individual wearing time is dependent on how long the pouch can remain intact without leaking.
Skin Care	
1. "When changing the system, skin care needs to be done as follows: a. Use lukewarm water only, without soap. b. Dry the skin well (the use of a hairdryer on a cool setting may be necessary if high humidity is present). c. Use an electric razor to shave abdominal hair under tapes and barriers; shave on a regular basis."	1. Cleaning is important for hygiene and skin integrity. a,b. Skin needs to be clean and dry for pouch tapes and barriers to adequately hold to the skin. c. Tapes and barriers adhere to abdominal hair and cause pain, as well as being a source of infection.
2. "Watch to see if any skin around the stoma has contact with ostomy contents."	2. It is sometimes difficult to obtain and maintain a good seal.
3. "If your skin has contact with ostomy contents, use a skin barrier paste around the stoma."	3. Skin barrier paste can fill in any dimpling or creases around the stoma to create a more uniform surface.
4. "Watch for the stoma to shrink in size in the first few weeks after surgery."	4. The stoma is largest immediately after surgery because of edema. The stoma may shrink in the first few days to weeks after surgery. After the first month, its size should not change.
5. "As the stoma shrinks, you need to resize the barrier around the stoma. To do this, use a stoma measuring guide to determine the general size of the stoma; cut the skin barrier to fit around the stoma."	5. Use of a pattern aids in uniform cutting of skin barriers and ensures a more contoured fit to the stoma.

Continued

CLIENT/FAMILY EDUCATION ■ How to Care for a Colostomy *Continued*

Instructions	Rationales
Diet	
1. "Gradually resume your regular diet."	1. There are no dietary restrictions unless the diet is restricted for other medical reasons. A balanced diet is essential for good healing and bowel function.
2. "Cautiously try foods that were problematic before surgery."	2. Foods that caused problems at one time might continue to cause problems.
Clothing	
1. "No change may be necessary."	1. Belts and close-fitting clothing will not harm the stoma.
Activities	
1. "Avoid lifting for 6–8 wk after surgery. Limit other activities per physician's order."	1. Activity limitations promote healing of abdominal muscles.
2. "Gradually resume all previous activities as tolerated."	2. There is no activity contraindicated for a client who has an ostomy.
Sexual Intercourse	
1. "Empty your pouch before sexual activity."	1. A clean pouch is more aesthetically pleasing in appearance.
2. "You may want to roll the pouch up and tape it to the abdomen."	2. This may prevent the pouch from getting in the way.
3. "You may want to wear a pouch cover (purchased or homemade)."	3. A pouch cover makes the pouch more aesthetically pleasing to the client and the sexual partner.
Travel	
1. "For day trips, carry an extra set of pouch equipment."	1–2. This prepares the client for any potential problem.
2. "For extended trips, carry several days' worth of equipment. You can call a local hospital to find an ostomy supply source."	
3. "When traveling by airplane, carry supplies on board in a carry-on case."	3. If the client's luggage is lost or does not arrive, the required items for ostomy care are available.

and proper functioning of the ostomy and the appliance. If the client is interested, the nurse can arrange for a visit from an ostomy volunteer or an enterostomal therapist. For information about other ostomy resources, the nurse or the client can contact the United Ostomy Association.

 Evaluation

The expected outcomes for all clients with diverticular disease include that the client

1. Verbalizes the need to include at least 15 g of bran in the daily diet
2. States what foods need to be avoided at all times
3. States what types of activities should be eliminated to avoid high intra-abdominal pressures
4. States the signs and symptoms of diverticulitis

In addition, the expected outcomes for clients with *diverticulitis* include that the client

5. Verbalizes the need to eliminate all fiber from the diet if active disease is present
6. Is afebrile and without abdominal distention, nausea, or vomiting
7. States that there is complete resolution of pain

COLORECTAL CANCER

OVERVIEW

Cancer of the small intestine is rare and therefore is not discussed in this text. Cancer of the colon, however, is the most common cancer in the United States among men *and* women when both groups are considered together (American Cancer Society [ACS], 1989). Cancer of the colon is second only to lung cancer as a cause of all deaths attributed to cancer in the United States (ACS, 1989). This disease is lethal in a significant number of cases because adequate screening tests are not available to detect the disease during its early stages and symptoms do not occur until later in the development of the tumor. Surgery is the only means to cure colon cancer at this time.

Pathophysiology

The malignant process begins within cells lining the bowel wall. Tumors occur in different areas of the colon in the following approximate proportions: 16% in the cecum and ascending colon, 8% in the transverse colon, 20% to 30% in the descending and sigmoid colon, and

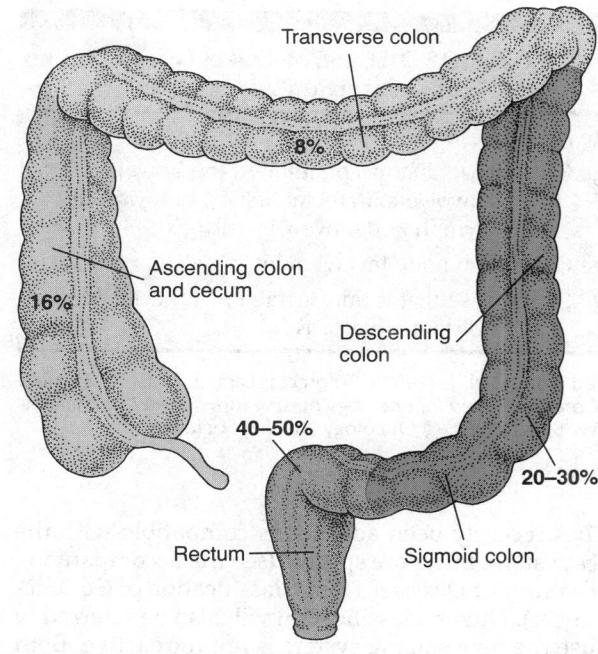

Figure 45–10

Incidence of cancer in relation to colorectal anatomy.

40% to 50% in the rectum (Knauer & Silverman, 1988) (Fig. 45–10). Almost all colorectal carcinomas develop from an adenomatous polyp (see Fig. 45–14). Tumors usually grow undetected until symptoms slowly and insidiously occur. Spread of the disease occurs by several methods. Locally, the tumor may spread deeper into the layers of the bowel wall, reaching the serosa and the mesenteric fat. The tumor may then begin to attach to other neighboring organs. It may enlarge into the lumen of the bowel or spread through the lymphatics or the circulatory system. Entry into the circulatory system occurs directly from the primary tumor through blood vessels in the bowel or via the lymphatics. After tumor cells enter the circulatory system, the cells most commonly travel to the liver. The second most common site for distant metastasis is the lung. Other metastatic sites include the adrenal glands, the kidneys, the skin, the bone, and the brain.

In addition to direct invasion and spread via the lymphatic and circulatory systems, colon tumors can also spread by peritoneal seeding during surgical resection of the tumor. The seeding occurs when a tumor is excised and cancer cells break off from the tumor into the peritoneal cavity.

Staging of the disease is important for determining prognosis and treatment. Several systems are used, but a uniform staging system has recently been approved in an effort to standardize the process worldwide. In the past, the most common staging classification used for colorectal carcinoma was the Dukes classification (see the accompanying Key Features of Disease: Dukes' Classification of Colorectal Cancer). The staging system

KEY FEATURES OF DISEASE ■ Dukes' Classification of Colorectal Cancer

Stage A	Disease confined to the bowel wall
Stage B	Disease that has penetrated the bowel to involve extrarectal tissues, but without lymph node involvement
Stage C	Lymph node involvement
Stage D	Disease that is unresectable, with evidence of distant metastasis

Adapted from Lind, J. (1987). Colorectal cancer. In C. R. Ziegfeld (Ed.), *Core curriculum for oncology nursing* (pp. 163–171). Philadelphia: W. B. Saunders. © Oncology Nursing Society.

KEY FEATURES OF DISEASE ■ TNM Classification of Colorectal Cancer

Primary Tumor (T)

TX	Primary tumor cannot be assessed
T0	No evidence of primary tumor
Tis	Carcinoma in situ
T1	Tumor invades submucosa
T2	Tumor invades muscularis propria
T3	Tumor invades through muscularis propria into subserosa, or into nonperitonealized pericolic or perirectal tissues
T4	Tumor perforates visceral peritoneum, or directly invades other organs or structures

Lymph Node (N)

NX	Regional lymph nodes cannot be assessed
N0	No regional lymph node metastasis
N1	Metastasis in 1 to 3 pericolic or perirectal lymph nodes
N2	Metastasis in 4 or more pericolic or perirectal lymph nodes
N3	Metastasis in any lymph node along course of a major named vascular trunk

Distant Metastasis (M)

MX	Presence of distant metastasis cannot be assessed
M0	No distant metastasis
M1	Distant metastasis

Stage Grouping

0	Tis	N0	M0
I	T1	N0	M0
	T2	N0	M0
II	T3	N0	M0
	T4	N0	M0
III	Any T	N1	M0
	Any T	N2	M0
	Any T	N3	M0
IV	Any T	Any N	M1

From American Joint Committee on Cancer. (1988). Beahrs, O. H., Henson, D. E., Hutter, R. V., Myers, M. H. (Eds.). *Manual for staging of cancer* (3rd ed.). Philadelphia: J. B. Lippincott.

that has recently been adopted is compatible with the Dukes system, but more specific (see the accompanying Key Features of Disease: TNM Classification of Colorectal Cancer). Dukes' classification will also be referred to because the new staging system is not retroactive. Both staging systems identify the location and amount of disease present.

According to Dukes' classification, stage A is the level of least disease and most favorable prognosis (with 80% to 90% 5-year survival rates). Dukes' stage B has a 60% 5-year survival rate (the nodes are not involved). Stage C has a 25% to 40% 5-year survival rate, and stage D has a less than 5% 5-year survival rate (Lind, 1987). The stage of the disease is identified at the time of surgery.

Complications related to the increasing growth of the tumor locally or through metastatic spread include bowel perforation with resulting peritonitis, abscess formation, and fistula formation to the urinary bladder or the vagina. The tumor may invade neighboring blood vessels and cause frank bleeding. A tumor growing into the bowel lumen can cause a gradual intestinal obstruction, with eventual complete blockage. Tumor extending beyond the bowel wall may place pressure on neighboring organs (uterus, urinary bladder, and ureters) and cause symptoms that mask those of the cancer.

Etiology

The exact cause of colorectal cancer is unknown. Diet and decreased bowel transit time (forward flow of stool) have been implicated as causative factors, and strict preventive guidelines are being promoted by a variety of health organizations (ACS, National Cancer Institute). Certain foods are suspected to contain chemical mutagens that are carcinogenic to the bowel. These foods also aid in decreasing bowel transit time, which would increase the exposure time of the bowel to carcinogens. A high-fat diet, particularly animal fat from red meats, increases bile acid secretion and anaerobic bacteria, which are thought to be carcinogenic within the bowel. Fried and broiled meats and fish also are thought to contain chemical mutagens that are carcinogenic. Diets with large amounts of refined carbohydrates that lack fiber decrease bowel transit time. Groups that typically adhere to diets that have less animal fat and are high in fruits and vegetables (e.g., Mormons, Seventh Day Adventists, and people living in Japan, Finland, and Africa) have demonstrated a decreased incidence of the disease.

Because almost all colorectal tumors develop from an

adenoma, the *primary* risk factor for colorectal cancer is the presence of an adenoma. There are three types of colorectal adenomas, namely, tubular, villous, and tubulovillous (see description of polyps later). Even though almost all colorectal cancers originate from adenomas, only 5% of all colorectal adenomas actually become malignant. Villous adenomas have the highest potential for malignancy. The factor that initiates the change from a benign adenoma to a malignant tumor is unknown. Familial polyposis is a hereditary disorder transmitted as an autosomal dominant trait; it is characterized by an early onset of multiple adenomatous polyps of the colon and rectum. The risk for cancer in clients with familial polyposis approaches 100% in the third and fourth decades of life.

Individuals who have had ulcerative colitis, particularly with a longer than 10-year history, are also at risk for colorectal cancer. The risk increases with younger age at onset and larger extent of colon involvement. There is also a two to three times greater risk of colon cancer if an immediate family member has this disease (Lind, 1987).

Incidence

Approximately 151,000 Americans will have been diagnosed with colorectal cancer in 1989, and 61,300 individuals are expected to have died of this cancer during this same year. It occurs with almost equal frequency in males and females. The majority of clients with colorectal cancer are older than 50 years of age, with the peak incidence occurring in the seventh and eighth decades of life (Schwesinger, 1990).

There is a high incidence in Western industrialized countries and a low incidence in Japan, Finland, and Africa. This is thought to be related to diet, because countries with a low incidence of colon cancer typically have diets high in fruits, vegetables, and fish and low in meat. Japanese individuals who immigrate to the United States have an increased incidence when compared with native Japanese. This is related to their change in diet after immigration to the United States (Miller, 1986).

PREVENTION

Prevention of this disease has been difficult because, even though groups at risk and possible contributing factors are being identified and studied, concrete preventive measures are still unknown. Because of the implication of dietary factors, guidelines have been established specifically to protect the public from colon cancer: (1) eat more cruciferous vegetables (cabbage family [e.g., broccoli, cauliflower, Brussels sprouts, cabbages, and kale]); (2) add more high-fiber foods (e.g., whole grains, fruits, and vegetables); (3) maintain ideal body weight; (4) eat less fat, particularly animal fat (ACS, 1985). Dietary indiscretions in these areas are

believed to be the components of Western diets that contribute to colorectal cancer. Efforts toward promoting awareness of and adherence to the guidelines are critical for the control of the disease.

Early detection efforts are also critical for control. ACS guidelines for early detection include a routine annual digital rectal examination beginning at age 40 years; an annual stool guaiac slide test beginning at age 50 years; and, after age 50 years, a sigmoidoscopy every 3 to 5 years after two negative sigmoidoscopy examinations performed 1 year apart.

The nurse is critical to achieving public awareness of and adherence to these guidelines. By actively providing education to the public and organizing or participating in early-detection clinics, the nurse has a major impact on the control of this disease. It is estimated that 75% of clients with colorectal cancer could be cured if the cancer were detected and treated early (Gomez et al., 1987). One easy and cost-effective approach to early detection is for clients to check their own stool samples for microscopic blood at home. Home test kits for stool guaiac reaction are available to facilitate the goal of early detection.

COLLABORATIVE MANAGEMENT

 Assessment

History

In taking a history from a client with cancer, the nurse obtains information including the client's *age* and *sex*, a *diet history*, and the *geographic location of residence*. The nurse questions the client with regard to major risk factors, such as a family history of *colorectal cancer* and a personal history of *ulcerative colitis, familial polyposis,* or *adenomas.*

Weight loss and a change in bowel habits are commonly reported by clients. Significant weight loss during a short time (e.g., 10 to 20 lb in 3 to 4 weeks) may be reported. Changes in bowel habits may be reported as diarrhea or constipation, with or without blood in stool. The nurse also assesses for pain or abdominal fullness, but these are usually late findings.

Physical Assessment: Clinical Manifestations

Rectal bleeding is the most common manifestation. Bleeding can range in color from dark maroon with clots mixed with stool, which represents upper colon bleeding, to bright red blood coating the stool, which indicates bleeding from the rectum or anal canal.

The nurse may observe clothing to be loose, indicating recent weight loss. The client who has experienced severe *weight loss* will be noticeably *cachectic*, with *loose skin* and *muscle wasting.*

The nurse observes for guarding or abdominal distention and palpates for a mass or distention, but these are usually late findings.

Psychosocial Assessment

The client often delays seeking health care. The primary reason is fear of cancer diagnosis. Most people fear that they have cancer or do not want to know that it is even a possibility. Cancer is commonly equated with pain and death. Many people are unaware of the advances in treatment of the disease and its side effects and of the increased survival rates. Unfortunately, early detection is critical to the control of colorectal cancer, and the delay in seeking health care can dramatically reduce the chance for survival and reinforce the client's and the family's fears.

Individuals who live healthy life styles and follow health guidelines may feel anger when clinical manifestations occur. These individuals may feel a sudden loss of control, helplessness, and shock. The diagnostic process used to confirm or negate the existence of cancer is generally extensive. The testing process can be long and tiresome, and it can increase the severity of the clinical manifestations or create additional ones. This can be extremely discouraging and tiring for the client and the family. The nurse enables the client to ventilate her/his feelings during this process.

Laboratory Findings

Routine complete blood counts (CBC) and blood chemistry testing may demonstrate an underlying anemia, which accounts for the malaise that the client is experiencing. These tests may show elevated alkaline phosphatase and bilirubin levels, which are indicative of hepatic metastasis.

A stool guaiac reaction test is done to confirm bleeding in the GI tract. When conducting this test, the nurse tells the client to *avoid* eating meat, peroxidase-containing foods (horseradish and beets), aspirin, or vitamin C for 48 hours before giving a stool specimen. The nurse assesses whether the client is taking phenylbutazone, corticosteroids, resperine, or analgesics and consults with the physician about prescribing other medications in place of these, or at least taking their ingestion into account in the guaiac test results. These foods and medications simulate bleeding when no true bleeding exists and lead to false positive guaiac testing results. Two separate stool samples are tested on 3 consecutive days. Negative results do *not* completely rule out the possibility of colon cancer.

Carcinoembryonic antigen (CEA) may be elevated in the presence of certain malignant and nonmalignant diseases. This test is helpful in determining the prognosis of the disease. It is often used to monitor the effectiveness of treatment and identify disease recurrence. CEA measurement, however, has *not* been helpful in screening for the detection of cancer.

Radiographic Findings

A barium enema may be performed to confirm the presence and identify the location of the tumor. This test may demonstrate an occlusion in the bowel where the tumor is decreasing in lumen size. Small lesions may not be identified by this test. A chest x-ray study and liver scan may be performed to locate distant sites of metastasis. Computed tomography (CT) helps confirm the existence of a mass and the extent of disease.

Other Diagnostic Tests

Sigmoidoscopy and colonoscopy are commonly done to identify smaller tumors and aid in determining the extent of the tumor mass. Two of three tumors can be seen via these tests, and biopsy of the mass can be performed (or even treatment conducted) at the same time.

 Analysis: Nursing Diagnosis

Common Diagnoses

The client with cancer of the colon has the following diagnoses:

1. Potential for injury related to possible metastasis
2. Potential for ineffective individual coping related to disturbance in self-concept

Additional Diagnoses

In addition, the client may have the following:

1. Pain related to tumor obstruction of the intestine, with possible pressure on other organs; the diagnostic work-up; and the surgical procedure
2. Ineffective family coping: compromised related to alteration in roles, life style changes, and fear of the client's death
3. Altered nutrition: less than body requirements related to the diagnostic work-up
4. Fear related to the disease process
5. Knowledge deficit related to the disease process, the diagnostic work-up, and the treatment plan
6. Altered sexuality patterns related to a disturbance in self-concept
7. Powerlessness related to the presence of life-threatening illness and its treatment

 Planning and Implementation

Potential for Injury

Planning: client goals. The goal is that the client will experience cure, increased survival, and increased quality of life.

Interventions: nonsurgical management

Radiation therapy. Preoperative radiation therapy may be administered to the client who has a large colorectal tumor. This therapy aids in creating more definite tumor margins, which facilitates resection of the tumor during surgery. Radiation can also be used postoperatively to decrease the risk of recurrence or as palliative measure to reduce pain, hemorrhage, bowel obstruction, or metastasis to the lung in advanced disease. The nurse explains the radiation therapy procedure to the client and the family and monitors for possible side effects (e.g., diarrhea and fatigue), implementing interventions to reduce side effects of the therapy (see References and Readings and Chap. 25 for care of clients undergoing radiation therapy).

Chemotherapy.   There is no cytotoxic regimen that promotes cure of colorectal cancer, except for tumors limited to the anal canal. Chemotherapy is generally used after surgical management to assist in controlling symptoms of metastasis and reduce metastatic spread. The drug typically used is fluorouracil (5-fluorouracil [5-FU]); it is given IV as a bolus or via intermittent continuous administration. Leucovorin (citrovorum factor) is given in conjunction with this agent to enhance its antitumor effect. Intrahepatic arterial chemotherapy is also administered to clients with liver metastasis. (Chapter 25 discusses the care of clients receiving these drugs.)

Interventions: surgical management.   Surgery is usually the primary treatment method for tumors located in the colon or rectum. It is the only therapy that can provide cure for the disease. A variety of surgical procedures are performed to remove colorectal cancer, all of which involve some type of colon resection. As shown in the accompanying Key Features of Disease, the specific type of surgery performed depends on the location of the tumor, the size of the tumor, and the overall condition of the client. Commonly, the segment containing the tumor is resected along with several inches of bowel beyond the margins of the tumor. An end-to-end anastomosis is then performed.

Depending on the location of the tumor and the condition of the surrounding bowel, a colostomy may be performed. The *colostomy* (or ostomy) involves the surgical creation of an opening between the colon and the abdominal surface from which stool will pass (called a stoma). The stoma may be located in the ascending colon, the transverse colon, the descending colon, or the sigmoid colon, depending on how much of the colon is resected (Fig. 45–11). A colostomy can also be temporary or permanent. A temporary colostomy is performed to remove the tumor and allow surrounding bowel to rest. Often, a tumor can cause bowel obstruction, with resulting inflammation. Temporary colostomy may be performed to allow the inflammation to resolve before reconnecting the edges of bowel. The client is rescheduled for surgery approximately 6 months after the initial surgery for closure of colostomy. The Hartmann procedure is often performed for tumors in the descending or sigmoid colon (see p. 1375). This procedure is commonly done when a colostomy is required at least temporarily and closure of the colostomy with anastomosis of the colon is planned.

For a tumor that is in the rectum, an *abdominal-perineal resection with permanent colostomy* may be performed; the stoma is in the descending or sigmoid colon. The entire rectum and support structure are removed and the anus is closed, resulting in a perineal wound. With advancements in surgical techniques, tumors lo-

KEY FEATURES OF DISEASE ■ Surgical Procedures Performed for Colorectal Cancers in Various Locations

Tumor Location	Procedures
Right-sided colon tumors	Right hemicolectomy for smaller lesions
	Right ascending colostomy or ileostomy for large, widespread lesions
	Cecostomy (opening into the cecum with intubation to decompress the bowel)
Left-sided colon tumors	Left hemicolectomy for smaller lesions
	Left descending colostomy for larger lesions (e.g., Hartmann's colostomy)
Sigmoid colon tumors	Sigmoid colectomy for smaller lesions
	Sigmoid colostomy for larger lesions (e.g., Hartmann's colostomy)
	Abdominal-perineal resection for large low sigmoid tumors (near the anus) with colostomy (the rectum and the anus are completely removed, leaving perineal wound)
Rectal tumors	Resection with anastomosis or pull-through procedure (preserves anal sphincter and normal elimination pattern)
	Colon resection with permanent colostomy
	Abdominal-perineal resection with colostomy

Adapted from Lind, J. (1987). Colorectal cancer. In C. R. Ziegfeld (Ed.), *Core curriculum for oncology nursing* (pp. 163–171). Philadelphia: W. B. Saunders. © Oncology Nursing Society.

cated in the rectum are more often being removed with the rectal sphinter left intact, avoiding creation of a stoma. These procedures have allowed normal bowel function to be maintained by the client.

Preoperative care.   The nurse assists the client in preparing for colon resection by reinforcing the physician's explanation of the planned surgical procedure. The client is told as accurately as possible what anatomic and physiologic changes will occur with surgery. Before evaluating the tumor and colon in surgery, the physician might not be able to determine if a temporary or a permanent colostomy will be necessary. If this is the case, the physician informs the client that a colostomy is a possibility. At times, the physician is certain that a permanent colostomy will be necessary, and the client is told this before surgery. If a colostomy is definitely

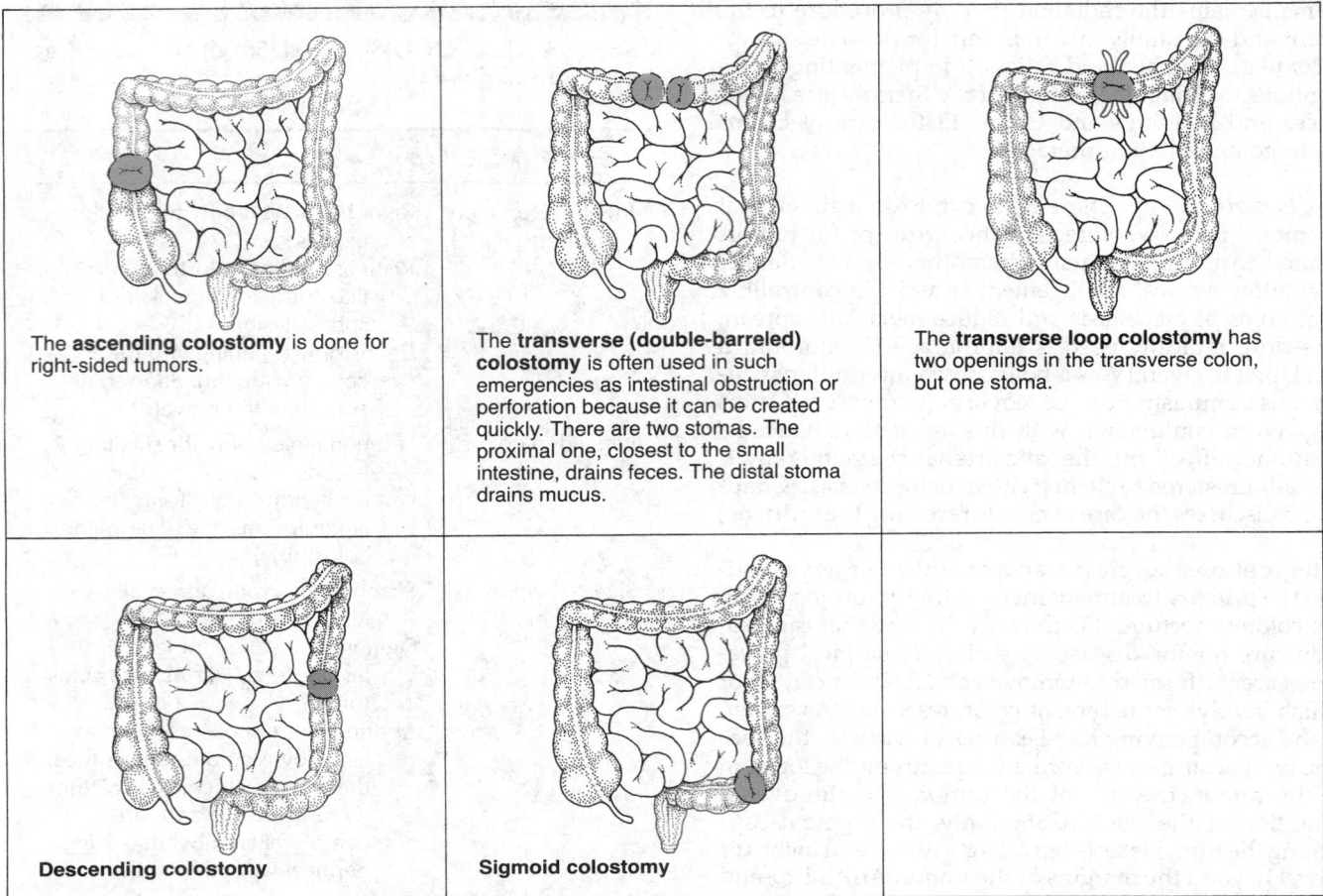

The **ascending colostomy** is done for right-sided tumors.

The **transverse (double-barreled) colostomy** is often used in such emergencies as intestinal obstruction or perforation because it can be created quickly. There are two stomas. The proximal one, closest to the small intestine, drains feces. The distal stoma drains mucus.

The **transverse loop colostomy** has two openings in the transverse colon, but one stoma.

Descending colostomy

Sigmoid colostomy

Figure 45–11

Types of colostomies.

planned, an enterostomal therapist is consulted to advise on optimal placement of the ostomy and instruct the client about the rationale and general principles of ostomies. Sexual dysfunction is a potential problem for men and women who undergo rectal surgery for cancer. The physician discusses this risk with the client, and the nurse supports the client regarding this concern. The nurse prepares the client for abdominal surgery with general anesthesia, as described in Chapter 18.

Thorough mechanical and pharmacologic cleaning of the bowel is done before colon surgery. This minimizes bacterial growth, thus assisting in the prevention of intraoperative infection. The nurse administers laxatives or enemas on the morning of surgery, or the day before surgery if the client is hospitalized. The nurse also administers antibiotics preoperatively. IV cephalothin (Keflin) or oral erythromycin (E-Mycin) and kanamycin (Kantrex) are administered the night before surgery. Clients are instructed to eat low-residue diets for a day or longer before bowel surgery to assist in minimizing colonic contents.

Postoperative care. Clients who have had colon resections without colostomies receive the same care as clients undergoing abdominal surgery (Chap. 20). At-

tention is given here to providing care for clients with a colostomy and a perineal wound.

Generally, the client who has had a colostomy returns from surgery with an ostomy pouch system in place. If there is no pouch system in place, the nurse keeps a petrolatum gauze dressing over the stoma to keep it moist, which is then covered with a dry sterile dressing. The nurse places a pouch system as soon as possible. The pouch system allows more convenient and acceptable collection of stool than a dressing. Table 45–2 describes the characteristics of a stoma. The nurse observes the stoma for any necrotic tissue, unusual bleeding, or dull coloring, which is indicative of poor circulation to the stoma. A small amount of bleeding at the stoma is common, but any appreciable bleeding is reported to the surgeon. The nurse also frequently checks the pouch system for proper fit and any signs of leakage. The colostomy should start functioning 2 to 4 days postoperatively. When the colostomy begins to function, the pouch may need to be emptied frequently for excess gas collection. It should be emptied when it is one-third to one-half full of stool. Stool is liquid immediately postoperatively, but becomes more solid, depending on where in the colon the stoma was placed.

The perineal wound is created by the removal of the

TABLE 45–2 Characteristics of a Stoma

A protrusion, or "bud," may rise above the skin surface, or the stoma may be flush with the skin.

Color ranges from red pink (a normal finding, owing to the high vascularity of the stoma) to pale pink (indicating low hemoglobin level and hematocrit values) to purple black (indicating compromised circulation).

The surface is that of moist mucous membrane, like the mouth or anus.

The stoma is painless; there are no pain receptors in the inner luminal lining.

The size of the stoma varies, depending on its location in the GI tract and the size of the lumen of the intestine at that location. Peristalsis may change the shape of the stoma throughout the day. It is larger immediately after surgery because of edema, and the size decreases in the days to weeks after surgery.

---

rectum, the anus, muscle, and fatty tissue. The hollow space eventually fills in with granulation tissue, with some realignment of internal organs to fill in the remaining space. There are three manners for closing the wound. The wound may be left open and a packing placed in the wound, which is left in place for 2 to 5 days. If this approach is used, wound irrigation and absorbent dressings are used until healing occurs. A second method of closure is partial closure through the use of sutures and Penrose drains, which are put in place for drainage of fluids that may collect within the wound. The third method is complete closure with placement of sump catheters through stab wounds alongside the perineal wound. These are left in place for 4 to 6 days, with one catheter used for irrigating the wound with sterile isotonic saline solution, and the other catheter connected to low continuous suction. Drainage of the perineal wound and cavity is important because of the possibility of infection and abscess formation. There is commonly copious serosanguineous drainage from the perineal wound. Healing of the perineal wound may take 6 to 8 months, and this can be a greater source of discomfort and require more care than the abdominal incision and ostomy. The client may experience phantom rectal sensations, which occur because sympathetic innervation for rectal control has not been interrupted. Occasionally, pain and itching may occur after healing. There is no physiologic explanation for this, but interventions may include use of antipruritic medications, such as benzocaine, and sitz baths. The nurse explains the physiology of perineal sensations to the client; continuously assesses for signs of infection, abscess, or other complications; and implements methods to promote wound drainage and comfort (see the accompanying Guidelines feature).

Cephalosporins, such cefalothin (Keflin), may be given intravenously postoperatively. If they are being given prophylactically, they are administered for only 2 days. If inflammation of the bowel was a problem, however, they are administered for several days.

Potential for Ineffective Individual Coping

Planning: client goals. The goal is that the client and the family will identify, develop, and utilize effective coping methods in dealing with the perceived changes and losses experienced.

Interventions: nonsurgical management. The client and the family are faced with the issues of the disease cancer, the possible loss of body functions, and altered body functions.

The nurse observes and identifies current methods of client and family coping, effective sources of support used in past crises, and present perceptions of the client and family regarding the client's health problem. The nurse encourages the client to verbalize feelings regarding the ostomy, acknowledging that feelings such as sadness, anger, loss, and depression are normal responses to this change in body function. It may be helpful to discuss colostomy as one aspect of the client's care, rather than the focus, just as defecation is only one aspect of the client's physiologic functioning. The nurse encourages the client to look at and touch the stoma. When the client is physically able, the nurse encourages client participation in colostomy care. The nurse assists the client and the family in formulating questions and verbalizing needs. The nurse observes whether the client has processed the necessary information and has learned the psychomotor skills for colostomy care. Client participation helps to restore control of life style, thus facilitating improved self-esteem.

■ Discharge Planning

Home Care Preparation

The nurse assesses all clients for their ability to perform incision care and to perform ADL with the constraint of activity limitations.

For the client who has undergone colostomy, the nurse reviews the home situation to aid the client in arranging for care. The client and the family must be aware of the need to keep ostomy supplies in an area (preferably the bathroom) where the temperature is neither hot nor cold, so that the ostomy products will function properly (e.g., skin barriers may become stiff or melt in extreme temperatures). No changes need to be made in sleeping accommodations. Some clients move into their own room or into twin beds. This can lead to physical and emotional distancing from the spouse and significant others. A rubber covering may initially be placed over the bed mattress if the client feels insecure about pouch system function.

Client/Family Education

Clients who have undergone a colon resection without colostomy receive instruction with regard to specific

GUIDELINES ■ Perineal Wound Care

Interventions	Rationales
Wound Care	
1. Irrigate the wound with normal saline and povidone-iodine (Betadine) or hydrogen peroxide solution as often as ordered by the physician, using meticulous sterile technique.	1. Irrigation aids in débridement and cleaning of the wound and promotes wound drainage.
2. Place an absorbent dressing (Kerlix or abdominal pad) over the wound.	2. Dressing promotes wound drainage and facilitates the collection of drainage.
3. Instruct the client that he/she may a. Use a feminine napkin as a dressing. b. Wear Jockey-type shorts rather than boxers. c. Shave perineal hair frequently.	3. These measures a. Decrease expense while providing adequate dressing for home use. b. Increase comfort while keeping the dressing in place. c. Promote comfort and possibly to prevent infection (controversial).
Comfort Measures	
1. Soak the wound area in a sitz bath for 10–20 min 3 or 4 times per day.	1. Use of a sitz bath promotes healing, wound cleaning, and comfort. Soaking for longer periods can result in vasodilation, causing vascular congestion or reflex vasoconstriction, which can increase discomfort. Soaking *does not replace irrigation.*
2. Administer pain medication as ordered and assess its effectiveness.	2. Pain medication provides comfort and aids the client in increasing activities, which can help the overall recovery process (perineal wound can cause great discomfort).
3. Instruct the client regarding permissible activities. The client should a. Assume a side-lying position in bed; avoid sitting for long periods. b. Use foam pads or a soft pillow to sit on *whenever* in a sitting position. c. *Avoid the use of air rings* or *rubber doughnut devices.*	3. Usual positioning may be uncomfortable. a. Buttock separation increases discomfort. b. These devices promote comfort during activities. c. These cause separation of buttocks.
Prevention of Complications	
1. Maintain fluid and electrolyte balance by monitoring intake and output and monitoring output from the perineal wound.	1. Monitoring identifies fluid and electrolyte imbalances.
2. Observe suture line integrity, watching for erythema, edema, bleeding, purulent drainage, unusual odor, and excessive or constant pain.	2. These are clinical manifestations of infection or abscess formation.

needs, similar to that given to other clients who have undergone abdominal surgery (Chap. 20). In addition to this information, the nurse teaches all clients with colon resections to watch for and report clinical manifestations of intestinal obstruction and perforation (e.g., cramping, abdominal pain, nausea, and vomiting).

Rehabilitation after ostomy surgery requires that the client and the family learn the principles of colostomy care and the psychomotor skills required to facilitate this care. Providing information is important, but the nurse must also allow adequate opportunity for the client to learn psychomotor skills involved in ostomy care. Sufficient practice time is planned for the client and the family so that they can handle, assemble, and apply all ostomy equipment. The nurse teaches the client and the family about the stoma; use, care, and application of the pouch system; skin protection; dietary control; control of gas and odor; potential problems and solutions; and tips on how to resume normal activities, including work, travel, and sexual intercourse (Table 45–3; see also Client/Family Education: How to Care for a Colostomy).

TABLE 45–3   Solutions to Special Problems in Ostomy Use

Problems	Solutions
Odor	
Foods	
Dairy products (boiled milk, eggs, and some cheese), fish, onion, garlic, coffee, alcohol, nuts, prunes, beans, cabbage, cucumber, asparagus, raddish, broccoli, turnips, peas, highly seasoned foods	Spinach, cranberry juice, yogurt, buttermilk, dark green vegetables (parsley is particularly helpful), increased vitamin C in food or vitamin preparations
Drugs	*Oral Medications*
Antibiotics, vitamins, iron	Chlorophyll tablets (Derifil) for fecal odors (absorb gas) Charcoal tablets Bismuth bicarbonate (0.6 g tid with meals) Bismuth subgallate (Devrom or Biscaps) 1 or 2 tablets with meals and 1 h.s.
	Pouch Preparations
	Odor-proof pouch or pouch with odor control mechanism Manufactured preparations (place small amounts in pouch): Banish II or Superbanish (United), Odor-Guard (Marlan), Ostobon (Pettibone Labs), activated charcoal, ostomy deodorant (Sween), Nilodor, Devko tablets (Parthenon Co.), D-Odor, M-9 (Mason Lab)
	Sodium bicarbonate solution (soaked cotton balls in pouch) Vanilla, peppermint, lemon, or almond extracts (put 10 drops into pouch or soak cotton balls) Favorite spice, cloves, or cinnamon (place ¼ tsp in pouch) Mouthwash (e.g., Cēpacol, Listerine) (several drops in pouch or soaked cotton balls in pouch)
	Cleaning Reusable Pouches
	Wisk and water (1 : 1 solution) Baking soda and water (1 : 1 solution) Household white vinegar and water (1 : 1 solution) Manufactured products: Uri-Kleen, Uni-Wash (United), Peri-Wash (Sween), Skin Care cleaner (Bard) Baking soda (after drying the pouch, powder inside with baking soda)

Table continued on following page

TABLE 45-3 **Solutions to Special Problems in Ostomy Use** *Continued*

Problems	Solutions
Flatulence	
Activities	
Eating fast and talking at same time, gum chewing, smoking, snoring, skipping meals, emotional upset	Avoid these activities; eat solids before taking liquids
Foods	**Pouch Adaptation**
Mushrooms, onions, beans, cabbage, Brussels sprouts, spinach, cheese, eggs, beer, carbonated beverages, fish, highly seasoned foods, some fruit drinks, corn, pork, peas, coffee, high-fat foods	Use pouches with gas or odor filters
Skin Irritation	
Allergy	
Erythema, erosion, edema, weeping, bleeding, itching, burning, stinging, irritation the same shape as allergic material	Creams: Sween cream, Unicare cream, or Hollister Skin Conditioning Cream (use small amount and rub in; tapes will adhere when dry)
Chemical Exposure	Powders (karaya gum, Stomahesive, cornstarch) used with skin gel (Skin Prep, Skin Gel)
Stool, urine, glues, solvents, soaps, detergents, proteolytic digestive enzymes	Antacids: aluminum hydroxide (Amphojel, Maalox) used with skin sealant (Skin Prep, Skin Gel)
	Skin sealant alone (for slightly reddened skin)
Epidermal Hyperplasia	Skin barriers: one application left on for 24 h or longer may clear irritations quickly
Increased formation of epidermal cells, causing generalized thickening of the outer layer of skin	Pastes (Hollister Premium, Stomahesive) used to fill in creases and spaces
	Hairdryer on cool setting to decrease moisture
Mechanical Trauma	Do not patch or tape leaks; correct leakage problem immediately
Pressure, friction, or stripping of skin (e.g., adhesives, tape, belts)	
Infection	**For Monilia**
Monilial infection (*Candida albicans*) indicated by pustular, reddened, weepy, white spots	Use nystatin (Mycostatin) powder, cover with skin sealant (Skin Prep or Skin Gel)
Radiation Therapy	
	Use drying agent (e.g., acroflavin)
	Place skin barrier (Stomahesive) over site

If the client has had a sigmoid colostomy performed, the client may benefit from colostomy irrigation to regulate elimination. The nurse discusses this technique with the client and the family to determine its feasibility and perceived worth (see the accompanying Guidelines feature). If irrigation is chosen as a method, the nurse teaches the client and the family how to perform colostomy irrigation (see the Client/Family Education feature on pp. 1390–1392). A variety of teaching tools may be used. Written instructions are helpful, because the client can take these home for future reference. Repetition is necessary while teaching the client these new

Text continued on page 1392

GUIDELINES ■ Determining Whether Irrigation of a Sigmoid Colostomy Should be Used As a Method of Elimination

Interventions	Rationales

1. Assess the client with regard to all of the following before irrigation is chosen as method:
  a. Presence of permanent sigmoid colostomy.
 	
  b. Client interest or desire.
 	
  c. Physical handicap or poor manual dexterity.
 	
  d. Inability to learn.
 	
  e. Lack of water supplies.
 	
  f. Ongoing intestinal medical problems.
  g. Active radiation therapy or chemotherapy.
 	
  h. History of irritable bowel habits (e.g., IBS).
2. Discuss the following considerations with the client and the family:
  a. Irrigation is *not* a medical necessity.
 	
  b. Irrigation can be initiated years after surgery; it need not be immediate.
  c. Prior bowel habits need to be considered.
 	
  d. Client may have the ability to control bowel evacuation to some extent *without* irrigation.
	1. Irrigation is not the method of choice for all clients.
	
	  a. Irrigation is used only with colostomy located in the sigmoid colon.
	  b. Client needs to be actively involved in irrigation for the procedure to be effective. Client may prefer natural evacuation through colostomy.
	  c. Client or the caregiver needs to have physical capability to perform irrigation independently.
	  d. Client or the caregiver needs to comprehend how to perform irrigation.
	  e. At least 500–1000 mL of water is necessary for irrigation procedure.
	  f. Irrigation may aggravate other disorders.
	  g. Irrigation may not control elimination time; radiation or chemotherapy may cause diarrhea; irrigation at this time may be fruitless and may actually add to fluid and electrolyte losses.
	  h. Irrigation may not control elimination.
	2. Clients should make an informed decision.
	  a. Evacuation through colostomy can occur naturally; irrigation is one method of management.
	  b. Client can take time to adjust to colostomy and to consider options for management.
	  c. If foods, activities, and psychologic factors caused varying elimination patterns before surgery, these may continue, and irrigation may not be successful in limiting evacuation to a convenient time.
	  d. Regular eating habits with occasional use of antidiarrheal medications and laxatives may control bowel elimination pattern, and irrigation may not be necessary.

Continued on following page

GUIDELINES ■ Determining Whether Irrigation of a Sigmoid Colostomy Should be Used As a Method of Elimination *Continued*

Interventions	Rationales

3. Discuss the advantages of irrigation, including
 	
  a. Client regains control of fecal elimination.
  b. Elimination occurs at a preferred time.
  c. Reduction of gas and odor is achieved.
  d. Client may not require a pouch.
	3. Clients and family need all available information to make an informed decision.

4. Discuss the disadvantages of irrigation, including
  a. Irrigation is time-consuming; it usually takes 45–60 min of bathroom time.
  b. Procedure may not eliminate spillage between irrigations.
 	
  c. There is danger of colon perforation.
	4. Disadvantages need to be discussed before irrigation is considered.
	  a. Client may not have the time to devote to irrigation.
	  b. If total control of drainage is the goal, client may not want to invest time in learning irrigation.
	  c. Catheter insertion too far into the colon or in the wrong direction can cause colon perforation.

CLIENT/FAMILY EDUCATION ■ Colostomy Irrigation

Instructions	Rationales

Irrigation Procedure
 	
1. "Assemble the necessary equipment:
  a. Irrigating kit with sleeve.
  b. Tubing with clamp.
  c. Cone.
  d. Container for solution.
  e. Skin care items.
  f. New pouch system ready for application."
	1. Most ostomy manufacturing companies produce irrigation kits that complement each pouch system. Kits may come with both irrigation catheter and cone; the cone is preferred owing to possible bowel perforation with catheter use.

2. "Remove the old pouch and dispose."	2. Removal allows placement of irrigating sleeve.
3. "Clean the stoma and the skin."	3. The stoma should be clearly visible.
4. "Apply the irrigating sleeve and place the end of the sleeve into the toilet."	4. The sleeve channels drainage into the toilet.
5. "Fill the irrigating container with 500–1000 mL of lukewarm water."	5. Lukewarm water helps prevent cramping.
6. "Suspend the irrigating container with the bottom of the container at shoulder level."	6. The height of the solution affects the rate of flow. *Continued*

CLIENT/FAMILY EDUCATION ▪ Colostomy Irrigation *Continued*

Instructions	Rationales
7. "Allow the solution to flow through the tubing to remove air from the tubing."	7. Air in the tubing will move into the bowel and be source of flatus and abdominal discomfort.
8. "Gently insert the irrigating cone or catheter into the stoma. The catheter is inserted 2–4 in into the stoma. Do not force. Slowly introduce the solution into the stoma."	8. Forcing the catheter could cause bowel perforation.
9. "Allow approximately 15–20 min to pass. When the majority of stool has passed, rinse the sleeve, dry the bottom, roll the sleeve up, and close the end. You may then go about other activities for next 30–45."	9. Adequate time should be allowed for complete evacuation.
10. "When evacuation of stool is complete, remove the irrigation sleeve, clean the stoma, and apply a new pouch system."	10. A pouch may be used between irrigations to control possible spillage.
11. "Clean the irrigating equipment, dry, and store."	11. Equipment can be reused as long as it is patent and clean.

Special Tips

1. "Irrigate at least once every 24 h."	1. Routine establishes bowel regularity and enables increased success in procedure outcome.
2. "You may wish to wear a small stomal covering instead of a pouch system between irrigations."	2. Stool drainage is anticipated between irrigations. Stoma must be kept moist to prevent tissue damage.
3. "If cramping occurs while you are irrigating, stop irrigating and wait. After cramping subsides, and you are ready to resume the procedure, try the following: slow down the flow of solution, lower the container, or warm the water."	3. Some cramping is normal and may be a sign that the bowel is ready to evacuate its contents. Too rapid administration of solution, too high pressure of solution because the container is too high, or use of water that is too cool can cause cramping.
4. "Make sure that air is out of the tubing before putting it into the stoma."	4. Air introduced into the bowel can also cause cramping.
5. "If water does not flow easily, try changing the position of the cone, checking the tubing for kinks and the level of the container, and relaxing with several deep breaths."	5. Opening of the cone may be blocked by bowel.
6. "If no returns occur, try gently massaging the abdomen or drinking warm liquids."	6. These activities may increase peristalsis.

Continued on following page

CLIENT/FAMILY EDUCATION ■ Colostomy Irrigation *Continued*

Instructions	Rationales
Approaches to Common Problems	

1. "If spillage occurs between irrigations, try
  a. Decreasing the rate of infusion
  b. Decreasing the amount of irrigant used
  c. Limiting how far the catheter is inserted into the bowel
  d. Allowing longer time for evacuation."
	1. Spillage can occur when too much solution enters the bowel or when there has been a change in diet.

2. "If your bowel retains the solution after irrigation, try
  a. Changing position.
  b. Walking around.
  c. Massaging your abdomen gently.
  d. Drinking something hot."
	2. These activities will increase peristalsis.

3. "If returns are less than usual, you may need to wear a pouch."	3. A pouch prevents spillage.
4. "If returns after irrigation are clear, decrease the irrigation frequency."	4. Clear returns indicate that evacuation occurred before irrigation.
5. "If you feel weak or faint during irrigaton, stop the procedure and lie down. When weakness subsides, change position to facilitate evacuation."	5. Rapid infusion or cold solution may cause temporary weakness, which should resolve within minutes.
6. "Call your physician if weakness does not resolve."	6. Fluid and electrolyte imbalance may be the problem, possibly the result of multiple irrigations.
7. "If you have had weakness during irrigation, which resolved quickly, use warmer water at a slower rate, and try inserting the cone or catheter less deeply in the stoma when you irrigate the next time."	7. This should prevent weakness from occurring if it is a result of cold solution, rapid irrigation, or deep penetration into the stoma.
8. "If weakness or faintness is a recurrent problem, notify your physician."	8. The cause should be identified and treated.

skills. Anxiety, fear, discomfort, and other distractions alter the client's and the family's ability to learn and retain information.

In addition to instructing the client about the clinical manifestations of obstruction and perforation, the nurse also teaches the client with a colostomy to report any fever or sudden onset of pain or swelling around the stoma.

Psychosocial Preparation

The diagnosis of cancer can be emotionally immobilizing for the client and the family. The treatment choice may be welcomed because it may provide hope for control of the disease. The nurse explores the client's reactions to the illness and perceptions of planned interventions. The client's reaction to ostomy surgery, which may include disfigurement, may involve feelings of being offensive to others; feelings of feeling dirty, with a reduced sense of value; and fear of rejection. The nurse allows the client to verbalize these feelings. By teaching the client how to physically manage the ostomy, the nurse assists the client in restoring self-esteem, which leads to solid relations with others. Inclusion of family and significant others in the rehabilitation process also helps to maintain relationships and raise the client's self-esteem.

Health Care Resources

There are several resources available that the nurse uses to complement the care provided, maintain continuity of care in the home environment, and provide for client needs that the nurse is not able to meet. These include the hospital social services department, an enterostomal therapy nurse, the United Ostomy Association, the American Cancer Society, a local home care agency, and a local pharmacy.

Social services department. The nurse makes a referral to the social worker who can provide further emotional counseling to the client and the family; aid in managing the financial concerns that the client and the family may have; and arrange home care or extended care (e.g., in a nursing home, group home, or hospice) as needed.

Enterostomal therapy nurse. An enterostomal therapy nurse is a registered nurse who has completed specialized training and is certified in ostomy nursing care. The nurse makes a referral to the enterostomal therapist to aid in preoperative teaching, evaluate and mark the stoma site, help with postoperative care and teaching, provide consultation for problems in care, and provide assistance with the discharge process. The enterostomal therapist may also conduct an outpatient clinic that would be available for ongoing client needs.

United Ostomy Association. The nurse provides information regarding this organization, which is a self-help group of people who have ostomies. Further literature, as well as the organization's publication (*Ostomy Quarterly*), can be obtained. Local chapters exist, and the nurse informs the client of the local group resource. This organization conducts a visitor program that provides specially trained visitors (who have an ostomy) to come and talk with clients. After obtaining the client's consent, the nurse makes a referral to the visitor program so that the visitor can see the client preoperatively, as well as postoperatively. Generally a physician's consent for visitation is also necessary (see Unit 13 Resources).

American Cancer Society. The local division of the ACS can provide necessary medical equipment and supplies, home care services, travel accommodations, and other resources for the client who is undergoing cancer treatment or ostomy surgery. The nurse informs the client and the family of the programs available through the local division.

Home care agency. The nurse makes a referral to a home care agency to provide for continuity of care. This resource will aid in physical care, teaching, and emotional support required when the client returns to the home environment.

Local pharmacy. The nurse informs the client and the family where and what ostomy supplies need to be purchased, considering price and location before making recommendations to the client.

 Evaluation

The nurse evaluates the care provided for the client with colorectal cancer. The expected outcomes include that the client

1. Attains and maintains a consistent bowel elimination pattern without blood in stool, diarrhea, or constipation
2. Verbalizes the diagnosis of cancer, defines cancer, and describes the treatment and its rationale
3. Verbalizes a beginning acceptance of the disease and starts to incorporate treatments into everyday life style
4. Demonstrates appropriate incision care and, if applicable, appropriate colostomy care with minimal assistance

OBSTRUCTION

OVERVIEW

Intestinal *obstruction* is a common and serious disorder that is caused by a variety of conditions. The obstruction can be *partial* or *complete* and can occur anywhere in the intestinal tract, although the ileum in the small intestine (the narrowest part of intestinal tract) is the most common site. Because obstruction is so common and is linked to so many other disorders, the nurse assesses for clinical manifestations of obstruction in all clients with GI disorders.

Pathophysiology

Partial and total obstruction can be either mechanical or nonmechanical (also termed paralytic, because it is a result of neuromuscular disturbance). *Mechanical* obstruction can be due to disorders outside the intestine (e.g., adhesions and hernias), disturbance inside the intestine (e.g., tumors, diverticulitis, and strictures), or blockage of the lumen of the intestine (e.g., by gallstone or intussusception).

Nonmechanical obstruction, also known as paralytic ileus or adynamic ileus, does not involve a physical obstruction in or outside the intestine. Instead, there is decreased muscular activity of the intestine, which results in a slowing of the movement of intestinal contents. Contents composed of ingested fluid and saliva; gastric, pancreatic, and biliary secretions; and swallowed air accumulate at the area of obstruction and above it. Intestinal distention results from the intestine's inability to absorb these contents and mobilize them down the intestinal tract. Increased peristalsis occurs in an effort to move intestinal contents forward; this stimulates more secretions, which leads to additional distention. Decreased absorption of the usual 7 to 8 L of electrolyte-rich fluid that normally enters the intestine in a 24-hour period and obstruction with increased secretion of fluids lead to fluid and electrolyte losses. The distended bowel can also impinge on arterial and venous blood flow in the abdomen, resulting in edema. High intestinal pressure can cause plasma to leak into the peritoneal cavity and fluid can follow.

ECF losses can range from 2 to 6 L within 2 to 3 days after a mechanical obstruction (McConnell, 1987). Hypovolemia, resulting from one or all of the above, ranges from mild to extreme (hypovolemic shock). Renal insufficiency and even death can occur as a consequence of severe hypovolemia.

Bacteria in intestinal contents lie stagnant in the obstructed intestine. This is not a problem unless the blood flow to the intestine is compromised. However, when the mechanical blockage is a so-called closed loop obstruction with blockage in two different areas or if there is a *strangulated* obstruction (obstruction with compromised blood flow) or an *incarcerated* obstruction (with compromised blood flow and necrosis), there is a great risk for peritonitis, with or without actual perforation. Bacteria without blood supply can form an endotoxin that, after release into the peritoneal or systemic circulation, can cause septic shock. In strangulated obstruction, there can also be a major blood loss into the intestine and the peritoneum.

The mortality is 10% for small bowel obstruction and 30% for large bowel obstruction. Strangulated small bowel obstruction has a mortality ranging from 20% to 75%. Strangulated large bowel has a 60% mortality rate (McConnell, 1987).

Specific fluid and electrolyte problems are dependent on the part of the intestine that is blocked. An obstruction high in the small intestine causes a loss of gastric hydrochloride, which can lead to *metabolic alkalosis*. An obstruction below the duodenum but above the large bowel results in loss of both acids and bases so that acid-base imbalance need not be significant. Obstruction at the end of the small intestine and lower, however, causes loss of base with fluids, thus risking *metabolic acidosis.*

Etiology

A mechanical obstruction can result from any of the following: adhesions; tumors; hernias; foreign bodies, such as gallstones and fecal impactions; strictures, resulting from Crohn's disease and radiation, or congenital strictures; intussusception (telescoping of a segment of intestine within itself) (Fig. 45–12); volvulus (twisting of intestine) (Fig. 45–12); fibrosis from disorders such as endometriosis; or vascular disorders, such as emboli and arteriosclerotic narrowing of mesenteric vessels.

Adhesions and hernias are the most common causes of mechanical obstruction in the small intestine. *Adhesions* are bands of granulation and scar tissue that de-

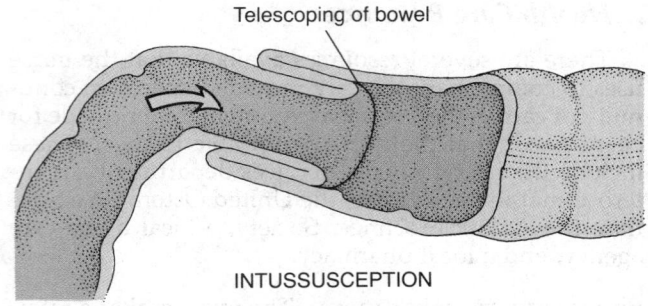
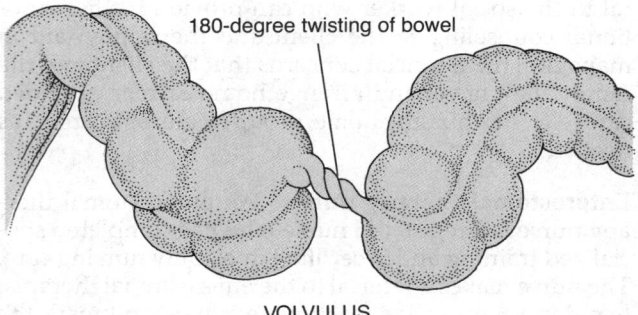

Telescoping of bowel

INTUSSUSCEPTION

180-degree twisting of bowel

VOLVULUS

Figure 45–12

Two types of mechanical obstruction.

velop after surgery. They commonly form after intestinal surgery, but usually do not cause obstruction. If obstruction does occur, it is more apt to happen many years after the surgery, when adhesions encircle the intestine and constrict the lumen. Adhesions rarely cause obstruction in the colon. The most common causes of colon obstruction are tumors, followed by diverticulitis and volvulus.

A *paralytic,* or adynamic, *ileus* is a nonmechanical obstruction, and it is the most common of all intestinal obstructions. It is caused by physiologic, neurogenic, or chemical imbalances associated with one or more of the following conditions: decreased peristalisis from trauma or toxin effect on autonomic intestinal control (as in abdominal surgery and trauma, hypokalemia, myocardial infarction, pneumonia, spinal injuries, peritonitis, or vascular insufficiency). Vascular insufficiency to the intestinal tract occurs when arterial or venous thrombosis or embolus decreases blood flow to the intestine. Vascular insufficiency can also occur when blood flow is reduced as a result of congestive heart failure or severe shock. Severe insufficiency of blood supply can result in infarction to surrounding organs.

Adynamic ileus can result from the handling of the intestines during abdominal surgery. It occurs to some degree after any abdominal surgical procedure, with intestinal function lost for a few hours to several days.

Incidence

Obstruction of the intestines occurs in all age groups. It is found in approximately 20% of all clients who are seen for acute abdominal pain (Brozenec & Rice, 1985). Because bowel obstruction occurs as a result of other disorders, statistics on the incidence of bowel obstruction are not readily available. Some statistics exist on the incidence of obstruction as a complication of specific disorders; for example, more than 50% of the obstructions in the large intestine result from malignant tumors (Brozenec & Rice, 1985). Volvulus obstruction occurs most commonly in elderly men as a result of constipation (Brozenec & Rice, 1985).

PREVENTION

Nonmechanical obstruction can be prevented by proper regulation of fluid and electrolyte balance. Limited manipulation of the intestines during abdominal surgery reduces the extent of diminished peristalsis. Nasogastric intubation and suction after abdominal procedures until intestinal function resumes also help limit the extent of a paralytic ileus, if the client does not become hypokalemic. Holding oral intake with or without nasogastric intubation after any trauma to the trunk of the body, after abdominal surgery, with spinal injuries, and during episodes of diverticulitis and exacerbations of Crohn's disease also helps prevent or limit the amount of decreased peristalsis and resulting distention.

Education of clients who are at risk for obstruction also helps identify obstruction early, limiting its sequelae. Individuals who should be instructed about the clinical manifestations of intestinal obstruction include all clients who have undergone abdominal surgery, clients with diverticulosis and diverticulitis, those with Crohn's disease or ulcerative colitis, clients with frequent constipation requiring enemas or disimpaction, clients with hernias, and those who have undergone radiation to the abdomen.

Persistent constipation, which is termed *obstipation*, and fecal impaction are common problems in the elderly, and this puts them at high risk for bowel obstruction. Constipation is problematic, because diet, activity, and medications affect normal elimination patterns. Elderly clients are likely to be taking medications that can contribute to constipation. They are also likely to have inadequate amounts of physical activity for promotion of bowel elimination. Ongoing nursing assessment of the elderly for effective bowel elimination patterns and education to optimize elimination can prevent obstruction from fecal impaction.

COLLABORATIVE MANAGEMENT

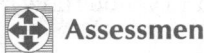 Assessment

History

The nurse obtains data from the client with a suspected or known intestinal obstruction, gearing questions to assessment factors that put an individual at risk for obstruction. The nurse assesses the *past medical his-*tory, specifically obtaining information about *abdominal or any surgery* and the date of the procedure, radiation therapy, and medical disorders, such as Crohn's disease, ulcerative colitis, diverticulosis, diverticulitis, gallstones, hernias, or tumors, always identifying the time of diagnosis and treatment. A *diet history,* recent occurrence of nausea or vomiting, and the time of the last bowel movement are also assessed.

Family history of colorectal cancer, along with a history of blood in stool or a change in bowel pattern, is also obtained by the nurse. This information is important because these might indicate a colon tumor, and tumors are the most common cause of mechanical obstruction of the colon and are often not diagnosed until the disease is advanced.

Physical Assessment: Clinical Manifestations

The client with *mechanical intestinal obstruction* most characteristically describes *cramping* in the mid-abdominal region that comes and goes. It occurs suddenly; it is more severe the higher the obstruction is. The client is relatively comfortable between episodes of cramping. Pain *decreases* as the obstruction worsens, unless strangulation or peritonitis occur.

On examination of the abdomen, the nurse may observe peristaltic waves. The nurse auscultates high-pitched bowel sounds (borborygmi) associated with the cramping, early in the obstructive process, as the intestine tries to push mechanical obstruction forward. In later stages of mechanical obstruction, the client has absent bowel sounds. *Abdominal distention,* caused by fatigue of the intestine, is the hallmark of intestinal obstruction. It can vary from relatively none to severe distention with taut, shiny skin and an umbilicus that rises higher in the abdomen as the distention increases.

Nausea and *vomiting* are common with mechanical obstruction, and vomitus varies in consistency, depending on the location of the obstruction. An obstruction above the ileum causes early and profuse vomiting, which initially contains partially digested food and chyme. As the intestine empties with vomiting, the contents become more watery, with bile and mucus. An obstruction below the ileum may not cause vomiting, or, if it does, the vomiting occurs in a different pattern and with different contents. The ileocecal valve in the large intestine tries to prevent regurgitation of intestinal contents below it. However, if the valve is unable to contain the intestinal contents, vomiting occurs. The vomitus from a mechanical obstruction in the large intestine is orange-brown, with a foul odor. The foul odor is the result of bacterial overgrowth in intestinal contents proximal to the obstruction or may actually be due to fecal contamination. Late stages of mechanical obstruction in the small intestine can also have this type of vomitus, also from bacterial overgrowth or fecal contents. Bacterial overgrowth can also cause the client to have *fecal breath.*

Obstipation is a characteristic manifestation of mechanical obstruction of the small and large intestines.

Early in the course of the obstruction, the bowel might evacuate remaining stool from below the obstruction; but, if complete obstruction occurs, neither stool nor gas is passed. Although obstipation is more characteristic of intestinal obstruction, diarrhea can occasionally occur.

In most types of *nonmechanical obstruction* (paralytic, or adynamic, ileus), the pain is described as a constant, diffuse discomfort. Colicky cramping is *not* characteristic of this type of obstruction. Pain associated with obstruction attributable to vascular insufficiency or infarction is usually severe. On auscultation of the abdomen, the nurse notes decreased bowel sounds in early obstruction and absent bowel sounds in later stages. Vomiting of gastric contents and bile is frequent, but it rarely has a foul odor and is rarely profuse. Obstipation may or may not be present. Shigultus (hiccups) is common with all types of intestinal obstruction.

Temperature with obstruction is rarely higher than 100° F (37.8° C). Temperature higher than this, with or without guarding and tenderness, and a sustained elevation in pulse not only associated with pain are indicative of strangulated obstruction or peritonitis.

Psychosocial Assessment

The nurse assesses the client's concerns and fears concerning the obstruction itself, the cause of the obstruction, and the diagnostic testing often necessary to determine the cause. Severe distention, pain, vomiting, and the abrupt presentation of obstructive manifestations are frightening. In addition to these uncomfortable symptoms, the client and the health care team are often initially unaware of the etiology of the obstruction. Fear of the unknown cause and the possibility of cancer is significant. Clients often become anxious when anticipating information about the results of diagnostic procedures. The nurse allows the client to verbalize fears and ask questions, which ensures that the client is kept informed of test results and treatment plans.

Laboratory Findings

There is no laboratory test that confirms a diagnosis of mechanical or nonmechanical obstruction. WBC counts are usually normal, unless there is a strangulated obstruction, in which case there may be leukocytosis. High obstruction in the small intestine is likely to show elevated serum venous carbon dioxide concentration and other values indicative of metabolic alkalosis. Obstruction in the large intestine is likely to show low serum venous carbon dioxide concentration and other values indicative of metabolic acidosis. Hemoglobin concentration and hematocrit are usually elevated, indicating dehydration.

Radiographic Findings

Flat-plate and upright x-ray films of the abdomen are obtained as soon as an obstruction is suspected, and their findings are considered valuable to the diagnostic process. Distention of loops of intestine with fluid and gas in the small intestine, with the absence of gas in the colon, gives evidence of an obstruction in the small intestine. However, x-ray findings are often normal when a small intestinal strangulated obstruction actually exists. Therefore, obstruction cannot be ruled out on the basis of x-ray findings.

Obstruction of the large intestine often shows gas distention of the colon on abdominal x-ray film. The presence of free air under the diaphragm on abdominal x-ray film is indicative of a perforated intestine.

Other Diagnostic Tests

Sigmoidoscopy, colonoscopy, or a barium enema may be done to determine the cause of the obstruction if the risk of perforation is not great. The examination chosen depends on the suspected location of the obstruction.

 ### Nursing Diagnosis

Common Diagnoses

The client with an intestinal obstruction most often has the following nursing diagnoses:

1. Altered (gastrointestinal) tissue perfusion related to obstructed intestine
2. Fluid volume deficit related to decrease in intestinal fluid reabsorption and loss of intestinal secretions secondary to obstruction and vomiting
3. Pain related to abdominal distention and increased peristalsis surrounding the obstruction

Additional Diagnoses

In addition, the client with intestinal obstruction may have

1. Potential for infection related to stagnant bacteria-rich intestinal contents and the risk of perforation
2. Ineffective breathing pattern related to elevation of the diaphragm from distention
3. Altered (gastrointestinal and renal) tissue perfusion related to impeded arterial and venous flow in the bowel
4. Altered nutrition: less than body requirements related to intestinal obstruction and NPO status
5. Decreased cardiac output related to decreased blood volume and impedence of arterial and venous flow in the bowel
6. Activity intolerance related to fluid and electrolyte imbalance and discomfort
7. Knowledge deficit related to the diagnostic work-up and the treatment regimen

⬛ Planning and Implementation ➡

Altered (Gastrointestinal) Tissue Perfusion

Planning: client goals. The goal is that the client will have return of effective peristalsis and usual pattern of bowel elimination, avoiding altered tissue perfusion.

Interventions. If the obstruction is partial and there is no evidence of strangulation, nonsurgical management is the treatment of choice. Decompression of the intestinal tract is commonly implemented at the same time as fluid and electrolyte balance is being restored.

Nonsurgical management. In addition to being placed on NPO status, all clients with intestinal obstruction of any type have a nasogastric tube or a nasointestinal tube inserted to decompress the bowel by draining fluid and air. This tube is attached to suction; the type of suction depends on what type of tube is inserted. Salem's sumps and Anderson's suction tubes are commonly used nasogastric tubes that sit distally in the stomach and are attached to *low continuous* suction. Continuous suction does not harm stomach mucosa with use of these particular tubes because an air vent is present.

Intestinal tubes, such as the Miller-Abbott, Cantor, and Harris tubes, are occasionally used in obstruction of the small intestine. These tubes are longer, extending into the small intestine, with mercury-filled balloons at the end of a lumen, which act as a bolus of food stimulating peristalsis and advancing down the intestinal tract (Fig. 45–13). The Cantor and Harris tubes are single-lumen tubes with mercury-filled balloons at the tips and suction ports within the same lumen, proximal to the tip. The Miller-Abbott tube has two separate lumenina for mercury and drainage. The nurse assists with progression of the tube by helping the client change position every 2 hours and by advancing the tube 3 to 4 in at specified times if ordered. These tubes are never taped to the nose until they reach a specified position in the intestine. As the tube is being inserted and advanced, it drains by gravity. The nurse monitors the drainage and if, drainage stops, obtains a physician's order to inject 10 mL of air. The nurse *does not irrigate* the nasointestinal tube with fluid. If ordered, low intermittent suction is attached to the suction lumen when the tube has stopped advancing. The accompanying Guidelines feature summarizes the nurse's role in caring for clients with nasointestinal tubes.

Use of nasointestinal tubes is avoided by many physicians because insertion of the mercury-filled lumen is often difficult and because the time it takes to insert the tube delays treatment. Insertion of this tube can also be uncomfortable for the client. Most clients, however, have at least a nasogastric tube in place in the presence of obstruction, unless obstruction is mild.

The nurse assesses the client with a nasogastric tube for proper placement of the tube, tube patency, and output at least every 4 hours and for skin integrity at the

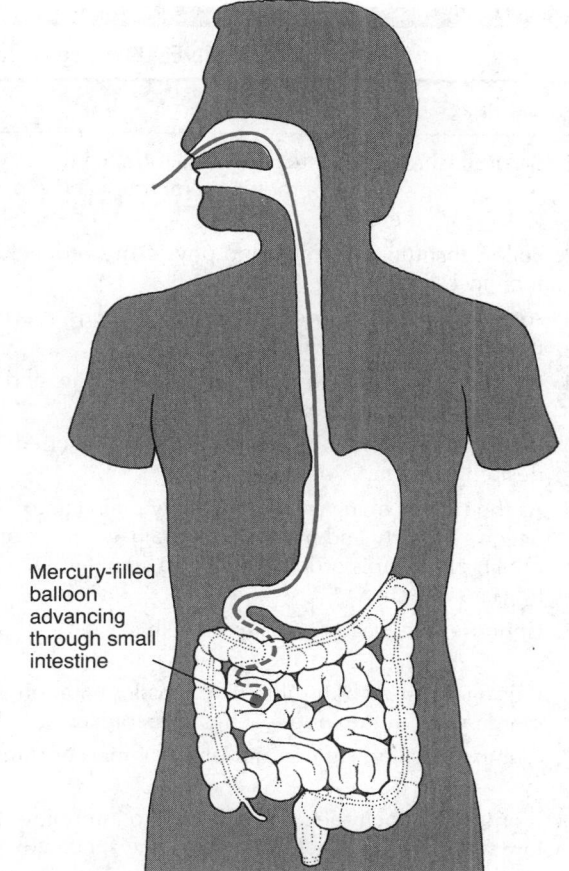

Mercury-filled balloon advancing through small intestine

Figure 45–13

A nasointestinal tube is passed down the intestinal tract. The mercury-filled balloon at the end of the lumen stimulates peristalsis.

point of insertion at least daily. Tape is removed daily and reapplied after the skin is washed and dried. The nurse assesses peristalsis during decompression by auscultating for bowel sounds every 4 hours, evaluating for flatus or bowel movements, and measuring abdominal girth at the same point each day. Clients are also assessed for nausea and asked to report this manifestation. If problems are noted with gastric tubes, the effect of nonfunctioning tubes is immediately determined. For example, nasogastric tubes often move out of optimal drainage position or become plugged. In this case, the nurse notes a decrease in gastric or intestinal output or stasis of contents in the tube. The nurse assesses the client for nausea, vomiting, increased abdominal distention, and placement of the tube. After appropriate placement is established, the contents are aspirated, and the tube is irrigated (usually with 30 mL of normal saline every 4 hours and as needed) to maintain patency.

Most types of nonmechanical obstruction respond to nasogastric decompression along with medical treatment of the primary disorder. Incomplete mechanical

GUIDELINES ■ Care of the Client with a Nasointestinal Tube

Interventions	Rationales
1. Before inserting a Cantor or Harris tube, fill the balloon bag's upper portion with mercury and aspirate all air from the bag.	1. Tubes vary with regard to filling with mercury before or after insertion.
2. Follow institutional policy and physician's orders for tube insertion.	2. Policies vary.
3. After the tube is inserted into the esophagus, place the client on his/her right side.	3. This position facilitates advancement of the tube through the pylorus.
4. If ordered, advance the tube 2–4 in at a time, and change the client's position.	4. Slow advancement decreases the possibility of kinks.
5. Do not secure the tube firmly until it has reached its desired position.	5. This inhibits advancement of the tube.
6. As the tube is being advanced, allow drainage to occur by gravity and monitor the drainage. If it stops, obtain physician's order to inject 10 cc of air. Do not irrigate with fluid.	6. The absence of drainage may indicate clogging of the tube.
7. Confirm tube placement on x-ray films.	7. Abdominal x-ray films are the only way to ensure that the tube has reached the small intestine.
8. If using Miller-Abbott tube, fill the balloon lumen with mercury when the tube reaches the stomach.	8. This procedure facilitates passage of the tube through the pylorus into the small intestine.
9. Clamp the balloon lumen and label it as mercury lumen.	9. Labeling prevents accidental mercury withdrawal through suction.
10. If ordered, attach the suction lumen to intermittent low suction when the tube reaches the specified destination.	10. Suction facilitates decompression, after the tube is in the proper position.
11. Keep client NPO and provide scrupulous mouth care every 2 h and prn.	11. Loss of GI contents can lead to dehydration.
12. When withdrawing the tube, remove the mercury from the balloon first, and pull the tube back 6 in/h.	12. Withdrawal should be done slowly to avoid separation of the balloon in the intestine.

obstruction can sometimes be successfully treated without surgical intervention. Obstruction caused by fecal impaction usually resolves after disimpaction and enema administration. Intussusception may respond to hydrostatic pressure changes during a barium enema.

Surgical management. *In all cases of complete mechanical obstruction and many cases of incomplete mechanical obstruction,* surgical intervention is necessary to relieve the obstruction. Strangulated or incarcerated obstruction is always complete and therefore always requires surgical intervention. An exploratory laparotomy of the abdomen is performed to locate the obstruction and to identify and treat the etiology. Specific procedures depend on the etiology and location of the obstruction. For example, if adhesions are the cause, they are lysed. Obstruction caused by tumor or diverticulitis in the colon requires colon resection with primary anastomosis if possible, or formation of a colostomy (see earlier). Obstruction caused by intestinal infarction may require an embolectomy or thrombectomy. Obstruction

caused by reduced blood flow may also require surgical resection of gangrenous bowel.

The nurse gives preoperative teaching as discussed in Chapter 18. All clients who require surgery for obstruction have nasogastric or intestinal intubation and suction before surgery if time permits. The nurse informs the client that nasogastric intubation and suction, along with NPO status, will continue for a few days postoperatively until peristalsis returns. The nasogastric tube may be weaned slowly before being completely removed to see if the client tolerates the absence of gastric decompression. This is done by first discontinuing suction to the tube, then clamping the tube for scheduled periods of time.

Fluid Volume Deficit

Planning client goals. The goal for this nursing diagnosis is that the client will retain and maintain a balanced systemic fluid volume.

Interventions: nonsurgical management. IV fluid replacement and maintenance are indicated for *all* clients with intestinal obstruction because all have some degree of vascular fluid loss from lack of normal reabsorption in the intestine, increased intestinal secretions around the blockage, nasogastric suction, and NPO status. Normal saline or a balanced salt solution with potassium is infused, based on electrolyte, BUN, and serum creatinine levels, as well as the overall condition of the client. Blood replacement may be indicated in strangulated obstruction because of blood loss into the bowel or the peritoneal cavity. The nurse monitors the client's vital signs and other measures of fluid status (e.g., urinary output, jugular veins, skin turgor, and mucous membranes). The nurse also assesses for edema from third spacing, as fluid is lost mostly from the vascular space into surrounding spaces (e.g., peritoneal cavity). Hyperalimentation (TPN) may be administered to improve the nutritional status of the client, especially if the client has had chronic nutritional problems. (Chapter 13 discusses the nursing care of clients receiving TPN.)

The client with intestinal obstruction is characteristically thirsty owing to fluid losses. The nurse provides frequent mouth care to help maintain moist mucous membranes. Lemon-glycerin swabs should be avoided because they can increase mouth dryness. A small amount of ice chips may be allowed if the client is *not* to undergo surgery; however, a physician's order should be obtained. These clients need to be monitored carefully with regard to intake and output to avoid electrolyte imbalance and false interpretation of gastric output measurements. Ice chips can provide more free water than electrolytes, also washing potassium and hydrochloric acid out of the nasogastric tube.

Broad-spectrum antibiotics are administered intravenously if strangulated or incarcerated obstruction is present.

Pain

Planning: client goals. The goal for this nursing diagnosis is that the client will have a reduction in discomfort while awaiting resolution of the obstruction. The abdominal distention commonly noted with intestinal obstruction can cause a great deal of discomfort, especially when severe. The colicky, crampy pain that comes and goes with mechanical obstruction and the nausea, vomiting, dry mucous membranes, and thirst that occur also contribute to client discomfort.

Interventions: nonsurgical management. It is essential that the nurse continuously assess the character and location of pain. If pain significantly increases or changes from a colicky, intermittent type to a constant discomfort, the nurse reports this immediately. Such changes could indicate perforation of the intestine or peritonitis. Narcotic analgesics are normally withheld in the diagnostic period so that clinical manifestations of perforation or peritonitis are not masked. The nurse

needs to explain to the client and the family the rationale for not giving analgesics. If an analgesic is ordered, it is most likely meperidine hydrochloride (Demerol), because morphine causes decreased intestinal motility, which may lead to nausea and vomiting.

The nurse assists the client to obtain a position of comfort and to change positions frequently to promote increased peristalsis. Semi-Fowler's positioning helps alleviate the pressure of abdominal distention on the chest, thereby not only making it a good comfort technique, but also facilitating adequate thoracic excursion and normal breathing patterns.

With nonmechanical obstruction, there is generally less discomfort than with mechanical obstruction. With both types of obstruction, discomfort is aggravated by ingesting food or fluids.

■ Discharge Planning

All clients with intestinal obstruction are hospitalized, with the length of stay depending on the etiology of the obstruction and the treatment necessary to relieve obstruction. If surgery is performed, a minimum of 1 to 2 weeks' hospitalization is required. Clients who have complicated obstruction, such as strangulation or incarceration, are at greater risk for peritonitis, sepsis, and shock; the hospital stay can range from weeks to months.

Clients with nonmechanical (adynamic) intestinal obstruction are less likely to require a lengthy hospitalization because of the obstruction alone. Adynamic obstruction responds to nasogastric intubation and suction within a few days.

Home Care Preparation

For the client who has had an intestinal obstruction, home care preparation is entirely dependent on the etiology of the obstruction and the treatment required. The nurse identifies what actions are necessary to prevent recurrent obstruction and what care is required with regard to the existing status of the obstruction's cause. Clients who have resolution of obstruction without surgical intervention are assessed for their ability to take preventive action independently to avoid obstruction. For example, if fecal impaction was the cause of the obstruction, the nurse assesses the client's ability to carry out a bowel regimen independently. For clients who have undergone surgery, the nurse evaluates their ability to function at home with the added tasks of incision care and possibly colostomy care.

Client/Family Education

The teaching plan for the client who has had an intestinal obstruction is dependent on the specific etiology and treatment. The nurse discusses the specific cause of obstruction and explains treatment of the obstruction and treatment of the cause. The nurse tells the client who had nonmechanical obstruction after surgery or trauma that, with return of motility to normal function, obstruction is resolved and no further treatment of the obstruction itself is necessary. These clients are instructed to report any abdominal pain or distention, nausea, or vomiting, with or without constipation, that could be indicative of recurrent obstruction. However, they should be reassured that recurrent adynamic ileus is not usually a problem. The client who has had mechanical obstruction resulting from fecal impaction needs to have a structured bowel regimen to prevent recurrence. The nurse instructs these clients to eat high-fiber diets and exercise daily. The administration of psyllium hydrophilic mucilloid (Metamucil) followed by at least 8 oz of water can be recommended to add bulk to the diet.

Clients who have surgery are taught incision care, drug therapy, and activity limitations specific to each individual. Drug therapy consists of an oral narcotic analgesic, such as oxycodone hydrochloride with acetaminophen (Percocet), to be taken as needed for incision discomfort.

Psychosocial Preparation

With resolution of obstruction, the client focuses on the cause and treatment necessary. Psychosocial preparation varies, depending on these two factors. Clients who had curative treatment of the underlying cause most likely require less support than clients who underwent treatment of obstruction related to a serious disease that will require further treatment. The nurse allows the client to express fears and concerns about the future and assesses the client's understanding and needs with regard to future treatment plans.

Home Care Resources

The need for follow-up appointments is dependent on the etiology and the treatment required for obstruction. If the client is at risk for fecal impaction, the nurse can arrange for a home care nurse to assess the GI function and dietary habits of the client on an ongoing basis. If the client needs assistance with incision or colostomy care, the nurse can arrange for the assistance of a home care nurse as needed.

 Evaluation

The nurse evaluates the client with intestinal obstruction on the basis of identified nursing diagnoses specific to each client's degree of illness. The expected outcomes include that the client

1. Has no abdominal distention, with normal bowel sounds
2. Has a formed bowel movement at least every 3 days
3. States that abdominal discomfort is resolved

TRAUMA

OVERVIEW

Approximately 25% of all deaths related to trauma are related to abdominal injuries (Trunkey et al., 1974). Clients with abdominal trauma can have injuries to one or various organs or body systems. Because the client with bowel trauma may have other abdominal injuries, it is more important for the nurse to focus on the risks of hemorrhage and peritonitis associated with abdominal trauma than pathologic changes in a specific organ. The client who has abdominal trauma often does not have a definitive diagnosis, even after examination by a health care provider. For these reasons, this discussion deals with care of the client who has experienced any type of abdominal trauma, not necessarily involving trauma to the bowel.

Abdominal injury is commonly divided into the two broad categories of blunt and penetrating trauma. Severe *blunt trauma* has an estimated mortality of 23% to 46% (Marx, 1983). Fifty per cent of all blunt trauma is a result of automobile accidents (Zuidema et al., 1985). Assaults and falls cause abdominal trauma, but less frequently than automobile accidents.

Penetrating abdominal trauma is usually associated with violence, most often with gunshot and stab wounds (Gibson, 1987). The mortality is 1% to 2% for stab wounds, and 5% to 15% for gunshot wounds (Cayten, 1984). The major cause of death is hemorrhage, which usually occurs before the client arrives at the hospital (Gibson, 1987).

In penetrating trauma, the liver and the small bowel are most commonly involved in stab wounds, and the small bowel is most often involved in gunshot wounds. Penetrating trauma is less likely to involve multiple organs than blunt trauma. However, a penetrating wound to the abdomen can also involve the thorax, the spine, and the retroperitoneum.

COLLABORATIVE MANAGEMENT

The nurse assesses for abdominal trauma by asking the client about the presence, location, and quality of pain. The abdomen is then inspected for contusions, abrasions, lacerations, ecchymosis, penetrating injuries, and symmetry. Assessment for abdominal trauma includes inspection and examination of the anterior abdomen, the flanks, the back, the genitalia, and the rectum.

For assessment of the abdomen, all of the client's clothes must be removed. Pneumatic garments (military anti-shock trousers [MAST]) are *not* removed unless aggressive fluid replacement has been given to the client, a surgical team is immediately available to intervene, and the attending physician orders it to be done. After pneumatic garments are removed, uncontrolled hemorrhage can occur. MAST have a constrictive effect on hemorrhage in the trunk and facilitate circulatory return to the heart. To perform an adequate inspection, the nurse turns the client while maintaining spinal immobilization. Ecchymosis may indicate internal bleeding. Ecchymosis around the umbilicus is known as Cullen's sign and may indicate retroperitoneal bleeding into the abdominal wall. Ecchymosis in either flank, known as Turner's sign, also is indicative of retroperitoneal bleeding. The nurse auscultates the abdomen for bowel sounds. Absent or diminished bowel sounds may be caused by the presence of blood, bacteria, or chemical irritant in the abdominal cavity. The nurse also auscultates for bruits in the abdomen, which indicate renal artery injury. The nurse percusses the abdomen next. Abnormal signs associated with abdominal trauma are resonance over the right flank with the client lying on the left side. This is known as Ballance's sign, which is found with a ruptured spleen. Resonance over the liver, which is normally dull, is due to free air, which is pathologic. Dullness over hollow organs that normally contain gas, such as the stomach, and the large and small intestines, may indicate blood or fluid. Light abdominal palpation is done to identify areas of tenderness, rebound tenderness, guarding, rigidity, and spasm. If the nurse palpates a mass, it may be blood or fluid collection.

Nursing interventions include placement of at least two large-bore IV catheters in the upper extremities. IV catheters in the lower extremities are not used to provide fluid if abdominal trauma has occurred, because if the vasculature in the abdomen is injured, fluid would pool in the abdomen and not aid in maintaining circulatory fluid balance. A central venous catheter may be inserted by the physician to assist with rapid fluid volume infusion. IV fluid consists of a balanced saline solution, crystalloids, and possibly blood. Arterial blood gas values; CBC; serum electrolyte, glucose and amylase, and BUN levels; liver enzyme levels; and clotting studies are performed and results monitored by the nurse. Hemoglobin level and hematocrit initially do not reflect true blood loss, and the values appear higher than they actually are because of hemoconcentration from volume loss. Serial hemoglobin level and hematocrit measurements are assessed to identify true blood loss. An elevated WBC count may be indicative of ruptured spleen. Elevation of serum amylase concentration may signal injury to the pancreas or the bowel. All laboratory work is compiled so that values can be compared and subtle changes noted. The client is also attached to a cardiac monitor in the emergency room. An indwelling catheter is inserted by the nurse, unless there is blood at the urinary meatus. Initially and hourly thereafter, urinary outputs are evaluated for bleeding and specific gravity. Urinalysis is performed, including assessment for blood and protein in the urine. If there is an open abdominal wound or evisceration, the nurse covers it with a sterile dry dressing, unless the physician orders otherwise. Unless contraindicated, as in case of concomitant skull

fracture, a nasogastric tube is inserted and kept in place to identify bleeding and to minimize the risk of vomiting and aspiration. Antibiotics may be administered to reduce the risk of peritonitis.

Clients with abdominal trauma undergo an exploratory laparotomy and repair of abdominal injuries immediately if the client has definite signs of peritoneal irritation, such as rebound tenderness, significant bleeding from a nasogastric tube or the rectum, active blood loss that cannot be associated with an injury outside the abdomen, evisceration, or a gunshot wound with possible peritoneal involvement. Most stab wounds require exploratory laparotomy, but as many as 25% are superficial and do not involve the peritoneum (Markovchick et al., 1985). Superficial stab wounds are explored and cleaned with local anesthetic, and the client does not require an exploratory laparotomy. Clients without obvious significant bleeding or definite signs of peritoneal irritation undergo abdominal radiography, peritoneal lavage, and CT.

If the client with known abdominal trauma has no definite clinical manifestations of active bleeding or abdominal injury, the client is admitted to the hospital for observation. Blunt trauma can cause active, but often not obvious, damage. The nurse assesses for abdominal or referred pain and nausea. Mental status; vital signs; clinical findings such as vomiting, guarding, rigidity, and rebound tenderness; skin temperature; bowel sounds; and urinary output are evaluated at least every 15 to 30 minutes in the early postinjury period and then hourly. Any change is reported immediately. It is more important for the nurse to recognize the high risk of an active abdominal injury and assess for general signs of abdominal injury (e.g., hemorrhage and peritonitis) than to attempt to identify the exact nature of the abdominal injury. Analgesics for pain are not given at this time so that clinical manifestations are not masked or overlooked. The nurse explains the rationale for this to the client and the family.

Before discharge from the hospital, all clients who have experienced abdominal trauma are taught the signs and symptoms of abdominal bleeding, regardless of whether they have had surgery. Clients are told to watch for and report any abdominal pain, nausea, vomiting, bloody or black stools, fever, weakness, or dizziness. Occasionally, hemorrhage can occur weeks after blunt abdominal trauma, despite medical evaluation and even hospitalization. Clients who undergo surgery or have exploration of wounds receive instructions on wound care before discharge from the hospital.

OBESITY

Obesity is defined as more than 20% increase in body weight for height and body build standards of ideal weight. The increased weight is due to deposition of fat in the body. Obesity results when caloric intake is greater than metabolic demands. The causes are multiple and include heredity, individual body build and metabolism, the presence of fat cells, and psychosocial factors. Traditional treatment combines dieting, exercise, psychosocial support, and behavior modification. In specific situations, medications for short-term appetite suppression are appropriate.

Jaw wiring is a drastic method for reducing food intake. Lipectomy, the excision of subcutaneous fat, can also be done. Both of these procedures have advantages and disadvantages, and they do not always result in permanent weight reduction.

Clients who do not respond to traditional measures may be considered for surgical procedures aimed at allowing permanent weight reduction. Three types of surgery are performed on the GI tract as treatments for obesity, namely, gastric bypass, gastroplasty (gastric stapling), and jejunoileal bypass. Clients who have any of these procedures performed must meet certain criteria before surgery. The criteria vary, depending on the individual hospital, but they typically include massive or morbid obesity (i.e., more than two times ideal weight) that has not responded to traditional weight reduction methods; absence of liver, cardiac, kidney, or inflammatory bowel disease; emotional stability and a commitment to comply with postoperative care; and age less than 50 years. Clients with health problems related to their obesity (e.g., hypertension and diabetes mellitus) are often considered for these procedures, and other criteria may be waived, depending on the perceived benefit of surgery. There are multiple complications and some uncertainties associated with all three procedures, and these are stressed to the client before surgery.

Jejunoileal bypass results in weight loss because the small intestine is shortened to allow less area for absorption. Postoperatively, *all* clients with jejunoileal bypass experience diarrhea, which lasts for months. The amount varies, the usual being 6 to 8 stools daily. Some clients have as many as 24 stools a day. Metabolic problems result, with potassium loss being the most common. Polyarthritis, malnutrition, renal failure, renal calculi, cholelithiasis, hepatic dysfunction, and cirrhosis can also occur after jejunoileal bypass, and many of the long-term effects are not known. If there is excessive weight loss, inadequate weight loss, or severe complications, revision of the bypass may be performed. Revision may be complete and involve returning the intestine to its previous anatomic position. Revision may also involve lengthening the bypass to decrease absorption further and cause more weight loss.

Gastric bypass and *gastroplasty* accomplish weight reduction by limiting the amount of food that can be ingested. Gastric bypass and gastroplasty have fewer associated complications; however, results have been variable and long-term effects are not known. Immediately postoperatively, the client has a nasogastric tube in place after either gastric bypass or gastroplasty. After gastroplasty, the nasogastric tube drains both the proximal pouch and the distal stomach. The nurse closely monitors the nasogastric tube for patency. The nurse *never* repositions the tube because this could cause disruption of the suture line. The nasogastric tube is removed on the third postoperative day if the client has bowel sounds and is passing flatus. The nurse gives the client 1 oz of water in a 1-oz medicine cup and instructs the client to sip it over 1 hour. Clear liquids are given to the client if water is tolerated, and 1-oz cups are used for each serving. Twenty-four to 48 hours after clear liquids are tolerated, puréed foods, juice, and soups thinned with broth, water, or milk are added to the client's diet. The client can increase the volume to 1 oz over 5 minutes or until satisfied, but the diet is limited to liquids for 8 weeks. Nausea, vomiting, or discomfort occurs if too much liquid is ingested. Before the client is discharged from the hospital, the nurse instructs the client to take liquid or chewable multivitamins daily and to drink high-protein liquids to promote wound healing.

POLYPS

OVERVIEW

Polyps in the GI tract are small growths covered with mucosa and attached to the surface of the intestine. Polyps are significant in that, although most are benign, some have the potential to become malignant.

Different types of polyps are identified by their tissue type. *Adenomas* always require medical consultation because of their malignant potential. Although only 5% of adenomas progress to cancer, almost all colorectal cancers develop from an adenoma (Schapiro, 1989). Adenomas are further classified as *villous* or *tubular*. Of these, *villous* adenomas are a greater cancer risk. *Familial polyposis* and *Gardner's syndrome* are inherited syndromes characterized by multiple colorectal polyps. Unless these syndromes are treated, the risk of colorectal cancer is almost 100% (Schapiro, 1989). Other types

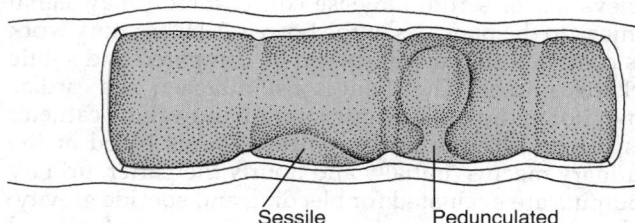

Sessile   Pedunculated

Figure 45–14

Pedunculated and sessile polyps. Pedunculated polyps, such as tubular adenomas, are stalk-like. Sessile polyps, such as villous adenomas, are broad based.

of polyps include *hamartomatous* and *hyperplastic* polyps. A hamartomatous polyp disorder, *Peutz-Jeghers* syndrome, is associated with a slight risk of cancer. Other types, however, are not.

In addition to being classified by their tissue type, polyps are described according to their appearance (Fig. 45–14). *Pedunculated* polyps are stalk-like, with a thin stem attaching them to the intestinal wall. They become elongated as peristalsis pulls them into the lumen of the intestine. *Tubular adenomas* tend to be *pedunculated.* Polyps attached to the intestinal walls by a broad base are described as *sessile. Villous adenomas* tend to be *sessile* in formation.

COLLABORATIVE MANAGEMENT

Polyps are usually asymptomatic and are discovered during routine diagnostic testing or tests for blood in stool. However, they can cause gross rectal bleeding, intestinal obstruction, or intussusception. Diagnostic studies involve a barium enema and proctosigmoidoscopy or colonoscopy to rule out cancer. Biopsies of polyps can be obtained or the entire polyp can actually be removed (polypectomy) with use of an electrocautery snare that fits through the sigmoidoscope or colonoscope. This often eliminates the need for abdominal surgery to remove a suspicious or definitely malignant polyp. Clients with familial polyposis or Gardner's syndrome most often require a total colectomy (colon removal) to prevent the development of cancer.

Nursing care focuses on client education regarding the significance of polyps, specific instructions on what clinical manifestations to watch for and report, and instruction on the need for ongoing monitoring by the health care team. Clients with a known benign polyp that does not need to be removed have routine sigmoidoscopic or colonoscopic examinations to monitor for any growth or change in the polyp or an increase in the number of polyps. If the client has had a polypectomy, follow-up is also needed via sigmoidoscopic or colonoscopic examinations because of the increased risk of having multiple polyps develop in clients who have had at least one polyp. Nursing care of clients after polypectomy of the colorectal area includes monitoring for abdominal distention and pain, rectal bleeding, mucopurulent rectal drainage, and fever. A small amount of blood might appear in the stool after a polypectomy, but this should be temporary. Care for clients who have total colectomy is described earlier.

HEMORRHOIDS

OVERVIEW

Hemorrhoids are unnaturally swollen or distended veins in the anorectal region that are common and not signifi-

cant, unless they cause pain or bleeding. These distended veins begin as part of the normal structure in the anal region. With limited distention, these veins function as a valve overlying the anal sphincter that assists in continence. Increased intra-abdominal pressure causes elevated systemic and portal venous pressure, which is transmitted to the anorectal veins. Arterioles in the anorectal region shunt blood directly to the distended anorectal veins, increasing the pressure. With repeated elevations in pressure from increased intra-abdominal pressure and engorgement from arteriolar shunting of blood, the distended veins eventually separate from the smooth muscle surrounding them. The result is prolapse of the hemorrhoidal vessels. Hemorrhoids are described as internal or external (Fig. 45–15). *Internal hemorrhoids,* which cannot be seen on inspection of the perineal area, lie above the anal sphincter. *External hemorrhoids* lie below the anal sphincter and can be seen on inspection of the anal region. Prolapsed hemorrhoids can become thrombosed or inflamed, or they can bleed.

The most common cause of repeated increased abdominal pressure resulting in hemorrhoids are straining at stool, pregnancy, and portal hypertension. The most common symptoms of hemorrhoids are bleeding and prolapse. Blood is characteristically bright red and is found on toilet tissue or outside the stool. Pain is also a common symptom and is often associated with thrombosis, especially if thrombosis occurs suddenly. Other symptoms include itching and mucous discharge.

COLLABORATIVE MANAGEMENT

Diagnosis is made by inspection, digital examination, and proctoscopy if necessary. Treatment is conservative and is aimed at reducing symptoms with a minimum of

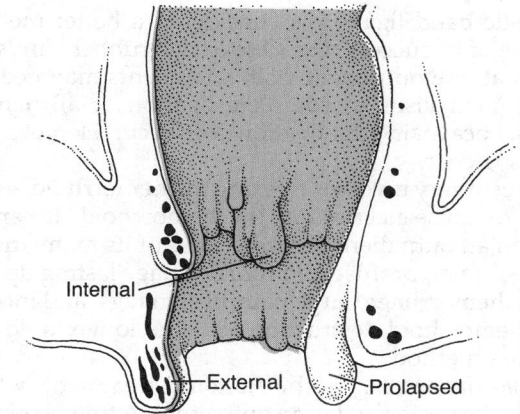

Figure 45–15

Internal, external, and prolapsed hemorrhoids. Internal hemorrhoids lie above the anal sphincter and cannot be seen on inspection of the anal area. External hemorrhoids lie below the anal sphincter and can be seen on inspection of the anal region. Hemorrhoids that enlarge, fall down, and protrude through the anus are called prolapsed hemorrhoids.

discomfort, cost, and time lost from usual activities. Local treatment and diet therapy are initiated when symptoms begin. Application of cold packs to the anorectal region for 3 to 4 hours at the onset of pain, followed by hot sitz baths 3 to 4 times a day, is often enough to relieve discomfort, even if the hemorrhoids are thrombosed.

Witch hazel soaks (e.g., Tucks) are also effective. Topical anesthetics, such as lidocaine (Xylocaine), are useful for severe pain. Dibucaine (Nupercainal) ointment, an OTC remedy, may be used for mild to moderate pain. This ointment, however, should be used only temporarily, because it could mask worsening symptoms and delay diagnosis of a severe disorder. If itching or inflammation is present, a steroid preparation such as hydrocortisone is prescribed. Diets high in fiber and fluids are recommended to promote regular bowel movement without straining. Stool softeners, such as docusate sodium (Colace), can be used temporarily. Irritating laxatives are avoided. Oral analgesics might be prescribed for thrombosed hemorrhoids. Conservative treatment should alleviate symptoms in 3 to 5 days. If symptoms continue or recur frequently, the client may require surgical intervention.

There are several types of surgical treatments that can be performed for symptomatic hemorrhoids. The type of intervention depends on the degree of prolapse, if there is thrombosis, and the overall condition of the client. Surgical methods include sclerotherapy, rubber band ligation, cryosurgery, and hemorrhoidectomy. Sclerotherapy is done by injecting a sclerosing agent into the tissues around the hemorrhoids to cause the vessels to obliterate. It can be done on an outpatient basis, without long-term pain. However, it can only be done for low-grade hemorrhoids, and there is a recurrence rate of greater than 50% (Knauer & Silverman, 1988).

Elastic band ligation is considered a better method because of its success rate. One or two rubber bands are put on at one outpatient visit, and clients may need to have repeat visits to complete ligation of all hemorrhoids. Local pain after ligation does occur. Hemorrhage can also occur.

Cryosurgery involves freezing the hemorrhoid with a probe to cause necrosis of the hemorrhoid. It can be done on an outpatient basis; because of its many disadvantages (e.g., profuse and foul drainage lasting up to 6 weeks, hemorrhage, large painful skin tags, and incomplete hemorrhoid destruction), it is no longer a widely accepted method.

Hemorrhoidectomy is the standard treatment, which can now be performed in an outpatient setting. Approximately 10% of clients with symptomatic hemorrhoids undergo hemorrhoidectomies (Smith, 1987). The most common problem after hemorrhoidectomy is pain, which is severe for 1 to 2 days after surgery. Urinary retention can also occur because of rectal spasms and anorectal tenderness. Hemorrhage is a rare but potential complication.

Nurses are typically involved in teaching clients with hemorrhoids about the need for adhering to high-fiber,

high-fluid diets to promote regular bowel patterns. Nurses can also teach the local treatments useful for clients with hemorrhoids. Clients who undergo any type of surgical intervention are monitored by the nurse for hemorrhage and pain postoperatively. All clients can have surgery on an outpatient basis, but clients requiring hemorrhoidectomy are likely to be hospitalized. These clients, in particular, require ongoing interventions for pain because of its severity. Appropriate nursing interventions include assisting clients to a side-lying position, keeping fresh ice packs over the dressing until packing is removed (if ordered by the physician), and using moist heat (as in sitz baths) three or four times a day after the first 12 hours postoperatively. Vasodilation from the sitz bath redirects blood to the rectal area, which might cause the client to feel faint. The nurse places an ice bag on the client's head during the sitz bath to prevent feelings of faintness. A flotation pad can be used under the buttocks for sitting. The client's first bowel movement postoperatively is painful. The administration of stool softeners, such as docusate sodium, is begun on the first postoperative day. Narcotic analgesics are administered before the client attempts to defecate, and the nurse stays near the client during the first defecation. All clients who have undergone hemorrhoidectomy are monitored for urinary retention. Measures to facilitate voiding, such as the administration of analgesics, provision of privacy, stimulation by running water, or spirits of peppermint in the commode, are provided as needed.

ANORECTAL ABSCESS

OVERVIEW

Anorectal abscesses most often result from obstruction of the ducts of glands in the anorectal region by feces, foreign bodies, or trauma. Stasis of obstructing contents occurs and results in infection that spreads into adjacent tissue. Most abscesses begin as cryptitis, which is a pocket of infection in an anal crypt.

Rectal pain is the first manifestation. There may be no clinical manifestations at the time of the first physical assessment, but clinical signs of local swelling, erythema, and tenderness on palpation are apparent within a few days after the onset of pain. A history of diarrhea before the rectal pain may be obtained from the client. If the abscess is a chronic condition, manifestations of discharge, bleeding, and pruritus (itching) may exist.

COLLABORATIVE MANAGEMENT

The diagnosis is usually made by physical examination and history. Anoscopy or sigmoidoscopy may be done to rule out concomitant disorders, such as anal fistulas.

Intervention for anorectal abscess requires surgical incision and drainage. Simple perianal and ischiorectal abscesses can often be incised under local anesthesia. More extensive abscesses may require incision under regional or general anesthesia in a hospital. Systemic antibiotics are given only for clients who are immunocompromised, diabetic clients, those with valvular disease or prosthesis, and those with extensive cellulitis. Incision and drainage in these clients are performed after antibiotic therapy.

Nursing interventions are focused on assisting the client to obtain and maintain comfort (before and after surgical intervention) and education regarding preventive measures, diet therapy for bowel regimens, and wound care. Preoperatively, witch hazel soaks (Tucks), local application of ice, or sitz baths may soothe the region. After incision and drainage of the abscess, narcotic analgesics are ordered.

In educating the client, the nurse stresses the need for careful cleaning of the anal region after bowel movements, trauma, or contact with any foreign body. This assists in the healing process of the existing abscess and also helps prevent recurrence of abscesses. The nurse educates the client about a diet high in fiber and fluids to assist with regular bowel patterns. Straining during bowel movements adds to discomfort of existing abscesses.

dyspareunia. The diagnosis is made by inspection and stretching of the perianal skin. If the client is having pain at the time of the examination, diagnostic testing is usually limited to inspection. However, if the client is not in severe pain, a digital examination and possibly a sigmoidoscopy are done. When painless or multiple fissures are present, a barium enema and sigmoidoscopy are performed to rule out an associated inflammatory bowel disorder. Management of an acute fissure is nonsurgical, with interventions aimed at local, symptomatic pain relief and softening of stool to reduce trauma to the area. Warm sitz baths and analgesia are recommended, along with use of bulk-producing agents, such as psyllium hydrophilic mucilloid (Metamucil), which help minimize pain associated with defecation. If fissures do not respond to medical management within several days to weeks, surgical excision of the fissure may be necessary under local anesthesia.

The nurse educates the client about the appropriate pain control measures. When nonsurgical management is initiated, the nurse instructs clients to notify the health care provider if pain is not relieved within a few days. The nurse instructs the client who undergoes surgery to continue with the same pain management and bowel regimen, including sitz baths and the administration of analgesics and bulk-forming agents. The nurse also instructs these clients to report any drainage or bleeding from the rectum to the health care provider.

ANAL FISSURE

OVERVIEW

An *anal fissure,* also called fissure in ano, is an elongated, ulcerated laceration between the anal canal and the perianal skin. Fissures can be primary or secondary, acute or chronic. *Primary fissures* are idiopathic with no known cause for their occurrence. *Secondary fissures* are associated with another disorder, such as Crohn's disease, tuberculosis, or leukemia, or are associated with trauma from a foreign body, child birth, or perirectal surgery. Constipated stool, diarrhea, or spasm of the anal sphincter are possible causes of fissures.

COLLABORATIVE MANAGEMENT

An acute anal fissure is superficial and resolves spontaneously or with conservative treatment. Chronic fissures, however, recur and often require surgical treatment. Pain during and after defecation is the most common symptom. Bleeding noted outside of the stool or on toilet tissue is the next most common symptom. Other symptoms associated with chronic fissures are pruritus, urinary frequency or retention, dysuria, and

ANAL FISTULA

OVERVIEW

An *anal fistula,* or fistula in ano, is an abnormal tract-like communication between the anal canal and the skin outside the anus. Most anal fistulas result from anorectal abscesses, which are caused by obstruction of anal glands (see earlier discussion of anorectal abscesses). However, fistulas can also be associated with tuberculosis, Crohn's disease, and ulcerative colitis (see earlier).

COLLABORATIVE MANAGEMENT

The client with anal fistula often has pruritus or purulent discharge. Diagnostic work-up includes digital examination, anoscopy or proctoscopy, and probing of the tract. A barium enema and sigmoidoscopy are performed when the fistula is not obviously due to an abscess to investigate the possibility of Crohn's disease or ulcerative colitis. The method of treatment depends on the cause. Fistulas attributable to local gland infection are surgically excised, along with excision of the infected area. A temporary colostomy may be performed at the time of this excision to allow the area to heal. Fistulas that are due to intestinal disorders such as Crohn's disease or ulcerative colitis are generally not treated surgically because of the high risk that the treatment will fail. In these clients, treatment of the primary disorder is the focus of care, with conservative management of the fistula.

Nursing care of clients with anal fistulas focuses on assisting the client in obtaining optimal skin integrity and adequate nutrition and fluid status to promote healing, replace fluid losses, and resolve or prevent infection. Several nursing measures are described under the heading Planning and Implementation for the client with Crohn's disease. The client who has a surgical excision of the fistula experiences pain for at least 1 or 2 days postoperatively. Nursing interventions focus on local management of pain with sitz baths and administration of systemic analgesics. Clients with Crohn's disease or ulcerative colitis also need to be educated on how to control their primary intestinal disorders, thus allowing for fistula healing and preventing development of new fistulas.

PARASITIC INFECTION

OVERVIEW

Parasites can enter and invade the GI tract and cause infections leading to varying degrees of illness. Parasites commonly enter through the mouth via fecal-oral transmission. Transmission commonly occurs via contaminated food or water, during sexual oral-anal practices, or via contact with feces from a contaminated person. Common parasites that cause infection in humans are *Entamoeba histolytica,* which causes *amebiasis* (amebic dysentery), and *Giardia lamblia,* which is responsible for *giardiasis.*

Humans are the only known hosts for *E. histolytica.* This organism occurs in cysts and trophozoites. Trophozoites die rapidly after they leave the body in stool. Cysts, however, can remain viable in the right type of environment for weeks or months. Humans who eliminate cysts are infectious. Flies have been found to be vectors for transmission of the cysts, and transmission is increased in areas that use human excrement for fertilizer. Amebiasis occurs worldwide but is most prevalent and severe in tropical areas, with prevalence rates as high as 40% in areas with poor sanitation, crowding, and poor nutrition (Goldsmith, 1988b). This disease is responsible for 40,000 to 100,000 deaths annually worldwide (Goldsmith, 1988b). The disease causes less severe symptoms and often goes undiagnosed in temperate climates. The organism has been reported to be in 2% to 5% of some of the populations in the United States (Goldsmith, 1988b).

E. histolytica either feeds on bacteria in the intestine or invades and ulcerates the mucosa of the large intestine. The parasite can be limited to the GI tract (intestinal amebiasis) or it can extend outside the intestines (extraintestinal amebiasis). Intestinal amebiasis can be present without any symptoms, or symptoms can range from mild to severe. Mild to moderate *E. histolytica* infestation causes clinical manifestations, including the passage of a few strongly odoriferous stools daily, possibly with mucus but without blood; abdominal cramping; flatulence; fatigue; and weight loss. There are characteristic remissions and recurrences. Severe amebic dysentery is manifested by frequent, more liquid, and odoriferous stools, with mucus *and* blood. Temperature up to 105° F (40.5° C), tenesmus, generalized abdominal tenderness, and vomiting can also occur. The ulcerations characteristic of invading amebiasis that occur in the colon can cause pain, bleeding, and obstruction. Ulcerations can also be localized in the rectum, resulting in formed stool with blood. Complications are rare, but include appendicitis and bowel perforation.

Extraintestinal ambiasis can occur without symptoms of intestinal infection. The most common is amebic liver abscess, which causes symptoms of fever, pain, and enlarged liver. Rupture of the abscess can occur. Death can result if the infection is not treated and complications occur.

COLLABORATIVE MANAGEMENT

Amebiasis is diagnosed by examination of stool for parasites. *E. histolytica* organisms are difficult to detect; therefore, there should be serial examinations of stool if the disease is suspected. Sigmoidoscopy may be done to detect ulcerations in the rectum or colon. Exudate obtained during this examination is examined for the parasite. WBC count can be as high as $20,000/mm^3$ with severe dysentery.

Treatment for all types of amebiasis mandate use of amebicide drugs. Metronidazole (Flagyl) and diloxanide furoate (Entamide) and tetracycline hydrochloride (Sumycine) are commonly given in combination. Clients with severe dysentery require IV fluids for replacement and maintenance of fluid volume and possibly opiates, such as diphenoxylate hydrochloride and atropine sulfate (Lomotil), to control bowel motility. Clients with extraintestinal amebiasis or severe dehydration are hospitalized. Clients with asymptomatic, mild, or moderate disease are treated with drug therapy as outpatients. All clients have at least three stools examined for parasites at 2- to 3-day intervals starting 2 to 4 weeks after drug therapy has been completed.

The nurse educates all clients about modes of parasitic transmission. Clients being treated for amebiasis are told that they can transmit this infection to others until the drugs effectively kill all parasites. They are taught to avoid any contact with stool, keep toilet areas clean, wash hands meticulously after any bowel movement, and maintain personal hygiene. Sexual practices that allow rectal contact should be avoided until drug therapy is completed. All household and sexual contacts should have stool examinations for parasites. The nurse also educates clients to avoid future contact with foods contaminated by flies or food and water that might be contaminated with feces. Prevention is the key to avoiding contact with parasitic organisms, and there is no drug that prevents the organism from entering and invading the human body.

G. lamblia is a protozoal parasite that causes superficial invasion, destruction, and inflammation of the mucosa in the small intestine. Like *E. histolytica, G. lamblia* also has a trophozoite and cyst form, and cysts can transmit the organism. Humans are host to this organism, but beavers and dogs may be reservoirs for infection. Modes of transmission are similar to those for amebiasis; however, giardiasis is much more prevalent in the United States, being the most common parasitic infection in this country. Prevalence rates up to 20% have been reported in lower economic groups (Goldsmith, 1988b). Giardiasis has also been found in travelers, campers, male homosexuals, and clients who are immunosuppressed.

Giardiasis affects only the intestinal system, causing no symptoms, acute diarrhea, chronic diarrhea, or malabsorption syndrome. The acute phase usually is self-limiting, lasting days or weeks. The chronic phase can last for years. Diarrhea is usually mild for both forms, but can be severe. As stools increase in frequency, they become more watery, greasy, frothy, and malodorous with mucus. Other common manifestations include weight loss and weakness. Malabsorption can occur with diarrhea that continues for longer than 3 weeks. Manifestations result from malabsorption of fat, protein, vitamin B_{12}, and lactase deficiency (see later discussion of malabsorption). Diagnosis of giardiasis is made by stool examination for parasites. Organisms may not be detected for at least 1 week after symptoms appear; therefore, multiple stool samples should be examined. Duodenal aspirate can also be examined for the parasite to make the diagnosis. Treatment is drug therapy, with tinidazole (Fasigyn) being the drug of choice and metronidazole (Flagyl) the alternative. Stools are examined 2 weeks after treatment is begun.

The nurse educates the client about modes of transmission and ways to avoid the spread of infection and recurrent contact with parasitic organisms. Clients are instructed to avoid stool from dogs and beavers and to use meticulous hand washing after contact with these animals. If a client is visiting an area where giardiasis is suspected to be problematic, some protection may be obtained by using iodine tablets or drops in small quantities of water. This is not effective if the water is cold.

HELMINTHIC INFESTATION

Helminths are worm-like animals; they are often parasitic and capable of causing infectious disease in humans. There are many species of helminths, and, for purposes of classification, they are divided into three general categories: *roundworms* (nematodes), *flukes* (trematodes), and *tapeworms* (cestodes). Helminths are typically capable of causing various degrees of GI symptoms in humans. Most often, they enter the human body through the skin or via the oral route with ingestion of food, water, or other substances contaminated with worms. Some helminths are able to gain access to the human body via insects, such as flies and mosquitoes. Helminths that are typically transmitted via insects are limited to tropical areas, however, and are not discussed here. Flukes (trematodes), which are passed to humans via snail-contaminated water, are also limited to tropical and subtropical areas outside the United States and are not discussed here.

Roundworms are commonly the cause of helminthic infections in the United States and worldwide. *Enterobiasis*, also called *pinworm* infection, is caused by *Enterobius vermicularis*, which is transmitted by oral ingestion of contaminated food, drink, or fomites. The most common symptoms of infection include nocturnal perianal pruritus, insomnia, and restlessness. The client might have vague GI symptoms, such as abdominal pain, nausea, vomiting, and diarrhea. However, many clients have no symptoms when infected with this organism. Diagnosis is made when eggs of the helminth are found on perianal skin or on cellulose tape that has been applied to perianal skin. Treatment includes preventing spread of the worms to others by having infected clients use meticulous hand washing after defecation and before meals. Drug therapy is indicated for all clients who have symptoms and in some clients who are infected but are not symptomatic. Household cohabitants of an infected client may be treated with drug therapy even if asymptomatic. Pyrantel pamoate (Antiminth) or mebendazole (Vermox) is given orally in one dose, which is repeated at 2 and 4 weeks. Infection with pinworms is curable and is not commonly associated with complications. It does, however, commonly recur.

Trichinosis is another helminthic disease caused by roundworms. It is much less prevalent in the United States, but is still estimated to cause more than 150,000 infectious cases annually, although most clients are asymptomatic (Goldsmith, 1988a). *Trichinella spiralis*, which lives in the intestine of humans, pigs, bears, and rats, is responsible for this disease. It is usually transmitted to humans when undercooked pork or pork products are ingested. Ingestion of other meats, such as ground beef, can also promote transmission if a common meat grinder was used for beef and pork. Incubation is 12 hours to 28 days after ingestion. Symptoms range from none to severe disease and rarely death. There are three stages of illness, including the intestinal stage, the stage of muscular invasion, and stage of convalescence. The intestinal stage is manifested most often by diarrhea, cramps, and malaise. During the stage of muscular invasion, there is fever, muscle pain, periorbital and facial edema, photophobia, conjunctivitis, pain on swallowing, dyspnea, coughing, and hoarseness. Vague muscle pain and malaise characterize the convalescence phase, which can last for several months.

Diagnosis is made by obtaining a history of ingesting raw meat. WBC and eosinophil counts are elevated 2 weeks after meat is ingested. Biopsy of skeletal muscle shows larvae of the *Trichinella* organism. Worms are rarely seen in feces. Treatment during the intestinal phase includes oral thiabendazole (Mintezol). Hospitalization is required during the stage of muscle invasion for the administration of high doses of corticosteroids.

Hookworms are also roundworms, but they differ from pinworms and *Trichinella* in that they typically initially enter the human body through the skin. Hookworm disease is caused by either *Ancylostoma duodenale* or *Necator americanus*. Hookworms infect one-fourth of the world population, but the disease is rare in areas outside the tropics or in areas with little rain (Goldsmith, 1988a). Worms are infective outside the body in warm, moist soil for up to 1 week. Transmission occurs when larvae penetrate through the skin. The organism can migrate to pulmonary capillaries via the blood stream and enter alveoli. Cilia carry the organisms up the respiratory tree to the pharnyx and the mouth, where they are swallowed and enter the GI tract. Hookworms probably also enter this system via ingestion of contaminated food. Early symptoms of hookworm disease include a pruritic, erythematous, raised vesicular inflammation of the skin. Infection in the GI tract may produce no symptoms or may cause anorexia, diarrhea, or mild abdominal and epigastric discomfort. Bleeding and anemia may occur when worms suck blood at sites of attachment in the GI tract. Symptoms of iron deficiency anemia, such as pallor, hair thinning, deformed nails, pica, and shortness of breath, may be present if blood loss is severe.

Diagnosis of hookworm infection is based on the presence of ova (eggs) in the feces. Occult blood is often present in stool. There may be low hemoglobin concentration and hematocrit values or low serum iron level and high iron-binding capacity, indicating hypochromic microcytic anemia. WBC counts and eosinophil counts are elevated. Treatment is given to all clients with symptoms and includes iron therapy and a diet high in protein and vitamins for at least 3 months after anemia is corrected. Pyrantel pamoate (Antiminth) or mebendazole (Vermox) is given for complete recovery.

Six different types of *tapeworms* (cestodes) commonly infect humans. They include beef, fish, dog, dwarf, pork, and rodent tapeworm. These infections generally cause no symptoms or occasional GI upset, such as nausea, diarrhea, or abdominal pain.

Transmission of tapeworms occurs via ingestion of undercooked beef, raw fish, and other contaminated food or water or via accidental swallowing of infected lice or fleas from dogs. Ingestion can also occur with accidental ingestion of arthropods, such as cockroaches, in stored foods or cereals. Diagnosis is made by laboratory examination of eggs found in stool (test of stool for ova and parasites). Drugs are administered for treatment. Niclosamide (Niclocide) can be given for all adult tapeworm infections.

The nurse uses enteric or universal precautions when in contact with any stool. All clients are taught to wash hands after defecation and before eating meals. Clients are also taught to avoid eating undercooked beef, fish, and pork and to avoid drinking water that may be contaminated. Care should be taken to keep one's mouth closed and to wash hands after petting dogs. All stored foods should be kept tightly closed to avoid contamination by cockroaches and other insects.

FOOD POISONING

Food poisoning is caused by ingestion of infectious organisms in food. It differs from gastroenteritis in that it is not directly communicable from person to person, incubation periods are shorter, and there is no acquired immunity after the illness. It is similar to gastroenteritis in that it causes diarrhea, nausea, and vomiting. Differentiating food poisoning and gastroenteritis is done by obtaining a good history of common food intake in groups that have common symptoms of acute diarrhea, nausea, and vomiting. Two common types of food poisoning are staphylococcal food poisoning and botulism, both of which are caused by bacterial toxins.

Staphylococcus grows in meats and dairy products. Symptoms of *staphylococcal food poisoning* include abrupt onset of vomiting, with some diarrhea usually 1 to 8 hours after the ingestion of contaminated food; however, symptoms may not occur for up to 18 hours after ingestion. There is no fever, but the client is weak. Diagnosis is made on when stool culture yields 100,000 enterotoxin-producing staphylococci. Treatment consists of giving oral or IV fluids to restore and maintain fluid and electrolyte balance. The illness is self-limiting, lasting approximately 2 days, and no drug therapy is indicated.

In contrast, *botulism* is a severe, life-threatening food poisoning, which has a high mortality (Grossman & Jawetz, 1986). It is commonly acquired from improperly processed canned foods such as home-canned vegetables, smoked meats, and vacuum-packed fish. The anaerobic organism *Clostridium botulinum* enters the blood stream from the intestines and blocks acetylcholine at neuromuscular junctions. Incubation is 24 to 96 hours, after which symptoms of diplopia, dysphagia, dysphonia, respiratory muscle paralysis, nausea, vomiting, and diarrhea or constipation can occur. Diagnosis is made on history and stool culture of *C. botulinum*. Serum may be positive for toxins. Treatment with trivalent botulism antitoxin (ABE) is given as soon as the diagnosis is made if the client is not hypersensitive to it. The client's stomach may be lavaged to stop absorption of toxin. All clients are hospitalized to observe for and treat respiratory paralysis. Nothing is given orally until swallowing and respiratory difficulties pass. IV fluids are administered as needed. Tracheostomy and mechanical ventilation is implemented if respiratory paralysis occurs. If ventilation can be maintained, the client can survive with no neurologic deficits after the illness.

To prevent botulism, the nurse teaches clients the importance of discarding cans of food that are punctured, swollen, or have defective seals. Containers for foods that are home canned must be sterilized by boiling for 20 minutes to destroy *C. botulinum* spores before canning.

Salmonellosis is a bacterial infection that is sometimes classified as a food poisoning because of its short incubation after ingestion of food contaminated with the organism. It can cause diarrhea, but it is communicated via the fecal-oral route from person to person, which differentiates it from other food poisonings discussed here. Symptoms occur 8 to 48 hours after contamination. In addition to diarrhea, a low-grade fever, nausea, vomiting, and abdominal pain may be present. Systemic infection can also occur. Diagnosis is made if *Salmonella* organism is found in stool culture. Treatment is symptomatic, and drug therapy is not usually indicated, unless the infection has causes septicemia. Ampicillin (Omnipen) is given if septicemia occurs. Clients without septicemia recover in 3 to 5 days, but all clients may be carriers of the bacteria for up to 1 year. The nurse instructs all clients with *Salmonella* and their contacts to wash their hands before meals and after defecating to avoid transmission of the organism.

All cases of botulism and salmonellosis need to be reported to local health departments. Staphylococcal food poisoning is reported if epidemic outbreaks occur.

MALABSORPTION SYNDROME

OVERVIEW

Malabsorption is a syndrome associated with a variety of disorders and intestinal surgical procedures in which one or multiple nutrients are not digested or absorbed.

The body requires absorption of proteins, carbohydrates, fats, and minerals for homeostasis. Normally, the absorption of protein and carbohydrates occurs in the small bowel. Pancreatic enzymes and enzymes from the stomach and the small intestine are required for protein breakdown and utilization. Carbohydrates also require pancreatic enzymes for digestion. The absorption of fat requires the presence of bile products, in addition to a pancreatic enzyme, along with adequate small bowel function and lymphatic integrity.

Physiologic mechanisms that occur with various disorders limit absorption of nutrients because of one or more of the following abnormalities: bile salt deficiencies, enzyme deficiencies, bacteria, disruption of the mucosal lining of the small intestine, alteration in lymphatic and vascular circulation, and decrease in gastric or intestinal surface area. The nutrient that is specifically malabsorbed depends on which abnormality exists and on the specific location of the abnormality in the intestinal tract.

Deficiencies of bile salts can lead to malabsorption of fats and fat-soluble vitamins. Bile salt deficiencies can result from decreased synthesis of bile in the liver, bile obstruction, or alteration of bile salt absorption in the small intestine. *Enzymes* normally found in the intestine split disaccharides (complex sugars) to monosaccharides (simple sugars). Examples of these enzymes are lactase, sucrase, maltase, and isomaltase. Lactase deficiency is the most common disaccharide enzyme deficiency. Without sufficient amounts of this enzyme, the body is not able to break down lactose, and consequently it is not absorbed. Lactase deficiency can be due to genetic transmission, or it can result from injury to intestinal mucosa from viral hepatitis, bacterial proliferation in the intestine, or sprue. Deficiencies of the other disaccharide enzymes are rare.

In addition to digesting carbohydrates, protein, and fat, pancreatic enzymes are necessary for absorption of vitamin B_{12}. With destruction or obstruction of the pancreas, or insufficient pancreatic stimulation, malabsorption of these nutrients occurs. Chronic pancreatitis, pancreatic carcinoma, resection of the pancreas, and cystic fibrosis can cause these malabsorption problems.

Loops of bowel can accumulate intestinal contents when there is a decrease in peristalsis, which can result in bacterial overgrowth. Bacteria at these sites break down bile salts, and fewer salts are available for fat absorption. These bacteria can also ingest vitamin B_{12}, contributing to vitamin B_{12} deficiency. This phenomenon can occur after a gastrectomy or with enteropathy, scleroderma, and diabetic enteropathy.

Disruption of the intestinal lining is responsible for the malabsorption that occurs with the following: celiac (nontropical) sprue, tropical sprue, Crohn's disease, and ulcerative colitis. In *celiac (nontropical) sprue*, absorptive surface area in the intestine is lost and there is malabsorption of *most* nutrients. Celiac sprue is thought to be due to a genetic immune hypersensitivity response to gluten or its breakdown products or to result from the accumulation of gluten in the diet with peptidase deficiency. Lactase deficiency can also occur because of intestinal mucosal damage.

Tropical sprue is caused by an infectious agent that has not been identified, but is thought to be bacterial. Mucosal changes occur in a more widespread manner than in celiac sprue. However, the changes are not as severe as in celiac sprue. Tropical sprue results in malabsorption of fat, folic acid, and vitamin B_{12} in later stages of the disease.

The inflammation in Crohn's disease interferes with the absorptive surface of cells absorbing bile salts and, therefore, leads to fat malabsorption. In ulcerative colitis, protein loss may occur.

Obstruction to lymphatic flow in the intestine can

lead to loss of plasma proteins, along with minerals (such as iron, copper, and calcium), vitamin B_{12}, folic acid, and lipids. Lymphatic obstruction can be caused by tumors, inflammation, radiation enteritis, Crohn's disease, lymphoma, Whipple's disease, congestive heart failure, and constrictive pericarditis. Interference with blood flow to the intestinal mucosa, which occurs in celiac and superior mesenteric artery disease, results in malabsorption.

With intestinal surgery, there is loss of surface area to facilitate absorption. Resection of the ileum results in vitamin B_{12}, bile salt, and other nutrient deficiencies. Gastric surgery is one of the most common causes of malabsorption and maldigestion.

Clinical manifestations of malabsorption are variable, but steatorrhea (greater than normal amounts of fat in the feces) is a common sign. Steatorrhea is a result of bile salt deconjugation, nonabsorbed fats, or bacteria in the intestine. Other clinical manifestations include weight loss, fatigue, decreased libido, easy bruising, anemia (with iron and folic acid or vitamin B_{12} deficiency), bone pain (with calcium and vitamin D deficiency), edema (caused by hypoproteinemia).

COLLABORATIVE MANAGEMENT

Laboratory studies reveal a decrease in mean corpuscular volume (MCV), mean corpuscular hemoglobin (MCH), and mean corpuscular hemoglobin concentration (MCHC), indicating hypochromic microcytic anemia due to iron deficiency. Increased MCV and variable MCH and MCHC are indicative of macrocytic anemia due to vitamin B_{12} and folic acid deficiencies. Low serum iron levels are present in protein malabsorption due to insufficient gastric acid for utilization of iron. Low serum cholesterol levels may result from decreased absorption and digestion of fat. Low serum calcium levels may be indicative of malabsorption of vitamin D and amino acids. Low levels of serum vitamin A (retinol) and carotene, its precursor, indicate a bile salt deficiency and malabsorption of fat. Serum albumin and total protein levels are low if protein loss occurs.

A lactose tolerance test result that shows less than 20% rise in blood glucose level over fasting blood glucose level is indicative of lactose intolerance. A monosaccharide test is done to validate or rule out lactase deficiency.

The xylose absorption test can reveal low urine and serum D-xylose levels if malabsorption in the small intestine is present, a common finding in celiac sprue.

The Schilling test measures urinary excretion of vitamin B_{12} to diagnose pernicious anemia and a variety of other malabsorption syndromes. The bile acid breath test is done to assess the absorption of bile salt.

Biopsy of the small intestine is performed via an oral endoscopic procedure to diagnose tropical sprue or celiac sprue.

Ultrasonography is used to diagnose pancreatic tumors and tumors in the small intestine that are causing malabsorption. X-ray films of the GI tract reveal pancreatic calcifications, tumors, or other abnormalities that cause malabsorption. Barium enema shows mucosal changes representative of celiac sprue or other abnormalities.

Intervention for most malabsorption syndromes focuses on avoiding dietary substances that aggravate malabsorption and supplementing nutrients. Surgical or nonsurgical management of the primary disease may be indicated. Drug therapy may also improve or resolve malabsorption. Examples of dietary management include a low-fat diet in gallbladder disease, severe steatorrhea, cystic fibrosis, and systemic scleroderma (progressive systemic sclerosis). A low-fat diet may or may not be indicated for pancreatic insufficiency because this disorder improves with enzyme replacement. Some clinicians believe that, with enzyme replacement, limitation of fat intake is not necessary. Dietary intake of fat is actually beneficial to the client because it has a high amount of calories. After a total gastrectomy, a high-protein, high-calorie diet and small, frequent meals are recommended. Lactose-free or restricted diets are available for clients with lactase deficiency and gluten-free diets are available for clients with celiac sprue.

Nutritional supplements are given on the basis of the specific deficiency. Common supplements include water-soluble vitamins, such as folic acid, vitamin B_{12}, and vitamin B complex; fat-soluble vitamins, such as vitamin A, vitamin D, and vitamin K; minerals, such as calcium, iron, and magnesium; or pancreatic enzymes. Examples of pancreatic enzyme supplements are pancrelipase (Pancrease) or pancreatin (Viokase).

Antibiotics are used to treat tropical sprue, Whipple's disease, and other disorders involving bacterial overgrowth. Tropical sprue is treated with trimethoprim and sulfamethoxazole (Bactrim, Septra). Bacterial overgrowth can be caused by a variety of disorders, but is often treated with tetracycline and metronidazole (Flagyl). Steroids are sometimes given in celiac disease to decrease inflammation.

Drug therapy is also used to control the clinical manifestations of the malabsorption disorder. Antidiarrheal agents, such as diphenoxylate hydrochloride and atropine sulfate (Lomotil), camphorated tincture of opium (paregoric), or kaolin with pectin (Kaopectate), are often used to control diarrhea and steatorrhea. Anticholinergics, such as belladonna, are often given before meals to inhibit gastric motility. IV fluids may be necessary to replenish fluid losses associated with diarrhea.

Nursing interventions include ongoing assessment for clinical manifestations of malabsorption and how these manifestations relate to activities and dietary intake. For example, clients with steatorrhea are monitored for fluid and electrolyte imbalances and are encouraged to take electrolyte-rich liquids liberally. (See earlier discussion of interventions for diarrhea.) The nurse teaches clients the rationale for dietary, drug, and surgical management and evaluates interventions on the basis of changes or resolution in clinical manifestations of nutritional deficiencies.

SUMMARY

Intestinal disorders are significant problems and are frequently encountered by the nurse. The clinical manifestations of the various intestinal disorders have commonalities yet subtle differences, which must be identified for each client. Clinical manifestations of a benign disorder, such as IBS, can resemble early manifestations of a life-threatening malignancy, such as cancer of the colon. Systematic use of nursing process is essential to identify appropriate nursing interventions.

Associated factors, such as diet and family history, have been identified for many of the disorders, yet no cause can be determined. Much work needs to be done to identify specific causes of these disorders.

IMPLICATIONS FOR RESEARCH

The association of diet with the causes and preventive tactics for a variety of intestinal disorders is striking. For example, high-fiber diets have been recommended to help prevent colorectal cancer, diverticular disease, and IBS. The ACS and other groups have put forth great efforts to inform the public about diet and its relation to disease. Much of the research and educational effort, however, has been relatively recent. Nursing research is needed to assess public knowledge of the association of diet and disease, public knowledge of what foods are recommended for various diets, dietary practices, and outcomes related to specific dietary practices.

With changes in the health care and reimbursement systems, care of intestinal disorders, as well as many other disorders, has shifted from the hospital to the home setting. Even the client with serious illness has hospitalization limited to the acute period of the illness. Fewer hospitalizations and earlier discharges have many possible implications for client outcomes, many of which are not known at this time. Clients need to be taught much more about actual and potential problems than ever before, because they are not in the hospital being monitored by the nurse.

Possible issues for nursing research include

1. What are the effects of public education programs on preventing GI disorders, such as colorectal cancer, diverticular disease, and IBS?

2. What are the effects of screening programs for occult blood in stool on the early detection of colorectal cancer?

3. What is the effect of nursing assessment on the recovery of clients with GI disorders?

4. What is the effect of nursing interventions on the recovery of clients with GI disorders?

5. What is the effect of surgical outpatient treatment on the recovery of clients with GI disorders?

6. What is the effect of early discharge from the hospital on the recovery of clients with GI disorders?

REFERENCES AND READINGS

American Cancer Society. (1985). *Taking control* (Publication No. 2019.05). New York: Author.

American Cancer Society. (1989). Cancer statistics, 1989. *Ca: A Cancer Journal for Clinicians, 39.*

American Public Health Association. (1980). *Control of communicable diseases in man* (13th ed.). Washington, D.C.: Author.

Barkin, J. S., & Flaxman, M. S. (1987). Diverticula of intestinal tract. In R. E. Rakel (Ed.), *Conn's current therapy 1987* (pp. 383–387). Philadelphia: W. B. Saunders.

Braunwald, E., Isselbacher, K. J., Petersdorf, R. G., Wilson, J., Martin, J. B., and Fauci, A. S. (Eds.). (1987). *Harrison's principles of internal medicine* (11th ed.). New York: McGraw-Hill.

Broadwell, D. C., & Jackson, B. S. (1982). *Principles of ostomy care.* St. Louis: C. J. Mosby.

Broadwill, D. C., & McGarity, W. C. (1981). Gastrointestinal disorders. In M. R. Kinney, C. B. Dear, D. R. Packa, & D. M. Voorman (Eds.), *AACN's clinical reference for critical care nursing* (pp. 697–739). New York: McGraw-Hill.

Brozenec, S. A., & Rice, H. V. (1985). Obstructive disorders. In L. Z. Cohen, N. Holmes, P. M. Shinehouse, & L. C. Moclock (Eds.), *Gastrointestinal disorders* (pp. 116–151). Springhouse, PA: Springhouse Corp.

Burkitt, D. (1984). Etiology and prevention of colorectal cancer. *Hospital Practice, 19,* 67–77.

Cahill, M. (Ed.). (1987). *Patient teaching.* Springhouse, PA: Springhouse Corp.

Caine, R. M., and Bufalino, P. M. (Eds.). (1987). *Nursing care planning guides for adults.* Baltimore: Williams & Wilkins.

Cape, R., Coe, R., & Rossman, I. (1983). *Fundamentals of geriatric medicine.* New York: Raven.

Cayten, C. G. (1984). Abdominal trauma. *Emergency Medical Clinics of North America, 2,* 799–821.

Cerrato, P. L. (1987, January). What to tell your patients about dietary fiber. *RN,* 63–64.

Chatton, M. J., & Ullman, P. M. (1986). Nutrition; nutrition and metabolic disorders. In M. A. Krupp, M. J. Chatton, & L. M. Tierney (Eds.), *Current medical diagnosis and treatment)* (pp. 799–823). Los Altos, CA: Lange Medical.

Cohen, L. Z., Holmes, N., Shinehouse, P. M., & Moclock, L. C. (Eds.). (1985). *Gastrointestinal disorders.* Springhouse, PA: Springhouse Corp.

Connor, S. F., D'Andrea, K. G., Piper, J. A., Shaughnessy,

M. E., Tonnelli, M. S., & Viner, H. F. (1984). *A comprehensive review manual for the nurse practitioner.* Boston: Little, Brown.

Dempsey, S., Nevidjon, B. M., & Wickham, R. (1985). Reviewing fundamental principles. In N. Holmes, P. Johnson, & P. M. Shinehouse (Eds.), *Neoplastic disorders.* Springhouse PA: Springhouse Corp.

Doering, K. (1987). Lower GI disorders. In P. M. Shinehouse (Ed.), *Gastrointestinal problems* (pp. 54–89). Springhouse PA: Springhouse Corp.

Ebersole, P., & Hess, P. (1985). *Toward healthy aging, human needs and nursing response.* St. Louis: C. V. Mosby.

Englert, D. M., & Storz, N. S. (1985). Nutritional disorders. In L. Z. Cohen, N. Holmes, P. M. Shinehouse, & L. C. Moclock (Eds.), *Gastrointestinal disorders* (pp. 52–85). Springhouse, PA: Springhouse Corp.

Ford, R. D. (Ed.). (1987). *Patient teaching manual.* Springhouse, PA: Springhouse Corp.

Gibson, D. E. (1987). Abdominal trauma. *Trauma Quarterly, 4:* 11–26.

Goldner, F. (1986). Answers to questions on diverticular disease. *Hospital Medicine, 22,* 23–47.

Goldsmith, R. S. (1988a). Infectious diseases: Helminthic. In S. A. Schroeder, M. A. Krupp, & L. M. Tierney (Eds.), *Current medical diagnosis and treatment* (pp. 924–954). Norwalk, CT: Appleton & Lange.

Goldsmith, R. S. (1988b). Infectious diseases: Protozoal. In S. A. Schroeder, M. A. Krupp, & L. M. Tierney (Eds.), *Current medical diagnosis and treatment* (pp. 896–923). Norwalk, CT: Appleton & Lange.

Gomez, J., Law, K. J., & Norris, J. (Eds.). (1987). *Nursing yearbook 87.* Springhouse, PA: Springhouse Corp.

Goroll, A. H., May, L. A., & Mulley, A. G. (1981). Management of diverticular disease. In A. H. Goroll, L. A. May, & A. G. Mulley (Eds.), *Primary care medicine.* Philadelphia: J. B. Lippincott.

Grossman, M., & Jawetz, E. (1986). Infectious diseases: Viral and rickettsial. In M. A. Krupp, M. Chatton, & L. M. Tierney (Eds.), *Current medical diagnosis and treatment* (pp. 834–857). Los Altos, CA: Lange Medical.

Heydanon, A. H. (1974). Intestinal bypass for obesity. *American Journal of Nursing, 74,* 1102–1104.

Hoppe, M. C., Descalso, J., & Kapp, S. R. (1983). Gastrointestinal disease: Nutritional implications. *Nursing Clinics of North America, 18,* 47–56.

Kayes, S. A. (1986). Stool culture. In P. Johnson & J. Rubin (Eds.), *Diagnostics* (2nd ed., p. 509). Springhouse PA: Springhouse Corp.

Kenney, R. (1982). *Physiology of aging.* Chicago: Year Book Medical.

Knauer, C. M., Carbone, J. V., & Silverman, S. (1986). Alimentary tract and liver. In M. A. Krupp, M. J. Chatton, & L. M. Tierney (Eds.), *Current medical diagnosis and treatment.* Los Altos, CA: Lange Medical.

Knauer, C. M., & Silverman, S. (1988). Alimentary tract & liver. In S. A. Schroeder, M. A. Krupp, & L. M. Tierney (Eds.), *Current medical diagnosis and treatment* (pp. 342–428). Norwalk, CT: Appleton & Lange.

Knezevich, B. A. (1986). Abdominal trauma. In Knezevich, B. A., *Trauma nursing: Principles and practices* (pp. 99–112). Norwalk, CT: Appleton-Century-Crofts.

Krugman, S., & Katz, S. L. (1981). *Infectious diseases of children* (7th ed.). St. Louis: C. V. Mosby.

Lanza, E., & Butrum, R. R. (1986). A critical review of food fiber analysis and data. *Journal of American Dietetic Association, 86,* 732–740.

Leonard, B. M. (1981). Giardiasis. In T. Leibrandt (Ed.), *Diseases* (pp. 421–422). Horsham, PA: Intermed Communications.

Levine, G. M. (1987). The malabsorption syndromes. In R. E. Rakel (Ed.), *Conn's current therapy 1987* (pp. 401–408). Philadelphia: W. B. Saunders.

Levine, M. M. (1981). Shigellosis. In P. F. Wehrle & F. H. Top (Sr. Eds.), *Communicable and infectious diseases* (9th ed.). St. Louis: C. V. Mosby.

Lind, J. (1987). Colorectal cancer. In C. R. Ziegfeld (Ed.), *Core curriculum for oncology nursing* (pp. 163–171). Philadelphia: W. B. Saunders.

Long, B. C., Roberts, R., & Brogswell, D. C. (1987). Interventions for persons with problems of intestinal elimination. In W. J. Phipps, B. C. Long, & N. F. Woods (Eds.), *Medical-surgical nursing concepts and clinical practice* (3rd ed., pp. 1525–1573). St. Louis: C. V. Mosby.

Markovchick, V. J., Moore, E. E., Moore, J., & Rosen, P. (1985). Local wound exploration of anterior abdominal stab wounds. *Journal of Emergency Medicine, 2,* 287–291.

Marx, J. A. (1983). Abdominal trauma. In P. Rosen (Sr. Ed.), *Emergency medicine, concepts and clinical practice.* St. Louis: C. V. Mosby.

McConnell, E. A. (1987). Meeting the challenge of intestinal obstruction. *Nursing '87, 17*(7), 34–41.

Mersheimer, W. L., Kazarian, K. K., & Dursi, J. F. (1977). A critical analysis of 51 patients with jejunoileal bypass. *Surgery, Gynecology, and Obstetrics, 145,* 847–852.

Miller, B. (1981). Jejunoileal bypass: A drastic weight control measure. *American Journal of Nursing, 81,* 564–568.

Miller, D. (1986) Cancer prevention: Steps you can take. In A. I. Holleb (Ed.), *The American Cancer Society cancer book* (pp. 15–40). Garden City, NY: Doubleday.

Mojzisik, C. M., & Martin, E. M. (1981). Gastric partitioning: The latest surgical means to control morbid obesity. *American Journal of Nursing, 81,* 569–572.

Padilla, G., & Grant, M. (1985). Quality of life as a cancer nursing outcome variable. *Advances in Nursing Science, 8,* 45–60.

Patras, A. Z., & Walsh, M. (1985). Inflammatory and infectious disorders. In L. Z. Cohen, N. Holmes, P. M. Shinehouse, & L. C. Moclock (Eds.), *Gastrointestinal disorders* (pp. 86–115). Springhouse PA: Springhouse Corp.

Raffensperger, E. B., Zusy, M. L., & Marchesseault, L. C. (1986). *Clinical nursing handbook.* Philadelphia: J. B. Lippincott.

Rainer, W. (1986). *Stoma therapy: An atlas and guide for intestinal stomas.* New York: Thieme.

Rakel, R. E. (Ed.). (1990). *Conn's current therapy 1990.*

Philadelphia: W. B. Saunders.

Reber, H. A., Roberts, C., Way, L. W., & Dunphy, J. E. (1978). Management of external fistulas. *Annals of Surgery, 188,* 460.

Root, H. D. (1965). Diagnostic peritoneal lavage. *Surgery, 57,* 633.

Ryan, S. A. (1981). Amebiasis. In T. Leibrandt (Ed.), *Diseases* (pp. 418–419). Horsham, PA: Intermed Communications.

Schapiro, R. (1989, May). Colonic polyps. In D. Hammond & A. Khazei (Co-Chair), *Colorectal cancer symposium.* Catholic Medical Center, Manchester, NH.

Schwesinger, W. H. (1990). Cancer of the large bowel. In R. E. Rakel (Ed.), *Conn's current therapy 1990* (pp. 483–486).

Seidel, H., Ball, J., Dains, J., & Benedict, G. (1987). *Mosby's guide to physical examination.* St. Louis: C. V. Mosby.

Shearman, D. J., & Finlayson, N. D. (1982). *Diseases of the gastrointestinal tract and liver.* New York: Churchill Livingstone.

Silen, W. (1987). Acute appendicitis. In E. Braunwald, K. J. Isserbacher, R. G. Petersdorf, J. Wilson, J. B. Martin, & A. S. Fauci (Eds.), *Harrison's principles of internal medicine* (11th ed., pp. 1304–1306). New York: McGraw-Hill.

Sleisenger, M., & Fordtran, J. (1983). *Gastrointestinal disease* (3rd ed.). Philadelphia: W. B. Saunders.

Smith, L. E. (1987). Hemorrhoids, anal fissures, and anorectal abscess and fistula. In R. E. Rakel (Ed.), *Conn's current therapy 1987* (pp. 392–395). Philadelphia: W. B. Saunders.

Spiro, H. M. (1983). *Clinical gastroenterology.* New York: Macmillan.

Spivak, J. L., & Barnes, H. V. (1983). Intestinal polyps. In J. L. Spivak & H. J. Barnes (Eds.), *Manual of clinical problems in internal medicine* (3rd ed., pp. 285–288). Boston: Little, Brown.

Spivak, J. L., & Barnes, H. V. (1983). Malabsorption. In J. L. Spivak & H. J. Barnes (Eds.), *Manual of clinical problems in internal medicine* (3rd ed., pp. 288–292). Boston: Little, Brown.

Spivak, J. L. & Barnes, H. V. (Eds.). (1983). *Manual of internal medicine* (3rd ed.). Boston: Little, Brown.

Swearingen, P. L., Sommers, M. S., & Miller, K. (1988). *Manual of critical care.* St. Louis: C. V. Mosby.

Thal, E. R. (1979). Evaluation of peritoneal lavage as local exploration in chest and abdominal stab wounds. *Journal of Trauma, 17,* 642.

Trunkey, D. D., Shires, G. T., & McClelland, R. (1974). Management of liver trauma in 811 consecutive patients. *Annals of Surgery, 179,* 722.

Whitney, E. N., Cataldo, C. B., & Rolfes, S. R. (Eds.). (1987). *Understanding normal and clinical nutrition* (2nd ed.). St. Paul, MN: West Publishing.

Williams, S. (1989). *Nutrition and diet therapy* (6th ed.). St. Louis: Times Mirror/Mosby College Publishing.

Wilson, R. (1981). Enteric infections. In P. F. Wehrle & F. H. Top (Sr. Eds.), *Communicable and infectious diseases* (9th ed.). St. Louis: C. V. Mosby.

Valentine, A. (1987). Early detection measures. In C. R. Ziegfeld (Ed.), *Core curriculum for oncology nurses* (pp. 65–68). Philadelphia: W. B. Saunders.

Wyngaarden, J., & Smith, L. (1988). *Cecil textbook of medicine* (17th ed.). Philadelphia: W. B. Saunders.

Zuidema, G. D., Rutherford, R. B., & Ballinger, W. F. (1985). *The management of trauma* (4th ed.). Philadelphia: W. B. Saunders.

ADDITIONAL READINGS

Bates-Jensen, B. (1989). Psychological response to illness: Exploring two reactions to ostomy surgery. *Ostomy/Wound Management, 23,* 24–30.

This article discusses denial and personal control, which are two responses to ostomy surgery. The nurse author presents a case study related to each response and suggests nursing interventions for clients manifesting denial or maladaptive attempts at personal control.

Bragg, V. (1989). Continent intestinal reservoir: Ileostomy option. *Ostomy/Wound Management, 23,* 32–41.

This article gives an overview of surgical procedures performed when removal of the colon and rectum is required. The continent intestinal reservoir was first introduced in 1969 by Kock. This reservoir has enabled clients to avoid an external appliance for collection of stool, thus avoiding potential problems with skin irritation and body image. The enterostomal therapist author provides an update on improvements that have been made in surgical technique and postoperative care for continent intestinal reservoir (CIR) clients.

Hassey, K. M. (1987). Radiation therapy for rectal cancer and the implications for nursing. *Cancer Nursing, 10,* 311–318.

This article discusses how radiation therapy is used for clients with rectal cancer. The nurse author provides guidelines for nursing assessment of these clients, as well as pertinent nursing diagnoses.

Lange, M. P., Thebo, L. M., Tiede, S. M., McCarthy, B., Dahn, M. S., Jacobs, L. A., & Park, A. (1989). Management of multiple enterocutaneous fistulas. *Heart and Lung, 18,* 386–391.

This article discusses the pathophysiology and clinical management of enterocutaneous fistulas. Effective management involves vigorous nutritional support and mechanical control via drainage collection and protection of the surrounding skin. The authors present a case report and illustrations to describe management techniques, care for surrounding skin, and vigorous nutritional support.

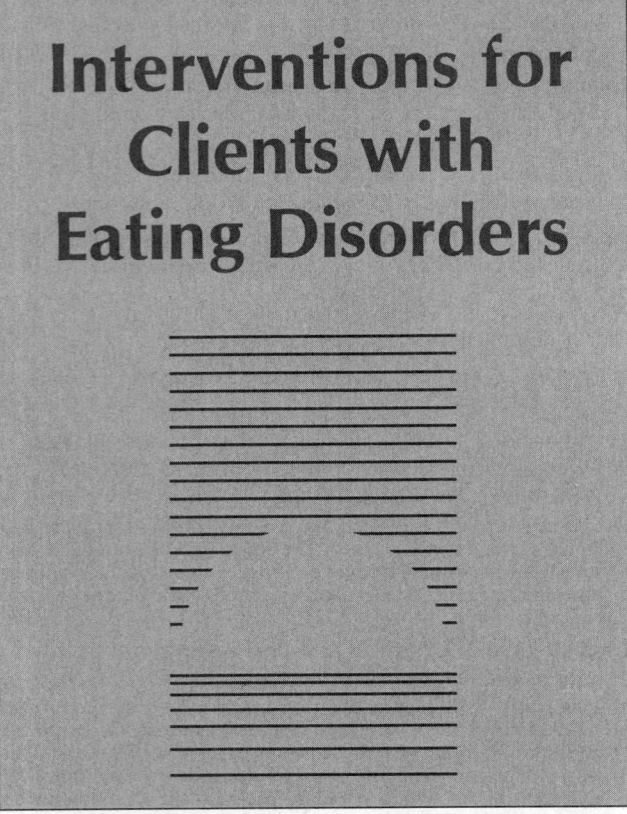

CHAPTER 46

Interventions for Clients with Eating Disorders

During the past several decades, health care professionals have found themselves challenged to accurately diagnose and treat two serious eating disorders: anorexia nervosa and bulimia nervosa. In the past 10 years, mass media coverage of the topic of eating disorders has educated and fascinated the lay public. Today's slimness-oriented culture creates a desire in even healthy individuals to suffer from a "mild case" of anorexia nervosa.

Anorexia nervosa is frequently misdiagnosed as a medical illness, and bulimia nervosa is often a hidden disorder. The medical-surgical nurse must be familiar with these syndromes because early diagnosis and intervention can eliminate years of suffering for the anorexic or bulimic individual. The nurse can be instrumental in assisting the interdisciplinary health care team, the client, and the family to identify the appropriate treatment approach.

ANOREXIA NERVOSA

OVERVIEW

Anorexia nervosa is a sometimes life-threatening illness that takes the form of indirect self-destructive behavior. It occurs primarily in females and most often has its onset during adolescence. It is a clinical syndrome of self-induced starvation. The anorexic* refuses to eat because of an intense fear of losing control of eating and thus becoming fat. She or he further suffers from a disturbed body image and continues to feel fat even when emaciated.

This disorder is not unique to the 20th century; it was first described in England in 1694 by R. Morton (1694/1985). In a speech delivered at Oxford in 1868 and published in 1874, Sir William Gull called the condition "hysterical apepsia" but later named it "anorexia nervosa." At about the same time, the syndrome was described in France by Professor Lasègue, who called it "hysterical anorexia (Lasègue, 1873/1985)."

Pathophysiology

Although the anorexic and family frequently search for a physical cause for the weight loss experienced, anorexia nervosa is a psychiatric rather than a medical illness. The anorexic often suffers medical sequelae from the effects of starvation and unhealthy behaviors such as purging (vomiting, laxative abuse, and diuretic

---

* The authors recognize that this term may be sensitive, but it is currently the acceptable term in the health literature.

abuse). It is crucial, however, to recognize that the medical problems are the results, not the cause, of the illness.

For many years, Russell's (1970) criteria have guided health care practitioners in diagnosing anorexia nervosa: (1) *self-induced starvation,* (2) *a morbid fear of fatness,* and (3) an abnormality in reproductive hormone functioning that leads to *amenorrhea in females* and *decreased sexual interest and function in males.* The presence of these hallmarks of the disorder alerts the nurse to the possibility that the client may suffer a psychiatric and not a medical condition. The American Psychiatric Association has outlined the features of anorexia nervosa in the *Diagnostic and Statistical Manual of Mental Disorders* (DSM-III-R). These criteria, which are listed in the accompanying Key Features of Disease, incorporate the three hallmark features plus additional criteria designed to differentiate anorexia nervosa from medical disorders. Diagnosis of anorexia nervosa is made based on these standardized criteria and not by doing extensive medical testing to eliminate all possible medical conditions.

Although the DSM-III-R provides the official criteria for diagnosis, the nurse may find the criteria given in the Key Features of Disease: Feighner's Diagnostic Criteria for Anorexia Nervosa helpful in providing even more specific identifying features of anorexia nervosa. The criterion requiring a 25% loss of original body weight for diagnosis was a source of some controversy among health care professionals, and the DSM-III-R criteria lowered this figure to 15%.

KEY FEATURES OF DISEASE ■ DSM-III-R Diagnostic Criteria for Anorexia Nervosa

A. Refusal to maintain body weight over a minimal normal weight for age and height, e.g., weight loss leading to maintenance of body weight 15% below that expected; or failure to make expected weight gain during period of growth, leading to body weight 15% below that expected.

B. Intense fear of gaining weight or becoming fat, even though underweight.

C. Disturbance in the way in which one's body weight, size, or shape is experienced, e.g., the person claims to "feel fat" even when emaciated, believes that one area of the body is "too fat" even when obviously underweight.

D. In females, absence of at least three consecutive menstrual cycles when otherwise expected to occur (primary or secondary amenorrhea). (A woman is considered to have amenorrhea if her periods occur only following hormone, e.g., estrogen, administration.)

Reprinted with permission from the *Diagnostic and statistical manual of mental disorders,* Third Edition, Revised. Copyright 1987 American Psychiatric Association.

KEY FEATURES OF DISEASE ■ Feighner's Diagnostic Criteria for Anorexia Nervosa

I. Age at onset less than 25 years

II. Accompanying weight loss of at least 25% of original body weight

III. A distorted, implacable attitude toward eating, food, or weight that overrides hunger, admonitions, reassurance, and threats

   A. Denial of illness, with a failure to recognize nutritional needs

   B. Apparent enjoyment in losing weight, with overt manifestation that food refusal is a pleasurable indulgence

   C. A desired body image of extreme thinness, with overt evidence that it is rewarding to the patient to achieve and maintain that state

   D. Unusual hoarding or handling of food

IV. No known medical illness that could account for the disorder and weight loss

V. No other known psychiatric disorder, particularly primary affective disorders, schizophrenia, and obsessive-compulsive and phobic neuroses (the assumption is made that even though it may appear phobic or obsessional, food refusal alone is not sufficient to qualify for obsessive-compulsive or phobic disease)

IV. Manifestation of at least two of

   A. Amenorrhea
   B. Lanugo hair
   C. Bradycardia (persistent resting pulse of 60 or less)
   D. Periods of overactivity
   E. Episodes of bulimia
   F. Vomiting (may be self-induced)

From Feighner, J. P., Robins, E., Guze, S. B., Woodruff, R. A., Wenokur, G., & Munoz, R. Diagnostic criteria for use in psychiatric research. *Archives of General Psychiatry, 26,* 57, Copyright 1972, American Medical Association.

Clinical manifestations such as amenorrhea, lowered body temperature, and bradycardia are indications of the body's efforts to protect itself and function on its limited food intake. To maintain vital functioning, the body attempts to decrease fuel requirements by lowering the core body temperature and decreasing the basal metabolic rate. The reduced core body temperature causes a decrease in enzyme production because enzyme production doubles with approximately every 10°F in temperature. The circulating norepinephrine level decreases, which causes a reduced heart rate. A decrease in blood pressure, as well as cold hands and feet with occasional cyanosis, may occur because of the reduced blood flow. Some anorexics have a covering of fine, downy lanugo hair, but the reason that it develops is not clear. Bone marrow function decreases, which results in anemia that is usually microcytic or normocytic. The gastrointestinal tract becomes more efficient and absorbs whatever it receives. There is evidence that gastric emptying time is decreased in the anorexic, although the full significance of this alteration is not clear. Changes in the endocrine system protect the body by stopping menses to preserve energy. Cessation of menses, or *amenorrhea*, prevents pregnancy, which would require thousands of stored calories to maintain. The changes in thyroid hormone levels account for the decreased metabolic rate mentioned earlier. A chronic state of anorexia nervosa can produce changes such as brown atrophy of the heart muscle, decreased liver function, chronic anemia, and osteoporosis (decreased bone mass).

The term *anorexia nervosa* is a misnomer. Anorexics do not experience a true loss of appetite until late in starvation; individuals experience the feeling of hunger but ignore it. As the illness progresses, food refusal continues and is accompanied by preoccupation with thoughts of food. It is not unusual for anorexics to be well educated in the area of nutrition. They may become gourmet cooks or "health food" advocates and insist that their families eat well while they continue to avoid food and lose weight.

The anorexic who controls weight by limiting nutritional intake is referred to as a *restrictor*. Some anorexics limit intake and also use laxatives and/or diuretics as purgatives to further decrease the effect of ingested calories. It is not unusual for anorexics to indulge in binge-eating and to purge by vomiting. These individuals are referred to as anorexics with bulimic features.

Etiology

The cause of anorexia nervosa is not fully understood. Many theories have been generated and discussed over the past century as anorexia nervosa has been studied and treated. The disorder appears to be the result of the interaction of many factors in a vulnerable person. The multifactorial concept of the illness blends many of the theories proposed. Theories of etiology are summarized in the accompanying Key Features of Disease. These causes can be considered to be factors contributing to the development of anorexia nervosa. Each individual is unique, so the degree of importance of each factor varies from person to person. Also, not every factor is a contributor in every case. However, Figure 46–1 shows several factors and suggests a rough estimate of how much each contributes to the development of anorexia nervosa. This figure may be viewed as a pie with pieces that vary in size according to the factor's importance.

Some researchers have suggested that anorexia nervosa is the result of a hormonal or hypothalamic dysfunction that predisposes an individual to the disorder. Others have identified a higher than expected incidence of affective illness, i.e., depression and manic-depressive illness, in families of anorexics. Further support of a genetic link is evidenced by the high incidence of ano-

KEY FEATURES OF DISEASE ■ Theories of the Causes of Anorexia Nervosa

Theory	Cause
Psychologic	Defense against anxiety, especially psychosexual issues
Social	Diet fads, cultural emphasis on slimness
Family	The *identified* client is the expression of an ill family
Biologic	Hypothalamic disorder
Learning	Anorexia behavior is the result of understandable behavior reinforcements
Developmental	Anorexia is a coping response to feeling overwhelmed by maturational crises

From Andersen, A. E. (1985). *Practical comprehensive treatment of anorexia nervosa and bulimia* (p.50). Baltimore: The Johns Hopkins University Press.

rexia nervosa in both of a pair of identical twins (i.e., 50% concordance rate) compared with that of dizygotic twins (7% concordance rate) (Garfinkel & Garner, 1982). Familial transmission related to genetics or to behaviors and attitudes is suggested in research that identifies a 6% risk factor for sisters of females with anorexia nervosa (Halmi et al., 1977). Kalucy et al. (1977) studied 56 families and found that 27% of the

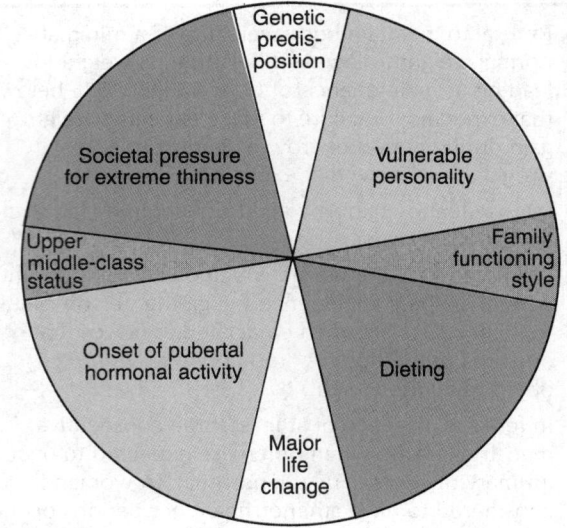

Figure 46–1

Factors contributing to the development of anorexia nervosa. (From Andersen, A. E. [1985]. *Practical comprehensive treatment of anorexia nervosa and bulimia*. Baltimore: The Johns Hopkins University Press.)

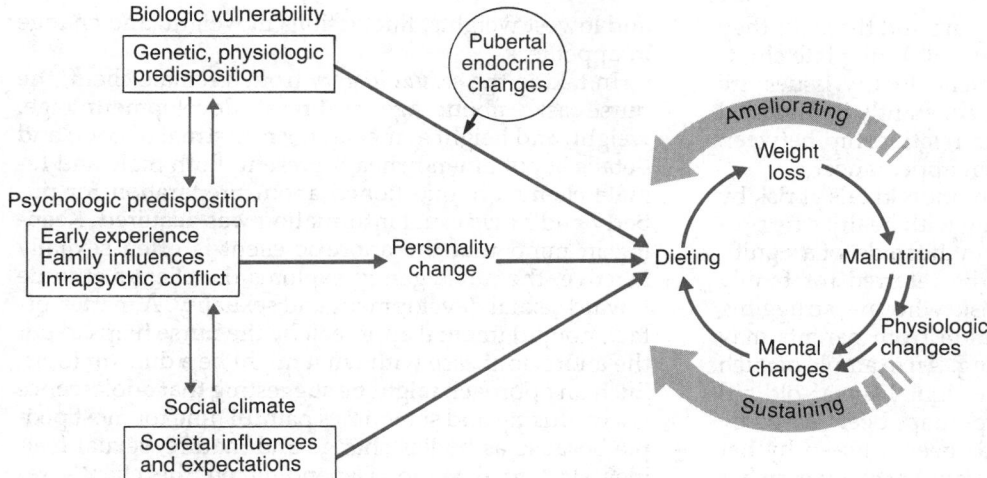

Figure 46–2

Biopsychosocial model for anorexia nervosa. (From Lucas, A. R. [1981]. Toward the understanding of anorexia nervosa as a disease entity. *Mayo Clinic Proceedings, 56,* 254.)

mothers and 16% of the fathers of anorexics had low weight during their own adolescence, anorexia nervosa, or weight phobias. This history of weight problems in parents of anorexics was identified again in 1980 by Crisp et al., who found a probable history of anorexia nervosa in 29% of first-degree relatives of individuals with diagnosed anorexia nervosa.

Because complete knowledge of the factors that cause anorexia nervosa is not available, it is important to remain open to the possibility that some factors may be disproved and new factors added. Until an etiology is confirmed, it is reasonable to proceed by characterizing this disorder as one arising from the interactions of the multiple factors. The biopsychosocial model for anorexia nervosa illustrated in Figure 46–2 shows the interrelationship of the factors and the resulting cycle of illness and consequences of illness-related behaviors.

Incidence

There is concern that the prevalence of anorexia nervosa is increasing. The incidence in the high-risk group of American girls, i.e., 12 to 18 years old, is estimated at 1 in 200 per year (0.5%) (Office of Research Reporting, 1983). Other investigators identify a prevalence of 1% among pre–college-age females (Crisp et al., 1976). Approximately 5% to 10% of the population with anorexia nervosa is male (Andersen, 1984). The disorder is infrequently diagnosed in older women or in children younger than 12 years of age. Anorexia nervosa is most commonly diagnosed in females from the middle and upper classes in the Western culture. This sociocultural difference in the prevalence of anorexia nervosa in England is further delineated by a study indicating that 1 in 100 girls aged 16 years and older who attend boarding schools have anorexia nervosa. The researchers report that only 1 in 550 girls of the same age who attend public schools suffer from this illness (Crisp et al., 1976).

Individuals who belong to professions or who participate in sports that demand low weight have an in-

creased risk of developing anorexia nervosa. Ballet dancers, models, jockeys, gymnasts, wrestlers, and actresses are examples. Morgan and Mayberry (1983) reported a 1.7% overall frequency of anorexia nervosa in dietitians. This statistic may reflect the interest of the anorexic in food and nutrition when choosing a profession rather than participation in the profession being a risk factor in and of itself.

Although the disorder may be increasing in prevalence, it is encouraging to note that the mortality rate for anorexia nervosa has decreased from 5% to 15% to 1% to 2% (Andersen, 1985). Death, when it occurs, is usually the result of starvation, intercurrent infection, or suicide.

PREVENTION

There is no easily identifiable approach to preventing anorexia nervosa. However, the nurse can educate the lay public about the disorder and its possible causes. Families can be encouraged to develop healthy eating patterns, e.g., eating in moderation from all food groups and avoiding an excess of concentrated fats or sweets. Parents can be taught to set examples for their children in their approach to eating and dieting. If a weight loss diet is necessary, it should be supervised by a health care professional. Fad diets should be avoided. Parents can be warned that perpetual dieting and constant verbalization of worries about weight are detrimental to their children. Parents can be urged to avoid such negative role modeling and to adopt healthy attitudes and behaviors in relation to food intake.

The self-esteem of the anorexic is usually quite low, and maintaining thinness is one way to maintain self-confidence. Regulating food intake and exercising strict self-discipline become a way of exerting control and of proving that there is one thing that she or he can do extremely well. Parents can help children to develop positive self-regard that is *not* related to weight and appearance by emphasizing from as early as the toddler stage the importance of who they are and the skills they have. This emphasis becomes crucial during late childhood and early adolescence when identity issues are prominent. The young person is constantly bombarded by media messages stressing the relationship between success and happiness and a slim appearance.

The nurse can assist families or individuals at risk by suggesting appropriate counseling with health care professionals. Families in conflict or in the midst of a significant change, e.g., divorce, can be referred for family counseling. Young people at risk who are struggling with identity issues and separation from parents may benefit from individual counseling. An example of such an individual might be an overweight 14-year-old girl from a wealthy family. She has perhaps been teased by peers because of her weight, has been advised by her mother to diet, and has had maturational changes in her body pointed out by her father. She feels unsure of herself and is worried about whether school performance meets her parent's standards even though she maintains an A average. This teen-ager will benefit from the nurse's assistance in making a referral to a mental health professional with whom the teen-ager can develop a relationship and explore psychosocial issues.

COLLABORATIVE MANAGEMENT

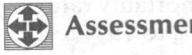 **Assessment**

History

Data collected by the nurse during history taking are invaluable in differentiating anorexia nervosa from medical illness. The client and family provide history data.

Demographic data that are collected are age, sex, socioeconomic status, education, and occupation. Educational history includes the highest grade achieved, the general level of performance, the attitude toward school work, and career plans.

A history of *medical problems* identifies both past and current diagnoses with information about each problem and how the diagnosis was made. The nurse gathers specific information about gastrointestinal symptoms such as nausea, vomiting, esophagitis, irritable bowel syndrome, and constipation. The client is asked to describe any difficulties or concerns about her or his physical functioning such as weakness, fatigue, intolerance to cold, change in sleep habits, swelling in any part of the body, and seizures.

The nurse pays special attention to the client's *weight history* and gathers data on current weight, height, and body build. The client is asked to describe the *onset of weight loss* by giving information about age and weight at the time and the reason for the weight loss, e.g., dieting, divorce of parents, break-up with boyfriend or girlfriend, or a medical illness. Further weight information needed for the history includes the client's highest

and lowest weights, fluctuations in weight, and change in appetite.

In taking the *sexual history* from a female client, the nurse asks about age at breast development; age, weight, and height at menarche; menstrual history; and details about amenorrhea if present. Both male and female clients are questioned about preparation for puberty and how sexual information was acquired. Keeping in mind that the anorexic client is often sexually inactive, the nurse gently explores the client's attitude toward sexual development and sexuality. A matter-of-fact, nonjudgmental approach by the nurse helps to put the anorexic at ease with what might be a difficult topic. Such an approach might be suggesting that adolescence is a confusing and sometimes painful time for most people because as bodies change and mature, sexual feelings start to develop. Depending on the client's response, the nurse might suggest further that adolescents sometimes are pressured by peers to explore these sexual feelings before they are ready or are pressured by parents not to acknowledge and explore issues of sexuality. It may be necessary to postpone some of the questions about sexual orientation and experiences until the client has established trust in the nurse.

Specific information is needed about the client's *attitudes and behavior related to food and weight.* The nurse asks about changes in appetite or denial of appetite, use of appetite-suppressing medication, self-induced vomiting, and frequency of weighing self. The client is asked to describe her or his typical pattern of eating, e.g., time of meals, amount of food eaten, variety of food intake, and preference for or avoidance of specific types of food. Information is sought about the use of laxatives and diuretics and about habits of hiding food or throwing food away. The nurse asks about preoccupation with thoughts of food, hoarding food, unusual handling of food (e.g., cutting it into extremely small pieces), feelings of guilt after eating, and fear of becoming fat. The client's knowledge of nutrition and calories, as well as interest in food preparation, is explored. The nurse inquires about the desire to lose more weight and asks the client to name the desired weight and to describe feelings related to the ability to lose weight. By asking, "How do you like the way you look?" and "Are you happy with the size of all your body parts?" the nurse can obtain information that helps to identify the presence of a perceptual distortion in body image (see Chap. 9 for additional information on body image).

The history of the client's *activity level* identifies the present level of activity and uncovers changes, e.g., more or less active than previously, previous and unhealthy behaviors such as compulsive exercise with a driven quality aimed at burning calories, or increased exercising at night when family members are asleep. The client is questioned about increased restlessness and change in strength and endurance related to weight loss.

A history of *psychiatric illness and treatment* includes diagnoses, dates and places of hospitalizations or outpatient treatment, and medications prescribed. *Personal data* are sought regarding the client's use of cigarettes, alcohol, or drugs (prescribed, over the counter, or illegal). The client and family are asked to describe the client's personality before the onset of weight loss and any changes perceived since that time. The nurse pays special attention to reports of a tendency toward perfectionism, self-criticism, and compulsiveness. The client is asked to describe her or his mood and any fluctuations, as well as the presence of anxiety or phobias. These questions assist the nurse in gathering data about the client's ability to describe mood and feelings to uncover the presence of *alexithymia*, or the inability to identify inner feelings, which is a feature of anorexia nervosa.

The *family history* comprises questions designed to identify parents' ages, education, careers, general health, and relationship with the client, e.g., very close to mother but cannot relate to father or vice versa. Age and sex of siblings and their relationships with the client are noted. Information is gathered about family functioning and conflict. The nurse asks about family history of psychiatric illness such as eating disorders, alcoholism, depression, or manic-depressive illness. The family's attitudes toward food and weight are explored, e.g., is anyone or has anyone been overweight or underweight? constantly dieting? teased about weight? Also important is the family's reaction to the client's illness, e.g., denying a serious problem, looking for a medical reason for the weight loss, blaming one's self or each other for the client's illness, or anger and disgust with the client.

Physical Assessment: Clinical Manifestations

Most clients with anorexia nervosa come to medical attention when *weight loss* is readily apparent. *Amenorrhea* may occur before excessive weight loss is noticed. As profound weight loss occurs, i.e., 15% or more of total body weight, physical assessment reveals signs of *hypothermia*, i.e., decreased core body temperature to 95° F (35° C) or lower. Other *vital signs* are also *lowered*, e.g., blood pressure may be as low as 60/40 mm Hg or the client may have orthostatic blood pressure changes (a drop in pressure when the client changes from lying to sitting or sitting to standing positions). The client's heart rate may range from 40 to 60 beats per minute, and the respiratory rate may be slow. The nurse carefully questions the client to determine if the weight loss has been slow and gradual. If so, the accompanying decrease in vital signs is probably not cause for alarm because the body has adjusted to the changes. The client may complain of intolerance to cold temperatures, dizziness, and weakness but is usually not in acute distress. Figure 46–3 summarizes the physical signs of anorexia nervosa.

Extremities are cool and sometimes cyanotic on examination. Although many anorexics do not purge by vomiting, the nurse observes for evidence of scars on the knuckles of the hands and calluses from digital pressure on the abdomen that indicate self-induced vomiting. An absence of such signs should *not* be interpreted as the absence of self-induced vomiting, however. The emaciated anorexic has *lost muscle mass and subcutaneous fat*, and a prominent bone structure is revealed. Severe emaciation, which creates the appearance of a skeleton covered with skin, e.g., a weight of 60 lb for a 5-ft, 5-in female, may be shocking to the nurse, and care is needed not to transmit this reaction to the client. The body may also be covered with fine *lanugo hair*, which may be especially evident on the extremities, the shoulders, and the face.

The *physical complications* that accompany anorexia nervosa vary with the degree of starvation and the method of weight control that has been used by the client. Food restrictors usually have fewer complications than anorexics who also use vomiting, laxatives, and diuretics to maintain low weight. Such behaviors lower potassium levels and may result in a state of *hypokalemic metabolic alkalosis*, which can cause seizure activity and cardiac dysrhythmias. A decreased potassium level can result from starvation as well as from purging, but in that case it is not as severe. The nurse is more likely to see *metabolic acidosis* with food restriction and starvation related to the conversion of fat to fatty acids and ketones (see Chap. 15 for a complete discussion of acid-base imbalances). The nurse observes for *tetany*, or intermittent tonic muscular contractions, which may result from *hypocalcemia*. *Hypophosphatemia*, when severe, may induce the clinical manifestations of paresthesia (abnormal tingling or prickling sensations), convulsions, coma, or death.

Other observations required of the nurse during physical assessment include a description of *edema* present anywhere on the body, e.g., 3+ pitting edema of ankles. The cause of this edema is not clear but is *not* usually related to kidney or liver failure. This symptom may become more prominent during refeeding. *Parotid gland tenderness and swelling* alert the nurse that the client probably practices self-induced vomiting. Other such indicators are *discolored tooth enamel* and excessive numbers of caries, which are the result of frequent exposure to gastric acids. Jaundice may indicate *abnormal liver function* and may be seen in older anorexics with a long history of illness.

Some practices of anorexics seem to protect them to some extent from the severe effects of starvation. Most anorexics take multiple vitamins, which counteract the effects of a vitamin-deficient diet and may protect against peripheral neuropathies and paresthesia. Anorexics who have high levels of regular exercise may be affected less by the loss of bone mass of *osteoporosis* secondary to estrogen deficiency and low calcium intake than are those individuals who do not exercise.

Psychosocial Assessment

The typical anorexic is a Caucasian, adolescent female or young adult from a middle-class to upper-class

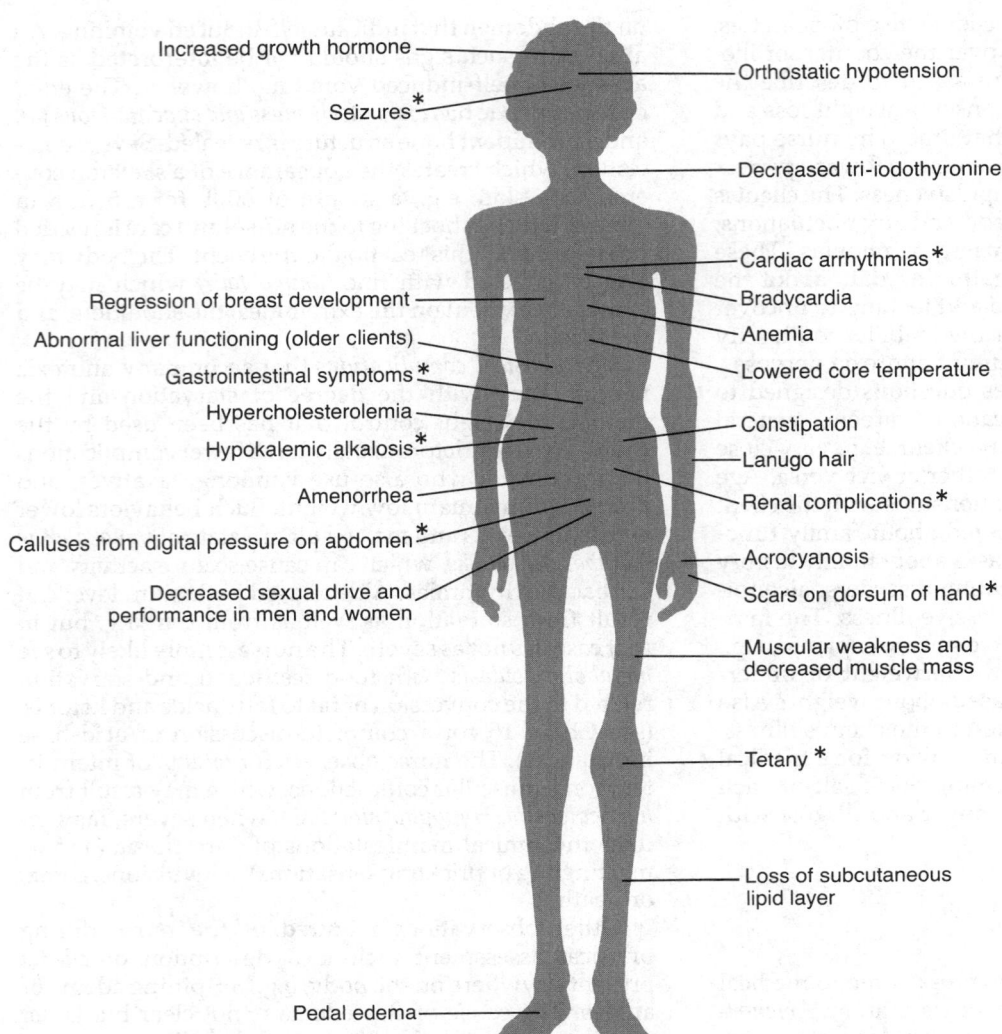

Increased growth hormone

Seizures*

Orthostatic hypotension

Decreased tri-iodothyronine

Cardiac arrhythmias*

Regression of breast development

Bradycardia

Abnormal liver functioning (older clients)

Anemia

Gastrointestinal symptoms*

Lowered core temperature

Hypercholesterolemia

Constipation

Hypokalemic alkalosis*

Lanugo hair

Amenorrhea

Renal complications*

Calluses from digital pressure on abdomen*

Acrocyanosis

Decreased sexual drive and performance in men and women

Scars on dorsum of hand*

Muscular weakness and decreased muscle mass

Tetany*

Loss of subcutaneous lipid layer

Pedal edema

Figure 46–3

Physical signs of anorexia nervosa and bulimia. (From Andersen, A. E. [1985]. *Practical comprehensive treatment of anorexia nervosa and bulimia.* Baltimore: The Johns Hopkins University Press.)

family who is a high achiever academically and exhibits a high level of motivation and compliance. Parents frequently describe their anorexic adolescent as having been a "perfect" child. Before the onset of illness, the adolescent was popular with peers and involved in social activities, frequently excelling in athletics. Although seemingly successful in facing the challenges of adolescence, the anorexic suffers from a sense of ineffectiveness and low self-esteem. Along with the physical symptom of weight loss, the nurse finds on psychologic assessment that the client has a severe distortion in body image. The anorexic's attitude toward the weight loss is significant to diagnosis in that the individual seems to enjoy losing weight and takes pride in extreme thinness. The anorexic does not see a thin, emaciated body in the mirror. Rather, she or he sees "fat thighs" or a "protruding stomach." Along with this distorted body image, the nurse may find that the client does not correctly perceive stimuli within the body, e.g., fails to recognize feelings of hunger and appetite.

The onset of illness frequently occurs when the client is struggling with the identity issues of adolescence. It may be triggered by an emotionally stressful situation such as a change in family structure or a move to a new city. Peer pressure may influence the onset of the illness, as when a group of adolescents begins to diet and one person continues to diet to extreme thinness.

Family dynamics frequently are a significant contributing factor to the illness. A tendency toward rigidity may lead to strong parental control and overinvolvement with the children. An intolerance for conflict leads to poor conflict resolution and communication difficulties. It is not unusual to see one parent dominate the other or to note that the anorexic is emotionally very close to one parent but somewhat distanced from the other. The anorexic desires parental approval and strives for perfection. The individual attempts to attain a sense of independence, achievement, and control over life while combating an unrealistic fear of failure. In the interview with the client and family, the nurse observes the interaction process and notes areas of tension or conflict, overprotectiveness, or family members' answering questions for others—especially parents' speaking for the adolescent.

A mental status examination is part of the psychologic assessment. During the mental status examination, the nurse identifies an alteration in the state of consciousness that may accompany starvation and an alteration in mood state such as depression. Questions are asked about feelings of self-worth and hopelessness, the ability to enjoy life, and suicidal thoughts (see Stuart & Sundeen, 1983, pp. 554–559, for a description of a full mental status examination). It must be noted, however, that depression reported by anorexics at low weight often resolves when weight is normal. The nurse also questions the client about obsessions, compulsions, phobias, and any unusual ideas about food. The anorexic may have peculiar ideas about what food does inside the body and sometimes outside the body, e.g., fear that the food will produce fat that will be deposited on the thighs, or fear that crumbs falling on one's self will cause absorption of calories and weight gain. When assessing for the presence of ritualistic behavior, the nurse may find that the client always goes through a certain fixed routine at mealtimes, such as sitting a certain way in a chair, using only certain utensils, or arranging food items in a certain way on the plate. The anorexic may have a self-imposed requirement of a set number of repetitions of a certain exercise for each calorie ingested. Standing or moving about constantly to burn more calories rather than sitting is another behavior seen in many anorexics.

Both male and female anorexics exhibit poor sexual adjustment. Delayed sexual development is noted in adolescents, and there is a decreased interest in sex among adult anorexics. The quality and number of social relationships tend to decline as the anorexic's preoccupation with food and body increases. The client and family are asked to describe changes in behavior such as decreased involvement with peers and family and changes in participation in school activities. The nurse might ask if the client does things with the family, e.g., family outings, watching television together, eating with family. Questions such as "Do you enjoy going to school dances or sports events?" and "Do you have a special boyfriend or girlfriend?" may illuminate a change in behavior.

Assessment of the client's strengths is not ignored. Positive coping skills are identified in both client and family. The anorexic's high motivation and desire for success are positive when used to regain health rather than maintain lower weight. Effective communication skills assist the anorexic in exploring issues with health care professionals. Chapter 6 discusses coping behaviors and skills and provides the nurse with additional information that is invaluable in planning nursing care that emphasizes and encourages positive coping behaviors.

Laboratory Findings

Abnormalities related to the client's blood such as profound anemia are revealed by a complete blood count with differential. The SMA-6 (6/60) (urea nitrogen, sodium, potassium, chloride, carbon dioxide, and glucose) and SMA-12 (12/60) (bilirubin, phosphate, calcium, total protein, albumin, alkaline phosphatase, uric acid, cholesterol, amylase, magnesium, aspartate aminotransferase [serum glutamic-oxaloacetic transaminase], and alanine aminotransferase [serum glutamic-pyruvic transaminase]) provide much useful information, especially about electrolyte balance and kidney function. Possible fluid and electrolyte abnormalities include hypokalemia, hypochloremia, metabolic alkalosis, and metabolic acidosis. Hypoglycemia may be severe in restrictors who fast for extended periods. An elevated blood urea nitrogen level indicates dehydration. Purging through vomiting, laxative abuse, or diuretic abuse can result in dehydration with hypokalemia, which may cause severe renal problems. A nephropathy related to low potassium levels can cause interstitial fibrosis and impaired renal function (Mitchell, 1986). Urinalysis with microscopic examination is indicated to assess for the presence of urinary tract infection. Endocrine studies identify low levels of luteinizing hormone, follicle-stimulating hormone, and estrogen in females, and decreased testosterone levels in males. Plasma cortisol levels may be elevated but do not generally indicate abnormal adrenal functioning. Cortisol levels that are measured again when the client is at normal weight usually are in the normal range. Because the dexamethasone suppression test is often false positive in anorexics, it is not recommended for use in identifying depression. Thyroid studies such as thyroxine (T_4), tri-iodothyronine resin uptake (T_3RU), and plasma tri-iodothyronine (T_3) often reveal a low-normal T_4 and a subclinical T_3 value. The anorexic's growth hormone level is usually normal or elevated. Males with anorexia nervosa are found to have growth retardation and arrested skeletal maturation related to starvation. Liver function tests often reveal abnormalities in the chronically ill client with anorexia nervosa that are related to starvation. The abnormalities may worsen as the client gains weight because of fatty degeneration during refeeding. Serum cholesterol levels are often elevated in the client with anorexia nervosa, whereas serum triglyceride levels are usually normal. The reasons for the noted abnormalities are not clear, but they often resolve after weight is gained. When they do not resolve, treatment is indicated.

Other Diagnostic Tests

A routine chest x-ray film is done and electrocardiography is indicated on admission to the hospital. However, more extensive medical tests are not indicated when the symptoms of the client suggest a diagnosis of anorexia nervosa. Symptoms that persist after the client returns to a healthy weight indicate the need for further diagnostic studies. Initially, however, efforts are directed at making an accurate diagnosis as promptly as possible so that costly, uncomfortable tests that prove to be negative are avoided. The hospital's consulting psychiatrist and/or psychiatric liaison nurse should be asked to evaluate the client as part of the process of establishing a diagnosis. These consultants may also assist in arranging for appropriate psychologic testing to be done by a psychologist. Such tests include the Minnesota Multiphasic Personality Inventory (MMPI), an intelligence quotient test (Wechsler's Adult Intelligence Scale [WAIS]), a perceptual distortion test, a depression scale, and, if available, an eating disorder scale such as the Eating Attitudes Test (EAT) developed by Garner and Garfinkel and the Eating Disorder Inventory (EDI) developed by Garner et al. (Fig. 46–4). Additional information on the purpose, methods, and meaning of results of psychiatric tests is available in psychology textbooks or psychiatric nursing texts.

 Analysis: Nursing Diagnosis

Common Diagnoses

Ten nursing diagnoses are common in the client and family when anorexia nervosa is present:

1. Altered nutrition: less than body requirements related to inadequate food intake
2. Pain (abdominal) related to refeeding
3. Potential fluid volume deficit related to self-imposed fluid restriction or purging behaviors
4. Fluid volume excess related to fluid retention during refeeding

---

INSTRUCTIONS

This is a scale that measures a variety of attitudes, feelings, and behaviors. Some of the items relate to food and eating. Others ask you about your feelings about yourself. THERE ARE NO RIGHT OR WRONG ANSWERS SO TRY VERY HARD TO BE COMPLETELY HONEST IN YOUR ANSWERS. RESULTS ARE COMPLETELY CONFIDENTIAL. Read each question and fill in the circle under the column which applies best to you. Please answer each question *very* carefully. Thank you.

	ALWAYS	USUALLY	OFTEN	SOMETIMES	RARELY	NEVER
1. I eat sweets and carbohydrates without feeling nervous	○	○	○	○	○	○
2. I think that my stomach is too big	○	○	○	○	○	○
3. I wish that I could return to the security of childhood	○	○	○	○	○	○
4. I eat when I am upset	○	○	○	○	○	○
5. I stuff myself with food	○	○	○	○	○	○
6. I wish that I could be younger	○	○	○	○	○	○
7. I think about dieting	○	○	○	○	○	○
8. I get frightened when my feelings are too strong	○	○	○	○	○	○
9. I think that my thighs are too large	○	○	○	○	○	○
10. I feel ineffective as a person	○	○	○	○	○	○
11. I feel extremely guilty after overeating	○	○	○	○	○	○
12. I think that my stomach is just the right size	○	○	○	○	○	○
13. Only outstanding performance is good enough in my family	○	○	○	○	○	○
14. The happiest time in life is when you are a child	○	○	○	○	○	○
15. I am open about my feelings	○	○	○	○	○	○
16. I am terrified of gaining weight	○	○	○	○	○	○
17. I trust others	○	○	○	○	○	○
18. I feel alone in the world	○	○	○	○	○	○
19. I feel satisfied with the shape of my body	○	○	○	○	○	○
20. I feel generally in control of things in my life	○	○	○	○	○	○

Figure 46–4

A portion of the Eating Disorder Inventory. (Adapted and reproduced by special permission of the Publisher, Psychological Assessment Resources, Inc., 16102 North Florida Avenue, Lutz, Florida 33549, from *The Eating Disorder Inventory*, by D. Garner, M. P. Olmstead, J. Polivy, Copyright, 1984. Further reproduction is prohibited without permission from PAR, Inc.)

5. Constipation related to decreased intake and/or laxative abuse

6. Anxiety related to increased food intake and consequent weight gain

7. Body image disturbance related to misperception of body size

8. Ineffective individual coping related to fears of loss of self-control and fatness

9. Potential for noncompliance (therapeutic recommendations) related to food refusal, vomiting, laxative abuse, overexercising, or decision to leave hospital against medical advice

10. Altered family processes related to difficulty in coping with client's illness and hospitalization

Additional Diagnoses

Anorexia nervosa is a complex disorder, and the client and family may present with many of the following nursing diagnoses:

1. Potential for decreased cardiac output related to alterations in rhythm caused by hypokalemia. (This can be a life-threatening problem. It is not common in restricting anorexia nervosa but may be seen in anorexia nervosa with bulimic features. See under the later heading Planning and Implementation in the section on bulimia nervosa.)

2. Knowledge deficit related to illness and/or treatment plan

3. Potential altered body temperature related to low weight

4. Potential for injury (fracture) related to low-estrogen condition and calcium deficiency with decreased bone mass

5. Activity intolerance or fatigue related to starved state and muscle weakness

6. Sleep pattern disturbance related to hyperactivity and nocturnal exercise habits

7. Potential for altered growth and development related to inadequate food intake

8. Potential for sexual dysfunction related to altered body function and psychosocial vulnerabilities

9. Sensory/perceptual alterations related to inability to recognize physical and emotional states of hunger and satiety or to identify emotions

10. Self-esteem disturbance related to overwhelming sense of ineffectiveness, issues of personal identity, and issues of role performance

11. Ineffective individual coping related to depressed mood

12. Potential for social isolation related to preoccupation with illness behaviors and thoughts of food

13. Ineffective family coping: compromised or disabling related to changes in family dynamics brought about by illness

14. Potential for altered health maintenance related to recurrent episodes of illness

Planning and Implementation

The following plan of care describes the general approach to managing the common diagnoses of the anorexic. A selected Client Care Plan accompanies the text. The diagnoses are grouped beginning with the physical and moving toward the psychosocial. Successful planning and implementation for all diagnoses require that

Text continued on page 1428

CLIENT CARE PLAN ■ The Client with Anorexia Nervosa

Goal/Outcome Criteria	Interventions	Rationales
Nursing Diagnosis 1: Altered Nutrition: Less Than Body Requirements Related to Inadequate Food Intake		
Client will develop an eating pattern that meets daily nutritional needs. ■ Eats all food presented by nurse.	1. Assist client to select foods from menu from all food groups. Allow for three food dislikes only.	1. The client may try to avoid some types of foods or entire food groups, e.g., meats, and needs advice and encouragement from the nurse to make healthy selections. Allowing the client to state three foods that need not be selected gives the client a sense of control. The three items should be specific, e.g., liver, beets, and applesauce, and decided on in advance, with a limit placed on the number of times that the food dislikes may be changed. *continued*

CLIENT CARE PLAN ■ The Client with Anorexia Nervosa *continued*

Goal/Outcome Criteria	Interventions	Rationales
	Nursing Diagnosis 1: Altered Nutrition: Less Than Body Requirements Related to Inadequate Food Intake	
	2. Make menu selections if the client refuses to do so or becomes distressed with the task.	2. Although preoccupied with thoughts of food, the anorexic may experience extreme distress at the prospect of having to select food that the staff will expect to be eaten. This task may be too stressful early in hospitalization and should not be insisted on.
■ Eats only food that is presented by nurse.	3. Teach the client, family, and friends the importance of eating only food that is presented by staff.	3. The client will be given a special diet to prevent complications and to determine body requirements for returning to and maintaining a healthy weight. When extra foods are eaten, the calorie count is inaccurate and does not reflect the true numbers of calories needed to gain weight.
	4. Sit with the client during and for 1 h after meals and snacks.	4. The client needs much encouragement and emotional support to eat all of the food presented without purging. The time after eating is also a time when the client needs support and someone with whom to talk.
	5. Maintain caloric count.	5. The client is expected to eat all food that is presented. However, this may not always occur, and a calorie count provides information on which to base decisions to increase the number of calories.

■ Experiences a weight gain of 2–4 lb/wk.
 ■ Does not engage in unhealthy behaviors to simulate weight gain.
	6. Weigh the client three times a week.
	   a. Keep a weight graph to document progress.
	   b. Ensure that the client wears only a hospital gown during weighing.
	   c. Prevent access to fluids before weighing.
	   d. Weigh the client at the same time of day, e.g., before breakfast.
	   e. Do unannounced spot weights periodically.
		6. Accurate weights are essential to decision-making but produce anxiety in the client, so only three per week are suggested. Clients may attempt to manipulate results, e.g., by placing objects in their pockets; weighing in the hospital gown eliminates this possibility. Clients may attempt to increase weight by ingesting large quantities of water just before they are weighed. A consistent time of day for weights provides consistent results. Unannounced weighing reveals an accurate weight if this is in question.

	7. Administer intravenous fluids as ordered.	7. Refusal of oral fluids and food puts the client at risk for dehydration and fluid imbalance. Temporary parenteral therapy corrects the situation.

Goal/Outcome Criteria	Interventions	Rationales
Nursing Diagnosis 1: Altered Nutrition: Less Than Body Requirements Related to Inadequate Food Intake		
	8. Administer tube feeding as ordered via nasogastric tube. a. Infuse slowly over several hours by using a pump. b. Remove feeding tube at night. c. Offer food by mouth for breakfast. d. Reinsert nasogastic tube if food is refused.	8. Tube feedings are a move away from normal eating and should be avoided unless absolutely necessary. Continuous infusion via pump avoids a bolus, which may cause abdominal distention. Bolus feeding also facilitates vomiting and so is to be avoided. Removing the tube each night provides for a more comfortable night of rest and allows for the reintroduction of food. The client may decide to take food by mouth rather than have a nasogastric tube reinserted.
Client will maintain a healthy weight. ■ Maintains weight within a 5-lb range set by treatment team.	1. Assist the health care team in setting a weight range, e.g., 122 – 127 lb, by using the appropriate chart.	1. A weight goal is set taking into consideration body build and height and weight at menarche. In general, weight to regain menses is approximately 10% higher than weight at onset. Final weight should be within 95% of ideal body weight.
	2. Reassure the client that the staff will not make her or him fat. The goal is a healthy weight.	2. The client needs constant reassurance that what is feared most will not happen. Emphasis is placed on improved health and not weight.
	3. Interrupt attempts on the client's part to bargain with staff members for a change in the goal weight range.	3. Anxiety related to attaining weight that is considered too high may drive the client to bargain or manipulate individual staff members. Weight range changes are made only as team decisions and not by individuals.
	4. Teach the client and the family the rationale for the weight range selected. a. Improved general health. b. Normal body functioning with establishment of a regular menstrual cycle. c. Relationship of body fat to menstruation and pregnancy. d. Continued amenorrhea at normal weight.	4. The client must be willing to maintain a healthy weight if general health is to be realized. Chronic conditions such as anemia or renal and hepatic dysfunction may develop when a starved state exists for an extended period. The female body requires about 24% fat composition to support the physiologic functions of menstruation and pregnancy. A desire for children may help to motivate a female client to maintain her goal weight range. However, attainment of healthy weight does not ensure a regular menstrual cycle. A year or more at normal weight may be necessary for the body to readjust.

continued

Goal/Outcome Criteria	Interventions	Rationales
Nursing Diagnosis 1: Altered Nutrition: Less Than Body Requirements Related to Inadequate Food Intake		
■ Agrees to have regular follow-up with a mental health professional.	5. Assist the client and the family to obtain appropriate psychiatric follow-up.	5. The client needs to develop a relationship with a mental health professional to resolve underlying conflicts and to learn new coping behaviors. Regular monitoring of weight is also necessary.
Nursing Diagnosis 2: Pain (Abdominal) Related to Refeeding		
Client will not experience abdominal pain. ■ Has minimal discomfort during refeeding.	1. Feed client a low-lactose, low-lipid diet for 1 wk. 2. Introduce milk products gradually during the second week. 3. Introduce lipids in the third week.	1–3. The level of enzymes required to digest lactose and lipids decreases when these substances are not ingested for a long time. After a period of starvation, enzyme production needs time to readjust. Introduction of milk products or fats before enzymes are regenerated causes indigestion and abdominal discomfort.
	4. Withdraw milk products and fats if cramping persists longer than 2 d and reintroduce after a 1-wk interval.	4. Severe cramping when lactose or lipids are introduced indicates that the body needs additional time to regenerate enzymes. Introduction of small quantities facilitates this regeneration.
	5. Administer medication for pain relief as ordered.	5. Some relief may be provided through the use of acetaminophen and antacids.

	6. Assist the client to develop strategies to decrease discomfort.
	  a. Teach relaxation techniques.
	  b. Provide diversionary activities.
		6. Increased tension increases pain. Therefore, techniques that promote relaxation result in decreased pain. Activities that distract also change the focus away from the pain sensation.

Nursing Diagnosis 3: Potential Fluid Volume Deficit Related to Self-Imposed Fluid Restriction or Purging Behaviors		

Client will experience correction of existing fluid volume deficit and will maintain an adequate fluid volume.
■ Maintains stable vital signs, intake and output, and specific gravity within normal ranges.
	1. Assess for signs of fluid volume deficit.
	  a. Low blood pressure.
	  b. Weak pulse.
	  c. Small volume of urinary output; very concentrated urine.
	  d. Presence of tenting of skin.
	  e. Dry skin and mucous membranes.
	  f. Dry mouth and complaint of thirst.
	  g. Lassitude.
		1. Rapid assessment and detection of a fluid volume deficit ensure rapid correction of the problem and prevention of shock and other sequelae.

■ Drinks 1000 mL of fluid/d.	2. Offer fluids orally each hour, approximately 100 mL.	2. The client may be helped to retain a sense of control by taking fluids orally rather than passively accepting intravenous fluids. The oral route is the safest and most natural and therefore the most desirable.

Goal/Outcome Criteria	Interventions	Rationales
Nursing Diagnosis 3: Potential Fluid Volume Deficit Related to Self-Imposed Fluid Restriction or Purging Behaviors		
	3. Maintain an accurate record of intake and output.	3. The intake and output record provides information used in making decisions to increase or decrease fluids offered and in assisting the assessment of kidney function. A balance of approximately 2000 mL intake and output is essential for normal cellular function, production of secretions, elimination of urine and feces, and maintenance of electrolyte balance.
	4. Teach the client the consequences of fluid volume deficit.	4. Anorexic clients frequently are intelligent and can understand explanations of physiologic functioning. When faced with facts about serious, immediate consequences of not taking fluids, they may decide to accept something to drink.
	5. Administer intravenous parenteral fluids as ordered.	5. When a state of dehydration exists or fluids have been refused for 24 h after admission to the hospital, intravenous fluids are indicated to increase fluid volume.
	6. Assess for the presence of edema.	6. Edema indicates too aggressive treatment of the volume deficit in a person whose body has adjusted to severe restrictions. The usual requirement of 2000 mL of fluid over a 24-h period may be excessive in an anorexic.

■ Does not decrease fluid volume by purging.	7. Monitor the client's behavior.
	  a. Observe client using the bathroom.
	  b. Interrupt purging by vomiting.
	  c. Inspect the environment and remove any diuretics or laxatives.
		7. Vomiting and the use of diuretics and laxatives all cause fluid loss and are to be avoided.

	8. Provide emotional support to the client.
	  a. Maintain a nonjudgmental attitude and approach if purging is detected.
	  b. Provide positive feedback for appropriate requests for support to avoid purging.
		8. The anorexic may use purging as a way of gaining control. In fact, the aorexic's behavior is out of control, e.g., restricting and/or purging. Structure coupled with an accepting, supportive attitude on the part of the nurse promotes relationship building. Positive feedback for healthy behaviors shows respect for the client and acknowledges strengths.

continued

CLIENT CARE PLAN ■ The Client with Anorexia Nervosa *continued*

Goal/Outcome Criteria	Interventions	Rationales
Nursing Diagnosis 4: Fluid Volume Excess Related to Fluid Retention During Refeeding		
Client will experience minimal occurrence of refeeding edema. ■ Maintains low-salt diet until edema resolves.	1. Provide a low-salt diet as ordered. 2. Teach the client about the relationship between salt intake and edema. 3. Instruct the client not to add salt to food while refeeding edema is evident.	1–3. Salt restriction is indicated because sodium chloride enhances fluid retention, which increases the likelihood of edema.
■ Complies with fluid restriction.	4. Restrict fluids to 1000–1500 mL/d for severe edema.	4. Restricting fluids and holding caloric intake constant for several days may be necessary to control severe refeeding edema.
■ Complies with directive to elevate feet.	5. Elevate the client's lower extremities.	5. Elevation decreases edema and discomfort from swelling in tissues.
	6. Instruct the client to remove rings from fingers.	6. Rings may have to be cut off if edema is severe. Left on, they may restrict blood flow and damage tissues, which results in pain.
	7. Assist the client in selecting nonrestrictive clothing without elastic arm, leg, or waist bands. 8. Instruct the client to wear soft, nonrestrictive footwear.	7, 8. Tight clothing on edematous tissue creates pain sensation and can restrict blood flow. Males may experience scrotal edema and be most comfortable in boxer shorts and "sweat" pants.
	9. Apply body lotion to affected areas.	9. Body lotion keeps skin soft and moist and prevents cracking as tissues expand.

the nurse assist the client in working on role relationships with health care professionals to establish trust. Therefore, psychosocial diagnoses must be viewed as high priority and addressed from the onset of treatment. Psychiatric nursing texts will assist the nurse in planning interventions for psychosocial problems that are not included in the care plan.

Altered Nutrition: Less Than Body Requirements

Planning: client goals. Two major goals for this nursing diagnosis are that the client will (1) develop an eating pattern that meets daily nutritional needs and (2) maintain a healthy weight.

Interventions: nonsurgical management. A healthy weight is determined for the client by using the Metropolitan Height and Weight Tables in Chapter 41. The data developed by Frisch and McArthur (1974) (Table 46–1) are also used when calculating the minimal weight needed for the onset or restoration of menses. Initial interventions are aimed at saving the person from death by starvation. Later interventions stress the return

to a healthy weight and normal body functioning, e.g., establishment of regular menstrual cycle.

Drug therapy. Because anorexics do not experience a true loss of appetite, appetite-stimulating medications are not indicated.

Diet therapy. An initial diet of 1200 to 1600 kcal is ordered. The nurse accepts the challenge of assisting the anorexic to eat "normally" by mouth. The number of calories is increased gradually to ensure a steady weight gain of 2 to 4 lb/week. Persistent refusal of food and fluid for 24 hours in a severely starved individual necessitates use of intravenous fluids. Liquid feedings via nasogastric tube may also be necessary depending on the extent of food refusal. Transfer to a psychiatric facility specializing in the treatment of eating disorders is considered when food refusal continues unabated or when purging behaviors persist after food consumption.

The nurse collaborates with the dietitian and client in selecting a diet for the anorexic that includes items from all food groups (see later text discussion of nursing diagnoses 3, 5, and 6 for suggestions for diets that reduce the

TABLE 46–1 Minimal Weight Necessary for the Onset or Restoration of Menstrual Cycles, by Height

Height		Menarch or Primary Amenorrhea			Secondary Amenorrhea		
		Minimal* Weight (10th Percentile)		Average Weight (50th Percentile)	Minimal† Weight (10th Percentile)		Average Weight (50th Percentile)
in	cm	lb	kg	kg	lb	kg	kg
53.1	135	66.7	30.3	34.9	74.6	33.9	38.9
53.9	137	68.6	31.2	36.0	76.8	34.9	40.1
54.7	139	70.6	32.1	37.0	79.0	35.9	41.2
55.5	141	72.6	33.0	38.0	81.2	36.9	42.4
56.3	143	74.4	33.8	39.0	83.4	37.9	43.5
57.1	145	76.3	34.7	40.1	85.6	38.9	44.7
57.9	147	78.3	35.6	41.1	87.8	39.9	45.8
58.7	149	80.3	36.5	42.1	90.0	40.9	47.0
59.4	151	82.3	37.4	43.1	92.2	41.9	48.1
60.2	153	84.3	38.3	44.2	94.4	42.9	49.3
61.0	155	86.2	39.2	45.2	96.6	43.9	50.4
61.8	157	88.2	40.1	46.2	98.8	44.9	51.5
62.6	159	90.2	41.0	47.2	101.0	45.9	52.7
63.4	161	92.2	41.9	48.3	103.2	46.9	53.8
64.2	163	93.9	42.7	49.3	105.4	47.9	55.0
65.0	165	95.9	43.6	50.3	107.6	48.9	56.1
65.7	167	97.9	44.5	51.4	109.8	49.9	57.3
66.5	169	99.9	45.4	52.4	112.0	50.9	58.4
67.3	171	101.9	46.3	53.4	114.0	51.8	59.6
68.1	173	103.8	47.2	54.4	116.2	52.8	60.7
68.9	175	105.8	48.1	55.5	118.4	53.8	61.8
69.7	177	107.8	49.0	56.5	120.6	54.8	63.0
70.5	179	109.6	49.8	57.5	122.8	55.8	64.1
71.3	181	111.8	50.8	58.5	125.2	56.9	65.3

* Equivalent to 17% fat/body weight.
† Equivalent to 22% fat/body weight.
Based on Frisch, R. E., & McArthur, J. W. (1974). *Science, 185,* 949–951. Reprinted with permission from Frisch, R. E. (1977). Food intake, fatness and reproductive ability. In R. A. Vigersky (Ed.), *Anorexia nervosa* (pp. 149–161). New York: Raven Press.

likelihood of refeeding edema, abdominal pain, and fluid volume deficit or excess). The client may experience anxiety when asked to select foods from a menu. The nurse assists the client in making decisions and sets firm limits regarding selecting items from each category on the menu. The client is not given a choice about the amount of food in each group to be eaten. When the client is extremely distressed by the process of food selection, the nurse makes all selections. Ultimately, the nurse assists the client in viewing diet as one way of regaining control. Selection and intake of a healthy diet provide a positive means for the client to eat, gain weight, and gain control over activities and behavior.

Prevention of complications. Introducing a diet of 1200 to 1600 kcal given in three meals and one or two snacks avoids painful abdominal distention and the

dangerous complication of gastric dilation. In gastric dilation, motility is lost and the stomach fills with food that does not pass through to the duodenum. The stomach contents must be evacuated to avoid rupture. Intravenous fluids are given temporarily until motility is restored.

Pain (Abdominal)

Planning: client goals. The goal for this nursing diagnosis is that the client will experience minimal abdominal discomfort during the refeeding period.

Interventions: nonsurgical management. Abdominal pain is usually the result of stomach distention, cramping from lactose intolerance, or difficulty with digestion of fats. Therefore, interventions are directed at assisting the client's body to adjust by introducing small amounts of food initially, i.e., 1200 to 1600 kcal, and by gradually including lactose and fats over the first few weeks of refeeding.

Drug therapy. Narcotic pain medications are never indicated because they contribute to the danger of decreased stomach and bowel motility. Acetaminophen (Tylenol) relieves minor abdominal discomfort. Antacids may provide some relief from a complaint of indigestion. The nurse encourages the client to tolerate symptoms without medications as much as possible because proper diet management will minimize distress in a few days.

Diet therapy. The client is given a low-lactose, low-lipid diet. Milk products and fats are introduced slowly during the second or third week of refeeding; they are withdrawn if cramping is severe and are reintroduced later. Abdominal pain related to stomach distention is avoided by initiation of a diet of 1200 to 1600 kcal, with gradual increases to ensure weight gain.

Potential Fluid Volume Deficit

Planning: client goals. The major goals related to this nursing diagnosis are that the client will (1) experience a correction of any existing fluid volume deficit and (2) maintain an adequate fluid volume during the treatment period.

Interventions: nonsurgical management. The client who has severely restricted food and fluid intake before hospitalization is assessed for fluid volume deficit by using the indicators of blood pressure, urinary output and concentration, and condition of skin and mucous membranes. Low blood pressure, small volumes of very concentrated urine (specific gravity of 1.020 to 1.025), tenting of skin, and dryness of membranes are often revealed. Fluids such as water, juice, soda, coffee, and tea are offered; milk products are avoided. The anorexic's body has made a gradual adjustment to a state of severely limited food and fluid intake. Therefore, fluids should be carefully introduced at a rate and in quantities that will not compromise the cardiovascular system and create a fluid volume overload.

Diet therapy. The nurse offers fluids hourly and maintains a strict record of intake and output. Intravenous fluids, such as normal saline, are used to replenish volume immediately if symptoms of impending shock are present. Intravenous fluids are also indicated if fluids are refused orally for 24 hours.

Prevention of complications. The nurse teaches the client about the consequences of inadequate fluid intake to increase the likelihood of the client's cooperation and to prevent the sequelae of volume deficit, as well as those related to intravenous parenteral fluid administration. Refer to Chapter 13 for more information on fluid volume deficit.

The nurse also monitors the client's behavior and assists the anorexic to avoid the use of usual coping behaviors of vomiting or using diuretics and laxatives, which deplete fluid volume. The nurse works with the client to identify new ways of coping such as asking for emotional support when the desire to purge is strong. Emphasis is placed on development of a nurse-client relationship that is viewed as an alliance to resolve or prevent problems.

Fluid Volume Excess

Planning: client goals. The major goal related to this nursing diagnosis is that the client will experience minimal refeeding edema.

Interventions: nonsurgical management. Refeeding edema is a common occurrence in the early days of nutritional rehabilitation and can cause discomfort. The client may complain of swelling in ankles, knees, fingers, and face. It is usually most severe in the lower extremities. The condition is annoying, but it does not appear to have a serious etiology such as kidney or liver failure. Interventions that prevent edema and provide increased comfort for the client are indicated.

Drug therapy. Diuretics are not recommended and are avoided unless serious complications such as heart failure appear.

Diet therapy. Refeeding edema responds well to a low-salt diet. A fluid restriction limiting the client to 1000 to 1500 mL/day is helpful with severe edema. The caloric intake is also held constant for several days.

Prevention of complications. Discomfort from the edema is the client's most frequent complaint. The nurse provides a comfortable chair and foot rest and encourages the client to keep the feet elevated for several hours a day. The nurse further cautions the client to remove rings from fingers and to avoid restrictive clothing or shoes. Older anorexics who have been chronically ill for several years seem to be most troubled by refeeding edema and may experience it for an extended time, sometimes for weeks. The nurse teaches the client to manage this prolonged edema.

Constipation

Planning: client goals. The primary goal for this diagnosis is that the client will establish a regular bowel elimination pattern without the use of laxatives.

Interventions: nonsurgical management. Normal physiologic bowel action is preferable to the use of cathartics. Chronic laxative abusers can find noncathartic ways to enhance elimination with teaching from the nurse. However, anxiety related to weight gain may prompt even the non–laxative-abusing anorexic to request laxatives or enemas and to exaggerate the extent of the problem. Interventions are sought that encourage physiologic bowel action and prevent complications such as fecal impaction.

Drug therapy. A bowel regimen that includes a bulk laxative (hydrophilic colloid) such as psyllium (Metamucil) and a stool softener such as docusate (Colace) given twice daily assists in the development of a regular bowel elimination pattern. Persistent constipation lasting longer than 3 or 4 days may be treated by using a cathartic suppository such as bisacodyl (Dulcolax). If this measure is ineffective, a sodium phosphate (Fleet) enema is suggested.

Diet therapy. The nurse collaborates with the dietitian to provide the starved anorexic with a diet that has an adequate fiber content (3 to 6 g daily). The fiber content of the diet for clients with bowel elimination problems may be gradually increased until it includes 12 to 18 g of fiber. An adequate fluid intake (at least 1500 mL/day) is essential. The dietitian will also include foods in the diet that enhance elimination, such as wheat bran, fresh fruits, fresh vegetables, and prunes or prune juice.

Other interventions. Physical activity enhances regular bowel elimination. Although the starved anorexic is restricted from rigorous exercise, walking around the unit is usually permitted. Warm fluids such as coffee, tea, or hot water, which stimulate the gastrocolic reflex, also help.

Prevention of complications. When the regular bowel regimen, suppositories, or enemas do not adequately relieve constipation, the nurse suspects a fecal impaction. Digital disimpaction may be necessary.

Anxiety

Planning: client goals. The major goal for this nursing diagnosis is that the client will demonstrate by verbalization and behavior control of the level of anxiety about eating and weight gain.

Interventions: nonsurgical management. The nurse is instrumental in assisting the anorexic to overcome anxiety so that it does not interfere with establishing a healthy eating pattern and consistent weight gain. Emotional support and encouragement are essential during mealtimes or when snacks are eaten. The nurse is present while food is eaten and interrupts statements on the client's part related to the number of calories being consumed or potential weight gain. The nurse guides the client through the meal with reminders to continue eating or to try an untouched food on the plate. Social conversation is encouraged unless the client uses talking as a means to avoid eating. In this case, the nurse discourages conversation during the meal. Although supportive measures are emphasized, introduction of antianxiety agents before meals may be necessary in the early stages of nutritional rehabilitation.

The nurse does not bargain with the client to ex-

change foods or to eliminate any of the presented items. The client is reminded that food is the "medicine" that will save her or his life and, therefore, the nurse holds firm in the expectation that all food presented will be eaten.

The time after meals or snacks is often one when the anorexic feels anxious about the number of calories consumed. The nurse provides emotional support and acceptance of the client's feelings.

Drug therapy. Extremely anxious clients who do not begin to eat despite supportive nursing interventions may require an antianxiety agent before meals are presented. A short-acting anxiolytic agent such as lorazepam (Ativan), 0.5 mg 1 hour before meals, may decrease anxiety enough so that the client makes the decision to eat.

Other interventions. Allowing the client to control some decisions may decrease anxiety. The nurse decides which decisions are negotiable and which are not. For example, after the menu is planned, it is not renegotiated. However, the time or place of the meal may be. The nurse might ask, "Do you want to have breakfast at 7 AM today?" or "Do you want to eat in your room or in the lounge this morning?" Allowing the client input into other non–food-related decisions may also decrease anxiety and increase cooperation. Another intervention that gives the client a sense of control is the use of deep breathing exercises and relaxation techniques.

Prevention of complications. The nurse maintains a calm demeanor that conveys to the client the message that the necessary support is available to prevent an uncontrolled feeling of anxiety. The nurse deflects rather than absorbs the client's anxiety and promotes feelings of safety and security. Parents, spouses, and friends are not permitted to be present during meals.

Body Image Disturbance

Planning: client goals. The goal for this nursing diagnosis is that the client will develop a realistic perception of body size.

Interventions: nonsurgical management. The anorexic client often has disturbances in self-concept related to personal identity, self-esteem, and role performance. The most common disturbance, however, is in the area of body image, which manifests itself in an inability to perceive body size and needs accurately. The client who overestimates the size of her or his own body or who expresses the belief that one part or all of the body is too large even when emaciated is encouraged by the nurse to express feelings about body size and function as well as self. The nurse points out misperceptions but does not argue with the client. For example, in response to a statement that the client's stomach is too large, the nurse acknowledges that the client's body is once more becoming stronger and healthier and is functioning in a more normal way. The client is given support, and affirmative statements are made related to an accurate perception of body size and function, e.g., positive feedback for a statement that the client feels hungry before a meal. The nurse assists the client in an ongoing way to accept the changes occurring in body size and function and provides an opportunity for communication of concerns and identification of strengths.

Ineffective Individual Coping

Planning: client goals. The major goal for this nursing diagnosis is that the client will demonstrate behaviors and statements that indicate self-control.

Interventions: nonsurgical management. The nurse concentrates efforts on assisting the client to use previously developed healthy coping measures and to learn new methods of coping. Collaboration with the hospital's consulting psychiatrist and/or psychiatric liaison nurse is essential in providing care related to the diagnosis. Individual therapy with one of these health professionals during the period of hospitalization enhances the supportive therapy provided by the nurse.

Drug therapy. The nurse explores with the client new ways of coping with the problems of everyday living. Unless a diagnosis of depression is made for which antidepressant therapy is indicated, the client is not given medication.

Diet therapy. The structure provided by the approach described for the first nursing diagnosis assists the client to stay in control of eating, thereby gaining self-confidence while exploring healthy ways of coping with problems that do not involve eating.

Psychotherapy. Individual therapy may begin with a psychiatrist, a psychologist, or the psychiatric liaison nurse while the client is an inpatient. It is essential that provisions be made for psychotherapy to continue after discharge from the hospital.

Support groups. Groups that are organized by recovering anorexics and/or families may be available to the client and family. These groups help clients and families to become better educated about anorexia nervosa. They also provide a support system during periods of extreme stress for the client and family. These groups are not psychotherapy groups and are usually not led by health professionals.

Occupational/recreational therapy. Many hospitals have occupational therapy departments that provide services for medical clients. If such services are unavailable, arrangements might be made with the inpatient psychiatric service to include the client in groups providing assertiveness training, relaxation techniques, creative expressions, art therapy, and dance therapy. The group setting provides a vehicle for interaction and socialization with others who can give feedback about the client's behaviors.

Potential for Noncompliance

Planning: client goals. Two major goals are that the client will (1) comply with the treatment plan and (2) continue to participate in a treatment program as recommended by the treatment team.

Interventions: nonsurgical management. The anorexic has developed behaviors over time that, although unhealthy, help her or him to cope with the problems of adolescence and life. The fear of fatness that is part of the illness contributes significantly to the maintenance of these unhealthy behaviors and makes the likelihood of noncompliance predictable. Interventions that increase the likelihood of compliance are those discussed for the preceding nursing diagnoses. There is no magic formula to solve the problem of noncompliance. Monitoring behavior and providing support are key nursing interventions, which, when combined with motivation on the client's part to move away from illness and toward health, can influence significantly successful completion of a treatment program. The psychiatric liaison nurse is an important resource for planning care with the nurse.

Noncompliance with treatment for anorexia nervosa can be life-threatening. The nurse teaches the client and family specifics related to the illness and treatment plan and emphasizes the consequences of noncompliance. Assistance is provided in finding an inpatient psychiatric program for treatment when indicated or in arranging appropriate outpatient psychiatric treatment. Anorexics are frequently treated during a crisis on a medical unit where ongoing treatment is not an option. The client and family may not understand that anorexia nervosa is a psychiatric illness and that many specialized programs are available to them. Such teaching and assistance with referral by the nurse may prevent serious complications and years of suffering for the client and family. The parents of a minor with anorexia nervosa that has reached a life-threatening stage may need information about placing their child in a psychiatric facility. This placement can be done even when the child does not want treatment. An adult whose illness has reached the life-threatening stage may also be committed for care to a psychiatric facility by two physicians who conclude that the client is a danger to herself or himself. Laws for such commitment vary from state to state, and the institution's legal department can provide the treatment team with such information.

Altered Family Processes

Planning: client goals. Two major goals related to this diagnosis are that the family will (1) demonstrate an understanding of the client's illness and (2) support the client by following the recommendations of the interdisciplinary health care team.

Interventions: nonsurgical management. Families are usually frightened for their anorexic member. They may be frustrated and angry about behaviors that they do not understand. They may feel guilty that perhaps they helped to cause the illness or that they cannot seem to stop it. The nurse assists family members to understand the illness and the method of treatment being implemented by the team. The nurse teaches the family the details of the emotional and physical manifestations of anorexia nervosa. Family members are assisted in gaining an understanding of the treatment approach and the rationale for specific interventions.

Families in considerable distress are assisted in making contact with the social worker responsible for the client's case. The social worker assesses the family dynamics and provides therapy as needed. If family therapy cannot be provided by the social worker, an outside referral may be necessary to support the family.

■ Discharge Planning

Home Care Preparation

The client with anorexia nervosa who has established a regular pattern of weight gain and whose behavior indicates a motivation to give up the illness may be discharged to home. Clients who verbalize a need for inpatient treatment or whose behavior makes it unlikely that outpatient treatment will be successful are transferred to a psychiatric facility for inpatient treatment. The ideal placement is a facility specializing in the treatment of eating disorders. It is absolutely essential for the client to have either inpatient or outpatient therapy arranged before being discharged from the medical unit.

Client/Family Education

During the client's hospital stay, the nurse focuses educational efforts on teaching the client and family to recognize and understand the physical, behavioral, and emotional characteristics of anorexia nervosa. The teaching plan is individualized to identify the problems specific to the client, e.g., food restriction, laxative abuse, hypothermia, hypokalemia, or distorted body image. Emphasis is placed on the importance of viewing anorexia nervosa as a psychiatric illness that is treated most effectively by mental health professionals through individual, group, and family therapy.

The client and family are taught to use food patterns and food exchanges by the nurse and dietitian. For the family whose anorexic member is returning home, the importance of eating together as a family is stressed. The client is encouraged to normalize both eating and family relationships. The family is cautioned not to use mealtimes to resolve family conflicts or to center on the anorexic and comment on eating behavior.

The nurse helps parents of teen-aged anorexics to set limits with their child that involve consequences for noncompliance. This teaching is done effectively by role modeling appropriate interventions for them, e.g., refusing to be drawn into discussions about the fairness of interventions. The anorexic must know with certainty that weight loss or refusal to attend outpatient psychotherapy sessions will result in action on the parents' part to admit the child for inpatient treatment.

Discharge teaching also includes information about the type and amount of exercise suggested for the client, which is particularly important if the anorexic has a history of overexercising.

Psychosocial Preparation

Whether the client is discharged to home with outpatient treatment or to an inpatient psychiatric setting, the client and family need much education and support. It is often difficult for clients and families to accept a psychiatric diagnosis because of the fear that they will be stigmatized and perhaps labeled as "crazy." They are encouraged to discuss their fears and concerns with the nurse to correct misconceptions about the illness and its treatment. The nurse emphasizes the availability of health care professionals and lay support groups. It is acknowledged that the illness is quite serious and that patience and hard work are necessary on the part of each family member. Families are encouraged to confront existing problems such as marital conflict and to seek treatment, which the nurse can help arrange.

Health Care Resources

If the client cannot return home for outpatient treatment, arrangements are made for appropriate inpatient treatment. The psychiatrist, psychiatric liaison nurse, or both provide information about inpatient facilities and assist the family in obtaining such treatment.

Some communities have anorexia nervosa organizations that offer support groups for clients and families. Hospitals with treatment programs may also provide such groups. These support groups do not take the place of individual or group psychotherapy for the client or of family therapy for the client and family. They do provide the opportunity for interaction with other individuals who have firsthand knowledge of the effects of anorexia nervosa and who can empathize and offer information about dealing with the illness.

The client and family may seek appropriate resource information from The National Anorexic Aid Society, Inc., as well as two other organizations: Anorexia Nervosa and Related Eating Disorders, Inc., and The National Association of Anorexia Nervosa and Associated Disorders, Inc.

 Evaluation

The nurse examines the effectiveness of the interventions described in the care plan to eliminate each problem identified. The outcome expectations for the client with anorexia nervosa related to the nursing diagnoses are that the client

1. Develops an eating pattern that meets daily nutritional needs
2. Maintains a healthy weight within a 5-lb range set by the health care team

3. Experiences minimal abdominal discomfort during refeeding
4. Ceases to use purging techniques to control weight
5. Maintains a fluid and electrolyte state that is reflective of normal balance
6. Experiences minimal evidence of and discomfort from refeeding edema
7. Verbalizes and behaves in manner that indicates decreased anxiety about food and weight and a sense of self-control and that reflects healthy coping strategies
8. Verbalizes a realistic and positive attitude toward body size and function
9. Verbalizes a willingness to receive treatment suggested by the health care team, e.g., inpatient or outpatient care

Additional outcome criteria are that the family members

1. Verbalize an understanding of anorexia nervosa as an illness and describe appropriate treatment modalities
2. Support the treatment team's recommendations for treatment
3. Verbalize a willingness to engage in family therapy as recommended by the treatment team

Treatment of the client with anorexia nervosa on a medical unit is a first step. If this treatment is successful in modifying the client's behaviors and obtaining cooperation with treatment plans, the outlook for the anorexic is optimistic. However, many of the client's and family's problems are not addressed adequately in this setting. The assistance of a psychiatric health professional is needed to identify and treat many of the problems mentioned earlier.

BULIMIA NERVOSA

OVERVIEW

Bulimia nervosa is an eating disorder that is characterized by episodes of binge-eating that recur, are uncontrolled, and involve the ingestion of a large amount of food in a short time. This binge-eating is usually followed by some form of purging behavior such as vomiting and/or the excessive use of laxatives or diuretics. The binge-eating usually results in feelings of depression and self-deprecating thoughts. Johnson and Connors (1987) reviewed research data and reported that about 50% of bulimics studied binge-eat daily or more often. Mitchell et al. (1981) gathered information from

40 bulimic clients about the frequency of binge-eating, the duration of a binge, and the number of calories consumed. These clients experienced an average of 11.7 binge-eating episodes a week, with a mean duration per episode of 1.18 hours. Foods chosen for a binge are frequently sweets or carbohydrates. The number of calories consumed during a binge-eating episode varies but is often high. Mitchell et al. (1985) reported a range of 1200 to 11,500 kcal per binge, with an average of 3415 kcal, in the 275 bulimic clients in their sample. The cost of a binge may range from a few dollars to more than $50 (Johnson et al., 1982). Most bulimics studied reported eating amounts of food in a binge that had far more calories than a normal meal. They tended to intersperse binge-purge episodes with periods of minimal food intake and did not eat normal meals. A common habit that was identified among bulimics was chewing and spitting out food without swallowing, but it has not received much attention in the literature (Mitchell et al., 1985).

Purging behavior is an attempt to regain a sense of control and to eliminate the calories ingested. After reviewing research related to purging behaviors, Johnson and Connors (1987) reported that vomiting was the preferred method of purging, with about 50% of the bulimics reporting at least daily vomiting and another 2.5% vomiting weekly or more often. Approximately 35% of the bulimics used laxatives at least weekly. Of the 40 clients in the Mitchell et al. (1981) sample, 37 reported vomiting an average of 11.7 times a week. The usual pattern was to terminate a binge with vomiting. Mitchell et al. (1985) gathered data on abnormal illness behaviors and found that 100% of their sample reported binge-eating, 88.1% indulged in self-induced vomiting, 60.6% abused laxatives, 33.1% abused diuretics, and 64.5% chewed and spit out food. In addition, the researchers found that more than one-third of their study population of 275 reported a history of problems with alcohol and other drugs.

Like the anorexic, the bulimic has an intense fear of fatness. This intense fear distinguishes the bulimic from individuals who binge-eat for pleasure or for reduction of stress.

Some controversy exists about whether bulimia nervosa is a separate syndrome from anorexia nervosa because the clinical manifestations of bulimia, i.e., binging and purging, occur in individuals at varied body weights ranging from starved to overweight. Figure 46–5 illustrates the overlapping nature of eating disorders and obesity. It shows that some clients with anorexia nervosa maintain low weight by food restriction alone, whereas others use purging behaviors to rid themselves of unwanted calories and may at times indulge in an eating binge. Normal-weight bulimics experiencing the binge-purge cycle frequently have a ± 10 lb weight fluctuation. The high-weight bulimic overlaps with the obese client who overeats but does not purge or have a morbid fear of fatness.

There is value in approaching bulimia nervosa as a

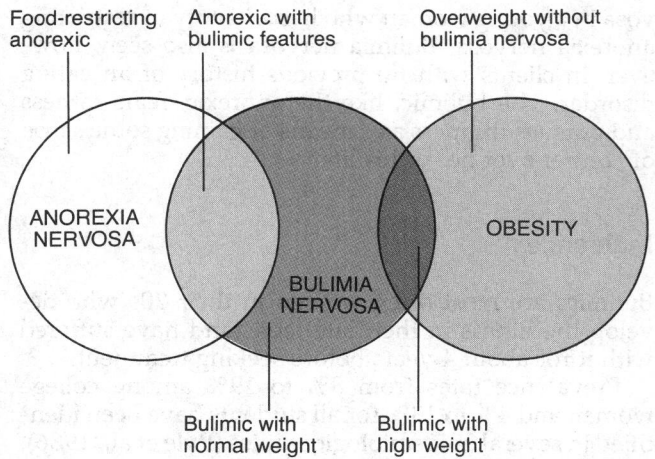

Food-restricting anorexic

Anorexic with bulimic features

Overweight without bulimia nervosa

ANOREXIA NERVOSA

OBESITY

BULIMIA NERVOSA

Bulimic with normal weight

Bulimic with high weight

Figure 46–5

Schematic representation of the overlapping relationship between eating disorders and obesity. (Adapted from Fairburn, C. [1982]. Binge-eating and bulimia nervosa. *SK&F Publications*, 1, 15.)

separate syndrome when the client is of normal weight or slightly overweight, because the problems related to impulse control seen in the bulimic require a different therapeutic approach from that used with anorexics. Treatments vary and include many psychotherapeutic approaches (Garner & Garfinkel, 1985; Root et al., 1986), as well as use of drugs (Garfinkel & Garner, 1987).

Like the anorexic, the bulimic may come to the attention of the medical community because of sequelae related to the disorder. It is critical to recognize the clinical manifestations of this psychiatric illness to avoid the misconception that there is a physically treatable origin. Accurate diagnosis can eliminate the extensive upper and lower gastrointestinal tract studies that are frequently done for the individual suffering from bulimia nervosa. The bulimic may be ashamed and embarrassed by purging behaviors and choose to undergo uncomfortable tests rather than to speak honestly with the health care professional.

Reports of bulimic behavior, especially binge-eating, date back to Gull's (1874) early case studies, which described the behavior in clients with anorexia nervosa. Descriptions of binge-purge behaviors continued to be reported mainly as they related to anorexia nervosa but became more frequent around 1940. Binge-eating in obese persons was first labeled as such by Stunkard in 1959. It was not until the 1970s that the high incidence of bulimic behaviors in normal-weight individuals was investigated and reported by Russell (1970) and others.

Pathophysiology

The bulimic secretly eats enormous quantities of food—often concentrated sweets or fats—very rapidly with-out appreciating the taste. The onset of a binge may be precipitated by a variety of factors such as hunger, boredom, anger, anxiety, or depression. The precipitant is not physiologic as in Prader-Willi syndrome, hypothalamic tumor, or increased metabolic demands related to hyperthyroidism or diabetes mellitus.

The diagnostic criteria for bulimia nervosa of the American Psychiatric Association are identified in the accompanying Key Features of Disease. These criteria are accepted and appropriate and guide decisions regarding diagnosis and treatment. The name of this disorder was changed in 1987 to bulimia nervosa when the DSM-III was revised. This change was made to distinguish the binge-purge symptoms, i.e., bulimia, from the disorder, i.e., bulimia nervosa. It was necessary because the symptoms occur in both anorexia nervosa and bulimia nervosa.

The term *bulimia* literally means "ox hunger." It implies that bulimics eat huge amounts of food because of a voracious appetite. However, most bulimics report they often eat for reasons unrelated to actual hunger. Although hunger may trigger a binge, it is probably sustained by other factors. Many bulimics do experience a weight gain on a low number of calories, e.g., 1000 to 1200, and this probably contributes to the problem of binging and purging. The bulimic feels hungry and deprived on such a restricted diet and gives in to the urge to binge. The bulimic also quickly finds that purging by vomiting is easier if large quantities of foods and fluids are ingested, and a vicious cycle begins.

The bulimic individual is aware that her or his eating pattern is abnormal and fears the actual loss of control over eating, i.e., an inability to stop eating once started. The bulimic may also experience difficulty with other types of impulse control, and alcohol or drug abuse, sexual promiscuity, or acts of stealing may result. The bulimic frequently suffers from depression and must be considered at risk for suicide.

KEY FEATURES OF DISEASE ■ DSM-III-R Diagnostic Criteria for Bulimia Nervosa

A. Recurrent episodes of binge-eating (rapid consumption of a large amount of food in a discrete period of time).

B. A feeling of lack of control over eating behavior during the eating binges.

C. The person regularly engages in self-induced vomiting, use of laxatives or diuretics, strict dieting or fasting, or vigorous exercise to prevent weight gain.

D. A minimum average of two binge eating episodes a week for at least 3 months.

E. Persistent overconcern with body shape and weight.

Reprinted with permission from the *Diagnostic and statistical manual of mental disorders*, Third Edition, Revised. Copyright 1987 American Psychiatric Association.

Etiology

It is possible to describe typical bulimic behavior but much more difficult to identify the cause. Research has shown that a high percentage of bulimics experience the onset of bulimic symptoms after undertaking a rigid diet (Fairburn & Cooper, 1984; Johnson et al., 1982; Pyle et al., 1981). Studies designed to identify factors that precipitate the binge-purge syndrome involve self-reporting by bulimics. Factors so identified are depression, loneliness, boredom, anger, interpersonal conflicts related to job or relationships, and issues of individuation and identity. The illness often starts in the late teens and coincides with loss or separation from family and friends.

The social pressure to be thin that is experienced by both sexes, but particularly women, is a major factor contributing to the development of bulimia nervosa. Biologic factors include a history of being at least slightly overweight and a vulnerability to fluctuation in mood state. Individuals at risk frequently have great conflict in their familial relationships, as well as personality traits that present difficulties with self-esteem and impulse control or self-discipline. The bulimic feels dysphoric, i.e., has a feeling of ill-being and dissatisfaction, and indulges in a binge, which temporarily relieves the feeling. The relief does not last long because the binge engenders feelings of guilt, shame, and self-disgust. The bulimic then attempts to undo the effects of the binge, regain control, and release tension through some form of purging behavior. Guilt and fear of discovery follow purging. A cycle is rapidly established that alternates between uncontrollable binging and purging and attempts at intense dietary restriction. Figure 46–6 illustrates the relationship between etiologic factors and pathways that end in a binge-purge cycle.

It is not unusual to find a diagnosis of bulimia ner-vosa in a young woman who has a history of restricting anorexia nervosa. Bulimia nervosa is also seen, however, in clients with no previous history of an eating disorder. The bulimic, like the anorexic, fears fatness and pursues thinness as a means of gaining some sense of control over her or his life.

Incidence

Bulimics are most often women in their 20s who develop the illness in their late teens and have suffered with it for about 4 years before seeking treatment.

Prevalence rates from 8% to 19% among college women and 4% to 13% for all students have been identified in several epidemiologic studies (Pyle et al., 1986). Bulimia nervosa in males has been reported at a prevalence rate of 1% to 6% (Pyle, 1985). A 1980 study of first-year female college students replicated in the same area in 1983 showed an increase of about 2% in bulimia nervosa over the 3-year period (Pyle et al., 1986). Hudson et al. (1985) reported that the prevalence of bulimia nervosa among adolescent and young adult females with diabetes mellitus equaled or exceeded that reported in age-matched populations of nondiabetic women. The combination of bulimia nervosa and diabetes mellitus creates the potential for serious health problems in the client.

PREVENTION

Health education aimed at counteracting the influence of social factors that contribute to the development and maintenance of eating disorders is essential in helping young women, and occasionally young men, avoid striving for a physiologically inappropriate weight. Sen-

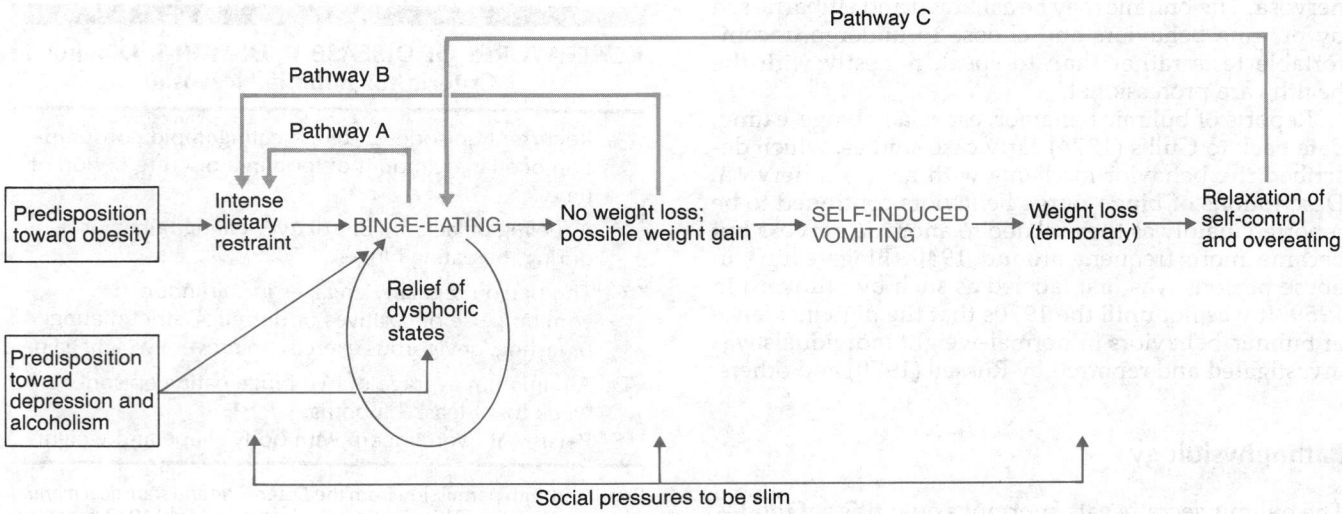

Figure 46–6

Etiologic factors and their relationship to the binge-purge cycle. (From Fairburn, C. [1982]. Binge-eating and bulimia nervosa. *SK&F Publications, 1,* 13.)

sitivity is needed when assisting overweight teen-agers and children to control weight and to develop healthy eating habits.

Early intervention with a mental health professional is indicated when the young person uses eating behaviors as a means of gaining control or coping with the problems of adolescence. The young person can be assisted in using direct methods to solve the developmental problems of individuation and identity formation rather than indirect methods such as abnormal eating behaviors. Such early intervention may prevent development of the disorder.

COLLABORATIVE MANAGEMENT

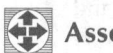 **Assessment**

History

Data are collected by the nurse from the client and family. The nurse is instrumental in gathering information that leads to an accurate diagnosis of this psychiatric illness and avoids costly and unnecessary medical tests.

The history gathered from the bulimic client is *similar to that gathered from the anorexic* (see earlier). Changes in the emphasis of questions are suggested. When gathering data about medical problems and clinical manifestations, the nurse emphasizes questions related to the *sequelae of vomiting and laxative abuse.* The nurse asks if the client has had diagnoses or treatment for *cardiac, renal,* or *gastrointestinal tract* difficulties. The client is questioned about a history of *seizures,* as well as about the use of *ipecac syrup* to induce vomiting.

The *weight history* uncovers any previous history of anorexia nervosa. The nurse gathers specific information about highest weight, lowest weight, and fluctuations in weight, e.g., how much weight is gained or lost, the time period, and how often fluctuations occur.

The client with bulimia nervosa may be *sexually active.* Information about the frequency and duration of sexually intimate relationships is sought, as well as information about the use of contraceptives and knowledge of birth control techniques. Reports from health care professionals treating clients with bulimia nervosa indicate that nearly 50% of these clients have suffered sexual abuse (Wooley & Wooley, 1986). Questioning about sexual abuse requires great care and sensitivity, and the nurse often postpones such discussion until a sense of trust is developed between client and nurse.

Questions about *attitudes and behaviors related to food and weight* are the same as those for anorexia nervosa. Information about *binges* should be specific and include the number of binges per day, the amount and type of food favored for binges, and the *method of purging.* Careful questioning by the nurse is needed to identify the client's *feelings* before, during, and after a binge-purge episode.

Information about *activity level* is obtained in the same way as for the anorexic. The bulimic may report decreased activity, which the nurse explores in more detail because it may be related to feelings of depression.

Careful attention is paid by the nurse to gathering data about *previous episodes of psychiatric illness.* Questions about previous treatment for an eating disorder, alcohol or drug abuse, anxiety disorder, depression, or suicide attempt are indicated.

If the client reports a history of alcohol or drug abuse, promiscuous behavior, or stealing, a *legal history* is taken by the nurse, which may reveal information about arrests and consequences such as probation, fines, or prison terms. Resulting difficulties related to school, work, or social or familial relationships are explored.

The *family history* questions are also those identified for the anorexic. The client is asked to describe the present living situation. The bulimic often lives away from the nuclear family. Important information is gathered by the nurse from both the client and the family about the family's knowledge of and attitude toward the eating disorder. The nurse asks about a history of any family therapy and the family's perception of their experience with it.

Physical Assessment: Clinical Manifestations

The client with bulimia nervosa presents with what looks like a normal, healthy body. However, bulimic practices create a high risk for serious physical complications. Figure 46–3 illustrates the *physical signs* seen in the client with bulimia nervosa. The starred items are particularly applicable to the bulimic. This figure shows a thin person because it is used to illustrate signs for both bulimia nervosa and anorexia nervosa, but the bulimic client is only slightly underweight, of normal weight, or overweight.

The physical assessment by the nurse may reveal complaints of *weakness, tiredness, constipation,* and *depression.* Such complaints, coupled with an *irregular pulse,* alert the nurse to a possible electrolyte imbalance resulting from practices of vomiting or laxative abuse. Ipecac syrup abuse can result in cardiotoxicity. These practices can lead to serious abnormalities in electrolyte levels, such as hypokalemia, and cardiac dysrhythmias, which can result in cardiac arrest and sudden death. The nurse uses data obtained from the electrocardiogram and laboratory tests to assess the immediate danger from such clinical manifestations (see under the later heading Laboratory Findings). The chronic hypokalemia that results from frequent vomiting, laxative abuse, and diuretic abuse can also cause kidney disturbances or damage. The nurse assesses for current evidence of *pain* or signs of *urinary tract infection* because these are often evident in bulimic clients who experience dehydration and ketonuria. Other serious complications of electrolyte imbalance considered by the nurse are *seizures* and *peripheral paresthesias,* i.e., pricking or tingling sensations on the skin.

The frequent practice of purging by vomiting causes *dry mouth* and *swelling of the parotid glands* with some tenderness but usually not pain. The nurse assesses the teeth for signs of frequent exposure to gastric acid, e.g., *loss of tooth enamel* and a *color change* to brown or gray, as well as evidence of *caries* and *periodontal disease.*

Gastrointestinal tract disturbances range from *esophagitis,* or inflammation of the esophagus, to the serious complication of *gastric dilation,* which is extreme expansion of the stomach caused by binge-eating. This gastric dilation has caused stomach rupture and even death. The nurse assesses the client for abdominal distention, listens for bowel sounds, and questions the client about abdominal pain. Abdominal distention with pain in the absence of bowel sounds signifies an emergency situation. Chronic laxative abuse can lead to permanent *loss of bowel reactivity* and prolapse of the rectum. Other signs of laxative abuse include recurrent abdominal pain, steatorrhea (fatty stools), and finger swelling or clubbing.

Dieting and purging cause fluctuations in fluid balance: episodes of *dehydration* alternate with rebound water retention. The nurse often detects in the bulimic an immediate weight gain, and also edema in hands and feet, related to *rebound fluid retention* after cessation of purging behavior. Proper fluid balance gradually returns after purging behaviors stop completely. The frequent fluctuations in weight may also interfere with the regularity of the menstrual cycle. Even at normal weight, the bulimic may have *irregular menses* or amenorrhea.

Skin integrity is assessed by the nurse who observes for tenting, which may be present if dehydration is severe. Scars on the knuckles of hands and calluses on the abdomen may indicate self-purging behaviors. Scars from cuts or burns may indicate self-mutilating behaviors or suicide attempts.

Psychosocial Assessment

The typical bulimic is a Caucasian female in her early to mid-20s of middle to upper socioeconomic status who frequently has problems with separation-individuation and identity formation related to family. The accompanying Key Features of Disease compares and contrasts features of anorexia nervosa and bulimia nervosa. It emphasizes the bulimic's greater awareness of inner states—both physiologic, such as hunger, and psychologic, such as depression. The bulimic's decreased ability to control urges and impulses can lead to difficulties in several areas besides food and weight. The bulimic has a poorly defined self-image and low self-esteem and is frequently sensitive to criticism while experiencing excessive need for approval. The bulimic tends to be an extroverted individual who is willing to discuss with the nurse feelings about the illness and psychologic distress. Bulimics may have hysterical, obsessional, borderline, or antisocial personality traits, which become emphasized during the illness. Hysterical clients may be self-dramatizing and emotionally labile, with outbursts of anger or crying spells. The bulimic with obsessional tendencies may be caught up in thoughts of food and planning all activities around binge-purge episodes. The client with borderline tendencies may have a serious

KEY FEATURES OF DISEASE ■ Differential Features of Anorexia Nervosa and Bulimia

Anorexia Nervosa	Bulimia
Rare vomiting or diuretic/laxative abuse	Vomiting or diuretic/laxative abuse
More severe weight loss	Less weight loss
Slightly younger	Slightly older
More introverted	More extroverted
Hunger denied	Hunger experienced
Eating behavior may be considered normal and source of esteem	Eating behavior considered foreign and source of distress
Sexually inactive	More sexually active
Obsessional features predominate	More hysterical or borderline features as well as obsessional features
Death from starvation (or suicide, in chronically ill)	Death from hypokalemia or suicide
Amenorrhea	Menses irregular or absent
More favorable prognosis	Less favorable prognosis
Fewer behavioral abnormalities	Stealing, drug and alcohol abuse, self-mutilation, and other behavioral abnormalities

From Andersen, A. E. (1985). *Practical comprehensive treatment of anorexia nervosa and bulimia* (p. 10). Baltimore: The Johns Hopkins University Press.

psychopathology that leads to various harmful practices such as shoplifting, inappropriate expression of anger or lack of control of anger, or acts of self-harm such as burning, cutting, or suicide gestures. The bulimic client with borderline features is often uncertain about issues of identity such as self-image, values, and loyalties and may have a pattern of unstable relationships. Clinical manifestations suggestive of antisocial personality traits in a bulimic client are excessive use of drugs or alcohol, promiscuous behavior, stealing, lying, and behavior problems at school or work. These examples are the extreme, and the nurse is careful not to draw quick conclusions about a client's behavior during the initial assessment nor to define behavior in a way that will label the bulimic.

The bulimic individual is usually aware that eating food serves to relieve emotional distress but also starts the cycle that leads to feelings of low self-esteem and depression. The bulimic feels the discomfort related to the eating disorder and is aware of personal mood state and can describe feeling depressed, demoralized, and hopeless. These feelings may lead to thoughts of suicide or to actual attempts, which initiate the client's first contact with health care providers.

The bulimic may experience relief from depression as well as help in controlling binge-eating by treatment with tricyclic antidepressants such as nortriptyline hydrochloride (Aventyl) and desipramine hydrochloride (Norpramin) or with monoamine oxidase inhibitors such as phenelzine sulfate (Nardil) and tranylcypromine sulfate (Parnate). The nurse's assessment includes questions about such prior or current treatment for depression and its effectiveness. The assessment reveals any suicide attempts, and questions are asked about the method used, the number of attempts, and what happened to prevent completion of the attempt to assess the lethality of the attempt. If cutting or burning is used in a nonlethal manner, the nurse assesses for evidence of a pattern of self-mutilating behavior that the client may use to relieve tension and decrease anxiety.

The nurse's assessment of the client's social pattern explores changes over time. Although the client may be outgoing and friendly, careful questioning reveals that the bulimic's social life is significantly affected by the illness. Social events where food is served may be avoided because of a fear of losing control and binging in public. Some bulimics find that they have no time for a social life because they work or go to school during the day and spend each evening, and perhaps all weekend, binging and purging. They tend to have few close friends, and their interpersonal relationships vary from superficial to dependent. As the illness becomes chronic, they become more isolated and withdrawn from relationships. They may describe a "false" sense of self and report that this is what they allow others to know of them but that it is different from their "real" self.

Family dynamics are assessed initially and in an ongoing manner to identify the extent of the client's support system as well as any conflictual relationships among family members. The nurse gathers information about the family's knowledge of the client's illness behaviors and their attitudes about them. The nurse determines what efforts have been made to help the client and by which family members. Intensely close or distant relationships are identified. The nurse observes family interaction and watches to see if family members speak for each other, and the nurse asks questions related to how the family members resolve conflicts and angry feelings. In this way, useful information about the relationship of bulimic episodes to a lack of conflict resolution may be gained. The nurse assesses how the family presents itself, e.g. as perfect, overprotective, or chaotic.

During the entire assessment, the nurse observes the client and identifies strengths, which provides a basis for forming a relationship and together planning nursing care. Some of these strengths may be communication skills, the ability to describe feelings, and a motivation to give up unhealthy behaviors and to learn new ways of coping with problems.

Laboratory Findings

The SMA-6 (6/60) and SMA-12 (12/60) give valuable information about electrolyte and fluid balance as well as kidney function. An elevated blood urea nitrogen level indicates dehydration. Dehydration associated with hypokalemia might predispose the client to develop serious renal problems. A complete blood count with differential reveals blood abnormalities such as anemia or a bleeding tendency if present. Endocrine studies usually reveal normal levels of luteinizing hormone and follicle-stimulating hormone and may show a prolactin elevation. Female bulimics who are amenorrheic or who have irregular menses may have low luteinizing hormone and low follicle-stimulating hormone levels and a low urinary estrogen level. A low testosterone level may be revealed in the male bulimic who reports a loss of interest in sex. Thyroid studies show normal levels of tyroxine, tri-iodothyronine resin uptake, and plasma tri-iodothyronine in most bulimics. These studies may help with regard to determining a differential diagnosis such as hyperthyroidism or Addison's disease. Bulimics, like anorexics, exhibit a high rate of dexamethasone nonsuppression when a dexamethasone suppression test is done (see Chap. 48). A urinalysis with microscopic analysis is ordered to screen for urinary tract infections. Any suspicion of drug or alcohol abuse justifies toxicologic screens of blood and urine.

Other Diagnostic Tests

An electrocardiogram is essential to the physical assessment of the bulimic client to screen for dysrhythmias that may be life-threatening and the result of hypokalemia or ipecac toxicity. A routine chest x-ray film is included in the assessment. Upper and lower gastrointestinal tract studies may be necessary if the client has seriously damaged the gastrointestinal tract by vomiting, which exposes the esophageal mucosa to acidic gastric contents, or by laxative abuse, which produces clinical manifestations of irritable bowel syndrome.

Psychologic testing is indicated and facilitated by collaboration with the hospital's consulting psychiatrist and/or psychiatric liaison nurse. The tests ordered for a bulimic client are similar to those suggested for the anorexic and are usually performed by a clinical psychologist (see under the heading Other Diagnostic Tests for anorexia nervosa). Involvement of psychiatric specialists is crucial if the bulimic client is admitted to the hospital as a result of a suicide attempt or if depression and suicidal thoughts are prominent in the client's presentation.

 Analysis: Nursing Diagnosis

Common Diagnoses

Eight nursing diagnoses are common in the client and family when bulimia nervosa is present:

1. Altered nutrition: more than body requirements related to increased food intake
2. Potential for decreased cardiac output related to alteration in rhythm caused by hypokalemia
3. Fluid volume excess related to edema with cessation of vomiting and laxative/diuretic abuse
4. Constipation related to chronic laxative abuse
5. Self-esteem disturbance related to overwhelming sense of ineffectiveness
6. Ineffective individual coping related to fears of loss of self-control and fatness
7. Potential for noncompliance (therapeutic recommendations) related to binging, vomiting, laxative abuse, or a decision to leave the hospital against medical advice
8. Altered family processes related to difficulty in coping with the client's illness and hospitalization

Additional Diagnoses

Clients with bulimia nervosa and their families may also have the following nursing diagnoses:

1. Knowledge deficit related to illness and/or treatment plan
2. Potential for injury related to binging and gastric dilation
3. Potential for altered patterns of urinary elimination related to chronic hypokalemia
4. Pain related to parotid gland swelling
5. Potential for injury related to alteration in integrity of tooth enamel caused by vomiting
6. Potential for injury related to seizure activity from electrolyte imbalance
7. Potential for fluid volume deficit related to purging behaviors
8. Potential for sleep pattern disturbance related to binging and purging episodes at night and/or depressed mood
9. Potential for social isolation related to binge-purge behaviors
10. Ineffective individual coping related to feelings of hopelessness and depressed mood
11. Potential for anxiety related to interruption of binge-purge cycle
12. Potential for violence: self-directed related to suicidal thoughts
13. Potential for sexual dysfunction related to psychosocial vulnerabilities
14. Potential for ineffective family coping: compromised or disabling related to changes in family dynamics brought about by illness
15. Potential for altered health maintenance related to recurrent episodes of illness

Planning and Implementation

A plan of care incorporating the common diagnoses for the client with bulimia follows. The nurse is referred to current psychiatric nursing texts for help in planning interventions for those psychosocial problems not covered in the care plan. Other chapters of this text provide helpful information related to interventions for physical problems not covered here.

Altered Nutrition: More Than Body Requirements

Planning: client goals. The goals for this nursing diagnosis are that the client will (1) develop a healthy eating pattern that does not exceed daily nutritional requirements and (2) maintain weight within a 5-lb range set by the health care team.

Interventions: nonsurgical management. The nurse teaches the client to eat adequate amounts of food from the four basic food groups. Nursing supervision provides emotional support and prevents binging behavior during the stressful period when the client is breaking the binge-purge cycle.

Drug therapy. Some experts in the treatment of bulimia advocate the use of a monoamine oxidase inhibitor such as tranylcypromine sulfate, which they believe decreases the client's urge to binge. Others prefer a supportive, behavioral approach without drugs to break the binge-purge cycle.

Diet therapy. The dietitian determines the client's daily nutritional needs related to basal metabolic rate and suggests the appropriate daily food pattern and number of calories to be used. It is not unusual for these requirements to be quite low for the bulimic, e.g., 1000 to 1200 kcal per day. Because this means that the ingestion of more than the required calories will cause weight gain, the bulimic frequently feels deprived with the small amount of food allowed and is tempted to binge and purge.

The nurse teaches the client to select the correct portion sizes and to think in terms of food patterns rather than counting calories. Bulimics are encouraged to eat slowly and to avoid bolting down their food without really tasting it. Most clients with eating disorders are not permitted to use diet foods and drinks while being treated. The exception is the bulimic who gains weight easily and can eat only a small number of calories, e.g., 1000, to maintain a constant weight. These clients may use artificial sweeteners and diet foods and drinks.

Exercise. The nurse teaches the client the importance of increasing the activity level and developing a regular exercise routine. Bulimics who gain weight on few calories find exercise to be particularly important because it allows for increased caloric intake. The client is cautioned to avoid extremes such over- or underexercising.

Potential for Decreased Cardiac Output

Planning: client goals. The main goal of this nursing diagnosis is that the client will not experience any life-threatening alteration in cardiac rhythm.

Interventions: nonsurgical management. Clients who purge by vomiting or using laxatives and diuretics are at risk for depleting potassium chloride and creating a state of hypokalemic metabolic alkalosis. The depletion of this electrolyte creates a situation that leads to low potassium levels and shrinkage of the effective arterial blood volume. Cardiac dysrhythmias and sudden cardiac arrest can result. (See Chap. 13 for more information on fluid and electrolyte imbalances.) The bulimic who habitually uses ipecac syrup to induce vomiting is also at risk because of its potential for causing cardiotoxicity. When a bulimic client is admitted to the hospital, the nurse is particularly alert for signs of an irregular pulse and/or blood volume depletion, e.g., orthostatic blood pressure changes and tachycardia when the client stands. The client's vital signs are taken on admission to the unit and frequently thereafter, usually every 3 to 4 hours. Blood chemistry tests done on admission reveal the extent of the electrolyte imbalance and guide decisions about interventions.

Drug therapy. Mild potassium depletion (3.0 to 3.4 mEq/L) in an otherwise asymptomatic client may be treated by using oral supplements. More serious electrolyte imbalance requires administration of intravenous sodium chloride solution with potassium.

Prevention of complications. The nurse's initial and ongoing assessments of the client's vital signs identify problems early and prevent serious complications. An electrocardiogram is done and a physician notified when an irregular pulse is detected by the nurse. Behaviors of the bulimic are monitored carefully to prevent purging, which may result in a serious electrolyte imbalance. If purging behaviors are discovered, the nurse's assessment and interventions are those previously identified.

Fluid Volume Excess

Planning: client goals. The goal for this nursing diagnosis is that the client will have minimal occurrence of edema and resulting discomfort.

Interventions: nonsurgical management. The nurse educates the client about the wide swings in fluid balance that result when a person uses vomiting and purgatives to control weight. The client is told to expect the presence of edema, especially in fingers, ankles, and face, and an initial weight gain when purging behaviors are discontinued. The weight gain may be significant,

e.g., 5 to 10 lb, and the nurse supports the client emotionally at this time to prevent resumption of purging behaviors out of fear of fatness. Reassurance is given that the client's body will readjust its fluid balance and that the edema will resolve.

Diet therapy. The nurse collaborates with the dietitian in selecting a low-sodium diet (2 g/day) to minimize fluid retention. The amount of fluid intake is limited to about 1000 mL daily while edema is severe.

Comfort measures. The client is encouraged to elevate the extremities to avoid fluid accumulation in tissues, which occurs when extremities are in a dependent position. The nurse encourages the client to select comfortable and nonconstricting clothing and footwear. The client is instructed to avoid wearing rings when swelling is present in fingers. Assuming a supine position with a cool compress over the face decreases discomfort from facial edema.

Constipation

The main goal for this nursing diagnosis is that the client will establish a regular pattern of elimination that does not depend on the use of laxatives. The nurse follows the care plan for the client with anorexia nervosa for detailed interventions and rationales.

Self-Esteem Disturbance

Planning: client goals. The goal of this nursing diagnosis is that the client will begin to develop a sense of effectiveness while in the hospital setting.

Interventions: nonsurgical management. The nurse realizes that the client's feelings of ineffectiveness and loss of self-esteem come from both a real and an imagined sense of failure. The client has failed to maintain control over eating behaviors. Frequently, however, the sense of failure comes from expectations from both self and family that are unrealistic or even impossible and may be long-standing. The nurse promotes the development of a trusting relationship with the client by interacting on an adult level, explaining hospital routine and expectations of all clients, teaching the client about bulimia nervosa, and helping the client to see that she or he is accepted as a person regardless of the symptoms of the illness. The nurse allows the client to have input into decisions regarding the plan of care while setting firm limits and providing structure related to interrupting unhealthy behaviors. The nurse assists the client in experiencing success in efforts to control eating and purging behaviors and encourages the client to keep a diary of feelings related to urges to binge or purge. Abilities and strengths of the client are identified, and opportunities are provided to use them in specific tasks or projects.

Diet therapy. The nurse incorporates the interventions described earlier for altered nutrition: more than body requirements, as well as teaches the client how to select daily menus from all food groups. The client is encouraged to eat slowly and to appreciate the taste and texture of food. Learning to maintain control over food selection and eating in a healthy way provide a vehicle for success and increase the client's sense of effectiveness.

Exercise. The value of a regular, moderate exercise program is stressed, and the client and nurse together develop an individualized plan. Emphasis is placed on the use of exercise to relieve tension.

Other interventions. The client is assisted to identify patterns of behavior and triggers for binging and purging. Alternative ways of expressing feelings are identified to help the client cope effectively with anxiety and stress. The nurse teaches problem-solving, assertiveness techniques, and communication skills and acts as a role model for the client by using "I" statements and effective communication techniques. Opportunities for role playing to practice new coping skills are provided. The client is given praise for learning and using adaptive coping skills and self-control. She or he is taught to reward and nurture herself or himself with activities that are enjoyable pastimes or hobbies and do not involve food.

Prevention of complications. The initiation of regular psychotherapy sessions with a mental health professional provides an opportunity for the client to further develop and maintain control over eating habits, to experience decreased anxiety, and to learn strategies for dealing with intense feelings and stress. The goal of increasing the client's sense of effectiveness, and by so doing increasing self-esteem and improving self-concept, may seem out of reach to the client. The nurse helps the client to realize that this goal is a long-term one that is achieved by accomplishing a series of small successes. It is emphasized that the process is enhanced by the development of a trusting therapeutic relationship with a mental health professional.

Ineffective Individual Coping

It is suggested that the care plan for the anorexic client with the nursing diagnosis ineffective individual coping be followed and adapted to the bulimic client. Much attention is given to the development of healthy coping skills. Clients who have multiple problems with impulse control, e.g., binge-eating, stealing, drug abuse, or promiscuity, require specialized care plans. Until appropriate inpatient or outpatient treatment is arranged, the nurse seeks assistance from the psychiatric liaison nurse in developing a care plan. Clients suffering from depression may also require treatment with an antidepressant medication. Input from psychiatric consultants is again required.

Potential for Noncompliance

The goals and interventions for this nursing diagnosis for the bulimic client are similar to those for the anorexic. Therefore, adaptation of the care plan for the client with anorexia nervosa is suggested.

The problem of noncompliance becomes particularly serious when the client is being treated with a monoamine oxidase inhibitor to interrupt the binge-purge cycle and treat symptoms of depression. The noncompliant client who binges on foods with a high tyramine content, e.g., aged cheese or chianti wine, may precipitate a hypertensive crisis (see Walsh, 1988, for a report of related research). The nurse improves the possibility of compliance significantly by teaching the client about drug-food interactions and by providing a list of foods to be avoided. It should be noted that after the bulimic's physical condition has stabilized and the binge-purge cycle has been interrupted, many experts recommend outpatient rather than inpatient treatment for this disorder. However, when depression with suicidal ideation is also diagnosed, inpatient psychiatric treatment is indicated.

Altered Family Processes

The nurse follows the care plan for the anorexic client with this nursing diagnosis and adapts it as necessary. For example, all references to anorexia nervosa are changed to bulimia nervosa, and the content of the teaching plan relates to bulimia nervosa. The differences in role expectations are addressed because the bulimic client is usually older than the anorexic and may be living alone or may be married with a husband and children. The nurse may collaborate with the social worker to educate the client and family and to gain their cooperation with the treatment plan.

■ Discharge Planning

Home Care Preparation

Home care preparation for the client with bulimia nervosa is the same as that for the client with anorexia nervosa, as described previously.

Client/Family Education

The educational needs of the bulimic client and family are addressed by the nurse throughout the course of hospitalization. At the time of discharge, the client and family can describe bulimia nervosa, identify the clinical manifestations of the disorder in the client, and identify appropriate interventions to increase healthy coping behaviors and to move the client away from bulimia nervosa toward wellness.

The nurse develops an individualized teaching plan to educate the client and family about the most appropriate treatment approach and the rationale for its use, e.g., inpatient versus outpatient psychiatric treatment, and individual, group, or family therapy.

An essential component of the plan is educating the client about the physical dangers of purging behaviors. Equally important is teaching the bulimic and family to identify the clinical manifestations that indicate an immediate need for medical intervention. Even though bulimics know about the danger of their purging behaviors, they may be unable to control them on their own. They may also have such serious medical sequelae to the behaviors that they are unable to seek help when needed; therefore, their family may have to intervene and transport them to a hospital.

Psychosocial Preparation

The client and family require assistance from the nurse to accept a psychiatric diagnosis and to plan for appropriate treatment. When the client is to be admitted directly from the medical unit to a psychiatric facility, the client and family need the opportunity to discuss their concerns and to ask questions about what to expect. When the client is to return home and have outpatient treatment for bulimia nervosa, both the client and family need the opportunity to discuss their expectations with regard to themselves and others, e.g., will the client allow family members to monitor meals and prevent either binging or vomiting, or will the client accept full responsibility for regulating behavior. The nurse enlists the help of the social worker and/or psychiatric liaison nurse in providing this assistance. The client and family are also encouraged to consider what they will tell friends, extended family, school authorities, or employers about the client's hospitalization and illness. The importance of family therapy is stressed, and the client and family are cautioned to expect that this initial period at home will be difficult for everyone as the bulimic gives up unhealthy coping methods and family members attempt to deal effectively with their interpersonal relationships.

Health Care Resources

The client's follow-up treatment for ongoing physical problems is arranged before discharge. The decision about inpatient or outpatient psychiatric treatment is also made before discharge from the medical unit. The client and family may receive information from the nurse about local resources for persons with eating disorders and their families. The nurse seeks such information from the state department of mental health and hygiene. Further information is obtained from the American Anorexia/Bulimia Association, Inc. These resources provide general information about the illness, as well as specific information about treatment programs and support groups in the area. Clients and families may benefit from involvement with groups established and maintained by individuals who are struggling with the same issues and problems.

 Evaluation

The nurse examines the client goals related to the identified nursing diagnoses to determine whether nursing interventions were effective in accomplishing outcome criteria. Specifically, the outcome criteria include that the client

1. Develops a healthy eating pattern and stops binge-eating
2. Maintains weight within a 5-lb goal weight range
3. Ceases all purging behaviors
4. Complies with interventions to minimize edema
5. Verbalizes an understanding of the consequences of purging behaviors
6. Establishes a bowel elimination pattern not dependent on laxatives
7. Experiences no cardiac dysrhythmias related to electrolyte imbalance while in the hospital
8. Verbalizes an understanding of fluid imbalance caused by binging and purging behaviors
9. Demonstrates an awareness of the relationship of feeling state to unhealthy eating behaviors
10. Develops healthy coping measures to deal with anxiety and fear of fatness
11. Sets realistic goals for self
12. Complies with treatment recommendations while on the medical unit and after discharge

The client who is able to make progress and accomplish outcome criteria successfully will be better prepared to continue efforts to eliminate this eating disorder and develop a more satisfying life style. Clients who are unable to meet outcome criteria may need the structure of an inpatient psychiatric program.

PICA

Pica is a condition in which people, especially children, eat nonfood substances, e.g., paint chips, dirt, pebbles, string, hair, or bugs. An iron or zinc deficiency can cause pica. Mental retardation is a predisposing factor.

The age at onset of pica is usually 12 to 24 months, and the disease usually remits in early childhood. However, pica may continue into adolescence and adulthood. Its cause is not fully understood. Adults with pica may have a long-standing history of the illness and benefit from assistance for both physical and emotional problems. Clients with chronic renal disease have been noted to eat odd items such as cornstarch or clothes starch.

Pica is considered to be a psychiatric diagnosis that is related to emotional deprivation rather than nutritional deficiencies. However, the nurse is alert for deficiencies in dietary intake such as milk, meat, and foods rich in iron and vitamin C and provides appropriate nutritional teaching. If deficiencies occur because of financial limitations, the nurse assists the client in obtaining help from appropriate state and federal agencies.

Clients also receive assistance from the nurse in dealing with emotional problems. The renal client may need help in accepting restrictions related to fluid and sodium intake. The individual may also be struggling with acceptance of a chronic illness, particularly if dependent on hemodialysis. The nurse asks specific questions about the nonfood substance ingested, such as what it is, how long the person has been eating it, how much is eaten each time, and how often the person eats it.

The client is told specifically to stop eating the substance, and the nurse explores with the client coping strategies to facilitate discontinuing this unhealthy behavior. Family members may be asked to provide emotional support and to encourage sound nutritional practices.

The assistance of a psychiatric health professional may be indicated. A long-standing habit may be difficult for the client to stop. Resolution of emotional issues may also mean resolution of pica.

SUMMARY

Anorexia nervosa and bulimia nervosa are serious psychiatric disorders that present a unique challenge to the medical-surgical nurse. The nurse may find it relatively easy to plan the nursing care required for clinical manifestations of a physical nature but extremely difficult to develop nursing interventions related to the client's emotional problems. It is possible and appropriate for the nurse to assist the client to develop healthy coping skills. However, the nurse must recognize that treatment of physical problems is only the beginning and that treatment for emotional problems will take an extended time because it involves the development of a therapeutic relationship. The nurse sets realistic goals with the client that can be accomplished in the medical setting. Long-term goals are identified along with an appropriate method for accomplishing them, e.g., individual or group psychotherapy and family therapy. The psychiatric liaison nurse is consulted for assistance with planning care and making appropriate referrals for psychiatric treatment.

Hospitalization of the anorexic or bulimic client on a medical unit provides the nurse with the opportunity to help define the client's disorder and to help resolve it by ensuring appropriate treatment. The client's perception of the quality of the nursing care and of the relationship with the nurse influences attitudes toward treatment and willingness to acknowledge the existence of the disorder and to accept further treatment.

IMPLICATIONS FOR RESEARCH

Although there is an abundance of research conducted by physicians on eating disorders, there is a dearth of nursing research. Nurses have participated in studies with physicians and have written numerous articles on eating disorders but have not conducted independent research projects. Nurses working in specialty units designed specifically to treat anorexia nervosa and bulimia nervosa and those whose clinic or private practice includes significant numbers of such clients have an opportunity to do valuable research. Validation of the effectiveness of nursing interventions is needed, which is accomplished through research. The discipline of nursing emphasizes the role of the nurse as educator. Research is needed to determine whether the teaching makes a significant difference in client outcomes. The following list identifies several research questions for which nurses can seek answers through research:

1. Does the use of one-to-one monitoring significantly influence weight gain and maintenance in the anorexic client?
2. Does educating the client about the consequences of purging behaviors significantly reduce the occurrence of such behaviors?
3. Do educational and support groups run by nurses for families of clients with eating disorders significantly alter the level of cooperation with treatment teams?
4. Does allowing menu selection by the client early in the course of treatment increase anxiety significantly?
5. Does nutritional teaching by the nurse significantly affect client outcome?
6. Do relaxation techniques and guided imagery effectively reduce binging and purging behaviors?
7. Is there a higher incidence of sexual abuse in the eating disorder population than in the general population?

REFERENCES AND READINGS

Akridge, K. (1989). Anorexia nervosa. *Journal of Obstetric, Gynecologic, and Neonatal Nursing, 18,* 25–30.

American Psychiatric Association. (1987). *Diagnostic and statistical manual of mental disorders* (3rd ed., revised). Washington, DC: Author.

Andersen, A. E. (1984). Anorexia nervosa and bulimia in adolescent males. *Pediatric Annals, 13,* 901–904, 907.

Andersen, A. E. (1985). *Practical comprehensive treatment of anorexia nervosa and bulimia.* Baltimore: The Johns Hopkins University Press.

Andersen, A. E., Morse, C. L., & Santmyer, K. S. (1985). Inpatient treatment for anorexia nervosa. In D. M. Garner & P. E. Garfinkel (Eds.), *Handbook of psychotherapy for anorexia nervosa and bulimia* (pp. 311–343). New York: Guilford.

Bowers, W. A. (1987). Medical complications of anorexia nervosa and bulimia: Implications for rehabilitation counselors. *Journal of Rehabilitation, 53,* 55–58.

Brownell, K. D., & Foreyt, J. P. (Eds.). (1986). *Handbook of eating disorders: Physiology, psychology, and treatment of obesity, anorexia, and bulimia.* New York: Basic Books.

Bruch, H. (1982). Anorexia nervosa: Therapy and treatment. *American Journal of Psychiatry, 139,* 1531–1538.

Cauwells, J. M. (1983). *Bulimia: The binge-purge compulsion.* Garden City, NY: Doubleday.

Crisp, A., Hsu, L., Harding, B., & Hartshorn, J. (1980). Clinical features of anorexia nervosa. *Journal of Psychosomatic Research, 24,* 179–191.

Crisp, A. H., Palmer, R. L., & Kalvey, R. A. (1976). How common is anorexia nervosa? A prevalence study. *British Journal of Psychiatry, 126,* 549–554.

Dresser, R. (1984). Legal and policy considerations in treatment of anorexia nervosa patients. *International Journal of Eating Disorders, 3,* 43–51.

Fairburn, C. (1982). Binge-eating and bulimia nervosa. *SK&F Publications, 1,* 1–19.

Fairburn, C. G. (1983). Bulimia: Its epidemiology and management. In A. J. Stunkard & E. Steltor (Eds.), *Eating and its disorders* (pp. 235–258). New York: Raven.

Fairburn, C. G., & Cooper, P. J. (1984). The clinical features of bulimia nervosa. *British Journal of Psychiatry, 144,* 238–246.

Feighner, J. P., Robins, E., Guse S. B., Woodruff, R. A., Jr., Wenokur, G., & Munoz, R. (1972). Diagnostic criteria for use in psychiatric research. *Archives of General Psychiatry, 26,* 57–63.

Flood, M. (1989). Addictive eating disorders. *Nursing Clinics of North America, 24,* 45–53.

Frisch, R. E., & McArthur, J. W. (1974). Menstrual cycles: Fatness as a determinant of minimum weight for height necessary for their maintenance or onset. *Science, 185,* 949–951.

Garfinkel, P. E., & Garner, D. M. (1982). *Anorexia nervosa: A multidimensional perspective.* New York: Brunner/Mazel.

Garfinkel, P. E., & Garner, D. M. (1987). *The role of drug treatment for eating disorders.* New York: Brunner/Mazel.

Garner, D. M. (1981). Body image in anorexia nervosa. *Canadian Journal of Psychiatry, 26,* 218–223.

Garner, D. M., & Garfinkel, P. E. (1985). *Handbook of psychotherapy for anorexia nervosa and bulimia.* New York: Guilford.

Garner, D. M., & Olmsted, M. P. (1984). *Manual for eating disorder inventory (EDI).* Odessa, FL: Psychological Assessment Resources.

Garner, D. M., Olmsted, M. P., Bohr, Y., & Garfinkel, P. E. (1982). The eating attitudes test: Psychometric features and clinical correlates. *Psychological Medicine, 12,* 871–878.

Gull, W. (1874). Anorexia nervosa (apepsia hysteria, anorexia hysteria). *Transactions of the Clinical Society of London, 7,* 22–28.

Halmi, K. A., & Falk, J. R. (1981). Common physiological changes in anorexia nervosa. *International Journal of Eating Disorders, 1,* 16–27.

Halmi, K., Goldberg, S., Eckert, E., Casper, R., & Davis, J. (1977). Pretreatment evaluation in anorexia nervosa. In R. A. Vigersky (Ed.), *Anorexia nervosa.* New York: Raven.

Hudson, J., Wentworth, S., Hudson, M., & Pope, H. (1985). Prevalence of anorexia nervosa and bulimia among young diabetic women. *Journal of Clinical Psychiatry, 46,* 88–89.

Johnson, C., & Connors, M. E. (1987). *The etiology and treatment of bulimia nervosa: A biopsychosocial perspective.* New York: Basic Books.

Johnson, C., Stuckey, M., Lewis, L., & Schwartz, D. (1982). Bulimia: A descriptive study of 316 cases. *International Journal of Eating Disorders, 11,* 1–16

Kalucy, R., Crisp, A., & Harding, B. (1977). A study of 56 families with anorexia nervosa. *British Journal of Medical Psychology, 50,* 381–395.

Kopeski, L. M. (1989). Diabetes and bulimia: A deadly duo. *American Journal of Nursing, 89,* 482–485.

Lasègue, C. (1985). On hysterical anorexia. In A. E. Andersen (Ed.), *Practical comprehensive treatment of anorexia nervosa and bulimia* (pp. 19–27). Baltimore: The Johns Hopkins University Press (Reprinted from *Archives of General Medicine,* 1873, 2, 367)

Mickley, D. W. (1988). Eating disorders. *Hospital Practice, 23,* 58–62.

Miles, M. W. (1988). Bulimia nervosa and gender identity: Symbols of a culture. *Holistic Nursing Practice, 3,* 56–66.

Mitchell, J. E. (1985). *Anorexia nervosa and bulimia: Diagnosis and treatment.* Minneapolis: University of Minnesota Press.

Mitchell, J. E. (1986). Bulimia: medical and physiological aspects. In K. D. Brownell & J. P. Foreyt (Eds.), *Handbook of eating disorders: Physiology, psychology, and treatment of obesity, anorexia, and bulimia.* New York: Basic Books.

Mitchell, J. E., Hatsukami, D., Eckert, E., & Pyle, R. L. (1985). Characteristics of 275 patients with bulimia. *American Journal of Psychiatry, 142,* 482–485.

Mitchell, J. E., Pyle, R. L., & Eckert, E. D. (1981). Frequency and duration of binge-eating episodes in patients with bulimia. *American Journal of Psychiatry, 138,* 835–836.

Mitchell, J. E., Pyle, R. L., Eckert, E. D., Hatsukami, D., & Lentz, R. (1983). Electrolyte and other physiological abnormalities in patients with bulimia. *Psychological Medicine, 13,* 273–278.

Mitchell, J. E., Pyle, R. L., & Miner, R. A. (1982). Gastric dilatation as a complication of bulimia. *Psychosomatics, 23,* 96–99.

Moodie, D., Salcedo, E. (1983). Cardiac function in adolescents and young adults with anorexia nervosa. *Journal of Adolescent Health Care, 4,* 9–14.

Morgan, G., & Mayberry, J. (1983). Common diseases and anorexia nervosa in British dietitians. *Public Health (London), 97,* 166–170.

Morton, R. (1985). *Phthisologica: Or a treatise of consumptions.* In A. E. Andersen (Ed.), *Practical comprehensive treatment of anorexia nervosa and bulimia* (pp. 11–13). Baltimore: The Johns Hopkins University Press. (Reprinted from *Phthisologica: Or a treatise of consumptions.* [pp. 4–10]. [1694]. London: Smith and Walford)

Office of Research Reporting, National Institute of Child Health and Human Development. (1983). *Facts about anorexia nervosa.* Bethesda: Author.

Pyle, R. L. (1985). The epidemiology of eating disorders. *Pediatrician, 12,* 102–109.

Pyle, R. L., Halvorson, P. A., Neuman, P. A., & Mitchell, J. E. (1986). The increasing prevalence of bulimia in freshman college students. *International Journal of Eating Disorders, 4,* 631–647.

Pyle, R. L., Mitchell, J. E., & Eckert, E. D. (1981). Bulimia: A report of 34 cases. *Journal of Clinical Psychiatry, 42,* 60–64.

Reighley, J. W. (1988). *Nursing care planning guides for mental health.* Baltimore: Williams & Wilkins.

Rigotti, N. A., Nussbaum, S. R., Herzog, D. B., & Neer, R. M. (1984). Osteoporosis in women with anorexia nervosa. *New England Journal of Medicine, 311,* 1601–1606.

Root, M. P. P., Fallon, P., & Friedrich, W. N. (1986). *Bulimia: A systems approach to treatment.* New York: W. W. Norton.

Roth, G. (1983). *Feeding the hungry heart: The experience of compulsive eating.* New York: Signet.

Roth, G. (1986). *Breaking free from compulsive eating.* New York: Signet.

Russell, G. F. M. (1970). Anorexia nervosa: Its identity as an illness and its treatment. In J. H. Price (Ed.), *Modern trends in psychological medicine* (Vol. 2, pp. 131–164). London: Butterworths.

Schultz, J. M., & Dark, S. L. (1982). Anorexia nervosa care plan. *Manual of psychiatric nursing care plans* (pp. 97–101). Boston: Little, Brown.

Silber, T. (1984). Anorexia nervosa: Morbidity and mortality. *Pediatric Annals, 13,* 851–859.

Stuart, G. W., & Sundeen, S. J. (1983). *Principles and practice of psychiatric nursing* (2nd ed.). St. Louis: C. V. Mosby.

Stunkard, A. J. (1959). Eating patterns and obesity. *Psychiatric Quarterly, 33,* 284–292.

Tolstrup, K., Brinch, M., Isager, T., Nielsen, S., Nystrup, J., Severin, B., & Olesen, S. (1985). Long-term outcome of 151 cases of anorexia nervosa. *Acta Psychiatrica Scandinavica, 71,* 380–387.

Walsh, B. T. (1988). *Eating behavior in eating disorders.* Washington, DC: American Psychiatric Press.

Walsh, B. T. Stewart, J. W., & Wright, L. (1982). Treatment of bulimia with monoamine oxidase inhibitors. *American Journal of Psychiatry, 139,* 1629–1630.

White, J. (1984). Bulimia: Utilizing individual and family therapy. *Journal of Psychosocial Nursing, 22,* 22–28.

Wooley, S., & Wooley, W. (1986). Ambitious bulimics: Thinness mania. *American Health, 10,* 68–74.

ADDITIONAL READINGS

Brockopp, D. Y., & Hall, S. Y. (1984). Eating disorders: A teen-age epidemic. *Nurse Practitioner, 9*(4), 32, 34–35.

This is an article coauthored by a registered nurse and a teen-ager concerned about the number of her friends suffering from eating disorders. It provides a brief overview of bulimia nervosa and anorexia nervosa, as well as nursing interventions appropriate for each disorder. Names and addresses of eight treatment programs in the United States are listed.

Keller, O. L. (1986). Bulimia: Primary care approach and intervention. *Nurse Practitioner, 11*(8), 42–51.

This article stresses the role of the nurse practitioner in identifying clients with bulimia nervosa and in providing education and counseling for them. It identifies emotional and physical manifestations of bulimia nervosa and appropriate interventions.

Robinson, R. G., Tortosa, M., Sullivan, J., Buchanan, E., Andersen, A., & Folstein, M. F. (1983). Quantitative assessment of psychologic state of patients with anorexia nervosa or bulimia: Response to caloric stimulus. *Psychosomatic Medicine, 45,* 283–292.

This reference describes a study undertaken on an inpatient unit that compared the psychologic state of bulimic and anorexic clients after ingestion of a liquid meal. Registered nurses (Tortosa and Sullivan) were investigators and played a major role in data collection.

CHAPTER 47

Interventions for Clients with Biliary, Pancreatic, and Hepatic Disorders

Disorders of the liver, the gallbladder, and the pancreas initially occur as single-organ processes. If the primary disorder is untreated, however, the inflammatory response may extend to other organs. The anatomic proximity of the liver, the gallbladder, and the pancreas, as well as the possibility of impeded flow of bile from the liver through the biliary ductal system, contributes to potential complications and multiorgan involvement in disease processes. Obstruction of bile flow by gallstones, edema, stricture, and tumors can cause inflammation of the gallbladder, the liver, or the pancreas, depending on the location of the obstruction in the biliary system. For example, gallstone impaction of the cystic duct causes cholecystitis (gallbladder inflammation), whereas gallstones lodged in the ampulla of Vater impede the flow of bile and pancreatic secretions, which results in pancreatitis (inflammation of the pancreas).

The pathologic changes in the liver, the gallbladder, and the pancreas can be broadly categorized as inflammatory, fibrotic, or neoplastic (see the accompanying Key Features of Disease). The disorders may develop insidiously or occur as acute life-threatening events with multiple complications.

BILIARY DISORDERS

CHOLECYSTITIS

OVERVIEW

Gallbladder disease is a common health care problem in the United States. *Cholecystitis* may occur as an acute or chronic inflammation of the gallbladder wall. Chronic inflammation may be complicated by an acute attack in the presence of an obstruction.

Pathophysiology

Acute cholecystitis usually develops in association with cholelithiasis (gallstones or calculous cholecystitis); gallstones or calculi lodge in the neck of the gallbladder or in the cystic duct. Gallstones interfere with or totally obstruct normal bile flow from the gallbladder to the duodenum, causing vascular congestion as a result of impeded venous return. Edema and congestion occur and contribute to the initial inflammatory process.

The second stage results when trapped bile is reabsorbed and acts as a chemical irritant to the gallbladder wall, producing a toxic effect. The presence of bile, in combination with impaired circulation, edema, and distention, causes ischemia of the gallbladder wall, resulting in tissue sloughing with necrosis and gangrene. Perforation of the gallbladder wall may occur. If the perforation is small and localized, an abscess may form.

KEY FEATURES OF DISEASE ■ Categories of Diseases of the Gallbladder, the Pancreas, and the Liver

Pathologic Change	Examples
Inflammatory	Cholecystitis Pancreatitis Hepatitis
Fibrotic	Chronic pancreatitis Hepatic cirrhosis
Neoplastic	Primary and metastatic carcinomas of the gallbladder, the pancreas, and the liver

Cholecystitis occurring in the absence of gallstones (acalculous cholecystitis) is believed to be due to bacterial invasion via the lymphatic or vascular route. *Escherichia coli* is the most common causative bacterium found. Streptococci and salmonellae are also seen.

Chronic cholecystitis results when inefficient bile emptying and gallbladder muscle wall disease persist. It may be caused by or lead to gallstone formation. In chronic cholecystitis, the gallbladder becomes fibrotic and contracted, which results in decreased motility and deficient absorption.

Pancreatitis and cholangitis (inflammation of the common bile duct) can occur as complications of cholecystitis attributable to the back-up of bile throughout the biliary tract.

Jaundice (the yellow discoloration of body tissues; icterus) can occur in acute cholecystitis, but is most commonly seen in the chronic phase of gallbladder inflammation. Impeded or obstructed bile flow caused by edema of the ducts or gallstones contributes to *extrahepatic* (outside the liver) *obstructive jaundice.* Jaundice in cholecystitis may also be caused by direct liver involvement. The inflammation of the liver's bile channels or bile ducts may cause *intrahepatic obstructive jaundice,* resulting in an increase in circulating levels of bilirubin, the principal pigment of bile. When the concentration of bilirubin in the blood becomes abnormally high (approximately three times the normal level), excess bilirubin collects in the tissues (the dermis and the epidermis), resulting in yellow discoloration of the skin. Excess bile salts also accumulate in the skin, causing pruritus (itching) and a burning sensation. Excess bilirubin in the blood collects in the connective tissue of the sclera (scleral icterus).

In obstructive jaundice, the normal flow of bile into the duodenum is blocked. Bilirubin is unable to reach the large intestine, where it is converted into urobilinogen, which accounts for the normal brown color of feces. As a result, clay-colored stools are seen. Water-soluble bilirubin is normally excreted by the kidneys in the urine. When an excess in circulating bilirubin occurs, the urine becomes dark and foamy because of the kidney's effort to clear the bilirubin.

(The reader is referred to later discussion of jaundice in hepatic and pancreatic disorders.)

Etiology

The exact etiology of cholecystitis is unknown. Other than gallbladder calculi formation, causes of acute cholecystitis include surgical trauma, inadequate blood supply, prolonged anesthesia, adhesion formation, edema, neoplasms, long-term dietary fasting, prolonged dehydration, gallbladder trauma, prolonged immobility, and excess narcotic use. Any condition that affects the regular filling or emptying of the gallbladder or causes "gallbladder shock" (a decrease in blood flow to the gallbladder) can result in acute cholecystitis. Cholecystitis has also been blamed on anatomic problems, such as twisting or kinking of the gallbladder neck or cystic duct, and pancreatic enzyme reflux into the gallbladder.

Incidence

A high incidence of biliary tract disease and cholecystitis is seen in individuals with sedentary life styles, a familial tendency to biliary disease, and obesity. Italian, Jewish, and Chinese ethnic groups, as well as insulin-dependent diabetics, are predisposed to gallbladder disease (Given & Simmons, 1984).

PREVENTION

Individuals who are obese and sedentary should be encouraged to consume a low-fat diet with small, frequent portions. A weight control regimen with a prescribed diet and an exercise program should also be initiated to assist in decreasing the risks of cholecystitis.

COLLABORATIVE MANAGEMENT

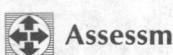 Assessment

History

The nurse obtains the client's height and weight and determines the *sex, age, race,* and *ethnic* group. If the client is female, the nurse ascertains the history of pregnancies or menopausal state and whether birth control pills, estrogen, or other hormone supplements are being taken. These may indicate risk factors for cholelithiasis, which can lead to cholecystitis.

The nurse questions the client about *food preferences* and determines if excessive fat and cholesterol are included in the diet. The client is asked if any foods are not tolerated and if gastrointestinal (GI) symptoms, such as flatulence, dyspepsia (indigestion), eructation (belching), anorexia, nausea, vomiting, abdominal pain, or discomfort, occur in relation to fatty food intake. The nurse asks the client to describe daily activity or exercise routines to determine if a sedentary life style exists. The client is asked if there is a *family history of gallbladder disease,* because there is a familial tendency for biliary tract diseases.

Physical Assessment: Clinical Manifestations

There is no typical presentation for clients with acute cholecystitis. Clinical manifestations vary in intensity and frequency. A careful history of all signs and symptoms must be taken because of their similarity to those of GI disorders. The nurse asks the client to describe the *pain,* including intensity and duration, precipitating factors, and relief measures, if any. The pain may be described as indigestion of varying intensity, ranging from a mild, persistent ache to a steady, constant pain in the right upper abdominal quadrant. The pain may radiate to the right shoulder or scapula. The abdominal pain of chronic cholecystitis may be vague and nonspecific.

The nurse asks the client if the pain typically occurs after a high-fat or high-volume meal or when assuming a recumbent position. The nurse also asks if *nausea, vomiting, dyspepsia* or heartburn, *flatulence* (excessive gastric or intestinal gas), *eructation,* or *feelings of abdominal heaviness* occur. These are common GI complaints with cholecystitis.

It is difficult to use abdominal palpation and percussion in assessing the client with acute cholecystitis. In acute inflammation, the gallbladder may be tender on palpation. With light palpation, tenderness increases on inspiration. *Guarding* and *rigidity,* as well as *rebound tenderness* (Blumberg's sign), are reliable indicators of peritoneal irritation. To elicit rebound tenderness, the client assumes a supine position and the nurse pushes his/her fingers deeply and steadily into the abdomen, then quickly releases the pressure. Pain that results from the rebound of the palpated tissue indicates peritoneal inflammation. Deep palpation below the liver border in the right upper quadrant may reveal *a sausage-shaped mass,* representing the distended, inflamed gallbladder. Percussion over the posterior rib cage intensifies localized abdominal pain.

In chronic cholecystitis, clients may develop insidious symptoms and may not seek medical treatment until such late symptoms as *jaundice, clay-colored stools,* and *dark urine* occur as a result of an obstructive process. *Steatorrhea* (fatty stools) occurs because of decreased fat absorption related to the lack of bile needed for the absorption of fats and fat-soluble vitamins in the intestine. As with any inflammatory process, the client may have an elevated temperature of 99° to 102° F (37° to 39° C), tachycardia, and dehydration from fever and vomiting.

Psychosocial Assessment

Impending surgical intervention or diagnostic procedures may provoke anxiety and fear in the client, and the nurse assesses for the presence of these feelings. The client may verbalize anxiousness related to the loss of income during the hospitalization and recovery period and may be worried about lack of health care insurance and large medical bills. The client may express concerns regarding child care and household responsibilities during hospitalization.

Laboratory Findings

There are no laboratory tests specific for gallbladder disease. Serum levels of alkaline phosphatase; aspartate aminotransferase (AST), also known as serum glutamic-oxaloacetic transaminase (SGOT); and lactate dehydrogenase (LDH) may be elevated, indicating abnormalities in liver function. The direct (conjugated) and indirect (unconjugated) serum bilirubin levels are elevated if an obstructive process is present. An increased white blood cell (WBC) count indicates inflammation. If there is pancreatic involvement, serum and urine amylase levels are elevated.

Radiographic Findings

If cholecystitis is suspected, the oral cholecystogram is the most frequently ordered diagnostic study to confirm biliary tract disease. Additional radiographic studies are done when cholelithiasis is suspected. If the gallbladder is not visualized during cholecystography or when only faint opacification occurs, inflammatory disease such as cholecystitis is suspected.

Other Diagnostic Tests

Technetium-labeled acetanilido iminodiacetic acid (^{99m}Tc HIDA) is also used to detect abnormal hepatobiliary function. The HIDA scan may have faster diagnostic capabilities than the oral cholecystography because the pretest fasting period required for the HIDA scan is 4 to 6 hours. Additionally, cholecystography is not performed if the serum total bilirubin level is greater than 1.8 mg/dL.

Ultrasonography of the gallbladder, a noninvasive procedure, is frequently used after an inconclusive oral cholecystogram or for emergency diagnosis of acute cholecystitis. Some physicians prefer to use the gallbladder ultrasound as a primary diagnostic measure and request it as a diagnostic test before the more invasive oral cholecystogram.

 Analysis: Nursing Diagnosis

The client with cholecystitis is typically admitted to the hospital for diagnostic work-up and surgical intervention.

Common Diagnoses

The most common nursing diagnosis for clients with acute or chronic cholecystitis is pain related to inflammation of the gallbladder and surrounding tissue.

Additional Diagnoses

The client may have the following additional nursing diagnoses:

1. Potential for altered (gastrointestinal) tissue perfusion related to the risk of obstruction by gallstones
2. Potential fluid volume deficit related to hypovolemia secondary to blood loss or excessive losses during nasogastric suction
3. Knowledge deficit related to prevention of acute attacks or postoperative treatment plan

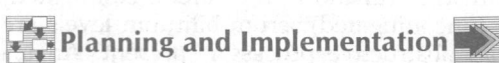
Planning and Implementation

The following plan of care includes interventions for pain.

Pain

Planning: client goals. The primary goal is that the client will experience relief of abdominal pain before or after surgical intervention.

Interventions. During the acute phase of cholecystitis, treatment measures are directed at resting the inflamed gallbladder in an effort to reduce the inflammatory process and reduce the pain. Nonsurgical interventions are implemented, but, if these are unsuccessful, the client requires surgery.

Nonsurgical management. Nonsurgical measures to relieve pain include diet therapy and drugs. The nurse consults with the physician and the dietitian when implementing these actions.

Diet therapy. In acute cholecystitis, food and fluids are withheld for clients experiencing mild nausea and vomiting to decrease stimulation of the gallbladder. For severe nausea and vomiting, decompression of the stomach is achieved by inserting a nasogastric tube and emptying the stomach contents. The nurse's role in caring for a client with a nasogastric tube is described in Chapter 45.

The client with chronic cholecystitis is encouraged to consume a low-fat diet to decrease stimulation of the gallbladder. Smaller, more frequent meals assist some clients in tolerating foods.

Drug therapy. Narcotic analgesics, such as meperidine (Demerol), are given to relieve abdominal pain and spasm. Antispasmodic agents, such as anticholinergics (e.g., propantheline bromide [Pro-Banthine]), may be used to relax the smooth muscles, preventing biliary contraction, which decreases secretions and assists in pain reduction. Antiemetics, such as prochlorperazine (Compazine), are often prescribed to provide relief from nausea and vomiting.

Surgical management. The usual surgical treatment of acute and chronic cholecystitis is cholecystectomy (the removal of the gallbladder). A complete Client Care Plan for clients undergoing cholecystectomy accompanies the text. The client usually has a drainage tube, such as Penrose's drain, positioned in the gallbladder bed to prevent fluid accumulation. The drainage is usually serosanguineous (serous fluid mixed with blood) and is bile stained in the first 24 hours postoperatively.

If the common bile duct is explored to assess for the presence of stones, a T tube drain is inserted surgically to ensure ductal patency (Fig. 47–1). Trauma to the common bile duct stimulates inflammation, which can impede bile flow and contribute to bile stasis. Nursing care of the client with a T tube is summarized in the Guidelines feature on page 1453.

Preoperative care. In addition to the usual preoperative care measures (Chap. 18), the nurse focuses teaching on aggressive measures to prevent respiratory complications. The nurse instructs the client in the importance of deep breathing, coughing, and turning. Clients are reluctant to take deep breaths after surgery because of increased muscle pain related to the high incision in the right subcostal area and the surgical manipulation near the diaphragm.

Clients who smoke are particularly susceptible to postoperative atelectasis (collapse of the lung's alveoli). The nurse instructs the client in the use of sustained maximal inspiration (SMI) devices, such as an incentive spirometer. The nurse stresses the importance of not smoking before surgery.

In an effort to minimize abdominal jarring during coughing, deep breathing, and turning, the nurse demonstrates the use of a folded bath blanket or pillow as a splinting device. The nurse also explains to the client the importance of early mobilization in preventing respiratory complications and warns the client to expect to get out of bed on the first postoperative day.

Postoperative care. Postoperative incision pain relief after cholecystectomy is usually achieved by intramuscular (IM) injection of meperidine (Demerol). Opiates, such as morphine, are generally not given because of the potential biliary ductal spasm. Relief of surgical pain is helpful in promoting preventive respiratory care measures. The client participates in coughing and deep breathing exercises more readily when pain is minimized. Therefore, the nurse plans the coughing and deep breathing exercises when pain relief is optimal.

Antiemetics may be necessary for episodes of postoperative nausea and vomiting. The nurse should administer the antiemetic early to prevent retching associated with vomiting to decrease the incidence of pain related to muscle straining.

The client receives nothing by mouth (NPO) for 24 to 28 hours postoperatively, and a nasogastric tube provides suction. When peristalsis returns, the nasogastric tube is removed, and a diet of clear liquids is begun. The diet is gradually advanced from clear liquids to solid

Goal/Outcome Criteria	Interventions	Rationales
Nursing Diagnosis 1: Pain Related to Inflammation of the Gallbladder and Obstructive Jaundice or Related to Surgical Removal of the Gallbladder		
Client will experience alleviation or reduction of postoperative abdominal pain. ■ States that pain is reduced or alleviated.	1. Assess the need for pain medication: narcotic or nonnarcotic analgesia. Administer IM injections of narcotic agents in the immediate postoperative period. Gradually reduce IM narcotic agents as pain relief and client toleration improve.	1. Pain medication is given on a prn schedule. Some patients are hesitant to request pain medication. Nurse must anticipate the need for analgesia in relation to increased activity and pulmonary toilet.
■ Identifies and utilizes alternative pain management techniques.	2. Instruct the client in alternative pain reduction methods (see Chap. 7). a. Teach the client to use a folded bath blanket or pillow to splint the abdominal incision when turning, moving, or coughing. b. Reposition the client to find a position of comfort (e.g., head of the bed elevated and side-lying position with knees to chest).	2. Use of abdominal splinting measures and comfortable positioning removes jarring movement and reduces tension in abdominal muscles.
■ Uses relaxation techniques.	3. Teach relaxation breathing exercises, as well as guided imagery techniques.	3. Anxiety may cause muscle rigidity and intensify pain. Slow, controlled breathing with the assistance of a nurse or family member can help the client relax tense muscles and ease mental tension, thereby promoting a reduction in pain.
Nursing Diagnosis 2: Potential for Ineffective Breathing Pattern Related to Painful Surgical Incision, Decreased Diaphragmatic Movement, or Anxiety		
Client will establish an effective breathing pattern. ■ Identifies ineffective breathing and increased respiratory effort.	1. Assess respiratory function. Monitor for shallow breathing pattern, guarded respiration with splinting, poor or weak cough, or decreased or adventitious breath sounds. a. Instruct the client to report feelings of dyspnea and changes in the breathing pattern.	1. Ongoing assessment of respiratory function can identify early complications.
■ Participates in preventive measures	2. Teach the importance of client participation in respiratory care. a. Instruct the client in the importance of early movement in bed with turning q 2 h and early ambulation. Assist the client as necessary. b. Teach the client to cough independently and deep breathe.	2. Client education and demonstrated participation can prevent complications such as atelectasis and pneumonia by mobilizing lung secretions.
	3. Consult with the respiratory therapist about the use of SMI devices. See Chapter 62 for more information on respiratory therapy.	3. Breathing devices can help prevent respiratory complications after surgery, particularly in obese and elderly clients and those who smoke.

continued

CLIENT CARE PLAN ■ The Client Undergoing Cholecystectomy *continued*

Goal/Outcome Criteria	Interventions	Rationales
Nursing Diagnosis 3: Potential for Infection Related to Dislodgment of T Tube with Bacterial Invasion of the Peritoneum (Peritonitis)		

Client will not develop a wound infection or peritonitis.
■ Participates in abdominal wound and T tube management.
	1. Assess for signs of inflammation.
	  a. Monitor the incision site for signs of infection. Inspect the T tube for dislodgment and changes in bile flow drainage. Report findings to the surgeon.
	  b. Instruct the patient to report increased incision tenderness or drainage, abdominal pain, or obvious T tube dislodgment.
	  c. Monitor temperature and report temperature above 100° F (37° C). Monitor WBC count daily, and report WBC count of greater than 10,000/mm³ to surgeon.
	  d. See Guidelines: Nursing Care of the Client with a T Tube and Client/Family Education: Home Care of the Client with a T Tube.
		1. Maintenance of T tube patency and early recognition of a wound infection can prevent serious complications, such as peritonitis and abdominal sepsis.

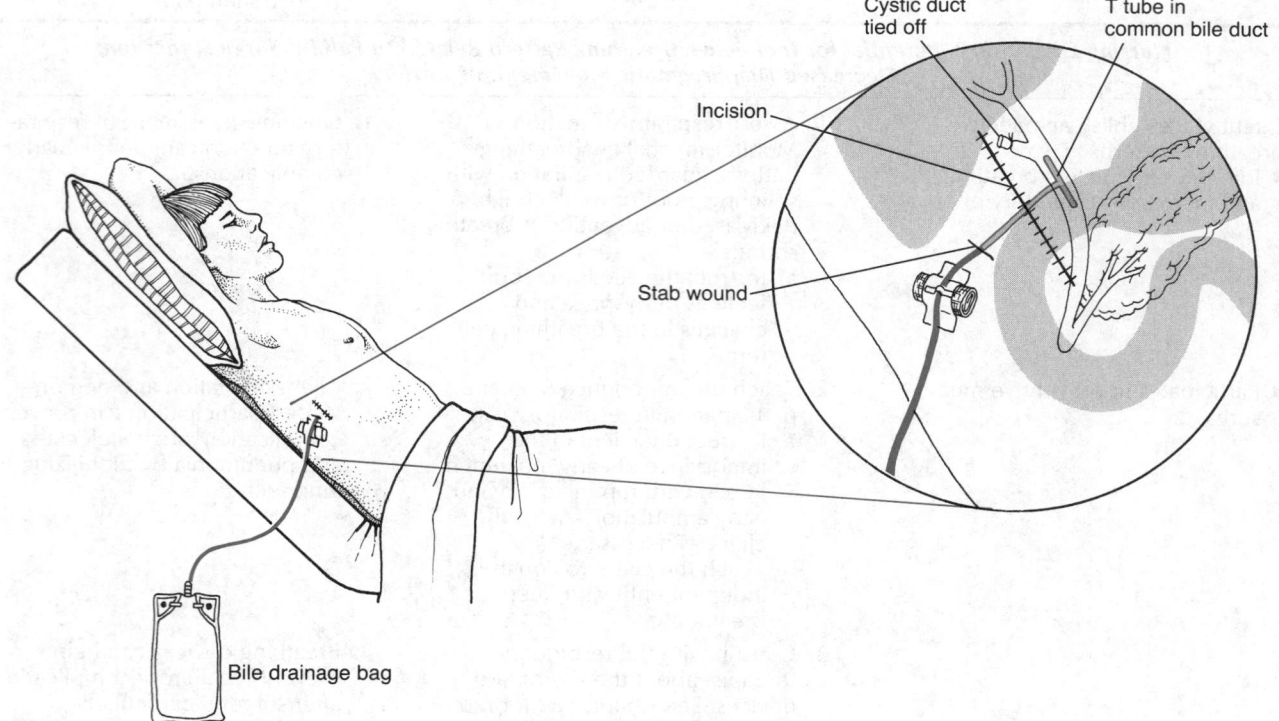

Cystic duct tied off

T tube in common bile duct

Incision

Stab wound

Bile drainage bag

Figure 47–1

T tube placement.

GUIDELINES ■ Nursing Care of the Client with a T Tube

Interventions	Rationales
1. Assess the amount, color, consistency, and odor of drainage at least q 4 h, then q 8 h. In the initial postoperative periods, expect bloody drainage, which changes to green-brown bile. Bile output will be 400 mL/d with a gradual decrease in amount. Report bile drainage amounts in excess of 1000 mL/d.	1. Close observation of bile flow is necessary to ensure patency of the bile duct and proper T tube placement. A decrease in bile flow in the early postoperative period may indicate obstruction or bile leakage into the peritoneal cavity. Excessive output may lead to a decrease in volume status with electrolyte imbalances.
2. Collect and administer excess bile output to the client by the nasogastric tube or give synthetic bile salts, such as dehydrocholic acid (Decholin).	2. Bile or bile salt replacement therapy is done to reduce excessive losses and prevent electrolyte imbalance.
3. Report sudden increases in bile output after a normally decreasing output pattern is established (9–10 d postoperatively).	3. Sudden increase may indicate ductal obstruction below the T tube site.
4. Assess for foul odor and purulent drainage, which indicate infection or extensive inflammation. Report changes in drainage to the physician.	4. Infection may require additional medical management with antibiotics.
5. Inspect the skin around the T tube insertion site for signs of inflammation, including redness, swelling, and erythema, and observe for frank bile leakage. Keep the dressing dry. (Utilize the hospital's procedure and provide drain care and dressing change per protocol. Site is usually cleaned and dressing changed daily.)	5. Bile drainage is irritating and excoriating to the skin. Bile leakage may indicate dislodgment of the T tube.
6. Keep the drainage system below the level of the gallbladder. Maintain the client in semi-Fowler's position.	6. This position allows for free-flowing bile drainage.
7. *Never* irrigate, aspirate, or clamp a T tube without a physician's order.	7. These precautions prevent disruption of the suture line by bile backflow.
8. Assess the drainage system for pulling, kinking, or tangling of tubing, especially when the client is positioned toward the right side. Assist the client with early turning and ambulation.	8. This allows for free-flowing bile drainage and prevents tube dislodgment.
9. When ordered by the physician, raise the drainage bag to the level of the abdomen (usually on the fourth or fifth postoperative day). Then, assess for feelings of fullness, nausea, or pain.	9. This helps to check for patency of the common bile duct.
10. Clamp the T tube for 1–2 h per physician's orders before and after meals. Assess the client's response for tolerance of food.	10. Clamping helps to check for digestion of foods.
11. Observe stools for return of brown color 7–10 d postoperatively.	11. As ductal edema subsides after surgical manipulation, the amount of bile is decreased and routed via the normal channel to the duodenum. The bile drainage decreases in the T tube drainage system and is channeled directly to the duodenum, where it is utilized for digestion of fats and fat-soluble vitamins.

foods as tolerated by the client. Within a few days, client resumes ingestion of solid foods.

The amount of fat allowed in the client's diet after cholecystectomy depends on the client's tolerance of fat. In the early postoperative period, if bile flow is reduced, a low-fat diet may be helpful to reduce discomfort and prevent nausea. Generally, a special diet is not required. The nurse advises the client to eat nutritious meals and avoid excessive dietary intake of fats. If the client is obese, a weight reduction program is recommended. The nurse consults with the physician and the dietitian in planning the appropriate diet.

■ Discharge Planning

Some clients with cholecystitis decide against surgical intervention and elect medical management with dietary control. Clients treated with diet and those who undergo cholecystectomy are discharged to home after hospitalization.

Home Care Preparation

The home environment is assessed with regard to the client's ability to procure foods and prepare meals. After cholecystectomy, clients usually need short-term assistance with procuring foods, preparing meals, and performing dressing changes. Clients who have undergone surgery need transportation to follow-up appointments with the health care provider.

Client/Family Education

The discharge teaching for the client and the family includes information on drug therapy, wound or drain care, activity restrictions, complication recognition, and medical follow-up, as for clients who have had abdominal surgery (see Chap. 20).

Diet therapy for clients who have had a cholecystectomy is based on the clients' tolerance of fats. A special diet may not be required, and, in this case, the nurse advises the client to eat nutritious, well-balanced meals. If the client has a poor tolerance of fats, the nurse recommends a low-fat diet and should provide the client and the family with a list of foods to avoid (see the accompanying Health Promotion/Maintenance feature). The dietitian may provide printed menu-planning guidelines. Some clients need to maintain a low-fat diet for 6 months or longer. They are advised to add fatty foods to the diet as tolerated.

If the client has problems tolerating three large meals a day, the nurse advises the client to try smaller, more frequent feedings. A weight reduction diet for obese clients is recommended, and appropriate dietary teaching is tailored to provide dietary guidelines and recommendations.

After cholecystectomy, the client is being discharged to home earlier after surgery today than in the past.

HEALTH PROMOTION/MAINTENANCE ■ Foods for Clients with Cholecystitis or Cholelithiasis to Avoid

Foods High in Cholesterol

Dairy Products

  Whole milk

  Ice cream

  Butter

  Cream

  Cheese

Other Foods

  Fried, fatty foods

  Rich pastries

  Gravies

  Nuts

  Chocolate

  Egg yolks

  Avocado

Gas-Forming Vegetables

  Cabbage

  Onions

  Broccoli

  Cauliflower

  Sauerkraut

  Radishes

  Cucumbers

  Beans

Many clients are sent home with drainage systems intact. The nurse instructs the client and one or more family members to inspect the incision wound and the T tube drainage site for signs and symptoms of inflammation, including redness, swelling, warmth, tenderness, excessive drainage, and an increase in incision pain, and to report these findings to the physician. The nurse provides the client with oral and written instructions for drainage tube care (see the accompanying Client/Family Education feature).

The client with cholecystitis who either refuses surgery or postpones surgery must be instructed on the signs of potential complications of chronic cholecystitis, including recurrent abdominal pain and jaundice. If these signs occur, the client must notify the physician for medical care and possibly surgery.

CLIENT/FAMILY EDUCATION ■ Home Care of the Client with a T Tube

Instructions	Rationales
1. "Wear loose fitting clothes."	1. This avoids irritation of the wound site and pressure on the tube.
2. "Wear clothes that are older to prevent ruining of good-quality clothes."	2. Bile leakage stains material.
3. "If staining occurs, soak the garment in a solution of detergent, baking soda, and bleach."	3. This usually removes the stain.
4. "Avoid baths. Take showers."	4. Running water will reduce the incidence of bacteria's entering the wound.
5. "Avoid heavy lifting and strenuous activity."	5. This prevents undue strain on the T tube wound site and the incision.
6. "Remove the dressing around the T tube every day. Hold the tube in place and wipe the skin around the tube with an alcohol wipe. Apply a precut dressing around the catheter, and tape it in place."	6. This prevents catheter infection.
7. "Empty the drainage bag at the same time each day. Allow the bile to flow from the bag's spout; do not disconnect the system."	7. Bile accumulates in the bag, and it needs to be emptied to avoid spillage.
8. "Watch the amount, color, and odor of drainage, and report any change in drainage, abdominal pain, nausea, or vomiting to the physician."	8. Change in the volume and character of drainage may indicate complications, such as obstruction.
9. "Coil the drainage tubing and secure it to the abdomen by taping or using a belt with hook and loop fasteners (Velcro). Keep the draining bag below the level of the T tube."	9. This position prevents strain on the T tube and prevents bile backflow into the common bile duct.
10. "Inspect the wound for signs of infection, including redness, swelling, warmth, abdominal firmness, pain, or purulent drainage at the tube site. Take your temperature and report a temperature of 100° F (87° C) or greater to the physician."	10. These are signs and symptoms of complications that require treatment.
11. "Return to the hospital for a cholangiogram."	11. If the cholangiogram indicates that the stones are resolved, the T tube will be removed.

Psychosocial Preparation

Discharge preparations often evoke anxiety for the client who has undergone surgery. Many are anxious about caring for wounds and drainage tubes. The fear of pain may be intense.

The nurse should include a supportive spouse or family member in postoperative teaching and discharge planning to provide reinforcement of information and to assist the client in adhering to the treatment plan.

Health Care Resources

A home care nurse may be required to provide support and follow-up nursing care and teaching in the home environment. The home care nurse assesses the client's adaptation to the treatment plan and evaluates

wound healing and T tube drainage system integrity. The need for further wound and skin care interventions is determined, and these are implemented by the home care nurse as needed.

 Evaluation

On the basis of the identified nursing diagnoses and health care (medical or surgical) interventions, the nurse evaluates the care of the client with acute or chronic cholecystitis. Expected outcomes include that the client

1. States that pain is alleviated and is nonrecurrent
2. Does not demonstrate manifestations of altered GI perfusion, such as increased abdominal pain, distention, or hypotension

3. Maintains adequate fluid volume
4. Complies with diet therapy, weight reduction program, or care of the incision if appropriate

CHOLELITHIASIS

OVERVIEW

Cholelithiasis is the most common disorder of the biliary tract. In more than 90% of the clients with cholecystitis, the cause of inflammation is bile stasis resulting from gallstone impaction of the cystic duct. Chronic cholecystitis occurs when repeated episodes of cystic duct obstruction result in chronic inflammation. Gallstones form in approximately 10% of the general population.

Pathophysiology

The exact cause of gallstones is not clearly understood. Contributing factors may include supersaturation of bile with cholesterol, excessive bile salt losses, decreased gallbladder-emptying rates, and changes in bile concentration or bile stasis within the gallbladder.

Gallstones may lie dormant within the gallbladder or may move to other areas of the biliary tree as the gallbladder empties and refills with bile. Stones may migrate and lodge within the gallbladder neck, the cystic duct, or the common bile duct, causing obstruction (Fig. 47–2). When bile cannot flow from the gallbladder, the stasis of bile and local irritation from the gallstones lead to cholecystitis (described earlier).

Cholangitis, usually associated with *choledocholithiasis* (common bile duct stones), involves infection of the bile ducts. *Ascending cholangitis,* the inflammation of the biliary tree, occurs after bacterial invasion of the ducts and can lead to life-threatening *suppurative* cholangitis when symptoms are not recognized quickly and pus accumulates in the ductal system.

The gallbladder provides an excellent environment for the production of gallstones. In particular, the gallbladder only occasionally mixes its normally abundant mucus and a highly viscous, concentrated bile. The constant temperature within the gallbladder also contributes to stone formation by delaying bile emptying, causing biliary stasis.

Gallstones are composed of substances normally found in bile, such as cholesterol, bilirubin, bile salts, calcium, and various proteins. Stones have been designated as cholesterol, mixed, or pigment stones. *Mixed stones* usually are composed of 50% cholesterol and account for almost 80% of all gallstones. When bile is supersaturated with cholesterol, precipitation of cholesterol crystals occurs, accounting for the high incidence of mixed stones.

Cholesterol stones are large and pale yellow and occur in groups or as a single stone. These stones form as a

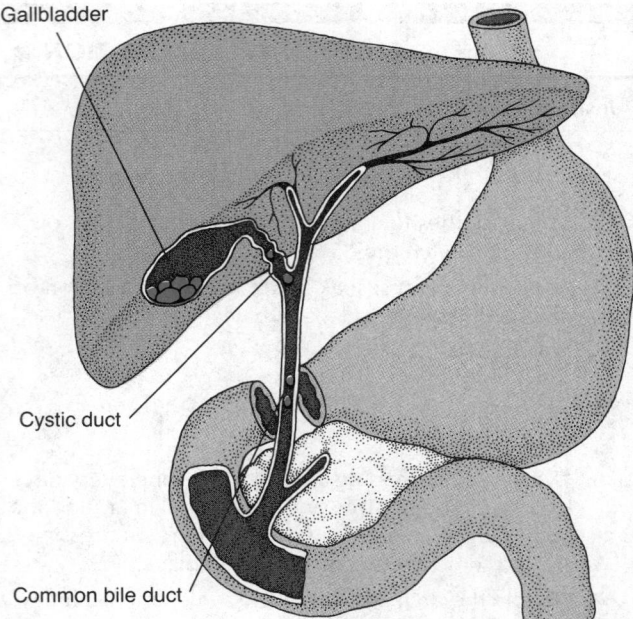

Figure 47–2

Gallstones within the gallbladder and obstructing the common bile and cystic ducts.

result of metabolic imbalances of cholesterol and bile salts. *Pigment stones* are small, are brown or black, and usually occur in clusters as a result of metabolic imbalances of unconjugated bilirubin.

Etiology

There appears to be a familial tendency toward the development of cholelithiasis, but this may be related to familial dietary habits (excessive dietary cholesterol intake) and sedentary life styles in some families. Gallstones are seen more frequently in obese individuals, probably as result of impaired fat metabolism.

Pregnancy tends to aggravate gallstone formation. Pregnancy and drugs such as estrogen and birth control pills alter hormone levels and delay muscular contraction of the gallbladder, causing a decreased rate of bile emptying. The incidence of gallstones is higher in women with multiple pregnancies. Combinations of causative factors increase the incidence of stone formation, especially in women. For example, an obese pregnant woman or an obese woman taking birth control pills may be at higher risk.

Cholelithiasis is seen with hemolytic blood disorders, with ileal disease (such as Crohn's disease), and after jejunoileal bypass surgery as a treatment for morbid obesity. Stone formation and cholecystitis are common in insulin-dependent diabetics.

Incidence

The incidence of cholelithiasis is four times higher in women than in men between the ages of 20 and 50 years. Male clients with cholelithiasis are usually 50 years of age or older. After age 50, the incidence of gallstones is equal in men and women. Cholelithiasis has been diagnosed in more than 20 million Americans, and 1 million new cases are reported yearly, equaling 10% to 20% of the adult population. Two-thirds of individuals with gallstones also experience chronic cholecystitis.

Caucasians and Native Americans, particularly the Navajo and Pima tribes, have a higher incidence of gallstones, although the disorder is also prevalent in Asian Americans and Blacks. The diagnosis of cholelithiasis is rated fifth among the causes of adult hospitalizations (Given & Simmons, 1984). Cholecystectomy is the third most common surgical procedure performed in the United States.

PREVENTION

As for clients with cholecystitis, the prevention of gallstones is aimed at the high-risk groups. A low-fat diet, weight reduction for obese clients, and an exercise program are useful preventive measures.

COLLABORATIVE MANAGEMENT

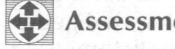 Assessment

History

The same historical data base may be obtained for clients with cholecystitis and cholelithiasis (see under History in discussion of cholecystitis). Additional information may be obtained if there is a prior client or family history of gallstones. The nurse asks the client if the type or color of the stones was identified and if any palliative *medical management* (e.g., dietary control and pain medication) or *surgical intervention* (e.g., cholecystotomy [surgical incision of the gallbladder]) was done.

Physical Assessment: Clinical Manifestations

The severity of *pain* and the presentation of symptoms in the client with cholelithiasis are dependent on the following factors: whether the stone is stationary or mobile, the size and location of the stone, the degree of obstruction, and the presence and extent of inflammation. Initially, the pain of cholelithiasis is usually a steady, mild ache located in the midepigastric area. It may increase in intensity and duration and may radiate to the right shoulder or back.

The severe pain of *biliary colic* is produced by ob-

struction of the cystic duct of the gallbladder. When a stone is moving through or is lodged within the duct, tissue spasm occurs in an effort to mobilize the stone through the small duct. This intense pain may be of such severity that it is accompanied by *tachycardia, pallor, diaphoresis,* and *prostration* (extreme exhaustion).

All of the clinical manifestations seen in acute or chronic cholecystitis may occur in cholelithiasis. Clients with chronic cholecystitis and acute ductal obstruction may experience the excruciating pain of biliary colic as well. The nurse may observe *jaundice* of the skin, the sclera, the upper palate, and oral mucous membranes on inspection. If gallstones occlude the common bile duct, prolonged severe inflammation and hepatic damage have occurred (see earlier discussion of jaundice).

A stone-filled gallbladder without accompanying ductal obstruction may be palpated as a painless, smooth, *sausage-shaped mass.* With possible ductal obstruction, deep palpation examination is deferred.

Psychosocial Assessment

Clients with cholelithiasis experience many of the same emotional feelings as those with cholecystitis, such as fear of pain, anxiety about diagnostic procedures or surgery, and financial worry.

Laboratory Findings

There are no specific laboratory tests for cholelithiasis. As in cholecystitis, the serum alkaline phosphatase, lactate dehydrogenase, AST, and direct and indirect bilirubin levels may be elevated. An elevated urinary bilirubin level is common in an obstructive process. If the common bile duct is obstructed, bilirubin does not reach the small intestine to be converted to fecal urobilinogen. Examination of a random stool specimen reveals absent or low levels of urobilinogen in the feces, indicating an obstructive process. If pancreatic involvement accompanies gallstone impaction, elevated serum and urine amylase levels are seen.

Radiographic Findings

Calcified gallstones are easily visualized on x-ray examination. An oral cholecystogram is diagnostic when the stones are radiopaque. Intravenous (IV) cholecystography is used in clients unable to absorb oral contrast agents. The gallbladder and ductal systems are outlined, and stones present are visualized.

Percutaneous transhepatic cholangiography is a fluoroscopic examination of the biliary ducts and may be used to diagnose obstructive jaundice and visualize stones located in the ducts.

Other Diagnostic Tests

Ultrasonography of the gallbladder is used to confirm the diagnosis of cholelithiasis and distinguish between obstructive and nonobstructive jaundice.

Analysis: Nursing Diagnosis

Common Diagnoses

The most common nursing diagnosis is pain related to inflammation of the gallbladder and obstructive jaundice or related to surgical removal of the gallbladder.

Additional Diagnoses

The client may also require care directed by one or more of the following nursing diagnoses:

1. Potential for infection related to risk of obstruction in the common bile duct of the gallbladder
2. Potential for altered (gastrointestinal) tissue perfusion related to risk of obstruction of the common bile duct
3. Potential for ineffective breathing pattern related to painful surgical incision, decreased diaphragmatic movement, or anxiety
4. Potential for infection related to dislodgment of T tube with bacterial invasion of the peritoneum (peritonitis)

 Planning and Implementation

The plan of care includes interventions for pain.

Pain

Planning: client goals. The goal for this nursing diagnosis is that the client will state that abdominal pain is minimized with treatment.

Interventions. Supportive treatment may be instituted for clients with cholelithiasis before surgical removal of the gallbladder and gallstones is performed.

Nonsurgical management. Some gallstones lie dormant and do not produce problems or cause pain. Acute pain occurs when the gallstones move into the duct or partially or totally obstruct the duct. Measures aimed at resting the inflamed gallbladder are the same as those discussed earlier for cholecystitis.

Diet therapy. In general, a low-fat diet must be adhered to in an effort to prevent further pain of biliary colic. If gallstones are causing an obstruction of bile flow, replacement of fat-soluble vitamins, such as vitamins A, D, E, and K, and administration of bile salts to facilitate digestion and vitamin absorption are implemented. The client has food and fluids withheld if nausea and vomiting are a problem.

Drug therapy. Pain caused by acute obstruction with gallstones requires narcotic analgesia with meperidine hydrochloride (Demerol). Antispasmodic or anticholinergic drugs, such as propantheline bromide (Pro-Banthine), may be given to relax smooth muscles and decrease ductal tone and spasm. Antiemetics are given to control nausea and vomiting.

Bile acid therapy has been effective in dissolving gallstones. Chenodiol (chenodeoxycholic acid [CDCA]; Chemix) successfully reduces cholesterol stones by maintaining a normal amount of cholesterol solubility in bile. Chenodiol may be effective in dissolving small stones, but larger stones usually cannot be dissolved. This treatment is generally reserved for elderly clients with mild or asymptomatic gallstone disease and those who are poor surgical risks. Unfortunately, it may take up to 2 years to dissolve gallstones. These drugs are expensive, and stones can recur if the client is not maintained on low drug doses for prolonged periods. The nurse observes for diarrhea, the common side effect of chenodiol therapy.

Obstructive jaundice in cholelithiasis, caused by impeded bile flow through the common bile duct as a result of the gallstone obstruction, may lead to excessive accumulation of bile salts in the skin. As a result, severe pruritus may occur. Cholestyramine (Questran) binds with bile salts in the intestine, forming an insoluble compound that is excreted in the feces, removing excessive bile salts and decreasing itching. The nurse administers the drug in powder form, which is mixed with fruit juices or milk and given before meals and at bedtime.

Alternative treatment measures. Extracorporeal shock wave lithotripsy is a noninvasive procedure that is being used as a treatment for gallstones in some settings. It involves the use of a machine, a lithotriptor, that generates powerful shock waves to shatter the gallstones (Fig. 47–3). The hour-long procedure includes repetition of up to 1500 shocks until the gallstone is completely fragmented. The minute particles are then able to travel through the biliary ductal system to be excreted via the intestines. Biliary lithotripsy is usually painless, although some clients experience mild pain as gallbladder spasms occur in an effort to expel the tiny stone fragments. The client requires minimal nursing care, and in the future this procedure may be performed on an outpatient (ambulatory) basis.

Percutaneous insertion of a transhepatic biliary catheter is performed under fluoroscopic guidance in an effort to decompress obstructed extrahepatic ducts so that bile can flow (Fig. 47–4). This procedure is primarily used for inoperable hepatic, pancreatic, or bile duct carcinoma, but may be used as a nonsurgical treatment alternative for biliary obstruction caused by gallstones and hepatic dysfunction secondary to obstructive jaundice and biliary sepsis in the *high-risk candidate* (see the Guidelines feature on p. 1460).

Surgical management. One of several procedures may be indicated in the surgical treatment of cholelithiasis. Cholecystotomy may be performed as an emergency procedure to remove gallstones. This procedure is often performed for elderly clients or those critically ill clients

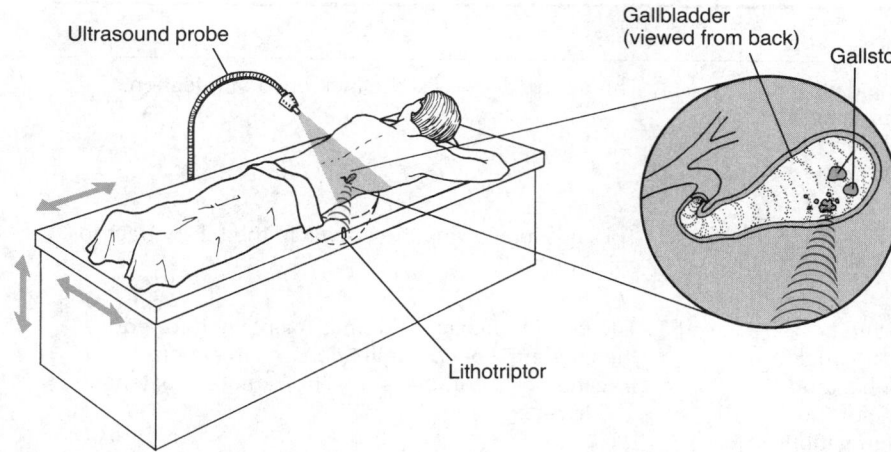

Ultrasound probe

Gallbladder
(viewed from back)

Gallstones

Lithotriptor

Figure 47 – 3

Biliary lithotripsy. With the assistance of a computer and an ultrasound monitor, the physician positions the client over a shock wave generator (lithotriptor) by means of a table that moves upward and downward, forward and backward, and side to side. When the client is positioned properly, the physician fires the lithotriptor, sloughing particles off the gallstones until they are completely fragmented and the fragments are able to pass through the biliary ductal system.

with life-threatening multisystem problems who may not withstand a prolonged surgical procedure. If the stones are located in the common bile duct, a *choledocholithotomy*, which is an incision into the common bile duct to remove stones, is required. If the common bile duct is explored, a T tube drain is inserted into the duct to ensure the patency until edema subsides and allows for collection of excessive bile drainage. A simple cholecystectomy is performed when stones are confined to the gallbladder. The common bile duct and adjacent ducts are explored for the presence of additional stones or stone fragments and crystals.

After cholecystectomy with T tube placement, drugs may be given to stimulate bile production and bile flow from the liver, promoting digestion and absorption of the fats, fat-soluble vitamins, and cholesterol in the duodenum. Hydrocholeretic drugs, such as dehydrocholic acid (Decholin, Cholin, Neocholin), and ketocholanic acids (Ketochol), which are synthetic bile salts, increase the solubility of cholesterol. This prevents the accumulation of cholesterol in bile, thereby decreasing the recurrence of biliary calculi and promoting drainage of (potentially infected) bile through the T tube drainage system.

A postoperative T tube cholangiogram can identify retained stones. Direct visualization of the biliary tract using an endoscope, termed *choledochoscopy*, enables the removal of calculi retained in the common bile duct. Choledochoscopy is performed through a T tube or an incision into the common bile duct. An instrument with a small basket-like attachment is used to snare the stone (Fig. 47 – 5). If this method fails, a fiberoptic endoscope is introduced into the duodenum. An incision into the papillae (papillotomy) allows the stone to pass into the duodenum.

The preoperative and postoperative nursing care measures for the client undergoing gallbladder surgical procedures are the same as those for cholecystectomy (see earlier). (Refer to Chap. 20 for general postoperative care.)

■ Discharge Planning

Most often, the client with cholelithiasis has surgery and is discharged to home postoperatively (see under Discharge Planning for cholecystitis). More frequently than in the past, the client is discharged with a T tube drainage system intact (see Client/Family Education: Home Care of the Client with a T Tube).

The nurse provides information to the client and the family about the potential occurrence of postcholecystectomy syndrome. The clinical manifestations of biliary tract disease occur after surgical intervention in up to 8% of clients undergoing cholecystectomy. Postcholecystectomy syndrome is caused by residual or recurring calculi or inflammation or stricture of the common bile

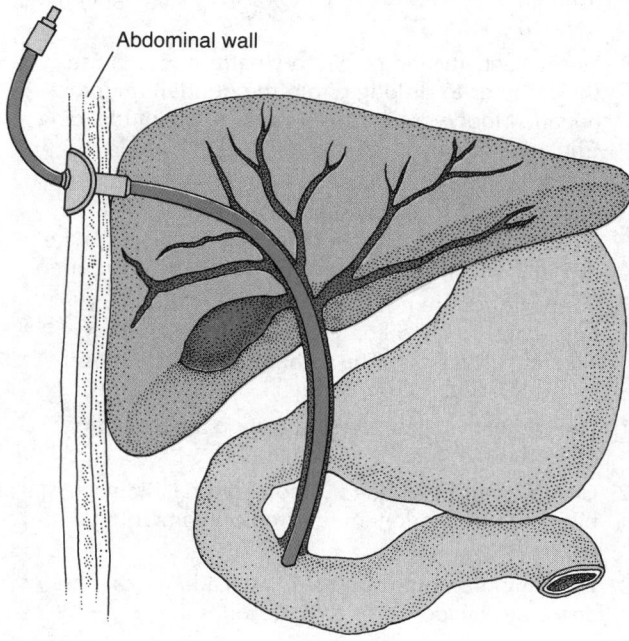

Abdominal wall

Figure 47 – 4

Transhepatic biliary catheterization.

GUIDELINES ■ Nursing Care of the Client with a Transhepatic Biliary Catheter

Interventions	Rationales
1. Change the catheter insertion site dressing daily, according to the hospital's policy. Recommended care includes cleaning the skin with hydrogen peroxide and applying antibiotic ointment and a small sterile dressing to the site.	1. This action decreases the incidence of infection.
2. During the first several days after catheter insertion, unclamp the catheter and allow it to drain into an internal drainage system.	2. This aids in allowing the edema in the biliary tract to subside.
3. Utilizing a three-way stopcock system located between the catheter and the drainage bag, irrigate the catheter twice daily with 5–20 mL of bacteriostatic saline. Check the physician's orders for the amount of solution and the frequency of irrigation. (Occlude the stopcock with a sterile cap when the irrigation procedure is complete.)	3. The closed drainage system is maintained to reduce the incidence of contamination and infection. Irrigation procedure ensures the catheter's patency.
4. Instruct the client that he/she may experience discomfort during irrigation. Observe for abdominal cramping or excessive pain; notify the physician.	4. Irrigation may irritate the liver bed and bile ducts, particularly if edema or cholangitis develops. The physician may decrease the amount of irrigation solution.
5. If pain is severe and abdominal rigidity develops, notify the physician immediately.	5. These symptoms may indicate an acute problem, such as intra-abdominal bleeding, small bowel perforation, or peritonitis. An emergency cholangiogram to evaluate the catheter's position is required.
6. Assess the client for decreasing jaundice. Stools should change from clay colored to normal brown; urine from dark and foamy to normal yellow. Monitor serum bilirubin test results for decreasing levels.	6. Improved client condition verifies proper catheter function.
7. Assess the client for fever, chills, and hypotension and report findings to the physician.	7. These signs indicate biliary sepsis caused by cholangitis, liver abscess, or catheter occlusion resulting from clots, tumors, or sediment. A cholangiogram is done to confirm.
8. Inspect the catheter for the presence of blood and notify the physician immediately.	8. Normal activity and respiratory pattern may cause the catheter to dislodge from the duodenum into a hepatic blood vessel, causing a backflow of bleeding. Cholangiography is indicated.
9. Assess the amount of drainage and report amounts in excess of 1500 mL during a 24-h period.	9. An excessive output may indicate retrograde flow of duodenal contents, causing excessive losses of bicarbonate, bile salts, and electrolytes. Appropriate fluid and electrolyte replacement therapy is required.
10. Inspect the skin sutures at the catheter's external transparent disk on the abdomen.	10. If the sutures are not intact, the catheter could slip out of position and float freely in the biliary tree or accidentally fall out. The catheter should be promptly reinserted under fluoroscopy.
11. Inspect the catheter for visualization of the drainage holes.	11. The catheter may be out of position, necessitating reinsertion.
12. Clamp the catheter and securely tape the external portion.	12. Clamping and securing promote internal drainage of bile into the duodenum (desired outcome of procedure).
13. Provide discharge instructions to the client or a family member, including a. Dressing care. b. Signs of catheter malfunction, infection, and dislodgment. c. Outpatient and cholangiography appointments.	13. Teaching promotes optimal home catheter care and decreases incidence of complications.

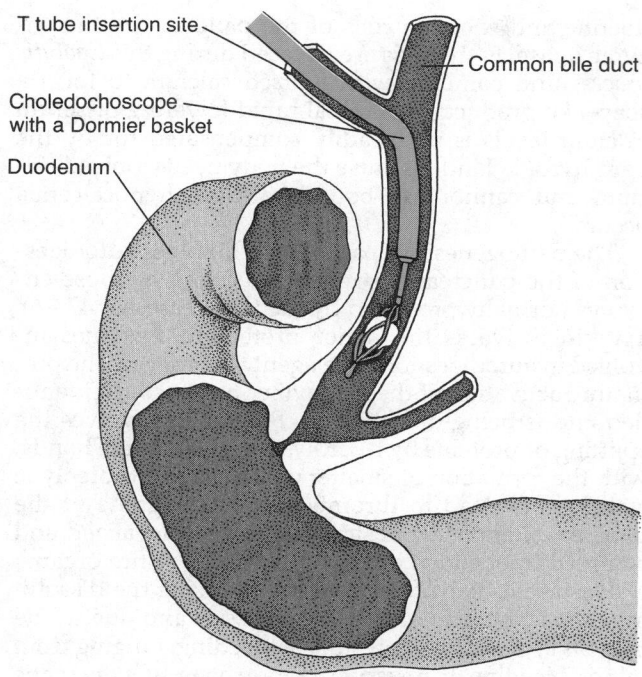

APPROACH THROUGH T TUBE INSERTION SITE

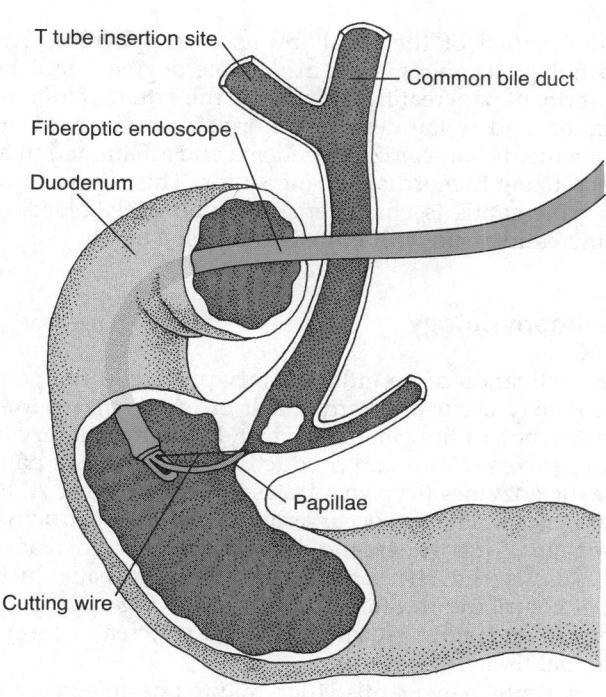

APPROACH THROUGH DUODENUM

Figure 47–5

Choledoscopic removal of gallstones.

duct. The nurse instructs the client to report symptoms of biliary tract disease to the physician, including jaundice of the skin or sclera, darkened urine, light-colored stools, pain, fever, or chills.

Evaluation

On the basis of the identified nursing diagnoses, the nurse evaluates the client with cholelithiasis. Expected outcomes include that the client

1. States that the pain is alleviated and is nonrecurrent

2. Does not demonstrate manifestations of infection, such as fever or increased abdominal pain

3. Does not demonstrate manifestations of altered tissue perfusion, such as increased abdominal pain, distention, or hypotension

CANCER

Primary cancer of the gallbladder is rare. Adenocarcinoma and squamous cell carcinoma of the gallbladder account for the majority of gallbladder cancers and typically infiltrate the liver and ducts, as well as the gallbladder. These rare gallbladder carcinomas appear more frequently in clients with pre-existing chronic cholecystitis and cholelithiasis.

Diagnosis of gallbladder cancer is difficult. Early symptoms are insidious in onset and similar to those of chronic cholecystitis and cholelithiasis. Characteristic signs and symptoms include anorexia, weight loss, nausea, vomiting, general malaise, jaundice, hepatosplenomegaly, and chronic, progressively severe epigastric or right upper quadrant pain. A moderately tender, irregularly shaped mass may be palpated. Often, gallbladder carcinoma is discovered during oral cholecystography for diagnosis of suspected cholecystitis or during cholecystectomy.

There is often a poor prognosis associated with cancer of the gallbladder. Surgical intervention is usually performed and may be extensive. Often, a bile drainage tube (transhepatic biliary catheter) may be inserted to relieve symptoms such as jaundice and itching (see Guidelines: Nursing Care of the Client with a Transhepatic Biliary Catheter).

PANCREATIC DISORDERS

ACUTE PANCREATITIS

OVERVIEW

Acute pancreatitis is a serious and at times life-threatening inflammatory process of the pancreas, resulting in *autodigestion* of the organ by its own enzymes. The pathologic changes occur in variable degrees; and the severity of pancreatitis depends on the extent of inflammation and tissue destruction, ranging from mild involvement characterized by edema and inflammation to necrotizing hemorrhagic pancreatitis. This severe form of pancreatitis is characterized by diffusely bleeding pancreatic tissue with fibrosis and tissue death.

Pathophysiology

The activation of an inflammatory process of the pancreas may occur after any insult or injury that causes obstruction of the pancreatic duct. Direct toxic injury to the pancreatic cells and production and release of pancreatic enzymes (trypsin, elastase, phospholipase A, lipase, and kallikrein) occur as a result of the obstructive damage. After pancreatic duct obstruction, increased pressure within the pancreas and the pancreatic ducts may contribute to ductal rupture, allowing spillage of trypsin and other enzymes into the pancreatic parenchymal tissue.

In acute pancreatitis, four major physiologic processes occur: the lipolytic process, proteolysis, necrosis of blood vessels, and inflammation. The hallmark of pancreatic necrosis is enzymatic fat necrosis of the en-

docrine and exocrine cells of the pancreas by the enzyme lipase. Fatty acids are released during this *lipolytic process* and combine with ionized calcium to form a soap-like product. This initial rapid lowering of serum calcium levels is not readily compensated for by the parathyroid gland. Because the body needs ionized calcium and cannot use bound calcium, hypocalcemia occurs.

The pathogenesis of pancreatitis involves autodigestion of the pancreatic parenchyma organ by those enzymes normally produced by the pancreas (Fig. 47–6). Trypsin activates the major proteolytic enzymes involved in autodigestion. The agent that triggers the premature activation of these enzymes has not been identified and is being investigated. *Proteolysis* involves the splitting of proteins by hydrolysis of the peptide bonds, with the formation of smaller polypeptides. Proteolytic activity may lead to thrombosis and gangrene of the pancreas. Pancreatic destruction may be localized and confined to one area or may involve the entire organ.

Elastase is activated by trypsin, causing the dissolving of elastic fibers of the blood vessels and ducts. The *necrosis of blood vessels* results in bleeding, ranging from minor bleeding to massive hemorrhage of pancreatic tissue. Another pancreatic enzyme, kallikrein, causes the release of vasoactive peptides, bradykinin and a plasma kinin known as kallidin, which contribute to

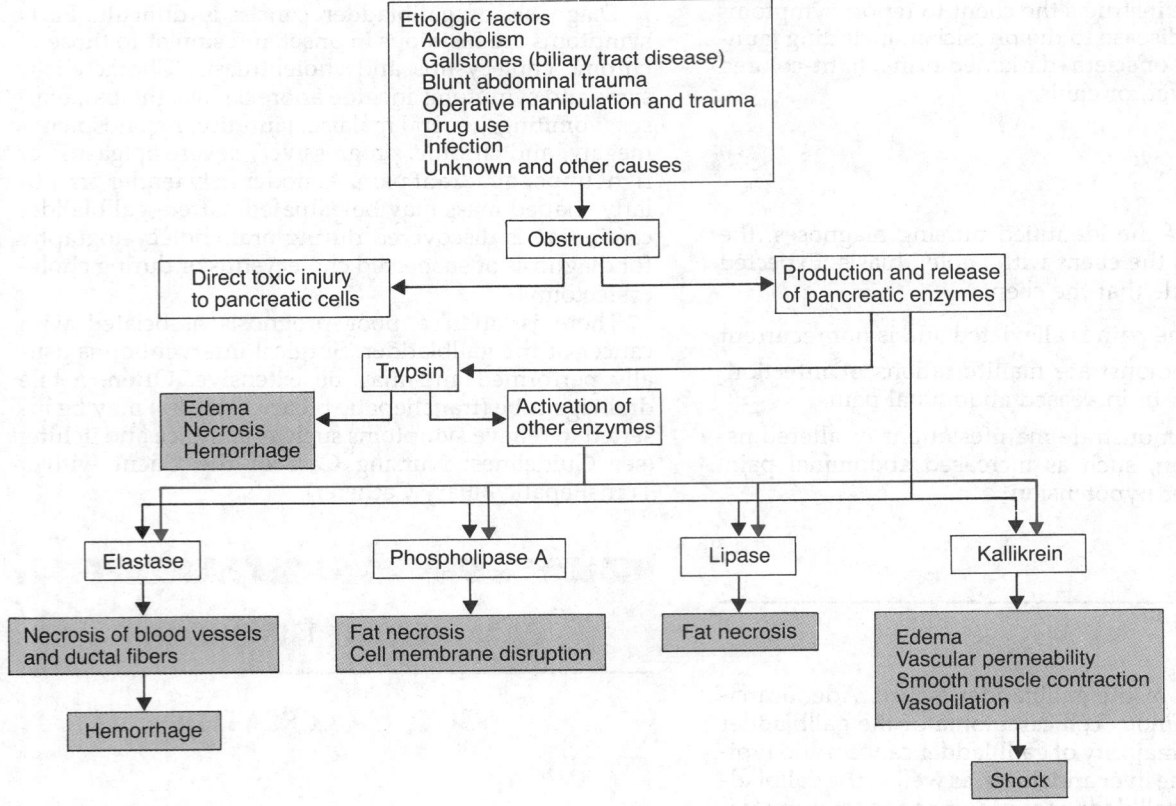

Figure 47–6

The process of autodigestion in acute pancreatitis.

vasodilation and increased vascular permeability, further compounding the hemorrhagic process. This massive destruction of blood vessels by necrosis may lead to generalized hemorrhage, with blood escaping into the retroperitoneal tissues. The client with *hemorrhagic pancreatitis* is critically ill, and extensive pancreatic destruction and shock may lead to death. The majority of deaths in those with acute pancreatitis result from irreversible shock.

The *inflammatory* stage occurs when leukocytes cluster around the hemorrhagic and necrotic areas of the pancreas. A secondary bacterial process may lead to suppuration of the pancreatic parenchyma or formation of an abscess (see later discussion of pancreatic abscess). Mild infected lesions may be absorbed. When these infected lesions are severe, calcification and fibrosis occur. If the infected fluid becomes walled off by fibrous tissue, a *pancreatic pseudocyst* is formed (see later).

Several theories have been developed to explain the triggering mechanisms leading to enzyme activation in acute pancreatitis. The *bile reflux,* or common channel, theory proposes that an obstruction of the common channel (the common bile duct and the main pancreatic duct channel) causes reflux of the bile into the pancreatic tissue, resulting in activation of the enzymes. Not all biliary tracts have this common channel, and, in these cases, the common bile and pancreatic ducts merge into the duodenum separately.

According to the hypersecretion-obstruction theory, rupture of the pancreatic duct occurs, with disruption or tearing of the cell membrane, allowing pancreatic secretion and enzymes to leak back into the parenchymal tissue.

The exact mechanism of *alcohol-induced* changes in pancreatitis is unclear. Alcohol appears to have a direct metabolic effect on the pancreas by stimulating hydrochloric acid and secretin production, which in turn stimulate exocrine functions of the pancreas. Alcohol also causes edema of the duodenum and the ampulla of Vater, obstructing the flow of pancreatic secretions. Alcohol may decrease the tone of the sphincter of Oddi and cause sphincter spasm with duodenal reflux.

According to the fourth theory, *reflux of duodenal contents* can occur from biliary tract disease; gallstones in the bile duct, causing the sphincter of Oddi to dilate; or generalized loss of tone caused by alcohol ingestion. Duodenal contents can enter the pancreatic duct through the weakened sphincter, activating the pancreatic enzymes.

The generalized abdominal pain of acute pancreatitis is related to peritoneal irritation. Ductal release of digested proteins and lipids into the peripancreatic tissues, along with stretching of the pancreatic tissue, causes the seepage of these substances into the mesentery. The resultant peritonitis stimulates the sensory nerves, contributing to intense pain in the back and flanks.

Mild *jaundice* occurs from swelling of the head of the pancreas, which impedes bile flow through the common bile duct. The bile duct may also be compressed by calculi or a pancreatic pseudocyst, with total bile flow obstruction, resulting in severe jaundice. Transient *hyper-*

glycemia from release of glucagon and decreased release of insulin results from damage to the pancreatic islet cells.

Left lung *pleural effusions* frequently develop in the client with acute pancreatitis. Amylase effusions probably occur when exudate containing pancreatic enzymes passes from the peritoneal cavity into the pleural cavity via the transdiaphragmatic lymph channels. The client is at risk for *adult respiratory distress syndrome* (ARDS). This severe form of pulmonary edema is caused by disruption of the alveolar-capillary membrane and is a serious complication of acute pancreatitis (see Chap. 62 for discussion of ARDS).

Coagulation defects are another major potential complication and may result in death. Complex physiologic changes in the pancreas cause release of necrotic tissue and enzymes into the blood stream, resulting in altered coagulation. *Disseminated intravascular coagulation* (DIC) involves hypercoagulation of the blood, with consumption of clotting factors and the development of microthrombi (see Chap. 67 for discussion of DIC).

Etiology

The exact cause of pancreatitis is not known. Many factors can cause injury to the pancreas. Most commonly cited are alcoholism and biliary tract disease with gallstones. Postoperative acute pancreatitis may occur iatrogenically as a result of trauma from surgical manipulation after biliary tract, pancreatic, gastric, and duodenal procedures, such as cholecystectomy, Whipple's procedure, or partial gastrectomy.

Other etiologic factors include pancreatic tumors, cysts, and abscesses; abnormal organ structure; penetrating gastric or duodenal ulcers, resulting in peritonitis; viral infections, such as with coxsackievirus B; and drug toxicities, including opiates, sulfonamides, thiazides, steroids, and oral contraceptives. The exact mechanism by which these and other drugs cause pancreatitis is unknown.

Blunt abdominal trauma, as well as metabolic disturbances (e.g., hyperparathyroidism and hyperlipidemia), has caused episodes of pancreatitis. Pancreatic inflammation has been reported after renal failure, fasciculitis (inflammation of fascia), renal transplantation, and endoscopic retrograde cholangiopancreatography (ERCP), a diagnostic procedure.

Heredity has been cited as a predisposing factor; in some cases, neurogenic or emotional factors have been involved. Frequently, the cause is never identified (i.e., idiopathic acute pancreatitis).

Incidence

In the United States the overall incidence of pancreatitis is less than 1% of the adult population; however, the diagnosis is often not recognized. Alcoholism is the most frequent cause of acute pancreatitis in the middle-aged male population. Episodes of pancreatitis usually occur after excessive alcohol consumption. These attacks are especially common during holidays and vacations. Steady, heavy alcohol intake over a period of 5 to 10 years is likely to produce pancreatitis. Women most frequently develop pancreatitis after cholelithiasis and biliary tract disturbances.

Death results in approximately 10% of clients with acute pancreatitis. With early diagnosis and treatment, mortality can be reduced. Death occurs at a higher rate in the elderly population and in those with postoperative pancreatitis. The prognosis for recovery is favorable for pancreatitis associated with biliary tract disease and poor if pancreatitis accompanies alcoholism. Mortality rises as high as 60% when necrosis and hemorrhage occur (Given & Simmons, 1984).

PREVENTION

Excessive alcohol intake is well documented as a major contributing factor in pancreatitis. Alcohol intake should be stopped immediately when acute pancreatitis is diagnosed. Clients with pancreatitis must be made aware that exacerbations commonly develop after holiday, vacation, or binge drinking. Cholelithiasis and cholecystitis should be medically or surgically treated as soon as possible to prevent potential extension of biliary tract dysfunction and pancreatic involvement.

COLLABORATIVE MANAGEMENT

 Assessment

History

When taking a history from a client with the medical diagnosis of acute pancreatitis, the nurse asks the client to state the reason for seeking medical treatment. Most often, the primary reason is relief of *abdominal pain*. The nurse asks the client if abdominal pain is related to excessive alcohol ingestion or occurs after eating a high-fat meal and explores the nature of the pain. The nurse asks the client about *alcohol intake*, including the amount of alcohol consumed over what period of time. The nurse questions the client to ascertain if there is a *family history of alcoholism, pancreatitis, or biliary tract disease*. The client is asked if any biliary tract problems, such as gallstones, have been experienced. The nurse determines if any *abdominal surgical interventions*, such as cholecystectomy, or diagnostic procedures, such as ERCP, have been performed recently.

The nurse assesses for the presence of *other medical problems* known to cause pancreatitis, including peptic ulcer disease, renal failure, vascular disorders, hyperparathyroidism, or hyperlipidemia. The client is asked if any recent viral infections have been experienced and to list all prescription and over-the-counter (OTC) drugs taken recently.

Physical Assessment: Clinical Manifestations

Clinical manifestations of acute pancreatitis vary widely and are dependent on the severity of the inflammation. A typical client is diagnosed after presenting with *abdominal pain*, the most frequent symptom. The nurse obtains in-depth data about the pain. The client often states that the pain has a sudden onset and is located in the mid-epigastric area or left upper quadrant, with radiation to the back; the pain is described as intense and continuous. The client may admit that the pain has been aggravated by eating a fatty meal, ingesting alcohol, or lying in a recumbent position. The nurse determines if the pain is relieved by positioning. Often, the client finds relief by assuming the fetal position (with knees drawn up to the chest and the spine flexed) or when sitting upright and bending forward.

The client may complain of *weight loss* with *nausea* and *vomiting*. When performing an abdominal assessment, the nurse may find the following on inspection: generalized *jaundice, discoloration of the abdomen and periumbilical area* (Cullen's sign), and *bluish discoloration of the flanks* (Turner's sign), caused by pancreatic enzyme leakage to cutaneous tissue from the peritoneal cavity. The nurse listens for bowel sounds; *absent or decreased bowel sounds* usually indicate paralytic (adynamic) ileus. On light palpation, the nurse finds *abdominal tenderness, rigidity,* and *guarding* from peritonitis. A *palpable mass* may be found if a pancreatic pseudocyst is present. *Pancreatic ascites* creates a dull sound on percussion.

The nurse takes and records vital signs frequently to assess for *elevated temperature, tachycardia,* and *decreased blood pressure.* The nurse utilizes these data to determine if complications are occurring. Respiratory complications, such as left lung pleural effusions, atelectasis, and pneumonia, commonly occur in acute pancreatitis. ARDS is a serious complication. The nurse performs a respiratory assessment, auscultating the lung fields for *adventitious sounds* or decreased aeration, and observes respirations for *dyspnea* or *orthopnea.*

The nurse assesses for any rapid changes in vital signs, which may indicate the life-threatening complication shock. *Hypotension* and *tachycardia* may occur as a result of frank pancreatic hemorrhage, excessive fluid volume shifting, or the toxic effects of abdominal sepsis from enzyme damage (see Chap. 17 for a discussion of shock). The nurse observes the client for *changes in behavior and sensorium* that may be related to alcohol withdrawal or indicate hypoxia or impending sepsis with shock.

Psychosocial Assessment

Excessive alcohol intake, particularly in men, is the most frequent cause of acute pancreatitis. Thus, the nurse gently explores the client's alcohol intake history. The nurse and the client discuss the intake of alcohol and reasons for overindulging. The nurse asks the client when increased drinking episodes occur and determines if binges occur during holidays, vacations, or weekends or revolve around particular activities, such as card playing or television viewing. The nurse also questions whether the client has recently experienced any traumatic event, such as the death of a family member or a job loss, which may have contributed to increased alcohol consumption.

Laboratory Findings

Diagnostic laboratory abnormalities are found in acute pancreatitis (see the accompanying Key Features of Disease). Elevated serum amylase and lipase levels provide the most reliable and direct evidence of pancreatitis and are considered the cardinal diagnostic signs of pancreatitis. Amylase levels should be obtained initially and are most reliable within the first 24 to 48 hours after the occurrence of acute abdominal pain. Levels may fluctuate throughout the course of the illness and may not be a reliable indicator of the severity of the disease process. Lipase levels remain elevated for a slightly longer period than serum amylase levels. Amylase levels in 2-hour urine collections also are elevated owing to the inflammatory process. If pancreatitis is accompanied by biliary dysfunction, serum bilirubin and alkaline phosphatase levels are elevated. Elevated serum glucose levels are also common in acute pancreatitis.

Decreased serum calcium and magnesium levels are seen with fat necrosis. Calcium levels may fall and remain decreased for 7 to 10 days. There is a poor prognosis if calcium levels consistently remain below 8 mg/dL.

Radiographic Findings

Computed tomography (CT) provides a reliable diagnosis of acute pancreatitis. This noninvasive technique may be used to rule out pancreatic pseudocyst or ductal calculi. Chest x-ray films may reveal hemidiaphragm elevation on the left side or pleural effusion.

Other Diagnostic Tests

Ultrasonography of the pancreas is used as a diagnostic tool in severe pancreatitis to help confirm an initial clinical impression, assess for degree of inflammatory resolution, or reveal common bile duct dilation from obstruction or gallstones.

 Analysis: Nursing Diagnosis

The client with acute pancreatitis may exhibit clinical manifestations varying from mild to life-threatening. The client is generally acutely ill, in acute distress and pain.

Common Diagnoses

The following two diagnoses occur commonly in clients with acute pancreatitis:

1. Pain related to pancreatic inflammation and enzyme leakage

---

KEY FEATURES OF DISEASE ■ Causes of Laboratory Diagnostic Abnormalities in Acute Pancreatitis

Abnormal Finding	Cause
Cardinal Diagnostic Tests	
Increased *serum* amylase	Pancreatic cell injury
Elevated *serum* lipase	Pancreatic cell injury
Elevated *urine* amylase	Pancreatic cell injury
Other Diagnostic Tests	
Elevated serum glucose	Pancreatic beta cell injury, resulting in impaired carbohydrate metabolism
Decreased serum calcium	Fatty acids combined with calcium; seen in fat necrosis
Elevated bilirubin	Hepatobiliary obstructive process
Elevated alkaline phosphatase	Hepatobiliary involvement
Elevated WBC count	Inflammatory response

2. Altered nutrition: less than body requirements related to treatment regimen

Additional Diagnoses

The client may have one or more additional diagnoses, including

1. Fluid volume deficit related to pancreatic hemorrhage and fluid loss into the abdominal cavity, GI fluid losses from a nasogastric tube, and sepsis
2. Ineffective breathing pattern related to complications of pleural effusion or ARDS
3. Potential for injury related to bleeding complications secondary to DIC and pancreatic hemorrhage
4. Potential for activity intolerance related to debilitation

---

CLIENT CARE PLAN ■ The Client with Acute Pancreatitis

Goal/Outcome Criteria	Interventions	Rationales
Nursing Diagnosis 1: Pain Related to Pancreatic Inflammation and Enzyme Leakage		
Client will experience reduction in acute abdominal pain.	1. Assess the client's verbal complaints of abdominal pain. Determine specific location and intensity of pain.	1. Pain of acute pancreatitis is often severe and diffuse.
■ Verbalizes reduction in abdominal pain with specific interventions.	2. Withhold food and fluids and keep environment free from food odors.	2. Goal of NPO status is to rest the pancreas. Food or fluid intake can activate the release of pancreatic enzymes, thereby increasing pain.
	3. Maintain the nasogastric tube for drainage or suction, as ordered.	3. Nasogastric drainage keeps the stomach empty and prevents the accumulation of gastric secretions, which stimulates pancreatic enzyme activity. Nasogastric decompression promotes comfort.
	4. Administer IM meperidine and assess its effectiveness in pain relief.	4. Meperidine is the drug of choice for pain relief in acute pancreatitis. It reduces spasms of the pancreatic duct and the spincter of Oddi.
	5. Administer antacids as ordered.	5. Antacids neutralize gastric acid to reduce production of pancreatic enzymes and reduce the incidence of gastric ulceration and bleeding.
	6. Position the client to promote comfort by turning the client to the side with the knees flexed. a. Teach the client to maintain a side-lying position independently.	6. This position reduces pressure and tension on the abdominal muscles.
	7. Restrict the client to bed rest and promote quiet and rest.	7. By keeping the client quiet and in bed, the metabolic rate and GI stimulation and secretion is reduced, thereby decreasing abdominal pain.
Nursing Diagnosis 2: Altered Nutrition: Less Than Body Requirements Related to Treatment Regimen		
Client will gain weight.	1. Assess the client's nutritional status. a. Weigh the client on admission and daily. Obtain the client's usual or preadmission weight.	1. Admissions weight and usual preadmission weight help to establish a baseline. a. Serial measurements indicate inappropriate trends in weight loss or gain.

5. Knowledge deficit related to illness, causative factors, and proposed treatment plan

 Planning and Implementation →

The plan of care focuses on the common nursing diagnoses identified in clients with acute pancreatitis (see the accompanying Client Care Plan).

Pain

Planning: client goals.   The major goal of this nursing diagnosis is that the client will experience pain relief and that chronic pain and inflammatory relapses will be prevented.

Interventions.   Abdominal pain is a prominent symptom of pancreatitis. The main focus of nursing care is aimed at reducing discomfort and pain by the use of

---

CLIENT CARE PLAN ■ The Client with Acute Pancreatitis *continued*

Goal/Outcome Criteria	Interventions	Rationales
Nursing Diagnosis 2: Altered Nutrition: Less Than Body Requirements Related to Treatment Regimen		
	b. On physical examination, inspect for signs of malnutrition, such as fragile, lackluster hair; sunken eyes with pale conjunctiva; dry, swollen oral mucous membranes; and smooth or coated tongue.	b. Physical assessment can provide valuable clues about the client's nutritional status.
	2. Maintain NPO status and nasogastric drainage until bowel sounds return and abdominal pain subsides.	2. Food and fluids are always withheld until relief of symptoms is obtained. The client's NPO status may further contribute to malnourished state.
	a. While the client is on NPO status, administer ordered IV fluid solution; add potassium chloride, multivitamin supplements, thiamine, and folate, as ordered.	a. IV fluids can provide hydration, electrolytes, and vitamins in early therapy.
	3. Consult with a nutritional support team or a dietitian regarding nutritional status and nutrition repletion program.	3. Early discussion of the client's nutrition aids in identifying nutritional deficits and determining whether intervention is needed.
■ Selects nutritious foods.	a. Teach the client what constitutes good nutritional intake. Reinforce the dietitian's nutrition plan.	a. When an oral diet is resumed, discharge teaching is crucial.
■ Identifies and avoids foods or fluids that stimulate the pancreas.	b. Assist the client in selecting foods and fluids that meet metabolic and nutritional needs.	b. Previous dietary habits may be unsatisfactory for the client's current needs for tissue regeneration and healing.
	c. Instruct the client to avoid caffeine, alcohol, and gas-forming foods and to avoid large, heavy meals.	c. Client *must* avoid foods that overstimulate the stomach and pancreas to prevent recurrence of symptoms.
	4. Institute alternate feeding methods if NPO status is prolonged.	4. Peripheral or central venous hyperalimentation may be required (see Chapter 13).

measures to decrease GI tract activity, thus decreasing pancreatic stimulation.

Nonsurgical management.   Pain relief by nonsurgical methods is attempted initially. These include fasting, drug therapy, and comfort measures.

Fasting.   In an effort to rest the pancreas and reduce pancreatic enzyme secretion, food and fluids are withheld in the acute period. Hydration is maintained intravenously.

Nasogastric drainage and suction may be necessary to decrease gastric distention and to suppress pancreatic secretion. This is accomplished by preventing gastric digestive juices from flowing into the duodenum. Because adynamic (paralytic) ileus is a common complication of acute pancreatitis, prolonged nasogastric intubation may be required. The nurse assesses for the presence of bowel sounds before the removal of the nasogastric tube and initiation of feedings.

Drug therapy.   Meperidine hydrochloride (Demerol) is the drug of choice for relieving abdominal pain associated with acute pancreatitis. Meperidine hydrochloride causes less incidence of spasm of the smooth musculature of the pancreatic ducts and the sphincter of Oddi than do opiate drugs, such as morphine. In mild pancreatitis, the pain usually subsides in 3 to 4 days; however, with severe, acute pancreatitis, the abdominal pain and tenderness may persist for up to 2 weeks. The nurse individualizes dosages and intervals of medication administration according to the severity of the disease and the symptoms.

Pancreatic stimulation is reduced by decreasing the release of secretin. The intestinal hormone stimulates the release of enzymes and bicarbonate from the pancreas when acidic chyme is present in the duodenum. Antacids administered orally or via a nasogastric tube that is clamped for 20 minutes neutralize gastric secretions. Histamine receptor–blocking drugs, such as ranitidine (Zantac) and cimetidine (Tagamet), are given to the client to decrease hydrochloric acid production so that pancreatic enzymes are not activated by an acid pH. These interventions also are useful in reducing the occurrence of GI erosion and bleeding. Anticholinergics, such as atropine and propantheline bromide (Pro-Banthine), are indicated to decrease vagal stimulation, decrease GI motility, and inhibit pancreatic enzyme and bicarbonate volume and concentration.

Comfort measures.   Helping the client to assume the fetal position (with legs drawn up to the chest) has been helpful in decreasing the abdominal pain of pancreatitis.

If the client has a nasogastric tube in place, the nurse provides frequent oral hygiene measures to keep mucous membranes moist and free from inflammation or crusting. Because of the drying effect of anticholinergic drugs and the absence of oral fluids, the mouth and oral cavity may be extremely dry and parched, causing considerable discomfort for the client.

Pain may also be substantially reduced by lowering the client's anxiety level. The nurse provides thorough explanations of procedures. The client is encouraged to express the emotions and responses he/she is experiencing. The nurse also provides reassurance and diversional activities, such as television, music, and reading material in an attempt to redirect attention away from pain.

Surgical management.   Surgical intervention in acute pancreatitis is usually not indicated. However, complications of pancreatitis, such as pancreatic pseudocyst or abscess, may require surgical drainage. If pancreatitis is caused by biliary tract obstruction, a laparotomy (abdominal exploration) for common bile duct exploration and release of obstruction may be indicated.

Preoperative care.   In addition to general preoperative care measures, the client usually has a nasogastric tube inserted and administration of IV fluids started. The nurse teaches the client to expect a pancreatic drainage tube and explains its care for the postoperative period.

Postoperative care.   When an abscess or pseudocyst is incised and drained under general anesthesia, drainage tubes are inserted, sutured in place, and connected to low suction (80 mmHg or less) to prevent further tissue erosion. The nurse monitors drainage tubes for patency by assessing for kinks in the tubes and maintaining the ordered drain suction pressure and system integrity. The drain output amount is recorded, and the character of the drainage is described. A sump-type drain is usually inserted. The nurse checks to make sure the drain is functioning, indicated by a hissing noise from the sump lumen. (Refer to Chap. 20 for further discussion on drainage devices.)

Meticulous skin care and dressing changes are provided. The nurse reports the first signs of redness or skin irritation to the physician, as pancreatic enzyme drainage is particularly excoriating to the skin. Skin barriers, such as a Stomahesive wafer around the drainage tube or aluminum paste, are applied to repel drainage from the skin. The nurse continually assesses for further deterioration of the tissue and consults an enterostomal therapist about measures to promote skin integrity, such as individualized ostomy appliances and topical ointments.

Altered Nutrition: Less Than Body Requirements

Planning: client goals.   The goal of nutritional therapy is that the client will have an optimal nutritional intake with a decrease in pancreatic stimulation.

Interventions: nonsurgical management.   The client is maintained on NPO status in the early stages of pancreatitis. If the client is severely nutritionally depleted, total parenteral nutrition (TPN) or hyperalimentation is indicated (see Chap. 13 for interventions related to TPN). If hyperalimentation is utilized for nutritional support, the nurse assesses for glucose intolerance by monitoring for elevated blood glucose levels. This is extremely important in clients with pancreatitis, because pancreatic dysfunction will affect the release of insulin.

When food is tolerated during the recovery phase, small, frequent, high-carbohydrate and high-protein feedings are given. Carbohydrates are not as stimulating to the pancreas as fats, which should be limited. Foods should be bland with little spice; caffeine-containing foods, such as tea, coffee, cola, and alcohol, should be avoided.

To boost caloric intake, liquid diet preparations, such as Ensure and Isocal, supplement the diet. If caloric intake is poor, a nasogastric tube may be required for enteral feedings. Fat-soluble and other vitamin and mineral replacement supplements may also be given.

■ Discharge Planning

Clients with acute pancreatitis are discharged to home after recovery from the acute episode.

Home Care Preparation

The home should require little special preparation, but home care measures must be individualized for each client's circumstances. Some clients with acute pancreatitis may be severely weakened from their acute illness and need to confine activity to one floor, limiting stair climbing and other strenuous activity until strength is regained.

Client/Family Education

Discharge education needs to be started early in the hospitalization period, but after acute episodes of pain have subsided. During acute pain, the client will not retain much of the information shared. The nurse assesses the client's and family members' knowledge of the disease, causative agents, and precipitating factors.

Goals of discharge planning education are aimed at preventing further episodes of pancreatitis and disease progression to a chronic state. The client is instructed to abstain from alcohol to prevent further pain attacks and extension of inflammation and pancreatic insufficiency. The client should be told that if alcohol is consumed, pain will be experienced and further autodigestion of the pancreas will lead to chronic pancreatitis and chronic pain.

The client should be instructed to notify the physician after discharge to home if acute abdominal pain or biliary tract disease (as evidenced by jaundice, clay-colored stools, or darkened urine) occurs, possibly indicating complications or disease progression.

Psychosocial Preparation

The client may require support after discharge if the hospital course was complicated. If alcohol consumption was associated with the pancreatitis, the client needs support to assess his/her use of alcohol and to abstain from further use.

Health Care Resources

Clients with acute pancreatitis require visits by a home care nurse if the hospital course was complicated. In these cases, home health care may be required for wound care and assistance with activities of daily living (ADL). The client requires medical follow-up with the primary care physician or clinic for monitoring of the disease process.

Evaluation

On the basis of the identified nursing diagnoses and health care interventions, the nurse evaluates the care of the client with acute pancreatitis. Expected outcomes include that the client

1. States that the acute abdominal pain has subsided and minimal discomfort is experienced
2. Maintains optimal weight and nutritional status
3. Maintains balanced fluid volume
4. Achieves independence in ADL

CHRONIC PANCREATITIS

OVERVIEW

Chronic pancreatitis is a progressive, destructive disease of the pancreas. Inflammation and fibrosis of the tissue contribute to pancreatic insufficiency and diminished function of the organ. Chronic pancreatitis usually develops after repeated episodes of alcohol-induced acute pancreatitis. It may also be associated with chronic obstruction of the common bile duct. Chronic pancreatitis may develop in the absence of a known acute disorder and is characterized by exacerbations and remissions.

Pathophysiology

Alcohol-induced chronic pancreatitis is also known as *chronic calcifying pancreatitis* (CCP). It is characterized by protein precipitates that plug the ducts and lead to ductal obstruction, atrophy, and dilation. As the protein plugging becomes diffuse, the epithelium of the ducts undergoes histologic changes, resulting in metaplasia (cell replacement) and ulceration. This inflammatory process causes fibrosis of the pancreatic tissue. Intraductal calcification and marked pancreatic parenchymal destruction develop in the late stages of chronic pancreatitis. Cystic sacs containing pancreatic secretions and enzymes form on the pancreas. The organ becomes hard and firm as a result of acinar cell atrophy and pancreatic insufficiency.

Chronic obstructive pancreatitis develops from inflammation, spasm, and obstruction of the sphincter of Oddi. Inflammatory and sclerotic lesions develop in the head of the pancreas and around the ducts, causing an obstruction and backflow of pancreatic secretions. (The reader is referred to the earlier discussion of acute pancreatitis and its complications.)

Pancreatic insufficiency in chronic pancreatitis is characterized by the loss of *exocrine function*. Pancreatic exocrine secretion is divided into two components: aqueous bicarbonate and enzymes. The aqueous component functions to neutralize the duodenal contents and pancreatic enzymes that are essential to normal digestion and absorption. Most clients with chronic pancreatitis have a decreased output of pancreatic secretion and bicarbonate. Pancreatic enzyme secretion must be reduced by more than 80% to produce steatorrhea resulting from severe malabsorption of fats. These characteristic stools are pale, bulky, and frothy and have an offensive odor. The action of colonic bacteria on unabsorbed lipids and proteins is responsible for the foul odor. On inspection of the stools, the fat content is visible. In severe chronic pancreatitis, stool fat output may exceed 40 g/day.

Fat malabsorption also contributes to weight loss and muscle wasting, or decrease in body muscle mass, and leads to general debilitation of the client. Protein malabsorption results in a "starvation" edema of the feet, legs, and hands caused by decreased levels of circulating protein.

The loss of pancreatic endocrine function is responsible for the development of frank diabetes mellitus in clients with chronic pancreatic insufficiency. (See Chap. 51 for a complete discussion of diabetes mellitus.)

The client with chronic pancreatitis may have pulmonary complications, such as pleuritic pain, pleural effusions, or pulmonary infiltrates. Pancreatic ascites may impede diaphragmatic excursion and decrease lung expansion, resulting in impaired ventilation. In the ill client with chronic pancreatitis, ARDS may develop.

Etiology

The cause of CCP is persistent excessive alcohol intake that results in repeated episodes of acute pancreatitis. The most common cause of chronic obstructive pancreatitis is cholelithiasis and biliary tract disease, which results in persistent inflammation. Other etiologic factors include pancreatic pseudocyst, postoperative ductal scarring, and cancer of the pancreas or duodenum. All of these factors can obstruct the pancreatic duct. Prolonged starvation and prolonged use of parenteral feedings as a method of nutritional support can result in pancreatic atrophy, causing pancreatic insufficiency.

Incidence

Alcohol-induced pancreatitis is predominantly found in men, but the incidence in women is increasing. In women, it occurs more frequently among those with biliary tract disease (cholecystitis and cholelithiasis). The age at occurrence of chronic pancreatitis is variable but is usually between 45 and 60 years (Given & Simmons, 1984).

PREVENTION

To prevent chronic exacerbations, alcohol consumption must be completely avoided. It is also recommended that the client abstain from coffee, tea, colas, and other caffeinated beverages. Antacids are helpful in preventing acid production, which stimulates the release of secretin and enhances pancreatic activity. Also recommended as a preventive measure is a bland, low-fat diet in small, frequent feedings with avoidance of all rich, fatty foods.

COLLABORATIVE MANAGEMENT

 Assessment

History

When obtaining a history from a client with chronic pancreatitis, it is helpful to ask the same questions as those asked of a client with acute pancreatitis. The nurse obtains more specific information regarding alcohol intake, including when alcohol was last ingested, the amount consumed, and the relationship to pain development. The nurse determines if the pain is always present and if it is intensified after alcohol ingestion.

Physical Assessment: Clinical Manifestations

Clinical manifestations of chronic pancreatitis differ from those of an acute inflammation. *Abdominal pain* is the major clinical manifestation. The client with chronic pancreatitis describes the pain as a continuous, burning, or gnawing dullness with periods of acute exacerbation. The pain is intense and relentless. The frequency of acute exacerbations may increase as the pancreatic fibrosis develops.

The nurse performs the same abdominal assessment as for clients with acute pancreatitis, but the findings may not be as significant. *Abdominal tenderness* is less intense. A *mass* may be palpated in the left upper quadrant, indicative of a pancreatic pseudocyst or abscess (see later). Massive *pancreatic ascites* may be present, producing dullness on abdominal percussion.

Because respiratory complications can accompany the condition, the nurse performs a respiratory assessment, auscultating the lung fields for *adventitious sounds* or decreased aeration, and observes respirations for *dyspnea* or *orthopnea*.

The client is asked to collect a random stool specimen, if able, or asked to describe his/her stools. The nurse inspects the specimen for the presence of *steatorrhea*. These foul-smelling fatty stools may increase in volume as pancreatic insufficiency progresses and lipase production decreases. The client may experience *weight loss, muscle wasting, jaundice, dark urine,* and the signs and symptoms of *diabetes mellitus.*

Psychosocial Assessment

Chronic persistent abdominal pain can cause the client with chronic pancreatitis to become dependent on narcotics for pain relief. Clients with chronic pain present problems for families and health care providers (see Chap. 7).

Clients with chronic pancreatitis require frequent, multiple admissions to health care settings during acute exacerbations of the illness. These can be demoralizing for clients and their families.

Laboratory Findings

In chronic pancreatitis, significant laboratory findings include elevated serum bilirubin, alkaline phosphatase, and amylase levels. Transient serum glucose elevations are common. Stool specimens may be examined for elevated levels of fat and trypsin.

Radiographic Findings

ERCP may reveal ductal system abnormalities, such as calcification or strictures, or may delineate the presence of pancreatic pseudocyst.

Other Diagnostic Tests

The only definitive diagnostic test for chronic pancreatitis is identification of calcification of pancreatic tissue in a biopsy specimen. The secretin test is often done to assess pancreatic exocrine function. Secretin is a hormone that stimulates hepatic and pancreatic secretion. In this test, the client swallows a double-lumen GI tube. The tip should reach the duodenum, with the proximal lumen port located in the stomach. Gastric and duodenal contents are aspirated before and after IV administration of secretin. Abnormally low volumes of enzymes and bicarbonate in the GI contents may indicate chronic pancreatitis. Abdominal ultrasonography is a helpful diagnostic tool, especially to reveal pseudocysts.

 Analysis: Nursing Diagnosis

Chronic pain, debilitated physical appearance, chemical dependence on drugs and alcohol, and frequent defecation typify the client with chronic pancreatitis. It is challenging to provide nursing care measures and interventions for these clients.

Common Diagnoses

Multiple nursing diagnoses are established for these clients and include

1. Chronic pain related to chronic pancreatic inflammation
2. Altered nutrition: less than body requirements related to chronic malabsorption or malnutrition from poor dietary intake
3. Diarrhea related to malabsorption of fat

Additional Diagnoses

As with any chronic illness, many potential problems develop that require individualized nursing interventions. The following represent possible additional nursing diagnoses:

1. Activity intolerance related to chronic illness and debilitated state
2. Noncompliance (dietary restrictions) related to persistent alcohol intake and poor dietary measures
3. Ineffective individual coping related to the stress of chronic illness, pain, and suffering
4. Potential impaired skin integrity related to steatorrhea
5. Ineffective breathing pattern related to pancreatic ascites, pleural effusions, or respiratory failure

 Planning and Implementation

Chronic Pain

Planning: client goals. The goal is that the client will experience an alleviation of or reduction in pain.

Interventions. The discomfort of chronic pancreatitis can be frequent, intermittent, or chronic, persisting in an unrelenting manner. The client may experience acute exacerbations after heavy alcohol intake.

Nonsurgical management. Drug therapy is the major intervention for the pain of chronic pancreatitis. In addition, the nurse acts to prevent the client from ingesting irritating substances that can precipitate pain. (See Chap. 7 for a thorough discussion of chronic pain management.)

The nurse medicates the client according to the assessment of level and intensity of pain and evaluates the effectiveness of the drug intervention. The client is experiencing pain and requires analgesia. Narcotic analgesia with meperidine hydrochloride (Demerol) is most frequently used, but narcotic dependency may become a problem. Pentazocine (Talwin), a nonnarcotic analgesic, has been utilized to relieve pain with success. (The reader is referred to earlier discussion of drug therapy for clients with acute pancreatitis for other pharmacologic treatment measures that are also indicated in chronic pancreatitis.)

If dependency on narcotics becomes a problem, behavior modification programs and drug and alcohol counseling by trained professionals are required. It is sometimes necessary to admit these clients to drug dependency programs.

Surgical management. Surgery is not a primary intervention for the treatment of chronic pancreatitis, but may be indicated for intractable abdominal pain, incapacitating relapses of pain, or complications, such as abscesses or pseudocysts.

The underlying pathologic changes determine the procedure indicated. An abscess or pseudocyst is incised and drained initially. *Cholecystectomy* or *choledochotomy* (incision of the common bile duct) is indicated if biliary tract disease is an underlying cause. If the pancreatic duct sphincter is fibrotic, a *sphincterotomy* (incision of the sphincter) is done in an effort to enlarge it.

In *pancreatojejunostomy*, the pancreatic duct is opened and anastomosed to the jejunum in an effort to relieve obstruction. This procedure relieves pain and preserves pancreatic tissue and function. The preoperative and postoperative care is similar to that for clients undergoing Whipple's procedure (see later). A partial pancreatectomy (resection of the pancreas) may be performed for clients with advanced pancreatitis or disabling pain. Vagotomy with gastric antrectomy is done to alter nerve stimulation and decrease pancreatic secretion (see Chap. 44 for a discussion of nursing care).

Altered Nutrition: Less Than Body Requirements

Planning: client goals. The goal is that the client will maintain an optimal nutritional intake in an effort to restore function and prevent complications of skin breakdown, debilitation with muscle wasting, and decreased energy.

Interventions: nonsurgical management. Protein and fat malabsorption results in significant weight loss and decrease in muscle mass in the client with chronic pancreatitis. The nutritional interventions for the client with acute pancreatitis are also relevant for clients in the chronic phase of pancreatitis.

Drug therapy. The client often limits food intake to avoid the recurrent pain, which is exacerbated by eating. For this reason, nutrition maintenance is often difficult to achieve and clients are provided with TPN, including vitamin and mineral replacement. Interventions are the same as those listed for clients with nutritional deficiencies in acute pancreatitis (see earlier).

Enzyme replacement. Pancreatic enzymes are essential dietary supplements. These are generally given with meals or snacks to aid in digestion and absorption of fat and protein. Drugs such as pancreatin (Viokase) and pancrelipase (Cotazym or Pancrease) are given in capsule, tablet, or powder form and contain amylase, lipase, and trypsin. The nurse mixes the powder form in applesauce or fruit juices to make it more palatable. Enzyme preparations should not be mixed with foods containing proteins because the enzymatic action dissolves the food into a watery substance. The nurse advises the client to wipe his/her lips with a wet towel to avoid skin irritation and breakdown that residual enzymes can cause.

The dosage of pancreatic enzymes depends on the severity of malabsorption and maldigestion. The nurse records the number of stools per day and stool consistency to monitor the effectiveness of enzyme therapy. If it is effective, the stools should become less frequent and less fatty.

Insulin therapy. If the client develops diabetes, insulin or oral hypoglycemic agents are given for control. Clients maintained on TPN are particularly susceptible to labile glucose levels and may require regular insulin additives to the solution. The nurse closely monitors blood glucose levels so that hyperglycemia is controlled and insulin shock is prevented. The use of bedside glucose monitoring meters, such as Accucheck II or Glucometers, allows for hourly assessment of levels during the critical insulin dosage adjustment period. Glucose levels should be checked at least every 2 to 4 hours.

Diarrhea

Planning: client goals. The goal for this diagnosis is that the client will experience a decrease in frequency and fat content of stools.

Interventions: nonsurgical management. Pancreatic insufficiency causes a decrease in the production of lipase, resulting in fat malabsorption in the bowel and fatty stools. These often large, gray-yellow, nonformed stools are greasy, frothy, and foul smelling. A yellow-orange oil-like leakage may seep from the rectum along with stools or may continually seep in the absence of stools in severe chronic pancreatitis. As pancreatic insufficiency progresses, steatorrhea increases, resulting in excoriation and skin care problems from frequent defecation.

Diet therapy. By adhering to the prescribed low-fat diet, the client assists in limiting fat intake, which can decrease the incidence of fatty stools. The nurse contacts the dietitian, who assists the client with in-hospital menu planning. The dietitian also supplies written dietary instruction for discharge, including a list of foods high in fat and protein content, which should be avoided. With chronic pancreatitis, the client may be hospitalized and require nutritional support with TPN or enteral tube feedings that do not contain fat. Because fat-soluble vitamins, such as vitamins A, D, E, and K, are not absorbed, replacement therapy must be included in the TPN solution or IV fluids or administered by oral supplements.

Skin care. The frequency of continent or incontinent defection poses challenging skin care problems. The client must be kept dry and the skin free from the abrasive fatty stools that are excoriating to the skin. The skin should be cleaned after each stool, and a soothing emollient, such as Sween products and other creams, should be applied. To prevent breakdown and maintain skin integrity, the nurse applies a barrier protection to the skin. Many products on the market, such as Sween ointments and zinc oxide cream, actively repel stool away from the skin. In the event of early breakdown, the nurse can apply a flexible hydroactive dressing (Duo-Derm) or a similar shield to the area. Preventive measures are important. If skin breakdown occurs, a vigorous regimen of skin care treatment must be instituted and maintained. These clients are often nutritionally depleted, and wound healing can be difficult.

■ Discharge Planning

Clients with chronic pancreatitis are discharged from the hospital with multiple, chronic health care needs requiring specialized and individualized discharge planning.

Home Care Preparation

The client with chronic pancreatitis is usually discharged to home, but some clients may require chronic care in an extended care setting.

If the client is discharged to home, the activity area should be limited to one floor until the client regains strength and activity can be increased. Toilet facilities must be easily accessible because of chronic steatorrhea and frequent defecation. If toilet facilities are not available in the immediate rest area, a bedpan or bedside commode must be obtained for the home.

Client/Family Education

Because there is no known curative treatment for chronic pancreatitis, client and family education is aimed at preventing further acute exacerbations of this chronic disease, providing chronic care, and promoting health maintenance.

The nurse instructs the client to avoid known precipitating factors, such as caffeinated beverages and irritating foods, particularly alcohol. The client should be firmly instructed to abstain from alcohol. The nurse elicits family participation in diet planning and food preparation arrangements. Diet instructions include bland, low-fat, frequent meals and avoidance of rich, fatty foods and caffeinated beverages. The nurse stresses the importance of dietary compliance and the need for increased nutritional intake to prevent acute exacerbations of this chronic illness. Written instructions are provided on diet and pancreatic enzyme replacement therapy.

The client and significant other or family members are instructed on the importance of adhering to the pancreatic enzyme replacement treatment. The client must take the prescribed enzymes with meals and snacks to aid in the digestion of food and promote the absorption of fats and proteins. The nurse instructs the client to take the enzymes at the beginning of the meal and to report to the physician any increase in the occurrence of foul-smelling, frothy, fatty stools, abdominal distention, and

cramping so that pancreatic enzyme replacement may be increased as needed. The client must also be instructed to report any skin excoriation or breakdown so that therapeutic interventions to promote skin integrity can be instituted.

Because the client with chronic pancreatitis experiences chronic pain, some clients may be discharged to home on injectable pain medication. In these cases, a reliable family member or significant other must be instructed in giving intramuscular (IM) injections. The nurse observes return demonstrations and actual IM injections given to the client during hospitalization. The client and family members must be able to state the desired effect of the drug, the schedule for drug administration, and potential side effects. The nurse provides written guidelines as reinforcement.

If the client develops diabetes mellitus as a result of chronic pancreatitis from endocrine dysfunction, management of elevated glucose levels after discharge from the hospital may require oral hypoglycemic agents or insulin injections. If this is the case, the client and the family require in-depth teaching concerning diabetes, its signs and symptoms, medical management, insulin administration, urine and blood glucose monitoring, and general care information (see Chap. 51 for discussion of diabetes).

Psychosocial Preparation

The client may fear recurrence of pain episodes. The nurse empowers the client by encouraging him/her to become active in health maintenance to assist in preventing recurrent pain.

Health Care Resources

Chronic illnesses are devastating to families. The high costs of medical insurance, medical treatment, and drug therapy cause serious financial problems. Often, the client with chronic pancreatitis is unable or unwilling to work. Financial counseling and social services assistance should be instituted during hospitalization. Vocational rehabilitation services can assist in training for a possible job change.

The client may require home care visits by nurses, depending on the severity of the chronic health problems and home maintenance and support needs. The home care nurse assesses the client for pain management, diet and alcohol abstinence compliance, effectiveness of pancreatic enzyme therapy, and psychosocial adaptation to chronic illness.

If alcohol consumption continues, the client is referred to a counselor or a self-help group, such as Alcoholics Anonymous.

 Evaluation

On the basis of the identified common nursing diagnoses, the nurse evaluates the care of the client with chronic pancreatitis. Expected outcome criteria include that the client

1. States that the pain of chronic pancreatitis is at a minimum or is relieved
2. Complies with diet restrictions and abstains from alcohol
3. Maintains adequate nutritional and fluid volume intake
4. States that there is a decrease in stool frequency

CARCINOMA

OVERVIEW

Pancreatic tumors are most often adenocarcinomas, occurring in the exocrine portion of the gland. Prognosis is poor, as pancreatic cancers are often fatal 1 to 3 years after discovery or onset of symptoms.

Pathophysiology

These highly malignant tumors usually originate from epithelial cells of the pancreatic ductal system. If the tumor is discovered in the early stages, the tumor cells may be localized within the glandular organ; however, this is highly unlikely. Most often, the tumor is discovered in the late stages of development and may be a well-defined mass or be diffusely spread throughout the pancreas.

The tumor may be a primary cancer or may result from metastasis from cancers of the lung, the breast, the thyroid, or the kidney or from skin melanoma. Primary pancreatic tumors are generally *adenocarcinomas* and grow in well-differentiated glandular patterns. Pancreatic adenocarcinoma grows rapidly and spreads to surrounding organs (stomach, duodenum, gallbladder, and intestine) by direct extension and invasion of lymphatic and vascular systems. This highly metastatic lesion may eventually invade the lung, the peritoneum, the liver, the spleen, and lymph nodes.

Clinical symptoms of pancreatic cancer depend on the location of the site of origin or metastasis. The *head of the pancreas* is the most common site of pancreatic carcinoma. These tumors are usually small lesions with poorly defined margins. Jaundice results from tumor compression and obstruction of the common bile duct and gallbladder dilation, causing the organ to enlarge.

Carcinomas of the body and tail of the pancreas are usually large and invade the entire tail and body. These tumors may be palpable abdominal masses, especially in the thin client. Because of metastatic spread via the splenic vein, metastasis to the liver may cause hepatomegaly (the liver is enlarged up to two to three times its normal size). Carcinomas of the body and tail spread more extensively than do pancreatic head carcinomas, with invasion of the retroperitoneum, the vertebral column, the spleen, adrenals, the colon, or the stomach.

Thrombophlebitis is a common sequela of pancreatic carcinoma. It is attributed to an increase in the levels of thromboplastic factors in serum. Necrotic products of the pancreatic tumor are believed to have thromboplastic properties, resulting in the blood's hypercoagulable state. *Migratory thrombophlebitis* is due to the client's confinement to bed and extensive surgical manipulation.

Etiology

The exact cause of pancreatic carcinoma is unknown. Research indicates that diabetes mellitus and chronic pancreatitis contribute to the likelihood of pancreatic carcinoma development. It is not clear whether the cancer is a sequela to these processes or whether the diseases are a result of the carcinoma.

As in the other types of cancer, potential predisposing factors include exposure to chemical carcinogens, cigarette smoking, and high-fat dietary intake. Investigation to delineate other risk factors is being conducted, including research on the role of coffee intake.

Incidence

Cancer of the pancreas is the fifth leading cause of cancer-related deaths in the United States (Silverberg & Lubera, 1989). It is 30% more common in men and has its highest rates of incidence between ages 70 and 79 years. It occurs 50% more frequently in Black than in Caucasian Americans, and the incidence is twice as high in smokers as in nonsmokers (American Cancer Society [ACS], 1987).

Workers with a high incidence of pancreatic carcinoma include engineers, coal workers, chemists, and other workers exposed to known chemical carcinogens, such as betanaphthylamine and benzidine.

PREVENTION

Because pancreatic carcinoma may develop after acute or chronic pancreatitis or diabetes mellitus, it is recommended that potential etiologic factors be avoided or treated. Clients should stop smoking, and intake of alcohol, coffee, and foods high in fat content should be restricted.

COLLABORATIVE MANAGEMENT

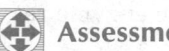 Assessment

History

When taking a history from a client with suspected pancreatic carcinoma, the nurse utilizes the same assessment questions as for clients with acute and chronic pancreatitis. The nurse questions the client about past medical diagnoses, including a *history of diabetes mellitus and pancreatitis*. The client is asked about *background information*, such as ethnic group, smoking history, coffee intake, and employment history to determine whether exposure to known environmental carcinogens has occurred. The nurse asks the client how long skin has been discolored if jaundice is present and determines if weight loss has occurred in the absence of a planned weight reduction program.

Physical Assessment: Clinical Manifestations

The client's first clue to the presence of pancreatic carcinoma may be the appearance of *jaundice,* which is a *late* sign. Jaundice appears as the initial sign in two-thirds of all cases because gallbladder and liver involvement are common. The green-gold skin color associated with obstructive jaundice progressively worsens as the tumor spreads. On noting the jaundice, the nurse asks the client if color changes have occurred in the stool and urine. As a result of the obstructive process, the *stool is clay colored* and *urine* is *dark and frothy.* The nurse inspects the skin for dryness and scratch marks, indicating *pruritus* from jaundice.

By the time jaundice appears, the pancreatic carcinoma is usually in an advanced stage. The nurse may be able to palpate the *enlarged gallbladder* and *liver.* In advanced cases, the pancreatic tumor may be palpated as a *firm, fixed mass* in the left upper abdominal quadrant or epigastric region.

The nurse questions the client about *abdominal pain,* which may be described as a vague, constant dullness in the upper abdomen and nonspecific in nature. Pain is a common early complaint in clients with pancreatic carcinoma. It is also present in the advanced stages of the disease. Pain may be related to eating or activity.

In addition, the nurse asks the client if he/she is experiencing pain in other areas of the body. Referred *back pain* may be caused by pressure on the nerve plexus, and some clients develop *leg* or *calf pain* with *swelling* and *redness* as a result of thrombophlebitis, a complication of pancreatic carcinoma.

The nurse weighs the client and determines the extent of weight loss and whether it has occurred rapidly. The nurse questions the client about food intake and intolerances. *Anorexia* accompanied by *early satiety, nausea, flatulence,* and *vomiting* are common.

The nurse performs a general abdominal assessment and, in particular, percusses the abdomen for dullness, which may indicate the presence of *ascites.* Pancreatic ascites occurs in the advanced stages of the disease process.

Psychosocial Assessment

The client with pancreatic carcinoma may be concerned with the sudden change in physical appearance. Profound weight loss and a cachectic appearance, coupled with jaundice discoloration, may provoke increased fear. The client may fear that his/her appearance affects relationships with family and friends. The nurse asks the client what fears are present to help in planning individualized care. Abdominal pain may be

constant and dull and related to activity and eating. There may be a fear of addiction to narcotics, which causes the client to refuse medication for pain.

The medical prognosis for most clients with pancreatic cancer is poor, and survival time is often limited. Families and clients feel profound grief and disbelief and require emotional counseling to help deal with diagnosis of this life-threatening disease.

Laboratory Findings

There are no specific blood tests to diagnose pancreatic carcinoma. Serum amylase levels, as well as alkaline phosphatase and bilirubin levels, are elevated. The degree of elevation depends on the acuteness or chronicity of the pancreatic and biliary damage. Elevated carcinoembryonic antigen levels occur in 80% to 90% of clients with pancreatic carcinoma. This test is helpful in providing early information about the presence of tumor cells. Biopsy of pancreatic tissue by needle aspiration reveals malignant cells.

Other Diagnostic Tests

CT is helpful in confirming the presence of a tumor and differentiating the tumor from a cyst. Ultrasound examinations do not distinguish pancreatic carcinoma from other pancreatic disorders. ERCP visualization and cytologic study of aspirate provides the most definitive diagnostic data. Aspiration of pancreatic ascites by abdominal paracentesis may reveal malignant cells and elevated amylase levels. When the secretin test is performed, duodenal or gastric aspirate may reveal a malignant cytologic finding (see earlier explanation of this procedure).

 Analysis: Nursing Diagnosis

Nursing interventions are based on the client's physical and emotional needs and also entail supportive care measures.

Common Diagnoses

Several nursing diagnoses commonly occur in clients with pancreatic carcinoma:

1. Pain related to tumor invasion
2. Altered nutrition: less than body requirements related to anorexia, flatulence, and vomiting
3. Impaired skin integrity related to pruritus secondary to altered skin pigmentation (jaundice) or pancreatic cutaneous fistula formation

Additional Diagnoses

The client may require individualized nursing care on the basis of one or more additional diagnoses, including

1. Potential for activity intolerance related to debilitated state

2. Fear related to life-threatening illness
3. Anticipatory grieving and hopelessness related to poor prognosis
4. Self-esteem disturbance related to profound weight loss and jaundice

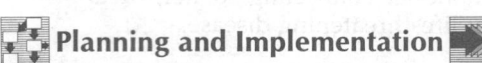 **Planning and Implementation**

Pain

Planning: client goals. The primary goal for this diagnosis is that the client will experience relief of pain and discomfort as a result of palliative care measures and therapeutic interventions.

Interventions. Management of the client with pancreatic carcinoma is geared toward preventing tumor spread and decreasing pain. These measures are not curative, only palliative. The cancers are often multifocal and recur despite treatment.

Nonsurgical management. As for other types of cancer, radiation or chemotherapeutic agents are employed to relieve pain. (See Chap. 25 for nursing interventions associated with these treatment modalities.)

Drug therapy. The nurse medicates the client with narcotic analgesics (meperidine hydrochloride [Demerol], morphine, hydromorphone hydrochloride [Dilaudid]) and provides comfort measures before the pain escalates and reaches a peak in an effort to keep the pain under control. Drug dependency is not a consideration because of the poor prognosis. High doses of narcotic analgesics may be needed for the intense abdominal and back pain in the late stages of the disease.

Chemotherapeutic interventions for pancreatic carcinoma have had limited success. Combining agents such as fluorouracil (5-fluorouracil [5-FU]) and carmustine (BCNU) has had better success than single-agent chemotherapy. The nurse provides the client with symptomatic relief and comfort measures for toxic side effects of chemotherapeutic agents (Chap. 25).

Radiation therapy. Intense external radiation therapy to the pancreas may provide the client effective pain relief by shrinking tumor cells, but does not improve survival rates. Implantation of radon seeds, in combination with systemic or intra-arterial administration of floxuridine (FUDR), has been used. The client may experience discomfort during and after the radiation treatments. Supportive nursing interventions for relief of symptoms is indicated.

Surgical management. The most effective management for pancreatic carcinoma is surgical intervention. The classic surgery, the *Whipple procedure* (or *radical pancreaticoduodenectomy*), involves extensive surgical manipulation and is used to treat cancer of the head of the pancreas. The procedure entails resection of the proximal head of the pancreas, the duodenum, a portion of the jejunum, the stomach (partial or total gastrectomy), and the gallbladder with anastomosis of the pancreatic duct (pancreatojejunostomy), the common bile duct (choledochojejunostomy), and the stomach (gastrojejunostomy) to the jejunum (Fig. 47–7). In addition, removal of the spleen (splenectomy) may also be done. As a palliative measure to relieve biliary obstruction in the likelihood of extensive tumor invasion, a simple surgical intervention, such as cholecystojejunostomy, may be done as a bypass procedure.

Preoperative care. The client with pancreatic carcinoma is a poor surgical risk owing to malnutrition and debilitation. A nasogastric tube is inserted, and the administration of IV fluids or hyperalimentation is started before surgery.

Postoperative care. In addition to routine postoperative care measures (Chap. 20), the client undergoing a radical pancreaticoduodenectomy requires intensive nursing care and is usually admitted to a surgical critical care unit. Table 47–1 lists potential complications of Whipple's procedure, for which the nurse assesses.

The monitoring of GI drainage and nasogastric tube patency is an important aspect of postoperative nursing care. Drainage tubes are strategically placed during surgery to remove drainage and secretions from the area and prevent stress on the anastomosis sites. The nurse assesses the tubes and drainage devices for undue stress or kinking and maintains drainage tubes in a dependent position. Suction gauge pressure is frequently checked by the nurse to keep the desired suction level. Most

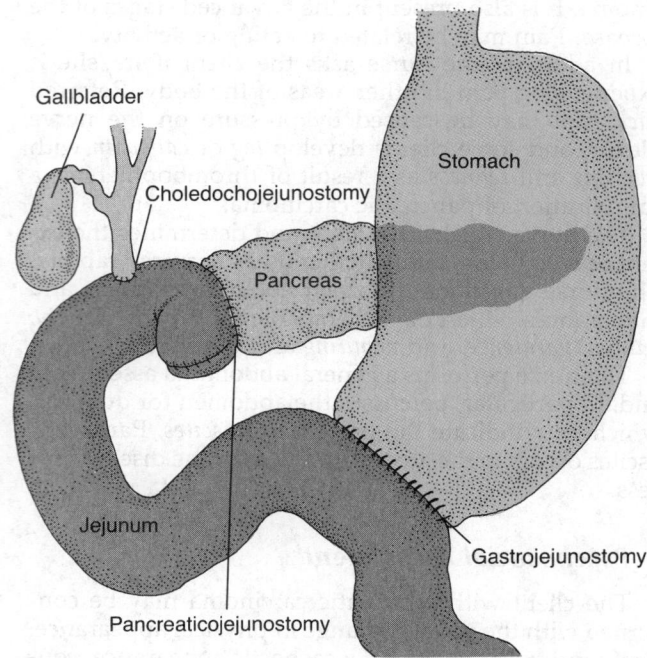

Figure 47–7

The three anastomoses that make up the Whipple procedure: choledochojejunostomy, pancreaticojejunostomy, and gastrojejunostomy.

TABLE 47–1   Potential Complications of Whipple's Procedure

Cardiovascular

Hemorrhage at anastomosis sites with hypovolemia
Myocardial infarction
CHF
Thrombophlebitis

Pulmonary

Atelectasis
Pneumonia
Pulmonary embolism
ARDS
Pulmonary edema

Gastrointestinal

Adynamic (paralytic) ileus
Gastric retention
Gastric ulceration
Bowel obstruction from peritonitis
Pancreatitis
Hepatic failure
Thrombosis to mesentery

Wound

Infection
Dehiscence
Fistulas—pancreatic, gastric, and biliary

Metabolic

Unstable diabetes mellitus
Renal failure

---

often, sump drains are used and connected to low suction (80 mmHg or less) to maintain drain patency.

The nurse monitors the drainage for color, consistency, and amount. The drainage should be serosanguineous; the appearance of clear, colorless, bile-tinged drainage or frank blood with an increase in output may indicate disruption or leakage of an anastomosis site.

The development of a *fistula* (an abnormal passageway) is the most common and most serious postoperative complication. Biliary, pancreatic, or gastric fistulas result from partial or total breakdown of an anastomosis site. The secretions that drain from the fistula contain bile, pancreatic enzymes, or gastric secretions, depending on which anastomosis site is ruptured. These secre-

tions, particularly pancreatic fluid, are corrosive and irritating to the skin, and internal leakage causes a chemical peritonitis. Peritonitis requires treatment with multiple antibiotics.

The nurse places the client in semi-Fowler's position to reduce suture line and anastomosis stress, as well as to optimize lung expansion. Gastric suture line stress can be minimized by maintaining nasogastric tube drainage at a low suction level to keep the remaining stomach (if a partial gastrectomy is done) or the jejunum (if a total gastrectomy is done) free of excess fluid build-up and pressure. The nasogastric tube is also used to reduce stimulation of the remaining pancreatic tissue.

If the nasogastric tube, usually a Salem sump tube, is obstructed, the nurse instills air first. If this method is not successful in keeping the drainage lumen open, irrigation with 10 to 20 mL of normal saline is gently performed.

Because the pancreaticoduodenectomy procedure is extensive and can take between 6 and 10 hours to complete, maintaining fluid and electrolyte balance can be difficult. These clients tend to have significant intraoperative blood loss and a tendency to bleed postoperatively. The intestine is exposed to air for long periods and evaporation of fluid occurs. Significant losses of fluid and electrolytes occur from nasogastric and drainage tubes. Additionally, these patients are usually malnourished and have low serum levels of protein and albumin. These substances maintain colloid osmotic pressure within the circulating system. Reduction in the osmotic pressure makes the client prone to "third spacing" of body fluids. For these reasons, the nurse closely monitors vital signs for decreased blood pressure and increased heart rate, decreased vascular pressures with a central venous line or pulmonary artery catheter (Swan-Ganz catheter), and decreased urinary output to detect early signs of hypovolemia and prevent shock. Maintenance of ordered IV volume replacement is important. The nurse monitors hemoglobin levels and hematocrit results to assess for blood loss and the need for blood transfusions and monitors electrolyte results for decreased serum levels of sodium, potassium, chloride, and calcium. IV fluid concentrations must be altered to correct these electrolyte imbalances. The nurse is alert for the development of the third spacing phenomenon, which is manifested by increased weight, fluid in the lungs, and pitting edema of the extremities and dependent edema in the sacrum and back, as well as an intake that far exceeds output. Nutritional repletion via hyperalimentation and the administration of albumin are helpful in promoting the shift of fluid from the interstitial space into the intravascular space.

After the Whipple procedure, transient hyperglycemia or hypoglycemia may occur in the immediate postoperative period owing to stress and surgical manipulation of the pancreas. The majority of the endocrine cells (islets of Langerhans responsible for insulin and glucose secretion) are located in the body and tail of the pancreas. Most clients have up to half of the gland remaining and do not develop diabetes; however, a large number of clients are diabetic before surgery. The nurse monitors serum glucose levels frequently during the early postoperative period and administers insulin injections as prescribed.

Altered Nutrition: Less Than Body Requirements

Planning: client goals. The goal is that the client will have optimal nutritional and caloric intake and maintain or gain weight.

Interventions: nonsurgical management. The client experiences anorexia with early satiety and, frequently, nausea and vomiting, making the oral intake of nutrition difficult to maintain. Management is geared toward providing optimal nutrition in the preoperative and postoperative periods.

Tube feedings. The client is often maintained nutritionally with enteral tube feedings as long as intestinal function is adequate. After tube feedings are tolerated, a small-lumen silicone feeding tube, such as a Dobhoff tube, is inserted to avoid the complications occurring with larger-lumen tubes, such as sinusitis and nasal irritation. Specific nutrients are provided by commercially prepared products chosen by the physician and the dietitian. Feedings are given by bolus or continuous infusion, depending on the client's tolerance and residual volumes.

Often, in the late stages of pancreatic carcinoma or during the Whipple procedure, a small catheter is inserted into the jejunum so that enteral feedings may be given. The *jejunostomy* feeding method is preferred to prevent reflux and to facilitate absorption. The feedings are initiated in low concentrations and volumes and are gradually increased as tolerated. The nurse delivers these feedings by tube feeding pump to maintain a constant volume and assesses for diarrhea frequency as a means to measure tolerance.

Total parenteral nutrition. For optimal nutrition, hyperalimentation by TPN may be required in addition to tube feedings or as a single measure to provide nutrition. When central venous access is required, a Hickman catheter may be necessary. Line care is an important nursing management measure to prevent catheter sepsis. Daily dressing changes and site observation are extremely important. Finger sticks to obtain blood for blood glucose measurements are performed to monitor the client's tolerance of dextrose in the solution and monitor pancreatic function. (Additional nursing care measures for the client receiving TPN are found in Chap. 13.)

Impaired Skin Integrity

Planning: client goals. The goal is that the client will maintain intact skin and experience relief from itching.

Interventions: nonsurgical management. Severe jaundice can cause skin care problems. Bile salt accumulation from increased skin pigmentation can contribute to severe pruritus. The nurse keeps the client's fingernails clipped so that aggressive scratching cannot result in disruption of skin integrity. If the scratching is uncontrollable, the client's hands may be wrapped with a protective covering. The nurse avoids using soap in the bath water and uses a soothing bath oil instead. Skin care is provided with emollient lotions to keep the skin soft and relieve itching. Special prescription ointments or lotions may be necessary. If itching is uncontrollable, diphenhydramine hydrochloride (Benadryl) can be given.

The drainage from gastric, pancreatic, or biliary fistulas, as well as leakage from around surgical drain sites, can be corrosive and disruptive to tissue integrity. (The reader is referred to the earlier discussion of skin care measures in acute pancreatitis.)

■ Discharge Planning

Carcinoma of the pancreas may be diagnosed after the client presents with abdominal pain and jaundice or recurrent chronic pancreatitis. These clients require discharge planning aimed at palliative care and emotional support.

Home Care Preparation

The stage of progression of pancreatic carcinoma and available home care resources dictate whether the client can be sent home or requires additional institutional care in a nursing home or hospice setting. Special home care preparations depend on the client's physical and activity limitations and should be tailored for each individual's needs.

Client/Family Education

When the client is sent home, many of the care measures are palliative and aimed at providing relief of symptoms and pain. Care measures and teaching information are similar to those for clients with chronic pancreatitis.

Psychosocial Preparation

The nurse provides emotional support for the client and the family to deal with issues related to this life-threatening illness.

The nurse assists family members to realistically and objectively ascertain the amount of physical care required for chronically ill clients. The family members must be told that their own physical and emotional health is at risk during this stressful period and that supportive counseling is indicated. If the family does not have a religious affiliation or a spiritual leader (e.g., a minister or a rabbi) to provide support, the nurse suggests alternative counseling options. Clients and their families may hesitate to seek support services. It may be appropriate for the nurse to institute an initial contact or appointment.

Health Care Resources

Regular home care nursing visits are scheduled to assist the client and the family. The visiting nurse provides physical, psychologic, and supportive care. The nurse recommends hospitalization if client care needs become excessive for the family or arranges for private duty nurses if indicated. The need for homemaking or resident care providers (nursing assistance) is determined by the nurse. Cancer support groups are also available to clients and families to provide information and emotional support (see Chap. 25).

 Evaluation

The nurse evaluates the plan of care for clients with pancreatic carcinoma according to established nursing diagnoses. Expected outcomes include that the client

1. States that pain is reduced or alleviated by prescribed medication or other pain relief measures
2. Utilizes psychologic support services
3. Maintains weight and receives optimal nutrition
4. Verbalizes that pruritus is decreased
5. Maintains intact skin integrity

ABSCESSES

Pancreatic abscesses consisting of infected, necrotic pancreatic tissue occur after severe acute pancreatitis, exacerbations of chronic pancreatitis, and biliary tract surgery. The development of a single abscess or multiloculated abscesses results from extensive inflammatory necrosis of the pancreas that is readily invaded by infectious organisms, such as *E. coli, Klebsiella, Bacteroides, Staphylococcus,* and *Proteus.*

Clients with pancreatic abscesses often appear more seriously ill than clients with pseudocysts. Clinical manifestations are similar; however, temperature in clients with abscesses may spike to as high as 104° F (40° C). Blood cultures are helpful in revealing the infective organism. Pleural effusions commonly accompany these abscesses. Ultrasonography and CT cannot differentiate between pancreatic pseudocysts and abscesses.

Pancreatic abscesses that are not surgically drained carry a 100% mortality. Drainage should be performed as soon as possible to prevent sepsis. Antibiotic treatment alone does not resolve the abscess. Mortality remains as high as 60%, even after surgical drainage, and many clients require multiple drainage procedures for recurrent abscesses.

PSEUDOCYSTS

Pancreatic pseudocysts develop as a complication of acute or chronic pancreatitis. Pseudocysts occur in pancreatitis caused by alcoholism, biliary tract disease, or abdominal and surgical trauma. Two per cent of all people with pancreatitis develop pseudocysts, and mortality is reported at approximately 15% (Given & Simmons, 1984).

Pancreatic pseudocysts, or false cysts, are named such because unlike true cysts they do not have an epithelial lining. Pseudocysts are encapsulated sac-like structures that form on or surround the pancreas. The pseudocyst wall is inflamed, vascular, and fibrotic. It may contain up to several liters of straw-colored or dark brown viscous fluid, the enzymatic exudate of the pancreas.

A pseudocyst can be palpated as an epigastric mass in approximately 50% of cases. The primary presenting symptom is epigastric pain radiating to the back. Other common clinical manifestations include abdominal fullness, nausea, vomiting, bloating, and jaundice. Pseudocysts are diagnosed, and their growth and resolution monitored, by serial abdominal ultrasound examination or CT.

Pseudocysts may spontaneously resolve or may rupture and produce hemorrhage. Other complications include obstruction involving other organs, abscess or fistula formation, and pancreatic ascites. Surgical intervention is required if the pseudocyst does not resolve within 6 weeks or if complications develop. Internal drainage is accomplished by surgically creating an opening (ostomy) between the pseudocyst and the stomach (cystogastrostomy), jejunum (cystojejunostomy), or duodenum (cystoduodenostomy). External drainage is provided by surgical insertion of a sump drainage tube to remove pancreatic secretions and exudate. Pseudocysts recur in approximately 10% of cases. Pancreatic fistulas are common postoperative occurrences, and skin breakdown from corrosive pancreatic enzymes presents a major nursing care challenge (see earlier discussion of acute pancreatitis).

LIVER DISORDERS

CIRRHOSIS

OVERVIEW

Cirrhosis is a chronic progressive liver disease. The term *cirrhosis* is derived from the Greek *kirrhos* (orange-colored or tawny). Cirrhosis may have an insidious development with a prolonged, destructive course. Hepatic cirrhosis, an end-stage process, is essentially an irreversible reaction to hepatic inflammation and necrosis.

Pathophysiology

Cirrhosis is characterized by diffuse fibrotic bands of connective tissue, which distort the liver's normal architectural anatomy. Extensive degeneration and destruction of hepatocytes (liver cells) occur. The liver, in its attempt to regenerate with new nodule formation, develops a disorganized lobular pattern. Flow alterations in the vascular system and lymphatic bile duct channels result from compression caused by the proliferation of fibrous tissue.

Classification

On the basis of morphologic changes in the regenerated liver nodules, cirrhosis has been classified as micronodular, macronodular, and mixed types. In *micronodular* cirrhosis, the liver tends to be enlarged; this form is seen in conditions in which the damaging agent persists (e.g., alcohol). It is characterized by small, regular, thick bands of connective tissue. Every liver lobule is involved, and the nodules do not vary in size. This is the hallmark of a continual destructive process. *Macronodular* cirrhosis results in a small, shrunken liver, which is not palpable. The liver is irregular in shape, multilobular, and characterized by bands of connective tissue of varying thicknesses. The nodules vary in size and shape. *Mixed* cirrhosis features both micronodular and macronodular disorganizational patterns of connective tissue.

Types

There are four main types of cirrhosis: Laënnec's, postnecrotic, biliary, and cardiac. *Laënnec's cirrhosis* is also known as alcohol-induced, nutritional, or portal cirrhosis. Alcohol has a direct toxic effect on liver cells, causing liver inflammation (alcoholic hepatitis), which usually precedes the onset of alcoholic cirrhosis. Metabolic changes in the liver induced by alcohol lead to fatty infiltration of the hepatocytes and scarring between the lobules. The liver becomes enlarged, with cellular degeneration and infiltration by fat, leukocytes, and lymphocytes (white blood cells). As the inflammatory process decreases, the destructive phase increases. Early scar formation is caused by fibroblast infiltration and collagen formation. Damage to the hepatic parenchyma progresses owing to malnutrition and repeated exposure to the hepatotoxin (alcohol, in the case of Laënnec's cirrhosis). If alcohol is withheld, the fatty infiltration is reversible. If alcohol abuse continues, widespread scar tissue formation and fibrosis infiltrate the liver as a result of cellular necrosis.

In early cirrhosis, the liver capsule is enlarged, firm, and hard. The regenerated nodules give the capsule a hobnailed, or bumpy, appearance. As the pathologic process of cirrhosis progresses, the liver shrinks in size, and the capsule is covered by fine nodules surrounded by gray connective tissue.

Postnecrotic cirrhosis occurs after massive liver cell necrosis. Broad bands of scar tissue cause destruction of liver lobules and entire lobes. Early hepatomegaly is replaced by a small liver with large nodules, representing macronodular structural changes throughout the organ. Postnecrotic cirrhosis occurs as a complication of acute viral hepatitis or after exposure to industrial or chemical hepatotoxins, such as carbon tetrachloride. This type of cirrhosis is suspected in clients who exhibit signs of chronic liver disease and do not have a history of excessive alcohol intake.

Biliary cirrhosis develops from chronic biliary obstruction, bile stasis, and inflammation. Diffuse hepatic fibrosis is characteristic. *Primary* biliary cirrhosis results from intrahepatic bile stasis. *Secondary* biliary cirrhosis is caused by obstruction of the hepatic or common bile ducts, which produces bile stasis in the liver. The accumulation of excessive hepatic bile leads to progressive fibrosis, hepatocellular destruction, and regenerated nodules. Severe obstructive jaundice is a key clinical manifestation in both types of biliary cirrhosis.

Cardiac cirrhosis, or vascular cirrhosis, is associated with severe right-sided congestive heart failure (CHF). It develops in long-standing CHF after cor pulmonale, constrictive pericarditis, and valvular insufficiency. (The reader is referred to Chap. 64 for discussion of these conditions.) The liver becomes enlarged and is congested with venous blood; it appears edematous and dark in color. The liver has served as a reservoir for large amounts of venous blood that the failing heart is unable to pump back into the systemic circulation. The increase in hepatic volume and pressure causes severe venous congestion, and the liver becomes anoxic, resulting in liver cell necrosis and fibrosis.

Complications

Common problems and complications associated with hepatic cirrhosis depend on the amount of damage the liver has sustained. The loss of hepatic function contributes to the development of metabolic abnormalities. Figure 47–8 presents altered body functions that result from impaired liver function. Liver cell degeneration may lead to portal hypertension, ascites, bleeding, esophageal varices, jaundice, portal-systemic encephalopathy (PSE) with hepatic coma, and hepatorenal syndrome.

Portal hypertension. Portal hypertension is a major complication of cirrhosis. It is defined as a persistent increase in pressure within the portal vein and develops as a result of increased resistance or obstruction to the flow of blood through the portal vein and its tributaries. The blood meets resistance to flow and seeks collateral venous channels around the high-pressure area.

Blood flow backs into the liver and the spleen, causing hepatomegaly and splenomegaly, respectively. Veins in the esophagus, the abdomen, and the rectum are dilated, accounting for esophageal varices, ascites, prominent abdominal veins (caput medusae), and hemorrhoids.

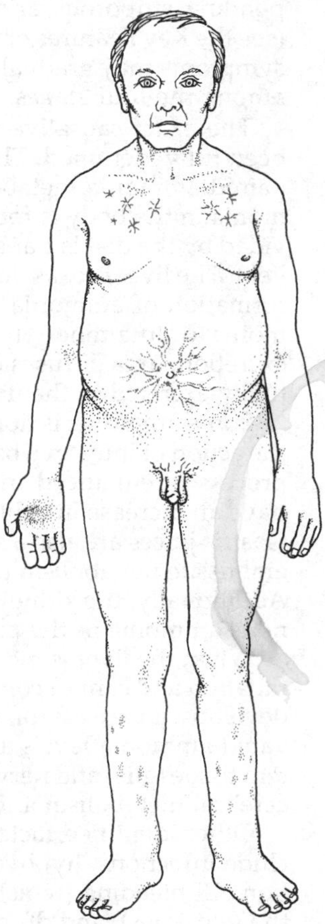

NEUROLOGIC FINDINGS
Asterixis
Portal-systemic encephalopathy
Paresthesias of feet
Peripheral nerve degeneration
Reversal of sleep-wake pattern
Sensory disturbances

GASTROINTESTINAL (GI)
FINDINGS
Abdominal pain
Anorexia
Ascites
Clay-colored stools
Diarrhea
Esophageal varices
Fetor hepaticus
Gallstones
Gastritis
GI bleeding
Hemorrhoidal varices
Hepatomegaly
Hiatal hernia
Hypersplenism
Malnutrition
Nausea
Small nodular liver
Vomiting

RENAL FINDINGS
Hepatorenal syndrome
Increased urine bilirubin

ENDOCRINE FINDINGS
Increased aldosterone
Increased antidiuretic hormone
Increased circulating estrogens
Increased glucocorticoids
Gynecomastia

IMMUNE SYSTEM DISTURBANCES
Leukopenia
Increased susceptibility to infection

CARDIOVASCULAR FINDINGS
Cardiac arrhythmias
Development of collateral circulation
Hyperkinetic circulation
Peripheral edema
Spider angiomas
Fatigue
Portal hypertension

PULMONARY FINDINGS
Dyspnea
Hydrothorax
Hyperventilation
Hypoxemia

HEMATOLOGIC FINDINGS
Anemia
Disseminated intravascular
   coagulation
Impaired coagulation
Splenomegaly
Thrombocytopenia

DERMATOLOGIC FINDINGS
Axillary and pubic hair changes
Increased skin pigmentation
Jaundice
Pruritus
Spider angiomas
Caput medusae
Palmar erythema
Ecchymosis

FLUID AND ELECTROLYTE
DISTURBANCES
Ascites
Decreased effective blood volume
Dilutional hyponatremia or
   hypernatremia
Hypocalcemia
Hypokalemia
Peripheral edema
Water retention

Figure 47 – 8

The clinical picture of a client with liver dysfunction. Signs and symptoms vary according to the progression of the disease. Early signs and symptoms are noted in color.

Ascites. *Ascites* is the accumulation of free fluid containing almost pure plasma within the peritoneal cavity. Increased hydrostatic pressure from portal hypertension results in venous congestion of the hepatic capillaries, causing plasma to leak directly from the liver surface and portal vein into the peritoneal cavity. The accumulation of plasma protein, primarily albumin, in the peritoneal fluid reduces the amount of circulating plasma protein in the blood. When this is combined with the liver's inability to synthesize albumin owing to impaired hepatocyte functioning, the effective serum colloid osmotic pressure is decreased in the circulatory system.

Another factor that contributes to ascites formation is *increased hepatic lymph formation.* The lymphatic system is unable to channel the increased amounts of lymph, and the resultant weeping of liver plasma ("liver sweat") occurs. Decrease of effective intravascular circulation from massive ascites may cause *renal vasoconstriction*, triggering the renin-angiotensin system. This causes sodium and water retention, which increases hydrostatic pressure and lymph formation, and the vicious circle of ascites formation continues.

Bleeding esophageal varices. Bleeding esophageal varices occur when fragile, thin-walled, distended esophageal veins are irritated and rupture. Variceal bleeding may be caused by any chemical irritant, such as alcohol, medications, or gastric acid reflux; mechanical trauma from abrasions by poorly chewed food particles or vomiting; or increased pressure in the esophagus caused by vigorous physical exercise, coughing, or retching and vomiting.

Varices most frequently occur in the distal (lower)

end of the esophagus, but can also occur in the proximal esophagus and stomach. The presence of gastric ulceration or erosion also puts the client at risk for frank hemorrhage from the stomach. Differentiation between gastric and esophageal bleeding can be determined by endoscopy if the client's condition permits time for a diagnostic procedure.

The client loses large volumes of blood from hematemesis (vomiting of blood) and may go into shock from hypovolemia. Bleeding esophageal varices are a medical emergency and require immediate medical intervention. (Refer to discussion of interventions for potential for injury related to hemorrhage later.)

Coagulation defects. In cirrhosis, there is a decrease in the synthesis of bile fats in the liver, preventing the absorption of fat-soluble vitamins (such as vitamin K). Without vitamin K, clotting factors II, VII, IX, and X are not produced in sufficient quantities, and the client is prone to bleeding and easy bruisability.

Jaundice. Jaundice found in hepatic cirrhosis is caused by one of two mechanisms: hepatocellular disease or intrahepatic obstruction (see the accompanying Key Features of Disease). *Hepatocellular jaundice* develops because the liver is unable to metabolize bilirubin. The liver's normal uptake of bilirubin from the blood is impaired, and altered conjugation and excretion result in excessive circulating bilirubin levels. *Intrahepatic obstructive jaundice* results from edema, fibrosis, or scarring of the hepatic bile channels and bile ducts, interfering with normal bile and bilirubin excretion. Hemolytic anemia is not related to cirrhosis, but can lead to jaundice. The red blood cell hemolysis that occurs in hemolytic anemia is responsible for increased bilirubin levels and subsequent jaundice.

Portal-systemic encephalopathy. PSE, also known as *hepatic encephalopathy* and *hepatic coma,* is a clinical disorder seen in end-stage hepatic failure and cirrhosis. PSE is manifested by neurologic symptoms, characterized by altered level of consciousness, impaired thinking processes, and neuromuscular disturbances.

The development of PSE may occur insidiously in chronic liver disease and go undetected until late stages. In acute liver dysfunction, the symptoms develop rapidly. Four stages of development (i.e., prodromal, impending, stuporous, and comatose) have been identified (see the Key Features of Disease on p. 1483). The client's symptoms may gradually progress to coma or fluctuate among the four stages.

The exact causative mechanisms for PSE have not been fully identified. The most probable etiology is impaired ammonia metabolism. The majority of the ammonia in the body is found in the GI tract. Protein provided by the diet is transported to the liver by the portal vein. The liver breaks down protein, which results in the formation of ammonia. The liver further converts ammonia to glutamine, which is stored, and then to urea for excretion; urea diffuses into the body fluids and is eventually excreted in the urine by the kidneys.

Some ammonia is normally formed in the GI tract by the action of intestinal bacteria on protein products. This process is enhanced in cirrhotic clients because they have an increase in coliform bacteria in the duodenum. Gastric juices are also a source of ammonia, and peripheral tissue metabolism produces a portion of ammonia. Additionally, the kidney may act as a source of endogenous ammonia in the presence of hypokalemia.

When the liver is incapable of adequate protein degradation and cannot convert ammonia to urea, the client develops an excess of circulating ammonia. The elevated ammonia levels are toxic to central nervous system tissue (glial and nerve cells), interfering with normal cerebral metabolism and function.

Other identified factors that may precipitate PSE include infections, hypovolemia, hypokalemia, constipation, GI bleeding (which causes a large protein load in the intestines), and drugs, such as hypnotics, narcotics, sedatives, analgesics, and diuretics. PSE may also occur after paracentesis or shunting procedures. Prognosis for PSE is dependent on the severity of the underlying cause, precipitating factors, and the degree of liver dysfunction.

Hepatorenal syndrome. The development of *hepatorenal syndrome* indicates a poor prognosis in the client with liver failure and is one of the primary causes of

KEY FEATURES OF DISEASE ■ Laboratory Diagnostic Differentiation of Jaundice

Test	Hepatocellular Jaundice	Obstructive Jaundice	Hemolytic Jaundice
Serum bilirubin			
Indirect (unconjugated)	Increased	Slightly increased	Increased
Direct (conjugated)	Increased	Moderately increased	Normal
Urine bilirubin	Increased	Increased	None
Urobilinogen			
Stool	Normal to decreased	None	Increased
Urine	Normal to increased	None	Increased

KEY FEATURES OF DISEASE ■ Manifestations of the
Four Stages of Portal-Systemic Encephalopathy

Stage I: Prodromal

Subtle manifestations that may not immediately be
     recognized
     Personality changes
     Behavior changes (agitation, belligerence)
     Emotional lability (euphoria, depression)
     Impaired thinking
     Inability to concentrate
     Fatigue, drowsiness
     Slurred or slowed speech
     Sleep pattern disturbances

Stage II: Impending

Continuing mental changes
     Mental confusion
     Disorientation to time, place, or person
     Asterixis (see Fig. 47–10)

Stage III: Stuporous

Progressive deterioration
     Marked mental confusion
     Stuporous, drowsy, but arousable
     Abnormal electroencephalogram tracing
     Muscle twitching
     Hyperreflexia
     Asterixis

Stage IV: Comatose

Unresponsiveness, leading to death in 85% of those
     clients progressing to this stage
     Unarousable, obtunded
     Response to painful stimulus
     No asterixis
     Positive Babinski's sign
     Muscle rigidity
     Fetor hepaticus (characteristic liver breath—musty,
          sweet breath odor)
     Seizures

death in end-stage cirrhosis. Progressive oliguric renal failure associated with hepatic failure results in functionally impaired kidneys with *normal* anatomic and morphologic features. This syndrome is manifested by a sudden decrease in urinary flow, elevated serum urea nitrogen and creatinine levels, with abnormally decreased urine sodium excretion, and increased urine osmolarity. Hepatorenal syndrome often occurs after clinical deterioration from GI bleeding or the onset of PSE. Drugs such as indomethacin (Indocin) and possibly acetaminophen (Tylenol) and aspirin (acetylsalicylic acid [ASA]) may precipitate renal failure when administered

to the client with cirrhosis. Hepatorenal syndrome is generally accompanied by elevated serum ammonia levels with an increase in jaundice and serum bilirubin levels, because the kidneys are not excreting these products in the urine. Hepatorenal syndrome may also complicate other liver diseases, including acute hepatitis, fulminant hepatic failure, and hepatic malignancy. Most clients die within 3 weeks of the onset of azotemia.

Etiology

The exact factors contributing to the development of cirrhosis have not been clearly defined. There tends to be a genetic component, with a familial tendency to develop cirrhosis, as well as a familial hypersensitivity to alcohol in some people. Many alcoholics do not develop cirrhosis, whereas others develop cirrhosis even when adequate nutrition is maintained.

The etiology varies with the type of cirrhosis. *Laënnec's cirrhosis* develops as the result of alcohol's hepatotoxic effect. Poor nutritional intake compounds the problem of a malnourished liver in most adults. *Postnecrotic cirrhosis* usually occurs after acute viral hepatitis, which may result from blood transfusions. It is seen after exposure to industrial or chemical hepatotoxins, such as carbon tetrachloride, arsenic, or phosphorus. *Biliary cirrhosis* occurs as the result of chronic biliary obstruction and inflammation. *Cardiac cirrhosis* is associated with prolonged hepatic venous congestion. Other causes of cirrhosis are being studied. Cirrhosis often develops as an idiopathic process.

Incidence

Cirrhosis of the liver is the fourth leading cause of death in clients between 35 and 54 years of age. It is the ninth most common cause of death among United States citizens (Silverberg & Lubera, 1989). Cirrhosis may occur at any age. More than 65% of all cases of cirrhosis are alcohol related, making Laënnec's cirrhosis the most common form of cirrhosis in the United States (Knauer & Silverman, 1988). This type of cirrhosis is more common in men than in women. Postnecrotic necrosis occurs more frequently in women and is the most common form worldwide. Mortality from cirrhosis occurs more frequently in men and the non-Caucasian population.

PREVENTION

To prevent alcohol-induced cirrhosis, clients with a familial tendency toward alcoholism should totally avoid alcohol, and their children should be instructed to avoid alcohol as well. Alcoholics with insidiously developing cirrhosis should abstain from alcohol immediately at the onset of any symptoms suggestive of cirrhosis to allow for regeneration of liver tissue and to decrease the incidence of further fat deposits in the liver.

Postnecrotic cirrhosis and biliary cirrhosis occur as sequelae to other physiologic insults. The best preventive measure is to seek medical treatment immediately for suspected viral hepatitis or other liver inflammations, exposure to industrial chemicals, and cholecystitis or cholelithiasis. The client follows the prescribed medical management for these problems.

Clients with frequent episodes of congestive heart failure should maintain their medication regimen and report any signs of right-sided heart failure to their physician immediately so that further treatment can be implemented (see Chap. 64).

COLLABORATIVE MANAGEMENT

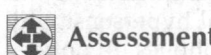 Assessment

History

The nurse obtains historical data from clients with suspected cirrhosis, including *age, sex, race,* and *employment history,* especially working conditions that may have exposed the client to harmful chemical toxins.

The nurse determines if there is a history of *alcoholism* in the family and asks the client to describe alcohol intake, including the amount consumed over what period of time. The client is asked about *previous medical conditions,* such as acute viral hepatitis, biliary tract disorders, viral infections, recent blood transfusions, or a history of heart failure or respiratory disorders.

Physical Assessment: Clinical Manifestations

Because cirrhosis has an insidious onset, many of the early signs and symptoms are vague and nonspecific. The client may have complaints of *generalized weakness, weight loss,* and *symptoms of a GI disorder,* such as loss of appetite, early-morning nausea and vomiting, dyspepsia, flatulence, and changes in bowel habits with constipation and bouts of diarrhea. The client may also complain of abdominal pain and liver tenderness, but these symptoms are often ignored by the client.

Many times, the presence of liver function abnormalities are detected when a physical examination or laboratory tests are done for an unrelated illness or problem. The development of late signs of advanced cirrhosis may trigger the client to seek medical treatment. *GI bleeding, jaundice, ascites,* and *spontaneous bruising* are indications of deteriorating liver function and represent complications of the disease.

The nurse thoroughly assesses the client with liver failure, as the disease process affects every body system (see Fig. 47–8). The clinical picture and clinical course vary from client to client, depending on the severity of the hepatic failure. When the nurse begins the assessment, an inspection may reveal obvious *yellowing of the skin and sclerae* (jaundice); *dry skin; rashes; purpuric lesions,* such as *petechiae* manifested as round, pinpoint red-purple lesions, or *ecchymosis,* large purple, blue, or yellow bruises; *warm and bright red palms of the hands*

(palmar erythema); and *vascular lesions* with a central red body and radiating branches, known as *spider angiomas* (telangiectasias, spider nevi, or vascular spiders), occurring on the nose, cheeks, the upper thorax, and shoulders.

When performing an assessment of the abdomen, the nurse keeps in mind that *hepatomegaly* occurs in 60% of all cases of early cirrhosis. The nurse palpates the right upper quadrant for an enlarged liver below the costal (rib cage) border. The nurse may also elicit the presence of hepatomegaly by percussing for dullness over the enlarged liver.

The nurse may readily assess the presence of massive ascites on inspection of the abdomen. The examination reveals a *distended abdomen with bulging flanks.* The *umbilicus may protrude* and dilated abdominal veins, or *caput medusae,* may radiate from the umbilicus. Ascites may cause other physical problems; for example, orthopnea and dyspnea from increased abdominal distention can interfere with lung expansion. The client may have difficulty in maintaining erect body posture, and *problems with balance* may affect walking. The nurse inspects and palpates for the presence of *inguinal or umbilical hernias,* which are prone to develop in clients with ascites because of increased intra-abdominal pressure.

Less ascites is often more difficult to detect, and advanced assessment techniques, such as the percussion test for shifting dullness and the presence of a fluid wave, may be performed. These techniques are generally used by the experienced clinician. *Abdominal girth* measurements are done to evaluate the progression of ascites (Fig. 47–9). To measure the client's abdominal

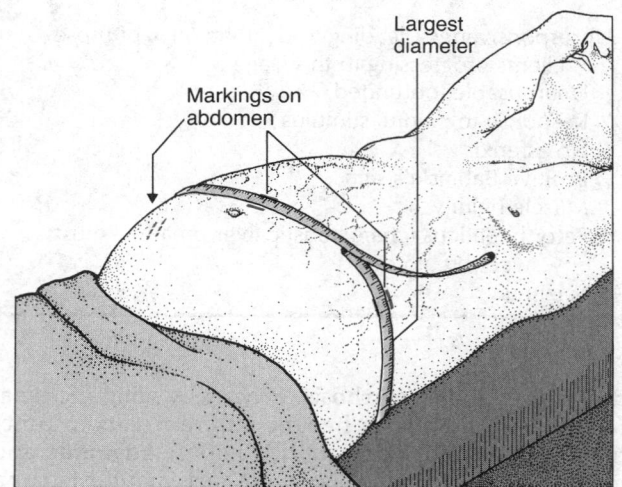

Figure 47–9

How to measure abdominal girth. With the client supine, the nurse brings the tape measure around the client and takes a measurement at the largest diameter of the abdomen. Before removing the tape, the nurse marks the client's abdomen along the sides of the tape on the client's flanks (sides) and midline to ensure that later measurements are taken in a consistent manner.

girth, the nurse asks the client to lie flat and pulls a tape measure around the largest diameter of the abdomen. The girth is measured during exhalation. The nurse marks the client's abdominal skin and flanks to ensure that the tape measure placement is the same on subsequent readings.

The nurse assesses nasogastric tube drainage (if present), vomitus, and stool for the *presence of blood.* This may be indicated by frank blood in the excrement or by positive *o*-toluidine test result for blood content (Hematest). Gastritis, stomach ulceration, or oozing esophageal varices may be responsible for the presence of blood or melanotic (black, tarry) stools.

Fetor hepaticus is the distinctive breath odor of chronic liver disease and PSE. It is characterized by a *fruity or musty odor,* which results from the damaged liver's inability to metabolize and detoxify mercaptan produced by bacterial degradation of methionine, a sulfurous amino acid.

Amenorrhea (absence of menstruation) may be a complaint in women, and men may exhibit *testicular atrophy, gynecomastia* (enlarged breasts), and *impotence* as a result of inactive hormones. Problems with the hematologic system caused by hepatic failure may be manifested by *bruising, petechiae,* and an *enlarged spleen.*

Continuous assessment of neurologic functioning must be done by the nurse. The development of PSE is manifested by neurologic changes, which the alert nurse should recognize (see Key Features of Disease: Manifestations of the Four Stages of Portal-Systemic Encephalopathy). These often *subtle changes in mentation and personality* frequently progress to the late condition of coma.

The nurse assesses for *asterixis* (liver flap or flapping tremor), a coarse tremor characterized by rapid, nonrhythmic extensions and flexions in the wrists and fingers. Asterixis also appears in the ankles, corners of the mouth, eyelids, and the tongue. Figure 47–10 illustrates the technique used to elicit asterixis during physical assessment. The nurse also inspects the extremities and the sacrum for the presence of peripheral, dependent edema.

Psychosocial Assessment

The client with hepatic cirrhosis may undergo subtle personality and behavior changes, such as agitation and belligerence; exhibit signs of emotional lability, euphoria, and depression; or experience sleep pattern disturbances as manifestations of the early stage of PSE.

A complete psychologic assessment and evaluation should be performed to distinguish PSE from alcohol withdrawal or underlying psychologic problems. The nurse gently questions the client to determine orientation and appropriate behaviors.

If the client with alcohol-induced cirrhosis is not compliant with the treatment plan, repeated hospitalizations are common. The nurse assesses the impact of the hospitalizations as interruptions in life style, particularly employment. The client may be unable to work and therefore be unable to pay health care costs. The nurse

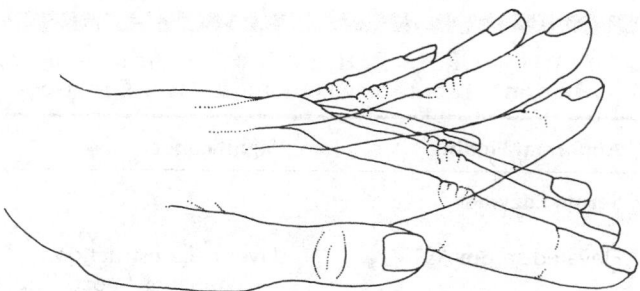

Figure 47–10

To elicit asterixis (flapping tremor), have the client extend the arm, dorsiflex the wrist, and extend the fingers. Observe for rapid, nonrhythmic extensions and flexions.

asks the client about financial capabilities to determine if referrals are needed for assistance. The nurse integrates this information with the neurologic assessment.

Laboratory Findings

Characteristic abnormalities of laboratory studies are found in liver disease (see the Key Features of Disease on p. 1486).

Liver enzyme levels are elevated in clients with hepatic disease. Elevated serum levels of aspartate aminotransferase (AST), also known as serum glutamic-oxaloacetic transaminase (SGOT); alanine aminotransferase (ALT), also known as serum glutamic-pyruvic transaminase (SGPT); and lactate dehydrogenase are present because these substances are released into the blood with the destruction of liver cells. Alkaline phosphatase levels are sensitive to mild extrahepatic or intrahepatic biliary obstruction and are therefore increased in cirrhosis.

Total serum bilirubin levels rise. Indirect bilirubin levels rise in cirrhosis owing to the failing liver's inability to conjugate bilirubin. Bilirubin is present in the urine in increased amounts, and fecal urobilinogen concentration is decreased in biliary tract obstruction, which occurs in biliary cirrhosis. Urine urobilinogen level is increased because of interference with the normal disposition of urobilinogen in hepatic dysfunction.

Total serum protein and albumin levels are decreased in severe or chronic liver disease owing to decreased synthesis by the liver. Serum globulins (alpha, beta, and gamma) are elevated because of the liver's increased synthesis of globulins by the reticuloendothelial system, indicating an immune response to hepatic disease.

Prothrombin time (PT) is prolonged because the liver has decreased synthesis of prothrombin, reflecting hepatocellular or obstructive biliary tract disease. Anemia may be reflected by altered complete blood count (CBC), with decreased hemoglobin level and hematocrit values.

KEY FEATURES OF DISEASE ■ Significance of Abnormal Laboratory Findings in Liver Disease

Abnormal Finding	Significance
Serum Enzymes	
Elevated serum AST	Liver cell destruction, hepatitis (most specific indicator)
Elevated serum ALT	Liver cell destruction, hepatitis
Elevated lactate dehydrogenase	Liver cell destruction
Elevated serum alkaline phosphatase	Obstructive jaundice, hepatic metastasis
Bilirubin	
Elevated serum total bilirubin	Liver cell disease
Elevated serum direct conjugated bilirubin	Hepatitis, liver metastasis
Elevated serum indirect unconjugated bilirubin	Cirrhosis
Elevated urine bilirubin	Hepatocellular obstruction, viral or toxic liver disease
Elevated urine urobilinogen	Hepatic dysfunction
Decreased fecal urobilinogen	Obstructive liver disease
Serum Proteins	
Increased serum total protein	Acute liver disease
Decreased serum total protein	Chronic liver disease
Decreased serum albumin	Severe liver disease
Elevated serum globulin	Immune response to liver disease
Other Tests	
Elevated serum ammonia	Advanced liver disease, PSE
Prolonged PT	Liver cell damage and synthesis of prothrombin

Another laboratory test is the determination of ammonia levels. Elevated ammonia levels occur in advanced liver disease and PSE because of a decreased conversion of ammonia to urea for excretion.

Radiographic Findings

Abdominal x-ray films may reveal liver size, gas, or cysts within the liver and the biliary tract; calcification of the liver; and massive ascites. The upper GI radiographic series examines the esophagus, the stomach, and the small bowel and may reveal the presence of esophageal varices or gastric or duodenal ulceration, which complicate the care of a client with cirrhosis. A barium swallow is a more specific examination of esophagus to assess for inflamed varices, but is not indicated during an acute episode of bleeding.

Angiographic studies may be required to identify actual arterial bleeding sites within the stomach.

CT is helpful in detecting small ascites, as well as providing information about the volume and character of fluid collections.

Other Diagnostic Tests

Esophagogastroduodenoscopy may be performed by the physician to directly visualize the upper GI tract to detect the presence of bleeding or oozing esophageal varices, stomach irritation and ulceration, or duodenal ulceration and bleeding. Injection sclerotherapy may be done during the endoscopic procedure to halt variceal bleeding as a palliative measure (see later). Radioisotope liver scans show abnormal hepatic thickening and identify liver masses. Liver biopsy is the definitive test for cirrhosis. Hepatic tissue biopsy reveals destruction and fibrosis of hepatic cells, indicative of cirrhosis. This examination is also diagnostic of hepatic malignancy and infection.

 Analysis: Nursing Diagnosis

The client with cirrhosis of the liver is admitted to the hospital in varying stages of the disease process and with the potential for life-threatening complications.

Common Diagnoses

The most common nursing diagnoses relate to potential complications for clients with severe cirrhosis of the liver.

1. Fluid volume excess related to ascites
2. Potential for injury (hemorrhage) related to portal hypertension (causing esophageal variceal bleeding), gastric ulcers, or altered coagulation
3. Potential for altered thought processes related to PSE with elevated ammonia levels

Additional Diagnoses

The client with cirrhosis may exhibit the following nursing diagnoses:

1. Altered nutrition: less than body requirements related to anorexia; nausea; and faulty absorption, metabolism, and storage of nutrients and vitamins
2. Ineffective breathing pattern related to ascites and decreased diaphragmatic excursion
3. Pain related to ascites or abdominal pressure
4. Potential for fluid volume deficit related to drastic removal of massive ascites, GI bleeding, or third spacing of fluid
5. Potential for infection related to decrease in white blood cells
6. Knowledge deficit related to unfamiliarity with pathophysiology and cognitive impairment
7. Potential impaired skin integrity related to pruritus secondary to jaundice, edema, and ascites
8. Altered (gastrointestinal) tissue perfusion related to hepatic blood flow alterations, ascites, edema, nutrition deficits, and blood loss
9. Sexual dysfunction related to altered hormonal function and decreased libido

 Planning and Implementation

The following plan of care includes interventions for the commonly occurring complications of the hepatic disease process.

Fluid Volume Excess

Planning: client goals. The goal for this nursing diagnosis is that the client will experience a decrease in extravascular and intra-abdominal fluid, such as abdominal ascites.

Interventions. During the early stages of ascites when fluid accumulations are minimal, interventions are aimed at preventing the accumulation of additional fluid and mobilizing the existing fluid collection. Nonsurgical treatment measures usually control ascites. However, if respiratory or abdominal functioning is compromised, surgical measures may be necessary.

Nonsurgical management. Supportive measures to control abdominal ascites include diet therapy, drugs, paracentesis, and comfort measures. The nurse elicits client compliance in adhering to the treatment plan.

Diet therapy. The client with abdominal ascites is usually placed on a low-sodium diet as an initial means to control fluid accumulation in the abdominal cavity. Daily sodium intake is restricted to 200 to 500 mg. The nurse explains the purpose of the diet and advises the client to eliminate table salt; salty foods, such as potato chips, pretzels, and snack foods; canned and frozen vegetables; and salted butter or margarine. The absence of

salt in low-sodium diets is distasteful to most people. The nurse provides the client with suggestions for alternative flavoring additives, such as lemon, vinegar, parsley, oregano, and pepper. The nurse consults the dietitian for information about additional flavoring substitutes and low-sodium products and diet instructions for the client.

The physician may limit the client's fluid intake. This measure is usually initiated when serum sodium levels fall. The kidneys retain sodium, and dilutional hyponatremia results, primarily from excessive fluid volume. Fluids, both IV and oral, are generally restricted to 1500 mL/day in an effort to reverse the fluid overload. The nurse calculates the amount of oral fluids the client is allowed on the basis of the anticipated IV intake.

Clients with cirrhosis have multiple dietary deficiencies. Vitamin supplements, such as thiamine, folate, and multivitamin preparations, are added to the IV fluids because of the liver's inability to store vitamins. When IV fluids are discontinued, the nurse administers vitamins in oral form.

Drug therapy. Diuretics, such as cholorothiazide (Diuril), are given to *increase* urinary sodium and water excretion to help reduce ascites. The primary goal of diuretic therapy is to reduce fluid accumulation and prevent cardiac and respiratory impairment. The nurse monitors diuretic therapy by assessing intake and output balances, weighing the client daily, measuring abdominal girths, and monitoring electrolyte levels. Serious electrolyte imbalances may accompany diuretic therapy. Hypokalemia (decreased potassium) and hyponatremia (decreased sodium) may occur as a result of treatment and precipitate serious side effects (see Chap. 13 for discussion of electrolyte imbalances).

Spironolactone (Aldactone) may be given as a potassium-sparing diuretic in an effort to decrease potassium depletion and to block the sodium-retaining action of aldosterone. Cirrhosis is often associated with increased levels of aldosterone in urine and plasma. Elevated plasma aldosterone levels can be attributed to increased adrenal secretion or a decreased metabolic degradation of this hormone. In addition, the nurse may give an oral or IV potassium supplement. More potent diuretics, such as furosemide (Lasix) or ethacrynic acid (Edecrin), are sometimes necessary to help rid the body of excess abdominal ascitic fluid.

These clients often require antacid therapy for GI disturbance. Because most antacids are high in sodium content, low-sodium antacids such as magaldrate (Riopan) and aluminum hydroxide gel (Amphojel) are given to these clients.

Paracentesis. If diet and drugs fail to control ascites, abdominal paracentesis is often indicated (see the accompanying Guidelines feature). The physician performs the procedure by inserting a trocar catheter into the abdomen to remove and drain ascitic fluid in the client's peritoneal cavity.

Paracentesis was once a primary treatment modality for ascites, but is currently utilized as a diagnostic tool to examine the ascitic fluid and as a palliative measure to

GUIDELINES ■ Nursing Care of the Client Undergoing Paracentesis

Interventions	Rationales
1. Explain the procedure to the client and provide answers to questions.	1. This prepares the client for the procedure and helps reduce anxiety.
2. Obtain vital signs, measure abdominal girth, and weigh the client.	2. Baseline data are collected for comparison with later findings.
3. Ask the client to void completely or drain Foley's catheter.	3. This decreases the incidence of inadvertent bladder injury by puncture during catheter insertion.
4. Position the client. Assist the client to sit in an upright position at the side of the bed with the feet propped on a stool. Support the client to maintain this position during the procedure.	4. Upright position allows the intestine to float posteriorly and helps prevent laceration during catheter insertion.

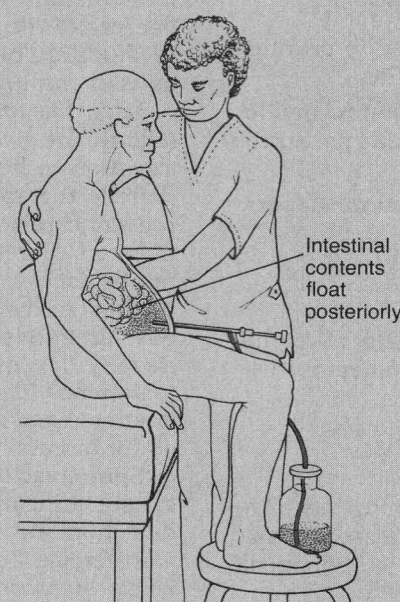

Intestinal contents float posteriorly

5. Monitor vital signs every 15 min during the procedure.	5. Excessive loss of abdominal ascites may cause hypovolemia and precipitate shock. (A drop in blood pressure may occur early in the procedure during initial volume loss.)
6. Measure the drainage and record on the intake and output record.	6. This assists in maintaining an accurate intake and output record.
7. Describe the collected fluid (e.g., clear, straw-colored, hazy, or cloudy). Send specimens for laboratory analysis.	7. The fluid is analyzed to aid in diagnosis.
8. After the physician removes the trocar catheter, apply a dressing to the puncture site. Assess for fluid leakage.	8. Sterile procedure prevents infection.
9. Position the client in bed and maintain bed rest until vital signs are stable and return to baseline values.	9. The client will be tired after the procedure. Stable vital signs indicate tolerance of the procedure.

relieve abdominal pressure, which causes severe respiratory and abdominal distress. To relieve acute symptoms, the physician slowly drains up to 2 to 3 L of ascitic fluid. The potential for hypovolemia with fluid volume deficit may occur with rapid ascites removal, as these clients have adjusted to the excess fluid volume in the abdomen. Rapid, drastic removal of the ascitic fluid leads to decreased abdominal pressure, which may contribute to possible massive vasodilation and shock. The nurse observes for impending signs of shock due to fluid shifting during and immediately after the procedure (see Chap. 17 on shock).

Repeated paracentesis procedures are contraindicated owing to the increased incidence of protein depletion, hypovolemia, and electrolyte imbalances (hypokalemic alkalosis), which can contribute to the development of PSE in the client with cirrhosis.

Comfort measures. Excessive ascitic fluid volume in the abdomen may cause the client to experience difficulty with respiration. The client may develop dyspnea as a result of increased intra-abdominal pressure, which limits thoracic expansion and diaphragmatic excursion. The nurse elevates the head of the bed to at least 30 to 45 degrees or as high as the client wishes in an effort to minimize shortness of breath. The nurse encourages the client to sit in a chair. This upright position, with the client's feet elevated to discourage dependent ankle edema, often relieves dyspnea.

When the nurse weighs the client, a standard upright bedside scale is utilized if the client can stand. Weighing the client on a bedscale requires the client to lie flat; this supine position can cause the client to feel increasingly short of breath and cause increased anxiety.

Surgical management. When medical management fails to control ascites, surgical intervention to divert ascites into the venous system is accomplished by the insertion of a shunt. This surgical bypass *shunting procedure* has a high mortality in clients with severe liver dysfunction, limiting its use as an effective treatment measure for ascites. These clients are poor surgical risks because of their susceptibility to infection, DIC, bleeding varices, and anesthesia reactions.

A peritoneovenous shunt, also known as a peritoneojugular or LeVeen's shunt (Fig. 47–11), operates by draining ascites through a one-way valve into a silicone rubber tube that terminates in the superior vena cava. A pressure gradient develops between the peritoneal cavity and the vena cava, facilitating the flow of ascites into the venous system through the valve. During inspiration, the diaphragm descends, increasing peritoneal fluid (ascites) pressure, and the pressure in the superior vena cava increases, creating the needed gradient. A difference of greater than 3 cmH$_2$O pressure is required to open the valve. The valve closes when the pressure is decreased.

After the insertion of the peritoneovenous shunt, the client is expected to lose weight and have a decrease in abdominal girth, improved urinary output, and increased renal excretion of sodium. These clinical improvements occur as a result of restored adequate peripheral circulation.

The Denver shunt, which has a subcutaneous pump that can be manually compressed, is often preferred for clients whose ascites contains large particles (common in neoplastic ascites). These particles can cause flow to become sluggish and result in a clotted shunt. Compressing the Denver shunt's pump helps to irrigate the tubing to maintain patency.

Preoperative care. The client with cirrhosis has many underlying medical problems; therefore, an optimal physical state is desired before surgery is performed. Electrolyte imbalances are corrected, and abnormal coagulation is treated with fresh frozen plasma and vitamin K. Packed red blood cells are made available for transfusion, because these clients have bleeding tendencies.

Figure 47–11

Peritoneovenous (LeVeen's) shunting for treatment of ascites.

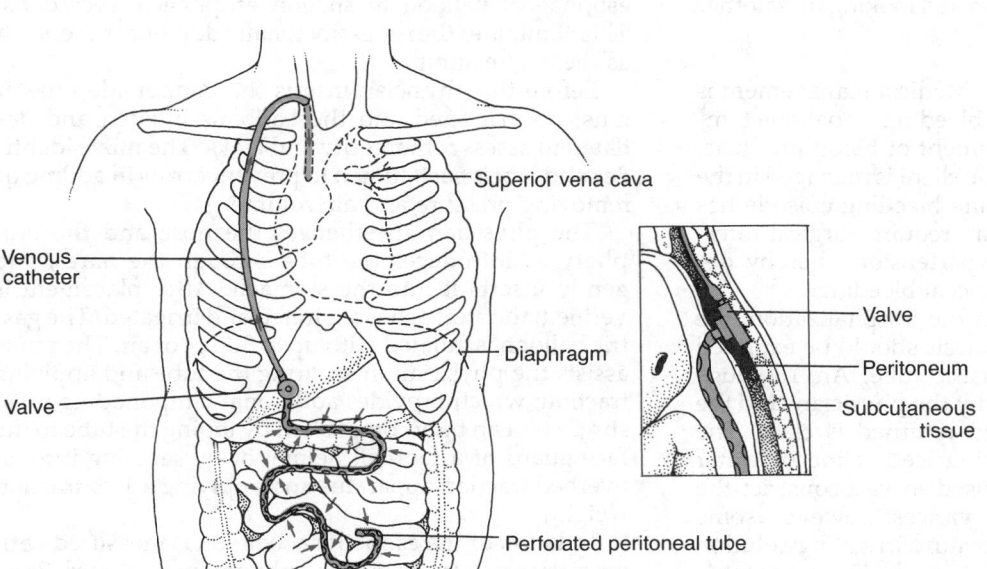

Superior vena cava

Venous catheter

Diaphragm

Valve

Perforated peritoneal tube

Valve

Peritoneum

Subcutaneous tissue

Postoperative care. The reader is referred to Chapter 20 for postoperative management. In addition, when caring for the client with a peritoneovenous shunt, the nurse must keep in mind that the ascites is routed into the venous system. This excess fluid results in vascular volume expansion and hemodilution. The nurse monitors the client's vital signs; an increase in blood pressure reflects an increase in volume. If the client has a central venous catheter in place, the nurse determines if the central venous pressure is elevated. Lung sounds are auscultated for the presence of crackles (rales), indicating excessive lung water. The nurse administers a diuretic, such as furosemide, to prevent pulmonary edema by mobilizing the body of excess fluid.

Results of coagulation studies (prothrombin time [PT]; partial thromboplastin time [PTT]) must be monitored by the nurse, who reports abnormal levels to the physician. Reabsorption of clotting factors in ascitic fluid may further inhibit an already altered clotting mechanism and lead to DIC and bleeding abnormalities (see Chap. 67 for further discussion of these complications). Daily weight, abdominal girth, and urinary output measurements are performed by the nurse to determine the effectiveness of the shunting procedure.

Potential for Injury

Planning: client goals. The primary goals are that the client will (1) experience relief from massive GI or esophageal variceal hemorrhage and (2) not have recurrent bleeding episodes.

Interventions. During the acute phase of bleeding, early interventions are based on identifying the source of bleeding and initiating treatment to halt it. Because massive esophageal bleeding can cause rapid blood loss, emergency interventions are initiated. If the client is a known alcoholic with a prior history of variceal bleeding, measures to treat the esophageal varices are initiated and valuable time is not wasted looking for another source of bleeding.

Nonsurgical management. Medical management is quickly initiated to control the bleeding by balloon tamponade, drug therapy, replacement of blood products, and injection sclerotherapy. The client is managed in the critical care unit. After the acute bleeding episode has been controlled, the client may require surgical intervention to decrease portal hypertension, thereby decreasing the risk of further variceal bleeding.

Gastric intubation. Early in the hospitalization, the client's complaints of hematemesis should be explored by the insertion of a nasogastric tube. An 18-gauge Salem's sump tube is inserted by the physician, and the stomach is lavaged until fluid returned is clear. The common practice of introducing iced saline or water lavage has historically been used to vasoconstrict the bleeding gastric ulceration or varices; however, some physicians prefer room temperature irrigating solution (see Chap. 45 for care of the client during nasogastric

lavage). Norepinephrine (Levophed) may be added to the solution to produce further constriction.

If the bleeding site has been identified by endoscopy as a gastric ulcer, medical treatment is initiated with drug therapy (antacids and histamine antagonists) and blood product replacement. If bleeding continues from the ulcer, surgical intervention is required (see Chap. 44 for the care of the client with gastric ulceration).

Esophagogastric balloon tamponade. If it is suspected that hematemesis has occurred as the result of bleeding esophageal varices, an esophagogastric tamponade tube is inserted (see the accompanying Guidelines feature). Bleeding varices are a medical emergency requiring immediate intervention. A primary early nursing concern is maintenance of a patent airway. The vomiting and accumulation of blood in the oropharynx may result in aspiration, occluded airway, and respiratory compromise. The nurse attempts to keep the client's oropharynx clear by suctioning secretions, turning the client's head, and keeping the head of the bed elevated during vomiting episodes to prevent aspiration.

The classic method of treating bleeding esophageal varices is by compressing the bleeding vessels with a Sengstaken-Blakemore tube (Blakemore tube). This tube has two balloons (Fig. 47–12). The large esophageal balloon compresses the esophagus when inflated and the smaller gastric balloon helps anchor the tube and exerts pressure against bleeding varices located in the distal esophagus and the cardia of the stomach. A third lumen terminates in the stomach and is connected to suction, allowing for aspiration of gastric contents and blood. A Salem sump is used in conjunction with the Sengstaken-Blakemore tube and is placed in the proximal esophagus to enable clearing of collected esophageal secretions, saliva, and blood.

Another esophagogastric balloon tube often used is the Minnesota tube (see Fig. 47–12). Similar to the Sengstaken-Blakemore tube, the Minnesota tube has an additional lumen (port), which is situated above the esophageal balloon to suction esophageal secretions. This eliminates the necessity for an additional tube, such as the Salem sump.

Before the physician inserts the tamponade tube, it must be inspected and the balloons inflated and deflated to assess for integrity and leaks. The nurse identifies and labels each lumen to prevent errors in adding or removing pressure and air volume.

The physician anesthetizes the nose and the oropharynx, introduces the tube through the nares, and gently inserts it into the stomach. After placement is verified, the stomach is aspirated and irrigated. The gastric balloon is inflated with up to 300 cc of air. The nurse assists the physician in securing the tube and applying traction, which provides additional tamponading pressure. This can be accomplished by taping the tube to the face guard of a football helmet or by securing it to an overbed traction apparatus and applying a 1-lb traction weight.

Inflation of the esophageal balloon is measured with mercury pressure by using a sphygmomanometer. Pres-

GUIDELINES ■ Nursing Care of the Client with an Esophageal Tamponade Tube

Interventions	Rationales
1. Assist the physician with tube placement. Before inflation of the gastric balloon, make sure a chest x-ray film is obtained and is available *immediately* on tube insertion.	1. Verification of tube placement is crucial before inflation to ensure that the gastric balloon is located in the cardia of the stomach and *not* in the esophagus. This verification procedure can prevent esophageal rupture with balloon inflation.
2. Elevate the head of the bed when the tube is in place.	2. This position enhances lung expansion and reduces portal blood flow, thereby permitting more effective compression of the varices.
3. Clearly label all lumina of the tamponade tube.	3. Labeling assists in prevention of inadvertent irrigations, accidental deflation, or excessive inflation of balloons.
4. Keep scissors at the bedside. Cut the tube and remove it immediately if signs of respiratory distress or airway obstruction occur.	4. Gastric balloon rupture is a rare complication. The tube may migrate upward to the laryngopharynx, causing airway obstruction and increasing the risk of suffocation and aspiration.
5. Apply gentle tension to the tube by securing the tube to the face guard of a football helmet or applying an overhead traction set-up with a 1-lb traction weight.	5. Securing the tube maintains the position of the gastric balloon against the cardioesophageal junction, reducing the risk of balloon migration.
6. Apply a cut gauze sponge around the tube under the client's nose.	6. The gauze prevents pressure on the nares and assists in preventing pressure necrosis.
7. Insert a drainage tube into the esophagus above the inflated balloon if the tamponade tube does not have an esophageal drainage port. If an esophageal drainage port is available, maintain drain patency.	7. The client cannot swallow and secretions collect in the esophagus and oropharynx proximal to the balloon. The additional suction port or drainage tube allows for suctioning of secretions and reduces the risk of aspiration.
8. Provide the client with frequent mouth care.	8. The client is unable to swallow and is maintained on NPO status. The oral cavity becomes dry and crusty, resulting in mucositis, halitosis, and discomfort for the client.
9. Restrain the client's hands loosely.	9. The prevents the client from disrupting the tube's placement.
10. Maintain the specified balloon pressures and volumes. (Esophageal balloon pressure is measured in millimeters of mercury; gastric balloon volume is measured in milliliters or cubic centimeters.) Release the pressure at specified intervals. (The client may experience substernal pressure when the esophageal balloon is inflated. This is a normal feeling.)	10. The pressure in the esophageal balloon compresses the varices to halt the bleeding. The pressure should be released intermittently to prevent or reduce the incidence of edema, ulceration, or necrosis to the esophagus.
11. Assess the client's sudden complaint of back and upper abdominal pain. Monitor vital signs for a drop in blood pressure and an increase in the heart rate. Report to the physician immediately.	11. These findings may indicate esophageal rupture. *This is a medical emergency!*

sure should be maintained between 20 and 25 mmHg. The nurse periodically checks the balloon pressures and volumes to prevent loss of pressure (with further bleeding or erosion) or rupture of the esophagus caused by overinflation. The esophagogastric balloon is usually removed after 48 hours of use. The nurse attaches the esophageal and gastric drainage lumina to low intermittent suction and monitors the amount and type of drainage.

Placement of the tamponade tube should halt variceal bleeding. After bleeding is controlled, the traction is released and the esophageal pressure is gradually de-

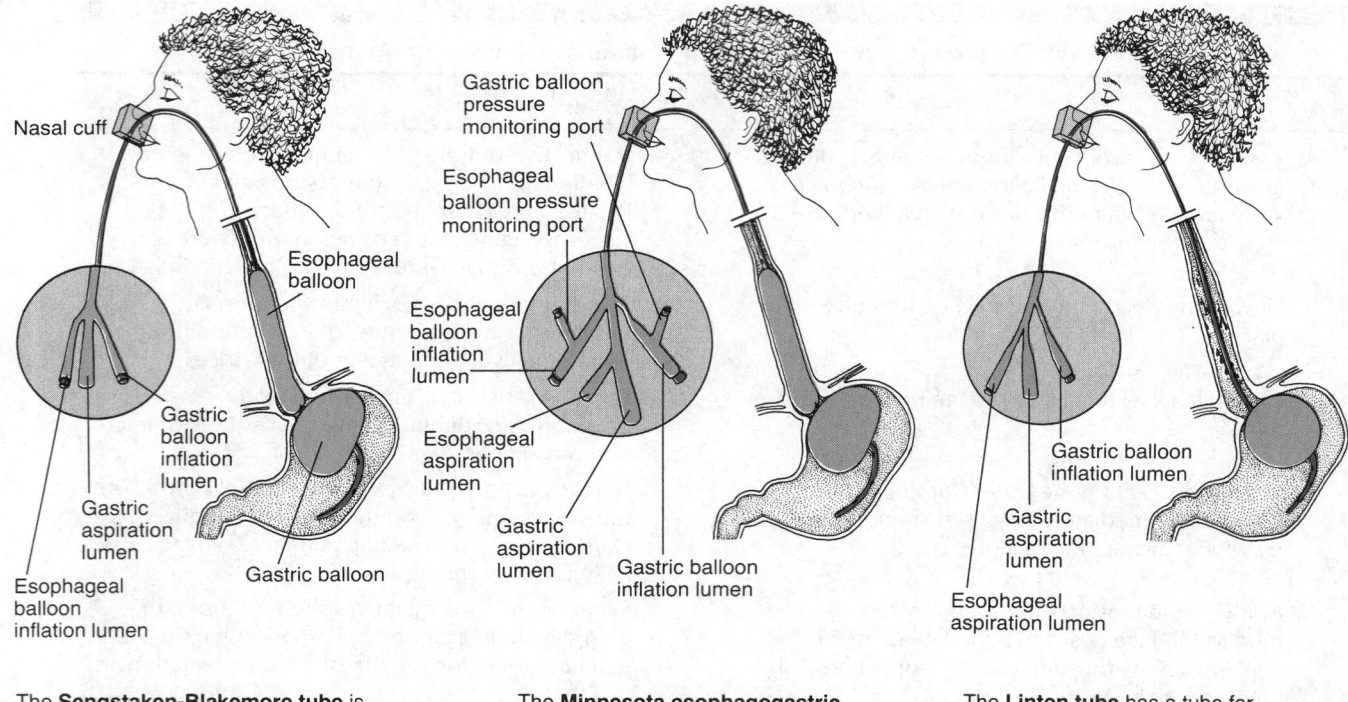

The **Sengstaken-Blakemore tube** is the best known. An additional tube must be placed in the proximal esophagus.

The **Minnesota esophagogastric tamponade tube** includes an esophageal aspiration lumen.

The **Linton tube** has a tube for esophageal aspiration but lacks an esophageal balloon.

Figure 47–12

Comparison of esophageal tubes.

creased. The gastric balloon is deflated, and the tube is removed. Another tube should be kept at the bedside for potential reinsertion if bleeding recurs.

The nurse should be alert for sudden respiratory compromise with acute distress caused by airway obstruction from upward esophageal balloon displacement. A pair of scissors is *always* secured at the bedside. In the event of tube dislodgment, the nurse cuts both balloon ports to allow for rapid balloon deflation and quickly removes the tube.

Blood transfusions. Massive hemorrhage requires replacement by blood products. Blood is drawn by the nurse or the physician to identify the client's blood type. Until the blood is available, the nurse administers large crystalloid (IV fluids) or colloid (plasma) volumes into large-bore IV access routes to maintain blood pressure.

The nurse rapidly administers packed red blood cells and fresh frozen plasma to replace blood volume and clotting factors. Trends in hemoglobin and hematocrit levels are monitored by the nurse and the physician, and additional blood products are transfused as indicated. If more than 10 units of blood are needed, non-cross-matched blood of the client's same type is transfused.

Vasopressin therapy. Vasopressin (Pitressin) is used in treating bleeding esophageal varices to control hemorrhage by lowering pressures within the portal blood flow system. Vasopressin causes contraction of smooth muscle in the vascular bed. By constricting preportal

splanchnic arterioles, vasopressin decreases blood flow to the abdominal organs, which reduces portal pressure and portal blood flow.

This drug is administered by infusion pump intravenously or through a catheter placed in the superior mesenteric artery. The IV route is indicated initially because of easy, rapid access. Insertion of a superior mesenteric artery catheter is an invasive procedure done under fluoroscopy. Both methods of infusing vasopressin have demonstrated effective short-term control of variceal bleeding, but recurrent hemorrhage is common. An initial bolus dose of 20 to 40 units of vasopressin in 100 to 200 mL of D_5W is given, followed by a continuous infusion of 200 units in 500 mL of D_5W at 0.2 to 0.4 unit/minute.

The nurse closely monitors the client for the occurrence of abdominal cramping and pallor caused by decreased abdominal blood flow and for cardiac arrhythmias evidenced by irregular heart beats. Vasopressin may precipitate acute angina or myocardial infarction in clients with coronary artery disease. Concurrent IV administration of nitroglycerin (Tridil), a vasodilator, may help prevent vasoconstriction of the coronary arteries during vasopressin therapy. The nurse reports these findings and the first complaint of chest pain to the physician. Vital signs and an electrocardiogram are obtained. The nurse should be prepared to discontinue the vasopressin infusion when necessary.

Injection sclerotherapy. The use of endoscopic injection sclerotherapy in bleeding esophageal varices is a primary treatment measure reserved for clients with repeated hemorrhagic episodes despite conservative medical management. This intervention was not utilized as often when surgical shunting procedures gained popularity. Because these shunting procedures have been found to be high risk, injection sclerotherapy is being advocated.

Before the examination, the nurse obtains baseline vital sign values and administers the ordered sedation, usually IV diazepam (Valium). The client's throat is sprayed with a topical anesthetic, such as benzocaine (Cetacaine).

Injection sclerotherapy is performed in conjunction with esophagogastric duodenoscopy. During the endoscopic examination, the physician introduces approximately 2 mL of a sclerosing agent (such as morrhuate sodium, sodium tetradecyl sulfate, or ethanolamine oleate) through a flexible injector (Fig. 47 – 13). After the sclerosing agent covers the inflamed and distended oozing varix or varices, it traumatizes the endothelial lining, causing thrombosis and eventual sclerosing (or hardening). After sclerosis, the esophageal veins have a white appearance (Fig. 47 – 13).

Bleeding from the varices should stop within 2 to 5 minutes. If it continues, a second injection attempt is made below the bleeding site. Prophylactic injection sclerotherapy may be done on other distended, nonbleeding varices.

Because the procedure is usually done during an acute bleeding episode, the nurse closely monitors the client's vital signs during this hour-long bedside or clinic procedure.

The client may complain of chest discomfort for 24 to 72 hours after the injection, which is noncardiac in origin and is relieved by analgesia. The nurse assesses the complaint of chest pain and administers pain medica-tion. Esophageal perforation and ulceration are other complications of the treatment, and these cause severe chest pain. The nurse reports acute changes to the physician immediately.

Because aspiration may occur and cause pneumonia and pleural effusion as complications, the nurse assesses lung sounds for decreased aeration and adventitious sounds. After injection sclerotherapy, nasogastric tubes should be utilized and inserted with caution. Some physicians prefer not to reinsert nasogastric tubes to decrease the risk of injury to the sclerosed esophagus.

Surgical management.   Portal-systemic shunts are considered a last-resort intervention for clients with portal hypertension and esophageal varices. The high mortality associated with shunting procedures occurs because clients with end-stage liver disease have coagulation abnormalities, are prone to infection, poorly tolerate anesthesia, and have ascites.

Surgical bypass shunting procedures are performed to decrease portal hypertension. This is accomplished by diverting a portion of the portal vein blood flow from the liver. The goal is to decrease the incidence of variceal bleeding, but maintain sufficient blood flow to the liver, reserving hepatocellular function. The shunting procedures most commonly employed are the portacaval and splenorenal shunts (Fig. 47 – 14). The purpose of the *portacaval shunt* is to divert the portal venous blood flow into the inferior vena cava to decrease portal pressure. The portal vein is anastomosed to the inferior vena cava. The *splenorenal shunting procedure* involves splenectomy with the anastomosis of the splenic vein and the left renal vein. There are variations of these procedures, such as the *mesocaval shunt,* in which the superior mesenteric vein is anastomosed to the inferior vena cava.

Portal-systemic decompression shunting procedures are not performed as frequently as they once were

Figure 47 – 13

Injection sclerotherapy.

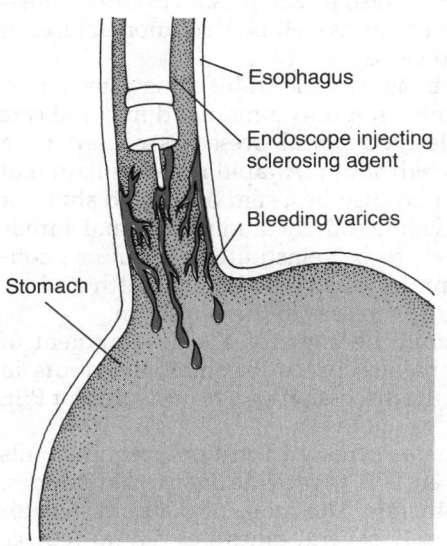

Esophagus

Endoscope injecting sclerosing agent

Bleeding varices

Stomach

Before

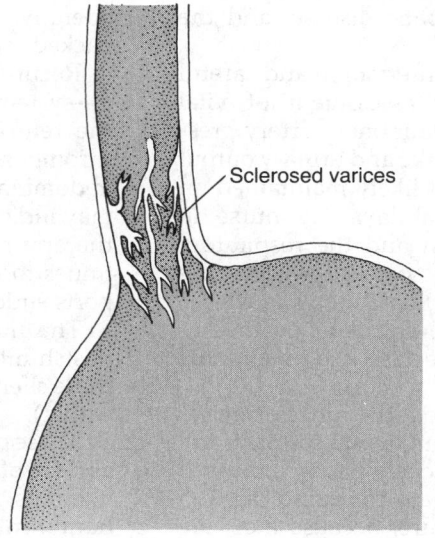

Sclerosed varices

After

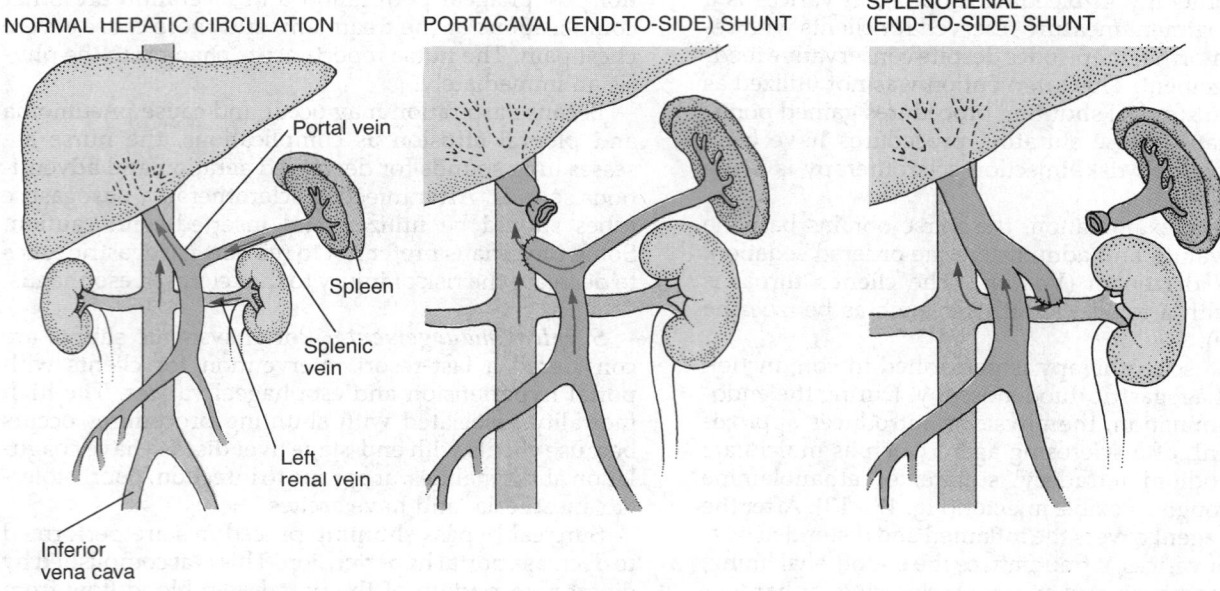

Figure 47–14

Surgical shunting diverts portal venous blood flow from the liver to decrease portal and esophageal pressure.

owing to the occurrence of complications, such as bleeding, PSE, shunt thrombosis, and infection. In general, a shunt may decrease the occurrence of variceal bleeding, but the survival time of the client is usually not prolonged.

Preoperative care. The client with hepatic cirrhosis has multiple underlying problems. The client with esophageal bleeding must be transfused before surgery with packed red blood cells and fresh frozen plasma to correct clotting deficiencies.

Postoperative care. The client is admitted to the critical care unit immediately after surgery. The extent of care required is dependent on the client's preoperative health status, the extent of hepatic disease, and the magnitude of the procedure.

The nurse provides constant observation and careful monitoring, including frequent assessment of vital signs, central venous pressure, pulmonary artery pressure (if indicated), and hourly intake and urinary output measures. These clients are most likely maintained on mechanical ventilation for several days. The nurse, in collaboration with the physician and the respiratory therapist, monitors respiratory status, protects the client's artificial airway (endotracheal tube), and checks the ventilator for correct settings. The usual postoperative care measures to prevent atelectasis and pneumonia should be instituted (Chap. 20).

During the postoperative period, the nurse exercises discretion in providing narcotic analgesia for pain and sedation, although the intubated client has an increased need for sedatives. These drugs are contraindicated in clients with chronic hepatic failure, because most are metabolized in the liver.

After these shunting procedures, clients are prone to develop oliguria (decreased urinary output) because they are often volume depleted (hypovolemic) as a result of uncompensated blood loss; excess fluid loss from prolonged exposure of the peritoneal space during surgery, resulting in fluid evaporation; the recurrence of ascites; preoperative fluid restriction; and diuretic therapy. The nurse administers the ordered fluid volume and assesses the effects of the volume by monitoring for increased blood pressure, decreased heart rate, and increased urinary output. The nurse reports excessive increases in the central venous pressure or pulmonary artery pressure after fluid challenge. Volume may be given in the form of fresh frozen plasma to correct postoperative coagulopathy, as well as IV solution boluses or packed red blood cells.

Recurrent esophageal variceal bleeding after a portal-systemic shunt is not uncommon and may indicate the return of elevated portal pressures caused by a thrombosed (clotted) shunt. A rapid reaccumulation of abdominal fluid may also be a sign of a failed shunt or may indicate excessive sodium administration. Diuretic therapy may need to be reinstituted. The nurse continues to measure the client's abdominal girth and reports sudden girth increases to the physician.

The nurse should be alert for the development of postshunt encephalopathy, as it commonly occurs in these clients (see the discussion of care measures for PSE earlier).

These clients have increased nutritional requirements and are often given TPN to provide the needed calories, vitamins, and minerals. The nurse also administers albumin intravenously several times per day to replace the albumin lost in ascites (see Chap. 13 for care associated with TPN and albumin administration).

Potential for Altered Thought Processes

Planning: client goals.   The goal is that the client will be able to clearly state factual information about the self and exhibit mental cognition at the pre–hospital admission level.

Interventions: nonsurgical management.   During the early stages of PSE in hepatic cirrhosis, interventions are focused on decreasing ammonia formation in an effort to decrease progressive cerebral dysfunction. The diseased liver is unable to convert ammonia to a less toxic form, and ammonia is carried by the circulatory system to the brain where high levels are toxic to normal cerebral function. The management of PSE aims to halt this process.

Because ammonia is formed in the GI tract by the action of bacteria on protein, nonsurgical treatment measures to decrease ammonia production include dietary limitations and drug therapy to reduce the bacterial breakdown. The nurse collaborates with the dietitian and the physician in planning and implementing these treatment measures.

Diet therapy.   The client with cirrhosis has increased nutritional requirements. The prescribed diet includes high-carbohydrate, moderate-fat, and high-protein foods. When the client has elevated serum ammonia levels and exhibits the signs of PSE, the diet is modified. The nurse aggressively limits the client's intake of dietary protein in an effort to reduce excessive breakdown of the protein by intestinal bacteria in the GI tract.

Low-protein foods are included in the client's diet, as well as simple carbohydrates, such as fruit juice. As the client's mental status deteriorates, proteins may totally be eliminated from the diet. When PSE fluctuates among the four stages, the nurse avoids giving the client foods high in protein content, such as meat, fish, poultry, eggs, and dairy products.

These clients often experience GI bleeding, resulting in the formation of increased amounts of ammonia as intestinal bacteria attempt to metabolize the blood cells. GI bleeding may precipitate hepatic coma (stage IV of PSE). These clients are maintained on NPO status with a nasogastric tube or an esophageal tamponade tube, depending on the source of the bleeding. Nutritional maintenance with IV TPN is required.

If mental status improves with treatment, protein is gradually added to the diet. The nurse consults the dietitian to assist in meal planning to limit dietary protein intake to 50 to 60 g/day.

Drug therapy.   Lactulose (Cephulac) is given to the client to promote the excretion of ammonia in the stool. Lactulose, a disaccharide with high molecular weight, is a viscous, sticky, sweet-tasting liquid that the nurse administers either orally or by nasogastric tube. When giving the drug orally, the nurse dilutes the lactulose with fruit juice to help the client tolerate the sweet taste. Lactulose retention enemas are often required when the client is unable to tolerate oral administration or when liquids are contraindicated in the upper GI tract.

Lactulose creates an acid environment in the bowel by keeping ammonia in its ionized state, resulting in a fall of the colon's pH from 7.0 to 5.0. This causes ammonia to leave the circulatory system and move into the colon, which reverses the normal passage of ammonia from the colon to the blood stream. The acid environment also discourages bacteria growth. Lactulose draws water into the bowel because of its high osmotic gradient, producing a laxative effect and facilitating evacuation of ammonia from the bowel.

The desired effect of lactulose is two to three soft stools per day with an acid fecal pH. In the acute phase of PSE, lactulose is administered in a dose of 20 to 30 g at 4-hour intervals until stools are achieved and then decreased to three or four times per day. As a retention enema, lactulose is given in a dose of 200 g diluted in 1000 mL of water at 4- to 6-hour intervals.

The nurse closely observes for watery diarrheal stools, which may signify excessive lactulose administration. The client may complain of intestinal bloating and cramping. The nurse also monitors daily for decreasing ammonia levels, reflecting a positive effect of drug therapy, and monitors for hypokalemia and dehydration, which can occur as a result of numerous stools.

Neomycin sulfate, a broad-spectrum antibiotic, is given to act as an intestinal antiseptic; it destroys normal flora in the bowel, which diminish protein breakdown and decrease the rate of ammonia production. Maintenance doses of neomycin are given orally, but it may also be administered as a retention enema.

Because constipation may lead to increased bacterial action on retained stool, with a resulting increase in ammonia levels, stool softeners should be included in the long-term treatment plan. Restriction of medications that are potentially toxic to the liver, such as narcotics, sedatives, or barbiturates, must be included in the plan of care.

Because the client with PSE exhibits progressive neurologic changes and is often confused, combative, uncooperative, or belligerent, the nurse may be required to give sedatives to prevent the client from self-harm or harming others. In such cases, the judicious use of drugs such as oxazepam (Serax) or diazepam (Valium) is warranted.

Levodopa (Dopar, Larodopa) has been used with some success in the treatment of chronic PSE. The use of levodopa (a precursor of dopamine and norepinephrine) is based on the theory that there are defective neurotransmitters in encephalopathy. Deficient dopamine and norepinephrine are replaced by false transmitters, the amine products from breakdown of dietary protein. The pathway for normal transmission is provided by synthetic levodopa.

Neurologic assessment.   The nurse continuously assesses the client for changes in level of consciousness and orientation. An individualized neurologic assessment is developed for each client, which includes assessment of simple tasks, such as name writing, bilateral handgrasping, and performing serial subtractions and additions.

The nurse also continuously assesses for the presence of asterixis (liver flap) and fetor hepaticus (liver breath). These signs are indicative of worsening encephalopathy.

■ Discharge Planning

If the client with hepatic cirrhosis survives life-threatening complications, she/he is usually discharged to home from the hospital after treatment measures have combated the acute medical problems. These chronically ill clients are frequently readmitted, and discharge planning is aimed at preventing rehospitalization.

Home Care Preparation

The nurse, the client, and the family identify any physical adaptations needed to prepare the home for convalescence. The client's rest area should be close to a bathroom because diuretic therapy increases the frequency of urination. If the client has difficulty reaching the toilet, additional equipment, such as urinals, bedpans, or bedside commodes, are required. If the client has an altered mental status and is incontinent of urine, special adult-sized incontinence pads or diapers may be helpful during the night.

If the client has undergone any surgical interventions, initial home activity may be limited and the client may be confined to one floor. It may be necessary to obtain a hospital bed for the client with chronic hepatic failure because of long-term problems. If the client experiences shortness of breath from massive ascites, elevating the head of the bed and maintaining the client in high Fowler's position may help alleviate respiratory distress. Alternatively, a reclining chair with foot elevator may be utilized.

Client/Family Education

The client is discharged to home with an individualized teaching plan. Important areas of concern include diet therapy, drug therapy, alcohol abstinence, complication recognition, and medical follow-up care. The client is given strict dietary instructions, depending on the problems identified. A typical client with hepatic cirrhosis requires the nurse and the dietitian to provide teaching information for a diet high in calories, protein, and vitamins. The dietitian can plan meals and menus with the client's favorite foods and provide lists of foods high in caloric, protein, and vitamin content. Some clients have certain food items restricted. The client with ascites requires a diet low in sodium content. The nurse advises the client to eat nutritious, well-balanced meals, but to limit the amount of or totally eliminate sodium in the diet. A list of foods high in sodium content, which should be eliminated in the diet, is prepared for the client; these include table salt, snack foods such as potato chips and pretzels, canned and frozen vegetables, and salted margarine and butter. The client and family members are instructed to read food labels and to avoid purchasing foods with high sodium content.

The client who develops PSE must avoid high-protein foods at home in an effort to decrease the incidence of progressive neurologic dysfunction. The client and the family are instructed by the nurse and the dietitian to modify the diet by limiting the ingestion of high-protein foods, such as meat, fish, poultry, eggs, and dairy products. If the client's nutritional intake is poor at home, supplemental liquid feedings and multivitamin supplements are required.

The client is often discharged while receiving drug therapy with diuretics. The client is provided with written instruction and prescriptions for the diuretic, as well as information about signs and symptoms of potential electrolyte imbalances, such as hypokalemia, which may result from diuretic therapy. The client may also be required to take a potassium supplement.

If the client has had problems with bleeding from gastric ulceration, he/she will be given antacids or an H_2 antagonist agent such as cimetidine (Tagamet). The nurse provides written guidelines and administration schedules for all medications to be taken at home.

The client is advised by the nurse to avoid all OTC medications and to consult the physician for follow-up medical care. The client is instructed to notify the physician immediately if any evidence of GI bleeding is noted, so that re-evaluation can be initiated quickly.

One of the most important aspects of discharge planning is stressing the need for alcohol abstinence. Avoiding alcohol can prevent further fibrosis of the liver by scarring and allow the liver to regenerate. It can also prevent gastric and esophageal irritation and reduce the incidence of bleeding, as well as prevent the occurrence of other life-threatening complications.

Psychosocial Preparation

The nurse includes a supportive spouse or other family member in discharge planning. After experiencing and surviving acute, life-threatening complications, the client may be extremely anxious and fearful about being discharged from the hospital. The family member can provide helpful reinforcement of information for the client, because the client's anxiety may block learning, and can help the client comply with the treatment plan. The client may require additional supportive therapy by counselors or a spiritual leader (e.g., rabbi or clergyperson) to help reduce fear and anxiety, as well as assisting in alcohol abstinence.

Health Care Resources

The client with chronic cirrhosis may require a home care nurse to assess the client's tolerance of dietary restrictions and to monitor the effectiveness of drug therapy or surgical shunt in controlling ascites.

Individual and group therapy sessions may be arranged to assist the client in dealing with abstinence from alcohol. The nurse may direct the client or family to self-help groups, such as Alcoholics Anonymous and Al-Anon.

 Evaluation

The nurse evaluates the care of the client with hepatic cirrhosis and complications of cirrhosis. On the basis of the identified nursing diagnoses, the expected outcomes vary from client to client, depending on disease progression. Generally, expected outcomes for the client with hepatic cirrhosis include that the client

1. States an understanding of the disease process and can list the negative effects that cirrhosis has on body functioning
2. Complies with the dietary plan and restrictions
3. Abstains from alcohol intake
4. Maintains cognitive function

HEPATITIS

OVERVIEW

Many factors are involved in the etiology of *hepatitis,* the widespread inflammation of liver cells. *Viral hepatitis,* the most prevalent type of hepatitis, occurs as a result of a infection caused by one of four categories of viruses: hepatitis A virus (HAV), hepatitis B virus (HBV), hepatitis C (non-A, non-B) virus, and recently described hepatitis delta virus (HDV), or delta agent.

Liver injury with inflammation can also develop after exposure to a number of pharmacologic and chemical agents by inhalation, ingestion, or parenteral (IV) administration. *Toxic and drug-induced hepatitis* can result from exposure to hepatotoxins, such as industrial toxins, alcohol, or medications used in medical therapies.

The client usually fully recovers from hepatitis, but may have residual liver damage. Although mortality from hepatitis is relatively low, fulminant hepatitis may result in death. Hepatitis may occur as a secondary infection during the course of infections with other viruses, such as cytomegalovirus, Epstein-Barr virus, herpes simplex virus, and varicella-zoster virus.

Pathophysiology

Pathologic Changes

After the liver has been exposed to causative agents, such as a virus, it becomes enlarged and congested with inflammatory cells, lymphocytes, and edema, resulting in right upper quadrant pain and discomfort. As the disease process continues and progresses, the liver's normal lobular pattern becomes distorted owing to widespread inflammation, necrosis, and hepatocellular regeneration. Pressure within the portal circulation increases as a result of the distortion, interfering with the blood flow into the hepatic lobules. Edema of the liver's bile channels results in intrahepatic obstructive jaundice.

Specific data on the pathogenesis of hepatitis A, hepatitis C, and delta hepatitis are limited. Investigational evidence suggests that clinical manifestations of acute HBV inflammation are determined by an immunologic response of the host (client). Immune complex–mediated tissue damage appears to contribute to the extrahepatic manifestations of acute hepatitis B. It is believed that circulating immune complexes are deposited in blood vessel walls and activate the complement system. Clinical responses include the development of an urticarial rash and arthritic joint pain.

The recovery phase of hepatitis is hallmarked by active phagocytosis and enzyme activity; damaged liver cells are removed, allowing for regeneration of the cells. Most clients recover normal hepatic function after a viral hepatic insult unless serious complications develop. Complete regeneration usually occurs within 2 to 3 months.

Sequelae

Failure of the liver cells to regenerate, with progression of the necrotic process, results in a severe, fulminant, frequently fatal form of hepatitis known as *fulminant hepatitis.* This form of massive hepatic necrosis is rare. *Chronic hepatitis* occurs as a sequela to hepatitis B or hepatitis C. Superimposed infection with delta hepatitis agent (HDV) in clients with hepatitis B surface antigen (HBsAg) may lead to the development of chronic active hepatitis and clinical deterioration. In some cases, fulminant hepatitis with death may result. In *chronic active hepatitis,* liver damage is progressive and is characterized by continuing hepatic necrosis, acute inflammation, and fibrosis. The client may be asymptomatic for long periods of the hepatic disease process, or the continued fibrosis may lead to liver failure, cirrhosis, and death. Chronic active hepatitis may be manifested by persistent clinical symptoms and hepatomegaly, the continual presence of HBsAg, and elevated, fluctuating serum levels of AST, bilirubin, and alkaline phosphatase levels for 6 to 12 months after the acute hepatitis episode. Liver biopsy is necessary to establish the diagnosis of chronic hepatitis.

In *chronic persistent hepatitis* and *chronic lobar hepatitis,* liver damage does not progress after the initial insult. These types of hepatitis result from infections with HBV and hepatitis C virus. In these nonprogressive disorders, development of cirrhosis is rare, and the recovery prognosis is good.

Most clients with chronic persistent hepatitis are asymptomatic, and physical findings are normal. Laboratory data may reveal a mild elevation of serum AST and alkaline phosphatase levels that may persist for up to 1 year.

KEY FEATURES OF DISEASE ■ Differential Features of the Four Types of Viral Hepatitis

Feature	Hepatitis A	Hepatitis B	Hepatitis C (Non-A, Non-B Hepatitis)	Delta Hepatitis
Synonyms	Infectious hepatitis Short-incubation hepatitis	Serum hepatitis Long-incubation hepatitis		
Diagnosis of acute disease	Anti-HAV IgM in serum	HBsAg in serum	Rule out other causes	Anti-HD titer increase
Incubation period	28–94 d	17–98 d		Same as for hepatitis B
High-risk groups	More common in young children and institutional settings	All age groups affected, especially drug addicts, clients undergoing long-term hemodialysis, and medical personnel	All ages; occurs after blood transfusions	Drug addicts
Season	Fall and early winter	All year	All year	All year
Transmission	Usually by fecal-oral route among persons living in close contact; ingestion of contaminated water or contaminated shellfish; also parenteral route	Usually by transfusion of blood and blood products or some other form of inoculation, especially parenteral drug abuse; also by fecal-oral route and sexual contact	Blood and body fluids	Co-infects with hepatitis B; nonpercutaneous, close personal contact
Clinical findings	Majority of type A infections mild and anicteric; symptoms similar to those of influenza	Changes similar to those of hepatitis A	Changes similar to those of hepatitis A	Changes similar to those of hepatitis A, but symptoms often more severe than those in hepatitis A and hepatitis B
	Fatigue, anorexia, low-grade fever, abdominal discomfort, arthralgias, rashes, enlarged tender liver, light stools, dark urine, jaundice	Tends to have more severe symptoms; sometimes requires hospitalization for extended periods		

Classification

Viral hepatitis. The four types of acute viral hepatitis vary by mode of transmission, manner of onset, and incubation periods (see the accompanying Key Features of Disease). The causative agent of *hepatitis A,* formerly known as *infectious* hepatitis, is probably a ribonucleic acid (RNA) virus of the enterovirus family. Hepatitis A is characterized by a mild course and often goes unrecognized. It is spread by the fecal-oral route by the oral ingestion of fecal contaminants. Sources of infection include contaminated water, shellfish caught in contaminated water, and food contaminated by food handlers infected with HAV. The virus may also be

KEY FEATURES OF DISEASE ■ **Differential Features of the Four Types of Viral Hepatitis** *Continued*

Feature	Hepatitis A	Hepatitis B	Hepatitis C (Non-A, Non-B Hepatitis)	Delta Hepatitis
	Elevated serum AST and ALT levels (early), hyperbili-rubinemia, abnormal liver function test results			
Virus in feces	2 wk before jaundice	Possible (suspected)	Not identified	Not identified
Virus in serum	During acute phase and incubation period	HBsAg is in serum throughout clinical course	Not identified	Present during entire phase of hepatitis B
Nosocomial problem	No	Yes	Yes	Yes
Mortality	Less frequent	More frequent	Unknown	Increased
Incidence of chronic active hepatitis as a complication	Low	Somewhat higher	Unknown	Yes
Associated with posttransfusion hepatitis	No	Rarely (causes 5%–8% of cases)	Yes (causes 90%–95% of cases)	No
Immune globulin (prophylaxis)	IG	HBIG or IG		*None* — only hepatitis B vaccine
Serologic test (specific antigen)	HA Ag	HBsAg, HB Ag	Not identified	HD Ag
Vaccine	No	Made from serum containing HBsAg	No	No
Antibody	Anti-HAV	Anti-HB$_3$m, anti-HBc, anti-HBe		Anti-HD

spread by oral-anal sexual activity and rarely by fecal shedding exposure in the hospital. In some cases, hepatitis A may be transmitted in the blood. The incubation period of hepatitis A is usually between 2 and 6 weeks, with an average of 4 weeks.

Hepatitis B was formerly known as *serum* hepatitis. HBV is a double-shelled particle containing deoxyribonucleic acid (DNA) composed of a core antigen (HBcAg), a surface antigen (HBsAg), and an independent protein (HBeAg) that circulates in the blood.

The primary mode of transmission of HBV is via the percutaneous route by contamination with blood and blood products. It may also spread via the mucous membranes by contact with infected body fluid, such as semen, saliva, or blood; direct contamination of an open wound; or handling of infected equipment and items. For these reasons, hepatitis B poses a major concern for health care professionals. Examples of situations in which transmission occurs include needle sticks (intentional or accidental); blood transfusion contamination of wounds, minor cuts, or abrasions; contamination of the mouth or the eye during wound irrigation or suc-

tioning; and oral surgery or dental procedures. Hepatitis B is also spread sexually and is especially prevalent in male homosexuals. The virus may also be spread by infected tattooing and ear-piercing equipment; contaminated, shared drug paraphernalia; kissing; and sharing such items as cups, toothbrushes, and cigarettes.

The clinical course of hepatitis B may be varied. It may have an insidious onset with mild signs and symptom or serious sequelae, such as fulminant hepatitis, chronic active or persistent hepatitis, cirrhosis, or hepatocellular carcinoma. The incubation period is generally between 40 and 180 days, but hepatitis B commonly develops 60 to 90 days after exposure.

The causative virus of *hepatitis C* is similar to HBV. It is transmitted through blood and blood products and has been identified in male homosexuals, being spread during sexual contact. Symptoms develop 40 to 100 days after exposure to the virus.

Delta hepatitis is caused by infection with HDV, a defective RNA virus that requires the helper function of HBV. HDV coinfects with HBV and requires its presence for viral replication. Delta agent can infect a client simultaneously with HBV or can superimpose infection on a client already infected with HBV. Superinfection may coexist with chronic hepatitis B and may develop into a chronic carrier state.

The duration of HDV infection is determined by the duration of the HBV infection. The HDV infection does not last longer than the HBV infection. However, chronic HDV infection appears to accelerate the progress of liver disease, causing additional damage to a liver that has already been compromised by chronic HBV infection.

The disease is primarily transmitted by nonpercutaneous routes, particularly close personal contact. In the United States and northern Europe, delta infection is most prevalent in persons exposed to blood and blood products (e.g., drug addicts and hemophiliacs).

Delta hepatitis can be introduced into a population through migration of people from endemic to nonendemic regions. Epidemics of severe hepatitis have occurred in remote South African villages as well as urban America owing to population migration and percutaneous contact.

Toxic and drug-induced (chemical) hepatitis. Two major types of toxic hepatitis have been recognized. *Direct toxic hepatitis* results in necrosis and fatty infiltration of the liver. Agents causing toxic hepatitis are generally systemic poisons or are converted in the liver to toxic metabolites. Persons with repeated, regular exposure to the offending agent or with a dose-related toxicity range develop direct toxic hepatitis.

For example, acetaminophen (Tylenol), a commonly used OTC analgesic, can cause severe hepatic necrosis when taken in large amounts in suicide attempts or accidental ingestion by children. Industrial toxins, such as carbon tetrachloride, trichloroethylene, and yellow phosphorus, have a direct toxic effect on the liver.

Idiosyncratic toxic hepatitis results in morphologic changes to the liver that are similar to those found in viral hepatitis. In idiosyncratic drug reactions, the occurrence of hepatitis is unpredictable and infrequent. It may occur at any time during or shortly after the exposure to the drug. Agents that result in idiosyncratic toxic hepatitis include halothane, an anesthetic agent; methyldopa (Aldomet), an antihypertensive drug; isoniazid (INH), an antituberculosis agent; and phenytoin (Dilantin), an anticonvulsant.

Treatment for toxic and drug-induced hepatitis is supportive, and withdrawal of the suspected agent is indicated at the first sign of a reaction. Chemical exposure of the liver to drugs and toxins has been responsible for the development of chronic active hepatitis and cirrhosis.

Etiology

Causes of hepatitis include viral infections; drugs, chemicals, and toxins; blood transfusion reactions from exposure to the hepatitis virus; hyperthyroidism; and

ingestion of ethyl alcohol, resulting in alcoholic hepatitis. Viral inflammation of the liver is the most common form of hepatitis. Hepatitis A is caused by HAV, and hepatitis B is due to infection with HBV. The viral agent responsible for hepatitis C has not yet been identified. The fourth type of viral hepatitis, delta hepatitis, occurs only in the presence of hepatitis B virus and is caused by HDV.

Routine screening of blood donors and the elimination of commercial blood sources have markedly decreased the incidence of hepatitis B after blood transfusion. However, the risk of viral hepatitis after a transfusion still remains a significant problem and is dependent on the method by which blood products are processed. Multiple pooled donor products carry the greatest risk.

Hepatitis B accounts for 5% to 10% of posttransfusion hepatitis; hepatitis C accounts for 90% of the posttransfusion hepatitis cases (Braunwald, 1987). At this time, there is not an acceptable serologic screening test to identify hepatitis C.

Incidence

Hepatitis A is the most common type of viral hepatitis, having recently regained the lead over hepatitis B (Altman, 1989). Its increased incidence is due to an epidemic among IV drug users. Poor hygiene is thought to be the most important cause of its transmission in this group.

Hepatitis B occurs primarily in young adults in the United States, with 75% of cases occurring between the ages of 15 and 39 years. The incidence of this infection has increased during the 1980s: approximately 300,000 new cases of hepatitis B occur in the United States each year; 59% of all cases occur in IV drug users, heterosexuals with multiple partners, and homosexual men; 3% of all cases are in health care workers (Altman, 1989).

Hepatitis C accounts for approximately 20% of all cases of viral hepatitis reported to the Centers for Disease Control (CDC) and is the most common cause of posttransfusion hepatitis (Keith, 1985).

Infection with the *delta agent* has a worldwide distribution; however, in the Mediterranean countries of northern Africa, southern Europe, and the Middle East, delta infection is endemic among people with hepatitis B. In southern Italy, approximately 90% of persons with acute HBsAg disease are infected with HDV (Schindler & Eastwood, 1987).

PREVENTION

Hepatitis A virus is almost always responsible for epidemics of viral hepatitis. To prevent spread of this virus in the community, increased sanitation and personal hygiene efforts in areas of high population density must be instituted. Improvements in water purification and sewage treatment systems must be made.

Prompt reporting of cases of hepatitis A to local

health departments is important. Officials must identify the infective source and infected persons so that spread of the virus can be controlled. This is especially important for food handlers and people involved in health and child care. Household spreading of the virus is common. Adequate sanitary practices at home are important—hand washing after toileting must be emphasized, and sharing of bed linens, towels, eating utensils, and glasses must be avoided.

In the hospital setting, clients admitted to the hospital with a diagnosis of hepatitis A are not a major source of hospital-acquired infections. By the time clients exhibit the symptoms of hepatitis and are identified, the chance of disease transmission is decreased. Hepatitis A is highly contagious during its 2- to 6-week incubation period and in the early stages of the disease when symptoms may be mild or nonexistent.

For hospitalized clients with hepatitis A who are fecally continent, it is not necessary to provide private rooms with bathrooms or to institute isolation precautions unless personal hygiene is poor. Use of gloves to handle fecally contaminated bedpans or bed linens is recommended. Frequent hand washing is essential for the client, the nurse, and other health care professionals.

Immune globulin (IG), formerly known as gamma globulin, is recommended as pre-exposure prophylaxis for people traveling to foreign countries with a high rate of hepatitis A or poor sanitation practices. For postexposure prophylaxis, IG is most effective when given within 2 weeks of exposure to the hepatitis A virus and can prevent hepatitis A if taken within the first 48 hours after exposure.

In the general population, *hepatitis B* is not readily transmitted. In the hospital setting, it is a major source of nosocomial infection. Health care professionals who have increased exposure to blood and blood products have up to a 30% risk of contracting HBV infection. Hospital environments are especially conducive to the transmission of HBV. Many potential situations expose nurses to the HBV, such as accidental needle punctures with contaminated needles; blood absorption into small cuts or abrasions on the hands; spraying of blood or infective secretions into the mouth or eyes; and contact during dressing changes, suctioning, or special procedures.

Universal precautions, which involve the use of barriers (e.g., gloves, goggles, and gowns) when in contact with blood, body fluids contaminated with visible blood, or select body fluids (cerebrospinal, synovial, pleural, peritoneal, and amniotic fluid) should be consistently used for all clients, regardless of the diagnosis. Universal precautions do not apply to feces, nasal secretions, sputum, sweat, tears, urine, or vomitus unless they contain visible blood. The risk of HBV transmission via these body fluids is extremely low or nonexistent. Therefore, as long as universal precautions are being adhered to, additional precautions for HBV are not necessary.

In addition to using barrier precautions, the nurse consistently makes an effort to prevent exposure to HBV

by *not* recapping, breaking, or bending used needles and by disposing of syringes and needles in puncture-resistant containers, which are located close to the area where they are used. Skin surfaces that are contaminated with blood or other fluids to which universal precautions apply should be washed immediately and thoroughly after the exposure.

Vaccinations to prevent hepatitis B infection are available for high-risk groups. Despite the availability of vaccines, most individuals at high risk have not been vaccinated. Individuals who should be vaccinated include users of illicit injectable drugs, sexually active homosexual males with multiple sexual partners, health care personnel who have frequent contact with blood, clients and staff in institutions for the mentally retarded, household and sexual contacts of HBV carriers, and clients who receive hemodialysis or frequent blood transfusions.

The hepatitis B vaccine (Hepatavax-B, Recombivax HB) is given in a series of three injections, with the second and third doses being given 1 and 6 months after the initial dose. The injections are relatively expensive, which probably accounts for failure of some individuals to be vaccinated. However, studies have also shown that health care providers do not know who should be vaccinated. Federal officials are considering broadening vaccination recommendations to include more of those at risk for hepatitis B.

Postexposure prophylaxis for hepatitis B is provided by hepatitis B immune globulin (HBIG) when there is percutaneous or mucous membrane exposure to HBsAg-positive blood. This is the prophylaxis of choice, although IG may also be given, because it contains antibodies against both hepatitis A and B, but in lesser concentrations than HBIG. IG is an acceptable alternative when HBIG is not available.

Because the exact viral agents for *hepatitis C* have not been identified, there are no established preventive measures or vaccination recommendations.

No product is available for prophylaxis to prevent *delta hepatitis* superinfection in hepatitis B. Infection with HDV can be prevented by vaccinating susceptible clients with the hepatitis B vaccine.

Case reporting to local health authorities for all types of *viral* hepatitis is mandatory.

COLLABORATIVE MANAGEMENT

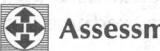 **Assessment**

History

When obtaining a history from the client with suspected viral hepatitis, the nurse asks the client if he/she has had *known exposure* to a person with HAV or HBV. The nurse determines if the client has had recent *blood transfusions* or undergoes *hemodialysis* for renal failure. The client is questioned about *social activities*, including sexual preference (bisexual or homosexual), IV drug use, recent ear piercing or tattooing, and living accommodations, such as crowded military barracks, correctional institutions, overcrowded apartments, or centers for mentally retarded persons.

The client's *employment history* is obtained. The nurse specifically questions the client about hospital employment, such as laboratory technicians; nurses in high-risk areas, such as operating rooms, emergency rooms, critical care units, or hemodialysis and pheresis units; or employees in a center for the mentally retarded.

The nurse asks the client about recent *travel* to a foreign country or an area with poor sanitation or water facilities. The client is questioned regarding ingestion of water from a possibly contaminated source or recent ingestion of shellfish, such as oysters.

Physical Assessment: Clinical Manifestations

The course and presentation of clinical manifestations for all four types of *viral* hepatitis are similar (see Key Features of Disease: Differential Features of the Four Types of Viral Hepatitis). The nurse assesses the client's general subjective complaints, determining if symptoms have occurred acutely (hepatitis A) or insidiously (hepatitis B and hepatitis C).

The client may verbalize feelings of *fatigue* and *loss of appetite*. The nurse explores further to assess if the client is experiencing *general malaise, weakness, myalgias* (muscle pain), arthritis-like *joint pain, dull headaches, irritability, depression, nausea,* and *vomiting*. The nurse asks the client if loss of appetite occurs late in the day, if greasy foods are tolerated, or if strong odors are offensive. Smokers may verbalize distaste for cigarettes.

The nurse palpates the right upper abdominal quadrant to assess for *liver tenderness* and *firmness*. The client may complain of *liver pain* with jarring movements. The skin, the sclerae, and mucous membranes are inspected for the presence of *jaundice*. The client may present for medical treatment only after jaundice appears, believing that other vague symptoms are related to an influenza-like syndrome.

Jaundice in hepatitis results from intrahepatic obstruction and is caused by edema of the liver's bile channels. *Dark urine* and *clay-colored stools* are often reported by the client as well. The nurse requests a urine and stool specimen for visual inspection and laboratory analysis. The nurse also inspects the skin for the presence of *rashes* in clients with suspected hepatitis B and hepatitis C. Irregular patches of erythema, redness, or pruritic urticarial hives may occur.

The client with hepatitis A may exhibit *fever*; temperature may range from 100° to 104° F (38° to 40° C). Fever may be low grade or absent with hepatitis B and hepatitis C.

The clinical picture in *toxic and drug-induced* hepatitis depends on the causative agent. Idiosyncratic reactions may result in clinical manifestations that are indistinguishable from those of viral hepatitis or may simulate extrahepatic bile duct obstruction symptoms, such as severe jaundice, rash, arthralgias, and fever.

Psychosocial Assessment

Viral hepatitis usually occurs as an acute illness, and its symptoms are often mild and abate rapidly or go undetected. The clinical manifestations of hepatitis B can persist for up to 6 months. Emotional problems for affected clients often center on their feelings of anger about being sick and feelings of being tired of experiencing fatigue. General malaise, inactivity, and vague complaints contribute to depression and despondency. These clients worry about long-term effects and complications.

Clients with viral hepatitis often feel guilty that they have exposed others to the virus. Infectious diseases such as hepatitis continue to have a social stigma attached to them. The client may feel embarrassed by the isolation and hygiene precautions that are imposed on clients in the hospital and that continue to be required at home. This embarrassment may cause the client to restrict social interactions. Self-imposed visitor restrictions may be instituted by the client for fear of spreading the virus to family and friends.

Family members sometimes experience fear of contracting the disease and may be standoffish to the client. The nurse allows the client and the family to verbalize these feelings and explores the reasons for these fears. Precautionary isolation measures evoke anxiety for the client and the family.

If transmission of hepatitis B is caused by generally unacceptable social behavior, such as illicit IV drug use or homosexual activity, the client may feel guilty and ashamed. Clients are unable to return to work until the results of blood tests for serologic markers are negative. The loss of wages and the cost of hospitalization for a client without insurance coverage may produce great anxiety and financial burden for the client and the family.

Laboratory Findings

The presence of hepatitis A and B is indicated by acute elevations in levels of liver enzymes, indicating liver cellular damage, and by specific serologic markers. Levels of ALT may be elevated to more than 1000 mU/mL and may rise to as high as 4000 mU/mL in severe cases of viral hepatitis. The AST levels may rise to 1000 to 2000 mU/mL. Alkaline phosphatase levels may be normal (30 to 90 IU/L) or mildly elevated. Serum total bilirubin levels are elevated to greater than 2.5 mg/dL and are consistent with the clinical appearance of jaundice. Elevated levels of bilirubin are also present in the urine.

The presence of HAV is established when HAV antibodies (anti-HAV) are identified in the serum. Ongoing inflammation of the liver by HAV is evidenced by the presence of immunoglobulin M (IgM) antibodies, which persist in the blood for 4 to 6 weeks. Previous infection is indicated by the presence of immunoglobulin G (IgG) antibodies. These antibodies persist in the serum and provide permanent immunity to HAV.

The presence of HBV is established if serologic testing confirms the presence of hepatitis B antigen-antibody systems in the blood. HBV is a double-shelled DNA virus consisting of an inner core and an outer shell. Antigens located on the surface or shell of the virus (HBsAg) are the most significant serologic marker, and their presence establishes the diagnosis of hepatitis B. As long as HBsAg is present in the blood, the client is considered to be infectious. Persistence of this serologic marker after 6 months or longer indicates a carrier state or chronic hepatitis. Normally, the HBsAg levels decline and disappear after the acute hepatitis B episode. The presence of antibodies to HBsAg (anti-HBs) in the blood indicates recovery and immunity to hepatitis B.

Hepatitis B early antigen (HBeAg) is detected in the serum about 1 week after the appearance of HBsAg. Its presence determines the infective state of the client. Clients who are positive for both HBsAg and HBeAg are more contagious than those who are HBsAg positive and HBeAg negative.

The presence of HDV can be confirmed by the identification of intrahepatic delta antigen or, more often, a rise in the anti-HD titer. Circulating hepatitis D antigen (HD Ag) is diagnostic of acute disease, but is detected only briefly in the serum.

Other Diagnostic Tests

Chronic hepatitis is diagnosed by percutaneous liver biopsy. The biopsy distinguishes between chronic active and chronic persistent hepatitis.

The finding of fatty infiltrates in liver biopsy specimens and inflammation with neutrophils is consistent with alcohol-induced hepatitis.

 Analysis: Nursing Diagnosis

The client with viral hepatitis can be mildly or acutely ill, depending on the severity of the inflammation. Except for hepatitis C, there is no specific treatment for viral hepatitis. Hepatitis C has recently been treated with interferon-alpha with success. The plan of care for all clients with viral hepatitis is based on measures to rest the liver, promote cellular regeneration, and prevent complications.

Common Diagnoses

Common nursing diagnoses have been established for planning client care.

1. Activity intolerance related to general malaise secondary to inflammatory process
2. Potential for infection related to transmission of viral hepatitis to others
3. Altered nutrition: less than body requirements related to anorexia, nausea, and vomiting

Additional Diagnoses

The client with viral hepatitis may also exhibit the following nursing diagnoses:

1. Anxiety related to hospitalization and illness
2. Pain related to inflammation of the liver
3. Diversional activity deficit related to social isolation
4. Knowledge deficit related to disease process and transmission
5. Potential impaired skin integrity related to jaundice and pruritus
6. Social isolation related to risk of transmission of infection

 Planning and Implementation

The plan of care is based on the common nursing diagnoses.

Activity Intolerance

Planning: client goals. The primary goal is that the client will gradually increase activity to the level of activity experienced before illness.

Interventions: nonsurgical management. During the acute stage of viral hepatitis, interventions are aimed at resting the inflamed liver to promote liver cell regeneration. Rest is an essential intervention to reduce the liver's metabolic demands and increase its blood supply. Treatment is generally supportive.

Physical rest. The nurse assesses the client's response to activity and rest periods. Strict bed rest may be indicated during the early icteric phase of hepatitis. The client is usually tired and expresses feelings of general malaise. Most often, complete bed rest is not required, but rest periods alternating with periods of activity are indicated and are frequently sufficient to promote hepatic healing.

The client's plan of care is individualized by the nurse and changes to reflect the severity of symptoms, fatigue, and results of liver function tests and enzyme determinations. Scheduled rest periods should be adhered to by the client and the nursing staff. Activities such as providing self-care, getting out of bed, and ambulating are gradually added to the activity schedule as tolerated.

Psychologic rest. Emotional and psychologic rest is essential for the client. Because bed rest and inactivity can be anxiety producing, the nurse includes diversional activities in the plan of care. If the client is interested, the nurse asks the client's family to bring in small craft projects; reading materials, such as magazines, books, and newspapers; or a portable radio. The hospital may provide television services or telephone access from each room. The nurse also encourages staff and family members to spend time in the client's room.

Potential for Infection

Planning: client goals. The goal is that the client will participate in the prevention of transmission of hepatitis by adhering to infection control measures.

Interventions: nonsurgical management. During the acute phase of hepatitis, the client, hospital staff, and family members must be acutely aware of disease transmission prevention. Interventions include strict adherence to blood and body fluid precautions (universal precautions). Use of gloves is recommended when there is a possibility of contact with feces of a client with hepatitis A (see the earlier discussion of prevention and Chap. 26).

Altered Nutrition: Less Than Body Requirements

Planning: client goals. The primary goal is that the client will have optimal intake of nutrients and calories to promote liver tissue healing.

Interventions: nonsurgical management. Supportive nutritional therapy is aimed at promoting hepatic cellular regeneration by providing a well-balanced diet. This is not always possible because of nausea and vomiting, anorexia, and general distaste for food. Treatment measures to increase nutritional intake are accomplished by diet therapy, drugs to control nausea, and general comfort measures.

Diet therapy. A special diet is usually not required. A diet high in carbohydrates and calories with moderate amounts of fat and protein may be recommended by the dietitian. Small, frequent meals are preferable to three standard meals with larger portions. The nurse determines the client's food preferences because those foods are tolerated better than randomly selected foods. The nurse encourages the client to prepare the dietary menu, selecting foods that are appealing. The dietitian is consulted to see if high-calorie snacks, such as milkshakes, are available.

Supplemental vitamins are given. If caloric intake is extremely poor, the nurse may be required to provide supplemental commercial feedings. If the client is unable to tolerate these orally, a feeding tube may be inserted for tube feedings.

The nurse can ask the client's family to prepare favorite foods from home and bring them to the hospital. Fried, fatty foods should be avoided. The family should be encouraged to prepare meals high in carbohydrates and proteins.

Drug therapy. Supportive treatment to relieve nausea may be accomplished by administering antiemetics, such as trimethobenzamide hydrochloride (Tigan) or dimenhydrinate (Dramamine). Prochlorperazine maleate (Compazine), a phenothiazine, is avoided because of its potential hepatotoxic effects.

Comfort measures. Some foods and smells may stimulate nausea. The nurse removes the source causing the nausea, if possible. In an effort to stimulate appetite, the nurse provides mouth care before meals. The meal may be more palatable when served outside the sleeping area, with the client sitting up in a chair at a table. This is often difficult to accomplish in the hospital, but should be encouraged at home. The nurse empties bedpans, urinals, and bedside commodes promptly and provides an air freshener for the room if tolerated by the client.

■ Discharge Planning

The client with viral hepatitis is discharged to home after hospitalization and is encouraged to continue the plan of care initiated in the hospital.

Home Care Preparation

If at all possible, the client should not share bathroom facilities at home unless he/she strictly adheres to personal hygiene measures. Individual washcloths, towels, and drinking and eating utensils, as well as toothbrushes and razors, must be clearly labeled and identified. The client must not prepare food for other family members.

Client/Family Education

The client and the family must be instructed to observe measures to prevent infection transmission (see earlier). Additionally, the nurse instructs the client with viral hepatitis to avoid alcohol and any nonprescription, OTC medications, particularly aspirin and sedatives, as these are hepatotoxic.

The client must determine patterns for rest based on physical tolerance of increased activity. The nurse encourages the client *not* to increase activity too strenuously to prevent fatigue. The client is encouraged by the nurse to eat small, frequent feedings of high-carbohydrate and low-fat foods. The dietitian is consulted to provide diet teaching and menu planning.

Clients are encouraged to follow precautionary measures and avoid sexual activity until it is determined that HBsAg testing results are negative.

Psychosocial Preparation

The client needs to increase social activities after being discharged to home, but may feel socially isolated because of the imposed isolation precautions in the hospital. The nurse provides psychologic reinforcement, as well as informative teaching, that the client can have normal contact with people as long as proper personal hygiene is maintained. Close personal contact, such as hugging and kissing, should be discouraged until HBsAg test results are negative.

Health Care Resources

Clients with viral hepatitis and their families may contact the local health department for information on infection control. Clients discharged to home with limited activity tolerance may need the assistance of a home care aide in performing ADL, particularly meals.

 Evaluation

On the basis of the nursing diagnoses and supportive health care interventions, the nurse evaluates the care of the client with viral hepatitis. Expected outcomes for the client with hepatitis A, hepatitis B, or hepatitis C include that the client

1. Adheres to physical and activity limitations
2. States which precautionary isolation measures are required and follows these measures
3. Complies with increased nutritional intake and has the return of full appetite
4. Seeks medical care for routine follow-up and laboratory analysis of serologic markers

By achieving the desired outcomes, the client with viral hepatitis usually exhibits full recovery from this viral insult.

FATTY LIVER

A *fatty liver* is caused by the accumulation of triglycerides and other fats in the hepatic cells. In severe cases, fat may constitute as much as 40% of the liver's weight and cause changes in liver function. Minimal, temporary fatty changes are usually reversible by eliminating the cause. The most common cause of fatty liver is chronic alcoholism. Other causes include malnutrition, diabetes mellitus, obesity, pregnancy, prolonged IV hyperalimentation, and exposure to large doses of drugs toxic to the liver. Fatty infiltration of the liver is believed to be the result of faulty fat metabolism in the liver and mobilization of fatty acids from adipose tissue.

Many clients with a fatty liver are asymptomatic. The most common, typical finding is hepatomegaly. Other symptoms include right upper abdominal pain, ascites, edema, jaundice, fever, and later signs of cirrhosis, depending on the severity of the fat infiltration and the longevity of the occurrence.

A liver biopsy confirms excess fat in the liver. Interventions are aimed at removing the underlying cause of the infiltration and dietary restrictions.

ABSCESSES

Hepatic abscesses are uncommon, but when a hepatic abscess does occur it carries a high mortality. The mortality may be as high as 60% for multiple abscesses (Knauer & Silverman, 1988).

Liver abscesses occur when the liver is invaded by bacteria or protozoa. These organisms destroy the liver tissue, producing a necrotic cavity filled with infective agents, liquefied liver cells and tissue, and leukocytes. The infectious necrotic tissue walls off the abscess from the healthy liver.

A *pyrogenic liver abscess* occurs when bacteria invade the liver. Infecting organisms include *E. coli, Klebsiella, Enterobacter, Salmonella, Staphylococcus,* and *Enterococcus.* Pyrogenic abscesses are generally multiple. The usual cause is acute cholangitis occurring as a complication of cholelithiasis. Pyrogenic liver abscesses may also result from liver trauma, abdominal peritonitis, and sepsis, or an abscess can extend to the liver after pneumonia or bacterial endocarditis.

The protozoan *Entamoeba histolytica* causes an *amebic hepatic abscess,* which may occur after amebic dysentery. These abscesses usually occur as a single abscess in the right hepatic lobe.

Clients with hepatic abscesses are generally quite ill. On occasion, an abscess is not diagnosed until autopsy. Clients with a pyrogenic liver abscess usually have a sudden onset of symptoms. Amebic abscesses generally cause a more insidious onset of symptoms. Common complaints include right upper abdominal pain with a palpable, tender liver; anorexia; weight loss; nausea and vomiting; fever and chills; shoulder pain; dyspnea; and pleural pain if the diaphragm is involved.

A hepatic abscess is usually diagnosed by liver scan. Hepatic arteriography differentiates an abscess from a malignancy. Blood cultures assist in identifying the causative organism in pyrogenic abscesses, and stool cultures may identify *E. histolytica.* With ultrasound guidance, a liver abscess may be aspirated percutaneously. Surgical drainage is indicated only for a single pyrogenic abscess or for an amebic abscess that fails to respond to long-term antibiotic treatment.

TRAUMA

The liver is the most common organ to be injured in clients with penetrating abdominal trauma of the abdomen (such as gunshot wounds, stab wounds, or rib fractures) and the second most commonly injured organ after blunt abdominal trauma. Damage or injury to the liver should be suspected whenever any upper abdominal or lower chest trauma is sustained. The liver is frequently injured by steering wheels in vehicular accidents. Common injuries to the liver include simple lacerations, multiple lacerations, avulsions, and crush injuries.

The liver is a highly vascular organ, receiving approximately 29% of the body's cardiac output. When hepatic trauma occurs, blood loss can be massive. The client may exhibit signs of hemorrhagic shock, such as hypotension; tachycardia; tachypnea; pallor; diaphoresis; cool, clammy skin; and confusion. A decreased hematocrit may confirm suspected blood loss. Clinical manifestations include right upper quadrant pain with abdominal tenderness, distention, guarding, and rigidity. Abdominal pain exaggerated by deep breathing and referred to the left shoulder (Kehr's sign) may indicate diaphragmatic irritation.

When hepatic and other abdominal organ trauma is suspected, an emergency peritoneal lavage is performed to confirm injury. If trauma is present, the lavage reveals gross blood or a high red blood cell count.

An exploratory laparotomy is done to identify and control the source and type of bleeding. Often, minor surgical interventions, such as suture placement, wound packing, decompression, or a combination of these procedures, are performed to halt bleeding. In some extensive hepatic injuries, hepatic lobe resection is required.

These clients require administration of multiple blood products, packed red blood cells, and fresh frozen plasma, as well as massive volume infusion to maintain adequate hydration. Postoperatively, the client with hepatic trauma is admitted to a critical care unit. The nurse monitors the client for persistent bleeding. CBC and coagulation studies must be closely monitored for trends in changes.

CANCER

Carcinoma of the liver usually develops as a metastatic process. Owing to the increased vascularity of the liver, the organ is a common site for metastasis from primary cancers of the esophagus, the stomach, the colon, the rectum, breasts, and lungs or from a malignant melanoma.

Primary hepatic carcinoma (cancer originating within the liver) is rare in the United States, with an annual incidence of fewer than 4 cases per 100,000 (Rustgi, 1988). However, in other parts of the world, such as Africa, it is one of the most common malignancies. The geographic variation probably reflects the prevalence of chronic hepatitis B infection in other countries. HBV is thought to be the primary carcinogen in as many as 80% of clients with primary hepatic cancer worldwide (Beasley & Hwang, 1984). Between 30% and 70% of clients with primary hepatic cancer also have cirrhosis, and the risk of hepatic cancer is 40 times greater in clients who have cirrhosis (Oberfield et al., 1989).

Primary hepatic cancer has also been associated with viral hepatitis, trauma, nutritional deficiencies, and exposure to carcinogens and hepatotoxins, such as aflatoxin, thorium dioxide, *Senecio* alkaloids, and the fungus *Aspergillus.*

The most common form of primary hepatic cancer is *hepatoma.* Signs and symptoms of hepatoma include jaundice, ascites, bleeding, and encephalopathy.

Clients with hepatic metastasis usually have elevated serum alkaline phosphatase levels. A nuclear radioisotope liver scan detects metastasis in many cases; however, ultrasonography with needle biopsy may be required to confirm the metastasis.

Surgical management is indicated for clients with a single metastatic lesion confined to one liver lobe. Hepatic lobe resection for surgical excision of metastasis has been successful for up to a 5-year survival rate.

Other treatments include high-dose chemotherapy to the liver and hepatic artery ligation to deprive the metastatic lesion of oxygen. Both of these treatments can be accomplished without systemic effect because of the unique portal vein circulation in the liver.

Hepatic chemotherapy employs a surgically implanted infusion pump, which enables controlled infusion for up to 14 days at a time.

TRANSPLANTATION

The client with end-stage liver disease that has not responded to conventional medical or surgical intervention is a potential candidate for liver transplantation. In the adult, diseases treated by liver transplant include end-stage cirrhosis from chronic active hepatitis or primary biliary cirrhosis; hepatic metabolic diseases, such as protoporphyria and Wilson's disease; Budd-Chiari syndrome (hepatic vein obstruction impairing blood flow out of the liver); and sclerosing cholangitis. Liver transplant is not performed for clients with malignant neoplasms, primarily because of tumor recurrence in immunosuppressed clients.

The potential transplant client undergoes extensive physiologic and psychologic assessment and evaluation by physicians and nurses to identify contraindications to the procedure. The client with severe end-stage disease with life-threatening complications, such as hepatorenal syndrome, repeated episodes of esophageal variceal bleeding, sepsis, severe cardiovascular instability with advanced cardiac disease, hypertension, diabetes mellitus, and severe hypoxemia, is not considered a candidate for transplant by the surgeon. Additional identified risk factors include portal vein thrombosis, advanced catabolic state, active alcoholism, age older than 55 years, primary and metastatic malignant disease, lack of knowledge and understanding of the procedure and required postoperative care measures, poor psychosocial support system, and psychologic instability.

After the client is identified as a candidate and a donor organ is procured, the actual liver transplant surgical procedure can take between 8 and 16 hours and up to 22 hours to complete. The procedure involves five anastomoses between recipient and donor organs, including the following vascular anastomosis sites: suprahepatic inferior vena cava, infrahepatic vena cava, portal vein, hepatic artery, and biliary tract. The biliary anastomosis site varies, depending on the client's extrahepatic biliary tract. Two common sites are end-to-end anastomosis between donor and recipient common bile duct and anastomosis between the donor common bile duct and the recipient jejunum.

The success of all transplants has greatly improved since the discovery of cyclosporine (cyclosporin A), an immunosuppressant drug. This drug is widely accepted as the primary agent to prevent rejection of the donor organ.

The rejection response after liver transplant most often occurs between the fourth and tenth postoperative days. Clinical manifestations of acute rejection include tachycardia, fever, right upper quadrant or flank pain, diminished bile flow through the T tube or change in bile color, and increasing jaundice. Laboratory findings include elevated serum bilirubin, transaminases, and alkaline phosphatase levels and increased prothrombin time.

If the rejection is not controlled by steroid administration, a rapid deterioration of liver function occurs. Multisystem organ failure, including respiratory and renal involvement, develops, along with diffuse coagulopathies and PSE. The only alternative for treatment is emergent transplantation.

Infection is another potential threat. Immunosuppressant therapy, which must be utilized to prevent and treat organ rejection, significantly increases the client's susceptibility to and risk of infection. Potential problems include respiratory infection, biliary tract inflammation, and sepsis from indwelling IV or central venous and Foley's catheters. The biliary anastomosis is prone to breakdown, obstruction, and infection. If leakage occurs or the site becomes necrotic or obstructed, an abscess can form, or peritonitis, bacteremia, and cirrhosis may develop. Other potential complications include hemorrhage, fluid and electrolyte imbalances, pulmonary atelectasis, acute renal failure, hypothermia, and psychologic maladjustment.

In the immediate postoperative period, the client who has undergone liver transplant is managed in the critical care unit and requires aggressive monitoring and care (see Chap. 20).

The nurse monitors the client's temperature and reports temperature greater than 100° F (38° C) and increased abdominal pain, distention, and rigidity, which are indicators of peritonitis. Nursing assessment also includes monitoring for a change in neurologic status that could indicate encephalopathy from a nonfunctioning liver; signs of coagulopathy (e.g., continuous bloody oozing from a catheter, drain, and incision sites; petechiae; or ecchymosis) are reported to the physician immediately, as they may indicate impaired function of the transplanted liver.

SUMMARY

Disorders of the biliary system are diverse and complex. Because the liver is vital to most life processes, even mild disorders of the biliary system can cause life-threatening alterations. The nurse needs a good understanding of biliary anatomy and physiology to appreciate the effects of these disorders on clients.

Many biliary disorders are the consequence of life style. Nurses must consistently assess the life styles of all clients they interact with. Nurses also need to find opportunities to explain risks of detrimental life styles and their relationship to biliary disease in an effort to prevent biliary disorders.

IMPLICATIONS FOR RESEARCH

Research in hepatobiliary and pancreatic disease has focused primarily on organ transplantation. Data concerning clients who have received a liver or pancreas transplant need to be reviewed and analyzed, especially with regard to life span improvements and prevention of organ rejection. Methods of infection control during the immediate postoperative period when the client is in a critical care setting need to be evaluated.

Questions that are appropriate for nursing research include

1. Does education for alcoholic clients result in a reduction in the rate of cirrhosis or pancreatic disease progression?

2. How can the nurse intervene to minimize the social isolation experienced by the client with hepatitis?

3. How can quality of life be measured in the posttransplantation client?

4. What additional measures can be taken by the nurse to prevent contamination of others by clients with hepatitis?

REFERENCES AND READINGS

General

American Cancer Society. (1987). *Cancer facts and figures— 1987*. New York: Author.

Bullock, B. L., & Rosendahl, P. P. (1984). *Pathophysiology, adaptations and alterations in function*. Boston: Little, Brown.

Gitnick, G. (Ed.). (1983). *Gastroenterology*. New York: Wiley Medical.

Given, B. A., & Simmons, S. J. (1984). *Gastroenterology in clinical nursing*. St. Louis: C. V. Mosby.

Granger, D. N., Barrowman, J. A., & Kvietys, P. R. (1985). *Clinical gastrointestinal physiology*. Philadelphia: W. B. Saunders.

Johnson, L. R. (1985). *Gastrointestinal physiology*. St. Louis: C. V. Mosby.

Jones, P. F. (1985). *Gastroenterology*. Chicago: Year Book Medical.

Nord, H. J., & Brady, P. G. (1982). *Critical care gastroenterology*. New York: Churchill Livingstone.

Orr, M. E. (1981). *Acute pancreatic and hepatic dysfunction*. New York: Wiley Medical.

Sherlock, S. (1985). *Diseases of the liver and biliary system*. Oxford: Blackwell Scientific.

Silverberg, E., & Lubera, J. A. (1989). Cancer statistics, 1989. *Ca: A Cancer Journal for Clinicians, 39*, 3–20.

Strange, J. M. (1983). The riddle of abdominal trauma. *RN, 46*(3), 43–46, 98, 100.

Taylor, D. L. (1983). Gallstones: Physiology, signs and symptoms. *Nursing '83, 6*(13), 44–45.

Thomson, N. A. (1983). Abdominal trauma. *Nursing '83, 13*(7), 26–33.

Biliary Disorders

Holland, P., & Hussain, I. (1989). Biliary lithotripsy: Nonsurgical treatment of gallstones. *Society of Gastrointestinal Assistants Journal, 3*, 158–162.

Pancreatic Disorders

Brasitus, T. A. (1982). Spotting and treating serious complications of pancreatic disease. *Geriatrics, 37*(7), 51–54.

Jeffres, C. (1989). Complications of acute pancreatitis. *Critical Care Nurse, 4*(9), 38–46.

Soergel, K. H. (1983). Acute pancreatitis. In M. H. Sleisinger & J. S. Fordtran (Eds.), *Gastrointestinal disease* (3rd ed., Vol. II). Philadelphia: W. B. Saunders.

Hepatic Disorders

Altman, L. K. (1989, August 1). As hepatitis B spreads, physicians reconsider vaccination strategy. *The New York Times.*, p. C3.

Beasley, R. P., & Hwang, L. Y. (1984). Hepatocellular carcinoma and hepatitis B virus. *Seminars in Liver Disease, 4*, 113–121.

Braunwald, E., Isselbacher, K. J., Petersdorf, R. G., Wilson, J. Martin, J. B., & Fauci, A. S. (Eds.). (1987). *Harrison's principles of internal medicine* (11th ed., Vol. II). New York: McGraw-Hill.

Dodd, R. P. (1984). Ascites: When the liver can't cope. *RN, 47*(10), 26–30, 70.

Dusek, J. L. (1984). Iced gastric lavage slows bleeding in gastric hemorrhage. *Critical Care Nurse, 4*(4), 8.

Epskin, M. (1985). Renal complications of liver disease. *Clinical Symposia, 37*(5), 3–33.

Gever, L. N. (1982). Lactulose: A crucial element in treating hepatic encephalopathy. *Nursing '82, 12*(8), 76–78.

Grimson, A. E. S., Westaby, D., Hegarty, J., Watson, A., & Williams, R. (1986). A randomized trial of vasopressin and vasopressin plus nitroglycerin in the control of acute variceal hemorrhage. *Hepatology, 6*, 410–413.

Gruber, M., & Nuwer, N. (1982). Treating esophageal varices with injection sclerotherapy. *American Journal of Nursing, 12*, 1214–1216.

Gullatte, M. M., & Foltz, A. T. (1983). Hepatic chemotherapy via implantable pump. *American Journal of Nursing, 83*, 1674–1676.

Keith, J. S. (1985). Hepatic failure: Etiologies, manifestations and management. *Critical Care Nurse, 5*(1), 60–86.

King, D. E. (1983). How to give your portal hypertension patient a fighting chance. *RN, 46*(7), 31–37.

Klopp, A. (1984). Shunting malignant ascites. *American Journal of Nursing, 84*, 212–213.

Knauer, C. M., & Silverman, S. (1988). Alimentary tract & liver. In S. A. Schroeder, M. A. Krupp, & L. M. Tierney (Eds.), *Current medical diagnosis & treatment* (pp. 342–428). Norwalk, CT: Appleton & Lange.

Oberfield, R. A., Steele, G., Gollan, J. L., & Sherman, D. (1989). Liver cancer. *Ca: A Cancer Journal for Clinicians, 39*, 206–218.

Patton, F. (1981). Hepatitis: Current concepts. *Critical Care Nurse, 1*(3), 20–30.

Quinless, F. W. (1985). Severe liver dysfunction. *Focus on Critical Care, 12*(1), 24–32.

Ricci, J. A. (1987). Alcohol induced upper GI hemorrhage: Case studies and management. *Critical Care Nurse, 7*(1), 56–65.

Rustgi, V. K. (1988). Epidemiology of hepatocellular carcinoma. In A. M. Di Bisceglie (moderator), Hepatocellular carcinoma. *Annals of Internal Medicine, 108*, 390–401.

Schiff L., & Schiff, E. R. (1987). *Diseases of the liver* (6th ed.). Philadelphia: J. B. Lippincott.

Schindler, M. S., & Eastwood, G. L. (1987). Delta hepatitis: A deadly corollary to hepatitis B. *Journal of Critical Illness, 2*, 91–100.

Schumann, D. (1983). Correction of ascites with peritoneovenous shunting: A study of clinical management. *Heart and Lung, 12*, 248–255.

Smith, S. L. (1985). Liver transplantation: Implications for critical care nursing. *Heart and Lung, 14*, 617–627.

Thompson, M. A. (1981). Managing the patient with liver dysfunction. *Nursing '81, 11*(11), 101–107.

U.S. Centers for Disease Control. (1988). Update: Universal precautions for prevention of transmission of human immunodeficiency virus, hepatitis B virus, and other bloodborne pathogens in health-care settings. *Morbidity and Mortality Weekly Report, 37*(24), 377–382.

Vargo, J. (1984). Viral hepatitis: How to protect patients and yourself. *RN, 47*(7), 22–27.

Vargo, R. L., & Rudy, E. B. (1989). Infection as a complication of liver transplant. *Critical Care Nurse, 9*(4), 52–62.

Vyas, G. N., Dienstag, J. L., & Hoofnagle, J. H. (1984). *Viral hepatitis and liver diseases*. Orlando, FL: Grune & Stratton.

Wimpsett, J. (1984). Trace your patient's liver dysfunction. *Nursing '84, 14*(8), 56–57.

Wiser, H. R., & Cooke, A. R. (1986). A five step approach to upper GI bleeding. *Journal of Critical Illness, 1*, 61–70.

ADDITIONAL READINGS

Anderson, F. D. (1986). Portal-systemic encephalopathy in the chronic alcoholic. *Critical Care Quarterly, 8*(4), 40–50.

This article discussed PSE and its clinical manifestations, theories of causation, and implications for nursing care, including identifying precipitating factors, eliminating and removing ammonia, and providing supportive therapy and care for the chronic alcoholic client.

Bagg, A. (1988). Whipple's procedure: Nursing guidelines. *Critical Care Nurse, 8*(5), 34–45.

Whipple's procedure is an extensive surgical procedure that is the classic operation for pancreatic cancer. This article discussed the anatomy and physiology of the pancreas, the assessment findings and diagnostic work-up for clients with cancer of the pancreas, and the surgical treatment itself. Preoperative and postoperative nursing management of clients undergoing this surgery was discussed, as well as potential complications. A care plan for the client undergoing Whipple's procedure was included.

Fain, J. A., & Amato-Vealey, E. (1988). Acute pancreatitis: A gastrointestinal emergency. *Critical Care Nurse, 8*(6), 47–63.

This article discussed the pathophysiology of acute pancreatitis, along with clinical manifestations, diagnostic work-up, and medical and nursing interventions for this disorder. Clinical problems pertinent to pancreatitis were identified, along with nursing interventions and their rationales. Actual and potential nursing diagnoses were identified separately.

Jermier, B. J., & Treloar, D. M. (1986). Bringing your patient through gallbladder surgery. *RN, 49*(11), 18–25.

This article was based on a case study of a client with cholelithiasis. Information on gallbladder function, diagnostic work-up, surgical intervention, and postoperative care was provided. Nonsurgical treatment for chronic cholecystitis was discussed.

LaSala, C. (1985). Caring for the patient with a transhepatic biliary decompression catheter. *Nursing '85, 15*(2), 53–55.

UNIT 13 RESOURCES

Nursing Resources

American Society for Parenteral and Enteral Nutrition (ASPEN), 8605 Cameron Street, Suite 500, Silver Spring, MD 20910. Telephone 301-587-6315.
See Unit 10 Resources for more information.

Certifying Council for Gastroenterology Board of Nurses and Associates, c/o Professional Examination Service, 475 Riverside Drive, New York, NY 10115.
Certifies nurses with experience in gastroenterology.

Enterostomal Therapy Nursing Certification Board (ENTCB), 2081 Business Center Drive, Suite 290, Irvine, CA 92715. Telephone 714-476-0268.
Certifies nurses with experience in enterostomal therapy.

International Association for Enterstomal Therapy (IAET), 2081 Business Center Drive, Suite 290, Irvine, CA 92715. Telephone 714-476-0268.
Promotes the education of clients, nurses, physicians, and allied health professionals in the biopsychosocial and sexual rehabilitation of persons with stomas, draining wounds, fistulas, pressure ulcers, vascular ulcers, and incontinence. Publishes the *Journal of Enterostomal Therapy*, regional newsletters, and *The Cost-Benefits of ET Nursing in Modern Healthcare Delivery*.

National Board of Nutrition Support Certification (NBSC), 8605 Cameron Street, Suite 500, Silver Spring, MD 20910. Telephone 301-587-6315.
See Unit 10 Resources for more information.

Society of Gastrointestinal Assistants, 1070 Sibley Tower, Rochester, NY 14604. Telephone 716-546-7241.

This article summarized the insertion procedure, care measures, and indications of malfunction for the transhepatic biliary decompression catheter, an effective nonsurgical approach to decompressing obstructed bile ducts. Concise discharge planning information was provided.

Maloney, J. P. (1986). Surgical interventions in the alcoholic patient with portal hypertension. *Critical Care Quarterly, 8*(4), 63–73.

This article provided general information about portal hypertension and specific medical management and surgical decompression procedures. Nursing care and interventions in the postoperative period, including routine concerns and strategies to monitor, prevent, and manage major complications were discussed.

Miller, H. D. (1988). Liver transplantation: Postoperative ICU care. *Critical Care Nurse, 8*(6), 19–31.

This article presented information on the history of liver transplantation, along with explanation and illustrations of the surgical procedure. Postoperative nursing care of the client was discussed as it relates to each physiologic system. The nurse-author has also included a sample care plan for the immediate postoperative period.

Other Resources

Alcoholics Anonymous (AA), 468 Park Avenue South, New York, NY 10016. Telephone 212-686-1100.

American Anorexia/Bulimia Association, Inc. (AA/BA), 133 Cedar Lane, Teaneck, NJ 07666. Telephone 201-836-1800.

American Cancer Society, 1599 Clifton Road NE, Atlanta, GA 30329. Telephone 404-320-3333.

American Dental Association, Council on Dental Care Programs, 211 East Chicago Avenue, 17th Floor, Chicago, IL 60611. Telephone 312-440-2500.

American Liver Foundation, 30 Sunrise Terrace, Cedar Grove, NJ 07009. Telephone 201-857-2626.

Anorexia Nervosa and Related Eating Disorders, Inc. (ANRED), PO Box 1012, Grove City, CA 93433. Telephone 24-hour hot line 805-773-4303.

The Living Bank International, PO Box 6725, Houston, TX 77265. Telephone 800-528-2971.

The National Anorexic Aid Society, Inc. (NAAS), PO Box 29461, Columbus, OH 43229. Telephone 614-436-1112.

The National Association of Anorexia Nervosa and Associated Disorders, Inc. (ANAD), Suite 2020, 550 Frontage Road, Northfield, IL 60093. Telephone 312-831-3438.

National Digestive Diseases Education and Information Clearinghouse, 1255 23rd Street NW, No. 275, Washington, DC 20037. Telephone 202-296-9610.

National Foundation for Ileitis and Colitis, 444 Park Avenue South, New York, NY 10016. Telephone 212-685-3440.

National Institute of Arthritis, Diabetes, and Digestive and Kidney Diseases, National Institutes of Health, Bethesda, MD 20892. Telephone 301-496-4000.

United Ostomy Association, 2001 West Beverly Boulevard, Los Angeles, CA 90057. Telephone 213-255-4681.

UNIT 14

Problems of Regulation and Metabolism: Management of Clients with Disruptions of the Endocrine System

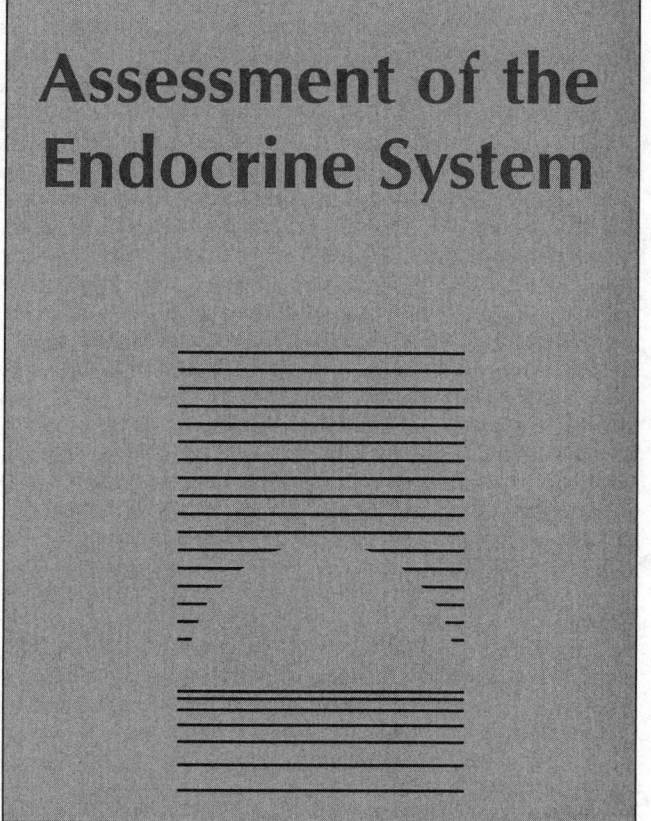

CHAPTER 48

Assessment of the Endocrine System

The endocrine system consists of the body's glands and their hormones (Table 48–1). The neuroregulatory mechanisms of the hypothalamus and the sympathetic nervous system are also key components in endocrine functions. The specific glands are the pituitary, thyroid, parathyroids, adrenals, islet cells of the pancreas, and gonads (see the illustration on p. 1515). An endocrine gland secretes a chemical substance called a hormone, which travels through the blood stream. Its effect, therefore, is widespread and occurs in distant parts of the body. Disorders of the endocrine system, although their causes may vary, are related to either an excess or a deficiency of one or more of the hormones produced by these glands, which regulate a wide variety of physiologic processes. The onset of the disorders can be slow and insidious or abrupt and life-threatening. The age at onset can range from infancy to old age. The observing and interviewing skills of the nurse are especially important because except for the thyroid and the testicles, the nurse cannot directly examine the endocrine glands. An appreciation of key concepts and the anatomy and physiology of the endocrine system, together with data obtained from the client history and *laboratory* diagnostic tests, is essential in assessment of the endocrine system.

ANATOMY AND PHYSIOLOGY REVIEW

The control of cellular function by any hormone depends on a series of reactions that begins with the synthesis of the hormone in the endocrine cell and ends with the feedback control systems acting on that cell. This series of reactions includes the integration of the neuroregulatory mechanisms to effect homeostasis. The central nervous system receives and reacts to various stimuli that are transmitted to the hypothalamus. The hypothalamus responds to the stimuli by the production and release of either releasing or inhibiting factors, which are transported via the portal system to the pituitary, where they stimulate or inhibit the release of specific tropic hormones. The anterior pituitary responds to these hormones by controlling the secretion of hormones from target organs or tissue. This type of control is demonstrated by the interaction of the hypothalamus and the anterior pituitary with a target organ, e.g., the thyroid, the adrenal cortex, and the gonads (Fig. 48–1). The range of the maintenance level of each hormone is well defined. Deviation from this range in either direction leads to pathologic conditions.

TABLE 48-1   Principal Hormones of Endocrine Glands

Gland	Hormones
Thyroid	Tri-iodothyronine
	Thyroxine
Adrenal	Cortisol
	Aldosterone
Ovary	Estrogen
	Progesterone
Testes	Testosterone
Parathyroids	Parathyroid hormone
Pancreas	Insulin
	Glucagon
Anterior pituitary	Thyroid-stimulating hormone (TSH)
	Adrenocorticotropic hormone (ACTH)
	Luteinizing hormone (LH)
	Follicle-stimulating hormone (FSH)
	Prolactin (PRL)
	Growth hormone (GH)
	Melanocyte-stimulating hormone (MSH)
Posterior pituitary	Vasopressin (antidiuretic hormone [ADH])
	Oxytocin

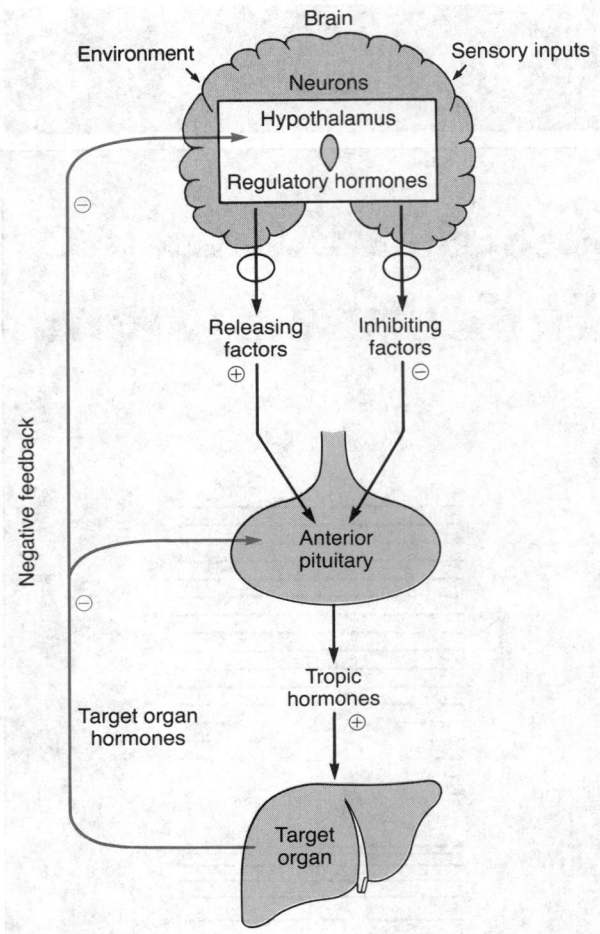

Figure 48–1

The feedback system of the hypothalamic–pituitary–target gland axis.

HYPOTHALAMUS AND PITUITARY GLAND

Structure

The hypothalamus plays a major role in regulating endocrine function. The *hypothalamus* consists of nervous tissue located beneath the cerebral hemispheres on each side of the third ventricle, with afferent and efferent fibers connecting it to the rest of the central nervous system. Blood from the internal carotid arteries flows to the superior hypophysial arteries through a capillary plexus in the median eminence to the infundibulum and then to a capillary plexus in the anterior pituitary. This venous portal system is called the hypothalamo hypophysial portal system. The *pituitary gland* is located in the sella turcica, an indentation of the sphenoid bone at the base of the brain. The gland is oval, has a diameter of approximately ⅓ in (1 cm), and is divided into two distinct lobes (Fig. 48–2). The largest lobe, which constitutes about 70%, is the anterior lobe, or *adenohypophysis;* the smaller part is the posterior lobe, or *neurohypophysis.*

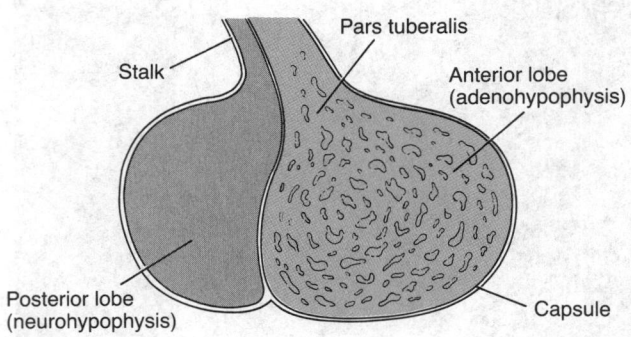

Figure 48–2

The two parts of the pituitary gland.

THE ENDOCRINE SYSTEM

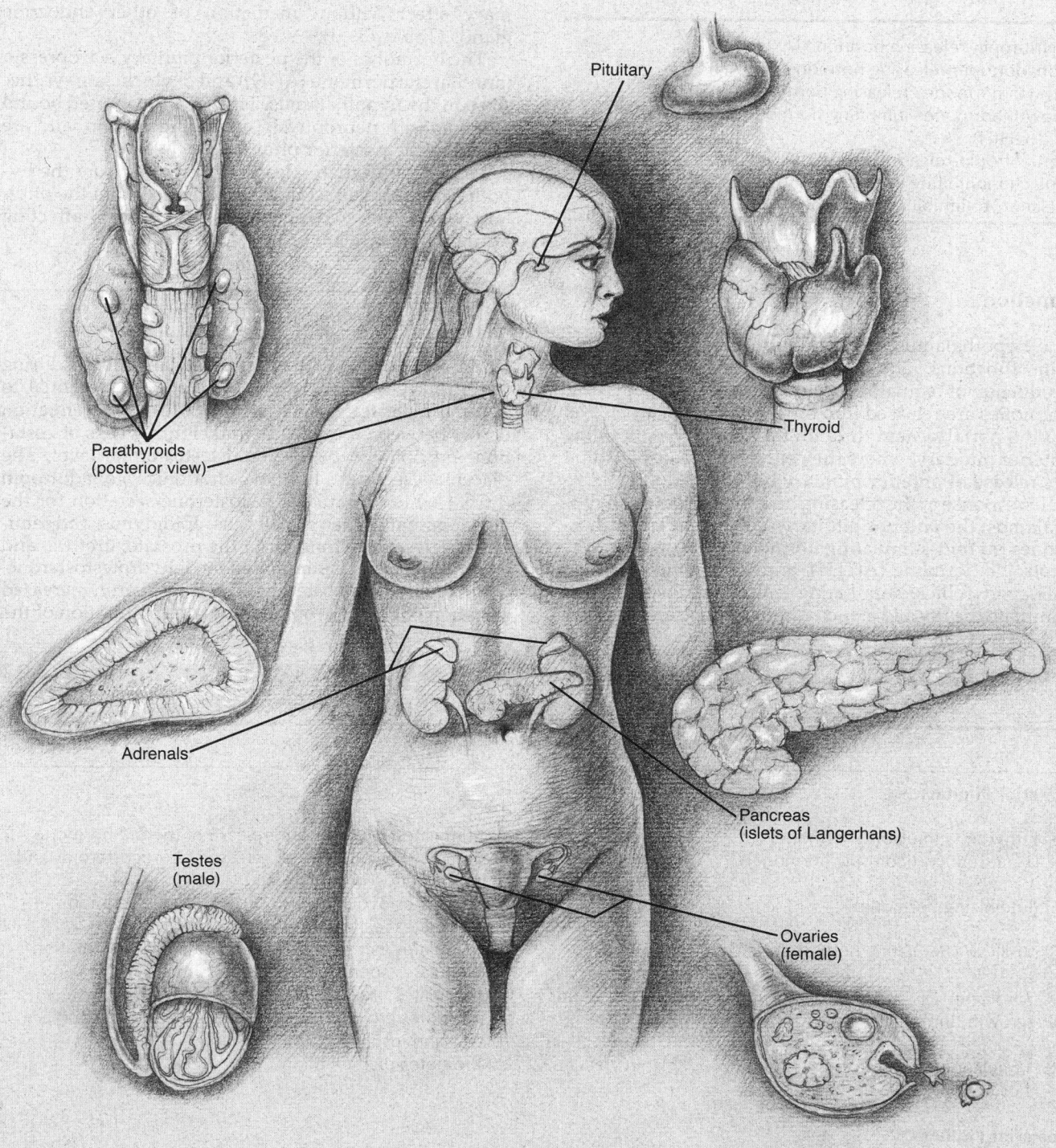

Pituitary

Thyroid

Parathyroids
(posterior view)

Adrenals

Pancreas
(islets of Langerhans)

Testes
(male)

Ovaries
(female)

TABLE 48-2 Hypothalamic Hormones

Thyrotropin-releasing hormone (TRH)
Gonadotropin-releasing hormone (Gn-RH)
Growth hormone–releasing hormone (GHRH)
Growth hormone–inhibiting hormone (somatostatin)
 (GHIH)
Corticotropin-releasing hormone (CRH)
Prolactin-inhibiting hormone (PIH)
Melanocyte-inhibiting hormone (MIH)

Function

The hypothalamus has both endocrine and nonendocrine functions. The endocrine function involves the production of regulatory hormones (Table 48–2). These hormones are released into the blood stream and travel via the portal system through the pituitary stalk to the anterior pituitary, where they either stimulate or inhibit the release of anterior pituitary hormones.

In response to the releasing hormones from the hypothalamus, the anterior pituitary secretes the tropic hormones thyroid-stimulating hormone (TSH), adrenocorticotropic hormone (ACTH), and luteinizing hormone (LH) and follicle-stimulating hormone (FSH), which stimulate the thyroid gland, adrenal cortex, and gonads,

respectively. Other pituitary hormones such as growth hormone (GH) and prolactin (PRL) produce their primary effect without mediation of other endocrine glands (Table 48–3).

The hormones of the posterior pituitary, vasopressin (antidiuretic hormone [ADH]) and oxytocin, are synthesized in the hypothalamus. They are transported bound together with neurophysin, a binding protein, and are stored in the posterior pituitary.

Factors other than releasing hormones from the hypothalamus can affect hormonal release from the pituitary gland. Selected hormones and factors affecting hormonal release are presented in Table 48–4.

GONADS

Undifferentiated gonads appear in the embryo during the fifth week of gestation and have the potential to become male testes or female ovaries. Differentiation occurs between the seventh and eighth weeks of gestation, precipitated by the fetal testosterone level. The placenta secretes human chorionic gonadotropin (hCG), which stimulates testosterone secretion for the development of the vas deferans, epididymis, and seminal vesicles. Development of the prostate, urethra, and external genitalia is stimulated by dehydrotestosterone, a metabolite of testosterone. During puberty, increased secretion of gonadotropins stimulates maturation of the

TABLE 48–3 Target Tissues and Actions of Pituitary Hormones

Hormone	Target Tissue	Action
Anterior Pituitary		
TSH (thyroid-stimulating hormone)	Thyroid	Stimulates synthesis and release of thyroid hormone
ACTH (adrenocorticotropic hormone)	Adrenal cortex	Stimulates synthesis and release of corticosteroids and adrenocortical growth
LH (luteinizing hormone)	Ovary	Stimulates ovulation and progesterone secretion
	Testes	Stimulates testosterone secretion
FSH (follicle-stimulating hormone)	Ovary	Stimulates estrogen secretion and follicle maturation
	Testes	Stimulates spermatogenesis
PRL (prolactin)	Mammary glands	Stimulates breast milk production
GH (growth hormone)	Bone and soft tissue	Promotes growth through lipolysis, protein anabolism, and insulin antagonism
MSH (melanocyte-stimulating hormone)	Melanocytes	Promotes pigmentation
Posterior Pituitary*		
ADH (antidiuretic hormone, or vasopressin)	Kidney	Promotes water reabsorption
Oxytocin	Uterus and mammary glands	Stimulates uterine contractions and ejection of breast milk

*These hormones are synthesized in the hypothalamus and are stored in the posterior pituitary gland. They are transported from the hypothalamus to the posterior pituitary while bound to neurophysins.

TABLE 48-4   Factors Affecting Release of Selected Hormones from the Pituitary

Hormone	Factor	Effect on Release
Vasopressin	Congestive heart failure	Increase
	Hemorrhage	Increase
	Diuretic use	Increase
	Opiate use	Increase
	Alcohol use	Decrease
	Chlorpropamide use	Increase
	Clofibrate use	Increase
	Surgical stress	Increase
	Hypoxia	Increase
	Prostaglandins	Increase
Growth hormone	High-protein diet	Increase
	Exercise	Increase
	Hypoglycemia	Increase
	Stress	Increase
	Levodopa use	Increase
	Hyperglycemia	Decrease
Prolactin	Stress	Increase
	Sucking at breast	Increase
	Estrogen use	Increase
	Use of dopamine antagonists	Increase
	Chlorpromazine use	Increase
Oxytocin	Sucking at breast	Increase
	Sexual activity (orgasm)	Increase
	Stress	Decrease

testes and external genitalia. A detailed description of the structure and functions of testes and ovaries is found in Chapter 52.

ADRENAL GLANDS

The adrenal glands are highly vascular, triangular bodies located in the retroperitoneal space at the superior poles of each kidney, as shown in the illustration on page 1515. Each gland is 1½ in (3.3 cm) long and weighs $\frac{1}{16}$ to $\frac{1}{8}$ oz (1.8 to 3.5 g). The adrenal glands consist of an outer portion called the *cortex* and an inner portion called the *medulla*, each with independent functions. The entire gland is surrounded by a tough connective tissue membrane called the *capsule*. The hormones of the adrenal glands have significant physiologic effects throughout the body.

ADRENAL CORTEX

Structure

The adrenal cortex is essential for maintenance of life-sustaining physiologic activities. It constitutes approxi-

mately 90% of the adrenal gland. The adrenal cortex consists of cells divided into three layers, or zones: the outer *zona glomerulosa,* the middle *zona fasciculata,* and the inner *zona reticularis* (Fig. 48–3). *Mineralocorticoids* are produced in the zona glomerulosa; *glucocorticoids, androgens,* and *estrogens* are produced in the zona fasciculata and zona reticularis. These hormones that are synthesized and secreted by the cortex are *steroids.*

Function

Mineralocorticoids

Aldosterone is the chief mineralocorticoid produced by the adrenal cortex. It plays a vital role in the maintenance of adequate extracellular fluid volume by promoting sodium reabsorption and potassium excretion in the distal convoluted tubules in the kidney. Aldosterone secretion is regulated primarily by the renin-angiotensin system but also by serum potassium ion concentration and ACTH.

Renin is produced by the juxtaglomerular cells of the renal afferent arterioles. Its release is stimulated by a decrease in extracellular fluid volume. Any factor that causes this decrease, such as blood loss, sodium loss, or changes in posture, can stimulate renin release. Renin

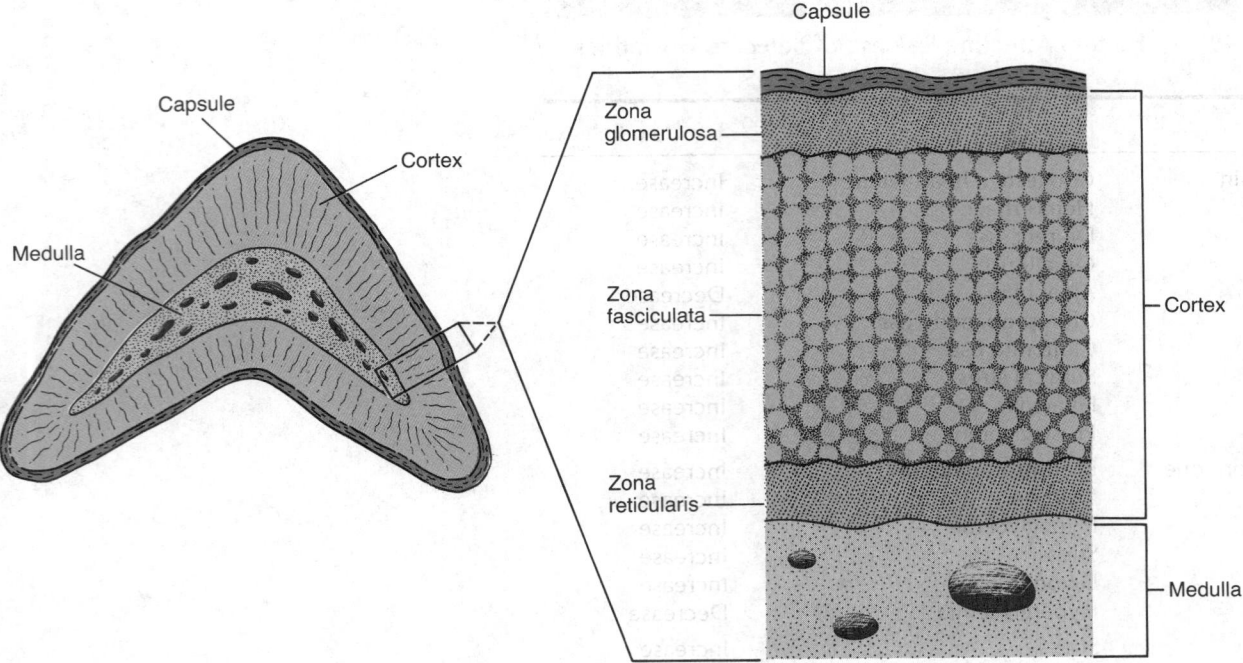

Figure 48 – 3

Structure of the adrenal glands.

acts on a plasma protein to yield angiotensin I, which undergoes a reaction catalyzed by a converting enzyme to form angiotensin II. In turn, angiotensin II stimulates the secretion of aldosterone. See Chapter 12 for further discussion of the renin-angiotensin system.

Serum potassium ion concentration also has a regulatory effect on aldosterone secretion. The adrenal cortex secretes aldosterone when the ratio of serum potassium ions to serum sodium ions increases. The increased serum potassium concentration directly stimulates the adrenals to release mineralocorticoids. *ACTH* has a weak effect on stimulation of aldosterone secretion. When ACTH is administered, a rapid rise in aldosterone occurs during the first hour of stimulation, after which secretion decreases rapidly to basal levels.

Glucocorticoids

The principal glucocorticoid that is secreted by the adrenal cortex is *cortisol.* Cortisol affects carbohydrate, protein, and fat metabolism. It also plays a role in the response to stress, maintains emotional stability, affects immune function, and has a permissive effect on other physiologic processes. The term *permissive effect* of glucocorticoids means that it (cortisol) must be present for other physiologic processes, such as catecholamine action and maintenance of normal excitability of the myo-

cardium, to occur. The many functions of glucocorticoids are summarized in Table 48 – 5.

The release of glucocorticoids is regulated primarily by the pituitary hormone ACTH and the hypothalamic corticotropin-releasing hormone (CRH). The release of CRH and ACTH is affected by (1) the serum concentration of free cortisol, (2) the diurnal sleep-wake cycle, and (3) stress. When levels of serum cortisol are low, the hypothalamus secretes CRH, which stimulates the ante-

TABLE 48 – 5 Functions of Glucocorticoid Hormones

Maintain blood glucose level by increasing hepatic gluconeogenesis and inhibiting peripheral glucose use

Increase lipolysis, releasing glycerol and free fatty acids

Increase protein catabolism

Degrade collagen and connective tissue

Increase the number of polymorphonuclear leukocytes released from bone marrow

Exert anti-inflammatory effects that decrease migration of inflammatory cells to sites of injury

Maintain behavior and cognitive functions

rior pituitary gland to release ACTH. ACTH then stimulates the adrenal cortex to secrete cortisol. Conversely, presence of adequate or elevated levels of circulating free cortisol inhibits the release of CRH and ACTH. This inhibitory effect is an example of a negative feedback system. Glucocorticoid release peaks in the morning and is at its lowest level 12 hours before and after each peak. Emotional, chemical, or physical stress results in the release of a large amount of glucocorticoids.

Sex Hormones

Small amounts of androgens and estrogens are secreted by the adrenal cortex. Adrenal secretion of these hormones is usually physiologically insignificant because the gonads—ovaries and testes—secrete large amounts of estrogens and androgens, respectively. However, the adrenal gland is the major source of androgens in the female.

ADRENAL MEDULLA

Structure

Embryonically, the adrenal medulla arises from the neural crest and is a sympathetic ganglion with glandular secretory cells instead of postganglionic neurons. Stimulation of the sympathetic nervous system results in the release of the adrenal medullary hormones or *catecholamines.* The catecholamines travel to all areas of the body via the blood stream and exert their effects on target cells. The adrenal medullary hormones are not essential for life, but they do have a role in the physiologic stress response.

Function

Two catecholamines are secreted by the adrenal medulla: *epinephrine* and *norepinephrine.* Normally, the adrenal medulla secretes 85% norepinephrine and 15% epinephrine. The effect of catecholamines varies depending on the specific receptor in the cell membranes of the target tissue. There are two types of receptors: alpha adrenergic and beta adrenergic. Both types of receptors are further classified as alpha$_1$- and alpha$_2$-receptors and beta$_1$- and beta$_2$-receptors. Norepinephrine acts primarily on alpha-adrenergic receptors, and epinephrine most often stimulates beta-adrenergic receptors.

The catecholamines exert actions on many target organs. Table 48–6 summarizes the effects of adrenal medullary hormone stimulation on body tissues and organs.

Activation of the sympathetic nervous system, with the subsequent release of adrenal medullary catecholamines, is an important component of the body's response to stress. Catecholamines are secreted in small amounts at all times for the maintenance of homeostasis. Severe physical or psychologic stress results in the secretion of larger amounts of catecholamines. This sympathetic activation results in the fight-or-flight re-

TABLE 48–6   Receptors and Effects of Adrenal Medullary Hormones on Selected Organs and Tissues

Organ or Tissue	Receptors	Effects
Heart	Beta$_1$	Chronotropic action Inotropic action
Blood vessels	Alpha Beta$_2$	Vasoconstriction Vasodilation
Gastrointestinal tract	Alpha, beta	Increased sphincter tone; decreased motility
Kidney	Beta$_2$	Increased renin release
Bronchioles	Beta$_2$	Relaxation; dilation
Bladder	Alpha Beta$_2$	Sphincter contractions Relaxation of detrusor muscle
Skin	Alpha	Increased sweating
Fat cells	Beta	Increased lipolysis
Liver	Alpha	Increased gluconeogenesis and glycogenolysis
Pancreas	Alpha Beta	Decreased glucagon and insulin release Increased glucagon and insulin release
Eyes	Alpha	Dilation of pupils

sponse, a state of heightened physical and emotional awareness.

THYROID GLAND

Structure

The *thyroid gland* is located anteriorly in the neck directly below the cricoid cartilage, as shown in the illustration at the beginning of this chapter. In the average adult, the thyroid weighs approximately ⅗ oz (18 g). It has two lobes joined by a thin isthmus, which lies on the trachea. The thyroid is an extremely vascular gland. Its blood supply comes from two pairs of arteries, the superior and the inferior arteries, which are branches of the external carotid and subclavian arteries, respectively. The right lobe has a greater blood supply and is often larger than the left lobe. The thyroid gland is innervated by the adrenergic and cholinergic nervous systems. Adrenergic stimulation arises from the cervical ganglia, and cholinergic stimulation comes from the vagus nerve.

The thyroid is composed of follicular and parafollicular cells. Follicular cells produce the thyroid hormones *thyroxine* (T_4) and *tri-iodothyronine* (T_3); parafollicular cells produce and secrete *thyrocalcitonin (calcitonin)*, which plays a role in calcium regulation.

Function

Approximately 99.5% of circulatory T_4 and T_3 is bound to plasma proteins, including prealbumin, albumin, and thyroid-binding globulin. T_3 has a more rapid and shorter-lived action than T_4. T_4 can be converted to T_3 after release from the thyroid gland. The cellular conversion of T_4 to T_3 is influenced by a number of factors. Stress, starvation, radiopaque dyes, beta-blockers, and propylthiouracil impair the conversion of T_4 to T_3, whereas cold temperatures appear to increase it.

Both hormones T_3 and T_4 increase the basal metabolic rate, which is associated with an increase in oxygen consumption and heat production. This effect is not seen in the brain, spleen, lungs, or testes. T_3 and T_4 also aid in growth and development. Table 48–7 summarizes thyroid hormone function.

Secretion of T_3 and T_4 is regulated by a hypothalamic–pituitary–thyroid gland axis or feedback mechanism. Pituitary secretion of TSH regulates thyroid hormone secretion and virtually every step of thyroid hormone metabolism. The circulating level of thyroid hormone is the major factor regulating the release of TSH. If the hormone levels are high, TSH release is inhibited. Low levels of thyroid hormone increase secretion of TSH. Thyroid hormones regulate the secretion of TSH at the level of the anterior pituitary. Secretion of TSH is also affected by the hypothalamic secretion of thyrotropin-releasing hormone (TRH). Cold and stress are two factors causing the hypothalamus to secrete TRH.

TABLE 48–7   Functions of Thyroid Hormones

Play an important role in fetal development, particularly neural and skeletal systems

Control metabolic rate of all cells

Promote sufficient pituitary secretion of GH and gonadotropins

Regulate protein, carbohydrate, and fat metabolism

Exert chronotropic and inotropic cardiac effects

Increase red blood cell production

Affect respiratory rate and drive

Increase bone formation and resorption

Act as insulin antagonists

The synthesis of thyroid hormones involves a series of steps. Sufficient dietary intake of protein and iodine is essential for production of thyroid hormones. Iodine is absorbed from the gastrointestinal tract as iodide, and the thyroid gland withdraws iodide from circulation. After its transport within the thyroid, iodide enters into a sequence of reactions resulting in the formation of T_4 or T_3. The hormones, bound to thyroglobulin, are stored in the follicular cells. With stimulation, T_4 and T_3 break off from thyroglobulin and are released into the circulation.

Calcitonin lowers serum calcium and serum phosphate levels by inhibiting bone resorption. The primary factor influencing calcitonin secretion is the serum calcium level. Low serum calcium levels suppress calcitonin release; elevated levels of serum calcium increase calcitonin secretion. Additional factors that cause increased calcitonin release are pregnancy, high-calcium diet, and increased gastrin secretion.

PARATHYROID GLANDS

Structure

The *parathyroid glands* consist of four small glands located close to, embedded in, or attached to the posterior surface of the thyroid gland. The parathyroid glands are composed of two types of cells: chief cells and oxyphil cells. The *chief cell* is the major cell of the parathyroid gland, and it synthesizes and secretes parathyroid hormone (PTH).

Function

PTH regulates calcium and phosphorus metabolism as a result of its effect on three target organs: bone, kidney, and gastrointestinal tract (Fig. 48–4). The bone is the primary reservoir of calcium in the body. PTH promotes

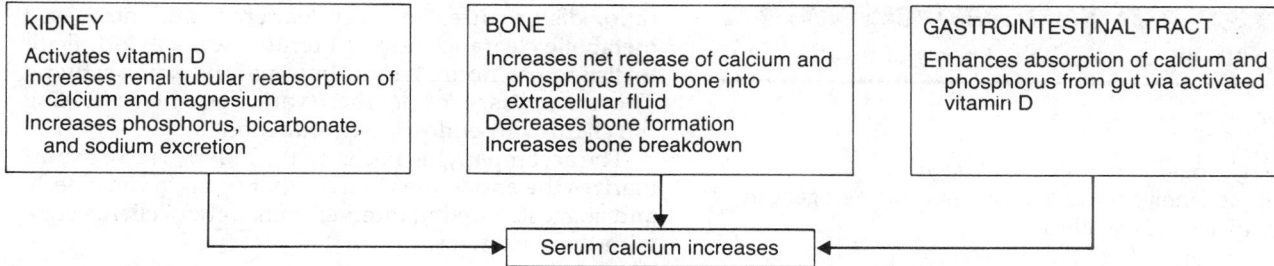

KIDNEY	BONE	GASTROINTESTINAL TRACT
Activates vitamin D Increases renal tubular reabsorption of calcium and magnesium Increases phosphorus, bicarbonate, and sodium excretion	Increases net release of calcium and phosphorus from bone into extracellular fluid Decreases bone formation Increases bone breakdown	Enhances absorption of calcium and phosphorus from gut via activated vitamin D

Serum calcium increases

Figure 48–4

Effects of parathyroid hormone on target organs.

increased bone resorption, which liberates calcium into the blood stream. In the renal tubules, PTH increases the reabsorption of calcium and magnesium, activates vitamin D, and promotes the excretion of phosphorus, bicarbonate, and sodium. In the presence of activated vitamin D, PTH increases the absorption of calcium and phosphorus from the gastrointestinal tract. The combined effect of these actions is to maintain normal serum calcium and phosphorus levels.

Calcium is the major controlling factor of PTH secretion. When the serum calcium level is elevated, secretion of PTH is decreased. PTH secretion increases in the presence of low serum calcium levels. Calcitonin and serum phosphate levels also affect PTH secretion, most likely because of their effect on serum calcium levels.

PANCREAS

Structure

The *pancreas* lies retroperitoneally behind the stomach and has both endocrine and exocrine functions. Its exocrine function is to secrete digestive enzymes through ducts that empty into the duodenum (see Chap. 47).

The *islets of Langerhans* are the cells that are involved in the endocrine function of the pancreas (Fig. 48–5). There are approximately 1 million islet cells throughout the pancreas. The islets of Langerhans are composed of three distinct cell types: alpha cells, which secrete *glucagon*; beta cells, which secrete *insulin*; and delta cells, which secrete *somatostatin*. Glucagon and insulin have a significant effect on carbohydrate, protein, and fat metabolism. The function of somatostatin, which is secreted not only in the pancreas but also in a number of tissues, including the brain and the gastrointestinal tract, is not totally understood. It is known to inhibit glucagon and insulin secretion in the pancreas.

Function

Glucagon

The primary physiologic function of glucagon is to increase blood glucose levels. Glucagon is stimulated by

a decrease in blood glucose levels and an increase in blood amino acid levels. It functions in conjunction with epinephrine, GH, and glucocorticoids to maintain blood glucose levels. The liver is the primary target organ of glucagon. In the liver, glucagon promotes glycogenolysis, the conversion of glycogen to glucose. In addition, it enhances amino acid transport from muscle and promotes gluconeogenesis, the conversion of amino acids and fatty acids to glucose. In metabolism of fats, glucagon enhances lipolysis and subsequent ketone formation.

Insulin

Insulin is primarily an anabolic hormone, promoting synthesis and storage in carbohydrate, protein, and fat metabolism (Table 48–8). Insulin lowers blood glucose levels by promoting glucose diffusion across cell membranes in most tissues. Basal levels of insulin are secreted continuously to control metabolism in the fasting state. Insulin secretion rises in response to an increase in blood glucose levels. Carbohydrates are the major stimuli for insulin secretion; however, amino acids may have a similar, but not as potent, effect.

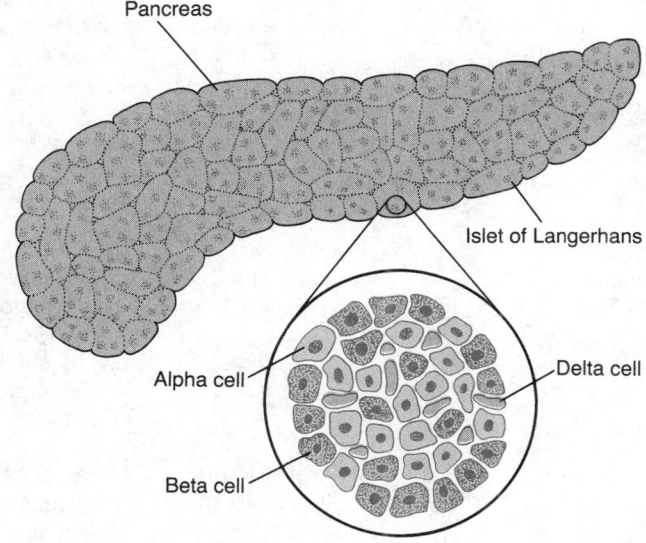

Figure 48–5

The islets of Langerhans of the pancreas.

TABLE 48–8 Anabolic Effects of Insulin

Effects on Liver

Promotes glycogen synthesis and storage
Inhibits glycogenolysis, gluconeogenesis, and ketogenesis
Increases triglyceride synthesis

Effects on Muscle

Promotes protein synthesis
Increases amino acid transport
Promotes glycogenesis

Effects on Fat

Increases fatty acid synthesis
Promotes triglyceride storage
Decreases lipolysis

ENDOCRINE CHANGES ASSOCIATED WITH AGING

Progress in the field of endocrinology in the elderly population has expanded dramatically in the last few years. There is considerable variation in the effects of aging on the endocrine system. A large number of age-related variables, such as acute and chronic illnesses; alterations in diet, activity, and lean body mass/fat ratio; disturbances in sleep patterns; and decreased metabolic clearance rate of hormones, make it difficult to distinguish normal from abnormal endocrine activity. The nurse must consider these variables when assessing the client with endocrine dysfunction.

The accompanying Focus on the Elderly feature summarizes the endocrine changes that occur in the elderly and suggests nursing interventions to help clients cope with these changes.

HISTORY

Developing a systematic approach to taking a history from the client with a suspected endocrine problem can be difficult because of the potential variety of clinical presentations.

Initially, the nurse focuses on the client's reason for seeking health care. Did the client's symptoms occur gradually or was the onset sudden? Has the client been treated for this problem in the past? How have the current symptoms interfered with activities of daily living? Such questioning provides valuable clues in identifying specific endocrine disorders. In addition, *age, sex,* and *past medical history* are essential baseline assessment data. Certain disorders, such as hyperosmolar states and the loss of ovarian function, are seen more frequently in older than in younger clients. Manifestations of endo-

---

FOCUS ON THE ELDERLY ■ Endocrine Changes Related to Aging

Structure	Change	Interventions	Rationales
Posterior pituitary	Increased secretion of antidiuretic hormone	1. Assess for dilute urine and polyuria. 2. Encourage fluid intake.	1, 2. To prevent complications, especially dehydration.
Gonads	Decreased ovarian function	1. Teach client signs and symptoms of estrogen. 2. Promote exercise and calcium intake.	1. To improve client's ability to cope with changes. 2. To slow bone loss and prevent complications related to osteoporosis.
Pancreas	Decreased glucose tolerance	1. Identify clients at risk: overweight, excess of fat in the diet, or little physical exercise. 2. Teach client signs and symptoms of hyperglycemia.	1. To avoid complications. 2. To improve client's recognition of hyperglycemia, which can occur after meals.
Thyroid	Decreased peripheral metabolism	1. Assess for signs of hypothyroidism, especially constipation, lethargy, dry skin, or mental deterioration.	1. To distinguish signs of hypothyroidism, which often resemble clinical features of aging.

crine disorders can be sex related, as in the case of the sexual effects of hyper- and hypopituitarism. A family history of endocrine dysfunction is obtained in the initial interview. The nurse notes any family history of obesity, growth and development difficulties, diabetes, infertility, and thyroid disorders. Changes in some general areas are helpful for the nurse to explore: energy levels, elimination patterns, nutritional status, sexual and reproductive functions, and physical appearance.

Changes in *energy levels* are associated with a number of endocrine problems, particularly those involving the thyroid and adrenal glands. The nurse asks the client if there has been a change in the ability to perform daily activities and assesses the current energy level. Has the client been sleeping longer or experiencing fatigue or generalized weakness? The nurse incorporates this information when planning activities and rest periods with the client.

Elimination patterns are affected by the endocrine system. The nurse questions the client about urinary frequency and amount. Does the client wake during the night to urinate (nocturia) or experience pain on urination? Information about frequency of bowel movements and consistency and color of feces may provide clues to problems in fluid balance. The nurse identifies the client's past pattern of elimination to determine deviations from the normal routine.

Changes in *nutritional status* or gastrointestinal tract disturbances may reflect a variety of endocrine problems. A history of nausea, vomiting, or abdominal pain is noted. An increase or a decrease in fluid or food intake may indicate specific disorders such as diabetes insipidus, in which thirst is seen, and primary adrenal hypofunction, in which salt craving occurs. It is often helpful for the nurse to ask the client to list the intake of all fluids and foods on a particular day to establish a dietary pattern.

Sexual and reproductive functions are greatly affected by disturbances in the endocrine system. The nurse asks the female client if there have been any changes in menstrual cycle, such as increased flow, duration, and frequency of menses or presence of pain or excessive cramping. Has the male client experienced impotence? The nurse determines if male or female clients have had a change in libido or a problem with fertility.

The nurse discusses any perceived changes in *physical characteristics* with the client. Identification of overt changes is accomplished during the physical assessment; however, clients may be able to describe subtle changes that might be missed. The nurse questions the client about changes in hair texture, hair distribution, facial contours, voice quality, body proportions, and secondary sexual characteristics. For example, the nurse might ask a male client if he is shaving less often or a female client if she has noticed an increase in the amount of facial hair. These changes may be associated with pituitary, thyroid, parathyroid, or adrenal dysfunction.

The information gathered from the history provides a basis for planning care. It is essential for the nurse to combine these data with physical, psychosocial, and laboratory findings for a comprehensive assessment of the endocrine system.

PHYSICAL ASSESSMENT

The nurse performs a thorough physical examination when assessing clients with suspected endocrine abnormalities. The physical assessment requires systematic inspection, as well as palpation and auscultation skills.

INSPECTION

Dysfunction of the endocrine system can result in characteristic physical changes because of its effect on growth and development, on the regulation of sex hormone levels, on fluid and electrolyte balance, and on the use of nutrients. It is important to note that many clinical findings can be associated with more than one endocrine disorder and that these findings may be related to another pathologic process. Initially, the nurse observes the client's general appearance. *Height, weight, fat distribution,* and *muscle mass* should be assessed in relation to age. It is important to remember that heredity and age may be responsible for significant deviations (e.g., short stature) rather than pathologic condition.

Skin abnormalities may reflect dysfunction of specific endocrine glands. The nurse observes skin color and notes areas of hypo- or hyperpigmentation. Bruising and/or petechiae are often seen in adrenocortical hyperfunction, and the location and size of the area affected should be documented. Skin over the finger joints, elbows, and knees and any scar tissue may show increased pigmentation in secondary hypofunction of the adrenal glands because of increased levels of ACTH and melanocyte-stimulating hormone. Vitiligo seen in primary hypofunction of the adrenal glands is due to destruction of melanocytes in the skin by an autoimmune process. This process results in areas of decreased pigmentation, most often on the face, neck, and extremities. Mucous membranes can exhibit increased areas of pigmentation. Any lesion, particularly one that is not healing properly, is identified, and the location, color, size, and distribution are noted.

The nurse examines the extremities and the base of the spine for the presence of *edema*, which might indicate a problem in fluid and electrolyte balance.

Hair distribution is assessed by the nurse. Hirsutism, excessive hair loss, and changes in hair texture can indicate endocrine gland dysfunction. The nurse inspects the client's *nails* for malformation and thickness or for brittleness, which may suggest thyroid gland difficulties.

When performing the physical assessment, it is important to have a systematic approach to avoid losing valuable data. Inspection of the client by using a head-to-toe approach is often effective. When examining the head, the nurse focuses on *abnormalities of facial structure, features, and expression,* such as prominent forehead or jaw, round or puffy face, dull or flat expression, and exophthalmos (protruding eyeballs and retracted upper lids). The nurse initially observes the lower half of the client's neck to observe the visible *enlargement of the thyroid gland.* Normally, thyroid tissue cannot be observed. Jugular vein distention may be noted when inspecting the neck and can indicate fluid overload (see Chaps. 12 and 13).

A visual examination of the trunk can provide symptoms of specific endocrine dysfunction. The nurse notes any abnormalities in *size and symmetry of the chest.* Truncal obesity, supraclavicular fat pads, and the presence of a buffalo hump can be symptoms of adrenocortical excess. Hormonal imbalance may result in change in *secondary sexual characteristics.* The nurse inspects the breasts (male and female) and pays particular attention

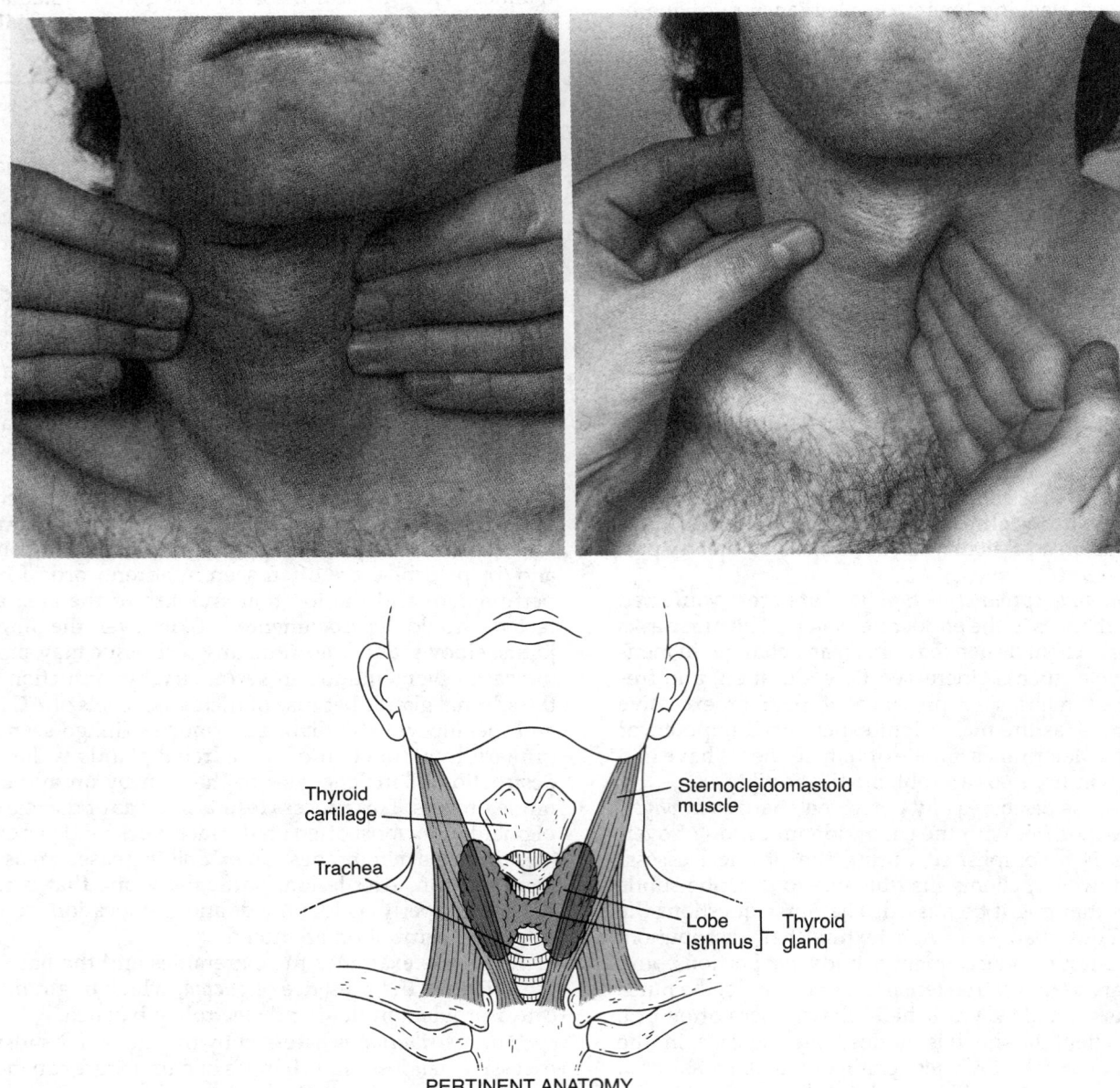

PERTINENT ANATOMY

Figure 48–6

Palpation of the thyroid glands. (Photographs from Swartz, M. H. [1989]. *Textbook of physical diagnosis: History and examination.* Philadelphia: W. B. Saunders.)

to size, symmetry, pigmentation, and presence of discharge. Striae, usually reddish purple, on the breasts and/or abdomen are frequently seen with adrenocortical excess.

Examination of the *genitalia* may reveal dysfunction in hormonal secretion. The nurse notes the size of the scrotum and penis in the male and the labia and clitoris in the female in relation to standards for the client's age. Distribution and quantity of pubic hair are often affected in hypogonadism, and the nurse documents any abnormalities.

AUSCULTATION

The nurse performs auscultation to establish baseline vital signs and to determine irregularities in cardiac rate and rhythm. A variety of endocrine disturbances can cause dehydration and volume depletion. Therefore, the nurse documents any difference in the client's *blood pressure* and *pulse* with the client in lying and standing or sitting positions (orthostatic vital signs). If an enlarged thyroid is palpated, the area of enlargement can be auscultated to determine the presence of bruits. Hypertrophy of the thyroid gland causes an increase in vascular flow, which may result in bruits.

PALPATION

The thyroid gland is one gland that is routinely palpated in the initial assessment. The thyroid gland is palpated to obtain information about its size, symmetry, and general shape and to identify the presence of nodules or their irregularities. Occasionally, the thyroid is not easily palpable. It is helpful if the client swallows during both inspection and palpation. The nurse offers the client sips of water to assist in swallowing during the examination.

The thyroid can be palpated with the nurse standing behind or in front of the client (Fig. 48–6). When palpating the thyroid gland from behind, the nurse asks the client to be seated and to lower the chin. The nurse places the thumbs of both hands on the back of the client's neck with the fingers curved around to the front of the client's neck and placed on either side of the trachea. The nurse asks the client to swallow. As the client does so, the nurse locates the isthmus of the thyroid and feels it rising upward. The nurse also identifies the anterior surface of the thyroid lobe. The nurse turns the client's head to the right, displaces the thyroid cartilage to the right with the fingers of the left hand, and palpates the right lobe with the right hand. The procedure is reversed for examining the left lobe.

To palpate the thyroid gland from the front, the nurse stands in front of the client and places the index and middle fingers of both hands below the cricoid on both sides of the trachea to palpate the thyroid isthmus. The nurse then moves the fingers laterally to identify the lateral lobes. The nurse asks the client to turn the head to the right and flex the head forward. With the right hand, the nurse displaces the thyroid cartilage to the left, the client's right. The nurse hooks the tips of the index and middle fingers of the left hand around the relaxed sternocleidomastoid muscle, then palpates the right lobe around the sternocleidomastoid muscle with the thumb and fingertips of the left hand. The procedure is reversed for examining the left lobe.

PSYCHOSOCIAL ASSESSMENT

Information obtained from the history and physical examination aids the nurse in identifying potential psychosocial problems. The nurse assesses the client's coping skills, support systems, and health-related beliefs. A number of endocrine disorders seriously affect the client's perception of self. For example, significant changes in body characteristics can occur in disorders of the pituitary, adrenal, and thyroid glands. Infertility, impotence, and other changes in sexual functioning may result from endocrine dysfunction. If the nurse recognizes a difficulty in coping with such changes, additional support from social or counseling services may be appropriate when planning care.

Clients with endocrine problems may require lifelong medication and follow-up care. The nurse assesses the client's readiness to learn and ability to carry out specific self-management skills. In addition, clients can be faced with financial difficulties resulting from a prolonged medical regimen or interruption of employment, and a referral to social services agencies may be needed.

DIAGNOSTIC ASSESSMENT

LABORATORY TESTS

STIMULATION/SUPPRESSION

Laboratory tests are an essential part of the diagnostic process for the client with suspected endocrine dysfunction. The highly specialized testing for specific disorders is found in the following chapters discussing these problems. However, there are some generalizations to be made concerning endocrine testing.

Measurement of individual hormones does not always allow a distinction between the normal and the abnormal. The broad normal range for some hormones makes it necessary to elicit responses based on stimulation or suppression tests. In suspected endocrine gland underactivity, it may be necessary to provide a stimulus to hormone production by the gland in question to see if it is capable of normal hormone production. This method is called *stimulation* testing. Measured amounts of selected hormones are given to stimulate the target gland to maximal production. Hormone levels are then measured and interpreted against a given norm. Failure of the hormone level to rise in the face of stimulation denotes hypofunction. *Suppression* tests are used when hormone levels are high or in the upper range of normal. Failure to suppress hormone production during standardized testing indicates hyperfunction. Further discussion of specific tests is in Chapters 49 and 50.

RADIOIMMUNOASSAY

Radioimmunoassay is a competitive binding assay in which labeled amounts of hormone compete with unlabeled hormone from the plasma or serum for binding sites on an antibody. The amount of unbound and bound hormone is measured by various techniques and identified as such. The unbound hormone is the active hormone.

URINE TESTS

In addition to the measurement of hormones in the blood, hormone levels in the urine are frequently measured. Because many of the endocrine hormones are secreted in a pulsatile fashion, measurement of a specific hormone in a 24-hour urine collection better reflects the overall function of certain glands such as the adrenal. The nurse must instruct the client in collecting a 24-hour urine sample. It is important to know that certain hormonal measurements require additives at the beginning of the collection. The nurse instructs the client not to discard the preservative from the container and to use caution when handling it because some solutions are caustic. The client is also reminded that this is a timed collection and that it should be collected for *exactly* 24 hours. Clients should be instructed to avoid taking any unnecessary medications during endocrine testing because drugs may interfere with the laboratory assays.

TESTS FOR GLUCOSE

Tests for functions of the islet cells of the pancreas include the standard 3-hour glucose tolerance test (GTT) and the 5-hour GTT. A simple fasting blood sugar and 2-hour postprandial blood sugar are usually used as screening tests for diabetes. The 3-hour GTT is used to detect diabetes mellitus when one of the screening tests has been abnormal. The 5-hour GTT is performed when reactive hypoglycemia is suspected. Reactive hypoglycemia occurs in response to excessive insulin production, usually after ingestion of a carbohydrate meal. Insulin levels, as well as blood glucose levels, are measured at intervals for 5 hours. The glycosylated hemoglobin or hemoglobin A_{1c} is a test that reveals what the average blood glucose level has been over a period of 2 to 3 months. Its primary use is in assessing overall control of glucose level in diabetes mellitus. See Chapter 51 for a discussion of diabetes mellitus.

RADIOGRAPHIC EXAMINATIONS

Anterior, posterior, and lateral skull films are frequently used for visualization of the sella turcica. Erosion of the sella can be seen and would indicate invasion of the wall from an abnormal growth. Computed tomography (CT) is used to determine the extent of growth of a macroadenoma or to find a microadenoma buried within the pituitary. CT scans are also used to determine the size and shape of other glands and nearby structures. Contrast media are sometimes used with these scans. Angiography and venography may reveal structural abnormalities such as aberrant blood vessels. Ultrasonography is useful, especially in the thyroid, for determining whether nodules or masses are solid or cystic.

OTHER DIAGNOSTIC TESTS

Needle biopsy is a method frequently used to determine the composition of thyroid nodules. It is a relatively safe, quick procedure done on an outpatient basis. It is done primarily to determine whether surgical intervention is necessary.

SUMMARY

Assessment of the endocrine system depends heavily on a comprehensive history and results of the diagnostic work-up. Physical assessment is accomplished primarily through inspection, except for the testicles and the thyroid, which can be palpated. During the history taking and the physical assessment, the nurse can often detect subtle clues indicating endocrine dysfunction. In addition, clients are often faced with a battery of diagnostic tests. The nurse assists clients in decreasing anxiety through education and emotional support.

REFERENCES AND READINGS

Bagdade, J. D. (1987). *The yearbook of endocrinology.* Chicago: Year Book Medical.

Besser, G. M., & Cudworth, A. G. (1987). *Clinical endocrinology: An illustrated text.* Philadelphia: J. B. Lippincott.

Brodde, O. E., & Wang, X. L. (1988). Beta-adrenoceptor changes in blood lymphatics and altered drug responsiveness. *Annals of Clinical Research, 20,* 311–323.

Carlson, H. E. (Ed.). (1983). *Endocrinology.* New York: Wiley Medical.

DeGroot, L. J., Besser, G. M., Cahill, G. F., Jr., Marshall, J. C., Nelson, D. H., Odell, W. D., Potts, J.T., Jr., Rubenstein, A. H., & Steinberger, E. (Eds.). (1989). *Endocrinology* (2nd ed., Vol. 3). Philadelphia: W. B. Saunders.

Felig, P., Baster, J. D., & Broadus, A. (Eds.). (1987). *Endocrinology and metabolism.* New York: McGraw-Hill.

Fischbach, F. (1988). *A manual of laboratory diagnostic tests* (3rd ed.). Philadelphia: J. B. Lippincott.

Greenspan, F. S., & Forsham, P. H. (1986). *Basic and clinical endocrinology* (2nd ed.). Los Altos, CA: Lange Medical.

Hershman J. M. (Ed.). (1980) *Management of endocrine disorders.* Philadelphia: Lea & Febiger.

Hobbie, W. L., & Swartz, C. L. (1989). Endocrine late effects among survivors of cancer. *Seminars in Oncology Nursing 5,* 14–21.

Krupp, M. A., & Chatton, M. J. (1984). *Current medical diagnosis and treatment.* Los Altos, CA: Lange Medical.

Malasanos, L., Barkauskas, V., & Stoltenberg-Allen, K. (1990). *Health assessment.* (4th ed.). St. Louis: C. V. Mosby.

Martin, C. R. (1985). *Endocrine physiology.* New York: Oxford University Press.

Mazzaferri, E. L. (Ed.). (1986). *Textbook of endocrinology* (3rd ed.). New York: Elsevier.

McDonald, E., Ruskoaho, H., Scheinin, M., & Virtanen, R. (1988). Therapeutic application of drugs acting on alpha-adrenoceptors. *Annals of Clinical Research, 20,* 298–310.

Metz, R., & Larson, E. B. (Eds.). (1985). *Blue book of endocrinology.* Philadelphia: W. B. Saunders.

Murthe, N. C. (1981). *Endocrinology—a nursing approach.* Boston: Little, Brown.

Sacktor, B. (Ed.). (1987). Endocrinology and aging. *Endocrinology and Metabolism Clinics of North America, 16,* 829–1059.

Segar, D. (1988). Toxic emergencies of endocrine and metabolic therapeutic agents. *Journal of Emergency Medicine, 6,* 527–537.

Tiwary, C. M. (1987). Neonatal screening for metabolic and endocrine diseases. *Nurse Practitioner, 12,* 28–35, 38, 41.

Widman, F. K. (1983). *Clinical interpretations of laboratory tests* (9th ed.). Philadelphia: F. A. Davis.

Wilson, J. D., & Foster, D. W. (Eds.). (1985). *Williams textbook of endocrinology* (7th ed.). Philadelphia: W. B. Saunders.

Wyngaarden, J. B., & Smith, L. H. (Eds.). (1988). *Cecil textbook of medicine* (18th ed.). Philadelphia: W. B. Saunders.

CHAPTER 49

Interventions for Clients with Disorders of the Pituitary and Adrenal Glands

Dysfunctions of the pituitary and adrenal glands are manifested by a wide variety of clinical findings. Pathology results from overabundance or insufficient amounts of specific hormone. Multiple etiologic factors cause hormone imbalance. The nursing challenges in caring for clients with disorders of the pituitary and adrenal glands are performing a careful assessment, educating clients, and providing psychosocial support.

A careful assessment involves obtaining a detailed history and performing a comprehensive physical examination to detect characteristic clinical findings. Clients with hormonal imbalance require extensive education to maintain health after discharge from the hospital. In addition, clients frequently undergo a variety of diagnostic tests necessitating specific instructions and explanations from the nurse. Psychosocial support is critical because adrenal and pituitary disorders may result in characteristic physical changes and drug dependence related to lifelong treatment. The nurse identifies difficulties in the client's coping skills and works with all members of the health care team to support the client.

Thorough understanding of the pathophysiology, etiology, and nursing management of specific disorders of the pituitary and adrenal glands provides the nurse with a comprehensive knowledge base to formulate a plan of nursing care and to meet the challenge of caring for these clients.

DISORDERS OF THE PITUITARY GLAND

Disturbances in pituitary function involve a deficiency or an excess of one or more of the pituitary hormones. Hormonal disturbance occurs as a result of a problem in the pituitary gland itself (primary pituitary dysfunction) or as a result of a hypothalamic dysfunction (secondary pituitary dysfunction).

Disorders of the Anterior Pituitary Gland

Growth, metabolic activity, and sexual development are regulated by the anterior pituitary gland. Hormones of the anterior pituitary gland, or adenohypophysis, have wide-reaching effects throughout the body when produced in insufficient or excessive amounts. These hormones include growth hormone (GH), prolactin (PRL), thyroid-stimulating hormone (TSH), adrenocorticotropic hormone (ACTH), follicle-stimulating hormone

(FSH), luteinizing hormone (LH), and melanocyte-stimulating hormone (MSH).

HYPOPITUITARISM

OVERVIEW

Hypopituitarism is a state in which there is a deficiency of one or more of the anterior pituitary hormones. Growth retardation (in children), metabolic abnormalities, and sexual immaturity result from such a deficiency. Partial or total failure of production of *all* of the anterior pituitary hormones results in a condition known as *panhypopituitarism.*

Pathophysiology

Complete absence of all anterior pituitary hormones is extremely rare. Most often, there is a marked decrease in one hormone and a lesser decrease in others. Deficiencies of ACTH and TSH are considered to be the most life-threatening. Absence of these hormones produces a state of insufficiency in their respective target glands, the adrenal glands and the thyroid. (See later section in this chapter for a discussion of adrenal hypofunction and Chap. 50 for a discussion of hypothyroidism.)

In hypopituitarism, the clinical entity that is seen most frequently is a decreased synthesis and secretion of the gonadotropins LH and FSH. Deficiency of LH and FSH in males results in testicular failure, with decreased testosterone production from the Leydig cells and decreased or absent spermatogenesis from the seminiferous tubules. Decreased testosterone production is responsible for delayed onset of puberty and for sterility in adult males. In females, deficiency or absence of gonadotropins results in ovarian failure, with the loss of follicular stimulation, ovulation, and formation and maintenance of the corpus luteum; in the adult sterility results. Deficiency of LH and FSH also results in the loss of or failure to develop secondary sex characteristics.

The absence of PRL in males is not clinically apparent. In females, a deficiency of PRL is one cause of failure to lactate in the postpartum period.

Deficiency in synthesis and secretion of GH is the second most frequently seen pathophysiologic alteration in hypopituitarism. In GH deficiency, there is a problem in synthesis, release, or use of GH or in the lack of tissue response to somatomedin. Somatomedin, a hormone produced in the liver under the direct stimulation of GH, is sometimes absent. Although GH is the stimulus, somatomedin directly promotes growth of bone and cartilage. GH or somatomedin deficiency in children causes growth retardation and short stature. Growth in the prenatal period is not affected by a deficiency in the fetus or the mother, as evidenced by normal birth length in these children. Absence of GH deficiency is not clinically apparent in the adult and can be diagnosed only on the basis of stimulation tests.

Etiology

The etiology of hypopituitarism is extremely varied. Nonsecreting *pituitary tumors* cause compression and destruction of pituitary tissue. Craniopharyngioma is the most common brain tumor causing hypopituitarism. Other causes of *primary hypopituitarism* include partial or total hypophysectomy (removal of the pituitary gland), radiation, infarction, metastatic disease, granulomatous process, and trauma. *Secondary hypopituitarism* may occur as a result of infection (e.g., meningitis), trauma, tumors, congenital defects, or infiltrative processes (e.g., sarcoidosis). *Idiopathic hypopituitarism* is usually associated with an isolated hormone deficiency. There are many cases in which no etiology can be defined.

Postpartum hemorrhage is the most common cause of pituitary infarction. This clinical entity is referred to as *Sheehan's syndrome*. The pituitary normally hypertrophies during pregnancy, and when hypotension results from hemorrhage, ischemia and necrosis of the gland occur. This condition may present in the immediate postpartum period or several years after delivery.

GH deficiency may be familial in origin, in which case the effect of GH or somatomedin on body tissue is impaired although adequate amounts of hormone are present. Severe malnutrition or rapid loss and depletion of body fat such as in anorexia nervosa has been known to impair function of the pituitary gland.

Incidence

The incidence of hypopituitarism is unknown and is difficult to determine because it can involve a deficiency of one or more hormones. Both hypopituitarism and panhypopituitarism are considered to be rare diseases.

PREVENTION

Safety issues are a factor in reducing head trauma, which might injure the pituitary or necessitate surgery leading to the development of hypopituitarism. The use of seat belts in motor vehicles, the use of helmets for motorcycles and bicycles, diving safety, and adequate protection during contact sports may decrease the risk of head injury. For congenital disorders, genetic counseling is of utmost importance.

COLLABORATIVE MANAGEMENT

 Assessment

Clinical features and symptoms of hypopituitarism vary depending on the severity of disease and the number of deficient hormones. The onset of symptoms usually occurs gradually. Assessment and nursing interventions focus on GH and gonadotropin deficiencies. (See the later section on adrenal hypofunction in this chapter and the section on thyroid hypofunction in Chap. 50 for assessment and intervention for these deficiencies.)

History

Gonadotropin (LH, FSH) deficiency results in *loss of secondary sex characteristics* in the adult male and adult female. Clients may be quite sensitive about questions relating to sexuality. The nurse is cognizant of the need to respect the privacy and dignity of the client when eliciting such information.

Adult male clients may report a loss of facial and body hair, episodes of impotence, and decreased libido. It may be helpful for the nurse to ask questions such as, "Has there been any change in your sexual functioning," so that the client notes a *discrepancy from past patterns.* When hypopituitarism occurs before puberty, male clients may complain of a lack of secondary sex characteristics or report an inability to initiate or maintain an erection. Adult female clients may experience *secondary amenorrhea.* The nurse asks the female client to describe her previous menstrual pattern, to identify recent changes, and to note the month when menstruation ceased. The nurse explores any difficulty the female client may have experienced in achieving pregnancy.

The nurse questions the client and family about a past medical history of *chronic renal failure; pancreatic, liver, and bone disease; diabetes mellitus; hypothyroidism;* and *administration of gonadal hormones,* because these conditions can cause growth retardation.

Nutritional defects, such as an inadequate supply of protein, carbohydrates, fats, vitamin D, calcium, or phosphorus, have also been identified as etiologic factors in growth retardation. Therefore, the nurse elicits information regarding past and current nutritional habits and notes a history of malnutrition, gastrointestinal malabsorption syndromes, or "failure to thrive" in infancy and childhood.

Physical Assessment: Clinical Manifestations

Neurologic manifestations of hypopituitarism often present as *visual disturbances.* During the physical assessment, the nurse evaluates the client's visual acuity, particularly peripheral vision. Bilateral temporal headaches are not an uncommon finding. Cranial nerves III, IV, and VI are sometimes affected by pituitary tumor growth, which results in diplopia and ocular muscle paralysis (see Chap. 32 for further discussion of neurologic assessment).

Gonadotropin deficiency results in characteristic physical changes. When examining the adult male, the nurse checks for a *decrease* or loss of *facial or body hair.* Examination of the extremities reveals a decrease in muscle mass and tone. *Testicular atrophy* is a common finding. In the prepubertal male, the nurse notes the *absence of secondary sex characteristics,* and gonad and penis size may appear small for the client's age. When

conducting the physical assessment of the adult female, the nurse observes any decrease or loss of axillary and pubic hair. Skin appears dry, and atrophy of the breast is noted. In the prepubertal female, there is a partial or complete absence of secondary sex characteristics; therefore, the nurse checks for breast development and presence of axillary and pubic hair. Clients may report painful intercourse because of decreased vaginal secretions and a decrease in libido.

GH deficiency does not cause appreciable clinical manifestations in the adult. Children appear to be normal at birth, but by 6 months of age, growth retardation is apparent. The nurse examines the client for an increase in truncal fat and delayed secondary tooth appearance.

Psychosocial Assessment

Hypopituitarism, particularly related to GH and gonadotropin deficiencies, produces marked changes in physical appearance. In the psychosocial assessment, the nurse focuses on the client's sense of body image and feelings of self-worth. An altered physical appearance can affect the client's self-esteem and may interfere with the development of interpersonal relationships.

In GH deficiency, decreased physical stature presents a number of developmental and social difficulties. The client's physical size may present limitations in performing activities of daily living (ADL). In social situations, clients with GH deficiency are sometimes viewed as being younger than their chronologic age and may not be accepted by their peers. Impaired growth is not normally accompanied by mental deficits, yet clients may report being spoken to as if they were children. The nurse attempts to elicit the client's feelings and experiences related to a small physical size.

The nurse assesses the client with gonadotropin deficiency for concerns relating to a change in physical appearance and determines the effect on the client's life style. Loss or absence of secondary sex characteristics are often profoundly disturbing to the client because sexual identity is a key element of an individual's self-concept. A client with a decrease in libido may report a serious strain in the relationship with the sexual partner.

Fertility difficulties cause emotional distress in individuals striving for parenthood. Emotional distress may be manifested by reports of depression, episodes of crying, and feelings of hopelessness and frustration.

Laboratory Findings

In hypopituitarism, there can be a wide variance in laboratory findings. When clinical suspicion of hypopituitarism exists, basal levels of some target organ hormones can be measured easily. Hormone assays are readily available for tri-iodothyronine and thyroxine from the thyroid and for testosterone and estradiol from the gonads. If levels of one or all of these hormones are low or in the low-normal range and there is a high clinical suspicion (e.g., client presents with a hypothalamic tumor), further evaluation is mandated. Basal levels of pituitary gonadotropins (LH and FSH) and TSH are sufficient if target organ function is demonstrated. ACTH levels may be normal or low, and PRL levels vary from low to high. GH levels are usually in the low to low-normal range. More sophisticated diagnostic evaluation in the form of stimulation tests may be necessary to assess pituitary reserve.

Radiographic Findings

Conventional x-ray films of the skull can define certain abnormalities of the sella turcica, including enlargement, erosion, and calcifications in the area of the sella. Computed tomography (CT) is used to define intrasellar and suprasellar lesions. Iohexol (Omnipaque), a water-soluble dye, is used in conjunction with a CT scan and has replaced pneumoencephalography in defining suprasellar lesions. Angiography is used routinely by some diagnosticians to rule out the presence of an aneurysm or congenital vascular malformations before any surgical intervention.

Other Diagnostic Tests

Magnetic resonance imaging is also used to define intrasellar and suprasellar lesions.

In some cases, pituitary reserve cannot be assessed without the use of stimulation tests. Cortisol deficiency may be life-threatening, and the ability of the pituitary to secrete ACTH in response to stress is essential for homeostasis. The insulin tolerance test is performed to assess ACTH and GH reserves. Regular insulin (0.05 to 1.0 units/kg of body weight) is administered to induce hypoglycemia, which acts as a stimulus for release of GH and ACTH.

Metyrapone is a drug that blocks the conversion of 11-deoxycortisol to cortisol. The hypothalamic-pituitary axis responds to the decreasing plasma cortisol level by increased production and release of ACTH. ACTH levels can be measured directly or indirectly by measuring the effect on the adrenal gland. The normal value for ACTH is less than 100 pg/mL.

Thyrotropin-releasing hormone (TRH) is given to stimulate production of TSH from the pituitary. PRL levels also rise in response to TRH. The normal value for PRL is less than 25 mg/mL.

Gonadotropin-releasing hormone (Gn-RH) is given to stimulate the production of LH and FSH. Normal results are based on a peak response occurring between 15 and 45 minutes after administration of Gn-RH.

 Analysis: Nursing Diagnosis

Common Diagnoses

The following nursing diagnoses are often seen in clients with hypopituitarism:

1. Body image disturbance related to lack or loss of hormones (FSH or LH) and to altered physical stature (GH)

2. Sexual dysfunction related to loss of testosterone or estrogen

3. Ineffective individual coping related to impaired self-concept

Additional Diagnoses

Clients with hypopituitarism may also have the following additional nursing diagnoses:

1. Self-esteem disturbance related to changes in physical appearance

2. Sensory/perceptual alterations (visual) related to compression by tumor

3. Knowledge deficit related to diagnosis and treatment

 Planning and Implementation

Body Image Disturbance

Planning: client goals.   The goal for this nursing diagnosis is that the client will experience an improvement in his or her body image.

Interventions: nonsurgical management.   In gonadotropin deficiency, an altered physical appearance, especially loss of secondary sex characteristics, can lead to a disturbance in self-concept. Clients are encouraged to verbalize feelings of concern or anxiety about body changes. The nurse stresses the role of hormone replacement, which usually corrects the loss of secondary sex characteristics. A major nursing role in gonadotropin deficiency is discussion and review of hormone replacement therapy (see the following section).

In GH deficiency syndromes, small physical size can affect the client's body image and performance of ADL. A common problem in clients with short stature is that they are not treated in accord with their chronologic age. Other individuals tend to respond to them based on how old they look, which is often many years younger than their actual age. It is important that the nurse relate to the client in the age-appropriate manner and encourage behaviors consistent with chronologic age. Promoting independence of clients who may have problems with ADL may enhance their self-concept.

Clients with isolated GH deficiency may be treated by administration of exogenous GH. Somatropin (Humatrope) should be used before closure of the epiphyses. It must be determined that short stature is the result of GH deficiency before initiation of therapy. Dosage and administration schedule are individualized for each client, and the route of administration is intramuscular injection. Somatropin can induce a state of insulin resistance. The nurse observes the client for the presence of hyperglycemia and glycosuria. Infrequently, headache, localized muscle pain, weakness, and a mild, transient edema have been observed during the course of therapy. Antibodies to GH have been observed in clients treated with somatropin. The long-term effects of antibody development are unknown at present, but they do not appear to limit growth. Clients being treated with somatropin should have periodic thyroid function studies because hypothyroidism is known to occur after initiation of therapy.

Sexual Dysfunction

Planning: client goals. The goal for this nursing diagnosis is that the client will achieve the personal desired level of sexual functioning.

Interventions: nonsurgical management. The nurse identifies the particular problems facing each client, including the effect that sexual dysfunction has had on the client's relationship with his or her sexual partner. Clients are instructed about hormone replacement therapy, which usually corrects the physiologic problems related to sexual activity.

Males with gonadotropin deficiency are treated with androgens (testosterone), and the most effective route of administration is intramuscular. The nurse instructs the client in self-administration. The initial dose may be as low as 50 mg, and the dosage is *gradually* increased to the usual maintenance level of 200 mg. Dosage often depends on age, with elderly clients requiring a lower amount of hormone replacement. Clients usually require testosterone injections every 4 to 6 weeks. Determination of the time interval between injections is based on clinical evaluation of the client and the recurrence of symptoms, e.g., impotence. Care must be taken not to institute testosterone therapy until the client's growth potential has been achieved because testosterone may cause premature closure of the bone epiphyses.

The nurse observes the client for side effects of testosterone therapy, which include gynecomastia (development of breast tissue in men) and baldness (if the client has an inherited tendency for balding). Prostatic hypertrophy may develop in older clients. Maximal effects of treatment include increases in penis size, libido, and muscle mass. Chest, facial, pubic, and axillary hair growth increases. The client's voice noticeably deepens, and bone size and strength increase. Clients usually report an increase in self-esteem and improved body image after therapy is initiated.

However, the therapy for achieving fertility in these clients, especially men, is difficult at best. Testosterone replacement is used for initial and long-term treatment of gonadotropin deficiency, but to restore or achieve fertility, parenteral gonadotropin administration is necessary. Testosterone therapy is discontinued because parenteral therapy cannot achieve the high levels necessary for spermatogenesis. Human chorionic gonadotropin (hCG), 5000 units, is administered intramuscularly three times per week for 4 to 6 months until testosterone levels are normal. hCG injections (3000 units) are continued three times per week to keep the testosterone level in the normal range. After the first 4 to 6 months of hCG therapy, Pergonal (75 units of LH and 75 units of FSH) is given intramuscularly three times per week.

Clients must receive the combined hCG and Pergonal treatment for at least 5 to 6 months. After 6 months of combined therapy, if testosterone levels and sperm counts remain low, therapy is usually discontinued. When therapeutic results are achieved, treatment is continued until conception occurs (Braunwald et al., 1987). The nurse's role in fertility treatment with hCG is education of the client about the course of therapy and support of the client and family because of the uncertainty of the treatment outcome.

Females who have reached the age of puberty receive hormone replacement with a combination of estrogen and progesterone administered in a cyclic manner, which causes withdrawal bleeding. Caution should be exercised in administering these hormones to clients who have not achieved full growth potential because they also may cause premature closure of the epiphyses. Clients must be aware of the possibility of developing hypertension or thrombophlebitis associated with estrogen therapy. In female clients who wish to become pregnant, clomiphene citrate (Clomid) is frequently used to induce ovulation.

Ineffective Individual Coping

Planning: client goals. The goal for this nursing diagnosis is that the client will develop coping responses to the physical and emotional features of GH deficiency.

Interventions: nonsurgical management. The nurse assists the client in identifying sources of support. Helping the client to see his or her particular strengths is the first step in promoting independence. The nurse includes the family when planning care, encourages the use of support groups, and suggests contacting individuals and families with the same diagnosis. Clients may also benefit from psychologic counseling to assist them in developing coping skills.

■ Discharge Planning

Home Care Preparation

The client with isolated gonadotropin deficiency does not require specific changes in the home environment. Clients with GH deficiency may need modifications in the home as a result of short stature. Most homes have kitchen and bathroom facilities that are built to accommodate individuals of average height. The nurse encourages the client to identify barriers in the home that may affect the ability to perform ADL. Simple adaptations, such as the use of tabletop telephones, stools, and stepladders, can greatly increase the independence of the client with GH deficiency.

Client/Family Education

Clients with hypopituitarism usually require hormone replacement therapy, which necessitates specific instruction about administration. Thyroid and adrenal replacement therapy is discussed under hypothyroidism and adrenal hypofunction, respectively. The nurse educates male clients with gonadotropin deficiency in intramuscular injection technique and emphasizes the importance of rotating injection sites. Testosterone replacement doses are prescribed by the physician on the basis of clinical evaluation and laboratory analysis. Once the maintenance dose is attained, clients are instructed to report any recurrence of symptoms, such as impotence and decreased libido, to the health care provider.

For fertility treatment, testosterone injections in the male client are stopped and hCG therapy is initiated. The nurse informs the client that he will again experience the symptoms of gonadotropin deficiency until the testicles respond to therapy by producing testosterone. The female client with gonadotropin deficiency must be aware of the side effects of estrogen therapy. Hypertension may occur, and the nurse recommends frequent blood pressure checks. Clients may be taught to monitor their own blood pressure. Another side effect of estrogen therapy is thrombophlebitis. Clients are instructed to report any pain in the legs, particularly the calves, to their health care provider. Periodic gynecologic and breast examinations are recommended for these clients for early identification of potential problems such as malignancy.

Clients receiving GH replacement and/or family members require instruction in intramuscular injection technique. Somatropin needs to be reconstituted before injection. The diluent is injected into the vial by aiming the stream against the glass wall, not directly into the powder. The vial is then *gently* rotated until the contents are dissolved. Clients should never shake the bottle because agitation decreases the effectiveness of the hormone preparation. The somatropin vial and diluent are stable when refrigerated (36° to 46° F) before reconstitution until the expiration date. After reconstitution, somatropin is stable for up to 14 days when refrigerated (*Physicians' Desk Reference*, 1990, p. 1216). The nurse reviews reported side effects of therapy, such as transient edema, headache, weakness, and localized muscle pain. Clients are instructed to test their urine for the presence of glucose because mild hyperglycemia has been known to occur with somatropin therapy.

Psychosocial Preparation

In clients with gonadotropin deficiency, target organ hormone replacement usually corrects physiologic problems associated with sexual activity and loss of secondary sex characteristics. The nurse must stress that changes occur *gradually*. Often clients anticipate a rapid resolution of symptoms and are disappointed when this does not occur. In the area of fertility, tropic hormones are used to stimulate the gonads. The nurse encourages a positive outlook but discusses the fact that conception does not always occur after initiation of therapy. Clients are encouraged to discuss their fears and concerns re-

garding fertility and can be referred to support groups if necessary.

In GH deficiency, the most important aspect of psychosocial preparation is to attempt to improve the client's self-concept and coping abilities. The nurse identifies the client's sources of support and strength and encourages the client to verbalize fears and anxieties. Ongoing professional counseling often helps the client to deal with stressors in daily life.

Health Care Resources

In both gonadotropin and GH deficiencies, clients must have ready access to the health care team. Questions about dosage and administration of replacement hormones often arise and need to be addressed promptly.

Clients with gonadotropin deficiency often experience stress related to infertility. Support groups in many geographic areas are specifically geared to discussing problems associated with infertility.

Clients requiring GH replacement are often faced with financial problems because somatropin is expensive therapy. If the client's health care insurance does not cover the cost, other avenues of financing need to be explored. The client's physician or social worker may be aware of other sources available to underwrite the cost.

 Evaluation

The following outcomes apply to the client with common nursing diagnoses for gonadotropin and GH deficiencies and include that the client

1. Improves body image
2. Participates in sexual activity as desired
3. Describes and complies with hormone replacement regimen
4. Demonstrates proper intramuscular injection technique
5. Identifies symptoms of inadequate hormone replacement
6. Identifies side effects of hormone replacement
7. Uses support groups if needed
8. Performs ADL independently
9. Develops relationships with peers

Clients meeting the stated outcomes will have a smoother adjustment period after discharge from the health care facility.

HYPERPITUITARISM

OVERVIEW

Hyperpituitarism is a pathologic state that occurs with pituitary tumors or hyperplasia not associated with the absence of the normal regulatory feedback mechanisms. These disorders usually arise from the somatotrophic (GH), lactotrophic (PRL), and corticotrophic (ACTH) cells located in the anterior pituitary (adenohypophysis). The major exception to this generalization is the overproduction of PRL that may be associated with tumors that produce other hormones such as GH or ACTH. Hypersecretion of ACTH is sometimes associated with increased secretion of MSH. Tumors producing TSH or LH and FSH are known to exist but are so rare that only a few cases have been documented.

Pathophysiology

A common reason for hyperpituitarism is the presence of a pituitary *adenoma*, a benign epithelial tumor. Adenomas are classified by size, degree of invasiveness, and the hormone secreted. An *invasive* pituitary adenoma involves a portion or all of the sella turcica. When there is no involvement of the sella turcica, the adenoma is termed *enclosed*. *Microadenomas* are less than 10 mm in diameter. Tumors larger than 10 mm are classified as *macroadenomas*.

Alterations in neurologic function may occur as adenomas grow and compress surrounding structures. Neurologic manifestations vary but may include visual defects, headache, and increased intracranial pressure. PRL-secreting tumors are the most frequently seen type of pituitary adenoma. Excess PRL inhibits the secretion of gonadal steroids and gonadotropins in males and females, which results in galactorrhea, amenorrhea, and infertility.

Overproduction of GH results in *gigantism* or *acromegaly* (Figs. 49–1 and 49–2). The onset of the disease may be insidious, and frequently the disorder has been present for years before the diagnosis is made. Early detection and treatment are essential to prevent irreversible changes in anatomic structure. The changes that occur in the soft tissues such as the face, hands, feet, and skin are to a certain extent reversible after treatment. The changes in the skeleton, however, are permanent. In gigantism, the age of onset of GH hypersecretion is *before* closure of the epiphyses and puberty, which causes rapid proportional growth in the length of all bones. In acromegaly, excess GH produces increased skeletal thickness, hypertrophy of the skin, and enlargement of visceral organs.

In adults, bony changes related to excess GH occur slowly and include cortical thickening, tufting of terminal phalanges (arrowhead fingertips), and bone cell proliferation. Degeneration of joint cartilage and hypertrophy of ligaments, vocal cords, and eustachian tube mucosa are common. Nerve entrapment occurs because of tissue overgrowth, and demyelination of peripheral nerves is also seen. In addition, GH is an insulin antagonist, and glucose intolerance is not an unusual occurrence.

Hypersecretion of ACTH results in overstimulation of the adrenal cortex, producing excessive amounts of glucocorticoids, mineralocorticoids, and androgens, which leads to the development of Cushing's disease (see later for a discussion of Cushing's disease).

Etiology

Most cases of hyperpituitarism are the result of hormone-secreting adenomas arising from their respective cell types. Hyperpituitarism can also occur because of hypothalamic dysfunction.

Most adenomas develop in clients without a family history of similar problems, but adenomas may be a part of a syndrome known as *multiple endocrine neoplasia*. As a familial disorder, it is passed on through an autosomal dominant trait and may include parathyroid and pancreatic tumors.

Incidence

The most common secretory tumors are prolactinomas, followed by GH-producing adenomas. Tumors secreting gonadotropin or TSH are the least common (Wilson & Foster, 1985). Of all tumors for which surgery is done, approximately 70% secrete one or more hormones. The

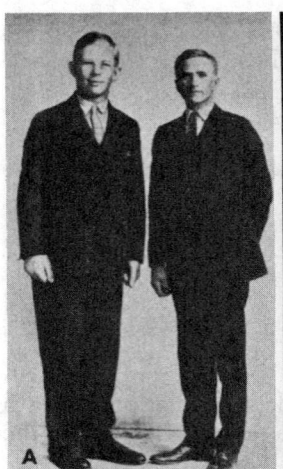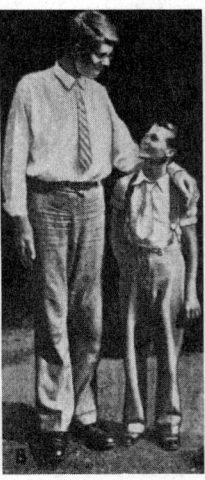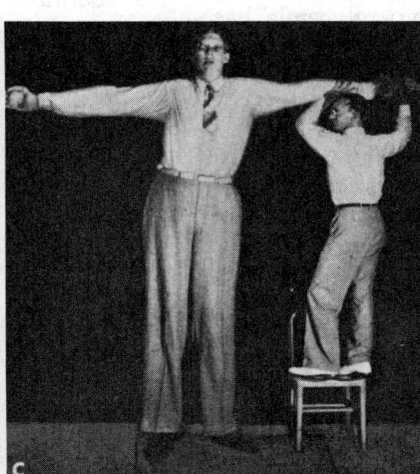

Figure 49–1

Clinical features of GH excess. Robert Wadlow, the "Alton giant," weighed 9 lb at birth but grew to 30 lb by 6 months of age. By his first birthday he had reached 62 lb. By the time of his death at age 22 from cellulitis of the feet, he was 8 ft 11 in tall and weighed 475 lb. (*A* and *B* from Fadner, F. [1944]. *Biography of Robert Wadlow.* Courtesy of Bruce Humphries, Publishers. *C*, Courtesy of C. M. Charles and C. M. MacBryde.)

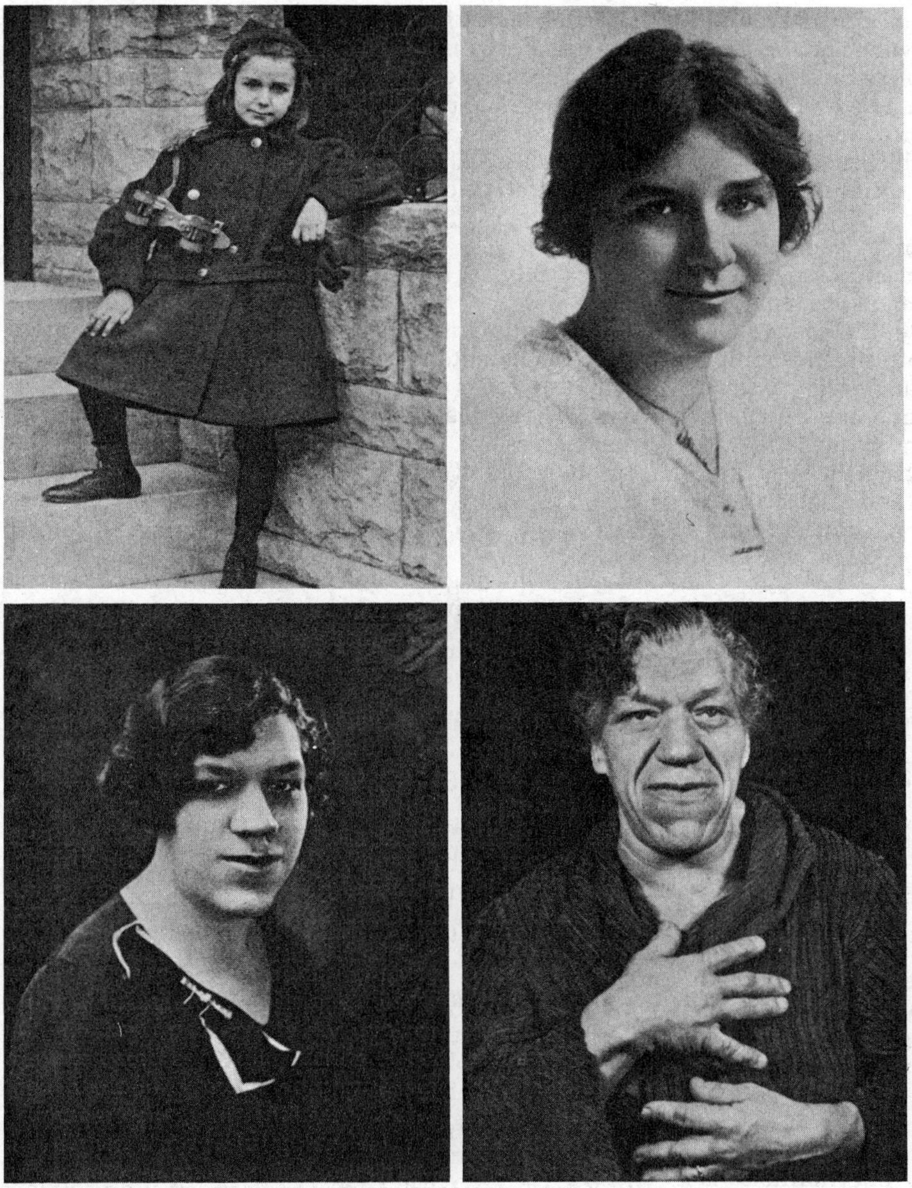

Figure 49–2

Progression of acromegaly. (From Mendeloff, A., & Smith, D. E. [Eds.]. [1956]. Acromegaly, diabetes, hypermetabolism, proteinuria and heart failure. Clinical Pathological Conference. *American Journal of Medicine, 20*, 133.)

occurrence of hyperpituitarism in the general population is rare.

COLLABORATIVE MANAGEMENT

Assessment

History

The symptoms of hyperpituitarism vary depending on the hormone produced in excess. The nurse obtains data from the client regarding *age, sex,* and *family history*. The nurse asks the client if there has been a change in hat, glove, ring, or shoe size. A change in energy level may occur, with the client reporting fatigue and lethargy. Individuals with excess GH describe *discomfort,*

such as backache and arthralgias. Complaints of visual difficulties and headaches should be noted.

Clients with hypersecretion of PRL often report difficulties in *sexual functioning*. The nurse asks the female client about *menstrual changes*, e.g., amenorrhea, irregular menses, or difficulty in achieving pregnancy, and about decreased libido or painful intercourse. Male clients may report decreased libido and impotence.

Physical Assessment: Clinical Manifestations

Initial manifestations noted in the hypersecretion of GH are changes in the *facial features* (increase in lip and nose size, prominent supraorbital ridge) and *enlarging head, hand, and foot size*. Prognathism, a projection of the jaw beyond the facial features, becomes marked, and the nurse assesses for difficulty in chewing and for dentures that no longer fit. *Arthritic changes* causing joint pain and decreased mobility are often noted. The nurse observes the distal phalanges for an arrowhead or tufted characteristic on x-ray films and a thickened appearance. Increased perspiration and oil secretion may be noted on the client's skin.

At the onset, both acromegaly and gigantism are characterized by increased metabolism and strength. As the diseases progress, these manifestations are replaced with lethargy and weakness. The nurse also assesses the client's vision. Other prominent features of this entity include *organomegaly* (cardiac or hepatic), *hypertension, dysphagia* because of an enlarged tongue, and a *deepening of the voice* because of hypertrophy of the larynx.

Hypersecretion of PRL (hyperprolactinemia) is frequently observed with hypogonadism and galactorrhea. Galactorrhea may be seen in either sex but is found predominantly in females.

Psychosocial Assessment

Clients with hyperpituitarism often present with dramatic changes in physical appearance. The nurse assesses the impact of these physical changes on the client's interpersonal relationships. Clients are encouraged to verbalize their feelings relating to body image. The nurse identifies the client's strengths and key supports, which may be incorporated into a plan of care.

In hyperpituitarism, clients may have fertility difficulties. In clients who are disturbed by an ability to conceive, the nurse identifies symptoms of emotional distress, such as crying and reports of depression. Irritability and hostility may be evident. Because intracranial lesions are often an etiologic factor in hyperpituitarism, clients may express fear of this diagnosis, as well as anxiety concerning subsequent surgery and prognosis.

Laboratory Findings

In hyperpituitarism, usually only one hormone is produced in excess, the most common being PRL, ACTH, or GH. Tumors producing LH or FSH are extremely rare. Elevated levels of any of these hormones demand further investigation. The level of LH and FSH is normally elevated in the postmenopausal and climateric adult.

Radiographic Findings

Radiographic evaluation in hyperpituitarism is identical to the diagnostic work-up for hyperpituitarism (see earlier).

Other Diagnostic Tests

Suppression tests are helpful in the diagnosis of hyperpituitarism. Dexamethasone suppression tests are used to test the suppressibility of ACTH from the pitui-

tary (see later discussion of diagnostic tests for Cushing's syndrome).

A glucose tolerance test for GH suppression is done by giving a standard amount of glucose (100 g orally or 0.5 g/kg body weight intravenously) and measuring GH levels serially for up to 120 minutes. Failure of GH levels to fall below 5 ng/mL indicates a positive result.

 ### Analysis: Nursing Diagnosis

In hyperpituitarism, there is an overproduction of one or more of the anterior pituitary hormones. The nursing diagnoses focus on excesses of PRL and GH. An excess of ACTH results in hypercortisolism (see later for further discussion). Overproduction of other anterior pituitary hormones (TSH, LH, and FSH) is extremely rare.

Common Diagnoses

The following common nursing diagnoses are seen in the client with hyperpituitarism:

1. Body image disturbance related to altered physical appearance
2. Sexual dysfunction related to PRL excess

Additional Diagnoses

The client with hyperpituitarism may also have the following additional nursing diagnoses:

1. Pain related to the presence of intracranial mass
2. Fear related to diagnosis and treatment (intracranial mass)
3. Ineffective individual coping related to impaired self-concept
4. Activity intolerance related to effects of excess GH, e.g., joint pain
5. Sensory/perceptual alterations (visual) related to tumor or compression of surrounding structures
6. Knowledge deficit related to diagnosis and treatment

 ### Planning and Implementation

Body Image Disturbance

Planning: client goals. The primary goal for this nursing diagnosis is that the client will experience an improvement in body image.

Interventions: nonsurgical management. The client with excess GH may have skeletal changes that cannot be reversed with treatment. Clients are encouraged to verbalize concerns and fears related to an altered physical appearance. The nurse helps the client to identify his or her strengths and positive characteristics, reinforcing the uniqueness and importance of each individual.

In the client with excess PRL, galactorrhea, gynecomastia, and difficulties in sexual functioning can cause disturbances in the client's body image and personal identity. The nurse reinforces that treatment may alleviate some of these symptoms but encourages the client to discuss feelings related to these changes.

Drug therapy. Bromocriptine mesylate (Parlodel) is the treatment of choice in clients with hyperprolactinemia. Bromocriptine is highly effective in decreasing PRL levels to normal in clients with microadenomas and by about 90% in clients with macroadenomas. Shrinkage of macroadenomas occurs in the majority of cases. Bromocriptine has been useful in treating clients with acromegaly by reducing GH levels and decreasing tumor size, especially when GH levels remain high after surgery or before the full effect of radiation therapy. Side effects of bromocriptine include postural hypotension, gastric irritation, nausea, headaches, abdominal cramps, and constipation. The nurse gives bromocriptine with a meal or snack to help alleviate some of these side effects. It is also helpful to start with a low dose and gradually increase it until the desired level (usually 7.5 mg/day) is reached. If pregnancy should occur during therapy with bromocriptine, the drug should be stopped immediately.

Radiation therapy. Radiation therapy is not a useful tool in the management of acute hyperpituitarism. Conventional radiation therapy regimens takes a long time to complete, and several years pass before any therapeutic effect is seen. Proton beam or alpha particle radiation is effective, but the response is slow. Side effects of radiation therapy include hypopituitarism, optic nerve damage, oculomotor dysfunction, and visual field defects (Wilson & Foster, 1985). Chapter 25 includes a discussion of nursing management for the client undergoing radiation therapy.

Interventions: surgical management. Surgical removal of a microadenoma or of the pituitary gland *(hypophysectomy)* is frequently done in the treatment of hyperpituitarism. A *transsphenoidal* approach to the pituitary gland is commonly used. Transsphenoidal hypophysectomy is microscopic surgery performed with the client under general anesthesia and in a semisitting position. The initial incision is made at the inner aspect of the upper lip, and the sella turcica is entered via the sphenoid sinus (Fig. 49–3). After the gland is removed, a muscle graft is taken, often from the anterior thigh, to pack the dura and to prevent leakage of cerebrospinal fluid (CSF). Nasal packing is done after the incision is closed, and a dressing is applied under the nose to prevent the packing from dislodging. If the tumor is inaccessible by this route, a *transfrontal craniotomy* may be indicated (see Chapter 33).

Preoperative care. The nurse reviews with the client that hypophysectomy will decrease hormone levels, relieve headaches, and possibly reverse changes in sexual functioning; body changes, visceral enlargement, and

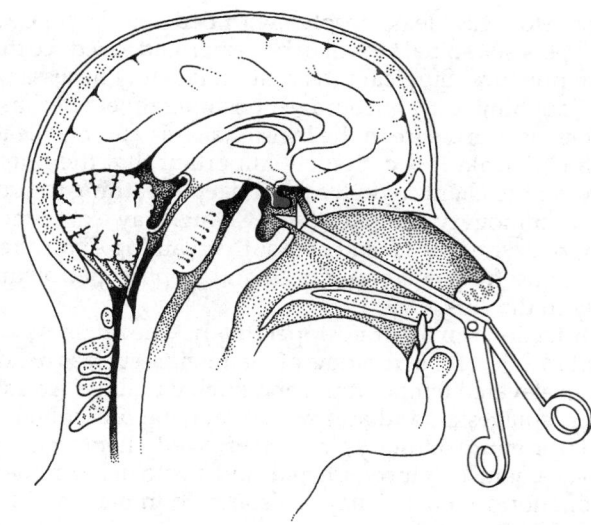

Figure 49–3

Transsphenoidal surgical approach to the pituitary gland. Selective adenomectomy leaves normal pituitary tissue undisturbed.

visual changes are not usually reversible. The nurse explains that nasal packing is present for 2 to 3 days postoperatively, which necessitates mouth breathing. A "moustache" dressing will be placed under the client's nose. Clients may experience headaches and some discomfort at the graft site on the thigh. The nurse reviews with the client that toothbrushing, coughing, sneezing, nose blowing, and bending are all avoided postoperatively because they can interfere with healing of the incision or can disrupt the muscle graft.

The nurse explains preoperative diagnostic tests, neuroradiologic examinations, endocrine testing, and visual field examinations to the client. Nasal and oral mucous membrane swabs for bacterial culture and sensitivity are obtained preoperatively.

Postoperative care. The nurse monitors the client's neurologic status and notes changes in vision, disorientation, change in level of consciousness, and decreased strength of extremities. The nurse observes the client for the occurrence of postoperative complications; e.g., transient diabetes insipidus can occur. The nurse monitors the intake of intravenous fluid, encourages fluid intake in response to thirst, and administers vasopressin when indicated. In diabetes insipidus, specific gravity measurements of urine are low, and clients are polyuric. A urinary catheter may be inserted for accurate measuring or urinary output, and daily weights are taken.

The nurse instructs the client to report any postnasal drip, which might indicate leakage of CSF. The head of the bed is elevated postoperatively. Nasal drainage is assessed for quantity and quality. Clear nasal drainage is tested for glucose, whose presence indicates that the fluid is CSF. If the client complains of persistent, severe headaches, CSF fluid may have leaked into the sinus area. Most CSF leaks resolve with bed rest. If the CSF leak persists, spinal taps may be performed to reduce the CSF pressure. Surgical intervention is rarely necessary.

Coughing is *not* encouraged postoperatively because it increases pressure in the incisional area and may lead to a CSF leak. It is extremely important that the nurse remind the client to do frequent deep breathing to prevent pulmonary complications. Clients may experience mouth dryness as a result of mouth breathing. The nurse performs frequent oral rinses and applies petroleum jelly to dry lips.

Infection can occur postoperatively. The nurse is particularly alert for symptoms of meningitis, such as headache, elevated temperature, and nuchal rigidity. Antibiotics, analgesics, and antipyretics may be prescribed.

If the entire pituitary gland is removed, clients require replacement of glucocorticoid and thyroid hormones. (Gonadotropin deficiency is also noted in male and female clients.)

Sexual Dysfunction

Planning: client goals. The primary goal for this nursing diagnosis is that the client will achieve a personal desired level of sexual functioning.

Interventions: nonsurgical management. The nurse identifies which specific problems the client is experiencing and encourages the client to discuss any effect that sexual dysfunction has had on the relationship with his or her sexual partner. Drug therapy with bromocriptine mesylate is effective in decreasing PRL levels in clients with PRL-secreting tumors. After PRL levels are decreased, normal gonadotropin function often returns. Clients requiring hypophysectomy for hyperpituitarism may experience sexual dysfunction as a result of gonadotropin deficiency after surgery. (See earlier for a discussion of hormone replacement in gonadotropin deficiency.)

■ Discharge Planning

Home Care Preparation

Clients with advanced acromegaly may experience arthritic changes. The nurse assesses the degree of mobility impairment and identifies appropriate adaptations, such as the use of ambulatory aids (cane or walker), and accessibility of bathroom facilities.

Client/Family Education

After transsphenoidal hypophysectomy, the nurse instructs the client to avoid activities that might interfere with healing.

Clients must avoid bending over from the waist to pick up objects or tie shoes. The nurse instructs the client to bend from the knees and then lower the body to the ground to retrieve fallen objects. Intracranial pressure increases when clients strain to have a bowel move-

ment. Measures to prevent constipation such as eating high-fiber foods, drinking additional fluids, and use of stool softeners or laxatives are instituted. Both bending and straining with defecation need to be avoided for up to 2 months after surgery.

The nurse encourages the client to use mouthwash or dental floss for 1 to 2 weeks until brushing of teeth can be resumed after the incision has healed. Transient numbness in the area of the incision and a decreased sense of smell are usual and lasts 3 to 4 months. Because of reduced sensation, the nurse advises the client to use a mirror to check gums for bleeding.

After hypophysectomy, hormone replacement may be required to maintain fluid balance (see later for discussion of vasopressin replacement). If the entire gland is removed, clients may require instruction in cortisol, thyroid, and gonadal insufficiency. The nurse instructs the client to report the return of any symptoms of hyperpituitarism immediately to the primary health care provider.

Psychosocial Preparation

After treatment, clients with hyperpituitarism may need to adhere to daily self-management regimens and frequent check-ups. The client may need to develop strategies to minimize stress to prevent alterations of hormone production.

Health Care Resources

Clients with decreased mobility related to acromegaly or those who have had recent surgery may require a home care nurse for maintenance of ADL. In addition, clients with hyperpituitarism must continue to have hormone levels monitored at regular intervals to detect recurrence of tumor at an early stage. Access to the physician and other health care team members is essential.

 Evaluation

The following expected outcomes are based on the common nursing diagnoses for hyperpituitarism and include that the client

1. Improves body image
2. Participates in sexual activity, as desired
3. Identifies activities to be avoided after transsphenoidal hypophysectomy
4. Identifies side effects of prescribed medications
5. Describes and complies with hormone replacement regimen (if applicable)
6. Identifies recurrence of symptoms of hyperpituitarism

Clients who meet these stated outcomes will have fewer problems with transition to the home after discharge from the health care facility and may be more likely to report problems to the health care team.

Disorders of the Posterior Pituitary Gland

Disorders of the posterior pituitary, or *neurohypophysis*, are directly related to a deficiency or excess of the hormone vasopressin (antidiuretic hormone [ADH]). Two disorders are associated with ADH deficiency or excess: diabetes insipidus and the syndrome of inappropriate antidiuretic hormone (SIADH). Knowledge of the pathophysiology, etiology, and clinical manifestations of diabetes insipidus and SIADH aids the nurse in making assessments that can lead to early detection and treatment.

DIABETES INSIPIDUS

OVERVIEW

Diabetes insipidus is a disorder of water metabolism caused by a deficiency of ADH. There is either a decrease in ADH synthesis or an inability of the kidney to respond appropriately to ADH.

ADH deficiency results in excretion of large volumes of dilute urine. Deficiency of ADH severely impairs the permeability of the distal tubules and collecting ducts of the kidneys to water. An excessive loss of free water occurs, and this results in polyuria.

Dehydration accompanying this massive diuresis results in an increase in plasma osmolality, which stimulates the osmoreceptors to relay a sensation or thirst to the cerebral cortex. Normally, thirst promotes increased fluid intake and aids in maintaining water homeostasis. However, if the thirst compensatory mechanism is inadequate or absent, dehydration persists and worsens.

ADH deficiency can be classified as nephrogenic, primary, secondary, or drug related. *Nephrogenic diabetes insipidus* is an inherited defect in which the renal tubules do not respond to the actions of ADH, which results in inadequate water reabsorption by the kidney. The amount of hormone is not deficient. *Primary diabetes insipidus* results from a defect in the pituitary gland related to familial or idiopathic causes. *Secondary diabetes insipidus* results from tumors in the hypothalamic-pituitary region, head trauma, infectious processes, surgical procedures (hypophysectomy), or metastatic tumors, usually from the lung or breast. Less frequently, it is caused by cerebrovascular hemorrhage, granulomatous disease, or cerebral aneurysm. *Drug-related ADH deficiency* is caused by lithium (Eskalith, Lithobid) and demeclocycline (Declomycin), which can interfere with the renal response to ADH.

COLLABORATIVE MANAGEMENT

In the process of assessing a client with diabetes insipidus, an increase in the frequency of urination and ex-

cessive thirst are key symptoms to note. A history of any of the known etiologic factors, such as recent surgery, head trauma, or medication use (e.g., lithium), is also noted. Although increased fluid intake usually prevents serious dehydration and volume depletion, clients deprived of fluids or clients who cannot increase their oral fluid intake may experience circulatory collapse caused by fluid loss and neurologic changes related to plasma hyperosmolality. Signs of dehydration such as poor skin turgor and dry or cracked mucous membranes or skin may be present in varying degrees (see Chap. 13 for further discussion of clients with dehydration).

Loss of free water produces characteristic changes in blood and urine studies (Wilson & Foster, 1985). The initial step in diagnosis is to measure a 24-hour fluid intake and output. The amount of the client's food and fluid is not restricted during this measurement. Urinary output must be more than 4 L during this period for the diagnosis of diabetes insipidus to be considered. The amount of urine excreted in a 24-hour period may vary from 4 to 30 L/day. Urine is dilute and therefore has a low specific gravity (less than 1.005) and low osmolality (50 to 200 mOsm/kg). Additional studies used for diagnosis are fluid deprivation and hypertonic saline tests. For nursing care of clients undergoing these special diagnostic tests, see the accompanying Guidelines feature.

Medical management is aimed at controlling the symptoms of the disease by various types of drug therapy. If only a partial deficit of ADH is present, effective control of symptoms can be achieved by the use of oral chlorpropamide (Diabinese) or clofibrate (Atromid S). These drugs augment the action of existing ADH and are believed to have a direct stimulating effect on the synthesis of ADH in the hypothalamus. When ADH deficiency is severe, ADH is replaced in amounts sufficient to maintain water homeostasis. For short-term therapy or when the dosage must be changed frequently, aqueous vasopressin is given subcutaneously or intramuscularly (Wilson & Foster, 1985). In long-term therapy, nasal sprays (lypressin or desmopressin) are preferred. However, ulceration of the mucous membranes, allergy, a sensation of chest tightness, and inhalation of the spray, which precipitates pulmonary problems, may be associated with the use of these sprays. If side effects occur or if the client develops an upper respiratory tract infection, sustained-action vasopressin (vasopressin tannate in oil) is administered intramuscularly (Table 49-1).

Nursing management is aimed at early detection of dehydration and maintenance of adequate hydration. Interventions include accurately measuring fluid intake and output, checking urine specific gravity, and recording daily weight. The nurse encourages the client to consume oral fluids approximately equal to the amount of urinary output. If fluids are administered intravenously, the nurse ensures the patency of the access line and pays meticulous attention to the amount infused each hour. Clients with permanent diabetes insipidus require lifelong vasopressin therapy, and the nurse must assess the client's ability to follow instructions and

GUIDELINES ■ Care of the Client Undergoing Special Tests for Diabetes Insipidus

Procedure	Purpose	Interventions	Rationales
Fluid deprivation	To identify the cause of polyuria.	1. Obtain baseline vital signs; then check them hourly. 2. Deprive client of fluid. 3. Observe client for violation of restriction.	1–3. To detect changes, especially postural hypotension or tachycardia.
		4. Measure urinary output, specific gravity, and osmolality hourly. 5. Weigh client hourly.	4, 5. To determine whether testing can proceed. Testing can proceed if urinary osmolality stabilizes for 3 samples and 3% weight loss is noted.
		6. Give 5 units of aqueous vasopressin (subcutaneously). 7. Continue hourly measurements.	6, 7. To trigger and detect changes in specific gravity and osmolality. Specific gravity and osmolality will increase with primary and secondary diabetes insipidus. No response is seen with nephrogenic diabetes insipidus.
Hypertonic saline test	To stimulate release of ADH.	1. Administer normal water load to client, followed by infusion of hypertonic saline. 2. Measure urinary output hourly.	1, 2. To detect ADH release. A sudden decrease is a sign of ADH release.

willingness to participate in health care. Clients using vasopressin preparations are also instructed to recognize recurrence of polyuria and polydipsia as signals for another dose of medication. All clients taking these preparations need to record daily weight measurements to identify weight gain. The nurse emphasizes using the same scale and weighing at the same time of day while wearing a similar amount of clothing. Clients with diabetes insipidus should wear a medical alert (Medic Alert) bracelet identifying the disorder and current medication.

SYNDROME OF INAPPROPRIATE ANTIDIURETIC HORMONE

OVERVIEW

SIADH occurs when ADH (vasopressin) is secreted in the presence of low plasma osmolality. A decrease in plasma osmolality normally inhibits ADH production and secretion. SIADH is also known as the Schwartz-Bartter syndrome.

Pathophysiology

In SIADH, the feedback mechanisms that regulate ADH do not function properly. ADH continues to be released in the face of plasma hypo-osmolality. Water is *retained*, which results in dilutional hyponatremia and expansion of extracellular fluid volume. The increase in plasma volume causes an increase in the glomerular filtration rate and inhibits the release of renin and aldosterone. The combined effect of these occurrences is to increase the loss of sodium in the urine, which further contributes to the hyponatremic state.

Etiology

SIADH is associated with a variety of pathologic conditions. Oat cell carcinoma of the lung; carcinoma of the pancreas, duodenum, and genitourinary tract; thymomas; Ewing's sarcoma; and Hodgkin's and non-Hodgkin's lymphoma are implicated in the development of this disorder. It appears that malignant cells synthesize, store, and secrete a substance that is physiologically identical to ADH. Nonmalignant pulmonary tissue can be responsible for ectopic ADH production; therefore, SIADH is sometimes seen in conjunction with viral and bacterial pneumonia, lung abscesses, active tuberculosis, pneumothorax, chronic obstructive pulmonary disease, mycoses, and positive-pressure ventilation. Central nervous system disorders such as trauma, cerebrovascular accidents, central nervous system infection, tumors, porphyria, and systemic lupus erythematosus may interfere with ADH regulatory mechanisms and result in SIADH. Certain endocrinopathies and pharmacologic agents have been identified as etiologic factors. Numerous drugs have an effect on ADH production and release, whereas others potentiate the effect of ADH on the renal tubules. Implicated drugs include exogenous ADH, chlorpropamide, vincristine, cyclophosphamide, carbamazepine, general anesthetic agents, narcotics, and tricyclic antidepressants.

Incidence

The actual incidence of SIADH is unknown, but it is one of the most common causes of hyponatremia. It is *associated* with a wide variety of disorders and drugs.

PREVENTION

Clients taking exogenous vasopressin for the treatment of diabetes insipidus must be wary of overdosage because excessive amounts can result in the development of SIADH. Monitoring weight daily and reporting acute

TABLE 49-1   Drugs Used in the Treatment of Diabetes Insipidus

Drug	Usual Daily Dosage	Interventions	Rationales
Vasopressin tannate in oil (Pitressin Tannate in Oil)	0.3–1 mL as needed (IM)	1. Warm medication by rolling it in the hands before administration. 2. Have client drink 1–2 8-oz glassfuls of water before administration.	1. To ensure consistency of hormone suspension in oil. 2. To reduce side effects.
Lypressin	4–8 sprays (5–10 pressor units) (nasal spray)	1. Monitor client for upper respiratory tract infections.	1. To maximize effectiveness. Effectiveness of nasal sprays is affected by these infections.
Desmopressin (DDAVP)	0.1–0.4 mL in single or divided doses (nasal spray)		
Aqueous vasopressin (Pitressin)	10–30 units in divided doses (SC, IM, nasal spray)	2. Instruct client to sit upright when spraying. 3. Instruct client to hold breath when using nasal spray. 4. Monitor client's fluid intake and output. 5. Have client space fluid intake during waking hours. 6. Monitor client frequently (q 3–4 h) for recurrence of symptoms. 7. Monitor client's weight.	2. To promote effective absorption in nasal mucosa. 3. To prevent pneumonia. 4. To guide dosage regulation. 5. To prevent nocturia. 6. To detect need for additional doses of these short-acting medications. 7. To detect water retention.
Clofibrate (Atromid S)	2 g in four doses (PO)	1. Watch for signs of SIADH.	1. To detect potentiation of vasopressin.
Chlorprompamide (Diabinese)	125–250 mg (PO)	1. Monitor client for signs and symptoms of hypoglycemia.	1. To detect this potentially severe side effect.

weight gain can lead to early identification of this problem.

COLLABORATIVE MANAGEMENT

 Assessment

History

The nurse determines the client's *age* and *sex.* It is essential that the nurse elicit information regarding the client's *past medical history*, which may be associated with the development of SIADH. Particular attention is paid to a history of recent trauma, cerebrovascular disease, tuberculosis or other pulmonary disease, cancer, and all past and current *medications.*

Physical Assessment: Clinical Manifestations

Initially, the symptoms of SIADH are related to retention of water. The most common complaints reported by clients include *gastrointestinal disturbances,* such as loss of appetite, nausea, and vomiting. The nurse weighs the client and documents any recent *weight gain.* The nurse checks the client's extremities for the presence of edema. In SIADH, free water, not salt, is retained and edema is not usually present.

Water retention and hyponatremia have an effect on *central nervous system* function. The client or family may report episodes of lethargy, headaches, uncooperativeness, hostility, and disorientation. A change in the client's *level of consciousness* is an early sign of SIADH. Neurologic symptoms can progress from lethargy and headaches to obtundation, seizures, and coma. The nurse assesses deep tendon reflexes, which are often decreased or sluggish.

Vital sign changes include *tachycardia* related to increased fluid volume and *hypothermia* related to central nervous system disturbance. (See Chap. 13 for further discussion of findings associated with hyponatremia.)

Psychosocial Assessment

A number of psychosocial changes can occur as a result of the water retention and hyponatremia. The nurse discusses a history of irritability, anxiety, and uncooperativeness with the client and family. These behaviors may have placed considerable strain on family relationships, and the nurse explains the physiologic basis of these effects to both the client and family.

Laboratory Findings

Extracellular fluid volume expansion affects electrolyte levels in the serum and the urine. Elevated urine sodium levels and specific gravity reflect an increased concentration of the urine. Serum sodium levels are decreased because of volume expansion and increased sodium excretion. Fluid retention causes changes in both plasma and urine osmolality. Plasma osmolality is decreased, and the urine is hyperosmolar in relation to the plasma.

Radiographic Findings

Chest x-ray films are helpful in diagnosing many of the pulmonary conditions associated with SIADH, including tuberculosis, pneumothorax, asthma, and pneumonia. Chest films are used to detect the carcinomas of the lung that secrete ectopic ADH. Computed tomography and/or x-ray films of the skull are used to detect head trauma or injury, which may cause the sudden release of stored ADH.

Other Diagnostic Tests

Radioimmunoassay of ADH is sometimes performed and is diagnostic of SIADH when levels are inappropriately elevated in relation to plasma osmolality. When plasma osmolality is normal or decreased, ADH hormone levels should be low.

 Analysis: Nursing Diagnosis

Common Diagnoses

The following common nursing diagnoses are seen in the client with SIADH:

1. Fluid volume excess related to compromised regulatory mechanism
2. Altered thought processes related to changes within the central nervous system

Additional Diagnoses

The following are additional nursing diagnoses for the client with SIADH:

1. Altered nutrition: less than body requirements related to anorexia, nausea, and vomiting
2. Constipation related to fluid restriction and decreased gastric mobility
3. Potential for injury related to altered level of consciousness and possibility of seizures
4. Knowledge deficit related to diagnosis and treatment

 Planning and Implementation

Fluid Volume Excess

Planning: client goals. The primary goal for this nursing diagnosis is that the client will have a restoration of fluid balance.

Interventions: nonsurgical management. Interventions to treat SIADH consist of restricting water intake, using diuretics to promote excretion of water, and administering drugs that interfere with the action of ADH.

Fluid restriction. Fluid restriction is essential in the management of the client with SIADH. In some cases, fluid intake may be kept as low as 500 to 600 mL/24-hour period. Measurement of intake and output, as well as of daily weights, provides a guide to determining the degree of fluid restriction necessary. A weight gain of 2 lb or more per day or a gradual increase over several days is cause for concern. Clients are often uncomfortable during fluid restriction. The nurse keeps mucous membranes moist by frequent oral rinsing and reminds the client not to swallow liquids that are used for this purpose. Rarely, hypertonic saline is used in the treatment of SIADH. Intravenous saline is given cautiously because it may contribute to the fluid overload already present and precipitate an episode of congestive heart failure.

Drug therapy. Diuretics are sometimes used in the treatment of SIADH, particularly if congestive heart failure results from fluid overload. When diuretics are utilized, the nurse must be aware of the potential effect of electrolyte losses; sodium loss can be potentiated, which further contributes to the clinical picture of SIADH.

Certain drugs, such as lithium (Eskalith, Lithobid) and demeclocycline (Declomycin), are associated with the development of diabetes insipidus. Their use has, therefore, been explored in the treatment of SIADH. Lithium has not been successfully used because of its toxic effects. Demeclocycline is more promising in the treatment of SIADH, but it has yet to be studied extensively (Wilson & Foster, 1985).

Altered Thought Processes

Planning: client goals. The goal for this nursing diagnosis is that the client will experience minimal neurologic dysfunction.

Interventions: nonsurgical management. Primary concerns for the client with SIADH who is experiencing an alteration in thought processes are neurologic monitoring and promotion of safety. Careful attention to changes in neurologic status is essential in the nursing care of these clients. The nurse attempts to detect subtle changes before neurologic symptoms progress to seizures or coma. The nurse checks the client's orientation to person, place, and time because disorientation may be present. Confusion is another neurologic symptom, and the nurse attempts to reduce environmental stimuli and to explain interventions in simple terms. Flow sheets containing serial information about the level of consciousness, motor and sensory neurologic assessments, and pertinent laboratory data are helpful in detecting trends. The frequency of neurologic checks varies depending on the status of the client. For example, for the client with SIADH who is hyponatremic but alert, awake, and oriented, neurologic checks every 4 hours are sufficient. For the client who has had a change in level of consciousness, neurologic checks should be done at least every hour.

■ Discharge Planning

Home Care Preparation

With treatment, symptoms of SIADH are not usually present at the time of discharge from the hospital, and extensive changes in the home environment are not usually required. The nurse considers the etiology of SIADH when planning the client's discharge. For example, if a malignancy has caused SIADH, clients may have undergone surgery, radiation, and/or chemotherapy necessitating significant modifications in the home.

Clients need to have a scale and a graduated container because clients with SIADH must continue to weigh themselves daily and to monitor intake and output.

Client/Family Education

If the condition of SIADH has not resolved by the time of discharge, the nurse reviews instructions with clients and families. Fluid restriction must be maintained at home; therefore, clients are taught to measure intake and output daily. Clients should also weigh themselves daily and report an acute weight gain (e.g., 6 lb over 3 days) to the physician or nurse following their progress. Attention must be given to over-the-counter preparations containing drugs that might contribute to the development of hyponatremia, such as aspirin and nonsteroidal anti-inflammatory agents.

Psychosocial Preparation

Many of the etiologic factors associated with the development of SIADH are chronic diseases. Often clients and families are faced with the diagnosis of a malignancy, chronic neurologic condition, or pulmonary disorder. Clients dealing with a chronic disorder need support from the entire health care team. Discussions about tests, medications, and progress aid in decreasing client anxiety.

Health Care Resources

Clients may require a home care nurse, usually as a result of needs caused by an underlying medical problem. The client with SIADH needs to communicate regularly with the health care team to relay any return of symptoms related to water retention and hyponatremia.

 Evaluation

On the basis of the identified common nursing diagnosis, the outcomes for SIADH include that the client

1. Maintains normal fluid volume (determined by balanced intake and output, stable vital signs, stable weight)
2. Remains oriented to person, place, and time
3. Remains free from injury
4. Describes and complies with fluid restriction regimen
5. Identifies the need for frequent oral rinsing
6. States the importance of recording daily weights and intake and output
7. States the importance of notifying the health care team of any acute weight change

The client with SIADH who meets the stated outcomes is prepared to be discharged to home. If the underlying etiology of SIADH is detected and treated, the client may be discharged with resolution of symptoms and no need for fluid restriction.

DISORDERS OF THE ADRENAL GLAND

Adrenal Hypofunction

OVERVIEW

Decreased production of adrenocortical steroids may occur because of inadequate secretion of ACTH, dysfunction of the hypothalamic-pituitary control mechanism, or complete or partial destruction of the adrenal glands. Manifestations may develop gradually or accelerate quickly when a stressful situation occurs. In acute adrenal insufficiency (adrenal crisis), manifestations may appear suddenly, without warning, and create a life-threatening situation.

Loss of the adrenal medulla, unlike that of the cortex, which secretes life-sustaining hormones, does not upset the maintenance of homeostasis because catecholamides are synthesized and released from other areas in the sympathetic nervous system.

Pathophysiology

Insufficiency of adrenocortical steroids causes defects associated with the loss of mineralocorticoid (aldosterone) and glucocorticoid (cortisol) action. Impaired secretion of cortisol results in decreased glyconeogenesis, with depletion of liver and muscle glycogen and thus hypoglycemia. Decreased glomerular filtration rate and gastric acid production also occur and lead to a reduction in urea nitrogen excretion, anorexia, and weight loss. Reduced aldosterone secretion causes disturbances in the clearance of potassium, sodium, and water by the kidney. Potassium clearance is decreased, which causes hyperkalemia; sodium and water clearance is increased, which causes hyponatremia and hypovolemia. Potassium retention also promotes the reabsorption of hydrogen ions, which can ultimately lead to metabolic acidosis.

The lower adrenal androgen levels may result in the decrease or loss of body, axillary, and pubic hair, especially in the female, in whom the adrenals are responsible for the major production of androgens. It is important to note that the *severity* of symptoms is related to the *degree* of deficiency in hormone secretion.

Acute adrenal insufficiency, or *addisonian crisis,* is a life-threatening event in a client whose physiologic requirement for glucocorticoid and mineralocorticoid hormones exceeds the available supply. In most cases, acute adrenal insufficiency is precipitated by a stressful event, e.g., surgery, trauma, or severe infection, and it also occurs in the client whose adrenal hormone output is already compromised. The pathophysiology of acute adrenal crisis is almost the same as that for chronic insufficiency. The one deviation is seen in the client presenting in acute adrenal crisis related to bilateral adrenal hemorrhage. These clients may have normal sodium and potassium levels because the time frame between the initial incident and presentation may be too short for a change to occur. However, unless intervention is initiated promptly, sodium levels will fall and potassium levels will rise rapidly. Intravascular volume depletion occurs secondary to the loss of mineralocorticoid, which results in more severe hypotension.

Emergency care for acute adrenal crisis is outlined in the accompanying Emergency Care feature.

Etiology

Adrenal insufficiency may be classified as being primary or secondary. *Primary* adrenal insufficiency, also referred to as *Addison's disease,* is frequently due to chronic destructive disease, resulting in the loss of the major adrenal hormones cortisol and aldosterone. *Idiopathic* (probably autoimmune) disease is now ranked as the leading cause of Addison's disease, followed by tuberculosis, infiltrative processes such as metastatic carcinoma and fungal lesions, acquired immunodeficiency syndrome (AIDS), and hemorrhage into the adrenal related to anticoagulant therapy or to gram-negative sepsis (Waterhouse-Friderichsen syndrome). Exogenous causes of adrenal insufficiency include adrenalectomy, abdominal radiation therapy, and the use of adrenal toxins such as mitotane (*o,p*-DDD).

Secondary adrenal insufficiency is a result of failure in the hypothalamic or pituitary portion of the adrenal axis, which causes decreased cortisol and adrenal an-

EMERGENCY CARE ■ Acute Adrenal Crisis

Interventions	Rationales
1. Before initiating treatment, obtain complete blood count and electrolyte, blood urea nitrogen, and plasma cortisol levels as ordered by physician.	1. To provide objective data for diagnosis.
2. Give an initial dose of hydrocortisone (Solu-Cortef), 100–300 mg IV; then infuse 100 mg/8 h, as ordered by physician.	2. To provide a loading dose and maintenance infusion. The output of adrenal glucose is 300 mg/24 h. The half-life of IV hydrocortisone is 60–90 min; 100 mg/8 h is needed to avoid a relapse.
3. Give concomitant doses of hydrocortisone, 50 mg IM every 12 h as ordered by physician.	3. To ensure constant source of glucocorticords in case of IV failure.

4. After resolution of crisis, adjust the dosage of medications as ordered by physician:
  a. Give oral glucocorticoids.
  b. Decrease the dosage of oral glucocorticoids over several days as maintenance levels are reached.
  c. Give supplemental mineralocorticoids as glucocorticoid dosage is tapered.
	4. To ensure adequacy of mineralocorticoid activity with minimal glucocorticoid dose.

drogen production with continued but sometimes decreased aldosterone secretion. Contributing causes of secondary disease include pituitary tumors, postpartum necrosis of the pituitary gland (Sheehan's syndrome), hypophysectomy, high-dose radiation therapy to the pituitary or other intracranial lesions, and high-dose, long-term glucocorticoid therapy causing adrenal gland suppression.

Incidence

In recent years, the incidence of adrenal hypofunction has increased as a result of improved diagnostic techniques, the use of newer drugs that may have cytotoxic action, and the increased use of high-dose glucocorticoids. Nonetheless, adrenal insufficiency is still considered to be rare. In the United States, most of the cases are due to autoimmune destruction of the adrenal gland, with a two- to threefold greater incidence in females than in males (Braunwald et al., 1987).

PREVENTION

One area in which preventive measures are of value is in avoidance of abrupt and sudden cessation of long-term, high-dose glucocorticoid therapy. If therapy is to be withdrawn, it must be done gradually, allowing time for pituitary production of ACTH and adrenal production of cortisol to return. In addition, prompt and adequate treatment of known infection of active tuberculosis would aid in the arrest of the disease before destruction of the gland is complete. Clients in high-risk groups should be monitored closely for the onset of symptoms of adrenal insufficiency.

COLLABORATIVE MANAGEMENT

 Assessment

History

While taking a history from the client with suspected adrenal hypofunction, the nurse asks pertinent questions regarding the presence of symptoms, as well as factors contributing to the etiology of adrenal hypofunction. The nurse questions the client about a change in activity level because *lethargy, fatigue,* and *muscle weakness* are often present. Questions about salt intake should be included because *salt craving* is often a symptom of adrenal hypofunction. Gastrointestinal problems, such as *anorexia, nausea, vomiting,* diarrhea, and abdominal pain, often occur. The nurse asks if the client has noticed weight loss over the past weeks or months. Female clients report menstrual changes related to weight loss, and males may experience impotence.

The *past medical history* aids in identifying potential etiologic factors in the development of adrenal hypofunction. The nurse asks if the client has had *radiation* to the *abdomen* or *head.* The nurse documents significant medical problems, such as *tuberculosis* or a history of *intracranial surgery.* All past and current medications are recorded, particularly a history of taking steroids, anticoagulants, or cytotoxic drugs.

Physical Assessment: Clinical Manifestations

The clinical manifestations of adrenal hypofunction vary from client to client, and the severity of symptoms is related to the degree of hormone deficiency. In primary adrenal hypofunction, plasma ACTH and mela-

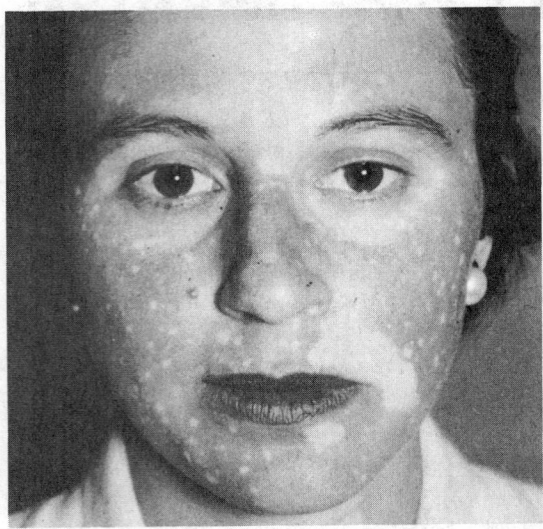
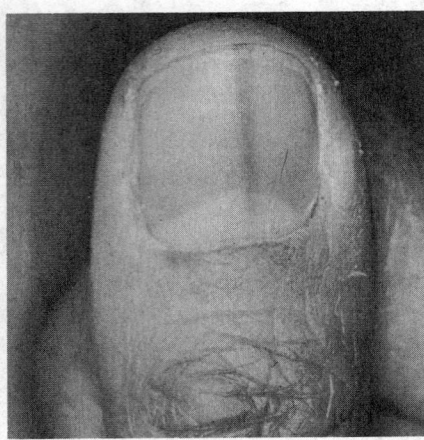

Figure 49–4

Increased pigmentation in primary adrenocortical insufficiency. (From Bondy, P. K., & Rosenberg, L. E. [1980]. *Metabolic control and disease* [8th ed.]. Philadelphia: W. B. Saunders.)

nocyte-stimulating hormone (MSH) levels are elevated because of the loss of the adrenal–hypothalamic–pituitary feedback system. Elevated MSH levels result in areas of *increased pigmentation* (Fig. 49–4). In primary disease with an autoimmune etiology, areas of decreased pigmentation may be found because of destruction of pigment-producing cells in the skin (melanocytes). The nurse assesses mucous membranes, surgical scars, areolae, skin folds, and the area over the knuckles on the hand for the presence of hyperpigmentation. While assessing the client's skin, the nurse may also detect a decreased amount of body hair. In secondary disease, there is no increase in skin pigmentation.

Cortisol hyposecretion may result in *hypoglycemia* because of impaired gluconeogenesis. The nurse assesses the client for symptoms of hypoglycemia, e.g., sweating, headaches, tachycardia, and tremors. In primary adrenal insufficiency, cortisol and aldosterone deficiencies result in *volume depletion*. The nurse observes the client for postural hypotension and symptoms of dehydration. A deficiency of aldosterone also affects electrolyte levels. Hyperkalemia can cause arrhythmias with an irregular heart rate.

Psychosocial Assessment

Depending on the degree of metabolic imbalance, clients may appear lethargic, apathetic, depressed, confused, or psychotic. The nurse observes the client and checks orientation to person, place, and time to detect these symptoms. Families may report that the client has a decreased energy level, is emotionally labile, and is forgetful. Such changes may seriously stress family relationships. The nurse assesses the client's ability for self-care and identifies sources of support.

Laboratory Findings

In adrenal hypofunction, laboratory findings may include low serum cortisol, decreased fasting blood glucose, low sodium, and elevated potassium levels, and increased serum blood urea nitrogen (BUN). In primary disease, an increased eosinophil count and an elevated ACTH level fail to rise during stimulation tests. Laboratory findings in hypofunction and hyperfunction of the adrenal gland are compared in the accompanying Key Features of Disease.

It is important to note that although basal cortisol and ACTH levels may be helpful, definitive stimulation studies are required to confirm a diagnosis of adrenal hypofunction.

Twenty-four-hour urine tests reflect steroid hormone secretion over a given time and can be a valuable diagnostic adjunct in adrenal disease. Urinary 17-hydroxycorticosteroids are the glycocorticoid metabolites, and 17-ketosteroid levels reflect the adrenal androgen metabolites. Both of these levels are in the low or low-normal range in adrenal hypofunction.

Radiographic Findings

Skull x-rays studies, CT, and arteriography may all be used to aid in the search for an intracranial lesion impinging on the pituitary gland, adenomas of the gland itself, aneurysms, or empty sella.

Noninvasive procedures of the adrenal such as CT scans may occasionally show atrophy of the gland. Although this is never considered to be diagnostic by itself, with other diagnostic criteria it may be of value in determining adrenal hypofunction.

Other Diagnostic Tests

An ACTH (Cosyntropin [Cortrosyn], synthetic ACTH) stimulation test is necessary for a definitive work-up for adrenal insufficiency. A rapid ACTH stimulation test may be administered as an outpatient test. Cosyntropin is given intramuscularly, and plasma cortisol levels are obtained at intervals, after the baseline, of 30 minutes and 1 hour. In primary insufficiency, the cortisol response is absent or markedly decreased; in secondary insufficiency, there is a decreased cortisol response. A longer ACTH stimulation test involves a continuous infusion of 50 units of ACTH in saline for 24 hours or an 8-hour infusion for 4 to 5 days, with simultaneously collected 24-hour urine samples. Levels of urinary 17-hydroxycorticosteroids and urinary free cortisol adrenal hormone (metabolites) are measured. In primary adrenal insufficiency, the response is low or absent; in secondary insufficiency, the value for 17-hydroxycorticosteroids fails to rise above 20 mg per total volume.

Metyrapone is a drug used to test the responsiveness of pituitary ACTH by blocking the hydroxylation of 11-desoxycortisol to cortisol. When the cortisol level falls, ACTH levels should rise appropriately.

An electrocardiogram is performed and can indicate an elevated potassium level. Characteristic changes include peaked T waves, widening of the QRS complex, and an increase in the PR interval.

 ### Analysis: Nursing Diagnosis

Common Diagnoses

The following common nursing diagnoses are frequently seen in the client with adrenal hypofunction:

1. Fluid volume deficit related to volume depletion secondary to adrenal insufficiency
2. Altered tissue perfusion related to hypovolemia

Additional Diagnoses

Additional diagnoses for the client with adrenal hypofunction include

1. Sleep pattern disturbance related to loss of diurnal rhythm
2. Potential for infection related to adrenal incapacity to respond to stress

3. Activity intolerance related to fatigue and muscle weakness
4. Altered nutrition: less than body requirements related to anorexia, nausea, and vomiting
5. Knowledge deficit related to treatment regimen
6. Ineffective individual coping related to disease process

 ### Planning and Implementation

Fluid Volume Deficit

Planning: client goals.   The goals for this nursing diagnosis are that the client will (1) experience a reduction in fluid volume deficit and (2) maintain an adequate fluid volume.

Interventions: nonsurgical management.   The nurse promotes fluid balance through careful monitoring to detect fluid deficit. Clients are weighed daily, and intake and output are recorded. The nurse checks vital signs every 1 to 4 hours, depending on the client's condition and the occurrence of arrhythmias or postural hypotension. Laboratory values are monitored to identify hemoconcentrations, e.g., increased hematocrit or BUN. Glucocorticoid and mineralocorticoid deficiencies should be completely corrected by replacement therapy. Cortisone and hydrocortisone are the most commonly used drugs to correct the glucocorticoid deficiency (Table 49-2). In the doses required for replacement therapy, there is insufficient mineralocorticoid effect to maintain electrolyte balance in clients with primary adrenal hypofunction. An additional hormone may then be required. The glucocorticoid replacement regimens vary, but generally divided doses are given, with two-thirds in the morning and one-third in the late afternoon to mimic the normal diurnal adrenal rhythm. Although the majority of clients do well on this regimen, others may not tolerate the dosage or may need more. The presence of hyperirritability, insomnia, and hypertension may indi-

---

KEY FEATURES OF DISEASE ■ **Laboratory Findings in Hypofunction and Hyperfunction of the Adrenal Gland**

Laboratory Test	Adrenal Hypofunction	Adrenal Hyperfunction
Sodium	Decreased	Increased
Potassium	Increased	Decreased
Glucose	Normal to decreased	Normal to increased
Calcium	Increased	Decreased
Leukocytes	Normal	Increased
Eosinophils	Increased	Decreased
Bicarbonate	Increased	Decreased
BUN	Increased	Normal
Cortisol	Decreased	Increased

TABLE 49-2 Replacement Hormones Used in the Treatment of Adrenal Hypofunction

Drug	Usual Daily Dosage	Interventions	Rationales

Cortisone
Hydrocortisone
Prednisone
	25–37.5 mg
	20–30 mg
	7.5–10 mg
		1. Instruct the client to take with meals or snack.
		2. Instruct the client to report the following signs or symptoms of excessive drug therapy:
		  a. Rapid weight gain.
		  b. Round face.
		  c. Fluid retention.
		3. Instruct the client to monitor levels of stress or exposure to stressful situations, such as:
		  a. Illness.
		  b. Family crisis.
		  c. Surgery.
			1. To prevent gastrointestinal irritation.
			2. To detect signs or symptoms of Cushing's syndrome, which indicate a need for dosage adjustment.
			
			3. To determine the need for dosage change. The usual daily dosage may not be adequate during periods of increased stress.

Fludrocortisone	0.05–1.5 mg	1. Monitor the client's blood pressure. 2. Instruct the client to report weight gain or edema.	1. To detect hypertension, which is a potential side effect. 2. To detect sodium-related fluid retention.

cate excessive glucocorticoid replacement dosage, but these symptoms should be thoroughly investigated before the dosage is decreased. Supplemental mineralocorticoids to maintain electrolyte balance are given in the form of fludrocortisone (Florinef). The average dose range is 0.1 to 0.2 mg daily, although as little as 0.1 mg three times a week is all some clients require. Overtreatment can result in hypertension, fluid retention, and congestive heart failure. The nurse monitors sodium and potassium levels closely when mineralocorticoid therapy is used. Adjustments in dosage may be necessary in extra warm weather when loss of sodium increases because of excessive perspiration.

Altered Tissue Perfusion

Planning: client goals. The goal for this diagnosis is that the client will maintain adequate perfusion to peripheral tissues.

Interventions: nonsurgical management. An alteration in peripheral tissue perfusion may occur in adrenal hypofunction related to hypovolemia. Replacement of fluids and hormone should correct the hypovolemia. Vital signs are monitored frequently to detect hypotension and tachycardia.

In the client with hypofunction of the adrenal gland, stress (both physical and emotional) may precipitate an adrenal crisis. In this instance, peripheral tissue perfusion becomes so impaired that vascular collapse and shock are inevitable without intervention. Careful nursing observation to detect decreasing blood pressure, cold, pale skin, and decreased urinary output leads to appropriate medical interventions and treatment of the crisis.

■ Discharge Planning

Home Care Preparation

The client with adrenal hypofunction does not usually require significant home or environmental changes unless there is another complicating problem. Clients require medication and need education concerning health maintenance.

Client/Family Education

Clients with adrenal hypofunction need to take hormone replacement for the rest of their lives. The nurse focuses on the dosage, administration, and side effects of the prescribed medication when educating the client and family. Instructions for the client taking cortisol replacement therapy are given in the accompanying Client/Family Education feature.

In clients with primary disease, supplemental mineralocorticoid may be needed to maintain electrolyte balance. Dietary sodium intake should remain constant after the requirements of mineralocorticoid replacement have been ascertained. A shift in either direction of sodium intake would necessitate a concomitant change in the mineralocorticoid replacement dosage. Abrupt decreases in sodium intake can precipitate adrenal crisis. In climates where temperatures vary from hot to cold, adjustment of the mineralocorticoid dosage may be necessary during the summer months. In hot weather, the body loses a large amount of sodium through perspiration. Fluid overload and hypertension can result from excess amounts of mineralocorticoid.

Occasionally, a female client with primary disease experiences muscle weakness and/or decreased libido.

These symptoms are usually due to the loss of adrenal androgens and can be treated with intramuscular injections of a small amount of testosterone.

Psychosocial Preparation

Clients must be aware of the fact that hormone replacement is a lifelong need. In addition, a diagnosis of adrenal insufficiency requires significant participation by the client in the health care regimen. The nurse aids the client in identifying potential emotional and environmental stressors and discusses possible strategies for reducing stress. Careful attention by the nurse to client and family education may alleviate anxiety often surrounding chronic illness.

Health Care Resources

A home care nurse should be contacted before the client is discharged from the hospital. Regular communication between the health care team in the hospital and the nurse in the home environment is important for consistency in managing the client with adrenal hypofunction.

 Evaluation

On the basis of the identified common nursing diagnoses, the expected outcomes include that the client

1. Maintains adequate fluid volume
2. Maintains adequate peripheral tissue perfusion

3. Describes and complies with the drug treatment regimen
4. Identifies symptoms of excess adrenal hormone replacement
5. Identifies situations that require an increase in adrenal hormone replacement dosage
6. Obtains and wears a medical alert bracelet or necklace
7. Demonstrates an ability to self-administer injections

The client with adrenal hypofunction who meets the stated outcomes has a smoother transition period after discharge and may exhibit less anxiety concerning hormone replacement therapy.

Adrenal Hyperfunction

OVERVIEW

Hypersecretion by the adrenal cortex may result in the production of excess amounts of glucocorticoids, which leads to *hypercortisolism* (e.g., Cushing's syndrome); excess amounts of mineralocorticoids, which leads to *hyperaldosteronism;* and excess amounts of androgens, which can be seen in generalized *cortical hyperplasia* or in the congenital and acquired enzyme deficiency states.

Hypersecretion by the adrenal medulla (in *pheochromocytoma*) results in excess secretion of catecholamines, of which 80% is epinephrine and the remainder, norepinephrine.

CLIENT/FAMILY EDUCATION ■ Instructions for Clients Taking Cortisol Replacement Therapy

1. "Take your medication in divided doses, the first dose in the morning and the second dose between 4 and 6 PM."

2. "Take your medication with meals or snacks."

3. "Weigh yourself daily."

4. "Increase your dosage as directed for increased physical stress or severe emotional stress, including surgery, dental work, influenza, fever, pregnancy, and family problems."

5. "Never skip a dose of medication. If you have persistent vomiting or severe diarrhea and cannot take your medication by mouth for 24–36 hours, call your doctor. If you cannot reach your doctor, go to the nearest emergency room. You may need an injection to take the place of your usual oral medication."

6. "Always wear your medical alert bracelet or necklace."

1. To mimic diurnal adrenal rhythm and prevent insomnia, which can occur when medications are taken late in the evening.

2. To prevent stomach irritation.

3. To detect weight gain or loss, which may signal need for dosage adjustment.

4. To maintain appropriate hormone levels in the face of stress-related hormonal changes.

5. To maintain the appropriate hormone level and prevent fluid loss.

6. To alert emergency personnel to the presence of adrenal hypofunction, which must be known to health care professionals.

HYPERCORTISOLISM

Pathophysiology

The metabolic effects in Cushing's syndrome are an exaggeration of the normal physiologic action of glucocorticoids, which causes widespread abnormalities. Adrenocortical hyperplasia that is caused by excessive stimulation by ACTH, of either pituitary or ectopic origin, results in the loss of normal diurnal rhythms; a decreased responsiveness of prolactin, thyrotropin, and gonadotropin to their respective releasing hormones; and abnormal sleep patterns. Although some of these changes are due to excessive amounts of glucocorticoids, others are linked with as yet undefined hypothalamic abnormalities. Clients with Cushing's syndrome exhibit alterations of nitrogen, carbohydrate, and mineral metabolism. An increase in total body fat results from a depressed turnover of plasma fatty acids, and a redistribution of bulk results in the typical centripetal (truncal) pattern. Moderate to marked increases in the breakdown of tissue protein and a marked increase in the urinary nitrogen level occur. These increases result in decreased muscle mass with a proximal myopathy, atrophic (thin) skin, decreased bone matrix and a loss of total skeletal calcium, and a loss of lymphoid tissue. High levels of corticosteroids kill lymphocytes, and organs that contain large numbers of these cells, such as the liver, spleen, and lymph nodes, shrink in size. Thus, the physiologic effectiveness of the antibody response to antigens is reduced. In most cases, there is evidence of increased androgen production with acne, hirsutism (increased hair growth), and, in rare instances, clitoral hypertrophy. Increased androgen production can also interrupt the normal pituitary-ovarian axis, thereby decreasing production of estrogens and progesterone from the ovary, causing oligomenorrhea (scant or infrequent menses).

Etiology

Cushing's syndrome is a clinical entity produced by an excess of cortisol, whether secreted by the adrenal cortex (endogenous) or administered as therapy for another clinical disorder (exogenous; iatrogenic). Excessive endogenous secretion of cortisol may be caused by increased production of ACTH by adenomas of the pituitary gland (Cushing's disease); ectopic production of ACTH by a tumor in the lung, gastrointestinal tract, or pancreas; or production by autonomously functioning adrenal adenomas of carcinomas. The majority of cases are due to bilateral adrenal hyperplasia that is caused by pituitary or nonendocrine tumors that produce excess ACTH (Wilson & Foster, 1985). Adrenal tumors are usually unilateral and are responsible for approximately 25% of all cases of Cushing's syndrome; in adults, approximately 50% of these tumors are classified as malignant. Adrenal carcinomas may also excrete large amounts of estrogens. At present, the most common cause of Cushing's syndrome in adults is the use of exogenous glucocorticoids or ACTH in the therapy of many clinical entities, including organ transplantation, as an adjunct in chemotherapy for various types of cancer, and in the treatment of many neurologic and cardiothoracic disorders (Braunwald et al., 1987).

Incidence

Hypercortisolism (i.e., Cushing's syndrome) caused by disease is relatively rare, affecting predominantly women by an 8:1 ratio compared with men. The average age of onset is between 20 and 40 years, but onset occurs up to age 60 years (Wyngaarden & Smith, 1988).

COLLABORATIVE MANAGEMENT

 Assessment

The clinical features present in hypercortisolism are a result of glucocorticoid excess. A thorough nursing history and physical assessment aid in detecting the clinical features that indicate this syndrome.

History

Clients with hypercortisolism present with varied complaints as a result of the widespread effect of excess cortisol in the body. The nurse asks the client about changes in *activity* or *sleep patterns*. The nurse asks if the client experiences *fatigue* and muscle weakness or is having difficulty sleeping at night.

Osteoporosis is a common occurrence in hypercortisolism. Clients are asked if they have *bone pain* or a *history* of *fractures*. The nurse questions clients about a history of frequent infections and easy bruising, which indicate hypercortisolism. Female clients may report a cessation of menses.

The nurse also collects data about the client's *past medical history*. Any history of *steroid* or *alcohol abuse* is noted because both can produce clinical and biochemical features of Cushing's syndrome.

Physical Assessment: Clinical Manifestations

The client with hypercortisolism presents with *characteristic physical changes* (Fig. 49–5). Changes in fat distribution may result in the appearance of a buffalo hump, centripetal obesity, supraclavicular fat pads, and a round face (moon face). The nurse observes the general appearance of the client and notes a large trunk with thin legs and arms, as well as the presence of generalized muscle wasting and weakness.

During the skin assessment, the nurse inspects the client for *characteristic skin changes* resulting from increased blood vessel fragility, such as bruises; thin,

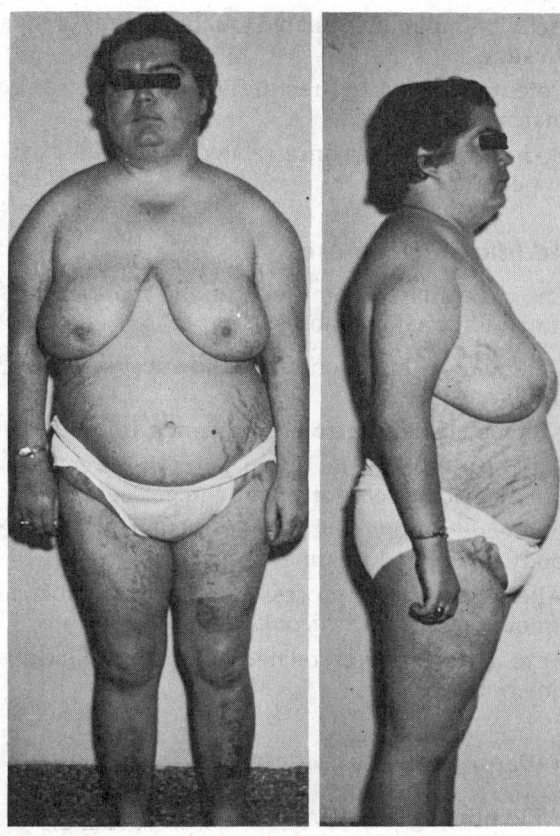

Figure 49–5

Characteristic changes in the client with adrenal hyperfunction. (From Bondy, P. K., & Rosenberg, L. E. [1980]. *Metabolic control and disease* [8th ed.]. Philadelphia: W. B. Saunders.)

translucent skin; and wounds that have not healed properly. Reddish-purple striae are often present on the abdomen and upper thighs. Excess cortisol secretion may result in a fine coating of hair over the face and body, and in acne. In the female client, the nurse observes for the presence of hirsutism and clitoral hypertrophy related to androgen excess. Increased production of androgen may also result in coarse, thin body hair and balding in the temporal area.

While assessing vital signs, the nurse notes elevated blood pressure. *Hypertension* is a common finding in clients with hypercortisolism.

Psychosocial Assessment

Cortisol hypersecretion can result in emotional lability. The nurse questions the client about recent mood swings, irritability, confusion, or depression. Clients can become neurotic or psychotic as a result of changes in blood cortisol levels. Because the client with hypercortisolism experiences a change in physical appearance, the nurse attempts to determine which physical characteristics particularly trouble the client by encouraging discussion.

Laboratory Findings

Plasma cortisol levels are elevated in hypercortisolism. Blood for cortisol assays should always be taken at the same time of day because levels vary throughout the day. Further diagnostic testing is done to confirm the diagnosis of hypercortisolism because an increase in cortisol level is seen in other situations such as acute illness and trauma. Plasma ACTH levels vary depending on the etiology of hypercortisolism. In ectopic (ACTH-producing) syndromes, the ACTH level is elevated. In Cushing's syndrome (primary disease of the adrenal gland), ACTH levels are low to immeasurable. Additional laboratory findings may include increased blood glucose level, elevated white blood cell and lymphocyte counts, increased sodium level, and decreased serum calcium and serum potassium levels.

Urine testing is performed to measure levels of free cortisol and adrenal metabolites of cortisol and androgens (17-hydroxycorticosteroids and 17-ketosteroids). Clients must be reminded to save *all* their urine for a 24-hour period. In hypercortisolism, basal levels of urinary free cortisol, 17-ketosteroids, and 17-hydroxycorticosteroids are all elevated, as are levels of urinary calcium, potassium, and glucose.

Other Diagnostic Tests

The overnight dexamethasone test, a suppression test, serves as an initial screening method for Cushing's syndrome. Clients must not take any medications for at least 2 days before the test. In particular, phenytoin (Dilantin) and phenobarbital interfere with test results. At midnight, the nurse administers 1.0 mg of oral dexamethasone and the following morning, the plasma cortisol level is measured. Normally, plasma cortisol levels are less than 5 mg/dL. If the plasma cortisol level is higher than 5 mg/dL, further definitive testing for Cushing's syndrome is necessary (Braunwald et al., 1987).

For the low-dose dexamethasone suppression test, if at all possible, the client must not take any medications for at least 2 days before this test, and no stressful procedures should be performed during the time of the test. Table 49–3 lists drugs that interfere with testing. A baseline 24-hour urine sample is collected on day 1. Dexamethasone, 0.5 mg, is administered every 6 hours on days 2 and 3, with concomitant 24-hour urine collections. The 24-hour urine collections are tested for 17-ketosteroids, 17-hydroxycorticosteroids, creatinine, and urinary free cortisol. Normally urinary 17-hydroxycorticosteroid excretion and free cortisol levels are suppressed, and Cushing's syndrome is ruled out. If these levels are not suppressed, an additional higher-dose dexamethasone test is performed.

The high-dose (8 mg) dexamethasone suppression test is used to distinguish between bilateral adrenocortical hyperplasia (e.g., Cushing's syndrome) and adrenocortical neoplasm as a cause of hypercortisolism. Clients must take no medication and avoid stressful procedures during the test. Dexamethasone, 2 mg, is given orally

TABLE 49–3   Some Drugs That Interfere with Tests for Urinary 17-Hydroxycorticosteroids and Urinary 17-Ketosteroids

Acetaminophen	Hydralazine
Acetazolamide	Iodides
Acetylsalicylic acid	Medroxyprogesterone
Amphetamines	Meperidine
Ascorbic acid	Meprobamate
Barbiturates	Metyrapone
Calcium gluconate	Mitotane
Carbon disulfide	Morphine
Chloral hydrate	Nalidixic acid
Chlordiazepoxide	Oral contraceptives
Chlormerodrin	Paraldehyde
Chlorothiazide	Penicillin
Chlorpromazine	Pentazocine
Chlorthalidone	Perphenazine
Colchicine	Phenobarbital
Corticotropin	Phenothiazines
Cortisone	Phenylbutazone
Dexamethasone	Promazine
Diazepam	Propoxyphene
Digitoxin	Quinidine
Digoxin	Quinine
Diphenhydramine	Reserpine
Diphenylhydantoin	Secobarbital
Erythromycin	Spironolactone
Estrogens	Testosterone
Fructose	Vitamin K
Glutethimide	

every 6 hours for 2 days, and two consecutive 24-hour urine samples are collected. Clients with bilateral adrenocortical hyperplasia suppress urinary 17-hydroxycorticosteroid excretion to 50% or less of the baseline control level.

The metyrapone test is used to assess the hypothalamic–pituitary–adrenal feedback responses. Metyrapone (Metopirone), 750 mg, is administered every 4 hours for 6 doses. Metyrapone lowers serum cortisol levels and therefore stimulates ACTH secretion. A normal response is an increase in ACTH and 11-deoxycortisol level. In clients with adrenal adenoma, no rise occurs.

 Analysis: Nursing Diagnosis

Common Diagnoses

The following common diagnoses are seen in clients with hypercortisolism (e.g., Cushing's syndrome):

1. Fluid volume excess related to sodium retention
2. Impaired skin integrity related to increased fragility of capillaries and skin, striae, and/or acne

3. Activity intolerance related to fatigue and/or muscle wasting
4. Potential for injury (fracture) related to loss of bone matrix
5. Body image disturbance related to altered physical appearance

Additional Diagnoses

The client may present with one or more of the following additional diagnoses:

1. Potential for infection related to suppression of the immune system
2. Knowledge deficit related to diagnosis and treatment
3. Altered nutrition: less than body requirements related to side effects of therapy (e.g., radiation)
4. Ineffective individual coping related to change in body image and treatment regimen
5. Altered thought processes related to increased amounts of glucocorticoids
6. Sexual dysfunction related to loss of libido and amenorrhea

 Planning and Implementation

Specific nursing interventions are used to address the problems identified by the nursing diagnoses. Preoperative and postoperative nursing care is an integral part of the management of the client with hypercortisolism because surgical intervention is usually required for relief of symptoms. The following plan of care for the client with hypercortisolism focuses on the common nursing diagnoses. By interfering with the production of excess glucocorticoids, drug therapy and surgical intervention can affect *all* of the identified nursing diagnoses.

Fluid Volume Excess

Planning: client goals.   The goal for this nursing diagnosis is that the client will have a restored fluid balance.

Interventions: nonsurgical management.   The nurse weighs the client daily and monitors the client's intake and output to assess the accumulation of excess fluid. Restriction of fluids is sometimes necessary to maintain fluid balance.

Drug therapy.   The majority of clients with hypercortisolism undergo surgical intervention. However, drugs that interfere with ACTH production or adrenal hormone synthesis may be used for palliation. Mitotane (Lysodren) is an adrenal cytotoxic agent that is used for inoperable adrenal tumors. Aminoglutethimide (Elipten, Cytadren) and metyrapone are adrenal enzyme inhibitors that decrease cortisol production. Metyrapone is more effective when used in combination with another agent, such as mitotane. Trilostane (Modrastane), also an enzyme inhibitor, has recently been introduced, but its effectiveness has been questioned. Less commonly, cyproheptadine (Periactin) is used to treat adrenal hyperfunction resulting from pituitary-related Cushing's disease by interfering with ACTH production. During drug therapy, the nurse assesses the client for symptoms of side effects or toxicity of specific agents.

Radiation therapy. Radiation may be used to treat hypercortisolism resulting from pituitary adenomas. In some instances, an ACTH-secreting adenoma becomes clinically apparent after bilateral adrenalectomy (e.g., Nelson's syndrome). Radiation applied internally (transsphenoidal implantation) or externally may help to prevent this syndrome. Radiation therapy is not always effective and may destroy normal tissue. The nurse notes any changes in the client's neurologic status, such as headache, elevated blood pressure or pulse, disorientation, and changes in pupil size or reaction. Clients may experience skin dryness, redness, flushing, or alopecia. The nurse reviews these possible side effects of radiation therapy with the client (see Chap. 25 for care of the client undergoing radiation therapy).

Interventions: surgical management. The surgical treatment of adrenocortical hypersecretion depends on the etiology of the disease. When adrenal hyperfunction is caused by increased pituitary secretion of ACTH, a transsphenoidal removal of a microadenoma may be attempted. Frequently, microadenomas cannot be localized, and *hypophysectomy* (surgical resection of the pituitary gland) is indicated. Hypophysectomy is performed via the transsphenoidal or transfrontal craniotomy route (see earlier for a discussion of hypophysectomy and Chap. 33 for nursing care of clients undergoing craniotomy).

If adrenal adenomas or carcinomas are the etiologic agents of hypercortisolism, an *adrenalectomy* (removal of the adrenal gland) is indicated. A unilateral adrenalectomy is performed when one gland is involved. A bilateral adrenalectomy is required in ectopic ACTH-producing tumors that cannot be treated by other means.

Preoperative care. Electrolyte imbalances are corrected before surgery, and the nurse monitors potassium, sodium, and chloride values. Clients with hypercortisolism are prone to developing complications such as infections and fractures. The nurse attempts to prevent infections by thorough hand washing and use of aseptic techniques. The occurrences of falls can be minimized by raising side rails of the bed and by encouraging the client to ask for assistance when getting out of bed. A high-calorie, high-protein diet is initiated before surgery. Clients having a bilateral adrenalectomy require lifelong glucocorticoid and mineralocorticoid replacement. In unilateral adrenalectomy, clients require glucocorticoid replacement for varying periods, possibly for 2 years after surgery. Preoperatively, the nurse ad-

ministers a glucocorticoid preparation to the client. The client continues to receive glucocorticoids throughout the operative procedure to prevent adrenal hypofunction. If hyperglycemia is present, it is controlled before surgery, and the nurse monitors blood glucose results.

Postoperative care. Clients undergoing an adrenalectomy are usually sent to an intensive care unit postoperatively. In the immediate postoperative period, the nurse assesses the client frequently to identify symptoms indicating cardiovascular collapse or shock. The nurse monitors serial vital signs and other hemodynamic parameters (central venous pressure, pulmonary wedge pressure), intake and output, daily weights, and serum electrolyte levels. Glucocorticoid preparations are administered as ordered. Hypotension, a rapid, weak pulse, and a decreasing urinary output indicate decreased tissue perfusion and impending shock. The nurse attempts to control discomfort and pain at the incision site by administering prescribed analgesics. The nurse assesses the client's response to pain medication and confers with the physician if a dose adjustment is necessary. Clients are encouraged to turn, cough, and deep breathe to prevent stasis of pulmonary secretions. Incisional dressings are changed or reinforced as necessary using aseptic technique (see Chap. 20 for postoperative care of the client).

Impaired Skin Integrity

Planning: client goals. The goal for this nursing diagnoses is that the client will maintain intact skin.

Interventions: nonsurgical management. The nurse assesses the client's skin frequently to detect reddened areas, excoriation, breakdown, and edema. If mobility is decreased, the nurse turns the client frequently and pads bony prominences to avoid skin breakdown. The nurse instructs the client to avoid activities that could result in skin trauma. Using a soft toothbrush and an electric razor may minimize tissue injury. Proper hygiene is important in preventing skin breakdown. Clients are instructed to keep the skin clean and to dry it thoroughly after washing. Excessive dryness may be prevented by using a moisturizing lotion when necessary. Adhesive tape frequently causes breakdown of the client's skin. If tape is necessary, it should be used sparingly, and extreme caution should be exercised when removing it. After venipuncture or arterial puncture, clients may experience an increase in bleeding because of blood vessel fragility. The nurse may need to exert pressure over the site for an additional time to prevent excess bleeding and ecchymosis.

Activity Intolerance

Planning: client goals. Clients with hypercortisolism experience activity intolerance as a result of fatigue, weakness, muscle wasting, and osteoporosis. The goals for this diagnosis are that the client will (1) conserve needed energy and (2) gradually increase activity level.

Interventions: nonsurgical management. Clients with hypercortisolism experience difficulty with ADL as a result of fatigue. They require frequent rest periods during the day. The nurse assists clients in identifying methods of conserving energy. A commode by the bedside and an elevated toilet seat are often useful aids. Working with the client, the nurse attempts to coordinate activities to provide quiet rest intervals during the day.

Potential for Injury (Fracture)

Planning: client goals. The primary goal for this diagnosis is that the client will not sustain a fracture as a result of osteoporosis.

Interventions: nonsurgical management. Hypercortisolism results in demineralization of bone, which, if it persists, may lead to osteoporosis. The nurse instructs the client about safety issues and dietary needs. Clients who develop osteoporosis are prone to developing fractures, frequently as a result of accidental falls or bumping against hard surfaces. The nurse instructs the client to call for assistance when ambulating. If needed, the nurse reviews the use of ambulatory aids (walkers or canes) with the client. Rooms should be kept free from extraneous objects that might cause a fall. When assisting with daily activities, the nurse prevents the client from bumping into side rails and other hard objects.

The nurse enlists the aid of the dietitian when counseling the client about diet therapy. A high-calorie diet is prescribed, including items from all the major food groups. Generous amounts of milk, cheese, yogurt, and green leafy and root vegetables add considerable amounts of calcium to the diet. The client who has osteoporosis needs to increase the amount of calcium and vitamin D in the diet. Substances containing caffeine and alcohol should be avoided.

Body Image Disturbance

Planning: client goals. Hypercortisolism results in characteristic body changes. The major goals for this diagnosis are that the client will (1) use cosmetic methods to enhance physical appearance and (2) verbalize realistic expectations about the physical appearance.

Interventions: nonsurgical management. Many physical features of hypercortisolism, such as the buffalo hump, supraclavicular fat pads, and truncal obesity, slowly improve after medical or surgical intervention has been instituted. In the interim, the nurse suggests clothing to minimize features that may be disturbing to the female client. The use of neck scarves may minimize the buffalo hump. Long-sleeved shirts and pants cover areas of bruising. If the client is experiencing hirsutism, shaving or the use of depilatories is recommended. The nurse encourages the client to discuss feelings related to physical changes and refers the client for further counseling if needed.

■ Discharge Planning

Home Care Preparation

The major consideration in planning home care is the degree of proximal muscle weakness and fatigue the client is experiencing. The client may need to limit activities such as climbing stairs if weakness and fatigue are severe. It may help to have a commode easily accessible, and the client may continue to require the use of ambulatory aids. Osteoporosis may be present; therefore, rooms should be free from clutter and extraneous objects to prevent accidental falls.

Client/Family Education

After bilateral adrenalectomy, the client depends on lifelong exogenous adrenal hormone replacement. Education of the client and family centers on compliance with the dosage regimen and side effects of the prescribed medication. Wearing a medical alert bracelet is essential.

Psychosocial Preparation

Clients need to know that many of the physical manifestations of hypercortisolism resolve with treatment. Measures to temporarily minimize the physical features were mentioned earlier. Drug therapy after adrenalectomy is a lifelong need, and clients must actively participate in their health care regimen. A knowledge of the client's health care beliefs is valuable in determining potential compliance with hormone replacement therapy.

Health Care Resources

Clients must have ready access to the health care team. A variety of situations call for a dosage change in hormone replacement and may require consultation with the primary physician or endocrine clinical nurse specialist. A home care nurse may be helpful for reinforcement of client/family education in the home environment.

 Evaluation

Expected outcomes for the client with hypercortisolism include that the client

1. Maintains fluid balance
2. Has intact skin
3. Increases activity tolerance
4. Remains free from injury
5. Improves body image

6. Describes and complies with drug regimen
7. Identifies symptoms of excess adrenal hormone replacement
8. Identifies situations that require an increase in adrenal hormone replacement dosage
9. Obtains and wears a medical alert bracelet or necklace.

(Outcomes 7 through 9 apply to the client who undergoes a bilateral adrenalectomy.)

HYPERALDOSTERONISM

OVERVIEW

In *hyperaldosteronism*, increased secretion of aldosterone by the adrenal glands results in a state of mineralocorticoid excess.

Primary hyperaldosteronism (Conn's syndrome) is due to excessive secretion of aldosterone from one or both adrenal glands. It is usually caused by the presence of an adenoma.

In *secondary hyperaldosteronism*, the continuous excessive secretion of aldosterone results from higher levels of angiotensin II because of high plasma renin activity, which can have a variety of causes. The principal causes are poor renal perfusion caused by a loss of effective blood volume, mechanical obstruction of the renal vessels, or, the major iatrogenic contributor, the use of thiazide diuretics.

Increased aldosterone levels primarily affect the renal tubular epithelial cells and cause sodium retention and potassium and hydrogen ion excretion from the extracellular fluid. Hypernatremia, hypokalemia, and alkalosis result. Sodium retention increases extracellular fluid volume, which elevates blood pressure and suppresses renin production. The elevated blood pressure may cause cerebrovascular accidents and renal damage. Peripheral edema occurs rarely because of the "renal escape mechanism," a point at which the proximal tubule decreases sodium reabsorption. However, no compensatory mechanism exists to stop or reverse the loss of potassium (see Chap. 15 for further discussion of electrolyte imbalances).

Hyperaldosteronism occurs more frequently in women than in men by a 3:1 ratio. It is most prevalent in the third to fifth decades of life.

COLLABORATIVE MANAGEMENT

Symptoms related to *elevated blood pressure* and *hypokalemia* are the most common presenting complaints. The nursing history may reveal a variety of nonspecific findings, such as headache, fatigue, muscle weakness, nocturia, and loss of stamina. Polydipsia and polyuria occur less frequently, and paresthesias may occur if potassium depletion is severe. Clients may note vision changes related to hypertension.

Diagnosis of primary hyperaldosteronism is based on laboratory studies and radiographic findings. Serum potassium levels are decreased, and sodium levels are elevated. Plasma renin levels are low, whereas aldosterone levels are elevated. Increased hydrogen ion secretion results in metabolic alkalemia (elevated blood pH). Urine studies demonstrate low specific gravity and elevated aldosterone levels. CT scans reveal the presence and location of adrenal adenomas.

Surgical management is the treatment of choice for hyperaldosteronism identified in its early stages. Adrenalectomy may be unilateral or bilateral. Surgery is not performed, however, until the client's potassium levels are within the normal range. The potassium-sparing diuretic and aldosterone antagonist spironolactone (Aldactone) and potassium supplements may be given to increase potassium levels before surgery. Clients may also benefit from a low-sodium preoperative diet, but no dietary restrictions are needed after surgery because aldosterone levels should return to normal. Clients undergoing unilateral adrenalectomy may require temporary glucocorticoid replacement, and those undergoing bilateral adrenalectomy require lifelong glucocorticoid replacement. Glucocorticoids are administered before surgery to prevent adrenal hypofunction. Clients receiving long-term replacement therapy should wear a medical alert identification. See the discussion of adrenalectomy under the heading Adrenal Hyperfunction for further postoperative care and client education.

When surgery is inadvisable, spironolactone therapy is continued to control the symptoms of hypokalemia and to control hypertension. Because spironolactone is a potassium-sparing diuretic, hyperkalemia can occur in clients taking the drug if they have impaired renal function or excessive potassium intake. The nurse advises the client to avoid taking potassium supplements and eating foods rich in potassium. Because hyponatremia can occur with spironolactone therapy, clients may require increased dietary sodium. The nurse instructs clients to note symptoms of hyponatremia such as dryness of the mouth, thirst, lethargy, and drowsiness. The nurse advises clients to avoid use of other potassium-sparing diuretics. The nurse alerts clients to report any additional side effects of spironolactone therapy, which include gynecomastia, diarrhea, drowsiness, headache, rash, urticaria, confusion, inability to maintain an erection, hirsutism, and amenorrhea.

PHEOCHROMOCYTOMA

OVERVIEW

Pheochromocytoma, the only well-defined disorder of catecholamine excess, is a catecholamine-producing tumor that arises in chromaffin cells. Pheochromocytomas usually present as solitary unilateral lesions, but approximately 10% present as bilateral lesions, and another 10% are found in the abdomen. Unilateral tumors are most frequently found on the right side (Wilson & Foster, 1985). Pheochromocytomas are most often benign but also exist in a malignant form (approximately 10% of all cases). The tumors produce and store catecholamines much the same as normal medullary tissue; however, little is known about the mechanism responsible for their excessive release of stored hormones.

Pheochromocytomas synthesize the catecholamines epinephrine and norepinephrine. Excess epinephrine and norepinephrine stimulate alpha- and beta-receptors and can have wide-ranging adverse effects. Alpha-receptor stimulation activates sweat glands, inhibits insulin secretion, and decreases intestinal blood flow. Stimulation of the beta-receptors results in tachycardia, peripheral vasodilation, bronchodilation, and increased myocardial contractility, glycogenolysis, and free fatty acid secretion. Postural hypotension results from decreased blood volume.

The cause of pheochromocytomas is unknown, but some are associated with inherited disorders such as neurofibromatosis and multiple endocrine neoplasia type II syndrome.

Pheochromocytomas are rare, seen in approximately 0.1% of the hypertensive population. They are slightly more common in women. Pheochromocytomas can occur from infancy to old age but often appear in the fourth and fifth decades of life. They are rare after the age of 60 years (Wilson & Foster, 1985).

COLLABORATIVE MANAGEMENT

The nursing history may reveal paroxysmal hypertensive episodes or "attacks," which vary in length from a few minutes to several hours. During these episodes, clients experience palpitations, severe headaches, profuse diaphoresis, flushing, and apprehension or a feeling of impending doom. Pain in the chest or abdomen, with nausea and vomiting, can also occur. The history may reveal certain stimuli, such as increased abdominal pressure, micturition, and vigorous abdominal palpation, that are known to provoke a hypertensive crisis. Clients may complain of heat intolerance, weight loss, and tremors.

Diagnostic tests include 24-hour urine collections for vanillylmandelic acid (VMA; a product of catecholamine metabolism), metanephrine, and free catecholamines, all of which have elevated levels in pheochromocytoma. Urinary creatinine levels should be measured for all urine samples to ensure adequacy of the sample. Basal plasma catecholamine levels are elevated after the client has been at rest for at least 30 minutes. The clonidine suppression test involves oral administration of clonidine, which blocks sympathetic nervous system activity. The drug suppresses plasma catecholamine levels in normal clients and in those with essential hypertension, but it has little effect on plasma catecholamines in clients with pheochromocytoma. Catecholamine stimulation of glycogenolysis and sup-

pression of insulin may cause hyperglycemia and glycosuria, revealed by blood and urine studies.

Once the diagnosis is established, CT of the adrenal glands is used to localize intra-adrenal tumors. Chest x-ray films and tomograms are useful in localizing lesions of the thoracic area. Arteriograms may be valuable in localizing intra-abdominal tumors.

Surgical interventions are the treatment of choice for pheochromocytoma. One or both adrenal glands are removed, depending on whether the tumor is unilateral or bilateral.

Preoperatively, the nurse focuses on adequate tissue perfusion, nutritional needs, and comfort measures. Hypertension is the hallmark of the disease, and the nurse monitors the client's blood pressure regularly and is careful to place the cuff on consistently the same arm with the client in lying and standing positions. The nurse identifies stressors that may precede a hypertensive crisis and attempts to minimize them. The nurse instructs clients not to smoke, not to drink caffeine-containing beverages, and not to change position suddenly. The nurse helps the client from a lying or sitting position to a standing position. The client's abdomen should not be palpated. A diet rich in calories, vitamins, and minerals should be provided.

Clients often benefit from preoperative hydration therapy because inadequate extracellular fluid volume increases the risk of intraoperative and postoperative hypotension. The nurse assesses the client's hydration status and notes symptoms of dehydration or fluid overload.

Because clients with pheochromocytoma can experience incapacitating headaches, the nurse provides a calm, restful environment. If available, a private, darkened room helps to promote rest. The nurse instructs the client to limit activity. If the client is sleeping, the nurse avoids interruptions if possible.

Stabilization of the client with alpha-adrenergic blocking agents is necessary before surgery because the client is at increased risk for hypertension during surgery. Use of anesthetic agents and manipulation of the tumor can produce a release of catecholamines. The short-acting alpha-adrenergic blocker phentolamine (Regitine) is used in an intravenous bolus or drip for a hypertensive crisis. Oral phenoxybenzamine (Dibenzyline) produces long-acting alpha-adrenergic blockade and is most suitable for preoperative management of hypertension and prevention of hypertensive crisis. It is also the drug of choice for long-term management of the client who is not a candidate for surgery. Drug dosages are adjusted gradually until blood pressure is controlled and no further hypertensive attacks occur. This adjustment normally takes 2 to 3 weeks, during which the contracted plasma expands and blood pressure in the supine position returns to normal. The alpha blocker prazosin (Minipress) is used less frequently for the preoperative client because its duration of action is much shorter.

Beta-receptor blocking agents should never be used in clients with a suspected or definitive diagnosis of pheochromocytoma until after alpha-adrenergic block-ade has been initiated, because these drugs may cause blood pressure to rise. After alpha-adrenergic blockade, low doses of propranolol (Inderal) may be used to treat tachycardia and arrhythmias.

Postoperative nursing care is similar to that for the client undergoing an adrenalectomy for adrenal hyper-function (see earlier). In addition, these clients must be closely monitored for hypotension related to the sudden decrease in catecholamine level and hypovolemia. Hemorrhage and shock are the potential complications, and the nurse administers plasma expanders and fluids as prescribed. The nurse monitors the client's vital signs frequently and carefully records fluid intake and output. If narcotics are administered, the nurse observes their effect on blood pressure.

Infrequently, tumors may not be operable because of disseminated malignancy or concurrent illness. Treat-ment in these cases is medical, with alpha- and beta-ad-renergic blocking agents, because these tumors do not respond well to chemotherapy or radiation therapy. For clients who are medically managed, self-measurement of blood pressure with home monitoring equipment is essential.

SUMMARY

Nursing care of clients with pituitary or adrenal dis-orders is complex and challenging. The hormones of the anterior pituitary gland regulate growth, metabolic ac-tivity, and sexual development. An excess or a defi-ciency of one or more of the anterior pituitary hormones can have widespread physiologic and psychologic ef-fects. Posterior pituitary dysfunction involves a defi-ciency or an excess of vasopressin, also known as the antidiuretic hormone (ADH). A decrease in the amount or effect of ADH results in diabetes insipidus. The syn-drome of inappropriate ADH results when ADH is se-creted in the presence of low plasma osmolality. Both disorders result in disturbances of fluid and electrolyte balance.

Disorders of the adrenal gland are caused by hypo- or hypersecretion of adrenal hormones. In hypofunction, decreased production of adrenocortical steroids has widespread effects on the body and may progress to a life-threatening situation. Hyperfunction of the adrenal gland results in a number of clinical entities, in particu-lar, Cushing's syndrome, hyperaldosteronism, and pheochromocytoma.

In pituitary and adrenal disorders, clients often un-dergo extensive diagnostic testing and surgical inter-vention. Hormone replacement is necessary in many instances, which requires extensive client education. Nursing interventions significantly influence the

client's clinical course and greatly affect the quality of life.

IMPLICATIONS FOR RESEARCH

There is ongoing research in the areas of pituitary and adrenal disorders. Etiologic factors of these disease pro-cesses are so diverse that it is difficult to identify a "cure" for them. In many instances, hormone replace-ment corrects problems seen in specific disorders, and research in this area is promising. With the advent of recombinant DNA therapy, hormone preparations (e.g., GH) may become available for more affected individ-uals.

Nursing research should focus on aiding individuals with pituitary and adrenal problems to adapt to changes that may occur in their lives. Priority areas for research include client education, body image, and, in certain diseases such as hypopituitarism or adrenal hypofunc-tion, prevention. Questions that may stimulate nursing research include

1. Do support groups assist clients in adjusting to their diagnosis (e.g., dwarfism, infertility)?
2. Does client education instituted in the hospital im-prove compliance after discharge?
3. Do nursing interventions to minimize physical changes related to pituitary and adrenal disorders have a positive effect on the client's body image?
4. What nursing interventions decrease the incidence of postoperative complications?

REFERENCES AND READINGS

Baer, C. L. (1988). Why does the patient have polyuria? *Nursing '88, 18*(10), 94–95.

Bagdade, J. D. (Ed.). (1987). *The yearbook of endocrinology.* Chicago: Year Book Medical.

Bergland, B. E. (1989). Pheochromocytoma presenting as shock. *American Journal of Emergency Medicine, 7,* 44–48.

Besser, G. M., & Cudeworth, A. G. (Eds.) (1987). *Clinical endocrinology: An illustrated text.* Philadelphia: J. B. Lippincott.

Braunwald, E., Isselbacher, K., Petersdorf, R., Wilson, J., Martin, J., & Fauci, A. (Eds). (1987). *Harrison's principles of internal medicine* (11th ed.) New York: McGraw-Hill.

Brunner, L. S., & Suddarth, D. S. (Eds.). (1986). *Lippincott manual of nursing practice* (4th ed.). Philadelphia: J. B. Lippincott.

Carlson, H. E. (Ed.). (1983). *Endocrinology.* New York: Wiley Medical.

Cohen, S., & Soloway, R. D. (Eds.). (1985). *Hormone-produc-*

ing tumors of the gastrointestinal tracts. New York: Churchill Livingstone.

Felig, P., Baster, J. D., & Broadus, A. (Eds.). (1987). *Endocrinology and metabolism* (2nd ed.) New York: McGraw-Hill.

Freidberg, S. R. (1986). Tumors of the brain. *Clinical Symposia, 38*(4), 2–32.

Garofano, C. D. (1981). Pituitary disorders: hypopituitarism. In *Diseases* (p. 811). Springhouse, PA: Springhouse Corp.

Garofano, C. D. (1981). Hyperpituitarism: Acromegaly and gigantism. In *Diseases* (p. 814). Springhouse, PA: Springhouse Corp.

Garofano, C. D. (1981). Diabetes insipidus. In *Diseases* (p. 816). Springhouse, PA: Springhouse Corp.

Garofano, C. D. (1984). Thyroid and adrenal crisis: Overcoming endocrine imbalance. In S. Williams & B. McVan (Eds.), *Nursing critically ill patients confidently* (2nd ed., pp. 147–156). Springhouse, PA: Springhouse Corp.

Garofano, C. D. (1984). Identifying posterior lobe dysfunction. In H. Hamilton & M. B. Rose (Eds.), *Endocrine disorders* (pp. 62–71). Springhouse, PA: Springhouse Corp.

Germon, K. (1987). Fluid and electrolyte problems associated with diabetes insipidus and syndrome of inappropriate antidiuretic hormone. *Nursing Clinics of North America, 22,* 785–796.

Gotch, P. M. (1981). Teaching patients about adrenal corticosteroids. *American Journal of Nursing, 81,* 78–81.

Greenspan, F. S., & Forsham, P. H. (1986). *Basic and clinical endocrinology* (2nd ed.). Los Altos, CA: Lange Medical.

Hartshorn, J., & Hartshorn, E. (1988). Vasopressin in the treatment of diabetes insipidus. *Journal of Neuroscience Nursing, 20,* 58–59.

Hershman, J. M. (Ed.). (1980). *Management of endocrine disorders.* Philadelphia: Lea & Febiger.

Ho, K. Y. (1988). Therapeutic applications of bromocriptine in endocrine and neurologic disease. *Drugs, 36,* 67–82.

Kaplan, S. A. (1982). *Clinical pediatric and adolescent endocrinology.* Philadelphia: W. B. Saunders.

Kessler, C. M. (1988). Protecting the adrenalectomy patient. *Nursing '88, 18*(12), 64.

Koppers, L. (1980). Pheochromocytoma: Critical care. *Critical Care Quarterly, 3*(2), 93–98.

Lancaster, L. E. (1987). Renal and endocrine regulation of water and electrolyte balance. *Nursing Clinics of North America, 22,* 761–772.

Lepshultz, L. I., & Howards, S. S. (Eds.). (1983). *Infertility in the male.* New York: Churchill Livingstone.

Martin, C. R. (1985). *Endocrine physiology.* New York: Oxford University Press.

Mazzaferri, E. L. (Ed.). (1986). *Textbook of endocrinology* (3rd ed.). New York: Elsevier Science.

McInerney, M. (1981). Prolactin producing pituitary adenomas. *Journal of Neurosurgical Nursing, 13,* 15–17.

Metz, R., & Larson, E. B. (Eds.). (1985). *Blue book of endocrinology.* Philadelphia: W. B. Saunders.

Motton, C., & Litwack, K. (1989). Practical points in the care of patients following transsphenoidal surgery. *Journal of Post Anesthesia Nursing, 4,* 109–111.

Murthe, N. C. (1981). *Endocrinology—nursing approach.* Boston: Little, Brown.

Physicians' Desk Reference. (1990). (44th ed.). Oradell, NJ: Medical Economics.

Sanford, S. J. (1980). Dysfunction of the adrenal gland: Physiologic considerations and nursing problems. *Nursing Clinics of North America, 15,* 481–498.

Schmike, R. N. (1980). Adrenal insufficiency. *Critical Care Quarterly, 3,* 19–28.

Shepple, N. A. (1988). A case study: Anesthesia for pheochromocytoma. *AANA Journal, 56*(2), 169–172.

Solomon, B. L. (1980). The hypothalamus and the pituitary gland: An overview. *Nursing Clinics of North America, 15,* 435–452.

Stachura, M. E. (1987). Human growth hormone use and potential abuse. *Hospital Formulary, 22*(1), 48–51, 55, 58–59.

Stukey, P., & Waters, H. (1989). Oncology alert for the home health nurse: Syndrome of inappropriate antidiuretic hormone. *Home Health Nurse, 6*(6), 26–30.

Tulchinsky, D., & Ryan, K. J. (Eds.). (1980). *Maternal-fetal endocrinology.* Philadelphia: W. B. Saunders.

Verbalis, J. G., & Robinson A. G. (1984). Hypopituitarism. *Emergency Medicine, 5,* 74–78.

Wilson, J. D., & Foster, D. W. (Eds.). (1985). *Williams textbook of endocrinology* (7th ed.). Philadelphia: W. B. Saunders.

Wyngaarden, J. B., & Smith, L. H. (Eds.). (1988). *Cecil textbook of medicine* (18th ed.). Philadelphia: W. B. Saunders.

Zucker, A. R., & Chernow, B. (1983). Diabetes insipidus and the syndrome of inappropriate antidiuretic hormone release. *Critical Care Quarterly, 6*(3), 63–74.

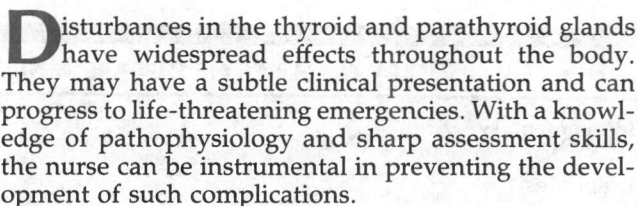

CHAPTER 50

Interventions for Clients with Disorders of the Thyroid and Parathyroid Glands

Disturbances in the thyroid and parathyroid glands have widespread effects throughout the body. They may have a subtle clinical presentation and can progress to life-threatening emergencies. With a knowledge of pathophysiology and sharp assessment skills, the nurse can be instrumental in preventing the development of such complications.

DISORDERS OF THE THYROID GLAND

HYPERTHYROIDISM

OVERVIEW

Hyperthyroidism occurs as a result of excessive thyroid hormone secretion. *Thyrotoxicosis* refers to the clinical signs and symptoms that appear when body tissues are stimulated by increased thyroid hormones. Thyroid hormones affect virtually all metabolic processes and many body organs; therefore, the clinical manifestations of hyperthyroidism are numerous and varied. Depending on the etiology, this disease may be transient or permanent. Interventions focus on blocking the effects or interfering with the excessive secretion of thyroid hormones, establishing normal or euthyroid function, and addressing the signs and symptoms the client may be experiencing.

Pathophysiology

In hyperthyroidism, the normal regulatory controls of thyroid hormone secretion are lost. In general, the action of thyroid hormones on most body systems is stimulatory. Excessive thyroid hormones produce a state of *hypermetabolism*, with increased sympathetic nervous system activity. Many of the signs and symptoms of hyperthyroidism (see the Key Features of Disease on p. 1560) result from the body's attempt to compensate for the hypermetabolic state. Increases occur in cardiac output, oxygen consumption, peripheral blood flow, and body temperature.

Excessive thyroid hormones directly stimulate the heart. Cardiac output and peripheral blood flow are increased owing to an increase in heart rate and stroke volume. A hyperdynamic circulatory state results from hypermetabolism and an increase in adrenergic responsiveness. Thyroid hormones appear to increase the number of beta-adrenergic receptor sites in the heart.

Elevated levels of thyroid hormones profoundly affect protein, carbohydrate, and lipid metabolism. Protein synthesis and degradation are increased, with degradation exceeding synthesis. Negative nitrogen balance results. In hyperthyroidism, glucose tolerance

KEY FEATURES OF DISEASE ■ Signs and Symptoms of Hyperthyroidism

Integumentary

Diaphoresis
Fine, soft, silky hair
Smooth, moist skin

Pulmonary

Dyspnea, with or without exertion

Cardiovascular

Palpitations
Chest pain
Increased systolic blood pressure
Widened pulse pressure
Tachycardia
Arrhythmias

Gastrointestinal

Weight loss
Increased appetite
Diarrhea

Musculoskeletal

Proximal muscle weakness

Neurologic

Blurred or double vision
Eye fatigue
Insomnia
Corneal ulcers or infections
Increased tears

Neurologic

Infected (red) conjunctiva
Photophobia
Eyelid retraction, eyelid lag
Globe lag
Hyperactive deep tendon reflexes
Tremors

Psychologic/Emotional

Decreased attention span
Restlessness
Irritability
Emotional lability
Manic behavior

Metabolic

Increased basal metabolic rate
Heat intolerance
Low-grade fever

Reproductive

Amenorrhea
Decreased menstrual flow
Increased libido

Other

Goiter
Wide-eyed (startled) appearance
Weakness, fatigue

---

may be slightly to markedly decreased. Mobilization, synthesis, and breakdown of triglycerides are increased, with a net effect of lipid depletion. A state of chronic nutritional and caloric deficiency results from the metabolic effects of excessive thyroid hormones.

Alterations occur in the secretion and metabolism of hypothalamic and pituitary and gonadal steroids. If hyperthyroidism is present before the onset of puberty, sexual development is delayed in both sexes. If hyperthyroidism develops after puberty, females experience menstrual irregularities and decreased fertility. An increase in libido occurs in both sexes.

Etiology

The causes of hyperthyroidism are numerous (see the Key Features of Disease on p. 1561). The most common cause is *Graves' disease* (toxic diffuse goiter), which is characterized by hyperthyroidism, enlargement of the thyroid gland (goiter), and exophthalmos (abnormal protrusion of the eyes). Graves' disease may be an autoimmune disorder. Immunoglobulins or antibodies known as thyroid-stimulating immunoglobulins (TSIs) stimulate enlargement of the thyroid gland and excessive thyroid hormone secretion. TSI activity is present in approximately 80% of clients with Graves' disease (Wilson & Foster, 1985).

Hyperthyroidism characterized by multiple thyroid nodules is termed *toxic multinodular goiter*. Affected individuals have usually had nontoxic multinodular goiter for years. The overproduction of thyroid hormone is usually milder than that seen in Graves' disease.

Incidence

Hyperthyroidism is a prevalent endocrine disorder, affecting females four times more frequently than males. Graves' disease is seen most commonly in women younger than 40 years of age. The exact incidence of Graves' disease is unknown. Toxic multinodular goiter usually occurs after the age of 50 years and is more common in women than in men.

EMERGENCY CARE: THYROID STORM

Thyroid storm (thyroid crisis) is a life-threatening event that occurs in a client with uncontrolled hyperthyroidism attributable to Graves' disease. Signs and symptoms of crisis develop quickly, and it is usually triggered by a major stressor, such as trauma or infection. In the past, thyroid storm occurred in clients undergoing thyroid surgery who were inadequately prepared. Today, antithyroid drugs, beta-blockers, steroids, and iodides are given before thyroid surgery, preventing thyroid crisis. Occasionally, if a large goiter is vigorously palpated, thyroid storm can be precipitated. It can develop when a critically ill individual is treated with radioactive iodine or when clients with a thyroid adenoma or nontoxic goiter are exposed to organic or inorganic iodine.

A rapid increase in the metabolic rate resulting from the discharge of excessive thyroid hormone causes the characteristic signs and symptoms. Fever, tachycardia, and systolic hypertension are present. Clients may experience gastrointestinal (GI) symptoms, such as abdominal pain, nausea, vomiting, and diarrhea. Typically, agitation, tremors, and anxiety are seen in thyroid storm. As it progresses, clients may exhibit restlessness, confusion, psychosis, and seizures, leading to a comatose state. Emergency measures are needed to prevent death. Emergency measures vary with the clinical presentation. After the determining cause or event has been identified, the primary concerns are maintaining airway patency, providing adequate ventilation, and stabilizing

KEY FEATURES OF DISEASE ■ Etiology of Hyperthyroidism

Etiology	Mechanism
Graves' disease (toxic diffuse goiter)	Probably autoimmune in nature. Immunoglobulins cause stimulation of the thyroid gland.
Toxic multinodular goiter	Multiple thyroid nodules, resulting in thyroid hyperfunctionings.
Thyroid adenoma	Autonomous functioning of adenoma of follicular cells.
Pituitary hyperthyroidism	Pituitary adenoma resulting in excessive TSH secretion.
Thyroiditis (radiation-induced)	T_3 and T_4 secretion increased before destruction of gland. Hyperthyroid state usually transient.
T_3 thyrotoxicosis	Increase in thyroid secretion of T_3. Cause unknown.
Factitious hyperthyroidism	Ingestion of excessive amounts of thyroid hormone.
Jodbasedow (iodine-induced)	Administration of iodine to an individual with endemic goiter, resulting in excessive production of thyroid hormone.
Struma ovarii	Dermoid tumor of the ovary that secretes thyroid hormone.
Thyroid carcinoma	Uncommon, usually occurs with large follicular carcinomas.
Trophoblastic tumors	Choriocarcinoma, hydatidiform mole, and embryonal carcinoma with high concentrations of chorionic gonadotropins that stimulate T_3 and T_4 secretion.

EMERGENCY CARE ■ Thyroid Storm

Interventions	Rationales
1. Maintain patent airway and adequate ventilation.	1. To alleviate the marked respiratory distress that may be present.
2. Give antithyroid drugs: propylthiouracil (PTU) 300–900 mg/d; methimazole (Tapazole) up to 60 mg/d.	2. To block synthesis, secretion, and peripheral effects of thyroid hormone.
3. Administer sodium iodide solution (2 g/d IV).	3. To stop release of thyroid hormone already in gland.
4. Give propranolol (Inderal) 1–3 mg IV. Give slowly over 3 min; client should be connected to a cardiac monitor and have a central venous pressure catheter in place.	4. To decrease excessive sympathetic stimulation if life-threatening arrythmias are present.
5. Give glucocorticoids: hydrocortisone 100–500 mg/d IV; prednisone 4–60 mg/d IV or IM.	5. To prevent the release of thyroid hormone from the gland.
6. Provide comfort measure, including a cooling blanket.	6. To make the client more comfortable. Increased metabolism causes diaphoresis and heat intolerance.
7. Monitor vital signs frequently.	7. To detect worsening of condition. Temperature may rise to 41°C (106°F); cardiac arrhythmias may be present.
8. Give nonsalicylate antipyretics.	8. To reduce fever safely. Acetylsalicylic acid (aspirin) can displace thyroid hormone from binding sites.

the hemodynamic status (see the accompanying Emergency Care feature).

COLLABORATIVE MANAGEMENT

 Assessment

History

The client's history provides essential information for the detection of hyperthyroidism. Because hyperthyroidism can affect numerous body systems, there are usually a wide array of subjective complaints.

The nurse obtains information regarding *age, sex,* and usual *weight.* The client may report recent weight loss and increased appetite. Clients may report diarrhea and are asked if there has been a noticeable change in the frequency and consistency of bowel movements.

A hallmark of hyperthyroidism is *heat intolerance.* The nurse determines whether the client has experienced diaphoresis or has noticed wearing less or lighter clothing in cold weather. Owing to the cardiovascular effects of hyperthyroidism, *palpitations* or *chest pain* may be reported. The nurse questions the client about changes in breathing patterns, as dyspnea, with or without exertion, can occur.

Visual difficulties in the hyperthyroid client result from ophthalmopathy (Fig. 50–1). The nurse questions the client about changes in vision, such as blurring, double vision, or eyes tiring easily.

The nurse inquires whether the client has noticed a change in his/her ability to perform activities of daily living (ADL). Complaints of fatigue, weakness, and insomnia are recorded.

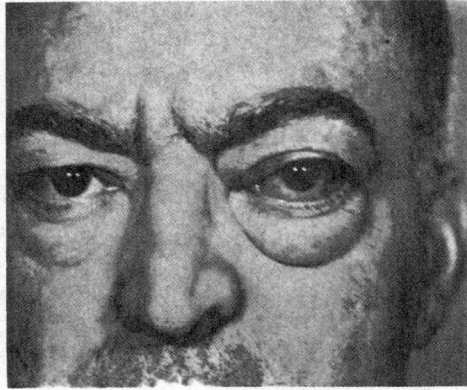

Figure 50–1

Ophthalmopathy. The client has proptosis, limited eye movement, and edema. (From Wilson, J., & Foster, D. [1985]. *Williams textbook of endocrinology* [7th ed.]. Philadelphia: W. B. Saunders.)

Females are asked about *changes in menses.* Amenorrhea or a decreased menstrual flow is not uncommon. An increase in libido is possible in affected persons of both sexes.

The client's previous medical history is also explored. A history of thyroid surgery or radiation therapy to the neck area can be significant in the hyperthyroid client, because some persons remain hyperthyroid after surgery and some persons are resistant to radiation therapy. The nurse asks about past or current medications, noting the use of thyroid hormone replacement or antithyroid drugs.

Physical Assessment: Clinical Manifestations

The nurse examines the general appearance of the client. Two types of ophthalmopathy are seen in hyperthyroidism. The first, seen in all forms of thyrotoxicosis, involves *eyelid retraction* and *eyelid lag,* in which the upper eyelid fails to descend promptly and steadily when the client gazes slowly downward. The second is *globe lag,* in which the upper eyelid pulls back faster than the eyeball is raised when the client gazes upward. The nurse asks the client to look down and up and observes the response.

Infiltrative ophthalmopathy, leading to *exophthalmos* (Fig. 50–2), is seen in Graves' disease. The wide-eyed or startled look is due to the accumulation of fluid in the extraocular muscles and retro-orbital fat, which pushes the globe forward. Pressure on the optic nerve may impair vision. Swelling and shortening of the muscles may result in problems with focusing. If the eyelid fails to close completely and the eye is unprotected, corneal ulcerations and infections can result. The nurse observes the client's eyes for excessive tearing, infected conjunctiva, and photophobia.

The thyroid gland is palpated to determine the presence of a mass or general enlargement. The nurse observes the size and symmetry of the gland. Goiter (enlargement of the thyroid gland) (Fig. 50–3) is present in

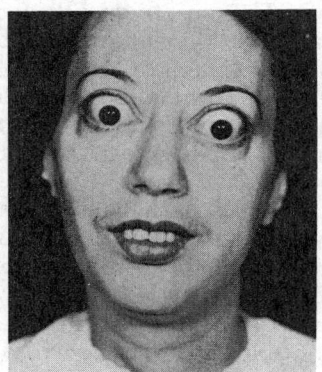

Figure 50–2

Exophthalmos. (From Wilson, J., & Foster, D. [1985]. *Williams textbook of endocrinology* [7th ed.]. Philadelphia: W. B. Saunders.)

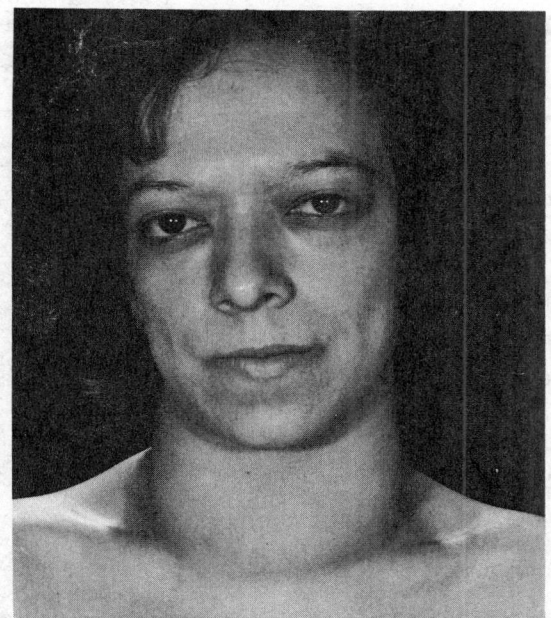

Figure 50–3

Goiter. (From Wilson, J., & Foster, D. [1985]. *Williams textbook of endocrinology* [7th ed.]. Philadelphia: W. B. Saunders.)

Graves' disease. The thyroid gland may increase to four times its normal size. If the thyroid is enlarged, bruits (turbulence from increased blood flow) may be auscultated. See Chapter 48 for discussion of thyroid palpation and auscultation.

Psychosocial Assessment

Clients with hyperthyroidism frequently experience emotional lability, irritability, decreased attention span, or manic behavior. Moods fluctuate, resulting in a chaotic emotional condition. Mild to severe hyperactivity often leads to a state of fatigue. The nurse asks the client if he/she has noticed crying or laughing inappropriately or if there has been difficulty concentrating on specific tasks. Often, the client's family report changes in mental or emotional status, and the nurse must include family members when identifying these problems.

Laboratory Findings

The diagnostic work-up for hyperthyroidism includes measurement of serum tri-iodothyronine (T_3) and thyronine (T_4), and T_3 resin uptake (T_3RU). Further evaluation may include thyrotropin-releasing hormone (TRH) stimulation test and thyroid suppression test. The laboratory findings in clients with hyperthyroidism are summarized in the accompanying Key Features of Disease.

Other Diagnostic Tests

A thyroid scan or radioactive iodine uptake (RAIU) test is employed to evaluate the position, size, and func-

KEY FEATURES OF DISEASE ■ Laboratory Findings in Hyperthyroidism

Test	Findings
Serum T_3	Increased
Serum T_4	Increased
Free T_3 and T_4	Increased
T_3RU	Increased
TRH stimulation test	Little or no TSH response
Thyroid suppression test	Fails to suppress RAIU or T_4 levels
TSH stimulation test (thyroid stimulation test)	No change
RAIU study	Increased
Thyroid antibodies	High titer of thyroglobulin antibodies

tioning of the thyroid gland. Radioactive iodine (RAI) (^{123}I) is given by mouth, and the uptake of iodine by the thyroid gland is measured. Normally, the thyroid has an uptake of 5% to 35% of the administered dose. In hyperthyroidism, the RAIU is increased. RAI not utilized by the thyroid is excreted by the kidney. The half-life of ^{123}I is short, and no radiation precautions are necessary. However, pregnancy should be ruled out before the scan is done. Any procedure that utilizes contrast material containing iodine should not be done for at least 4 weeks before RAIU. The administration of any medication containing iodine should be discontinued for 1 week before the scan.

Ultrasonography of the thyroid gland can be used to determine size of the thyroid gland and evaluate masses or nodules. The nurse reassures the client that this procedure is painless; it takes approximately 30 minutes to perform.

An electrocardiogram (ECG) may show tachycardia, atrial fibrillation, and alterations in P and T wavelengths.

 ### Analysis: Nursing Diagnosis

Common Diagnoses

The following nursing diagnoses are frequently seen in the client with hyperthyroidism:

1. Potential for decreased cardiac output related to hypermetabolic state
2. Altered nutrition: less than body requirements related to increased caloric demand secondary to hypermetabolic state
3. Potential for sensory/perceptual alterations (visual) related to infiltrative ophthalmopathy

Additional Diagnoses

Clients with hyperthyroidism may also have the following nursing diagnoses:

1. Ineffective individual coping related to emotional lability
2. Activity intolerance related to increased metabolic rate
3. Altered thought processes related to decreased attention span and emotional lability
4. Diarrhea related to increased metabolic activity
5. Knowledge deficit related to diagnosis and treatment

 ### Planning and Implementation

Potential for Decreased Cardiac Output

Planning: client goals. The goal for this nursing diagnosis is that the client will have cardiovascular function return to his/her baseline level.

Interventions. Clients with hyperthyroidism can have increased systolic blood pressure, a widened pulse pressure, tachycardia, and arrhythmias; therefore, nonsurgical management is directed toward interfering with the effect of thyroid hormone on peripheral tissues and decreasing the secretion of thyroid hormone. Surgery may be necessary when nonsurgical interventions are unsuccessful.

Nonsurgical management. The nurse monitors the client's pulse, blood pressure, and temperature at least every 4 hours. The client is instructed to report any palpitations, dyspnea, vertigo, or chest pain immediately. The nurse minimizes client discomfort from the clinical effects of hyperthyroidism. Activity intolerance and fatigue are common. Clients are encouraged to rest, and the nurse provides as quiet an environment as possible. Frequent bed linen changes, sponge baths, and a cool environment decrease discomfort caused by diaphoresis and heat intolerance.

Drug therapy. The most frequently employed antithyroid drugs are the thionamides, including propylthiouracil (PTU) and methimazole (Tapazole). Their action is to block thyroid hormone synthesis (Table 50–1).

Iodine preparations may be used in the treatment of hyperthyroidism to inhibit synthesis and release of thyroid hormone.

Lithium carbonate also inhibits thyroid hormone release. Its side effects, such as depression, nephrogenic diabetes insipidus, tremors, nausea, and vomiting, limit the use of this drug. It may be prescribed when a client cannot tolerate other antithyroid drugs.

Beta-adrenergic blocking drugs, such as propranolol (Inderal), aid in decreasing the diaphoresis, anxiety, tachycardia, and palpitations experienced by clients with hyperthyroidism.

Radioactive iodine therapy. In RAI therapy, ^{131}I is

TABLE 50–1   Antithyroid Drugs Used in the Treatment of Hyperthyroidism

Drug	Usual Daily Dosage	Interventions	Rationales
Propylthiouracil (PTU)	100–150 mg PO	1. Give at 8-h intervals around the clock.	1. To maintain suppression of hormone.
Methimazole (Tapazole)	5–15 mg PO	1. Monitor vital signs. 2. Weigh the client weekly. 3. Observe for sore throat, fever, headache, and skin eruptions.	1–3. To detect adverse reactions, which may necessitate discontinuation of drug use.
Strong iodine (Lugol's) solution	6 drops in ½ glassful of liquid PO	1. Give in fruit juice or water. 2. Observe for fever, sore mouth, severe GI distress, and burning mouth and throat.	1. To improve taste 2. To detect signs of iodism, which may necessitate discontinuation of drug use.
Potassium iodide (SSKI)	900–1800 mg tablet 0.9–2.4 mL of solution 20–60 mL of syrup PO	1. Dilute solution in a glassful of water. 2. Instruct the client to take tablets after meals. 3. Encourage fluid intake. 4. Observe for rash, fever, epigastric pain, brassy taste, nausea, and vomiting.	1. To improve taste. 2. To enhance absorption. 3. To liquefy respiratory secretions. 4. To detect side effects, which may necessitate discontinuation of drug use.
Lithium carbonate	Individualized, 900–1200 mg PO	1. Observe for signs of hypothyroidism. 2. Instruct the client to drink 10–12 glassfuls of fluid a day. 3. Instruct the client to maintain normal sodium intake.	1. To detect drug-induced thyroid enlargement. 2. To prevent dehydration. 3. To prevent retention of drug caused by reduced sodium intake.
Propranolol (Inderal)	30 mg in divided doses PO	1. Weigh the client daily. 2. Measure intake and output. 3. Instruct the client to take with food. 4. Instruct the client to avoid smoking. 5. Monitor the client's pulse.	1,2. To detect congestive heart failure, as manifested by increased weight and decreased intake and output. 3. To enhance absorption. 4. To promote drug effect, which is reduced by smoking. 5. To detect tachycardia, a sign of hyperthyroidism.

administered orally. The dosage depends on the size of the thyroid and the degree of radiosensitivity of the gland. The thyroid gland picks up the RAI, and some of the cells that synthesize thyroid hormone are destroyed by the local radiation. A decrease in thyroid hormone level causes a subsequent decrease in the symptoms of hyperthyroidism. Relief of symptoms does not occur until 6 to 8 weeks after treatment. In the interim, clients may require propranolol administration.

RAI therapy usually entails one dose and can be performed on an outpatient (ambulatory) basis. Unless the dosage is extremely high, clients require no radiation precautions. The nurse reassures the client that the radioactivity quickly dissipates. Occasionally, a client requires a second or even a third dose. One of the most frequent complications is the development of hypothyroidism, which can occur several years after treatment. In this instance, clients need lifelong thyroid hormone replacement.

RAI therapy is contraindicated in pregnant women, because ^{131}I crosses the placenta and can adversely affect the fetal thyroid gland.

Surgical management. Antithyroid drugs and RAI therapy have become the treatment of choice for clients with hyperthyroidism. Clients who have large goiters causing tracheal or esophageal compression or who are unresponsive to antithyroid drugs may be candidates for surgery to remove all or part of the thyroid gland. Removal of the thyroid tissue results in a decrease in the excessive amount of thyroid hormones. In a subtotal thyroidectomy, part of the thyroid gland is removed. The remaining thyroid gland tissue may then be capable of synthesizing a sufficient amount of thyroid hormones. In a total thyroidectomy, the entire thyroid gland is removed. This surgery is indicated in certain types of thyroid cancer.

Preoperative care. If at all possible, clients should be euthyroid before thyroid surgery. The euthyroid state is achieved by the administration of antithyroid drugs to decrease the secretion of thyroid hormone and iodine preparations to decrease the size and vascularity of the gland, diminishing the risk of hemorrhage. Preoperatively, cardiac problems should be under control. Clients with hyperthyroidism are often not at optimal weight, and special attention to adequate nutrition with a high-protein, high-carbohydrate diet is essential.

The nurse instructs the client to perform coughing and deep breathing exercises and demonstrates how to support the neck when coughing or moving. Placing both hands behind the neck reduces the strain on the suture line that occurs with movement. The nurse explains that the client may experience hoarseness for a few days as a result of the endotracheal tube placement during surgery.

Clients are often afraid of thyroid surgery, perhaps because the incision is in the neck area. Preoperatively, the nurse identifies areas of client concern and reassures the client by calmly providing information about the surgery and postoperative care that is appropriate for the client's age and educational level.

Postoperative care. Care of the client recovering from thyroidectomy is summarized in the accompanying Client Care Plan. Initially vital signs are monitored every 15 minutes until they are stable, then every 30 minutes. The frequency of vital signs evaluation is increased or decreased on the basis of changes in the client's condition.

The nurse assesses the client's level of discomfort. Sandbags or pillows are used to support the client's head and neck. When the client is awake, he/she is placed in semi-Fowler's position. The nurse attempts to decrease tension on the suture line when positioning the client. Pain medications are administered when needed.

Humidification of the air is necessary to promote easier respiration and to liquefy thick respiratory secretions. The nurse assists the client to cough and deep breathe every 30 minutes to 1 hour and suctions oral and tracheal secretions when necessary.

The complications that may arise from thyroid surgery include hemorrhage, respiratory distress, parathyroid gland injury (resulting in hypocalcemia and tetany), and damage to laryngeal nerves. After surgery, the neck dressing is inspected. A drain is usually in place, and clients normally have a moderate amount of serosanguineous drainage. The nurse is alert for the development of hemorrhage, particularly during the first 24 hours after surgery. Hemorrhage may be manifested by bleeding at the incision site or by respiratory distress caused by tracheal compression.

Respiratory distress can also result from swelling, tetany, or laryngeal stridor. Equipment for emergency tracheostomy should be easily available, preferably at the client's bedside. The nurse checks that oxygen and suctioning equipment are nearby and in working order. In some instances, nurses are instructed to remove clips or sutures when medical assistance is unavailable.

The parathyroid glands can be damaged or their blood supply impaired during thyroid surgery. Hypocalcemia and tetany result when parathyroid hormone (PTH) levels decrease. The nurse notes client complaints of tingling around the mouth or of the toes and fingers and muscular twitching as signs of calcium deficiency. Additional later signs of hypocalcemia are positive Chvostek's and Trousseau's signs (see later). Calcium gluconate or calcium chloride for intravenous (IV) administration should be kept at the client's bedside. The care of clients with hypocalcemia is discussed in Chapter 13.

If laryngeal nerve damage occurs during surgery, hoarseness and a weak voice can result. The nurse assesses the client's voice at approximately 8-hour intervals and notes any changes. Clients are reassured that hoarseness is usually temporary.

Altered Nutrition: Less Than Body Requirements

Planning: client goals. The goals for this nursing diagnosis is that the client will maintain his/her normal weight or gain weight gradually if the client's weight is below normal.

CLIENT CARE PLAN ■ The Client Recovering from Thyroidectomy

Goal/Outcome Criteria	Interventions	Rationales

Nursing Diagnosis 1: Ineffective Airway Clearance Related to Hemorrhage or Edema at Surgical Site or Damage to Recurrent Laryngeal Nerves or Injury to Parathyroid Glands

Goal/Outcome Criteria	Interventions	Rationales

Client will not experience postoperative respiratory difficulty.
■ Has negative Chvostek's and Trousseau's signs.
■ Has no signs of respiratory distress, such as cyanosis, tachypnea, and noisy respirations.
■ Does not hemorrhage.
■ Has no or temporary hoarseness.
	1. Identify potential problems relating to respiratory functions.
	  a. Inspect neck dressings every hour during the initial postoperative period, then q 4 h.
	  b. Maintain the client in semi-Fowler's position with an icebag to reduce swelling.
	  c. Monitor the amount of drainage and frequency of dressing reinforcement.
	  d. Ask the client to speak q 2 h, noting changes in tone or hoarseness.
	  e. Check with the client regarding sensation of tightness around the incision site.
	  f. Assess for the presence of Chvostek's and Trousseau's signs.
	  g. Identify the presence of numbness or tingling of extremities.
	  h. Monitor serum calcium levels.
	  i. Keep emergency tracheostomy suction equipment, oxygen, suture removal kit, and IV calcium readily available.
	  j. Monitor the client for signs of respiratory distress, cyanosis, tachypnea, and noisy respirations.
		1. To detect and prevent respiratory problems. Surgery in the neck area can result in airway obstruction, primarily owing to postoperative edema. In addition, damage to laryngeal nerves during thyroid surgery can cause closure of the glottis. Hypocalcemia, resulting from parathyroid gland damage or removal, can cause tetany and laryngospasm.

Nursing Diagnosis 2: Potential for Decreased Cardiac Output Related to Hemorrhage

Goal/Outcome Criteria	Interventions	Rationales

Client will maintain cardiac output necessary for adequate tissue oxygenation.
■ Remains alert and oriented.
■ Does not hemorrhage.
■ Has vital signs stabilized to preoperative levels.
■ Does not develop tachycardia or cardiac arrhythmias.
	1. Identify changes in cardiovascular status.
	  a. Monitor vital signs every 15 min in the initial postoperative period, then q 1–4 h.
	  b. Monitor cardiac rhythm, noting tachycardia or irregularity.
	  c. Check dressing for excessive bleeding. Check on front, back, and sides of neck, feeling behind neck.
	  d. Identify changes in level of consciousness or orientation.
	  e. Administer fluids as ordered.
		1. To detect hypovolemia, hypertension, and eventual shock related to excessive blood loss.

continued

CLIENT CARE PLAN ■ The Client Recovering from Thyroidectomy *continued*

Goal/Outcome Criteria	Interventions	Rationales
Nursing Diagnosis 3: Pain Related to Surgical Incision		

Client will experience minimal pain and discomfort.
■ States that pain relief is satisfactory after interventions.
	1. Assist the client in maintaining correct head and neck position.
	  a. Place the client in semi-Fowler's position with sandbags or pillows to support the neck.
	  b. Place fluids and call light within easy reach of the client.
	  c. Teach the client to support the head and neck.
	  d. Maintain a quiet environment, decreasing stress.
		1. To decrease tension on the suture line.

■ Uses comfort measures to reduce pain.	2. Assess level of discomfort.	2. To determine the need for interventions. Severe pain is uncommon after thyroidectomy, but discomfort occurs owing to difficulty in positioning the head and neck.
	3. Administer pain medication.	3. To reduce pain.
	4. Monitor response to pain medication.	4. To determine the effectiveness of medication in reducing pain.

Interventions: nonsurgical management. The nurse obtains a baseline weight and monitors the client's weight daily. Clients are encouraged to eat frequent high-calorie, high-protein, and high-carbohydrate meals. A referral to the dietitian is recommended, because snacks and additional supplements to the diet are often necessary.

Potential for Sensory/Perceptual Alterations (Visual)

Planning: client goals. The primary goal for this nursing is that the client will have no further decrease in vision or injury to the eye structures.

Interventions: nonsurgical management. The infiltrative ophthalmopathy of Graves' disease is not influenced by the medical therapy for hyperthyroidism. Treatment of this type of ophthalmopathy is symptomatic. If the symptoms are mild, the nurse instructs the client to elevate the head of the bed at night and use an eye lubricant (artificial tears). If photophobia (sensitivity to light) is present, dark glasses or eyepatches are often helpful. For clients who cannot close their eyelids completely, the nurse may recommend gently taping the eyes closed with a nonallergenic tape. In severe cases, it may be necessary to suture the eyelids closed. These actions are geared to prevent further irritation to the eye and are sufficient to prevent vision loss and injury in the majority of clients.

In severe cases, short-term steroid therapy is given to reduce swelling and halt the infiltrative process. Predni-sone (Deltasone) is usually administered in high doses (often 120 mg/day) and is tapered in accordance with the client's response. The nurse discusses the necessity of gradually reducing the prednisone and reviews its side effects with the client. Diuretics may also be given to decrease periorbital edema. In extreme cases, if loss of sight or damage to the eyeball is possible, surgical intervention (orbital decompression) may be necessary.

■ Discharge Planning

Home Care Preparation

Clients are often still experiencing symptoms of hyperthyroidism on returning home. Most antithyroid medications and RAI therapy do not provide immediate relief of symptoms. If heat intolerance is a problem, clients need a cool environment and benefit from the use of a fan or air conditioner. Continuing weakness and fatigue interfere with the client's ADL. The nurse assists the client in identifying a support person who can be of assistance after discharge from the hospital.

Client/Family Education

Clients and their families require education concerning the prescribed medical regimen and its potential side effects. PTU and methimazole have short half-lives. The nurse reviews this concept when stressing the importance of taking these medications consistently. Allergic reactions occur infrequently, but include the development of a rash and pruritus. PTU can cause agranulocytosis. The nurse instructs the client to report any temperature elevation, sore throat, or symptom of infection to the health care team immediately. White blood cell counts are monitored at daily intervals to detect a decrease in number. The nurse reviews the signs and symptoms of hyperthyroidism and instructs the client to report an increase or recurrence of symptoms to the physician. In addition, certain treatments, such as RAI therapy, can result in hypothyroidism. The nurse discusses symptoms of hypothyroidism (see later) and the need for thyroid hormone replacement if this occurs. Clients are reminded of the need for medical follow-up, as hypothyroidism can occur several years after RAI therapy.

If the client has had surgery, the sutures are usually removed on the third or fourth postoperative day. Clients are instructed to inspect the incision area and to report redness, tenderness, drainage, or swelling to a member of the health care team.

Psychosocial Preparation

Clients may continue to be emotionally labile as a result of hyperthyroidism when discharged to home. The nurse explains the reason for emotional lability to the client and the family and reassures them that it will improve with continued treatment. The nurse aids the client in identifying coping skills, support systems, and potential stressors. If the surgical scar is visible and concerns the client, the nurse discusses the use of clothing and jewelry to hide the scar.

Health Care Resources

A visiting nurse or home care aide is helpful for the client who is having difficulty with ADL. Quick access to the health care team is important if the client has questions regarding medications or symptoms.

 Evaluation

The expected outcomes are based on the common nursing diagnoses and include that the client

1. Maintains normal cardiovascular function
2. Maintains or attains ideal body weight
3. Has no further deterioration of visual acuity
4. Identifies side effects of prescribed medications
5. Identifies signs and symptoms of hyperthyroidism and hypothyroidism

HYPOTHYROIDISM

OVERVIEW

Signs and symptoms of *hypothyroidism* (see the accompanying Key Features of Disease) are the result of inade-

quate peripheral tissue thyroid hormone levels. Hypothyroidism can occur throughout the life span. A thorough knowledge of the manifestations of hypothyroidism aids in early detection. Clients usually require lifelong thyroid hormone replacements; therefore, client education is an extremely important part of nursing care.

Pathophysiology

When the production of thyroid hormones is inadequate, the thyroid gland enlarges in an attempt to compensate. *Goiter* is the term used to describe this type of enlargement of the thyroid gland. Simple or nontoxic goiter is the most common form seen in hypothyroidism. Endemic goiter occurs in areas where the soil and water are deficient in iodine. Iodine is necessary for synthesis and secretion of thyroid hormones.

Low levels of thyroid hormone result in an overall decrease in the basal metabolic rate, affecting virtually every body system. There is a general slowing of many metabolic processes; achlorhydria (decreased production of hydrochloric acid by the stomach), reduced GI motility, decreased heart rate, impairment of neurologic function, and decreased heat production result.

Insufficient amount of thyroid hormone causes abnormalities in lipid metabolism, with an increase in cholesterol and triglyceride levels. This increase is associated with the development of atherosclerosis and subsequent cardiac disease in the hypothyroid client.

A characteristic pathophysiologic change in hypothyroidism for unknown reasons is an accumulation of *hydrophilic proteoglycans*, primarily hyaluronic acid, in the interstitial space. This causes an increase in interstitial fluid and the characteristic mucinous edema *(myxedema)* seen in hypothyroidism (Fig. 50-4).

Adequate amounts of thyroid hormone are necessary for optimal erythropoiesis. Anemia is frequently seen with thyroid deficiency. Vitamin B_{12} deficiency and iron and folate deficiencies may also occur.

Etiology

The majority of cases of hypothyroidism occur as a result of thyroid surgery and RAI treatment of thyrotoxicosis. Glandular disease (e.g., chronic thyroiditis), thyroid or metastatic cancer, and idiopathic thyroid atrophy are additional causes of hypothyroidism.

Other causes of simple goiter include genetic defects that prevent the metabolism of iodine; diets consisting mainly of large amounts of goitrogens (thyroid stimulants), such as turnips, cabbage, spinach, and seafood; medications containing large amounts of iodine (e.g., para-aminosalicylic acid, phenylbutazone, and lithium); and, rarely, PTU.

KEY FEATURES OF DISEASE ■ **Signs and Symptoms of Hypothyroidism**

Integumentary

Cool, pale or yellowish, dry, coarse, scaly skin
Thick, brittle nails
Dry, coarse, brittle hair
Decreased hair growth, with loss of eyebrow hair

Pulmonary

Hypoventilation
Pleural effusion
Dyspnea

Cardiovascular

Bradycardia
Arrhythmias
Enlarged heart
Decreased exercise or activity tolerance
Hypotension

Gastrointestinal

Anorexia
Slight weight gain
Constipation
Abdominal distention

Musculoskeletal

Muscle aches and pains
Delayed contraction and relaxation of muscles

Neurologic

Slowing of intellectual functions
    Slowness or slurring of speech
    Impaired memory
    Inattentiveness
Lethargy
Somnolence
Confusion
Hearing loss
Paresthesias (numbness and tingling of extremities)
Decreased tendon reflexes

Psychologic/Emotional

Apathy
Agitation
Depression
Paranoia
Withdrawal
Maniac behavior

Metabolic

Decreased basal metabolic rate
Decreased body temperature
Cold intolerance

Reproductive

Women
    Changes in menses, such as amenorrhea or
        prolonged menses
    Infertility
    Anovulation
    Decreased libido
Men
    Decreased libido
    Impotence

Other

Periorbital edema
Facial puffiness
Facial coarseness
Nonpitting edema of the hands and feet
Hoarseness
Goiter
Thick tongue
Increased sensitivity to narcotics and tranquilizers
Blank expression
Weakness, fatigue
Decreased urinary output
Anemia
Easy bruising

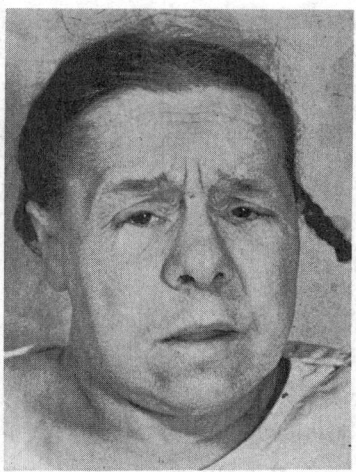

Figure 50–4

Myxedema. (From Wilson, J., & Foster, D. [1985]. *Williams textbook of endocrinology* [7th ed.]. Philadelphia: W. B. Saunders.)

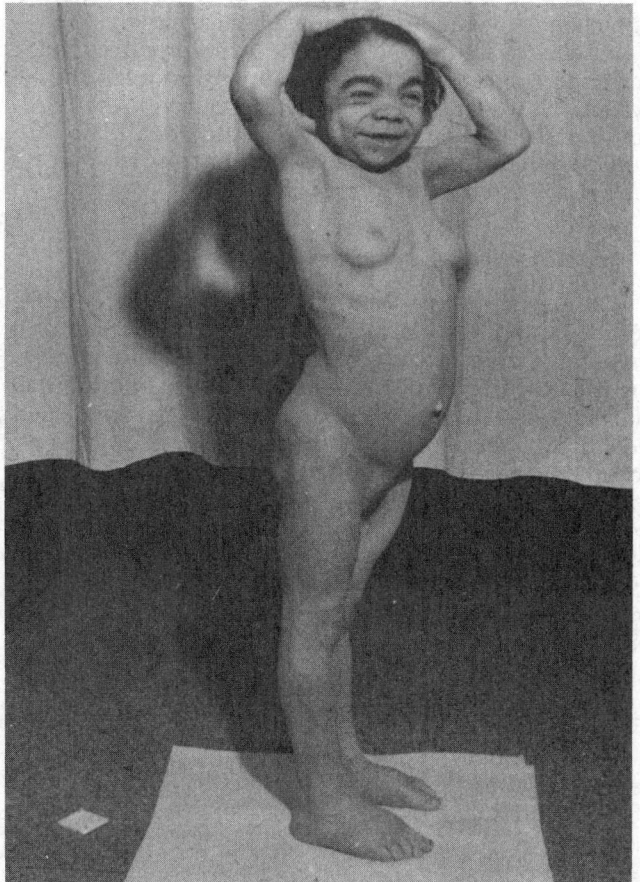

Figure 50–5

This 33-year-old, untreated, adult cretin exhibits characteristic features: dwarfism (height 44 in, in this case), underdeveloped breasts, protuberant abdomen, umbilical hernia, wizened facial features, and scant axillary and pubic hair. (Courtesy of Dr. Norman Schneeberg, Philadelphia, PA.)

Congenital hypothyroidism, or *cretinism*, (Fig. 50–5) most commonly results from thyroid gland dysgenesis (failure of the thyroid gland to develop properly). Enzymatic defects may cause impaired synthesis of thyroid hormone, which can also cause congenital hypothyroidism.

Impaired synthesis of thyroid hormone can result from overuse of antithyroid medications, such as PTU and methimazole.

Pathologic changes within the thyroid gland itself cause decreased thyroid hormone levels; this is termed *primary* hypothyroidism. Inadequate pituitary production of TSH can cause a *secondary* hypothyroidism. Pituitary tumors, metastatic disease, infarction, radiation, granulomatous processes, or trauma can cause hypopituitarism, resulting in hypothyroidism. Disorders of the hypothalamus (infections, trauma, congenital defects, tumors, or infiltrative processes) have the potential to interfere with TSH release owing to problems with TRH production or transport to the pituitary. Hypothyroidism resulting from decreased TRH production in the hypothalamus is termed *tertiary*.

Incidence

Hypothyroidism occurs four times more frequently in women than in men. Most cases of hypothyroidism occur in those 30 to 60 years of age. The incidence of congenital hypothyroidism is approximately 1 in 4000 births (Wilson & Foster, 1985).

PREVENTION

Endemic goiters frequently occur in individuals living in iodine-deficient areas. Iodization of salt or other food products has virtually eliminated this problem in the United States, but it remains a preventable health problem in other areas of the world.

Congenital hypothyroidism cannot usually be prevented. However, the associated physical and mental retardation can be minimized with early detection and treatment.

EMERGENCY CARE: MYXEDEMA COMA

Myxedema coma is a rare, but serious, presentation of hypothyroidism. Myxedema coma can be precipitated by acute illness, rapid withdrawal of thyroid medication, anesthesia, use of sedatives or narcotics, surgery, or hypothermia. The mortality with myxedema coma is extremely high. It is manifested by coma, hypotension, hypothermia, respiratory failure, hyponatremia, and hypoglycemia. Treatment should be instituted as quickly as possible and should be based on the clinical presentation and history without waiting for confirmation by laboratory data (see the accompanying Emergency Care feature).

EMERGENCY CARE ■ Myxedema Coma

Interventions	Rationales
1. Maintain a patent airway.	1. To prevent respiratory acidosis and carbon dioxide narcosis.
2. Replace fluids.	2. To maintain a stable hemodynamic state.
3. Give levothyroxine sodium IV.	3. To increase thyroid hormone levels.
4. Administer glucose IV.	4. To correct hypoglycemia, if present.
5. Administer corticosteroids.	5. To correct adrenocortical hypofunction.
6. Check temperature frequently.	6. To detect correction of hypothermia.
7. Monitor blood pressure.	7. To detect worsening of hypotension.
8. Cover the client with warm blankets.	8. To increase body temperature.

COLLABORATIVE MANAGEMENT

 ### Assessment

History

A decrease in thyroid hormone produces a variety of signs and symptoms related to decreased metabolic activity. The nurse asks the client if there has been any change in *sleep habits.* Clients usually report an increase in time spent sleeping, sometimes up to 14 to 16 hours/day. Clients may also complain of generalized weakness, anorexia, muscle aches, and paresthesias. *Constipation* is common, and the nurse asks the client about the frequency and consistency of bowel movements. Hypothyroid clients often experience cold intolerance and should be asked if they have required more blankets at night or sweaters and extra clothing in warm weather.

Both male and female clients may identify a *decrease in libido.* In addition, the nurse asks the female client with hypothyroidism if she has had difficulty conceiving or any changes in menses. Males can experience impotence and fertility problems.

The nurse questions the client regarding the *medical history.* Current or previous use of medications such as lithium, aminoglutethimide, sodium or potassium perchlorate, thiocyanates, or cobalt can impair synthesis of thyroid hormone. Clients with a history of hyperthyroidism may have had surgical, radioactive, or medical (drugs) treatment, which may have damaged the thyroid gland and resulted in hypothyroidism. It is important to determine if the client is taking any narcotics or tranquilizers. Hypothyroid individuals have an increased sensitivity to these types of drugs as a result of metabolic dysfunction.

Physical Assessment: Clinical Manifestations

Initially, the nurse observes the client's *overall appearance.* When inspecting the face, the nurse notes coarse features, the presence of edema around the eyes and face, and a blank facial expression (see Fig. 50–4). A thick tongue is also characteristic of hypothyroidism. The client's overall muscle movement is slow.

A decrease in thyroid hormone levels produces characteristic clinical manifestations in almost every body system. However, some of these clinical manifestations could occur in a euthyroid client. Additional data obtained from the psychosocial assessment and laboratory testing are essential in identifying hypothyroidism.

Psychosocial Assessment

The symptoms of hypothyroidism cause major difficulties in psychosocial functioning. Complaints of depression or mania are often given as the reason for seeking medical attention. Family members often bring the client for the initial encounter with a member of the health care team. Clients may be too lethargic, apathetic, or somnolent to recognize changes in their condition. Family members may report that the client has withdrawn from them, but this can also occur as a result of hearing loss. The nurse assesses the client's attention span and memory, both of which can be impaired by hypothyroidism. Paranoia and agitation may be additional findings.

Laboratory Findings

The laboratory findings in hypothyroidism are in direct contrast to those in hyperthyroidism (see the accompanying Key Features of Disease).

 ### Analysis: Nursing Diagnosis

Common Diagnoses

The following nursing diagnoses are frequently seen in the hypothyroid client:

1. Decreased cardiac output related to bradycardia, decreased stroke volume, and arteriosclerotic coronary artery disease

2. Ineffective breathing pattern related to hypoventilation and respiratory acidosis

3. Altered thought processes related to increased interstitial edema and water retention

Additional Diagnoses

1. Constipation related to decreased motility of the GI tract

2. Impaired physical mobility related to weakness, fatigue, and muscle aches

3. Impaired skin integrity related to extreme dryness of skin

4. Sexual dysfunction related to decreased libido or infertility

5. Body image disturbance related to changes in physical appearance

6. Altered nutrition: more than body requirements related to decreased metabolic rate

7. Knowledge deficit related to diagnosis and treatment

 Planning and Implementation

Decreased Cardiac Output

Planning: client goals. The goal for this nursing diagnosis is that the client's cardiovascular function will remain stable.

Interventions: nonsurgical management. Clients with hypothyroidism can have decreased blood pressure, bradycardia, and arrhythmias. The nurse monitors blood pressure and heart rate and rhythm. Clients are closely observed for signs of hemodynamic compromise, such as hypotension, decreasing urinary output, and mental status changes. If the hypothyroidism has been chronic, clients may have cardiovascular disease.

The nurse instructs the client to report episodes of chest pain or discomfort immediately to the health care provider.

Hypothyroid clients require lifelong replacement of thyroid hormone. A variety of thyroid preparations are available. Synthetic hormone preparations are usually prescribed; the most commonly utilized is levothyroxine sodium (Synthroid, Levoid, Levothroid). Drug therapy is initiated cautiously, particularly in the client with known cardiovascular problems. The nurse observes the client closely for chest pain and dyspnea when initiating thyroid replacement therapy. The starting dosage of thyroid hormone is usually low and is increased every 2 to 3 weeks until the desired response is obtained. The dosage and the time required for relief of symptoms vary with each individual. Replacement therapy does relieve the clinical manifestations associated with hypothyroidism. The nurse monitors the client for signs and symptoms of hyperthyroidism that can occur with replacement therapy.

Ineffective Breathing Pattern

Planning: client goals. The goal for this nursing diagnosis is that the client will maintain normal respiratory function.

Interventions: nonsurgical management. The nurse observes and records the rate and depth of respirations. The lungs are auscultated, and the nurse notes any abnormalities, such as a decrease in breath sounds. In severe hypothyroidism, significant respiratory distress can occur, necessitating ventilatory support. Severe respiratory distress is usually associated with myxedema coma.

Sedating a hypothyroid client can contribute to respiratory difficulties and should be avoided, if at all possible. When a tranquilizer or sedative is needed, the dosage should be reduced because hypothyroidism

---

KEY FEATURES OF DISEASE ■ Laboratory Findings in Hypothyroidism

Test	Findings
Serum T_3	Decreased
Serum T_4	Decreased
Free T_3 and T_4	Decreased
T_3 RU	Decreased
TRH stimulation test	Delayed or poor TSH response in secondary hypothyroidism; elevated in primary hypothyroidism
Thyroid suppression test	No change in RAIU or T_4 levels
TSH stimulation test (thyroid stimulation test)	Elevated TSH in primary hypothyroidism
RAIU	Decreased
Thyroid antibodies	Normal thyroglobulin

increases sensitivity to these drugs; the nurse carefully observes for signs of respiratory compromise.

Altered Thought Processes

In hypothyroidism, there is a general slowing of all intellectual functioning.

Planning: client goals. The goal is that the client's thought processes will improve to normal levels.

Interventions: nonsurgical management. The nurse notes the presence and severity of symptoms, such as lethargy, drowsiness, memory deficit, inattentiveness, and difficulty in communicating. With thyroid hormone treatment, symptoms should clear, and mentation usually returns to normal levels in the adult client within 2 weeks. In the interim, the nurse orients the client to person, place, and time; explains all procedures slowly and carefully; and provides a safe environment. Family members often have difficulty tolerating these symptoms in the client. They are encouraged to accept the client's mood changes and mental slowness as manifestations of the disease, which should improve with therapy.

■ Discharge Planning

Home Care Preparation

Clients with hypothyroidism do not usually require environmental changes in the home as a result of their disease. If symptoms have not cleared before discharge from the hospital, clients may need extra heat or clothing owing to cold intolerance. Activity intolerance and fatigue might necessitate one-floor living for a short time.

Client/Family Education

Most of the education needed by hypothyroid individuals centers around the prescribed hormone replacement therapy. The nurse emphasizes that lifelong administration of medication is needed. A review of the signs and symptoms of hyperthyroidism and hypothyroidism is necessary for the client and the family. They can identify the need to seek medical interventions for dosage adjustment with this information. The nurse reviews the name, dosage, administration frequency, and side effects of the prescribed medication. All clients should wear medical alert (Medic Alert) identification, because thyroid hormone preparations potentiate and interact with many other drugs. The contraindications to the use of all over-the-counter (OTC) medications should be discussed with the client and the primary caretaker.

Clients are instructed to maintain a well-balanced diet, with adequate fiber and fluid intake, to prevent constipation. The nurse stresses the importance of adequate rest periods before resuming a full schedule of daily activities. Family members are encouraged to voice their concerns to the health care providers. The nurse discusses the necessity for follow-up care.

Psychosocial Preparation

The time required for resolution of the symptoms of hypothyroidism varies from client to client. The most important aspect of psychosocial preparation is to educate the family to be tolerant of any mental dullness or slowness. The nurse encourages the family to orient the client frequently and explain everything clearly and simply. Eventually, clients should exhibit interest in the environment, work, family, and friends.

Health Care Resources

Clients often require a support person to stay with them immediately after discharge from the hospital. They may need more attention initially than a visiting nurse or home care aide can provide. Contact with the health care team is necessary for follow-up and identification of potential problems.

 Evaluation

The expected outcomes are based on the common nursing diagnoses and include that the client

1. Maintains normal cardiovascular function
2. Maintains normal respiratory function
3. Experiences improvement in mental status and thought processes
4. Identifies the time of administration, dosage, and side effects of prescribed medication
5. Identifies signs and symptoms of hyperthyroidism and hypothyroidism

THYROIDITIS

Thyroiditis is an inflammation of the thyroid gland. There are three types: acute, subacute, and chronic. Chronic thyroiditis, or Hashimoto's disease, is the most common.

Acute suppurative thyroiditis is uncommon. It is caused by bacterial invasion of the thyroid gland. Symptoms include neck tenderness, pain, elevated temperature, malaise, and dysphagia. It is treated symptomatically and usually responds to antibiotic therapy.

Subacute granulomatous thyroiditis results from a viral infection of the thyroid gland, occasionally occurring after an upper respiratory tract infection. It is characterized by fever, chills, dysphagia, and muscle and joint pain. The pain can radiate to the ears and the jaw. On palpation, the gland feels hard and moderately enlarged. Thyroid function can remain normal, although hyperthyroidism or hypothyroidism may develop.

Clients with mild subacute thyroiditis are managed with rest, fluids, and acetylsalicylic acid (aspirin). In more severe cases, corticosteroids are given to reduce inflammation.

Chronic thyroiditis (Hashimoto's disease) affects females more frequently than males and occurs most commonly in the third to fifth decades. It is believed to be an autoimmune disease. The thyroid becomes infiltrated with antithyroid antibodies and lymphocytes, resulting in glandular destruction. Serum thyroid hormone levels are low, and TSH secretion is increased. TSH causes an increase in thyroid function and may maintain a euthyroid state for some time, but hypothyroidism eventually develops.

Clinical manifestations of Hashimoto's disease include dysphagia and painless enlargement of the gland. Diagnosis is based on the presence of circulating antithyroid antibodies and characteristic needle biopsy findings of the thyroid gland. Serum thyroid hormone levels, TSH levels, and RAIU vary, depending on the progress of the disease.

Clients are given thyroid hormone to prevent hypothyroidism and suppress TSH secretion, thereby decreasing gland size. If the goiter does not respond to thyroid hormone administration, is disfiguring, or compresses other structures, surgery (subtotal thyroidectomy) is necessary. Nursing interventions focus on promoting client comfort and providing education regarding hypothyroidism, medications, and surgery, if needed.

THYROID CANCER

There are four distinct histologic types of thyroid cancer: papillary, follicular, medullary, and anaplastic. The initial clinical manifestation of thyroid cancer is a solitary, painless nodule in the thyroid gland. Additional signs and symptoms depend on the presence and location of metastasis.

Papillary carcinoma, the most common type of thyroid cancer, is found more frequently in women and in individuals less than 40 years of age. It is a slow-growing tumor and can be present for years before metastasis to the regional lymph nodes occurs. If the tumor is localized to the thyroid gland, prognosis is good with a partial or total thyroidectomy.

Follicular carcinoma constitutes approximately 25% of all thyroid cancers. It primarily affects individuals older than 50 years of age. Follicular carcinoma invades blood vessels and metastasizes to bone and lung tissue. It rarely spreads to regional lymph nodes, but can adhere to the trachea, neck muscles, great vessels, and skin, resulting in dyspnea and dysphagia. When the tumor involves the recurrent laryngeal nerves, clients may experience hoarseness. This type of tumor has a fair prognosis if metastasis is minimal at the time of diagnosis.

Medullary carcinoma arises from the parafollicular thyroid tissue. It accounts for 5% to 10% of all thyroid cancers and is more common in those older than 50 years of age. Metastasis occurs via regional lymph nodes and invasion of surrounding structures. This tumor often occurs as part of multiple endocrine neoplasia (MEN) type II, a familial endocrine disorder. With medullary carcinoma, excessive secretion of calcitonin, adrenocorticotropic hormone, prostaglandins, and serotonin may be seen.

For papillary, follicular, and medullary carcinomas, surgery is the treatment of choice. A partial or total thyroidectomy is performed, with a modified radical neck dissection if regional lymph nodes are involved. Postoperatively, clients are given suppressive doses of thyroid hormone. The therapy is continued for 3 months and then withdrawn. An RAIU study is then performed. If there is RAI uptake, clients are treated with ablative amounts of RAI. If recurrent thyroid cancer does not respond to RAI, a course of chemotherapy is initiated.

Anaplastic carcinoma is a rapid-growing, extremely aggressive tumor. It directly invades adjacent structures, causing symptoms of stridor, hoarseness, and dysphagia. The prognosis with anaplastic carcinoma is poor, with death occurring on the average of a year after diagnosis. This type of tumor may be treated with palliative surgery, radiation, or chemotherapy.

Clients with a diagnosis of thyroid cancer experience considerable anxiety and stress. The nurse obtains baseline data from the client relating to knowledge of the disease, coping skills, and family relationships. The client's response to a diagnosis of cancer is individual, and the nurse encourages verbalization of fears and a discussion of the illness (see Chap. 25).

DISORDERS OF THE PARATHYROID GLANDS

HYPERPARATHYROIDISM

OVERVIEW

The function of the parathyroid glands is to maintain calcium and phosphate homeostasis. PTH acts directly on the kidney and bone and indirectly alters the absorption of calcium from the GI tract through its effect on vitamin D (Fig. 50–6). Serum calcium concentration is normally maintained within a narrow range, whereas serum phosphate levels vary more widely.

Pathophysiology

Increased levels of PTH act directly on the kidney, causing increased tubular resorption of calcium and in-

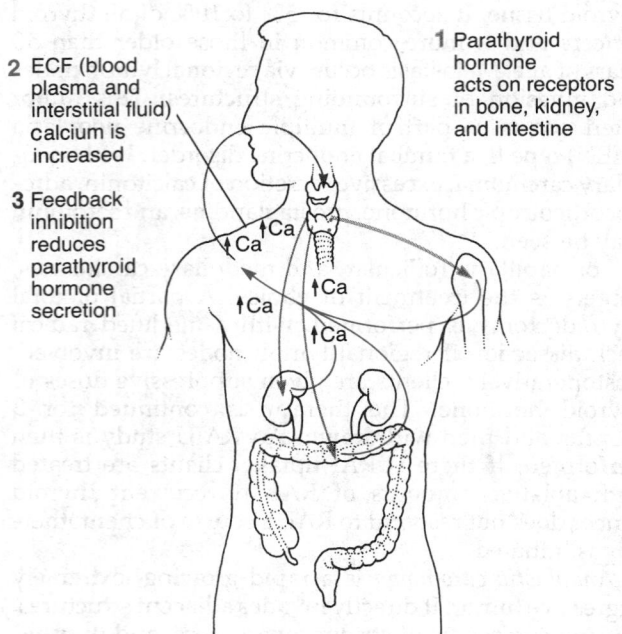

1 Parathyroid hormone acts on receptors in bone, kidney, and intestine

2 ECF (blood plasma and interstitial fluid) calcium is increased

3 Feedback inhibition reduces parathyroid hormone secretion

Figure 50-6
Physiologic actions of parathyroid hormone. ECF, extracellular fluid.

creased phosphate excretion; these contribute to hypercalcemia and hypophosphatemia. Metabolic acidosis, urinary alkalosis, and hypokalemia result from increased bicarbonate excretion and decreased acid excretion. In this environment, renal calculi frequently develop. In the bone, excessive PTH increases bone resorption owing to decreased osteoblastic activity and increased osteoclastic activity. This results in the release of calcium and phosphorus into the circulation and decalcification of bone. When the normal solubility of calcium in the serum is exceeded, calcium is deposited in soft tissues. This usually occurs in only long-standing hypercalcemia (serum calcium level of 11.5 to 12 mg/dL or greater). Hypertension may be seen in acute hypercalcemia, probably owing to vasoconstriction, whereas in chronic hypercalcemia, the hypertension is due to renal damage. The ECG shows a shortening of the QT interval from the onset of systole to the onset of repolarization.

Etiology

Although the exact triggering mechanism is unknown, *primary* hyperparathyroidism results when one or more hyperfunctioning glands is unresponsive to the normal feedback of serum calcium. The most common presentation (in approximately 80% to 85% of the cases) is a benign, autonomous adenoma in *one* of the glands. Hyperplasia in *all four* of the parathyroid glands is present in the remainder of cases of primary hyperparathyroidism. Genetic factors are occasionally associated with a familial form of the disease with autosomal dominant inheritance. Previous radiation therapy to the neck has

been found to be a common denominator in a large number of clients with primary disease. Carcinoma of the parathyroid glands is quite rare and represents less than 3% of the cases of primary hyperparathyroidism.

Secondary hyperparathyroidism is a response to the hypocalcemia in chronic renal disease and in vitamin D deficiency, which results in hyperplasia of the glands. Eventually, the hyperplastic glands develop *autonomous function* and no longer respond to the normal feedback when serum calcium levels are corrected. This stage is termed *tertiary* hyperparathyroidism.

Hypercalcemia is also seen in cases of *ectopic* hyperparathyroidism. Production of a *PTH-like* substance from nonparathyroid tissue is seen in carcinoma of the lung, the kidney, or the GI tract. This substance keeps the parathyroid glands from responding to the increased calcium levels.

Incidence

The advent of automated multitest screening, including the measurement of serum calcium levels, has greatly increased the detection of primary hyperparathyroidism. The incidence increases dramatically after the age of 50 years in both sexes and is two to four times greater in females.

COLLABORATIVE MANAGEMENT

 Assessment

History

The nurse initiates history taking from a client with suspected hyperparathyroidism by eliciting a thorough *family history.* Primary hyperparathyroidism occurs in a number of familial syndromes, such as MEN. The nurse questions the client regarding relatives who have had ulcer disease, bone disease, kidney stones, or any form of endocrine disorders. Mothers whose newborns developed tetany are prime suspects for primary hyperparathyroidism. The nurse questions the client regarding the use of *prescription and OTC drugs.* Thiazide diuretics and excessive vitamin D intake can produce hypercalcemia. The nurse inquires about the client's symptoms. These include headache, drowsiness, flank pain, muscle weakness, GI disturbance, or depression. The nurse asks the client whether he/she has experienced bone fractures, recent weight loss, or arthritis. Information about the use of *radiation treatment* to the head or neck for another medical problem is also obtained.

Physical Assessment: Clinical Manifestations

Assessment of the client with hyperparathyroidism is limited to history taking. No obvious physical manifestations occur, especially in the milder forms of the disorder. Palpation and auscultation of the neck are not helpful in diagnosis. In clients with long-standing disease, the nurse may observe a waxy pallor of the skin and bone deformities in the extremities and back.

Most commonly primary hyperparathyroidism is discovered incidentally when hypercalcemia is identified by multiple screening tests. These clients usually have moderate hypercalcemia and are either asymptomatic or have vague symptoms, such as headache or fatigue, which are not easily associated with this disorder. Clinical features can be divided into those related to the effects of excessive PTH and those directly related to the hypercalcemia. *Excessive PTH* results in *renal calculi* (kidney stones) and *nephrocalcinosis,* a deposition of calcium in the soft tissue of the kidney. Trauma or urinary tract obstruction by stones predisposes to recurrent infections and impaired renal function. Nephrocalcinosis is seen in long-standing, severe hypercalcemia and, when present, is usually associated with a significant reduction of tubular and renal glomerular function.

Bone lesions are due to *enhanced bone resorption* and result in pathologic fractures, bone cysts, and osteoporosis in advanced cases (Fig. 50–7). *GI manifestations,* e.g., anorexia, nausea, vomiting, epigastric pain, constipation, and weight loss, are encountered frequently, particularly with the high levels of serum calcium. *Hypergastrinemia* (increased serum gastrin levels) is the result of hypercalcemia and probably accounts for the increased incidence of associated peptic ulcer disease. Varying degrees of fatigue and lethargy may also be seen and become more severe as the serum calcium levels increase. The clinical course in clients with calcium levels greater than 12 mg/dL includes *organic psychosis* with mental confusion, leading to coma and death if untreated. The *tendon reflexes* in hypercalcemia may be decreased.

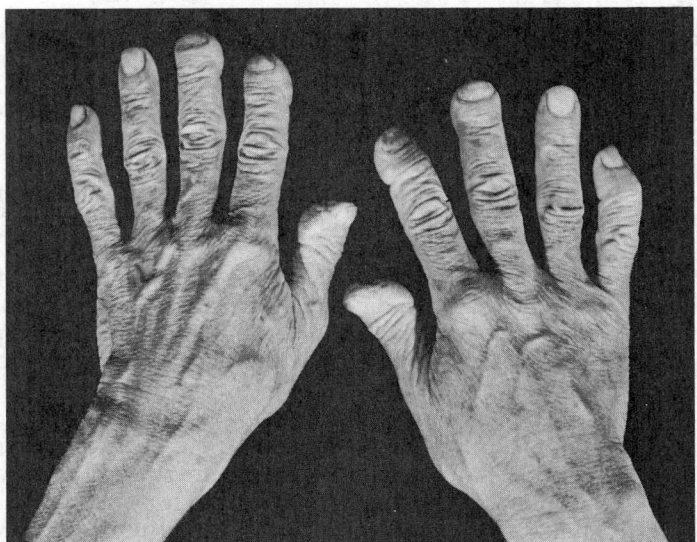
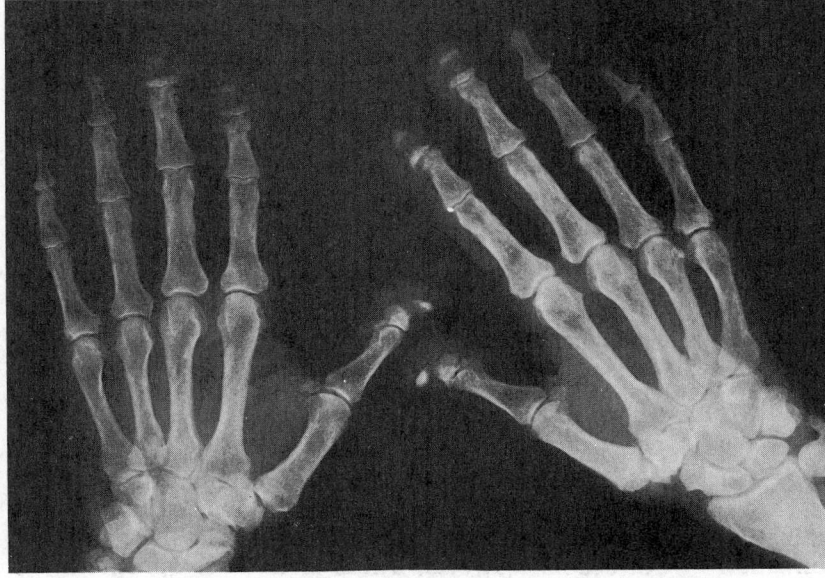

Figure 50–7

Extensive bone erosion resulting from untreated long-standing hyperparathyroidism. Note the absence of bone at the tips of some fingers, resulting in digital clubbing. (From Wilson, J., & Foster, D. [1985]. *Williams textbook of endocrinology* [7th ed.]. Philadelphia: W. B. Saunders.)

Psychosocial Assessment

Clients with hyperparathyroidism exhibit symptoms associated with hypercalcemic effects on the central nervous system. The nurse asks the client if he/she has experienced any drowsiness or lethargy. The client's family may describe personality changes, recent memory loss, or emotional lability. The nurse explains that these symptoms may be the result of hypercalcemia and will resolve when the underlying cause is treated.

Laboratory Findings

Serum PTH, calcium, and phosphorus measurements and urinary cyclic adenosine monophosphate (cAMP) determinations are the diagnostic tests most frequently employed in detecting hyperparathyroidism (see the accompanying Key Features of Disease).

Radiographic Findings

Radiographic tests are employed to demonstrate the presence of renal calculi, nephrocalcinosis, and bone lesions, such as cysts or fractures. Generalized bone demineralization, subperiosteal resorption in long bones, and a "salt-and-pepper" appearance of the skull can be seen in chronic hyperparathyroidism.

Localization studies are usually employed when an adenoma has not been found or when all four of the glands are not identified on initial surgical exploration. They include arteriography, in which radiopaque dye is injected into the thyroid arteries. Computed tomography (CT) may be helpful in locating adenomas in the mediastinum and chest if the lesions are large enough.

Other Diagnostic Tests

Selective venous catheterization of the thyroid veins with sampling of the blood may show PTH levels higher in a specific area, thus localizing the adenoma to one side or pole of the thyroid.

Ultrasonography may be useful in locating large adenomas in other areas of the neck.

 Analysis: Nursing Diagnosis

Common Diagnoses

The client with hyperparathyroidism often has potential for decreased cardiac output related to cardiac arrhythmias.

Additional Diagnoses

Clients with hyperparathyroidism may also have the following diagnoses:

1. Potential for injury (bone fractures) related to osteoporosis
2. Potential for altered patterns of urinary elimination related to hypercalciuria and renal calculi formation

---

KEY FEATURES OF DISEASE ■ Laboratory Findings in Hyperparathyroidism

Test	Findings
Serum calcium	Elevated in primary hyperparathyroidism
Serum phosphorus	Decreased
Serum PTH	Increased
Urinary cAMP	Increased

3. Impaired physical mobility related to bone and joint pain
4. Knowledge deficit related to diagnosis and treatment

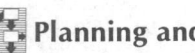 **Planning and Implementation**

Potential for Decreased Cardiac Output

Planning: client goals. The primary goal is that the client will maintain normocalcemia, thereby reducing the risk of cardiac dysfunction.

Interventions: nonsurgical management. In clients who are not candidates for surgical intervention, the most frequently employed therapy to reduce serum calcium levels is hydration and the administration of furosemide (Lasix), a diuretic that increases the excretion of calcium by the kidney. IV saline in large volumes promotes calcium excretion with the increased clearance of sodium by the kidney.

The nurse monitors intake and output every 2 to 4 hours during hydration therapy. The client is instructed to report any nausea, vomiting, increased lethargy, or palpitations, which can result from hypercalcemia. The nurse observes for changes in blood pressure, rate or rhythm of the pulses, and increasing confusion or irritability. Clients may require continuous cardiac monitoring. Administration of large volumes of saline may lead to congestive heart failure in clients with compromised renal and cardiac function. Calcium levels must be closely monitored, and any precipitous drop reported immediately to the physician. Sudden drops in calcium levels may cause tingling sensations and numbness in muscles.

Drug therapy. When hydration and furosemide administration are insufficient to reduce the hypercalcemia, or it becomes necessary to discontinue the IV fluids, oral phosphates can be added. Phosphates work by inhibiting bone resorption and interfere with calcium absorption. IV phosphates are only used when the serum calcium levels need to be lowered rapidly.

Calcitonin decreases skeletal calcium release and increases the renal clearance of calcium. Calcitonin is not effective when used alone because of its short duration of action. However, if it is given in conjunction with glucocorticoids, the therapeutic effects are greatly enhanced.

Mithramycin, a cytotoxic antibiotic, is the most effective and potent pharmacologic agent used to lower serum calcium levels. A single dose of 10 to 15 μg/kg of body weight is sufficient to lower serum calcium levels within 48 hours in most clients with hypercalcemia, regardless of the etiology. However, the toxic effects of the drug limit its use to two or three doses. Thrombocytopenia and renal and hepatic toxicity can be seen in some cases after only one dose. Liver function studies, blood urea nitrogen and creatinine concentrations, and complete blood count (CBC) should be closely monitored, along with the serum calcium level.

All IV antihypercalcemic agents are given with an infusion pump at a slow rate. The nurse observes the client for side effects, such as nausea and bleeding, or allergic reactions, such as rash, hives, edema, or dyspnea.

Interventions: surgical management. A diagnosis of primary hyperparathyroidism related to adenoma or hyperplasia can only be made at the time of surgery. All four of the glands must be identified by the surgeon. If one gland is enlarged and the rest are normal or subnormal in size, a biopsy is done, a diagnosis of adenoma is confirmed, and the enlarged gland is completely removed. The remaining three glands, which have been nonfunctioning owing to overproduction of PTH by the adenoma, require several days to several weeks to return to normal function. During this critical period, hypocalcemic crisis can occur.

Preoperative care. Before surgery, clients are stabilized and calcium levels decreased to near normocalcemia. If mithramycin has been used to lower serum calcium levels, serologic studies should be done to determine bleeding and coagulation times and CBC should be performed to ascertain bone marrow function.

The nurse explains the procedure to the client and advises that coughing and deep breathing exercises should be performed postoperatively. The nurse demonstrates neck support by having the client place both hands behind the neck to assist in elevating the head. The client is advised that talking may be painful for the first day or two postoperatively. The client is usually hospitalized for an average of 5 days.

Postoperative care. Immediately postoperatively, a serum calcium level is obtained, and levels are monitored every 4 hours until the initial calcium levels stabilize. The nurse checks vital signs and identifies any change in status. The neck dressing is checked for abnormal amounts of drainage or bleeding. Some serosanguineous drainage (approximately 1 to 5 mL) is normal. The nurse observes the client for signs of respiratory distress, which may be due to compression of the trachea by hemorrhage. Swelling of adjacent tissues may also contribute to respiratory distress. Emergency equipment, including suction, oxygen, and tracheostomy equipment, should be available at the client's bedside. Removal of clips from the incision may be necessary if severe swelling occurs.

The nurse monitors signs and symptoms of hypocalcemia. Tingling and twitching may be noted in the extremities and face. The nurse checks for Trousseau's sign by inflating a blood pressure cuff above the level of the systolic pressure and maintaining the pressure for 2 minutes. The hand is observed for carpal spasm (Fig. 50–8) when the cuff is released. A spasm lasting longer than 5 seconds is considered a positive sign. Chvostek's sign is elicited by tapping the facial nerve anterior to the earlobe just below the zygomatic arch or tapping the cheek between the zygomatic arch and the corner of the mouth. A positive response ranges from simple twitching of the corner of the mouth to include all muscles on that side of the face. Positive responses for either sign signal potential for tetany.

Damage to the recurrent laryngeal nerve is rare; however, the nurse assesses the client for changes in voice patterns and hoarseness that does not seem to be resolving.

When hyperparathyroidism is due to hyperplasia, usually three and a half of the glands are removed and the remaining portion of the fourth gland is tagged to make it easy to find if future surgery is necessary. If all four glands are removed, a small portion of a gland may be implanted in the forearm where it produces PTH and maintains calcium homeostasis. Should all of these maneuvers fail, and the client becomes permanently hypoparathyroid, lifelong treatment with calcium and vitamin D is necessary (see earlier).

■ Discharge Planning

Home Care Preparation

If the client has any residual effects of hyperparathyroidism, such as bone fractures or osteoporosis, the

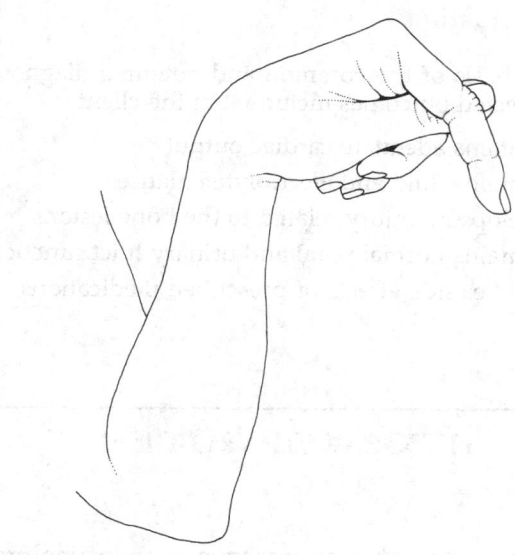

Figure 50–8
Carpal spasm.

nurse counsels the client about making the home safer by removing small or scatter rugs or clutter in passageways or areas frequently used for work or recreation. Provision should be made for the safe use of bathroom facilities with the use of grab bars, bathtub grips, and nonslip tub decals. The nurse advises immediate family, relatives, or friends to check with the client on a frequent basis to assist with any needs as they arise.

Client/Family Education

Clients and their families need to understand the action and dosages of prescribed medications, if any are necessary. When surgery has been successful, no medication is required. Follow-up calcium determinations are necessary to ascertain that calcium homeostasis is maintained, and postoperative medical evaluation ensures proper healing of the incision. Only if surgical hypoparathyroidism occurs is medication necessary. Treatment of hypocalcemia is discussed later under the heading Hypoparathyroidism.

Psychosocial Preparation

Normally, clients who may have experienced irritability, confusion, or lethargy attributable to their hypercalcemia recover before discharge from the hospital or shortly thereafter. The nurse advises the client and the family that there may be some lingering symptoms, but that these will clear within a short time.

Health Care Resources

If the client is experiencing lingering effects of bone disease, home care services may be useful in obtaining equipment devised to make ADL easier, such as a bedside commode or a walker or wheelchair.

 Evaluation

On the basis of the common and potential diagnoses, the expected outcomes include that the client

1. Maintains adequate cardiac output
2. Maintains fluid and electrolyte balance
3. Develops no injury related to the bone lesions
4. Maintains normal renal and urinary tract functions
5. Identifies side effects of prescribed medications

HYPOPARATHYROIDISM

OVERVIEW

Hypoparathyroidism is an uncommon endocrine problem in which pathologic findings are directly related to lack of PTH secretion or to decreased effectiveness of PTH on target tissue. Whether the problem is lack of PTH secretion or ineffectiveness of PTH on tissues, the result is the same: hypocalcemia.

Iatrogenic hypoparathyroidism is the most common form. It is inadvertently caused by removal of all viable parathyroid tissue during total thyroidectomy or surgical removal of hyperplastic parathyroid glands.

Idiopathic hypoparathyroidism is a rare condition, which can occur spontaneously in children and adults. An autoimmune basis is suspected because of its association with adrenal insufficiency, hypothyroidism, diabetes mellitus, pernicious anemia, gonadal failure, and certain skin disorders (e.g., vitiligo). Antiparathyroid antibodies have been found in a significant number of affected clients.

Hypomagnesemia may be a cause of hypoparathyroidism. Hypomagnesemia is seen in alcoholism, malabsorption syndromes, renal disease, and malnutrition. It causes impairment of PTH secretion and may interfere with PTH effects on target organs (bones and kidneys).

Resistance to PTH, or *pseudohypoparathyroidism,* is a rare hereditary disorder characterized by unresponsiveness of bone, renal tubules, and intestines to PTH, resulting in hypocalcemia and elevated serum phosphate levels.

In pseudohypoparathyroidism, the nurse may observe short stature; facial roundness; a short, thick neck; obesity; and shortened metacarpals and metatarsals, usually the fourth (Fig. 50–9). There may be evidence of mild to moderate mental retardation.

COLLABORATIVE MANAGEMENT

Assessment of the client with suspected hypoparathyroidism begins with a thorough history. The nurse questions the client regarding any neck surgery or radiation therapy to the head or neck area. These factors are known to be involved in development of the disorder. The nurse questions the client about the signs and symptoms of hypoparathyroidism, which may range in severity from mild paresthesias to tetany. Perioral tingling and numbness and tingling sensations in the hands and feet reflect mild to moderate hypocalcemia. Severe muscle cramps, carpopedal spasms, and convulsions (in which there is no loss of consciousness or incontinence) reflect a more severe form of the disorder. Mental changes that the client or caregiver may notice range from irritability to frank psychosis.

Physical assessment for hypoparathyroidism may reveal characteristic metacarpal, phalangeal, carpal, and elbow flexion, which can signal an impending attack of tetany (see Fig. 50–8). The nurse checks for Chvostek's sign and Trousseau's sign (see earlier); positive responses indicate potential tetany. A parkinsonian-like syndrome may be evident, and the nurse may discover the presence of cataracts, denoting chronic hypocalcemia. Bands or pits may encircle the crowns of the teeth, indicating enamel hypoplasia. The roots of teeth may be defective.

Laboratory and other diagnostic tests include elec-

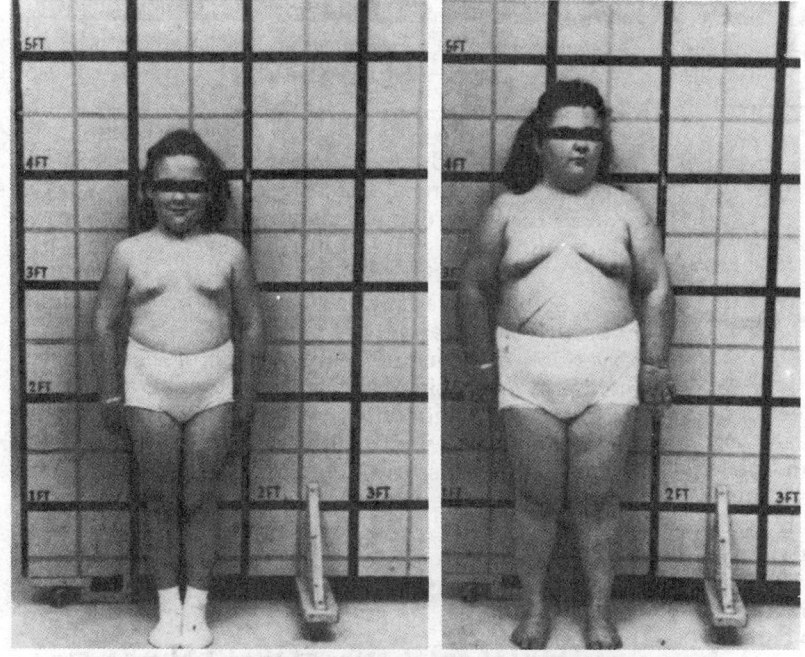

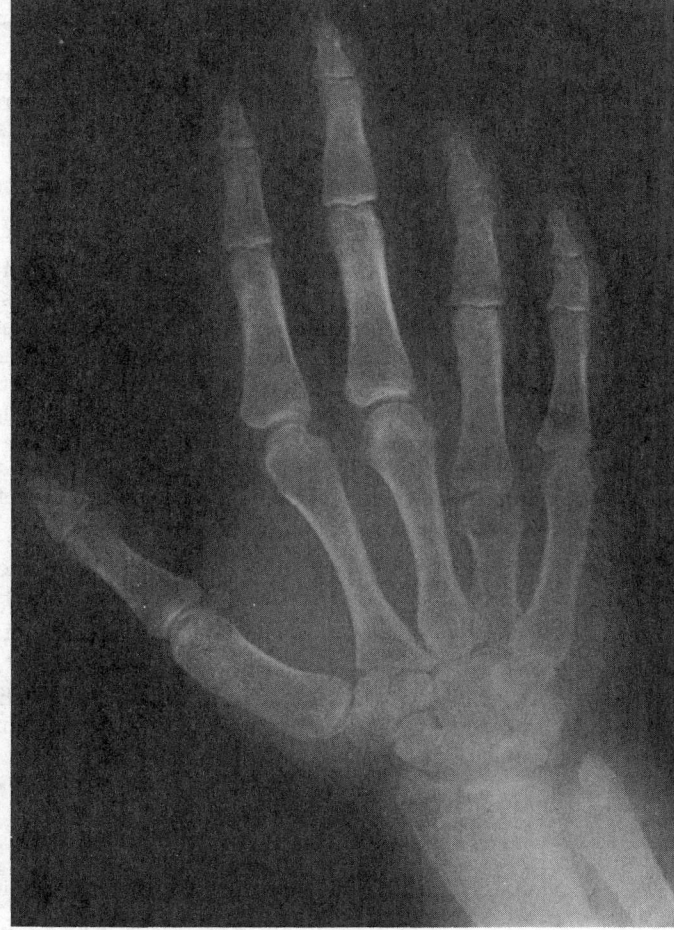

Figure 50–9

Clinical and radiographic features of pseudohypo-parathyroidism. Note the short fourth finger in the x-ray film. (From Wilson, J., & Foster, D. [1985]. *Williams textbook of endocrinology* [7th ed.]. Philadelphia: W. B. Saunders.)

KEY FEATURES OF DISEASE ■ Laboratory Findings in Hypoparathyroidism

Test	Findings
Serum calcium	Decreased
Serum phosphorus	Increased
Serum PTH	Decreased
Urinary cAMP	Decreased

troencephalography, blood tests, and CT. Electroencephalographic changes in hypoparathyroidism are nonspecific and revert to normal with correction of hypocalcemia. Serum calcium, phosphate, magnesium, and vitamin D levels and urinary cAMP level may be employed in the diagnostic work-up for hypoparathyroidism (see the accompanying Key Features of Disease). CT may be useful in demonstrating intracranial and basal ganglia calcification, which indicates chronic hypocalcemia.

Medical management of hypoparathyroidism focuses on immediate and long-term correction of hypocalcemia, vitamin D deficiency, and hypomagnesemia. In acute and severe hypocalcemia, IV therapy with calcium chloride or calcium gluconate is administered as a 10% solution of calcium chloride or calcium gluconate and is given over 10 to 15 minutes. Acute vitamin D deficiency is treated with calcitrol (Rocaltrol) in doses of 0.5 to 2.0 μg/day. Acute hypomagnesemia is corrected by administering 50% magnesium sulfate in 2-mL doses (up to 4 g/day) intramuscularly or in an IV solution. Long-term oral therapy for hypocalcemia involves administration of elemental calcium (0.5 to 2.0 g/day in divided doses) as lactate, gluconate, or carbonate. Long-term oral therapy for vitamin D deficiency is 50,000 to 400,000 units of ergocalciferol daily. Dosage is adjusted to keep the client's calcium level in the low-normal range (slightly hypocalcemic) sufficient to prevent symptoms of hypocalcemia. It must also be low enough to prevent hypercalciuria, which can lead to stone formation.

Nursing management includes measures to ensure compliance with the prescribed medication regimen and to alleviate anxiety. The client is encouraged to eat foods that are high in calcium but low in phosphorus. Milk and cheese products need to be avoided because of their high phosphorus content. The nurse stresses to clients and caretakers that therapy for hypocalcemia is lifelong. The nurse advises the client of the necessity of wearing some form of identification, such as a Medic Alert emblem and wallet card. Clients with severe hypocalcemia may be extremely anxious when leaving the protective atmosphere of the hospital. The nurse reassures the client that as long as he/she adheres to the prescribed regimen, the calcium level will remain in a range sufficiently high to prevent any crisis.

SUMMARY

Astute nursing judgment and care can have a significant impact on the clinical outcome of the client with disorders of the thyroid and parathyroid glands. Nursing interventions are geared toward preventing complications; providing client education; and, if necessary, aiding the client in adapting to changes in life style. In hyperthyroidism and hyperparathyroidism, surgical intervention is frequently employed. Nurses are instrumental in decreasing client anxiety preoperatively and in detecting potential problems postoperatively. Caring for clients with thyroid and parathyroid dysfunction is rewarding, because, in most instances, adequate treatment reverses the clinical course of the disease.

IMPLICATIONS FOR RESEARCH

The hormones of the thyroid and parathyroid glands affect so many body functions that research regarding their efficacy in many clinical situations continues to expand. Osteoporosis is one clinical problem for which hormone replacement is being investigated as a treatment regimen. Age-related bone loss may result from changes in plasma levels of calcitonin, PTH, and vitamin D metabolites. Research utilizing these agents in treatment is ongoing. A decrease in injuries and hospital visits are two potential benefits for the elderly client.

As clients age, their need for thyroid hormone decreases. Currently, investigators are looking at optimal doses of thyroid hormone replacement, depending on the age of the client.

The following are potential nursing research topics relating to the client with dysfunction of the thyroid or parathyroid gland:

1. Is antithyroid drug therapy cost effective when compared with other treatment regimens (e.g., ^{131}I)?
2. What is the effect of client education on compliance with thyroid replacement therapy?
3. What are the effects of diet and exercise on clients who have osteoporosis and are receiving hormone replacement?

REFERENCES AND READINGS

Avioli, L. V. (1987). Primary hyperthyroidism recognition and management. *Hospital Practice, 22*(9), 69–74.

Bagdade, J. D. (1987). *The yearbook of endocrinology.* Chicago: Year Book Medical.

Besser, G. M., & Cudworth, A. G. (Eds.). (1987). *Clinical*

endocrinology: An illustrated text. Philadelphia: J. B. Lippincott.

Bybee, D. E. (1987). Saving lives in thyroid crisis. *Emergency Medicine, 19*(16), 20–30.

Carlson, H. E. (Ed.). (1983). *Endocrinology.* New York: Wiley Medical.

De Groot, L. J. (Ed.). (1984). *The thyroid and its diseases.* New York: Wiley.

Felig, P., Baster, J. D., & Broadhaus, A. (Eds.). (1987). *Endocrinology and metabolism.* New York: McGraw-Hill.

Greenspan, F. S., & Forsham, P. H. (1986). *Basic and clinical endocrinology* (2nd ed.). Los Altos, CA: Lange Medical.

Hershman, J. M. (Ed.). (1980). *Management of endocrine disorders.* Philadelphia: Lea & Febiger.

Ingbar, S. H., & Braverman, L. E. (Eds.). (1986). *Werner's the thyroid* (5th ed.). Philadelphia: J. B. Lippincott.

Kini, S. R. (1987). *Guides to clinical aspiration biopsy thyroid.* New York: Igaku-Shoin.

Lazarus, J. H., & Hall, R. (Eds.). (1988). *Hypothyroidism and goitre.* Philadelphia: Balliere Tindall.

Martin, C. R. (1985). *Endocrine physiology.* New York: Oxford University Press.

Mazzaferri, E. L. (Ed.). (1986). *Textbook of endocrinology* (3rd ed.). New York: Elsevier Science.

McMillan, J. Y. (1988). Preventing myxedema coma in the hypothyroid patient. *Dimensions in Critical Care Nursing, 7,* 136–145.

Metz, R. M., & Larson, E. B. (Ed.). (1985). *Blue book of endocrinology.* Philadelphia: W. B. Saunders.

Murthe, N. C. (1981). *Endocrinology—a nursing approach.* Boston: Little Brown.

Papazoglou, N., Kelermenos, N., & Andriopoulos, J. (1987). Vasospastic angina with hyperthyroidism. *Heart and Lung, 16,* 437–438.

Sacktor, B. (Ed.). (1987). Endocrinology and aging. *Endocrinology and Metabolism Clinics of North America, 16,* 829–1075.

Sarsany, S. L. (1988). Thyroid storm. *RN, 51*(7), 46–48.

Sherwood, L. M. (1988). Diagnosis and management of primary hyperparathyroidism. *Hospital Practice, 23*(3), 9–10.

Stein, P. P., et al. (1988). Factitious thyrotoxicosis: Searching for the source of this disorder. *Consultant, 28*(6), 64–65.

Van Middlesworth, L. (1989). Effects of radiation on the thyroid gland. *Advances in Internal Medicine, 34,* 265–284.

Vaughn, E., & Baker, K. L. (1989). Continued bone disease and symptoms post-parathyroidectomy. *AANA Journal, 16*(1), 45–46.

Wilson, J., & Foster, D. (Eds.). (1985). *Williams textbook of endocrinology* (7th ed.). Philadelphia: W. B. Saunders.

Wyngaarden, J. B., & Smith, L. H. (Eds.). (1988). *Cecil textbook of medicine* (18th ed.). Philadelphia: W. B. Saunders.

CHAPTER 51

Interventions for Clients with Diabetes Mellitus

OVERVIEW

Diabetes mellitus is a genetically and clinically heterogeneous group of chronic systemic disorders of various causes, affecting the metabolism of carbohydrate, protein, and fat. Diabetes mellitus can potentially affect every body organ and system, can cause long-term complications, and, if untreated, can be life-threatening. Although no cure has yet been found, great progress has been made in controlling diabetes with medical advances such as methods for self-monitoring of blood glucose levels; improved diabetes medications; improved nutrition, diet, and exercise guidelines; and, most importantly, education of the individual with diabetes mellitus.

Diabetes affects millions of people and requires billions of dollars for health care each year. The number of people affected by some form of diabetes in the United States is estimated at 11 million, or 6% of the population. Diabetes is ranked third as cause of death from disease, preceded only by heart disease and cancer. The money spent on health care related to the treatment of diabetes and dollars lost because of clients' absenteeism from work or inability to work totalled $20.4 billion dollars in 1987. This amounted to 3.6% of all U.S. health care costs (American Diabetes Association, 1987).

Diabetes can also be a personal financial burden, and thus an additional stressor, for affected clients and their families. To provide proper care, nurses must be aware not only of the physical effects of diabetes, but also of the financial, psychologic, and emotional stresses related to diabetes.

PATHOPHYSIOLOGY

THE ROLE OF INSULIN

Insulin is an anabolic hormone made in the beta cells of the islets of Langerhans in the pancreas and plays a key role in allowing the cells of the body to store carbohydrates. It affects several crucial activities in the cell that alter the permeability of cell membranes to allow entrance of glucose, free fatty acids, and amino acids. Insulin also acts as a catalyst to stimulate enzymes and chemicals necessary for cell function and energy production.

Proinsulin (composed of alpha-, beta-, and C-peptide chains) is stored in granules inside the beta cell in the pancreas until the beta cells evacuate the substance into the extracellular space, where it is absorbed into the passing blood vessels (Fig. 51–1). After the proinsulin is released, it is routed through the liver. There, the C-peptide chain is cleaved and excreted by the kidneys, leaving activated insulin (a polypeptide hormone). Acti-

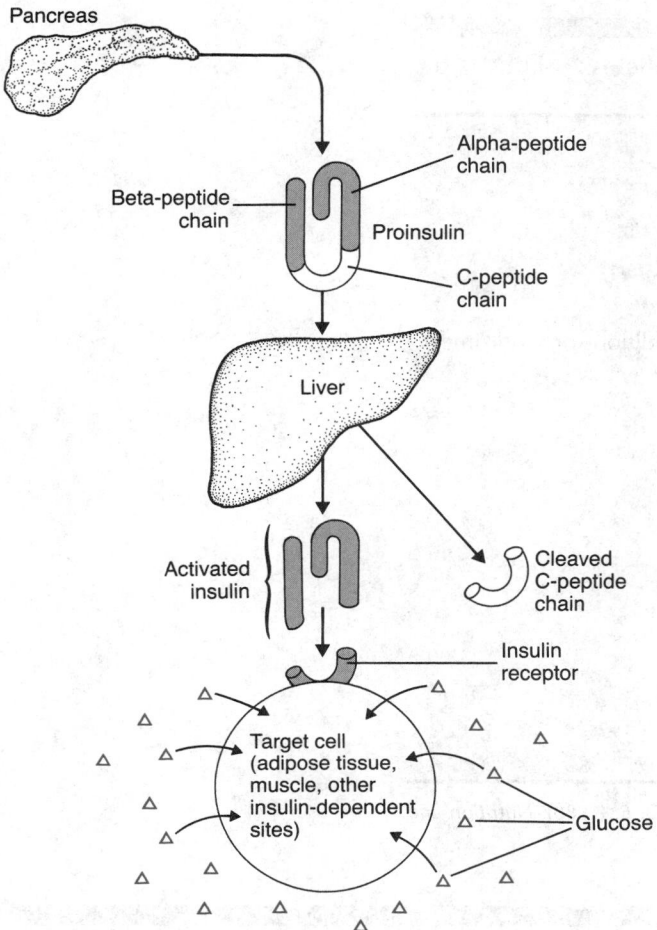

Pancreas

Alpha-peptide chain

Beta-peptide chain

Proinsulin

C-peptide chain

Liver

Activated insulin

Cleaved C-peptide chain

Insulin receptor

Target cell (adipose tissue, muscle, other insulin-dependent sites)

Glucose

Figure 51–1

Proinsulin, secreted by and stored in the beta cells of the islets of Langerhans in the pancreas, is transformed by the liver into activated insulin. Insulin attaches to receptors on target cells, where it promotes glucose transport into the cells through the cell membranes.

vated insulin then functions to promote glucose transport across the cell membrane. Most of the glucose is stored as glycogen; other glucose is stored in muscle, is converted to fat in adipose tissue, and is used for energy.

CLASSIFICATION

Diabetes and glucose intolerance are classified as shown in the accompanying Key Features of Disease: Classification of Diabetes Mellitus and Glucose Intolerance. The primary focus of this chapter is on type I, or insulin-dependent diabetes mellitus (IDDM), and type II, or non–insulin-dependent diabetes mellitus (NIDDM), diabetes. The accompanying Key Features of Disease: Differential Features of Type I and Type II Diabetes Mellitus gives the differential features of IDDM and NIDDM. IDDM (type I) and NIDDM (type II) affect the largest segments of the diabetic population, with IDDM

affecting 10% to 15% and NIDDM affecting 85% to 90%.

Type I: Insulin-Dependent Diabetes Mellitus

IDDM (type I) can be associated with deficiency in the amounts of insulin produced, malfunctioning insulin receptor sites, and/or disruption of the glycolytic pathway, which ultimately produces energy for the body to sustain life. Regardless of the specific physiologic etiology, when insulin is absent (as in IDDM), glucose is prevented from entering the cells and the cells are in a state of starvation while an excess of glucose is present in the blood.

The body perceives this cell starvation as a crisis and begins to secrete counterregulatory hormones (glucagon, epinephrine, norepinephrine, growth hormone, and cortisol). These counterregulatory hormones attempt to maintain the body's homeostasis by speeding up the availability of glucose by using alternative sources of energy by the following processes:

Lack of insulin

↓

Decreased glycogenesis (decreased conversion of glucose to glycogen, a process normally promoted by insulin)

↓

Increased glycogenolysis (increased production of glucose from glycogen, a process normally opposed by insulin)

↓

Increased gluconeogenesis (increased formation of glucose from noncarbohydrates such as amino acids, a process stimulated by glucocorticoids)

↓

Decreased glycolysis (decreased breakdown of glucose to carbon dioxide and water)

↓

Increased lipolysis (increased breakdown of fats to ketones to provide an alternative energy source when glucose is unavailable, a process [known as ketogenesis] modulated by insulin)

IDDM is diagnosed by a fasting plasma glucose (fasting blood sugar [FBS]) level of 140 mg/dL or greater in addition to two or more plasma glucose readings of greater than 200 mg/dL, usually with ketones present in both blood and urine. This presence of excessive amounts of glucose in the blood (hyperglycemia) causes a series of fluid and electrolyte imbalances that ultimately result in several classic symptoms known as the "three polys": polyuria, polydipsia, and polyphagia. *Polyuria* (frequent and excessive amount of urination) is

KEY FEATURES OF DISEASE ■ Classification of Diabetes Mellitus and Glucose Intolerance

Diabetes mellitus
  Insulin-dependent diabetes mellitus
  Non–insulin-dependent diabetes mellitus
    Nonobese diabetes mellitus
    Obese diabetes mellitus
    Maturity-onset diabetes of the young (MODY)
  Malnutrition-related (type J) diabetes mellitus (MRDM)
  Other types of diabetes mellitus (associated with certain conditions or syndromes)
    Pancreatic disease–associated diabetes mellitus
    Hormonally associated diabetes mellitus
    Drug- or chemical-induced diabetes mellitus
    Abnormalities related to insulin or its receptors
    Diabetes mellitus caused by certain genetic syndromes
    Miscellaneous diabetes mellitus

Impaired glucose tolerance (IGT)
  Nonobese diabetes mellitus
  Obese diabetes mellitus
  Diabetes mellitus associated with certain other conditions

Gestational diabetes mellitus (GDM)

Statistical risk classes
  Previous abnormality of glucose tolerance (prev AGT)
  Potential abnormality of glucose tolerance (pot AGT)

Modified from Kinney, J. M., Jeejeebhoy, K. N., Hill, G. L., & Owen, O. E. (1988). *Nutrition and metabolism in patient care.* Philadelphia: W. B. Saunders.

KEY FEATURES OF DISEASE ■ Differential Features of Type I and Type II Diabetes Mellitus

Feature	Type I	Type II
Former names	Juvenile, growth-onset, ketosis-prone	Adult, maturity-onset, ketosis-resistant
Age of onset	Usually under 30 yr of age; occurs at any age	Peak incidence — 5th decade; may occur at younger ages
Symptoms	Usually abrupt; thirst, polyuria, weight loss	Frequently none or thirst, fatigue, visual blurring, vascular or neural complications
Nutritional status	Usually nonobese	60% to 80% obese
Coma syndrome	Diabetic ketoacidosis	Hyperosmolar state; ketosis rarely with infection or stress
Endogenous insulin and C-peptide	Negligible to absent	Normal levels, but low in relation to blood sugar
Lipid abnormalities	Frequent cholesterol and LDL elevations; hyperlipidemia in ketoacidosis	Triglyceride (VLDL) and LDL cholesterol increased
Insulin	All patients dependent on insulin	Required for 20% to 30%
Sulfonylurea	No response	Effective for majority
Diet	Mandatory	Mandatory; diet alone may control blood sugar

From Kinney, J. M., Jeejeebhoy, K. N., Hill, G. L., & Owen, O. E. (1988). *Nutrition and metabolism in patient care.* Philadelphia: W. B. Saunders.

a result of an osmotic gradient developed in the kidneys owing to the presence of excessive glucose. The resulting dehydration stimulates the thirst mechanism, and *polydipsia* (excessive thirst) occurs; frequent fluid intake is the outcome. Because the cells are not receiving any food, the starvation mechanism results in *polyphagia* (excessive eating). In spite of the ingestion of vast amounts of food, the person remains in a state of starvation until adequate insulin is available to facilitate movement of the glucose into the cells. People with diabetes could literally starve, even when excessive glucose is present in the blood stream.

When cells cannot take up glucose as fuel to use for the generation of energy, alternative fuel sources are used. One alternative fuel source is the breakdown products of fatty acids, ketone bodies. Limited amounts of these ketone bodies can be used successfully by cells to generate energy. However, because these ketone bodies represent *incomplete* (and abnormal) degradation products of free fatty acids, they are not further metabolized and thus they accumulate in the blood and other extracellular fluids when insulin is not available. Some of these excessive ketone bodies are cleared from the body by kidney filtration and by evaporation through exhaled air. These processes are responsible for the presence of measurable amounts of ketones in the urine and for the "fruity" odor of the breath in clients experiencing ketoacidosis.

Because ketone bodies are acid products, when they accumulate in the blood they increase the concentration of free hydrogen ions and lower the pH, creating an acidemia of metabolic origin (see Chap. 15). As the blood pH decreases, the concentration of both hydrogen ions and carbon dioxide increases. These products stimulate the central chemoreceptors in the respiratory control areas of the brain, causing an increase in the rate and depth of respiration in an attempt to compensate for the acidemia. This type of breathing pattern is known as Kussmaul's respiration.

Potassium (K) levels are also adversely affected by metabolic acidosis. Because of the increased loss of fluids and the shift of potassium from intracellular to extracellular fluid, excessive amounts of potassium are lost in the urine. Serum potassium levels may be elevated (hyperkalemia), low (hypokalemia), or even normal, depending on the severity of dehydration.

Other minerals, such as calcium (Ca), magnesium (Mg), and phosphates, are lost as well, although the consequences to the body's functioning are less immediate.

IDDM was formerly known as juvenile-onset diabetes and brittle diabetes.

Diabetic ketoacidosis (DKA) is the most acute state of type I diabetes and is characterized by severe hyperosmolarity of body fluids, hypotension, and coma (Fig. 51–2). These symptoms are triggered by lack of insulin and excessive accumulation of ketones, causing large amounts of glucose and ketones to circulate in the body.

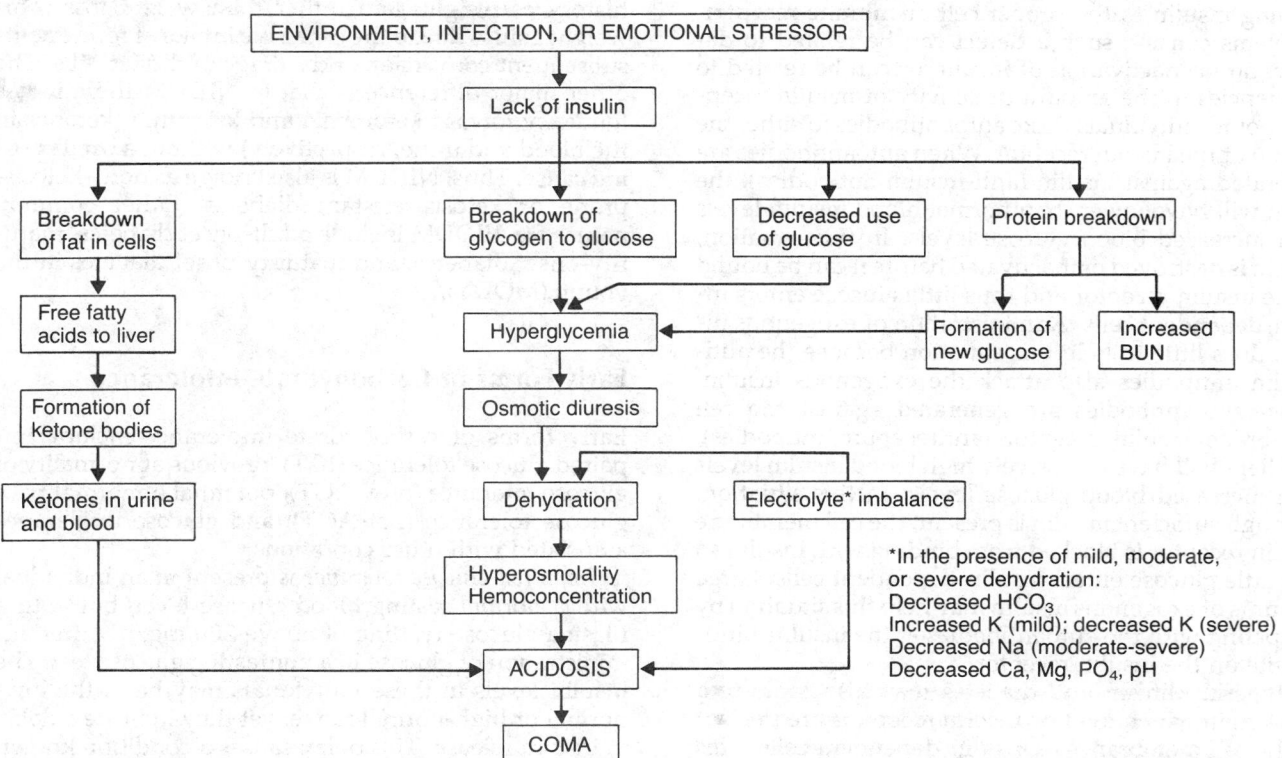

Figure 51–2

Pathophysiology of diabetic ketoacidosis.

The body attempts to rid itself of the excessive glucose and ketones in the urine, further perpetuating the hyperosmolar state and intracellular dehydration. The excessive ketones in the blood cause extreme acid build-up that severely inhibits the metabolic processes and the ability of the body to rid itself of metabolic by-products. Circulation is also compromised by loss of fluid volume, which results in low blood pressure and hypoxia (lack of oxygen to the cells). Hence, the body cells are deprived of the necessary food and fuel to sustain life, and the individual lapses into a comatose state.

Type II: Non–Insulin-Dependent Diabetes Mellitus

NIDDM (type II) appears to have several different mechanisms that induce the diabetic condition. In NIDDM, the beta cells of the pancreas remain able to synthesize and release insulin. For some clients, the amount of insulin secreted may be insufficient compared with the insulin need. This situation may result from decreased insulin production, excessive carbohydrate intake, or an increase in hepatic glucose production. Clients with this type of NIDDM often respond well to oral agents that stimulate the pancreas to increase synthesis and release of insulin.

Other clients with NIDDM may actually have higher than normal blood levels of insulin while manifesting symptoms of diabetes. NIDDM has as its basic defect an interference with some aspect of the process involved in binding insulin to the proper cell membrane receptor. Problems causing such a defect can be related to destruction or inactivation of insulin or can be related to deficiencies in the amount or activity of insulin receptors. Some individuals make autoantibodies to either the insulin or the insulin receptor. When autoantibodies are generated against insulin (anti-insulin antibodies), the client will have lower than normal blood insulin levels with increased blood glucose levels. In this situation, insulin is destroyed or inactivated before it can be bound to the insulin receptor and thus little glucose enters insulin-dependent cells. Administration of exogenous insulin does little to help this situation because the anti-insulin antibodies also attack the exogenous insulin. When autoantibodies are generated against the cell membrane insulin receptor (antireceptor antibodies), the client will have excessively high blood insulin levels with increased blood glucose levels. In this situation, although sufficient insulin is present, the cell membrane insulin receptor is blocked from binding with insulin so that little glucose enters insulin-dependent cells. Large amounts of exogenous insulin may help this situation by competing with the autoantibodies at the insulin-binding site on the insulin receptor.

Hyperinsulinism and diabetes may also indicate a problem in which too few insulin receptors are present on the cell membranes of insulin-dependent cells. This problem may be referred to as "insulin-resistant diabetes" (because additional insulin appears to intensify the problem rather than to resolve it) or "downregula-tion of insulin receptor sites" (because the cell itself appears to regulate the actual number of receptor sites it synthesizes and makes available for activity). The causes of this phenomenon are complex and appear to be related to the cell's biologic homeostatic tendencies.

In NIDDM, the body first responds to food intake by delayed secretion of insulin, followed by an overrelease of insulin. The person thus feels extremely hungry and is sometimes nervous and shaky until more food is ingested. This condition of delayed insulin release may be a precursor to complete loss of ability to produce insulin.

The increase in insulin level in people with NIDDM may also be a result of excessive food intake related to other physical or environmental stressors, such as peripheral resistance to insulin, obesity, or persistent overwhelming stress.

Eighty per cent of the NIDDM population are overweight. Inheritance of the disease occurs in an autosomal dominant manner.

Diagnostic criteria include an elevated fasting plasma glucose level (> 140 mg/dL). If the fasting plasma glucose level is less than 140 mg/dL, diagnosis can be confirmed by two or more plasma glucose levels above 200 mg/dL when taken at subsequent time periods of 30 minutes, 1 hour, and 2 hours. If the fasting plasma glucose level is 140 mg/dL or higher, only one other reading needs to be above 200 mg/dL.

The classic symptoms of IDDM—polyuria, polydipsia, and polyphagia—also occur in NIDDM. A major difference in symptoms between IDDM and NIDDM is that, in a majority of the NIDDM population, there is a history of weight gain rather than weight loss. This weight gain is due to the excessive intake of food and its subsequent conversion and storage in the fat cells. The other major difference is that in NIDDM there is less tendency toward ketonemia and ketonuria (ketones in the blood and urine, respectively) without a predisposing cause. Thus, NIDDM is also known as non–ketosis-prone or ketosis-resistant diabetes. Other common names for NIDDM include adult-onset diabetes, maturity-onset diabetes, and maturity-onset diabetes in the young (MODY).

Early Forms of Carbohydrate Intolerance

Early forms of carbohydrate intolerance include impaired glucose tolerance (IGT), previous abnormality of glucose tolerance (prev AGT), potential abnormality of glucose tolerance (pot AGT), and glucose intolerance associated with other conditions.

Impaired glucose tolerance is present in an individual with a normal fasting blood glucose level, but with a plasma glucose reading of above 200 mg/dL after administration of glucose in a nonfasting glucose test. The insulin levels in these individuals may be in the low-normal or high-normal range, yet they indicate a delay in insulin release. This delay causes a condition known as *reactive hypoglycemia*. This results from the body's response to the delayed release of insulin by releasing more insulin than is necessary. With this excessive insulin release, there is a drop in blood glucose level because of the rapid movement of glucose into the cells.

Previous abnormality of glucose tolerance refers to a previous diagnosis. It describes the person who was previously assessed as having some abnormal blood glucose readings, but who currently has a normal glucose tolerance test (GTT) result. The previous abnormal reading could have been associated with a heart attack, a severe burn, pregnancy, or situations of extreme stress.

Potential abnormality of glucose tolerance describes high-risk individuals, such as those who are overweight, women with a history of multiple stillbirths or miscarriages, women who have borne babies weighing more than 9 lb, or individuals with a strong family history of diabetes. This is a retrospective diagnosis, except in a few individuals who have a known genetic predisposition, such as an identical twin of a diabetic person or a child of diabetic parents.

Gestational diabetes mellitus develops during preg- nancy and may revert to IGT or prev AGT after the pregnancy. It is possible that a woman with GDM will progress to frank IDDM or NIDDM, particularly if she is overweight.

CHRONIC COMPLICATIONS

All diabetic clients exhibit diabetes-associated complications to some degree. Some complications are related to increased build-up of sugars within the cell. The most common complications are organ pathologic alterations that occur as a result of changes in and around the small and large blood vessels. The complications may be a result of microangiopathy or macroangiopathy (see the accompanying Key Features of Disease). Although all diabetics have these vascular-based complications, the degree of pathologic changes and the rate at which they occur are related to control of the blood glucose levels.

KEY FEATURES OF DISEASE ■ Pathologic Course of the Chronic Complications of Diabetes Mellitus

Complication	Body System	Pathologic Course
Microangiopathic complications		
Neuropathy	Neurologic	Numbness or tingling ↓ Extensive numbness or severe pain
Nephropathy	Genitourinary (kidney)	Dilation of renal pelves and tubules ↓ Protein leakage ↓ Sclerosis ↓ Renal failure
Retinopathy	Sensory (eye)	Blurring of vision due to hyperglycemia ↓ Leakage of vessels ↓ Hemorrhage ↓ Formation of new blood vessels ↓ Complete occlusion of vision
Macroangiopathic complications	Cardiovascular	Silent myocardial infarction ↓ Complete vascular collapse
	Peripheral vascular	Ulcerations ↓ Fulminating infections ↓ Gangrene ↓ Amputation

The more closely the client's blood glucose levels are maintained within the normal range, the more slowly the pathologic processes occur.

Increased blood glucose levels result in an imbalance of substances used for making the matrix between cells. Enzyme systems, such as aldose reductase, are induced to convert glucose to other, non–insulin-dependent sugar forms, such as sorbitol and fructose, in an attempt to lower the actual blood glucose level (Fig. 51–3). These other sugar forms, sorbitol and fructose, accumulate within as well as between cells. The intracellular accumulation of sorbitol causes intracellular edema, lens opacities, and intracellular osmolar alterations that adversely affect cell function.

Microangiopathy. Extracellular accumulation of glucose and these other sugar forms causes a thickening of the basement membranes between tissues and around blood vessels. This thickening increases the distance over which nutrients and waste products must diffuse. As a result, the microcirculation, especially at the capillary level, is impaired. Thus, many cells and tissues receive marginal to inadequate nutrients (including oxygen) and tend to retain toxic products of cellular metabolism longer, which increases the likelihood of cellular damage. Most of the long-term complications of

diabetes mellitus are related directly or indirectly to this pattern of altered exchange and nutrition at the cellular level and are first evident in highly vascular oxygen-dependent tissues.

Neuropathy. Even though nerve fibers themselves do not contain a separate blood supply, their health and continued function are dependent on diffusion of nutrients from the extracellular fluid. Inadequate microcirculation in tissues near nerve axons and dendrites contributes to inadequate nutrition of these nerve components and eventual nerve dysfunction. In addition, some sorbitol also accumulates in nerve tissue, further diminishing both sensory and motor nerve function.

Neuropathy is common among diabetic clients. The signs and symptoms vary widely, depending on which specific nerves are involved (see the accompanying Key Features of Disease). This nerve damage has many direct and indirect consequences for the diabetic client. Not only do some tissues, such as skeletal muscle, atrophy when motor innervation is impaired, but the loss of sensory acuity to painful stimulation decreases the diabetic client's perception of discomfort and reduces the likelihood of instituting protective responses. As a result, the diabetic client may experience more tissue damage whenever an injurious situation exists simply be-

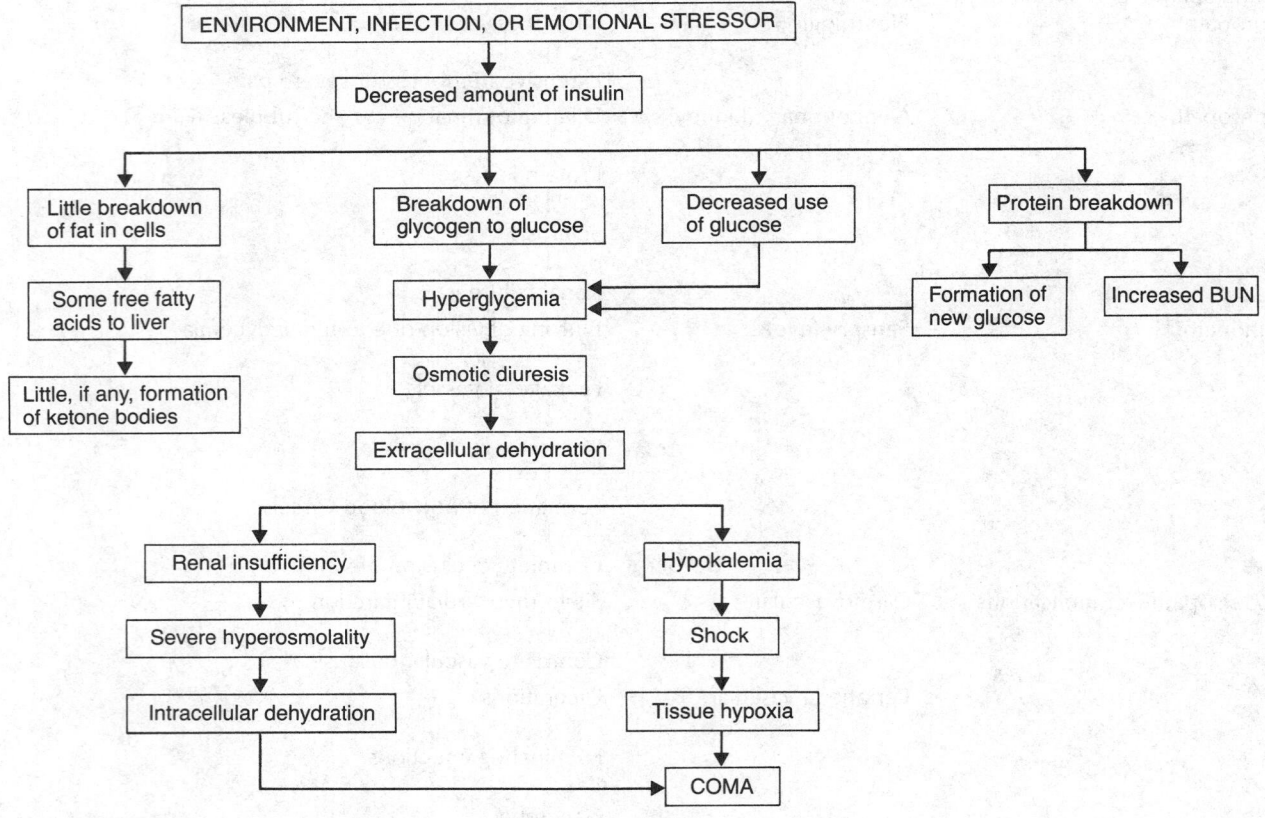

Figure 51–3

The alternative glycolytic pathway used in diabetes mellitus leads to microangiopathy.

KEY FEATURES OF DISEASE ■ Signs and Symptoms of Neuropathic Complications of Diabetes Mellitus

Complication	Signs and Symptoms
Amyopathy	
Nerve damage, leading to pain, weakness, and a wasting away of the muscles of the thighs, the pelvic girdle, and the hands	Wasted muscle mass Weakened response to resistance
Autonomic Neuropathy	

A variety of conditions caused by damage to the nerves in the autonomic nervous system:
  Impotence
  Frigidity
  Postural hypotension
  Gastroparesis (bloating and feeling of fullness in the upper GI tract)
  Diarrhea (an outcome of pockets of infection occurring in areas of flaccid intestine)
  Vesical atony or neurogenic bladder (inability of the muscles of the bladder to function properly)
  Cardiorespiratory arrest
  Gustatory sweating (increase in salivation)
  Anhidrosis (inability to perspire)
	Lack of perspiration in a hot environment
	Sexual dysfunction
	Bloating
	Nocturnal diarrhea
	Bladder distention
	Tachycardia

Carpal Tunnel Syndrome	
Pressure on the nerve going through the canal at the base of the wrist, resulting in loss of functioning of the affected hand	Weak grasp or numbness
Mononeuropathy	
An affliction of the spinal or cranial nerves	Pain Sensory loss or weakness Abnormal reflexes
Neuroarthropathy (Charcot's Joint)	
Pain, inflammation, and deterioration of the joints of the foot	Discomfort in ankles Enlarged ankles Flat feet
Polyneuropathy	

Damage to a variety of nerves, resulting in
  Weakness
  Pain
  Glove-and-stocking paresthesia
  Sensory loss
  Reflex loss
	Abnormal neurologic findings
	Altered vibratory sense
	Decreased perception of sharp and dull sensation
	Reflexes decreased or absent

Radiculopathy	
Sensory loss and pain along the dermatomes of the skin	Altered responses to sharp and dull sensation

cause he/she does not feel the pain associated with the injurious situation and does not take action to stop or limit the injury. For example, because of diminished pain perception, the client with peripheral neuropathy may not be aware of a thorn in the sole of the food until obvious manifestations of infection are present.

Nephropathy. Microangiopathy in the kidneys can cause complications involving the renal pelvis, tubules, and glomeruli. Renal disease can progress from mild proteinuria to renal failure. The treatment of end-stage renal disease (ESRD) is similar to that of ESRD in nondiabetics (see Chap. 59), except that the diabetic client may require changes in insulin dosage because insulin is excreted more slowly.

Retinopathy. Microvascular changes in the retina develop over time, with as many as 80% of clients who have had diabetes for 20 years exhibiting some degree of retinopathy. Diabetes is the leading cause of blindness in the United States.

The two most common types of diabetic retinopathy are background retinopathy and proliferative retinopathy. In *background retinopathy*, microaneurysms develop in the retinal vessels, causing the formation of hard exudates. These changes may progress to a more serious type, *proliferative retinopathy*, in which there is formation of new blood vessels, termed *neovascularization*. The new vessels can cause retinal detachment and hemorrhage into the vitreous cavity. Permanent blindness can occur.

Diabetic clients should have yearly eye examinations with dilated pupils by an ophthalmologist because there are no symptoms of early retinal changes.

Two treatments of diabetic retinopathy are laser photocoagulation and vitrectomy. *Laser photocoagulation* uses thermal energy to obliterate new vessels and to seal capillary leaks. *Vitrectomy* is a surgical procedure to remove vitreous hemorrhage, to arrest neovascularization, and to halt retinal detachment.

Macroangiopathy. Macroangiopathy is a disease of larger blood vessels characterized by atherosclerotic changes. These changes are more frequently found in clients with NIDDM than in those with IDDM. The process of atherosclerosis is similar to that in nondiabetic persons, except that it is accelerated by factors that are poorly understood. Complications of macroangiopathy include cardiovascular disease, coronary artery disease, and peripheral vascular disease.

Diabetic clients with these problems are treated in the same manner as nondiabetic individuals. The reader is referred to Chapters 64 and 65 for further discussion.

Lower-extremity involvement. Microvascular and macrovascular changes and neuropathies can cause changes in the lower extremities of the diabetic client. These complications can lead to compromised circulation, resulting in infection, gangrene, and even necessity for amputation. Decreased sensation from loss of sensory nerve function can lead to trauma or uncontrolled

infections, resulting in gangrene. Amputation may be necessary if infections cannot be reversed. Proper care of the feet (see later) is critical in reducing the need for amputations.

ETIOLOGY

A variety of etiologic factors are responsible for the syndromes of type I and type II diabetes mellitus (see the accompanying Key Features of Disease).

Type I diabetes (IDDM) is most frequently associated with the destruction of beta cells in the islets of Langerhans. This destruction is attributed to genetic predisposition; an infectious process, most commonly owing to mumps or a coxsackievirus B4 (HLA-DR4 gene); or a primary autoimmune response associated with the HLA-DR3 gene. Theoretically, the presence of one of these genes causes a defect in the immune system, which in turn causes increased susceptibility to viral infections. In the autoimmune response, circulating antibodies cause beta cell destruction, resulting in a lack of available insulin (Davidson, 1986).

IDDM is usually diagnosed when clients are younger than 30 years of age. They frequently exhibit the classic symptoms of hyperglycemia, ketosis, and even ketoacidosis. Although the clinical onset is thought to be sudden, the pathologic changes that cause decreased insulin availability may have occurred over an extended period of time.

After the acute episode, or the appearance of early symptoms leading to the diagnosis, there may be a period of *remission* in which the body appears to be able to make some insulin again. This period, when individuals are secreting some of their own insulin, is referred to as the "honeymoon period." No solid scientific research evidence has documented what really occurs during this period.

Any illness, extreme emotional stress, or growth spurts appear to aid in further destruction of the beta cells and may shorten the remission. Eventually, the person becomes *completely dependent on exogenous insulin.*

Type II diabetes (NIDDM) is often diagnosed in individuals older than 30 years of age and is relatively slow in onset. The two factors most frequently associated with NIDDM are the *aging process* and *obesity.* The obese client with NIDDM is resistant to the development of diabetic ketoacidosis and is insulin resistant.

Heredity is also a major factor. The rates of transmission from parent to child range from 80% to 90% (Cotran et al., 1989). There is a strong association of NIDDM and hypertension and heart disease.

INCIDENCE

It is estimated that, in the United States, approximately 3% of the population have abnormally high blood glucose concentrations, and probably half of these have

KEY FEATURES OF DISEASE ■ **Etiologic Factors in Type I and Type II Diabetes Mellitus**

Type I	Type II
Genetic Factors	
HLA antigens (particularly DR3 and DR4)	Not associated with HLA antigens
Heredity	
Unknown: <50%	Unknown: 90%–100% concordance in monozygotic twins
Autoimmunity	
Strong autoimmune basis	No strong autoimmune basis
Presence of islet cell antibodies	Some positive islet cell antibodies
Environmental Factors	
Associated with viral infections	Obesity
	Decreased physical activity

diabetes mellitus. The prevalence of type I diabetes (IDDM) is estimated to be 0.2% of the population. In adults aged 20 to 74 years, diabetes is considered the leading cause of new cases of blindness. Each year, more than 2 million adults are hospitalized because of diabetes. Other figures reported by the American Diabetes Association (1987) reveal that this disease results in 20,000 leg and foot amputations annually, predominantly because of gangrene. Women are affected two times more often than men. Black Americans are two times more likely, and Hispanic Americans five times more likely, to develop this disease than other groups in the United States. The incidence is higher for people whose income is less than poverty levels. Because diabetic individuals have high risk of heart disease, stroke, renal failure, and severe nerve damage, it is not surprising to find that one-half of the heart attacks and three-quarters of the strokes are due to the complications of this disease. ESRD is the cause of death for 20% of those people with type I diabetes and for 1% to 4% of those with type II diabetes.

PREVENTION

There is no known way to prevent diabetes, except diabetes resulting from secondary causes (e.g., surgical removal of the pancreas, use of steroids). Although diabetes is predominantly an inherited disease, environmental factors appear to influence whether the specific type of diabetes occurs earlier or later in life. Meticulous prenatal care, prevention of obesity, pre-

vention of illnesses, or reduction of environmental stressors may lead to the delay of the occurrence of overt signs and symptoms of the disease. Susceptibility to primary diabetes increases with advancing age, especially if the individual has a strong family history of diabetes or related diseases, such as heart attacks and strokes.

Evidence of the effectiveness of measures to prevent the pathologic changes that result in morbidity and mortality is mounting. Although prevention or control of hypertension is a major factor, the first line of prevention is *hyperglycemic control.* Correction of hyperglycemia gives the individual the best chance of preventing, or at least delaying, the complications associated with diabetes. The major components in preventing hyperglycemia are meal planning, exercise, and medications as needed. Education can help a person manage diabetes. Education should stress an appropriate self-care plan that results in a healthier individual in spite of the presence of a chronic condition.

EMERGENCY CARE

Three emergencies can arise in diabetes care: DKA, hyperglycemic hyperosmolar nonketotic syndrome (HHNKS), and hypoglycemia.

DKA, characterized by hyperglycemia and acidemia, occurs when the insulin present is inadequate to the extent that very little glucose enters the cell. Oxidation of fatty acids becomes the main energy-generating process. Excessive oxidation of fatty acids leads to the synthesis of ketone bodies called *ketoacids* (acetone,

KEY FEATURES OF DISEASE ■ Differential Features of Diabetic Ketoacidosis and Hyperglycemic Hyperosmolar Nonketotic Syndrome

	Diabetic Ketoacidosis	Hyperglycemic Hyperosmolar Nonketotic Syndrome
Onset	Gradual or sudden	Gradual
Precipitating Factors	Infection, other stressors, stopping insulin	Infection, other stressors, poor fluid intake
Manifestations	Thirst, nausea, vomiting, abdominal pain, fatigue, polyuria to anuria, blurred vision	Polyuria, fatigue
	Elevated temperature; signs of dehydration; Kussmaul's respiration; fruity odor to breath; flushed face; rapid, thready pulse; soft, sunken eyeballs; hypotension; coma	Decreased temperature; lethargy, confusion, coma, seizures, hemiplegia, rapid pulse, dehydration
Laboratory Findings		
Serum glucose	Usually 400–800 mg/dL	Usually >800 mg/dL
Osmolarity	About 320 mOsm/L	>350 mOsm/L
Serum acetone	Large	Nondetectable or small
Serum HCO_3	10 mEq/L or less	17 mEq/L
Arterial pH	About 7.07 (low)	About 7.26
Serum Na	Low, normal, or high	Normal to high
Serum K	High, normal, or low	Low
Serum P	High, but total (whole blood) is low	Not known
Anion gap	Increased	Normal
BUN	Normal to slight elevation	High

acetoacetate, and β-hydroxybutyrate).

HHNKS, characterized by hyperglycemia without an accompanying acidemia, occurs when the amount of insulin present is inadequate to prevent hyperglycemia but adequate to allow glucose to be used as fuel for energy generation. Excessive oxidation of fatty acids does not occur.

Hypoglycemia occurs if there is too much insulin. (See the accompanying Key Features of Disease and Emergency Care feature for differential features of and emergency care for DKA and HHNKS, respectively.)

DIABETIC KETOACIDOSIS

The presentation of DKA may vary in severity. The person may walk into the physician's office or may arrive in the emergency room completely comatose.

Goals of treatment for this acute condition are rehydration, restoration of electrolyte balance, and reduction of blood glucose levels. Regular insulin is administered subcutaneously or intravenously during DKA to assist in transporting glucose into the cells. Fluids are administered intravenously, usually at 150 to 200 mL/hour as tolerated by the client. Blood glucose levels should not be lowered faster than 50 to 100 mg/dL per hour. If the blood glucose levels are decreased too quickly or the fluids are administered too swiftly, cerebral edema could result. It is possible in the treatment of DKA that the client can change from a hyperglycemic state to a hypoglycemic state without becoming conscious. The nurse is responsible for monitoring the various physiologic changes. Reporting responses to early signs of DKA may avert further progression of the acidotic state.

HYPERGLYCEMIC HYPEROSMOLAR NONKETOTIC SYNDROME

In HHNKS much the same process occurs as in diabetic ketoacidosis, except there is not the excessive formation of ketones (Fig. 51–4). Hence, people experiencing HHNKS do not usually manifest Kussmaul's respirations or elevated levels of serum and urinary ketones, as in diabetic ketoacidosis. The hyperosmolar state in HHNKS can still lead to serious volume depletion and shock, and the individual's life can be in jeopardy.

HHNKS does not occur frequently, but as people are living longer, the likelihood of its occurrence is much greater. Most individuals experiencing this hyperosmo-

EMERGENCY CARE ■ Diabetic Ketoacidosis and Hyperglycemic Hyperosmolar Nonketotic Syndrome*

Interventions	Rationales
1. Per physician's orders, administer insulin loading dose (50–100 units of regular insulin) followed by 5–10 units/h via IV infusion pump.	1. To decrease risk of hypoglycemia and hypokalemia.
2. Replace fluid and electrolytes with normal saline or ½ normal saline (0.9% or 0.45% NaCl solution) IV.	2. To correct hypovolemia and electrolyte imbalance, especially potassium.
3. Assess blood glucose level.	3. To determine the need for continued insulin therapy. Goal is to achieve plasma glucose level of 250 mg/dL or less.
4. Check vital signs.	4. To detect fever, shock, tachycardia, and Kussmaul's respirations.
5. Assess skin turgor.	5. To determine degree of dehydration.
6. Assess level of consciousness.	6. To ascertain worsening status.
7. Monitor intake and output.	7. To assess renal status.
8. Monitor central venous pressure.	8. To determine degree of hypovolemia.
9. Implement cardiac monitoring.	9. To detect cardiac arrhythmias.
10. Administer bicarbonate only if blood pH < 7.0.	10. To correct severe acidosis.

* The emergency treatment of HHNKS is similar to that of DKA, except that there is a need for increased fluid replacement and assessment for fluid overload in HHNKS and a need for less insulin.

lar state are conscious or in various levels of semiconsciousness. The mortality rate is greater in HHNKS than in DKA because of misdiagnosis, delayed diagnosis, and other complications in elderly clients.

The nurse assists in monitoring the serum levels of potassium and other electrolytes while administering replacements as ordered. Assessing levels of consciousness and aiding in the fluid replacement while keeping the airway patent and the skin intact are primary nursing responsibilities.

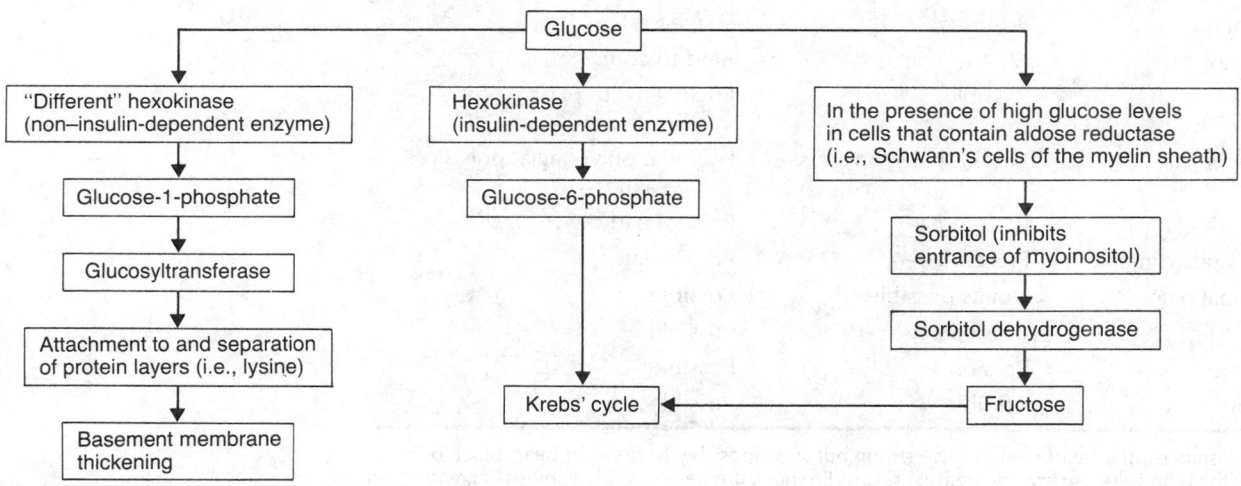

Figure 51–4

Pathophysiology of hyperglycemic hyperosmolar nonketotic syndrome.

HYPOGLYCEMIA

Symptoms of hypoglycemia occur when the brain signals the body that it is not receiving the amount of glucose to which it has become accustomed. *Hypoglycemia* has been called a variety of names, including insulin reaction, insulin shock, and low blood sugar. The clinical manifestations may be adrenergic (sweating, palpitations, pallor, irritability, angina, anxiety, tremulousness, hunger, piloerection) or neuroglycopenic (blurred vision, diplopia, headache, slurred speech, weakness, inability to make decisions, agitation, seizures, unconsciousness, confusion). However, some patients remain alert and have few symptoms at a glucose level of 40 mg/dL (2.2 mmol/L), whereas others become comatose at this same glucose level.

Some symptoms of hypoglycemia may be confused with hyperglycemic responses, such as headache, nausea, irritability, and coma (see the accompanying Key Features of Disease). Symptoms reportedly occur if the blood glucose levels fall below normal levels (plasma glucose level < 60 mg/dL) or rapidly change from one level to another (e.g., 400 to 250 mg/dL during a few hours).

Treatment depends on the level of hypoglycemia. Plasma glucose levels of 40 to 60 mg/dL respond to ingestion of food such as milk or crackers (40 to 80 kcal). People with plasma glucose levels of 20 to 40 mg/dL respond better when simple sugar is given, such as 10 to 15 g (20 to 40 kcal) of honey, table sugar, or juice. This should usually be followed in 10 to 15 minutes by a well-balanced meal. In the hospital, 50% dextrose solution (D$_{50}$W) by IV push is the treatment of choice for the client in seizure or the unconscious person with low plasma glucose levels. Although the more severe form of hypoglycemia is not usually experienced in type II diabetes, it can occur. Capillary blood glucose monitoring and level of consciousness can indicate the client's responsiveness to treatment. Overtreatment (continuing to treat until symptoms subside) is discouraged. If one is in doubt as to whether hypoglycemia or hyperglycemia is occurring, treatment for hypoglycemia is administered until a measurement of capillary blood glucose can be done.

Glucagon is an alternative treatment for the uncon-

KEY FEATURES OF DISEASE ■ Differential Features of Hypoglycemia and Hyperglycemia

Feature	Hypoglycemia	Hyperglycemia
Temperature	Below normal	Above normal
Pulse	Rapid, strong*	Rapid, thready
Respirations	Little change	Deep and rapid
Blood pressure	Initially hypertensive	Hypotensive
Skin	Cool, clammy	Warm, dry
Dehydration	Not present	Present
Eyes	Pupils dilated	Globes soft
Perspiration	Profuse†	Decreased
Consciousness	Alert to coma	Alert to coma
Seizures	Possible	Possible (with plasma glucose levels of 1000 mg/dL)
Symptoms	Weak, shaky, anxious	Polyuria, polyphagia, polydipsia, weakness
Hunger	Present early	Present early
Nausea and vomiting	Present later	Present later
Abdominal pain	Not as possible	Possible
Staggering gait	Possible	Possible
Headache	Possible	Possible
Irritability	Possible	Possible

* In a few instances, the heart beat may be strong but slow (possibly because of heart block or other reasons, as the blood glucose level decreases and insulin shock progresses. With diabetes of greater than 5 yr duration, there may be a decreased epinephine response and the pulse may be rapid and weaker and is less of an indicator of the hypoglycemic state.

† May be decreased in person with neuropathy.

scious client. Glucagon is the drug of choice for the person at home and can be used in the hospital as well if a vein cannot be found for IV glucose administration. Nursing responsibilities are to assist the client to detect and treat hypoglycemic episodes. Clients should be taught to carry glucose tablets or solution as well as a card or medallion that identifies them as diabetic.

COLLABORATIVE MANAGEMENT

 Assessment

History

History taking from the client who has diabetes may be delayed, depending on the person's level of consciousness. Accompanying family members may provide the general information needed, including *age, sex, race, usual weight* (before becoming noticeably ill), *height,* and *dietary intake* (24-hour food history for 3 days, if possible). The nurse finds out if the diabetes was diagnosed earlier and whether it was identified as type I or II. The nurse also inquires about the specific symptoms and how long the *symptoms were present*. If the person is taking any *diabetes medication,* the nurse asks for the name, dosage, and last time taken. The person is asked what sites are used for insulin injection. The nurse questions the client about hypoglycemic reactions: "What symptoms usually occur? What treatment was used? How did it work?" Other questions concern types of *stressors* related to work, home, or family and presence of other *illnesses.* The nurse notes any other medications, vitamins, minerals, analgesics, and laxatives used. The client is asked what *type of monitoring* is being used for blood, urine, or both, and the names of the products and equipment. The *past history* (major illnesses, childhood illnesses, surgical operations, social habits, and immunizations) should be obtained. Of particular importance in the person with diabetes is a *family history* of diabetes, heart disease, and stroke and the individual's history of obesity and, for women, history of stillbirths, miscarriages, and babies weighing more than 9 lb. The nurse also asks the person if he/she has been participating in any kind of *exercise program* and, if so, what type of program.

Questions to guide the nurse in assessing complications may include the following: Has the individual noticed floaters, double or blurry vision, halos around lights, or blind spots? When walking or exercising, has the client experienced intermittent claudication (increased cramping in the legs when walking, but decreased discomfort when resting)? Has the client observed numbness, change in color, coldness, tingling, or pain in the extremities? If diarrhea is present, is there fecal incontinence? Does this just occur at night? Are there any problems with voiding? Is there a problem in passing urine? Is urine retained in the bladder, which causes an abnormal fullness? Is eating associated with a feeling of fullness, followed by bloating and gas? If these complications can be detected early, it may be possible to arrest, slow, or reverse their development.

Nurses should also ascertain information regarding the person's or family's concerns, expectations, and special needs. General information that is not disease specific should not be forgotten in the attempt to determine all the diabetes-related data.

Physical Assessment: Clinical Manifestations

The nurse assesses *skin turgor* to determine the state of dehydration. The *level of consciousness* is determined by the client's orientation and response to stimulation. *Vital signs,* including blood pressure, are noted. The presence of acetone in the breath may be detected.

The nurse observes the diabetic client for manifestations of complications (see the accompanying Key Features of Disease). These complications include signs of retinopathy, neuropathy (including decreased sensation, decreased reflexes, and positional blood pressure changes), and decreased vascular flow as evidenced by decreased pulse rate and signs of circulation deficits. Decreased temperature of the skin, as well as weak pulse (e.g., posterior tibial and dorsalis pedis), demonstrates *peripheral vascular deficits. Neuropathy* is assessed by determining the reflexes, the vibratory senses, and the responses to sharp and dull sensations. *Retinopathy* is assessed by the nurse skilled in ophthalmoscopic assessment. Tortuosity of the vessels, beading of the vessels, pinpoint hemorrhages, or exudates on the retinal surface may be noted.

Psychosocial Assessment

The nursing assessment should include the following to give a true picture of the emotional and psychosocial status and identify special needs: how clients with diabetes visualized themselves before the diagnosis and their current perception, and whether they can see themselves as capable of performing specific tasks and functions. The nurse needs to check basic mathematics capabilities and reading levels to make sure that clients are able to understand and perform the self-care techniques. The nurse determines how clients interact with family members and people at work or school. The nurse aids the client to identify times when and places where they feel more stressed, as well as support people and services. Because stress can adversely affect blood glucose levels, psychosocial adjustment is extremely important for diabetes control.

Studies note that cognitive depression is an ongoing, recurrent problem in clients with diabetes (Kovacs et al., 1985; Wysocki et al., 1989). Clients with diabetes recognize the threats of the disease to their life style and life span. Depression is especially frequent in older dia-

KEY FEATURES OF DISEASE ■ Clinical Manifestations of the Complications of Diabetes Mellitus

Early Manifestations	Early to Middle Manifestations	Late Manifestations
Polyuria, polyphagia, polydipsia	Lipodystrophy	Retinopathy, leading to partial or complete visual loss
Blurring of vision	*Candida albicans* infection	Neuropathy, leading to dysfunction, pain, or loss of sensation
Sores that do not heal properly	Necrobiosis lipoidica Ulcers of extremities	Microangiopathy, peripheral ischemia
Tiredness, lethargy	Xanthomas	Macroangiopathy, leading to cardiovascular disease, stroke, or necessity for amputation
Dry, itchy skin	Diabetic dermopathy	Severe skin disease
Urinary tract infection	Proteinuria	Nephropathy, ESRD

betics, and grieving occurs as complications develop (Papatheodorou, 1983). Clients sense a loss of function, a loss of freedom, or a loss of control related to these complications.

Laboratory Findings

Initial laboratory tests should include electrolyte studies; determination of blood glucose, blood urea nitrogen (BUN), serum creatinine, microalbuminuria, and glycosylated hemoglobin (Hb A_{1c}) levels; pH; and partial pressure of carbon dioxide (PCO_2). Table 51–1 explains the rationales for performing these studies. Tests for urinary ketones should also be done initially. Table 51–2 presents normal blood glucose values and explains the interpretation of abnormal findings. The accompanying Guidelines feature describes nursing care of the client undergoing blood glucose testing.

TABLE 51–1 Rationales for Performing Laboratory Tests in Diabetes Mellitus

Test*	Rationales
Serum electrolytes (K and Na)	To determine biochemical imbalances that interfere with electrical innervation of muscles and proper cardiovascular function.
Blood glucose	To determine the severity of glucose deprivation in cells.
BUN and serum creatinine	To determine the extent of kidney dysfunction or damage.
Microalbuminuria	To detect early renal damage.
Glycosylated hemoglobin or 7- to 10-d fructose amine test or glycosylated serum protein	To evaluate hyperglycemic state by giving mean glucose level during previous 2–3 mo.
pH and PCO_2 values	To determine the severity of diabetic ketoacidosis; the higher the level of osmolarity, the lower the level of consciousness.

* Other laboratory values may indicate immediate medical intervention for underlying infections or conditions. These include liver function test results, Ca and Mg levels, lipid studies (levels of cholesterol, triglycerides, high-density lipoproteins, low-density lipoproteins, and very-low-density lipoproteins), and cardiac enzyme levels (lactate dehydrogenase, creatine kinase, and aspartate aminotransferase [serum glutamic-oxaloacetic transaminase]) that indicate cardiac functioning and globulin levels. An abnormal lactate dehydrogenase level might indicate the presence of a silent myocardial infarction that may have triggered the overt symptoms of diabetes.

TABLE 51–2 Normal Values and Significance of Abnormal Findings in Blood Glucose Tests

Test	Normal Plasma Glucose Values	Significance of Abnormal Findings
Fasting blood glucose	70–100 mg/dL	*Elevations > 140 mg/dL* are diagnostic of diabetes mellitus.
2-h postprandial blood glucose	<140 mg/dL	*Elevations > 140 mg/dL* indicate the need for further testing (when used for screening) or changes in therapy (when used for evaluation of treatment).
Oral glucose tolerance test (OGTT)		*Elevations of 2 values* (one of which is 2-h value) *>200 mg/dL* are diagnostic of diabetes mellitus.
Fasting	<140 mg/dL	
½ h, 1 h	<115 mg/dL	
2 h	<200 mg/dL	
3 h	<140 mg/dL	
Intravenous glucose tolerance test (IGTT)	Same as for OGTT.	Same as for OGTT.

Other Diagnostic Tests

Other diabetes-related tests include retinal photographs (the best way to document retinal status) and nerve conduction studies. Nerve conduction tests are administered when abnormalities such as tingling, numbness, or pain are observed; retinal studies are performed when a diagnosis of type II diabetes is made or 5 years after diagnosis of type I diabetes. Fluorescein angiography is used to assess the patency of retinal vessels and to find areas possibly contributing to macular edema. Other studies would be done to assess specific organs affected. For example, excretory urography (in-travenous pyelography) may be done to assess kidney function. A yearly multitest chemical profile, including Hb A_1 or Hb A_{1c} level, is done, and microalbuminuria tests are done annually in specially equipped laboratories to detect early damage. Tests for blood glucose levels should be performed daily.

 ### Analysis: Nursing Diagnosis

The nurse uses information from the assessment to identify appropriate nursing diagnoses. These diag-

---

GUIDELINES ■ Nursing Care of the Client Undergoing Blood Glucose Testing

Test	Interventions
Fasting blood glucose	Instruct the client to fast after midnight.
2-h postprandial blood glucose	Measure 2 h after high-carbohydrate meal or intake of 75- to 100-g sugar load.
OGTT	Instruct the client to eat an unrestricted diet including 200–300 g of carbohydrates daily for 3 d before the test.
	Instruct the client to fast after midnight. Obtain a fasting blood glucose value.
	Give a glucose load and take blood and urine samples at intervals of ½ h, 1 h, 2 h, up to 5 h.

noses are affected by a variety of psychologic, social, and biologic factors and by whether the diabetes is newly diagnosed or has been present for some time.

Common Diagnoses

The following diagnoses are commonly noted in clients with diabetes mellitus:

1. Knowledge deficit related to lack of exposure to or unwillingness to learn about diabetes and its treatment
2. Potential for infection related to an elevation in blood glucose levels
3. Sensory/perceptual alterations related to less-than-optimal physiologic functioning
4. Ineffective individual coping and ineffective family coping related to denial, anger, or anxiety
5. Altered nutrition: more than body requirements and altered nutrition: less than body requirements related to food intake needs
6. Sexual dysfunction related to perceived (or actual) alterations in physiologic functioning

Additional Diagnoses

This following list reflects some of the major diagnoses that could potentially occur during the lifetime of a client with diabetes mellitus. Because the disease affects virtually every organ and system of the body, the list is not exhaustive.

1. Pain and chronic pain related to numbness secondary to less-than-optimal vascular supply or neurologic complications
2. Altered patterns of urinary elimination related to bladder dysfunction secondary to nephropathy or neuropathy
3. Colonic constipation, bowel incontinence, and diarrhea related to bowel dysfunction secondary to neuropathy
4. Potential for infection and impaired tissue integrity related to a less-than-optimal circulatory response secondary to peripheral vascular deficits
5. Anxiety related to unknown expectations secondary to the diagnosis of diabetes
6. Fear related to a perceived lack of control such as might occur if the client is concerned about the potential of having a hypoglycemic reaction
7. Altered thought processes related to confusion or irritability secondary to diabetes
8. Anticipatory grieving and dysfunctional grieving related to perceived loss of body function secondary to diabetes
9. Altered role performance related to noncoping responses if one or more family members have diabetes

10. Self-esteem disturbance related to self-perception of a person with a chronic, potentially life-threatening illness
11. Potential for injury related to less-than-optimal physiologic functioning

 Planning and Implementation

The interventions are based on the common nursing diagnoses. Additional interventions might be necessary for alterations that might occur with this disease. Care for complications depends on the body organ or system affected (see elsewhere in the text).

Knowledge Deficit

Planning: client goals.   The goals for this nursing diagnosis are that the client will (1) be able to describe important aspects of diabetes care (capillary blood glucose and urine ketone monitoring, diet, exercise, stress management, and medications) that will help to safely attain and maintain normoglycemia and (2) implement self-care on the basis of this knowledge.

Interventions: nonsurgical management.   The nurse teaches the client about treatment measures that will become an important part of the individual's daily life style. Adequate education allows these daily tasks to become well integrated into the daily life style and facilitates self-management. The self-care of the person with diabetes can be complicated. Teaching these procedures should be made as simple as possible so that the client is not overwhelmed. Education is geared to different levels of learning (see the accompanying Health Promotion/Maintenance feature).

The following measures not only help the individual prevent hyperglycemia and hypoglycemia, but also give the individual a feeling of control over the disease, which in turn leads to a sense of well-being.

Capillary blood glucose monitoring.   Monitoring for elevated glucose levels in the body was for many years accomplished by daily urine testing at home, and blood glucose testing was done in the physician's office or the hospital. However, urine testing for glucose is more accurate for children than adults, and even for children urine testing is inaccurate because of variable renal thresholds and range of blood glucose values, which may give a negative urine test result. The major problem is the variability of the *renal threshold* (the point of glucose concentration at which the kidney excretes glucose in the urine). The normal renal threshold for adults is a plasma glucose level of 160 to 180 mg/dL (Marble et al., 1985), but some adults have plasma glucose levels of 250 to 300 mg/dL before glucose is noted in the urine. Moreover, the aging process or kidney damage causes the renal threshold to rise so that the test results correlate even more poorly with blood glucose values. The urine test results can also be altered by the amount of fluid ingested, timing errors, or medications taken for

HEALTH PROMOTION/MAINTENANCE ■ Levels of Diabetic Education

	Initial Education	Continuing Education
Definition	Provides the basic or initial "lifesaving" education for people with diabetes and their families	Provides in-depth education and counseling to assist people with diabetes and their families to incorporate diabetes into their life style and to control it
Content Areas		
Nutrition	Basic nutrition and meal planning, with an emphasis on a diet that is 55%–60% carbohydrate, 30% or less fat, and 12%–15% protein; low in salt, alcohol, and caffeine; and high in fiber	Nutritional management in relation to life style
Exercise	Guidelines for safe physical activity and for adjusting food and/or insulin intake	Individualization of exercise program
Medication	An understanding of insulin, how it works, how it is administered, where to buy it, and how to store it	Metabolic control of insulin and how to integrate insulin therapy into life style For diabetic persons taking oral hypoglycemic drugs: the doses, effects, and side effects of the drugs
Monitoring	Daily self-monitoring of glucose levels Blood glucose monitoring preferred, but teaching of how to test urine for ketones required	Test result interpretation and appropriate actions Relationship of glycosylated hemoglobin to diabetes management
Acute complications	Hypo- and hyperglycemia prevention, recognition, and treatment	What to do during illness
Psychosocial adjustment	Discussion by clients and families of the emotional impact of having diabetes	Specific problems such as compliance with treatment regimen or depression
Health habits	Care of feet, teeth, and skin Use of alcohol and tobacco Drug abuse Need for regular check-ups and eye examinations	
Long-term complications	Discussion of complications such as kidney disease and cardiovascular disease	
Community resources	Information about resources for special needs	
Benefits and use of health care system	Assistance for the client to acknowledge the need for planned care and continuing education	

Information compiled and modified from American Diabetes Association Task Group on Goals for Diabetic Education. (1989). *Goals for diabetic education* (pp. 1–26). Alexandria, VA: American Diabetes Association.

other purposes. Some tests are more accurate than others. Arguments exist about whether to use the first- or the second-voided urine test. The second-voided test result is closer to the actual blood glucose level at a particular time, but the first-voided urine test gives an indication of the glucose excreted in the urine over a period of time.

The introduction of the mechanically released lancing device for capillary blood glucose monitoring and the availability of visually or machine-read strips have revolutionized diabetes monitoring. Capillary blood glucose monitoring is now recommended for all people with diabetes mellitus. Through capillary blood glucose monitoring, individuals who are unsure about blood glucose control can easily master techniques of self-management. These techniques include consistent monitoring of blood glucose levels and using past blood glucose patterns to determine future needs, under the direction of the physician, of course.

There are a variety of test strips and easy-to-use machines available for blood glucose monitoring. The choice of testing device depends on the cost, ease of use, availability of service, and, most importantly, the client's ability to discriminate color changes. Hence, clients need to be assessed for color blindness. Supplies for blood glucose monitoring include a lancing device to pierce the finger, control solutions to check the testing techniques and the accuracy of the machine, and the machine itself. Third-party reimbursement is available for most people, because it is now recognized that capillary blood glucose monitoring is more cost effective than treating the complications of the disease. All tests have a time period that must be strictly followed. Machine-read strips give results in specific numbers, which may be influenced by the amount of blood on the strip, the calibration of the machine, or environmental conditions (presence of heat, cold, or moisture). Most machines display numbers, but others have voice readouts, memories that can be displayed, or capabilities for graphic displays on a computer.

Visually impaired clients have special needs. Some glucose monitors report blood glucose level by sound. Instruments in which one can put the test strip and place a finger to get a drop of blood on the test strip are also available. This allows visually impaired people to maintain independence by monitoring their own blood specimens.

Some machine procedures are easier to follow than others, but the accuracy of the machines is not significantly different. The nurse supplies the information on which the client can base a decision and instructs the client to choose a machine on the basis of cost, ease of use, availability of service, and ability to discriminate color. The accompanying Client/Family Education feature presents instructions for the use of a blood glucose monitor.

How frequently clients need to monitor capillary blood glucose varies. Those who require or depend on insulin may need to test as often as four times daily. Long-term control of diabetes mellitus is also being achieved by laboratory monitoring with glycosylated hemoglobin, fructose amine, or glycosylated serum protein tests administered by the physician. These test results indicate what the blood glucose levels have been over the previous 60 to 120 days (the life of a red blood cell). A well-managed client will have values of approximately 7% or less. Higher levels (8% to 12%) suggest poor compliance. An ambient plasma glucose level of 120 mg/dL is equivalent to an Hb A_{1c} value of approximately 6%, and a plasma glucose level of 250 mg/dL is reflected in an Hb A_{1c} value of 12%.

Urine testing for ketone bodies. Urine testing is recommended for identifying ketonuria. Nurses should teach people with type I and type II diabetes to test for ketones when their capillary blood glucose level is greater than 250 mg/dL, when they are ill or under prolonged emotional stress, or when they are initiating an exercise program. Individuals with type II diabetes might be unable to compensate in their insulin-making ability during these times. Detection sticks or tablets are available. The nurse instructs the client to report the presence of ketones in the urine (1) if ketones persist even with normal blood glucose levels or (2) if ketones in the urine are accompanied by hyperglycemia and do not respond to an intervention by a prescribed management protocol. Freshly voided urine should be used for testing for ketone bodies.

Diet therapy. A well-balanced meal plan must be determined for each individual, whether that individual has type I or type II diabetes. Individualized programs are based on usual dietary intake, weight/height ratios, cultural norms, and daily schedule. The fewer changes made in usual dietary habits, the more likely it is that the meal plan will be followed. Some clients can achieve diabetes control by diet alone.

Meal planning is perhaps the most important part of diabetes management. Although it is more difficult if an individual's schedule includes swing shifts or evening or night schedules, 24-hour management can be programmed for a variety of life styles.

The basic principles of meal planning include determining the person's activity pattern, finding out what is eaten and when, and coordinating activity and eating patterns with the time of medication administration and duration of action of the medication (if medication is necessary). Meals should be nutritious and composed of 55% to 60% carbohydrate, 12% to 15% protein, 30% or less fat, and vitamins and mineral content in accordance with the recommended dietary allowances (RDA). Meals should be free from concentrated sweets and should include a moderate amount of fiber. Ideally, daily food intake should be divided into three meals and a number of snacks. A bedtime snack is desirable to coordinate with the time action of the medication during the night.

The nurse, in collaboration with the physician and the dietitian, conducts the nutritional assessment and

CLIENT/FAMILY EDUCATION ■ How to Use a Blood Glucose Monitor

Instructions	Rationales
1. "Wash your hands in warm water."	1. Hands must be clean and warm to prevent infection and to facilitate getting a large drop of blood.
2. "Select the side of your finger pad as a puncture site."	2. It is usually less uncomfortable to pierce the side of the finger than the end of the finger.
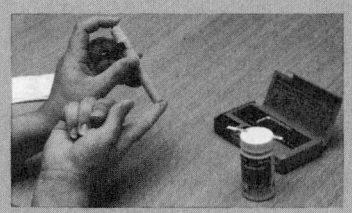	
3. "Hold your hand in a relaxed position to collect a drop of blood on the test strip."	3. It is easier to obtain a drop of blood if the finger is relaxed (this improves vasodilation).
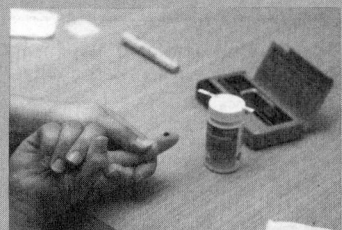	
4. "Start timing the procedure as soon as a drop of blood touches the test strip or as soon as the monitor beeps."	4. This achieves the most accurate chemical response of the blood on the test strip.
5. "At the time indicated, blot or wipe the test strip exactly as directed by the manufacturer."	5. The strip must be wiped or blotted exactly as the company directs when the monitor or elapsed time indicates. Alteration of this procedure affects the accuracy of the results.
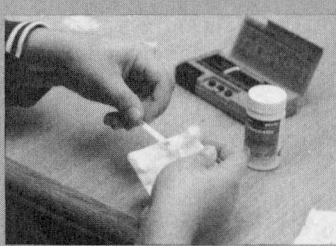	
6. "Insert the test strip into the monitor and note the blood glucose reading."	6. Note carefully if the machine's directions indicate a longer waiting period for higher blood glucose values. Variations in time also affect accuracy of the results.
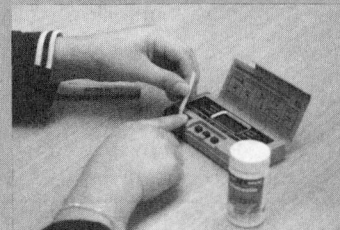	

Continued

CLIENT/FAMILY EDUCATION ■ How to Use a Blood Glucose Monitor (Continued)

Instructions	Rationales
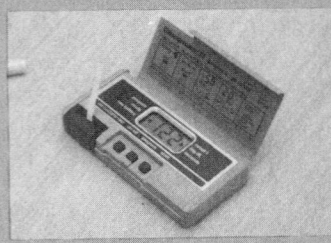 7. "Clean the monitor as directed by the manufacturer." 8. "Calibrate the monitor regularly as indicated by the manufacturer."	7. An uncleaned "window" of the machine affects the accuracy of the results. 8. Calibrate the machine as indicated (by the enclosed strip or the hard plastic strips and/or the glucose solutions) at the recommended times and frequency. This assists in maintaining the accuracy of the machine's functioning.

Note: Placement of the strip into the machine varies with the product. Some machines now require no blotting or wiping and have shorter countdowns. It is important that the procedure be done accurately, with a sufficient amount of blood, and with exact timing.

Photographs courtesy of Jonas McKoy, University of North Carolina at Chapel Hill School of Nursing.

HEALTH PROMOTION/MAINTENANCE ■ Exchange System of Diet Therapy

Food Group*	Food Content			Calories (kcal)	Examples of Equivalents
	Carbohydrate (g)	Protein (g)	Fat (g)		
Starch or bread	15	3	Trace	80	1 slice of bread, ½ bagel, ½ hamburger bun, ¾ c of cereal
Meat					
Lean		7	3	55	¼ c of cottage cheese, 1 oz of lean beef
Medium-fat		7	5	75	1 oz of ground beef, ¼ c of tuna
High-fat		7	8	100	1 tbsp of peanut butter, 1 oz of cheddar cheese, 1-oz hot dog
Vegetable, nonstarchy	5			2	½ c of carrots, tomatoes, asparagus, etc.
Fruit	15				1 apple, ½ banana, ½ grapefruit
Milk					
Skim	12	8	Trace	90	1 c of skim milk, 1 c of yogurt
Low-fat	12	8	5	120	
Whole	12	8	8	150	
Fat			5	45	1 tsp of butter or margarine, 1 strip bacon, 2 tbsp of salad dressing

* Clients can exchange foods within one group to obtain variety in food intake.

makes recommendations about specific dietary programs.

A variety of meal planning programs are available. The most common is the exchange system (see the Health Promotion/Maintenance feature on p. 1604). This system is based on six food groups (starch or bread, meat, vegetable, fruit, milk, and fat); the person is given a prescription for how many items from each food group are to be eaten at a meal or snack. Other programs are the point, constant carbohydrate, and total available glucose (TAG) systems. The point system is a program in which 75 kcal equals 1 point. After the individual's suggested caloric level and life style are determined, a point total is given to each meal or snack, representing part of the total day's needs. Determinations are made in line with RDA guidelines. Educational emphasis is on total nutrition, not just the points needed per meal or snack, so that appropriate choices of food can be made at the appropriate times (see the accompanying Health Promotion/Maintenance feature, below).

The client's ability to use any kind of list must be assessed. Too often, the person's lack of understanding or inability to comply may be overlooked, or clients are given the exchange lists or point totals without sufficient explanation of the reasons for the nutritional choices. The goal is to guide the ingestion of the correct number of calories, distributed throughout the day, to meet the needs of daily activity and to aid the person in maintaining normal blood glucose levels.

At times, the nurse will be asked about alcohol, the use of dietetic foods, and the use of artificial or low-calorie sweeteners. Moderate consumption of alcohol is permitted. The American Diabetes Association recommendations permit no more than two glassfuls of dry wine or equivalent amount of alcohol from other beverages per day. Metabolism of alcohol is not insulin dependent. Alcohol is utilized similarly to fat, and it prevents glycogenolysis (the process whereby glycogen is converted into glucose), which is especially needed at the time of hypoglycemia.

The nurse should relate that dietetic foods are more expensive, and fresh fruits and vegetables and other protein sources are more economical. The nurse also stresses that many of the dietetic foods may not have

HEALTH PROMOTION/MAINTENANCE ■ 1500-Calorie Meal Plan*

Meal	Exchange System	Point System	Examples
Breakfast	1 bread	1 point	Slice of toast
	1 fat	½ point	1 tsp of margarine
	1 meat	1 point	Egg (poached)
	1 fruit	1 point	Orange
	1 milk	1 point	1 c of skim milk
Snack	½ meat	½ point	½ slice (½ oz) of low-fat cheese
	1 bread	1 point	½ slice of bread
Lunch	2 breads	2 points	2 slices of bread
	1 meat	1 point	1 oz of chicken
	1 vegetable	½ point	½ c of green beans
	1 fat	½ point	1 tsp of mayonnaise
	1 fruit	1 point	1 apple
Snack	½ meat	½ point	⅙ c of cottage cheese
	1 bread	1 point	4 crackers
Supper	1 bread	1 point	½ c of potatoes
	2 meats	2 points	2 oz of lean meat
	2 vegetables	1 point	½ c of green beans
			½ c of spinach
	1 fruit	1 point	½ c of mixed fruit
	1 milk	1 point	1 c of skim milk
Snack	½ meat	½ point	½ oz of low-fat cheese
	1 milk	1 point	1 c of skim milk

* A sample 1500-kcal meal plan comparing the exchange system and the point system.

sugar, but may be higher in calories or fats than products containing sugar. Sweeteners should also be used in moderation. Testing by the Food and Drug Administration (FDA) has demonstrated that when sweeteners are used in moderate amounts, side effects are not considered a threat.

Concentrated sweets are discouraged because they are absorbed into the blood stream faster than insulin action allows glucose into the cell. The client should be encouraged to increase the intake of soluble fiber, such as in legumes, oats, and barley (to aid in decreasing the absorption of glucose); increase the intake of insoluble fiber, such as in wheat and corn bran (to increase stool bulk); decrease fat intake; and consider the choice and timing of protein intake—remembering that it is the most slowly absorbed food component.

The nurse helps the client plan the distribution of food intake to coordinate periods of greater activity with greater caloric intake of food or the peak action of the medication. For overweight people, the body is better able to digest smaller amounts of food, spaced throughout the day, than a large meal three times a day.

Exercise. Exercise is an important part of the management regimen. Ideally, an exercise prescription should be part of every management program. Regular exercise improves physical fitness, which may help to reduce the incidence of heart disease, stroke, and hypertension. It improves the efficiency of circulation and helps the client to reduce or maintain weight, as needed. During moderate exercise, glucose stored in muscles is used first, followed by glucose in the blood. Blood glucose levels remain low after exercise until the muscles replenish their glucose stores.

Before beginning an exercise program, the client should have a complete physical examination and ask the physician to help develop a safe exercise program. Assessment includes considerations of the time to do the exercise, the individual's cardiovascular and retinal status, and the individual's personal choice of exercise. After participation in such a program has been medically approved, the nurse directs the individual to choose one or more exercises on the basis of interest and capability.

Each individual should determine his/her target heart rate zone. This is the range of the number of pulse beats per minute that each person should use as a goal to reach while exercising. The nurse teaches the client how to ascertain a pulse rate correctly. The person should try to maintain a pulse rate between the upper and lower limits to reach the maximal aerobic benefit from exercise.

Target Heart Rate

Lower limit = 220 − age × 65%
Upper limit = 220 − age × 80%

It is also helpful to show clients a chart listing the target pulse rates according to age categories.

Aerobic exercises are continuous activities with the purpose of getting the heart rate into the target zone. Low-impact aerobics, walking, and swimming are considered the best choices. Usual activity burns off 2 kcal/minute; moderate activity burns off closer to 5 kcal/minute; heavy activity, such as cross-country skiing, has the potential to burn off 10 or more kcal/minute. For a nonathletic person, walking in place (at home), inside a shopping mall, or outside is the most frequently recommended exercise. If the individual has some problems with feet, legs, or back, swinging the arms while sitting in a chair can give some aerobic activity to the body.

The minimal exercise time recommended is 30 minutes three times a week or 20 minutes five or six times a week. The duration and frequency of exercise can be increased if the client desires. For weight loss, exercise must be extended to 45 minutes to 1 hour on a daily basis.

Exercise may be restricted for a person with retinopathy until the condition of the eyes is stabilized—and then, the head is not to be positioned lower than the heart in any of the exercises performed. Moreover, for clients with blood glucose levels higher than 250 mg/dL, exercise acts as a stressor, causing the blood glucose levels to become more elevated. Exercise is contraindicated for these clients. Similarly, if the client with type I diabetes has urinary ketones along with elevated blood glucose levels, exercise should be omitted and attention given to diabetes control (either contacting the physician or proceeding with a protocol to prevent diabetic ketoacidosis).

General instructions by the nurse should include telling the client to stop exercising and contact the health care provider if any pain is experienced, to warm up gradually and to cool down by continuing to move until the pulse rate has dropped to below 100 beats per minute, and, most importantly, to begin the exercise program gradually. The older the person is, the slower the person should start (beginning with 3 to 5 minutes the first few days, with gradual increases until the goal time is reached). Exercise should not be performed at the peak time of insulin actions, and the client should preferably exercise no sooner than 20 minutes to an hour after mealtime. The nurse ensures that the client is able to perform urine ketone testing. The nurse instructs the client to take a blood glucose measurement before, during, and 30 minutes after exercising or if the person has symptoms of hypoglycemia to help determine the effect of exercise on the body, especially when the client is beginning an exercise regimen. Insulin should not be administered in the extremity being exercised because the insulin will be absorbed much faster than normally in that extremity. Clients should be instructed to *always* carry simple sugar such as hard candy to take for symptomatic hypoglycemia and food for early signs and symptoms of hypoglycemia or during times of extra activity. The client should carry an emblem or card identifying himself/herself as diabetic and should exercise with a partner if possible. The client should wear comfortable shoes.

Stress management. Methods of dealing with stressors include exercise (low-impact aerobic activity), behavior conditioning and relaxation techniques, problem-solving skills, techniques learned in assertiveness training, and time management skills. Taking responsibility for one's thoughts and actions may also alleviate stress. Use of support systems and biofeedback are important in helping the client become better able to overcome obstacles and thus reduce stress to help control blood glucose levels. For more information on stress and its management, see Chapter 6.

Drug therapy. Medications are indicated when blood glucose levels can no longer be controlled by di-

TABLE 51-3   Oral Hypoglycemic Agents

Drug	Usual Daily Dosage	Mean Half Life (h)	Duration of Activity (h)	Interventions	Rationales
First-Generation Sulfonylureas					
Short Acting					
Tolbutamide (Orinase)	0.5–3.0 g in divided doses	7	6–12	1. Give 30 min before eating.*	1. To obtain best time action.
Intermediate Acting					
Acetohexamide (Dymelor)	0.25–1.5 g in single or divided doses	6	12–18	1. Use cautiously in elderly and clients with renal impairment.	1. To prevent hyperresponsiveness.
Tolazamide (Tolinase)	0.1–1.0 g in single or divided doses	7	12–24	1. Observe for GI upset, rash, photosensitivity, and hypoglycemia.*	1. To detect side effects.
Long Acting					
Chlorpropamide (Diabinese)	0.1–0.75 g in single dose	35	24–72	1. Instruct the client to avoid alcohol ingestion.	1. To prevent disulfiram (Antabuse) effects: headache, nausea, and sweating.
				2. Use cautiously in elderly and clients with renal impairment.	2. To prevent hyperresponsiveness.
Second-Generation Sulfonylureas					
Intermediate Acting					
Glipizide (Glucotrol)	2.5–40.0 mg in single or divided doses	4	12–24	1. Administer 30 min before eating.	1. To decrease postprandial hyperglycemia.
Glyburide (DiaBeta, Micronase)	1.25–20.0 mg in single or divided doses	10	16–24	1. Give with breakfast or first meal.	1. To avoid GI upset.

* Intervention should be done for all oral hypoglycemic agents.

etary measures, exercise, and stress management. Oral hypoglycemic agents are given if the disease cannot be controlled by diet. If these drugs are not effective, insulin is administered.

Oral hypoglycemic agents. Oral hypoglycemic agents (sulfonylurea drugs) help to lower blood glucose levels (Table 51–3). All of the hypoglycemic agents are believed to enhance insulin secretion. They are also thought to enhance the number or sensitivity of the receptor sites on the cell for its interaction with insulin and may have postreceptor effects.

The nurse first informs the client of the purpose and side effects of these drugs (see Table 51–3). The client should be reminded that oral hypoglycemic agents should not be considered a cure, but a biochemical means to enhance the use of insulin in the body. The nurse emphasizes that clients must adhere to dietary and exercise protocols, along with taking the medication. Clients should be alerted that certain drugs prolong or enhance the effects of oral hypoglycemic agents and can cause hypoglycemia or hyperglycemia. The use of nonprescription (over-the-counter) drugs should be avoided unless approved by the physician. Table 51–4 lists drugs that affect blood glucose levels.

The nurse educates the client about self-administration and observes for possible side effects, including gastrointestinal (GI) symptoms, hypoglycemia, and rashes. A disulfiram (Antabuse) reaction (flushed sensation, nausea, and perspiration) occurs in individuals ingesting alcohol while taking chlorpropamide. In extremely rare cases, oral hypoglycemic agents may have hematologic effects on bone marrow. Chlorpropamide, along with tolbutamide, has also been known to have an indirect effect on antidiuretic hormone secretion. The nurse reports any problems in kidney function or a history of kidney problems; if a positive history of kidney disease is determined, chlorpropamide and acetohexamide are discontinued or not considered drugs of choice. Their use might result in prolonged hypoglycemia, especially if renal shutdown occurs.

Insulin. Exogenous insulin is necessary for the management of type I diabetes and for some type II disease when glucose control by other means (diet, exercise, stress management, and oral hypoglycemic agents) fails or during periods of extreme stress (illness or surgery).

Table 51–5 lists the characteristics of the types of insulin available. The therapeutic duration of action of insulin varies, as shown in Table 51–5. In addition, the effectiveness of insulin action depends on the absorption by the individual person. Factors affecting absorption include injection site (abdominal area is best), whether the client has taken a hot shower (increases absorption), whether the muscle area is exercised (increases absorption), the blood glucose level, whether the client is dehydrated (delays absorption), and whether the client is cold (delays absorption). Thus, it is extremely important that nurses educate clients to accurately monitor and record their blood glucose test results so that the appropriate insulin type and schedule of administration can be used.

TABLE 51–4 Drugs That Affect Blood Glucose Levels

Drugs That Increase the Metabolism of Oral Hypoglycemic Agents

Digitoxin

Drugs That Decrease the Effects of Oral Hypoglycemic Agents

Beta-adrenergic blocking agents

Diazoxide

Drugs That Increase the Risk of Hypoglycemia

Chloramphenicol

Clofibrate

Dicumarol

Fenfluramine hydrochloride

Insulin

Isoniazid

Monamine oxidase inhibitors

Nonsteroidal anti-inflammatory agents

Oxyphenbutazone

Probenecid

Sulfonamides

Drugs That Increase the Risk of Hyperglycemia

Calcium channel blockers

Corticosteroids

Estrogen

Nicotinic acid

Oral contraceptives

Phenothiazides

Phenytoin

Sympathomimetics

Thiazides and diuretics

Thyroid products

Insulin treatments of people with diabetes vary. The decision to divide the insulin into multiple doses per day is made if the client experiences midafternoon hypoglycemia and early morning hyperglycemia, if the individual is having difficulty maintaining normoglycemia, or if the client simply desires greater flexibility in life style. Decisions to divide the insulin and administer it in doses proportionate to individual needs are based on laboratory data, self-monitoring of blood glucose levels, and observations often contributed by nurses.

The nurse teaches clients about the use of various

TABLE 51–5   Insulin Preparations

Type	Source	Therapeutic Effect			Pharmacologic Duration (h)
		Onset (h)	Peak (h)	Duration (h)	
Short Acting					
Regular (Insulin Injection)					
Iletin II R	Pork (purified)	½	2–4	4–6	6–8
Iletin II R	Beef (purified)	½	2–4	4–6	6–8
Iletin I R	Beef/pork mix	½	2–4	4–6	6–8
Humulin R	DNA biosynthetic	½	2–3	3–6	4–6
Humulin BR*	DNA biosynthetic	½	2–3	3–6	4–6
Velosulin	Pork (purified)	½	2–3	4–6	6–8
Velosulin Human	Semisynthetic	½	1–3	3–6	4–6
Regular	Pork (purified)	½–1	2½–5	4–6	6–8
Novolin R	Human	½–1	2–4	3–6	4–6
Semilente (Prompt Insulin Zinc Suspension)					
Iletin I S	Beef/pork mix	1–2	3–8	8–10	16
Iletin S/H	Human	1–2	3–8	8–10	16
Semilente	Beef	½–1	5–10	8–10	16
Intermediate Acting					
NPH (Isophane Insulin Suspension)					
Iletin II N	Beef or pork	1–2	6–12	12–14	20–24
Iletin I N	Beef/pork mix	1–2	6–12	12–14	20–24
Humulin	DNA biosynthetic	1–2	6–12	10–12	16–20
Insulatard NPH	Pork	1–2	6–12	12–14	20–24
Insulatard NPH/H	Semisynthetic	1–2	4–10	10–12	16–20
NPH	Beef	1–1½	6–12	12–14	20–24
Novolin N	Human	1–2	4–10	10–12	14–18
Lente (Insulin Zinc Suspension)					
Iletin II L	Pork (purified)	1–3	6–12	14–16	20–24
Iletin I L	Beef/pork mix	1–3	6–12	14–16	20–24
Iletin II L/H	Human	1–3	4–12	12–18	16–20
Lente	Beef	1–2	8 + 2	14–16	24+
Novolin L	Human	2½	4–12	12–18	16–20
NPH and Regular Insulin Premixed Insulins					
Mixtard (30% R/70% N)†	Pork (purified)/ human mix	½+	2–4/8±	6–8/12–14	8+/18–24
Novolin Mix 30% R/70% N		½+	2–4/8±	6–8/12–14	8+/18–24

Table continued on following page

TABLE 51–5 Insulin Preparations *Continued*

Type	Source	Therapeutic Effect			Pharmacologic Duration (h)
		Onset (h)	Peak (h)	Duration (h)	
Long Acting					
Ultralente (Extended Insulin Zinc Suspension)					
Iletin I U	Beef/pork mix	4–6	Minimal	24–36	24–36
Iletin II U/H	Human	4–6	Minimal	18–20	20–30
Ultralente	Beef	4–6	Minimal	24–36	24–36
Humulin Ultralente	Human	4	Minimal	18–20	20–30
PZI (Protamine Zinc Insulin Suspension)					
Protamine, zinc, and Iletin II (pork)	Pork (purified)	4–6	Minimal	36–72	24–36
Protamine, zinc, and Iletin II (beef)	Beef (purified)	4–6	Minimal	36–72	24–36
Protamine, zinc, and Iletin I	Pork/beef mix	4–6	Minimal	36–72	24–36

* Available in a buffered form for pump use only.
† Initard 50% R/50% N is being evaluated by the FDA.

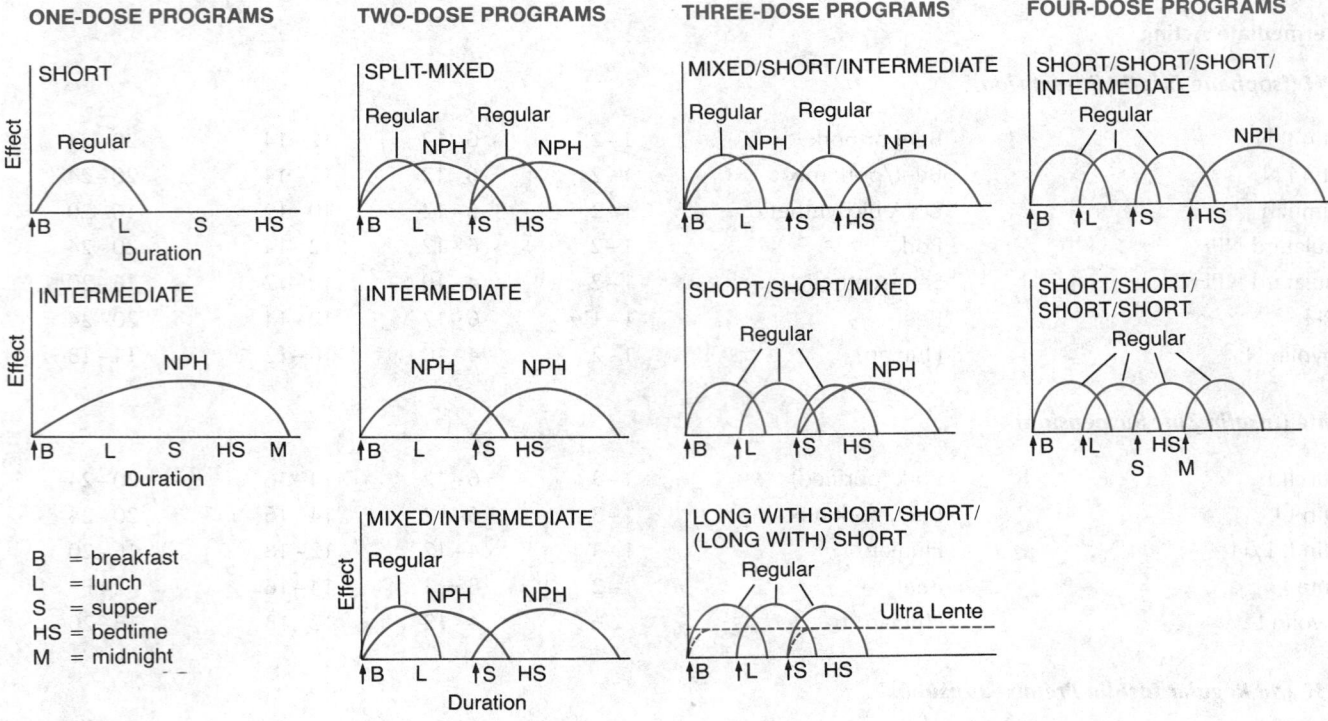

Figure 51–5

Insulin regimens. One injection a day of short-acting or intermediate-acting insulin may be enough to control blood glucose levels. However, split doses (two, three, or four injections of the daily dose) or split mixed doses (a mixture of short- and longer-acting insulins) may give better control.

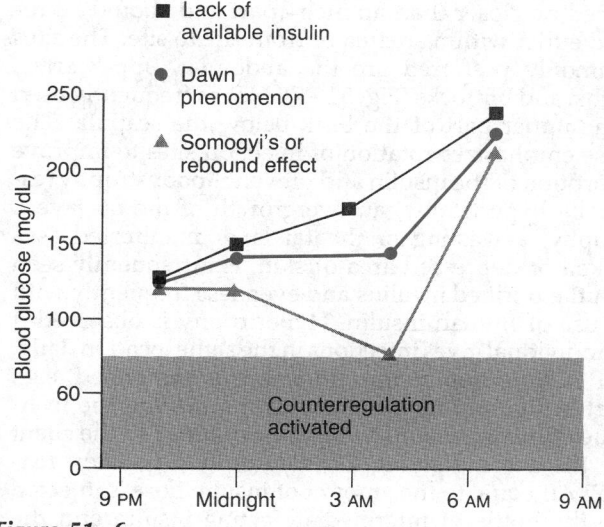

Legend:
- ■ Lack of available insulin
- ● Dawn phenomenon
- ▲ Somogyi's or rebound effect

Figure 51–6

Three blood glucose phenomena seen in diabetic clients.

insulin management programs, as well as the program prescribed by the physician. There are several alternatives (such as variations in the use of mixtures of insulin or the use of combinations of short-acting, intermediate-acting, and/or long-acting insulins) that should be described and explained (Fig. 51–5).

Multidose programs have become much more popular since the advent of self-monitoring of blood glucose levels. The mixed/short/intermediate three-dose program—i.e., mixture before breakfast, short-acting insulin before supper, and intermediate-acting insulin before bedtime—has proved effective.

Since the advent of self-monitored blood tests, three phenomena have been noticed to occur in blood glucose levels (Fig. 51–6). There may be a lack of insulin to cover blood glucose needs during the night; the "dawn phenomenon" might occur, with early morning rises in blood glucose levels between 4 and 6 AM caused by growth hormone secretions; and the Somogyi or rebound effect can occur when there is an imbalance of food, diabetes medication, and activity, with a physio-

---

GUIDELINES ■ Subcutaneous Insulin Administration

Interventions*	Rationales
1. Wash your hands.	1. Washing minimizes the spread of bacteria.
2. Inspect the bottle for the type of insulin and expiration date.	2. One must ascertain that the correct drug is being used and that it is not out of date.
3. Roll the bottle of insulin between the palms of your hands.	3. The insulin should be mixed and at room temperature.
4. Wipe the top of the bottle with an alcohol swab.	4. The bottle top should be clean to prevent contamination of the needle and the insulin.
5. Remove the needle cover and pull back the plunger to draw air into the syringe. The amount of air should equal the insulin dose. Put the needle in the bottle and inject the air.	5. This makes it easier to withdraw insulin.
6. Turn the bottle and syringe upside down in one hand and draw up the insulin dose into the syringe.	6. Inverting the bottle facilitates drawing up the drug into the syringe.
7. Remove air bubbles in the syringe by tapping on syringe or injecting insulin back into the bottle; redraw the correct amount.	7. Presence of air bubbles prevents injection of the full dose.
8. Remove the needle from the bottle and select a site for injection (one that has not been used in the past month).	8. Sites need to be rotated to ensure proper absorption of insulin.
9. Clean the site with an alcohol swab. Pinch up the area of skin, and insert the needle at a 90-degree angle. Push the needle all the way in and inject the insulin.	9. The tip of the needle should reach the fatty tissue layer.
10. After insulin is injected, pull the needle straight out quickly.	10. Discomfort is minimized.
11. Dispose of the syringe and needle without recapping in a puncture-proof container (plastic, metal, or heavy cardboard).	11. Contamination from used needles is prevented.

* These interventions may be implemented by the nurse, the client, or a family member or friend.

logic response to hypoglycemia resulting in secretion of counterregulatory hormones that cause a rapid elevation of blood glucose levels.

A nighttime lack of insulin or the dawn phenomenon usually necessitates the administration of more insulin earlier in the evening or at bedtime. With Somogyi's phenomenon, contrary to what the blood glucose finding is on awakening, less insulin should be given the evening before or more food eaten at bedtime.

A simple way to rule out the Somogyi phenomenon is for the nurse, in consultation with the physician or in accordance with medical protocol, to educate the client to increase food intake at bedtime. If Somogyi's response is present, the morning blood glucose levels will be lower rather than higher. Another way to determine if there is a lack of insulin, a dawn phenomenon, or Somogyi's response would be to obtain and record blood glucose levels between 1 and 3 AM.

Insulin must be administered by injection because it is inactivated by gastric juices. Methods of insulin administration have become varied, but subcutaneous (SC) injection by needle and syringe is still the most common method (see the Guidelines feature on p. 1611).

Insulin requires special storage. If the vial of insulin has been opened, it may be kept at room temperature for 3 months, unless drug package information states that refrigeration is needed. All *unopened* insulin should be refrigerated.

The nurse or the client is taught to insert the needle into areas of subcutaneous tissue. Injections should be spaced no closer than an inch apart and should be rotated either within an area or from site to site. The sites commonly preferred are the abdomen, upper arms, thighs, and buttocks (Fig. 51–7). Not as frequently used is the upper part of the back below the scapula. The nurse emphasizes rotation of injection sites to improve absorption of the insulin and prevent lipodystrophy (especially hypertrophy, an overgrowth of the fat layer). Atrophy, a wasting of the fat layer manifested as a sunken or depressed area of skin, is infrequently seen with the purified insulins and even less frequently with the use of human insulin. Hypertrophy is observed if the individual gives injections in the same location daily.

If SC injection of mixed insulins is prescribed, e.g., short-acting and intermediate-acting insulin, the technique of mixing insulins must be explained to the client (see the accompanying Client/Family Education feature). Air equal to the amount of insulin dose is injected into the bottle of intermediate-acting insulin and the short-acting type. The amount of short-acting insulin is withdrawn from the bottle first to avoid contamination with intermediate-acting insulin, which would render it unreliable for use in emergency situations, such as DKA. After the short-acting insulin is in the syringe, the intermediate-acting insulin can be withdrawn from its bottle.

Insulin infusion pumps are at present the most sophisticated way of administering insulin (Fig. 51–8). The machine automatically administers a small amount of insulin or a dose infused at the basal rate (often equal to about half of the 24-hour total) every few seconds. Automatically or with manual activation, depending on

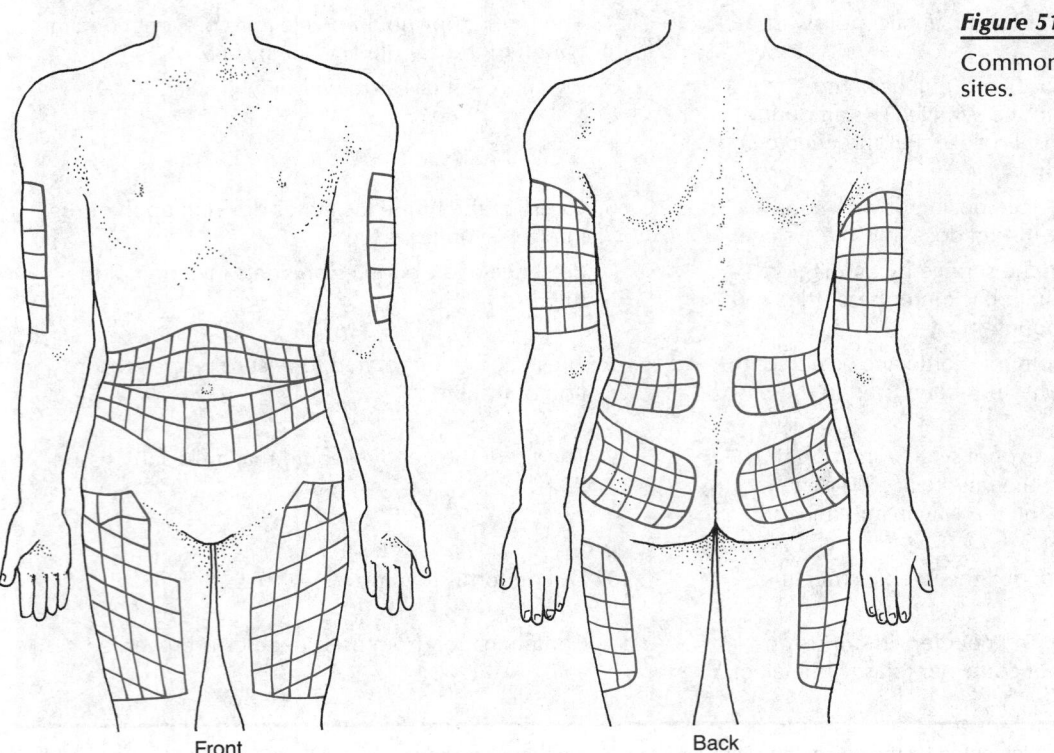

Figure 51–7

Common insulin injection sites.

Front

Back

CLIENT/FAMILY EDUCATION ■ **How to Mix a Prescribed Dose of 10 Units of Regular Insulin and 20 Units of NPH Insulin**

1. "Inject 20 units of air into the NPH insulin suspension bottle. The amount of air injected is equal to the dose of insulin desired. Always inject air into the longer-acting insulin first."

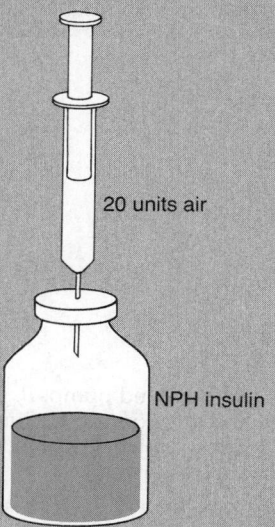

20 units air

NPH insulin

2. "Inject 10 units of air into the regular insulin. The amount of air injected is equal to the dose of insulin desired."

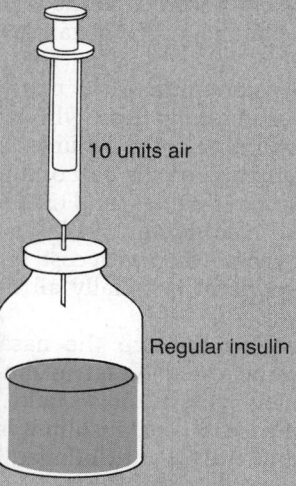

10 units air

Regular insulin

3. "Withdraw 10 units of regular insulin. Be sure that it is free from bubbles. Always withdraw the shorter-acting insulin first."

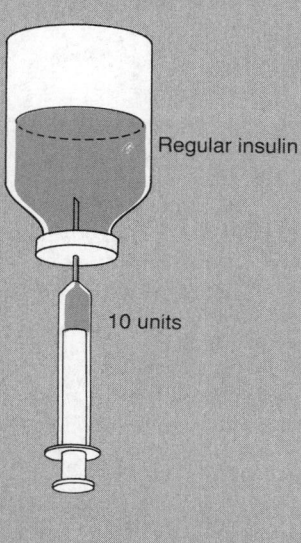

Regular insulin

10 units

4. "Withdraw 20 units of NPH insulin with the same syringe, being careful not to inject any short-acting insulin into the bottle (a total of 30 units is now in the syringe)."

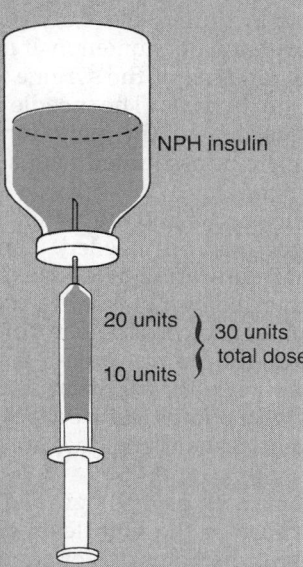

NPH insulin

20 units
10 units
} 30 units total dose

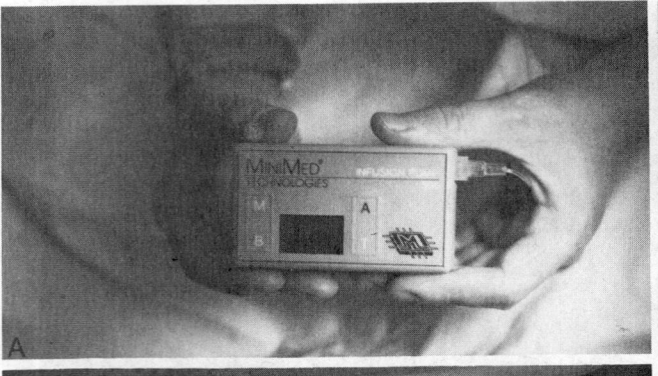

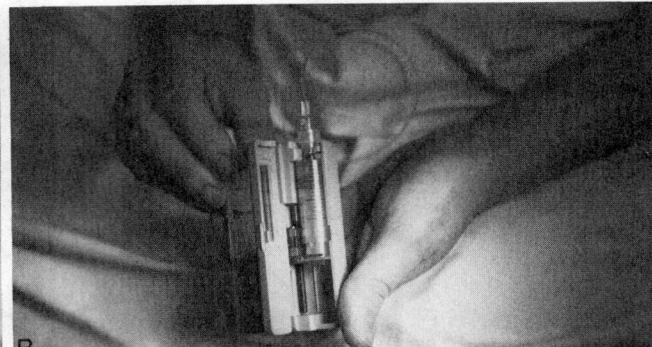

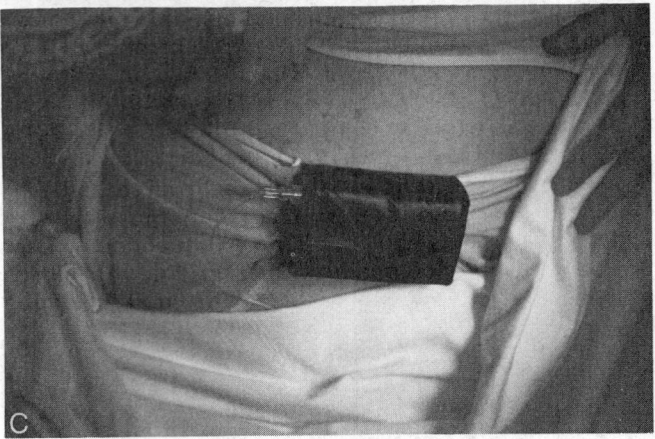

Figure 51–8

Insulin infusion pump. *A,* The MiniMed pump. *B,* Components of the pump-syringe and infusion set. *C,* Pump in place. (Courtesy of Jonas McKoy, University of North Carolina at Chapel Hill School of Nursing.)

the wishes of the wearer of the machine, bolus doses are injected by activating a pre-entered program or pressing a button before any large food intake (e.g., at meals) or for supplements of insulin when elevated blood glucose levels are determined (e.g., during illness). Some machines can be programmed to automatically give an increased amount of insulin during the early morning hours for coverage of the dawn phenomenon, if needed. The insulin container is replaced or the syringe is filled and replaced every 1 to 3 days. The needle site is changed every 1 to 3 days. (Use of the pump for longer periods in one site seems to be associated with a higher incidence of skin infection.)

Each night, the insulin supply and the battery should be checked and changes made as needed. The nurse instructs the client that showering is allowed if the pump is thoroughly protected by a plastic bag and tape. Sexual activity, swimming, and contact sports often necessitate the removal of the pump, unless it can be placed or protected in such a manner that it and the needle are not injured. Most pumps feature a lock mechanism, so that inadvertent mishandling does not change the pump program.

Screening of the client, both psychologic and procedural, is necessary because of the high level of client participation required and the potential for administering an excessive dose of insulin at one time. The use of insulin pumps necessitates more frequent self-monitoring of glucose levels (several times daily). This ensures that the proper amount of insulin is being administered because the tight blood glucose control achieved with an insulin pump makes the symptoms of hypoglycemia more difficult to recognize. Hypoglycemia can result when the pump tubing becomes kinked, halting the flow of insulin to the body, and DKA can develop rapidly.

Although the infusion pump has many benefits, educating and supporting the person who is using this machine is time-consuming for the nurse. Use of the pump requires participation on the part of the person in education plus the motivation to spend time learning to use the machine and also money ($4,000). Insurance reimbursement helps somewhat with cost, but, at most, partial third-party payment is usually all that can be expected.

Insulin administration through the nasal mucous membranes is now being tested. Nasal insulin is self-administered immediately before food intake. Unfortunately, the detergent base of nasal insulin is irritating to the nasal mucosa, and the amount inhaled cannot be verified. These problems must be resolved before nasal insulin is approved for routine use.

Implantable insulin pumps—another experimental alternative for insulin delivery—are implanted surgically, usually in the peritoneal cavity, where insulin can be absorbed in a manner similar to normal absorption from the pancreas. These pumps are programmed to release specific amounts of insulin at specific times in

NURSING RESEARCH

Implanted Insulin Pumps May Contribute to a Client's Sense of Well-being.

Meize-Grochowski, A. R. (1989). Experiences with diabetes mellitus and implantable insulin pump therapy: A summary of interview data. *The Diabetes Educator, 15*, 50–55.

Few studies on the use of the insulin pump have looked at the psychologic or social effects of its use. This qualitative study used a semistructured interview to examine the concerns of diabetic clients about their diagnosis and their feelings about using the pump. Twenty-three subjects in the United States and Europe participated in the study.

Concerns about having diabetes most often cited were related to fear of the unknown, especially the development of complications in the future. Present concerns were related to the development of hypoglycemia. Most subjects desired to use the pump to gain better control of their diabetes. Most thought that its use had minimal effects on their social life and expressed feelings of well-being.

Critique. The results of this study are not generalizable because of the small sample size and the investigational nature of the pump when this study was conducted. Cultural and physiologic variations of subjects were not examined in detail.

Possible nursing implications. Nurses can use information from this study concerning client feelings about using the pump to counsel clients considering its use. Nurses can also develop other research studies to determine what exactly enhances client feelings of well-being—use of the pump, increased knowledge of diabetes, or increased sense of control.

response to readings by the pump's glucose sensor. Preoperative and postoperative nursing care must be as meticulous as for any surgical procedure. If the pump is working adequately, blood glucose level documentation, carefully monitored by the nurse, will indicate no need for additional exogenous injections of insulin, except for refilling the pump's reservoir every 2 to 4 weeks. Unfortunately, researchers working with the implantable pump have thus far been unable to overcome the body's "walling off" of the implanted glucose sensor, so external blood glucose testing is still needed.

A third experimental means of insulin delivery, the artificial pancreas, is a computerized glucose monitor and controller. This large machine is programmed to administer insulin or glucose (in an amount depending on the weight of the client, the lumen size of the tubing, and the desired ranges of blood glucose levels) through plastic tubing and a flexible needle. It has been found useful during surgery, labor and delivery, and dialysis procedures and for some management problems. Its availability is limited at this time.

Interventions: surgical management

Pancreas transplants. Pancreas transplants are reasonably successful, although rejection remains a problem. Transplants are classified as segmental (from living donors) or whole pancreas (from cadavers). Transplants result in normalization of blood glucose levels and some reversal of previous pathologic changes. Pancreas transplants are usually carried out in conjunction with a kidney transplant, especially because most of this work is still experimental.

Potential for Infection

Planning: client goals. The goal for this diagnosis is that the client will remain free from infection.

Interventions: nonsurgical management. Diabetic clients have an increased potential for infection if the blood glucose levels are elevated above normal levels. Hyperglycemia leads to decreased phagocytosis, decreased fibroblast activity, and an increase in platelet adhesiveness.

Any infection could lead to elevated blood glucose levels. Dental disease and skin infections, especially of the feet and toes, are more likely to occur if hyperglycemia exists. The nurse encourages daily hygiene measures, including flossing of teeth, bathing, and inspecting the skin for breakdown. The goal is to prevent complications, such as ulcers or gangrene. The nurse encourages early treatment of complications and routine preventive visits (every 6 months for dental examinations, once a year for ophthalmic examinations, and once a year for total physical assessment). This routine can prevent problems and enable early detection of disease.

Sensory/Perceptual Alterations

Planning: client goals. The goals for this nursing diagnosis are that the client will (1) compensate for sensory loss and (2) prevent injury related to sensory loss.

Interventions: nonsurgical management. The diabetic client may feel altered sensation, pain, or numbness in the foot or hand. These changes can have serious consequences because the client is unable to feel normal warning signs of excessive cold or heat or of trauma. The accompanying Client/Family Education feature gives instructions for foot care.

Ineffective Individual Coping; Ineffective Family Coping

Planning: client goals. The goal is that the client and the family will develop effective coping mechanisms.

Interventions: nonsurgical management. Chronic illness and its treatment stress the family and an individual to the limits. Developing effective coping mecha-

CLIENT/FAMILY EDUCATION ■ Instructions for Foot Care

"Inspect your feet daily. Report any cuts, blisters, and other signs of injury or infection to your health care provider."

"Keep your feet clean, dry, and protected from injury."

"Bathe your feet in warm—not hot—water, and do *not* soak your feet, because soaking will dry them out."

"Cut your toenails straight across; have ingrown toenails, calluses, or corns treated by a podiatrist."

"Wear properly fitting shoes and cotton socks when walking; never walk barefoot."

"Use warm blankets or socks to warm your feet; do not use a heating pad or hot water bottle."

"Use lubricating cream or lotion for dry feet; use powder if your feet are moist."

"Elevate your feet one or two times a day to aid circulation."

nisms aids the individual to attain and maintain health to enhance quality of life. Without good coping mechanisms, the individual would not be able to consistently take prescribed medications, eat properly, exercise, practice good hygiene measures, or seek resources to assist with psychologic adjustment, if needed.

Organization is an important coping mechanism needed for self-care of persons with diabetes. Clients are taught methods of placing supplies, medicine, and the meal plan in conspicuous places to remind the person to follow the prescribed program. Keeping exercise clothes at the bedside reminds the person with diabetes, when returning home from school or work, that it is time to work out. Another coping mechanism might be taking 5 minutes a day to "regroup" (e.g., sit back in a chair and relax, thinking about positive things that had occurred that day or pleasant thoughts that would assist in allowing both the mind and body to become relaxed).

Learning to become appropriately assertive is another coping mechanism, and future planning helps put the disease and its treatment in perspective to life's goals. The nurse asks the client to list goals and state how to get what one wants out of life without injuring others in the process. Clients are also asked to list their strengths and weaknesses. The client should be assisted to say things in an efficient way, get the things done that need to be done, and explain disturbing feelings.

The nurse also instructs the person in time management. This assists in scheduling activities so that deadlines do not become stressful situations and sleep is not lost because of fear of failure. Other helpful activities include keeping a log of the relaxation periods and perceptions before and after the relaxation session. Reviewing problem-solving strategies demonstrated by

the nurse aids the person in improving her/his problem-solving skills. These activities and others are helpful in increasing the coping mechanisms in one's life and thereby decreasing the stressors, which, if allowed to go unharnessed, lead to an elevation of blood glucose levels.

When the diagnosis is initially learned, it often causes great disruption in the daily schedule and dynamics among family members, such as spouse, siblings, and even extended family members living under the same roof. Some family members may become so focused on the person with diabetes that other family members feel neglected or they disregard their own needs. This intense focus on the "sick person" might be a distraction from other family problems or needs, but ultimately creates further problems.

It is a good idea to encourage a prearranged family time when all family members come together and spend about 30 minutes each week discussing concerns and communicating with each other. The purpose of getting the family members together is to allow discussion of feelings about diabetes and its effect on the family, to coordinate family interaction, and to enhance communication.

Increased family communication may be the best deterrent to potential depression. When inadequate or disturbed family relationships are identified, nurse referrals to a family therapist or other counselor may be appropriate.

Altered Nutrition: More Than Body Requirements; Altered Nutrition: Less Than Body Requirements

Planning: client goals. The goal for these diagnoses is that the client will attain the ideal body weight while meeting the caloric demands of activity.

Interventions: nonsurgical management. Too much or too little insulin may lead to weight gain or weight loss. Poor self-perception may lead to decreased eating or increased eating. Frustration with lack of control of blood glucose levels may also lead to either of these responses.

Dietary intake that is *more than body requirements* may be caused by a previously obese state, may be self-induced, or may be stimulated by imbalance between body needs and medication levels. To reverse this phenomenon, the nurse supports the client as the physician directs the gradual decreasing rather than increasing of insulin administration. Some individuals, after noticing the higher blood glucose levels, might go ahead and eat what they want and try to purge themselves later to keep the blood glucose level down. This binging and purging behavior is detrimental, and control may be difficult to attain unless the person is willing to modify this behavior and alter eating patterns. Weight loss procedures may also be needed. Fad diets and trendy approaches to quick weight loss should be discouraged in those with diabetes.

Weight loss is encouraged for many individuals with type II diabetes. A standard decrease in caloric intake is 500 kcal less than the daily caloric need, or 10 to 15 kcal/kg for women and 15 to 20 kcal/kg for men (see the accompanying Guidelines feature to learn how to calculate caloric needs). Basic behavior modification and aerobic exercise (e.g., walking) complete the program. The goal is a loss of 0.5 lb to not more than 2 lb of weight per week. If the weight loss is more than 2 lb per week, the caloric intake should be increased so that such a limit may be realized.

Nutrition that is *less than body requirements* may be more evident before the actual diagnosis of type I diabetes. During the replenishment phase (i.e., replacing nutritional stores relative to the body's needs for height, weight, and activity), the first few days after the initial diagnosis and treatment of diabetic ketoacidosis, a greater number of calories are required. The person's appetite should be the guide. After replenishment has been completed and caloric requirements have stabilized, daily levels of intake are determined.

In adolescents and adults, observing food intake could become an obsession to the point that a person's self-perception might be altered. An excessive attention to food intake could even lead to the development of eating disorders, e.g., anorexia nervosa. The nurse counsels people to consider their meal plan as a guide and to become so familiar with it that choices are automatic. As a result, the mind is not constantly centered on food. Family members should be cautioned not to nag about food intake and to provide a nonstressful environment at mealtimes. The potential for either bulimia or anorexia nervosa is increased when the person feels unable to control hyperglycemia or to control environmental stressors. If the person does become anorexic or bulimic, the nurse directs him/her to appropriate resources (see Chap. 46 for further information on eating disorders).

The nurse assists the client in determining both short- and long-term goals. This helps the client feel more in control and increases chances of success. Gradually increasing or decreasing weight as needed, along with participating in exercise programs, aids in preventing complications related to food intake.

Sexual Dysfunction

Planning: client goals.   The goal for this diagnosis is that the client will maintan or achieve a desired level of sexual functioning.

GUIDELINES ■ How to Calculate Caloric Needs*

Procedure	Example
Method 1†	
For Women	
	In a normally active, small-framed, 5 ft 4 in, postmenopausal woman, the calculation is as follows:
1. Start by assuming 100 lb of body weight for the first 5 ft of height.	1. 100 lb
2. Add 5 lb for each inch above 5 ft, or subtract 5 lb for each inch below 5 ft.	2. + (4 × 5) = 120 lb
3. To account for body frame, add 10% of the total in step 2 for a large frame, or subtract 10% for a small frame to arrive at *estimated body weight*.	3. − (120 − 10%) = 108 lb
4. To determine *basic caloric need*, multiply the estimated body weight from step 3 by 10.	4. × 10 = 1080 kcal
5. To account for activity level	
a. Add 3 kcal/lb of estimated body weight to basic caloric need for an inactive woman.	
b. Add 5 kcal/lb of estimated body weight to basic caloric need for a normally active woman.	5. + (108 × 5) = 1620 kcal
c. Add 8–10 kcal/lb of estimated body weight to basic caloric need for a very active woman.	
6. To account for menopausal status, subtract 25% from the total in step 5 for a postmenopausal woman.	6. − (1620 × 25%) = 1215 kcal

Continued

GUIDELINES ■ How to Calculate Caloric Needs* *Continued*

Procedure	Example
For Men	In a very active, large-framed, 5 ft 11 in man, the calculation is as follows:
1. Start by assuming 106 lb of body weight for the first 5 ft of height.	1. 106 lb
2. Add 6 lb for each inch above 5 ft, or subtract 6 lb for each inch below 5 ft.	2. $+ (11 \times 6) = 172$ lb
3. To account for body frame, add 10% of the total in step 2 for a large frame, or subtract 10% for a small frame to arrive at *estimated body weight.*	3. $+ (172 + 10\%) = 189.2$ lb
4. To determine *basic caloric need,* multiply the estimated body weight from step 3 by 10.	4. $\times 10 = 1892$ kcal
5. To account for activity level	
a. Add 3 kcal/lb of estimated body weight to basic caloric need for an inactive man.	
b. Add 5 kcal/lb of estimated body weight to basic caloric need for a normally active man.	
c. Add 8–10 kcal/lb of estmated body weight to basic caloric need for a very active man.	5. $+ (9 \times 189.2) = 3594.8$ kcal
Method 2‡	In a normally active, 120-lb adult, the calculation is as follows:
1. Convert body weight from pounds to kilograms by multiplying by 0.45.	1. $120 \times 0.45 = 54$ kg
2. To determine *caloric need,* multiply weight in kilograms by 30 for a normally active person, by 35–40 for a very active person, or by 25 for an inactive person.	2. $\times 30 = 1620$ kcal

* These methods are a starting point. Caloric needs should be fine-tuned to account for individual variations.
† This method can be used when the client's height is known, but weight is not.
‡ This less precise method can be used when the client's weight is known.

Interventions: nonsurgical management. The nurse responds to questions concerning sexuality in an objective manner and knows when to refer the client to other resources. The misinformed client often becomes sexually dysfunctional because of increased anxiety about sexual performance. The nurse includes various aspects of human sexuality as part of the total health care education program.

The nurse takes a sexual history using an assessment tool (see Chap. 10). The questions should identify whether sexual dysfunction is present and its type. The nurse asks if the client is orgasmic and if intercourse is painful. The nurse asks male clients if retrograde ejaculation has occurred (the urine is cloudy without burning after sexual activity) or if an erection is attained and maintained. If the male client has heard that impotence is associated with diabetes, he might naturally assume that he will become impotent. The anxiety about this concern could lead to sexual dysfunction.

Possible alteration of the autonomic nervous system, indirectly related to glycemic control, may actually lead to physiologically based sexual dysfunction. If the process is directly related to diabetes, the incidence in males should be the same as in females. However, there is a higher incidence of sexual dysfunction in males (50%, in the form of impotence) than in females (35%). Sexual dysfunction in males includes nonpsychogenic impotence, retrograde ejaculation, and inability to maintain an erection. Females experience difficulty in vaginal lubrication during stimulation and reduction in the frequency of orgasm. The statistics reveal that 50% of impotence is psychologic and the other 50% is physiologic.

Screening for sexual dysfunction in males can be accomplished to differentiate between psychologic and physiologic dysfunction (Chap. 10).

If physiologic dysfunction is still suspected, a tumescence study may be performed. For this test, the hospitalized individual has electrodes placed on the penis and the readings are obtained while the individual sleeps. If the results are abnormal, the client is given choices of interventions. One method involves the insertion of a rigid, semirigid, or inflatable penile prosthesis. Another technique requires the use of a vacuum-evacuated test tube (Vacutainer). After blood has been pulled into the corpus cavernosum penis by the vacuum pump, a tight Velcro cuff is placed at the base of the penis, preventing the return flow. Another intervention is the injection of papaverine hydrochloride, a vasoactive drug, into the corpus cavernosum penis. This is a self-injecting procedure that requires 10 minutes for response and lasts 50 to 60 minutes. If a surgical implant is considered, the decision should be made by the client and the sexual partner. Postsurgical counseling by the nurse assists in the adjustment of the couple. (Chapter 55 includes nursing interventions and information regarding penile implants.) Clients often choose the option of learning alternative methods of achieving sexual satisfaction.

■ Discharge Planning

Both the person with diabetes and the family members have much learning and adjusting to do. Although only limited education and accommodation occur in the hospital, the initial introduction influences the further learning and adjustment that takes place at home and later.

The nurse encourages the client to follow the guidelines for optimal physical and mental health. These guidelines include (1) take time daily for self-examination, both physically and mentally; (2) make and keep routine appointments: dentist every 6 months, ophthalmologist once a year, family physician for a full physical once a year, and specialists every 3 months, unless problems indicate otherwise; (3) observe the timing, amount, and content of food intake; (4) have an adequate intake of fluid; (5) exercise routinely; (6) follow medication regimen, if medication is prescribed; and (7) take time to relax and enjoy one's self. The nurse recommends that the person have a method of self-evaluation at least once a month that would indicate whether stress levels have increased or health care practices have diminished.

Home Care Preparation

Before the client is discharged from the hospital, the nurse must help the client plan to obtain supplies needed immediately, including the prescribed medication and equipment for taking the medication and monitoring blood glucose levels. Some hospitals do not allow clients to take home unused equipment or medication,

so arrangements must be made for the client to obtain these and continue the program without interruption after discharge from the hospital. Clients should be instructed to purchase equipment or medication similar to that used in the hospital to avoid confusion. Other teaching should include where and how to obtain supplies, where to place the supplies in the home, a schedule for the use of supplies, and the disposal of used supplies.

Adequate predischarge preparation makes the return home safer. The nurse discusses the daily schedule to be followed at home. This assists the physician in fine-tuning the medical regimen to fit the person's life style. The nurse also indicates to the person that return to normal activity is possible. The concept to support is that a person can have diabetes mellitus and still be "healthy."

Providing information about resource people is important. It is essential for the person to know whom to contact in case of emergency and to identify and educate another person to administer the glucagon. Guidance is given to family members to assist them in taking supporting rather than controlling roles. The nurse also gives guidance in appropriate meal planning and special instructions for carrying extra food and supplies whenever extra activity, such as family outings, sexual activity, and travel, is involved.

Any diabetic client, but especially the elderly person living alone, needs some special home care preparation. A neighbor contact should be established, and someone should telephone the client daily, especially during the first few weeks at home. During the early adjustment period, there is a greater possibility of hypoglycemia. During this period of psychologic and physical adjustment, arrangements need to be made to assist the individual who lives alone. If the individual is impaired by retinal surgery or an amputation, living quarters should be cleared of things that could easily be knocked over or cause the individual to fall or be injured.

Client/Family Education

The teaching plan includes much information and should be broken down into segments of basic or initial education and in-depth continuing education. Clients should receive information about meal planning, taking medications (what to take and when), monitoring care, recognizing untoward symptoms (and when to call the health care provider), and controlling the diabetes during illness (see the accompanying Client/Family Education feature). Some guidance should be given regarding returning home and to the community (see the earlier discussion of interventions for knowledge deficit). The nurse stresses the importance of regular follow-up with appropriate specialists.

Monitoring self-care is a must. Recording the results of blood glucose and urinary ketone tests is crucial, as these indicate whether changes are needed for the normalization of blood glucose levels. Clients need to be reminded to take their records of dietary intake, daily exercise routine, medication regimen (amount of drug

CLIENT/FAMILY EDUCATION ■ Instructions for Sick Days

"When you are ill, you need to take extra care to control your diabetes by these measures:

"Notifying your doctor.

"Taking your medication even if you do not feel like eating.

"Monitoring your blood glucose at least every 2 h.

"Testing for ketones in your urine if your serum glucose levels are greater than 250 mg/dL.

"Drinking an adequate amount of fluids—about 8 oz each hour.

"Drinking clear liquids, fruit juices, or regular soft drinks to replace carbohydrate in your diet when you cannot eat your usual meals.

"Treating your symptoms (e.g., diarrhea, nausea, vomiting, and fever) as directed by your physician or diabetes educator.

"Resting."

and number of times taken), and blood glucose monitoring results (and ketone testing results) with them when visiting the physician. Analysis of records can help the physician make judgments about changes in the type of medication and its strength or dosage.

Recognizing untoward signs and symptoms, along with record-keeping, can assist in decision-making. The nurse ascertains whether the client can differentiate between hyperglycemia and hypoglycemia (see earlier). If the person does not learn to respond to the warning signs or symptoms, there is a greater possibility that a diabetic emergency will occur.

Preparation for returning to the home and the community includes proper education for adequate hygiene measures and instructions regarding exercise, job training, and rehabilitation. The listing of daily hygiene measures might be posted on the bathroom mirror. Exercise time and location should be preplanned. The exercise prescription should include choices of exercise, target zone for pulse rate, a schedule for progression of exercise, and the duration of daily exercises to reach the weekly exercise time goal. The prescription should also include the symptoms and signs of too much or too intensive exercise. In most cases, there should be few restrictions, if any, on returning to a usual life style. Reintegrating into society and becoming physically active support the goals of medical and nursing management.

Psychosocial Preparation

Fear of actual or perceived loss is perhaps the first reaction of the individual with a diagnosis of diabetes. This fear may remain until the person recognizes that those with diabetes can maintain an active life style and

may even improve their general health. As the person recognizes and shares the learned health care information with her/his family, the whole family has the potential to become healthier.

Fear of loss becomes worse when complications occur. The nurse assists the client in developing plans for readjustment, even though this may be difficult.

Fear of having a severe insulin reaction and "making a fool of one's self," fear of being different, and fear of loss of control or self-concept disturbances are three of the greatest fears encountered in the person who has diabetes. Education helps to alleviate these fears.

Clients should be directed toward getting involved in their own care and controlling their diabetes. Clients can learn to identify situations that are stress-producing and can learn methods of stress management. Engaging in self-care can be a positive factor for many and can counteract the helplessness and disappointment initially felt on learning that they have a chronic disease. For many clients, this self-care is seen as a challenge and an opportunity to keep themselves healthy. For some, it becomes a challenge not to let the disease hinder them, and their own control of the disease and life style changes actually boost their self-esteem and make them feel more confident.

Health Care Resources

The community health nurse and the home care agency may play important roles in ongoing health maintenance or the immediate rehabilitation process. If there is any doubt about a person's home environment or the person's ability to use community resources, contact needs to be made with a community health nurse or a home care agency. The initial home visit determines whether information learned in the hospital setting has been translated correctly into the home setting. Further planning at this time may assist in the client's adjustment to the home and the community. The home care nurse assesses for complications that may require special services or resources, including vocational rehabilitation, services for the blind, or financial assistance.

The American Diabetes Association and the Juvenile Diabetes Foundation offer other services in addition to promoting public awareness and supporting research endeavors. The American Diabetes Association has literature and continuing education classes. Local diabetic organizations may offer support groups, camps, and other activities (e.g., hiking and skiing) that are supervised by health care professionals. Support groups provide interaction with others with the same disease and help the person not to feel alone. Continuing education is essential and is offered through diabetes centers, hospitals, clinics, and voluntary health associations (see Unit 14 Resources).

Evaluation

Achievement of expected outcomes is measured by attainment of the nursing goals or the goals designated by an individual program. The expected outcomes for the client with diabetes include that the client

1. States the overall goal for diabetes therapy
2. Describes the times for eating, the amounts of food to be eaten, and the choices that would be most conducive to achieving proper nutrition and normoglycemia
3. States the duration of action and side effects of the medication taken
4. Demonstrates the correct procedure for injection or insulin infusion pump
5. Demonstrates the correct procedure for testing the blood for glucose and the urine for ketones
6. Adheres to a process of record-keeping
7. Complies with an exercise regimen
8. Describes resources to assist with rehabilitation, if or when needed
9. Maintains or achieves the desired level of sexual functioning
10. Remains free from infections
11. Maintains daily practices of appropriate foot care

SUMMARY

Managing diabetes is not easy, and many factors are involved in achieving optimal blood glucose level control. The medical regimen needs to be one that gives 24 hours of glycemic coverage, but equally important is the nurse's role in educating the individual to follow through on the prescribed regimen in the safest manner. The goal is to integrate the regimen into the individual's life style so it becomes automatic and the person can resume normal living. Nurses must make sure that individuals with diabetes are familiar with how their activity level and daily care may affect blood glucose levels and to respond promptly to any warning signs and symptoms. They must be knowledgeable in giving supportive care in the hospital, offering education to prepare the person and the family for resumption of home and work routines, providing direction to varied resources in the community, and counseling to assist the person and the family in the emotional adjustment to a chronic, potentially life-threatening condition.

IMPLICATIONS FOR RESEARCH

Research is still needed to find a cure and prevention for this syndrome. More and more is being learned each year. Pancreas transplants or an implanted artificial pancreas with internal glucose sensors may be curative. Prevention may be accomplished by immunization or by genetic surgery. Although methods for educating clients, delivering insulin, monitoring, and record-keeping assist in preventing hypoglycemia and diabetic ketoacidosis, further improvements are needed. The challenge for the health care professionals is to motivate individuals, year after year, to take good care of themselves and sustain good health so they may benefit from new research findings when made available.

Nursing research should be directed to improve efforts and skills in education of participating individuals and their families. It should also be directed to determine ways to assist people to adjust to diabetes. Nurses should continue in their contributions to improved methods of delivering insulin, monitoring, record-keeping, and developing products for self-care. Ultimately, the nurse's goal is to find the best and safest methods to help people who have diabetes to stabilize blood glucose levels, blood pressure, fluid volume, and electrolyte balance, with limited side effects or complications, while maintaining quality of life.

Questions for further research include

1. Is piercing the skin perceived as less painful if the lance or needle is visualized or not visualized?
2. If supervised foot care is instituted in the hospital, is adherence to foot care at home improved?
3. Will the use of micro-needles and lack of dead space in the syringe influence the decision to draw up one or another insulin first in mixed administration?
4. Is education by one-to-one contact or by small group interaction better in assisting the client to adjust to the diagnosis of diabetes?
5. Does relaxation training, introduced early in the diabetes management program, assist a person to stabilize blood glucose levels even after counterregulatory hormone responses have become impaired?

REFERENCES AND READINGS

American Diabetes Association. (1986). *Third party reimbursement for people with diabetes mellitus.* Alexandria, VA: Author.

American Diabetes Association. (1987). *Direct and indirect cost in diabetes mellitus.* Alexandria, VA: Author.

American Diabetes Association. (1988). *Meeting the standards.* Alexandria, VA: Author.

American Diabetes Association Task Group on Goals for Diabetic Education. (1989). Goals for diabetic education (pp. 1–26). Alexandria, VA: American Diabetes Association.

Anderson, J. W., Story, L. J., Zettwock, N. C., Gustafson, N. J., & Jefferson, B. S. (1989). Metabolic effects of fructose supplementation in diabetic individuals. *Diabetes Care, 12,* 337–344.

Andreoli, T. E., Carpenter, C. C. J., Plum, F., & Smith, L. H.,

Jr. (1990). *Cecil essentials of medicine* (pp. 496–505). Philadelphia: W. B. Saunders.

Barmann, K. A. & Domas, M. E. (1989). A multidisciplinary approach: Assuring quality care of the diabetic client. *Journal of Nursing Quality Assurance, 3*(2), 19–25.

Bliss, M. (1982). *The discovery of insulin.* Chicago: University of Chicago Press.

Bookchin, R. M., & Gallop, P. M. (1968). Structure of hemoglobin A_{1c}. *Biochemical and Biophysical Research Communications, 32*, 86–93.

Broadstone, V. L., Cyrus, J., Pfeifer, M. A., & Greene, D. A. (1987). Diabetic peripheral neuropathy. Part I: Sensorimotor neuropathy. *The Diabetes Educator, 13*, 30–35.

Brown, S. A. (1988). Effects of educational interventions in diabetic care: Meta-analysis of findings. *Nursing Research, 37*, 223–230.

Cotran, R. S., Kumar, V., & Robbins, S. L. (1989). *Robbins' pathologic basis of disease* (4th ed.). Philadelphia: W. B. Saunders.

Davidson, M. B. (1986). *Diabetes mellitus: Diagnosis and treatment* (Vols. 1 & 2, 2nd ed.). New York: Wiley.

Diabetes in America, diabetes data compiled 1984 (DHEW Publication No. 85–1468). (1985). Washington, DC: U.S. Government Printing Office.

Drass, J. A., Muir-Nash, J., Boykin, P. C., Turek, S. M., & Baker, K. L. (1989). Perceived and actual level of knowledge of diabetes among nurses. *Diabetes Care, 12*, 351–356.

Dunning, D. (1989). Diabetes now—safe travel tips for the diabetic patient. *RN, 52*(4), 51–55.

Friedman, E. A., & Peterson, C. M. (1986). *Diabetic nephropathy: Strategy for therapy.* Boston: Martinus Nijhoff.

Gavin, J. F. (1988). Diabetes and exercise. *American Journal of Nursing, 88*, 178–180.

Gordon, E. E., & Kabadi, U. M. (1976). The hyperglycemic, hyperosmolar syndrome. *American Journal of the Medical Sciences, 271*, 252–268.

Guthrie, D. W., & Guthrie, R. A. (1986). Diabetes mellitus: An update. In D. A. Zschoche (Ed.), *Mosby's comprehensive review of critical care* (3rd ed., pp. 523–537). St. Louis: C. V. Mosby.

Guthrie, D. W., Guthrie, R. A., & Hinnen, D. (1976) Double voided and single voided specimens. *Diabetes Supplement, 25*, 335.

Hernandez, C. G. (1989). The pathophysiology of diabetes mellitus: An update. *The Diabetes Educator, 15*, 162–170.

Hoffman, R. G., Speelman, D. J., Hinnen, D. A., Conley, K. L., Guthrie, R. A., & Knapp, R. K. (1989). Changes in cortical function with acute hyperglycemia in type I diabetes. *Diabetes Care, 12*, 193–197.

Kopeski, L. M. (1989). Diabetes and bulimia. A deadly duo. *American Journal of Nursing, 89*, 482–485.

Kovacs, M., Feinberg, T. L., Paulauska, S., Finkelstein, R., Pollack, M., & Crouse-Novek, M. (1985). Initial coping responses and psychosocial characteristics of children with insulin dependent diabetes mellitus. *Journal of Pediatrics, 6*, 827–834.

Maillard, L. C. (1912). Action of amino acids on sugar formation. *Comptes Rendus Academy of Sciences, 164*, 66.

Marble, A., Krall, L. P., Bradley, R. F., Christlieb, A. R., & Soeldner, J. S. (1985). *Joslin's diabetes mellitus* (12th ed., p. 348). Philadelphia: Lea & Febiger.

Mazze, R. S., Lucido, D., & Shamoon, H. (1984). Psychological and social correlates of glycemic control. *Diabetes Care, 7*, 360–366.

National Commission on Diabetes. (1975). *Report of the National Commission on Diabetes to the Congress of the United States* (DHEW Publication No. 76–1019). Washington, DC: U.S. Government Printing Office.

National Diabetes Control Project. (1990). *The physical guide to nine complications of diabetes mellitus.* Atlanta, GA: Center for Diabetes Control.

National Diabetes Data Group. (1979). Classification and diagnosis of diabetes mellitus and other categories of glucose intolerance. *Diabetes, 28*, 1039–1057.

Papatheodorou, N. H. (1983). The psychosocial aspects of aging in diabetics [Special issue]. *The Diabetes Educator, 9*, 49–53.

Schneider, S. J. (1986). Exercise and physical training in the treatment of diabetes mellitus. *Comprehensive Therapy, 12*(1), 49–56.

Spiro, R. G., & Spiro, J. J. (1971). Effect of diabetes on the biosynthesis of the renal glomerular basement membrane: Studies on the glucosyltransferase. *Diabetes, 20*, 641.

Teza, S. L., Davis, W. K., & Hiss, R. G. (1988). Patient knowledge compared with national guidelines for diabetes care. *The Diabetes Educator, 14*, 207–211.

VanSon, A. (1982). *Diabetes and patient education: A daily nursing challenge.* New York: Appleton-Century-Crofts.

Wiles, P. G., Stickland, M. H., Birtwell, A. S., & Wales, J. K. (1988). Laboratory, nurse and patient assessment of Glucostix blood glucose reagent strips. *Diabetic Medicine, 5*, 791–794.

Winegrad A. L., & Greene, D. A. (1976). Diabetic polyneuropathy: The importance of insulin deficient hyperglycemia and alterations in myoinositol metabolism in its pathogenesis. *New England Journal of Medicine, 295*, 1416.

Wysocki, T., Huxtable, K., Linscheid, T. R., & Wayne, W. (1989). Adjustment to diabetes mellitus in preschoolers and their mothers. *Diabetes Care, 12*, 524–529.

Zagoria, R. B. (1982). Your right to work. *Diabetes Forecast, 35*(3), 20–23.

ADDITIONAL READINGS

Haire-Joshu, D., et al. (1986). Diabetes: Controlling the insulin balance. *American Journal of Nursing, 11*, 1239–1258.

Four articles were written about different aspects of diabetes management and care. One article compared type I and type II diabetes. The second article reviewed diabetes-related medications. Another article centered on intense insulin therapy. The last article discussed diabetes control.

Fox, M. A., Cassmeyer, V., Eaks, G. A., Hamera, E., O'Connell, K., & Knapp, T. (1984). Blood glucose self-monitoring usage and its influence on patients' perceptions of diabetes. *The Diabetes Educator, 12,* 27–31.

This is a descriptive study that reported on the assessment of a group of subjects to determine if blood glucose monitoring influenced their perception of their disease. Using the blood glucose monitors has been reported to make people more aware of their disease.

Guthrie, D. W., & Guthrie, R. A. (1991). *Nursing management of diabetes mellitus.* (3rd ed.). New York: Springer.

This text was designed for the undergraduate student and the hospital- or clinic-based nurse. It covers numerous topics that would be useful in a variety of client care settings. One chapter addresses the education process necessary to improve self-management techniques for the person who has diabetes.

Guthrie, D. W., Guthrie, R. A., & Walters, J. F. (1984). Dealing with diabetes. In *Endocrine disorders* (pp. 125–149). Springhouse, PA: Springhouse Corp.

A chart demonstrated the process of development of diabetic keto-acidosis. Nursing diagnoses were also included.

Guthrie, D. W., Hinnen, D. H., & DeShetler, E. (Eds.). (1988). *Diabetes education: A core curriculum for health professionals.* Chicago: American Association of Diabetes Educators.

A major guide to assist health care professionals to study about the education and care of the person with diabetes includes sentence outlines, study questions, one or two case studies, and recommendations for further study. Continuing education unit programs are being developed to accompany this curriculum guide.

Jackson, R. L., & Guthrie, R. A. (1986). *The physiological management of diabetes in children.* New York: Medical Examination.

Although the title refers to children, this program was opened to adults in the 1970s. What was working for children was effective in adults. This book contains considerable research to support the discussion on the "need for control." Dr. Jackson was one of the early pioneers in the field and was, early on, able to attain and maintain a high degree of controlled blood glucose levels in those individuals so treated.

Mecklenburg, R. S., Benson, E. A., Benson, J. W., Fredlund, P. N., Guinn, T., Metz, R. J., Nielsen, R. L., & Sannar, C. A. (1984). Acute complications associated with insulin infusion pump therapy: Report of experience with 161 patients. *JAMA, 252,* 3265–3269.

Diabetes control improved substantially, but 42% of the population experienced one or more acute complications (diabetic keto-acidosis or hypoglycemia). The article indicates that the infusion pump is helpful, but is not without problems.

Shichiri, M., Asakawa, J., Yamasaki, Y., Kawamori, R., & Abe, H. (1986). Telemetry glucose monitoring device with needle-type glucose sensor: A useful tool for blood glucose monitoring in diabetic individuals. *Diabetes Care, 9,* 298–301.

A sensor transmitter converts signals generated by a glucose sensor to audio signals in the process of continuously calculating the glucose concentrations in the subcutaneous tissues. This information is significant as this device is one step closer to either a portable external or an implanted internal unit combined with an insulin infusion pump that is complete with sensor, power, and insulin release.

UNIT 14 RESOURCES

Nursing Resources

American Association of Diabetes Educators, 500 North Michigan Avenue, Suite 1400, Chicago, IL 60611. Telephone 312-661-1700.

National Certification Board for Diabetes Educators, 500 North Michigan Avenue, Suite 1400, Chicago, IL 60611. Telephone 312-661-1700. Certifies nurses with experience in diabetic client education.

Other Resources

American Diabetes Association, National Service Center, 1660 Duke Street, Alexandria, VA 22314. Telephone 800-232-3472.

Human Growth Foundation, 7777 Leesburg Pike, Falls Church, VA 22043. Telephone 800-451-6434.

A support and education resource for clients with growth disorders.

International Diabetes Federation, 40 Washington Street, Brussels, Belgium 1050.

Joslin Diabetes Center, One Joslin Place, Boston, MA 02215. Telephone 617-732-2415.

Juvenile Diabetes Foundation International, 60 Madison Avenue, New York, NY 10010. Telephone 212-889-7577.

Little People Research Fund, 80 Sister Pierre Drive, Towson, MD 21204. Telephone 301-494-0055.

Turner's Syndrome Society, 3539 Tonka Road, Minnetonka, MN 55345. Telephone 612-938-3118.

UNIT 15

Problems of Reproduction: Management of Clients with Disruptions of the Reproductive System

CHAPTER 52

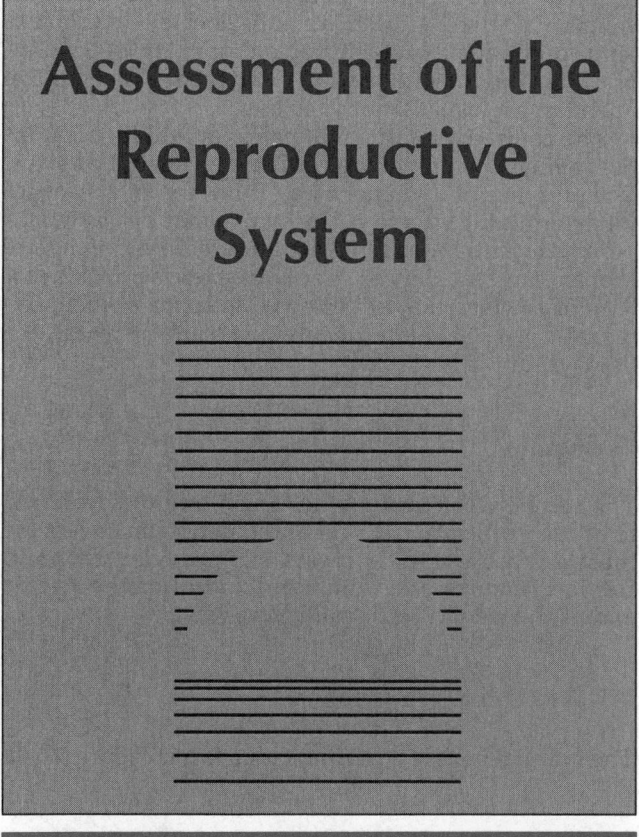

Assessment of the Reproductive System

The assessment of the male and female reproductive systems is an important component of health care. Reproduction and sexuality (discussed in Chap. 10) are becoming less difficult or less sensitive areas to be assessed as individuals become more comfortable discussing these subjects. Still, certain clients are hesitant and uncomfortable with talking about these topics and wait until symptoms are intolerable or disease is advanced before seeking health care.

In many instances, the nurse first collects assessment data from the client with a reproductive system disorder. Often, the nurse must convey confidentiality and respect before the client volunteers personal data. To be effective, the nurse must be comfortable with his or her own sexuality and be nonjudgmental of other variations in sexual practices.

This chapter provides a theoretical base for understanding the male and female reproductive systems as a foundation for nursing assessments.

ANATOMY AND PHYSIOLOGY REVIEW

FEMALE REPRODUCTIVE SYSTEM

Females begin to develop secondary sex characteristics at a wide range of ages. The average girl begins pubertal development at age 11 years. Normally, young girls exhibit the beginning of breast buds and pubic hair between 8 to 14 years of age. Development of secondary sex characteristics is completed in from 1.5 to 6 years. Delayed puberty may be due to a familial history of late growth; a low percentage of body fat; abnormalities of the pituitary, ovaries, or hypothalamus; congenital structural abnormalities; or chronic illnesses, such as diabetes mellitus and renal disease. Female sexual precocity is defined as the onset of puberty before age 8 years.

EXTERNAL GENITALIA

The region of the external female genitalia (Fig. 52–1), or *vulva*, is the area from the mons pubis to the anal opening.

Mons Pubis

The *mons pubis* is a fat pad that covers the symphysis pubis and protects it during coitus. The mons becomes prominent and covered with hair during puberty. Within an average of 3 years from the onset of puberty, the female has developed an adult, triangular distribution of coarse, curly hair that extends from the mons downward to the labia majora and inner thighs.

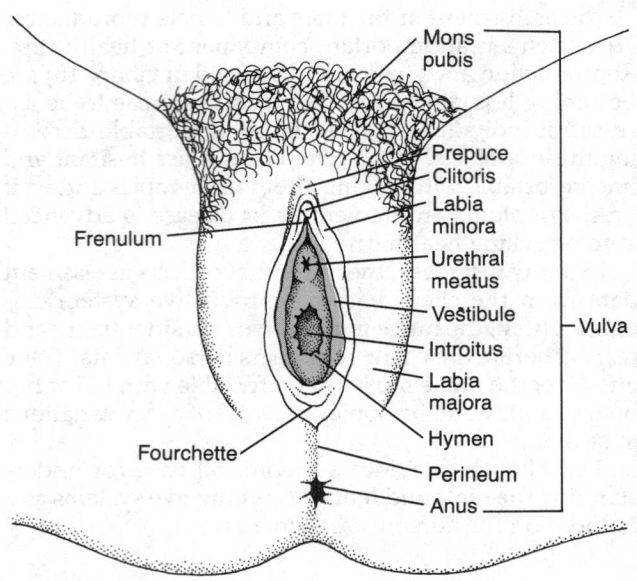

Figure 52–1

External female genitalia.

Labia Majora

The *labia majora* are two vertical folds of adipose tissue that extend posteriorly from the mons to the perineum. Because fatty tissue deposits vary among individuals, the size of the labia majora varies. The skin over the labia majora is usually darker than the surrounding skin and is highly vascular. The labia become prominent during puberty and develop hair on the outer surfaces. The labia majora protect inner vulval structures and enhance sensual arousal.

Labia Minora

The labia majora surround two thinner, vertical folds of reddish epithelium, the *labia minora*. The labia minora are highly vascular and have a rich nerve supply. Emotional or physical stimulation produces marked swelling and sensitivity. Numerous sebaceous glands in the labia minora lubricate the entrance to the vagina.

Each side of the anterior labia minora divides into two branches. The pairing of the outer branches forms the *prepuce* (hood of the clitoris), and the union of the inner branches forms the *frenulum*. Projecting through these branches is the *clitoris*, a small, cylindrical organ, which is homologous with the penis, that is composed of erectile tissue and a high concentration of sensory nerve endings. During sexual arousal, the clitoris becomes larger and increases sexual tension. The tissue formed at the merger of the posterior ends of the labia minora folds is called the *fourchette*.

Vestibule

The *vestibule* is a longitudinal fossa (a lower area) between the labia minora, clitoris, and fourchette. This area contains Bartholin's glands and the openings of the urethra, Skene's glands (paraurethral glands), and the vagina. The two Bartholin's glands, located deeply posterior on both sides of the vaginal opening, secrete lubrication fluid during sexual excitement. Their ductal openings are usually not visible.

The connective tissue that partly or wholly occludes the vaginal opening in the vestibule is called the *hymen*. The presence of hymenal tissue is not the sole measure for determining virginity. The hymen may be elastic and permit distention, or it may rupture before coitus. The hymen can tear during strenuous exercise, masturbation, or the insertion of tampons. In some women, hymenal tags remain after the hymen tears; in others, the tissue disappears.

Perineum

The area between the fourchette and the anus is referred to as the *perineum*. The skin of the perineum covers the muscles, fascia, and ligaments that provide support to pelvic structures and voluntary control of the vagina and of the urinary and anal sphincters.

INTERNAL GENITALIA

The internal female genitalia are shown in Figure 52–2.

Vagina

The *vagina* is a collapsible hollow tube extending from the vestibule to the uterus. In addition to being the channel for the passage of the menstrual flow, the vagina allows reception of the penis during intercourse and passage of the fetus during childbirth. The opening of the vagina in the vestibule is called the *introitus*. Squamous epithelium and abundant blood vessels line the thin, muscular walls of the vagina that are transversely rugate during the female's reproductive years and highly distensible. Normally, the anterior and posterior vaginal walls lie in contact with each other. There are few sensory nerve endings in the lower vaginal segment near the introitus, which allows the vagina to be relatively insensitive to distention.

The amounts of glycogen and lubricating fluid that are secreted by the vaginal epithelium are influenced by ovarian hormones. *Döderlein's bacilli*, the normal vaginal flora, interact with the secreted glycogen to produce lactic acid and maintain an acid pH (4.0 to 5.0) in the vagina. The acidity reduces the vagina's susceptibility to infection. Estrogen deprivation occurring during postpartum periods, lactation, and menopause causes the

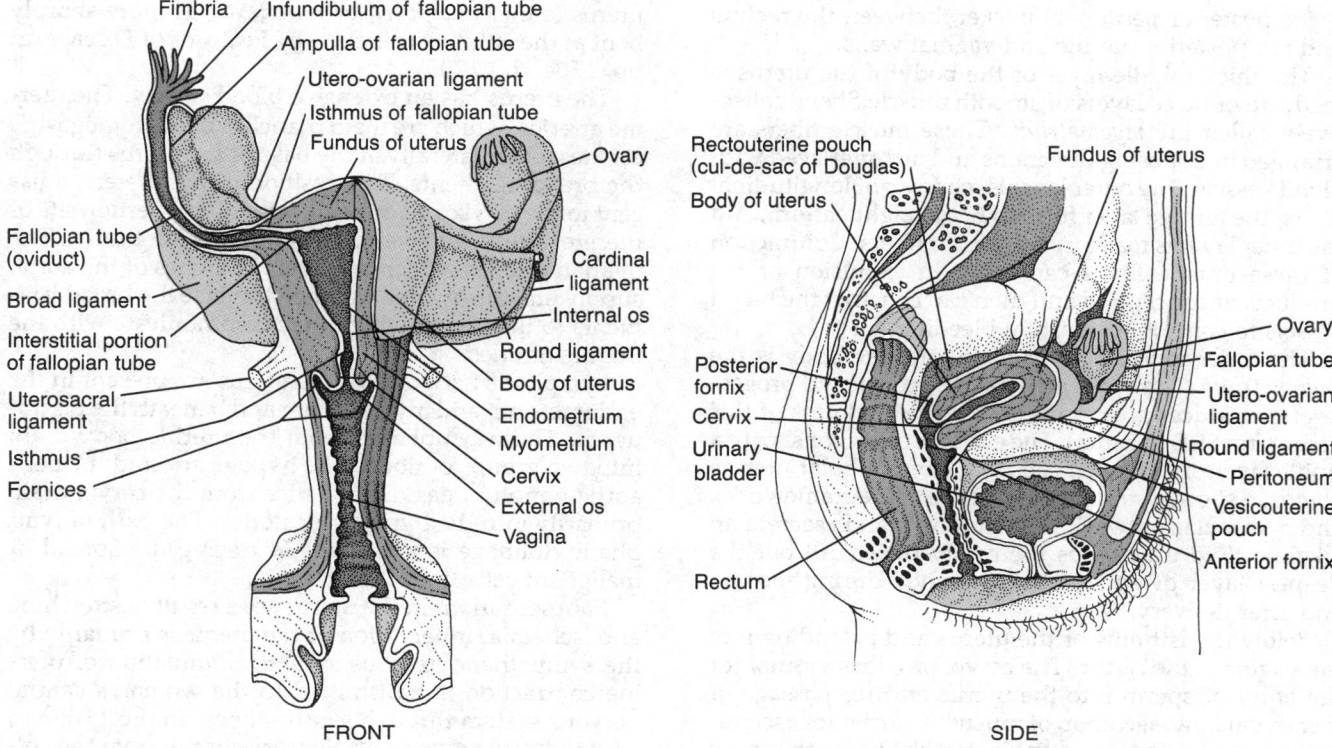

Fimbria
Infundibulum of fallopian tube
Ampulla of fallopian tube
Utero-ovarian ligament
Isthmus of fallopian tube
Fundus of uterus
Ovary
Fallopian tube (oviduct)
Broad ligament
Interstitial portion of fallopian tube
Uterosacral ligament
Isthmus
Fornices
Cardinal ligament
Internal os
Round ligament
Body of uterus
Endometrium
Myometrium
Cervix
External os
Vagina

FRONT

Rectouterine pouch (cul-de-sac of Douglas)
Body of uterus
Fundus of uterus
Posterior fornix
Cervix
Urinary bladder
Rectum
Ovary
Fallopian tube
Utero-ovarian ligament
Round ligament
Peritoneum
Vesicouterine pouch
Anterior fornix

SIDE

Figure 52–2

Internal female genitalia.

vaginal wall to become dry and thinner and the rugae to become smoother. When ovarian function resumes after a pregnancy, it promotes rethickening of the vaginal tissue.

Connective tissue forming the *vesicovaginal septum* separates the anterior wall of the vagina from the urethra and bladder. The posterior wall of the vagina is separated from the rectum by the *rectovaginal septum*. At the upper end of the vagina, the uterine cervix projects into a cup-shaped vault of thin vaginal tissue. This recessed pocket around the cervix, called the *fornix*, permits palpation of the internal pelvic organs. It is divided into four areas: anterior, posterior, and right and left fornices. The length of the vagina in the area of the posterior fornix (7 to 10 cm [about 2 to 3 in]) is approximately 2.5 cm (about 1 in) longer than that in the area of the anterior fornix. The posterior fornix is clinically significant because it provides access into the peritoneal cavity (through the cul-de-sac of Douglas) for diagnostic or surgical purposes.

Uterus

The *uterus* is a flat, thick-walled, muscular organ attached to the upper end of the vagina. In the nonpregnant woman, the inverted pear-shaped organ is located within the true pelvis, between the bladder and the rec-

tum. Functionally, the uterus responds to hormonal stimulation and prepares to receive, nurture, and finally expel the products of conception.

The size of the uterus depends on the woman's developmental stage and obstetric history. In a woman who has never been pregnant, the average uterine dimensions are $7.5 \times 5.0 \times 2.5$ cm ($3\frac{1}{2} \times 2 \times 1$ in). In a woman who has carried a fetus, the uterus may be larger.

Anatomically, the uterus is described as having two major sections, the *body* (or *corpus*) and the *cervix*. These two areas are separated by a constricted region called the *isthmus*. The upper segment of the uterine body, between the insertion sites of the fallopian tubes, is referred to as the *fundus*. Although the uterus is a hollow organ, its walls are in such close approximation in the nonpregnant state that its cavity is merely a slit. These walls are composed of three layers. The outer layer, the *peritoneum*, separates the uterus from the abdominal cavity. The peritoneum covers the anterior section of the uterus above the bladder and all of the posterior aspect of the uterus (except the portion of cervix extending into the vagina). The lateral uterine segments are the sites of attachment of the *broad ligaments*. The pouch that is formed by the peritoneum, where it lines the anterior uterus and reflects to the top of the bladder, is called the *vesicouterine pouch*. The *rectouterine pouch* (also referred to as the *cul-de-sac of Douglas* or the *posterior cul-de-sac*) is the posterior peritoneal pocket, between the rectum and the posterior uterine and vaginal walls.

The thick middle layer of the body of the uterus is made up of three layers of smooth muscle fibers, collectively called the *myometrium.* These muscle fibers are arranged in opposing directions and are interlaced with blood vessels. The outer layer is made up of longitudinal fibers, the middle layer forms a figure eight pattern, and the inner layer is made up of circular fibers. Contraction of these muscle fibers can result in expulsion of the products of conception and then can constrict the blood vessels to control postpartum bleeding.

The inner mucosal layer of the uterine body is the *endometrium.* The cyclic activity of estrogen and progesterone produces great variation in the thickness of this tissue (from 0.5 to 5 mm). The endometrium consists of a single layer of epithelial cells that cover tubular uterine glands, a spongy stroma (connective tissue framework), and a vascular network. The uterine glands secrete an alkaline fluid that keeps the cavity moist. All but the deepest layer of endometrium is shed during menses and after delivery.

Below the isthmus of the uterus and extending into the vagina is the *cervix.* The cervix provides a canal for the entry of sperm into the uterus and for passage of menstrual flow; secretion of mucus; a barrier for ascending vaginal bacteria; and sphincter-like fibers that hold the products of conception in the uterine cavity or that stretch to permit vaginal delivery.

The cervical portion of the uterus is approximately 2.5 cm (1 in) long. The upper boundary, the *internal os,* is approximately at the level where the peritoneal covering of the anterior uterus deflects over the bladder. The lower boundary, the *external os,* projects into the vaginal fornix. In the nonpregnant woman, the cervix around the external os is usually smooth, firm, and pink. A woman who has borne a child would have a small, transverse slit-like external os. The *endocervical canal* connects the internal os with the external os and provides access from the vagina to the uterine cavity.

The cervical tissue contains only about 10% muscle fibers. Its elastic ability comes from the predominance of collagen, blood vessels, and elastic tissue. The outer cervix is covered with a single flat layer of squamous epithelium. The mucosa of the cervical canal is a single layer of high, ciliated, columnar epithelium with numerous cervical glands. These glands secrete watery to tenacious mucus in response to the ovarian hormones. The *squamocolumnar junction,* where the two types of epithelial cells meet, is usually just inside the external cervical os. Neoplastic changes occur most frequently in the cells at this junction. Cells obtained by scraping the squamocolumnar junction are used in the Papanicolaou smear.

Most commonly, when a nonpregnant woman is standing, the axis of the uterus is tilted anteriorly *(anteverted),* with the body of the uterus resting on the bladder and the cervix directed toward the sacrum. Other nonpregnant women may demonstrate a uterus that is in the midposition or retroverted. A malpositioned

uterus, either *anteflexed* or *retroflexed,* is more sharply bent at the isthmus (see the Key Features of Disease on pp. 1704 and 1705).

The uterus has an extensive blood supply. The uterine arteries, which are main branches of the hypogastric arteries, enter laterally at the base of the uterus through the broad ligaments. The position of the ureters, adjacent to the cervix and crossing under the insertion site of uterine artery and vein, is important surgically. The ovarian arteries, which are direct branches of the aorta, supply first the ovaries and then traverse the broad ligaments to the uterus where they communicate with the uterine arteries.

Lymphatic networks of the uterus are present in the endometrium and myometrium and beneath the peritoneum. These lymphatics from the uterine body drain into two groups of nodes, the hypogastric and the periaortic lymph nodes. Lymphatics from the cervix drain primarily into the hypogastric nodes. The path of lymphatic drainage is important in tracing the spread of malignant cells from the uterus.

Pain sensations in the uterus are a result of stretching and ischemia. Innervation of the uterus is primarily by the sympathetic nervous system. Stimulation of uterine contraction is transmitted to the woman's central nervous system through sensory fibers in the 11th and 12th thoracic nerve roots. Sensory stimuli from the cervix and upper vagina pass through the pelvic nerves and are received at the second, third, and fourth sacral nerves.

The normal uterus is partially mobile in the pelvis, especially in the anteroposterior plane. The uterus is supported by ligaments and muscles of the pelvic floor. The *broad ligaments* attach to the lateral walls of the uterus, between the insertion of the fallopian tubes and the pelvic floor. Broad ligaments, i.e., folds of peritoneum, divide the pelvis into anterior and posterior cavities. The upper boundary consists of three folds that almost completely cover the fallopian tube, the round ligament, and the utero-ovarian ligament. The thick portion at the base of each broad ligament is also called the *cardinal ligament.*

The *round ligaments* extend outward on each side of the uterus and downward through the inguinal canal, and they terminate in the upper portion of the labia majora. They are a combination of connective tissue and smooth muscle.

The two *uterosacral ligaments* are composed of smooth muscle, connective tissue, and a peritoneal covering. They attach to either side of the posterior cervix and extend posteriorly, around the rectum, to the fascia over the second and third sacral vertebrae. These ligaments exert posterior traction on the cervix and hold the body of the uterus in its anterior position.

Fallopian Tubes

The *fallopian tubes,* or *oviducts,* insert into the upper lateral portion of the body of the uterus and extend laterally to a site near the ovaries. Functionally, the fallopian tubes provide a duct between the ovaries and the uterus for the passage of ova and sperm. Fertilization of the ovum most frequently occurs in the fallopian tubes.

Each tube, about 8 to 14 cm long (3⅛ to 5½ in), is covered by one of the peritoneal folds of the broad ligament. The tubes are made up of smooth muscle cells with a mucosal lining of ciliated and secretory columnar epithelial cells. The lining is arranged in longitudinal folds. Rhythmic contractions of the musculature of the tubes vary in response to the ovarian cycle. The tubal contractions and the current that is produced by the movement of the cilia transport the ovum to the uterus.

The fallopian tubes are divided into four anatomic sections: the *interstitial portion*, the *isthmus*, the *ampulla*, and the *infundibulum*. The interstitial portion is embedded in the uterine musculature and leads outward from the uterine cavity. Outside the body of the uterus is the isthmus, the narrow portion of the oviduct. The ampulla is a wider area that extends from the isthmus distally to the infundibulum. The infundibulum is a funnel-like expansion of the distal end of the tube. Fimbriated ends of the infundibulum open through the peritoneum into the abdominal cavity. One of the fringe-like fimbriae at the end of each fallopian tube is considerably longer than the others. This projection nears the ovary and facilitates capture of a released ovum.

Ovaries

The *ovaries* are a pair of almond-shaped organs, approximately 3 × 2 × 1 cm (1⅛ × ⅞ × ⅜ in), that are situated near the lateral walls of the upper pelvic cavity. The dimensions of the ovaries vary among women. After menopause, the ovaries are significantly smaller. Functionally, these small organs are responsible for the development and release of *ova* and for the production of at least four types of hormones: *estrogens, progesterone, androgens,* and *relaxin*. Adequate amounts of these steroidal sex hormones are necessary for normal female growth and development and for maintenance of a pregnancy.

In a female infant at the time of birth, about 2 million oocytes (immature ova) are found in undeveloped follicles of the ovaries. Significant oocyte degeneration occurs throughout the female's life span, so that by adulthood the surviving oocytes number in the thousands. Of these, only a small percentage are actually ovulated. During the reproductive years, selected ova mature and make their way to the surface of the ovaries. The cyclic maturation of a dominant follicle, the *graafian follicle,* and the release of the ovum are referred to as *ovulation* (see later).

The appearance of the ovaries varies with age. In the young woman, the surface of the ovary is a smooth, dull white. After follicles appear on the surface and rupture, scarring produces a roughened, pitted appearance.

Each ovary is attached to the uterus, just beneath the insertion of the fallopian tube, by the utero-ovarian ligament and the *mesovarium* portions of the broad ligament. The ovarian arteries, veins, and nerves reach the ovaries through these ligaments.

The ovary is not covered by the peritoneum, which allows an ovum to be released within the pelvic cavity and potentially retrieved by the fimbriated ends of the fallopian tubes. The ovarian body is composed of two layers: the inner layer, or *medulla,* and the outer portion, or *cortex.* Follicles and ova in various stages of development are contained in the cortex. As the follicles develop, the epithelial cells that surround the oocyte increase in number and begin to secrete fluid that accumulates in an enclosed cavity. Two layers of theca cells begin to form from the ovarian cells around the follicle. *Theca cells* line the follicles and are the principal site of production of the steroid *estrogen.*

Granulosa cells are an epithelial layer inside of the theca cells. Just before ovulation, this layer becomes quite vascular. After a mature follicle ruptures, a *corpus luteum* forms in the cavity. *Progesterone* is secreted by the corpus luteum in the postovulatory phase of the ovarian cycle.

MENSTRUATION AND MENOPAUSE

Normal Menstrual Cycle

Menstruation is the cyclic shedding of the endometrial lining of the uterus. The term *menarche* refers specifically to the female's first menstruation and is one sign of puberty. The average girl begins to menstruate between the ages of 12 and 13 years, with a normal range of between 10 to 16 years. A young girl's age at menarche correlates with that of her mother.

The occurrence of cyclic menstruation and of reproduction depends on maturation of the *hypothalamic-pituitary-ovarian-uterine axis*. Normally, this cycle is not achieved for the first 1 to 2 years after menarche. The first menstrual cycles are typically anovulatory and irregular.

The *menstrual cycle* is under a feedback control system of three interrelated cycles: the *hypothalamic-pituitary cycle*, the *ovarian cycle*, and the *uterine (or endometrial) cycle*. The relationship of these cycles is illustrated in Figure 52–3.

The idealized menstrual cycle is 28 days; however, 29- to 30-day cycles are more typical, and variations are normal. The first day of the menstrual cycle is calculated as the first day of monthly menstrual bleeding. The menstrual flow is referred to as the *menses*. Ovulation occurs approximately 14 days before the beginning of the next menstrual cycle. Regular menstrual cycles indicate normal sex hormone production and the occurrence of ovulation. Variations in the length of a woman's menstrual cycle occur in response to variations in the length of the preovulatory stage versus the postovulatory stage.

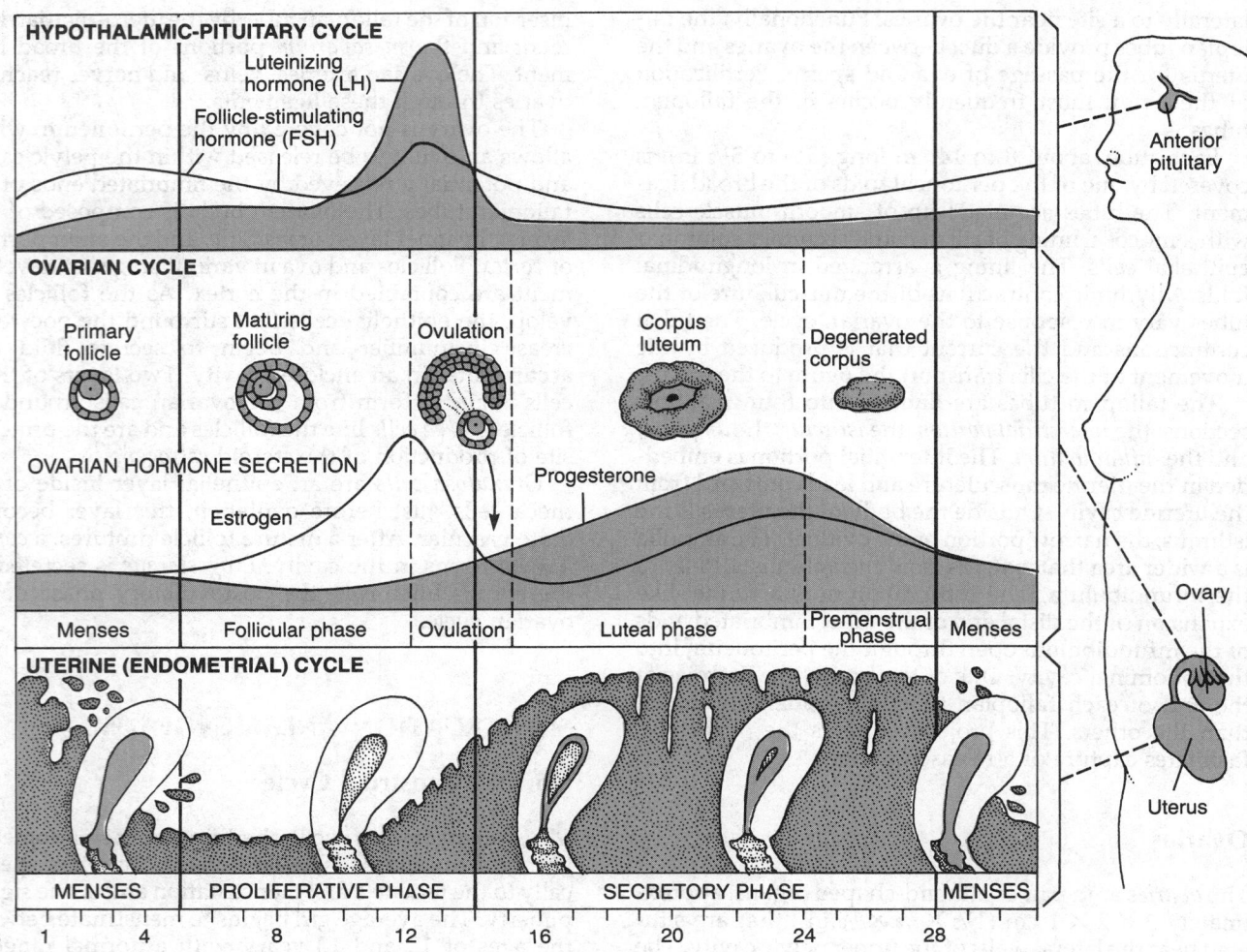

HYPOTHALAMIC-PITUITARY CYCLE

Luteinizing hormone (LH)

Follicle-stimulating hormone (FSH)

Anterior pituitary

OVARIAN CYCLE

Primary follicle | Maturing follicle | Ovulation | Corpus luteum | Degenerated corpus

OVARIAN HORMONE SECRETION

Estrogen

Progesterone

Ovary

Menses | Follicular phase | Ovulation | Luteal phase | Premenstrual phase | Menses

UTERINE (ENDOMETRIAL) CYCLE

Uterus

MENSES | PROLIFERATIVE PHASE | SECRETORY PHASE | MENSES

Days 1 4 8 12 16 20 24 28

Figure 52–3

Interrelationships of the events of the menstrual cycle.

Hypothalamic-Pituitary Cycle

The hypothalamus regulates the release of neurohormonal secretions in response to the blood levels of ovarian steroids. Low levels of estrogen and progesterone at the end of the menstrual cycle stimulate the hypothalamic release of *gonadotropin-releasing factor* and *prolactin-inhibiting factor*. In response to the neurohormones, the anterior pituitary gland releases *follicle-stimulating hormone* (FSH) and *luteinizing hormone* (LH). This release initiates the follicular stage of the menstrual cycle, corresponding to the growth of the graafian follicle and proliferation of the lining of the uterus.

Oral contraceptives act on the hypothalamus to inhibit the releasing factors and, therefore, inhibit ovulation and alter the endometrium. Numerous external factors, such as emotional stress, may also affect the hypothalamus and interfere with the monthly rhythm, which causes a period of *amenorrhea*, or absence of menstrual flow.

Ovarian Cycle

Day 1 of the menstrual cycle (concurrent with the onset of menses) is the first day of the *follicular, or pre-ovulatory, phase* of the ovarian cycle. At the beginning of this phase, the ovaries are under the influence of both FSH and a small amount of LH, which are released by the anterior pituitary into the blood stream. Initially, 20 follicles or more may begin to develop in the ovary, but typically only one will eventually mature and become the graafian follicle. Each of the developing follicles secretes estrogen, which enhances its own development. The dominant follicle produces the major portion of estrogen.

The high serum level of estrogen acts as a negative feedback mechanism to the hypothalamus and causes it to suppress FSH secretion from the pituitary. Decreased secretion of FSH causes all follicles but the dominant one to regress. At the same time, the elevated estrogen level causes an increase in the amount of LH to be released. A preovulatory LH surge completes the maturation of the dominant follicle and causes it to thin and swell. The ovum, surrounded by the follicular fluid, is released from the ruptured follicle within approximately 24 hours of the LH surge. Ovulation occurs on approximately day 14 of the idealized cycle. About 25% of women experience one-sided pain in the lower abdomen at the approximate time of ovulation. This pain, called *mittelschmerz,* corresponds to the release of the follicular fluid from the ovulating ovary and is thought to be caused by peritoneal irritation.

Immediately after ovulation, the ruptured follicle collapses in on itself. Cells that fill the space accumulate a yellow pigment and become the *corpus luteum.* The granulosa cells become larger and vascularized and use cholesterol from low-density lipoproteins in the plasma to synthesize progesterone. The luteinized theca cells secrete estrogen in the corpus luteum.

The *luteal phase* of the cycle corresponds to the secretory phase of the uterine cycle (see next section). The corpus luteum secretes the maximal level of steroids at about 8 days after ovulation. Unless a pregnancy occurs, the corpus luteum begins to rapidly degenerate 10 to 12 days after ovulation. Its life span is about 14 days, which is the average length of time from ovulation to menses. The corpus luteum is completely resorbed before the menses. Connective tissue replaces the luteinized cells and forms scar-like tissue called the *corpus albicans.* The decreased levels of estrogen and progesterone stimulate the hypothalamus to repeat the menstrual cycle by releasing gonadotropin-releasing factor.

It is important for some women to be able to determine the time of ovulation. If conception is to occur, fertilization must take place within hours of ovulation. Basal body temperature charts are useful to determine when ovulation has occurred. During the follicular (preovulatory) phase, the woman's temperature remains at a relatively constant low level. After ovulation, the effects of progesterone on the hypothalamus cause the woman's temperature to rise to a higher level (Bobak et al., 1989). The abrupt temperature rise is characteristic of the rupture of the follicle.

Uterine (Endometrial) Cycle

The endometrial lining of the uterus reflects the effects of the ovarian steroids in four stages: menstruation, proliferative phase, secretory phase, and premenstrual phase. In direct response to the withdrawal of progesterone, *menstruation* occurs from days 1 through 5 of the cycle, when the upper layers of the endometrium are shed. Although there is great variation in the duration of the flow (2 to 8 days) and in the normal amount of blood lost (25 to 60 mL), the average duration is 5 days and the average blood loss is approximately 50 mL. The discharge also includes mucus and epithelial cells. A woman typically experiences the same duration of flow each month.

The *proliferative phase* of the uterine cycle, days 5 to 14 in the idealized cycle, corresponds to the follicular phase of the ovarian cycle. Estrogen promotes the rapid thickening of the endometrium. The vascular supply to the endometrium increases and forms a loose capillary network.

After ovulation (approximately day 14), the combined effects of estrogen and progesterone begin the *secretory phase.* At the beginning of the secretory phase, the three layers of the endometrium become easily defined. The glandular secretions and edema in the stroma (framework) of the endometrium begin to increase. As the secretory stage continues, the endometrium becomes quite vascular and rich in glycogen. The arteries that branch from the portion of the endometrial lining closest to the myometrium become spiraled or coiled. At this point in the menstrual cycle, the endometrium is ideal for implantation of a fertilized ovum.

The last stage, or *premenstrual phase,* occurs in response to regression of the corpus luteum in the ovary. About 2 to 3 days before the onset of menstruation, the stroma of the endometrium begins to disintegrate. With the loss of fluids and secretions in the tissue, the arteries and glands collapse. Constriction of the arteries causes the upper portion of the endometrium to become ischemic and to slough off. Through an unknown mechanism, the arteries then relax and cause small hemorrhages from the smaller arterioles. The onset of menstrual bleeding and endometrial tissue loss begins the cycle again.

The Climacteric and Menopause

Menopause is the biologic end of reproductive ability, but the term applies only to the *last menstrual period.* The phase of a woman's life from the initial decline in the amount of estrogen produced by the ovaries to cessation of symptoms produced by this phenomenon is called the *climacteric.* Lay terminology for this phase is the *change of life.* Menopause is only one sign of the climacteric.

During a woman's life span, follicles in the ovary atrophy continuously. The progressive decline in the number of follicles that are able to produce estrogen in response to pituitary hormones causes the woman (usually between 40 and 50 years of age) to begin to notice physical changes in her body. The levels of estrogen and progesterone diminish gradually until the effect of these hormones on the endometrial lining of the uterus is absent. At the same time, the low levels of the ovarian hormones continue to stimulate the hypothalamus-pituitary axis. The anterior pituitary secretes high levels of FSH and LH after menopause has occurred.

For a time, the inner core of the ovary produces androstenedione (a weak male hormone) and testosterone. Eighty per cent of the androstenedione is produced by the adrenal glands. When the ovarian core ceases to function, the adrenal cortices are the only source of steroids. The production of androstenedione is significant, especially after menopause, because it is converted to a form of estrogen, *estrone,* in body fat. Consequently, women with greater percentages of body fat have higher estrone levels after menopause.

During the climacteric, a woman experiences irregular menstrual and ovarian cycles. Often, the ovary fails to ovulate. The menstrual flow may be lighter or heavier during the period of irregular cycles. The actual date of menopause cannot be determined until at least 1 year has passed without menses.

Decreased amounts of estrogen affect multiple sites in the body. The uterus, cervix, and ovaries, as well as the labia and the clitoris, shrink in size. The low estrogen levels cause the vagina to narrow and shorten. The vaginal mucosa becomes thin and dry, which makes intercourse uncomfortable.

Muscular support to the pelvis becomes more relaxed. The loss of tone in addition affects bladder support.

Bone density is of concern after decreased estrogen production. Estrogen is needed by bone tissue for calcium uptake. It also increases the metabolism of vitamin D that is needed for absorption of calcium from the intestines. With decreased calcium uptake, bone density decreases. The reduction in the amount of bone mass is called *osteoporosis* (see Chap. 30).

One of the most common symptoms occurring during the climacteric is *hot flushes ("hot flashes")*, which are caused by vasomotor instability. Their etiology is not clear, but it is thought that surges of FSH and LH on the hypothalamus cause vasodilation and increased heat production.

BREASTS

The female *breasts* are a pair of mammary glands that develop in response to secretions from the hypothalamus, pituitary gland, and ovaries. Functionally, the breasts are an accessory of the reproductive system meant to nourish the infant after delivery. *Lactation* is the secretion of *colostrum* (precursor of mature milk) or mature milk from the breasts.

The breasts are located between the second and sixth ribs, between the edge of the sternum and the midaxil-

lary line. About two-thirds of the breast diameter is over the greater pectoral muscle and one-third is superficial to the anterior serratus muscle.

The structure of a mature female breast is shown in Figure 52-4. The *nipple* rises from the center of the pigmented *areola*, which is usually located slightly lateral to the midline of each breast. *Montgomery's glands* are small, round sebaceous glands that appear as elevations on the areola and that are thought to secrete a fatty substance that protects the nipple during breastfeeding.

Breast tissue has three principal components: a network of glandular and ductal tissue, fibrous tissue, and fat. The proportion of each component of breast tissue depends on genetic factors, nutrition, age, and obstetric history. The breast is supported by *Cooper's suspensory ligaments* attached to underlying muscles.

Each mature breast is composed of 15 to 25 *lobes* that are arranged radially around the breast and are separated by fat. Each lobe is composed of several *lobules* that consist of large numbers of *alveoli.* Alveoli are saclike structures that are lined with epithelium. The epithelial lining synthesizes and secretes the components of breast milk in response to *prolactin,* which is released by the anterior pituitary. Each alveolus is connected, by way of an individual small duct, to a single larger duct from the lobule. The ducts from the lobules, the *lactiferous ducts*, combine to form one duct from each lobe that ends at the nipple openings. The surfaces of the alveoli and the ducts are covered with myoepithelial cells that contract in response to tactile or autonomic stimulation. Just before the ducts open at the nipples, they expand into reservoirs called *ampullae* or *lactiferous sinuses.* There should be no nipple discharge or milk production unless the woman is pregnant or is nursing a child.

The abundant blood supply to the breasts is from branches of the internal mammary and lateral thoracic arteries. The veins of the breast connect with the superior vena cava. Much of the lymph drains through an extensive network that is radial to the axilla (Fig. 52-5). Depending on the location of a lesion, lymph may spread malignant cells directly into the infraclavicular nodes, deeply into the chest or abdomen, or into the

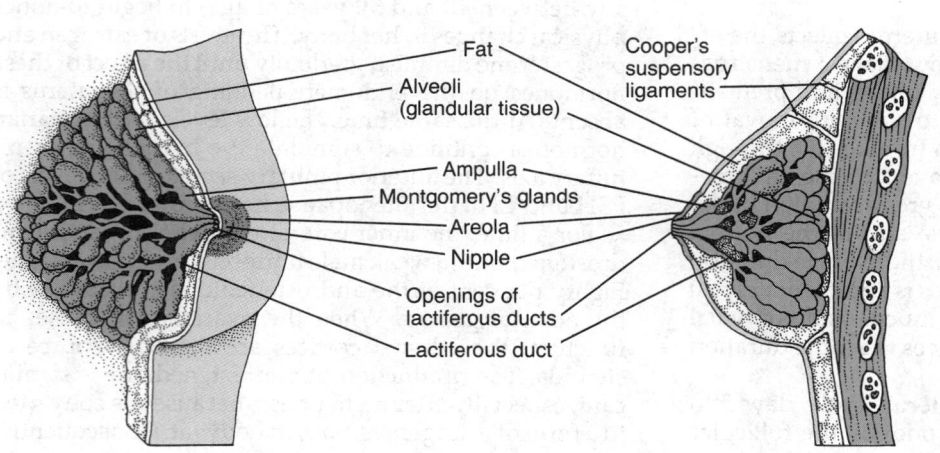

Fat
Alveoli (glandular tissue)
Ampulla
Montgomery's glands
Areola
Nipple
Openings of lactiferous ducts
Lactiferous duct

Cooper's suspensory ligaments

Figure 52-4

Structure of the mature female breast.

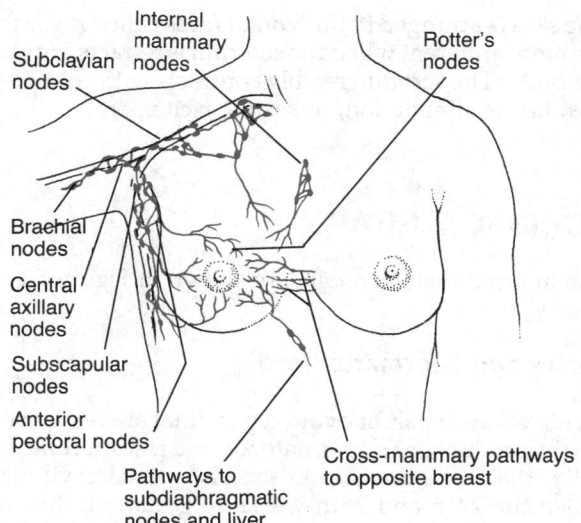

Figure 52–5

Lymphatic drainage of the female breast.

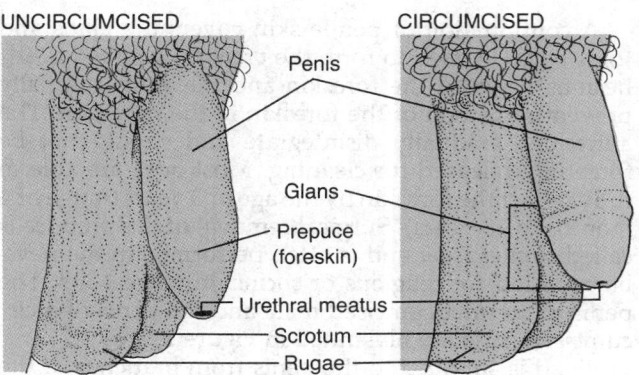

Figure 52–6

External male genitalia.

opposite breast. Lymphatic drainage from the axillary nodes empties into the jugular and subclavian veins. This short route allows cancerous cells to move rapidly into the general circulation and to metastasize to the lungs, pelvis, vertebrae, and brain.

The breasts may not develop symmetrically during puberty. By adulthood, both breasts are usually symmetric in size and contour, although it is not unusual for the breast on the woman's dominant side (on the basis of right- or left-handedness) to appear larger because of the more developed pectoral muscle base.

In many women, the breasts become slightly larger and tender during the premenstrual period. The tissue may also feel nodular at this time. The breasts respond to the increasing levels of estrogen and progesterone 3 to 4 days before menses by increasing vascularity, inducing growth of the ducts and alveoli, and promoting water retention. After menstruation, the cellular growth regresses, the ducts and alveoli decrease in size, and water retention subsides.

MALE REPRODUCTIVE SYSTEM

EXTERNAL GENITALIA

The external male genitalia (Fig. 52–6) undergo multiple changes during puberty. The first visible sign of pubescence is enlargement of the scrotum and testes, which typically occurs between the ages of 11 and 13.5 years. As the boy develops, pubic hair grows in a diamond-shaped pattern, pigmentation increases over the genital area, and the penis enlarges. Complete sexual maturity is usually achieved within 2 to 5 years, the average being about 3 years. At maturity, the male can impregnate a female.

These changes occur in response to a rise in the level of testosterone produced in the body. The release of *gonadatropin-releasing factor* from the male's hypothalamus stimulates the anterior pituitary to secrete *LH* and *FSH*. As the levels of the gonadotropins increase, the amount of testosterone significantly increases. Other signs of puberty that relate to testosterone production are the growth of axillary hair, the lengthening and thickening of the vocal cords, increased sebaceous gland activity, and a general increase in muscle mass and body size.

As the postadolescent male ages, testosterone production remains relatively constant. There is only a slight and gradual reduction of testosterone in the older adult male. The lower testosterone levels contribute to a decrease in muscle mass, loss of skin elasticity, postural changes, and changes in sexual performance.

Penis

The *penis* is the male organ for urination and copulation. The *root* of the penis is attached to the anterior pubic arch by a continuation of fascia, a triangular suspensory ligament, and muscle tissue, and consists of the posterior ends of the three erectile columns from the body of the penis. The *corpus* or *body* is the pendulous, soft-tissue portion that extends from the attached root to the *glans penis,* the distal end of the penis. Engorgement of the highly vascular, erectile columns with blood during sexual excitement causes the penis to expand and elongate and to become firm and erect. A ridge of tissue forms where the glans expands and meets the corpus, called the *corona* of the glans. The glans tissue surrounds the slit-like opening of the urethral meatus. The male urethra serves as the pathway for the exit of both urine and semen.

The penis is covered by thin skin that is loosely attached to the underlying fascia, which allows the penis to enlarge during erections. The skin is darker than the rest of the body and has hair only at the base of the penis, near its root.

A continuation of penile skin covers the glans and folds back on itself to form the *prepuce* or *foreskin*. Adhesions between the foreskin and the glans normally prevent retraction of the foreskin in the newborn. The adhesions gradually disintegrate and should not be forcefully released for cleaning. Most boys are able to fully retract the foreskin by the age of 3 years (range of 4 months to 13 years). Surgical removal of the prepuce is called *circumcision* and is often performed in the newborn period for religious or sociocultural reasons. The penis of an uncircumcised male and the penis of a circumcised male are illustrated in Figure 52–6.

Blood is supplied to the penis from branches of the internal pudendal artery. The skin of the penis also receives blood from the external pudendal and femoral arteries. Afferent arteries bring blood into the meshwork of the erectile columns during sexual excitement (causing *tumescence,* or swelling). At the same time, outflow of blood is partially stopped. After orgasm and ejaculation, the decrease in sexual tension causes the arteries to contract. Blood is drained by the venous plexus of efferent veins, which causes a reduction in the size and firmness of the penis *(detumescence).* At the end of detumescence, the penis has returned to its flaccid state.

Lymphatic drainage of the penis is through the inguinal nodes. The superficial inguinal and subinguinal nodes are carefully palpated when a penile lesion is noted.

The penis is richly innervated through branches of the sympathetic and parasympathetic nervous systems and by nerves of cerebral origin. Parasympathetic fibers, originating at sacral spinal levels S-2, S-3, and S-4, provide sensory innervation of the penile skin and allow the smooth muscle of the arteries to relax. Parasympathetic stimulation allows blood to flow freely into the cavernous spaces. Sympathetic fibers, which are especially evident in the corpus spongiosum, are rooted at the lumbar spinal segments. They control the rhythmic muscle contractions that lead to the ejaculation of semen and constrict the smooth muscle of the arteries to allow blood to flow from the erectile bodies. The cerebral cortex is thought to be responsible for most of the erogenous stimulation.

Scrotum

The *scrotum* is a thin-walled, fibromuscular sac that is suspended below the pubis bone, posterior to the penis. The pouch protects the testes, epididymis, and vas deferens in a position that is relatively cooler than one inside the abdominal cavity. Normal spermatogenesis requires a controlled temperature. The slightly lower temperature, about 2° C less than body temperature, is optimal for sperm production and viability. The left side of the scrotum usually hangs about a centimeter (³/₈ in) lower than the right side.

Scrotal skin is darkly pigmented and contains multiple sweat and sebaceous glands, plus few hair follicles.

The skin is arranged in horizontal folds called *rugae* that are more apparent when the scrotum is retracted toward the body. The scrotum readily contracts with cold, exercise, tactile stimulation, or sexual excitement.

INTERNAL GENITALIA

The internal male genitalia are shown in Figure 52–7.

Testes and Spermatic Cord

The *testes* are a pair of ovoid organs that are responsible for the production of spermatozoa and testosterone. Initially, the testes develop in the abdominal cavity; between the 24th and 35th weeks of gestation, they descend into the scrotum through the inguinal canal. Each testis is approximately 4 cm (1⁵/₈ in) long and 2.5 cm (1 in) wide. The scrotal ligament provides the only attachment to the scrotum and allows the testis to be mobile within the scrotal cavity.

Each testis is suspended in the scrotum by the *spermatic cord,* which provides vascular, lymphatic, and nerve supports to the testis (Fig. 52–8). The cord also covers the *epididymis* and a portion of the *vas deferens.* The cord and testes are encircled by layers of spermatic fascia and cremaster muscle. There are sympathetic nerve fibers on the arteries in the cord, and sympathetic and parasympathetic fibers on the vas deferens. When the testes sustain a trauma, these autonomic nerve fibers transmit excruciating pain and a sickening sensation.

Each testis is divided into approximately 250 lobes by fibrous septa. Two or three hair-like *seminiferous tubules,* each about 60 cm (23⁵/₈ in) long, are tightly coiled within each lobe of the testis. The tubules unite as they leave each lobe and combine in a network of canals, called the *rete testis.* Eight to 20 efferent ductules emerge from this network and connect the internal testis with the epididymis.

The seminiferous tubules are the functional unit of the testes and consist of germinal epithelial cells and *Sertoli's cells.* FSH stimulates Sertoli's cells to develop sperm. Sertoli's cells appear to nurture spermatids during cell division and appear to be attached to the spermatocytes. They aid in transformation of spermatids to more mature gametes by helping to break down the cytoplasm. When the sperm enter the lumen of the seminiferous tubule, they are still not fully mature.

The normal ejaculate of 3.5 mL (range of 1.5 to 6 mL) of semen contains between 50 and 150 million sperm. This number is remarkable when it is remembered that only one sperm can penetrate and fertilize an ovum. The large number of spermatozoa in the testicular fluid make up only 1% of the total volume of the ejaculate.

Leydig's cells are found in small groups within the interstitial tissue surrounding the seminiferous tubules. They secrete the major male hormone, *testosterone,* in response to stimulation by LH from the anterior pitui-

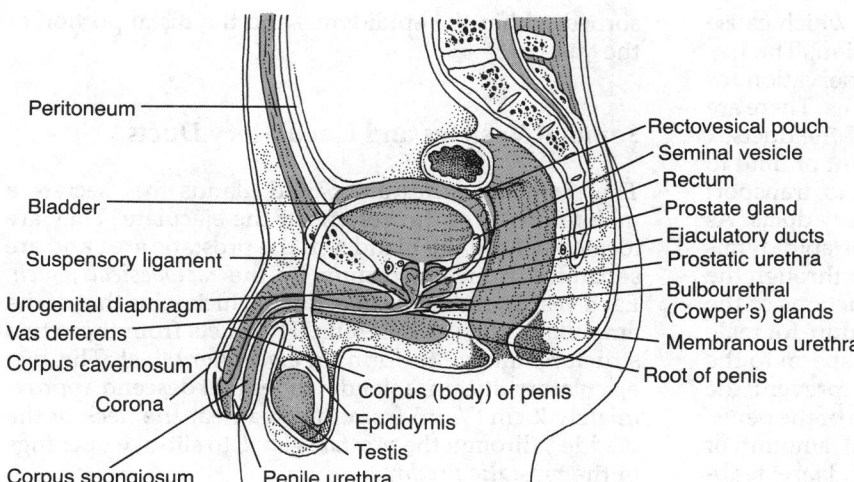

Peritoneum

Bladder

Suspensory ligament

Urogenital diaphragm

Vas deferens

Corpus cavernosum

Corona

Corpus spongiosum

Rectovesical pouch

Seminal vesicle

Rectum

Prostate gland

Ejaculatory ducts

Prostatic urethra

Bulbourethral (Cowper's) glands

Membranous urethra

Root of penis

Corpus (body) of penis

Epididymis

Testis

Penile urethra

Figure 52–7

Internal male genitalia.

tary. Testicular production of testosterone is regulated by a negative feedback control system on the hypothalamus. As serum testosterone levels rise, neurofeedback to the hypothalamus slows its secretion of the gonadotropin-releasing factor.

It is important to note that lymphatics of the testes drain into the abdomen and if enlarged, are not palpable. Lymphatics from scrotal and penile surfaces drain into the inguinal nodes, which can be palpated if enlarged. When these nodes are enlarged or tender, an inflammatory or possibly malignant lesion may be present (Bates, 1987).

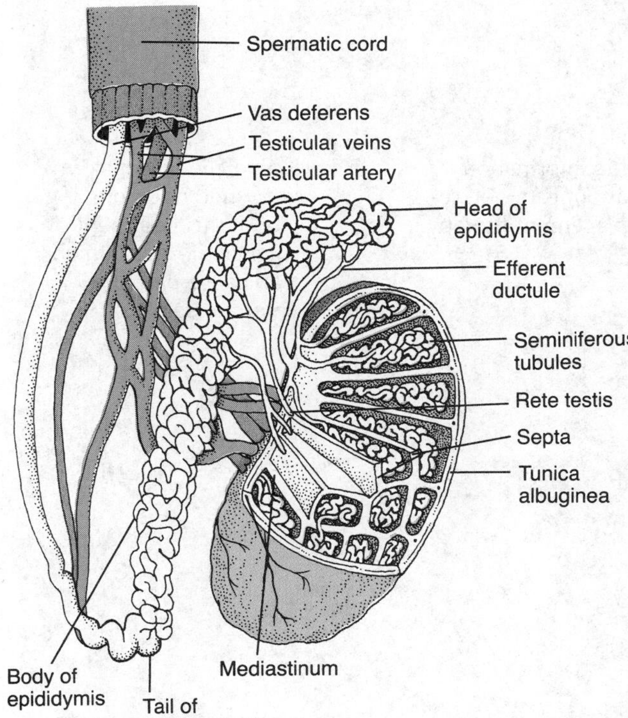

Epididymis

The *epididymis* is the first portion of a ductal system used to transport sperm from the ductules of the testes to the urethra; it also aids in maturation of the sperm. Comma-shaped and lying posterolateral to one side of each testis, the epididymis is described in three anatomic sections: head, body, and tail. The *head* of the epididymis attaches to the posterior aspect of the testis. The *body* descends against the lateral wall of the testis. At the lower border of the testis, the *tail* folds back over on itself and ascends toward the spermatic cord, merging gradually into the vas deferens and providing storage for sperm.

Vas Deferens

The *vasa deferens,* or *ductus deferens,* are firm, muscular tubes about 45 cm (17¾ in) long that continue from the tail of each epididymis. Each ductus leaves the spermatic cord at the deep inguinal ring and continues under the peritoneum toward the posterior abdominal wall. Crossing over the lateral bladder and then between the ureters, both ducts descend behind the bladder to the area of the prostate. The terminal end of the vas deferens enlarges to form an *ampulla,* which serves as a major reservoir for sperm and tubular fluids. The ampulla of each vas deferens merges with a duct from the seminal vesicle to form the ejaculatory ducts at the base of the *prostate gland.* Sperm from the vas deferens and nutritive secretions from the seminal vesicles are transported through the ejaculatory duct to mix with prostatic fluids in the prostatic urethra.

The cremaster muscle envelops the vas deferens and the testes within the spermatic cord. The ductus is heav-

Spermatic cord

Vas deferens

Testicular veins

Testicular artery

Head of epididymis

Efferent ductule

Seminiferous tubules

Rete testis

Septa

Tunica albuginea

Body of epididymis

Tail of epididymis

Mediastinum

Figure 52–8

Structure of the testis and the epididymis.

ily innervated by autonomic nerve fibers, which cause the expulsive contractions during ejaculation. The hypogastric and pelvic nerves provide the innervation for the contractile movements of the vas deferens. There are also sensory neurons in the outer layers of the ducts.

Although the vas secretes a small amount of fluid to support the sperm, its main function is to transport sperm from the epididymis to the ejaculatory ducts. As opposed to movement of sperm through the epididymis by ciliary action, the sperm are transported through the vas deferens by means of peristaltic contractions of the ducts. Thus, a *vasectomy*, the surgical procedure for male sterilization, prevents only the passage of sperm to the ejaculatory ducts. A vasectomy does not prevent the production of sperm, does not limit erection of the penis, and does not significantly alter the total amount of semen. Unexpelled sperm degenerate and are reab-

sorbed within the epididymis and the distal portion of the vas.

Seminal Vesicles and Ejaculatory Ducts

The *seminal vesicles* are paired glands that secrete a major portion of the volume of the ejaculate. They are located behind the bladder in the prostatic area and are separated from the rectum by the *rectovesical pouch*. Each vesicle ends in a small duct, which joins that of the ampulla of the vas deferens. The ducts from these two structures merge to form an *ejaculatory duct*. The two ejaculatory ducts are slender tubes that descend approximately 2 cm (¾ in) from the area near the neck of the bladder, through the *prostate gland*, to slit-like openings in the *prostatic urethra*.

FOCUS ON THE ELDERLY ■ **Reproductive Changes Related to Aging**

Structure	Change(s)	Interventions	Rationales
Women			
Pubic hair	Becomes gray, thinner	Discuss changes with client (applies to all structures for both women and men).	To help prevent problems with body image (applies to all structures for both women and men).
Labia majora, clitoris	Decrease in size		
Breasts	Become flabby and fibrous and hang lower on the chest wall; nipples less erectile		
Vaginal walls	Become dry, smoother, thinner	Provide information about estrogen replacement therapy.	To enable client to make informed decisions about this treatment of vaginal dryness, which can cause painful intercourse.
Uterus	Decreases in size		
Endometrium	Atrophies		
Ovaries	Decrease in size, with marked convolution		
Pelvic ligaments and connective tissue	Lose tone and elasticity		
Men			
Pubic hair	Becomes gray, thinner		
Scrotum	Becomes more pendulous, has fewer rugae		
Prostate	Likely to enlarge; ureteral obstruction can occur	Teach client signs of ureteral obstruction.	To detect enlargement or obstruction, which may indicate the presence of cancer.

Each seminal vesicle is a tortuous, 15-cm-long (6-in-long) structure, with numerous outpouchings, that coils to a 4-cm (1⅝-in) length. The connective tissue of the walls of the vesicle contains opposing layers of smooth muscle fibers, lined with secretory epithelial cells. Its blood supply is from the same artery as that supplying the vas deferens. When the muscles of the seminal vesicles contract during orgasm, the glands secrete a thick, mildly acidic mucus into the ejaculatory ducts. Motor innervation to the vesicles is primarily from sympathetic nervous system fibers.

Seminal vesicle fluid makes up 40% to 60% of the semen. A large percentage of the viscous fluid is *fructose,* which is nutritive for the sperm. Smaller percentages of *fibrinogen* and *prostaglandins* aid in the process of fertilization of the ovum. The vesicles secrete this fluid into the ejaculatory ducts shortly after the sperm has been emitted from the vas deferens and the prostate has released its secretions. Contractions of the seminal vesicles forcefully expel its mucoid fluid, which pushes the sperm and prostatic secretions forward in the urethra. Thus, the first fraction of semen is richer in sperm and prostatic secretions than the last fraction.

Prostate Gland

The *prostate gland* is the largest accessory gland of the male reproductive system. It is a chestnut-shaped, glandular, and fibromuscular organ. Functionally, it secretes a milky alkaline fluid that adds bulk to the semen, enhances sperm motility, and neutralizes female acidic vaginal secretions. During *emission,* the first stage of the male orgasm, the smooth muscle of the prostate gland contracts and secretes its fluid at the same time as does the vas deferens. Fluid from the prostate gland contributes 20% to 30% of the total ejaculate. The average pH of the combined secretions of semen is approximately 7.5, whereas secretions from the vagina normally have a pH of 3.5 to 4.0. Sperm need a surrounding fluid pH of 6.0 to 6.5 before they become optimally motile.

The prostate gland, approximately 15 cm (6 in) long, is situated between the neck of the bladder and the *urogenital diaphragm,* which is a musculomembranous structure composed of fascia, the urethral sphincter, and perineal muscles. The prostate is separated from the anterior wall of the rectum by a thin fascial sheath that is part of the rectovesical septum. The prostate should not project more than 1 cm (⅜ in) into the rectal lumen.

The *prostatic portion of the urethra* descends through the prostate gland from the internal urethral orifice at the neck of the bladder to the urethral sphincter in the urogenital diaphragm. There is controversy about the names of the anatomic divisions of the prostate, but most refer to a *median lobe* and two *lateral lobes.* Most of the glandular tissue, composed of numerous follicles, is located posterior and lateral to the prostatic urethra. The follicles join into 20 to 30 excretory ducts that open into *prostatic sinuses* on each side of the posterior prostatic urethra.

The arterial blood supply to the prostate is derived from the pudendal, vesical, and rectal arteries; veins form a venous plexus around the sides and base of the prostate. Most lymph vessels of the prostate terminate in the internal iliac and sacral lymph nodes. The nerve supply is derived from the inferior hypogastric nerves.

As men age the prostate becomes more significant clinically. At birth, the gland is small. With puberty, the prostate rapidly enlarges to the normal adult size. By age 50 or 60 years, about 80% of men have an enlarged prostate, or benign prostatic hypertrophy, which can cause urinary problems (Johnson et al., 1984).

Prostatic function depends on adequate levels of testosterone. Without the sex hormones, the prostate becomes smaller and more fibrous.

Bulbourethral (Cowper's) Glands

Semen is ejaculated through the prostatic urethra, the membranous urethra, and the penile urethra. The *membranous urethra* is the component of the urethra that is below the prostate gland in the urogenital diaphragm. The *bulbourethral glands* are two yellow, pea-sized glands that are located posterior to the membranous urethra within the muscle of the urethral sphincter. They are connected to the penile portion of the urethra by ducts that descend approximately 3 cm (1¼ in) through the fascia of the urogenital diaphragm and the bulb of the corpus spongiosum.

The bulbourethral glands secrete an alkaline mucus into the penile urethra during emission. The mucus mixes with the sperm and other glandular secretions to form the semen. The bulbourethral glands contribute about 5% to 6% of the total ejaculate. The alkalinity of the mucus further protects the sperm against the relative acidity within the urethra.

The filling of the internal urethra stimulates the pudendal nerve roots in the sacral spinal cord. In response, the nervous system causes further rhythmic contractions of the internal genitals and contractions that compress the bases of the three penile erectile bodies. The rhythmic, increased pressure in the ducts and the urethra causes *ejaculation* of the semen through the penile urethra (urinary meatus), which is the second phase of the male orgasm.

REPRODUCTIVE CHANGES ASSOCIATED WITH AGING

The functional capacity of the reproductive system depends on age for both the male and the female. Until puberty, the reproductive system is primordial. As the individual continues to age, hormones produced by the gonads affect the normal functioning of many of the other body systems, as described in the accompanying Focus on the Elderly feature.

HISTORY

DEMOGRAPHIC DATA

Data related to culture, race, and age allow the nurse to assess the client's risk of developing certain diseases. Many of the data interrelate with the socioeconomic history and can lead to certain inferences, which should be further validated in the interview. During the course of the interview, the client is likely to provide information about concerns other than that expressed in the chief complaint. Because physical examination of the reproductive system is of a highly personal nature, the time spent in collecting these data allows the nurse to convey respect and professionalism.

Cultural influences and expectations account for variations in acceptable gender-related and sexual identity. The child's attitude and behavior regarding the meaning and use of the genitals begin in infancy and are modeled after significant adults' behavior. Religious dictates often parallel those of a specific culture and strongly affect sexual activity. Specific sexual practices, the acceptable number of partners, contraceptive use, and specific treatments to terminate a pregnancy, end future fertility, or remove barriers to infertility are often guided by religious beliefs.

Race often has an epidemiologic influence on particular diseases. The incidence of cancer of the reproductive system and associated death rates are higher for Black than for Caucasian Americans (American Cancer Society, 1988). Black females are generally more advanced in the development of secondary sex characteristics than Caucasian women of the same age (Bates, 1987). Axillary hair appears at an earlier age in Blacks than in Caucasians; Asian persons have finer, more sparse pubic hair than persons of other races.

The nurse considers the client's *age* in evaluating the reproductive system. The age at which secondary sex characteristics develop needs to be compared with the established normal ranges for males or females.

PERSONAL AND FAMILY HISTORY

Health habits of the client, such as diet, sleep, and exercise patterns, are important for the nurse to assess. Low levels of body fat may be related to ovarian dysfunction. It is also necessary to determine the client's alcohol, tobacco, and drug use because libido, spermatogenesis, and potency can be affected (Bobak et al., 1989).

The client's personal medical history gives data concerning his or her general health. The occurrence of certain *childhood illnesses* is particularly related to the reproductive system. Females need to be screened for sufficient rubella titers and should be treated if necessary to prevent possible teratogenic effects on their un-

born children. Mumps or smallpox in the postpubertal male may cause *orchitis* (painful inflammation and swelling of the testes) and occasionally leads to testicular atrophy and sterility.

Major adult illnesses or chronic illnesses may severely affect reproductive function. *Endocrine disorders* are likely to affect the hypothalamus–pituitary–gonadal axis of the male or female. Almost any disease that disturbs metabolism or nutrition may depress ovarian function and cause amenorrhea. Hypothalamic-pituitary failure disorders can cause delayed development or regression of secondary sex characteristics. A history of infertility and failure of ovulation is associated with a greater risk of developing endometrial cancer. Some *pre-existing cancers* increase a woman's risk of developing other reproductive system cancers. Chronic *nervous system, respiratory system,* or *cardiovascular system disorders* can alter the sexual response. Some *drugs* such as antihypertensives, narcotics, monoamine oxidase inhibitors, methyldopa, and histamine antagonists may impair fertility (Olds et al., 1988). Radiation and prolonged use of corticosteroids, exogenous estrogen or testosterone, and chemotherapeutic agents can cause reproductive system dysfunction.

Past *severe infections* can alter a person's reproductive ability. Pelvic inflammatory disease or ruptured appendix followed by peritonitis can cause strictures or adhesions in the fallopian tubes and pelvic scarring. *Salpingitis* is most frequently caused by *Neisseria gonorrhoeae.* Unfortunately, infertility is a common sequela of tubal infection. In the male, infections or prolonged fever may damage sperm production or cause obstruction of the seminal tract, which leads to infertility. The nurse explores a history of *surgeries, serious injuries, current medications,* and *allergies* because each can affect reproductive structure or function.

A *genitoreproductive history* is completed for both the male and female client. With a female client, the nurse asks questions about her menses: age of menarche, cycle frequency and duration, amount of flow, spotting between periods, dysmenorrhea (painful periods), premenstrual symptoms, and the date of her last normal menstrual period. If she is of menopausal age, the nurse determines the date of her last menstrual period and the presence of climacteric symptoms. All women should be interviewed about the possibility of vaginal discharge, history and treatment of sexually transmitted diseases, the date and the result of her last Papanicolaou's (Pap) smear, breast self-examination practices, and douching practices. It is also necessary to take an obstetric history of postpubertal women. If the woman has ever been pregnant, the nurse inquires as to the outcome of the pregnancies. In addition, information is collected about the date and mode of deliveries or termination of the pregnancy; complications during pregnancy, labor, and delivery; birth weight and gestational age of the infants; and the condition of the infants at birth and at present. Sexual activity, satisfaction with sexual response, any occurrence of pain or bleeding with sexual intercourse, and contraceptive use are evaluated. Questions about monthly breast self-examinations determine whether the client has observed pain, discomfort, lumps, or discharge from the nipples, and whether these occurred at specific times during the menstrual cycle.

For male clients, testicular changes and self-examination practices, problems with urination, discharge from the penis, rectal problems, history and treatment of sexually transmitted diseases, and symptoms related to hernias are evaluated. For postpubertal men, the nurse inquires as to sexual functioning. Prior reproductive history and contraceptive use, current problems or changes in sexual response, and any occurrence of impotence provide additional data to direct the physical examination.

The *family history,* including parents, grandparents, siblings, spouse, and children, helps to determine the client's risk of developing conditions that affect reproductive system functioning.

The age and course of puberty of the parents often correspond to those of the child. A seeming delay or precocious development of secondary sex characteristics may be a familial pattern.

The current age and state of health of the living members of the extended family are of interest. Also, the cause and age at death of specific members may be important. The evidence of family members' having significant diseases, such as diabetes, cardiovascular disease, hypertension, renal disease, cancer, or complications of pregnancy, allows the nurse to better interpret the client's presenting symptoms. For example, daughters of women who were given DES (diethylstilbestrol) to control bleeding during pregnancy have an increased risk of infertility and reproductive tract carcinomas.

The occurrence of multiple pregnancies, genetic disorders, or congenital anomalies within the extended family may predispose the future offspring of the client to the same problems.

DIET HISTORY

A *diet history* is often critical for correct interpretation of presenting symptoms of the reproductive system. Fatigue and lack of sexual interest may be associated with poor diet and anemia. *Obesity* raises a person's risk of developing breast and uterine cancer. A *dietary recall* for a recent 24-hour period is valuable to estimate the quality of the diet. High-fat diets have been linked with cancer of the breast and prostate.

The nurse needs to compare the client's height, weight, and body build with the dietary recall. Clients may be hesitant to divulge practices such as binging, purging, anorexic behaviors, or excessive exercise, although these practices may affect the reproductive system. There seems to be a certain level of body fat and weight necessary for the onset of menses and the maintenance of regular menstrual cycles. A decreased amount of body fat is associated with insufficient estrogen for the maintenance of normal ovulatory cycles.

In addition, women have special dietary needs. The diet of women who use oral contraceptives should reflect increased sources of folic acid and vitamins B_6, B_{12}, and C. Heavy bleeding associated with menses, particularly in women who have intrauterine devices, may necessitate oral iron supplements. All women need to be aware of the female body's need for calcium. Although adequte calcium intake throughout life is optimal, it is especially important during the pre- and postmenopausal periods. With the decreased production of estrogen during the climacteric, a woman's bone density decreases, which predisposes her to osteoporosis and fractures.

SOCIOECONOMIC STATUS

The *social history* of the client provides insight into the whole person. Included within this sphere are birthplace, childhood environment, position in the family, education and job history, marital status, financial situation, existence of stressors, religion, leisure time activities, and support systems. All can influence the health of the reproductive system. Single women and women who have never had children have significantly higher rates of ovarian and breast cancer than do multiparous women. Early age at first intercourse and multiple sex partners are associated with an increased risk of cervical cancer. Religious beliefs may dictate contraceptive practices for a couple. Stress has long been associated with menstrual and ovulatory irregularities. The nurse asks about *leisure time activities* that have a high risk of injury to the reproductive system. For example, men who lounge for long periods in hot tubs or saunas often experience decreased sperm production. Women who are long distance runners have reduced percentages of body fat and a higher risk of menstrual irregularities.

The client's choice of *occupation* may directly affect the reproductive system. Men and women who are routinely exposed in their work to potential *teratogenic* substances (i.e., agents capable of producing birth defects in offspring) have a higher incidence of abnormal sperm morphology and low sperm counts, or of spontaneous abortion (miscarriage). Those who work around certain chemicals, radiation, and heavy metals are at risk. Trauma and exposure to extremely high temperatures in the workplace are potential causes of male infertility. In addition, exposure to some industrial agents, such as cadmium, may be related to the development of carcinomas of the reproductive system.

It is necessary for the nurse to assess the *educational level* of the client to be able to individualize health teaching. Lay language for body parts and function is commonly used when discussing the reproductive system. It is important for the nurse to be familiar with such terms and to be unaffected by their use. Clients may try to evoke a particular response in the nurse by use of certain words, or they may have no other terminology to express the problem. The nurse who responds with shock or disdain displays a judgmental attitude that hinders successful data gathering. Health care professionals can use some of these instances as teaching opportunities to provide more appropriate terminology.

The client's general satisfaction with life and the support systems available often have a direct relationship to the current health problem. Questions designed to elicit information about daily routines often give insight into perception of the quality of life and outlook for the future.

CURRENT HEALTH PROBLEM

If a client seeks medical attention for a problem related to the reproductive system, the nurse asks additional questions to explore the chief complaint. Most complaints from males or females concern pain, bleeding, discharge, masses, or reproductive functioning.

Pain related to reproductive system disorders may be confused with gastrointestinal or urinary tract problems. The client needs to describe the type of pain, its intensity, when and where it occurs, its duration, what exacerbates it or gives relief, and the relationship to menstrual, sexual, urinary, or gastrointestinal function. Reproductive system disorders can be multifaceted, so it is imperative not to assume that the first diagnosis is the only diagnosis.

Heavy *bleeding* or a lack of bleeding may be of concern to the client. The possibility of pregnancy is considered in any sexually active woman presenting with amenorrhea. Any bleeding after the menopause needs to be evaluated. The character of abnormal bleeding and amount of blood from the vagina or penis are noted in the client's words. The nurse asks when the bleeding occurs in relation to certain events, such as the menstrual cycle or menopause, intercourse, trauma, or strenuous exercise. Because multiple factors may cause bleeding, sources other than the genital tract must be considered. The nurse determines the onset and duration of bleeding, the interval between bleeding episodes, and precipitating factors of the bleeding. The character of the bleeding should be described in terms of the amount of blood, color, consistency, and change in the nature of the flow. The presence of associated symptoms needs to be noted, such as pain, cramping or abdominal fullness, change in bowel habits, urinary difficulties, and weight changes.

Discharge from either the male or the female reproductive tract can cause severe irritation of the surrounding tissues, itching, pain, embarrassment, and anxiety. The nurse asks about the amount, color, consistency, odor, and chronicity of the discharge. Other symptoms may be associated with a discharge and need to be evaluated. Medications (such as antibiotics) and clothing (wearing tight jeans, noncotton underwear, for example) may also initiate or exacerbate genital discharge. Many types of discharge are caused by sexually transmitted diseases. The localization of venereal disease in the body depends on the client's sexual practices. The nurse questions the client about sores, bleeding, itching,

and pain related to the genitals and orifices used by the client during intercourse. It is often helpful to determine if the client's sexual partner displays any symptoms. Many clients attempt relief measures, such as using over-the-counter preparations or douching, before seeking health care. Questions that raise this possibility may give important data.

Masses in the breasts or testes need to be evaluated after discovery by the client. Some masses change in character or size, and the client can often relate these changes to menstrual cycles or trauma. The nurse inquires as to associated symptoms, such as tenderness, heaviness, pain, dimpling, and tender lymph nodes.

For information on reproductive dysfunction, see Chapters 54 and 55.

PHYSICAL ASSESSMENT

FEMALE REPRODUCTIVE SYSTEM

Examination of the breasts, axillae, and lymph nodes often precedes that of the anterior thorax in a complete physical examination. Inspection of the female genitalia and the pelvic examination are usually done at the end of the physical examination. The client often is more apprehensive about these portions of the examination than any other segment. Pain or lack of privacy during previous pelvic or breast examinations may prevent the client from relaxing. The nurse can show the equipment that is going to be used, along with three-dimensional models to demonstrate the assessment procedures. Relaxation and breathing techniques can be taught during this time to assist the client's sense of control. The client is informed about what is going to be done and what she may expect to feel as the examination proceeds. This information allows her to incorporate learned coping mechanisms more successfully than if she were not expecting any discomfort. If the client displays signs of pain or exceptional concern during the procedures, the nurse should stop and make adjustments in his or her assessment plan or techniques. A support person may also be of benefit to the client during the examination.

An annual pelvic examination is recommended for women older than 20 years, as well as for younger sexually active girls. A pelvic examination is indicated to assess menstrual irregularities, unexplained abdominal pain, vaginal discharge or infection, appropriateness of desired contraceptive, rape trauma, and physical changes in the vagina, cervix, uterus, and adnexa. The woman should not douche for at least 24 hours before the pelvic examination because douching may prevent accurate evaluation of smears, cultures, and cytologic data.

Before the pelvic and breast examination, the client is

asked to empty her bladder and to undress completely. The woman is adequately draped to protect modesty throughout the examination. If the client is not wearing a gown, a small towel, placed over the breasts, can be used under the larger drape. Drapes are removed only over the region that is being examined and are replaced when that area has been examined. Drapes that prevent eye contact between the examiner and the client dehumanize the client and prevent successful assessment of the client's comfort during the examination. Mirrors are suggested to facilitate client teaching. The examination is performed in a room that has adequate lighting for body inspection, a comfortable temperature, and assurance of privacy.

BREAST EXAMINATION

The physical examination of the reproductive system begins with the breasts (see Chap. 53 for discussion).

ABDOMINAL EXAMINATION

After the breast examination, the examiner generally completes the thorax and cardiovascular examinations and then inspects, auscultates, and palpates the *abdomen.* The client's arms should be at her sides or over her chest to allow for better relaxation of the abdominal muscles. In the gynecologic examination, the health care provider palpates for symptomatic and asymptomatic abdominopelvic masses. A mass can be of reproductive, gastrointestinal, or urinary tract origin. Careful history taking, combined with the physical examination, can usually determine the origin of a mass. Gynecologic masses, such as ovarian and adnexal masses, can be further differentiated from lesions on the body of the uterus during the bimanual portion of the pelvic examination.

EXAMINATION OF THE EXTERNAL GENITALIA

After the abdominal examination, the client is readied for the inspection of the external genitalia and the pelvic examination. The woman is assisted to the lithotomy position and is asked to place her arms at her sides or over her chest. Her buttocks should extend slightly beyond the edge of the table with her thighs abducted. Drapes and mirrors should be used according to the client's wishes. All equipment should be ready for the vaginal and speculum examination and cytologic studies. Adequate lighting is necessary for careful inspection of the external genitalia and cervix.

The initial inspection and palpation of the *external genitalia* provide an assessment of age-appropriate development. Hair color and distribution over the symphysis pubis and vulva give an indication of the woman's age and hormonal functioning. Pubic hair is

inspected for the presence of lice or scabies. The nurse wears gloves to protect against possible disease and potential cross-contamination from other clients. The client is informed that the genitalia will be touched and separated. The skin and mucosa of the vulva are inspected in a systematic pattern from anterior to posterior for signs of inflammation, infestation, swelling, lesions, or discharge. The paraurethral glands (Skene's glands) are barely visible on either side of the urethral meatus. If infection is suspected, the urethra should be gently "milked" at this time by inserting the index finger into the vagina and pressing its pad against the anterior vaginal wall as the finger is being withdrawn. This procedure usually produces no pain or discharge unless there is inflammation or infection present. The openings of the ducts from the Bartholin's glands cannot be visualized, but the area just outside the lower vaginal orifice is carefully palpated to assess for their inflammation, tenderness, or swelling. Any discharge elicited from these ducts should be cultured because these structures are often involved in gonorrhea infections.

In older women or those who have had difficult deliveries, it is also important to assess *perineal support and the strength of the vaginal walls.* The labia are separated and the client strains downward while the nurse observes any bulging of the anterior or posterior vaginal walls that respectively would indicate a cystocele or rectocele.

PELVIC EXAMINATION

Pelvic Examination with a Speculum

Internal examination of the vagina and cervix is first done manually with the index finger to locate the cervix and to determine its size, consistency, and dilation of the external cervical os. This procedure also allows the examiner to gauge the size of the speculum that is appropriate for the introitus and to predetermine the placement angle of the speculum for visualization of the cervix. Sterile gloves are used for the internal vaginal examination. Water is used if a lubricant is necessary when cytologic or other studies are planned.

After the correct speculum is determined, it should be warmed and lubricated with warm water. The examiner's fingers can ease insertion of the speculum, by pressing down on the perineal body just inside of the vaginal orifice (Fig. 52–9, step 1). The closed speculum should be inserted in an oblique position, with the pressure exerted toward the posterior vaginal wall. The examiner's fingers are removed, and the closed blades of the speculum are rotated to a horizontal position as it is inserted to its full length (Fig. 52–9, step 2). The blades are opened, and the speculum is maneuvered to enable visualization of the cervix. The blades are then locked in place by tightening the thumb screw of the speculum (Fig. 52–9, step 3).

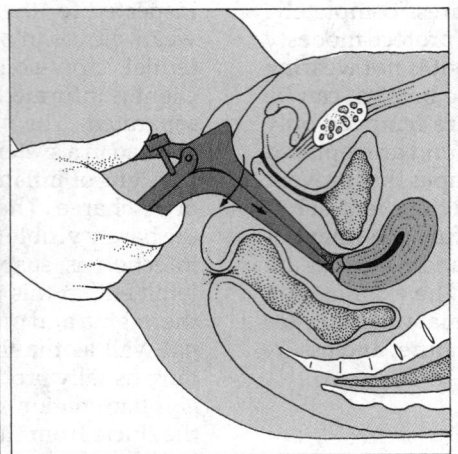

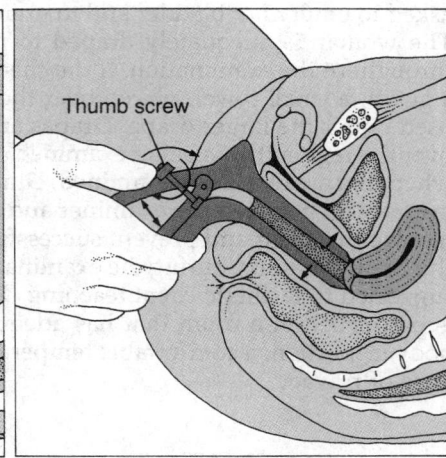

1. With the speculum blades positioned vertically, the nurse presses down on the perineal body just inside the vagina as the speculum is inserted.

2. The nurse removes the fingers from the vagina while continuing to insert the closed blades of the speculum to their full length and rotating them into a horizontal position.

3. The nurse opens the blades and maneuvers the speculum for optimal visualization of the cervix, then tightens the thumb screw to lock the blades in place.

Thumb screw

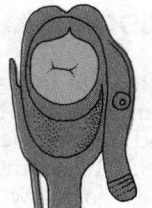

View of the cervix through the speculum

Figure 52–9

Internal examination of the cervix.

The cervix is inspected for color, shape, and dilation of the os; erosions; nodules; masses; discharge; and bleeding. Herpes simplex virus, syphilis, and carcinomas can produce characteristic lesions on the cervix. Specimens are obtained from the cervix, endocervix, and vaginal pool for cytologic studies (see under the later heading Papanicolaou's Test). After completion of the cervical examination, the thumb screw of the speculum is loosened and the blades are slowly withdrawn. The vaginal tissue is inspected for lesions or inflammation during the withdrawal of the speculum.

Bimanual Examination

After withdrawal of the speculum, the examiner proceeds with a bimanual examination. Using a new sterile glove and lubricant, the examiner stands and inserts one or two fingers of one hand into the client's vagina (Fig. 52–10). The examiner exerts pressure primarily against the posterior vaginal wall and checks for masses or tenderness. The cervix and fornix around the cervix are identified. The opposite hand of the examiner is placed on the client's abdomen between her umbilicus and symphysis pubis. Lifting the cervix and uterus with the pelvic hand toward the abdominal hand traps the uterus between them, which allows for examination of the

uterus and adnexa. The size, shape, consistency, and mobility of the uterus are assessed, as well as any tenderness or masses. To palpate each ovary and adnexa, the examiner presses the abdominal hand into the right or left lower quadrant. The fingers in the fornix are used to palpate the ovaries and adnexa against the opposite hand. Obesity or tense abdominal muscles may prevent the examiner from locating the ovaries. A normal ovary is somewhat tender and is assessed for size, shape, consistency, and degree of tenderness. Any mass on the ovary or adnexa is carefully palpated for its size, position, shape, consistency, and mobility. In the premenopausal woman, ovarian cysts may be quite painful and recurrent. An ovarian cyst less than 5 cm (2 in) in diameter is usually functional and responds to hormonal influence. Cysts that are larger than 6 cm (2⅜ in) in diameter are possible neoplasms. Any palpable structure in the adnexa of postmenopausal women suggests cancer because the ovaries 3 to 5 years after menopause are normally atrophied and nonpalpable.

Rectovaginal Examination

A rectovaginal and rectal examination is the last segment of the pelvic examination. The examiner relubricates the glove and places the middle finger in the rec-

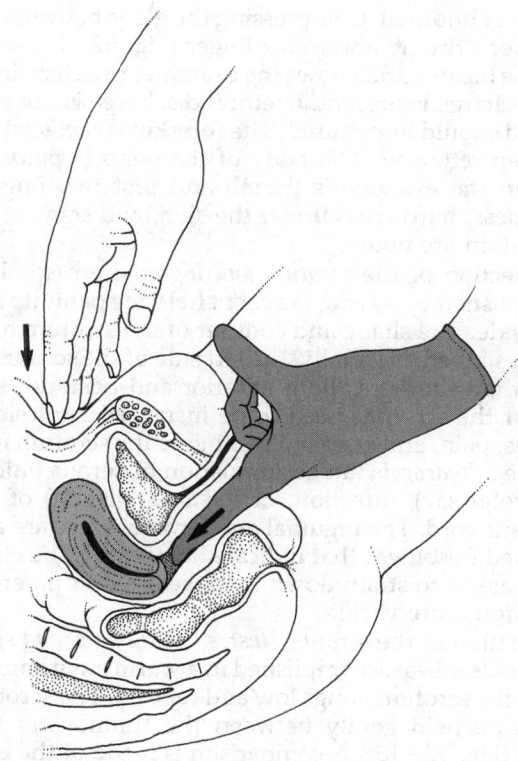

Figure 52-10
Bimanual pelvic examination.

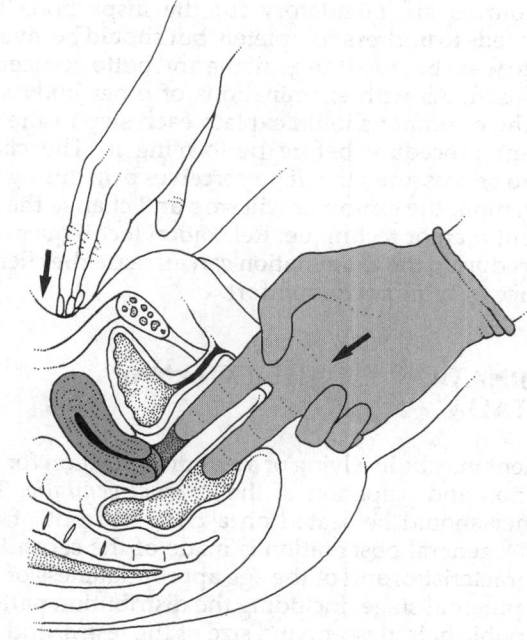

Figure 52-11
Bimanual rectovaginal examination.

tum and the index finger in the vagina (Fig. 52–11). Insertion of the rectal finger is facilitated if the client strains and relaxes the anal sphincter. The procedure for the bimanual examination is repeated. The posterior vaginal and uterine walls are palpated through the rectal mucosa. This examination is especially helpful in assessing a retroflexed or retroverted uterus. An assessment of the tissue structure between the vagina and the rectum can be made by palpating between the two fingers. Care is taken to avoid cross-contamination between the rectum and the vagina. The examiner's finger is slowly removed from the rectum, and any fecal material that remains on the glove should be tested for occult blood.

After the pelvic examination, the perineal area is gently wiped to remove secretions, fecal material, and lubricant. After the foot of the examining table is raised, the client's feet are lowered from the stirrups at the same time to reduce strain on the perineal muscles and lumbosacral ligaments. Nurses should be aware that some clients experience orthostatic hypotension if they sit up too quickly. The nurse evaluates the client for signs of dizziness before letting her get off the examining table. The client may need to clean herself further and is provided with appropriate supplies, including perineal napkins or minipads. The nurse allows the client adequate time and privacy for dressing and is available to answer questions and provide support.

MALE REPRODUCTIVE SYSTEM

Unless a client seeks health care for a genital tract problem, inspection and palpation of the male genitalia and rectum are often "forgotten" or ignored during routine physical examinations. Male clients are often embarrassed and anxious when the reproductive system is assessed. The concern is compounded when the examiner is a woman. The client may be concerned about discomfort, the developmental stage of his genitalia, or the likelihood of an erection during the examination. If the client does have an erection, the examiner should assure him that this is a normal response to a tactile stimulus and should continue the examination.

The examination of the male genitalia is an excellent time for teaching the client about contraceptives, testicular self-examination, and the need for regular prostate examinations. Testicular cancer is one of the most common cancers in young males and can be treated effectively if it is found early. Prostate cancer is common in older men but has a favorable prognosis if diagnosed early. Annual rectal and prostate examinations are currently recommended for men older than 40 years of age, although there is debate about the overall effectiveness of this practice for detecting localized disease.

The examiner wears gloves to protect from possible infection. The room for the examination should offer the client privacy and a comfortable temperature. Proper light sources are mandatory for the inspection. The client needs to undress completely but should be given a gown to wear because the genitalia and buttocks need to be exposed. As with examinations of other body systems, the examiner should explain each step of the assessment procedure before performing it. The client needs to be reassured that if he perceives pain during the examination, the examiner will stop and change the assessment plan or technique. Relaxation techniques and support during the examination can increase the client's tolerance of minimal discomfort.

EXAMINATION OF THE EXTERNAL GENITALIA

The client may be in a lying or a standing position for the inspection and palpation of the *external genitalia*. The examiner should be seated on a chair in front of the client. A general observation is made of the secondary sex characteristics and of the age appropriateness of the developmental stage, including the distribution pattern of the pubic hair, descent and size of the testes, and the size of the scrotum and the penis. Pubic hair is inspected for the presence of lice or scabies.

The skin of the *penis* is inspected for intactness; the dorsal vein should be apparent. Any lesions or ulcers on the penis are noted and may be scraped for cytologic study. If the client has not been circumcised, he is asked to retract the foreskin. This should be accomplished easily, unless the client has developed *phimosis* (a tight prepuce that cannot be retracted). The glans penis is inspected for possible inflammation, fungal infection, syphilic chancres, and carcinomas. *Smegma*, a white, cheesy secretion from the sebaceous glands in the glans, may accumulate under the prepuce. This secretion will not be present in the circumcised male. The glans should also be inspected for the placement of the urinary meatus. Positions other than at the distal end of the

glans are abnormal. Compressing the glans between the examiner's thumb and index finger (Fig. 52 – 12) separates the meatus and allows the examiner to determine if any discharge is present. Urethral discharge is not normal and should be cultured. The foreskin is replaced if it has been retracted. The body of the penis is palpated between the examiner's thumb and first two fingers; tenderness, hard areas under the skin, and signs of inflammation are noted.

Inspection of the *scrotum and inguinal areas* is best accomplished by having the client hold the penis up and to the side. The shape and contour of the scrotum need to be described. Normally, the left side of the scrotum is lower than the right. Both anterior and posterior surfaces of the scrotum need to be inspected for lesions, nodules, pain, and edema. Swelling of the scrotum may indicate a *hydrocele* (an accumulation of serous fluid in the scrotal sac), infection, or *torsion* (twisting) of the spermatic cord. The inguinal and femoral areas are also inspected for bulges that indicate herniation. The client can be asked to strain down to make areas of potential herniation more visible.

Palpation of the *scrotum, testes, epididymis, and spermatic cords* is best accomplished in a warm environment so that the scrotum hangs low and relaxed. The scrotum should be held gently between the thumb and two fingers (Fig. 52 – 13). A comparison is made of the contents of each side of the scrotal sac. Each testis is located and examined for size, shape, symmetry, tenderness, nodules, and consistency. The normal testis has smooth borders, is somewhat sensitive to light palpation, and feels rubbery. Males should be taught self-examination

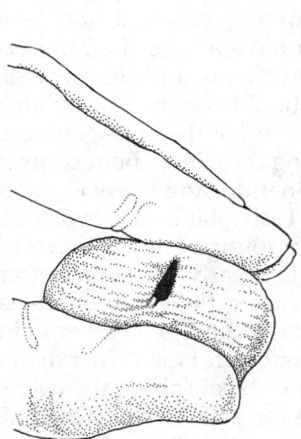

Figure 52 – 12

Compression of glans penis.

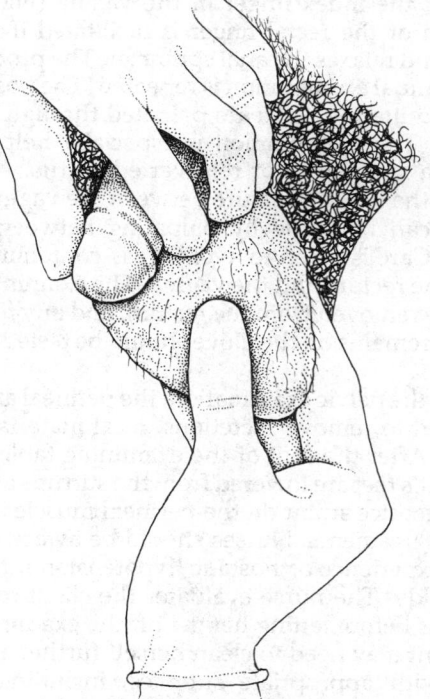

Figure 52 – 13

Palpation of the scrotum.

of the testes (see Chap. 25) and encouraged to perform it monthly. The epididymis can be palpated on the posterior surface of the testis and is examined for size, shape, and tenderness. In clients with infection of the epididymis, its outline will be indistinguishable from that of the testis. The spermatic cord can be palpated along its length between the epididymis and superficial inguinal ring; nodules and swelling are noted and further evaluated. Varicose veins of the spermatic cord (varicocele) feel like a ''bag of worms'' above the testis. If any swelling of the scrotum is observed, the swollen area should be transilluminated. The examining room needs to be darkened for this procedure, and the beam from the penlight is directed through the scrotal swelling from the posterior surface of the scrotum. The light transmits a red glow if the swelling contains a serous fluid. Blood and solid tissue do not transmit the light.

EXAMINATION FOR INGUINAL HERNIA

Palpation for *inguinal hernias* is carried out with the client standing in front of the examiner. The examiner uses the right index finger to examine the client's right side, and the left index finger to examine the left side. To provide sufficient mobility of the examining finger, the fingertip is placed low on the scrotal sac and the loose skin of the sac is directed toward the inguinal canal. The slit-like opening of the external inguinal ring is located by following the direction of the spermatic cord. If possible, the examiner gently introduces the finger into the canal, asks the client to cough or bear down, and is alert for a tapping or pushing sensation against the finger.

EXAMINATION OF THE RECTUM AND PROSTATE

The final assessment of the male reproductive system includes an examination of the *rectum* and *prostate gland*. Ambulatory clients are best examined by having them stand and lean over the examining table. The man is asked to turn his feet inward to relax his buttocks and to provide better accessibility to the anus during the examination. If a client cannot tolerate this position, he can be directed to lie on his side with his top leg flexed. If a pelvic mass is suspected, a lithotomy position permits a bimanual examination.

Proper lighting is necessary for visualization of the anus and surrounding tissue. The examiner notes any lesions, ulcerations, masses, or fissures. Sexual practices of certain clients may increase the risk of developing venereal disease.

To examine the prostate, the pad of a well-lubricated, gloved index finger is pressed against the anus. The finger is slowly inserted, as the sphincter relaxes, in the direction of the umbilicus and is rotated to palpate the anterior rectal wall. The posterior surface of the prostate gland should be felt extending less than 1 cm (3/8 in) into the rectum (Fig. 52–14). The client is informed that he

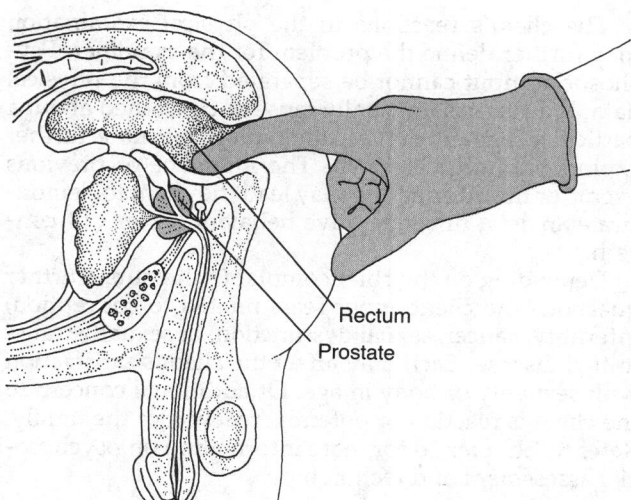

Figure 52–14
Rectal examination of the prostate.

may feel an urge to urinate as the prostate is being examined but that he will not do so. The examiner notes the size of the lateral prostate lobes and their contour, consistency, and mobility. The prostate should feel firm (the consistency has been equated to that of a pencil eraser), smooth, and slightly mobile. It should be nontender across its diameter. The examining finger is extended further to attempt to palpate the *seminal vesicles,* which are palpable only if inflamed. If any discharge is secreted from the penis during palpation of the prostate and seminal vesicles, it should be cultured and examined microscopically. The examining finger is withdrawn, and any fecal material is tested for occult blood.

PSYCHOSOCIAL ASSESSMENT

In addition to the physical assessment, the psychosocial assessment may suggest some contributory factors to the client's illness. The data gathered during the social history provide information on the client's sources of support, strengths, and likely reactions to illness or dysfunction.

Events in a client's personal history and a client's beliefs may negatively influence the ability to enjoy a satisfactory sexual life. These factors may include sexual trauma inflicted during childhood or adulthood, punishment or reproach for masturbation, psychologic trauma, descriptions of reproductive organs or function as ''dirty,'' and cultural influences, such as female passivity during intercourse.

The client's reactions to the physical examination may further define the problem for the examiner. Psychosocial input cannot be separated from the physical data. If a client is unusually tense or concerned about a particular segment of the examination, the nurse further explores nonphysical data. The influence of previous events or misinformation may lead the client to demonstrate anxiety, uncooperative behavior, or lack of concern.

Depending on the chief complaint, the nurse further questions the client about fears related to conception, infertility, cancer, sexual dysfunction, or sexually transmitted disease. Each may affect the client's satisfaction with sexuality or body image. Of additional concern to the client is reaction or potential reaction of the family. Refer to Chapter 10 for more information on psychosocial assessment and techniques.

DIAGNOSTIC ASSESSMENT

An accurate diagnosis of both male and female reproductive system disorders requires the addition of various diagnostic studies to enhance the physical examination and historical data.

LABORATORY TESTS

PAPANICOLAOU'S TEST

Papanicolaou's test, or Pap smear, is a cytologic study that has proved to be an effective tool to detect precancerous and cancerous cells among those shed by the cervix. Health care providers vary in their recommendations for routine Pap tests. Many suggest that the test be performed annually during routine physical examinations. Women in high-risk groups (see Chap. 54) should be advised to have semiannual examinations. The American Cancer Society advises all asymptomatic women older than 20 years of age, and those younger than 20 years if they are sexually active, to have a Pap test at least every 3 years after they have had two negative tests 1 year apart.

Cytologic examinations can also be used to detect viral, fungal, and parasitic disorders. Examination of cells from the vaginal walls can be used to evaluate the function of steroid hormones.

Client preparation. The Pap test should be scheduled between the client's menstrual periods so that the menstrual flow does not interfere with the test interpretation. The woman should not douche, use vaginal medications or deodorants, or have sexual intercourse for at least 24 hours before the test.

At the time of the examination, the woman is placed in the lithotomy position. Relaxation techniques, including concentration on breathing patterns or a visual focus point, may be valuable for the apprehensive client. All steps of the examination should be explained to the client before performing them.

Procedure. A speculum, lubricated with warm water, is inserted into the vagina. The cervix is visualized and then scraped with a curved, wooden spatula (Fig. 52–15). Exfoliated cells are obtained from the cervix, endocervix, and vaginal pool. The specimens are immediately transferred from the wooden spatula to glass slides and are either sprayed with or immersed in a fixative

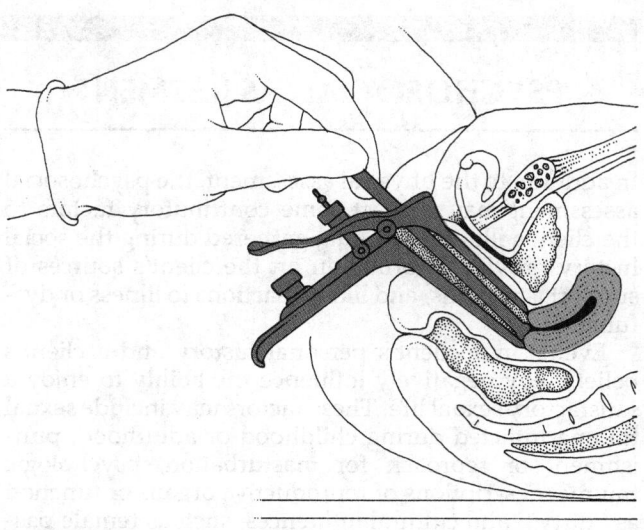
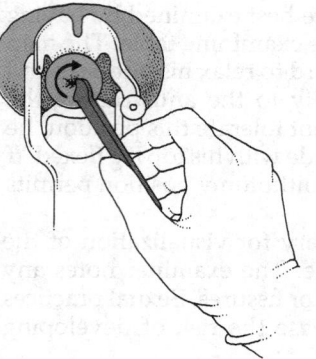
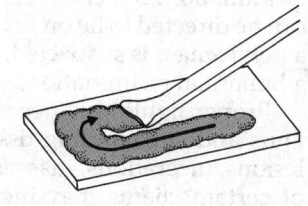

1. Through a vaginal speculum, the nurse takes a scraping of exfoliated cells from the cervix, endocervix, and vaginal pool with a wooden spatula.

2. The nurse immediately transfers the specimens to a glass slide and applies a fixative solution.

Figure 52–15

Procedure for obtaining a cervical smear (Pap test).

TABLE 52–1   Classification of Papanicolaou's Test Results

Current Descriptive Terminology

Normal

Metaplasia

Inflammation

Minimal atypia, koilocytosis

Mild dysplasia

Moderate dysplasia

Severe dysplasia, carcinoma in situ

Invasive carcinoma

Papanicolaou's Classification

Class 1: absence of atypical or abnormal cells

Class 2: atypical cytologic results but no evidence of malignancy

Class 3: cytologic results suggestive of, but not conclusive for, malignancy

Class 4: cytologic results strongly suggestive of malignancy

Class 5: cytologic results conclusive for malignancy

solution. If the smear is allowed to dry on the slide before the fixative has been applied, diagnosis will be inaccurate. The slides are sent to a laboratory where they are interpreted.

Papanicolaou's classification of the cytologic findings and the descriptive terminology currently preferred by clinicians are given in Table 52–1.

Follow-up care. The client should be provided with a perineal pad after the procedure to protect her clothes from any bleeding from the cervix. The results of the test are shared with the client in person, by telephone, or by letter. If a woman's smear has demonstrated atypical cells, she should be encouraged to have follow-up testing.

BLOOD STUDIES

Pituitary Gonadotropin

Determinations of the quantitative levels of follicle-stimulating hormone (FSH), luteinizing hormone (LH), and prolactin are helpful in the differential diagnosis of male and female reproductive tract disorders. The serum levels are measured by the radioimmunoassay method. There are no dietary restrictions before the test. Table 52–2 gives the normal values and the significance of abnormal findings.

Steroid Hormones

The radioimmunoassay technique is available to detect estrogen, progesterone, and testosterone levels at any given time in the female menstrual cycle and for the adult male (see Table 52–2).

Serologic Tests

Serologic blood studies detect antigen-antibody reactions that occur in response to foreign organisms. This form of diagnostic testing is of benefit only after an infection has become well established. Serologic testing can be used in the evaluation of exposure to organisms causing syphilis and rubella and to type 2 herpes simplex virus. Results may be read as "nonreactive," "weakly reactive," or "reactive." A single titer is not as revealing as serial titers, which can detect the rise in antibody reactions as the body continues to fight the intruder.

VDRL

The VDRL (Venereal Disease Research Laboratory) test is used to detect, confirm, and follow cases of syphilis. This type of nontreponemal antigen test is not absolutely specific or sensitive for syphilis, but it is economical and highly indicative. Some acute and chronic conditions that cause false-positive results are tuberculosis, infectious mononucleosis, recent smallpox vaccination, rheumatoid arthritis, systemic lupus erythematosus, subacute bacterial endocarditis, and hepatitis.

The results of a test vary with the stage of syphilis. During the first week after a chancre appears, the test result is usually negative because the body has not had enough time to produce a sufficiently elevated amount of antibody. The serologic test result is usually positive 1 to 3 weeks after the chancre appears. If the primary syphilis is treated, the serologic titers almost always return to nonreactive levels within 6 months. During the secondary stage of syphilis, the titers are quite high and remain so for up to 2 years after treatment. The VDRL cannot effectively detect tertiary syphilis.

The results of the VDRL are read qualitatively. The normal range is classed as "nonreactive." A titer of 1:8 or greater indicates the presence of syphilis. A titer above 1:32 can indicate the second stage.

Treponema pallidum *Immobilization Test and Fluorescent Treponemal Antibody Absorption Test*

The treponemal antibody test (treponemal immobilization test [TPI]; fluorescent treponemal antibody absorption test [FTA-ABS]) is specific to *Treponema pallidum*; however, it is more expensive and time-consuming than the VDRL. Samples are usually sent to special laboratories for analysis. This test yields few false-positive results and is used to confirm or rule out the

TABLE 52–2 Normal Values and Significance of Abnormal Findings in Common Laboratory Tests Used in Assessment of the Reproductive System

Test	Normal Values	Significance of Abnormal Findings
Serum Studies		

Follicle-stimulating hormone (FSH)	Men 4–25 mIU/mL
	Women
	  Follicular phase 5–20 mIU/mL
	  Midcycle 15–40 mIU/mL
	  Luteal phase 5–11 mIU/mL
	  Postmenopause 40–200 mIU/mL
		Decreased levels indicate possible
		  Infertility
		  Anorexia nervosa
		  Neoplasm
		Elevations indicate possible
		  Turner's syndrome

Luteinizing hormone (LH)	Men 6–23 mIU/mL
	Women
	  Follicular phase 5–30 mIU/mL
	  Midcycle 75–150 mIU/mL
	  Luteal phase 5–40 mIU/mL
	  Postmenopause 35–120 mIU/mL
		Decreased levels indicate possible
		  Infertility
		  Anovulation
		Elevations indicate possible
		  Ovarian failure
		  Turner's syndrome

Prolactin	Men 7–18 ng*/mL
	Women 6–24 ng/mL
		Elevations indicate possible
		  Galactorrhea (breast discharge)
		  Pituitary tumor
		  Disease of hypothalamus or
		    pituitary gland
		  Hypothyroidism

Estradiol	Men 0.5–5 ng/dL
	Women
	  Follicular phase 2–20 ng/dL
	  Midcycle 12–40 ng/dL
	  Luteal phase 10–30 ng/dL
	  Postmenopause 1–5 ng/dL
		*Elevations of estradiol, total
		  estrogens, and estriol in men*
		  indicate possible
		  Gynecomastia
		  Decreased body hair
		  Increased fat deposits
		  Feminization

Total estrogens	Men 4–14 ng/dL
	Women
	  Follicular phase 40–103 ng/dL
	  Midcycle 75–139 ng/dL
	  Luteal phase 47–113 ng/dL
		*Elevations of estradiol, total
		  estrogens, and estriol in women*
		  indicate possible
		  Uterine cancer
		  Precocious puberty
		  Cystic breast disease
		  Corpus luteum cysts

Estriol	Men and nonpregnant women
	  <0.5 ng/dL
		*Decreased levels of estradiol, total
		  estrogens, and estriol in women*
		  indicate possible
		  Amenorrhea
		  Climacteric
		  Impending abortion
		  Hypothalamic disorders

Progesterone	Men <1 ng/mL
	Women
	  Follicular phase 0.2–0.6 ng/mL
	  Midcycle 0.3–3.5 ng/mL
	  Luteal phase 6.5–32 ng/mL
		Decreased levels in women indicate
		  possible
		  Inadequate luteal phase
		  Amenorrhea
		Elevations in women indicate
		  possible
		  Ovarian luteal cysts

Testosterone	Men 300–1100 ng/dL
	Women 25–90 ng/dL
		Decreased levels in men indicate
		  possible
		  Hypogonadism
		  Klinefelter's syndrome

TABLE 52–2   Normal Values and Significance of Abnormal Findings in Common Laboratory Tests Used in Assessment of the Reproductive System *Continued*

Test	Normal Values	Significance of Abnormal Findings
Serum Studies		
		Hypopituitarism
		Orchidectomy
		Elevations in women indicate possible
		Adrenal neoplasm
		Polycystic ovaries
		Ovarian tumors
Urine Studies		
Total estrogens	Men 5–18 µg/24 h	*Elevations* indicate possible
	Women	Testicular tumors
	Follicular phase 4–25 µg/24 h	Adrenal tumors
	Midcycle/luteal phase 22–105	Ovarian tumors
	µg/24 h	Pregnancy
		Decreased levels indicate possible
		Ovarian dysfunction
		Intrauterine death
Pregnanediol	Men 0.1–0.2 mg/24 h	*Elevations* indicate possible
	Women	Luteal ovarian cysts
	Follicular phase 0.5–1.5 mg/24 h	Ovarian neoplasms
	Luteal phase 2–7 mg/24 h	Adrenal disorders
	Menopause 0.2–1 mg/24 h	*Decreased levels* indicate possible
		Amenorrhea
17-Ketosteroids	Men (20–50 yr) 5–26 mg/24 h	*Elevations* indicate possible
	Women (20–50 yr) 3–16 mg/24 h	Cushing's syndrome
		Increased androgen or cortisol production
		Severe stress
		Decreased levels indicate possible
		Addison's disease
		Hypopituitarism

* 1 ng = 1 billionth of a gram.

diagnosis of syphilis after a positive VDRL result. The test results may remain positive long after treatment.

URINALYSIS FOR STEROID HORMONES

Twenty-four-hour urine samples can be screened for levels of total estrogens and pregnanediol (urinary by-product of progesterone) (see Table 52–2).

MICROSCOPIC STUDIES

Wet Prep (Wet Smears)

Secretions from the vaginal pool can be obtained at the beginning of a speculum examination. Specimens can also be obtained from the vaginal walls, labia, or vulva during the examination. The specimens are placed on glass slides and are treated with a wet preparation such as saline or potassium hydroxide (KOH). The slides are examined under a microscope to confirm or rule out the presence of a pathogen. Table 52–3 presents the common types of wet preparations used to diagnose selected vaginal problems.

Cultures

Cultures are used to identify pathogenic organisms and to determine the appropriate antibiotic therapy. Specimens for culture analysis are obtained from any discharge or orifice of the male or female reproductive system. When a nonspecific bacterial infection is sus-

TABLE 52–3 Wet Preparations Used for the Diagnosis of Common Vaginal Problems

Wet Preparation	Problems
Normal saline	Cervicitis Trichomoniasis Nonspecific vaginitis
Potassium hydroxide (KOH)	Candidiasis (*Candida albicans, Monilia*) *Gardnerella* vaginitis
Gram's stain	*Haemophilus* vaginitis
Tzanck's test	Herpes simplex virus (HSV type 2) infection

pected, routine bacteriologic cultures and antibiotic sensitivity studies are ordered.

The culture to detect *Neisseria gonorrhoeae* is one of the most important in evaluating the reproductive system. The culture is the only means of confirming the diagnosis of gonorrhea in asymptomatic women. To collect the specimen, the female client is prepared for a speculum examination, and any excess mucus is wiped from the cervix. A sterile cotton-tipped swab is inserted into the endocervical canal and is moved from side to side. It is important to leave the swab in the endocervix long enough for it to absorb secretions (approximately 30 seconds). Specimens from male clients can be taken directly from any penile discharge. Additional specimens from males or females can also be obtained from the urethra, rectum, and oropharynx. The swab is then rolled in a Z-shaped pattern on a medium that is selective for the growth of gonococcus and that inhibits the growth of the usual contaminants. The Z-shaped pattern is cross-streaked with a sterile wire loop to help isolate the *N. gonorrhoeae* colonies. The plates are then incubated in a carbon dioxide–rich atmosphere.

Tests for Acquired Immunodeficiency Syndrome

Routine laboratory tests are of little diagnostic value in detecting acquired immunodeficiency syndrome (AIDS). One screening test that is approved by the U.S. Food and Drug Administration is ELISA (enzyme-linked immunosorbent assay), which tests for the presence of the AIDS antibody in blood. The test detects the presence of only the antibodies, not the virus. Five to 10 mL of venous blood is taken from the client after consent has been obtained. If the client is a blood donor, signed consent is not required, and 10 to 100 mL is obtained from the donated blood. If the first sample is reactive, it is retested because false-positive results can occur ("Recommendation for Assisting," 1985).

The procedure that confirms the presence of human T cell lymphotrophic virus type III (HTLV III) is the Western blot. The virus protein is separated on a gel and is then incubated and treated with antihuman antibody detector. A positive reaction confirms a high probability of exposure to the virus (Kee, 1987). For further discussion, see Chapter 27.

RADIOGRAPHIC EXAMINATIONS

GENERAL X-RAY STUDIES

A *KUB* (kidney, ureter, and bladder) is an x-ray film of the abdomen that shows these structures and is used in the assessment of either male or female reproductive system disorders. Pelvic masses, calcified tumors or fibroids, dermoid cysts, and metastatic bone changes are evident on this x-ray film. Urologic studies may enhance the film by use of contrast media. No specific client preparation is needed.

Bone scans, intravenous pyelograms, barium enemas, and chest films are also included in the work-up of the client with suspected metastatic cancer. They help to determine the extent of the metastasis and obstruction or displacement of the organs.

COMPUTED TOMOGRAPHY

Computed tomography scans for reproductive system disorders primarily involve the abdomen and the pelvis. They are useful to detect and evaluate masses and lymphatic enlargement from metastasis. This scan can differentiate solid tissue masses from cystic or hemorrhagic structures.

HYSTEROSALPINGOGRAPHY

A *hysterosalpingogram* is an x-ray study of the cervix, uterus, and fallopian tubes that is done after the injection of a contrast substance. It is useful in infertility work-ups to evaluate tubal anatomy and patency and uterine abnormalities, such as fibroids, tumors, and fistulas. The study can also provide data as to the cause of repeated abortions, dysmenorrhea, and postmenopausal bleeding. The study should not be attempted for at least 6 weeks after abortion, delivery, or dilation and curettage. Other contraindications to the test include reproductive tract infection or severe systemic illness. There is a significant incidence of false-positive and false-negative interpretations.

Client preparation. The examination should be scheduled in a radiology department for the 24th day after the end of the client's normal menses. The scheduling is important to prevent the accidental flushing of a fertilized ovum from the fallopian tube or the exposure of a fetus to radiation.

The client prepares herself by taking a cathartic the evening before the test, followed by an enema on the morning of the examination, to reduce distortion of the x-rays by gas shadows.

The date of her last menstrual period is confirmed on the day of the examination and is recorded in the progress notes. A consent form needs to be signed by the woman. Because discomfort is anticipated during the examination, the woman may be premedicated with analgesics or nonsteroidal anti-inflammatory agents. She should be informed that she may experience some nausea and vomiting, abdominal cramping, or faintness. The nurse provides support and assistance with relaxation techniques.

Procedure. The client is placed in the lithotomy position with the cervix visualized through a speculum. A radiopaque oil or water-soluble dye is injected by the radiologist through the cervix to fill and highlight the interior of the cervix, uterus, and fallopian tubes. If the fallopian tubes are patent, the contrast material spills into the peritoneal cavity. Usually, only two or three films are taken to show the path and distribution of the contrast medium.

Follow-up care. The client may experience pelvic pain after the study and should receive medications accordingly. She may also experience referred shoulder pain because of irritation of the phrenic nerve by the dye. The woman is given a perineal pad after the test to prevent the soiling of clothes from dye draining from the cervix. The woman should contact her physician if bloody discharge continues for 4 days or more and to report any signs of infection, such as lower quadrant pain, fever, malodorous discharge, and tachycardia.

MAMMOGRAPHY

Mammography is an x-ray study of the soft tissue of the breast. Mammograms are used to assess differences in the density of the breast tissue. They are especially helpful in the evaluation of breasts that have poorly defined masses, multiple masses or nodules, nipple changes or discharge, skin changes, and pain. Mammography can detect many cancers that are not palpable by physical examination; however, some actual cancers are evaluated as benign by mammography.

In young women's breasts, there is little difference in density between normal glandular tissue and malignant tumors, which makes the mammogram less useful for discovery and diagnosis of breast masses in these women. In older women, the higher percentage of fatty tissue appears lighter than do neoplasms. Cancer and cysts may have the same density, but cysts usually have smooth borders and neoplasms often have starburst-shaped margins.

Client preparation. There are no dietary restrictions before the mammogram. The woman is asked not to use creams, powders, or deodorant on the breasts or underarm areas before the study because the aluminum

chlorhydrate can mimic calcium clusters. If there is any possibility of pregnancy, the test should be rescheduled. The purpose of the examination and its anticipated discomforts should be explained. The nurse provides a cover gown and adequate privacy for the client to undress above the waist. The client also needs appropriate support and may need time to express her concerns about the mammogram and the presence of any lumps. Because this is a time when the client is anxious about the health of her breasts, it is an excellent opportunity to teach or reinforce self-examination of the breasts.

Procedure. The client is positioned next to the x-ray machine with one breast exposed. A film plate and the platform of the machine are placed on opposite sides of the breast to be examined. As much breast tissue as possible is included between the plates. The woman may experience some discomfort when the breast is compressed during the positioning and the test. The test takes approximately 15 minutes; however, the client is asked to wait until the films are developed in case a view needs to be repeated. Mammography usually requires two low-dose x-ray views of each breast: a view from the side and a view from above each breast. Mammograms of small breasts are not as effective as those of larger breasts because there is not sufficient breast tissue to compress in the x-ray views.

Follow-up care. The client needs to understand that repeating one or more breast views does not imply that she has breast cancer. It is important to have a physician speak to the client to interpret the films as soon as possible after the test.

XEROMAMMOGRAPHY

The *xeromammogram* provides an x-ray image of the breast for which a much lower dose of radiation is used than that for the traditional low-dose mammogram. This dose is made possible by the use of a special selenium-coated plate that is placed under the breast to be x-rayed. The xerogram is photoelectrically recorded on paper, without the use of film. Its use has gradually been gaining in popularity because the high-contrast effect of the picture is easier to read and often more accurate. Xerography is used for the same indications as low-dose mammography and has the same client preparation and follow-up care.

OTHER DIAGNOSTIC STUDIES

ENDOSCOPIC STUDIES

Colposcopy and Colpomicroscopy

The colposcope and colpomicroscope allow three-dimensional magnification and intense illumination of epithelium that is suspected of being diseased. Colposcopy is suited for inspection of the cervical epithelium, vagina, and vulvar epithelium. The use of this procedure can locate the exact site of precancerous and malignant lesions for biopsy, and it is an effective tool to screen women at high risk for developing vaginal changes because of DES exposure (Nelson et al., 1984).

Client preparation.   The woman is placed in the lithotomy position and is given the same support as that for a pelvic examination. She should not have douched or used vaginal preparations before the examination. The relatively painless procedure is explained in advance, and the instrument is shown to the client.

Because this procedure provides the opportunity for accurate site selection for tissue biopsy, the client should also be prepared for the latter test. Materials required for cytologic studies and biopsy should be readily available.

Procedure.   The cervix, or vaginal site, is located through a speculum examination. Lubricants other than water should not be used. Cells in the area may be stained or left unstained to enhance visualization. The cervix is cleaned of secretions and is moistened with normal saline, which allows vascular patterns and the junction between the columnar epithelium and the squamous epithelium to be better visualized. Acetic acid, 3%, applied to the cervix acts as a mucolytic agent to draw moisture from the tissue and to accentuate important morphologic features. The colposcope or colpomicroscope is then used to inspect the area in question.

Follow-up care.   The woman is assisted after the procedure as with a pelvic examination and is provided with supplies to clean the perineum. She is also given a perineal pad to absorb any dye or discharge. If procedures other than direct visualization were done, follow-up care needs to be revised appropriately.

Culdoscopy

Culdoscopy, a type of endoscopy, is the simplest procedure for direct visualization of the pelvic viscera in women. As a highly accurate diagnostic tool, it is used in an attempt to avoid surgical intervention. Culdoscopy is useful to rule out ectopic pregnancy and to evaluate ovarian disorders and pelvic masses. It can also provide data in some cases of infertility or unexplained pelvic pain.

Client preparation.   The procedure and its associated discomforts are explained to the woman before the examination. The woman is assisted to a knee-chest position, which provides the best view of the pelvis. She will need support to maintain this position during the procedure. Most culdoscopies are done with only light sedation and a local anesthetic in the vaginal cul-de-sac.

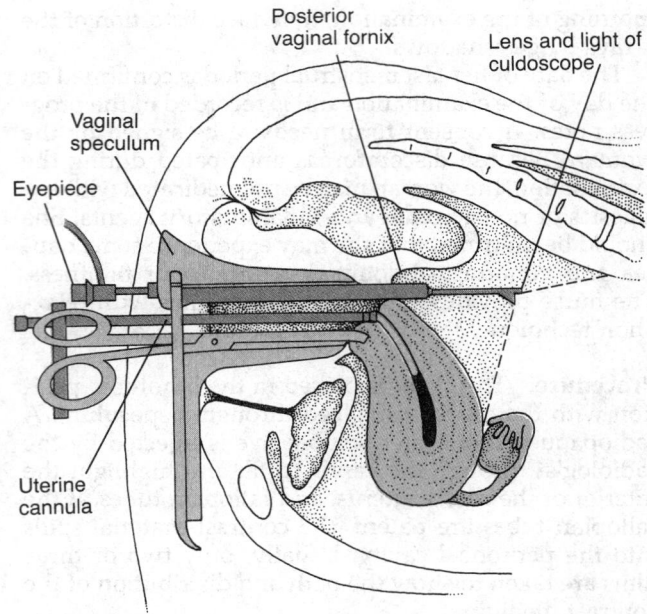

Figure 52–16

Culdoscopy.

Additional teaching may instruct the client to forcefully exhale on removal of the culdoscope to remove some intraperitoneal air and to minimize referred shoulder pain.

Procedure.   With the client in the knee-chest position, the posterior vaginal wall is retracted. After the cervix is stabilized, the culdoscope, a tubular instrument with a lamp and a lens near its tip, is inserted through an incision in the posterior vaginal fornix (Fig. 52–16). The instrument provides a detailed view of the posterior cul-de-sac and pelvic contents. After the examination, the site heals easily without sutures.

Follow-up care.   The client may experience severe shoulder pain when she first sits up. This pain is caused by air irritating the phrenic nerve of the diaphragm. The client is advised not to douche or have intercourse for approximately 2 weeks after the procedure.

Laparoscopy

Laparoscopy (pelvic peritoneoscopy) can be used as a diagnostic tool to explore the pelvic cavity. In addition to the indications previously given for culdoscopy, laparoscopy is used as a route for surgical procedures such as tubal sterilization, ovarian biopsy, cyst or graafian follicle aspiration (to retrieve ova for in vitro fertilization), lysis of adhesions around the fallopian tubes, and retrieval of "lost" intrauterine devices. Laparoscopy is preferable to laparotomy for minor surgical procedures because it requires only a small infraumbilical incision and involves less discomfort and hospitalization.

Client preparation. The procedure, risks (associated with the use of general anesthesia; occurrence of postoperative shoulder pain; rare complications of infection or electric burns) (Dugan, 1985), and anticipated discomforts are explained to the client. The procedure can be performed with the client under regional or general anesthesia. Clients should expect mild discomfort from the incision site and may experience referred shoulder pain from phrenic nerve irritation.

Procedure. The client is anesthetized and is placed in the lithotomy position. A straight drainage catheter is inserted into the bladder, and the abdomen is prepared. The operating table is placed in a slight Trendelenburg's position to cause the intestines to fall away from the pelvis. The cervix is held with a cannula to allow for movement of the uterus during laparoscopy (Fig. 52–17). A needle is inserted below the umbilicus to infuse carbon dioxide into the pelvic cavity, which distends the abdomen and permits better visualization of the organs. A trocar and cannula are inserted into an infraumbilical incision. After they are in place in the abdominal cavity, the trocar is removed and the laparoscope is inserted. The surgeon can thus visualize the pelvic cavity and reproductive organs. Further instrumentation is possible through a second small incision. The laparoscope is removed at the end of the procedure, and the abdomen is deflated. The incision is usually closed with absorbable sutures and is dressed with an adhesive bandage.

Follow-up care. The client receives postoperative care similar to that of other clients after general anesthesia but is usually discharged on the day of the surgery. The discomfort from the incision is usually alleviated by oral analgesics. The greatest discomfort is due to referred shoulder pain caused by residual gas in the peritoneal cavity. Most of these sensations disappear within 48 hours. Clients are instructed to change their own dressing and to observe the wound for signs of infection or hematoma. They should be advised to shower, not bathe in a tub, until the umbilical incision has healed. Strenuous activity should be avoided for the first week after the procedure.

Hysteroscopy

Hysteroscopy is an endoscopic examination that permits visualization of the interior of the uterus and the cervical canal. The hysteroscope includes a lens with fiberoptic lighting in conjunction with an aqueous solution of carbon dioxide as the medium to distend the uterus. Hysteroscopy can be used for removal of intrauterine devices and as a complement to other diagnostic tests for infertility and unexplained bleeding.

Client preparation. The client is informed of all aspects of the procedure and is given the same preparation as that for a pelvic examination. The procedure is best performed 5 days after menses have ceased to eliminate the possibility of pregnancy. The client is placed in the lithotomy position and is anesthetized with a pericervical or spinal block.

Procedure. After the client is anesthetized, the cervix is dilated. The hysteroscope is inserted through the cervix. Because a medium is used to distend the uterus, an opportunity is provided for cells to be pushed through the fallopian tubes and into the pelvic cavity. Hysteroscopy is contraindicated in clients with suspected cervical or endometrial cancer, in clients with infection of the upper genital tract, and in pregnant clients.

Follow-up care. If the client has had spinal anesthesia, she should remain in a flat position for 8 hours after the procedure. The client may experience some cervical and uterine cramping and should be treated with analgesics. Care is the same as that after a pelvic examination.

Culdocentesis

Culdocentesis, although not an endoscopic study, provides data on the character of fluid in the pelvic cavity. *Culdocentesis* is the needle aspiration of fluid from the posterior cul-de-sac to determine the presence or absence of free blood (presence may indicate ruptured ectopic pregnancy) or pus (presence may indicate infection, e.g., pelvic inflammatory disease) (Kuczynski, 1986). Usually, no anesthesia is required for insertion of the aspiration needle through the vaginal fornix. The amount of information obtainable from this procedure is limited, and a negative result is inconclusive.

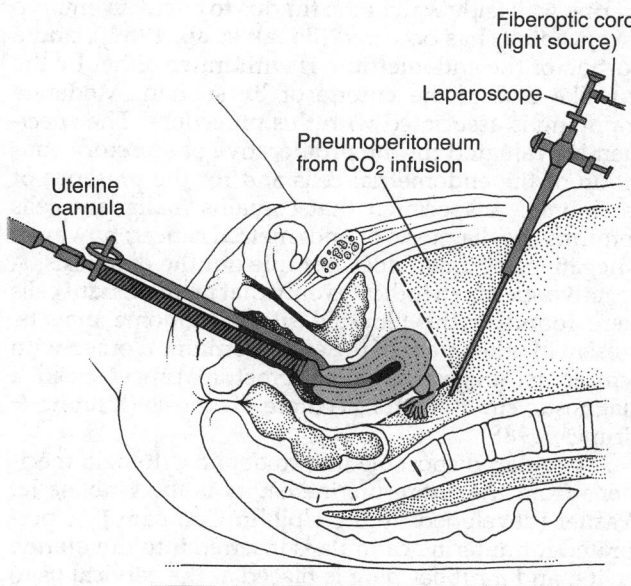

Figure 52–17
Laparoscopy.

BIOPSY STUDIES

Cervical Biopsy

In a *cervical biopsy*, cervical tissue is removed for cytologic study. A biopsy should definitely be performed in a client with an identifiable cervical lesion, regardless of the cytologic findings. The biopsy is usually performed in conjunction with colposcopy as a follow-up to a suggestive Pap test. The type and extent of the biopsy vary. If a lesion is clearly visible with the use of a colposcope, a punch biopsy may be used to extract a small column of tissue. Cervical tissue specimens should include a portion of the squamous-columnar epithelial junction because most cervical malignancies occur in this area. Punch biopsy can be done as an office procedure without the use of anesthesia because the cervix has few pain receptors. When no lesions are visible or when the Pap smear indicates malignancy, an inverted cone biopsy (*conization*) of the cervix is advised. This procedure requires anesthesia and operating room capabilities because of the increased risk of complications.

Client preparation. The client should be scheduled for the biopsy in the early proliferative phase of the menstrual cycle, when the cervix is least vascular. The procedure that is selected should be explained to the client. Because a biopsy is done to evaluate potentially malignant cells, most women become anxious and need time to discuss their feelings and fears. The use of relaxation techniques may facilitate the woman's comfort. The client is placed in the lithotomy position and is prepared in the same way as for a pelvic examination. Further preparation depends on the type of procedure to be performed.

Procedure. The client is anesthetized according to the needs of the chosen procedure. The cervix is visualized, and the tissue sample obtained by needle punch or conization (removal of a cone-shaped tissue specimen with a cold knife scalpel). All specimens are immediately placed into a formalin solution. Cauterization of the biopsy site with a silver nitrate stick usually is sufficient to control light bleeding from the punch biopsy.

Follow-up care. The type of anesthesia that was used for the procedure determines the type of immediate postoperative care provided by the nurse. The client should be advised to rest for 24 hours and to avoid lifting of heavy objects. A tampon, used as postoperative packing, should be left in place for 8 to 24 hours. Although some oozing is considered to be normal, the client needs to be advised to report any excessive bleeding (more than the amount of normal menstrual flow). She should also be taught about and know to report any signs of infection. Perineal care is encouraged with antiseptic solution rinses and frequent changing of the perineal pad. The client is advised to minimize her potential for constipation by drinking fluids, eating a high-fiber diet, and getting light exercise. Douching, use of tampons, and sexual intercourse should be avoided until healing of the biopsy site is complete (about 2 weeks).

Endometrial Biopsy and Aspiration

Both *endometrial biopsy* and *aspiration* are techniques to obtain cells directly from the lining of the uterus in women at risk for cancer of the endometrium. Endometrial biopsy is also of significant value for assessment of functional menstrual disturbances (especially anovulatory bleeding) and infertility (corpus luteum function).

When menstrual disturbances are evaluated, the biopsy is generally done in the immediate premenstrual period to serve as an index of progesterone influence and ovulation. A biopsy done in the last half of the menstrual cycle (approximately days 21 and 22) is used to evaluate corpus luteum function and the presence or absence of a persistent secretory endometrium. Postmenopausal women may have biopsies done at any time.

Client preparation. Menstrual data need to be obtained from the client and included on the specimen slip for the pathologist. The client is given the same preparation as that for a pelvic examination but is advised that she may experience some cramping when the cervix is dilated. Relaxation and breathing techniques and analgesia are often of value.

Procedure. An endometrial biopsy is often done as an office procedure with or without anesthesia. After the uterus is sounded (measured) and the cervix is sufficiently dilated, the curette or intrauterine cannula is inserted into the uterus.

If a curette is used, it is pressed firmly against the uterine wall (side wall in the fundus to avoid an embryo if conception has occurred [Bobak et al., 1989]), and a portion of the endometrium is withdrawn either by the cup-like end of the curette or by suction. Moderate cramping is associated with this procedure. The specimen is evaluated for the proliferative or secretory condition of the endometrial cells and for the presence of carcinoma. A specimen that contains malignant cells confirms the diagnosis of endometrial cancer; however, a negative specimen does not rule out the diagnosis. A negative specimen indicates only that no malignant cells were found at the biopsied site. Carcinoma may be present in other areas of the endometrium. Women with symptoms suggestive of endometrial cancer need a diagnostic curettage for accurate diagnosis (Kaunitz & Grimes, 1988).

A popular, disposable unit to obtain cytologic specimens from the entire uterine cavity is the Gravlee Jet Washer (developed by the Upjohn Company). A perforated intrauterine cannula is inserted into the uterine cavity, and a rubber plug is placed at the cervical os to create an air-tight system. A reservoir filled with isotonic saline and an empty collecting syringe are attached to the end of the cannula. When the plunger of the syringe is pulled, a negative pressure is created in the uterus. Saline is drawn from the reservoir, and the entire uterine cavity is irrigated. During the process, cells and small tissue fragments are dislodged and collected in the syringe. The negative pressure that is created in the uterus prevents potentially malignant cells from being forced into the fallopian tubes.

Follow-up care. The client should be allowed to rest on the examining table until cramping has subsided. She is allowed to clean the perineum and is given a perineal pad. Any signs of infection or excessive bleeding should be reported to the physician. The woman should refrain from intercourse or douching until all discharge has ceased.

Breast Biopsy and Aspiration

Figure 52–18 shows three types of breast biopsy. An *incisional* breast biopsy is the surgical removal of tissue from a breast mass. An *excisional* biopsy removes the mass itself for histologic evaluation. *Aspiration* biopsy is the removal of fluid or tissue from the breast mass through a large-bore needle. Any breast mass needs to be further evaluated for the possibility of cancer. Fibrocystic lesions, as well as fibroadenomas and intraductal

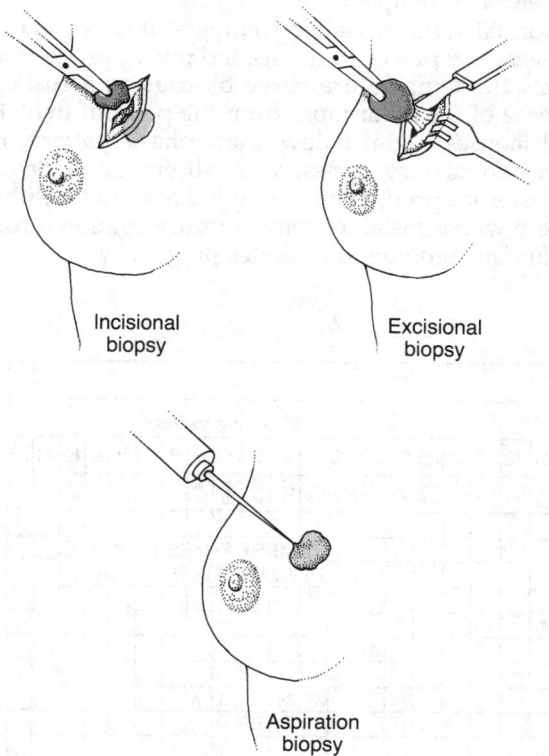

Incisional biopsy

Excisional biopsy

Aspiration biopsy

Figure 52–18

Breast biopsy techniques.

papillomas, can be differentiated by biopsy. Histologic examination should also be done on any discharge from the breasts.

Client preparation. The instructions to the client depend on the type of biopsy that she is to have and the type of anesthesia required. The woman should be prepared to expect sensations of pulling or probing during the procedure.

Procedure. Aspiration biopsy is often performed in outpatient settings without anesthesia. The mass is located by palpation of the breast. The needle is then directed into the lump, and the contents are aspirated into the syringe. The contents are placed on a slide for Papanicolaou's evaluation. Fluid from benign cysts may appear clear to dark green-brown; bloody fluid suggests cancer. If no fluid is aspirated, the tumor is said to be solid and should be examined by incisional biopsy.

Incisional or excisional biopsies are performed in a day surgery or hospital setting with local or general anesthesia. The tumor specimen that is obtained is evaluated by the frozen section technique.

Follow-up care. Postoperative discomfort is usually mild and controlled with analgesics. The incisional site should be assessed for bleeding and edema. A properly supportive brassiere should be continuously worn by the woman for 1 week postoperatively. The woman should avoid cold temperatures to prevent nipple contractions that can cause stress on the incision. Numbness around the biopsy site may last 2 to 3 months.

Needle Biopsy of the Prostate

A *needle aspiration biopsy* of the prostate gland is done to retrieve cells for histologic study when prostatic cancer is suspected. The procedure is often done at the same time as cystoscopy with the client under the same anesthesia. Needle biopsies can also be done without or under local anesthesia.

Client preparation. Preparation for the procedure depends on the technique to be used to puncture the gland. Client teaching provides data on the expected discomforts. Breathing and relaxation techniques can also be taught and used during the examination. Because this procedure is to evaluate prostatic cells for potential malignancy, the man will need support and time to discuss his fears. Preparation for a transrectal biopsy involves the use of cleaning enemas and prophylactic antibiotics to reduce the risk of bacterial contamination of the blood stream or prostatic tissue. Local anesthesia is used at the site of transperineal biopsy.

Procedure. The client is placed in the same position as that for a rectal examination. After the local anesthetic is injected for the transperineal biopsy, the examiner's finger is placed in the rectum to help guide the needle to the prostate. In the transrectal biopsy, the needle is placed against the examining finger and then inserted into the rectum to the prostate. Once at the site, the needle is advanced through the rectal mucosa and into the prostate gland. The aspiration may be repeated several times to get a satisfactory specimen.

Follow-up care.   Sepsis is a potential life-threatening complication of transrectal biopsy. Any signs of infection or septic shock must be immediately reported. The man also needs reinforcement on the importance of continuing the prophylactic antibiotics.

ULTRASONOGRAPHY

Ultrasonography as a diagnostic technique is becoming routine for assessing reproductive problems. There is no exposure to radiation, and it is considered to be safe for use during pregnancy. It can be used to locate escaped intrauterine devices and to monitor the progress of tumor regression after medical treatment. Ultrasonography is especially helpful in obese clients when bimanual examinations are not satisfactory to make a differential diagnosis.

Client preparation.   There are no specific preparations for this study, although a full bladder is needed to visualize the uterus or to make the location of other structures more distinct.

Procedure.   After the client's abdomen is exposed, an oil or gel is applied to the area to be scanned to provide better transmission of the sound waves from the transducer through the client's skin. The transducer is moved in a linear pattern across the abdomen to outline and define soft-tissue masses and to differentiate tumor types, ascites, and encapsulated fluid. The client is often interested in the oscilloscope screen and appreciates a brief explanation of the landmarks and structures visualized.

Follow-up care.   There are no side effects of ultrasonography and no specific interventions required for follow-up care.

INFERTILITY STUDIES

Basal Body Temperature Charting

A *basal body temperature chart* is a simple graph that plots the woman's morning body temperature as an indication of ovulatory function (Fig. 52–19). It is important for the client to take her temperature every morning at the same time, before getting out of bed, talking, or moving, so that the temperature can be determined at total rest. The basal body thermometer, if used, is similar to a standard oral thermometer except that the markings between degrees are given in tenths rather than fifths. The temperature is recorded on a graph that plots the degrees Fahrenheit for each day of the menstrual cycle. The chart should be kept for 4 months or more to be able to identify recurring patterns. The charts are useful in planning optimal times for intercourse and are an integral tool for infertility assessment, including scheduling of other diagnostic work-ups and treatment. The woman should indicate on the chart the days when intercourse occurred and any reasons for a nonovulatory elevated temperature.

Normally, the basal body temperature is lower in the preovulatory phase. In the second phase, progesterone affects the temperature curve by causing a sustained increase of 0.4° F or more from the point of ovulation until menses begin. A low, monophasic pattern indicates anovulatory cycles, with absent or inadequate progesterone production. A graph that shows a biphasic pattern with a sustained temperature elevation through the first missed period indicates pregnancy.

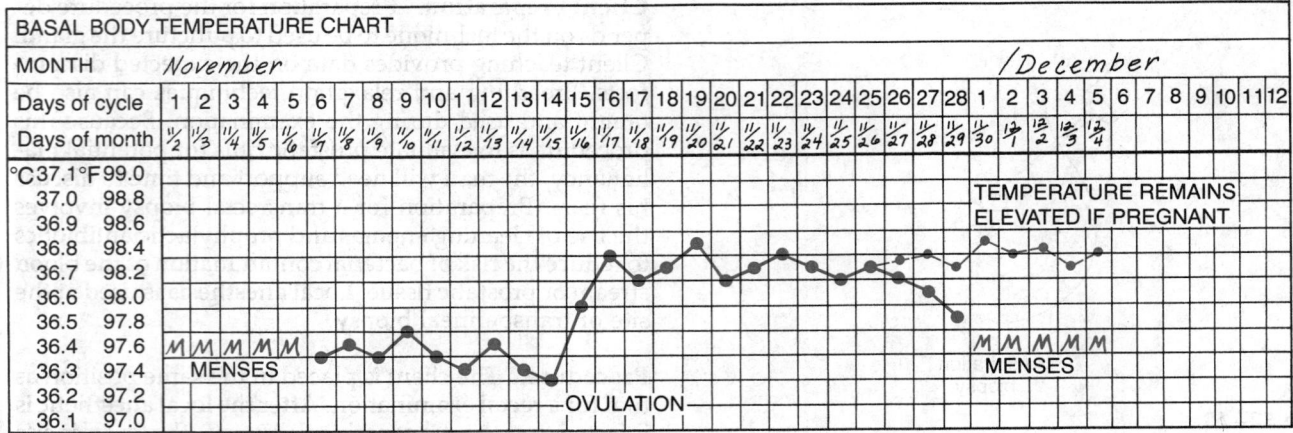

Figure 52–19

Basal body temperature charting.

Fern Test (Cervical Mucus Arborization Test)

Cervical mucus under the influence of increasing estrogen production has a high concentration of sodium shortly before ovulation. Thus, when drying it forms crystal patterns resembling fern fronds. The characteristic ferning is seen in dried cervical mucus only when there is adequate production of estrogen. After ovulation and the secretion of progesterone, this pattern is inhibited or completely abolished, even though estrogen is still being produced. During pregnancy, when there is continuous progesterone influence, this pattern does not occur. The cervical mucus of a menopausal woman does not show ferning because of the absence of sufficient estrogen.

Client preparation.   The client should not douche before the examination. She is placed in a lithotomy position for a speculum examination, and the cervix is swabbed clean.

Procedure.   A sample of mucus from the endocervical canal is obtained and smeared on a glass slide. If the sample is spread too thinly or if blood is present in the specimen, ferning will not be able to occur. The slide is allowed to completely air-dry before it is read under a microscope. A positive fern test indicates a predominant estrogen state. The ferning test can be helpful in determining ovulation by inspecting the cervical mucus smear after the last date ovulation would have been expected to occur in a menstrual cycle.

Follow-up care.   No special nursing care is required after the fern test.

Spinnbarkeit Test

The cervical mucus responds to the effects of estrogen and progesterone during the menstrual cycle. The *spinnbarkeit test* evaluates the stretchability of the endo-

cervical mucus. At the beginning of the menstrual cycle, the mucus is scant, viscid, and sticky. By midcycle, the watery mucus is copious, clear, slippery, and stretchable. The midcycle mucus has been compared to raw egg white and exhibits the characteristic spinnbarkeit. This physiologic phenomenon assists sperm transport through the cervix.

Client preparation.   Women may already notice the increased amount and the stretchability of the vaginal discharge at midcycle. The mucus specimen may be obtained with a sponge forceps from the cervix during a pelvic examination. Gentle opening of the forceps demonstrates the presence or absence of the spinnbarkeit. An alternative method is to transfer the mucus to a glass slide and apply a coverslip. The coverslip is then raised to observe the stretchability of the mucus (Fig. 52–20). At midcycle, the mucus stretches for at least 5 cm (2 in) into a string or thread without breaking. After midcycle, with progesterone being dominant, the mucus tends to become thick and cloudy. Therefore, the absence of stretchable strings is a good indicator that ovulation has occurred.

Follow-up care.   There is no special nursing care required after this test.

Sims-Huhner Test

The *Sims-Huhner test* (postcoital cervical mucus test; PK test) provides both male and female reproductive assessment data.

Client preparation.   Usually, the test is scheduled on or within 24 hours of the day that ovulation is predicted. The couple is advised to abstain from intercourse for 48 hours before the test. Intercourse needs to take place about 6 to 8 hours before the woman is to be examined. The woman needs to be advised not to tub bathe or douche after intercourse for this test.

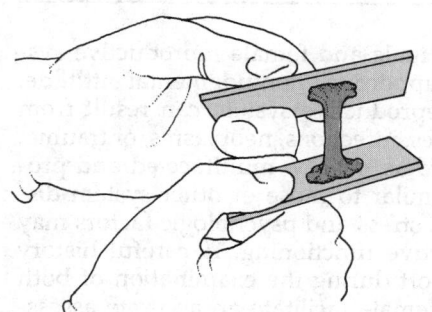 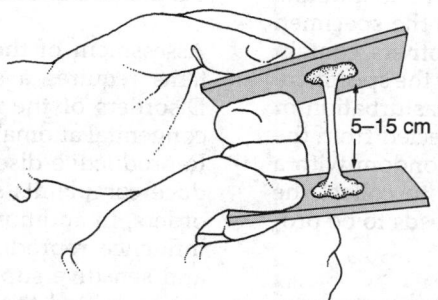 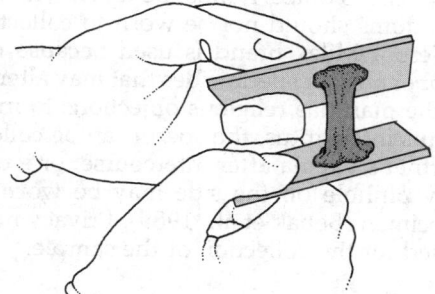

At the beginning of the cycle, the mucus is sparse and quite cloudy.

By the middle of the cycle, mucus is abundant and clear. Spinnbarkeit—stretchiness—is at its peak. The mucus is extremely slippery.

At the end of the cycle, the mucus once again becomes thick and cloudy and may appear whitish or yellow.

Figure 52–20

Spinnbarkeit testing.

Procedure. After the couple has had intercourse, the woman is prepared for a pelvic examination, and the cervix is exposed with a nonlubricated speculum. A sample of endocervical mucus and a vaginal pool specimen are obtained and examined separately under a microscope. A cervical mucus sperm count should show 5 to 20 sperm per high-power field. Ideally, the mucus should show midcycle changes. Four hours after intercourse, approximately 50% of the sperm are still active. The number of active sperm normally decreases to 25% by 12 hours after intercourse. If the sperm are all immotile, the cervix could have been examined too late after intercourse. Results of this test are invariably abnormal when there is cervical infection or during the early menstrual cycle when the mucus is scanty and thick. A single abnormal test result is not conclusive. Poor results may be attributed to poor coital technique, low sperm count, inadequate seminal fluid, poor cervical mucus quality, or scheduling the test on the wrong day of the menstrual cycle.

Follow-up care. There is no special nursing care required after the postcoital test.

Semen Analysis

Semen analysis includes assessment of sperm motility and morphology and of the volume and density of the ejaculate. An analysis from a single ejaculate is not conclusive; analysis should be performed on at least two different occasions.

Client preparation. The male should abstain from intercourse for at least 48 hours before the test; however, abstinence for longer than 5 days decreases the quality and motility of the sperm in the ejaculate. Because the sperm are sensitive to heat and cold and have decreased motility over time, the male should collect the specimen in the physician's office. Unless there are religious sanctions against masturbation, the client is asked to masturbate to orgasm and to collect the specimen in a small clean glass jar. If the specimen is not collected at the physician's office, it must be taken within 1 to 2 hours. Condoms should not be worn to collect the specimen unless a Milex brand is used because others contain rubber and/or spermicides that may alter the specimen. If the man has religious objections to masturbation or coitus interruptus, the sperm can be collected from the partner's vagina after intercourse, or a condom with a tiny pinhole on the side may be worn to collect the specimen (Bobak et al., 1989). Privacy needs to be provided for the collection of the sample.

Procedure. Sperm are analyzed under a microscope in the laboratory. The total volume of the ejaculate should be from 2 to 6 mL. Within each milliliter, there are approximately 20 million sperm. A normal sperm count, done within 2 hours after ejaculation, should show 60% to 70% of the sperm to be motile and at least 70% of them to appear normal.

Progesterone (Progestin) Withdrawal Test

The *progesterone withdrawal test* is an aid to the diagnosis of anovulation as a cause for amenorrhea. It provides data on the ability of the ovaries to secrete estrogen and on the quality of the endometrial lining of the uterus.

The client is given a pregnancy test and after a negative result, she is given 5 to 10 mg of short-term oral progestin daily for 5 days. If there has been previous estrogen stimulation from the ovaries, the endometrial lining will slough in the next 2 to 5 days as the hormonal levels fall. If the endometrium is not influenced by estrogen, proliferation does not occur and withdrawal bleeding cannot take place. Withdrawal bleeding indicates that progesterone is not already being produced in the body (such as from a pregnancy or corpus luteum cyst). If there was an endogenous source of progesterone, the administration of this additional amount would have no effect and the endometrium would be maintained. A positive progesterone withdrawal test is highly indicative of anovulation. This condition is related to either the failure of the pituitary to secrete LH or the ovary's inability to respond to the LH.

Estrogen/Progesterone Withdrawal Test

A combined *estrogen/progesterone withdrawal test* is an additional means to determine the etiology of amenorrhea in the client who does not have withdrawal bleeding after the progesterone withdrawal test.

The woman is given 0.02 to 0.05 mg of ethinyl estradiol orally for 21 days, followed by progestin, 5 to 10 mg orally for 7 days. Withdrawal bleeding after the conclusion of this regimen indicates that the woman does have an endometrial base but that it has not been adequately proliferated by estrogen in previous cycles. Withdrawal bleeding signifies a positive test result.

SUMMARY

Assessment of the male and female reproductive systems requires a supportive, nonjudgmental attitude. Disorders of the reproductive system can result from congenital anomalies, infections, neoplasms, or trauma. Reproductive disorders may be multifaceted and produce complaints similar to those of other system disorders. In addition, stress and psychologic factors may influence reproductive functioning. A careful history and sensitive support during the examination of both the male and the female facilitate an accurate assessment.

Many reproductive system disorders cannot be evaluated or treated by examining just one member of a couple. A dysfunction or disease in one client affects the other, as in the transmission of venereal disease or in infertility.

REFERENCES AND READINGS

American Cancer Society. (1988). *Cancer facts and figures—1988.* New York: Author.

Anderson, J. E. (1978). *Grant's atlas of anatomy* (7th ed.). Baltimore: Williams & Wilkins.

Bates, B. (1987). *A guide to physical examination and history taking.* Philadelphia: J. B. Lippincott.

Bobak, I. M., Jensen, M. D., & Zalar, M. K. (1989). *Maternity and gynecologic care* (4th ed.). St. Louis: C. V. Mosby.

Boulton, J. M. (1982). *Diagnosis and management of renal and urinary diseases.* Oxford: Blackwell Scientific.

Droegemueller, W., Herbst, A. L., Mishell, D. R., Jr., & Stenchever, M. A. (1987). *Comprehensive gynecology.* St. Louis: C. V. Mosby.

Dugan, K. A. (1985). Diagnostic laparoscopy under local anesthesia for evaluation of infertility. *Journal of Obstetric, Gynecologic, and Neonatal Nursing, 14,* 363–366.

Eddy, D. (1986). *The value of mammography for women under 50.* New York: American Cancer Society.

Graham, E. A. (1986). Menstruation and menopause. In J. Griffith-Kenney (Ed.), *Contemporary women's health: A nursing advocacy approach* (pp. 435–448). Menlo Park, CA: Addison-Wesley.

Grimes, J., & Burns, E. (1987). *Health assessment in nursing practice* (2nd ed.). Boston: Jones & Bartlett.

Guyton, A. C. (1986). *Textbook of medical physiology* (7th ed.). Philadelphia: W. B. Saunders.

Johnson, D. E., Swanson, D. A., & von Eschenbach, A. C. (1984). Tumors of the genitourinary tract. In Smith, D. R. (Ed.), *General urology* (11th ed.). Los Angeles: Lange Medical.

Kaunitz, A. M., & Grimes, D. A. (1988). The woman over 50: Endometrial sampling in older women [Special issue]. *Contemporary Obstetrics and Gynecology, 31,* 85.

Kee, J. L. (1987). *Laboratory and diagnostic tests with nursing implications* (2nd ed.). Norwalk, CT: Appleton & Lange.

Kuczynski, H. J. (1986). Support for the woman with an ectopic pregnancy. *Journal of Obstetric, Gynecologic, and Neonatal Nursing, 15,* 306–310.

LaCamera, D. J., Masur, H., & Henderson, D. K. (1985). Symposium on infections in the compromised host. The acquired immunodeficiency syndrome. *Nursing Clinics of North America, 20,* 241–256.

Lee, P., Geoffrey, A. P., & Kaminski, P. F. (1988). Accuracy of Papanicolaou smears: Art or science? *Journal of Reproductive Medicine, 33,* 795–798.

Lowdermilk, D. L. (1986). Reproductive surgery. In J. Griffith-Kenney (Ed.), *Contemporary women's health: A nursing advocacy approach* (pp. 604–621). Menlo Park, CA: Addison-Wesley.

Moore, K. L. (1985). *Clinically oriented anatomy.* Baltimore: Williams & Wilkins.

Neeson, J. D., & May, K. A. (1986). *Comprehensive maternity nursing: Nursing process and the childbearing family.* Philadelphia: J. B. Lippincott.

Nelson, J. H., Averette, H. E., & Richert, R. M. (1984). *Dysplasia, carcinoma in situ, and early invasive cervical carcinoma.* New York: American Cancer Society.

Olds, S. B., London, M. L., & Ladewig, P. A. (1988). *Maternal newborn nursing* (3rd ed.). Menlo Park, CA: Addison-Wesley.

Oxorn, J. A., McDonald, P. C., & Gant, N. F. (1987). *Williams obstetrics* (18th ed.). Norwalk, CT: Appleton-Century-Crofts.

Recommendation for assisting in the prevention of prenatal transmission of human T lymphotrophic virus type III/lymphadenopathy associated with acquired immunodeficiency syndrome. (1985). *Morbidity and Mortality Weekly Report, 34,* 721.

Rudy, E. B., & Gray, V. R. (1986). *Handbook of health assessment* (2nd ed.). Norwalk, CT: Appleton-Century-Crofts.

Schlossberg, L., & Zuidema, G. D. (1977). *The Johns Hopkins atlas of human functional anatomy.* Baltimore: The Johns Hopkins University Press.

Seidel, H. M., Ball, J. W., Dains, J. E., & Benedict, G. W. (1987). *Mosby's guide to physical examination.* St. Louis: C. V. Mosby.

Smith, D. B. (1989). Discussing sexuality. *Oncology Nursing Forum, 16*(1), 106.

Staite, A. (1989). Cervical cytology in general practice. *New Zealand Nursing Journal, 82*(1), 18–19.

Szydlo, V. L. (1988). Approaching a male adolescent about a pelvic exam. *American Journal of Nursing, 88,* 1052–1056.

Tilkian, S. M., Conover, M. B., & Tilkian, A. G. (1987). *Clinical implications of laboratory tests* (4th ed.). St. Louis: C. V. Mosby.

Whitley, N. A. (1985). *A manual of clinical obstetrics.* Philadelphia: J. B. Lippincott.

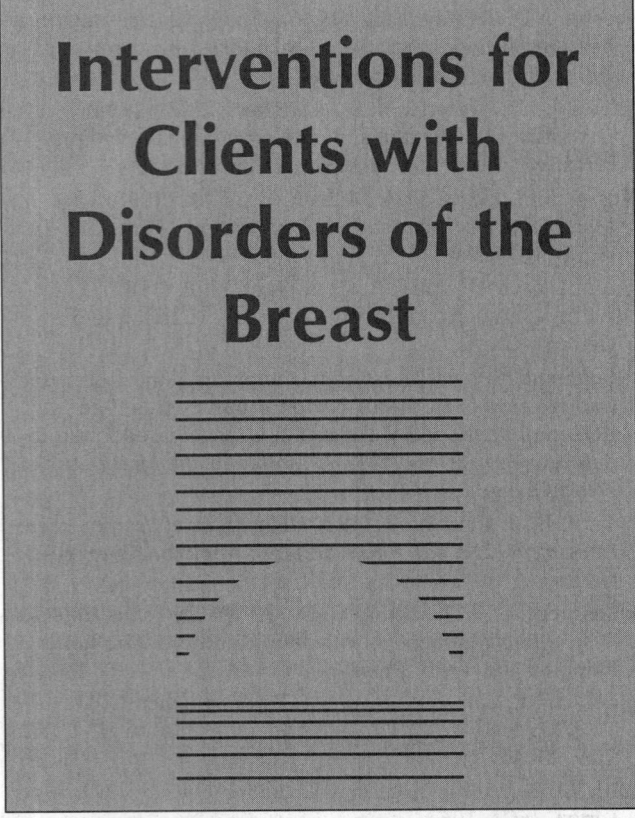

CHAPTER 53

Interventions for Clients with Disorders of the Breast

The discovery of a lump in a woman's breast, whether made by herself or her physician, is often perceived as a sentence of death. Even if the woman is aware that 90% of all breast lumps are benign, she may think that the lump is breast cancer. This reaction, full of fear and apprehension, accompanies the woman throughout the period of diagnosis, decision-making, and treatment, no matter what the final outcome. Whether the etiology of the disease proves to be benign or malignant, whether the care ends after diagnosis, treatment, or death, the nurse must be aware of both the physiologic and emotional factors involved to be effective in nursing care.

SCREENING FOR BREAST MASSES

The American Cancer Society (ACS) and the National Cancer Institute have established guidelines for breast cancer screening (see Chap. 25, Table 25–2). The nurse must be familiar with these guidelines to work effectively with clients.

Breast Self-Examination

The goal of screening for breast cancer is early detection. Breast self-examination (BSE), used in conjunction with mammography and professional examination, has been found to be extremely effective in detecting early breast cancer. Women who practice BSE present with smaller tumors and have earlier stage disease, thus improving their prognosis (Foster et al., 1978). It is recommended that all women older than the age of 20 years practice BSE. Unfortunately, although the majority of women have heard of BSE, only about 50% practice it regularly (Philip et al., 1986) (see the accompanying Nursing Research feature). Whether the client seeks health care because she has found a breast lump, because she needs a routine physical examination, or because she has an unrelated health problem, the nurse's encounter with her provides an excellent opportunity to assess and teach BSE. It is erroneous to assume that most women who practice BSE do so competently and regularly. Most women prefer this type of individualized instruction to learning from pamphlets and magazines. Women who are taught by a health care professional on an individual or group basis practice BSE more often, more proficiently, and more confidently.

Before beginning to teach the hands-on aspect of BSE, it is important to assess the psychologic factors influencing the client's motivation to practice BSE. Lack of knowledge about the technique is not the only reason that women fail to perform BSE regularly. Many women do not understand the benefits of early detection. The fact that treatment for breast cancer is more successful the earlier the disease is found should be stressed. It is also important that the client develop confidence in her ability to detect changes early and understand that a yearly breast examination by her physician cannot substitute for her practicing BSE. The method of BSE that is

NURSING RESEARCH

Knowing About Breast Self-Examination Does Not Necessarily Increase Frequency of Its Performance.

Redeker, N. C. (1989). Health beliefs, health locus of control, and the frequency of practice of breast self examination in women. *Journal of Obstetric, Gynecologic, and Neonatal Nursing, 18,* 45–51.

BSE is recommended as an inexpensive method of detection of breast lesions at any stage, but many women do not practice BSE monthly or even at regular intervals.

This study examined the relationship of health beliefs, health locus of control, and the frequency of performing BSE in 48 mothers of preschool children. Instruments used in the survey included the Stillman health beliefs instrument and the Multidimensional Health Locus of Control Scale. Data were analyzed by using discriminant function analysis, canonical correlation, and analysis of variance. The combined variables of health beliefs, internal health locus of control, religion, and occupation accounted for 80% of the variance in nonpractice and more than 73% of that in high practice. Thirty-eight of the 48 subjects reported practicing BSE, but only 15 reported practice of 9 to 12 times a year (high practice).

Critique.   Generalizability is limited because of the small nonrandom sample size and exploration of multiple variables. The effectiveness of BSE was not explored.

Possible nursing implications.   Nurses have a role in educating the public about the benefits of BSE and can motivate women to practice this health care behavior. Providing information is not sufficient motivation for practice, but this article suggests that personal instruction, encouragement, and reinforcement of the learned behavior may be useful. Teaching in a group situation may also increase perceived susceptibility to breast cancer and may motivate women to perform BSE regularly.

KEY FEATURES OF DISEASE ■ Risk Factors for Breast Cancer

Significant Risk Factors

Female sex

Age greater than 50 yr

Family history of breast cancer (mother or sister)

History of previous breast cancer

Less Significant Risk Factors

History of endometrial cancer

Obesity

Nulliparity

First pregnancy after age 30 yr

Early menarche

Late menopause

Member of Caucasian group

European-Jewish descent

Residence in North America or northern Europe

High-fat diet

Heavy use of alcohol

Cigarette smoking

recommended by the ACS is given in Chapter 25 as a Client/Family Education feature (see p. 574–575). One problem with a health care practice such as BSE is that it detects but does nothing to prevent breast cancer, in contrast to diet modification and heart disease, for example. Therefore, the asymptomatic woman, when choosing whether to do BSE, may think, "What's the use? It won't keep me from getting breast cancer." Again, it is helpful to emphasize the advantages of early detection in terms of outcome and to help the client review her risk factors to demonstrate her level of vulnerability. To be motivated to practice BSE, she must believe that there are benefits and that the barriers to practicing are minimal. Without dealing with these issues, teaching alone increases only knowledge and not the practice.

Also before teaching the technique, the nurse discusses the client's fears, beliefs, and concerns about breast disease and BSE with her, including an assessment of risk factors for breast cancer and a history of prior breast problems (see the accompanying Key Features of Disease). Proper timing for BSE should be discussed also. Premenopausal women should examine their breasts 1 week after the menstrual period. At this time, hormonal influence on breast tissue is minimal, which reduces fluid retention and tenderness. Postmenopausal women should identify a monthly event with which to correlate BSE, such as the first day of the month or payday. In addition to being able to relate the need for monthly BSE, the client should be able to discuss the need for a yearly professional examination and the mammogram recommendations appropriate for her age, as shown in Table 25–2.

The setting in which BSE is demonstrated should be private and, because little clothing is worn, warm. The woman should be asked to undress from the waist up and should be provided with a gown and sheet. Before teaching the actual technique for BSE, the nurse assesses the client's technique by asking her to demonstrate her own method. If she is unsure or does not have a history of performing BSE, the nurse can slowly lead her through the examination while explaining the reasons for the different techniques and answering questions. It is also helpful to point out different findings at this time, especially those that might be perceived as abnormal by the client. For example, nodular breast tissue may normally feel lumpy, which conjures up visions of widespread cancer in the unknowledgeable woman. Placing her hand directly on the involved area and showing her precisely what is normal for her build self-confidence. Another area that should be pointed out is the inframammary ridge, the area of the breast where the skin folds under the breast. This thickened area may be perceived as a lump instead of a normal finding. In thin or small-breasted women, the ribs may be mistaken for masses. The client should be shown how to follow the rib to the sternum to be sure that it is bone and not breast tissue. The hands-on technique should also be used to demonstrate two other aspects of the examination: the amount of pressure needed and the correct position of the hands. The fingers should press deeply enough through the tissue to detect the underlying ribs. Teaching models of both normal and abnormal breasts are available and may be helpful. The difference in examining the breasts, especially in large-breasted women, with the arm overhead while lying down as opposed to having the arm by the side should also be demonstrated. This difference shows her the advantage of using the correct method, which spreads the tissue over the chest wall for more effective palpation.

Professional Examination

The professional examination has been shown in a major study to be effective in detecting more than 55% of breast cancers (Baker, 1982). Many nurses find themselves in a position not only to teach BSE but also to have responsibility for the professional examination. This examination may be done before or after the BSE session, and the same guidelines apply of providing a private, warm setting, maintaining dignity, and allowing time for discussion. Taking a breast history is vital. Results are recorded on a breast evaluation form, which becomes a part of the client's record (Fig. 53–1). This record helps the nurse establish the relative risk for breast disease and the need for follow-up diagnostic tests, such as mammograms, and teaching.

CLIENT'S NAME ______ Sex ______ Race ______ Age ______

Weight ______ Ideal Weight ______ Marital Status ______

HISTORY	Yes	No	Comments
Family history of breast cancer			
Personal history of breast cancer			
Previous mammograms			
Previous biopsy (findings)			
Nipple discharge			
Hormone use (specify)			
BSE Practice			
High-fat diet			
ETOH/smoking			
Current medications (list)			

Age at menses ______ Age at menopause ______

COMMENTS

PHYSICAL FINDINGS

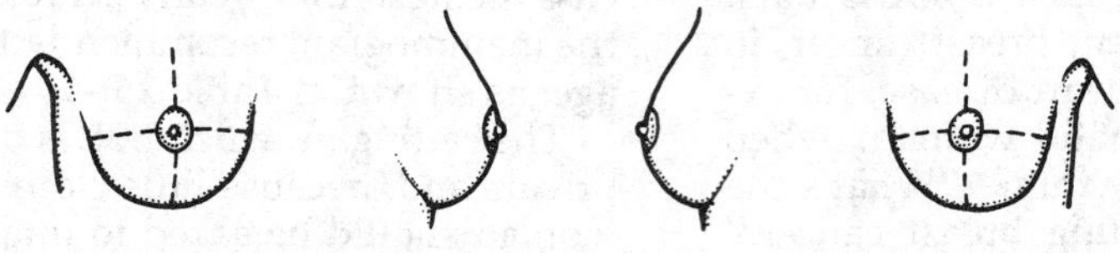

Mammogram Report ______

Biopsy/Cytology Results ______

BSE Return Demonstration ______

Plan ______

CLIENT EDUCATION ______

Figure 53–1

A breast evaluation form.

The first step of the physical assessment is the visual examination. The woman is unclothed from the waist up and first sits with her hands by her sides. The breasts are inspected for symmetry and size, skin changes, and nipple changes. It is important to remember that many women have one breast that is larger than the other and that inverted nipples are not uncommon. The client can usually state whether these findings are normal for her. Symmetry is an important concept because any change that occurs on one side and not the other is more likely to indicate a problem. While the arms are by the side and are relaxed, the axillae can be palpated. If it is necessary to move the arms away from the body, the woman should rest her arm on the nurse's to prevent flexion of the underlying muscles. The axilla and area beneath the clavicle should be palpated deeply for enlarged lymph nodes. The woman is then asked to raise her hands over her head. This exposes the sides and underneath portions of the breast for inspection. Finally, she is asked to place her hands on her hips and press, thus flexing the pectoral muscles. This action accentuates skin dimpling or masses. The remainder of the examination is done with the client lying supine. A pillow or rolled sheet should be placed under the examined breast and the arm on that side raised above the head. Each breast is palpated separately while the other breast remains covered. If the woman has identified a problem in one breast, the other "normal" breast should be examined first to establish a baseline for comparison. To ensure complete coverage of the breast tissue, the examiner should palpate in a vertical pattern, in a horizontal pattern, or in concentric circles, which covers every inch of the breast tissue. Finally, the nipple should be compressed to detect the presence of a discharge. If there has been history of a discharge, the client is often able to express the discharge more successfully than the examiner and can be asked to do so.

If, during the examination, the nurse discovers a suspicious area or discharge, consultation with or referral to a physician should be made and follow-up ensured. Follow-up usually involves mammography.

BENIGN DISORDERS

Seventy per cent of all breast lumps are found to be benign (Townsend, 1980). The risk of different breast diseases is related to age, and, for that reason, breast diseases are discussed in an age-related format, followed by a discussion of breast cancer.

FIBROADENOMA

Fibroadenomas are the most common cause of breast lumps during the teen-age years, although they may occur into the 30s. A fibroadenoma is a solid, benign mass of connective tissue that is unattached to the surrounding breast tissue. It is usually discovered by the client herself, and usually by accident because these women are too young to be practicing BSE regularly. Although the immediate fear is that of breast cancer, in fact only 0.2% of these masses prove to be malignant. At presentation, the lump is characteristically firm, hard but not cystic, easily movable, and clearly delineated from the surrounding tissue. It is not usually painful or sore and does not change with the menstrual cycle. Fibroadenomas are usually located in the upper outer quadrant of the breast, and it is not unusual for more than one to be present. The physician may recommend follow-up without treatment to observe the mass for 3 months if the client is younger than 25 years old. If she is older, the physician may attempt needle aspiration to establish whether the lump is cystic or solid. If the lump is solid, it is usually excised on an outpatient basis by using local anesthesia.

FIBROCYSTIC BREAST DISEASE

OVERVIEW

Fibrocystic breast disease (FBD), also called cystic disease or dysplasia, is the most common breast problem of women in their 20s. The disease may proceed through several clinical stages or may present in only one form.

The first stage, common between the late teens and early 20s, is characterized by premenstrual bilateral fullness and tenderness, especially in the outer upper quadrant. Symptoms usually resolve after menstruation and then recur before the next menstrual period in a cyclic fashion.

In the second stage, which usually occurs in the late 20s and throughout the 30s, bilateral multicentric nodular areas that feel like small marbles can be felt and accompany the fullness and soreness. The examiner cannot place the fingers around the masses and often cannot distinguish their borders. The woman with these findings is frequently advised to have a baseline mammogram because physical examination is difficult in the presence of these nodules.

In the third stage, which generally occurs between the ages of 35 and 55 years, microscopic or macroscopic cysts develop. These cysts generally appear suddenly and are associated with pain, tenderness, or burning. They are usually three-dimensional, smooth, mobile, and well delineated. Although the cysts may recede somewhat before menstruation, they do not disappear completely. Mammography is generally indicated, and aspiration may be performed. Biopsy is indicated if the aspirated fluid is bloody, if no fluid is aspirated, if the mammogram shows suspicious findings, if a mass remains palpable after aspiration, or if the cytology report of the aspirated fluid reveals malignant cells.

Although the cause of FBD is unknown, the disorder appears to be related to normal fluctuations in progesterone and estrogen levels during the menstrual cycle. FBD is a disease of the reproductive years. Symptoms usually resolve after menopause in the absence of estrogen supplementation. Risk factors include nulliparity or low parity, late age of birth of first child, and late menopause (Parazzini et al., 1984).

COLLABORATIVE MANAGEMENT

Medical management is generally symptomatic. Hormonal manipulation has been the primary means of pharmacologic intervention. Oral contraceptives have been used to suppress oversecretion of estrogen. Progestins are used to correct luteal insufficiency. Danazol (Danocrine) suppresses ovarian function and suppresses estrogen stimulation of breast tissue. Bromocriptine (Parlodel) can be used to increase progesterone secretion in women with borderline hyperprolactinemia (Norwood, 1990).

Medical management may also include the use of E and B complex vitamins. Diuretics may be prescribed to decrease premenstrual fluid engorgement. Clients may be counseled to avoid the use of caffeine.

The nursing role includes encouraging the client to continue prescribed medical interventions and monitoring the effectiveness of these interventions. The nurse suggests supportive measures, such as the use of mild analgesics or limiting salt intake before menses, as an attempt to decrease swelling. The nurse suggests that the client wear a well-padded, supportive brassiere to decrease tension on ligaments. Local application of ice or heat can be suggested to provide temporary relief of pain. The nurse promotes the practice of BSE and teaches the procedure when necessary. Emotional support for the client with FBD is an essential component of care.

DUCTAL ECTASIA

Ductal ectasia is a benign breast problem that is usually seen in women approaching menopause. The disease is caused by dilation and thickening of the collecting ducts in the subareolar area. These ducts become distended and filled with cellular debris, which begins an inflammatory response. Two clinical signs result from these changes: a mass develops that feels hard, has irregular borders, and may be tender; and a greenish-brown nipple discharge, enlarged axillary nodes, and redness and edema over the site of the mass are noted. These masses are often difficult to distinguish from breast cancer. Because the risk for developing breast cancer is increased in this age group, accurate diagnosis is vital. A microscopic examination of the nipple discharge is performed to detect any atypical or malignant cells, and the affected area is excised. As with FBD, nursing care is directed at alleviating the anxiety that is associated with the threat of breast cancer and at supporting the woman through the diagnostic and treatment procedures.

INTRADUCTAL PAPILLOMA

Intraductal papilloma, like ductal ectasia and breast cancer, occurs primarily in the 40- to 55-year-old age group. It is caused by a benign process in which the epithelial lining of the duct forms a papilloma, a pendulated outgrowth of tissue. As the papilloma grows, it causes trauma and erosion within the duct and results in a serosanguineous or serous nipple discharge. A mass may be palpable, and the area may be tender. Diagnosis is aimed first at ruling out the possibility of breast cancer. Microscopic examination of the nipple discharge and surgical excision of the mass and ductal area are usually indicated.

PROBLEMS OF THE LARGE-BREASTED WOMAN

As much as our society emphasizes the aesthetic attributes of large breasts, women with excessive breast tissue experience difficulties and discomforts. Fashion is directed at the small-breasted figure, so clothes are often hard to find and feel attractive in. The breast size may be disproportionate to the rest of the body, which adds to the problems of fitting clothes. Brassieres are expensive and may have to be special ordered, and the straps create large dents in the shoulders. In addition, many large-breasted women experience fungal infections under the breasts because it is difficult to keep this area dry and exposed to air. Backaches from the added weight are also common. The only alternative for this condition, if well-fitting brassieres do not help and being overweight is not part of the problem, may be surgery. Breast reduction surgery involves the removal of excess breast tissue, repositioning the nipple, and repositioning the resulting skin flaps to produce the optimal cosmetic effect. This operation is a major surgical procedure, and the decision to have it done is usually made after years of living with the discomforts of excessive breast size. The nurse may be involved in the decision-making stage by listening to the client verbalize her feelings and by providing information as appropriate. The postoperative diagnoses and goals are consistent with those found for the woman undergoing reconstructive surgery.

GYNECOMASTIA

Gynecomastia is a benign condition of breast enlargement in males. Usually, this enlargement is bilateral, but enlargement is asymmetric in about 10% (Lucas, 1987). The condition is caused by proliferation of the glandular tissue, including the mammary ducts and ductal stroma. In many men, it is difficult to distinguish gynecomastia from breast enlargement related to excess adipose tissue. Etiologic factors of gynecomastia include drugs; aging; obesity; underlying diseases causing estrogen excess, such as malnutrition, liver disease, or hyperthyroidism; and androgen deficiency states, such as age or chronic renal failure. Men with abnormal breast findings, especially a breast mass, are carefully evaluated for the risk of breast cancer (see next section).

CANCER

Breast cancer is the second leading cause of breast masses. When a lump is detected, there is a risk of 20% that it will be breast cancer (Baker, 1982). Because of the high incidence of the disease, almost every woman has had a close personal association with another woman having the disease. Thus, most women have strong reactions to the threat of breast cancer. These reactions greatly influence a woman's health habits, including BSE and her readiness to seek care when a suspicious area is discovered. Until prevention (through research) becomes an option, early detection is the key to better treatment and survival. Statistics support the advantages of early detection and treatment. Localized breast cancer is associated with a 90% 5-year survival rate, whereas the 5-year survival rate for regional disease drops to 60% (ACS, 1989).

OVERVIEW

Pathophysiology

There are many pathologic types of breast cancer, but the most common, causing more than 80% of cases, is infiltrating ductal carcinoma. As the name implies, the disease originates in the mammary ducts, specifically growing in the epithelial cells lining these ducts. The rate of cancer growth varies and partially depends on hormonal influences. Estimates of the time it takes for a cancer cell to divide and result in a lesion large enough to be clinically palpable range from 5 to 9 years. As long as the cancer remains within the duct, it is considered to be *noninvasive*. The cancer is classified as *invasive* when it penetrates the tissue surrounding the duct. Once invasive, the cancer grows into the tissue around it in an irregular pattern, which is the reason that, once palpable, the lesion is felt as an irregular, poorly defined mass. As the tumor continues to grow, fibrosis develops around the cancer. This fibrosis may cause shortening of Cooper's ligaments and thus the characteristic skin dimpling that is seen with more advanced disease. The tumor also invades the lymphatic channels, blocking skin drainage and causing skin edema and an orange peel appearance of the skin (peau d'orange). Invasion of

the lymphatic channels carries tumor cells to the lymphatic nodes, including those in the axillary region. For this reason, pathologic examination of the axillary nodes is imperative for staging the disease. Eventually, the tumor replaces the skin itself, and ulceration of the overlying skin occurs. Metastases result from seeding of the cancer cells into the blood and lymph systems, which permits spread of these cells to distant sites. The most common sites of metastatic disease from breast cancer are bone, lungs, brain, and liver. The course of metastatic breast cancer is related to the site affected and the function impaired. Chapter 25 further describes the pathophysiology of cancer.

Less than 1% of all cases of breast cancer occur in males. Symptoms are similar to those of female breast cancer and include a mass, bloody nipple discharge, or significant axillary lymph node enlargement. Treatment and response rates of male breast cancer parallel those of females at a similar stage at diagnosis (Bezwada et al., 1987).

Etiology

There is no known etiologic agent responsible for breast cancer. This disease probably results from multiple factors, the presence of which are known to increase a woman's risk for developing the disease. Although being female is the greatest risk factor, some women are at greater risk than others. For every 100 people diagnosed with breast cancer, only 1 is a male.

As mentioned, as age increases, so does risk. More than 85% of cases are diagnosed after the age of 45 years, and 65% after the age of 50 years. Women with a familial history, particularly a mother or sister with breast cancer, have a threefold risk increase. A history of previous breast cancer, nullparity, late age at birth of first child, and late menopause are also considered to heighten risk (Levine & Lippman, 1984). Other genetic and environmental risk factors are listed in Key Features of Disease: Risk Factors for Breast Cancer.

Incidence

Approximately 140,000 new cases of breast cancer are diagnosed each year in the United States (ACS, 1989). The incidence of breast cancer has risen, but longer survival has helped to stabilize the mortality rate. Breast cancer has relinquished its place to lung cancer as the leading cause of death from cancer in women. Unfortunately, this change is not due to a decrease in deaths from breast cancer but to a rapid rise in deaths from lung cancer. Breast cancer is still responsible for one of four cancers in women. It is estimated that 1 of every 10 women will be diagnosed with the disease.

PREVENTION AND EARLY DETECTION

Until recent years, public health education related to reducing mortality from breast cancer focused on early detection. Then, the discovery of risk factors related to life style has added the dimension of prevention to early detection of the disease. Life style changes, such as eating low-fat diets, ceasing to smoke, and moderating alcohol intake, may decrease a woman's risk for developing breast cancer.

Although research has shown that the above-mentioned factors influence a woman's risk for breast cancer, many myths about the causes of breast disease remain. Many women erroneously believe that trauma to the breast, either accidental or by manipulation during self-examination or lovemaking, may cause breast cancer. Nulliparity and a negative history for breast-feeding increase a woman's risk only slightly. Women should be counseled that neither they nor any other risk factor alone is responsible for causing cancer. Conversely, many women believe that a breast lump is benign if it is sore and that a professional examination once a year adequately substitutes for their own self-examination. These misconceptions, whether they produce an inordinate amount of fear or false assurance, must be explored with the client before continuing through the detection process.

COLLABORATIVE MANAGEMENT

 Assessment

History

The initial history may be taken after a mass has been discovered but before positive diagnosis has been made, or at the time the woman is seen for treatment of an identified cancer. The history should focus on three major areas: risk factors, events related to the breast mass, and health maintenance practices. *Age, sex, race, marital status, weight,* and *height* should be recorded. Marital status and identification of the client's primary support person provide information regarding those to be included in the woman's care, teaching, and support. Specific information on a *personal and family history of breast cancer* should be obtained. In addition to increasing her own risk, these factors also affect any sister's or daughter's risk and should be incorporated into later counseling. The *hormonal history* should include whether she has reached or has any symptoms of menopause, age at first menarche, age at menopause, age at first child's birth, and number of children. It is believed that prolonged hormonal stimulation (i.e., by early menses and/or late menopause) increases a woman's risk, as do birth of first child after the age of 30 years and nulliparity.

The second area of assessment focuses on the *history of the breast mass* and reveals not only the course of the disease but also data related to health care–seeking practices and health-promoting behaviors. Knowledge of how, when, and by whom the mass was discovered and of the interval between discovery and seeking care is crucial. If the woman found the mass, was it discovered through BSE or by accident? The answer to this question might alert the nurse to the need for discussion and teaching regarding BSE, regardless of whether the mass is found to be malignant. What was the time interval between discovery and seeing the practitioner? If there was a delay, what caused it? These questions are linked to the psychosocial assessment but also provide data on the length of time that the tumor has been present. The diagnostic procedures done, directed at diagnosing this problem and others in the past, are also important to note. Finally, a review of systems focusing on the most common areas of metastases should be taken.

The third area, that of *health maintenance practices,* should be evaluated. In addition to questioning the client about the knowledge, practice, and regularity of BSE, a *mammographic history* should be taken. The existence of previous mammograms allows the physician to compare current with past mammograms and to facilitate diagnosis. A brief *diet history,* in which the client is asked to recall a typical day's menu and alcoholic intake per week, provides information on the average intake of fat and alcohol. The nurse asks the client what types of medications she uses, specifically questioning her about hormonal supplements and remembering that estrogen can be administered not only orally but also vaginally. Postmenopausal use of estrogen creams intravaginally is not uncommon and should be considered to be a major source of estrogen.

Physical Assessment: Clinical Manifestations

The approach to physical assessment has been discussed earlier in this chapter under the headings Breast Self-Examination and Professional Examination. In addition, specific information on the breast mass must also be noted. The *mass* should be described in the chart in terms of location, shape, size, consistency, and fixation to the surrounding tissues. Any *skin changes,* such as dimpling, peau d'orange, increased vascularity, nipple retraction, or ulceration, may indicate advanced disease and need to be documented. The examination of the axillary and supraclavicular areas needs to be thorough by palpating deeply for *enlarged lymph nodes* and noting their presence and location in the client's record. The presence of *pain* or *soreness* in the affected breast should be evaluated. After gathering this information, a diagram drawn on the chart (see Fig. 53–1) will be helpful for others involved in the client's care.

Psychosocial Assessment

The woman with potential or diagnosed breast cancer faces two major issues: the fear of cancer and the threat to body image. A woman's previous experience with cancer, and especially with other women with breast cancer, influences her reactions to the disease. The nurse asks the client whether she has known anyone with breast cancer and what types of experiences she has had with cancer in general. It is important to explore her feelings about the disease because her choices of treatment, her recovery, and her ability to learn are greatly influenced by these emotions. Often, her perception of her situation is influenced by outdated information. Perhaps she knew someone who had had a radical radical mastectomy 30 years ago and associates breast surgery with the chest deformity and lymphedema that that woman experienced. Dispelling misconceptions by providing current information can affect her attitude in a positive way.

The nurse also assesses the client with breast cancer for problems related to sexuality. Three critical areas of distress contribute to the psychosexual morbidity of clients with breast cancer: psychologic distress, physiologic distress, and relational distress. These three areas are described in detail in the accompanying Key Features of Disease.

The need for additional resources is also evaluated at this time. Will extra psychologic counseling be needed? Are there financial concerns that need to be discussed with social services? Will her spouse, family, or friends support her throughout this period, and how much support and teaching do they need? Answers to these types of questions provide guidelines in establishing goals and in planning nursing care.

Laboratory Findings

The diagnosis of breast cancer relies primarily on pathologic examination of tissue from the breast mass. No serum-based laboratory test aids the physician with this diagnosis. After the presence of cancer is established, laboratory tests, including pathologic examination of the lymph nodes, help to detect possible metastases. Elevated liver enzyme levels indicate possible liver metastases, and increased serum calcium and alkaline phosphatase levels suggest bone metastases.

Radiographic Findings

Mammography is the most sensitive tool for screening for breast cancer (Fig. 53–2). Its use, however, must be combined with BSE for optimal early detection and with the professional examination for full interpretation of the findings. These three methods together create an effective program that detects breast cancer as early as possible. Mammography's uniqueness results from its ability to reveal preclinical lesions, masses too small to be palpated manually (Fig. 53–3). Client preparation and the procedure for mammography are discussed in Chapter 52.

KEY FEATURES OF DISEASE ■ Three Critical Areas of Distress That Contribute to Psychosexual Morbidity of Breast Cancer Clients

Psychologic

Coping strategies
Self-esteem index
Body image
Investment in fertility

Physiologic

Stage of disease
Pain
Physical limitations
Treatment-related complications

Relational

Single or partnered
Stability/support of interaction
History of sexual satisfaction
Flexibility in relation to new ideas
Role responsibility

From Schain, W. (1988). The sexual and intimate consequences of breast cancer. *CA: A Cancer Journal for Clinicians, 38*(3), 159.

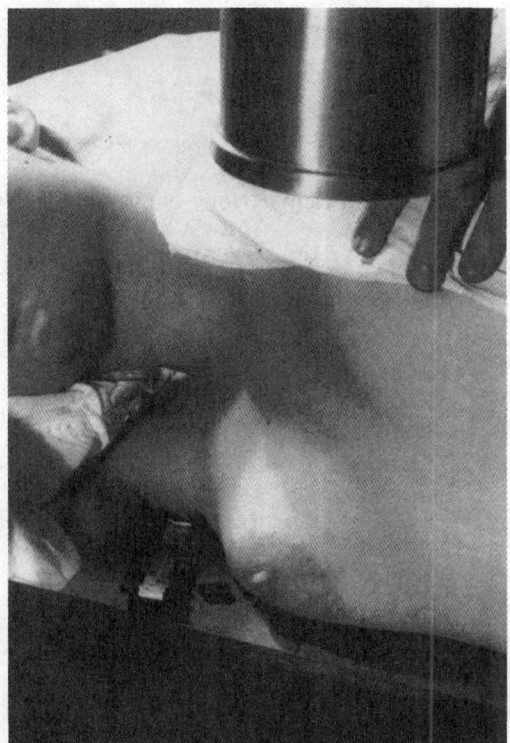

Figure 53–2

A client undergoing mammography, the most sensitive tool for screening for breast cancer. (From Egan, R. L. [1988]. *Breast imaging: Diagnosis and morphology of breast diseases.* Philadelphia: W. B. Saunders.)

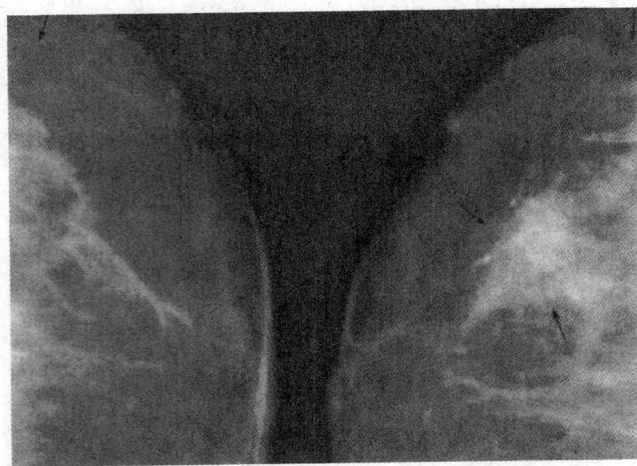

Figure 53-3

The well-defined light area in this mammogram is carcinoma. The tumor was found on routine follow-up of cancer of the other breast. The client had no symptoms of disease. (From Egan, R. L. [1988]. *Breast imaging: Diagnosis and morphology of breast diseases.* Philadelphia: W. B. Saunders.)

KEY FEATURES OF DISEASE ■ Stages of Breast Cancer

Stage	Tumor Size	Involvement of Lymph Nodes	Metastases	
I	Smaller than 2 cm	None or movable	None evident	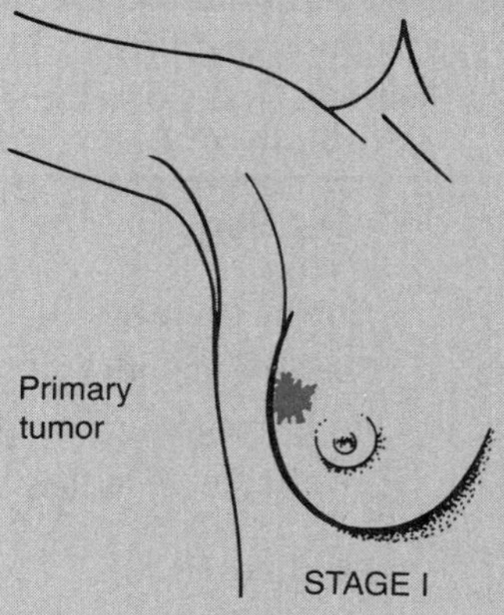 Primary tumor / STAGE I
II	2–5 cm	None or movable	None evident	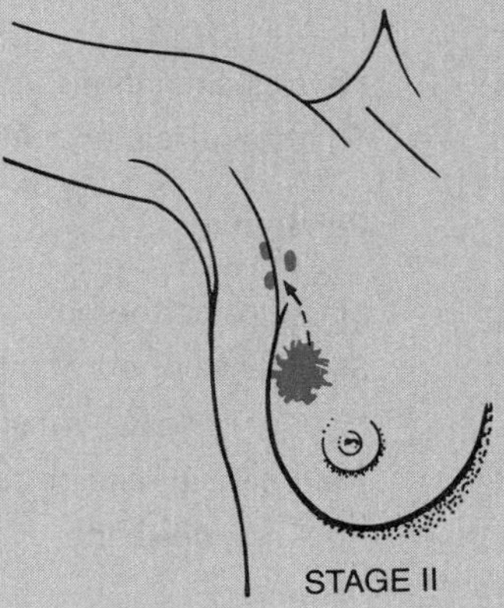 STAGE II

Other radiographic procedures may be used preoperatively to rule out metastases. A chest x-ray film is routine to screen for lung metastases. Bone, liver, and brain scans and resonance imaging are sensitive for detecting distant metastases.

Other Diagnostic Tests

Additional diagnostic and screening techniques include thermography and ultrasonography of the breast. It was hoped that thermography would be an effective screening tool because it has the advantage of avoiding exposure to radiation. Unfortunately, its sensitivity in detecting nonpalpable lesions is less than that of mammography. Ultrasonography is not used as a screening tool but may be used after a palpable lesion is found to distinguish between solid and cystic masses.

Pathologic examination of the breast tissue is the key to positive diagnosis in breast cancer. Breast tissue is obtained by one of several types of biopsies (see Chap. 52 for discussion of breast biopsy).

Several other tests are useful for establishing the stage of disease after the diagnosis of breast cancer is made. These tests include a pathologic examination of the lymph nodes on the affected side. Women with four or fewer involved nodes have a better prognosis than those with more than four. The level of the axilla in which the affected nodes are discovered is also prognostic; the higher the level, the worse the prognosis. As mentioned earlier, a variety of procedures related to specific sites of possible metastases also help to establish the stage or progression of the breast cancer. The accompanying Key Features of Disease explains the four stages of breast cancer.

KEY FEATURES OF DISEASE ■ Stages of Breast Cancer *Continued*

Stage	Tumor Size	Involvement of Lymph Nodes	Metastases	
III	Larger than 5 cm Smaller than 2 cm 2–5 cm	None Axillary nodes Supraclavicular or intraclavicular	None evident	
IV	Any size	Present or not	Distant metastases present	

After the breast cancer has been removed, hormonal receptor status of the tumor is evaluated. This information is used to plan the appropriate course of therapy and is somewhat prognostic. A tumor that contains receptors capable of binding with circulating hormones, specifically estrogen and progesterone, is said to be estrogen receptor (ER) positive. More postmenopausal women (70%) are found to be ER positive than premenopausal women (Levine & Lippman, 1984). Women with ER-positive tumors are found to respond better to adjuvant therapy and have an overall improved survival rate. The receptor status also predicts which women will respond to hormonal manipulation in treating the disease.

In addition, the tumor cells are examined for specialization or differentiation. Well-differentiated tumors tend to be less aggressive than poorly differentiated ones. Thus, a woman with a well-differentiated breast cancer has a better prognosis than the woman with a poorly differentiated tumor.

Analysis: Nursing Diagnosis

The woman with breast cancer is usually admitted to the health care facility with a positive diagnosis of the mass established through an outpatient biopsy. The practice of admitting a woman with a suspicious lesion and using general anesthesia for a biopsy, frozen section, and possible mastectomy has been largely abandoned. Women who have an interval between biopsy and treatment in which they actively participate in the choice of treatment are found to cope more effectively after surgery, no matter what treatment is chosen. The nursing diagnoses specific for any given client depend on that treatment. Because the modified radical mastectomy continues to be the treatment of choice in more than 60% of cases, the following diagnoses focus on the issues concerned with that procedure. Diagnoses and interventions related to caring for the client with advanced cancer are found in Chapter 25.

Common Diagnoses

The common diagnoses seen in the client with breast cancer include

1. Anxiety related to the diagnosis of cancer
2. Potential for injury related to metastases

Additional Diagnoses

In advanced breast cancer, the following additional diagnoses may apply:

1. Anticipatory grieving related to loss
2. Knowledge deficit related to adjunctive therapy
3. Pain related to metastases

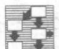 Planning and Implementation

Anxiety

Planning: client goals. The major goals related to this diagnosis are that the client will (1) experience an appropriate level of anxiety and (2) cope effectively throughout the treatment period as demonstrated by her participation in the decision-making process, discussion of her concerns, and increased knowledge related to self-care measures.

Interventions: nonsurgical management. The anxiety for the woman with breast cancer begins the moment the lump is discovered. The level of anxiety felt may be related to past experiences and personal associations that she has with the disease. Many women also have an intuitive feeling about the diagnosis even before it has been established. The clinical likelihood that the lesion is or is not cancer is irrelevant to her level of fear. The nurse assesses and deals with the woman's perceptions of her own situation and personal level of anxiety. If possible, the nurse should attempt to allow time for ventilation of these feelings, even if a diagnosis has not been established.

After the mass has been diagnosed as cancer, many women feel a partial sense of relief to be dealing with a known entity. A feeling of shock or disbelief may predominate. It is difficult to accept a diagnosis such as cancer when one feels basically well. Clients and their families deal in individual ways with the mix of feelings including shock, disbelief, and grief. Some may want to read and discuss any available information. Others may want to know as little as possible and resent attempts at teaching. Whereas one woman may want to talk at length about her concerns, another may want to be alone. Flexibility is the key to nursing care; the nurse adjusts the approach to care as the client's emotional state changes. An integral part of the plan to meet these emotional needs is the use of outside resources. Most health care professionals view the role of groups such as Reach to Recovery to be one of support in the postoperative period, but it is often helpful to suggest these groups in the preoperative phase.

The physicians working with breast cancer clients may also have other clients willing to make a preoperative visit. These resource people may be chosen on the basis of individual concerns. The woman who is worried especially about the side effects of radiation may benefit more from talking to someone who has been so treated than from talking to the nurse about second-hand experiences.

In addition to Reach to Recovery, clients may seek formal community support groups or informal groups such as Encouragement, Normalcy, Counseling, Opportunity, Reaching Out, Energies Revived (ENCORE). These informal groups are reached through the health care provider or by word of mouth.

Potential for Injury

Planning: client goals.   The primary goal for this diagnosis is that the woman will remain free from metastases or recurrence.

Interventions.   There has been significant controversy in the past years regarding the treatment of breast cancer. Until about 1950 the radical radical mastectomy was considered to be the treatment of choice. Gradually, the modified radical procedure became popular. Evidence that has supported less traumatic procedures with comparable survival rates has been presented. Figure 53–4 summarizes the factors influencing the choice of treatment approaches that a physician uses after a positive diagnosis by breast biopsy. Because of the various options, the woman with breast cancer often faces difficult decisions.

Nonsurgical management.   For women with late-stage breast cancer, nonsurgical treatment may be the only alternative. If the disease is at a late stage, such as stage IV, with the presence of confirmed metastases, or if the client cannot withstand a major surgical procedure, the tumor may be removed with local anesthesia, and follow-up treatment may include chemotherapy and sometimes radiation. In cases in which the tumor is attached to the skin or the underlying muscle, resection may be impossible. Again, follow-up therapy for those women involves radiation, usually in conjunction with chemotherapy.

Surgical management.   The various types of breast surgery are shown in the illustration on page 1675. Although controversy exists regarding the best treatment for a malignant mass, most experts agree that the mass itself should be removed. This removal helps to prevent local recurrence. Removal of the axillary lymph nodes, for staging purposes, is usually recommended also. The treatment that ensues is termed conservative or surgical. *Conservative treatment* of breast cancer is an option for treating early disease, such as stage I or II, and usually involves *lumpectomy* or simple mastectomy followed by radiation. Studies have indicated that this approach offers 5- and 10-year survival and local recurrence rates at least equivalent to those of the modified radical mastectomy (Fisher et al., 1985). The cosmetic results have been found to be good to excellent, and other long-term problems are comparable to more radical procedures. For many women, the psychologic benefits of avoiding breast removal are significant and lead them to choose this option. The modified radical mastectomy continues to be favored by many surgeons, although consumer requests and new evidence have increased acceptance of less radical procedures.

The *modified radical* mastectomy differs from the *radical radical* mastectomy in that the pectoral muscles and

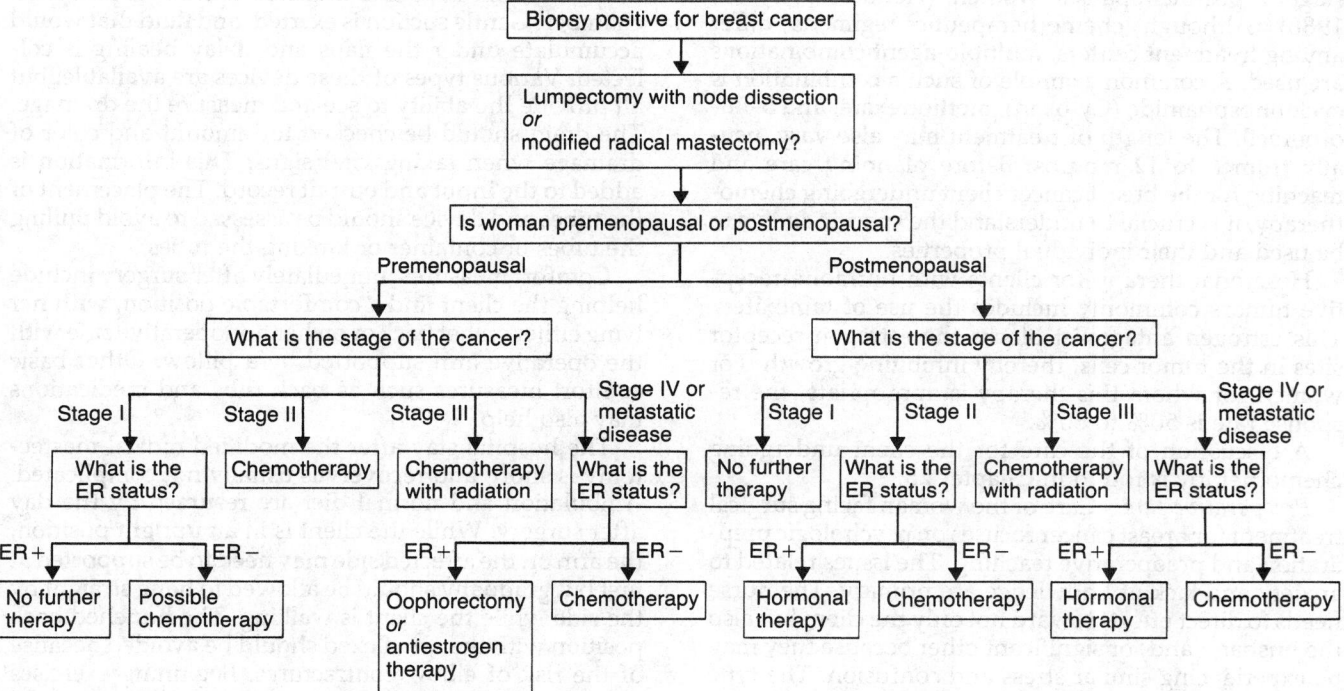

Figure 53–4

Treatment approaches after diagnosis of breast cancer. Because of the many approaches, the woman with breast cancer faces difficult decisions.

nerves remain intact. Thus, the breast tissue and skin and the axillary nodes are removed and the underlying muscles are left in place. The incision is from the mid-chest to the axilla, as shown in the figure on p. 1675. If reconstruction is to follow the procedure, the plastic surgeon may recommend a different location for the incision and may elect to use skin flaps or implants to create a breast mound at the time of the original procedure.

The use of carbon dioxide laser procedures in place of cutting and cauterizing for mastectomies is an option that is becoming more available. Advantages of laser use include less blood loss and faster recuperation (Wang, 1987).

Adjuvant therapy. The decision whether to follow the original procedure with chemotherapy, radiation, or hormonal therapy is based on the stage of the disease, age and menopausal status of the client, client preferences, and hormone receptor status, as shown in Figure 53–4. The purpose of adjuvant therapy is to decrease the risk of recurrence for the client who has no evidence of but is at risk for metastases, or to prolong survival after metastases occur. Chemotherapy is recommended for premenopausal women with negative nodes who are ER negative or have positive nodes. Postmenopausal women who have positive nodes and are ER negative also receive chemotherapy but receive hormonal treatment in addition if ER positive. A review indicated benefits of chemotherapy in premenopausal women with early breast cancer (stage I) and of hormonal therapy for stage I postmenopausal women (Henderson et al., 1988). Although chemotherapeutic regimens differ among treatment centers, multiple-agent combinations are used. A common example of such a combination is cyclophosphamide (Cytoxan), methotrexate, and 5-flu-orouracil. The length of treatment may also vary, usually from 6 to 12 months. Before planning care and teaching for the breast cancer client undergoing chemotherapy, it is crucial to understand the specific agents to be used and their individual properties.

Hormonal therapy for clients with hormone-receptive tumors commonly includes the use of tamoxifen. This estrogen antagonist blocks the estrogen receptor sites in the tumor cells, thereby inhibiting growth. For women for whom this therapy is appropriate, the response rate is 50% to 60%.

A discussion of the care for the client undergoing chemotherapy is found in Chapter 25.

Preoperative care. Care of the woman facing surgical treatment for breast cancer focuses on psychologic preparation and preoperative teaching. The issues related to anxiety and lack of knowledge are primary. The nurse needs to direct efforts toward not only the client but also the husband and/or significant other because they may be experiencing similar stress and confusion. The type of procedure should be reviewed. The discussion may be initiated with open-ended questions such as, "What type of surgery are you having tomorrow? Can you explain what will happen?" This questioning facilitates assessment of the level of knowledge and provides an opening for additional explanations as needed. The client should be knowledgeable about the type of procedure; specific postoperative information such as the presence of a drainage device, location of the incision, any mobility restrictions, length of hospital stay, and possibility of additional therapy; and the basic pre- and postoperative information needed by any surgical client (see Chap. 18).

The level of anxiety related to the cancer was discussed earlier (see the previous nursing diagnosis). It is important to deal with the threat to body image before the surgery to correct misconceptions about postoperative appearance and to begin adjustment to changes in the postoperative period.

Postoperative care. Postoperative and discharge care of the woman undergoing mastectomy is given in the Client Care Plan on pages 1676 to 1679. Before the woman returns from surgery, the nurse places a sign over the client's bed to warn the staff to avoid taking blood pressure, giving injections, or drawing blood from the affected arm. Return from the recovery room occurs as soon as vital signs return to baseline and if no complications have occurred. On the client's return, nursing care is directed at maintaining physiologic stability and comfort. Vital signs are usually ordered on a schedule of decreasing frequency, such as every 30 minutes for two times, every hour for two times, and then every 4 hours. During these checks, the nurse assesses the dressing for bleeding. After a modified radical mastectomy, two drainage tubes are usually placed and may be sutured under the skin flaps and attached to a small collection chamber. Gentle suction is exerted, and fluid that would accumulate under the flaps and delay healing is collected. Various types of these devices are available, but all provide the ability to see and measure the drainage. The drain should be checked for amount and color of drainage when taking vital signs. This information is added to the input and output record. The placement of the tubes and device should be assessed to avoid pulling the tubes or container or kinking the tubes.

Comfort measures immediately after surgery include helping the client find a comfortable position, with her lying either on her back or on her nonoperative side with the operative arm supported by a pillow. Other basic comfort measures such as back rubs and medications may also help.

The hospital stay after the modified radical mastectomy is short, and recovery is usually not complicated. Ambulation and normal diet are resumed by the day after surgery. While the client is in an upright position, the arm on the affected side may need to be supported at first but gradually should be allowed to hang straight by the side while the client is walking. The hunched back position with the arm flexed should be avoided because of the risk of elbow contractures. Beginning exercises that do not stress the incision can usually be started almost immediately. These exercises include squeezing the affected hand around a soft, round object (a ball or rolled washcloth) and flexion/extension of the elbow. The progression to more strenuous exercises depends on

Text continued on page 1679

SURGICAL MANAGEMENT OF BREAST CANCER

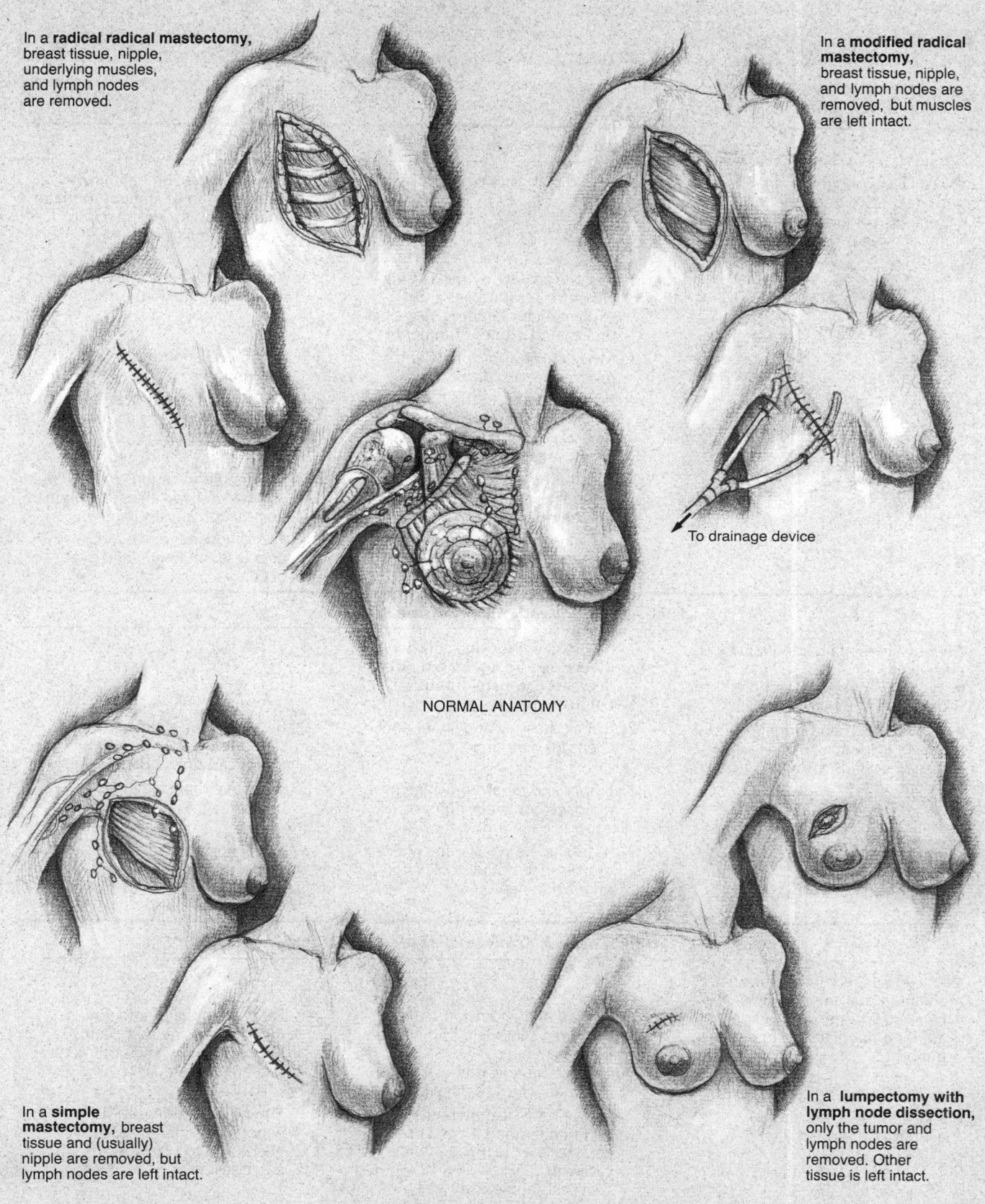

In a **radical radical mastectomy,** breast tissue, nipple, underlying muscles, and lymph nodes are removed.

In a **modified radical mastectomy,** breast tissue, nipple, and lymph nodes are removed, but muscles are left intact.

To drainage device

NORMAL ANATOMY

In a **simple mastectomy,** breast tissue and (usually) nipple are removed, but lymph nodes are left intact.

In a **lumpectomy with lymph node dissection,** only the tumor and lymph nodes are removed. Other tissue is left intact.

CLIENT CARE PLAN ■ Postoperative and Discharge Care of the Woman Undergoing Mastectomy

Goal/Outcome Criteria	Interventions	Rationales
Nursing Diagnosis 1: Pain		
Client will experience minimal pain or unnecessary discomfort. ■ Remains comfortable and without physical signs or complaints of pain.	1. Assess pain and identify possible causes. 2. Reduce anxiety by reorienting client to surroundings and explaining procedures, dressings, drains, and other equipment. 3. Medicate as appropriate with ordered medications. 4. Position client on the back or the unaffected side, with the arm on the side of surgery elevated slightly on a pillow. 5. Check drains and dressings for constriction, position, and functioning. 6. Explain potential for phantom sensations of missing breast.	1. Thorough assessment allows identification of and appropriate intervention for the specific cause of pain. 2. Anxiety and fear of the unknown decrease the pain threshold. 3. Pain medications decrease perception of pain. 4. Elevation of the arm decreases swelling, which would cause discomfort. 5. Impeded circulation or swelling under skin flap caused by drain obstruction causes pain. 6. Prior knowledge of event decreases anxiety when event occurs.
Nursing Diagnosis 2: Altered Tissue Perfusion		
Client will maintain adequate tissue perfusion. ■ Maintains normal blood pressure, pulse, and urinary output. ■ Remains alert and oriented. ■ Shows evidence of minimal bleeding on dressing and from wound.	1. Assess client for signs of shock (decreased BP, increased pulse, decreased urinary output, confusion). 2. Check dressing and sheet under client for bleeding. 3. Empty and record drainage in drainage container. Report excessive amounts. 4. Assess operative site for swelling or presence of fluid collection under skin flaps.	1. These signs indicate shock. 2. Bleeding may stain dressing or seep under dressing and be unnoticed unless bed is checked. 3. Excessive drainage indicates hemorrhage. 4. Collection of fluid under skin flaps disrupts healing and may indicate malfunctioning drainage device or bleeding.
Nursing Diagnosis 3: Impaired Physical Mobility		

Client will experience return of mobility to preoperative level.
■ Demonstrates exercises appropriate for immediate postoperative period.
 	
■ Demonstrates appropriate exercises after discharge.
	1. Flexion and extension of fingers and wrist can begin immediately postoperatively.
	  a. Encourage gentle use of arm for activities of daily living.
	2. Consult physical therapist to recommend and teach appropriate exercises (with surgeon's consent).
	  a. Teach home exercises, as shown in Client/Family
		1. Early use of hand and arm muscles and joints prevents muscle atrophy and contractures and enhances fluid return.
		
		2. The physical therapist has expertise to identify specific needs and to plan specific exercises.

CLIENT CARE PLAN ■ Postoperative and Discharge Care of the Woman Undergoing Mastectomy *continued*

Goal/Outcome Criteria	Interventions	Rationales
Nursing Diagnosis 3: Impaired Physical Mobility		
	Education: Instructions for Postmastectomy Exercises. ■ Hand wall climbing ■ Pulley exercise ■ Rope turning b. Exercises should be done 3–5 times a day and not beyond the point of discomfort. c. Review the exercises with the client.	
	3. Inform client about Reach to Recovery and contact the organization with the client's permission to arrange an in-hospital visit.	3. Reach to Recovery will provide written materials on exercises that are safe to perform at home.
■ Stands upright with shoulders back and the operative arm hanging straight.	4. Encourage upright posture with shoulders held back and the arm by the side while walking and standing.	4. The tendency is to hold the arm bent across the waist and to stoop over, which results in elbow and shoulder contractures.
Nursing Diagnosis 4: Potential for Infection		
Client will have an incision that remains free from infection. ■ Has a wound that is free from purulent drainage and is without redness, swelling, and heat. Remains afebrile.	1. Assess for signs of infection and swelling.	1. Infection and collection of serosanguinous fluid delay wound healing and disrupt adhesion of skin flaps.
■ Identifies measures to reduce risk of infection. ■ Has an incision that heals without signs of infection or swelling.	2. Teach client measures to reduce risk of infections. a. Avoid taking blood pressure, drawing blood, and giving injections. b. Avoid injury to the arm, such as burns, scratches, and scrapes. c. Treat injuries immediately to avoid infection.	2. Injury and infection in operative arm increase risk of lymphedema related to removal of lymph nodes. a–c. Same as for no. 2.
	d. Encourage client to look at the incision before discharge and explain signs of infection, including redness, heat, swelling, and wound discharge.	d. Discharge usually occurs before complete healing. Client or some other responsible person must monitor wound healing.
	e. Instruct client to notify physician if swelling, redness, or pain occurs.	e. Early intervention may prevent disruption of skin flaps.
	f. Instruct client to avoid use of creams and ointments on incision and to avoid use of deodorant under affected arm.	f. Chemical irritation may lead to infection.
	g. Encourage client to bathe or shower if wound is healed and drains are removed.	g. Same as for no. 2.

continued

CLIENT CARE PLAN ■ Postoperative and Discharge Care of the Woman Undergoing Mastectomy *continued*		
Goal/Outcome Criteria	**Interventions**	**Rationales**

Nursing Diagnosis 5: Body Image Disturbance		

Client will maintain a positive body image.
■ Discusses the impact of the loss of the breast on body image.
■ Demonstrates knowledge and use of prostheses.
	1. Encourage verbalization of concern about body changes.
	2. Discuss use of temporary and fitting of permanent prostheses.
	  a. Assess brassiere for nonbinding, nonwired structure.
	  b. Advise client that the usual time for fitting of a permanent prosthesis is 6–8 wk postoperatively.
	  c. Provide information about sources of permanent forms (such as department stores, medical supply stores, specialty shops) and the need to be fitted by person with experience.
	  d. Inform client that insurance should cover the cost if need is validated by the physician.
		1. Verbalization decreases anxiety and allows validation of feelings.
		2. Maintaining outward appearance promotes positive feelings.
		  a. Pressure impairs blood supply to healing tissue.
		  b. Permanent prostheses can be permanently fitted after swelling resolves and wound healing is complete.
		  c. Specific information encourages client to undergo fitting to obtain the prosthesis.
		
		  d. Reducing concerns about cost encourages the client to obtain a prosthesis.

■ Demonstrates knowledge of breast reconstruction.	3. Encourage client to discuss options for breast reconstruction with the physician.
	  a. Encourage client to discuss feelings about possible breast reconstruction.
		3. Options for breast reconstruction will vary.
		
		  a. Client may have ambivalent feelings about reconstruction and need an objective listener.

Nursing Diagnosis 6: Impaired Social Interaction		
Client will maintain relationships with significant other, family, and friends. ■ Client verbalizes satisfaction with relationships. ■ Significant other demonstrates support and verbalizes concerns.	1. Encourage verbalization of concerns about possible changes in relationships. 2. Allow significant other to verbalize concerns. Provide information and support.	1. Verbalization of concerns decreases anxiety. 2. Client's significant other's reactions to breast cancer and treatment may severely threaten relationship.

Nursing Diagnosis 7: Knowledge Deficit Related to Postdischarge Care		
Client will understand postdischarge care. ■ Returns for follow-up visits. ■ Can explain plans for follow-up therapy.	1. Provide written and oral information about appointment dates and times and reasons for follow-up care. 2. Explain and provide written information about follow-up therapy based on the physician's individualized recommendations.	1. Written reinforcement enhances compliance. 2. Follow-up care is based on each client's needs. The nurse collaborates with the physician to ensure the accuracy of information.

CLIENT CARE PLAN ■ Postoperative and Discharge Care of the Woman Undergoing Mastectomy *continued*

Goal/Outcome Criteria	Interventions	Rationales
Nursing Diagnosis 7: Knowledge Deficit Related to Postdischarge Care continued		

■ Resumes role in family and with friends.	3. Allow client to express concerns about resuming previous roles.
	  a. Discuss appropriateness of roles as related to physical abilities.
	  b. For premenopausal women, provide information about childbearing after breast cancer treatment.
		3. Role issues are individual and discussion will enhance planning.
		  a. Roles may need to be modified because of physical limitations.
		  b. Pregnancy and lactation are possible after surgery, radiation, and chemotherapy. Pregnancy after breast cancer does not adversely affect survival.

	4. Assess need for professional intervention.	4. Ongoing counseling may be needed for support and therapy for clients at risk.
■ Resumes sexual activity or relationship.	5. Initiate discussion related to sexual activity. a. Advise that client may resume sexual activity when she feels comfortable. To avoid trauma to operative area, she may prefer woman-on-top position.	5. Client may be reluctant to initiate questions but needs this information before discharge.

the subsequent procedures planned, such as reconstruction, and the surgeon's orders. Typical instructions for postmastectomy exercises are given in the Client/Family Education feature on pages 1680 and 1681.

The amount of wound drainage will continue to be measured, although measurements of general fluid intake and output are usually discontinued by the first postoperative day. Observation of the wound for signs of swelling and infection is necessary throughout the hospital stay. When wound drainage is minimal, usually within 3 or 4 days, the drainage tubes are removed by the physician. The client should be reassured that these tubes lie just under the skin and that removal may be uncomfortable but not painful.

As soon as the woman is fully ambulatory, eating well, and has had the drain removed without subsequent swelling or infection, she will be discharged to continue recuperation at home.

Reconstruction. With reconstruction after mastectomy becoming increasingly available, women should have this option presented before treatment begins. The nurse assesses the client's attitude about this by asking about plans for restoring appearance postoperatively. Although reconstruction is not appropriate for some clients and others may not be interested in it, all should have information about indications and contraindications, advantages and disadvantages, and typical postoperative recovery discussed with them by the surgeon. If reconstruction is chosen, the surgeon should be aware of this preoperatively so that the surgeon's plans can be coordinated with those of the plastic surgeon.

There are several available procedures for restoring the appearance of the breast, as shown in Table 53-1. Reconstruction may begin during the original operative procedure or may be done later in one to several stages. Some of the more common techniques include using a flap of skin and tissue from the abdomen, back, or hip to create a breast mound; placement of a silicone prosthesis; or use of progressive tissue expanders to slowly create a pocket under the mastectomy site for placement of a permanent implant. A new nipple may be created by using tissue from the other nipple or from similar body tissue such as the labia or inner thigh.

Nursing care of the woman undergoing breast reconstruction is given in the Client Care Plan on page 1684.

■ Discharge Planning

The client who has undergone breast surgery can be discharged to the home setting unless other physical disabilities exist. Even without support in the home, she is usually able to function alone without difficulty.

Home Care Preparation

Alterations of the home environment specifically for the client after breast surgery are usually not necessary. If fatigue is a major problem and the home has two stories, limiting activities to one level may help. Activities involving stretching or reaching for heavy objects

CLIENT/FAMILY EDUCATION ■ Instructions for Postmastectomy Exercises

Hand Wall Climbing

"Face the wall and put the palms of your hands flat against the wall at shoulder level. Flex your fingers so that your hands slowly 'walk' up the wall. Stop when your arms are fully extended. Then slowly 'walk' your hands back down the wall until they return to shoulder level."

Pulley Exercise

"Drape a 6-foot-long rope over a shower curtain rod or over the top of a door. If you use a door for this exercise, have someone put a nail or hook at the top of the door so that the rope does not slip off. Grab the ends of the rope, one in each hand, and extend your arms out to your sides until they are straight. Pull down—keeping your arms straight—with your left arm to raise your right arm as high as you can. Then pull down with your right arm to raise your left arm as high as you can."

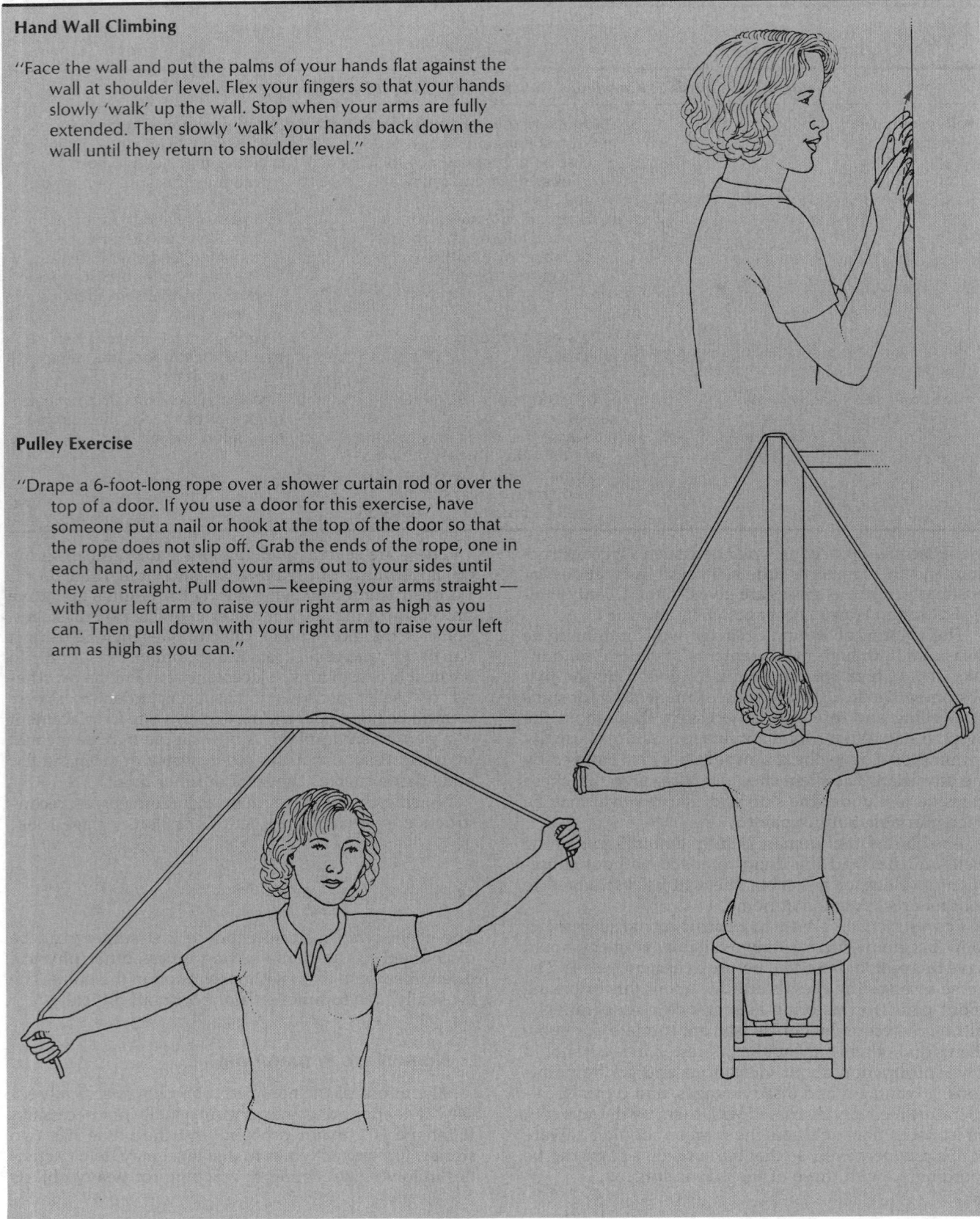

Rope Turning

"Tie a rope to the knob of a closed door. Hold the other end of the rope and step back from the door until your arm is almost straight out in front of you. Swing the rope in a circle. Start with small circles and gradually increase to larger circles as you become more flexible."

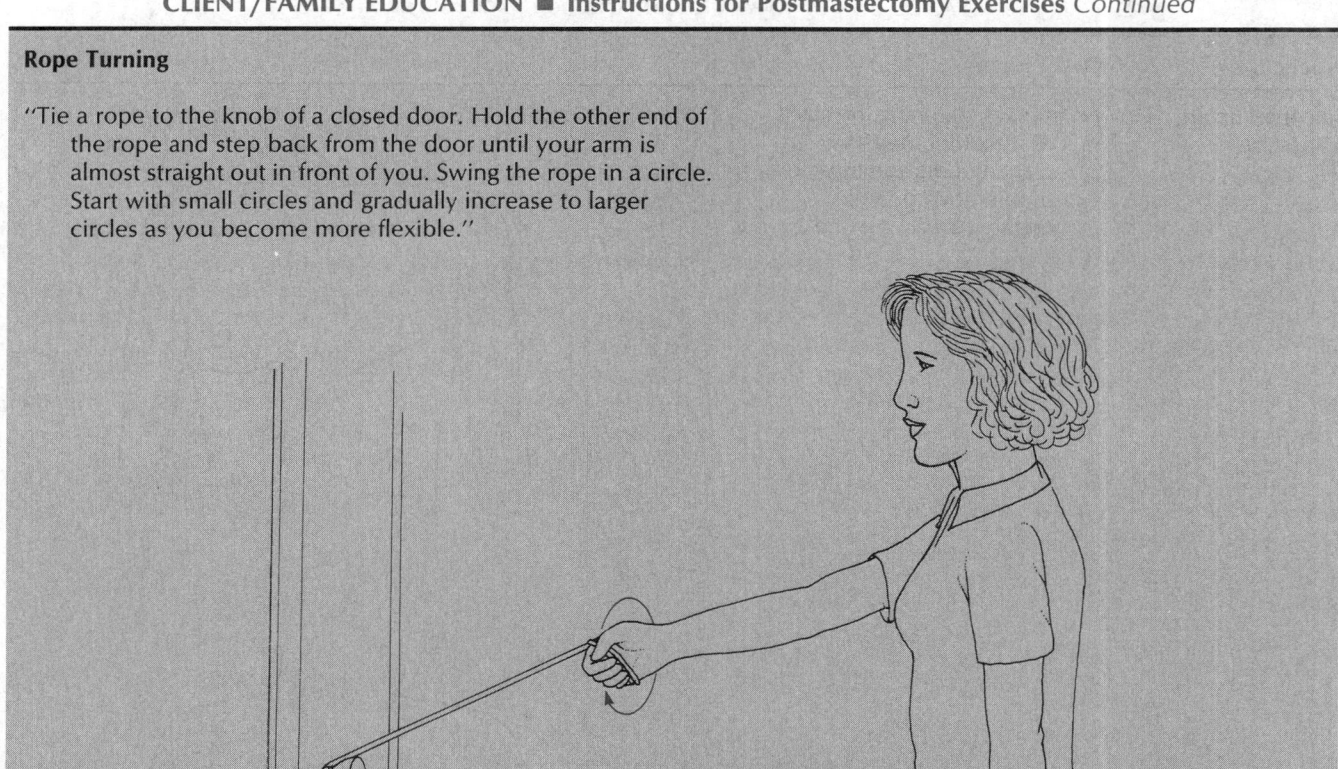

should be avoided. This restriction can be discussed with a family member who can perform these tasks or place the objects within easy reach of the client.

Client/Family Education

The teaching plan for the client after surgery includes (1) measures to optimize a positive body image, (2) information to enhance interpersonal relationships and roles, (3) exercises to regain full range of motion, (4) measures to prevent infection of the incision, and (5) measures to avoid injury, infection, and subsequent swelling of the affected arm.

The nurse takes the opportunity to explain incisional care. A light dressing may be worn to prevent irritation. No lotions or ointments should be used on the area, and use of deodorant under the affected arm should be delayed until healing is complete. Although swelling and redness of the scar itself are normal for the first few weeks, swelling, redness, increased heat, and tenderness of the surrounding area indicate infection and should be reported to the surgeon. The nurse asks the client to have a family member bring a loose-fitting, nonwired brassiere to try before discharge, to be used with a soft cotton- or polyester fiber–filled form supplied by the hospital or by Reach to Recovery. This form

is usually worn until the incision is completely healed and the physician approves the fitting of a more sophisticated prosthesis, usually 6 to 8 weeks after discharge. After going home, the client should be encouraged to dress in street clothes, not pajamas, to further enhance a positive self-image.

Exercises that began in the hospital should continue at home. A physical therapist may be consulted to plan a program of strengthening and range-of-motion exercises in the home setting. It should be emphasized that reaching and stretching exercises should continue only to the point of pain or pulling, never higher. ENCORE, a YWCA program, is appropriate for women as early as 3 weeks postoperatively and includes exercise to music, exercise in water, and psychologic support. Precautions or limitations specific to plans for future procedures such as reconstruction may be prescribed by the surgeon before discharge.

Information needed to help the client avoid infection and subsequent edema of the affected arm after mastectomy should be provided. The client should avoid having blood pressure taken, having injections, and having blood taken from the arm on the side of the mastectomy. Common practices, such as wearing a mitt when using the oven, wearing gloves when gardening, and treating cuts and scrapes appropriately, should be used. If

TABLE 53–1   Breast Reconstruction Procedures

Procedure	Description	
Silicone implantation	An implant matching the size of the other breast is placed under the muscle of operative side to create a breast mound.	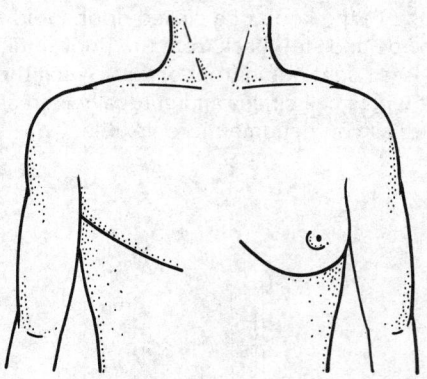
		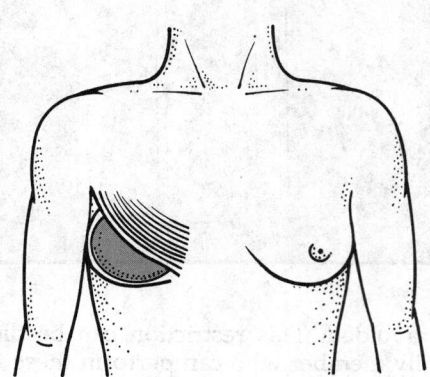
Tissue expansion	A tissue expander is placed under the muscle and gradually expanded with saline to stretch the overlying skin and create a pocket. After several weeks, the tissue expander is exchanged for a silicone implant.	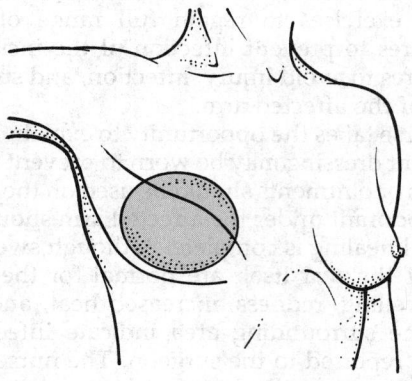

TABLE 53–1   Breast Reconstruction Procedures *Continued*

Procedure	Description
Autogenous procedures	A flap of skin, fat, and muscle is transferred from the donor site to the operative area. The flap contains an appropriate amount of fat to match the other breast and is similar in appearance to breast tissue. A blood supply is established by reanastomosing vessels from the operative area to those with the flap when possible. A new nipple may be created by using similar tissue, such as the other nipple or labia or thigh tissue.

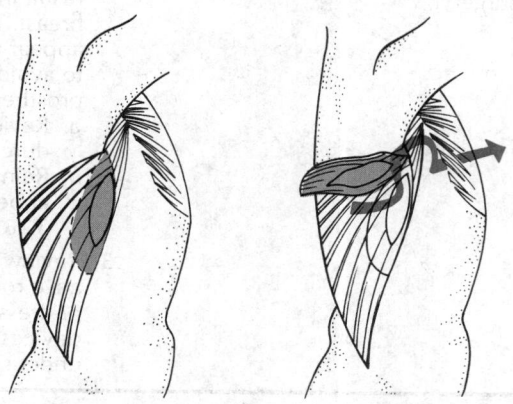

Latissimus dorsi musculocutaneous flap

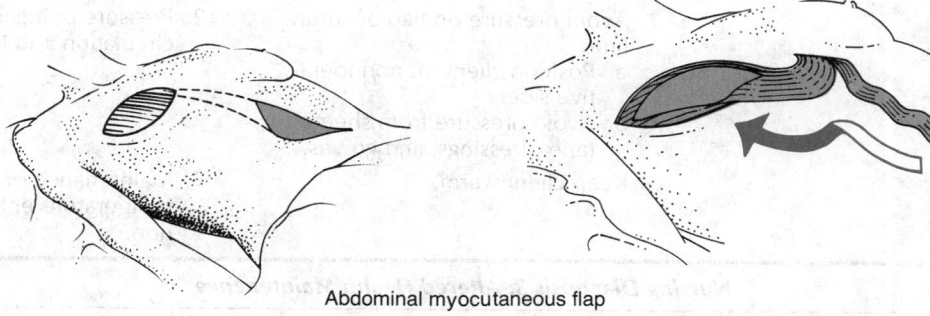

Abdominal myocutaneous flap

edema that is unrelated to a specific injury occurs, the arm should be elevated when possible and special attention should be paid to the above-mentioned warnings. A detailed review of this information is presented in the earlier Client Care Plan: Postoperative and Discharge Care of the Woman Undergoing Mastectomy.

Psychosocial Preparation

Concerns about appearance after surgery are common and are often a threat to one's self-concept as a woman. After a modified radical mastectomy, any woman can benefit from an explanation of the expected postoperative appearance. Usually, the actual result is much less terrifying than what she has imagined. The chest wall is fairly smooth and has a horizontal incision from the axilla to the mid-chest area. The scar may be red and raised at first, but these characteristics diminish within the first few months. After this explanation, the nurse encourages the woman to look at her incision before she leaves the hospital and offers to be present when she does so.

CLIENT CARE PLAN ■ The Woman Undergoing Breast Reconstruction

Goal/Outcome Criteria	Interventions	Rationales
Nursing Diagnosis 1: Knowledge Deficit Related to Preoperative and Postoperative Care		

Client will demonstrate knowledge of surgical procedure.
■ Verbalizes goals of surgery.
■ Explains schedule for procedures.
■ States specific restrictions related to surgery.
	1. Assess knowledge of and expectations about surgery.
	
	2. Explain that surgery may not result in duplication of opposite breast. The purpose may be to appear normal when dressed and to avoid the inconvenience of a prosthesis.
	  a. Review schedule for procedures.
	  b. Reinforce that optimal appearance may not occur for 3–6 mo postoperatively.
	
	3. Review usual pre- and postoperative routine, including presence of dressings and use of drainage devices to avoid fluid collection under skin flaps.
		1. Client may have unrealistic expectations, which should be discussed to maximize postoperative satisfaction.
		2. Implants and skin flaps gradually assume the desired position and shape.
		
		3. Understanding routines encourages cooperation and enhances recovery.

Nursing Diagnosis 2: Altered Tissue Perfusion Related to Transferred Tissue for Breast Reconstruction		

Client will have viable incision and skin flap.
■ Develops no infection.
■ Has normal tissue perfusion.
	1. Assess incision and flap for
	  a. Signs of infection (redness, drainage, odor).
	  b. Signs of poor perfusion (blanching, duskiness, decreased capillary refill).
	2. Avoid pressure on flap or suture lines.
	  a. Position client on nonoperative side.
	  b. Avoid pressure from sheets, tape, dressings, and gowns.
	3. Keep client warm.
		1. Monitoring for signs of impaired perfusion allows early intervention to prevent loss of viability.
		
		2. Pressure points decrease circulation and threaten viability.
		
		3. Maintenance of normal body temperature enhances circulation.

Nursing Diagnosis 3: Altered Health Maintenance		

Client will understand discharge instructions to optimize results of surgery.
■ Follows instructions.
	1 Advise gradual return to daily activities except
	  a. Avoid heavy lifting.
	  b. Avoid sleeping on stomach.
	  c. Do not participate in contact sports or in activities that increase the risk of trauma to the chest.
	  d. Minimize pressure on the breast during sexual activity.
	  e. Refrain from driving until advised by physician.
	2. Advise client to ask at the 6-wk postoperative visit when full activity can be resumed.
	3. If implants have been inserted, teach proper method of breast massage (consult with physician).
	4. Review BSE and the need to continue this practice on a regular basis.
		1. Trauma and pressure to the breast mound may cause skin flap necrosis or infection.
		
		2. The schedule for return to normal activity differs according to the operative technique used.
		3. Regular breast massage enhances expansion and prevents capsule formation.
		4. Women with breast cancer history are at increased risk for cancer in the other breast.

Much of one's body image is a reflection of how others respond. Therefore, the response of the client's family and partner to the surgery will be crucial in determining the effect on self-concept. These people may also need the support of the nurse. They may have concerns about their ability to accept the changes and need to discuss these feelings with an objective listener. They may need help with communicating their feelings, both negative and positive, with their loved one. Involving them in teaching may also help reinforcement and increase retention. Sexual concerns should be discussed before discharge. The client may be embarrassed to broach the topic, so the nurse should be sensitive to possible concerns and approach the subject first. For women of childbearing age, the issues related to childbearing may be a concern.

Health Care Resources

Resources available to the client after discharge from the hospital involve personal support and/or community programs. After discharge, the client's spouse or significant other may need aid in planning support for home responsibilities. For example, the husband may feel stress because of an assumption of additional duties at home and work. Exploring temporary relief resources for child care, cleaning, or cooking may be helpful until the woman regains her previous energy level. Discussing the need for ongoing emotional support is also beneficial to both client and spouse or significant other. Leaving the hospital and appearing normal do not end the anxiety and fear that the client may feel. Identification of a support person with whom the client or couple can explore these feelings and discussion of the need to ventilate feelings enhance personal and family recovery.

Reach to Recovery and ENCORE, as mentioned, are two examples of community resources that provide support and information to women with breast cancer. Reach to Recovery will provide a volunteer who visits the client in the hospital or at home. She brings a personal message of hope, written information, and a soft, temporary breast form. Some communities have additional resources such as support groups and exercise classes.

Evaluation

The processes of care planning and implementation are important, but it is only through evaluation that practice can improve. The process of evaluation is based on the identified nursing diagnoses. The expected outcomes for the client with breast cancer are that she

1. Demonstrates the correct method of BSE
2. Practices BSE on a monthly basis
3. Complies with guidelines for mammography and professional examination
4. Follows a low-fat, low-alcohol diet, abstains from smoking, and stays within her recommended weight range
5. Participates in the decision-making process during the diagnostic period
6. Demonstrates an appropriate level of anxiety as shown by her ability to sleep, an absence of physical signs of anxiety, and verbal confirmation of feeling calm
7. States that she feels positive about her self-image
8. Maintains positive interpersonal relationships with family and friends
9. Regains full range of motion of the affected arm
10. Remains free from arm edema or infection
11. Describes and complies with the adjuvant therapy regimen

SUMMARY

Most breast diseases are benign, occurring throughout the life cycle. Fibroadenomas and fibrocystic disease are common in females in the early to middle adult years; ductal ectasia and intraductal papilloma occur in women older than the age of 40 years. Breast cancer affects primarily women older than 50 years, with less than 1% occurring in men. Breast disorders can affect the client's self-esteem and life style and can cause physical discomfort, anxiety and psychologic stress, and even death.

The emphasis of nursing interventions should be teaching women that early detection of any breast lump is important. Screening through BSE, professional examination, and mammography is the most effective approach for this early detection. After diagnosis of cancer, nursing care is focused on meeting physiologic and emotional needs that are present.

IMPLICATIONS FOR RESEARCH

Nursing care of the client with breast cancer focuses on both physiologic and psychologic needs during the stages of detection, diagnosis, and treatment. The following research questions are relevant for detection:

1. What is the effect of health care professionals' attitudes toward cancer on teaching BSE?
2. How do different health care settings affect nurses' knowledge and beliefs about breast cancer and prevention?

3. What is the best approach for teaching BSE?

Examples of research questions related to diagnosis and treatment include

1. What should be included on tools to identify the women at high risk for psychologic difficulties?

2. What are the physiologic parameters that could be measured to assess psychologic stress?

3. What effect does early referral and counseling have on clients' well-being once they are identified to be at high risk for emotional distress?

REFERENCES AND READINGS

Abramowicz, M. (1985). Cancer chemotherapy. *Medical Letter, 27,* 13–20.

American Cancer Society. (1989). *Cancer facts and figures— 1989.* New York: Author.

Ashraf, J., & Fentiman, S. (1986). Conservative treatment of early breast cancer. *British Journal of Hospital Medicine, 35,* 263–365.

Baden, W. F., & Thorton, D. R. (1980). *Primary health care for obstetricians and gynecologists* (pp. 115–119). Baltimore: Williams & Wilkins.

Baker, L. H. (1982). Breast Cancer Detection Demonstration Project: Five-year summary report. *CA: A Cancer Journal for Clinicians, 32,* 194–225.

Bezwada, W. R., Hesdorffer, C., Dansey, R., de Moor, N., Derman, D. P., Browde, S., & Lange, M. (1987). Breast cancer in men. Clinical features, hormone receptor status, and response to therapy. *Cancer, 60,* 1337–1340.

Beadle, G. F., Silver, B., Botnick, L., Hellman, S., & Harris, J. R. (1984). Cosmetic results following primary radiation therapy for early breast cancer. *Cancer, 54,* 2911–2918.

Berger, G. S., & Keith, L. G. (1982). Screening for breast cancer and cost-effectiveness of thermal diagnostic techniques. *Progress in Clinical and Biological Research, 107,* 839–849.

Berger, K., & Bostwick, J. (1984). *A woman's decision: Breast care, treatment, and reconstruction.* St. Louis: C. V. Mosby.

Bishop, H. M., & Blamey, R. W. (1979). A suggested classification of breast pain. *Postgraduate Medical Journal, 55,* 59–60.

Brownson, R. D., Blackwell, C. W., Pearson, D. K., Reynolds, R. D., Richens, J. W., Jr., & Papermaster, B. W. (1988). Risk of breast cancer in relation to cigarette smoking. *Archives of Internal Medicine, 148,* 140–144.

Clarke, D. E., & Sandler, L. S. (1989). Factors involved in nurses' teaching breast self-examination. *Cancer Nursing, 12,* 41–46.

Consensus Conference. (1985). Adjuvant chemotherapy for breast cancer. *JAMA, 254,* 3461–3463.

d'Angelo, T. M., & Gorrell, C. R. (1989). Breast reconstruction using tissue expanders. *Oncology Nursing Forum, 16,* 23–27.

deHaes, J. C. J. M., & Welvaart, K. (1985). Quality of life

after breast cancer surgery. *Journal of Surgical Oncology, 28,* 123–125.

Devitt, J. E. (1985). Management of nipple discharge by clinical findings. *American Journal of Surgery, 149,* 789–792.

Dunn, C. F. (1988). Hormonal therapy for breast cancer. *Cancer Nursing, 88,* 288–294.

Duttenhaur, J. (1987). The role of radiation therapy in the treatment of breast cancer. *Journal of the Medical Association of Georgia, 76,* 349–353.

Edgar, L., Shamian, J., & Patterson, D. (1984). Factors affecting the nurse as a teacher and practicer of breast self-examination. *International Journal of Nursing Studies, 21,* 255–265.

Ellerhorst-Ryan, J. M., Turba, E. P., & Stahl, D. L. (1988). Evaluating benign breast disease. *Nurse Practitioner, 13(9),* 13, 16, 18.

Fisher, B., Bauer, M., Margolese, R., Poisson, R., Pilch, Y., Redmond, C., Fisher, E., Wolmark, N., Deutsch, M., Montague, E., et al. (1985). Five-year results of a randomized clinical trial comparing total mastectomy and segmental mastectomy with or without radiation in the treatment of breast cancer. *New England Journal of Medicine, 312,* 665–673.

Fisher, B., Redmond, C., Fisher, E. R., Bauer, M., Wolmark, N., Wickerham, D. L., Deutsch, M., Montague, E., Margolese, R., & Foster, R. (1985). Ten-year results of a randomized clinical trial comparing radical mastectomy and total mastectomy with or without radiation. *New England Journal of Medicine, 312,* 674–681.

Forrest, A. P. M. (1986). Advances in the management of carcinoma of the breast. *Surgery, Gynecology, and Obstetrics, 163,* 89–100.

Foster, R. S., Lang, S. P., Costanza, M. C., Worden, J. K., Haines, C. R., & Yates, J. W. (1978). Breast self examination practices and breast cancer stage. *New England Journal of Medicine, 299,* 265–270.

Gates, C. C. (1988). The "most-significant-other" in the care of the breast cancer patient. *CA: A Cancer Journal for Clinicians, 38,* 146–153.

Georgiade, G. S. (1984). Immediate reconstruction of the breast following modified radical mastectomy for carcinoma of the breast. *Clinics in Plastic Surgery, 11,* 383–388.

Goodson, W. H., III, Mailman, R., Jacobson, M., & Hunt, T. K. (1985). What do breast symptoms mean? *American Journal of Surgery, 150,* 271–274.

Gottschalk, L. A., & Hoigaard-Martin, J. (1985). The emotional impact of mastectomy. *Psychiatry Research, 17,* 153–167.

Hartrampf, C. R., Black, P. W., & Beagle, P. H. (1987). Breast reconstruction following mastectomy. *Journal of the Medical Association of Georgia, 76,* 328–334.

Hassey, K. M. (1988). Pregnancy and parenthood after treatment for breast cancer. *Oncology Nursing Forum, 15,* 439–444.

Henderson, I. C., Mouridsen, H., Abe, O., & Early Breast

Cancer Trialists' Collaborative Group. (1988). Effects of adjuvant tamoxifen and of cytotoxic therapy on mortality in early breast cancer. *New England Journal of Medicine, 319,* 1681–1992.

Hislop, T. G., & Threlfall, W. J. (1984). Oral contraceptives and benign breast disease. *American Journal of Epidemiology, 120,* 273–280.

Hopkins, M. B. (1986). Information-seeking and adaptational outcomes in women receiving chemotherapy for breast cancer. *Cancer Nursing, 9,* 256–262.

Huguley, C. M. (1987). Screening for breast cancer. *Journal of the Medical Association of Georgia, 76,* 310–313.

Jamison, R. N., Burish, T. G., & Wallston, K. A. (1987). Psychogenic factors in predicting survival of breast cancer patients. *Journal of Clinical Oncology, 5,* 768–772.

Johnson, B. L., & Gross, J. (1985). *Handbook of oncology nursing.* New York: Wiley.

Levine, R. M., & Lippman, M. E. (1984). *Breast cancer management: Recent advances and recommendations* (pp. 215–239). Chicago: Year Book Medical.

Lierman, L. M. (1988). Sensory and physical alteration after mastectomy. *Health Care Women International, 9*(4), 263–279.

Lucas, L. M., Kumar, K. L., & Smith, D. L. (1987). Gynecomastia. A worrisome problem for the patient. *Postgraduate Medicine, 82,* 73–76, 79–81.

Mamon, J. A., & Zapka, J. G. (1985). Improving frequency and proficiency of breast self-examination: effectiveness of an education program. *American Journal of Public Health, 75,* 618–624.

McDonald, H. D. (1988). Reconstruction of the breast. In M. E. Lippman, A. S. Lichter, & D. N. Danforth (Eds.), *Diagnosis and management of breast cancer* (pp. 468–485). Philadelphia: W. B. Saunders.

Miller, A. B., Chamberlain, J., & Tsechkovski, M. (1985). Self-examination in the early detection of breast cancer. *Journal of Chronic Diseases, 38,* 527–540.

Mushlin, A. I. (1985). Diagnostic tests in breast cancer: Clinical strategies based on diagnostic probabilities. *Annals of Internal Medicine, 103,* 79–85.

Nail, L., Jones, L. S., Giuffre, M., & Johnson, J. E. (1984). Sensations after mastectomy. *American Journal of Nursing, 84,* 1121–1123.

Neeson, J. D., & Stockdale, C. R. (1981). *The practitioner's handbook of ambulatory OB/GYN.* New York: Wiley.

Nettles-Carlson, B. (1989). Early detection of breast cancer. *Journal of Obstetric, Gynecologic, and Neonatal Nursing, 18,* 373–381.

Norwood, S. L. (1990). Fibrocystic breast disease. *Journal of Obstetric, Gynecologic, and Neonatal Nursing, 19,* 116–121.

O'Malley, M. S., Fletcher, S. W., & Bruce, L. A. (1985). Physicians and the teaching of breast self-examination: Implications from a survey at a university teaching hospital. *American Journal of Public Health, 75,* 673–675.

Parazzini, F., La Vecchia, C., Franceschi, S., Decarli, A.,

Gallus, G., Regallo, M., Liberati, M., & Tognoni, G. (1984). Risk factors for pathologically confirmed benign breast disease. *American Journal of Epidemiology, 120,* 115–122.

Pastides, H., Kelsey, J. L., LiVolsi, V. A., Holford, T. R., Fischer, D. B., & Goldenberg, I. S. (1983). Oral contraceptive use and fibrocystic breast disease with special reference to its histopathology. *Journal of the National Cancer Institute, 71,* 5–9.

Paulus, D. D. (1987). Imaging in breast cancer. *CA: A Cancer Journal for Clinicians, 37,* 133–150.

Philip, J., Harris, W. G., Flaherty, C., & Joslin, C. A. (1986). Clinical measures to assess the practice and efficiency of breast self-examination. *Cancer, 58,* 973–977.

Pilnik, S. (1979). Clinical diagnosis of benign breast diseases. *Journal of Reproductive Medicine, 22,* 277–289.

Powell, R. W. (1987). The surgical management of breast cancer. *Journal of the Medical Association of Georgia, 76,* 315–321.

Raina, S., Rush, B. F., Jr., Blackwood, J. M., & Lazaro, E. J. (1985). Trends in the management of breast cancer. *Journal of Surgical Oncology, 28,* 117–122.

Rosenburg, L., Miller, D. R., Kaufman, D. W., Helmrich, S. P., Stolley, P. D., Schottenfeld, D., & Shapiro, S. (1984). Breast cancer and oral contraceptive use. *American Journal of Epidemiology, 119,* 167–176.

Rust, D. L., & Kloppenborg, E. M. (1990). Don't underestimate the lumpectomy patient's needs. *RN, 53*(3), 59–64.

Rutledge, D. N. (1987). Factors related to women's practice of breast self-examination. *Nursing Research, 36,* 117–121.

Schain, W. S. (1988). The sexual and intimate consequences of breast cancer treatment. *CA: A Cancer Journal for Clinicians, 38,* 154–161.

Schain, W. S., Wellisch, D. K., Pasnau, R. O., & Landsverk, J. (1985). The sooner the better: A study of psychological factors in women undergoing immediate versus delayed breast reconstruction. *American Journal of Psychiatry, 142,* 40–46.

Schatzkin, A., Jones, D. Y., Hoover, R. N., Taylor, P. R., Brinton, L. A., Ziegler, R. G., Harvey, E. B., Carter, C. L., Licitra, L. M., Dufour, M. C., et al. (1987). Alcohol consumption and breast cancer in the epidemiologic follow-up study of the first National Health and Nutrition Examination Survey. *New England Journal of Medicine, 316,* 1169–1173.

Sheahan, S. L. (1984). Management of breast lumps. *Nurse Practitioner, 9,* 19–22.

Silverman, D. C., Edbril, S., Gartrell, N., Wise, S., Botnick, L., Liao-Rosenblatt, E., & Huntley, B. (1985). A pilot study of women's attitudes towards breast-conserving surgery with primary radiation therapy for breast cancer. *International Journal of Psychiatry in Medicine, 15,* 381–391.

Smith, R. E. (1987). Dietary fat and breast cancer. *Cancer Detection and Prevention, 10,* 193–196.

Taylor, S. G. (1986). Adjuvant treatment of breast cancer. *Current Concepts in Oncology, 8,* 2–6.

Townsend, C. M. (1980). Breast lumps. *Clinical Symposia, 32*, 3–32.

Urban, J. A. (1986). Breast cancer 1985: What have we learned? *Cancer, 57*, 636–643.

Wang, Y. (1987). Laser operations for breast cancer. *International Surgery, 72*, 208–210.

Ward, C. M. (1985). Cosmetic and reconstructive surgery of the breast. *British Medical Journal, 290*, 1337–1339.

Willett, W. C., Stamfer, M. J., Colditz, G. A., Rosner, B. A., Hennekens, C. H., & Speizer, F. E. (1987). Moderate alcohol consumption and the risk of breast cancer. *New England Journal of Medicine, 316*, 1174–1180.

Wright, J. C. (1985). Update on cancer chemotherapy: General considerations and breast cancer, part II. *JAMA, 77*, 691–703.

ADDITIONAL READINGS

Northouse, L. L., & Swain, M. A. (1987). Adjustments of patients and husbands to the initial impact of breast cancer. *Nursing Research, 36*, 221–225.

This article discusses a study of 50 breast cancer clients and their husbands and focuses on their psychologic reactions to the diagnosis of cancer. The results revealed that not only the women but also their spouses experienced significant stress and difficulty in performing normal daily responsibilities. The need for support for both partners is emphasized, and research implications are discussed.

Rudolph, A., & McDermott, R. J. (1987). The breast physical examination: Its value in early cancer detection. *Cancer Nursing, 10*, 100–106.

The physical examination of the breast by the professional is the focus of this article. A review of the literature is provided, with information on the value, sensitivity, specificity, and predictive value of the procedure. Because the professional examination is often the nurse's responsibility, the article is useful for nurses in all settings.

Taylor, S. E., Lichtman, R. R., Wood, J. V., Bluming, A. Z., Dosik, G. M., & Leibowitz, R. L. (1985). Illness-related and treatment-related factors in psychological adjustment to breast cancer. *Cancer, 55*, 2506–2513.

The authors interviewed 78 women who were treated for breast cancer to determine factors that affect adjustment to the disease. Several were identified, including prognosis and type of surgery. These factors provide a beginning profile of the woman at high risk for psychologic difficulties after diagnosis and treatment.

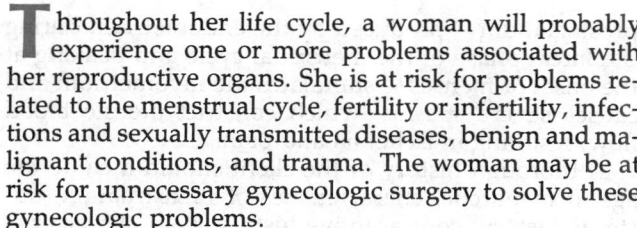

CHAPTER 54

Interventions for Clients with Gynecologic Disorders

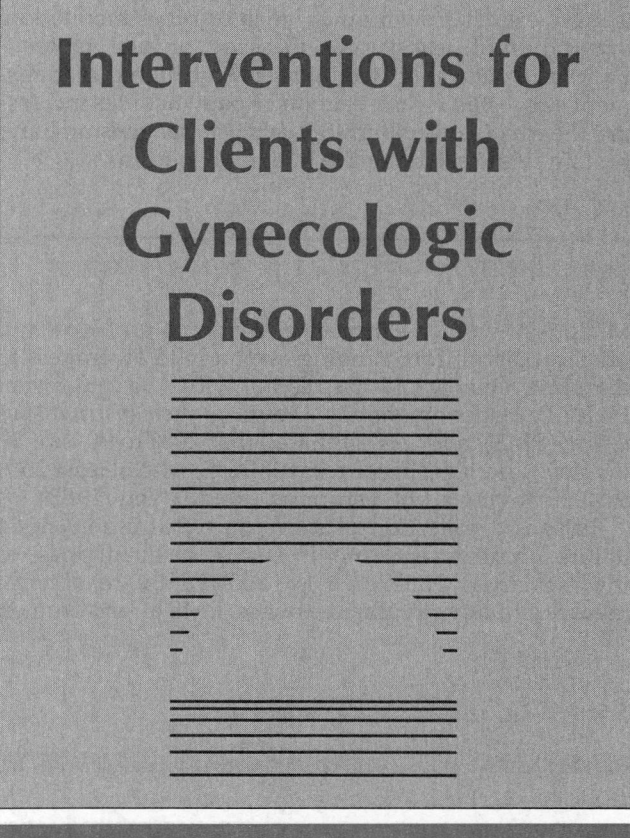

Throughout her life cycle, a woman will probably experience one or more problems associated with her reproductive organs. She is at risk for problems related to the menstrual cycle, fertility or infertility, infections and sexually transmitted diseases, benign and malignant conditions, and trauma. The woman may be at risk for unnecessary gynecologic surgery to solve these gynecologic problems.

Nurses can play an important role in assessing gynecologic disorders by being sensitive to the client's complaints and by encouraging discussion about menstrual or other reproductive problems. Educating women about their bodies, helping them to recognize when professional help should be sought, and providing them with knowledge to make an informed decision about treatments are major goals for nurses working with female clients in any setting.

MENSTRUAL CYCLE DISORDERS

Almost all women experience a problem associated with their menstrual cycle at some time during their reproductive years. Whether a woman seeks professional help depends on the severity of the problem, as well as its perceived significance. Women may seek counseling, advice, or care for their menstrual problems from nurses.

PRIMARY DYSMENORRHEA

Dysmenorrhea, or painful menstrual flow, is one of the most common gynecologic problems, reportedly affecting as many as 80% of all women to some degree and incapacitating as many as 10% (Wilson, 1984). Dysmenorrhea is usually classified as primary or secondary; the former is not associated with pelvic pathologic changes, whereas the latter usually begins with an underlying disease condition.

Primary dysmenorrhea usually occurs after ovulation is established and is characterized by spasmodic lower abdominal pain that begins with the onset of menstrual flow and lasts 12 to 48 hours. The pain often radiates to the lower back and thighs, and nausea and vomiting frequently occur. Less common symptoms include headache, syncope, nervousness, fatigue, diarrhea, bloating, and breast tenderness. Primary dysmenorrhea occurs more frequently in obese women, nulliparas, older adolescents, and college-aged women (Graham, 1986). The symptoms usually become increasingly severe until about age 27 years or after pregnancy.

Most researchers believe that the cause of primary dysmenorrhea is increased uterine prostaglandin production and release. It is thought that an excess of prostaglandin—produced by the endometrium during the luteal phase of the menstrual cycle and peaking at the onset of menses—stimulates the myometrium and causes severe spasms, which constrict uterine blood flow, resulting in ischemia and pain.

A thorough history of the client should include the age at menarche, characteristics of menstruation, obstetric history, contraceptive history, pain characteristics, and previous therapy. Clients should be asked whether they have any conditions suggestive of pelvic problems. Assessment of emotional factors—the individual woman's response to dysmenorrhea, her attitudes about menstruation, and the extent to which dysmenorrhea is perceived to disrupt her life—provides essential data for planning care.

Interventions for primary dysmenorrhea include prevention, therapeutic measures, and education and support and are tailored to each woman's needs. Currently recommended for pain relief is the prescription of prostaglandin synthetase inhibitors (Table 54–1). The three prescription drugs approved for dysmenorrhea by the U.S. Food and Drug Administration are ibuprofen (Motrin), naproxen sodium (Anaprox), and mefenamic acid (Ponstel). Additionally, numerous over-the-counter ibuprofen products (e.g., Advil and Nuprin) are available. Aspirin is a mild prostaglandin synthetase inhibitor and may relieve mild dysmenorrhea.

Ovulation inhibitors that decrease prostaglandin activity are also used to treat primary dysmenorrhea. Oral contraceptives, especially combination agents, may be used for women who desire contraception as well as pain relief.

Other interventions that may alleviate or prevent pain include acupressure, use of sedatives and narcotics, aerobic exercise, swimming, yoga or other meditation, application of heat or cold, massage, orgasm, biofeedback, and relaxation techniques. Nutritional management suggested for prevention of pain includes increasing the intake of vitamin B_6, calcium, magnesium, and protein while reducing the intake of sodium.

PREMENSTRUAL SYNDROME

Millions of women experience emotional problems and physical discomfort, ranging from a mild awareness to disabling symptoms, associated with the menstrual cycle. The phenomenon is known as *premenstrual syndrome* (PMS), and it is estimated that 70% to 90% of all women experience some form of PMS, with at least 20% to 40% having a life disruption (Reid & Yen, 1983).

PMS is a collection of symptoms that are cyclic in nature, occurring each month during the luteal phase of the menstrual cycle; this is followed by relief with menses and a symptom-free phase. PMS affects women

TABLE 54–1 Prostaglandin Synthetase Inhibitor Drugs Used in the Treatment of Dysmenorrhea

Drug	Usual Daily Dosage*	Interventions	Rationales
Ibuprofen (Motrin)	300–400 mg, PO prn, tid, or qid	1. Give with meals or milk. 2. Avoid use in pregnancy. 3. Watch for rash or pruritus. 4. Use with caution if activities require alertness.	1. These measures decrease or prevent GI upset. 2. Safety has not been established. 3. Drug may cause dermatologic reactions. 4. Drug may cause dizziness or drowsiness.
Naproxen sodium (Anaprox)	550 mg PO first dose, 275 mg q 6–8 h prn	1. Same as for ibuprofen.	1. Same as for ibuprofen.
Mefenamic acid (Ponstel)	500 mg PO first dose, 250 mg q 6 h prn	1. Same as for ibuprofen.	1. Same as for ibuprofen.
Aspirin (acetylsalicylic acid)	325–600 mg q 4 h prn PO	1. Same as 1 and 2 for ibuprofen. 2. Watch for bruising or bleeding. 3. Watch for tinnitus.	1. Same as 1 and 2 for ibuprofen. 2. Agent may increase bleeding time. 3. Overdose is possible.

*Drugs are usually taken for 2 to 3 d, beginning at the onset of menstrual flow. They are no more effective if taken before the onset of menses.

of all races, socioeconomic levels, and educational levels. It seems to be more prevalent in women 30 to 40 years of age, and the severity increases with aging until menopause. Women are more at risk for PMS after pregnancy, childbirth, and tubal ligation; during the perimenopausal years; and with major life stresses.

Symptoms vary greatly from woman to woman and affect many body systems (see the accompanying Key Features of Disease).

The etiology of PMS is not well understood. Neuroendocrine mechanisms seem to be involved, but whether there is a single syndrome or several is not known. The symptoms appear only in the luteal phase of the menstrual cycle and disappear with menopause. Theories that have been reported in the literature include estrogen-progesterone imbalance; vitamin and mineral deficiencies (e.g., vitamin B$_6$ and magnesium); hypoglycemia (resulting from altered carbohydrate intolerance in the luteal phase); fluid retention (caused by high levels of aldosterone); increased prolactin levels in the luteal phase; and psychosomatic and stress-related factors (Schroeder & Lesh, 1986).

There is no reported objective means of diagnosing PMS. Assessing the timing of the symptoms is as critical as noting the type of symptoms. The most effective and readily available assessment tool is a menstrual chart. The woman should be instructed to keep a chart for at least three consecutive cycles, showing the length of the menstrual cycle, the duration of bleeding, and occurrence of symptoms. If the woman has PMS, the symptoms recur during the luteal phase (from ovulation to menstruation), followed by a symptom-free time (at least 7 days). When taking a menstrual history, it is also important to assess to what extent the woman feels that the activities of daily living (ADL) are disrupted by the symptoms. Often, reassurance that the symptoms are legitimate and that other women share these problems can facilitate education about PMS.

Management is focused on eliminating the uncomfortable symptoms. Management is highly individualized, as each woman may describe different symptoms; however, one of the most important interventions is education. Each woman needs information about her body, especially the menstrual cycle, so that she can begin to understand the physiologic basis for PMS. Women need to express their feelings and discuss their experiences with PMS; self-help groups and support groups are helpful resources (see Unit 15 Resources). These groups also encourage significant others to participate, as PMS usually affects not only the woman but her family and friends as well. For example, increased family conflict, communication problems with family and friends, and decreased family cohesion have been reported (Brown & Zimmer, 1986) (see the accompanying Nursing Research feature). Stress management is encouraged, and both relaxation and exercise are important methods of stress reduction (see Chap. 6).

Diet and nutrition are also important in managing PMS. If hypoglycemia is a problem, the nurse instructs the woman to eat six small meals a day and to limit her

KEY FEATURES OF DISEASE ■ Clinical Manifestations of Premenstrual Syndrome

Dermatologic

Acne
Urticaria
Herpes

Respiratory

Sinusitis
Asthma
Rhinitis
Colds

Urologic

Oliguria
Cystitis
Enuresis
Urethritis

Ophthalmologic

Conjunctivitis
Styes
Glaucoma

Neurologic

Headaches
Migraine
Syncope
Vertigo
Numbness of hands and feet
Epilepsy (if susceptible)

Metabolic

Edema
Breast tenderness

Emotional/Psychologic

Depression
Irritability
Tension
Panic attacks
Change in libido
Mood swings
Anxiety

Behavioral

Lowered work performance
Food cravings
Alcohol and drug over-indulgence
Confusion
Sleeplessness
Lack of coordination
Suicide
Lethargy
Child abuse
Assaultive behavior

Other

Allergies
Hypoglycemia
Joint pain
Backache
Palpitations
Water retention

intake of sugar, red meats, alcohol, coffee, tea, and chocolate. Eliminating caffeine can also help reduce irritability. Salt and sodium intake should be limited if edema is a problem. Vitamin B$_6$, 100 to 300 mg/day, has been suggested for relief of depression. Vitamin E, 600 IU/day, and magnesium, 300 to 500 mg/day, have been shown to decrease breast tenderness (Schroeder & Lesh, 1986; Sloane, 1985).

NURSING RESEARCH

How Do Men Cope with Premenstrual Syndrome in Their Partners?

Cortese, J., Brown, M. A. (1989). Coping responses of men whose partners experience premenstrual symptomatology. *Journal of Obstetric, Gynecologic, and Neonatal Nursing, 18,* 405–412.

The number of women in the United States with severe premenstrual symptoms is estimated to be 3–7 million. The effects of this problem on family functioning and relationships are a concern to health care providers. Men's coping strategies with this health issue are not well documented.

This exploratory study was designed to describe and categorize coping strategies used by partners of women with premenstrual symptoms. Eighty-six female subjects and their partners were included in the sample that was recruited from a variety of sources, including clinics, newspaper advertisements, and PMS mailing lists. Two instruments were developed for the study and were used in an interview format. First, the women were given a score based on the Premenstrual Symptomatology Inventory and the group was divided into high- and low-symptom groups. Then the men were interviewed to identify coping strategies. Coping strategies were rank ordered by frequency before being analyzed by discriminant analysis.

The coping response with the greatest discriminating ability was "tried to learn more about the symptom." The results included a wide variety of multiple coping responses. Those identified as not helpful or harmful included "get angry" or "hit her," although these were infrequently reported.

Critique. This study was well designed, and the instruments were tested for content validity and reliability. Many questions for further study were identified.

Possible nursing implications. When planning care for women with PMS, the nurse needs to consider the needs of the male partner as well. Providing information about PMS is recommended, either through written information or by including the male in appointments to discuss coping strategies.

Drug therapy is still controversial, but studies have shown that some treatments have been somewhat effective. Diuretics such as hydrochlorothiazide (Hydro-Diuril), 50 mg/day orally for 10 days before menstruation, can provide relief for some women. Women may need to increase their intake of potassium if they are receiving this therapy. Progesterone is used to relieve physical and psychologic symptoms. Natural progesterone is preferable to synthetic progesterone, necessitating the drug to be specially made by a pharmacist at the time it is prescribed. The route of administration is by rectal or vaginal suppository or intramuscular (IM) injection. Daily dosages range from 200 to 800 mg (suppository) to 50 mg (IM) from ovulation to menstruation.

Long-term side effects are unknown at this time. Bromocriptine mesylate (Parlodel), 2.5 mg two or three times a day with meals during the luteal phase, has been effective for treatment of breast symptoms. The side effects (lightheadedness and hypotension) may not be well tolerated. Meprobamate (Equanil), 200 mg twice a day for 10 days before menstruation, has been effective in the relief of tension (Martin, 1985; Wilson, 1984).

AMENORRHEA

Amenorrhea, or the absence of menstrual periods, has been classified as *primary,* menstruation that has failed to occur by age 16 years, and *secondary,* menstruation that has started, but has since stopped and has not recurred for at least 3 months. Primary amenorrhea is often associated with anomalies of the reproductive tract and usually has a poor prognosis for fertility. Secondary amenorrhea is probably due to a functional disorder and has a better prognosis for fertility. Amenorrhea can cause a woman much distress and concern.

Menstruation is a complex series of events that rely on the interplay of the hypothalamic, pituitary, ovarian, and endometrial functions. Dysfunction related to any of these four factors may cause amenorrhea (see the Key Features of Disease on p. 1693, left column). Primary amenorrhea is relatively uncommon. Congenital factors are responsible for about two-thirds of the cases and the remaining one-third is caused by ovarian, pituitary, or hypothalamic disease. Pregnancy, lactation, and menopause are the most common physiologic causes of secondary amenorrhea.

Assessment of amenorrhea includes questions about family history, because girls tend to start menstruation within 2 years of the age when their mothers started. Other factors that should be considered when assessing primary amenorrhea include a family history of genetic abnormalities, ambiguous genitalia at birth, the development of secondary sex characteristics, nutritional habits, past surgery, and emotional stress. Physical assessment is extremely important in evaluating primary amenorrhea. Certain factors associated with anomalies of the genital tract or hormonal causes, such as short stature, lack of breast development, lack of pubic and axillary hair, and abnormality of external genitalia, should be noted.

Diagnosis can also be aided by pelvic examination, chromosomal studies, determination of serum prolactin levels, and hormone withdrawal tests. Progesterone, 10 mg/day orally for 7 days, is given to stimulate withdrawal bleeding that usually indicates normal function of the hypothalamus, the pituitary gland, the ovary, and the uterus. Abnormal test results or dysfunction of these organs must be investigated further.

Assessments for secondary amenorrhea are similar to those for primary amenorrhea, but additional factors must be considered. Menstrual and obstetric histories are important. Questions about possible sexual activity and symptoms of pregnancy must be asked. A medical history may identify a systemic disease as a cause of amenorrhea. The nurse needs to ask questions about current eating habits and past history of dieting because both obesity and starvation (e.g., anorexia nervosa) can result in amenorrhea. Strenuous exercise associated with competitive athletics, such as long-distance running, can cause stress or a reduction of body fat, resulting in amenorrhea. Hormone deficiencies, such as those associated with menopause that can cause hot flashes and vaginal dryness, need to be assessed. Women should be questioned about their ingestion of drugs (e.g., oral contraceptives, phenothiazines, and antihypertensives). The nurse also needs to be alert for signs of galactorrhea (watery or milky breast secretions in nonbreastfeeding or nulliparous women) and hirsutism (un-

usual hair growth in women), both of which are related to polycystic ovary disease.

The nurse's role in implementing care is primarily to present information about amenorrhea in easily understandable terms and to answer questions about tests and treatments. Counseling and emotional support are also important nursing interventions. Amenorrhea may be a threat to a woman's self-concept; she usually needs to ventilate feelings about sexuality and/or fertility.

Interventions for specific causes of amenorrhea must be based on the woman's individual needs. Medical and surgical management of amenorrhea is directed at the underlying causes and includes hormone replacement, corrective surgery, ovulation stimulation, and periodic progesterone withdrawal. Conservative therapy is usually recommended instead of surgery for both primary and secondary amenorrhea.

KEY FEATURES OF DISEASE ■ Some Causes of Amenorrhea

Primary

Congenital anomalies, such as Turner's syndrome
Hypothalamic and pituitary disorders, such as delayed puberty
Systemic disease
    Thyroid and adrenal dysfunction
    Diabetes
    Extreme malnutrition
Ovarian disease
Malformations of the reproductive tract

Secondary

Pregnancy
Menopause
Lactation
Cervical stenosis
Asherman's syndrome
Polycystic ovary disease
Pituitary tumor or insufficiency
Psychogenic stress
Excessive physical activities
Medications
    Antihypertensives
    Birth control pills
    Phenothiazines
Nutritional disorders
    Obesity
    Anorexia nervosa
    Sudden weight loss
Ovarian disease, failure, or destruction

POSTMENOPAUSAL BLEEDING

Postmenopausal bleeding (vaginal bleeding occurring after a 12 months' cessation of menses after the onset of menopause) is a symptom rather than a diagnosis. It is considered serious and should be evaluated, as gynecologic cancer occurs in 20% to 40% of the women who experience postmenopausal bleeding.

Postmenopausal bleeding can be caused by numerous benign and malignant conditions (see the accompanying Key Features of Disease, below), but the three most common causes are atrophic vaginitis, cervical polyps, and endometrial abnormalities. *Atrophic vaginitis* is a condition in which the vaginal mucosa is thin and dry and is easily traumatized by intercourse and infec-

KEY FEATURES OF DISEASE ■ Some Causes of Postmenopausal Bleeding

Benign

Estrogen therapy
Endometrial hyperplasia
Cervical polyps
Uterine fibroids
Atrophic vaginitis
Cervical erosion

Malignant

Endometrial cancer
Cervical cancer
Ovarian cancer
Vaginal cancer
Tubal cancer

tion, causing spotting. *Cervical polyps* are usually soft, red, oval tissue masses that appear within the cervical canal and bleed spontaneously or after intercourse.

The most serious cause of postmenopausal bleeding is *endometrial hyperplasia*, a precursor of endometrial cancer. Bleeding is caused by declining ovarian function that leads to prolonged estrogen stimulation, producing the hyperplasia that eventually breaks down and bleeds. Estrogen stimulation can also be caused by estrogen replacement therapy.

Because many women who report postmenopausal bleeding need medical or surgical interventions, assessment is the nurse's major focus. An accurate assessment of menstrual and family history is the initial step. Questions include the age at menopause, the frequency and amount of bleeding, previous bleeding episodes, the use of medications (especially estrogen-only [unopposed estrogen] replacement therapy), and whether gastrointestinal (GI) or genitourinary symptoms have been experienced. The nurse also needs to identify the woman who is at high risk for endometrial cancer (i.e., women who are obese, hypertensive, or diabetic, or who have never had children).

Urine and stool specimens can be collected and tested for blood to rule out other sources of bleeding. Often, blood specimens are drawn for hemoglobin or hematocrit determinations, because clients are often anemic as a result of excessive bleeding. The nurse can prepare the woman for physical and pelvic examinations, including a Papanicolaou's test (Pap smear), which are usually done to evaluate the cause of bleeding.

Nursing interventions focus on providing information and support for diagnostic and treatment procedures directed at the specific causes of bleeding. Endometrial biopsy can be used to evaluate the presence of malignancy (Chap. 52). A dilation and curettage (D & C) procedure may also be used diagnostically to rule out malignancy (see later discussion of dysfunctional uterine bleeding). Atypical hyperplasia is frequently treated with a hysterectomy (see later discussion of uterine leiomyomas), and malignancy is usually treated with a combination of surgery, radiation therapy, and chemotherapy (see later discussion of endometrial cancer).

Medical treatment for a woman receiving unopposed estrogen therapy may include the monthly administration of a progesterone daily for the last 10 days of the estrogen therapy (days 16 to 25) or a one time IM progesterone injection. This treatment can decrease the abnormal endometrial proliferation and is suggested for the prevention of endometrial and breast cancer.

Treatment of atrophic vaginitis is the administration of estrogen via vaginal, oral, transdermal, or subdermal route (see the accompanying Client/Family Education feature for client instructions). Women who use the vaginal estrogen cream need to be aware that it can cause systemic effects. Women who take estrogen may be at risk for gallbladder disease, hypertension, breast cancer, and endometrial cancer. All women need to be counseled that any postmenopausal bleeding should be considered abnormal and should be evaluated.

CLIENT/FAMILY EDUCATION ■ Instructions for the Client Taking Estrogen Replacement Therapy

For All Types of Estrogen Replacement Therapy

"Call your doctor if you have pain in your calves or groin, if you suddenly get short of breath, if you have abnormal vaginal bleeding, if you feel a lump in your breast, if you have a severe headache, or if you feel weak or numb in your arms or legs."

"Use sunscreen if you are in the sun for a prolonged period."

"You should keep appointments for check-ups as your physician advises."

For Oral Therapy

"Take one pill a day for the first 25 days each month."

"If you feel nauseated or have intestinal upset, you should take your medication with food."

For Transdermal or Subdermal Administration

"You should rotate sites for the patches or injections to avoid skin irritations."

"Change the patches twice a week, according to your prescribed schedule."

For Vaginal Therapy

"Use an applicator to insert suppository or cream daily as prescribed."

"You may need to wear a minipad to protect clothing from soiling or staining by the drug."

ENDOMETRIOSIS

OVERVIEW

Endometriosis is usually a benign disease characterized by implantation of endometrial tissue outside the uterine cavity. The tissue is commonly found on the ovaries and the cul-de-sac and less commonly on other pelvic organs and structures (Fig. 54–1). A *chocolate cyst* is an area of endometriosis inside an ovary.

Endometrial tissue located outside the endometrium responds similarly to the endometrium to hormonal stimulation and goes through the same cyclic changes. Bleeding occurs at the site of implantation, and the blood is trapped in the tissues and causes scarring and adhesions as it is reabsorbed. Endometriosis progresses slowly; it regresses during pregnancy and at menopause. Rarely does endometriosis become a malignant disease.

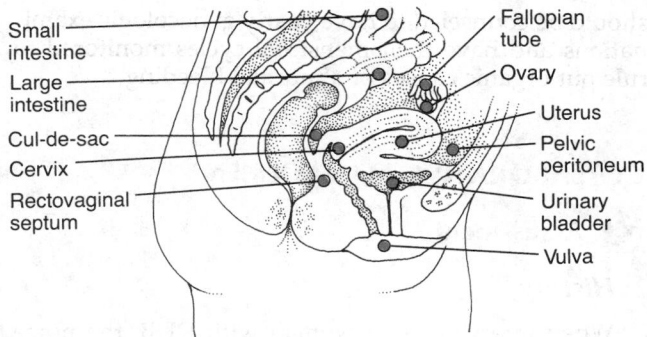

Small intestine
Large intestine
Cul-de-sac
Cervix
Rectovaginal septum
Fallopian tube
Ovary
Uterus
Pelvic peritoneum
Urinary bladder
Vulva

Figure 54–1

Common sites of endometriosis.

The cause of endometriosis is unknown. The most accepted theories of causation are *transportation* and *formation*. There are two transportation theories: implantation and vascular and lymphatic dissemination. The *implantation* theory holds that endometrial tissue flows back through the fallopian tubes during menstruation and then implants on pelvic structures. The *vascular and lymphatic dissemination* theory proposes that endometrial glands are transported through the vascular and lymphatic system to foreign locations. This latter theory may explain implantation in areas outside the pelvis, such as the lungs and the kidneys. Formation theories propose that endometrial tissue develops spontaneously outside the uterus.

Endometriosis occurs most frequently in women in their 30s and 40s; rarely does it appear before age 20 years. It is most common in nulliparous women and in those whose mothers had endometriosis. The disease occurs less frequently among Black women (Thorn, 1986).

COLLABORATIVE MANAGEMENT

The nursing assessment should be as detailed as possible and should include the client's menstrual history, sexual history, and characteristics of bleeding. Pain is the most common symptom of endometriosis, although as many as 30% of women are asymptomatic (Garner & Webster, 1985). The peak of pain usually occurs just before the menstrual flow, and pain is usually located in the lower abdomen, causing many women to feel a sense of rectal pressure. The degree of pain is not related to the extent of the endometriosis, but it is related to the site. Often, women with minimal disease have more severe pain than women with extensive disease. Other symptoms include dyspareunia (painful intercourse), painful defecation, sacral backache, hypermenorrhea (excessive, prolonged, or frequent bleeding), and infertility. A pelvic examination may reveal pelvic tenderness, nodular uterosacral ligaments, and fixed or limited movement of the uterus. Psychosocial assessment may reveal anxiety because of uncertainty about the diag-

nosis. The woman may also have concerns about her self-concept if she is infertile and desires to become pregnant.

Diagnostic studies include blood tests (erythrocyte sedimentation rate and white blood cell count) to rule out pelvic inflammatory disease (PID) and ultrasonography to confirm or delineate pelvic masses that could be endometriosis. Laparoscopy is the key diagnostic procedure for pelvic endometriosis. The endometrial implants are seen as brown or blue-black nodules or multiple tiny hemorrhagic foci that are referred to as "powder burn spots" (Garner & Webster, 1985, p. 13). Examination of tissue specimens obtained during laparoscopy can confirm the diagnosis.

Medical (hormonal) and surgical management may be employed, depending on the symptoms, the extent of disease, and the desire for childbearing.

Medical management involves the use of mild analgesics or prostaglandin synthetase inhibitors for pain relief. Two hormonal therapies are also used to relieve pain by suppressing ovulation. In the first, *pseudopregnancy* is induced with oral contraceptives and/or progesterone. A 6-month course of a low-dose estrogen oral contraceptive is usually given, followed by cyclic oral contraceptive use or therapy with progesterone alone. The second hormonal treatment causes ovarian suppression, or *pseudomenopause*, by using *danzol* (Danocrine), an antigonadotropin testosterone derivative. This therapeutic approach is the current choice of many practitioners, but it is expensive (> $100/month) and may cause undesirable side effects, such as acne, hirsutism, weight gain, decreased breast size, and hot flashes.

Other nonsurgical interventions that have been used with some success for pain relief include the application of a heating pad to the abdomen or sacrum, relaxation techniques, yoga, and biofeedback. These approaches may decrease muscle tissue hypoxia and hypertonicity and relieve ischemia by increasing blood flow to the affected areas.

Surgical management of endometriosis for a woman who wishes to remain fertile is conservative and involves removal of endometrial implants and adhesions. A carbon dioxide laser may also be used to treat endometriosis by vaporizing adhesions and endometrial implants (Tulandi, 1986). If childbearing is not desired, the uterus and ovaries may be removed.

Nursing management is aimed at reduction of pain, restoration of sexual function that was impaired by dyspareunia, alleviation of anxiety related to the clinical manifestations of the disease and the uncertainty of the diagnosis, elimination of the client's knowledge deficit regarding the disease or its treatment, alleviation of fear related to the possibility of laparoscopy or surgery, and prevention of self-esteem disturbance related to infertility. Several organizations such as the Endometriosis Society and RESOLVE (an organization for infertile couples) offer additional information on endometriosis that may be helpful in planning care. Nursing care for gynecologic surgery can be found in the discussion of benign and malignant neoplasms (see later).

DYSFUNCTIONAL UTERINE BLEEDING

OVERVIEW

Dysfunctional uterine bleeding (DUB) is abnormal bleeding that is excessive or abnormal in amount or frequency without predisposing anatomic or systemic conditions. DUB is responsible for 50% to 75% of the complaints of abnormal bleeding reported by women seeking gynecologic care.

Pathophysiology

Normally, the menstrual cycle represents a series of complex hormonal events related to balanced hypothalamic, pituitary, ovarian, and uterine functions. Menses, the sloughing of the endometrial lining, is an expected result. DUB occurs when there is a breakdown of these functions, causing hormonal imbalance.

Etiology

The mechanism of DUB is unknown, but several theories have linked DUB with endometrial or myometrial dysfunction. Excessive fibrinolytic activity in the endometrium and changes in prostaglandin production in the uterus have also been suggested as causes.

Generally, DUB is bleeding in the absence of ovulation related to ovarian dysfunction. Estrogen stimulation of the endometrium is prolonged, and it grows past its hormonal support, causing bleeding and desquamation.

Anovulatory DUB during the reproductive years is associated with polycystic ovary disease, stress, extreme weight changes, and long-term drug use (e.g., of anticholinergics, reserpine, morphine, and oral contraceptives). Ovulatory causes of DUB are uncommon and are related to a dysfunctional corpus luteum and irregular maturation and shedding of the endometrium.

Incidence

DUB most often occurs at either end of the span of reproductive years, when ovulation is becoming established or when it is becoming irregular at menopause. DUB accounts for about 20% of the complaints of abnormal bleeding among adolescents and for half of such complaints among women older than 50 years (Martin, 1985).

PREVENTION

DUB is not known to be preventable. Half of the adolescents who have DUB because of anovulatory cycles have abnormal bleeding cycles as adults. These clients should be counseled to have yearly gynecologic examinations and have their menstrual cycles monitored to rule out organic causes of abnormal bleeding.

COLLABORATIVE MANAGEMENT

 Assessment

History

When interviewing a woman with DUB, the nurse must take a *complete menstrual history*. The history should also include questions about *illnesses*, variations in *weight* or *diet, exercise, drug ingestion*, and the presence of *pain*. An adolescent's history should focus on the irregularity of menstrual cycles, whereas the history for women in their reproductive years should focus on the other menstrual complaints.

Physical Assessment: Clinical Manifestations

Physical assessment for adolescents is usually limited to general examination. A pelvic examination is done only if bleeding persists or is severe enough to cause anemia. If a pelvic examination is performed, a pediatric speculum should be used and the presence of a support person, such as a parent or friend, often is helpful in performing the examination successfully.

Physical assessment of the adult woman includes a general examination to observe for symptoms of *anemia* or *systemic disease*, such as renal or hepatic disease, *obesity, undernutrition, abnormal hair growth* related to hormonal dysfunction, and evidence of *abdominal pain or masses*. An examination that includes inspection of the external genitalia and bimanual pelvic and rectal examination is essential to identify or rule out lesions or tenderness.

Psychosocial Assessment

The woman experiencing DUB may be anxious or concerned about the irregularity of bleeding. She may be apprehensive and fearful about having uncontrolled hemorrhage and have fears related to sexual or childbearing abilities. DUB can be a threat to a woman's sexual identity because menstruation often is tied to gender identity. The nurse assesses the woman's feelings about menstruation and gynecologic bleeding by asking about her reactions to bleeding during menstruation and at other times in the menstrual cycle.

Laboratory Findings

Investigative procedures for adult women are usually aimed at ruling out other causes of bleeding and include complete blood count and platelet number determination to identify chronic blood loss, urinalysis to check for infection, examination of a stool specimen for occult blood, cytologic examination and biopsy of any suspicious lesions, and a Pap smear to detect malignancy. Pregnancy tests are done routinely. Serum progesterone or urinary pregnanediol determinations may be ordered to assess ovulation unless this has been demonstrated by basal temperature studies.

Radiographic Findings

Hysterosalpingography may be ordered if other diagnostic measures have been inconclusive and bleeding persists.

Other Diagnostic Tests

Ultrasonography is not usually ordered for clients with DUB unless a pelvic mass is felt on examination. Endometrial biopsy by suction aspiration or D & C (see later) is usually done if bleeding is from the uterine cavity. These are important procedures for women older than 40 years, who are more at risk for endometrial cancer.

 Analysis: Nursing Diagnosis

Care of the woman with DUB is a challenge to the health care team. Assessment data are used to identify nursing diagnoses that are relevant for each woman.

Common Diagnoses

The common diagnoses for the woman with abnormal bleeding are

1. Anxiety related to an unknown cause of abnormal bleeding
2. Fear related to lack of knowledge about treatments (hormonal therapy and surgery) for abnormal uterine bleeding
3. Potential for self-esteem disturbance related to abnormal bleeding as a threat to sexual identity

Additional Diagnoses

Some women may have the following diagnoses:

1. Potential for activity intolerance related to weakness and fatigue secondary to anemia
2. Sexual dysfunction related to abnormal uterine bleeding
3. Powerlessness related to infertility secondary to anovulation
4. Pain related to DUB or its surgical treatments

 Planning and Implementation

The care plan focuses on the common diagnoses for the woman with DUB.

Anxiety

Planning: client goals. The major goals are that the woman will (1) experience an increase in psychologic comfort and (2) use effective coping mechanisms to manage anxiety during the diagnostic stage of care.

Interventions: nonsurgical management. Nursing measures include assessing the level of anxiety; providing reassurance and comfort before and during diagnostic procedures; assessing the woman's usual coping mechanisms (e.g., crying or talking) and support systems (e.g., husband or mother); and explaining alternative behaviors (e.g., relaxation or distraction techniques) if coping mechanisms do not reduce anxiety (see Chap. 6). The nurse can convey empathic understanding by using touch, encouraging expression of feelings, and listening.

Fear

Planning: client goals. The major goal is that the woman will be less fearful of treatment by being able to (1) explain the purpose of therapy, (2) understand the reasons for and take medications correctly, and (3) describe what she can expect before and after the surgery.

Interventions. Nonsurgical management is usually the treatment of choice, although surgery may be needed to treat the problem. The nurse counsels the client about treatment.

Nonsurgical management. The majority of women can be treated successfully with hormonal manipulation. For women with anovulatory DUB who are not contemplating pregnancy, medroxyprogesterone or combination oral contraceptives are prescribed. Women with ovulatory DUB who have inadequate progesterone levels may be treated with supplemental progesterone (10 to 20 mg/day on days 16 to 25 of each month). Nursing interventions include explaining the desired and side effects of these drugs and making sure that the woman understands the dosage and administration schedule.

Surgical management. D & C may be performed as a diagnostic procedure, but it is generally not used therapeutically, except for women who have profuse bleeding and for long-standing cases if hormonal therapy has not been successful.

A D & C can be performed as an inpatient or outpatient (ambulatory) procedure, with local, regional, or general anesthesia. A speculum is inserted in the vagina to enable visualization of the cervix; the cervical os is dilated and a curette is used to scrape out the endometrium to check for possible causes of bleeding or to remove the bleeding tissue.

Preoperative care. The nurse assesses the woman's understanding of the preoperative procedures before implementing them. Perineal shave, vaginal douche, and enema are uncommon, but the woman is usually restricted to nothing by mouth (NPO) for 6 to 8 hours before surgery. The nurse can teach the client what to expect after surgery and encourage the woman and her family or other support persons to ask questions (see Chap. 18 for a discussion of preoperative care).

Postoperative care. Immediate postoperative care includes checking vital signs frequently until they are stable, assessing vaginal bleeding (there should be no more than one saturated pad every 4 hours), assessing the need for pain relief, offering nourishments as ordered, and encouraging ambulation as tolerated. The woman is usually discharged to home after her condition is stable (see Chap. 20 for a discussion of postoperative care).

Potential for Self-esteem Disturbance

Planning: client goals. The major goals are that the woman will (1) express confidence in being able to continue role-related responsibilities, (2) verbalize feelings about having children (if this is a concern), and (3) discuss bleeding problems in relation to her role as a woman.

Interventions: nonsurgical management. Nursing care focuses on providing a private environment in which the woman feels comfortable in discussing feelings and expectations about menstruation and abnormal bleeding as they relate to her feminine role and her ability to become pregnant. The nurse encourages questions about treatments, progress, and prognosis; provides reliable information; and clears up misconceptions. The nurse also supports the woman as she shares her concerns and assists her in resolution and grief work by providing encouragement and realistic alternatives.

■ Discharge Planning

Home Care Preparation

Because DUB is usually treated on an outpatient basis, no special home care preparation is necessary.

Client/Family Education

The woman with mild or moderate DUB is usually treated with hormones. If she is taking oral contraceptives, she should take one pill a day for 21 or 28 days, beginning on the first day of the menstrual cycle. Medroxyprogesterone is taken on days 16 to 25 of each month. Monthly withdrawal bleeding is expected with both therapies.

If the woman has a D & C, postoperative instructions are given, regardless of whether the procedure was done on an inpatient or outpatient basis (see the accompanying Client/Family Education feature).

Psychosocial Preparation

A woman with DUB is probably relieved to know the cause of her abnormal bleeding does not involve ana-

---

CLIENT/FAMILY EDUCATION ■ Instructions for the Woman Who Has Undergone Dilation and Curettage

"Take your temperature once a day for the next 2 d. If your oral temperature is more than 100°F (38°C), call the clinic or your physician."

"Avoid sexual intercourse, tub bathing, and the use of tampons for 2 wk to allow healing and prevent infection."

"Slight bleeding is normal. However, if bleeding is as heavy as in your normal menstrual period, or if bleeding lasts more than 2 wk, call the clinic or your physician."

"You can use a heating pad or hot water bottle to relieve abdominal cramping if it occurs."

"You can take mild analgesics, such as acetaminophen (Tylenol), for abdominal pain."

---

tomic or systemic conditions. She may need support and encouragement from health care providers and significant others to continue treatments during the months of hormonal management before bleeding is controlled.

Health Care Resources

Usually no specific equipment is needed for treatment of DUB. Local support groups or counseling may be suggested for women who continue to have psychosocial problems after treatment.

 Evaluation

On the basis of the identified nursing diagnoses, the nurse evaluates the care of the woman with DUB. The expected outcomes are that the client

1. Verbalizes decreased anxiety about the abnormal bleeding
2. Describes and complies with the hormonal therapy as ordered
3. States an understanding of preoperative and postoperative procedures
4. Verbalizes confidence in herself in relation to her feminine role

---

INFLAMMATIONS AND INFECTIONS

Vaginal discharge and itching are two of the most common complaints of gynecologic clients. Women with these complaints may need information from health care providers about the normal vaginal physiology, causes of symptoms, and methods of treatment. The nurse must be well informed about these topics to provide comprehensive care to clients with vaginal infections.

The infections discussed may be considered sexually transmitted diseases because their causative organisms may be transmitted to sexual partners; however, they can develop without sexual contact, and sexual partners may not always become infected. Other sexually transmitted diseases, such as gonorrhea, syphilis, chlamydial infection, herpes simplex virus infection, and acquired immunodeficiency syndrome (AIDS), are discussed in Chapter 27.

SIMPLE VAGINITIS

Simple vaginitis is an inflammation of the lower genital tract. Vaginitis can develop whenever there is a disturbance of the balance of hormones and bacterial interaction in the vagina caused by changes in the normal flora; alkaline pH; insertion of foreign bodies, such as tampons or condoms; chemical irritations, such as from douches or sprays; and medications, especially antibiotics.

Assessment of simple vaginitis is usually made by asking questions regarding the symptoms, performing a pelvic examination, and laboratory testing of vaginal smears (Table 54–2). The nurse is nonjudgmental and reassuring while making these assessments because the client may be embarrassed or afraid to discuss her symptoms.

Interventions for simple vaginitis are dependent on the causes and the specific vaginal infection (see the Key Features of Disease on p. 1700). Good health habits of the woman can be beneficial to treatment, so it is important that she gets enough rest and sleep, observes good nutritional habits, gets regular exercise, and uses good personal hygiene. Popular but not scientifically tested hygiene practices to prevent vaginitis are perineal cleaning (wiping front to back) after urinating or defecating, wearing cotton underwear, avoiding strong douches and feminine hygiene sprays, and avoiding tight-fitting pants. If antibiotics are prescribed, it has been suggested that eating yogurt or taking *Lactobacillus* culture (Lactinex) tablets may help restore the natural flora (Döderlein's bacilli) of the vagina (Scherger & Sullivan, 1986; Schober, 1986; Sloane, 1985).

Client education should focus on preventive measures and on information about infection transmission (see the Client/Family Education feature at the top of p. 1701).

CANDIDA ALBICANS INFECTION

Candida albicans infection, also known as candidiasis, moniliasis, and yeast infection, is the most common

---

TABLE 54–2   Important Points in the Assessment of the Client with Simple Vaginitis

History

Onset of symptoms

Characteristics and color of discharge

Odor of discharge

Associated symptoms
  Itching
  Dysuria
  Others

Type of contraceptive use

Recent antibiotic use

Sexual activity

History of previous vaginal infection

Hygiene practices
  Douching
  Tampon use

Physical Examination

Abdomen
  Palpation for tenderness or pain

External genitalia
  Inspection for erythema, edema, excoriation, odor, and discharge

Vaginal examination
  Speculum examination to visualize the vagina and the cervix
  Note the source of discharge or inflammation

Laboratory Tests

Wet smear
  Saline
  Potassium hydroxide

Nitrazine paper to test vaginal pH

---

form of vaginitis. Symptoms appear in women during the reproductive years, usually developing in the premenstrual period. Etiology is unknown, but a change in the vaginal pH encourages growth of this gram-positive fungus, which is commonly found on the skin and in the digestive tract. Recurrences are frequent. Predisposing factors include pregnancy; diabetes; oral contraceptive use; frequent douching; antibiotic therapy, especially tetracycline; and poor hygiene. Candidiasis is not usually considered a sexually transmitted disease (Schober, 1986).

TRICHOMONAS VAGINALIS INFECTION

Trichomonas vaginalis is a parasitic protozoan that is considered to cause sexually transmitted disease be-

KEY FEATURES OF DISEASE ■ Etiology, Transmission, Assessment, and Drug Therapy of Common Vaginal Infections

Etiology	Sexual Transmission	Assessment		Drug Therapy
		Physical Findings	*Laboratory Findings*	
Candida albicans infection	Unlikely	Odorless, white or yellow, cheesy discharge Patches on vaginal walls and cervix Inflamed vaginal walls and cervix Itching	Hyphae and spores visible on potassium hydroxide wet slide Vaginal pH 4.5	Miconazole nitrate (Monistat), clotrimazole (Gyne-Lotrimin), or nystatin (Mycostatin) vaginal creams or suppositories for 7 d
Trichomonas vaginalis infection	Yes	Green, yellow, or white, frothy, foul-smelling discharge Itching Strawberry spot on cervix	Flagellated, pear-shaped protozoa on saline wet slide Vaginal pH 7.45	Oral metronidazol (Flagyl), single 2-g dose for client and sexual partners
Gardnerella vaginalis infection	Yes	Gray-white discharge Fishy odor Itching Normal vaginal mucosa 10%–40% asymptomatic	"Clue" cells on examination of saline wet slide Positive "whiff" test Vaginal pH 5–5.5	Oral metronidazole, 500 mg qid for 7 d, or ampicillin or tetracycline
Cervicitis	Yes	Mucopurulent discharge from endocervix Pelvic pain, postcoital, intermenstrual bleeding Cervix may be inflamed and bleed when touched	Need to rule out herpes and gonorrhea Vaginal pH 4.5	Dependent on diagnosis (see Chap. 56)
Atrophic vaginitis	No	Pale, thin, dry mucosa Itching No odor Scant white or pink discharge Dyspareunia, postcoital bleeding	Parabasal cells Leukocyte predominance Vaginal pH 6.0	Topical conjugated estrogen cream ½ to 1 application at night for 7 nights, then twice weekly

cause infection is more prevalent in sexually active women. As many as 60% to 70% of the male sexual partners of affected women, however, are asymptomatic (Schober, 1986). *T. vaginalis* infection frequently occurs in women aged 16 to 35 years, and symptoms usually appear during or immediately after menstruation. Although the initial source of infection is unknown, predisposing factors include a nonacidic vaginal pH, pregnancy, illness, a crash diet, and GI disturbances. Transmission of the organisms is also theo-

retically possible through shared bathing facilities, washcloths, and douching equipment (King, 1984).

GARDNERELLA VAGINALIS INFECTION

Gardnerella vaginalis infection is a common form of vaginitis that has been responsible for almost all cases of what has previously been referred to as nonspecific vag-

CLIENT/FAMILY EDUCATION ■ Instructions for the Client with a Vaginal Infection

"Your risk of getting vaginal infections increases if you have sex with more than one person."

"When you have a vaginal infection, do not have sexual intercourse, or at least make sure that your partner wears a condom."

"Sexual partners may need treatment for infection."

"The only way to identify what infection you have is to be examined by a physician or a nurse and to get the results of laboratory tests."

"Take your medicine as prescribed, not just until your symptoms go away."

initis. *G. vaginalis* infection is one of the most contagious and most common sexually transmitted infections. It is a benign infection that does not invade the vaginal mucosa.

CERVICITIS

Cervicitis is an infection of the endocervix that is most often caused by sexually transmitted diseases, particularly chlamydiosis, gonorrhea, trichomoniasis, and herpes simplex virus infection.

ATROPHIC VAGINITIS

Atrophic vaginitis occurs in postmenopausal women as a result of a lack of endogenous estrogen production. The vaginal mucosa becomes thin, pale, dry, and susceptible to infection.

VULVITIS

Vulvitis is an inflammatory condition of the vulva that is associated with symptoms of pruritus (itching) and burning sensation. The vulvar skin is sensitive to hormonal, metabolic, and allergic influences, and symptoms can be caused by systemic conditions, by direct contact with irritants, or by extension of infections from the vagina.

The most common skin disease affecting the vulva is contact dermatitis, which can be caused by an irritant such as feminine hygiene sprays, fabric dyes, soaps and detergents, and allergens. Primary infections that affect the vulva include herpes genitalis and condyloma acuminatum (veneral warts) (see Chap. 56). Secondary in-

fections of the vulva are caused by organisms responsible for the numerous types of vaginitis, including candidiasis in diabetic women. Pediculosis pubis (crab lice infestation) and scabies (itch mite infestation) are common parasitic infestations of the skin of the vulva. Other causes of vulvitis include atrophic vaginitis (see earlier), vulvar kraurosis (a postmenopausal disorder causing dryness and atrophy), vulvar leukoplakia (postmenopausal atrophy and thickening of vulvar tissues), cancer, and urinary incontinence.

Assessment of the woman usually identifies symptoms of itching and burning sensation. Erythema, edema, and superficial skin ulcers may also be present. Some women may develop an itch-scratch-itch cycle, in which the itching leads to scratching that causes excoriation that then must heal. As healing takes place, itching occurs again, which leads to further scratching. If the cycle is not interrupted, the condition can become chronic, causing the vulvar skin to become white and thickened (leathery). This skin is dry and scaly and cracks easily, increasing the woman's chances of infection.

Medical treatment of vulvitis depends on the cause. Nursing interventions to relieve itching include the following: Wet compresses (Burow's solution diluted 1 : 20) can be applied to the affected area for 30 minutes several times a day, followed by cool air drying with a hair dryer. Other helpful measures include sitz baths for 30 minutes several times a day or the application of prescribed topical medications, such as hydrocortisone or fluorinated corticosteroids (betamethasone valerate [Valisone] or fluocinolone acetonide [Synalar]).

Oral antibiotics can be prescribed if infection is the underlying cause. Removal of any irritant or allergen should be accomplished, such as by changing detergents. Treatment for pediculosis and scabies can be instituted if appropriate. This entails the application of lindane (1% gamma-benzene hexachloride [Kwell]) lo-

CLIENT/FAMILY EDUCATION ■ Instructions for the Prevention of Vulvitis

"You should wear cotton underwear."

"Avoid wearing tight clothing, such as pantyhose or tight jeans, because these can cause chafing. You can also get hot and sweaty, which can cause an infection."

"Always wipe front to back after having a bowel movement or urinating."

"Do not douche or use feminine hygiene sprays."

"If your sexual partner has an infection of his sex organs, you should not have intercourse with him until he has been treated."

"You are more likely to get an infection if you are pregnant, have diabetes, take oral contraceptive drugs, or are menopausal."

tion, shampoo, or cream to the affected area as directed; cleaning affected clothes, bedding, and towels; and disinfecting the home environment (lice cannot live more than 24 hours away from the body) (Sloane, 1985).

If the vulvitis is chronic or severe, laser therapy (see under the later heading Interventions in the section on cervical cancer) or "skinning" vulvectomy (see later discussion of vulvar cancer) may be performed.

Preventive measures that may be helpful are discussed in the Client/Family Education feature at the bottom of page 1701.

until 1980, when it was found to be related to menstruation and tampon use. Other conditions that have been associated with TSS include surgical wound infection, nonsurgical focal infections, postpartum conditions, and nonmenstrual vaginal conditions. Young women, aged 15 to 19 years, appear to be more at risk than women older than 30 years, as one-third of the cases of TSS have been in this adolescent group (Colls, 1985).

The pathophysiology of TSS is not understood clearly. Certain strains of *Staphylococcus aureus* produce

TOXIC SHOCK SYNDROME

Toxic shock syndrome (TSS) is not a new disease, although it was infrequently recognized by physicians

---

KEY FEATURES OF DISEASE ■ CDC Criteria for Toxic Shock Syndrome

Fever (temperature >102° F)

Diffuse rash, resembling sunburn

Peeling of skin—primarily soles of feet and palms of hands—1–2 wk after onset of illness

Hypotension (systolic blood pressure <90 mmHg or orthostatic syncope)

Involvement of three or more of the following:
Gastrointestinal system: vomiting, diarrhea at onset
Musculoskeletal system: severe aching or serum creatinine phosphatase level twice the normal level
Kidneys: BUN or creatinine twice the normal level; elevated serum levels of white blood cells in absence of urinary tract infection
Liver: total bilirubin, aspartate aminotransferase (serum glutamic-oxaloacetic transaminase), and alanine aminotransferase (serum glutamic-pyruvic transaminase) twice the normal levels
Hematologic system: platelet levels below normal
Central nervous system: disorientation, alteration in consciousness in absence of fever or hypertension
Mucous membranes: hyperemia of vaginal walls, the throat, or the conjunctiva of the eye

Negative laboratory test results for the following:
Rocky Mountain spotted fever, measles, scarlet fever, and throat, blood, and cerebrospinal fluid cultures

Data from *Toxic shock syndrome: Assessment of current information and future research needs: Report of a study.* (1982). Division of Health Sciences Policy, Division of Health Promotion and Disease Prevention, Institute of Medicine. Washington, DC: National Academy Press.

CLIENT/FAMILY EDUCATION ■ Instructions for the Prevention of Toxic Shock Syndrome

Tampon Use

"Wash your hands before inserting a tampon."

"Do not use a tampon if it is dirty."

"Insert the tampon carefully to avoid injuring the delicate tissue in your vagina."

"Change tampons every 3–6 h."

"Do not use superabsorbent tampons."

"Use sanitary napkins at night."

"Call your physician if you suddenly develop a high fever, vomiting, or diarrhea."

"Do not use tampons at all if you have had toxic shock syndrome."

"Not using tampons almost guarantees that you will not get toxic shock syndrome."

Vaginal Sponge Use

"Wash your hands before inserting the sponge."

"Use only clean water to wet the sponge."

"Do not use the sponge if it is dirty."

"Do not use the sponge during your menstrual period."

"Do not use the sponge for more than 30 h at a time."

"Call your physician if you get two or more symptoms of toxic shock syndrome."

Diaphragm Use

"Wash your hands before inserting the diaphragm."

"Remove the diaphragm within 24 h after intercourse."

"Do not use the diaphragm during your menstrual period."

"After you take out the diaphragm, wash it with mild soap, rinse it, and dry it. Store it in a clean, dry place."

a toxin that has been associated with the symptoms of TSS. Numerous theories have been reported to explain the mechanism of *S. aureus* absorption in the development of TSS. It has been suggested that the vagina is highly susceptible to the toxin released by *S. aureus.*

In menstrually related TSS, the theories about the mechanisms of absorption focus on tampon use. Possible explanations include the following: toxins readily cross the vaginal mucosa; highly absorbent tampons rub vaginal walls and cause ulceration that allows transport of the toxins; prolonged or continued tampon use can cause chronic vaginal ulcerations through which *S. aureus* is absorbed; and plastic tampon inserters can cause ulceration through which toxins are transported (Colls, 1985). Use of the diaphragm, cervical cap, and vaginal contraceptive sponge has also been linked to cases of TSS.

Influenza-like symptoms for the first 24 hours are common. The abrupt onset of a high fever associated with a headache, sore throat, vomiting, diarrhea, generalized rash, and hypotension are often present. The most common clinical manifestations are skin changes (initially a rash similar to a severe sunburn that changes to a macular erythema similar to a drug-related rash). Because not all women experience all these clinical manifestations, the criteria established by the Centers for Disease Control are used in epidemiologic studies to verify cases of TSS (see the Key Features of Disease on p. 1702).

Nurses may be involved in the prevention as well as treatment of TSS. Management in the outpatient setting is focused on client education and prevention. Instructions for prevention of TSS related to tampon, vaginal sponge, and diaphragm use are outlined in the Client/Family Education feature on page 1702. Primary treatment in the acute care setting includes fluid replacement because dehydration and electrolyte imbalance result from vomiting and diarrhea. Antibiotics (oxacillin, nafcillin, and cephalosporin) are administered if the penicillin-resistant strain of *S. aureus* is responsible for TSS. Other measures may include administering transfusions for low platelet counts, corticosteroids to treat skin changes, and drugs such as naloxone hydrochloride (Narcan) to treat hypotension. The vagina may or may not be washed out with a local vaginal disinfectant, such as a dilute iodine solution, to decrease the number of toxins in the vagina that could be absorbed into the systemic circulation (Sloane, 1985; Wager, 1983).

PELVIC INFLAMMATORY DISEASE

PID refers to an infectious process that may involve one or more pelvic structures and can cause ectopic pregnancy and infertility. The rising incidence of sexually transmitted diseases in the United States has increased the occurrence of PID (see Chap. 56). The primary causes of PID are *Neisseria gonorrhoeae* and *Chlamydia trachomatis.*

PROBLEMS RELATED TO PELVIC SUPPORT TISSUES

UTERINE DISPLACEMENT

Normally, the uterus lies in the midline of the pelvis and is freely movable. The cervix is located posteriorly in the vagina, and the body of the uterus has a slight degree of anterior flexion (Fig. 54–2). Variations from this position can result from congenital or acquired weakness of the pelvic support structures (see the Key Features of Disease on pp. 1704 and 1705). The most common variation is posterior displacement of the uterus, or retroversion. The uterus is tilted posteriorly, and the cervix rotates anteriorly. Other variations include retroflexion, anteversion, and anteflexion.

The woman with uterine displacement may be asymptomatic, or she may report a history of backaches, secondary amenorrhea, infertility, dyspareunia, or feelings of pelvic pressure or heaviness.

If symptoms are uncomfortable, several interventions may be implemented. To correct a mildly retroverted uterus, a woman may assume a knee-chest position for a few minutes several times a day. A vaginal *pessary,* a device placed in the vagina to hold the uterus in correct position, may be prescribed. A pessary that is inserted correctly should not be felt by the woman. However, the vaginal mucosa may be irritated, and measures to keep the vaginal pH at 4.0 to 4.5 should be implemented. For example, commercially prepared douches or solutions of 1 tbsp of vinegar to 1 qt of water can be used twice a week.

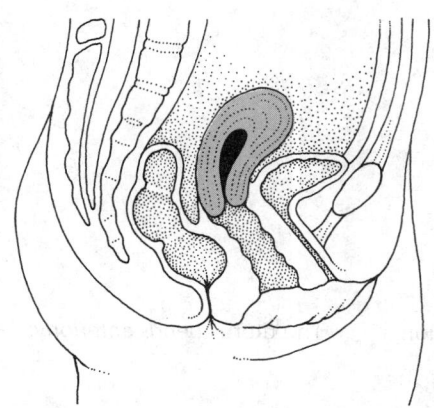

Figure 54–2

Normal position of the uterus.

KEY FEATURES OF DISEASE ■ Types of Uterine Displacement

Minor Displacements

Retroversion   The uterus *tilts posteriorly,* and the cervix rotates anteriorly.

Retroflexion   The uterus *bends posteriorly.*

Anteversion   The uterus *tilts anteriorly.*

Anteflexion   The uterus *bends anteriorly.*

KEY FEATURES OF DISEASE ■ Types of Uterine Displacement *Continued*

Prolapse

Grade I	The uterus bulges into the vagina, but the cervix does not protrude through the entrance to the vagina.
Grade II	The uterus bulges further into the vagina, and the cervix protrudes through the entrance to the vagina.
Grade III	The body of the uterus and the cervix protrude through the entrance to the vagina. The vagina is turned inside out.

UTERINE PROLAPSE

A more serious type of displacement is uterine prolapse. Three stages of prolapse have been described according to the degree of descent of the uterus (see the accompanying Key Features of Disease). Prolapse of the uterus can be caused by congenital defects, persistent high levels of intra-abdominal pressure related to heavy physical labor or exertion, or any other cause that weakens the pelvic supports. The incidence of prolapsed uterus is higher in Caucasian and Japanese women (Nichols & Randall, 1983). Prolapse is often a complication of childbirth injuries, occurring many years later, but it is also found in elderly nulliparas.

Certain data may alert a nurse that a client may have a prolapsed uterus. These assessment findings include a feeling that the client relates ("something is in my vagina"), dyspareunia, backache, a feeling of heaviness or pressure in the pelvis, and bowel or bladder problems (if cystocele or rectocele is also present). A pelvic examination may reveal a protrusion of the cervix when the woman is asked to bear down.

Interventions are based on the degree of prolapse.

Conservative treatment, such as the use of pessaries, is preferred to surgical treatment when possible. Vaginal hysterectomy with repair is the usual surgical procedure (see later discussion of uterine leiomyomas). Before surgical intervention, the woman should be questioned about her desire for future childbearing (surgery could be delayed) and her desire for coital activities (surgery will probably shorten and narrow the vagina, possibly causing painful intercourse).

Whenever the uterus is displaced, other structures, such as the bladder, the rectum, and the small intestine, are affected and can protrude through the vaginal walls.

CYSTOCELE

A *cystocele* is a protrusion of the bladder through the vaginal wall and is due to weakened pelvic structures (Fig. 54–3). This protrusion can be caused by obesity, advanced age, childbearing, or genetic predisposition. The development of a cystocele is more noticeable in the postmenopausal years when estrogen loss also weakens tissue supports and can cause relaxation of the supports.

Assessment findings may include difficulty in emptying the bladder, urinary frequency and urgency, urinary tract infection, and stress urinary incontinence (loss of urine during stressful activities such as laughing, coughing, sneezing, or lifting heavy objects). A pelvic examination reveals a significant bulge of the anterior vaginal wall when the woman is asked to bear down. Diagnostic tests that may be ordered are cystography (to show the presence of bladder herniation), measurement of residual urine by catheterization, or urine culture and sensitivity testing (which may reveal infection caused by urine retention).

Medical management is usually conservative if the woman is asymptomatic or has mild symptoms. A pessary may be recommended to support the bladder in some patients. Estrogen therapy for the postmenopausal woman may be prescribed to prevent atrophy and weakening of vaginal walls. Kegel's exercises may help strengthen perineal muscles. The nurse can teach the woman to tighten and relax her perineal muscles by pressing the buttocks together and holding the position for at least 5 seconds. The exercise should be repeated frequently throughout the day. An alternative exercise is having the woman try to stop the flow of urine after she has started urinating, holding the position for a few seconds before letting the urine flow again.

Surgery may be recommended for severe symptoms. An *anterior colporrhaphy* (anterior repair) is a procedure to tighten the pelvic muscles for better bladder support. The procedure is performed through a vaginal surgical approach. Nursing care of a woman having an anterior repair is similar to that for a woman having surgery for urologic disorders (Chap. 58) or vaginal hysterectomy (see later).

Postoperatively, a woman should be instructed to limit her activities, not to lift anything heavy (> 20 lb), to avoid strenuous exercises, and to avoid sexual intercourse for 6 weeks. The importance of keeping the follow-up appointment should be stressed.

RECTOCELE

A *rectocele* is a protrusion of the rectum through a weakened vaginal wall (see Fig. 54–3). It can develop as a result of the pressure of a baby's head during a difficult delivery, a traumatic forceps delivery, or a congenital defect of the supporting tissues. Symptoms usually do not appear until the woman is older than 35 years of age.

The woman's history may reveal symptoms of constipation, hemorrhoids, fecal impaction, and feelings of rectal or vaginal fullness. A pelvic examination may show a bulge of the posterior vaginal wall when the woman is asked to bear down. A rectal examination reveals the presence of a rectocele. A barium enema also confirms the presence of a rectocele.

Medical management is focused on promoting bowel elimination. A high-fiber diet, stool softeners, and laxatives are usually ordered. The surgical procedure that

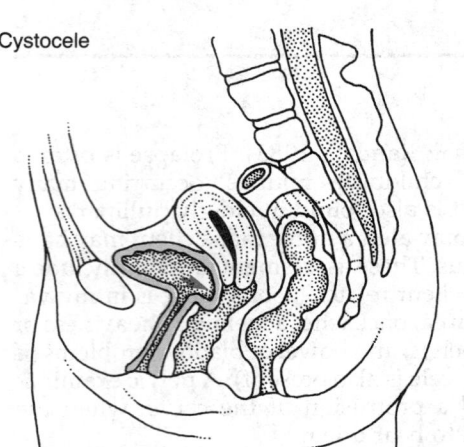

Cystocele

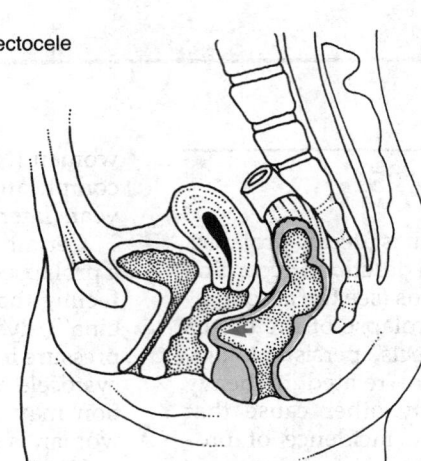

Rectocele

Figure 54–3

In cystocele, the urinary bladder is displaced downward, causing bulging of the anterior vaginal wall. In rectocele, the rectum is displaced, causing bulging of the posterior vaginal wall.

strengthens pelvic supports and reduces the bulging is *posterior colporrhaphy* (posterior repair). If both a cystocele and rectocele are present, an anterior *and* posterior colporrhaphy (anterior and posterior repair) is performed.

The nursing care of a woman having a posterior repair is similar to care after rectal surgery (Chap. 45). Postoperatively, the woman is usually given a low-residue diet to prevent bowel movements and allow time for the incision to heal. The woman should be informed not to strain when she does have a bowel movement, so that she does not put pressure on the suture line. Bowel movements are often painful, and clients may need pain medication before having a bowel movement. Postoperative instructions for clients having a posterior repair are similar to those for anterior repair.

FISTULAS

Fistulas are abnormal openings between two adjacent organs and are infrequent complications of gynecologic surgery. The types of vaginal fistulas include urethrovaginal (urethra), vesicovaginal (bladder), and rectovaginal (rectum) (Fig. 54–4). Trauma is the primary cause of fistulas, although they can result from complications of surgery, obstetric complications, spread of malignancy, or radiation therapy for cancer.

Symptoms depend on the location of the fistula. A fistula should be considered as a possible cause if a woman's history includes the following complaints: urine, flatus, or feces leaking into the vagina; irritation or excoriation of the vulva and vaginal tissues; unpleasant odor (fecal or urine) in vagina; and complaints of feeling wet or dribbling in the vagina.

Women who have fistulas may be embarrassed to seek help until symptoms are severe. Often they withdraw from social activities or from relationships with significant others as the symptoms become more difficult to manage.

Management depends on the location of the fistulas.

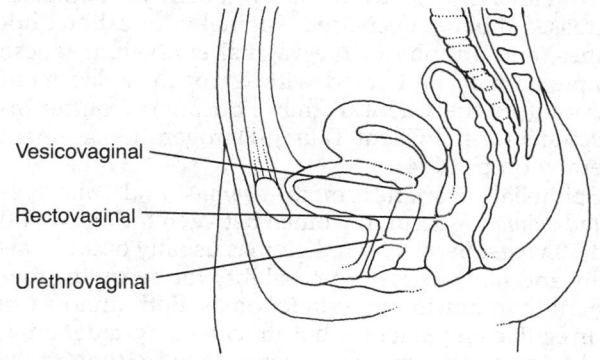

Figure 54–4
Sites of vaginal fistulas.

Surgery is not recommended if infection or inflammation is present and, even if performed, may not be successful. Nursing care is focused on assisting the woman with the frequent and time-consuming perineal hygiene — sitz baths, perineal cleaning with mild unscented soap and water, and low-pressure douching with commercial deodorizing solutions or homemade solutions (1 tsp of nonchlorine household bleach to 1 qt or 1 L of water). The woman may need to wear sanitary napkins or undergarments (such as Depend), depending on the leakage of urine or feces. The application of deodorizing powders, the use of heat lamps for irritated areas, and the application of vitamins A and D ointment to excoriated tissues may be beneficial.

If the fistula is repaired surgically, postoperative care is aimed at preventing infection and avoiding stress on the repaired area (low-residue diet and stool softeners for 2 weeks after rectovaginal fistula repair). Nursing care and postoperative teaching are similar to the care and teaching of the client who has a cystocele or rectocele repair (see earlier).

BENIGN NEOPLASMS

OVARIAN MASSES

An enlarged ovary may indicate that a disturbance in the ovulatory cycle has led to the development of functional ovarian cysts or benign or malignant ovarian neoplasms. It is important for the nurse or other health care provider to get as detailed a history as possible from a woman with an enlarged ovary. Nurses should be alert for symptoms related to pressure from the enlargement on other organs, such as urinary frequency, constipation, dyspareunia, or a heavy feeling in the lower abdomen or pelvis. Some women complain of abdominal discomfort or an increase in their abdominal girth (clothes are too tight in the waist). Women may complain of menstrual irregularities, infertility, or masculinizing effects from hormone imbalance. Women should be questioned about previous occurrences of cancer of the breast or reproductive organs.

Most laboratory testing is done to rule out other conditions, such as pregnancy, infection, or cancer. Ultrasonography is somewhat useful in visualizing ovarian masses, and scans can differentiate solid tumors, cysts, and ascites.

FUNCTIONAL OVARIAN CYSTS

Functional ovarian cysts can occur in a woman of any age but are rare after menopause. *Follicular cysts* are usually found in young menstruating females. These cysts are nonneoplastic and do not grow without hormonal influences. A cyst can develop when a mature follicle fails to rupture or an immature follicle fails to reabsorb follicular fluid during the second half of the menstrual cycle. The cyst is usually small (<6 to 8 cm [2⅜ to 3⅛ in]) and may be asymptomatic unless it ruptures. Rupture of a follicular cyst or torsion (twisting) may cause acute, severe pelvic pain. The pain usually resolves after several days of bed rest and the administration of mild analgesics. If the cyst does not rupture, it usually disappears within two or three menstrual cycles without medical intervention. If the cyst does not shrink, oral contraceptive pills may be prescribed for one or two cycles to depress ovulation, resulting in shrinking of the cyst. Follow-up care is necessary when the cyst is managed conservatively to confirm that it has disappeared.

If the cyst is larger than 6 to 8 cm (2⅜ to 3⅛ in), a neoplasm may be suspected, and further evaluation by ultrasound or laparoscopy is necessary. Larger cysts are often associated with menstrual irregularities.

Surgery is recommended only before puberty, after menopause, or when cysts are larger than 8 cm (3⅛ in). A *cystectomy* (removal of the cyst) is recommended instead of an *oophorectomy* (removal of the ovary). Nursing care is similar to care of the client having a tubal ligation (see later).

Corpus luteum cysts occur after ovulation and are often associated with increased secretion of progesterone. The cysts are usually small, averaging 4 cm (1½ in), and are purplish red owing to hemorrhage within the corpus luteum. Corpus luteum cysts are associated with a delay in the onset of menses and irregular or prolonged flow. They may also be accompanied by unilateral low abdominal or pelvic pain that is usually described as dull or aching. If the cyst ruptures, intraperitoneal hemorrhage can occur.

Corpus luteum cysts may disappear in one or two menstrual cycles or with suppression of ovulation. The treatment is the same as for follicular cysts.

Theca-lutein cysts are the least common of the functional cysts. They are associated with hydatidiform mole (molar pregnancy), occurring in 50% of these complicated pregnancies. Theca-lutein cysts develop as a result of prolonged stimulation of the ovaries by excessive amounts of human chorionic gonadotropin (hCG).

Theca-lutein cysts regress spontaneously within 3 months with the removal of the molar pregnancy or source of excessive hCG, and no other treatment is usually required.

Polycystic ovary, or *Stein-Leventhal*, *syndrome* results when elevated levels of luteinizing hormone (LH) cause hyperstimulation of the ovaries, which produces multiple cysts on one or both ovaries. High levels of estrogen are produced by these cysts and are unopposed by postovulatory progesterone. Endometrial hyperplasia or even carcinoma may result.

A typical client is obese, is hirsute, has irregular menses, and may be infertile because of anovulation. Treatment of polycystic ovary syndrome depends on which disorder is of greatest concern to the woman. The best treatment is the administration of oral contraceptives because they inhibit LH production. A woman who is older than 35 years and no longer desires childbearing may be advised to have a bilateral salpingo-oophorectomy (removal of both tubes and ovaries) and hysterectomy (removal of the uterus). Women who desire fertility can be treated with drugs such as clomiphene citrate (Clomid) to stimulate ovulation.

OTHER BENIGN CYSTS AND TUMORS

Dermoid cysts are the most common germ cell tumors and are benign in more than 99% of cases. These cysts are the most common ovarian tumors of childhood, although they can develop in a female of any age.

Dermoid cysts may contain hair, sebaceous material, teeth, and other calcifications. They are usually asymptomatic unless they grow large and put pressure on other organs, such as the bladder or the bowel. The cysts develop bilaterally in 10% to 25% of cases. They are often attached to the ovary by a pedicle (stalk).

Management of dermoid cysts is by cystectomy, for if they are not removed, they usually continue to grow and rupture, causing hemorrhage and infection.

Fibromas are the most common benign, solid ovarian neoplasms. These pearly white tumors of connective tissue origin have a low potential for becoming malignant. Fibromas can range in size from a small nodule to a mass weighing more than 50 lb. The average size is 6 cm (2⅜ in), slightly smaller than a tennis ball. Ninety per cent of fibromas are unilateral and, on examination, feel firm, have a slightly irregular contour, and are mobile. Fibromas greater than 6 cm (2⅜ in) may be associated with ascites and may cause feelings of pelvic pressure or abdominal enlargement. The neoplasm is usually asymptomatic, unless rupture or torsion occurs. Fibromas often occur postmenopausally.

Management of a solid ovarian neoplasm is surgical removal of the tumor. Oophorectomy may be performed for borderline tumors (when there is a question of possible malignancy). Nursing care of a woman having an oophorectomy is similar to care of a woman having a tubal ligation (see later). When both ovaries are removed, surgical menopause occurs in a premenopausal woman. As a result, a woman frequently experiences decreased libido, decreased vaginal lubrication, hot flashes, and atrophy of the vaginal epithelium. These symptoms may be treated with estrogen replacement therapy (see the Client/Family Education feature: Instructions for the Client Taking Estrogen Replacement Therapy on p. 1694).

Epithelial ovarian tumors—*serous* and *mucinous cystadenomas*—occur in women between the ages of 30 and 50 years. Serous cystadenomas usually occur bilaterally and have a greater probability for becoming malignant than mucinous cystadenomas. Both tumors can be irregular and smooth, but mucinous cystadenomas tend to grow to large size—some to more than 45 kg (100 lb).

Management of cystadenomas is usually by unilateral salpingo-oophorectomy, because it is often impossible to tell whether the tumor is benign or malignant. Small cystadenomas may be removed by cystectomy, but the larger ones are difficult to resect from the ovary.

UTERINE LEIOMYOMAS

OVERVIEW

Leiomyomas, also called myomas and fibroids, are the most frequently occurring pelvic tumors. They are benign, slow-growing solid tumors. It is estimated that at least 20% to 30% of all women will develop leiomyomas sometime in their lives (Droegemueller et al., 1987).

Pathophysiology

Leiomyomas initially develop from the uterine myometrium. As they grow, fibroids stay attached to the myometrium by means of a pedicle. Leiomyomas are classified according to their position in the layers of the uterus and their anatomic position. The most common types of leiomyomas are intramural, submucosal, and subserosal (Fig. 54–5). *Intramural* leiomyomas are contained in the uterine wall within the myometrium. *Submucosal* leiomyomas protrude into the cavity of the uterus. *Subserosal* leiomyomas protrude through the outer surface of the uterine wall. Subserosal leiomyomas may grow laterally and extend to the broad ligament *(intraligamen-*

tous fibroid). Although most fibroids develop within the uterine wall, 5% to 10% may appear in the cervix *(cervical fibroids).* Rarely, a fibroid breaks off the pedicle and attaches to other tissues *(parasitic fibroid).*

Etiology

The etiology of leiomyomas is not precisely known. Leiomyomas are usually a result of a localized proliferation of smooth muscle cells in their initial stages. It has been suggested that the stimulus for proliferation may be physical or mechanical and may operate at points of maximal stress within the myometrial layer of the uterine wall. Because there are multiple points of stress owing to the contractions of the uterine muscle, multiple fibroids develop.

Growth of leiomyomas may be related to estrogen stimulation because fibroids often enlarge during pregnancy and diminish in size after menopause.

Incidence

It is not clear why leiomyomas develop in some women and not in others. The incidence in Black women is three times higher than in Caucasian women (Meyers, 1986). Fibroids are more common in women in their older reproductive years and postmenopausally, with the average age being older than 50 years (Droegemueller et al., 1987).

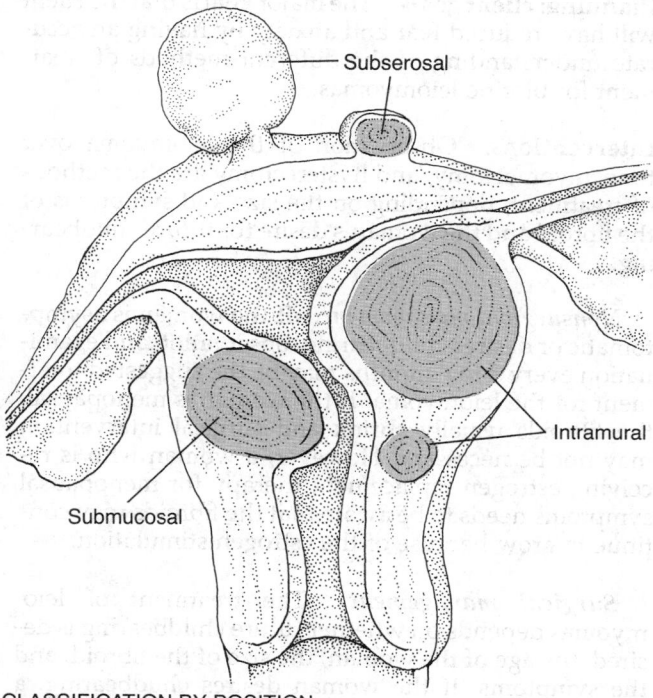

CLASSIFICATION BY POSITION
WITHIN UTERINE LAYERS

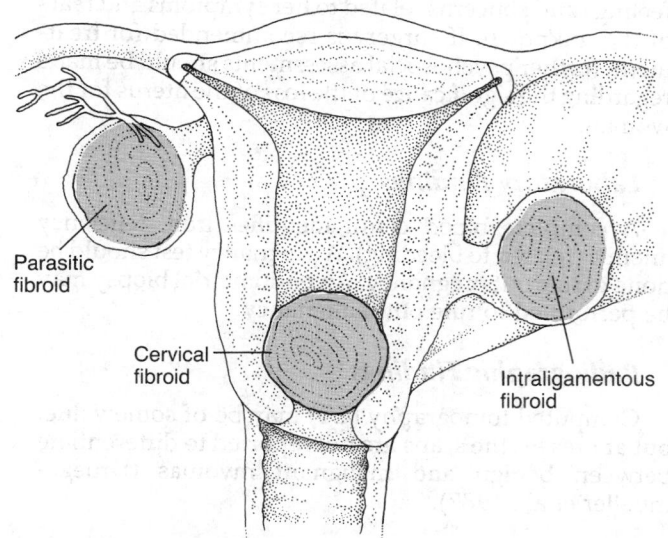

CLASSIFICATION BY ANATOMIC POSITION

Figure 54–5

Classification of uterine leiomyomas.

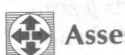 COLLABORATIVE MANAGEMENT

Assessment

History

Although the majority of women are asymptomatic, *abnormal bleeding* is the most common complaint. Black women and postmenopausal women older than 50 years are at risk for leiomyomas and should be questioned about the presence of abnormal bleeding. The bleeding may be only an increase in menstrual bleeding, or it may be continuous.

Physical Assessment: Clinical Manifestations

Pain is usually not a complaint, although *acute pain* may occur with torsion of the fibroid on the pedicle. A woman may complain of a feeling of *pelvic pressure, constipation,* or *urinary frequency or retention.* These symptoms result when an enlarged fibroid presses on other organs. She may also notice that her abdomen has increased in size with or without noticeable weight gain. Dyspareunia and infertility have also been associated with leiomyomas.

Abdominal, vaginal, and rectal examinations usually establish the presence of a uterine enlargement that indicates a leiomyoma. However, other types of lesions should be ruled out by other diagnostic procedures.

Psychosocial Assessment

A woman who is asymptomatic may be fearful that she has a malignancy. She may be anxious or concerned about abnormal bleeding or her failure to conceive. She may also be concerned if surgical procedures are recommended for treatment. The nurse assesses the woman's feelings and concerns related to her symptoms and fears of the unknown. If surgery is recommended for treatment, further psychosocial assessments should be made regarding the significance of the loss of the uterus for the woman.

Laboratory Findings

A complete blood count identifies iron deficiency anemia (related to bleeding). A pregnancy test should be done to rule out pregnancy. An endometrial biopsy may be performed to rule out malignancy.

Radiographic Findings

Computed tomography (CT) may be of some value, but at present the scans are not reported to differentiate between benign and malignant myomas (Droegemueller et al., 1987).

Other Diagnostic Tests

Ultrasonography may be useful in ruling out other causes of pelvic masses, including ovarian masses and pregnancy. Culdoscopy or laparoscopy may also be of value in differentiating a uterine fibroid from ovarian masses.

 Analysis: Nursing Diagnosis

Common Diagnoses

Common diagnoses in women with leiomyomas are fear and anxiety related to an uncertain diagnosis and potential surgical treatment.

Additional Diagnoses

The woman with leiomyomas may also have the following diagnoses:

1. Pain related to leiomyoma
2. Anticipatory grieving or dysfunctional grieving related to perceived or actual loss of the uterus or reproductive function
3. Potential for sexual dysfunction related to dyspareunia
4. Ineffective individual coping related to depression in response to surgery

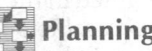 Planning and Implementation

The care plan focuses on the common diagnoses.

Fear; Anxiety

Planning: client goals. The major goal is that the client will have reduced fear and anxiety by having an accurate understanding of the different methods of treatment for uterine leiomyomas.

Interventions. Observation of the leiomyoma over time, myomectomy, and hysterectomy are the methods of treatment, depending on the size and symptoms of the fibroid and the woman's desire for future childbearing.

Nonsurgical management. If the woman is asymptomatic or desires childbearing, observation and examination every 3 to 6 months may be the suggested treatment for the leiomyoma. If the woman is menopausal, the fibroids usually shrink and surgical intervention may not be necessary. However, a woman who is receiving estrogen replacement therapy for menopausal symptoms needs to be aware that the fibroids may continue to grow because of the estrogen stimulation.

Surgical management. The treatment of leiomyomas depends on whether future childbearing is desired, the age of the woman, the size of the fibroid, and the symptoms. If the woman desires childbearing, a *myomectomy* (the removal of leiomyomas with preservation of the uterus) is possible, regardless of the size, number, or location of the fibroids. Myomectomy is usually performed in the proliferative phase of the menstrual cycle to minimize blood loss and to avoid the possibility of interrupting an unsuspected pregnancy. One-fourth of the women who undergo a myomectomy subsequently undergo a hysterectomy, primarily owing to recurrence of leiomyomas. The rate of conception after myomectomy ranges from 40% to 50% (Droege-mueller et al., 1987). Nursing care is similar to that of a woman having a hysterectomy.

A hysterectomy is the usual surgical management in the older woman who has multiple symptomatic leiomyomas. An abdominal hysterectomy is usually performed for leiomyomas greater in size than a 12-week pregnancy. The uterus is removed through a midline (vertical) or a horizontal incision. A uterus that has smaller fibroids may be removed via a vaginal hysterectomy. The uterus is removed through the vagina without an incision. In both vaginal and abdominal hysterectomies, the uterus is removed from the supporting ligaments, which are then attached to the vaginal cuff so that normal depth of the vagina is maintained (Table 54–3).

Preoperative care. The woman is assessed carefully to make sure she understands all the options for surgery, the advantages and risks of having surgery, preoperative and postoperative procedures, and convalescence needs. With this information, the woman can make an informed decision about consenting to surgery.

The nurse is responsible for psychologic, as well as physiologic, preparation of the woman scheduled for a hysterectomy. Preoperative teaching may be done on an individual basis or in groups. Routine preoperative procedures that may need to be explained include surgical preparation (douche, enema, abdominal-mons or perineal shave); laboratory tests for baseline data (blood tests, chest x-ray, electrocardiogram, and urinalysis); and preoperative medications, such as diazepam (Valium), atropine, and prophylactic antibiotics. The woman may need preparation for postoperative measures, including turning, coughing, and deep breathing exercises, early ambulation, and the need for pain relief.

Psychologic assessment is essential. The first topic that needs to be explored is the significance of the loss of the uterus for the woman. She may feel a great loss if she wishes to retain her childbearing ability, relates her uterus to her self-image and femininity, or feels that her sexual function is related to her uterus. Often, a woman has misconceptions about the effects of hysterectomy, associating it with masculinization and weight gain, for example, and these need to be identified so that correct information can be provided. A woman's support system needs to be assessed to see if she has adequate support. Often, the woman fears rejection by her husband or sexual partner, and inclusion of the partner in teaching sessions should be encouraged.

Postoperative care. Postoperative care of the woman having an abdominal hysterectomy is similar to that of any client having abdominal surgery (see Chap. 20). Interventions that are specific for abdominal hysterectomy include assessing vaginal bleeding (there should be less than one saturated pad in 4 hours), assessing abdominal bleeding at the incision site (a small amount is normal), checking the incision for intactness, providing Foley's catheter care for 24 to 48 hours, and offering pain medications or a heating pad for the abdominal pain (see the accompanying Client Care Plan). Specific interventions for a vaginal hysterectomy include assessment of vaginal bleeding (there should be less than one saturated pad in 4 hours), Foley's or suprapubic catheter care, and perineal care (sitz baths, heat lamps, or ice packs). Abdominal sutures or clips are removed by the fifth postoperative day, whereas vaginal sutures are usually absorbed.

The nurse must be aware of complications associated with hysterectomies (Table 54–4). Older women are more at risk for all complications, particularly pulmonary embolism. Obese women are more at risk for thromboembolism.

Psychologic complications can occur with both abdominal and vaginal procedures. Depression is the most frequent reaction reported. Other reactions are perceived loss of femininity and decreased libido. Loss of femininity may be the problem if a woman, who before surgery was interested in her appearance, afterwards has no interest, even when she is feeling better. Decreased sexual desire is usually temporary if it occurs and is usually related to discomfort.

■ **Discharge Planning**

Home Care Preparation

Discharge planning begins early in the postoperative period. The woman is usually discharged to her home

---

TABLE 54–3   Surgical Techniques Used to Remove the Uterus

Type of Procedure	Description
Total hysterectomy	All of the uterus is removed. The procedure may be vaginal or abdominal.
Subtotal hysterectomy	All of the uterus, except the cervix, is removed. This procedure is rarely performed.
Panhysterectomy	Total abdominal hysterectomy and bilateral salpingo-oophorectomy. The uterus, ovaries, and fallopian tubes are removed abdominally.
Radical hysterectomy	All of the uterus is removed abdominally. The lymph nodes, the upper third of the vagina, and the surrounding tissues (parametrium) are also removed.

CLIENT CARE PLAN ■ The Client Undergoing Total Abdominal Hysterectomy

Goal/Outcome Criteria	Interventions	Rationales
Nursing Diagnosis 1: Pain Related to the Surgical Procedure		
Client will experience relief of pain. ■ States that pain is reduced or eliminated.	1. Monitor the client for the presence of pain. 2. Administer prescribed analgesics before pain or discomfort becomes severe. Discuss the effectiveness of medications with the client; document their effectiveness. 3. Encourage relaxation and slow-breathing techniques to minimize pain. 4. Use nonpharmacologic methods of relieving discomfort, such as back rubs, position changes, guided imagery, and application of a heating pad. 5. Keep the client's environment quiet to promote rest.	1. Pain assessment aids in proper management. 2. Pain relief is provided. 3, 4. These techniques decrease pain. 5. Pain increases fatigue.
Nursing Diagnosis 2: Potential Fluid Volume Deficit Related to Abnormal Loss Secondary to Postoperative Bleeding or Decreased Intake Secondary to NPO Status		
Client will not become dehydrated. ■ Does not exhibit signs of dehydration or signs of excessive bleeding.	1. Assess the client for dehydration status (e.g., poor skin turgor and dry mucous membranes). 2. Monitor vital signs. 3. Administer and regulate IV fluids and electrolytes as prescribed until the client is no longer NPO; then encourage oral intake. 4. Monitor intake and output and urine specific gravity. 5. Assess postoperative bleeding q 2–4 h by noting amount of drainage on the dressing or perineal pad. 6. Review CDC values.	1. These indicate fluid volume deficit. 2. Hypotension and tachycardia may signal dehydration; decreased blood pressure, decreased pulse rate, and poor quality of respirations are associated with internal bleeding. 3. An adult usually requires 2000–3000 mL of fluid per day. 4. Specific gravity is elevated when dehydration persist. The usual urinary output is 1500 mL/day. 5. More than 1 saturated pad per hour may indicate excessive bleeding. 6. Decreased hemoglobin level and hematocrit may indicate bleeding.
Nursing Diagnosis 3: Potential for Infection Related to Surgery		
Client will not develop infection. ■ Exhibits no signs and symptoms of infection.	1. Monitor the use of antibiotic therapy, if ordered. 2. Assess for indications of infection. 3. Maintain aseptic techniques when doing wound care; use good hand-washing technique before making assessments. 4. Encourage the client to consume a diet high in protein and calories when oral intake is resumed. 5. Assess the wound for signs of infection (redness, edema, ecchymosis, drainage, and lack of approximation). 6. Assess vital signs, especially temperature.	1. Antibiotics prevent infection. 2. Early detection allows prompt treatment. 3. These techniques reduce access of organisms to the client. 4. A positive nitrogen balance enhances wound healing. 5. Early detection of deviations may prevent further impairment. 6. These may indicate early signs of infection.

CLIENT CARE PLAN ■ The Client Undergoing Total Abdominal Hysterectomy *continued*

Goal/Outcome Criteria	Interventions	Rationales
Nursing Diagnosis 4: Potential for Injury Related to Sequelae of Immobility		
Client will experience no adverse sequelae to immobility. ■ Does not exhibit signs of urinary, respiratory, circulatory, or GI complications.	1. Monitor intake and output at least every nursing shift: Output should be 1500 mL/d; intake should be 2000–3000 mL/d. 2. Assess breath sounds and respiratory rate. Teach or coach the client in coughing, deep breathing, and use of incentive spirometry. 3. Check for Homan's sign. 4. Assist with range-of-motion (leg) exercises. Assist with ambulation. Help the client to change positions. 5. Assess bowel sounds and function. 6. Medicate for pain and promote comfort measures.	1. This aids in maintaining optimal hydration and detecting urinary problems. 2. These measures detect and prevent respiratory complications. 3. This sign may indicate thromboembolic processes. 4. These promote circulation. 5. Detection of GI problems and promotion of peristalsis is important. 6. These promote mobility.
Nursing Diagnosis 5: Potential Body Image Disturbance and Altered Role Performance Related to Changes Caused by Hysterectomy		
Client will maintain positive self-concept. ■ Verbalizes her preceptions of past, present, and future role expectations. ■ Does not demonstrate or verbalize a negative self-attitude.	1. Assess the meaning of the loss of uterus or reproductive function and the client's emotional investment in this loss. 2. Encourage the client to share feelings with significant others. 3. Allow the client to ventilate feelings and grieve. 4. Identify strengths and resources (support systems).	1. The nurse needs to understand the client's self-concept to plan care. 2. Responses of others to the loss can affect the client's response. 3. Grief reactions should be expected. 4. Support can facilitate adaptation to an altered self-concept.
Nursing Diagnosis 6: Potential for Ineffective Individual Coping Related to Depression		
Client will cope well with her condition. ■ Verbalizes feelings about her emotional state. ■ Identifies positive patterns of coping and accepts the support of others.	1. Assess the client's perception of the situation. 2. Assess the client's coping mechanisms. 3. Assist the client to develop or use existing support systems. 4. Assess factors that cause or contribute to ineffective coping. 5. Teach constructive problem-solving techniques. 6. Refer the client for counseling if appropriate.	1. Causative factors need to be identified from the client's perspective. 2. Past methods of successful coping may be useful now. 3. Inadequate support can have negative effects on coping. 4. Successful interventions depend on identifying causative factors. 5. Various approaches to coping can be utilized. 6. Some problems may be beyond the scope of the nurse generalist.

setting in 4 to 7 days. Whether she had an abdominal or a vaginal hysterectomy, she should be told to avoid or limit stair climbing for 1 month. She should also avoid tub baths and sitting for long periods of time (which causes pooling of blood in the pelvic vessels). The woman should avoid strenuous activity or lifting anything weighing more than 4.5 to 9.0 kg (10 to 20 lb). Some physicians restrict driving a car for 2 weeks or longer.

Client/Family Education

The teaching plan for the woman who has had a hysterectomy includes information about the physical changes to be expected, exercise and activities, diet, sexual activity, complications, and follow-up care. The physical changes include cessation of menses, inability to become pregnant, weakness and fatigue in the con-

TABLE 54–4 Postoperative Complications of Abdominal and Vaginal Hysterectomies

Abdominal

Intestinal obstruction (paralytic ileus)
Thromboembolism
Atelectasis
Pneumonia
Wound dehiscence

Vaginal

Hemorrhage
Urinary tract complications
Wound infection

valescence period, and no menopausal symptoms unless the ovaries are also removed. Moderate exercise, such as walking, is encouraged, but active sports, such as jogging and aerobic exercise, should be avoided for at least 1 month. The client should be advised to consume foods that aid in healing tissues, such as foods high in protein, iron, and vitamin C. The client should avoid sexual intercourse for 3 to 6 weeks. The first coital activity may cause some tenderness or pain because the vaginal walls are tight and need to be stretched out. Water-soluble lubricants may be used to decrease discomfort. The client should be taught the signs of complications, particularly infection. An appointment for follow-up medical care should be scheduled 4 to 6 weeks postoperatively.

Psychosocial Preparation

Women who have had a hysterectomy need information about emotional reactions that can occur. Generally, a woman who has completed her childbearing, works, or has interests outside the home; has no misconceptions about the effects of hysterectomy; and has support from her family, especially her husband or sexual partner, has a positive adjustment to her surgery. Reactions may be different after vaginal and abdominal procedures because women who have had a vaginal hysterectomy have no external focus (no obvious change in body image) for their feelings.

Reactions can occur 3 months to 3 years after surgery. Women identified as being high at risk for psychologic problems may need long-term follow-up care or referral. Women may need to be counseled about signs of depression. Intermittent sadness is normal, but continued feelings of low self-esteem or loss of interest or pleasure in usual activities and pastimes is not normal and should be evaluated. The incidence of psychologic reactions often decreases after the nurse provides written materials and discusses with the client and her sig-

nificant others the positive forces in her life (Drummond & Field, 1984).

Health Care Resources

Usually, no special equipment or home resources are needed for a woman who has had a hysterectomy. Financial assistance may be needed, and referral to the hospital's department of social services may be indicated if the woman has no insurance coverage. Referral for psychologic or sexual counseling may be needed if potential problems are assessed before discharge from the hospital.

 Evaluation

On the basis of the identified nursing diagnoses, the nurse evaluates the care of the woman who has had surgery for treatment of leiomyomas. The expected outcomes are that the client

1. States an understanding of the reproductive system and the changes that occur after hysterectomy (without misconceptions)
2. Recovers without signs of complications
3. Demonstrates a positive psychologic adjustment to surgery as evidenced by the absence of depression and the presence of a positive self-concept
4. Resumes sexual activities at her previous level of satisfaction

BARTHOLIN'S CYSTS

Bartholin's cysts are one of the most common disorders of the vulva. The cysts result from obstruction of a duct. The secretory function of the gland continues, and the fluid fills up the obstructed duct. The cause of the obstruction may be infection, congenital stenosis or atresia, thickened mucus near the ductal opening, or mechanical trauma, such as lacerations or episiotomy.

The woman may be asymptomatic if the cyst is small, but a history may reveal complaints of dyspareunia, inadequate genital lubrication, or feeling a mass in the perineal area. A large cyst usually causes constant localized pain and may cause difficulty with walking or sitting. A physical examination of the vulva reveals a swelling immediately beneath the skin in the posterior portion of the vulva (Fig. 54–6). The cyst may appear brown or sanguineous, depending on its contents. Usually, the cyst is unilateral and ranges from 1 to 10 cm (³⁄₈ to 4 in) in size.

If the cyst is draining, the fluid should be sent to the laboratory for culture (gonorrhea, aerobic, and anaerobic cultures) and sensitivity testing. If the woman is older than 40 years, a specimen of the cyst should be sent for pathologic examination to rule out malignancy. If the woman is asymptomatic, no interventions are

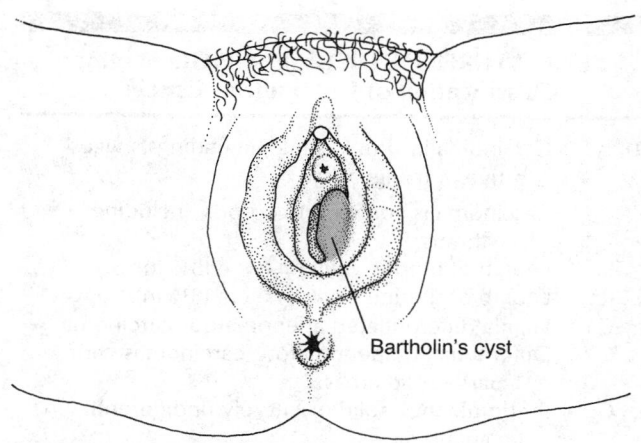

Figure 54-6

Bartholin's cyst.

necessary. If the cysts are symptomatic, surgical treatment by simple incision and drainage may provide temporary relief; however, cysts tend to recur as the opening of the duct becomes obstructed again. Usually, a permanent opening for drainage is established. *Marsupialization* (formation of a pouch that is a new duct opening) is accomplished under local, regional, or general anesthesia. Any postoperative discomfort may be relieved by administration of analgesics and sitz baths. Antibiotics may be given prophylactically.

BARTHOLIN'S ABSCESSES

Bartholin's cysts may become infected. Abscesses are formed when bacteria *(Escherichia coli, N. gonorrhoeae, S. aureus, Streptococcus, T. vaginalis,* or *Mycoplasma hominis)* enter the duct, resulting in infection that closes the duct.

A history may reveal complaints of perineal discomfort, dyspareunia, low-grade fever, swelling of the labia, purulent discharge, or difficulty with sitting or walking. A pelvic examination reveals an extremely tender mass on the side of the vaginal opening that may be swollen and red. The abscess usually ruptures spontaneously within 72 hours of formation. Drainage may be expressed from the abscess and sent to the laboratory for culture.

Interventions for the woman with an abscess include bed rest, administration of analgesics or application of moist heat (sitz baths or hot wet packs) to the vulva. Broad-spectrum antibiotics, such as tetracycline (500 mg four times a day for 7 or 10 days by mouth), may be given. Incision and drainage of the abscess may provide temporary relief.

Total excision of the Bartholin's glands may be performed in women older than 40 years when cancer is suspected or for repeated infections with abscess formation. Postoperative interventions include application of

heat lamps, ice packs, or sitz baths several times a day for comfort and promotion of healing; administration of analgesics for pain, if needed; prophylactic administration of antibiotics; and assessment of the incision for signs of healing or infection.

CERVICAL POLYPS

Cervical polyps are pendunculated (on stalks) tumors arising from the mucosa and extending to the opening of the cervical os. The etiology is unknown, although polyps are a result of a hyperplastic condition of the endocervical epithelium. They may also be due to inflammation. Polyps are the most common benign neoplastic growth of the cervix. Cervical polyps are most common in multiparous women older than 40 (Droegemueller et al., 1987).

A woman may be asymptomatic, or a history may reveal complaints of premenstrual or postmenstrual bleeding or bleeding after coitus. A speculum examination may reveal small (< 1 to 4 cm [⅜ to 1½ in]), single or multiple polyps that are bright red; have a soft, fragile consistency; and may bleed when touched.

Polyp removal is easily accomplished as an office procedure. The base of the polyp can be grasped with a clamp, twisted off, and sent to the pathology laboratory for evaluation. If bleeding occurs at the site of removal, electrocautery or chemical cautery usually stops the bleeding. Postprocedure instructions may include the avoidance of tampon use, douches, and sexual intercourse for a week or until healing has taken place.

MALIGNANT NEOPLASMS

ENDOMETRIAL CANCER

OVERVIEW

Endometrial cancer (cancer of the uterus) is the most frequently occurring reproductive cancer (Meyers, 1986). It is a slow-growing tumor associated with the menopausal years, is asymptomatic in its early development, and has a good prognosis in 80% to 90% of cases (Swearingen, 1986).

Pathophysiology

Adenocarcinoma of the endometrium accounts for 90% of all endometrial cancers. It arises from the glandular component of the endometrial mucosa and may be preceded by endometrial hyperplasia. The initial growth of the cancer is within the uterine cavity, followed by extension into the myometrium and the cervix. Spread

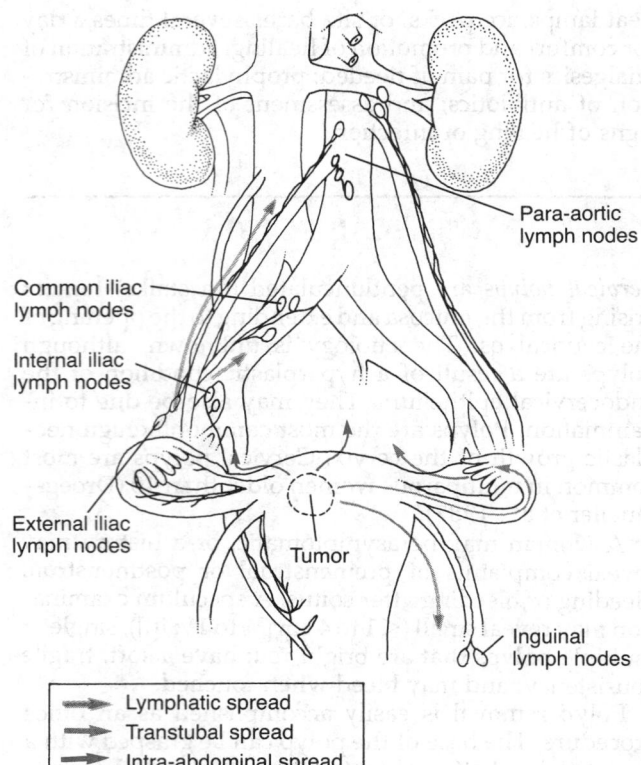

Figure 54–7

Extrauterine spread of endometrial cancer. (Reproduced by permission from Droegemueller, W., Herbst, A. L., Mishell, D. R., Jr., & Stenchever, M. A., *Comprehensive gynecology*, St. Louis, 1987, The C. V. Mosby Co.)

	KEY FEATURES OF DISEASE ■ FIGO Staging Classification of Endometrial Cancer
0	Carcinoma in situ. Histologic findings suggestive of malignancy.
I*	Carcinoma is confined to corpus, including isthmus.
Ia	Length of uterine cavity ≤8 cm (3⅛ in).
Ib	Length of uterine cavity >8 cm (3⅛ in).
G1	Highly differentiated adenomatous carcinoma.
G2	Differentiated adenomatous carcinomas with partly solid areas.
G3	Predominantly solid or entirely undifferentiated carcinoma.
II	Carcinoma has involved corpus and cervix but has not extended outside uterus.
III	Carcinoma has extended outside uterus but not outside true pelvis.
IV	Carcinoma has extended outside true pelvis or has involved bladder or rectal mucosa. Bullous edema does not make a case stage IV.
IVa	Spread to adjacent organs.
IVb	Spread to distant organs.

* Stage I is subgrouped by grade.

outside the uterus occurs through lymphatic spread to the ovaries and parametrial, pelvic, inguinal, and para-aortic lymph nodes; by hematogenous (spread by blood) metastasis to the lungs, liver, or bone; and by transtubal or intra-abdominal spread to the peritoneal cavity (Fig. 54–7).

A clinical staging system has been developed by the International Federation of Gynecology and Obstetrics (FIGO) for identifying the pattern and extent of spread (see the accompanying Key Features of Disease).

Etiology

Estrogens are primary stimulants of endometrial proliferation. This hormone may be necessary for the development of some endometrial cancers (Weiss, 1984).

The risk factors associated with GTD and other gynecologic cancers are summarized in the Key Features of Disease on page 1717.

Risk factors associated with endometrial cancer include obesity; diabetes mellitus; history of uterine polyps; sterility; nulliparity; polycystic ovary disease; estrogen stimulation, including unopposed menopausal estrogen replacement therapy; late menopause (after age 52 years); postmenopausal bleeding; and family history of uterine cancer.

Incidence

The National Cancer Institute (NCI) estimated that 34,000 new cases of endometrial cancer would be diagnosed in 1989 (American Cancer Society [ACS], 1989). This means that about 1 of every 100 women in the United States will develop endometrial cancer. The estimated death rate for endometrial cancer in 1989 was 4000 (ACS, 1989). Endometrial cancer occurs more frequently in Caucasian women than in Black women and typically in postmenopausal women, aged 50 to 65 years.

PREVENTION

There is no practical method of screening asymptomatic or low-risk women. Yearly pelvic examinations with Pap smears are recommended, even though the Pap test is only about 50% effective in detecting endometrial cancer. A woman who is in the high-risk category may need to have a yearly endometrial biopsy done. Women who are receiving estrogen replacement therapy should take estrogen on a cyclic basis and take the lowest effective dose (≤0.625 mg). A progestational agent is administered during the last 7 to 10 days of the menstrual cycle.

KEY FEATURES OF DISEASE ■ Risk Factors for Cancers of the Female Reproductive System

Risk Factor	Endometrial Cancer	Cervical Cancer	Ovarian Cancer	Vulvar Cancer	Vaginal Cancer	Fallopian Tube Cancer	Gestational Trophoblastic Disease
Age	After 40 yr, Peak incidence in 60s	CIS: 25–40 yr; Invasive 40–60 yr	Infrequent before 35 yr; range usually is 40–65 yr	After 40 yr, peak 60–70 yr	Most after 50 yr; adenocarcinoma 14–30 yr	After 50 yr, range 18–80 yr	After 40 yr, under 20 yr
Family history	Increased risk		Increased risk				
Personal history	Uterine cancer, diabetes, hypertension		Breast, bowel, or endometrial cancer	Cervical cancer, diabetes	DES exposure in utero; Vulvar or cervical cancer	Ovarian or uterine cancer, infertility	Previous molar pregnancy (3%–5%)
Race	Caucasian	Black, Native American	Caucasian				Asian
Mother's age at birth		<18 yr	>30 yr				
Body size	Obesity			Possibly obesity			
Socioeconomic class		Low		Low			Low
Marital status		Divorced, separated	Never married				
Parity	Nulliparity	Multiparity	Nulliparity		Multiparity	Nulliparity	
Estrogen use	Prolonged use >3.5 yr menopausally	Possibly long-term birth control pill use					
Smoking		Possibly					
Infection	Possibly sexually transmitted diseases	Possibly sexually transmitted diseases, papillomavirus infection		Possibly sexually transmitted diseases, papillomavirus infection	Sexually transmitted diseases, herpesvirus type 2 and papillomavirus infection	PID, chronic salpingitis	Exposure to infectious agents

COLLABORATIVE MANAGEMENT

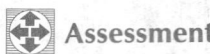 **Assessment**

History

The nurse notes the presence of risk factors (see earlier).

Physical Assessment: Clinical Manifestations

The primary symptom of endometrial cancer is *postmenopausal bleeding.* In addition, the woman may complain of a watery, serosanguineous vaginal discharge, low back or abdominal pain, and low pelvic pain (caused by pressure of the enlarged uterus). A pelvic examination reveals the presence of a palpable uterine mass or uterine polyp. The uterus is enlarged if the cancer is in an advanced stage.

Psychosocial Assessment

Before a diagnosis is made, the woman may deny that the symptoms are related to cancer. During the diagnostic phase, the woman may express fears and concerns about having a malignancy. After the diagnosis is confirmed, the woman may express disbelief, anger, depression, anxiety, or withdrawal behaviors. The woman needs support from significant others, as well as the health care team, to move to acceptance of the diagnosis.

The client may also express anxiety or fears about the proposed treatments. For example, she may fear being radioactive with radiation therapy and may have concerns about changes in appearance related to chemotherapy (loss of hair) or altered body image if surgery is performed.

Laboratory Findings

A complete blood count, liver function tests (aspartate aminotransferase [serum glutamic-oxaloacetic transaminase, or SGOT], alkaline phosphatase, and bilirubin determinations), renal function tests (serum blood urea nitrogen [BUN] and creatinine determinations), and blood glucose tests are usually done as part of the investigative procedure for diagnosing endometrial cancer.

Radiographic Findings

Chest radiography is done to rule out lung metastasis. Other tests that may have specific applicability to certain clients include intravenous pyelography (IVP) (excretory urography) to check the function of the ureters; barium enema to rule out metastasis to those organs; CT of the pelvis to identify the origin and spread of the tumor; lymphangiography to evaluate lymph node involvement; and liver and bone scans to evaluate distant spread.

Other Diagnostic Tests

Fractional D & C (scraping individual sections of the uterus) and endometrial biopsy are the definitive diagnostic procedures for endometrial cancer. Other tests that may be useful for some clients include proctosigmoidoscopy (visualization of the distal sigmoid colon, the rectum, and the anal canal with an endoscope); ultrasonography; and hysteroscopy (examination of the uterus via an endoscope).

 Analysis: Nursing Diagnosis

Common Diagnoses

The following diagnoses are common for the woman with endometrial cancer:

1. Anxiety and fear related to lack of knowledge of treatment procedures for endometrial cancer
2. Body image disturbance secondary to diagnosis of cancer or treatment

Additional Diagnoses

Diagnoses for the woman with endometrial cancer may also include

1. Dysfunctional or anticipatory grieving related to anticipated or actual loss
2. Potential for sexual dysfunction related to cancer or treatment

 Planning and Implementation

The care plan is based on the common nursing diagnoses.

Anxiety; Fear

Planning: client goals. The major goal is that the client will demonstrate reduction in anxiety and fear with increased understanding of the different types of treatment for endometrial cancer.

Interventions. Nonsurgical (radiation therapy and chemotherapy) and surgical interventions may be used alone or in combination, depending on the stage of the cancer.

Nonsurgical management. Radiation therapy (external and internal) is used if the stage of cancer is hard to determine and in combination with surgery for stage II and III cancers. Radiation therapy is usually done for 6 weeks preoperatively to destroy cancer cells in the pericervical lymphatics and to inhibit recurrence. If intracavitary radiation therapy (IRT) is done, an applicator is positioned within the woman's uterus through the vagina while she is anesthetized (Fig. 54–8). After the correct position of the applicator is confirmed by radiog-

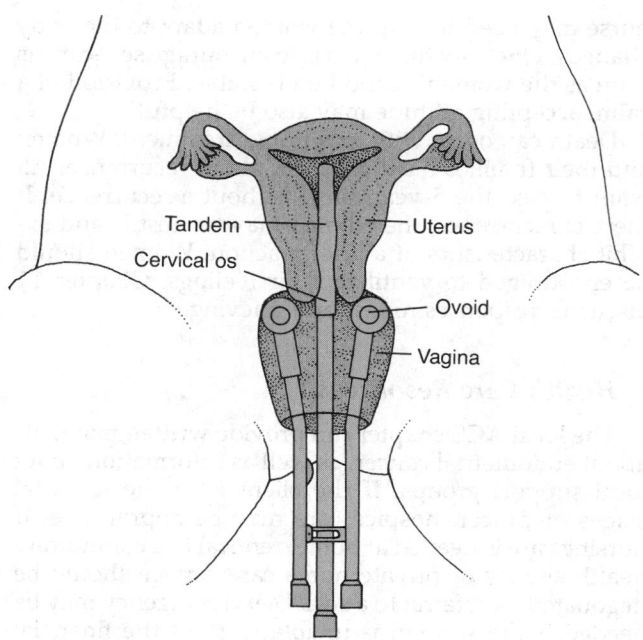

Figure 54-8

Intrauterine placement of applicator for intracavitary radiation therapy. Radiation sources are inserted into the tandem and ovoids.

raphy, the woman is taken to the hospital room and a radiologist places a radioactive isotope in the applicator, which remains for 1 to 3 days. Before the implant, the client is instructed on postoperative activities, such as deep breathing and leg exercises. While the implant is in place, the woman is strictly isolated, usually in a private room. She is restricted to bed rest on her back with the head of the bed flat or slightly elevated (< 20 degrees). Movement in bed is restricted to prevent dislodgment of the radioactive source. A Foley catheter is inserted into the bladder to prevent dislodgment, which can be caused by a full bladder or attempting to void. The nurse carefully assesses the skin for breakdown over bony pressure points. The woman is usually on a low-residue diet (to prevent bowel movements that could dislodge the implant), and fluid intake is encouraged (to prevent stasis of urine and possible infection). Medications that are usually given include antiemetics, broad-spectrum anti-infectives (to prevent bladder infections), tranquilizers (to help the client relax), analgesics, heparin (to prevent thromboembolism), and antidiarrhea medications (to prevent bowel movements).

Radiation precautions should be practiced while the implant is in place. The nurse should organize care so that minimal time is spent at the bedside. Care should be given as far away from the radioactive source as possible and behind lead shields as much as possible. Nurses who are pregnant or attempting pregnancy are usually not assigned to these clients. Visitors are restricted to brief visits, and pregnant women and children younger than 18 years old should not be allowed to visit. Further

discussion of nursing care for the client with intracavitary implants may be found in Chapter 25.

External radiation therapy may also be used in all stages of endometrial cancer, although it is usually used in combination with surgery, preoperatively or postoperatively. Depending on the extent of the tumor, external radiation is given on an outpatient basis for 4 to 6 weeks. The lateral extension of the tumor in the parametrium and pelvic wall nodes are irradiated. Nursing care for the client receiving external radiation is discussed in Chapter 25. Specific instructions for the woman having external radiation for endometrial cancer include watching for signs of skin breakdown, especially in the perineal area, no sunbathing, and no bathing over the markings outlining the treatment site. The woman also needs to know that cystitis and diarrhea are common complications, as are nutritional problems that result from alteration in taste and anorexia.

Chemotherapy is used to treat advanced and recurrent disease. Chemotherapeutic agents that have been used to treat endometrial cancer include doxorubicin (Adriamycin), cisplatin, cyclophosphamide (Cytoxin), 5-fluorouracil, and vincristine (DiSaia & Creaseman, 1984). Most agents are used in combination, and the length of treatment and dosage is determined by the woman's response. Chapter 25 discusses nursing interventions for clients receiving chemotherapy.

Progestational therapy is used for stage I and II cancers that are estrogen dependent and for stage IV cancer when palliative treatment may be needed. The hormones frequently used are medroxyprogesterone (Depo-Provera) and megestrol acetate (Megace). Tamoxifen, an antiestrogen, is also used. The progestational agents do not cause acute side effects, but nausea and vomiting and hot flashes are associated with tamoxifen.

Surgical management.   A total abdominal hysterectomy and bilateral salpingo-oophorectomy is usually performed for stage I tumors without cervical involvement. A radical hysterectomy is performed for stage II cancer. Nursing care is essentially the same as that for hysterectomy (see earlier), except that the woman's hospitalization is usually longer and her convalescence period may be extended.

Body Image Disturbance

Planning: client goals.   The goal is that the client will state that she has a more positive body image.

Interventions: nonsurgical management.   Women need to discuss their concerns about the presence of cancer and the potential for recurrence. The nurse provides emotional support and tries to create an atmosphere that encourages the woman to ask questions or express her fears and concerns. Significant others should be included in discussions when possible.

Reactions to radiation therapy vary. Some women may feel radioactive or "unclean" after treatments.

They may exhibit withdrawal behaviors. The nurse needs to provide information that will clear up misconceptions.

Women who have chemotherapy may be upset if alopecia (loss of hair) occurs. Women should be warned of this possibility before treatment starts. Often, wigs, scarves, or turbans can be worn until regrowth occurs. (See Chap. 25 for discussion of psychosocial responses to cancer and its treatment.)

■ Discharge Planning

Home Care Preparation

Home care after surgery for endometrial cancer is the same as for the woman who has had a hysterectomy (see earlier discussion of uterine leiomyomas). Women who are receiving chemotherapy or external radiation therapy are usually treated on an outpatient basis, which may mean that a woman and her family have to plan daily activities around trips to the clinic or physician's office.

If there is recurrence of the tumor and cure is not likely, the client and her family need to think about terminal care and whether the woman can be cared for in the home.

Client/Family Education

For the woman who has had a hysterectomy for endometrial cancer, the teaching plan is the same as that for the woman who has had a hysterectomy for uterine leiomyomas (see earlier). After intracavitary radiation implant, the teaching plan includes the following information: Side effects should be reported to the physician, including vaginal bleeding, rectal bleeding, foul-smelling discharge, abdominal pain or distention, or hematuria. The high dose of radiation causes sterility. Vaginal shrinkage can occur. Vaginal dilators can be used with water-soluble lubricants for 10 minutes/day until sexual activity resumes (in 10 days to 6 weeks). The woman is not radioactive nor will her partner "catch" cancer from engaging in sexual intercourse. Vaginal douching may decrease inflammation. A normal diet may be resumed. Any medications prescribed should be explained in terms of dosage, schedule of administration, effects, and side effects. The woman should understand the importance of keeping appointments for follow-up care.

Psychosocial Preparation

Often, women experience emotional crises because of the physical effects of the treatments. Radical hysterectomy may be seen as mutilating, and chemotherapy may also affect the woman's body image if hair loss occurs. A woman may exhibit a grief reaction to this perceived change in body image. The feelings of loss depend on the visibility of the loss, the function of the loss, and the amount of emotional investment. The

nurse may need to help the woman adapt to the body changes. One way to do this is to encourage self-care as soon as the woman's condition is stable. Provision of a calm, accepting attitude may also be helpful.

Death can occur with or without treatment. Women and their families have concerns about recurrence. All want to pass the 5-year mark without a recurrence. If there is recurrence, the woman may be hostile and exhibit characteristics of a grief reaction. Women should be encouraged to ventilate their feelings. Chapter 11 discusses responses to loss and grieving.

Health Care Resources

The local ACS chapter can provide written materials about endometrial cancer, as well as information about local support groups. If the client is in the terminal stages of cancer, hospice care may be appropriate. If nursing care is needed at home, referral to a community health agency or private home care service should be negotiated. A referral to a social services agency may be needed if the woman is unable to meet the financial demands of treatment and long-term follow-up.

 Evaluation

On the basis of the identified nursing diagnoses, the nurse evaluates the care of the woman who has been treated for endometrial cancer. The expected outcomes are that the client

1. Does not experience recurrence or metastasis
2. Demonstrates a decrease in pain
3. Accepts body image changes and exhibits adaptation to her situation
4. Verbalizes feelings of grief
5. Resumes normal sexual activities or identifies alternative ways to reach previous levels of satisfaction
6. Demonstrates a decrease in anxiety level by stating an understanding of endometrial cancer and its management
7. Resumes prior activities and relationships with minimal difficulty

CERVICAL CANCER

OVERVIEW

Cervical cancer is the third most frequently occurring reproductive cancer, after endometrial and ovarian cancers. Death rates for cervical cancer have dropped 50% in the past 20 years, primarily owing to the availability of Pap tests for screening of premalignant cervical changes. However, cervical cancer is still the second most common cause of death related to reproductive cancers (Silverberg & Lubera, 1987).

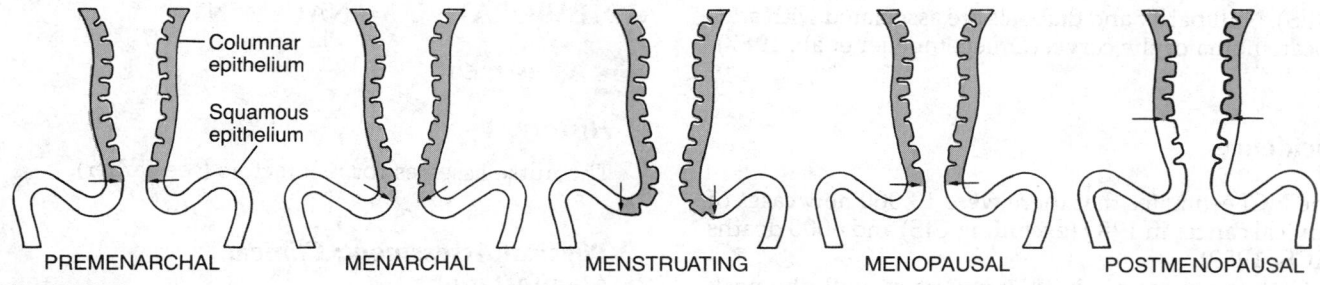

Figure 54-9

Location of the transformation zone at various stages of adult development.

Pathophysiology

Cervical cancer may be described as preinvasive or invasive. *Preinvasive* cancer is limited to the cervix, whereas *invasive* cancer is in the cervix, as well as other pelvic structures. Preinvasive lesions usually originate in the area called the *transformation zone* (Fig. 54-9). This area includes the squamocolumnar junction, which is located near the external cervical os where squamous and columnar (glandular) epithelium changes normally occur. Abnormal squamous epithelium can also be found in this zone, and these cells have the potential to develop into invasive carcinoma.

These premalignant changes can be described on a continuum from dysplasia—the earliest premalignant change—to carcinoma in situ (CIS)—the most advanced premalignant change (Fig. 54-10). Preinvasive cancers can also be described using the term *cervical intraepithelial neoplasia* (CIN) and classified according to severity: CIN I is mild dysplasia. CIN II is moderate dysplasia. CIN III is severe dysplasia to CIS.

Squamous cell cancers spread by direct extension to the vaginal mucosa, the lower uterine segment, the parametrium, the pelvic wall, the bladder, and the bowel.

Metastasis is usually confined to the pelvis, but distant metastases can occur through lymphatic spread and, rarely, via the circulatory system to the liver, the lungs, or bones.

Etiology

The cause of squamous cell cervical cancer is unknown, but numerous factors have a potential role in carcinogenesis. Droegemueller and associates (1987) described an association with early and frequent sexual contact and with viral infections of the cervix, such as with herpes simplex virus type 2, cytomegalovirus, and papillomavirus, but studies have not yet shown a definite relationship.

Risk factors associated with cervical cancer include low socioeconomic status; race (occurrence is twice as high for Black women); early age at first sexual contact or first pregnancy; multiple sexual partners; early marriage; prostitution; male factors, such as having intercourse with men whose previous wives had cervical cancer; use of oral contraceptives; cigarette smoking; vitamin A and C deficiencies; occurrence of venereal diseases; and intrauterine exposure to diethylstilbestrol

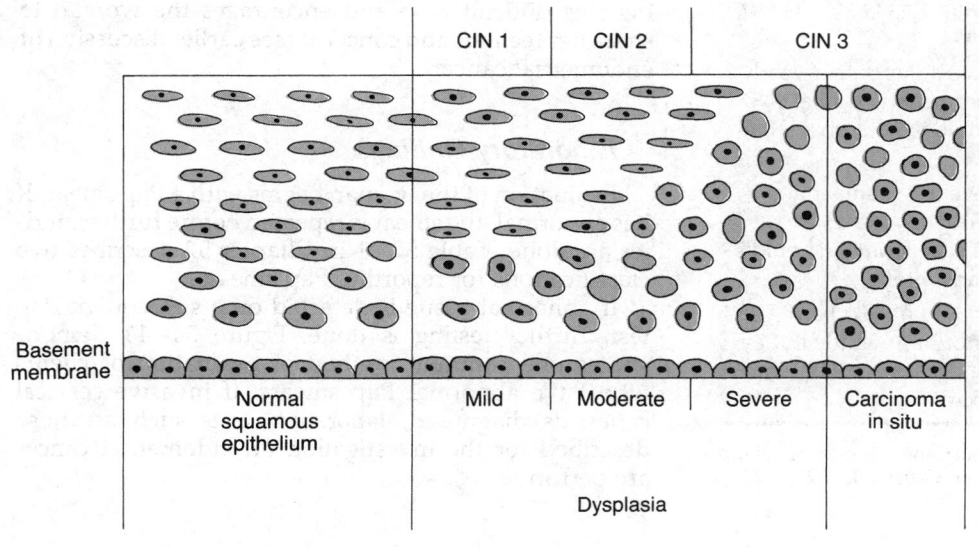

Figure 54-10

Continuum of cervical premalignant lesions from dysplasia to carcinoma in situ. (Reproduced by permission from Droegemueller, W., Herbst, A. L., Mishell, D. R., Jr., & Stenchever, M. A., *Comprehensive gynecology*, St. Louis, 1987, The C. V. Mosby Co. Modified from Richart, R. M. [1976]. *Canadian Journal of Medical Technology, 38,* 177.)

(DES). Nulliparity and diabetes are associated with adenocarcinoma of the cervix (Droegemueller et al., 1987).

Incidence

The NCI estimates that there were 13,000 new cases of cervical cancer in 1989 (excluding CIS) and 6000 deaths (ACS, 1989).

CIN occurs mainly in young women, with the peak incidence of dysplasia occurring in clients in their mid-20s; CIS, about 30 years; and invasive cancer, in the late 40s. Cervical adenocarcinoma occurs most often in women in their 50s, and no relationship to sexual transmission or viral infection has been found (Droegemueller et al., 1987).

PREVENTION

The Pap smear is a reliable, inexpensive screening tool. It has been used to screen large numbers of women for premalignant and malignant lesions of the cervix and is probably responsible for the decline in incidence of invasive cervical cancer.

The ACS recommendations for Pap smears (see the accompanying Health Promotion/Maintenance feature) have not been agreed on by all health care providers. Most gynecologists still recommend yearly Pap tests for women who have not had hysterectomies and yearly pelvic examinations for women older than 40 years.

HEALTH PROMOTION/ MAINTENANCE ■ American Cancer Society Recommendations for Pap Smears

Women should begin having Pap smears at age 20 yr or earlier if they are sexually active.

Women aged 25–35 yr should have a Pap smear yearly until the results of two tests are negative. After two negative test results, these women should have Pap smears every 3 yr.

Women aged 36–60 yr should have a Pap smear at least every 3 yr, and more frequently if they are at high risk for cervical cancer. These women should have a pelvic examination yearly after age 40 yr.

Women older than 60 yr of age should have a Pap smear at least every 3 yr, or more frequently if they are at high risk for cervical cancer. These women should have a yearly pelvic examination.

From Fink, D.J. (1988). Change in American Cancer Society check-up guidelines for detection of cervical cancer. *Cancer, 38,* 127–128.

COLLABORATIVE MANAGEMENT

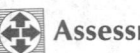 Assessment

History

The nurse assesses for risk factors (see earlier).

Physical Assessment: Clinical Manifestations

The woman who has preinvasive cancer is often asymptomatic. The classic symptom of invasive cancer is *painless vaginal bleeding.* The bleeding may start as spotting between menstrual periods or after coitus or douching. As the malignancy grows, the bleeding increases in frequency, duration, and amount. It may become continuous.

The woman may also complain of a watery, blood-tinged *vaginal discharge* that may become dark and foul smelling as the disease progresses. *Leg pain* (along the sciatic nerve) or unilateral swelling of a leg may be a late symptom or may indicate recurrent disease. Other signs of recurrence may include unexplained weight loss, pelvic pain (caused by pressure of the tumor on the bladder or the bowel), dysuria, hematuria, rectal bleeding, chest pain, or coughing.

A physical examination may not reveal any abnormalities, although a speculum examination may identify late-stage disease. Diagnostic testing must be relied on if the woman has an abnormal Pap smear.

Psychosocial Assessment

A woman who has an abnormal Pap smear may express fears of having cancer and be concerned with death or dying. She may be anxious until the diagnosis of cancer is made and the extent of the lesion is determined. After the diagnosis is confirmed, the woman may demonstrate grief. She may have concerns about treatment alternatives. The nurse provides support during this difficult time and encourages the woman to share her feelings and concerns (see earlier discussion of endometrial cancer).

Laboratory Findings

Evaluation of the woman begins with a Pap smear. If it is abnormal, the smear is repeated before further studies are done. Table 52–1 in Chapter 52 describes two classifications for reporting Pap smears.

If abnormal tissue is detected on a subsequent Pap test, further testing is done. Figure 54–11 demonstrates one common method of evaluation of clients who have abnormal Pap smears. If invasive cervical cancer is diagnosed, laboratory tests such as those described for the investigation of endometrial cancer are performed.

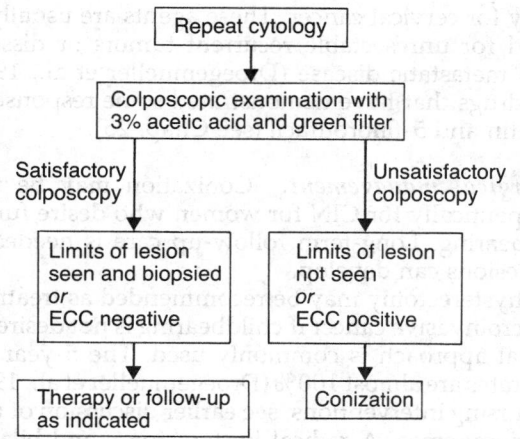

Figure 54-11

One method of evaluating women who have abnormal Pap smear results. (Reproduced by permission from Droegemueller, W., Herbst, A. L., Mishell, D. R., Jr., & Stenchever, M. A., *Comprehensive gynecology*, St. Louis, 1987, The C. V. Mosby Co.)

Radiographic Findings

If invasive cancer is diagnosed, chest radiography and other studies applicable to the specific circumstances are done to assess the extent or metastasis of the cancer (see earlier discussion of endometrial cancer).

Other Diagnostic Tests

A colposcopic examination is performed to view the transformation zone, where dysplasia, CIN, and CIS

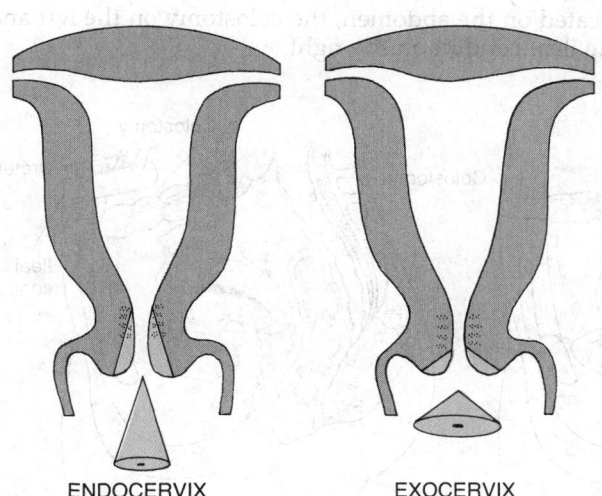

ENDOCERVIX   EXOCERVIX

Figure 54-12

Conization biopsy for CIN of the endocervix and cervix. (Reproduced by permission from DiSaia, Philip J., & Creasman, William T., *Clinical gynecologic oncology*, ed. 3, St. Louis, 1989, The C. V. Mosby Co.)

usually originate. If abnormal tissue is recognized, multiple biopsies of the cervical tissue are performed (see Chap. 52).

An endocervical curettage (scraping of the endocervix from the internal to the external os) is usually performed as well. This procedure is uncomfortable, and the nurse may need to encourage the woman to use relaxation or breathing exercises to cope with the cramping and pain. Bleeding may occur after the biopsies for up to 2 weeks.

Conization is the definitive treatment for microinvasive cervical cancer. The procedure is done when the lesion cannot be visualized by colposcopic examination. A cone-shaped area of cervix is removed surgically (Fig. 54-12) and sent to the laboratory to determine the extent of the malignancy. Risks associated with conization include hemorrhage, uterine perforation, incompetent cervix, cervical stenosis, and risk of preterm labor in future pregnancies.

Analysis: Nursing Diagnosis

Common Diagnoses

The following diagnoses are common to the woman with cervical cancer:

1. Anxiety and fear related to lack of knowledge about treatment of cervical cancer
2. Body image disturbance and altered role performance secondary to diagnosis of cancer

Additional Diagnoses

Depending on the extent of malignancy and type of treatment selected, the following diagnoses may be appropriate:

1. Dysfunctional grieving or anticipatory grieving related to the loss of a body part or changes in body function
2. Potential for sexual dysfunction related to cancer or its treatments

Planning and Implementation ➡

Nursing care of the client with cervical cancer is similar to that of the client with endometrial cancer (see earlier); the only interventions discussed are those that differ from those for endometrial cancer.

Anxiety; Fear

Planning: client goals. The major goal is that the client will demonstrate reduced fear and anxiety about treatments of cervical cancer after receiving informaion about surgical and nonsurgical treatments.

Interventions. Management of cervical cancer depends on the extent of spread and may include surgery, radiation therapy, chemotherapy, or other nonsurgical treatments.

Nonsurgical management of cervical intraepithelial neoplasia. Laser therapy is an outpatient procedure that is used whenever all the boundaries of the lesion are visible under colposcopic examination and the endocervical curettage findings are normal. In *laser therapy,* the invisible beam is directed to the abnormal tissues, where energy from the beam is absorbed by the fluid in the tissues, causing them to vaporize. There is usually minimal bleeding associated with the procedure. The woman may have a slight vaginal discharge, and healing occurs in 6 to 12 weeks.

Cryosurgery is another common treatment of CIN. In *cryosurgery,* a probe is placed against the cervix to cause freezing of the tissues and subsequent necrosis. No anesthesia is required, although the woman may experience slight cramping. The woman has a heavy watery discharge for several weeks after the procedure, and she should avoid intercourse and use of tampons while discharge is present because the cervix is fragile.

Nonsurgical management of invasive cancer of the cervix. Most women with cervical cancer are treated with radiation. For cancer that has extended beyond the cervix but not to the pelvic wall, radiation therapy is as effective as a radical hysterectomy. Intracavitary and external radiation therapies are used in combination, depending on the extent and location of the lesion. Intracavitary implants are usually used for lesions that have extended beyond the pelvic wall (Roberts & Morley, 1984). Nursing care related to radiation therapy is presented in the earlier discussion of endometrial cancer and in Chapter 25.

Chemotherapeutic agents generally have performed poorly for cervical cancer. These agents are usually reserved for unresectable recurrent tumors or disseminated metastatic disease (Droegemueller et al., 1987). Two drugs that have demonstrated some response are cisplatin and 5-fluorouracil (see Chap. 25).

Surgical management. Conization may be used therapeutically for CIN for women who desire further childbearing. Long-term follow-up care is needed, as new lesions can develop.

A hysterectomy may be recommended as treatment of microinvasive cancer if childbearing is not desired. A vaginal approach is commonly used. The 5-year survival rates are almost 100% (Droegemueller et al., 1987). For nursing interventions, see earlier discussion of uterine leiomyomas. A radical hysterectomy and bilateral lymph node dissection (see Table 54–3) is as effective as radiation for treating cancer that has extended beyond the cervix but not to the pelvic wall. The 5-year survival rates are approximately 80% (Droegemueller et al., 1987).

Pelvic exenteration. One of the most radical surgical procedures is the pelvic exenteration. It is performed for recurrent cancers if there is no evidence of tumor outside the pelvis and no lymph node involvement. There are three types of exenteration: anterior, posterior, and total (Fig. 54–13). *Anterior* exenteration is the removal of the uterus, ovaries, fallopian tubes, vagina, bladder, urethra, and pelvic lymph nodes. *Posterior* exenteration is the removal of the uterus, ovaries, fallopian tubes, descending colon, rectum, and anal canal. *Total* exenteration is a combination of anterior and posterior procedures. When the bladder is removed, urine is diverted through an ileal conduit (intestinal pouch), and a colostomy is created for passage of feces. The stomas are located on the abdomen, the colostomy on the left and the ileal conduit on the right.

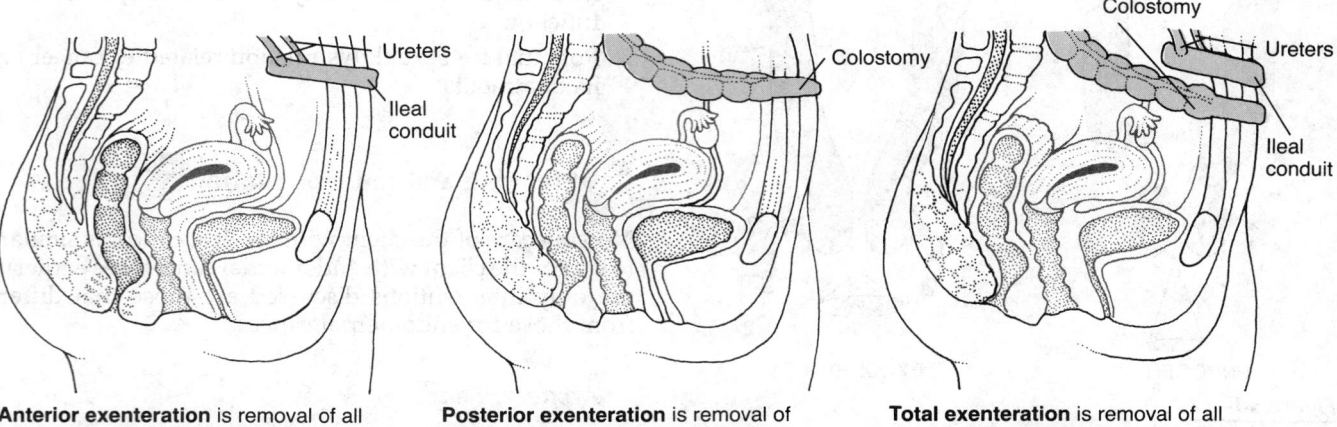

Anterior exenteration is removal of all pelvic organs except the descending colon, rectum, and anal canal. Urine is diverted into an ileal conduit.

Posterior exenteration is removal of all pelvic organs except the bladder. A colostomy is created for the passage of feces.

Total exenteration is removal of all pelvic organs with creation of an ileal conduit and a colostomy.

Figure 54–13

Pelvic exenteration.

Preoperative care. Nursing care of the woman scheduled for exenteration includes assessment of preoperative anxiety, concerns about the impact on sexual function, and the ability to adjust to her altered body image. Significant others should be involved in discussions about postoperative expectations. Physical preparation includes selection of stoma sites, extensive bowel preparation, and extensive radiographic and laboratory tests to rule out spread of cancer outside the pelvis. The client should be taught about postoperative recovery in a critical care unit, pain management, the presence of numerous intravenous and arterial catheters, and nasogastric suction. The reader is referred to Chapters 45 and 58 for preoperative care and teaching of clients with colostomy and ileal conduit, respectively.

Postoperative care. The woman usually goes to a critical care unit for the first 3 to 4 days because of the risks of serious complications resulting from the massive tissue resection. Nursing concerns in this period include assessment for cardiovascular complications, such as hemorrhage and shock; pulmonary complications, such as atelectasis and pneumonia; fluid and electrolyte imbalances, such as metabolic acidosis or alkalosis; renal or urinary complications; and pain. Nursing interventions include assisting with deep breathing and coughing hourly, observing for dehydration, monitoring urinary output and specific gravity, administering narcotic analgesics, and monitoring parenteral nutrition.

After the woman's condition is stable, she returns to the regular postoperative unit, and the usual postoperative interventions continue (see Chap. 20), with the addition of colostomy and ileal conduit care. Nursing concerns in the recovery period include assessment of late cardiovascular complications, such as deep vein thrombosis, and pulmonary emboli; GI complications, such as paralytic ileus; wound infections; wound dehiscence or evisceration; and pain. Nursing interventions include the administration of prophylactic heparin and the use of antiembolism stockings for the prevention of thrombosis, continual auscultation of the lungs, assessment for the presence of bowel sounds and identification of abdominal distention, assessment for signs of wound infection, administration of antibiotics, and pain management with a gradual withdrawal of narcotic analgesics.

After the dressings are removed, perineal irrigations may be implemented. Irrigation is with a solution of one-half normal saline and one-half hydrogen peroxide applied with an Asepto syringe, followed by drying of the perineum with a heat lamp (25 watt at a distance of 18 in) or hair dryer (using cool air). Sitz baths may be ordered as tolerated. The reader is referred to Chapters 45 and 58 for postoperative care of clients with colostomies and urinary diversions, respectively.

■ Discharge Planning

Home Care Preparation

The client is usually in the hospital several weeks postoperatively and not infrequently is discharged to a convalescent nursing center for continued recovery and care. When the client returns home, she will need assistance. She will not be able to engage in strenuous activities associated with most household work for up to 6 months. The family may need to consider outside help if there is no one in the family who can assume household responsibilities.

No special equipment is needed in the home, although an "eggcrate" mattress may be placed on the bed to prevent skin breakdown and to increase comfort, as the woman spends more time in bed. Colostomy and ureterostomy bags and equipment for changing these can be purchased in local pharmacies.

Client/Family Education

The teaching plan for the woman who has had an exenteration includes the following topics: The client is thoroughly taught how to manage new functions with equipment (colostomy and ileal conduit) and to perform ADL and self-care. The perineal opening may drain for several months to a year. The client can wear sanitary napkins (minipads or maxipads) if they are beltless (so as not to interfere with the stomas). The woman may need help in adjusting her diet to maintain high nutritional requirements for healing while selecting foods that are tolerated. The woman should understand the effects, dosages, and side effects of all medications prescribed. Sexual function will be different after exenteration (even if an artificial vagina is constructed) and counseling about alternatives to intercourse may be needed by the couple. Even with vaginal reconstruction, the use of vaginal dilators is necessary to achieve good sexual function. Physical activities may be limited during convalescence. If walking is not permitted, range-of-motion exercises should be encouraged. Follow-up care is important, and women should be counseled about keeping all follow-up appointments. Information about late complications (e.g., infection and bowel obstruction) is needed so that the woman can seek medical care promptly.

Psychosocial Preparation

Usually, by the end of the first postoperative week, the woman begins expressing grief about her mutilated body. At first she may deny changes by refusing to look at the wound or stoma sites. Later, she may become depressed or withdrawn or even angry or hostile. She may then move to reality testing by asking questions about her care, watching the nurses do wound care, and becoming actively involved in self-care.

The woman may have mood swings, and the nurse should be alert when the woman becomes depressed so that interventions can be implemented to reorient the woman to other activities. The woman needs intense emotional support if she is to adapt to her altered body image and functions.

Unless the woman has a vaginal reconstruction after anterior or total pelvic exenteration, she is not able to have vaginal intercourse. The nurse must assess the need for sexual counseling by listening for cues about altered perceptions of body image and anxiety about her sexual partner's response. Further sexual counseling may be needed to provide information on alternative methods of sexual gratification.

Health Care Resources

Resources for the woman who has cervical cancer are similar to those discussed for the woman with endometrial cancer (see earlier).

 Evaluation

On the basis of the identified nursing diagnoses, the nurse evaluates the care of the woman who has been treated for cervical cancer. The expected outcomes are that the client

1. Does not have recurrence or metastasis of cancer
2. Demonstrates reduction in anxiety level by stating an understanding of cervical cancer and its treatment options
3. Demonstrates a decrease in pain
4. Accepts body image changes and exhibits adaptation to her altered self-concept
5. Verbalizes feelings of grief
6. Recovers without complications from surgery or radiation therapy
7. Verbalizes an understanding of the effects of surgery or radiation therapy on sexual function and resumes sexual activities that are satisfying

---

OVARIAN CANCER

OVERVIEW

Ovarian cancer is the leading cause of death from female reproductive malignancies. Death rates have risen during the past 4 decades, and it is now projected that 1 of every 70 women will develop ovarian cancer sometime in her life (Barber, 1984). Survival rates continue to be low because ovarian cancer is poorly detected in its early stages.

Eighty-five per cent of ovarian cancers are epithelial tumors, with the most common type of tumor being serous adenocarcinoma. These tumors grow rapidly, spread fast, are often bilateral, and have the worst prognosis of all epithelial tumors. The cancer spreads by several mechanisms: direct spread to other organs in the pelvis that are in close proximity to the ovary (e.g., uterus, bladder, and colon); distal spread through lymphatic drainage (via para-aortic and iliac lymph nodes to the rest of the pelvis, the abdomen or the liver, the lung, or bones); and peritoneal seeding (malignant spread of free-floating cells usually after the development of ascites).

The etiology of ovarian cancer is not precisely known. Suggested etiologic theories include a familial association; an environmental association related to products of industry in countries such as the United States and those of Western Europe; and a hormonal association, as evidenced by increased incidence with menopause, nulliparity, and breast cancer and decreased incidence with oral contraceptive use.

Risk factors include a family history of ovarian cancer; history of breast, bowel, or endometrial cancer; nulliparity; infertility; and a history of dysmenorrhea or heavy bleeding. Diets high in animal fat have recently been linked to ovarian cancer (DiSaia & Creaseman, 1984; Droegemueller et al., 1987).

Ovarian cancer ranks second to endometrial cancer in incidence, with an estimated 20,000 new cases in 1989. The death rate from ovarian cancer was estimated to be 12,000 in 1989 (ACS, 1989). The incidence increases in women older than 40 and peaks at 50 to 55 years. Ovarian cancer is more frequently seen in Caucasian women than in Black women. (Droegemueller et al., 1987).

There is no effective means of prevention, other than removal of healthy ovaries. This is not a practical option when less than 2% of women get ovarian cancer. Women can be informed about risk factors and can be encouraged to have yearly physical examinations, particularly after the age of 40 years.

COLLABORATIVE MANAGEMENT

Women may complain of abdominal pain or swelling or have vague symptoms of abdominal discomfort, such as dyspepsia, indigestion, gas and distention, or other mild GI disturbances. The woman may have a history of ovarian imbalance, such as evidenced by premenstrual tension, heavy menstrual flow, or dysfunctional bleeding.

The only sign may be an abdominal mass, and this may be noticed only after it reaches a size of 15 cm (6 in). Most pelvic examinations do not identify abnormalities; however, an enlarged ovary found postmenopausally should be evaluated as if it were malignant.

The woman who is diagnosed with ovarian cancer has concerns similar to those described for women with endometrial cancer (see earlier). Because the malignancy is usually diagnosed in an advanced stage, fears of death and dying are frequently present and may be more of a concern than the proposed treatments.

Cytologic examination has limited application, as a Pap smear is abnormal in only 20% to 30% of women, even in advanced cases. Diagnosis is dependent on surgical exploration. Usually a complete laboratory work-up is done before exploratory surgery, including a complete blood count, urinalysis, and liver studies if ascites occurs.

The level of ovarian antibody designated as CA 125 may be elevated if ovarian cancer is present. This test may be useful to monitor a woman's progress after treatment but may not be as useful for diagnostic purposes (Droegemueller et al., 1987).

Ultrasonography, IVP, CT, and radiography are used in detecting ovarian tumors (see earlier discussion of endometrial cancer). In addition, a barium enema and an upper GI radiographic series can be performed to rule out tumor in the adjacent structures. Magnetic resonance imaging (imaging of the physiologic and pathologic states of the human body, including tumor) is being studied as a method to measure and evaluate tumors. This technique shows promise for early diagnosis of ovarian cancer, as it identifies soft-tissue lesions inaccessible to other imaging techniques (Droegemueller et al., 1987).

Exploratory laparotomy is performed to diagnose and stage ovarian tumors. Ovarian cancer is the only neoplasm that is staged when it is removed (see the accompanying Key Features of Disease).

Nursing care of the woman who is diagnosed with ovarian cancer is similar to that of the woman with endometrial or cervical cancer (see earlier). The options for treatment include chemotherapy, intraperitoneal therapy, immunotherapy, radiation therapy, and surgery, depending on the extent of the cancer.

Chemotherapeutic agents are usually used postoperatively for all stages of ovarian cancer, although their purpose is usually palliative for stage IV tumors. Alkylating agents (melphalan, cyclophosphamide, and chlorambucil) have been used as single agents for treating ovarian cancer; however, they have been shown to increase the woman's chance of getting leukemia within 8 years of treatment (Droegemueller et al., 1987). Combinations of agents seem to obtain higher response rates, especially if cisplatin is one of the drugs used.

Chemotherapy is usually administered every 3 to 4 weeks for 1 week and can be administered on an inpatient or an outpatient basis (see Chap. 25).

Intraperitoneal therapy is the instillation of chemotherapeutic agents into the abdominal cavity. It is believed that the cytoxic effects of the drugs on the tumor are increased (Droegemueller et al., 1987). Radioactive colloids have also been injected into the abdomen to increase survival rates. A primary beta-emitter, ^{32}P, is injected through a catheter placed during surgery. After instillation, the woman is asked to turn frequently for 1½ to 2 hours to facilitate the distribution of the radioactive colloids throughout the peritoneal cavity (e.g., turning to the right, to the left, head down, feet down, prone, and supine).

Immunotherapy, also used to treat ovarian cancer, alters the immunologic response of the ovary and promotes tumor resistance.

External radiation therapy (see Chap. 25) is also used postoperatively if tumors have invaded other organs. It may be given with chemotherapy or alone.

A total abdominal hysterectomy and bilateral salpingo-oophorectomy is the surgical procedure for all stages of ovarian cancer. In stage III and IV cancer, the goal is to remove as much tumor as possible, because it

---

KEY FEATURES OF DISEASE ■ FIGO Staging Classification of Ovarian Cancer

I   Growth limited to the ovaries.
  Ia Growth limited to one ovary, no ascites. No tumor on the external surface; capsule intact.
  Ib Growth limited to both ovaries; no ascities. No tumor on the external surfaces; capsules intact.
  Ic Tumor either stage Ia or Ib, but with tumor on surface of one or both ovaries, or with capsule ruptured, or with ascites present containing malignant cells, or with positive peritoneal washings.

II   Growth involving one or both ovaries with pelvic extension.
  IIa Extension and/or metastases to the uterus and/or tubes.
  IIb Extension to other pelvic tissues.
  IIc Tumor either stage IIa or IIb, but with tumor on surface of one or both ovaries, or with capsule(s) ruptured, or with ascites present containing malignant cells or with positive peritoneal washings.

III Tumor involving one or both ovaries with peritoneal implants outside the pelvis and/or positive retroperitoneal or inguinal nodes. Superficial liver metastasis equals stage III. Tumor is limited to the true pelvis but with histologically proven malignant extension to small bowel or omentum.
  IIIa Tumor grossly limited to the true pelvis with negative nodes but with histologically confirmed microscopic seeding of abdominal peritoneal surfaces.
  IIIb Tumor of one or both ovaries with histologically confirmed implants of abdominal peritoneal surfaces none exceeding 2 cm in diameter. Nodes are negative.
  IIIc Abdominal implants greater than 2 cm in diameter and/or positive retroperitoneal inguinal nodes.

IV   Growth involving one or both ovaries with distant metastases. If pleural effusion is present, there must be positive cytologic findings to allot a case to stage IV. Parenchymal liver metastasis equals stage IV.

---

has spread to adjacent organs. Nursing care of the woman is similar to care of the woman having hysterectomy for uterine leiomyomas (see earlier).

A second-look procedure (laparoscopy or laparotomy) is performed, usually after 1 year of chemotherapy, to confirm the absence or presence of tumor or to remove residual tumor if it was too large to be removed at the time of the first operation (Barber, 1984). Nursing care is similar to care required after any major abdominal surgery.

The woman who is faced with the diagnosis of advanced ovarian cancer may be concerned about dying. She needs to be encouraged to ventilate her feelings regarding her diagnosis. Realistic assurance can be provided, as well as accurate information about treatments. Often, providing the woman with information about ovarian cancer and its treatment decreases her fears. Providing continuity of care, with at least one regular caregiver, may be helpful. The woman should be encouraged to use her support system, including family, friends, and spiritual leader (e.g., rabbi or clergyperson). A visit from another woman who has survived a similar disease may decrease fears.

If there is recurrence, the woman may deny symptoms at first or express feelings of anger and grief. The family is often fearful of the outcome. The nurse needs to provide encouragement and support during this difficult time and help the family and the woman work through their grief and prepare for death.

VULVAR CANCER

OVERVIEW

Vulvar cancer represents only 4% of all gynecologic malignancies, even though it ranks fourth in occurrence. Vulvar cancer is slow growing, stays localized for a long time, and metastasizes late.

Ninety per cent of vulvar cancers are squamous cell carcinomas. The other 10% consist of adenocarcinomas, sarcomas, and Paget's disease. Most vulvar cancers develop in the absence of premalignant changes in the epithelium, but occasionally they develop and spread similarly to cancer of the cervix. The first change is usually vulvar atypia or mild dysplasia (vulvar intraepithelial neoplasia [VIN] I), followed by moderate dysplasia (VIN II) and severe dysplasia or carcinoma in situ (VIN III) until the lesion becomes invasive. Vulvar cancer can spread directly to the urethra, the vagina, or the anus and through the lymphatic system to the inguinal, femoral, and deep iliac pelvic nodes (Fig. 54–14).

The cause of vulvar cancer is unknown. There is no proven relationship to sexually transmitted diseases, although a history of condylomata acuminata (venereal warts) may be present. Obesity, hypertension, diabetes, and granulomatous disease of the vulva have been suggested as possible causes, but no scientific data support these suggestions. Vulvar cancer occurs frequently in women who have had cancer of the cervix or the vagina (Droegemueller et al., 1987).

More than 50% of the cases of vulvar cancer occur in women older than 60 years. It seldom occurs before age 40 years, although studies have found premalignant changes in women in their 20s and 30s. This increase may be linked to the increase in sexually transmitted infections (Droegemueller et al., 1987). Vulvar cancer is more prevalent in women of lower socioeconomic status (DiSaia & Creaseman, 1984).

The prognosis for vulvar cancer is related to the stage of the cancer and whether cancer is present in the lymph nodes.

COLLABORATIVE MANAGEMENT

Women with vulvar lesions are likely to complain of irritation or itching in their perineal area. Sometimes they describe a "sore that will not heal." Bleeding is a late symptom. Women usually try to treat themselves before seeking medical help, and often a lesion has been present for months. Embarrassment has been suggested as the reason older women delay seeking medical attention.

Pelvic examinations usually reveal multifocal lesions, the majority developing on the labia. The lesions may be whitish or reddish, and the vulvar skin may be excoriated owing to irritation.

The woman may be anxious or fearful about the diagnosis of cancer. She may have fears that her partner will reject her because of the diagnosis, or she may have fears about disfigurement related to surgery. The nurse needs to assess the woman's past experiences in coping with stressful situations and whether she has the psychologic resources to cope with the present crisis.

A Pap smear and colposcopic examination of the vulva (see earlier discussion of cancer of the cervix) may aid in diagnosis. A toluidine test may be used to identify abnormal cells for biopsy. A 1% aqueous solution of toluidine blue is applied to the vulva and allowed to dry. Then a 1% acetic acid solution is applied. Biopsy of the areas that remain blue is performed. The test chemical stains nuclei in the superficial epithelium, where cells do not normally contain nuclei; an abnormal finding does not necessarily indicate malignancy, because ulcerations also stain.

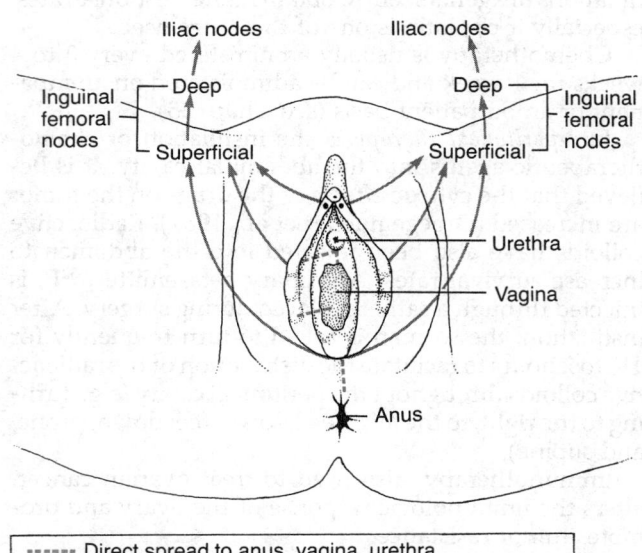

----- Direct spread to anus, vagina, urethra
—— Lymphatic spread to femoral, inguinal, iliac nodes

Figure 54–14

Spread of vulvar cancer. (Reproduced by permission from Droegemueller, W., Herbst, A. L., Mishell, D. R., Jr., & Stenchever, M. A., *Comprehensive gynecology*, St. Louis, 1987, The C. V. Mosby Co.)

A biopsy of the lesion is necessary for diagnosis. This is easily accomplished with a Keyes dermal punch (a device that removes a disk of tissue). Depending on the site of the lesion, one or more biopsies may be done.

Nursing care of the client with vulvar cancer is similar to that of one who has endometrial cancer; only the interventions that differ are discussed. Management of vulvar cancer depends on the extent of the spread and may include laser therapy, chemotherapy, radiation therapy, and surgery.

If a woman has premalignant vulvar lesions, laser therapy may be used (see earlier discussion of cervical cancer). The treatment is usually done on an outpatient basis; local, regional, or general anesthesia is used. Healing occurs over several weeks, and usually the lesions are removed without scarring.

Chemotherapy in the form of a topical application of 5-fluorouracil has been used to treat carcinoma in situ successfully. However, the treatment causes severe vulvar edema and pain and is not often used.

External radiation therapy (see earlier discussion of endometrial cancer and Chap. 25) may be used postoperatively to the deep pelvic nodes. Radiation treatments cause ulceration and dermatitis that can be uncomfortable for the woman.

Several surgical procedures are effective for the treatment of vulvar cancer. A local wide excision may be used to remove the abnormal area (for CIS). A simple vulvectomy (removal of vulva, the labia majora, the labia minora, and possibly the clitoris) may also be performed for CIS, but this disfiguring surgery is used less frequently today. Instead, a *skinning vulvectomy*—the removal of superficial vulvar skin (without removal of the clitoris), and replacement of removed skin with split-thickness grafts—is performed (Fig. 54–15). Sexual function is less affected, and the appearance of the vulva is less changed.

For invasive cancer, the surgery most often recommended is the *modified radical* or *radical vulvectomy* (see Fig. 54–15) (removal of the entire vulva—skin, labia, clitoris, subcutaneous tissues, and possibly inguinal and femoral node dissection), depending on node involvement.

The woman needs a complete explanation of the extent of the surgical procedure to be performed and information about preoperative and postoperative procedures (see Chaps. 18 and 20). Specific preoperative procedures for vulvectomy may include abdominal or perineal shave, enema, douche, and insertion of an indwelling catheter into the bladder.

Postoperatively, the woman can expect suction drains (Hemovacs) in the inguinal or vulvar areas for wound drainage for 7 to 10 days. An air mattress or eggcrate mattress may be placed on the bed to prevent pressure sores and increase comfort. A bed cradle can be used to keep linens off the incision site. The client usually wears antiembolism stockings to prevent thromboembolism and leg edema. Nursing care is focused on wound healing. Dressings over the incision are usually changed frequently because of the amount of wound

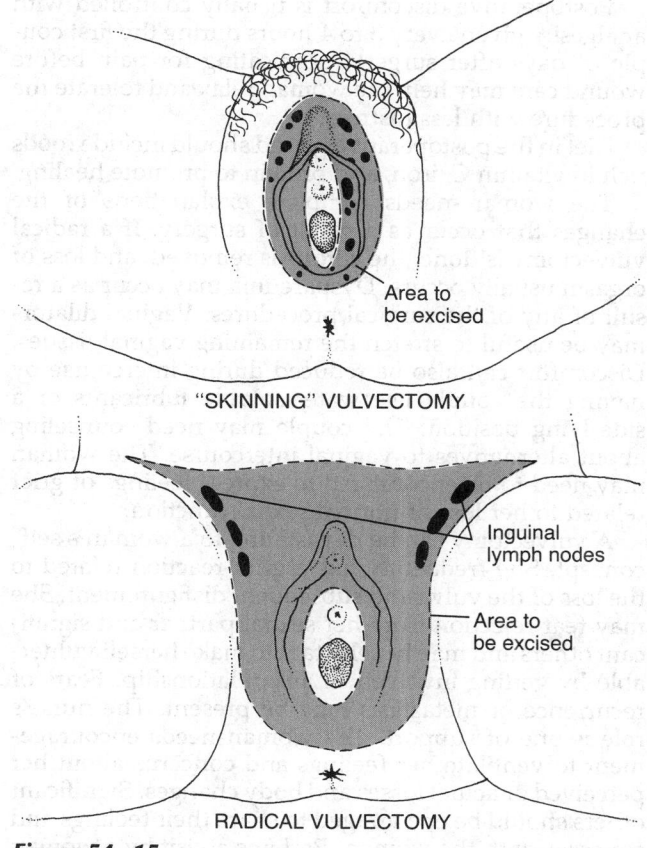

Figure 54–15
Vulvectomy.

drainage and the risk of infection. Wound complications, such as infection or dehiscence, frequently occur after vulvectomies; subsequently, the healing process may take up to 6 months. Meticulous wound care is necessary and usually involves débridement. A solution of half-strength hydrogen peroxide is used to clean the wound, followed by cleaning with normal saline. These solutions may be applied with an Asepto bulb syringe or a waterpick (on low speed). The wound is then dried with a heat lamp or air dried with a hair dryer (using cool air). Wound care is usually done three or four times a day.

The Foley catheter remains in the bladder for 7 to 10 days to prevent ureteral stenosis and incontinence. After the catheter is removed, the urine stream may be deflected down the leg owing to edema or even be uncontrolled. Having the woman stand while voiding may decrease the incidence of these annoying problems. Stool softeners can be given to prevent straining and decrease discomfort related to bowel movements. Perineal care or sitz baths may be done after voidings or bowel movements to prevent contamination of the incision site.

Postoperative discomfort is usually controlled with analgesics given every 3 to 4 hours during the first couple of days after surgery. Medicating for pain before wound care may help the woman relax and tolerate the procedure with less distress.

Diet in the postoperative period should include foods rich in vitamin C, iron, and protein to promote healing.

The woman needs complete explanations of the changes that occur as a result of surgery. If a radical vulvectomy is done, the clitoris is removed, and loss of orgasm usually occurs. Dyspareunia may occur as a result of any of the surgical procedures. Vaginal dilators may be useful to stretch the remaining vaginal tissues. Discomfort can also be reduced during intercourse by having the couple use water-soluble lubricants or a side-lying position. The couple may need counseling about alternatives to vaginal intercourse. The woman may need to be encouraged to express feelings of grief related to her loss of normal sexual function.

A vulvectomy can be devastating to a woman's self-concept. She frequently has a grief reaction related to the loss of the vulva and subsequent disfigurement. She may fear rejection from her sexual partner and significant others and may be reluctant to make herself vulnerable by getting involved in any relationship. Fears of recurrence or metastasis may be present. The nurse's role is one of support. The woman needs encouragement to ventilate her feelings and concerns about her perceived or actual losses and body changes. Significant others should be encouraged to share their feelings and concerns with the woman. Perhaps a visit by a woman who has successfully recovered from similar surgery would be beneficial.

VAGINAL CANCER

OVERVIEW

Primary invasive *vaginal cancer* is rare, accounting for less than 2% of all gynecologic cancers. Usually, vaginal cancer is an extension of cervical, endometrial, or vulvar cancers. Most vaginal cancers are squamous cell carcinomas that develop in the upper one-third of the vagina. They most frequently occur in women older than 50 years, with 90% of the cases found postmenopausally. Adenocarcinoma of the vagina is found in females between the ages of 14 and 30 years and is associated with intrauterine exposure to DES as a result of maternal ingestion during pregnancy.

The cause of vaginal cancer is unknown. Predisposing factors that have been associated with the development of vaginal cancer include repeated pregnancies, sexually transmitted disease (especially syphilis and herpesvirus type 2 and papillomavirus infections), and prior radiation (Droegemueller et al., 1987).

The spread of vaginal cancer depends on the location of the tumor. Upper vaginal lesions spread in the same manner as cervical cancer, whereas lower lesions spread similarly to vulvar cancer. Because of the rich lymphatic drainage in the vaginal area, metastasis can occur early.

COLLABORATIVE MANAGEMENT

Premalignant lesions (vaginal intraepithelial neoplasia) are usually asymptomatic. An abnormal Pap smear is the most common presenting problem. Uncommon or late symptoms include pain, foul-smelling vaginal discharge, painless vaginal bleeding, pruritus, or urinary symptoms attributable to the pressure of the lesion on the bladder.

A pelvic examination may reveal a lesion. Premalignant changes are diagnosed through colposcopic examination and biopsy (see earlier discussion of cervical cancer).

Both nonsurgical and surgical interventions may be used to treat women with vaginal cancer. Noninvasive malignancy and early-stage vaginal cancers may be treated nonsurgically with a variety of techniques. Laser therapy (see earlier discussion of cervical cancer) may be used. The abnormal tissues are stained with an iodine solution to identify the areas for treatment. A vaginal discharge may be present several days after treatment, and healing normally takes a few weeks. Close follow-up is necessary: a Pap smear and colposcopic examination every 4 months for 1 year, then every 6 to 12 months.

Local application of 5-fluorouracil cream to the vagina daily for 1 week is another treatment. This chemotherapeutic agent is irritating to the skin, and often zinc oxide ointment is recommended for application to the vulvar area. The treatment is repeated in 3 to 4 weeks, and follow-up is the same as that for laser therapy.

Radiation therapy can be used for all stages of vaginal cancer. IRT (see earlier discussion of endometrial cancer) is usually used alone for treatment of cancer limited to the vaginal wall, and external radiation therapy is combined with IRT for treatment of cancer that extends beyond the vaginal wall. Complications of radiation therapy include vaginal stenosis and adhesions and vaginal discharge. Women need to use vaginal dilators after treatment, and assessment for sexual dysfunction is suggested (see earlier discussion of vulvar cancer).

Chemotherapy may be used for recurrent disease, although there is no effective therapy.

A local wide excision may be performed for localized lesions. A partial or total vaginectomy (removal of part or all of the vagina) may be done for invasive disease. Vaginectomy affects sexual function. Without reconstruction surgery, vaginal intercourse is impossible. The woman and her sexual partner need counseling about alternative activities for achieving sexual satisfaction. A radical hysterectomy or pelvic exenteration (see earlier) may also be performed, depending on the extent of the cancer.

Preventive measures for vaginal cancer are to avoid prescription of DES during pregnancy and to continue to have Pap screening and pelvic examinations after menopause on a regular basis.

FALLOPIAN TUBE CANCER

OVERVIEW

Fallopian tube cancer is the rarest of gynecologic cancers, with an incidence of less than 1%. It occurs in women older than age 50 years, with 80% to 90% of the cancers resulting from metastasis from ovarian and endometrial cancers.

The cause of squamous cell fallopian tube cancer is unknown. It has been suggested that PID and chronic salpingitis may be associated with adenocarcinomas of the fallopian tubes (Droegemueller et al., 1987). Nulliparity and infertility have also been cited as risk factors.

The initial lesion is confined to the lumen of the tube. From there it invades the serosa and spreads intraperitoneally to the bowel, the omentum, and the peritoneum. Lymphatic spread is to the para-aortic and retroperitoneal lymph nodes.

COLLABORATIVE MANAGEMENT

Women are usually asymptomatic until the tumor is in a late stage. In 50% of the cases, bleeding is present. Other symptoms include clear vaginal discharge, lower abdominal pain or distention, and feelings of pressure. A history of abnormal bleeding, adnexal pain, and watery vaginal discharge in a postmenopausal woman may suggest fallopian tube cancer, and further evaluation is needed.

Diagnosis is rare preoperatively. A Pap smear has reportedly been abnormal in only 10% of cases. A mass may be felt on examination in about 60% of cases in late stages. Abdominal x-rays, ultrasound, or CT scan may be used to confirm a mass.

Chemotherapy may be used postoperatively in later stages or for recurrence. The lesions have responded to alkylating agents (see Chap. 25). External radiation therapy has also been used postoperatively for late-stage tumors. The usual treatment for cancer limited to the fallopian tube is a total abdominal hysterectomy and bilateral salpingo-oophorectomy with omentectomy (removal of the connective tissues covering these organs). Care of the woman with fallopian tube cancer is similar to that described for cancer of the ovary.

PROBLEMS RELATED TO PREGNANCY

GESTATIONAL TROPHOBLASTIC DISEASE

OVERVIEW

Gestational trophoblastic disease (GTD) includes benign and malignant tumors that develop from the trophoblast of the human pregnancy. They are neoplasms of placental origin that produce hCG, which can be measured to predict the status of GTD.

Hydatidiform mole is a benign degenerative process of the placenta in which the chorionic villi degenerate into edematous, cystic vesicles. They can be partial (incomplete) or complete (classic). A *partial mole* is a rare molar pregnancy characterized by the presence of embryonic tissue or membranes, some swollen chorionic villi, and trophoblastic hyperplasia. A *complete mole* has no embryonic tissues present, and all chorionic villi are swollen. A complete mole may develop after fertilization of an "empty" egg, as studies have shown that only paternal chromosomes are present (Droegemueller et al., 1987).

Choriocarcinoma is at the other end of the GTD spectrum and is the most malignant of the GTDs. Choriocarcinoma can develop after a molar pregnancy, spontaneous abortion, or normal pregnancy. Choriocarcinoma proliferates profusely and has widespread metastases to organs such the vagina, the vulva, the lungs, the brain, the liver, and the kidneys.

The etiology of GTD is unknown, but there is a higher incidence reported in women of lower socioeconomic status (possibly related to dietary factors). The incidence in the United States is low (1 per 1500 to 2000 women), whereas the incidence is much higher in Asian women (1 per 100 to 125 women) (Gilbert & Harmon, 1986; Porter, 1985). Increased incidence of hydatidiform mole has been reported in women older than 40 and in women who have had a previous molar pregnancy (3% to 5%) (Droegemueller et al., 1987).

COLLABORATIVE MANAGEMENT

Vaginal bleeding, often brownish, 6 to 8 weeks after a missed period is present in 90% of the cases of hydatidiform mole. Uterine size is usually greater than it should be for the date of gestation in about 50% of cases. Other symptoms include pregnancy-induced hypertension before 24 weeks' gestation, hyperemesis gravidarum, passage of grape-like cysts, lack of fetal heart tone, absence of fetal movement or inability to palpate fetal parts, and hyperthyroidism (rare).

Diagnosis is usually by ultrasound—a snowstorm pattern is usually present—and serial hCG titers—levels of hCG are greater than 100,000 mU/mL, which is the normal level at 10 to 14 weeks' gestation.

A suction curettage may be performed to remove the hydatidiform mole from the uterus. Oxytocin may be administered to keep the uterus contracted and prevent hemorrhage. The woman is given oral contraceptives (or diaphragm use) to defer pregnancy for at least 1 year. Serial hCG titers are monitored weekly until they are normal for two values, then monthly for 1 year. The woman should also have a chest x-ray during the diagnostic phase and have it repeated if it was abnormal or if hCG titers stop falling or start to rise. Pelvic examinations should be performed every 2 weeks until findings are normal, then every 3 months.

Assessment and diagnosis of choriocarcinoma are usually accomplished by determining hCG titers after a hydatidiform mole has been removed. A plateau or rise in titer should be evaluated further. Chest x-rays, electrocardiograms, CT scans of the brain, and ultrasound can be used to rule out metastases to other parts of the body. After GTD is diagnosed as choriocarcinoma, staging is done to determine the extent of the disease and whether metastasis is present. The most common site for metastasis is the lung. A prognostic classification of GTD is presented in the accompanying Key Features of Disease.

Methotrexate and dactinomycin (actinomycin D) are effective in the treatment of choriocarcinoma. Treatments are usually given intravenously daily for 5 days every 2 weeks, and women are usually hospitalized for these treatments. Treatment continues until a negative

---

KEY FEATURES OF DISEASE ■ Classification for Prognosis of Metastatic Gestational Trophoblastic Disease

Good Prognosis

No prior chemotherapy

Serum hCG level <40,000 mU/mL

Symptoms present for <4 mo

No metastasis to liver or brain

Poor Prognosis

Prior chemotherapy

Serum hCG level >40,000 mU/mL

Symptoms present for >4 mo

Presence of liver or brain metastases

Data from Droegemueller, W., Herbst, A. L., Mishell, D. R., Jr., & Stenchever, M. A. (1987). *Comprehensive gynecology*. St. Louis: C. V. Mosby.

---

hCG titer is obtained, then one additional course of therapy is given. Follow-up usually includes weekly serum hCG titers until three negative titers are obtained, followed by monthly titers for 1 year. Women with nonmetastatic disease may be completely cured.

Women who have metastatic disease are treated with multiagent chemotherapy. A hysterectomy may also be performed. Radiation may be given for liver or brain metastasis. Follow-up is similar to that for nonmetastatic disease, except that chest x-rays are repeated more frequently (every 3 months) during the first year.

Emotional support is important for the woman who has GTD. Even if the woman is cured, it takes more than a year for her life to get back to normal. She may need to ventilate her feelings and concerns about her prognosis, loss of pregnancy, or fertility. She and her family need support as they address their grief. The nurse may need to refer the woman and her family to support groups or for counseling for problems that may affect their relationships.

ABORTION

SPONTANEOUS ABORTION

Spontaneous abortion is the termination of pregnancy from natural causes before viability of the fetus. Viability has various definitions, but it is usually reached by 24 weeks' gestation and a fetal weight of 600g or more (Bobak & Jensen, 1987).

Abortions or miscarriages usually occur before 16 weeks of gestation, with the majority occurring before the eighth week of pregnancy. More than half of the spontaneous abortions are caused by defects in fetoplacental development (Bobak & Jensen, 1987).

Nursing assessments are related to the specific type of spontaneous abortion experienced by the woman (see the Key Features of Disease on pp. 1733 and 1734).

For *threatened* abortion, management usually consists of bed rest followed by restriction of activities. Women should avoid stress and orgasms. Approximately 50% of women who have symptoms of threatened abortion eventually lose the pregnancy (Bobak & Jensen, 1987).

In the case of *inevitable* abortion, the woman may also complain of low back pain. The products of conception pass. If the fetus and placenta are expelled, the loss becomes a *complete* abortion. The cervix then closes, and the bleeding becomes minimal. If there is no infection or hemorrhage, there is usually no further intervention after a pelvic examination has been performed. On the other hand, if some of the products of conception are retained (an *incomplete* abortion), a D & C or vacuum aspiration is usually performed to remove the remaining tissue.

A *missed* abortion is one in which the fetus dies and is retained in utero for a period of time. Usually, a missed abortion terminates spontaneously, but if this has not

KEY FEATURES OF DISEASE ■ Characteristics of Spontaneous Abortion

Type	Status of Cervical Os	Bleeding	Status of Fetus	Status of Placenta	Cramping
Threatened	Closed	Minimal	Retained	Retained	Mild
Inevitable	Dilated	Moderate or heavy	Not yet passed	Not yet passed	Moderate
Incomplete	Dilated	Heavy	Passed	Retained	Severe

Continued

KEY FEATURES OF DISEASE ■ Characteristics of Spontaneous Abortion *Continued*

Type	Status of Cervical Os	Bleeding	Status of Fetus	Status of Placenta	Cramping
Complete	Partially dilated	Minimal	Passed	Passed	Mild
Missed	Closed	None or slight	Retained	Retained	None

occurred in 4 weeks, pregnancy should be terminated by a method appropriate for the length of gestation. If fetal parts are retained longer than 5 weeks after the end of the first trimester, disseminated intravascular coagulation and uncontrolled hemorrhage can occur.

Nursing management after spontaneous abortion includes physiologic and psychosocial interventions. The nursing priorities are to prevent hemorrhage and infection; assess uterine involution; and administer medications as ordered, including oxytocics, analgesics, antibiotics, and Rh$_o$ (D) immune globulin (RhoGAM) if the woman is Rh negative and previously unsensitized.

Women need to be informed that they have an increased chance of having a subsequent abortion if they become pregnant. The risks of subsequent abortions range from 24% to 50% (Gilbert & Harmon, 1986).

Preventive measures that should be discussed include encouragement to abstain from alcohol consumption and smoking during pregnancy; to avoid taking any medications, especially known teratogenic drugs; and to avoid exposure to x-rays. Measures that decrease the chances of contracting an infection — eating a well-balanced diet, avoiding fatigue, and avoiding crowds or people who have infections — should also be discussed.

Spontaneous abortion is often a crisis for the woman and her family and/or significant others. They may need help in managing their grief from the loss of the fetus. A woman may need counseling about the etiology of abortions, especially if she expresses guilt feelings about causing the loss.

INDUCED ABORTION

Induced abortion is the purposeful termination of pregnancy. Reasons for the interruption of pregnancy include the preservation of the life or health of the mother; avoidance of the birth of a child with a severe developmental or hereditary disorder; and voluntary abortion performed after rape or because of the mother's mental incompetence, inability of the mother to care for or support the child, and failure to use or failed contraception, resulting in an unwanted pregnancy.

Procedures to terminate pregnancy include vacuum aspiration, dilation and evacuation, D & C, and intra-amniotic and extra-amniotic instillations (prostaglandins [PGs], hypertonic saline, and urea). First-trimester abortions by vacuum aspiration or suction curettage are usually performed as outpatient procedures in clinics or physician's offices.

Before the procedure, certain assessments should be made: Are there physical or psychosocial risks in continuing the pregnancy? Has the woman explored alternatives to abortion? What does the woman know about the abortion procedure? Can she make an informed decision to have the procedure? What are the father's feelings about the pregnancy and the decision to terminate it? Does the woman have an adequate support system? Are any medical conditions present? Was any method of birth control used?

Preabortion procedures include a pregnancy test, accurate assessment of uterine size and gestational age, and laboratory tests, including hematocrit and hemoglobin determinations, Rh-negative antigen screening, serologic testing, and blood typing. The woman should be given an explanation of the specific procedure to be done and what she may expect to experience during the procedure.

If the procedure is an early abortion, the woman usually receives paracervical block anesthesia before the cervix is dilated. The contents of the uterus are then either aspirated or scraped out (vacuum aspiration or suction curettage). Nursing care after the procedure includes checking the woman's vital signs until they are stable and assessing bleeding and cramping. If bleeding is heavy, an oxytocic drug can be administered. The woman is usually ready to leave the office or clinic within 2 to 4 hours after the procedure. The woman should have someone take her home, rather than driving herself.

The most common second-trimester abortion procedure is the administration of PGs, either $PGF_{2\alpha}$ intra-amniotic injection or PGE_2 vaginal suppository. Both procedures are performed in an inpatient setting. PGs stimulate uterine contractions, causing labor and delivery of the uterine contents about 16 hours after administration. Often, placental passage is incomplete, and a D & C may be performed to remove the retained tissue. Common side effects of prostaglandins are nausea, vomiting, diarrhea, and transient elevated temperature. Expulsion of a fetus with signs of life can occur (Schneider, 1984).

The other second-trimester abortion procedure is the transabdominal intrauterine injection of hypertonic saline. Amniocentesis is performed, and 200 mL of amniotic fluid is removed and replaced with the saline solution. The fetus dies within an hour and is usually aborted within 24 hours.

Nursing care of a woman having a second-trimester abortion includes providing comfort measures and peri-

---

CLIENT/FAMILY EDUCATION ■ Discharge Instructions for the Client Who Has Undergone an Abortion

"Call your physician if any of the following occur:
1. Temperature above 100° F
2. Excessive, bright red bleeding with clots (more than on the heaviest day of your normal menstrual period)
3. Heavy bleeding lasting more than 2 wk.
4. Foul-smelling vaginal discharge
5. Severe or prolonged abdominal pain or cramping
6. No menstrual period within 8 wk."

"Avoid douching, using tampons, and having sexual intercourse for 3 wk."

"Avoid strenuous activities for 2 wk."

"Decide on a birth control method before your next menstrual period."

"Return for a follow-up visit in 2 wk."

---

neal hygiene; administering medications for nausea, diarrhea, or pain; and coaching the woman to use breathing and relaxation techniques during labor.

Postabortion nursing care for women having either a first- or second-trimester abortion includes assessing the woman's level of comfort with her decision to abort. Rh_o (D) immune globulin should be given if the woman is Rh negative. The client is given discharge instructions (see the accompanying Client/Family Education feature). Referral to postabortion support groups may be necessary.

ECTOPIC PREGNANCY

OVERVIEW

An *ectopic pregnancy* is one in which the fertilized ovum is implanted outside the uterine cavity (Fig. 54–16). About 95% implant in the fallopian tubes.

Most ectopic pregnancies are caused by obstruction of the tubes or delayed passage of the fertilized ovum. Common causes of tubal obstruction are PID, chronic salpingitis, and other bacterial infections. The tubes become narrower, and often peristalsis is impaired, thus favoring tubal implantation. The embryo attaches to the wall of the tubes, and, as the embryo grows, the wall thickens. However, the tube cannot enlarge as the muscular uterus can, and it becomes distended; the risk of rupture increases. It is likely to occur approximately 6 to 8 weeks after implantation.

Risk factors for ectopic pregnancy include the use of an intrauterine device for contraception, PID, or previous tubal ligation. Women who are older than 35 years

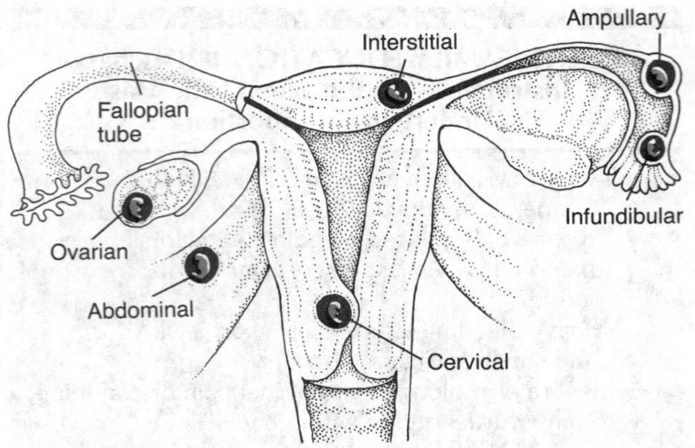

Figure 54-16

Common sites of ectopic implantation.

or who are non-Caucasian have an increased chance of having an ectopic pregnancy. Women who have had one ectopic pregnancy have about a 5% to 10% chance of having a subsequent one.

COLLABORATIVE MANAGEMENT

Ectopic pregnancies are frequently misdiagnosed because numerous vague symptoms can occur. Often, the presenting symptom is pain early in pregnancy. This pain can be localized or general; if it is a sharp pain, rupture should be suspected. Vaginal bleeding, if present, is usually dark brown or red. Three-fourths of the women report missing a menstrual period. If internal bleeding is present and has extended to the level of the diaphragm, the woman may experience shoulder pain. Cullen's sign (a blue discoloration of the skin around the umbilicus) is a late sign of intraperitoneal hemorrhage.

A pelvic examination may detect a local mass or adnexal tenderness. A serum or urine pregnancy test to measure the beta-subunit of hCG can be performed to help confirm the diagnosis.

Ultrasound may be used to identify a gestational sac in the uterus and thus to rule out ectopic pregnancy. Culdocentesis can also be used to diagnose ectopic pregnancy. A needle is inserted in the posterior vagina into the cul-de-sac, and fluid is aspirated from the peritoneal cavity. A ruptured ectopic pregnancy may be indicated if nonclotting blood is aspirated. A laparoscopy can be done if all other diagnostic tests are inconclusive. Visualization of the tubes can confirm an ectopic pregnancy.

For a ruptured ectopic pregnancy, control of hemorrhage is the management priority. The nurse needs to monitor vital signs and observe for shock or hemorrhage while preparing the woman for surgery. The type of surgery depends on the amount of tubal damage and the site of the ectopic pregnancy. If the ectopic pregnancy

has ruptured, a laparotomy is usually performed to control the hemorrhage and remove the ectopic pregnancy. If the damage is severe, a salpingectomy (surgical removal of the tube) is performed. However, current, more conservative management for a less severely damaged ruptured tube and for an unruptured ectopic pregnancy is a laparotomy and small incision into the tubes at the site of implantation with removal of the trophoblastic tissue. Postoperative care is similar to that of any client having tubal surgery (see earlier). Steroids are usually given to decrease inflammation and reduce incidence of adhesions (Osguthorpe, 1986). If adhesions develop or there is scar tissue, reconstructive surgery may be an option (see later).

Emotional support for the woman and her partner is also a nursing priority. These couples may have feared for the life of the woman, and they may be experiencing feelings of guilt or blame or other symptoms of grief. The nurse listens to their concerns about future pregnancies and possibly diminished fertility and encourages the couple to share their feelings.

STERILIZATION

OVERVIEW

Tubal ligation is a surgical procedure in which a female is sterilized by occluding the fallopian tubes to prevent the passage of the ovum.

A woman needs to be fully informed about sterilization before she gives consent for the procedure. The Department of Health and Human Services has set up the following guidelines for federally funded sterilizations to ensure that a woman understands the procedure (U.S. Laws):

1. An explanation of the risks, benefits, and alternatives to the procedure

2. A statement that describes sterilization as a permanent, irreversible method of birth control

3. A statement that a 30-day waiting period is required between giving consent and the sterilization

4. The consent forms in the woman's native language, or provision for interpretation

Although a husband's consent is not required in most states, many physicians request his consent (Lowdermilk, 1986).

COLLABORATIVE MANAGEMENT

Preoperatively, the nurse should assess the woman's reasons for sterilization, such as the desire for no more pregnancies. The woman should be asked to think about the irreversibility of the procedure and what she would

POMEROY'S TECHNIQUE

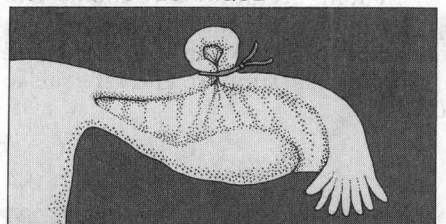
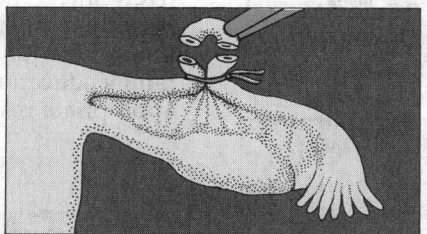
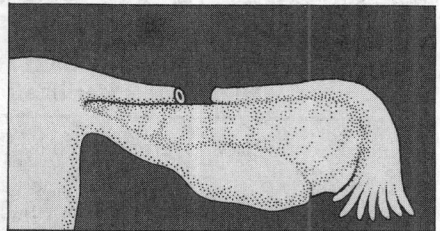

1. The tube is tied.

2. A section of the resulting loop is removed.

3. The sutures dissolve, and the ends of the tube pull apart.

FIMBRIECTOMY

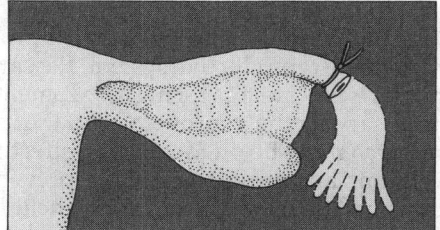

The fimbriated end is removed and the remaining end of the tube is ligated.

ELECTROCAUTERIZATION

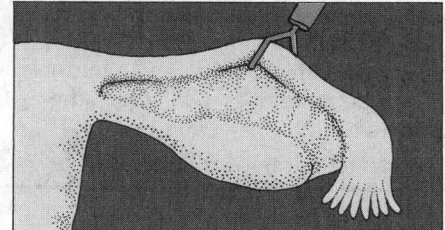

The tube is sealed by an electrocautery —a device that "melts" tissue.

RING TECHNIQUE

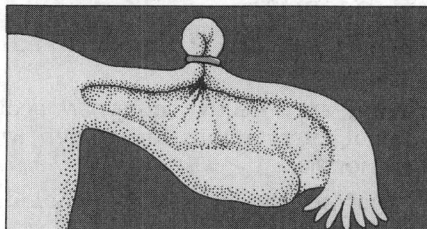

A ring is placed around a loop of the tube to occlude it.

CLIP TECHNIQUE

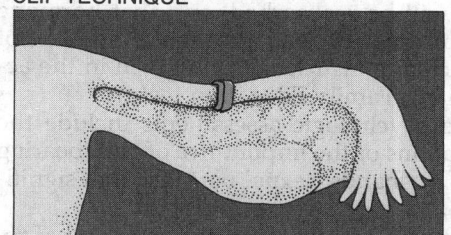

A clip is placed around the tube to occlude it.

Figure 54–17

Sites and methods of tubal occlusion.

do if she later got divorced, remarried, or lost a child now living.

Nursing care depends on the type of procedure performed and when it is performed. *Postpartum* sterilization is performed within 24 to 48 hours of a vaginal delivery or at the time of a cesarean delivery and is usually an inpatient procedure. *Interval* procedures are performed at least 6 weeks after a delivery and any time thereafter. Sterilization can also be performed after abortions.

Sterilization can be performed through several surgical approaches: laparotomy (subumbilical incision 5 to 7.5 cm [2 to 3 in] long), minilaparotomy (suprapubic incision 2 to 3 cm [¾ to 1⅛ in] long), laparoscopy (laparoscope inserted through a subumbilical incision with a second incision above the symphysis pubis), and colpotomy (incision in the posterior vagina).

After the tubes are visualized, they can be cut, tied, clipped, or cauterized. Figure 54–17 illustrates the various sites and methods of tubal occlusion. The most popular postpartum method is the Pomeroy technique, in which the tubes are tied and resected. Failure rates are

low (0.4%), and this method is reported to have higher potential for reversibility than other surgical methods (Saidi & Zaine, 1980). Fimbriectomy, or removal of the fimbriated end, is almost totally irreversible. Electrocautery is the most popular interval method. Although failure rates are low (0.1% to 2.0%), the potential for reversibility is also low owing to the destruction of the tubes. Procedures using rings or clips have a high potential for reversibility, but failure rates are also higher (2.9% to 11.2%) (Saidi & Zainie, 1980).

The woman needs to know that all these procedures can be performed on an outpatient basis and under local, regional, or general anesthesia. Preoperative preparation includes ensuring that the woman consumes nothing by mouth the night before surgery, administering preoperative medications, and performing skin preparation, which may include shaving of the pubic hair.

Postoperative recovery is usually swift. The woman can usually return to normal activities within 24 to 48 hours after surgery. Abdominal discomfort may be experienced, and mild analgesics may be administered.

CLIENT/FAMILY EDUCATION ■ Discharge Instructions for the Client Who Has Undergone Sterilization

"Keep the incision covered with a bandage for several days."

"You may take showers as you normally do."

"Do not use tampons if vaginal bleeding occurs."

"You can resume sexual intercourse after about a week or after any bleeding has stopped."

"If you have any abdominal pain that is not relieved by mild analgesics, such as acetaminophen (Tylenol), or if you have any abdominal tenderness, unusual bleeding, or a temperature over 99.6° F, call the clinic or your physician."

"Return to have your stitches removed in 5–7 d."

Deep breathing exercises should be done frequently during the first postoperative day. The woman should be taught that she will continue to menstruate and ovulate (the ovum will be reabsorbed) and that hormone production is not affected. Sexual responses should not be affected. Discharge instructions are given in the accompanying Client/Family Education feature.

Postoperative psychologic assessments include the woman's perceptions of the importance of childbearing and attitudes of husbands, sexual partners, and significant others.

There has been an increase in requests for tubal reconstruction for reversal of tubal ligations. For various reasons, women who have been sterilized surgically are desiring to attempt to get pregnant again. Tubal reanastomosis is a procedure that reconnects the tubes under magnification and with microsurgical techniques. Success rates depend on the condition of the tube, the length of the remaining segments of the tubes, and the location of the previous occlusion surgery. Pregnancy rates after reconstruction surgery reportedly range from 0 to 83%, but a rate less than 50% is most often reported (Saidi & Zainie, 1980). Microsurgical techniques have also been used for treatment of infertility when there is some type of tubal obstruction or adhesions.

SUMMARY

Gynecologic disorders occur throughout the life cycle. They can be related to the menstrual cycle, infections, trauma, benign and malignant conditions, and fertility. Problems of the reproductive system can interfere with a woman's life style and cause physical discomfort, psychologic distress, and even death. The nurse can effec-tively intervene by making accurate assessments and providing nursing care, which includes specific prevention advice or management interventions, client and family education, psychosocial support, and referrals to appropriate resources.

IMPLICATIONS FOR RESEARCH

Nursing research is needed for all problems related to the female reproductive system. Research conducted by nurses who are practicing in women's health care is necessary for the improvement of that care. The focus of research must be on identifying effective nursing interventions and ways to improve preventive health care practices. Suggestions for study include

1. What are the specific psychologic and physiologic impacts of PMS on women?

2. Is stress management the most effective coping strategy for PMS?

3. What is the effect of nutritional and other therapeutic modalities on PMS?

4. What are effective nonpharmacologic and nutritional interventions for women with primary dysmenorrhea?

5. What health care practices should be promoted to prevent vaginal infections?

6. Is long-term use of Kegel's exercises effective in preventing problems related to pelvic supports?

7. What nursing interventions are effective in decreasing psychologic complications of hysterectomy?

8. What are effective interventions for complications related to radiation, surgery, and chemotherapy for gynecologic cancers?

9. What are the long-term psychologic effects of pregnancy termination?

REFERENCES AND READINGS

Menstrual Cycle Disorders

Ball, K. A. (1988). Laser endometrial ablation treatment of dysfunctional uterine bleeding. *AORN Journal, 48,* 1153–1164.

Bernhard, L. A. (1982). Endometriosis. *Journal of Obstetric, Gynecologic, and Neonatal Nursing, 11,* 300–304.

Brown, M. A., & Zimmer, P. A. (1986). Personal and family impact of premenstrual symptoms. *Journal of Obstetric, Gynecologic, and Neonatal Nursing, 15,* 31–86.

Carpenito, L. J. (1989). *Nursing diagnosis: Application to clinical practice* (3rd ed.). Philadelphia: J. B. Lippincott.

Dalton, K. (1978). *Once a month.* London: Fontana.

Dawood, M. Y. (1983). Dysmenorrhea. *Clinical Obstetrics and Gynecology, 26,* 719–727.

Dewhurst, J. (1983). Postmenopausal bleeding from benign causes. *Clinical Obstetrics and Gynecology, 26,* 769–776.

Ellerhorst-Ryan, J. M., Turba, E. P., & Stahl, D. L. (1988). Evaluating benign breast disease. *Nurse Practitioner, 13*(9), 13, 16, 18.

Fogel, C. I. (1981a). The gynecological triad: Discharge, pain, and bleeding. In C. I. Fogel & N. F. Woods (Eds.), *Health care of women: A nursing perspective* (pp. 220–256). St. Louis: C. V. Mosby.

Fortier, K. J. (1986). Postmenopausal bleeding and the endometrium. *Clinical Obstetrics and Gynecology, 29,* 440–445.

Garner, C. H., & Webster, B. H. (1985). Endometriosis. *Journal of Obstetric, Gynecologic, and Neonatal Nursing, 14*(Suppl.), 10–20.

Graham, E. A. (1986). Menstruation and menopause. In J. Griffith-Kenney (Ed.), *Contemporary women's health* (pp. 435–448). Menlo Park, CA: Addison-Wesley.

Halban, J. (1924). Metastatic hysteroadenosis. *Weiner Klinische Wochenschrift, 37,* 1205.

Hansen, A. M., & Immordino, K. F. (1984). The diagnostic evaluation and therapy of secondary amenorrhea. *Journal of Obstetric, Gynecologic, and Neonatal Nursing, 13,* 180–184.

Hanson, F. (1986). Amenorrhea. In C. Havens, N. Sullivan, & P. Tilton (Eds.), *Manual of outpatient gynecology* (pp. 89–99). Boston: Little, Brown.

Martin, P. L. (1985). *Handbook of office gynecology.* Orlando, FL: Grune & Stratton.

Masterson, B. J. (1986). Perimenopausal bleeding. *American Family Physician, 33,* 233–240.

Meldrum, D. R. (1983). Perimenopausal menstrual problems. *Clinical Obstetrics and Gynecology, 26,* 762–768.

Murata, J. (1989). Primary amenorrhea. *Pediatric Nursing, 15,* 125–129.

Parisi, V., & Majewski, M. (1986). Abnormal uterine bleeding. In C. Havens, N. Sullivan, & P. Tilton (Eds.), *Manual of outpatient gynecology* (pp. 77–87). Boston: Little, Brown.

Reid, R. L., & Yen, S. S. (1983). The perimenopausal syndrome. *Clinical Obstetrics and Gynecology, 26,* 710–718.

Sampson, J. A. (1921). Perforating hemorrhagic (chocolate) cysts of the ovary. *Archives of Surgery, 3,* 245.

Schroeder, L., & Lesh, G. (1986). Premenstrual syndrome. In C. Havens, N. Sullivan, & P. Tilton (Eds.), *Manual of outpatient gynecology* (pp. 125–139). Boston: Little, Brown.

Sheppard, B. L. (1984). The pathology of dysfunctional uterine bleeding. *Clinics in Obstetrics and Gynecology, 11,* 227–236.

Sloane, E. (1985). *Biology of women* (2nd ed., pp. 83–110). New York: Wiley.

Spellacy, W. N. (1983). Abnormal bleeding. *Clinical Obstetrics and Gynecology, 26,* 702–709.

Swearingen, P. L. (1986). *Manual of nursing therapeutics* (pp. 431–447). Menlo Park, CA: Addison-Wesley.

Thorn, S. (1986). Endometriosis. In C. Havens, N. Sullivan, & P. Tilton (Eds.), *Manual of outpatient gynecology* (pp. 73–76). Boston: Little, Brown.

Tilton, P. (1986a). Dysmenorrhea. In C. Havens, N. Sullivan, & P. Tilton (Eds.), *Manual of outpatient gynecology* (pp. 109–116). Boston: Little, Brown.

Tulandi, T. (1986). Salpingo-ovariolysis: A comparison between laser surgery and electrocautery. *Fertility-Sterility, 45,* 489.

Wilson, M. A. (1984). Menstrual disorders: Premenstrual syndrome, dysmenorrhea, amenorrhea. *Journal of Obstetric, Gynecologic, and Neonatal Nursing, 13,* 11–19.

Inflammation and Infection

Colls, J. P. (1985). Toxic shock syndrome: In perspective. *NAACOG Update Series, 3*(17), 1–8.

Centers for Disease Control. (1984). Counsel carefully about sponge, toxic shock, CDC advises. *Contraceptive Technology Update, 5*(3), 29–40.

Centers for Disease Control. (1989). 1989 sexually transmitted diseases treatment guidelines [Special issue]. *Morbidity and Mortality Weekly Report, 38.*

Hyde, L. (1983). Toxic shock syndrome associated with diaphragm use. *Journal of Family Practice, 16,* 616–620.

King, J. (1984). Vaginitis. *Journal of Obstetric, Gynecologic, and Neonatal Nursing, 13,* 41–48.

Miles, P. A. (1984). Sexually transmitted diseases. *Journal of Obstetric, Gynecologic, and Neonatal Nursing, 13,* 102–123.

Scherger, J., & Sullivan, N. (1986). Vulvovaginitis. In C. Havens, N. Sullivan, & P. Tilton (Eds.), *Manual of outpatient gynecology* (pp. 3–12). Boston: Little, Brown.

Schober, M. (1986). Gynecologic and urinary problems. In J. Griffith-Kenney (Ed.), *Contemporary women's health* (pp. 589–601). Menlo Park, CA: Addison-Wesley.

Toxic shock syndrome: Assessment of current information and future research needs: Report of a study. (1982). Division of Health Sciences Policy, Division of Health Promotion and Disease Prevention, Institute of Medicine. Washington, DC: National Academy Press.

Wager, G. (1983). Toxic shock syndrome: A review. *American Journal of Obstetrics and Gynecology, 146,* 93–102.

Problems Related to Pelvic Support Tissues

Henderson, J. S., & Taylor, K. H. (1987). Age as a variable in an exercise program for the treatment of simple urinary stress incontinence. *Journal of Obstetric, Gynecologic, and Neonatal Nursing, 16,* 266–272.

Nichols, D. H., & Randall, C. L. (1983). *Vaginal surgery* (2nd ed.). Baltimore: Williams & Wilkins.

Benign and Malignant Neoplasms

American Cancer Society. (1989). *Cancer facts and figures—1989.* New York: Author.

Barber, H. R. K. (1984). Ovarian cancer: Diagnosis and surgical management. In A. A. Forastiere (Ed.), *Gynecologic cancer* (pp. 47–66). New York: Churchill Livingstone.

Benedet, J. L., & Sanders, B. H. (1984). Carcinoma in situ of the vagina. *American Journal of Obstetrics and Gynecology, 148,* 695–700.

Chamorro, T. (1985). Radical gynecologic surgery. *NAACOG Update Series, 3*(7), 1–8.

Christiano, M. Y. (1981). Hysterectomy. In E. D. Smith (Ed.), *Women's health care: A guide for patient education* (pp. 122–127). New York: Appleton-Century-Crofts.

Cramer, D. W., Welch, W. R., Hutchinson, G. B., Scully, R. E., & Ryan, K. J. (1984). Dietary animal fat in relation to ovarian cancer risk. *Obstetrics and Gynecology, 63,* 833.

DiSaia, P. J., & Creaseman, W. T. (1984). *Clinical gynecological oncology* (2nd ed.). St. Louis: C. V. Mosby.

Droegemueller, W., Herbst, A. L., Mishell, D. R., Jr., & Stenchever, M. A. (1987). *Comprehensive gynecology.* St. Louis: C. V. Mosby.

Drummond, J., & Field, P. (1984). Emotional and sexual sequelae following hysterectomy. *Health Care for Women International, 5,* 261–271.

Fink, D. A. (1988). Change in American Cancer Society check-up guidelines for detection of cervical cancer. *Cancer, 38,* 127–128.

Krakoff, I. (1987). Cancer chemotherapeutic agents. *CA: A Cancer Journal for Clinicians, 37,* 2–20.

Lalinec-Michaud, M., & Engelsmann, F. (1985). Anxiety, fear and depression related to hysterectomy. *Canadian Journal of Psychiatry, 30,* 44–47.

Lowdermilk, D. L. (1981a). Reproductive surgery. In C. I. Fogel & N. F. Woods (Eds.), *Health care of women: A nursing perspective* (pp. 157–209). St. Louis: C. V. Mosby.

Lowdermilk, D. L. (1981b). Reproductive malignancy. In C. I. Fogel & N. F. Woods (Eds.), *Health care of women: A nursing perspective* (pp. 301–333). St. Louis: C. V. Mosby.

Lowdermilk, D. L. (1985a). Cancer risk factors and prevention. *NAACOG Update Series, 2*(19), 1–8.

Lowdermilk, D. L. (1985b). Nursing perspectives related to intracavitary radiation therapy. *NAACOG Update Series, 3*(18), 1–8.

Lowdermilk, D. L. (1986). Reproductive surgery. In J. Griffith-Kenney (Ed.), *Contemporary women's health* (pp. 604–621). Menlo Park, CA: Addison-Wesley.

Marcus, S. L. (1961). Multiple squamous cell carcinoma involving the cervix, vagina and vulva—the theory of multicentricity. *American Journal of Obstetrics and Gynecology, 80,* 802.

Meyers, M. (1986). The enlarged uterus. In C. Havens, N. Sullivan, & P. Tilton (Eds.), *Manual of outpatient gynecology* (pp. 51–56). Boston: Little, Brown.

Ozols, R. F., Myers, C. F., & Young, R. C. (1984). New investigational techniques in ovarian cancer. In A. A. Forastiere (Ed.), *Gynecologic cancer* (pp. 177–195). New York: Churchill Livingstone.

Porter, L. L. (1985). Gestational trophoblastic disease. *NAACOG Update Series, 3*(12), 1–8.

Roberts, J. A., & Morley, G. W. (1984). The staging and surgical therapy of cervical carcinoma. In A. A. Forastiere (Ed.), *Gynecologic cancer* (pp. 47–66). New York: Churchill Livingstone.

Rostad, M. E. (1988). The radical vulvectomy patient: Preventing complications. *Dimensions of Critical Care Nursing, 7,* 289–294.

Silverberg, E., & Lubera, J. (1987). Cancer statistics. *CA: A Cancer Journal for Clinicians, 37,* 2–20.

Stanfill, P. H. (1982). The psychosocial implications of hysterectomy. *Journal of Obstetric, Gynecologic, and Neonatal Nursing, 11,* 318–320.

Taylor, K. (1986). Adnexal masses. In C. Havens, N. Sullivan, & P. Tilton (Eds.), *Manual of outpatient gynecology* (pp. 57–71). Boston: Little, Brown.

Tilton, P. (1986b). Diseases of the vulva. In C. Havens, N. Sullivan, & P. Tilton (Eds.), *Manual of outpatient gynecology* (pp. 39–43). Boston: Little, Brown.

Wabrek, A. J., & Gunn, J. L. (1984). Sexual and psychological implications of gynecologic malignancy. *Journal of Obstetric, Gynecologic, and Neonatal Nursing, 13,* 371–376.

Webb, C., & Wilson-Barnett, J. (1983). Self-concept, social support and hysterectomy. *International Journal of Nursing Studies, 20,* 97–107.

Weiss, N. S. (1984). Epidemiology of endometrial cancer: A review of hormonal and non-hormonal risk factors. In A. A. Forastiere (Ed.), *Gynecologic cancer* (pp. 199–214). New York: Churchill Livingstone.

Problems Related to Pregnancy

Adasczik, J. P. (1981). Sterilization by tubal ligations. In E. D. Smith (Ed.), *Women's health care: A guide for patient education* (pp. 76–89). New York: Appleton-Century-Crofts.

Bobak, I. M., & Jensen, M. D. (1987). *Essentials of maternity nursing* (2nd ed.), pp. 170–175, 817–823). St. Louis: C. V. Mosby.

Cooper, D. C. (1988). Ectopic pregnancy. *American Journal of Nursing, 88,* 842.

Fogel, C. I. (1981b). Abortion. In C. I. Fogel & N. F. Woods (Eds.), *Health care of women: A nursing perspective* (pp. 524–538). St. Louis: C. V. Mosby.

Gilbert, E. S., & Harmon, J. S. (1986). *High risk pregnancy and delivery nursing perspectives* (pp. 157–207). St. Louis: C. V. Mosby.

Gomel, V. (1980). The impact of microsurgery in gynecology. *Clinical Obstetrics and Gynecology, 23,* 1301–1310.

Henshaw, S. K., & O'Reilly, K. (1983). Characteristics of abortion patients in the United States, 1979–1980. *Family Planning Perspectives, 15,* 5–16.

Kuczynski, H. J. (1986). Support for the woman with an ectopic pregnancy. *Journal of Obstetric, Gynecologic, and Neonatal Nursing, 15,* 306–309.

Pritchard, J. A., & McDonald, P. C. (1980). *Williams obstetrics* (16th ed.). New York: Appleton-Century-Crofts.

Saidi, M. H., & Zainie, C. M. (1980). *Female sterilization: A handbook for women.* New York: Garland STPM Press.

Schneider, T. B. (1984). Voluntary termination of pregnancy. *Journal of Obstetric, Gynecologic, and Neonatal Nursing, 13,* 77–83.

Supreme Court of the United States Syllabus. (1973). *Roe et al. v. Wade.* District Attorney of Dallas County, January 22, 1973.

U. S. Laws, Statutes. (1974). Sterilization of persons in federally assisted family planning projects. *Federal Register, 39*(78), 13872–13873.

ADDITIONAL READINGS

Celeste, S. M., & Smith, M. D. (1986). Gestational tropho-blastic neoplasms. *Journal of Obstetric, Gynecologic, and Neonatal Nursing, 15,* 11–16.

This article provides a comprehensive overview of GTD, which is described as one of the most curable malignancies, but also one of the most emotionally devastating diseases. A crisis theory framework is suggested to identify nursing diagnoses and plan specific nursing interventions. Nurses who provide care to women with GTD will find this information essential.

Foley, S. F. (1987). Preventive gynecologic nursing in an inpatient setting. *Journal of Obstetric, Gynecologic, and Neonatal Nursing, 16,* 160–166.

This article describes a screening program done by nurses, which offers gynecologic examinations and health care teaching and counseling to female clients. Although the nursing role described is a specialist one, the article identifies ways that nurses in general practice, especially gynecologic care, can incorporate women's health care teaching and counseling.

Heitkemper, M. N., Shaver, J. F., & Mitchell, E. S. (1988). Gastrointestinal symptoms and patterns across the menstrual cycle in dysmenorrhea. *Nursing Research, 37,* 108–113.

This study compared women with and without dysmenorrhea in describing GI functional indicators during the menstrual cycle. A convenience sample of 34 women, aged 19 to 37 years, was studied for two menstrual cycles. Participants answered the Menstrual Distress Questionnaire and completed a GI health survey. Results showed that women with dysmenorrhea had more complaints of looser stools and stomach pain and decreased food intake during menses. This information can be used by nurses in planning therapeutic interventions for women with dysmenorrhea.

Jenkins, B. (1988). Patients' reports of sexual changes after treatment for gynecological cancer. *Oncology Nursing Forum, 15,* 349–354.

Twenty sexually active women were studied after surgery and radiotherapy for endometrial and cervical cancer. They answered questions about frequency of intercourse, orgasm, and feelings of enjoyment and desire. Results showed statistically significant negative changes at the 95% level for these four variables. The study also found that 59% of the women received no sexual counseling before or after treatment. Radiotherapists were responsible for the counseling that was provided; none was reportedly given by nurses. The study reported that 88% of the women wanted sexual discussions initiated by a physician or a nurse. The findings have implications for client teaching.

O'Laughlin, K. M. (1987). Changes in bladder function in the woman undergoing radical hysterectomy for cervical cancer. *Journal of Obstetric, Gynecologic, and Neonatal Nursing, 15,* 380–385.

Radical hysterectomy can cause temporary or permanent bladder dysfunction postoperatively. This article describes the four major types of dysfunction—hypertonia of bladder muscle, loss of sensation of bladder fullness, difficulty initiating urination, and bladder hypotonia. Nursing interventions that can prevent these problems or help women adapt to them are discussed.

Osguthorpe, N. C. (1986). Ectopic pregnancy. *Journal of Obstetric, Gynecologic, and Neonatal Nursing, 16,* 36–41.

Ectopic pregnancy is the leading cause of maternal mortality in the first trimester, and women who have had a ruptured ectopic pregnancy have only a 33% chance of having a live baby in future pregnancies. This article presents an overview of ectopic pregnancy, including the etiology, signs and symptoms, treatment, and nursing management. The nurse's role is described as one in which prevention and education are as important as identification and management of ectopic pregnancy.

Walton, J., & Youngkin, E. (1987). The effects of a support group on self-esteem of women with premenstrual syndrome. *Journal of Obstetric, Gynecologic, and Neonatal Nursing, 16,* 174–178.

This article reports the findings of a descriptive study that explored the effects of support groups on the self-esteem of women with PMS. A revised Coopersmith Self Esteem Inventory was administered to a group of women who participated in a support group and to a group that did not. No statistical significances were found, but women in the support group reported that they benefited from the experience. Areas for further nursing research were identified.

Webb, C. (1986). Professional and lay support for hysterectomy patients. *Journal of Advanced Nursing, 11,* 167–177.

The purpose of this study was to identify social support of women having a hysterectomy. Interviews were conducted with 50 women in one hospital setting, with half of them getting information about their surgery and half receiving no information. Follow-up interviews were conducted 3 months after surgery. Significant differences were found between the groups in their feelings about their hospital treatment. No significant differences were found in the level of satisfaction, health, and resumption of activities after the hysterectomies. One group identified as needing more social support were full-time housewives, as they are more likely to be isolated from other support sources.

Yasko, J. M., & Greene, P. A. (1987). Coping with problems related to cancer and cancer treatment. *CA: A Cancer Journal for Clinicians, 37,* 106–125.

This article outlines suggestions for clients coping with and living with different aspects of cancer therapy, including anemia, bleeding due to thrombocytopenia, constipation, diarrhea, difficulty in swallowing, dry mouth, and fatigue. Additionally, suggestions are given to help families and clients cope with hair loss, infection, pruritus, loss of appetite, stomatitis, nausea and vomiting, pain, respiratory problems, sexual and reproductive problems, skin reactions, taste alterations, and urinary tract problems. This information is invaluable to nurses working with cancer clients.

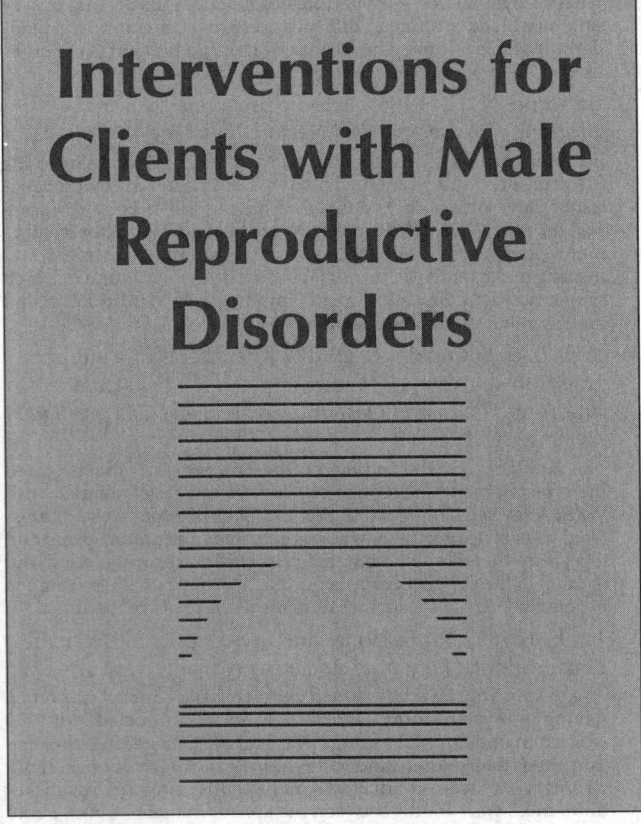

CHAPTER 55

Interventions for Clients with Male Reproductive Disorders

In spite of the heightened awareness about sexuality and reproduction, clients with reproductive disorders or sexual dysfunction are often reluctant to ask questions or tell anyone about their problems. They may have never discussed their sexuality with anyone, much less a stranger, or they may feel that their sexual preferences or practices will not be accepted. They may feel that the private sexual aspect of their lives may be disclosed or discussed without permission. For these reasons, some clients do not seek help from health care professionals until they are acutely symptomatic.

Although sexuality and reproduction are closely linked, they are not the same. Nurses need to be knowledgeable about the anatomy and physiology of male reproductive function so they can instruct their clients about the impact a disease process or treatment modality has on the male reproductive ability. Nurses need to include the client and his spouse, sexual partner, or significant other in the decision-making process and to make referrals to other health care professionals as necessary.

A variety of disorders affect or have the potential to affect the client's reproductive function. Nurses must be especially sensitive to and supportive of affected clients and their significant others. Nursing diagnoses and nursing interventions for the client with reproductive disorders are based on the professional nurse's acceptance of each client's sexuality.

BENIGN PROSTATIC HYPERPLASIA

OVERVIEW

The prostate gland is the major accessory sex gland of the male. It is frequently a site of infection and benign and malignant neoplasms, all of which can cause problems with urinary elimination.

Pathophysiology

In a young adult male, the prostatic capsule is thin and is attached to the underlying tissue. As a male ages, the glandular units in the prostate begin to undergo tissue hyperplasia (an abnormal increase in the number of cells), resulting in prostatic hypertrophy. Although *prostatic hypertrophy* is the more common term used to describe this phenomenon, *prostatic hyperplasia* is the correct term for the pathologic process.

When the prostate gland enlarges, it extends upward, into the bladder, and inward, narrowing the prostatic urethral channel, and obstructs the outflow of urine by encroaching on the bladder opening (Fig. 55–1). In response to this outlet resistance, the bladder is affected in several ways (Fig. 55–2). First, the bladder may become hyperirritable, which produces urgency and frequency.

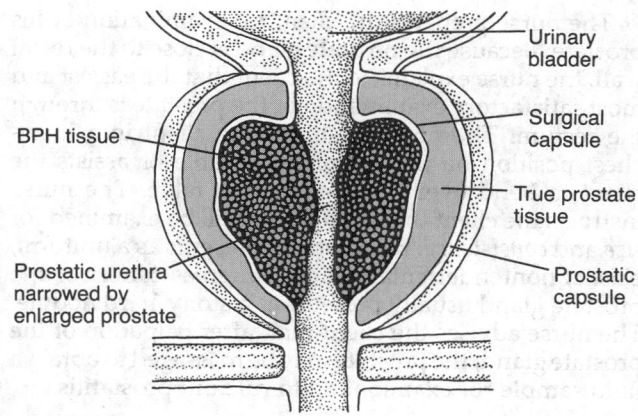

Figure 55–1

Benign prostatic hyperplasia grows in an inward direction, causing narrowing of the urethra.

As the bladder tries to compensate for its increased workload, muscles in the bladder wall hypertrophy (trabeculation) and may develop cellules and diverticula. If allowed to continue, this obstruction of urine flow can also result in a gradual dilation of the ureters (hydroureter) and kidneys (hydronephrosis). The enlarged prostate may also obstruct the bladder neck or the prostatic urethra, causing urinary retention or incomplete bladder emptying. Urinary stasis can result in urinary tract infections.

Etiology

The exact etiology of benign prostatic hyperplasia (BPH) remains unknown. Because the development of BPH is almost a universal condition in older men, several theories have been examined: the effect of chronic inflammation of the prostate gland, the role of general metabolic and nutritional factors (diet), and the possible contribution of atherosclerosis. Demographic data, such as race, and social factors, such as socioeconomic status and heredity, have been examined as predictors for the development of BPH. Although these theories continue to be investigated, it is thought that BPH results from a systemic hormonal alteration. Support for this theory is based on the observation that aging is a factor in the development of BPH, as is the presence of testicular androgen. It has been documented that BPH does not occur in men who have been castrated before puberty (testicular androgen is absent); men with BPH experience a regression of their disease after bilateral orchiectomies (testicular androgen is removed); and in animal models BPH can be reproduced by treatment with the potent androgen hormone dihydrotestosterone (Freed, 1986).

Incidence

The incidence of BPH consistently increases with age. Characteristically, BPH is a disease of men older than 40

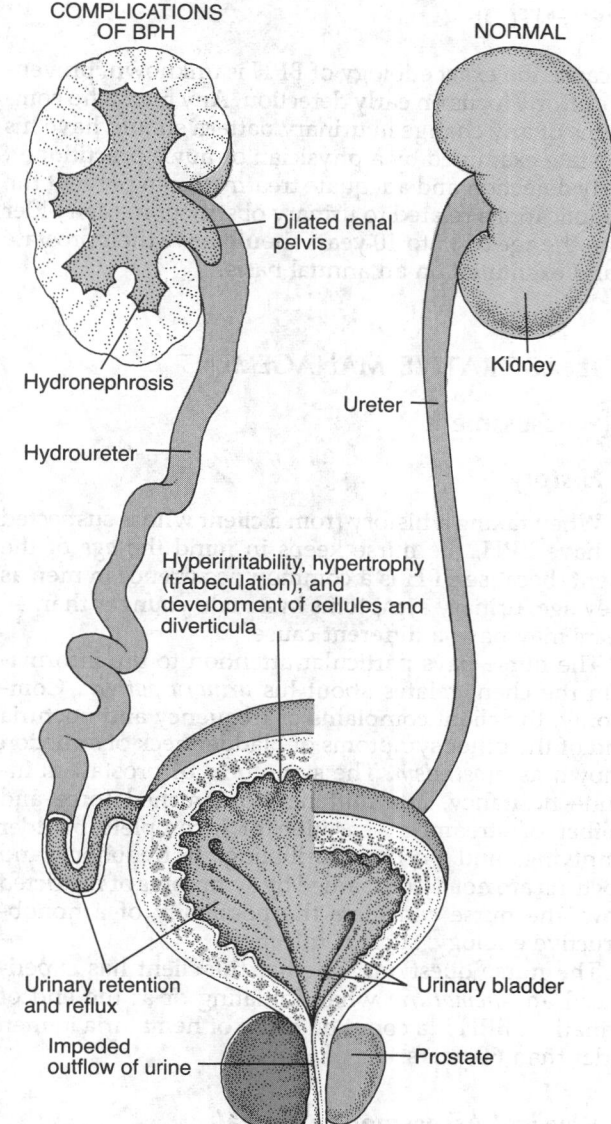

Figure 55–2

Potential complications of benign prostatic hypertrophy. Right side of illustration shows a normal male urologic system. Left side shows potential complications.

years of age, with an increase in incidence occurring with each decade of life. Studies of male autopsies revealed that the incidence of BPH in men older than 50 years of age was 50%, rising to 75% in men older than 80 years (Berry et al., 1984).

Worldwide, BPH seems to be most common in Caucasians (Iceland, Europe, and the United States). The reported incidences of BPH in Black and in Caucasian men in the United States are similar. The incidence of BPH in Asian countries, such as China and Japan, is lower than that in Caucasian or Black populations (Fay, 1983).

PREVENTION

Because the exact etiology of BPH is unknown, preventive efforts focus on early detection. Any man who complains of any change in urinary pattern should have his prostate examined by a physician or nurse practitioner. Early detection and adequate treatment can prevent the complications related to urinary obstruction. Men older than the age of 35 to 40 years should have their prostate gland examined on an annual basis.

COLLABORATIVE MANAGEMENT

 Assessment

History

When taking a history from a client who is suspected to have BPH, the nurse keeps in mind the *age* of the client. Because BPH is a common occurrence in men as they age, urinary symptoms in a male younger than 40 years may have a different cause.

The nurse pays particular attention to the information the client relates about his *urinary pattern*. Commonly, the client complains of frequency and nocturia and of the other symptoms of bladder neck obstruction known as *prostatism*. The symptoms of prostatism include hesitancy, intermittency, diminished force and caliber of stream, a sensation of incomplete bladder emptying, and postvoid dribbling. If frequency and nocturia are not accompanied by symptoms of restricted flow, the nurse considers the possibility of a nonobstructive etiology, such as infection.

The nurse questions whether the client has experienced any *hematuria* when initiating or at the end of urination. BPH is a common cause of hematuria in men older than 60 years.

Physical Assessment: Clinical Manifestations

The nurse performs a physical examination of the client, paying particular attention to the *abdomen*. The nurse observes the client for evidence of any *nutritional deficiencies, edema, pruritus, pallor,* or *ecchymoses,* indicating that the client may have renal insufficiency from long-standing obstruction.

The nurse instructs the client to void before his physical examination. Then the nurse inspects, palpates, and percusses the client's abdomen for any evidence of a *distended bladder.* Normally, the bladder must contain 150 mL of urine to allow its palpation and percussion. A bladder with a larger amount of urine may be visible on inspection. An enlarged bladder may be palpated as a mass in the lower abdomen. If suprapubic pressure on the mass results in a feeling of urgency, the nurse may be able to ascertain that the mass is a distended bladder. The nurse needs to remember that the bladder of an obese client is best identified through percussion rather than inspection or palpation.

The nurse prepares the client for examination of his prostate. Because the prostate gland is close to the rectal wall, the nurse explains to the client that the easiest and most satisfactory examination of the prostate is through the rectum. The nurse positions the client in a knee-chest position on the examination table or assists the client to bend over the examination table. The nurse instructs the client that his *prostate* will be examined for *size* and *consistency.* BPH usually presents as a uniform, elastic, nontender enlargement, whereas cancer of the prostate gland usually presents as a stony-hard nodule. The nurse advises the client that, after palpation of the prostate gland, the prostate may be massaged to obtain a fluid sample for examination to rule out prostatitis.

Psychosocial Assessment

Because BPH is commonly associated with aging, the nurse pays close attention to the impact that this diagnosis has on the client and his self-image. The client may think of BPH as an "old man's disease," and the diagnosis of BPH may threaten his self-image. The nurse is aware that some of the interventions for the treatment of BPH can result in a reproductive or erectile dysfunction and investigates the effect that these ramifications have on the client's sexuality. The nurse includes the client's significant other in any pretreatment counseling.

Laboratory Findings

Common laboratory tests include a urinalysis and urine culture to detect any urinary abnormality or evidence of urinary tract infection. Urinalysis includes tests for glucose, protein, occult blood, and pH levels. If an infection is present, the urinary pH may be alkaline, and the specimen may contain white blood cells (WBCs), red blood cells (RBCs), or pus.

Blood studies that are desirable at the time of the client's initial evaluation include a complete blood count to evaluate any evidence of infection or anemia, blood urea nitrogen and serum creatinine determinations to evaluate the client's renal function, and a serum acid phosphatase measurement if a prostatic malignancy is suspected.

If fluid was expressed during the prostatic examination, it is sent to the laboratory for microscopic examination and cultures.

Radiographic Findings

Common radiologic studies utilized in the work-up of the client with suspected BPH include radiography of the kidneys, the ureters, and the bladder (KUB) (an abdominal flat-plate x-ray) and intravenous pyelography (IVP) (excretory urography). A flat-plate x-ray film of the abdomen demonstrates the placement of the urinary tract in the abdomen. The IVP provides particularly useful information about the structure and function of the urinary tract. This study also provides information about bladder emptying and postvoid urinary retention, any evidence of upper urinary tract obstruction, hydronephrosis, calculi, masses, or any defect in bladder filling.

Other Diagnostic Tests

Urodynamic studies play an important role in the diagnosis and evaluation of clients with bladder neck obstruction. Urodynamic flow studies include flow rate analysis and assessment of residual urine. Flow rate analysis, or flowmetry, is simply a way of assessing the activity of the bladder and the outlet during the emptying phase of micturition.

A cystourethroscopic examination (visual examination of the interior of the bladder, the bladder neck, and the urethra with a cystoscope) is necessary to study the presence and effect of bladder neck obstruction. This procedure is most frequently done in an outpatient setting.

Residual urine determination is commonly done by catheterizing the client immediately after he voids or, because the client always voids before cystourethroscopy, residual urine may be measured at that time. Chapter 57 describes these studies.

 Analysis: Nursing Diagnosis

Common Diagnoses

The common diagnoses for clients with BPH are potential for injury and potential for infection related to urinary obstruction.

Additional Diagnoses

Some clients may also have

1. Pain related to urinary obstruction
2. Sexual dysfunction related to urinary obstruction
3. Anxiety related to urinary obstruction

 Planning and Implementation

The plan of care is based on the common nursing diagnoses.

Potential for Injury; Potential for Infection

Planning: client goals. The major goal is that the client will not experience any complications from the treatment of urinary retention.

Interventions. The only effective treatment for the relief of the symptoms caused by BPH has been surgical, although attempts at medical management have been made.

Nonsurgical management. A variety of hormonal agents, estrogens and androgens, alone or in combina-

tion, have been utilized in attempts to alter BPH and its effects on voiding. Hormonal manipulation of the client has not been successful, because the exact relationship between hormones and prostate growth is not fully understood.

Some nonsurgical measures that may help to minimize obstructive symptoms include those that cause the release of prostatic fluid, such as prostatic massage, frequent intercourse, and masturbation. These measures are particularly helpful for the client whose urinary obstructive symptoms are the result of an enlarged prostate with a large amount of retained prostatic fluid.

Clients are instructed to avoid drinking large amounts of fluid in a short time, to avoid alcohol and diuretics, and to void as soon as the urge is felt. These measures are aimed at preventing overdistention of the bladder, which may result in loss of detrusor muscle tone. Clients should also avoid any medications that can cause urinary retention, such as anticholinergics, antihistamines, and decongestants.

Surgical management. Because the vast majority of men (especially those older than 60 years) have some evidence of BPH, the mere presence of the condition may not require surgical intervention. In assessment of the client to confirm the need for surgical intervention, some or all of the following criteria should be present: acute urinary retention; chronic urinary tract infections secondary to residual urine in the bladder; hematuria; hydronephrosis; and bladder neck obstruction symptoms that are worrisome to the client, such as urinary frequency and nocturia. The goals of surgical interventions for the client with BPH are to relieve the symptoms associated with bladder neck obstruction and to improve the quality of the client's life by allowing him to void at normal intervals while retaining adequate urinary control and normal sexual functioning.

The client's general physical condition, the size of the prostate gland, and the client's preference must be considered when planning surgical interventions for the client with BPH.

The client is thoroughly evaluated for any other diseases common in the older population, such as cardiovascular disease, chronic obstructive pulmonary disease, diabetes, or renal disease. Any renal impairment resulting from hydronephrosis from bladder neck obstruction should be resolved by inserting a Foley catheter, with close monitoring of the client's intake and output and serum electrolyte and creatinine levels until renal status has improved. In some cases, a thorough work-up and evaluation of the medical condition of the client may indicate that surgery would carry too great a risk for the client. For these clients, relief of bladder neck obstruction may be achieved by permanent tube drainage.

In addition, clients with BPH are at high risk for urinary tract infection from residual urine in the bladder, invasive procedures such as cystourethroscopy, or the insertion of indwelling Foley's catheters. Each client must be assessed for the presence of urinary tract infection and have any infection resolved before surgical intervention for BPH.

There are several possible surgical procedures for removing the hypertrophied portion of the prostate gland (Fig. 55–3). All approaches remove the hyperplastic tissue and leave the prostatic capsule. The transurethral approach is a closed procedure; the others are considered open procedures owing to the need for a surgical incision. The choice of procedure depends on the size of the prostate gland, the location of the enlargement, whether surgery on the bladder is also needed, and the age and physical condition of the client.

A *transurethral resection of the prostate* (TURP) is per-

formed by means of a resectoscope (an instrument similar to a cystoscope, but with a cutting and cauterizing loop) inserted through the urethra. A TURP is performed when the major enlargement exists in the medial lobe of the prostate that directly surrounds the urethra and there is a relatively small amount of tissue to be removed. The enlarged portion of the prostate gland is then resected in small pieces (prostate chips). The advantages of a TURP are that it is safer for the client who is at high risk for surgery, a surgical incision is not necessary, and hospitalization and convalescence are usually shorter than with any other type of prostatectomy. The disadvantage of a TURP is that, because only small

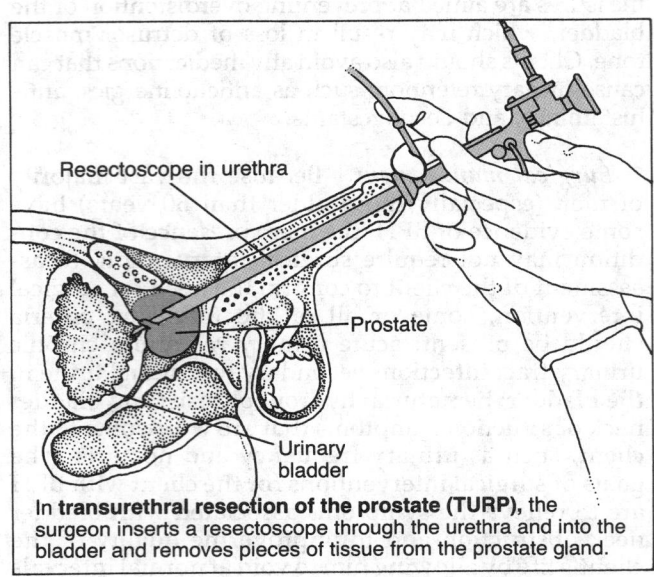

In **transurethral resection of the prostate (TURP)**, the surgeon inserts a resectoscope through the urethra and into the bladder and removes pieces of tissue from the prostate gland.

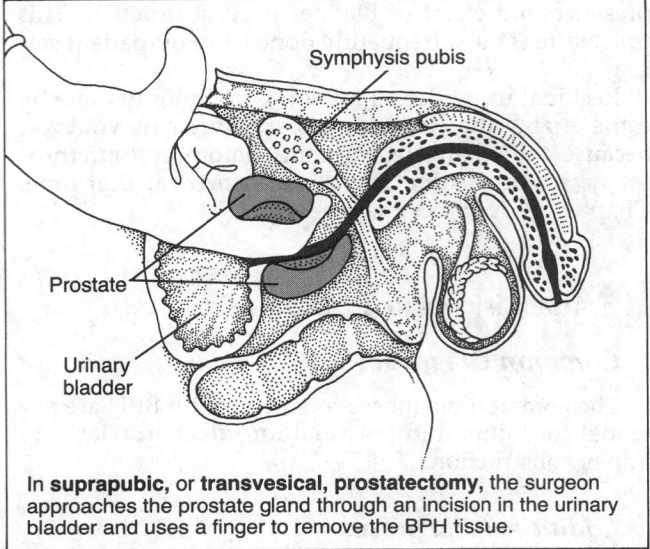

In **suprapubic**, or **transvesical**, **prostatectomy**, the surgeon approaches the prostate gland through an incision in the urinary bladder and uses a finger to remove the BPH tissue.

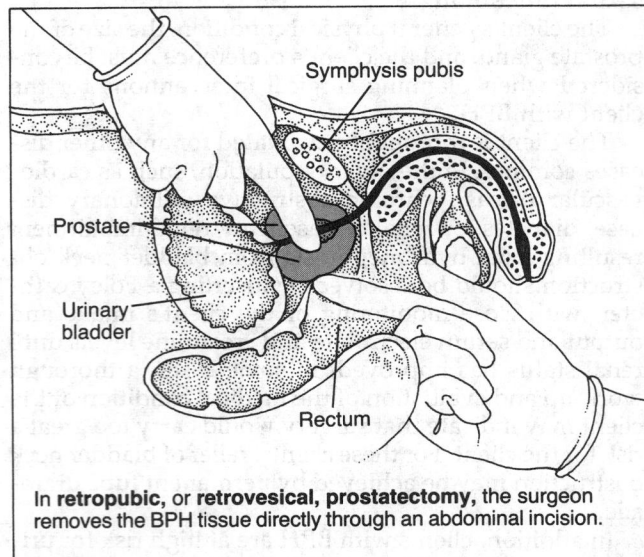

In **retropubic**, or **retrovesical**, **prostatectomy**, the surgeon removes the BPH tissue directly through an abdominal incision.

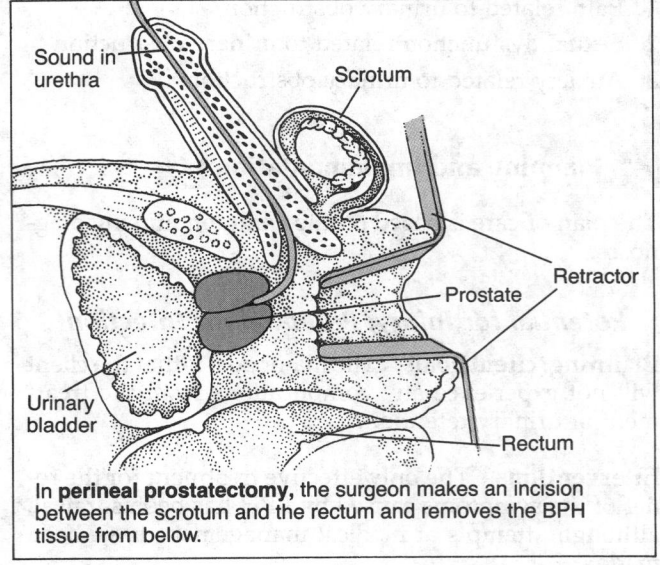

In **perineal prostatectomy**, the surgeon makes an incision between the scrotum and the rectum and removes the BPH tissue from below.

Figure 55–3

Prostatectomy procedures.

pieces of the gland are removed, prostatic tissue may grow back, resulting in recurrent urinary obstruction and necessitating additional TURPs. There is also the possibility of urethral trauma from the resectoscope, with resultant urethral strictures.

Suprapubic, or *transvesical, prostatectomy* is performed when the prostate is larger than the surgeon believes can be removed transurethrally or if coexisting bladder abnormalities can be treated concurrently. The surgeon makes a low, horizontal abdominal incision just above the symphysis pubis and exposes the bladder. The bladder is then distended with fluid, and a small incision is made in the bladder wall. The prostate gland is enucleated through the bladder cavity and any bladder disease is treated at this time. The ability to treat bladder problems is the major advantage of this surgical approach, because an incision is made into the bladder to reach the prostate. Disadvantages of a suprapubic prostatectomy are that it requires an abdominal incision and an incision into the bladder, the client also has a suprapubic tube in place postoperatively, the surgery is more painful, and convalescence is longer than with a TURP.

Retropubic, or *extravesical, prostatectomy* is utilized when the prostate is too large to be resected via the transurethral approach, but no coexisting bladder abnormalities are identified. With this technique, the surgeon makes an abdominal incision above the symphysis pubis to expose the prostate gland. A small incision is made in the prostate gland, and the gland is enucleated. Therefore, the difference between the suprapubic and the retropubic approaches is the bladder incision.

Perineal prostatectomy is used primarily to remove enlarged prostate glands that are filled with calculi; to treat prostatic abscesses that have not responded to conservative treatment; to repair complications, such as lacerations in the prostatic capsule that may have occurred during a different type of prostatectomy; or to treat clients who are poor surgical risks. For a perineal prostatectomy, the client is placed in an exaggerated lithotomy position in which the knees are positioned on the chest. The surgeon makes a U-shaped incision between the ischial tuberosities, the scrotum, and the rectum. The prostatic capsule is then opened and enucleated. This type of prostatectomy provides direct anatomic approach to the prostate gland. The major disadvantage of perineal prostatectomies is the loss of sexual potency resulting from damage to the pudendal nerve. Clients with peripheral vascular disease or chronic pulmonary problems do not tolerate the exaggerated lithotomy position and are not candidates for a perineal prostatectomy. Other disadvantages of this procedure include a greater risk for infection, the possibility of damage to the client's rectum and anal sphincter, and the possibility of urinary incontinence.

Preoperative care. Preoperatively, the client is thoroughly evaluated for the need for surgical intervention and the appropriate type of surgical procedure. The client may have many fears and misconceptions about prostatic surgery, such as automatic loss of sexual func-

tioning or permanent incontinence. The nurse assesses the client's anxiety, corrects any misconceptions about the surgery, and provides accurate information to the client and his family. Regardless of the type of surgery, the nurse informs the client and his family about anesthesia (see Chap. 19). The client may have concurrent medical problems that put him at risk for complications of general anesthesia and may be advised to have spinal anesthesia. Spinal anesthesia may be used for any of the procedures and is the most commonly used type of anesthesia for TURP. The client is awake; therefore, it is easier to assess for hyponatremia, fluid overload, and water intoxication.

Another topic for the nurse to include in the preoperative teaching plan for the client and his family is urinary catheters. After prostatic surgery, all clients have an indwelling urethral (Foley's) catheter. The nurse instructs the client that he may also have continuous bladder irrigation (CBI) or traction on his catheter, but this may not be known until return from the postanesthesia recovery room. The nurse also instructs the client preoperatively that it is normal for his urine to be blood tinged and for him to pass blood clots and tissue debris both while the catheter is in place and immediately after its removal.

Postoperative care. After TURP, a three-way Foley's catheter with a 30- to 45-mL retention balloon is inserted through the urethra into the bladder. The catheter is pulled down into the prostatic fossa to help provide hemostasis. The surgeon may apply traction on the client's catheter by pulling the catheter taut and taping it to the client's abdomen or thigh. If the catheter is taped to the client's thigh, the nurse instructs him to keep his leg straight.

The nurse informs the client that, because of the large diameter of the Foley catheter and the pressure that the retention balloon exerts on the internal sphincter of the bladder, he will continually feel the urge to void. The nurse instructs the client that this is a normal event and not a complication. It is important for the nurse to instruct the client not to try to void around the catheter, which causes the bladder muscles to contract and may result in painful bladder spasms. The nurse assures the client that medication can be given to keep him comfortable.

A continuous irrigation with normal saline or another solution ordered by the physician may be utilized to keep the catheter free of obstruction and to facilitate detection of obstruction or other complications. Continuous irrigation is used to irrigate the catheter, not the bladder. The irrigation is kept at a rate sufficient to maintain a colorless or light-pink drainage return and to prevent bladder distention. For the nursing care of the client undergoing CBI, see the accompanying Guidelines feature. The continuous irrigation is usually discontinued 24 to 48 hours after TURP. The Foley catheter may be removed 2 to 3 days later.

When the catheter is removed, the client may have some burning on urination and experience some frequency, dribbling, and leakage. These symptoms are

GUIDELINES ■ Care of the Client Undergoing Continuous Bladder Irrigation

Interventions	Rationales
1. Use only normal saline for irrigation of the bladder.	1. The irrigating fluid must be isotonic to the blood to prevent complications, such as hemolysis. It is possible for some of the irrigating fluid to be absorbed through bleeding blood vessels.
2. Monitor the color of the output, and adjust the rate accordingly.	2. If the output is bloody, the rate should be increased, as the dilution of blood aids in the prevention of clot formation.
3. Instruct the client to remain on bed rest with bathroom privileges, especially if his urine is bloody.	3. Bed rest promotes hemostasis.
4. Monitor the client's ouput frequently for any evidence of obstruction: external obstruction (kinks, client lying on tubing) or internal obstruction (clot or tissue fragments, bladder spasms occluding drainage of fluid from the bladder).	4. If the bladder becomes distended with fluid, it can cause severe discomfort and damage the surgical incision or surgical site.
5. If the catheter is obstructed, turn off the CBI and hand irrigate the catheter with a 60-mL irrigating syringe.	5. To accurately measure the amount of fluid to instill with hand irrigation, the CBI should be stopped to prevent overdistention of the bladder. Hand irrigation provides the negative pressure needed to aspirate clots or tissue fragments obstructing the client's catheter.
6. Notify the client's physician if the obstruction is not resolved after hand irrigation.	6. Medical interventions may be needed to resolve the obstruction.

normal and will subside. The client may also pass clots and tissue debris for several days after the TURP. The nurse instructs the client to increase his fluid intake to a minimum of 3000 mL/day, which helps to decrease the dysuria and to keep the urine clear. By the time of discharge (2 to 5 days postoperatively), the client should be voiding 150 to 200 mL of clear yellow urine every 3 to 4 hours. Usually, postoperative pain is minimal and analgesics may not even be required.

The nurse is aware that clients who undergo open prostatectomies are at risk for postoperative bleeding or hemorrhage. Bleeding is most common within the first 24 hours postoperatively and may not occur until the client has returned to his hospital room. Bladder spasms or movement may initiate bleeding from previously controlled vessels. This bleeding may be arterial or venous, but venous bleeding is more common. The nurse monitors the client's urinary output every 2 hours and his vital signs every 4 hours. If the bleeding is arterial, the nurse notices that the client's urinary drainage is bright red or "ketchupy" with numerous clots. The nurse also monitors the client's blood pressure to identify any decrease. The nurse keeps in mind that, if the client's bleeding is arterial, surgical intervention is necessary to clear the bladder of clots and stop the arterial bleeding.

If the client's bleeding is venous, his urinary output is burgundy, with or without any change in vital signs. The nurse informs the client's surgeon of any of the signs and symptoms of bleeding. The surgeon may apply traction on the client's catheter for a few hours, which may control venous bleeding. The nurse assesses the success of this procedure to stop the bleeding and is aware that the traction on the client's catheter is quite uncomfortable and increases the risk of bladder spasms. The nurse monitors the client's pain closely.

With a retropubic prostatectomy, the urinary sphincter muscles are seldom damaged, the bladder is not entered, and there should be no urinary drainage on the abdominal dressing. The nurse notifies the client's surgeon if there is any urinary or purulent drainage, fever, or increased pain, as these symptoms may indicate a serious complication, such as a deep wound infection or pelvic abscess.

If the client has had a suprapubic prostatectomy, he has a suprapubic catheter in place in addition to a Foley catheter. Each catheter is connected to a closed drainage system and drains the bladder via gravity. The nurse is aware that catheter traction is not effective for the client who experiences postoperative bleeding after a suprapubic prostatectomy. This client needs brisk, continuous irrigation via his catheter. If the client has CBI, he is instructed to remain in bed until the irrigation is discontinued. If the CBI does not control the postoperative bleeding, the client needs surgical intervention.

If the client has a suprapubic catheter in place, the urethral catheter is generally removed between the third and fifth postoperative days. After the removal of the urethral catheter, the nurse clamps the suprapubic catheter and the client attempts to void. After urination, the nurse checks the residual urine in the bladder by unclamping the suprapubic tube. When the client consistently empties his bladder and the residual urine in the bladder is 75 mL or less, the suprapubic catheter is then removed. An antimicrobial ointment is applied daily to the site. The client with a suprapubic catheter in place is at increased risk for bladder spasms. This client also needs to have his incision dressing observed and changed more frequently than the client who does not have an incision drain, as the dressing becomes saturated with urine until the incision heals. If the suprapubic drain is not connected to gravity drainage, the nurse may enclose the drain with an ostomy bag to accurately measure the output and to prevent any skin problems or breakdown.

With the perineal approach to prostatectomy, the client has an incision dressing and may or may not have an incision drain. The use of rectal thermometers and rectal tubes and enemas are contraindicated because of the possibility of causing trauma or bleeding.

■ Discharge Planning

Home Care Preparation

Unless the client experiences a complication of surgery, such as a wound infection or an unusual problem with voiding, he does not have a dressing or indwelling catheter.

Client/Family Education

After any type of prostatectomy, some clients, and especially those who have had TURP, may have some temporary loss of control of urination or a dribbling of their urine. The nurse assures the client and reinforces that these symptoms are almost always temporary and will resolve. The nurse assists the client and his significant other in devising ways to keep his clothing dry until sphincter control returns. The nurse instructs the client to contract and relax his sphincter frequently to re-establish urinary control. Condom catheters are not used except in extreme cases, as they may give the client a false sense of security and delay his urinary control.

CLIENT/FAMILY EDUCATION ■ Postprostatectomy Care

Instructions	Rationales
1. "Eat and drink what you like, but use alcohol, soft drinks, and spicy foods in moderation."	1. To prevent irritation of remaining prostatic tissue.
2. "Drink 12 to 14 glassfuls of water during the day, preferably before 8 PM."	2. To keep urine flowing freely.
3. "During the first 2–3 wk after you leave the hospital, avoid strenuous activities such as driving, riding in a car for more than 20–25 min, walking more than ½ mile, climbing stairs quickly, lifting objects weighing more than 8 lb, having sexual intercourse, or engaging in sports."	3. To prevent injury.
4. "If you notice blood in your urine, go to bed and rest quietly, drink more fluids, and call your physician if the bleeding persists."	4. To prevent excessive bleeding. It is normal to have some intermittent bleeding and to pass occasional clots or pieces of tissue.
5. "If you have a desk-type job, do not return to work until 2–3 wk after you leave the hospital. If your job is more strenuous, do not return to work until 4 wk after you leave the hospital."	5. To prevent injury.
6. "After you leave the hospital, call your physician to schedule a follow-up appointment. Before you see your physician again, write down any questions you want to ask."	6. To ensure healing.

The nurse provides specific instructions for each client on the basis of the type of surgical procedure he had and any further interventions he may need in the future. Discharge instructions for a client undergoing surgery on his prostate gland are given in the Client/Family Education feature on page 1749.

Psychosocial Preparation

The client who undergoes prostatic surgery may need emotional support. The client who undergoes a perineal prostatectomy is at risk for permanent sexual dysfunction. The nurse informs the client of the options, such as a penile prosthesis, available to treat impotence (see later discussion of impotence).

Health Care Resources

Clients may be referred to a suppprt group such as Impotence Anonymous (see Unit 15 Resources).

 Evaluation

Evaluation measures the extent to which the client's goals are met and the effectiveness of nursing interventions. For nursing diagnoses of actual or potential problems related to urinary obstruction, the expected outcomes are that the client

1. Has resolution of the urinary obstruction without any infection or permanent complications
2. No longer experiences any pressure or pain
3. Reports a decrease or absence of anxiety about urinary retention
4. Exhibits a return to his previous level of sexual function or, if the client is not able to return to this functional level because of postsurgical complications (such as retrograde ejaculations or impotence), demonstrates psychosocial adjustment to this limitation

It is imperative that the nurse include the client and his family in the evaluation process. The client and his family should identify which nursing interventions were most influential in helping him achieve the expected outcomes and provide suggestions for changing interventions that were not useful.

PROSTATE CANCER

OVERVIEW

Prostate cancer is the most common cancer among American men and the third leading cause of cancer deaths. Black men develop prostate cancer twice as frequently as Caucasian men, tend to develop cancer of the prostate at an earlier age, have more advanced disease at the time of diagnosis, and have a higher mortality than Caucasian men. On the other hand, Hispanic and Asian men have a lower incidence of prostate cancer than Caucasian men and a lower mortality, implying cultural, genetic, or life style variables (American Cancer Society [ACS], 1990).

The etiology of prostate cancer remains unclear, but two factors influence its development. First, there must be an intact hypothalamic–pituitary–testicular pathway (men who were castrated before puberty have little risk of developing prostate cancer). Second, the advancing age of the client also increases his risk of prostate cancer. Cancer of the prostate is rare in men younger than 50 years, but increases with each decade, 73 years being the average age at diagnosis (ACS, 1990).

Dietary fat is thought to promote the development of the tumor. Several viruses, including cytomegalovirus and herpesvirus type 2, are found more frequently in cancerous prostatic tissue than in noncancerous tissue (Crawford & Dawkins, 1986).

The relationship between BPH and cancer of the prostate is controversial. Although some researchers believe that BPH and cancer of the prostate are unrelated diseases, others believe that cancer is more likely to occur within or adjacent to any proliferative cell population.

Ninety-five per cent of cancers of the prostate are adenocarcinomas, arising from the epithelial cells of the prostate, and are usually located in the posterior lobe or outer portion of the prostate gland (Fig. 55–4). The remaining types of prostatic neoplasms are classified as nonepithelial carcinomas and include ductal carcinomas, transitional cell carcinomas, squamous cell carcinomas, and sarcomas.

Knowledge about the growth and spread of adenocarcinoma of the prostate is important to enable effective treatment. Prostate cancer is one of the slowest growing of all malignancies, and it metastasizes in a fairly predictable pattern. The common sites of meta-

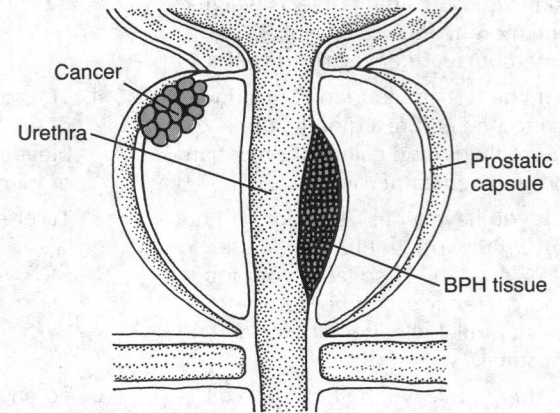

Figure 55–4

The prostate gland with cancer and BPH. Note that cancer normally arises in the periphery of the gland, and BPH occurs in the center of the gland.

static spread are the prostatic and perivesicular lymph nodes; the pelvic lymph nodes; the bone marrow; and the bones of the pelvis, the sacrum, and the lumbar spine. Metastatic involvement of the visceral organs tends to occur late in the natural history of the disease. The organs that are the most common sites for metastatic prostate cancer are the lungs, the liver, the adrenals, and the kidneys.

COLLABORATIVE MANAGEMENT

As with any cancer, accurate staging of the disease is necessary for treatment planning and monitoring the clinical course of the disease (see the accompanying Key Features of Disease). As in BPH, the first symptoms that the client may experience are related to bladder neck obstruction, such as difficulty in initiating urination, re-

current bladder infections, and urinary retention. At times, a client may be undergoing intervention for BPH and is found to have cancer of the prostate. Bone pain is a symptom of a more advanced stage of prostate cancer, and the client who has symptoms of urinary obstruction and bone pain is most likely to have metastatic disease at the time of diagnosis.

The digital rectal examination remains the standard procedure for diagnosing cancer of the prostate (see Chap. 52, Fig. 52–15). A prostate that is found to be stony hard and with palpable irregularities or indurations is suspected to be malignant.

When the diagnosis of cancer of the prostate is suspected, it is necessary to obtain a biopsy for confirmation. Prostatic ultrasonography may be utilized to isolate the area of the prostate for biopsy. One of several procedures may be used to obtain the biopsy specimen, the most common being needle core or aspiration biop-

---

KEY FEATURES OF DISEASE ■ TNM Classification for Prostate Carcinoma

Primary Tumor (T)

TX   Primary tumor cannot be assessed.

T0   No evidence of primary tumor.

T1   Tumor is incidental histologic finding.
    T1a   Three or fewer microscopic foci of carcinoma.
    T1b   More than three microscopic foci of carcinoma.

T2   Tumor is present clinically or grossly, limited to the gland.
    T2a   Tumor ≤ 1.5 cm in greatest dimension with normal tissue on at least three sides.
    T2b   Tumor > 1.5 cm in greatest dimension or in more than one lobe.

T3   Tumor invades the prostatic apex or into or beyond the prostatic capsule, bladder neck, or seminal vesicle, but is not fixed.

T4   Tumor is fixed or invades adjacent structures other than those listed in T3.

Regional Lymph Nodes (N)

NX   Regional lymph nodes cannot be assessed.

N0   No regional lymph node metastasis.

N1   Metastasis in a single lymph node, ≤ 2 cm in greatest dimension.

N2   Metastasis in a single lymph node, > 2 cm but not > 5 cm in greatest dimension, or multiple lymph nodes, none > 5 cm in greatest dimension.

N3   Metastasis in a lymph node > 5 cm in greatest dimension.

Distant Metastasis (M)

MX   Presence of distant metastasis cannot be assessed.

M0   No distant metastasis.

M1   Distant metastasis.

Histopathologic Grade (G)

GX   Grade cannot be assessed.

G1   Well differentiated, slight anaplasia.

G2   Moderately well differentiated, moderate anaplasia.

G3–4   Poorly differentiated, or undifferentiated, marked anaplasia.

Stage Grouping

Stage	T	N	M	G
0	T1a	N0	M0	G1
	T2a	N0	M0	G1
I	T1a	N0	M0	G2, G3–4
	T2a	N0	M0	G2, G3–4
II	T1b	N0	M0	Any G
	T2b	N0	M0	Any G
III	T3	N0	M0	Any G
IV	T4	N0	M0	Any G
	Any T	N1, N2, N3	M0	Any G
	Any T	Any N	M1	Any G

From American Joint Committee on Cancer. (1988). Beahrs, O. H., Henson, D. E., Hutter, R. V. P., & Myers, M. H. (Eds.). *Manual for staging of cancer* (3rd ed., p. 181). Philadelphia: J. B. Lippincott.

sies. For a *perineal needle biopsy*, the client is placed in a lithotomy position. The biopsy needle is inserted through the perineum into the prostate gland, and a sample or core of tissue is removed.

A *transrectal needle biopsy* is performed in the same manner as a perineal needle biopsy, except that the biopsy needle is inserted into the prostate gland through the rectal wall (Fig. 55–5). Because most prostate cancers are adjacent to the rectal wall, this method is the most commonly used.

If the client has bladder obstruction resulting from an enlarged prostate gland, a *transurethral biopsy* may be performed. For this procedure, the biopsy needle is inserted through the urethra into the prostate gland to obtain the tissue specimen. This type of biopsy is the least accurate, and its use is limited to those clients who have urinary obstruction.

Usually, needle biopsies are performed in the outpatient (ambulatory) setting with local anesthesia. Dressings are not required at the biopsy site. The nurse instructs the client to report any complication, such as bleeding or fever, to his physician.

Another procedure utilized for obtaining a prostatic tissue specimen is an *open perineal biopsy*. In this type of biopsy, a small incision is made in the perineum between the scrotum and the anus. This method is the most accurate of all biopsy techniques because the prostate gland is exposed, the area in question is clearly identified, and multiple tissue specimens can be obtained.

A dressing is placed over the incision for 24 to 48 hours or until any drainage stops. The nurse instructs the client to report any complications such as bright red bleeding, fever or urinary retention to his physician.

After the diagnosis of prostate cancer is made, the client undergoes radiographic and blood studies to ascertain the extent of his disease. Common tests include computed tomography (CT) of the pelvis and abdomen to assess the status of the pelvic and para-aortic lymph nodes and a bone scan to ascertain any evidence of metastatic disease. Hepatomegaly or abnormal results of liver function studies indicate a need for further evaluation for the presence of any liver metastasis. The levels of prostate-specific antigen (PSA), a glycoprotein found in prostatic tissue and seminal plasma, can be elevated in clients with carcinoma of the prostate, BPH, prostatic infarction, and prostatitis, but not in healthy men or those with carcinomas other than prostate carcinoma. A client with an elevated PSA level should have a decrease in the PSA level a few days after surgery. An increase in the PSA level at postoperative visits indicates that the disease has recurred. The vast majority of clients with advanced prostate cancer have elevated levels of serum acid phosphatase. Approximately 90% of clients with prostate cancer metastatic to the bone have elevated alkaline phosphatase levels.

Management of prostate cancer includes surgery and radiation therapy for localized disease and hormonal manipulation and combination chemotherapy for metastatic disease. Management is based on the extent of the disease and the physical condition of the client. The client may undergo surgical procedures for biopsy of the tumor, for the staging and removal of the tumor, or for palliation to control the spread of his disease or relieve distressing symptoms.

The surgical approaches for prostatectomy in the client with prostate cancer are the same as for the client with BPH (see earlier), but in the majority of cases, the surgical procedure is much more extensive and includes a pelvic lymphadenectomy. Clients who have stage 0 cancer of the prostate require only close follow-up by their physician. Repeat of needle biopsies or TURPs, if the client has recurring obstruction, should be part of the screening.

Clients with stage I or II disease may undergo a *radical* prostatectomy via a suprapubic, retropubic, or perineal approach. In this type of prostatectomy, instead of only enucleating the prostate gland as with BPH, the entire gland is removed along with the prostatic capsule, the cuff at the bladder neck, the seminal vesicles, and the regional lymph nodes. The remaining urethra is then anastomosed to the bladder neck (Fig. 55–6). The removal of tissue at the bladder neck allows the seminal fluid to travel upward into the bladder rather than down the urethral tract, resulting in retrograde ejaculations. The client is sterile, but his ability to have an erection and an orgasm should not be impaired.

The surgeon advises clients who undergo radical perineal prostatectomy that they may have an erectile dysfunction or impotence after the surgery. This is directly related to any damage done to the pudendal nerve

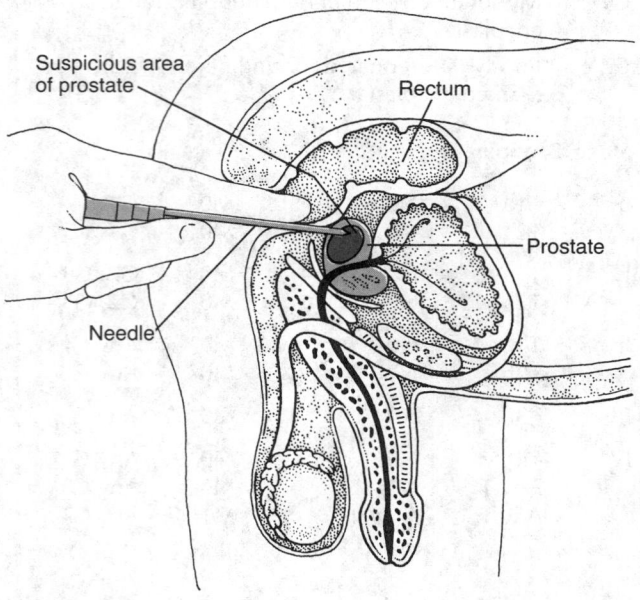

Figure 55–5

Transrectal biopsy of the prostate gland.

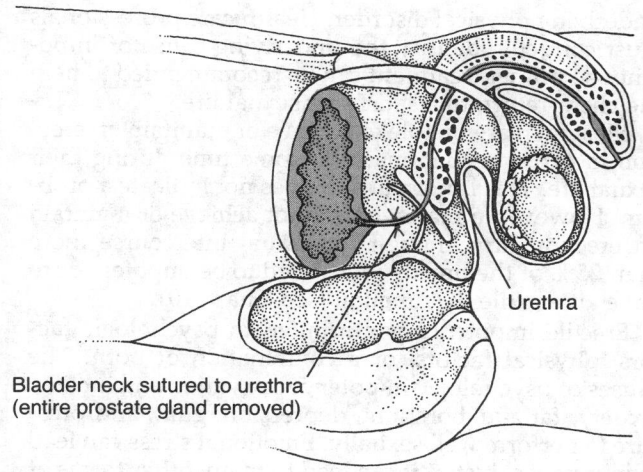

Figure 55–6

After total removal of the prostate (total prostatectomy), the bladder neck is sutured to the urethra.

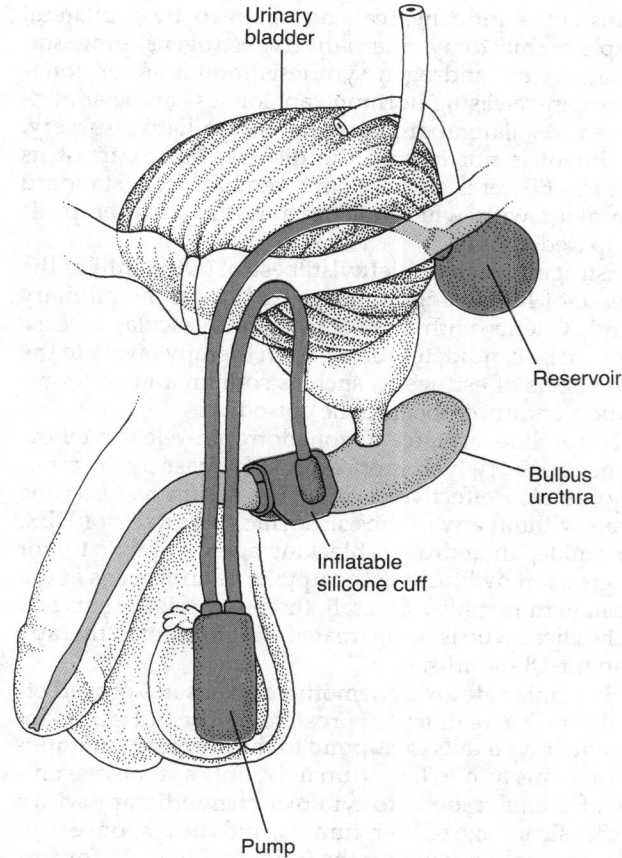

Figure 55–7

An artificial urinary sphincter is a fluid-filled system with a silicone cuff that surrounds the urethra and functions as a urinary sphincter. A pump is placed in the scrotum, and a fluid reservoir is placed in the abdomen. When the pump is squeezed, fluid leaves the urethral cuff and flows into the reservoir, allowing the client to empty his bladder.

(which is necessary for erection and orgasm) during the surgery. Because the internal and external sphincters of the bladder lie close to the prostate gland, another complication of radical prostatectomies can be urinary incontinence.

The nurse teaches the client perineal exercises to help facilitate the return of urinary continence after a radical prostatectomy or after the removal of the Foley catheter. The exercises consist of contracting and relaxing the perineal and gluteal muscles in several different ways. Some of the different exercises the client is taught are the following: tighten the perineal muscles for 3 to 5 seconds as if to prevent voiding, then relax; then bear down as if having a bowel movement; then relax and repeat the exercise. The client is instructed to inhale through pursed lips while tightening the perineal muscles and to exhale when he relaxes. Other exercises that help the client to regain urinary control are to hold an object, such as a pencil, in the fold between the buttock and the thigh, or to sit on the toilet with his knees apart while voiding and start and stop his stream several times.

If the client is unsuccessful in recovering urinary continence, an artificial urinary sphincter may be surgically implanted (Fig. 55–7). Artificial sphincters are more successful for males than females, possibly owing to the difference in urethral length.

After the implantation of the sphincter, the nurse instructs the client to report any complications, such as fever, pain on inflation of the device, edema or cellulitis in the genitalia, or the recurrence of incontinence, indicating a possible mechanical malfunction in the system.

External beam radiation therapy plays an important role in the treatment of prostate cancer. It is used as an alternative curative treatment to surgery for locally contained tumors; as an adjunct to radical prostatectomy

when surgical margins or regional lymph nodes are found to have evidence of malignancy postoperatively; and for palliation of the client's symptoms. Palliative radiation therapy has been effective in relieving pain caused by skeletal metastases and in relieving ureteral or bladder neck obstruction.

Interstitial radiation therapy, or radioactive seed implantation, with ^{198}Au or ^{125}I may be a treatment option for some clients. Clients who may be candidates for interstitial radiation therapy include those with limited local tumors who have had no previous treatment and those who have had external radiation or surgery and have small areas of tumor remaining (refer to Chap. 25 for further discussion of radiation therapy).

Because prostate cancer is a hormone-dependent cancer, clients with extensive tumors or those with metastatic disease are usually managed by androgen deprivation. Manipulating the hormonal environment in the client may be accomplished in two ways. The testosterone influence can be removed by a bilateral simple orchiectomy; alternatively, estrogens, progestational agents, androgen synthesis inhibitors, or gonadrotropin-releasing hormone analogues can be administered. A bilateral orchiectomy is a palliative surgery; the intent is not to cure the disease, but to arrest its spread. Bilateral orchiectomy remains the standard treatment with which all other hormonal therapy is compared.

Estrogens such as diethylstilbestrol (DES) inhibit the release of luteinizing hormone (LH) from the pituitary gland. Clients with significant cardiovascular disease may not be candidates for estrogen therapy owing to the side effects of estrogens, such as sodium and water retention and thromboembolic episodes.

Leuprolide acetate, a gonadotropin-releasing hormone agonist (which suppresses LH release by the pituitary), is also effective in reducing serum testosterone levels without any of the estrogenic side effects of DES. Flutamide, an androgen-blocking agent, inhibits tumor progression by blocking the uptake of androgens at the prostate tumor sites. Overall, the prognosis for survival of the client who is being treated with hormonal therapy is about 18 months.

Systemic cytotoxic chemotherapy has not proved effective in the treatment of prostate cancer and is used for the client who fails to respond to the hormonal manipulation of his tumor. Unfortunately, only a small percentage of clients respond to cytotoxic chemotherapy with a partial shrinkage of their tumors, and the response usually lasts only a few months (refer to Chap. 25 for further discussions of chemotherapy).

Nursing management of the client with prostate cancer always includes the client's spouse or sexual partner. Clients with prostate cancer may require nursing interventions in a wide variety of settings, such as the physician's office, the hospital, the radiation therapy department, the oncologist's office, or the client's home, and at any stage of the disease process. Major quality-of-life issues facing the client with prostate cancer include sexuality, body image, and the impact of the cancer diagnosis on his life.

IMPOTENCE

OVERVIEW

An erection is an involuntary reaction in response to sexual stimulation and excitement. *Impotence*, the inability to achieve or maintain an erection, is caused by a variety of disorders. It was once believed that 90% of impotence was of psychologic origin. It is now believed that at least 50% of the men with impotence have an

underlying physical disorder. Health care professionals must correctly identify the underlying cause of impotence so proper treatment can be recommended to help the client return to a satisfying sexual life.

Most men are unable to achieve or maintain an erection in certain situations or at some time during their sexual life. This is normal and does not indicate a problem. However, a man who cannot achieve or maintain an erection firm enough for sexual intercourse more than 25% of the time is considered to be impotent or to have an erectile dysfunction (see Chap. 10).

Erectile impotence is attributed to psychologic factors, physical factors, or a combination of both. The causes of psychologic impotence are varied and include anxiety, fatigue, boredom, depression, guilt, and pressure to perform well sexually. Emotional stress can lead to impotence, just as it can lead to many other forms of illness. Persistent psychologic impotence also can be triggered by one incident of sexual failure. A man who is worried about achieving an erection may not be able to relax and may find it difficult to achieve an erection.

Physiologic impotence is caused by a physical disorder, such as an injury, a disease, a hormonal imbalance, or surgery (see the accompanying Key Features of Disease). Diabetes mellitus is one of the most common causes of physical impotence (see Chap. 51). Impotence occurs in 50% to 60% of diabetic men of any age.

COLLABORATIVE MANAGEMENT

Assessment begins with a sexual and medical history. The client with psychologic impotence usually reports acute onset, selectivity, periodicity, nocturnal erections and emissions, an ability to masturbate, an ability to have an erection and to function sexually under certain circumstances, and retention of testicular sensitivity. The client with physical impotence usually reports a gradual loss of erectile function, some degree of erectile dysfunction in all sexual circumstances, and absence of nocturnal erections and emissions. The nurse also gathers data about the presence of common causes of impotence. The nurse investigates whether there is a family history of impotence or a family history of any physiologic or psychologic conditions that may contribute to erectile dysfunction. The nurse gathers information about any of the symptoms associated with diabetes or hypertension.

A complete physical assessment of the client, emphasizing the cardiovascular, neurologic, endocrine, and genitourinary systems, is performed. The nurse monitors the client's blood pressure for any evidence of hypertension.

Psychosocial assessment helps to identify psychologic factors that cause and perpetuate erectile dysfunction.

Laboratory studies usually include a complete blood count, renal function tests, liver function tests, serum electrolyte determinations, urinalysis, and culture and

KEY FEATURES OF DISEASE ■ Common Causes of Physiologic Impotence

Pathologic Causes

Diabetes mellitus
Thyroid disorders
Adrenal disorders
Hypothalamic – pituitary – gonadal disorders
Decreased testosterone secretion
Multiple sclerosis
Amyotrophic lateral sclerosis
Alzheimer's disease
Stroke
Arteriosclerosis
Pelvic fracture
Hypertension
Brain or spinal cord injury

Iatrogenic Causes

Prostatectomy or other surgery of the prostate, the
     bladder, or the rectum
Cystectomy
Abdominoperineal resection
Pelvic irradiation
Sympathectomy
Antihypertensive drugs
Narcotics
Barbiturates
Tranquilizers
Monoamine oxidase inhibitors and other antidepressants
Estrogens
Antihistamines

Other Causes

Alcohol, tobacco, and illicit drugs
Normal changes of aging
     Loss of tissue elasticity
     Decreased levels of circulating testosterone

sensitivity testing of urine to rule out any genitourinary disease. Cholesterol and triglyceride levels are examined to assess the client for arteriosclerosis. A glucose tolerance test is usually done to rule out diabetes mellitus. Serum follicle-stimulating hormone, LH, and testosterone levels are measured to rule out a hypothalamic – pituitary – gonadal cause.

Other diagnostic tests include IVP and CT of the pelvis to rule out genitourinary disease or malignancy, which may interfere with erection. Urethrography may also be ordered to rule out any urethral strictures (see Chap. 57 for assessment of urologic problems). Doppler ultrasound arterial flow studies of the penile arteries may be done to determine whether the client has penile

vascular disease, one of the causes of organic impotence. The nocturnal penile tumescence test is used to record and measure nocturnal erections to help distinguish physiologic and psychologic impotence. Depending on his age, a man usually has three or four erections, each lasting about 20 to 30 minutes, during a night's sleep. If the client experiences normal erections during sleep, erectile dysfunction while awake is most likely psychologic.

Management of impotence may be medical, surgical, or psychosocial, depending on its cause.

Nonsurgical management focuses on the underlying cause of the problem. The client may need psychosocial intervention, changes or adjustments in medications that he may be taking, or control of any underlying disease. The client with psychogenic impotence is referred, with his partner, to a sexual therapist (see Chap. 10). If a medication is found to be the cause of impotence, a change of medication may be implemented. However, depending on the client's illness, this may not be possible and the client's erectile dysfunction may be managed surgically. If an underlying disease causes the impotence, interventions are aimed at controlling the disease. Impotence resulting from hypothalamic – pituitary – gonadal dysfunction may be reversed with proper hormonal therapy, such as testosterone replacement or the administration of gonadotropin-releasing factor, or pituitary gonadotropins.

Surgical management may be employed for clients who are impotent because of physical causes. Clients with insufficient blood flow to the penis may be able to have an arterial bypass or other vascular procedures to correct their erectile dysfunction. Other clients may be candidates for a penile prosthesis if they meet the following criteria: irreversible physiologic impotence demonstrated by history and diagnostic testing, strong desire to sexually satisfy himself or his partner, the presence of some penile sensation, and the absence of any prostatic and genitourinary problems.

The types of penile prostheses available are the semirigid type, the self-contained type, and the inflatable type (Fig. 55 – 8). The semirigid and self-contained types are easier to insert, are less expensive, and necessitate fewer days in the hospital than implantation of the inflatable type.

The semirigid prosthesis consists of two silicone rods, which simulate a normal erection. These rods are implanted into the corpora cavernosa via a perineal or dorsal penile incision. This type of prosthesis has no moving parts that could break or malfunction, but the penis remains in a constant state of semierection which may be unacceptable to the client or his sexual partner.

The self-contained type of prosthesis is a newer variation of the semirigid type. Like the semirigid prosthesis, it is totally contained in the penis, but allows the penis to hang in a more natural position. A self-contained prosthesis consists of a cylinder, a pump, and a reservoir filled with fluid. By pumping the prosthesis behind the head of the penis, fluid is transferred from the reservoir

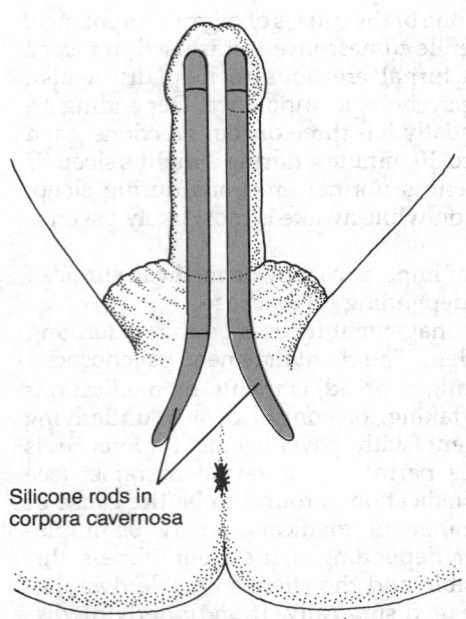

Semirigid penile prostheses consist of rods inserted into the corpora cavernosa via a perineal or dorsal penile incision. The penis remains in a constant state of semierection.

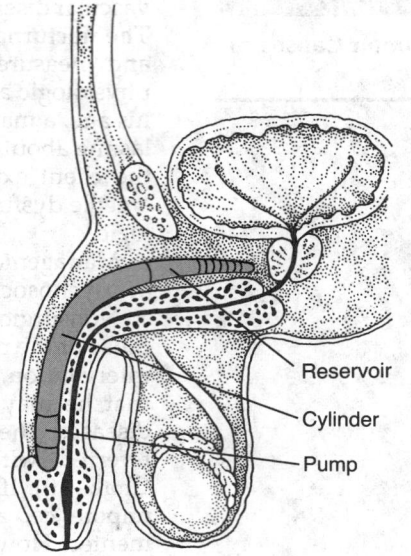

Self-contained penile prostheses consist of a pump, a cylinder, and a reservoir, all in a single unit. The client squeezes the pump just below the head of the penis to fill the cylinder and achieve erection.

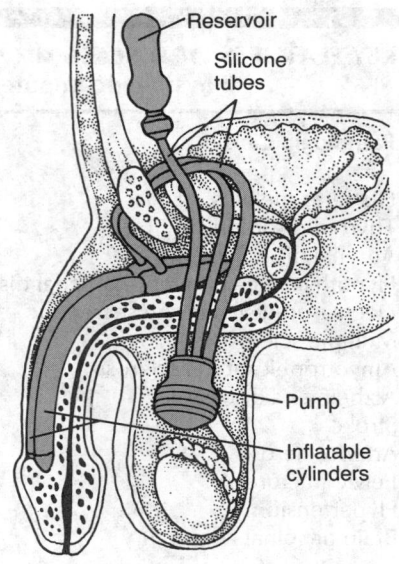

Inflatable penile prostheses consist of two hollow silicone cylinders, an abdominal reservoir, and a scrotal pump. The client squeezes the pump to fill the cylinders and achieve erection.

Figure 55–8

Penile prostheses.

in the rear portion of the device to the part of the device in the shaft of the penis. The cylinder then becomes enlarged and produces an erection. When an erection is no longer desired, the fluid is returned to the reservoir by pressing a release valve located behind the pump.

The inflatable type of prosthesis consists of two hollow silicone cylinders, a reservoir, and a pump. The cylinders are surgically implanted into the corpora cavernosa, the reservoir containing radiopaque fluid is placed under the abdominal fascia, and the pump is placed in the scrotum. When the pump in the scrotum is compressed, the fluid flows from the reservoir into each cylinder, causing an erection. A one-way valve keeps the fluid in the cylinders until a release valve in the pump is compressed, allowing the fluid to return to the reservoir. This type of prosthesis simulates natural erections and flaccidity, but mechanical problems may occur, and this type of prosthesis costs more than the others.

Postoperatively, the nurse observes the client with a penile prosthesis for complications, such as shock, atelectasis, pneumonia, fever, deep vein thrombosis, signs of wound infection, and urinary retention. Before discharge from the hospital, instructions for home care are given (see the accompanying Client/Family Education feature).

TESTICULAR CANCER

OVERVIEW

Although malignant tumors of the testis are rare and represent less than 2% of all cancers in men, testicular cancer is the third leading cause of cancer death in young men. Testicular cancer strikes young men at a productive time of life and thus has significant economic, social, and psychologic impact on the client and his family. However, with the advent of combination chemotherapy, testicular cancer, which once had a high death rate, has become one of the most curable cancers.

Pathophysiology

Primary testicular cancers fall into two major groups: *germinal* tumors arising from the sperm-producing germ cells and *nongerminal* tumors arising from the other structures in the testes. Germinal tumors are the most

---

CLIENT/FAMILY EDUCATION ■ Home Care After Penile Implant Surgery

Instructions	Rationales
1. "In the first 3–4 wk after surgery, you may have some itching caused by the sutures. This is normal. The sutures will dissolve completely in about 2 wk, and the incision itself should heal in 3–4 wk."	1, 2. To reduce client anxiety about normal postoperative events.
2. "During the first few weeks after surgery, you will have pain or discomfort where the prosthesis has been implanted. The pain usually starts to subside in a few weeks, but in some men it lasts longer. This is normal. The pain or discomfort will decrease. If your prosthesis is an inflatable or a self-contained inflatable one, you will experience pain temporarily as the prosthesis is inflated. This too is normal, and this pain will decrease."	
3. "You may shower or bathe the day after you leave the hospital."	3. To encourage return to normal daily hygiene measures.
4. "You do not need to wear a dressing, but you may want to. If so, place a piece of gauze over the incision and tape it in place with strips of surgical tape.."	4. To reduce irritation from rubbing of sutures on clothing.
5. "If you have a temperature of 101° F or greater, call your physician or report to the nearest emergency room."	5. To detect infection so that antibiotics can be administered promptly.
6. "Do not return to work until your incision has healed properly, usually within 2–4 wk."	6–8. To prevent injury
7. "Do not have sexual intercourse until 4–6 wk after injury."	
8. "Do not be afraid of normal physical activity, but be careful not to overdo it, especially in the first 2 wk. During this time, avoid driving, riding in a car for more than 20–25 min, walking more than ½ mile, climbing stairs quickly, lifting objects weighing more than 8 lb, or playing golf, tennis, or other sports."	
9. "After you leave the hospital, call your physician to schedule a follow-up appointment. At your follow-up visit, your physician will tell you how to use your prosthesis."	9. To ensure healing and restoration of function.

---

common type of testicular tumors, accounting for more than 95% of the cases (Mustofi & Price, 1973).

Germinal Tumors

Germinal tumors of the testis are classified into two broad categories: seminoma and nonseminoma (see the accompanying Key Features of Disease).

The most common type of testicular tumor is the *seminoma*. Clients with pure seminomatous tumors have the most favorable prognoses because the tumors generally remain localized and metastasize late. In most clients with seminomatous testicular tumors, seminomas are diagnosed when they are confined to the testicles and retroperitoneal lymph nodes. These tumors also respond extremely well to radiation therapy. Clients with early-stage seminomas have about a 95% 5-year survival rate with surgery (orchiectomy) and radiation therapy (National Institutes of Health [NIH], 1989).

Nonseminomatous germ cell tumors include three types: embryonal carcinoma, teratoma, and choriocarcinoma. These tumors are made up of cells that are not as sensitive to treatment with radiation therapy. Therefore, they are treated with surgery or chemotherapy, depending on the extent of the disease at presentation (NIH, 1989). *Pure embryonal carcinomas* are commonly found in young men between the ages of 19 and 26 years. Embryonal carcinoma tends to spread earlier than seminoma and most commonly first affects retroperitoneal lymph nodes. This type of tumor may also spread via the blood stream to other sites in the body, such as the lung or the liver. Pure *teratomas* rarely occur. They are usually found mixed with other types of testicular tumors. *Choriocarcinoma* is a lethal type of nonseminomatous cancer, which spreads rapidly throughout the body. Clients with choriocarcinoma almost always have metastatic disease when they are initially diagnosed, as choriocarcinoma spreads via the hematogenous route rather than via the lymphatic system.

KEY FEATURES OF DISEASE ■ Classification of Testicular Tumors

Germinal (Germ Cell) Tumors

Seminoma

Nonseminoma

    Embryonal carcinoma

    Teratoma

    Choriocarcinoma

Nongerminal (Non–Germ Cell) Tumors

Interstitial cell tumor

Androblastoma

Testicular cancers with a *mixture of cell types* are also common. Almost any combination of germ cell tumors is possible, but the most common combination is embryonal carcinoma and teratoma (*teratocarcinoma*). Twenty-four per cent of all testicular cancers are teratocarcinomas.

Nongerminal Tumors

The remaining 5% of testicular tumors arise from the nongerminal elements in the testes, such as the interstitial cells or cells that compose fibrous or vascular networks. Nongerminal testicular neoplasms are classified as either interstitial cell tumors or androblastomas (testicular adenomas).

Interstitial cell tumors, which arise from the Leydig cells (the cells that secrete testosterone into the blood stream), are rare and usually benign. These tumors often secrete an excessive amount of androgenic hormones, which causes young boys with such tumors to undergo an early puberty. *Androblastomas* (testicular adenomas) are also rare and usually benign. They sometimes secrete estrogen, which accounts for the feminization and gynecomastia (breast enlargement) occasionally seen in these clients.

Etiology

The etiology of testicular cancer is unknown. The risk of testicular tumors is reported to be higher in males who have an undescended testis (cryptorchidism). In cryptorchid males, the testicular cancer usually develops in the undescended testis (80%), and there is a 25% chance of developing cancer in the normally descended testis. Seminoma is the most common type of testicular cancer associated with cryptorchidism. The undescended testis undergoes gradual involution and degeneration over time, which may contribute to tumor development. It is not known why the normally descended testis is at risk

for development of cancer. Brothers and close male relatives of clients with testicular cancer have a 6% greater risk of testicular cancer than the general population.

Although a history of trauma or infection is common in clients who develop testicular cancer, these have not been established as causes of testicular cancer and may be coincidental findings at the time of the testicular examination. Therefore, it is important that the client with a history of trauma or infection be examined by a physician or nurse practitioner after the acute episode subsides to rule out the existence of a tumor.

Testicular cancer is rarely bilateral. There is only a 0.07% increased chance that a client with a tumor in one testis will develop another primary testicular tumor in the other testis. In rare instances, leukemias, lymphomas, plasmacytomas, and metastatic carcinomas may involve the testes. A client with bilateral testicular tumors is more likely to have metastatic disease to the testes than bilateral primary testicular tumors.

Incidence

The incidence of testicular cancer in the United States is 2 to 3 per 100,000 males (ACS, 1990). This cancer is the most common solid tumor diagnosed in men between the ages of 15 and 40 years and is the leading cause of cancer death in men 25 to 34 years of age. Testicular cancer can occur during infancy and middle age (after age 50); however, the peak incidence is between the ages of 18 and 40 years (ACS, 1990). Testicular cancer is most frequently found in Caucasians and is rare in Blacks. The incidence of testicular cancer is also low in Asia and New Zealand (Javadpour, 1980).

PREVENTION

Early diagnosis of testicular cancer is the key to successful treatment. The average time interval from the client's discovery of the lump in his testis to a physical examination by a health care professional is estimated to be approximately 5 months. Another delay in correct treatment for some clients can occur if there is an initial misdiagnosis of epididymitis, venereal disease, or musculoskeletal disorder. Any man who complains of scrotal or testicular enlargement, pain, heaviness, or a pulling or dragging sensation in the scrotum or groin should have his testes examined by a physician or nurse practitioner to verify the presence or absence of a mass. Any scrotal or testicular mass that does not transilluminate is assumed to be malignant until proved to be benign. Other causes of testicular symptoms are given in the accompanying Key Features of Disease on page 1759.

The major risk factor for testicular cancer is a cryptorchid or undescended testis. Before the age of 3 years, cellular differences between the undescended and the normal testis cannot be detected. Between the ages of 3 and 8 years, the normal testis begins to grow and de-

KEY FEATURES OF DISEASE ■ Common Benign Causes of Testicular Symptoms

Orchitis (infection or inflammation of the testis)
Epididymitis (infection or inflammation of the epididymis)
Torsion (twisting of the testicle, usually during trauma)
Hydrocele (accumulation of fluid in the scrotum)
Varicocele (engorgement of the veins in the scrotum)

velop, but the undescended testis does not. The undescended testis gradually involutes and degenerates; this can lead to cancer. If the cryptorchid testis is surgically transferred to the scrotum (see later discussion of orchidopexy for cryptorchidism) before the child reaches 2 to 3 years of age, the testis develops normally. The majority of testicular tumors in cryptorchid males occur in individuals who have never had an orchidopexy performed or who had the procedure after they were 6 years old. (It is therefore recommended that cryptorchid males who did not undergo orchidopexy at an early age have a prophylactic unilateral orchiectomy.) Nurses in obstetric and pediatric settings should screen all male infants and children for this easily reversible condition.

There is a need for teaching the public how to perform a testicular self-examination (TSE). Community health nurses should institute local education and screening programs in the school systems, in boys' and men's clubs, and in the military to help with the early diagnosis of testicular cancer. Nurses in hospital settings should teach TSE to clients who may be at risk for testicular cancer. The technique is performed as described in Chapter 25.

COLLABORATIVE MANAGEMENT

 Assessment

History

When taking a history from a client with a suspected testicular tumor, it is important for the nurse to keep the risk factors in mind. Basic but important data to collect are *age* and *race,* because the disease occurs most frequently in Caucasian males between the ages of 15 and 40 years. Other risk factors to be alert for include a history or presence of an *undescended testis* and a *family history* of testicular cancer.

In addition to information about the client, the nurse assesses the client's family situation. Is the client married? Does the client have children? Does he want children in the future? Depending on the treatment plan chosen, would he be interested in sperm storage in a sperm bank? If the client has one healthy testis, he can function sexually and may not have any reproductive dysfunction. If the client undergoes a retroperitoneal

NURSING RESEARCH

Study Finds That Few College Men Practice Testicular Self-Examination.

Reno, D. R. (1988). Men's knowledge and health beliefs about testicular cancer and testicular self-examination. *Cancer Nursing, 11,* 112–117.

This study used an adapted version of the Health Belief Model as a framework to examine men's knowledge and beliefs about testicular cancer and TSE.

A convenience sample of 126 college males enrolled in a midwestern state university were administered a questionnaire designed to measure factual knowledge, beliefs about the benefits of TSE, and beliefs about susceptibility to testicular cancer. Statistical analyses included descriptive statistics, the chi-square test, Pearson's product moment correlation coefficient, and the Mann-Whitney U test.

Only 12 subjects were found to practice TSE. Of the 114 who did not practice TSE, 87% had not heard about it, but said they would practice it if taught how to do it. The findings suggested a relationship between perceived susceptibility and benefits and whether TSE was practiced.

Critique. The small convenience sample does not allow for generalizability to other populations without further replications with different samples.

Possible nursing implications. The findings of this study suggest that TSE information should be provided to young men to encourage routine practice of this health care behavior, just as breast self-examination is taught to young women. Nurses in settings in which male clients are seen can promote this health care practice by providing information on testicular cancer and how to perform self-examination.

lymph node dissection or chemotherapy, he may become sterile because of treatment effects on the sperm-producing cells or surgical trauma to the sympathetic nervous system, resulting in retrograde ejaculations.

Physical Assessment: Clinical Manifestations

Physical examination of the testes should be performed as described in Chapter 52. A thorough examination of the lymph nodes and abdomen should also be performed. The presence of any *palpable lymphadenopathy, abdominal masses,* or *gynecomastia* usually indicates metastatic disease. The nurse should also examine the chest for any evidence of pulmonary metastasis. Chapter 60 describes physical assessment of the respiratory system.

Psychosocial Assessment

Because the diagnosis of testicular cancer occurs during the client's most productive years, the nurse pays close attention to the psychosocial ramifications of the disease. Even if the cancer is detected at an early stage and the client is cured after orchiectomy, he may be afraid that he is sexually handicapped. Even if the client's disease is arrested with surgery, radiation, or chemotherapy, he may think of himself as less than a whole man. These fears can disrupt the psychosocial and sexual development of the young male, as well as threaten the identity of adult males. The client may be afraid that he will not be able to perform sexually, will no longer be sexually attractive or desirable, and will face rejection. Feelings of sexual inadequacy may be denied, repressed, or displaced, causing increased stress on his personal and work relationships. It is important that the nurse perform a psychosocial assessment of these clients on a routine basis, because problems may arise at any time, and make referrals to other resources as appropriate. The reader is referred to Chapter 10 for a further assessment of the client's sexuality.

Laboratory Findings

An important diagnostic indicator for the client with a testicular mass is the presence of any serum or urinary marker proteins (tumor markers) that are often produced by testicular cancers. *Benign* testicular tumors *never* cause an elevation in the levels of any of these marker proteins.

The primary tumor markers for testicular cancer are alpha-fetoprotein (AFP) and the beta subunit of human chorionic gonadotropin (hCG-β). Approximately 90% of clients with nonseminomatous testicular tumors (embryonal carcinoma, teratoma, or choriocarcinoma) initially have elevated serum levels of AFP, hCG-β, or both. Clients with pure seminoma do not have an elevated AFP level, and only 10% have a slightly elevated hCG-β level, and this resolves after orchiectomy.

If a client has a diagnosis of seminoma and also has an elevated AFP level, he must have his tumor specimen re-examined for evidence of a component of nonseminomatous cancer. This step is necessary because the treatments differ for seminomatous and nonseminomatous tumors.

AFP and hCG-β determinations are also utilized to evaluate responses to therapy for testicular cancer and to document the presence of residual or recurrent disease. With effective treatment, the levels of abnormal markers fall. The persistence of elevated levels of markers after orchiectomy is substantive evidence that the client has metastatic disease, even if results of clinical staging procedures (x-ray films and scans) are normal. The reappearance of the tumor markers heralds a recurrence of the cancer. Therefore, marker levels must be monitored regularly during the follow-up of clients treated for testicular cancer.

Radiographic Findings

After the diagnosis of testicular cancer, the client should have a CT scan of the abdomen and the chest, or chest tomograms, to identify any small lesions not apparent on conventional x-ray films or physical assessment.

Clients with pure seminoma undergo bipedal lymphangiography as part of the staging work-up to assess for any evidence of retroperitoneal lymph node involvement. Lymphangiograms are also valuable in determining the extent of radiation therapy.

Other Diagnostic Tests

After a mass has been discovered, the client undergoes an orchiectomy. The standard surgical approach is the inguinal orchiectomy (the total removal of the testicle through an inguinal incision) (see the accompanying Client Care Plan for appropriate nursing care). A biopsy, the usual diagnostic procedure with most other masses or tumors, is contraindicated for testicular tumors because of the possible risk of disseminating tumor cells along the spermatic cord or into the scrotal sac. If the testicular mass is malignant, a transscrotal biopsy may increase the risk of local recurrence of the cancer.

Surgical implantation of a gel-filled silicone prosthesis into the scrotum can usually be performed at the time of the orchiectomy or at a later date if the client so desires. The nurse needs to assure the client that this surgery does not impair fertility or sexual function and the client cosmetically appears to have two testes.

 Analysis: Nursing Diagnosis

Common Diagnoses

The following diagnoses are commonly found in the man with testicular cancer:

1. Knowledge deficit related to treatment
2. Sexual dysfunction related to treatment

Additional Diagnoses

Depending on the extent of malignancy and the type of treatment selected, the following diagnoses may be appropriate:

1. Dysfunctional grieving or anticipatory grieving related to loss of a body part or changes in body function
2. Body image disturbance and altered role performance related to diagnosis of cancer

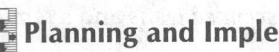 **Planning and Implementation**

Knowledge Deficit

Planning: client goals. The major goal is that the client will demonstrate an understanding of the nonsurgical and surgical treatments of a testicular cancer.

Interventions. A combination of nonsurgical and surgical management is often necessary to prevent the occurrence of metastatic disease or to provide relief from

CLIENT CARE PLAN ■ The Client Undergoing Orchiectomy

Goal/Outcome Criteria	Interventions	Rationales
Nursing Diagnosis 1: Knowledge Deficit Related to Orchiectomy for Suspected Testicular Cancer		
Client verbalizes an understanding of the surgical procedure. ■ States how the surgery will be performed. ■ States why levels of tumor markers are determined preoperatively and in follow-up care.	1. In addition to the topics covered in the standard preoperative care plan, the client undergoing an orchiectomy for suspected testicular cancer needs information on the following: a. Surgery via the inguinal approach is preferred instead of the scrotal approach when testicular cancer is suspected, because the latter increases the risk of metastases. b. AFP and hCG-β levels are elevated in clients with testicular tumors. These tumor markers are evaluated preoperatively and during follow-up.	1. To increase understanding of the surgical treatment.
Client discusses the impact of the surgery on his sexuality. ■ Verbalizes concerns about body image and sexuality.	1. Encourage the client to verbalize his feelings regarding body image and sexuality. a. Teach the client about the impact of orchiectomy on sexual drive, sexual function, and fertility. Because the client has a remaining functional testis, he is able to function sexually. b. Remind the client that he may need additional treatment in the future. c. Inform the client that a silicone gel–filled prosthetic testis can be inserted at the time of orchiectomy or at a later date.	1. To elicit concerns that client will no longer be sexually attractive or that he will be impotent or sterile and to alleviate anxiety.
Client understands his discharge instructions. ■ Verbalizes an understanding of instructions, schedules a follow-up examination, and knows how to get in touch with the physician.	1. Include the following in discharge teaching: a. General postoperative instructions. b. Emphasis on the need for follow-up examinations. c. Information on support groups (see Unit 15 Resources).	1. To prevent complications and facilitate recovery.

symptoms associated with metastatic disease and cause tumor regression. The nurse provides information about the different interventions that are used to treat testicular cancer.

Nonsurgical management. Nonsurgical management of the client at high risk for metastatic disease or of the client with metastatic disease consists of chemotherapy and radiation therapy.

Chemotherapy. Combination chemotherapy may be used as adjuvant therapy for nonseminomatous testicular tumors or as primary treatment when there is evidence of metastatic disease. Combination chemotherapy is dramatically effective in treating nonseminomatous testicular cancer, particularly if cisplatin (Platinol) is used. This agent is necessary in any successful combination chemotherapy regimen for treating testicular cancer. Other drugs commonly used in combination with cisplatin are bleomycin sulfate (Blenoxane), vinblastine sulfate (Velban), etoposide (VP-16-213), dactinomycin (actinomycin D), cyclophosphamide (Cytoxan), and doxorubicin (Adriamycin). The specific combination of drugs; the route of administration; and the frequency, cycling, and duration of treatment can vary considerably from client to client, depending on the extent of the disease and the particular protocol being followed by the physician. Chapter 25 discusses the nursing care of the client receiving chemotherapy.

Radiation therapy. After orchiectomy, external beam radiation therapy is the treatment of choice for clients with pure seminomatous testicular cancer (stage II disease) because of the marked radiosensitivity of this type of testicular cancer. If radiation therapy is administered, a staging lymphangiogram is used to determine the treatment portals. Preservation of reproductive function is another advantage of using radiation therapy instead of radical lymph node dissection, because surgical dissection of the sympathetic ganglia is avoided. To preserve reproductive function, the client undergoing radiation therapy to the retroperitoneal lymph nodes should have his remaining testis shielded with lead cups. Normally, the client's sperm count returns to the pretreatment level 24 to 30 months after the completion of the radiation treatment. Even though the client's remaining testis is shielded with a lead cup, it is not uncommon for the client to have transient oligospermia, or decreased sperm count, owing to radiation scatter. Clients who develop metastases outside the lymphatic system may still be cured with radiation therapy if the area of involvement is limited. However, if there is extensive lymphatic involvement, or involvement of the visceral organs, combination chemotherapy similar to that for nonseminomatous testicular cancer is used. Chapter 25 discusses the nursing care for the client receiving external radiation therapy.

Surgical management. A unilateral orchiectomy is used for diagnosis and primary surgical management of the client with a testicular tumor (see earlier). Additional surgical management of clients with testicular cancer is a radical retroperitoneal lymph node dissection. Radical retroperitoneal lymph node dissections are performed to accurately stage the disease and to debulk or reduce the tumor volume so that chemotherapy or radiation therapy is more effective.

A *radical retroperitoneal lymph node dissection* involves the removal of the retroperitoneal nodes in the iliac and lumbar regions. Because the blood supply and the lymphatic vessels of the testes and kidneys are directly related, an extensive midline incision from the xiphoid process to the pubis is necessary. After mobilization of the colon, the perinephric nodes are removed, along with the nodes near the aorta and both renal hila. The node dissection also includes the inguinal area on the affected side. During the lymphadenectomy, the sympathetic ganglia around the lower lumbar lymphatics are dissected. This removal of the sympathetic ganglia abolishes peristalsis in the ductus deferens and contractions of the seminal vesicles. This disruption results in sterility because the client's ejaculate no longer contains sperm. This surgery, however, usually does not interfere with the client's ability to have a normal erection and does not affect his ability to experience orgasm.

The postoperative needs of the client should be anticipated and planned for preoperatively. The nurse informs the client and his family about what to expect postoperatively. The surgical incision for a retroperitoneal lymph node dissection is quite extensive. Depending on the extent of the dissection and the need for surgical exploration, the client may have not only a midline incision but also a transthoracic incision or a combination of the two incisions (thoracoabdominal). The nurse should be aware and inform the client that radical retroperitoneal lymph node dissections are relatively long operations, lasting from 6 to 14 hours. It is also routine for clients to go to a critical care unit immediately postoperatively. The nurse needs to assure the client and the family that a long operation and subsequent admission to the critical care unit does not necessarily indicate problems or that the client is in a life-threatening situation. Clients undergoing radical retroperitoneal lymph node dissections need close and frequent observation, which is most expertly done by nurses in a critical care unit.

Because of the length of the surgery, the manipulation of the abdominal and retroperitoneal viscera, and the loss of a major part of the lymphatic fluid, nodes, and channels, the nurse observes and assesses the client for any of the complications of major abdominal surgery (see the accompanying Client Care Plan). Expected problems for which the nurse intervenes are pain related to surgical incisions, immobility related to prolonged maintenance of surgical positioning and postoperative pain, and injuries related to any invasive catheters or tubes.

The hospitalization for a client having a radical retroperitoneal lymph node dissection is 10 to 14 days or longer. Client and family education (see the accompanying feature) regarding care after discharge is offered during this time.

Sexual Dysfunction

Planning: client goals. The major goals for this diagnosis are that the client will (1) identify potential or actual alterations in reproductive function and (2) identify alternate methods of meeting reproductive needs.

Interventions: nonsurgical management. There is an increased incidence of oligospermia and azoospermia in clients with testicular cancer at the time of diagnosis. It has been speculated that this may be due to the disease process itself and to stress. However, the exact reasons are unknown. The client may not discover that he is oligospermic or azoospermic until he has a presurgery sperm count. This discovery of infertility occurs when the client is trying to cope with the diagnosis of cancer and its consequences and can become an additional major stressor for an already anxious client and family. If the client does have an adequate sperm count he may be interested in sperm storage in a sperm bank before undergoing treatment. Male cancer clients who are not candidates for sperm storage in a sperm bank

CLIENT CARE PLAN ■ The Client Recovering from Retroperitoneal Lymph Node Dissection

Goal/Outcome Criteria	Interventions	Rationales
Nursing Diagnosis 1: Potential for Injury Related to Surgery		

Client will not experience shock
■ Has no signs or symptoms of shock.
	1. Assess the client for signs and symptoms of shock q 2–4 h if the client is stable, and every 15 min if unstable.
	  a. Monitor vital signs.
	  b. Monitor urinary output.
	  c. Monitor skin color and temperature.
	  d. Notify the physician immediately of any signs or symptoms of shock.
		1. To detect neurogenic shock from prolonged anesthesia and hypovolemic shock from loss of lymphatic fluid secondary to lymph node dissection. The client is at high risk for both types of shock.

Client will not experience any wound complications.
■ Has temperature within normal limits.
■ Experiences wound healing.
	1. Assess the wound for potential complications.
	  a. Monitor the dressing for drainage.
	  b. Inspect the incision, which is extensive (from ribs to pelvis) and may drain moderately, often through an incision drain (Penrose's or Jackson-Pratt drain).
	2. Monitor the client's temperature.
		1, 2. To detect infection or dehiscence.

Client will not experience any electrolyte imbalance.
■ Has electrolyte values within normal limits.
	1. Monitor fluid intake and output closely.
	  a. IV intake.
	  b. Urinary output.
	  c. Nasogastric output.
		1. To detect electrolyte imbalance attributable to large fluid shift secondary to the procedure. Recording the client's output (especially nasogastric drainage) is important for calculating the amount of replacement fluid and electrolytes needed. The client is at risk for urinary retention from prolonged anesthesia.

CLIENT/FAMILY EDUCATION ■ Home Care After Testicular Surgery

Instructions	Rationales
1. "After you leave the hospital, call your physician to schedule a follow-up appointment."	1. To ensure healing and detect complications.
2. "If any of the following occur before your follow-up appointment, call your physician: chills or fever, increasing tenderness or pain around the incision, drainage from the incision, or opening of the incision."	2. To allow prompt interventions for complications.
3. "Do not lift anything heavier than 20 lb and do not climb stairs. Ask your doctor when you can resume these activities. After 1 wk you should be able to resume most of your normal activities."	3. To prevent injury.
4. "Each month, perform TSE on the remaining testis."	4. To detect metastases or new primary tumors.
5. "Continue to make follow-up appointments with your doctor for at least 3 years. Your physician will probably have your urine and blood checked during follow-up visits."	5. To detect recurrence.

may select from other options, such as donor insemination, adoption, or not fathering children. It is essential that the nurse initiate client education about reproduction, fertility, and sexuality in the pretreatment phase. The nurse begins by reviewing normal reproductive function and explains the effects that cancer and its treatment may have on reproductive function. The nurse reviews various reproductive options with the client and gives the client general information on sperm banks and artificial insemination (see the accompanying Client/Family Education feature). The sperm bank facility provides comprehensive information on the semen collection and storage procedures, the storage contract, costs, and the insemination process.

When preparing the client for the collection and storage of sperm, the nurse assumes the role of client advocate and keeps in mind the effect of the cancer diagnosis on the client. The psychologic benefit of having stored sperm may be important for the client and influence his response to treatment. Knowing that the potential for being a father still exists may help the client cope with other assaults to his masculinity, such as alopecia or erectile dysfunction.

It is important that the client arrange for semen storage as soon as possible after diagnosis. It is essential that the sperm collection be completed before the client begins radiation therapy or chemotherapy or undergoes a radical retroperitoneal lymph node dissection. After radiation therapy or chemotherapy has been implemented, the client may be at increased risk for producing mutagenic sperm, which may not be viable or could result in fetal abnormalities.

The recommended number of samples to optimize the chances of later fertilization is three to six ejaculates, collected 2 to 4 days apart. This procedure could delay the client's treatment for as long as 1 month, especially if the client is still recovering from surgery and multiple procedures or tests. The client's diagnosis (e.g., acute leukemia, sarcoma, advanced lymphoma, or testicular cancer) and his physical condition may not allow the client to postpone treatment, making sperm storage an unfeasible reproductive option.

■ Discharge Planning

The client is hospitalized for approximately 3 to 5 days after an orchiectomy. However, the period of hospitalization may need to be extended if the client must undergo additional surgery or chemotherapy. Because it may not be known until after the orchiectomy whether the client has cancer or what type of testicular cancer he has, or if he needs additional surgery or treatment with radiation therapy or chemotherapy, discharge planning may need to be deferred until the postoperative period.

Home Care Preparation

After a unilateral orchiectomy, unless the client has a wound complication, he should be discharged without a dressing on his inguinal incision (unless he chooses to wear one to prevent his clothing from rubbing on his sutures and producing irritation). Because his sutures are intact at the time of discharge from the hospital, he is told that they will be removed in the physician's office 10 to 14 days postoperatively.

Because the hospitalization for a radical retroperitoneal lymph node dissection is 10 to 14 days or longer, the client usually has his sutures removed before discharge from the hospital. His incision should be healed, so he should not require a dressing.

Client/Family Education

The nurse emphasizes to the client who has had an orchiectomy or radical retroperitoneal lymph node dissection the importance of scheduling a follow-up visit with the physician who will examine his incision for healing and complications. The nurse instructs the client to notify the physician if any of the following symptoms occur before his scheduled appointment: chills, fever, increasing tenderness or pain around the incision, drainage, or dehiscence of the incision. These symptoms may indicate the presence of an infection and require medical attention. The client is instructed by the nurse that he will be able to resume most of his usual activities within 1 week after discharge from the hospital, except lifting heavy objects (> 20 lb) or stair climbing. The nurse instructs the client to ask his physician when strenuous activities may be resumed.

The client who has had an orchiectomy is instructed that he may make arrangements with his physician to have a silicone prosthesis inserted into his scrotum if a prosthesis was not inserted at the time of the orchiectomy.

CLIENT/FAMILY EDUCATION ■ **Information on Sperm Banking**

"You may want to investigate sperm storage in a sperm bank as a way to preserve your sperm for future use."

"No one knows how long sperm can be stored successfully, but pregnancies have occurred using sperm that have been stored longer than 10 yr."

"You should check with the sperm bank facility to see how much it costs to process and store the sperm and if payment must be made when the service is provided."

"You also need to see if your health insurance company will reimburse you for the sperm collection and storage."

"Usually, you have to collect the semen specimen at the facility because sperm need to be processed 30–60 min after ejaculation when they are the most viable and motile."

"The facility will provide specific instructions for collection of the sperm."

"Most facilities will store any or all successful specimens collected."

The nurse also instructs the client about the importance of performing monthly TSE on his remaining testis and to schedule follow-up examinations with his physician. The client who has had testicular cancer should have determinations of urinary and serum levels of tumor markers checked and CT or magnetic resonance imaging performed as part of his routine follow-up for a minimum of 3 years.

Depending on the pathologic findings and the stage of the client's cancer, he may need to undergo further treatment. This information may not be available when the client is discharged from the hospital. If it is known that the client needs further surgery, he and his family need information about the future surgery. If it is known that the client must undergo radiation therapy or chemotherapy, he needs education about his radiation therapy and chemotherapy regimen (see Chap. 25).

Psychosocial Preparation

The client who undergoes treatment for testicular cancer may need emotional support. If permanent sterility occurs and sperm storage was not feasible, the man may need to be counseled about other options for reproduction.

Health Care Resources

The client may be referred to agencies or support groups such as RESOLVE or the American Fertility Society (see Unit 15 Resources).

 Evaluation

On the basis of the identified nursing diagnoses, the nurse evaluates the care of the man who has been treated for testicular cancer. The expected outcomes are that the client

1. Does not have recurrence of cancer or metastases
2. Accepts body image changes and exhibits adaptation to his altered self-concept
3. Verbalizes feelings of grief
4. Recovers from surgery, chemotherapy, or radiation therapy without complications
5. Verbalizes an understanding of the effects of surgery or radiation therapy on sexual function and identifies alternative methods of meeting reproductive needs

COMMON PROBLEMS AFFECTING THE TESTES AND ADJACENT STRUCTURES

Problems that develop inside the scrotum usually occur as a mass or as scrotal edema. Some problems produce pain, whereas others do not. Figure 55–9 shows some of

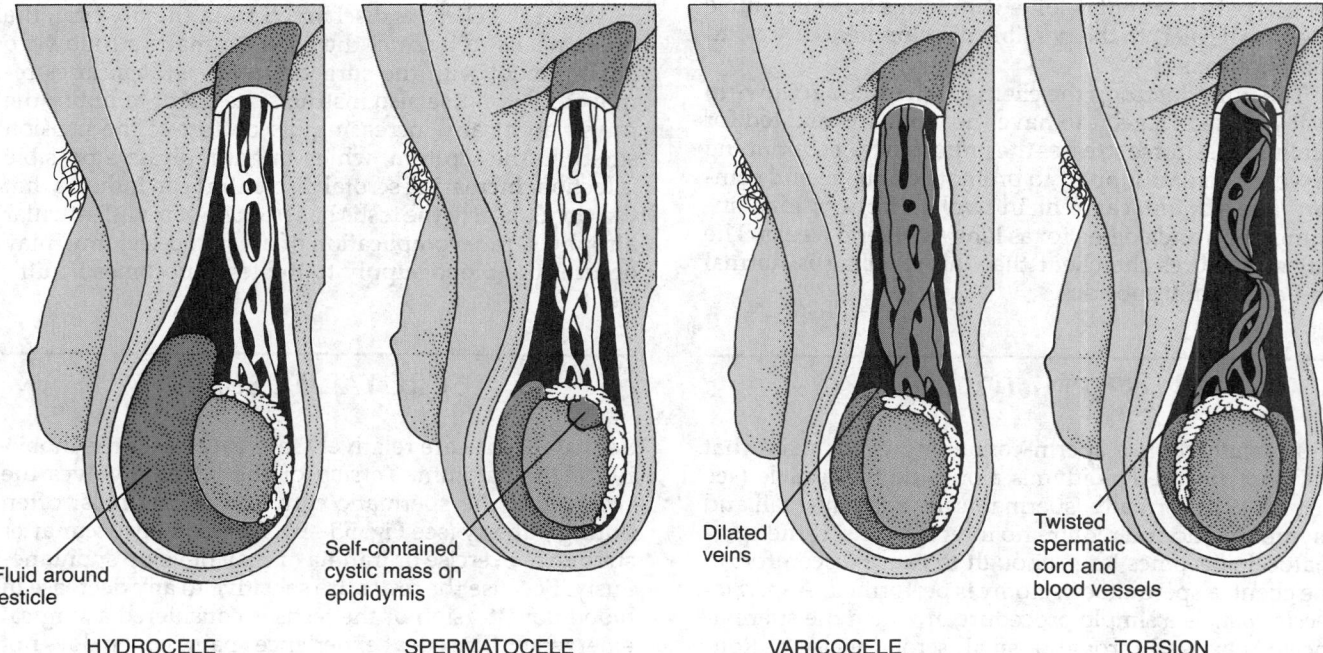

Figure 55–9

Common problems affecting the testes and adjacent structures.

the most frequent conditions found in the male: hydrocele, spermatocele, varicocele, and scrotal trauma.

HYDROCELE

A *hydrocele* (see Fig. 55–9) is a cystic mass, usually filled with straw-colored fluid, which forms around the testis. It is the result of a disorder in the lymphatic drainage of the scrotum, causing a swelling of the tunica vaginalis, which surrounds the testes. Unless the swelling becomes large and uncomfortable or begins to compromise the circulation to the testis, no treatment is necessary.

A hydrocele may be aspirated via a needle and syringe or surgically removed. To surgically correct a hydrocele, an incision is made in the scrotum and the hydrocele is removed. The client may or may not return from the operating room with a drain at the incision site. Normally, hydrocelectomies are performed on an outpatient basis, but, if the client requires hospitalization, it is for only 1 or 2 days. The nurse instructs the client that if an incision drain is present, there is usually some serosanguineous drainage for the first 24 to 48 hours after surgery. The nurse also instructs the client about the importance of wearing a scrotal support. The scrotal support keeps the scrotal dressing in place and keeps the scrotum elevated, which helps to prevent edema.

Clients vary considerably in the degree of pain experienced with this surgery. The nurse assesses and observes the client for pain every 2 to 3 hours in the immediate postoperative period. Moderate incision pain is expected for approximately 24 hours after surgery and should markedly decrease within 1 or 2 days. If the client's pain does not resolve within this time, the nurse needs to be alert to the possible development of wound complications.

The nurse instructs the client to schedule a follow-up visit with his surgeon to have the wound evaluated for healing. The nurse stresses the importance of continuing to wear a scrotal support to promote drainage and comfort. The scrotum can remain swollen from residual inflammation and edema for as long as several weeks. The nurse reassures the client that this swelling is normal and eventually subsides.

SPERMATOCELE

A *spermatocele* is a sperm-containing cystic mass that develops on the epididymis alongside the testicle (see Fig. 55–9). Normally, spermatoceles remain small and asymptomatic and require no interventions. If the spermatocele becomes large enough to cause discomfort to the client, a spermatocelectomy is performed. A *spermatocelectomy* is a simple procedure in which the spermatocele is excised through a small scrotal incision. Routinely, no incision drain is used, as drainage and swelling are minimal.

VARICOCELE

A *varicocele* is a cluster of dilated veins posterior to and above the testis (see Fig. 55–9). Varicoceles can be diagnosed by scrotal palpation, particularly when the client performs a Valsalva maneuver. The scrotum feels "worm-like" when palpated. Varicoceles can be either unilateral or bilateral, but most are unilateral and on the left side of the scrotum. In many cases, varicoceles are asymptomatic and require no treatment. In a few men, varicoceles are painful and require surgical removal. Varicoceles can also cause infertility in some men. It is generally believed that the increase in scrotal temperature resulting from the venous stasis near the testis is the etiology of the altered spermatogenesis.

Surgical removal of the varicocele (a *varicocelectomy*) is usually performed through an inguinal incision, in which the spermatic veins are ligated in the cord, or through an incision adjacent to the superior iliac spine, in which the spermatic veins are ligated in the retroperitoneal space.

A varicocelectomy may be done on an outpatient basis, or the client may be hospitalized for 1 or 2 days.

The nurse is aware that persistent venous congestion of the scrotum is common after this type of surgery because of the changed circulation in the area and explains this to the client preoperatively. To promote drainage of the scrotum, a rolled towel is placed under the scrotum while the client is in bed. The nurse may also apply ice to the scrotum if necessary. Any intervention that facilitates drainage and decreases swelling from the area promotes relief. The nurse instructs the client about the importance of wearing a scrotal support while ambulating.

When the client is discharged from the hospital, the nurse needs to instruct the client to make a follow-up appointment with the surgeon to have the sutures removed. The nurse also instructs the client to notify the physician of any increasing discomfort at the incision site or in the scrotum, which might indicate a possible infection. Increasing scrotal discomfort can indicate that the circulation to the testis has been impaired. Testicular atrophy, a rare complication of a varicocelectomy, may occur if the blood supply to the testis becomes insufficient.

SCROTAL TRAUMA

Scrotal injuries are relatively rare because of the mobility of the scrotum. *Torsion* of the testes involves the twisting of the spermatic cord and occurs most often during puberty (see Fig. 55–9). Torsion may occur after strenuous exercise or trauma or may develop spontaneously. Because the testes are sensitive to any decrease in blood flow, torsion of the testis is considered a surgical emergency. The client experiences pain, which does not subside with scrotal elevation. In addition to pain, the client usually complains of nausea and vomiting.

In addition to caring for the physical needs of the client with an injury to his scrotum, the nurse must be attuned to the psychosexual needs of these clients. Of primary concern to the male client with an injury to his external genitalia are his masculinity and sexuality. The nurse must be ready to use crisis intervention techniques and knowledge of sexuality to assist the client to adjust to the injury to the genital area.

CRYPTORCHIDISM

An undescended testis (*cryptorchidism*) is mainly a pediatric problem. Three per cent of full-term male infants and 20% of premature infants have an undescended testis. In approximately 80% of cases, the undescended testis descends spontaneously during the infant's first year. If an adult is found to have bilateral cryptorchidism, an orchidopexy (surgical placement of the testicle into the scrotum) is performed not only for cosmetic and psychosexual reasons but also to prevent the adverse effect of body temperature on spermatogenesis and primarily to reduce the risk of testicular cancer and to facilitate its early detection.

For an *orchidopexy*, the client is placed in a supine position, the surgeon makes an inguinal incision, and the spermatic cord is released from the surrounding fascia to obtain maximal length. The surgeon then creates a dartos pouch and places the testis between the skin and the dartos muscle of the scrotum. The tunica albuginea of the testis is sutured to the dartos muscle of the scrotum. The inguinal incision and the scrotal incision (if there is one) are then closed, and a dressing is applied. If there is an incision in the scrotum, it is also covered with a dressing, and the client should be instructed to wear a scrotal support.

PROBLEMS AFFECTING THE PENIS

CARCINOMA OF THE PENIS

Carcinoma of the penis represents less than 1% of all malignancies in men in the United States. Epidermoid carcinoma is the most common cancer of the penis. In countries where circumcision is not practiced, such as India, China, or African countries, it represents approximately 12% of all cancers (ACS, 1990).

Carcinoma of the penis usually occurs as a painless wart-like growth or ulcer on the glans under the prepuce (foreskin) and may initially be mistaken for a veneral wart (see Chap. 56). It may appear as a reddened lesion with plaque. Small lesions involving only the skin may be controlled by excisional biopsy. When the lesion is not curable by excisional biopsy or radiation therapy, a penectomy (partial or total removal of the penis) may be required. When the lesion is limited to the glans, a partial penectomy is performed. For a partial penectomy, the client is placed in a lithotomy position, and a tourniquet is applied around the penis. An incision is made to amputate a portion of the corpora cavernosa and corpus spongiosum. The urethra is anastomosed to the skin, and a dressing is applied. The client has a Foley catheter in place for 3 to 5 days after the surgery until the edema surrounding the urethra subsides. The nurse assesses the dressing for drainage, which should be minimal, and the catheter for patency every 4 hours for the first postoperative day.

A total penectomy is required when the lesion has penetrated the shaft of the penis or when the tumor has recurred after a partial penectomy or radiation therapy. For a total penectomy, the client is placed in a lithotomy position, and an incision is made from the pubic bone, encircles the penis, and extends into the perineum. The bases of both corpora cavernosa are exposed and excised, and the penis is amputated. An incision drain is placed in the wound before it is sutured. Clients who undergo a total penectomy also have a perineal urethrotomy (anastomosis of the urethra to the skin in the perineum) for urinary drainage. After a total penectomy, the nurse observes the incision dressing every 2 to 4 hours during the first 24 to 48 hours postoperatively. There may be a moderate amount of serosanguineous drainage from the wound from the incision drains.

The nurse caring for the client with a penectomy must be aware that, regardless of how accepting he may appear preoperatively, the client may experience severe emotional problems after the surgery. If the client undergoes a partial penectomy, he must adjust to considerable changes in body image and sexuality. The nurse encourages the client to verbalize his feelings about the loss of his penis. If the client undergoes a total penectomy, he is no longer able to have penile-vaginal or penile-anal intercourse and is not able to urinate in a standing position. It is difficult for most clients to accept the possibility that death can result from the lesion on the penis, especially because these clients are rarely experiencing any systemic cancer symptoms and are otherwise healthy. It is important for the nurse to help the client realize that the removal of his penis may save his life. The nurse needs to be aware of the possibility of suicide attempts, as the client's penis may be more important to him than his life. The nurse may be the one to detect the need for professional psychologic assistance for the client or his significant other. Early interventions by the nurse can make a tremendous difference in the client's or significant other's well-being.

Circumcision in infancy almost eliminates the possibility of penile cancer, as it is chronic irritation and inflammation of the glans penis that predisposes uncircumcised men to penile cancer. Because of the ongoing controversy about neonatal circumcision, it is important for nurses to teach both mothers and men that strict personal hygiene is the preventive measure against penile cancer.

PHIMOSIS

Phimosis is a condition in which the prepuce is constricted so that it cannot be retracted over the glans. Because there is a recent trend away from routine circumcision of newborns, the nurse needs to instruct new mothers, male children, and adult men in the importance of cleaning the prepuce. Phimosis is corrected by circumcision.

PROBLEMS RELATED TO CIRCUMCISION

Circumcision (the surgical removal of the prepuce from the penis) in the adult male is usually done for medical reasons, such as to correct phimosis and to eliminate the infections that frequently occur as a result of this condition.

When a circumcision is performed on an adult, one of two surgical procedures is used. For either method, the client is in a supine position. In the first procedure, the prepuce is pulled forward and clamped distal to the tip of the glans. The prepuce is then excised, the clamp is removed, and sutures are applied in the foreskin around the base of the glans (corona) to prevent bleeding. In the second method, the outer and inner surfaces of the prepuce are incised and dissected away without cutting the larger blood vessels in the prepuce. The two surfaces of the prepuce are approximated and sutured. A nonadhesive (Telfa or petrolatum [Vaseline]) dressing may or may not be applied after either procedure.

Normally, the client is discharged from the hospital on the same day of the circumcision. If the client has a dressing, the nurse instructs him to soak in a warm bath and allow the dressing to float off the next day. If the dressing falls off before the next day, the client is instructed not to replace it. The nurse informs the client that the sutures will be absorbed and need not be removed. The client is informed that there are no residual or side effects of this surgery and that he should be able to resume his normal activities within 1 week and sexual intercourse may be resumed after 1 to 2 weeks.

The client may be discharged with a prescription for barbiturate sleeping medication to be taken for several nights postoperatively. The nurse instructs the client that barbiturate sleeping medication suppresses the rapid eye movement phase of sleep, so that normal nocturnal erections do not occur. This prevents any tension on the sutures by an erection. Nonbarbiturate sleeping medications do not have this inhibiting effect on the nocturnal erection pattern. It is important that the nurse explain the relationship between barbiturate sleeping medication and nocturnal erections because the client may not comply with the instructions to take the medication, especially if he is not having any difficulty sleeping.

The nurse also instructs the client to notify his physician if he has any wound complications, such as swelling at the incision area or drainage, and to schedule a postoperative office visit.

PRIAPISM

Priapism is an uncontrolled and long-maintained erection without sexual desire, which causes the penis to become large, hard, and painful. Priapism affects the two corpora cavernosa; the corpus spongiosum and glans penis are not affected.

Priapism can occur from neural, vascular, or pharmacologic causes. Some of the common causes are thrombosis of the veins of the corpora cavernosa (usually resulting from trauma), leukemia, sickle cell anemia, diabetes, and malignancies. Sickle cell disease causes priapism by the accumulation of erythrocytes within the corporal bodies. Leukemia may cause priapism because the increase in the number of WBCs permits persistent engorgement of the corporal bodies. Malignancies may also infiltrate the corporal bodies, causing persistent engorgement. Priapism can also be the result of an abnormal neurogenic reflex, and priapism associated with psychotropic medications, antidepressants, and antihypertensives has been documented.

Priapism is considered a urologic emergency because the circulation to the penis may be compromised, and the client may not be able to void with an erect penis. The goal of medical intervention is improvement of the venous drainage of the corpora cavernosa. Conservative measures involve prostatic massage, sedation, and bed rest. Meperidine is usually administered immediately because of its hypotensive effect. Warm enemas may be administered to cause venous dilation and thus increase the outflow of the trapped blood. Urinary catheterization is required if the client is unable to void.

If conservative therapy is unsuccessful, treatment may proceed to aspiration of the corpora cavernosa with a large-bore needle or surgical intervention. The priapism should be resolved within the first 24 to 30 hours to prevent penile ischemia, gangrene, fibrosis, and impotence. If a cause of priapism is identified, treatment is directed toward that underlying cause.

It is important for the nurse who is caring for the client with priapism to be sensitive to his emotional needs. The client may be uncomfortable and in crisis, but at the same time embarrassed by his erection and loss of control. It is imperative that the nurse assure the client that he or she understands that the client is not in control of his erection and provide him with privacy.

PROBLEMS RELATED TO VASECTOMY

A *vasectomy* (Fig. 55–10) is an elective procedure for a man who wants a permanent method of contraception (although a small percentage of vasectomies are successfully reversed with a surgical procedure called a vasovasotomy). The procedure is routinely performed in an outpatient setting or in the urologist's office with local anesthesia.

The client is placed in a supine position. The vas deferens is palpated in the upper part of the scrotum, and an incision is made into the scrotal skin. The vas is

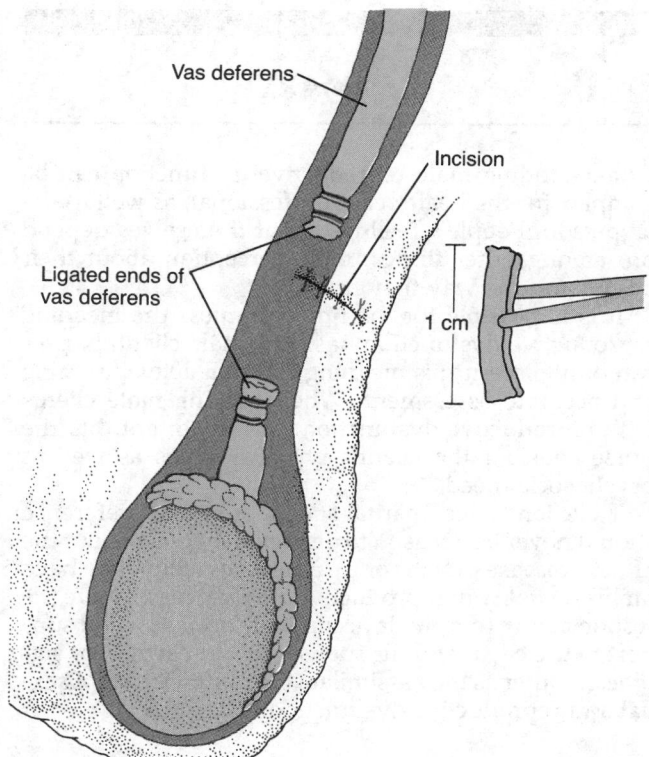

Figure 55–10

Vasectomy.

brought out through the incision and resected, the ends are ligated, and the incision is sutured. The procedure is then repeated on the other side. The nurse instructs the client that he may resume sexual intercourse whenever it is comfortable, but, because viable sperm are still in the ampulla of the vas, the client is instructed to continue to use another means of contraception until follow-up semen analyses document that the client is azoospermic or infertile.

The nurse instructs the client that complications after a vasectomy are rare. Any scrotal pain and swelling are usually relieved by the administration of aspirin or acetaminophen and the application of ice in the immediate postoperative period. The nurse instructs the client that he may find wearing Jockey shorts or a scrotal support increases comfort.

INFECTIONS

PROSTATITIS

A number of inflammatory conditions can affect the prostate gland. The most common is abacterial prostatitis. *Abacterial prostatitis* can occur after a viral illness or can result from a sudden decrease in sexual activity,

especially in young males. In many instances an exact etiology for the perineal discomfort cannot be found. It can be related to psychosexual problems. *Prostodynia* is a term sometimes used to describe this condition. *Bacterial prostatitis* is usually associated with urethritis or an infection of the lower urinary tract.

Organisms are believed to reach the prostate via the blood stream or the urethra. The most common organisms are *Escherichia coli, Enterobacter, Proteus,* and group D streptococci.

Acute bacterial prostatitis may be manifested by fever, chills, dysuria, urethral discharge, and a boggy, tender prostate. Gentle palpation of the prostate usually results in a urethral discharge, which is evidenced by WBCs in the prostatic secretions.

The client with chronic prostatitis usually complains of backache, perineal pain, mild dysuria, and urinary frequency; hematuria may be present. The prostate may feel irregularly enlarged, firm, and slightly tender when palpated. Complications of prostatitis are epididymitis (inflammation of the epididymis) and cystitis (inflammation of the bladder). A rare complication is a prostatic abscess. The client with either acute or chronic bacterial prostatitis is likely to experience urinary tract infections. He may have a decrease in sexual function because of discomfort.

Early diagnosis and treatment of prostatitis with antimicrobials such as carbenicillin indanyl sodium (Geocillin) or the newer quinolones can help prevent an abscess. The nurse instructs the client about the importance of utilizing comfort measures, such as sitz baths, and taking prescribed antibiotics on schedule, stool softeners to prevent straining and any rectal irritation of the prostate during a bowel movement, and any analgesics that may be used for symptomatic relief.

The nurse instructs the client with chronic prostatitis as to the long-term nature of the problem. Because prostatitis could cause other urinary tract infections, the nurse teaches the client about the importance of increasing fluid intake and long-term antibiotic therapy (for 30 days). Trimethoprim diffuses into the prostatic fluid, so it is the antibiotic of choice for the client with chronic prostatitis. The nurse instructs the client about activities that drain the prostate (intercourse, masturbation, and prostatic massage), which may help in the management of chronic prostatitis.

EPIDIDYMITIS

Epididymitis is an infection of the epididymis, which may result from an infection of the prostate. It used to be a frequent complication of gonorrhea. Epididymitis can also occur as a complication of long-term use of an indwelling Foley's catheter, prostatic surgery, and occasionally cystoscopic examination. In men younger than 35 years of age, the major cause of epididymitis is *Chlamydia trachomatis.* The infective organism passes upward through the urethra and the ejaculatory duct, and then along the vas deferens to the epididymis.

The client with epididymitis usually complains of pain along the inguinal canal and along the vas deferens and then pain and swelling in the scrotum and the groin. If epididymitis is untreated, the epididymis becomes swollen and painful and the client's temperature may become elevated. The client may develop pyuria and bacteriuria, with resultant chills and fever. An abscess may develop, necessitating an orchiectomy.

The nurse instructs the client with epididymitis to remain in bed with his scrotum elevated on a towel to prevent traction on the spermatic cord, to facilitate venous drainage, and to relieve pain. The client may be given antibiotics until all acute symptoms of inflammation are gone. If the epididymitis is chlamydial or gonorrheal in origin, the client's sexual partners must also be treated with antibiotics.

Other comfort measures that the client may find effective include the intermittent application of cold compresses or ice to the scrotum and sitz baths. The nurse instructs the client to avoid lifting, straining, or sexual activity until the infection is under control (which may take as long as 4 weeks). In a client with this condition, there must always be the suspicion of a testicular tumor, especially if the condition does not resolve in a week or two. Ultrasound is frequently employed to rule out an abscess or tumor. Clients with recurrent or chronic painful conditions may require an epididymectomy (the excision of epididymis from the testicle).

ORCHITIS

Orchitis is acute testicular inflammation. It may be the result of trauma or infection. The infection may be caused by the direct spread of bacteria through the urethra or from an infection elsewhere in the body, such as pneumonia, tuberculosis, gonorrhea, syphilis, or mumps. It is rare that the testes alone are involved; usually both the testes and the epididymis are involved (epididymo-orchitis).

Orchitis may be unilateral or bilateral. If the orchitis is bilateral, the client is at increased risk for sterility because of the testicular atrophy and fibrosis that occur during healing.

The signs and symptoms of orchitis are the same as those of epididymitis (scrotal pain and edema). In addition, the client may experience nausea and vomiting and pain radiating to the inguinal canal. The treatment of orchitis is the same as for epididymitis: bed rest with scrotal elevation, application of ice, and administration of analgesics and antibiotics.

Mumps orchitis, which occurs in approximately 20% of males who develop mumps after puberty, is usually bilateral, with the orchitis symptoms developing 4 to 6 days after the parotitis. Any postpubertal male who has not had mumps and is exposed to or contracts mumps is usually given gamma globulin. Although gamma globulin does not prevent mumps, the clinical course of the disease is likely to be less severe, with fewer complications. Childhood vaccination against mumps is an important preventive measure.

SUMMARY

Understanding male reproductive dysfunction can be complex for the health care professional, as well as the layperson. People's feelings about themselves depend on, among other things, their perception about their bodies and the way they function.

It is impossible for the nurse to guess the meaning reproductive dysfunction has for a male client. Nurses can only discern this meaning through active listening and accurate assessment. When helping male clients with reproductive dysfunction, it is important that the nurse consider the client's physical needs as well as psychosocial needs.

The client's age, marital status, or sexual preference should never be a reason to omit explanations about the effect a disease process or treatment modality may have on his sexuality or reproductive ability. Nurses have the responsibility to provide accurate information and support to the client and his spouse, sexual partner, or significant other as they assimilate the ramifications of sexual and reproductive dysfunction.

IMPLICATIONS FOR RESEARCH

Male reproductive dysfunction lends itself readily to nursing research. Because of its physiologic and psychologic components, nursing research on male reproductive dysfunction can be conducted in a wide variety of settings. Nursing research is necessary to develop a sound knowledge base from which to direct our teaching and practice. Some questions to investigate include

1. What do clients need to know about surgery on the male genitalia?
2. What are nurses' attitudes and beliefs related to men with reproductive dysfunction?
3. What are the factors influencing sexual activity after a prostatectomy?
4. What is the psychologic impact of testicular or prostate cancer on the client and his family?
5. What are men's knowledge and beliefs about testicular or prostate cancer screening?
6. What nursing interventions promote self-esteem in the client with a reproductive dysfunction?
7. What are the predictors for the client's and his sexual partner's acceptance of penile prosthetic devices?

Answers to such questions will provide nurses with the knowledge necessary to improve the quality of life for clients and will provide the framework for further study.

REFERENCES AND READINGS

American Cancer Society. (1987). *Proceedings of the Workshop on Psychosexual and Reproductive Issues Affecting Patients with Cancer—1987*. San Antonio: Author.

American Cancer Society. (1990). *Cancer facts and figures—1990*. Atlanta: Author.

American Urological Association. (1987). *Fifth Annual Video Teleconference—Medical and surgical management of male erectile dysfunction*. Bellaire, TX: Author.

Bachers, E. S. (1985). Sexual dysfunction after treatment for genitourinary cancers. *Seminars in Oncology Nursing, 1*(1), 18–24.

Berry, S. J., Coffee, D. S., Walsch, P. C., & Ewing, L. L. (1984). The development of human benign prostatic hyperplasia with age. *Journal of Urology, 132*, 474–479.

Blackmore, C. (1988). The impact of orchidectomy upon the sexuality of the man with testicular cancer. *Cancer Nursing, 11*, 33–40.

Blesch, K. S. (1986). Health beliefs about testicular cancer and self-examination among professional men. *Oncology Nursing Forum, 13*(1), 29–33.

Cozad, K. (1988). Impotence: Psychosocial aspects, evaluation, methods, and treatment. *Urologic Nursing, 9*(2), 10–12.

Crawford, E. D., & Dawkins, C. A. (1986). Diagnosis and management of prostate cancer. *Hospital Practice, 21*, 159–174.

DePauw, A. P. (1986). Prostatic malignancy: Early diagnosis for optimal treatment. *Hospital Medicine, 22*, 117–136.

Dixon, D., & Moore, R. A. (1952). Tumors of the male sex organs. In *Atlas of tumor pathology* (fascicle 31b;32, series 1). Washington, DC: Armed Forces Institute of Pathology.

Draller, M. J. (1980). Cancer of the testis: An overview. *Urologic Clinics of North America, 7*, 731–733.

Durie, B. (1987). Drugs and sexual function. *Nursing Times, 83*(32), 34–35.

Einhorn, L. (1980). Chemotherapy of metastatic seminoma. In L. Einhorn (Ed.), *Testicular tumors: Management and treatment*. New York: Masson.

Fay, R. (1983). Prostatic obstruction in Chinese population. In F. Hinman, Jr. (Ed.), *Benign prostatic hypertrophy* (pp. 27–29). New York: Springer-Verlag.

Freed, S. Z. (1986). Genitourinary disease in the elderly. In I. Rossman (Ed.), *Clinical geriatrics* (3rd ed., pp. 352–363). Philadelphia: J. B. Lippincott.

Fisher, S. G. (1983). The psychosexual effects of cancer and cancer treatment. *Oncology Nursing Forum, 10*(2), 63–67.

Fisher, S. G. (1985a). The sexual knowledge and attitudes of oncology nurses: Implications for nursing education. *Seminars in Oncology Nursing, 1*(1), 63–68.

Fisher, S. G. (1985b). Sexuality as a variable in oncology nursing research. *Oncology Nursing Forum, 12*(1), 87–89.

Frank-Stromberg, M. (1985). Sexuality and the elderly cancer patient. *Seminars in Oncology Nursing, 1*(1), 49–55.

Gault, P. (1981). Taking your part in the fight against testicular cancer. *Nursing '81, 11*(5), 47–50.

Gillenwater, J. Y., Grayhack, J. T., Howards, S. S., & Duckett, J. W. (Eds.) (1987). *Adult and pediatric urology* (Vol. 2). Chicago: Year Book Medical.

Glasgow, M., Halfin, V., & Althausen, A. F. (1987). Sexual response and cancer. *CA: A Cancer Journal for Clinicians, 36*, 322–328.

Goodman, M. (1988). Concepts of hormonal manipulation in the treatment of cancer. *Oncology Nursing Forum, 15*, 639–647.

Heinrich-Rynning, T. (1987). Prostatic cancer treatments and their effects on sexual functioning. *Oncology Nursing Forum, 14*(6), 37–62.

Holmes, P. (1987). New treatments for impotence. *Nursing Times, 83*(34), 42–43.

Hubbard, S., & Jenkins, J. (1983a). An overview of current concepts in the management of patients with testicular tumors of germ cell origin—part I: Pathophysiology, diagnosis, and staging. *Cancer Nursing, 10*, 39–47.

Hubbard, S., & Jenkins, J. (1983b). An overview of current concepts in the management of patients with testicular tumors of germ cell origin—part II: Treatment strategies by histology and stage. *Cancer Nursing, 10*, 125–139.

Javadpour, N. (1980). *Principles and management of urologic cancer*. Baltimore: Williams & Wilkins.

Johnson, D. (Ed.). (1972). *Testicular tumors* (pp. 1–32). London: Henry Kimpton.

Kaempfer, S. H., Hoffman, D. J., & Wiley, F. (1983). Sperm banking: A reproductive option in cancer therapy. *Cancer Nursing, 10*, 31–38.

Kaempfer, S. H., Wiley, F. M., Hoffman, D. J., & Rhodes, E. A. (1985). Fertility considerations and procreative alternatives in cancer care. *Seminars in Oncology Nursing, 1*(1), 25–34.

LaFollette, S. S. (1987). Radical retropubic prostatectomy. Campbell and Walsh techniques. *AORN Journal, 45*, 57–69.

Lerner, J., & Khan, Z. (1982). *Mosby's manual of urologic nursing*. St. Louis: C. V. Mosby.

Lewis, S., & Collier, P. (1983). *Medical-surgical nursing: Assessment and management of clinical problems*. New York: McGraw-Hill.

Libman, E., Creti, L., & Fichten, C. S. (1987). Determining what patients should know about transurethral prostatectomy. *Patient Education and Counseling, 9*, 145–163.

MacElveen-Hoehn, P. (1985). Sexual assessment and counseling. *Seminars in Oncology Nursing, 1*(1), 69–75.

MacElveen-Hoehn, P., & McCorkle, R. (1985). Understanding sexuality in progressive cancer. *Seminars in Oncology Nursing, 1*(1), 56–62.

McConnell, E. A., & Zimmerman, M. F. (1983). *Care of patients with urologic problems*. Philadelphia: J. B. Lippincott.

Mustofi, F. K. (1977). Testicular tumors: Recent results in cancer research. In E. Grunderman & W. Vahlensieck (Eds.), *Tumors of the male genital system* (pp. 176–195). Berlin: Springer-Verlag.

Mustofi, F. K., & Price, E. B., Jr. (1973). *Atlas of tumor pathology* (fascicle 8, series 2). Washington, DC: Armed Forces Institute of Pathology.

National Institutes of Health. (1989). *National Cancer Institute research report: Progress in treatment of testicular cancer* (DHHS Publication No. NCI 89–654). Washington, DC: U.S. Government Printing Office.

Peckham, M. J., & McElwain, T. J. (1975). Testicular tumors. *Clinical Endocrinology and Metabolism, 4,* 665–692.

Pinch, W. J., Nilges, A., & Schnell, A. (1988). Testicular self-examination: Reaching the college male. *Journal of American College Health, 37,* 131–132.

Reno, D. R. (1988). Men's knowledge and health beliefs about testicular cancer and testicular self-examination. *Cancer Nursing, 11,* 112–117.

Rous, S. (1988). *The prostate book—sound advice on symptoms and treatment.* New York: W. W. Norton.

Rudolf, V. M., & MacEwen Quinn, K. L. (1988). The practice of TSE among college men: Effectiveness of an educational program. *Oncology Nursing Forum, 15,* 45–48.

Sandella, J. A. (1983). Programmed instruction: cancer care. Cancer prevention and detection: testicular cancer. *Cancer Nursing, 6,* 468–486.

Saxton, D., Pelikan, P., Nugent, P., & Hyland, P. (1983). *The Addison-Wesley manual of nursing practice.* Menlo Park, CA: Addison-Wesley.

Schäufele, B. (1988). Teaching testicular self-examination. *Professional Nurse, 3,* 409–411.

Schwarz-Appelbaum, J., Dedrick, J., Jesunius, K., & Kirchner, C. (1984). Nursing care plans: Sexuality and treatment of breast cancer. *Oncology Nursing Forum, 11*(6), 16–24.

Shipes, E., & Dehr, S. (1982). Sexuality and the male cancer patient. *Cancer Nursing, 9,* 375–380.

Silverberg, E., & Lubera, J. (1987). Cancer statistics 1987. *CA: A Cancer Journal for Clinicians, 37,* 1–19.

Smith, D. B. (1989). Sexual rehabilitation of the cancer patient. *Cancer Nursing, 12,* 10–15.

Tarpy, C. C. (1985). Birth control considerations during chemotherapy. *Oncology Nursing Forum, 12*(2), 75–78.

Turocillo, P. (1988). Testicular cancer: A historical review and current update. *AUAA Journal, 8*(3), 19–22.

Waterhouse, J., & Metcalfe, M. C. (1986). Development of the sexual adjustment questionnaire. *Oncology Nursing Forum, 13*(3), 53–59.

Webb, C. (1987). Sexual healing. *Nursing Times, 83*(32), 28–30.

Williams, H. A., Wilson, M. E., Hongladarom, G., & McDonell, M. (1986). Nurses' attitudes toward sexuality in cancer patients. *Oncology Nursing Forum, 13*(2), 39–43.

Wilson, M. E., & Williams, H. A. (1988). Oncology nurses' attitudes and behaviors related to sexuality of patients with cancer. *Oncology Nursing Forum, 15,* 49–53.

Woods, N. F. (1984). *Human sexuality in health and illness.* St. Louis: C. V. Mosby.

Yarbro, C. H., & Perry, M. C. (1985). The effect of cancer therapy on gonadal function. *Seminars in Oncology Nursing, 1*(1), 3–8.

ADDITIONAL READINGS

Kaker, S. R. (1990). Epididymitis in the young adult male. *Nurse Practitioner, 15*(5), 10–18.

This article discusses epididymitis, or inflammation of the scrotum, which is an increasing cause of infertility in men ages 18 to 35. The etiology and pathology of epididymitis are described, particularly in relation to sexually transmitted diseases. Diagnostic tests and treatments are specified. This information is important in helping nurses to identify this infection early to prevent infertility problems.

Mason, D. R. (1989). Erectile dysfunction: Assessment and care. *Nurse Practitioner, 14*(12), 23–34.

Erectile dysfunction or impotence is a common sexual problem for men. This article discusses the organic and psychogenic causes of impotence. In addition, assessment and management including medical, surgical, and counseling treatments for impotence are described. This article is a valuable resource for nurses working with male patients who are at risk for erectile dysfunction.

CHAPTER 56

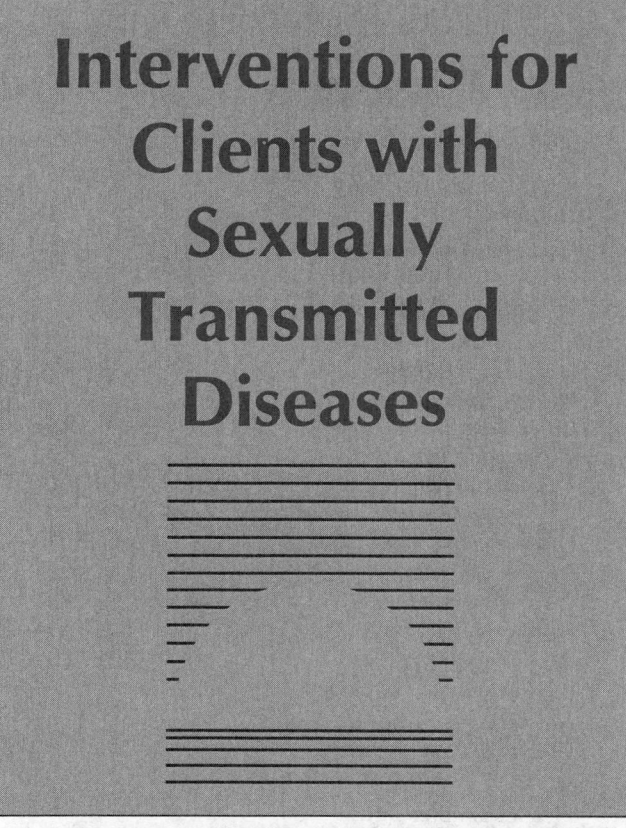

Interventions for Clients with Sexually Transmitted Diseases

Sexually transmitted diseases (STDs) are defined as diseases caused by organisms that have been transmitted to an individual through anal, oral, or vaginal intercourse. Some organisms that cause these diseases are transmitted *only* through sexual contact, whereas others can be transmitted in other ways, including parenteral exposure to infected blood, intrauterine transmission to the fetus, and perinatal transmission from mother to neonate.

Historically, five classic diseases were known to be sexually transmitted: syphilis, gonorrhea, chancroid, lymphogranuloma venereum (LGV), and granuloma inguinale. By 1989 the list of STDs had grown (Table 56–1) because of improved diagnostic techniques, an increased number of organisms and systemic diseases that can be sexually transmitted, and changes in sexual attitudes and practices.

The prevalence of STDs is a major health concern because treatment is costly and the incidence is high in minority populations of low socioeconomic and educational attainment (Centers for Disease Control [CDC], 1989b). STDs also cause complications that can contrib-

TABLE 56–1   Sexually Transmitted Diseases

Acquired immunodeficiency syndrome and human
   immunodeficiency virus infections

Chancroid

Syphilis

Lymphogranuloma venereum

Genital herpes simplex virus infections

Genital warts

Gonococcal infections

Chlamydial infections

Nongonococcal urethritis

Mucopurulent cervicitis

Epididymitis

Pelvic inflammatory disease

Sexually transmitted enteritis

Sexually transmitted proctitis

Trichomoniasis

Candidal infections

Bacterial vaginosis

Viral hepatitis

Cytomegalovirus infections

Ectoparasitic infections
   Pediculosis pubis
   Scabies

From Centers for Disease Control. (1989b). 1989 sexually transmitted diseases treatment guidelines [Special issue]. *Morbidity and Mortality Weekly Report, 38*(Suppl. 8), 1–43.

KEY FEATURES OF DISEASE ■ Complications Caused by Sexually Transmitted Organisms

Complication	Causative Organisms
Salpingitis, infertility, and ectopic pregnancy	*Neisseria gonorrhoeae* *Chlamydia trachomatis* *Mycoplasma hominis*
Reproductive loss (abortion/miscarriage)	*Neisseria gonorrhoeae* *Chlamydia trachomatis* Herpes simplex virus *Mycoplasma hominis* *Ureaplasma urealyticum* *Treponema pallidum*
Puerperal infection	*Neisseria gonorrhoeae* *Chlamydia trachomatis*
Perinatal infection	Hepatitis B virus Human immunodeficiency virus Human papillomavirus *Neisseria gonorrhoeae* *Chlamydia trachomatis* Herpes simplex virus *Treponema pallidum* Cytomegalovirus Group B streptococcus
Cancer of genital area	*Chlamydia trachomatis* Herpes simplex virus Human papillomavirus
Male urethritis	*Mycoplasma hominis* Herpes simplex virus *Neisseria gonorrhoeae* *Chlamydia trachomatis* *Ureaplasma urealyticum*
Vulvovaginitis	Herpes simplex virus *Trichomonas vaginalis* Bacteria causing vaginosis *Candida albicans*
Cervicitis	*Neisseria gonorrhoeae* *Chlamydia trachomatis* Herpes simplex virus
Proctitis	*Neisseria gonorrhoeae* *Chlamydia trachomatis* Herpes simplex virus *Campylobacter jejuni* *Shigella* species *Entamoeba histolytica*
Hepatitis	*Treponema pallidum* Hepatitis A virus
Dermatitis	*Sarcoptes scabiei* *Phthirus pubis*
Genital ulceration or warts	*Chlamydia trachomatis* Herpes simplex virus Human papillomavirus *Treponema pallidum* *Haemophilus ducreyi* *Calymmatobacterium granulomatis*

ute to severe physical and emotional suffering, including infertility, ectopic pregnancy, cancer, and death. Complications caused by sexually transmitted organisms are noted in the accompanying Key Features of Disease.

Cases of the classic STDs are reportable to local health authorities, but newer STDs such as genital herpes and chlamydial infections may or may not be reported, depending on local statutory requirements. In the past, efforts by federal and local public health departments have resulted in decreasing the incidence of gonorrhea and syphilis. Nurses have played a major role in these efforts through counseling, case finding, and treatment. With the advent of newer STDs, the nurse must continue to work with other health care professionals for control of these diseases. This control is based on education of clients at risk about modes of transmission, detection of clients who are asymptomatic or who are symptomatic but are unlikely to seek treatment, effective assessment and treatment of infected clients, and treatment and counseling of sexual partners of infected clients.

Nurses in advanced practice in a variety of community settings, in collaboration with physicians, are primarily responsible for diagnosing and treating clients with STDs. However, nurses in secondary and tertiary care settings also have a responsibility to recognize clients who are at risk or who have symptoms of STDs and to provide care to those clients who may be hospitalized with complications related to STDs. Information in this chapter is provided to assist the nurse in caring for clients with STDs.

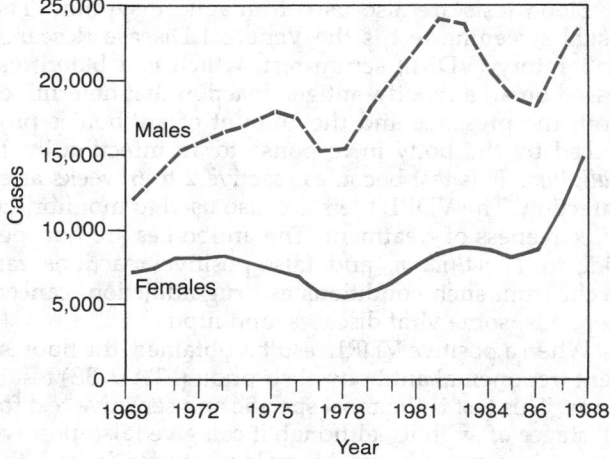

Figure 56–1

Primary and secondary syphilis cases, by sex, in the United States, 1969–1988. (From Centers for Disease Control. [1989a]. Summary of notifiable diseases, United States, 1988. *Morbidity and Mortality Weekly Report, 37*[54].)

ACQUIRED IMMUNODEFICIENCY SYNDROME

Acquired immunodeficiency syndrome (AIDS) is a disease caused primarily by infection with the human immunodeficiency virus (HIV). AIDS is a disorder of immunoregulation affecting the body's ability to fight disease. AIDS can be transmitted by semen, vaginal secretions, blood and blood products, and breast milk that are infected with HIV. Persons at risk include sexually active men who are bisexual or homosexual with multiple sexual partners, sexual partners of both sexes of persons at risk for AIDS, intravenous drug users, persons with hemophilia or other conditions requiring blood transfusions, and infants born to women who are infected with HIV.

Because AIDS affects the immune system, a detailed discussion of it is presented in Chapter 27.

INFECTIONS ASSOCIATED WITH ULCERS

SYPHILIS

OVERVIEW

Syphilis is one of the classic STDs. It ranks third in incidence behind gonorrhea and chickenpox among reportable communicable diseases in the United States. The use of new techniques for diagnosis and treatment, particularly the discovery of penicillin, has resulted in a decline in the incidence of syphilis since 1941. However, in 1988, the highest number of cases was reported since 1949 (Fig. 56–1). This rise has been associated with increased drug abuse and prostitution (Smith et al., 1990).

The primary population that is infected with syphilis consists of young adults in their early 20s. The incidence of syphilis in Caucasian homosexual males has declined since 1982, but rates for all males outnumber those for women by a ratio of 2:1 (see Fig. 56–1). There has been a rise in incidence in low-income, inner-city, heterosexual minority populations. The increased incidence of congenital syphilis reflects a rise in syphilis in heterosexuals and a lack of use of health care services by mothers of infected infants (CDC, 1989a).

The causative organism of syphilis is *Treponema pallidum*. It is a spirochete with a slender, spiral shape that resembles a corkscrew. Nonpathogenic members of the *Treponema* family are found in the mouth, intestinal tract, and genital areas of humans and animals. The organisms can be seen only with a dark-field microscope. *T. pallidum* is susceptible to dry air or to any known disinfectant. The organisms die within hours at temperatures of 41° to 42° C and are not airborne. The infection is usually transmitted by sexual contact, but transmission can occur through close body contact and kissing as well.

Primary

The chancre is the first lesion of syphilis, developing at the site of inoculation or entry of the organism between 10 and 90 days after exposure. Chancres have been found on the genitalia, on the lips and in the oral cavity, on the anus and in the rectum, on the nipples, and on the fingers and hands. During this highly infectious stage, the chancre begins as a small papule. Within 3 to 7 days, it breaks down into its characteristic appearance: a painless, indurated, smooth weeping lesion. Regional lymph nodes enlarge, feel firm, and are not tender. Without treatment, the chancre usually disappears within 6 weeks; however, the organism will have disseminated throughout the body by means of the blood stream.

Secondary

Secondary syphilis develops from 6 weeks to 6 months after the onset of primary syphilis. Secondary syphilis is a systemic disease because the spirochetes circulate throughout the blood stream. Symptoms include malaise, low-grade fever, headache, muscular aches and pains, and sometimes a sore throat. These symptoms are frequently mistaken for those of influenza. A generalized rash develops; unlike any other rash, it involves the palms and soles of the feet. Although there is no typical appearance of the rash, it has a tendency to evolve sequentially from papules to squamous papules to pustules. Other skin lesions can include psoriasiform rashes, wart-like lesions, and mucous patches. The lesions are highly contagious and should not be touched with the bare skin. The rash subsides spontaneously in 4 to 12 weeks, but 25% of clients have recurrences within 6 months.

Early and Late Latent

After the second stage, there is a period of latency. According to the CDC, *early latent* syphilis occurs during the first year after infection, and infectious lesions can recur. *Late latent* syphilis is disease of more than 1 year's duration after infection. This stage of syphilis is noninfectious except to the fetus of a pregnant woman. Clients with latent syphilis may or may not have reactive serologic tests.

Late

Late syphilis develops after a highly variable period, from 4 to 20 years. This stage develops in untreated cases and can mimic almost any pathologic condition. Manifestations of late syphilis include benign lesions, or *gummas*, of the skin, mucous membranes, and bones; cardiovascular syphilis, usually in the form of aortitis and aneurysms; and neurosyphilis, which includes central nervous system involvement.

COLLABORATIVE MANAGEMENT

Assessment of the client presenting with symptoms of syphilis begins with a history, which should include a sexual history (see Chap. 10), information about the lesions noticed, and whether previous testing or treatment for syphilis has occurred (Table 56–2). The client should be asked about allergic reactions to drugs, especially penicillin. A physical examination, including inspection and palpation, is then done to identify manifestations of syphilis. Women frequently have the chancre on areas that are invisible to them, e.g., the vagina or cervix. These women may present with complaints of inguinal lymph node enlargement, the location that drains the area of the vagina and cervix. Also, they may state a history of sexual contact with a male with an ulcer that they noticed during the encounter. Men usually discover the chancre on the penis or scrotum.

After the physical examination, a specimen of the chancre is obtained and examined under a dark-field microscope. Diagnosis of primary or secondary syphilis is confirmed if *T. pallidum*, the characteristic spirochete, is present. If the first slide is negative, the procedure should be repeated in 3 days because many conditions can cause a false-negative result (Neeson & Stockdale, 1981).

Blood tests are also used to diagnose syphilis. The usual screening test is the Venereal Disease Research Laboratory (VDRL) serum test, which is a blood test based on an antibody-antigen reaction that determines both the presence and the amount of antibodies produced by the body in response to an infection by *T. pallidum*. This test becomes reactive 2 to 6 weeks after infection. The VDRL titers are also used to monitor the effectiveness of treatment. The antibodies are not specific to *T. pallidum*, and false-positive reactions can occur from such conditions as drug addiction, cancer, hepatitis, some viral diseases, and lupus.

When a positive VDRL result is obtained, the fluorescent treponemal antibody absorption (FTA-ABS) test is done. This test is the most specific and sensitive test for all stages of syphilis, although it can give false-positive results in cases of lupus. Many laboratories do both the VDRL and the FTA-ABS on all samples for syphilis. In some cases, an FTA-ABS is reactive when the VDRL is nonreactive. (See Chap. 52 for further discussion of serologic tests.)

TABLE 56–2 Data Collection for the Client with a Sexually Transmitted Disease

---

History

The chief complaint.

Thorough description of the history of the present illness. (Describe major symptoms by quality, quantity, precipitating and palliative factors, radiation, associated symptoms, and chronology of events. Self-care treatments and use of prescribed or over-the-counter medicine should be noted.)

Major adult health problems.

Sexual history (type and frequency of sexual activity, number of contacts, past history of STDs, potential sites of infection, sexual preference).

Allergies.

General women's health (date of last menstrual period, date of last Papanicolaou's (Pap) smear, pattern of contraception).

Physical Examination of the External Genitalia

1. Inspection.
2. Palpation (refer to a physical assessment text for more detail).

Laboratory Tests

Saline wet preparation (*Trichomonas* and *Gardnerella*).

Whiff test (*Gardnerella*).

Potassium hydroxide preparation (*Candida*).

Urinalysis (U/A).

Gonorrhea culture.

Cervical culture.

Herpes cervical culture.

Pap smear.

Complete blood count.

Venereal Disease Research Laboratory (VDRL), fluorescent treponemal antibody absorption test (FTA-ABS).

Herpes simplex virus type 1 and 2 antibodies.

From Smith, L. S., Lauver, D., & Gray, P. A., Jr. (1989). Sexually transmitted disease. In C. I. Fogel & D. Lauver (Eds.), *Sexual health promotion* (p. 460). Philadelphia: W. B. Saunders.

Management of syphilis is by antibiotic therapy. Several antibiotics can be used, but the drug of choice is penicillin (Table 56–3). Allergic reactions to the antibiotic occur frequently, and the nurse should be alert for these signs and symptoms. The client who has never had penicillin previously should be skin tested before receiving a penicillin injection. All clients who have re-

ceived injections of antibiotics remain at the health care facility for at least 30 minutes so that signs of a severe and immediate allergic reaction can be detected. Thus, if this type of reaction does occur, treatment can begin immediately. The most severe reaction that can occur is anaphylaxis. All nurses working in clinics where injections of penicillin are given should be familiar with the symptoms and treatment of anaphylaxis, which are discussed in more detail in Chapter 27.

The Jarisch-Herxheimer reaction may follow antibiotic therapy for syphilis and is due to the rapid release of products from the disruption of the cells of the organism. Onset occurs within 2 hours after therapy, with a peak at 4 to 8 hours. Symptoms include generalized aches and pain at the injection site, vasodilation and hypotension, and a rise in temperature. These symptoms do not always occur and generally are benign. This reaction may be treated symptomatically with analgesics and antipyretics.

Nursing interventions are based on assessments and medical treatments. Nursing diagnoses for clients with syphilis as well as STDs in general are given in Table 56–4.

Clients should be informed about treatment, including side effects, possible complications of untreated disease, and the need for follow-up care. Adequate treatment of all sexual partners is needed as soon as possible, and the client needs to furnish accurate information for this follow-up. The client is informed that the disease must be reported to the local health authority and that all information will be held in strict confidence. Information seeking and teaching should take place in a setting that offers privacy and encourages open discussion.

The client should be urged to comply with the treatment regimen, especially if oral antibiotics are included. The nurse stresses the contagiousness of the disease and discusses frankly the role of the client in preventing spread to sexual partners (see the Client/Family Education feature on p. 1779).

The emotional responses to syphilis vary and may include feelings of shame, fear, depression, and anxiety. Guilt related to the client's infecting others or anger related to the client's being infected by a partner may also be present. The nurse encourages the client to discuss these feelings or refers the client to other resources such as psychotherapy groups, self-help support groups, or STD clinics if further psychosocial interventions are necessary.

GENITAL HERPES SIMPLEX

OVERVIEW

Two types of herpes simplex virus (HSV) have been identified as affecting the genitalia: type 1 (HSV 1) and type 2 (HSV 2). Most nongenital lesions such as cold sores are caused by HSV 1, whereas HSV 2 causes most

TABLE 56–3 Drugs Used in Treatment of Syphilis

Drug	Usual Daily Dosage	Interventions	Rationales
Early Syphilis (Less Than 1 yr Duration)			
Benzathine penicillin G	2.4 million units IM in one dose	1. Give deep IM injection. 2. Assess client for rashes, itching, chills, and fever. 3. Skin test client before giving penicillin. 4. Have client remain in clinic or office for 30 min after injection.	1. To increase absorption of drug. 2, 3. To prevent complications of allergic reactions. 4. To detect signs of severe allergic reaction.
or Tetracycline	500 mg qid PO for 2 wk	1. Assess client for rashes, nausea, and diarrhea. 2. Encourage fluid intake. 3. Have client take drug on an empty stomach.	1. To detect drug side effects. 2. To decrease esophageal irritation. 3. To increase absorption of drug.
or Doxycycline	100 mg bid PO for 2 wk	1. Do not give with iron or antacids.	1. To avoid inhibition of absorption of drug.
Syphilis (More Than 1 yr Duration)			
Benzathine penicillin G	2.4 million units IM once a week for 3 wk (total 7.2 million units)	Same as for early syphilis	
or Tetracycline	500 mg qid PO for 4 wk	Same as for early syphilis	
or Doxycycline	100 mg bid PO for 4 wk	Same as for early syphilis	
Neurosyphilis			
Aqueous crystalline penicillin G	12–24 million units IV daily (divided doses) for 10–14 d	See benzathine penicillin G for early syphilis	
or Aqueous procaine penicillin G	2.4 million units IM daily for 10 d	See benzathine penicillin G for early syphilis	
plus Probenecid	500 mg qid PO for 10 d	1. Give with food. 2. Encourage fluid intake (10 glasses a day).	1. To avoid gastrointestinal upset. 2. To prevent formation of kidney stones.
may be followed by Benzathine penicillin G	2.4 million units IM weekly for 3 wk	See benzathine penicillin G for early syphilis	

Modified from Centers for Disease Control. (1989b). 1989 sexually transmitted diseases treatment guidelines [Special issue]. *Morbidity and Mortality Weekly Report, 38*(Suppl. 8), 5–12.

TABLE 56-4   Selected Nursing Diagnoses for Clients with Syphilis and Other Sexually Transmitted Diseases

Potential for injury related to the disease process

Ineffective individual coping related to guilt, shame, or anger

Noncompliance related to treatment and/or partner follow-up

Sexual dysfunction related to fear of transmission

Impaired skin integrity related to the presence of chancre or rash

Knowledge deficit related to the mode of transmission, disease process, or need for treatment

Impaired social interaction related to social stigma

Pain related to STD

Anxiety related to possible infertility as a result of having an STD

Self-esteem disturbance related to having an STD

of the genital lesions. However, either type can produce oral or genital lesions through oral-genital contact (Miles, 1984).

The incubation period is 2 to 20 days, with the average period being 1 week (Smith et al., 1990; Miles, 1984). Many people are asymptomatic during the primary infection, but if symptoms occur, they are usually most severe during this first infection (Miles, 1984).

A tingling sensation may be felt in the skin 1 to 2 days before an outbreak. This sensation is followed by the appearance of vesicles (blisters) in a characteristic cluster on the penis, scrotum, vulva, perineum, vagina, cervix, or perianal region. The vesicles rupture spontaneously in a couple of days and leave painful erosions. These lesions can become extensive, and other symptoms such as headaches, fever, and general malaise may be present. Urination may be painful, and urinary retention may require catheterization. Lesions resolve within 2 to 6 weeks.

After the lesions heal, the virus remains in a dormant state in the nerve ganglia, specifically in genital herpes, the sacral ganglia. Periodically, the virus may activate, and episodes of infection recur. These recurrences may

CLIENT/FAMILY EDUCATION ■ Safe Sex Practices

Instructions	Rationales
1. "The only effective way to prevent acquiring STDs is to abstain from all forms of sexual contact."	1. To acknowledge an alternative for nonsexually active persons.
2. "Do not have sexual contact with a lot of different partners, partners you do not know well, prostitutes, or other people who have a lot of sexual partners."	2-8. To reduce the risk of STD for those who are sexually active.
3. "Do not have sexual contact with people who have a genital discharge, genital warts, genital herpes lesions, or other suspicious lesions."	
4. "Do not have sexual contact with persons who have HIV or hepatitis B infections."	
5. "Avoid oral-anal sex to prevent enteric infections."	
6. "Avoid genital contact with oral cold sores."	
7. "Use condoms and diaphragms in combination with spermicides."	
8. "If you are at high risk for getting an STD, be sure to get periodic examinations for the presence of STDs."	

Modified from Centers for Disease Control. (1989b). 1989 sexually transmitted diseases treatment guidelines [Special issue]. *Morbidity and Mortality Weekly Report, 38*(Suppl. 8), 1-43.

be stimulated by many factors, including stress, fever, sunburn, menses, and sexual activity (Miles, 1984). Recurrences are not usually caused by reinfection. In general, these episodes of recurrent infection are less severe and shorter than the primary infection; they may not even occur at all. Occasionally, HSV infection may become active without producing apparent clinical manifestations. However, there is *viral shedding*, and the client is infectious.

COLLABORATIVE MANAGEMENT

The diagnosis of genital herpes is usually based on the history and physical examination of the client and is confirmed through viral culture. Cultures are most accurate if specimens are obtained within 48 hours of the outbreak of the blisters.

Management of HSV focuses on decreasing pain and promoting comfort, promoting healing without secondary infection, decreasing viral excretions, and preventing transmission of the infection. Treatment is usually symptomatic (see accompanying Guidelines feature).

Acyclovir is an antiviral drug that is used to treat genital herpes. The drug is not a cure, but it partially controls signs and symptoms and accelerates healing. Topical therapy is not as effective as oral therapy. The CDC recommends acyclovir, 200 mg orally five times a day for 7 to 10 days, for the first infection. Recommended treatment for recurrent episodes is acyclovir, 200 mg orally five times a day for 5 days, or 800 mg twice a day for 5 days. Most recurrent episodes do not benefit from treatment, but therapy for severe recurrent disease may be beneficial if started within 2 days of the appearance of lesions.

Clients who have frequent (more than six in a year) recurrences may benefit from daily treatment with acyclovir, 200 mg two to five times a day. Long-term safety (more than 3 years) of this treatment is unknown. Clients receiving continuous therapy should stop after 1 year for reassessment of the recurrence rate (CDC, 1989b).

Long-term complications of genital herpes include the risk of developing cervical cancer, the risk of neonatal transmission, and an increased risk of acquiring HIV infections (CDC, 1989b; Smith et al., 1990). An association between HSV 2 infections and cervical cancer has been demonstrated (Rapp, 1981), especially in women

---

GUIDELINES ■ Interventions for Symptomatic Relief of Genital Herpes

Interventions	Rationales
1. Administer oral analgesics as prescribed.	1–5. To decrease pain and promote comfort.
2. Apply topical steroids to lesions.	
3. Apply local anesthetic sprays or ointments as prescribed.	
4. Apply ice packs or warm compresses to lesions.	
5. Administer sitz baths 3 or 4 times a day.	
6. Encourage an increase in fluid intake.	6–9. To prevent dysuria or to relieve retention of urine.
7. Encourage frequent voidings.	
8. Pour water over genitalia while voiding or encourage voiding while sitting in a tub of water or standing in a shower.	
9. Catheterize as necessary.	
10. Encourage genital hygiene and encourage keeping the skin clean and dry.	10–13. To prevent infection.
11. Wear gloves when applying ointments.	
12. Inform client to avoid sexual activity when lesions are present.	
13. Inform client that condoms should be used during all sexual exposures.	

with recurrent infections. Women with genital herpes should be encouraged to have an annual Papanicolaou's (Pap) smear. The risk of transmission to the neonate is greater in a pregnant woman who has a primary infection than in one who has recurrent herpes. Women who have active lesions at the onset of labor should be delivered by cesarean section to avoid neonatal infection.

Nursing management must include client counseling and education about the infection and the potential for recurrent episodes. Advice about sexual activity is extremely important. Clients should be told to abstain from sexual activity while lesions are present. Condom use during all sexual exposures should be encouraged because of the increased risk of HIV infections and because HSV infections can be transmitted during viral shedding even when lesions are not present (see accompanying Client/Family Education feature). The risk of fetal infection should be emphasized to all clients. Women who have genital herpes need to inform their maternity care provider of their history during future pregnancies.

Psychologic responses to the diagnosis of genital herpes need to be assessed. Many clients are initially shocked and search frantically for a cure or some assur-

ance that the disease can be managed. Feelings of disbelief, uncleanliness, isolation, and loneliness have been reported by infected clients. Clients also have reported anger at their partners for transmitting the infection or fear of rejection by partners because they have the infection (Breslin, 1988; Smith et al., 1990). The nurse helps clients cope with the diagnosis of genital herpes by being sensitive and supportive during assessments and interventions. Social supports should be encouraged and referrals to support groups such as HELP may be beneficial (see Unit 15 Resources).

LYMPHOGRANULOMA VENEREUM

LGV has a worldwide distribution, but it is found primarily in South America, the West Indies, Southeast Asia, India, and Africa. Cases in the United States usually occur in clients who have visited these countries, such as military personnel and other travelers.

LGV is caused by serotypes of Chlamydia trachomatis. The incubation period is 3 to 30 days. The primary lesion is transient and painless and is not usually noticed by the client. The lesion usually appears on the penis in

---

CLIENT/FAMILY EDUCATION ■ Proper Use of Condoms

Instructions	Rationales
1. "Use latex condoms rather than natural membrane condoms."	1. To maximize protection against HIV infection and other viral STDs.
2. "Keep condoms in a cool, dry place, out of direct sunlight."	2. To prevent decomposition.
3. "Do not use condoms that are in damaged packages or that are brittle or discolored."	3. To avoid use of unreliable condoms.
4. "Always handle condoms with care."	4. To prevent puncture.
5. "Put condoms on before any genital contact. Hold condom by the tip and unroll it on the penis. Leave space at the tip to collect semen."	5. To prevent exposure to fluids that may be infectious.
6. "If you use lubricant with condoms, make sure that it is water based."	6. To avoid breakage that can be caused by petroleum- or oil-based lubricants.
7. "You can use condoms that contain spermicide."	7. To provide some additional protection against STDs.
8. "If a condom breaks, replace it immediately."	8–10. To avoid reduction in protection.
9. "After ejaculation, withdraw the penis carefully to prevent the condom from slipping off."	
10. "Never use a condom more than once."	

Modified from Centers for Disease Control. (1989b). 1989 sexually transmitted diseases treatment guidelines [Special issue]. *Morbidity and Mortality Weekly Report, 38*(Suppl. 8), p ix.

men and on the vaginal wall in women; however, sores may also be located in the mouth and rectum. Lesions vary in form from herpes-like blisters to ulcers, vesicles, papules, or pustules. Within 1 to 2 weeks after the appearance of the primary lesion, secondary signs of infection appear. Lymphadenopathy is present, and symptoms of headache, malaise, arthralgia, and anorexia may occur. Lymphadenopathy can recede or develop into abscesses. Complications of the infection can cause chronic lymphadenopathy, fistulas, rectal strictures, and proctitis. Systemic involvement can also cause carditis, arthritis, and pneumonia.

The usual treatment of LGV is doxycycline, 100 mg orally twice a day, or tetracycline, 500 mg orally four times a day, for at least 3 weeks. Incision and drainage of infected lymph nodes are contraindicated, but the nodes may be aspirated by needle. Surgical intervention may be required for late complications such as strictures and fistulas.

CHANCROID

Although *chancroid* has a worldwide distribution, it is most common in tropical and subtropical countries. Recent spread of the causative organism *Haemophilus ducreyi* has made chancroid an important STD in the United States. This rise is particularly troublesome because the open lesions of chancroid have been associated with increased infection rates for HIV (CDC, 1989b).

The incubation period for chancroid varies from 1 to 14 days. A tender papule appears at the site of inoculation. This lesion rapidly breaks down to form an irregularly shaped, deep ulcer that has a purulent discharge and bleeds easily. Complications include inguinal adenitis, balanitis, phimosis, and urethral fistulas. Chancroids are different from chancres caused by syphilis in that the former are soft and painful. Transmission of the disease is through contact with the ulcer or with the discharge from the infected local lymph glands during sexual relations.

Treatment consists of erythromycin, 500 mg orally four times a day for 7 days, or ceftriaxone, 250 mg intramuscularly in a single dose. Clients should be followed until ulcers heal. Client education is similar to that for the client with syphilis. Sexual contacts must be located and treated whether or not they are symptomatic.

GRANULOMA INGUINALE

Granuloma inguinale is endemic in parts of Africa, Southeast Asia, southern India, and New Guinea. Incidence in the United States, Japan, and Europe is rare. It is more common in dark-skinned persons and in gay men than in the general population (Smith et al., 1990).

The causative organism is *Calymmatobacterium granulomatis.* A papule appears at the site of inoculation after 1 to 12 weeks. This lesion ulcerates and others are formed; they grow together, becoming a spreading ulcer

on the genitalia. Left untreated, these lesions can be mutilating. Although pregnancy may accelerate the disease, there is no evidence of transmission to the fetus.

Treatment is administration of antibiotic: tetracycline, 500 mg orally four times a day for at least 10 days or until lesions heal. Clients need long-term follow-up on a yearly basis because these lesions may be precancerous (Smith et al., 1990).

The nurse's responsibility in client management of LGV, chancroid, and granuloma inguinale is similar to that for clients with other STDs. An adequate history is taken by the nurse. The client is asked about physical signs and travel abroad. In addition, information about sexual partners is obtained.

The nurse explains the correct way to take prescribed medications and stresses the importance of taking the entire amount prescribed. Possible side effects and what to do if they occur are described. The nurse also provides information on the disease: how it is acquired; how it is spread; and the prognosis, with and without adequate treatment.

INFECTIONS OF EPITHELIAL SURFACES

CONDYLOMATA ACUMINATA

OVERVIEW

Condylomata acuminata, also referred to as *venereal warts* or *genital warts,* are caused by certain types of human papillomavirus (Sonstegard et al., 1982). Genital warts are sexually transmitted and often are seen with other STDs such as gonorrhea and trichomoniasis. Sites commonly affected include the urinary meatus, vulva, labia majora, vagina, cervix, penis, scrotum, anus, and perineal area. The infection is exacerbated in pregnant women and the elderly (Lucas, 1988). The incubation period is usually 1 to 3 months (Margolis, 1984). Genital warts are believed to be highly contagious and have been reported in more than 50% of sexual partners of infected persons.

The genital warts are initially single, small papillary growths that grow into large cauliflower-like masses. Some women also experience a profuse, foul-smelling vaginal discharge. Bleeding may occur. If there are only a few warts, they may regress spontaneously without treatment.

Genital warts are strongly associated with genital dysplasia and carcinoma. A biopsy should be done for atypical, pigmented, or persistent warts (CDC, 1989b).

COLLABORATIVE MANAGEMENT

The diagnosis of condylomata is made by examination of the lesions, which will appear wart-like. To rule out the presence of other infections such as syphilis and gonorrhea, a VDRL test and gonorrheal culture are obtained. Wet mounts are done if vaginitis is present, and a Pap smear is obtained to assess cervical abnormalities. If lesions bleed easily or appear to be infected, a biopsy may be done to rule out other pathologic conditions. Colposcopy (see Chap. 54) is recommended to assess lesions that are not visible to the naked eye.

The goal of management of condylomata is to remove the warts and to treat the symptoms. No therapy has been shown to eradicate human papillomavirus; therefore, recurrences after treatment are likely. Treatment of choice for external warts is cryotherapy (see Chap. 54) with liquid nitrogen or a cryoprobe. Clients need to be informed that this treatment does not require anesthesia and usually does not cause scarring. Extensive warts have been treated with the carbon dioxide laser (see Chap. 54) or surgery.

Podophyllum resin, 10% to 25% in compound tincture of benzoin or trichloroacetic acid (80% to 90%), may be applied to external warts as an alternative therapy. Podophyllum resin is teratogenic, and its use is contraindicated in pregnancy (CDC, 1989b). Before its application, the surrounding skin or tissues are covered with petrolatum (Vaseline) or a paste of baking soda and water for protection from the caustic effects of the treatments. These treatments are left in place for 1 to 4 hours, after which they are washed off. Treatment may be repeated weekly if necessary. Side effects of these treatments include nausea, diarrhea, lethargy, paralysis, and coma.

Electrocautery or surgical removal may also be used to treat external warts. The type of surgery depends on the site of the warts, such as a cone biopsy for cervical lesions and "skinning" vulvectomy for vulvar lesions (see Chap. 54 for discussion of these procedures).

Effective management includes treatment of sexual partners. Also, intimate sexual contact should be avoided until external lesions are healed.

Nursing management focuses on client education about the mode of transmission, incubation period, treatment, and complications. Use of condoms is recommended to help reduce transmission (see earlier Client/ Family Education: Proper Use of Condoms). Clients need to know that recurrence is likely and that repeated treatments may be necessary. Women who have had codylomata should be encouraged to have an annual Pap smear. As with other STDs, emotional support for the client is needed, and referral for counseling may help.

GONORRHEA

OVERVIEW

Gonorrhea continues to be the most reported communicable disease in the United States (CDC, 1989b). The incidence of gonorrhea is highest among sexually active individuals between the ages of 15 and 34 years. This bacterial infection occurs in men and women, and infants can be infected during childbirth. The causative organism is *Neisseria gonorrhoeae*, a gram-negative diplococcus. *N. gonorrhoeae* cannot survive long outside of the host and cannot be transmitted by inanimate objects such as towels and toilet seats. Transmission is by direct sexual contact (vaginal intercourse or orogenital or anogenital contact) and through an infected birth canal to the neonate.

The initial symptoms of gonorrhea may appear 3 to 10 days after sexual contact with an infected person. The infection can be asymptomatic in both males and females, but women have asymptomatic, or silent, infections more often than men. If symptoms are present, males most likely notice dysuria and a penile discharge that can be either profuse, yellowish-green fluid or scant, clear fluid. The urethra is the site most commonly affected, but infection can extend to the prostate, seminal vesicles, and the epididymis. Women may report a change in vaginal discharge, urinary frequency, or dysuria. The cervix and urethra are the most common sites of infection, but upward spread can cause pelvic infection (pelvic inflammatory disease [PID]), endometritis, salpingitis, and pelvic peritonitis.

Anal manifestations may include anal itching and irritation, rectal bleeding or diarrhea, and painful defecation. Oral manifestations are related to pharyngeal infection. Symptoms are seldom noted but may include a sore throat, ulcerated lips, tender gingivae, and vesicles in the oropharynx.

Figure 56–2 shows common sites of gonococcal infections.

Asymptomatic clients may present to the health care facility for routine physical examination or for hospital admission or preoperative examinations and may be found to have positive culture results for gonorrhea. Other clients may come to the health care facility because his or her sexual partner has been diagnosed with the infection and assessment for transmission is needed.

COLLABORATIVE MANAGEMENT

A history should include a medical history, especially allergies to drugs such as penicillin, and a sexual history. A nonjudgmental approach in eliciting information should be used, and assumptions about sexual orientation should be avoided. These techniques may decrease the client's anxiety and embarrassment about having an STD.

Physical assessment of the client includes inspection for lesions, rashes, and discharges from the urethra, vagina, and rectum. Palpation of affected areas may reveal tenderness. Fever may be present, especially in complicated infections. Positive diagnosis involves laboratory tests.

Identification of gonorrhea in males can be made with smears of the discharge that has been swabbed on a glass slide, dried, and stained with Gram's stain. The presence of gram-negative diplococci is diagnostic for gonococcal urethritis. Smears do not confirm the diag-

THROAT

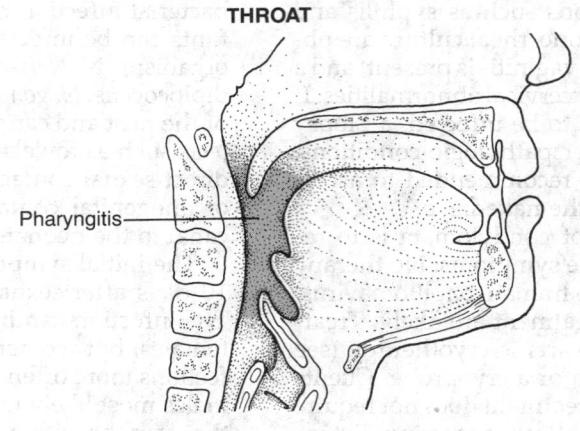

Pharyngitis

PELVIC/GENITAL

MEN

WOMEN

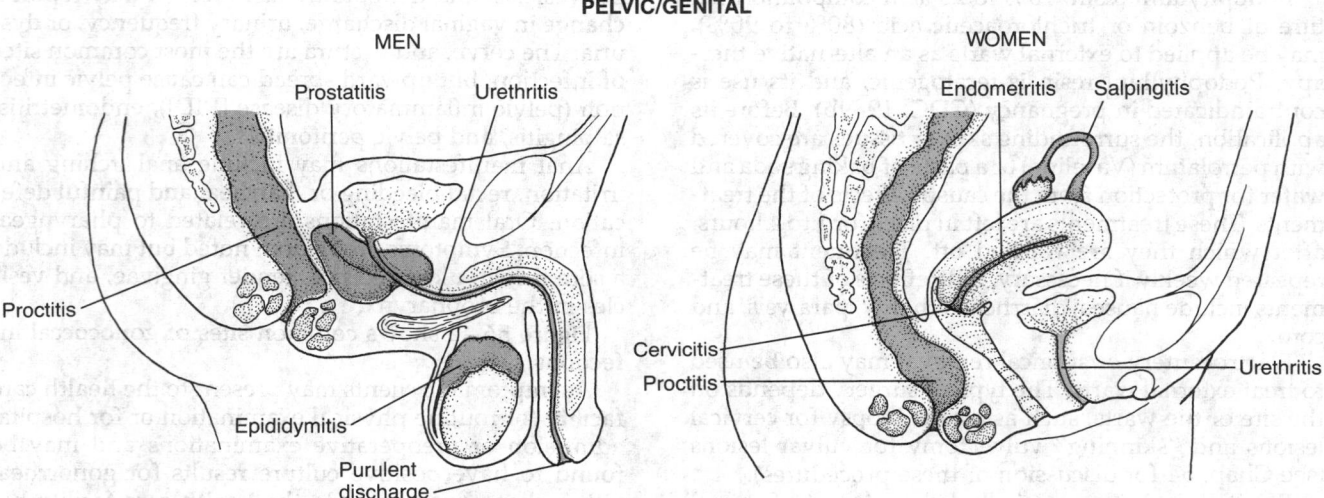

Prostatitis

Urethritis

Endometritis

Salpingitis

Proctitis

Cervicitis

Proctitis

Urethritis

Epididymitis

Purulent discharge

Figure 56–2

Some areas of involvement with gonorrhea in men and women.

nosis in women because the female genital tract normally harbors organisms that resemble *N. gonorrhoeae.* Cultures provide a more definitive diagnosis and are the most reliable method to confirm a diagnosis. A specimen is obtained from the male urethra or female cervix, and a Thayer-Martin culture medium is inoculated and placed in a carbon dioxide–rich environment. Depending on the history given by the client, cultures may also be obtained from the throat and rectum. After 24 to 48 hours, the culture is examined for the presence of gram-negative diplococci.

All clients with gonorrhea should be tested for syphilis and should be offered HIV testing because they may have been exposed to these STDs. Sexual partners who have been exposed in the last 30 days should be examined and have cultures done.

Treatment of uncomplicated gonorrhea is with antibiotics. Treatment is influenced by the increasing numbers of organisms that have become resistant to antibi-

otics, especially penicillin and tetracycline. Treatment is also influenced by the high frequency of chlamydial infections found in clients with gonorrhea. In the past, penicillin was the drug of choice; today, a number of antibiotics are effective against gonorrhea (Table 56–5). The treatment recommended by the CDC is ceftriaxone, 250 mg intramuscularly in a single dose, plus doxycycline, 100 mg orally two times a day, for 1 week. This combination appears to be effective for all mucosal gonorrhea infections; treatment failure is rare. Sexual partners need to be treated as well. The client should be advised to return for a follow-up examination if symptoms persist after treatment. Reinfection is usually the cause of this infection and indicates a need for more education of the client and sexual partner.

Gonorrheal infections can become systemic and develop into disseminated gonococcal infection. Symptoms develop abruptly and include fever; chills; skin lesions on distal parts of extremities; and arthritis-like

TABLE 56–5   Drugs Used to Treat Gonorrhea

Drug	Usual Daily Dosage	Interventions	Rationales
Ceftriaxone	250 mg IM once	1. Give deep IM injection in outer upper quadrant of gluteus maximus. 2. Watch for fever, chills, and nausea.	1. To avoid local irritation and increase absorption. 2. To detect allergic reactions.
plus			
Doxycycline	100 mg bid PO for 7 d		See Table 56–3
or			
Spectinomycin	2 g IM once		See ceftriaxone
plus			
Doxycycline	100 mg bid PO for 7 d		

Modified from Centers for Disease Control. (1989b). 1989 sexually transmitted diseases treatment guidelines [Special issue]. *Morbidity and Mortality Weekly Report, 38*(Suppl. 8), 21–27.

joint involvement with or without swelling, heat, or erythema. Meningitis and endocarditis occur rarely. Hospitalization for these clients is recommended for the initial treatment, especially if endocarditis or meningitis is suspected. Treatment is with intravenous antibiotic therapy using ceftriaxone, 1 g every 24 hours. If symptoms resolve within 24 to 48 hours, the client may be discharged to home to continue oral antibiotic therapy for at least 1 week. If meningitis or endocarditis is present, therapy may be continued for 2 to 4 weeks.

If the client with gonorrhea is a pregnant woman, the effect of the disease and treatment needs to be discussed. The nurse reassures the woman that if the disease is adequately treated, the fetus should not be affected. Untreated gonorrhea can cause eye infections in newborns (ophthalmia neonatorum) and can cause permanent blindness. Prophylactic treatment with drugs such as silver nitrate (1%), tetracycline (1%), or erythromycin (0.5%) instilled into eyes of newborns within 1 hour of birth can prevent this problem. Almost all states require this treatment.

Nursing diagnoses are similar to those described for clients with syphilis. Interventions focus on client education about transmission and treatment of gonorrhea. Clients must understand why medications should be taken for the prescribed time for maximal effectiveness. The possibility of reinfection should be discussed. Clients should avoid sexual activity until the infection is cured. Male clients should be told to wear condoms if abstinence is not possible, and female clients should be told to make sure that their partner uses condoms. Clients need to know that gonorrhea is a reportable disease. All sexual contacts need to be examined, cultured, and treated if necessary.

When a positive diagnosis of gonorrhea is made, the client may have feelings of shame and guilt. Clients also may see the disease as a punishment for promiscuity or "unnatural" sex acts. Clients may believe that getting gonorrhea (or any STD) is a risk that they must take to pursue their desired life style (Whelan, 1988). Such feelings can impair relationships with sexual partners. The nurse encourages expression of feelings during assessments and teaching sessions. Privacy for client teaching and maintenance of confidentiality of medical records are important interventions in meeting psychosocial needs of these clients.

CHLAMYDIAL INFECTIONS

OVERVIEW

Chlamydia trachomatis was the most commonly transmitted bacteria in the United States in 1988 (CDC, 1989a). The disease is not reportable, but 4 million acute infections are estimated annually (Loucks, 1987). In males, about one-half of the cases of nongonococcal urethritis and epididymitis are caused by *C. trachomatis*. In women, about 40% of PID is caused by *C. trachomatis*, and 8% to 12% of pregnant women have the infection. Transmission to the newborn can occur during vaginal delivery, with resulting neonatal eye infections and pneumonia. An estimated 155,000 infants are infected with *C. trachomatis* yearly (Loucks, 1987).

C. trachomatis invades the columnar epithelial tissues in the reproductive tract and causes clinical manifestations similar to those of gonorrheal infections. The incubation period ranges from 1 to 3 weeks (Smith et al., 1990), but the pathogen may be present in the genital tract for months or years without producing symptoms.

In men, the primary symptom is nongonococcal urethritis, accompanied by dysuria, frequency of urination, and a mucoid discharge that is more watery and less copious than a gonorrheal discharge. Some men have the discharge only in the morning when arising. Complications include epididymitis, prostatitis, infertility, and Reiter's syndrome.

In contrast, up to 75% of women (CDC, 1989b) may have no symptoms. Some have a mucopurulent cervicitis with symptoms of a change in vaginal discharge, dysuria, urinary frequency, and soreness in the affected area. Complications include salpingitis, PID, ectopic pregnancy, and infertility.

COLLABORATIVE MANAGEMENT

A complete history, including medical, menstrual, and sexual history, should be obtained from the client. Clients should be questioned about the presence of symptoms, history of STDs, and whether sexual partners are having suspicious symptoms or have a history of STDs. The nurse needs to remember that many women with chlamydial infections are asymptomatic, and a history may reveal only risk factors associated with *C. trachomatis*. These factors include pregnancy, sexual activity during adolescence, use of a nonbarrier method of birth control, and a history of multiple sexual partners. As with all interviews concerning sexual behavior, the nurse is more effective if a nonjudgmental approach is used and if privacy and confidentiality are provided.

Diagnosis of chlamydial infections is usually made by excluding gonorrhea on a urethral Gram's stain and culture. The presence of polymorphonuclear leukocytes and the absence of gram-negative intracellular diplococci may suggest a chlamydial infection. Absolute diagnosis may be made with a tissue culture from the endocervix and urethra of a female client and from the urethra of the male client. The cultures require special media and are expensive. Many laboratories are not equipped to do these tests; therefore, routine cultures may not be performed in all health care settings (Bourcier & Seidler, 1987). Screening asymptomatic women who are at high risk for having chlamydial infections is strongly encouraged by the CDC (CDC, 1989b) (see the accompanying Nursing Research feature).

Two tests that can be performed easily, less expensively, and more quickly than cultures are the Chlamydiazyme, an enzyme-linked immunoassay, and the Microtract, a direct fluorescent antibody test (Bourcier & Seidler, 1987). Both tests use urogenital secretions for specimens. Chlamydiazyme depends on antigen-antibody reactions that are read by using a spectrophotometer. A reading of optical density that is equal to or more than 0.1 is considered to be positive. Microtract examines stained urogenital secretions under a fluorescent microscope. The sensitivity of all available laboratory tests is less than 100%, and false-negative results are possible. For these reasons, test results should be interpreted with caution.

The treatment of choice for chlamydial infections is

NURSING RESEARCH

Many College Women May Have Asymptomatic Chlamydial Infections.

Woolard, D. G., Larson, J., & Hudson, L. (1989). Screening for *Chlamydia trachomatis* at a university health service. *Journal of Obstetric, Gynecologic, and Neonatal Nursing, 18*, 145–149.

The most common bacterial STD in the United States is infection with *C. trachomatis*. This infection is often asymptomatic but can lead to complications of infertility and ectopic pregnancy. This study was done to determine the frequency of occurrence of *C. trachomatis* infection in female college students at a midwestern university family planning clinic. The study was also conducted to identify clinical signs and symptoms that could be reliable diagnostic indicators of the presence of *C. trachomatis*.

A nonprobability convenience sample of 419 female clients was used in this retrospective study. All participants were asked to give a complete history and were given a physical examination, including a pelvic examination, during which culture specimens for Pap smears and gonorrhea were collected in Chlamydiazyme culture media. Clinical signs and self-reporting of symptoms were also documented.

C. trachomatis infection was reported for 12.6% of the sample. Clinical signs of infection were not found to be diagnostic indicators because 53 women who had positive test results denied having symptoms. Six women reported symptoms but tested negatively. No statistical differences between women with positive and those with negative test results occurred in relation to birth control method. Women who tested positively had more sexual partners than women who tested negatively, and this finding was statistically significant. The study indicates that routine screening for chlamydial infection is needed.

Critique. The findings of the study have limited generalizability to other populations. The historical data about sexual partners may have been unreliable, depending on the women's memory and perceptions of past events.

Possible nursing implications. Nurses in all settings need to educate women about chlamydial infections. Women need to be taught that the infection is often asymptomatic, but that clinical symptoms of increased vaginal discharge, burning with urination, and bleeding between periods should be evaluated by a health care provider. Routine pelvic examinations with screening for *C. trachomatis* should be encouraged.

doxycycline, 100 mg two times a day, or tetracycline, 500 mg four times a day, for 7 days. For clients who are allergic to these drugs or who are pregnant, erythromycin, 500 mg four times a day, for 7 days, is recommended. Sexual partners should be tested for *C. trachomatis* and treated if infection is present.

Client education is an important nursing intervention. Information about the mode of transmission, incu-

CLIENT/FAMILY EDUCATION ■ Oral Antibiotic Therapy for STDs

Instructions	Rationales
1. "It is important that you take your medicine the number of times a day and for the specific number of days prescribed."	1. To provide the most effective treatment.
2. "Your sexual partner must be tested and may have to be treated."	2. To prevent reinfection.
3. "Return to the clinic (health care setting) for your follow-up appointment after completing your antibiotic treatment."	3. To assess for the need for further treatment.
4. "Call the clinic if you have any questions or concerns."	4. To decrease concerns and increase compliance with treatment.
5. "Do not engage in sexual intercourse until after your antibiotic therapy is completed. If your partner is being treated, you can resume sexual intercourse after 48 hours if you use condoms."	5. To avoid reinfection.
6. "Drink at least 8–10 glasses of fluids a day while taking your antibiotic."	6. To decrease esophageal irritation and prevent renal complications.
7. "Do not take antacids containing calcium, magnesium, or aluminum."	7. To prevent decreased absorption of antibiotic.
8. "Take your antibiotic on an empty stomach unless your physician allows you to take it with food."	8. To prevent gastrointestinal upset and prevent interference with absorption.

bation period, signs and symptoms, treatment, and possible complications of untreated or inadequately treated infection should be discussed. (See the accompanying Client/Family Education feature for client instructions for antibiotic therapy, and refer to the earlier Client/Family Education: Safe Sex Practices for additional client teaching.) Psychosocial support is similar to that discussed in the section on gonorrhea.

BACTERIAL SEXUALLY TRANSMITTED DISEASE SYNDROMES

PELVIC INFLAMMATORY DISEASE

OVERVIEW

Acute PID is considered to be the major gynecologic health problem in the United States (Faulkner & Soman, 1986). PID is an infectious process that may involve one or more pelvic structures, although the most common site is the fallopian tube. In fact, many practitioners use the term PID and salpingitis synonymously for acute infections. PID is one of the leading causes of infertility and is being related to the rise of the number of ectopic pregnancies reported in the United States (Prepas, 1985). Chronic PID is a term no longer commonly used because pelvic infections are not chronic; subsequent infections are also primary infections, and the long-term effects of acute infections such as adhesions are not infectious processes.

Pathophysiology

Acute PID is a complex disease in which organisms from the lower genital tract migrate from the endocervix through the endometrial cavity to the fallopian tubes. The spread of infection to other organs of the upper genital tract occurs by way of direct contact with mucosal surfaces or through the fimbriated ends of the tubes to the ovaries, parametrium, and peritoneal cavity (Fig. 56–3). Resultant infections include endometritis (infection of the endometrial cavity), salpingitis (inflammation of the fallopian tubes), oophoritis (ovarian infec-

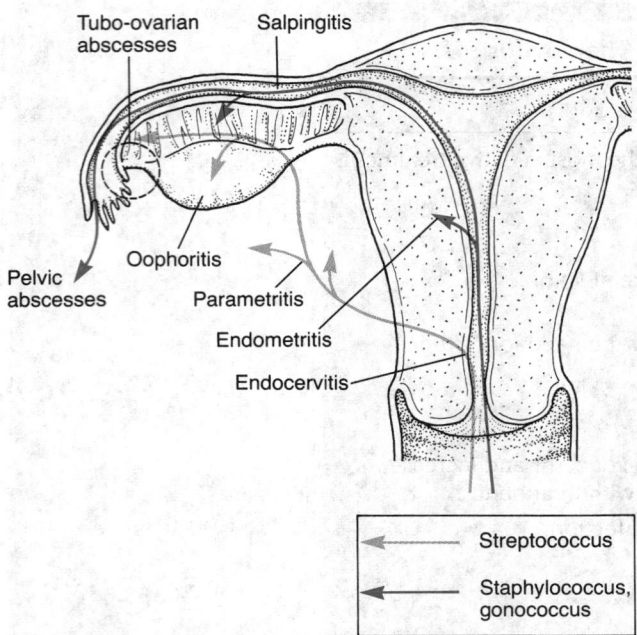

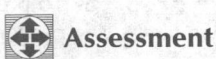

Figure 56–3

Spread of PID.

tion), parametritis (infection of the parametrium), and peritonitis (infection of the peritoneal cavity). These conditions cause adhesions and strictures of the fallopian tubes and can cause sterility.

Etiology

Three sexually transmitted organisms are most often responsible for PID: *N. gonorrhoeae, C. trachomatis,* and *Mycoplasma hominis,* with *Chlamydia* being the most common cause of acute PID in the United States (Faulkner & Soman, 1986). In addition to these bacteria, staphylococcus, streptococcus, and other aerobic and anaerobic organisms have been identified in clients with PID. These organisms most likely invade the pelvis from an ascending infection from the vagina or cervix. Infections have been spread during sexual intercourse and childbirth (including post partum), and after abortion. Rarely do infections result from transperitoneal spread from a ruptured appendix or intra-abdominal abscess.

Sexually active women who have multiple sexual partners may have an increased risk for PID. Other factors that increase a woman's chance of developing PID include use of an intrauterine device for contraception and a history of PID. Questionable risk factors are nulliparity, low socioeconomic status, non-Caucasian ethnic origin, and divorced or separated marital status (Faulkner & Soman, 1986).

Incidence

The incidence of PID is on the rise. Accurate incidence rates are unavailable because PID is not a reportable disease, but it is estimated that at least 13 in 1000 women between the ages of 14 and 34 years will develop PID yearly (Faulkner & Soman, 1986).

Younger women are at higher risk for developing PID, with two-thirds of all cases found in women younger than 25 years (Faulkner & Soman, 1986).

PREVENTION

Clients who are identified at high risk for PID may need to be counseled about both their increased risk for developing PID and the early signs of PID that can lead to early diagnosis and treatment.

Women who use oral contraceptives may be at lower risk for developing acute PID. Barrier methods such as condoms, diaphragms, and spermicidal foams and jellies have been shown to provide some protection against PID (Faulkner & Soman, 1986). Good perineal hygiene (e.g., wiping from front to back and frequent pad changes) should be taught to women who are at risk, especially those who recently had gynecologic surgery, experienced childbirth, or had an abortion.

COLLABORATIVE MANAGEMENT

Assessment

History

The nurse obtains a complete medical, family, menstrual, obstetric, and sexual history, including a history of previous episodes of PID or other infections. The nurse also assesses for contraceptive use, especially the intrauterine device, history of reproductive surgery, and other risk factors previously identified. Symptoms of acute PID most often develop during or after menstruation.

Physical Assessment: Clinical Manifestations

The examination may reveal lower abdominal tenderness with rigidity or rebound pain. One of the most frequent symptoms of acute PID is lower abdominal pain and tenderness. Other symptoms may include chills, fever, malaise, purulent vaginal discharge, tachycardia, dysuria, and irregular vaginal bleeding. A pelvic examination may reveal uterine or cervical tenderness with motion and swollen adnexa (tubes and ovaries). Characteristics of vaginal and cervical discharges, if present, should be noted.

Psychosocial Assessment

The woman who presents with symptoms of PID is usually anxious and fearful of the examination and unknown diagnosis. She may need much reassurance and support during the physical examination because she is likely to be quite tender and wish to avoid further pain. Explanations of what is taking place often help to promote cooperation during the examination.

If the PID is associated with an STD, the woman may be embarrassed or have guilt feelings about having this infection. The nurse uses a nonjudgmental approach in making assessments and encourages expression of feelings and concerns.

Laboratory Findings

Laboratory tests include the following:

1. Cultures of the cervix, urethra, and rectum to evaluate the presence of *N. gonorrhoeae* or *Chlamydia*
2. White blood cell count and erythrocyte sedimentation rate, which may be elevated but are not sensitive enough for sole diagnosis of PID
3. Gram-stained examination of endocervical secretions, which may show the presence of *N. gonorrhoeae*
4. Pregnancy testing, for the presence of human chorionic gonadotropin, which may indicate an ectopic pregnancy rather than PID in women presenting with acute pelvic pain

Other Diagnostic Tests

Ultrasonography has been more accurate in assessing pelvic abscesses than in assessing enlargements and abscesses related to ovaries and tubes. Laparoscopy is the most definitive test and gives an immediate, accurate diagnosis through direct inspection of the tubes and ovaries.

Culdocentesis is a technique that is performed to aspirate peritoneal fluid or pus from the cul-de-sac. Culturing this fluid may assist in the diagnosis of PID.

 Analysis: Nursing Diagnosis

Common Diagnoses

The following diagnoses are common for the woman with PID:

1. Pain related to PID
2. Anxiety related to possible infertility as a result of PID

Additional Diagnoses

In addition, some women may have the following diagnoses:

1. Self-esteem disturbance related to guilt of having PID (associated with sexual transmission)
2. Chronic pain after acute PID episode

3. Sexual dysfunction related to PID
4. Knowledge deficit related to risks, prevention, symptoms, treatment, and effects of PID

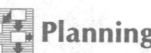 **Planning and Implementation**

The following care plan focuses on the common nursing diagnoses for the woman with PID.

Pain

Planning: client goals.   The goal is that the client will have a reduction or alleviation of pain.

Interventions.   Medical (pain management and antibiotic therapy) and surgical management may be used, depending on the symptoms and the extent of the disease.

Nonsurgical management.   Pain management of PID is based on the severity of the symptoms. Relief measures include offering analgesics, using sitz baths, and applying heat to the lower abdomen or back. Bed rest in semi-Fowler's position promotes drainage that may provide pain relief as well.

Treatment of the infection relieves pain, and a variety of antibiotics are used (Table 56–6). Inpatient therapy initially involves a combination of several intravenous antibiotics for 4 to 5 days, followed by oral antibiotic therapy for 7 to 10 days. Outpatient therapy combines oral and/or intramuscular antibiotics given once, followed by oral therapy for 10 to 14 days.

Two-thirds to three-fourths of women with uncomplicated PID are treated on an outpatient basis with oral antibiotics. The main concern is that these women be re-evaluated and re-examined 48 to 72 hours after antibiotic therapy is started. If the infection has not responded to treatment, hospitalization for intravenous antibiotic therapy and further evaluation may be necessary.

Surgical management.   In a small number of clients, the pain and tenderness may not be relieved by antibiotic therapy. For these clients, a laparotomy may be performed to remove an abscess or a pelvic mass. A laparotomy is usually performed through a subumbilical incision that is several inches long to provide better access to the tubes.

Preoperative care.   Preoperatively, the nurse provides information about hospital routines and procedures. Procedures for a laparotomy are similar to those for tubal surgery (see Chap. 54).

Postoperative care.   The postoperative care of the woman with PID is similar to that of a woman after tubal sterilization. One difference is that the woman with PID may have a wound drain in place for drainage of abscess fluid that may not have been completely removed dur-

TABLE 56–6 Drugs Used in the Treatment of Acute Pelvic Inflammatory Disease*

Drug	Usual Daily Dosage	Interventions	Rationales
Inpatient Treatment			
Regimen A			
Cefoxitin	2.0 g qid IV for 4 d	1. Assess client for rash, itching, and hypotension. 2. Observe IV site for signs of redness, heat, and tenderness.	1. To detect adverse reactions. 2. To detect phlebitis.
plus			
Doxycycline	100 mg bid IV or PO for 4 d	1. Do not give with iron or antacids.	1. To avoid inhibition of drug absorption.
followed by			
Doxycycline	100 mg bid PO for 10–14 d	2. Assess client for rashes, nausea, and diarrhea. 3. Encourage fluid intake.	2. To detect side effects. 3. To decrease esophageal irritation.
Regimen B			
Clindamycin	900 mg tid IV	1. Observe client for rash and urticaria. 2. Observe client for hypotension, dyspnea, and restlessness. 3. Observe client for diarrhea. 4. Observe IV site for redness, heat, and tenderness.	1. To detect adverse reactions. 2. To detect anaphylactic reaction. 3. To avoid pseudomembranous colitis. 4. To detect phlebitis.
plus			
Gentamicin	2.0 mg/kg IV once followed by 1.5 mg/kg tid for 4 d	1. Encourage oral intake of fluids. 2. Observe IV site for redness, heat, and tenderness. 3. Measure fluid intake and output.	1. To prevent irritation to renal tubules. 2. To detect phlebitis. 3. To detect oliguria or anuria.
then			
Doxycycline	100 mg bid PO for 10–14 d	See 1–3 above for doxycycline	
or			
Clindamycin	450 mg 5 times a day PO for 10–14 d	1. Give with 8 oz of water. See 1–4 above for clindamycin	1. To decrease esophageal irritation.
Outpatient Treatment			
Cefoxitin	2.0 g IM once	1. Give deep IM injection in outer upper quadrant of gluteus maximus. 2. Watch for fever, chills, and nausea. 3. Tell client that injection may be painful.	1. To avoid local irritation and to increase drug absorption. 2. To detect allergic reactions. 3. To prepare client for discomfort related to inflammatory reaction.

TABLE 56–6   Drugs Used in the Treatment of Acute Pelvic Inflammatory Disease* *Continued*

Drug	Usual Daily Dosage	Interventions	Rationales
plus			
Probenecid	1 g PO once	1. Give with food.	1. To avoid gastrointestinal upset.
		2. Encourage fluid intake (10 glasses a day).	2. To prevent formation of kidney stones.
or			
Ceftriaxone	250 mg IM once	1. Give deep IM injection in outer upper quadrant of gluteus maximus.	1. To avoid local irritation and to increase drug absorption.
		2. Watch for fever, chills, and nausea.	2. To detect allergic reactions.
followed by			
Doxycycline	100 mg bid PO for 10–14 d	See 1–3 above for doxycycline	

* These are examples of combinations of drugs recommended by the CDC. No single drug is active against all the pathogens causing PID. Modified from Centers for Disease Control. (1989b). 1989 sexually transmitted diseases treatment guidelines [Special issue]. *Morbidity and Mortality Weekly Report,* 38(Suppl. 8), 32–33.

ing surgery. Drainage should be measured and recorded (see Chap. 20 for care of wound drains).

Anxiety

Planning: client goals. The major goal is that the client will use effective coping mechanisms to reduce anxiety about infertility.

Interventions: nonsurgical management. Infertility is the most common complication of PID and affects at least 15% to 25% of women who have had at least one episode of PID (Torrington, 1985). Nursing interventions are aimed at assessing the woman for her knowledge of PID and its relation to infertility, and for verbal and nonverbal clues of anxiety about this potential problem. If anxiety is present, the nurse tries to provide an atmosphere in which the woman feels comfortable in expressing her feelings and in asking questions. Emotional support from significant others should be encouraged. Providing information about the advantages of early diagnosis and treatment—possibly limiting damage to one area of the pelvis—and the advances in surgery for infertility may reassure the woman.

■ Discharge Planning

Home Care Preparation

No special home care preparation is necessary for women who are treated for PID.

Client/Family Education

Client teaching focuses on providing information about PID: identification of recurrences (persistent pain, dysmenorrhea, low backache, fever) and meticulous perineal hygiene. A woman needs to be counseled to contact her sexual partner for examination and possible treatment of an STD. She also needs to be reminded about follow-up care and must be counseled about the complications that can occur after an episode of PID (increased risk for ectopic pregnancy and infertility and development of chronic pelvic pain). If contraceptive measures are desired, methods that may prevent future episodes of PID such as oral contraceptive pills and barrier methods should be discussed.

Young women need to understand the factors that are associated with their life style—sexual intercourse with multiple partners, potential for recurrence of PID, and use of certain contraceptive methods (e.g., intrauterine devices)—that place a woman at risk for other episodes of PID.

Psychosocial Preparation

A woman who has PID may exhibit feelings of guilt about having a condition that may have been transmitted to her sexually. These guilt feelings may affect her relationships with significant others. She may also have concerns about future fertility if PID has caused major damage or scarring of the fallopian tubes and other reproductive organs. The nurse provides emotional support and allows time for the woman to express her feelings.

Health Care Resources

If infertility is a result of PID, the woman may need referral to a clinic specializing in infertility treatment and counseling. The woman can also contact support groups for infertile couples that exist in many local communities.

 Evaluation

On the basis of the identified nursing diagnoses, the expected outcomes of care for the woman with PID are that she

1. Reports that the pain is relieved and that she feels more comfortable
2. Relates that anxiety about future infertility has decreased
3. Describes the risk factors, signs and symptoms, treatment modalities, and effects of PID
4. Resumes usual sexual activities without discomfort
5. Expresses her feelings about having an infection that was likely caused by a sexually transmitted organism

VAGINAL INFECTIONS

Vaginal infections are associated with discharge and are frequent and recurring problems for sexually active women. Common causes of vaginal infection are *Trichomonas vaginalis, Candida albicans,* and bacteria that produce vaginosis, or *Gardnerella*-associated vaginitis. These infections can be spread by sexual contact. Males can develop these infections, but they usually do not present with symptoms and often are not treated unless the female partner has trichomoniasis. Because these infections are usually seen in women, assessments and interventions are discussed with other causes of vaginitis in Chapters 52 and 54.

OTHER SEXUALLY TRANSMITTED DISEASES

SCABIES

Scabies is caused by a mite, *Sarcoptes scabiei.* Scabies is usually transmitted by close body contact with infected persons or by contact with contaminated bed linens and clothes. The presenting symptom is a rash that can erupt on the genitalia, buttocks, and various parts of the body,

including behind the knees, under the arms, and between the fingers and toes. Itching is present and may worsen at night.

Diagnosis may be confirmed by microscopic examination of mites or their eggs, although these can be hard to find. Usually diagnosis is made by history and location of skin lesions. Treatment consists of lindane (1%), 1 oz of lotion or 30 g of cream (Kwell), applied thinly to all areas of the body from the neck down. This application is washed off in 8 hours. Lindane may be neurotoxic and should not be used by pregnant women and children younger than 2 years of age. For these clients, crotamiton (10%) can be applied to the same areas of the body as lindane for 2 nights and washed off after the second application (CDC, 1989b).

Clients should be informed that itching may continue for several weeks, even after successful treatment. Clothing and bed linens should be machine washed and dried (hot cycle) or dry cleaned. Sexual partners and close household contacts should be treated. Retreatment may be necessary in 1 week if live mites are still present.

PEDICULOSIS PUBIS

Crab lice, or *Pediculus pubis,* can cause infections that usually result from close body contact with an infected person but can be through contact with infested bed linen or clothes. Itching is the main symptom.

Diagnosis is made when the adult lice or eggs (nits) are found attached to pubic hair. Treatment is with lindane (1%) shampoo applied for 4 minutes and then rinsed off thoroughly. The pregnant or lactating woman may use permethrin (1%) cream rinse (Nix) or pyrethrins and piperonyl butoxide. These treatments should be applied to the affected areas and washed off after 10 minutes. Clients should be rechecked in 1 week if symptoms persist. Retreatment may be necessary.

Clients should be informed that bed linens and clothing worn within the last 2 days may be contaminated. These articles should be machine washed and dried (hot cycle) or dry cleaned. Clients also should be informed that sexual partners should also be treated.

SUMMARY

The nurse's primary role in prevention of STDs is one of educating the client, the family, the client's sexual partners, and the community about the necessity of practicing safe and responsible sex. Nurses can provide information to clients about ways of changing sexual behaviors that put them at risk, modes of transmission and how to reduce those risks, physical and psychosocial manifestations of infections, treatments, and possible complications. Information alone may not be enough to produce changes in sexual behavior; guidelines such as those described in this chapter should be provided.

Having an STD affects many aspects of a client's life and often the client expresses a feeling of being out of control. Nurses can assist clients in controlling their lives by helping them to develop positive coping strategies to deal with emotional feelings and fears.

IMPLICATIONS FOR RESEARCH

Research in STDs occurs in two major areas: identification of causative organisms and testing of treatment modalities.

Nursing research in this area is needed for improvement of care to clients with STDs. Research must focus on identifying effective nursing interventions and ways to improve preventive health practices. Suggestions for study include

1. How can a client be motivated to comply with treatment and partner follow-up?

2. How can the client be motivated to practice safe sex for all sexual encounters?

3. Is there a pattern for how different sociocultural subgroups react to STDs?

4. What are effective stress re-education and other coping strategies for clients with STDs?

5. What are the long-term psychologic effects of chronic STD infections?

6. What is the most effective method of teaching clients about risk assessment?

7. For which at-risk groups should routine screening of asymptomatic clients be performed for selected STDs?

REFERENCES AND READINGS

AIDS [Special issue] (1988). *Nursing Clinics of North America, 23,* 863–973.

Andrist, L. C. (1988). Taking a sexual history and educating clients about safe sex. *Nursing Clinics of North America, 23,* 959–973.

Bourcier, K. M., & Seidler, A. J. (1987). Chlamydia and condylomata acuminata: An update for the nurse practitioner. *Journal of Obstetric, Gynecologic, and Neonatal Nursing, 16,* 17–22.

Breslin, E. (1988). Genital herpes simplex. *Nursing Clinics of North America, 23,* 907–916.

Campbell, C., & Herten, R. (1981). VD to STD: Redefining venereal disease. *American Journal of Nursing, 81,* 1629–1634.

Centers for Disease Control. (1987). *Sexually transmitted disease statistics 1987, issue 136.* Atlanta: Author.

Centers for Disease Control. (1989a). Summary of notifiable diseases, United States, 1988. *Morbidity and Mortality Weekly Report, 37* (54).

Centers for Disease Control. (1989b). 1989 sexually transmitted diseases treatment guidelines [Special issue]. *Morbidity and Mortality Weekly Report, 38*(Suppl. 8), pp. 1–43.

Daly, J. A. (1985). *Haemophilus ducreyi. Infection Control, 6,* 203–205.

Dirubbo, N. (1987). The condom barrier. *American Journal of Nursing, 87,* 1306–1309.

Enterline, J. A. (1989). Condylomata acuminata (venereal warts). *Nurse Practitioner, 14*(4), 8–16.

Faulkner, S., & Soman, M. (1986). Pelvic inflammatory disease. In C. Havens, N. Sullivan, & P. Tilton (Eds.), *Manual of outpatient gynecology* (pp. 29–38). Boston: Little, Brown.

Felman, Y. M. (1986). *Sexually transmitted diseases.* New York: Churchill Livingstone.

Felman, Y., & Nikitas, J. A. (1981). Nongonococcal urethritis: A clinical review. *JAMA, 245,* 381–386.

Fogel, C. I. (1988). Gonorrhea: Not a new problem but a serious one. *Nursing Clinics of North America, 23,* 885–897.

Fogel, C. I., & Nettles-Carlson, B. (1987). Gonorrhea in women: A serious health problem. *Health Care of Women International, 8*(1), 75–86.

Freeman, P. E. (1980). Gonorrhea. *Journal of Emergency Nursing, 6*(3), 17–22.

Goddard, J. (1989). The many manifestations and implications of herpes virus infection. *Nursing RSA, 4*(3), 23–24.

Goldmeier, D., & Barton, S. (1987). *Sexually transmitted diseases.* London: Springer-Verlag.

Kee, J. L. (1987). *Laboratory and diagnostic tests with nursing implications* (2nd ed.). Norwalk, CT: Appleton & Lange.

Kramer, M. A., Arul, S. O., & Curran, J. W. (1980). Self-reported behavior patterns of patients attending a sexually transmitted disease clinic. *American Journal of Public Health, 70,* 997–999.

Loucks, A. (1987). Chlamydia: An unheralded epidemic. *American Journal of Nursing, 87,* 920–922.

Lucas, V. A. (1988). Human papillomavirus infection: A potentially carcinogenic sexually transmitted disease (condylomata acuminata, genital warts). *Nursing Clinics of North America, 23,* 917–935.

Lutz, R. (1986). Stopping the spread of sexually transmitted disease. *Nursing '86, 16*(3), 47–50.

Margolis, S. (1984). Genital warts and molluscum contagiosum. *Urology Clinics of North America, 11,* 163–170.

Miles, P. A. (1984). Sexually transmitted diseases. *Journal of Obstetric, Gynecologic, and Neonatal Nursing, 13*(Suppl.), 1025–1235.

Neeson, J. D., & Stockdale, C. R. (1981). *The practitioner's handbook of ambulatory OB/GYN.* New York: Wiley.

Prepas, R. (1985). Pelvic inflammatory disease. *NAACOG Update Series, 3*(1), 1–8.

Rapp, F. (1981). Summary of discussion I of conference of early cervical neoplasia. *Gynecology and Oncology, 112* (Suppl.), S88–S89.

Rein, M. F. (1984). Nosocomial sexually transmitted diseases. *Infection Control, 5,* 117–122.

Ridenour, N. (1980). Chlamydia. *Nurse Practitioner, 5*(5), 45–48.

Roberts, A. (1982). The pox and the people: A history of venereal diseases and sexual attitudes. *Nursing Times, 78*(28), 1177–1185.

Shattuck, J. C. (1988). Pelvic inflammatory disease: Education for maintaining fertility. *Nursing Clinics of North America, 23,* 899–906.

Silver, P. S., Auerbach, S. M., Vishniavsky, N., & Kaplowitz, L. G. (1986). Psychological factors in recurrent genital herpes infection: Stress, coping style, social support, emotional dysfunction, and symptom recurrence. *Journal of Psychosomatic Research, 30,* 163–171.

Smith, L. S. (1988). Ethnic differences in knowledge of sexually transmitted disease in North American black and Mexican-American migrant farmworkers. *Research in Nursing and Health, 11,* 51–58.

Smith, L. S., Lauver, D., & Gray, P. A., Jr. (1990). Sexually transmitted disease. In C. I. Fogel & D. Lauver (Eds.), *Sexual health promotion* (pp. 459–484). Philadelphia: W. B. Saunders.

Sonstegard, L., Kowalski, K. M., & Jennings, B. (Eds.). (1982). *Women's health: Ambulatory care* (Vol. 1, pp. 141–166). New York: Grune & Stratton.

Stamm, W. E., Harrison, H. R., Alexander, E. R., Cles, L. D., Spence, M. R., & Quinn, T. C. (1984). Diagnosis of *Chlamydia trachomatis* infections by direct immunofluorescence staining of genital secretions. A multicenter trial. *Annals of Internal Medicine, 101,* 638–641.

Sun, I. (1986). *Sexually related infectious diseases: Clinical and laboratory aspects.* Chicago: Field, Rich and Associates.

Thompson, E., & Washington, A. E. (1983). Epidemiology of sexually transmitted *Chlamydia trachomatis* infections. *Epidemiologic Review, 5,* 96–119.

Torrington, J. (1985). Pelvic inflammatory disease. *Journal of Obstetric, Gynecologic and Neonatal Nursing, 14*(Suppl.), 21s–31s.

Wardell, D. W. (1988). Chronic exposure to sexually transmitted diseases. *Nursing Clinics of North America, 223,* 947–957.

Wasley, G. D. (1985). Treponemal diseases of man. *Nursing Times, 81*(17), 34–35.

Whelan, M. (1988). Nursing management of the patient with *Chlamydia trachomatis* infection. *Nursing Clinics of North America, 23,* 877–883.

Willcox, R. R. (1981). Sexual behavior and sexually transmitted disease patterns in male homosexuals. *British Journal of Venereal Disease, 57,* 167–169.

ADDITIONAL READINGS

Enterline, J. A., & Leonardo, J. P. (1989). Condylomata acuminata (veneral warts). *Nurse Practitioner, 14*(4), 8–17.

This article discusses the STD condylomata acuminata and its relationship to cervical carcinoma. Information about the clinical signs and symptoms, etiology, and pathogenesis is given. Diagnosis and treatment are discussed as well. Nursing considerations for patient counseling are identified so that compliance with treatment and follow-up is enhanced.

Nettina, S. L., & Kauffman, F. H. (1990). Diagnosis and management of sexually transmitted genital lesions. *Nurse Practitioner, 15*(1), 20–39.

Genital lesions are often caused by STD. This article discusses clinical manifestations, differential diagnosis, and treatment of these diseases, including herpes genitalis, syphilis, LGV, chancroid, genital warts, granuloma inguinale, and molluscum contagiosum. The article includes a comprehensive table that nurses may find useful for comparing incubation periods, clinical signs and symptoms, diagnostic tests, and treatment among these STDs.

UNIT 15 RESOURCES

Nursing Resources

American Board of Urologic Allied Health Professionals (ABUAHP), 407 Strawberry Hill Avenue, Stamford, CT 06902. Telephone 203-323-1227.

See Unit 16 Resources for more information.

American College of Nurse-Midwives (ACNM), 1522 K Street NW, Suite 1000, Washington, DC 20005. Telephone 202-289-0171.

Serves as an advocate for Certified Nurse-Midwives. Promotes certified nurse-midwifery nationally and internationally. Promotes health of mothers and infants in underdeveloped areas of the world. Provides technical assistance to Certified Nurse-Midwives. Conducts research. Sponsors seminars, continuing education workshops, and an annual conference. Publishes the *Journal of Nurse-Midwifery* (bimonthly), *Quickening* (newsletter), and special reports. Certifies nurse-midwives and accredits nurse-midwifery educational programs.

American Urological Association Allied, 6845 Lake Shore Drive, PO Box 9373, Raytown, MO 64133. Telephone 816-358-3317.

Association of Nurses in AIDS Care (ANAC), 10141 Liberty Road, Randallstown, MD 21133. Telephone 301-922-1446; 215-750-1684.

See Unit 8 Resources for more information.

Association for Practitioners in Infection Control, 505 East Hawley Street, Mundelein, IL 60060. Telephone 312-949-6052.

See Unit 7 Resources for more information.

Nurses Association of the American College of Obstetricians and Gynecologists (NAACOG), 409 12th Street SW, Washington, DC 20024. Telephone 202-638-0026.

Promotes high standards of obstetric, gynecologic, and neonatal nursing practice, education, and research. Publishes the *Journal of Obstetric, Gynecologic, and Neonatal Nursing* (JOGNN; bimonthly), *NAACOG Newsletter* (monthly), *Standards for Obstetric, Gynecologic, and Neonatal Nursing*, and many other publications.

NAACOG Certification Corporation, Suite 1058, 645 North Michigan Avenue, Chicago, IL 60611. Telephone 312-951-0207.

Certifies nurses working in the obstetric, gynecologic, and neonatal nursing specialties.

Other Resources

American Cancer Society, 1599 Clifton Road NE, Atlanta, GA 30329. Telephone 404-320-3333.

American Fertility Society, 1608 13th Avenue South, Suite 101, Birmingham, AL 35205. Telephone 205-933-8494.

Provides referrals to infertility specialists.

Division of Sexually Transmitted Diseases, Center for Prevention Services, Centers for Disease Control, Department of Health and Human Services, U.S. Public Health Service, Atlanta, GA 30333. Telephone 404-639-3534.

ENCORE (Encouragement, Normalcy, Counseling, Opportunity, Reaching Out, Energies Revived), National YWCA, Health Promotions Department, 726 Broadway, New York, NY 10003. Telephone 212-475-5990.

Endometriosis Society, PO Box 164453, Milwaukee, WI 53202. Telephone 414-355-2200.

HELP (Herpes Resource Center), PO Box 100, Palo Alto, CA 94302. Telephone 415-328-7710.

HELPhiladelphia, PO Box 13193, Philadelphia, PA 19101. Telephone 215-735-4878.

Impotence Anonymous, PO Box 1257, Maryville, TN 37802. Telephone 615-983-6064.

National Center for PMS and Menstrual Disorders, 15 Smith Road, Bedford, NH 03102.

National Institute of Allergy and Infectious Diseases (NIAID), Building 10, Bethesda, MD 20892. Telephone 301-496-4000.

National Organization for Nonparents, 806 Riestertown Road, Baltimore, MD 21208.

National PMS Society, PO Box 11467, Durham, NC 27703.

OURS (Organization for a United Response), 3148 Humbolt Avenue South, Minneapolis, MN 55408. Telephone 612-827-5709.

Provides information for clients interested in adoption.

PMS Action, PO Box 9326, Madison, WI 53715. Telephone 608-833-4767.

Reach to Recovery, American Cancer Society, 1599 Clifton Road NE, Atlanta, GA 30329. Telephone 404-320-3333.

RESOLVE, PO Box 474, Belmont, MA 02178. Telephone 617-484-2424.

Provides education and support for infertile clients.

Rocky Mountain PMS Society, PO Box 16453, Salt Lake City, UT 84116. Telephone 801-584-2105.

U.S. Public Health Service AIDS Hot Line, 800-342-AIDS.

Problems of Excretion: Management of Clients with Disruptions of the Urinary System

CHAPTER 57

Assessment of the Urinary System

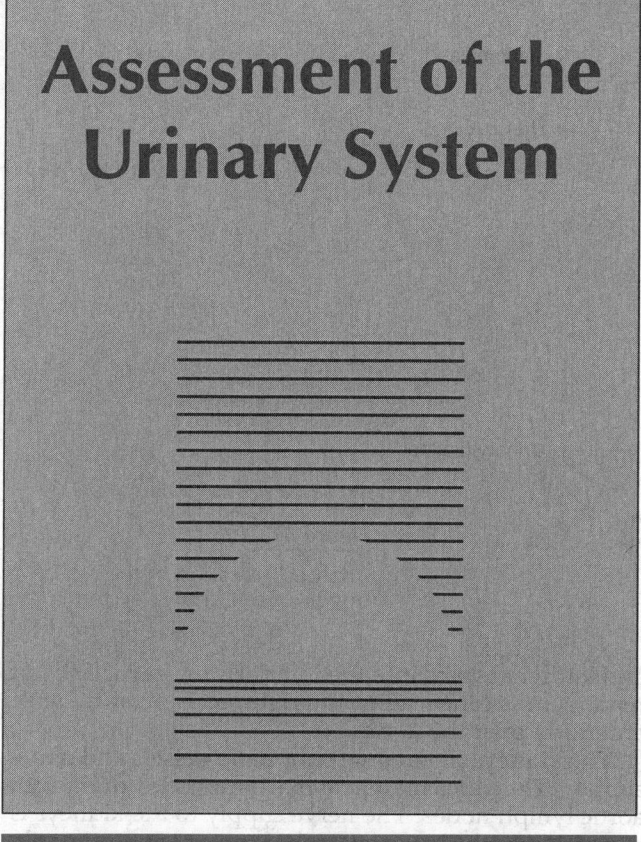

The urinary system is composed of the kidneys, the ureters, the urinary bladder, and the urethra. The kidneys filter metabolic waste products from the blood and excrete these wastes in excessive body water. The ureters, bladder, and urethra provide a drainage route for the excretion of urine. The integrity and functional status of the urinary tract are critical to the maintenance of overall homeostasis and health. Structural or functional alterations in any part of the urinary tract may be life-threatening.

ANATOMY AND PHYSIOLOGY REVIEW

KIDNEYS

STRUCTURE

Gross Anatomy

There are usually two kidneys located in the retroperitoneal space; one kidney is on either side of the vertebral column (Fig. 57–1). The kidneys lie in an oblique position. When the client is in a supine position, the kidneys are located between the twelfth thoracic and third lumbar vertebrae; in Trendelenburg's position, the kidneys may ascend to the tenth intercostal space; in a standing position, the kidneys may descend to the top of the sacroiliac crest. The adult kidney is 4 to 5 in (11 to 13 cm) long, 2 to 3 in (5 to 7 cm) wide, and about 1 in (2.5 to 3.0 cm) thick; the weight is about 5 oz (150 g). The left kidney is slightly longer and narrower than the right kidney.

The kidneys are surrounded by several layers of tissue; these tissues protect and anchor the kidneys in position. The outer surface of the kidney is a layer of fibrous tissue called the renal capsule. The *renal capsule* is surrounded by layers of perirenal fat and Gerota's fascia. External to these protective layers are the muscles of the back, flank, and abdomen, as well as layers of fat, subcutaneous tissue, and skin. The capsule covers all aspects of the kidney, except the *hilum,* which is the area from which the renal artery, the renal vein, and the ureter exit. The upper poles of each kidney are partially protected by the lower portion of the rib cage.

The gross structural components of the kidney are more easily appreciated when the kidney is bisected (Fig. 57–2). Lying beneath the capsule is the parenchyma. The renal *parenchyma* is the functional tissue of the kidney and is composed of distinct structural units, the cortex and the medulla. The renal *cortex* is in direct contact with the capsule; the *medulla,* or medullary tissue, is deeper into the kidney below the cortex. The medullary tissue is in the form of *pyramids,* which are

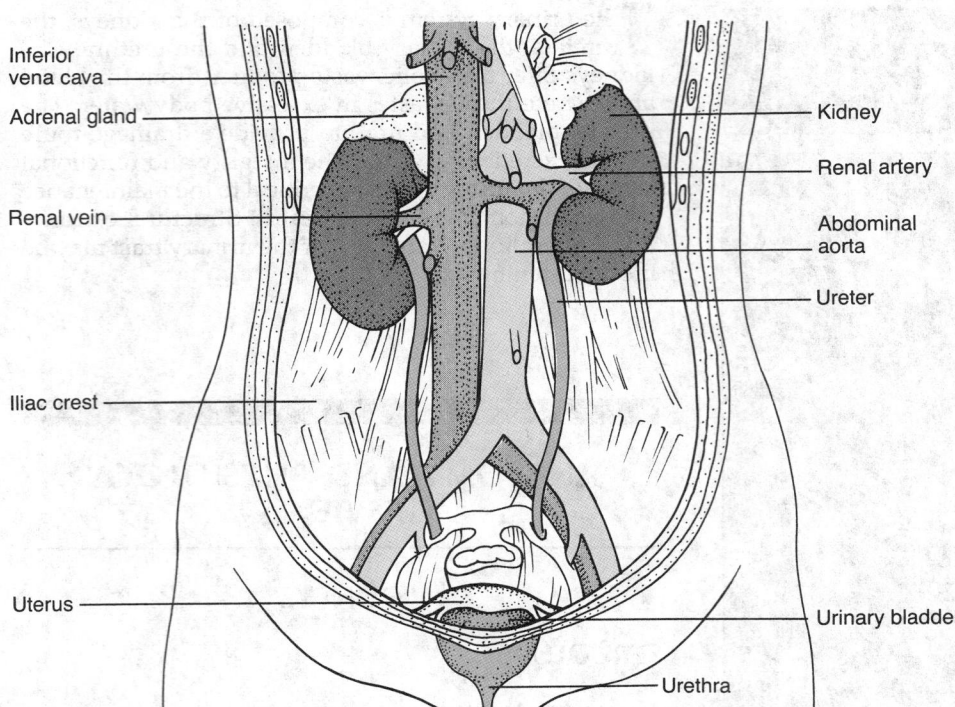

Inferior vena cava
Adrenal gland
Renal vein
Iliac crest
Uterus
Kidney
Renal artery
Abdominal aorta
Ureter
Urinary bladder
Urethra

Figure 57–1

Anatomic location of the organs of the urinary system.

spread in the shape of a fan. There are 12 to 18 pyramids per kidney. Separating the pyramids are the renal *columns* (columns of Bertin), or cortical tissue, that descend into the interior of the kidney. The tip of each pyramid is called the *papilla*. The papillae funnel formed urine into the collecting system.

The innermost aspect of the kidney is the renal pelvis. The *renal pelvis* is a small basin that funnels urine from the parenchyma into the ureter. Structurally, the *minor calyx* cups the papilla of each pyramid; several minor calyces merge together to form a *major calyx*. The major calyces merge to form the renal pelvis. The renal pelvis narrows into the ureter; the point of juncture is a narrowing called the ureteropelvic (UP) junction.

The blood supply to the kidneys is delivered by a single *renal artery*, which is a major branch of the abdominal aorta. The *right renal artery* is longer and extends below the inferior vena cava to deliver blood into the right kidney. The *left renal artery* is shorter, as the aorta is closer to the left kidney. Each renal artery separates into segmental arteries that supply the anterior and posterior portions of the kidney. These segmental arteries branch into progressively smaller arteries supplying all areas of the renal parenchyma. The kidneys receive 20% to 25% of the total cardiac output. Renal blood flow varies widely within a range of approximately 600 to 1300 mL/minute (Brenner et al., 1986).

The renal venous system in general is parallel to the arterial system. Renal venules in the cortex become progressively larger and finally return blood via the right and left renal veins into the inferior vena cava. The left renal vein is longer than the right, as it must traverse anteriorly over the aorta.

The kidneys have some lymphatic vessels and nerve supply. The renal parenchyma lymphatics drain into aortic lymph nodes. The nerve supply to the kidneys is derived from the lesser splanchnic nerves and primarily influences renal circulation.

Microscopic Anatomy

The *nephron* is the functional unit of the kidney (see the illustration on p. 1803). There are 1 to 1.25 million nephrons per kidney; each nephron is capable of functioning as an independent unit. Structurally, the nephrons are contained within the renal cortex and the renal medulla. There are two types of nephrons: cortical and juxtamedullary. In the cortical nephrons, all vascular and tubular components are within the renal cortex. In the juxtamedullary nephrons, the vascular components are near the corticomedullary junction and the tubular components are in the medulla.

The nephron has two major components: a vascular system and a tubular system. The vascular component of the nephron comprises the afferent arteriole, the glomerulus, and the efferent arteriole. The arterial blood supply of the nephron is delivered via the renal artery into the afferent arteriole. The *afferent arteriole* is the smallest, most distal portion of the renal artery. From

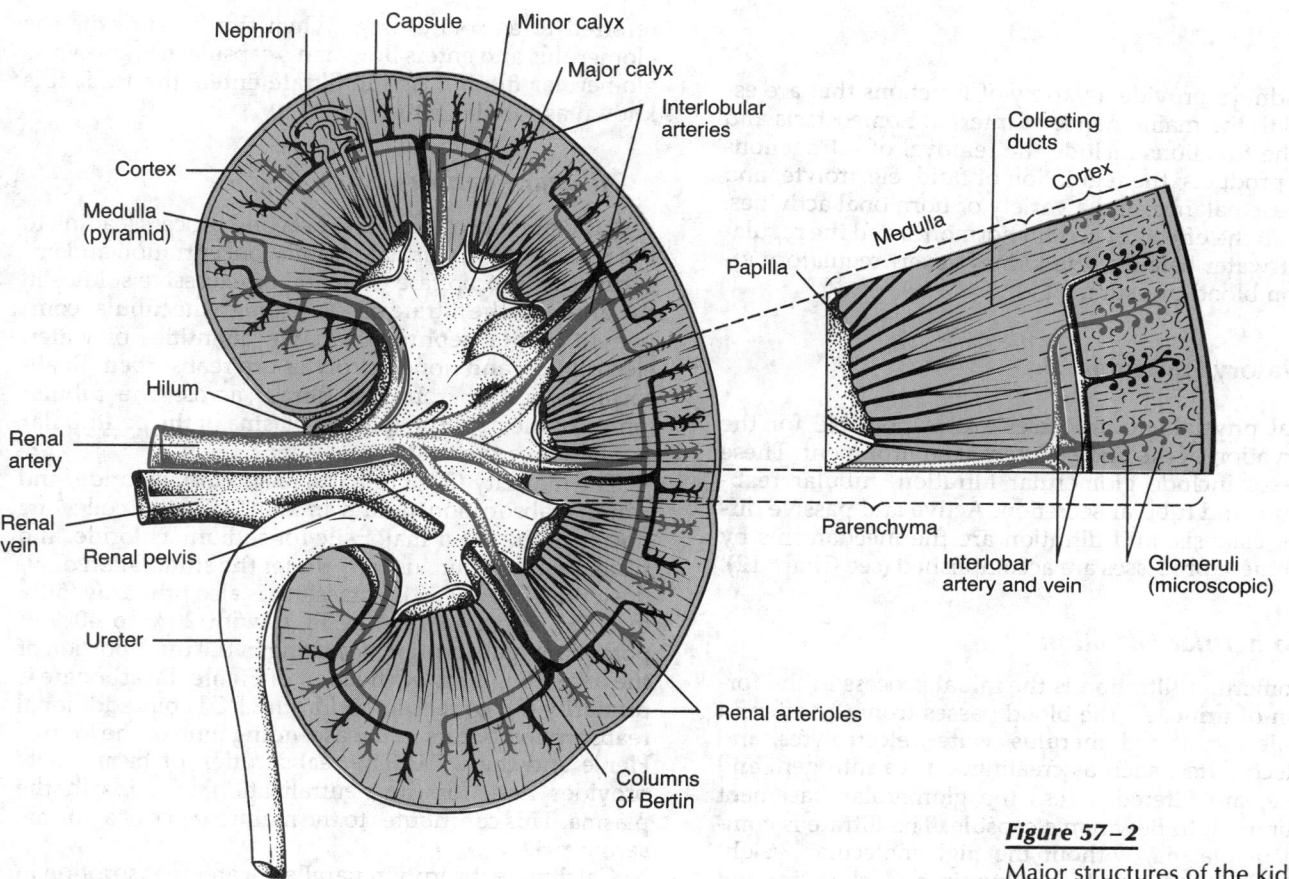

Figure 57–2

Major structures of the kidney.

the afferent arteriole, blood is delivered into the glomerulus. The *glomerulus* is a series of specialized capillary loops. Blood exits from the glomerulus via the *efferent arteriole*. From the efferent arteriole, blood exits into one of two additional capillary systems: the *peritubular capillaries* or the *vasa recta*.

The tubular component of the nephron begins with *Bowman's capsule*, a sac-like structure that concavely surrounds the glomerulus. The tubular tissue of Bowman's capsule narrows into the *proximal convoluted tubule* (PCT), a structure that twists and turns, finally straightening into the descending limb of the loop of Henle. The *descending limb of the loop of Henle* dips in the direction of the medulla, but forms a hairpin loop and redirects toward the cortex. As the loop of Henle changes direction, two segments are identified in the *ascending limb of the loop of Henle:* these are the thin and thick segments of the loop of Henle. From the thick segment of the ascending limb of the loop of Henle, the *distal convoluted tubule* (DCT) is identified. The DCTs of several nephrons terminate in one of many *collecting ducts,* which are located in the renal parenchyma. The collecting ducts pass through the papillae and empty into the calyceal system of the renal pelvis.

A series of specialized cells are located in the afferent arteriole, the efferent arteriole, and the DCT and are known as the *juxtaglomerular apparatus* (JGA). The cells in the afferent arteriole and the efferent arteriole are called the *juxtaglomerular cells* (JGCs). These cells store renin, a hormone that participates in the regulation of blood flow, glomerular filtration rate (GFR), and systemic blood pressure. The cells in the DCT are known as the *macula densa* and contain receptors sensitive to volume and pressure changes. The macula densa of the DCT lies adjacent to the JGCs of both afferent and efferent arterioles. When there is a decrease in blood flow or blood volume through the arterioles or an alteration in the sodium ion concentration of the tubular filtrate, the JGCs release renin (Guyton, 1986).

The microscopic anatomy of the nephron can be described owing to advances in electron microscopy. The glomerular capillary wall has three distinct layers: the endothelium, the basement membrane, and the epithelium. The capillary loops of the glomerulus also contain mesangial cells, which provide some structural support. Cells that line the endothelium and epithelium are separated by pores or slits through which certain molecular substances may pass. The tubular lumen is lined with cells of varying sizes and characteristics. These variations are responsible for promoting or delaying molecular movement. The glomeruli and tubules are surrounded by tissue known as the interstitium.

FUNCTION

The kidneys provide a variety of functions that are essential to the maintenance of internal homeostasis and life. The functions include the removal of nitrogenous waste products; the regulation of fluid, electrolyte, and acid-base balance; and a variety of hormonal activities. Through the effects of certain hormones and the regulation of water balance, the kidneys exert regulatory effects on blood pressure.

Regulatory Functions

Several physiologic processes are responsible for the preservation of the body's internal environment. These processes include glomerular filtration, tubular reabsorption, and tubular secretion. Active and passive diffusion, osmosis, and filtration are the mechanisms by which these processes are accomplished (see Chap. 12).

Glomerular Filtration

Glomerular filtration is the initial process in the formation of urine. As the blood passes from the afferent arteriole into the glomerulus, water, electrolytes, and nonelectrolytes, such as creatinine, urea nitrogen, and glucose, are filtered across the glomerular basement membrane into Bowman's capsule. The filtrate is composed of plasma, without the high-molecular-weight protein molecules such as albumin and globulin, and without red blood cells (RBCs).

The creation of a net positive pressure is responsible for glomerular filtration. The hydrostatic pressure (blood pressure) is the primary force promoting the ultrafiltration of the blood. The forces that oppose glomerular filtration are the plasma oncotic pressure of the blood in the glomerulus and the tubular filtrate pressure of the filtrate in Bowman's capsule. When the hydrostatic pressure exceeds the sum of the two opposing pressures (plasma oncotic and tubular filtrate pressures), a net pressure in favor of filtration exists.

The ability of the kidneys to autoregulate renal blood pressure and renal blood flow promotes a relatively constant GFR. The smooth muscle fibers of the afferent and efferent arterioles are responsible for this autoregulation. Although increased systemic blood pressure could greatly increase GFR, vasodilation of the afferent arteriole decreases the blood pressure in the kidney and thus maintains a fairly constant GFR. Similarly, with a relatively low systemic blood pressure, the vasoconstriction of the smooth muscles of the efferent arterioles raises the renal blood pressure, allowing glomerular filtration to continue without major alteration. Approximately 180 L of glomerular filtrate are formed each day. If all glomerular filtrate were excreted as urine, death would promptly ensue from massive fluid and electrolyte depletion. Actually, only about 1 to 2 L is excreted each day as urine. Electrolytes and nonelectrolytes are transported into the glomerular filtrate by a mechanism

referred to as solute drag. When the filtrate exits the glomerulus and enters Bowman's capsule, it is known as glomerular filtrate. As the filtrate enters the PCT, it is known as tubular filtrate.

Tubular Reabsorption

Tubular reabsorption is the second process leading to the restoration of normal plasma concentration and ensuring the appropriate excretion of excessive solutes in the urine. As the filtrate passes through the tubular component of the nephron, variable quantities of water, electrolytes, and nonelectrolytes are reabsorbed. Reabsorption occurs from the filtrate across the tubular lumen of the nephron into the plasma of the peritubular capillaries or the vasa recta.

The majority (50% to 75%) of sodium, chloride, and water reabsorption occurs in the PCT; the collecting ducts are the other major site for sodium, chloride, and water reabsorption, usually under the stimulation of aldosterone (Fig. 57–3). Potassium is also primarily (50% to 70%) reabsorbed in the PCT, with 20% to 40% of potassium reabsorption occurring in the thick portion of the ascending limb of the loop of Henle. Bicarbonate is primarily (75%) reabsorbed in the PCT, but additional reabsorption occurs in the ascending limb of the loop of Henle and the DCT. The reabsorption of bicarbonate provides base for the neutralization of acids in the plasma. This contributes to the maintenance of a normal serum pH.

Calcium reabsorption parallels water reabsorption in the PCT: in the thick ascending limb of the medullary nephron loop of Henle, calcitonin influences calcium reabsorption; in the thick ascending limb of the cortical nephron loop of Henle, parathyroid hormone (PTH) influences calcium reabsorption. A small percentage of calcium is reabsorbed in the DCT; excessive calcium is excreted in the urine through the effect of PTH, which increases calcium transport to the urine.

Almost all phosphate is reabsorbed in the PCT. Numerous hormones, calcium, magnesium, and vitamin D are being investigated for their potential role in mediating phosphate reabsorption.

Magnesium is primarily (66%) reabsorbed in the thick ascending limb of the loop of Henle; a smaller percentage (20% to 30%) is reabsorbed in the PCT. Small quantities of urea nitrogen are reabsorbed. Almost all glucose is reabsorbed, and no creatinine is reabsorbed.

Tubular Secretion

Tubular secretion is a third process involved in the formation of urine. Tubular secretion, in addition to glomerular filtration, is a method by which substances may move from the plasma into the tubular filtrate. During tubular secretion, molecules pass from the peritubular capillaries across capillary membranes into the cells that line the tubules. A constant exchange of molecules and corresponding chemical reactions permit the removal of

WHAT HAPPENS IN THE NEPHRON (THE KIDNEY'S FUNCTIONAL UNIT)

Blood enters the afferent arteriole on its way to the glomerulus for filtration. In the glomerulus, hydrostatic pressure and other forces promote the filtration of water, electrolytes, and other substances out of the capillaries and into the space within Bowman's capsule. The blood components remaining in the capillaries are returned to the systemic circulation through the efferent arteriole and the peritubular capillary network. Meanwhile, the filtered substances—known as filtrate—pass through the proximal convoluted tubule, the loop of Henle, and the distal convoluted tubule and are altered by tubular reabsorption and tubular secretion. The final filtrate that remains after passage through the tubules is excreted through the collecting duct as urine.

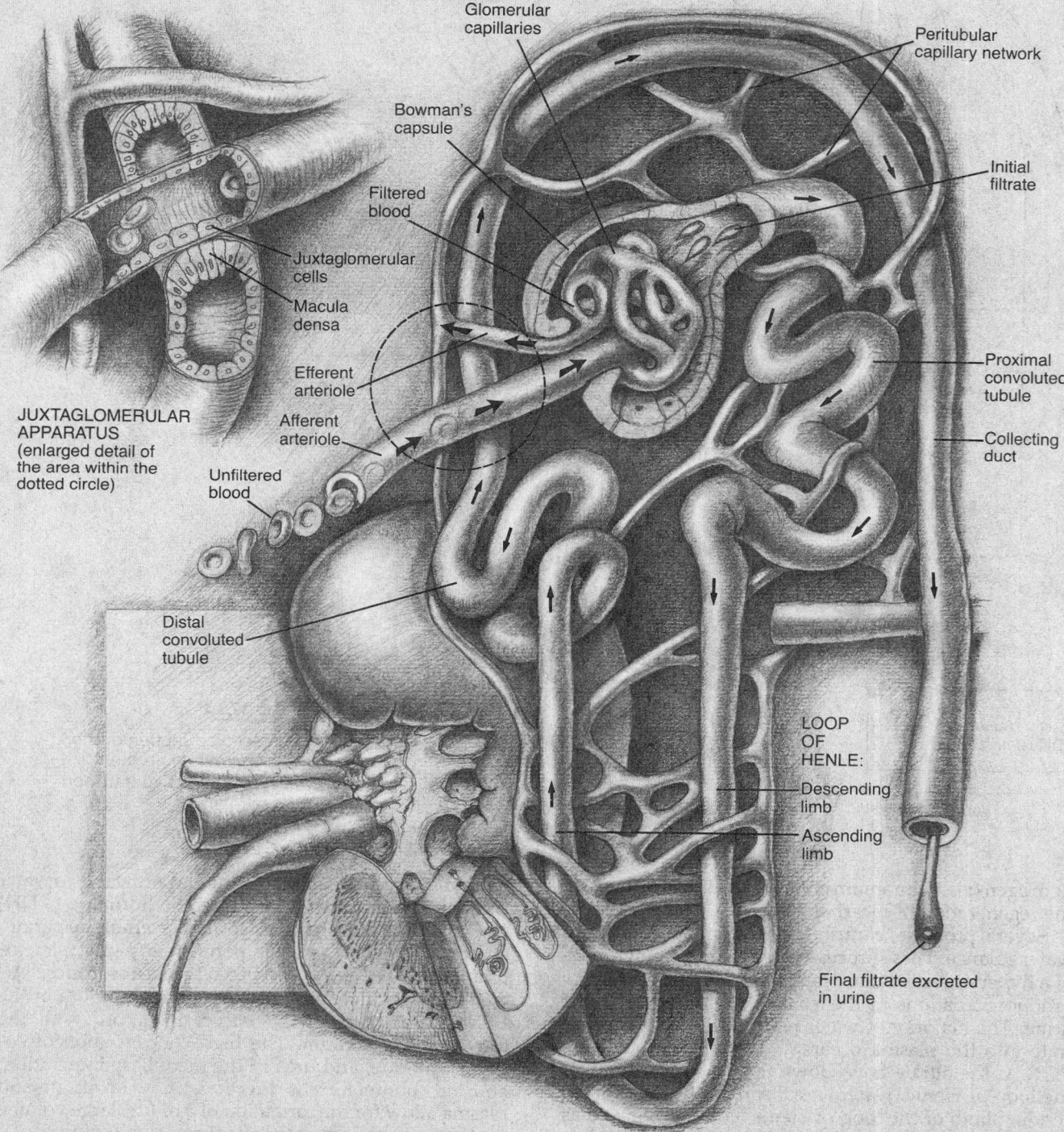

Glomerular capillaries

Peritubular capillary network

Bowman's capsule

Initial filtrate

Filtered blood

Juxtaglomerular cells

Macula densa

Efferent arteriole

Proximal convoluted tubule

Afferent arteriole

Collecting duct

JUXTAGLOMERULAR APPARATUS (enlarged detail of the area within the dotted circle)

Unfiltered blood

Distal convoluted tubule

LOOP OF HENLE:

Descending limb

Ascending limb

Final filtrate excreted in urine

The specialized cells of the juxtaglomerular apparatus—juxtaglomerular cells in the afferent and efferent arterioles and macula densa in the distal convoluted tubule—regulate the flow of blood into and out of the nephron by dilating or constricting as they sense changes in blood volume and pressure. Dilation of the afferent arteriole together with constriction of the efferent arteriole increases glomerular capillary blood volume and hydrostatic pressure to promote filtration and increase urinary output. Constriction of the afferent arteriole with dilation of the efferent arteriole promotes the opposite effect: decreased filtration and decreased urinary output.

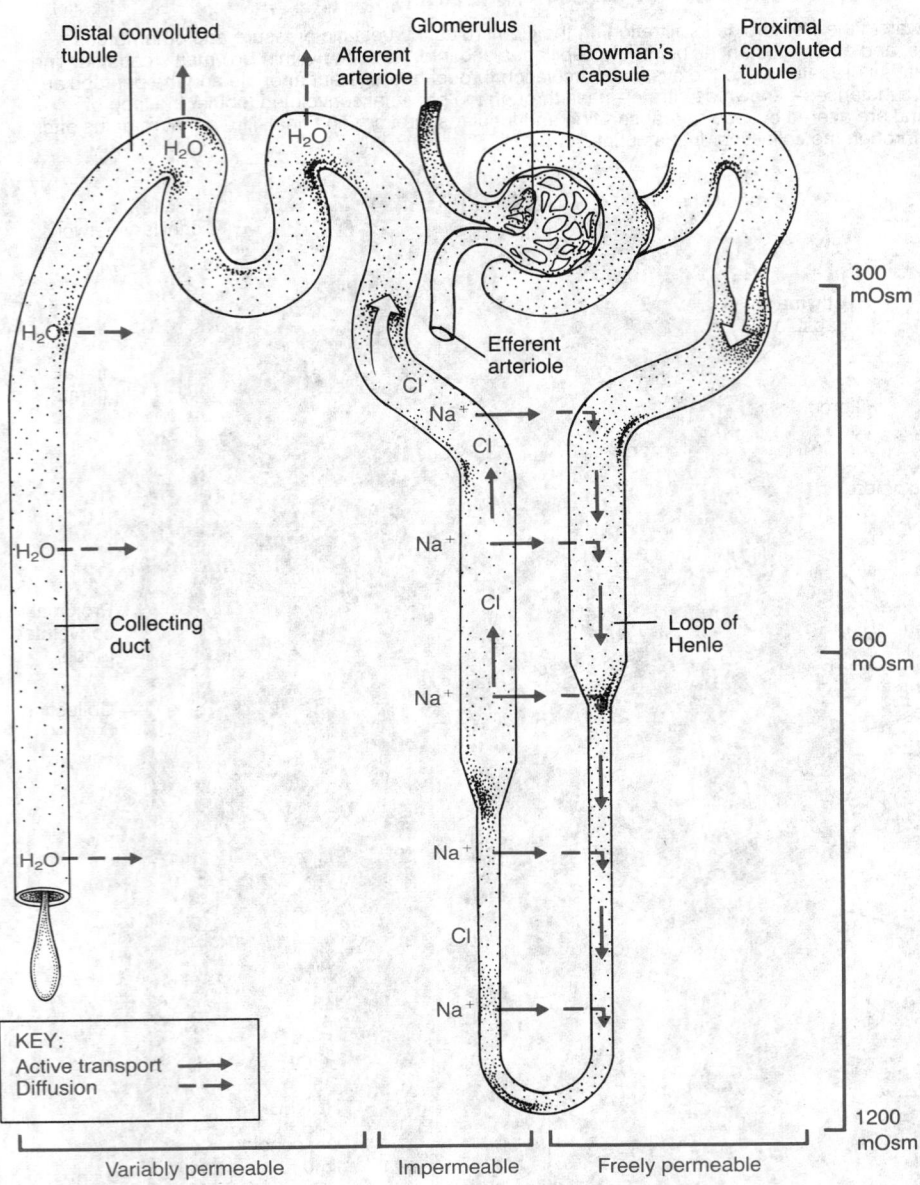

Figure 57–3

Microscopic function of the nephron unit. Note the diffusion and active transport of electrolytes.

KEY:
Active transport →
Diffusion - →

hydrogen (via ammonium chloride) and potassium, and the regeneration of bicarbonate.

Several processes contribute to the renal regulation of water balance. These processes include the maintenance of a hypertonic medullary interstitium and the ability to produce variations in the volume or concentration of urine. The majority of water reabsorption from the filtrate into the plasma occurs as it passes through the PCT. As the filtrate flows down the descending limb of the loop of Henle, water is reabsorbed. In the thin ascending limb of the loop of Henle, chloride, as well as sodium, is actively reabsorbed, but the thin ascending limb is not permeable to water. Consequently, the interstitial tissue fluid of the medulla is hypertonic.

As the filtrate continues to flow through the tubule and enters the DCT, water reabsorption occurs because the membrane is potentially permeable to water. The membrane of the DCT may be made permeable to water through the influence of antidiuretic hormone (ADH) (vasopressin); aldosterone also alters membrane permeability. ADH increases the permeability of the membrane to water and enhances water reabsorption. Aldosterone promotes the reabsorption of sodium in the DCT; water reabsorption occurs in accord with the movement of sodium. The high concentration of sodium, chloride, and urea in the medullary interstitium and the countercurrent directional flow of filtrate and plasma allow for the formation of a dilute, large volume of urine or a concentrated, smaller volume of urine.

Hormonal Functions

The kidneys produce several hormones that significantly affect physiologic well-being. These hormones include erythropoietin, active vitamin D, renin, prostaglandins (PGs), and kinins. In addition, the kidneys have a role in the breakdown and excretion of insulin.

Erythropoietin

Erythropoietin is believed to be produced in the renal parenchyma, but a specific site has yet to be identified. Essentially, erythropoietin is responsible for stimulating bone marrow to produce RBCs. The lack of RBC production and resulting anemia are believed to be primarily due to a deficit of erythropoietin; however, there is a shortening of the life span of RBCs in clients who are uremic. The potential effects of inhibitory factors on erythropoiesis and RBC survival are being explored (Anagnostou & Kurtzman, 1985). As the renal parenchymal mass decreases, erythropoietin production decreases. Recombinant DNA techniques have permitted the reproduction of erythropoietin in the laboratory. The recombinant DNA production of erythropoietin has enabled the exogenous administration of this necessary hormone to treat the anemia of chronic renal failure.

Active Vitamin D

A series of metabolic changes are necessary for vitamin D, a hormone, to achieve an active form. These metabolic conversions take place in the skin through exposure to ultraviolet light and in the liver. Vitamin D is converted to an active form in the kidney; the active form of vitamin D is 1,25-dihydroxycholecalciferol ($1,25[OH]_2D_3$). Active vitamin D is necessary for the gastrointestinal (GI) absorption of calcium from ingested foods and thus is critical in the regulation of calcium balance. Active vitamin D also promotes renal and bone reabsorption of calcium and phosphorus. In addition to active vitamin D, PTH helps to regulate serum calcium and phosphorus levels. Together, these hormones promote GI absorption of calcium from foods, reabsorption and storage of calcium in the bone, or urinary calcium excretion. Because calcium and phosphorus levels have an inverse relationship, alterations in the level of one electrolyte result in changes in the concentration of the other.

Renin

Renin, a hormone stored in the JGCs of the afferent and efferent arterioles of the nephron, assists in the regulation of blood pressure. The release of renin occurs when there is a decrease in blood flow or blood volume or a decrease in the sodium concentration of the tubular filtrate, which is detected through the receptors of the JGA. The release of renin stimulates the production of angiotensin I through conversion of angiotensinogen in the liver. *Angiotensin I* is then converted to angiotensin II via a converting enzyme, angiotensinase. *Angiotensin II* is a powerful vasoconstricting agent, and its production results in increased systemic blood pressure. In addition, angiotensin II stimulates the release of aldosterone by the adrenal cortex. *Aldosterone*, a mineralocorticoid, promotes increased reabsorption of sodium in the distal tubule of the nephron. Therefore, more water is reabsorbed and blood pressure is increased owing to increases in intravascular volume expansion. This system of blood pressure regulation is referred to as the renin-angiotensin-aldosterone system and influences the autoregulatory blood pressure processes within the nephron, as well as systemic blood pressure when renal blood flow is diminished.

Prostaglandins

PGs are substances produced in a variety of tissues, including the renal cortex and the renal medulla. PGs are formed from the metabolism of arachidonic acid, which is derived from fatty acids. In general, the PGs have either vasoconstricting or vasodilating properties. Specific PGs produced in the renal cortex are PGE_2 and prostacyclin (PGI_2); these facilitate the regulation of glomerular filtration, vascular resistance, and renin production. Within the medulla, PGE_2 acts on the distal tubule and collecting tubule to inhibit ADH, decrease membrane permeability, and promote sodium and water excretion. Although considerable research on the role and functions of the PGs is in progress, there is general agreement that the renal PGs counter the effects of ADH and promote urinary excretion of water (Beck et al., 1987). Clinically, clients taking nonsteroidal anti-inflammatory drugs (NSAIDs) may experience PG inhibitory effects and acute renal failure.

Kinins

The kinins represent a variety of enzymes that influence arteriolar dilation and capillary permeability. Bradykinin is an example of an activated kinin. In the kidney, the effects of kinin stimulation include vasodilation and urinary sodium and water excretion, as well as the production of PGs.

URETERS

STRUCTURE

Each kidney has a single *ureter*, which is a hollow tube-like structure connecting the renal pelvis with the urinary bladder. The ureter is about ½ in (2 to 8 mm) in diameter and about 12 in (30 cm) in length. The ureters are within the retroperitoneal space.

The diameter of the ureter narrows in three distinct areas. In the upper third of the ureter, the point of narrowing is known as the UP junction. In the distal third, the ureter narrows as each ureter arches toward the anterior abdominal wall traversing beneath the iliac vessels. The third point of narrowing occurs as the ureter enters the posterior wall of the urinary bladder at an oblique angle. This distal portion of the ureter is referred to as the *ureterovesical junction* (Fig. 57–4).

The ureter is composed of three layers: an inner lining of mucous membrane (urothelium), a middle layer of

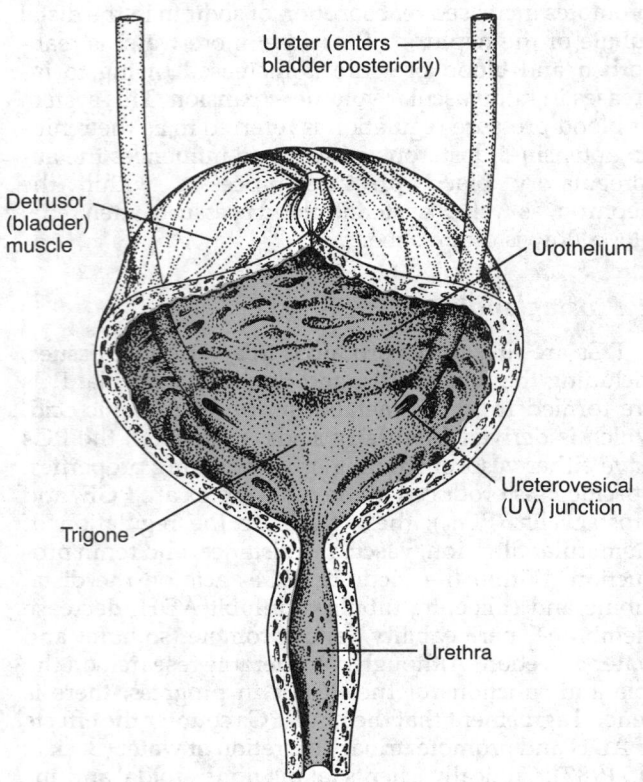

Figure 57–4

Gross anatomy of the urinary bladder.

smooth muscle fibers, and an outer layer of fibrous tissue. The outer layer of the ureter contains the blood supply. The blood supply to the ureters is derived primarily from the ureteral artery, a branch of the renal arteries. Branches from other vessels, such as the aorta and internal spermatic, iliac, uterine, vaginal, hemorrhoidal, and superior vesical arteries, may also supply the ureter. The middle layer of tissue contains longitudinal and circular muscle fibers, under the control of a variety of nerve pathways from the sacroiliac branches. Ureteral peristalsis is regulated by branches of the sacroiliac nerves.

FUNCTION

The primary function of the ureters is to propel urine from the renal pelvis into the urinary bladder. Peristaltic contractions of the smooth muscle fibers of the middle layer of the ureter are responsible for the transport of urine from the kidney to the bladder.

URINARY BLADDER

STRUCTURE

The *urinary bladder* is a muscular sac that provides a reservoir for urine. The urinary bladder is in the poste-

rior peritoneal cavity near the pelvic floor. In males, the urinary bladder is anterior to the rectum. In females, the urinary bladder is anterior to the vagina. The bladder is directly behind the pubic symphysis, the point of connection for the pelvic bone structures. The urinary bladder is composed of the *fundus,* the rounded sac portion, and the *bladder neck,* a portion of the posterior urethra.

The urinary bladder has an inner lining of epithelial cells known as the *urothelium,* a middle layer of three types of smooth muscle known as the *detrusor muscle,* and an outer lining. The *trigone* is an anatomic landmark on the inner aspect of the posterior urinary bladder formed by the points of ureteral entry on the posterior bladder wall (UV junctions) and the urethra (see Fig. 57–4).

The *internal urethral sphincter* is composed of the smooth muscle of the bladder neck that encircles the urethra. The *external urethral sphincter* is composed of skeletal muscle that surrounds the urethra. In males, the external sphincter surrounds the urethra at the base of the prostate gland. In females, the external sphincter is at the base of the bladder. The urinary bladder receives blood supply from the internal iliac arteries.

FUNCTION

The primary function of the urinary bladder is to provide a site for the temporary storage of urine. Thus, the urinary bladder functions to provide continence and enable micturition (voiding). In addition, the lining of the urinary bladder is described as having a resistance to bacteria.

The bladder functions to achieve continence during bladder filling through the combination of detrusor muscle relaxation and external and internal sphincter contraction. As the bladder fills with urine, neuroreceptors transmit stimuli to fibers in segments of spinal sacral nerves S-2, S-3, and S-4.

Continence is maintained by the interaction of nerves that control the muscles of the bladder, the urethra, and the pelvic floor and factors that provide for closure of the urethra. During the period of bladder filling, the sympathetic nervous system fibers dominate and override detrusor muscle contraction. These control centers are located in the cerebral cortex and nuclei in the pons and the sacral part of the spinal cord. For urethral closure to be adequate for continence, the mucosal surfaces must be in contact and adhesive. Contact depends on structural and functional integrity of the nerves and muscles of the bladder, the urethra, and the pelvic floor. Adhesion depends on adequate secretion of mucus-like substances.

Micturition is a reflex under the control of parasympathetic fibers that stimulate detrusor muscle (bladder) and internal sphincter contraction with the simultaneous relaxation of the external sphincter and muscles of the pelvic floor. When the detrusor muscle contracts, the UV portion of the ureter is closed and the normally round bladder assumes the shape of a funnel. After bladder continence is learned, control of voiding is voluntary as a result of a learned response controlled by the cerebral cortex and the brain stem.

URETHRA

STRUCTURE

The *urethra* is a narrow tube-like structure lined with mucous membrane and epithelial cells. The *urethral meatus* is the terminal point of the urethra, the external opening.

In the male, the urethra is about 6 to 8 in (15 to 20 cm) long. The urethral meatus is located at the tip of the penis. The male urethra is composed of three sections: The *prostatic urethra* is about 1½ in (3.75 cm) long and traverses the prostate gland after exiting the urinary bladder. The *membranous urethra* is about ½ in (1.25 cm) long and traverses the wall of the pelvic floor. The *cavernous urethra* is external and extends through the length of the penis.

In the female, the urethra is about 1½ in (3.75 cm) long. The urethra exits the urinary bladder through the pelvic floor. The urethral meatus in females is located slightly posterior to the clitoris and directly anterior to the vagina and rectum.

FUNCTION

The major function of the urethra is to serve as a conduit for the elimination of urine from the body. There is general agreement that the flushing of urine promotes bacterial removal.

URINARY SYSTEM CHANGES ASSOCIATED WITH AGING

Structural and functional changes occur in the kidney as a result on the aging process (see the accompanying Focus on the Elderly feature). Although gross changes are not always readily apparent, microscopic alterations occur and are clinically relevant.

The overall size of each kidney may decrease slightly owing to a decrease in the mass of the renal cortex. Presumably, these changes are related to alterations in renal blood flow. The renal medulla appears not to be affected by perfusion changes associated with aging. Consequently, the juxtamedullary nephrons are generally preserved. Within the nephron, a thickening of the glomerular and tubular basement membranes is observed on microscopic examination. Both the number of

---

FOCUS ON THE ELDERLY ■ Changes in the Urinary System Related to Aging

Change	Interventions	Rationales
Bladder capacity decreases	1. Encourage the client to use toilet, bedpan, or urinal at least q 2 h. 2. Respond as soon as possible to the client's indication of need to void.	1, 2. To prevent episodes of urinary incontinence.
Tendency to retain urine develops	1. Observe the client for signs and symptoms of urinary tract infection, such as confusion (or increased confusion) and urinary frequency (dysuria is *not* a common finding in the elderly).	1. To detect infection and underlying urinary retention.
Nocturia increases	1. Ensure adequate nighttime lighting. 2. Ensure the availability of toilet, bedpan, or urinal.	1. To prevent injury. 2. To prevent episodes of urinary incontinence.
Urinary sphincter weakens	1. Respond as soon as possible to the client's indication of need to void. 2. Provide thorough perineal care after each voiding.	1. To prevent episodes of urinary incontinence. 2. To prevent skin irritation.

glomeruli and their surface area decrease with aging. The length of the tubules decreases proportionately.

Age-related changes also affect the functioning of the kidney. GFR decreases with aging, more rapidly after age 45 years. In younger persons, the removal of one kidney results in hypertrophy of the kidney that remains. However, in older persons, this does not occur because alterations in blood flow develop with aging and the blood vessels become thickened and more rigid, preventing hypertrophy. Tubular changes occur as well, as demonstrated by the inability to concentrate urine. As a result, when plasma osmolality varies, renal compensatory responses may be ineffective. Excretion and regulation of solutes (e.g., acids, bicarbonate, and sodium) remain effective, but less efficient; several more hours may be required for homeostasis to occur. Changes in renal endocrine function occur as well; there is a decrease in renin production and activation of vitamin D.

The aging process may also affect the elasticity of the detrusor muscle, causing decreased bladder capacity and urinary retention. When the elderly individual feels the urge to void, the bladder may need emptying immediately, as the urinary sphincter often becomes weaker with age. Nocturia is common because of muscle weakness and the kidneys' decreased ability to concentrate urine.

HISTORY

DEMOGRAPHIC DATA

Age and sex are important in the overall history of the client with suspected genitourinary tract dysfunction. Some renal and urologic conditions are directly related to *age* of the individual at the time of onset. Several examples illustrate the relation of age to pathologic changes: The sudden onset of hypertension in persons older than age 50 years is suggestive of a secondary cause, perhaps a renovascular cause, of the hypertension. Clinical evidence of polycystic kidney disease typically occurs in clients in their 40s or 50s. Persons with insulin-dependent diabetes mellitus are most likely to demonstrate manifestations of renal insufficiency such as proteinuria; proteinuria usually occurs within 16 to 21 years after the diagnosis of the insulin-deficient state. In men older than 50 years of age, alterations in urinary patterns suggest prostatic disease.

Anatomic variations related to *sex* differences similarly suggest the potential for specific renal and urologic disorders. For example, men rarely have urinary tract infections unless there are structural abnormalities, such as ureteral reflux or prostatic involvement. On the other hand, women, who have a shorter urethra, frequently

experience cystitis, because of easier bacterial passage into the bladder.

PERSONAL AND FAMILY HISTORY

The personal and family history of the client with a suspected urologic problem is significant, as some disorders are genetically transmitted or have a familial inheritance pattern. It is important to elicit information about parents, parents' siblings, grandparents, or the client's siblings who have had a *history of renal problems.* Terms used in the past for renal disease include Bright's disease, nephritis, and nephrosis; clients may use them to describe the diseases of the kidney as they were known by parents or grandparents in the earlier part of the 20th century.

Alport's disease is a fairly uncommon renal disorder that is transmitted by a chromosomal defect from mothers to their male offspring. Familial characteristics include male deafness and death from renal failure. Polycystic kidney disease is a much more common cause of chronic renal failure and is transmitted to children as a result of autosomal genetic defects of the parent of either sex.

The nurse inquires about any previous renal or urologic disorders, including *infections,* or *urologic surgical interventions.* A history of any *chronic health problems,* such as diabetes mellitus, arthritis, or high blood pressure, is important in renal or urologic assessment. Over time, these conditions or related treatments may cause deterioration of renal function. For example, type I diabetes mellitus results in end-stage renal disease in about 50% of cases; type II diabetes mellitus may also result in renal failure. Medications prescribed for the treatment of arthritis may cause injury to renal tissue. Hypertension, particularly if untreated or uncontrolled, can result in nephrosclerosis and subsequently renal failure.

When the client reports no known history of renal or urologic disorders, the nurse inquires about the results of previous physical examinations, such as may have been performed for school, employment, insurance eligibility, or military induction. Occasionally, comments such as "protein in the urine" or "albumin in the urine" prompt recall of problems not readily remembered as renal. Recall of these physical examinations may also prompt the client to remember a previous diagnosis of high blood pressure, which could suggest a correlation with current problems. Questioning about health problems associated with pregnancy may also reveal a history of proteinuria, high blood pressure, or urinary tract infections.

Exposure to chemical or environmental toxins in occupational or other settings and travel to geographic regions with a variety of viral, bacterial, parasitic, or fungal microorganisms may also contribute significant historical data. Recent physical injuries, trauma, or sexual contacts may also provide information significant to the urologic assessment.

DIET HISTORY

Exploration of the diet history of the client with known or suspected renal or urologic disorders is necessary and should include the *usual dietary intake* of the individual. The nurse seeks information that describes any *recent changes in the dietary pattern*. Excesses of certain foods, such as dairy products, or deletion of certain categories of foods needs to be noted. The diet history includes fluid intake as well as food items. Changes in appetite, alterations in taste acuity, or inability to discriminate tastes are also important components of the diet history, as these symptoms are associated with the accumulation of nitrogenous waste products from renal failure. In addition, if the client has decided to follow a certain diet for weight reduction, the details of the diet plan need to be described. Some diets, such as those with a high protein intake, can result in transient renal problems. If the person prone to form calculi ingests a diet high in calcium-containing products, new stone formation may occur. Changes in thirst or fluid intake patterns might also result in alterations in urinary output, prompt an increased tendency for stone formation, or yield other manifestations of urologic disorders.

SOCIOECONOMIC STATUS

The socioeconomic status of the client may reveal that lack of available financial resources or health insurance has influenced health care practices. Individuals with limited income or no health insurance often forego attention to physical ailments by ignoring symptoms or their potential significance because they lack funds to pay for diagnosis and/or treatment. They are also often unable or reluctant to follow medical advice by having prescriptions filled and frequently do not keep follow-up appointments. Consequently, poor control of diseases such as high blood pressure and diabetes mellitus may contribute to the development of renal disease.

In addition, Blacks have a higher incidence, greater prevalence, and more severe effects of high blood pressure, resulting in increased incidence of target organ damage. Although racial differences in blood pressure are not seen in children, after age 17 years, blood pressure in Blacks is consistently reported to be higher than in Caucasians. Proposed reasons for this increased vulnerability in Blacks include genetic and physiologic variations, as well as health system access limitations for prevention, detection, and follow-up (Saunders, 1987).

The client's educational level may be related to the amount of information that he/she has regarding diseases and their symptoms. Lack of knowledge may prevent the client from seeking medical care or adhering to treatment regimens. Other problems related to socioeconomic status or educational level may be seen in the urinary tract infections that recur because of inadequate treatment or lack of follow-up to ensure eradication. Lack of knowledge or limited financial resources may

result in clients' not obtaining antibiotic medications or not completing the course of medication. The lack of money to pay for nutritious foods or the lack of knowledge or motivation to select healthful foods may inhibit full recovery.

The language used by persons of various socioeconomic or cultural groups may be quite different from that of the health care professional. Terms that health care professionals use in making inquiries about urinary symptoms and alterations in urinary function may have absolutely no meaning to the client. When obtaining a history, the nurse needs to listen to and explore the terms used by the client. Using the terms or language of the client may assist in gaining a more complete and thorough description of the problems being experienced. The use of a familiar language, even though it may be slang or colloquial, may also benefit the client by helping to decrease embarrassment or discomfort when discussing bodily functions.

MEDICATION HISTORY

The nurse identifies all prescription and over-the-counter (OTC) medications taken by the client, including drugs taken routinely and those taken as needed. The nurse inquires about the length of time an agent has been taken and whether any recent changes in prescribed medications have occurred. The prescribed medications for chronic health problems, such as diabetes mellitus, hypertension, cardiac disorders, hormonal replacements, and arthritis, are potential causes of renal dysfunction. Antibiotics, such as gentamicin (Garamycin), taken for infectious processes may also produce sudden renal dysfunction.

In addition, the nurse solicits information about OTC medications or agents, including vitamin and mineral supplements and replacements, laxatives, and analgesics. The nurse seeks to identify any medications used for control of symptoms such as swelling, joint aches and pains, and constipation, as these medications could influence renal function. Chronic analgesic intake, particularly involving combination agents, could affect renal function. The nurse asks the client to describe in as much detail as possible the specifics of medication intake.

CURRENT HEALTH PROBLEM

The nurse elicits from the client a complete list of perceived current health problems. It is important to describe all concerns, as some renal and urologic disorders have symptoms related to other body systems or occurring as generalized problems. Common concerns that prompt a client to seek health care attention include discomfort associated with urination or sudden changes in the appearance or quantity of urinary output.

Specifically, the nurse inquires about any changes in

the appearance of the urine, the pattern of urination, ability to initiate or control voiding, or other unusual symptoms. Alterations in appearance include changes in the color, odor, or clarity of the urine. Urine that is reddish, dark brown or black, greenish, or any deviation from the usual yellowish, straw-colored urine usually prompts the client to seek health care assistance. Typically, urine has a mild but distinctive odor suggestive of ammonia. An increase in the intensity or a change in the quality of the odor suggests the presence of infection. Similarly, a decrease in clarity may suggest the presence of infection.

Pattern changes to be elicited include waking during the night to void, a change in frequency (an increase or decrease in the number of times per day that urine is passed), or an increase or decrease in the quantity of urine. Several terms may be used to describe the quantity of urine produced. Although the client generally does not have information about the specific quantity of urine produced, an understanding of these terms assists in the interpretation of data. *Oliguria* refers to a decrease in urinary output; specifically, the term describes a urinary output of 100 to 400 mL/24 hours. *Anuria* refers to the absence of urinary output; specifically, the term describes a urinary output of less than 100 mL/24 hours. Less precise definitions guide the use of the term polyuria. *Polyuria* means an increase in urinary output. Because the usual 24-hour urinary output is about 1500 mL, polyuria is urinary output greater than this amount.

The nurse also inquires about any difficulties encountered in initiating the flow of urine, whether burning or other discomfort is associated with the urinary flow, or if there is a decrease in the force of the urinary stream in males. Specific terms describe these sensations. *Hesitancy* refers to difficulties in initiating the flow of urine. *Dysuria* describes any discomfort associated with the passage of urine. *Urgency* refers to sensations experienced when there is a sudden need to void and may be associated with a loss of urinary continence.

The nurse inquires about any loss of urinary continence. Situations that increase intra-abdominal pressure, e.g., coughing or sneezing, may result in involuntary passage of urine. Clients may also report persistent dribbling of urine.

The onset of pain in the flank, lower abdomen or pelvic region, or the perineal area is of great concern to the client and usually prompts the client to seek assistance. The nurse inquires about the onset and duration of pain, its location, and its association with any activity or event. The pain may be sharp or dull, localized or diffuse. The pain associated with renal or ureteral irritation is often severe and spasmodic; when the pain radiates into the perineal area, groin, scrotum, or labia, it is described as *renal colic.* This pain is usually associated with distention of the ureter, or spasm, occurring with obstruction as may occur with passage of a stone. Pain associated with the descent of a stone through the ureter is excruciating and can result in a dramatic presentation. As a result of sympathetic nervous system stimulation, clients may exhibit a shock-like condition, with pallor,

diaphoresis (profuse perspiration), and hypotension. In addition, the client may have GI symptoms, such as nausea, vomiting, or diarrhea, because of the proximity of nerve tracts associated with the kidneys, ureters, and internal abdominal organs.

The recent onset of upper respiratory tract problems, generalized musculoskeletal discomfort, or GI problems may be related to systemic conditions that could influence renal function. GI symptoms, such as anorexia, nausea, and vomiting, are classic manifestations of uremia, but could be present with other pathologic conditions as well. Because the kidneys are in proximity to the GI organs and nerve pathways are similar, nausea, vomiting, diarrhea, and other GI symptoms may be a part of the client's presenting history. These *renointestinal reflexes* commonly complicate the detailed description of the problem.

Uremia refers to the clinical symptoms associated with the accumulation of nitrogenous waste products in the blood, an effect of renal failure. These symptoms include anorexia, nausea and vomiting, muscle cramps, and pruritus (itching). In addition, fatigue and lethargy, as well as other systemic manifestations, occur with uremia. Because the effects of renal failure result in changes in all body systems, a thorough listing of the client's current health problems may be most informative.

PHYSICAL ASSESSMENT

The physical assessment of the client with known or suspected renal or urologic disorders includes an assessment of general appearance, a general review of body systems, and specific consideration of the organs and functions of the urinary tract.

The nurse assesses the *general appearance* of the client, noting a yellowish skin color and the presence of any rashes, ecchymoses, or other discoloration. The skin and tissues are also assessed for evidence of *edema.* With renal disorders, edema may be detected in the pedal, pretibial, presacral, and periorbital tissues. In addition, the nurse auscultates the lungs to determine the presence of fluid. Weight and blood pressure measurements are obtained. The nurse assesses the client's general *level of consciousness,* noting deficits in concentration, use of thought processes or memory, dysarthria (the inability to speak clearly and distinctly), and level of alertness. The nurse observes the client's gait and hand coordination.

ASSESSMENT OF THE KIDNEYS, URETERS, AND BLADDER

Assessment of the kidneys, ureters, and bladder is performed in conjunction with abdominal assessment procedures. The traditional order of inspection, percussion, palpation, and auscultation is altered for the abdominal assessment. Auscultation should precede percussion and palpation. The rationale is based on the need to auscultate for abdominal bruits before enhancing bowel sounds as a result of abdominal palpation or percussion.

INSPECTION

The nurse initiates physical assessment of the abdomen by inspecting the abdomen and the flank regions with the client in both supine and sitting positions. The nurse observes for asymmetry or discoloration. The specific anatomic landmark to be inspected in the flank region is known as the *costovertebral angle* (CVA). The CVA is defined by the lower portion of the rib cage and the vertebral column.

AUSCULTATION

After inspection, the nurse listens to the aorta and renal arteries for the presence of a bruit. A *bruit* is the audible sound produced when the volume of blood or the diameter of the blood vessel is changed. The presence of a bruit over a renal artery is usually associated with blood flow through a narrowed vessel. Auscultation of the right and left renal arteries is performed at the midclavicular line. When a bruit is detected by auscultation, a thrill may also be present. A *thrill* is a palpable sensation of blood flow that is similar to a rippling pulse.

PALPATION

After auscultation, the examiner proceeds to lightly palpate all quadrants of the abdomen. The examiner verbally identifies areas of tenderness or discomfort and examines these areas after nontender areas are explored. With severe bladder distention, the outline of the bladder may be identified as high as the umbilicus. When severe bladder distention is present, abdominal palpation to locate and examine the kidneys produces discomfort and may be impossible. Although the ureters are not palpable, a spasm of the ureteral musculature results in flank or low abdominal pain that is severe, excruciating, and similar to colic. The sensations spread to the scrotum in males and the labia in females.

Palpation of the kidneys requires special training and practice under the guidance of a qualified practitioner and is usually reserved for nurses in advanced practice roles (Fig. 57–5). The procedure is briefly described, but the reader is cautioned against attempting palpation without appropriate guidance. If tumor or aneurysm is suspected, palpation may result in harm to the client.

Because the kidneys are deep, posterior structures, palpation is more readily accomplished in thinner individuals. When the kidneys are of normal size and position, only the lower poles are palpable. In persons with a well-developed abdominal musculature or in the pres-

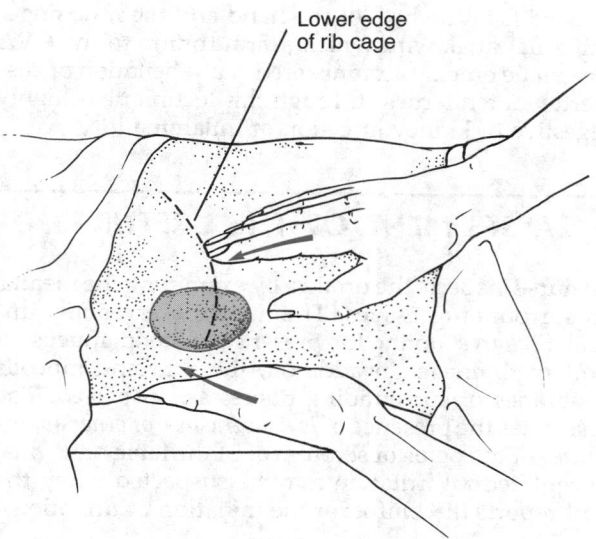

Figure 57–5

Advanced technique for palpation of the kidney.

ence of significant adipose tissue or abdominal fluid, palpation of the kidneys may be difficult or impossible. To palpate the right kidney, the nurse places one hand under the right flank and the other hand over the abdomen below the lower right part of the rib cage. The lower hand raises the flank and the upper hand depresses the anterior abdomen, as the client is asked to take a deep breath. The procedure is repeated on the left side. The left kidney is deeper and more difficult to palpate.

If the kidneys are enlarged because of polycystic kidney disease or the presence of other renal masses, palpation should be gentle to avoid increasing the client's discomfort. Palpation of a transplanted kidney is more easily accomplished. The nurse palpates the transplanted kidney in the lower right or lower left abdominal quadrant.

PERCUSSION

A distended urinary bladder sounds dull when percussed. After gently palpating to determine the general outline of the distended bladder, the nurse places the pads of the fingers of one hand on the skin of the lower abdomen. Using the fingertips of the other hand as a striking hammer, the nurse gently thumps those fingertips over the top of the fingers of the other hand. The fingers in contact with the abdomen are moved in the direction of the umbilicus until dull sounds are no longer produced.

Inflammation or infection in the kidney, the renal capsule, or the adjacent fascia is characteristically demonstrated as discomfort or a constant, dull ache. If the client has not identified flank pain or tenderness, the nurse percusses the nontender CVA. For percussion of the CVA, the client assumes a sitting, side-lying, or supine position. The nurse positions the hand into a clenched fist. The heel of the hand and the little finger form a flat area, with which a firm thump to the CVA area can be quickly administered. The elicitation of costovertebral tenderness through this technique is highly suggestive of kidney infection or inflammation.

ASSESSMENT OF THE URETHRA

The nurse inspects the urethra by examining the meatus and surrounding tissues. The nurse observes any unusual *discharge,* noting the presence of blood, mucus, or purulent drainage. In addition, the skin and mucous membranes of surrounding tissues are inspected. The nurse notes the presence of *lesions, rashes, or other abnormalities* of the penis or scrotum or of the labia or vaginal orifice. Urethral irritation may be suspected when the client reports discomfort at the initiation of urination.

PSYCHOSOCIAL ASSESSMENT

Emotional responses to concerns about the urologic system may include embarrassment, fear, anxiety, anger, guilt, or sadness. For most adults, the lessons of childhood include general privacy with regard to habits associated with urination or sexual activity. Childhood experiences, such as difficult toilet training or bed-wetting, may evoke emotional responses and memories previously forgotten. In addition, language skills may not be sufficiently developed for the client to clearly express specific concerns. Any of these responses may prompt the client to delay seeking health care.

Emotional responses to problems of change in the structure or function of the urologic system may occur because of concerns related to general anxieties about body image, fear of sexual dysfunction, or fear of death. For example, exploration of one's body is a common childhood activity. These memories are often recalled with feelings of guilt or shame. Thus, symptoms of the urogenital system may be irrationally linked to natural childhood activities and result in fears of sexual dysfunction. Similarly, adult sexual practices outside the tradition of the monogamous heterosexual couple may also evoke anxieties and other emotional responses.

Other memories, such as those related to the deaths of relatives or friends, often provoke a fear of death. Particularly if there is a history of polycystic kidney disease or diabetes mellitus in the family, the client may recall that these individuals died or suffered with the disease. These past experiences are easily internalized and thus become a great source of anxiety. These memories may represent events of the immediate or distant past.

DIAGNOSTIC ASSESSMENT

LABORATORY TESTS

BLOOD UREA NITROGEN

Blood urea nitrogen (BUN), less frequently called serum urea nitrogen, measures the renal excretion of urea nitrogen; the normal BUN level is 5 to 15 mg/dL. Urea nitrogen is a by-product of the hepatic metabolism of protein. The primary source for the production of urea nitrogen is food sources of protein, which undergo biotransformation by the liver. The kidneys filter urea nitrogen from the blood and excrete the nitrogenous waste in urine. Therefore, BUN levels indicate the renal clearance of this nitrogenous waste product. Because other factors may influence the BUN level, an elevation of BUN does not always represent renal disease. For example, dehydration and decreased renal perfusion or a diet excessively high in protein may result in an elevated BUN value. In addition, blood is a protein. Therefore, in any situation in which there is blood in body tissues, e.g., a massive bruise or retroperitoneal bleeding, the reabsorption of the blood protein will be processed by the liver, resulting in an increased BUN level. The role of the liver in production of urea nitrogen is also important to consider. The liver must function properly to produce urea nitrogen; when liver and renal dysfunction are both present, urea nitrogen levels are not increased. Therefore, the BUN level is not always elevated with renal disease and is not the most reliable indicator of renal function. However, an elevated BUN level is highly suggestive of renal dysfunction.

SERUM CREATININE

Serum creatinine is a measurement of the end product of phosphocreatine metabolism. Phosphocreatine metabolism occurs in skeletal muscles and results in the production of creatinine. Creatinine, also a protein waste product, is filtered by the kidneys and excreted in urine. Because muscle metabolism and the amount of muscle mass are relatively constant, the serum creatinine level is an excellent indicator of renal function. The metabolism of muscle is minimally influenced by other factors, such as hydration. If there is muscle disease, measurement of the enzyme creatine kinase indicates a problem not necessarily related to renal disease.

Serum creatinine level is expressed as a range of normal to allow for variances in muscle mass in individuals. For adult men, the normal serum creatinine value is 0.8 to 1.7 mg/dL; for adult women, the normal serum creatinine value is 0.6 to 1.0 mg/dL. Men generally have a larger muscle mass than women, but there are exceptions.

An elevation in the serum creatinine level is indicative of renal disease. There is no other pathologic condition that results in an increase in serum creatinine level. In persons who increase muscle mass with exercise, the serum level may increase slightly. As long as renal function is normal, the increased amount of creatinine produced is excreted in the urine. It is also important that the nurse understand that the serum creatinine level is not increased until at least 50% of the renal function is lost. Therefore, any elevation is significant.

RATIO OF BLOOD UREA NITROGEN TO SERUM

The ratio of BUN to serum creatinine level is used to determine whether factors such as dehydration or lack of renal perfusion are causing the elevated BUN level. Normally, the ratio of BUN to creatinine is approximately 10 to 20 : 1. When an intravascular fluid volume deficit or hypoperfusion exists, the BUN level rises more rapidly than the serum creatinine; consequently, the ratio of BUN to serum creatinine is increased. Similarly, if liver failure, fluid volume excess, or starvation with limited dietary protein intake exists, the BUN/serum creatinine ratio decreases. Generally, these variables are considered potentially correctable; thus, restoration of the BUN/serum creatinine ratio is reflective of normalization of renal function.

ANALYSIS OF URINE

Urinalysis (Routine)

Urinalysis is a usual component of any complete physical examination, but is particularly informative for clients with suspected renal or urologic disorders. The urinalysis specimen is ideally collected at the first morning voiding, usually by voiding; specimens obtained at other times may not provide sufficient concentration or acidity. The specimen may be collected by a variety of techniques, such as by voiding, clean catch technique, or catheterization (see the accompanying Guidelines feature).

The urinalysis provides information regarding acidity or alkalinity; the presence or absence of various waste products or compounds, sediment, or microorganisms; and an indication of concentration or dilution (Table 57–1).

pH

Normally, the pH of the urine is 4.5 to 8.0. Values less than 7 are considered acidic; values greater than 7 are alkaline; 5.5 to 6.0 is considered average. Diet, freshness of the specimen, infection, and renal function influence the acidity or alkalinity of urine.

Protein foods, such as meats and eggs, produce an acid load when metabolized. Consequently, persons who consume a high-protein diet are expected to produce a more acidic urine. Diets that are high in certain fruits and vegetables result in a more alkaline urine.

Urine that is allowed to stand unrefrigerated or urine in which urea-splitting bacteria are present becomes more alkaline. *Escherichia coli* is an exception to the urea-splitting bacteria; its presence results in an acidic urine. The breakdown of the urea into ammonia causes the urine to be more alkaline. An alkaline urine promotes cellular disintegration; thus, abnormal urinary sediment (e.g., RBCs) may be missed if the specimen is not analyzed promptly.

During systemic processes in which there is acidosis or alkalosis (metabolic or respiratory), it is expected that the kidneys will respond appropriately to maintain a normal serum pH. With respiratory acidosis (retention of volatile acids), the kidneys increase the excretion of hydrogen ions, contributing to a more acidic urinary pH. With respiratory alkalosis (loss of volatile acids), the kidneys conserve hydrogen and the urine becomes alkalotic. During metabolic alkalosis, systemic processes produce an excess of bicarbonate; therefore, the renal response expected is an alkaline urine attributable to excretion of bicarbonate. Yet, the kidneys have an obligatory load of hydrogen to excrete, and this results in a more acidic urine than expected. With metabolic acidosis, systemic processes produce an excess of hydrogen, and available bicarbonate is being utilized as a blood buffer. The urine is expected to be acidic, if the kidneys are properly excreting the increased acid load. However, renal failure is one of the most frequent causes of metabolic acidosis (bicarbonate deficit), and the failure of the kidneys to excrete hydrogen and conserve bicarbonate results in a urine that is less acidic than expected. Chapters 14 and 15 discuss acid-base balance and imbalance.

Color, Odor, and Turbidity

The color of urine is pale yellow ranging to amber. The basic yellowish color of urine derives from urochrome pigment. Variations in color may result from increased levels of urochrome or other pigments, changes in the concentration or dilution of the urine, or medication. Usually, urine smells faintly like ammonia because of the breakdown of urea. A foul odor suggests infection or may be the result of ingestion of certain foods or drugs. Turbidity is a description of cloudiness. Normally, the urine is clear, and there is no cloudiness or haziness on visual inspection. An increase in turbidity occurs with infection, the presence of sediment, or high levels of urinary protein.

Specific Gravity

The specific gravity of urine measures the relative concentration, or density, of urine in relationship to water. The specific gravity of water is 1.000. The normal specific gravity of urine is 1.010 to 1.030. If renal function is normal, a change in the specific gravity of urine

Collection	Indications	Interventions	Rationales
Voided urine	Random urinalysis or urinary electrolyte determinations	1. Collect a specimen first voided in the morning. 2. Send the specimen to the laboratory as soon as possible. 3. Refrigerate the specimen if a delay is unavoidable.	1. Urine is more concentrated at that time. 2. Rapid analysis prevents alkalinization. 3. Refrigeration delays alkalinization.
Clean catch specimen	Urine for culture and sensitivity testing	1. Explain the purpose of the procedure to the client. 2. Instruct the client in self-cleaning before voiding. 　a. Instruct the female client to separate the labia and use the sponges and solution provided to wipe with three strokes over the urethra. The first two wiping strokes are over each side of the urethra; the third wiping stroke is centered over the urethra (from front to back). 　b. Instruct the male client to retract the foreskin of the penis, if present, and to similarly clean the urethra, using three wiping strokes with the sponge and solution provided (from the head of the penis downward). 3. Instruct the client to initiate voiding after cleaning. The client then stops and resumes voiding into the container. Only 1 oz (30 mL) or more is needed; the remainder of the urine may be discarded into the commode. 4. Ensure that the client understands the procedure. 5. Assist the client as needed.	1. The procedure is used to remove any surface secretions or bacteria and to rid distal secretions or bacteria from the inside of the urethra. 2. Correct technique is needed to obtain a valid specimen. 3. This method clears the urethral tract via flushing, and fresh, uncontaminated urine is obtained. 4, 5. Understanding and assistance ensure proper collection.

GUIDELINES ■ **Collection of Urine Specimens** *Continued*

Collection	Indications	Interventions	Rationales

Catheterized specimen	Essential for diagnosis and/or treatment when other methods are not possible	1. For nonindwelling (straight) catheters:
		  a. Avoid routine use.
		  b. Follow the hospital's procedures for catheterization technique.
		2. For indwelling catheters:
		  a. Clean the injection port cap of the catheter drainage tubing with an appropriate antiseptic. Povidone-iodine or alcohol is acceptable.
		  b. Apply a clamp to the drainage tubing, distal to the injection port.
		  c. Insert a sterile needle and syringe into the port and aspirate the quantity of urine required.
		  d. Inject the urine sample into a sterile specimen container.
		  e. Remove the clamp to resume drainage.
			1. Bacterial entry should be minimized.
			
			2. Surface contamination should be prevented.

24-h urine collection	Quantitative analysis of electrolytes, nonelectrolytes, hormones, or medications	1. Instruct the client carefully. 2. Provide written materials to assist in instruction. 3. Place signs appropriately. 4. Inform all personnel and/or family caregivers. 5. On initiation discard urine and note time. 6. 24 h later ask the client to empty bladder and *save* urine to add to container.	1. An accurate and complete collection is necessary. 2–4. These aids enhance memory and understanding. 5, 6. A 24-h collection is needed.

occurs when there is a need to excrete more or less water to normalize the serum. An increase in specific gravity occurs with insufficient fluid intake or the presence of ADH. ADH production is normally increased with stress, surgery administration of anesthetics and certain drugs, and decreased renal perfusion. In each of these situations, the expected renal response is to resorb water and decrease urinary output. Consequently, the urine produced is more concentrated. A decrease in specific gravity occurs with increased fluid intake and the use of

diuretics. In each of these situations, the normal renal response is to excrete more water; thus urinary output is increased. As renal function deteriorates, the specific gravity becomes fixed and does not vary with changes in plasma osmolality.

Glucose

Glucose is filtered at the glomerulus and reabsorbed in the PCT in the nephron. Usually, when the blood

TABLE 57-1 Normal Findings and Significance of Abnormal Findings in Urinalysis

Characteristic	Normal Findings	Significance of Abnormal Findings
Color	Pale yellow	*Dark amber* indicates concentrated urine. *Very pale yellow* indicates dilute urine. *Dark red or brown* indicates blood in the urine; *brown* also may indicate increased urinary bilirubin level. *Other color changes* may result from diet or medications.
Odor	Specific aromatic odor, similar to ammonia	*Foul smell* indicates possible infection and/or dehydration.
Turbidity	Clear	*Cloudy urine* indicates infection or sediment.
Specific gravity	Usually 1.015–1.025; possible range 1.010–1.030	*Changes* reflect a disturbance in the concentrating and diluting function of the tubules. Specific gravity is influenced by many factors. Specific gravity may become fixed in renal insufficiency.
pH	6; possible range 4.6–8.0	*Changes* are caused by diet, medications, infection, acid-base imbalance, and altered renal function.
Glucose	None or < 15 mg/dL	*Presence* may indicate decreased tubular reabsorption capacity or hyperglycemia that exceeds this capacity.
Ketones	None	*Presence* reflects incomplete metabolism of fatty acids, as in diabetes mellitus.
Protein	2–8 mg/100 mL	*Increased levels* may indicate stress, infection, strenuous exercise, or glomerular disorders.
Red blood cells	1 or 2 per high-power field	*Increased levels* are normal with indwelling or intermittent catheterization or menses, but may reflect tumor, stones, or glomerular disorders.
White blood cells	1–3 per high-power field	*Increased levels* may indicate infectious or inflammatory processes.
Bilirubin	None	*Presence* suggests hepatic or biliary disease or obstruction.

TABLE 57–1 Normal Findings and Significance of Abnormal Findings in Urinalysis *Continued*

Characteristic	Normal Findings	Significance of Abnormal Findings
Casts	A few or none, composed of RBC or WBC, protein, or tubular cell casts	*Increased levels* indicate presence of bacteria or protein, which is seen in severe renal disease.
Crystals	None	*Presence* of normal and/or abnormal crystals may indicate that the specimen has been allowed to stand.
Bacteria	< 1000 colonies/mL	*Increased levels* indicate need for urine culture to determine the presence of urinary tract infection.

glucose level rises above a certain level (>150 to 180 mg/dL), the renal threshold for reabsorption is exceeded and glucose is excreted in the urine; thus glucose is considered a threshold substance. The presence of glucose in the urine may result from elevated blood glucose level (hyperglycemia) or a decrease in the renal threshold. Variations in the renal threshold for glucose occur in individuals who have had diabetes mellitus for a number of years. It is possible that their serum glucose level may be high (e.g., ≥400 mg/dL), and glucose may still not be present in the urine.

Ketones

Ketones are a by-product of the incomplete metabolism of fatty acids. Normally, there are no ketones in urine. Ketones are produced when there is a deficiency of insulin and when alternative metabolic pathways are utilized to convert fat sources to glucose and provide cellular energy. There are three types of ketones: acetone, acetoacetic acid, and beta-hydroxybutric acid. Consequently, when ketones are in the serum, glomerular filtration results in a partial urinary excretion of the ketones.

Protein

Protein, such as albumin, is not normally present in the urine. The glomerular membrane is semipermeable to small molecules; protein molecules are too large to pass through this semipermeable membrane. When permeability of the glomerular membrane is increased, the protein molecules pass through and are excreted in the urine. An increased glomerular membrane permeability may be the result of infection or inflammation and associated immunologic mechanisms. Certain systemic processes result in the production of abnormal proteins, such as globulin or others. These proteins are not detected with routine urinalysis procedures; urine protein electrophoresis or other tests are necessary to detect these unusual proteins.

Protein in the urine may occur transiently with infection, stress, certain medications (e.g., gold), or strenuous exercise. A random finding of proteinuria followed by a series of negative findings does not imply renal disease. When protein is detected in the urine, further investigation must take place to ensure that renal dysfunction is not present. If infection is suspected to be the cause of the proteinuria, urinalyses after eradication of the infection should yield a negative result for the presence of protein. Persistent proteinuria needs further investigation. Usually, a 24-hour urine collection for total protein determination is indicated. Protein in the urine is associated with glomerular disease, usually as a result of immunologic mechanisms.

Sediment

Urinary sediment refers to abnormal particles present in the urine. These include cells, bacteria, crystals, and casts. Types of *cells* abnormally present in the urine may include tubular cells (from the tubule of the nephron), epithelial cells (from the urothelial lining of the urinary tract), RBCs, and white blood cells (WBCs). One or two RBCs or WBCs per high-power field are considered within the range of normal. *Bacteria* are not normally present in the urine; one or two bacteria per high-power field on microscopic examination are not of concern. *Crystals* in the urine come from various salts; these particles may be from components of the diet, drug administration, or disease. The salts may be composed of calcium, oxalate, phosphate, magnesium, urea, or other substances. Certain drugs, such as the sulfates, also can produce crystals. *Casts* are structures formed around other particles. There may be casts of cells, bacteria, or protein. When casts are formed, there is a clumping or agglutination of the element and gelatinous substances form the surrounding structure, a cast. Casts are described in reference to the type of element in the structure or the stage of degeneration. Casts may be termed RBC cast, WBC cast, tubular cell cast, or other type. The degeneration of casts refers to the stage of breakdown of the internal element. Terms used to describe casts include *granular* (coarse or fine) and *waxy*.

Urinary Electrolytes

A sample of urine may also be collected by voiding or catheter aspiration for analysis of urinary electrolytes, such as sodium or chloride. Normally, the amount of sodium excreted in the urine is nearly equal to that consumed. Urinary sodium levels are measured to assist with the differential medical diagnosis of acute tubular necrosis (ATN) and other potential renal disorders, such as prerenal azotemia from volume depletion or cardiac pump failure. The amount of urinary sodium excreted provides information about how well the tubules are functioning to conserve (reabsorb) sodium. For example, when there is intravascular volume depletion, the renal tubules are expected to reabsorb sodium from the tubular filtrate in an attempt to restore intravascular volume. Consequently, the amount of urinary sodium is low (<10 mEq/L). If tubular damage is already present, whether it is due to toxins, prolonged ischemia, or other reasons, the tubules do not reabsorb sodium. Thus, urinary sodium levels of 40 mEq/L or greater suggests that ATN is present. The calculation of the *fractional excretion of sodium*, a comparison of sodium excreted with sodium filtered, is more informative than a random urinary sodium determination. However, clinicians continue to report that neither test is absolutely reliable in differentiating ATN from prerenal azotemic states.

Information about the amount of urinary sodium excreted is important in considering treatment options. For example, if intravascular volume is low, fluid replacement is indicated. However, if ATN has already occurred, the administration of fluids may precipitate hypervolemia, heart failure, or pulmonary edema. On the other hand, the administration of fluids and diuretics may convert oliguric acute renal failure into a nonoliguric form and more rapidly normalize renal function (Pru & Kjellstrand, 1985).

Urine Osmolality

Osmolality is a measurement of the concentration of particles in solution and, in this case, the concentration of solutes in urine. These solutes include both electrolytes and nonelectrolytes, such as glucose, urea, and creatinine. The kidneys excrete or reabsorb water to maintain a plasma osmolality in the range of 275 to 295 mOsm/L. When the plasma osmolality is decreased, the release of ADH is inhibited; without ADH, the distal tubule and collecting ducts are not permeable to water. Therefore, water is excreted, not reab-

sorbed. When the plasma osmolality is increased, ADH is produced. With ADH production, the distal tubule is made permeable to water; consequently, water is reabsorbed and less urine is excreted. Thus, increased urine osmolality reflects a concentrated urine with less water than solutes. In addition, a decreased urine osmolality value reflects a dilute urine with more water than solutes. The urinary osmolality can vary from 300 to 1200 mOsm/L, depending on the clinical status of the client and the functional status of the kidneys. The fixed acids and other wastes that are continually produced constitute a solute load that must be excreted via urine on a regular basis; this is referred to as obligatory solute excretion. If the client has lost excessive fluids, the renal response is to conserve water, preserve plasma osmolality, and excrete a small-volume, highly concentrated urine. Although many factors, such as diet, medications, and activity, can influence the urine osmolality, it is considerably more accurate than the bedside urine specific gravity measurement, which also measures the ability of the tubules to concentrate urine.

Urine for Culture and Sensitivity

A sample of urine may be collected and submitted for culture to identify the number and the types of pathogens present. The presence of clinical symptoms or unexplained bacteria in a urinalysis specimen are indications for urine culture and sensitivity. After the culture is incubated in the laboratory for 24 to 48 hours, the colonies are inoculated onto plates with various antimicrobial agents. Those antibiotics to which the microorganisms are sensitive and/or resistant are reported to guide decisions about needed therapy. A clean catch or catheter-derived specimen is always preferred for culture and sensitivity testing.

Twenty-four–Hour Urine Collection

Twenty-four–hour urine collections are used to complete a quantitative and qualitative analysis of one or more substances. Twenty-four–hour collections are requested for measurement of urinary creatinine or urea nitrogen, sodium, chloride, calcium, catecholamines, or other components (Table 57–2). When collecting a 24-hour urine specimen, it is essential that *all* urine be collected. If small quantities must be removed from the collection for other analytic purposes, such as urine culture and sensitivity testing, the amount removed is measured and appropriately documented.

To collect urine for a defined period, such as 24-hours, the nurse instructs the client to empty the bladder. The time is noted, and this is referred to as the start time. From the start time until the defined period has elapsed, all urine produced is collected, measured, and stored in a specific container, depending on the reason for the urine collection. It is important that the urine be free from fecal contamination. Twenty-four hours after the start time (for 24-hour collection), the client is in-

TABLE 57–2 Normal Values and Significance of Abnormal Findings in 24-Hour Urine Collections

Component	Normal Values	Significance of Abnormal Findings
Creatinine (clearance)	0.8–2.0 g/24 h Men, 1–2 g/24 h Women, 0.6–1.8 g/24 h	*Increased levels* indicate glomerular dysfunction caused by renal disease, shock, or hypovolemia.
Urea nitrogen	6–17 g/24 h	*Increased levels* commonly result from high-protein diet, dehydration, trauma, or sepsis.
Sodium	40–180 mEq/24 h	*Decreased levels* are seen in hemorrhage, shock, and hyperaldosteronism. *Increased levels* are common with diuretic therapy, excessive salt intake, and hypokalemia.
Chloride	110–254 mEq/24 h	*Decreased levels* are seen in certain renal diseases.
Calcium	50–300 mg/24 h	*Increased levels* are commonly seen with calcium renal stones and hypercalcemia. *Decreased levels* indicate hypocalcemia.
Total catecholamines	110–254 mEq/24 h	*Increased levels* occur with hypertension, pheochromocytoma, neuroblastomas, stress, or strenuous exercise.

structed to again empty the bladder; this urine is included in the 24-hour collection. The urine collection should be refrigerated or stored on ice to prevent changes in the urine.

The collection of urine for a 24-hour period is often more difficult than it would seem. In clients who are hospitalized, the cooperation of staff, family and visitors, and the client is essential. All persons who might forget and discard collected urine contribute to sources of error during the collection process. Signs in the bathroom, client and family instruction, and repeated diligence in remembering to save the urine are helpful.

Creatinine Clearance

Creatinine clearance is a measurement of GFR and is the best indication of overall renal function. GFR is calculated through the measurement of creatinine clearance. In essence, the amount of creatinine cleared, or filtered into the urine, is quantified in the urine excreted in a defined period of time; the time period is usually 24

hours. The calculation requires comparison with the serum creatinine level.

Because age, sex, height, and weight influence the expected amount of creatinine to be excreted, these variables are considered in the calculation. Although nurses generally do not calculate the creatinine clearance, the ability to interpret its significance and meaning is necessary for care planning and client education.

The formula for the calculation of creatinine clearance is as follows:

$$\text{Creatinine clearance} = \frac{U \times V}{P}$$

U = creatinine in urine (mg/dL)

V = volume of urine (mL/24 hours)

P = creatinine in plasma (mg/dL)

The rate of creatinine clearance is expressed as milliliters per minute per 1.72 m² of body surface area. The above formula is also corrected for estimated variations in surface area.

The normal creatinine clearance for adult males is in the range of 95 to 135 mL/minute; for adult females, the normal range is 85 to 125 mL/minute. Usually, an adult male excretes about 1.0 to 2.0 g of creatinine into the urine, and adult females excrete about 0.6 to 1.8 g of creatinine in 24 hours. Knowledge about the total grams of creatinine excreted into the urine collection assists in determining the adequacy of the collection. A shortened, simplified method of estimating creatinine clearance may be used to estimate overall renal function, until a 24 collection is made and creatinine clearance can be calculated. In this method, the formula is as follows:

$$\text{Creatinine clearance} = \frac{140 - \text{age}}{\text{plasma creatinine (mg/dL)}}$$

For females, the number obtained is multiplied by 0.85 (85%) to correct for a smaller muscle mass. This formula is easily used to quickly estimate the percentage of renal function that remains. It is useful to identify persons at high risk for acute renal failure, to quantify the percentage of renal function remaining for individuals with chronic renal disease, and to serve as a guide for dosage modifications for medications requiring renal excretion.

The use of this formula is particularly important for elderly clients, as GFR, and thus creatinine clearance, diminishes with aging. Persons aged 70 years and older experience a predictable decrease in creatinine clearance, even though there is often minimal increase in the serum creatinine level. The decrease in renal clearance of creatinine represents a decrease of overall function and consequently an increase in susceptibility to nephrotoxic agents. Antibiotics (especially the aminoglycosides, such as gentamicin [Garamycin] and tobramycin [Nebcin]), NSAIDs (such as indomethacin [Indocin]), and radiopaque contrast media (used for many radiologic and angiopathic procedures) increase the elderly client's susceptibility to acute renal failure. When coupled with the loss of tubular concentrating ability that occurs with aging, dehydration, or lack of ability to conserve water, nephrotoxin exposure increases the vulnerability of the client with renal insufficiency to the development of renal failure.

The typical elderly client takes multiple prescribed and OTC drugs, most of which depend on a high level of renal function for excretion. Because there is a compromise in the creatinine clearance ability of the kidneys, the elderly individual is more readily susceptible to toxic effects of drug therapy and drug interactions. The physician, the pharmacist, and the nurse practitioner can use a formula based on age to estimate the client's individual clearance and modify drug dosages accordingly. The staff nurse may calculate the creatinine clearance to determine whether dosage changes should be recommended if the need is not detected by the physician.

RADIOGRAPHIC EXAMINATIONS

A variety of radiographic, radionuclide imaging, and other special procedures are used to diagnose structural and functional abnormalities within the genitourinary system (Table 57-3). As with other diagnostic tests, the nurse explains the procedures thoroughly to the client.

KIDNEYS, URETERS, AND BLADDER

Radiographic examination of the kidneys, ureters, and bladder (KUB) is a plain film of the abdomen taken without any client preparation except an explanation. The KUB demonstrates gross anatomic features by identifying whether the client has two kidneys, ureters, and a bladder. It may show whether obvious stones or obstructions are present in the urinary tract. This test identifies only gross features (shape, size, and relationship to other parts of the urinary tract); further tests are required for definitive diagnosis of functional or structural abnormalities. The nurse instructs the client that there is no discomfort or risk from the procedure. The nurse informs the client that the films will be taken while the client lies in a supine position. No specific preparation or postprocedure care is required.

INTRAVENOUS PYELOGRAPHY (EXCRETORY UROGRAPHY)

Client preparation. Client preparation considerations for the intravenous pyelogram (IVP), also known as the excretory urogram, include assessment of iodine sensitivity, determination of risk of contrast media–induced renal failure, and bowel preparation procedures to promote adequate visualization. The nurse asks the client whether there is a history of iodine sensitivity through known prior reactions or a sensitivity to shellfish. For persons at high risk for the development of acute renal failure after the administration of the contrast media, the IV administration of mannitol (Osmitrol) may be prescribed after injection of the contrast agent.

Specific procedures to ensure that films provide adequate visualizations vary, depending on the preferences of the radiologist. Some radiologists recommend that the client not fast and thus fluid intake is allowed. Other radiologists recommend that the client preparation for an IVP include a light evening meal then fasting from midnight on the night before the procedure. When fluid is not allowed, the contrast medium is not diluted; when fluid intake is permitted, the risk of dehydration is minimized. The risk of dehydration is greatest in clients with a serum creatinine level greater than 1.5 mg/dL. Many physicians request that IV fluid administration be initiated to ensure that hydration is maintained and nephrotoxic potential is decreased in the dehydrated client. The development of contrast materials that are less hypertonic and nephrotoxic may decrease the risk of complications from this test in persons with renal insufficiency; however, assessment to prevent and detect acute renal failure from contrast media must continue. The elderly client is most at risk for dehydration and other toxic effects of this procedure.

Bowel preparation to remove fecal contents, fluid,

TABLE 57–3 Common Radiologic and Special Diagnostic Tests for Clients with Disorders of the Urinary System

Test	Purpose	Comments
Radiography of kidneys, ureters, and bladder (plain film of abdomen)	To screen for the presence of two kidneys To measure kidney size To detect gross obstruction	
Intravenous pyelography (excretory urography)	To measure kidney size To detect obstruction To assess parenchymal mass	Radiopaque contrast media may cause an allergic (hypersensitivity) reaction in iodine-sensitive clients. Contrast agent is also hypertonic and increases the risk of acute renal failure in adults with serum creatinine levels greater than 1.5 mg/dL, diabetes mellitus, multiple myeloma, or dehydration. These complications can be prevented by parenteral fluid administration, use of mannitol, and daily monitoring of serum creatinine levels.
Nephrotomography	To assess various planes of kidney tissue for cysts, tumors, or calculi	Same as for IVP.
Computed tomography	To measure the size of the kidneys To evaluate contour to assess for masses or obstruction	Contrast media may provoke acute renal failure (as in IVP). May be performed without contrast media and still obtain adequate visualization. See comments for IVP for high-risk persons and preventive measures.
Cystography and cystoscopy	To identify abnormalities of bladder wall and the urethral and ureteral occlusions To treat small obstructions or lesions via fulguration, lithotripsy, or removal with stone basket	Instrumentation of the urinary tract produces risk for infection. Monitor for infection for 48–72 h after the procedure.
Voiding cystourethrography	To outline bladder contour and detect urinary reflux from vesicourethral junctions	Risk for infection is similar to that in cystography because urinary catheterization is required. Monitor for postprocedure infection.
Renal arteriography	To identify vascular abnormalities within each kidney and adjacent aorta	Contrast media may provoke acute renal failure (as in IVP). Essential for diagnosis and treatment of some vascular abnormalities, such as renal artery stenosis. Monitor for bleeding and decrease in renal function after the procedure.
Ultrasonography	To identify the size of the kidneys or obstruction in the kidneys or lower urinary tract May detect tumors or cysts	Minimal risk to client. Good alternative to IVP.

and air is necessary to permit adequate outlining of the lower poles of the kidneys, the ureters, and the bladder. Preparatory procedures vary, but usually include the administration of laxatives. Enemas are sometimes prescribed, but are also controversial because of the air and fluid introduced if there is inadequate expulsion of fecal contents.

Procedure. For the IVP, a radiopaque contrast medium is intravenously injected. As blood (with the contrast medium) circulates into the renal vasculature and is filtered by the glomeruli, the contrast medium is excreted in the urine. A series of films are taken at various times after injection. As a result, an outline of the kidneys, the ureters, and the bladder is produced as urine containing the contrast medium is excreted. Consequently, the IVP provides information about the number, size, and location of the kidneys; contrast uptake adequacy and rate of excretion; the number, size, location, and patency of the ureters; and the size, location, and nature of the urinary bladder.

Follow-up care. After IVP, the nurse monitors the client for alteration in renal function. The nurse encourages fluid intake orally or administers parenteral fluids at the prescribed rate to minimize the potential for renal deterioration. Serum creatinine levels are monitored, as elevations may be due to contrast media–induced acute renal failure. An elevation of the serum creatinine level may occur despite normal urinary output.

NEPHROTOMOGRAPHY

Client preparation. Nephrotomograms are taken at the same time as the IVP. If previous IVP studies were performed, the client is informed that this procedure will take longer and that more films will be obtained. The physical preparation for tomograms is similar to that for the IVP, including assessment for iodine sensitivity and elevated serum creatinine levels.

Procedure. The procedure for obtaining tomograms is similar to that for the IVP. Tomograms provide images of different planes of tissue, demonstrating any abnormalities present at varying depths.

Follow-up care. The follow-up care for the client who has nephrotomograms is the same as that after an IVP. The risk for contrast media–induced acute renal failure is similar. The nurse ensures adequate hydration and monitors the serum creatinine level and urinary output.

COMPUTED TOMOGRAPHY

Client preparation. The nurse informs the client that computed tomography (CT) is performed to provide three-dimensional information about the structures of the abdomen, including the kidneys, the ureters, the bladder, and surrounding tissues. CT is usually performed after other diagnostic procedures and yields definitive information about tumors, cysts, abscesses, or other masses, as well as obstruction or some vascular abnormalities. The preparation of the client includes a bowel preparation with laxatives or an enema, and a light meal the evening before the procedure. The client is then given nothing by mouth (NPO) after midnight on the night preceding the examination.

Procedure. The CT scan is performed in a special room, usually located in the radiology or nuclear medicine department. An IV injection of radiopaque contrast media may be administered before the initiation of imaging procedures. The use of contrast media may be eliminated in persons at risk for contrast media–induced acute renal failure, but the images produced will be less distinct. Tomograms (images obtained from cross-sectional angles) are obtained at various levels.

Follow-up care. No special follow-up care is required after CT.

CYSTOGRAPHY AND CYSTOURETHROGRAPHY

Client preparation. The preparation of the client who requires a cystography or cystourethrography begins with an explanation of the nature of the procedure. The client needs to know that a urinary catheter is temporarily required to instill the contrast medium, which is necessary for visualization of the lower urinary tract.

Procedure. In both cystography and cystourethrography, contrast medium is instilled into the bladder via a urethral catheter. After bladder filling, a variety of films are obtained from anterior, posterior, and oblique positions. For the voiding cystourethrogram (VCUG), the client is requested to void and films are taken during the voiding. VCUG is obtained to determine whether vesicoureteral reflux is present. The cystogram is often indicated in cases of trauma when urethral or bladder injury is suspected.

Follow-up care. The follow-up care of the client involves monitoring for the development of infection as a result of urinary catheterization. The contrast medium is not nephrotoxic, as it is not injected into the blood stream. Because pelvic or urethral trauma may be present, the nurse monitors the client for changes in urinary output, such as might result from disruption of urinary tract patency.

RENAL ARTERIOGRAPHY (ANGIOGRAPHY)

Client preparation. The nurse informs the client that arteriography is performed to assess the arterial blood supply of the kidneys. The nurse explains that before the examination a bowel preparation is given to remove fecal contents, gas, and fluid. A light evening meal is given, and the client is then maintained on NPO restrictions the night before the procedure. The client also signs a form indicating informed consent. Because renal arteriography is done to explore suspected causes of severe hypertension or bleeding from trauma, the client needs to know that information obtained is diagnostic and that subsequent corrective procedures, potentially surgical intervention, may be involved.

Procedure. The injection of a radiopaque contrast medium into the renal arteries requires entry into the arterial vasculature, usually the femoral artery in the groin. After sedation, skin preparation, and draping, a local anesthetic is injected. An arterial puncture is performed through which the angiographic catheter is inserted. The movement of the catheter into the abdominal aorta and the orifices of the renal arteries is guided by fluoroscopic examination. When the tip of the catheter is positioned at the renal arteries, contrast medium is injected into each artery, and films are taken at specified time intervals. The speed of the distribution of the contrast media is noted, along with any areas of vascular narrowing. Arterial blockage is noted when there is failure of contrast media uptake. Extravasation of contrast media into surrounding tissue is indicative of vessel rupture, such as might be present after trauma.

Follow-up care. Bleeding from the catheter insertion site and contrast medium–induced acute renal failure are the two most common complications of renal arteriography. The nurse monitors the site of catheter insertion for signs of bleeding or swelling. Vital signs are measured and recorded according to the individual hospital's policy. A typical protocol specifies vital signs determinations every 15 minutes for 1 hour, every 30 minutes for 2 hours, every hour for 4 hours, and then every 4 hours. Distal pulse rates are checked, and their sudden absence may reflect hematoma formation or embolization. Hemoglobin and hematocrit levels are measured closely for 24 hours after the procedure, usually every 6 hours. The period of absolute bed rest (to prevent bleeding) after arteriography varies with the physician's and the hospital's preference. In general, bed rest for 24 hours is prescribed. When variations are allowed, absolute bed rest is maintained for at least 6 hours. After 6 hours and if there is no evidence of bleeding, the client may be permitted to stand to void or use a bedside commode.

The serum creatinine level is measured for several days after the arteriogram to determine if any deterioration in renal function has occurred as a result of the procedure. For some persons with renal insufficiency, the administration of contrast media may provoke an episode of acute renal failure sufficient to require short-term dialysis. Because the test is utilized to provide definitive information that may permit interventions to restore blood flow and thus preserve renal function,

many clients are willing to accept the risk of short-term dialysis to prevent the need for permanent dialysis.

OTHER DIAGNOSTIC STUDIES

CYSTOSCOPY

Client preparation. Preparation of the client for cystoscopy includes a complete description of and reasons for the procedure. The nurse is usually required to complete a preoperative check list as described in Chapter 18. The client may be requested to sign a consent form, or operative permit. Cystoscopy may be performed for diagnostic or treatment purposes. Indications for diagnostic cystoscopy include examination for bladder or urethral trauma and identification of causes of urinary tract obstruction from stones or tumors. Cystoscopy for surgical treatment may be indicated to remove bladder tumors or an enlarged prostate gland. Cystoscopy may be done under general or local anesthesia with sedation. The age of the client and the expected duration of the procedure are considered in the decision about anesthesia. The client receives a light evening meal and is placed on NPO restrictions after midnight on the night preceding the cystoscopy. Bowel preparation with laxatives or enemas may be administered the evening before the procedure.

Procedure. The cystoscopic examination is performed in a specially designed cystoscopic examination room. If it is performed in a surgical suite under general anesthesia, traditional surgical support personnel are present, including an anesthesiologist or nurse anesthetist, circulating and scrub nurses, and a surgical assistant. Increasingly, the procedure is performed in outpatient settings, such as a clinic or urologist's office.

The client is assisted onto a table and into the lithotomy position. After the administration of anesthesia, skin cleaning, and draping, a cystoscope is inserted via the urethra into the urinary bladder. If visualization of the urethra is also indicated, a urethroscope is utilized. Commonly, examinations include the use of both the cystoscope and the urethroscope.

Follow-up care. After cystoscopic examination with general anesthesia, the client is returned to a postanesthesia recovery unit. If local anesthesia and sedation were administered, the client is returned directly to the hospital room. Clients having cystoscopic examinations as outpatients are transferred to an area for monitoring before discharge to home. The client is monitored for maintenance of airway and breathing; alterations in vital signs, including temperature; and changes in urinary output. Bleeding and infection are the major complications for which the nurse observes. After cystoscopy, a catheter may or may not be present. The urine is frequently tinged pink but gross bleeding is not expected. Bleeding, or the presence of clots, may result in catheter obstruction and a decrease in urinary output. Fever, with or without chills, and an elevated WBC count suggest that infection is present.

RETROGRADE PROCEDURES

Client preparation. The client is prepared for retrograde procedures (retrograde pyelography, retrograde cystography, and retrograde urethrography) in a manner similar to that required for the cystoscopic examination. The nurse explains that the retrograde examination of the ureters and pelvis (pyelogram), bladder (cystogram), and urethra (urethrogram) involves the direct injection of radiopaque contrast medium into the lower urinary tract. By directly instilling the contrast medium to obtain an outline of the structures desired, the contrast medium does not enter the blood stream. Consequently, the client is not at risk for the development of contrast medium–induced acute renal failure or an allergic response.

Procedure. Retrograde films are obtained during the cystoscopic examination. After the placement of the cystoscope, catheters are placed into each ureter and contrast medium is instilled into each ureter and renal pelvis. The catheters are removed, and films are taken to outline these structures as the contrast medium is excreted. The procedure identifies any obstruction or structural abnormality. For retrograde cystoscopy or urethrography, contrast medium is instilled similarly into the bladder or the urethra, also to identify structural abnormalities, such as fistulas, diverticula, or tumors.

Follow-up care. After retrograde procedures, the client is monitored for the development of infection as a result of instrumentation of the urinary tract. Because these procedures are performed during cystoscopic examination, the follow-up care is the same as that described earlier for cystoscopy.

RENAL BIOPSY

Client preparation. The nurse explains that a biopsy of the kidney is performed to determine the reason for unexplained renal dysfunction. The client is requested to indicate informed consent by signing an operative permit. Often, a biopsy is performed when proteinuria or hematuria develops without obvious reason. There are two options for obtaining the tissue required for renal biopsy: a percutaneous (closed) biopsy and a surgical (open) biopsy. Factors to be considered in the selection of the type of procedure include the presence of only one kidney, the ability of the client to participate cooperatively, and whether abdominal surgical exploration is necessary. If a percutaneous biopsy is selected, the client must have two kidneys, be able to breathe comfortably in a prone position for 30 to 45 minutes, and be able to suspend breathing on request for several seconds.

An open renal biopsy is performed when the client has only one kidney, if the client cannot participate by suspending breathing, if the client is unable to tolerate a prone position, or when a malignancy is suspected. If abdominal surgery is necessary for other reasons and a renal biopsy is also needed, the nephrologist may request the surgeon to perform the biopsy, thus eliminating a second procedure via the percutaneous route. If an open biopsy is performed, client preparation is as for general surgery and anesthesia (see Chap. 18).

Procedure. For the percutaneous biopsy, the client is maintained on NPO status for 4 to 6 hours before the procedure. The left kidney is selected for biopsy because it is closer to the skin and is not adjacent to the liver. The exact position of the kidney is determined via fluoroscopic or ultrasonic examination. For some clients, the nephrologist may locate the kidney before the biopsy and then insert the biopsy needle using landmarks identified by the images produced. This is referred to as a blind technique. For other clients, the closed biopsy is performed under fluoroscopic or ultrasonic examination. Because preferences and training of nephrologists vary, the biopsy technique varies. During the closed biopsy, the client is placed in a prone position. A roll of padding is placed under the client's abdomen to angle the kidney closer to the skin. The skin is prepared and draped, and a local anesthetic is injected. The depth of the kidney is identified by the insertion of a thin-gauge spinal needle. Movement of the spinal needle with breathing helps to determine that the capsule of the kidney has been located. A specially designed trocar is inserted in the path established by the spinal needle. A specimen of tissue is then obtained by inserting the biopsy needle through the trocar and capsule into the renal cortex. Ideally, three specimens of tissue are obtained.

Follow-up care. After a closed biopsy, the major risk to the client is the potential for bleeding from the biopsy site. For 24 hours after the biopsy, the nurse monitors vital signs, urinary output, hemoglobin levels, and hematocrit (as for postarteriography protocols). The client must be on strict bed rest lying in a supine position with a back roll for additional support for at least 6 hours after the biopsy. The head of the bed may be elevated, and oral intake of food and fluids may be resumed. After 6 hours and if there is no evidence of bleeding, the client may be permitted to have limited bathroom privileges. The urine may be tinged with blood for 24 hours after the biopsy; there should not be obvious blood clots in the urine.

After the percutaneous renal biopsy, the client may experience some local discomfort. If aching originates at the biopsy site and begins to radiate to the flank and around the front of the abdomen, an onset of bleeding should be suspected. This typical pattern of discomfort with bleeding occurs because blood in the perirenal tissues and musculature increases the pressure on local nerve tracts. If bleeding occurs, administration of fluid, packed RBCs, or both may be required to restore blood pressure. Generally, a small amount of bleeding creates sufficient pressure to compress bleeding sites; this is termed *tamponade effect*. If tamponade does not occur and bleeding becomes extensive, surgical intervention for hemostasis or even nephrectomy may be necessary. If no bleeding occurs, the client can resume general activities after 24 hours. The nurse instructs the client to avoid lifting heavy objects, exercise, or other strenuous activities for 1 to 2 weeks after the biopsy.

For the follow-up care of a client undergoing an open renal biopsy, refer to Chapter 20 for general postoperative care.

RENOGRAPHY

Client preparation. The nurse explains to the client that a kidney scan is performed to provide general information about the nature of renal blood flow. The nurse instructs the client about the injection of the radionuclide and provides reassurance that there is generally no danger from the small amount of radioactive material present in the agent.

Procedure. For a kidney scan, the radionuclide is injected intravenously. After injection of the agent, its uptake in the renal parenchyma is measured by a scintillator. A specially designed camera records the emissions, or scintillations, provided by the radionuclide. In this manner, an image is produced. Simultaneously, the rate and location of the emissions are recorded by computer, and information about the nature of renal blood flow or glomerular filtration is provided. Specific types of radionuclides provide varying information. A kidney scan demonstrates only the relative amount of radionuclide uptake (renal blood flow) into each kidney, thus providing primarily structural information. On the other hand, the *renogram* provides some functional information by noting the amount of radionuclide excreted and thus measuring glomerular filtration and tubular secretion, in addition to perfusion.

Follow-up care. In general, no specific follow-up care is required. If the client is able, urination into a commode is acceptable, as there is a small amount of radioactive material present to be excreted. If the client is incontinent, the nurse changes the bed linens promptly and wears gloves to prevent unnecessary skin contact.

ULTRASONOGRAPHY

Client preparation. The nurse informs the client that ultrasonography of the abdomen is without discomfort or risk. The nurse explains that by applying sound waves to structures of different densities, images of these structures may be reproduced. Consequently, the sonograms (echograms) provide information about the size and nature of the kidneys, the ureters, the bladder, and, to a certain extent, the tissues surrounding these structures. The ultrasound scan is informative in identi-

fying obstruction in the urinary tract, tumors, cysts, and other masses and does not require administration of potentially harmful nephrotoxic agents.

Procedure. The client is usually placed on a table in a prone position. A gel that promotes the conduction of sound waves is applied to the skin over the back and flank areas. A transducer, in contact with and moving across the skin, delivers sounds waves and measures the echoes; images of the internal structures are reproduced.

Follow-up care. No special follow-up care is required after abdominal ultrasonography.

URODYNAMIC STUDIES

Urodynamic studies are procedures to describe the processes of voiding. These studies include tests of bladder capacity, pressure, and tone; studies of urethral pressure and urinary flow; and examination of the function of voluntary muscles of the perineum. These tests are often used in conjunction with excretory urography or cystoscopic procedures as part of the overall evaluation of problems with urinary flow.

Cystometrography

Client preparation. The nurse explains that the purpose of cystometrography is to determine the effectiveness and sensitivity of the bladder wall (detrusor) muscle. With these measurements of the quality of the detrusor muscle, determinations about bladder capacity, bladder pressure, and voiding reflexes may be made. The client is informed that a urinary catheter may be required temporarily during the procedure.

Procedure. Initially, the client is requested to void normally; measurements of the amount, rate of flow, and time of voiding are recorded. A urinary catheter is then inserted to measure the residual bladder urine volume. The cystometer is attached to the catheter, and fluid is instilled via the catheter into the bladder. The point at which the client notes a feeling of the urge to void is recorded, as well as when the client notes a strong urge to void. Readings of bladder capacity and bladder pressure are recorded graphically. The client is requested to void when the bladder instillation is complete (about 500 mL). The urinary residual after voiding is noted, and the catheter is removed. Electromyography (EMG) of the perineal muscles may also be performed during the cystometric examination (see later).

Follow-up care. The client is monitored for the development of infection as might follow any instrumentation of the urinary tract. The nurse measures and records the client's temperature, notes the characteristics and amount of urinary output, and observes the WBC count for an increase, indicative of infection.

Urethral Pressure Profile

Client preparation. The nurse explains to the client that a urethral pressure profile is potentially informative about the nature of urinary incontinence or urinary retention. The client is informed that a urinary catheter may be temporarily placed during the procedure.

Procedure. A special catheter with pressure-sensing capabilities is inserted into the urinary bladder. As the catheter is slowly withdrawn, variations in the pressure of the smooth muscle of the urethra are recorded.

Follow-up care. As with other studies involving instrumentation of the urinary tract, the client is monitored for the development of infection.

ELECTROMYOGRAPHY

Client preparation. The nurse explains that EMG of the perineal muscles may be useful in evaluating the quality of the voluntary muscles involved in voiding. This information may assist in identifying methods of improving continence. The client should be informed that some temporary discomfort accompanies the placement of the electrodes.

Procedure. In EMG of the perineal muscles, electrodes are placed in either the rectum or the urethra to measure muscle contraction and relaxation (see Chap. 29).

Follow-up care. After completion of EMG, the nurse administers analgesics to promote client comfort. The discomfort is usually mild and of short duration.

SUMMARY

The nurse assesses the client with potential or actual problems of the urinary system and pays special attention to the history and physical examination findings. The nurse also provides information and emotional reassurance during the frequently difficult period of urologic diagnostic work-up. A variety of diagnostic tests provide information about the structure and function of the urinary tract. These diagnostic tests may pose increased risks for the client with confirmed renal deterioration. The nurse prepares the client for diagnostic tests and assists in helping the client to understand their purpose.

REFERENCES AND READINGS

Anagnostou, A., & Kurtzman, N. (1985). The anemia of chronic renal failure. *Seminars in Nephrology, 5,* 115–127.

Beck, T., Levenson, D. J., & Brenner, B. M. (1987). Renal prostaglandins and kinins. In M. H. Maxwell, C. R. Kleeman, & R. G. Narins (Eds.), *Clinical disorders of fluid and electrolyte metabolism* (pp. 343–370). New York: McGraw-Hill.

Brenner, B. M., Zatz, R., & Ichikawa, I. (1986). The renal circulations. In B. M. Brenner & F. C. Rector (Eds.), *The kidney* (3rd ed.). Philadelphia: W. B. Saunders.

Cella, J. H., & Watson, J. (1989). *Nurse's manual of laboratory tests.* Philadelphia: F. A. Davis.

Chadwick, A. T. (1989). BVI 2000: A noninvasive technique to assess bladder function. *Journal of Neuroscience Nursing, 21,* 256–257.

Dunn, M. J. (1984). Clinical effects of prostaglandins in renal disease. *Hospital Practice, 19*(3), 99–113.

Fine, E. J., Axelrod, M., & Blaufox, M. D. (1985). Physiologic aspects of diagnostic renal imaging. *Seminars in Nephrology, 5,* 188–207.

Fritz, M. (1988). Noninvasive bladder volume measurement. *Urologic Nursing, 9,* 8–9.

Guyton, A. C. (1986). *Textbook of medical physiology* (7th ed.). Philadelphia: W. B. Saunders.

Hjelm-Karlsson, K. (1989). Comparison of oral, written, and audio-visually based information as preparation for intravenous pyelography. *International Journal of Nursing Studies, 26,* 53–68.

Keyes, J. L. (1985). *Fluid, electrolyte and acid-base regulation.* Monterey, CA: Wadsworth.

Lee, D. B., & Kurokawa, K. (1987). Physiology of phosphorus metabolism. In M. H. Maxwell, C. R. Kleeman, & R. G. Narins, *Clinical disorders of fluid and electrolyte metabolism* (4th ed.). New York: McGraw-Hill.

Matteson, M. A., & McConnell, E. S. (1988). *Gerontological nursing: Concepts and practice.* Philadelphia: W. B. Saunders.

Pru, C., & Kjellstrand, C. (1985). Urinary indices and chemistries in the differential diagnosis of prerenal failure and acute tubular necrosis. *Seminars in Nephrology, 5,* 224–233.

Re, R. N. (1987). The renin-angiotensin systems. *Medical Clinics of North America, 71,* 877–895.

Rebensen-Piano, M. (1989). The physiologic changes that occur with aging. *Critical Care Nursing Quarterly, 12*(1), 1–14.

Saunders, E. (1987). Hypertension in blacks. *Medical Clinics of North America, 71,* 1013–1029.

Stark, J. L. (1988). A quick guide to urinary tract assessment. *Nursing '88, 18*(7), 56–58.

Wilkinson, G. B. (1988). Clean catch. Urodynamic studies: A balloon as a teaching device. *Urologic Nursing, 9,* 18–19.

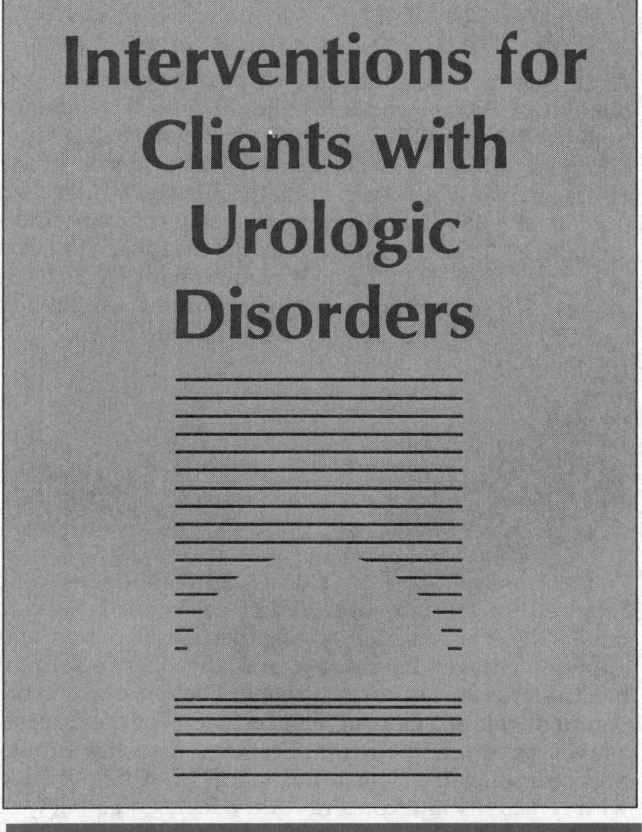

CHAPTER 58

Interventions for Clients with Urologic Disorders

Disorders of the structure or function of the kidneys, ureters, bladder, or urethra originate from a variety of problems, including congenital defects and hereditary disorders, infections, immunologic responses, pathologic degeneration, obstructions, tumors, and trauma. In addition, although some disorders derive from multifactorial causes, other problems have an undetermined etiology. Structural and functional abnormalities of the genitourinary system may have serious, life-threatening sequelae if appropriate diagnostic and treatment procedures are not implemented. Nursing interventions are directed toward prevention, detection, and management of urologic disorders.

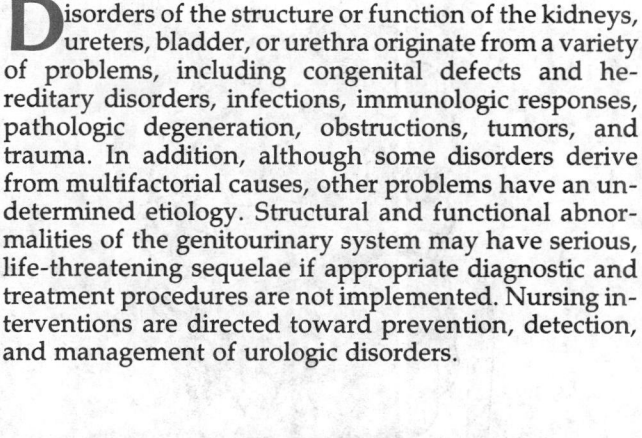

CONGENITAL DISORDERS

POLYCYSTIC KIDNEY DISEASE

OVERVIEW

Polycystic kidney disease (PKD) is an inherited kidney disorder that was initially described in the 17th century. The pattern of familial transmission and the overall effects of the disease demonstrated at the end stage were first published in a 1957 report of 242 clients (Dalgaard, 1957). PKD is one of the most common inherited disorders, occurring 5 times as often as cystic fibrosis and 10 times more often than sickle cell anemia; yet, the general public is much more aware of these other disorders.

Pathophysiology

PKD is a disorder of the renal parenchyma that occurs bilaterally. Although it has been traditionally viewed as a kidney disease, there is a considerable incidence of cysts occurring in other tissues, such as the liver and the cerebral and cardiac blood vessels. Research efforts have been directed toward exploration of the possible relationship of these multiple findings. One theory being investigated is that the disorder involves the extracellular matrix that is responsible for cellular support.

In the kidney, the nephron is the primary site of pathophysiologic damage. Cysts develop in both the glomeruli and the tubules. These small cysts become progressively larger and more diffusely distributed. The glomerular and tubular membrane is damaged; glomerular filtration, tubular reabsorption, and tubular secretion are less effective as the cysts become filled with tubular filtrate.

Over a period of years, the renal parenchymal tissue is replaced by these nonfunctioning cysts, which are frequently described as appearing like a cluster of grapes (Fig. 58–1). The kidneys are grossly enlarged, and each

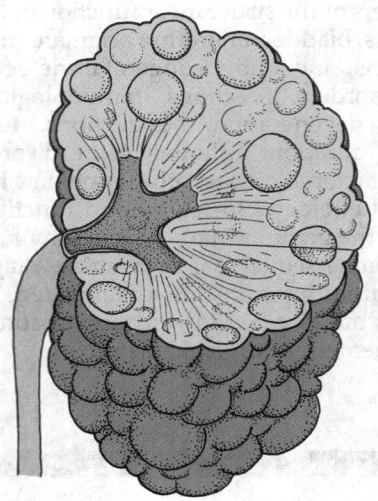

Figure 58-1

Polycystic kidney.

cystic kidney may grow to the size of a football. The polycystic kidneys may enlarge to two or three times their normal size; consequently, other abdominal organs are displaced and considerable discomfort results. In addition, the cysts fill with fluid and are prone to infection, rupture, and bleeding.

In the liver, cysts may result in the alteration of liver functions. In the brain, spontaneous rupture of vascular cysts, called *berry aneurysms,* may result in the sudden death of individuals with previously undiagnosed PKD.

High blood pressure is also present in more than 50% of persons with PKD. The hypertension may be present before actual diagnosis of the PKD. The reason for the development of hypertension is not known.

Etiology

Adult PKD is transmitted genetically in an autosomal dominant pattern. Because the gene resulting in PKD is not located on the sex chromosomes, men and women have an equal chance of getting the disease. Therefore, children of persons with PKD have a 50% probability of inheriting the gene causing the disease. The gene responsible for causing PKD has been identified as occurring on chromosome 16; however, the specific gene has not been determined.

Incidence

PKD affects approximately 400,000 to 600,000 Americans. It is the cause of end-stage renal disease for one of every eight Americans (about 10%) requiring chronic dialysis or renal transplantation (Gabow, 1986).

Although PKD is transmitted genetically at conception, clinical evidence of the disease does not usually appear until the third or fourth decade of life, or later.

The age at onset of clinical symptoms or laboratory evidence of decreased renal function varies considerably. Yet, if the gene is present, the disease will eventually develop if the person lives long enough.

PREVENTION

At the present time, there is no way to prevent the development of PKD. For adult children who have one or both parents with PKD, genetic counseling and evaluation have limited use. Because clinical evidence of the disease may not be present until the 30s, the 40s, or even the 50s, the childbearing years are past for many individuals. There are reports of prenatal diagnosis (Reeders et al., 1986) of PKD through recombinant DNA techniques. These methods now have limited availability and applicability but may be useful in the future.

COLLABORATIVE MANAGEMENT

 Assessment

History

The family history is an essential component to be explored for a client suspected of having or known to have PKD. Factors such as whether either parent was known to have the disease and the client's current health status are important to elicit. The age at which the parent developed clinical manifestations of the disease, as well as any related complications, may have prognostic significance. This information must be obtained with sensitivity and concern for the fears and anxiety of the client about the course of the unknown or suspected disease.

Specific information to be gathered during the history include the following: *family history of kidney disease, specifically PKD; family history of sudden death from a stroke-like phenomenon; problems with constipation; change in the color of the urine or frequency of urination; history of high blood pressure;* and *history of headaches.*

Physical Assessment: Clinical Manifestations

The nurse inspects the abdomen of the client with PKD. A protruding and *distended abdomen* is common as the size of the polycystic kidneys increases and pushes the abdominal contents forward. The palpation of polycystic kidneys is more readily accomplished because they may be two or three times their normal size. The nurse proceeds with gentle palpation because the polycystic kidneys and nearby tissues may be quite *tender* and *uncomfortable.* In addition to abdominal discomfort, the client may experience *flank pain;* the flank discomfort may be reported as a dull ache or as sharp and intermittent. Sharp, intermittent pain in the flank or abdominal region may be the result of a ruptured cyst. The dull and aching pain may be from increased kidney size with distention or because of infection within the cyst. When a cyst ruptures, the client may notice bright red or cola-colored urine. If the urine is cloudy or smells foul or if there is dysuria, an infection should be suspected. Because of the frequent concurrence of berry aneurysms in clients with PKD, a *severe headache* with or without neurologic or vision alterations deserves particular attention. As renal function deteriorates, the client may present with increasing *hypertension*, evidence of *edema*, or obvious *uremic symptoms* such as anorexia, nausea, vomiting, pruritus, and fatigue. Refer to Chapter 59 for a discussion of the symptoms of uremia.

Psychosocial Assessment

As a familial transmitted disease, complex psychosocial responses and concerns may be present. Usually, the person with PKD has known about the illness for a period of years. In addition, the client has frequently had direct experience with the effects and consequences of the disease in other close family members. The person may have had a parent who died as a result of the disease or other siblings or parents who required dialysis or transplantation. As the family history is obtained, the nurse listens carefully for spoken and unspoken messages. Expressions of mood or tone may be reflected in a change in the volume or pitch of the voice; feelings of anger, resentment, hostility, futility, sadness, or anxiety may thus be detected and explored further by the nurse. The focus of these feelings may be one or both parents or the diagnosis and treatment process. In addition, feelings of guilt and concern for the client's own children may also be present and further complicate the adjustment process.

Laboratory Findings

Urinalysis usually reveals proteinuria. Hematuria is also a frequent finding and may be gross as well as microscopic. The presence of bacteria in the urine suggests that infection may be present. The cysts are a frequent site for the development of infection. A urine sample for culture and sensitivity testing should be obtained if there is clinical or laboratory evidence of potential infection. Elevation of the serum creatinine and blood urea nitrogen (BUN) levels occurs as renal function deteriorates. Creatinine clearance as measured with the 24-hour urine assay also decreases with increasing renal insufficiency. The renal management of sodium may include sodium wasting or sodium retention. Serum levels of sodium generally reflect water balance; consequently, the serum sodium level appears normal, or low, depending on the overall water balance.

As renal insufficiency progresses to end-stage disease, electrolyte abnormalities also develop. These changes include hyperkalemia, hypocalcemia, hyperphosphatemia, hypermagnesemia, and metabolic acidosis (bicarbonate deficit). Hemoglobin and hematocrit values also decrease as a result of reduced erythropoietin production.

Radiographic Findings

Diagnostic studies include intravenous pyelography (IVP) (excretory urography), computed tomography (CT), and renal arteriography. The use of contrast media, as necessary for IVP and arteriography, introduces an element of risk for the individual with decreased renal function (i.e., elevated serum creatinine level). These tests may thus contribute to worsening renal function. Administration of contrast media should be avoided if other available diagnostic tests are equally informative. CT can be performed without contrast media and still provides adequate detail and delineation of structure.

Other Diagnostic Tests

Renal ultrasonography (echography) provides diagnostic evidence of PKD with minimal risk for a majority of cases. Yet, this method is not always informative for individuals with a single cyst, or for those with small renal cysts.

Fetal testing for prenatal identification of PKD is not generally available but is limited to certain research projects. Currently, the scientific and medical research community is searching for simple, conclusive methods to identify the genetic markers responsible for this disease.

 Analysis: Nursing Diagnosis

Hospitalizations of the client with PKD are most often related to gross hematuria, cyst infection, or uremia. Analysis of assessment data may suggest the following nursing diagnoses.

Common Diagnoses

The client with PKD typically has these common nursing diagnoses:

1. Pain related to pressure on abdominal organs and tissues or related to ruptured cysts
2. Body image disturbance related to abdominal enlargement
3. Fluid volume excess related to sodium and water retention
4. Anxiety and ineffective (individual and family) coping related to diagnosis and treatment uncertainties

Additional Diagnoses

In addition to the common diagnoses, some clients may also have the following nursing diagnoses, some of which are directly related to decreasing renal function and the development of renal failure:

1. Potential for injury related to excessive bleeding
2. Potential for infection related to the presence of cysts
3. Constipation related to abdominal organ displacement

4. Activity intolerance related to fatigue and anemia
5. Altered nutrition: less than body requirements related to anorexia, hypogeusia (lack of or change in taste), nausea, and vomiting
6. Sexual dysfunction related to discomfort and hormonal changes (decreased testosterone and/or estrogen levels)
7. Knowledge deficit related to treatment options and interventions

Planning and Implementation

The nursing care plan for the client with PKD addresses the common nursing diagnoses. Many of the additional nursing diagnoses just listed would be common in clients with end-stage renal failure. The reader is referred to Chapter 59 for the nursing care for clients with end-stage renal disease.

Pain

Planning: client goals. The goal for this diagnosis is that the client will achieve a state of comfort that allows maximal rest or continuation of desired activities.

Interventions. Nursing interventions directed toward the management of the discomfort associated with PKD require that the nurse considers a variety of interrelated factors. These factors include the client's pain history, meaning and interpretation of the pain experience, and etiologic considerations.

Nonsurgical management. Nonsurgical strategies for promoting comfort include chemical, physical, and psychosocial approaches. A combination of strategies may be most effective.

Drug therapy. Analgesics such as acetaminophen (Tylenol) may be prescribed to promote comfort; however, aspirin-containing compounds should be avoided to prevent increased potential for bleeding. If infection of the renal cysts is the cause of the discomfort, appropriate antibiotics are prescribed. Monitoring of renal function through assay of daily serum creatinine levels is necessary to prevent the development of nephrotoxicity resulting from antibiotic therapy.

Other pain relief measures. Application of dry heat to the abdomen or flank may promote comfort when renal cysts are infected. The nurse teaches the client methods of enhancing relaxation and promoting comfort with the use of deep breathing, guided imagery, or other relaxation strategies. The overall goal is one of self-management of discomfort. See Chapter 7 for a discussion of pain management strategies.

Surgical management. Nephrectomy, or kidney removal, is the surgical procedure performed when pain, infection, or bleeding from polycystic kidneys cannot be controlled by medical management. The decision to re-move a single, or even both, polycystic kidneys is a difficult one. Even with diseased kidneys, usually some production of erythropoietin and urine provides physiologic benefits. Therefore, a decision to proceed with nephrectomy, or bilateral nephrectomy, is often delayed until other treatment options have been exhausted.

Preoperative care. Preoperative care includes the administration of blood and fluids to achieve hemodynamic stabilization. Because the presence of blood provides an excellent medium for the proliferation of bacteria, the preoperative administration of antibiotics is to be expected. Preoperative care of a client undergoing a nephrectomy is discussed in Chapter 59.

Postoperative care. Postoperative care of the client undergoing a nephrectomy is discussed in Chapter 59.

Body Image Disturbance

Planning: client goals. The goal for this diagnosis is that the client will state that he or she accepts the alteration in body contour.

Interventions: nonsurgical management. The nurse provides supportive counseling and education to assist in the achievement of the desired goal. The client is encouraged to ventilate and verbalize any feelings or frustrations associated with the alteration in body image. The nurse explains that changes in abdominal contour may represent a variety of concerns related to the overall disease process, such as the possible fear that the disease is worsening. Further, the nurse reassures the client that these concerns are a normal part of the adjustment process.

In addition, the nurse assists the client in recognizing and planning for appropriate responses and methods of coping with the responses of friends and relatives who do not understand the reason for changes in the body configuration. Women may be falsely regarded as being in the early stages of pregnancy. Men may endure the jokes and taunts of friends and colleagues who comment about the "middle-age spread." The nurse helps the client to avoid the shock and surprise of these comments by assisting the client to prepare in advance a simple statement of explanation about the change in body contour.

The nurse refers the client for dietary counseling if the client is overweight. Dietary restrictions to modify body weight need to be closely supervised to prevent further compromise of overall renal function and general health.

Fluid Volume Excess

Planning: client goals. The goal for this nursing diagnosis is that the client will achieve control of blood pressure without edema and/or the worsening of renal function. The client's knowledge and understanding of the prescribed and recommended therapy are critical to achievement of this goal.

Interventions: nonsurgical management. Interventions for clients with fluid volume excess related to the effects of PKD include educational strategies for promotion of self-management techniques and understanding. Control of fluid volume in these clients is related to sodium retention and secondary fluid volume retention. In the early stages of the disease, regulation of blood pressure and fluid volume is primarily through restriction of excess dietary sodium intake, but fluid volume intake is not restricted. However, when the disease progresses to renal failure, oliguria usually requires restriction of fluid volume intake, in addition to sodium restriction.

Drug therapy. Medications prescribed for control of fluid volume excess include antihypertensive agents and diuretics. Antihypertensive agents include vasodilators, such as hydralazine (Apresoline), beta-blockers such as propranolol (Inderal), and centrally acting agents such as methyldopa (Aldomet). The reader is referred to Chapter 59 for an overview of antihypertensives used for clients with renal insufficiency. Mild diuretics may be used for persons with mild renal insufficiency. As renal function deteriorates, as measured by the 24-hour urine assay for creatinine clearance, more potent diuretics may be required. It is common to use an agent such as furosemide (Lasix), which acts in the loop of Henle, singly or in combination with an agent such as metolazone (Zaroxolyn), which enhances diuresis in persons with advanced renal insufficiency. The mechanism for this enhanced action is unknown. The nurse monitors all sources of fluid gain and loss, with particular attention to urinary output and daily weights. The nurse explains the relationship of blood volume and blood pressure, as well as the purpose and desired effects of the prescribed medications, to the client. The client or significant other should be taught how to measure and record blood pressure. In addition, the nurse assists the client in establishing a schedule for self-administering medications, blood pressure record-keeping, and monitoring of daily weights. The nurse helps the client and/or significant other to understand and recognize potential side effects of the specific medications prescribed. Written materials, such as medication teaching cards and booklets, should be made available to facilitate the client's understanding.

Diet therapy. A low-sodium diet is frequently prescribed to control the hypertension that accompanies PKD in the majority of people. Some clients may experience a salt-wasting phenomenon, however, and may not require a sodium-restricted diet. In addition, as renal insufficiency progresses, limitation of protein intake may be prescribed in an effort to retard the development of renal failure. The nurse assists the client and significant other to understand the recommended diet plan and offers supplemental information to clarify the rationale for the prescribed diet. The nurse works closely with the dietitian to ensure that adequate understanding by the client has occurred.

Prevention of complications. The nurse helps the client to gain understanding of the importance of self-monitoring practices, such as measurement of blood pressure and body temperature. With the increased fluid volume because of failure of adequate sodium and water excretion, there is considerable potential for long-term effects on the heart and on cardiovascular function. The control of high blood pressure, through self-monitoring, medications, and diet therapy, are important preventive measures. Long-term control of hypertension is important to preserve renal and cardiovascular function. The client who alertly detects cloudy or foul-smelling urine, measures temperature, and contacts a physician demonstrates actions that will help prevent further renal deterioration. These activities are useful in identifying problems such as hypertension and infection.

Anxiety; Ineffective (Individual and Family) Coping

Planning: client goals. The major goal for these nursing diagnoses is that the client will use effective methods of coping with the anxiety surrounding the diagnosis of a chronic disease.

Interventions: nonsurgical management. Interventions for the client with anxiety include counseling, support, and education about health maintenance activities. The development of a relationship that promotes communication and trust is an essential aspect of intervention. The nurse listens to what the client says and the tone and method of delivering those expressions. The nurse elicits information from the client about previous anxiety-provoking situations and methods used to cope. The nurse helps the client to identify internal strengths and external resources that may offer assistance with coping. The nurse does not judge or minimize the expressed concerns of the client or significant other. Rather, the nurse identifies opportunities to clarify and provide information to assist the client and significant other in attaining a realistic perspective based on factual information. The nurse provides written materials and referrals to nurse specialists, support groups, and other health care professionals.

■ Discharge Planning

Home Care Preparation

Client care needs at home relate to maximizing knowledge for self-care. Preservation or restoration of the ability to maintain optimal nutrition, elimination, activity, and mobility is the primary objective. If renal function has deteriorated and the client requires dialysis, a wide variety of needs related to vascular or peritoneal catheter access care, routines and requirements of outpatient therapy, emergency and disaster preparedness, dietary and fluid prescriptions, modification of medications, and many other aspects of care need to be discussed. See Chapter 59 for a discussion of home care for the client with renal failure.

Client/Family Education

The nurse instructs the client and family or significant other about measuring and monitoring blood pressure and body weight; dietary and fluid prescriptions; the use of antihypertensive and diuretic medications; methods of preventing constipation; and symptoms indicating the development of uremia.

The ability of the client and significant other to measure and record blood pressure accurately should be evaluated by using the client's own equipment. Periodic rechecking of accuracy by the client and/or significant other should be encouraged. In addition to the accurate measurement of blood pressure, the client and significant other should understand the relationship of blood pressure control and regulation to diet and medication therapy. The client is instructed to measure weight daily, using the same scale and wearing the same amount of clothing. Records of blood pressure measurements and weights should be available for discussion with the physician, nurse, or dietitian.

Dietary recommendations generally require limitation of foods that have a high sodium content. The client should know to avoid the addition of salt at the table or during food preparation. Foods with a high sodium content, such as processed foods, "fast" foods, potato chips, pretzels, pickles, ham, bacon, and sausage, should be consumed in moderation. The use of salt substitute agents, many of which are composed of potassium chloride, should be avoided; the labels of seasoning agents should be inspected carefully for sodium and potassium content. The nurse provides basic explanations about the prescribed dietary modifications. References and resource materials are used to reinforce the explanations. The nurse may also initiate a referral for nutritional counseling. As renal function decreases, the dietary protein allowance will also be decreased. The restriction of dietary protein helps to preserve renal function.

The nurse explains the importance of medications that are prescribed to control high blood pressure. Control of blood pressure is important to the overall health of the client, particularly in relationship to cardiovascular function. Because many antihypertensive agents have unpleasant side effects, the client should be encouraged to communicate freely and openly about all new and unusual physical or psychologic responses. Habits and patterns related to appetite, sleep, sexual function, daily activity, and emotional and cognitive processes may change as a result of antihypertensive side effects. Other agents may be prescribed to control blood pressure without bothersome side effects. Clients should know that other medications may be available for prescription when side effects result in avoidance of the medication.

The nurse teaches the client about methods to pre-vent the development of constipation. The nurse includes in the teaching plan information about adequate fluid intake, the role of dietary fiber, and the need for regular exercise to achieve regular bowel elimination. The nurse explains that as the polycystic kidneys increase in size, pressure on the large intestine may further impede normal peristalsis. Consequently, the client should know that these recommendations for bowel management may change. Further, when renal failure develops, the nurse assists the client in learning how the bowel management program needs to be modified. These modifications require consideration of the mode of dialysis selected and the need to avoid excessive fluid volume and hyperkalemia. The client may also be advised about the appropriate use of stool softeners and bulk agents, including the monitored use of laxatives, which may be necessary to prevent complications related to chronic constipation.

Finally, the nurse reviews the symptoms that are considered to be evidence of uremia or that suggest the need to initiate dialysis. Symptoms of nausea and vomiting, anorexia, hiccups, fatigue, lethargy, muscle cramps, and itching may be clinical evidence that the need for dialysis is developing. The nurse encourages the client and significant other to not deny the presence of these symptoms or rationalize their presence on the basis of some other explanation such as being caused by influenza. The nurse emphasizes the need to report these symptoms to the client's nephrologist for evaluation and further treatment as needed.

Psychosocial Preparation

Concerns related to future or current needs for dialysis and transplantation may be overwhelming, even though the client may have anticipated this outcome for years. The statement that one actually needs dialysis or transplantation creates a new reality that must be confronted. Thus, the process of adjustment begins anew. Referral to dialysis support groups may help the individual to cope effectively with this new challenge.

Health Care Resources

Local chapters of the National Kidney Foundation and the American Association of Kidney Patients may provide a resource for client support.

 ### Evaluation

The nurse evaluates the effectiveness of the interventions on the basis of the outcomes expected for the identified nursing diagnoses, which include that the client

1. Demonstrates the ability to measure blood pressure
2. Relates the significance of sodium intake, antihypertensive medications, and presence of edema to overall control of PKD

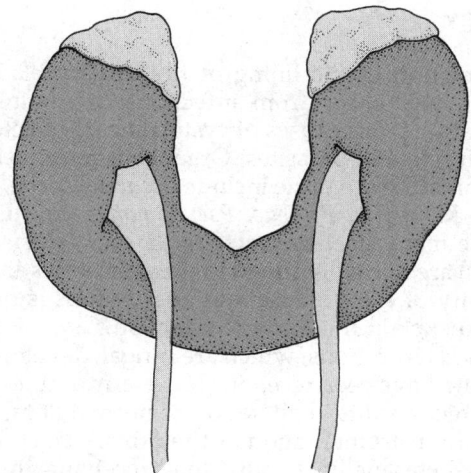

Figure 58–2

Horseshoe kidney: fusion of lower poles of both kidneys.

3. Describes methods of enhancing comfort
4. Relates strategies for effectively coping with anxiety, stress, and changes in body image
5. Describes methods of maintaining a regular pattern of bowel elimination
6. Modifies activity to ensure a balance of rest and exercise
7. Seeks appropriate medical assistance for the development of symptoms that may indicate the onset of uremia

HORSESHOE KIDNEY

A *horseshoe kidney* is a congenital deformity in the structural development of the kidney. During embryonic development of the kidneys, the renal masses fuse. The fusion usually occurs at the lower poles, and a single structure, shaped like a horseshoe, results (Fig. 58–2). Ureteral displacement and twisting may also occur and result in increased risk for infection and stones (Brenner & Rector, 1986). Therefore, the nurse instructs the client to increase fluid intake to 2 to 3 L/day. Kidney function is usually normal.

INFECTIOUS DISORDERS

Normally, the urinary system is a sterile body system in which a sterile body fluid (urine) is excreted. *Urinary tract infection* (UTI) is a commonly used phrase referring to infections in this sterile system. Infections within the urinary tract are described in reference to the primary structure or site of the infectious process (e.g., bladder, thus cystitis). More than 10^5 (100,000) organisms per milliliter are required to meet the definition of UTI, if the specimen is obtained by the clean catch technique.

A number of terms are used to describe infections of the urinary tract; these should be understood and used correctly. For acute infections in the lower urinary tract, terms include *urethritis*, *cystitis*, and *prostatitis*. For acute infections of the upper urinary tract, the correct term is *acute pyelonephritis*.

There is considerable debate about the importance of UTIs in terms of their potential to result in end-stage renal disease. Kunin (1985) described severe deterioration of renal function as rare without the presence of one or more predisposing factors such as anatomic abnormalities, pregnancy, obstruction, reflux, calculi, or diabetes mellitus. Increasing attention has been directed toward the significance of asymptomatic bacteriuria and the potential for increased susceptibility to symptomatic UTIs. Kidney, bladder, and prostate gland infections may produce similar symptoms. Therefore, identification of the site or locus of infection, as well as the specific bacterial species, is especially important for treatment and for maintenance of long-term health. In addition, interest is increasing in the role of an autoimmune response that may be responsible for the damage of pyelonephritis (Kunin, 1987).

CYSTITIS

OVERVIEW

Cystitis refers to an inflammation of the urinary bladder. More commonly, cystitis is the term used to refer to symptomatic lower UTIs caused by bacterial invasion. Other forms include noninfectious cystitis (caused by chemicals or radiation) and interstitial cystitis (an inflammatory process of unknown etiology).

Pathophysiology

The lining of the urinary bladder is composed of urothelial cells, which produce mucin, a substance that helps to maintain the integrity of the lining and to prevent cellular inflammation and damage. The usual acid pH of urine and the constant downward and outward flow of urine also contribute to the maintenance of mucosal integrity.

The anatomic configuration of the components of the urinary tract both prevent and potentially contribute to the development of UTIs. Urine is a sterile product resulting from ultrafiltration of blood in the glomeruli of the nephrons. As such, the urinary tract is considered to be a sterile body system; yet, the external opening via the urethra is a potential entry point for contaminating pathogens. In females, the urethra is only 1 to 1½ in (2.5 to 3.8 cm) long. In addition, the urethra is close to the vagina and the rectum. Each of these body orifices contains a normal flora of bacteria that may readily inoculate the urethra and bladder. In males, the usual length of the urethra is about 6 to 8 in (15 to 20 cm), and this length is believed to contribute to the rarity of UTIs in men. The frequent outward flow of urine through the length of the urethra is a constant and effective barrier to bacterial entry. Yet, the prostate gland, which encircles the urethra as it exits the urinary bladder, may serve as a reservoir of bacteria and contribute to bladder colonization and infection. Infections within the prostate gland are more common in older men, probably because of stasis of fluid caused by prostatic hypertrophy. In addition, their prostatic fluid is deficient in antibacterial characteristics.

The term cystitis is often used to refer to a symptomatic UTI. In addition, there may be the mistaken use of the term cystitis to describe a urethritis syndrome in which there are similar symptoms. The typical symptoms associated with cystitis are pain or burning with urination, frequency or urgency associated with the initiation of urination, or incontinence, with or without retention. In bacterial cystitis, bacteria are cultured from urine specimens. To further complicate matters, the client may have significant bacteriuria without symptoms (asymptomatic bacteriuria).

There is considerable discussion about the possibility of a relationship of cystitis (bladder infections) to the development of renal parenchymal damage, i.e., kidney disease and possible kidney failure. In persons with normal renal and genitourinary structure and function, i.e., without obstruction, stones, urinary reflux, neurogenic bladder, or diabetes mellitus, cystitis-induced renal failure is unlikely (Kunin, 1985).

A urine specimen obtained properly, without contamination, should contain less than 10,000 colony-forming units (CFU)/mL. Thus, colony counts of less than 10,000 CFU/mL are not considered to be significant. Significant bacteriuria is defined as more than 100,000 CFU/mL. However, urine *cultures* that demonstrate more than 10,000 CFU/mL are also considered to be significant because bacteria are in the process of multiplying. When another urine culture is obtained within 6 hours, bacterial multiplication is confirmed. Variable growth rates of bacterial species, alterations in urinary pH, and flow rate contribute to the variable multiplication rate. Alteration in urinary flow occurs in persons with reflux, a neurogenic bladder, or other conditions resulting in stasis of urine. These factors greatly increase the potential for growth of bacteria. One study (Stark & Maki, 1984) suggested that although this criterion for significant bacteriuria may apply to the uncatheterized population, for persons with indwelling catheters a lower level of colonization, i.e., less than 10^5 CFU/mL, may be significant and contribute to the high morbidity in nosocomial UTIs.

Etiology

Inflammation of the lining of the urinary bladder, or cystitis, may occur from infectious or noninfectious causes. Infectious causes of cystitis include bacteria, viruses, fungi, and parasites. Organisms most frequently contaminating the urine include *Escherichia coli, Enterococcus, Klebsiella, Proteus, Pseudomonas,* and *Candida.* Because many of these bacteria (*E. coli, Klebsiella,* and *Proteus*) are normally found in the gastrointestinal tract, proximity of the urethral and anal orifices is often offered to explain the route of infection.

Candida infections, which are fungal, develop in persons who have been receiving long-term antibiotic therapy, which results in alteration of normal flora, or who have had instrumentation of the urinary tract. Persons with diabetes mellitus, individuals receiving glucocorticosteroids or other immunosuppressive agents, or others with decreased resistance to infection are also at risk of developing *Candida* UTIs or bacteremia (Kunin, 1987).

Noninfectious cystitis may result from chemical exposure, such as to drugs, e.g., cyclophosphamide, or from radiation therapy. Immunologic responses, as seen with systemic lupus erythematosus, may also result in cystitis. In other cases, as in interstitial cystitis, the cause is generally unknown but may be an autoimmune response.

A number of hypotheses about the development of UTIs have been proposed over the years. These include postdefecation and/or postvoiding wiping habits in women, frequency and vigor of sexual intercourse, irritation from bubble bath, masturbation, and use of vaginal diaphragms. To date, studies are generally inconclusive or nonexistent for the implication of these factors. Pregnancy with increasing parity, diabetes mellitus, and aging are factors that are documented as contributing to the development of symptomatic UTIs. The use of indwelling urinary catheters is a major contributor to the development of nosocomial UTIs. For clients with acute retention, spinal cord injury, or a neurogenic bladder, intermittent catheterization is recommended (Kunin, 1987). Because of the potential of multiple contributing factors and the lack of confirmatory studies, it is unclear which specific factors contribute to the development of cystitis. The importance of recurrent infections, particularly in women, is another area of controversy that remains to be resolved. Some evidence is accumulating that women with recurrent infections may have increased morbidity, either because of the effects of the repeated infections or the residual scars that develop from the inflammation (Kunin, 1985). Similarly, there is increasing evidence that more women have had urinary reflux than previously believed.

In men, aging and the increased frequency of prostate disease over the age of 50 years contribute to the development of UTIs. Male clients rarely have cystitis unless there is prostate disease or a structural abnormality of the urinary tract. Normally, prostatic fluid has antibacterial qualities; this property decreases with aging. Instrumentation, e.g., a urinary catheter, contributes significantly to the development of bacteriuria, regardless of gender.

Incidence

Documentation of the frequency of occurrence of cystitis is not readily obtained. Some clinicians have suggested that women have an increased incidence of cystitis because of the shorter urethra and/or proximity of the urethra to the rectum and vagina. These hypotheses have not been supported by research; however, a shorter than normal urethra in females has been shown to increase the incidence of episodes of cystitis. In postmenopausal women, decreased estrogen production and resultant vaginal atrophy may contribute to urethritis and trigonitis. In addition, infections recur in the same individual.

PREVENTION

Prevention begins with the identification of persons at risk for the development of cystitis. Preventive interventions are recommended to eliminate risk factors, such as unnecessary instrumentation. Routine mass screening is not recommended. Populations that may be appropriately screened include hospitalized clients, pregnant women, diabetic individuals, and renal transplant recipients. It is imperative that any effort at prevention include attention to adequate treatment, follow-up, and early identification of recurrences or infections that are resistant to therapy. Because some of the frequently identified contributing factors are subject to much debate and there is a lack of confirmatory studies, educational efforts about avoidance techniques and/or behavioral changes may be counterproductive (Kunin, 1987). Common sense suggests that front-to-back wiping techniques by women may decrease the likelihood of developing infections and thus should be included in client education efforts. Similarly, in individuals who are prone to urethritis or UTIs, prevention of problems may be enhanced by the avoidance of known irritants, such as bubble bath and nylon undergarments. Inadequate hydration contributes to decreased flow of urine, and thus encouraging adequate fluid intake may assist in the prevention of UTIs, particularly in individuals at greatest risk. The Client/Family Education feature under Discharge Planning summarizes the measures for prevention of UTI.

For urinary catheter care, the Centers for Disease Control (CDC) has issued guidelines for the prevention of UTIs. Included among these guidelines are the following: (1) catheterize only when necessary, (2) use aseptic technique and sterile equipment, (3) maintain a closed system, (4) use an intermittent irrigation technique only when necessary, (5) emphasize hand washing and education of health care personnel. Some individuals or institutions may continue to use povidone-iodine (Betadine) or antibiotic ointments at the urethral meatus in persons with indwelling catheters. This practice has become outdated and is no longer recommended; studies have consistently demonstrated that these practices contribute to increased bacterial colonization and development of resistant organisms (Daifuku & Stamm, 1986).

COLLABORATIVE MANAGEMENT

 Assessment

History

The *age* and *sex* of the client are important factors to be identified when obtaining the history. In addition, the nurse inquires about the presence of known *risk factors* such as a history of prior UTIs as a child or an adult, other renal or urologic problems such as stones, and health problems such as diabetes mellitus.

When obtaining a history from a person presenting with symptoms of cystitis, the nurse considers the sensitivity of the client when discussing organs and functions associated with urination, bowel movements, and sexual functioning. The nurse begins to take the history by encouraging the client to explain the problem in his or her own words. By listening to the words and terms used to describe the nature of the problem, the nurse assesses the person's level of understanding about basic anatomy.

Physical Assessment: Clinical Manifestations

Specific information to be assessed includes the following: *pain or discomfort with urination, a feeling of urgency about the need to void, difficulty in initiating urination, feelings of incomplete bladder emptying, voiding in only small amounts, increased frequency of voiding,* or *complete inability to urinate.* Other information to be obtained includes any *change in urine color, clarity, or odor,* such as that occurring with the presence of *blood* or *mucus* in the urine, and the presence of *other abdominal or back discomfort.*

In the *elderly* client, the typical clinical manifestations are not usually present. The client, especially a female client, generally does not experience dysuria. *Confusion,* or increased confusion in the client who is already confused, may be the first indication of a UTI. Frequency or hesitancy usually accompanies this finding.

The nurse inspects the lower abdomen and palpates the urinary bladder to detect *distention.* In addition, the urethral meatus should be inspected to determine whether surrounding tissues are inflamed or whether any skin lesions are present. The nurse ensures that the privacy of the client is maintained through the use of drapes; the nurse also wears gloves.

For the male, the *prostate gland* should be palpated via rectal examination for size, alteration in contour, and any evidence of tenderness. The physician or advanced nurse practitioner performs this assessment.

Psychosocial Assessment

Female clients often have their first episode of cystitis in young adulthood. Commonly, the client is concerned with her developing sexual identity and may be beginning to be sexually active. Feelings of embarrassment and/or guilt about sexual activity may cause the client to delay seeking treatment. In addition, the client may have concerns that she has contracted a sexually transmitted disease.

In males, any alteration in the urinary tract results in concerns about sexual functioning. Regardless of age, all men who are sexually active are concerned that impotency will develop. The possibility of acquiring a sexually transmitted disease is also a concern for men with cystitis.

Laboratory Findings

The urinalysis, preferably obtained by the clean catch method, reveals the presence of bacteria and usually white blood cells. In addition, red blood cells may be present. A urine culture and sensitivity assay demonstrates the type of microorganism and the number of colonies present. A clean catch urine sample is preferred; if use of this method is not possible, it may be necessary to obtain the specimen via catheterization. To be classified as a UTI, the colony count must be higher than 100,000 colonies per high-power field. A colony count of less than 100,000 but more than 10,000 requires another specimen analysis. In addition, the white blood cell count may be elevated; the differential white blood cell count typically shows "a shift to the left," which indicates that the number of immature white cells is increasing in response to the infectious organisms. Consequently, the number of bands, or immature white cells, is elevated.

Radiographic Findings

The diagnosis of cystitis is usually based on the history, the clinical examination, and laboratory data. If urinary retention and obstruction to urinary outflow are detected, IVP, abdominal ultrasonography, or CT provides images to determine the site of obstruction.

Other Diagnostic Tests

Cystoscopy is often performed if there is urinary retention; frequently, the cystoscopic examination reveals bladder or urethral abnormalities that may be contributing to the development of the cystitis. Retrograde pyelography accompanies the cystoscopic examination; through the retrograde injection of contrast media into the urinary collecting system, outlines and images of the drainge tract may be obtained. Areas of obstruction or malformation are thus identifiable. If prostate enlargement is detected during the digital rectal examination, further definition of the problem is needed via cystoscopy.

 Analysis: Nursing Diagnosis

Analysis of assessment data typically results in the following nursing diagnoses.

Common Diagnoses

The client with cystitis usually has the following common diagnosis: pain related to inability to void, burning with urination, or bladder spasm.

Additional Diagnoses

In addition to the common diagnosis, some clients may also have

1. Altered thought processes related to the infectious process
2. Knowledge deficit related to methods of prevention and/or treatment protocols

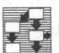 **Planning and Implementation**

The nursing care plan for the client with cystitis addresses the common nursing diagnosis. The reader is referred to later sections for discussion of nursing care of clients with urinary incontinence.

Pain

Planning: client goals. The goal for this nursing diagnosis is that the client will achieve a level of comfort that allows for uninterrupted rest and sleep and the ability to urinate without pain or burning.

Interventions. Nursing interventions to promote comfort include a variety of strategies such as chemical and physical measures and techniques to promote coping and understanding.

Nonsurgical management. Interventions for management of the discomfort accompanying cystitis include the use of medication and fluid administration. Local comfort measures to the perineal area may also provide relief.

Drug therapy. Medications prescribed to promote comfort in the client with cystitis include analgesics, urinary antiseptics such as nitrofurantoin (Furadantin, Macrodantin) and trimethoprim (Proloprim, Trimpex), and anticholinergics such as propantheline bromide

TABLE 58-1 Antiseptics Used in the Treatment of Cystitis

Drug	Usual Daily Dosage	Indications	Interventions	Rationales
Quinolones				
Nalidixic acid (NegGram)	1 g qid PO for 1-2 wk	Acute or chronic UTIs (especially gram-negative bacterial infections)	1. Use with caution in persons with decreased renal or liver function. 2. Ensure adequate fluid intake.	1. Drug is metabolized in the liver and is excreted via the kidneys. 2. Adequate fluids promote drug excretion.
Cinoxacin (Cinobac Pulvules)	1 g bid-qid PO for 1-2 wk	Acute or chronic UTIs		
Norfloxacin (Noroxin)	400 mg bid PO for 7-10 d	People allergic to penicillins, cephalosporins, and sulfonamides		
Methenamines				
Methenamine (Urised)	1 g qid PO	Chronic bacteriuria; not effective for urea-splitting bacteria	1. Maintain urinary pH at 5-5.5. 2. Avoid using with urine-alkalinizing agents. 3. Ensure adequate hydration.	1, 2. Drug is bactericidal only in acidic urine.
Methenamine mandelate (Mandelamine)	1 g qid PO			
Methenamine hippurate (Hiprex; Urex)	1 g bid PO			3. Adequate fluids promote drug excretion.
Nitrofurantoins				
Nitrofurantoin (Furadantin; Macrodantin)	50-100 mg qid PO	UTIs (acute or recurrent); not effective in persons with creatinine clearance less than 30-40 mL/min	1. Give with foods or milk. 2. Advise client of pending change in color of urine; urine will be brown or orange.	1. Absorption of drug is enhanced by food. 2. Drug is highly soluble in urine and results in color change.

(Pro-Banthine). The anticholinergic agents (antispasmodics) decrease bladder spasm and promote complete bladder emptying. Table 58-1 summarizes the drugs used in cystitis. Antibiotics are prescribed if there is a systemic infection, as evidenced by fever and/or increased serum white blood cell count. The nurse instructs the client about self-administration of medications. It is important to stress appropriate spacing throughout the day to promote maximal blood levels. The nurse also emphasizes that the entire prescription needs to be taken. If the medication will change the color of the urine, the nurse informs the client to expect this occurrence.

Diet therapy. Dietary intake should represent intake from all food groups and include an adequate number of calories for the increased metabolic processes associated with infection. Fluid intake needs to be at least 2 to 3 L/per day. This amount of fluid intake ensures adequate flushing of the collecting system but does not dilute the antibiotic levels within the serum excessively. Cranberry juice has been long believed to be useful in preventing infections of the urinary tract. Kunin (1987) reported studies demonstrating that large quantities are required and that the probable effect is from the increased fluid intake.

Other pain relief measures. A warm sitz bath may

provide comfort and some relief of local symptoms. The bath may be taken two or three times a day for 20 minutes.

Surgical management. Surgical interventions for clients with cystitis may include endourologic procedures for the management of retention if a bladder or urethral calculus is the cause. Preoperative and postoperative care of the client receiving cystoscopic examination is described in Chapter 57. During cystoscopic examination, stone manipulation or pulverization allows for removal of the obstruction.

■ Discharge Planning

Home Care Preparation

The client with cystitis, uncomplicated with problems such as prostatitis or acute urinary retention, usually does not require hospitalization. Preparation for self-management at home should include assurance of provision for activities of daily living (hygiene, grooming, dressing, rest and sleep, and elimination), nutrition, and exercise. The client should have a means of having prescriptions for medications filled. Transportation for follow-up appointments with the physician is crucial for completion of a successful course of therapy.

Client/Family Education

The nurse's assessment of the client's overall knowledge about factors contributing to the development of the cystitis provides a beginning from which further teaching interventions may be planned. The nurse assesses the client's level of understanding as provided from the client's description of the problem.

The nurse instructs the client and family or significant other about the need to complete the prescribed medication regimen; to consume a liberal fluid intake; to obtain adequate rest, sleep, and nutrition; to avoid known irritants; to practice proper hygiene; to keep follow-up appointments; and to seek prompt medical care if recurrences are suspected.

The prescribed medications usually include a urinary antiseptic and an antibiotic. The nurse explains the dosage schedule of the medications and emphasizes the need to establish a round-the-clock pattern to achieve adequate blood levels and the need to not skip doses. It is important to stress that the entire antibiotic prescription must be taken, even if symptoms subside, to prevent recurrent infections. The nurse offers techniques of remembering the medication schedule, such as the use of a daily calendar or the association of medications with usual activities such as mealtimes. The nurse explains that the color of the urine may change as a result of the effect of the urinary antiseptic prescribed. The accompanying Client/Family Education feature gives instructions for the prevention of primary and recurrent UTIs.

CLIENT/FAMILY EDUCATION ■ Prevention of Urinary Tract Infection

Instructions	Rationales
To Prevent Primary Infection	
1. "Drink 2 to 3 L of fluid every day."	1. To dilute and flush foreign substances, including microorganisms, from the urinary tract.
2. [For women] "Clean your perineum (the area between the legs) from front to back."	2. To prevent transfer of bacteria, especially *E. coli*, from the rectum to the urethra or vagina.
3. [For women] "Avoid irritating substances like bubble bath, nylon underwear, and scented toilet tissue. Wear cotton underwear."	3. To prevent inflammation, which promotes infection.
4. "If you experience burning when you urinate, if you have to urinate frequently, or if you find it difficult to begin urinating, notify your physician or other health care provider right away, especially if you have a chronic medical condition such as diabetes."	4. To prevent systemic infection through early detection of local infection.
5. "Empty your bladder as soon as you feel the urge to urinate."	5. To prevent urinary stasis or retention, which can lead to infection.
To Prevent Recurrent Infection	
1. "Take your medication even after the symptoms go away."	1. To maintain a therapeutic drug level.
2. "Schedule a follow-up appointment for 10–14 days after you finish taking your medication. At your follow-up visit, another urine sample will be taken for culture."	2. To ensure that infection has resolved.

Psychosocial Preparation

Fear and anxiety are common manifestations of the emotional concern experienced by clients with new or recurrent episodes of cystitis. Particularly for clients who have frequent recurrences, the concern associated with a sudden flare of cystitis may significantly alter life style, particularly with regard to planning for social and leisure time activities. Of course, clients may also associate symptoms of discomfort with sexual activities and experience feelings of guilt and embarrassment. The generally widespread belief, based on myth, that intercourse and cystitis (so-called honeymoon cystitis) are related has not been proved. Although a variety of factors seem to suggest a link between sexual intercourse and UTIs, it is difficult to design studies to yield conclusive data. Kunin (1987) suggested that other factors such as age, pregnancy, use of a diaphragm, and urethral or periurethral colonization with uropathogens may be most significant.

Health Care Resources

Educational materials about cystitis may be obtained from medical, health education, or community libraries that have special collections for clients with health-related concerns. In addition, the National Kidney Foundation chapters and affiliates have some basic pamphlets and brochures that explain the problem. The Interstitial Cystitis Foundation, located in Los Angeles, provides a newsletter and ongoing mailings of items of interest for clients with this type of cystitis.

 Evaluation

The nurse evaluates the effectiveness of the interventions on the basis of the outcomes expected for the identified nursing diagnoses, which include that the client

1. Describes methods of promoting comfort
2. Demonstrates understanding about the method of self-administration of medications
3. Identifies strategies of preventing reinfection or recurrence through liberal fluid intake, detection of symptoms, and prompt seeking of medical attention

URETHRITIS

Urethritis is an inflammation of the urethra. In males, urethritis presents with burning and/or difficulty with urination and usually a discharge from the urethral meatus of the penis. The most common cause of urethritis in males is gonorrhea. Nonspecific urethritis may be caused by *Ureaplasma, Chlamydia,* or *Trichomonas vaginalis.*

In females, urethritis mimics cystitis of bacterial ori-

gin. It is sometimes referred to as the *pyuria-dysuria syndrome,* the *frequency-dysuria syndrome, trigonitis syndrome,* or *urethral syndrome.* The client experiences painful urination, difficulty with urination, or both. Internal discomfort in the lower abdomen may also be present. The presence of pus cells (pyuria) without significant bacteriuria is an important diagnostic consideration because an infection may be present elsewhere in the urinary tract and the client may be asymptomatic. Low-level bacteriuria may result in the later development of significant bacteriuria, i.e., UTI. Therefore, the presence of pyuria-dysuria warrants a thorough evaluation for the long-term physical and mental health of the client. The role of irritation caused by sexual intercourse has been implicated but not confirmed (Kunin, 1987).

PYELONEPHRITIS

OVERVIEW

Pyelonephritis is a term that has evolved in meaning over recent years. Pyelonephritis has been used to refer to a bacterial infection of the renal pelvis. With improved diagnostic techniques and more precise understanding about the nature of the inflammatory response, pyelonephritis now refers to the active presence of microorganisms or the effects remaining from previous infections within the kidney.

Pathophysiology

The pelvis of the kidney is a basin of small capacity that collects urine produced in the nephrons. The flow of urine from the collecting ducts is into the minor and major calyces, which merge into the collecting basin known as the *renal pelvis.* In pyelonephritis, microorganisms enter the renal pelvis and activate the inflammatory response, which results in mobilization of white blood cells, specifically polymorphonuclear leukocytes and monocytes. As with any inflammatory response, local edema results. The tissue involved in this inflammatory response begins near the papillae but may extend into the renal cortex.

As the inflammatory process subsides, fibrosis or scar tissue develops. The calyces become blunted, and scars develop in the interstitial tissue. Repeated infectious episodes produce additional scar tissue. When fibrosis of this tissue occurs, tubular reabsorption and secretion become impaired. Consequently, renal function is diminished (Fig. 58–3).

Complications associated with acute pyelonephritis include renal abscess, perinephric abscess, and emphysematous pyelonephritis. *Emphysematous pyelonephritis* refers to the presence of gas in the collecting system, originating from gas-producing bacteria such as *E. coli* and *Pseudomonas.* It is commonly present in persons with diabetes mellitus and ureteral obstruction.

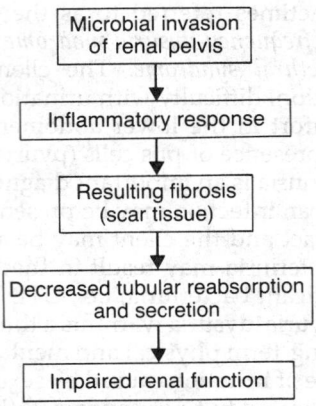

Figure 58–3

Pathophysiology of pyelonephritis.

Etiology/Incidence

Pyelonephritis is generally classified as acute or chronic. *Acute* pyelonephritis may occur as a result of bacterial contamination via the urethra or from instrumentation. *Chronic* pyelonephritis may be idiopathic or may occur in association with reflux or obstruction. The mechanism of reflux or obstruction leading to chronic pyelonephritis is often due to the presence of stones, obstruction, or neurogenic impairment involving the voiding mechanism. Pregnancy, diabetes mellitus, and chronic renal calculi pose an increased risk of developing acute and/or chronic pyelonephritis. For persons with diabetes mellitus, the development and progression of autonomic neuropathy and subsequent bladder atony promote an increased tendency to develop acute and/or chronic pyelonephritis. Similarly, in individuals with chronic stone disease, the calculi provide a site for ongoing infection and subsequent development of renal scarring in the pelves.

Introduction of microorganisms into the normally sterile urinary tract may be via the urethra (ascending route), after instrumentation, or by hematogenous spread. The ascending route of bacterial entry is commonly associated with the movement of bacteria that are found on the skin surface into the urethra and then their upward migration. An ability to adhere to the cells lining the urinary tract is one explanation offered for this ascending route of infection. The hematogenous spread of bacteria results in deposition of bacteria in the kidney and subsequently in the urine, even when the original site of entry of bacteria into the body is not related to the urinary tract. Thus, bacteremia may result in a UTI. Instrumentation of the urinary tract, especially indwelling urinary catheters, is a common cause of UTIs. Bacteria that cause pyelonephritis are most often one of the following: *E. coli, Klebsiella, Enterobacter, Pseudomonas, Serratia,* and *Morganella.* The exact incidence of pyelonephritis is not known.

PREVENTION

The prompt detection of acute pyelonephritis may prevent sequelae and progression into a chronic health problem. In persons at high risk for this development of pyelonephritis, prevention is directed toward the elimination of factors that may contribute to this development. Structural alterations of the urinary tract, the presence of foreign bodies, and mechanical drainage difficulties may be such factors and yet be difficult to modify. Persons with diabetes mellitus or chronic renal stone disease or pregnant individuals have particularly high risk factors for the development of pyelonephritis. Prevention is aimed at early detection, adequate treatment, and thorough follow-up to ensure eradication of the infection in a prompt and timely manner.

COLLABORATIVE MANAGEMENT

 Assessment

History

The history of the client with known or suspected pyelonephritis is extremely important. Recurrences of the disease are frequent and may result in deterioration of renal function. The nurse elicits whether *previous experiences* with pyelonephritis are known to the client, or whether similar symptoms have been present in the past. A history of *UTIs, diabetes mellitus, stone disease,* or *other structural or functional abnormalities of the genitourinary tract* should be elicited. For female clients, it is important to determine if UTIs have been associated with pregnancy.

Physical Assessment: Clinical Manifestations

The nurse assesses the client for information about the following: *flank or abdominal discomfort, general malaise or fatigue,* and *chills and fever.* The client may also have burning, urgency, or frequency of urination. The nurse inspects and percusses the right and left flanks of the client to assess for asymmetry and tenderness. The specific anatomic landmark to be assessed is known as the costovertebral angle (CVA); this area is the angle formed by the vertebral column and the lower portion of the rib cage. The upper thirds of the right and left kidneys lie beneath the lower portion of the rib cage.

The nurse inspects each CVA to determine the presence of any enlargement or asymmetry, edema, or erythema, which may be manifestations of inflammation. If there is no local tenderness to light palpation in either CVA, the nurse firmly percusses each area (see Chap. 57). A response of tenderness or discomfort is considered to be positive evidence of infection or inflammation.

Psychosocial Assessment

As with any disorder associated with the genitourinary tract, the client may have feelings of anxiety, embarrassment, or guilt. The nurse listens carefully to the client's descriptions of the nature of the problem for evidence of generalized anxiety or specific fears. In addition, the nurse helps the client to minimize any embarrassment during the assessment process. Feelings of guilt, often associated with sexual habits or practices, may be masked through denial mechanisms, such as delay in seeking treatment or vague, nonspecific responses to specific or direct questions. The nurse encourages the client to "tell his or her own story" in language that is familiar and comfortable. This approach is extremely valuable to the development of rapport and trust from which more in-depth interviewing may proceed.

Laboratory Findings

A urinalysis demonstrates the presence of white blood cells and bacteria; the urine should be analyzed by Gram's stain procedures to determine whether gram-positive or gram-negative organisms are responsible. The urine sample for culture and sensitivity testing, obtained by the clean catch method, provides specific information on the bacterial species and the susceptibility or resistance of the specific organism to various antibiotics. Blood cultures should also be examined for the presence of specific pathogenic microorganisms. Nonspecific serologic tests include the C-reactive protein and erythrocyte sedimentation rate, which are often elevated in the presence of infection.

In individuals with recurrent episodes of pyelonephritis or upper UTIs, more specific testing of bacterial antigens and antibodies may help to determine whether the same organism is responsible for the recurrent infections.

Radiographic Findings

Radiographic examination of the kidneys, ureters, and bladder (KUB) and IVP are procedures done initially to determine whether stones or obstructions are present. For many clients, a cystourethrogram is also indicated, at least for the first episode of pyelonephritis. These radiographic procedures define the structures of the urinary tract and identify any structural defects. Specific defects to be identified include (1) the presence of foreign bodies, such as stones; (2) obstruction to the outflow of urine, such as tumors or prostate enlargement; and (3) the reflux of urine, associated with incompetent ureterovesical valve closure.

Other Diagnostic Tests

Several other diagnostic tests are the topic of research investigations, including the examination of antibody-coated bacteria in urine, certain enzymes such as lactate dehydrogenase isoenzyme 5, and radionuclide scintillation methods (e.g., the gallium scan). The examination of urine for the presence of antibody-coated bacteria is not a useful index for therapy decisions; its primary value is apparently for identifying which individuals may need long-term antibiotic therapy. The presence of high-molecular-weight enzymes in the urine, such as lactate dehydrogenase isoenzyme 5, is also not specific; these enzymes are present with any process associated with renal tissue deterioration. The gallium scan is useful for identification of active pyelonephritis or abscesses in the perinephric region.

 ## Analysis: Nursing Diagnosis

The client with acute or chronic pyelonephritis may exhibit one or more of the following nursing diagnoses.

Common Diagnoses

The primary common diagnosis is pain (flank and abdominal) related to the inflammatory/infectious process.

Additional Diagnoses

In addition to the common nursing diagnosis, the client may also have the following:

1. Knowledge deficit related to medical diagnosis and therapy
2. Noncompliance with follow-up diagnostic and therapeutic procedures
3. Activity intolerance related to fatigue and debilitation associated with the infection
4. Fear related to the development of chronic renal failure as a result of recurrences of infection

 ## Planning and Implementation

The nursing care plan for the client with pyelonephritis addresses the common nursing diagnosis of pain.

Pain

Planning: client goals. The goal is that the client will state that he or she has achieved a state of comfort that allows for adequate rest, nutrition, and activity.

Interventions. Interventions for clients with pyelonephritis include nonsurgical and surgical methods. Surgical interventions may become necessary if structural defects require correction to restore proper drainage or if the infection cannot be controlled.

Nonsurgical management. Nonsurgical interventions include use of medications, diet and fluid therapy, and educational counseling to ensure understanding about the treatment recommendations.

Drug therapy. Analgesic and urinary antiseptic medications are prescribed to provide comfort; antibiotics are prescribed to definitively treat the infection, which is the source of the discomfort. Initially, the antibiotics prescribed are appropriate for a broad spectrum of bacteria, those that are most commonly responsible for pyelonephritic infections. When the reports of urine and blood culture sensitivity are obtained, antibiotic prescriptions may be altered (see Table 58–1).

Diet therapy. The nutritional intake for the client with pyelonephritis needs to represent an adequate number of calories and a balance from all food groups. The recommended amount of fluid intake is 2 to 3 L/day.

Surgical management. Surgical interventions for clients with pyelonephritis may become necessary to correct structural abnormalities that may be causing urinary reflux or obstruction of urinary outflow, or to eradicate the source of intractable infection. These surgical procedures may be one of the following: pyelolithotomy (removal of a stone from the renal pelvis), nephrectomy (removal of the kidney), ureteral diversion, or reimplantation of ureter to restore the bladder drainage mechanism. A pyelolithotomy is indicated for removal of a large calculus in the renal pelvis that contributes to blockage of urinary flow and to the development of infection. The availability and success of a variety of noninvasive techniques that result in stone crushing, such as extracorporeal shock wave lithotripsy and percutaneous ultrasonic pyelolithotomy, have decreased the frequency of surgical intervention. Surgical excision of an entire kidney is considered to be a last resort, reserved for situations in which all other measures to eradicate the infection have failed. For clients with incompetent ureterovesical valve closure or dilated ureters, ureteroplasty (repair or revision) or ureteral reimplantation (through another site in the posterior bladder wall) may be attempted to preserve renal function and eliminate infections.

Preoperative care includes the administration of antibiotics, usually intravenously, so that sterile blood culture results are achieved or adequate blood levels of antibiotics are present. Other aspects of preoperative care include client education about the nature and purpose of the proposed surgical intervention, the expected outcome, and expectations of how the client can participate in the process. The specific preoperative and postoperative nursing care for the client undergoing these surgical interventions is discussed later in this chapter.

■ Discharge Planning

Home Care Preparation

The client with pyelonephritis frequently requires hospitalization that may include medical or surgical in-

tervention or both. If no surgery is performed, the client's home care requirements may include assistance with self-care, nutrition, and medication administration. If surgical intervention is necessary, the client may require assistance with care of the incision, with personal activity, and with transportation for follow-up medical appointments.

Client/Family Education

After assessment of the client's and family's understanding of pyelonephritis and the suggested treatment, the nurse instructs the client and family about medication administration (purpose, timing, frequency, duration, and possible side effects); the role of nutrition and adequate fluid intake; the need for a balance between rest and activity, including any limitations after surgical intervention; and the symptoms of disease recurrence.

The nurse advises the client about the need to take the complete prescription of antibiotics. Also, the nurse encourages the client to report any side effects or unusual symptoms to the prescribing physician rather than suspend taking the prescribed medications. The nurse refers the client and family for nutritional counseling as needed, because many clients have special nutritional requirements, such as those caused by diabetes mellitus or pregnancy.

Psychosocial Preparation

Pyelonephritis, whether acute or chronic, provokes fear and anxiety in the client and family. The severity of the acute process and its potential for development into a chronic process are quite frightening. Both the client and the family require emotional reassurance that treatment and attention to preventive measures are important and can be accomplished.

Health Care Resources

The client may need a community health nurse for a short time to help at home with administration of medications or nutrition. Housekeeping services may also be of assistance while the client is regaining strength.

Evaluation

The nurse evaluates the effectiveness of the interventions on the basis of the outcomes expected for the identified nursing diagnoses, which include that the client

1. Demonstrates methods of enhancing comfort
2. Describes the role of antibiotics and the method of self-administration of medications to promote eradication of bacteria
3. Explains and offers techniques to be used to ensure that adequate nutrition and fluids are obtained
4. Describes the plan for posttreatment follow-up, including knowledge of the symptoms of recurrence

RENAL ABSCESS

An *abscess* is a collection of fluid and cells resulting from the inflammatory response to bacteria. An abscess may occur within the renal parenchyma (renal abscess), in the region of the renal and Gerota's fascia (perinephric abscess), or in the flank region. An abscess should be suspected when fever and symptoms are not relieved promptly in response to antibiotic therapy. Diagnosis of a renal or perirenal abscess is readily accomplished via ultrasonography or CT. Arteriography and radionuclide scintillation methods (e.g., gallium scan) may also be diagnostic. Symptoms of a renal abscess include fever, flank pain, and general malaise. Local edema may be observed. Drainage procedures, by surgical incision or needle aspiration, are often necessary. In addition, appropriate broad-spectrum antibiotics are prescribed.

RENAL TUBERCULOSIS

Tuberculosis of the kidney is sometimes referred to as *granulomatous nephritis*. After invasion by *Mycobacterium tuberculosis,* usually by a blood-borne route, an inflammatory response is activated and results in formation of scar tissue (granuloma) that replaces renal parenchyma. Clinically, clients may have urinary frequency, dysuria, hypertension, hematuria and/or proteinuria, and renal colic. Skin test or chest x-ray film evidence of tuberculosis may not be present. In 1982, the CDC reported that tuberculosis of the genitourinary tract involved 2.3% of the 25,520 newly reported cases of tuberculosis. Treatment of renal tuberculosis includes chemotherapy and surgical excision of diseased tissue. As with treatment of pulmonary tuberculosis, there is debate about short-course versus long-course therapy.

Individuals with current or previous pulmonary tuberculosis who develop symptoms of unexplained fever, hematuria, and sterile pyuria are at high risk for the presence of renal tuberculosis. The diagnosis is made through urine culture of three clean catch, first-morning specimens (Kunin, 1987). Other genitourinary sites for tuberculosis include the prostate, epididymis, ureters, testes, bladder, and seminal vesicles.

URINARY INCONTINENCE

OVERVIEW

Incontinence of urine can result from a multitude of factors, including the aging process. Incontinence is one of the most disturbing problems of the urinary system because it may cause social isolation and other life style changes. Incontinence is a significant problem for family caregivers and may cause them to seek alternative care arrangements for the client, such as a long-term care setting or a nursing home. Chronic incontinence may also be a costly problem for the health care industry because maintaining skin integrity is difficult. Even with increasingly sophisticated diagnostic and treatment methods, long-term management of the client with incontinence is a tremendous nursing challenge.

Pathophysiology

The pathophysiology of urinary incontinence is complex. Yet, there is a simple approach to understanding the various possibilities. Problems exist when the bladder (site of storage) fails to contract at the appropriate time or when it contracts inappropriately. Similarly, the urethra (site of outlet) may open or close inappropriately.

In males, urinary continence is achieved through the combined effects of the smooth muscle fibers of the bladder (the detrusor muscle), the smooth muscle fibers of the prostatic urethra, and the striated muscle fibers of the external sphincter. In females, urinary continence is related to the effects of the pelvic, bladder, and urethral musculature, the integrity of the structural components of the genitourinary tract, and integrated neuromuscular control. The parasympathetic nerves innervate the bladder, the bladder neck is supplied by the sympathetic nerves, and the urethral sphincters are supplied by the somatic nerves. The voluntary containment of urine is a learned response and is controlled by the cerebral cortex and brain stem.

In general, loss of urinary continence is the result of bladder pressure exceeding urethral resistance. Various mechanisms may result in this situation. Consequently, the problem of urinary incontinence is categorized into several types on the basis of the pathophysiologic mechanism involved. These general types of incontinence include stress incontinence, urge incontinence, overflow incontinence, functional incontinence, and total incontinence. The causes of the five types of urinary incontinence are summarized in the accompanying Key Features of Disease.

Stress incontinence occurs when the resistance of the urethra is overcome by the pressure in the bladder. The problem of stress incontinence occurs because of the weakness of the urethra and surrounding muscles and tissues, not the bladder. Typically, the client is in an upright position and is involved in an activity that produces coughing, sneezing, or laughing, which results in an increase in intra-abdominal pressure sufficient to overcome the weakened resistance of the urethra and surrounding muscles. It is also a common occurrence in females who have had vaginal deliveries or who are postmenopausal. Women who are nulliparous may also have stress incontinence, possibly because of tissue changes associated with aging and/or hormonal changes of menopause.

Changes in the urethrovesical angle influence the development of stress incontinence. The urethrovesical angle is normally 90 degrees, so that the urethra exits in a straight line from the middle portion of the base of the

KEY FEATURES OF DISEASE ■ **Differential Features of the Five Types of Urinary Incontinence**

Type of Incontinence	Cause	Associated Factors
Stress	Weakness of urethra and/or surrounding muscles and tissues Alteration in urethrovesical angle	Laughing Coughing Sneezing Obesity Multiple pregnancies Estrogen level decreases
Urge	Hypertonic bladder with stimulation of detrusor muscle	Bladder stones UTIs Spinal cord lesions Emotional stress
Overflow (paradoxical)	Bladder pressure exceeds urethral resistance	Bladder overfilling Autonomic neuropathies (e.g., of diabetes mellitus) Bladder neck obstruction (e.g., by fecal impaction or benign prostatic hypertrophy)
Functional	Physical and environmental factors Psychologic causes	Lack of access to, availability of, or assistance in reaching toilet facilities Depression and regression
Total	Neurologic disorders	Multiple sclerosis Parkinson's disease Cerebrovascular accident (stroke)

urinary bladder. Therefore, the intra-abdominal pressure is distributed equally over both structures, the bladder and the urethra. Continence is maintained because urethral resistance and bladder pressure are balanced. When the urethra exits from the *posterior* wall of the bladder, intra-abdominal forces are applied directly on the urinary bladder. Consequently, the bladder pressure exceeds the urethral resistance.

Factors that contribute to the development of stress incontinence include abdominal muscle wall weakness, increased intra-abdominal pressure, a short urethra, or general loss of abdominal muscle or perineal muscle tone. Abdominal muscle wall weakness may develop from multiple pregnancies, aging, a history of surgical procedures, and obesity. Increased intra-abdominal pressure occurs with laughing, coughing or sneezing, obesity, excess abdominal fluid, or tumors. Menopause and surgically induced estrogen deficiency seem to promote stress incontinence because of the loss of tissue turgor and tone that is associated with lower estrogen levels.

Urge incontinence involves a strong feeling of the need to urinate. It is commonly associated with a hypertonic bladder and occurs because of detrusor muscle stimulation. The detrusor muscle is the smooth muscle in the urinary bladder that relaxes during bladder filling. When the detrusor muscle is stimulated through the sacral spinal S-2, S-3, and S-4 segments or local irritation, contraction occurs and urination results. Bladder irritation may be caused by stones, infection, spinal cord lesions, or other factors. This sudden contraction may be also associated with psychologic causes.

Overflow incontinence occurs when bladder pressure exceeds urethral resistance, usually because of overfilling of the bladder. It is sometimes referred to as *paradoxical incontinence*. Sphincter integrity may be intermittently returned as the overflow of urine restores balance. Urinary retention with overflow is associated with neuropathy or bladder neck obstruction. The autonomic neuropathy of diabetes mellitus, spinal cord injuries involving defects of the lower motor neurons of S-2, S-3, or S-4, or postsurgical sphincter neurologic deficits may result in overflow incontinence. Obstruction of the bladder neck may occur as a result of benign prostatic hypertrophy or fecal impaction. Clients who are unable to perceive bladder filling or to respond to a full bladder experience overflow incontinence.

Functional incontinence refers to incontinence resulting from physical, environmental, or psychologic causes. These problems may include difficulty in reaching or lack of adequate assistance in getting to toilet facilities, as well as depression or regression. Increased assistance by caregivers, attention to environmental constraints such as adequate privacy, psychotherapy, and/or use of medications may help.

Total incontinence occurs as the result of neurologic disease with dysfunction of the nerves controlling the urinary bladder. The degenerative neurologic diseases, such as multiple sclerosis, Alzheimer's disease, and Parkinson's disease, or cerebrovascular accidents may also result in total incontinence.

Etiology

The causes of urinary incontinence are multiple, and it is rarely possible to identify a single cause in one client. Incontinence may have reversible or nonreversible etiologies. Reversible causes are correctable; nonreversible causes are permanent but may be improved with treatment. The basis for the incontinence may also be considered organic or functional.

Reversible causes of urinary incontinence include such conditions as symptomatic infections; fecal impaction; medications such as sedatives, anticholinergics, diuretics, and adrenergic agents; acute confusion; vaginal and urethral atrophy in women; prostatic enlargement; and maladaptive emotional responses.

Nonreversible organic causes of urinary incontinence include congenital defects, traumatic or surgical effects, and a neurogenic bladder, as well as those resulting in stress incontinence, urge incontinence, and overflow incontinence. Psychologic problems such as depression, regression, or other emotional responses may also result in urinary incontinence. Urinary incontinence may result from structural or functional defects of the bladder or the sphincters. In addition, injuries of the spinal cord, brain stem, or cerebral cortex may result in urinary incontinence (see Chap. 22 for a discussion of incontinence in clients with spinal cord and head injuries).

Congenital defects resulting in urinary incontinence include exstrophy of the bladder and spina bifida. These problems are identified in infancy, and corrective surgical interventions are usually initiated.

Surgical and traumatic causes of urinary incontinence typically involve procedures or events that necessitate surgical interventions in the lower pelvic structures, areas that are richly supplied by complex nerve pathways. Radical urologic and gynecologic procedures associated with prostate or pelvic malignancies may result in postsurgical urinary incontinence. Trauma in which there is injury to the sacral segments (S2-4) of the spinal cord also results in problems with continence. These problems may be characterized as resulting from failure of the bladder to contract when appropriate.

Inappropriate bladder contraction may result from disorders of the brain and nervous system, and bladder irritation from chronic infection, stones, chemotherapy, or radiation therapy may also cause urinary incontinence. Failure of bladder contraction accompanies the autonomic neuropathy associated with diabetes mellitus and syphilis.

Incontinence is typically associated with the aging process. Although many elderly persons experience urinary incontinence, numerous factors other than age contribute to this problem. Factors contributing to urinary incontinence in the elderly are given in the accompanying Key Features of Disease. An elderly individual may have decreased mobility from disease, neurologic dysfunction, or musculoskeletal degeneration. In the hospital setting, the older client is placed in bed and may be restrained with a Posey vest, which further limits mobility.

Multiple medications can contribute to changes in mental status or mobility in the elderly. Vision and hearing impairments may also prevent the client from locating a call bell to notify the nurse that he or she needs to void. The nurse assesses for these factors and minimizes them if possible to prevent urinary incontinence.

KEY FEATURES OF DISEASE ■ Factors Contributing to Urinary Incontinence in the Elderly*

Medications

Central nervous system depressants, such as narcotic analgesics, decrease level of consciousness and the urge to void.
Diuretics cause frequent voiding, often of large amounts of urine.

Disease

Cerebrovascular accidents and other neurologic disorders decrease mobility, sensation, and/or cognition.
Arthritis decreases mobility and causes pain.
Parkinson's disease causes muscle rigidity and an inability to initiate movement.

Depression

Depression decreases energy that is necessary to maintain continence.

Inadequate Resources

Products that help clients manage incontinence are often costly.
No one may be available to assist the client to the bathroom or help with incontinence products.

*These factors are in addition to the physiologic changes of aging given in Chapter 57.

Incidence

Urinary incontinence affects millions of people in the United States. Exact figures are not known, but estimates consistently are reported that suggest urinary incontinence to be a significant problem. For individuals in nursing homes or other long-term care institutions, the incidence of incontinence of urine is estimated at 50% or higher. For noninstitutionalized persons, urinary incontinence is estimated to be present in 5% to 15% of the population. Urinary incontinence occurs more frequently in women than in men and is not necessarily associated with the aging process.

Incontinence in women may occur after one or more pregnancies. In nulliparous women who do not have other risk factors for the development of incontinence, problems usually occur after the onset of menopause, presumably because of estrogen deficiency. Obesity, particularly in women, contributes to the development of incontinence. Males rarely experience urinary incontinence unless there is prostate disease or spinal cord injury.

PREVENTION

The prevention of urinary incontinence may be influenced by the elimination of known risk factors. Achievement or maintenance of an ideal body weight by obese individuals may assist in preventing urinary incontinence. The use of pelvic exercises (e.g., the Kegel exercises, which are explained later) by postpartum women may prevent later problems. Appropriate and complete treatment of bladder infections, as well as avoidance of common bladder irritants such as caffeine and alcohol, may also prevent incontinence.

COLLABORATIVE MANAGEMENT

 Assessment

History

The nurse obtains from the client information about the nature of the onset and circumstances surrounding the urinary incontinence. The specific information to be obtained includes *sex, age, voiding patterns and changes* (e.g., decreases in quantity or increases in frequency), *whether incontinence occurs during sleep or intermittently throughout the day, whether the onset is recent or long ago, contributing factors* (e.g., coughing, sneezing), *perceptions of bladder fullness, presence of warning signals* (e.g., bladder spasm), *history of pregnancies or surgical procedures, menstrual pattern versus menopause, medication history* (including prescription and over-the-counter agents), and *stresses or concerns associated with work, family, or financial affairs.*

Other significant information may be related to *previous or concurrent health problems,* such as past urologic surgical procedures or urologic or spinal cord trauma, a history of diabetes mellitus, or a neurologic disease process such as Parkinson's disease, Alzheimer's disease, or multiple sclerosis.

Physical Assessment: Clinical Manifestations

The nurse assesses the urinary bladder for evidence of distention or discomfort. When the nurse detects a *distended bladder,* percussion produces a tympanic sound. The nurse gently palpates the distended bladder to determine whether tenderness is increased or whether loss of urine occurs. If the client has a full bladder and can stand, the nurse requests that he or she induce straining by coughing or bearing down while standing.

For female clients, the nurse inspects the external genitalia to determine whether there is apparent *urethral or uterine prolapse* or *cystocele.* The nurse describes the color, consistency, and odor of any secretions from the genitourinary orifices. In males, the nurse also inspects the urethral meatus for the presence of any *discharge,* noting the color or other characteristics.

The specially skilled nurse or physician performs a digital rectal examination of both male and female clients. The technique of digital rectal examination may provide information about the integrity of the *nerve supply* to the bladder. The nurse determines if there is tactile sensation in the anorectal area by noting whether the rectal sphincter is relaxed or contracted on digital insertion. Positive tactile sensation and a rectal sphincter that contracts suggest that the nerve supply to the bladder is intact because the nerve supply of both areas is similar. The nurse also notes the presence of a fecal impaction, as well as whether the male has prostate enlargement.

Psychosocial Assessment

The nurse proceeds gently in conducting the history and physical and psychosocial assessment of the client with urinary incontinence. Often, the client experiences embarrassment in discussing this problem. Incontinence often jeopardizes personal self-concept, body image, and self-esteem, as well as relationships with significant others. Urinary incontinence may alter sexual relationships and sexual expression.

Laboratory Findings

The possibility of an associated UTI should be assessed by urinalysis. A urinalysis that shows more than one or two red or white blood cells per high-power field or the presence of bacteria indicates a potential infection. A urine culture result is positive if the colony count is 100,000 CFU/mL. A count of 10,000 CFU/mL suggests that a urine culture that should be repeated at least twice to confirm that an acute infectious process is not in progress.

Analysis: Nursing Diagnosis

The nurse carefully analyzes the assessment data to make the appropriate nursing diagnosis, which include the following.

Common Diagnoses

The common diagnoses for the client with incontinence include the following (because there are multiple possible etiologic factors, they are not listed):

1. Stress incontinence
2. Urge incontinence
3. Reflex incontinence
4. Total incontinence

Additional Diagnoses

In addition to the common diagnoses, the client may also have the following:

1. Social isolation related to fear of embarrassment
2. Potential impaired skin integrity related to frequent contact with urine
3. Body image disturbance related to odor, need to alter clothing selections, or need to wear continence briefs or supplies
4. Functional incontinence related to physical, environmental, or psychologic factors

 ## Planning and Implementation

The nursing care plan for the client with urinary incontinence addresses the common nursing diagnoses. The additional diagnoses may be avoided if interventions for the common diagnoses are successful.

Stress Incontinence

Planning: client goals. The goal is that the client will have a reduction in stress incontinence.

Interventions. Interventions for clients with urinary incontinence include education, exercise, medications, protective or collection devices, and surgery.

Nonsurgical management. Most interventions for incontinence involve a significant amount of client participation. In addition, the ongoing availability of a nurse to provide encouragement, clarification, and support is extremely valuable for maximizing the effects of drugs, exercise, and other interventions.

Drug therapy. Prescription of medications for stress incontinence is based on an understanding of the pathophysiology of stress incontinence and an application of the pharmacologic properties of the agents. Because the problem in stress incontinence is bladder pressure ex-

ceeding urethral resistance, medications may be prescribed to increase the resistance of the urethra. Examples include ephedrine sulfate (Efedron), which is an adrenergic agent, and amitriptyline hydrochloride (Elavil), which is a tricyclic antidepressant, each of which stimulates urethral sphincter resistance. Beta-adrenergic blocking agents, such as propranolol hydrochloride (Inderal), increase outlet resistance. These medications can have potent effects on the cardiovascular system and thus must be used cautiously, especially in elderly clients.

Diet therapy. A dietary plan to encourage weight reduction is indicated to assist obese clients with stress incontinence, which is aggravated by increased abdominal pressure from obesity. Alcohol and caffeine are bladder stimulants and should be avoided. The nurse provides support for nutritional counseling and may refer the client to nutritional specialists or dietitians.

Exercise therapy. Exercise therapy for female clients with stress incontinence is designed to strengthen the muscles of the pelvic floor (circumvaginal muscles). This exercise, known as circumvaginal muscle or Kegel exercise, encourages systematic contraction of these muscles and requires regular practice and implementation. The muscles are strengthened by these frequent and repeated contractions. The muscles are held in contraction for 3 seconds and then released for 3 seconds. The exercise (10 contractions per minute) is repeated several times a day. The goal is to strive for 20 contractions per minute. Determining whether the exercise is being practiced effectively is difficult. Consequently, a device has been designed to assist individuals in learning to correctly implement the technique through the use of a perineometer and pelvic floor stimulator. The client inserts an intravaginal balloon, which is inflated with a hand-controlled inflation pump. To monitor the pelvic muscle contractions, the client observes the pressure gauge to note the level and effectiveness of the contractions. Special instruction in the correct use of the instrument is required and is available through incontinence clinics. Nursing research is beginning to examine the best procedure for and effectiveness of exercise therapy (see the accompanying Nursing Research feature).

Other therapy. Behavior modification, psychotherapy, and electrical devices for inhibition of bladder contraction may be of assistance.

Surgical management. Stress incontinence may be surgically corrected in certain situations. The surgical procedures are used for women and are designed to (1) restore the normal urethrovesical angle (Pereyra's procedure, Marshall-Marchetti-Krantz operation) or (2) increase the length of the urethra (anterior urethropexy). For both men and women, stress incontinence may be treated by the implantation of an artificial urinary sphincter.

Preoperative care. The nurse prepares the client for surgical intervention by providing instruction and clarification about events surrounding the surgery.

Postoperative care. After surgery, the nurse assesses

NURSING RESEARCH

How Effective Are Circumvaginal Exercise Devices and Regimens?

Dougherty, M., Bishop, K., Mooney, R., & Gimotty, P. (1989). The effect of circumvaginal muscle (CVM) exercise. *Nursing Research, 38*, 331–334.

CVM exercise has been widely recommended to decrease urinary incontinence in women. This study examined the effects of CVM exercise with an intravaginal resistance device, exercise without the device, and the use of the device without exercise. The researchers found that there was a significant difference among the groups, but a large variance was demonstrated.

Critique. Incontinence is generally more frequently associated with the older woman than the young woman. For this study, the researchers used 48 healthy women of reproductive age. The women were compliant with the exercise regimen. In view of the selected sample, the findings cannot be generalized to any other population, especially elderly women.

Possible nursing implications. The researchers posed questions that need to be considered when the nurse is educating a client in the technique of CVM exercise. There is no standard prescription for the number of repetitions and frequency of the exercise, and no widely accepted method to ensure consistency of muscle contractions. More research in the area is needed to validate the need and most effective technique for the use of CVM exercise. Further studies need to be conducted to validate the effectiveness of exercise with and without the resistance device.

and intervenes with the client to prevent and/or detect complications. An indwelling urinary catheter is placed during surgery. The catheter is secured with adhesive tape to prevent unnecessary movement or traction on the bladder neck (Marshall et al., 1986). The reader is referred to Chapters 18 through 20 for a thorough discussion of preoperative and postoperative care after general surgery.

Urge Incontinence

Planning: client goals. The goal is that the client will use techniques to prevent or manage urge incontinence.

Interventions: nonsurgical management. Medications, bladder training, and external devices (see under the later heading Total Incontinence) are the primary interventions available for management of urge incontinence.

Drug therapy. Medications that are prescribed for urge incontinence are designed to control the hypertonic bladder that contracts involuntarily as a result of irritant stimulation. Categories of medications that may yield this effect include anticholinergic agents, such as oxy-

butynin chloride (Ditropan). These agents have the effect of inhibiting the cholinergic fibers that stimulate bladder contraction. Anticholinergic agents are contraindicated in individuals with glaucoma, gastric atony, or urinary retention because these conditions worsen with further nerve inhibition. Other agents that are prescribed for urge incontinence include smooth muscle relaxants, such as flavoxate (Urispas), and calcium channel blockers, such as verapamil hydrochloride (Calan). Antihistamine combinations, such as Ornade, are effective in some individuals, but their exact mechanism of action is unknown.

Bladder training. Bladder training programs may be useful in treating urge incontinence in which typically the bladder volume is small and cerebral awareness is intact. Clients with urge incontinence lack either the time to respond to the urge or the warning of the need to void. By establishing a preset pattern for voiding, such as every half-hour or every hour initially, the bladder capacity may be increased. Over time, the interval between voidings is lengthened, and incontinence is avoided.

Reflex Incontinence

Planning: client goals. The goal for the client with overflow incontinence is that the client will achieve continence.

Interventions. Interventions for the client with overflow incontinence caused by obstruction of the bladder outlet may include surgery to relieve the obstruction. For overflow incontinence related to detrusor muscle inadequacy, the most effective method of treatment is intermittent catheterization. Medications have not generally been proved effective (Gray & Dougherty, 1987).

Drug therapy. Medications prescribed for the treatment of overflow incontinence may include cholinergics, such as bethanechol chloride (Urecholine), which increase bladder pressure, and/or alpha-adrenergic blocking agents, which decrease urethral resistance.

Bladder training. The Credé method, the Valsalva maneuver, and double-voiding techniques assist in promoting bladder contraction. In the Credé method, the client is instructed in external compression of the urinary bladder, which manually assists in bladder emptying. The Valsalva maneuver uses breathing techniques to increase intrathoracic and intra-abdominal pressure, which then is directed toward the bladder during exhalation. With the technique of double voiding, the client empties the bladder and then consciously attempts a second bladder emptying.

Total Incontinence

Planning: client goals. The goal is that the client will use methods of urine containment or collection that will ensure dryness.

Interventions: nonsurgical management. Nonsurgical interventions include the use of external devices, incontinence pads and briefs, and urinary catheters.

Devices. Applied devices include intravaginal devices for women and urethral clamps for men. The intravaginal devices include the pessary, which must be removed before voiding, and the balloon, which is deflated before voiding. The *pessary* is a device that provides support to the uterus and helps to maintain a correct angle of urethral exit from the bladder (see Chap. 54 for further discussion of pessaries). For men, the penile clamp is applied externally to compress the urethra and to prevent the leakage of urine. See also the discussion of artificial sphincters in Chapter 55.

Incontinence pads and briefs. Incontinence pads and briefs are designed to collect urine and keep the client's skin and clothing dry. A variety of types and sizes of pads are available. Briefs include those with elastic legs (e.g., Attends) and those without elastic legs (e.g., Bard and Curity). Some absorbent liners are worn inside a brief or panty; these liners are either flat or contoured (e.g., Aqua-Gel). There are also undergarments with their own straps that may be worn directly under the clothing (e.g., Depend). A major concern with the use of incontinence pads is the risk of development of skin breakdown.

Urinary catheters. Use of a urinary catheter for the control of incontinence may involve intermittent catheterization or indwelling catheter placement. The technique of intermittent self-catheterization is preferable because there is decreased likelihood of infection. Techniques of self-catheterization are well established and can be learned fairly easily. Indwelling urinary catheters should be used minimally, temporarily, and only when all other alternatives have been tried and have been unsuccessful. An indwelling urinary catheter is appropriate for clients with skin breakdown who need a dry environment for healing, clients who are terminally ill and deserve comfort, and clients who are acutely or critically ill and need careful measurement of urinary output.

■ Discharge Planning

Discharge planning for the client with urinary incontinence must take into consideration the personal, physical, emotional, and social resources of the client. The personal resources for self-care of particular significance include limitations in mobility, vision, and/or manual dexterity. The nurse considers who the primary caregiver will be and what circumstances or factors exist in the environment that will influence the effectiveness of the plan.

Home Care Preparation

If the client is to be discharged to his or her own home, the environment is assessed for barriers that im-

pede access to the toileting facilities. In addition, environmental hazards that might slow walking or contribute to injury should be eliminated, such as small area rugs (throw rugs), tables or chairs with legs that extend into the walking area and that promote tripping, and waxed or polished floors that are slippery. If stairs are necessary for access to a bathroom, hand railings should be installed and stairs should be kept free from peripheral items. Toilet seat extenders may help to provide the appropriate level of seating so that maximal abdominal pressure may be applied to encourage voiding. Portable commodes may be obtained for homes in which ambulatory access to toilets is impractical or impossible. Physical and occupational therapists are valuable adjunctive resources for assisting with home care preparation.

Client/Family Education

The nurse teaches the client and family about the cause and treatment options available for the management of the identified type of urinary incontinence. The teaching plan should address the prescribed medications (purpose, dosage, method and route of administration, and expected and potential side effects). The nurse teaches the client and family about the importance of weight reduction and dietary modification to assist with interventions to control urinary incontinence. Because many clients seek to control incontinence by limiting fluid intake, the nurse emphasizes the importance of adequate fluid intake to overall kidney and health maintenance. The nurse also explains, demonstrates when possible, and obtains a return demonstration of the indicated exercises. When external devices or incontinence pads are needed, the nurse describes the possible options, discusses advantages and disadvantages of each, and helps the client to make a selection that considers life style and resources. For clients who will use intermittent catheterization, the nurse demonstrates the technique to the client and/or caregiver; return demonstrations are necessary to evaluate that the technique is correct.

Psychosocial Preparation

The personal embarrassment that is experienced by the incontinent individual is potentially devastating in terms of self-esteem, body image, and interpersonal relationships. Clients who cannot achieve urinary continence seek personal isolation and avoid any situation that might produce personal embarrassment. The client who suffers with urinary incontinence fears having wet clothing and a noticeable odor; everyone is anxious about the unpredictability of incontinence. Individuals who are incontinent often think that no one else has the same problem. They are embarrassed to seek help, and even when resources are identified, they must be assisted to feel comfortable in using the resources available. Purchasing supplies in the local drugstore or grocery store is often a major threat to personal exposure and privacy.

Society values adult behaviors; urinary incontinence

is associated with early childhood behaviors. The nurse assists in psychosocial preparation by accepting and acknowledging the personal concerns of the client and caregiver. These concerns must never be minimized or made to seem trivial. Although adults who are continent may not view the incontinent person negatively, the incontinent adult experiences negative thoughts toward self. The nurse helps the client to learn methods of controlling or managing the fear or anxiety. As the client learns the specifics of the plan that will allow for control of urinary incontinence, the confidence for resumption of psychosocial interactions should return.

Health Care Resources

For the client who returns home, referral to home care agencies for assistance with personal care may be appropriate. Referral to continence clinics that specialize in individual evaluation and treatment may also be helpful. In many continence clinics, nurses collaborate with physicians to evaluate and manage clients. The treatment plan is highly individualized; supplies and products are custom selected. Clients benefit emotionally from education and from the support of others who experience similar concerns. Help for Incontinent Persons (HIP) and the Simon Foundation for Continence publish newsletters that contain informative articles written with simple, easy to understand explanations.

 Evaluation

The nurse evaluates the effectiveness of the interventions on the basis of the outcomes expected for the identified nursing diagnoses, which include that the client

1. Describes the type of urinary incontinence experienced
2. Demonstrates knowledge of proper use of medications and correct procedures for self-catheterization or care of an indwelling urinary catheter
3. Demonstrates effective use of the selected exercise or bladder training programs
4. Selects and appropriately uses incontinence devices and products

IMMUNOLOGIC DISORDERS

OVERVIEW

Glomerulonephritis refers to an inflammatory process that involves the glomeruli. *Acute glomerulonephritis*, which is also referred to as *acute nephritic syndrome*, is one of several clinical syndromes in which the primary site of pathology is the glomerulus. Other syndromes that involve the glomerulus include rapidly progressive glomerulonephritis, chronic glomerulonephritis, and the nephrotic syndrome . This particular classification of these glomerular disorders is an attempt to describe the type of clinical presentation and probable prognosis. As such, any of the syndromes may involve prior infectious processes or multisystem disease. Also, immunologic response mechanisms are implicated in the pathogenesis of the disorders.

ACUTE GLOMERULONEPHRITIS

Pathophysiology

The pathophysiology of acute glomerulonephritis is initiated by activation of immunologic response mechanisms in the client. The antigen that activates the immune system may be endogenous or exogenous. Endogenous antigens include those that may already be present in the glomerulus or other tissues such as the nasopharynx, blood vessels, or joints; exogenous antigens are derived most typically from infections, including viruses, bacteria, fungi, and parasites. The formation of antibodies in response to antigenic stimulation results in several events causing glomerular injury.

Two mechanisms of antigen-antibody reaction have been described as causing the glomerular injury. In one response, the antigen-antibody complexes circulate and are deposited in the glomerular tissue. In the second mechanism, the immune complexes form directly in the glomerular tissue as a result of local interaction. Regardless of the mechanism responsible for initiating the injury to the glomerulus, the immune system responds via humoral and cellular activity.

The immune complexes are deposited in the mesangium and in the subendothelium and subepithelium of the walls of the glomerular capillary membrane. Additional injury results from activation of complement and release of vasoactive substances and other mediators of immunity. Disruption of cell membranes, local edema, movement of macrophages and neutrophils to the site of inflammation, and activation of platelets are some of the major responses promoting the local injury. With injury to the glomerular membrane, red blood cells and protein molecules may move into Bowman's capsule.

Etiology

Many causes of acute glomerulonephritis have been reported. Most of these causes are described as postinfectious or related to multisystem diseases already present. Primary and secondary causes of acute glomerulonephritis are listed in the accompanying Key Features of Disease.

KEY FEATURES OF DISEASE ■ Primary and Secondary Causes of Acute Glomerulonephritis

Primary (immune response to pathogens)

Group A beta-hemolytic streptococcus
Staphylococcal or pneumococcal bacteremia
Syphilis
Visceral abscesses
Bacterial endocarditis
Hepatitis B
Infectious mononucleosis
Measles
Mumps
Cytomegaloviral infection
Any parasitic, fungal, or viral infection (potentially)

Secondary (related to systemic disease)

Systemic lupus erythematosus
Progressive systemic sclerosis
Thrombocytopenic purpura
Postpartum renal failure
Henoch-Schönlein purpura
Goodpasture's syndrome
Wegener's granulomatosis
Polyarteritis nodosa
Hemolytic-uremic syndrome

Incidence

The exact incidence of acute glomerulonephritis is unknown, but it is twice as common in males as females. The reader is referred to sections of the book where multisystem diseases are discussed.

PREVENTION

Specific procedures to prevent acute glomerulonephritis are not known. Because of the frequent association of the syndrome with infectious causes, early recognition with prompt, appropriate treatment of the infectious disorder may diminish the severity of an immunologic response. The adequacy of renal blood flow and the integrity of the host's immune system are other factors that may influence prevention and/or development.

COLLABORATIVE MANAGEMENT

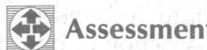 Assessment

History

The nurse inquires about *recent infectious processes*, particularly of the *skin* or *upper respiratory tract*. The nurse seeks information about *recent travel* or other activities during which exposure to viruses, bacteria, fungi, or parasites may have occurred. *Recent illnesses, surgery,* or other *invasive procedures* may suggest situations in which infectious processes could have been present. The nurse also inquires about any *known systemic diseases*, such as systemic lupus erythematosus (SLE), which could be the cause of the acute glomerulonephritis.

Physical Assessment: Clinical Manifestations

The nurse inspects the skin for evidence of any lesions or recent incisions. The nurse examines the face, eyelids, hands, and other peripheral tissues for *edema; blood pressure* is measured and recorded because systolic and diastolic hypertension is frequently present. The nurse questions the client about any changes in the pattern of urination and notes any *change in urine color,* which might be described as *smoky, reddish brown,* or *cola colored.* The nurse asks the client about *dysuria* or a *decrease in the amount of urine* produced. The nurse also inquires about any *difficulty in breathing, nocturnal or exertional dyspnea,* or *orthopnea.* It is important to measure the *weight* of the client because changes in urinary output may result in fluid retention. The nurse assesses the cardiovascular system for evidence of fluid overload. Lung fields and heart sounds are assessed for *crackles* and an S_3 *heart sound,* respectively. The nurse also inspects the client for *neck vein engorgement.* The client may manifest fatigue, lack of energy, anorexia, nausea, and/or vomiting if uremia from renal failure is present.

Psychosocial Assessment

The nurse assesses the client for the type of emotional reaction to the alteration in renal function. The nurse expects anxiety and fear, as well as sadness or grief. The nurse listens carefully to the questions and comments of the client to determine the mood and attitude regarding the onset of the disease process. The nurse assesses the availability of family, friends, and persons significant to the client because these resources may be quite supportive during the period of illness.

Laboratory Findings

The urinalysis report reveals the presence of red blood cells and protein. Microscopic examination of an early morning specimen of urine is preferred because the urine is most acidic and formed elements are more intact. Further microscopic examination, usually performed personally by the physician or consulting nephrologist, often reveals red blood cell casts. Leukocytes, white blood cell casts, granular casts, or waxy casts may be present in the urine. There is usually a positive urinary sediment assay.

The glomerular filtration rate (GFR), as measured by the 24-hour urine test for creatinine clearance, may be decreased to 50 mL/minute. Yet, serum creatinine levels may be within the normal range (0.6 to 1.0 mg/dL for women; 0.8 to 1.7 mg/dL for men), or at the upper limits of the normal range. BUN levels are increased. A 24-hour urine collection for total protein assay is also obtained. The 24-hour protein excretion value of persons with acute glomerulonephritis may be expected to be between 500 mg and 3 g.

Blood, skin, and/or throat cultures are obtained if indicated on the basis of the history or clinical examination. If oliguria is present, the client may also have hyperkalemia, hypocalcemia, and dilutional hyponatremia, which are all signs of renal insufficiency.

Other serologic tests to be done include the following: antistreptolysin O titers; complement levels for C3, C4, and total complement; hepatitis B surface antigen and hepatitis B surface antibody; and antinuclear antibodies. Antistreptolysin O titers are increased after group A beta-hemolytic streptococcus infections. Complement levels are decreased when the complement system is activated; a variety of causes may be implicated, such as SLE and postinfectious factors. A seropositive report for hepatitis B antigen or antibody may suggest the hepatitis B virus as the etiology. The presence of antinuclear antibodies suggests an autoimmune response, with SLE as only one possibility.

Radiographic Findings

There are no specific radiographic tests to confirm acute glomerulonephritis. These studies, such as renal ultrasonography, might be prescribed to rule out urinary tract obstruction or to confirm the presence of two kidneys. Confirmation of the presence of two kidneys and their location is essential before percutaneous renal biopsy.

Other Diagnostic Tests

A percutaneous renal biopsy may be performed for precise diagnosis of the pathologic condition. The specific morphology is determined by use of light microscopy, immunofluorescent stains, and electron microscopy. These procedures identify the type of cellular proliferation (light microscopy), the presence of immunoglobulins (immunofluorescence), and the specific type of tissue deposits (electron microscopy). A tissue diagnosis often assists in determining diseases potentially responsive to immunosuppressive therapy. The biopsy also assists in determining the prognosis.

 Analysis: Nursing Diagnosis

Clients with acute glomerulonephritis may have very mild or very serious effects of the illness. Some clients may be managed as outpatients, whereas others require hospitalization. The nursing diagnoses identified are those that would be present with the more serious manifestations of the disorder.

Common Diagnoses

The common diagnoses experienced by the client with acute glomerulonephritis include the following:

1. Altered nutrition: less than body requirements related to increased metabolic demands and anorexia
2. Potential for activity intolerance related to fatigue, fluid volume excess, and loss of energy
3. Fluid volume excess related to oliguria

Additional Diagnoses

In addition to the common diagnoses, the client may also experience the following:

1. Knowledge deficit related to new diagnostic tests and therapeutic procedures
2. Anticipatory grieving or anxiety related to unknown prognosis

 Planning and Implementation

Altered Nutrition: Less Than Body Requirements

Planning: client goals. The goal for this nursing diagnosis is that the client will achieve a state of nutrition that permits maximal healing and prevents further deterioration.

Interventions: nonsurgical management. Interventions for the management of nutritional deficits in persons with acute glomerulonephritis include strategies to promote dietary intake with as few limitations as possible. If nutritional intake is diminished as a result of azotemia and/or uremic symptoms, dialysis may be necessary to permit the attainment of nutritional needs (see Chap. 59 for nursing care associated with dialysis treatments).

The dietary plan is prescribed to provide for adequate caloric and nutrient intake from all food groups. The plan varies depending on whether oliguria is present. For a client with a "normal" urinary output, the diet is not modified; the client is encouraged to consume foods representing the various food groups and to eat those items that have the most appeal.

For clients with oliguria, a variety of limitations of the usual diet may be necessary. Fluid intake is restricted. The usual fluid allowance is that equal to the urinary output for 24 hours plus 500 mL to account for the insensible fluid losses. Also, when oliguria is present, there is usually urinary retention of sodium and potassium and elevation of the BUN level. Restriction of potassium and protein intake is necessary to prevent hyperkalemia and additional uremic manifestations of the elevated BUN.

In addition, a low-sodium diet and antihypertensive medications may be needed to control hypertension and edema. Because sodium content significantly influences the taste and appeal of food for many clients, the sodium restriction may be minimized to encourage the client to eat. Nausea, vomiting, or anorexia may indicate that uremia is interfering with the maintenance of nutrition. If dietary control of sodium intake is not adequate to control hypertension, antihypertensive agents will be needed. If uremic symptoms or fluid volume excess cannot be controlled, dialysis will be necessary. Plasmapheresis may also be attempted; steroids are generally not helpful.

The nurse assesses the client's interest in eating and ability to eat and notes food preferences and intolerances. The nurse offers to assist with or to provide meticulous and frequent oral hygiene to improve taste and to remove the unpleasant mouth odors that accompany uremia. The nurse initiates a referral to a dietitian if needed.

Potential for Activity Intolerance

Planning: client goals. The goal for this diagnosis is that the client will obtain adequate rest and sleep to permit resumption of usual activities.

Interventions: nonsurgical management. The nurse intervenes to encourage and promote a restful environment by eliminating unnecessary intrusions, by spacing activities, and by coordinating necessary assessments and treatments to facilitate conservation and maintenance of energy. The nurse demonstrates techniques of energy conservation, which may be accomplished by alternating active periods with rest periods. The client also needs to minimize emotional stress to achieve optimal rest and potential for healing. The nurse encourages the client to practice relaxation techniques and to participate in diversional activities.

Fluid Volume Excess

The goals and interventions for the client with excess fluid volume are discussed in Chapter 59.

■ Discharge Planning

Home Care Preparation

The nurse assists the client and family or significant other to examine the home environment in preparation for discharge from the hospital. Major preparations are not usually required because the client is expected to be able to assume responsibility for self-care processes related to hygiene and bathing, grooming and dressing, toileting, and feeding. If other coexisting health problems or systemic illnesses are present, home care assistance may be necessary. The nurse helps the client to identify potential needs for food purchase and meal preparation, laundry, and housekeeping. Clients who live alone may need temporary assistance during the period of recuperation.

Client/Family Education

The nurse instructs the client and family or significant other about the purpose and desired effects of prescribed medications, the dosage and route of administration, and potentially adverse side effects. The nurse ensures that the client and family demonstrate understanding of dietary or fluid modifications, including methods of detecting fluid retention. The nurse advises the client to measure weight and blood pressure daily. The nurse encourages the client to perform regular exercise, as tolerated, and to schedule defined periods for extra rest and sleep. If short-term dialysis is required for control of fluid volume excess or uremic symptoms, the nurse instructs the client about peritoneal or vascular access care, as well as dialysis schedules and routines.

Psychosocial Preparation

The nurse helps the client to prepare emotionally for a period of recuperation in which the client's ability to meet self-expectations may be decreased. By advance discussion, the client may gain a more realistic perspective about the temporary modifications needed because of the effects of the illness on his or her ability to maintain usual activities. Similarly, the nurse encourages the client to accept help from significant others without excessive feelings of inadequacy, dependency, or loss of self-esteem.

Health Care Resources

The nurse assesses the need for health care resources depending on the age, social support structure, and physical and emotional needs of the client. Home nursing care, physical and occupational therapy, and social services agencies are potential resources to be considered. In addition, community centers providing programs for adults and elderly persons may be useful.

 Evaluation

The nurse evaluates the care of the client with acute glomerulonephritis on the basis of the identified nursing diagnoses. Outcomes expected include that the client

1. Demonstrates an understanding of the importance of regular and balanced periods of rest and activity
2. Demonstrates knowledge of medications, including administration (dosage, route, and frequency) and potential and expected side effects
3. Adheres to the dietary and fluid intake modifications as necessary
4. Accepts the need for temporary dialysis as needed
5. Copes with temporary limitations to personal life style and interpersonal relationships

CHRONIC GLOMERULONEPHRITIS

OVERVIEW

Chronic glomerulonephritis, which is also referred to as *chronic nephritic syndrome*, is one of several syndromes involving the glomeruli. Chronic glomerulonephritis is a diagnostic name given to known and unknown causes of renal deterioration or renal failure that develop over a period of years. In many instances, the cause of the disease is not known because the kidneys are atrophied and tissue is not available for biopsy and/or diagnosis.

The exact pathogenesis of chronic glomerulonephritis is not known. The changes in the renal parenchyma are believed to be due to the effects of hypertension, intermittent or recurrent parenchymal infections and inflammation, and altered metabolism and hemodynamics.

In chronic glomerulonephritis, kidney tissue atrophies and the functional mass of nephrons decreases significantly. The cortex of the parenchyma is thinned, but the calyces and pelves are normal. Tissue obtained by renal biopsy in the late stages of atrophy may reveal hyalinization of the glomeruli, loss of tubules, and fibrosis of the interstitium. Immunofluorescent examination and electron microscopy may reveal residual effects of immune complex deposition.

The loss of nephrons, which are the functional units of the renal parenchyma, results in decreased glomerular filtration. Commonly, hypertension with sclerosis of renal arterioles is present. In addition, the glomerular injury results in proteinuria because of increased permeability of the glomerular basement membrane. Eventually, chronic glomerulonephritis results in end-stage renal disease and uremia (see Chap. 59 for the pathophysiology of chronic renal failure). The progression is slow and insidious and may occur over 10 to 30 years or longer.

The exact cause of chronic glomerulonephritis is often not known. The renal manifestations of systemic diseases such as SLE, amyloid disease, or diabetes mellitus become similar to those of chronic glomerulonephritis. In end-stage renal disease, tissue differentiation is usually not possible.

Chronic glomerulonephritis is the primary cause of end-stage renal disease resulting in the need for dialysis or transplantation. It is reported to be the etiology for chronic dialysis in 35% to 40% of the 80,000 persons requiring these treatments.

Current evidence suggests that after glomerular injury has occurred, progression of the disease is predictable and difficult to prevent. In some situations, early recognition and treatment may yield remission or delay progression. Consistent follow-up by clients to control hypertension, to modify dietary protein and phosphate intake, and to avoid nephrotoxic agents and salt depletion may delay the onset of end-stage renal disease.

COLLABORATIVE MANAGEMENT

The client is questioned about previously identified health problems, including systemic diseases and prior renal or urologic disorders. The nurse solicits information about childhood infectious diseases, such as streptococcal infections, and recent exposures to infections. The nurse inquires about the client's perception of overall health status and notes increasing fatigue and lethargy. Information about the client's pattern of voiding is elicited—whether the frequency of voiding has increased and the quantity of urine produced has decreased. The nurse asks the client about changes in the color, odor, or clarity of the urine. Because edema can result from oliguria and fluid volume excess, the nurse inquires about the level of general comfort and whether the client experiences dyspnea at rest or with exertion. The nurse asks about the client's ability to pursue activities such as reading, job-related functions, or other processes requiring mental concentration. Changes in memory or ability to concentrate occur with the accumulation of waste products that accompanies renal failure. Alterations in mental functioning may be manifested through a report of an inability to concentrate or remember, frequent interruptions of the conversations of others, and generalized irritability.

The nurse inspects the skin for a yellowish color, ecchymoses, and rashes or eruptions and examines it for texture while noting areas of dryness and breaks in the skin that may have occurred from scratching. The nurse assesses the cardiovascular and peripheral tissues for evidence of fluid retention by measuring blood pressure and weight and by auscultating the heart to describe rate, rhythm, and the presence of an S_3 heart sound. The nurse auscultates the lung fields to detect the presence of rales or crackles and observes the rate and depth of the breathing pattern. The nurse inspects the neck veins to identify venous engorgement and checks for edema in the pedal, pretibial, and presacral tissues. The nurse notes whether there is slurred speech, ataxia, tremors, or asterixis (flapping tremor, or the inability to maintain a fixed posture). Urinary output may decrease in quantity. Gross visual changes in urine are not usual unless there is an associated UTI. The above-mentioned findings suggest the onset of uremia from renal failure.

The urinalysis commonly reveals proteinuria, usually less than 2 g in a 24-hour collection. The specific gravity of the urine is usually fixed at a constant level of dilution, around 1.010. There may be red blood cells and casts (hyaline, waxy, or granular) in the urine, which suggests chronic renal disease processes.

The GFR, as measured by creatinine clearance, is decreased from the normal range of 105 ± 20 mL/minute. With end-stage renal disease, the creatinine clearance value is less than 5 to 10 mL/minute. The serum creatinine level is elevated and varies depending on the individual's muscle mass. Serum creatinine levels are usually above 6 mg/dL but may be as high as 30 mg/dL or more. The BUN value is increased and varies in relation to the dietary protein intake; BUN levels are often between 100 and 200 mg/dL.

Serum electrolytes also reveal the deterioration of renal function. Sodium retention commonly occurs, but dilution of the plasma results in an apparently normal serum sodium level (136 to 145 mEq/L) or a dilutional hyponatremia (less than 136 mEq/L). When oliguria develops, potassium retention occurs; hyperkalemia is present when levels exceed 5.5 mEq/L. Hyperphosphatemia develops, and levels are higher than 4.7 mg/dL. Serum calcium levels are usually at the lower end of the normal range (8.0 to 10.5 mg/dL) or are slightly below normal. A base deficit is noted by the decrease in serum CO_2 or CO_2-combining power to less than 24 to 32 mEq/L. Respiratory compensation for this metabolic acidosis (base deficit) is accomplished by hyperventilation to lower the PCO_2 of arterial blood. The pH of arterial blood is between 7.35 and 7.45 if respiratory compensation is present. Metabolic acidemia, a pH of less than 7.35, signifies inadequate respiratory compensation for metabolic acidosis.

In clients with chronic glomerulonephritis, the kidneys appear to be quite small when observed by radiography (KUB) or IVP. Similarly, the kidneys are small when measured by ultrasonography or CT.

The renal biopsy (percutaneous or open) is rarely performed for end-stage renal disease because the kidneys are too small to obtain tissue. In the early stages, when proteinuria or hematuria is initially identified, a renal biopsy is an important diagnostic test. Changes noted include an increase in the number and types of cells infiltrating the glomerular tissue, deposition of immune complexes, and sclerosis of the vessels.

The nursing diagnoses for the client with chronic glomerulonephritis depend on the stage of renal deterioration that is present. Treatment for end-stage renal disease may be conservative, consisting of diet, fluid, and medication therapy to temporarily control the symptoms of uremia. Eventually, the client requires dialysis or transplantation to prevent death from the numerous potential systemic effects of uremia. The nursing care for the client with end-stage renal disease requiring dialysis or transplantion is discussed in Chapter 59.

NEPHROTIC SYNDROME

Nephrotic syndrome represents a clinical entity that is usually a consequence of severe proteinuria. The alteration of the glomerular membrane that allows the loss of protein into the urine may result from many different etiologies. Often, the disorder is immunologically mediated. The causes of nephrotic syndrome may be primary glomerular disease, neoplastic disease, multisystem disease (e.g., diabetes mellitus, SLE, and amyloidosis), or exposure to pathogens (viral, bacterial, or fungal).

The primary feature of this syndrome is severe proteinuria — more than 3.5 g of protein in 24 hours. Clients diagnosed as having nephrotic syndrome also often have hypoalbuminemia, hyperlipidemia, and edema. Renal vein thrombosis is often reported to occur concurrently, either as an etiology or as a result of the nephrotic syndrome. The tendency for thromboembolic phenomena is not clearly understood, but abnormalities in clotting studies may be detected. The nephrotic syndrome may progress to end-stage renal disease, but this progression is not considered to be an inevitable consequence.

Treatment of clients with the nephrotic syndrome varies depending on the specifics of the glomerulopathy identified by analysis of the renal biopsy. Some immunologic processes may respond to steroids or cytotoxic agents. Dietary modification is also frequently prescribed. If the GFR is normal, a normal dietary intake of protein is recommended, but the high-biologic-value proteins should be emphasized. If the GFR is decreased, dietary protein intake is decreased (Glassock et al., 1986). Mild diuretics and dietary sodium restriction may be prescribed to control edema and hypertension. The nurse assesses the client to ensure that intravascular volume depletion does not occur and lead to hemodynamic changes and possible acute renal failure. The effects of hyperlipidemia in nephrotic syndrome on the development of atherosclerosis is unclear, as are the effects of dietary modifications.

DEGENERATIVE DISORDERS

Degenerative disorders resulting in alterations of renal function are usually associated with the pathophysiologic effects of a multisystem disorder. Because the renal parenchyma is extremely vascular, many of these disorders occur as a sequela to changes in the renal vasculature.

NEPHROSCLEROSIS

Nephrosclerosis refers to changes in the nephron, specifically the afferent and efferent arterioles and the glomerular capillary loops. The changes that occur include thickening of the vessel walls and narrowing of the lumen of the vessel. As a result, renal blood flow is decreased and interstitial tissue changes occur. Over time, ischemia and fibrosis develop. Nephrosclerosis is associated with benign essential hypertension or malignant hypertension and the effects of atherosclerosis. A history of diabetes mellitus is also common. The effects of essential hypertension on renal vasculature may be controlled with adequate blood pressure control. When malignant hypertension occurs, with systolic pressures in the range of 200 to 250 mmHg and diastolic pressures higher than 120 mmHg, ischemia and necrosis may develop quickly. The changes associated with malignant hypertension may be reversible or may progress to end-stage renal disease within a period of months or years.

Treatment for clients with nephrosclerosis is aimed at controlling high blood pressure and preserving renal function. Although many antihypertensive agents may adequately lower the blood pressure, one key to long-term adherence to the prescribed therapy is the individual's response to the medications. The nurse inquires about medication tolerance and the presence of unusual or bothersome side effects. Agents that produce unusual fatigue, drowsiness, or impotence are often not taken. In addition, the cost of some medications may be prohibitive for some clients. Doses of medications that must be taken several times a day are often missed, and thus blood pressure control may be erratic and inadequate.

RENAL ARTERY STENOSIS

Pathologic processes affecting the renal arteries may result in severe narrowing of the lumen and drastically reduced blood flow to the renal parenchyma. Uncorrected renal artery stenosis results in ischemia and atrophy of renal tissue. Renal artery stenosis is suspected when there is a sudden onset of hypertension, particularly in individuals older than 50 years of age. In addition, clients with high blood pressure but with a negative family history for hypertension may be considered as potential candidates for renal artery stenosis.

Two types of processes have been identified as resulting in renal artery stenosis: atherosclerosis and fibromuscular hyperplasia. Atherosclerotic changes in the renal artery are frequently associated with corresponding disease of the aorta and other major vessels; changes in the renal artery are usually within a centimeter of the point at which the renal artery and the aorta meet. Fibromuscular changes of the vessel wall occur throughout the length of the renal artery between the aortic junction and the points of branching into the renal segmental arteries.

Diagnosis of renal artery stenosis is accomplished by use of renal arteriography and measurement of renal vein renin levels. The renal arteriogram provides visualization of the renal vasculature and offers critical information for invasive treatment procedures. A comparison of renal vein renin levels may offer information on which kidney is producing more renin and thus worsening the high blood pressure. Excellent visualization of the type of defect is critical.

In addition to the precise location of the defect and the extent of narrowing, the overall condition of the client and the size of the atrophied kidney influence decisions about the choice of therapeutic intervention. Renal artery stenosis may be treated by use of medications (to control high blood pressure) and percutaneous transluminal balloon angioplasty or renal artery bypass surgery. Medications may control high blood pressure but may not preserve kidney function over the years. In young and middle-aged adults, a lifetime of treatment with multiple agents for high blood pressure may be a difficult management plan; there is also concern for preservation of renal function. Clients with compromised renal blood flow and renal function require procedures to restore blood flow and to preserve renal function. Two procedures are currently available: balloon angioplasty and renal artery bypass surgery. The balloon angioplasty technique is considered to be less risky and requires much less time for recovery than renal artery bypass surgery (see Chap. 65 for a discussion of balloon angioplasty). Renal artery bypass surgery is a major procedure and requires 2 months or more for convalescence. This surgery may be performed for either one or both renal arteries. A synthetic graft is inserted and redirects blood flow from the abdominal aorta through the graft into the renal artery beyond the area of stenosis. Technically, the process is similar to other arterial bypass procedures, as are discussed in Chapter 64. For clients with renal artery stenosis, the diagnostic and treatment alternatives present tremendous decisional conflict. Often, clients have deterioration of renal function, as noted by elevated serum creatinine levels and decreased creatinine clearance. Therefore, these clients are at increased risk for developing acute renal failure from the administration of radiopaque contrast agents and possible intraoperative hypotensive episodes. On the other hand, no treatment means that dialysis is probably inevitable.

DIABETIC NEPHROPATHY

Diabetes mellitus is the identified cause of end-stage renal disease in 25% or more of clients requiring chronic dialysis or renal transplantation. Diabetic nephropathy occurs as a result of type I diabetes mellitus (insulin dependent, ketosis prone) and type II diabetes mellitus (non–insulin dependent, non–ketosis prone). For clients with type I diabetes mellitus, end-stage renal disease is expected within 5 years after the onset of proteinuria. Proteinuria is usually present within 16 to 21 years after the development of diabetes mellitus. For clients with type II diabetes mellitus, the development of diabetic renal manifestations is less predictable and is influenced by a number of variables, including the extent, duration, and effects of atherosclerosis and hypertension and the effects of autonomic neuropathy, which promotes bladder atony, urinary stasis, and UTIs. Immunologic response mechanisms have also been implicated in glomerular basement membrane thickening and in other changes observed in clients with diabetic renal disease. Investigations continue to explore whether the defects are from genetic or metabolic disturbances.

Diagnosis of renal disease from diabetes mellitus is often presumptive, given the history and clinical examination of the client. If funduscopic examination of the retina demonstrates capillary leakage and fibrosis, glomerular changes are usually concurrent; therefore, a renal biopsy is not necessary. Proteinuria may be mild, moderate, or severe, as in nephrotic syndrome. Persons with diabetes mellitus are always considered to be at risk for the development of renal failure; nephrotoxic agents (such as radiopaque contrast media or aminoglycosides) and dehydration must be avoided if possible. Clients with worsening renal function may begin to have frequent hypoglycemic episodes and a decrease in their need for insulin or oral antihyperglycemic agents. The nurse explains to the client that the kidneys metabolize and excrete insulin. Consequently, when renal function is deteriorating, the insulin is available longer and less insulin is needed. Unfortunately, many clients believe that the diabetes mellitus is improving, but their renal function is actually deteriorating. The result is often end-stage renal disease requiring chronic dialysis or transplantation.

OBSTRUCTIONS

UROLITHIASIS

OVERVIEW

Urolithiasis refers to the presence of stones in the urinary tract, in particular, when stones pass into the lower urinary tract or are formed in the bladder. The term *nephrolithiasis* is used more specifically to describe stones that are formed in the renal parenchyma. Formation of stones in the ureter is referred to as *ureterolithiasis*. Stones form anywhere in the urinary tract depending on a variety of factors. The formation of renal or urologic stones is one of the most common urologic problems for adults.

Pathophysiology

The exact mechanism of formation of renal or urologic calculi is not known. Because of the renal mechanisms for excretion of calcium, phosphate, and other crystals, it is generally believed that conditions that limit or promote excretion influence the formation of calculi. The supersaturation of the filtrate with a particular element is believed to be the primary factor contributing to calculi formation. The acidity or alkalinity of the urine, urinary stasis, and other substances (e.g., pyrophos-

phate, magnesium, and citrate) that may inhibit crystallization are other factors contributing to the formation of calculi.

Calculi may be formed from calcium, phosphate, oxalate, uric acid, struvite, and cystine crystals. The vast majority of stones contain calcium as one component of the stone complex, such as calcium phosphate or calcium oxalate. Uric acid stones derive from purine metabolism; struvite stones result from urea-splitting bacteria and contain magnesium, phosphate, and ammonium; and cystine stones originate from cystine crystals as a result of a hereditary renal tubular defect. When the solute load of a particular element to be excreted is increased, the conditions are conducive to supersaturation. For example, the effects of prolonged immobility are well documented as a cause of calcium mobilization from bone. Increased levels of serum calcium result in an increased solute load to be excreted. If fluid intake is inadequate, supersaturation is more likely to occur, and stone formation through calcium complexing has an increased probability of occurring. The calcium complex often serves as a nidus (breeding site) for additional deposition, and eventually a stone forms.

The pH of the urine may promote stone formation or stone dissolution. Uric acid and cystine stones tend to form in acidic urine; struvite and calcium phosphate stones tend to form in alkaline urine. Calcium oxalate stone formation is not influenced by the pH of urine. The pathophysiology of stone formation is complex. It is essential that the type of stone produced be analyzed for mineral content. The causes and treatments of the different types of renal stones are given in the accompanying Key Features of Disease.

Stones formed in the kidney that pass into the ureter commonly lodge in the ureteropelvic angle, the aorto-iliac bend, or the ureterovesical angle. When the stone occludes the ureter and blocks the flow of urine, the ureter dilates. An enlargement of the ureter is referred to as *hydroureter*. The pain associated with ureteral spasm is excruciatingly severe and may cause the client to develop shock. In addition, the client may manifest hematuria as a result of damage to the urothelial lining. If the obstruction is not removed, urinary stasis may result in infection and subsequently impair renal function on the side of the blockage. As the blockage persists, the client may develop *hydronephrosis*, or enlargement of the kidney.

Etiology

The etiology of nephrolithiasis is unknown, although a variety of hypotheses have been suggested. Presently, the question is whether a single explanation is possible in view of the variety of presentations and responses. Pak (1986) described the potential causes of hypercalciuria as (1) absorptive (increased intestinal calcium absorption), (2) renal (impaired renal tubular reabsorption of calcium), (3) combined (increased formation of active vitamin D and hypophosphatemia), and (4) resorptive

KEY FEATURES OF DISEASE ■ Causes and Treatments of Renal Stones

Stone Type	Cause	Dietary Interventions	Rationales
Calcium phosphate	Supersaturation of urine with calcium and/or phosphate	1. Decrease intake of foods high in calcium, such as milk and other dairy products. 2. Increase intake of meats, eggs, fish, plums, and cranberries.	1. To reduce urinary calcium content. 2. To make urine acidic.
Calcium oxalate	Supersaturation of urine with calcium and/or oxalate	1. Avoid oxalate sources, such as spinach.	1. To reduce urinary oxalate content. Urinary pH is not a factor.
Uric acid (urate)	Excess dietary purine Gout (primary or secondary)	1. Decrease intake of purine sources, such as organ meats, gravies, red wines, and sardines. 2. Avoid citrus fruits and citrus juices, milk and milk products, and potatoes.	1. To reduce urinary purine content. 2. To make urine alkaline.
Struvite (magnesium ammonium phosphate)	Urea splitting by bacteria	1. Limit high-phosphate foods, such as dairy products, red and organ meats, and whole grains. 2. Increase intake of eggs, fish, plums, and cranberries.	1. To reduce urinary phosphate content. 2. To make urine acidic.
Cystine	Hereditary cystine crystal formation	1. Avoid citrus fruits and citrus juices, milk and milk products, and potatoes.	1. To make urine alkaline.

(primary hypoparathyroidism). In the absorptive category, three different types have been identified and may or may not be associated with calcium intake. In the renal category, tubular defects in the nephron are proposed as a major cause of stone formation. Tubular defects may be inherited or may be associated with a familial tendency. In clients who are immobile, the lack of weight bearing on the long bones of the skeleton results in the release of stored calcium. The increase in plasma calcium level may promote an environment conducive to stone formation.

Proper fluid intake is necessary to ensure adequate hydration and to decrease the potential for precipitation of crystals. Excess vitamin D intake and primary hyperparathyroidism are also potential causes of stone forma-

tion because each results in excess plasma calcium levels. Vitamin D promotes calcium absorption in the gastrointestinal tract. In hyperparathyroidism, the excess parathyroid hormone stimulates the release of calcium stored in the bone. A dietary intake high in calcium is not believed to result in renal calculi unless a stone-forming tendency or renal tubular defect already exists. Urinary stasis, urinary retention, and dehydration all contribute to a stone-forming environment. Similarly, medications containing calcium, e.g., calcium carbonate, are not associated with the formation of kidney stones unless the client already has a tendency to form calculi. Diuretics have the potential to result in volume depletion and thus could enhance conditions promoting the formation of stones.

Clients with gout are at risk for the development of uric acid stone formation. With a chronically elevated serum uric acid level, the substance crystallizes and deposits in the urinary system.

Incidence

The incidence of renal or urologic stones in the adult population is relatively high. The rate of kidney stones is 4.5 per 1000 (Collins, 1988). Some regions of the United States seem to have higher frequencies of stone disease, i.e., the southern and midwestern states. Stone disease is more common in men than in women and tends to occur in young adults or early middle adulthood. The recurrence rate is at least 50% within 5 to 10 years (Coe & Favus, 1986). Stone disease in Black persons is uncommon.

PREVENTION

Primary prevention of stone formation involves avoiding immobility and fluid-depleted states. Immobility increases the concentration of solutes; fluid depletion reduces the potential for solubility and excretion. Together, these two factors contribute to an environment conducive to stone formation. Secondary prevention refers to measures taken to prevent recurrences of stone formation. For some clients, prevention is not possible because the problem represents a tubular defect. For others, especially clients with gout, preventive measures include a fluid intake of at least 3000 mL/day, possible dietary modifications, or alterations in urinary acidification or alkalinization through medication, diet, and fluid intake prescriptions.

COLLABORATIVE MANAGEMENT

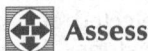 Assessment

History

The nurse inquires about a *previous personal or family history* of renal or urologic stones and the *diet history*. If the client has a history of stone formation, the nurse asks whether chemical analysis of the stone was performed and what preventive measures the client follows. In addition, the nurse obtains historical information about any surgical, invasive, or noninvasive treatments required to eliminate the stone.

Physical Assessment: Clinical Manifestations

The nurse obtains information specifically describing the client's current status, including the *presence, location, and duration of the pain;* whether other symptoms such as *nausea and vomiting* or *chills and fever* are present; and information about *changes in the pattern of*

urination. Flank pain suggests localization of the calculi in the kidney or upper ureter; pain in the flank that radiates abdominally or into the scrotum and testes or the vulva suggests that calculi are in the ureters or bladder. Gastrointestinal symptoms, such as nausea and vomiting, develop as a result of sympathetic and parasympathetic nerve stimulation associated with ureteral peristalsis and spasm. Ureteral spasm, or *colic,* is usually intermittent but is *extremely* severe and is present when the ureter is in spasm and the stone is unable to pass through. The pain is a *dull ache* when the stone is lodged and immobile, and there is no spasm.

The nurse observes the *color, amount, clarity,* and *odor* of the client's urine. Blood may make the urine appear *smoky or rusty;* increased *turbidity and odor* are associated with infectious processes. *Oliguria or anuria* suggests that obstruction is present, possibly at the bladder neck or urethra. Obstruction of the urinary tract is an emergency and must be managed immediately to preserve kidney function.

The nurse examines the client to detect *bladder distention.* The physical examination may reveal pale, ashen, diaphoretic skin, and the client suffering with excruciating pain. The nurse measures temperature, pulse rate, respiratory rate, and blood pressure, which are moderately elevated with pain; temperature and pulse are elevated with infection. Blood pressure may decrease markedly if the severe pain causes shock.

Psychosocial Assessment

The nurse assesses the client with urolithiasis to determine the emotional response to the problem. For the client with stone disease, anxiety about pain control is a major concern. If the client has had prior episodes of urolithiasis, there are memories of the pain and anticipatory anxiety. The nurse assesses the client's memories about the pain, identifies specific concerns, and elicits information about previous methods of coping with the discomfort. The client may also experience concern about the future, such as whether the stone disease and related pain may interfere with work or other personal goals. The client may also fear that chronic kidney failure may result.

Laboratory Findings

The urinalysis report may include findings of red blood cells, white blood cells, and bacteria. Red blood cells are most likely the result of direct trauma caused by the calculi on the endothelial lining of the ureter, bladder, or urethra. White blood cells and bacteria may be present as a result of urinary stasis. The urine culture reveals the number of CFU present; sensitivity studies of the culture identify antibiotic effectiveness. Microscopic examination of the urine may allow identification of crystals from which stones could grow. The white blood cell count is elevated with infection; the differential count indicates an increased number of immature white blood cells, such as bands, if the infection is recent and acute. Increases in the serum calcium, serum phosphate, or serum uric acid levels suggest that excess minerals are present and contributory to the stone formation. The pH of the urine is also measured.

Radiographic Findings

The presence of stones in the urinary tract may be evident by KUB, IVP, or tomography. The primary purpose of these radiographic procedures is to confirm the presence and location of the stones. IVP is useful for identifying whether urinary tract obstruction is present. Because of the risk of contrast media–induced acute renal failure, other diagnostic tests may be chosen for high-risk individuals (the elderly and persons with diabetes mellitus, multiple myeloma, or elevated serum creatinine levels). CT produces more precise images to identify the size and location of calculi or obstruction of the urinary tract.

Other Diagnostic Tests

Renal ultrasonography uses imaging techniques derived from sound waves to reproduce structures of varying density. Solid structures, such as calculi, are extremely dense; therefore, the images produced of stones are quite obvious. The presence of small calculi and their exact location may not be as precise as desired with renal ultrasonography.

 Analysis: Nursing Diagnosis

Common Diagnoses

The nursing diagnoses are derived from assessment data and include the following common diagnoses:

1. Pain related to the presence and/or movement of the stone
2. Potential for infection related to urinary stasis and the presence of a foreign object (e.g., hydronephrosis)
3. Potential for injury related to the risk of urinary obstruction

Additional Diagnoses

Additional diagnoses for the client with urolithiasis include

1. Anxiety related to potential for severe discomfort
2. Knowledge deficit related to prevention of recurrences

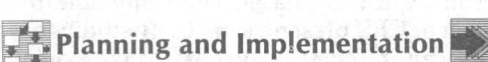 Planning and Implementation

Pain

Planning: client goals. The goal for this nursing diagnosis is that the client will achieve sufficient comfort to allow adequate rest and relaxation.

Interventions. Nonsurgical interventions include provision of analgesics during diagnostic and therapeutic procedures. It is hoped that the client will be able to expel the stone without invasive procedures, but surgery or other interventions may be necessary.

Nonsurgical management. Nonsurgical interventions include drug therapy and strict monitoring of urine to determine stone excretion.

Drug therapy. Medications prescribed to control the pain of calculi in the urinary tract include narcotic analgesics and spasmolytic agents. Narcotic agents such as morphine sulfate are generally administered intravenously to ensure prompt and adequate absorption. In addition, control of pain is more effective when medications are given at regularly scheduled intervals instead of as needed. The spasmolytic agents include oxybutynin chloride (Ditropan) and propantheline bromide (Pro-Banthine). These agents are also extremely important for the relief and control of pain.

Other measures. The nurse provides other comfort measures such as assistance with hygiene and bathing, mobility, or toileting. Changes of bed linens and periodic back rubs to promote relaxation, comfort, and rest are offered. The nurse checks the client frequently, including the measurement of vital signs, because shock may occur as a result of the severe pain. Vital signs are checked at least hourly until the severe pain subsides. The nurse helps the client to exercise through ambulation (assisted if necessary) or sitting in a chair at regular intervals.

Surgical management. Various endourologic, surgical, and other procedures may be used to remove the stones that are too large to pass spontaneously. These procedures include cystoscopy with stone basketing, percutaneous nephrostomy, and lithotripsy, i.e., the application of energy waves (sound or shock waves) via nephrostomy, cystoscopy, or extracorporeal techniques. The decision about the mode of therapy selected depends greatly on the size and location of the stones. In general, nonsurgical methods are attempted initially; most stones can be managed without surgical intervention.

For stones within the kidney pelvis or upper portion of the ureter, removal options include percutaneous nephrostomy, with or without lithotripsy; extracorporeal shock wave lithotripsy; and general surgical procedures such as nephrolithotomy, pyelolithotomy, or pyeloureterolithotomy. Surgical procedures for stone removal are summarized in the accompanying Key Features of Disease.

Preoperative care. The nurse prepares the client for the selected procedure by giving information describing details related to how, when, and where the procedure is performed, as well as what to expect before and after the procedure. The client receives nothing by mouth and also receives preoperative bowel preparation. Refer to Chapter 18 for a complete discussion of routine preoperative care.

Percutaneous nephrostomy involves a small incision

KEY FEATURES OF DISEASE ■ Surgical Procedures for Urinary Stone Removal

Procedure	Location of Stone	Presence and Type of Surgical Incision
Cystoscopy (use of endoscope through urethra to visualize stone, with special attachment to extract stone)	Bladder or lower ureter	No incision
Percutaneous nephrostomy (use of endoscope to visualize stone, with special attachment to extract stone)	Kidney	Small flank incision
Percutaneous ultrasonic lithotripsy (use of sound waves directed by probe inserted via cystoscopy or nephrostomy to break up stone)	Bladder, ureter, or kidney	No incision for cystoscopy Small flank incision for nephrostomy
Extracorporeal shock wave lithotripsy (use of sound waves while client's flank area is under water)	Kidney or upper ureter	No incision
Pyelolithotomy (direct visualization and removal of stone)	Renal pelvis	Large flank incision
Nephrolithotomy (same as for pyelolithotomy)	Kidney	Large flank incision
Pyeloureterolithotomy (same as for pyelolithotomy)	Ureter	Large flank or lower abdominal incision

in the flank and the introduction of an endoscope to visualize the interior of the renal pelvis. After visualization, the stone may be extracted by using a forceps or by basketing. Subsequently, a nephrostomy tube is placed to ensure urine drainage.

Percutaneous ultrasonic lithotripsy is a procedure in which sound waves are directed by an ultrasonic probe inserted via nephrostomy or cystoscopy to break up stones and to allow urinary elimination of fragments. The route of insertion depends on the site of the stone. A percutaneous route via nephrostomy is selected for calculi in the renal pelvis or upper ureter. A transurethral route via cystoscopy is required for calculi in the middle or lower ureter or bladder. Percutaneous ultrasonic lithotripsy is performed with the client under general or epidural anesthesia.

For extracorporeal shock wave lithotripsy, there is no incision. The client is allowed nothing by mouth for 8 hours before the procedure and receives epidural or general anesthesia. The client is positioned in a chair sling that provides support during submersion in the water bath. He or she is positioned so that the shock waves are directed toward the stone, which is visualized by fluoroscopy. During the procedure, cardiac rhythm is monitored by electrocardiography, and the shock waves are administered in synchrony with the R wave. Five hundred to 1500 shock waves are administered in 30 to 45 minutes; continuous electrocardiographic monitoring for ectopy and fluorscopic observation for stone disintegration are maintained. After lithotripsy proce-

dures, the urine may be strained to ensure elimination of stone fragments.

Pyelolithotomy, nephrolithotomy, and pyeloureterolithotomy are procedures that require a surgical incision and general anesthesia. Potential sites for the incision include the lumbar flank and abdomen. The pyelolithotomy involves a direct incision into the renal pelvis to remove the stone. With a nephrolithotomy, the renal parenchyma is incised for removal of the calculus. In a pyeloureterolithotomy, the ureter is surgically incised to remove the calculus. Because these procedures involve dissection through major muscle tissues, the period of postoperative healing is extended; 4 to 8 weeks or longer is required for convalescence.

Postoperative care. The nurse follows routine procedures for assessment of the client who has received anesthesia. Chapters 19 and 20 discuss routine operative and postoperative care for general surgery.

After a nephrolithotomy, the nurse inspects the flank for the presence of a nephrostomy tube. Leakage of urine around the nephrostomy tube may promote skin breakdown or allow bacterial entry. The drainage is frequently tinged with blood immediately after the operation. Frank bleeding is not expected. The nurse changes the dressings as necessary to prevent infection and to maintain a dry skin. Urinary output is measured hourly for 24 hours. An indwelling urinary catheter may be placed in addition to the nephrostomy drainage tube. The presence of large amounts of urine in the dressings makes accurate fluid intake and output records difficult.

Weighing the dressings is an option, but this is often inconvenient. A more practical and satisfactory solution is to monitor fluid status through measurement of blood pressure and daily weights.

After a pyelolithotomy, one or two Penrose drains are placed to facilitate removal of fluid that may be present around the site of incision. The drainage may also be blood tinged initially, but it becomes clear and generally colorless within 24 hours. The nurse changes these dressings frequently as necessary to maintain dry skin. An indwelling urinary catheter may also be placed; urinary output is measured hourly for the first 24 hours.

After a pyeloureterolithotomy, one or more Penrose drains are placed. If a flank incision was selected, the drains are in that region. If a lower abdominal incision was made, one or more drains are placed near that incision. In either case, a ureteral stent catheter is placed to ensure patency of the incised ureter. A *ureteral stent* is a hollow piece of tubing that has a narrower diameter than the ureter into which it is placed. It is placed to prevent closure of the ureter. The ureteral stent catheter and indwelling urinary catheter are usually removed within 3 to 5 days after the surgery. The nurse turns the client frequently to inspect the flank region for redness, swelling, or abnormal drainage. The nurse ensures that drainage catheters (ureteral, urethral, and/or nephrostomy) and dressings are secure, dry, and intact. Urinary output from each catheter is measured hourly and recorded separately for each site of drainage to account for adequate drainage from each kidney. These outputs are then totaled for explanation of overall urinary output.

Potential for Infection

Planning: client goals. The goals are that the client will (1) have no new infectious process and (2) be free from previously acquired infections.

Interventions: nonsurgical management. Control of infections before invasive and noninvasive procedures is critical to prevent the development of urosepsis. Nonsurgical interventions include the administration of appropriate antibiotics for elimination or prophylaxis of infection and the maintenance of adequate nutrition and fluid intake.

Drug therapy. Broad-spectrum antibiotics, such as the aminoglycosides (e.g., gentamicin) and cephalosporins (e.g., cephalexin [Keflex]), are prescribed initially for treatment of infections occurring with urologic stone disease. The broad coverage includes activity against gram-negative bacilli. After the results of the culture and sensitivity studies are obtained, more specific antibiotics are selected. Culture and sensitivity studies are done 48 hours after the initiation of antibiotic therapy and again 48 hours after the conclusion of the prescribed course of therapy. In addition, blood levels of antibiotics are measured to ensure that appropriate levels of the antibiotic have been obtained. If the desired blood level of antibiotic is exceeded, toxicity and renal damage may result. If the blood level of antibiotic is inadequate, bactericidal or fungicidal effects will not be achieved. New clinical evidence of an infectious process, such as chills, fever, or altered mental status, warrants the collection of a urine sample for culture and sensitivity tests.

Diet therapy. The diet of the client ideally includes adequate caloric intake representing a balance of all food groups. In addition, the nurse encourages the client to consume 2 to 3 L of fluid per day. The nurse discourages an excessive fluid intake (more than 3 L) because serum dilution of antibiotic levels and more rapid urinary excretion of the drug may result.

Potential for Injury

Planning: client goals. The goal is that the client will remain free from urinary obstruction.

Interventions: nonsurgical management. Measures to prevent urinary obstruction from stone disease include a high intake of fluids (3 L or more per day) and attention to changes in voiding pattern or volume. Nonsurgical interventions depend on the type of stone formation occurring. Medications, dietary modification, and fluid intake are the major strategies available.

Drug therapy. Drugs prescribed for prevention of obstruction depend on the type of problem promoting the stone formation and the type of stone being formed. Hypercalciuria is the most prevalent abnormality associated with the formation of stones; there are several types of hypercalciuria. The drug treatment prescribed depends on the nature of the disorder. Medications may include thiazide diuretics (e.g., chlorothiazide [Diuril] or hydrochlorothiazide [Hydrodiuril]), orthophosphate, and sodium cellulose phosphate. For clients with hyperoxaluria, drug prescriptions may include allopurinol (Zyloprim) and/or vitamin B_6 (pyridoxine). Allopurinol may also be prescribed for hyperuricuria. Antibiotics, such as the penicillins, and acetohydroxamic acid may be prescribed for clients with struvite stones. Medications such as 50% sodium citrate may be prescribed to alkalinize the urine.

Diet therapy. As with medications, dietary modification needs to be individualized on the basis of the type of stone formed. The nurse consults with the dietitian to plan the appropriate diet for the client. If the client forms stones containing calcium (calcium phosphate or calcium oxalate), the diet is modified to limit calcium-containing foods. With limitation of dairy foods and others high in calcium, the dietary calcium intake will be approximately 400 to 500 mg/day. In some clients who decrease their dietary calcium intake, oxalate production increases. Consequently, sources of oxalate intake may also need to be limited. Oxalate is found in dark green foods like spinach; absorption of oxalate increases when calcium intake decreases. For clients who form uric acid stones, a reduced intake of foods containing purines, such as boned fish and organ meats, is encouraged. Rich foods, such as organ meats, red wines, and gravies, need to be avoided (see Key Features of Disease: Causes and Treatments of Renal Stones for a summary of dietary modifications).

Other measures. The client is encouraged to ambulate frequently to promote passage of the calculi. A liberal fluid intake of at least 3 L/day assists in preventing dehydration, promotes the flow of urine, and decreases the chances of crystals' precipitating into stones. The pH of the urine is checked daily, and the urine is strained by using filter paper for collection of passed stone fragments.

■ Discharge Planning

Preparation for discharge after treatment for urologic stone disease may be minimal or complex. The age and general health status of the client, as well as the type of treatment intervention, influence the client's discharge planning.

Home Care Preparation

If the client has the support of family or a significant other, the nurse includes those persons in the assessment and planning for home care. In many instances, no additional home care is necessary. The nurse may suggest that home care assistance be considered by clients who live alone, or whose families or significant others are not available or able to provide the needed supportive care.

Client/Family Education

The nurse instructs the client and family about medications to combat infection or alter the pH of the urine. The client is advised to self-administer the entire prescription of antibiotics to ensure eradication of urinary pathogens. The client is also instructed in the use of urinary reagent strips to test the pH of the urine; urinary pH testing should be done daily. The client is advised to resume usual activities of daily living and to balance regular exercise with sleep and rest. The client may return to work within 2 to 6 weeks after surgery, depending on personal tolerance and the physician's directives. On the basis of the type of stone-forming process, if identified, the nurse instructs the client to consume a diet that minimizes calcium-containing or other foods (such as organ meats) that are known to promote calculus formation. Regardless of the cause of stone formation, a nutritious, balanced diet is encouraged. The intake of at least 3 L of fluid per day is encouraged. The nurse instructs the client about the rationale for preventing dehydration and promoting urine flow. Drains and catheters are removed before discharge. The nurse instructs the client to keep the incision line dry until after the sutures are removed and the skin is intact. The nurse also instructs the client about the symptoms of recurrent infection, such as fever, chills, and general malaise. The nurse explains the purpose, method, and duration of administration of prescribed medications, including route, frequency, and expected and undesired side ef-

fects. The nurse teaches the client to shower, to avoid a tub bath, and to use a clean towel to pat dry a healing incision. The nurse also instructs the client about symptoms of recurrent UTI and wound infection.

Psychosocial Preparation

The nurse helps the client to prepare emotionally for resumption of self-care and health maintenance through provision of information pertinent to the client's needs and concerns. The client often experiences tremendous anxiety and fear that a stone and its related pain may recur in the future. In addition to anxiety about the pain, the thought of the need for repeated surgical interventions is a factor of tremendous concern. Although the memories of the pain are blunted over time, the intensity of the experience is not forgotten. The client should obtain reassurance from knowledge of preventive and health promotion activities designed to prevent recurrence. Psychosocial preparation is generally enhanced when clients know what to expect and what actions to take should unexpected developments arise.

Health Care Resources

Health care resources that may be of interest to the client include the National Kidney Foundation, including local chapters and affiliates. This organization has literature written specifically for client education. Other resources include hospital and community libraries and clinical nurse specialists, who provide education and counseling.

Evaluation

The nurse evaluates the care of the client with renal or urologic stone disease and expects that the following outcomes are attained. The client

1. Demonstrates knowledge about preventive health actions related to dietary modification, fluid intake, and medication administration
2. Can follow self-care routines necessary to return of usual activities of daily living
3. Demonstrates knowledge of the symptoms of infection and of the presence of an obstruction of urine flow
4. Describes measures to minimize discomfort and to seek medical attention as appropriate

---

HYDRONEPHROSIS/HYDROURETER/ URETHRAL STRICTURE

OVERVIEW

Hydronephrosis and hydroureter are disorders that are usually associated with obstruction of the outflow of urine. Urethral strictures also obstruct outflow. Prompt recognition and treatment are crucial for preventing permanent renal damage.

In *hydronephrosis*, the kidney becomes enlarged as urine accumulates in the pelvis and the calyceal system. The capacity of the renal pelvis is normally 5 to 8 mL. Therefore, obstructions within the pelvis or the ureteropelvic junction quickly result in renal pelvic distention. As the volume of urine grows, the calyces dilate and the medulla endures increasing pressure. Over time, which may be a matter of hours, extensive damage to the vasculature and the renal tubules can result (Fig. 58–4).

In *hydroureter*, the pathophysiologic effects are similar but the level of obstruction is lower in the urinary tract. The ureter is most likely to become obstructed at the point of the iliac vessel's crossing or the ureterovesical entry. Consequently, dilation of the ureter proximal to the point of obstruction results in enlargement as the urine continues to accumulate (see Fig. 58–4).

With *urethral stricture*, the point of obstruction is the most distal in the urinary tract. Consequently, bladder distention occurs before hydroureter and hydronephrosis. The pathologic sequelae may be similar, however, if treatment is not promptly implemented.

In urinary tract obstruction, pressure builds up directly on tissue, which can cause structural damage. In addition, within the nephron, the tubular filtrate pressure increases as drainage through the collecting system is impaired. With the increase in tubular filtrate pressure, the force opposing glomerular filtration is enhanced. Consequently, glomerular filtration decreases or ceases and renal failure results. Nitrogenous waste products (BUN, creatinine, and uric acid) are retained in the serum; electrolytes (sodium, potassium, chloride, phosphorus, and calcium) are not excreted; and renal regulation of acid-base balance is impaired.

Disorders with the potential to cause hydronephrosis or hydroureter include tumors, stones, trauma, congenital structural defects, and retroperitoneal fibrosis. Therefore, the treatment of these disorders can prevent the development of hydronephrosis and hydroureter. When treatment is initiated promptly, there is an increased likelihood that permanent renal damage will not occur. The specific time needed to prevent permanent damage is uncertain and depends on the underlying renal status of the client. For some clients, permanent damage may occur within less than 48 hours; for others, several weeks of obstruction may transpire before permanent damage is detected. Pregnancy may result in ureteral dilation as the uterus enlarges and presses forward onto the ureter and bladder. Urethral stricture is most likely the result of chronic inflammation and resulting stricture formation from scar tissue. The urologic disorders that can lead to chronic renal failure are given in the accompanying Key Features of Disease.

COLLABORATIVE MANAGEMENT

The nurse obtains the history from the client with known or suspected hydronephrosis or hydroureter and focuses on known renal or urologic disorders. A history of childhood urinary tract problems may signal that structural defects are present and not previously identified. The nurse inquires about the client's pattern of urination and seeks specific information such as the amount, frequency, color, clarity, and odor of urine. The nurse questions the client about recent flank or abdominal pain. Chills, fever, and malaise may be present if a UTI exists.

The nurse inspects each flank area to identify asymmetry, which may occur if a renal mass is present. The abdomen is gently palpated to identify any areas of tenderness. The nurse measures blood pressure, pulse rate, respiratory rate, and temperature; the nurse weighs the client. The nurse palpates and percusses the urinary bladder to detect distention. Gentle pressure on the abdomen may result in leakage of urine, which is a manifestation of a full urinary bladder, and possible obstruction of the bladder/urethral junction.

The urinalysis may show bacteria or white blood cells if infection is present. With prolonged urinary tract obstruction, microscopic examination of the urine may demonstrate the presence of tubular epithelial cells. The chemical analysis of serum is normal unless decreased glomerular filtration has occurred; with decreased GFR, serum creatinine and BUN levels increase. Serum electrolyte levels may also be altered and indicate hyperka-

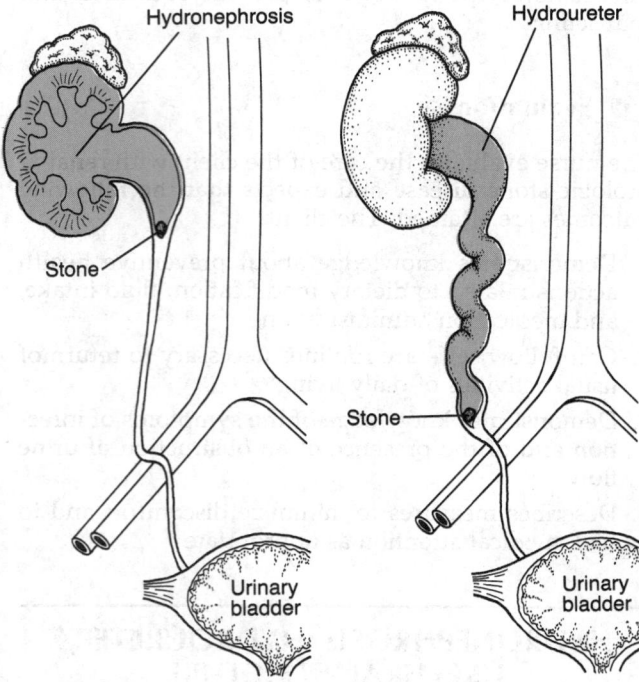

Figure 58–4

Hydronephrosis is caused by obstruction in the upper part of the ureter; hydroureter is caused by obstruction in the lower part of the ureter.

KEY FEATURES OF DISEASE ■ Urologic Disorders That Can Cause Chronic Renal Failure

Congenital Disorders

Adult polycystic kidney disease
Reflux nephropathy

Infectious or Obstructive Disorders

Chronic pyelonephritis
Neurogenic bladder
Bilateral nephrocalcinosis

Incontinence

Diversions resulting in frequent infections of the upper
    urinary tract

Glomerular Disorders

Chronic glomerulonephritis
Rapidly progressing glomerulonephritis
Nephrotic syndrome (variable)

Degenerative Disorders

Nephrosclerosis (essential hypertension)
Renal artery stenosis
Diabetic nephropathy
Atheroembolic disease

Neoplastic Disorders

Renal carcinoma with nephrectomy in clients with a
    solitary kidney
Multiple myeloma

Traumatic Disorders

Bilateral renal pedicle injury resulting in bilateral
    nephrectomy

lemia, hyperphosphatemia, hypocalcemia, and metabolic acidosis (bicarbonate deficit).

IVP demonstrates ureteral or renal pelvis dilation. Obstruction of urinary outflow can also be demonstrated by ultrasonography (renal echography) or CT.

Urinary retention and potential for infection are the primary problems resulting from hydronephrosis, hydroureter, and urethral stricture. Methods of correcting obstruction related to stone disease are discussed earlier in this chapter. Additional interventions for treatment of obstruction related to trauma, tumor, or structural abnormality are discussed in those sections. Failure to treat the cause of urinary obstruction may lead to infection and result in renal failure.

TUMORS

BENIGN TUMORS

Benign growths of the urinary tract include *cysts* and *benign tumors* of the renal parenchyma or urinary bladder. Because malignant growths may occur within cystic structures, thorough evaluation is essential. A simple renal cyst grows out of renal parenchymal tissue, usually the cortical tissue. The cyst is filled with fluid and as it enlarges can result in local tissue destruction. Many cysts are not symptomatic and are discovered accidently during fluoroscopic examination or during autopsy.

The exact etiology of a renal cyst is unknown. Cysts are usually considered to be an embryonic developmental defect. Similarly, the etiology of benign tumors is unknown. There are no accurate figures to indicate the incidence of renal cysts. There are no known methods to prevent the development of renal cysts or benign tumors.

Diagnosis of a simple cyst of the kidney involves the use of IVP, ultrasonography, and/or CT. If the cyst appears to be filled with fluid at urographic examination, ultrasonography is generally recommended. If the cyst appears to be more dense, a CT scan is done. Treatment may consist of percutaneous aspiration of a fluid-filled cyst or surgical exploration with potential for total or subtotal nephrectomy.

RENAL CELL CARCINOMA

OVERVIEW

Renal cell carcinoma is also referred to as *adenocarcinoma* or *hypernephroma*. The last term is outdated but frequently used.

Pathophysiology

As with other malignant neoplasms, the healthy functional tissue of the kidney is replaced and displaced by the growth of abnormal, nonfunctional cells. Although the exact mechanism of development is not known, it is generally believed that the tumor cells originate in the proximal convoluted tubules of the nephron. The reader is referred to Chapter 24 for a discussion of the pathophysiology of cancer.

Pathophysiologic effects commonly associated with renal cell carcinoma include fever, anemia, erythrocytosis, hypercalcemia, liver dysfunction, and other miscellaneous hormonal effects. The cause of the fever is unknown, but pyrogens produced by the tumor cells have been suggested. The anemia and the erythrocytosis may appear to be contradictory. There is some blood loss from hematuria, but the amount lost is not considered to be consistent with the degree of anemia. Erythrocytosis may originate from erythropoietin production from the tumor cells. The production of parathyroid hormone from the tumor cells may be the cause of the hypercalcemia; other hormone alterations include increased renin levels, potentially accounting for the hypertension, and increased human chorionic gonadotropin levels, which are accompanied by decreased libido and changes in secondary sex characteristics. The cause of changes in liver function studies is not known.

Renal tumors are categorized into four stages. Stage I involves tumors that are within the capsule of the kidney; the renal vein, perinephric fat, and adjacent nodes have no tumor. Stage II tumors extend beyond the capsule but are within Gerota's fascia; the renal vein and nodes are not involved. Stage III tumors extend into the renal vein and/or nodes. Stage IV tumors include invasion of adjacent organs or metastasis to distant tissues (Garnick & Richie, 1986).

Complications include metastasis and urinary tract obstruction. Metastasis is usually via blood or lymph to the liver, lungs, long bones, or other kidney. Direct tumor invasion surrounding the ureter may result in hydroureter and urinary tract obstruction.

Etiology

The exact etiology of renal cell carcinoma is unknown. There are links between this type of cancer and tobacco use, as well as exposure to chemicals such as lead, phosphate, and cadmium. Other studies seek to explore the possibility of genetic transmission and the meaning of observed chromosome translocations.

Incidence

Renal malignancies account for approximately 3% of reported cancers. The 5-year survival rates for 1979 to 1984 for Caucasians and Blacks, respectively, were 51% and 53% (American Cancer Society, 1989).

COLLABORATIVE MANAGEMENT

 Assessment

History

The nurse asks the client about general perceptions of overall health and ability to pursue activities of daily living. Specific information to be obtained includes the following: *age, sex,* presence of *known risk factors such as smoking or environmental exposures, history of weight loss, changes in color of urine, abdominal or flank discomfort,* and *fever. Hematuria,* a late sign, is frequently observed, and urine may appear smoky or cola colored.

Physical Assessment: Clinical Manifestations

The nurse inspects the flank areas of the client and notes *asymmetry* or obvious protrusions. An *abdominal*

mass may be detected through palpation; palpation techniques should be gentle. The nurse inspects the *skin* for pallor, increased areolar pigmentation of the nipples, and gynecomastia. *Muscle wasting, weakness,* generally *poor nutritional status,* and *weight loss* may also be found. *Blood in the urine* may also be grossly observable as bright red flecks or clots. With microscopic evidence of hematuria, the urine may appear smoky or cola colored. Hematuria may even be absent on microscopic examination. The nurse inquires about the nature of the discomfort; terms used to describe the pain typically include *dull* and *aching.* If bleeding into the tumor occurs, the pain may be more intense. All of these symptoms tend to occur later in the disease process.

Psychosocial Assessment

Anxiety and fear are responses to be expected in clients with known or suspected renal neoplasms. The client may also have denied or minimized the presence of symptoms and thus guilt feelings related to a delay in seeking medical attention are common. The client may fear that death from the cancer may occur or that kidney failure could result. Anxieties about potential effects of treatment such as chemotherapy or radiation represent other concerns. Chapter 25 describes the psychosocial concerns of the client with cancer.

Laboratory Findings

The urinalysis may reveal the presence of red blood cells. Hematologic studies reveal decreased hemoglobin and hematocrit values, increased erythrocyte sedimentation rate, hypercalcemia, and increased levels of adrenocorticotropic hormone, human chorionic gonadotropin, cortisol, and renin. Increased parathyroid hormone levels may also be detected.

Radiographic Findings

Detection of renal masses may occur incidentally through surgical explorations, IVP, or other fluoroscopic procedures of the abdomen. Nephrotomograms are useful for further delineation if a mass is apparent during IVP procedures. Subsequently, delineation of the mass and surrounding structures is accomplished via CT. Staging of the degree of localization or the extent of spread of the tumor is best accomplished via renal arteriography and renal venography.

 Analysis: Nursing Diagnosis

Common Diagnoses

The common diagnoses in the client with renal cancer include

1. Potential for injury related to possible metastases or recurrence of cancer
2. Anxiety and fear related to diagnostic and therapeutic options

Additional Diagnoses

Additional diagnoses may include

1. Pain related to the tumor mass
2. Knowledge deficit related to diagnostic and treatment procedures
3. Altered patterns of urinary elimination related to urinary tract obstruction
4. Altered nutrition: less than body requirements related to increased metabolic demands
5. Activity intolerance related to discomfort and weakness
6. Anxiety and fear of dying or the dying process

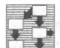 ## Planning and Implementation

Potential for Injury

Planning: client goals.   The goal for this nursing diagnosis is that the client will not experience metastasis or recurrence of the cancer.

Interventions.   Interventions to manage the potential for injury include prevention of known risk factors by smoking cessation or minimization of occupational exposure and early detection through regular physical examination. Surgery is usually the treatment of choice.

Nonsurgical management.   Chemotherapy for renal cell carcinoma has had limited effectiveness. A variety of agents, used singly and in combination, have been studied. Interleukin-2 has been approved by the U.S. Food and Drug Administration for expanded clinical trials. To date, chemotherapeutics and hormonal agents (e.g., progesterone and estrogen) have not been effective for control of tumor cell growth.

Surgical management.   Renal cell carcinoma is treated surgically by radical nephrectomy. In a *radical nephrectomy,* the entire kidney and adjacent adrenal gland, renal artery and vein, and surrounding Gerota's fascia are removed.

Preoperative care.   The nurse advises the client about routines associated with surgical intervention. The nurse explains the probable site of incision and the presence of postoperative dressings, drains, or other equipment. The nurse teaches the client about the need for postoperative breathing, exercises of the lower extremity, and early ambulation to prevent complications. The nurse also assures the client that pain management will be provided. Chapter 18 describes preoperative care of clients in detail.

Postoperative care.   In conducting the postoperative assessment, the nurse observes the abdomen for distention from bleeding and symptoms of adrenal insufficiency. The nurse observes bed linens under the client, who is in a supine position, because bleeding may be present. Hypotension, decreases in urinary output, and alterations in the level of consciousness may accompany hemorrhage or adrenal insufficiency. A decrease in blood pressure is one of the earliest manifestations of both hemorrhage and adrenal insufficiency. However, with hypotension, urinary output also decreases immediately. In adrenal insufficiency, there is a large loss of water and sodium in the urine; consequently, a large urinary output is followed by hypotension and subsequent oliguria (less than 400 mL/24 hours or less than 25 mL/hour). Intravenous replacement of fluids and packed red blood cells may be prescribed.

It is expected that the second kidney will provide adequate renal function. The nurse assesses the urinary output hourly for the first 24 hours postoperatively; a urine flow of 30 to 50 mL/hour is acceptable. Flow rates of less than 25 to 30 mL/hour suggest a decrease in renal perfusion. Hemoglobin level, hematocrit, and white blood cell count are measured every 6 to 12 hours postoperatively. Temperature, pulse rate, and respiratory rate are monitored at least every 4 hours; careful measurement and recording of fluid intake and output are also critical. The client is weighed daily. Frequently, the client is cared for in a critical care unit for 24 to 48 hours postoperatively to monitor for bleeding and/or adrenal insufficiency. A Penrose drain is placed near the site of incision, usually the abdomen, to ensure that residual fluid is removed. Because of the discomfort associated with lung expansion, the client is prone to develop atelectasis. The onset of fever, chills, thick sputum, or decreased breath sounds may suggest that pneumonia has developed.

Postoperatively, narcotic analgesics, such as meperidine (Demerol), hydromorphone (Dilaudid), and morphine sulfate, are given parenterally to provide adequate comfort. Acute pain control is more effectively achieved when sedatives such as promethazine hydrochloride (Phenergan) or hydroxyzine pamoate (Vistaril) are used in combination with the narcotic analgesic. Concerns about respiratory depression and a potential for addiction are usually not warranted. The site of the surgical incision, in which the major muscle groups associated with breathing and movement are involved, necessitates the liberal use of analgesic agents. The nurse expects that these medications may be required for 3 to 5 days. When food and fluids may be consumed orally, oral analgesic agents may be considered for pain management.

One or more antibiotics may be prescribed for intraoperative and postoperative prophylaxis. Usually, these agents are given as single-dose prescriptions. The need for additional antibiotics is based on clinical and laboratory evidence of the development of infection. Steroid replacements may be necessary if adrenal insufficiency is present.

Radiation therapy may follow radical nephrectomy if either presumed total removal or known incomplete removal has not been effective in altering the 5-year survival statistics. As for chemotherapy, studies continue for the identification of an adjuvant therapy to accompany surgical intervention.

Anxiety; Fear

Planning: client goals. The goal for these diagnoses is that the client will state that she or he is less anxious and fearful after nursing interventions.

Interventions: nonsurgical management. Interventions to manage the anxiety and fear include the provision of reassurance, explanations, and opportunities for verbalization of concerns. The nurse educates and counsels the client about all aspects of the diagnostic and treatment regimen. When encouraging the client to verbalize concerns, fears, and expectations, the nurse provides factual information and clarifies misconceptions. The process of staging for extent of metastatic spread of the carcinoma requires time, during which anxiety is heightened. The nurse listens to verbalizations by the client to identify particular persons who could assist in providing support. The client's or the hospital's clergy or religious leader may be of assistance.

■ **Discharge Planning**

The nurse explores with the client and family or significant other the anticipated needs for posthospital care. Resources such as home care assistance and social services personnel and transportation requirements should be considered. The age and overall health status of the client are other variables that may influence the discharge planning process.

Home Care Preparation

Preparation for home care varies depending on the availability of family, friends, or significant others to provide assistance during the immediate posthospitalization period. Shortened postoperative hospital stays result in the discharge of clients who may be considerably weakened by surgery or other treatment. Client may be limited to climbing stairs once a day for a week or so. If so, preparations for providing a place to rest, bathroom facilities, or preparation of meals may be required.

Client/Family Education

The nurse instructs the client and family or significant other about proper care of the surgical incision. In most instances, the incision requires no specific local care. If a dressing is placed over the incision, it should be changed at least daily or when drainage is present. Showering is permitted as soon as the client is able. Some clients prefer a light dressing to protect the site from the irritation of clothing. The nurse advises the client to obtain regular exercise and rest periods; driving and climbing stairs may not be permitted for 1 to 2 weeks postoperatively. Lifting of heavy objects, major physical activities associated with housework, and participation in sports should be avoided for 4 to 6 weeks. The nurse explores specific recommendations about the resumption of activities with the surgeon because individualized recommendations are often necessary.

Psychosocial Preparation

The nurse assists the client in preparing emotionally for discharge from the hospital by discerning the areas of concern and anxiety in the individual client. Because the client's perceptions of concerns and potential problems vary from person to person, the nurse determines areas in which more intensive education and counseling are required. The nurse assesses the client and the significant other's need for information and the level of information requested. For some clients, in-depth information is necessary to allay anxiety. For others, minimal information to comply with the recommendations is the coping strategy. The client may worry about the loss of the other kidney and a need for chronic dialysis or may fear death from the disease process. Refer to Chapter 25 for further discussion of the psychosocial effects of a diagnosis of cancer.

Health Care Resources

The American Cancer Society affiliates and chapters provide educational materials and programs to support the therapeutic plan. Oncology clinical nurse specialists also provide educational counseling and support during the pre- and postoperative and convalescent periods.

 Evaluation

The nurse evaluates the effectiveness of the interventions on the basis of outcomes expected for the nursing diagnoses. Expected outcomes include that the client

1. Verbalizes appropriate postoperative self-care measures related to hygiene, activities, exercise, and care of the incision
2. Demonstrates willingness to participate in the plan of care through self-administration of medications, attendance at outpatient chemotherapy or radiation therapy visits, and attendance at follow-up medical visits
3. Demonstrates a decrease in anxiety and an ability to cope with concerns
4. Experiences no postoperative complications such as atelectasis, hemorrhage, or adrenal insufficiency
5. Demonstrates comfort and ability to mobilize adequately

UROTHELIAL CANCER

OVERVIEW

Urothelial cancer refers to malignancies of the urothelium, which is the lining of transitional cells in the renal pelvis, ureters, urinary bladder, and urethra. Most urothelial tumors occur in the urinary bladder; consequently, *bladder cancer* is a general term that is sometimes used to describe this pathologic condition.

Pathophysiology

Staging classification for bladder cancer is given in the accompanying Key Features of Disease. Pathophysiologically, the urothelium is described initially according to the presence of a dysplasia. The exact type of cellular alteration is nonspecific in the first stages. In the second stage of cell growth, the superficial lesions are said to be flat or papillary; the lesions may be either high or low grade. The third stage refers to local invasion of tissues, e.g., the bladder wall or ureters. The fourth stage represents metastasis into the lymphatics or vasculature. The effects of cellular and tissue invasion from tumor include local inflammation, ischemia, hemorrhage, and obstruction. If the bladder cancer is untreated, death results from hemorrhage or renal failure from urinary tract obstruction.

Etiology

A variety of etiologic agents have been associated with the development of bladder cancer. Active and passive consumption of cigarette smoke is highly linked with the development of bladder cancer. Various environmental and occupational agents have been implicated and studied to determine the potential for bladder cancer after exposure. To date, the lack of ability to quantify and compare among and between studies the amount and specific type of agent limits the ability to identify specific etiologic agents. Chemicals that have been studied and implicated, but not confirmed, include dyes, metals, paints, rubber by-products, and organic chemicals. Coffee and artificial sweeteners have also been explored for the risk for inducing bladder cancer. Studies are weakly positive and not believed to indicate a significant influence on the development of bladder cancer. Other factors that are associated with the development of bladder cancer include chronic infections, bladder stones, and chronic abuse of phenacetin-containing analgesics.

Incidence

The incidence of bladder cancer was estimated at 47,000 new cases in the United States in 1989, affecting males about three times more often than females. About 7% of new cancer diagnoses in males and about 3% of new cancer diagnoses in females are bladder cancer diagnoses. It is the 5th most common cancer in males and the 10th most common cancer in females. Persons living in northern states demonstrate a greater frequency of development of bladder cancer than those living in southern states. The frequency of onset increases after the fifth or sixth decade of life.

PREVENTION

On the basis of the available studies, exposure to cigarette smoke would appear to be the single most influential factor contributing to the development of bladder cancer. Consequently, if one were to consider methods to prevent bladder cancer, it would seem that efforts to curtail exposure to cigarette smoke would be a helpful preventive action. Risks are also associated with certain occupations, such as rubber and leather working and those in which workers are exposed to certain dyes (American Cancer Society, 1989).

KEY FEATURES OF DISEASE ■ Staging Classification for Bladder Cancer

Primary Tumor (T)

TX	Primary tumor cannot be assessed
T0	No evidence of primary tumor
Tis	Carcinoma in situ: "flat tumor"
Ta	Noninvasive papillary carcinoma
T1	Tumor invades subepithelial connective tissue
T2	Tumor invades superficial muscle (inner half)
T3	Tumor invades deep muscle or perivesical fat
T3a	Tumor invades deep muscle (outer half)
T3b	Tumor invades perivesical fat
T4	Tumor invades any of the following: prostate, uterus, vagina, pelvic wall, abdominal wall

Lymph Node (N)

NX	Regional lymph nodes cannot be assessed
N0	No regional lymph node metastasis
N1	Metastasis in a single lymph node, 2 cm or less in greatest dimension
N2	Metastasis in a single lymph node, more than 2 cm but not more than 5 cm in greatest dimension, or multiple lymph nodes, none more than 5 cm in greatest dimension
N3	Metastasis in a lymph node more than 5 cm in greatest dimension

Distant Metastasis (M)

MX	Presence of distant metastasis cannot be assessed
M0	No distant metastasis
M1	Distant metastasis

Adapted from American Joint Committee on Cancer. (1988). Beahrs, O. H., Henson, D. E., Hutter, R. V. P., & Myers, M. H. (Eds). *Manual for staging of cancer* (3rd ed.). Philadelphia: J. B. Lippincott.

COLLABORATIVE MANAGEMENT

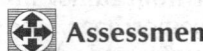 **Assessment**

History

The nurse inquires about the client's perception of general health. The nurse documents the *sex* and *age* for the client with known or suspected bladder cancer. The nurse inquires about active and passive exposure to *cigarette smoke* and describes the *occupation* of the client in detail for detection of potentially harmful environmental agents.

Physical Assessment: Clinical Manifestations

The nurse observes the overall appearance of the client and notes skin color and general nutritional status. The nurse inspects, percusses, and palpates the abdomen to detect evidence of asymmetry, tenderness, and bladder distention. The nurse asks the client specifically to describe the following: *change in color, frequency, or amount of urine* and any *abdominal discomfort*. The nurse also observes the urine for any changes in color or clarity. The *hematuria* that is associated with bladder cancer is usually *painless*. A *burning sensation during voiding, dysuria, frequency,* and *urgency* are potential symptoms because infection or obstruction may also be present.

Psychosocial Assessment

The nurse assesses the client's emotional response to known or suspected bladder cancer and notes anxiety, fear, sadness, anger, or guilt. Early symptoms are painless, and many clients deny the presence of hematuria because it is often intermittent. Consequently, the client may experience guilt and or self-anger about delays in seeking medical attention. The nurse assesses the client's personal methods of coping and the degree of support evident from family or significant others. Social interaction and active role relationships with others may provide support and motivation for coping with convalescence.

Laboratory Findings

Cytologic examinations of urine demonstrate the presence of abnormal cells.

Radiographic Findings

Cystoscopy with retrograde pyelography is the primary diagnostic method for evaluation of painless hematuria. IVP is particularly informative in delineating obstructions, especially at the ureterovesical junction. The CT scan is useful for demonstrating tumor invasion of surrounding tissues.

Other Diagnostic Tests

Flow cytometry is a diagnostic test in which the cells of the bladder epithelium are analyzed for deoxyribo-

nucleic acid (DNA) and ribonucleic acid (RNA) content. After several bladder irrigations, a collection of irrigant undergoes preparation to produce a suspension of cells. The cells are stained; some stains are specific for DNA, others stain RNA. The detection of cells with abnormal DNA staining reflects the presence of bladder cancer. Currently, the primary application of flow cytometry is for long-term follow-up of clients at high risk for bladder cancer or of those receiving conservative treatment.

Another informative study is ultrasonography, which demonstrates masses but is less valuable for tumor staging.

 Analysis: Nursing Diagnosis

Analysis of the assessment data provides the basis for the determination of the most common and additional nursing diagnoses.

Common Diagnoses

The common diagnoses include

1. Potential for injury related to metastasis or recurrence
2. Anxiety related to concern for body image, body functioning, and fear of death

Additional Diagnoses

Other possible diagnoses include

1. Knowledge deficit related to proposed diagnostic and treatment procedures
2. Fear related to possible death
3. Altered nutrition: less than body requirements related to increased metabolic needs

 Planning and Implementation

The nurse implements a plan designed to meet the individual needs of the client. The age, sex, and overall health status of the client are factors to be considered in the development of the plan. Because anxiety was just discussed for renal cell carcinoma, the following plan of care is for potential for injury.

Potential for Injury

Planning: client goals. The goal is that the client will not experience recurrence or metastasis.

Interventions. The usual therapy for the client with bladder cancer involves a variety of surgical procedures. Chemotherapy and radiation therapy are frequently adjunctive treatments but are rarely used alone. Refer to Chapter 24 for the care of the client receiving chemotherapy or radiation therapy.

Nonsurgical management. Specific chemotherapeutic agents for bladder cancer include thiotepa, cisplatin, doxorubicin (Adriamycin), and mitomycin (mitomycin C). Thiotepa and mitomycin may be instilled directly into the bladder (Baer & Williams, 1988). Radiation therapy may also be prescribed for treatment of bladder cancer.

Surgical management.   The client needs a means of diversion of urine because the cancerous bladder must be removed. Techniques for urinary diversion include the following: partial (segmental) or complete cystectomy, cutaneous ureterostomy and cutaneous ureteroureterostomy, ileal conduit (Bricker's procedure), colon conduit, ureterosigmoidostomy or ureteroileosigmoidostomy, and the continent internal ileal reservoir (Kock's pouch). Other techniques of removing smaller bladder tumors include cystoscopy with fulguration and open loop resection with fulguration. Urinary diversion procedures used for bladder cancer are described and illustrated in the accompanying Key Features of Disease.

In a *partial cystectomy*, a portion of the urinary bladder is removed. In general, this procedure is reserved for treatment of a solitary isolated bladder tumor. A *complete cystectomy*, also called a *radical cystectomy*, is usually performed for clients with a large, invasive bladder tumor or with a pelvic tumor that extends into the bladder. Extensive surgical dissection for removal of the bladder and adjacent muscles and tissues occurs with a complete cystectomy, and permanent urinary diversion is required.

In the *cutaneous ureterostomy*, one ureter is brought to the surface of the skin for the purpose of diverting urine. The urine is collected in an externally worn appliance or pouch, similar to that worn for an ileostomy, as shown in Chapter 45. For the *ureteroureterostomy*, one ureter is surgically joined to the other and a single cutaneous stoma is formed. The *bilateral cutaneous*, or *double-barrelled, ureterostomy* is a variation of these procedures in which the ureters lie side by side on the skin surface.

The *ileal conduit* is known by a variety of names, including ureteroileal urinary conduit, ileal bladder, ileal loop, Bricker's procedure, and ureteroileostomy. The ileal conduit is constructed by isolation of a portion of ileum from the small intestine. One end is closed, the segment is thoroughly irrigated, and the vascular, neural, and lymphatic supplies remain intact. One or both ureters may be surgically inserted into the isolated portion of ileum. Then, the open end of the ileum is brought to the surface of the skin. Urine exits from the ileal conduit into a pouch worn on the skin. The colon conduit is constructed similarly, but a portion of the sigmoid colon is isolated and brought to the surface of the skin for urinary diversion. A colon conduit results in fewer problems with stoma stricture and renal deterioration from infection compared with an ileal conduit. An exterior pouch for collection of urine is required with the colon conduit. Although the ileal conduit is more common than the colon conduit, neither procedure is as common as in the past. However, many clients still have functioning ileal and colon conduits, and surgical revision is usually not indicated or desired.

The *ureterosigmoidostomy* involves the surgical diversion of the ureters into the sigmoid. Urine empties into the rectum, and there is no control of urinary outflow. For the *ureteroileosigmoidostomy*, the ureters are diverted into a portion of the ileum that is isolated and anastomosed to the sigmoid. Urine exits by the rectum, and continence is not possible.

The *continent internal ileal reservoir (Kock's pouch)*, initially reported in 1982, represents a major advance in the treatment of clients with bladder cancer requiring cystectomy, or others with cutaneous urinary diversions. Many individuals have been treated with the Kock pouch after cystectomy or have had ileal conduits converted to the continent reservoir. Kock's pouch is created from a segment of ileum that has been isolated; the supply of blood and nerves remains intact. The pouch is created, and the ureters are implanted into the side of the pouch. Special nipple valves connect the pouch to the exterior of the skin and prevent reflux of urine into the renal pelvis from the points of ureteral entry into the pouch. Eventually, the client learns to catheterize the pouch and enjoys urinary continence without an exterior collecting device (Grieg, 1986).

Preoperative care.   The preoperative care for the client having a urinary diversion procedure includes discussion about the type of diversion and the selection of a site for the stoma. The goal is that the client will have a positive attitude about body image and a positive self-image. The nurse intervenes with educational counseling to ensure accurate understanding about self-care practices, methods of pouching, control of urine drainage, and minimization of odor. The site selected for the stoma should be visible and should avoid folds of skin, bones, and scar tissue. Ideally, the waistline or belt area of the client is avoided. The nurse prepares the client for the number and type of drains that will be present postoperatively.

Postoperative care.   Postoperatively, if a partial cystectomy was performed, the client has an indwelling Foley's catheter and a Penrose drain in the suprapubic region. If a complete cystectomy was performed, the urinary drainage is diverted via cutaneous ureterostomy or other ureteral diversion procedure.

After cutaneous ureterostomy or ureteroureterostomy, an external pouch covers the ostomy to collect the urine drainage. The location of the cutaneous ureterostomies may be on either side of the abdomen or side by side. For the ileal and colon conduits, the stoma is located below the waistline and usually to either side of midline. An external pouch collects urine from the diversion. Edema in the ileal stoma postoperatively may result in decreases in urinary output. The nurse assesses the client to prevent conduit distention. The larger diameter of the colon conduit decreases the likelihood of postoperative edema's impairing urinary output.

For the ureterosigmoidostomy or ureteroileosigmoidostomy, the client has some continence. Urine exits via the rectum with bowel movements and with the passage of flatus. Excoriation of the anal skin tissue can become a problem. Additional problems associated with this procedure involve long-term electrolyte abnormalities because of the ability of the intestinal mucosa to absorb

Text continued on page 1876

KEY FEATURES OF DISEASE ■ Urinary Diversion Procedures Used in the Treatment of Bladder Cancer

Diversion Procedure	Purpose	Site of Urinary Excretion
Ureterostomy Cutaneous ureterostomy	Diverts urine directly to the skin surface via a ureteral skin opening	Skin stoma; requires pouch

Cutaneous ureteroureterostomy

KEY FEATURES OF DISEASE ■ Urinary Diversion Procedures Used in the Treatment of Bladder Cancer *Continued*

Diversion Procedure	Purpose	Site of Urinary Excretion
Bilateral cutaneous ureterostomy		
Conduits Ileal (Bricker's) conduit	Collects urine in a portion of the intestine, which is then opened onto the skin surface as a stoma	Skin stoma; requires pouch

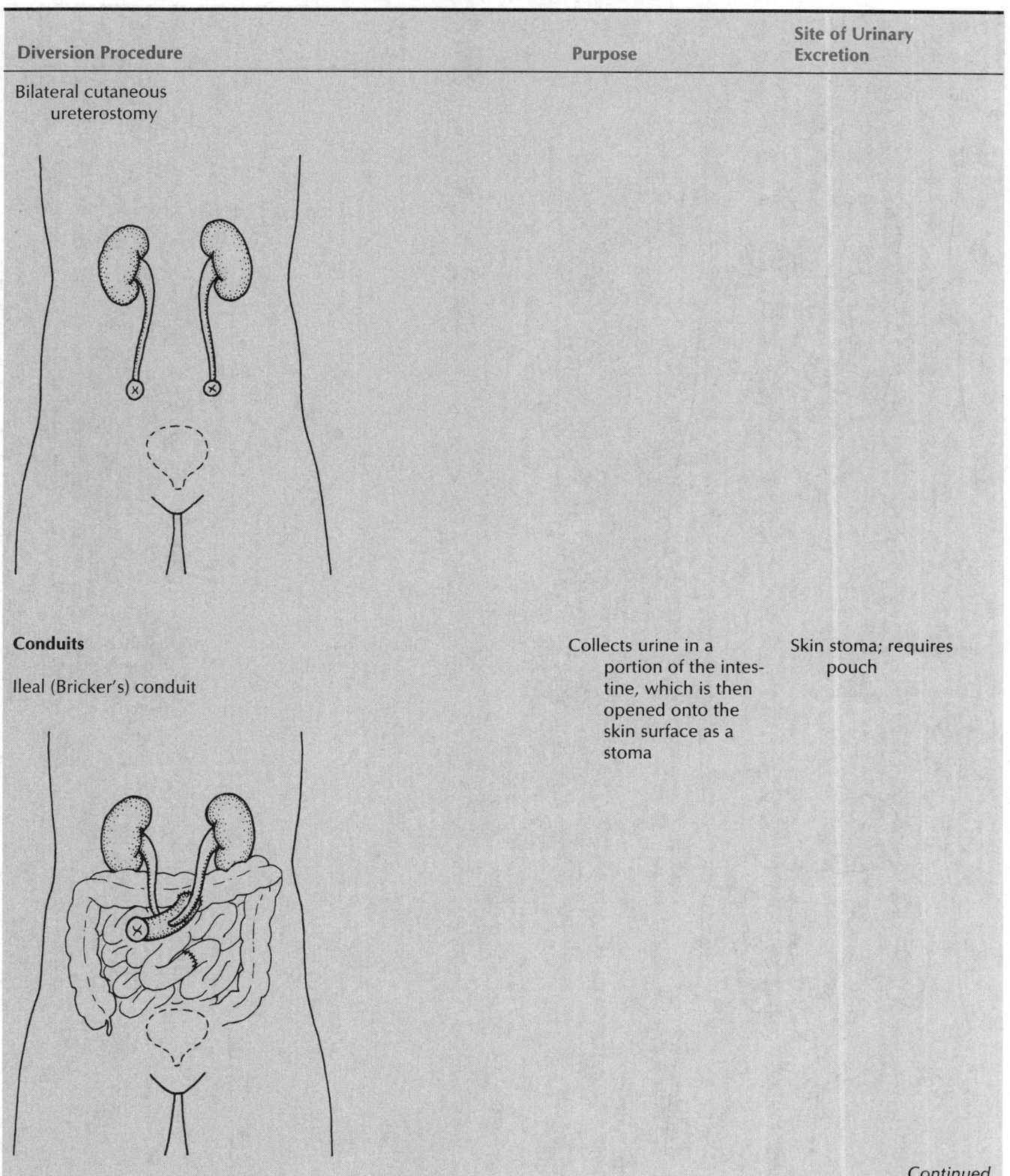

Continued

KEY FEATURES OF DISEASE ■ **Urinary Diversion Procedures Used in the Treatment of Bladder Cancer** *Continued*

Diversion Procedure	Purpose	Site of Urinary Excretion
Colon conduit		
Sigmoidostomy Ureterosigmoidostomy	Diverts urine to the large intestine	Anus, with bowel movements; client has urinary incontinence

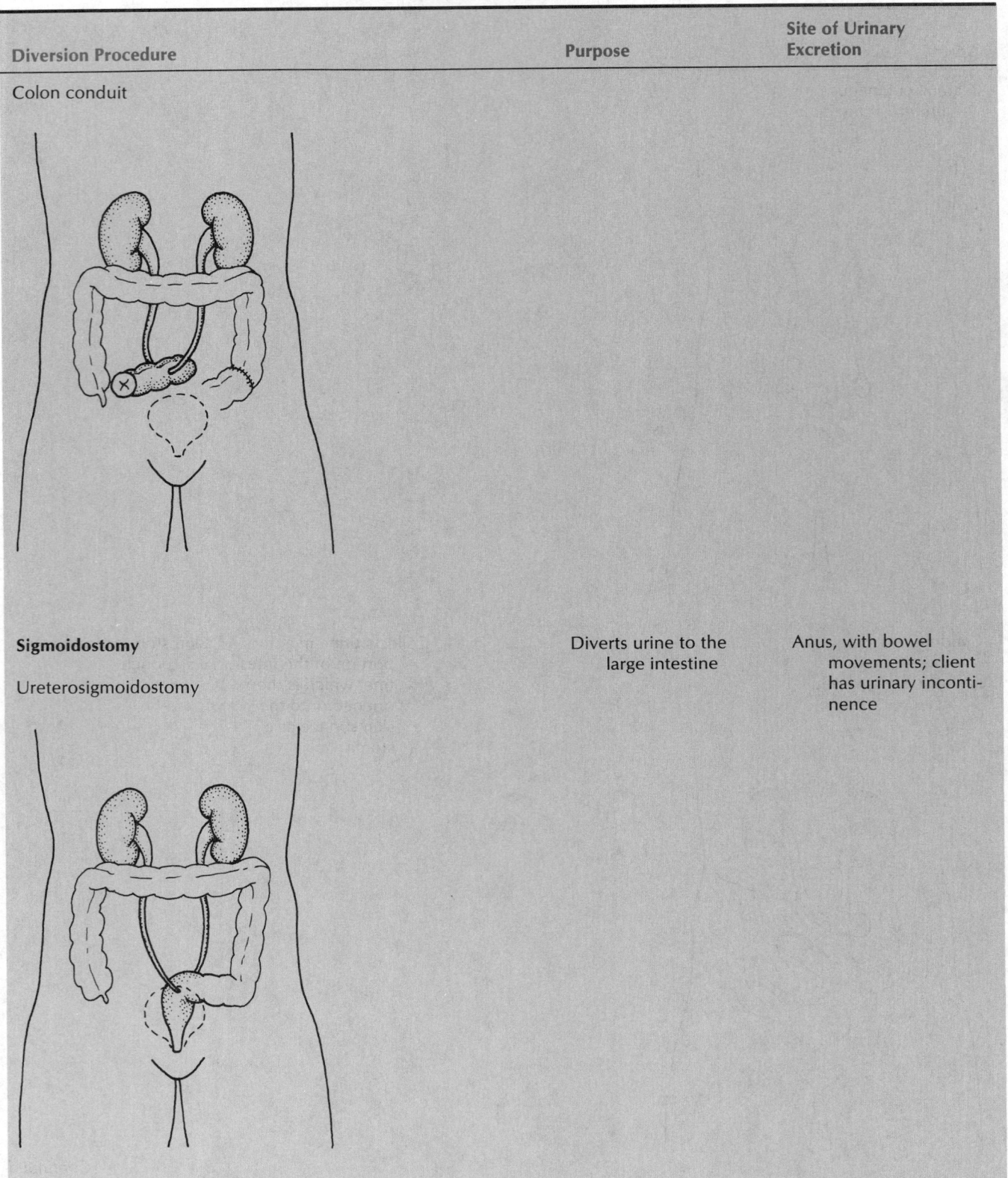

KEY FEATURES OF DISEASE ■ Urinary Diversion Procedures Used in the Treatment of Bladder Cancer *Continued*

Diversion Procedure	Purpose	Site of Urinary Excretion
Ureteroileosigmoidos-tomy		
Ileal Reservoir Continent internal ileal reservoir (Kock's pouch)	Diverts urine to a surgically created pouch or pocket that functions as a bladder	Stoma, via catheter

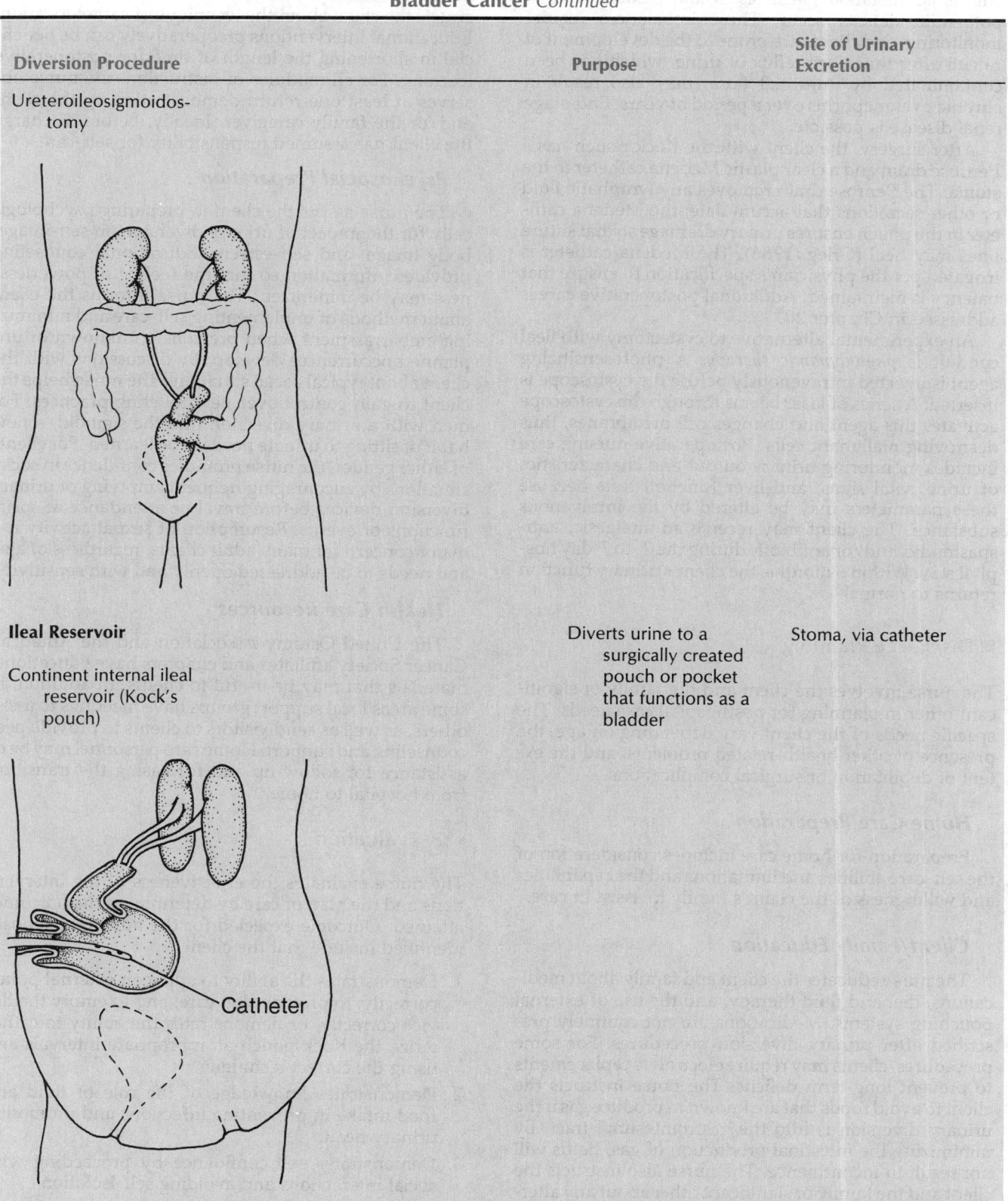

electrolytes from the urine. Sodium, chloride, and hydrogen are absorbed; bicarbonate is lost, and hyperchloremic metabolic acidosis results. Consequently, potassium deficits occur. These imbalances require monitoring, and clients are prone to the development of calculi after time. The reflux of urine, which has been contaminated by intestinal flora, may also result in chronic pyelonephritis over a period of years. End-stage renal disease is possible.

After surgery, the client with the Kock pouch has a Penrose drain and a clear plastic Medena catheter in the stoma. The Penrose drain removes any lymphatic fluid or other secretions that accumulate; the Medena catheter in the pouch ensures urinary drainage so that suture lines may heal (Grieg, 1986). The Medena catheter is irrigated per the physician's specification to ensure that patency is maintained. Additional postoperative care is addressed in Chapter 20.

An experimental alternative to cystectomy with ileal conduit is *photodynamic therapy*. A photosensitizing agent is injected intravenously before the cystoscope is inserted. A series of laser beams through the cystoscope activates this agent and changes cell membranes, thus destroying malignant cells. Postoperative nursing care includes monitoring urinary output and characteristics of urine, vital signs, and liver function tests because these parameters may be altered by the intravenous substance. The client may receive an analgesic, antispasmodic, and/or antibiotic during the 2- to 7-day hospital stay. Within 3 months, the client's urinary function returns to normal.

■ Discharge Planning

The nurse involves the client and the family or significant other in planning for posthospital care needs. The specific needs of the client vary depending on age, the presence of other health-related problems, and the extent of debilitation or surgical complications.

Home Care Preparation

Preparation for home care includes consideration of the self-care abilities and limitations and the capabilities and willingness of the client's family to assist in care.

Client/Family Education

The nurse educates the client and family about medications, diet and fluid therapy, and the use of external pouching systems. Medications are not routinely prescribed after urinary diversion procedures. For some procedures, clients may require electrolyte replacements to prevent long-term deficits. The nurse instructs the client to avoid foods that are known to produce gas if the urinary diversion is into the gastrointestinal tract. By minimizing the intestinal production of gas, flatus will not result in incontinence. The nurse also instructs the client and the family or significant other about any alterations in self-care activities that may have occurred as a result of the urinary diversion. The nurse demonstrates external pouch application, including local skin care, pouch care, methods of adhesion, and drainage mechanisms. If a Kock pouch has been created, the nurse instructs the client about the technique of catheterization. Educational interventions preoperatively can be beneficial in shortening the length of time for postoperative learning. For all modules of instruction, the nurse observes at least one return demonstration by the client and/or the family caregiver. Ideally, before discharge the client has assumed responsibility for self-care.

Psychosocial Preparation

The nurse assists the client in preparing psychologically for the impact of urinary diversion on self-image, body image, and self-esteem. Educational counseling provides information so that the feeling of powerlessness may be minimized. The nurse informs the client about methods of implementing self-care and minimizing embarrassment when previously unknown or unplanned occurrences develop. By discussions with the client about typical social situations, the nurse helps the client to gain control over new toileting practices. For men with a urinary diversion into the sigmoid, a new habit of sitting to urinate needs to be learned. For clients of either gender, the nurse promotes confidence in social situations by encouraging frequent emptying of urinary diversion devices before travel or attendance at social functions or events. Resumption of sexual activity is a major concern for many adult clients, regardless of age, and needs to be addressed openly and with sensitivity.

Health Care Resources

The United Ostomy Association and the American Cancer Society affiliates and chapters have educational materials that may be useful to clients. In addition, in some areas local support groups have meetings to assist others, as well as send visitors to clients to provide peer counseling and support. Home care personnel may be of assistance for follow-up and for easing the transition from hospital to home.

 Evaluation

The nurse evaluates the effectiveness of the interventions and the plan of care by determining the outcomes attained. Outcome expected for the nursing diagnoses identified include that the client

1. Demonstrates the ability to apply an external pouch correctly, to provide skin care, and to empty the device correctly, or demonstrates the ability to catheterize the Kock pouch at appropriate intervals and using the correct technique

2. Demonstrates knowledge of the role of fluid and food intake in preventing infections and promoting urinary health

3. Demonstrates self-confidence by proceeding with social interactions and avoiding self-isolation

4. Improves self-esteem and body image during adjustment phase

TRAUMA

RENAL TRAUMA

OVERVIEW

Trauma to one or both kidneys is always a concern when there are penetrating wounds or blunt injuries to the back, flank, or abdomen.

Pathophysiology

The pathophysiologic effect of trauma to the kidneys usually occurs as a result of decreased renal perfusion and thus ischemia. Injuries to the kidney are described as minor, major, or pedicle injuries. Figure 58–5 illustrates the common types and locations of minor and major kidney injuries. Ureteral and/or renal pelvic injury may cause diffuse abdominal pain, local collections of urine, and infection.

Minor injuries to the kidney include contusions, small lacerations, and disruption of the integrity of the parenchyma and the calyx (forniceal disruption). With a contusion, one or both kidneys sustain a bruise as a result of major impact. Small blood vessels may be damaged, resulting in some hematuria. One or more small lacerations may result in small, localized hematomas. There may also be a small hematoma at the site of forniceal disruption.

MINOR TRAUMA

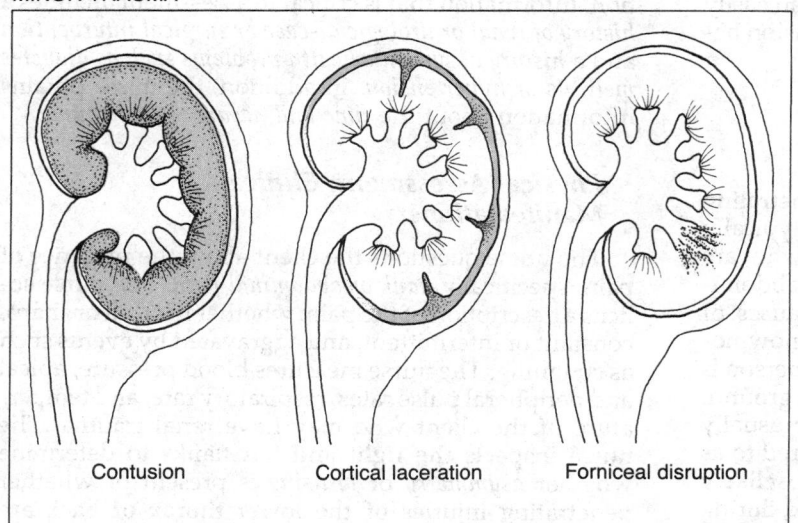

Contusion   Cortical laceration   Forniceal disruption

PEDICLE INJURY

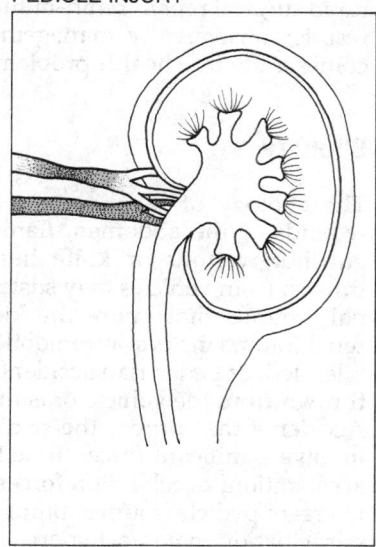

MAJOR TRAUMA

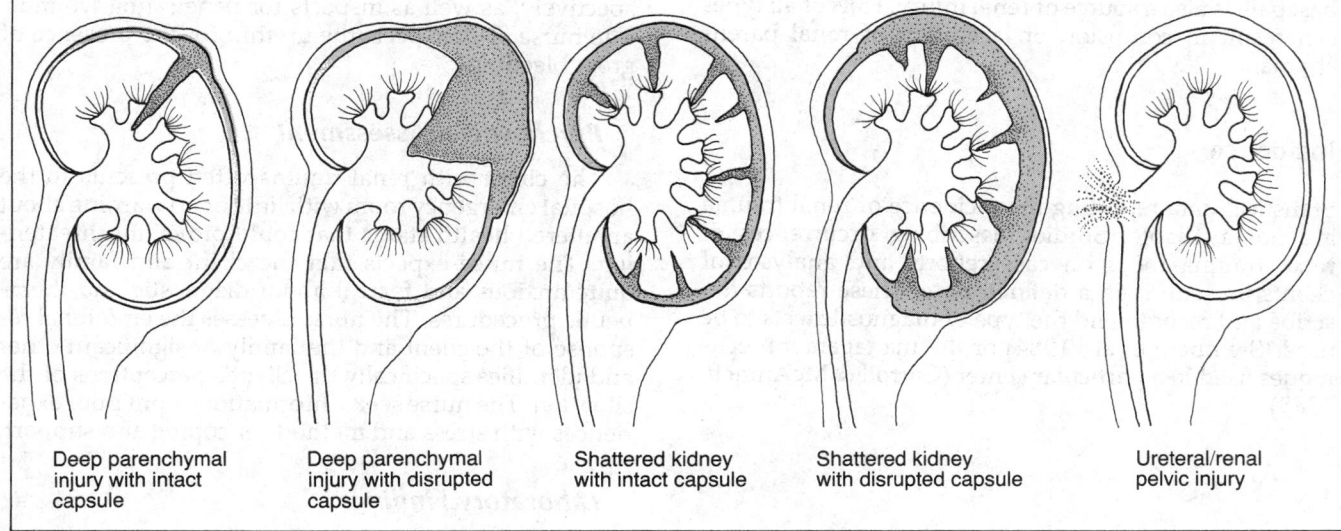

Deep parenchymal injury with intact capsule

Deep parenchymal injury with disrupted capsule

Shattered kidney with intact capsule

Shattered kidney with disrupted capsule

Ureteral/renal pelvic injury

Figure 58–5

Common types and locations of renal trauma.

Major injuries to the kidneys involve lacerations to the cortex, medulla, or one of the segmental branches of the renal artery or vein. Deep parenchymal injuries may extend throughout the kidney and result in hematomas that are contained within the capsule or that disrupt the capsule. Other parenchymal injuries involve the cortex and cause shattering of tissue, with either an intact or a disrupted capsule resulting from the hematoma. A major injury to the kidney is most likely to follow a penetrating abdominal, flank, or back wound. Bleeding is extensive and surgical exploration is often required. Because of the hemorrhage, hypoperfusion of renal parenchyma can produce renin-induced hypertension for either short- or long-term periods.

Pedicle injuries involve a laceration or disruption of the renal artery and/or renal vein. Hemorrhage is extensive and rapid; death may ensue quickly unless diagnosis and intervention are promptly initiated. Even with rapid surgical repair, renin-induced hypertension easily results; consequently, management of hypertension becomes a lifetime health problem.

Etiology

The etiology of renal trauma is diverse. Penetrating wounds of the abdomen, flank, or back are typically gunshot wounds or knife injuries. Clients who are thrown from vehicles may sustain penetrating abdominal wounds that injure the kidneys. Blunt causes of renal trauma include automobile, motorcycle, snowmobile, sled, or pedestrian accidents in which the person is thrown from the vehicle or is thrown from the ground. Accidents that propel the person into the air usually involve significant force; these forces are referred to as acceleration/deceleration forces and are the most likely to create pedicle injuries. Blunt trauma suffered during participation in contact sports, such as football, soccer, rugby, hockey, skiing (snow or water), basketball, and baseball, is also a source of renal injury. Falls of all types can result in contusion or laceration of renal parenchyma.

Incidence

Statistical data reporting the incidence of renal trauma are not available. Studies describing occurrences of renal trauma focus on case reports and analyses of clients presenting in a defined time. These reports describe and recommend the type of diagnostic tests to be used (Steinberg et al., 1984) or the management techniques used in a particular center (Carroll & McAninch, 1985).

PREVENTION

Renal trauma may be prevented by the exercise of some common sense practices and avoidance of certain high-risk behaviors. Common sense practices include use of

motor vehicle seat belts and appropriate caution when riding or driving motorcycles. Hitchhiking or walking along roadways increases the probability of being a pedestrian accident victim. For contact sports, conditioning and wearing protective pads may lessen the opportunities for injury. For clients with a solitary kidney, actions to prevent renal trauma can be lifesaving.

COLLABORATIVE MANAGEMENT

 Assessment

History

The nurse obtains a history of the client's personal health status and the events surrounding the trauma from the client or whoever has the necessary information. Information that is critical to assessment includes a *history of renal or urologic disease or surgical intervention* and a *history of systemic health problems such as diabetes mellitus or hypertension.* In addition, the nurse obtains information about the *time and nature of the trauma.*

Physical Assessment: Clinical Manifestations

The nurse questions the client about the presence of pain, specifically *flank or abdominal pain.* The nurse solicits a description of the pain: whether it is dull or sharp, constant or intermittent, and aggravated by events such as coughing. The nurse measures blood pressure, apical and peripheral pulse rates, respiratory rate, and temperature of the client who may have renal trauma. The nurse inspects the right and left flanks to determine whether *asymmetry* or *bruising* is present or whether penetrating injuries of the lower thorax or back are present. Similarly, the nurse inspects and percusses the abdomen for *ecchymoses* and *abdominal distention,* respectively, as well as inspects for penetrating wounds. The nurse also inspects the urethra for the presence of gross bleeding.

Psychosocial Assessment

The client with renal trauma often presents to the hospital emergency room with little or no warning about an altered health status that could prove life-threatening. The nurse expects that the client and family are quite anxious and fearful about diagnostic and therapeutic procedures. The nurse assesses the emotional response of the client and the family or significant other and identifies specifically the client's perceptions of the situation. The nurse seeks information about prior experiences with stress and methods of coping and support.

Laboratory Findings

The urinalysis commonly reveals the presence of hemoglobin or red blood cells that results from rupture of small or large renal blood vessels. Microscopic examination of the urine may also show red blood cell casts, which suggest tubular damage. The hemoglobin level and hematocrit are decreased with blood loss; the white blood cell count is increased with inflammatory processes, as might be the situation if the trauma had occurred several days previously.

Radiographic Findings

Fluoroscopic procedures performed for assessment of renal trauma include IVP, renal arteriography, and CT. IVP provides information on the number of kidneys present and the integrity and patency of the collecting system. Renal arteriography also demonstrates the number of kidneys present, but more specifically it describes the blood supply to each kidney. With pedicle injuries, contrast media extravasates from the ruptured vessels, and the renal parenchyma is not shown by nephrogram. The CT scan yields information also about the location of the injury and vascular and tissue integrity. Intracapsular and extracapsular hematomas are readily observable on the CT scan.

Other Diagnostic Tests

Renal ultrasonography is an alternative diagnostic procedure to IVP that allows the avoidance of radiopaque contrast media in clients with elevated serum creatinine levels.

 Analysis: Nursing Diagnosis

Common Diagnoses

The common diagnosis for the client with renal trauma includes

1. Altered (renal) tissue perfusion related to bleeding

Additional Diagnoses

In addition, some clients may experience one or more of the following:

1. Anxiety related to sudden onset of need for diagnostic and therapeutic interventions
2. Pain related to bruising or surgical incisions
3. Altered patterns of urinary elimination related to changes in renal perfusion
4. Post trauma response related to fear and anxiety associated with the precipitating events
5. Potential for infection related to loss of tissue integrity or exposure to pathogens

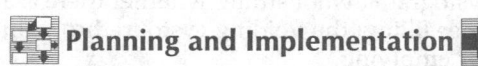 **Planning and Implementation**

Altered (Renal) Tissue Perfusion

Planning: client goals. The goal is that the client will have preserved renal function by ensuring adequate renal perfusion.

Interventions. Interventions for clients with altered renal tissue perfusion include medical and surgical interventions to restore intravascular volume and/or to ensure perfusion.

Nonsurgical management. Nonsurgical interventions for the client with altered renal tissue perfusion include medications for vascular support and fluid administration for restoration of fluid volume depletion.

Drug therapy. Medications, such as dobutamine (Dopamine), are prescribed for support of renal perfusion. This agent promotes peripheral vasoconstriction and elevates blood pressure. Low doses of dobutamine also enhance renal blood flow.

Fluid therapy. Fluid administration to restore circulating blood volume is critical for renal tissue perfusion. Crystalloid solutions, such as 0.9% sodium chloride, D_5 0.45% sodium chloride, and Ringer's solution, replace water and some electrolytes. Crystalloid solutions are usually readily available and are an initial replacement solution. When significant bleeding has occurred, whole blood or packed red cell replacement is necessary to restore oxygen-carrying capacity derived from hemoglobin. Plasma volume expanders such as dextran or albumin help to re-establish plasma oncotic pressure and to minimize fluid shift from the intravascular space to the interstitial fluid space. During fluid resuscitation or restoration efforts, the nurse administers the fluid at the prescribed rate and monitors the client for evidence of hemodynamic stability. The nurse monitors vital signs frequently, as often as every 5 to 15 minutes. In addition, the nurse measures and records urinary output hourly. Urinary output should be no less than 25 to 30 mL/hour. Specific urinary flow guidelines may be detailed by the physician.

Surgical management. Surgical interventions for the client with renal trauma may include nephrectomy and partial nephrectomy. For clients with major vascular tearing, the kidney may be surgically removed, repaired through revascularization techniques, and then reimplanted into the client. The repair of kidney tissue outside of the client is referred to as *bench surgery*. A transplantation of one's own kidney is referred to as *autotransplantation*. The care of the postnephrectomy client is described earlier in this chapter. Renal transplantation is discussed in Chapters 25 and 59.

■ Discharge Planning

Discharge planning for the client with urinary trauma involves the client and the family or significant other. Appropriate follow-up care and evaluation may be major components of the discharge plan.

Home Care Preparation

Clients who experience minor trauma may be evaluated in the emergency room or an urgent care center and released. These clients must be prepared to monitor and care for themselves, perhaps with the assistance of a family member or friend. If major traumatic injury results in hospitalization, preparation for home care may require more elaborate planning to include home nursing care (skilled or from a nursing assistant), physical or occupational therapy, and/or other appropriate services.

Client/Family Education

The nurse instructs the client and family about the nature of the effects of the injury and how to assess for the presence of infection or other complications, such as the onset of bleeding or the development of urinary retention. The nurse instructs the client to observe the pattern and frequency of urination and to note whether the color, clarity, and amount of urine produced appear normal. The nurse instructs the client to seek medical attention if these characteristics change significantly. The client is told to seek attention if there is a feeling of bladder distention or inadequate bladder emptying, which suggests that there is obstruction to urinary outflow. The client is advised that the presence of chills, fever, lethargy, and/or cloudy, foul-smelling urine may suggest the presence of a UTI. The nurse informs the client that these symptoms must not be ignored and that medical care should be sought promptly.

Psychosocial Preparation

Injuries to the organs of the urinary tract may result in considerable fear and anxiety. Concerns include loss of normal excretory ability and potential impairment of sexual functioning. In addition, there may be concerns related to body image changes, particularly if drainage catheters or surgical repairs are required. The nurse reassures the client in the form of education about the treatment and the client's responsibilities for self-care. When the client must participate in new self-care practices, the nurse reassures the client through reinforcement of learning that self-care is possible. In addition, the nurse suggests potential resources for additional follow-up and supportive care.

Health Care Resources

Health care providers with whom contact has been made during the acute stage of illness may be considered as resources during the recovery stage. In addition, home care personnel may provide additional or supplemental support. In some areas, there are specific support groups for victims of traumatic injury. A support group for a required therapy, e.g., ureterostomy, may be an appropriate recommendation, even if the therapy is expected to be short term.

◢ Evaluation

The nurse evaluates the care of the client with renal trauma and expects that the client

1. Demonstrates normal urinary output, patterns, and characteristics
2. States evidence suggesting the presence of a UTI or urinary retention
3. Describes self-care measures appropriate for activity and maintenance of nutrition

URETERAL TRAUMA

Ureteral trauma is rare unless there is a wound penetrating the abdomen. Because the ureters lie deep within the abdomen, covered and surrounded by multiple layers of tissue, blunt trauma to the abdomen is unlikely to harm them. Ureteral injury during surgical procedures performed deep within the pelvis is not uncommon. Procedures that increase the risk of ureteral injury are gynecologic procedures in the pelvis, surgeries for colon resection, and vascular surgical repairs such as with resection of an abdominal aortic aneurysm. When penetrating abdominal wounds have occurred, renal trauma is often readily apparent and ureteral trauma can be missed. Clinical manifestations of ureteral trauma include fever, vague flank or abdominal pain, urine at the drain site or from the vagina, and hematuria or anuria. IVP or cystoscopy reveals the presence of a urinoma, a collection of urine that has pooled in tissue. Techniques of repair include ureteroplasty (resection and anastomosis) and/or the temporary placement of ureteral stent catheters.

BLADDER TRAUMA

Bladder trauma occurs because of blunt or penetrating injury to the lower abdomen. Penetrating lower abdominal wounds may occur as a result of a stabbing, gunshot wound, or other trauma that results in objects piercing the abdominal wall. A fractured pelvis in which bone fragments puncture the bladder is the most common cause of bladder trauma. Blunt trauma of the bladder occurs with compression of the abdominal wall and the bladder. A seat belt over the bladder may provide sufficient compression to cause bladder injury, especially if the bladder is full or distended.

Clients with a penetrating bladder wound often have anuria and hematuria. Diagnostic tests include cystography and voiding cystourethrography. If renal or ureteral trauma is suspected, IVP is scheduled before cystography to prevent any leakage of bladder contrast medium from masking the outlines of the kidneys or ureters. The cystogram demonstrates whether there is a defect in bladder filling; the voiding cystourethrogram defines bladder emptying.

Bladder trauma, other than a simple contusion, requires surgical intervention. Surgical interventions include procedures to repair the anterior or posterior bladder wall and respective peritoneal membrane. Fracture stabilization usually precedes bladder repair. In general, repairs of the bladder are accomplished by closure procedures. The client with an anterior bladder wall injury commonly has a Penrose drain and Foley's catheter in place postoperatively; clients with a posterior bladder wall injury have a Penrose drain and Foley's or suprapubic catheter in place postoperatively. In some instances, vaginal or rectal fistulas may also require repair.

SUMMARY

Nurses provide clients experiencing urologic disorders with direct care as well as with assistance in gaining the knowledge and skills to promote self-care. The nursing care is guided by goals of prevention, detection, and management. Through assessment of the client's physical and psychosocial responses to the actual or potential disorder, the nurse plans interventions to achieve the desired outcomes. Evaluation of progress made with the care plan occurs continuously.

Urologic disorders are potentially life-threatening. Some urologic disorders require prompt and effective detection to prevent death or to ensure a healthful outcome. Many urologic disorders result in some degree of chronic disability and require the client and family to acquire knowledge and skills for effective management. These disorders may alter normal physical functions, body image, and self-image, as well as modify interpersonal relationships and the preferred life style. The cyclic nature of acuity and chronicity for many of the urologic disorders presents enormous challenges to the nurse who cares for clients with these problems.

IMPLICATIONS FOR RESEARCH

The opportunities for research related to the nursing care of clients with urologic disorders are unlimited. The problem of urinary incontinence results in physical and psychosocial responses that alter individual and family functioning. Although nursing research has begun to describe how individuals and families manage urinary incontinence, specific questions need to be answered.

The following are possible questions for nursing research:

1. Are interventions for urinary incontinence the same in all ethnic, cultural, and age groupings?
2. What interventions to manage urinary incontinence are the most effective and efficient?
3. What role does client education play in the prevention and management of urinary incontinence?
4. What interventions are the most effective in preventing cystitis?

REFERENCES AND READINGS

Congenital Disorders

Brenner, B. M., & Rector, F. C. (Eds.) (1986). *The kidney* (3rd ed.). Philadelphia: W. B. Saunders.

Dalgaard, O. Z. (1957). Bilateral polycystic disease of the kidneys: A follow-up of 284 patients and their families. *Acta Medica Scandinavica, 328*(Suppl.), 1–255.

Gabow, P. A. (1986). Polycystic kidney disease: New research findings may lead to prevention. *Kidney '86, 2*(3), 4–5.

Reeders, S. T., Zerres, K., Gal, A., Hogenkamp, T., Propping, P., Schmidt, W., Waldherr, R., Dolata, M. M., Davies, K. E., & Weatherall, D. J. (1986). Prenatal diagnosis of autosomal dominant polycystic kidney disease with a DNA probe. *Lancet, 2,* 6–8.

Infectious Disorders

Baer, C. L. (1989). Investigating dysuria. *Nursing '89, 19,* 108–110.

Conway, J. (1989). Taking a look at lower UTIs . . . urinary tract infections. *Journal of Urological Nursing, 8,* 641–643.

Daifuku, R., & Stamm, W. E. (1986). Bacterial adherence to bladder urothelial cells in catheter-associated urinary tract infection. *New England Journal of Medicine, 314,* 1208–1213.

Does cranberry juice help in urinary infection? (1988). *Nurses Drug Alert, 12,* 87.

Kunin, C. M. (1985). Does kidney infection cause renal failure? *Annual Review of Medicine, 36,* 165–176.

Kunin, C. M. (1987). *Detection, prevention and management of urinary tract infections* (4th ed.). Philadelphia: Lea & Febiger.

Preshlock, K. (1989). Detecting the hidden UTI. *RN, 52*(5), 65–66, 68–69.

Sawyer, D. L. (1989). Potential for infection: A nursing diagnosis for the patient with an indwelling catheter. *Focus on Critical Care, 16,* 47–52.

Schaeffer, A. J., & Chmiel, J. (1983). Urethral meatal colonization in the pathogenesis of catheter-associated bacteriuria. *Journal of Urology, 130,* 1096–1099.

Stark, R. P., & Maki, D. G. (1984). Bacteriuria in the catheterized patient: What quantitative level of bacteriuria is relevant? *New England Journal of Medicine, 311,* 560–564.

Wong, E. S. (1982). Guideline for prevention of catheter-associated urinary tract infections. In *Guidelines for the prevention and control of nosocomial infections.* (DHHS Publication No. PB 84-923402-LL). U.S. Public Health Service. Atlanta: Centers for Disease Control.

Urinary Incontinence

Gray, M., & Dougherty, M. C. (1987). Urinary incontinence—pathophysiology and treatment. *Journal of Enterostomal Therapy, 14,* 152–162.

Hahn, K. (1988). Think twice about urinary incontinence. *Nursing '88, 18*(8), 65–67.

Marshall, V. F., Vaughan, E. D., Jr., & Parnell, J. P. (1986). Suprapubic vesicourethral suspension (Marshall-Marchetti-Krantz) for stress incontinence. In P. C. Walsh, R. F. Gittes, A. D. Perlmutter, & T. A. Stamey (Eds.), *Campbell's urology* (5th ed., pp. 2711–2717). Philadelphia: W. B. Saunders.

McCormick, K. A. (1988). Urinary incontinence in the elderly. *Nursing Clinics of North America, 23,* 135–137.

Newman, D. K. (1989). The treatment of urinary incontinence in adults. *Nurse Practitioner, 14*(2), 21–22, 24, 26+.

Ouslander, J. G., Krane, R. J., & Abrams, I. B. (1982). Urinary incontinence in elderly nursing home patients. *JAMA, 248,* 1194–1198.

Weigel, J. W. (1988). Urinary incontinence. *Journal of Enterostomal Therapy, 15,* 24–29.

Immunologic Disorders

Glassock, R. J., Adler, S., Ward, H. J., & Cohen, A. H. (1986). Primary glomerular diseases. In B. M. Brenner & F. C. Rector, Jr. (Eds.), *The kidney* (3rd ed., pp. 929–1013). Philadelphia: W. B. Saunders.

Steinberg, A. D. (1986). The treatment of lupus nephritis. *Kidney International, 30,* 769–787.

Schwab, T. R., & Donadio, J. V. (1985). Serology in renal disease: A review. *Seminars in Nephrology, 5,* 179–187.

Degenerative Disorders

Fitzsimmons, S. C., Agodoa, L., Stiker, L, Conti, F., & Striker, G. (1989). Kidney disease of diabetes mellitus: NIDDK initiatives for the comprehensive study of its natural history, pathogenesis, and prevention. *American Journal of Kidney Diseases, 13,* 7–10.

Morgensen, C. E., & Schmitz, O. (1988). The diabetic kidney: From hyperfiltration and microalbuminuria to end-stage renal failure. *Medical Clinics of North America, 72,* 1465–1492.

Teutsch, S., Newman, J., & Eggers, P. (1989). The problem of diabetic renal failure in the United States: An overview. *American Journal of Kidney Diseases, 13,* 11–13.

Obstructions

Brennan, C. (1989). Lithotripter treatment of kidney stones in outpatient surgery. *Journal of Post Anesthesia Nursing, 4,* 170–171.

Chapman, C. J., Bailey, R. R., Janus, E. D., Abbott, G. D., & Lynn, K. L. (1985). Vesicoureteric reflux: Segregation analysis. *American Journal of Medical Genetics, 20,* 577–584.

Coe, F. L., & Favus, M. J. (1986). Disorders of stone formation. In B. M. Brenner & F. C. Rector, Jr. (Eds.), *The kidney* (3rd ed., pp. 1403–1442). Philadelphia: W. B. Saunders.

Collins, J. G. (1988). *Prevalence of selected chronic conditions, United States, 1983–85. Advance data (155), May 24* (DHHS Publication No. [PHS] 88–1250). Washington, DC: U. S. Government Printing Office.

Guidos, B. (1988). Preparing the patient for home care of the percutaneous nephrostomy tube. *Journal of Enterostomal Therapy, 15,* 187–190.

Lorentz, W. B., & Browning, M. C. (1986). Vesicoureteral reflux, proteinuria, and renal failure. *Journal of Urology, 135,* 559–561.

Pak, C. Y. C. (1986). New developments in the diagnosis and management of patients with renal stone disease. *Mediguide to Nephrology, 1*(2), 1–7.

Reid-Czarapata, B. J. (1988). Post ESWL positioning . . . extracorporeal shock wave lithotripsy. *Urologic Nursing, 9,* 14–15.

Slader, S. (1988). Lasertripsy of urinary calculi. *Laser Nursing, 2,* 9–12.

Stone, L. A. (1988). Ureteroscopy: Treatment for distal ureteral stone. *Point of View, 25,* 16–17.

Thomsen, H. S. (1985). Vesicoureteral reflux and reflux nephropathy. *Acta Radiologica Diagnosis, 26,* 3–13.

Tumors

American Cancer Society. (1989). *Cancer facts and figures—1989.* Atlanta: Author.

Baer, C. L., & Williams, B. R. (1988). *Clinical pharmacology and nursing.* Springhouse, PA: Springhouse Corp.

Bellinger, M. F. (1989). The history of urinary diversion and unidiversion. *Journal of Enterostomal Therapy, 16,* 39–41.

Brinkso, V. (1989). Preventing infection in the continent urinary reservoir. *Journal of Urological Nursing, 8,* 624–625.

Garnick, M. B., & Richie, J. P. (1986). Renal neoplasia. In B. M. Brenner & F. C. Rector, Jr. (Eds.), *The kidney* (3rd ed., pp. 1533–1550). Philadelphia: W. B. Saunders.

Glassock, R. H., Adler, S. G., Ward, H. J., & Cohen, A. H. (1986). Primary glomerular diseases. In B. M. Brenner & F. C. Rector, Jr. (Eds.), *The kidney* (3rd ed., pp. 929–1013). Philadelphia: W. B. Saunders.

Grieg, B. J. (1986). Interventions of the ET nurse with the continent urinary Koch pouch patient. *Journal of Enterostomal Therapy, 13,* 226–231.

Koch, M. O. (1989). Bladder substitution with intestine: Past and present. *Journal of Urological Nursing, 8,* 610–617.

Shipes, E. (1989). Nursing care of patients with CUR: Continent urinary reservoir. *Journal of Urological Nursing, 8,* 595–609.

Trauma and Other Disorders

Carroll, P. R., & McAninch, J. W. (1985). Operative indications in penetrating renal trauma. *Journal of Trauma, 25,* 587–593.

Frevele, G. (1989). Urinary tract injuries due to blunt trauma. *Physician Assistant, 13,* 123–126, 128–130, 135–140+.

Kidd, P. (1989). Genitourinary trauma patients. *Topics in Emergency Medicine, 9,* 71–87.

Steinberg, D. L., Jeffrey, R. B., Federle, M. P., & McAninch, J. W. (1984). The computerized tomography appearance of renal pedicle injury. *Journal of Urology, 132,* 1163–1164.

Tuberculosis in the United States. Statistics: States and cities. (1984). (DHHS Publication No. [CDC] 04-8247). Department of Health and Human Services, U.S. Public Health Service. Atlanta: Centers for Disease Control.

Weiskittel, P., & Sommers, M. S. (1989). The patient with lower urinary tract trauma. *Critical Care Nurse, 9,* 53–65.

Additional Readings

Kidd, P. A. (1989). Action stat! Ruptured bladder. *Nursing '89, 19*(1), 33.

This concise article provides the clues that should make a nurse expect that the client in the case study has a ruptured bladder, including pelvic pain, blood at the urinary meatus, and an urge to void with pain. The author explains the emergency interventions and assessment skills necessary to prevent shock and possible death.

Tootla, J., & Easterling, A. (1989). P. D. T.—destroying malignant cells with laser beams. *Nursing '89, 19*(11), 48–49.

This article describes the purpose and nursing care associated with an experimental alternative to cystectomy for clients with bladder cancer. Photodynamic therapy involves the introduction of laser beams through a cystoscope. The major precaution for the client after surgery is the need to avoid sunlight for 3 months because the client experiences photosensitivity.

Wyman, J. F. (1988). Nursing assessment of the incontinent geriatric outpatient population. *Nursing Clinics of North America, 23,* 169–187.

This is one of several articles in the issue on incontinence in the elderly. Incontinence is not always present in an older individual, and this article provides tips on how to determine the type of incontinence that the client may have.

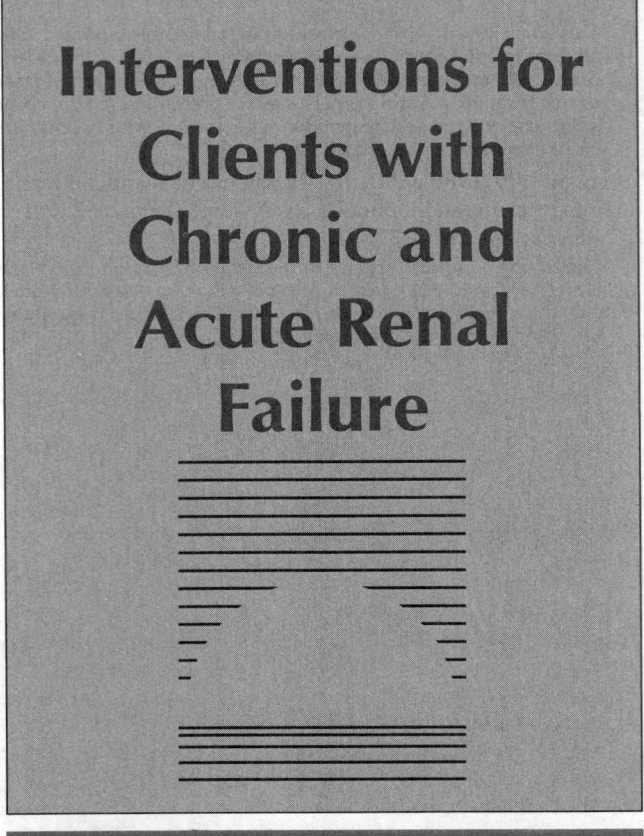

CHAPTER 59

Interventions for Clients with Chronic and Acute Renal Failure

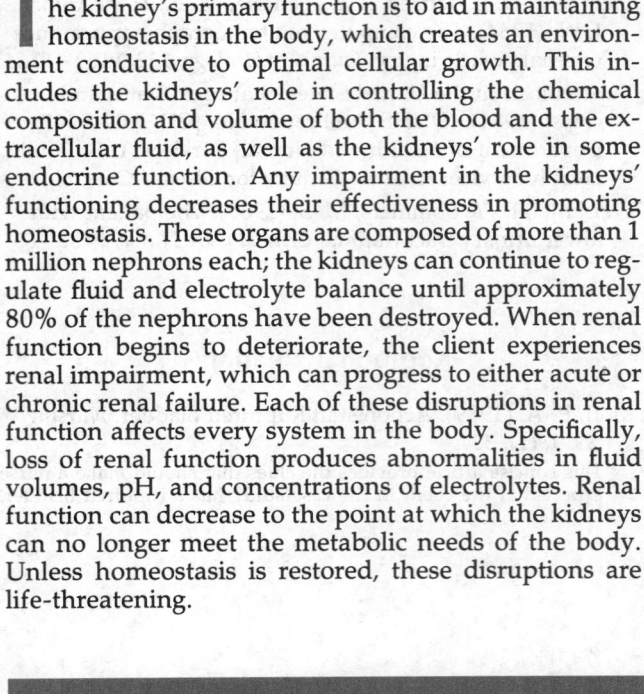

The kidney's primary function is to aid in maintaining homeostasis in the body, which creates an environment conducive to optimal cellular growth. This includes the kidneys' role in controlling the chemical composition and volume of both the blood and the extracellular fluid, as well as the kidneys' role in some endocrine function. Any impairment in the kidneys' functioning decreases their effectiveness in promoting homeostasis. These organs are composed of more than 1 million nephrons each; the kidneys can continue to regulate fluid and electrolyte balance until approximately 80% of the nephrons have been destroyed. When renal function begins to deteriorate, the client experiences renal impairment, which can progress to either acute or chronic renal failure. Each of these disruptions in renal function affects every system in the body. Specifically, loss of renal function produces abnormalities in fluid volumes, pH, and concentrations of electrolytes. Renal function can decrease to the point at which the kidneys can no longer meet the metabolic needs of the body. Unless homeostasis is restored, these disruptions are life-threatening.

CHRONIC RENAL FAILURE

OVERVIEW

Chronic renal failure (CRF) is a condition in which the kidney ceases to remove metabolic wastes and excessive water from the blood. When this disease progresses to end-stage renal disease, the kidney impairment is not reversible. The signs, symptoms, and physiochemical changes that occur in CRF are frequently referred to as *uremia*. Early in the course of CRF, the clinical manifestations may be controlled by dietary and fluid restrictions. An artificial means of replacing kidney function must be instituted when the functioning of both kidneys is significantly compromised and cannot sustain life.

Pathophysiology

Stages

The client's progression toward end-stage renal disease begins with a usually gradual decrease in renal function. The progression toward renal failure is summarized in the accompanying Key Features of Disease. Initially, there is a *diminished renal reserve.* At this stage, the reduction in functioning occurs without any accumulation of metabolic wastes. The unaffected kidney may compensate for decreasing function in the diseased kidney.

The next stage in the progression toward renal failure is *renal insufficiency.* This can be mild (40% to 80% of normal function), moderate (15% to 40%), or severe (2% to 20%) (Bricker & Kirschenbaum, 1984). In renal

---

KEY FEATURES OF DISEASE ■ Progression Toward Chronic Renal Failure

Stage I: Diminished Renal Reserve

Renal function is reduced, but no accumulation of metabolic wastes occurs.

The healthier kidney compensates for the diseased kidney.

Stage II: Renal Insufficiency

Metabolic wastes begin to accumulate in the blood because the unaffected nephrons can no longer compensate.

The degree of insufficiency is determined by decreasing GFR and is classified as mild, moderate, or severe.

Treatment is medical.

Stage III: End-Stage Renal Disease

Excessive amounts of metabolic wastes accumulate in the blood.

The kidneys are unable to maintain homeostasis.

Treatment is by dialysis.

---

insufficiency, metabolic wastes begin to accumulate in the blood because the healthier kidney tissue can no longer compensate for the loss of function in the diseased kidney. Serum levels of blood urea nitrogen (BUN), creatinine, uric acid, and phosphorus are increasingly elevated, depending on the degree of renal function loss. In this stage, careful medical management of fluid volume, electrolyte concentrations, dietary intake, and medication administration can partially compensate for the loss of renal function and limit the progression of renal disease in some clients.

Ultimately, the client enters *end-stage renal disease.* Excessive amounts of nitrogenous wastes, such as BUN and creatinine, accumulate in the blood, and the kidneys are unable to maintain homeostasis. Initially, severe fluid and electrolyte imbalances occur, and, unless some form of dialysis is begun, this condition can be fatal.

Pathologic Alterations

Renal dysfunction results in multiple pathologic occurrences, including disruptions in the glomerular filtration rate (GFR), abnormalities of urine production and water excretion, electrolyte imbalances, and metabolic anomalies. The kidneys are able to maintain an effective *glomerular filtration rate* until approximately 70% to 80% of renal function is lost. This is explained by Bricker's hypothesis (Bricker & Kirschenbaum, 1984), which describes two types of nephrons: those affected by the pathologic process and those that remain free from disease. Homeostasis is maintained by the hypertrophy of the disease-free nephrons until late in the course of renal failure. When less than 20% of the nephrons are functional, the GFR is altered, despite the hypertrophy of the remaining nephrons. This occurs

because the hypertrophied nephrons can only maintain the excretion of solutes or waste products by decreasing water reabsorption. This results in *hyposthenuria* (the loss of urine concentrating ability) and *polyuria* (increased urinary output). Both hyposthenuria and polyuria are early signs of CRF and, if untreated, can cause severe dehydration. As the disease progresses, the ability to dilute the urine becomes increasingly diminished, which results in urine with a fixed osmolality. This state is called *isosthenuria.* As the renal function continues to diminish, an increased concentration of urea occurs in the urine, and urinary output decreases. When renal function reaches this level, the serum BUN rises dramatically, and the client is at risk for fluid overload owing to loss of adequate urinary output. Thus, the client with CRF may be dehydrated or experience fluid overload, depending on the degree of renal compromise.

Metabolic Alterations

Renal failure also causes disturbances in BUN and creatinine excretion. *Creatinine* is derived from creatine and phosphocreatine, which are present in skeletal muscle. The normal rate of creatinine excretion depends on muscle mass, physical activity, and diet. Creatinine is partially excreted by the renal tubules, and a decrease in renal function leads to a build-up of serum creatinine. Urea is the primary product of protein metabolism and is excreted by the kidneys. The *blood urea nitrogen* level normally varies directly with dietary protein intake. The presence of increased concentrations of BUN and creatinine in the blood is called *azotemia* and is one of the classic indications of renal failure.

An important method for determining renal function is *creatinine clearance.* Clearance is the rate at which a specific substance is excreted by the kidneys relative to its plasma concentration. The creatinine clearance is the rate at which the kidneys remove creatinine from the plasma and is measured in milliliters per minute (the formula for calculating creatinine clearance is found in Chap. 57). The body's production of creatinine is not affected by other metabolic processes, such as diet. Therefore, the GFR can be accurately estimated by monitoring the creatinine clearance of the kidneys. As renal function and glomerular filtration diminish, creatinine clearance also decreases and the serum creatinine level rises. Mild renal disease is indicated by a clearance of 50 to 80 mL/minute and a serum creatinine level of 1.5 to 2.0 mg/dL. A client with severe or end-stage renal disease typically has a creatinine clearance of 0 to 10 mL/minute and a serum creatinine level of 6.5–12.0 mg/dL or higher (Lancaster, 1984).

In addition to alterations in BUN and creatinine removal, there can also be wide variations in sodium excretion in a client with renal failure. Early in CRF, the client is particularly susceptible to hyponatremia (sodium depletion), because, although a diminishing number of nephrons are reabsorbing sodium at their maximal ability, there is an obligatory loss of sodium in urine production. Thus, the polyuria often seen in early renal failure also causes sodium depletion. In the later stages of renal failure, the kidney's ability to excrete sodium decreases as the urine production decreases. As a result, hypernatremia can occur with only modest increases in dietary sodium intake and can lead to severe fluid and electrolyte imbalances (see Chap. 13).

The kidney is the primary organ responsible for potassium excretion. Any increase in potassium load during the later stages of renal disease can lead to hyperkalemia (excessive potassium retention). Normal serum potassium levels of 3.5 to 5.0 mEq/L are maintained until the 24-hour urinary output falls below 500 mL with a decreased GFR. There is little warning of impending hyperkalemia until serum levels reach 7 to 8 mEq/L, and then severe electrocardiographic (ECG) changes may rapidly progress to cardiac arrest and death. Causes of hyperkalemia in renal failure include ingestion of potassium in medications, failure to restrict potassium in the diet, blood transfusions, and excessive bleeding or hemorrhage. (See Chap. 13 for further discussion of hyperkalemia.)

Other pathologic occurrences caused by renal dysfunction include numerous metabolic disruptions, such as changes in pH, calcium and phosphorus imbalances, and vitamin D insufficiency. In the early stages of renal disease, loss of functioning nephrons causes little change in blood pH because the remaining nephrons increase their rate of acid excretion. As the loss of nephrons continues, the kidneys are unable to compensate and acid excretion is restricted, resulting in *metabolic acidosis* (see Chap. 15).

Numerous factors contribute to acidosis in renal failure. First, the kidney develops an inability to excrete excessive hydrogen ions. Normally, renal tubular cells secrete hydrogen ions into the tubular lumen for excretion, but ammonia and bicarbonate are required for excretion to take place. In renal failure, the kidney's ability to produce ammonia is decreased, and the normal reabsorption of filtered bicarbonate does not occur. This results in a build-up of hydrogen ions that contributes to the acidotic state. As renal failure advances and acid retention increases, respiratory compensation is essential to maintain a blood pH compatible with life. The respiratory system compensates for the decreased pH by increasing the rate and depth of breathing to excrete carbon dioxide through the lungs. This pattern of breathing is called *Kussmaul's respirations* and usually only occurs in clients with advanced, untreated renal failure. The serum bicarbonate level is used to measure metabolic acidosis, with a level less than 15 mEq/L indicating the need for treatment (Lancaster, 1984).

As described in Chapter 12, there is a complex, balanced reciprocal relationship between calcium and phosphorus, which is influenced by vitamin D. Vitamin D facilitates calcium absorption in the intestines, and the kidney is responsible for final activation of vitamin D.

In renal failure, phosphorus retention occurs and contributes to the disruption in calcium metabolism. Plasma calcium and phosphorus have a reciprocal relationship. If the calcium level increases, the phosphorus level decreases; the reverse is also true. Normally, excessive dietary phosphorus is excreted by the kidneys in the urine. Parathyroid hormone (PTH) controls the amount of phosphorus in the blood and causes tubular reabsorption or excretion of phosphorus as needed by the body. One of the initial effects of decreased renal function is decreased phosphorus excretion owing to a diminished GFR. As plasma phosphorus levels increase, calcium levels decrease. This results in a chronic stimulation of PTH, which causes hypertrophy of the parathyroid gland. This hyperparathyroidism leads to resorption of surface bone, or demineralization, to obtain additional calcium to compensate for the elevated plasma phosphorus concentration. The problem of hypocalcemia is compounded because decreased renal function also causes decreased production of vitamin D. Thus, there is less calcium absorbed in the intestines in the absence of sufficient vitamin D.

The pathologic process caused by hypocalcemia and phosphorus retention is called *renal osteodystrophy*. The skeletal demineralization resulting from hyperparathyroidism may be manifested as bone pain, pseudofractures, sclerosis of the spine, demineralization of parts of the skull, osteomalacia, resorption of bone, and the loss of the lamina dura in the teeth. Metastatic calcifications, crystals formed from excessive calcium phosphate, may precipitate to various parts of the body. When the plasma concentration of the calcium-phosphorus product (serum calcium concentration × serum phosphorus concentration) exceeds 70 mg/100 mL, the crystals may lodge in the kidneys, the heart, the lungs, the joints, the eyes, and the brain (Lancaster, 1984).

Cardiac Alterations

CRF also causes numerous disruptions in the cardiovascular system. The more common manifestations include anemia, hypertension, congestive heart failure (CHF), and pericarditis. Anemia is the primary hematologic abnormality in clients with renal failure. This anemia has multiple causes, such as decreased erythropoietin level, decreased red blood cell (RBC) survival time resulting from uremia, deficiencies in iron and folic acid, and gastrointestinal (GI) bleeding attributable to poor coagulation.

Hypertension is found in the majority of clients with CRF. The blood pressure elevation is the result of fluid and sodium overload and the malfunction of the renin-angiotensin-aldosterone system. The retention of sodium and water in renal disease causes circulatory overload, which leads to elevated blood pressure. The second cause of hypertension is the malfunction of the renin-angiotensin system (see Chaps. 12 and 13). In renal failure, the kidneys fail to recognize the increase in renal blood flow and continue to produce renin, resulting in severe hypertension that is difficult to treat.

Many clients with renal failure have some form of myocardial dysfunction. CRF causes an increased workload on the heart because of anemia, hypertension, and fluid overload. Left ventricular dysfunction and CHF are common manifestations of late end-stage renal disease (Leaf & Cotran, 1985). Uremia itself may cause uremic cardiomyopathy, which is the result of effects of uremic toxins on the myocardium. CHF is also common in these clients because of the presence of hypertension and frequently coronary artery disease.

Pericarditis occurs in approximately 30% to 50% of clients with renal disease (Lancaster, 1984). This inflammation of the pericardium can lead to pericardial effusion, cardiac tamponade, and death if it is not carefully treated. In the client with CRF, the pericardial sac may become inflamed and irritated by uremic toxins or infection. Manifestations of the disease include a pericardial friction rub that can be heard on auscultation, low-grade fever, chest pain, and a decreased blood pressure.

Etiology

The etiology of chronic renal failure is complex and multifaceted. More than 100 different disease processes can cause progressive loss of renal function (see the accompanying Key Features of Disease). These disorders are divided into two basic categories: morphologic and etiologic. *Morphologic* diseases affect the renal system itself. The disorders in this category attack glomeruli, tubules, renal blood vessels, and the urinary outflow tract. The most common of the glomerular diseases is glomerulonephritis. Acute glomerulonephritis is an inflammatory process involving both kidneys. Acute glomerulonephritis can completely resolve or progress to chronic glomerulonephritis and eventually renal failure. Chronic glomerulonephritis can occur in clients with no previous history of renal disease. In its chronic form, glomerulonephritis is a progressive inflammatory disease that causes sclerosis, scarring, and atrophy of the kidneys. In the later stages, the client experiences

KEY FEATURES OF DISEASE ■ Causes of Chronic Renal Failure

Morphologic

Glomerular Disease

Glomerulonephritis
Basement membrane disease
Goodpasture's syndrome
Intercapillary glomerulosclerosis

Tubular Disease

Chronic hypercalcemia
Chronic potassium depletion
Fanconi's syndrome
Heavy metal (lead) poisoning

Vascular Disease of the Kidney

Ischemic disease of the kidney
Bilateral renal artery stenosis
Nephrosclerosis
Hyperparathyroidism

Urinary Tract Disease

Obstructive nephropathy

Congenital Anomalies

Hypoplastic kidneys
Medullary cystic disease
Polycystic kidney disease

Etiologic

Infection

Pyelonephritis
Tuberculosis

Systemic Vascular Disease

Intrarenal renovascular hypertension
Extrarenal renovascular hypertension

Metabolic Renal Disease

Amyloidosis
Gout (hyperuricemic nephropathy)
Diabetic nephropathy
Milk-alkali syndrome
Sarcoidosis

Connective Tissue Disease

Progressive systemic sclerosis
Systemic lupus erythematosus
Polyarteritis

progressive renal insufficiency and eventually end-stage renal disease.

Another group of morphologic disorders results from urinary tract disease. Obstructive nephropathy is the most common cause of reversible renal insufficiency. If the obstruction is removed in time, renal function can return to normal and renal failure may be avoided. Obstructions in the urinary tract can cause backflow of urine and lead to obstructive nephropathy. The area of obstruction can be anywhere from the urethral meatus to the renal calyx. Obstructions can be caused by calculi, neoplasms, anomalies of the bladder neck or urethra, prostatic enlargement, or urethral stricture. Depending on the site of obstruction, the condition may involve one or both kidneys. When urinary outflow is blocked, the retained urine eventually causes pressure in the kidneys, which leads to renal hypoxia and, in time, atrophy of renal tissue. In addition, urinary stasis leads to precipitation of solutes that can cause renal calculi (kidney stones), which can further compromise renal function. Obstructive nephropathy can be insidious, and the symptoms are subtle.

The second category of renal disorders is *etiologic* disease. Etiologic diseases are those that originate outside the kidneys, such as infection, systemic vascular diseases, immunologic disorders, metabolic diseases, and congenital anomalies. In the group of systemic vascular diseases, benign essential hypertension is the most common cause of CRF. The onset of intrarenal renovascular disease caused by benign hypertension usually occurs between 30 and 50 years of age. The client may exhibit only elevated blood pressure with little apparent renal compromise for as long as 20 or 30 years. Eventually, as a result of the progressive vascular disease in this type of hypertension, gradual shrinking and scarring of the kidneys occur.

Metabolic diseases form another group of etiologic disorders. The most common metabolic disorder involving renal disease is diabetes mellitus. The diabetic nephropathy seen in diabetic clients leads to pathologic structural changes in renal arteries and arterioles, glomeruli, tubules, and interstitial tissues. These pathologic changes occur gradually and are manifested initially by mild proteinuria. Over a period of years, the proteinuria becomes more severe and moderate hypertension and edema appear. As renal function slowly decreases, azotemia develops, with increasing edema and severe hypertension. These clients usually require some form of dialysis to sustain life and are sometimes poor risks for renal transplantation because the diabetes can cause the same pathologic changes in the grafted kidney (see Chap. 58 for discussion of urologic disorders and Chap. 51 for more information on diabetic nephropathy).

Incidence

The number of clients with CRF is continually growing in the United States as a result of the increasing ability to prolong life indefinitely with technical replacements for renal function. Clients with end-stage renal disease require hemodialysis, peritoneal dialysis, or transplantation to survive. Before 1973, many people with end-stage renal disease were unable to afford the expensive long-term treatment and consequently died from the disorder. Since 1973, the federal government has paid all expenses for treatment of clients with chronic renal disease through Medicare funding. As a result, in 1985 there were more than 80,000 people with end-stage renal disease undergoing some form of dialysis, compared with only 300 in 1965 (Battelle Human Affairs Research Centers, 1985). The total cost of care for these clients has risen dramatically from $242 million in 1974 to more than $3 billion in 1984 (Battelle Human Affairs Research Centers, 1985). The rapid expansion of this area of medicine requires all nurses to be familiar with the disease and the routine methods of treatment.

In 1985, the National Kidney Dialysis and Kidney Transplantation Study collected and analyzed a variety of data concerning selected clients with CRF throughout the United States (Battelle Human Affairs Research Centers, 1985). The most common cause of CRF was glomerulonephritis, followed by hypertensive renal disease. The demographic statistics from this study showed that the majority of clients with CRF are middle aged, with a relatively even distribution of male and female.

PREVENTION

A variety of conditions can adversely affect renal function or aggravate already existing renal insufficiency. Systemic diseases, such as untreated infections, hypertension, and diabetes, can lead to CRF if they are not properly managed. Untreated or inadequately treated infections, especially streptococcal infections, can lead to glomerulonephritis, which is the most common cause of CRF. Any type or source of infection, including infection causing sore throats or influenza-like symptoms and wound infection, in clients with renal insufficiency should be brought to a physician's attention immediately. The organisms should be cultured, and the client should be treated with a full course of appropriate antibiotics to prevent disease spread to the kidneys. Appropriate antihypertensive therapy for clients with hypertension can control progression of the renal impairment to end-stage disease.

Diabetes mellitus can lead to diabetic nephropathy, which adversely affects all renal structures. The arteriosclerotic vascular changes in the kidney as a result of diabetes cause changes in glomeruli, tubules, and interstitial tissues. The onset and severity of the disease can vary widely. Careful management of the diabetes itself can postpone for many years, if not prevent, end-stage renal disease. Thus, in these clinical situations, irreversible damage to the kidneys can be prevented by appropriate treatment of the primary disorder.

COLLABORATIVE MANAGEMENT

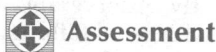 Assessment

History

When taking a history from a client with suspected renal failure, the nurse should remember the clinical manifestations of CRF. The nurse notes the client's *age* and *sex*. The nurse takes accurate *weight* and *height* measurements and inquires about usual weight or recent weight gain, because any recent weight gain or edema may indicate cardiovascular overload and fluid retention caused by inadequately functioning kidneys.

The nurse also obtains a complete history of *current and past medical conditions* and *medications*. Information on current medical problems and recent past medical conditions may help indicate the cause of renal dysfunction. Medical problems, such as those underlying throat infections or influenza, can lead to glomerulonephritis. A history of prostatic enlargement can reflect obstructive renal disease. Information concerning *long-term diseases* is also obtained, because illnesses such as hypertension, diabetes, systemic lupus erythematosus, cancer, tuberculosis, and many others can contribute to decreased renal function. In addition, the nurse questions the client about any *family history of renal disease*, which could indicate a congenital abnormality. The *medications* the client is currently using, both prescription and over the counter, are documented by the nurse. Many medications are nephrotoxic and can cause renal damage (see later).

The nurse examines the client's *dietary or nutritional habits* and discusses any *GI problems* that may be present. A change in the taste of foods often accompanies renal failure. Excessive consumption of foods high in salt and protein can contribute to electrolyte imbalance and accelerate the build-up of metabolic wastes that is already present in these clients. In addition, excessive fluid intake in renal failure can contribute to cardiovascular overload, resulting eventually in peripheral edema, pulmonary edema, and CHF. The nurse specifically assesses the client for a history of *GI problems*, such as nausea, vomiting, anorexia, diarrhea, or constipation. These manifestations could be the result of the build-up of nitrogenous and other metabolic wastes that the body is unable to excrete because of renal malfunction.

The client is questioned about his/her current *energy level* and any recent *injuries* or *bleeding*. Weakness, drowsiness, and shortness of breath are also typically noted in renal failure and can indicate neurologic degeneration or impending pulmonary edema. The nurse asks the client specifically about abnormal bleeding or bruising. This could be indicative of decreased erythrocyte production, thrombocytopenia, and a resulting defect in platelet production.

The nurse discusses the client's *urinary elimination* in detail. The frequency of urination, the appearance of the urine, and any difficulty starting or controlling urination should be described. This information can help identify the stage of renal dysfunction and possibly assist in determining the cause of the renal damage. Lastly, the nurse questions the client about her/his *daily routine* and *environment.* The nurse asks if the client has made any recent changes in his/her daily routine as a result of physical limitations possibly caused by decreasing renal function.

Physical Assessment: Clinical Manifestations

CRF is a multisystem disease, and the clinical manifestations reflect how each system is disrupted by the lack of adequate renal function (see the accompanying Key Features of Disease). The nurse must be aware that the clinical manifestations of CRF or uremia may be explained by changes in fluid volume and the chemical composition of the body fluids. These changes result from the loss of homeostasis when kidneys are diseased.

The disruption of homeostasis leads to specific *cardiovascular abnormalities*, which include hypertension, anemia, and abnormal bleeding. In CRF, the nurse assesses the client for signs of the kidneys' diminished ability to excrete salt and water. The resulting circulatory fluid overload, if untreated, can lead to hypertension, peripheral edema, CHF, and pulmonary edema. Blood pressure elevations are further compounded by the altered functioning of the renin-angiotensin-aldosterone system in renal disease. Anemia in CRF is caused by decreased erythrocyte production and shortened RBC life spans. The nurse notes indicators of anemia, which include pallor, weakness, lethargy, and possible shortness of breath and dizziness. Another disruption of the cardiovascular system is abnormal bleeding. The nurse observes for easy bruising, mucous membrane bleeding in the nose and of the gums, abnormal vaginal bleeding, and GI bleeding (often demonstrated by black tarry stools [melena]).

The *respiratory manifestations* of CRF vary widely among clients. The client may have breath that smells like urine and occasionally deep sighing, yawning, or shortness of breath. The nurse may observe a more serious disruption, with severe acidosis manifested by extreme hyperventilation or Kussmaul's respirations. A few individuals have hilar pneumonitis or *uremic lung.* In these clients, the nurse assesses for thick sputum, minimal coughing, increased respiratory rate, and, if pneumonitis is present, an elevated temperature.

The *neurologic manifestations* of CRF are numerous and can vacillate widely relative to serum electrolyte levels. The nurse may note weakness and lassitude, with periods of extreme drowsiness, but these manifestations can alternate with excitement and insomnia. The nurse observes for shortened attention span and peripheral neuropathies with numb, weakened extremities, particularly the hands. Neurologic disruptions can also cause headaches and muscle twitching, which progresses to convulsions and coma in severe cases.

The *gastrointestinal disruptions* of uremia can range

KEY FEATURES OF DISEASE ■ Clinical Manifestations of Chronic Renal Failure

Cardiovascular

Hypertension
Anemia
Edema
CHF
Pericarditis
Abnormal bleeding
Uremia

Respiratory

Deep sighing
Kussmaul's respirations
Breath that smells of urine
Hilar pneumonitis
Shortness of breath
Pulmonary edema

Neurologic

Headache
Weakness
Drowsiness
Insomnia
Muscle twitching
Convulsions
Coma
Shortened attention span
Peripheral neuropathy

Gastrointestinal

Anorexia
Nausea
Vomiting
Unpleasant or metallic taste
Constipation
Diarrhea
GI bleeding

Genitourinary

Change in urination frequency
Hematuria
Change in urine appearance
Proteinuria

Integumentary

Uremic frost
Yellow pallor
Dry skin
Pruritus
Purpura
Ecchymosis

from mild discomfort to dehydration and even hemorrhagic shock. The nurse may frequently observe anorexia, nausea, and vomiting in clients with renal failure, but the cause of these problems is uncertain. Constipation or diarrhea is also typical in these individuals. These problems are produced by nervous system disruptions, drug therapies, and changes in diet and fluid intake. The normal flora of the oral cavity is altered in uremia. The mouth normally contains the enzyme urease that hydrolyzes urea. The ammonia generated from this reaction contributes to breath that smells like urine and may also cause uremic stomatitis (mouth inflammation). Ulcerations may occur in the GI tract, causing erosion of blood vessels. The blood loss caused by these erosions may result in melena or progress, in more serious cases, to hemorrhagic shock from severe GI bleeding.

The *genitourinary findings* in renal failure reflect the kidneys' decreasing functioning. Initially, there are changes in the amount, frequency, and appearance of the urine. Chronic renal disease causes hematuria and proteinuria, and the urine may become cloudy with heavy sediments. In end-stage renal disease, the urine may become more dilute and clearer, which reflects a diminished GFR in the diseased kidney. The nurse must be aware that the actual urinary output in an individual with CRF varies with the amount of remaining renal function. The client experiencing end-stage renal disease usually is oliguric (scant urinary output or <500 mL/day), and after dialysis therapy is initiated, may become anuric (no urinary output or <75 mL/day) as the treatment removes excessive body fluid (Bricker & Kirschenbaum, 1984).

There are several *dermatologic manifestations* of CRF. In uremia, the skin becomes pale yellow owing to an accumulation of urochrome pigments. A crust of urea crystals, from evaporated perspiration, is sometimes seen on the face and eyebrows and is known as *uremic frost*. The nurse seldom sees uremic frost in the hospital setting, unless the client has avoided medical care before admission and has severe untreated renal failure. One of the most uncomfortable problems of uremia is severe pruritus (itching). The cause is unknown, but it is usually treated with an oily skin lotion to decrease skin dryness and with antihistamine drug therapy. Other skin problems for which the nurse assesses include ecchymosis, purpura, and occasionally drug-induced rashes.

Psychosocial Assessment

CRF and its treatment disrupt more aspects of a client's life than almost any other illness. Nurses are in a unique position to evaluate and assist the client with newly diagnosed renal failure with these adjustments.

Psychosocial assessment and support are part of the nurse's role from the time that CRF is first diagnosed. Initially, the nurse questions the client concerning her/his understanding of the diagnosis and its implications regarding treatment regimens (e.g., diet, medication, and dialysis). The nurse assesses for any signs of anxiety and any coping mechanisms used by the client or family members. The nurse provides continuity of care whenever possible to establish a consistent nurse-client relationship to decrease anxiety and promote discussions of client and family concerns. As the nurse-client relationship develops, the nurse encourages the client to discuss current problems or concerns. Some of the psychosocial aspects that are altered by CRF include family relations, social activity, work patterns, body image, and sexual activity.

Laboratory Findings

CRF results in serious disruptions of a large number of laboratory values (see the accompanying Key Features of Disease). The following values are routinely monitored in these clients: serum sodium and potassium levels, pH, serum phosphorus level, hemoglobin level, hematocrit, blood urea nitrogen level, serum and urinary creatinine concentrations, creatinine clearance, serum calcium level, and urinalysis. The causes of alterations in the above-mentioned laboratory values are discussed under the heading Pathophysiology.

In the early stages of renal insufficiency, the urinalysis provides some key indicators of kidney function. Urinary creatinine level is measured from a 24-hour urine collection. This value, along with the serum creatinine level, is used to determine the creatinine clearance of the kidneys. A routine urinalysis is also useful in the early stages of renal failure, as diseased kidneys produce abnormal urine. The urinalysis may show excessive protein, glucose, RBCs, and white blood cells (WBCs), and a decrease in urine osmolality. As renal failure progresses, the urinary output may decrease dramatically and make frequent examinations of urine impractical.

Monitoring the serum BUN and creatinine levels is essential in the client with renal failure. Urea nitrogen is the end-product of protein metabolism, and excessive urea is excreted by the kidneys. Unfortunately, renal function is not the only factor that affects the level of BUN. The normal serum ratio of BUN to creatinine is approximately $20:1$. When only the BUN level increases, this usually indicates dehydration or excessive protein intake. When both the BUN and creatinine levels increase in proportion and the $20:1$ ratio remains constant, this situation can indicate renal failure.

Radiographic Findings

Several radiographic tests are used in the evaluation of the kidneys in cases of suspected renal dysfunction or failure. The tests performed depend on the specific clinical manifestations and the suspected cause of renal dysfunction. Flat-plate radiography, or radiographic examination of kidneys, ureters, and bladder (KUB), is often done initially to identify the kidneys' size, shape, and position and any calcifications that may be present. From this initial x-ray film, general problems can be identified, such as bilaterally small kidneys associated with chronic renal diseases or enlarged kidneys that may indicate an acute inflammatory process.

Radiographic techniques using injected radiopaque contrast material can be particularly useful because of the kidneys' ability to concentrate the dye. Unfortunately, contrast material is contraindicated in many clients because some dyes are nephrotoxic and may further damage already compromised kidneys. Computed tomography (CT) can be done with or without contrast material. The procedure done without contrast material can make CT safer than the radiographic tests that require dye. The CT scan also provides a more exact multidimensional image of the kidney than a KUB x-ray film and can show anatomic structures not seen with other techniques.

Another radiographic test that always requires contrast media is intravenous pyelography (IVP), which is also known as intravenous excretory urography. IVP is used to visualize the renal parenchyma, calyces, pelves, ureters, and the urinary bladder by intravenous (IV) injection of contrast dye that is excreted by the kidneys. This test is particularly useful in evaluating renal problems caused by trauma, surgery, congenital anomalies, prostate gland enlargement, renal calculi, renal masses, or urinary tract obstruction. IVP is also a valuable test of approximate renal function. Typically, prompt, clear visualization indicates adequate renal function.

Aortorenal angiography allows the visualization of the whole arterial, venous, and capillary systems surrounding the kidneys. This test also requires the injection of IV contrast media and carries the same risks of nephrotoxic and allergic reactions as IVP. Renal angiography is indicated in clients with suspected renovascular hypertension, renal artery stenosis, renal aneurysms, arteriovenous fistula, and other vascular malformations.

Other Diagnostic Tests

The other diagnostic studies used to evaluate clients with suspected renal failure are ultrasonography, magnetic resonance imaging (MRI), and renal biopsy. Ultrasound is utilized for renal evaluation in cases of suspected obstructive uropathy, acute renal failure (ARF), and inflammatory processes, and for evaluation of transplant function. This is a noninvasive technique, with no known side effects, that uses echo patterns to produce an image of the functioning organ. MRI provides a three-dimensional image of parts of the body. It is a noninvasive procedure that requires no ionizing radiation. Thus, it is appropriate for clients with renal disease who are especially sensitive to radiopaque dyes. MRI allows visualization of the kidneys, the renal blood vessels, and postrenal structures. This test can locate renal carcinoma or abnormal growths anywhere in the genitourinary system. In addition, MRI has been able to differentiate between acute transplant rejection and acute tubular necrosis (ATN).

Renal biopsy is used to make an exact histologic diagnosis in a variety of renal disorders. The major uses of renal biopsy are in clients with suspected glomerulone-

Text continued on page 1897

KEY FEATURES OF DISEASE ■ Laboratory Values in Renal Failure

Test	Normal Range	Values in Renal Failure	Comments
Tests to Evaluate Removal of Nitrogenous Wastes			
Serum creatinine	0.6–1.0 mg/dL (women) 0.8–1.7 mg/dL (men)	*In chronic renal failure:* May increase by 0.5–1.0 mg/dL every 1–2 yr. May be as high as 15–30 mg/dL *before* symptoms of CRF are present. *In acute renal failure:* Gradual increase of 1–2 mg/dL every 24–48 h. May increase from 1–6 mg/dL in 1 wk or less.	Consistently elevated levels indicate decreased renal function. Serum creatinine levels are used to evaluate the effectiveness of dialysis treatments.
Blood urea nitrogen	5–15 mg/dL	*In chronic renal failure:* May reach 180–200 mg/dL *before* symptoms develop. *In acute renal failure:* Often increases by 10–20 mg/dL at same pace as serum creatinine level. May reach 80–100 mg/dL within 1 wk.	Increases are dependent on protein intake and other factors (see text). Rate of increase is controlled by limiting protein intake. This intervention is believed to decrease the rate of onset of systemic uremic symptoms, such as anorexia, nausea, and vomiting. Elevations have multiple causes, including diminished renal function, excessive protein intake, sepsis, GI bleeding, and tissue catabolism.
Electrolyte Studies			
Serum sodium	136–145 mEq/L	Normal or decreased.	Clients with renal failure retain sodium. With associated water retention, serum sodium levels *appear* normal. With *excessive* water retention, serum sodium levels *appear* decreased, owing to hemodilution. Assess the client for evidence of fluid volume excess: edema, weight

KEY FEATURES OF DISEASE ■ Laboratory Values in Renal Failure *Continued*

Test	Normal Range	Values in Renal Failure	Comments
Electrolyte Studies			
			increase, or elevation of diastolic blood pressure.
			Limit fluid intake.
			Avoid excessive sodium intake.
			Monitor for signs of hypernatremia: dry skin, excessive thirst, dry mucous membranes, elevated body temperature, and flushed skin.
			Client may need diuretics or dialysis.
Serum potassium	3.5–5.0 mEq/L	Increased.	Advise the client to avoid salt substitutes and limit potassium-containing foods.
			Monitor for rapidly increasing serum potassium levels in ARF.
			ECG changes occur with serum potassium levels of ≥7.0.
			Monitor for signs of hyperkalemia: dizziness, weakness, cardiac irregularities, muscle cramps, diarrhea, and nausea.
			May require administration of sodium polystyrene sulfonate (Kayexalate).
Serum phosphorus (phosphate)	2.5–4.0 mg/dL	Increased.	Short-term increases have potential to cause rapid decrease in serum calcium level and cardiac rhythm disturbances.
			Long-term increases demineralize bones of calcium and enhance fracture potential.
			Phosphate-binding medications help control hyperphos-

Continued

KEY FEATURES OF DISEASE ■ Laboratory Values in Renal Failure *Continued*

Test	Normal Range	Values in Renal Failure	Comments
Electrolyte Studies			
			phatemia and prevent calcium depletion.
Serum calcium	8.0–10.5 mg/dL	Decreased.	Decreases in ARF may necessitate replacement.
			Decreases in CRF may be only slight and may or may not necessitate replacement. As the serum phosphorus level increases, the serum calcium level decreases.
			Chronic calcium deficiency leads to renal osteodystrophy.
			Control of phosphorus excess is usually essential before calcium replacement is initiated.
			Monitor for signs and symptoms of hypocalcemia: abdominal cramps, hyperactive reflexes, tingling in fingertips, and spasms in feet and wrists.
Serum magnesium	1.5–2.5 mEq/L	Increased.	Advise the client to avoid compounds containing magnesium (e.g., laxatives).
Serum carbon dioxide combining power (bicarbonate)	22–28 mEq/L (venous)	Decreased.	Replace bicarbonate. Monitor respiratory rate and depth. Monitor for decreased orientation.
Tests of Acid-Base Balance			
Arterial blood pH	7.34–7.45	Decreased (in metabolic acidosis) or normal.	The respiratory system attempts to compensate by hyperventilation (increased rate and depth of respiration).
			Values are normal if blood buffers and lungs can compensate.

KEY FEATURES OF DISEASE ■ Laboratory Values in Renal Failure *Continued*

Test	Normal Range	Values in Renal Failure	Comments
Tests of Acid-Base Balance			
			Monitor breathing rate and depth. Monitor level of consciousness.
Arterial blood bicarbonate	20–26 mEq/L	Decreased.	Provide replacement PO, IV, or via hemodialysis or peritoneal dialysis.
Arterial blood PCO_2	32–45 mmHg	Decreased.	Monitor for respiratory fatigue (client breathes more rapidly and deeply to "blow off" carbon dioxide).
			Monitor changes in consciousness level to detect carbon dioxide retention.
Other Blood Studies			
Hemoglobin	12–15 g/dL (women) 14–16.5 g/dL (men)	Decreased.	Decreased levels indicate anemia.
			Monitor for pallor, weakness, lethargy, dizziness, and possible shortness of breath.
Hematocrit	37%–45% (women) 42%–50% (men)	Decreased to 20%.	Same as for hemoglobin.
Urinalysis*			
Specific gravity	1.010–1.030	Usually decreased and fixed.	Reflects inability of the tubules to produce a concentrated or dilute urine in response to changes in plasma osmolality.
			Monitor for fluid volume deficit or excess.
pH	4.6–8.0	May be fixed. pH does not change with dietary changes.	Collect a freshly voided specimen for testing.
Glucose	Detectable in urine when blood level is 160–180 mg/dL	Increased.	The renal threshold is often increased; therefore, the blood glucose level may be >160–180 mg/dL before glucose is detectable in the urine.

Continued

KEY FEATURES OF DISEASE ■ Laboratory Values in Renal Failure *Continued*

Test	Normal Range	Values in Renal Failure	Comments
Urinalysis*			
			Monitor *blood* glucose levels.
Protein	2–8 mg/dL	Increased.	Increases may be an incidental and benign finding. Transient increases occur with extreme exercise, fever, stress, or infection. Persistent proteinuria requires 24-h collection for determination of total quantity excreted. Persistent proteinuria may indicate a serious renal problem.
			Instruct the client regarding the need for follow-up.
			Instruct the client in the correct procedure for collection of 24-h specimen.
Occult blood	No RBCs or occasionally 2 or 3 RBCs per high-power field No hemoglobin	More than 2 or 3 RBCs per high-power field. Detectable hemoglobin.	Hemoglobin is detectable when hemolysis of RBCs has occurred. Intact RBCs are only detectable with microscopic examination. Collect a freshly voided specimen for testing.
WBCs	4 or 5 per high-power field	Increased in urinary tract infection.	Often indicates need for urine culture.
Bacteria	Less than 1000/mL	Increased in the presence of infection, with or without an increase in WBCs.	Obtain urine culture.
Casts	None, or occasional hyaline cast	Casts present.	Casts may be a benign occurrence or may signify that some renal injury or disease is present.
			Collect a freshly voided specimen for direct microscopic examination.
Creatinine clearance	100–180 L/24 h	Decreased.	Change reflects decreases in GFR.

KEY FEATURES OF DISEASE ■ Laboratory Values in Renal Failure *Continued*

Test	Normal Range	Values in Renal Failure	Comments
Urinalysis*			
			Creatinine clearance is determined from a 24-h urine collection and serum creatinine studies.

* Urine may become cloudy with heavy sediment. Urinary output and appearance vary, depending on remaining renal function.

phritis, nephrotic syndrome, renal involvement with systemic diseases, hereditary renal diseases, ARF, and in the management of renal transplants.

 ### Analysis: Nursing Diagnosis

The client with CRF has usually experienced a progressive degeneration of renal function and is frequently hospitalized for evaluation and modification of the treatment plan. The focus of care is to control symptoms and prevent complications.

Common Diagnoses

These diagnoses are applicable to all clients with renal failure:

1. Fluid volume excess related to the inability of the kidney to maintain body fluid and electrolyte balance

2. Altered nutrition: less than body requirements related to necessary dietary restrictions and altered taste sensations

3. Anxiety related to lack of knowledge about procedures and diagnostic tests and lack of understanding of the disease process

Additional Diagnoses

The client may also exhibit one or more of the following diagnoses:

1. Decreased cardiac output related to fluid excess, drug therapy, and excessive blood loss

2. Impaired physical mobility related to renal osteodystrophy, peripheral neuropathy, paresis or paralysis, or coma

3. Constipation related to decreased fluid intake and decreased dietary bulk

4. Diarrhea related to electrolyte imbalance, fear, and anxiety

5. Altered oral mucous membrane related to parotid gland changes, limited fluid intake, and elevated levels of uremic toxins

6. Activity intolerance related to chronic fluid overload and fatigue

7. Sleep pattern disturbance related to fluid retention, CHF, and uremia

8. Ineffective individual coping related to the stress of chronic illness

9. Potential for injury related to increased susceptibility to bleeding, falls, and pathologic fractures

10. Self-esteem disturbance related to changes in body image and role performance

11. Chronic pain related to nausea, vomiting, pruritus, muscle cramps, and paresthesias

12. Impaired skin integrity related to pruritus, irritation, and possibly uremic frost

13. Altered thought processes related to irritation or depression of the central nervous system associated with uremia

14. Knowledge deficit related to lack of information about the disease process, care regimen, and follow-up care

15. Sexual dysfunction related to decreased libido and impotence

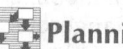 ### Planning and Implementation

The plan of care for clients with renal failure focuses on the common nursing diagnoses.

Fluid Volume Excess

Planning: client goals. The goals for this nursing diagnosis are that the client will (1) achieve and maintain an acceptable fluid and electrolyte balance and (2) minimize the risk of complications from fluid and electrolyte imbalances.

Interventions: nonsurgical management. The nonsurgical management of the client with CRF includes drug therapy, diet therapy, hemodialysis, and peritoneal dialysis.

Drug therapy. Managing drug therapy in clients with renal disease is a complex clinical problem. The nurse must be acutely aware of the use of each drug, its side effects, and its site of metabolism. It is most important to avoid certain medications and to adjust the dosage of others according to the degree of remaining renal metabolism. As the client's renal function decreases, adjustments in the medication's dosage are repeatedly required. The nurse assesses the client for side effects and signs of drug toxicity and notifies the physician as appropriate.

A number of medications are routinely administered to clients with renal failure (Table 59–1). Nurses administering these medications should understand the rationale for administration and the nursing interventions for each drug. Many of these clients have some degree of cardiac disease and may require cardiotonic drugs, such as digoxin and digitoxin. The nurse must be aware that clients with decreased renal function are particularly susceptible to digoxin toxicity because the drug is excreted by the kidneys. The nurse caring for clients with CRF who are receiving any digitalis derivative, including digoxin, monitors for signs of digitalis or digoxin toxicity, such as nausea, vomiting, anorexia, visual disturbances, restlessness, headache, fatigue, confusion, cardiac irregularities, bradycardia (pulse rate < 60 beats per minute), or tachyarrhythmias. In addition, serum levels of electrolytes, such as potassium, must be closely monitored in any client receiving cardiotonic medications.

All individuals with renal dysfunction are given some type of vitamin and mineral supplement. As a result of the severely restricted diet that these clients must adhere to, they are deficient in many vitamins. The nurse must avoid giving the client these supplements before hemodialysis because they will be dialyzed out of the body and the client receives no benefit.

Antacids, such as aluminum hydroxide gel, are used to bind phosphorus in clients with renal failure because, with decreased renal function, the metabolism of calcium and phosphorus is disrupted. Individuals with renal disease should avoid all antacids containing magnesium. The kidney's decreased ability to metabolize this material predisposes these persons to dangerous levels of magnesium retention. In clients taking aluminum-based phosphate binders for prolonged periods, the nurse monitors for signs of hypophosphatemia, including muscle weakness, anorexia, malaise, tremors, bone pain, and negative calcium balance. Finally, the nurse usually administers stool softeners or laxatives to clients with CRF because these individuals have a minimal fluid intake and many of their medications, including aluminum hydroxide antacids, cause constipation.

In addition to the drugs used to treat renal failure, other medications require special consideration in clients with renal failure; these include antibiotics, narcotics, antihypertensives, diuretics, insulin, and heparin. Many antibiotics are safe for clients with renal failure, but those excreted primarily by the kidney require dosage modification. Prophylactic antibiotic treatment is routinely given to clients with CRF before any dental procedures to prevent endocarditis, which may result if oral bacteria enter the blood stream. The antibiotic used and the protocol vary with the client's needs and the physician's preference. Narcotics should also be used cautiously in clients with renal failure because the effects often last much longer than in people with healthy kidneys. Uremic clients are particularly sensitive to the respiratory depressant effects of these drugs. Because narcotics are metabolized by the liver and not the kidneys, the dosage recommendations are often the same regardless of the level of renal function. The nurse is responsible for monitoring these clients closely after narcotic administration and evaluating the need for additional administration on the basis of the client's individual reaction to the drug.

Most clients with CRF have some degree of hypertension, and, as a result, many of these individuals receive antihypertensives. Antihypertensive drugs are used carefully in clients with renal disease to avoid severe hypotension. Many clients with long-standing hypertension develop renal insufficiency. Some antihypertensives are metabolized by the kidneys and require careful dosage adjustment according to each client's renal function. Included in this group are methyldopa (Aldomet) and hydralazine hydrochloride (Apresoline). Other blood pressure medications not metabolized by the kidneys are preferable for these clients. These drugs include propranolol (Inderal), clonidine hydrochloride (Catapres), and prazosin (Minipress).

Diuretics are frequently used in clients in the early stages of renal insufficiency. The diuresis produced by these drugs is useful in treating fluid overload in clients that still have some urinary output. The nurse must maintain careful intake and output records for these clients. As kidney function diminishes, these drugs can become increasingly nephrotoxic and are seldom used in clients with end-stage renal disease after dialysis has been initiated.

An estimated 25% of the population undergoing hemodialysis are diabetic, and thousands of additional people are diabetic and in various stages of renal insufficiency (Kosier & Thompson, 1985). As renal disease progresses, the diabetic individual requires a decrease in insulin dosage because insulin is partially metabolized by the kidneys. Frequent blood glucose determinations should be obtained to evaluate insulin needs because urinary glucose measurements may be inaccurate owing to the renal disease.

Hemodialysis. Hemodialysis is one type of treatment for renal failure (Table 59–2). Hemodialysis is required only when the kidney's function decreases to a life-threatening level. The purpose of this therapy is to remove from the body excessive fluids and waste products that would normally be removed by the kidneys. Hemodialysis involves circulating the client's blood through a semipermeable membrane that acts as an artificial kidney.

Procedure. The principles of hemodialysis are based on the transfer of toxins and fluid removal, which are accomplished by diffusion. *Diffusion* is the movement of

TABLE 59-1 Drugs Used in the Treatment of Renal Failure

Drug	Indications	Interventions	Rationales
Cardiotonics			
Digoxin Digitoxin	Decreased stroke volume Decreased strength of cardiac contractions	1. Monitor for signs of digoxin toxicity and hypokalemia. 2. Monitor for bradycardia (pulse <60 beats per minute). 3. Give after dialysis.	1. Digoxin remains in the body longer when renal function is impaired. 2. This is a symptom of digoxin toxicity. 3. Effective levels of digoxin are reduced during dialysis.
Vitamins and Minerals			
Folic acid	Dietary supplement	1. Usually give after dialysis.	1. Water-soluble vitamins are removed during dialysis.
Ferrous sulfate	Anemia	1. Monitor for constipation. 2. Note change in stools, which normally become blackish green.	1. This is a frequent and uncomfortable side effect associated with oral iron supplements. 2. Color is caused by the presence of unabsorbed iron and is harmless.
Calcium gluconate	Dietary supplement	1. Give only when serum phosphorus levels are normal.	1. Calcium supplements may cause a *decrease* in the serum phosphorus levels because these two minerals exist in the blood in a balanced *reciprocal* relationship.
Phosphate Binders			
Aluminum hydroxide gel (Amphojel, Alternagel, Alu-Cap) Aluminum carbonate gel (Basaljel)	Phosphate binder; prevention of renal osteodystrophy	1. Monitor for constipation, which occurs frequently. 2. Monitor for signs of hypophosphatemia.	1. This is a frequent side effect of many drugs that bind phosphorus. 2. Drugs can prevent intestinal absorption of phosphorus to the extent that the client develops hypophosphatemia.
Stool Softeners and Laxatives			
Docusate sodium (Colace) Bisacodyl (Dulcolax)	Prevention of constipation caused by limited fluid intake, iron, supplements, and phosphate binders	1. Observe for abdominal cramps and diarrhea.	1. These indicate drug overdose.

Table continued on following page

TABLE 59–1 Drugs Used in the Treatment of Renal Failure *Continued*

Drug	Indications	Interventions	Rationales
Antihypertensives			
Hydralazine hydrochloride (Apresoline) Methyldopa (Aldomet) Metoprolol tartrate (Lopressor) Prazosin (Minipress) Propranolol (Inderal) Clonidine hydrochloride (Catapres)	Hypertension	1. Monitor for hypotension. 2. Avoid giving before dialysis.	1. These drugs decrease peripheral resistance and lower the diastolic and mean arterial blood pressures, which could cause the client to experience hypotension. 2. Blood pressure drops during and immediately after dialysis. If these agents are given just before dialysis, the client is at greater risk for hypotension.
Diuretics			
Osmotic Diuretics (Act on Proximal Convoluted Tubule)			
Mannitol Urea	Causes rapid diuresis (e.g., after contrast media infusion)	1. Measure fluid intake and output.	1. Severe dehydration is possible.
Thiazide and Thiazide-like Diuretics (Act on Cortical Diluting Site of Ascending Limb of Loop of Henle)			
Chlorothiazide (Diuril) Hydrochlorothiazide (HydroDiuril) Chlorthalidone (Hygroton) Metolazone (Zaroxolyn)	Hypertension CHF with edema	1. Observe for signs and symptoms of electrolyte imbalance.	1. Common complications of this therapy include hypokalemia and hypercalcemia.
Loop Diuretics (Act on Ascending Limb of Loop of Henle)			
Furosemide (Lasix) Bumetanide (Bumex) Ethacrynic acid (Edecrin)	Hypertension CHF Edema (when creatinine clearance is <25–50 mL/min)	1. Observe for orthostatic hypotension. 2. Monitor for possible hyponatremia and hypokalemia.	1. Rapid fluid volume depletion may occur. 2. These agents increase excretion of both sodium and potassium.
Potassium-Sparing Diuretics (Act on Distal Convoluted Tubule)			
Spironolactone (Aldactone) Triamterene (Dyazide)	Primary aldosteronism Hypertension (with other drugs to decrease potassium loss)	1. Observe for signs and symptoms of electrolyte imbalance.	1. Hyperkalemia with cardiac manifestations is a common complication of this drug therapy.

TABLE 59–2   A Comparison of Hemodialysis and Peritoneal Dialysis

Hemodialysis	Peritoneal Dialysis
Advantages	
More efficient clearance	Easy access; fewer hemodynamic complications
Short time needed for treatment	
Complications	
Disequilibrium syndrome	Protein loss
Muscle cramps	Peritonitis
Hemorrhage	Hyperglycemia
Air embolus	Respiratory distress
Hemodynamic changes (hypotension, cardiac arrythmias, and anemia)	Bowel perforation
Contraindications	
Hemodynamically unstable	Extensive peritoneal adhesions
	Peritoneal fibrosis
	Recent abdominal surgery
Access	
Vascular access route	Intra-abdominal catheter
Procedure	
Complex	Simple
Specially trained registered nurses required	Special training not needed
Nursing Implications	
Vascular access care	Abdominal catheter care
Restrict diet	More flexible diet

molecules from an area of higher concentration to an area of lower concentration. The rate of diffusion is affected by numerous factors: diffusion during dialysis occurs more rapidly when the membrane pores are large, there is a large surface area of membrane, the temperature of the solutions is higher, and there is a greater difference in the solute concentrations. Molecules that are too large, such as blood, cannot pass through the membrane (see Chap. 12 for discussion of diffusion).

When hemodialysis is initiated, blood and dialysate are pumped past opposite sides of an enclosed semipermeable membrane. The dialysate is a balanced mix of electrolytes and fluid that closely resembles human plasma. On the other side of the membrane is the client's blood, which contains metabolic waste products, excessive fluid, and excessive electrolytes. During hemodialysis, the waste products move from the blood into the

dialysate because of the difference in their concentrations. Excessive fluid is also removed from the blood into the dialysate. Electrolytes can move in either direction as needed and take some fluid with them. This process continues as the blood and the dialysate are circulated past the membrane for a fixed length of time or until equilibrium is achieved.

The components of a hemodialysis system include a dialyzer, dialysate, vascular access routes, and a hemodialysis machine. The artificial kidney, or *dialyzer*, is manufactured in a number of different designs (Fig. 59–1). All dialyzers have essentially four components: a blood compartment, a dialysate compartment, a semipermeable membrane, and an enclosed structure that supports the membrane. *Dialysate* is made from clear water and chemicals and is free from any metabolic waste products or drugs. Bacteria and other microorganisms are too large to pass through the membrane,

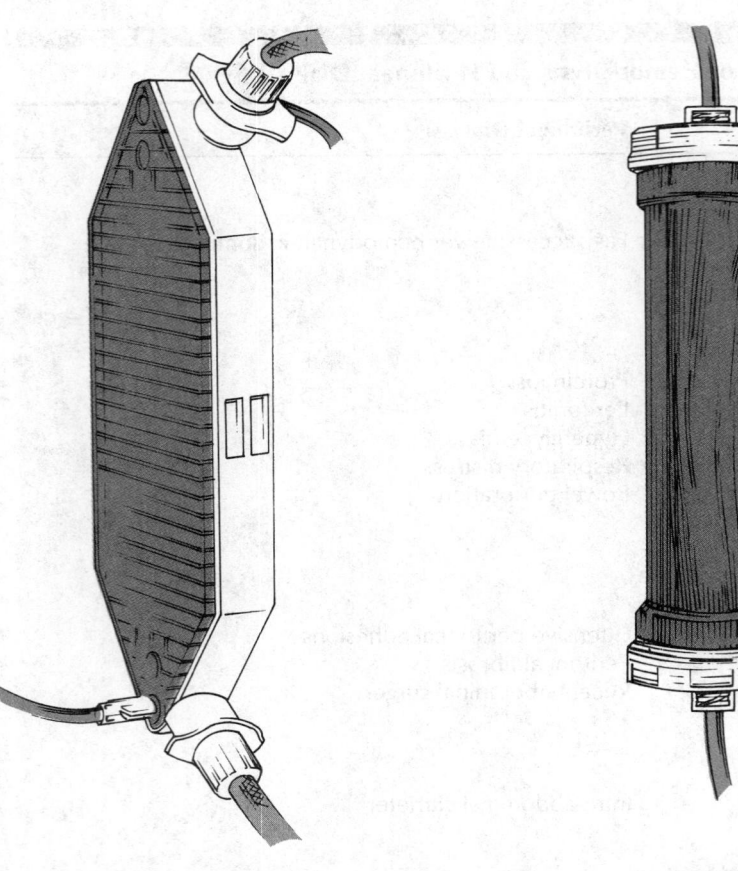

PLATE DIALYZER

HOLLOW FIBER
DIALYZER

Figure 59–1

Artificial kidneys (dialyzers)
used in hemodialysis.

thus dialysate does not need to be sterile. The water used in dialysate must meet specific standards, and water treatment systems are used to ensure a safe water supply. The dialysate's composition may be altered according to the client's needs to treat electrolyte imbalances, such as an increase or decrease in sodium and potassium content. During hemodialysis, the dialysate is warmed to approximately 100° F (37.8° C) to increase the efficiency of diffusion and prevent a decrease in the temperature of the client's blood.

An essential function of a hemodialysis machine is monitoring for a variety of potential problems, including changes in dialysate temperature, the presence of air in the blood tubing, a blood leak in the dialysate compartment, and changes in the pressures in the blood and the dialysate compartments. If any of these problems is detected, an alarm alerts the nurse. The monitoring systems exist to protect the client from life-threatening complications that can result if these technical problems are not corrected.

Discussion of the many different models of hemodialysis machines is beyond the scope of this text, but all of them function, in principle, as illustrated in Figure 59–2. Figure 59–3 shows one type of hemodialysis machine.

Anticoagulation with heparin is necessary during hemodialysis treatments to prevent blood clots from forming in the dialyzer and the blood tubing. Heparin, a short-acting anticoagulant, inhibits the tendency of blood to clot when it comes in contact with foreign surfaces. There is considerable variability among individuals in their anticoagulation response and elimination of heparin. The heparin dosage should be adjusted on the basis of each client's need. In addition, heparin remains active in the body for 4 to 6 hours after administration. This situation places the client at risk for hemorrhage during and immediately after dialysis treatments. The client must avoid any invasive procedures during that time. Thus, the nurse has a primary responsibility to closely monitor clients for any signs of bleeding or hemorrhage. Clotting tendencies can be monitored by whole blood clotting times (Lee-White clotting test) or activated partial thromboplastin times during and after hemodialysis. Protamine sulfate is used as an antidote to neutralize heparin's anticoagulant activity when necessary.

Vascular access routes. To perform hemodialysis, a vascular access route is required (Table 59–3). Dialysis treatments necessitate the easy availability of a large amount of blood flow, at least 200 to 300 mL/minute,

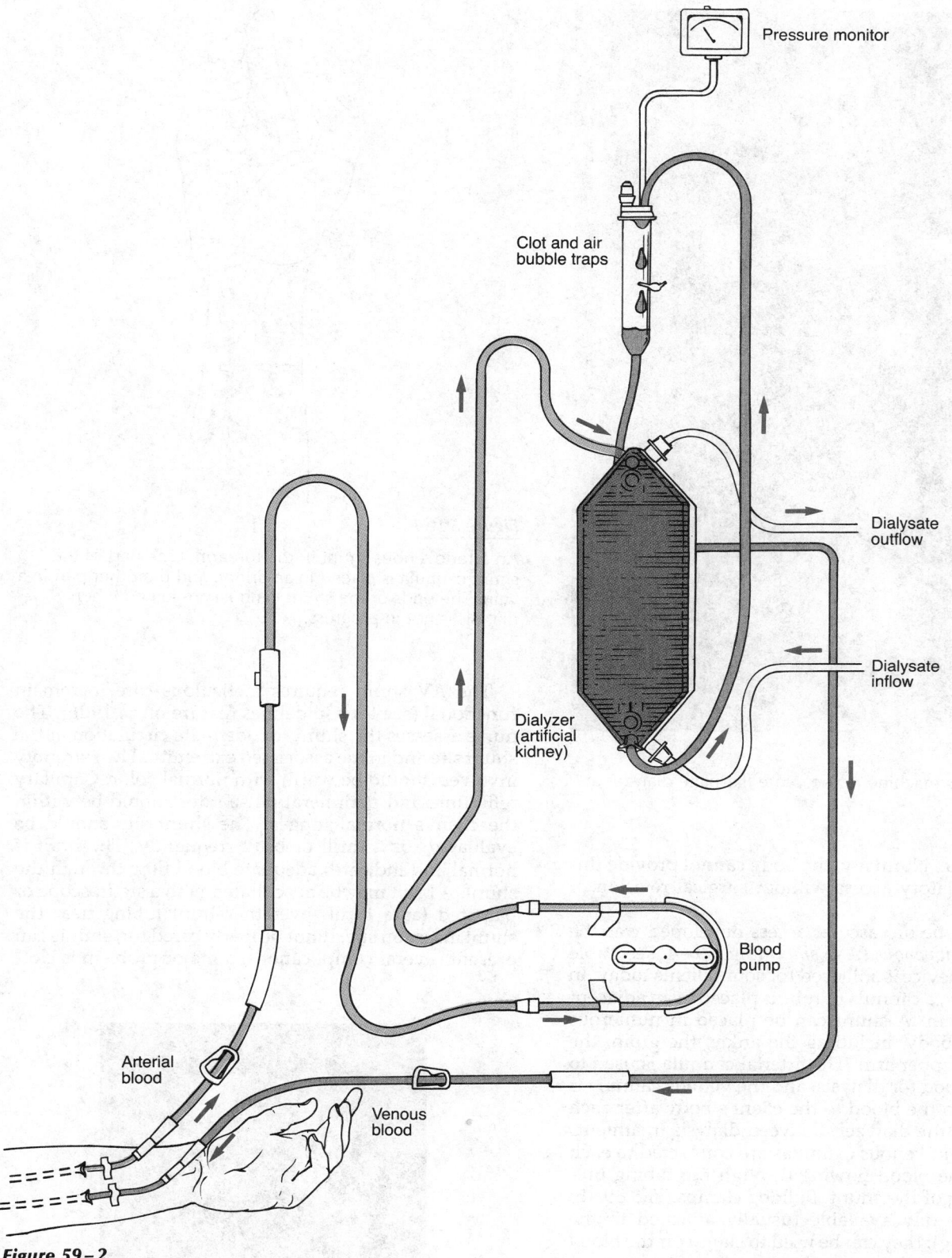

Pressure monitor

Clot and air
bubble traps

Dialysate
outflow

Dialysate
inflow

Dialyzer
(artificial
kidney)

Blood
pump

Arterial
blood

Venous
blood

Figure 59–2

A hemodialysis circuit.

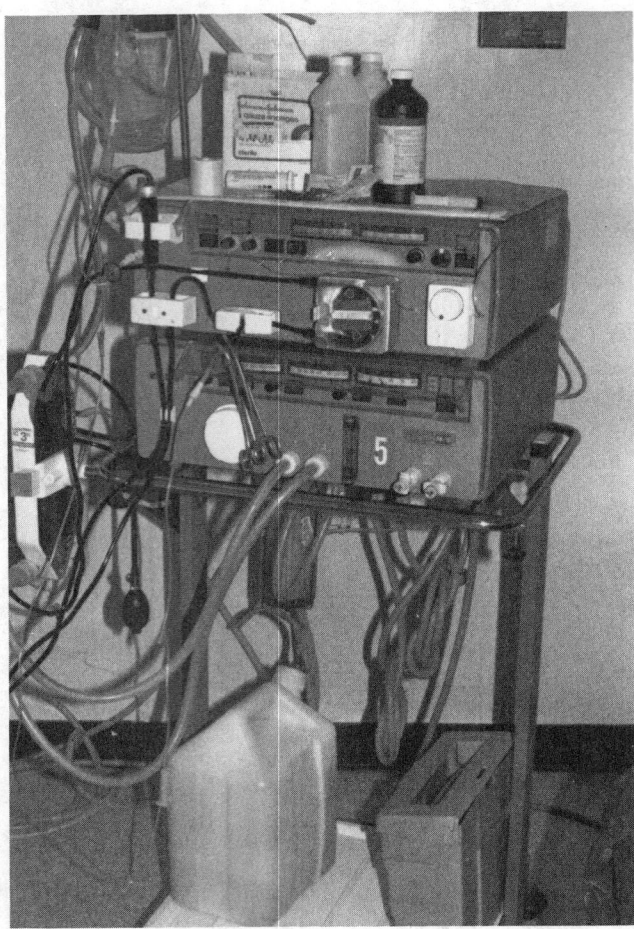

Figure 59–3

A hemodialysis machine in use. Note flat-plate dialyzer at left.

for a long time. Normally, the body cannot provide this type of circulatory access without surgical revision of blood vessels.

The first type of vascular access developed was the external *arteriovenous* (AV) *shunt* (Fig. 59–4; see Table 59–3). This device is still used for some clients today. In this technique, a cannula or tube is placed in an adjacent artery and vein. A shunt can be placed in numerous areas of the body, including the ankle, the groin, the wrist, or the upper arm. The arterial cannula is used to obtain the blood for dialysis, and the venous cannula is used to return the blood to the client's body after each pass through the dialyzer. Between dialysis treatments the arterial and venous cannulas are connected to each other, and the blood flowing through the tubing prevents clotting of the shunt. Bulldog clamps (Fig. 59–5) should be readily available (usually attached to the shunt dressing); they can be used to clamp off the blood flow if the shunt becomes disconnected. The average life span of an external AV shunt is only 6 to 9 months, which makes its use impractical for clients undergoing long-term dialysis unless no other access is available.

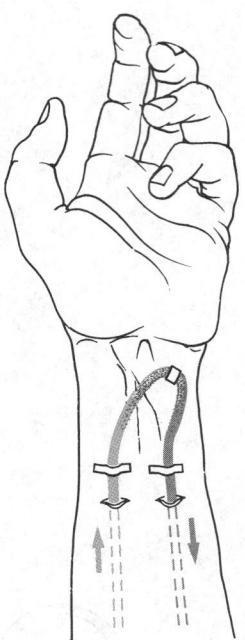

Figure 59–4

An arteriovenous shunt in the forearm. One part of the shunt cannula is placed in an artery, and the other part in a vein. The ends of the shunt cannula are joined when dialysis is not in progress.

The AV shunt requires meticulous care to remain functional (see the Guidelines feature on p. 1906). The nurse assesses the shunt for adequate circulation at the shunt site and in the associated extremity. The extremity involved should be warm with normal color. Capillary refill time and peripheral pulse rates should be within the client's normal ranges. The shunt site should be evaluated for a thrill or bruit frequently. The bruit is normal and indicates adequate blood flow through the shunt. A bruit may be auscultated with a stethoscope or palpated (as a thrill) over the shunt tubing near the shunt insertion site. If not properly cared for, shunts can present several complications; a major problem is clot-

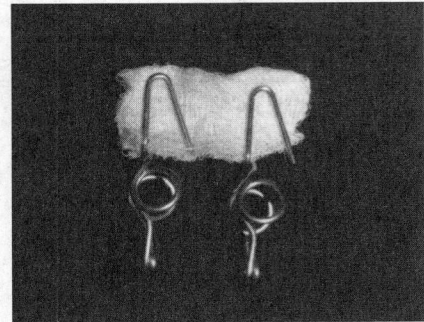

Figure 59–5

Bulldog clamps.

TABLE 59–3   A Comparison of External and Internal Access for Hemodialysis

External Access (AV Shunt)	Internal Access (AV Fistula)
Advantages	
No needle puncture necessary for dialysis or blood tests.	Provides adequate blood flow for dialysis indefinitely.
Possible to use access soon after surgery.	Decreased incidence of infection.
	Seldom clots.
	More freedom of movement.
	No external dressing required.
Disadvantages	
High incidence of infection.	Needle insertions required for hemodialysis and blood tests.
Increased incidence of clotting.	
Decreased mobility for client.	Infiltration of needles during hemodialysis can cause hematomas.
Indications	
As a temporary hemodialysis access in ARF clients awaiting transplant, and initial management of rapid-onset CRF.	CRF requiring long-term hemodialysis.
Insufficient development of the vascular system for an internal access.	
Complications	
Blood loss if access is dislodged.	Prolonged bleeding postdialysis necessitating pressure at needle sites.
Skin erosion around catheter site.	
Temporary access.	Aneurysm in fistula.
	Cannot be used for 6–12 wk after surgery (alternate access required).
	Ischemia below fistula (steal syndrome).
	CHF from increased blood flow in venous system.
Nursing Implications	
Keep a dressing over the shunt site.	Do not take blood pressure measurements or do venipunctures in the fistula arm.
Draw blood for laboratory tests from the shunt.	
Keep the shunt site dry.	Palpate pulses below fistula for indications of ischemia.
Do not take blood pressure measurements in shunt arm.	Palpate for bruit over fistula.
Palpate for bruit at shunt site.	

ting. The signs of clotting are an absence of bruit or thrill, the cooling of the blood temperature in the cannula, and darkness and separation of blood in the cannula. Shunts can be declotted at the bedside by the physician with a nurse's assistance. Another more common complication in clients with shunts is infection. The nurse observes for signs of shunt infection, which include redness, tender-ness, pain, swelling, and unusual bleeding, or drainage around the shunt site. To avoid infection at the shunt site, the nurse uses sterile technique when cleaning the area.

In some situations, clients with CRF may briefly re-quire a more easily inserted temporary external vascular access, such as a subclavian or femoral vein dialysis

GUIDELINES ■ Arteriovenous Shunt Care

Interventions	Rationales
1. Remove old dressing.	1. The dressing should be changed daily and whenever it becomes soiled to prevent infection.
2. Use cotton swabs to clean around shunt sites with hydrogen peroxide.	2. Hydrogen peroxide facilitates removal of old crusts and blood that might serve as a medium for bacteria.
3. Assess area for signs of infection or clotting.	3. Early recognition of infection indicates treatment with antibiotics and limits systemic involvement. A clotted shunt requires immediate declotting. The earlier this is identified, the more likely it is that the shunt can be saved.
4. Apply an antiseptic solution, such as povidone-iodine, around each site.	4. An antiseptic barrier prevents bacteria from invading the shunt.
5. Cover with a sterile gauze dressing and tape. The dressing should not bind the shunt too tightly.	5. A dressing protects the area from infection. It should not constrict blood flow, which could cause the shunt to clot.
6. Always keep bulldog clamps near the shunt. They are usually placed on the edge of the dressing.	6. In case of accidental separation of the shunt, the bulldog clamps are used to clamp each side of the catheter to avoid excessive blood loss.

catheter. Insertion of these catheters is a comparatively quick, sterile procedure that can be performed at the client's bedside. Refer to the later discussion of dialysis for fluid volume deficit in clients with ARF.

The majority of clients undergoing long-term hemodialysis have an internal *AV fistula* (Fig. 59–6; see Table 59–3). This fistula is formed by the anastomosis of an artery to a vein. This process increases the blood flow through the vessels to 250 to 400 mL/minute, which is the amount required for dialysis to be effective. The most commonly used vessels are the radial or brachial artery and the cephalic vein. A fistula must mature for 6 to 12 weeks after surgery to permit arteriolization of the venous walls. During this time, the increased pressure of the arterial blood flow into the vein encourages the vessel walls to thicken. This increases their strength and suitability for repeated cannulation. To obtain access to a fistula, the nurse must cannulate it or insert two needles, one toward the venous blood flow and one toward the arterial blood flow. This allows the hemodialysis machine to draw the blood out of the arterial needle and return it through the venous needle. The client may require a temporary AV shunt or subclavian catheter to provide dialysis treatments until the fistula is ready for use.

The three most commonly used types of fistulas are the simple vascular fistula, the bovine (cow) graft, and the polytetrafluoroethylene (PTFE) graft. The simple fistula that is created by the anastomosis of a vein to an artery is the most commonly used vascular access route. Another type is the bovine graft. This is usually a loop graft obtained from a bovine carotid artery and anastomosed to the vein and artery of the client. The bovine graft is used most often in individuals with natural vessels that could not form a fistula. The third type of fistula is a PTFE graft. The PTFE graft is made of synthetic material (Gore-Tex) and has several advantages over a bovine graft, including numerous different sizes and ready availability at a low cost.

Several precautions must be observed to ensure the functioning of an internal AV fistula. First, the nurse assesses for adequate circulation in the fistula and in the distal portion of the extremity. The nurse checks the fistula for a bruit or a thrill by auscultation or palpation over the access vessel. Blood pressure measurements should not be taken in the extremity with the fistula unless absolutely necessary because the repeated compression can result in the loss of the fistula. In addition, the fistula cannot be used for administration of IV fluids and no venipunctures should be done in the arm used for hemodialysis access.

Complications can occur regardless of the type of fistula. The most common problems include thrombosis, infection, aneurysm formation, ischemia, and high-output heart failure. Thrombosis, or clotting, is the most frequent complication. Some individuals are more prone to clotting than others and may be given anticoagulants. Declotting a fistula can sometimes be performed at the client's bedside, but surgical intervention is often required. The majority of infections that occur in clients undergoing long-term hemodialysis involve the vascular access. The most common organism causing infection is *Staphylococcus aureus*, which can be introduced via punctures for dialysis access. The nurse can limit the incidence of these infections by careful sterile technique before needle cannulation. Aneurysms can form in any

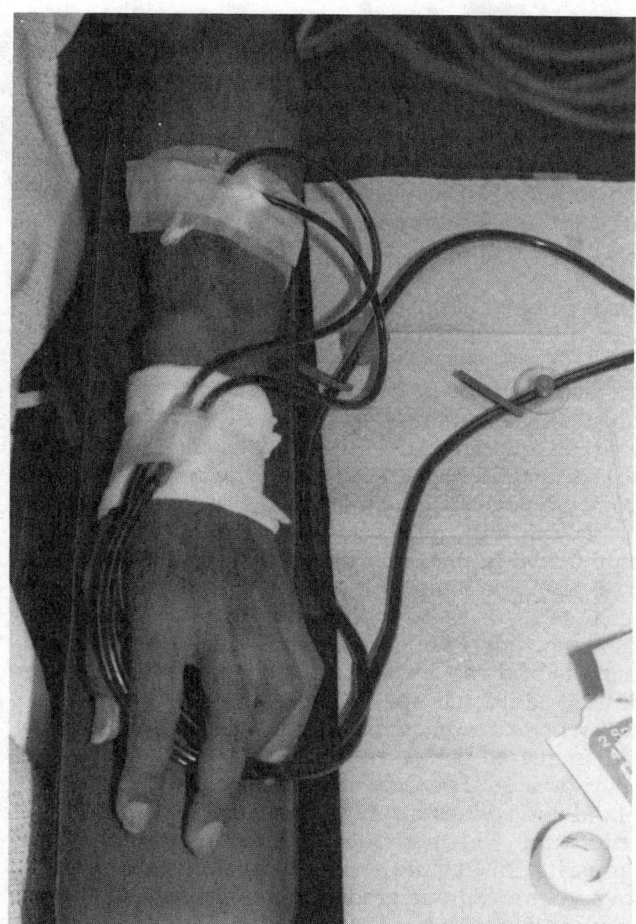

Figure 59 – 6

A cannulated AV fistula.

internal fistula and are caused by repeated needle punctures at the same site. Aneurysms that appear to be increasing in size require surgical repair and may cause the loss of the fistula's function. Ischemia occurs in a small number of clients with vascular accesses when the formation of the fistula causes a decrease in arterial blood flow to areas distal to the fistula. Ischemic symptoms vary from cold or numb fingers to gangrene. If the collateral circulation is inadequate, the fistula may have to be ligated and placed in another area to preserve circulation in the extremity. Finally, the shunting of blood directly from the arterial system to the venous system, through the fistula, can cause high-output heart failure in clients with a limited cardiac reserve. This occurs rarely and may necessitate revision of the fistula to decrease the blood flow and limit the arterial shunt.

The duration and frequency of hemodialysis treatments depend on the amount of metabolic waste to be cleared, the clearance capacity of the dialyzer, and the amount of fluid to be removed. Most dialyzers provide sufficient clearance to limit the total number of hours of dialysis to 12 per week. This is usually divided into three 4-hour treatments per week, or two 6-hour treatments per week. If an individual gains large amounts of fluid

weight, a longer treatment time may be required to remove the fluid without hypotension or severe side effects.

Postdialysis nursing care. The client should be closely monitored by the nurse in the immediate postdialysis period and for several hours for any side effects from the treatment. The more common clinical manifestations of complications include hypotension, headache, nausea, malaise, vomiting, dizziness, and muscle cramps. The nurse obtains vital signs and weight for comparison with predialysis measurements. The blood pressure and weight are expected to be reduced owing to fluid removal. Excessive hypotension may require rehydration with IV fluids, such as normal saline. The client may also have an elevated temperature because the dialysis machine warms the blood slightly. If the temperature is elevated excessively, sepsis is suspected and blood for cultures should be drawn. As discussed earlier, the heparinization required for hemodialysis increases the clotting time and thus the risk for excessive bleeding. All invasive procedures must be avoided for 4 to 6 hours after dialysis, and the individual is continuously monitored by the nurse for signs of hemorrhage during the dialysis and for 1 hour after dialysis.

Complications. A complication that is seen in some clients is dialysis *disequilibrium syndrome.* This syndrome is seen during hemodialysis and sometimes after the dialysis treatment has been completed. The cause is unknown, but it is hypothesized to be due to the rapid decrease in BUN levels during hemodialysis. These changes in urea levels can cause cerebral edema, which leads to increased intracranial pressure. This results in neurologic complications, including headache, nausea, vomiting, restlessness, decreased level of consciousness, convulsions, coma, and death. Early recognition by the nurse of the signs of the syndrome and appropriate treatment with anticonvulsant medications and barbiturates may prevent a life-threatening situation.

Infectious disease transmitted by blood transfusion constitutes another serious complication associated with long-term hemodialysis. The chronic anemia caused by renal failure and exacerbated by hemodialysis requires frequent blood transfusions. As a result, hepatitis has long been a problem for clients undergoing hemodialysis, and the number of cases has been increasing yearly. Transmission of the hepatitis B virus can occur through use of contaminated needles or instruments, via entry of contaminated blood through open wounds in the skin or mucous membranes, or through transfusion of blood contaminated with the virus. The incubation period for acute hepatitis is 6 weeks to 6 months. Thus, the nurse continuously monitors the client undergoing hemodialysis who is receiving frequent transfusions for signs of hepatitis virus infection (see Chap. 47).

Acquired immunodeficiency syndrome (AIDS) has become a new and deadly threat to clients undergoing hemodialysis. Before the introduction of routine blood screening for AIDS, the disease could be transmitted by transfusions of blood or blood products. Since the advent of blood screening, the supply of blood for transfusion is considered safe. Despite this progress, an unknown number of clients may have already been infected with the human immunodeficiency virus (HIV). It can take 5 years or more after HIV infection for the clinical manifestations of AIDS to become apparent. Thus, individuals who have been undergoing hemodialysis and receiving frequent transfusions during the past 10 years are at risk for AIDS. The nurse routinely caring for these clients should be aware of the signs of HIV infections and consistently use precautions when handling any blood products or when contact with the client's blood is possible (Chap. 27 discusses AIDS).

Client selection.   When CRF can no longer be managed with conservative therapies, such as diet, medication, and fluid restriction, maintenance dialysis is begun. Before CRF progresses to end-stage renal disease, the concepts of dialysis are introduced, and the nurse initiates teaching. After the client understands the necessity for dialysis, a vascular access is created in preparation for initiation of hemodialysis therapy.

Any individual may be accepted for hemodialysis therapy. Duration of survival with hemodialysis is dependent on the client's age, the cause of renal failure, and the presence of other diseases, such as hypertension and diabetes, at the beginning of therapy. Medicare coverage of treatment of CRF does not limit access to hemodialysis on the basis of financial status. General guidelines for appropriate client selection for hemodialysis include the presence of fatal, irreversible renal failure when other therapies are unacceptable, absence of illnesses that would prevent or seriously complicate hemodialysis, expectation of rehabilitation, and the individual's acceptance of the treatment regimen.

Clients may receive hemodialysis treatments in any of several settings, depending on individual needs. They may be dialyzed in an acute care (hospital-based) center if they have recently begun treatment or have complicating conditions that require close medical and nursing supervision. Many CRF clients may be transferred for longer-term maintenance to a hemodialysis center in the community when they no longer require intensive supervision. Ideally, stable clients begin in-home hemodialysis after they are prepared to manage the treatment independently. In-home hemodialysis necessitates a consistent partner to administer the therapy and manage the dialysis machine. In addition, a water treatment system must be installed in the home to provide a safe, clean water supply for the dialysis process.

In-home hemodialysis offers the least disruptive form of therapy and allows for the most individual adaptation of the hemodialysis regimen to the client's life style. Unfortunately, many clients cannot participate in home dialysis because of lack of a reliable partner. In addition to the client who is undergoing in-home dialysis, the individual (partner) who performs the in-home dialysis also requires nursing intervention in the form of home visits by a nurse trained in dialysis techniques or regular visits to a dialysis center where a nurse would provide physical assessment and client teaching. Regardless of the site of therapy, the client needs ongoing nursing support and intervention to maintain this complex and lifesaving treatment.

Peritoneal dialysis.   Peritoneal dialysis is an alternative method of dialysis used by clients with chronic and acute renal failure (see Table 59–2). This dialysis takes place within the individual's peritoneal cavity.

Procedure.   The surgical insertion of a siliconized rubber catheter (Tenckhoff's catheter) into the abdominal cavity is required to allow the infusion of dialyzing fluid (Fig. 59–7). Approximately 1 to 2 L of fluid is infused by gravity into the peritoneal space during approximately 20 minutes. The fluid dwells in the cavity for a time ordered by the physician (usually 20 minutes) and is then allowed to flow out of the body by gravity into a drainage bag. The dialyzing fluid takes with it excess fluid and metabolic waste products that have accumulated in the client's body. The entire process of infusion, "dwell time," and outflow is considered one exchange. It takes 40 L of fluid exchange to complete what is considered one dialysis procedure. This method is simple and can be performed by any skilled nurse without additional specialized training. This process uses an open system, which leaves the client vulnerable to an increased risk of infection.

The process of peritoneal dialysis occurs via a transfer of fluid and solutes from the blood stream through the peritoneum. The peritoneal membrane is large and porous. It allows solutes, which carry fluid with them, to move via an osmotic gradient from an area of higher concentration in the body to an area of lower concentration in the dialyzing fluid. The peritoneal cavity is rich in capillaries and provides a ready access to the blood supply. The fluid and waste products dialyzed from the client move through the blood vessel walls, the interstitial tissues, and the peritoneal membrane and are removed when the dialyzing fluid is drained from the body. The efficiency of peritoneal dialysis can be affected by numerous situations, such as changes in the peritoneal membrane's permeability caused by infection or irritation and changes in capillary blood flow resulting from vasoconstriction, vascular disease, or decreased perfusion of the peritoneum. Thus, peritoneal dialysis is much less efficient than hemodialysis and takes four to five times longer to obtain the same effect.

The major difference in the composition of *dialysate* used for peritoneal dialysis and that used for hemodialysis is the glucose concentration. Hemodialysis uses hydraulic positive pressure to increase ultrafiltration, but peritoneal dialysis depends on osmotic pressure to produce ultrafiltration. Increasing the glucose concentration in peritoneal dialysis fluid increases the concentration of active particles that cause osmosis. This also increases the rate of ultrafiltration and the amount of fluid removed. Commercial solutions are 1.5%, 2.5%, and 4.25% glucose. The higher the glucose concentration, the greater is the amount of fluid that is removed from the client during an exchange. The percentage of

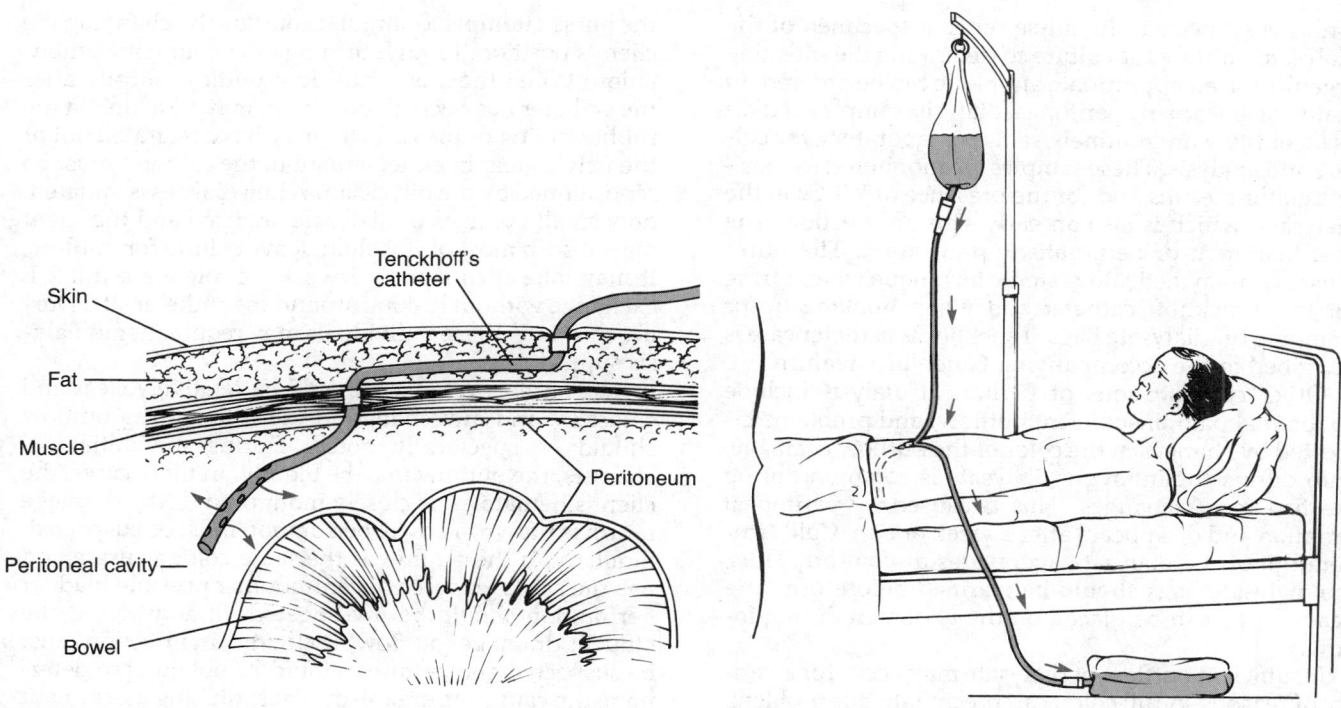

Figure 59–7

Manual peritoneal dialysis via an implanted abdominal catheter (Tenckhoff's catheter).

glucose in the dialysis solution is ordered by the physician and is based on each client's needs.

The medications for clients undergoing peritoneal dialysis are similar to those given to individuals undergoing hemodialysis. Multivitamin supplements are needed and must be administered daily. These clients also need regular supplements of folate and iron because the diseased kidneys are unable to maintain sufficient levels of folate and iron. In addition, owing to the kidneys' inability to secrete phosphorus, clients undergoing peritoneal dialysis also require phosphate binders to prevent calcium wasting and bone disease. As in hemodialysis, heparin is given during peritoneal dialysis. However, in this form of dialysis, the heparin is added to the dialysate bag and infused through the catheter into the peritoneum. This prevents catheter obstruction by fibrin clots and does not result in systemic anticoagulation for the client. These individuals are susceptible to infections in the form of peritonitis. Prophylactic antibiotics are often added to the dialysate to prevent this complication.

There are three types of peritoneal dialysis: intermittent, continuous ambulatory, and continuous cycling. *Intermittent peritoneal dialysis* (IPD) can be performed manually or with the aid of a cycling machine. The client usually requires approximately 40 hours/week of dialysis. Manual dialysis is performed by the nurse in an acute care setting. The nurse individually initiates dialysate infusion and times infusion, dwell time, and outflow. Automated IPD involves the use of a cycler that controls these functions automatically during a period

of 8 to 10 hours while the client sleeps. The machine has numerous safety monitors and alarms and is used for clients undergoing longer-term peritoneal dialysis.

Continuous ambulatory peritoneal dialysis (CAPD) is an outpatient dialysis therapy. The client performs self-dialysis 24 hours/day, 7 days/week. The client infuses the dialysate into the peritoneal cavity where it remains for 4 to 8 hours. During this time, the dialysate bag is usually attached to the catheter and is carried in the client's clothing until it is used for outflow. The old bag is then removed, and a new one replaces it to repeat the process. With the use of disposable CAPD bags and tubing, the empty bag can be disconnected between infusions. CAPD requires no machine or partner and encourages client independence. In addition, it closely resembles renal function because it is a continuous process.

Continuous cycle peritoneal dialysis (CCPD) uses a cycling machine for exchanges at night while the client sleeps. The final exchange of the night is left to dwell through the day and is drained the next evening as the process is repeated. CCPD offers the advantage of 24-hour dialysis, as in CAPD, but involves less frequent violation of the sterile catheter system.

Complications.   A number of complications are seen relatively frequently, but often can be treated or prevented with careful nursing care. The major complication of peritoneal dialysis is *peritonitis.* This infection of the peritoneum is manifested by fever, rebound abdominal tenderness, abdominal pain, general malaise, nausea, vomiting, and cloudy dialysate outflow. When peritonitis is suspected, the nurse sends a specimen of the dialysate outflow for culture to determine the infecting organism so an appropriate antibiotic can be ordered. In many facilities using peritoneal dialysis, samples of dialysate outflow are routinely sent to a laboratory for culture and analysis. These samples are monitored for positive culture results and for the presence of WBCs in the dialysate, which is also an early sign of infection. The best treatment of peritonitis is prevention. The nurse must maintain meticulous sterile technique when caring for the Tenckhoff catheter and when hooking up or clamping off dialysate bags. Tenckhoff's catheter care is described in the accompanying Guidelines feature.

Other complications of peritoneal dialysis include abdominal pain, insufficient outflow, and problems indicated by changes in the color of the outflow drainage. Pain during the inflow of dialysate is common during the first few exchanges. This is caused by peritoneal irritation and disappears after a week or two. Cold temperature of the dialysate aggravates discomfort. Thus, the dialysate bags should be warmed before use, or a heating pad can be placed on the abdomen during inflow.

Insufficient outflow of dialysate may occur for a variety of reasons. A full colon can precipitate this problem, and a high-fiber diet, stool softeners, and rectal suppositories can prevent its occurrence. Because outflow drainage is by gravity, the drainage bag should be lower than the client's abdomen. If drainage is still inadequate,

the nurse attempts to stimulate outflow by changing the client's position through turning or encouraging ambulation. When there is insufficient outflow shortly after the catheter has been placed, there may be a kink in the rubber tubing or the catheter may have migrated out of the pelvic area. In either situation, the catheter must be repositioned by the physician. When dialysis is initiated, only small volumes of dialysate are used and the client may absorb most of this fluid, leaving little for outflow. It may take clients up to 2 weeks to tolerate a full 2-L exchange without leaking around the catheter site. During this time, these individuals may require hemodialysis support.

The outflow drainage should be relatively clear and colorless, and any change in the color of the outflow should be specifically noted. During the initial exchanges, the outflow may be bloody. In these cases, the client's hematocrit is closely monitored. If the drainage return is brown, a bowel perforation must be suspected. Similarly, if the outflow is the same color as urine and has the same glucose concentration, a possible bladder perforation should be investigated. In addition, if the effluent drainage (outflow) is cloudy, an infection must be suspected and cultures should be obtained to determine the causative organism. Thus, nursing assessment of the peritoneal dialysis outflow is essential to the well-being of these clients.

Nursing care during peritoneal dialysis. In the hospital setting, peritoneal dialysis is routinely initiated and

---

GUIDELINES ■ Peritoneal Dialysis Catheter Care

Interventions	Rationales
1. Mask yourself and your client. Wash your hands.	1. This decreases the risk of airborne contamination and prevents cross-contamination.
2. Put on sterile gloves. Remove the old dressing. Remove the contaminated gloves.	2. The dressing should be changed daily and whenever it becomes soiled to prevent infection. Gloves should be worn while removing contaminated dressings to avoid cross-contamination.
3. Assess area for signs of infection, such as swelling, redness, or discharge around the catheter site.	3. Early recognition of infection facilitates treatment by antibiotics and limits systemic involvement.
4. Use *aseptic technique.*	4. Peritonitis is a constant threat to anyone receiving peritoneal dialysis. The best protection is strict aseptic technique.
a. Open the sterile field on a flat surface and place two precut 4 × 4 in gauze pads on the field.	a. Movement of microorganisms into insertion site is inhibited.
b. Place three cotton swabs soaked in povidone-iodine on the field. Put on sterile gloves.	b. Povidone-iodine solution provides an antiseptic barrier against bacteria.
5. Use cotton swabs to clean around the catheter site. Use a circular motion starting from the insertion site and moving away toward the abdomen. Repeat with all three swabs.	5. Aseptic technique is maintained by avoiding contamination of the already cleaned area nearest the catheter.
6. Apply precut gauze pads over the catheter site. Tape only the edges of the gauze pads.	6. This method prevents infection while allowing the skin around the catheter to breathe.

monitored by the nursing staff. Before the treatment, the nurse measures baseline vital signs, including evaluation of blood pressure, apical and radial pulse rates, rectal temperature, quality of respirations, and breath sounds. The client is weighed, always on the same scale, before beginning the procedure and at least every 24 hours while receiving treatment. Baseline laboratory value determinations, such as electrolyte and glucose levels, are also essential and are repeated every 4 to 8 hours during treatment.

During peritoneal dialysis, the nurse constantly monitors the client. Vital signs are taken regularly and recorded on a flow sheet. For the first few exchanges, the nurse records the vital signs every 15 minutes. The nurse also performs an ongoing assessment of the client for signs of respiratory distress, pain, or discomfort. In addition, the abdominal dressing around the catheter exit site must be regularly checked for wetness. The nurse also monitors dwell time and initiates outflow. The physician orders the dwell time on the basis of the client's needs for fluid removal and electrolyte balance.

Dwell time usually ranges from 20 to 45 minutes. An extended dwell time increases the risk of hyperglycemia from glucose absorption. The outflow should be a continuous stream after the clamp is completely open. Changing the client's position may be necessary to facilitate outflow. The nurse should have the client turn from side to side or sit upright if the outflow is slow to start. The total amount of outflow should be accurately recorded after each exchange. It is of primary importance that the nurse maintain accurate intake and output records during peritoneal dialysis. The inflow of dialysate is considered intake, and the outflow is considered output. The difference between the inflow and the outflow is the amount of fluid removed during dialysis when outflow is sufficient. When outflow is less than inflow, the difference is equal to the amount absorbed or retained by the client during dialysis and should be counted as intake.

Client selection. Clients can select either hemodialysis or peritoneal dialysis for the treatment of CRF (see Table 59–2). Peritoneal dialysis may be preferred for some clients. For individuals who are hemodynamically unstable and those who cannot tolerate systemic anticoagulation, peritoneal dialysis is less hazardous than hemodialysis. Any client with no vessels available for hemodialysis access undergoes peritoneal dialysis. In addition, some clients with a new AV fistula receive peritoneal dialysis while waiting for the access to mature for hemodialysis. Peritoneal dialysis is also often the treatment of choice in the elderly and pediatric populations because it offers more flexibility if frequent changes in the client's status occur.

There are some situations in which peritoneal dialysis cannot be performed. This relatively rare situation is usually caused by peritoneal adhesions or intra-abdominal surgery that has occurred in the peritoneal cavity. In these cases, the peritoneal membrane's surface area has been reduced too much to allow for adequate dialysis exchange. In other circumstances, peritoneal membrane

fibrosis may occur after repeated infections, which decreases membrane permeability despite adequate surface area. The nurse obtains a careful history and performs a physical examination to determine if any potential problems would make peritoneal dialysis difficult.

Interventions: surgical management. Renal transplantation is considered a viable alternative for treatment of end-stage renal disease. Transplantation is not a permanent cure for loss of renal function. Renal transplantation and dialysis are life-sustaining treatments for end-stage renal disease. It is up to each individual to determine which type of therapy is best suited to his/her physical condition and life style.

Preoperative care. The major barrier to successful renal transplantation after a suitable donor kidney is available is the body's ability to identify and reject tissue that is not its own. This immunologic process attacks the transplanted kidney and renders it nonfunctional. To overcome immunologic contraindications, in-depth tissue typing is done on all candidates for transplantation. These studies include simple ABO blood group typing for compatible blood transfusions and human leukocyte antigen (HLA) studies, as well as other tests. The HLAs have become the principal histocompatibility system used to match transplant recipients with compatible donors. The more similar the antigens of the donor are to those of the recipient, the more likely it is that the transplant will be successful and immunologic rejection will be avoided. Research is ongoing in immunology, and new information in this area could increase the success rate of organ transplants in the future (see Chaps. 23 and 27 for discussion of immunity and organ transplantation).

Candidates for transplantation must be free from medical problems that could increase the risks associated with the procedure. The usual age range for clients undergoing transplantation is 4 to 60 years old. In clients older than 60 years of age, the risk of complications increases, and older clients are considered carefully on an individual basis. A thorough body systems assessment of the client is performed before she/he is considered for transplantation. The process of transplantation can place a life-threatening stress on the cardiac system in individuals with advanced, uncorrectable cardiac disease. Thus, these individuals are usually excluded from consideration for a transplant.

In addition, long-standing disease in the pulmonary system also increases the risk of morbidity and mortality owing to respiratory tract infections after transplantation. Clients with diseases of the GI system may require treatment before consideration for transplantation. Problems such as peptic ulcer disease and diverticulosis can be severely aggravated by the high dosages of steroids used after transplantation. The urinary system must be completely evaluated to ensure its ability to manage normal urine flow. Many clients with end-stage renal disease have not used their lower urinary tract for extended periods, and ureteral or bladder abnormalities may require surgical correction before a renal transplant. Metabolic diseases, such as diabetes mellitus, gout, or hyperparathyroidism, cause even greater risks. These clients can still accept a renal transplant, but careful observation and management are necessary to limit complications.

Other conditions that may also complicate transplantation include malignancy and inflammatory disease. Clients with a recent history of malignancy are usually treated with dialysis because of the shortage of donor organs, the possibility that the cancer could attack the transplanted kidney, and the limited life expectancy of these individuals. In addition, the immunosuppressive agents used after transplantation increase the risk of cancer recurrence. If more than a year has passed since eradication of the cancer, the client can again be considered for transplantation. Other complicating conditions are considered on an individual basis, depending on the client's current health status. Renal transplantation can be considered for the majority of clients with end-stage renal disease and may prove to be the optimal therapy for many people.

The sources of donor kidneys are limited to living related donors and cadaver donors. The available kidneys are matched on the basis of immunologic similarity between the donor and the recipient. Clients and donors do not need to be matched for age, race, or sex. The size of the kidney is seldom a problem, except in the youngest pediatric clients, because pediatric cadaver kidneys hypertrophy to accommodate adult needs within a few months and adult kidneys can be placed in a child's abdominal cavity. Organs from *living related donors* provide the highest rates of renal graft survival (90%). Donors are usually at least 18 years old because of legal age requirements and are seldom older than 65 years of age. General physical criteria for donors include the absence of systemic disease and infection, no history of cancer, the absence of hypertension and renal disease, and adequate renal function as evidenced by diagnostic studies. In addition, living related donors must express a clear understanding of the associated surgery and a willingness to give up a kidney. Some transplant centers also require a psychiatric evaluation to determine the motivation of the donor.

The *cadaver donor* is usually a child or young adult who has been the victim of trauma or other cerebral injury. The individual must be diagnosed as brain dead by a physician, on the basis of specific criteria, which may vary from state to state. Cadaver donors must meet all the physical criteria that living related donors meet, and the deceased's family must give written consent to organ donation in the absence of a signed uniform donor card. These cards express the individual's wish to serve as a donor, but transplant centers still request agreement from the next of kin. The brain dead individual's body is kept functioning by technical means until immediately before the kidneys are removed. The kidneys are then specially preserved and transplanted immediately to recipients waiting in another operating room or in another hospital. The success rate of cadaver transplants has improved greatly during the previous 10 years to approximately 70%.

The surgical team is a group of medical specialists trained in transplant procedures. The team includes operating room nurses (circulating and scrub nurses), clinical nurse specialists, and preoperative nurses, as well as transplant surgeons and nephrologists. The role of the preoperative nurse includes teaching about the procedure and postoperative care, in-depth client assessment, coordination of diagnostic tests, and development and implementation of treatment plans. The transplant recipient usually requires dialysis within 24 hours of the surgery. In addition, the recipient often receives a blood transfusion before surgery. The current research favors donor-specific transfusions, in which blood from the kidney donor is transfused into the recipient. This has resulted in increased graft survival, especially of organs from living related donors.

Procedure. The donor nephrectomy procedure varies with cadaver and living related donors. The cadaver donor nephrectomy is conducted as a sterile autopsy in the operating room. All arterial and venous vessels are carefully preserved. After removal, the kidneys are preserved and transferred to a transplant center. Cadaver donors are not transferred to transplant centers because preservation techniques can maintain the kidney's viability after removal from the body. The technique for kidney removal from a living related donor requires greater surgical care and is a delicate procedure lasting 3 to 4 hours. A flank incision is used, and care is taken to avoid scarring. Usually, donors experience more pain than recipients. They also need special nursing care and support for the psychologic adjustment to loss of a body part.

The transplant surgery usually takes 4 to 5 hours. The transplanted kidney is placed in the anterior iliac fossa instead of the usual anatomic position. This allows easier anastomosis of the ureter and the renal artery and vein. The position also minimizes postoperative pain. The recipient's own nonfunctioning kidney may be removed at this time or during a previous separate operation. The client is then taken to the postanesthesia recovery room, and then, when stable, to the surgical critical care unit within the transplant center.

Postoperative care. Postoperative care of the renal transplant recipient is similar to that of any client who has undergone abdominal surgery. Nursing care includes ongoing physical assessment, with an emphasis on renal function evaluation. The transplant recipient requires particularly close attention because the immunosuppressive drug therapy to prevent tissue rejection causes impaired healing and an increased susceptibility to infection. To promote graft success, careful urologic management is essential. These clients always have an indwelling (Foley) catheter for accurate urinary output measurements. The urine color is carefully monitored (usually hourly). Initially, the urine is pink and bloody, but it gradually returns to normal during several days to several weeks, depending on renal function.

Occasionally, a three-way Foley catheter may be used for bladder irrigation to decrease the incidence of blood clot formation, which could increase pressure in the bladder and jeopardize the graft. Care of Foley catheter is performed regularly to minimize contamination of the catheter; the individual hospital's policy is adhered to. The catheter is removed as soon as possible to avoid infection, usually 3 to 7 days postoperatively. The nurse is also responsible for obtaining daily urine tests, including urinalysis, glucose determinations, presence of acetone, culture, and specific gravity measurement.

During the postoperative period, the renal graft function can result in either oliguria or diuresis. Oliguria may occur as a result of ATN, rejection, and other complications. To increase urinary output, diuretics and osmotic agents, such as mannitol, are administered. Careful monitoring of the individual's fluid status is essential. Fluid overload could cause hypertension, CHF, and pulmonary edema. Daily weight measurement, frequent blood pressure readings, and careful intake and output measurements are required to evaluate fluid status.

Instead of oliguria, the client may have diuresis. The nurse carefully monitors fluid intake and output. The nurse also observes for electrolyte imbalances, such as hypokalemia and hyponatremia. Dehydration from excessive diuresis may cause hypotensive episodes. The nurse strives to prevent this situation, because decreased blood pressure also decreases the oxygen and blood supply to the transplanted kidney, which can threaten graft survival.

Complications. Unfortunately, numerous potential complications are associated with transplant surgery. Vascular complications nearly always require surgical intervention. Stenosis of the renal artery is detected by identification of hypertension, a bruit over the artery anastomosis site, and decreased renal function. The involved artery must be surgically resected and the kidney anastomosed to another artery. Other vascular problems include vascular leakage or thrombosis, both of which require an emergency nephrectomy. Wound complications, such as hematomas, abscesses, and lymphoceles, can become a medium for infection, as well as place external pressure on the new kidney. Genitourinary tract complications also often necessitate surgical intervention. These problems can include ureteral leakage, ureteral fistula, ureteral obstruction, calculus formation, bladder neck contracture, scrotal swelling, and graft rupture.

The most common and the most threatening complication of renal transplantation is rejection. In rejection, a reaction occurs between the antigens in the transplanted kidney and the antibodies and cytotoxic T cells in the recipient's blood. These immunologic substances treat the new kidney as a foreign invader and cause tissue destruction, thrombosis, and eventual necrosis of the kidney. There are three types of rejection—hyperacute, acute, and chronic (see the accompanying Key Features of Disease). *Hyperacute rejection* occurs immediately after the transplant surgery. There is no treatment of this type of rejection, and, after recognition of the problem,

---

KEY FEATURES OF DISEASE ■ A Comparison of Hyperacute, Acute, and Chronic Posttransplant Rejection

Hyperacute Rejection	Acute Rejection	Chronic Rejection
Onset		
Within 48 h after surgery	1 wk to 2 yr postoperatively (most common in first 2 wk)	Occurs gradually during a period of months to years
Clinical Manifestations		
Increased temperature	Oliguria or anuria	Gradually increase BUN and serum creatinine levels
Increased blood pressure	Increased temperature	Fluid retention
Pain at transplant site	Increased blood pressure	Changes in serum electrolyte levels
	Enlarged tender kidney	
	Lethargy	
	Changes in urinalysis and blood chemistry values	
Treatment		
Immediate removal of the transplanted kidney	Increased dosages of immunosuppressive drugs	Conservative management until dialysis is required

the rejected kidney is removed quickly to prevent further complications. Accelerated rejection, which occurs 24 to 48 hours after surgery, is another form of hyperacute rejection. This type of rejection is now rare because of advances in tissue typing and cross-matching of donor and recipient.

Acute rejection differs from hyperacute rejection in that it does not occur until 1 week to 2 years after surgery. Nearly all transplant clients have at least one or two episodes of acute rejection. These occur most commonly 7 to 14 days after transplantation. Most of these episodes can be stopped with early recognition and immediate administration of increased dosages of immunosuppressive drugs. Occasionally, the rejection process cannot be reversed and eventually causes the failure of the transplanted kidney. All nurses caring for clients with renal transplants need to be aware of the clinical manifestations of acute rejection and report any symptoms of rejection immediately. The most common manifestations include oliguria or anuria, temperature greater than 100° F (37.8° C), enlarged and tender kidney, fluid retention, increased blood pressure, chronic fatigue, and changes in urinalysis and blood chemistry values.

Finally, *chronic rejection* occurs much more slowly than acute or hyperacute rejection. Chronic rejection can occur during a period of months or years. The clinical manifestations include gradually increasing BUN and serum creatinine levels, as well as fluid retention and changes in serum electrolyte levels. There is no treatment of chronic rejection, and the client is conservatively managed until renal function deteriorates to the point at which dialysis is required.

Immunosuppressive drug therapy. The success of renal transplantation depends on being able to change the client's immunologic response so that the new kidney is not rejected as a foreign organ. The role of the nurse caring for these clients includes administration and knowledge of the immunosuppressive drugs that protect the transplanted organ. These drugs include corticosteroids, antilymphocyte preparations, monoclonal antibodies, and cyclosporine (cyclosporin A); these are representative of the numerous immunosuppressive agents.

Corticosteroids are widely used after transplantation and act as anti-inflammatory agents to prevent the movement of leukocytes into tissue during rejection. They also limit antibody production and block antigen-antibody complex formation. The nurse must constantly be aware of the numerous side effects of corticosteroids, such as infections, GI bleeding, ulcers, pancreatitis, delayed wound healing, diabetes mellitus, psychosis, cataracts, fluid and electrolyte imbalance, and hypertension. Prednisone (Deltasone) and methylprednisolone (Medrol) or methylprednisolone sodium succinate (Solu-Medrol) are typically used.

Antilymphocyte preparations are made from the sera of animals and cover the antigens of the graft, making them unrecognizable to lymphocytes. The nurse must monitor for side effects, including fever, chills, joint

pain, phlebitis, infection, and anaphylaxis. These drugs can be given intravenously or intramuscularly, but can only be used for short-term immunosuppression. Monoclonal antibodies, such as muromonal-CD3 (OKT3), are more specific antilymphocyte drugs that react with the antigen on the T cell and destroy those cells. These preparations require particularly meticulous nursing assessment because they are given intravenously and reactions frequently occur with the first administration. Reactions are seldom seen with later doses. The clinical manifestations of a reaction include fever, chills, dyspnea, and chest pain. These antibodies are also effective in reversing rejection episodes.

Cyclosporine is a newer drug used to prevent and treat rejection of renal transplants. It works by interfering with T cell growth and can be given orally, intramuscularly, or intravenously. This drug is toxic to the body, and nursing responsibilities require observing for nephrotoxicity, hepatotoxicity, and potential malignancy, especially lymphoma. In addition, the nurse closely monitors the blood levels of the drug to ensure that they are therapeutic, but not toxic.

Altered Nutrition: Less Than Body Requirements

Planning: client goals. The goals for this nursing diagnosis are that the client will (1) maintain an adequate nutritional status; (2) maintain ideal body weight for age, height, and body build; (3) maintain serum laboratory values within safe levels; and (4) comply with the prescribed dietary regimen.

Interventions: nonsurgical management. The nutritional requirements of the client with renal failure vary according to the degree of decrease in renal function and the type of dialysis performed, if any (see the accompanying Health Promotion/Maintenance feature). The dietary restrictions for these clients are based on these principles: regulation of protein intake; limitation of fluid intake; restriction of potassium, sodium, and phosphorus intake; administration of appropriate vitamin and mineral supplements; and provision of adequate caloric intake. The diet prescribed for each client should also consider the nutritional needs dictated by age, height, and body build; level of activity; and remaining renal function.

All clients with decreased renal function must limit their protein consumption to some degree. Because the accumulation of the waste products from protein metabolism is the primary cause of uremia, protein in the diet is restricted on the basis of the degree of renal insufficiency and the severity of the symptoms associated with nitrogen retention. The GFR is often used as an indicator of renal function and, thus, a guide to safe levels of protein consumption in the client. An individual with a severely reduced GFR who is not undergoing dialysis usually is permitted 0.55 to 0.60 g of protein per kilogram of body weight (e.g., 40 g of protein daily for a 70-kg [150-lb] adult). The client receiving dialysis requires more protein because of losses incurred as a result

HEALTH PROMOTION/MAINTENANCE ■ **Dietary Restrictions for the Client with Renal Failure**

Dietary Component	With Chronic Uremia	With Hemodialysis	With Peritoneal Dialysis
Protein	0.55–0.60 g/kg of body weight per day	1.0–1.3 g/kg of body weight per day	0.8–1.5 g/kg of body weight per day
Fluid	1500–3000 mL/d	700 mL/d plus amount of urinary output	Restriction based on fluid weight gain and blood
Potassium	70 mEq/d	70 mEq/d	Usually no restriction
Sodium	1–3 g/d	1–2 g/d	Restriction based on fluid weight gain and blood pressure
Phosphorus	700 mg/d	700 mg/d	800 mg/d

of the therapy. These clients usually are allowed 1.0 to 1.3 g of protein per kilogram daily. Approximately three-fourths of the protein should be of high biologic value, such as milk, meat, or eggs. If protein intake is inadequate, a negative nitrogen balance develops and causes muscle wasting. The serum albumin and BUN levels are used to monitor the adequacy of protein consumption. Decreases in serum albumin levels indicate inadequate protein intake and malnutrition. Excessive protein intake can cause dramatic increases in BUN levels in clients with diminished renal function.

The nurse closely monitors fluid and sodium intake in clients with renal failure. In clients with little or no urinary output, fluid and sodium retention can cause edema, hypertension, and CHF. In other clients who still have urinary output, the kidneys may be unable to conserve sodium, and sodium intake must replace urinary losses. The client's current status of fluid and sodium retention can be estimated by monitoring body weight and blood pressure. In nondialyzed uremic clients, sodium is limited to 1 to 3 g daily and fluid intake to approximately 1500 to 3000 mL, depending on urinary output. In oliguric individuals receiving dialysis, the sodium restriction is 1 to 2 g daily, and fluid intake is limited to about 700 mL, plus the amount of urinary output.

Potassium and phosphorus retention requires constant attention by the nurse caring for the client with renal disease. The control of phosphorus levels is begun early in renal failure to avoid osteodystrophy. Serum phosphorus levels are monitored regularly, and clients are given aluminum hydroxide gel to bind the phosphorus. Most clients with kidney disease already restrict their protein intake, and, because high-protein foods are high in phosphorus, their phosphorus consumption is also reduced. Potassium intake is carefully monitored by the nurse, as hyperkalemia can cause dangerous cardiac arrhythmias. The client's serum potassium level is monitored frequently, and individuals with advanced CRF should limit their potassium intake to 70 mEq/day. Chapter 12 lists foods high in potassium, sodium, and phosphorus.

Most clients with renal failure require vitamin and mineral supplementation. Low-protein diets are usually deficient in vitamins, and water-soluble vitamins are removed from the blood during dialysis. In addition, anemia is a chronic problem in clients with renal failure owing to the limited iron content of low-protein diets and decreased erythropoietin production by the kidneys. Calcium and vitamin D supplements may also be required if individual serum levels and bone status warrant. Clients with CRF should receive a daily multivitamin supplement to meet these needs.

Clients undergoing peritoneal dialysis require a slightly different diet from those undergoing hemodialysis. Protein is lost with the dialysate in peritoneal dialysis. The major nutritional problem for these clients is compensating for this loss. In many cases, 100 to 120 g of protein daily is recommended. The amount of sodium restriction varies with fluid weight gain and blood pressure. There is usually no need to restrict dietary potassium because the dialysate is potassium free. The potassium restriction, if any, is determined by the client's serum potassium level.

The nurse plays a vital role in managing the client's diet. In collaboration with the dietitian, nurses provide teaching and perform ongoing assessments of the client's comprehension of and compliance with dietary regimens. The nurse can help clients adapt the diet to their budget, ethnic background, and food preferences to maximize caloric intake within the diet's restrictions.

Anxiety

Planning: client goals. The goal for this nursing diagnosis is that the client will display reduced anxiety by an absence of physical cues indicating increased anxiety, an ability to describe the renal failure process, and an awareness of the purpose and procedures for all treatments and tests.

Interventions: nonsurgical management. The nurse has the most frequent contact with the client with CRF after he/she is hospitalized. Thus, nurses should perform an ongoing assessment of the client's anxiety level to determine the level of nursing intervention that is required by the individual client. This assessment includes observing the individual's behavior for physical cues indicating anxiety (e.g., anxious facial expression or gestures and increased pulse rate). In addition, the nurse evaluates the client's support systems, such as evidenced by the involvement of family and friends during the hospital stay.

Unfamiliar settings and situations and lack of knowledge about treatments and tests can increase the client's anxiety level. The nurse caring for the client explains all procedures, tests, and treatments. The nurse identifies the client's knowledge deficits concerning normal renal function and renal failure. Evaluating the client's current knowledge avoids needless repetition during teaching sessions. The nurse provides instruction appropriate to the client's needs and ability to understand. By explaining the disease process, the nurse enhances the individual's acceptance and decreases anxiety.

Finally, the nurse encourages the client to ask questions and discuss fears about her/his diagnosis of renal failure. An open atmosphere that allows for discussion can decrease the client's anxiety level. Nurses also facilitate discussions with family members concerning the client's prognosis and the potential impact on the client's life style. This allows the nurse to provide support to the family and may also facilitate discharge planning.

■ Discharge Planning

Home Care Preparation

The nurse plays a vital role in the long-term care and support of the client with CRF. As the client's renal disease progresses, the client is seen on an ongoing basis by a physician and may have frequent hospitalizations. It is appropriate for the nursing staff to provide ongoing health care teaching about the diet in renal disease and the pathophysiology of renal disease. As a result of such instruction, the client may be more compliant with dietary restrictions and the required medical regimen.

As CRF approaches end-stage renal disease, a course of treatment must be chosen: hemodialysis, peritoneal dialysis, or transplantation. For each of these forms of treatment, the client must learn the relevant information and procedures.

Treatment with hemodialysis necessitates a working knowledge of the dialysis machine and the care of the client's vascular access. If the individual chooses in-home hemodialysis, preparations for installation of the appropriate equipment, including a water treatment system, must be made. Usually, a nurse makes home visits to facilitate the client's transition from the hemodialysis center to the home. Regardless of whether the treatment is provided at home or in a hemodialysis center, the nurse provides ongoing physical assessment and health care teaching to promote maximal independence at home.

The client receiving peritoneal dialysis has less fre-

quent contact with the nursing staff after discharge from the hospital than the client undergoing hemodialysis. For peritoneal dialysis, the client needs extensive training in the procedures. In addition, the client also needs assistance in obtaining equipment and the numerous supplies required by this therapy.

Finally, the nurse plays a vital role in the long-term care of the client with a renal transplant. Usually, this client is discharged from the hospital 3 to 4 weeks after surgery. Meticulous maintenance of prescribed immunosuppressive drug therapy is essential for the survival of the renal graft. Thus, the nurse facilitates the client's acceptance and understanding of this regimen as a part of his/her daily life.

Client/Family Education

Health care teaching is a primary function for nurses caring for clients with any form of renal disease. As the severity of the decreasing renal function increases, clients and family members are instructed in all aspects of diet therapy, necessary drug therapy, and associated renal pathologic changes. When an individual requires a more advanced form of therapy, such as dialysis or transplantation, the teaching focuses on the chosen therapeutic intervention.

Hemodialysis is the most complex form of therapy for the client and family to understand. Even if the client receives hemodialysis in a dialysis center instead of at home, the individual is usually expected to have some knowledge of the hemodialysis machine. The client or a family member must be taught to adequately care for the vascular access. If the client plans to have in-home dialysis, a partner is required. Both the client and the partner must be completely educated in the entire process of hemodialysis and must be able to perform it independently before the client is discharged from the hemodialysis center or hospital hemodialysis unit.

Peritoneal dialysis also requires extensive client health care teaching. This instruction can be done with the client alone or with a family member if the client is unable to perform the procedures. The entire peritoneal dialysis procedure must be mastered by the individual. The nurses providing the instruction must emphasize sterile technique because peritonitis is the most common complication of peritoneal dialysis performed at home.

The individual receiving a renal transplant also requires extensive health care teaching. The nurse is largely responsible for this instruction, which includes information about medication regimens, side effects of immunosuppression, clinical manifestations of rejection, and changes in diet and activity level.

Psychosocial Preparation

The nurse provides psychologic support for the client and the family. The nurse's goal is to facilitate adjustment to the diagnosis of renal failure and eventual acceptance of the treatment regimens.

Often, during the early stages of treatment of CRF

(from several weeks to 6 months), the treatment, usually some form of dialysis, relieves the uremic symptoms. Clients feel better physically, their mood may be happy and hopeful, and they tend to overlook the inconvenience and discomfort of the frequent dialysis therapies. The nurse should realize that this is temporary and utilize the time to initiate health care teaching. It is important for the nurse to stress that, although the client's uremic symptoms have diminished, the client will not return to her/his previous state of well-being. The client and the family may have looked on dialysis as a cure instead of a required lifelong treatment modality.

Next, the client enters a phase of discouragement and disillusionment, which may last a few months to a year. The difficulties of incorporating dialysis into daily life are staggering, and clients frequently become disappointed and depressed as these become apparent. During this time, the individual is likely to struggle against the idea of having to be permanently dependent on a disruptive therapy. The fear of rejection by hospital staff and family members reinforces feelings of helplessness and dependence. Some people retreat into complete or partial denial of the disease and the need for treatment. They may say that they do not need dialysis or may not comply with medication administration and dietary restrictions. Nurses who work with these individuals need to monitor any maladaptive behaviors that could contribute to noncompliance and suggest psychiatric referrals as appropriate. Nurses and family members should focus on the positive aspects of the treatments. Health care education should be continued by the nursing staff, but with the client as an active participant and decision-maker.

Finally, the client with CRF enters a phase of acceptance. The prospect of a chronic illness may be devastating for some people, and each individual reacts differently. This long-term adaptation requires the client to adjust to continuous change depending on current physical status and treatment method.

After the clients have accepted the chronicity of their disease, they usually attempt to return to the type of life they led before the disease occurred. Resuming the level of activity that existed before the disease is impossible. The nurse and other health care professionals can help clients to establish realistic individual goals that allow them to lead active, productive lives.

Health Care Resources

Professionals from various disciplines can be used as health care resources for the client with renal failure. Home care nurses are often required to monitor the client's status and evaluate maintenance of the prescribed treatment regimen (hemodialysis or peritoneal dialysis). Social services personnel are usually involved because of the complex process of applying for financial aid to pay for the required medical care. Physical and occupational therapists often work with these individuals, depending on their needs. Finally, individuals with CRF are routinely followed by a physician, usually a nephrologist.

 Evaluation

Nurses caring for clients with CRF evaluate each individual's progress on the basis of the common nursing diagnoses. The expected outcomes include that the client

1. Achieves and maintains appropriate fluid volume
2. Maintains serum electrolyte levels within a normal range for that client
3. Complies with the prescribed dietary regimen
4. Maintains an adequate nutritional status
5. Displays a reduction in anxiety

ACUTE RENAL FAILURE

OVERVIEW

Acute renal failure (ARF) is the rapid deterioration of renal function associated with an accumulation of nitrogenous wastes in the body (azotemia) that is not due to extrarenal factors. This situation differs from the much more gradual decline in renal function seen in CRF. Numerous renal insults can cause ARF, but the acute syndrome, unlike the chronic condition, is usually reversible.

Pathophysiology

The rapid decline in renal function characteristic of ARF results in the build-up of nitrogenous wastes. This causes a progressive elevation of the serum BUN and creatinine levels. The normal serum BUN/creatinine ratio is approximately 20:1. When the BUN rises faster than the serum creatinine level, and the 20:1 ratio is not maintained, the cause is usually related to protein catabolism or volume depletion. When both the BUN and creatinine levels rise and the 20:1 ratio remains constant, renal failure is present.

The types of ARF are prerenal, intrarenal, or postrenal (see the accompanying Key Features of Disease). *Prerenal* ARF occurs when the blood flow is diminished before reaching the kidneys, leading to ischemia in the nephrons. This can be reversed by establishing normal intravascular volume, blood pressure, and cardiac output. Prolonged hypoperfusion can lead to severe ischemic injury and intrarenal failure. *Intrarenal* ARF results from histologic damage to the kidney itself attributable to inflammatory or immunologic processes. These disease processes include acute glomerulonephritis, vasculitis, hepatorenal syndrome (associated with cirrhosis), and ATN. *Postrenal* ARF is characterized by an obstruc-

KEY FEATURES OF DISEASE ■ Causes of the Three Types of Acute Renal Failure

Pathologic Change	Causes
Prerenal	

Decreased blood flow to the kidneys leading to ischemia in the nephrons. Prolonged hypoperfusion can lead to tubular necrosis and ARF.	Conditions that cause decreased cardiac output
	  Shock
	  CHF
	  Pulmonary embolism
	  Anaphylaxis
	  Pericardial tamponade
	  Sepsis

Intrarenal	
Actual tissue damage to the kidney caused by inflammatory or immunologic processes.	Exposure to nephrotoxins Acute glomerulonephritis Vasculitis Hepatorenal syndrome ATN
Postrenal	
Obstruction of the urinary collecting system anywhere from the calyces to the urethral meatus. Obstruction of the bladder must be bilateral to cause postrenal failure unless only one kidney is functional.	Urethral or bladder cancer Renal calculi Atony of bladder Prostatic hyperplasia or cancer Cervical cancer

tion of the urinary collecting system anywhere from the calyces to the urethral meatus. Obstruction above the bladder must occur bilaterally to cause ARF, unless only one kidney is functional. Chronic overdistention of the bladder can lead to ARF as a result of obstructive uropathy. Obstructions, such as renal calculi and urethral strictures, can also cause ARF.

After a client's renal function has been compromised, the phases of ARF commence. These phases include the onset of ARF, oliguria, diuresis, recovery, and convalescence. The *onset phase* begins with the precipitating event and continues until oliguria is observed. This initial phase can last hours or several days. *Oliguria* can last 1 week to several weeks. The clinical manifestations are rising BUN and serum creatinine levels, urinary output of less than 400 mL/24 hours, low urine specific gravity, low urinary sodium level, and traces of protein, RBCs, and casts in the urine. In some cases, individuals do not experience significant oliguria, but may instead progress directly to the diuretic phase. After the urinary output exceeds 400 mL/24 hours, the *diuretic,* or *high-output, phase,* begins. The diuresis can result in an output of up to 10 L/day of dilute urine. This phase usually occurs 2 to 6 weeks after onset and continues until the BUN level ceases to rise. *Recovery* begins when the BUN level starts to fall and lasts until the BUN level reaches normal limits. Normal renal tubular function is re-established during this phase. Adequate clearance of urea and creat-

inine also returns. The final phase of ARF is *convalescence.* In this phase, the client begins to return to his/her normal activities, but he/she functions at a lower energy level and has less stamina than before the illness. Regular monitoring of renal function is required to detect any residual renal insufficiency that may occur.

Etiology

Many different types of renal insults can lead to reduced renal function. Severe hypotension, from excessive blood loss, results in hypoperfusion of blood to the kidneys and can lead to prerenal ARF. Cardiac disease or heart failure also results in decreased renal perfusion. Dehydration causes decreased intravascular volume and thus decreases the blood supply to the kidneys. This can cause the client to be oliguric, or even anuric, if the dehydration is severe. Other conditions that precipitate ARF include disseminated intravascular coagulation; obstruction by thrombi, uric acid crystals, or other obstructing precipitates; acute hemolytic transfusion reactions; severe hypertension; and complications of infection (e.g., pyelonephritis), acute glomerulonephritis, vasculitis, and hepatorenal syndrome, which is associated with cirrhosis. (The reader is referred to other chapters for discussion of these disorders.)

The most common cause of ARF is *acute tubular necrosis.* Tubular necrosis is primarily caused by histologic damage in the nephrons attributable to ischemia or nephrotoxicity, leading to an abrupt decline in renal function. The kidneys normally receive 1200 mL/minute of blood, or 20% to 25% of the cardiac output. Renal perfusion is reduced when vascular volume decreases or when the blood pressure declines. Prolonged periods of hypoperfusion can lead to nephrologic damage and ATN. Tubular necrosis can also be caused by ingestion of nephrotoxic drugs or other materials. Substances that are toxic to the kidneys include numerous antibiotics, analgesics, heavy metals, and vascular and renal contrast media (Table 59-4). When any of these or other renal toxins are taken under conditions of dehydration and reduced renal perfusion, their nephrotoxic effects may be accentuated.

TABLE 59-4   Some Nephrotoxic Substances

Drugs

Antibiotics/Anti-infectives	*Other Drugs*
Amphotericin	Penicillamine
Colistimethate	Phenacetin
Methicillin	Phenazopyridine
Polymyxin B	hydrochloride
Rifampin	Quinine
Sulfonamides	
Tetracycline	**Other Substances**
hydrochloride	
Vancomycin	*Organic Solvents*
Aminoglycosides	Carbon tetrachloride
	Ethylene glycol
Gentamicin	
Kanamycin	*Nondrug Chemical Agents*
Neomycin	
Netilmicin sulfate	Radiographic contrast dye
Tobramycin	Pesticides
	Fungicides
Antineoplastics	Myoglobin (from break-
	down of skeletal
Cisplatin	muscle)
Cyclophosphamide	
Methotrexate	*Heavy Metals and Ions*
Other Drugs	Arsenic
	Bismuth
Acetaminophen	Copper sulfate
Captopril	Gold salts
Fluorinated anesthetics	Lead
Indomethacin	Mercuric chloride
Lithium	Mercury
Mercurial diuretics	Uranium

Incidence

The incidence of ARF depends largely on the underlying disease process. Severe hypotension leading to ATN is the most common cause of ARF. Prerenal hypovolemia is the second most common cause of renal insufficiency. Other causes of ARF (see earlier) are each responsible for a small percentage of renal failure cases (Van Stone, 1984).

The mortality of clients with ARF is high, with most studies finding that only about 50% of individuals with the disease survive (Van Stone, 1984). The rate of survival is not affected by the age of the client. The highest mortality occurs with trauma and surgery, and ARF caused by nephrotoxic substances is associated with the lowest rates. ATN results in more deaths than any other type of renal disease, but the prognosis depends on the underlying disease process. The prognosis for ARF attributable to obstruction or glomerulonephritis is much better. Complications during the course of ARF can vastly increase the incidence of mortality. Infection is the most serious and most common complication. The combination of renal disease and the infectious process results in a high mortality. The lungs and the pulmonary system are the most frequent sites of infections.

PREVENTION

Nurses have an essential role in the prevention of ARF. The nurse is often the first to note the signs of impending renal dysfunction by careful physical assessment and close monitoring of laboratory values. Prompt recognition and correction of extrarenal problems usually restore renal function before tissue damage can occur. Careful physical assessment is required to evaluate the client's fluid status. If the individual has vascular volume depletion, he/she has decreased urinary output, postural hypotension, and tachycardia. Prompt fluid resuscitation can prevent intrarenal problems that can lead to renal tissue damage and renal failure. The nurse also monitors laboratory values for any changes that could reflect compromised renal function. When renal tubular damage occurs, the earliest sign is a decrease in urine concentrating ability. This is reflected by dilute urine with a decreased specific gravity and inappropriately high urinary sodium and chloride levels. Other laboratory values that are helpful in monitoring renal function include serum electrolyte levels, serum BUN and creatinine levels, and urinalysis.

Nurses must also be aware of nephrotoxic substances that the client may ingest (see Table 59-4). Orders for nephrotoxic drugs should be questioned, and the ordered dose validated before the client receives the drug. Antibiotics are the most likely drug group to have nephrotoxic side effects. If an individual must receive a potentially nephrotoxic drug, the nurse's responsibility is to monitor the client's laboratory values closely for any clinical manifestations of renal dysfunction.

COLLABORATIVE MANAGEMENT

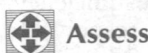 **Assessment**

History

The accurate diagnosis of ARF, its type, and etiology largely depends on a detailed history. A history taking must include questions relating to the potential causes of ARF. The nurse questions the client carefully and examines the hospital chart concerning exposure to nephrotoxins, recent surgery or trauma, transfusion, or other factors that could precipitate renal ischemia. In some situations, ARF must be differentiated from chronic end-stage renal disease. In these cases, the nurse focuses on inquiring about known *renal diseases; systemic diseases,* such as diabetes mellitus, systemic lupus erythematosus, and other connective tissue diseases; and chronic malignant hypertension. To identify possible acute glomerulonephritis, the interviewing nurse includes questions about *acute illnesses,* such as influenza, colds, gastroenteritis, sore throats or pharyngitis, and other seemingly minor infections. Reversible prerenal azotemia can be suspected after massive hemorrhage or shock, burns, CHF, or any situation in which the client experiences intravascular volume depletion. Postrenal azotemia can also be identified by the nurse's focusing on any history of *obstructive disease processes* that would be manifested as difficulty in starting the urine stream, changes in the amount or appearance of the urine, narrowing of the urine stream, nocturia, urgency, or symptoms of renal calculi. The nurse also notes any history of *malignant carcinoma* that could cause bilateral obstruction. The nurse must be responsible for obtaining or validating a detailed history when ARF is suspected, because of the widely varied causes and the potentially reversible nature of the illness.

Physical Assessment: Clinical Manifestations

The clinical manifestations of ARF are numerous (see the accompanying Key Features of Disease). The specific signs and symptoms noted in a client with suspected ARF depend on the type of renal insult: prerenal, intrarenal, or postrenal. Prerenal factors that result in renal hypoperfusion cause hypotension, tachycardia, decreased urinary output, decreased cardiac output and decreased central venous pressure (CVP), and lethargy. The general clinical appearance of an individual with prerenal failure is similar to that of a client with heart failure or dehydration, depending on the etiology of the renal compromise. Intrarenal failure usually involves damage to either the glomeruli or the tubules. Tubular involvement is most often in the form of ATN. When intrarenal failure is suspected, the nurse assesses for *decreased urinary output,* recent *hypotension,* elevated

---

KEY FEATURES OF DISEASE ■ **Clinical Manifestations of Acute Renal Failure**

Cardiovascular	Gastrointestinal
Chest Pain	Nausea
Tachycardia	Vomiting
Hypotension	GI bleeding
Decreased cardiac output	Constipation
Decreased CVP	Diarrhea
Peripheral edema	Flank pain
Cardiac irritability with tall T waves on ECG	
	Genitourinary
Respiratory	Decreased urinary output
	Hematuria
Shortness of breath	Changes in urine stream
Pulmonary edema	Difficulty starting urination
Friction rub	Dysuria
	Urgency
	Incontinence
Neurologic	
	Integumentary
Lethargy	
Somnolence	Ecchymosis
Tremors	Yellow pallor
Headache	
Mental confusion	
Muscle cramps	
Generalized weakness	
Seizures	
Flaccid paralysis	
Coma	

CVP, and tachycardia. The clinical manifestations of postrenal failure reflect some obstruction in the lower urinary tract. In these clients, the nurse monitors for *oliguria* or *intermittent anuria,* severe uremia, lethargy, and reports of changes in the character of the urine stream or difficulty starting urination. The nurse caring for any client at risk for ARF must also be aware of these additional clinical manifestations that may occur with the onset of any type of ARF: *nausea, vomiting, headaches, weight gain, peripheral edema,* and *tremors.* If ARF progresses without treatment, later manifestations may include severe peripheral edema, friction rub, and cardiac irritability with tall T waves on ECG.

Psychosocial Assessment

Clients and their families may require emotional support when ARF is diagnosed. The individual who is alert and understands the severity of the diagnosis may be anxious. The nurse constantly assesses the client's anxiety level and his/her ability to cope with this stressful situation. The nurse explains every procedure and answers questions as completely as possible to decrease the individual's anxiety and promote cooperation. If the client is critically ill, the family must be evaluated and their ability to cope with the situation should also be assessed by the nurse.

Laboratory Findings

The numerous alterations in laboratory values in the client with ARF are similar to those occurring in CRF (see the earlier discussion of laboratory findings in chronic renal failure and Key Features of Disease: Laboratory Values in Renal Failure). The oliguric phase of ARF has many of the same abnormalities in laboratory values as CRF. The diagnostically definitive increase in the BUN and serum creatinine levels with a consistent 20 : 1 ratio occurs in both diseases. The alterations in the serum levels of electrolytes (potassium, sodium, calcium, and phosphorus) in ARF are also consistent with those occurring in the chronic disease. In addition, clients with ARF also display progressive anemia as renal function deteriorates. The decreased hemoglobin level and hematocrit are gradually reversed when renal function improves. Analysis of the urine in ARF is necessary to examine osmolality, specific gravity, and urinary sodium concentration. In the majority of clients with oliguric ARF, the urine specific gravity is greater than 1.020, urine osmolality is greater than 600 mOsm/L, and the urinary sodium level is less than 20 mEq/L.

Individuals who develop high-output renal failure have lost their urine concentrating ability and demonstrate different laboratory values than clients in the oliguric state. In the high-output stage of ARF, both urine specific gravity and osmolality are low. A urinalysis may show WBCs, RBCs, tubular cells, and a variety of casts. In oliguric clients, urinary concentrations of sodium and chloride are low; in high-output failure, the levels are elevated. This salt wasting and loss of urinary acidification result in severe hyponatremia with a reduced urine pH. Clients with high-output renal failure can experience a rapidly increasing serum osmolality as they become increasingly dehydrated owing to diuresis. Thus, the nurse must constantly monitor the urinary output and facilitate appropriate fluid replacement.

In addition, metabolic acidosis may develop in the client with ARF. This is measured by arterial blood gas determinations that identify arterial pH levels, normally 7.34 to 7.45. Nurses monitor individuals with ARF for respiratory compensation for the acidosis or decreased pH. This is reflected by a low PCO_2 (less than 35 mmHg), a pH within normal limits, and a PO_2 level greater than 80 mmHg. When clients fail to adequately compensate for metabolic acidosis caused by decreased renal function, the nurse notes a serum pH of less than 7.34.

Radiographic Findings

Radiographic studies are useful in determining the etiology of ARF (see also under the heading Radiographic Findings for CRF). A flat-plate x-ray film of the abdomen should be obtained to determine the size of

the kidneys. The x-ray film may reveal small kidneys suggestive of chronic failure or enlarged kidneys possibly caused by hydronephrosis. This film may also illustrate obstructing calculi in the renal pelvis, the ureters, or the bladder. CT with contrast dye can be done to examine the renal vasculature, the patency of the ureters, and the renal parenchyma. IVP (also known as excretory urography) and/or ultrasonography can also be used to determine kidney size and the patency of the ureters. Aortorenal angiography may be used to examine renal blood vessels. This may reveal any occlusion of major renal vessels by thrombus, embolus, or stenosis. Cystoscopy or retrograde pyelography can be used in some cases to identify possible obstructive lesions in the urinary tract.

Other Diagnostic Tests

Renal biopsy is occasionally performed if the primary etiology is uncertain or if an immunologic disease is suspected. Renal biopsies are also performed to determine the reversibility of the renal failure if ARF has persisted for an extended period. Although the nurse cannot usually perform these diagnostic studies, he/she is responsible for the client's preparation before the test and for follow-up care. In addition, the nurse must be aware of all test results and understand how they may affect the client's treatment regimen. These diagnostic studies are discussed in Chapter 57.

 Analysis: Nursing Diagnosis

The client with ARF requires meticulous nursing care. A detailed nursing care plan should be written to meet the needs of clients with this complex disease. The nursing care needs and interventions for the client with CRF as described earlier apply to the client with ARF as well, with a few modifications. As discussed earlier, the client with ARF may pass from an oliguric phase (in which fluid and electrolytes are retained) to the high-output phase. While in the oliguric phase, the diagnostic procedures and care described for the client with CRF also apply to the client with ARF. If the client moves to the high-output phase, hypovolemia and electrolyte loss are the problems. As a result, the client with high-output failure needs a care plan that focuses on fluid replacement and sodium supplementation. These examples of output variation reflect the continually changing nature of ARF and the need to constantly update the nursing care plans to reflect the client's movement through the stages of the disease process.

Common Diagnoses

The common diagnosis for ARF is fluid volume deficit related to diuresis in high-output renal failure.

See under Common Diagnoses and Additional Diagnoses for CRF for other nursing diagnoses that also apply to the client with ARF.

Planning and Implementation ➡

Fluid Volume Deficit

For more information on specific interventions for clients with either dehydration (fluid volume deficit) or overhydration (fluid volume excess), see Chapter 13.

Planning: client goals.   The goals are that the client will (1) maintain a stable fluid volume with fluid intake balancing fluid losses and (2) maintain safe serum electrolyte levels.

Interventions: nonsurgical management.   The following interventions are utilized in the nonsurgical management of ARF: drug therapy, diet therapy, peritoneal dialysis or hemodialysis, and hemofiltration.

Drug therapy.   As in clients with CRF, clients with ARF receive numerous drugs and, as a result, present a particular challenge in nursing care. Drug metabolism is altered in all individuals with renal dysfunction owing to the kidney's decreased ability to excrete medications. The nurse must be especially careful in administering medications to these clients and be knowledgeable about the site of drug metabolism. In addition, the nurse must constantly monitor for possible interactions among the numerous drugs the client with ARF is receiving. Refer to the earlier discussion of drug therapy for fluid volume excess in clients with CRF and Table 59–1 for a description of the medications used in ARF and CRF.

In clients with oliguric ARF, fluid challenges and diuretics are frequently used to promote renal perfusion. When oliguric renal failure is suspected, the client should be fully evaluated before the administration of diuretics because these medications alter laboratory test results. After diagnostic laboratory test specimens of blood and urine have been obtained, a controlled fluid challenge of IV normal saline is rapidly infused. At this time, mannitol or a strong loop (high-ceiling) diuretic, such as furosemide (Lasix), is usually given to potentiate the diuretic response. The physician may order dopamine in a small continuous infusion to restore renal perfusion and increase blood pressure. Frequently, these clients require CVP monitoring or measurement of pulmonary arterial pressures via a Swan-Ganz catheter for a more exact evaluation of their hemodynamic status. They also require constant nursing supervision to assess the response to fluid and drug administration. The nurse must carefully monitor the individual for signs of possible fluid overload.

Diet therapy.   Individuals with ARF often have a high rate of catabolism. This hypercatabolic state results in the breakdown of muscle for protein, which leads to an increase in azotemia and an even more elevated serum BUN level. If the client with ARF has adequate dietary intake (see earlier discussion of interventions for altered nutrition: less than body requirements in clients with CRF), hyperalimentation (total parenteral nutrition [TPN]) can be avoided. The nurse constantly assesses the individual's oral intake to make certain that she/he is consuming enough calories. Unfortunately, many clients with ARF are unable to eat sufficient food because of the acuity of their condition. In those cases, some form of TPN must be initiated to avoid catabolism. TPN is administered intravenously, and the solutions may be formulated to meet the client's individual needs. Owing to the labile status of the client with ARF, the nurse constantly monitors the serum electrolyte concentrations and facilitates revisions in the hyperalimentation solution as needed.

In addition to TPN, IV fat emulsion (Intralipid) infusions are often used in clients with ARF to provide a nonprotein source of calories. IV lipids are an emulsion of fats from soybean, safflower, or cottonseed oil, with egg yolk phospholipid, soybean phospholipid, or lecithin serving as the emulsifying agent (Mars & Treloor 1984). IV lipids are used because of their high caloric content. In uremic clients, fat emulsions can be used in place of glucose to avoid the problems associated with excessive sugars.

Dialysis.   The techniques, advantages, and disadvantages of hemodialysis and peritoneal dialysis are discussed earlier. These procedures can be implemented for individuals with ARF, if necessary. The indications for dialysis in ARF are symptoms of uremia, persistent hyperkalemia, persistent acidosis, severe fluid overload, severe hyponatremia, pericarditis, the presence of dialyzable toxins, and the need for prophylaxis (Bricker & Kirschenbaum, 1984).

The problem with performing hemodialysis for clients with ARF is that they are often too unstable to tolerate the surgery needed for a shunt placement and there is not enough time for a fistula to mature. In these situations, a temporary external vascular access, such as a femoral vein dialysis catheter or a subclavian dialysis catheter, is utilized. Cannulation of the femoral vein for hemodialysis access is a sterile procedure that can be performed quickly at the client's bedside. Single-needle dialysis must be performed through Y-shaped tubing because there is only one vascular access route that serves as both the arterial infusion and venous outflow sites. A femoral vein dialysis catheter has one major disadvantage — the catheter cannot be left in place between dialysis treatments without immobilizing the client. The repeated recannulation of the catheter may cause hematoma formation and make repeated use of the vein impossible.

The subclavian vein can also be cannulated for temporary hemodialysis access. It is often preferred to femoral vein cannulation because the catheter can be left in place between dialysis treatments. This is also a disadvantage because the longer the catheter is left in place, the greater is the chance of infection. The subclavian dialysis catheter (Fig. 59–8) is inserted at the bedside. A physician performs the sterile procedure, and then the catheter is covered with a sterile dressing. The placement of the catheter is checked on a chest x-ray film before its use. This type of dialysis catheter also necessitates single-needle dialysis.

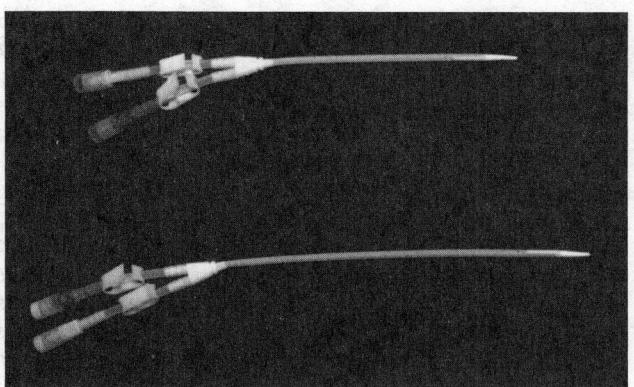

Figure 59-8

Subclavian dialysis catheters. These catheters are radio-paque polyurethane tubes that can be used for subclavian dialysis access. The *Y*-shaped tubing allows arterial outflow and venous return through a single catheter.

Hemofiltration. Continuous arteriovenous hemo-filtration (CAVH) provides an alternative to hemodialysis and peritoneal dialysis for clients with ARF. Numerous other terms refer to essentially the same process: slow continuous ultrafiltration, diafiltration, and Amicon filtration. CAVH is used to treat hypervolemia and toxic solute accumulation in individuals in whom conventional forms of dialysis may not be advisable. Other indications for CAVH include clients with severe fluid and electrolyte problems, such as clients with burns or pulmonary edema; clients with CRF and concomitant

acute renal disease; and sometimes clients with drug intoxication.

Hemofiltration necessitates a vascular access and entails a process similar to that for hemodialysis, with several important differences. The most common vascular accesses used in CAVH are femoral or subclavian catheters and, occasionally, AV shunts. As shown in Figure 59-9, tubing from the catheter is attached to a filter. The filters used in CAVH are smaller, but similar to the hollow-core, fiber-filled filters used in hemodialysis. The tubing then moves from the filter to a container used to collect the filtered fluid. Finally, the tubing returns to the catheter to complete the circuit. The catheter utilized as an access has a Y-shaped connector with a venous and an arterial side, as in hemodialysis. Blood flow is driven by blood pressure and gravity. No blood pump is used. Thus, blood circulates at a much slower rate than in hemodialysis, which avoids hypotension and extreme shifts in fluid volume and electrolyte levels. As a result, the client is unlikely to experience dialysis disequilibrium syndrome. Hemofiltration also represents a process closer to that of normal renal functioning in that it is continuous, and a typical treatment may last 2 to 5 days. CAVH does not require any specialized or expensive equipment and can be carried out by the nursing staff in a critical care setting. This makes the whole process more accessible and less expensive for the client.

The nursing responsibilities during CAVH include close, constant monitoring of the client's status, as well as the functioning of the hemofiltration circuit. The nurse monitors vital signs every 15 minutes during the first hour of treatment, then hourly, and notes any signs

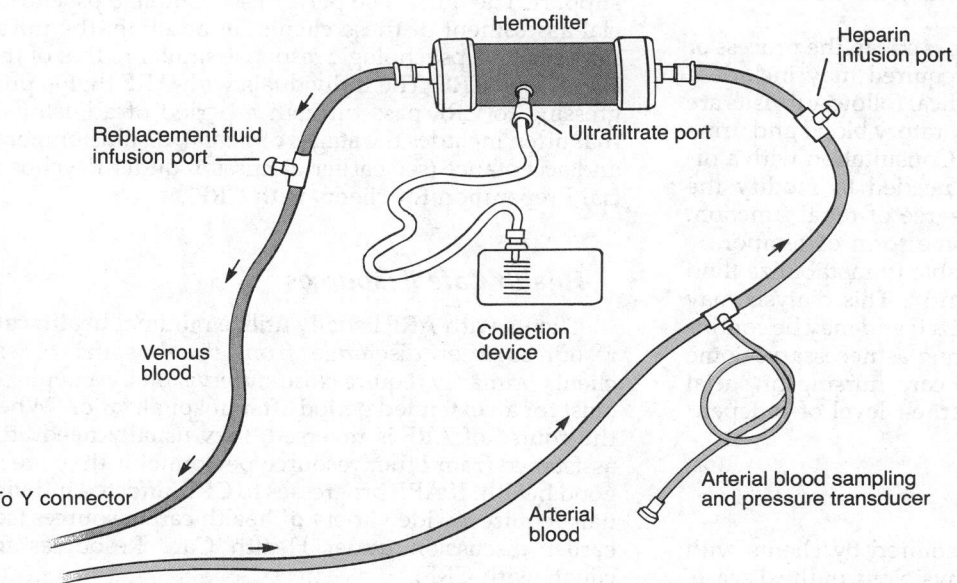

Figure 59-9

The tubing circuit used for continuous arteriovenous hemofiltration.

of hypotension. The nurse also observes the amount and color of the filtered drainage, or *ultrafiltrate,* in the collection container and notes any change. The dialysis catheter or shunt site must be assessed for signs of infection, and the dressing must be changed daily. These clients require frequent monitoring of their laboratory values, especially electrolyte levels. The nurse must review the laboratory test results carefully and be certain that samples for laboratory analysis are obtained as needed. Finally, although these individuals do receive heparin during CAVH, clotting of the filter and the tubing is still possible. The nurse monitors the client's clotting ability by doing modified whole blood clotting time (Lee-White clotting test) hourly or by frequently obtaining a PTT. If clots begin to form in the hemofilter or the tubing, they must be changed before CAVH can continue. The nurse is also aware of other potential complications, including sepsis, bleeding attributable to heparinization, hypotension and shock due to decreased intravascular volume, and rupture of the hemofilter membranes. The nursing care of the client receiving CAVH includes continuous monitoring, accurate assessment, and a thorough knowledge of the expected course in ARF.

■ Discharge Planning

Home Care Preparation

The posthospital care for a client with ARF may vary widely, depending on the status of the disease when the client is discharged from the hospital. If the client's renal failure is resolving, the follow-up care is provided largely by his/her physician, usually a nephrologist. In contrast, in some clients, ARF results in permanent renal damage that eventually leads to end-stage renal disease. In these cases, the posthospital care may be as extensive and multifaceted as for any other individual with CRF (see earlier under Discharge Planning for the client with CRF).

If a client's acute renal disease is still in the process of resolving, the follow-up care required may include a variety of services. Frequent medical follow-up visits are necessary, as well as routine laboratory blood and urine tests to monitor renal function. Consultation with a dietitian or nutritionist may be needed to modify the client's diet according to the degree of renal function. Some individuals may need some form of temporary dialysis until their kidneys are able to metabolize fluid and waste products independently. This dialysis may begin while the client is hospitalized and may be continued at a dialysis center for as long as necessary. Some clients may also require home care nursing or social work assistance, depending on their level of independence and family support.

Client/Family Education

The health care education required by clients with ARF centers around the pathophysiology of the disease,

clinical manifestations of progressive renal failure, and necessary treatments. Individuals with ARF and their families should be aware of the basic pathophysiology and precipitating factors of ARF. This health care teaching begins while the client is in the hospital, and the nursing staff is primarily responsible for the client's instruction. The nurse also instructs the client concerning the clinical manifestations of a decrease in renal function. This knowledge allows clients to monitor themselves after discharge from the hospital and encourages them to seek medical care when it is indicated. Clients and their families are also taught about all treatments that are needed by the individual after discharge from the hospital. The health care teaching varies with each client's degree of renal function, and the nurse tailors the instruction to the individual client's needs and ability to comprehend.

Psychosocial Preparation

While preparing the client with ARF for discharge from the hospital, the nurse assesses the individual's psychosocial status. These clients often display anxiety about the status of their renal function. The nurse must be particularly aware of the sources of their increasing anxiety and take steps to decrease it if possible. If the individual's renal function is improving and the ARF has been reversed, the nurse should provide health care teaching concerning the pathophysiology of ARF. To decrease the client's anxiety, the nurse assures the client that, after ARF is reversed, optimal renal function gradually returns over a period of weeks. The nurse instructs the client about the clinical manifestations of decreasing renal function. In addition, the nurse encourages the individual to notify the physician immediately if any problems occur.

In contrast, if the client's ARF is progressing to CRF, the nurse must provide a different form of psychosocial support. The nurse also performs a complete psychosocial assessment of these clients. In addition, the nurse may expect a psychologic response similar to that of the client with CRF. The individuals with ARF that is progressing to CRF pass through a period of adjustment that often includes the stages of denial, disillusionment, and acceptance (see earlier discussion under Psychosocial Preparation for clients with CRF).

Health Care Resources

Clients with ARF usually utilize minimal health care resources after discharge from the hospital. These clients primarily require close supervision by a nephrologist for an extended period after hospitalization. When the course of ARF is reversed, they usually need little assistance from other resource personnel if they are in good health. If ARF progresses to CRF, affected individuals require a wide variety of health care resources (see earlier discussion under Health Care Resources for clients with CRF).

Evaluation

Nurses caring for clients with ARF evaluate each individual's progress by an examination of the common nursing diagnoses. The expected outcomes are that the client

1. Maintains appropriate fluid volume
2. Maintains serum electrolyte levels within a normal range for that client

SUMMARY

Renal failure is a multifaceted disorder, and the nurse must be familiar with the pathophysiology and possible treatment plans. Every system in the body and, thus, every aspect of client care are affected. Accurate assessment of the clinical symptoms and laboratory findings is essential. In addition, the nurse educates the client about her/his disease and the associated therapies.

The treatment modalities for chronic and acute renal failure require skilled nursing care throughout the disease process. Initial regimens for clients with either type of renal failure necessitate that nurses manage fluid and dietary restrictions. As the disease progresses, the nurse may participate in preparing the client for hemodialysis, peritoneal dialysis, or hemofiltration, depending on the client's status. When the disease progresses to end-stage renal disease, renal transplantation may be performed. The client requires specialized nursing care preoperatively and postoperatively that includes immunosuppression and protective isolation (see Chaps. 26 and 27). Thus, nurses play a vital role in moving every client with renal failure toward homeostasis and survival.

IMPLICATIONS FOR RESEARCH

The client could benefit from further nursing research that would investigate the physiologic and psychologic aspects of renal failure. Some of the topics that require further nursing research include client compliance with treatment regimens, coping methods utilized by clients with renal disease, and stressors in individuals receiving dialysis therapy. The following nursing questions are appropriate to investigate when considering the special needs of the client with renal failure:

1. Is it possible to improve compliance in clients with renal failure by modifying health care beliefs by providing additional education and/or by enlisting help from family and friends?

2. Is there a relationship between the physiologic and psychologic stressors identified by clients undergoing hemodialysis versus peritoneal dialysis?

3. Are the physiologic and psychologic stressors identified by clients with renal failure consistent with the stressors identified by individuals with other chronic illnesses?

4. What coping methods are most effective and/or most commonly used by clients with renal insufficiency, those with end-stage renal disease undergoing hemodialysis, and those with end-stage renal disease receiving peritoneal dialysis?

REFERENCES AND READINGS

Abels, L. (1986). *Critical care nursing: A physiologic approach.* St. Louis: C.V. Mosby.

Amaro, J., Cohen, B., Lange, P., & Persijn, G. (1983). Renal transplantation: Pediatric recipients. *Dialysis and Transplantation, 12,* 88–91.

Battelle Human Affairs Research Centers. (1985). National kidney dialysis and kidney transplantation study: A summary of results. *Contemporary Dialysis and Nephrology, 6*(9), 41–47.

Beer, J. (1988). Treatment of anaemia in chronic renal failure. *Nursing Times, 84*(47), 55–57.

Bauers, C. M. (1983). A review of the end stage renal disease program. *Nephrology Nurse, 5*(4), 17–22.

Binkley, L. (1984). Keeping up with peritoneal dialysis. *American Journal of Nursing, 84,* 729–733.

Birdsall, C. (1986). How do you manage peritoneal dialysis? *American Journal of Nursing, 86,* 592–596.

Bricker, N., & Kirschenbaum, M. (Eds.). (1984). *The kidney: Diagnosis and management.* New York: Wiley Medical.

Brown, R. O. (1983). Nutritional support in acute renal failure. *American Association of Nephrology Nurses and Technicians Journal, 10*(5), 25–29.

Burbige, E. (1984). Hepatorenal syndrome. *Hospital Medicine, 20*(12), 32–36.

Butler B. (1985). Dietary phosphorus. *Journal of Nephrology Nursing, 2*(2), 69–70.

Butler, B. (1985). Nutritional assessment in end stage renal disease. *Journal of Nephrology Nursing, 2,* 36–37.

Carbone, V. (1987). Continuous ambulatory peritoneal dialysis procedures. *Critical Care Nurse, 7*(4), 74–80.

Cerilli, J. (1984). Current status of renal transplantation. In G. M. Abouns (Ed.), *Current status of clinical organ transplantation.* Boston: Martinus Nijhoff.

Chambers, J. K. (1983). Bowel management in dialysis patients. *American Journal of Nursing, 83,* 1051–1052.

Chambers, J. K. (1987). Fluid and electrolyte problems in renal and urologic disorders. *Nursing Clinics of North America, 22,* 815–825.

Coleman, E. A. (1986). When the kidneys fail. *RN, 49*(7), 28–37.

Coleman, S. (1985). Aluminum bone disease. *Journal of Nephrology Nursing, 2,* 125–126.

David-Kasden, J. (1984). An alteration in body image in the hemodialysis population. *Journal of Nephrology Nursing, 1,* 25–28.

Doenges, M. E., Jeffries, M. F., & Moorhouse, M. F. (1984). *Nursing care plans: Diagnoses in planning patient care.* Philadelphia: F. A. Davis.

Eddins, B. (1985). Chronic self-destructiveness as manifested by noncompliance behavior in the hemodialysis patient. *Journal of Nephrology Nursing, 2,* 194–198.

End stage renal disease patient profile tables—1986. (1988). *Contemporary Dialysis and Nephrology, 9*(5), 46–48.

Epstein, F. H., & Brown, R. S. (1988). Acute renal failure: A collection of paradoxes. *Hospital Practice, 23*(1), 171–194.

Fleming, L. M., & Kane, J. (1984). Step-by-step guide to safe peritoneal dialysis. *RN, 47*(2), 44–47.

Foulks, C. J. (1988). Nutritional evaluation of patients on maintenance dialysis therapy. *American Nephrology Nurses' Association Journal, 15,* 13–17.

Fuchs, J., & Schreiber, M. (1988). Patient's perceptions of CAPD and hemodialysis stressors. *American Nephrology Nurses' Association Journal, 15*(5), 282–285.

Gharbieh, P. A. (1988). Renal transplant: Surgical and psychologic hazards. *Critical Care Nurse, 8*(6), 58–70.

Goodinson, S. (1988). Emergency dialysis in acute renal failure: Basic principles. *Nursing (London), 3*(32), 44–48.

Gurklis, J. A., & Menke, E. M. (1988). Identification of stressors and use of coping methods in chronic hemodialysis patients. *Nursing Research, 37,* 236–239.

Hahn, K. (1987). The many signs of renal failure. *Nursing '87, 17*(8), 34–41.

Harwood, C. H., & Cook, C. V. (1985). Cyclosporine in transplantation. *Heart and Lung, 14,* 529–540.

Howard, S. (1989). How do I ask? Requesting tissue or organ donations from bereaved families. *Nursing '89, 19*(1), 70–73.

Hulman, P., & Wolfson, M. (1988). Acute renal failure. *Hospital Medicine, 24*(11), 68–89.

Irwin, B. C. (1983). Renal transplantation advances in immunology—A nursing perspective. *American Association of Nephrology Nurses and Technicians Journal, 10*(4), 11–15.

Kadas, N. (1986). Reducing fluid overload without hemodialysis. *RN, 49*(5), 27–31.

Kaplan, A., Sosler, G., & Longnecker, R. (1985). Use of the Hemasite device in patients with multiple access failures. *Dialysis and Transplantation, 14*(5), 288–296, 309.

Kaplan, L. J. (1985). Ophthalmic manifestations of renal disease. *Journal of Nephrology Nursing, 2,* 74–76.

Kiely, M. A. (1984). Continuous arteriovenous hemofiltration. *Critical Care Nurse, 4*(4), 39–43.

Kosier, J. H., & Thompson, A. (1985). Supervising the hemodialysis client in self medication in the home. *Home Health Care Nurse, 3*(3), 31–36.

Kutner, N. G. (1983). Renal rehabilitation: A state of the art review. *American Association of Nephrology Nurses and Technicians Journal, 10*(6), 13–18.

Lancaster, L. E. (1984). *The patient with end stage renal disease.* New York: Wiley.

Lane, T., Strophal, V., & Waldorf, P. (1983). Standards of care for the CAPD patient. *Home Health Care Nurse, 1*(1), 48–58.

Leaf, A., & Cotran, R. (1985). *Renal pathophysiology* (3rd ed.). New York: Oxford University Press.

Lee, D. (1983). General aspects for consideration in renal transplant patients. *Nephrology Nurse, 5*(5), 15–16.

Levinsky, N. G. (1985). Acute kidney failure: Prerenal, renal or postrenal? *Hospital Practice, 20*(3), 68G–68J, 68N, 68Q–68R.

Lubkin, I. M. (1986). *Chronic illness: Impact and interventions.* Boston: Jones & Bartlett.

Luckenbaugh P. R. (1983). An overview of nursing diagnosis and suggestions for use with chronic hemodialysis patients. *Nephrology Nurse, 10*(7), 58–61.

Macliver, C. (1989). Polycystic kidney disease. *Nursing Times, 85*(6), 52–54.

Mailloux, L. U. (1983). Hypertension: Achieving control in patients with renal disease. *Consultant, 23*(11), 97–99, 104, 113.

Mars, D. R., & Treloor, D. (1984). Acute tubular necrosis—pathophysiology and treatment. *Heart and Lung, 13,* 194–202.

Martin, K. (1985). Terminating dialysis: A case study and public health policy analysis. *American Nephrology Nurses' Association Journal, 12,* 347–351.

Maxwell, M. (1984). The kidney. *Nursing Mirror, 158*(1), 31–34.

Miller, C. A., & Evans, D. (1987). CNS manifestations of acute renal failure. *Critical Care Nurse, 7*(3), 94–95.

Mitz, M., Di Benedetto, M., Klingbeil, G., Melvin, J., & Piering, W. (1984). Neuropathy in end-stage renal disease secondary to primary renal disease and diabetes. *Archives of Physical Medicine and Rehabilitation, 65,* 235–238.

Monahan, R. S., & Levin, A. (1988). Choosing to end dialysis: Standards for nursing care. *American Nephrology Nurses' Association Journal, 15,* 229–232.

Mooney, J. O., Taylor, S., & Ulrich, B. (1985). Care of the renal transplant patient receiving cyclosporine. *Journal of Nephrology Nursing, 2,* 274–276.

Moore, S., Ecklund, D. K., Trommeter, C., & Bohac, C. (1988). Protocol for nutritional intervention for the adult chronic hemodialysis patient. *Contemporary Dialysis and Nephrology, 9*(5), 16–24, 48–50.

Nace, G. S. (1985). Preventing adverse drug reactions in patients with renal failure. *Journal of Nephrology Nursing, 2,* 30–31.

Nace, S. G. (1985). Use of analgesic medications in patients with renal failure. *Journal of Nephrology Nursing, 2,* 185–186.

Nogueira, H., & Cutler, R. E. (1985). Anemia in chronic renal failure. *Dialysis and Transplantation, 14,* 483–484.

Norris, M. (1989a). Action STAT! Dialysis disequilibrium syndrome. *Nursing '89, 19*(4), 33.

Norris, M. (1989b). Acute tubular necrosis: Preventing complications. *Dimensions of Critical Care Nursing, 8*(1), 716–726.

Nova, G. (1987). Dialyzable drugs. *American Journal of Nursing, 87,* 933–941.

Outcome criteria and nursing diagnosis in ESRD patient care planning—section 1: Conservative management. (1987). *American Nephrology Nurses' Association Journal, 14,* 36–39.

Outcome criteria and nursing diagnosis in ESRD patient care planning—section 2: Peritoneal dialysis. (1987). *American Nephrology Nurses' Association Journal, 14,* 131–139.

Outcome criteria and nursing diagnosis in ESRD patient care planning—section 3: Renal transplantation. (1987). *American Nephrology Nurses' Association Journal, 14,* 197–212.

Outcome criteria and nursing diagnosis in ESRD patient care planning—section 4: Hemodialysis. (1987). *American Nephrology Nurses' Association Journal, 14,* 213–221.

Palmer, J. C., Koorejian, K., London, J. B., Dechert, R. E., & Bartlett, R. H. (1986). Nursing management of continuous arteriovenous hemofiltration for acute renal failure. *Focus on Critical Care, 13*(5), 21–30.

Parker, K., Howel, M., Healy, K., Petrides, C., Owens, A., Powell, E., Rosson, Z., Royal, E., Simmons, C., & White, B. (1985). Nursing intervention based on the health belief model and compliance in patients on chronic dialysis. *Journal of Nephrology Nursing, 2,* 144–151.

Pierce, P. (1983). Caring for patients with renal osteodystrophy. *American Association of Nephrology Nurses and Technicians Journal, 10*(3), 49–55.

Plawecki, H., Brewer, S., & Plawecki, J. (1987). Chronic renal failure. *Journal of Gerontological Nursing, 13*(12), 14–17, 34–35.

Pullman, T. N., Coe, F. L., Netter, F. H., & McKinsey, M. E. (1984). Pathophysiology of chronic renal failure. *Clinical Symposia, 36*(3), 3–32.

Ragozzino, M. W., Field, B. D., Beaulieu, M. D., Brady, M. D., & Deluca, S. A. (1987). Magnetic resonance imaging. *American Family Physician, 35,* 107–114.

Rambaks, I. (1985). Post transplant hypertension. *Journal of Nephrology Nursing, 2,* 115–118.

Rehan, A. (1985). Hemodialysis emergencies. *Emergency Medicine, 17*(1), 138–152.

Richard, A. B., Robbins, K. C., & Rovelli, M. A. (1985). Renal transplantation: Nursing management of the recipient. *AORN Journal, 41,* 1022–1036, 1038, 1040–1041.

Rickus, M. A. (1987). Sexual concerns of the femalepatient: Research study and analysis. *AmericanNephrology Nurses' Association Journal, 14,* 192–195.

Rivers, R. (1987). Nursing the kidney transplant patient. *RN, 50*(8), 46–53.

Sasdelli, M., Vagnoli, E., Candi, P., & Duranti, E. (1986). Comparison of hemodialysis and hemofiltration in patients with high vascular instability. *Dialysis and Transplantation, 15,* 49–50.

Schreiber, W. K., & Huber, W. (1985). Psychological situation of dialysis patients and their families. *Dialysis and Transplantation, 14,* 696–698.

Scott, J. (1983). Dietary management of chronic renal disease. *The Australian Nurses Journal, 13*(4), 29–30, 52.

Shurr, M., Roy, C., & Atcherson, E. (1984). CAPD: Dialysis 365 days a year. *Journal of Nephrology Nursing, 1,* 20–24.

Snyder, T. E. (1989). An exercise program for dialysis patients. *American Journal of Nursing, 89,* 362–364.

Soloman, J. (1986). Does renal failure mean sexual failure? *RN, 49*(8), 41–43.

Southby, J. R., & Moore, J. B. (1983). Nursing diagnosis for a child with end stage renal disease. *American Association of Nephrology Nurses and Technicians Journal, 10*(4), 23–27.

Stark, J. L. (1985). Combating acute tubular necrosis. *Nursing Life, 5*(4), 33–40.

Stark, J. L., Reiley, P., Osiecki, A., & Cook, L. (1984). Attitudes affecting organ donation in the intensive care unit. *Heart and Lung, 13,* 400–404.

Steinhiser, S. A., & Plawecki, H. M. (1987). OKT3 for the treatment of patients with acute renal allograft rejection. *American Nephrology Nurses' Association Journal, 14,* 127–129.

Strangio, L. (1988). Believe it or not: Peritoneal dialysis made easy. *Nursing '88, 18*(1), 43–46.

Strupp, T. (1988). Postshock resuscitation of the trauma victim: Preventing and managing acute renal failure. *Critical Care Nursing Quarterly, 11*(2), 1–9.

Tietze, M. (1983). Human sexuality—Female nurses' responses to their male hemodialysis patients. *American Association of Nephrology Nurses and Technicians Journal, 10*(4), 19–22.

Ulrich, S. P., Canale, S. W., & Wendell, S. A. (1986). *Nursing care planning guides: A nursing diagnosis approach.* Philadelphia: W. B. Saunders.

Vanherwegham, J., Dhaene, M., Goldman, M., Stolear, J., Sabot, J., Waterlot, Y., Serruys, E., & Thayse, C. (1986). Infections associated with subclavian dialysis catheters: The key role of nurse training. *Nephron, 42*(2), 116–119.

Van Stone, J. C. (1984). *Dialysis and the treatment of renal insufficiency.* New York: Grune & Stratton.

Williams, V., & Perkins, L. (1984). Continuous ultrafiltration: A new ICU procedure for the treatment of fluid overload. *Critical Care Nurse, 4*(4), 44–49.

Winkelman, C. (1985). Hemofiltration: A new technique in critical care nursing. *Heart and Lung, 14,* 265–271.

Winslow, K. (1985). Hemodialysis shunts. *Journal of Emergency Nursing, 11*(3), 157–158.

Worsman, R. (1988). Haemodialysis: A fragile lifeline. *Nursing Times, 84*(42), 31–32.

Wright, T. R., & Purcell, T. (1987). Uremic pneumonitis: Case report and literature review. *Topics in Emergency Medicine, 8*(4), 65–74.

Yanitski, A. F. (1983). Compliance of the hemodialysis patient. *American Association of Nephrology Nurses and Technicians Journal, 10*(2), 11–16.

ADDITIONAL READINGS

Fuches, J., & Schreiber, M. (1988). Patient's perceptions of CAPD and hemodialysis stressors. *American Nephrology Nurses' Association Journal, 15,* 282–285.

The purpose of this study was to identify and compare the stressors perceived by clients receiving CAPD and hemodialysis. The Stressor Assessment Scale was administered to a population of 60 patients. The results found that clients undergoing CAPD and hemodialysis report similar numbers and intensity of stressors. When nurses teach clients about the various treatment modalities available for end-stage renal disease, the nurse needs to explain that certain stressors are more common in the dialysis population or the CAPD group. This knowledge could influence which treatment alternative the client chooses.

Gurklis, J., & Menke, E. (1989). Identification of stressors and use of coping methods in chronic hemodialysis patients. *Nursing Research, 37,* 236–239.

These nurse researchers explored the relationships among treatment-related stressors, coping methods, and length of time on hemodialysis. The Hemodialysis Stressor Scale and the Jalowiec Coping Scale were completed by 68 subjects. The results of this study indicated that length of time receiving hemodialysis was significantly related to problem-oriented coping. The length of time receiving dialysis was not significantly related to the total coping scores and the physiologic and psychosocial stressors. The results of this study could encourage nurses to identify and support clients who are more likely to have difficulty with the stresses of chronic hemodialysis.

Miles, M., & Fraumen, A. (1988). Public attitudes toward organ donation. *Dialysis and Transplantation, 17,* 74–76.

This study conducted by nurse researchers consisted of a random telephone survey of 585 North Carolina residents concerning public attitudes about organ donation. The relationship between demographic variables and agreement to organ donation was analyzed. Only slightly more than half of the respondents were in favor of organ donation. This study indicated that nurses should promote more public and client education concerning the benefits of organ donation.

UNIT 16 RESOURCES

Nursing Resources

American Board of Urologic Allied Health Professionals (ABUAHP), 407 Strawberry Hill Avenue, Stamford, CT 06902. Telephone 203-323-1227.
Certifies nurses with experience in urology.

American Nephrology Nurses' Association (ANNA), North Woodbury Road, PO Box 56, Pitman, NJ 08071. Telephone 609-589-2187.

American Urological Association Allied, 6845 Lake Shore Drive, PO Box 9373, Raytown, MO 64133. Telephone 816-358-3317.

Board of Nephrology Examiners, Nursing and Technology (BONENT), PO Box 4085, Madison, WI 53719. Telephone 608-238-4553.
Certifies nurses with experience in hemodialysis and peritoneal dialysis. Publishes *BONENT Directions* (quarterly).

Enterostomal Therapy Nursing Certification Board (ENTCB), 2081 Business Center Drive, Suite 290, Irvine, CA 92715. Telephone 714-476-0268.
Certifies nurses with experience in enterostomal therapy.

International Association for Enterostomal Therapy (IAET), 2081 Business Center Drive, Suite 290, Irvine, CA 92715. Telephone 714-476-0268.
See Unit 13 Resources for more information.

Nephrology Nursing Certification Board, North Woodbury Road, PO Box 56, Pitman, NJ 08071. Telephone 609-589-2152.
Certifies nurses with experience in nephrology.

Other Resources

American Cancer Society, 1599 Clifton Road NE, Atlanta, GA 30329. Telephone 404-320-3333.

American Council on Transplantation, 700 North Fairfax Street, Suite 204, Alexandria, VA 23314. Telephone 703-836-4301.

American Kidney Fund, 7315 Wisconsin Avenue, 203E, Bethesda, MD 20814. Telephone 800-638-8299.

American Society of Nephrology (ASN), 6900 Grove Road, Thorofare, NJ 08086. Telephone 609-848-1000.

Help for Incontinent Persons, PO Box 544, Union, SC 29379.
Publishes *Resources Guide of Continence Products and Services,* as well as a newsletter, *The HIP Report.*

National Association of Patients on Hemodialysis and Transplantation (NAPHT), 211 East 43rd Street, New York, NY 10017. Telephone 212-867-4486.

National Kidney Foundation, 30 East 33rd Street, New York, NY 10016. Telephone 212-889-2210.

Simon Foundation for Continence, Wilmette, IL 60091. Telephone 800-237-4666.
Publishes a newsletter, *The Informer.*

United Network for Organ Sharing (UNOS), 3001 Hungary Spring Road, Richmond, VA 23228. Telephone 804-289-5380.

UNIT 17

Problems of Oxygenation: Management of Clients with Disruptions of the Respiratory System

CHAPTER 60

Assessment of the Respiratory System

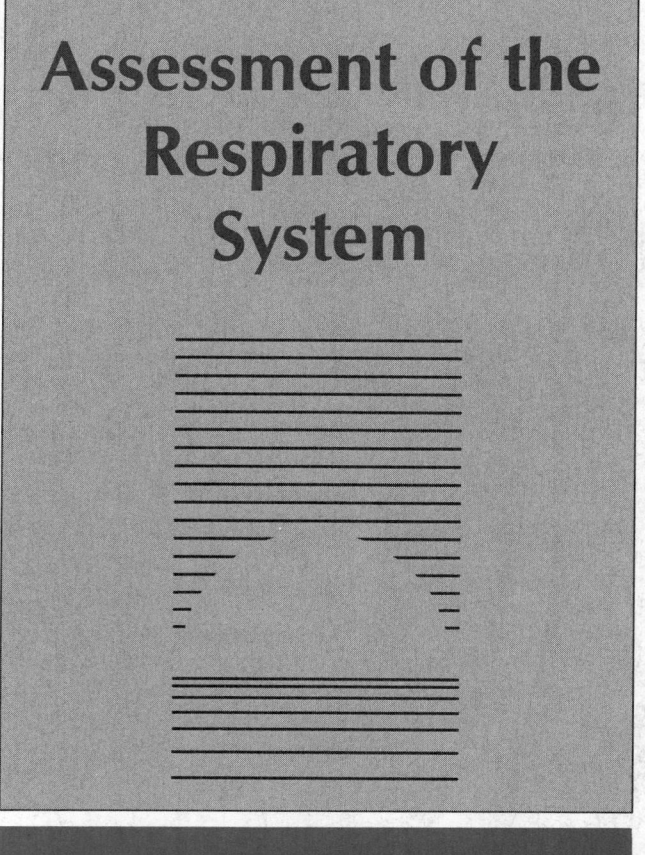

Respiratory disease currently ranks as the sixth leading cause of death in the United States. As individuals with these chronic respiratory impairments live longer because of advances made in diagnosis, treatment, and management, the nurse will be confronted with planning and implementing care of increasing numbers of clients with various respiratory disorders. An adequate knowledge base pertaining to anatomy, physiology, and pathophysiology of the respiratory system is essential for the nurse to meet this challenge.

ANATOMY AND PHYSIOLOGY REVIEW

STRUCTURE AND FUNCTION

The major purpose of the respiratory system is to provide oxygen for the combustive process of metabolism and to remove carbon dioxide, the waste product of metabolism, from the body. The respiratory tract performs several secondary functions, including maintenance of acid-base balance, production of speech, and maintenance of body water and heat balance. Divided into the upper and lower respiratory tracts, this complex system makes respiration, and, ultimately, the support of all other vital functions, possible.

UPPER RESPIRATORY TRACT

The upper airways consist of the nose, sinuses, pharynx, and larynx (Fig. 60–1). The *nose,* a rigid structure that is bony in the upper one-third and cartilaginous in the lower two-thirds, contains two passages that are separated in the middle by the *septum.* The septum and interior walls of the nasal cavity are lined with mucous membrane, as is the rest of the respiratory tract. The *nostrils (anterior nares),* or external openings into the nasal cavities, are lined with skin and hair follicles *(vibrissae),* which are the first defense mechanisms of the respiratory system. The *posterior nares,* called the *choanae,* are openings from the internal nose into the nasopharynx.

Three major bony projections called *turbinates,* or *conchae,* arise from the lateral walls of the internal portion of the nose (see Fig. 60–1). Turbinates increase the total surface area for filtering, heating, and humidifying inspired air before it passes into the nasopharynx. Thus, inspired air entering the nose is *filtered* first by vibrissae in the nares. Particles that are not filtered in the nares are then filtered and trapped in the mucous layer of the turbinates and are passed posteriorly by cilia to the oropharynx, where they are swallowed. Inspired air is *humidified* by contact with the mucous membrane and is *warmed* by heat from the vascular network.

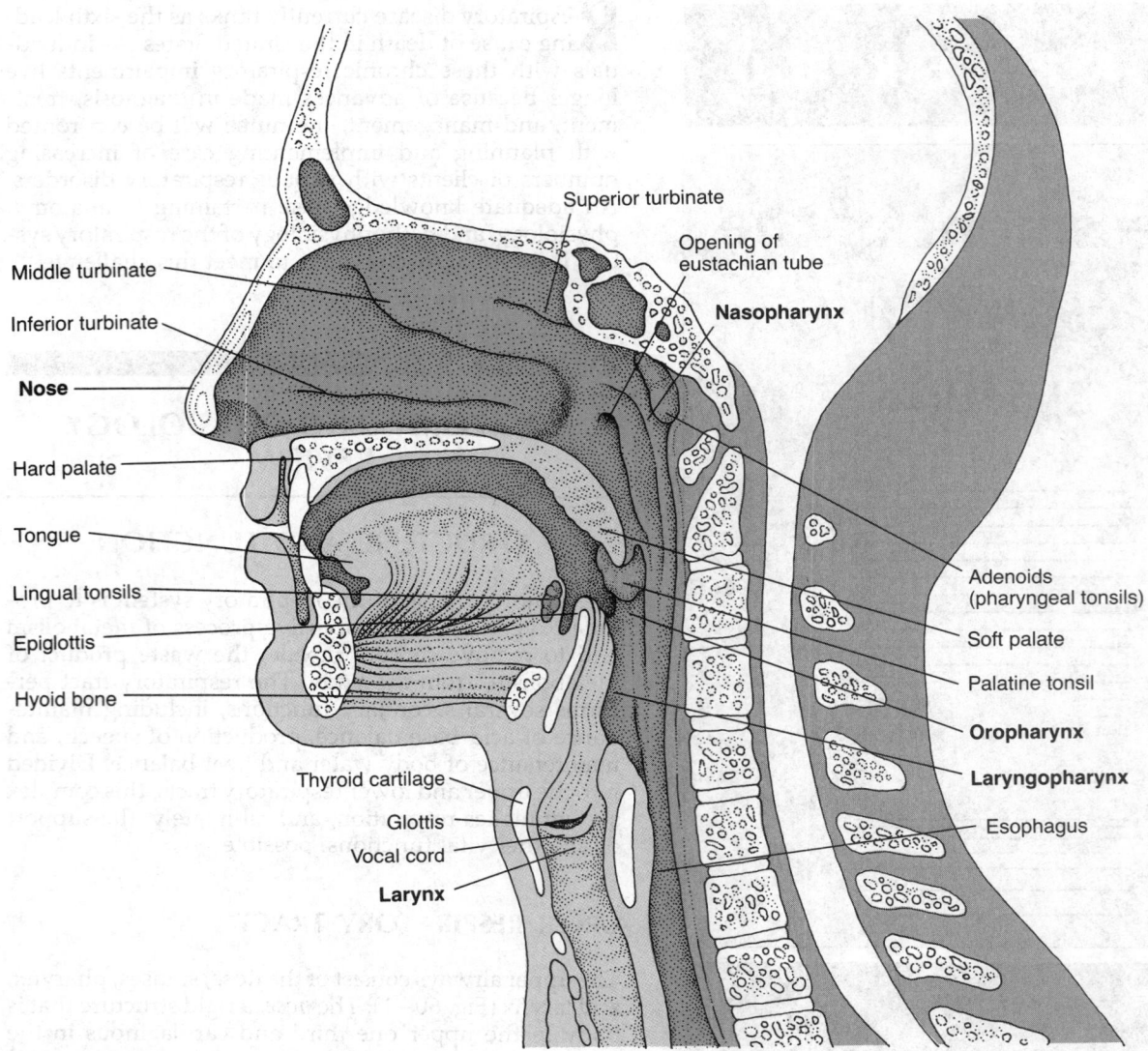

Superior turbinate

Opening of
eustachian tube

Nasopharynx

Middle turbinate

Inferior turbinate

Nose

Hard palate

Tongue

Lingual tonsils

Epiglottis

Hyoid bone

Adenoids
(pharyngeal tonsils)

Soft palate

Palatine tonsil

Oropharynx

Laryngopharynx

Esophagus

Thyroid cartilage

Glottis

Vocal cord

Larynx

Figure 60–1

Structures of the upper respiratory tract.

The nose also serves as the organ of smell because olfactory receptors are located in the roof of the nose and in the superior turbinate.

The paranasal *sinuses* are air-filled cavities within the hollow bones that surround the nasal passages and are lined with ciliated epithelium. The four paranasal sinuses are the frontal, maxillary, ethmoid, and sphenoid (Fig. 60–2). The function of the sinuses is to provide resonance during speech.

The *pharynx,* or *throat,* is located behind the oral and nasal cavities and is divided into the nasopharynx, oropharynx, and laryngopharynx. Located behind the nose, the *nasopharynx* lies above the soft palate and contains the adenoids and the eustachian tube. The *adenoids* (pharyngeal tonsils) are located in the back of the throat in the roof of the nasopharynx and serve as an important defense mechanism by guarding against invasion by

organisms entering the nose and mouth. The eustachian tube connects the nasopharynx with the middle chamber of the ear and opens during swallowing to equalize the pressure across the middle ear.

The *oropharynx* is located behind the mouth, below the nasopharynx, and extends from the soft palate to the base of the tongue. Located on the anterolateral borders of the oropharynx are the *tonsils,* which, with the adenoids, guard the body against invasion by organisms entering the nose and throat. The center for swallowing and the gag reflex is located in the oropharynx, which allows food to be propelled into the esophagus while simultaneously closing off the larynx to prevent aspiration of food into the lower airways.

Located behind the larynx, the *laryngopharynx* extends from the base of the tongue to the esophagus. The entire pharynx serves as a passageway for the respira-

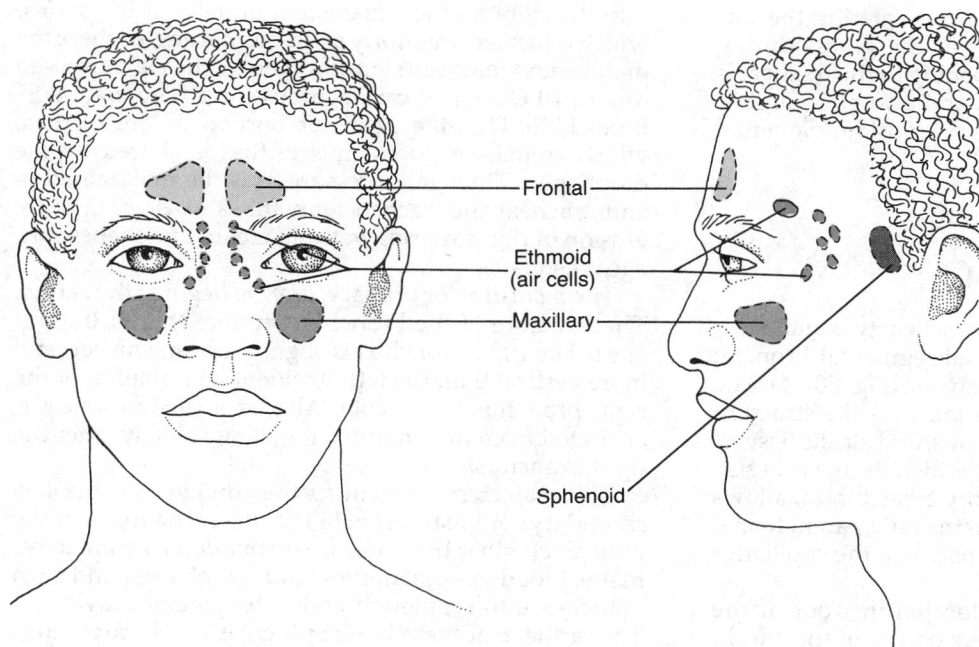

Figure 60-2

The paranasal sinuses.

tory and digestive tracts because both food and air must pass through it before reaching the appropriate destination. The laryngopharynx serves as the critical dividing point in separating solids and fluids from air. At this point, the passageway bifurcates into the larynx and the esophagus.

The larynx is located above the trachea, just below the pharynx at the root of the tongue. The *larynx*, or *voice box*, is composed of several cartilages (Fig. 60-3). The *thyroid* cartilage is the largest and is commonly referred to as the Adam's apple. The *cricoid* cartilage,

which contains the vocal cords, lies below the thyroid cartilage and is the only complete ring of cartilage in the airway. The cricothyroid membrane lies below the level of the vocal cords and joins the thyroid and cricoid cartilages. This site is used in an emergency to provide access to lower airways (cricothyroidotomy). The two *arytenoid* cartilages, to which the posterior ends of the vocal cords are attached, are used with the thyroid cartilage in vocal cord movement.

The *epiglottis* is a leaf-shaped, elastic structure that is attached along one edge to the top of the larynx. Its

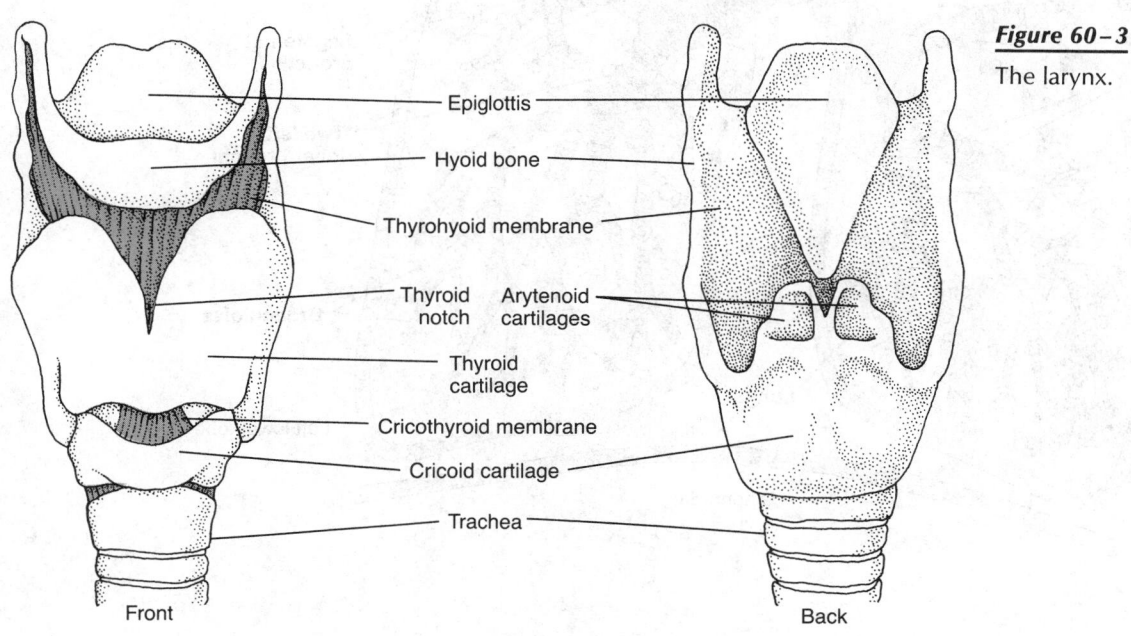

Figure 60-3

The larynx.

hinge-like action prevents food from entering the tracheobronchial tree by closing over the glottis during swallowing. The *glottis,* or the opening to the trachea, is located between the vocal cords and also plays an important role in coughing, which is the most fundamental defense mechanism of the lungs.

LOWER RESPIRATORY TRACT

The lower airways consist of the trachea; two mainstem bronchi; lobar, segmental, and subsegmental bronchi; bronchioles; alveolar ducts; and alveoli (Fig. 60–4). The tracheobronchial tree is an inverted tree-like structure consisting of muscular, cartilaginous, and elastic tissues. This system of bifurcating tubes, which decrease in size from the trachea to the respiratory bronchioles, allows for the passage of gas to and from the lung parenchyma, where gas exchange takes place between the capillaries and the alveoli.

The *trachea,* or *windpipe,* is located in front of the esophagus, beginning at the lower border of the cricoid cartilage of the larynx and extending to the level of the sixth or seventh thoracic vertebra. The trachea branches into the right and left mainstem bronchi at the *carina,* which is located anteriorly at the sternal angle where the manubrium joins the sternum. The trachea is composed of 6 to 10 C-shaped cartilaginous rings. The open portion of the C is the posterior portion of the trachea, which contains smooth muscle that is shared by the esophagus. Thus, low pressure must be maintained in endotracheal and tracheostomy tubes so as not to cause erosion of this posterior wall and create a tracheoesophageal fistula.

The *mainstem,* or primary, *bronchi* begin at the carina. The structure of the bronchi resembles that of the trachea. The right bronchus is slightly wider, shorter, and more vertical than the left. Accidental intubation of the right bronchus is possible. Also, if a foreign object is aspirated from the pharynx, it will most likely enter the right bronchus.

The mainstem bronchi further divide into the five secondary, or lobar, bronchi that enter the lobes of the lung. Each lobar bronchus is surrounded by connective tissue, blood vessels, nerves, and lymphatics, and each branches into segmental and subsegmental divisions. The cartilage of these lobar bronchi is nearly circumferential and resists collapse. The bronchi are lined with ciliated, mucus-secreting epithelium. These *cilia* serve to

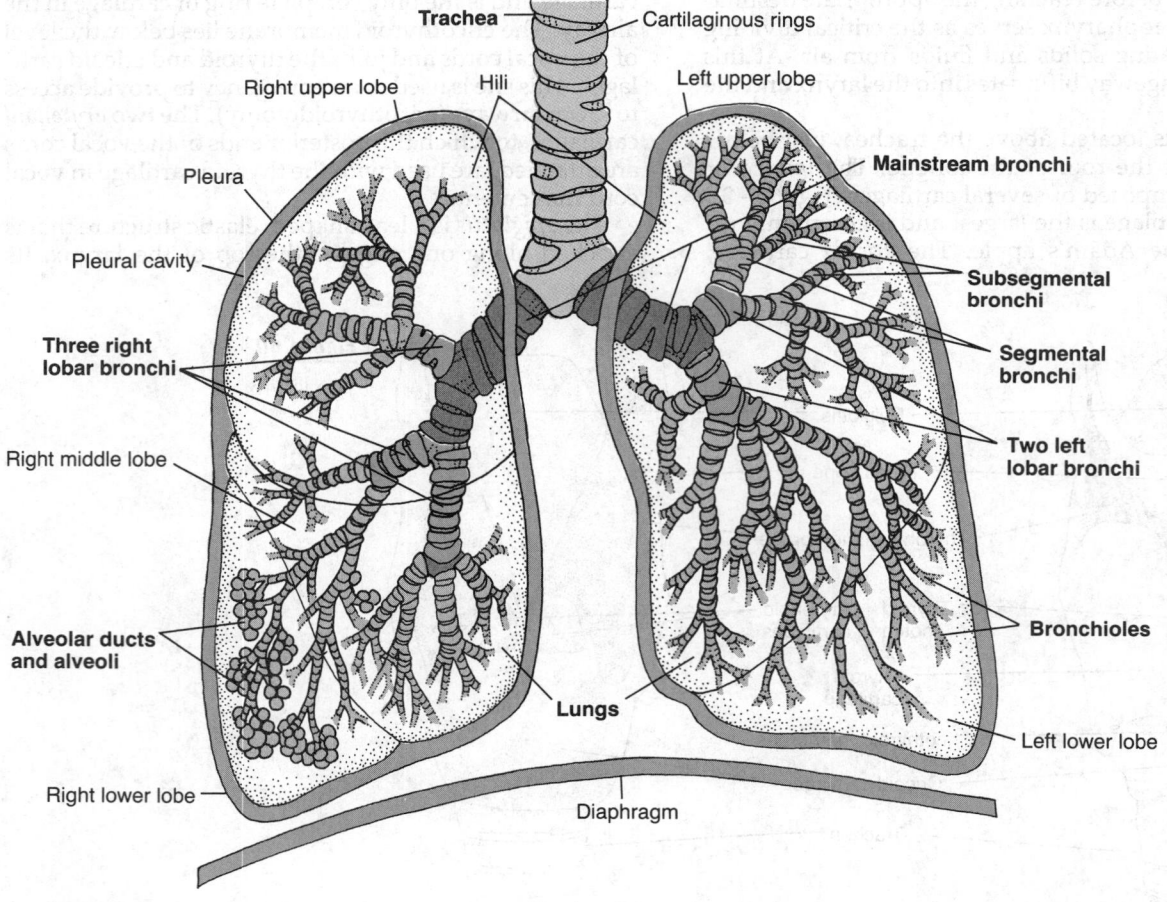

Figure 60–4

Structures of the lower respiratory tract.

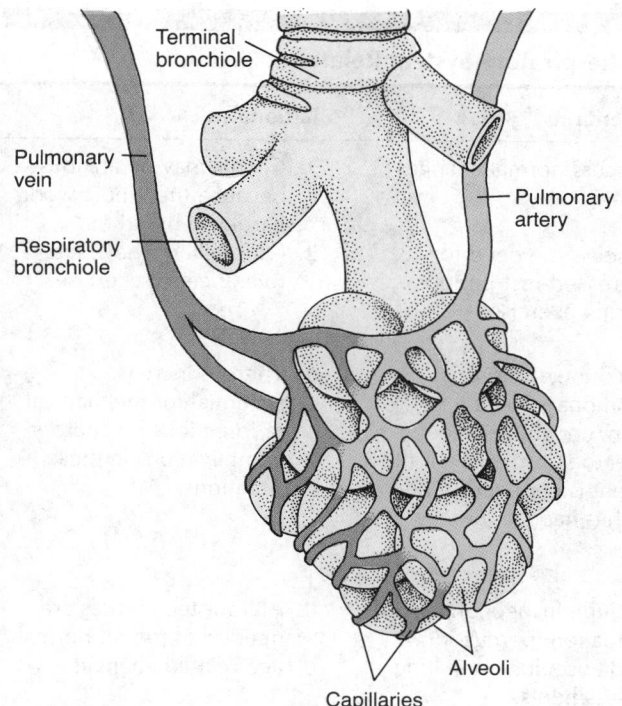

Figure 60–5

The terminal and respiratory bronchioles.

propel mucus up and away from the lower airway to the trachea, where it can be expectorated or swallowed.

The *bronchioles*, branching from the secondary bronchi, subdivide into smaller and smaller tubes: the terminal and respiratory bronchioles (Fig. 60–5). These terminal and respiratory tubes, which are less than 1 mm in diameter, have no cartilage and therefore depend entirely on the elastic recoil of the lung for patency. The terminal bronchioles contain no cilia and do not participate in gas exchange.

Alveolar ducts, which resemble a bunch of grapes, branch from the respiratory bronchioles. From these ducts, alveolar sacs arise that contain clusters of *alveoli*, the basic units of gas exchange. It is estimated that the lungs contain about 300 million alveoli surrounded by pulmonary capillaries (see Fig. 60–5). Because these microscopic alveoli are so numerous and share common walls, the surface area for gas exchange is quite extensive in the lungs. In fact, it is estimated that in the healthy adult, this surface area is approximately the size of a tennis court (Boyda, 1985). Certain cells located in the walls of the alveoli secrete *surfactant,* a phospholipid protein that reduces the surface tension in the alveoli and prevents their collapse and ultimately *atelectasis* (lung collapse).

The *lungs,* which are composed of millions of alveoli with their related ducts, bronchioles, and bronchi, are located in the pleural cavity in the thorax (see Fig. 60–4). The lungs are elastic, cone-shaped organs extending from the diaphragm (the major muscle of inspiration) at the base to just above the clavicles at the apex. The right

lung, which is larger than the left, is divided into three lobes: upper, middle, and lower. The left lung, which is somewhat narrower than the right to accommodate the heart, is divided into two lobes. All five lobes of the lungs are further divided into segments that correspond to the segmental bronchi. The *hilum* is the point at which the primary bronchus, pulmonary blood vessels, nerves, and lymphatics enter each lung.

Composed of two surfaces, the *pleura,* a continuous smooth membrane, totally encloses the lung. The *parietal* pleura lines the inside of the thoracic cavity, including the upper surface of the diaphragm. The *visceral* pleura covers the lung surfaces, including the major fissures between the lobes. A thin fluid layer, which is produced by the cells lining the pleura, lubricates these opposing surfaces, thereby allowing them to glide smoothly during respirations.

Two separate systems, the pulmonary and the bronchial, provide the circulation of blood to the lungs. The *bronchial* arteries, arising from the thoracic aorta, are part of the systemic circulation and do not participate in gas exchange. This system carries the blood supply to meet the metabolic demands of the conducting airways from the trachea to the terminal bronchioles. The *pulmonary* circulation is composed of a highly vascular network. Oxygen-depleted blood travels from the right ventricle into the pulmonary artery, which eventually branches into arterioles and venules that form the capillary networks. The capillaries are enmeshed around and through the alveoli, the site of gas exchange (see Fig. 60–5). After oxygen diffusion, oxygenated blood returns through the pulmonary venous circulation to the left atrium to be pumped throughout the systemic circulation.

RESPIRATORY CHANGES ASSOCIATED WITH AGING

Consequences of the inevitable process of aging vary with each individual and ultimately affect all body systems. The changes in the respiratory system that are associated with aging—decreases in vital capacity and diffusing capacity and increases in residual volume—are influenced by a lifetime exposure to environmental stimuli (e.g., cigarette smoke, air pollutants, and industrial fumes and irritants) and heredity. Respiratory disease is a major cause of acute illness and chronic disability in the elderly. Although respiratory function declines with increasing age, there is little difficulty with the demands of ordinary activity. However, with exercise, the sedentary elderly client often complains of feeling breathless. Respiratory changes that occur in the aged are described in the accompanying Focus on the Elderly feature.

It is difficult to differentiate the normal changes related to aging and the pathologic changes associated with respiratory disease or exposure to pollutants. In addition, abnormalities of the neuromuscular and cardiovascular systems that occur with aging may result in

FOCUS ON THE ELDERLY ■ Changes in the Respiratory System Related to Aging

Structure	Change	Interventions*	Rationales
Chest wall	Anteroposterior diameter increases. Slope changes. Progressive kyphoscoliosis occurs. Decreased mobility occurs. Osteoporosis is possible.	1. Discuss normal changes of aging. 2. Discuss the need for increased rest periods during exercise.	1. Clients may be anxious because they must work harder to breathe. 2. Older clients have less tolerance for exercise.
Alveoli	Alveolar membranes thicken. Diffusion capacity decreases. Elastic recoil decreases. Dilation of bronchioles and alveolar ducts occurs. Ability to cough decreases.	3. Encourage vigorous pulmonary toilet (i.e., turn, cough, and deep breathe), especially if the client is confined to bed or has had surgery.	3. There is increased potential for mechanical or infectious respiratory complications in these situations.
Lungs	Residual volume increases. Decreased capacity results in less efficient oxygen and carbon dioxide exchange. Elasticity decreases.	4. Include inspection, palpation, percussion, and auscultation in lung assessments. 5. Assess the client's respiration for abnormal breathing patterns. 6. Encourage frequent oral hygiene.	4. All four techniques are needed to detect normal age-related changes. 5. Periodic breathing patterns can occur (e.g., Cheyne-Stokes). 6. Oral hygiene aids in removal of secretions.
Pharynx and larynx	Muscles atrophy. Vocal cords become slack. Laryngeal muscles lose elasticity and cartilage.	7. Have face-to-face conversations with clients when possible.	7. Voices of clients may be soft and difficult to understand.
Pulmonary artery	Increased vascular resistance to blood flow through pulmonary vascular system occurs. Risk of hypoxia increases.	8. Assess the client's level of consciousness.	8. Clients can become confused during acute respiratory conditions.

* Interventions 1–6 apply to all structures; 7 and 8 are specific for those structures.

abnormal respiration even if the lungs are normal. Adequate functioning of both of these systems is essential for the pulmonary system to perform its various functions.

and diagnostic findings. Many of the diagnostic studies that are relevant to respiratory disorders, e.g., pulmonary function tests, use these data for determining predicted normal values.

PERSONAL AND FAMILY HISTORY

The nurse questions the client about the *past medical history*, including childhood illnesses (e.g., asthma, pneumonia, croup, eczema, frequent upper respiratory tract infections, hay fever, allergies, and communicable diseases), adult illnesses (e.g., pneumonia; chronic sinusitis; tuberculosis, including the date of the last tuberculin test and reaction; diabetes; hypertension; and heart disease), immunizations (influenza and pneumococcal

HISTORY

DEMOGRAPHIC DATA

The biographical or identifying data, consisting of at least *age, sex,* and *race,* can affect the client's physical vaccine [Pneumovax]), operations, injuries, and hospitalizations (including date of last chest x-ray film and pulmonary function test). The circumstances of some chest injuries and operations may suggest that they are related to the present illness. For example, a foreign body lodged in the lung may cause recurrent coughing or development of a pulmonary abscess.

The nurse obtains information about the client's *home and living conditions,* such as the type of heat used (e.g., gas heater, woodburning stove, fireplace, kerosene heater) and exposure to environmental irritants (e.g., noxious fumes, chemicals, animals, and air pollutants), either in the home or in the workplace.

Habits pertaining to *smoking* are essential for the nurse to obtain for comprehensive respiratory assessment. The nurse questions the client about use of cigarettes, cigars, pipe tobacco, and marijuana. Information on the client's association with smokers on a daily basis is also important. If the client smokes, it is vital for the nurse to obtain information on how long the client has smoked, how many packs a day, and, if the client has quit, how long ago he or she stopped smoking. Smoking history is documented in pack-years (number of packs per day multiplied by number of years smoked). The nurse assumes a nonjudgmental attitude when questioning the client about smoking because of the guilt the client may harbor about this habit.

Questions about *travel* and *area of residence* may elicit data about exposure to certain diseases. For example, histoplasmosis is found in the middle United States, the Mississippi and Missouri River valleys, and Central America. Coccidioidomycosis is found predominantly in the western and southwestern United States, Mexico, and portions of Central America.

Current and past medication use is significant information for the respiratory history. The client is questioned about medications that are taken for breathing problems and also about other drugs that are taken for other conditions. It is also important to determine what over-the-counter medications, such as antihistamines, decongestants, cough syrups, inhalants, and nasal sprays and/or drops, the client may be using. Home remedies must be assessed also. The client is questioned about past medication use and why it was discontinued. For example, a client may have used numerous bronchodilator metered-dose inhalers but may prefer one particular drug for relieving shortness of breath. Aspirin-induced asthma (the symptom complex of acetylsalicylic acid sensitivity, nasal polyps, and asthma) has been recognized for many years as a syndrome found in a significant number of adult asthmatics.

Eliciting data about *allergies* is extremely important and relevant to the respiratory history. The nurse determines if the client has any known allergies to foods, dust, molds, pollen, trees, grass, flowers, animal dander, or medications. The client is questioned about the specific allergic response: e.g., Does he or she wheeze, cough, sneeze, or experience rhinitis after exposure to the allergen?

The *family history* is obtained to rule out any genetically transmitted respiratory disorders or disorders in which genetic factors may operate, such as cystic fibrosis, asthma, allergies, tuberculosis, pneumonia, kyphoscoliosis, emphysema, and cancer of the lung.

DIET HISTORY

An evaluation of the client's diet history may reveal allergic reactions after ingestion of foods containing certain preservatives, such as various benzoic acid derivatives including tartrazine (a component of FD&C Yellow No. 5), which is used as a coloring agent in foods and beverages. Preservatives such as sulfites are widely used to maintain the freshness of vegetables in restaurant salads, to prevent discoloration of dried fruit and uncooked potatoes, and to preserve processed fruits, vegetables, and juices. These preservatives are also used in the production of wine and beer. Signs and symptoms range from rhinitis, chest tightness, weakness, shortness of breath, urticaria, and severe bronchospasm to loss of consciousness.

SOCIOECONOMIC STATUS

A thorough *occupational history* is particularly relevant for the assessment of the respiratory client because the incidence of occupational pulmonary diseases, including pneumoconiosis, toxic lung injury, and hypersensitivity disease, continues to increase annually. The occupational history includes exact dates of employment and a brief description of what the job entails. Exposure to industrial dusts (both organic and inorganic) and/or noxious chemicals found in smoke and fumes may cause respiratory disease in coal miners, stonemasons, cotton handlers, welders, potters, plastic and rubber manufacturers, printers, farm workers, and steel foundry workers.

An assessment of the client's *hobbies and leisure activities* may reveal that such seemingly innocent pastimes as painting, ceramics, or woodworking may be exposing the person to harmful irritants.

CURRENT HEALTH PROBLEM

The *chief complaint* is a single sentence, or a brief statement, in the client's own words describing the reason for seeking help. If there is more than one problem, they are listed in order of the client's priorities.

After the client's chief complaint has been determined, the nurse explores the *history of the present illness.* This analysis includes the following: onset, duration, location, frequency, progressing and radiating patterns, quality and number of symptoms, aggravating and relieving factors, associated signs and symptoms, and treatment.

Whether the pulmonary problem is acute or chronic,

the client's chief complaint will probably include cough, sputum production, chest pain, shortness of breath, and/or shortness of breath on exertion.

Cough is the cardinal sign of respiratory disease. The nurse asks the client how long the cough has persisted (e.g., 1 week, 3 months) and if it occurs at a specific time of the day (e.g., on awakening in the morning) or in relation to any physical activity. The nurse also determines whether the cough is productive or nonproductive, congested, dry, tickling, or hacking.

An important symptom that is associated with coughing is *sputum production.* The color, consistency, and amount of sputum produced are noted because the type of sputum produced suggests the underlying pathologic process. Sputum may be clear, white, tan, gray, or, if infection is present, yellow or green. Voluminous, pink, frothy sputum is characteristic of pulmonary edema. Pneumococcal pneumonia is often associated with rust-colored sputum, and foul-smelling sputum is often found in anaerobic infections such as lung abscess. The presence of blood in the sputum may be noted as streaks in clients with an acute respiratory tract infection; clients with tuberculosis, pulmonary infarction, or tumors may expectorate grossly bloody sputum *(hemoptysis).*

Sputum can be quantified by describing its production in terms of a measuring device such as a teaspoon, tablespoon, one-half cup, and cup. The nurse should remember, however, that normally, the tracheobronchial tree can produce up to 3 oz (90 mL) of sputum per day. The nurse determines if sputum production is increasing, which may result from external stimuli (such as an irritant in the work setting) or from internal causes (such as chronic bronchitis or a lung abscess).

A detailed description of *chest pain* helps to differentiate among pleural, musculoskeletal, and cardiac pain. The lungs have no pain-sensitive nerves, but the ribs, muscles, parietal pleura, and tracheobronchial tree do. Because of its purely subjective nature, pain must be analyzed in relation to the characteristics described in the history of the present illness.

The perception of *shortness of breath* is also subjective and varies among individuals. A client's perception may not be consistent with the severity of the presenting problem. For that reason, the nurse determines the onset (slow or abrupt), duration (number of hours, time of day), relieving factors (repositioning, medication, activity cessation), and evidence of audible sounds (wheezing, stridor). An attempt at quantifying dyspnea is made by the nurse, who also determines if this symptom interferes with activities of daily living (ADL). For example, is the client short of breath while dressing, showering, shaving, or eating? Does dyspnea on exertion occur after the client walks one block or after climbing one flight of stairs? Table 60–1 correlates dyspnea classifications with ADL.

The nurse inquires about paroxysmal nocturnal dyspnea and orthopnea, which are commonly associated with chronic pulmonary disease and/or left ventricular failure. The client is questioned about recent weight loss and night sweats, both of which may indicate tuberculosis or an underlying pathologic condition of a different body system. The nurse determines if the client experiences regurgitation symptoms, such as indigestion and heartburn. Regurgitation syndrome, the aspiration of gastric contents into the lungs, can contribute to pulmonary disease.

PHYSICAL ASSESSMENT

NOSE AND SINUSES

The nose and sinuses are examined by inspection and palpation. The nurse inspects the client's external nose for deformities or tumors, and the nostrils for symmetry of size and shape. *Nasal flaring,* which may indicate increased respiratory effort, is noted.

The interior nose is examined with the client's head tilted back for easier observation. A nasal speculum and nasopharyngeal mirror may be used for a more thorough examination of the nasal cavity; however, for a routine nursing assessment, a penlight is sufficient. Using the penlight, the nurse inspects the internal mucous membranes, nasal septum, and inferior and middle turbinates for *color, swelling, drainage,* and *bleeding.* The mucous membrane of the nose normally appears redder than the oral mucosa, but it may appear pale, engorged, and bluish gray in clients with allergic rhinitis. The nurse checks the nasal septum for evidence of bleeding, perforation, or deviation. Some degree of septal deviation is common in most adults and appears as an S shape, inclining toward one side or the other. A *perforated septum,* which is indicated if the light shines through the perforation into the opposite nostril, is often found in cocaine abusers. *Nasal polyps,* which are a frequent cause of obstruction, appear as pale, shiny, gelatinous structures attached to the turbinates.

The nurse palpates the nose and paranasal sinuses to detect *tenderness* or *swelling.* Only the frontal and maxillary sinuses are readily accessible to clinical examination because the ethmoid and sphenoid sinuses lie deep within the skull (see Fig. 60–2). Using the thumbs, the nurse checks for sinus tenderness by pressing upward on the frontal and maxillary areas; both sides are assessed simultaneously. Tenderness in these areas suggests inflammation or acute sinusitis.

Transillumination of the sinuses may also be used to detect sinusitis. This procedure requires a darkened room and a penlight. Normally, the nurse would see a faint glow of light through the bone outlining the sinus. Transillumination is absent or decreased when acute sinusitis is suspected. X-ray films of the sinuses are used as a more definitive tool for detecting inflammation or acute sinusitis.

TABLE 60–1   Correlation of Dyspnea Classification with Performance of Activities of Daily Living

Classification	ADL Key
CLASS I: No significant restrictions in normal activity. Employable. Dyspnea occurs only on more than normal or strenuous exertion.	4: No breathlessness, normal.
CLASS II: Independent in essential ADL but restricted in some other activities. Dyspneic on climbing stairs or on walking on inclines but not on level walking. Employable for only sedentary job, or under special circumstances.	3: Satisfactory, mild breathlessness. Complete performance possible without pause or assistance, but not entirely normal.
CLASS III: Dyspnea commonly occurs during usual activities, such as showering or dressing, but client can manage without assistance from others. Not dyspneic at rest; can walk for more than a city block at own pace but cannot keep up with others of own age. May stop to catch breath part way up a flight of stairs. Is probably not employable in any occupation.	2: Fair, moderate breathlessness. Must stop during activity. Complete performance possible without assistance, but performance may be too debilitating or time-consuming.
CLASS IV: Dyspnea produces dependence on help in some essential ADL such as dressing or bathing. Not usually dyspneic at rest. Dyspneic on minimal exertion; must pause on climbing one flight, walking more than 100 yards, or dressing. Often restricted to home if lives alone. Has minimal or no activities out of home.	1: Poor, marked breathlessness. Incomplete performance; assistance necessary.
CLASS V: Entirely restricted to home and often limited to bed or chair. Dyspneic at rest. Dependent on help for most needs.	0: Performance not indicated or recommended; too difficult.

PHARYNX, TRACHEA, AND LARYNX

Examination of the mouth and pharynx begins with inspection of the external structures of the mouth. The reader is referred to Chapter 42 for complete physical assessment of the oral cavity.

Using a tongue depressor, the nurse presses down one side of the tongue at a time (to avoid stimulating the client's gag reflex) to visualize the structures of the posterior pharynx. As the client says "ah," the nurse notes the rise and fall of the soft palate and uvula and observes for *color* and *symmetry,* evidence of *mucopurulent discharge* (postnasal drainage), *edema* or *ulceration,* and *tonsillar enlargement.*

The neck is usually examined together with the trachea. The neck is inspected for symmetry and masses and for use of accessory neck muscles in breathing. Lymph nodes are palpated for *size, shape, mobility, consistency,* and *tenderness.* Tender nodes are usually movable and suggest inflammation. Malignant nodes, on the other hand, are often hard and fixed to the surrounding tissue.

The client's trachea is inspected for *swelling, bruises,* and *alignment* and is palpated for *deviation, tenderness,* and *masses.* Palpation is accomplished by gently placing the fingers on the trachea because firm palpation may elicit coughing and/or gagging. The trachea is located in the area of the sternal notch. The spaces between each side of the trachea and the ends of the notch should be equal. Many lung disorders cause the trachea to deviate from the midline. Masses push the trachea away from the affected area, whereas atelectasis causes a pull toward the affected area.

The larynx is usually examined by a specialist with a laryngoscope. The nurse may observe an *abnormal voice,* especially hoarseness.

LUNGS AND THORAX

Physical assessment of the lungs and thorax involves inspection, palpation, percussion, and auscultation. A thorough assessment of the chest is vital for formulating nursing diagnoses and planning care for the client.

Before examination of the thorax, the nurse must become familiar with anatomic landmarks. Localization of physical assessment findings depends on accurate numbering of the ribs, intercostal spaces, and vertebrae and on accurate identification of imaginary lines drawn on the chest (Fig. 60–6).

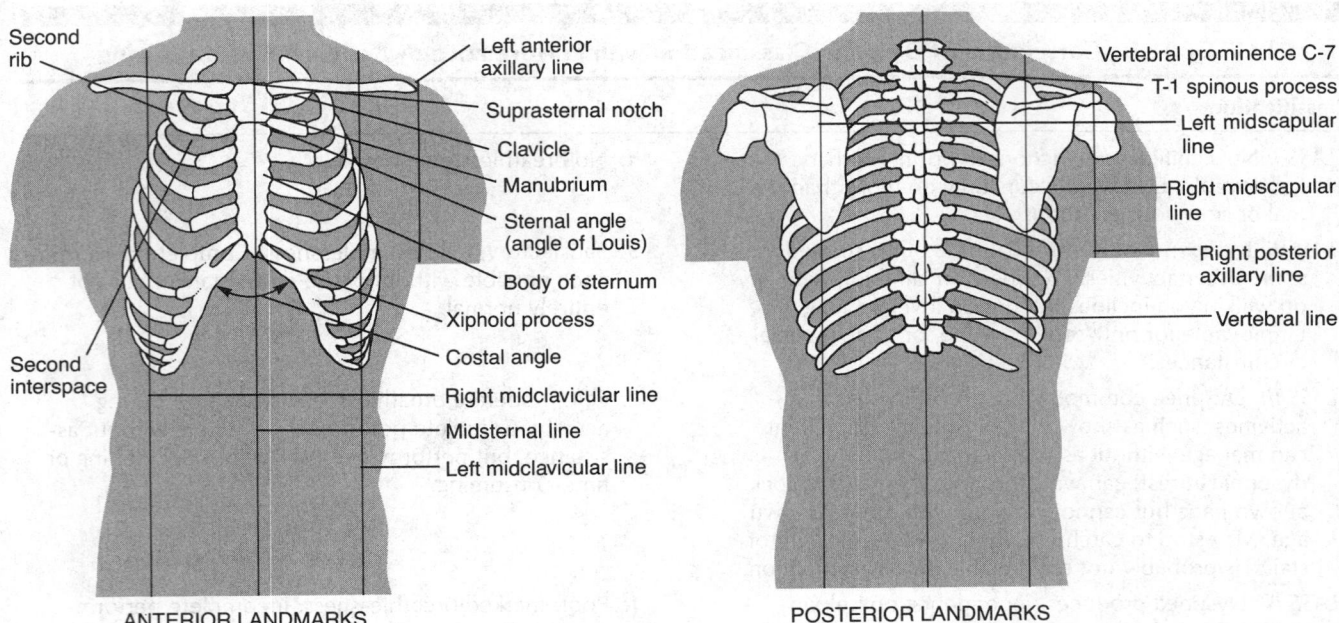

ANTERIOR LANDMARKS

Second rib
Left anterior axillary line
Suprasternal notch
Clavicle
Manubrium
Sternal angle (angle of Louis)
Body of sternum
Xiphoid process
Costal angle
Right midclavicular line
Midsternal line
Left midclavicular line
Second interspace

POSTERIOR LANDMARKS

Vertebral prominence C-7
T-1 spinous process
Left midscapular line
Right midscapular line
Right posterior axillary line
Vertebral line

Figure 60–6

Anterior and posterior thoracic landmarks.

INSPECTION

Inspection of the chest begins with assessment of the posterior thorax, with the client in a sitting position if possible. The client should be undressed to the waist and draped for privacy and warmth. The chest is observed by comparing one side with the other. The nurse works from the top (apexes of the lungs) and moves downward (toward the bases). The posterior thorax is inspected for *skin color and condition, scars, lesions, masses,* and *spinal deformities* such as kyphosis, scoliosis, and lordosis (described in Chap. 30).

The nurse notes the rate, rhythm, and depth of respirations, as well as symmetry of movement. The nurse observes the type of breathing exhibited by the client, such as *pursed-lip* or diaphragmatic breathing and use of accessory muscles. When the nurse observes the quality of respirations, the inspiratory-to-expiratory ratio is noted, which is normally 1:2. A prolonged expiratory phase indicates obstruction of air outflow and is frequently seen in clients with COPD.

The nurse notes the client's chest configuration and compares the anteroposterior (AP) diameter with the lateral diameter. This ratio normally ranges from 1:2 to about 5:7, depending on the client's body build. The ratio of the AP to the lateral diameter approximates 1:1 in the client with emphysema, and the client has the typical barrel-chested appearance.

The nurse observes for normal upward and outward symmetric movement of the chest on inspiration. An *impaired movement* or *unequal expansion,* which may indicate underlying disease of the lung or pleura, is noted. Normally, the ribs slope downward. However, clients with air trapping in the lungs caused by chronic asthma and/or emphysema have little or no slope to the ribs; i.e., the ribs are more horizontal.

The nurse also checks for *abnormal retractions of the interspaces during inspiration,* which indicate airflow obstruction. These retractions may be due to fibrosis of the underlying lung, severe acute asthma, emphysema, or tracheal or laryngeal obstruction. *Abnormal bulging of the interspaces on expiration* results from forced prolonged expiration, as in asthma or emphysema, or it may result from a loss of thoracic structure, as with multiple rib fractures.

PALPATION

Palpation of the chest follows inspection to assess symmetry of respiratory movement, to assess observable abnormalities, to identify areas of tenderness, and to elicit *vocal* or *tactile fremitus* (vibration). Palpation of respiratory or diaphragmatic excursion (see under the later heading Percussion) or expansion is a more sensitive assessment method than inspection.

In *palpation,* the nurse's thumbs are placed posteriorly on the spine at the level of the ninth ribs; the fingers are extended laterally around the rib cage. As the client inhales, both sides of the chest should move upward and outward together in one symmetric movement; the nurse's thumbs thus move apart. On exhalation, the thumbs should come back together as they return to the midline. *Splinting* or *decreased movement on one side* (unilateral expansion) may be due to pleuritic pain, trauma, or pneumothorax (air in the pleural cavity). *Respiratory lag* or *impairment of thoracic movement* may also indicate the presence of a lung mass, pleural fibrosis, atelectasis, pneumonia, or lung abscess.

The thorax is palpated for any abnormalities found on inspection, e.g., masses, lesions, bruises, and swelling, and for tenderness, particularly if the client has reported pain. *Crepitus,* or subcutaneous emphysema, is a crackling sensation felt beneath the fingertips and should be noted, especially around a wound site. Crepitus indicates that air is trapped within the tissues.

Vocal fremitus is a vibration of the chest wall that is produced when the client speaks; when perceived by palpation, it is termed *tactile fremitus.* To elicit tactile fremitus, the nurse places the palm or the base of the fingers against the client's chest wall and instructs the client to say "99" or "1, 2, 3." The vibrations are compared (with the same hand) from one side of the chest to the other, moving from the apexes to the bases of the lung. Palpable vibrations are transmitted from the tracheobronchial tree, along the solid surface of chest wall, to the nurse's hand. Symmetry of the vibrations and areas of enhanced, diminished, or absent fremitus should be noted. Fremitus is decreased if the transmission of sound waves from the larynx to the chest wall is slowed, such as when the pleural space is filled with fluid (pleural effusion), air (pneumothorax), or solid tissue (pleural thickening). Fremitus is increased over large bronchi because of their proximity to the chest wall. Disease processes such as pneumonia or lung abscesses that decrease the distance that vibrations must travel to reach the chest wall also result in increased tactile fremitus.

PERCUSSION

Percussion is used to assess for pulmonary resonance, boundaries of organs, and diaphragmatic excursion. *Percussion* involves tapping the chest wall, which sets the underlying tissues into motion and produces audible sounds. The nurse places the distal joint of the middle finger of the less dominant hand firmly on the surface to be percussed. No other part of the nurse's hand should touch the client's chest wall because such touching dampens the vibrations. The plexor (in this case, the tapping finger of the dominant hand) is used to deliver quick, sharp strikes to the distal joint of the positioned finger. The nurse maintains a loose, relaxed wrist while delivering the blows with the *tip* of the plexor or middle finger, not the finger pad (Fig. 60–7). The nurse repeats this technique two or three times and listens to the intensity, pitch, quality, and duration of the sound produced.

Percussion produces five distinguishable notes, which assist the nurse in determining the density of the underlying structures, i.e., whether the lung tissue contains air or fluid or is solid. The five percussion notes elicited are described in Table 60–2. Percussion of the thorax is done over the rib interspaces because percussing the sternum, ribs, and/or scapulae would indicate the solid nature of bone. Percussion penetrates only 2 to 3 in (5 to 7 cm), so deeper lesions are not detected with this technique.

Figure 60–8 shows the correct sequence for percussion and auscultation. The percussion technique begins with the client sitting in an upright position; the posterior thorax is assessed first. The nurse proceeds systematically, beginning at the apexes and working toward the bases and remembering that the apex of the lung rises about ¾ to 1½ in (2 to 4 cm) above the clavicle anteriorly. Posteriorly, there is approximately a 2-in (5-cm) width of lung tissue at the apex. While percussing the posterior chest, the nurse assesses the client's *diaphragmatic excursion:* The distance that the diaphragm moves during inspiration and expiration may be measured by noting the difference in the level of dullness percussed at rest from the level of dullness percussed at

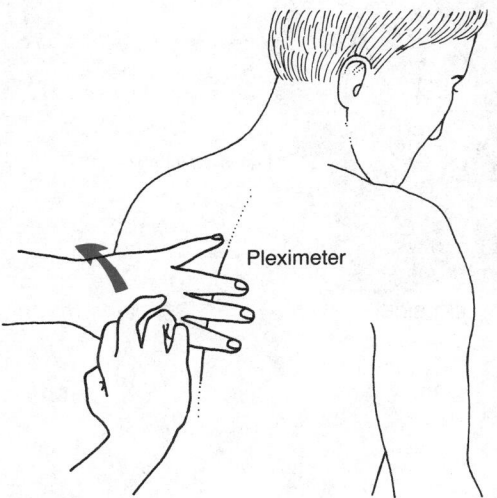

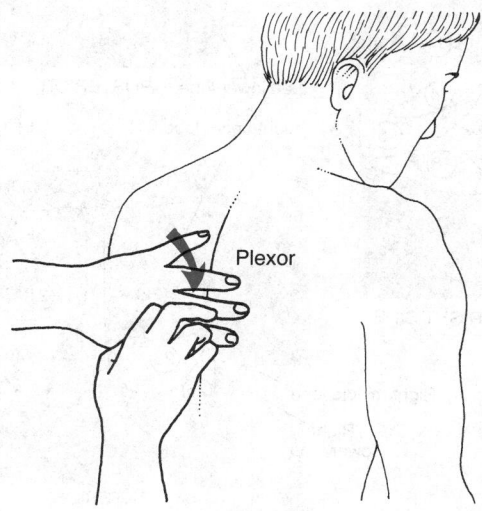

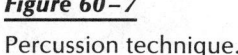

Figure 60–7

Percussion technique.

TABLE 60-2 Characteristic Features of the Five Percussion Notes

Note	Pitch	Intensity	Quality	Duration	Findings
Resonance	Low	Moderate to loud	Hollow	Long	Resonance is characteristic of normal lung tissue.
Hyperresonance	Higher than resonance	Very loud	Booming	Longer than resonance	Hyperresonance indicates the presence of trapped air, so it is commonly heard over an emphysematous and/or asthmatic lung and occasionally over a pneumothorax.
Flatness	High	Soft	Extreme dullness	Short	An example location is the sternum. Flatness percussed over the lung fields may indicate a massive pleural effusion.
Dullness	Medium	Medium	Thud-like	Medium	An example location is over the liver and kidneys. Dullness can be percussed over atelectatic lung or consolidated lung.
Tympany	High	Loud	Musical, drum-like	Short	Examples are the cheek filled with air and the abdomen distended with air. Over the lung, a tympanic note usually indicates a large pneumothorax.

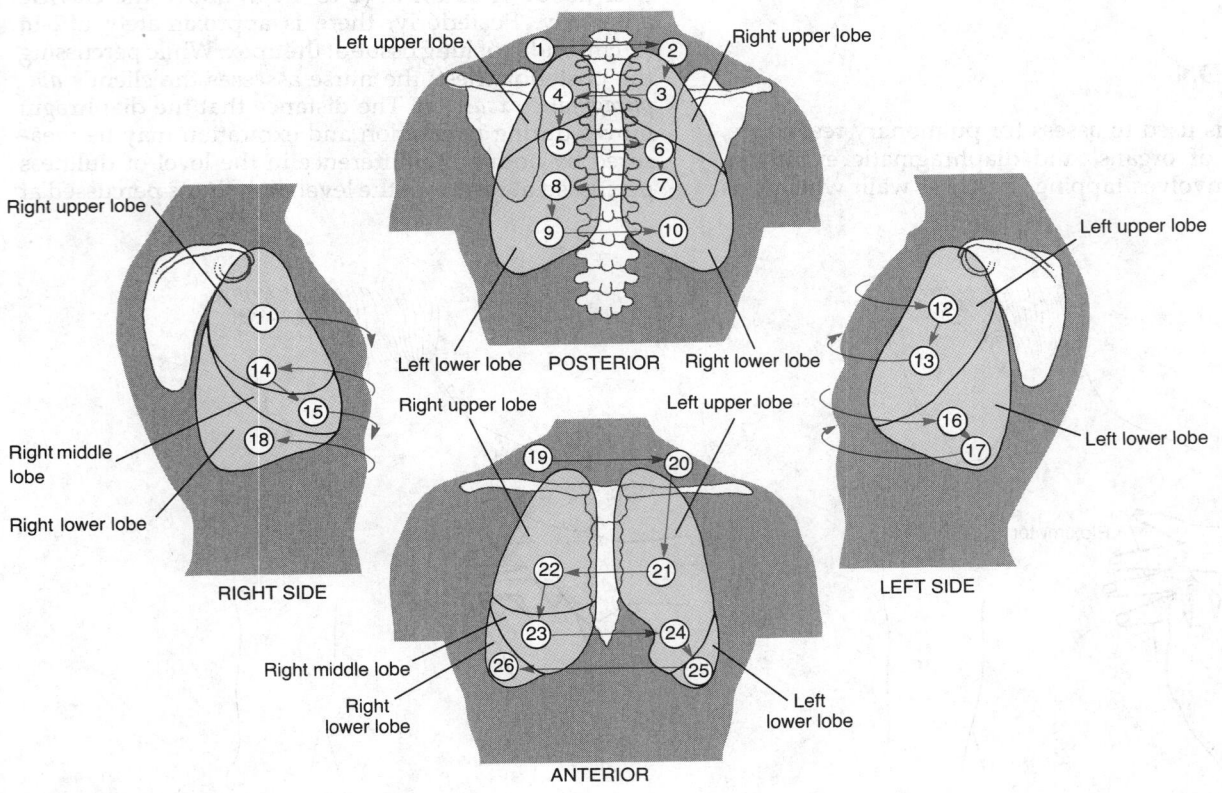

Figure 60-8

Sequence for percussion and auscultation.

full inspiration. The client is instructed to take a deep breath and hold it while the nurse percusses downward until dullness identifies the lower border of the lung. Normal resonance of the lung stops at the diaphragm, where the sound becomes dull, and this site is marked. The client is instructed to exhale deeply and again stop breathing while the nurse percusses to the area of dullness of the diaphragm. This location is noted. The nurse repeats the procedure on the opposite side and notes the difference. The difference between the two markings and/or sounds is the diaphragmatic excursion, which may range from 1 to 3 in (3 to 8 cm). The diaphragm is normally higher on the right side because of the location of the heart and liver. The range of motion of the diaphragm should be equal on both sides of the chest but may be decreased in clients with pleurisy or emphysema.

The nurse continues assessment of the thorax with percussion of the anterior chest. Boundaries of organs such as the heart and liver can be percussed anteriorly by noting the change in percussion notes; i.e., the percussion note changes from resonance of the normal lung to dullness at the borders of the heart and liver. If a dull percussion note is noted over lung tissue, the nurse expects fluid or solid material to be replacing the normal air-containing lung (e.g., as in clients with pneumonia, pleural effusion, fibrosis, or atelectasis).

AUSCULTATION

Auscultation is the final and most reliable assessment technique and includes listening for normal breath sounds, adventitious (abnormal) sounds, and voice sounds. Auscultation provides information about the flow of air through the tracheobronchial tree and enables the nurse to identify the presence of fluid, mucus, or obstruction in the respiratory system. The nurse uses the diaphragm of the stethoscope for auscultation because it is designed to detect high-pitched sounds.

The auscultation procedure begins with the client sitting in an upright position. The nurse uses a systematic approach and works from the apexes of the lungs to the basal segments (see Fig. 60–7). Auscultation is performed on the posterior, anterior, and lateral thorax. Using the diaphragm of the stethoscope pressed firmly against the client's chest wall because clothing can distort and/or muffle sounds, the nurse instructs the client to breathe slowly and deeply with an open mouth. The nurse listens to a full respiratory cycle and notes the quality and intensity of the breath sounds and then observes for adventitious sounds and their locations. The nurse observes the client for signs of lightheadedness and/or dizziness caused by hyperventilation during auscultation and allows the client to breathe normally for a few minutes.

Normal Breath Sounds

Normal breath sounds are produced as air vibrates while passing through the respiratory passages from the larynx to the alveoli. Breath sounds are identified by their location, intensity, pitch, and duration (i.e., ratio of inspiration to expiration). Normal breath sounds are known as vesicular, bronchovesicular, and bronchial (or tubular). Figure 60–9 illustrates normal breath sounds and their location. The nurse describes these sounds as decreased, diminished, or absent.

Vesicular breath sounds are low-pitched, soft, breezy sounds resembling wind blowing through the trees. The inspiratory phase is longer and more audible than the expiratory phase; expiration is heard as a puff. There is no perceptible pause between inspiration and expiration. Vesicular sounds are normal breath sounds that are heard over most of the peripheral lung fields, with the exception of the area between the scapulae posteriorly or above the sternum anteriorly.

Bronchovesicular breath sounds are a mixture of vesicular and bronchial sounds. The sound is harsh and moderate in pitch and intensity, with inspiration equal to expiration in duration. Bronchovesicular sounds are heard over the thorax where the bronchi are closest to the chest wall, i.e., anteriorly near the mainstem bronchi at the level of the first and second intercostal spaces and in the intrascapular region posteriorly. Bronchovesicu-

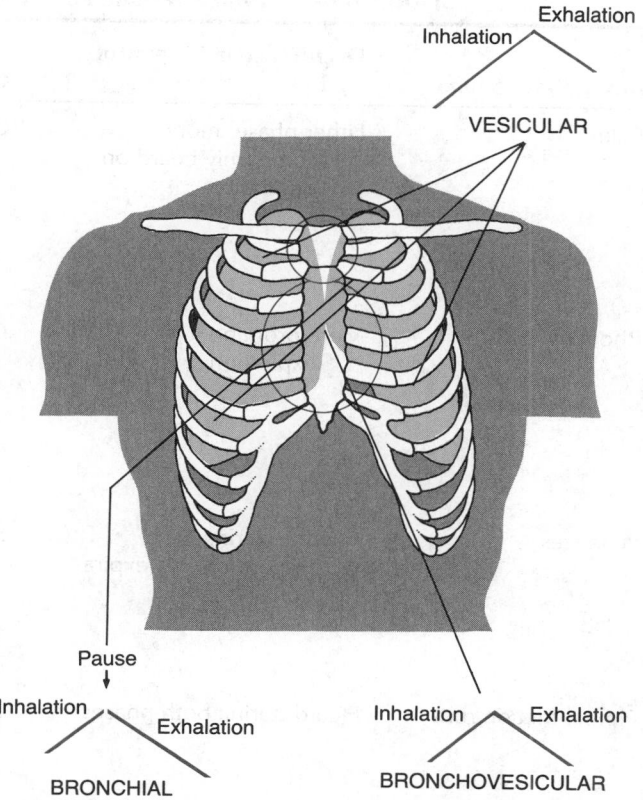

Figure 60–9

Location of normal breath sounds. I, inspiration; E, expiration.

lar breath sounds are also audible elsewhere, when they indicate an abnormality and may be the result of pulmonary consolidation, normal aging, chronic airway disease, or other pathologic condition.

Bronchial breath sounds are also called *tubular* sounds because they resemble the sound produced by wind going through a long tube. The bronchial breath sound is loud, harsh, or coarse, with a blowing, hollow quality. The expiratory phase is prolonged and longer than the inspiratory phase, and there is a distinguishable pause between the two phases. Bronchial breath sounds are normally heard over the trachea. When these sounds are heard peripherally, they become abnormal sounds and are due to transmission of centrally generated bronchial sounds to an area of increased density such as in clients with atelectasis, tumor, or pneumonia.

Adventitious Breath Sounds

Adventitious sounds are abnormal breath sounds that are superimposed on normal sounds that indicate pathologic changes in the tracheobronchial tree. Table 60–3 classifies and describes the adventitious sounds: *rales,*

rhonchi, wheezes, and *pleural friction rubs.* Various subclassifications of these categories exist. The terminology that is used to describe adventitious sounds varies among respiratory care practitioners. The nurse is encouraged to document exactly what is heard on auscultation instead of relying on numerous labels. Adventitious sounds vary in pitch, intensity, duration, and phase of the respiratory cycle in which they occur.

Voice Sounds

If during the physical assessment of the lungs and thorax the nurse has discovered abnormal findings, the client is assessed for vocal resonance. Auscultation of voice sounds through the normally air-filled lung produces a muffled, unclear sound because sound vibrations travel poorly through air. Vocal resonance is increased when the sound must travel through a solid or liquid medium as in clients with a consolidated lung, pneumonia, atelectasis, pleural effusion, tumor, or abscess. *Bronchophony* is the abnormally loud transmission of voice sounds through an area of increased density. For assessment of bronchophony, the client repeats the

---

TABLE 60–3 Characteristic Features of the Four Adventitious Breath Sounds

Adventitious Sound	Occurrence in Respiratory Cycle	Character	Findings
Rales	Either phase; more commonly heard on inspiration	Crackling, discontinuous sounds caused by air passing through moisture in alveoli or bronchioles. Sounds like hair being rolled between fingers near the ear.	Atelectasis Interstitial fibrosis Pulmonary edema Bronchitis Pneumonia Tuberculosis
Rhonchi	More prominent on expiration	Continuous musical, coarse, rattling sounds caused by fluid, secretions, or obstruction in large airways. Likely to change with coughing or suctioning.	Chronic bronchitis Pneumonia Tumors Chronic lung diseases
Wheezes	Audible during both inspiration and expiration	Squeaky, musical sounds associated with air rushing through narrowed small airways. May be heard without a stethoscope.	Bronchospasm (as in asthma) Edema Tumors Secretions
Pleural friction rubs	Heard during both phases	Rough, grating, scratching sounds caused by inflamed surfaces of the pleura rubbing together. Often associated with pain on deep inspirations.	Pleurisy Tuberculosis Pulmonary infarction Pneumonia Lung cancer

number "99" while the nurse systematically auscultates the thorax. *Whispered pectoriloquy* is much more sensitive than bronchophony and is perceived by having the client whisper the number sequence "1, 2, 3." Normally, whispered words sound faint and indistinct; if heard loudly and distinctly, the nurse suspects pulmonary consolidation and correlates this assessment with other findings. *Egophony*, another form of abnormal vocal resonance, has a high-pitched, bleating, nasal quality. The nurse instructs the client to repeat the letter "E" and auscultates the thorax. Egophony exists when this letter is heard as a flat, nasal sound of *A* through the stethoscope, which indicates an area of consolidation, pleural effusion, or abscess.

PSYCHOSOCIAL ASSESSMENT

The nurse assesses aspects of the client's life style that may have a significant impact on respiratory function. Some respiratory conditions may be exacerbated by stress. The nurse questions the client about present life stresses and the coping patterns used to reduce stress. Chronic respiratory illnesses such as COPD may cause changes in family roles and relationships, social isolation, financial problems, and unemployment and/or disability. By discussing coping mechanisms, the nurse assesses the client's reaction to these psychosocial stressors and discovers maladaptive behaviors and strengths. For instance, the client may react to stress by becoming dependent on family members, by withdrawal, or by noncompliance with treatment. After completing the psychosocial assessment, the nurse assists the client in determining the support systems available to help the client cope with respiratory impairment. (See the accompanying Nursing Research feature.)

DIAGNOSTIC ASSESSMENT

LABORATORY TESTS

Several laboratory tests are relevant to the care of clients with respiratory disorders. Table 60–4 summarizes these diagnostic studies that the nurse correlates with the history and assessment findings to form nursing diagnoses, formulate care plans, and implement client teaching. The reader is referred to Chapter 14 for more detail regarding the tests used to assess acid-base balance. (Also, see Chap. 66 for more information on the complete blood count.)

NURSING RESEARCH

Educational Support May Increase Feelings of Well-being in Clients with COPD.

Hunter S. M., & Hall, S. S. (1989). The effects of an educational support program on dyspnea and the emotional status of COPD clients. *Rehabilitation Nursing, 14,* 200–202.

COPD is a debilitating disease that may limit activities and affect psychologic well-being. Clients are often afraid to exert themselves because of fears of dyspnea and can become depressed. Nurses need proven nursing measures to assist clients with attaining the highest possible level of the quality of life.

The study was conducted to determine if a support group and educational program would be beneficial in decreasing the number of dyspneic episodes and in improving the mental status of COPD clients.

A pre- and posttest design was used for the study. A questionnaire about dyspneic episodes, medications, and other measures used to improve breathing was filled out weekly by the eight subjects. All clients were administered the Profile of Moods State during the first and fifth weeks of the 5-wk course. Weekly educational sessions were conducted to teach breathing exercises and conservation of energy. Small group sessions were also conducted to discuss clients' feelings and how to cope with changes in life style.

t tests of this profile's scores revealed no significance among the paired comparisons. Clients did report that they felt better about coping, although they reported no change in dyspnea.

Critique. Results of this study have limited generalizability because of the small sample size from a single population. No physiologic measures for dyspnea were taken, so the reports are subjective.

Possible nursing implications. Nurses need to teach COPD clients to help themselves improve their quality of life. Providing support and education are two ways in which clients can be assisted in coping with their chronic disease.

RADIOGRAPHIC EXAMINATIONS

STANDARD RADIOGRAPHY

Chest x-ray films are taken for clients with respiratory disorders to evaluate the present status of the chest and to provide a baseline for comparison of future changes. The diagnostic intent of the test helps to determine the type that will be ordered, which includes anteroposterior (AP), front to back; posteroanterior (PA), back to front; or right (RL) or left (LL) lateral side views. Chest x-ray films can be used to assess pathologic changes in the lung such as those occurring in clients with pneumonia, atelectasis, pneumothorax, and tumor. The presence of pleural fluid and the position and placement of

TABLE 60–4 Normal Findings and Significance of Abnormal Findings in Common Laboratory Tests Used in Respiratory Assessment

Test	Normal Values	Significance of Abnormal Findings
Blood studies		
Complete Blood Count		
Red blood cells	3.6–5.0 million/mm³ (women) 4.2–5.5 million/mm³ (men)	*Decreased levels* indicate possible chronic infections or anemia.
Hemoglobin	12–15 g/dL (women) 14–16.5 g/dL (men)	*Decreased levels* indicate possible anemia. *Elevations* indicate possible COPD or hypoxemia related to late-stage pulmonary emphysema.
Hematocrit	30%–45% (women) 42%–50% (men)	See Hemoglobin entry.
White blood cells, total	4500–11,000/mm³	*Decreased levels* indicate possible anemia. *Elevations* indicate possible acute infections, pneumonia, meningitis, tonsillitis, or emphysema.
Differential		
Neutrophils	50%–70% of total	*Elevations* indicate possible acute infection (influenza, pneumonia) or COPD. *Decreased levels* indicate possible viral disease.
Eosinophils	1%–3% of total	*Elevations* indicate possible COPD, asthma, or allergies.
Basophils	<0.5% of total	*Elevations* indicate possible inflammation.
Lymphocytes	20%–40% of total	*Elevations* indicate possible viral infection, pertussis, or infectious mononucleosis.
Monocytes	2%–6% of total	See Lymphocytes entry; also tuberculosis or anemia.
Arterial Blood Gases		
PO_2	>80 mmHg	*Decreased levels* indicate possible COPD, chronic bronchitis, cancer of the bronchi and lungs, cystic fibrosis, respiratory distress syndrome, anemias, or atelectasis (respiratory alkalosis).
PCO_2	32–45 mmHg	*Decreased levels* indicate possible hypoxia. *Elevations* indicate possible COPD, pneumonia, anesthesia effects, or use of narcotics (respiratory acidosis).
pH	7.35–7.45	*Elevations* indicate possible metabolic or respiratory alkalosis. *Decreased levels* may indicate possible acidosis.
HCO_3^-	20–26 mEq/L	*Elevations* indicate possible respiratory acidosis. *Decreased levels* indicate possible respiratory alkalosis.
SO_2	95%–100%	*Decreased levels* indicate possible impaired ability of hemoglobin to release oxygen to tissues.
Sputum Studies		
Gram's stain	Negative	Presence of gram-positive or gram-negative bacteria indicates the microorganism that is causing respiratory infection.
Culture and sensitivity	Negative	Presence of microorganisms indicates possible respiratory infections (e.g., pneumonia or bronchitis).
Acid-fast stain	No acid-fast bacilli	Presence of bacilli indicates possible tuberculosis.
Cytologic tests	Negative	Presence of abnormal cells indicates possible malignancy.

an endotracheal tube can also be detected by chest radiography. However, these films have limitations; they may appear normal even in a severe form of certain diseases, such as chronic bronchitis, asthma, and emphysema.

Sinus and facial x-ray films are taken to assess the fluid levels in the sinus cavities to assist in the diagnosis of acute and/or chronic sinusitis.

BRONCHOGRAPHY

Bronchography involves the instillation of a liquid contrast medium into the trachea followed by x-ray films of the bronchial tree (see the summary of the procedure in the accompanying Guidelines feature).

TOMOGRAPHY

Tomography is valuable in the assessment of the client with a respiratory disorder because pulmonary densities, tumors, and lesions can be demonstrated. *Positron*

emission tomography is useful for studying ventilation-perfusion relationships in the lung. *Computed tomography* (CT) provides cross-sectional views of the thorax and produces a three-dimensional assessment of the lungs and thorax. CT can be used with or without an intravenously injected contrast agent. Nursing interventions for care of the client undergoing CT include education of the client about the procedure and determination of the client's sensitivity to the contrast medium.

OTHER DIAGNOSTIC STUDIES

MAGNETIC RESONANCE IMAGING

Magnetic resonance imaging (MRI) is the most advanced diagnostic imaging tool available. It assists in the diagnosis of respiratory system disorders by providing information about the type and condition of the tissues being imaged along any plane inside the body: vertically, horizontally, or diagonally. This noninvasive procedure requires little client preparation other than the removal of all metal objects. Individuals with pace-

---

GUIDELINES ■ Care of the Client Undergoing Special Diagnostic Tests for Respiratory Disorders

Procedure	Purpose	Interventions	Rationales
Bronchography	To diagnose abnormalities of the bronchi, such as narrowing, dilation, or obstruction. Dye is instilled into the trachea, and the chest is tilted at various angles to assist the flow of contrast medium. X-ray films are then taken.	1. Allow the client nothing by mouth for several hours before the test.	1. To prevent aspiration of gastric contents.
		2. Assess the client for allergies to iodine, contrast media, or local anesthetics.	2. To prevent allergic reactions.
		3. Administer pretest medications (atropine, diazepam) as ordered.	3. To decrease the amount of secretions and to reduce anxiety.
		4. Assess the client for fears concerning the procedure. Assure the client that he or she will be monitored for any respiratory problems.	4. To reduce fears about not being able to breathe during the procedure.
		5. After the procedure, allow the client nothing by mouth until the gag reflex returns.	5. To prevent aspiration of gastric contents.
		6. Encourage coughing and fluid intake.	6. To promote expectoration of secretions and facilitate the removal of dye.
		7. Assess vital signs frequently for 24 h. Assess the client for bleeding.	7. To detect changes such as dyspnea. Slight temperature elevation is normal.

continued

GUIDELINES ■ Care of the Client Undergoing Special Diagnostic Tests for Respiratory Disorders *Continued*

Procedure	Purpose	Interventions	Rationales
Bronchoscopy	To assess airway anatomy for tumors, obstruction, and atelectasis. To assist in diagnosis of tuberculosis or cancer by biopsy of lesions. To remove thick secretions, mucous plugs, or foreign bodies. A flexible fiberoptic bronchoscope is inserted through the mouth, nose, endotracheal tube, or tracheostomy tube. The procedure may be done in the operating room or radiology department. Oxygen administration and cardiac monitoring are usually used.	1. Follow interventions 1–3 for bronchography. 2. Prepare the client for topical anesthetic administration into the oropharynx. 3. Remove the client's dentures if present. 4. After the procedure, monitor the client's vital signs for 15 min until stable. 5. After the procedure, allow the client nothing by mouth until the gag reflex returns. 6. Discourage smoking, talking, and coughing for several hours.	1. See rationales 1–3 for bronchography. 2. To decrease anxiety related to numbness of the throat and gagging. 3. To prevent injury. 4. To detect respiratory distress and signs of complications related to the procedure. 5. To prevent aspiration of gastric contents. 6. To decrease throat irritation.
Laryngoscopy	*Direct:* To detect or remove lesions or foreign bodies in the larynx or to diagnose cancer by removing tissue for biopsy or samples for culture. A fiberoptic laryngoscope is used. *Indirect:* To assess the function of the vocal cords or to obtain tissue for biopsy. Observations are made during rest and phonation by using a laryngeal mirror, head mirror, and light source.	1. Follow interventions 1–7 for bronchography. 2. For indirect laryngoscopy, assist the client to sit in an upright position and encourage normal breathing. 3. After the procedure, administer lozenges or gargles as ordered.	1. See rationales 1–7 for bronchography. 2. To facilitate passsage of the laryngeal mirror into the mouth. 3. To relieve sore throat.
Mediastinoscopy	To inspect and remove samples for biopsy of lymph nodes that drain the lung. To detect metastasis of lung cancer. To obtain tissue for biopsy for diagnosis of tuberculosis or sarcoidosis. The procedure is done in the operating room with the client given local or general anesthesia; a suprasternal incision is used.	1. Explain preoperative measures and the procedure to the client. 2. Postoperatively, assess the client for bleeding, pneumothorax, and vocal cord paralysis. 3. Assess the client for pain and administer analgesics as ordered.	1. To decrease anxiety. 2. To detect complications of the procedure. 3. To decrease discomfort.

makers, aneurysm clips, inner-ear implants, cardiac valves, or metallic foreign objects in the body are not candidates for MRI. The nurse informs the client of possible claustrophobia and discomfort from lying inside the magnet's small cylinder on a hard, cool table. In addition, the client is informed that the noises that are heard during the examination are the natural, rhythmic sounds of radio frequency pulses, which may range from barely audible to quite noticeable.

ENDOSCOPIC EXAMINATIONS

Endoscopic diagnostic studies that are performed to assess respiratory disorders include bronchoscopy, laryngoscopy, and mediastinoscopy. These procedures are summarized in the Guidelines feature on pages 1947 and 1948.

PULMONARY FUNCTION TESTS

Pulmonary function tests evaluate the lungs' ability to maintain ventilation and the effects of ventilation and oxygenation on the cardiopulmonary circulatory system. The overall evaluation of the lungs requires multiple pulmonary function studies that vary in complexity and sophistication. Such studies measure pulmonary volumes and capacities, flow rates, diffusion capacity, gas exchange, airway resistance, and distribution of ventilation. These results are interpreted by comparing the client's results with normal results, which are predicted according to age, sex, height, and weight.

Pulmonary function tests are useful in the screening of persons for pulmonary disease even before the onset of signs or symptoms. Serial testing gives objective data that may be used as a guide to treatment (e.g., improvement in pulmonary function can support a decision to continue or discontinue specific therapy). Preoperative evaluation of clients with pulmonary function tests may identify individuals at risk of developing postoperative pulmonary complications. One of the most common reasons for performing such tests is to determine the cause of breathlessness. When performed while the client exercises, pulmonary function tests help to determine if dyspnea is caused by a pulmonary or a cardiac dysfunction, or by muscle deconditioning. These tests are also useful for evaluating the effect of occupation on pulmonary function and any related disability for legal purposes.

Client preparation.   The nurse prepares the client for pulmonary function tests by explaining the purpose and value of the tests for planning the client's care. The client is advised not to smoke before testing. According to institutional policy and procedure, the nurse withholds bronchodilator medication 4 to 6 hours before the test. Many individuals with respiratory impairment fear further breathlessness and are usually anxious before

these "breathing tests." The nurse helps to alleviate apprehension by explaining to the client what is expected during and after the testing.

Procedure.   Pulmonary function tests can be performed at the client's bedside or in the respiratory laboratory. The client is asked to breathe through the mouth only. A nose clip is used to prevent air from escaping. The client is asked to perform different breathing maneuvers while measurements are obtained. Table 60–5 describes the most frequently used pulmonary function tests and their purpose.

Follow-up care.   Because numerous breathing maneuvers are performed during pulmonary function tests, the nurse observes the client for increased dyspnea and/or bronchospasm after completion of such studies. The nurse notes whether bronchodilator medication was administered during testing and alters the client's medication schedule as indicated.

THORACENTESIS

Thoracentesis is the aspiration of pleural fluid or air from the pleural space. This procedure is used for diagnosis or treatment. Pleural fluid may be drained to relieve pulmonary compression and resultant respiratory distress caused by cancer, empyema, pleurisy, or tuberculosis. Aspiration of the pleural fluid and subsequent bacteriologic examination can assist in diagnosis of respiratory disease. To assist in further assessment of the parietal pleura, thoracentesis is usually followed by a pleural biopsy (see under later heading Percutaneous Lung Biopsy). Thoracentesis also allows for the instillation of medications into the pleural space, which may be necessary to prevent further fluid formation in certain cases of pleural effusion caused by lung cancer.

Client preparation.   Adequate client preparation is essential before thoracentesis to ensure the client's participation during the procedure and to prevent complications. The client is told to expect a stinging sensation from the local anesthetic and a feeling of pressure when the needle is inserted. The nurse reinforces the importance of the client's remaining immobile (avoiding coughing, deep breathing, or sudden movement) during the procedure to avoid puncture of the visceral pleura or lung.

Figure 60–10 illustrates the appropriate positions for thoracentesis. The nurse properly positions and supports the client. These positions widen the intercostal spaces and permit easy access to the pleural cavity. Pillows are used to make the client comfortable and to provide physical support.

Before the procedure, the nurse checks the client's history for hypersensitivity to local anesthetic agents. The entire chest or back is exposed, and the aspiration site is shaved if necessary. The actual site varies, de-

TABLE 60-5 Characteristics and Purposes of Pulmonary Function Tests

Test	Purpose
FVC (forced vital capacity) records the maximal amount of air that can be exhaled after maximal inspiration.	FVC gives an indication of respiratory muscle strength and ventilatory reserve. FVC is often reduced in COPD because of air trapping.
FEV₁ (forced expiratory volume in 1 s) records the maximal amount of air that can be exhaled in the first second of expiration.	FEV_1 is effort dependent and declines normally with age. This measure provides an estimate of the amount of obstruction of the client's breathing.
FEV₁/FVC is the ratio of expiratory volume in 1 s to FVC.	This ratio provides a much more sensitive indication of obstruction to airflow. This ratio is the hallmark of obstructive pulmonary disease.
FEF₂₅%₋₇₅% records the forced expiratory flow over the 25%–75% volume (middle half) of the FVC.	This measure provides a more sensitive index of obstruction in the smaller airways.
FRC (functional residual capacity) records the amount of air remaining in the lungs after normal expiration. FRC is an anatomic measurement of lung compartment and requires use of the helium dilution technique.	Increased FRC indicates hyperinflation or air trapping, which may result from obstructive pulmonary disease. FRC is normal or decreased in restrictive pulmonary diseases.
TLC (total lung capacity) records the amount of air in the lungs at the end of maximal inhalation.	Increased TLC indicates air trapping associated with obstructive pulmonary disease. Decreased TLC indicates restrictive disease.
RV (residual volume) records the amount of air remaining in the lungs at the end of a full, forced exhalation.	RV is increased in obstructive pulmonary disease such as emphysema.
DLCO (diffusing capacity for carbon monoxide) is a comparison of the amount of carbon monoxide (milliliters per minute) exhaled with the amount inhaled.	This measure reflects the movement of gas across the alveolar capillary membrane into the alveolar blood. DLCO is reduced whenever the alveolar-capillary membrane is diminished, as occurs in emphysema, pulmonary hypertension, and pulmonary fibrosis. It is increased with exercise and in conditions such as polycythemia and congestive heart disease.

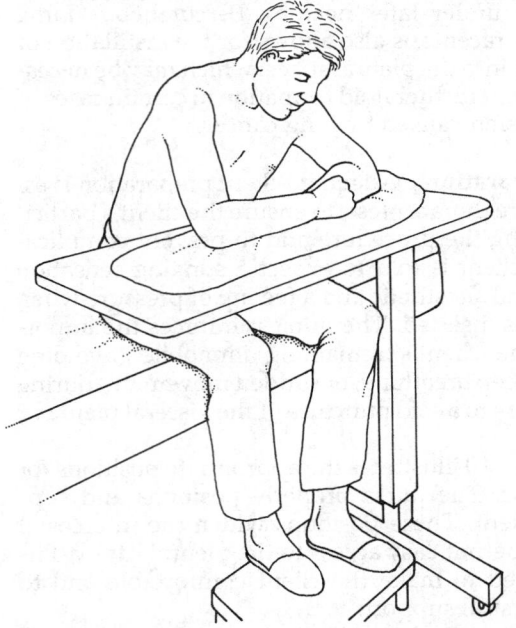

Sitting on the edge of a bed with the feet supported. The arms and shoulders are elevated, and the head is resting on the overbed table, which is padded with pillows or bath blankets.

Sitting in bed in semi-Fowler's position with the arm on the side on which the procedure will be performed raised above the head.

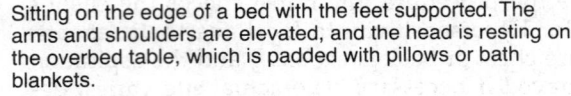

Figure 60-10

Positions for thoracentesis.

pending on volume and location of the effusion, which is determined by radiography and physical findings such as percussion.

Procedure. Thoracentesis is usually done at the bedside. After draping the client and cleaning the skin with a germicidal solution, the physician uses an aseptic technique and injects a local anesthetic into the intercostal space. The nurse keeps the client informed of the procedure while observing for shock, pain, nausea, pallor, diaphoresis, cyanosis, tachypnea, and dyspnea. The physician advances the thoracentesis needle with a syringe attached into the pleural space. Gentle suction is applied as the fluid in the pleural space is slowly aspirated. A vacuum collection bottle is sometimes necessary to remove larger volumes of fluid. To prevent hypovolemic shock and circulatory collapse, no more than 1200 mL of fluid is removed at one time. After the needle is withdrawn, pressure is applied to the puncture site, followed by the application of a small sterile dressing.

Follow-up care. After thoracentesis, a chest x-ray film is taken to rule out possible pneumothorax and subsequent mediastinal shift that can occur. The nurse monitors vital signs and auscultates breath sounds while noting absent or diminished sounds on the affected side. The puncture site and dressing are observed for leakage. The nurse assesses for other complications after thoracentesis, such as reaccumulation of fluid in the pleural space, subcutaneous emphysema, pyrogenic infection, and tension pneumothorax. The client is encouraged to breath deeply to promote lung re-expansion. The nurse documents the procedure and notes the client's tolerance, volume and character of fluid removed, location of the puncture site, and respiratory assessment before, during, and after the procedure.

PERCUTANEOUS LUNG BIOPSY

A *percutaneous lung biopsy* is performed to obtain tissue for pathogenic analysis by culture or cytologic examination. Needle biopsies are done to identify pulmonary lesions, granulomas, parenchymal changes, and the etiology of pleural effusions.

Client preparation. The nurse prepares the client for this nonoperative procedure by explaining what to expect before and after the biopsy. Clients undergoing percutaneous lung biopsy may have predetermined ideas about the outcome. The terms "biopsy" and "cancer" may be closely associated in the client's mind, so the nurse explores the client's feelings and fears before and after the procedure. Analgesics and sedatives may be given before the procedure to reduce discomfort and anxiety. The nurse informs the client that discomfort is minimized by a local anesthetic but that the client may experience a sensation of pressure during insertion of the needle and aspiration of the tissue.

Procedure. This test may be performed in the client's room or in the radiology department with fluoroscopic monitoring. The positioning of the client for percutaneous needle biopsy is similar to that for thoracentesis. After the skin is cleaned with an antibacterial agent, a local anesthetic is administered. Under sterile conditions, a spinal-type needle is inserted through the skin into the pleural space, and fluid is aspirated and tissue is obtained for microscopic examination. A dressing is applied to the site after the procedure.

Follow-up care. After percutaneous lung biopsy, the nurse monitors the client's vital signs and breath sounds every 4 hours for the first 24 hours. Signs of respiratory distress (e.g., dyspnea, pallor, diaphoresis, and tachypnea) are reported. Pneumothorax is the major complication after needle biopsy, so a chest x-ray film is taken after the procedure. The nurse has the necessary equipment available for chest drainage if needed.

SKIN TESTS

Skin tests are used in combination with other diagnostic data to diagnose various infectious diseases (such as tuberculosis), viral diseases (such as mononucleosis and mumps), and fungal diseases (such as coccidioidomycosis and histoplasmosis). An assessment of allergic hypersensitivity and the status of the immune system can be demonstrated by skin testing. Exposure to the allergen or organism used in testing produces a specific reaction (delayed hypersensitivity reaction) of the client's immune system. For further discussion, the reader is referred to Chapters 23 and 27.

Client preparation. The nurse explains the purpose of skin testing and the procedure to the client to ensure cooperation and to alleviate anxiety. The client is questioned about a history of hypersensitivity to any of the local antigens used or a previous reaction to skin tests. The nurse also informs the client what is expected after testing is completed; e.g., the client is warned not to scratch the testing site so as not to cause infection and/or abscess formation. The client is also instructed to refrain from washing the infection sites that have been circled with a marking pen for identification.

Procedure. The actual procedure depends on the specific purpose of the test and on institutional policy. An intradermal injection technique causes a wheal to be formed after injection of the antigen. It is vital that the nurse perform the procedure correctly because incorrect antigen administration is responsible for erroneous results. The nurse ensures that the chosen test site is free from excessive body hair, dermatitis, and/or blemishes. A severe anaphylactic response can result in clients who are hypersensitive to the test antigens. The nurse must recognize and be prepared to treat reactions as described in Chapter 27.

Follow-up care.   Interpretation of the reaction at injection sites is done 24 to 72 hours after administration of the test antigen. If testing is done as an outpatient procedure, the nurse instructs the client when to return to have the results read. The nurse documents the amount of induration (hard swelling) in millimeters and the presence of erythema and vesiculation (formation of small blister-like elevations).

SUMMARY

An assessment of the respiratory system involves thorough history taking; physical examination by use of inspection, palpation, percussion, and auscultation; psychosocial assessment; and an evaluation of diagnostic studies. After analyzing the data collected, the nurse can identify any actual or potential health problems and formulate nursing diagnoses. Assessment, as the first step in the nursing process, provides the necessary information that the nurse needs to plan and implement care for clients with respiratory disorders.

REFERENCES AND READINGS

American College of Chest Physicians and American Thoracic Society's Joint Commission on Pulmonary Nomenclature. (1975). Pulmonary terms and symbols. *Chest, 67*, 583–593.

Bates, B. (1987). *A guide to physical examination* (3rd ed.). Philadelphia: J. B. Lippincott.

Boyda, E. K. (1985). *Respiratory problems.* Oradell, NJ: Medical Economics.

Brody, J. S., & Snider, G. L. (Eds.). (1985). *Current topics in the management of respiratory diseases.* New York: Churchill Livingstone.

Burggraf, V., & Stanley, M. (1989). *Nursing the elderly* (pp. 129–134). Philadelphia: J. B. Lippincott.

Burton, G., & Hodgkin, J. E. (Eds.). (1984). *Respiratory care — a guide to clinical practice.* Philadelphia: J. B. Lippincott.

Carnevali, D. L., & Patrick, D. M. (1986). *Nursing management for the elderly* (2nd ed., pp. 80–82). Philadelphia: J. B. Lippincott.

Clemente, C. D. (Ed.). (1985). *Gray's anatomy of the human body* (30th ed.). Philadelphia: Lea & Febiger.

Emanuelsen, K. L., & Densmore, M. J. (1981). *Acute respiratory care.* Bethany, CT: Fleschner Publishing.

Epstein, J., & Gaines, J. (1983). *Clinical respiratory care of the adult patient.* Bowie, MD: Robert J. Brady.

Ganong, W. F. (1985). *Review of medical physiology* (12th ed.). Los Altos, California: Lange Medical.

Guyton, A. C. (1986). *Textbook of medical physiology* (7th ed.). Philadelphia: W. B. Saunders.

Hamilton, H., & Rose, M. B. (Eds.). (1984). *Respiratory disorders.* Springhouse, PA: Springhouse Corp.

Kee, J. L. (1987). *Diagnostic tests with nursing implications* (2nd ed.). Norwalk, CT: Appleton & Lange.

Keller, C., Solomon, J., & Reyes, A. V. (1984). *Respiratory nursing care.* Englewood Cliffs, NJ: Prentice-Hall.

Lubkin, I. M. (1986). *Chronic illness — impact and interventions.* Boston: Jones & Bartlett.

Luce, J. M., Tyler, M. L., & Pierson, D. J. (1984). *Intensive respiratory care.* Philadelphia: W. B. Saunders.

Messenger, M. A. (1982). Pulmonary function tests: The telephone connection. *Respiratory Therapy, 12*, 27–29.

Seidel, H., Ball, J., Dains, J., & Benedict, G. (1987). *Mosby's guide to physical examination.* St. Louis: C. V. Mosby.

Steffl, B. M. (Ed.). (1984). *Handbook of gerontological nursing.* New York: Van Nostrand Reinhold.

Stevens, S. A., & Becker, K. L. (1988). How to perform a picture perfect respiratory assessment. *Nursing '88, 18*(1), 57–63.

Traver, G. A. (1973). Assessment of thorax and lungs. *American Journal of Nursing, 73*, 466–471.

Tse, C. S. T. (1982). Food products containing tartrazine. *New England Journal of Medicine, 306*, 681–682.

Williams, S., & McVan, B. (Eds.).(1985). *Respiratory care.* Springhouse, PA: Springhouse Corp.

Williams, T. F. (Ed.). (1984). *Rehabilitation in the aging.* New York: Raven.

CHAPTER 61

Interventions for Clients with Upper Respiratory Tract Disorders

Problems of the upper airway are common occurrences during one's life span. The nurse encounters clients with diseases of the upper respiratory system in homes, clinics, physicians' offices, emergency rooms, or hospitals. These diseases can be acute or chronic, emergent or scheduled, self-limiting or terminal. The nursing priority for the client with problems of the upper airway is to *ensure a patent airway.*

This chapter discusses problems of the nose, pharynx, and larynx. Emergency nursing care for the client with an upper airway obstruction is included. Critical care texts and emergency manuals should be consulted for further information.

DISORDERS OF THE NOSE AND SINUSES

RHINITIS

OVERVIEW

Rhinitis is the inflammation of the nasal cavities, and it is the most common disorder to affect the nose and accessory nasal sinuses. The etiology of rhinitis often involves an interplay of viruses, bacteria, and allergens.

Acute rhinitis may be caused by allergens or a virus. *Allergic rhinitis,* frequently called hay fever, is commonly initiated by sensitivity reactions to allergens, especially plant pollens. *Acute* episodes tend to be seasonal: they disappear after a few weeks and recur at the same time the following year. *Chronic,* or perennial, rhinitis presents intermittently or continuously when an individual is exposed to certain allergens, such as dust, animal dander, wool, and foods (e.g., seafood). Rhinitis can also occur after excessive use of nose drops or sprays *(rhinitis medicamentosa),* as a rebound effect causing nasal congestion. Decreasing or discontinuing the drug is the treatment for this condition.

In both acute and chronic allergic rhinitis, the offending substance causes a release of vasoactive mediators, e.g., histamine, serotonin, bradykinin, and prostaglandins, which induces vasodilation and increased capillary permeability. Edema and swelling of the nasal mucosa result, and the client complains of headache, nasal irritation, sneezing, nasal congestion, rhinorrhea (watery drainage from the nose), and itchy, watery eyes. Chapter 27 describes the physiologic mechanisms that occur in allergic reactions in detail.

Acute viral rhinitis (coryza, or the common cold) is caused by one or more of more than 30 viruses. It usually spreads from one person to another via droplet nuclei from sneezing or coughing and is most contagious in the first 2 to 3 days after symptoms appear. The condition is self-limiting unless complications such as otitis media, sinusitis, bronchitis, or pneumonia occur. These complications are most likely seen in elderly or immunosuppressed individuals, especially when these individuals live in crowded conditions or in group settings such as a long-term care facility. In addition to the clinical manifestations that are found in clients with allergic rhinitis, clients with viral infections often present with fatigue; a sore, dry throat; and, at times, a low-grade fever with chills.

COLLABORATIVE MANAGEMENT

Management of the client with any type of rhinitis includes symptomatic relief and client education. Drugs, including antihistamines and decongestants, are commonly given but must be used with caution in the elderly because of side effects such as vertigo, hypertension, urinary retention, and insomnia. These medications work by causing vasoconstriction and subsequently decreasing edema. Antipyretics are administered if fever is present in the client with viral rhinitis.

The nurse teaches the client with viral rhinitis the importance of proper rest (10 to 12 hours a day) and an adequate fluid intake of at least 2000 mL/day. The client is instructed to avoid individuals who are susceptible to becoming infected for the first few days after symptoms occur. Thorough hand washing is also an important precaution, especially after cleaning the nose or sneezing. Antibiotic therapy may be prescribed to prevent secondary bacterial infection, but these agents do not kill the offending virus. An uncomplicated cold typically subsides within 7 days.

The client with allergic rhinitis undergoes allergy testing to determine the causative factors, and hyposensitization (desensitization) may help to prevent future episodes. The client may be able to avoid the offending substance. Chapter 27 discusses allergies and their treatment.

SINUSITIS

OVERVIEW

Sinusitis is the inflammation of the mucous membranes of one or more sinuses (see Chap. 60, Fig. 60–2). *Acute sinusitis* is the obstruction of the flow of secretions from sinuses that subsequently become infected. The disorder frequently accompanies or follows acute or allergic rhinitis, or it can result from a deviated nasal septum, polyps, tumors, chronically inhaled air pollutants, or cocaine abuse. In *chronic sinusitis*, the mucous membrane becomes permanently thickened from prolonged or repeated inflammation or infection.

Infection, most commonly caused by *Streptococcus pneumoniae, Haemophilus influenzae,* and *Bacteroides* species, develops in the maxillary and frontal sinuses most frequently. The clinical manifestations of sinusitis include nasal swelling and congestion, headache, facial pressure and pain, low-grade fever, and purulent or bloody nasal drainage.

COLLABORATIVE MANAGEMENT

The treatment for sinusitis includes the use of broad-spectrum antibiotics, analgesics for pain and fever (e.g., acetaminophen [Tylenol]), and decongestants (e.g., phenylephrine [Neo-Synephrine]). If this combination is not successful in facilitating the flow of sinus secretions, surgical intervention may be necessary.

Antral irrigation, also known as antral puncture and lavage, is a surgical procedure that can be performed in a physician's office or a clinic. After the area is anesthetized, a large-gauge needle is inserted under the inferior turbinate of the nose and into the maxillary sinus on the affected side. Fluid or pus from the sinus is withdrawn. If no purulent material is present, the sinus is irrigated with saline. Irrigation is contraindicated in the presence of infection because osteomyelitis may result.

If antral irrigation is not successful, other surgical procedures may be used to open the sinus cavities in clients with chronic sinusitis. In the Caldwell-Luc procedure, an opening is made in the anterior wall of the maxillary sinus under the upper lip. The infected contents are removed, and a "window" is made in the anterior portion of the inferior turbinate. The sinus is packed with gauze for 48 hours, and the client has difficulty eating for the first few days. The nurse carefully provides oral hygienic care to prevent injury to the surgical incision and teaches the client to avoid chewing on the affected side or wear dentures until the incision heals. The client is also instructed to avoid the Valsalva maneuver (no coughing, blowing the nose, or straining at stool) for at least 2 weeks to prevent bleeding.

The ethmoid sinuses are opened via an external approach for better visualization and preservation of nerves. The surgical incision is made along the side of the nose from the middle of the eyebrow. Nasal polyps may also be removed by using this procedure.

The surgical procedure for the frontal sinuses differs from that for the other areas in that the diseased tissue of the sinus can be removed and the sinus obliterated. The osteoplastic flap procedure requires the replacement of the sinus mucosal lining with subcutaneous fat obtained from the client's abdomen. The client usually experiences minimal sinus pain, but the abdomen is tender for several days. Nasal packing is not necessary for this type of sinus surgery.

NASAL SEPTAL DEVIATION

A slight deviation of the nasal septum is present in most adult individuals and causes no symptoms. Major deviations may obstruct the nasal passages and/or interfere with sinus drainage. *Nasoseptoplasty* or *submucous resection* (SMR) may be required to straighten the septum when chronic symptoms or discomfort occurs. The surgeon removes the deviated section of the cartilage and bone; the amount resected depends on the type and degree of deformity present. Nursing care for this client is similar to that for the client with a rhinoplasty, which is described in the next section of this chapter.

FRACTURE OF THE NOSE

OVERVIEW

Nasal fractures commonly occur from minor injuries that are received during falls or participation in sports, or from trauma related to violence or motor vehicle accidents. If the bone or cartilage is not displaced, no serious complications result from the fracture. Displacement, however, can cause airway obstruction and cosmetic deformity.

COLLABORATIVE MANAGEMENT

During the assessment, the nurse notes that the nose is deviated to one side and/or has a malaligned bridge. Blood or clear fluid (cerebrospinal fluid) may drain from one or both nares, which indicates a possible skull fracture. Radiographic examination is not always reliable.

Simple, closed reduction of the fracture with the use of local anesthesia within the first 24 hours after injury is the treatment of choice. After this period, the fracture is more difficult to reduce because of edema formation.

For severe fractures or those that do not heal properly, a *rhinoplasty* may be performed. This procedure is surgical reconstruction of the nose, primarily for cosmetic improvement. The client returns from surgery with packing in both nostrils to prevent bleeding and to provide a splint for the nose. The ½-in gauze that is used is typically treated with an antibiotic ointment such as bacitracin or the combination of polymyxin B sulfate, neomycin sulfate, and hydrocortisone (Cortisporin) to decrease the odor of old blood and to reduce the risk of infection. A "moustache" dressing pad, usually a folded 2 × 2 in gauze pad, is placed under the nose and is changed as necessary by the nurse or client. A splint or cast may cover the nose for additional alignment and protection (Fig. 61–1).

Postoperatively, the nurse monitors the client for edema formation and bleeding and checks vital signs every 4 hours for the first 24 hours. The nurse pays particular attention to how often the client swallows. Repeated swallowing may indicate posterior nose bleeding; the nurse checks the pharynx with a penlight for bleeding, and, if it is present, notifies the physician immediately.

The client is kept in semi-Fowler's position and is instructed to move slowly and to rest as much as possible. Ice may be applied to the nose to decrease swelling

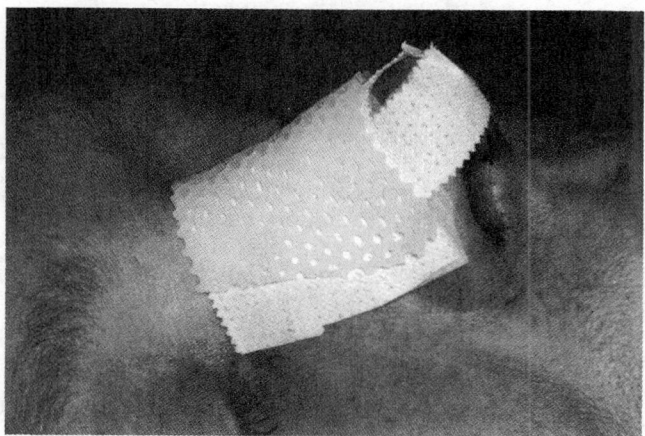

Figure 61–1

A basic rhinoplasty dressing including an Aquaplast cast. (From Johnson, C. M., Jr., & Toriumi, D. M. [1990]. *Open structure rhinoplasty.* Philadelphia: W. B. Saunders.)

and bleeding. Cool compresses applied to the eyes or face may prevent excessive discoloration. The nurse offers fluids frequently but allows the client to select what food he or she desires.

The client is instructed to avoid the Valsalva maneuver, such as coughing or straining at stool, for the first few days after removal of the packing to prevent bleeding. Laxatives or stool softeners may be administered to facilitate defecation. Aspirin should be avoided during this time as well to prevent the possibility of bleeding. The client may be given prophylactic antibiotics to prevent infection postoperatively; the nurse reinforces the need for the client to take all of the medication as prescribed. Clients need to understand that edema and discoloration usually last for several months.

CANCER OF THE NOSE AND SINUSES

OVERVIEW

Tumors of the nasal cavities and sinuses are relatively uncommon and may be benign or malignant. Malignant lesions of these areas occur at all ages but are more common between the fifth and seventh decades of life. Men are affected more than women. Carcinomas of these areas metastasize early, and there is progressive invasion of the neck and cervical lymph nodes, with eventual spread to distant areas such as the lung and liver.

The onset of sinus malignancies is insidious, and symptoms are frequently interpreted by clients as representing sinusitis. Therefore, most clients have relatively advanced disease when they are first diagnosed. Detection and diagnosis are often delayed because the symptoms mimic those of common upper respiratory tract illnesses. Persistent nasal obstruction, drainage, bloody discharge, and pain that do not improve after treatment of sinusitis should lead to suspicion of nasal and/or sinus malignancy.

COLLABORATIVE MANAGEMENT

Treatment of malignancies of the nose and sinuses consists of surgical resection, radiation therapy, and chemotherapy. These procedures are described in detail in Chapter 25 under the heading Collaborative Management. Radical surgery is often required because of the danger of recurrence and the extent of the invasive tumor. The exact procedure performed depends on the amount of tissue to be removed.

The nurse provides general postoperative care including maintenance of a patent airway, tracheostomy care, and care of the client with a nasogastric tube (Chaps. 20, 44, and 62). The nurse provides meticulous mouth care for the client and monitors for alterations in comfort. The general care of the client undergoing a radical procedure for nasopharyngeal malignancy is similar to the care of the client undergoing radical neck dissection, as discussed under the later heading Cancer in the section Disorders of the Larynx.

Nursing management of clients requiring such extensive surgery is complex and involves collaborating with other health care professionals. Each member of the multidisciplinary team (e.g., speech therapy, nutrition, dentistry, psychology, and medicine) assists the client in adjusting to the numerous changes imposed by the surgical procedure. The reader is referred to the later heading Discharge Planning for the client with laryngeal cancer for additional information about psychosocial adaptation, home care preparation, client/family education, and health care resources for these clients.

NASAL POLYPS

Nasal polyps are benign grape-like clusters of mucous membrane and loose connective tissue. Polyps typically occur bilaterally and are often caused by irritation to the mucosa of the nose or sinuses from allergies or infection (chronic sinusitis). If polyps become too large, airway obstruction may result.

Nasal polyps are removed surgically (polypectomy) with the use of either local or general anesthesia. The nurse observes the client for postoperative bleeding. The nostrils are usually packed with gauze for 24 hours postoperatively. Nasal polyps tend to recur.

HYPERTROPHY OF THE TURBINATES

The passage of air through the nostrils may be obstructed by hypertrophy of the turbinates. Medical management of hypertrophied turbinates includes using inhaled steroids such as beclomethasone (Becon-

EMERGENCY CARE ■ Nosebleeds

Interventions	Rationales
1. Position the client to sit leaning forward.	1. To prevent blood from entering the stomach.
2. Reassure the client and attempt to keep him or her quiet.	2. To reduce anxiety.
3. Apply direct pressure to the nose for 3–5 min.	3, 4. To stop the bleeding.
4. Apply ice or cool compresses to the nose and face if possible (may require a second person to assist).	
5. Instruct the client not to blow his or her nose for several hours after the bleeding stops.	5. To prevent recurrence.
6. If nasal packing is necessary, pack the nose loosely with one small gauze pad rather than a piece of cotton.	6. To prevent adherence of cotton to mucous membranes.
7. Seek medical assistance if these measures are ineffective.	7. To prevent possible shock.

ase, Vancenase) and flunisolide (Nasalide). These nasal aerosols do not cause systemic side effects and are used for their anti-inflammatory action. The nurse teaches the client how to use these drugs properly. If medication is not successful in treating this problem, surgical removal of hypertrophied tissue may be necessary.

EPISTAXIS

OVERVIEW

Epistaxis (nosebleed) is a fairly common problem because of the rich capillary network within the anterior portion of the nose. Nosebleeds may occur as a result of trauma, hypertension, blood dyscrasias (e.g., leukemias), inflammation, tumor, decreased humidity, excessive nose blowing, and nose picking. Men are usually affected more than women, and the elderly tend to bleed most often from the posterior portion of the nose.

COLLABORATIVE MANAGEMENT

If a nosebleed occurs, the nurse keeps the client quiet, positions the client to sit forward if possible, and applies direct pressure to the nose for 3 to 5 minutes. In addition, cold compresses or ice applied directly to the nose or face constricts blood vessels and decreases bleeding. The client is instructed not to blow his or her nose for several hours after bleeding subsides. The nurse may loosely pack the affected nares with a small gauze pad during the application of pressure and/or after the bleeding stops. The accompanying Emergency Care feature summarizes the first aid interventions for this problem.

If the nosebleed does not respond to the described interventions, medical attention is needed. The physician may need to cauterize the affected capillaries with silver nitrate or electrocautery, followed by a local or postnasal packing. Postnasal packing is a large gauze packing with a string attached that is threaded through the nose and out through the mouth. The string is taped to the cheek to prevent its movement. This procedure is uncomfortable and may cause airway obstruction. The nurse observes the client for respiratory function and tolerance of the packing. Humidification and oxygen, as well as bed rest and antibiotics (to prevent infection), may be prescribed. After the packing is removed by the physician, petroleum jelly may be applied to the nares for lubrication.

DISORDERS OF THE PHARYNX AND TONSILS

PHARYNGITIS

OVERVIEW

The throat is one of the first barriers to an infectious organism that may attack the respiratory system. Thus, infection is the most common cause of pharyngeal dysfunction. *Pharyngitis* is an infection of the mucous membranes of the pharynx. It usually precedes or occurs simultaneously with acute rhinitis or sinusitis. Individuals who are most at risk are those who are exposed to pollutants such as cigarette smoke or gaseous fumes.

Acute pharyngitis has multiple causes, usually bacteria or viruses (see the accompanying Key Features of Disease). The most common bacterial organism causing pharyngitis is group A beta-hemolytic streptococcus, but 90% of all adult cases are caused by a virus. The acute inflammation is usually part of an upper respiratory tract disorder. The incidence of streptococcal infections rises between late fall and spring, especially in cold climates. Recently, *Mycoplasma*, *Neisseria gonorrhoeae*, and *Chlamydia* have been identified as causal agents in

KEY FEATURES OF DISEASE ■ Causes of Pharyngitis

Bacterial Causes

Streptococcus
Staphylococcus
Haemophilus influenzae
Pneumococcus
Corynebacterium diphtheriae

Viral Causes

Adenovirus
Rhinovirus
Epstein-Barr virus
Cytomegalovirus
Influenza virus
Parainfluenza virus
Herpesvirus
Coxsackievirus A
Echovirus

Other Causes

Chlamydia
Mycoplasma pneumoniae
Candida
Physical and chemical causes
  Alcohol
  Tobacco
  Heat
  Irritants
  Dehydration
  Trauma

pharyngitis. Previously, infections caused by these organisms were classified under viral infections or those of unknown cause.

COLLABORATIVE MANAGEMENT

Pharyngitis is characterized by soreness and dryness in the throat, pain, difficulty in swallowing (dysphagia), and fever. During the physical examination, it is often difficult to differentiate viral from bacterial pharyngitis. Clients with viral sore throats are more likely to complain of a gradual onset, rhinorrhea, headache, mild hoarseness, and a low-grade fever. The manifestations of a bacterial infection are abrupt onset, dysphagia, arthralgias, myalgias, malaise, and temperature higher than 101° F (38.3° C). When inspecting the mucous

KEY FEATURES OF DISEASE ■ Differential Features of Acute Viral and Bacterial Pharyngitis

Feature	Viral Pharyngitis	Bacterial Pharyngitis
Temperature	Low-grade or no fever	High fever (above 101° F [38° C], and usually 102°–104° F [38.5°–40° C])
Ear manifestations	Retracted and/or dull tympanic membrane	Retracted and/or dull tympanic membrane
Throat manifestions	Scant or no tonsillar exudate Slight erythema of pharynx and tonsils	Severe hyperemia of pharyngeal mucosa, tonsils, and uvula Erythema of tonsils with yellow exudate
Neck manifestations	Possible lymphadenopathy	Anterior cervical lymphadenopathy and tenderness
Skin manifestations	No rash	Possible scarlatiniform rash Possible petechiae on chest and/or abdomen
Dysphagia	Present	Present
Associated symptoms	Cough Rhinitis Hoarseness Malaise	No cough Sudden onset of chills, malaise, and headache
Laboratory data	Complete blood count usually normal White blood cell count usually lower than 10,000/mm³ Negative throat culture results	Complete blood count abnormal White blood cell count usually higher than 12,000/mm³ Throat culture results positive for beta-hemolytic streptococcus

membranes of the throat that is infected with either virus or bacteria, the nurse may observe a mild to severe hyperemia (redness), with or without enlarged erythematous tonsils and with or without exudate. Nasal discharge varies from thin and watery to purulent. Cervical lymphadenopathy may be present in either viral or bacterial pharyngitis. Clinical studies indicate that streptococcal (bacterial) infections are more often associated with enlarged erythematous tonsils with exudate, temperature higher than 101° F (38° C), purulent nasal discharge, and cervical lymphadenopathy. Differential features of acute viral and bacterial pharyngitis are summarized in the Key Features of Disease above.

Viral pharyngitis is communicable for 2 to 3 days and usually subsides within 3 to 10 days after onset. Bacterial pharyngitis, such as group A streptococcal infection, however, can lead to dangerous medical complications (see the Key Features of Disease to the right). The two most serious complications, acute glomerulonephritis and rheumatic fever, occur in 1% to 3% of cases. Rheumatic fever typically develops 3 to 5 weeks after an acute streptococcal infection. The client may experience fever, painful and/or swollen joints, rash, subcutaneous nodules, a cardiac murmur, and involuntary irregular movements (choreiform). Acute glomerulonephritis generally occurs 7 to 10 days after the acute infection, with sudden onset of hematuria, proteinuria, and, less commonly, edema and hypertension.

Throat cultures are important to differentiate viral from group A beta-hemolytic streptococcal infection. A cotton swab is rubbed over each tonsillar area and the posterior pharynx to obtain a specimen (Fig. 61–2, part 1). The cotton swab is then streaked on a blood agar plate (see Fig. 61–2, part 2), which is incubated for 24 hours. Recently, an easier and faster method for determining the type of infection has been developed. The test uses latex agglutination for group A streptococcal antigen and requires 10 minutes to provide results. This test is a rapid, accurate tool for obtaining immediate results so that clients can be treated at the initial visit. This rapid test can significantly increase the rate at which treatment starts, which decreases the incidence of sequelae of streptococcal infection. Throat culture results are not entirely accurate; about 10% are false-negative results and 20% are false-positive results.

A complete blood count is done when the client's

KEY FEATURES OF DISEASE ■ Complications of Group A Streptococcal Infection

Rheumatic fever	Sinusitis
Acute glomerulonephritis	Mastoiditis
Peritonsillar abscess	Bronchitis
Retropharyngeal abscess	Pneumonia
Otitis media	Scarlet fever

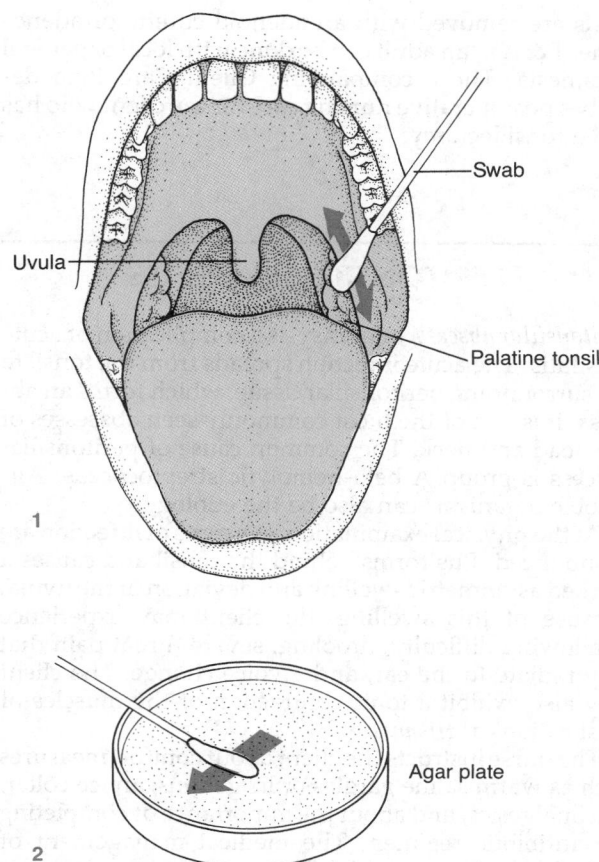

Figure 61–2

Throat culture technique.

condition is severe or not improving. The client may exhibit extremely high fevers, lethargy, or signs and symptoms of complications. A complete blood count may also be done to rule out other causes of pharyngitis. In a viral infection, the white blood cell count is usually normal or low, but it may be moderately elevated. In bacterial pharyngitis, the white blood cell count is usually elevated.

When taking a history, the nurse inquires about the client's recent exposure to environmental toxins or contacts within the last 10 days with an individual who has been ill. Of particular importance is whether the client has been ill with symptoms of a cold or upper respiratory tract infection recently or in the past. It is essential to document previous streptococcal infections that the client has experienced. The nurse documents a history of rheumatic fever, valvular heart disease, streptococcal infections, or penicillin allergy. Because diphtheria (*Corynebacterium diphtheriae*) can cause pharyngitis, the nurse questions and documents whether the client has had a diphtheria immunization.

The nurse determines and documents if the onset of illness was slow and insidious, as with viral pharyngitis, or abrupt, as with bacterial pharyngitis. The nurse asks the client if he or she has experienced any nasal or aural symptoms such as rhinorrhea, sneezing, coughing, or ear pain. These symptoms are frequently associated with pharyngitis. The nurse asks questions that will assist in determining whether the pharyngitis is viral or bacterial. The client is asked if he or she is experiencing high fevers, chills, malaise, and/or general aching of the muscles or joints.

In managing the client, the nurse teaches the difference between viral and bacterial (group A beta-hemolytic streptococcus) pharyngitis. Most sore throats in adults are viral and do not require the use of antibiotics. Viral pharyngitis usually resolves in 3 to 10 days with symptomatic care. The treatment plan includes rest, increased fluid intake, analgesics for pain, warm saline throat gargles, and throat lozenges containing mild anesthetics.

The management of bacterial pharyngitis involves the use of antibiotics and the supportive care provided for viral pharyngitis. The antibiotic typically chosen for streptococcal infection is penicillin G or V, 250 mg orally every 6 hours for 10 days. If the client is allergic to penicillin, erythromycin (E-Mycin), 250 mg four times a day, may be given. The nurse counsels the client on the importance of completing the entire 10-day dosage of antibiotics, even if symptoms have subsided. The entire course is needed to eradicate the organism and to prevent complications such as rheumatic fever or glomerulonephritis. If the client cannot tolerate the medication, he or she should be instructed to notify the nurse or physician immediately. If compliance is a concern or the client cannot swallow pills, long-acting benzathine penicillin, 1.2 million units, can be administered intramuscularly to eradicate the organism. The nurse tells the client that if he or she is not improving or if after completion of the antibiotic the symptoms are still present, the client needs to be re-evaluated.

The client is instructed about how to take an oral temperature reading. This reading should be taken in the morning and in the evening until convalescence is complete. The client is not contagious after 24 hours of treatment. Family members or significant others who develop a sore throat need to be evaluated, and a throat culture may need to be done.

TONSILLITIS

OVERVIEW

Tonsillitis is an inflammation of the tonsils and the lymphatic tissue that are located on each side of the oropharynx. The tonsils consist of lymphatic tissue that is shaped like a small almond. Each tonsil is covered by a mucous membrane. These lymphatic tissues filter microorganisms, thus functioning as a protective mechanism for the respiratory and gastrointestinal tracts.

Tonsillitis is a contagious airborne or food-borne infection. Acute or chronic tonsillitis can occur in any age group, but 5- to 10-year-old children are affected most often. The infection is usually more severe when it occurs in adolescents or adults.

The acute form usually lasts from 7 to 10 days. Acute tonsillitis is usually caused by a bacterial organism; the most common organism is *Streptococcus*. Other bacterial pathogens include *Staphylococcus aureus, H. influenzae,* and pneumococcus. Viruses can also cause tonsillitis. Chronic tonsillitis usually results from an acute infection that did not resolve or from recurrent infections.

COLLABORATIVE MANAGEMENT

Acute tonsillitis begins with the sudden onset of a mild to severe sore throat. Other symptoms that can accompany the sore throat are fever, muscle aches, chills, dysphagia, pain in the ears, headache, anorexia, and malaise. On physical examination, the tonsils are swollen and red with pus; white or yellow exudate can cover the tonsils. Pressing a tonsil may produce purulent drainage. The uvula may be edematous and inflamed, and cervical lymph nodes are usually tender and enlarged.

Diagnostic studies should be done to rule out other causes of the sore throat and fever (such as acute pharyngitis). The following diagnostic studies are performed for a client with suspected tonsillitis: complete blood count, throat culture and sensitivity studies, Monospot test, and chest x-ray film if respiratory complications are suspected. The white blood cell count is typically elevated if a bacterial infection is present. The throat culture and sensitivity studies identify the bacteria and the appropriate antibiotic for treatment.

Systemic antibiotics (usually penicillin or erythromycin [E-Mycin]) are given for 7 to 10 days. Warm saline throat gargles, analgesics, antipyretics, and lozenges with topical anesthetic ingredients may provide symptomatic relief.

The surgical removal of the tonsils and adenoids has become a controversial issue. Each individual client must be evaluated to determine the optimal time for surgery, if it is indicated, and for any contraindications to the procedure.

The indications for a tonsillectomy and adenoidectomy (T&A) include (1) recurrent acute infections or chronic infections that have not responded to antibiotic therapy; (2) peritonsillar abscess; (3) tonsils that are malignant; (4) hypertrophy of the tonsils or adenoids that obstructs the airway; and (5) diphtheria carriage, because the tonsils are the source of infection. The indication for surgery becomes stronger if there is evidence of repeated group A beta-hemolytic streptococcal infections.

Surgery is not indicated if the client is experiencing an acute tonsillar infection (except with an acute peritonsillar abscess), has active tuberculosis, or has a blood dyscrasia such as purpura, aplastic anemia, hemophilia, or leukemia.

The surgical procedure most commonly performed to remove the tonsils is dissection and snare. However, some surgeons still use the guillotine method. The ade-

noids are removed with an adenoid curette or adenotome. T & A in an adult can be done with local or general anesthesia. The accompanying Client Care Plan describes postoperative nursing care for the client who has had a tonsillectomy.

PERITONSILLAR ABSCESS

Peritonsillar abscess, or quinsy, is a complication of acute tonsillitis. The acute infection spreads from the tonsil to the surrounding peritonsillar tissue, which forms an abscess. It is one of the most commonly seen abscesses of the head and neck. The common cause of peritonsillar abscess is group A beta-hemolytic streptococcus. Anaerobic organisms can also be the etiology.

At the physical examination, the signs of infection are pronounced. Pus forms behind the tonsil and causes a marked asymmetric swelling and deviation of the uvula. Because of this swelling, the client may experience swallowing difficulty, drooling, severe throat pain that may radiate to the ear, and a voice change. The client may also exhibit a tonic contraction of the muscles of mastication, or *trismus.*

The nurse instructs the client about comfort measures such as warm saline gargles or irrigations, an ice collar, and analgesics, and about the importance of completing the antibiotic regimen. The medical management of PTA remains controversial. The treatment plan includes incision and drainage of the abscess plus antibiotic therapy. After the healing process is complete, a tonsillectomy may be performed to prevent recurrence. However, studies have shown success with outpatient management through perimucosal needle drainage.

DISORDERS OF THE LARYNX

LARYNGITIS

OVERVIEW

Laryngitis can be defined as an inflammation of the mucous membranes lining the larynx and may or may not include edema of the vocal cords. It is commonly associated with upper respiratory tract infections, and can be an entity itself or a symptom of a related disease process. As either, it is an illness that accounts for more absences from work than any other illness. Etiologic factors include exposure to irritating inhalants and pollutants including chemical agents, tobacco, alcohol, and smoke; overuse of the voice as in lecturing, cheering, and singing; and inhalation of volatile gases such as glue, paint thinner, and butane.

Goal/Outcome Criteria	Interventions	Rationales

Nursing Diagnosis 1: Pain Related to Surgery and Swelling

Goal/Outcome Criteria	Interventions	Rationales
Client will experience minimal or no pain. ■ Verbalizes experiencing little or no pain.	1. Administer analgesics as needed (prn), as ordered by physician.	1. To keep client as comfortable as possible.
	2. Apply an ice collar.	2. To decrease inflammation or swelling and consequent pain.
	3. Offer oral fluids (e.g., ice-cold drinks, ice chips, gelatin, Popsicles) when the client is awake, alert, and responding appropriately.	3. To soothe the throat.
	4. Instruct the client to modify intake as follows:	
	a. To drink at least 2–3 L/d unless fluids are restricted.	4. a. To prevent dehydration.
	b. To gradually progress from intake of fluids to cereals and eggs to a soft diet.	4. b. To allow the throat to adjust gradually after surgery.
	c. Not to drink acidic fluids (e.g., fruit juices), hot foods, rough foods (e.g., crackers), or highly seasoned foods for the first postoperative week.	4. c. To prevent irritation.
	5. Teach the client proper oral hygiene.	5. To prevent infection.
	6. Teach the client about the overall harmful effects of smoking, including throat irritation.	6. To prevent irritation.
	7. Reinforce the importance of resting and not engaging in vigorous exercise or other strenuous activities.	7. To allow the body time to heal.

Nursing Diagnosis 2: Potential for Injury Related to Possible Ineffective Airway Clearance

Goal/Outcome Criteria	Interventions	Rationales
Client will maintain a patent airway. ■ Demonstrates effective air exchange by normal respiratory rate and rhythm.	1. If the client had general anesthesia, place a pillow under the shoulder and place the client partially face down or partially prone, with the head to the side. Leave the artificial airway in place until the swallowing reflex has returned.	1. To facilitate drainage and to keep the airway clear.
	2. If the client had local anesthesia, elevate the head to approximately 45 degrees.	2. To prevent the tongue from blocking the airway.
	3. Assess respiratory rate and rhythm and observe for tachypnea or dyspnea.	3, 4. To detect an ineffective airway.
	4. Assess the client for central and peripheral cyanosis.	
	5. Monitor vital signs every 5 min until they are stable, then every 15 min for the first hour if stable, then every hour for the first 24 h.	5. To detect hemorrhage
	6. Instruct the client not to cough or clear the throat.	6–8. To prevent injury or bleeding.
	7. Provide tissues and an emesis basin with which to collect secretions.	
	8. Use extreme care if suction must be used to clear secretions.	

continued

CLIENT CARE PLAN ■ The Client with a Tonsillectomy continued

Goal/Outcome Criteria	Interventions	Rationales
Nursing Diagnosis 3: Altered (Cerebral, Renal, Peripheral) Tissue Perfusion Related to Potential Hemorrhage		

Client will not experience hemorrhage.
■ Has no signs of bleeding.
■ Has vital signs within normal limits.
■ Has hemoglobin and hematocrit values within normal postoperative limits for a tonsillectomy and adenoidectomy.
	1. Monitor vital signs every 5 min until they are stable, then every 15 min for the first hour if stable, then every hour for the first 24 h.
	2. Notify the physician if any of the following occur:
	  a. Increased pulse rate.
	  b. Decreased blood pressure.
	  c. Restlessness.
	  d. Bright red drainage.
	3. Reinforce that the client should not cough or clear the throat.
	4. Monitor and document the amount of blood lost through secretions.
	5. When the client is ready for discharge, instruct the client and family about the signs and symptoms of and potential for bleeding. Instruct them to notify the physician immediately if any of these signs or symptoms occur.
		1. To detect hemorrhage.
		
		2. To treat decreased cardiac output.
		
		3. To prevent bleeding.
		
		4. To detect hemorrhage.
		
		5. To detect complications.

COLLABORATIVE MANAGEMENT

Clinical manifestations include acute hoarseness, dry cough, and dysphagia. Complete voice loss (aphonia) may also occur. Diagnosis is determined by client history and laryngeal examination. The practitioner is aided by the use of a laryngeal mirror to visualize the larynx and to differentiate inflammation, polyps, edema, and tumor growth. Further examination of the larynx includes radiography of the neck, computed tomography (CT) of the neck, and laryngoscopic examination. Most clients presenting to their private physician, nurse practitioner, or the emergency department are referred to an ear, nose, and throat specialist for any suspected disorder other than acute laryngitis.

Nursing management is aimed toward relief of present symptoms and the introduction of preventive measures. Treatment for laryngitis consists of steam inhalations, voice rest, cool liquids, and topical throat lozenges. Antibiotic therapy and bronchodilators may be necessary in instances in which sinusitis and bronchitis are also present. The main role of the nurse is to communicate with the client and family about immediate acute care therapies and to provide additional information related to prevention and avoidance of alcohol, tobacco, and pollutants.

Preventive therapy is aimed toward making the client and family aware of the hazards of tobacco and alcohol abuse. The nurse plays the role of educator by reviewing these hazards. The nurse also emphasizes the activities that place an added strain on the larynx such as singing and cheering. The nurse stresses to the client that recurrent bouts of laryngitis require further medical evaluation.

PARALYSIS

OVERVIEW

Laryngeal paralysis may result from injury, trauma, metallic poisons, or a disease process that has affected either the laryngeal nerves or the vagus nerve. Dysfunctional innervation causing laryngeal paralysis can occur in clients experiencing neurologic disorders. Damage to the vagus nerve or medulla may lead to innervation dysfunction. The location of the recurrent laryngeal nerve subjects the nerve to vulnerability in disorders involving the esophagus or thyroid.

Vocal paralysis can be unilateral or bilateral. When only one vocal cord is involved, the airway remains patent but voice use may be affected. Many surgical procedures have been used to improve the voice in these clients, including the injection of Teflon into the affected cord so that it will swell and protrude toward the unaffected cord, which leads to better approximation. Paralysis of both vocal cords usually results from a traumatic injury or a massive cerebrovascular accident. Symptoms of bilateral vocal cord paralysis include dyspnea, hoarseness, stridor, and a weak voice.

COLLABORATIVE MANAGEMENT

Management is aimed toward astute nursing observations for clinical decompensation, as evidenced by signs and symptoms of upper airway obstruction (see under the later heading Upper Airway Obstruction for discussion). The nurse is aware that dyspnea and stridor in these clients may lead to an inadequate airway and thus to an emergency tracheostomy.

Treatment is aimed toward providing a patent airway. The nurse examines these clients frequently for possible aspiration of liquids because of the paralysis. Frequent chest x-ray films and chest auscultation are used to rule out aspiration. Positioning the client in Fowler's position is vital to prevent aspiration.

NODULES AND POLYPS

Nodules occurring on the vocal cords usually appear at the point at which the cords come together forcibly. *Nodules* are hypertrophied fibrous tissue that result from overuse of one's voice and may appear after an infectious process. The populations most affected are teachers, coaches, sports fans, and singers. Polyps occur most commonly in adults who smoke, have many allergies, and live in a dry climate. Vocal cord *polyps* are chronic edematous masses. Both nodules and polyps are painless to the client but produce hoarseness because of the loss of approximation of the vocal cords (Fig. 61–3).

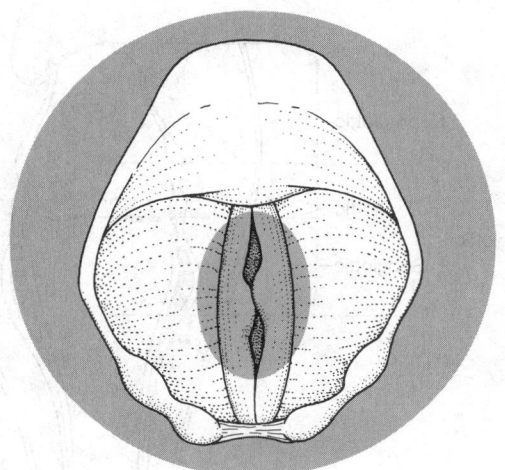

Figure 61–3

Vocal cord nodules and polyps prevent approximation of the vocal cords. Hoarseness results.

Nursing management of the client with vocal cord nodules or polyps is aimed at education of the client and family. The nurse instructs the client about the hazards of tobacco use and the importance of voice rest. Conservative treatment includes voice rest, humidification, speech therapy to help reduce the intensity of the spoken word, and treatment of underlying allergies. If hoarseness is not relieved, excision of the nodules or polyps must be done with direct laryngoscopy which is described in Chapter 60 in the Guidelines feature. If both cords are involved, one cord is usually allowed to heal before an excision is performed on the other cord.

Postoperative recovery involves 10 to 14 days of complete voice rest to promote healing. The nurse ensures alternative methods of communication such as a slate board, pen and paper, magic slate, or alphabet board. The nurse reports to the nursing staff the plan of care for this client. Placing signs on the client's door, over the bed, and on the intercom system helps to implement this important nursing intervention.

EDEMA

Acute laryngeal edema is a potential medical emergency that requires *immediate* recognition by the nurse. Etiology includes anaphylaxis, acute laryngitis, inflammation, trauma, difficult intubation, and radiation to the neck area. Symptoms include hoarseness, dyspnea, and the classic laryngeal stridor.

Nursing management consists of maintaining a patent airway and alleviating the client's anxiety. Inadequate inhalation is extremely frightening to the client and family and causes anxiety. Procedures to be performed should be explained to the client in simple terms and by using visual aids when appropriate. A gentle approach with clients experiencing air hunger is most effective during the period of anxiety.

The nurse alerts the physician and/or respiratory therapist about the need for probable endotracheal intubation or emergency tracheostomy. The use of epinephrine by inhalation may be instituted to decrease edema. The nurse must be aware of the drug's possible side effects such as tachycardia, hypotension, and dry mouth. Corticosteroids may also be used to reduce laryngeal edema and to increase air exchange. Arterial blood gas assays may be ordered by the physician and should be reviewed by the nurse to discover abnormalities. Laryngeal edema related to blunt trauma to the larynx must be further evaluated for possible injuries involving the head and neck areas.

TRAUMA

Laryngeal *trauma* can consist of crushing injuries, fractures, or intrinsic injuries. Intrinsic injuries can be caused by prolonged endotracheal intubations (endotracheal tubes and nasogastric tubes), which cause a fracture between the esophagus and trachea and therefore create an esophagotracheal (E-T) fistula. Symptoms of trauma to the larynx include hoarseness and aphonia. Edema and bleeding (hemoptysis) may occur depending on the exact cause of the trauma. A tracheostomy may be necessary.

Nursing management of the injuries consists of assessment and frequent monitoring of vital signs (every 30 to 60 minutes), including respiratory status. The nursing priority is to establish a patent airway. If the client is having respiratory difficulty as evidenced by tachypnea, anxiety, sternal retraction, nasal flaring, and stridor, the nurse stays with the client and instructs other trauma team members to prepare for a tracheostomy. Examination of the larynx determines the nature of the injury. Lacerations of the mucous membranes, cartilage exposure, and paralysis of the cords all require specific treatment modalities. If the cricoid cartilage is lacerated, it needs immediate repair because it is the only completely circular cartilage. When damage occurs to this cartilage, the larynx closes and a tracheostomy must be performed. If the trauma to the larynx is extensive, a total laryngectomy may be necessary (see under the heading Surgical Management in the later section on cancer of the larynx). Repair of the larynx, if it is feasible, is done as soon as possible to prevent laryngeal stenosis.

CANCER

OVERVIEW

Cancers of the head and neck account for more than 4% of all carcinomas. More than 80% of all head and neck cancers are squamous cell carcinomas arising from the mucosal epithelium. Only a small number of these cancers are laryngeal, but the incidence of resulting disability from laryngeal cancer is high. The cure rate for cancer of the larynx is excellent when the disease is limited to the vocal cords.

Pathophysiology

Of the tumors affecting the larynx, 90% are squamous cell (mucosal epithelial) in origin. Pathogenesis of these tumors is usually related to injury. These tumors are fast seeding and have a high rate of recurrence. Most of these tumors present as malignant ulcerations with underlying filtration. Spread is predominantly to areas like muscle and bone, although cartilage and bone act as barriers in the early stages. Dissemination through the lymphatic system can occur in the early stages. If metastasis occurs, it is most common in the lungs. Metastasis to the larynx *from* other primary sites is rare.

The development of malignancy in laryngeal mucosa is a process requiring several years and takes place in a step-like manner, similar to that seen in bronchial epithelium and the uterine cervix. When laryngeal mucosa is subjected to an irritating substance such as cigarette smoke or mechanical trauma such as voice abuse, the mucosa responds by transforming itself into a tougher mucosa (squamous metaplasia), by increasing the mucosal thickness (acanthosis or hyperplasia), or by developing a keratin layer (keratosis). When the irritating substance contains a carcinogen, these benign protective changes may be accompanied by epithelial atypia or dysplasia. These atypical lesions take the form of white, patchy lesions or red, velvety patches. Documentation suggests that even though most laryngeal carcinoma is diagnosed with reference to white, patchy mucosal lesions, the red patches are overlooked and are actually a late stage of laryngeal carcinoma. The red layer is seen after the white patch has sloughed away.

Growth and spread of laryngeal carcinoma depend on the site of the primary tumor (Fig. 61–4). Anatomic barriers of the larynx and surrounding structures are present in the glottic area, but fewer barriers exist in the subglottic and supraglottic areas.

Etiology

The exact etiology of laryngeal carcinoma is unknown; however, numerous risk factors have been identified as contributing to the likelihood of an individual's developing laryngeal cancer. The two most important risk factors are tobacco use and alcohol abuse, and especially the combination of the two. The relative risk for smokers has been calculated to be as high as 39 times greater than for that for nonsmokers. Other risk factors include voice abuse, chronic laryngitis, exposure to industrial chemicals or toxins or to radiation, and heredity.

Incidence

The frequency of occurrence of carcinoma of the larynx is increasing. It is estimated that in the United States

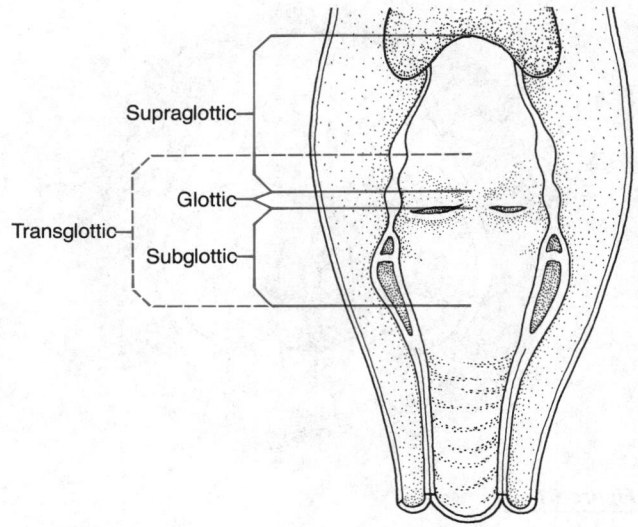

Figure 61–4

Sites of primary laryngeal tumors.

KEY FEATURES OF DISEASE ■ Differential Features of the Three Types of Laryngeal Cancer

Cancer Type	Areas Affected	Clinical Manifestations
Supraglottic (extrinsic)	Epiglottis, false cords	Usually no *early* warning Throat discomfort followed by hoarseness
Glottic (intrinsic)	True vocal cords	Hoarseness (early sign)
Subglottic	Below vocal cords	Throat discomfort Feeling of a lump in the throat

there are more than 11,500 cases of laryngeal carcinoma and more than 3700 related deaths every year. The National Cancer Institute reported that there were 8.5 cases per 100,000 males and 1.3 cases per 100,000 females in the United States during the period of 1973 to 1976. When this cancer does appear in females, it is usually at an early age (fourth to fifth decades of life). Laryngeal cancer represents 2.3% of all malignant tumors in males and 0.4% of all malignant tumors in females, excluding basal and squamous cell carcinomas of the skin. In the United States, there is 1 laryngeal cancer to every 10 lung cancers (Thawley et al., 1987).

The incidence of laryngeal cancer peaks in the sixth and seventh decades of life. Approximately 60% of clients with laryngeal cancers are diagnosed when the tumor is limited to the larynx. Tumor locations in the larynx are divided as follows: 40% supraglottic, 59% glottic, and 1% subglottic. The Key Features of Disease above differentiates the three types of laryngeal cancer by location.

PREVENTION

Prevention is aimed toward minimizing risk factors. Public awareness of the warning signs of cancer is a nursing priority. The early warning signs for all head and neck cancers are summarized in the Key Features of Disease below. Education of clients and families in of-

KEY FEATURES OF DISEASE ■ Early Warning Signs of Head and Neck Cancers

Color changes in the mouth and tongue to white, gray, dark brown, or black

A sore that does not heal in 2 wk

A lump in the mouth or neck

Persistent or unexplained bleeding

Numbness of the mouth or lips

Persistent or recurrent low-grade pain in the ears or face

Hoarseness

fice and clinic settings should include provision of information on risk factors associated with all cancers and those specific to laryngeal carcinomas. The nurse stresses the hazards of tobacco abuse, i.e., smoking and chewing. Treatment is aimed at prevention and early recognition of tumors. Laryngeal cancer is a potentially curable disease *if* it is discovered early. Untreated cancer of the larynx is inevitably a fatal disease; 90% of untreated clients die within 3 years.

Singers, cheerleaders, sports fans, orators, teachers, and others who continually strain their vocal cords must be cautioned against voice abuse. Clients who have a history of chronic laryngitis and who continue to abuse the larynx (such as with tobacco, alcohol, voice strain, or exposure to environmental pollutants) should be taught that they are in the risk group for developing laryngeal carcinoma.

COLLABORATIVE MANAGEMENT

 Assessment

History

When taking a history from a client with laryngeal cancer, the nurse keeps the risk factors for the disorder in mind. The nurse is aware that the client may have difficulty in speaking because of hoarseness and/or pain. Data collection includes *age* and *sex* because the problem occurs most frequently in males in the sixth and seventh decades of life.

The nurse questions the client about the risk factors of *tobacco* and *alcohol use* and a past history of *recurrent acute laryngitis* or *chronic laryngitis.* The nurse also takes a thorough life style history to ascertain if the client has been exposed to certain environmental pollutants (dust from woodworking, asbestos, mustard gas, diethyl sulfate). A family history of cancer is noted. In addition to the above-mentioned information about the client, the nurse assesses the client's socialization. For example, what is the client's occupation? Does it require continual oral communication? Will the client need retraining in other vocational areas or can this job be resumed after surgery and/or radiation treatment?

Physical Assessment: Clinical Manifestations

The client with laryngeal carcinoma usually presents to the physician's office or clinic with the symptom of *persistent hoarseness.* Hoarseness occurs because of a lack of approximation of the vocal cords during phonation. When tumor growth prevents the cords from coming together completely, hoarseness occurs. Vocal cord tumors are the earliest form of laryngeal cancer. They are easy to treat and do not metastasize at the same rate as tumors at other sites. The nurse stresses the necessity of evaluation for anyone who has a history of hoarseness for a period of 3 weeks or longer.

Other symptoms include sore throat for many weeks, painless mass in the neck, feeling of a lump in the throat, dysphagia, change in voice quality, burning in the throat when drinking citrus juices or hot liquids, dyspnea, weight loss, or loss of appetite. Pain is usually *not* an early presenting symptom. These symptoms are usually due to a more advanced form of laryngeal cancer and may involve lymph nodes and the thyroid.

The nurse uses the techniques of inspection and palpation while performing the physical examination. The nurse who is specially trained can perform a laryngeal examination, which includes the use of the laryngeal mirror and the laryngoscope. Masses may be visualized by inspection, or the nurse may palpate the neck area for tumor growth and node involvement.

Psychosocial Assessment

The typical client with laryngeal carcinoma is a man in the fifth to seventh decades of life who has a long-standing history of cigarette and/or alcohol abuse. The nurse assesses his daily activities of living including number of packs of cigarettes smoked per day. The nurse asks the client if he drinks alcohol and if he does, how much per day. Questions of this nature may be uncomfortable for both the client and the nurse but are a necessary part of the psychosocial examination.

The nurse also assesses the problems that arise that are related to the risk factors. Nutrition may be poor because of alcohol intake, and liver function may be subsequently impaired. Lack of sensation and mental alertness could cause multiple problems during the course of this disease process, including lack of cultural awareness of disease process and outcomes, need for self-care of a tracheostomy if one is needed, difficulty with comprehension of educational instruction, and continual abuse of alcohol and tobacco.

Laboratory Findings

The routine diagnostic laboratory tests are performed, including a complete blood count and SMA-12 (12/60). The nurse should be alert to a decrease in hemoglobin and hematocrit values and an increase in alkaline phosphatase levels. These changes indicative of, but are not specific for, malignancies. Renal and liver function tests are usually performed to rule out metastatic disease and to evaluate the client's ability to metabolize therapeutic agents if chemotherapy is needed.

Radiographic Findings

X-ray studies are used to locate the tumor. In addition, x-ray films of the skull, sinuses, neck, and chest are taken to identify possible metastasis or the extent of tumor invasion. CT of the neck and larynx is done to help evaluate and stage laryngeal tumors. CT may or may not include the use of contrast media.

Other Diagnostic Tests

The newest diagnostic test is magnetic resonance imaging. This technique can differentiate normal tissue from diseased tissue with a greater degree of sensitivity than CT. Clients with a definitive diagnosis of laryngeal cancer have further scanning to detect possible metastatic disease. The brain, bone, and liver may be scanned.

Other diagnostic tests include direct and indirect laryngoscopy and laryngeal biopsy. Direct and indirect laryngoscopy is summarized in Chapter 60 in the Guidelines feature. Laryngeal biopsies are performed at the time of the laryngoscopy to confirm the diagnosis and to determine the tumor type and localization.

 Analysis: Nursing Diagnosis

Common Diagnoses

Three nursing diagnoses are common in most clients with laryngeal carcinomas:

1. Potential for injury related to possible metastasis and subsequent obstructed airway
2. Anxiety related to fear of the unknown
3. Body image disturbance related to treatment

Additional Diagnoses

In addition to the most common diagnoses, the client may present with one or more of the following diagnoses:

1. Ineffective airway clearance related to tumor growth and/or metastasis to surrounding structures
2. Pain related to tumor pressure on surrounding tissues and nerves
3. Altered nutrition: less than body requirements related to dysphagia, anxiety, or metastatic process
4. Impaired verbal communication related to tumor growth and associated aphonia or hoarseness
5. Ineffective individual coping related to altered body image, communication method, and/or socialization
6. Impaired social interaction related to body image disturbance

7. Impaired adjustment related to self-care of tracheostomy, alternative communication methods, and body image disturbance

8. Knowledge deficit related to treatment regimen

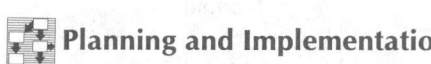 **Planning and Implementation**

The following plan of care of the client with laryngeal cancer focuses on the common nursing diagnoses.

Potential for Injury

Planning: client goals.   The major goals for this nursing diagnosis are that the client will (1) maintain a patent airway and (2) be free from metastasis.

Interventions.   After a diagnosis of laryngeal carcinoma is confirmed, the physician outlines the available treatment modalities for each client. The family or significant other should be included in this conference. The primary goal is to remove or eradicate the cancer while preserving as much normal function as possible. Modalities may be used alone or in combination. Many factors are considered when planning treatment, such as general physical condition, nutritional status, age, and effects of the tumor on body function. The client's ability to manage his or her own care postoperatively should be considered before extensive surgery is undertaken.

Nonsurgical management.   Positioning the client to obtain optimal air exchange is essential. The nurse educates the client and family about the use of Fowler's and semi-Fowler's positions to assist airway patency. It may be easier for the client to spend most of the waking hours in a reclining chair where he or she can breathe and eat more comfortably. Depending on the size and location of the tumor and metastasis, if any, the client may need close observation for possible aspiration of liquids and solid foods.

Monitoring of the client's respiratory effort is an important nursing function. Respiratory rate, arterial blood gas values, and pulmonary function tests are additional measures that are used to assess respiratory status. Signs of respiratory distress may indicate narrowing of the airway related to tumor growth.

Radiation therapy may be the treatment of choice if the cancer is limited to a small area, usually one cord. Treatment of early cancers with radiation offers a 90% cure rate. Therapy with 5000 to 7000 rads or more is usually used. The physician may opt for radiation alone, before or after surgery, or in combination with radical surgery. The most common treatment plan is to use radiation preoperatively, perform surgery to remove the tumor, and use radiation again 3 to 6 weeks postoperatively. This treatment plan has proved to be the most effective. The nurse must remember that radiation therapy causes ineffective tissue healing, and for this reason may not be used preoperatively in certain clients. Care

of clients undergoing radiation therapy is described in Chapter 25.

Chemotherapy is typically not used alone for cancers of the head and neck; it remains under clinical investigation for these cancers. At times, it is used as adjuvant therapy to surgery or radiation. The most commonly used chemotherapeutic agents for cancer of the neck include methotrexate (Mexate), vincristine sulfate (Oncovin), bleomycin sulfate (Blenoxane), and cisplatin (Platinol). Multiple-drug regimens have been reported to achieve higher response rates. Chapter 25 includes a detailed discussion of the care of clients receiving chemotherapy.

Surgical management.   Surgical intervention for cancer of the larynx can include a small tumor excision or radical neck surgery and tracheostomy. A total laryngectomy is favored for infiltrative laryngeal tumors that involve vocal cord paralysis and for tumors that do not respond to radiation therapy. If the lymph nodes are involved, a radical neck dissection (on the lesion side) is performed in conjunction with removal of the larynx. This procedure includes removal of all tissue from the lower edge of the mandible to the clavicle and from the anterior edge of the trapezius to the midline, except for the carotid arteries, the vagus, hypoglossal, and phrenic nerves, and trunks of the brachial plexus. Dissection routinely involves the sternocleidomastoid muscle, the jugular vein, the eleventh cranial nerve, the submaxillary salivary gland, and surrounding soft tissue. Because the eleventh cranial nerve is severed, shoulder drop will be present. Neck exercises can help the client to ease the shoulder drop by increasing the use of other muscle groups.

Other surgical procedures performed for cancer of the larynx include laser surgery, transoral cordectomy, laryngofissure with partial laryngectomy, hemilaryngectomy, and supraglottic laryngectomy (Table 61-1).

Preoperative care.   Preoperatively, the nurse actively educates the client and family. The actual surgical procedure is explained by both the physician and the nurse; explanations are also given for cosmetic repair (if needed), rehabilitation plans, tracheostomy care (if one is planned), compensatory methods of communication, suctioning, critical care environment including use of ventilators and critical care routines, and nutritional support, such as feeding tubes. Chapter 18 describes general preoperative assessment and education in detail.

Postoperative care.   The client usually spends the immediate postoperative period in the surgical critical care unit where the nurses provide individualized care. The nurse monitors the client's vital signs, airway patency, and level of comfort. The nurse is also alert to the possibility of postoperative hemorrhage and other general complications of anesthesia and surgery, as described in Chapter 20.

In the immediate postoperative period, the client is placed on a ventilator. On the next morning, the client typically receives a tracheostomy collar with humidifi-

TABLE 61-1 Surgical Procedures for Laryngeal Cancer

Procedure	Description	Resulting Voice Quality
Carbon dioxide laser surgery	Tumor reduced or destroyed by laser beam through laryngoscope	Normal
Transoral cordectomy	Tumor (early lesion) resected through laryngoscope	Normal (high cure rate)
Laryngofissure	One true cord removed (early lesion)	Normal (high cure rate)
Supraglottic partial laryngectomy	Hyoid bone, false cords, and epiglottis removed Radical neck dissection on affected side performed (extrinsic lesion)	Normal
Hemilaryngectomy or vertical laryngectomy	One true cord, one false cord, and one-half of thyroid cartilage removed	Hoarse voice
Total laryngectomy	Entire larynx, hyoid bone, strap muscles, one or two tracheal rings removed Radical neck dissection usually performed	No voice

cation to help liquefy mucous secretions. Tracheostomy secretions remain blood tinged for 1 to 2 days. Any increase in bleeding or the presence of blood clots should be reported to the physician immediately. Aseptic technique is always used when suctioning the trachea via the laryngectomy or tracheostomy tube. The laryngectomy tube has a larger lumen and is shorter than the tracheostomy tube. Because the client cannot verbalize with either of these tubes, the nurse provides a magic slate or paper and pencil for communication.

Positioning of the client in semi-Fowler's or Fowler's position helps with oxygenation and airway patency. The nurse reinforces the proper technique for use of the incentive spirometer and offers the spirometer to the client every 1 to 2 hours while the client is awake. This device helps to expand the lungs, to facilitate movement of secretions, and to prevent atelectasis in the lower airways. The client may be able to expectorate most of the tracheostomy secretions, or suction may be needed to clear the tracheostomy tube. The nurse can include the client in his or her own care by providing a catheter for suctioning secretions and a mirror. Thus, the client can have some control over his or her care. The nurse provides a clean environment for the catheter unless oral surgery was also performed. Chapter 62 describes tracheostomy care in detail under the section on chronic obstructive pulmonary disease.

Suctioning of the tracheostomy is done frequently in the immediate postoperative period (every 30 to 60 minutes), and then every 2 hours or as necessary. The nurse monitors vital signs every hour for the first 24 hours, then every 2 hours until the client is stable. After the client is transferred from the critical care unit, vital signs can be monitored every 4 hours or as per hospital policy.

Hemorrhage is a possible postoperative complication for all clients undergoing surgery. However, it is not common in clients who have had a laryngectomy. The use of a Hemovac or other surgical drain in the neck area is favored over pressure dressings to prevent bleeding because the dressings can compromise the blood supply to the skin flaps protecting the structure of the neck. The Hemovac is used as a closed suction apparatus and blood receptacle for 72 hours postoperatively (Fig. 61-5; see also Chap. 20, Fig. 20-5). The nurse checks the Hemovac frequently to ensure drainage and records the amount of bloody drainage at least every 8 hours.

A nasogastric or feeding gastrostomy/jejunostomy tube is placed postoperatively. For the first 48 hours, the client receives intravenous fluids and/or total parenteral nutrition (see Chap. 13). After that, he or she receives nutrients via the nasogastric tube or the gastrostomy/jejunostomy tube, depending on the preference of the surgeon. The nutritional support team assesses the client preoperatively and may be consulted about diet therapy after surgery.

The nasogastric tube (most commonly used) usually remains in place for about 10 days after surgery. At this time, if the client is to receive nutrition by mouth, he or she is assessed for swallowing ability. The nurse is supportive during this time. Reassuring the client with a total laryngectomy that he or she will not choke and staying with the client while the client swallows are essential during the first few swallowing attempts.

If the client has had a subtotal horizontal or supraglottic laryngectomy, the fear of choking, especially on fluids, is quite real. This client has only the true vocal cords to act as a defense in swallowing. The nurse, speech and language pathologist, or both teach the client the procedure for supraglottic swallowing, which consists of the following: (1) clearing the throat, (2) inhaling, (3) placing food into the mouth, (4) bearing down (Valsalva's maneuver), (5) swallowing, (6) coughing, (7) swallowing again, and (8) breathing. A chart detailing the eight steps can be helpful for the client to review.

The multidisciplinary team should initiate rehabilita-

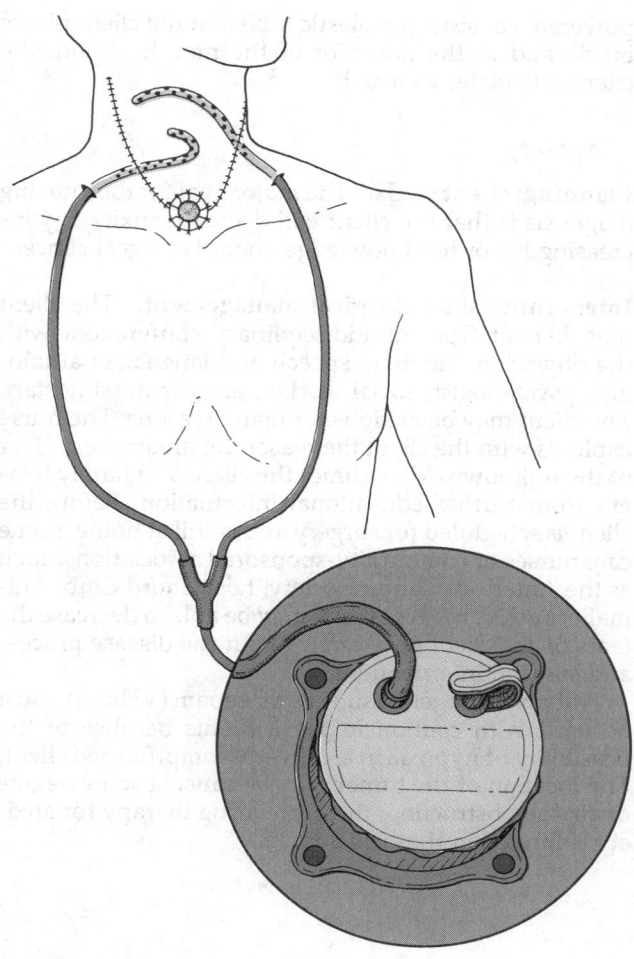

Figure 61–5

Use of Hemovac drainage device as a closed suction apparatus and blood receptacle after laryngectomy.

tive therapy preoperatively. The principles of speech therapy should be discussed with the client and family early in the course of the proposed treatment plan. The client and family need to be aware that the client's voice will sound different after surgery, depending on the type of surgery performed (see Table 61–1).

The usual speech rehabilitation plan consists initially of use of an artificial larynx followed by learning esophageal speech. About 3 months after the laryngectomy or 6 months after surgery with radiation, a tracheo-esophageal fistula may be performed. If the neck tissue is not healed well enough for the use of an external artificial larynx, an extra oral artificial larynx is introduced. Vocal rehabilitation is aimed at developing the most effective communication system for each individual client.

Alternative speech methods include esophageal speech and use of a tracheoesophageal prosthesis or external speech aids. Teaching of esophageal speech is attempted with most clients. This process is started as soon as the esophageal suture is healed. The client with

a partial laryngectomy has the least difficulty with normal speech and improves in a few days. Esophageal speech should be attempted by all clients having a total laryngectomy. Esophageal speech is produced by the eructation of swallowed air through the cricopharyngeal muscle. The voice produced is a monotone; it cannot be raised or lowered and carries no pitch.

To master esophageal speech, the client must learn to draw air into the esophagus at the time of inspiration. Gastrointestinal bloating may occur because of the swallowing of air for speech. Antacids may help to diminish this distention.

The client needs support and encouragement from the hospital team and the family while relearning to speak. This process can be time-consuming and necessitates concentration each time the client speaks. The client must have adequate hearing, or esophageal speech will be difficult because the client uses his or her mouth to shape the words as he or she hears them. Fifteen English language consonants require the use of vocal cords; the remaining 10 can be formed by shaping the mouth. A hearing aid may also be needed for hearing-impaired clients.

Esophageal speech also helps to strengthen the respiratory and abdominal musculature, which aids the client in expectorating secretions and in breathing. The nurse reinforces the techniques of esophageal speech frequently throughout the client's hospital stay. Having a laryngectomee from one of the local self-help organizations visit the client and family is quite beneficial.

The client may feel reserved and socially isolated because of the change in voice and disfigurement after surgery. The nurse and family must make all attempts to ease the client into a more familiar environment. Encouragement and positive reinforcement, along with feelings of acceptance and caring, make it much easier for the client. Psychologic family counseling sessions beginning in the hospital can also be useful.

A tracheoesophageal prosthesis is used for clients who, for whatever reason, cannot benefit from pure esophageal speech. A fistula is created between the trachea and the esophagus, either at the time of the laryngectomy or later (Fig. 61–6). The surgeon places a catheter in the fistula and usually sutures the catheter to the neck. After the fistula heals, a silicone prosthesis, such as the Blom-Singer trapdoor prosthesis or the Panje voice button (Fig. 61–7), is inserted in place of the catheter. The client covers the opening of the prosthesis with the finger or opens and closes the opening with a special valve to divert air from the lungs, through the trachea, into the esophagus, and out of the mouth. Speech is produced by lip and tongue movement, not by the prosthesis itself.

External esophageal prostheses are mechanical devices such as a vibrator—an electronic artificial larynx that is used externally on the skin. Many different artificial larynges are available. Most contain a battery-powered device that is placed against the side of the neck. The air inside the mouth is vibrated and the client articulates as usual. Another external device, also battery

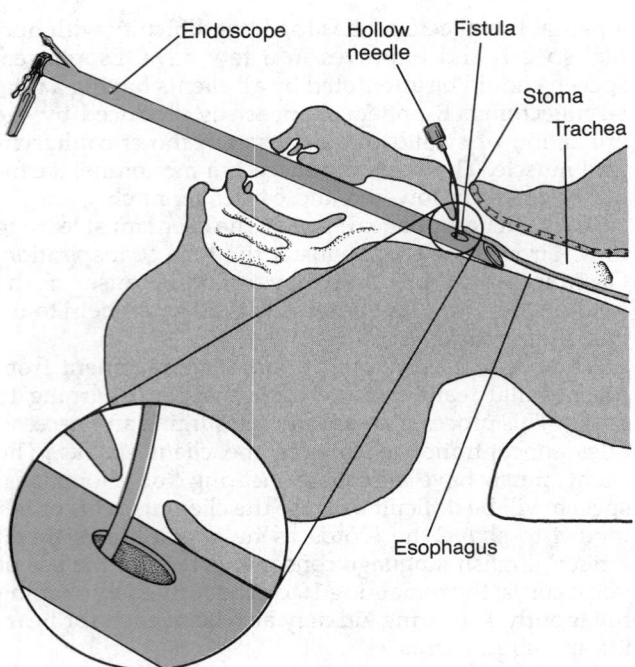

Figure 61–6

One method of creating a tracheoesophageal fistula.

powered, consists of a plastic tube that the client places inside and to the posterior of the mouth. Again, the client articulates as usual.

Anxiety

Planning: client goals. The major goal for this nursing diagnosis is that the client will decrease anxiety by increasing his or her knowledge about laryngeal cancer.

Interventions: nonsurgical management. The client may benefit from multidisciplinary conferences with the physician, dietitian, speech and language pathologist, psychologist, social worker, and/or nursing staff. The client may be anxious for many reasons. The nurse explores with the client the reason for anxiety, e.g., fear of the unknown. Many times the client and family benefit from further educational information. Before the client is scheduled for surgery and is still at home, home care nurses or community-sponsored associations, such as the American Cancer Society, Lost Chord Club, Animalio, and New Voice Club, may be able to decrease the fears of the client and family about the disease process and surgical interventions.

Antianxiety agents, such as diazepam (Valium), must be used with caution in these clients because of the possibility of hypoxia in an already compromised client. The location of the tumor may be causing some degree of airway obstruction; therefore, drug therapy for anxiety is limited in these clients.

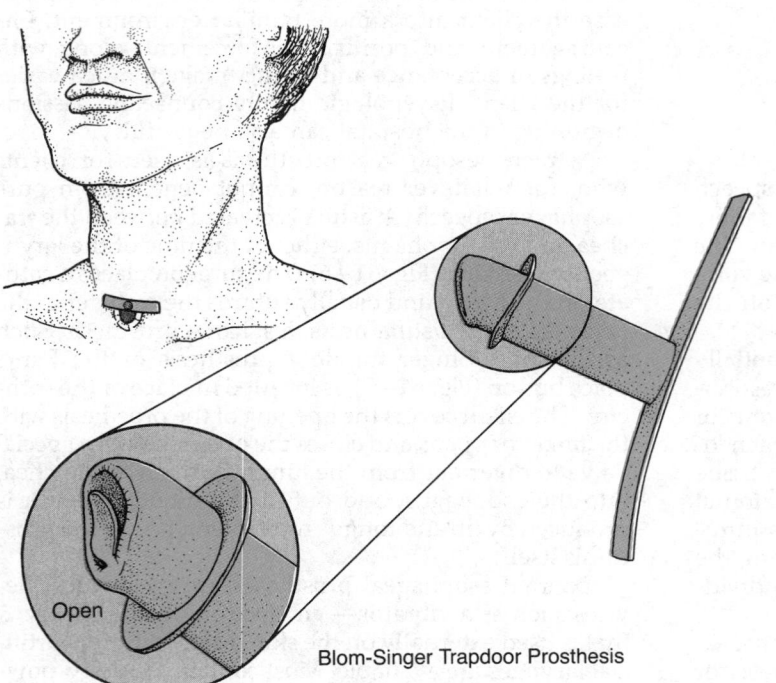

Blom-Singer Trapdoor Prosthesis

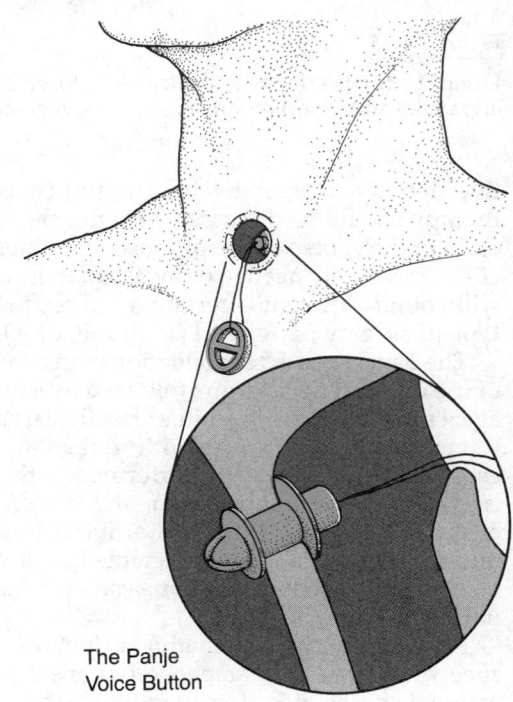

The Panje
Voice Button

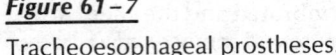

Figure 61–7

Tracheoesophageal prostheses.

Body Image Disturbance

Planning: client goals.   The goal for this nursing diagnosis is that the client will state that he or she accepts body image changes and returns to an active life style within the limits of the disease process.

Interventions: nonsurgical management.   The client with a total laryngectomy and/or a radical neck dissection experiences a permanent change in body image because of deformity and the presence of a neck stoma or tube. The client may not have any voice or may have permanent hoarseness. The nurse helps the client to set realistic goals, starting with involvement in self-care. Alternative communication methods are taught so that the client can communicate in the hospital and after discharge. To cover the stoma and neck and shoulder changes related to surgery, the nurse suggests that the client wear loose-fitting, high-collar shirts or sweaters (turtleneck), and jewelry. For women, cosmetics may aid in covering any disfigurement, although most surgeons try to place the surgical incisions in the client's natural skin fold lines. Chapter 9 discusses body image in detail, including additional nursing interventions.

■ Discharge Planning

Home Care Preparation

The client with a radical neck dissection and laryngectomy is usually ready to be discharged from the hospital at the end of 2 weeks. By this time, the client should be able to provide his or her own tracheostomy care, should have learned esophageal speech, and should feel comfortable with the extended plan of care.

The client and family may feel more comfortable about discharge if the community health nurse has made at least one visit to the home. The multidisciplinary team should assess the client's specific discharge needs.

Health Care Resources

Clinic or physician follow-up visits are scheduled early after discharge. The nurse informs the client and family of community organizations that can offer support, supplies, and friendships. The International Association of Laryngectomees, a voluntary organization that sponsors the Lost Chord Club or New Voice Club, can offer information to the client on any of the prosthetic devices now available and can also provide support to the client and family, as well as be an important contact for the nurse.

Client/Family Education

The client and family or significant other are taught how to care for the stoma or tracheostomy or laryngectomy tube, depending on the type of surgery performed. The nurse teaches the clean suctioning technique and

reviews the client's plan of care if chemotherapy or radiation therapy is scheduled for a later date. Incision and stoma care, including cleaning and inspection for signs of infection, is reviewed with the client and family before discharge. The client is reminded that swimming is prohibited if a stoma or a tube is present and that showers should be taken with caution so as not to allow water onto the neck area. To shield the stoma, a protective cover, or stoma guard, may be worn. Humidity of air in the home can be increased by using a humidifier, growing houseplants, and/or placing pans of water in various rooms.

The selected method of alternative communication that began in the hospital setting is continued in the home setting, as discussed earlier under the heading Potential for Injury. The nurse recommends that the client wear a medical alert (Medic Alert) bracelet and carry a card for identification as a laryngectomee, or total neck breather. These cards are provided by local chapters of the International Association of Laryngectomees and tell the reader what to do to provide an airway or to resuscitate the client (Fig. 61–8).

The accompanying Client/Family Education feature summarizes the highlights of education for the client being discharged after laryngeal cancer surgery.

Psychosocial Preparation

The client going home with a permanent stoma or laryngectomy tube experiences an alteration in body

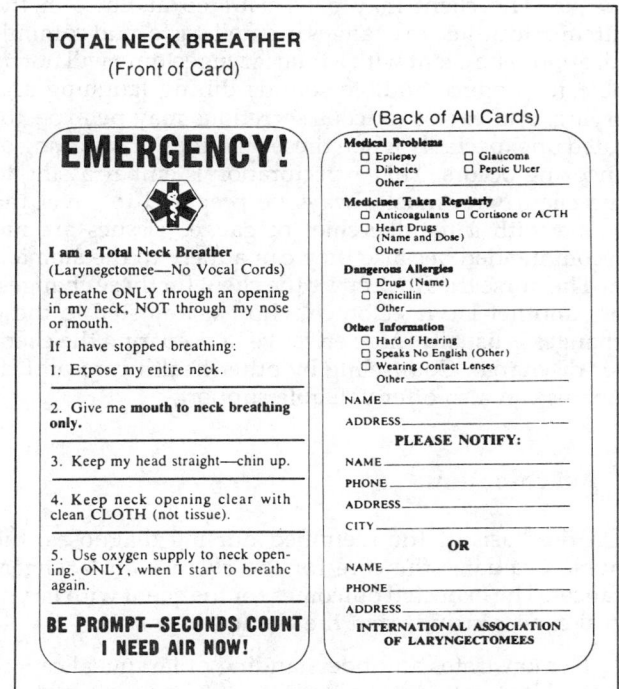

Figure 61–8

Emergency wallet card for identification of laryngectomees.

CLIENT/FAMILY EDUCATION ■ Care of the Laryngectomee at Home

Instructions	Rationales
1. "Avoid swimming and be careful when showering or shaving. Keep shaving creme and small hairs away from your incision."	1. To prevent water and other substances from entering the stoma and causing airway obstruction.
2. "Lean forward and cover the stoma when coughing, sneezing, or laughing."	2. To prevent uncontrolled expulsion of secretions.
3. "Wear a stoma guard or loose clothing to cover the stoma."	3. To protect the stoma from foreign substances.
4. "Clean the stoma with mild soap and water, being careful not to get water into it. Use a small amount of petroleum jelly around the stoma for lubrication."	4. To prevent crusting of secretions and subsequent tissue irritation.
5. "Use a humidifier, pans of water, and/or houseplants to increase the humidity in your home."	5. To substitute for the nose and pharynx, where air is usually warmed, filtered, and humidified. The laryngectomee inhales through the stoma.
6. "Carry a medical emergency card and wear a Medic Alert bracelet."	6. To inform emergency personnel that the client is a neck breather and requires an alternative method to maintain an airway.

---

image. The nurse stresses the importance of returning to a normal life style within the limitations of the disease process. About one-half of clients with this condition return to full-time employment. The remainder work part-time or apply for disability income. Most clients can resume many of their usual activities within 4 to 6 weeks. The client may get frustrated at times in the attempt to adjust to changes in smell, taste, and communication. The client with a total laryngectomy will not be able to produce audible sounds during laughing and crying, and excess mucous secretions may be expectorated unexpectedly when these emotions or coughing or sneezing occurs. This expectoration is embarrassing to the client who must always be prepared to cover the stoma with a handkerchief or gauze. Tissues are not recommended because they can adhere to the stoma.

The nurse tries to prepare the client for these changes, but another laryngectomee who has adjusted to these changes is usually more effective in preparing the client for discharge. Counseling by other health care professionals can also offer valuable support.

 Evaluation

On the basis of the identified nursing diagnoses, the nurse evaluates the care for the client with laryngeal cancer. The expected outcomes for the client with laryngeal cancer include that the client

1. Demonstrates an understanding of laryngeal cancer and its treatment
2. States that levels of anxiety are reduced
3. Maintains a patent airway

4. Uses proper body positioning, incentive spirometry, and suctioning for self-care
5. Resumes as normal a life style as possible through vocal rehabilitation
6. States acceptance of body image changes

OTHER UPPER RESPIRATORY TRACT DISORDERS

MONONUCLEOSIS

OVERVIEW

Mononucleosis is an acute, infectious, systemic process thought to be caused by the Epstein-Barr virus, which is a member of the herpesvirus family. The disease is common in the adolescent to young adult population between the ages of 15 to 25 years. College students experience a higher incidence than the general population. Mononucleosis is mildly contagious and is spread by close intimate contact. The incubation period is from 2 to 6 weeks after exposure to an infected individual.

COLLABORATIVE MANAGEMENT

The clinical course can vary from the client's being asymptomatic to severe systemic involvement. The test for heterophil antibody titer (Monospot) detects the presence of the agglutinating antibody. The test result is positive usually after 2 weeks of illness. Because the testing technique of each laboratory varies, the nurse must check with that particular laboratory for the titer value that is considered to be positive.

A throat culture is performed to rule out any superimposed beta-hemolytic streptococcal infection, which can occur in 10% to 15% of clients with mononucleosis. Values for liver function tests such as lactate dehydrogenase (LDH), serum glutamic-oxaloacetic transaminase (SGOT) (aspartate aminotransferase), serum glutamic-pyruvic transaminase (SGPT), and alkaline phosphatase may be elevated but usually return to normal after the client has recovered from the infection. The white blood cell count may be normal or reduced in the early stage of the disease, as in any other viral infection. As the disease progresses, the count may rise to between 10,000 and 20,000/mm^3, with more than 50% lymphocytes. There may be 10% to 15% of lymphocytes that appear in atypical form. If complications such as thrombocytopenia occur, the platelet count can fall below 140,000/mm^3, or in *severe* cases, below 1000/mm^3.

In taking a history from the client, the nurse is aware of the clinical manifestations that the client may be experiencing. The client may complain of a sore throat, temperature of 101° to 103° F (38.3° to 39.4° C), chills, diaphoresis, malaise or fatigue, headache, generalized aches and pains, tender lymphoadenopathy, and anorexia. The client may experience these symptoms for up to 2 weeks, but fatigue may last for several months. At the physical examination, the client may have the following signs: generalized lymphadenopathy with anterior and posterior cervical areas involved; a grayish-white exudate on tonsils; pharyngeal inflammation and swelling; a red, raised rash on the trunk and extremities; abdominal discomfort; moderate enlargement of the spleen in 50% of clients; liver enlargement (hepatomegaly) in 15% of clients; and jaundice in less than 5% of clients.

Mononucleosis is a self-limiting viral illness, and therefore antibiotics are not effective. Nursing interventions are supportive with symptomatic care and client education. The client can relieve the sore throat by use of saline throat gargles; aspirin can be used for fever, headaches, pain, and myalgias. Bed rest for the first 3 to 5 days and during febrile periods is recommended.

Client education plays an important role. Family members or significant others who have intimate contact are at risk of developing mononucleosis. Most clients return to their normal activities within 3 to 4 weeks. Because the spleen may rupture, it is important that the client does not engage in heavy lifting, intense exercise, or contact sports. This activity restriction is generally for 4 to 6 weeks, depending on the client. If liver function test results are elevated, the client should be counseled to avoid drinking alcohol until the values return to normal. If the client exhibits jaundice, no alcohol should be consumed for 6 to 12 months. The client is instructed to seek immediate medical attention if abdominal pain develops because the spleen can rupture. The client needs to have a thorough understanding of the disease process so that complications can be prevented.

DIPHTHERIA

Diphtheria is a serious infection that is caused by toxin from *Corynebacterium diphtheriae*. Immunizations have caused a decrease in the incidence of this disease, which was once the leading cause of death in children. Diphtheria is a highly contagious disease that is transmitted by direct contact or by contaminated articles. The major source of infection is asymptomatic carriers who incubate the disease. Clients who are at the greatest risk are those who live in crowded conditions, such as city slums and migrant farm camps, and individuals who are inadequately immunized.

The clinical symptoms include sore throat, hoarseness, temperature of 101° to 103° F (38.3° to 39.4° C), a productive cough, and rhinitis. During the physical examination, the nurse may assess cervical lymphadenopathy; tachycardia; a thick, grayish membrane covering the oral cavity; and malodorous breath. The nurse should be aware that during the acute phase, airway obstruction can occur because of inflammation and edema. Other serious complications are myocarditis and cranial or peripheral nerve paralysis. In view of these possible serious complications, the client should be hospitalized for treatment.

Diagnosis is made by throat culture. The treatment plan includes use of penicillin and the diphtheria antitoxin. Family members or significant others should be evaluated for the presence of the disease and a throat culture obtained from each person.

NECK TRAUMA

Injuries to the neck are most often caused by a knife, gun, or traumatic accident. Neck trauma can involve multiple body systems, including cardiovascular, respiratory, gastrointestinal, and neurologic. The reader is referred to a critical care and/or emergency textbook for more in-depth information.

The final outcome of this type of injury depends on the initial assessment and management. The nurse's first priority in the management of neck trauma is assessment for a patent airway. The nurse must be prepared to assist in emergency procedures (emergency intubation or cricothyroidotomy, which is discussed later under the heading Upper Airway Obstruction) to establish a patent airway. The nurse then assesses the cardiovascular system for signs of internal or external bleeding, and impending shock (see Chap. 17 for interventions for clients in shock).

Gastrointestinal injuries usually involve the esophagus and occur in conjunction with other neck injuries. The nurse observes the client for clinical manifestations such as pain and tenderness, oral bleeding, crepitus, and resistance of the neck to range of motion. An initial neurologic assessment needs to be performed by the nurse to provide a baseline for observation of any changes, including mental status, sensory level, and motor function. The reader is referred to the specific areas of the text describing these problems.

FACIAL TRAUMA

The client experiencing major facial trauma usually presents to the emergency or trauma department of a hospital. The nurse's *first* intervention is to establish a patent airway, and if one is not present, to prepare for emergency tracheotomy or cricothyroidotomy. After ensuring airway patency, the nurse assesses the degree of bleeding. Trauma care involves many nursing personnel. When the client arrives at the trauma center, key personnel have specific duties, including controlling hemorrhage, establishing an airway, and assessing for the extent of injury. (For a more detailed account of trauma care, consult a specialized trauma book.)

The signs and symptoms of shock may be present and alert the nurse to the need for early fluid resuscitation (see Chap. 17). Additional findings on assessment may include edema of soft tissue or leakage of cerebrospinal fluid through the ears and/or nose, which indicates skull fracture or neurologic damage of some type.

Head and neck trauma requires the nurse to be astute in the areas of trauma and critical care nursing. Time is the key factor in stabilizing the client and in providing the client with the optimal environment for rehabilitation and plastic surgery for facial deformities or scars. Early treatment and response of the appropriate services, including the trauma team, maxillofacial surgeon, general surgeon, plastic surgeon, and dentist, optimize the client's posttrauma recovery period.

UPPER AIRWAY OBSTRUCTION

OVERVIEW

Upper airway obstruction is a life-threatening emergency that can be defined as any significant interruption in airflow through the nose or mouth and into the lungs. Early recognition by the nurse is essential for preventing further complications including respiratory arrest.

COLLABORATIVE MANAGEMENT

Prompt nursing and medical care is essential for preventing a partial airway obstruction from quickly progressing to a complete obstruction. A client with a partial obstruction (e.g., caused by minimal edema; infection) may have few symptoms. Unexplained or persistent recurrent symptoms need to be evaluated. The nurse explains to the client that even though the symptoms seem to be vague, further evaluation is necessary. Diagnostic procedures such as chest x-ray, laryngoscopic examination, and CT may be needed to rule out potentially life-threatening conditions such as tumors, foreign bodies, or infectious processes. Upper airway obstruction can be a frightening experience for the client and family. The nurse remains calm and provides support for the client while acting quickly to help alleviate and/or prevent further obstruction.

The upper airway can be obstructed by many of the disease processes already discussed in this chapter, such as laryngeal edema, peritonsillar abscess, laryngeal carcinoma, and tumor growth. Neurologic problems such as those associated with a cerebrovascular accident and thick secretions can also cause airway obstruction. Loss of protective reflexes and the tone of the pharyngeal muscles can result in the tongue's falling posteriorly and occluding the airway.

Injury from smoke inhalation, tracheal and laryngeal trauma, foreign body aspiration, and anaphylaxis are also acute airway obstruction processes that require immediate nursing and medical interventions.

Nursing assessment for the client with upper airway obstruction consists of observing the client for signs of

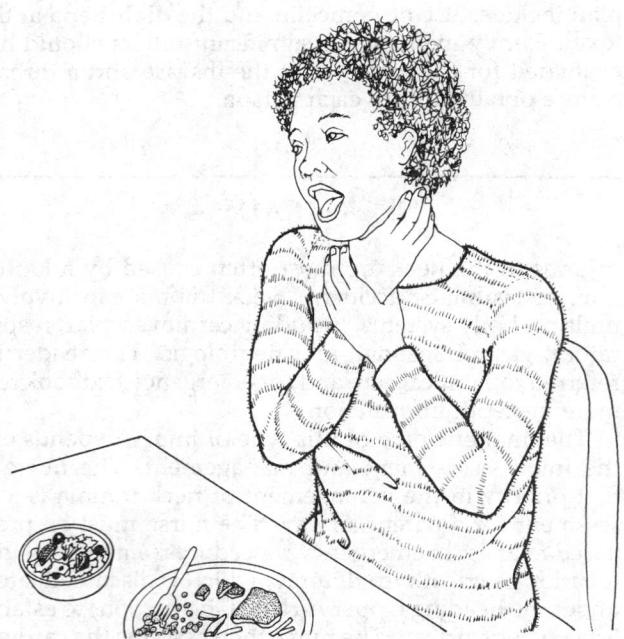

Figure 61–9

The universal distress signal for airway obstruction.

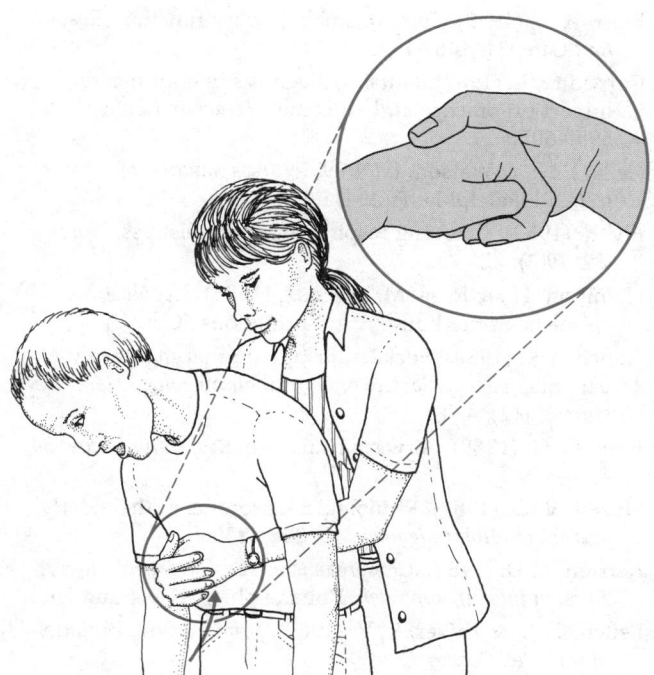

With the **conscious victim standing or sitting,** place your fist between the victim's lower rib cage and navel. Wrap the palm of your other hand around your fist. A quick inward, upward thrust expels the air remaining in the victim's lungs and with it the foreign body. If the first thrust is unsuccessful, repeat several thrusts in rapid succession until the foreign body is expelled or until the victim loses consciousness.

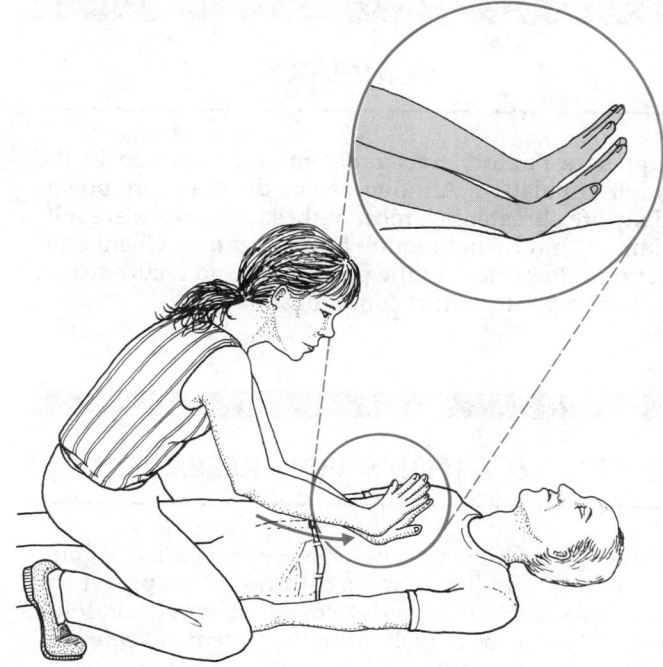

With the **unconscious victim lying supine,** straddle the victim's thighs. Place your hands one over the other as shown, with the heel of the bottom hand just above the victim's navel. Quickly thrust inward and upward, toward the victim's head.

Figure 61–10

The Heimlich maneuver for relief of upper airway obstruction caused by a foreign body.

increasing anxiety, sternal retractions, seesawing chest, abdominal movements, a feeling of impending doom related to actual air hunger experienced by the client, and the universal distress signal for airway obstruction (Fig. 61–9).

Nursing management consists of assessing the situation to diagnose the cause of the obstruction. If the cause is due to the tongue's falling back or to the accumulation of secretions, the nurse places the head and neck in a slightly hyperextended position (see intervention 4 in the feature entitled Emergency Care: Adult Cardiopulmonary Resuscitation, in Chap. 64), and/or uses suction for secretions. If the airway is obstructed because of the presence of a foreign body, the nurse uses the Heimlich maneuver, as outlined in Figure 61–10.

Upper airway obstruction may lead to the need for adjuncts to breathing. Emergency procedures such as a cricothyroidotomy, endotracheal intubation, or tracheotomy may be necessary. Cricothyroidotomy is considered to be a life-saving emergency procedure and is usually performed outside the hospital or in the emergency department. A *cricothyroidotomy* consists of making a stab wound at the cricothyroid membrane, between the thyroid cartilage and the cricoid cartilage ring (see Chap. 60, Fig. 60–3). Any hollow tube can be placed through this opening to keep the new airway open until a tracheotomy tube can be inserted or a tracheotomy performed. This procedure is an emergency one, done when it is the *only* way to make a patent airway for the client. An alternative method to making an incision is to insert a 14-gauge needle into the cricoid space to allow air into and out of the lungs by bypassing the obstruction.

Endotracheal intubation is the insertion of a tube into the trachea via the nose (nasotracheal) or mouth (orotracheal). The most common use of endotracheal intubation is to administer general anesthesia to the client undergoing surgery.

A tracheotomy can be performed as an emergency procedure or as a scheduled surgery. A *tracheotomy* consists of a surgical incision into the trachea for the purpose of establishing an airway. *Tracheostomy* is the stoma (tracheal), or opening, that results from the tracheotomy. Chapter 62 discusses the use of endotracheal and tracheostomy tubes in detail and the nursing care associated with each (under the heading Impaired Gas Exchange in the section on chronic obstructive pulmonary disease).

SUMMARY

Upper respiratory tract problems are common in the adult population. Although some disorders are potentially life-threatening, most of these conditions are self-limiting and do not require hospitalization. Client education is important in the prevention and recurrence of upper respiratory tract conditions.

IMPLICATIONS FOR RESEARCH

Although multiple viruses have been identified as causative factors for the common cold, no cure or preventive immunization has been developed. Research continues to identify the best methods for treatment of acute viral and allergic rhinitis.

Possible questions for nursing research include

1. What role does emotional stress play in the onset of allergic rhinitis?

2. How can the nurse be most effective in helping a client with a total laryngectomy accept the accompanying changes in body image?

3. What is the role of stressors such as humidity and emotional stress in the onset of acute and chronic sinusitis?

REFERENCES AND READINGS

Bates, B. (1987). *A guide to physical examination and history taking* (4th ed.). Philadelphia: J. B. Lippincott.

Buist, A. S. (1989). Tests of small airways function. *Respiratory Care, 34,* 446–454.

Carpenito, L. (1987). Nursing diagnosis in critical care: Impact on practice and outcomes. *Heart and Lung, 16,* 595–605.

Cella, J. H., & Watson, J. (1989). *Nurses' manual of laboratory tests.* Philadelphia: F. A. Davis.

Ely, E. (1989). Grunting respirations: Sure distress. *Nursing '89, 19*(3), 72–73.

Hamilton, H., & Rose, M. B. (Eds.). (1985). *Neoplastic disorders.* Springhouse, PA: Springhouse Corp.

Hancher, K. (1988). Social adjustment of laryngectomy patients. *Journal: Society of Otorhinolaryngology Head-Neck Nurses, 6*(2), 4–8.

Irvin, C. G. (1989). Airways challenge. *Respiratory Care, 34,* 455–469.

Janzen, V. D. (1987). Rhinological disorders in the elderly. *Journal of Otolaryngology, 15,* 228–230.

Kersten, L. D. (1989). *Comprehensive respiratory nursing: A decision making approach.* Philadelphia: W. B. Saunders.

Leitch, C. J., & Tinker, R. V. (1987). *Primary care.* Philadelphia: F. A. Davis.

Lockhart, J. S., & Griffin, C. (1986). Action stat! Epistaxis. *Nursing '86, 16*(11), 33.

Matthewson, H. S. (1988). Quinolones: Antibacterial agents for respiratory diseases. *Respiratory Care, 33,* 357–360.

Rebensen-Piano, M. (1989). The physiologic changes that occur with aging. *Critical Care Nursing Quarterly, 12*(1), 1–14.

Springhouse drug reference. (1989). Springhouse, PA: Springhouse Corp.

Thawley, S. E., Panje, W. R., Batsakis, J. G., & Lindberg, R. D. (Eds.). (1987). *Comprehensive management of head and neck tumors.* Philadelphia: W. B. Saunders.

CHAPTER 62

Interventions for Clients With Lower Respiratory Tract Disorders

PNEUMONIA

OVERVIEW

Pneumonia is an inflammatory process that results in edema of interstitial lung tissue and extravasation of fluid into alveoli, thus causing hypoxemia. It is a condition that primarily affects the terminal gas-exchanging portions of the lung. Although at one time pneumonia was a major cause of death, antibiotics have reduced mortality significantly.

Pathophysiology

Pneumonia is an infection of the pulmonary tissue, including the interstitial spaces, the alveoli, and often the bronchioles. The pneumonic process begins when pathogens successfully penetrate the airway mucus and multiply in the alveolar spaces. To do this, they must survive the lung's many defenses against microbial invasion, including the branching airway system, the mucociliary transport system, and alveolar macrophages. As the pathogenic organisms multiply, edematous fluid forms and other evidence of inflammation becomes apparent. White blood cells migrate into the alveoli and cause thickening of the alveolar wall. Fluid fills the alveoli, which protects the organisms from phagocytosis and facilitates the movement of organisms to other alveoli. In this way, the infection spreads. Blood flow to the involved portions of the lung is enhanced, which is followed by vascular sludging and diminished capillary blood flow. The products of inflammation are drained by the lymphatic system and can overflow into the venous circulation. If the invading organisms obtain access to the blood stream, septicemia results.

The edema of inflammation stiffens the lung, thus causing decreased compliance and a decline in the vital capacity (VC) of the lung. Decreased production of surfactant further reduces compliance and leads to *atelectasis,* or alveolar collapse. In addition, the pneumonic process causes a shunt-type ventilation-perfusion defect. Because bronchi and alveoli are partially occluded, arterial oxygen tension falls. Venous blood coming into the lungs passes through the underventilated area and returns unoxygenated to the left side of the heart. Therefore, a shunt results. Eventually, the mixing of oxygenated and unoxygenated blood leads to arterial hypoxemia.

Systemically, fever results from the infection itself. Phagocytes release a chemical called endogenous pyrogen when ingesting particles. When this substance is carried by the blood to the hypothalamus, the body temperature is raised. An individual may develop shaking chills in an attempt to increase heat production and raise the metabolic rate. An increase in metabolic demand causes secondary tachypnea with tachycardia.

Blood pressure may be lowered as a result of peripheral vasodilation and decreased circulating blood volume secondary to dehydration. Cardiac function may be compromised by hypoxemia and enhanced metabolism. Congestive heart failure or shock may result, and cardiac irritability may be enhanced because of inadequate tissue oxygenation, thus causing arrhythmias.

Infection may cause the breakdown of red blood cells and may block their maturation. In response, marginated polymorphonuclear neutrophils (PMNs) mobilize, and the splenic reserve of PMNs is exhausted, which results in an elevated white blood cell count. If the bone marrow cannot produce white blood cells at the rate at which they are needed, immature PMNs are released.

Fever and tachypnea cause water loss through the skin and respiratory tract, which subsequently results in dehydration. Conversely, the pulmonary infection may cause the body to retain fluid through the mechanism of inappropriate antidiuretic hormone (ADH) (vasopressin) release. In this case, the client becomes overloaded with water. Loss of potassium and other electrolytes occurs, triggered by dehydration, antidiuretic hormone abnormalities, or vomiting and diarrhea.

The extent of pulmonary involvement after the microbial invasion depends on the defenses of the host. In an immunocompromised host, bacteria can multiply. Tissue necrosis results when multiplying anaerobic organisms form an abscess that perforates the bronchial wall. Pneumonia may present as diffuse patches throughout both lungs (bronchopneumonia), or it may cause consolidation, or solidification, in one lobe.

Community-acquired pneumonias are those caused by *Mycoplasma pneumoniae*, *Streptococcus pneumoniae*, *Legionella pneumophila*, and viruses. Hospital-acquired pneumonias include those caused by *Staphylococcus aureus*, *Klebsiella pneumoniae*, *Pseudomonas aeruginosa*, and fungi (see the Key Features of Disease on pp. 1979–1981).

Etiology

In general individuals develop pneumonia when their defense mechanisms are unable to combat the virulence of the invading organisms. Risk factors are given in the Key Features of Disease at the top of page 1982. Certain environments predispose young and otherwise healthy individuals to develop pneumonia. For example, dormitory settings or communal living situations can promote an epidemic spread of organisms. The pneumonia may develop after an upper respiratory tract infection or influenza virus infection. Several types of organisms cause pneumonia, including bacteria, viruses, mycoplasmas, fungi, rickettsiae, protozoa, and helminths. The incidence of fungal pneumonias is increasing in immunosuppressed and critically ill clients; these pneumonias are not communicable. Examples of fungal agents include *Histoplasma*, *Aspergillus*, and *Candida*.

Noninfectious causes of pneumonia include inhalation of toxic gases, chemicals, and smoke; and aspiration of water, food, fluid, and vomitus. Because nosocomial infections are prevalent in hospitals, the very ill, immunosuppressed client is at high risk.

Incidence

Pneumonia remains a leading cause of death in the United States, ranking fifth, as does influenza. It accounts for more than 10% of hospital admissions and occurs in about 5% of clients who are admitted with other diagnoses. Pneumonia is the most frequent cause of death by infection among clients aged 65 years or older, and it is the third leading cause of death from any cause in clients older than age 85 years (Fedullo & Swinburne, 1985). Mortality is highest in individuals with underlying chronic diseases secondary to respiratory complications, which are summarized in the Key Features of Disease at the bottom of page 1982.

During late fall and winter, a higher incidence of pneumonia is likely because this illness frequently follows viral infection.

PREVENTION

Prevention is aimed at reducing the cause of infection. In the elderly, particularly, influenza is a major cause of pneumonia. Therefore, the influenza vaccine is highly recommended for clients older than 65 years of age and for younger people with chronic cardiac disease, severe diabetes, or impaired immune defenses. High-risk clients are identified during hospitalization or other institutionalization as candidates for the vaccine. The influenza vaccine should be given annually to maintain immunity against new pathogenic strains. High-risk clients should also receive the pneumococcal vaccine, which is given once in a lifetime and provides immunity to several strains of pneumococcus.

Client education is an important factor in the prevention of pneumonia. All clients at risk should be taught effective airway clearance techniques such as coughing, deep breathing, turning, and ambulating. Clients with chronic lung disease should be taught in addition to avoid sources of infection and to clean home respiratory equipment according to specified guidelines. Avoidance of indoor pollutants such as dust, smoke from woodburning stoves, and aerosols should also be stressed. The consequences of smoking should be addressed, and clients should be given information on local support groups for smoking cessation if desired.

Clients who are at high risk for the development of any infection because of impaired immunity should be taught infection avoidance, sensible nutrition, adequate fluid intake, and a balance of rest and activity. In the hospital setting, nurses follow strict hand washing techniques to avoid the spread of nosocomial infection. In addition, respiratory therapy equipment is well maintained and is decontaminated daily.

When feeding immobile or comatose clients, the

KEY FEATURES OF DISEASE ■ Differential Features of Community-Acquired and Hospital-Acquired Pneumonias

Etiology	Population at Risk	Clinical Presentation	Diagnostic Indications	Antibiotic Treatment	Complications of Disease
Community-Acquired Pneumonias					
Mycoplasma pneumoniae					
Acquired by droplet infection Occurs where people live and work Occurs in 10%–35% of those infected in the community	Adolescents and young adults in all seasons	Gradual onset Fatigue, headache, myalgia Temperature of less than 102° F (38.9° C), chills, anorexia Hacking, nonproductive cough Pharyngitis Possible rhonchi or rales on auscultation Wheezing and bronchospasms	Chest x-ray film: peripheral infiltrates Often unilateral presentation in the lower lobes Elevated erythrocyte sedimentation rate Elevated white blood cell count	Tetracycline Erythromycin	Pericarditis Myocarditis Arthritis Polyneuritis Meningoencephalitis
Streptococcus pneumoniae (pneumococcus)					
Gram-positive bacterium Most common type in the community Follows influenza where people are in close contact	Middle-aged and elderly clients with history of previous infections Occurs in late fall and winter	Acute onset Severe, shaking chills Tachypnea, shortness of breath, pleuritic chest pain, temperature of higher than 102° F (38.9° C) Cough with expectoration of rusty or green purulent sputum Chest dull to percussion Crackles, bronchial breath sounds Possible confusion in the elderly	Chest x-ray film: one or more areas of alveolar consolidation Elevated white blood cell count	Penicillin G	Shock, pleural effusion Pericarditis Superinfections Otitis media

Continued

Etiology	Population at Risk	Clinical Presentation	Diagnostic Indications	Antibiotic Treatment	Complications of Disease
Legionella pneumophila					
Gram-negative bacterium	Middle-aged and elderly men	Acute onset	Chest x-ray film: multilo-bar consolidation	Erythromycin	Respiratory failure
Spread by airborne route	Smokers, alcohol abusers	Malaise, myalgia		Rifampin	Mortality 20%–25%
Found in contaminated air-handling systems	Clients with chronic diseases and impaired immunity	Headache, temperature higher than 102° F (38.9° C)			
	All seasons	Dyspnea, vomiting, diarrhea			
		Central nervous system symptoms			
		Bradycardia			
Viruses					
Influenza A virus	Adults	Occurs shortly after viral symptoms arise	Chest x-ray film: intersti-tial pattern	Symptomatic treatment	Pericarditis
Adenovirus	Elderly persons with chronic bronchopul-monary, cardiac, or metabolic disorders	Begins as acute coryza in many clients			Endocarditis
Varicella-zoster virus		Bronchitis and pleurisy in some clients; gastrointestinal symptoms in others			Bronchopneumonia
Tagavirus (rubella)	Pregnant women				Superimposed bacterial infection
Paramyxovirus	Late fall and winter	Presentation as acute illness, with anxiety and agitation; fever, tachypnea, periph-eral cyanosis			
Herpes simplex virus					
Cytomegalovirus		Productive cough, with possibly bloody sputum			
Epstein-Barr virus					
Accounts for 50% of all pneumonias transmitted by droplet infection					
Hospital-Acquired Pneumonias					
Staphylococcus aureus					
Gram-positive bacterium acquired via blood	Hospitalized compro-mised clients	Insidious onset	Chest x-ray film: patchy areas	Methicillin	Effusions
		Variable pulse		Nafcillin	Pneumothorax

Organism	Risk (Clients)	Signs and Symptoms	X-ray	Treatment	Complications
or aspiration Cause of nosocomial infections in hospital settings	Clients with history of viral infection Drug abusers, clients undergoing dialysis, and diabetics at high risk Postsurgical clients	Productive cough with yellow, blood-streaked sputum Fever, pleuritic chest pain Necrotizing infection with lung destruction Prolonged recovery	X-ray visualization: pleural involvement common Multiple nodular lesions and necrotization often present		Lung abscess Meningitis
Klebsiella pneumoniae (Friedländer's bacillus) Gram-negative bacillus Cause of nosocomial infections, especially in the critically ill	Clients with chronic lung disease Chronically ill clients, alcoholics Elderly men Diabetics	Sudden onset High fever, chills, pleuritic chest pain Productive cough with gray, green, or brick red sputum Rapid destruction of lung tissue	Chest x-ray film: involvement of more than one lobe Lobar consolidation	Cefazolin Tobramycin Gentamicin	Lung abscess Pericarditis Mortality 20%–50%
Pseudomonas aeruginosa Gram-negative bacterium Most common cause of hospital-acquired infection Associated with use of mechanical ventilation	Hospitalized clients using respirators or respiratory equipment Clients being given antibiotics Clients with pre-existing lung disease Tracheostomized clients Immunosuppressed clients	Gradual onset Confusion Apprehension Bradycardia Cyanosis Productive cough with green sputum with foul odor	Chest x-ray film: multiple infiltrates	Gentamicin Carbenicillin Tobramycin	High mortality Possible lung infarction
Fungi Candida Histoplasma Coccidioides Blastomyces Cryptococcus Aspergillus	Neutropenic individuals Clients being given antibiotics and steroids	Erratic fever Chest pain Hemoptysis Productive cough	Chest x-ray film: infiltration, consolidation, cavitation, and empyema	Amphotericin B	Vascular infarction High mortality

---

KEY FEATURES OF DISEASE ■ Risk Factors for Pneumonia

Altered level of consciousness

Prolonged immobility, especially bed rest

Age more than 65 yr

Chronic disease, such as chronic obstructive pulmonary disease (COPD), diabetes mellitus, or heart disease

Inadequate nutrition

Impaired swallowing or gag reflex

Aspiration of fluid, food, or other substance

Immunosuppression, by either disease or drug

Tracheal intubation

Smoking

Air pollution

---

nurse raises the head of the bed to prevent aspiration during feeding. Frequent repositioning of the immobile and/or elderly client prevents the development of atelectasis.

COLLABORATIVE MANAGEMENT

 Assessment

History

In preparing to take the history from the client who may have pneumonia, the nurse considers risk factors that are consistent with infection. The following essen-

---

KEY FEATURES OF DISEASE ■ Common Complications of Pneumonia

Atelectasis	Collapse of one or more lobes of the lung
Pleural effusion	Collection of fluid in the pleural space (usually sterile fluid that resolves)
Lung abscess	Collection of purulent material in lung parenchyma
Pleurisy	Pain caused by friction between layers of pleura; quite common
Pericarditis	Inflammation or infection of pericardium resulting from hematogenous spread of offending organism
Endocarditis	Inflammation or infection of endocardium resulting from hematogenous spread of offending organism

---

tial data are collected from the client or from a family member if the client is too dyspneic. The *age* of the client is important to note because the incidence of pneumonia is quite high in the elderly. The living, work, or school *environment*, as well as recent changes in environment, is pertinent for etiology. *Diet, exercise,* and *sleep routines* are discussed. The nurse asks the client about the use of *cigarettes* and *alcohol* because these factors pose an enhanced risk for atelectasis. The client's past and current use of *medications* is important information to obtain. Also, any past history of drug addiction or intravenous drug use should be known. The nurse lists the client's past illnesses, particularly those with a respiratory origin such as chronic pulmonary diseases, tuberculosis, and acute episodes of asthma or bronchitis. The nurse also inquires about the client's *recent medical history,* particularly whether the client has been exposed to influenza or pneumonia or has experienced a recent viral episode. A history of any rashes, insect bites, or exposures to animals is also important to note.

The nurse asks if the client has any past or current history of *neurologic deficits,* particularly those causing immobility or diaphragmatic paralysis. If the client has chronic respiratory problems, the nurse asks whether respiratory equipment is used in the home. It is essential to determine whether the client's cleaning regimen is adequate to prevent infection. The nurse also notes prior inoculations with influenza or pneumococcal *vaccine.* Finally, the nurse observes the client's *current symptoms or clinical manifestations.* If pneumonic infection is present, the client may have chest or pleuritic pain, myalgia, headache, chills, fever, diarrhea, dyspnea, and/or sputum production.

Physical Assessment: Clinical Manifestations

In assessing the client with a possible pulmonary infection, the nurse first observes the *general appearance* of the individual. The client may present with flushed cheeks, bright eyes, and an anxious expression. If the illness has been present for several days, the client may wince with pain or hold his or her side when coughing. The chest may have severe muscular weakness from sustained coughing. During this initial observation, the nurse may note dyspnea.

The nurse observes the client's breathing pattern, position, and use of accessory muscles. The acutely compromised client is uncomfortable in a lying position and sits upright, balancing with the hands. The presence of cyanosis of the lips and nail beds is noted, as well as the presence of diaphoresis, which indicates that greater effort is needed to breathe. Chest expansion may be diminished or unequal on inspiration. The nurse auscultates the lungs for *adventitious sounds* such as rales, rhonchi, and wheezes, which are likely. Bronchial breath sounds are heard over areas of density or consolidation. Sound waves are easily transmitted over consolidated tissue. Crackling rales are likely to be heard when there is fluid in interstitial and alveolar areas. Breath sounds may be decreased when airflow is decreased because of bronchial obstruction; muscular weakness; or pleural effusion, tumors, or pleural disease. *Tactile fremitus* is increased over areas of pneumonia, and percussion is dulled in these areas. For further discussion of these respiratory assessment techniques, the reader is referred to Chapter 60. The character of the client's *cough* is observed, as well as the type of *sputum* produced. It is essential to assess the amount, color, and presence of odor because these characteristics offer diagnostic clues about the offending pathogen.

When taking *vital signs,* the nurse notes not only the rate but the quality of the pulse. A weak, thready pulse indicates dehydration or impending shock. In evaluating the vital signs, comparison with baseline values is important because the client who has pneumonia is likely to be hypotensive with orthostatic changes. In addition, fever and chills may be present, so evaluation of temperature is an important aspect of the initial assessment.

Mental status is assessed by the nurse because changes in mental status frequently occur with hypoxemia, particularly in the elderly. A neurologic examination is performed to determine any neurologic causes of muscle weakness, which may impair respiratory mechanics.

The *skin* of the client is inspected for the presence of rashes, which may occur with *Mycoplasma* infection, cytomegalovirus infection, or Rocky Mountain spotted fever. In the last infection a rash is accompanied by mental status changes. The client with legionnaires' disease or other viral infections may experience gastrointestinal symptoms such as nausea, diarrhea, and abdominal pain.

Psychosocial Assessment

The client with pneumonia experiences pain, fatigue, and often dyspnea, which promotes anxiety. The nurse assesses anxiety by looking at the client's facial expression and general tenseness of facial and shoulder muscles. A client's rapid talking may be an indication of anxiety. The nurse listens to the client carefully and uses a calm, slow approach as he or she proceeds with the assessment process.

Laboratory Findings

Examinations of sputum from the client with pneumonia are important for making a specific diagnosis. These samples are obtained easily from the client who can cough into a specimen container. Extremely ill clients who often acquire pneumonia in the hospital setting may require nasotracheal suctioning by the nurse or suctioning via a tracheostomy or endotracheal tube. In these situations, the nurse obtains a sputum specimen via the use of a sputum trap while suctioning. Other methods for obtaining sputum include transtracheal aspiration and bronchoscopy (see Chap. 60).

These methods are more likely to be used for the comatose client.

A complete blood count (CBC) is done to determine leukocytosis, which is commonly seen with infectious processes. Blood cultures may be performed to determine if the organism has invaded the blood stream. Urine may be examined for hematuria, pyuria, or the presence of protein, which may occur in the septic client with pneumonia.

Values for arterial blood gases (ABGs) are obtained to determine baseline arterial oxygen and carbon dioxide levels and the need for supplemental oxygen. Serum electrolyte, blood urea nitrogen, and creatinine levels are also assessed. Clients with pneumonia may develop a rising blood urea nitrogen value, which is often the result of an increased catabolic rate and a diminished glomerular filtration rate. Electrolyte changes occur with dehydration, which is the result of fever and malaise.

Radiographic Findings

The chest x-ray film is an essential tool for diagnosis of pneumonia because it indicates the severity of the pneumonic process. Infiltrates, consolidation, tumors, and effusions are visualized on the film.

 Analysis: Nursing Diagnosis

Clients with pneumonia present with difficulty in breathing, pulmonary congestion, and fatigue. Age, immune status, and the presence of chronic respiratory diseases or other chronic illnesses have an impact on the severity of the illness.

Common Diagnoses

Regardless of the cause of pneumonia, three nursing diagnoses are common in the client with pneumonia:

1. Ineffective airway clearance related to inflammation and increased secretions
2. Ineffective breathing pattern related to tachypnea
3. Activity intolerance related to fatigue

Additional Diagnoses

Some clients present with one or more additional diagnoses:

1. Anxiety related to dyspnea
2. Hyperthermia related to the infectious process
3. Pain related to excessive coughing
4. Fluid volume deficit related to fever
5. Impaired gas exchange related to Shunt-type ventilation-perfusion defect
6. Altered nutrition: less than body requirements related to anorexia

7. Knowledge deficit related to the disease process
8. Sleep pattern disturbance related to discomfort
9. Altered thought processes related to hypoxemia

 Planning and Implementation

Ineffective Airway Clearance

Planning: client goals. The major goals for this nursing diagnosis are that the client will (1) maintain a patent airway, (2) facilitate the removal of mucous plugs and secretions, and (3) remain free from aspiration.

Interventions: nonsurgical management. The client with pneumonia is encouraged to cough and deep breathe at least every 2 hours. The incentive spirometer may be used to facilitate deep breathing in the alert client. Because many clients experience pain with coughing, the nurse splints the client's chest with a firm pillow. Chest physical therapy techniques such as postural drainage and percussion may facilitate airway drainage and movement of secretions. Secretions are expectorated more easily if they are liquefied. Therefore, the nurse offers the client warm fluids and encourages a total fluid intake of 3000 mL/day unless otherwise contraindicated by renal or cardiac disease. The client with pneumonia is usually easily fatigued, with exercise causing hypoxia. Therefore, the bedridden client should be assisted with changes in position every 2 hours. If the client can tolerate sitting in a chair, the nurse assists him or her with this activity because it helps to further mobilize secretions. The nurse offers small frequent meals to conserve the client's energy and to promote nutrition for healing.

The client with a weak cough and weak pulmonary musculature may be unable to expectorate sputum. In this situation, the nurse performs nasotracheal suctioning. If the client is hypoxemic, the nurse asks the client to take several deep breaths or oxygenates the client with 100% oxygen via an Ambu bag before, during, and immediately after the suctioning. After coughing, suctioning, or other activity, the client is assessed for increased dyspnea, tachycardia, or arrhythmia. Skin color, particularly of the lips and nail beds, is continually assessed for cyanosis, which indicates oxygen depletion. For the client who expectorates productively, mouth care is given frequently, and lips are lubricated as necessary because the oral cavity and lips can become quite dry. Ice chips should be kept at the bedside.

All clients are not hospitalized for pneumonia. It is common for clients to be treated with antibiotics on an outpatient basis. This milder form of infection may be termed *walking pneumonia.*

Drug therapy. The use of mucolytic agents (e.g., acetylcysteine [Mucomyst]) and expectorants (e.g., iodides) has been found to be of marginal value in the treatment of pneumonia. However, bronchodilators may be valuable when there is a significant degree of bronchospasm. Bronchodilators are frequently given via the aerosol route. Commonly used drugs are metaproterenol sulfate (Alupent), isoetharine (Bronkosol), and terbutaline sulfate (Brethine). Inhaled steroid preparations are generally not used with acute pneumonia except in the presence of bronchial asthma or respiratory failure.

Antibiotic therapy is given for all types of pneumonia except viral. The appropriate antibiotic is determined by the results of the sputum Gram's stain. Penicillin G is the antibiotic of choice for pneumococcal pneumonia. Drugs that are effective for other bacterial strains are erythromycin (E-Mycin, ERYC), clindamycin (Cleocin), cephalosporins, and other penicillins. The hospitalized client is usually given these medications via the intravenous route.

Oxygen therapy. Clients may be given oxygen via a Venturi mask or nasal cannula. The prescription for oxygen is based on the degree of hypoxemia. ABG analysis determines the need for oxygen therapy. Most clients are managed with intermediate flow rates of 4 to 6 L/minute, or up to 40% oxygen via a Venturi mask. Higher concentrations of oxygen (more than 2 to 3 L/minute) are avoided in clients with chronic obstructive pulmonary disease (COPD) because the low arterial oxygen level is this client's primary drive to breathe. If the client's condition continues to deteriorate while nasal or mask oxygen is given more aggressive therapy is required. Intubation and mechanical ventilation may be necessary for the client in respiratory failure. These modalities are discussed in detail under the later heading Collaborative Management in the section on COPD.

Ineffective Breathing Pattern

Planning: client goals. The primary goal for this diagnosis is that the client will have improved ventilation as evidenced by adequate chest expansion, clear lung fields on auscultation, and elimination of fatigue and dyspnea.

Interventions: nonsurgical management. The nurse monitors the client's rate and depth of respirations and notes the use of accessory muscles and pursed-lip breathing. If the client is coughing frequently but nonproductively, the nurse assists the client in conserving energy and using respiratory muscles more effectively. The client is placed in an upright position with the head of the bed elevated. Many clients are comfortable sitting on the side of the bed and leaning over the bedside table with the elbows forward. This position allows for enhanced chest expansion. The nurse auscultates the chest anteriorly and posteriorly to assess the degree of pulmonary congestion and to determine the client's baseline. The nurse helps the client to take several slow, deep breaths and then to cough. The client is encouraged to take slow deep breaths, or to take several pursed-lip breaths, between periods of coughing. The client further conserves energy and coughs more productively by using diaphragmatic breathing techniques (described under the later heading Collaborative Management in the section on COPD).

The client's level of anxiety is a major factor in the use of energy and consequently the experience of dyspnea. Therefore, the nurse alleviates anxiety and promotes effective breathing patterns by caring for the client in an unhurried manner and listening to the client carefully. When teaching to cough or deep breathe, it is helpful to demonstrate each activity for the client and to help the client into the desired position. The nurse also assists the client in splinting the chest with a pillow when coughing.

After the client completes the coughing and breathing regimen, the nurse auscultates the chest to assess the effectiveness of these procedures. In addition, the client is given a mild analgesic to alleviate pain and to promote comfort. The nurse assesses the ABGs for hypoxemia and hypercapnia because analgesics may depress respiration. Cough suppressants are given with caution if the client is experiencing an irritating, nonproductive cough, which depletes energy.

Activity Intolerance

Planning: client goals. The major goal for this nursing diagnosis is that the client will be able to perform self-care and other daily activities. In addition, the client should be able to walk for short periods without experiencing dyspnea or tachycardia.

Interventions: nonsurgical management. The client with pneumonia tires quite easily. A balanced rest and activity regimen should be planned on the basis of the client's feeling of fatigue and the extent of hypoxemia. If supplemental oxygen is ordered, it should be used continually, particularly during periods of increased energy use such as bathing or walking for short periods. It is important that the nurse allow the client to perform self-care activities as slowly as the client feels it is necessary.

The nurse instructs the client not to rush through morning activities because rushing is likely to increase hypoxemia, dyspnea, and fatigue. The nurse works with the physical therapist to teach the client muscle-strengthening exercises if the client has had a significant period of bed rest. As the client increases his or her level of activity, the nurse continually assesses the physiologic response by noting skin color changes, pulse rate and regularity, and blood pressure. Activity is gradually increased daily, so that by the time of discharge, the client can ambulate for short periods.

■ Discharge Planning

Home Care Preparation

No special structural changes are needed in the home. If the home consists of more than one story, the client may prefer to stay on the first floor for a few weeks because stair climbing may increase fatigue and dyspnea. Bath and hygiene needs may be met by using a bedside commode if a bathroom is not located on the first level.

Client/Family Education

Before discharging the recovering client with pneumonia, the nurse emphasizes to the client and family or significant others the importance of rest and a gradual increase in activity to avoid fatigue. In addition, the client is instructed to maintain natural resistance to infection with proper nutrition and adequate fluid intake. The client is warned to avoid chilling and exposure to others with upper respiratory tract infections or viruses. The client and family are made aware of the fact that one episode of pneumonia increases susceptibility to recurrent infections.

The client is taught about all medications that will be continued at home. The nurse provides written instructions as necessary. It is important that the client understand the rationale for antibiotic therapy. The client is given instructions to continue use of the incentive spirometer and to perform deep breathing and coughing exercises four times a day for 6 to 8 weeks. The client is also instructed to notify the physician if he or she experiences chills, fever, dyspnea, hemoptysis, increasing fatigue, or other respiratory complications.

Psychosocial Preparation

The prolonged convalescent phase of the disease process, particularly in the elderly client, can be frustrating and perhaps depressing. Fatigue, weakness, and residual cough can last for weeks. The client may fear that he or she will never return to a "normal" level of functioning. It is important that the nurse prepare the client for the course of the disease and offer reassurance so that complete recovery will occur.

Health Care Resources

Clients who smoke are taught that this is a risk factor for pneumonia. The nurse provides information on smoking cessation classes through the American Lung Association (ALA) and American Cancer Society. Clients can also be given information booklets on pneumonia provided by the ALA. If the client has not already been vaccinated against influenza or pneumococcal pneumonia, he or she should be encouraged to take this preventive measure.

 Evaluation

On the basis of the identified nursing diagnoses, the nurse evaluates the care of the client with pneumonia. The expected outcomes are that the client

1. Maintains a patent airway
2. Does not experience dyspnea

3. Is not hypoxic
4. Performs self-care and other daily activities independently
5. Walks for short periods without experiencing dyspnea or tachycardia
6. Describes and complies with the medication regimen

ACUTE BRONCHITIS

OVERVIEW

Acute bronchitis is an inflammation of the bronchi that is associated with increased production of mucus. The larynx and the trachea may also be inflamed, causing tracheobronchitis or laryngotracheobronchitis. The individual experiences production of excessive mucus and cough. Most persons suffer from these infections many times throughout life.

Pathophysiology

When the conducting airways are assaulted by chemical agents or microorganisms, they respond by inducing an inflammatory response. The typical sequence of this response includes vasoconstriction followed by vasodilation, and transudation of fluid into interstitial spaces and into the luminal surface of the airways. PMNs migrate from the capillaries into the mucous exudate and change it to the characteristically yellow-green sputum of tracheobronchitis. Ulceration of the mucosa may develop, with exfoliation of bronchial epithelial cells, and bleeding may occur. This bleeding results in blood-tinged mucus. The extent of injury depends on the distribution of the noxious agent and/or organism and its concentration at various levels of the tracheobronchial tree.

Etiology

A wide variety of agents can produce acute bronchitis, including noxious gases, particulate irritants, and various microorganisms. Some common infecting organisms are *Streptococcus, Staphylococcus, Haemophilus,* and *P. aeruginosa.* Infection of the trachea and bronchi commonly occurs after upper respiratory tract viral syndromes.

In adults, the most common cause of acute bronchitis is exacerbation of chronic bronchitis. In the elderly, predisposing underlying conditions such as chronic bronchitis or emphysema combined with an aging immune system account for the onset of acute disease. Other clients who are prone to develop the disease are those with immunoglobulin deficiencies, ciliary dyskinesia, or cystic fibrosis. Any individual with a defect in mucous secretion or in the mucociliary transport system is prone to the development of acute bronchitis. Because smoke causes bronchial irritation and ciliary paralysis, smokers are also at risk.

Incidence

Acute bronchitis occurs commonly and severely in the elderly, as well as in infants and children. It is frequently associated with viral infections, so it may be more prevalent in late fall and winter months.

PREVENTION

Many of the preventive measures that were specified for pneumonia also apply to acute bronchitis because the condition may be associated with pneumonia, particularly in the elderly, or in those with chronic respiratory diseases. Clients who are at risk are cautioned to avoid crowds, especially during influenza season, and to be inoculated with influenza and pneumococcal vaccines. Smokers are made aware of the relationship between smoking and bronchitis and can be given information on smoking cessation groups from the American Heart Association and the ALA. Booklets on bronchitis are also available from the ALA. If the cause of bronchitis is inhalation of noxious gases or particulate material, clients are cautioned to avoid exposure to these substances.

COLLABORATIVE MANAGEMENT

 Assessment

History

In assessing the client with an episode of acute bronchitis, *age* and the presence of *chronic lung disease* are important to note because they are major risk factors. The nurse also inquires as to the use of *medications,* particularly steroids, bronchodilators, or antibiotics that are being taken for an ongoing chronic condition or recent infection. The client's use of *cigarettes* and *alcohol* is recorded, as well as the client's recent sleep, rest, and *activity* regimen. The nurse ascertains whether the client has been exposed to influenza or has experienced a *recent viral episode* or infection. Because environmental exposure to noxious gases or particulate material predisposes an individual to bronchitis, the nurse questions the client about exposure to forms of *environmental pollution.* Finally, the nurse lists the symptoms that brought the client to the hospital or physician's office. Symptoms commonly reported are dyspnea, increased irritability and anxiety, fatigue, sleep disturbance, chest tightness, chest fullness, wheezing, and coughing.

Physical Assessment: Clinical Manifestations

The client with acute bronchitis is assessed for *dyspnea;* the nurse observes the client's breathing pattern, color, and position. A pulmonary examination is performed, including auscultation for *adventitious sounds* and percussion for *abnormal dullness* (see Chap. 60 for a further explanation of techniques). The *amount, color, quantity, and quality of sputum* are observed, as well as the *frequency of coughing.* The nurse assesses *vital signs* and notes temperature elevation with tachycardia. Confusion and mental status changes occur frequently in the elderly, which indicate hypoxemia.

Psychosocial Assessment

The client with acute bronchitis is likely to be dyspneic and consequently anxious and irritable. The nurse assesses the client's behavior and observes facial and shoulder muscle tension and speech patterns. It is helpful for the nurse to assist the client into a comfortable position and to talk slowly and calmly.

Laboratory Findings

As with pneumonia, sputum cultures are important for determining the causative organism so that the client can receive appropriate antibiotics. In addition, a CBC with differential count is done. ABGs may be assayed if the client appears to be hypoxemic and to need supplemental oxygen.

Other Diagnostic Tests

In the presence of obstructive disease, severe hypoxemia, and dyspnea, pulmonary function studies are done to gather baseline information and are repeated later to assess the response to treatment. Chest x-ray films may also be taken to follow the course of the disease.

 ## Analysis: Nursing Diagnosis

Common Diagnoses

The following nursing diagnoses are common in clients with acute bronchitis:

1. Ineffective airway clearance related to increased production of mucus
2. Impaired gas exchange related to airway obstruction

Additional Diagnoses

In addition to the common diagnoses, the client with acute bronchitis may present with one or more of the following diagnoses:

1. Pain related to excessive coughing
2. Altered thought processes related to decreased cerebral oxygenation

3. Hyperthermia related to the infectious process
4. Sleep pattern disturbance related to excessive coughing
5. Fatigue related to excessive coughing
6. Knowledge deficit related to disease and treatment regimen

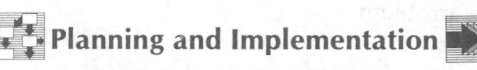 ## Planning and Implementation

Ineffective Airway Clearance

Planning: client goals. The major goals for this nursing diagnosis are that the client will (1) maintain a patent airway and (2) facilitate the removal of mucous plugs.

Interventions: nonsurgical management. The client with bronchitis is assisted with coughing and breathing techniques that help him or her to maximize expectoration of secretions while conserving energy (see Figs. 62–21 and 62–22). The client who is not educated in these techniques becomes extremely fatigued because of the frequent coughing that is triggered by bronchial irritation. In addition, the client with airway congestion benefits from postural drainage and chest physical therapy techniques (see Fig. 62–24). If the client's illness is not complicated by cardiac or renal failure, a fluid intake of 2000 to 3000 mL/day is encouraged. This intake assists in liquefaction of secretions and in the maintenance of fluid balance. A humidifier in the room and aerosol treatments are frequently ordered to further liquefy secretions and provide maximal bronchodilation. For the client who cannot break the cough cycle related to bronchial irritation, cough suppressants are given with caution. Antibiotic therapy may also be prescribed for identified pathogens or prophylactically to prevent further respiratory complications. Inhaled bronchodilators may be used to facilitate an open airway and clearance of secretions.

Impaired Gas Exchange

Planning: client goals. The major goals for this nursing diagnosis are that the client will (1) achieve arterial oxygen saturation and arterial carbon dioxide levels within the normal range and (2) prevent the development of perfusion abnormalities related to patches of atelectasis.

Interventions: nonsurgical management. After the administration of pulmonary treatment measures, including chest physical therapy, postural drainage, and coughing and deep breathing, the nurse assesses the client's lung fields for adventitious sounds and diminished sounds. Chest x-ray results assist the nurse in determining the effectiveness of treatment while the client is hospitalized. The presence of unilateral or bilateral infiltrates indicates perfusion abnormalities in those areas. An assessment of ABG results by the nurse and physician results in an accurate determination of the oxygen prescription and respiratory treatment regimen for the hypoxemic client.

■ Discharge Planning

The client with bronchitis is frequently discharged to the home environment if there are no other severe underlying pulmonary problems.

Home Care Preparation

Before the client is discharged to the home setting, the nurse helps the client to identify sources of indoor pollution. The client is advised to avoid using detergents and cleaners that produce noxious gases or fumes. Woodburning stoves are a source of pollution and bronchial irritation. If this type of stove is the client's primary source of heat, the client is assisted in developing heating alternatives. The client is warned that frequent use of fireplaces may be a source of irritation. The client and family are instructed to remove dust particles that settle on furniture, rugs, blinds, and baseboards. If dust is a significant irritant for the client, scatter rugs over wood floors are more desirable than wall-to-wall carpeting. Before the client returns home, it is advisable that filters on heating and air-conditioning systems be checked and replaced as necessary to prevent the dissemination of dust and particulate matter in the home.

Client/Family Education

The client recovering from bronchitis is instructed to increase activity gradually to avoid fatigue. It is advisable to avoid crowds, chilling, and exposure to others with upper respiratory tract infections or viruses. The client is instructed to avoid smoking because smoke is irritating to the tracheobronchial tree. The nurse clarifies the relationship between smoking and bronchitis or other related pulmonary diseases. The nurse also makes recommendations about the work environment if noxious stimuli inhaled in the work setting are the precipitating cause of the illness. The nurse reviews the client's medications, which may include oral antibiotics, bronchodilators, inhaled bronchodilators, and inhaled steroids. It is important that the client understand the purpose, timing, and side effects of medications. Clients frequently have difficulty in using metered-dose bronchodilator inhalers, so the nurse asks the client to demonstrate the use of this before discharge (see the Client/Family Education feature entitled How to Use an Inhaler Correctly, in the section on COPD). The client is also instructed to maintain adequate hydration to liquefy secretions. The nurse reviews the prescribed coughing and deep breathing techniques and provides written materials if available.

Psychosocial Preparation

The client who has experienced dyspnea is anxious that this situation may recur. Therefore, the client and family are reassured about the prevention of future episodes. Elderly clients generally have a longer recovery period from acute bronchitis. Therefore, the nurse makes a special effort to repeat the information that is provided at discharge several times with the client and family members. Written materials and time schedules for medications are essential. The client with underlying pulmonary disease may continue to have dyspnea. To reduce anxiety, the nurse talks slowly and uses demonstration as the primary teaching technique.

Health Care Resources

The ALA is an excellent resource for clients with bronchitis. Through this organization, clients can be provided with information on bronchitis, smoking cessation classes, and exercise classes for clients with other pulmonary diseases. The American Cancer Society and local hospitals also present classes for smoking cessation, but the ALA is likely to disseminate this information.

 Evaluation

The nurse evaluates the care of the client with acute bronchitis on the basis of the identified nursing diagnoses. The expected outcomes are that the client

1. Demonstrates appropriate coughing and deep breathing techniques
2. Breathes comfortably without the use of accessory neck muscles
3. Describes and complies with the medication regimen
4. States that dyspnea is alleviated
5. Describes potential environmental hazards and avoids them
6. States the risk factors that are associated with bronchitis and avoids them

CHRONIC OBSTRUCTIVE PULMONARY DISEASE

OVERVIEW

COPD is actually a group of diseases including emphysema, chronic bronchitis, and asthma (see the accompanying illustration). It is also referred to as chronic obstructive lung disease (COLD) and chronic airflow limitation (CAL). Usually, asthma, chronic bronchitis, and emphysema are not seen as distinct clinical conditions. Instead, they coexist in most clients, although one disease may predominate.

These disorders are chronic and are characterized by progressive limitation of the flow of air into and out of

WHAT HAPPENS IN COPD

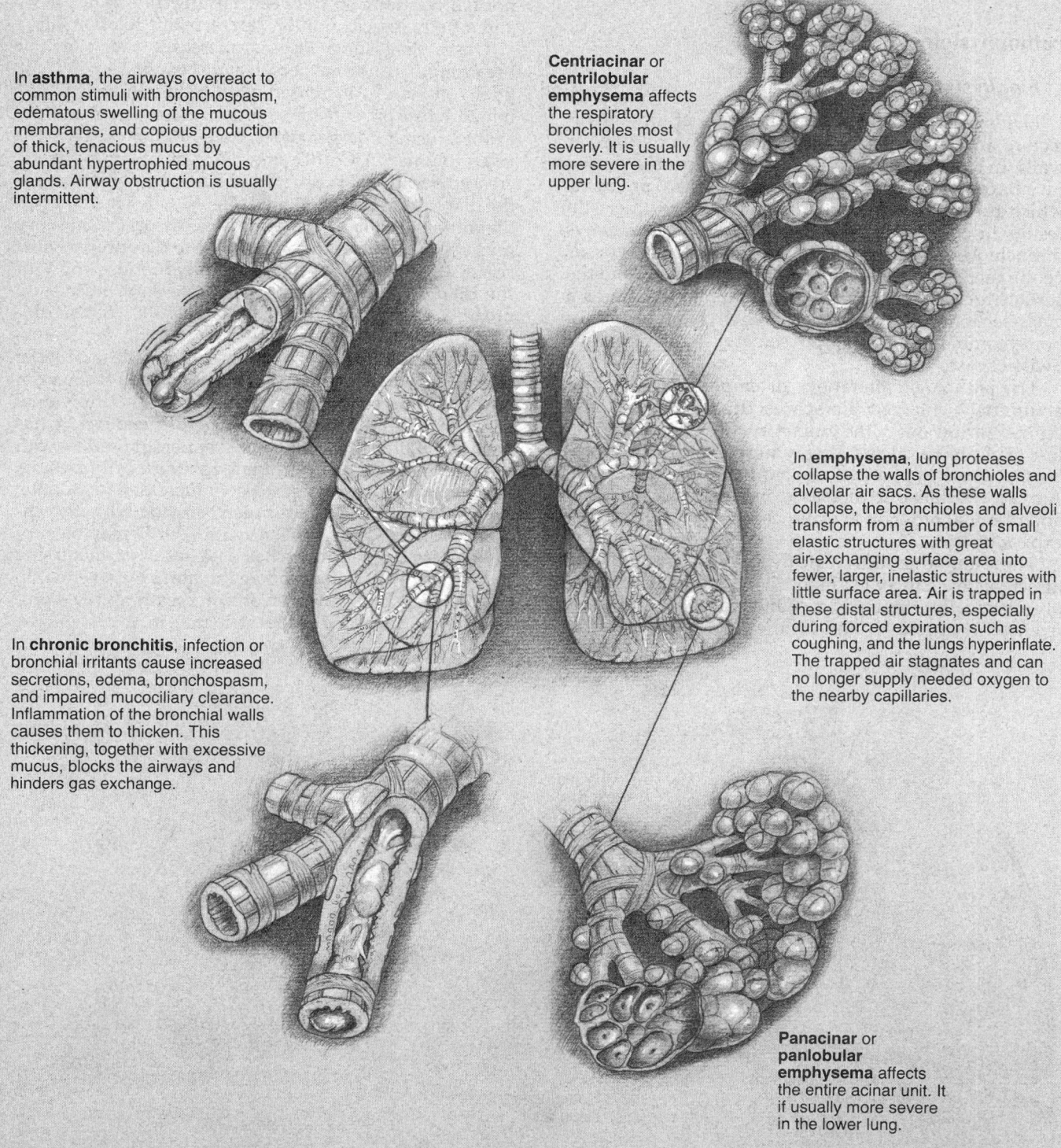

In **asthma**, the airways overreact to common stimuli with bronchospasm, edematous swelling of the mucous membranes, and copious production of thick, tenacious mucus by abundant hypertrophied mucous glands. Airway obstruction is usually intermittent.

Centriacinar or **centrilobular emphysema** affects the respiratory bronchioles most severly. It is usually more severe in the upper lung.

In **emphysema**, lung proteases collapse the walls of bronchioles and alveolar air sacs. As these walls collapse, the bronchioles and alveoli transform from a number of small elastic structures with great air-exchanging surface area into fewer, larger, inelastic structures with little surface area. Air is trapped in these distal structures, especially during forced expiration such as coughing, and the lungs hyperinflate. The trapped air stagnates and can no longer supply needed oxygen to the nearby capillaries.

In **chronic bronchitis**, infection or bronchial irritants cause increased secretions, edema, bronchospasm, and impaired mucociliary clearance. Inflammation of the bronchial walls causes them to thicken. This thickening, together with excessive mucus, blocks the airways and hinders gas exchange.

Panacinar or **panlobular emphysema** affects the entire acinar unit. It if usually more severe in the lower lung.

the lungs. COPD is characterized by elevated airway resistance, irreversible lung distention, and ABG imbalance. COPD eventually leads to pulmonary insufficiency, pulmonary hypertension, and cor pulmonale.

Pathophysiology

Emphysema

Emphysema is identified by alteration of lung architecture and is characterized by destruction of alveolar walls. In emphysema, the alveolar destruction is caused by abnormalities of lung enzymes, called *proteases,* which break down elastin. This abnormality in elastin results in collapse or narrowing of the small airways (bronchioles and the walls of the small air sacs, or alveoli), thereby decreasing the number of alveoli and the surface area of the pulmonary membrane. Whereas a cross-section of normal lung parenchyma looks like a honeycomb, that of an emphysematous lung looks like Swiss cheese.

The pathologic alterations of emphysema result in abnormally enlarged air spaces (hyperinflation) and limited airflow out of the lung. Airway enlargement and loss of elastic recoil and airway support structures combine to cause trapping of stagnant air and obstruction. Airway resistance is increased because of respiratory and terminal bronchiole walls, especially during forced expiration.

These abnormalities create two serious problems that affect gas exchange: (1) blood flow and airflow to the alveolar walls where gas exchange takes place are uneven or mismatched, and (2) the work of pushing air through narrowed, obstructed airways becomes increasingly more difficult.

Some alveoli have an adequate supply of blood but little air, whereas others get an adequate supply of fresh air but not enough blood. Gas exchange depends on the normal relationship between airflow and blood flow, and a pathologic condition can alter this relationship.

Obstructive lung disease increases the work of breathing. The normal person at rest uses 10% of VC for tidal volume. An increased work of breathing is determined when oxygen consumption is increased and the client is using a larger percentage of vital capacity for tidal volume. In COPD, the work of breathing is increased because of the hyperinflated lung, which causes the diaphragm to be flattened (Fig. 62–1). The flattened diaphragm requires the use of accessory respiratory muscles during expiration, when the diaphragm must rise against gravity. A healthy individual uses 65% of the diaphragm and 35% of the accessory muscles to breathe; individuals with COPD use 30% of the diaphragm and 70% of the accessory muscles to breathe. Predominant use of the accessory muscles for tidal breathing increases the COPD client's need for oxygen and gives the sensation of air hunger. The individual reacts by initiating inspiration before expiration has been completed. The result is a dyspneic individual with an inefficient and uncoordinated pattern of breathing. In severe cases, the oxygen cost of increased ventilation exceeds the additional oxygen provided by the increased effort. Thus, a client with COPD may be supplying less oxygen to tissues as a result of increasing pulmonary ventilation and aggravating hypoxemia. In addition, such increased work of breathing may produce extra carbon dioxide at a rate in excess of the

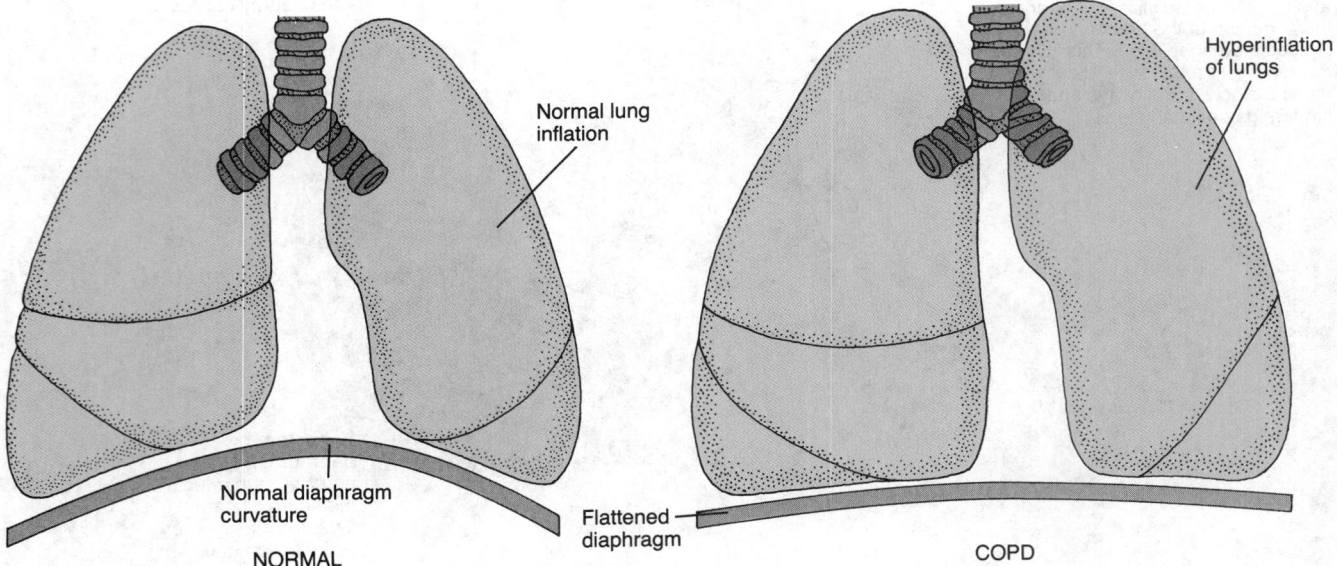

Figure 62–1

Comparison of normal diaphragm shape and lung inflation with those in the client with COPD.

client's ability to eliminate it, which aggravates hypercapnic acidosis.

Emphysema is classified according to patterns of destruction and dilation of the gas-exchanging units (acini) of the lung. The patterns of emphysema may exist alone or in combination in the same lung. Each acinus—defined as all structures distal to the terminal bronchiole—is composed of respiratory bronchioles, which divide into alveolar ducts, which in turn divide into alveolar sacs. *Panacinar*, or *panlobular*, *emphysema* (PLE) involves destruction of the alveoli in the pulmonary acinus until only a few strands of tissue and blood vessels remain. Panacinar emphysema is a diffuse disease that is usually more severe in the lower lung area. In *centriacinar*, or *centrilobular*, *emphysema* (CLE), fenestrations selectively develop in respiratory bronchioles and allow spaces to develop as tissue walls disintegrate. Although centrilobular emphysema is a diffuse disease process that commonly affects the upper portions of the lung most severely, one may encounter extreme variability in damage to the acini within the same lung segment.

Chronic Bronchitis

In *chronic bronchitis*, infection and bronchial irritants contribute to cause increased secretions, edema, bronchospasm, and impaired mucociliary clearance. Diffuse airway obstruction occurs because of inflammatory changes in bronchial walls, which causes them to thicken and impinge on the airway lumen. This thickening, together with production of excessive mucus, obliterates some of the smaller air passages and narrows larger ones. Occasionally, these changes occur at the level of segmental bronchi and therefore produce increased airway resistance at this point. Chronic bronchitis hinders airflow and gas exchange in part because of mucous plugs and secondary infections. As a result, the arterial blood oxygen concentration (arterial PO_2) falls and the arterial blood carbon dioxide concentration (arterial PCO_2) increases, which leads to respiratory acidosis. Chapters 14 and 15 discuss respiratory acidosis in detail.

Asthma

Bronchial asthma can be defined as intermittent airway narrowing caused by three processes: constriction of bronchial smooth muscle, excess production of mucus, and mucosal edema. Asthma, like bronchitis, affects the airways, not the air sacs, and may be reversible. Therefore, asthma does not typically lead to emphysema; however, asthma may coexist with emphysema and bronchitis. In the adult, asthma usually presents as a *chronic* long-term illness that can occur at any time. *Acute* asthma is discussed thoroughly in pediatric nursing textbooks. Asthma characteristically occurs as attacks that are separated by symptom-free intervals, but it may also occur on a continuous basis. The airways of an individual with asthma are overreac-

tive and ready to respond to various stimuli. In adult asthmatics, changes in the environment within the airways precipitate a wheezing episode. Because the treatment for asthma is aimed at preventing wheezing episodes, it is vital to understand the mechanisms by which environmental stimuli cause bronchoconstriction. The more common nonallergic agents or stimuli that cause bronchoconstriction are exercise, fog, odors, smoke, aerosols, and dust. Pollen, mold spores, and animal danders usually produce bronchoconstriction only in the truly allergic asthmatic. Emotional excitement and anxiety are not causes of asthma but may aggravate or even initiate an episode of wheezing.

Inhaled agents stimulate the contraction of airway smooth muscle by different mechanisms. After the agent is inhaled, it is in contact with several different cells within the airway lumen before it can reach the airway smooth muscle itself. Some agents cause bronchoconstriction by directly stimulating the smooth muscle. However, the direct effects of many environmental stimuli are likely to be dissipated within a short distance of the airway lumen. These agents, then, are more likely to cause smooth muscle contraction *indirectly* by affecting neural pathways, mediated by activation of afferent nerve endings and the ultimate release of bronchoconstrictor substances.

Three neural pathways have been studied in environmentally induced bronchoconstriction. The *muscarinic pathway*, the most studied, involves reflex activation of the parasympathetic efferent nerves that innervate the smooth muscle. When these nerves are activated, they release acetylcholine, which directly causes contraction of airway smooth muscle. Another neural pathway involves *alpha-adrenergic* activity. This pathway was suggested on the basis of the observation that alpha-adrenergic blockage can inhibit exercise-induced bronchoconstriction. However, adrenergic nerves are not prominent in the vicinity of airway smooth muscle. The third possible neural pathway is the stimulated *release of* bronchoconstrictor *peptides* from airway afferent nerve endings that are activated by retrograde stimulation via an axonal reflex.

The nonneural mechanisms of bronchoconstriction involve humoral cells: macrophages, eosinophils, and mast cells. *Macrophages* are present throughout the tracheobronchial tree. By contact with one of the environmental stimuli, macrophages can be activated to stimulate the release of platelets that have potent contractile effects on airway smooth muscle.

Eosinophils are likewise present in the lumina of the airways and occur in increased numbers in clients with asthma. The exact role of eosinophils remains unknown, but it is believed that they secrete bronchoconstrictor sulfadeopeptide leukotrienes.

There is indirect evidence to suggest the role of *mast cells* in bronchoconstriction. The drug cromolyn sodium (Intal) causes mast cell stabilization. The other line of evidence supporting the action of mast cells in the response to environmental stimuli comes from measurements of histamine and the chemotactic factor in venous blood, which are thought to be released from mast cells after an inhalation challenge.

Bronchiectasis

Bronchiectasis is an uncommon, chronic respiratory disorder in which one or more bronchi are abnormally and permanently dilated. It is sometimes classified as part of COPD, but it tends to be the result of frequent childhood respiratory infections. Management is similar to that for adult clients with COPD.

Complications of COPD

Among complications of COPD, acute *respiratory infections* cause increased production of mucus, increased bronchial smooth muscle irritability, and edema of the involved mucosa. Airflow is limited, the work of breathing increases, and dyspnea ensues. A bacterial cause cannot be identified in most acute respiratory illnesses. Therefore, even in the absence of adequate supportive data, severely compromised clients are treated with antibiotics. Some physicians prescribe antibiotics on an as needed basis for the client to self-medicate according to changes in sputum appearance.

In a client with worsening dyspnea, consideration must be given to the presence of *cardiac failure* and *cor pulmonale*. These problems are difficult to detect because the clinical signs of cor pulmonale are generally obscured by those of the underlying COPD. Symptoms include fatigue, weakness, and increasing dyspnea. An enlarged, tender liver; warm cyanotic extremities with bounding pulses; cyanotic facies; distended neck veins; cardiac enlargement; lower sternal or epigastric pulsations; gastrointestinal disturbances; and dependent edema may be noted during the physical examination. COPD places a heavy workload on the heart, especially the right side, which is responsible for pumping blood into the lungs. As the disease progresses, the amount of oxygen in the blood decreases, which causes important blood vessels in the lung to constrict. To pump blood through these narrowed vessels, the right side of the heart must generate high pressures. In response to this heavy workload, the right chambers of the heart enlarge and thicken, which causes right-sided heart failure, or cor pulmonale.

Cardiac dysrhythmias occur fairly frequently in clients with COPD. They may be due to hypoxemia, other cardiac disease, drug effects, or respiratory acidosis (discussed in Chaps. 14 and 15).

Status asthmaticus is another complication of bronchial asthma. It is a severe, potentially life-threatening acute episode of bronchospasm that tends to intensify once it begins. The client presents to the emergency room of the hospital with extremely labored breathing and wheezing that is audible without a stethoscope. Accessory muscle use and neck vein distention are common. If the condition is not reversed, the client can experience cor pulmonale, pneumothorax, and eventually cardiac and/or respiratory arrest. Immediate administration of intravenous fluids, bronchodilators, and oxygen is initiated in an attempt to reverse the acute condition. When wheezing diminishes, medical management is similar to that for any client with COPD.

Etiology

Cigarette Smoking

Beyond any question, cigarette smoking is *the* most important risk factor. A careful smoking history should include the age at which the client started to smoke, the number of packs smoked daily, an estimate of the amount of each cigarette or other tobacco smoked, and the type of cigarette or other tobacco smoked. This information helps to quantify the tobacco exposure. The harmful effects of tobacco result in part because the inhaled smoke stimulates excess release of elastase protease from cells that are normally found in the lung. The elastase protease breaks down elastin, the major structural protein of the lung. In addition, oxidants that are found in tobacco inactivate a significant number of the protease inhibitors that are present, thereby decreasing the amount of active antiprotease available. Smoking also paralyzes the cilia and therefore impairs mucociliary clearance.

Family History

It has been known for a number of years that emphysema and chronic bronchitis may occur in families more often than would be expected by chance. However, in some individuals a genetic defect results in decreased levels of an antiprotease called alpha$_1$-antitrypsin. The client with emphysema that is associated with alpha$_1$-antitrypsin deficiency is frequently young, has rapidly progressive obstructive pulmonary disease, and may have obstructive pulmonary disease in the absence of smoking. The emphysema that is associated with alpha$_1$-antitrypsin deficiency results from a lack of anti–neutrophil elastase protection in the lower respiratory tract. Alpha$_1$-antitrypsin is the principal inhibitor of neutrophil elastase, an omnivorous protease that can destroy alveolar walls.

In alpha$_1$-antitrypsin deficiency, the fragile alveolar walls have little protection against the elastase released by the neutrophils in the lower respiratory tract. The disease progresses slowly but can be markedly accelerated by cigarette smoking or other lung irritation. As part of the inflammatory response to tobacco smoke, an increased number of inflammatory cells are present in the lungs of smokers. These cells may result in an increased amount of elastase being present in the lung. In addition, tobacco smoke can oxidize the alpha$_1$-antitrypsin in the lung, which further contributes to the imbalance between levels of elastase and levels of alpha$_1$-antitrypsin. The net result can be excess levels of elastase, which leads to destruction of alveolar walls and the development of emphysema. Panlobular emphysema is typically seen in clients with alpha$_1$-antitrypsin deficiency.

Air Pollution

At the present time, it appears that the effect of air pollution is additive to tobacco exposure, but alone it plays only a relatively small role in nonsmokers.

Incidence

More than 17 million Americans are thought to have COPD. Since 1968, COPD has been the fastest rising major cause of death in the United States (ALA, 1983). In 1983, an estimated 62,000 Americans died of chronic pulmonary disease. It is responsible for a greater limitation of activity than any other major disease category; 40% more persons with emphysema reported limitation of activity than did those with heart disease (ALA, 1983).

PREVENTION

COPD can best be prevented by avoiding its primary cause—cigarette smoking. This measure is particularly important because there is no known cure for COPD. In individuals with a genetic predisposition (alpha$_1$-antitrypsin deficiency) to COPD, it becomes even more critical that they do not smoke. The nurse should be aware that avoiding smoking almost always prevents COPD from developing and that cessation of smoking slows the disease process. If a person can stop smoking before serious COPD develops, the rate at which lung function deteriorates returns to normal. Unfortunately, some lung damage is irreversible. The nurse should not minimize the importance of smoking cessation but yet should be cognizant of the difficulty that this may pose for the client. Teaching the client about the various programs to assist the client to quit smoking may be more beneficial than just telling the client to stop. The nurse refers individuals who are not comfortable in group settings to self-help booklets or videotapes produced by the ALA.

Clients in whom COPD manifests itself predominantly as asthma need to know how to prevent airway irritation. The nurse instructs the client to keep the home environment as free from dust as possible. If that is not possible, the client's bedroom must be kept dust-free. If the client is the individual responsible for cleaning, he or she should be instructed to wear a mask when cleaning. The nurse reminds the client to use air conditioning and to keep cooling and heating vents clean. Clients with asthma also need to avoid pet dander. If the client is particularly close to a pet, he or she might first try to bar the pet from the bedroom before giving the pet away. The client should be instructed to avoid using any sprays (e.g., for hair, deodorant, cleaning, and air freshener). The client needs to avoid all irritating fumes, such as gasoline, paint, ammonia, and chlorine, as well as smoke from a fireplace. Clients are informed to avoid occupational exposure to dusts and fumes and to avoid air pollution, including smoke-filled rooms. The nurse provides the client with the phone number of the Air Pollution Control Index, which is sponsored by the National Weather Bureau. Finally, clients with COPD can best prevent acute respiratory tract infections and exacerbations of their disease by getting influenza and pneumococcal immunizations.

COLLABORATIVE MANAGEMENT

 Assessment

History

If the nurse develops a systematic process for assessing the client with COPD, significant findings are less likely to be overlooked. The nurse begins by asking the client to discuss his or her *chief complaint*. The nurse pays particular attention to the client's ability to answer questions. Can he or she give lucid answers and state them in complete sentences? Or is breathlessness so severe that one- or two-word answers are given to the questions. After the chief complaint has been discussed, the nurse proceeds to the classic symptoms of COPD.

Cough, dyspnea, and *wheezing* are the three classic symptoms of COPD, although they occur in various combinations and intensity. When eliciting a history from a client with COPD, the nurse questions the client about each of these symptoms. *Early* symptoms of COPD include mild shortness of breath and a slight cough in the morning. The nurse determines the client's coughing pattern by asking when, if ever, he or she is troubled by coughing and how the cough sounds—dry, hacking, barking, or loose. The nurse tries to determine whether the client's cough is related to cigarette smoking or irritants. The cough may be productive or nonproductive of sputum. The client is asked if sputum is clear or colored and how much is expectorated per day. The client is asked to recall the time of day when most sputum is expectorated. Smokers typically cough when they get up in the morning; nonsmokers generally do not. When irritants trigger coughing, it usually occurs during exposure to the substances. The client is asked if sputum production is increasing; the sputum is usually clear. During acute respiratory tract infections, shortness of breath and coughing may be much more problematic. The sputum usually turns from clear to yellowish or greenish as a result of the infection. Episodes of wheezing are likely to occur, especially during or after colds or other respiratory tract infections.

The nurse always asks the client about *activity tolerance* and dyspnea at each visit or at each hospital admission. The client is asked to compare his or her activity level and shortness of breath compared with those of a month ago and a year ago. Likewise, the nurse elicits from the client any difficulty with *eating* and *sleeping*.

Many clients sleep in a semisitting position because breathlessness prevents them from lying down. The client is weighed at admission, and this weight is compared with previous weights. Clients with COPD have increased metabolic requirements associated with the increased work of breathing. The increased metabolic requirements plus bothersome dyspnea often result in the client's not eating balanced meals. The nurse asks the client to recall a typical day's meals and fluid intake. The nurse determines if the client uses any breathing maneuvers during dyspneic episodes and asks for a demonstration.

The nurse obtains a thorough *smoking history*, if appropriate. The number of packs smoked per day times the number of years smoked helps to quantify the client's cigarette use. Knowing the tar and nicotine content of the brand of cigarettes likewise aids in quantifying the smoking history.

The nurse asks the client to list current *medications*, including over-the-counter preparations. Questioning the client to determine knowledge of the actions and side effects of the drugs may point out opportunities for client education. The nurse also asks if the client has a readily available written *emergency plan* for respiratory emergencies. Although many clients think that they know this information, they should be reminded that during an emergency they may not be able to recall telephone numbers, names of people to contact, and doses of medications.

Physical Assessment: Clinical Manifestations

The nurse is pivotal in assessing the client with COPD throughout the course of the disease. The nurse inspects the chest to determine the *breathing rate and pattern*. Clients with respiratory muscle fatigue breathe with rapid, shallow respirations. Three breathing patterns are commonly seen in clients with respiratory muscle fatigue. In *abdominal paradox*, the diaphragm is nonfunctional so that inspiration is accomplished by the intercostal and abdominal accessory muscles. *Respiratory alternans* is diaphragmatic breathing alternating with abdominal paradox. In *asynchronous breathing*, the chest wall motion is unorganized. It has been suggested that respiratory alternans may serve to rest the diaphragm, whereas asynchronous breathing reflects the uncoordinated activity of fatigued muscles (Larson & Kim, 1987). The nurse checks the client for a *barrel chest* by noting the ratio between the anteroposterior diameter of the chest and its lateral diameter; the normal ratio is 1:2, but in individuals with COPD the ratio can be 1:1. The nurse observes the client's breathing to determine the use of accessory muscles and abnormal retractions. The nurse observes the client for cyanosis, capillary refill, and clubbing of the fingernails, which indicate decreased arterial oxygen levels.

When a client presents with a *predominant* diagnosis of chronic bronchitis or pulmonary emphysema, the nurse may expect the classic "blue bloater" or "pink puffer" manifestations. The bronchitic client typically has a cyanotic, or blue-tinged, appearance, a stocky build, and a complaint of excessive sputum production (blue bloater). By contrast, the client with emphysema appears cachectic with little or no change in skin color. This client most often complains of chronic cough and shortness of breath (pink puffer).

The nurse auscultates the chest to determine the depth of inspiration and to ascertain whether the breath sounds are unusual. A silent chest may be an ominous sign of airflow obstruction.

The nurse performs a systematic palpation of the client's anterior chest, feeling for areas of tenderness and abnormal retractions or moves. The nurse palpates for symmetric chest expansion. Respiratory assessment is detailed in Chapter 60.

Because of the likelihood of cardiac complications, the nurse determines *heart rate* and *rhythm*. The nurse asks the client to recall if he or she has had swelling of the feet and ankles and assesses for the presence of *edema*.

Psychosocial Assessment

Like any chronic disease, COPD tends to affect all aspects of a person's life: social, economic, and psychologic. COPD can plague a client in two ways: friends may avoid the client because of annoying coughs, repulsive sputum, or dyspnea; and the client may impose a self-isolation because dyspnea interferes with his or her ability to socialize with friends. The nurse questions the client about interests and hobbies to determine stimulation. The client should be cautioned about building or refinishing old furniture because this activity may expose the client to harsh chemical irritants.

The nurse questions the client about home conditions. The nurse determines if the client lives near a constant source of air pollution, such as a chemical factory or a freeway. Crowded living conditions facilitate the transmission of communicable respiratory conditions. Exposure to animals may precipitate allergic or asthmatic attacks.

The nurse assesses the client's ability to cope with chronic disease. Anxiety and fear related to episodes of dyspnea have a direct impact on the client's ability to participate in a full life. Local chapters of the ALA sponsor support groups. Various hospitals and physicians' offices likewise offer group support. The nurse should be knowledgeable about these resources and how to arrange access to them.

The client's economic status may be affected by the disease. A client may have had to retire early or stop working altogether. If the client is the breadwinner, severe COPD may dictate a role reversal with the spouse or mate. This change may have a deleterious impact on the client's self-image. If the client is still employed, the nurse questions him or her about exposure on the job to cigarette smoke or to other substances that may irritate the respiratory system.

Laboratory Findings

ABG assays are done initially to identify abnormalities of ventilation, oxygenation, and acid-base status. The nurse compares serial ABG results to determine the client's status and to guide in making clinical decisions. As COPD progresses, the amount of oxygen in the blood decreases and that of carbon dioxide increases.

Clients who exhibit signs of an acute respiratory tract infection have sputum samples collected for culture. A bacterial cause cannot be identified in most acute respiratory illness, but *Haemophilus influenzae* and *S. pneumoniae* are commonly isolated from the sputum of clients with COPD.

Radiographic Findings

Chest roentgenograms are taken routinely to rule out other chest diseases and to determine the progress of clients with respiratory tract infections. Chest x-ray films usually show marked overinflation, a flattened diaphragm, and decreased lung markings. Chest x-ray films may not be helpful in diagnosing early or moderate COPD.

Other Diagnostic Tests

COPD is classified from mild to severe and is diagnosed by pulmonary function tests. Airflow rates and lung volume measurements help to distinguish airway disease (obstructive disease) from restrictive patterns that are typical of interstitial lung disease. The three major components of pulmonary function tests are measurements that determine lung volumes, flow volume curves, and diffusion capacity, performed before and after bronchodilator agent is inhaled. In the client with asthma, an improvement in abnormal variables is usually observed after inhalation of a bronchodilator. However, if no reversibility is demonstrated after bronchodilator treatment, diagnosis of asthma is not excluded.

The three *lung volume measurements* most relevant to COPD are *vital capacity* (VC), *residual volume* (RV), and *total lung capacity* (TLC). VC is the maximal volume of air that can be forcibly expelled after inhaling as deeply as possible. Not all of the air in the lungs can be removed when VC is measured. The amount remaining is called the RV. The TLC is the combination of the VC and RV. Although most of the measured lung volumes or capacities change to some degree with COPD, RV usually increases quite markedly. This increase reflects the trapped, stagnant air remaining in the lungs. Typical pulmonary function findings in COPD are given in the accompanying Key Features of Disease.

Flow volume curves are used to measure the ability to move air into and out of the lung. The rate of airflow out of the lungs during a rapid, forceful, and complete expiration from TLC to RV provides an indirect measure of the flow-resistive properties of the lung. The amount exhaled — the *forced expiratory volume* — in the first second is called FEV_1, and the total volume exhaled is the *forced vital capacity* (FVC). FEV_1 can also be expressed as a percentage of the FVC. As the disease progresses, the ratio of FEV_1 to FVC becomes smaller. A diagnosis of COPD is based primarily on the FEV_1. FEV_1 is independent of expiratory effort and thus serves as a tool in diagnosing or evaluating COPD when compared with other measurements, which depend more on the client's cooperation.

KEY FEATURES OF DISEASE ■ Pulmonary Function Findings in COPD

Test	Findings
Residual Volume (RV): The volume of gas remaining in the lungs after a maximal expiration.	Loss of elastic recoil causes RV to be increased in emphysema and chronic bronchitis because of the narrowing and obstruction of airways.
Total Lung Capacity (TLC): The total amount of gas in the lungs at the end of a maximal inspiration.	TLC is increased in emphysematous clients because of loss of elastic recoil. TLC is normal in clients with chronic bronchitis.
Vital Capacity (VC): The maximal amount of gas that can be expired after a maximal inspiration.	VC may be normal or decreased in the client with COPD.
Forced Vital Capacity (FVC): VC that is produced from a maximal forced expiratory effort.	FVC is often increased in COPD clients secondary to air trapping.
Forced expiratory volume (FEV): Volume of air that is exhaled during a specified time (in seconds) while measuring FVC.	FEV mainly reflects resistance in large airways and is usually reduced.
Functional residual capacity (FRC): The amount of gas remaining in the lungs at the end of a tidal expiration.	FRC is increased in clients with chronic bronchitis if obstruction is severe.
Diffusion Capacity (DC): Measure of carbon monoxide uptake across the alveolar capillary membrane.	The DC value is decreased in severe emphysema. Chronic bronchitis has little effect on DC.

The *diffusing capacity* of the lung is a measure of the lung's ability to conduct a gas from the alveoli to the capillary blood. The gas most suitable for measuring the lung's diffusing capacity is carbon monoxide, which has diffusing characteristics similar to those of oxygen. A number of factors can cause the diffusing capacity to decrease. In emphysema, the decrease is the result of the destruction of alveolar walls, which leads to a significant decrease in surface area for diffusion of oxygen into the blood. In asthma, even though lung volumes are increased, the diffusion capacity is usually normal.

Analysis: Nursing Diagnosis

Most often, an individual with COPD is admitted to the hospital because of decompensation or exacerbation of the disease. Often, the exacerbation is due to a respiratory tract infection. In addition, many other hospitalized clients have a secondary medical diagnosis of COPD. Within the list of 10 most frequently used diagnosis-related groups, 3 are related directly to COPD.

Common Diagnoses

The nursing diagnoses that are common in most clients with COPD include

1. Impaired gas exchange related to airflow limitation, respiratory muscle fatigue, and production of mucus
2. Ineffective airway clearance related to inadequate cough and/or excessive production of mucus
3. Anxiety related to dyspneic episodes and/or asthmatic attacks

Additional Diagnoses

In addition, some clients may have the following diagnoses, depending on the progression or stage of their disease:

1. Altered nutrition: less than body requirements related to increased work of breathing
2. Knowledge deficit related to self-care techniques and medication regimen
3. Activity intolerance related to imbalance between oxygen supply and demand
4. Ineffective individual and/or ineffective family coping related to chronic disease situations (e.g., loss of health, loss of job, changes in life style)
5. Hopelessness related to decreased health state
6. Self-esteem disturbance related to decreased health state
7. Total self-care deficit related to dyspnea and weakness
8. Sexual dysfunction related to episodes of breathlessness
9. Sleep pattern disturbance related to nocturnal dyspnea
10. Social isolation related to activity intolerance
11. Fatigue related to decreased arterial blood oxygen concentration and subsequent dyspnea

Planning and Implementation

The following plan of care for COPD clients focuses on the common nursing diagnoses. The care plan may include additional nursing diagnoses when it is individualized to meet a particular client's needs (see the accompanying Client Care Plan).

Impaired Gas Exchange

Planning: client goals. Two major goals for this nursing diagnosis are that the client will (1) use a breathing pattern that does not lead to tiring and (2) achieve VC and ABG measurements that are optimal for that client's health.

Interventions: nonsurgical management. Before any interventions can be implemented, the client must be assessed to determine his or her breathing pattern—rate, rhythm, depth, and use of accessory muscles—and to determine the level of tiring in relation to the breathing pattern. The COPD individual relies more on accessory muscles than the diaphragm for ventilation. These muscles are less efficient, and consequently there is increased work of breathing. The nurse determines if there are any contributing factors to the increased work of breathing such as a respiratory tract infection. The interventions are aimed at improving the individual's breathing efforts and at decreasing the work of breathing by the judicious use of bronchodilators and corticosteroids, energy conservation, and dyspnea management.

Drug therapy. Three main classes of drugs are used in the management of COPD: bronchodilators, corticosteroids, and cromolyn sodium. Table 62–1 summarizes these drugs. The bronchodilators are divided into methylxanthines and sympathomimetics. Theophylline and aminophylline are the two major drugs in the methylxanthine group. These drugs act to increase the levels of adenosine 3',5'-cyclic phosphate (cAMP), the body's own natural bronchodilator. Aminophylline is usually given intravenously at a loading dose of 6 mg/kg of body weight infused over 20 to 40 minutes. The maintenance dose is 0.5 mg/kg in otherwise healthy, nonsmoking adults. Theophylline (Theo-Dur) is useful in managing moderate to severe bronchospasms, and, like aminophylline, is considered to be a first-line drug. The initial dose is 400 mg/day for adults, with the dose increased by 25% at 3-day intervals until maximal doses are achieved and symptoms are relieved. Theophylline is well absorbed orally, with peak serum concentrations in 1 to 2 hours. Adjustments in dosage are guided by the signs and symptoms of toxicity, which include nausea, vomiting, and restlessness. The therapeutic level of theophylline is a narrow range: 10 to 20 μg/mL. Achiev-

CLIENT CARE PLAN ■ The Client with Chronic Obstructive Pulmonary Disease

Goal/Outcome Criteria	Interventions	Rationales
Nursing Diagnosis 1: Impaired Gas Exchange Related to Airflow Limitation, Respiratory Muscle Fatigue, and Production of Mucus		
Client will breathe without tiring. ■ Demonstrates modified breathing techniques that facilitate ventilatory capacity.	1. Assess client and ventilation: 　a. Weakness or tiring in relation to attempts to breathe. 　b. Breathing pattern, rate, rhythm, and depth; chest expansion; presence of respiratory distress (shortness of breath, wheezing, or dyspnea); nasal flaring; pursed-lip breathing; prolonged expiratory phase; use of accessory muscles. 　c. VC measurements: TLC, RV, FEV_1, and functional residual capacity, as ordered.	1. Information is gained about the effectiveness of the treatment plan and the need for its modification.
	2. Instruct client in techniques of breathing such as: 　a. Pursed-lip breathing. 　b. Diaphragmatic breathing. 　c. Relaxation therapy. 　d. Coughing and deep breathing.	2. Breathing techniques facilitate exhalation of stagnant, trapped air and are beneficial during dyspneic episodes.
	3. Assist client in maintaining proper body positioning during dyspneic episodes. 　a. Sitting up and leaning on over-bed table. 　b. Sitting up and resting with elbows on knees. 　c. Standing and leaning against wall.	3. Use of accessory muscles is facilitated by supporting arms and shoulders, and thoracic cavity is enlarged for increased lung expansion.
	4. Maximize the effect of medical interventions by proper sequencing of respiratory treatments and by judicious use of bronchodilators and steroids (in any form: intravenous, oral, inhaled).	4. Work of breathing is reduced by decreasing inflammatory process and through bronchodilation.
	5. Assess the quality and quantity of sputum: color, consistency, amount, and odor.	5. These characteristics may indicate pulmonary infection.
■ Modifies behavior to conserve energy.	6. Refer the client to rehabilitation programs for general body exercises.	6. Exercises improve overall muscle function and allow more efficient use of oxygen by the muscles.
	7. Formulate a plan with the client for pacing activities of daily living. 　a. Encourage sitting for most activities, such as peeling potatoes or talking on the telephone. 　b. Teach the client to always breathe during an activity and never to hold his or her breath. 　c. Be aware that activities involving arms consume the most energy. 　d. Plan rest periods during more strenuous activities.	7. Pacing conserves energy that is needed for breathing.

continued

CLIENT CARE PLAN ■ The Client with Chronic Obstructive Pulmonary Disease *continued*

Goal/Outcome Criteria	Interventions	Rationales

Nursing Diagnosis 1: Impaired Gas Exchange Related to Airflow Limitation, Respiratory Muscle Fatigue, and Production of Mucus

Goal/Outcome Criteria	Interventions	Rationales

	8. Evaluate nutritional state of the client and offer support.
	  a. Compare baseline weight to present weight.
	  b. Evaluate laboratory data: serum total protein and albumin levels.
	  c. Assist the client in choosing foods that are easy to chew and swallow and that are high in calories.
	  d. Assist the client by cutting food and feeding if the client tires easily.
	  e. Suggest that the client eat small, frequent meals.
		8. Eating consumes energy needed for breathing; clients who have increased work of breathing have higher calorie requirements.

Nursing Diagnosis 2: Ineffective Airway Clearance Related to Inadequate Cough and/or Excessive Production of Mucus

Goal/Outcome Criteria	Interventions	Rationales

Client will maximize airway clearance.
■ Demonstrates controlled cough and postural drainage.
	1. Assess the client's ability to mobilize secretions; if inability is identified:
	  a. Teach a method of controlled cough.
	  b. Use suction as necessary to remove secretions.
	  c. Teach use of postural drainage and chest physiotherapy.
	  d. Note characteristics of sputum.
		1. Secretions that can obstruct airways and/or lead to respiratory complications are removed and/or mobilized.

	2. Frequently (at least once every 8 h) auscultate the chest for quality of breath sounds and the presence of adventitious sounds.	2. Auscultation provides vital information on the client's respiratory status.
	3. Administer bronchodilators, mucolytics, and expectorants if ordered; observe the client for a therapeutic response; monitor the theophylline level as indicated.	3. These medications dilate the airways and assist in expectorating mucus.
	4. Provide hydration of at least 2 L/d if not medically contraindicated.	4 Hydration provides an excellent method of liquefying secretions without the side effects of medication.
	5. Administer vaporization therapy and perform postural drainage with percussion as ordered (at least 1 h before meals; provide oral hygiene after treatment).	5. Therapy aids in mobilizing secretions.

■ Identifies the importance of adequate fluid intake and of the need to receive influenza and pneumococcal vaccination.	6. Instruct the client on prevention of infection. Stress the following:
	  a. Avoidance of crowded rooms or contact with individuals with known cases of influenza or colds.
	  b. Avoidance of irritants such as tobacco smoke.
		6. These measures help to prevent life-threatening complications of COPD.

CLIENT CARE PLAN ▪ The Client with Chronic Obstructive Pulmonary Disease *continued*

Goal/Outcome Criteria	Interventions	Rationales
Nursing Diagnosis 2: Ineffective Airway Clearance Related to Inadequate Cough and/or Excessive Production of Mucus **continued**		
	c. Importance of receiving pneumococcal and influenza vaccines. d. Importance of recognizing changes in sputum characteristics.	
Nursing Diagnosis 3: Anxiety Related to Dyspneic Episodes and/or Asthmatic Attacks		
Client will manage anxiety. ▪ Identifies factors that elicit anxious behaviors.	1. Identify in writing various factors that elicit an anxious response.	1. Clarification gives the client control over the situation, builds confidence, and thus may decrease anxiety.
	2. Help the client to formulate a plan for coping with anxiety.	2. A plan prepares the client for episodes of anxiety.
▪ Identifies activities that tend to decrease anxious behaviors.	3. Help the client to formulate a plan for coping with dyspneic and wheezing episodes.	3. Symptom flare-ups may trigger anxiety; having a clear-cut plan gives the client confidence in knowing exactly what to do.
	4. Allow the client to verbalize feelings.	4. Verbalization tends to prevent or help to decrease anxiety.
	5. Refer the client for professional counseling if necessary.	5. Counseling assists the client with self-analysis and coping techniques.

	6. Teach the client various interventions for anxiety, such as
	   a. Relaxation techniques.
	   b. Biofeedback.
		6. Interventions decrease stress, which results in diminishing anxiety.

ing a therapeutic level can be challenging because various conditions influence the serum concentrations. See Table 62–2 for a review of these factors. Sustained-release forms of theophylline (e.g., Theo-Dur) maintain a continuous concentration of the drug and are appropriate for clients who awaken at night with shortness of breath.

The sympathomimetic drugs or adrenergic bronchodilators are drugs that mimic the sympathetic nervous system. These drugs cause bronchodilation through activation of the enzyme adenylate cyclase, which converts adenosine triphosphate (ATP) to cAMP. These drugs are rapidly metabolized and hence are short acting. In choosing the specific drug, the beta-adrenergic activity of each drug should be considered. Beta-adrenergic receptors are located in both the lung and the heart. Beta$_1$-receptors are located in the heart, whereas beta$_2$-receptors are located in the lung. For the most part, the more selective beta$_2$-adrenergic drugs (e.g. metaproterenol [Alupent], terbutaline [Brethine], and albuterol [Proventil]) generally do not stimulate the heart

directly and have a slower onset of action and longer duration. Many of the sympathomimetics can be administered in an inhaled form. The Client/Family Education feature on page 2003 outlines the correct use of an inhaler.

Corticosteroid preparations reduce inflammation in the throat and lungs but also act to stimulate cAMP production and hence bronchodilation. Steroids may be given by the intravenous, oral, or inhalation route. The decision to prescribe systemic steroids must be made with great care because the majority of clients must take them indefinitely. The side effects are usually related to long-term use, with adrenal suppression being the most potentially hazardous. Other side effects include gastrointestinal upset and peptic ulcers, drug-induced diabetes mellitus, weight gain, abnormal fat distribution, osteoporosis, fluid retention, and psychoses. Various methods have been used to minimize these side effects. Alternate-day therapy minimizes adrenal suppression. A dosage total for 2 days of the steroid is given every other day. Clients need to be instructed and reminded to

TABLE 62–1 Drugs Used in the Treatment of COPD

Drug	Usual Daily Dosage	Interventions	Rationales
Bronchodilators Methylxanthines Aminophylline	IV: Loading dose: 6 mg/kg Maintenance dose: 0.5 mg/kg	1. Observe the client for nausea and vomiting, palpitations, dizziness and restlessness. 2. Space doses equally throughout a 24-h period. 3. Administer with food, such as milk and crackers. 4. Instruct the client to take medication even when feeling good.	1. To detect toxicity. The drug has a narrow therapeutic range of 10–20 μg/mL. 2. To ensure even coverage throughout the day. 3. To prevent gastrointestinal irritation. 4. To maintain a therapeutic level.
Theophylline (Slo-Phyllin, Theo-Dur)	Initially: 400 mg/d, increased by 25% at 3-d intervals until maximal oral dose of 13 mg/kg/d in 3 or 4 divided doses	Same as for aminophylline.	Same as for aminophylline; sustained-release preparations give better coverage than do regular preparations, which makes them ideal for clients who awaken at night with shortness of breath.
Sympathomimetics (adrenergics; beta stimulants) Isoetharine (Bronkosol)	Nebulizer: 0.5 mL diluted 1:3 with saline	1. Observe the client for tachycardia, palpitations, headache, and blood pressure alterations.	1. To detect side effects. The drug stimulates beta-adrenergic receptors in the heart and lungs.
Epinephrine (Adrenalin)	SC or IM: 0.2–0.5 mL of 1:1000 solution; may repeat in 10–15 min IV: 0.1–0.25 mL of 1:1000 solution	1. Observe the client for anxiety, tremors, and palpitations. 2. Assess the client for a history of hypertension, hyperthyroidism, and ischemic heart disease.	1. To detect side effects. The drug is fast acting, with an onset of about 20 min. 2. To detect possible contraindications.
Isoproterenol HCl (Isuprel HCl)	Inhalation: 1 or 2 puffs 4–6 times/d	1. Monitor the client for palpitations.	1. To detect severe cardiac arrhythmias, especially with IV administration.
Terbutaline (Brethine)	PO: 5 mg q 8 h SC: 0.25 mg, not to exceed 0.5 mg q 4 h	1. Monitor the client for palpitations and tachycardia.	1. To detect these infrequent side effects. The drug has a more selective beta$_2$ action, a slower onset, and a longer duration than other sympathomimetics.

TABLE 62–1   Drugs Used in the Treatment of COPD *Continued*

Drug	Usual Daily Dosage	Interventions	Rationales
Metaproterenol (Metaprel, Alupent)	Inhalation: 1 or 2 puffs tid PO: 20 mg tid	1. Instruct the client to use the bronchodilator inhaler before the steroid inhaler (if ordered). 2. Teach the client the correct method of using the inhaler and observe the client's technique.	1. To open the airways with the beta$_2$ agent to facilitate deeper penetration of the steroid. 2. To ensure proper inhalation. Sequencing the steps of using an inhaler can be tricky for children and the elderly. Two critical variables are the speed of inhalation and the duration of breath holding.
Albuterol (salbutamol, Proventil)	Inhalation: 1 or 2 puffs q 4–6 h PO: 2–4 mg q 6–8 h	1. Observe the client for fine finger tremors.	1. To detect side effects of this selective beta$_2$ agent.
Corticosteroids Prednisone (Deltasone) Methylprednisolone (Solumedrol)	PO, IV: Dosage varies	1. Instruct the client about the side effects of long-term steroid use such as a. Hyperglycemia. b. Osteoporosis. c. Increased fat production. d. Immunologic impairment. e. Reduced inflammatory response. f. Increased gastric acidity. 2. Instruct the client to take medication with food. 3. Instruct the client to never discontinue steroid use suddenly.	1. To warn client of possible side effects, many of which are irreversible but must be treated. 2. To minimize gastric irritation. 3. To prevent adrenal crisis and shock.
Beclomethasone (Vanceril)	Inhalation: 1–4 puffs tid–qid	1. Observe the client's mouth for oral candidiasis. 2. Instruct the client in the proper sequencing of sympathomimetic and steroid inhalers, if appropriate, and observe the client's technique. 3. Instruct the client to drink 8 oz of water after inhaling steroids.	1. To detect this complication of inhaled steroids. 2. To promote optimal distribution of the steroid. 3. To wash away excess medication from the back of the throat and thus to minimize the growth of candida.

Table continued on following page

TABLE 62-1 Drugs Used in the Treatment of COPD *Continued*

Drug	Usual Daily Dosage	Interventions	Rationales
Cromolyn sodium (Intal)	1 or 2 puffs qid	1. Observe the client for maculopapular rash and urticaria.	1. To detect rare side effects.
		2. Instruct the client that cromolyn is a prophylactic drug.	2. To encourage the client to seek other treatment during an acute attack.
		3. Inform the client that an optimal response may not occur before 2 mo of daily use.	3. To promote continued use while the drug takes effect.

never suddenly stop taking a steroid because they could easily experience shock.

Steroid drugs may be administered via aerosol. Most often, if clients require 30 mg or less of a steroid, it can be administered via the aerosol route, or in combination with the oral form to decrease oral steroid needs. The major advantage of the aerosol route is equivalent or greater bronchodilation and protection with fewer systemic side effects. However, when switching from an oral to an aerosol form, it is best to continue the oral dose and to slowly decrease the dosage. One additional side effect of steroid aerosols is *Candida* infection of the oropharynx. The nurse performs a daily oral assessment and looks for a bright, fire red or cherry red color of the mouth. This side effect can be minimized if the client is instructed to gargle and drink 8 oz of water after aerosol use. If the individual is also using a bronchodilator aerosol preparation, he or she should be instructed to use the bronchodilator first, followed by the steroid aerosol. Sequencing the aerosols in this manner serves to dilate the large airways, thereby allowing a greater portion of the steroid preparation to reach the peripheral airways.

Cromolyn sodium (Intal) can be used prophylactically in asthmatic clients whose symptoms are not controlled adequately by bronchodilators. It is not useful during acute attacks. The desired effects of cromolyn are to reduce the severity of asthmic attacks and to enhance the effects of concomitantly administered bronchodilators and steroids. Cromolyn probably acts by strengthening the mast cell membrane to prevent release of histamine and thereby decreases bronchospasm in the allergic asthmatic. Cromolyn is administered via inhaler, usually four times a day.

The Food and Drug Administration believes that individuals should have ready access to certain bronchodilator drug products. However, these preparations have a potential for abuse, particularly when taken in conjunction with prescription products. Clients are counseled that over-the-counter preparations contain active ingredients and are to be respected. The three principal ingredients in most nonprescription bronchodilator products are epinephrine, ephedrine, and theophylline, along with other additives. The nurse asks if the client routinely uses over-the-counter preparations and cautions the client about the potential for their abuse.

TABLE 62-2 Factors That Influence Serum Theophylline Levels

Factors That Increase Levels	Factors That Decrease Levels
Age	
More than 55 yr	Less than 9 yr
Diseases	
Cirrhosis or other liver abnormalities	
Congestive heart failure	
Alcoholism	
Upper respiratory tract infections	
Drugs	
Caffeine	Isoproterenol (Isuprel)
Allopurinol (Zyloprim)	Rifampin (Rifadin)
Erythromycin (E-Mycin)	Phenobarbital
Cimetidine (Tagamet)	Phenytoin (Dilantin)
Oral contraceptives	
Other factors	
	Cigarette smoking

Oxygen therapy. Oxygen (O_2) is a potent *drug* that is used to treat hypoxemia and relieve symptoms of hypoxia (decreased tissue oxygenation). Because symp-

CLIENT/FAMILY EDUCATION ■ How To Use an Inhaler Correctly

Instructions	Rationales
1. "Before each use, remove the cap and shake the inhaler, according to the instructions in the package insert."	1. To ensure correct mixture of medication.
2. "Breathe out fully."	2. To ensure distribution of medication throughout lungs on inhalation.
3. "Place the mouthpiece at your lips or well into your mouth; aim at the back of your throat."	3, 4. To promote inhalation of all of the medication dose.
4. "As you begin to breathe in deeply through your mouth, press the canister of the inhaler down firmly to release one dose. Continue to breathe in until your lungs are completely filled."	
5. "Remove the inhaler from your mouth, but hold your breath for at least 10 seconds, then breathe out slowly."	5. To ensure distribution of medication throughout lungs.
6. "Wait several minutes before using the inhaler again if your physician has ordered a second inhalation."	6. To allow the first inhalation to open airways so that the second can penetrate more deeply.

toms of hypoxia are difficult to measure for every system in the body, hypoxemia (a low level of arterial PO_2) is measured by ABG analysis. These blood gases are the best tool for determining the need for oxygen therapy and for evaluating its effects. *Hypoxemia* is defined as an arterial PO_2 of 55 mmHg or less with an oxygen saturation of 85% or less. The need for oxygen can also be determined by noninvasive monitoring such as the widely used pulse oximetry. The *pulse oximeter* uses waves of light and a sensor placed on the client's finger or ear to measure oxygen saturation, which is then displayed on the monitor.

Oxygen therapy is used for both acute and chronic conditions. In either case, the goal of oxygen therapy is to use the lowest fraction of inspired oxygen (FIO_2) to produce the most acceptable oxygenation without the development of harmful side effects. Although oxygen improves the arterial PO_2, it does not cure the condition or arrest the disease process.

The amount of oxygen that is required by a client is extremely precise. Prescribed doses of oxygen must not be changed without close monitoring of symptoms and ABG levels. Precise delivery of oxygen is warranted because high levels of FIO_2 can be fatal to the COPD client, who depends on a hypoxic drive to breathe. On the other hand, insufficient levels of FIO_2 result in deleterious effects of hypoxemia. Only in an emergency situation does the nurse deliver 100% FIO_2 regardless of the client's clinical status. After the client is stable, the correct FIO_2 is titrated to meet the client's oxygen needs.

Indications.   Oxygen therapy is indicated in conditions associated with decreased arterial PO_2 levels, decreased cardiac output, decreased blood oxygen-carrying capability, and increased oxygen demand. *Decreased arterial PO_2 levels* (hypoxemia) are found in numerous clinical situations, most of which are due to ventilation-perfusion mismatching and respond well to

oxygen therapy. Examples include pulmonary edema and pulmonary emboli. *Decreased cardiac output* results in decreased oxygen delivery to tissues. Clinical examples include myocardial infarction, hypotension, and congestive heart failure. *Decreased blood oxygen-carrying capability* occurs in various types of anemia. Insufficient amounts or quality of hemoglobin cannot carry enough oxygen to the cells. Clinical examples are sickle cell anemia, hemorrhagic shock, and hemolytic anemia. *Increased oxygen demand* may result in hypoxemia. Conditions that increase oxygen demand include sepsis, hyperthyroidism, and sustained fever.

Hazards.   Oxygen therapy is associated with several hazards. It is important for the nurse to understand these hazards so that early signs and symptoms may be detected. Oxygen itself does not burn, but it supports *combustion*. Therefore, a fire burns more readily in the presence of oxygen. The nurse takes special precautions during administration of oxygen, including posting a sign on the door of the room for the client receiving this therapy. In the client's room, smoking is prohibited and all electrical equipment must be grounded. Frayed cords must be repaired because they can cause a spark that can ignite a flame. The presence of any type of flammable solution containing alcohol or oil is prohibited when oxygen is in use.

Oxygen-induced hypoventilation is another hazard of oxygen therapy. This situation is seen in the client whose principal respiratory drive is hypoxia, namely, the COPD client.

In COPD, the carbon dioxide level gradually rises over time, and the central chemoreceptors are no longer sensitive to high carbon dioxide levels. Instead, the peripheral chemoreceptors found in the carotid and aortic arch bodies become the major stimulus for breathing. These chemoreceptors are sensitive to low levels of arterial PO_2. When an arterial PO_2 level of 60 mmHg or less occurs, the chemoreceptors signal the brain to increase the respiratory rate or depth, which results in a hypoxic drive to breathe. When the client with COPD receives oxygen therapy, the arterial PO_2 level increases, and the hypoxic drive to breathe is eliminated. The client experiences respiratory depression that may lead to apnea. A system that delivers precise FIO_2, such as a nasal cannula or Venturi's mask, is warranted for any client with COPD. The nurse closely monitors a client with COPD who receives oxygen for the first time. Signs and symptoms of hypoventilation are seen during the first 30 minutes of oxygen administration, and "pinking up," related to high arterial PO_2 levels, occurs before apnea begins.

The occurrence of *oxygen toxicity* is determined by the concentration of oxygen delivered (FIO_2) and the duration of therapy. The general guideline is *oxygen concentrations of greater than 50% administered continuously for more than 24 to 48 hours may damage the lungs*. The precise FIO_2 value and length of time needed for lung damage to occur vary based on the degree of lung disease present before oxygen therapy is started. Nevertheless, prolonged exposure to high levels of oxygen results in acute lung injury; therefore, the pathophysiology and clinical manifestations are the same as those for adult respiratory distress syndrome (ARDS) (see ARDS discussion later in this chapter). Initial symptoms are tracheobronchitis, nonproductive cough, substernal chest pain, gastrointestinal upset, and dyspnea. As exposure to high levels of oxygen continues, the symptoms become more severe and are accompanied by decreased VC, decreased compliance, and hypoxemia. Prolonged exposure to high levels of oxygen causes structural damage to the lungs. Atelectasis, pulmonary edema, pulmonary hemorrhages, and hyaline membrane formation result. Mortality depends on the ability to correct the underlying disease process and to decrease the FIO_2 delivered.

Oxygen toxicity is difficult to treat; hence, it is best to avoid using high levels of oxygen unless they are absolutely necessary. The addition of positive end-expiratory pressure (PEEP), which is a modality found on the mechanical ventilator, may help to decrease FIO_2 requirements. When high levels of oxygen are required, nursing interventions focus on identification of the client at risk. The nurse asks the client about signs and symptoms of oxygen toxicity because the client on mechanical ventilation may be unable to volunteer this information. Close monitoring of ABGs as well as of the response to changing levels of FIO_2 is needed. The lowest level of FIO_2 must be used and decreased as soon as the client's clinical condition allows.

Absorption atelectasis occurs in the client receiving high levels of oxygen. Normally, nitrogen plays a large role in the maintenance of patent airways and alveoli. When high levels of oxygen are delivered, (1) nitrogen is washed out, (2) the oxygen diffuses from the alveoli into the pulmonary circulation, and (3) the alveoli collapse. Collapsed alveoli cause atelectasis, which is detected by auscultation as decreased or tubular breath sounds. The

nurse monitors the client closely for these findings, every 1 to 2 hours initially.

Delivery systems. Oxygen can be delivered by numerous systems. The nurse must understand the rationale for the type of oxygen delivery system used for a particular client and be able to use the equipment properly. The type of delivery system chosen depends on the following.

1. Concentration of oxygen required by the client
2. Concentration of oxygen achieved by a delivery system
3. Importance of accuracy and control of oxygen concentration
4. Client's comfort
5. Expense to client
6. Importance of humidity

Oxygen delivery systems are classified according to the rate at which oxygen is delivered. There are two systems: low-flow systems and high-flow systems. Low-flow systems do not provide enough oxygen to meet the total inspiratory effort of the client. Part of the tidal volume is supplied by inspiring room air. The concentration of oxygen received depends on respiratory rate and tidal volume. In contrast, high-flow systems provide a flow rate that is adequate to meet the entire inspiratory effort and tidal volume of the client regardless of the respiratory pattern. High-flow systems are used for critically ill clients.

Low-flow oxygen delivery systems include the nasal cannula, the simple face mask, the partial rebreather, and the nonrebreather mask. Table 62–3 compares low-flow oxygen delivery systems and provides appropriate nursing interventions for each. These systems are inexpensive, easy to use, and comfortable for the client. A major disadvantage is that the oxygen concentration is extremely variable and unpredictable, depending on the client's ventilator pattern. High tidal volumes entrain larger volumes of more room air gas (21%) and lower the FIO_2; small tidal volumes entrain smaller volumes of room air gas and increase the FIO_2 delivered.

The *nasal cannula* is the most frequently used device and is preferred for the client with COPD (Fig. 62–2). Flow rates of 1 to 6 L/minute are used. The FIO_2 obtained per liter is quite variable and depends on the client's minute ventilation. However, an approximate FIO_2 of 24% to 40% can be achieved. Flow rates of higher than 6 L/minute will not significantly increase oxygenation because the anatomic reserve (oral and nasal cavities) is full; however, they increase mucosal irritation. When delivering oxygen by nasal cannula, an effective oxygen concentration can be delivered to both nose breathers and mouth breathers. The nasal cannula is frequently used for the COPD client and for long-term maintenance of clients with other illnesses. The COPD client who retains carbon dioxide should never receive oxygen at a rate higher than 2 to 3 L/minute. The nasal prongs are placed in the nostrils, with the openings fac-

TABLE 62–3   Comparison of Low-Flow Oxygen Delivery Systems

System	FIO$_2$ Delivered	Interventions	Rationales
Nasal cannula	24%–40% FIO$_2$ at 1–6 L/min. 1 L = 4% FIO$_2$ added + 21% for room air.	1. Ensure that prongs are in the nares properly 2. Provide water-soluble jelly to nares. 3. Assess the patency of the nostrils. 4. Assess the client for changes in respiratory rate. 5. Suggest to physician to switch the client from a mask to the nasal cannula during eating.	1. A poorly fitting nasal cannula leads to hypoxemia and skin breakdown. 2. This substance prevents mucosal irritation related to the drying effect of oxygen. 3. Congestion or a deviated septum prevents effective delivery of oxygen through the nares. 4. The respiratory pattern affects the amount of oxygen delivered. A different delivery system may be needed. 5. Use of the cannula prevents hypoxemia during eating.
Simple face mask	40%–60% FIO$_2$ at 5–10 L/min. Flow rate must be set at least 5 L/min to flush mask of carbon dioxide.	1. Mask must fit well. 2. Assess skin and provide skin care to the area covered by the mask. 3. Monitor the client closely for risk of aspiration. 4. Provide emotional support to the client who feels claustrophobic.	1. Poor-fitting mask reduces the FIO$_2$ delivered. 2. The mask and bag may cause skin breakdown. 3. The mask limits the client's ability to clear the mouth, especially if vomiting occurs. 4. Emotional support decreases anxiety, which contributes to a claustrophobic feeling.
Partial rebreather mask	At liter flow to maintain bag two-thirds full in inspiration. At 6–15 L/min provides FIO$_2$ of 70%–90%.	1. Make sure that the reservoir does not twist or kink, which results in a deflated bag. 2. Adjust the flow rate to keep the reservoir bag inflated (two-thirds full during inspiration).	1. Deflation results in decreased oxygen delivered and rebreathing of exhaled air. 2. The flow rate is adjusted to meet the pattern of the client.
Nonrebreather mask	60%–100% FIO$_2$ at liter flow to maintain bag two-thirds full.	1. Interventions as for partial rebreather mask; this client requires close monitoring to ensure proper functioning. 2. Make sure that valves and rubber flaps are patent, functional, and not stuck. Remove mucus or saliva.	1. As for partial rebreather mask. 2. Valves should open during expiration and close during inhalation to prevent dramatic decrease in FIO$_2$. Suffo-

Table continued on following page

TABLE 62-3 Comparison of Low-Flow Oxygen Delivery Systems *Continued*

System	FIO₂ Delivered	Interventions	Rationales
			cation can occur if the reservoir bag kinks or if the oxygen source disconnects.
		3. Closely assess client on increased FIO₂ via nonrebreather mask. Intubation is the only way to provide more precise FIO₂.	3. The client may require intubation.

ing the client. Water-soluble jelly may be applied to the nares to prevent mucosal drying. When a flow rate of higher than 2 L/minute is needed, humidification is added by using a bubble humidifier (Fig. 62-3).

A *simple face mask* is used to deliver oxygen concentrations of 40% to 60% for short-term oxygen therapy or in an emergency (Fig. 62-4). A minimal flow rate of 5 L/minute is needed to prevent rebreathing of exhaled air. Special attention is given to skin care and to proper fitting of the mask so that FIO₂ levels are maintained.

A *partial rebreather mask* provides an FIO₂ of 70% to 90%, with flow rates of 6 to 15 L/minute. It consists of a mask with a reservoir bag but no flaps, as seen in Fig. 62-5. The client first rebreathes one-third of the ex-

haled tidal volume, which is high in oxygen, thus providing a high FIO₂. The flow rate is adjusted so that the reservoir bag deflates only slightly during inspiration.

A *nonrebreather mask* provides the highest FIO₂ of the low-flow systems and can deliver an FIO₂ of 90% to 100%, depending on the client's ventilatory pattern. The nonrebreather mask, delivering high FIO₂, is most frequently used in the client with deteriorating respiratory status who may require intubation. The nonrebreather mask has a one-way valve between the mask and the reservoir, and two flaps over the exhalation

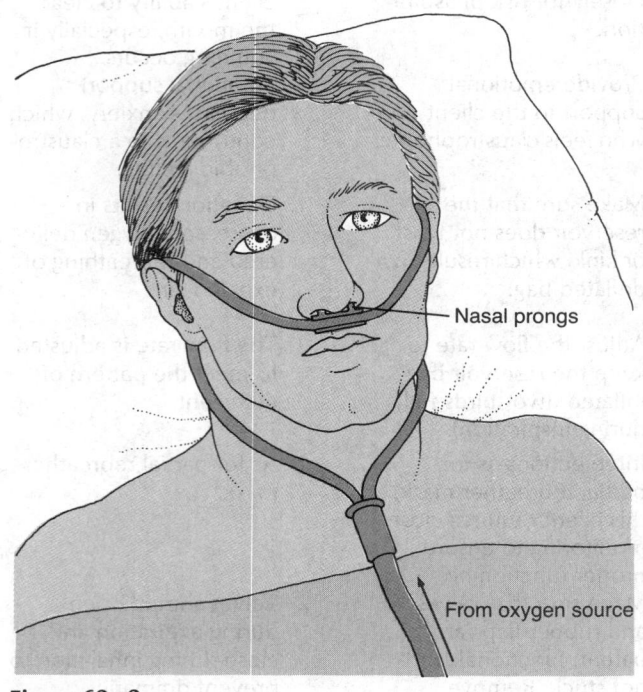

Figure 62-2
Nasal cannula.

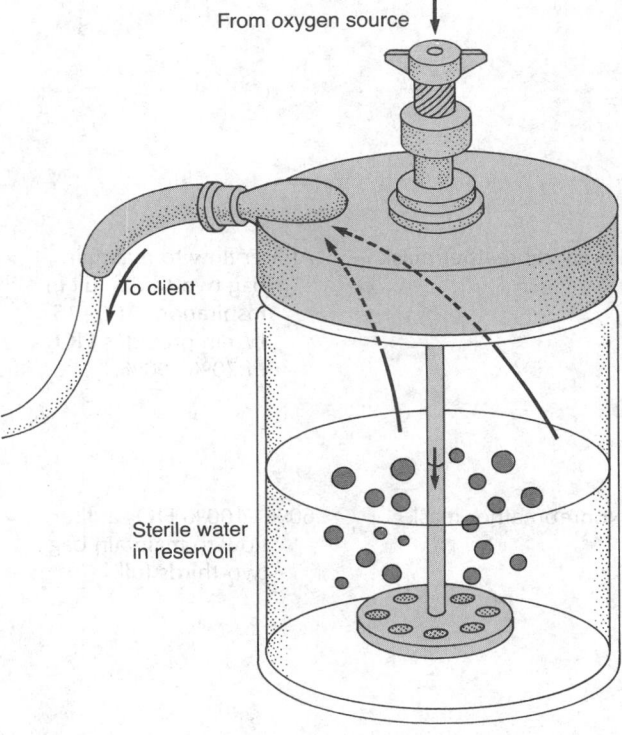

Figure 62-3
Bubble humidifier bottle used with oxygen therapy.

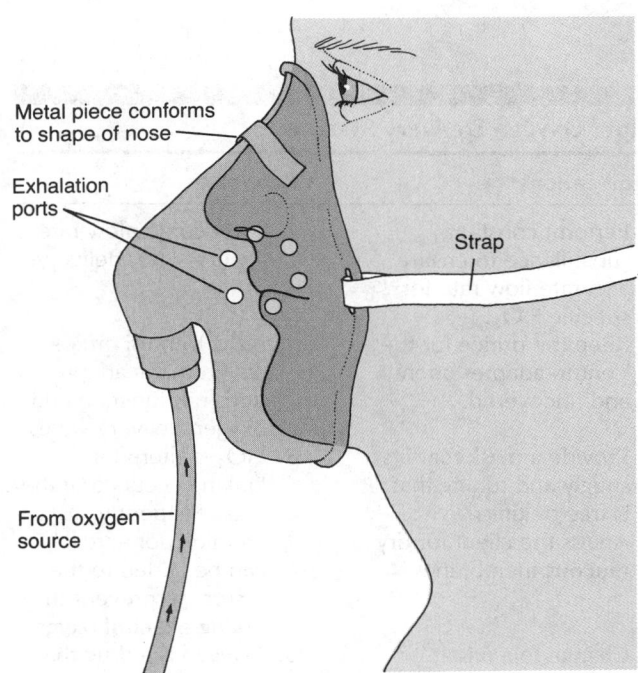

Figure 62-4

Simple face mask used to deliver oxygen.

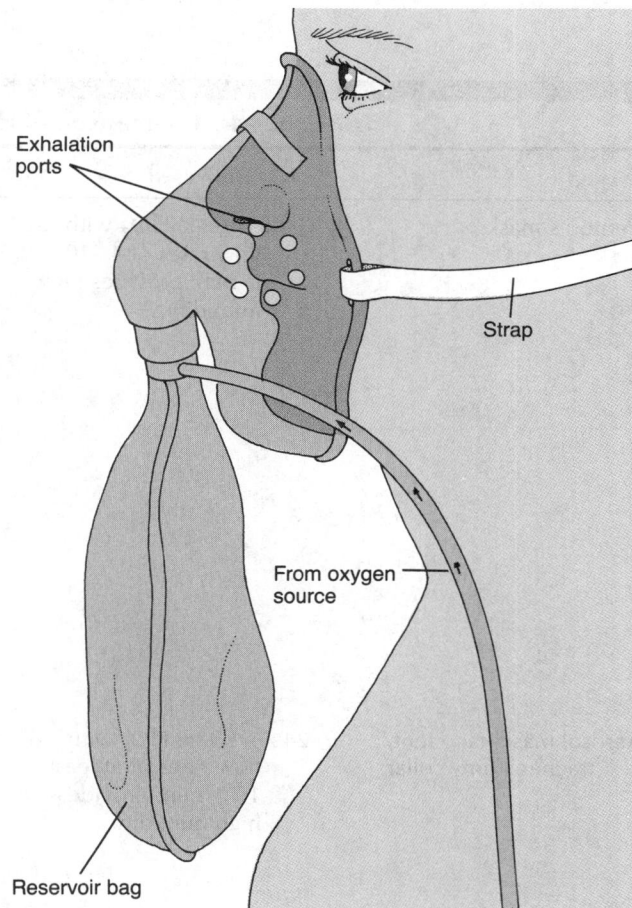

Figure 62-5

Partial rebreather mask.

ports. The valve allows the client to draw his or her entire oxygen from the reservoir bag, and the flaps prevent air from entering from the exhalation ports. During exhalation, air leaves through these ports while the one-way valve prevents exhaled air from entering the reservoir bag. It is crucial for the nurse to ensure that the valve and flaps are intact and functional during each breath.

High-flow systems consist of the Venturi mask, the aerosol mask, the face tent, the tracheostomy collar, and the T piece. Table 62-4 compares high-flow oxygen delivery systems and provides appropriate nursing interventions for each. All of these devices deliver a consistent and accurate FIO_2 that meets the client's inspiratory effort when the mask fit is proper. A high-flow system provides oxygen concentrations of 24% to 100% at 8 to 15 L/minute.

The *Venturi mask* delivers the most *accurate* FIO_2. Its operation is based on a mechanism that entrains a specific proportional amount of room air for each liter flow of oxygen. (Each FIO_2 setting has its own FIO_2/room air ratio.) An adapter is located between the bottom of the mask and the gas source (Fig. 62-6). Adapters with holes of different size allow only specific amounts of air to mix with the oxygen. Precise delivery of FIO_2 results. Each adapter also stipulates the flow rate with which it is to be used, e.g., to deliver 24% of oxygen, the flow rate must be 4 L/minute. This delivery system is the best one for the COPD client.

The *aerosol mask, face tent, tracheostomy collar,* and *T piece* all require a flow rate of at least 10 L/minute and are often used to administer high humidity. Each system delivers an FIO_2 that ranges from 21% to 100%, which is regulated by a dial on the humidification source. A face tent fits over the client's chin with the top extending halfway across the face. The FIO_2 rate varies but the face tent is useful for facial trauma and burns instead of a tight-fitting mask. The T piece attaches to an endotracheal or tracheostomy tube. An aerosol mask is used for the client who requires high humidity after extubation or upper airway surgery, or for the client who has thick secretions. The tracheostomy collar can be used to deliver high humidity and the desired FIO_2 to the client with a tracheostomy. A special adapter, called the T piece, is used to deliver any desired FIO_2 to the client with a tracheostomy, laryngectomy, or endotracheal tube (Fig. 62-7). The flow rate is regulated so that the aerosol does not disappear on the exhalation side of the T piece.

Nursing management.   Regardless of the type of oxygen delivery system used, the nurse must understand the indications, advantages, and disadvantages of each. The nurse prevents skin irritation from the mask and oxygen by checking for pressure points and signs of irritation every 2 to 4 hours. The elastic band may need

TABLE 62–4 Comparison of High-Flow Oxygen Delivery Systems

System	FIO₂ Delivered	Interventions	Rationales
Venturi's mask	24%–100% FIO$_2$ with flow rates of 4–10 L/min; provides high humidity.	1. Perform constant surveillance to ensure accurate flow rate for specific FIO$_2$. 2. Keep the orifice for the Venturi adapter open and uncovered. 3. Provide a mask that fits snugly and tubing that is free of kinks. 4. Assess the client for dry mucous membranes. 5. Change to a nasal cannula during mealtimes.	1. An accurate flow rate ensures FIO$_2$ delivery. 2. If the Venturi orifice is covered, the adapter does not function and oxygen delivery varies. 3. FIO$_2$ is altered if kinking occurs or if the mask fits poorly. 4. Humidity or aerosol can be added to the system to prevent the drying effect of oxygen. 5. Oxygen is a drug that needs to be given continuously.
Aerosol mask, face tent, tracheostomy collar	24%–100% FIO$_2$ with flow rates of at least 10 L/min; provides high humidity.	1. Assess that aerosol mist escapes from the vents of the delivery system during inspiration and expiration. 2. Empty condensation from the tubing. 3. Keep the aerosol water container full.	1. Humidification should be delivered to the client. 2. Emptying prevents the client from being lavaged with water and promotes an adequate flow rate. 3. Adequate humidification is ensured.
T piece	24%–100% FIO$_2$ with flow rates of at least 10 L/min; provides high humidity.	1. Empty condensation from the tubing. 2. Keep the exhalation port open and uncovered. 3. Position the T piece so that it does not pull on the tracheostomy or endotracheal tube. 4. Make sure the humidifier creates enough mist. A mist should be seen during inspiration and expiration.	1. Condensation interferes with flow rate and may drain into the tracheostomy if not emptied. 2. If the port is occluded, the client can suffocate. 3. The weight of the T piece pulls on the tracheostomy and causes pain or erosion of skin at the insertion site. 4. An adequate flow rate is needed to meet the inspiratory effort of the client. If not, FIO$_2$ is decreased.

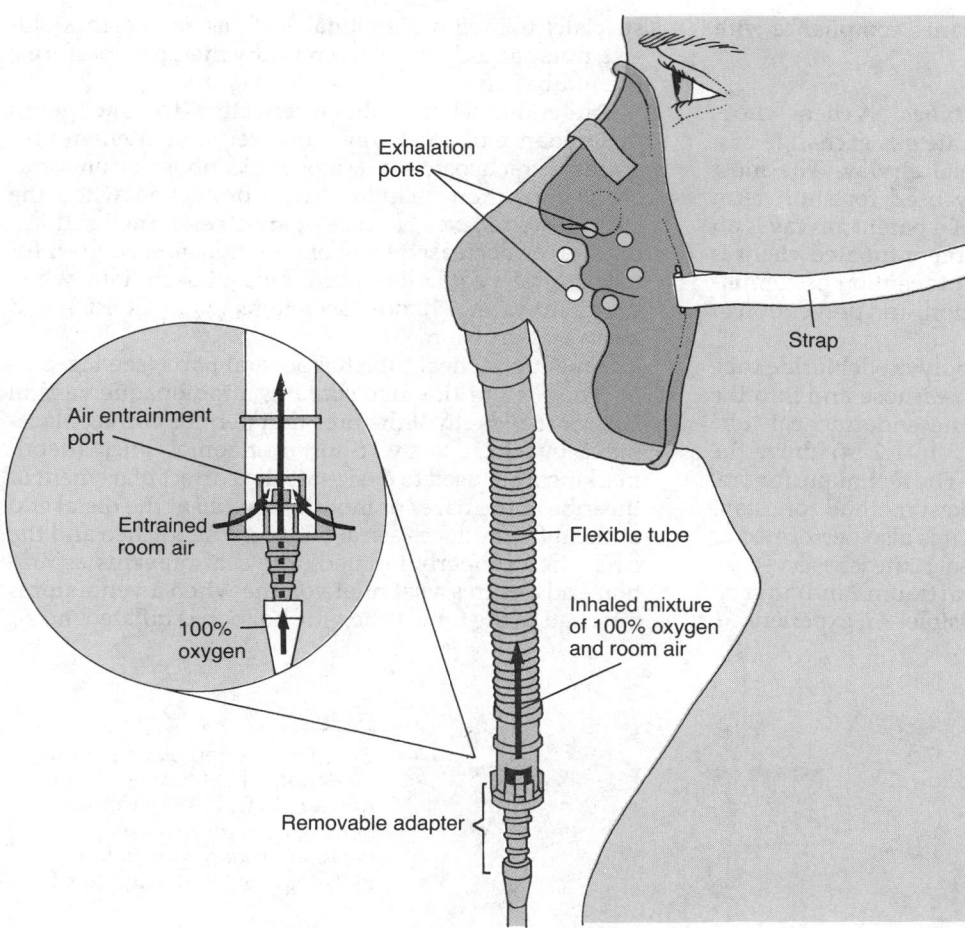

Figure 62–6

Venturi's mask for accurate oxygen delivery.

to be padded or its position frequently changed to prevent skin breakdown. The drying effects of oxygen are relieved by lubricating the affected areas with water-soluble jelly. All tubing is positioned so that it does not pull on the client's face, nose, or artificial airway, if present.

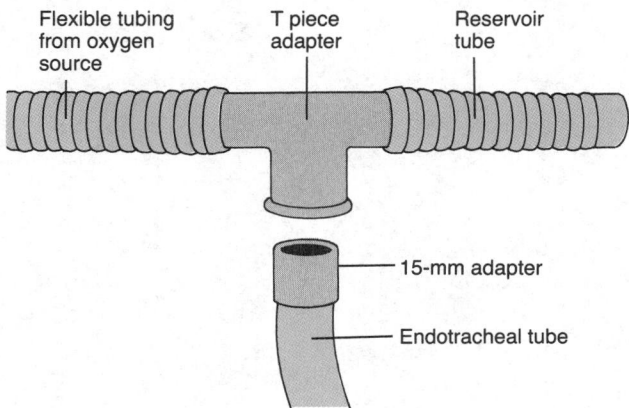

Figure 62–7

T piece apparatus for attachment to endotracheal tube.

The nurse also ensures the proper use and maintenance of the oxygen delivery equipment. When a mask is used, it should fit securely over the nose and mouth so that oxygen does not escape from the top or sides of the mask. If humidification is needed, the nurse ensures that a constant mist of humidification escapes from the vents of the delivery system during inspiration and expiration. A sufficient amount of water must be kept in the humidification bottle and an adequate flow rate must be maintained so that proper humidification is delivered to the client (see Fig. 62–3). Condensation often forms in the tubing and is removed as needed by disconnecting the tubing and emptying the water into an appropriate receptacle. The fluid should never be drained back into the humidification bottle to prevent bacterial contamination.

If the client requires a mask but is able to eat, the nurse requests an order for a nasal cannula at an appropriate liter flow for mealtimes only. The mask is replaced after the meal is completed. A flow rate of 1 L/minute delivers 4% FIO_2. Therefore, 6 L via a nasal cannula delivers 44% FIO_2 (20% to 21% room air plus 24% by oxygen supplementation).

The nurse documents the client's response to oxygen therapy, including clinical appearance, ABG results, and exercise tolerance. Ongoing teaching and reassurance are given to the client to enhance compliance with oxygen therapy.

Intubation with endotracheal tubes. A client who is no longer able to maintain adequate gas exchange or a patent airway requires an artificial airway. The most common type of artificial airway used for short-term establishment and maintenance of a patent airway is an endotracheal tube. The goal for the intubated client is maintenance of a patent airway, prevention of complications from endotracheal intubation, and prevention of infection.

An *endotracheal tube* is a long polyvinylchloride tube that is passed through the mouth or nose and into the trachea (Fig. 62–8). The tip of the endotracheal tube rests approximately 2 to 3 cm (0.8 to 1.2 in) above the carina when properly positioned. The technique for oral intubation is the easiest and quickest method for establishment of an airway; therefore, it is also performed as an emergency procedure. The nasal route is reserved for elective intubation, for facial or oral trauma and surgery, or when oral intubation is not possible. An experienced,

specially trained professional, such as an anesthesiologist, nurse anesthetist, or respiratory therapist, performs the intubation.

An endotracheal tube is effective for short-term maintenance of an airway. Long-term maintenance requires a tracheostomy. Major indications for endotracheal intubation include airway protection when the client loses reflexes because of anesthesia, medications, disease, or decreased level of consciousness; a need for mechanical ventilation; suctioning of secretions when the client cannot handle secretions (as in COPD); and airway obstruction.

An endotracheal tube has several parts (see Fig. 62–8). The *shaft* of the tube contains a radiopaque vertical line for the length of the tube that permits correct placement by chest x-ray. Short horizontal lines (depth markings) are used to designate the correct placement of the tube at the nares or mouth. The *cuff* at the distal end of the tube produces a seal between the trachea and the cuff when properly inflated. The seal prevents aspiration and ensures a set tidal volume when a ventilator is attached to the tube. When the balloon is inflated, no air

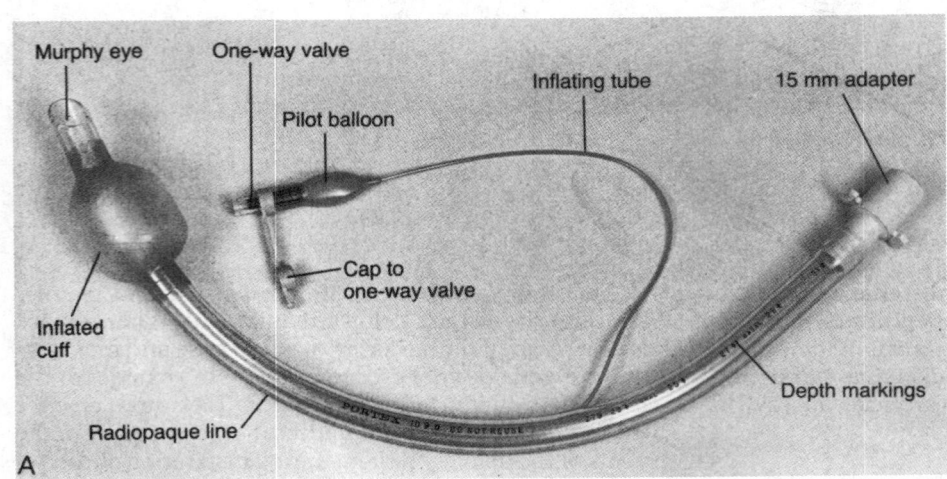

Murphy eye · One-way valve · Inflating tube · 15 mm adapter · Pilot balloon · Cap to one-way valve · Inflated cuff · Radiopaque line · Depth markings · PORTEX · A

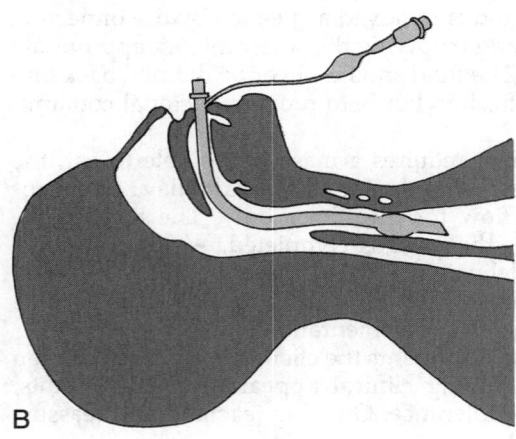

B

Figure 62–8

Components and placement of an endotracheal tube. (*A* from Kersten, L. D. [1989]. *Comprehensive respiratory nursing: A decision making approach.* Philadelphia: W. B. Saunders.)

can pass through the cuff to the vocal cords, nose, or mouth; therefore, the client is unable to talk when the cuff is inflated. The *pilot balloon* with a one-way valve permits air to be inserted into the cuff yet prevents air from escaping. The balloon provides a general guideline for the absence or presence but not the actual amount of air in the cuff. The *universal adapter,* which is 15 mm in diameter, enables attachment to a ventilator or to other types of oxygen delivery system. The *size* of the tube is indicated on the adapter or shaft of the tube. Adult sizes range from 5 to 10 mm. Size 8.5 to 9.0 is commonly used for men; size 7.5 to 8.0 (smaller sizes), for women.

It is important for the nurse to know the proper mechanism to summon personnel responsible for intubation to the bedside and to explain the procedure to the client as much as possible. Basic life-support measures, such as establishment of a patent airway and the administration of 100% oxygen via a resuscitation (Ambu) bag with face mask, are crucial to the client's survival. The coordination to perform resuscitation via a bag and mask device can be cumbersome; therefore, practice is necessary.

The code (or "crash") cart, respiratory equipment box, and suction equipment are placed at the bedside. The nurse's role is to maintain a patent airway until the client is intubated. During intubation, the nurse continuously monitors for changes in the client's vital signs, signs of hypoxia, arrythmias, and aspiration. The nurse also ensures that intubation attempts last no longer than 30 seconds. After 30 seconds, oxygen is provided to prevent hypoxia and potential cardiopulmonary arrest.

Immediately after an endotracheal tube is inserted, its placement must be verified. To do this, the nurse assesses the client for bilateral equal breath sounds and bilateral equal chest excursion, and air is felt emerging from the endotracheal tube. If these findings are not present, the endotracheal tube may be in the right mainstem bronchus. In this case, breath sounds and chest wall movement are absent or diminished on the left side.

The stomach is auscultated to rule out esophageal intubation. If the endotracheal tube is in the stomach, breath sounds are louder over the stomach than over the chest, and abdominal distention is noted. The *absence* of bilateral equal breath sounds requires reintubation. Ongoing close attention to chest wall movement and breath sounds is necessary until tube placement is verified by a chest x-ray film.

Stabilization of the endotracheal tube at the mouth or nose is performed by the nurse. The tube is marked at the level it touches the mouth or nare. Two people are then required to secure the tube at this position. Securement of the tube is done through a head halter technique with tape. Ongoing care requires that the tube is switched to the opposite side of the mouth daily. This maneuver helps to prevent pressure on and necrosis of the lip and mouth area, to prevent nerve damage, and to facilitate thorough inspection and cleaning of the mouth. One person stabilizes the tube at the correct position and prevents head movement while the other person applies the tape as shown in the accompanying Guidelines feature. After the procedure is completed, the presence of bilateral equal breath sounds, as well as correct tube placement, is verified. Care of the airway is discussed in the next section on tracheostomy. An oral airway may be needed to prevent the client from biting an oral endotracheal tube.

Assessment of tube placement, the presence of bilateral equal breath sounds, and chest wall movement is incorporated into all nursing care activities of the intubated client, at least every hour. Care is taken to prevent pulling or tugging on the tube when the client is turned, suctioned, or disconnected from the ventilator. Tubing from the ventilator is supported by special adapters to allow the client to move without tugging on the tubing. If a client coughs frequently, tries to speak, or is out of synchrony with the ventilator, extra stress is placed on the endotracheal tube and may cause dislodgement of the tube. Head flexion moves the tube closer to the carina; head extension moves the tube away from the carina. Rotation of the head also causes movement of the tube. Mouth secretions and tongue manipulations can loosen the tape and allow malposition of the tube. To prevent accidental movement of the tube or extubation, the client may need to have soft wrist restraints applied. The rationale for restraints must be explained to both the client and the family to decrease anxiety and ensure their cooperation. Other facets of nursing care for the client with an endotracheal tube are the same as those for tracheostomy, as described in the next section.

The endotracheal tube is removed when the indication for intubation has resolved; i.e., the client has a patent airway and is able to mobilize secretions effectively. The removal of the endotracheal tube is called *extubation.*

Before extubation, the nurse explains the procedure to the client. An oxygen delivery system such as a mask or a cannula is set up at the bedside along with suctioning equipment, tissues, and equipment for reintubation (usually found in the respiratory emergency box). The client is then hyperoxygenated and hyperinflated, and both the endotracheal tube and oral cavity are suctioned thoroughly. The person performing the extubation must be proficient in intubation (or personnel capable of performing an intubation must be present) in case the client needs an emergency intubation.

During the extubation process, the cuff is deflated and the tube is removed during peak inspiration. The client is instructed to take deep breaths and to cough. A large amount of oral secretions that have accumulated in the back of the throat is expected. An oxygen mask or cannula is placed on the client, usually at an FIO_2 10% higher than the level maintained during the intubation process.

Postextubation monitoring is essential. The nurse monitors the client's vital signs every hour initially, with a special focus on respiratory pattern and any signs and symptoms of respiratory distress. The client usually experiences hoarseness and a sore throat for a few days after extubation. The client is instructed to sit in a semi-

GUIDELINES ■ How to Tape an Oral Endotracheal Tube

1. If the client is alert, instruct her or him not to move and to keep the head in the midline position while you tape the tube. Provide reassurance as follows:
   a. State that taping the tube takes about 5 min.
   b. Emphasize that the procedure will not interfere with breathing or cause pain.
2. To make a halter, cut two strips of tape, one 65 cm (26 in) long and the other 15–20 cm (6–8 in) long.
3. Lay the 65-cm (26-in) length flat with the adhesive side up. Place the 15-cm (6-in) length sticky side down in the middle of the longer strip. The sticky sides of the tape are apposed so that the hair bordering the client's posterior neck area does not stick to the halter.

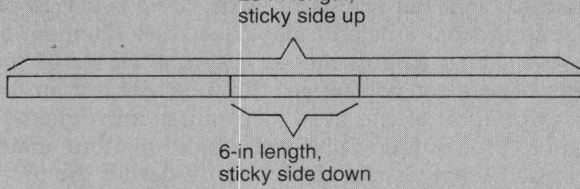

26-in length, sticky side up

6-in length, sticky side down

4. Place the halter under the client's neck.

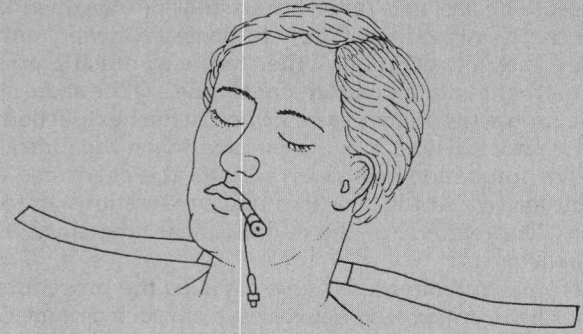

5. Split or tear each tape end lengthwise to the point at which the endotracheal tube exists from the mouth.
   a. Be careful not to tear the tape too far. The halter will not fit if the tape is torn to a point beyond the mouth.
   b. Trim excess tape with scissors, as needed.

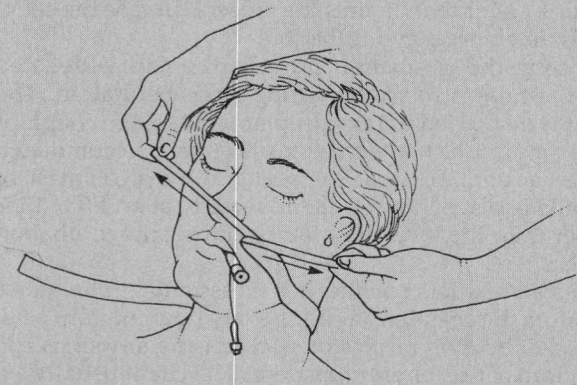

6. Prepare the skin by applying benzoin to the face and

tube where tape contact is anticipated. Properly prepared skin surfaces are vital for tape adhesion and adequate tube stabilization. Whenever possible
   a. Allow at least 1 min for the benzoin to dry before tape application. Fan the skin with a package of 4 × 4 in gauze pads if necessary, to reduce drying time.
   b. For diaphoretic skin, wash with soap and water and dry before benzoin application.
7. To tape one side of the face
   a. Wrap the top split end beneath the nose and across the opposite cheek.

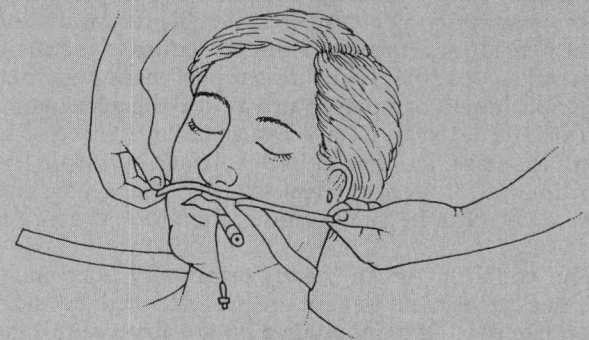

   b. Wrap the bottom split end around the tube.

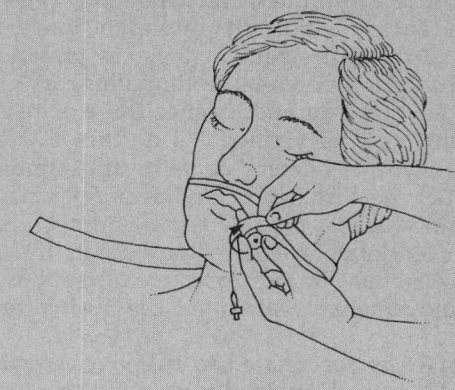

8. Repeat step 7 with the other end of the tape.
9. When you are finished wrapping the tube, fold a ¼-in end of tape back on itself to make a pull tab. This pull tab facilitates later tape removal.

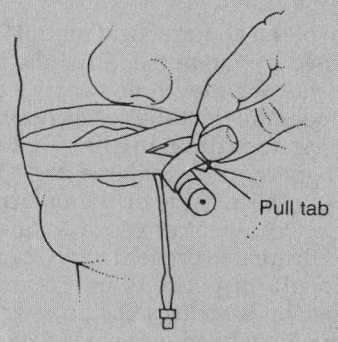

Pull tab

Modified from Kersten, L. D. (1989). *Comprehensive respiratory nursing: A decision making approach*. Philadelphia: W. B. Saunders.

Fowler position, to take deep breaths every ½ hour, and to limit speaking in the immediate period after extubation. These measures facilitate gas exchange and decrease laryngeal edema and vocal cord irritation. The client is also closely observed for signs of upper airway obstruction. Early signs of obstruction are mild dyspnea, coughing, and inability to expectorate secretions. If these signs occur, the nurse notifies the physician who evaluates the need for reintubation. The nurse is especially concerned if the client develops stridor, which is a late sign of a narrowed airway. *Stridor* is a high-pitched, crowing noise heard during inspiration and is caused by laryngospasm or edema above or below the glottis. Racemic epinephrine, a topical aerosol vasoconstrictor, is given and reintubation is performed.

Intubation with tracheostomy tubes. A *tracheotomy* is the surgical incision into a trachea. The resulting *tracheostomy* is the opening, or stoma, that is made during surgery, and a *tracheostomy tube* is inserted into the stoma. A tracheostomy is performed for various reasons; however, the use of a tracheostomy implies that an artificial airway is needed for a prolonged period. A tracheostomy is done after an endotracheal tube has been in place for about a month; however, if prolonged intubation is anticipated, the physician may perform a tracheostomy a week after an endotracheal tube has been placed.

Indications for tracheostomy include

1. Prolonged intubation or mechanical ventilation
2. Acute upper airway obstruction when oral or nasal intubation is not possible (if there is facial or nasal obstruction, trauma, or burns)
3. Chronic obstructive airway diseases such as obstructive sleep apnea
4. Retention of secretions, especially in clients with COPD
5. Facilitation of the weaning process (decreased dead space and length of tube makes breathing and expectoration of secretions easier)
6. Airway protection for large aspirations
7. Prophylaxis against airway obstruction, such as with facial burns, radical neck surgery, radiation to the neck area, and various neurologic surgeries that may alter the ability to protect the airway
8. Laryngectomy

Intubation procedure. A tracheostomy is usually an elective procedure that takes approximately 20 minutes to perform. The procedure can be performed in the operating room or at the bedside with the client under local or general anesthesia. An emergency tracheostomy is reserved for the client who cannot be intubated with an oral endotracheal tube because of facial trauma, burns, or airway obstruction. During the operation, the neck is extended while the endotracheal tube is still in place. A horizontal incision is made below the cricothyroid cartilage, followed by a second vertical incision that

is made through the second, third, and fourth tracheal rings (Fig. 62–9). There can be variations on the second type of incision depending on the surgeon's preference. After the incision is made, the endotracheal tube is quickly removed and the tracheostomy tube is inserted. The tracheostomy tube is secured in place by sutures and tracheostomy ties. The tracheostomy cuff is inflated and an x-ray film taken to ensure proper placement.

Postoperative nursing care focuses on ensuring a patent airway and confirming the presence of bilateral equal breath sounds. The three major complications that arise in the immediate postoperative period include bleeding, infection at the tracheostomy site, and subcutaneous emphysema and pneumothorax. A small amount of bleeding is to be expected for the first few days; however, a constant oozing warrants surgical intervention or ligation of blood vessels. To prevent infection, sterile technique is used for suctioning and tracheostomy care; the stoma site is closely watched for purulent drainage, redness, pain, or cellulitis. If a tracheostomy dressing is used, it must be kept clean and dry; a moist dressing provides an excellent medium for bacterial growth. Early detection and prevention of a local infection are important because it can lead to a more diffuse pulmonary infection. Care is also taken to prevent oxygen or ventilator tubing from pulling on the tracheostomy. Minimizing manipulation and traction on the tracheostomy prevents tissue breakdown, erosion, and infection. In addition, the client is not allowed to eat or drink initially, and the cuff is inflated to prevent aspiration.

The neck and chest areas are assessed for subcutaneous emphysema (air bubbles under the skin) or unequal breath sounds, which may reflect a pneumothorax (monitoring for these complications continues while the tracheostomy tube is present). As a safety measure, a

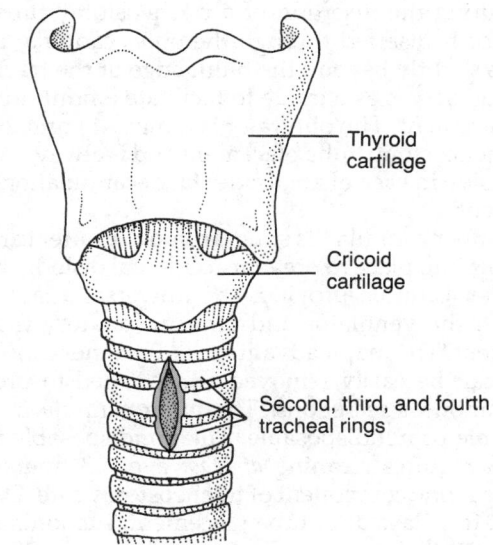

Thyroid cartilage

Cricoid cartilage

Second, third, and fourth tracheal rings

Figure 62–9

Vertical tracheal incision for a tracheostomy.

tracheostomy set of the same size and tracheostomy insertion tray is kept at the bedside for an emergency intubation.

Although these physical complications are potentially life-threatening, addressing the psychologic concerns of the client is an important aspect of nursing care. The tracheostomy tube feels different from the endotracheal tube. The client needs reassurance that the tube is supposed to feel different but that an adjustment to this difference generally occurs quickly. Many people find the tracheostomy tube to be more comfortable than the endotracheal tube. A means of communication via a writing tablet, magic slate, or hand signals, as well as a call light within reach, is essential to promote communication and to decrease the client's frustration.

Types of tracheostomy tubes. A variety of tracheostomy tubes are available, the one that is used depending on the specific needs of the client. A tracheostomy tube is similar to an endotracheal tube but is shorter (it is usually 2 to 6 in [5 to 15 cm] long). In contrast to an endotracheal tube, the tracheostomy tube has associated with it a high risk of infection, but it is more comfortable and allows the client to eat. A tracheostomy can be temporary or permanent (laryngectomy). A tracheostomy tube is available in various sizes and types of materials and may be disposable or nondisposable. In addition, a tracheostomy tube can have a cuff or can be cuffless.

Most clients in the acute care setting have a *double-lumen tracheostomy* tube, which has three major parts: the outer cannula, the inner cannula, and the obturator (Fig. 62–10). The outer cannula fits into the stoma and keeps the airway open. The flange, or face plate, of the outer cannula anchors the tube in the trachea and has small holes on both sides that allow the tube to be secured with tracheostomy ties. The face plate also indicates the size and type of tube.

The obturator is a plastic or metal tube with a blunted end. During the insertion of a tracheostomy tube, the obturator is inserted through the outer cannula; its tip extends slightly beyond the blunt edge of the tracheostomy and serves as a guide to facilitate a nontraumatic tube placement. The obturator is removed immediately after tracheostomy tube placement and is always kept at the bedside in case of an accidental decannulation (displacement).

The inner cannula fits snugly into the outer cannula and locks into place to prevent accidental dislodgement. The inner cannula provides the universal adapter for use with the ventilator and other respiratory therapy equipment. The major advantage of the inner cannula is that it can be easily removed and cleaned to prevent encrustation of secretions. The inner cannula may be disposable or nondisposable. The nondisposable inner cannula requires cleaning *at least* every 8 hours; this cleaning is one component of tracheostomy care. During the first few days after tube placement, suctioning and cleaning of the cannula may be needed every 30 to 60 minutes.

An alternative to the double-lumen tracheostomy

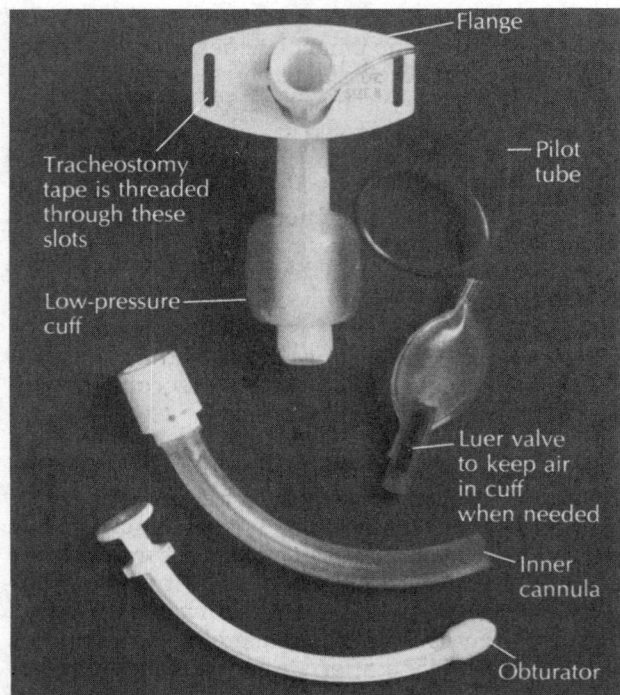

Figure 62–10

Metal tracheostomy tube and obturator. (Reproduced courtesy of Shiley, Inc., Irvine, CA.)

tube is the *single-lumen tracheostomy tube* (Fig. 62–11). The single-lumen tube requires less tracheostomy care but is reserved for the client with minimal secretions, for short-term use, or for special circumstances according to hospital protocol. The single-lumen tracheostomy tube is longer and has different diameter sizes compared with the double-lumen tracheostomy tube.

The single- or double-lumen tracheostomy tube may have a cuff or may be cuffless. The cuffless tube is for long-term airway patency in the client with an intact swallow and gag reflex. A tracheostomy tube with a cuff should have the cuff inflated to prevent a large aspiration of blood, secretions, and gastric contents, and to facilitate mechanical ventilation; otherwise, the cuff should be deflated. The inflated cuff can interfere with glottic function and swallowing ability and is the major cause of complications for the client with a tracheostomy. When a cuff is present, a pilot balloon attached to the outside of the tube indicates the presence or absence of air in the cuff; however, it does not reflect whether the correct amount of air is present.

A fenestrated tracheostomy tube is a special type of tube that has a precut opening (fenestration) in the posterior wall of the outer cannula. This type of tube is used to facilitate speech and helps to wean the client from the tracheostomy tube (Fig. 62–12). It may or may not have a cuff.

When the inner cannula is in place, the fenestration is covered and the tube functions as a normal double-lumen tracheostomy tube. When the inner cannula is

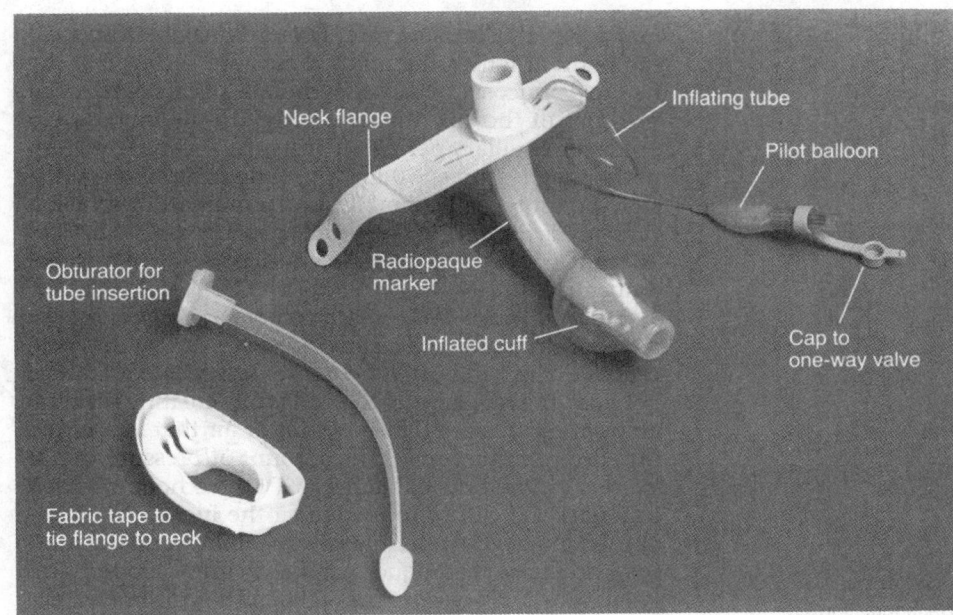

Figure 62-11

Single-lumen tracheostomy tube (Portex). (Photograph from Kersten, L. D. [1989]. *Comprehensive respiratory nursing: A decision making approach.* Philadelphia: W. B. Saunders.)

removed, air can pass through the fenestration, the vocal cords, and the mouth. When the cuff (if present) is deflated, the client can then breathe through the fenestration as well as the tracheal stoma. The tube can be plugged with a short decannulation cannula (which comes with the tracheostomy tube), thus allowing the client to breathe through the fenestration, the deflated cuff, and the upper airways. The client can then cough, speak, and become accustomed to breathing through the upper air passages again. If the client has trouble with any of these maneuvers, the fenestration must be assessed by the physician for proper placement and patency, and the tube should not be capped until the problem is corrected.

A fenestrated tracheostomy tube is often used to ensure that the client can tolerate breathing normally through the upper air passages for several days before the tracheostomy tube is removed (Fig. 62-13). The most important point to remember with a fenestrated tube is to ALWAYS DEFLATE THE CUFF BEFORE THE TUBE IS CAPPED WITH THE DECANNULATION CANNULA. Otherwise, the client will suffocate.

A *metal tracheostomy tube* is used for a permanent tracheostomy or laryngectomy. The most popular types of metal tubes are the Jackson and the Holinger tubes. This type of tube is often used for home care because it can be cleaned and reused indefinitely. Like the double-lumen tracheostomy, the metal tube has an inner cannula, an outer cannula, and an obturator, but it is cuffless. The metal tracheostomy tube is rarely used today in the acute care setting because it is rigid and causes necrosis and discomfort. The metal causes irritation and

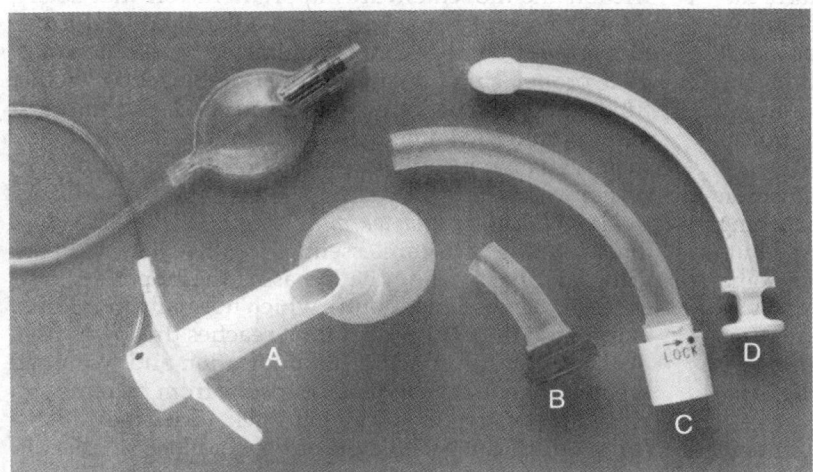

Figure 62-12

The Shiley fenestrated low-pressure cuffed tracheostomy tube, showing the outer cannula with a fenestration above the cuff (A); decannulation cannula used to plug the tracheostomy tube (B); inner cannula (C); and obturator (D). (Reproduced courtesy of Shiley, Inc., Irvine, CA.)

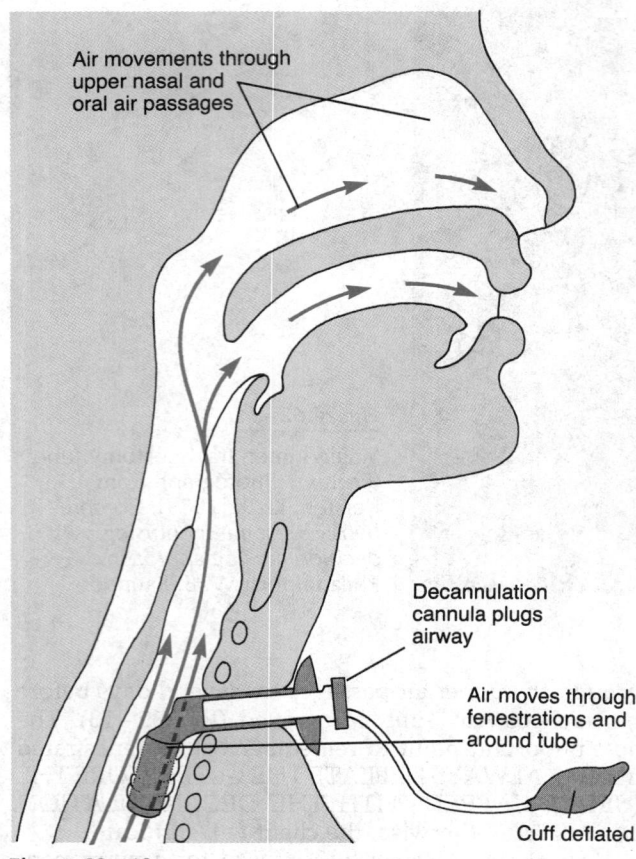

Air movements through upper nasal and oral air passages

Decannulation cannula plugs airway

Air moves through fenestrations and around tube

Cuff deflated

Figure 62–13

Breathing through a fenestrated tracheostomy tube with a cannula in place and the cuff deflated.

stimulates mucus production, and the tube does not have a 15-mm universal adapter that facilitates use with a manual resuscitator bag or mechanical ventilator.

The *talking tracheostomy tube* (such as the Pitt Trach Speaking Tube [National Catheter Corporation] and Communitrach [Implant Technologies, Inc.]) provides a means of communication for the client using a ventilator on a long-term basis. In these types, a standard tracheostomy tube with an extra air channel allows speaking with the cuff inflated. For the client who has a permanent tracheostomy, a speaking valve, such as the Olympic Trach-Talk or Passy-Muir Tracheostomy Speaking Valve, can be used to facilitate communication.

Another device that can be used for the transition from mechanical ventilation to spontaneous breathing is a *tracheostomy button.* A variety of tracheostomy buttons can be used to maintain the patency of the stoma and to facilitate spontaneous breathing in the client who can expectorate secretions adequately. The Kistner tracheostomy tube and Olympic tracheostomy button are examples of this type of device. They both must be carefully fitted and sized to work properly.

Prevention of tissue damage. Prevention of tissue damage from the cuff of the tracheostomy tube is a major aspect of nursing care. Tissue damage can occur at the point at which the inflated cuff presses against the tracheal mucosa. Mucosal ischemia occurs when the pressure of the cuff that is exerted on the mucosa exceeds the capillary perfusion pressure. Arterial capillary perfusion pressure is 30 mmHg, venous capillary perfusion pressure is 18 mmHg, and lymphatic perfusion pressure is 5 mmHg. Therefore, a cuff pressure of 14 to 20 mmHg is believed to reduce the incidence of tracheal damage.

Most cuffs are designed to receive a high volume of air while maintaining a low pressure on the tracheal mucosa. The cuff is inflated to provide an adequate seal between the trachea and the cuff while creating the least amount of pressure. The amount of air that is inserted into the cuff determines the amount of pressure that is exerted on the tracheal mucosa. Two methods are used to inflate the cuff while reducing the incidence of tracheal damage: the minimal leak technique and the minimal occlusive technique. After the cuff is properly inflated, the cuff pressure is checked. The cuff pressure is then checked every 8 hours and anytime air is added to or removed from the cuff. The cuff pressure is checked by a manometer device and is maintained at 14 to 20 mmHg. If a higher pressure is needed, the physician is notified. Cuff pressure should not exceed 20 mmHg, or 25 cmH$_2$O, except in rare situations. There is no need to deflate the cuff routinely. The cuff is deflated only as needed to allow the client to speak or to check whether the cuff is overinflated. Manufacturers provide guidelines for safe volumes allowed for each tracheostomy size.

Although a high cuff pressure causes tracheal damage, other factors contribute to the severity of tracheal damage sustained. The condition of the client determines, to a degree, the susceptibility to tissue damage. The client who is malnourished, hypotensive, dehydrated, hypoxic, or receiving corticosteroids is unable to promote adequate tissue healing and is prone to further tissue damage.

The duration of intubation, the extent and technique of suctioning, and the stabilization of the tube against friction and movement are important factors that determine the extent of tracheal mucosa damage. Therefore, local airway damage can be minimized by maintenance of a proper cuff pressure, proper stabilization of the tube, judicious suctioning only as needed, and the prevention and/or immediate treatment of malnutrition, hemodynamic instability (low blood pressure), or hypoxia.

Humidification and warming of air. Humidification and warming of air are essential for any client with an artificial airway. The tube bypasses the upper air passages of the nose and mouth, which normally humidify, warm, and filter the air before it reaches the lower part of the respiratory tract. If humidification and warming are not done, tracheal damage results from extremes in air temperature; in addition, thick, dried secretions form, which can occlude the airway or block smaller air passages and cause atelectasis and pneumonia. To prevent these complications, a humidification source is provided to the client who has an artificial airway. A fine mist should be seen emerging from the tracheostomy collar or T piece apparatus during inspiration and expiration. To increase the amount of humidification delivered, a warming device is attached to the humidification source. A temperature probe is placed in the tubing circuit so that the temperature is constantly monitored and maintained at 98.6° to 100.4° F (37° to 38° C), but no greater than 104° F (40° C). The nurse monitors the temperature by feeling the tubing during client care or by checking the temperature probe. Humidification can also be given by parenteral or enteral routes. A liberal fluid intake helps to mobilize secretions and facilitate their removal. Close monitoring of intake and output is needed, and special attention is warranted for the client with conditions for which fluid intake is restricted.

Suctioning. Suctioning maintains a patent airway by removal of secretions from clients who cannot cough or expectorate. This sterile procedure promotes gas exchange and prevents pneumonia. The Guidelines feature on pages 2019 and 2020 describes the interventions and rationales for the suctioning procedure. Suctioning is never performed unless needed. Indications for suctioning include audible, noisy expiration; restlessness; increased pulse and respiratory rates; presence of mucus in the artificial airway; an expressed need for suctioning by the client; and increased peak airway pressure on the ventilator.

Suctioning is associated with several complications, which can be avoided by using meticulous nursing care. *Hypoxia* is the major complication. Hypoxia is caused by (1) ineffective oxygenation before, during, and after suctioning; (2) use of a catheter that is too large for the endotracheal tube; (3) prolonged suctioning time; (4) excessive suction pressure; (5) frequent suctioning; and (6) removal of the client's air while removing secretions.

Hypoxia is prevented by hyperventilation with 100% oxygen from an oxygen delivery device (Ambu bag or oxygen mask) for at least 3 minutes before, during, and after suctioning and after the instillation of saline to loosen secretions, if needed. If the client is able to take deep breaths (is not using a ventilator), the nurse instructs the client to deep breathe three times instead of using the device. If possible, simultaneous monitoring of heart rate and/or rhythm or use of a pulse oximeter is helpful in assessing tolerance of the suctioning procedure. The client is assessed for signs and symptoms of hypoxia, which include increased heart rate, increased blood pressure, and onset of arrhythmias. The client with minimal cardiopulmonary reserve may experience hypotension, bradycardia, onset of arrhythmias, or oxygen desaturation (a reading below 90% on the pulse oximeter). If these signs and symptoms occur, the suctioning procedure must be immediately terminated and the client is manually resuscitated until baseline parameters are achieved.

Hypoxia is also prevented by using a catheter of the correct size. The suction catheter size should not exceed one-half of the size of the endotracheal lumen. In adults, the standard catheter size is 12 or 14 French. Adequate size facilitates efficient removal of secretions without causing hypoxemia.

Tissue trauma is the second major complication of suctioning. The mucosa of the respiratory tract is extremely fragile, and damage is caused by frequent suctioning, prolonged suctioning time, and excessive suction pressure. (These factors also contribute to hypoxia.) Tissue trauma is prevented by suctioning only when indicated. The catheter is lubricated with water or water-soluble lubricant before insertion, and suction is applied only during the withdrawal of the catheter. Use of a twirling motion during withdrawal prevents the catheter from grabbing the mucosa. In addition, suction is applied for only 10 to 15 seconds. This time frame can be estimated by the nurse's holding a breath and counting to 10 or 15 during the suctioning procedure. When the nurse needs to breathe, the client also needs to breathe, and the suctioning procedure ends. The suction pressure is tested before suctioning and is set between 80 and 120 mmHg. Higher pressures result in significant mucosal trauma and hypoxia.

The third complication of suctioning is the increased risk of *infection.* Each time the catheter is passed into the trachea, bacteria may be introduced. Strict sterile technique is used for suctioning and for all equipment including suction catheters, gloves, and water (Fig. 62–14). The endotracheal tube or tracheostomy tube is always suctioned first, after which the mouth is suctioned. Suctioning equipment that has been used in the mouth is never used for suctioning an artificial airway. The mouth is contaminated with bacteria, which could be introduced into the lower parts of the lungs and cause pneumonia (see Guidelines: Endotracheal and Tracheal Suctioning).

The last complication of suctioning is *vagal stimulation and bronchospasm.* Vagal stimulation results in severe bradycardia, hypotension, heart block, ventricular tachycardia, or asystole. If vagal stimulation occurs, the nurse stops suctioning immediately and oxygenates the client manually with 100% oxygen. Bronchospasm can be triggered when the catheter passes into the airway; it is difficult to provide ventilation with a resuscitation bag, and the client may require a bronchodilator to relieve respiratory distress.

Tracheostomy care. Tracheostomy care is performed by the nurse to keep the tracheostomy tube and the stoma free from secretions and mucus to prevent infection and to maintain a patent airway when the client is unable to cough or expectorate secretions. Tracheostomy care is performed at least every 8 hours and as needed, as described in detail in the Guidelines feature on page 2021. In the acute care setting, suctioning is used before tracheostomy care is performed to remove any excess secretions. The extent of tracheostomy care varies depending on the type of tracheostomy tube. For example, the client with a nondisposable inner cannula has it removed and cleaned; the client with a disposable inner cannula has a new inner cannula inserted and the

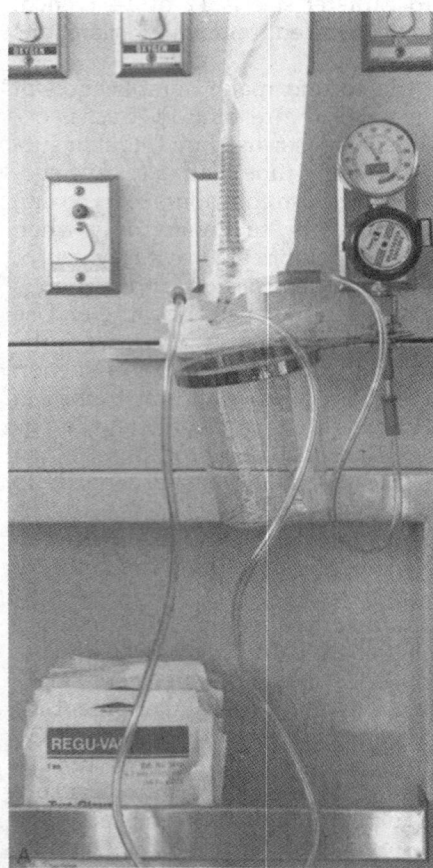

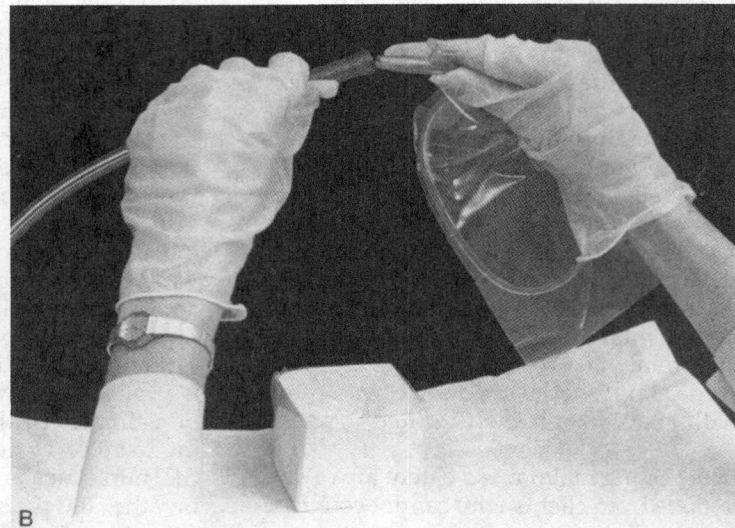

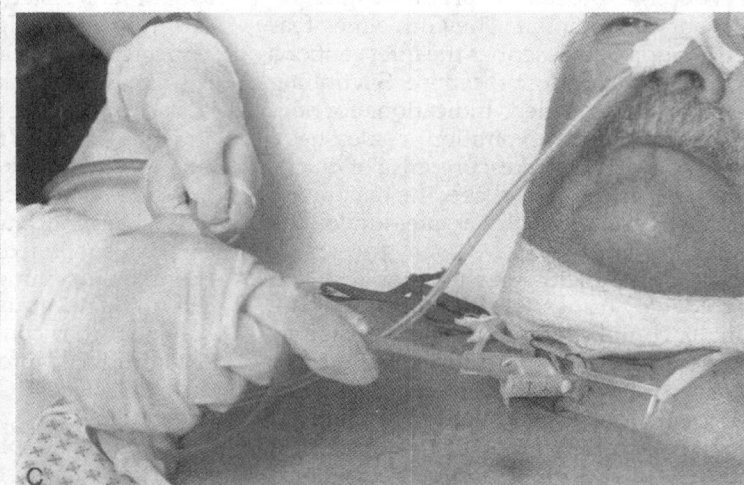

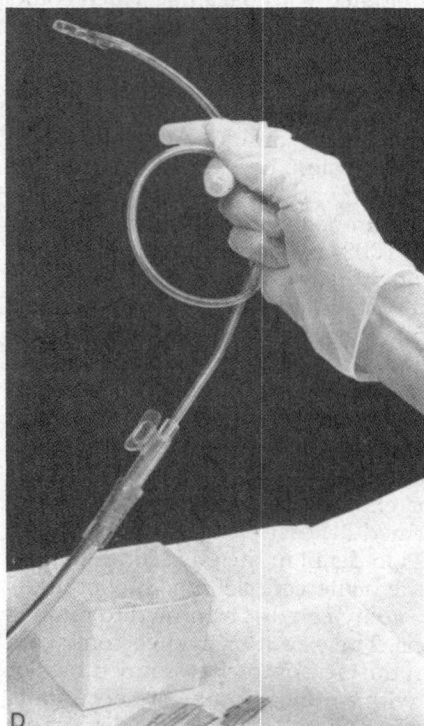

Figure 62–14

Sterile technique for suctioning. *A*, Bedside suction canister, tubing, and tonsil tip (also called Yankauer's pharyngeal suction tip) attached to wall vacuum. *B*, Attaching a suction catheter to the suction source. *C*, Suctioning by passing a catheter through a tracheostomy tube. *D*, Holding the catheter with one hand away from the client to prevent possible contamination between suctioning passes. (From Kersten, L. D. [1989]. *Comprehensive respiratory nursing: A decision making approach.* Philadelphia: W. B. Saunders.)

GUIDELINES ■ Endotracheal and Tracheal Suctioning

Interventions	Rationales
1. Assess the need for suctioning.	1. Routine suctioning causes mucosal damage, bleeding, or bronchospasm.

2. Assemble the following equipment:
  a. Suction kit, which normally includes
    ■ 2 sterile gloves.
    ■ 1 sterile suction catheter (adult size 14).
    ■ Sterile container for sterile water (ready to use or cap removed so that it can be poured later).
  b. Sterile saline.
  c. Self-inflating resuscitator bag connected to oxygen meter at 15 L/min.
  d. Suction source with connecting tube.
	2. Proper equipment facilitates infection control standards.

3. Wash hands.	3. Use of antiseptic soap in the hospital setting decreases the chance of contamination.

4. Explain the procedure to the client.
  a. Explain that sensations such as shortness of breath and coughing are to be expected.
  b. Explain that the procedure causes discomfort but is short.
	4. Information helps the client to prepare for the procedure and facilitates cooperation.

5. Check the suction source. Occlude the suction source and adjust the pressure dial to 80–120 mmHg.	5. Excessive or inadequate suction creates hypoxemia; mucosal trauma occurs with excessive pressure.
6. Place a towel or barrier over the client's chest (optional).	6. The barrier protects the gown and the client from secretions that are expectorated from the artificial airway.
7. Open the suction kit and put on sterile gloves.	7. Two gloves prevent contamination and exposure to the client's secretions.
8. Pour sterile water into the sterile container using the nondominant hand.	8. The nondominant hand is no longer sterile, is considered to be clean, and can be used to touch the tubing connection, ventilator, or client during the procedure.
9. With the sterile dominant hand, remove the sterile catheter from wrapping. Keep it coiled to prevent touching nonsterile objects.	9. The catheter must remain sterile. If the catheter is contaminated, it must be thrown away to prevent infection.
10. Hold the catheter in the sterile dominant hand and place the connecting tubing in the clean nondominant hand.	10. The nondominant hand is used to control suction tubing and to regulate suction.
11. Lubricate the catheter tip in sterile saline solution. Occlude the control valve of the catheter while the tip is immersed in the sterile saline solution.	11. Lubrication facilitates catheter insertion and reduces tissue trauma.
12. Don goggles or protective eyewear (varies by institution).	12. Use of goggles is in accordance with universal precautions.

13. Preoxygenate the client with 100% oxygen for 30 s to 3 min to prevent hypoxemia (at least three hyperinflations).
  a. Try to keep breaths synchronized with client's breathing pattern.
  b. Whenever possible, have a second person use the Ambu bag while the other person suctions.
	13. The length of reoxygenation varies depending on the client's pulmonary status, the effectiveness of inflation, and the oxygen delivery device used.
	  a. Synchrony facilitates comfort.
	
	  b. A two-person technique improves the efficiency of the procedure, especially if the client is using a ventilator.

14. Quickly insert the catheter into the trachea through the endotracheal or tracheal tube until resistance is met. Do not apply suction during insertion.	14. Keeping suction off and moving quickly avoid hypoxia and tissue trauma.

Continued

GUIDELINES ■ Endotracheal and Tracheal Suctioning *Continued*

Interventions	Rationales

15. Withdraw the catheter 1–2 cm (0.4–0.8 in) and begin to apply suction for 10–15 s by occluding the control valve with the thumb of clean hand.
  a. *Never suction longer than 10–15 s.*
  b. Use intermittent suction.
  c. Use a twirling motion of the catheter during withdrawal.
	15. This technique prevents hypoxia and ensures that the procedure is done within 15 s.

16. Hyperoxygenate the client with 100% oxygen for at least 1–5 min or until baseline heart rate and oxygen saturation are within normal limits.	16. Variable time is needed to return the client to baseline arterial PO_2 values.
17. Suction as needed following steps 12–15 but do not use the same catheter for more than three insertions.	17. This action prevents excessive suctioning and its side effects, as well as prevents cross-contamination.
18. Instill 3–5 mL of sterile saline.	18. Saline provides humidification to loosen secretions and facilitate their removal.
19. Suction the mouth as needed and provide mouth care after endotracheal suction is completed. A catheter that has been used for the mouth is contaminated and should *never* be used for endotracheal suctioning.	19. The client may have a large amount of oral secretions that needs removal.
20. Discard suctioning material following institutional policy and procedure.	20. Discarding contaminated equipment appropriately prevents contact with other clients.
21. Wash hands and replenish suctioning materials at the bedside.	21. Suctioning equipment must be available for emergency situations.

22. Document the procedure.
  a. The client's tolerance of the procedure.
  b. The type, amount, and consistency of secretions.
	22. Document provides guidelines for assessment and effectiveness of interventions.

old one discarded; the client with a single-lumen tracheostomy tube requires stoma care only. No matter what type is used, every client requires stoma care and assessment to determine whether tracheostomy ties are to be changed. Usually, the tracheostomy tie is changed once a day; hook and loop (Velcro) ties may be changed only as needed (Fig. 62–15). In either case, a properly secured tie allows space for only one finger to be placed between the tie and the neck. After tracheostomy care is completed, an assessment of the tracheostomy site, type of drainage, and tolerance of the procedure is documented.

Bronchial and oral hygiene. Bronchial and oral hygiene measures are used to promote a patent airway and help to prevent infection in a client who cannot cough or expectorate secretions. Turning and repositioning the client every 1 to 2 hours, getting the client out of bed, and encouraging ambulation all promote lung expansion and gas exchange and facilitate mobilization of secretions.

Frequent oral hygiene is important not only to ensure a patent airway, but also to prevent bacterial growth and to promote client comfort. Gloves are worn to protect the client and the nurse from cross-contamination. The use of glycerine swabs and mouthwash is discouraged because both further dry the mouth mucosa, change its pH, and therefore promote bacterial growth. Instead, a toothette that has been dipped in water or saline is best used for mouth care because it promotes granulation and healing. Hydrogen peroxide solutions can help to remove crusted material, but these should be avoided in the client with granulation tissue because hydrogen peroxide breaks down new tissue.

During mouth care, the nurse closely examines the mucosa for ulcers (e.g., as in herpes simplex), bacterial or fungal (candidal) growth, or other infections. The physician is notified of abnormalities so that appropriate local medications can be ordered. Application of lip balms or water-soluble jelly can prevent cracked lips and further skin breakdown and can help keep the client comfortable. Providing mouth care is a simple method of promoting client comfort and aesthetics. Offering an opportunity for the client or family member to do mouth care encourages participation in care and decreases the sense of helplessness.

Measures to promote emotional well-being. While providing physical care to the client, the nurse must be cognizant of the psychologic impact of the tracheos-

GUIDELINES ■ Tracheostomy Care

During this procedure, the nurse must ensure that the tracheostomy tube is secured at all times to prevent dislodgement. This procedure can be done with two people; one person changes the ties while the other person secures the tube. If the one-person technique is used, the old tracheostomy ties must remain intact until the new ties have been secured.

1. Assemble the following equipment:
   a. Equipment for suctioning.
   b. Scissors.
   c. Sterile water.
   d. Sterile gloves.
   e. Tracheostomy kit, which includes
      - Containers for sterile water and peroxide.
      - Sterile precut tracheostomy dressing.
      - Tracheostomy ties.
      - Pipe cleaners.
      - Tracheostomy brush.
      - Cotton-tipped swabs.
      - Forceps.
      - 4 × 4 in gauze pads.

2. Wash hands.

3. Explain the procedure to the client and assist the client to a comfortable position that facilitates easy access to the tracheostomy.

4. Suction the tracheostomy tube.

5. Remove old dressings and excess secretions.

6. Open the tracheostomy kit and pour a solution of one-half strength hydrogen peroxide and sterile water in equal amounts into one bowl; pour sterile water into the other bowl.

7. Put on sterile gloves.

8. Remove the inner cannula and clean it.
   a. Immerse the inner cannula in the hydrogen peroxide solution.
   b. Use the tracheostomy brush and pipe cleaners to clean secretions from the inside inner cannula.
   c. Rinse the inner cannula in the bowl of sterile water; pat it dry.
   d. Reinsert the inner cannula into the outer cannula; ensure that the locking mechanism is engaged; reconnect the ventilator or oxygen source.
   e. If client is using a ventilator, replace the inner cannula with an extra one or an adapter so that the client continues to use the ventilator while tracheostomy care is accomplished.

9. Clean the stoma site and then the tracheostomy plate with half-strength hydrogen peroxide solution followed by sterile water and then dry them; ensure that none of the solution enters the stoma.

10. Change tracheostomy ties if they are soiled.
    a. Velcro ties can be used according to the manufacturer's directions.
    b. Use tracheostomy ties from the tracheostomy kit.
       - Cut a hole ¾ in from one end of each tape.
       - Pass a short length of tape with the hole through one end of the cannula's flange loops.
       - Take the other end of the tie and thread it all the way through the hole and pull firmly. Repeat on the opposite side.
       - Bring the ties around the side of the neck and tie them in a square knot.
       - Tie in a square knot (not a bow) that allows one finger to be placed between the tape and the neck. The knot must be in a visible place on either side of the neck. The position of the knot is rotated to the other side with each tie change to prevent skin breakdown and pressure.

11. Place a new tracheostomy dressing if desired. Cut gauze pads are not used because loose fragments may fall into the stoma.

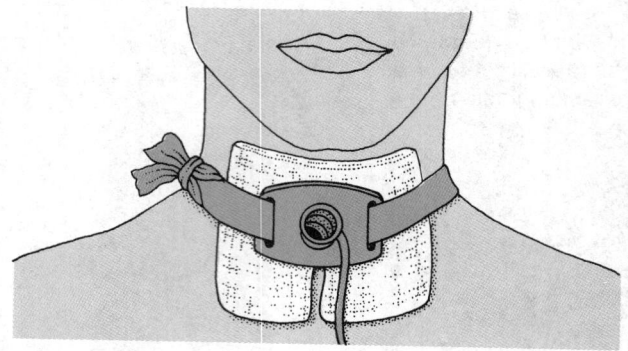

Figure 62–15

Placement of precut gauze and tie around a tracheostomy tube.

tomy tube. The nurse acknowledges the client's frustration in communicating. When speaking to the client, the nurse uses a normal tone and loudness of voice; the tracheostomy tube has altered the client's ability to speak but has not altered the client's ability to hear or understand. A means of communication is established that is easy for the client to use. Items such as a communication board with pictures and letters, a magic slate, or a note pad can decrease the frustration associated with communicating needs. (The nurse phrases questions that require "yes" or "no" responses.) The client is cautioned not to nod or shake the head because these movements cause the tube to move and the tracheal mucosa to be irritated.

Inability to talk is the major stressor of the intubated client; therefore, every effort should be made to facilitate speech as soon as possible. After the client is stable and does not aspirate, the cuff can be deflated while a finger occludes the stoma so that a few words can be spoken. A fenestrated tube can replace a standard tube so that speech and breathing through the upper air passages are facilitated.

Detection and management of complications. While providing care to the client with a tracheostomy, the nurse is alert to potential problems and complications. Possible problems include tube displacement or accidental decannulation, airway obstruction, aspiration, cuff leak or rupture, and tissue damage.

Tube displacement occurs easily if the tube is too long for the client or if the client has a short, large neck. In either case, the tube can slip into the right mainstem bronchus or into the subcutaneous tissue, which results in unequal breath sounds or chest excursion, or subcutaneous emphysema. The tube must then be repositioned. The incidence of tube displacement is highest shortly after a tube is inserted.

A tracheostomy tube can also be dislodged when the client coughs or pulls out a tube that is not properly secured. Dislodgement occurs if the tracheostomy ties are loose or if there is excessive moving or pulling of the tube. If decannulation occurs of a tracheostomy tube that has been in place for less than 7 days, the stoma

closes because a track has not formed. The client is provided with supplemental oxygen and ventilation via a manual resuscitation mask. The physician is notified immediately to reinsert the tube. In a tracheostomy stoma that is older than 7 days, a track has formed that allows a patent airway. The client's neck is slightly extended to open the stoma as much as possible and supplemental oxygen is supplied if tube dislodgement occurs after 7 days.

A second problem encountered in the tracheostomy client is *airway obstruction*. This obstruction can be due to encrusted secretions, malposition of the tube in the stoma, or herniation of the cuff over the distal opening of the tracheal tube; herniation occurs when the cuff is overinflated. Humidification, suctioning, proper alignment of the tube, and proper cuff inflation can prevent these problems.

Aspiration is a major problem in the client with a tracheostomy tube. The client at risk for aspiration is one who has a swallowing problem, who has decreased mental status, who has gastrointestinal problems, or who is receiving tube feedings, especially when given through a large-bore nasogastric tube. Further, any client with an inflated cuff may experience swallowing difficulties and aspiration. The cuff balloons into the esophagus and interferes with effective swallowing. To avoid aspiration, the following precautions are observed: the head of the bed is elevated at all times, especially when tube feedings are being given; the position of the feeding tube is checked and assessment for residual feeding is performed at least every 4 hours; and frequent assessments for abdominal distention are performed and measures are taken for its prevention. The tube-fed client is switched to a small-bore feeding tube that is placed in the duodenum, or a jejunostomy tube is placed to prevent aspiration; also, the cuff is kept inflated at all times. Aspiration can be verified via a swallowing test or a methylene blue test. During the latter test, a small amount of blue dye is added to food or the tube feeding. A positive result occurs when secretions that are suctioned from the tracheostomy are blue, which indicates that aspiration has occurred. When the client is allowed to eat, swallowing exercises may be helpful. Solid or soft foods are less likely to be aspirated than liquids; therefore, the diet is adjusted accordingly.

Aspiration can also occur if the cuff is underinflated or has ruptured. In either case, symptoms are easily recognized. Air is felt or is seen escaping through the stoma, nose, or mouth; bubbling secretions are noticed in the mouth and the client can talk. For the client who is using a ventilator, the set tidal volume is not delivered, which causes the low tidal volume alarm to sound. To correct the problem, the nurse inflates the cuff with air until a minimal air leak is achieved. If the leak continues despite insertion of air, the cuff has ruptured or is defective and the tracheostomy tube must be replaced. A tracheostomy tube is not routinely changed; it is changed only if there is a problem with the tube or if a different type or size of tube is desired (e.g., a fenestrated tube).

Displacement, airway obstruction, aspiration, and cuff problems can occur *any* time the client has a tracheostomy tube; however, most major complications of a tracheostomy are associated with *prolonged* use of a cuffed tube. These serious complications include the following: tracheomalacia; trachea stenosis; tracheoesophageal (TE) fistula; and trachea–innominate artery fistula (Table 62–5).

Weaning. The process of weaning the client from a tracheostomy tube entails a gradual decrease in the tube size and ultimate removal of the tube. First, the cuff is deflated as soon as the client can tolerate it; this change allows the client to breathe through the stoma as well as the upper air passages. An uncuffed tube gradually replaces a cuffed tube, and the tube size is decreased. When a small tube is in place (usually a No. 4), the tube may be plugged so that all the air must go through the upper airway and none through the tube. When this is tolerated, the tube is removed and a dressing is applied over the stoma, which then gradually heals on its own. A small scar remains. A fenestrated tracheostomy that is capped can also be used to facilitate the weaning process.

Mechanical ventilation. Mechanical ventilation to support and maintain clients has become more widely used. Once restricted to critical care units, clients using mechanical ventilators are now found not only on medical-surgical units but also in the home setting. The nurse has a pivotal role in the coordination of care and the prevention of complications.

Indications. Mechanical ventilation is initiated when the respiratory system cannot provide adequate ventilation (i.e., a normal arterial PCO_2 level) or adequate oxygenation (i.e., a normal arterial PO_2 level), or it is not able to maintain an effective breathing pattern. The work of breathing is excessive and the client becomes fatigued, as with COPD. Each of these functions may be affected alone or in combination. The lungs can no longer supply adequate amounts of oxygen to the tissues and/or remove carbon dioxide sufficiently. The respiratory dysfunction may be a component of a myriad of diseases, but the major underlying disturbances involve a dysfunction in the nervous system, the intrapulmonary tissue, or the muscles and skeletal structures surrounding the thoracic cage. Because of these disturbances, respiratory failure ensues and mechanical ventilation is warranted. The goals of mechanical ventilation are to improve oxygenation, to improve ventilation, and to decrease the amount of oxygen and work needed to accomplish an effective breathing pattern. Mechanical ventilation is used to support the client until lung function returns to normal and/or the acute episode has passed. A ventilator does not cure diseased lungs; it supports lungs until they are healthy enough to resume the process of breathing. Therefore, it is important that the nurse remember why the client is using the ventilator so that aggressive attempts to correct the underlying cause of the respiratory failure are always at the forefront of management plan. After normal oxygenation, ventilation, and respiratory muscle strength are achieved, mechanical ventilation can be discontinued.

Types of ventilators. A wide variety of ventilators are available. The ventilator selected depends on the severity of the disease process, the client's acuity level, hospital policies, and the length of time that ventilator support is required. There are two major types of ventilators: negative-pressure ventilators and positive-pressure ventilators.

The *negative-pressure ventilator* provides a noninvasive method of ventilation. The iron lung, widely used during the poliomyelitis epidemic, is the prototype for the negative-pressure ventilator. The client is placed in an air-tight apparatus that encompasses either the chest area or the entire body and leaves the head exposed. During inspiration, with the expansion of the chest wall, negative pressure is generated in the chest cavity. Because of the pressure gradient created, air rushes from the atmosphere (high pressure) into the thoracic cavity (low pressure). At a preset time, negative pressure ceases and expiration occurs. This type of ventilator, therefore, creates pressure gradients that mimic normal physiologic respiration.

Updated versions of the iron lung include the cuirass, poncho, and body wrap. These ventilators are used for clients with neuromuscular disease, central nervous system disorders, spinal cord injuries, and COPD. Often, clients with these diseases use negative-pressure ventilation for home nighttime ventilatory support so that their muscles can rest. Advantages are that an artificial airway is not required and that the newer models are lightweight and easy to use. Disadvantages are that nursing care is difficult because the ventilator encloses the client, who may find it uncomfortable if the machine is not in synchrony with the client's inspiratory effort. In addition, the client must be able to clear his or her oral secretions and must have compliant lungs to benefit from this mode of ventilation.

Although negative-pressure ventilation is not frequently used in the hospital setting, it is an emerging trend in the home care environment. Further refinement may also enhance its use in the acute care setting as a noninvasive means of ventilatory support (Fig. 62–16).

The *positive-pressure ventilator* is the most widely used ventilator in the acute care setting. During inspiration, a pressure is generated that pushes air into the lungs and expands the chest. An endotracheal tube or tracheostomy is needed for this type of ventilation. Positive-pressure ventilators are classified according to the mechanism that ends inspiration and starts expiration. Inspiration is terminated or cycled in three major ways: pressure cycled, time cycled, and volume cycled.

The *pressure-cycled ventilator* pushes air into the lungs until a preset airway pressure is reached. Tidal volumes and time are variable, and minimal alarms are available. Pressure-cycled ventilators are often used for short periods, such as in the postanesthesia care unit and for respiratory therapy. The most common examples are the Puritan-Bennett PR-1 and PR-2 (Fig. 62–17) and the Bird Mark 7 and 8.

TABLE 62–5 Signs and Symptoms, Management, and Prevention of Serious Complications of Tracheostomy

Complications	Signs and Symptoms	Management	Prevention
Tracheomalacia: Constant pressure exerted by cuff causes tracheal dilation and erosion of cartilage.	An increased amount of air is required in the cuff to maintain the seal. A larger tracheostomy tube is required to prevent an air leak at the stoma. Food particles are seen in tracheal secretions. The client does not receive tidal volume on the ventilator. Increased coughing and choking are seen while the client eats. The methylene blue test result is positive.	No special management is needed unless bleeding occurs.	Use an uncuffed tube as soon as possible. Monitor cuff pressure and air volumes closely and detect changes.
Tracheal stenosis: Narrowed tracheal opening is due to scar formation from irritation of tracheal mucosa by the cuff.	Stenosis usually seen after the cuff is deflated or the tracheostomy tube is removed. The client has increased coughing; inability to expectorate secretions; or difficulty in breathing or talking.	Tracheal dilation or surgical intervention is used.	Prevent pulling of and traction on the tracheostomy tube. Properly secure the tube in the midline position. Maintain proper cuff pressure.
Tracheoesophageal fistula: Excessive cuff pressure causes erosion of the posterior wall of trachea. A hole is created between the trachea and the anterior esophagus. The client at highest risk also has a nasogastric tube present.	Similar to tracheomalacia. Food particles are seen in tracheal secretions. Increased air in cuff is needed to achieve a seal. There is a positive methylene blue test result. The client has increased coughing and choking while eating. The client does not receive the set tidal volume on the ventilator.	Oxygen is given manually by mask to the client to prevent hypoxemia. The Dobhoff or a small soft tube is used instead of nasogastric tube for tube feedings. The client with a nasogastric tube is monitored closely, and assessment is done for tracheoesophageal fistula and aspiration.	Maintain cuff pressure. Monitor the amount of air needed for inflation and detect changes. Progress to deflated cuff or cuffless tube as soon as possible.
Trachea-innominate artery fistula: A malpositioned tube causes its distal tip to push against the lateral wall of the tracheostomy. Continued pressure causes necrosis and erosion of the innominate artery. THIS IS A MEDICAL EMERGENCY.	The tracheostomy tube pulsates in synchrony with the heart beat. There is exsanguination from the stoma. This is a life-threatening complication.	The tracheostomy tube is removed immediately. Direct pressure is applied to the innominate artery at the stoma site. Emergency surgery is done for repair.	Correct tube size, length, and midline position. Prevent pulling or tugging on tracheostomy tube. Immediately notify physician of pulsating tube.

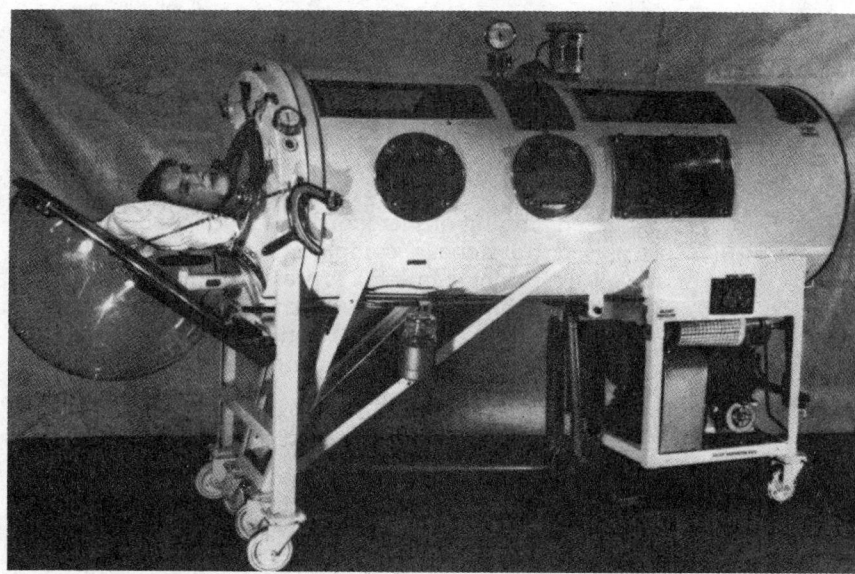

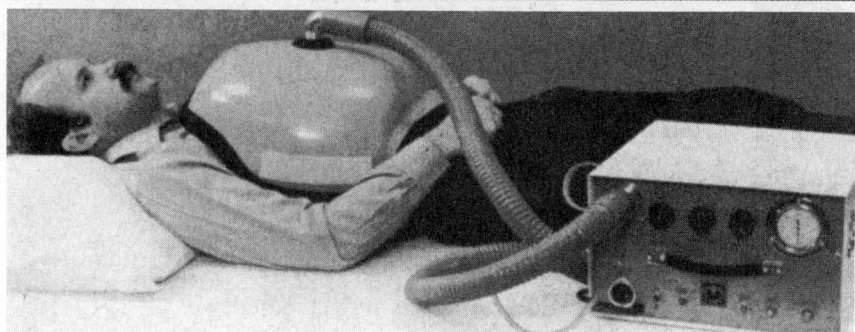

Figure 62–16

Two negative-pressure ventilators: the Emerson Iron Lung (top) and the Lifecare Chest Shell (bottom). (Top photograph reproduced courtesy of J. H. Emerson Co., Cambridge, MA; bottom photograph from Hill, N. [1986]. Clinical applications of body ventilators. *Chest, 90*[6], 900.)

The *time-cycled ventilator* pushes air into the lungs until a preset time has elapsed. Tidal volume and pressure are variable depending on the characteristics of the client and the ventilator. The time-cycled ventilator is used primarily in pediatric and neonatal populations. Examples of these ventilators are the Bird Babybird, Siemens Servo 900, 900B, and 900C, the Monaghan 225, and the Puritan-Bennett PR-2.

The *volume-cycled ventilator* pushes gas into the lungs until a preset volume is delivered. A constant tidal volume is delivered regardless of the pressure that is needed to deliver the tidal volume. There is, however, a pressure limit that is set to prevent excessive pressure from being exerted on the lungs. The advantage of this type of ventilator is that a constant tidal volume is delivered regardless of the changing compliance of the lungs and chest wall or the airway resistance found in the client or ventilator. Examples of volume-cycled ventilators are the Bear I and II (Fig. 62–18), Puritan-Bennett MA-1 and MA-2, and Monaghan 225/SIMV.

The microprocessor ventilator is the most sophisticated of the volume-cycled ventilators. A computer, or microprocessor, is built into the ventilator to allow ongoing monitoring of ventilatory functions, alarms, and client parameters. The ventilator often has components of volume-, time-, and pressure-cycled ventilators

present. The microprocessor ventilator is more responsive to clients who have severe lung disease, who require prolonged weaning trials, and who may not be able to be ventilated via older volume-cycled ventilators.

Two newer modes of ventilation, pressure support and continuous flow (flow-by), are modalities that are available only in microprocessor ventilators. Both modalities decrease the work of breathing and are often used for weaning clients from mechanical ventilation. Examples of the microprocessor ventilator are the Bear IV and V, Puritan-Bennett 7200, and Siemens Servo C and Servo D.

Ventilator settings. The volume-cycled ventilator is the most widely used ventilator in the hospital setting. Regardless of the type of volume-cycled ventilator used, the settings are universal (Fig. 62–19). It is important for the nurse to understand the normal ventilator settings so that appropriate monitoring and care of the client are ensured.

Tidal volume (TV) is the volume of air that the client receives with each breath; it can be measured on either inspiration or expiration. The normal tidal volume is 10 to 15 mL/kg of body weight. Adding a zero to the kilogram weight of the client gives a general idea of tidal volume that is selected.

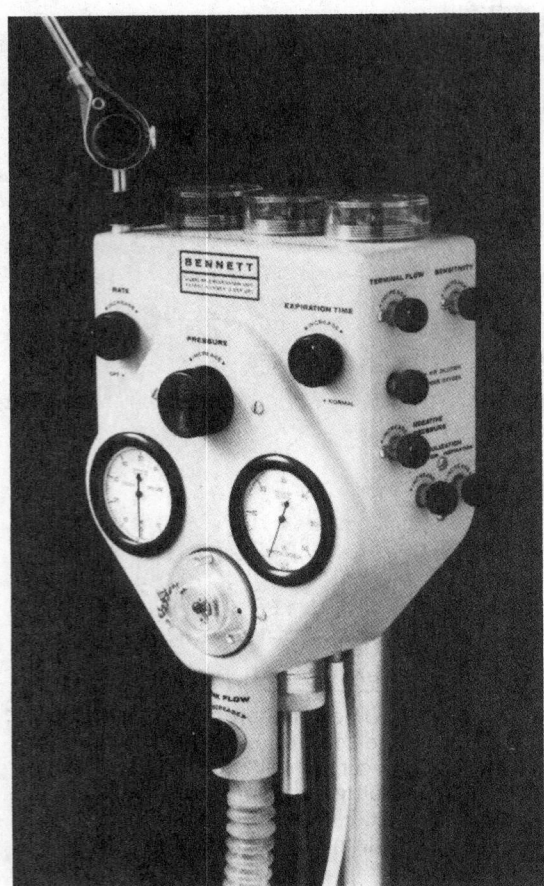

Figure 62–17

Puritan-Bennett PR-2 pressure-limited ventilator. (Photograph reproduced courtesy of Puritan-Bennett Corp., Overland Park, KS.)

Rate or breaths per minute (BPM) is the number of ventilator breaths delivered per minute. It is usually set at 10 to 14 breaths per minute. *Fraction of inspired oxygen* (FIO_2) is the oxygen concentration that is delivered to the client. The FIO_2 is determined by the arterial blood gas value and the client's condition. Ventilators can provide 21% to 100% FIO_2, depending on the client's needs.

The oxygen that is delivered to the client is warmed to body temperature (98.6° F [37°C]) and is humidified to 100%. *Humidification* and *warming* are necessary because the upper air passages of the respiratory tree that normally warm, humidify, and filter air are bypassed by the endotracheal tube or tracheostomy tube. Humidification and warming are needed to prevent mucosal damage and to facilitate clearance of secretions.

Sighs may be used to prevent atelectasis in special circumstances. Sighs are volumes of air that are 1½ to 2 times tidal volume delivered at 6 to 10 times per hour. *Peak airway (inspiratory) pressure* (PIP) provides an indication of the pressure that is needed by the ventilator to deliver a set tidal volume. The peak airway pressure

measurement appears on the manometer on the front of the ventilator. Peak pressure is read as the highest pressure indicated by the manometer needle during inspiration. Monitoring trends in PIP reflect changes in compliance (elasticity) of the lungs and resistance in the ventilator and/or client. An increased PIP reading means increased airway resistance (bronchospasm), increased amount of secretions, pulmonary edema, or decreased pulmonary compliance (lungs and/or chest wall are harder to inflate). A pressure limit is set by a dial on the ventilator to prevent barotrauma (lung damage from excessive pressure). When the limit is reached, the high-pressure alarm sounds and the remaining volume is not given.

The term *modes of ventilation* describes the way in which the client receives breaths from the ventilator. There are five types of modes of ventilation. *Controlled ventilation* is the least used method. During this mode, a

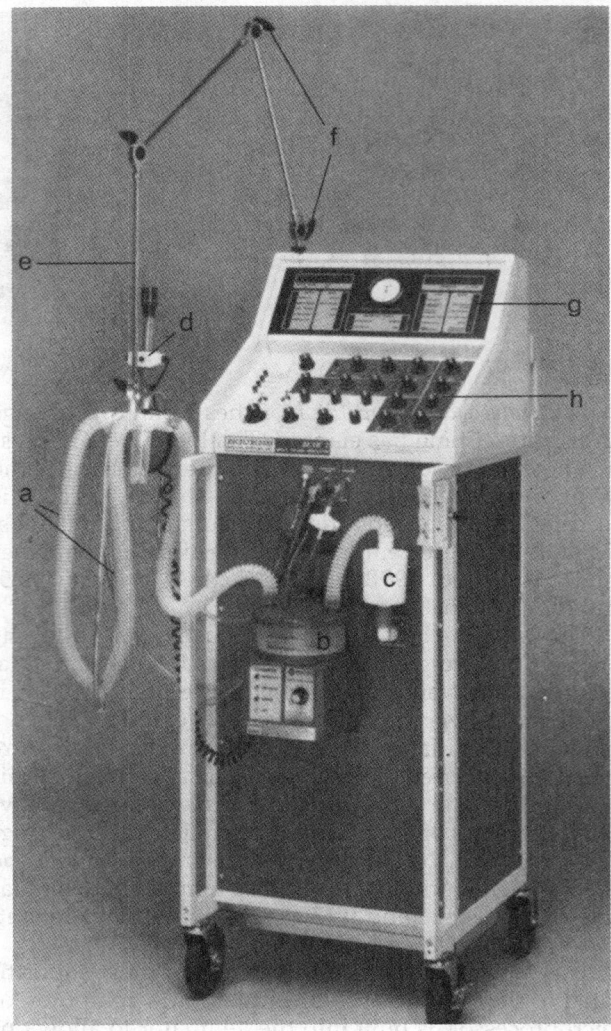

Figure 62–18

Bear II Adult Volume Ventilator. (Photograph reproduced courtesy of Bear Medical Systems, Inc., Riverside, CA.)

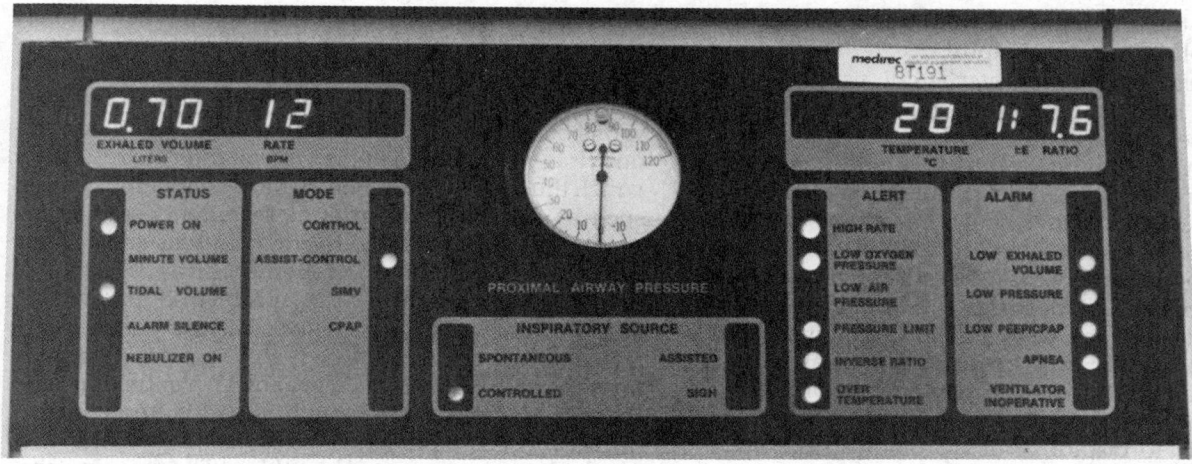

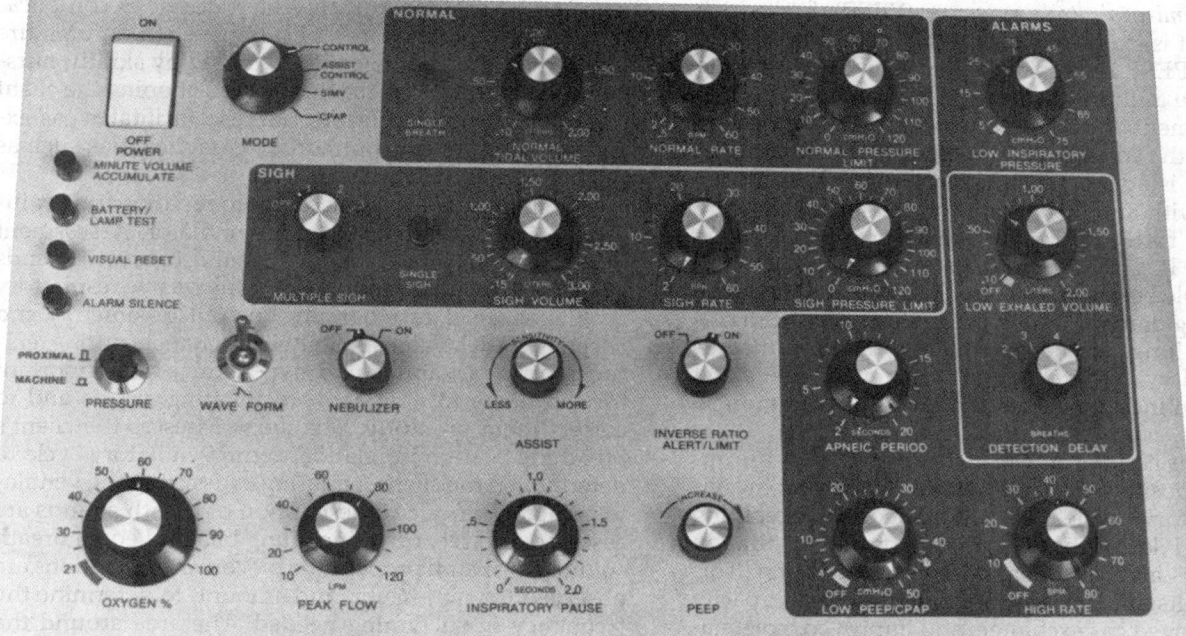

Figure 62–19

Display signals and alarms (top) and control panal (bottom) of a typical ventilator. (From Kersten, L. D. [1989]. *Comprehensive respiratory nursing: A decision making approach.* Philadelphia: W. B. Saunders.)

set tidal volume and a set rate are delivered to the client regardless of the client's inspiratory effort. If the client attempts to initiate a breath, the efforts are blocked by the ventilator. This maneuver results in the client's "fighting" the ventilator. Clients with central nervous system dysfunction, those who are paralyzed, and those with flail chest are the rare clients for whom this mode is used.

Assist-control mode (AC) is the most commonly used mode of ventilation. It is used mainly as a resting mode, in which the ventilator takes over the work of breathing for the client. A preset tidal volume and respiratory rate are set on the ventilator; therefore, if the client does not

breathe, a minimal ventilatory pattern is established. The ventilator is also programmed to respond to the client's inspiratory effort if the client does initiate a breath. In this case, the ventilator delivers a preset tidal volume while allowing the client to control the rate of breathing.

One major disadvantage of AC is that if the client's respiratory rate increases, the ventilator continues to deliver a preset tidal volume with each breath. The client may then hyperventilate, and respiratory alkalosis occurs. Causes of hyperventilation such as pain, anxiety, or uncompensated metabolic acidosis must be corrected. If measures to correct hyperventilation are not effective, the synchronized intermittent mandatory ventilation (SIMV) may be helpful.

Synchronized intermittent mandatory ventilation is similar to AC in that a preset tidal volume and respiratory rate are set on the ventilator; therefore, if the client does not breathe, a minimal ventilatory pattern is established. In contrast to AC, SIMV allows the client to breathe at his or her own rate and tidal volume between the ventilator breaths. Therefore, respiratory alkalosis is less likely to occur than with AC. SIMV can be used as a primary ventilatory mode or as a weaning modality. When SIMV is used as a weaning mode, the number of mechanical breaths (SIMV breaths) is decreased, and the client gradually assumes spontaneous breathing. The mandatory ventilator breath is delivered when the client is ready to inspire, which promotes synchrony between the ventilator and the client.

Positive end-expiratory pressure (PEEP) is positive pressure that is exerted during the expiratory phase of ventilation. PEEP improves oxygenation by enhancing gas exchange and preventing atelectasis. It is indicated for the treatment of persistent hypoxemia that does not improve with an acceptable oxygen concentration. Often PEEP is added when the arterial PO_2 value remains low with an FIO_2 of 60% or greater.

The need for PEEP indicates a severe gas exchange disturbance. It is important to lower the FIO_2 delivered when possible because prolonged use of a high FIO_2 can result in lung damage. PEEP prevents alveoli from collapsing; the lungs are kept partially inflated so that alveolar capillary gas exchange is facilitated. The effect should be an increase in arterial blood oxygenation so that the FIO_2 can be decreased.

Continuous positive airway pressure (CPAP) is the application of positive airway pressure throughout the entire respiratory cycle for spontaneously breathing clients. CPAP keeps the alveoli open during inspiration and prevents alveolar collapse during expiration. This process results in increased functional residual capacity (FRC), improved gas exchange, and improved oxygenation. CPAP is used primarily as a weaning modality. During CPAP, no ventilator breaths are delivered; the ventilator delivers oxygen and provides monitoring and an alarm system. The respiratory pattern is determined by the client's efforts. Normal levels of CPAP are 5 to 15 cmH_2O, adjusted to promote adequate oxygenation. If no pressure is set on the ventilator, the client receives no positive pressure. The client is essentially using the ventilator as a T piece with alarms.

Nursing management. The decision to use mechanical ventilation for a client involves a complex decision-making process. Both physical and psychologic concerns of the client and family must be addressed. Frequently, the mechanical ventilator causes anxiety for the client and family. Therefore, the nurse carefully explains the purpose of the ventilator and the sensations that might be felt, as well as encourages the client and family to express their concerns. The nurse acts as the coach who both physically and psychologically helps and supports the client and family through this experience. In emergency situations, these explanations may not be accomplished until the life-threatening process has been controlled.

When caring for a ventilated client, the nurse's responsibility is to the client first and the ventilator second. It is vital that the nurse understands the reason for which the client requires mechanical ventilation. Causes such as excessive amounts of secretions, sepsis, and trauma all require different interventions to facilitate ventilator independence. In addition, an appreciation of the client's chronic health problems, particularly COPD, right-sided heart failure, cardiac disease, anemia and malnutrition, is essential. These problems may impede weaning from mechanical ventilation and therefore warrant close monitoring and intervention.

Weaning is the process of going from ventilatory dependence to spontaneous breathing. The weaning process can be prolonged if the client develops complications. Many of these complications, such as pressure ulcers or malnutrition, can be avoided by skillful nursing care. For example, turning and positioning the client not only promotes comfort, but also facilitates gas exchange and prevents pulmonary complications such as pneumonia and atelectasis.

The first goal of nursing care is to monitor and evaluate the client's response to the ventilator. Assessment includes taking vital signs and listening to breath sounds every 30 to 60 minutes initially, noninvasive respiratory monitoring (e.g., capnography and pulse oximetry), and checking ABG values. Vital signs change during episodes of hypercapnea and hypoxemia. It is important for the nurse to note any precipitating causes and to correct them promptly. The nurse assesses the client's breathing pattern in relation to the ventilatory cycle to determine if the client is fighting or assisting the ventilator. The presence and description of breath sounds are assessed and recorded, including bilateral equal breath sounds, to ensure proper tube placement. Secretions are observed for type, color, and amount, to determine the frequency of suctioning needed. The area around the endotracheal tube or tracheostomy site is assessed at least every 4 hours for color, tenderness, skin irritation, and drainage. Continuous noninvasive monitoring provides the nurse with a barometer to guide the client's activities such as weaning, physical or occupational therapy, and self-care. These activities can be paced so that oxygenation and ventilation are adequate. Interpretation of ABG values is essential for the nurse to evaluate and suggest ventilator settings that help the client. Although the physician prescribes specific ventilator changes, the nurse assesses and evaluates the client's response to those changes. Because the nurse spends more time with the client, the nurse is most likely to be the first person to recognize slight changes in the vital signs, fatigue or distress in the client, or changes in the ABG values. The nurse then promptly confers with the physician and implements the appropriate interventions.

While monitoring and evaluating the client's clinical status, the nurse also serves as an excellent resource for addressing the psychologic needs of the client and family. Anxiety can play a major role in the tolerance of mechanical ventilation. Therefore, skilled and sensitive nursing care is needed to promote psychologic well-being and to facilitate synchrony with the ventilator. Communication can be frustrating and anxiety-producing because the client cannot speak. The client and family may panic because they prematurely believe the client has lost his or her voice. They must be reassured that the endotracheal tube prevents speech but that it is a temporary situation. Alternative, creative methods of communication must be individualized to meet the client's needs. Magic slates, writing paper, computers, and tracheostomy tubes that permit talking are potential means of facilitating communication. Finding a non-stressful means for communication is important because the client often experiences feelings of isolation related to the inability to speak. Anticipation of the client's needs, easy access to frequently used belongings, and a nursing call light within reach are effective ways to give the client a sense of control over the environment. In addition, the client is not isolated from participation in self-care.

The second goal of nursing care is directed toward safe management of the ventilator system. Ventilator settings are ordered by the physician and include the following: tidal volume, respiratory rate, FIO$_2$, mode of ventilation (AC, SIMV, CPAP), and any adjunctive modes such as PEEP, pressure support, or continuous flow. Nursing responsibilities are to perform and document ventilator checks according to the standards of the unit or hospital and to respond promptly to emergency situations as indicated by alarms. During a ventilator check, the nurse compares the ventilator settings ordered by the physician with the actual settings. The level of water in the humidifier and the temperature of the humidification system are checked to ensure that they are within normal limits. Extremes in temperature cause damage to the mucosa of the airways. Any condensation in the ventilator tubing is removed by draining water into drainage collection receptacles, which should be emptied frequently. Moisture and water are never allowed to enter the humidifier to prevent bacterial contamination.

Mechanical ventilators have alarm systems that warn the nurse of a problem with either the client or the ventilator. Alarm systems must be activated and functional at all times. It is crucial for the nurse to recognize emergency situations and to intervene promptly so that complications are prevented. If the cause of the alarm cannot be determined, the client receives manual ventilation with an Ambu bag until the problem is corrected. The two major alarms on a ventilator indicate either a high pressure or a low exhaled volume. The accompanying Guidelines feature presents nursing interventions for various causes of ventilator alarms.

Ensuring proper functioning of the ventilator also includes care of the endotracheal tube or tracheostomy tube. Maintenance of a patent airway is accomplished through suctioning only as needed. Indications for suc-

tioning in the ventilated client include the presence of secretions, increased PIP, the presence of rhonchi, and decreased breath sounds.

Careful maintenance of the endotracheal tube or tracheostomy tube also ensures a patent airway. Frequent assessment of tube position is warranted, especially for the client whose airway is attached to heavy ventilator tubing that may pull on the tracheostomy or endotracheal tube. The ventilator tubing should be positioned to allow the client to move yet prevent pulling on the endotracheal or tracheostomy tube. The endotracheal tube can move and slip into the right mainstem bronchus. To detect minimal changes in the tube's position, the nurse marks the level at which the tube touches the mouth or nose. Mouth care is done frequently to promote adequate oral hygiene and to prevent the tape that holds the tube from loosening.

The *final goal* in providing nursing care of the client receiving mechanical ventilation is prevention of complications. Most of these complications are due to the positive pressure from the ventilator. Nearly every body system is affected.

Cardiac complications of mechanical ventilation include hypotension and fluid retention. Hypotension is caused by the application of positive pressure to the lungs. Positive pressure decreases venous return to the right side of the heart, decreases cardiac output, and is clinically reflected as hypotension. Hypotension is most frequently seen in the client who is dehydrated or requires high PIP to be ventilated. Fluid retention occurs because of decreased cardiac output. The kidneys receive less blood flow and stimulate the aldosterone–angiotensin–renin system to retain fluid. In addition, humidified air via the ventilator system can contribute to fluid retention. The nurse monitors the client's fluid intake and output, weight and hydration, and signs of hypovolemia.

The lungs experience barotrauma and acid-base abnormalities. *Barotrauma,* or damage to the lungs by positive pressure, includes pneumothorax, subcutaneous emphysema, and pneumomediastinum. Clients at risk for barotrauma have COPD or blebs or require high pressures to ventilate the lungs (decreased compliance or "stiff" lungs, as seen in ARDS). Another pulmonary complication from mechanical ventilation is ABG abnormalities, which can be corrected by appropriate ventilator changes and correction of fluid and electrolyte abnormalities.

The gastrointestinal system also sustains complications from mechanical ventilation. Stress ulcers occur in approximately 25% of clients on mechanical ventilation. Prophylactic antacids, sucralfate (Carafate), and histamine blockers such as cimetidine (Tagamet) and ranitidine (Zantac) are often instituted as soon as the client is intubated. The nurse administers these medications as well as suggests therapeutic strategies for stress management, as discussed in Chapter 6.

Malnutrition is a prevalent problem in clients receiving mechanical ventilation. Because many other acute or life-threatening events are occurring simultaneously,

GUIDELINES ■ Nursing Interventions for Various Causes of Ventilator Alarms*

Cause	Interventions
High-Pressure Alarm	
Sounds when peak inspiratory pressure reaches the set alarm limit (usually 10–20 mmHg above the client's baseline PIP).	
There is an increased amount of secretion in airways.	Apply suction as needed.
The client coughs, gags, or bites on oral ETT.	Insert oral airway to prevent biting on ETT. Provide emotional support to decrease anxiety.
The client is anxious or fights the ventilator.	Explain all procedures to the client. Provide sedation or paralyzing agent per the physician's order.
Airway size decreases related to wheezing or broncho-spasm.	Auscultate breath sounds. Consult with the physician for management of broncho-spasm.
Pneumothorax occurs.	Auscultate breath sounds. Consult with the physician regarding a new onset of decreased breath sounds or unequal chest excursion, which may be due to a pneumothorax.
The artificial airway is displaced; the ETT may have slipped into the right mainstem bronchus.	Assess the chest for unequal and equal breath sounds and chest excursion. Obtain a chest x-ray film as ordered to evaluate the position of the ETT. After the proper position is verified, tape the tube securely in place.
Obstruction in tubing occurs because the client is lying on the tubing or there is water or a kink in the tubing.	Assess the system, moving from the artificial airway toward the ventilator. Empty water from the ventilator tubing and remove any kinks.
There is increased PIP associated with deliverance of a sigh.	Adjust the pressure alarm.
Decreased compliance of the lung is noted; a trend of gradually increasing PIP is noted over several hours or a day.	Evaluate the reasons for the decreased compliance of lungs. Increased PIP occurs in ARDS.
Low Exhaled Volume Alarm	
Sounds when there is a leak in the ventilator circuit or in the artificial airway of the client.	
A leak in the ventilator circuit prevents breath from being delivered.	Assess all connections and all ventilator tubing for disconnection.
The client stops spontaneous breathing in the SIMV or CPAP mode.	Evaluate the client's tolerance of the mode.
A cuff leak occurs in the ETT tracheostomy tube.	Evaluate the client for a cuff leak. A cuff leak is suspected when the client is able to talk (air escapes from the mouth) or when the pilot balloon on the artificial airway is flat (see section on tracheostomy tubes).
The exhalation valve on Bear I or II is wet.	Keep exhalation part horizontal. Unsnap and check the membrane for dampness. If the sensor is wet, gently dab dry and resnap.

* PIP, peak inspiratory pressure; ETT, endotracheal tube; ARDS, adult respiratory distress syndrome; CPAP, continuous positive airway pressure; SIMV, synchronized intermittent mandatory ventilation.

nutrition is often neglected. Malnutrition is an extreme problem for these clients and a major reason that clients cannot be weaned from the ventilator. In clients with malnutrition, the respiratory muscles lose their mass and strength. The diaphragm, which is the major organ of inspiration, is affected early in this process. When the diaphragm and other muscles of respiration are weakened, an ineffective breathing pattern emerges, fatigue occurs, and the client cannot be weaned from the ventilator. A balanced diet via the parenteral or enteral route is essential whenever a ventilator is used. Furthermore, nutrition for the client with COPD requires that special attention be given to the percentage of carbohydrates in the client's diet. During metabolism, carbohydrates are broken down to glucose to produce energy (ATP), carbon dioxide, and water. Excessive carbohydrate loads increase carbon dioxide production, which the COPD client may be unable to exhale. Hypercapnic respiratory failure results. Enteral or parenteral formulas with a higher fat content (Intralipid, Pulmocare) can be an alternative source of calories to combat this problem.

Another important aspect of nutritional support is electrolyte replacement. Electrolytes also have a major impact on the efficiency of respiratory muscle function. Specifically, calcium, magnesium, and phosphorus levels must be closely monitored and deficiencies replenished. All three electrolytes are important in respiratory muscle contraction and function and can easily be added to the nutritional regimen.

Infections are always a potential threat for the client using a ventilator. The endotracheal or tracheostomy tube bypasses the body's normal process of filtering and warming air and provides direct access for bacteria to enter the lower parts of the respiratory system. Usually within 48 hours, the artificial airway is colonized with bacteria. An environment is established in which pneumonia can develop. Pneumonic infections are associated with prolonged hospitalization and increased morbidity. Special emphasis must therefore focus on prevention of infections through strict adherence to infection control standards, especially during hand washing, suctioning, and care of the tracheostomy or endotracheal tube. Ongoing pulmonary hygiene, including chest physiotherapy, postural drainage, and turning and positioning, is implemented by the nurse to prevent pneumonia.

Overall muscle deconditioning can occur because of immobility. Getting out of bed, ambulating with assistance, and performing exercises with the nurse, physical therapist, and/or occupational therapist not only improve muscle tone and strength, but also boost the client's morale, facilitate gas exchange, and promote oxygen delivery to all muscles.

The final complication of mechanical ventilation is ventilator dependence. Ventilator dependence can be psychologic or physiologic but more often has a physiologic basis. The older client, especially one who has smoked or who has an underlying lung dysfunction like COPD, is at risk for ventilator dependence. The longer a client uses a ventilator, the more difficult the weaning

process. The respiratory muscles fatigue and are unable to assume breathing. Attempts are made to optimize all major body systems and to exhaust every method of weaning before a client is declared unweanable. The client's quality of life, goals, and values are discussed. In accordance with this discussion, arrangements are made for home ventilation, nursing home placement, or withdrawal of life support (in terminal cases).

Breathing techniques. Diaphragmatic or abdominal and pursed-lip breathing maneuvers are beneficial interventions for managing dyspneic episodes. If the individual learns the techniques shown in the accompanying Client/Family Education feature and uses them during all activities, the amount of stagnant air in the lung is minimized and the client gains confidence in managing dyspnea. In diaphragmatic breathing, the client attempts to *consciously* increase diaphragmatic excursion. To teach the client this maneuver, the nurse instructs him or her to lie comfortably on the back with the knees bent. This position allows the abdomen to relax. The client is instructed to place his or her hands or a book lightly on the abdomen to create resistance; the client then breathes using abdominal muscles. The client is performing the technique correctly if the abdomen rises and falls during breathing. Pursed-lip breathing is a technique that uses the mild resistance of partially opposed lips to prolong exhalation and to increase airway pressure, thereby delaying dynamic compression of airways and minimizing the effects of air trapping. Many clients with COPD have learned this technique on their own. The client is instructed to close the mouth and breathe in through the nose, taking a normal breath. The client then purses the lips as done to whistle and breathes out slowly through the mouth. The exhalation through pursed lips should take at least twice the time it took to breathe in. Pursed-lip breathing can be used during diaphragmatic or abdominal breathing. Both of these breathing techniques are best taught when a client is free from dyspnea.

Positioning. The nurse and client can use various positioning maneuvers to assist in alleviating dyspnea. (Fig. 62–20). If the client is in bed, the nurse assists him or her to sit up on the edge of the bed. The client's arms are folded and positioned by resting them on an overbed table that has been propped up with two or three pillows. This position allows the client to fully expand the chest while conserving energy by supporting his or her arms and upper body. This position is particularly helpful for the client who is having an acute attack and who is tired but too short of breath to lie back.

Another helpful position can be used in almost any location. The client sits forward on a chair, spreads the feet a shoulder-width apart, and then places the elbows on the knees. This position allows the client to relax the arms and hands while supporting the shoulders. COPD clients use a greater proportion of their accessory muscles for breathing. Supporting the thorax, therefore, allows these muscles to work better.

CLIENT/FAMILY EDUCATION ■ Instructions for Breathing Exercises

Diaphragmatic or Abdominal Breathing

1. "Lie on your back with your knees bent."
2. "Place your hands or a book on your abdomen to create resistance."
3. "Begin breathing from your abdomen while keeping your chest still. You can tell if you are breathing correctly if your hands or the book rises and falls accordingly."

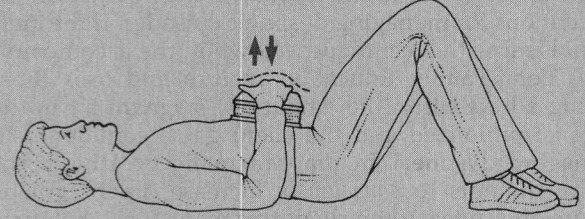

Pursed-Lip Breathing

1. "Close your mouth and breathe in through your nose."
2. "Purse your lips as you would to whistle. Breathe out slowly through your mouth, without puffing your cheeks. Spend at least twice the amount of time it took you to breathe in. Use your abdominal muscles to squeeze out every bit of air you can."
3. "Remember to use pursed lip breathing during any physical activity. Always inhale before beginning the activity and exhale while performing the activity. Never hold your breath."

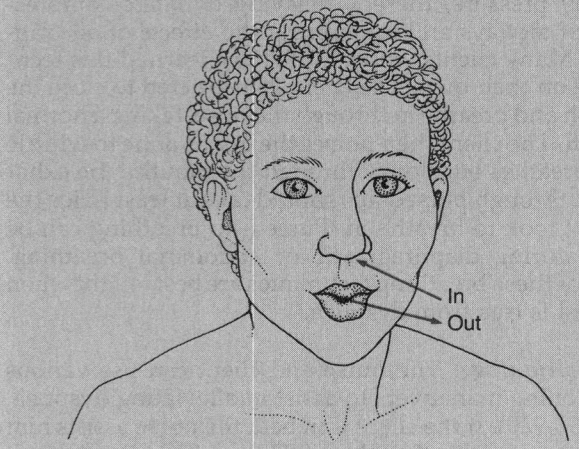

The last position can be used when an individual is walking. If the client becomes short of breath, he or she is taught to lean the back and hips against a wall or other support and spread the feet comfortably apart. The client then slumps the shoulders forward and relaxes the arms.

Exercise conditioning. Dyspnea creates a vicious circle. Clients suffering from exercise-induced shortness of breath respond by limiting their activity, even their basic activities of daily living. Table 60–1 in Chapter 60 summarizes the correlation between dyspnea and the performance of daily activities. Over time, the muscles of respiration and the general large muscle groups weaken and become less efficient in their use of oxygen. The end result is increased dyspnea with lower activity levels. Exercise conditioning in pulmonary rehabilitation programs can be done in several ways: conditioning of the general large muscle groups (indirect) or retraining of the respiratory muscles (direct). The *indirect approach* is accomplished through any general exercise program (see the Nursing Research feature on p. 2034) and improves pulmonary function by its effect on overall cardiopulmonary fitness and reconditioning of large muscle groups. Two techniques that are currently used work *directly* on the respiratory muscles. *Isocapnic hy-*

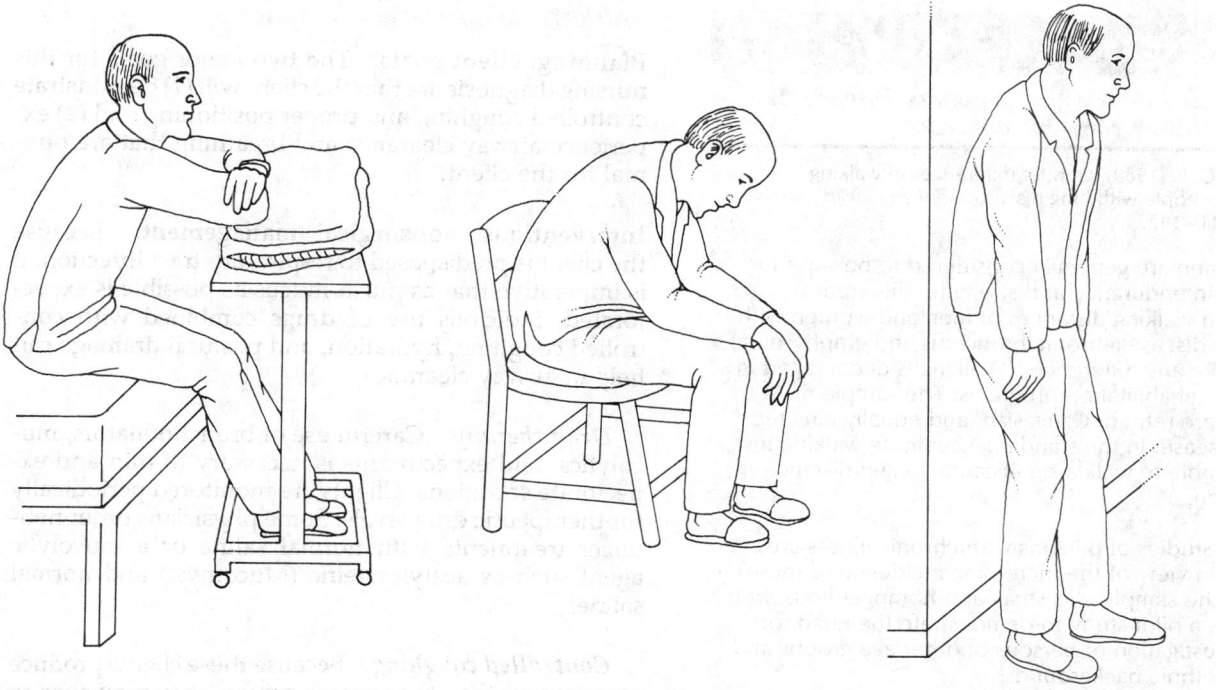

Sitting on the edge of a bed with the arms folded and placed on two or three pillows positioned over a nightstand.

Sitting in a chair with the feet spread a shoulder-width apart and leaning forward with the elbows on the knees. Arms and hands are relaxed.

Standing with the back and hips against a wall and the feet about 12 in (30 cm) from the wall. Shoulders are relaxed and bent slightly forward.

Figure 62–20
Alternative positions to assist COPD clients with breathing.

hyperventilation is designed to increase endurance. Individuals hyperventilate into a machine that controls concentrations of oxygen and carbon dioxide. In *resistive breathing,* individuals breathe against a set resistance. Theoretically, resistive breathing trains respiratory muscles for both strength and endurance. Currently, retraining of the respiratory muscles is done predominantly in research settings. In all likelihood, neither the indirect or the direct approach will be found to be superior; instead, a combination of the two will most likely achieve maximal benefits.

Energy conservation. Energy conservation is the planning and pacing of activities for maximal client tolerance and minimal client discomfort. The nurse or physical or occupational therapist begins by first describing a client's typical daily schedule. Then, each activity is divided into its constituent parts, and it is determined if that task can be performed in a different way or at a different time of the day. Activities are spread out over the day with rest periods between activities. Clients are reminded to avoid working with their arms raised. Activities that involve the arms decrease exercise tolerance because the accessory muscles of respiration are then used to stabilize the shoulders. Many activities that involve the arms can be done while sitting at a table and leaning on elbows. The nurse reminds the client to ad-

just work heights because improper working height causes back strain and fatigue. The best work height for a table top is 5 cm (2 in) below the bent elbow. Rapid, jerky arm motions cause shortness of breath and fatigue and put an extra strain on the heart. Clients should be reminded to keep arm motions smooth and flowing. Long-handled dust pans, sponges, and feather dusters minimize bending and reaching. The nurse gives suggestions to the client about the organization of work spaces so that items that are used most often are within easy reach. Measures such as dividing clothes for laundry or groceries into small parcels that can be handled easily, using disposable plates to save washing time, or letting dishes dry in the rack also conserve energy. The nurse suggests that clients straighten bedcovers before getting out of bed for easier bedmaking. Clients are instructed that the key to any activity is to remember to avoid holding his or her breath and to always exhale while performing any activity.

Diet therapy. The increased work of breathing raises the calorie requirements for individuals with COPD, and many clients become nutritionally compromised. These individuals lose total body mass and respiratory muscle mass accompanied by a loss of respiratory muscle strength. A referral to a dietitian may be indicated. In the hospital setting, clients may need assist-

Thompson, C. L. (1989). Gender differences in walking distances of people with lung disease. *Applied Nursing Research, 2,* 141–142.

NURSING RESEARCH

Women and Men with Pulmonary Disease Can Both Meet Exercise Goals.

In sports, men are generally considered to be superior to women in endurance and strength. This study investigated walking distances of men and women with pulmonary disease (chronic bronchitis and emphysema) to determine any differences. Walking is encouraged in pulmonary rehabilitation programs. The sample of 31 subjects were retired, Caucasian, and equally affected by their disease. In the standard 12-minute walking test, men were able to walk a significantly longer distance than women.

Critique. Studies of persons with chronic illness are important in view of the increasing incidence of these diseases. The sample was small and homogeneous, but it served as a pilot study to demonstrate the need for further investigation of persons of other age groups and of various ethnic backgrounds.

Possible nursing implications. When teaching clients about pulmonary rehabilitation, nurses need to realize that expectations and goals for women should be different from those for men. Women with pulmonary disease can be reassured that they are successfully meeting their goals even if they cannot walk as far as men.

ance in completing menus; the nurse reminds them to choose foods that are easy to chew. Nursing staff may need to feed the client if he or she tires easily. Most clients do not expend the energy to feed themselves when they are working to breathe. Many times an individual does not have the urge to eat. If this is the case, it is imperative to try various interventions to deal with the anorexia. Sucking on hard candy or chewing gum before meals to begin salivation and stimulate taste buds may help. The nurse offers to assist the client with oral hygiene before meals. The nurse explores the types of high-calorie foods that the client likes, such as butter, mayonnaise, peanut butter, and cream cheese. Dietary supplements such as Pulmocare are designed to provide nutritional supplements specifically for clients with pulmonary illnesses. The biggest meal of the day should be planned for the time when the client is most hungry. Shortness of breath during mealtimes can be handled by stressing the need to rest before meals, particularly if the client is preparing the meal. The nurse suggests the use of pursed-lip breathing and abdominal breathing to alleviate the dyspnea. The use of oxygen by nasal cannula (prongs) during meals and for 10 minutes after meals may have a significant effect on alleviating dyspnea.

Ineffective Airway Clearance

Planning: client goals. The two major goals for this nursing diagnosis are that the client will (1) demonstrate controlled coughing and proper positioning and (2) experience airway clearance and breathing that are optimal for the client.

Interventions: nonsurgical management. Because the client is predisposed to respiratory tract infection, it is imperative that as much mucus as possible is expectorated. Judicious use of drugs combined with controlled coughing, hydration, and postural drainage can help in airway clearance.

Drug therapy. Careful use of bronchodilators, mucolytics, and expectorants is necessary to thin and expectorate secretions. Clients are monitored periodically for therapeutic drug levels. Some physicians order nebulizer treatments with normal saline or a mucolytic agent such as acetylcysteine (Mucomyst) and normal saline.

Controlled coughing. Because these clients produce more mucus than the average person, they may need to perform a specific coughing maneuver, especially at certain times of the day. On arising early in the morning, the client should cough to get rid of the mucus that collected during the night. Coughing to expectorate mucus before mealtimes may facilitate a more pleasant meal, and coughing before bedtime may ensure that the lungs are clear for an uninterrupted night's sleep. To cough effectively the client sits in a chair or on the side of a bed. The feet are not allowed to dangle. The nurse instructs the client to turn his or her shoulder inward and to bend the head slightly downward, hugging a pillow against the stomach. After the fifth deep breath, the client slowly bends forward while producing two or three strong coughs without taking any breaths between coughs. As the client returns to a sitting position, he or she should take a comfortable deep breath. The entire coughing procedure should be repeated at least twice.

Postural drainage and chest physiotherapy (PT). Chest physiotherapy with postural drainge is a technique that assists in mobilizing secretions from peripheral to central airways, in re-expanding lung tissue, and in promoting efficient use of the respiratory muscles. Chest physiotherapy combines chest percussion with vibration to loosen the secretions (Fig. 62–21). Postural drainage is the use of specific positions (Fig. 62–22) to enlist the force of gravity in removing bronchial secretions. Postural drainage and chest physiotherapy are most beneficial in clients with excessive amounts of mucus.

Hydration. Unless hydration is medically contraindicated because of congestive heart failure or cor pulmonale, individuals with COPD must drink extra liquid,

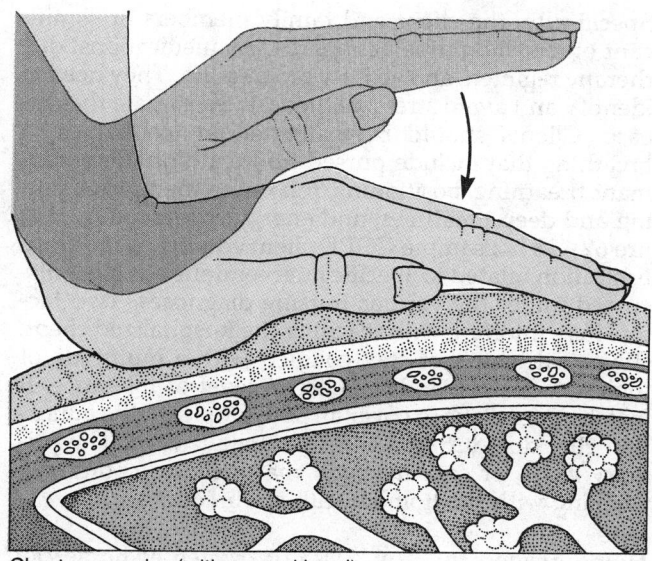

Chest percussion (with cupped hand)

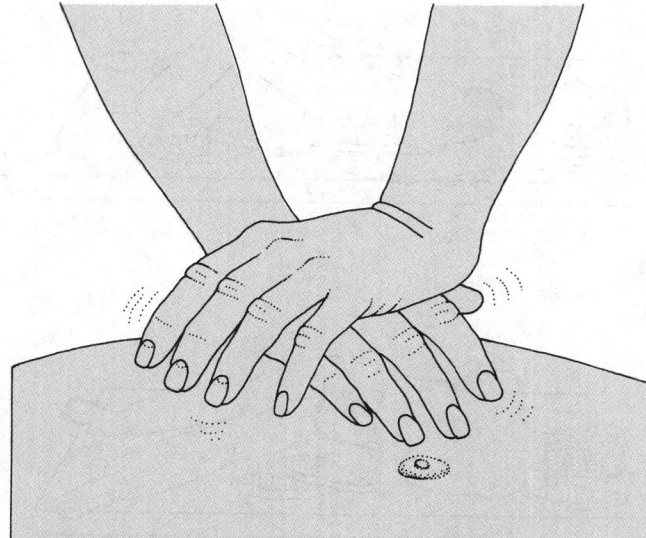

Chest vibration

Figure 62-21

Percussion and vibration techniques in chest physiotherapy.

a total of 2 to 3 L, to keep the secretions liquefied. If the client lives in a dry climate or if the home is unusually dry, the client should be encouraged to buy a humidifier.

Prevention of secondary infection. Individuals with excessive mucus, particularly clients with chronic bronchitis, have a propensity to develop respiratory tract infections. Prevention via vaccination with pneumococcal and influenza vaccines should be stressed.

Anxiety

Planning: client goals. The two goals for this nursing diagnosis are that the client will identify (1) factors that elicit anxious behaviors and (2) activities that tend to decrease anxious behaviors.

Interventions: nonsurgical management. Anxiety plays a major role in clients with emphysema and chronic bronchitis. In clients with asthma, emotional upset can trigger or aggravate wheezing episodes. If a client's symptoms are worsened because of anxiety, it is important that the client understand this effect and have a clear plan prepared in advance for dealing with the anxiety. Having this plan gives the client confidence in knowing exactly what to do, which often helps to reduce anxiety. The nurse counsels clients to think of themselves not as asthmatics but as persons who have asthma. This distinction is an important one because it allows focusing on the person, not just on the disease. The client should be encouraged and allowed to discuss his or her feelings with the nursing staff and other members of the health care team. Counseling, if recom-

mended, should be viewed by the client as a positive suggestion; in no way should the client view this need as a failure to cope. The client should be made to feel that talking with a professional counselor can make a big difference in the course of the disease.

Other alternative psychologic approaches should be explored by the nurse. Relaxation techniques have been used as a method of teaching clients to relax so that they can control dyspneic episodes. Biofeedback has been used so that clients can determine the impact of various stimuli on their symptoms. Ultimately, the client learns to relax and control these stimuli to avoid the aggravating symptoms. The nurse and the client together develop a written plan that states exactly what the client should do if symptoms flare. This method is one way to reduce the anxiety associated with wheezing and dyspnea and gives the client confidence to manage symptoms. Relaxation techniques are described in detail in Chapter 6.

■ Discharge Planning

Home Care Preparation

The COPD client is usually discharged to his or her previous home setting. However, most clients can benefit from a structured pulmonary rehabilitation program, and the nurse often plays a vital role in these programs. Pulmonary rehabilitation programs vary in composition. However, the overall goal of such programs is to increase a person's ability to compensate for and live with COPD. Most programs may have one or more of the following interventions: education, exercise condi-

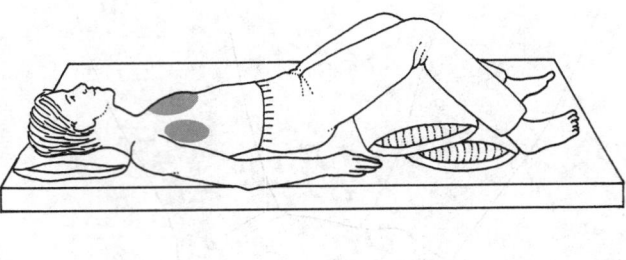

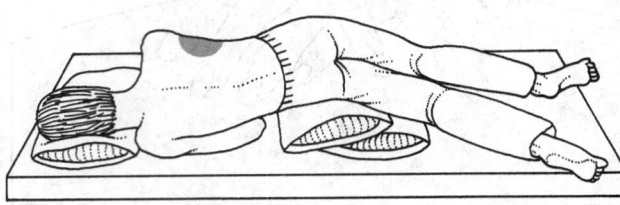

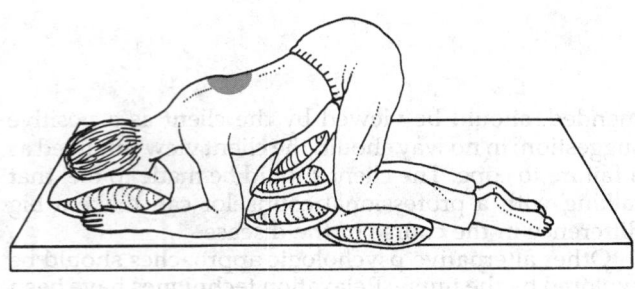

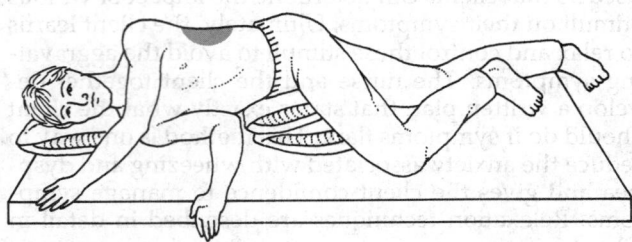

Figure 62–22

Positions for postural drainage of respiratory secretions.

tioning, energy conservation, breathing retraining, bronchial hygiene, psychologic counseling, and vocational training. Individuals with COPD should be referred to a pulmonary rehabilitation program before illness becomes severe because clients with the least severe functional abnormality benefit the most.

Client/Family Education

Clients with a chronic, disabling disease such as COPD need to know as much about the disease as possible so that they can better manage it and themselves.

Specifically, the client and family members or significant others should be able to discuss medications, diet therapy regimen, and activity progression. They need to identify and avoid stressors that can exacerbate the disease. Clients should be instructed in techniques of breathing that include pursed-lip breathing, diaphragmatic breathing, positioning, relaxation therapy, coughing and deep breathing, and energy conservation, Figure 62–23 is a sample COPD client education checklist. Education related to specific interventions has been discussed under the various nursing diagnoses. Two factors may interfere with teaching the hospitalized client: shortened length of stay coupled with a multitude of topics to discuss, and the client's level of tolerance. It may be unrealistic to cover all of the topics in the education checklist during a single hospitalization. The primary nurse or case manager may need to coordinate teaching with the home health or clinic staff.

Home oxygen therapy. Use of oxygen at home can benefit some clients on a long-term basis. As with other therapies, the decision of whether to use home oxygen must be made with calculated analysis. Continuous oxygen therapy may severely limit a client's mobility and be counterproductive to an exercise or rehabilitation schedule. A client may sometimes benefit by using oxygen only during periods of exercise or while sleeping. Continuous, long-term administration of oxygen can reverse tissue hypoxia, polycythemia, and decreased pulmonary vascular resistance; it can also improve cognitive ability and well-being.

Specific criteria must be met for oxygen therapy to benefit the client. First, the client must be clinically stable and optimally treated before the need for home oxygen is determined. For Medicare to cover the cost of continuous oxygen therapy, the client must have severe hypoxemia, which is defined as an arterial PO_2 value of less than 55 mmHg on room air at rest or an arterial oxygen saturation value of less than 85% on room air at rest (ABG or pulse oximetry). A variation of this criterion is an arterial PO_2 value of 56 to 59 mmHg or an arterial oxygen saturation value of 86% to 89% with a secondary diagnosis of symptomatic congestive heart failure, "p" pulmonale as seen on an electrocardiogram, or erythrocytosis with a hematocrit of 56%. Specific criteria are also established for coverage of nocturnal oxygen and portable oxygen therapy. Medicare guidelines are continually changing; therefore, it is important for the nurse to be aware of these criteria and the documentation that is required to meet the standards.

After the need for home oxygen therapy is verified, the nurse begins a teaching plan about oxygen therapy. A durable medical equipment company is selected to deliver oxygen equipment and a community health nursing referral is made for follow-up care in the home. A re-evaluation of the need for oxygen therapy is made about 4 to 6 weeks after the client's discharge from the health care facility.

The nurse teaches the client about the equipment that is needed for home oxygen therapy: (1) the oxygen

Checklist for COPD Client Education

The Client Has Received the Following Education: Date   Signature

A. Basic anatomy and physiology of the respiratory system   _____   _____
   1. Structures composing the respiratory system
   2. Functions of the respiratory passageways
B. Pathophysiology related to condition   _____   _____
   1. Name of lung disease
   2. Generalized physiologic effects
   3. Generalized psychosocial effects
C. Medications   _____   _____
   1. Medication safety
   2. Name of each medication
   3. Action of each medication
   4. Dosage
   5. How to take each medication
   6. Recognition of side effects
   7. Importance of carrying a medication list and a medical alert
      (Medic Alert) bracelet or card
D. Respiratory therapy interventions and bronchial hygiene   _____   _____
   1. Proper care and cleaning of home equipment
   2. Sequence of treatments
   3. Adequate hydration
   4. Postural drainage and chest physiotherapy
   5. Prevention of respiratory tract infection:
      a. Avoid exposure to persons with respiratory tract infections
         and crowds
      b. Signs and symptoms of respiratory tract infection
      c. Use of prescribed antibiotics with as needed (prn) schedule
      d. Influenza immunization; pneumococcal immunization
      e. Use of measures to promote oronasal hygiene
E. Management of dyspnea   _____   _____
   1. Controlled cough maneuver
   2. Pursed-lip breathing
   3. Diaphragmatic breathing
   4. Positioning techniques
   5. Stress management and relaxation techniques
F. Adaptation of a daily routine   _____   _____
   1. Daily schedule of graded exercises
   2. Walking exercise on level ground
   3. Stair climbing
   4. Activities of daily living: adjust activities according to individual
      fatigue patterns
G. Nutrition   _____   _____
   1. Type of diet prescribed
   2. Basic four food groups: meat, dairy, grain, fruit and vegetables:
      2:2:4:4 ratio
   3. Low salt intake
H. Control of environment   _____   _____
   1. Environmental problems related to pulmonary disease
   2. Ways to make the environment conducive to living with
      pulmonary disease
      a. Avoid irritants
      b. Use mask when exposed to dusts
      c. Stay indoors with air conditioning operating when air
         quality is poor
      d. Check air quality telephone recording (telephone number:
         _____)   *Continued*

Figure 62–23

Checklist for education of the client with COPD.

Checklist for COPD Client Education *Continued*

The Client Has Received the Following Education: Date   Signature

I. Smoking
   1. Rationale for smoking cessation
   2. Suggest ways to stop smoking
J. Body image and human sexuality
   1. Alterations in self-esteem and body image related to pulmonary disease
   2. Communication in human relationships
   3. Alterations in sexual relationships related to pulmonary disease
K. Available community resources
   1. Discharge planning; referral to home care professionals
   2. Available community services: Meals on Wheels; American Lung Association; American Heart Association; American Cancer Society

Figure 62–23

Continued

source, (2) the oxygen delivery device, and (3) the humidification source. The nurse discusses the sources of oxygen delivery available. Home oxygen is provided in one of three ways: compressed gas in a tank or a cylinder; liquid oxygen in a reservoir; or an oxygen concentrator. Compressed gas in an oxygen tank (green) is the most common type of oxygen source. The small E tank is available for transporting the client; the large H cylinder is used as a stationary source (Fig. 62–24). An oxygen

tank is economical, and pure oxygen can be delivered at a wide range of flow rates. The second type of home oxygen, liquid oxygen, is oxygen gas that has been liquefied by cooling to −300° F (−147° C); thus, a concentrated amount of oxygen is available in a container similar to a thermos bottle. This container is lightweight and easy to carry. This type of oxygen lasts longer than oxygen in a conventional tank of the same size; however, it is expensive, and the oxygen evaporates if it is

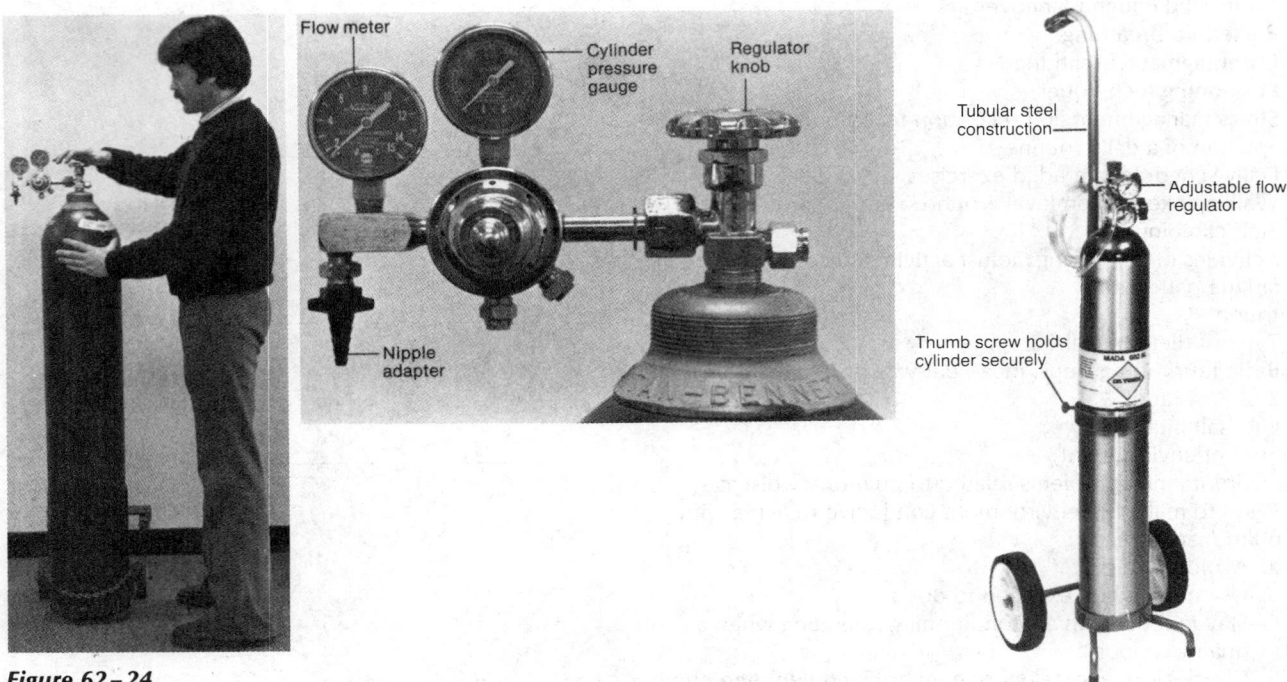

Figure 62–24

Comparison of a large H oxygen cylinder (left and center), with stand, regulator, and flowmeter, and a small E cylinder (right). (Left and center photographs from Kersten, L. D. [1989]. *Comprehensive respiratory nursing: A decision making approach.* Philadelphia: W. B. Saunders; right photograph reproduced courtesy of Mada Medical Products, Inc., Carlstadt, NJ.)

not used continuously. The last type of home oxygen source is the oxygen concentrator (Fig. 62–25), which is an electrical machine that removes nitrogen, water vapor, and hydrocarbons from room air. Oxygen is concentrated from the 21% FIO_2 in room air and is delivered at more than 90%. The concentrator is the least expensive of the systems but is not portable and is often noisy. Humidification is rarely needed for any of these systems. Nevertheless, humidification may help when a flow rate of higher than 2 L/minute is required, the client has a tracheostomy, or mechanical ventilation is used (see Fig. 62–3).

The most common type of oxygen delivery device used with any of these systems is the nasal cannula (see Fig. 62–2). There are several modified versions of the nasal cannula for the home setting. These devices use less oxygen, reduce nasal drying, are cosmetically appealing, and offer a financial saving when used properly.

While providing discharge planning and teaching, the nurse is also sensitive to the psychologic adjustment of the client to oxygen therapy. The client is encouraged to share feelings and concerns. The client may be concerned about social acceptance by and misconceptions of friends who may view the client differently because a

cannula is worn. The client must realize that compliance with oxygen therapy is important so that normal activities of daily living and events that bring enjoyment can be continued.

Tracheostomy care.   Home care of the client with a tracheostomy is similar to the care in the acute care setting. The client with a tracheostomy learns to perform self-care and manages the tube independently and effectively. Teaching is individualized, and tracheostomy care is planned so that it is easily integrated into the client's life style. In general, clean technique is taught, and the importance of clean equipment and storage area is stressed.

The client and family are encouraged to participate as soon as possible in various aspects of tracheostomy care. For example, the first activity might be to allow the client or family member to manually ventilate the client (with an Ambu bag) during suctioning. Time must be given for the client to adjust to the change in body image from the tracheostomy. Teaching is provided in several sessions, which permits adequate time to learn and practice the new skills and to ask questions.

The major aspects of teaching tracheostomy care to the client and/or family include the following: purpose and parts of the tube; equipment needed; care for the skin around the tube; removal, cleaning, and replacement of the inner cannula; suctioning of the tracheostomy tube; changing the tracheostomy ties; humidification and infection control measures; and safety measures.

In the home setting, tracheostomy care is done once a day if secretions are minimal. The same procedure that was used in the hospital is followed, except that clean technique is sufficient and gloves and a tracheostomy kit are not needed. Instead, a clean bowl with a half-strength solution of hydrogen peroxide and tap water is used to clean the tracheostomy tube. The inner cannula is cleaned with a pipe cleaner and is then rinsed with running tap water. Tracheostomy ties are changed as needed. Cotton-tipped applicators and 4 × 4 in gauze pads are used to clean around the stoma site.

Suctioning may be needed in the home setting, but the client can usually mobilize secretions by coughing if proper hydration, respiratory medications, and positioning are followed. When suctioning is required, clean technique is practiced and the client takes three or four deep breaths, which is sufficient for preoxygenation and postoxygenation in the spontaneously breathing client. The client or family member needs reassurance that shortness of breath and coughing are common during the suctioning procedure. Special red rubber suction catheters can be cleaned in hot soapy water, rinsed, and reused. Humidification is needed to prevent encrustation of secretions; humidification in the home is provided by a room humidifier and strategically located smaller humidifiers.

The tracheostomy tube and tape are changed as needed according to the physician's guidelines. The client, family member, or significant other changes the

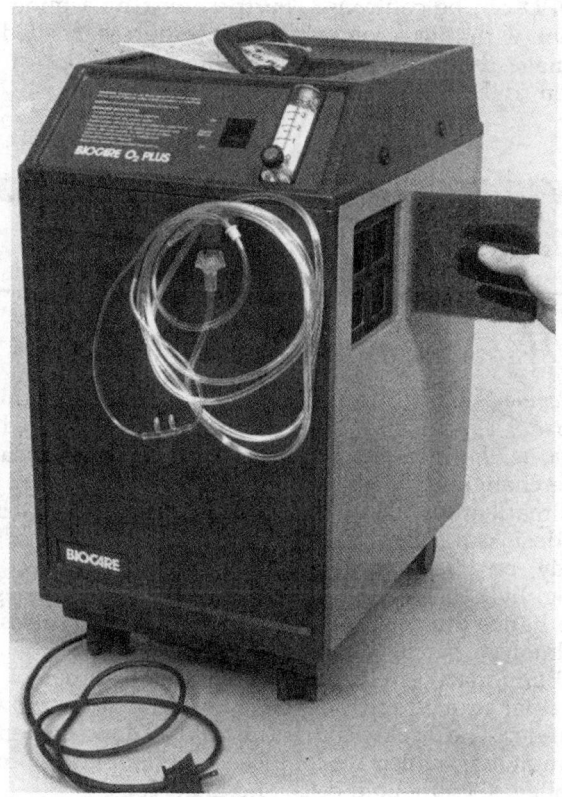

Figure 62–25

Oxygen concentrator for long-term use. (Photograph from Kersten, L. D. [1989]. *Comprehensive respiratory nursing: A decision making approach*. Philadelphia: W. B. Saunders.)

tube. The client takes several deep breaths after the tube is replaced and determines whether adequate ventilation and air movement are present. This procedure is simple in the home because the tube is cuffless and is inserted into a well-established track.

Several safety measures are important for the client with a tracheostomy. Otherwise, the client is able to continue with usual activities, hobbies, and work. Care is taken to avoid areas with excessive dust, fumes, aerosols, smoke, and powder. The opening of the tracheostomy can be covered with a scarf, lint-free cloth covering, or crocheted bib to protect the lungs against foreign materials such as hair, dust, or food. This protection offers a cosmetic benefit as well as filters and warms air that enters the tracheostomy. Extremes in temperatures are avoided because they can be irritating to the tracheal mucosa. A medical alert (Medic Alert) bracelet is helpful for identification of the client as a neck breather in an emergency situation.

To augment teaching sessions, video tapes and teaching guides are available to meet educational goals of the client. A visiting community health nurse is helpful to ensure proper follow-up and to help the client prevent complications. A durable medical equipment company is contacted that provides equipment to the home and often brings the equipment to the hospital so that the client can become accustomed to it. Finally, a community support group can provide ongoing educational and social opportunities and can serve as a forum for the client to share concerns and coping strategies.

Psychosocial Preparation

The client with COPD faces a lifelong disease with remissions and exacerbations. The nurse explains to both the client and the family that the client may experience periods of anxiety, depression, and ineffective coping. The client may also have self-directed anger, particularly if he or she was a smoker and recognizes that smoking caused the disease.

Financial concerns often increase the client's anxiety and interfere with disease management. The client's condition may worsen to the point that he or she cannot work. Disability benefits through Social Security or private disability insurance plans can help ease the financial burden. Medicare or other health insurers may assist with payment for home oxygen therapy and nebulizer treatments. The nurse collaborates closely with the hospital social worker or discharge planner to help the client make the necessary arrangements.

Health Care Resources

The nurse provides appropriate referrals as necessary. Home care visits may be warranted, particularly if the client is being sent home and must use oxygen therapy for the first time. Referral to assistance programs such as Meals on Wheels can be extremely helpful. The nurse provides the client with a listing of various support groups and Better Breathing groups sponsored by the ALA. If the client is having difficulty with smoking cessation and indicates the need for assistance, the nurse makes the appropriate referrals.

 Evaluation

The nurse evaluates the care of the COPD client on the basis of the identified nursing diagnoses. The expected outcomes include that the client

1. Demonstrates breathing techniques of pursed-lip breathing and abdominal or diaphragmatic breathing
2. Describes and complies with the ordered drug regimen
3. Identifies various methods of conserving energy
4. States positioning techniques to use during dyspneic episodes
5. States the need to increase or maintain fluid intake
6. Demonstrates the controlled coughing maneuver
7. States the need to avoid irritants, particularly cigarette smoke
8. States methods of alleviating anxiety and fear

By meeting the desired outcomes, the progression of COPD can be controlled. Furthermore, by arming the client with the knowledge and resources needed to manage the disease, the client can better control the often frightening episodes of dyspnea.

SARCOIDOSIS

OVERVIEW

Sarcoidosis is just one of a group of diseases within a broader classification of pulmonary diseases called *interstitial lung disease.* Interstitial lung disease is used interchangeably with the term *fibrotic lung disease.* The hallmark of sarcoidosis is noncaseating granuloma. Sarcoidosis can occur in almost any organ or tissue of the body, but the granulomas most frequently affect the lung, liver, spleen, lymph nodes, eyes, small bones of the hands and feet, and skin. This section focuses on pulmonary sarcoidosis.

Pulmonary sarcoidosis is a chronic disorder of the alveolar structure that develops over time in a stepwise manner. The disease is characterized by development of granulomas, which are composed of lymphocytes, macrophages, epithelioid cells, and giant cells.

The development of the fiberoptic bronchoscope has allowed researchers to sample the epithelial fluid of the lower respiratory tract to investigate the alveolitis of clients with active disease. This test confirms that pulmonary sarcoidosis is a disease that is associated with an intense cellular immune response in the alveolar structure.

The current concept of the development of pulmonary sarcoidosis involves the activation of T lymphocytes; the stimulus for this activation is unknown. The stimulus causes normal resident immune cells (the T lymphocytes) to recruit additional immune cells, probably by releasing chemotactic factor, to attract blood monocytes to the lung. Monocytes are precursors of macrophages, epithelioid cells, and multinucleated giant cells, which compose the granuloma. *Alveolitis* is the term that describes this process. The term is used specifically to refer to the accumulation of inflammatory immune cells in the lung.

The presence of T lymphocytes and macrophages and the substances that they secrete leads to disorder of the cellular arrangement in the lung. Individual cell shapes are also altered. It is believed that the T lymphocytes are primarily responsible for granuloma formation and that the activated macrophages are primarily responsible for interstitial fibrosis (because of their ability to recruit and increase the number of fibroblasts). The fibrosis results in a loss of lung compliance and a loss of functional ability to exchange gases. Cor pulmonale (right-sided cardiac failure) is often present because the heart can no longer pump against the noncompliant, fibrotic lung.

In the United States, sarcoidosis affects Black persons 10 times more frequently than Caucasian. The overall prevalence is similar in women and men, but it is twice as common in women of childbearing age compared with women of other ages. A distinctive feature of sarcoidosis is its age distribution: most cases develop between 20 and 40 years of age.

COLLABORATIVE MANAGEMENT

Indications for treatment vary. If the client is asymptomatic with no abnormalities in pulmonary function, no treatment is given. If pulmonary function is reduced and there are pulmonary infiltrates, the client is administered corticosteroids (e.g., prednisone). A daily maintenance dose of 10 to 15 mg may be needed. After the symptoms resolve, the maintenance dose may be reduced and eventually withdrawn, but relapses may occur.

PULMONARY TUBERCULOSIS

OVERVIEW

In 1900, tuberculosis (TB) was the leading cause of death in the United States and Europe. Although the incidence has declined markedly, it remains a worldwide problem. Continuous assessment and intervention to prevent the spread of the disease must continue. The increasing numbers of homeless individuals in U.S. cities and of individuals who have acquired immunodeficiency syndrome (AIDS) present new challenges to the control and eradication of TB.

Pathophysiology

TB is a highly communicable disease that is typically caused by *Mycobacterium tuberculosis.* The tubercule bacillus is transmitted via aerosolization, i.e., an airborne route. When an infected person coughs, laughs, sneezes, or sings, droplet nuclei are produced and may be inhaled by others. When the tubercle bacillus reaches a susceptible site (bronchi or alveoli), it multiplies freely. An exudative response occurs, causing a nonspecific pneumonitis. With the development of acquired immunity, further multiplication of bacilli is controlled in the majority of initial lesions. The lesions typically resolve and leave little or no residual. A small percentage of individuals who are initially infected develop the disease (5% to 15%). Cell-mediated, or type IV, immunity develops 2 to 10 weeks after infection and is manifested by a significant reaction to a tuberculin test, inflammation, and necrosis. A primary infection may be microscopic in size and may never appear on an x-ray film. The process of infection occurs in the following way: the granulomatous inflammation that is created by the tubercle bacillus becomes surrounded by collagen, fibroblasts, and lymphocytes. In the center of the lesion (Ghon's tubercle), necrosis, which is called *caseation necrosis,* occurs.

After this development, areas of caseation localize and undergo resorption, hyaline degeneration, and fibrosis. These necrotic areas may calcify (calcification) or may liquefy (liquefaction). If the latter occurs, the liquid material then empties into a bronchus, and the evacuated area becomes a cavity (cavitation). Bacilli continue to proliferate in the necrotic cavity wall. The evacuated material leads to endobronchial spread of disease into new areas of the lung; this process can be a recurring one. A lesion may also progress by direct extension if bacilli multiply rapidly and there is a marked exudative response. These lesions may extend through the pleura, which results in tuberculous pleural effusion with a small number of organisms. Similarly, pericardial effusions may also occur.

If a large number of organisms enter the blood stream, disseminated disease, which is called *miliary tuberculosis,* or *hematogenous tuberculosis,* occurs. Typically, many tiny, discrete nodules scattered throughout the lung are visualized on an x-ray film. If disseminated disease occurs through blood-borne foci, the brain, meninges, liver, kidney, and bone marrow are commonly involved.

Initial infection is seen more often in the middle or lower lobes of the lung. The regional lymph nodes, particularly the hilar and paratracheal nodes, are commonly involved. There is usually an asymptomatic interval after infection that lasts for years, or less commonly, decades before clinical symptoms develop. The upper lobes are the most common site of reinfection. The TB classification that has been adopted and revised by the ALA (1981) is given in the accompanying Key Features of Disease.

Etiology

The organism *M. tuberculosis* is nonmotile, nonsporulating, and an acid-fast rod that secretes niacin. The tubercle bacillus is transmitted via aerosolization.

Individuals who are most commonly infected are those having *repeated* close contact with an infected person who has not yet been diagnosed with TB. After the infected person has received chemotherapy for 2 to 3 weeks, the risk of transmission is greatly reduced.

Incidence

At the beginning of the 20th century, TB was the leading cause of death in the United States. However, figures for 1981 reveal that TB accounts for 0.8% of deaths in the United States. The greatest proportion of new cases originates in cities in which the prevalence of poverty and homelessness is high. Non-Caucasian males are affected more than Caucasian males or females. Research has also revealed that there is a higher incidence of TB and positive reactors to tuberculin tests among Hispanic immigrants than among those born in the United States (Perez-Stable et al., 1986). Those at high risk for acquiring TB are those who live in substandard housing with large groups of people, the elderly, alcoholics, drug abusers, and persons with AIDS or AIDS-related complex. These individuals often have poor health and/or are immunocompromised.

PREVENTION

Because the untreated individual is likely to infect others, public health professionals can prevent the spread of the disease by locating the individual's contacts. When contacts have been identified, these individuals are assessed with a tuberculin test and chest x-ray film to determine infection with TB. Health care workers who may be exposed to individuals with untreated TB are at high risk of becoming infected, but close, frequent, prolonged exposure presents the greatest risk. If the area of reaction to the tuberculin test is greater than 10 mm in diameter, the person is assumed to be infected. However, they should be assessed after infection by taking a yearly chest x-ray film. One year of chemotherapy with isoniazid is usually recommended. In addition, individuals in a high-risk group may receive preventive chemotherapy.

The infected client should be instructed to cover the mouth and nose when coughing and to wear a mask when in contact with crowds until chemotherapy is effective in eliminating the infection. Health care workers should prevent infection to themselves by wearing masks in the presence of individuals who are coughing and whose diagnosis is not yet confirmed.

COLLABORATIVE MANAGEMENT

 Assessment

History

Early detection of TB depends on subjective findings rather than presentation of symptoms. TB has an insidious onset, and many clients do not become aware of symptoms until the disease is well advanced. A thorough history includes assessment of *past exposure to TB.* The nurse inquires about the client's *country of origin* and *travel* to foreign countries in which there is a high incidence of TB. It is important to note whether the client has had *prior tests for TB* and what the results were. In addition, the nurse asks whether the client has had *bacille Calmette-Guérin* (BCG) *vaccine,* a vaccine containing attenuated tubercule bacilli that is given routinely in many foreign countries to produce increased resistance to TB. Anyone who has received BCG will have a positive skin test and should be evaluated for TB with a chest x-ray film.

Physical Assessment: Clinical Manifestations

Typically, the client with TB presents with progressive *fatigue, lethargy, nausea, anorexia, weight loss, irregular menses,* and *low-grade fevers,* which may have oc-

---

KEY FEATURES OF DISEASE ■ American Lung Association Classification of Tuberculosis

0   No TB exposure, not infected

1   TB exposure, no evidence of infection

2   TB infection, no disease

3   TB: current disease (persons with completed diagnostic evidence of TB: both a significant reaction to tuberculin skin test and clinical and/or x-ray evidence of TB)

4   TB: no current disease (persons with previous history of TB or with abnormal x-ray films but no significant tuberculin skin test reaction or clinical evidence)

5   TB: suspect (diagnosis pending) (used during diagnostic testing of suspect persons, for no longer than a 3-mo period)

curred for weeks to months. Fever may also be accompanied by *night sweats.* The client finally notices a *cough* and the production of mucoid and mucopurulent *sputum,* which is occasionally streaked with blood. Chest tightness and a dull, aching chest pain may accompany the cough. The physical examination of the chest does not provide conclusive evidence of tuberculosis. The nurse may hear dullness with percussion over involved parenchymal areas, bronchial breath sounds, rales, and increased transmission of spoken or whispered sounds. Partial obstruction of a bronchus because of endobronchial disease or compression by lymph nodes may produce localized wheezing.

Psychosocial Assessment

The client with TB is usually not anxious because of dyspnea, as dyspnea is uncommon unless there is a massive pleural effusion. However, the client may be aware of an ill-defined anxiety or nervousness associated with this altered state of wellness. The nurse considers this possibility in the initial interview and explains slowly the purpose of every aspect of the diagnostic work-up. If the individual does not speak English, an interpreter should be involved in the client's first encounter with the health care agency.

Laboratory Findings

Sputum culture of *M. tuberculosis* confirms the diagnosis. Usually, three samples are obtained for an acid-fast smear. After the start of chemotherapy, sputum samples are obtained again to determine the effectiveness of therapy. Most clients have negative cultures after 3 to 6 months.

The tuberculin test (Mantoux's test) result is the most reliable determinant of infection with TB. A small amount of intermediate-strength purified protein derivative (PPD) is given intradermally in the forearm. An area of induration measuring 10 mm or more in diameter 48 to 72 hours after injection indicates exposure to TB. A positive reaction does not mean that active disease is present but indicates exposure to TB or the presence of inactive (dormant) disease.

The chest x-ray film is essential for detecting old or new lesions after they are large enough to be seen. This examination is routinely performed for all individuals with a positive PPD. Caseation and inflammation may be visualized on the film if the disease is active.

 Analysis: Nursing Diagnosis

Common Diagnoses

The following nursing diagnoses are most commonly seen in the client with TB:

1. Potential for injury related to possible spread of infection

2. Altered nutrition: less than body requirements related to nausea and/or drug therapy
3. Anxiety related to diagnosis and physical alterations

Additional Diagnoses

Other nursing diagnoses that may occur are

1. Ineffective airway clearance related to sputum production
2. Pain related to lung infection
3. Total self-care deficit related to fatigue and lethargy
4. Sleep pattern disturbance related to night sweats and coughing
5. Fatigue related to infection, coughing, and weight loss
6. Knowledge deficit related to the disease and its treatment

 Planning and Implementation

Potential for Injury

Planning: client goals. The goal for this diagnosis is that the client will be compliant with the treatment regimen to prevent the spread of disease.

Interventions: nonsurgical management. Chemotherapy is the most effective method for managing the disease and preventing transmission. Active TB is treated with a combination of drugs to which organisms are susceptible. Therapy is continued until the disease is under control. Use of multiple-drug regimens destroys organisms as quickly as possible and minimizes the emergence of drug-resistant organisms. In the United States, a 9-month regimen consisting of isoniazid (INH) (Hyzyd) and rifampin (Rifadin) is frequently used. Ethambutol (Myambutol) and streptomycin may be added for the initial 2 to 8 weeks of treatment. Isoniazid may also be combined with one or more of the following: streptomycin, ethambutol, and pyrazinamide.

The major role of the nurse is to teach clients the necessary information about drug therapy. The nurse recognizes that the client who is anxious may not absorb information well. The nurse repeats the information and enlists the assistance of family members if available. The use of teaching aids that are available through the ALA is also helpful. The client should be able to describe the treatment regimen and major side effects for which to call the health care agency and physician. TB is almost always treated outside of the hospital so that the client is convalescing in the home setting. In this setting, respiratory isolation is not necessary because family members have already been exposed. The client is instructed to cover his or her mouth and nose when coughing or sneezing. Possible complications of TB include hemorrhage and pleurisy; either complication may indicate recurrence of tuberculous activity, and the client and family should be made aware of these complications. Alcoholic clients may have a tendency to be noncompliant with medication and therefore may be at risk for recurrence of symptoms. These clients can be referred to clinics for treatment of alcoholism or other appropriate agencies.

The client is instructed to have examinations of sputum every 2 to 4 weeks until two sputum culture results are negative. When results are negative, the client is considered to be noninfectious and can usually return to former employment. He or she should avoid excessive exposure to silicone or dust because these substances can cause further lung damage.

The hospitalized client with TB is also instructed to cover his or her mouth and nose when coughing. The staff wear masks when caring for the client if the client is coughing—also known as respiratory precautions (see Chap. 26). Gowns are indicated only in case of gross contamination of clothing. Hands are always thoroughly washed after caring for the client.

Altered Nutrition: Less Than Body Requirements

Planning: client goals. Nausea and anorexia are commonly experienced by clients with TB, especially when they are receiving chemotherapy such as rifampin and isoniazid. Therefore, the goal is that the client will have adequate nutrition to maintain body weight or to prevent further weight loss.

Interventions: nonsurgical management. Nausea may be prevented by taking the daily dose of the chemotherapeutic drug at bedtime. Antinausea drugs such as prochlorperazine (Compazine) may also prevent this symptom. The nurse instructs the client about the need for adequate nutrition, including the basic four food groups, to promote healing. Increasing the intake of foods that are rich in iron, protein, and vitamin C is recommended.

Anxiety

Planning: client goals. The goal for this diagnosis is that the client will state that anxiety is reduced after interventions are initiated.

Interventions: nonsurgical management. The client with TB notices changes in physical stamina, which may be frightening. The client also faces concerns about the prognosis of the disease. The nurse is realistic in offering a positive outlook for the client if he or she complies with the medication regimen and suggests that fatigue will diminish as the treatment progresses. The nurse listens carefully to the client's concerns throughout the treatment and responds in a supportive manner. The client's return to work and the usual daily routines is likely to reduce anxiety.

■ Discharge Planning

Home Care Preparation

Most clients with TB are managed outside of the hospital. However, clients may be diagnosed with TB while in the hospital if pneumonia is suspected or other possible complications exist. Discharge may be delayed if the living situation is considered to lead to high risk or if the client is likely to be noncompliant. A consultation with the social service worker in the hospital and/or the community health nurse agency may ensure the client's discharge to the appropriate environment with continued supervision.

Client/Family Education

The client is instructed to follow the drug regimen exactly as prescribed and to always have a supply of the medication on hand. Side effects and ways to minimize them are also stressed to ensure compliance. The nurse reminds the client with TB that the disease is not communicable 2 to 3 weeks after drug therapy is initiated. However, the client must continue with the prescribed medication for 9 to 12 months as ordered.

If the client has experienced weight loss and severe lethargy, he or she should gradually resume usual activities. Proper nutrition with foods from the basic four food groups must be maintained to prevent recurrence.

Psychosocial Preparation

The nurse forewarns the client with TB that society may associate a stigma with the disease by relating it to substance abusers and homeless people. Not everyone who has TB is a member of one of these groups. Family members and other support groups in the community (e.g., religious organization) can present a positive attitude to help the client overcome possible negative reactions.

Health Care Resources

The client needs to receive follow-up care by a physician for at least 1 year during active treatment. In addition, the ALA, an organization that uses volunteers, can provide free information to the client about the disease and its treatment. Alcoholics Anonymous and other health care resources for clients with alcoholism are available as well if needed. The nurse assists the client who abuses drugs to locate an appropriate drug treatment program.

 Evaluation

The nurse evaluates the care for a client with TB on the basis of the identified nursing diagnoses. The expected outcomes include that the client

1. Complies with the treatment regimen and follow-up care
2. Maintains body weight via adequate nutritional intake
3. States that anxiety about disease and treatment has been reduced
4. Returns to the usual level of activity before treatment is discontinued (within 1 year)

LUNG ABSCESS

OVERVIEW

A *lung abscess* is a localized area of lung destruction caused by liquefaction necrosis, which is usually related to pyogenic bacteria. Clients who present with this problem often have a history of pneumonia, possibly complicated by aspiration of oropharyngeal contents. Other causes of aspiration leading to abscess include alcoholism that causes loss of consciousness; seizure disorders or other neurologic defects; and disorders of swallowing. An obstruction of a bronchus may cause a necrotizing process in the distal lung that eventually becomes an abscess. Formation of multiple abscesses and cavities occurs commonly in clients with TB or fungal infections of the lung. Immunosuppressed individuals, such as clients receiving chemotherapy or clients with a disease such as leukemia, are particularly susceptible to fungal infection.

COLLABORATIVE MANAGEMENT

The client's recent history of influenza, pneumonia, febrile illness, cough, and sputum production is noted. In addition, the nurse inquires about the color and odor of the sputum and the presence of any pleuritic chest pain (a stabbing pain, especially when taking a deep breath). Physical assessment of the client often reveals a febrile client who appears pale and fatigued. Auscultation of breath sounds may reveal decreased sounds in the involved area of the lung as well as dullness on percussion. Bronchial breath sounds and rales are heard over the site of the lesion. A chest x-ray film and sputum samples are the most valuable diagnostic tools. If the physician is unable to obtain sputum, transtracheal aspiration via suction may be done to obtain a sample so that sputum can be cultured and the appropriate organism identified.

Nursing diagnoses and interventions that were identified for the client with pneumonia also apply to the client with a lung abscess. The client may be taking more than one antibiotic, so the nurse also observes for oral overgrowth with *Candida albicans* and provides frequent mouth care.

PULMONARY EMPYEMA

OVERVIEW

Empyema refers to a collection of pus in the pleural space. The most common cause of empyema is pulmonary infection or lung abscess. Pneumonia or lung abscess can spread across the pleura or obstruct lymph nodes and cause a retrograde flood of infected lymph into the pleural space. In addition, an intrahepatic or subphrenic abscess can spread through the diaphragm's lymphatic system. Thoracic surgery and chest trauma are common predisposing conditions in which bacteria is introduced directly into the pleural space. Incomplete evacuation from the pleural space of blood that has accumulated because of trauma presents a culture medium for empyema.

COLLABORATIVE MANAGEMENT

Important history findings include recent febrile illnesses (including pneumonia), chest pain, dyspnea, cough, and trauma. The character and color of the sputum are noted. Physical assessment includes observation of chest symmetry and chest wall motion because the client with pleural effusion may have diminished chest wall motion. The nurse auscultates and percusses the lungs and assesses for fremitus. If an effusion is present, the client may have decreased breath sounds, decreased or absent fremitus, and a flat percussion note. Compression of lung tissue adjacent to the effusion is likely to produce bronchial breath sounds over the area, egophony, and whispered pectoriloquy. Some clients present with fever, chills, and weight loss. Night sweats may also occur. If there is cardiorespiratory compromise, the client may be hypotensive. There may be a displacement of the PMI (point of maximal impulse) on auscultation of the heart because of a mediastinal deviation.

Major diagnostic studies include the chest roentgenography thoracentesis. A pleural fluid sample is obtained and analyzed for appearance, odor, red blood cell count, white blood cell count and differential, glucose and protein levels, lactate dehydrogenase (LDH), and pH; Gram's and acid-fast stains of smears and cytologic studies are also done. An exudative process is indicated if the protein concentration is higher than 3.0 g/100 mL of pleural fluid. Empyema fluid is thick, opaque, and intensely foul-smelling.

Therapy for empyema is based on emptying the empyema cavity, re-expanding the lung, and controlling the infection. Usually, the client is treated with antibiotics appropriate for the isolated pathogen. In addition, closed-chest drainage is used to promote lung expansion (see Figs. 62–26 through 62–29). One or more chest tubes are placed in the inferior parts of the empyema sac. Underwater seal drainage is used without suction initially, but negative pressure may be added if the lung fails to expand. The tube is removed over a period of weeks. Open thoracotomy and decortication may be needed for thick pus or marked pleural thickening. Nursing considerations are the same as those for clients with a pleural effusion, pneumothorax, and infection.

LUNG CANCER

OVERVIEW

Lung cancer is the leading cause of cancer-related mortality. It is essentially incurable with forms of therapy other than surgical intervention. Advances in treatment of small cell carcinoma of the lungs have resulted in a survival rate of 10% to 20% of clients with disease confined to the thorax. However, because lung cancer often metastasizes before symptoms are noticed, therapy is often palliative rather than curative. Only 9% of clients with lung cancer are alive 5 years after the diagnosis is made. Therefore, the nurse has a major role in public education aimed at prevention.

Pathophysiology

Bronchogenic carcinoma spreads chiefly through direct extension and lymphatic dissemination. Lymphatic spread is predominantly by embolism and to a lesser extent by continuity of growth. Cancer originating in the periphery of the lung remains contained for a longer period than cancer originating in a major bronchus. The bodies of the lower thoracic and upper lumbar vertebrae and other bones are common sites of metastases. Pulmonary tumors also frequently metastasize to the adrenal glands. Other metastatic sites include the central nervous system and the liver.

The four major cell types of lung cancer differ greatly in their characteristics, treatment, and prognosis. These tumor types are summarized and differentiated in the accompanying Key Features of Disease.

Etiology

As early as the 1930s, evidence suggested a correlation between smoking and the development of lung cancer. Research has consistently confirmed that smoking plays a predominant role in the development of the disease, with lung cancer occurring 10 times more commonly in smokers than in nonsmokers. Cigarette smoke may be inhaled actively (by actually smoking a cigarette) or pas-

sively (by inhaling smoke created by others who are smoking). Both types of inhalation are positively correlated with the development of lung cancer. Active smoking is the primary risk factor associated with the development of lung cancer, and the amount of active cigarette smoking positively correlates with the frequency and intensity of pathologic changes. Cigarette smoke that is inhaled passively—so-called sidestream smoke—contains many of the carcinogens that are found in actively inhaled tobacco smoke. Groups at high risk for the development of lung cancer secondary to passive smoking are those heavily exposed to passive smoke in the workplace; e.g., persons who work in bars and restaurants. It is believed that the historically higher incidence of lung cancer in males is related to higher numbers of male smokers. Current evidence suggests that this gap between the sexes is closing, most probably related to the fact that increasing numbers of women are smoking. Lung cancer risk is also influenced by other factors such as age at which smoking started, degree of inhalation, and number of years of smoking.

Other influential factors in the development of lung cancer include atmospheric and industrial pollution. It is logical that the incidence of lung cancers is higher in industrial areas. In addition, coal tar, radioactive ore, asbestos, nickel, silver, arsenic, and certain plastics have been proved to be carcinogenic. Clients with chronic respiratory diseases are also at higher risk of developing lung cancer. An individual who smokes *and* has one or more of the predisposing factors is at the greatest risk for the disease.

Little evidence for inherited influences exists for bronchogenic carcinoma. However, evidence for adenocarcinoma and alveolar cell carcinoma suggests the presence of familial factors. These factors do not seem to be related to smoking and are found in families with other tumors, AIDS, or inheritable disorders of the lung. Research has shown that there may be a link between vitamin A deficiency in the diet and the development of lung cancer.

Incidence

Lung cancer is recognized as a worldwide problem. It commonly occurs in both sexes and in industrialized as well as underdeveloped nations, but it is more prevalent in highly industrialized areas. Males in the United Kingdom have the highest incidence. Incidence and mortality rates for males in the United States are also high and are increasing for women. Estimates for 1987 in the United States are 136,000 deaths from lung cancer (92,000 male and 44,000 female). Of all cancer deaths in men, 36% are due to lung cancer; the corresponding figure for women is 20% (Oleske, 1987).

Incidence and mortality rates for lung cancer were higher for Caucasians than for non-Caucasians in the United States until 1960. Since then, the mortality rates for non-Caucasian males has exceeded that of Cauca-

KEY FEATURES OF DISEASE ■ Differential Features of the Four Major Types of Lung Cancer

Type	Approximate Incidence	Characteristics	Treatment
Small cell (oat cell)	20%	Centrally located most malignant type spread via the lymphatic and circulatory systems. There is a high frequency of early extrathoracic spread. Survival rate is poor, usually not more than 2 yr with treatment.	Most cancers respond to chemotherapy. Surgical resectability is poor.
Epidermal (squamous cell)	30%	Cancer arises in pleural periphery and generally extends centrally, with subsequent involvement of mainstem bronchi. Cavitation may develop in lung to tumor. Client presents with chest pain, cough, dyspnea, and hemoptysis. Growth rate is slow with metastases being uncommon. If metastasis does occur, the spread is to lymph, adrenal glands, and liver (in that order).	Surgical resectability is good if stage I or II. The response to chemotherapy and radiation therapy is poor, but these methods may be used for palliation.
Adenocarcinoma	30%	Lesions generally remain in the periphery where they originate. Cancer often arises in previously scarred or fibrotic lung tissue. The incidence in smokers is high, with an increasing incidence in women. Client often presents with cough, chest pain, dyspnea, and pleuritic pain. Growth is slow. Metastasis to other organs is possible.	Surgical resectability is good if localized stage I or II. Radiation therapy is used for palliation. Clients have a moderately good response to chemotherapy.
Large cell anaplastic carcinoma	11%	Cancer is often located peripherally but tends to form larger tumor masses than adenocarcinoma. Cavitation is common. Growth is slow. Metastasis may occur to the kidneys, liver, and adrenal glands (in that order).	Surgical resectability is poor if involvement is widespread. Better prognosis if stage I or II. Chemotherapy has limited use, and radiation therapy is palliative.

sian males. Smoking is identified as a contributing factor. Lung cancer mortality and incidence are also influenced by environmental factors such as employment in a hazardous workplace and poor nutrition. In Caucasian and Black males studied, the incidence of lung cancer is inversely related to socioeconomic status.

Among women, a higher incidence is found in upper-income and lower-income groups. Caucasian males in the Northeast have a high lung cancer mortality, but the highest rates are along the Gulf of Mexico, particularly in Louisiana and along the southeast Atlantic coast. High lung cancer rates for non-Caucasian males tend to be in urban areas of the South. The impact of industrial factors on the geographic variation in lung cancer rates is pronounced. Mortality among Caucasian males is pronounced in countries with significant paper, chemical, and petroleum industries (Oleske, 1987).

PREVENTION

Because smoking is the predominant cause of lung cancer, clients are encouraged to quit or reduce smoking. Many people begin smoking as adolescents, so education should begin with children in elementary school. A number of adult smoking cessation programs, which include the method of hypnosis, are available in most geographic areas. Nonsmokers are encouraged to avoid sidestream smoke. Clients should also be warned to avoid exposure to asbestos and other occupational carcinogens. To prevent vitamin A deficiency, daily consumption of green and yellow vegetables is encouraged. Nurses should emphasize the warning signals of and risk factors for lung cancer (see the accompanying Key Features of Disease). Individuals with a family history of lung cancer or those with warning signals are encouraged to avoid risks and to seek frequent medical examinations.

COLLABORATIVE MANAGEMENT

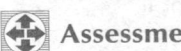 **Assessment**

History

The nurse asks extensive questions about the *presence of risk factors*, including smoking and contact with materials in the workplace. A detailed history of the duration, frequency, and intensity of exposure is elicited.

KEY FEATURES OF DISEASE ■ **Warning Signals Associated with Lung Cancer**

Change in respiratory pattern

Persistent cough

Blood-streaked sputum

Rust-colored or purulent sputum

Frank hemoptysis

Chest pain or chest tightness

Shoulder, arm, or chest wall pain

Recurring episodes of pleural effusion, pneumonia, or bronchitis

Dyspnea

Hoarseness

Fever associated with one or two other signs

In obtaining the history, the nurse is alert to vague subjective complaints that have persisted longer than normally expected. *Hoarseness* is an early sign of lung cancer that occurs because of recurrent laryngeal nerve invasion. In addition, the nurse asks whether positional changes affect hoarseness because a recumbent position often exacerbates this sign. The nurse explores the issue of *pain* because vague discomfort to severe pain occurs at any stage of tumor development. The nurse assesses for any ill-defined sensation of fullness, tightness, or pressure in the chest, which may suggest obstructive pain; there may also be a pleuritic pain accompanying inspiration, or a piercing chest pain. Subscapular pain radiating to the arm commonly occurs because of tumor extension in advanced disease.

Physical Assessment: Clinical Manifestations

Sputum quantity and quality are assessed. If infection or necrosis is present, sputum may be purulent and quite productive. Tumor invasion of vascular spaces causes production of bloody sputum. The nurse also elicits any history of fever to determine whether infection is present.

The nurse assesses *breathing patterns.* Rapid, shallow breathing suggests pleuritic chest pain and an elevated diaphragm. The nurse assesses for labored or painful breathing. An obstructive breathing pattern may be evident; expiration is prolonged and labored and alternates with periods of shallow breathing. Inspiratory efforts may alter in advanced disease. The nurse assesses for abnormal retractions, stridor, or use of accessory muscles, which indicates obstruction by the tumor. The nurse also observes for asymmetry of diaphragmatic movement on inspiration. Dyspnea may be present because of bronchial obstruction or pressure in the carina, mediastinum, or trachea. The client's level of dyspnea at rest and with activity is assessed, and the nurse notes the coping mechanisms that the client uses to control it.

Palpation of the chest wall may reveal areas of tenderness or masses. Changes in tactile fremitus may be detected and indicate areas of consolidation. Fremitus is decreased or absent when the bronchus is obstructed or the pleural space is occupied by a tumor. Palpation of the trachea may reveal deviation related to a thoracic mass.

Percussion of the chest wall may reveal areas of dullness or obvious masses. When diaphragmatic excursion is percussed, resonance usually occurs around the 10th rib. In the presence of a pleural effusion, an unusually high diaphragmatic level may be detected.

The nurse *auscultates* the chest to determine changes in breath sounds directly related to the presence of a tumor. The occurrence of decreased or absent breath sounds is an ominous sign. Rhonchi or wheezes indicate partial obstruction of airflow in passages that are narrowed by tumors. Absent breath sounds indicate impairment of air passages caused by obstruction by a tumor or replacement of lung tissue with a solid tumor.

Auscultation of vocal fremitus (i.e., bronchophony, pectoriloquy, and egophony) reveals changes in the sound normally heard. Increased loudness or sound intensity indicates consolidation or compression of the pleural tissue by tumor involvement. Auscultation of a pleural friction rub suggests an inflammatory response to an invading tumor.

In assessing the *cardiac status* of the individual, the nurse notes that distant heart sounds may indicate tamponade related to an extended tumor. Murmurs may be auscultated if tumors extend to cardiac valve leaflets. Arrhythmias may be evident as a result of hypoxemia; cyanosis of lips and fingertips may also be observed.

The *skin* of the individual with lung cancer may be ecchymotic because of low-grade chronic disseminated intravascular coagulation (DIC) (see Chap. 65). The client may have experienced weight loss because of a difficulty in swallowing or the activity of the disease process.

Lethargy and somnolence may occur with superior vena cava syndrome leading to increased intracranial pressure. Therefore, the nurse performs a baseline neurologic assessment. Bowel and bladder tone may be affected by tumor spread to the spine and spinal cord, as well.

Psychosocial Assessment

The client with lung cancer is undoubtedly quite frightened by the onset of symptoms. If dyspnea is a part of the initial presentation, the client is typically extremely anxious. The nurse is sensitive to this situation by talking slowly, assessing the client's apprehension, and listening carefully to the client's concerns. If the nurse and health care team can succeed in alleviating the dyspnea and pain, a relationship of trust is likely to develop.

It is important to involve the family and/or significant others in this relationship. Loved ones can help to alleviate the client's anxiety and act as a liaison between the staff and the client. The dyspneic client cannot tolerate increased emotional stress because it increases oxygen consumption. The family and/or significant other can reduce the client's stress by anticipating the client's needs as much as possible and interpreting these needs for others.

Fear of death is a common concern for any client with cancer. The nurse assesses the stages of grieving as the client progresses through them and adapts care accordingly. Chapter 11 discusses grief and loss in detail.

Laboratory/Radiographic Findings

No specific laboratory tests, except for cytologic analysis of sputum, assist in diagnosis. Frequently, pulmonary lesions are seen on the chest x-ray film, but tomograms and computed tomography scans are used for clear visualization of lesions. Bronchoscopy may also be done to visualize centrally located lesions and to obtain sputum specimens and tumor cells (by bronchial brushings) for cytologic studies and biopsies.

In addition, percutaneous needle biopsy, direct surgical biopsy, scalene node biopsy, and mediastinoscopy may be performed if chest x-ray studies and/or bronchoscopy cannot be used to visualize the lesion.

 Analysis: Nursing Diagnosis

Common Diagnoses

Three nursing diagnoses are common in clients with lung cancer:

1. Pain related to tumor pressure
2. Ineffective airway clearance related to tumor obstruction
3. Impaired gas exchange related to tissue destruction

Additional Diagnoses

In addition to the common diagnoses, the client may present with one or more of the following diagnoses:

1. Activity intolerance related to dyspnea, fatigue, and weight loss
2. Altered nutrition: less than body requirements related to the active disease process (increased metabolism)
3. Altered tissue perfusion related to metastases
4. Decreased cardiac output related to arrhythmias
5. Impaired skin integrity related to immobility
6. Ineffective family coping related to disease, treatment, and/or prognosis
7. Ineffective individual coping related to disease and treatment process
8. Knowledge deficit related to disease and treatment regimen
9. Anxiety and fear related to diagnosis and treatment

 Planning and Implementation

Pain

Planning: client goals. The major goal for this nursing diagnosis is that the client will experience a reduction or alleviation of pain.

Interventions: nonsurgical management. The client with lung cancer experiences chest pain, and possibly subscapular pain radiating to the arm. Pleuritic pain, which is a stabbing pain that worsens with deep breathing, may also occur. The nurse administers the prescribed analgesic so that the client obtains relief. Parenteral or oral meperidine HCl (Demerol) may be given, or an intravenous morphine drip may be used for more severe pain in clients with advanced disease.

Ineffective Airway Clearance

Planning: client goals. The two major goals for this nursing diagnosis are that the client will (1) breathe without dyspnea or discomfort and (2) maintain a patent airway.

Interventions: nonsurgical management. When clients have copious secretions, they may benefit from the use of humidifiers and vaporizers, which provide moisture to loosen the secretions. If the client has underlying COPD, which frequently occurs with lung cancer, beta-agonists may provide symptomatic relief. In moderately advanced disease, postural drainage and chest physiotherapy can help. Because the client with lung cancer fatigues easily, the client receiving therapy is often most comfortable in a semi-Fowler position or in a reclining chair. Clients can be relieved of dyspnea with supplemental oxygen, use of a morphine drip, and positioning, which facilitates comfort and drainage of secretions. The severely dyspneic client may be more comfortable sitting in a lounge or reclining chair. The nurse and physician work closely to provide a formula for relief of pain and dyspnea. Additional interventions for the client with COPD can be found earlier under the heading Collaborative Management in the section on COPD.

Impaired Gas Exchange

Planning: client goals. The major goal of the nursing diagnosis is that the client will be adequately oxygenated, as evidenced by decreased dyspnea and decreased signs of hypoxemia.

Interventions. The hypoxemic client is evaluated frequently by the nurse, as often as every 2 hours if warranted. Skin color, as well as the color of lips and nail beds, is noted. The nurse also assesses for signs of respiratory distress, such as dyspnea and use of accessory muscles for breathing. The client who is in obvious distress is further evaluated by ABG studies.

Nonsurgical management. If the client is hypoxemic, the nurse provides supplemental oxygen via mask or nasal cannula as ordered. Even if the client is not overtly hypoxemic, oxygen may be used as needed to relieve dyspnea and anxiety in the lung cancer client (see under the earlier heading Oxygen Therapy in the section on COPD for associated nursing care). If the client is experiencing bronchospasm, bronchodilators (as used with asthmatic clients) and corticosteroids may be given to decrease bronchospasm, inflammation, and edema. The reader is referred to the earlier heading Drug Therapy in the section on COPD for further information on these medications.

Chemotherapy. Because of the frequency of metastasis on presentation and the inevitability of metastasis for most clients, chemotherapy is frequently used for bronchogenic carcinoma. The advantage of using chemotherapeutic agents is that they provide a more continuous method of promoting tumor regression, whereas the usefulness of surgery and radiation therapy is limited to a specific time frame.

Current evidence suggests that small cell carcinomas respond more favorably to chemotherapy, which is thus more widely accepted for this type of cancer. Many agents are active against pulmonary malignancies. See Chapter 25 for further discussion of chemotherapeutic agents and associated nursing care.

Immunotherapy. Many clients with lung cancer are immunoincompetent, so therapy is directed toward building a strong cell-mediated type of immune response, which favorably affects the course of the disease. Evidence suggests that solid tumors as well as leukemias and lymphomas respond to immunotherapy. In body systems that are affected, immunotherapy is active in preventing a recurrence after the disease has been minimized by surgery, chemotherapy, radiation therapy, or a combination of modalities.

Active immunotherapy, either specific or nonspecific, is the most popular approach. This modality implies that the client's own immune response is stimulated against the tumor. Tumor extracts, irradiated whole tumor cells, or cells killed by other methods are used. Nonspecific immunotherapy refers to the use of the immune adjuvants to produce a general immune response. Many agents are available, but the most commonly used are BCG vaccine and levamisole. Side effects include localized reactions at the injection site, nausea, malaise, influenza-like symptoms, hepatitis, and anaphylactic reactions (see also Chap. 25 for additional information).

Radiation therapy. Radiation is widely used for localized intrathoracic lung cancers if the tumor is not resectable. Preoperative irradiation is not widely used. Postoperatively, radiation has been successful in reducing residual pleural or mediastinal disease. Radiation can achieve relief from such symptoms as hemoptysis, obstruction of the bronchi and great veins (superior vena cava syndrome), cough, and dysphagia related to esophageal compression. Brain and bone metastases are also treated palliatively with radiation therapy.

Surgical management. Surgery is the treatment of choice for tumors that can be resected or removed. It is not indicated for small cell carcinomas because of their characteristic widespread metastasis. Total resection of a non–small cell primary bronchogenic lesion is undertaken to effect a cure. If complete resectability is not possible, surgery removes the bulk of the tumor and decreases the possibility of metastatic extension. Most clients who survive bronchogenic carcinomas for 5 years have resectable tumors.

The choice of surgical procedure depends on the extent of malignant disease and the functional capacity of the client.

Laser therapy. Lasers are used palliatively to relieve endobronchial obstructions in clients with benign or malignant tumors that are accessible by bronchoscopy.

The obstructive portion of the tumor is destroyed to facilitate oxygenation. Lasers do not produce systemic or toxic effects and are tolerated well by most clients.

Thoracotomy.   A thoracotomy is an opening into the thoracic cavity to locate tumors, to perform a biopsy, or to locate sources of bleeding or injury. A thoracotomy is most often performed to remove all or a portion of the lung. Three types of incisions can be made in performing this surgery. A *posterolateral thoracotomy* is one in which the incision is begun in the submammary fold of the anterior chest, drawn below the scapular tip and along the course of the ribs, and then curved posteriorly and upward as far as the spine of the scapula. An *anterolateral thoracotomy* involves an incision below the breast and above the costal margins. This incision extends from the anterior axillary line and then turns downward to avoid the axillary apex. A *median sternotomy* is a straight incision from the suprasternal notch to below the xyphoid process. The sternum must be transected with an electric or air-driven saw.

Pneumonectomy.   A pneumonectomy is the removal of the entire lung. This procedure is most often indicated for bronchogenic carcinoma. Less frequent indications for this type of surgery include extensive unilateral TB, extensive unilateral bronchiectasis, multiple lung abscesses, and rare varieties of malignant tumors. When a pneumonectomy is performed, the mainstem bronchus is severed and sutured at its bifurcation. The pulmonary artery and veins are also ligated. When the lung is removed, the pleural cavity on the affected side is an empty space. After a pneumonectomy, closed-chest drainage is not usually used because it is helpful for serous fluid to accumulate in the space to prevent an extensive mediastinal shift.

Lobectomy.   The resection of a single pulmonary lobe can be curative for many carcinomas that grow within a single lobe. When the tumor is confined to a single lobe and easily resectable, the procedure to remove it is defined as a *simple lobectomy.* When carcinomas grow within or compress a lobar bronchus, they are removed by using a "sleeve technique" or a bilobectomy. In the former surgery, the resection is extended to the mainstem bronchus and is followed by a bronchial anastomosis. In the latter case, the resection includes the adjacent lobe. After lobectomy, the remaining lung tissue expands to fill in the portion of lung space previously occupied by lung tissue. A chest tube is usually inserted for postoperative closed drainage.

A *segmental resection* involves removing one or more lung segments, which are division of lobes. A *wedge resection* is the removal of small localized areas of disease. These two procedures may be used if the client is unable to tolerate a lobectomy or pneumonectomy. However, lobectomy and pneumonectomy are the procedures offering the best survival rates for lung cancer.

Postoperative management of clients who have a lobectomy or any type of chest surgery other than a pneumonectomy requires *closed-chest drainage* to drain air and blood that may accumulate in the pleural space. A chest tube is a drain that is placed in the pleural space so that the lung can expand. The chest tube also prevents air and fluid from returning to the chest. The drainage system consists of one or more chest tubes or drains, a collection container placed below the chest level, and a water seal to keep air from entering the chest. The tip of the tube that is used to drain air is usually placed anteriorly near the lung apex. The tube that drains liquid is placed laterally near the base of the lung. After lung resection, two tubes — anterior and posterior — are used. After a pneumonectomy, a tube is usually not used. Sometimes, a clamped tube is inserted for only a day to allow the empty side of the chest to fill with fluid and create adhesions that reduce a mediastinal shift toward the affected side.

The chest tube is connected to about 6 ft of tubing that leads to a collection bottle placed several feet below the chest, which allows the client to turn and move easily. The position of the bottle takes advantage of gravity and allows for drainage of the pleural space. The chest tube opens into the chest wall so that air can move in and out during breathing. The water seal mechanism of the chest tube is necessary so that air does not enter the pleural space. Therefore, the end of the tubing is placed beneath the surface of a solution (sterile saline). A water seal is created that closes the open end of the system from the atmosphere. When the positive pressure in the lungs during exhalation pushes air out of the pleural space through the tubing, it bubbles into the saline.

The most simple closed drainage system is one in which the drainage tubing leads to a *single bottle* that serves as both a collection container and a water seal (Fig. 62–26). The drainage tubing is connected to a rigid straw inserted through a stopper into a sterile glass bottle so that the straw is submerged about 2 cm (¾ in). A vent is placed through the stopper so that incoming pleural air cannot build up, and further air entry is prevented. The system is checked routinely to ascertain that the water seal is intact, the air vent is open, and the connections are tight. The nurse tapes the tubing junctions to prevent disconnections. The amount and type of drainage are assessed by the nurse frequently. If the bottle is not marked, a strip of tape is placed on the bottle as a baseline before drainage begins. The nurse notes the

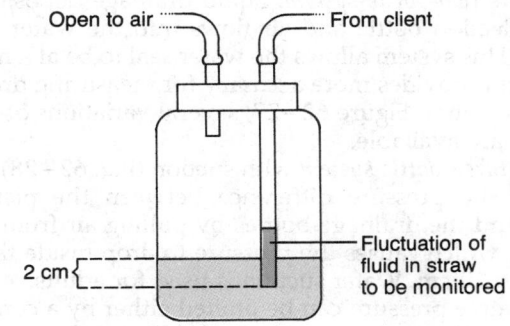

Figure 62–26

A one-bottle chest drainage system.

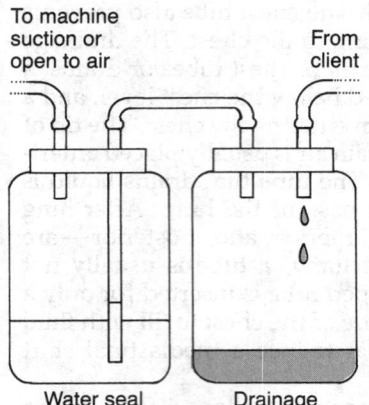
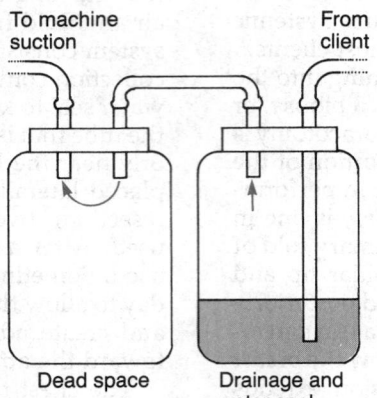
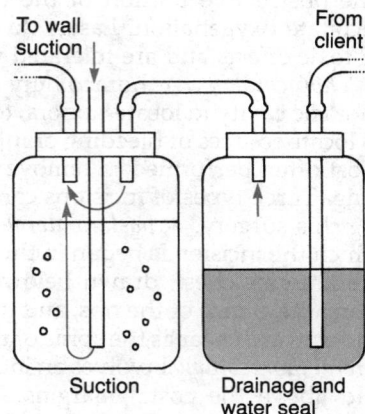

Figure 62–27

Two-bottle chest drainage systems.

initial level of solution. Immediately after surgery, the amount of drainage is checked hourly; more than 100 mL/hour is considered to be a large amount. After the first 24 hours following surgery, drainage is assessed at the end of each 8-hour shift. The water seal is also assessed. Bubbling from the straw when the client exhales or coughs indicates an air leak.

In addition, the nurse checks for rising and falling of fluid in the straw as the client breathes in and out. These fluctuations provide a continuous manometer of the pressure changes in the pleural space and are a reliable indication of overall respiratory effort. Fluctuations of 5 to 10 cm (2 to 4 in) during normal breathing are common. The absence of fluctuations could mean that the tubing is obstructed by a kink, the client is lying on the tubing, or dependent fluid has filled a loop of tubing. Expanded lung tissue can also block the chest tube eyelets during expiration, thus interfering with pressure changes that would push the fluid column back down into the straw. Another explanation is that no more air is leaking into the pleural space. In this case, the fluctuations disappear and the fluid level creeps up in the water seal straw. The one-bottle system has a limitation in that as drainage fills the bottle, there is more resistance to drainage.

In the *two-bottle system,* liquid drainage deposits in the collection bottle and air flows into the water seal bottle. This system allows the water seal to be at a fixed level and provides more accuracy for measuring drainage. As seen in Figure 62–27, several variations of this system are available.

The *three-bottle system* with suction (Fig. 62–28) enhances the pressure difference between the pleural space and the drainage bottles by pulling air from the bottles, which causes the pressure to drop inside them by 15 to 20 cm. Water suction is used for adults.

Negative pressure can be limited either by a control device in the suction or by the addition of a control bottle. The control bottle contains a long straw with the upper end open to the atmosphere and the lower end

submerged in sterile saline. The open straw provides another place where air can enter. When suction is added, air is pulled down into the control straw. If the straw is submerged to a depth of 20 cm, the amount of negative pressure that is required to pull air to the bottom of the straw where it bubbles out into the solution is 20 cmH$_2$O. The depth of the control straw under water determines the maximal suction level on the system. Increasing the suction source causes more bubbling, but it cannot increase the effective suction because the outside air offsets any further air removal. The control straw must bubble continuously for the expected degree of suction to be reached. The nurse checks the fluid level in the control bottle and adds saline when necessary. The addition of suction, therefore, causes bubbling in the water seal and prevents fluctuations. The water seal straw stays at a fixed level.

Other commercial chest drainage units duplicate or modify the one-, two-, or three-bottle systems. The *Pleur-evac system* is one of the most popular systems that use a one-piece disposable, molded plastic unit with

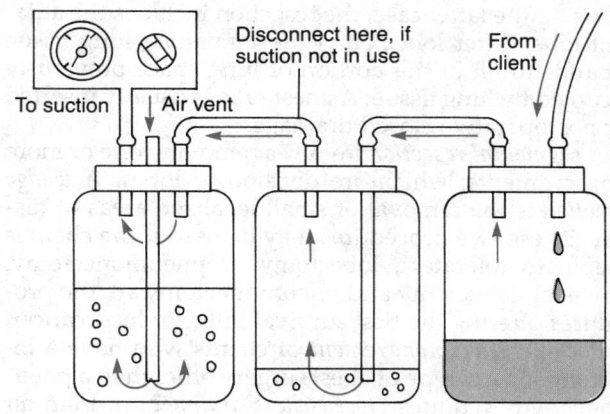

Figure 62–28

A three-bottle chest drainage.

three chambers. This system operates on the same principle as the three-bottle system. From right to left, the system contains chambers for drainage, a water seal, and suction control (Fig. 62–29).

■ Discharge Planning

Home Care Preparation

The client with lung cancer and his or her family usually have significant needs on discharge. The nurse works with the family to determine whether the family needs the help of a community health nurse or a nursing assistant or housekeeper. Before discharge of the client, the nurse communicates with the client and physician about the need for oxygen in the home.

Client/Family Education

The nurse reviews with the client and family any limitations of physical activity and prescribes an acceptable activity level. Instruction on coping with dyspnea is provided, as well as positions that facilitate easier breathing such as leaning forward and sitting in a chair. The nurse instructs the family to call the physician when the prescribed pain medications are not effective in providing comfort to the client and when the client is not receiving adequate relief from dyspnea.

Psychosocial Preparation

Psychosocial preparations differ depending on the prognosis of the client. The client with resectable carcinoma of the lung can be encouraged to have an optimistic outlook and to gradually resume normal activities. The nurse continues to help the client and family with their fear of death and anxiety related to the cancer diagnosis, as well as the client's uncertainty about future health status.

The client whose prognosis is poor is one who, with the family, is facing death. The nurse helps by supporting the client's feelings. Family members facing the loss of their loved one also benefit from the nurse's continued support and understanding. Chapter 11 discusses nursing interventions for persons experiencing loss and grief.

Health Care Resources

For the client dying of lung cancer, a referral to a hospice program may be beneficial. The hospital social worker can make these arrangements. Through this type of program, the family may be able to be supported in the home with periodic visits from home case workers, or the client may be placed in a hospice outside of the home. The American Cancer Society may also be able to provide assistance, with support groups for clients and families and the use of equipment such as a hospital bed. Chapter 25 describes health care resources for clients with cancer.

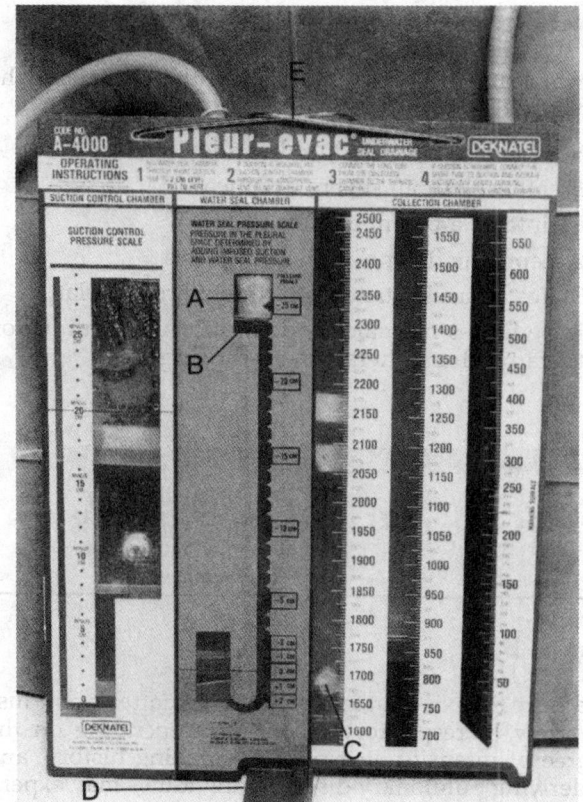

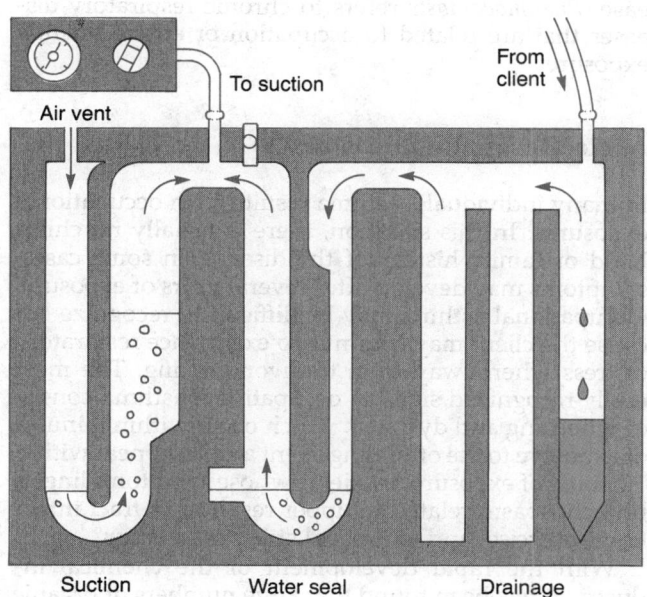

Suction control   Water seal   Drainage collection

Figure 62–29

The Pleur-evac drainage system, a commercial three-bottle chest drainage device. Top photograph shows a float valve (A); well indicator (B); self-sealing diaphragm for drainage sampling (C); floor stand (D); and hooks from which to hang the unit (E). (Top photograph from Kersten, L. D. [1989]. *Comprehensive respiratory nursing: A decision making approach.* Philadelphia: W. B. Saunders.)

Evaluation

In evaluating the care of the client with lung cancer, the nurse expects that the client

1. States that pain is reduced or alleviated
2. Breathes without severe dyspnea
3. Maintains a patent airway
4. Accepts the diagnosis and prognosis
5. States an understanding of the treatment plan
6. Experiences no major complications from radiation therapy, chemotherapy, and/or surgery

OCCUPATIONAL PULMONARY DISEASE

OVERVIEW

Exposure to toxic dust and particulate matter may cause a variety of respiratory disorders. Depending on the degree of intensity of exposure, smoking history, and underlying pulmonary disease, individuals may experience acute reversible effects or chronic pulmonary disease. *Pneumoconiosis* refers to chronic respiratory diseases that are related to occupation or environmental exposure.

Acute Occupational Diseases

In many individuals, asthma results from occupational exposures. In this situation, there is usually no childhood or family history of the disease. In some cases, symptoms may develop after several years of exposure. Occupational asthma may be difficult to recognize because the client may continue to experience respiratory distress when away from the work setting. The most easily recognized signs of occupational asthma consist of wheezing and dyspnea, which occur within minutes of exposure to the offending agent and disappear within 12 hours of exposure. In clients whose symptoms linger, bronchospasm related to upper respiratory tract infections, exercise, and emotional stress may occur.

With the rapid development of the chemical industry, it has been found that large numbers of organic and nonorganic substances can cause asthma via direct bronchial irritation. Aside from chemical irritants, enzymes that are used in food processing, detergents, and pharmaceutical industries may be asthma-inducing agents. Plant- and animal-derived materials may also be sources of irritation.

Byssinosis is an occupational pulmonary disease of textile workers that is caused by excessive inhalation of certain vegetable fiber dusts. It is characterized by chest tightness, coughing, wheezing, and dyspnea, which are especially prominent on the first day back to work after a break in exposure, such as a holiday or a weekend. Evidence suggests that chronic pulmonary damage results from prolonged exposure. However, the chest tightness, dyspnea, and decline in expiratory flow are completely reversible in many individuals.

Acute symptoms may be caused by working with the dusts of a variety of cereal grains. Acute conjunctivitis, rhinitis, and pharyngitis, as well as a hypersensitivity pneumonitis, may be presenting symptoms. Workers who complain of cough and dyspnea often show no pulmonary function abnormalities. It is believed that symptoms result from a relatively benign hypersecretory condition of the bronchial mucosa without a high risk of disability.

Excessive exposure to irritant gases such as ammonia, sulfur dioxide, chlorine, ozone, and nitrogen dioxide may produce an acute respiratory illness called *toxic pneumonitis*. Exposure may cause inflammation or edema of any portion of the respiratory tract. This condition may be fatal if not treated immediately.

Both transient *pleural effusions* and recurrent attacks of *pleurisy* are recognized with increased frequency among workers who are exposed to asbestos. In addition, asbestos exposure may cause exudative or hemorrhagic effusions. Exposure to talc and zeolite dusts is associated with benign pleural effusions.

Chronic Occupational Diseases

Silicosis is a chronic fibrosing disease of the lungs that is produced by excessive inhalation of free crystalline silica dust. Mining and quarrying are associated with a high incidence of silicosis. Hazardous exposure to silica dust also occurs in foundry work, tunneling, sandblasting, pottery making, stone masonry, and the manufacture of glass, tile, and bricks. The finely ground silica that is used in soaps, polishes, and filters is especially dangerous.

Chronic silicosis results from exposure to low concentrations of silica dust for 20 years or more. The disease is characterized by the formation of selective nodules in the pulmonary parenchyma. This process may be accompanied by progressive massive fibrosis.

Uncomplicated, or simple, silicosis is often entirely asymptomatic and causes only mild ventilating restriction and evidence of fibrosis on an x-ray film. Clients with chronic complicated disease experience significant dyspnea on exertion, marked reduction in lung volume, and massive fibrosis causing obstructive problems. Malaise, anorexia, and weight loss may be present with an outcome of respiratory failure.

Asbestosis is a term that refers to diffuse interstitial fibrosis caused by exposure to asbestos. There is generally a considerable latency period between initial exposure and the onset of clinical manifestations of fibrosis, often 10 to 20 years. Individuals who are at risk for asbestosis are asbestos miners and millers and those employed in the building trade and shipyards, such as loggers, insulation workers, pipe fitters, steam fitters, sheet metal workers, and welders. Because of its harmful effects, the use of asbestos for new insulation has been markedly curtailed since 1975. Asbestos causes a diffuse pleural thickening with diaphragmatic calcification. Pulmonary function abnormalities usually indicate a restrictive ventilatory defect. Removal of the worker from exposure does not necessarily prevent the effects of the disease. The chances of arresting the disease are best in its early stages. Frequent respiratory infections are common in this disease.

Talcosis is a pulmonary fibrosis that occurs after years of exposure to high concentrations of talc dust. Significant exposures can occur during the manufacture of paints, ceramics, asphalt, roofing materials, cosmetics, and rubber goods. The clinical picture of the client closely resembles that of asbestosis.

Two different respiratory diseases can develop from chronic excessive inhalation of coal dust: *coal workers' pneumoconiosis* and *chronic bronchitis*. The clinical picture of these illnesses is similar to that of silicosis.

Berylliosis is sarcoidosis with a defined cause, which is exposure or sensitivity to beryllium. The typical exposure history includes involvement in an operation in which metals are heated to fumes (e.g., welding, burning, or casting) or are machined to dust. Clients with berylliosis have a higher likelihood of progression to advanced irreversible disease than those with sarcoidosis of unknown etiology.

COLLABORATIVE MANAGEMENT

Prevention is extremely important for avoiding pulmonary disability caused by dust-related disease. Use of masks and the provision of adequate ventilation are stressed. When assessing the client who presents with respiratory distress, the nurse ascertains whether symptoms are acute or chronic. If the client is having an allergic reaction, avoidance of the allergen is stressed.

Nursing interventions for clients experiencing occupational pulmonary disorders are based on the fact that restrictive pulmonary disease is present, i.e., there are deficits in chest wall compliance, vital capacity, and total lung volume. These deficits are related to the fibrotic process, which restricts lung expansion. Most nursing diagnoses that are appropriate for clients with COPD, as delineated earlier in this chapter, apply to these clients. Clients who are hypoxemic require supplemental oxygen. In addition, respiratory therapies to promote sputum clearance are essential.

RIB FRACTURE

Rib fractures most frequently result from direct blunt chest trauma. The fifth through ninth ribs are most often injured by blunt trauma. Direct force applied to the ribs tends to fracture them and drive the bone ends into the thorax. Thus, there is a potential for intrathoracic injury such as pneumothorax or pulmonary contusion.

The ribs are the most commonly injured component of the thoracic cage, and often significant injury results. The client usually experiences pain with movement and splints the chest defensively. Thoracic splinting results in impaired ventilation and inadequate clearance of tracheobronchial secretions. If the client has pre-existing pulmonary disease, there is an increased incidence of atelectasis and pneumonia related to the rib fracture.

The fractured ribs unite spontaneously and are generally not splinted by tape or other materials. The primary consideration for the client is to decrease pain so that adequate ventilatory status is maintained. Intercostal nerve block may be used if pain is severe. Potent analgesia that causes respiratory depression is avoided.

FLAIL CHEST

OVERVIEW

Flail chest is frequently associated with high-speed vehicular accidents. It is more common in older clients because their declining agility predisposes them to vehicular accidents, pedestrian accidents, and falls. It is associated with a high mortality rate (40%) and is one of the most critical of the chest injuries.

Flail chest (paradoxical respiration) is the inward movement of the thorax during inspiration, with outward movement during expiration. It usually involves one hemothorax and is the result of rib fractures secondary to blunt chest trauma. Flail chest occurs when, because of a fracture of two or more adjacent ribs, a loose segment of chest wall is left and the movement of this segment becomes paradoxical to the expansion and contraction of the rest of the chest wall. Gas exchange is significantly impaired as is the ability to cough and clear secretions. The defensive splinting that occurs as a result of the rib fracture further reduces the client's ability to exert the extra effort required for breathing.

COLLABORATIVE MANAGEMENT

The nurse assesses the client with a flail chest for paradoxical chest movement, dyspnea, cyanosis, tachycardia, and hypotension. Anxiety is usually associated with the experience of pain and dyspnea.

Interventions for flail chest include the administration of humidified oxygen, pain management, promotion of lung expansions through deep breathing and positioning, and secretion clearance via coughing and tracheal aspiration. Psychosocial support is given to this extremely anxious client by explaining all procedures, talking slowly, and allowing the client the time to verbalize feelings and concerns.

The client with a flail chest may be managed conservatively with vigilant respiratory care or may require mechanical ventilation if complications such as respiratory failure or shock ensue. ABG values are monitored closely. If the client becomes severely hypoxemic and hypercapnic, he or she is intubated and a ventilator with PEEP is used (see the earlier section on COPD). If there is a pulmonary contusion or underlying pulmonary disease, the potential for respiratory failure increases. The client's vital signs and fluid and electrolyte balance are monitored closely so that hypovolemia and/or shock can be treated immediately. If the client has a pulmonary contusion, central venous pressure is determined, and fluids are administered accordingly.

TENSION PNEUMOTHORAX

OVERVIEW

Tension pneumothorax, one of the most rapidly developing complications of blunt chest trauma, occurs as a result of an air leak in the lung or chest wall. Air that is forced into the thoracic cavity causes complete collapse of the affected lung. The air that enters the pleural space during expiration does not exit during inspiration. As a result, air progressively accumulates under pressure, compresses the mediastinal vessels, and interferes with venous return. Because this process leads to rapid filling of the heart, the situation is quickly fatal if not promptly detected and treated. Typical causes of tension pneumothorax are blunt chest trauma in which the parenchymal injury has failed to seal and mechanical ventilation with PEEP.

COLLABORATIVE MANAGEMENT

Assessment findings with pneumothorax include tracheal deviation to the unaffected side, respiratory distress, unilateral absence of breath sounds, distended neck veins, and cyanosis. On percussion, there is also a hypertympanic sound over the affected hemothorax. Pneumothorax is detectable on a chest x-ray film. ABG assays demonstrate hypoxia and respiratory alkalosis.

Initial treatment for a tension pneumothorax includes inserting a large-bore needle into the second intercostal space in the midclavicular line of the affected side. After this lifesaving measure is completed, it can be followed by the placement of a chest tube into the fourth intercostal space of the midaxillary line and attachment of the tube to a water seal drainage system until the lung reinflates.

HEMOTHORAX

Hemothorax is one of the most common problems encountered following blunt chest trauma. A *simple hemothorax* is defined as blood loss of less than 2000 mL into the thoracic cavity. Bleeding is frequently caused by injuries to the lung parenchyma, such as pulmonary contusions, or lacerations, which are often associated with rib and sternal fractures. Massive intrathoracic bleeding in blunt chest trauma generally stems from the heart, great vessels, or major systemic arteries such as the intercostal arteries.

Physical assessment findings vary with the size of the hemothorax. If a hemothorax is small, the client may be asymptomatic. If the hemothorax is larger, the client experiences respiratory distress. In addition, breath sounds are diminished on auscultation. The percussion note on the involved side is dull. Blood in the pleural space is visualized by a chest x-ray film.

Interventions are aimed at evacuating the blood in the pleural space to normalize pulmonary function and to prevent infection related to blood accumulation. Anterior and posterolateral chest tubes are inserted to evacuate the pleural space and to reduce the rush of clotted blood. Chest tube drainage is carefully monitored, and chest x-ray films are evaluated serially.

PNEUMOTHORAX

Any thoracic injury that allows accumulation of atmospheric air in the pleural space results in a rise in intrathoracic pressure and a reduction in vital capacity depending on the amount of pulmonary collapse produced. Pneumothorax is often caused by blunt chest trauma and is associated with some degree of hemothorax.

Assessment findings include diminished breath sounds on auscultation, hyperresonance percussion, and prominence of the involved hemithorax, which moves poorly with respirations. In addition, the client may have pleuritic pain, tachypnea, and subcutaneous emphysema. A chest film is used for diagnosis. Interventions are the same as those described for a tension pneumothorax.

TRACHEOBRONCHIAL TRAUMA

Most tears of the tracheobronchial tree are the result of severe blunt trauma, primarily involving the mainstem bronchi. Injuries to the cervical trachea usually occur at the junction of the trachea and cricoid cartilage. These injuries are frequently caused by striking the anterior neck against the dashboard during a vehicular accident. Clients with lacerations of the trachea develop massive air leaks, which produce pneumomediastinum and extensive subcutaneous emphysema. Upper airway obstruction may also occur and produce severe respiratory distress and inspiratory stridor. Major cervical tears are managed by cricothyroidotomy or tracheostomy below the level of injury. The client is assessed for hypoxemia via assays of ABGs, and oxygen is administered appropriately. Depending on the degree of injury, the client may require mechanical ventilation. Frequent assessment of vital signs is essential because the client is likely to be hypotensive and in shock. The nurse continues to assess for subcutaneous emphysema and auscultates lungs to assess for further complications every 1 to 2 hours initially. Decreased breath sounds or wheezing may indicate further obstruction, atelectasis, or pneumothorax. Care of the client with a tracheostomy and mechanical ventilation is discussed earlier under the heading Collaborative Management in the section on COPD.

PULMONARY CONTUSION

Pulmonary contusion is the *most* common, potentially lethal chest injury seen in the United States. After a contusion, respiratory failure can develop over time rather than instantaneously. This condition most frequently follows injuries that are caused by the rapid deceleration that occurs during vehicular accidents. The contusion is characterized by interstitial hemorrhage, which is almost invariably associated with intra-alveolar hemorrhage. The resulting interstitial edema causes a decrease in pulmonary compliance. The client usually becomes hypoxemic and dyspneic. The bronchial mucosa becomes irritated, and the client has increased bronchial secretions. Clients who may be initially asymptomatic can develop respiratory failure. They present with hemoptysis, decreased breath sounds, rales, and wheezes. The chest x-ray film of the client with a contusion may show a hazy opacity in the lobes or parenchyma. If there is no disruption of the parenchyma, resorption of the lesion often occurs without treatment. Treatment includes maintenance of ventila-

tion and oxygenation. Central venous pressure is monitored closely, and fluid intake is restricted accordingly. Colloid and steroid use remains controversial. The client in obvious respiratory distress may require mechanical ventilation with use of PEEP to inflate the lungs. A vicious circle occurs in which more muscular effort is required for ventilation because of the flailing chest and the client becomes progressively hypoxemic. When the client attempts to compensate, he or she tires easily, becomes less efficient in breathing, and becomes more fatigued and hypoxemic. Flail chest may also be associated with pulmonary contusion that is associated with parenchymal damage. The sequela to this situation is the likely development of adult respiratory distress syndrome (ARDS).

ADULT RESPIRATORY DISTRESS SYNDROME

OVERVIEW

ARDS is a form of acute respiratory failure that is characterized by dyspnea, hypoxemia, decreased pulmonary compliance, and the presence of pulmonary infiltrates. It is caused by a diffuse injury of the lung, which leads to increased extravascular lung fluid. It usually occurs after a catastrophic event in individuals with no previous pulmonary disease. The mortality rate is higher than 50%.

Despite diverse etiologies leading to injury of the lung in ARDS, no common pathway has been found in the development of ARDS. In some forms of ARDS, the pathophysiology is understood, whereas in many others it is not.

The major site of injury in the lung is the alveolar capillary membrane, which is normally permeable to only small molecules. The balance between the Starling forces of osmotic and hydrostatic pressures plus the effectiveness of lymph flow serves to keep the interstitium of the lung relatively dry. It is believed that one etiology for the development of ARDS is serious nervous system injury. Trauma, cerebrovascular accidents, tumors, and sudden increases in cerebrospinal fluid pressure may produce ARDS. Massive sympathetic discharge may lead to systemic vasoconstriction with redistribution of large volumes of blood into the pulmonary circuit, which produces marked elevation of hydrostatic pressure, probably causing lung injury. Processes that produce cerebral hypoxia such as shock and ascent to high altitudes may operate by a similar mechanism.

It is known that some factors produce ARDS by direct injury to the lung. For example, aspiration of gastric contents leads to mechanical obstruction or produces an acid burn to the airway when the pH is less than 2.5. In such a direct injury, rapid necrosis of the alveolar type I pneumocyte occurs and the injured capillary endothelium allows protein and cellular elements to escape from the intravascular space. Similarly, radiation, near drowning, and inhalation of toxic gases injure the alveolar and capillary endothelium. In addition, trauma and other processes such as sepsis, drowning, and burns cause the release of thromboplastins, which form fibrin clots in the peripheral blood. The clots, together with platelets and leukocytes, are filtered out in the lung. In many cases of ARDS, especially after trauma, production of plasminogen activation inhibitors by the liver is enhanced. Fibrinolysis is prevented and microemboli remain in the lung. Disseminated intravascular coagulation plays a role in some clients.

Other significant changes occur in the alveoli and respiratory bronchioles. The type II pneumocyte is responsible for producing surfactant. Therefore, surfactant activity is reduced in ARDS either because of destruction of the type II pneumocyte or because of inactivation of surfactant. Consequently, the alveoli become unstable and tend to collapse unless they are filled with fluid from the interstitial space. These alveoli can no longer participate in gas exchange. As a result, interstitial edema forms around terminal airways, which are compressed and obliterated. Lung volume is thus further reduced, and there is even less compliance. As the leak expands, fluid, protein, and blood cells collect in the interstitium and alveoli. Lymph channels are compressed and ineffective. Poorly ventilated alveoli receive blood, thus increasing the shunt fraction and resulting in hypoxemia and ventilation-perfusion mismatching.

A number of factors have been associated with causing ARDS. Some major causes include shock, trauma, pulmonary infections, inhalation of toxic gases, pulmonary aspiration, drug ingestion, hemolytic disorders, and multiple blood transfusions.

The incidence of ARDS is unknown. About 1980, it was estimated that 150,000 cases of ARDS occurred in the United States per year. It is likely that the incidence has increased because of the improved treatment of other forms of catastrophic illness (Brandsetter, 1986).

A major goal in the prevention of ARDS is the recognition of clients who are at high risk of developing the syndrome. Clients with witnessed aspiration of gastric contents are at the greatest risk (Brandsetter, 1986). Therefore, vigilant assessment and monitoring of *elderly* clients receiving tube feeding and of clients with neurologic deficits and altered swallowing and gag reflexes are essential. In addition, clients who are treated for underlying pulmonary problems, pneumonia, disseminated intravascular coagulation, burns, and fractures should be observed carefully for the increasing dyspnea and hypoxemia that are characteristic of ARDS. Clients who are admitted for shock and receive multiple blood transfusions are also at high risk. For this same reason, clients who have undergone cardiopulmonary bypass surgery have a predisposition for the development of ARDS.

COLLABORATIVE MANAGEMENT

The nurse assesses the client's respirations and notes whether increased work of breathing is evident, as indicated by hyperpnea, grunting respiration, cyanosis, pallor, and intercostal or suprasternal retraction. The presence of diaphoresis and mental status change is noted. Auscultation of the lungs may reveal no abnormal sounds because the edema of ARDS occurs first in the interstitial spaces and not in the airways. Vital signs are monitored frequently to assess for hypotension, tachycardia, and arrhythmias.

The primary laboratory study for establishing the diagnosis of ARDS is a lowered arterial PO_2 value, which is determined by ABG measurements. The client with ARDS is poorly responsive to high concentrations of oxygen. A widening alveolar oxygen gradient develops, with increased shunting of blood. This gradient is assessed by providing the client with 100% oxygen by mask and measuring ABGs after 20 minutes. A large difference between the predicted and actual alveolar oxygen tension indicates shunting. Sputum cultures are obtained to isolate any organisms causing an infection that must be treated. Because mortality depends on aggressive therapy, sputum may be obtained through a bronchoscopy and transtracheal aspiration.

The chest x-ray film shows the diagnostic diffuse haziness or "whited-out" appearance of the lung. An electrocardiogram is done to rule out cardiac abnormalities and usually reveals no specific changes. The placement of a Swan-Ganz catheter is a diagnostic tool in that in the client with ARDS, the pulmonary capillary wedge pressure is usually normal. This situation differs from that in the client with cardiogenic pulmonary edema, in which the pulmonary capillary wedge pressure is higher than 12 mm Hg.

Clients with ARDS usually require endotracheal intubation and mechanical ventilation with PEEP and continuous positive airway pressure. Sedation may be necessary for adequate ventilation. Because one of the side effects of PEEP is the development of tension pneumothorax, the nurse assesses lung sounds frequently and maintains a patent airway with suctioning. The reader is referred to discussions of intubation and mechanical ventilation under the heading Collaborative Management in the section on COPD.

Corticosteroids are used in the treatment of ARDS and have theoretical benefit in that they may impair neutrophil mobilization. However, their efficacy has not been determined. Antibiotics are used to treat infections with organisms that have been identified by culture.

The optimal type of fluid therapy for the client with ARDS remains unknown. Several researchers have recommended the use of colloids for more effective intravascular volume expansion. However, the value of colloid therapy has not been proved. Researchers and clinicians agree that fluid volume should be titrated to maintain adequate cardiac output and tissue perfusion. Judicious diuresis may help to decrease extravascular lung fluid.

Clients with ARDS are at risk for the development of malnutrition, which further compromises the respiratory system. An altered immune response as well as an altered ventilatory response to hypoxemia may occur with undernourished clients. Diaphragmatic functioning is also altered. Therefore, enteral nutrition in the form of tube feeding or parenteral nutrition in the form of hyperalimentation is instituted.

PULMONARY EMBOLISM

OVERVIEW

A *pulmonary embolism* (PE) results when a thrombus breaks loose from an attachment in the lower extremity (usually) and blocks a branch of the pulmonary artery. Widespread pulmonary vasoconstriction occurs, which impairs ventilation and perfusion and produces life-threatening hypoxemia and the potential for pulmonary ischemia and infarction.

An embolism is a process that is characterized by the release or entry of a solid, liquid, or gaseous substance into the vascular system. The embolus is then carried to a smaller vessel or bifurcation, where it lodges and obstructs circulation. Any type of substance can cause an embolism, but a thrombus is the most common absorbable type. Fat, air, and calcium emboli are also absorbable.

A pulmonary embolism occurs when a thrombus that has formed in a deep vein detaches and travels to the heart (as in deep venous thrombosis). There, it travels through the vena cava and the right side of the heart and lodges at a bifurcation in a pulmonary artery. Platelets accumulating behind the embolus trigger the release of serotonin and thromboxane A_2, two potent vasoconstrictors. Widespread pulmonary vasoconstriction impairs ventilation and perfusion, which causes unoxygenated blood to be shunted into the arterial circulation to produce hypoxemia. To compensate, the client increases respiratory effort. This hyperventilation creates a state of hypercapnia and respiratory alkalosis. Later, metabolic acidosis occurs when the kidneys fail to excrete enough hydrogen ions. The result of sustained pulmonary hypertension is increased venous pressure, engorged neck veins, hepatomegaly, cerebral congestion, and myocardial dysfunction. Cardiac output is also reduced, causing ischemia to every major organ.

Clients who are prone to pulmonary embolism are also prone to the development of deep venous thromboses. Risk factors include prolonged immobilization, surgery, obesity, pregnancy, congestive heart failure, advancing age, and prior history of thromboembolism. In addition, clients who have had strokes, malignancies (particularly of the lungs), and major trauma are at risk.

Pulmonary embolism occurs more frequently than any other type of embolus. It affects about 600,000 persons a year in the United States and may be even more common than statistics indicate. Pulmonary embolism secondary to deep venous thrombosis is the most common type of pulmonary embolism.

Nursing interventions that help to prevent pulmonary embolism are those that also prevent venous stasis. These interventions include initiating passive and active range-of-motion exercises for the extremities of immobilized and postoperative clients; ambulating postoperative clients soon after surgery; using antiembolism and pneumatic compression stockings postoperatively; avoiding the use of tight garters, girdles, and constricting clothing; and preventing pressure under the popliteal space (such as with a pillow).

Clients who may be immobilized for a prolonged period after surgery or who are restricted to bed rest may be given low-dose subcutaneous heparin therapy to prevent hypercoagulability. Elderly clients are particularly at risk. Adequate fluid intake and the avoidance of oral contraceptives are also preventive measures.

COLLABORATIVE MANAGEMENT

The nurse assesses the client for dyspnea accompanied by anginal and pleuritic pain that is exacerbated by inspiration. These symptoms are found in 80% of clients diagnosed with a pulmonary embolism. The nurse also notes whether the client is coughing and producing sputum, especially blood stained. A cough is typical, but hemoptysis is not. The lungs are auscultated for adventitious sounds. Breath sounds may be normal, but rales occur in 50% of clients with pulmonary embolism. Hyperresonance may be heard on percussion. Vital signs are assessed for tachycardia with shallow respirations. These changes occur as a compensatory effort to increase oxygenation. A low-grade fever may also be present. The nurse assesses for distended neck veins, syncope, and cyanosis because they are associated with massive emboli. Heart sounds may reveal an S_3 or S_4 sound with an accentuated and delayed pulmonic component of S_2.

ABG studies are performed to detect hypoxemia, but this alone is not sufficient evidence to diagnose pulmonary embolism. A client with a small embolism may not be hypoxemic. A chest x-ray is typically done, but in one-fourth to one-third of affected clients, no abnormality is found.

A ventilation-perfusion lung scan is one of the most important studies to determine pulmonary embolism. Pulmonary angiography may be done if lung scans are inconclusive. An electrocardiogram is done; typically, findings are usually abnormal but nonspecific and transient. T wave changes and ST segment abnormalities develop in almost 50% of clients, but left axis and right axis deviations occur with equal frequency. Electrocardiographic signs of cor pulmonale can be found in 25% to 35% of clients. Clients with suspected pulmonary embolism are often examined with Doppler ultrasound stethoscope or by impedance plethysmography to document the presence of deep venous thrombosis and to support a diagnosis of pulmonary embolism.

Most often, the client is managed by medical interventions. If these measures are not successful, surgery may be performed. Oxygen therapy is important for the client with pulmonary embolism. The client who is severely hypoxemic may be placed on a mechanical ventilator and monitored closely by following ABG levels. In less severe cases, oxygen may be administered via a nasal cannula or mask. The client's vital signs and urinary output are assessed at least every 1 to 2 hours. The nurse performs a careful cardiac assessment at least every 4 hours to determine arrhythmias, distended neck veins, and pedal or sacral edema. Homans' sign is assessed as well. The lungs are auscultated for the presence of rales and adventitious sounds. Lips and nail beds are assessed for cyanosis.

Anticoagulants are routinely used to keep the embolus from enlarging and to prevent the formation of new clots. The initial protocol is usually an intravenous loading dose of 5000 units of heparin, followed by a continuous or intermittent infusion of 1000 units per hour. The client's activated partial thromboplastin time (aPTT) is monitored every 30 minutes initially, and then every 4 hours to ascertain that it is 2½ times that of control time, or that a therapeutic drug level has been achieved.

Heparin therapy usually lasts 5 to 7 days. About 3 to 4 days before it is discontinued, most clients are given oral anticoagulants such as warfarin (Coumadin). Particular clients at high risk may take warfarin indefinitely. The client taking this drug is monitored so that prothrombin time is maintained at 1½ to 2 times the control value. Chapter 65 further discusses the use of anticoagulants and associated nursing care.

When a client cannot maintain adequate vital signs and urinary output despite medical therapy, an embolectomy may be necessary. When an embolism involves 60% to 70% of the pulmonary vascular tree, embolectomy may be the only effective treatment. *Embolectomy* involves surgical removal of the embolus or emboli from the pulmonary arteries. Other procedures that may be done to prevent further complications are vein ligation, to prevent the embolus from traveling to the heart, and vena cava plication, or insertion of an umbrella filter to trap emboli that might enter the heart. These surgeries are performed via thoracotomy, as described under the heading Collaborative Management in the earlier section on lung cancer. The vena cava plication procedure is further discussed in Chapter 65.

INFLUENZA

Influenza ("flu") is an acute viral respiratory infection that can occur in adults of all ages. Because it is highly contagious, influenza epidemics are common and can lead to complications such as pneumonia or death, especially in elderly and immunocompromised individuals. Influenza may be caused by one of several viruses, usually referred to as A, B, and C. The client with this disorder typically complains of severe headache, muscular aches, fever, chills, fatigue, weakness, and anorexia. Clinical manifestations that are associated with the respiratory system, such as a sore throat, cough, and rhinorrhea (watery discharge from the nose), generally follow the initial symptoms for a week or more. Most individuals continue to complain of general malaise for 1 to 2 weeks after the acute episode has resolved.

Treatment of influenza is symptomatic because antibiotics are ineffective against viral infections. The nurse recommends that the client remain in bed for several days, drink a copious amount of fluids, and take acetaminophen (Tylenol) or aspirin, two tablets every 4 hours, for fever and achiness. Saline gargles may ease the throat pain, and antihistamines may reduce the rhinorrhea. Other palliative measures are the same as those for clients with acute rhinitis.

During the past two decades, vaccinations for the prevention of influenza have been developed and widely administered. With advanced refinement of the vaccine, allergic reaction is rare. The vaccine is altered every year based on the specific viral strains that are likely to pose a problem during the influenza season, i.e., in late fall and winter. It is highly recommended that persons older than 65 years of age and those with chronic illness or immune compromise receive the vaccine each year, typically during October or November.

SUMMARY

The client with a disorder of the lower respiratory tract can be extremely ill from an acute or chronic problem. With a growing elderly population, pneumonia and lung cancer are increasing in frequency and often lead to death, even with prompt treatment. The nurse must be familiar with the numerous modalities to sustain breathing or lessen the work of breathing and must be prepared to handle respiratory emergencies and complications while allaying a client's anxiety and fear.

IMPLICATIONS FOR RESEARCH

Although many technologic advances have been made in the area of mechanical ventilation, only a few vaccines are available for the prevention of the multiple respiratory infections that are seen in individuals of all ages. The increase in diseases that cause immunosuppression adds to the susceptibility to infections and associated complications, e.g., TB and pneumonia. Research needs to focus in this area, as well as in the area of lung cancer and occupational diseases.

Questions that nursing needs to address include

1. What is the effect of teaching about risk factors and warning signs of lung cancer on the morbidity and mortality of the disease?
2. Do diaphragmatic breathing and chest physiotherapy increase the arterial PO_2 of the client with COPD?
3. How can the nurse be most effective in reducing dyspnea in the client with a lower respiratory tract disorder?
4. How can the nurse be most effective in reducing anxiety and fear in the client experiencing dyspnea?

REFERENCES AND READINGS

Chronic Obstructive Pulmonary Disease

American Lung Association. (1983). *Facts in brief about lung disease.* New York: Author

American Thoracic Society. (1987). Standards for the diagnosis of patients with chronic obstructive pulmonary disease. *American Review of Respiratory Disease, 136,* 235–236.

Au, J., & Ziment, I. (1986). Drug therapy and dosage adjustment in asthma. *Respiratory Care, 31,* 415–418.

Bauer, L. E. (1989). Discharge of a patient with chronic respiratory failure. Part 2. *Home Healthcare Nurse, 1*(4), 10–12.

Belman, M., Thomas, S., & Lewis, M. (1986). Resistive breathing training in patients with chronic obstructive pulmonary disease. *Chest, 90,* 662–669.

Berlauk, J. F. (1986). Prolonged endotracheal intubation vs. tracheostomy. *Critical Care Medicine, 14,* 742–745.

Bernstein, I. (1985). Cromolyn sodium. *Chest, 87*(Suppl.), 68–72.

Bishop, M. J. (1989). Mechanisms of laryngotracheal injury following prolonged tracheal intubation. *Chest, 96,* 185–186.

Blaufuss, J. A., & Wallace, C. J. (1987). Two negative pressure ventilators: current clinical application and nursing care. *Critical Care Nursing Quarterly, 9*(4), 14–30.

Carroll, P. (1986). Caring for ventilator patients. *Nursing '86, 16*(2), 34–40.

Carroll, P. F. (1989). Good nursing gets COPD patients out of hospitals. *RN, 52*(7), 24–28.

Chronic obstructive pulmonary disease: The source may be treatable. (1988). *Emergency Medicine, 20*(9), 59–60.

Cosenza, J., & Norton, L. (1986). Secretion clearance: State of the art from a nursing perspective. *Critical Care Nurse, 6*(4), 23–27.

Davis, L. (1986a). Managing the patient with advanced chronic obstructive pulmonary disease. Part 1. *Hospital Medicine, 22*(1), 127–151.

Davis, L. (1986b). Managing the patient with advanced chronic obstructive pulmonary disease. Part 2. *Hospital Medicine, 22*(2), 70–94.

Egglund, E. (1987). Teaching the ABC's of C.O.P.D. *Nursing '87, 17*(1), 60–64.

Feinsilver, S. H. (1988). Respiratory failure in asthma and COPD. *Emergency Medicine, 21*(7), 90, 93–94, 96.

Flenly, D. (1985). Long-term home oxygen therapy. *Chest, 87,* 99–103.

Gift, A., Plaut, M., & Jacox, A. (1986). Psychologic and physiologic factors related to dyspnea in subjects with chronic obstructive pulmonary disease. *Heart and Lung, 15,* 595–600.

Goodnaugh, S. (1985). The effects of oxygen and hyperinflation on arterial oxygen tension after endotracheal suctioning. *Heart and Lung, 14,* 11–17.

Grossbach, I. (1986a). Troubleshooting ventilator and patient-related problems. Part 1. *Critical Care Nurse, 6*(4), 58–65.

Grossbach, I. (1986b). Troubleshooting ventilator and patient-related problems. Part 2. *Critical Care Nurse, 6*(5), 64–74.

Hahn, K. (1989). Sexuality and COPD. *Rehabilitation Nursing, 14,* 191–195.

Hahn, L. (1987). Slow-teaching the C.O.P.D. patient. *Nursing '87, 17*(4), 34–41.

Heffner, J., Miller, K., & Sahn, S. (1986). Tracheostomy in the intensive care unit: Part 1. Indications, technique, management. *Chest, 90,* 269–274.

Hill, N. (1986). Clinical applications of body ventilators. *Chest, 90,* 897–905.

Hoffman, L. (1987). Airway management for the critically ill patient. *American Journal of Nursing, 87,* 39–53.

Howard, J., Davis, J., & Roghmann, K. (1987). Respiratory teaching of patients: How effective is it? *Journal of Advanced Nursing, 12,* 207–214.

Howland, J., Nelson, E., Barlow, P., McHugo, G., Meier, F., Brent, P., Laser-Wolston, N., & Parker, H (1986). Chronic obstructive pulmonary disease, impact on health education. *Chest, 90,* 233–238.

Irwin, M. M., & Openbrier, D. R. (1985). A delicate balance: Strategies for feeding ventilated COPD patients. *American Journal of Nursing, 85,* 274–280.

Johnson, A. P. (1988). The elderly and COPD. *Journal of Gerontological Nursing, 14*(12), 20–24, 35–36.

Kersten, L. D. (1989). *Comprehensive respiratory nursing: A decision making approach.* Philadelphia: W. B. Saunders.

Kim, M., & Larson, J. (1987). Ineffective airway clearance and ineffective breathing patterns: Theoretical and research base for nursing diagnosis. *Nursing Clinics of North America, 22,* 125–133.

Kirby, R. R. (1988). Best PEEP: Issues and choices in the selection and monitoring of PEEP levels. *Respiratory Care, 33,* 569–580.

Lareau, S., & Larson, J. (1987). Ineffective breathing pattern related to airflow limitation. *Nursing Clinics of North America, 22,* 179–189.

Larson, J., & Kim, M. (1987). Ineffective breathing pattern related to respiratory muscle fatigue. *Nursing Clinics of North America, 22,* 207–221.

Mapp, C. (1988). Trach care: Are you aware of all the dangers? *Nursing '88, 18*(7), 34–43.

Nett, L. M., Morganroth, M. J., & Petty, T. (1987). Weaning from the ventilator: Protocols that work. *American Journal of Nursing, 87,* 1173–1184.

Norton, L. C. (1988). Weaning the long-term ventilator dependent patient: Common problems and management. *Critical Care Nurse, 9*(1), 42–52.

Openbrier, D. R., & Corey, M. (1987). Ineffective breathing pattern related to malnutrition. *Nursing Clinics of North America, 22,* 225–246.

Openbrier, D.R., Fuoss, C., & Mall, C. (1988). What patients on home oxygen therapy want to know. *American Journal of Nursing, 88,* 198–202.

Rashkin, M., & Davis T. (1986). Acute complications of endotracheal intubation—relationship to reintubation, route, urgency, and duration. *Chest, 89,* 165–167.

Riegel, B., & Forshee, T. (1985). A review and critique of the literature on preoxygenation for endotracheal suctioning. *Heart and Lung, 14,* 504–518.

Schulthesis, A. (1989). When and how to extubate in the recovery room. *American Journal of Nursing, 89,* 1040–1045.

Sheppard, D. (1986). Mechanisms of bronchoconstriction from nonimmunologic environmental stimuli. *Chest, 90,* 584–586.

Traver, G. A. (1988). Measures of symptoms and life quality to predict emergent use of institutional health care resources in chronic obstructive airway disease. *Heart and Lung, 17,* 698–697.

Vasbinder-Dillon, D. (1988). Understanding mechanical ventilation. *Critical Care Nurse, 8*(7), 42–56.

Winters C. (1988). Monitoring ventilator patients for complications. *Nursing '88, 18*(6), 38–41.

Other Lower Respiratory Tract Disorders

Brandsetter, R. D. (1986). The adult respiratory distress syndrome. *Heart and Lung, 15,* 155–165.

Carr, D. T. (1988). Lung cancer: Pitfalls and controversies in diagnosis and treatment. Part 2. *Consultant, 28*(5), 33–38, 40, 45.

Chatburn, R. L. (1988). Similarities and differences in the management of acute lung injury in neonates (IRDS) and in adults (ARDS). *Respiratory Care, 33,* 539–556.

Engelking, C. (1987a). Lung cancer: Chemotherapy. *American Journal of Nursing, 87,* 1438–1439, 1440–1441.

Engelking, C. (1987b). Lung cancer: The language of staging. *American Journal of Nursing, 87,* 1434–1437.

Fedullo, A. J., & Swinburne, A. J. (1985). Relationships of patient age to clinical features and outcome for in-hospital treatment of pneumonia. *Journal of Gerontology, 40*(1), 29–33.

Gerdes, L. (1987). Recognizing the multisystemic effects of embolism. *Nursing '87, 17*(12), 34–41.

Goldhaber, S. (1986). Pulmonary embolism, diagnostic and therapeutic options. *Consultant, 26*(2), 124–128, 137–138.

Harwood, K. V. (1987). Non-small cell lung cancer: Issues in diagnosis staging and treatment. *Seminars in Oncology Nursing, 3,* 183–193.

Hinton, L. H. (1986). Hidden chest trauma in the head injured patient. *Critical Care Nurse, 6*(4), 51–57.

Idell, S. (1989). The deadly danger of ARDS . . . adult respiratory distress syndrome. *Emergency Medicine, 21*(7), 67–68, 70, 72.

Ingersoll, G. L. (1989). Respiratory muscle fatigue research: Implications for clinical practice. *Applied Nursing Research, 2*(1), 6–15.

Kronenberg, R. S. (1989). Asbestos inhalation and cigarette smoking make a lethal combination. *Occupational Health and Safety, 58*(3), 50–53, 55–56, 68.

Littleton, M. T. (1989). Complications of multiple trauma. *Critical Care Nursing Quarterly, 1*(1), 75–84.

Lung abscess: Possible causes. (1989). *Hospital Medicine, 23*(11), 135–137, 141.

Majors, M. (1988). Nutritional support of the mechanically ventilated patient. *Critical Care Nursing Quarterly, 11*(3), 50–61.

Martin, L. (1988). Acute respiratory failure. Part 1. *Hospital Medicine, 24*(12), 58, 60, 63–65.

Matheson, M. (1987). Thoracic Trauma. *Current Reviews for Recovery Room Nurses, 8,* lesson 22, 171–175.

Matthewson, H. S. (1988). Quinolones: Antibacterial agents for respiratory diseases. *Respiratory Care, 33,* 357–360.

McDonald, S., & Ma, M. (1987). Identifying compliance incentives for screening and treatment of tuberculosis. *Journal of Community Health Nursing, 4*(3), 131–143.

Metheney, N., Esenberg, P., & Spies, M. (1986). Aspiration pneumonia in patients fed through nasoenteral tubes. *Heart and Lung, 15,* 256–261.

O'Byrne, C. (1985). Postoperative care and complications in the thoracotomy patient. *Critical Care Quarterly, 7*(4), 53–58.

Oleske, D. M. (1987). The epidemiology of lung cancer: An overview. *Seminars in Oncology Nursing, 3,* 165–173.

O'Mara, S. R. (1986). Lung carcinoma. *Critical Care Quarterly, 9*(3), 1–11.

Perez-Stable, E. J., Slutkin, G., Paz, E.A., & Hopewell, P. C. (1986). Tuberculin reactivity in United States and foreign-born Latinos: Results of a community-based screening program. *American Journal of Public Health, 76,* 643–646.

Torbeck, G. S., Werhane, M. J., & Shawfnagel, D. E. (1987). Treatment of tuberculosis in a nurse managed clinic. *Heart and Lung, 16,* 30–33.

Ward, J. J. (1989). Lung sounds: Easy to hear, hard to describe. *Respiratory Care, 34,* 17–19.

White, E. (1987). Home care of the patient with advanced lung cancer. *Seminars in Oncology Nursing 3,* 216–221.

ADDITIONAL READINGS

Benedict, S. (1989). The suffering associated with lung cancer. *Cancer Nursing, 12,* 34–40.

This article explores in depth the problems with which a client with lung cancer has to cope. Physical complications associated with the disease and its treatment, as well as the psychosocial sequelae, are discussed, with implications for nursing practice.

Nield, M., Kim, M. J., & Patel, M. (1989). Use of magnitude estimation for estimating the parameters of dyspnea. *Nursing Research, 38,* 77–80.

This complex physiologic study applied an established physiologic methodology in the examination of variables associated with the sensation experienced by clients with dyspnea. The formula presented quantifies the sensation for comparison among dyspneic persons.

Sommers, M. S. (1988). Blood gas interpretation: Application to ARDS and COPD. *Journal of Intravenous Nursing, 11,* 299–307.

Because acid-base imbalances are often difficult to determine from clinical and laboratory data, this article reviews how to interpret ABG values in the typical client with two common adult respiratory disorders. The primary difference is that in COPD, the body attempts to compensate for respiratory acidosis by retaining bicarbonate, as evidenced by the ABG profile.

Unit 17 Resources

Nursing Resources

American Association of Critical-Care Nurses (AACN), One Civic Plaza, Suite 330, Newport Beach, CA 92660. Telephone 714-644-9310.

American Association of Critical-Care Nurses Certification Corporation, One Civic Plaza, Suite 315, Newport Beach, CA 92660. Telephone 714-644-9310.
Certifies nurses with experience in critical care.

American Thoracic Society, Section on Nursing, 1740 Broadway, New York, NY 10019. Telephone 212-315-8700.

Enterostomal Therapy Nursing Certification Board (ENTCB), 2081 Business Center Drive, Suite 290, Irvine, CA 92715. Telephone 516-928-4215.
Certifies nurses with experience in enterostomal therapy.

International Association for Enterostomal Therapy (IAET), 2081 Business Center Drive, Suite 290, Irvine, CA 92715. Telephone 516-928-4215.
See Unit 13 Resources for more information.

Other Resources

Alcoholics Anonymous, PO Box 459, Grand Central Station, New York, NY 10163. Telephone 212-686-1100.

American Academy of Allergy and Immunology, 611 East Wells Street, Milwaukee, WI 53202. Telephone 414-272-6071.

American Cancer Society, 1599 Clifton Road NE, Atlanta, GA 30329. Telephone 404-320-3333.

American College of Allergists, 800 East Northwest Highway, Suite 101, Mount Prospect, IL 60056. Telephone 800-842-7777.

American Lung Association, 1740 Broadway, New York, NY 10019. Telephone 212-315-8700.

Asthma and Allergy Foundation of America, 1717 Massachusetts Avenue NW, No. 305, Washington, DC 20036. Telephone 800-7ASTHMA.

International Association of Laryngectomees, 1599 Clifton Road NE, Atlanta, GA 30329. Telephone 404-329-7651.

National Institute of Allergy and Infectious Diseases (NIAID), Building 10, Bethesda, MD 20892. Telephone 301-496-4000.

National Jewish Center for Immunology and Respiratory Medicine, 1400 Jackson Street, Denver, CO 80206. Immunologic diseases hot line 800-222-LUNG.

UNIT 18

Problems of Oxygenation: Management of Clients with Disruptions of the Cardiovascular System

CHAPTER 63

Assessment of the Cardiovascular System

ANATOMY AND PHYSIOLOGY REVIEW

HEART

The leading cause of death in industrialized nations is heart disease. In the United States, cardiovascular disease is the major cause of disability and death in approximately 1 million people per year (American Heart Association [AHA], 1989). However, the rate of rise of heart disease has declined in the general population because of improved technology for early diagnosis and treatment and increased public awareness of the importance of proper nutrition, exercise, and cessation of smoking.

This chapter examines the normal structure and function of the cardiovascular and lymphatic systems, including changes that occur during a client's lifetime. The various diagnostic tools to help the nurse assist the adult client in achieving and maintaining optimal health and wellness are also reviewed.

STRUCTURE

The human *heart* is a cone-shaped, hollow, muscular organ between the lungs and is approximately the size of an adult fist (Figs. 63–1 and 63–2). The heart rests on the diaphragm and tilts forward and to the left in the client's chest. The apex of the heart is rotated anteriorly. This small organ must pump continuously during basal metabolic conditions and periods of stress or strenuous physical activity. In a normal healthy adult at rest, the heart pumps between 70 and 80 beats per minute, propelling oxygen-enriched blood into the arterial system. With each beat, when the client is in a normal resting state, the heart pumps approximately 2 oz of blood, which is about 5 qt/minute or 75 gal/hour (Crouch, 1985; Tilkian & Daily, 1986). During strenuous physical activity, the heart can double the amount of blood pumped to meet the increased oxygen needs of the peripheral tissues.

The heart is encapsulated by a protective covering called the *pericardium*, which consists of two layers: the visceral pericardium, or inner layer, and the parietal pericardium, or outer layer. The *visceral pericardium* is a thin transparent tissue that adheres to the heart muscle itself. The *parietal pericardium* is a tough, fibrous layer that attaches to the great vessels, the manubrium and xiphoid process of the sternum (anteriorly), the diaphragm (inferiorly), and the vertebral column (posteriorly). Between the visceral and parietal pericardial layers is the pericardial space, which is filled with 5 to 20 mL of thin pericardial fluid. The pericardial fluid serves two purposes: to lubricate the heart's surfaces and to alleviate friction between the heart's surfaces as the heart pumps.

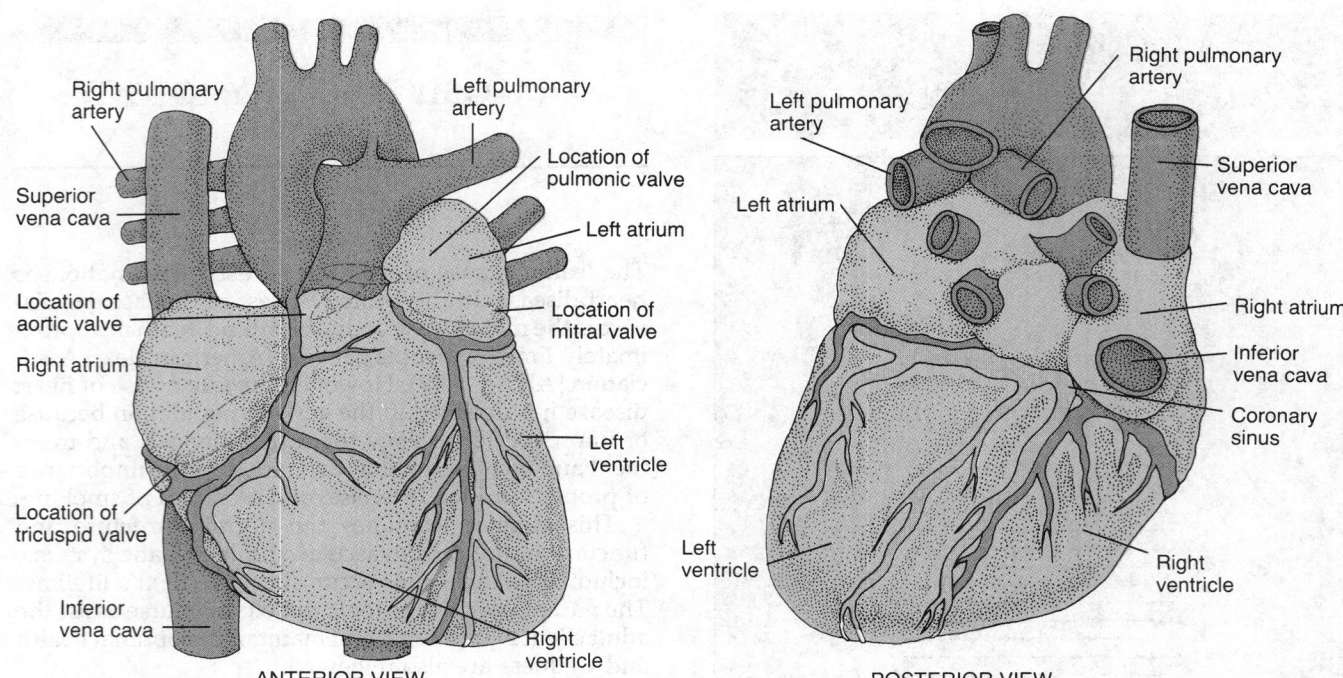

Figure 63 – 1

Surface anatomy of the heart.

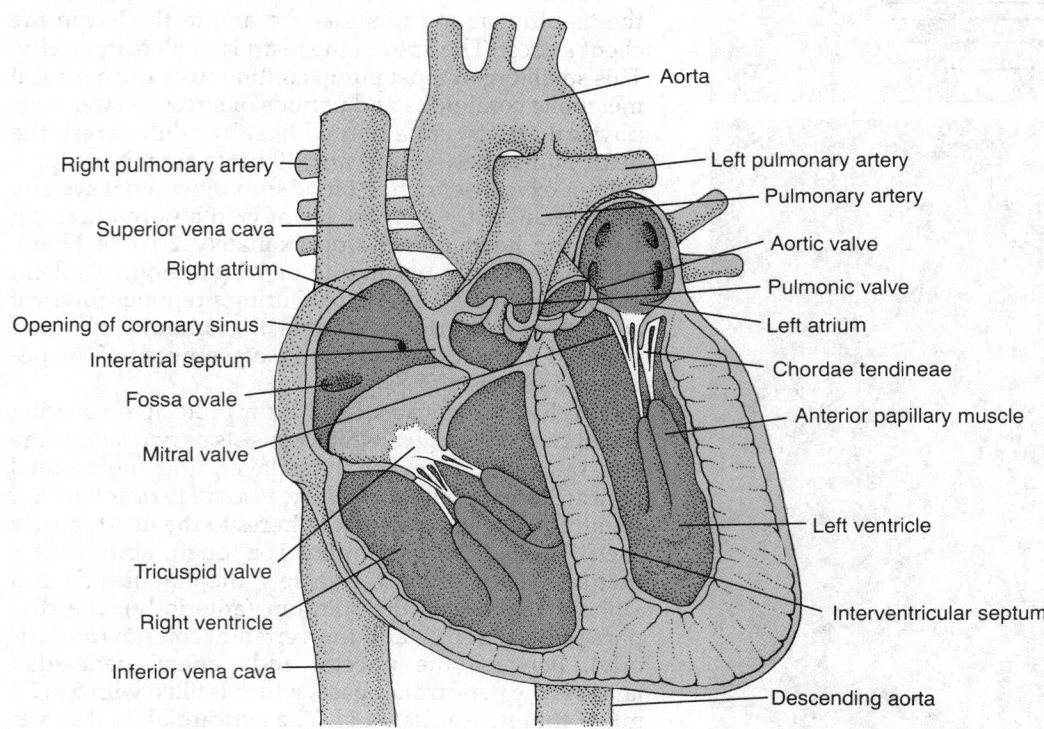

Figure 63 – 2

Cross-section of the heart.

The cardiac muscle tissue is composed of three layers: the epicardium, the myocardium, and the endocardium. The *epicardium*, the outer surface, is structurally a thin transparent tissue, the same as the visceral pericardium. The *myocardium*, the middle layer, is composed of striated muscle fibers interlaced together into bundles. This layer is responsible for the heart's contractile force. The innermost layer, the *endocardium*, is composed of endothelial tissue. This tissue lines the inside of the chambers of the heart and covers the four heart valves.

A muscular wall, known as the *septum*, separates the heart into two halves: right and left. Each half has an upper chamber called an *atrium* and a lower chamber called a *ventricle*. The right and left atria are referred to as the receiving chambers because they serve as reservoirs for blood before emptying into the ventricles. The interatrial septum separates the two atria. The ventricles are referred to as the distributing chambers because they eject blood into the vascular system. The interventricular septum separates the right and left ventricles.

The right atrium is a thin-walled structure that receives deoxygenated blood from all the peripheral tissues by way of the superior and inferior venae cavae and from the heart muscle by way of the coronary sinus. Deoxygenated blood that is received by the right atrium is called venous return. Approximately 15% to 20% of venous return is actively propelled by the right atrium into the right ventricle during atrial systole, or contraction. The remaining 75% to 80% of this venous return flows from the right atrium through the opened tricuspid valve to the right ventricle during ventricular diastole, or filling.

Blood flow through the cardiac chambers can be described by Poiseuille's law, which states that the flow rate of a fluid through a tube is proportional to pressure differences and the diameter of the tube in relation to the length of the tube and the viscosity of the fluid. Fluids flow from an area of higher pressure to one of lower pressure. Blood flows from the venous system (superior and inferior venae cavae and coronary sinus), which averages about 8 to 10 mmHg of pressure, into the right atrium, which averages about 0 to 5 mmHg of pressure. Although the right ventricle is relaxed during diastole, blood flows to this chamber because of the continued lower pressure.

The right ventricle is a flat muscular pump located behind the sternum. Because of the way the heart is oriented in the chest, this chamber is the anteriormost part of the heart. The right ventricle receives venous blood from the right atrium during ventricular diastole. The passive filling of blood and the additional ejected volume of blood generate enough pressure (about 25 mmHg) to close the tricuspid valve and open the pulmonic valve to propel blood into the pulmonary artery and then into the lungs. Structurally, the right ventricle is crescent shaped, with an outer wall that is approximately 5 mm thick (Fig. 63–3). The workload of the right ventricle is light compared with that of the left ventricle because the pulmonary system is a low-pressure system, which imposes less resistance to flow.

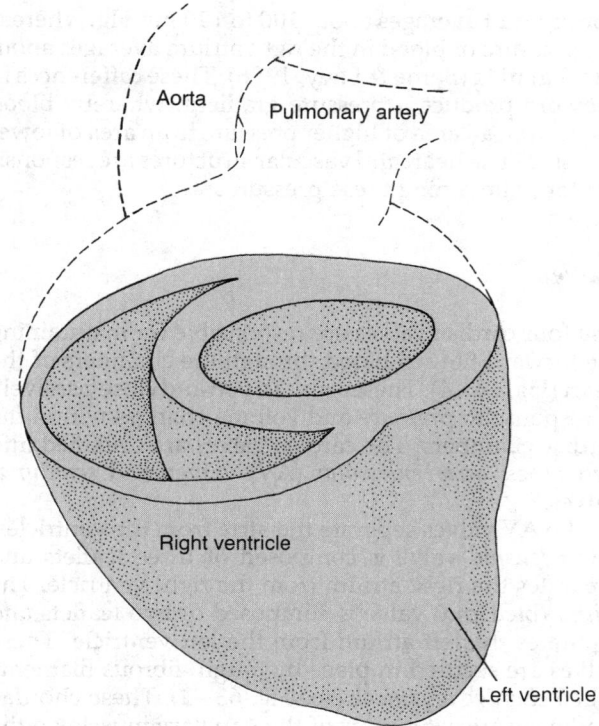

Figure 63–3

Size and shape of the right ventricle with respect to the left ventricle.

After blood is reoxygenated in the lungs, the left atrium receives this blood from the four pulmonary veins. Blood flows freely into the left atrium, then through an opened mitral valve into the left ventricle during ventricular diastole because the pressure in both chambers averages about 0 to 5 mmHg. When the left ventricle is about 75% to 80% full, the left atrium contracts the remaining 15% to 20% of blood volume to generate enough pressure (about 120 mmHg) to close the mitral valve and open the aortic valve. Blood is propelled into the aorta and into the systemic arterial circulation. Blood flow through the heart is shown in the illustration on page 2071.

The left ventricle is ellipsoid and is the largest and most muscular chamber of the heart (see Fig. 63–3). Its wall measures about 8 to 15 mm thick and is two to three times the thickness of the right ventricular wall. The left ventricle must generate a higher pressure than the right ventricle because it must contract against a high-pressure systemic circulation, which imposes a greater resistance to flow. If pressure rises in the circulatory system (as with hypertension), creating greater resistance, the left ventricle must generate a higher pressure, thus increasing its workload.

Blood flows from the aorta, is propelled throughout the systemic circulation to the various tissues of the body, and returns to the right atrium because of pressure differences. The pressure of blood in the aorta in a young adult averages about 100 to 120 mmHg, whereas the pressure of blood in the right atrium averages about 0 to 5 mmHg (Berne & Levy, 1986). These differences in pressure produce a pressure gradient, whereby blood flows from an area of higher pressure to an area of lower pressure. The heart and vascular structures are responsible for maintaining these pressures.

Valves

The four cardiac valves are responsible for maintaining the forward flow of blood through the chambers of the heart (Fig. 63–4). These valves open and close passively in response to pressure and volume changes within the cardiac chambers. The cardiac valves are classified into two types: *atrioventricular* (AV) valves and *semilunar* valves.

The AV valves separate the atria from the ventricles. The *tricuspid* valve is composed of three leaflets and separates the right atrium from the right ventricle. The *mitral* (bicuspid) valve is composed of two leaflets and separates the left atrium from the left ventricle. These valves are secured in place by tough, fibrous filaments called *chordae tendineae* (see Fig. 63–2). These chordae tendineae are extensions of the papillary muscle on the ventricular walls. During ventricular diastole, the valves act as funnels, facilitating the flow of blood from the atria to the ventricles. During ventricular systole, the papillary muscles and the chordae tendineae work together to keep the AV valves closed and to prevent them from reversing or prolapsing into the atria. There is some degree of overlapping of the valve leaflets during closure to prevent the backflow (regurgitation) of blood into the atria. Some clinical conditions, such as myocardial infarction (MI) or myocardial trauma, may damage the chordae tendineae or the papillary muscles, which

may allow this backward flow of blood into the atria during ventricular systole.

The semilunar valves are structurally different from the AV valves; each consists of three cup-like cusps, or pockets, around the inside wall of the artery that prevent blood from flowing back into the ventricles during ventricular diastole (see Fig. 63–2). During ventricular systole, these valves are open to permit blood flow into the pulmonary artery and aorta. There are two semilunar valves: *pulmonic* and *aortic* valves; each named for the arteries in which they are located. The pulmonic valve separates the right ventricle and the pulmonary artery. The aortic valve separates the left ventricle and the aorta.

Circulation

The heart muscle receives blood to meet its metabolic needs by way of the coronary arterial system (Fig. 63–5). The coronary arteries originate from an area on the aorta just beyond the cusps of the aortic valve. This area is the first branch from the aorta and is known as the sinuses of Valsalva.

There are two main coronary arteries: the *left coronary artery* (LCA) and the *right coronary artery* (RCA). The LCA arises from the left sinus of Valsalva and bifurcates, or divides into two branches: the left anterior descending (LAD) and the circumflex coronary artery (CCA). The LAD branch descends toward the anterior wall and apex of the left ventricle, supplying blood to the anterior wall of the left ventricle, the anterior ventricular septum, the anterior papillary muscle, and portions of the right ventricle. In addition, the LAD branch usually supplies the anterior apex of the left ventricle and portions of the posterior apex.

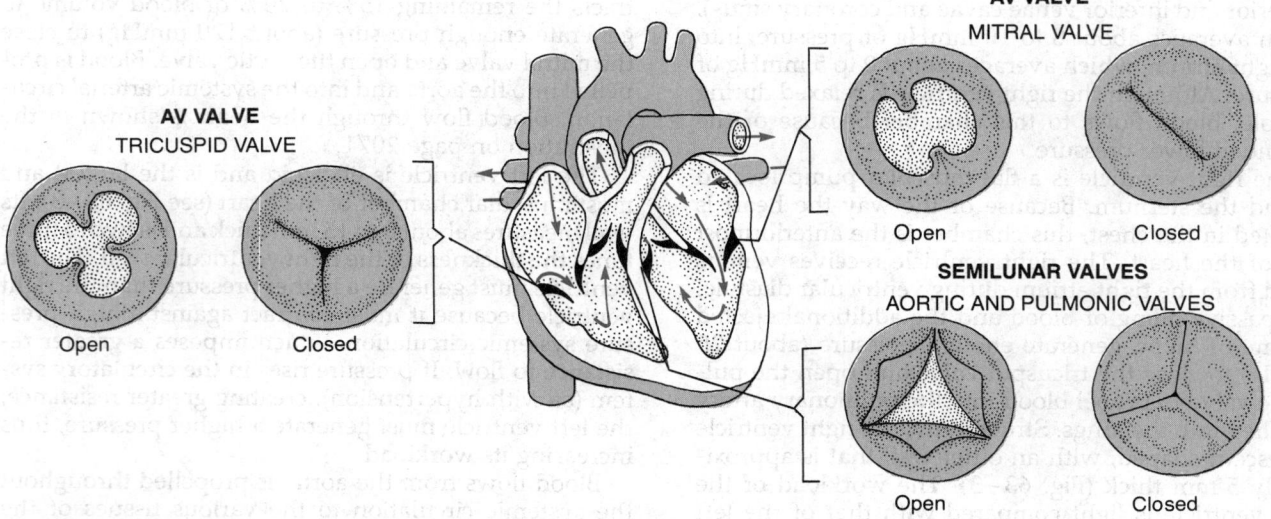

Figure 63–4

The valves of the heart.

HOW BLOOD FLOWS THROUGH THE HEART

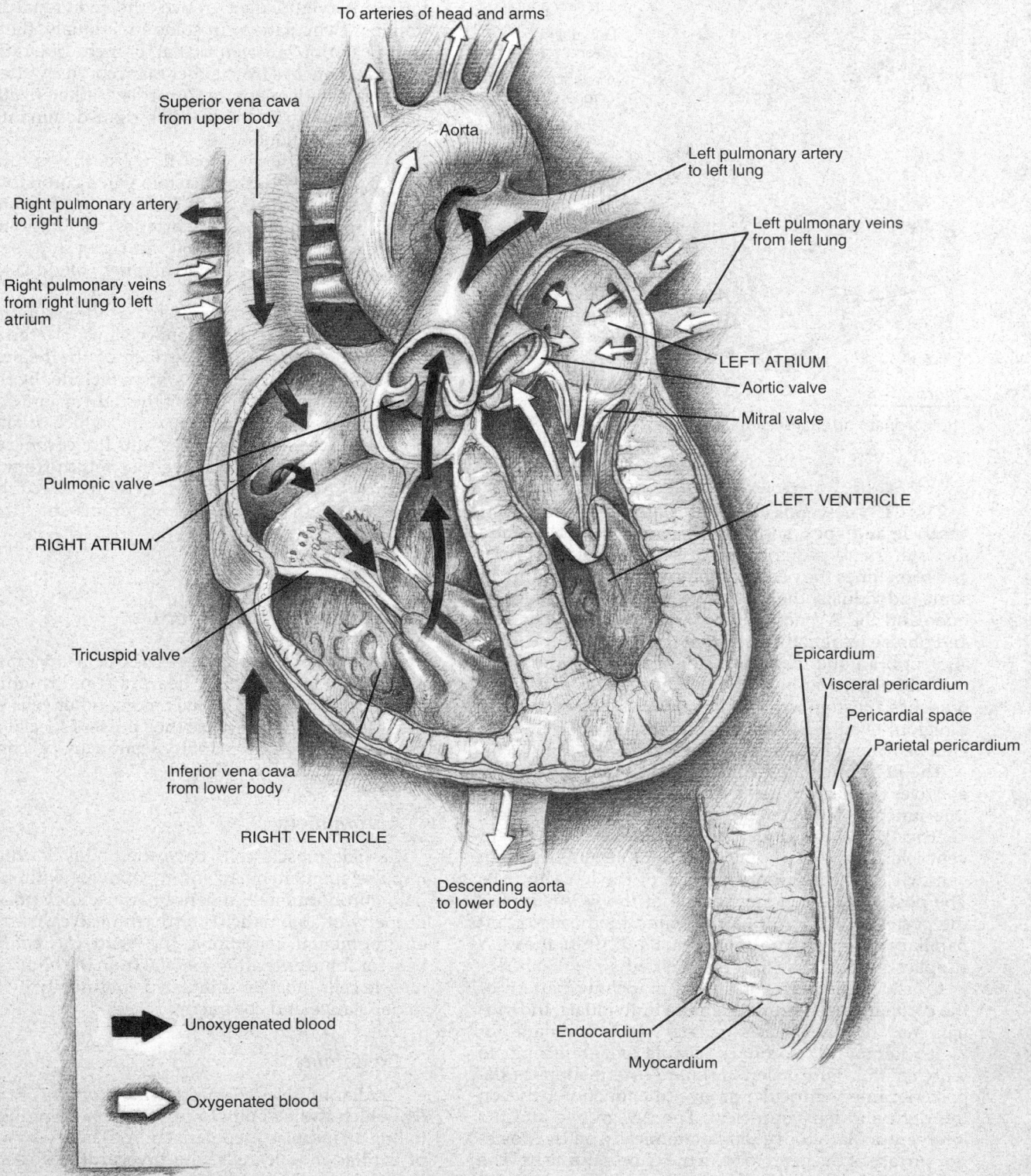

To arteries of head and arms

Superior vena cava from upper body

Aorta

Left pulmonary artery to left lung

Right pulmonary artery to right lung

Left pulmonary veins from left lung

Right pulmonary veins from right lung to left atrium

LEFT ATRIUM

Aortic valve

Mitral valve

Pulmonic valve

LEFT VENTRICLE

RIGHT ATRIUM

Tricuspid valve

Epicardium

Visceral pericardium

Pericardial space

Parietal pericardium

Inferior vena cava from lower body

RIGHT VENTRICLE

Descending aorta to lower body

Endocardium

Myocardium

➡ Unoxygenated blood

⇨ Oxygenated blood

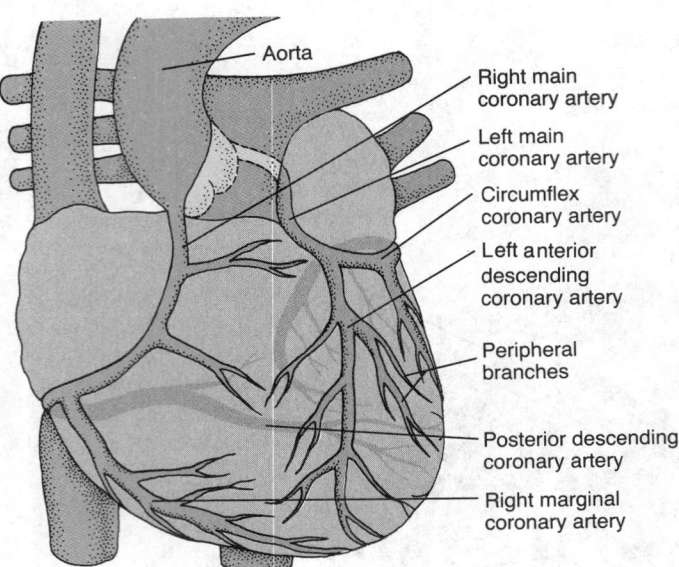

Figure 63–5

The coronary arterial system.

The CCA descends toward the lateral wall of the left ventricle and apex, supplying blood to the left atrium, the lateral and posterior surfaces of the left ventricle, and sometimes the posterior interventricular septum. In some individuals, the CCA supplies the sinoatrial (SA) node and the AV node. Peripheral branches (diagonal and obtuse marginal) arise from the LAD and the CCA and form an abundant network of vessels throughout the entire myocardium. Sometimes, these peripheral branches anastomose, which maintains blood supply to a region, even if the main blood vessel supplying the area becomes blocked.

The RCA originates from the right sinus of Valsalva; encircles the heart, passing through the right AV groove (the junction between the right atrium and the right ventricle); and descends toward the apex of the right ventricle. The RCA supplies the right atrium, the right ventricle, and the inferior portion of the left ventricle. The posterior descending branch of the RCA supplies the posterior wall of the septum and the posterior left papillary muscle. In most individuals (> 50%), the RCA supplies the SA node and the AV node.

Considerable variation in the branching pattern of the coronary arteries exists among individuals. Individuals may be classified as having "right dominant" or "left dominant" coronary circulation, referring to whether the right or left coronary artery supplies the posterior interventricular groove (the junction between the right and left ventricles). The AV groove and the interventricular groove join anatomically on the posterior surface of the heart to form the crux of the heart. The location of the crux of the heart is important because this is the area where the AV node is located. If the RCA turns at the crux of the heart and descends into the posterior interventricular groove, the circulation is right dominant, which occurs in most individuals. If the CCA reaches the crux of the heart and descends into the posterior interventricular groove, the individual has left dominant circulation. In some individuals, there is no true posterior interventricular branch, but rather peripheral branches from either main coronary artery supply the posterior septum. A cardiac catheterization can determine if an individual has right dominant or left dominant circulation.

Coronary artery blood flow to the myocardium occurs primarily during diastole when coronary vascular resistance is minimized. To maintain adequate blood flow through the coronary arteries, the diastolic blood pressure must be at least 60 mmHg or autoregulatory mechanisms are activated to maintain blood flow to the myocardium.

The coronary venous system has three subdivisions, which converge at the coronary sinus, a large venous channel on the posterior surface of the heart. These subdivisions of the venous system include the thesbian veins, which drain portions of the right atrium and right ventricle; the anterior cardiac veins, which drain a large portion of the right ventricle; and the coronary sinus, which receives myocardial venous return from the left ventricle and the other subdivisions. Deoxygenated blood from these subdivisions drains into the right atrium.

Electrophysiologic Properties

The electrophysiologic properties of heart muscle are responsible for regulating heart rate and rhythm. Cardiac muscle cells are unique among other cells in other tissues of the body because they possess special properties: automaticity, excitability, conductivity, contractility, and refractoriness.

Automaticity

Cardiac muscle cells have the ability to initiate an impulse spontaneously and repetitively without external neurohormonal influence because they possess the property of automaticity, or rhythmicity. Under proper environmental conditions, the heart can continue to beat for some time after removal from the body. Skeletal muscle cells must be stimulated continually by a nerve to depolarize and contract.

Excitability

Cardiac muscle cells possess the property of *excitability*, which is the ability to respond to a stimulus by initiating an impulse (depolarization). There are two types of cardiac muscle cells: the myocardial working cells (excitatory cells) located throughout the myocardium, and the pacemaker cells located in specialized tissue known as the conduction system of the heart. Myocardial working cells differ from pacemaker cells in that pacemaker cells do not need a stimulus to initiate depolarization, which occurs spontaneously. Excitability of cardiac cells can be affected by medications, hormones, electrolytes, infection, and oxygen supply.

Like the neurons, cardiac muscle cells have a membrane potential capable of changing its electrical charge, depending on the ion concentration within the cell (intracellular) and outside the cell (extracellular). Differences in ionic concentrations of sodium and potassium, intracellularly and extracellularly, create electrical and concentration gradients, which permit ionic movement across the semipermeable cell membrane.

In the resting state of the cardiac muscle cell, the inside of the cell is more negatively charged than the outside. A lowered concentration of positive ions occurs because the cell membrane allows movement of potassium out of the cell yet remains relatively impermeable to sodium. This resting membrane potential results from differences in the distribution of sodium and potassium ions. Although these ions are present both in and out of the cell, there is a greater concentration of potassium ion intracellularly, whereas the sodium ions have a greater extracellular concentration.

When the cardiac cell is stimulated, it changes the electrical potential of the cell membrane (transmembrane potential), which is known as an *action potential* (Fig. 63–6). There are two phases of the action potential: depolarization and repolarization. Clinically, the action potentials of cardiac cells are reflected on the electrocardiogram (ECG) (see Chap. 64).

After depolarization is initiated, the cell undergoes the following changes: an increase in cell membrane permeability to sodium (spontaneously by pacemaker cells or in response to a stimulus by myocardial working cells), a rapid influx of sodium ions, and an efflux of potassium ions from the cell. The electrical current that results from these changes in ionic concentration shifts the intracellular electrical potential from negative to positive. When the concentration of sodium ions reaches a critical level, an electrical impulse is generated. The impulse is propagated to adjacent cells throughout the heart as a wave of depolarization, likened to the ripples generated when a pebble is dropped into water.

Repolarization is the phase when the cell returns to its normal resting state. For this process to occur, the cell must undergo the following changes: a decrease in cell membrane permeability to sodium; an efflux of sodium ions from the cell; and a rapid efflux of potassium ions, promoting the return of the resting membrane potential. There is an active ion transport system on the cell membrane called the *sodium-potassium pump*, which maintains and monitors the balance of concentrations of sodium and potassium ions.

Other ions play a role in the action potential. These ions include calcium, chloride, and magnesium. During the plateau phase of the action potential, there is an increased cell membrane permeability to calcium. Calcium is the major ion that catalyzes a chemical interaction with the contractile elements (actin and myosin

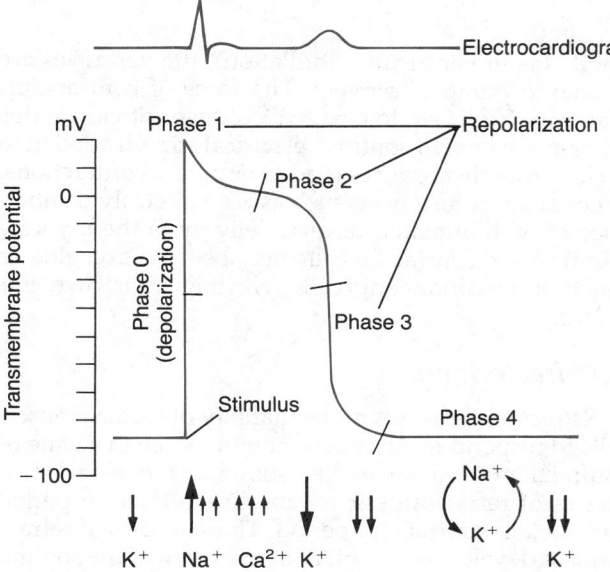

Figure 63–6

Action potential of a single myocardial cell. Exchange of ions across the cell membrane occurs at different points of the action potential. At rest, the inside of the cardiac cell is more negatively charged than the outside of the cell, and the cell membrane is more permeable to potassium (K^+) than to sodium (Na^+) ions. With a sufficient electrical stimulus, the cell membrane becomes more permeable to Na^+ (phase 0). As Na^+ enters the cell, the inside of the cell becomes positively charged (phase 1). Calcium (Ca^{2+}) ions also enter the cell and contribute to the positive potential. K^+ exists in the cell (phases 2 and 3), making the cell membrane less permeable to Na^+ ions. The resting period (phase 4) of the cell allows K^+ to regain dominance over Na^+ diffusion and establish equilibrium before another stimulus is elicited.

filaments) within the cell, resulting in contraction of myocardial muscle fibers.

Conductivity

Conductivity refers to the ability of the cardiac muscle cells to transmit electrical impulses along their cell membranes. Specialized tissue along the conduction system of the heart contains pacemaker cells, which propagate the electrical impulse from cell membrane to cell membrane. Adjacent myocardial working cells are joined by intercalated disks, which facilitate rapid conduction throughout the myocardium.

Contractility

Contractility refers to the ability of cardiac muscle cells to respond to an impulse by contracting. When these cardiac muscle cells are stimulated, the heart contracts maximally as a whole unit (all-or-none law). The myocardial muscle fibers must contract simultaneously to produce efficient pumping, enough to maintain normal blood pressure. If the muscle fibers contract randomly (as in ventricular fibrillation), the ventricles are unable to pump effectively. The force of contractions may vary from beat to beat, which does not violate this all-or-none law. In contrast, electrical stimuli applied to skeletal muscle produces graded or partial contractions. In certain circumstances (such as with electrolyte imbalance or with impaired oxygen delivery to the myocardium), these contractile cells may become excitable or function as conducting cells, eliciting their own impulses.

Refractoriness

Refractoriness refers to the inability of cardiac muscle cells to respond to successive stimuli while in a state of contraction from an earlier stimulus. There are two phases of refractoriness: an absolute refractory period and a relative refractory period. These phases of refractoriness develop as a result of inactivation of the sodium channels. During the absolute refractory period, cardiac muscle cells do not respond to any stimuli. This phase begins during depolarization and extends to the first part of repolarization, until the sodium channels are open to transport sodium ions necessary for depolarization.

The relative refractory period occurs during the final stages of repolarization, when the sodium channels begin to open for transport of sodium. During this short period, a stronger-than-normal stimulus can initiate a cardiac impulse and cause the heart to contract. After the resting state of the cell is attained (when sodium channels are restored), the cell is no longer refractory and can conduct action potentials.

The refractory periods of the cells of the atria are shorter than those of the cells of the ventricles, which means that the cells of the atria can contract faster. The absolute refractory period of the cells of the atria is about 0.15 second, whereas the absolute refractory period of the cells of the ventricles is 0.25 to 0.30 second (Braunwald, 1988).

This property of refractoriness of the myocardium prevents tetanic contractions, the uncontrolled rapid cardiac contractions (e.g., ventricular fibrillation), which would prove fatal without immediate intervention. Cardiac muscle does not exhibit tone, as skeletal muscle does. Therefore, refractoriness is a protective mechanism of the myocardium to preserve heart rhythm.

Conduction System

The cardiac conduction system (Fig. 63–7) is composed of atypical cardiac muscle myofibrils that have abundant sarcoplasm, which is rich in glycogen. This specialized tissue has the capability of rhythmic electrical impulse formation and can conduct impulses much more rapidly than other cells located in the myocardium. The SA node, located at the junction of the right atrium and the superior vena cava, is considered the main regulator of heart rate. The SA node is composed of pacemaker cells, which spontaneously initiate impulses at a rate of 60 to 100 per minute, and myocardial working cells, which transmit the impulses to surrounding atrial muscle.

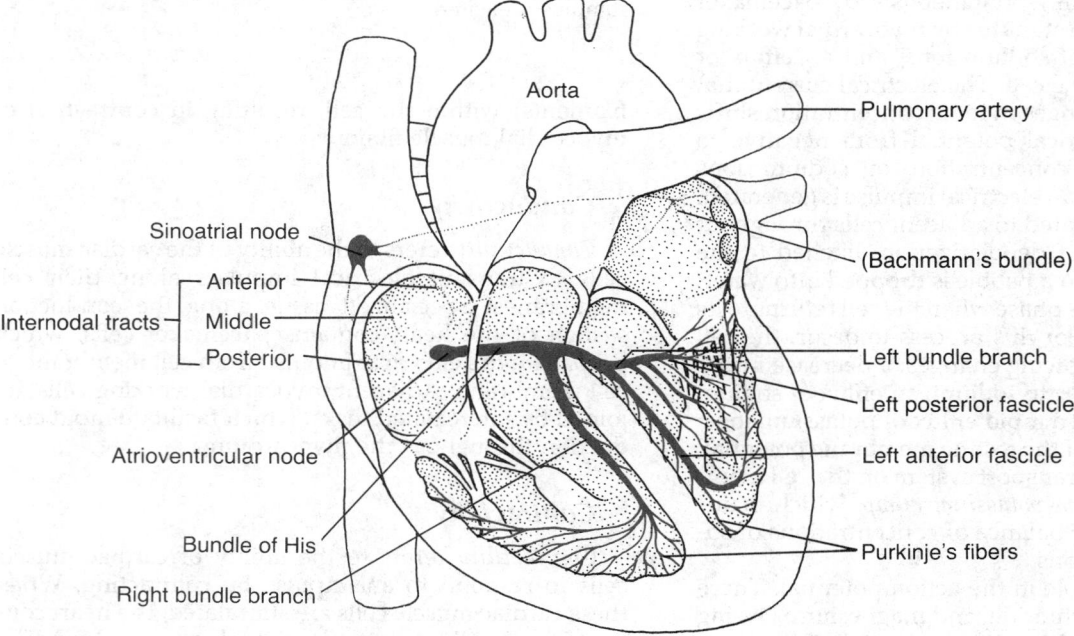

Figure 63–7

Conduction system of the heart.

Conduction of the impulse(s) throughout the atria occurs by way of internodal tracts. These tracts, referred to as the anterior, middle, and posterior, composed of Purkinje-like fibers and myocardial cells, are routed throughout the right atrium. An interatrial tract called Bachmann's bundle extends from the anterior nodal tract to the left atrium.

The three internodal tracts merge at the AV node, also called the junctional or nodal area, where the atrial and ventricular tissues meet. Cells in the junctional area are capable of initiating an electrical impulse should the SA node fail to elicit an electrical impulse. The junctional or nodal cells can initiate impulses at a rate of 40 to 60 per minute.

The AV node contained in the junctional area is located anatomically on the right side of the interatrial septum in front of the coronary sinus. After the impulse reaches the AV node, conduction of the impulse is delayed 0.07 to 0.10 second before reaching the ventricles. This physiologic delay allows the atria to contract completely before the ventricles are stimulated and contract.

The bundle of His is a continuation of the AV node and runs in the inferior border of the membranous portion of the interventricular septum. When the bundle of His reaches the muscular portion of the interventricular septum, it divides into the right and left bundle branches.

The right bundle branch (RBB) extends down the right side of the interventricular septum under the endocardium to the anterior papillary muscle of the right ventricle, where it fuses with the Purkinje fiber system. The common left bundle branch (LBB) divides after a short distance into a long, thin anterior branch (the left anterior descending) and a shorter, thicker posterior branch (the posterior descending). The anterior descending fascicle extends anteriorly down the left side of the interventricular septum to the anterior papillary muscle of the left ventricle. The posterior descending fascicle courses to the posterior papillary muscle of the left ventricle. These three fascicles subdivide to ramify over respective ventricles just under the endocardium in terminal branches.

The Purkinje fibers are the terminal branches of the conduction system and are responsible for carrying the wave of depolarization to both ventricular free walls. The Purkinje fibers can act as an intrinsic pacemaker, but their discharge rate is only 20 to 40 beats per minute. Thus, these intrinsic pacemakers seldom initiate an impulse, except when there is complete AV block and complete absence of AV nodal impulses.

An impulse from the SA node initiates the process of depolarization and hence the activation of all myocardial cells. Depolarization occurs in the right atrium first, followed by the left atrium. Activation of the atria occurs normally in 0.11 second or less.

After both atria are depolarized, the impulse travels to the junctional area, activating this region, including the AV node. The AV node delays the impulse by 0.07 to 0.10 second before the impulse continues its course to the bundle of His (Braunwald, 1988).

From the bundle of His, the impulse travels down toward the right and left bundle branches. The ventricular septum is activated first because the impulse travels from the left side to the right side.

The impulse continues to activate the length of the bundle branches into the Purkinje fiber network, which depolarizes the free walls of the ventricles simultaneously. Activation of the ventricles moves from the apex of the heart upward toward the base of the heart to complete the process of depolarization.

The process of depolarization within the ventricular walls progresses from the endocardium to the epicardium. Repolarization is a passive process not involving the conduction system of the heart. Repolarization of the atria occurs from the endocardium to the epicardium (Braunwald, 1988). However, repolarization in the ventricles follows the reverse order such that the first cells to depolarize are the last to repolarize.

Sequence of Events During the Cardiac Cycle

The phases of the cardiac cycle are generally described in relation to changes in pressure and volume in the left ventricle during ventricular filling (diastole) and ventricular contraction (systole) (Fig. 63–8). *Diastole,* the longer of the two phases of the cardiac cycle, consists of relaxation and filling of the atria and ventricles, whereas *systole* consists of the contraction and emptying of the atria and ventricles. If the client has a heart rate of 75 beats per minute, diastole lasts about 0.53 second and systole about 0.27 second.

Cardiac muscle contraction results from the release of large numbers of calcium ions from the sarcoplasmic reticulum, which diffuse into the myofibril sarcomere (the basic contractile unit of the myocardial cell). Calcium ions promote the interaction of actin and myosin protein filaments, causing a linking and overlapping of these filaments. As the protein filaments slide over or overlap each other, cross-bridges or linkages are formed, which act as force-generating sites. The sliding of these protein filaments of multiple myofibril sarcomeres causes shortening of the sarcomeres, producing myocardial contraction.

Relaxation of the cardiac muscle occurs when calcium ions are pumped back into the sarcoplasmic reticulum, causing a decrease in the number of calcium ions around the myofibrils. This reduced number of ions causes the protein filaments to disengage or dissociate, the sarcomere to lengthen, and the muscle to relax.

Atrial Systole

The right and left atria contribute 15% to 20% of additional blood volume before ventricular systole, which is termed *atrial kick* (Braunwald, 1988). This additional volume of blood does not make a major contri-

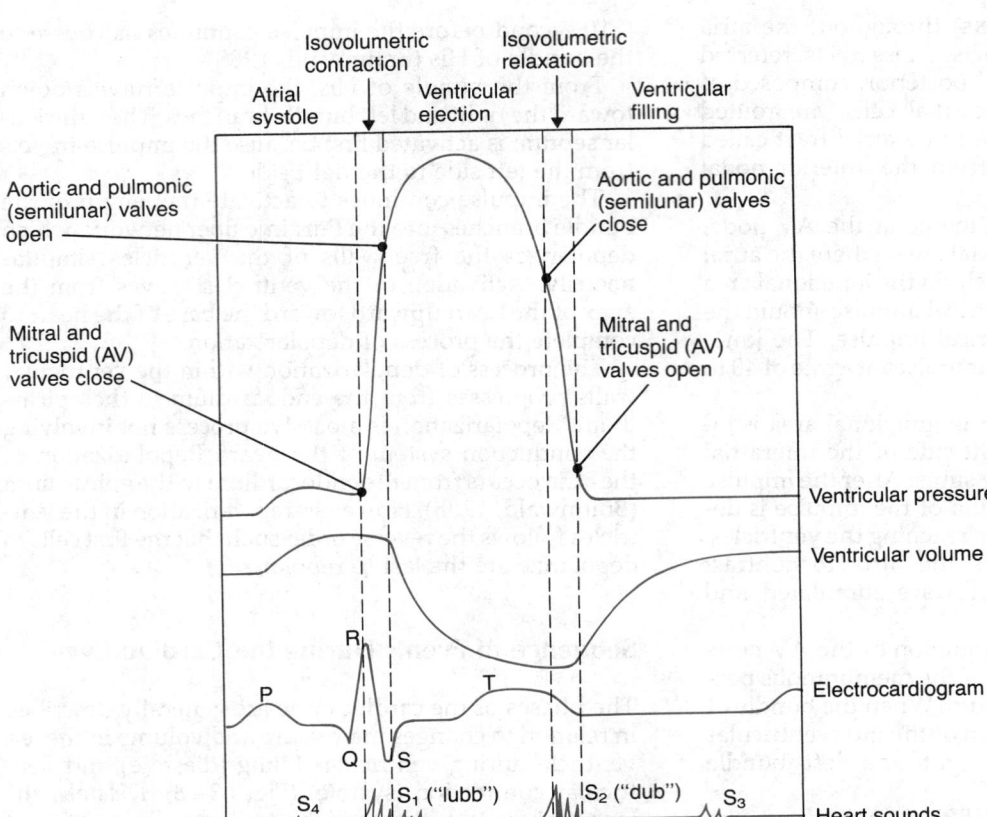

Figure 63–8

Events of the cardiac cycle.

bution to the normal pumping action of the heart, although some clients with aortic stenosis may depend on this volume of blood to provide a more effective cardiac output.

Ventricular Systole

Ventricular systole begins during the isovolumetric contraction phase when all four valves are closed. Closure of the AV valves marks the beginning of systole and creates the first heart sound (S_1). Blood volume and muscle fiber length remain constant (isometric), while myocardial tension and intraventricular pressure increase to generate a pressure greater than aortic root and pulmonic pressures. The higher pressures in the aortic root and pulmonary artery are the result of the previous systoles that just ejected blood into the aorta and pulmonary artery. When right and left intraventricular pressures exceed aortic and pulmonic pressures, the aortic and pulmonic valves open and maximal ventricular ejection commences. The ventricles pump blood into the

systemic and pulmonic circulations. The rate of ejection of blood slows and blood continues to be ejected from the ventricles, until ventricular relaxation ensues, resulting in a rapid decrease in intraventricular pressure. The semilunar valves close in response to the pressure changes when pressures from the aorta and the pulmonary artery push blood back toward the ventricles. Closure of the aortic and pulmonic valves creates the second heart sound (S_2) and marks the beginning of ventricular diastole.

Ventricular Diastole

Isovolumetric ventricular relaxation (diastole) occurs on closure of the semilunar valves, and ventricular pressure continues to decrease. During this brief period, all four valves are again closed; ventricular pressure is higher than atrial pressure. Blood collects in the atria, generating enough pressure so that the AV valves eventually open when ventricular pressure falls to its low diastolic level. After the tricuspid and mitral valves open, blood rapidly fills the ventricles, causing intraventricular pressures to rise. This rapid ventricular filling phase (protodiastole) lasts approximately the first third of diastole. As ventricular pressure rises, ventricular filling slows. This resultant slowing of blood, when all four chambers of the heart are relaxed and blood flows passively from the atria to the ventricles, is termed *diastasis*.

Mechanical Properties

The electrical and mechanical properties of cardiac muscle determine the function of the cardiovascular system. The heart is able to adapt to various pathophysiologic conditions (e.g., stress, infections, and hemorrhage) to maintain adequate blood flow to the various body tissues. Blood flow to the tissues is measured clinically as the cardiac output. Cardiac output is dependent on the relationship between heart rate and stroke volume; it is the product of these two variables and the basic determinant of heart function.

$$\text{Cardiac output} = \text{heart rate} \times \text{stroke volume}$$

Cardiac Output and Cardiac Index

Cardiac output is the volume of blood ejected by each ventricle into the pulmonic and systemic circulation per minute. The ejection of blood is a result of the synchronized, rhythmic contraction of the myocardium. Normally, cardiac output in the adult ranges from 4 to 8 L/minute (Braunwald, 1988; Gardner & Woods, 1989). Because cardiac output requirements vary according to an individual's body size, the cardiac index is calculated to adjust for size differences. The *cardiac index* can be determined by dividing the cardiac output by the body surface area and is based on the assumption that cardiac output is more proportional to body surface area than to body mass.

$$\text{Cardiac index} = \frac{\text{cardiac output}}{\text{body surface area}}$$

Body surface area is determined by the client's height and weight using the DuBois scale (Fig. 63–9). The normal range of cardiac index is 2.8 to 3.3 L/minute per square meter of body surface area, thus adjusting for the client's body size and variability in cardiac function (Braunwald, 1988).

The volume of blood ejected during each ventricular contraction is referred to as *stroke volume*. More specifically, it is the difference between the amount of blood in the ventricle at the end of diastole and the residual ventricular volume at the end of systole.

$$\text{Stroke volume} = \text{end-diastolic volume} - \text{end-systolic volume}$$

Several variables influence stroke volume and, ultimately, cardiac output. These variables include heart rate, preload, afterload, compliance, contractility, and synergy of contraction.

Heart Rate

Heart rate refers to the number of times the ventricles contract per minute. The normal resting heart rate for an adult is between 60 and 100 beats per minute (AHA, 1989). Rate is extrinsically controlled by the autonomic nervous system and is able to provide for rapid adjustments necessary to regulate cardiac output. The parasympathetic system exerts an inhibitory effect on rate, whereas the sympathetic system imposes an excitatory effect. Both of these systems in conjunction with circulating endogenous catecholamines, such as norepinephrine, epinephrine, and dopamine, mediate and control heart rate (Fig. 63–10).

Other factors, such as the central nervous system (CNS) and baroreceptor (pressoreceptor) reflexes, influence the effects of the sympthetic and parasympathetic nervous systems on heart rate. Pain, fear, and anxiety can cause an increase in heart rate. When the baroreceptors are stimulated, reflex changes can influence heart rate. The baroreceptor reflex acts as a negative feedback system. Afferent branches from the CNS located in the aortic arch, the carotid sinus, and other areas sense and regulate pressure in the arteries and regulate the resistance of blood vessels in the periphery. If a client experiences hypotension, the baroreceptors in the aortic arch and carotid sinus sense a lessened pressure in the blood vessels, thus the receptors are stimulated less. With the baroreceptors receiving less stimulation, a signal is relayed to the parasympathetic system to have less inhibitory effect on the SA node, which results in a reflex increase in heart rate.

Other factors are involved in regulating and mediating heart rate. These factors include body temperature, medications, hormones, arterial blood gas tensions, and electrolyte concentrations.

Preload

Preload refers to the degree of myocardial fiber stretch at the end of diastole just before contraction. The stretch imposed on the muscle fibers is a result of the volume contained within the ventricle, or its end-diastolic volume. Preload is determined by ventricular (end-diastolic) volume.

An increase in ventricular volume increases muscle fiber length and tension, thereby enhancing contraction and improving stroke volume. This length-tension relationship was first described by Starling and associates in 1914. The length-tension relationship, namely Starling's law of the heart, states that, when a muscle fiber is stretched, it yields a measurable change in developed muscle tension up to a critical length. Any further increases in excess of the critical length do not correspond to an increase in stroke volume or developed tension

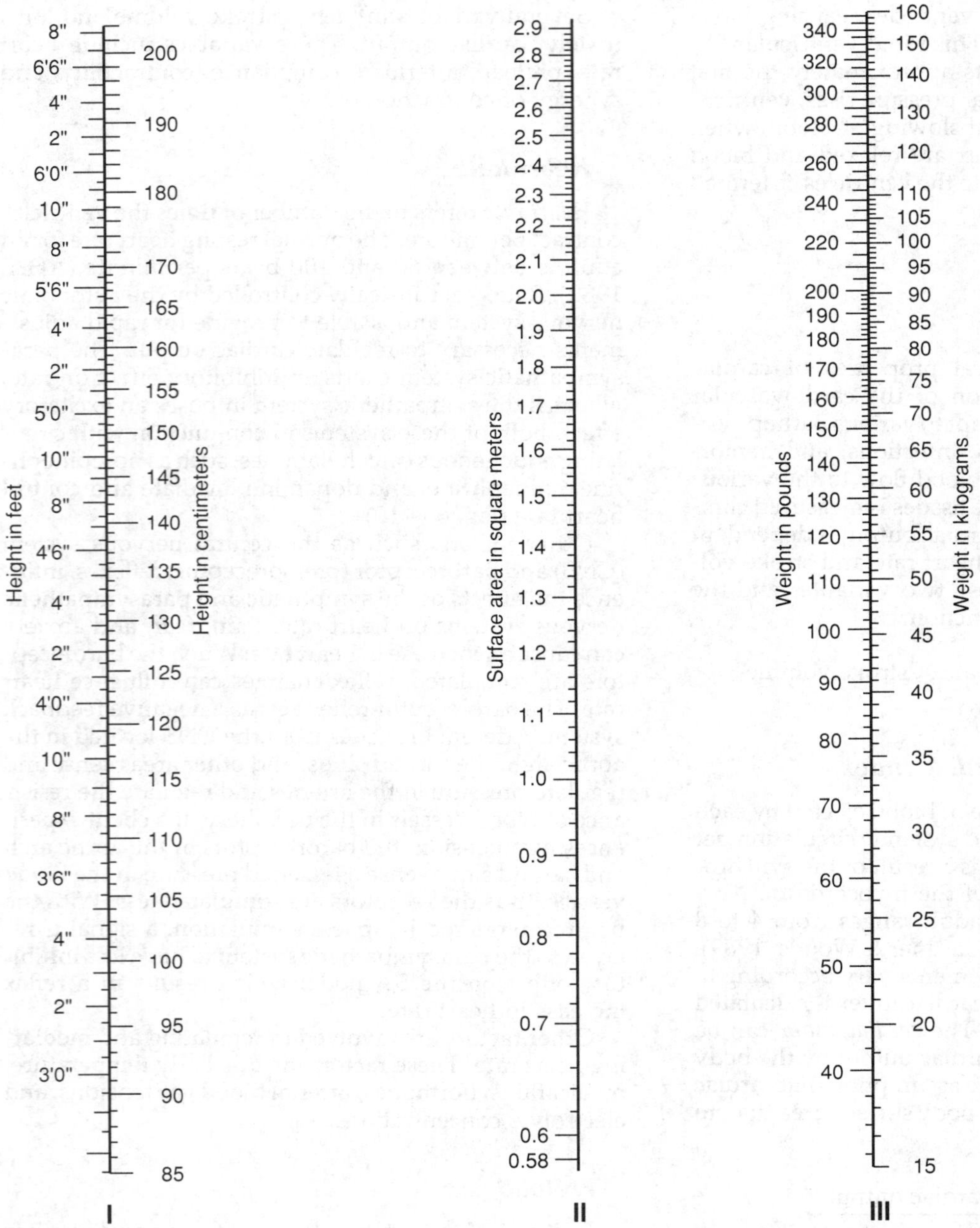

Height in feet | Height in centimeters | Surface area in square meters | Weight in pounds | Weight in kilograms

I   II   III

Figure 63–9

DuBois' body surface chart. To find the body surface area of the client, the nurse locates the height in inches (or centimeters) on scale I and the weight in pounds (or kilograms) on scale II. A straight-edged ruler is placed between those two points, which will intersect scale III and determine the client's surface area. (From DuBois, E. F. [1936]. *Basal metabolism in health and disease*. Philadelphia: Lea & Febiger. Copyright 1920 by W. M. Boothby and R. B. Sandiford.)

and may result in a decrease in stroke volume. A ventricular function curve can be drawn if the length-tension relationship is expanded to include the muscle fibers of the entire ventricle (Gardner & Woods, 1989) (Fig. 63–11).

Afterload

Another determinant of stroke volume is afterload. *Afterload* is the amount of tension developed by the ventricles during systole to open the aortic and pul-

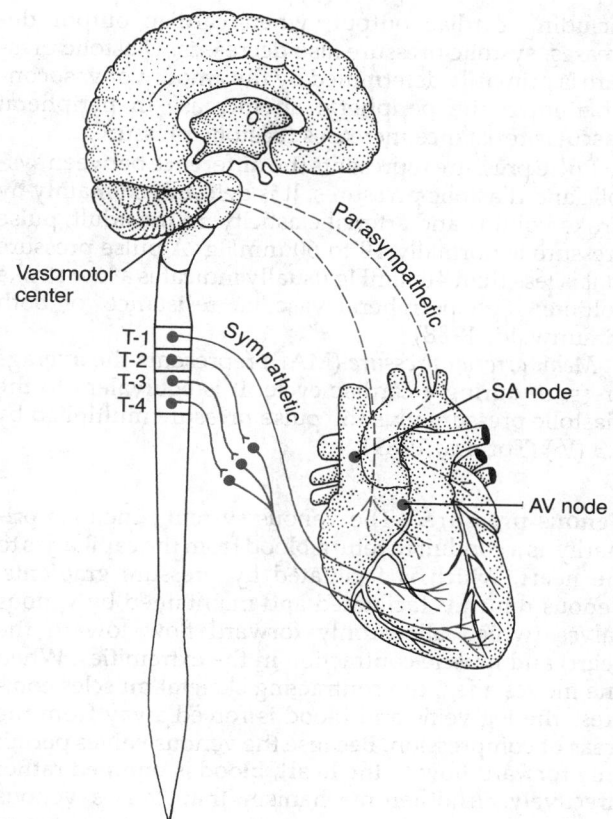

Figure 63–10

Influence of the autonomic nervous system on the heart.

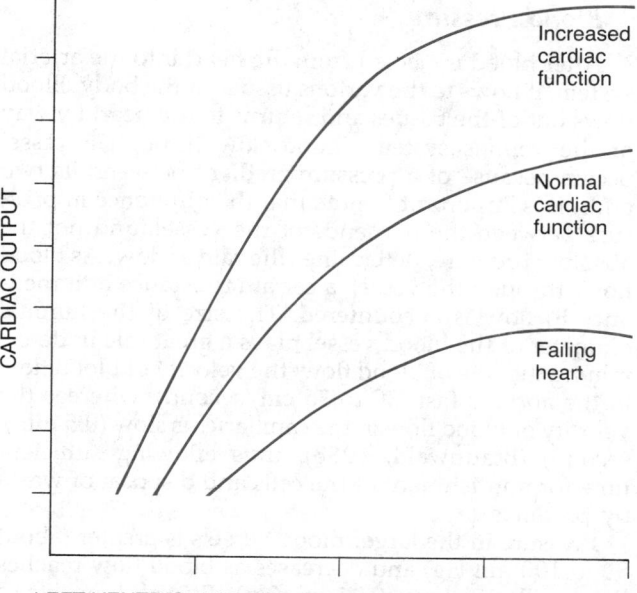

Figure 63–11

Length-tension ventricular function curves.

monic valves and to eject blood into the pulmonary artery and aorta and into the peripheral vessels. The amount of resistance is directly related to the function of arterial pressure and the diameter of the ventricle. Afterload increases with intraventricular pressures, an enlarged ventricle, or a thinner-than-normal muscle wall. Impedance is the peripheral component of afterload, which is the pressure that the heart must overcome to open the aortic valve. The amount of impedance depends on aortic compliance and total peripheral vascular resistance, a combination of blood viscosity and arteriolar constriction. A decrease in stroke volume can result from an increase in impedance without the benefit of compensatory mechanisms.

Compliance

Compliance refers to the distensibility of the ventricles. Compliance is the relationship between end-diastolic volume and end-diastolic pressure expressed as a change in volume resulting from a given change in pressure. Both preload and afterload can be affected by altered compliance in the ventricles or the peripheral vessels.

In a ventricle or a vessel with normal compliance, large increases in end-diastolic volume can occur with relatively minor increases in end-diastolic pressure. However, if the distensible ventricle or vessel is stretched to its capacity, small increases in volume elicit markedly higher pressures. In MI, the compliance of the affected ventricle is lowered; therefore, small increases in volume incur major increases in pressure, such that maximal distention occurs with smaller volumes.

Contractility

Contractility also affects ventricular function. Myocardial contractility occurs independently of the fiber length and refers to the force of contractions generated by the myocardium under given loading conditions. The myocardium has an inherent property to alter its contractile force and velocity.

Synergy of Contraction

Synergy of contraction is the contraction of the myocardium in a synchronized, uniform fashion to obtain a maximal ejection of blood. Certain pathologic changes cause an asynchrony of contraction, which results in decreased flow and interferes with the ejection of blood, thereby reducing the cardiac output.

Six variables (heart rate, preload, afterload, compliance, contractility, and synergy of contraction) provide important indices for assessing cardiac function. Alterations in any one or a combination of these variables can either augment or compromise cardiac performance.

Blood Pressure

After blood is ejected from the heart into the arterial system, it flows to the various tissues of the body. Blood flows out of the tissues and returns to the heart by way of the venous system. Blood flow through a vessel occurs because of a pressure gradient between its two ends. It is important to note that the difference in pressure between the two ends of the vessel, and not the absolute pressure, determines the rate of flow. As blood flows through the vessel, a certain resistance or impedance to flow is encountered. The size of the luminal diameter of the blood vessel plays a great role in determining the rate of blood flow: the velocity of blood flow in the aorta is fast (30 to 35 cm/second), whereas the velocity of blood flow in the capillaries is slow (0.5 mm/second) (Braunwald, 1988), thus allowing sufficient time for nourishment of the cells and disposal of waste by-products.

Pressure in the larger blood vessels is greater (about 80 to 100 mmHg) and decreases as blood flow reaches the capillaries (about 25 mmHg). By the time blood enters the right atrium, blood pressure is approximately 0 to 5 mmHg.

Arterial pressure. The blood pressure in the arterial system is determined primarily by the quantity of blood flow or cardiac output and the resistance in the arterioles.

Blood pressure = cardiac output
$$\times \text{ peripheral vascular resistance}$$

Therefore, any factor that increases cardiac output or total peripheral vascular resistance increases blood pressure. In general, blood pressure is maintained at a relatively constant level so that an increase or decrease in total peripheral vascular resistance is associated with a decrease or an increase in cardiac output, respectively. Three mechanisms mediate and regulate blood pressure: the autonomic nervous system by way of chemoreceptors and baroreceptors and other impulses transmitted to the vasomotor center excites or inhibits sympathetic nervous system activity; the kidneys sense a change in blood flow, which activates the renin–angiotensin–aldosterone mechanism; and the endocrine system releases various hormones (catecholamines, aldosterone, kinins, serotonin, and histamine) to stimulate the sympathetic nervous system at the tissue level.

Systolic blood pressure represents the highest pressure occurring in an artery with each contraction of the heart; *diastolic* blood pressure represents the lowest pressure during the relaxation phase of the heart. In the adult, systolic pressure is normally 90 to 140 mmHg and diastolic pressure is normally 60 to 90 mmHg (AHA, 1989). Blood pressure is expressed as a fraction: systolic/diastolic.

Systolic pressure is affected by a number of factors, including cardiac output; when cardiac output decreases, systolic pressure also decreases. Diastolic pressure is primarily determined by the amount of vasoconstriction in the periphery; an increase in peripheral vascular resistance increases diastolic pressure.

Pulse pressure represents the difference between systolic and diastolic pressures. It is determined mainly by stroke volume and arterial elasticity. In the adult, pulse pressure is normally 40 to 60 mmHg. A pulse pressure that is less than 40 mmHg usually indicates a low stroke volume, high peripheral vascular resistance, or both (Braunwald, 1988).

Mean arterial pressure (MAP) represents the average pressure during a cardiac cycle. It is equivalent to the diastolic pressure plus the pulse pressure multiplied by 0.3 (⅓) (Tortora, 1989).

Venous pressure. The venous system functions primarily as a conduit to return blood from the capillaries to the heart, which is facilitated by pressure gradients. Venous return is facilitated and maintained by venous valves (which allow only forward flow toward the heart) and muscle contraction in the extremities. When one moves a leg, the contracting skeletal muscles compress the leg veins and blood is forced away from the areas of compression. Because the venous valves permit only forward flow to the heart, blood is pumped rather effectively. Another mechanism that causes venous pressure to change is that every time one inhales or inspires, intrathoracic pressure decreases, facilitating venous return. Venous blood is also drawn into the atrium during ventricular contraction, which creates a negative pressure in the atrium relative to the pressure in the venae cavae.

Capillary pressure. Movement of blood into and out of the capillaries is determined largely by the balance between hydrostatic or filtration pressures in the capillary and plasma oncotic pressure. Capillary pressure at the arterial end is 20 to 25 mmHg and at the venous end is 10 to 15 mmHg (Crouch, 1985; Landau, 1980; Tilkian & Daily, 1986).

If the capillary hydrostatic pressure rises or if the integrity of the capillary endothelium is impaired, fluid moves out of the vascular system into the interstitial fluid space. In contrast, if the capillary hydrostatic pressure falls, fluid moves into the capillaries from the interstitial spaces to re-expand blood volume.

FUNCTION

The function of the cardiovascular system is twofold: (1) to pump oxygenated blood into the arterial circulation to transport and deliver nutrients to the various tissues of the body, and (2) to receive deoxygenated blood in the venous system and deliver it to the pulmonary system for reoxygenation. The cardiovascular system can adapt readily to changes that occur internally or externally by way of the autonomic nervous system (see Fig. 63–10). Regulation is controlled by balancing the sympathetic and parasympathetic nervous systems. Changes in sympathetic and parasympathetic activities are responses to messages sent by the sensory receptors in the various tissues of the body. These receptors, including the baroreceptors, the chemoreceptors, and the stretch receptors, respond differently to biochemical and physiologic changes of the body.

Baroreceptors have been identified in the walls of most of the large thoracic and neck arteries, specifically in the arch of the aorta and at the origin of the internal carotid arteries. These receptors are stimulated when the arterial walls are stretched by an increased blood pressure. Impulses from these baroreceptors inhibit the vasomotor center, located bilaterally in the reticular substance of the lower one-third of the pons and the upper two-thirds of the medulla. Inhibition of this center results in a drop in blood pressure.

Several chemoreceptors have been identified in the bifurcations of the carotid arteries and along the aortic arch. These small specialized collections of tissue, 1 to 2 mm in size, are called the *carotid* and *aortic bodies*, respectively. They contain specialized receptors that are sensitive primarily to hypoxemia (a decrease in arterial PO_2). The carotid chemoreceptors send impulses along Hering's nerves; the aortic chemoreceptors send impulses along the vagus nerves; when stimulated, the CNS stimulates a vasoconstrictor response (Berne & Levy, 1986).

The chemoreceptors are also stimulated to a certain extent by hypercapnia (an increase in arterial PCO_2) and acidosis (a decreased pH). However, the direct effect of carbon dioxide on the CNS is 10 times as strong as the effect it produces by stimulating the chemoreceptors.

Stretch receptors are found primarily in the terminal portions of the venae cavae and the right atrium. These receptors are sensitive to pressure or volume changes. When a client is hypovolemic, the stretch receptors in the blood vessels sense a reduced volume or pressure and elicit fewer impulses to the CNS; this stimulates the sympathetic nervous system to increase heart rate and to constrict the peripheral blood vessels.

The renal system helps to regulate cardiovascular activity. When renal blood flow or pressure decreases, the kidneys tend to retain sodium and water. Blood pressure tends to rise because of fluid retention and because of activation of the renin–angiotensin–aldosterone mechanism (Berne & Levy, 1986). Vascular volume is also regulated by the release of antidiuretic hormone (vasopressin) from the posterior pituitary gland.

Other factors can influence the activity of the cardiovascular system. Emotional factors, such as excitement, pain, or anger, stimulate the sympathetic nervous system. Exercise or inactivity, such as prolonged bed rest, can augment or compromise the effects of the cardiovascular system. Body temperature can affect the metabolic needs of the tissues, thereby influencing the delivery of blood: in hypothermia, tissues require fewer nutrients, whereas in hyperthermia, the metabolic requirement of the tissues is greater.

VASCULAR SYSTEM

The purpose of the vascular system is to provide conduits for blood to travel from the heart to nourish the various tissues of the body, to carry away cellular wastes to the excretory organs, to allow lymphatic flow to drain tissue fluid back into the circulation, and to return blood to the heart for recirculation. This system of conduits is dependent on an efficient heart and patent blood vessels to regulate and maintain systemic and regional blood flow and temperature. The vascular system is divided into the arterial system and the venous system.

BLOOD VESSELS

Structure

Blood vessels constitute the vascular system (Fig. 63–12). Blood expelled by the heart is carried by the arteries, which branch into arterioles, which divide to form capillaries, where the exchange of nutrients to the tissues occurs. The branching pattern of blood vessels of the vascular system is such that large vessels divide into smaller vessels, which subdivide into even smaller vessels until the blood reaches the capillaries. The joining of blood vessels leaving the capillary follows a reverse pattern, with smaller vessels converging into larger blood vessels. In the arterial system, blood moves from a system of larger conduits to a network of smaller blood vessels, whereas in the venous system, blood travels from the capillaries to the venules and to the larger system of veins, eventually returning in the venae cavae to the heart for recirculation.

Blood vessels vary in size and wall thickness according to their function and position in the vascular system. All blood vessels (arteries and veins), except capillaries, are composed structurally of three distinct layers of tissue: the tunica intima, the tunica media, and the tunica adventitia (Fig. 63–13). The innermost layer, the *tunica intima*, consists of a single layer of endothelial cells resting on a layer of connective tissue. The internal elastic membrane separates the intima from the media. The *tunica media* is a relatively thick layer of smooth muscle cells, connective tissue, and elastic fibers arranged in a circular fashion. The external elastic membrane separates the media from the adventitia. The outer layer, the *tunica adventitia*, is composed of connective tissue with collagen and elastic fibers. It provides a major portion of the total strength of the blood vessel. The intima and the inner aspect of the media receive nutrients by diffusion from the lumen. There are small nutrient vessels known

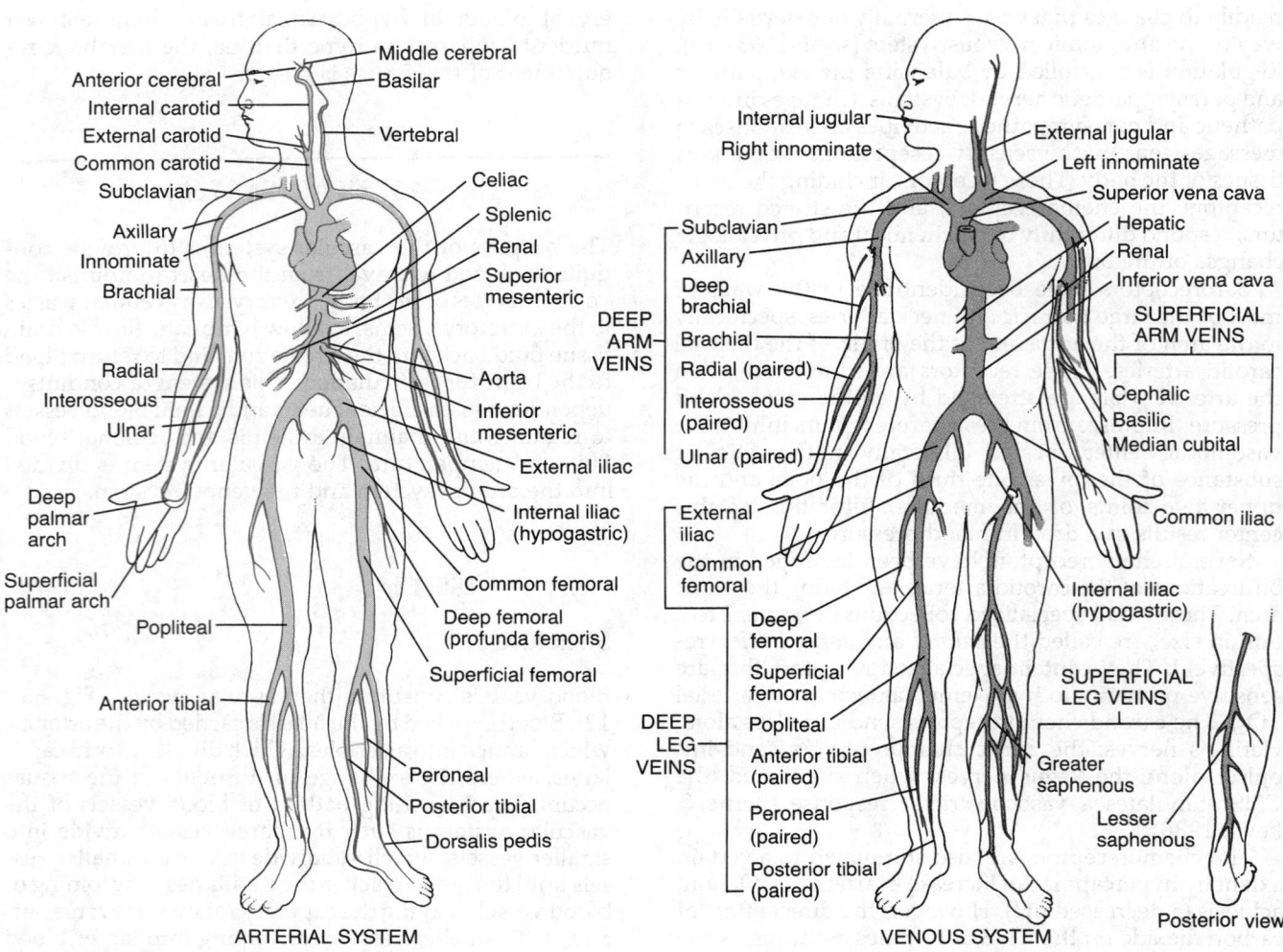

Figure 63–12

Anatomy of the arterial and venous systems.

as vasa vasorum that penetrate the outer portion of the media and the adventitia.

Structurally, deep veins have a thinner medial layer, which renders them distensible and collapsible. However, superficial veins of the extremities have relatively thick medial walls composed primarily of smooth muscle. This medial layer is able to hypertrophy in response to increases in pressures within the vessels. These changes are seen in the saphenous veins used as arterial bypass grafts. Veins are also equipped with valves, which permit unidirectional blood flow to the heart. Venous valves are generally found in the smaller, distal veins of the extremities. A few venous valves have been identified in the femoral veins, whereas the common iliac veins and venae cavae are valveless.

In the peripheral tissues, the capillaries bridge the arterial system and the venous system, providing for exchanges between the interstitial spaces and the blood (Fig. 63–14). Capillaries have two components: a single layer of endothelial cells and connective tissue fibers.

Function

As mentioned earlier, blood flow through a vessel occurs because of a pressure gradient between its two ends; fluid flows from a high-pressure area to a low-pressure area. The rate of blood flow through a vessel is determined by four factors: vessel size, viscosity of blood, metabolic autoregulation, and autonomic nervous system control.

Vessel Size

The size of the blood vessel is important because the quantity of blood that flows through a vessel in a given period of time is equal to the velocity (rate) of flow times the cross-sectional area. As the aorta and large proximal arteries progressively divide and arterial vessels become smaller in diameter, the total cross-sectional area of the vessels becomes progressively larger.

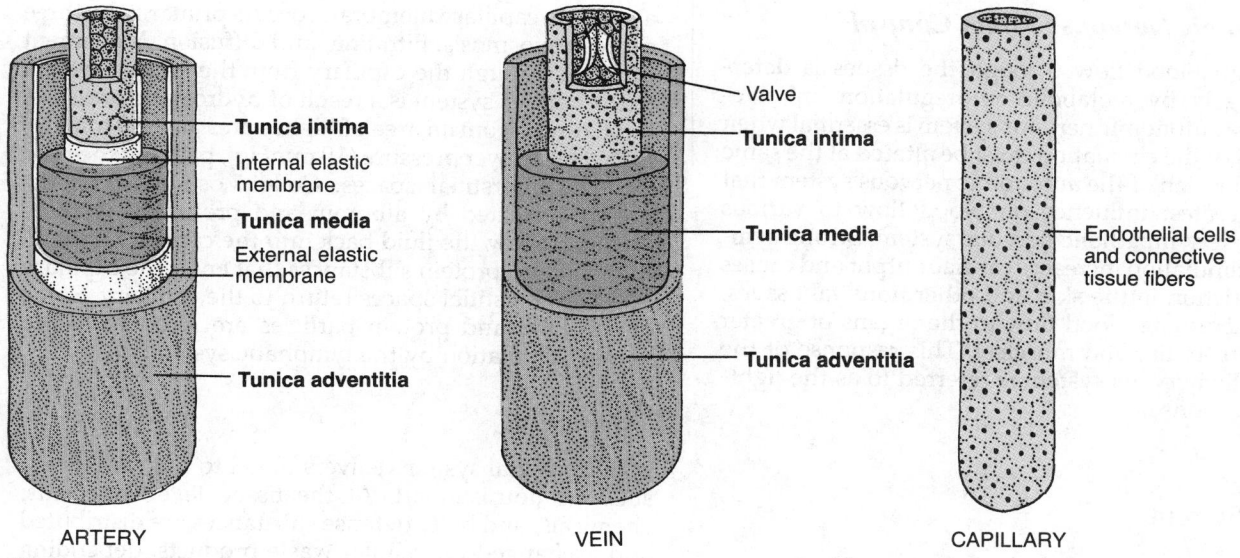

Figure 63–13

Microscopic anatomy of an artery, a vein, and a capillary.

The velocity of blood flow varies inversely with the cross-sectional areas of the lumina. Velocity of blood flow through a capillary is slower than through the aorta, allowing adequate time for the exchange of nutrients across the capillary membranes. The cross-sectional area of veins is about four or more times that in the adjacent arteries; thus, flow in the veins is reduced. Poiseuille's law relates blood flow through a blood vessel to the change in pressure, the luminal diameter, the length of the vessel, and the viscosity of blood (Berne & Levy, 1986; Tilkian & Daily, 1986). Of these factors, the size of the lumen of a blood vessel plays a greater role in determining the velocity of blood flow.

Blood vessels have the capacity to expand (*vasodilation* or venodilation) or contract (*vasoconstriction* or venoconstriction), affecting the flow of blood. Nerve impulses from the autonomic nervous system and hormonal stimulation can influence blood flow to the tissues by stimulating the vasomotor tone of the blood vessel. However, the metabolic needs of the tissues are the main determinants of the amount of vasoconstriction and local blood flow.

Viscosity of Blood

A direct correlation exists between the hematocrit and the viscosity of blood. When hematocrit increases to greater than 55% in the adult client, viscosity rises precipitously (Braunwald, 1988). With a greater viscosity, blood flow decreases and the tendency for blood to clot is enhanced, thereby further impairing blood flow.

Metabolic Autoregulation

The term *autoregulation* refers to the regulation of blood flow through a tissue in response to its need for nutrients and oxygen independent of any influence by the autonomic nervous system. The mechanism of autoregulation is not fully understood, but it appears that the level of oxygen concentration in the tissues is an important factor. Studies have shown that the arteries respond to increased oxygen concentration by constricting and to decreased levels of oxygen by dilating (Lane & Winslow, 1987).

Another metabolic factor that may influence local blood flow is the availability of amino acids, glucose, and fatty acids to the tissues relative to their internal needs (Lane & Winslow, 1987). The greater the rate of metabolism or decreased availability of nutrients, the greater is the rate of formation of vasodilator substances, such as lactic acid or bradykinin. These substances may diffuse or circulate back, causing vasodilation of the precapillary sphincters, meta-arterioles, and arterioles.

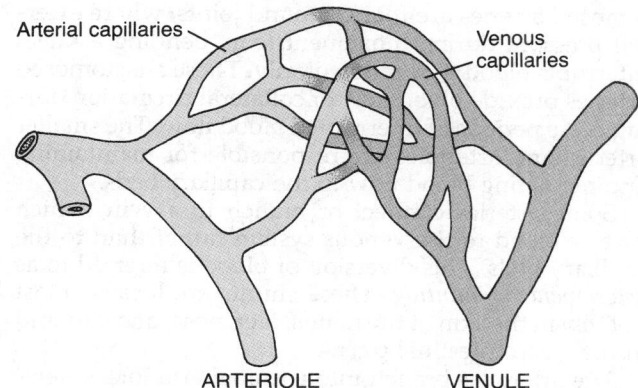

Figure 63–14

Capillary bed.

Autonomic Nervous System Control

Although blood flow through the tissues is determined largely by metabolic autoregulation, involvement of the autonomic nervous system is essential when large parts of the circulation must be altered at the same time. The branch of the autonomic nervous system that has the greatest influence on blood flow to various organs is the sympathetic nervous system. Strong sympathetic stimulation increases cardiac output and causes vasoconstriction in the skin and other nonvital tissues, thereby increasing blood flow to the organs of greater need (heart, brain, and muscles). This response of the sympathetic nervous system is referred to as the fight-or-flight response.

Arterial System

Structure

The high-pressure blood vessels of the arterial system may be classified according to their size, wall structure, or function (conductive or distributive). Arteries are referred to as conductive or distributive vessels, because they provide a continuous flow of blood from the heart to the periphery. The large, or conductive, arteries follow relatively straight routes and have few branches. Conductive arteries include the aorta, the common and external iliac arteries, the femoral arteries, and the popliteal arteries. These conductive arteries tend to be most affected by atherosclerosis. The distributive arteries divide from the conductive arteries and have multiple branches. Distributive arteries include the mesenteric arteries of the abdomen, the internal iliac arteries, and the deep femoral vessels. Some arteries have features of both conductive and distributive vessels; these include the anterior and posterior tibial arteries. The structure and function of the vasculature of the cerebrum, the abdomen, and the viscera are discussed as they relate to each body system. Some arteries branch into arterioles, which measure less than 0.5 mm in diameter, whereas some arteries anastomose with other arteries. The anastomosed arteries are found around joints, where external pressure during movement (e.g., bending a knee) interrupts blood flow momentarily. These anastomosed arteries provide blood flow or collateral circulation during these periods of interrupted blood flow. The smaller arteries and arterioles are responsible for maintaining and regulating blood flow to the capillary beds.

Some arteries connect or branch to a vein, which diverts blood to the venous system rather than to the capillary beds. This diversion of blood is referred to as *arteriovenous shunting*. These shunts are located most notably in the skin of the hands, feet, nose, and ears and in the gastrointestinal tract.

The arterioles branch into terminal arterioles (metaarterioles), which join with the capillary or capillaries and ultimately join with venules, forming the capillary network (see Fig. 63–14). The exchange of nutrients across the capillary membrane occurs primarily by three processes: osmosis, filtration, and diffusion. Movement of fluids through the capillary from the arterial system to the venous system is a result of hydrostatic pressure; fluid moves from an area of higher pressure (30 mmHg) to that of a lower pressure (10 mmHg), pushing the fluid into the interstitial spaces. Colloid osmotic (oncotic) pressure created by albumin and protein substances works to draw the fluid back into the capillary. Not all the fluid and protein substances that enter the capillary and the interstitial spaces return to the capillary. Some of the fluid and protein particles are rerouted to the venous circulation by the lymphatic system.

Function

The arterial system delivers blood to the various tissues for nourishment. At the tissue level, nutrients, chemicals, and body defense substances are distributed and exchanged for cellular waste products, depending on the needs of the particular tissue. The arteries transport the cellular wastes to the excretory organs, such as the kidneys, the liver, and the lungs, to be reprocessed or removed. The arteries also contribute to tissue temperature regulation. Blood can be either directed toward the skin to promote heat loss or diverted away from the skin to conserve heat.

Venous System

Structure

The venous system is composed of a series of veins that course adjacent to the arterial system. In addition, there is a second venous circulation that is superficial and runs parallel to the subcutaneous tissue of the extremity. These two venous systems are connected by communicating veins, which provide a means for blood to travel from the superficial veins to the deep veins. Blood flow is directed toward the deep venous circulation.

The venules collect blood from the capillaries and the terminal arterioles. Venules also serve as a location where white blood cells enter into and exit from the body tissues.

Venules branch into veins, which are called low-pressure blood vessels. Veins are also referred to as capacitance or reservoir vessels because they have a high degree of compliance. These vessels have the ability to accommodate large shifts in volume with minimal changes in venous pressure. This flexibility allows the venous system to accommodate the administration of intravenous (IV) fluids and blood transfusions, blood loss, and dehydration. The venous system can contain approximately 50% to 60% of the body's total blood volume. In both the superficial and deep venous systems, all veins, except for the smallest and largest, have valves directing blood flow back to the heart, preventing retrograde flow.

Function

The primary function of the venous system is to provide for the return of blood from the capillaries to the right side of heart for circulation. It also acts as a reservoir for a large portion of the blood volume. In contrast to the arterial system, which consists of a high-pressure, laminar flow system through relatively rigid conduits, the venous system consists of a low-pressure, intermittent flow system through collapsible tubes working against the effects of gravity.

Several factors can facilitate or hinder venous return to the heart. These factors include the pressure changes that occur during normal respiration: During the inspiratory phase, there is an increase in intra-abdominal pressure and a decrease in intrathoracic pressure, resulting in an increase in venous return in the veins of the chest, the abdomen, and the upper extremities. Lower-extremity flow to the heart is augmented during the expiratory phase.

Another important factor that facilitates venous return is the musculovenous pump. The contracting muscles of the extremities squeeze blood from the veins toward the heart. Competent venous valves prevent the escape of blood in the reverse direction (retrograde flow).

On the other hand, gravity exerts an increase in hydrostatic pressure (blood pressure) when the client is in an upright position, which acts to impede venous return. When the client is recumbent, the hydrostatic pressure is lessened, and thus there is less hindrance of venous return to the heart.

Lymphatic System

The lymphatic system, an auxiliary venous system, consists of an elaborate and extensive capillary network that serves to collect lymph (which has the same consistency as plasma, except it contains more albumin than globulin) from the various organs and tissues. Lymph is collected from the intercellular fluid, travels to the plexuses and collecting channels, is transported to the blood stream, and empties into the venous system (Fig. 63–15).

Structure

The lymphatic system begins with dead-end vessels resembling capillaries lying near the veins. The vessels of the lymphatic system are similar in structure to veins, but contain many more valves. It is postulated that the larger lymph vessels are innervated by the CNS. These vessels are located near other blood vessels throughout the body, except in the CNS.

The lymphatics begin as small, thin, vein-like vessels and merge into larger lymphatic vessels. Lymph nodes (small, oval bodies of lymphoid tissue) are situated along the path of these collecting vessels and serve as

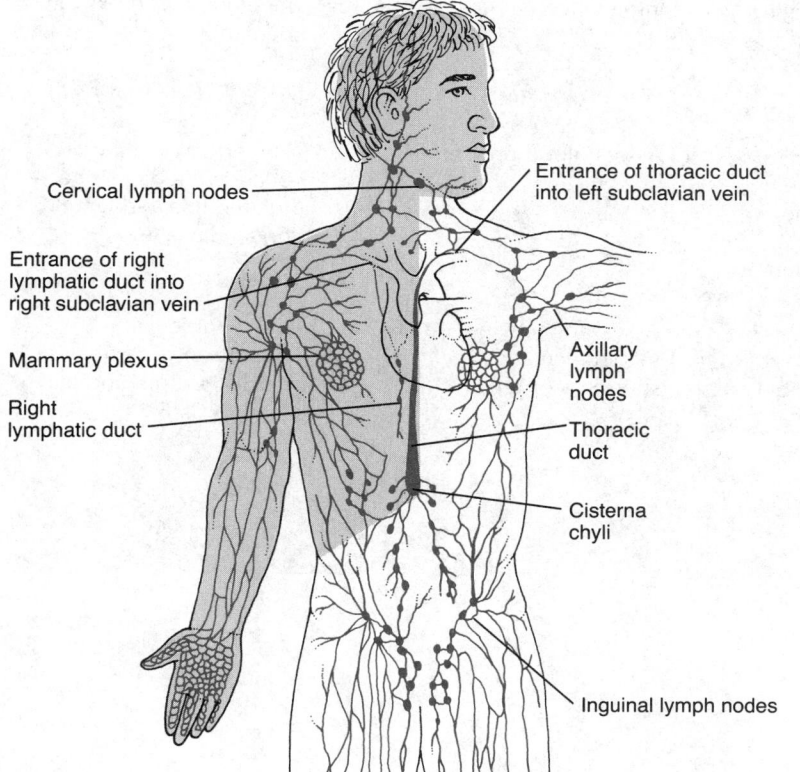

Cervical lymph nodes

Entrance of right lymphatic duct into right subclavian vein

Mammary plexus

Right lymphatic duct

Entrance of thoracic duct into left subclavian vein

Axillary lymph nodes

Thoracic duct

Cisterna chyli

Inguinal lymph nodes

Figure 63–15

The lymphatic system. Lymph in the shaded area returns to the circulatory system through the right lymphatic duct. Lymph in the rest of the body returns through the thoracic duct.

FOCUS ON THE ELDERLY ■ Changes in the Cardiovascular System Related to Aging

Structure/Function	Change	Interventions	Rationales
Cardiac valves	Thicken and stiffen owing to lipid accumulation, degeneration of collagen, and valve fibrosis.	1. Assess heart sounds for murmurs.	1. Systolic ejection murmurs are common in the elderly owing to valve thickening and stiffness.
Conduction system	Decrease in number of pacemaker cells and increase in fibrous tissue and fat in the SA node. Few muscle fibers in the atrial myocardium and bundle of His.	1. Assess ECG and heart rhythm for arrhythmias or heart rate less than 60 beats/min.	1. SA node may lose its inherent rhythm.
Left ventricle	Increases in size.	1. Assess ECG for longer PR and QT intervals.	1. Conduction time increases.
	Becomes stiff and less distensible. Longer ejection phase and delay in early diastolic filling to compensate for stiff ventricle, allowing heart to more effectively "empty."	2. Assess for activity intolerance.	2. Ventricular changes result in decreased stroke volume, ejection fraction, and cardiac output; the heart is less able to meet increased oxygen demands.
		3. Assess heart rate at rest and with activity.	3. Maximal heart rate with exercise is decreased.
Blood flow in coronary vessels	Distribution changes, with more blood flowing to venous vessels and sinusoids and less flowing to coronary arteries.	1. Assess for activity intolerance.	1. Heart is less able to meet increased oxygen demands.
Aorta and large arteries	Thicken and become stiffer and less distensible. Systolic blood pressure increases to compensate for stiff arteries.	1. Assess blood pressure.	1. Hypertension may occur, which must be treated to avoid target organ damage.
	Systemic vascular resistance increases as a result of less distensible arteries, so the left ventricle pumps against greater resistance contributing to left ventricular hypertrophy.	2. Assess for activity intolerance and shortness of breath.	2. Left ventricular hypertrophy decreases cardiac output and may lead to CHF.

FOCUS ON THE ELDERLY ■ Changes in the Cardiovascular System Related to Aging *Continued*

Structure/Function	Change	Interventions	Rationales
Baroreceptors	Become less sensitive.	1. Assess blood pressure with the client lying and sitting or standing. 2. Assess for dizziness when client changes from a lying to a sitting or standing position. 3. Teach clients to change positions slowly.	1–3. Orthostatic (postural) changes occur owing to ineffective baroreceptors. Changes may include drop in blood pressure of 10 mmHg or more, dizziness, or fainting.

filters. The larger lymphoid tissues, which function as collecting and filtering chambers, include the cisterna chyli, the thoracic duct, and the right lymphatic duct. The lymphoid organs, which are the sites of lymphocyte production, include the tonsils, the thymus, the walls of the intestine, and the spleen. The circulating lymphocytes remove foreign substances from the lymph before it is emptied into the venous system.

Lymph from the legs and the left side of the body empties into the thoracic duct and left subclavian vein. The right lymphatic duct and the right subclavian vein serve as collecting chambers for lymph draining from the right thorax, the right arm, and the right side of the head.

Function

The importance of the lymphatic system cannot be overstated. One of its functions is to develop, maintain, and repair the immune system. The lymphatics collect microorganisms in the interstitial spaces and carry them to the lymph nodes, where the macrophages and lymphocytes engulf the microorganisms.

Digested fat particles (chylomicrons) are reabsorbed by the lymph capillaries (lacteals) of the small intestine of the digestive tract. The lymphatics also collect fluid and proteins from the interstitial spaces and transport them back to the veins; this function helps in preventing edema.

CARDIOVASCULAR CHANGES ASSOCIATED WITH AGING

A number of physiologic changes in the cardiovascular system occur with advancing age (see the accompanying Focus on the Elderly feature). The changes are most often noticeable when elderly clients are stressed, because their hearts cannot meet increased metabolic demands.

HISTORY

The nurse obtains a thorough history, which includes demographic data, personal and family history, diet, socioeconomic status, and a functional health pattern assessment. Information relative to risk factors and symptoms of cardiovascular disease are the focus of the history.

DEMOGRAPHIC DATA

Demographic data include the client's *age, sex,* and *ethnic origin. Height* and *weight* of the client are included. Throughout the aging process, the incidence of conditions such as coronary artery disease (CAD) and valvular disease increases (Braunwald, 1988; Coodley, 1985; Epiopoulos, 1987). Information about the client's ethnic background can be important because some disease conditions may be more prevalent in specific ethnic groups. For example, high blood pressure is more prevalent in Black individuals. However, ethnicity may imply life style or personal habits that may be modifiable. It is also known that, with increasing age, men have a greater incidence of CAD than women (Braunwald, 1988). Women who are postmenopausal have a lower incidence of CAD than men.

Age, sex, and ethnic background, as well as a family history of cardiovascular disease, are considered non-modifiable or uncontrollable risk factors for cardiovascular disease (Braunwald, 1988). Clients identified with any one or combination of modifiable risk factors (e.g., high blood pressure, excessive weight, and excessive blood cholesterol level) are especially important to work with because altering risk factors known to be modifiable or controllable can reduce the risk of heart disease.

PERSONAL AND FAMILY HISTORY

Major illnesses, such as diabetes mellitus, renal disease, anemia, high blood pressure, stroke, gout, bleeding disorders, collagen diseases, chronic pulmonary diseases, heart disease, and thrombophlebitis, must be noted, especially if any have particular influence on the client's cardiovascular status. Previous hospitalizations may have included treatment for injuries, operations, and diagnostic testing (e.g., ECG and cardiac catheterization) in either an inpatient or an outpatient (ambulatory) setting. It is important that the client be specifically asked about *streptococcal infections* and *rheumatic fever;* these conditions may lead to valvular abnormalities of the heart. In addition, the nurse inquires about any known *congenital heart defects.*

Clients are asked about any known *sensitivity to penicillin* or any drugs that may be administered in an emergency, such as lidocaine hydrochloride. A thorough assessment of all prescription *drugs* and over-the-counter drugs is imperative. The nurse specifically asks female clients if they are taking oral contraceptives. There is an increased incidence of MI and cerebrovascular accident in older women who take oral contraceptives, but only if they smoke, have diabetes, or have hypertension (Mishell, 1989).

A *family history* includes information about the age and health status, as well as deaths, of immediate family members (i.e., parents, sibling, spouse, and children). Information on the extended family, including grandparents or grandchildren, may also be elicited. This information can be recorded in a narrative outline or as a diagram with the client's history.

DIET HISTORY

A diet history may include intake during a 24-hour period and any dietary restrictions or supplements. The type of foods selected by the client should be examined for any excesses in sodium, sugar, cholesterol, and fat. These elements have been associated with CAD and high blood pressure. A diet history also examines the client's attitudes toward food, knowledge level of essential and nonessential dietary elements, and willingness to make changes in the diet. Cultural beliefs and economic status can influence the client's choice of food items and must be considered before changes are made in the diet regimen. Spouses or significant others who are responsible for shopping and cooking are included in the discussion of diet to ensure institution of suggested changes.

SOCIOECONOMIC STATUS

Social history includes information about the client's domestic situation, such as marital status, number of children, household members, living environment, and occupation. Support systems can also be identified.

Information about the client's occupation includes the type of work performed and the requirements to do the specified job. Does the job involve lifting of heavy objects? Is the job emotionally stressful? What does a day's work entail? Has there been any recent change in how long it takes to get a day's work completed? Are there any recent changes that inhibit or delay the client's work? Socioeconomic history also includes life style habits. Life style habits that are specific risk factors for heart disease include cigarette smoking, alcohol intake, illicit drug intake, physical inactivity, obesity, weight changes, and emotional stress. These factors are considered to be modifiable or controllable risk factors.

Cigarette smoking is a major risk factor for cardiovascular disease, specifically CAD and peripheral vascular disease (AHA, 1989). Three compounds in cigarette smoke, tar, nicotine, and carbon monoxide, have been implicated in the development of CAD. The smoking history should include the number of cigarettes smoked daily, the duration of this smoking habit, the age of the client when smoking started, and the pattern of inhaling. Typically, the smoking history is recorded as pack-years, which is the number of packs per day multiplied by the number of years.

Physical inactivity is also considered a significant risk factor in the development of CAD. Routine aerobic exercise is thought to confer protection from complications of CAD and to lower blood pressure. However, rigorous physical activity such as marathon running has been associated with sudden death in individuals, even those without a history of cardiovascular disease.

With regard to *emotional stress* and its relationship to cardiovascular disease, researchers have identified individuals with type A personalities as being more vulnerable to development of heart disease (Braunwald, 1988). Type A personalities are highly competitive, experience time-urgency, and are impatient. Although there is a positive correlation between individuals identified as having type A personalities and heart disease, conclusive proof remains elusive. It is known, however, that emotional stress (through its influence on the CNS) has direct effects on the cardiovascular system, including increased oxygen requirements by the heart.

CURRENT HEALTH PROBLEM

Inquiring about the client's major symptom(s) helps the nurse to establish priorities in nursing care and management. Information obtained about any symptom must include the time and manner of onset, duration, chronology and frequency, location, quality, intensity, associated symptoms, and precipitating or aggravating factors. Major symptoms identified by clients with cardiovascular disease include the following: chest pain or discomfort, dyspnea, fatigue, palpitations, weight gain, syncope, and extremity pain.

CHEST PAIN

Chest pain or discomfort, a cardinal symptom of cardiac disease, can result from ischemic heart disease, pericarditis, and aortic dissection. Chest pain can also originate from other conditions, such as pleurisy, pulmonary embolus, hiatal hernia, and, more commonly, anxiety. Nurses must thoroughly evaluate the nature and characteristics of the client's chest pain. Because chest pain resulting from myocardial ischemia is life-threatening and can lead to serious complications, the cause of chest pain should be considered ischemic (reduced or obstructed blood flow to the myocardium) until proved otherwise.

When assessing for chest pain, the nurse uses alternative terms such as discomfort, heaviness, or indigestion to elicit information from the client. Often, clients deny a true pain in the chest, but admit to discomfort or a feeling of indigestion, thus understating the significance of the event (see the accompanying Nursing Research feature). The client may also use other descriptors, such as aching, choking, strangling, tingling, squeezing, or constricting.

The nurse assesses when the pain was first noticed (onset). Did the pain begin suddenly or develop gradually over time (manner of onset)? How long did the pain last (duration)? If the client has repeated chest pain episodes, the nurse assesses how long the pain usually lasts (chronology and frequency). Is this pain different from any other episodes of pain? The nurse asks the client to describe what activities he/she was doing at the time it first occurred (e.g., eating dinner, watching television, arguing, or running) (precipitating factors). The client can point to the area where the chest pain occurred. Did the pain stay in one specific area or did it radiate (location)? If the client makes a tight fist over the center of the chest, this is referred to as Levine's sign, a classic sign that strongly indicates that the chest pain is a result of ischemia.

In addition, the client may describe how the pain feels and whether it is sharp or dull (quality). To understand how severe the pain is, the nurse may ask the client to grade the pain from 1 to 10, with the higher numbers indicating a more severe pain (intensity). The client may also report other signs and symptoms that occur at the same time (associated symptoms), such as dyspnea, diaphoresis, nausea, and vomiting. Other factors that need to be addressed are those that may have made the chest pain worse (aggravating factors) or made the pain less intense (relieving factors). It is imperative that the nurse address these areas to ascertain the origin of the client's chest pain. When the possibility of myocardial ischemia has been ruled out, questions to determine other causes can be asked.

After obtaining the history of the client's cardiac status, the client may be classified according to the New York Heart Association's Functional Classification (Table 63–1). The four classifications (I, II, III, and IV) depend on the degree to which ordinary physical activities (routine activities of daily living [ADL]) are affected by heart disease.

NURSING RESEARCH

Clients in Coronary Care Units Are Not Reporting Chest Pain.

Schneider, A. C. (1987). Unreported chest pain in a coronary care unit. *Focus on Critical Care, 14*(5), 21–24.

The client's subjective report of chest pain is a key indicator of myocardial ischemia. Nurses caring for clients in coronary care units (CCUs) need to know when clients are experiencing chest pain, so they can intervene to prevent MI or extension of myocardial damage. This descriptive study was done to assess the extent of unreported chest pain of clients in CCUs. Nineteen clients with documented or suspected MIs were interviewed within the first 48 hours after transfer from a CCU. Fourteen described one or more episodes of chest pain that they did not report to the CCU staff at the time of the occurrence. Reasons for not reporting the pain were that (1) the pain was not considered severe enough; (2) the client did not want to bother the staff or complain; (3) the client waited to see if the pain went away on its own; (4) there was a misunderstanding in communication (one client, who was experiencing "burning" in his chest, did not report its presence because staff wanted to know about chest "pain"); (5) no particular reason was given.

Critique. The sample in this study was small and was representative of clients in only one unit and one hospital. However, the finding that the majority of these clients did not report chest pain is significant. The study should be repeated in other CCUs.

Possible nursing implications. Nurses need to teach all clients at risk for myocardial injury the physiologic significance of chest discomfort. Nurses should emphasize that any abnormal feeling in the chest, the arms, the back, or the jaw is significant, and it need not be painful. Nurses should also frequently ask clients about the presence of chest discomfort in case clients are not reporting it.

DYSPNEA

Dyspnea is a symptom that can occur from both cardiac and pulmonary disease. *Dyspnea* is described as difficult or labored breathing and is associated with changes in activity. More often, clients report shortness of breath with exertion with cardiac disease, unless they have end-stage heart disease. Clients with pulmonary disease usually report shortness of breath at rest and with an increase in activity, such as walking.

There are several different types of dyspnea. When obtaining the client's history, the nurse ascertains what factors precipitate and relieve dyspnea, what level of

---

TABLE 63–1 New York Heart Association Functional Classification of Cardiovascular Disability

Class I

Clients with cardiac disease but without resulting limitations of physical activity.

Ordinary physical activity does not cause undue fatigue, palpitation, dyspnea, or anginal pain.

Class II

Clients with cardiac disease resulting in slight limitation of physical activity.

They are comfortable at rest.

Ordinary physical activity results in fatigue, palpitation, dyspnea, or anginal pain.

Class III

Clients with cardiac disease resulting in marked limitation of physical activity.

They are comfortable at rest.

Less than ordinary physical activity causes fatigue, palpitation, dyspnea, or anginal pain.

Class IV

Clients with cardiac disease resulting in inability to carry on any physical activity without discomfort.

Symptoms of cardiac insufficiency or of the anginal syndrome may be present even at rest.

If any physical activity is undertaken, discomfort is increased.

Excerpted from *Diseases of the heart and blood vessels — nomenclature and criteria for diagnosis,* 6th edition, Boston, Little, Brown and Company, copyright 1964 by the New York Heart Association, Inc.

---

activity produces dyspnea, and what the assumed body position was when dyspnea first occurred.

Dyspnea that is associated with exertional activity, such as climbing stairs, is referred to as *dyspnea on exertion.* This is usually an early symptom of heart dysfunction (congestive heart failure [CHF]).

Another symptom that the client may describe is dyspnea that occurs in the lateral recumbent position. This symptom is referred to as *orthopnea* and usually indicates a more advanced stage of heart failure. A client may use several pillows at night to elevate the head and prevent nighttime breathlessness. The severity of orthopnea is measured by the number of pillows needed to provide restful sleep. Orthopnea is relieved within a matter of minutes by sitting up or standing.

Paroxysmal nocturnal dyspnea occurs when the client is sleeping. When the client is in a lateral recumbent position, blood from the splanchnic beds and lower extremities is redistributed to the venous system, thereby increasing venous return. This increase in blood volume returning to the heart elevates pulmonary venous and pulmonary arterial pressures. A diseased heart is unable to compensate for the increased intravascular volume and is ineffective in pumping the additional fluid into the circulatory system, and thus pulmonary congestion results. Clients awaken abruptly and sit upright with their legs dangled over the bedside to relieve the dyspnea. It may take as long as 20 minutes before the client obtains relief, which can be quite distressing.

FATIGUE

Fatigue may be described as the inability to complete routine ADL. The client may indicate that a certain activity takes longer to complete. Fatigue in itself is not diagnostic of heart disease. Nevertheless, in clients with heart disease, fatigue may result from nocturia, insomnia, and exertional and nocturnal dyspnea. Fatigue that occurs after mild activity and exertion is usually indicative of an inadequate cardiac output (low stroke volume). Clients often require one or two naps during the day.

PALPITATIONS

A feeling of fluttering in the chest or an unpleasant awareness of the heart beat is referred to as *palpitations.* Palpitations may result from a change in heart rate or rhythm or from an increase in the force of heart contractions. Rhythm disturbances that may cause palpitations include paroxysmal atrial tachycardia, premature contractions, or sinus tachycardia. Palpitations that occur during or after strenuous physical activity, such as running or swimming, may indicate overexertion or possibly heart disease. Some noncardiac factors that may precipitate palpitations include anxiety, stress, fatigue, insomnia, and ingestion of caffeine, nicotine, or alcohol.

WEIGHT GAIN

A sudden increase in weight of 2.2 lb (1 L of fluid) can be the result of an accumulation of excessive fluid in the interstitial spaces, commonly known as *edema.* It is possible, however, for weight gains of up to 10 to 15 lb (4 to 7 L of fluid) to occur before any associated edema occurs (Mason et al., 1980). Clients with heart disease who are receiving diuretic therapy must be taught to weigh themselves daily. Normally, basal body weight varies little on a daily basis; thus, small, yet subtle, changes in weight can be detected early.

Peripheral edema and weight gain are clinical indicators of right-sided heart failure. Other causes may include fluid overload caused by saline excess and venous obstruction from an injury. Edema may be localized to a specific area, and measurements of the girth of parts can be assessed. Generalized edema is referred to as *anasarca.*

SYNCOPE

Syncope refers to a transient loss of consciousness. The most common cause is decreased perfusion to the brain. Any condition that suddenly reduces the cardiac output, resulting in decreased cerebral blood flow, could potentiate a syncopal episode. Conditions such as cardiac rhythm disturbances (ventricular dysrhythmias or Stokes-Adams attack) or valvular disorders (aortic or subaortic stenosis) may potentiate this symptom.

Near-syncope refers to dizziness with an inability to remain in an upright position. Circumstances that lead to dizziness or syncope must be explored.

Syncope in the aging client may result from hypersensitivity of the carotid sinus bodies, located in the neck arteries. Pressure applied to the carotid arteries, by way of turning the head, shrugging the shoulders, shaving, or buttoning a shirt, stimulates a vagal response. A decrease in blood pressure and heart rate usually results, but an exaggerated response may produce syncope.

EXTREMITY PAIN

Extremity pain may result from two conditions: ischemia from atherosclerosis or venous insufficiency of the peripheral blood vessels. Clients who report an aching sensation in their legs associated with an activity such as walking have intermittent claudication. Extremity pain is usually relieved by resting or elevating the affected extremity. Leg pain that results from prolonged standing or sitting is related to venous insufficiency either from incompetent valves or venous obstruction.

PHYSICAL ASSESSMENT

A thorough physical assessment serves as the foundation for the nursing data base and the formation of nursing diagnoses. Any changes noted during the client's hospital course can be compared with this initial data base. Vital signs (blood pressure, pulse rate, and respiration rate) are evaluated when the client is admitted to the hospital and every 4 hours until the condition of the client improves. Assessment is a dynamic process and, depending on the condition of the client, may need to be done more frequently or perhaps once per nursing shift.

GENERAL APPEARANCE

Examination begins with the client's general appearance. The following areas are assessed: the *general build and appearance* of the client, as well as *skin color, distress level, level of consciousness, presence of shortness of breath, position,* and *verbal responses.*

Clients with chronic heart failure may appear malnourished, thin, and cachectic. Latent signs of severe heart failure are ascites, jaundice, and anasarca as a result of prolonged congestion of the liver. Heart failure may result in fluid retention, and clients may have engorged neck veins and edema.

CAD is suspected in clients with yellow lipid–filled plaques on the upper eyelids (xanthelasma) or earlobe creases. Clients with poor cardiac output and decreased cerebral perfusion may have mental confusion, memory loss, and slowed verbal responses.

INTEGUMENTARY SYSTEM

Assessment and evaluation of the integumentary system is determined by the *color, turgor, mobility, texture, and temperature* of the skin. The best areas to assess circulation include the nail beds, mucous membranes, and the conjunctival mucosa because the blood vessels are located near the surface of the skin. If there is normal blood flow or adequate perfusion of a given area, it appears pink, perhaps rosy in color, and warm to touch. Decreased flow is depicted as cool, pale-looking, and moist skin. Pallor (pale skin) is characteristic of anemia and can be seen in areas such as the nail beds, the palms, and the conjunctival mucous membranes.

A bluish discoloration of the skin and mucous membranes is referred to as *cyanosis.* Cyanosis results from an increased amount of deoxygenated hemoglobin.

In central cyanosis, there is decreased oxygenation of the arterial blood in the lungs, which manifests as a bluish tinge of the conjunctivae and the mucous membranes of the mouth and tongue. Central cyanosis may indicate impaired lung function or a right-to-left shunt found in congenital heart conditions or ventricular septal defect.

As a result of impaired circulation, there is a marked desaturation of hemoglobin in the peripheral tissues, which produces a bluish discoloration of nail beds, earlobes, lips, and toes. Peripheral cyanosis occurs in severe heart disease when blood flow to the peripheral vessels is decreased by peripheral vasoconstriction. The clamping down of the peripheral blood vessels is the result of a low cardiac output or an increased extraction of oxygen from the peripheral tissues. Peripheral cyanosis localized in an extremity is usually a result of arterial or venous obstruction.

The temperature of the skin can be assessed for symmetry by touching different areas of the client's body (e.g., arms, hand, legs, and feet) with the dorsal surface of the hand or fingers. Decreased blood flow results in a decrease in temperature to the dermis. There are several clinical conditions in which skin temperature is lowered, including CHF, peripheral vascular disease, and shock.

EXTREMITIES

The hands, arms, feet, and legs must be assessed for *skin changes, vascular changes, clubbing, capillary filling,* and *edema.* Skin mobility and turgor are affected by the fluid status of the client. Dehydration and aging reduce skin turgor, and edema decreases skin mobility. Vascular changes of an affected extremity may include paresthesia, muscle fatigue and discomfort, numbness, pain, poikilothermy (coolness), and loss of hair distribution from a reduced blood supply. Clubbing of the fingers and toes results from chronic oxygen deprivation in these tissue beds. Clubbing is characteristic in clients with advanced chronic obstructive pulmonary disease, congenital heart defects, and cor pulmonale. Clubbing can be identified by assessing the angle of the nail bed. The angle of the normal nail bed is 160 degrees; with clubbing, the angle of the nail bed increases to greater than 180 degrees and the base of the nail becomes spongy. Figure 63–16 describes assessment of clubbing using the Schamrath method.

Capillary filling of the fingers and toes is an indicator of peripheral circulation. Pressing or blanching the nail bed of a finger or toe produces a whitening effect; when pressure is released, a brisk return of color should occur in the nail bed. If color returns within 3 seconds, peripheral circulation is considered intact. If the capillary refill time exceeds 3 seconds, the lack of circulation may be due to arterial insufficiency from atherosclerosis or spasm.

Edema is an accumulation of fluid in the interstitial spaces. The location of edema helps the nurse to determine its potential cause. Bilateral edema of the legs may be seen in clients with heart failure or with chronic venous insufficiency. Abdominal and leg edema can be seen in clients with heart disease and cirrhosis of the liver. Edema may also be noted in dependent areas, such as the sacrum, when a client is confined to bed. Edema can be graded, as described in Chapter 13. The nurse should document the location as precisely as possible (e.g., mid-tibial or sacral) and the number of centimeters from an anatomic landmark. Localized edema in one extremity may be the result of venous obstruction (thrombosis) or lymphatic blockage of the extremity (lymphedema).

BLOOD PRESSURE MEASUREMENT

The measurement of arterial blood pressure is done by the method of sphygmomanometry (see the accompanying Guidelines feature). This technique of measurement is described in greater detail in nursing skills books.

The normal blood pressure in adults older than 45 years of age ranges from 90 to 140 mmHg for systolic pressure and 60 to 90 mmHg for diastolic pressure (AHA, 1989). A blood pressure that exceeds 140/90 mmHg increases the workload of the left ventricle and oxygen consumption. A blood pressure less than 90/60 mmHg may be inadequate in providing proper and sufficient nutrition to the cells of the body.

POSTURAL BLOOD PRESSURE

Clients may report dizziness or lightheadedness when they move from a flat supine position to sitting or standing at the edge of the bed. Normally, these symptoms

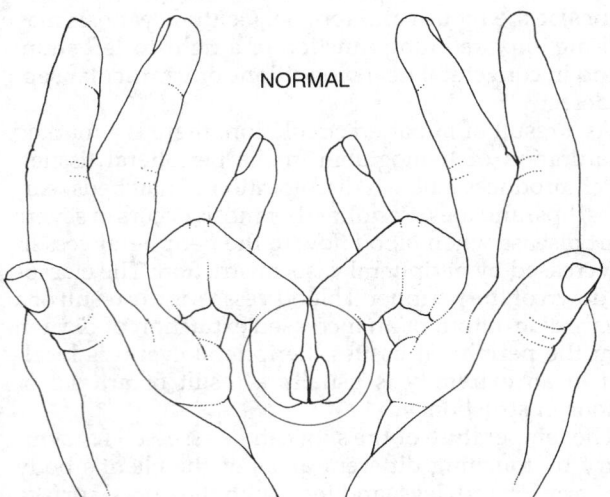
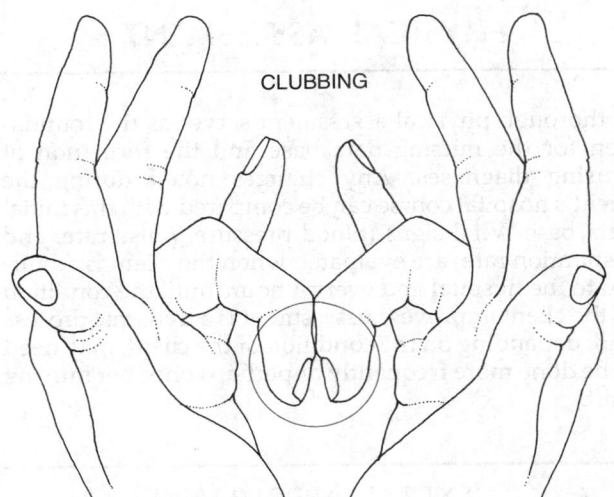

Figure 63–16

Assessment of clubbing by the Schamrath method. The client places the fingernails of the ring fingers together and holds them up to a light. If the examiner can see a diamond shape between the nails, there is no clubbing. Clubbing is identified by the absence of the diamond shape.

GUIDELINES ■ Tips for Accurate Blood Pressure Measurement

Select the proper cuff size:
>   Adult cuff size is 12 to 14 cm wide and 30 cm long.
>   Pediatric cuff size is 8 to 10 cm wide and 26 cm long.
>   Larger adult cuff size is 18 to 20 cm wide.

Ensure that equipment is properly assembled and calibrated:
>   Cuff bladder should be intact inside the cuff.
>   Sphygmomanometer should be calibrated to 0 mmHg every few months to ensure reliability.
>   Cuff must be placed above the area to be auscultated (e.g., if right arm used, the cuff is placed above the brachial artery).

Follow these steps to ensure correct blood pressure measurement and recording:
>   After the brachial or radial pulse is palpated, the cuff is inflated 30 mmHg above the level at which those pulses disappear. The cuff is released slowly to palpate the systolic pressure. The cuff is reinflated and systolic and diastolic pressures are auscultated. The auscultated pulses are referred to as Korotkoff's sounds.
>   Measurements should be recorded on both arms to rule out dissecting aortic aneurysm, coarctation of the aorta, vascular obstruction, and possibly errors in measurement. Subsequent readings should be done on the extremity with the highest pressure.
>   If arms are inaccessible (after amputation or mastectomy) pressures can be obtained using the client's thigh or calf. The popliteal artery or posterior tibial artery, respectively, is auscultated.
>   The nurse obtains and records blood pressure with the client in different positions, including supine, sitting, and standing.
>   The position of the client and the site used to obtain the blood pressure are recorded.

are transient and pass quickly; however, when these symptoms become pronounced, it may be due to postural (orthostatic) hypotension. Three conditions can cause postural hypotension: extracellular volume (saline) depletion from diuretic therapy; decreased vascular tone, leading to inadequate vasoconstricting properties; and autonomic insufficiency, which interferes with the nervous system control of heart rate.

It is important to note the position of the client (supine, sitting, or standing), the blood pressure in each position, and the pulse or heart rate in each position. With a change in position (supine to sitting), the normal fluctuation of blood pressure and heart rate is to increase slightly (about 5 mmHg for systolic and diastolic pressures and 5 to 10 beats per minute in heart rate). After changing the postural position (moving from supine to sitting) of the client, a time delay of 1 to 3 minutes should be permitted before auscultating a blood pressure and palpating the radial pulse. The cuff should remain in proper position on the client's arm. Any signs or symptoms of client distress should be observed and recorded. If the client is unable to tolerate the position change, he or she is returned to the previous position of comfort. Postural hypotension is defined as a blood pressure fall of more than 10 to 15 mmHg of the systolic pressure or a fall of more than 10 mmHg of the diastolic pressure *and* a 10% to 20% increase in heart rate; changes must be noted in both the blood pressure and the heart rate (Braunwald, 1988).

To differentiate between extracellular volume deficit and decreased vascular tone, it is important to obtain an accurate history from the client. Both of these conditions exhibit the same manifestations of postural hypotension. With extracellular volume depletion, both heart rate and vasoconstricting properties behave appropriately, but, because of depletion of extracellular fluid, these reflexes are unable to increase and maintain systolic pressure and thus a fall in blood pressure occurs. With decreased vascular tone, there is an increase in heart rate, but an inadequate vasoconstricting response and thus a fall in blood pressure. These two conditions can occur together, complicating the clinical picture.

As a client ages, the autonomic nervous system may lose the ability to rapidly compensate for gravitational effects of position change. With autonomic insufficiency, there is no increase in heart rate when the client moves to an upright position. Autonomic insufficiency can also occur from the effects of some cardiac drugs, including digoxin, calcium channel blockers, and beta-adrenergic blockers, that inhibit increases in heart rate.

PARADOXICAL BLOOD PRESSURE

Paradoxical blood pressure is defined as an exaggerated decrease in systolic pressure by more than 10 mmHg (normal is 3 to 10 mmHg) during the inspiratory phase of the respiratory cycle (Braunwald, 1988). It is sometimes referred to as pulsus paradoxus. Certain clinical conditions, including pericardial tamponade, constrictive pericarditis, and pulmonary hypertension, that potentially alter the filling pressures in the right and left ventricles may produce a paradoxical blood pressure. During inspiration, the filling pressures normally decrease slightly, but, with decreased fluid volume in the ventricles because of these pathologic conditions, there is an exaggerated or marked reduction in cardiac output.

A paradoxical blood pressure can be assessed by inflating the cuff approximately 20 mmHg above the systolic pressure. The cuff is slowly deflated by 1 to 2 mmHg/second until the first Korotkoff's sound is noted. This occurs at expiration, and sounds disappear during inspiration. The cuff is deflated until sounds are heard equally during both inspiration and expiration. The difference between these sounds determines the degree of paradox. If sounds during inspiration and expiration are more than 10 mmHg apart, pulsus paradoxus is present.

PULSE PRESSURE

The difference between the systolic and diastolic values is referred to as *pulse pressure*. A normal pulse pressure is 30 to 40 mmHg (Kennedy, 1988). This value can be used as an indirect measure of the client's cardiac output. An increased pulse pressure may be seen in clients with slow heart rates (bradycardia), aortic regurgitation, atherosclerosis, hypertension, and aging. Decreased pulse pressure results from increased peripheral vascular resistance and decreased stroke volume in clients with heart failure or cardiogenic shock. Decreased pulse pressure can also be seen in clients who are hypovolemic (e.g., owing to hemorrhage) or who have mitral stenosis or regurgitation.

VENOUS AND ARTERIAL PULSATIONS

Observations of the venous pulsations in the neck are used to assess the adequacy of blood volume and central venous pressure (CVP). Jugular venous pressure (JVP) can be assessed to estimate the filling volume and pressure on the right side of the heart (see the accompanying Guidelines feature). The right internal jugular vein is usually used to estimate JVP because this vessel contains fewer valves than the left.

JVP is normally 3 to 10 cm (Bates, 1987). Increases in JVP are caused by conditions such as right ventricular failure, tricuspid regurgitation or stenosis, pulmonary hypertension, cardiac tamponade, constrictive pericarditis, and hypovolemia.

Hepatojugular reflux is determined by positioning the client with the head of the bed elevated to 45 degrees and locating the internal jugular vein. The right upper abdomen is compressed for 30 to 40 seconds. If a sudden distention of the neck veins is noted, it is usually indicative of right-sided heart failure.

Assessment of arterial pulsations gives the nurse information about vascular integrity and circulation. All major peripheral pulses, including the temporal, carotid, brachial, radial, ulnar, femoral, popliteal, posterior tibial, and dorsalis pedis, need to be assessed for presence or absence, amplitude, contour, rhythm, rate, and equality. Examination of the peripheral arteries is done in a head-to-toe approach with a side-to-side comparison (Fig. 63–17).

A *hypokinetic pulse* is a weak pulsation indicative of a narrow pulse pressure. It is seen in clients with hypovolemia, aortic stenosis, and decreased cardiac output.

A *hyperkinetic pulse* is a large, bounding pulse caused by an increased ejection of blood. It is seen in clients with a high cardiac output (with exercise or thyrotoxicosis) or with increased sympathetic system activity (with pain, fever, or anxiety).

Pulsus alternans is a condition in which a weak pulse alternates with a strong pulse, despite a regular heart rhythm. It is seen in clients with severely depressed cardiac function. Clients may be asked to hold their breath to exclude any false readings. Palpation of the brachial or radial arteries may be used to assess this condition but is more accurately assessed by auscultation of blood pressure.

Pulsus biferiens (twice beating) occurs when the first peak of the pulsation is caused by the pulse pressure and the second peak is caused by reverberations from the peripheral circulation. It is seen in clients with aortic stenosis and aortic regurgitation.

Auscultation of the carotid arteries is necessary to assess for bruits. Using the bell of the stethoscope over the skin of the carotid artery with the client holding her/his breath, the nurse can assess for the absence or presence of sounds. Normally, there are no sounds if the carotid artery has uninterrupted blood flow. A *bruit* (swishing blood sound) can be heard with a narrowed carotid artery. A bruit may develop when the internal diameter of the vessel is narrowed by 50% or more (Fahey, 1988). A bruit does not indicate the severity of disease in the carotid arteries. Severity of disease is determined by Doppler's flow studies and arteriography.

LUNGS

Assessment of the respiratory system involves observing the shape and symmetry of the chest and respiratory movements. For further information on pulmonary assessment, refer to Chapter 60. The rate and character of respirations are noted and recorded. Normally, the adult client breathes at a rate of 12 to 20 breaths per minute (Bates, 1987).

In normal respiratory movement, the inspiratory phase (active phase) is shorter than expiration (passive

GUIDELINES ■ How to Assess Jugular Venous Pressure and Central Venous Pressure

1. Place the client in a supine position.
2. Raise the head of the bed to approximately 30 to 45 degrees.
3. Shine a light across the client's neck (tangential lighting) to highlight the pulsations of the internal jugular vein.
4. To differentiate the internal jugular vein from the carotid artery, occlude the internal jugular with a fingertip at its base, then release. This maneuver easily eliminates the pulse wave in the internal jugular vein.

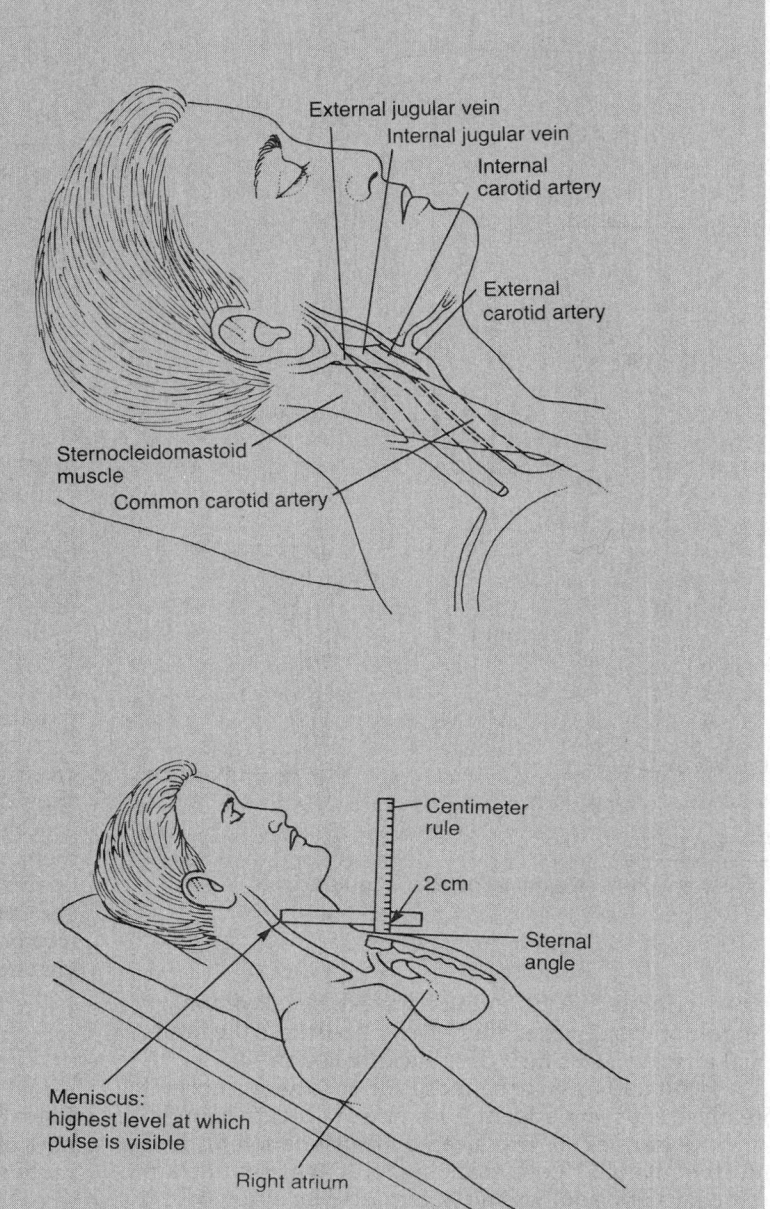

5. Locate the meniscus (the highest point at which pulsations of the internal jugular vein can be seen).
6. Locate the sternal angle (angle of Louis), which can be felt as a notch at the top of the sternum. It is roughly 4 cm above the right atrium.
7. With a centimeter rule, measure the vertical distance from the sternal angle to the meniscus of the internal jugular vein. The reading in centimeters equals the JVP, which generally does not exceed 4 cm.
8. To calculate CVP, add 4 cm to JVP.

phase). If muscles are used during expiration, it indicates forced expiration, which is a potentially early sign of CHF. Another early sign of heart failure is tachypnea, a rapid respiratory rate (> 24 breaths per minute).

A sudden, unexplained dyspnea may be due to pulmonary emboli or pulmonary infarction. Shallow respirations may indicate pain from pericarditis or pleurisy. Cheyne-Stokes respirations are often seen in aging clients with severe heart failure. These respirations are characterized by a cycle of shallow breathing that increases in rate and depth followed by a decrease in rate and depth and periods of apnea of notable duration. Cheyne-Stokes respirations are a common finding in clients with anemia and anoxic encephalopathy.

Noting the amount and color of sputum is important as well. Any sign of pink, frothy sputum (hemoptysis)

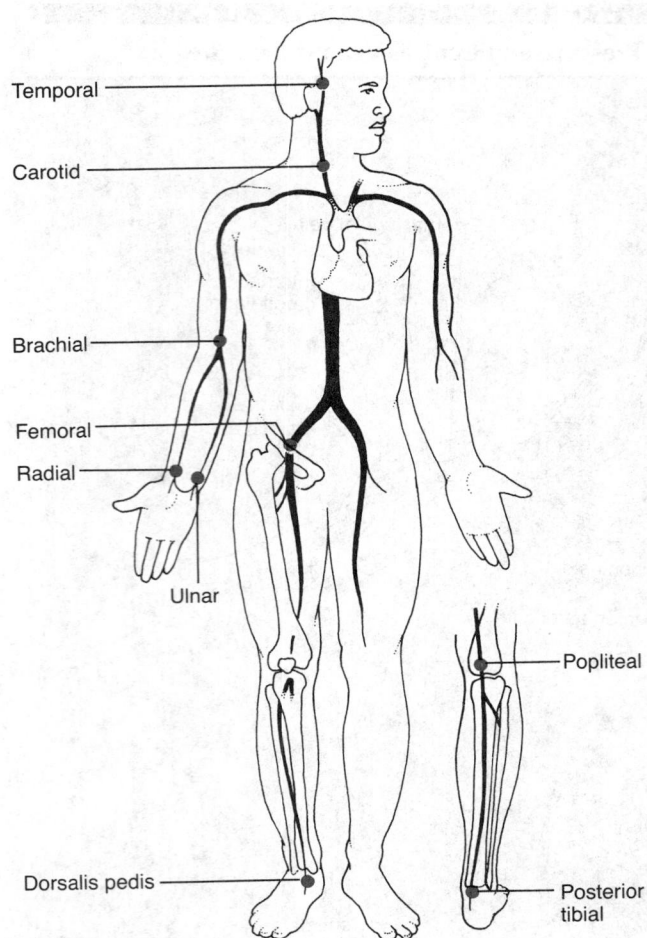

Figure 63–17

Pulse points for assessment of arterial pulses.

may be indicative of pulmonary edema. Pulmonary congestion from heart failure may also irritate the bronchial airways, causing a dry, hacking cough.

Auscultation of lung sounds is done to assess normal breath sounds and adventitious or extra breath sounds. Crackles or rales are produced by transudation of fluid into the alveoli. These crackling, crepitant sounds are best heard at peak inspiration and may be a sign of left ventricular failure. Crackles may also result from primary pulmonary conditions, such as atelectasis from prolonged bed rest and the effects of narcotics.

Wheezes are caused by movement of air through narrow bronchial tubes and sound like high-pitched, continuous musical sounds. Usually, wheezes are heard at the beginning of expiration but, as obstruction of the airways worsens, can be heard throughout the respiratory cycle. Wheezes can occur in clients with CHF.

Rhonchi have a coarse, rumbling sound similar to a snoring sound of someone sleeping. Although related to wheezes, rhonchi are caused by movements of air

through narrowed airways filled with fluid or secretions. These sounds are heard during inspiration or expiration.

ASSESSMENT OF THE PRECORDIUM

Assessment of the precordium is done by the techniques of inspection, palpation, percussion, and auscultation. It is helpful to have the client in a supine position with the head of the bed slightly elevated for the client's comfort. Some clients may require greater elevation of the head of the bed (to 45 degrees) for ease and comfort in breathing.

INSPECTION

Cardiac examination is usually done in a systematic order beginning with inspection. The chest should be inspected from the side, at a right angle, and downward over areas of the precordium where vibrations are visible. Cardiac motion is of low amplitude and sometimes the inward movements are more easily detected by the naked eye.

Seven precordial areas should be examined (Fig. 63–18). Any prominent precordial pulsations should be noted. Movement over the aortic, pulmonic, and tricuspid areas is abnormal. Pulsations in the mitral area are considered normal and are referred to as the *apical impulse*, or point of maximal impulse. The apical impulse should appear in the mitral area, the fifth intercostal space medial to the mid-clavicular line. If visible, movement of the apical impulse should appear with a rapid upstroke and downstroke no larger than the size of a quarter. If the apical impulse appears in more than one intercostal space and has shifted lateral to the mid-clavicular line, it may indicate left ventricular hypertrophy.

PALPATION

Palpation is done with the fingers and the most sensitive part of the palm of the hand for detecting precordial motion and thrills, respectively. The nurse palpates the seven precordial areas, starting with the aortic area. Turning the client on his/her left side brings the precordium closer to the surface of the chest and may be helpful in achieving maximal tactile sensitivity. When palpating for heaves or thrills, several factors should be considered, including the location, amplitude, duration, distribution, and timing in relation to the cardiac cycle.

The apical impulse must be assessed according to the above-mentioned factors. The apical impulse is localized (<3 cm) and is usually felt in only one intercostal space. It is associated with left ventricular contraction and can be felt after the first heart sound. The duration of the apical impulse is brief (<0.08 second), and the

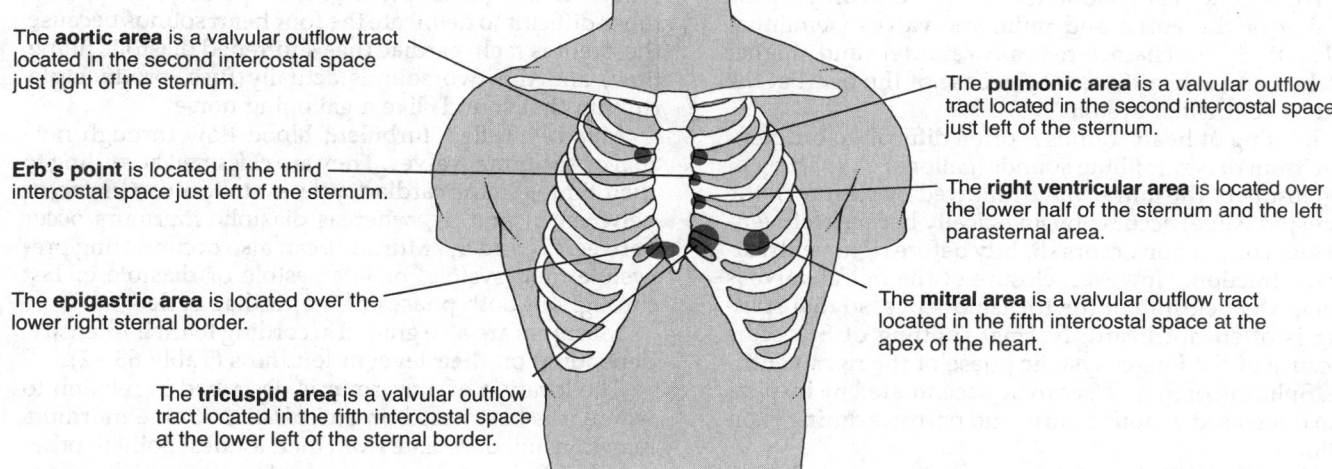

The **aortic area** is a valvular outflow tract located in the second intercostal space just right of the sternum.

The **pulmonic area** is a valvular outflow tract located in the second intercostal space just left of the sternum.

Erb's point is located in the third intercostal space just left of the sternum.

The **right ventricular area** is located over the lower half of the sternum and the left parasternal area.

The **epigastric area** is located over the lower right sternal border.

The **mitral area** is a valvular outflow tract located in the fifth intercostal space at the apex of the heart.

The **tricuspid area** is a valvular outflow tract located in the fifth intercostal space at the lower left of the sternal border.

Figure 63–18

Areas for myocardial inspection, palpation, and auscultation.

amplitude is palpated as an instantaneous "tap." If the nurse is unable to locate the apical impulse, rolling the client on his/her left side helps to determine the actual presence of the impulse, but not its size or position. A sustained and displaced apical impulse indicates left ventricular enlargement.

An abnormal forceful thrust accompanied by a sustaining outward movement felt over the left anterior chest is usually indicative of left ventricular enlargement. An outward systolic lift along the left sternal border extending from the fourth to the fifth intercostal space represents right ventricular enlargement. Heaves or lifts are terms that imply pulsations associated with valvular diseases or pulmonary hypertension. Thrills are vibrations that are associated with abnormal heart valve function (mitral regurgitation, tricuspid regurgitation, and pulmonic stenosis).

PERCUSSION

The technique of percussion is done to determine the size of the myocardium. With the client in the supine position, percussion of the heart is begun at the anterior axillary line in the fifth intercostal space on the chest using the middle finger of both hands. By striking one finger against the other on the surface of the chest, sounds are produced. Sounds produced over specific anatomic regions by percussion include dullness (heart and liver), tympany (stomach and intestine), flatness (muscle), resonance (normal lung), and hyperresonance (abnormal lung, such as in emphysema). Percussing the cardiac region produces a dull sound. If cardiac dullness exceeds the left mid-clavicular line, to the right of the sternum, and extends below the fifth intercostal space, cardiac enlargement or dilation is suggested. Cardiac size is usually determined by chest roentgenography.

AUSCULTATION

Auscultation is a method to evaluate heart rate and rhythm, cardiac cycle (systole and diastole), and valvular function. The technique of auscultation requires a good-quality stethoscope and extensive clinical practice. Evaluating heart sounds should be done in a systematic order; examination may begin at the aortic outflow tract area and progress to the apex of the heart, using the diaphragm of the stethoscope. The diaphragm of the stethoscope is used for high-frequency sounds and is useful in listening to the first and second heart sounds and high-frequency murmurs. Progression from the apex to the base of the heart can be done using the bell of the stethoscope. The bell is able to screen out high-frequency sounds and is useful in listening for low-frequency gallops (diastolic filling sounds) and murmurs.

All areas in Figure 63–18 should be auscultated, except for the epigastric area. Auscultation should be performed every 4 to 8 hours to check for heart rate and rhythm, murmurs, extrasystolic sounds, and rubs.

Heart Sounds

Normal Heart Sounds

The first heart sound (S_1) is closure of the mitral and tricuspid valves (AV valves). When auscultated, the first heart sound is softer, longer, and of a lower pitch and is best heard at the lower left sternal border or the apex. S_1 marks the beginning of ventricular systole. On the ECG, it occurs right after the QRS complex.

The first heart sound can be accentuated or intensified in conditions such as exercise, hyperthyroidism, or mitral stenosis. A decrease in sound intensity occurs in clients with mitral regurgitation and CHF.

The second heart sound (S_2) is caused mainly by the closing of the aortic and pulmonic valves (semilunar valves). S_2 is characteristically shorter and higher pitched and is heard best at the base of the heart at the end of ventricular systole.

Splitting of heart sounds is often difficult to differentiate from diastolic filling sounds (gallops). A splitting of S_1 (closure of the mitral valve followed by closure of the tricuspid valve) occurs physiologically because left ventricular contraction occurs slightly before right ventricular contraction. However, closure of the mitral valve is louder than closure of the tricuspid valve, so that splitting is often not heard. Normal splitting of S_2 occurs because of the longer systolic phase of the right ventricle. Splitting of S_1 and S_2 can be accentuated by inspiration (increased venous return) and narrows during expiration.

Abnormal splitting of S_2 is referred to as paradoxical splitting, which is characteristic of a wider split heard on expiration. Paradoxical splitting of S_2 is heard in clients with severe myocardial depression, causing early closure of the pulmonic valve or delay in aortic valve closure. Such conditions include MI, LBB block, aortic stenosis, aortic regurgitation, and right ventricular pacing (Braunwald, 1988).

Gallops and Murmurs

Diastolic filling sounds (S_3 and S_4) are produced when blood enters a noncompliant chamber during the two phases of rapid ventricular filling (protodiastole and diastasis). The third heart sound (S_3) is produced during the rapid filling phase of ventricular diastole when blood flows from the atrium to a noncompliant ventricle. The sound arises from vibrations of the valves and supporting structures. The fourth heart sound (S_4) occurs as blood enters the ventricles at the end of ventricular diastole. S_3 is termed *ventricular gallop*, and S_4 is referred to as *atrial gallop*. These sounds can be caused by decreased compliance of either or both ventricles. Left ventricular diastolic filling sounds are best heard with the client on her/his left side, using the bell of the stethoscope at the apex and the left lower sternal border during expiration. Right ventricular diastolic filling sounds are heard best on inspiration along the left sternal border.

It probably is a normal finding if an S_3 is heard in children or young adults up to 30 years of age (Kennedy, 1988). An S_3 gallop in clients older than 40 years of age is considered an abnormal finding and represents a decrease in left ventricular compliance. S_3 can be detected as an early sign of heart failure, ventricular septal defect, or ruptured papillary muscle.

An atrial gallop (S_4) may be heard in clients with hypertension, anemia, ventricular hypertrophy, MI, aortic or pulmonic stenosis, and pulmonary emboli. It may also be heard with advancing age because of a stiffened ventricle.

The auscultation of both S_3 and S_4, called a *summation*, or *quadruple, gallop*, is an indication of severe heart failure. If the quadruple rhythm is present, it is sometimes difficult to delineate the four heart sounds because the client is tachycardiac (has shortened diastolic filling time) and the two sounds actually fuse, producing a rhythm that sounds like a galloping horse.

Murmurs reflect turbulent blood flow through normal or abnormal valves. They are classified according to their timing in the cardiac cycle: systolic murmurs occur between S_1 and S_2, whereas diastolic murmurs occur between S_2 and S_1. Murmurs can also occur during presystole, mid-systole, or late systole or diastole or last throughout both phases of the cardiac cycle.

Murmurs are also graded according to their intensity, depending on their level of loudness (Table 63–2).

The location of a murmur is described in relation to where it is best heard on auscultation. Some murmurs may transmit or radiate from their loudest point to other areas, including the neck, the back, and the axilla. Configuration of a murmur is described as crescendo (increases in intensity) or decrescendo (decreases in intensity). The quality of murmurs can be further characterized as harsh, blowing, whistling, rumbling, or squeaking.

Pericardial Friction Rub

A pericardial friction rub originates from the pericardial sac and occurs with the movements of the heart during the cardiac cycle. Rubs are usually transient and are a sign of inflammation, infection, or infiltration. Pericardial friction rubs may be heard in clients with pericarditis as a result of MI and cardiac tamponade.

The three phases of cardiac movement, atrial systole, ventricular diastole, and ventricular systole, can produce three components of a rub. Usually, only one or two components can be heard. With each movement, a short, high-pitched scratchy sound is produced; the loudest component is heard in systole. Rubs are best heard with the client sitting upright or leaning forward. The pericardial friction rub is accentuated with inspiration.

TABLE 63–2 Grading of Heart Murmurs

Grade I	Very faint
Grade II	Faint, but recognizable
Grade III	Loud, but moderate in intensity
Grade IV	Loud and accompanied by a palpable thrill
Grade V	Very loud, accompanied by a palpable thrill, and audible with the stethoscope partially off the client's chest
Grade VI	Extremely loud, may be heard with the stethoscope slightly above the client's chest

PSYCHOSOCIAL ASSESSMENT

The heart, to many clients, is the symbol of their existence and longevity. When a client has a heart-related illness, whether acute or chronic, it is perceived as a major life crisis. Clients and families confront a situation that presents not only the possibility of death but also fears about pain, disability, lack of self-esteem, physical dependence, and changes in family role dynamics. Formerly adequate support systems may no longer be effective. Disequilibrium is created, and adaptations must occur to re-establish a sense of balance. In the face of these stressful circumstances, clients and families attempt to regain a sense or feeling of control, which is referred to as *coping.*

Coping behaviors vary from client to client. Clients who feel helpless to meet the demands of the situation may exhibit behaviors such as disorganization, fear, or anxiety. A common and normal coping response is denial, which is a defense mechanism to protect from the actual conditions of threat. Prolonged denial, however, can be maladaptive.

DIAGNOSTIC ASSESSMENT

LABORATORY TESTS

Assessment of the client with cardiac dysfunction includes the examination of the blood for abnormalities to establish a diagnosis, to detect concurrent disease, and to assess risk factors. Normal values are listed in Table 63–3.

SERUM CARDIAC ENZYMES

Events leading to cellular injury cause a release of enzymes from intracellular storage, and circulating levels of these enzymes are dramatically elevated. Acute MI can be confirmed by abnormally high levels of enzymes or isoenzymes in the serum.

Creatine Kinase

Creatine kinase (CK) is an enzyme specific to cells of the brain, the myocardium, and skeletal muscle. The appearance of CK in the blood indicates muscle necrosis or injury, and CK levels follow a predictable rise and fall during a specified period of time. Cardiac specificity must be determined by measuring isoenzyme activity. There are three isoenzymes of CK: CK-MM is the predominant muscle isoenzyme; CK-MB, myocardial muscle; and CK-BB, the brain. CK-MB activity is most specific for MI and shows a predictable rise and fall during a period of 3 days, with a peak of activity occurring approximately 24 hours after the onset of chest pain. Percutaneous transluminal angioplasty and intracoronary streptokinase infusion may also result in elevated levels of CK-MB. Early, high CK-MB activity is indicative of successful reperfusion of the coronary artery and can be differentiated from MI by its peak at approximately 12 to 14 hours after symptom onset (Packa & Norris, 1987; Pantaleo, 1981).

Lactate Dehydrogenase

Lactate dehydrogenase (LDH) is widely distributed in the body and is found in the heart, the liver, the kidney, the brain, and the erythrocytes. LDH elevation starts within 12 to 24 hours after an MI, reaches a peak between 48 and 72 hours, and falls to normal in 7 days. Because LDH is not specific to the myocardial cell, assessment of isoenzymes and patterns of elevation are necessary for confirmation of MI. There are five isoenzymes for LDH, of which LDH_1 and LDH_2 are cardiac specific. If the serum level of LDH_1 is higher than the concentration of LDH_2, the pattern is said to have flipped, signifying myocardial damage (Packa & Norris, 1987).

Another enzyme that may be assessed to monitor the presence and progression of an acute cardiovascular event is aspartate aminotransferase (serum glutamic-oxaloacetic transaminase). Like LDH, it is not specific to cardiac muscle tissue.

SERUM LIPIDS

Elevated lipid levels are considered a CAD risk factor. Cholesterol, triglycerides, and the protein components of high-density lipoproteins (HDL) and low-density lipoproteins (LDL) are evaluated to assess a client's degree of risk for CAD. A serum cholesterol level greater than 260 mg/dL gives a client a three times greater risk for CAD than a serum level of 200 mg/dL (Pantaleo, 1981).

Each of the lipoproteins contains varying proportions of cholesterol, triglyceride, protein, and phospholipid. HDL contains mainly protein and 20% cholesterol, whereas LDL is predominantly cholesterol. Elevated LDL levels are positively correlated with CAD, whereas elevated HDL levels are negatively correlated and may be a protective factor, as HDL converts cholesterol to a less active form.

A nonfasting blood sample for measurement of serum cholesterol is acceptable; however, if triglycerides are to be evaluated, measurement should be obtained after a 12-hour fast.

TABLE 63–3 Normal Values and Significance of Abnormal Findings in Laboratory Tests Used in the Assessment of the Cardiovascular System

Test	Normal Range	Significance of Abnormal Findings
Serum Cardiac Enzymes		
Creatine kinase	Women, ≤2.5 U, or 5–35 IU/L Men, ≤4.3 U, or 5–50 IU/L	*Elevations* indicate possible brain, myocardial, and skeletal muscle necrosis or injury.
CK-MM (CK$_3$)	95–100% of total CK	*Elevations* occur with muscle injury.
CK-MB (CK$_2$)	0–5% of total CK	*Elevations* occur with myocardial injury or after percutaneous transluminal angioplasty and intracoronary streptokinase infusion.
CK-BB (CK$_1$)	0%	*Elevations* occur with brain tissue injury.
Lactate dehydrogenase	80–120 Wacker units or 70–207 IU/L	*Elevation* occurs with injury to heart, liver, kidney, brain, and erythrocytes.
LDH$_1$	16–33% of total LDH	*Elevation* occurs higher than LDH$_2$ with myocardial damage.
LDH$_2$	28–40% of total LDH	
LDH$_1$/LDH$_2$ ratio	<1.0	*Elevation* occurs with myocardial damage.
Serum Lipids		
Total lipids	400–1000 mg/dL	*Elevation* indicates increased risk for coronary artery disease (CAD).
Cholesterol	Women, mean of 170–230 mg/dL (range increases with age) Men, mean of 140–215 mg/dL (range increases with age)	*Elevation* indicates increased risk for CAD.
Triglycerides	Women, mean of 90–130 mg/dL (range increases with age) Men, mean of 100–150 mg/dL (range increases with age)	*Elevation* indicates increased risk for CAD.
Plasma high-density lipoproteins	Women, mean of 55–60 mg/dL (range increases with age) Men, mean of 45–50 mg/dL (range increases with age)	*Elevations* may protect against CAD.
Plasma low-density lipoproteins	Women, mean of 105–150 mg/dL (range increases with age) Men, mean of 105–145 mg/dL (range increases with age)	*Elevation* indicates increased risk for CAD.
HDL/LDL ratio	3:1	*Elevated ratios* may protect against CAD.

BLOOD COAGULATION TESTS

Blood coagulation tests evaluate the ability of the blood to clot and are important in clients with a greater tendency to form thrombi (e.g., clients with atrial fibrillation, prosthetic valves, or infective endocarditis) or those clients in whom anticoagulation is employed (e.g., during cardiac surgery, after thrombolysis, and during treatment of established thrombus).

Prothrombin Time

Prothrombin time is used when initiating and maintaining therapy with oral anticoagulants, such as warfarin; it measures the activity of prothrombin, fibrinogen, and factors V, VII, and X.

Partial Thromboplastin Time

Partial thromboplastin time is assessed in clients receiving heparin; it measures deficiencies in all coagulation factors, except factors VII and XIII.

ARTERIAL BLOOD GASES

Arterial blood gas determinations are frequently evaluated in the client with cardiovascular disease, as determination of tissue oxygenation, carbon dioxide removal, and the acid-base status is essential to appropriate intervention and treatment. Complete discussion of these variables can be found in Chapter 14.

SERUM ELECTROLYTES

Fluid and electrolyte balance is essential for normal cardiovascular performance (see Chap. 12). Cardiac manifestations occur when there is an imbalance. Cardiac effects of hypokalemia (low serum potassium level) include increased electrical instability, ventricular arrhythmias, the appearance of U waves on ECG, and an increased risk of digitalis toxicity. The effects of hyperkalemia (high serum potassium level) on the myocardium include asystole and ventricular arrhythmias.

Cardiac manifestations of hypocalcemia (low serum calcium levels) are ventricular arrhythmias, prolonged QT interval, and cardiac arrest. Hypercalcemia (high serum calcium levels) shortens the QT interval and causes AV block, digitalis hypersensitivity, and cardiac arrest.

Serum sodium values reflect water balance and may be decreased, indicating a water excess in clients with heart failure.

COMPLETE BLOOD COUNT

The erythrocyte (red blood cell) count is usually decreased in rheumatic fever and subacute infective endocarditis, whereas it is increased in heart diseases characterized by inadequate tissue oxygenation (e.g., right-to-left shunts).

Decreased hematocrit and hemoglobin levels (e.g., caused by hemorrhage or hemolysis from prosthetic valves) indicate anemia and can manifest as angina or aggravate heart failure. Vascular volume depletion with hemoconcentration (e.g., hypovolemic shock and excessive diuresis) results in an elevated hematocrit.

The leukocyte (white blood cell) count is elevated after MI and in the various infectious and inflammatory diseases of the heart (e.g., infective endocarditis and pericarditis). Chapter 66 discusses the complete blood count.

RADIOGRAPHIC EXAMINATIONS

CHEST RADIOGRAPHY

Routinely, posteroanterior and left lateral views are taken to determine the size, silhouette, and position of the heart. In acutely ill clients, a simple anteroposterior view is taken at the bedside. Cardiac enlargement, pulmonary congestion, cardiac calcifications, and placement of central venous catheters, endotracheal tubes, and hemodynamic monitoring devices are all assessed on x-ray films.

CARDIAC FLUOROSCOPY

Fluoroscopy is a simple x-ray examination that reveals the action of the heart. Continuous visual observation of the heart, lungs, and vessel movement on a luminescent x-ray screen in a darkened room is provided. Fluoroscopy is used to place and position intracardiac catheters and IV pacemaker wires and can be helpful in identifying abnormal structures, calcifications, and tumors of the heart. In critically ill clients, fluoroscopy can be performed at the bedside for placement of intracardiac catheters or IV pacemaker wires. The client preparation and follow-up are dependent on the procedure. Commonly, fluoroscopy is used in conjunction with cardiac catheterization, and the client is taken to a special cardiac catheterization room (see later discussion of cardiac catheterization).

ANGIOGRAPHY

Angiography of arterial vessels, or *arteriography*, is an invasive diagnostic procedure that involves fluoroscopy and x-ray studies. This procedure is performed when an arterial obstruction, narrowing, or aneurysm is suspected. Selective arteriography is performed to evaluate specific areas of the arterial system. For example, coronary arteriography, which is performed during left-sided cardiac catheterization, assesses arterial circulation within the heart (see later in this section). Angiography can also be performed on arteries in the extremities, mesentery, or cerebrum.

Client preparation. The radiologist explains the procedure and the risks to the client before the client signs a consent form. Because this procedure involves injection of contrast medium into the arterial system, the risks are serious. They include hemorrhage, thrombosis, embolism, and death. The client is told to expect a warm sensation when dye is injected during the procedure. The nurse assesses the client for any allergies to contrast medium, iodine-containing substances such as seafood, or local anesthetics. The nurse also shaves and scrubs the area that will be catheterized with an antiseptic skin preparation. Most often, the femoral artery in a groin area is used. Vital signs are documented and pedal pulses are marked and described in nursing progress notes.

Procedure. The client is placed in a supine position on an x-ray table in the radiology department. A radiologist usually performs this procedure and begins by injecting a local anesthetic into the tissue surrounding the artery being catheterized. Contrast medium is injected via this catheter, and fluoroscopy and x-ray studies are done.

Follow-up care. After the procedure, the client is restricted to bed rest in the supine position for 8 to 12 hours. The extremity that was catheterized should not be flexed during this time. A pressure dressing or bandage is kept in place over the injection site, with or without a sandbag over the dressing. The nurse assesses the insertion site for bloody drainage or hematoma formation, assesses distal pulses, and compares skin temperature in the affected extremity with that in the opposite extremity. Vital signs are assessed at the time of every dressing, pulse, and temperature check, the first set being obtained immediately after the client is transferred from the radiology department. These assessments continue every 15 minutes for 1 hour, then every 30 minutes for 2 hours, followed by every 4 hours or prn. The radiologist is called immediately if bleeding or changes in vital signs occur.

DIGITAL SUBTRACTION ANGIOGRAPHY

Digital subtraction angiography (DSA) combines x-ray detection methods and a computerized subtraction technique with fluoroscopy for visualization of the cardiovascular system without interference from adjacent structures, such as bone or soft tissue.

Client preparation. DSA involves injection of dye into the venous system. Therefore, before the procedure, the nurse assesses the client for a history of allergies to contrast medium.

Procedure. A radiologist injects dye into the venous system via the superior vena cava. As the contrast medium circulates through the heart and the arterial system, a fluoroscopic image intensifier displays the vessels and focuses the image. A computer then converts the images to numbers, and the first image obtained before the injection of the dye is subtracted from the postinjection images.

Follow-up care. Because DSA does not involve an arterial puncture and because little contrast dye is used, nursing care after the procedure is not as extensive as that after cardiac catheterization. The nurse monitors the client for vital signs and assesses the injection site for bleeding or discomfort.

OTHER DIAGNOSTIC STUDIES

ELECTROCARDIOGRAPHY

A routine part of every cardiovascular evaluation, the ECG is one of the most valuable diagnostic tests. Various forms are available: resting ECG, continuous ambulatory ECG (Holter's monitoring), and exercise ECG (stress test) (see later discussion of ambulatory ECG and exercise ECG). The resting ECG provides information regarding cardiac dysrhythmias, myocardial ischemia, the site and extent of MI, cardiac hypertrophy, electrolyte imbalances, and the effectiveness of cardiac drugs. The normal ECG pattern of one cardiac cycle is illustrated in Figure 63–19. Further discussion about interpretation and evaluation of normal and abnormal patterns may be found in Chapter 64.

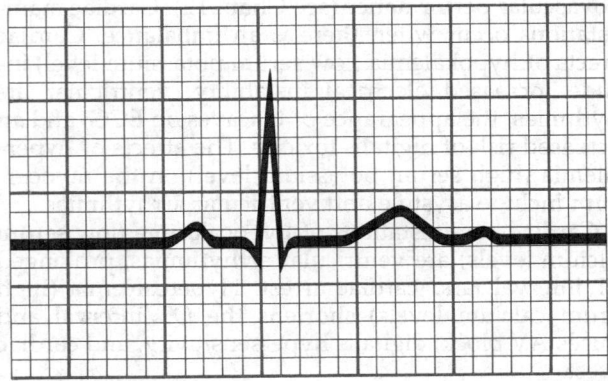

Figure 63–19

Normal ECG pattern.

The ECG graphically records electrical current generated by the heart. This current is measured by electrodes placed on the skin and connected to an amplifier and strip chart recorder (Fig. 63–20). In the standard 12-lead ECG, five electrodes attached to the arms, legs, and chest measure current from 12 different views, or leads: three bipolar limb leads, three unipolar augmented leads, and six unipolar chest leads. The bipolar limb leads (leads I, II, and III) have positive and negative poles and measure the difference in electrical activity between two selected limbs (Fig. 63–21). The unipolar augmented leads (aVR, aVL, and aVF) have only a positive pole and measure the electrical potential between the center of the heart and each limb (Fig. 63–22). The unipolar precordial leads (V_1 to V_6) have only a positive pole and measure the electrical activity of the heart in the horizontal plane (Fig. 63–23).

Client preparation. The nurse explains the purpose and procedure of the ECG and informs the client that the test is safe and painless. The client is requested to lie as still as possible during the test.

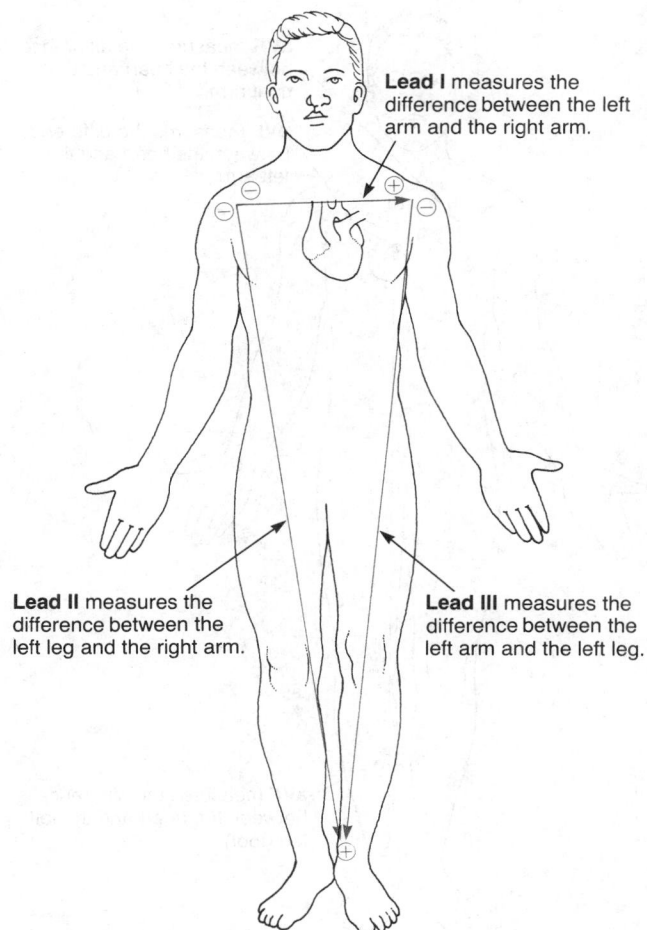

Lead I measures the difference between the left arm and the right arm.

Lead II measures the difference between the left leg and the right arm.

Lead III measures the difference between the left arm and the left leg.

Figure 63–21

Standard limb leads.

Procedure. The ECG is performed with the client in a supine position with the chest exposed. Electrode sites selected are clipped of hair. Before applying the electrodes, the skin is cleaned with an alcohol swab to reduce skin oils and to improve electrode contact. Electrode paste, gel, or saline pads are applied to the electrode sites if metal plates or suction cups are used. To ensure good contact between the skin and the electrodes for the limb leads, the electrodes should be placed on a flat surface above the wrists and the ankles. A total of 10 electrodes are used for a standard ECG and are attached to lead wires that connect to the ECG machine. The 12-lead ECG reading is obtained by selecting the indicators on the machine. No specific follow-up care is warranted.

Ambulatory Electrocardiography

Ambulatory ECG (also called Holter's monitoring) allows continuous recording of heart activity during an extended period (usually 24 hours) while the client is per-

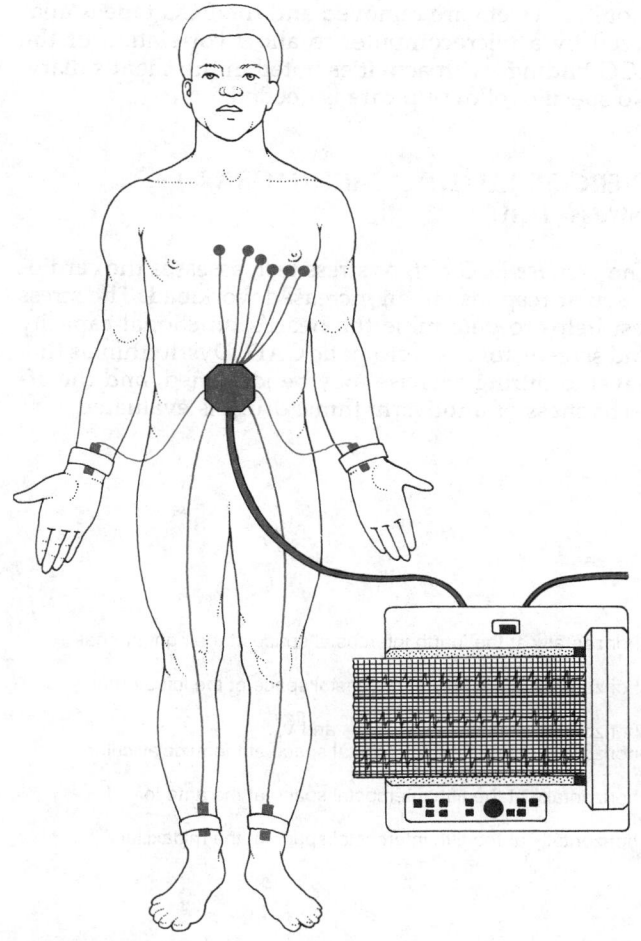

Figure 63–20

Placement of electrodes for 12-lead ECG.

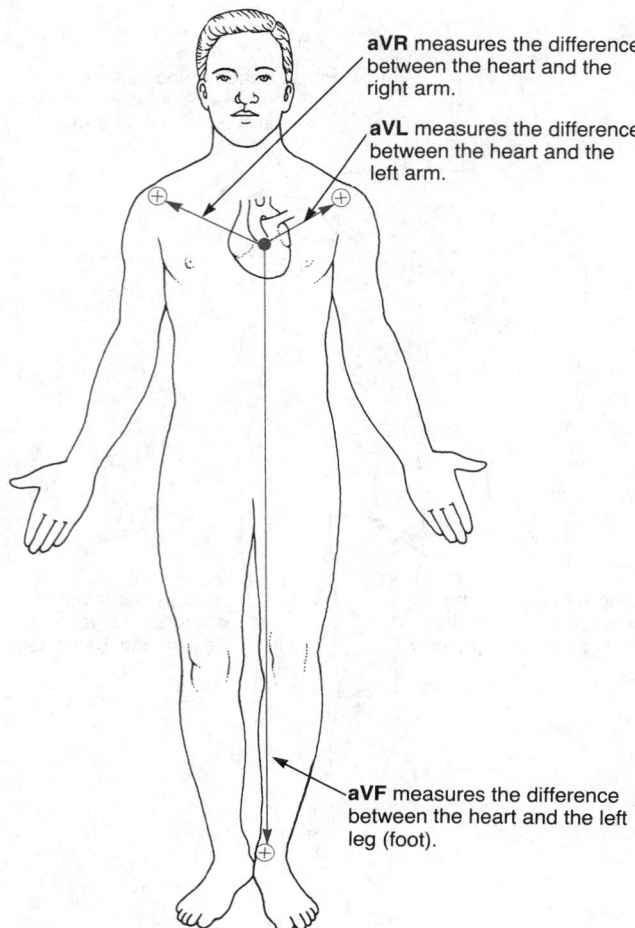

aVR measures the difference between the heart and the right arm.

aVL measures the difference between the heart and the left arm.

aVF measures the difference between the heart and the left leg (foot).

Figure 63–22

Unipolar augmented leads.

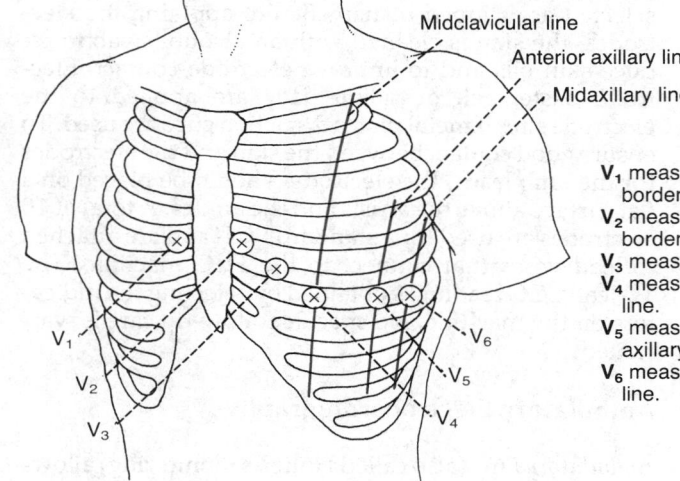

Midclavicular line

Anterior axillary line

Midaxillary line

Figure 63–23

Unipolar precordial leads.

forming ADL. This ambulatory ECG allows for assessment and correlation of dyspnea, chest pain, CNS symptoms (such as lightheadedness and syncope), and palpitations with actual cardiac events and the client's activities.

Client preparation.   The client is instructed to keep a diary in which to note the time of activities, such as eating, sleeping, walking, and working, and to record any symptoms, such as chest pain, lightheadedness, fainting, or palpitations. The client should be informed to avoid operating heavy machinery, using electric shavers and hairdryers, and bathing or showering, as these activities may interfere with the ECG recorder.

Procedure.   The client has electrodes placed on the chest and attached to the Holter's monitor, which is a small portable ECG tape recorder about the size of a transistor radio. The monitor is worn in a sling or holder around the chest or waist. The client is encouraged to go about his/her normal daily activities and keep the written diary as accurately as possible. After the monitoring period, which is usually 24 hours, the electrodes and monitor system are removed and the ECG tape is analyzed by a microcomputer to allow correlation of the ECG findings with activities noted in the client's diary. No specific follow-up care is needed.

EXERCISE ELECTROCARDIOGRAPHY (Stress Test)

The *exercise ECG test*, or stress test, assesses the cardiovascular response to an increased workload. The stress test helps to determine the heart's functional capacity and screens for asymptomatic CAD. Dysrhythmias that develop during exercise may be identified, and the effectiveness of antidysrhythmic drugs is evaluated.

V_1 measures horizontally at the fourth intercostal space at the right sternal border.

V_2 measures horizontally at the fourth intercostal space at the left sternal border.

V_3 measures horizontally midway between V_2 and V_4.

V_4 measures horizontally at the fifth intercostal space at the midclavicular line.

V_5 measures horizontally at the fifth intercostal space at the anterior axillary line.

V_6 measures horizontally at the fifth intercostal space at the midaxillary line.

Client preparation.   Because risks are associated with exercising, the client must be adequately informed about the purpose, the procedure, and the risks involved and a written consent obtained. Anxiety and fear are common before stress testing, and the nurse needs to assure the client that the procedure is performed in a controlled environment with prompt nursing and medical attention available. The nurse instructs the client to get plenty of rest the night before the procedure. The client should not eat anything after going to bed, or at least not within 2 hours before the test. The client should not smoke or drink alcohol- or caffeine-containing beverages on the day of the test. The physician should be consulted about stopping any heart medications. The client is advised to wear comfortable, loose clothing and rubber-soled, supportive shoes. The nurse instructs the client to tell the physician if any symptoms, such as chest pain, dizziness, shortness of breath, or an irregular heart beat, are experienced during the test.

A resting 12-lead ECG is done, as well as cardiovascular history and physical examination, before the stress test to check for any ECG abnormalities or medical factors that may preclude the test.

Emergency supplies such as cardiac drugs, a defibrillator, and other equipment necessary for resuscitation are available in the room in which the stress test is performed. The nurse assisting the physician and client during the test should be proficient in using resuscitation equipment because adverse signs and symptoms of cardiac disease are not uncommon during this test.

Procedure.   Electrodes are placed on the client's chest and attached to a multilead monitoring system. Baseline blood pressure, heart rate, and respiration rate are noted. Two major modes of exercise available for stress testing are bicycle ergometry or treadmill walking. A bicycle ergometer is a device equipped with a wheel operated by pedals that can be adjusted to increase the resistance to pedaling. The treadmill is a motorized device that has an adjustable conveyor belt; it can reach speeds of 1 to 10 miles/hour and can also be adjusted from a flat position to a 22-degree gradient.

After the client is instructed in the use of the bicycle or shown how to walk on the treadmill, the exercise is started. During the test, the client's blood pressure and ECG are closely monitored by a physician, a nurse, or an appropriately trained individual. The client exercises until one of the following occurs: a predetermined heart rate is reached and maintained; signs and symptoms, such as chest pain, fatigue, extreme dyspnea, vertigo, hypotension, or ventricular dysrhythmias, appear; or significant ST segment depression occurs.

Follow-up care.   After the test, the ECG and blood pressure continue to be monitored until the client has completely recovered. The client may continue to experience the aforementioned signs and symptoms (e.g., chest pain, hypotension, and fatigue). After the client has recovered, she/he can return home. The nurse advises the client to avoid taking a hot shower for 1 to 2 hours after the test, as this may precipitate hypotension. If the client continues to have chest pain or ventricular dysrhythmias or appears medically unstable, she/he is admitted to a coronary care unit for observation.

ECHOCARDIOGRAPHY

As a noninvasive, risk-free test, echocardiography is easily performed at a client's bedside or on an outpatient basis. *Echocardiography* uses ultrasound to assess cardiac structure and mobility, particularly the valves. Echocardiograms are used to help assess and diagnose cardiomyopathy, valvular disorders, pericardial effusion, left ventricular function, ventricular aneurysms, and cardiac tumors.

Client preparation.   There is no special preparation for this test; the client is informed that the test is painless and takes 30 to 60 minutes to complete. The nurse instructs the client to lie quietly during the test and assists the client to lie slightly on his/her left side with the head of the client elevated 15 to 20 degrees.

Procedure.   A small transducer lubricated with gel to facilitate movement and conduction is placed on the client's chest at the level of the third or fourth intercostal space near the left sternal border. The transducer transmits high-frequency sound waves and receives them back from the client as they are reflected from different structures. These echoes are usually videotaped simultaneously with the client's ECG and can be recorded on graph paper for a permanent copy.

There are two echocardiographic techniques: the *M mode* and the *two-dimensional* (cross-sectional) technique. The M, or motion, mode uses a narrow beam of sound, producing an "icepick" view of the cardiac structures. The two-dimensional mode transmits a wider sound beam and produces images with both motion and shape. Regardless of which technique is used, after the images are taped, cardiac measurements that require several images can be obtained. Some routine measurements are chamber size, ejection fraction, and flow gradient across the valves. There is no specific follow-up care.

PHONOCARDIOGRAPHY

Phonocardiography is the graphic recording of heart sounds during auscultation and can be helpful in determining the exact timing and characteristics of extra heart sounds and murmurs.

A phonocardiography machine simultaneously records the pulse wave, ECG, and heart sounds graphically. A pressure-sensitive transducer is applied to the selected pulse (e.g., apical or carotid artery), and the ECG is obtained through standard limb leads. A special microphone, used in the same manner as a stethoscope, is applied to the various areas for auscultation on the client's chest. Client preparation and follow-up care are similar to those for echocardiography.

NUCLEAR CARDIOGRAPHY

The use of radionuclide techniques in cardiovascular assessment is called *nuclear cardiology*. Using radioactive tracer substances, cardiovascular abnormalities can be viewed, recorded, and evaluated. These studies are useful for detecting MI and decreased myocardial blood flow and for evaluating left ventricular ejection.

Client preparation. The nurse tells the client that the tests are relatively noninvasive and the radiation exposure and risks are minimal. The client is informed that the test involves the IV injection of small amounts of radioisotope. Written consent is obtained.

Procedure. The most common tests in nuclear cardiology include technetium (^{99m}Tc) pyrophosphate scanning, thallium imaging, and gated cardiac blood pool scanning.

Technetium pyrophosphate scanning. A small dose of ^{99m}Tc pyrophosphate is injected into the client's antecubital vein. The client then waits 2 hours while the renal system clears the unbound technetium. A gamma-scintillation camera scans the heart to identify the areas of increased uptake of the radioisotope. The radioisotope accumulates in damaged myocardial tissue and is referred to as a hot spot. This test helps to detect acute MI and define its location and size but does not show an old infarction.

Thallium imaging. A small dose of ^{201}Tl is injected into the client's antecubital vein. The imaging of the heart is done within 4 to 10 minutes with a gamma-scintillation camera, as the normal blood supply and intact cells rapidly take up this radioisotope, whereas necrotic or ischemic tissue does not and appears as cold spots on the scan.

Thallium imaging is performed with the client at rest or during an exercise test. Performing the thallium imaging during an exercise test may demonstrate perfusion deficits not apparent at rest. The stress test procedure is performed (see earlier). After the client reaches maximal activity level, a small dose of ^{201}Tl is injected intravenously, and the client continues to exercise for approximately 1 to 2 minutes. The scanning is then done.

This test, performed either with the client at rest or during an exercise test, is used to assess myocardial scarring and perfusion, to detect the location and extent of an acute or chronic MI, to evaluate graft patency after coronary bypass surgery, and to evaluate antianginal therapy, thrombolytic therapy, or balloon angioplasty.

Gated cardiac blood pool scanning. This test utilizes a computer to analyze ventricular function. ECG

leads are attached to the client, and the ECG is synchronized with a computer and a gamma-scintillation camera. A small amount of ^{99m}Tc (attached to either human serum albumin or autologous red blood cells) is injected intravenously. After 3 to 5 minutes, the scanning begins. The computer constructs an average cardiac cycle that represents the summation of several hundred heart beats.

Left ventricular function, including the contractile state (areas of decreased, absent, or paradoxical movement) of the left ventricle and the ejection fraction, can be evaluated.

Follow-up care. The client may complain of fatigue, depending on which test is performed, or discomfort at the antecubital injection site. If a stress test was paired with the ^{201}Tl study, the nurse needs to be aware of the same follow-up care as for the stress test (see earlier).

CARDIAC CATHETERIZATION

The most definitive, but most invasive, test in the diagnosis of cardiac disease is cardiac catheterization. Cardiac catheterization may include studies of the right or left side of the heart and the coronary arteries. There are many indications for cardiac catheterization (Table 63–4).

Client preparation. Many clients express a great deal of anxiety and fear regarding cardiac catheterization. The nurse assesses the client's physical and psychosocial readiness and knowledge level.

The nurse explains the purpose of the procedure and informs the client how long the procedure usually takes, who will be present while it is going on, and what kind

---

TABLE 63–4 **Indications for Cardiac Catheterization**

To confirm suspected heart disease including CAD, myocardial disease, valvular disease, and valvular dysfunction

To determine the location and extent of the disease process

To assess
  Stable, severe angina unresponsive to medical management
  Unstable angina pectoris
  Uncontrolled heart failure, ventricular dysrhythmias, or cardiogenic shock associated with acute MI, papillary muscle dysfunction, ventricular aneurysm, or septal perforation
  Whether cardiac surgery is necessary

To evaluate
  Effects of medical treatment on cardiovascular function
  Percutaneous transluminal coronary angioplasty or coronary artery bypass graft patency

of physical environment it is done in (e.g., catheterization laboratory). The client is also informed as to certain temporary sensations that may be experienced during the procedure, such as palpitations (as the catheter is passed up to the myocardium); a feeling of heat or hot flash (as the dye is injected into either side of the heart); and a desire to cough (as the dye is injected into the right heart). The nurse may elect to use written, illustrated materials or videotapes to assist the client's understanding.

The risks of cardiac catheterization are usually explained by the cardiologist and vary with the procedures to be performed and the client's physical status (Table 63–5). Coronary arteriography has the most risk of complications, including MI, cerebrovascular accident, arterial bleeding, thromboembolism, lethal dysrhythmias, or death. Right-sided heart catheterization has the least risk. A written informed consent from the client is obtained.

The client may be admitted to the hospital before the catheterization procedure. Standard preoperative tests are performed, which usually include chest radiography, complete blood count, urinalysis, and 12-lead ECG. The client receives nothing by mouth after midnight or has only a liquid breakfast if the catheterization is to take place in the afternoon. The catheterization sites are shaved, and an antiseptic skin preparation is done.

TABLE 63–5   Complications of Cardiac Catheterization

Right-Sided Heart Catheterization

Thrombophlebitis

Pulmonary embolism

Vagal response

Left-Sided Heart Catheterization and Coronary Arteriography

MI

Cerebrovascular accident

Arterial bleeding or thromboembolism

Dysrhythmias

Right- or Left-Sided Heart Catheterization*

Cardiac tamponade

Hypovolemia

Pulmonary edema

Hematoma or blood loss at insertion site

Reaction to contrast medium

---

* In addition to those cited for each procedure.

Nursing assessment includes taking the client's vital signs, auscultation of heart and lungs, and evaluation of peripheral pulses. The client is questioned as to any prior history of allergy to iodine-containing substances (e.g., seafood or contrast agents), as an antihistamine may be given to a client with a positive history. A mild sedative is given before the procedure.

Procedure. The client is taken to the cardiac catheterization laboratory and is placed supine on an x-ray table. The client is securely strapped to this table and informed of this precaution, as the table will turn like a cradle during the procedure. The client is given a local anesthetic at the injection site. The client is instructed to report any angina or chest pain or other symptoms to the staff. During the procedure, the client may also experience nausea or hot flashes during the injection of contrast medium or discomfort and pain at the insertion site if the anesthetic wears off.

Right-sided heart catheterization. A catheter is inserted through the femoral vein to the inferior vena cava or through the basilic vein to the superior vena cava. The catheter is advanced through either the inferior or the superior vena cava and, guided by fluoroscopy, is advanced through the right atrium, through the right ventricle, and, at times, into the pulmonary artery (Fig. 63–24). Intracardiac pressures (right atrial, right ventricular, pulmonary artery, and pulmonary artery wedge pressures) are obtained, and blood samples are withdrawn. Contrast dye or medium is usually injected to detect any cardiac shunts or regurgitation from the pulmonic or tricuspid valves.

Left-sided heart catheterization. The left-sided heart catheterization is more invasive. The catheter is passed in a retrograde direction to reach the heart, which is performed by advancing the catheter from the femoral or brachial artery up the aorta, across the aortic valve, and into the left ventricle (Fig. 63–25). The catheter may also be passed from the right side of the heart through the atrial septum, using a special needle to puncture the septum. Intracardiac pressures and blood samples are obtained. The pressures of the left atrium, the left ventricle, and the aorta and mitral and aortic valve status are evaluated. In addition, contrast dye is injected into the ventricle and using cineangiograms (rapidly changing films); left ventricular motion is filmed. Ventriculography can evaluate ventricular function, and calculations are made of end-systolic volume, end-diastolic volume, stroke volume, and ejection fraction.

Coronary arteriography. The technique is the same as for left-sided heart catheterization. The catheter is advanced into the aortic arch and positioned selectively in the right or left coronary arteries. Injection of contrast medium permits visualization of the coronary arteries. By assessing the flow of dye through the coronary ar-

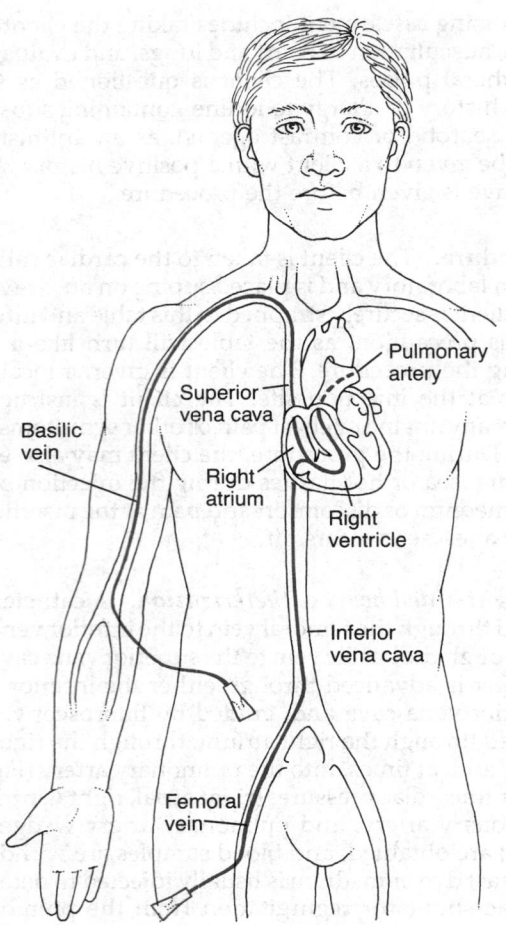

Figure 63–24

Right-sided heart catheterization. The catheter is inserted into the femoral vein and advanced through the superior vena cava (or if into an antecubital or basilic vein through the inferior vena cava), right atrium, and right ventricle and into the pulmonary artery.

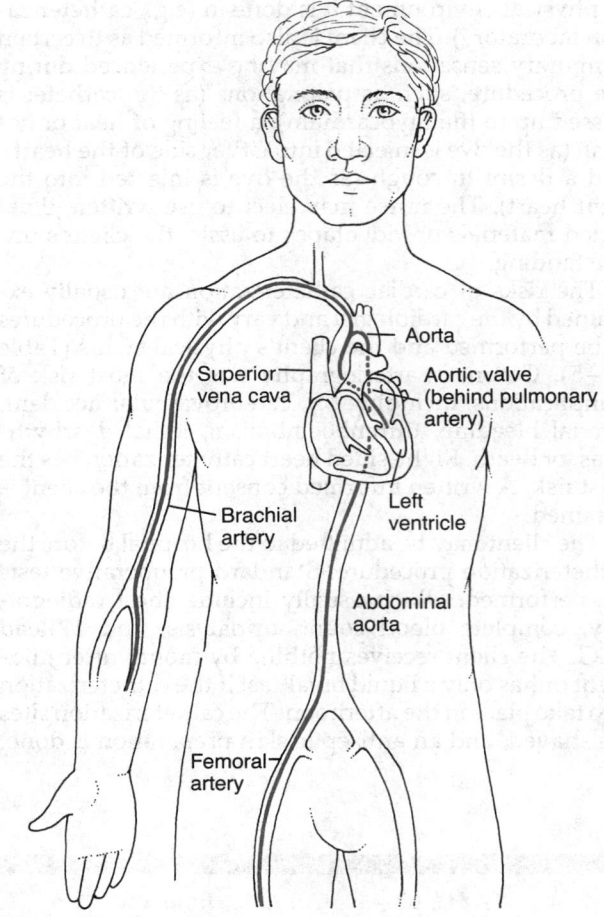

Figure 63–25

Left-sided heart catheterization. The catheter is inserted into the femoral artery or the antecubital artery. The catheter is passed through the ascending aorta, through the aortic valve, and into the left ventricle.

teries, information about the site and severity of coronary lesions is obtained.

Follow-up care. After the catheterization, the client is restricted to bed rest for 8 to 12 hours; the client is supine, with the insertion site extremity nonflexed. A pressure dressing or bandage may be present over the insertion site. The nurse has many postcatheterization responsibilities. Vital signs are monitored every 15 minutes for 1 hour; then every 30 minutes for 2 hours or until vital signs are stable; then every 4 hours. The nurse observes the insertion site for bloody drainage or hematoma formation. Peripheral pulses in the affected extremity, as well as skin temperature and color, are monitored with every vital sign check. A 5- or 10-lb sandbag or a C clamp may be applied over the insertion site to ensure hemostasis.

The nurse must be constantly vigilant regarding the complications of cardiac catheterization (see Table 63–

5). The nurse assesses the client's complaints of pain and discomfort at the insertion site, chest pain, nausea, or feelings of lightheadedness. Carefully monitoring the client's cardiac rhythm and pulse rate and auscultating heart sounds detects any dysrhythmias. The nurse may administer pain medication for insertion site discomfort as ordered.

If the client experiences chest pain, lethal dysrhythmias, or dramatic change in peripheral pulses in the affected extremity, the nurse reports these findings to the physician immediately and provides immediate medical and nursing interventions.

HEMODYNAMIC MONITORING

Hemodynamic monitoring provides quantitative information about vascular capacity, blood volume, pump effectiveness, and tissue perfusion. In the early 1970s, hemodynamic monitoring was introduced at the bedside in the critical care unit and in the cardiac catheterization laboratory to permit measurement of several cardiac indices: CVP, pulmonary artery pressure (PAP) and pulmonary artery wedge pressure (PAWP), and cardiac output. Bedside monitoring may also include systemic intra-arterial pressure measurement.

Central Venous Pressure

CVP directly reflects right atrial pressure or pressure in the superior vena cava and indirectly reflects right ventricular filling pressure (preload). The CVP is determined by the interaction of venous tone, central venous volume (blood returning to the heart), and the pumping ability of the heart.

Client preparation. CVP is measured in the superior vena cava or the right atrium by a water manometer (in centimeters of water) or by a pressure transducer (in millimeters of mercury). Water manometers are more commonly used on medical-surgical units, whereas pressure transducers are used strictly in units with the electrical monitoring equipment. Normally, the CVP ranges from 3 to 8 cmH$_2$O or 2 to 6 mmHg (Gardner & Woods, 1989). A CVP less than 3 cmH$_2$O may indicate hypovolemia (saline depletion), vasodilation, or increased myocardial contractility. Conversely, an elevated CVP may reflect increased circulatory blood volume, vasoconstriction, and decreased contractility. An elevated CVP is seen in clinical states such as tricuspid insufficiency, right-sided heart failure, positive-pressure breathing with a ventilator, cardiac tamponade, and chronic obstructive pulmonary disease. Clients with acute MI of the left ventricle may experience left ventricular pump failure, which may lead to right-sided heart failure. In this instance, an elevated CVP represents a late sign of left-ventricular failure.

Procedure. Insertion of a CVP catheter is achieved percutaneously or by venous cutdown through a central or peripheral vein. Acceptable insertion sites include the medial basilic, lateral cephalic, internal or external jugular, and subclavian veins. Selection of the appropriate site depends on the skill of a qualified clinician (usually a physician) inserting the catheter, the physical structure and age of the client, thoracic deformities, and clinical circumstances. Written consent is necessary because clients and families must be informed of the indications and the possible complications of infection and air embolism.

The selected site is cleaned with an antiseptic or antibacterial solution. Lidocaine may be used for local anesthesia. With aseptic technique, the catheter is inserted into the vein and is threaded through the venous vessel until the distal end of the catheter rests in the right atrium or superior vena cava. Placement of the catheter should be verified by chest radiography. The catheter is secured in place by a skin suture and is attached to a three-way stopcock to an IV set-up and a water manometer or pressure transducer.

Obtaining central venous pressure readings. To obtain a CVP reading, the zero point on the manometer must be placed at the correct position, the phlebostatic axis (see the accompanying Guidelines feature). CVP readings can be obtained with the client supine with the head of the bed elevated up to 20 degrees as long as the zero point on the manometer is adjusted to the phlebostatic axis.

High CVP readings may indicate hypervolemia, right-sided heart failure, pericardial tamponade, or constrictive pericarditis. A low CVP reading may indicate hypovolemia.

In addition to pressure measurements, central venous catheters are used to administer fluids, blood derivatives, and medications and to obtain blood samples.

Follow-up care. An occlusive dry dressing covers the insertion site. The dressing and IV tubing are changed every 24 hours, and the insertion site is inspected for signs of infection: redness, swelling, drainage, and heat.

Pulmonary Artery and Pulmonary Artery Wedge Pressures

Client preparation. PAP and PAWP measurements are obtained in critically ill clients to evaluate left ventricular function. PAP is more useful than CVP in assessing the function of the left ventricle. The data derived from serial measurements are used to guide and evaluate therapy.

Procedure. A balloon-tipped catheter (Gould's or Swan-Ganz catheter) is inserted percutaneously through a large vein by a physician. The balloon is inflated and advances with the flow of blood through the tricuspid valve, into the right ventricle, past the pulmonic valve, and into a branch of the pulmonary artery. The balloon is deflated after the catheter tip reaches the pulmonary artery. Waveforms can be visualized on the oscilloscope as the pulmonary artery catheter is advanced (Fig. 63–26). The management and care of clients with pulmonary artery catheters can be found in texts dealing with critical care nursing.

Obtaining pulmonary artery pressure measurements. PAPs (systolic/diastolic and mean) are obtained by a transducer and pressure monitor. These pressures are dependent on blood flow to the lungs and the state of the lung tissue. Normal PAP is 25/9 mmHg, with a mean of 15 mmHg (Beller, 1981). When the balloon is inflated by the nurse, the catheter wedges into a branch of the pulmonary artery. The tip of the catheter is able to sense transmitted pressures of the left atrium, which reflects left ventricular end-diastolic pressure (LVEDP). PAWP closely approximates left atrial pressure and LVEDP in clients with normal left ventricular function, with normal heart rates, and without mitral valve disease. The PAWP is a mean pressure and is

GUIDELINES ■ How to Obtain a Central Venous Pressure Reading

1. Determine the phlebostatic axis (the level of the right atrium).
   a. Position the client supine.
   b. Palpate the fourth intercostal space at the sternum.

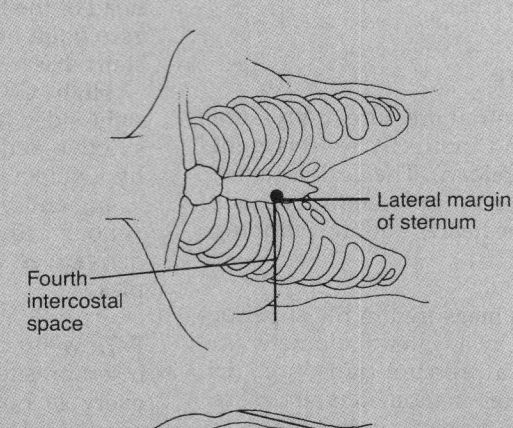

Lateral margin of sternum

Fourth intercostal space

   c. Follow the fourth intercostal space to the side of the client's chest.
   d. Determine the midway point between anterior and posterior.
   e. Find the intersection between the midway point and the line from the fourth intercostal space, and mark it with an **X** in indelible ink. This is the phlebostatic axis.

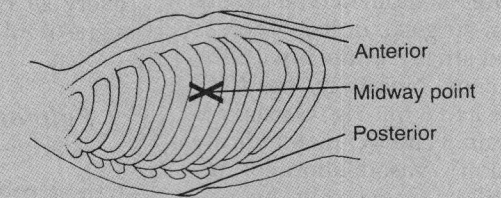

Anterior

Midway point

Posterior

2. Position the water manometer so that the zero mark or the air-fluid interface is at the same height as the **X**.

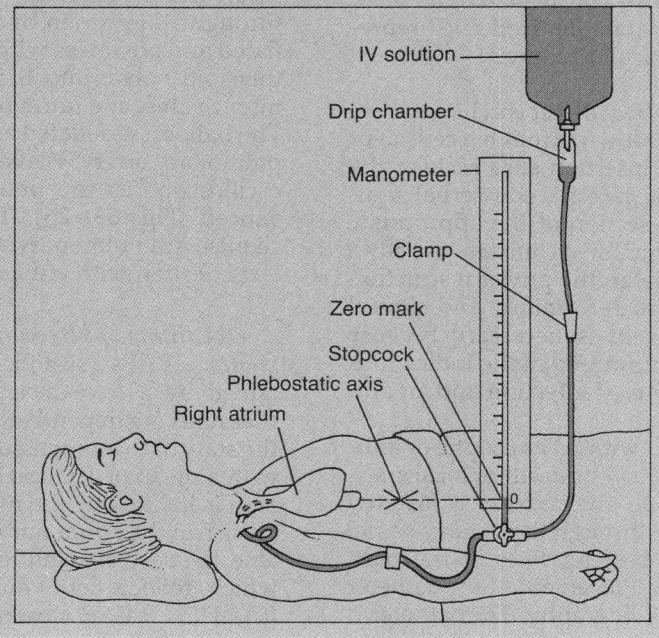

IV solution

Drip chamber

Manometer

Clamp

Zero mark

Stopcock

Phlebostatic axis

Right atrium

GUIDELINES ■ How to Obtain a Central Venous Pressure Reading *Continued*

3. Turn the stopcock as shown to fill the manometer with IV fluid.

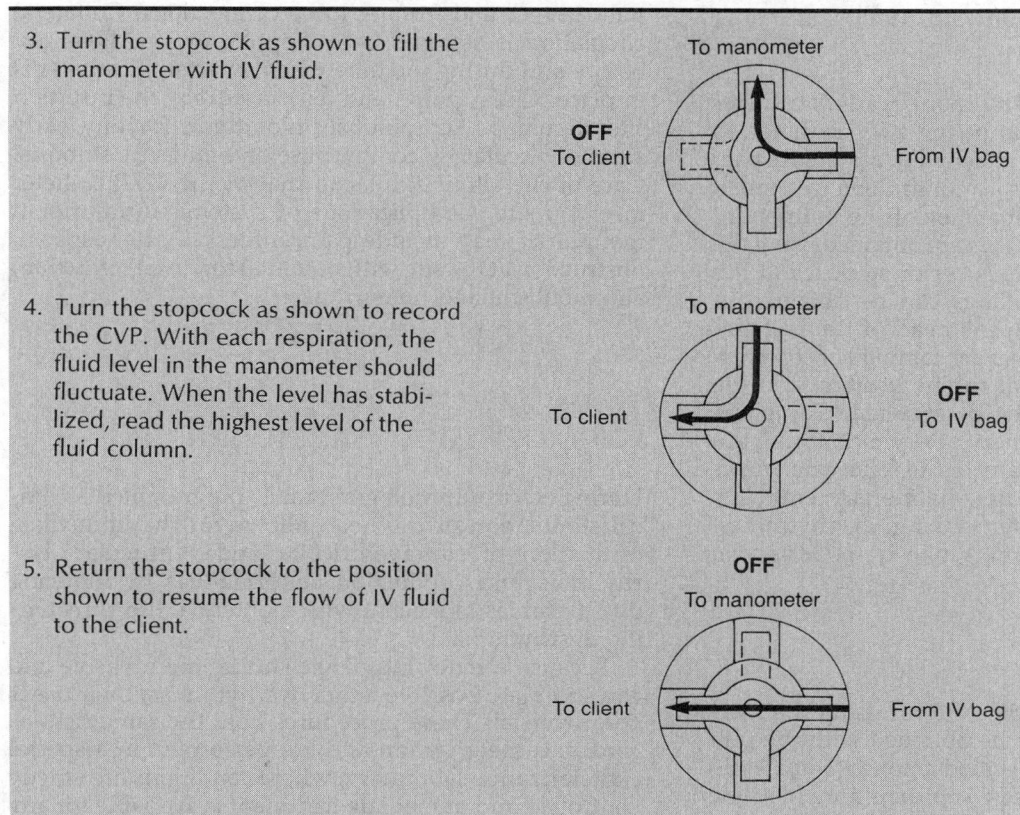

To manometer

OFF
To client

From IV bag

4. Turn the stopcock as shown to record the CVP. With each respiration, the fluid level in the manometer should fluctuate. When the level has stabilized, read the highest level of the fluid column.

To manometer

To client

OFF
To IV bag

5. Return the stopcock to the position shown to resume the flow of IV fluid to the client.

OFF
To manometer

To client

From IV bag

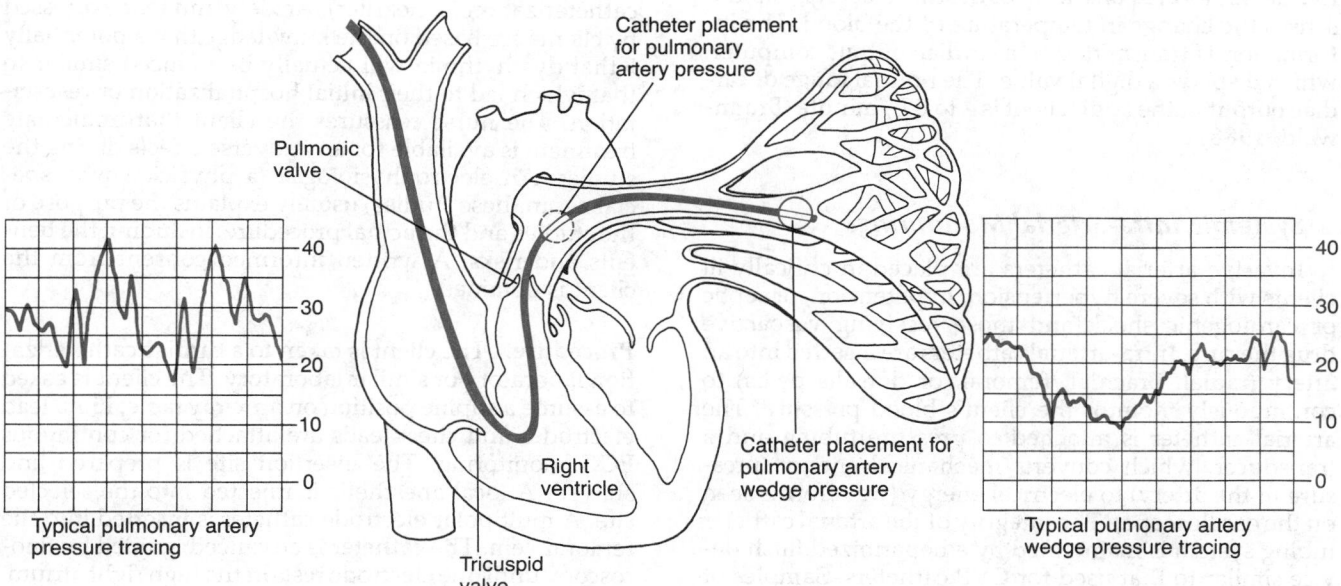

Catheter placement for pulmonary artery pressure

Pulmonic valve

Right ventricle

Tricuspid valve

Catheter placement for pulmonary artery wedge pressure

Typical pulmonary artery pressure tracing

Typical pulmonary artery wedge pressure tracing

Figure 63–26

Cardiac pressure waveforms can be visualized on the oscilloscope.

normally between 4 and 12 mmHg. For clients who have undergone coronary artery bypass, the expected range is 8 to 16 mmHg (Braunwald, 1988; Gardner & Woods, 1989).

Follow-up care. Care of the pulmonary artery catheter and the site is similar to that of the CVP catheter. A heparinized flush solution is attached to a pressure bag, and a flush device delivers a continuous yet small amount of fluid to maintain patency of the pulmonary artery catheter. Pressure readings are obtained using the air-fluid interface of the transducer or stopcock at the phlebostatic axis. These readings can be obtained in most critically ill clients with the head of the bed elevated up to 20 degrees; however, comparison of pressure measurements in the flat supine position and the elevated position needs to be determined. Complications associated with pulmonary artery monitoring are uncommon but may include any of the following: infection, pulmonary artery rupture, pulmonary embolus, pulmonary infarction, catheter kinking, dysrhythmias, air embolism, intracardiac trauma, and systemic venous thrombosis.

Cardiac Output

The measurement of cardiac output using the thermodilution method can also be obtained with the pulmonary artery catheter. A specified amount (5 or 10 mL) of iced or room-temperature IV solution (normal saline or dextrose in water) is injected in one of the lumina (proximal port) of the catheter. The solution mixes with the blood in the right atrium and travels with the flow of blood through the heart, where the temperature-sensitive device located on the tip of the catheter registers and senses the change in temperature of the blood. The information is transmitted to a cardiac output computer, which displays a digital value. The normal range of cardiac output in the adult client is 4 to 8 L/minute (Braunwald, 1988).

Systemic Intra-arterial Monitoring

Invasive arterial catheters are placed in critically ill clients with severe hypertension, hypotension, or septic or cardiogenic shock and those receiving vasoactive drug therapy. Intra-arterial catheters are inserted into an artery (radial, brachial, femoral, or dorsalis pedis) to continuously monitor the client's blood pressure. The arterial catheter is attached to pressure tubing and a transducer, which converts mechanical energy (pressure in the artery) to electrical energy (waveforms seen on the oscilloscope). The integrity of the arterial catheter tubing system is maintained by a heparinized flush device similar to that used for CVP catheters. Samples of arterial blood can be obtained from the catheter to determine arterial blood gas tensions or serial electrolyte or drug level determinations.

Frequent assessment of the arterial site and system is necessary to observe for bleeding around the intra-arterial catheter and for any loose connections. Collateral circulation is assessed by a Doppler or an Allens test before and during the time when an arterial catheter is in place. Color, pulse, and temperature at the insertion site should be scrupulously monitored for any early signs of circulatory compromise or venous thrombosis. Care of the site is similar to that of the CVP catheter insertion site. Complications of systemic intra-arterial monitoring may include pain, infection, arteriospasm, obstruction at the site with potential for distal infarction, air embolism, and hemorrhage.

ELECTROPHYSIOLOGIC STUDIES

During electrophysiologic studies, programmed electrical stimulation of the heart allows for the immediate evaluation of supraventricular and ventricular dysrhythmia and conduction abnormalities by inducing dysrhythmias in a client with a potential life-threatening dysrhythmia.

Because electrophysiologic studies are invasive and can stimulate possible lethal dysrhythmias, their use is controversial. These procedures hold the same risks as cardiac catheterization and are performed in a special catheterization laboratory, where conditions are strictly controlled and immediate treatment is available for any adverse effects.

Client preparation. The preparation for these clients parallels preparation for the client undergoing cardiac catheterization (see earlier). Anxiety and fear expressed by clients are based on the knowledge that a potentially lethal dysrhythmia will actually be induced similar to that which led to their initial hospitalization or resuscitation. The nurse reassures the client that immediate treatment is available for any adverse effects during the studies. An electrophysiologist (a physician who specializes in these studies) usually explains the purpose of the studies and the actual procedure, including the benefits and risks. A written informed consent from the client is obtained.

Procedure. The client is taken to a cardiac catheterization laboratory or similar laboratory. The client is asked to assume a supine position on an x-ray table. Limb lead electrodes and chest leads are attached for continuous ECG monitoring. The insertion site is prepared and shaved. A local anesthetic is injected into the selected site. A multipolar electrode catheter is inserted into the femoral vein. The catheter is advanced, guided by fluoroscopy until one electrode rests in the high right atrium, one adjacent to the bundle of His, and one in the right ventricle. An additional electrode may be placed in the coronary sinus.

During electrophysiologic studies, the conduction time can be measured: the AH interval (conduction time from the low right atrium through the His bundle) and the HV interval (conduction time from the proximal His bundle to the ventricular myocardium). By pacing the heart and measuring these intervals and refractory periods (the response of cardiac tissue to premature stimulus), dysrhythmias can be evaluated.

The client may experience back discomfort during the procedure, as she/he must remain supine for 2 to 6 hours, as well as pain at the insertion site as the anesthetic wears off. The client needs to be advised to tell the staff of any symptoms she/he is experiencing. During the rapid pacing, the client is aware of the rapid heart beat and states that he/she is experiencing palpitations. Clients may also experience chest pain or loss of consciousness if they become hypotensive.

Follow-up care. The follow-up care is the same as that for the client who has undergone cardiac catheterization. The nurse may provide comfort measures to alleviate back discomfort. If the client lost consciousness during the procedure and received electrical cardioversion or defibrillation, the client may complain of chest discomfort over the area where the electrical current was applied. The nurse assesses the skin for any signs of redness, swelling, or burns. In addition, the client might describe a loss of memory of the events during the procedure, and the nurse needs to provide reassurance and explain the events of the procedure in careful detail.

SUMMARY

The purpose of the cardiovascular system is to provide the tissues with metabolic substrates and nutrients; remove waste products; transport hormones, gases, and immunologic substances; promote fluid and electrolyte homeostasis; and regulate body temperature. Nurses must be knowledgeable about the pathophysiologic mechanisms of the cardiovascular system to understand, recognize, and manage clients with cardiovascular disease. This chapter focuses on the normal structure and function of the cardiovascular and lymphatic systems, including changes that occur with age.

The nursing management of a client with cardiovascular disease includes physical and psychosocial assessment and evaluation. Various diagnostic tests are also performed.

REFERENCES AND READINGS

Almerda, D., Bradford, J. M., Wenger, N. K., King, S. B., & Hurst, J. W. (1983). Return to work after coronary bypass surgery. *Circulation, 68*(Suppl. 2), 205–213.

Alpert, J. S. (1985). Coronary vasomotion, coronary thrombosis, myocardial infarction, and the camel's back. *Journal of American College of Cardiology, 5,* 617–618.

American Heart Association. (1989). *Heart facts* (pp. 1–3). Dallas, TX: Author.

American Nurses' Association Division on Medical-Surgical Nursing Practice and American Heart Association Council on Cardiovascular Nursing. (1981). *Standards of cardiovascular nursing practice.* Kansas City: American Nurses' Association.

Bates, B. (1987). *A guide to physical examination and history taking* (4th ed.). Philadelphia: J. B. Lippincott.

Berger, H., & Zaret, B. (1981). Nuclear cardiology. *New England Journal of Medicine, 305,* 855–865.

Berne, R. M., & Levy, M. N. (1986). *Cardiovascular physiology* (5th ed.). St. Louis: C. V. Mosby.

Braunwald, E. (Ed.). (1988). *Heart disease: A textbook of cardiovascular medicine* (3rd ed.). Philadelphia: W. B. Saunders.

Brunner, L. S., & Suddarth, S. D. (1986). *The Lippincott manual of nursing practice* (4th ed.). Philadelphia: J. B. Lippincott.

Buja, L. M., & Willerson, J. T. (1981). Clinicopathologic correlates of acute ischemic heart disease syndromes. *American Journal of Cardiology, 47,* 343–356.

Clark, S. (1988). Ineffective coping: Patient and family. In L. S. Kern (Ed.), *Cardiac critical care nursing.* Rockville, MD: Aspen Publishers.

Coodley E. L. (1985). *Geriatric heart disease.* Littleton, MA: PSG Publishing.

Crouch, J. E. (1985). *Functional human anatomy* (4th ed.). Philadelphia: Lea & Febiger.

Cunningham, S. G. (1987). Nonpharmacologic management of high blood pressure. *Cardiovascular Nursing, 23*(4), 18–22.

Eliopoulos, C. (1987). *Gerontological nursing.* Philadelphia: J. B. Lippincott.

Epstein, S. E., & Palmeri, S. T. (1984). Mechanisms contributing to precipitation of unstable angina and acute myocardial infarction: Implications regarding therapy. *American Journal of Cardiology, 54,* 1245–1252.

Fahey, V. A. (1988). *Vascular nursing.* Philadelphia: W. B. Saunders.

Fitzgerald, S. T. (1989). Occupational outcomes after treatment for coronary heart disease: A review of the literature. *Cardiovascular Nursing, 25*(1), 1–6.

Froelicher, E. S. (1989). Exercise testing. In S. L. Underhill, S. L. Woods, E. Froelicher, & C. J. Halpenny (Eds.), *Cardiac nursing* (2nd ed., pp. 418–430). Philadelphia: J. B. Lippincott.

Gardner, P. E., & Woods, S. L. (1989). Hemodynamic monitoring. In S. L. Underhill, S. L. Woods, E. S. Froelicher, & C. J. Halpenny (Eds.), *Cardiac nursing* (2nd ed., pp. 451–482). Philadelphia: J. B. Lippincott.

Kennedy, G. (1988). Clinical cardiac assessment. In L. S.

Kern (Ed.), *Cardiac critical care nursing* (pp. 1–31). Rockville, MD: Aspen Publishers.

Gilbert, C. J., & Ashtar, M. (1980). Right heart catheterization for intracardiac electrophysiologic studies: Implications for the primary care nurse. *Heart and Lung, 9,* 85–92.

Gillis, C., & Gortner, S. R. (1986). Improving recovery from cardiac surgery: The UCSF/Stanford/Sequoia Family Heart Study. *Nursing Research, 35,* 125.

Gotto, A. M., & Farmer, J. A. (1988). Risk factors for coronary artery disease. In E. Braunwald (Ed.), *Heart disease: A textbook of cardiovascular medicine* (3rd ed., pp. 1153–1190). Philadelphia: W. B. Saunders.

Harrell, J. S. (1988). Age-related changes in the cardiovascular system. In M. A. Matteson & E. S. McConnell (Eds.), *Gerontological nursing* (pp. 193–217). Philadelphia: W. B. Saunders.

Johnson, W. T. M., Salenga, G., & Lee, W. (1986). Arterial intimal embrittlement: A possible factor in atherogenesis. *Atherosclerosis, 59,* 161–171.

Josephson, M. E., & Seides, S. F. (1979). *Clinical cardiac electrophysiology techniques and interpretations.* Philadelphia: Lea & Febiger.

Kauffman, S., & Lemberg, L. (1979). Exercise stress testing in the patient with coronary artery disease. *Heart and Lung, 8,* 148–152.

Kennedy, G. (1988). Clinical cardiac assessment. In L. S. Kern (Ed.), *Cardiac critical care nursing* (pp. 1–31). Rockville, MD: Aspen Publishers.

Kirkendall, W. M., Feinleib, M. D., & Fries, E. D. (1988). *Recommendations for human blood pressure determination by sphygmomanometers.* Dallas, TX: American Heart Association.

Landau, B. R. (1980). *Essential human anatomy and physiology* (2nd ed.). Glenview, IL: Scott, Foresman.

Lane, L. D., & Winslow, E. H. (1987). Oxygen consumption, cardiovascular response, and perceived exertion in healthy adults during rest, occupied bedmaking, and unoccupied bedmaking activity. *Cardiovascular Nursing, 23*(6), 31–36.

McGrath, M. A., Verhaeghe, R. H., & Shepherd, J. T. (1980). The physiology of limb blood flow. In J. L. Juergens, J. A. Spittell, Jr., & J. F. Fairbairn, II (Eds.), *Peripheral vascular diseases.* (pp. 83–105). Philadelphia: W. B. Saunders.

Mason, D., Demaria, A., & Berman, D. (1980). *Principles of noninvasive cardiac imaging echocardiography and nuclear cardiology.* New York: Le Jacq Publishing.

Michaelson, C. R. (1983). *Congestive heart failure.* St. Louis: C. V. Mosby.

Mishell, D. R. (1989). Correcting misconceptions about oral contraceptives. *American Journal of Obstetrics and Gynecology, 161,* 1385–1389.

Newton, K. (1989). Cardiac catheterization. In S. L. Underhill, S. L. Woods, E. S. Froelicher, & C. J. Halpenny (Eds.), *Cardiac nursing* (2nd ed., pp. 431–450). Philadelphia: J. B. Lippincott.

New York Heart Association Criteria Committee. (1964). *Diseases of the heart and blood vessels: Nomenclature and criteria for diagnosis* (6th ed.). Boston: Little, Brown.

O'Connor, A. M. (1983). Factors related to the early phase of rehabilitation following aortocoronary bypass surgery. *Research Nurse Health, 6,* 107–116.

Packa, D. R., & Norris, B. W. (1987). Conceptualization in cardiovascular nursing research. *Cardiovascular Nursing, 23*(5), 25–29.

Pagana, K. D., & Pagana, T. J. (1982). *Diagnostic testing and nursing implications.* St. Louis: C. V. Mosby.

Pantaleo, N. (1981). Thallium myocardial scintigraphy and its uses in the assessment of coronary artery disease. *Heart and Lung, 106,* 61–71.

Sanderson, R. (1983). Diagnostic techniques. In R. Sanderson & C. Kurth (Eds.), *The cardiac patient: A comprehensive approach* (2nd ed.). Philadelphia: W. B. Saunders.

Shabetai, R., & Adolph, R. J. (1980). Principles of cardiac catheterization. In N. O. Fowler (Ed.), *Cardiac diagnosis and treatment* (3rd ed., pp. 106–185). Hagerstown, MD: Harper & Row.

Tilkian, A. G., Daily, E. K. (1986). *Cardiovascular procedures: Diagnostic techniques and therapeutic procedures.* St. Louis: C. V. Mosby.

Tortora, G. (1989). *Principles of human anatomy* (5th ed.). New York: Harper & Row.

Underhill, S. L. (1989). History-taking and physical examination of the patient with cardiovascular disease. In S. L. Underhill, S. L. Woods, E. S. Froelicher, & C. J. Halpenny (Eds.), *Cardiac nursing* (pp. 242–274). Philadelphia: J. B. Lippincott.

Zeluff, G. W., Cashion, W. R., & Jackson, D. (1980). Evaluation of the coronary arteries and myocardium by radionuclide imaging. *Heart and Lung, 9,* 344–349.

CHAPTER 64

Interventions for Clients with Cardiac Disorders

Each normal heartbeat is the result of an electrical stimulus and a mechanical response. When the cardiac muscle cells are strong and able to respond to the electrical stimulation, depolarization and repolarization are coupled with the mechanical responses of contraction (systole) and relaxation (diastole). The electrical impulse usually originates in specialized cells of the right atrium and conducts rapidly through a network of fibers to stimulate the contraction of myocardial cells of the right and left ventricles in a rhythmic fashion. These chambers are responsible for pumping blood to the lungs for oxygenation and to the body tissues and organs for cellular nutrition.

Primary cardiac dysfunction may result from a number of causes, such as impaired or obstructed blood flow to the cardiac muscle (coronary artery disease [CAD]) structural defects or infections within the valves, or inflammatory conditions of the heart. Any of these disorders can cause electrophysiologic abnormalities that result in disturbances of cardiac rhythm—dysrhythmias. The danger of dysrhythmias is that they can affect the pumping efficiency of the heart. The client with cardiac dysfunction is therefore evaluated closely by continuous monitoring of selected electrocardiographic (ECG, which in this chapter also refers to electrocardiogram and electrocardiography) leads and by intermittent ECG. Because ECG to detect rhythm disturbances is an important part of the care of clients with cardiac dysfunction, this chapter discusses rhythm disturbances recorded on 12-lead ECGs and single-lead monitor tracings.

DYSRHYTHMIAS

OVERVIEW

Any disorder of the heartbeat is termed *dysrhythmia.* Historically, the term *arrhythmia* has been used in the literature; however, arrhythmia means absence of rhythm. Dysrhythmia, which means disorder of the rhythm, is more accurate. The two terms may be used interchangeably; however, the more accurate term dysrhythmia is used here.

Dysrhythmias, which impair cardiac output and thus cellular nutrition, result from an alteration in the order or speed of conduction of electrical impulses. Dysrhythmias may consist of slow impulse formation, resulting in bradycardias (heart rate < 60 beats per minute), or rapid impulse formation, resulting in tachycardiacs (heart rate > 100 beats per minute). A delay in impulse conduction may result in atrioventricular (AV) nodal blocks or intraventricular conduction delays (bundle branch blocks). Premature, or ectopic, beats result in an irregular rhythm related to irritable cardiac cells (premature atrial, junctional, or ventricular contractions). Failure to produce an impulse may result in a pause in the conduction rhythm (sinus pause, ventricular standstill, or asystole), in which case another site in the conduction system may override the natural pacemaker of the heart and assume the activity of regular impulse formations (junctional or ventricular escape rhythms).

The most life-threatening result of cardiac dysrhythmias is sudden cardiac death. Sudden cardiac death can have either of two causes: a dysrhythmia or myocardial failure. Although sudden death related to dysrhythmias occurs most often in clients with previously diagnosed heart disease, in 20% of clients experiencing cardiac arrest, death is the first manifestation of heart disease (American Heart Association [AHA], 1987). Therefore, identification of clients at high risk for sudden death and early recognition through continuous monitoring of selected ECG leads enable prompt identification and treatment of potentially life-threatening dysrhythmias.

ELECTROCARDIOGRAM INTERPRETATION AND RECOGNITION OF NORMAL SINUS RHYTHMS

Chapter 63 describes the principles underlying ECG. This chapter focuses on how to recognize normal sinus rhythms and dysrhythmias on ECG and single-lead monitor tracings.

The heart's electrical activity is represented in all ECG lead tracings by P, Q, R, S, and T waves. Each of these waves represents some part of the cardiac cycle and is evaluated on the ECG for its presence and shape. Some of these waves, when observed in combination with another, represent an interval that is measured in

fractions of a second to determine the duration of a particular event in the cardiac cycle. The PR interval and the QRS complex are examples (Fig. 64–1).

ECG waves are measured in amplitude (voltage) and duration (time). Amplitude is measured on the ECG by a series of horizontal lines (Fig. 64–2). Each horizontal line is 1 mm apart and represents 0.1 mV. (The amplitude of the wave reflects only its electrical force, and not the muscular strength of the contraction.) The duration of a wave is measured by a series of vertical lines, also 1 mm apart. The time interval between each vertical line is 0.04 second. If an interval measures three small blocks, its duration is 0.12 second (0.04 second × 3 blocks = 0.12 second). Every fifth horizontal and vertical line is inscribed boldly.

ECG paper is divided into 3-second segments by lines along the margin (Fig. 64–3). From one line to the next is 3 seconds of time, provided that the monitor is set on the standard speed of 25 mm/second. Therefore, two 3-second segments equal 6 seconds of time.

The heart rate may be estimated by counting the number of complexes (P waves for atrial rate, QRS complexes for ventricular rate) in 6 seconds and multiplying that number by 10 to get the rate for a full minute. For example, if seven QRS complexes are identified in a 6-second strip, the estimated ventricular rate for 1 minute is 70 (see Fig. 64–3). For accuracy, this method should be used when the rhythm of the waveforms is regular.

Another method of estimating the heart rate is to count the number of small blocks from one wave to the next (P to P for atrial rate, R to R for ventricular rate). That number is divided by 1500 (because there are 1500 small blocks in 1 minute). The quotient is the rate of

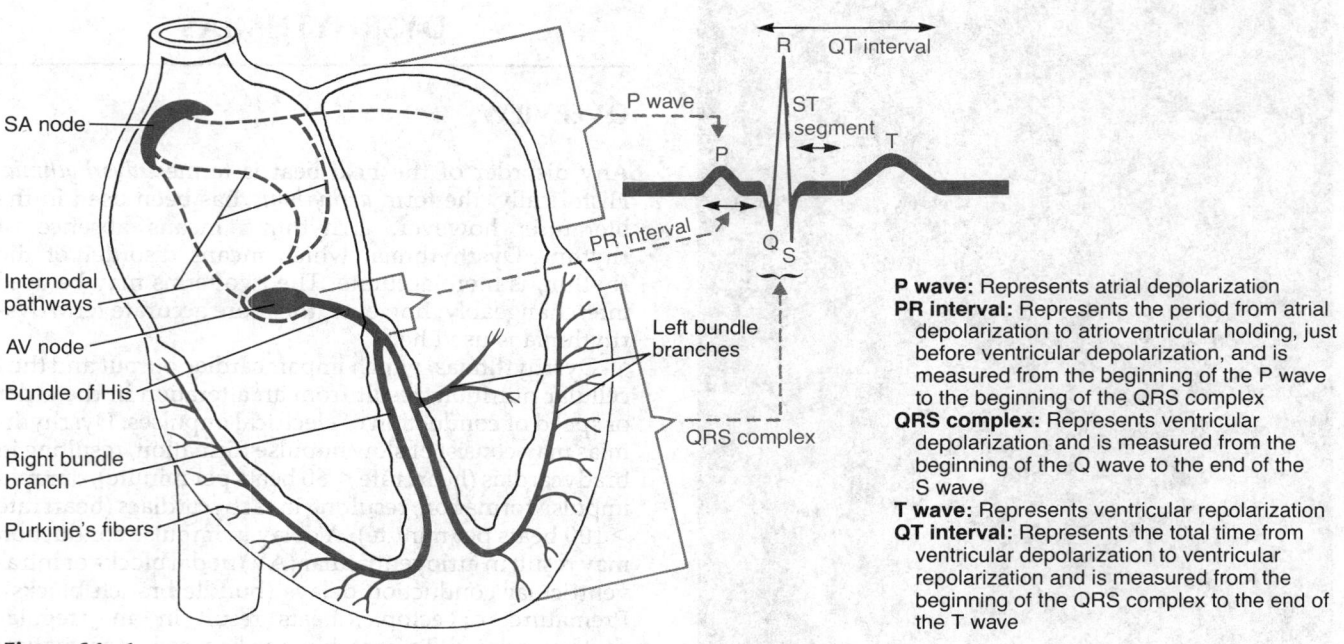

P wave: Represents atrial depolarization

PR interval: Represents the period from atrial depolarization to atrioventricular holding, just before ventricular depolarization, and is measured from the beginning of the P wave to the beginning of the QRS complex

QRS complex: Represents ventricular depolarization and is measured from the beginning of the Q wave to the end of the S wave

T wave: Represents ventricular repolarization

QT interval: Represents the total time from ventricular depolarization to ventricular repolarization and is measured from the beginning of the QRS complex to the end of the T wave

Figure 64–1

Significance of the components of an ECG tracing.

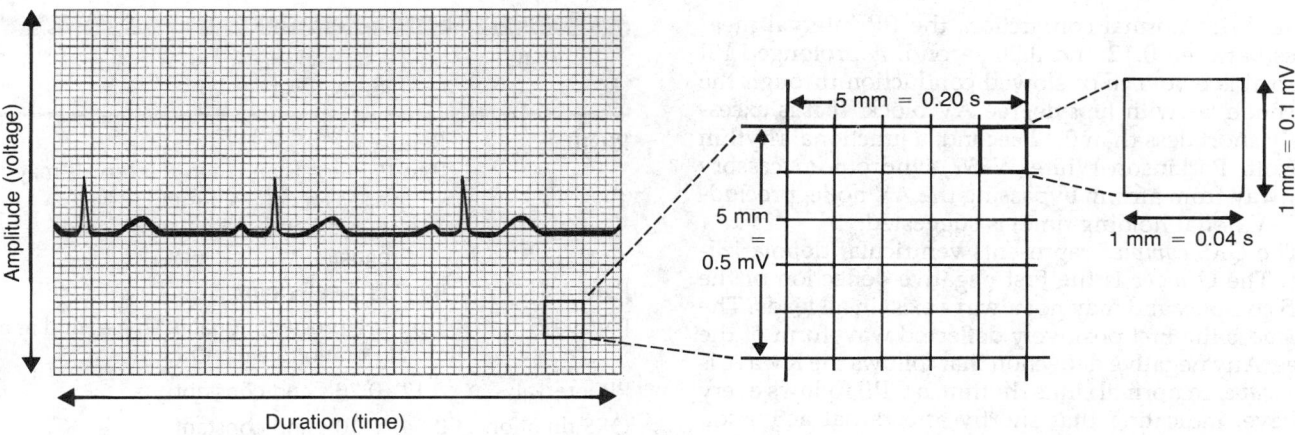

Figure 64–2

ECG waveforms are measured in amplitude (voltage) and duration (time).

those impulses for 1 minute. For example, there are 20 small blocks from one R wave to the next. Dividing 20 by 1500 yields 75 (see Fig. 64–3). Therefore, the ventricular rate is 75 beats per minute. For accuracy, this method should be reserved for regular rhythms. Commercially prepared rate rulers are sometimes used in estimating the heart rates of regular rhythms.

When irregular rhythms are observed, it is best to obtain the rate with a 60-second apical pulse by auscultation. Palpating the pulse peripherally may reveal a pulse deficit, sometimes seen with irregular rhythms. A *pulse deficit* is an identified difference between the apical pulse rate and the radial pulse rate. This occurs in irregular rhythms because all beats may not perfuse equally to result in a palpable pulse.

The *P wave* represents the electrical activity of sinoatrial (SA) node impulse formation and the depolarization of the atria. P waves in normal sinus rhythm are usually rounded, are identical in appearance, and occur in a regular pattern at a rate of 60 to 100 times per minute. All P waves in normal sinus rhythm must be equally spaced from each other for the rhythm to be described as regular. The rhythm is still considered regular if there is no more than 3 mm (three small blocks on ECG paper) in variation. If P waves are not present, or if they have different shapes from other P waves, it implies that the SA node is not firing or that a different focus from an ectopic impulse is firing. The term *ectopic* refers to a stimulus originating from outside of the normal cardiac conduction system from the atrial, junctional, or ventricular tissue. However, in the case of differently shaped P waves, it refers to ectopic atrial foci.

The *PR interval* represents the amount of time for atrial impulse formation (P wave), atrial depolarization, and AV nodal impulse holding time. It is measured from the beginning of the P wave to the beginning of the QRS

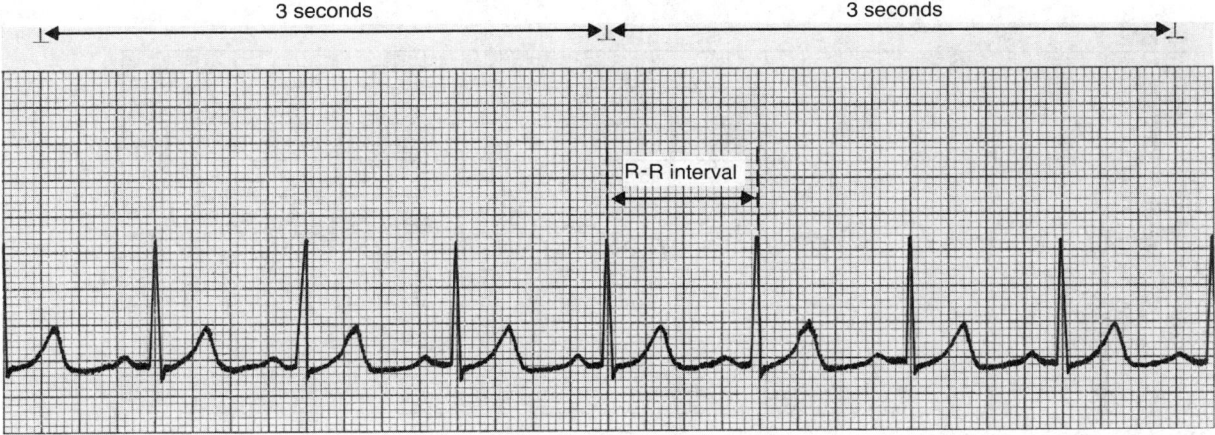

Figure 64–3

Each segment between the dark lines (above the monitor strip) represents 3 s, when the monitor is set at a speed of 25 mm/s.

wave. With normal conduction, the PR interval measures between 0.12 and 0.20 second. A prolonged PR interval is evidence of slowed conduction through the AV node, as with first-degree AV block. If it is excessively short, less than 0.12 second, a junctional rhythm or Wolff-Parkinson-White (WPW) syndrome (accessory pathway from atrium bypassing the AV node, precluding AV nodal holding time) is suggested.

The *QRS complex* represents ventricular depolarization. The *Q wave* is the first negative deflection of the QRS complex and may not always exist in all leads. The *R wave* is the first positively deflected waveform of the three. Any negative deflection that follows the R wave is an *S wave*. In normal sinus rhythm, a QRS follows every P wave, indicating that shortly after atrial activation comes ventricular activation. In normal sinus rhythm, the ventricular rate equals the atrial rate and is usually between 60 and 100 beats per minute. The QRS interval is measured from the beginning of the Q wave (or R wave, if no Q wave exists) to the end of the S wave. A normal QRS interval measures between 0.04 and 0.10 second in duration. When the ventricles are conducting the impulse in a delayed or abnormal fashion, as with bundle branch blocks or aberrantly conducted beats (conducted abnormally, originating from outside of the His bundle system), the duration of the QRS interval is abnormal, lasting longer than 0.12 second. Table 64–1 summarizes the characteristics of normal sinus rhythm.

The *ST segment* is the interval between ventricular depolarization and the beginning of ventricular repolarization. Normally, this segment is isoelectric, meaning it is neither elevated nor depressed, because the positive and negative forces are equally balanced during this period. However, elevated or depressed ST segments may indicate an abnormality in the initial repolarization phase. This is usually a result of myocardial ischemia or injury (see Fig. 64–31). Digitalis therapy can also influence the ST segment (Fig. 64–4). It should be emphasized that to fully analyze the ST segment, a standard 12-lead ECG, rather than a single-lead monitoring unit, must be employed. The continuous single-lead moni-

TABLE 64–1   Characteristics of a Normal Sinus Rhythm

Rhythm:	Regular
	P-to-P intervals and R-to-R intervals may vary as much as 3 mm (3 small squares) and still be considered regular
Rate:	60–100 beats/min
P waves:	They are present, equal in shape, and at a 1:1 ratio to each QRS
PR interval:	0.12–0.20 s and constant
QRS duration:	0.04–0.10 s and constant
QT interval:	Usually less than 0.40 s

Example

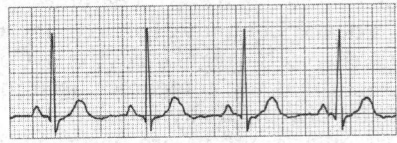

Rhythm:	Regular
Rate:	Atrial—70 beats/min
	Ventricular—70 beats/min
P waves:	Present, equal, and occur at a 1:1 ratio to each QRS
PR interval:	0.16 s
QRS interval:	0.08 s
QT interval:	0.40 s

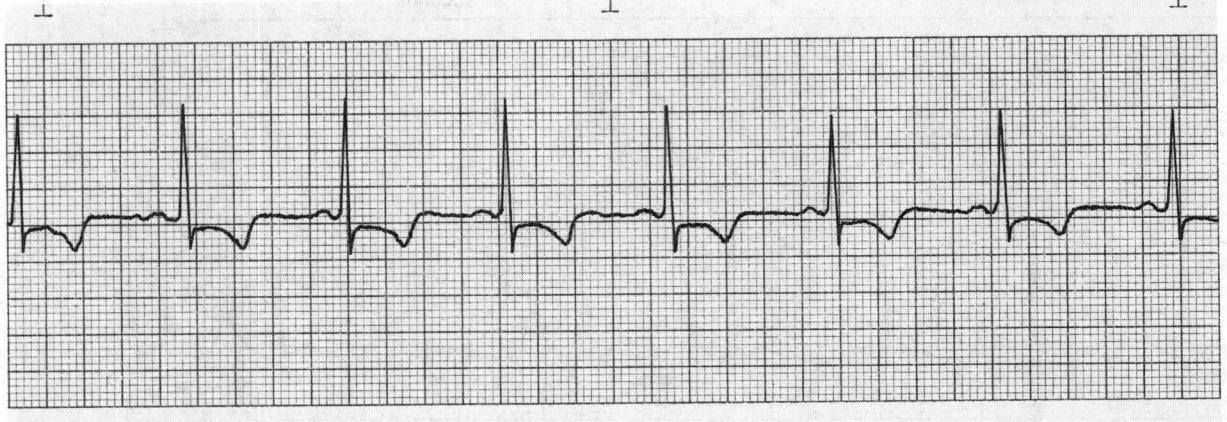

Figure 64–4

ST segment changes commonly seen in clients receiving digitalis therapy; changes include depression of ST segments, as either a straight line or a sagging contour, and T wave lowering or inversion.

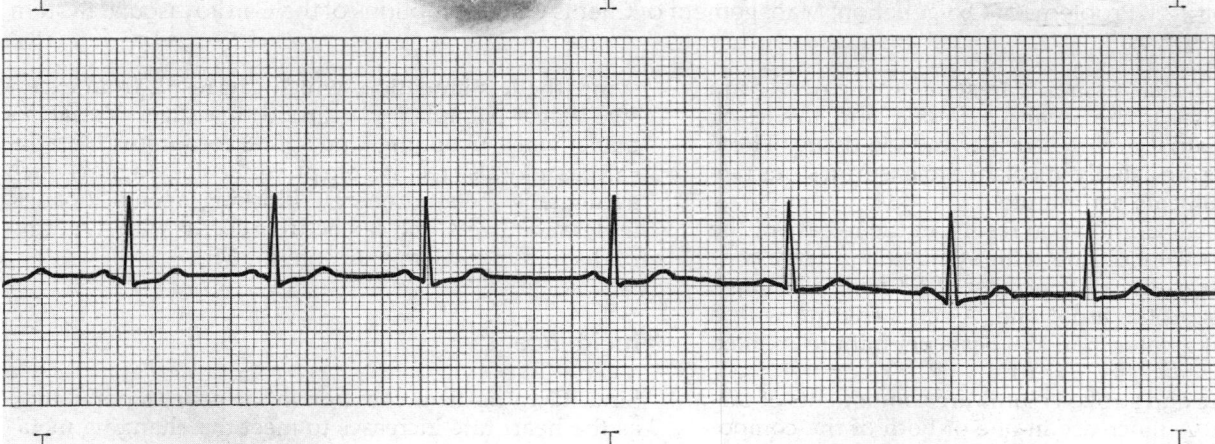

Figure 64–5

Sinus arrhythmia, considered normal.

toring, which is usually used in critical care, telemetry, or cardiac rehabilitation units, provides valuable data for dysrhythmia recognition. If ischemia or injury to the myocardium is suggested by ST segment abnormalities on single-lead monitors, a 12-lead ECG provides much more information, such as the location of the ischemic wall.

The *T wave* represents ventricular repolarization. It always follows the wave representing ventricular depolarization, the QRS. Thus, it is important to differentiate it from other waveforms that are similar in appearance, such as the P waves. Stimuli (either endogenous premature ventricular beats or exogenous pacing stimuli) occurring on the T wave of the previous beat can result in ventricular irritability in the form of ventricular tachycardia or ventricular fibrillation, especially in the presence of recent myocardial infarction (MI) or electrolyte imbalance.

The *QT interval* is the total time from ventricular depolarization to ventricular repolarization. It is measured from the beginning of the QRS complex to the end of the T wave. The normal duration of a QT interval varies with the heart rate. The slower the rate, the longer the QR interval is. It seldom exceeds 0.40 second in normal sinus rhythm. However, some medications (procainamide hydrochloride [Pronestyl], quinidine, and amio-

darone [Cordarone]) and electrolyte deficiencies (potassium or magnesium deficit) can prolong the QT interval, predisposing the client to a sometimes fatal type of ventricular tachycardia called torsades de pointes (see Fig. 64–20).

Sinus arrhythmia is a normal variation of sinus rhythm that is characterized by an irregular rhythm. The irregularity is related to the speeding up and slowing down of the discharges from the SA node in response to intrathoracic pressure changes, which accompany respirations. Children are noted to have more dramatic sinus arrhythmia than adults. In either case, it is considered normal (Fig. 64–5).

Fast and Slow Sinus Rhythms

OVERVIEW

Pathophysiology

The heart is supplied by both sympathetic and parasympathetic nerves. Sympathetic nerves are distributed mainly to the SA node, the AV node, and atrial and

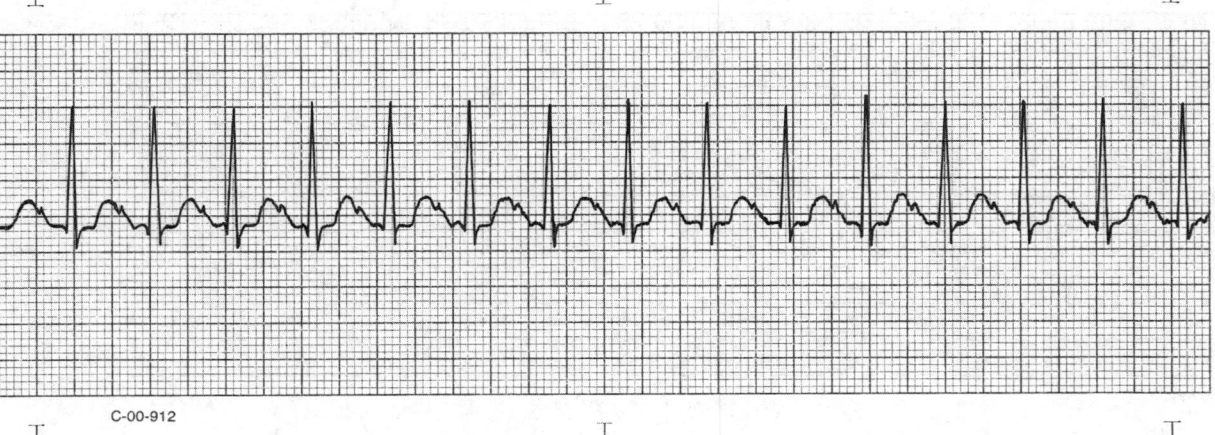

C-00-912

Figure 64–6

Sinus tachycardia.

ventricular muscle tissues. Parasympathetic nerves are also distributed to the SA and AV nodes and, to a lesser extent, the atrial and ventricular muscle tissue. These two systems are usually in balance to ensure a sinus rate of 60 to 100 beats per minute.

Sympathetic domination results in the release of the hormone norepinephrine at the sympathetic nerve endings, which results in the increase of SA node discharge, thus increasing the atrial rate. A sinus rhythm with a heart rate of greater than 100 beats per minute is called *sinus tachycardia* (Fig. 64–6).

Heart rate and stroke volume are components of cardiac output. An increase in one or both of the components increases the cardiac output. Sympathetic stimulation and circulating catecholamines increase not only the heart rate, but also the stroke volume. Therefore, cardiac output is greatly enhanced in these states. However, rapid heart rates shorten diastolic filling time, which can lead to diminished cardiac output and coronary insufficiency.

If the balance of sympathetic and parasympathetic systems is dominated by parasympathetic stimulation, a decrease in SA node discharge occurs, decreasing the atrial rate. A sinus rhythm with a rate of less than 60 beats per minute is called *sinus bradycardia* (Fig. 64–7).

Etiology

Central nervous system–mediated sympathetic stimulation can be caused by anxiety, pain, fright, or stress. Any condition that requires the heart to beat faster in compensation for a decreasing stroke volume (e.g., fever, alcohol ingestion, hypovolemia, heart failure, hyperthyroidism, and anemia) increases the heart rate in an attempt to maintain cardiac output at a constant volume.

Sinus bradycardia often occurs in well-conditioned athletes because the strong heart muscle is extremely efficient in providing an adequate stroke volume, while not requiring a higher heart rate for adequate cardiac output. Sinus bradycardia may also be caused by para-

sympathetic stimulation, which can result from excessive vagal stimulation (carotid massage, Valsalva's maneuvers, suctioning, and spinal cord injury). Bradycardias may also result from pharmacologic agents, such as digitalis, beta-adrenergic blocking agents, opiates, and tranquilizers, and can occur in clients with hypothyroidism, hyperkalemia, or inferior MIs.

Incidence

Sinus tachycardia is common in the general population as the heart rate increases to meet the changing metabolic demands of the body. Sinus tachycardia occurs in approximately 35% to 43% of patients with acute MI (Woods, 1982). In clients with a history of angina, a shortened diastolic filling time occurring with tachycardias can lead to symptoms of coronary insufficiency.

Sinus bradycardia occurs in approximately 25% of clients with MI (Woods, 1982) and is usually associated with inferior MIs.

A syndrome characterized by alternating bradycardia and tachycardia is called *sick sinus syndrome.* The underlying pathologic process is fibrosis of the conduction system. The bradycardia is usually accompanied by symptoms such as dizziness, weakness, and syncope. It has often been documented in the elderly population and is usually the reason for pacemaker implantation.

Premature Beats and Ectopic Rhythms

OVERVIEW

Pathophysiology

Occasionally, a small area of the heart becomes much more excitable than normal and causes an abnormal impulse to fire early. A depolarization wave spreads outward from the irritable area and initiates a premature

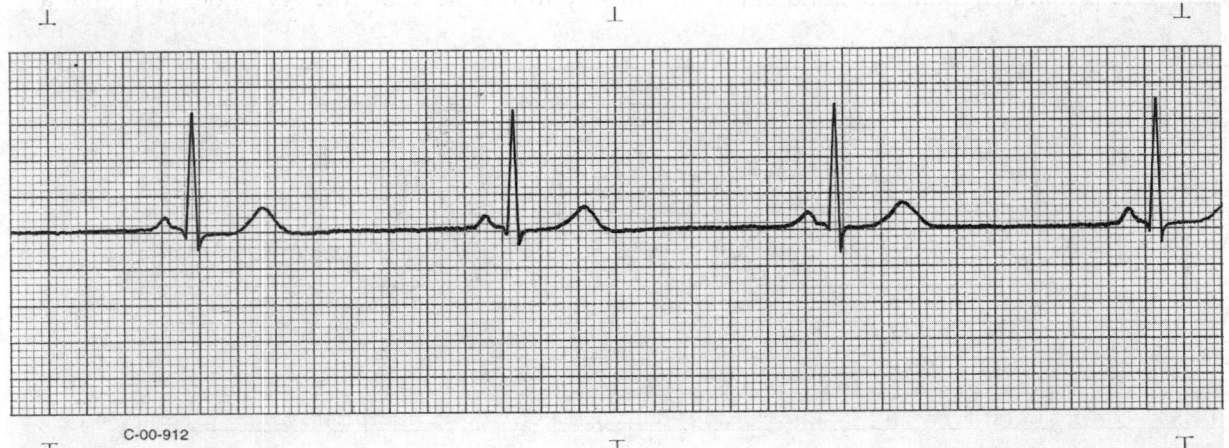

C-00-912

Figure 64–7

Sinus bradycardia.

contraction of the heart. The focus at which the abnormal impulse is generated is called an *ectopic focus*; the focus may be generated by the atrial, junctional, or ventricular tissue. These beats are termed premature atrial contractions (PACs), premature junctional contractions (PJCs), or premature ventricular contractions (PVCs), respectively (Fig. 64–8).

As an isolated occurrence, the premature contraction is not threatening. However, an increase in premature beats could be a precursor of more irritability in that particular area of the heart. For instance, an increase in the frequency of PACs may precede atrial tachycardia, atrial flutter, or atrial fibrillation. Likewise, frequent PVSs may be precursors of more life-threatening

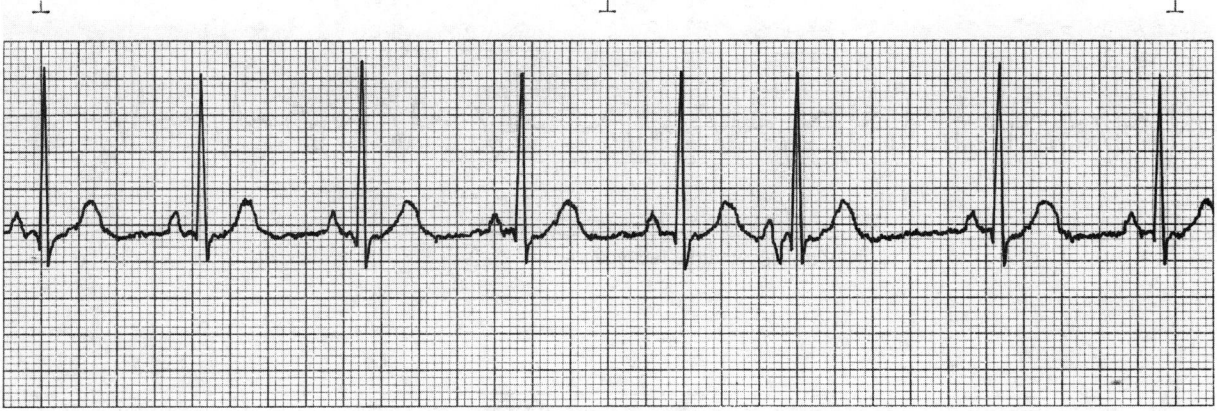

Premature atrial contraction

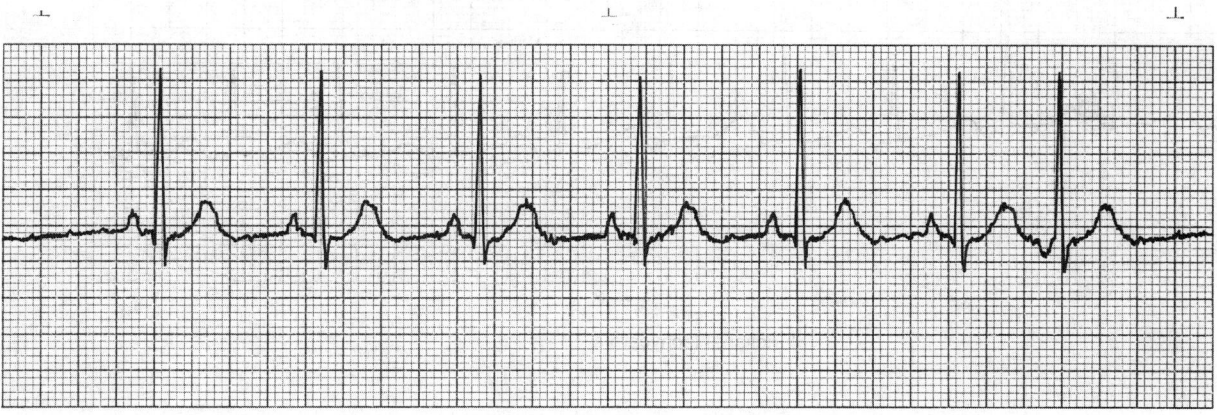

Premature junctional contraction

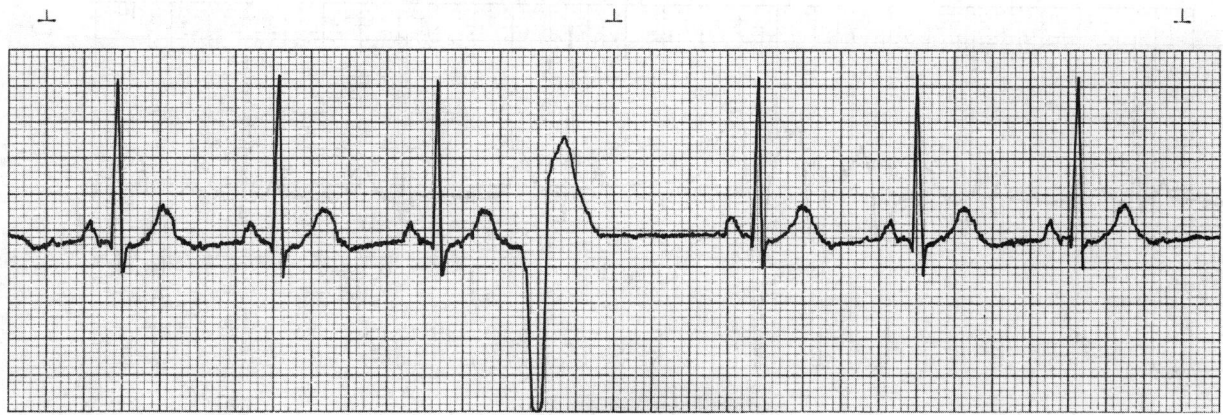

Premature ventricular contraction

Figure 64–8

Premature beats.

rhythms, such as ventricular tachycardia and ventricular fibrillation.

When premature beats increase in frequency, an ectopic or irritable focus is developing excessive excitability. The automatic cell (atrial, junctional, or ventricular) becomes so irritable that it establishes rhythmic rapid discharges overriding the rhythm of the SA node. Thus,

the ectopic focus becomes the pacemaker of the heart by circuitous repetitive depolarization and tachycardia (Fig. 64–9). Note that to call any of these rhythms tachycardia, the rate must exceed 100 beats per minute.

At times, a tachycardia consisting of a narrow QRS interval is observed, yet evidence of atrial P waves may not be observable. In these cases, the term *supraventric-*

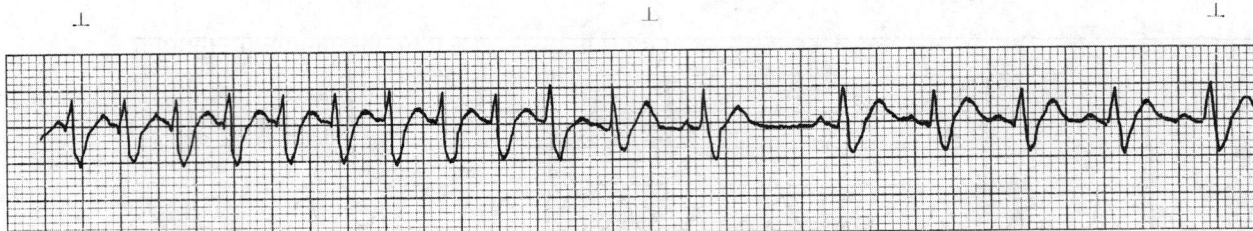

Paroxysmal atrial tachycardia

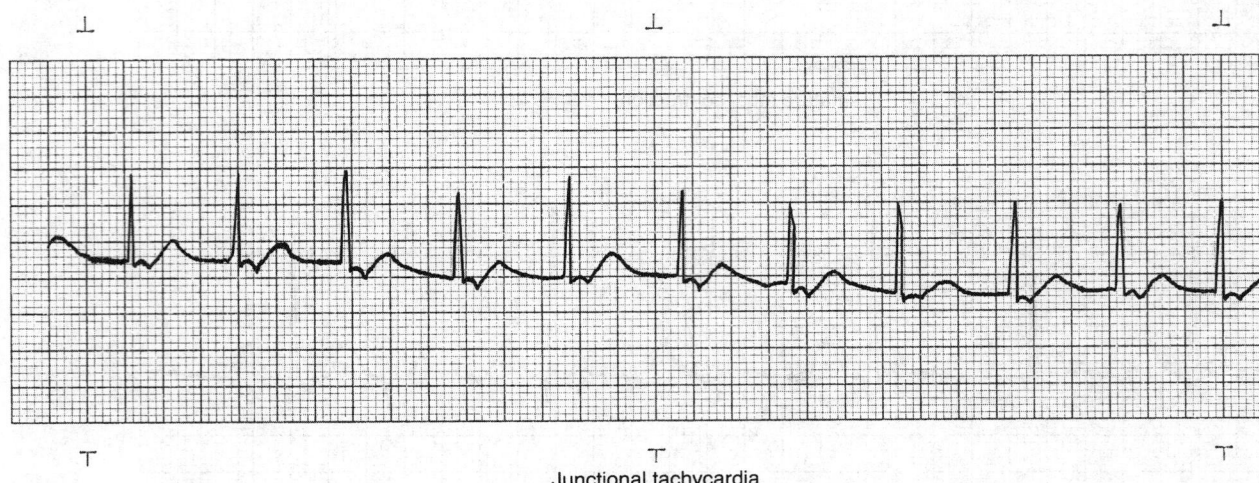

Junctional tachycardia

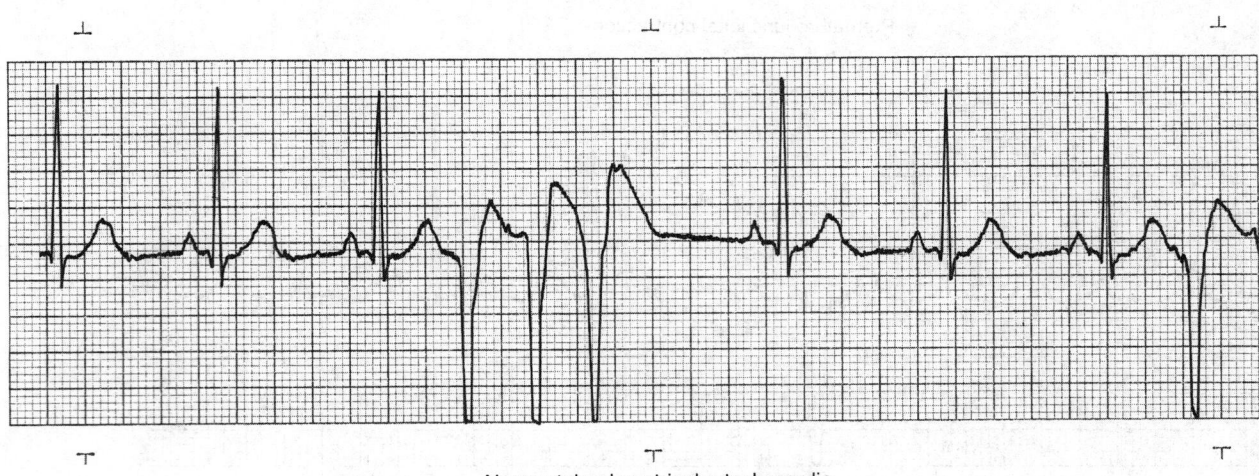

Nonsustained ventricular tachycardia

Figure 64–9

Ectopic rhythms.

ular tachycardia is used to signify a tachycardia originating from above the ventricles, from either the atrial or junctional tissue.

Etiology

The usual cause of an ectopic focus is an irritable area of cardiac muscle resulting from local ischemia (too little coronary blood flow to the cardiac tissue), digitalis toxicity, increased catecholamine release, edema at the tissue level, hypoxia, electrolyte imbalance, overuse of stimulants (e.g., caffeine or nicotine), lack of sleep, anxiety, or stretching of the myocardial fibers (as seen in fluid overload, heart failure, or valvular disorders).

Incidence

Supraventricular premature beats (atrial or junctional in origin) have been documented in healthy women (Romhilt et al., 1984) and men without significance. Paroxysmal (starts and stops suddenly) atrial tachycardia is common in younger persons, often in the absence of heart disease. It is uncommon in older individuals, yet may complicate acute MI (Sokolow & McIlroy, 1981). Sustained or nonsustained tachycardias increase the metabolic demands of the heart while shortening the diastolic filling time of the coronary arteries. This is a major detriment in clients whose coronary blood flow is already compromised.

The most common cause of premature ventricular beats in older persons is cardiac disease. It is the most common dysrhythmia noted during MI, occurring in approximately 80% of cases (Woods, 1982). However, ventricular ectopy has been documented in both healthy athletes and healthy sedentary subjects (Palatini et al, 1985). The likelihood of sudden death is enhanced in patients with ventricular premature beats caused by cardiac disease, especially if the premature beats occur in multifocal patterns or are frequent, early, in pairs, or associated with short or long runs of ventricular tachycardia (Sokolow & McIlroy, 1981). Hypertensive clients with left ventricular hypertrophy have an increased incidence of ventricular dysrhythmias (Le Heuzey & Guize, 1988).

Atrial Flutter and Fibrillation

OVERVIEW

Pathophysiology

There are two basic theories of atrial fibrillation and flutter (Fig. 64–10). The first is that single or multiple ectopic foci emit many impulses one after another in rapid succession. The second is that a circus movement occurs, in which the impulse travels around and around through the heart, never stopping.

The atrial rate in atrial flutter is usually 200 to 350 times per minute; however, the AV node blocks many of those impulses from entering the ventricles. Instead of evidence of the SA node's discharging, a saw-toothed baseline representing the flutter from the atrial tissues is a hallmark of the dysrhythmia.

In atrial fibrillation, numerous (> 350) chaotic waves travel over the surface of the atria, all at the same time. This results in complete incoordination of atrial contraction, so that effective atrial pumping ceases. Thus, overall cardiac output is diminished because of the elimination of the atrial kick. In controlled atrial fibrillation, the ventricular rate is less than 100 beats per minute. In uncontrolled atrial fibrillation, the ventricular rate is greater than 100 beats per minute. The characteristics of atrial fibrillation include no identifiable P waves and an irregular ventricular response.

Etiology

Atrial flutter and atrial fibrillation can occur with atrial ischemia or in any condition in which the atrial chambers become stretched or compressed, as in fluid overload, mitral valve stenosis, or heart failure.

Incidence

Atrial flutter is less common than atrial fibrillation. It is most commonly seen in persons older than 40 years of age who have ischemic heart disease and in clients with chronic obstructive pulmonary disease with or without pre-existing cardiac disease. Atrial fibrillation is the most common cardiac dysrhythmia (Sokolow & Massie, 1988). It occurs in clients who have hypertension, mitral valve prolapse, cardiomyopathy, or pericarditis, or after excessive alcohol intake.

Escape Rhythms

OVERVIEW

Pathophysiology

As discussed earlier, the cardiac impulse begins in the SA node and its rate of rhythmic discharge is greater than that of any other part of the heart. Therefore, the SA node controls the overall rate of the heart under normal circumstances. In abnormal conditions (as when strong stimulation of the vagus nerve causes acetylcholine to be released, decreasing the rate of the SA node discharge), other parts of the heart can provide an escape beat or a series of escape beats until the SA node resumes the function of providing regular rhythmic impulses. These escape impulses may originate in the AV nodal area or the Purkinje fibers in the ventricles if the SA node fails to discharge.

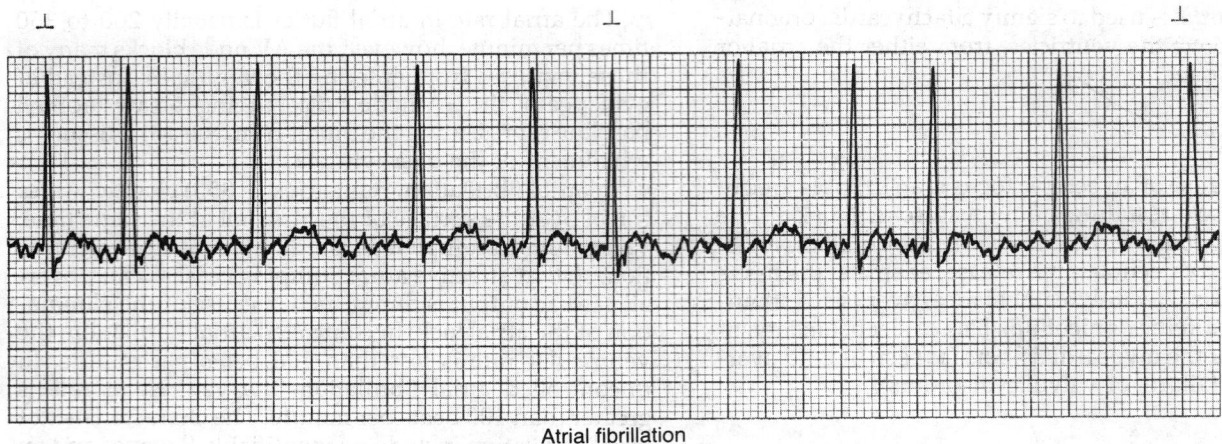

Atrial fibrillation

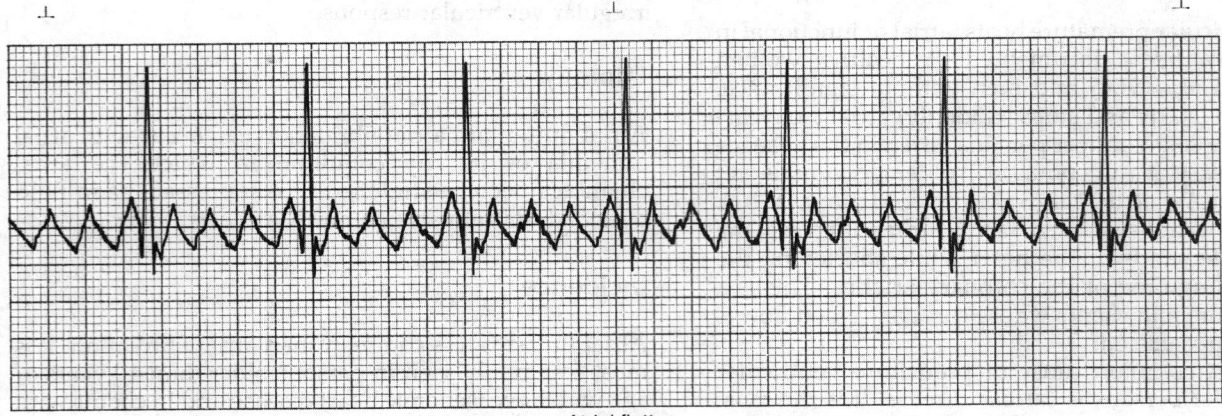

Atrial flutter

Figure 64–10

Atrial flutter and atrial fibrillation.

If the AV node assumes the rhythmic impulse formation, the rhythm would be known as a *junctional escape* rhythm (Fig. 64–11). The intrinsic rate of the junctional tissue is 40 to 60 times per minute. The rhythm is regular; P waves are absent, near, during, or after the QRS; and the QRS width is within normal limits, because the impulse travels through the bundle of His to the bundle branches.

Sometimes, the automaticity of junctional tissue is enhanced by metabolic abnormalities related to hypoxia, ischemia, and associated digitalis therapy. The resultant junctional rhythm is then called an *accelerated*

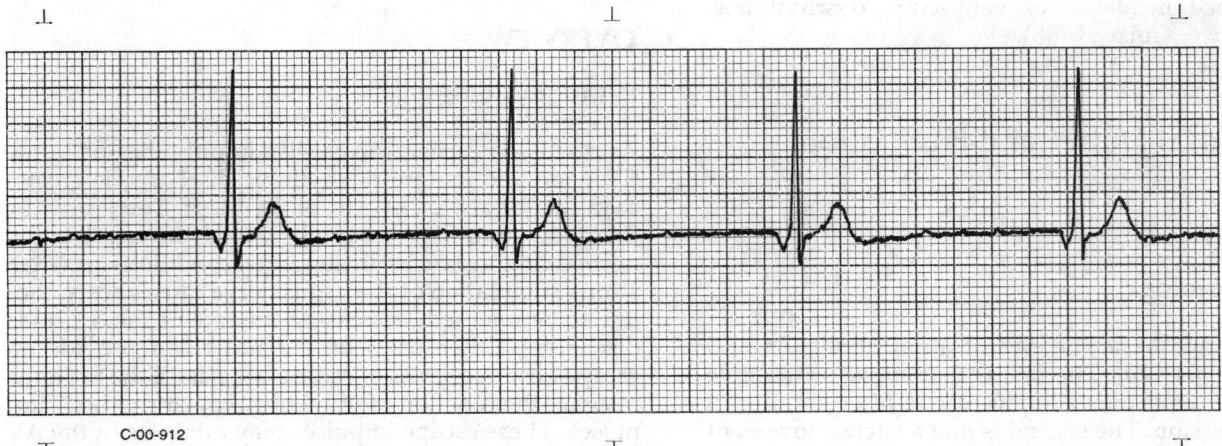

C-00-912

Figure 64–11

Junctional escape rhythm.

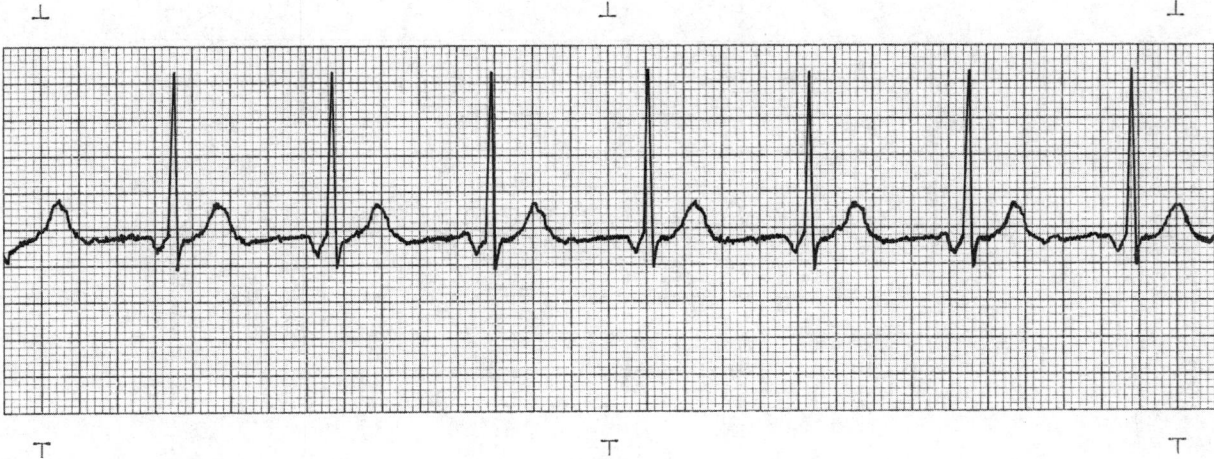

Figure 64–12

Accelerated junctional rhythm.

junctional rhythm because it exceeds the intrinsic junctional rate of 40 to 60 beats per minute and occurs at a rate of 60 to 100 beats per minute. This rhythm is usually temporary and well tolerated (Fig. 64–12).

If the SA node and the AV node both fail to produce an impulse, the Purkinje fibers may assume the rhythmic impulse formation. In this case, the intrinsic rate of the Purkinje fibers is between 15 and 40 times per minute. This is known as a *ventricular escape* rhythm, also called an idioventricular rhythm (Fig. 64–13). The rhythm is regular, P waves are absent, and QRS width is greater than 0.12 second in duration because the impulse originated outside of the His bundle system.

Etiology

Vagal stimulation with carotid massage, Valsalva's maneuvers, and prolonged suctioning results in pauses in sinus node discharge and promotes the development of escape rhythms. Hyperkalemia or digitalis toxicity may also promote the development of escape beats or escape rhythms.

Incidence

Junctional rhythms are seen in approximately 19% of clients with MIs (Woods, 1982).

Conduction Delays and Blocks

Delays in conduction can occur at the AV nodal area (AV blocks), within the bundle branches, or both.

ATRIOVENTRICULAR BLOCKS

OVERVIEW

Pathophysiology

Occasionally, transmission of the impulse is blocked at a critical point in the conduction system. One of the most

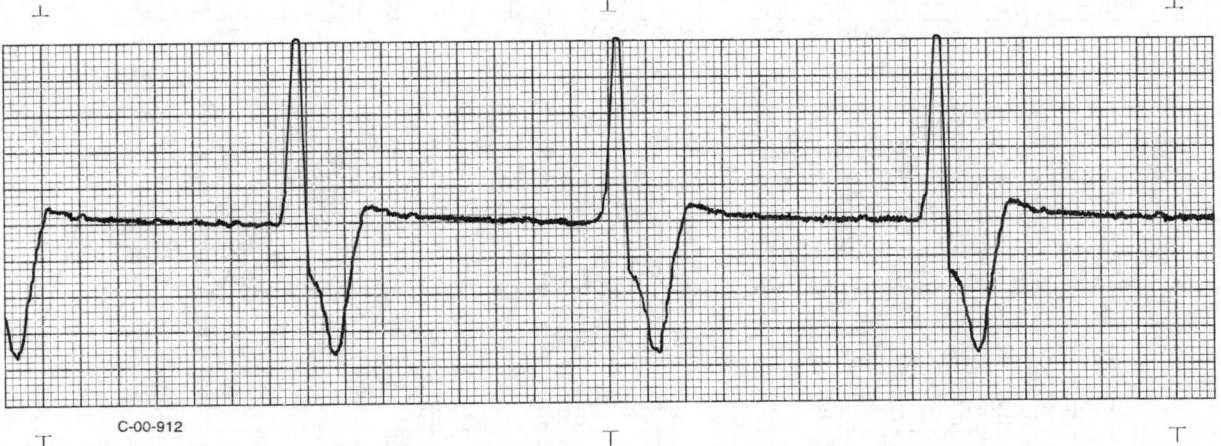

C-00-912

Figure 64–13

Ventricular escape rhythm (idioventricular).

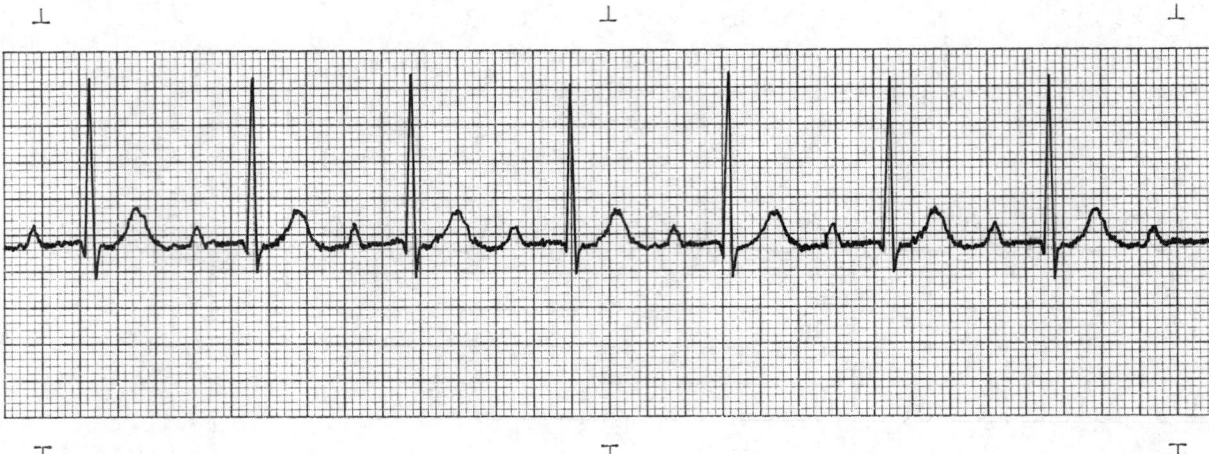

Figure 64–14

First-degree AV block.

common of these points is between the atrium and the ventricles. This condition is called *AV block*.

AV blocks may be categorized as first-, second-, or third-degree blocks, in order of their severity of conduction delay. *First-degree AV block* is characterized by a prolonged PR interval, which is not a block at all. Every impulse from the SA node reaches the conduction system in the ventricles, however, in a delayed fashion. The PR interval reflects this delay by measuring greater than 0.20 second and remains constant from beat to beat (Fig. 64–14).

There are two types of *second-degree AV block*, namely Mobitz's type I (or Wenckebach's) and Mobitz's type II (Fig. 64–15). In Mobitz's type I block, the PR interval progressively lengthens, with shortening of the R-to-R interval, until a beat is blocked. Mobitz's type I block is often transient and does not progress. In many cases, it is well tolerated by clients. In Mobitz's type II

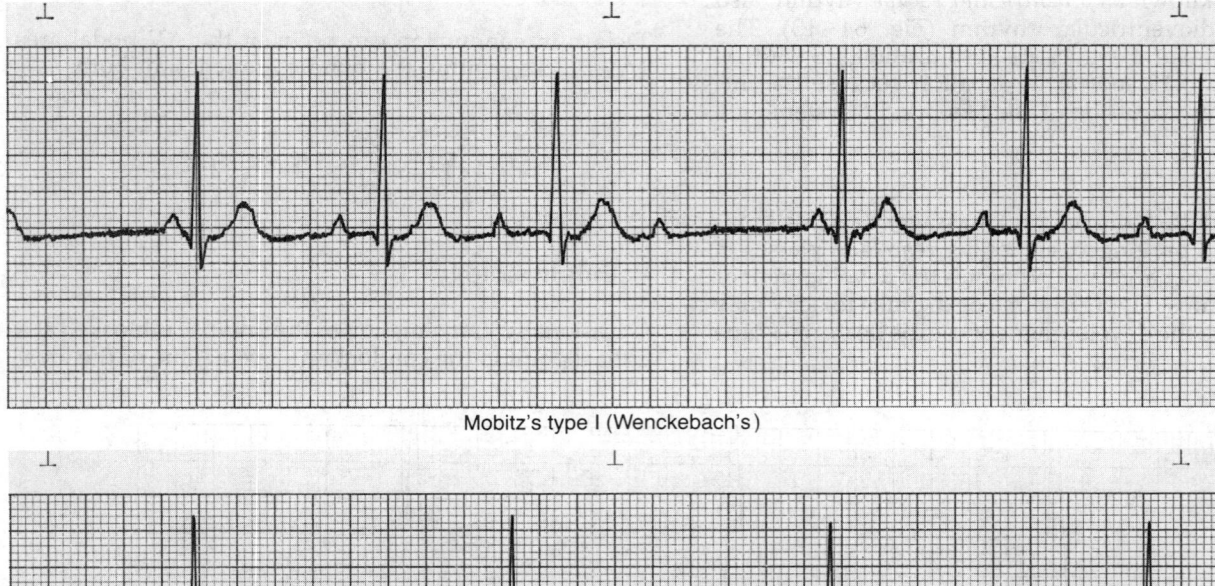

Mobitz's type I (Wenckebach's)

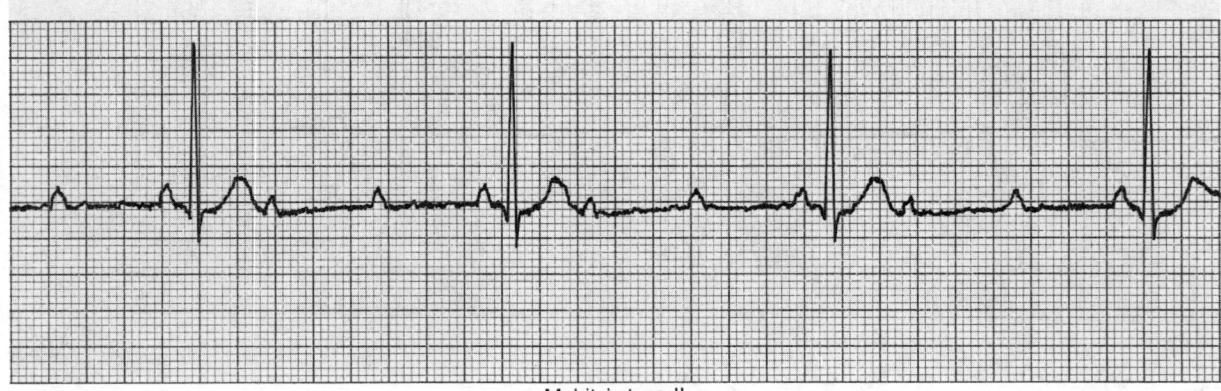

Mobitz's type II

Figure 64–15

Second-degree AV blocks.

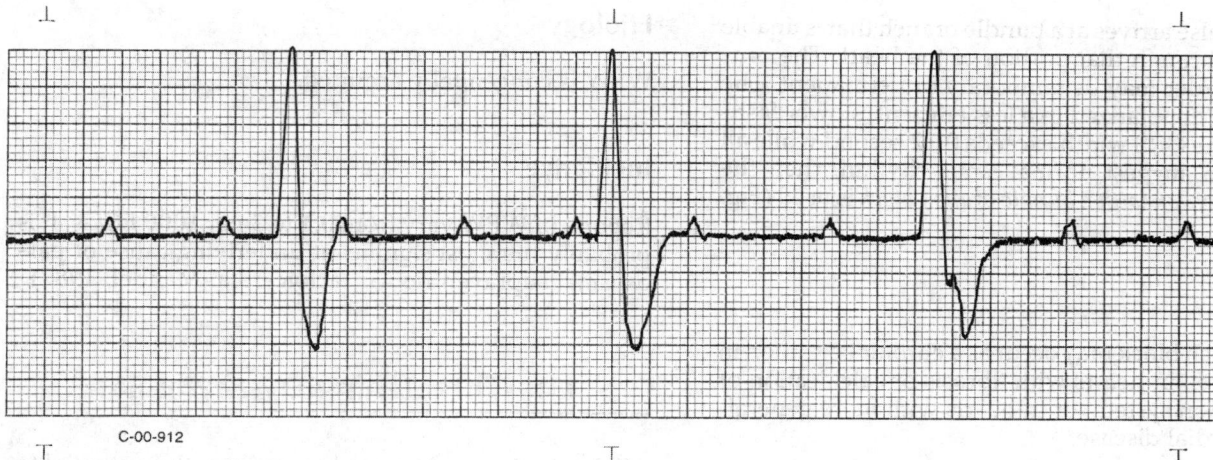

C-00-912

Figure 64–16

Complete heart block.

block, the PR interval is constant, and beats are abruptly blocked. Mobitz's type II block more often progresses to third-degree block. Even if it appears to be well tolerated by the client, it is considered an ominous sign, especially when it occurs with acute ischemia.

Third-degree AV block is also known as complete heart block. In this block, none of the sinus node impulses are able to conduct through the AV node to penetrate the ventricles. The rhythm strip shows evidence of SA node discharge with regular P waves at a rate of 60 to 100 per minute, but there is no relationship of P waves to the QRS complex. The rate of the ventricular rhythm and the width of the QRS complex is related to the level of the block. If the escape impulse originates at the top of the bundle of His, the ventricular rate between 40 and 60 beats per minute may be well tolerated by the client. If the escape originates from the bundle of His or below, the rate is slower and less dependable, with a regular ventricular escape rhythm between 15 and 40 beats per minute (Fig. 64–16).

Etiology

First-degree block and Mobitz's type I second-degree block may occur in clients with heightened vagal tone,

and in clients taking digoxin, calcium channel blockers, or beta-blockers. They can also occur in clients with ischemia, infarctions, or inflammatory heart disorders.

Mobitz's type II second-degree block and third-degree block are most always due to ischemia or degeneration of the conduction system.

Incidence

First-degree AV block is commonly seen in elderly clients with or without cardiac disease. First-degree AV block also occurs in up to 13% of clients with an acute MI (usually inferior), 75% of whom subsequently develop second- or third-degree block (Lie & Durrer, 1980).

BUNDLE BRANCH BLOCKS

OVERVIEW
Pathophysiology

Another common point for conduction delay is within the bundle branch system. It occurs when a supraven-

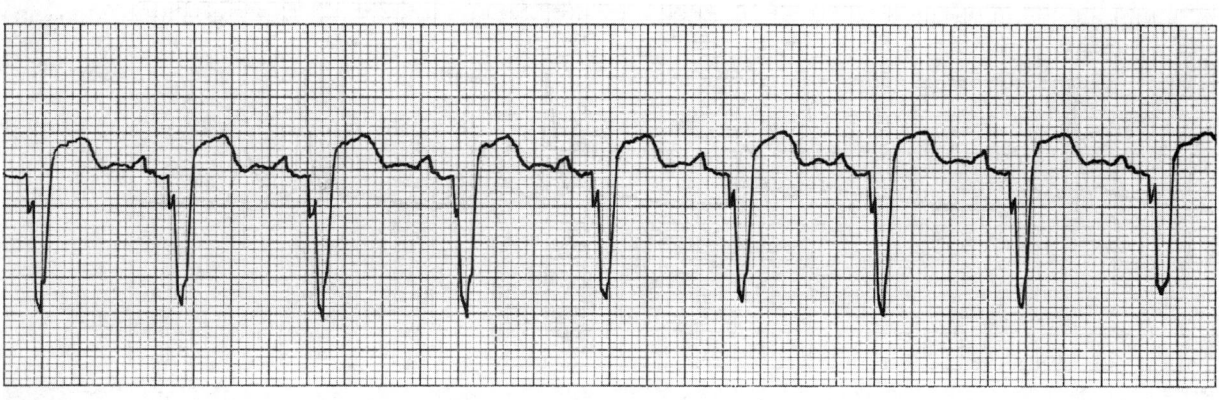

Figure 64–17

Bundle branch block.

tricular impulse arrives at a bundle branch that is unable to conduct through that portion of the heart. The conduction disorder may be temporary or permanent. The heart is then depolarized in a less efficient, slower fashion. When the QRS width exceeds 0.12 second while all other criteria suggest normal sinus rhythm, then the term *sinus rhythm with a bundle branch block* is used (Fig. 64–17).

Etiology

Bundle branch block may occur as a chronic condition in normal hearts, in hearts with fibrosis or calcification of the conduction system, or in hearts with more generalized myocardial disease.

Incidence

Bundle branch blocks are commonly seen in normal hearts; however, they more commonly occur with heart disease, such as ischemic heart disease, inflammatory disease, or aortic valve disease.

PRE-EXCITATION SYNDROMES
OVERVIEW
Pathophysiology

Accessory pathways bypassing the AV node (precluding AV holding time) can conduct impulses originating in the atrium to the ventricles in an unusually rapid fashion. The most common of the pre-excitation syndromes is *Wolff-Parkinson-White syndrome*. In WPW, the PR interval is less than 0.12 second in duration and the QRS complex has a slurred initial portion called the delta wave (Marriott, 1987) (Fig. 64–18). The greatest danger in WPW is the development of atrial dysrhythmias. With the bypassing of the AV node, rapid atrial dysrhythmias quickly conduct to the ventricles, resulting in life-threatening ventricular dysrhythmias.

Etiology

WPW is congenitally acquired.

Incidence

Reports of WPW vary from 0.1 to 3 per 1000 ECGs. It is probably the most significant underlying cause of paroxysmal supraventricular tachycardia (Mandel, 1987).

Life-Threatening Dysrhythmias

All dysrhythmias discussed so far have the potential to be life-threatening, depending on their symptoms and the clinical context. However, some dysrhythmias are considered malignant in that they can result in immediate death if not promptly detected and treated.

The life-threatening dysrhythmias include sustained ventricular tachycardia, ventricular fibrillation, and asystole. They are categorized as life-threatening because of the lack of cardiac output accompanying each. If cardiac output is compromised for a period of 4 to 10 minutes, brain damage or death follows. If one of these dysrhythmias occurs, the performance of cardiopulmonary resuscitation (CPR) may sustain the client until treatment of the dysrhythmia is available.

SUSTAINED VENTRICULAR TACHYCARDIA
OVERVIEW
Pathophysiology

Nonsustained ventricular tachycardia consists of three or more consecutive PVCs in a row. *Sustained ventricular tachycardia* consists of a repetitive, rapid ventricular

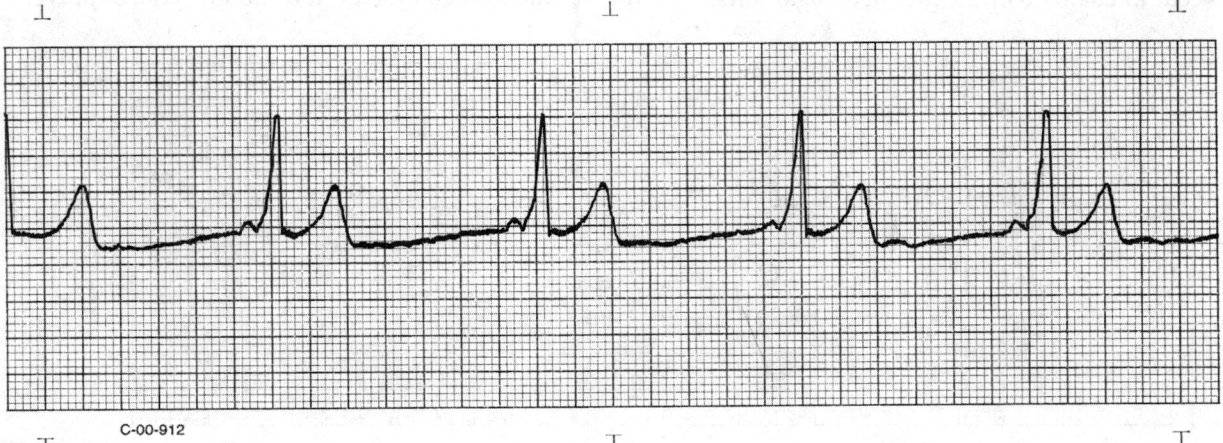

C-00-912

Figure 64–18

Wolff-Parkinson-White syndrome.

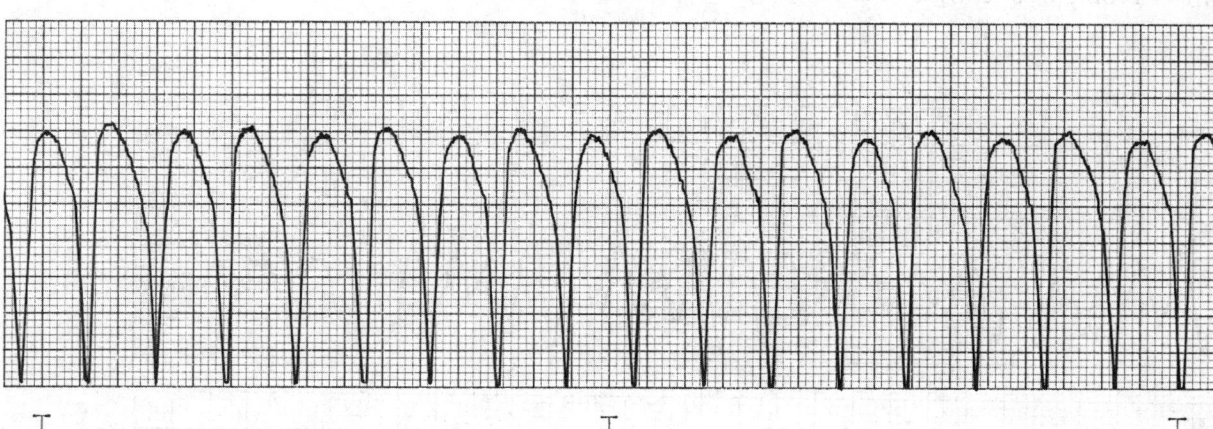

Figure 64–19

Ventricular tachycardia.

rhythm that compromises cardiac output and diastolic filling time. The dominant features of ventricular tachycardia include a mainly regular rhythm, a rate between 150 and 200 beats per minute, and a QRS interval measuring greater than 0.12 second in duration. P waves, as evidence of atrial impulses, if they occur, are usually not distinguishable, as they may be hidden in the rapid firing of the ventricles (Fig. 64–19). Some cases of ventricular tachycardia are accompanied by palpable pulses and stable blood pressure, and the client does not lose consciousness. However, most cases of sustained ventricular tachycardia are accompanied by loss of consciousness and can be considered precursors to ventricular fibrillation.

One type of ventricular tachycardia is termed *torsades de pointes* ("twisted points") and occurs in the setting of prolonged QT interval (Fig. 64–20).

Etiology

Ventricular tachycardia can be the result of myocardial ischemia or infarction, digitalis toxicity, mitral valve prolapse, cardiomyopathy, myocarditis, hypokalemia, prolonged QT interval (often associated with the administration of antiarrhythmic agents), or excessive circulating catecholamines.

Incidence

Approximately 28% of clients with acute MIs experience ventricular tachycardia (Woods, 1982), but it also occurs frequently in clients with cardiomyopathy or mitral valve prolapse. It is commonly associated with a high mortality because it frequently results in a more lethal dysrhythmia, ventricular fibrillation.

VENTRICULAR FIBRILLATION

OVERVIEW

Pathophysiology

The ultimate and most life-threatening result of ventricular irritability is *ventricular fibrillation*. When the ventricles fibrillate, they no longer contract simultaneously.

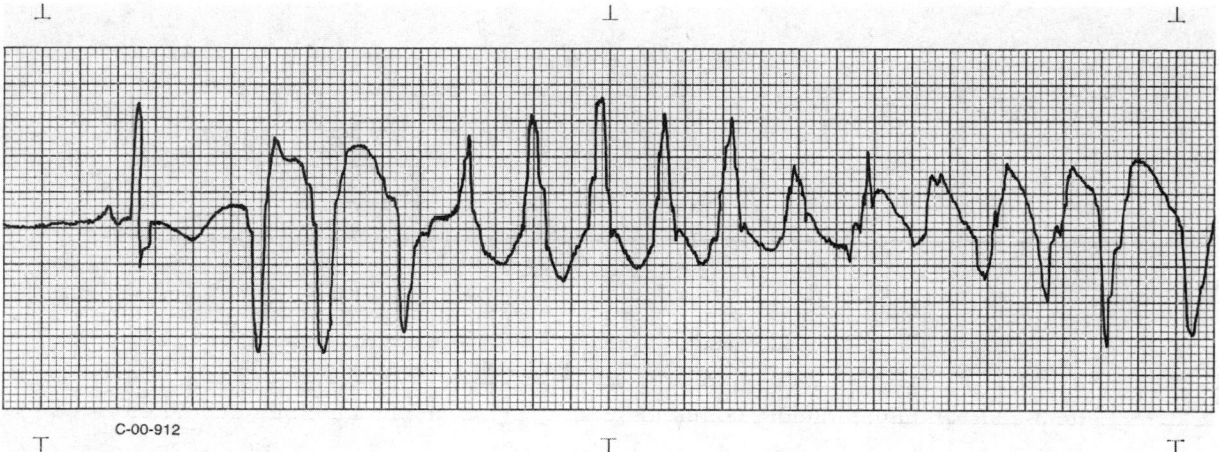

C-00-912

Figure 64–20

Torsades de pointes, a type of ventricular tachycardia that can result from a prolonged QT interval.

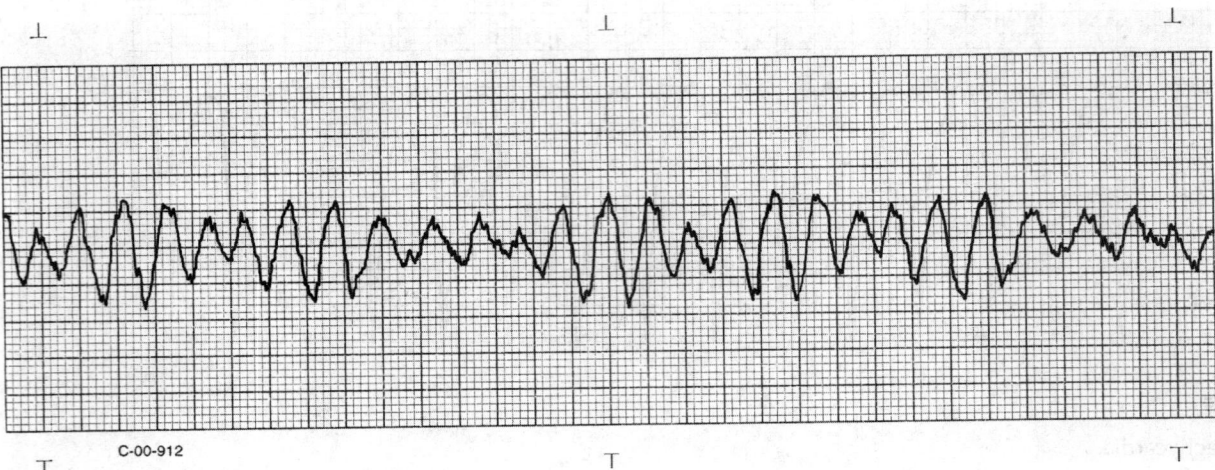

C-00-912

Figure 64–21

Ventricular fibrillation.

Asynchronous chaotic impulses result in the absence of cardiac output and pulse, and P waves and QRS complexes are not present on the monitor pattern. The client quickly loses consciousness when this occurs, sometimes with seizure activity (Fig. 64–21).

Etiology

Coronary artery disease is the most common cause of ventricular fibrillation, the most common terminal event in sudden cardiac death (Surawicz, 1985). In coronary artery disease, ventricular fibrillation can be initiated by a single PVC or by the rapidly firing single focus of ventricular tachycardia. It can be caused by ischemia, infarction, hypoxia, hypothermia, acidosis, or electrolyte imbalance.

Incidence

All clients admitted to the hospital with the diagnosis of MI are at risk for ventricular fibrillation. Ventricular fibrillation that occurs less than 48 hours after acute MI

commonly recurs and has a poor prognosis (Campbell, 1983). More than 40% of patients with documented ventricular fibrillation outside of the hospital can be successfully resuscitated if CPR is provided promptly and followed by advanced cardiac life support ("Standards and Guidelines," 1986).

ASYSTOLE

OVERVIEW
Pathophysiology

When no electrical impulse is generated from the heart, no mechanical or muscular response can be expected. This absence of impulse is termed *asystole*. It is characterized by a straight line on the cardiac monitor (Fig. 64–22). There is no evidence of atrial or ventricular activity. Thus, there is no cardiac output. If the cause is reversible, electrical pacing may be instituted to provide the impulse that is missing endogenously. Fine ventricu-

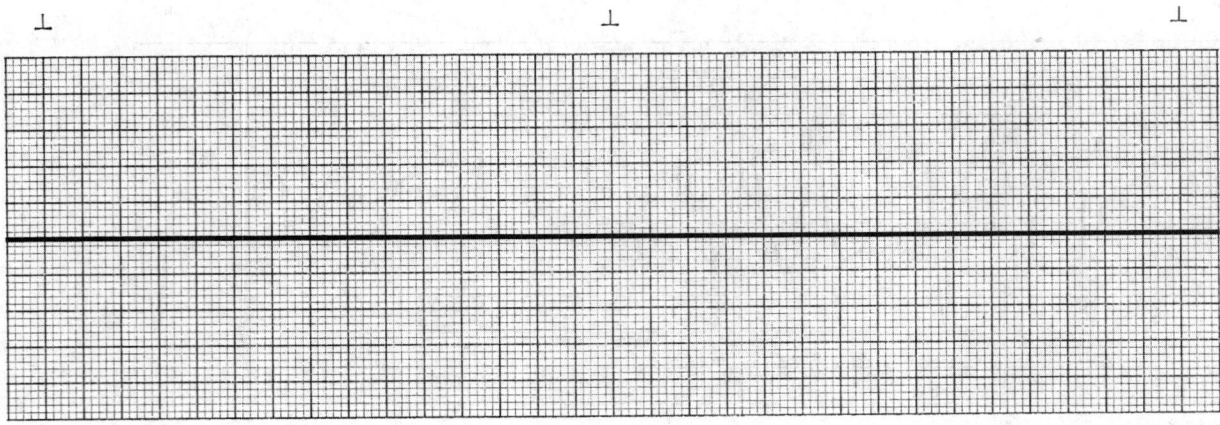

Figure 64–22

Asystole.

lar fibrillation can sometimes appear to be similar to asystole on ECG tracings. Because the treatment of asystole differs greatly from the treatment of ventricular fibrillation, observing the dysrhythmia in two different leads is recommended.

Etiology

Asystole is usually the result of extensive myocardial ischemia from prolonged periods of inadequate coronary perfusion. It can also be caused by severe metabolic disorders, such as hyperkalemia and acidosis. Rarely, parasympathetic stimulation can result in asystole.

Incidence

Asystole is an extremely rare cardiac disorder, which can be accurately described as an arrhythmia, rather than a dysrhythmia, because no rhythm exists. After it has been identified, prompt treatment is necessary to avoid death.

PREVENTION OF DYSRHYTHMIAS

Clients who have bradycardia, especially those with CAD, should be cautioned to avoid Valsalva's maneuvers. Health care providers should avoid vagal stimulation of clients with bradycardia. Procedures that cause vagal stimulation include suctioning, enema administration, rectal temperature checks, and rectal examinations.

Clients who have premature beats and ectopic rhythms are cautioned to avoid smoking, consumption of caffeine and alcoholic beverages, and stress. All clients at risk for ischemic heart disease should be taught how to treat anginal attacks promptly with rest and nitroglycerin to limit the ischemic period, during which ventricular dysrhythmias often occur. Clients at risk for electrolyte imbalance, such as those taking diuretics, should be monitored for hypokalemia and given potassium supplements as needed.

COLLABORATIVE MANAGEMENT OF DYSRHYTHMIAS

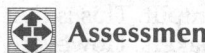 Assessment

History

When taking a history from a client with suspected or validated dysrhythmias, the nurse assesses for the following: *history of cardiac arrest, CAD, heart failure, congenital defects, rheumatic fever, use of cardiac medications or diuretics,* or *supplemental electrolyte therapy.* The nurse inquires about *subjective complaints,* such as palpitations, shortness of breath, chest pain, weakness, diz-

ziness, confusion, blackouts, or diaphoresis. If episodes of these symptoms were experienced in the past, clarification as to the length, frequency, and tolerance of each episode is necessary. Activities that precipitate, exacerbate, or relieve the episodes, if any, may be noted, including medications. The nurse also asks about symptoms associated with caffeine or alcohol intake and smoking.

Physical Assessment: Clinical Manifestations

The emphasis of the physical assessment is on the impact of the dysrhythmia on left ventricular function. Measurements that reflect left ventricular function include the following: *heart rate and rhythm, blood pressure,* or assessment of *cerebral, coronary, and renal perfusion.* The nurse assesses for clinical effects of dysrhythmias on left ventricular function by evaluating *hypotension, confusion, chest pain, shortness of breath,* and *oliguria.* The nurse assesses the *apical and radial pulses* for a full minute for any irregularity, which may occur in clients with premature beats, escape beats after pauses, atrial fibrillation, or second-degree AV blocks. Should the apical pulse differ from the radial pulse, a pulse deficit exists and may suggest that not all beats are perfusing peripherally, as seen sometimes with PVCs or severe heart failure.

Psychosocial Assessment

Some dysrhythmias occur only during an acute event, such as an MI, but others may be chronic. Chronic or recurrent dysrhythmias often cause the client to fear that he/she may become incapacitated or even die if it recurs or cannot be controlled. The nurse assesses the client for fear related to possible recurrence and frustration related to management difficulties.

Laboratory Findings

Elevated or low levels of serum potassium, calcium, and magnesium can cause dysrhythmias. Hypokalemia is a common cause of ventricular premature beats and rhythms. Hyperkalemia can cause bradycardia, and, at high potassium levels, ventricular fibrillation can occur. Hemoglobin level and hematocrit may indicate anemia, which can cause sinus tachycardia. Arterial blood gases are evaluated to assess for hypoxemia and acid-base imbalance, both of which can cause ventricular dysrhythmias. Serum levels of digoxin and quinidine may be elevated in clients who take these drugs, with dysrhythmias occurring as a result.

Radiographic Findings

A chest x-ray film is obtained to assess for congestive heart failure (CHF) or hypertrophy, either of which can cause a dysrhythmia.

Other Diagnostic Tests

A 12-lead ECG and bedside telemetry or ambulatory (Holter's) monitoring are usually used to assess for the frequency and type of dysrhythmia. Holter's monitoring is often instituted for 24 hours, which permits continuous transmission and storage of the ECG.

If dysrhythmias cannot be assessed during usual activity, an exercise tolerance (stress) test may be performed to assess for a dysrhythmia associated with stress, ischemia, or both. Echocardiography, nuclear scanning, and, if necessary, cardiac catheterization may also be performed to assess for other possible causes, such as valve disorders or ischemia.

If clients are suspected of having dysrhythmias, yet the type or cause cannot be determined by the tests described, electrophysiologic studies are conducted. These studies are done in a laboratory where emergency equipment is available. A special catheter is used to introduce electrodes under sterile conditions for simultaneous cardiac pacing and recording. A variety of rhythms may be induced for the identification of the cells responsible for the dysrhythmia.

 Analysis: Nursing Diagnosis

Common Diagnoses

The most common nursing diagnosis that occurs in clients with dysrhythmias is decreased cardiac output related to electrical and mechanical malfunction.

Additional Diagnoses

The following diagnoses may also occur in clients with dysrhythmias:

1. Altered (cardiopulmonary, cerebral, renal, peripheral, and gastrointestinal) tissue perfusion related to decreased cardiac output
2. Activity intolerance related to imbalance between oxygen supply and demand

 Planning and Implementation

The plan of care for clients with cardiac dysrhythmias is focused on the nursing diagnoses. Because dysfunction in impulse formation or impulse conduction can dramatically affect the cardiac output, attempts should be made to minimize the occurrence of the dysrhythmia and the clinical symptoms associated with decreased cardiac output. With the more serious, life-threatening dysrhythmias, cardiac output ceases completely, resulting in inadequate tissue perfusion and death, if not promptly treated.

Decreased Cardiac Output

Planning: client goals. The major goal for this nursing diagnosis is that the client will have a cardiac rhythm, either natural or paced, that is substantial enough to support adequate cardiac output.

Interventions. Treatment of dysrhythmias is specific to the type of dysrhythmia, the cause, the effect it has on the client's cardiac output, and the risk it presents to the client (see the accompanying Key Features of Disease).

Nonsurgical management. Noninvasive medical interventions that may be used to terminate dysrhythmias, such as supraventricular tachycardia, include carotid massage and Valsalva's maneuvers. When stretch receptors within the carotid sinus are stimulated, the blood pressure and heart rate decrease via vagal influence. Nursing responsibilities during these activities are mainly supportive. The nurse obtains the client's heart rate, rhythm, and blood pressure and, if possible, a cardiac rhythm strip from the monitor before, during, and after the event; these are important in determining the effect of the therapy.

Drug therapy. Pharmacologic therapy administered for the control of dysrhythmias often includes drugs from one or more of the four classes of antidysrhythmic agents (Table 64–2). They are grouped into classes on the basis of the effect they have on the cardiac muscle. Class I antidysrhythmics depress the rate of depolarization and decrease the conduction velocity by impeding the flow of sodium into the cell during depolarization. Eamples of class I antidysrhythmics include lidocaine (Xylocaine), procainamide (Pronestyl), and quinidine.

Class II antidysrhythmics control dysrhythmias associated with too much sympathetic stimulation by depressing depolarization of the cardiac action potential. An example of a class II antidysrhythmic includes the beta-blocker propranolol (Inderal).

Class III antidysrhythmics lengthen the absolute refractory period and act on the myocardium by prolonging the action potential. Examples of class III antidysrhythmics include bretylium tosylate (Bretylol) and amiodarone.

Class IV antidysrhythmics impede the flow of calcium into the cell during depolarization, thereby depressing activity of the SA and AV nodes, prolonging conduction in the AV node, and increasing AV node refractoriness. Calcium channel blockers are class IV antidysrhythmic agents.

Temporary pacing. Temporary pacing is a nonsurgical intervention that is employed to provide an electrical stimulus to the right atrium, right ventricle, or both when a stimulus does not exist or, if it does, the rate is too slow to provide adequate cardiac output. This is the most common use of temporary pacemakers. However, atrial tachycardias, such as atrial flutter, may be terminated by rapid atrial pacing, also called atrial overdrive pacing.

One method of temporary pacing includes the use of fluoroscopy to thread a catheter through a vein to the right side of the heart under sterile conditions. This is referred to as temporary endocardial pacing, because

Text continued on page 2137

KEY FEATURES OF DISEASE ■ Common Dysrhythmias and Their Treatment

Dysrhythmia	Treatment
Sinus tachycardia	Correction of the underlying problem (fever, hypovolemia, pain, anxiety) Beta-adrenergic blockade (propranolol) if increased catecholamine secretion is the underlying problem
Sinus bradycardia	Treatment necessary only if the client is symptomatic (has hypotension, diaphoresis, or altered level of consciousness): 　Atropine 　Pacemaker 　Avoidance of parasympathetic stimulation, such as prolonged suctioning, and stimulation of the gag reflex.
Premature beats and ectopic rhythms	
Supraventricular beats	Quinidine Digitalis Propranolol Verapamil Sedatives
Supraventricular rhythms	Digitalis Verapamil Propranolol Vagal stimulation with carotid massage Valsalva's maneuver Synchronized cardioversion if the above measures are unsuccessful
Premature ventricular beats and ventricular tachycardia	Restoration of electrolyte balance Lidocaine bolus and infusion Procainamide bolus and infusion Class I and II antiarrhythmics
Atrial flutter	Atrial overdrive pacing Cardioversion
Atrial fibrillation	Digitalis Quinidine Procainamide Verapamil Cardioversion
Escape rhythms	Correction of the underlying cause if the client is symptomatic: 　Atropine 　Isuprel 　Pacemaker
Conduction delays	
First-degree AV block	Withholding digitalis Atropine if associated with symptomatic bradycardia
Second-degree AV block (Mobitz's type I)	Atropine if associated with symptomatic bradycardia
Second-degree AV block (Mobitz's type II)	Isuprel Pacemaker
Third-degree AV block	Isuprel Pacemaker
Pre-excitation syndromes	Vagal maneuvers Verapamil Propranolol Quinidine Disopyramide

Continued

KEY FEATURES OF DISEASE ■ Common Dysrhythmias and Their Treatment *Continued*

Dysrhythmia	Treatment
	Cardioversion
	Pacing
	Amiodarone
	Catheter or surgical ablation
Life-threatening dysrhythmias	
Sustained ventricular tachycardia	Lidocaine
	Procainamide
	Cardioversion
	CPR if client is unconscious
Ventricular fibrillation	CPR
	Defibrillation
	Epinephrine
	Lidocaine
	Procainamide
	Bretylium
Asystole	CPR
	Epinephrine
	Pacemaker

TABLE 64–2 Common Antidysrhythmic Drugs

Drug	Usual Daily Dosage	Interventions	Rationales
Class I Drugs			
Quinidine	200–400 mg q, 4–6 h PO, 6–10 mg/kg IV slowly, may be given IM	1. Monitor blood pressure. 2. Watch for diarrhea, nausea, or vomiting and administer with food if these occur. 3. Monitor for widening QRS, prolonged QT interval, heart block, and onset or increase of PVCs.	1. Hypotension is a common side effect. 2. Diarrhea is common during early therapy. Diarrhea and other GI symptoms often improve when quinidine is administered with food. 3. All of these are toxic side effects, which necessitate stopping quinidine administration.
Procainamide (Pronestyl)	250–750 mg q 4–6h PO, 100 mg q 5–15 min IV for total of 1 g	1. Monitor blood pressure. 2. Monitor for widened QRS and prolonged QT or PR. 3. Monitor for joint pain and fever.	1. Hypotension is a common side effect. 2. These are toxic side effects, which may necessitate stopping procainamide administration. 3. Lupus-like syndrome is common with long-term therapy.
Disopyramide (Norpace)	100–200 mg q 6 h PO	1. Monitor blood pressure.	1. Hypotension is a common side effect.

TABLE 64–2   Common Antidysrhythmic Drugs *Continued*

Drug	Usual Daily Dosage	Interventions	Rationales
		2. Watch for shortness of breath and weight gain.	2. Disopyramide can cause CHF in a client with CAD.
Lidocaine (Xylocaine)	1 mg/kg IV bolus followed by 1–4 mg/min infusion	1. Watch for confusion, paresthesias, slurring of speech, drowsiness, or seizure activity.	1. CNS adverse effects predominate; they may require decrease in dosage or discontinuation of infusion.
Mexiletine hydrochloride (Mexitil)	200–400 mg q 6–8 h PO, 250–500 mg q 12 h IV	1. Monitor blood pressure and heart rate. 2. Assess for tremors, blurred vision, dizziness, ataxia, or confusion. 3. Administer with food.	1. Hypotension and bradycardia commonly occur. 2. CNS adverse reactions predominate. 3. This helps prevent GI distress.
Tocainide (Tonocard)	400–800 mg q 8 h PO	1. Administer with food. 2. Assess heart rate. 3. Teach client to report shortness of breath, wheezing, chest pain, or cough.	1. This helps prevent GI distress. 2. Bradycardia may occur. 3. Pulmonary fibrosis is a serious side effect, which necessitates discontinuation of drug.
Flecainide acetate (Tambocor)	100 mg bid PO, maximum dose 400 mg/d	1. Monitor Holter's ECG for increase in arrhythmias.	1. Drug can induce arrhythmias.
Class II Drugs			
Propranolol (Inderal)	10–80 mg qid PO, 0.5–1 mg IV push slowly	1. Monitor heart rate and blood pressure. 2. Assess for shortness of breath or wheezing.	1. Bradycardia and decrease in blood pressure are expected effects. 2. Beta-blocking effects on lungs can cause bronchospasm.
Class III Drugs			
Bretylium tosylate (Bretylol)	5–10 mg/kg IV push repeated q 15–30 min, up to 30 mg/kg/d; 1–2 mg/min by infusion	1. Observe cardiac monitor for PVCS, increase in heart rate, and other arrhythmias. 2. Monitor blood pressure. 3. Maintain the client in a supine position for several days.	1. PVCs and increase in heart rate commonly occur within a few minutes to 1 h after drug is started. 2. Hypertension may occur in first hour after drug is administered, followed by significant hypotension 3. Orthostatic hypotension is a significant problem until tolerance to the drug develops.

Table continued on following page

TABLE 64–2 **Common Antidysrhythmic Drugs** *Continued*

Drug	Usual Daily Dosage	Interventions	Rationales
		4. When the client begins to sit up or get out of bed, raise the head of bed slowly, and advise the client to make position changes slowly.	4. Client could become dizzy and faint.
		5. Anticipate vomiting during administration.	5. This is a common side effect.
Amiodarone hydrochloride (Cordarone)	800–1200 mg q d PO for 1 wk, then 200–800 mg q d PO	1. Assess the client's knowledge of treatment regimen and side effects.	1. Drug has major side effects, which make noncompliance a problem; clients may be on drug 1 ½–3 mo before full clinical effects are apparent.
		2. Monitor blood pressure, heart rate, and cardiac rhythm when initiating therapy.	2. Bradycardia, hypotension, and worsening of arrhythmia can occur.
		3. Teach clients to report any muscle weakness, tremors, or difficulty with ambulation.	3. These are common side effects, which usually develop in the first week of treatment.
		4. Teach clients to report shortness of breath, cough, pleuritic pain, or fever.	4. These may indicate drug-induced pulmonary toxicity.
		5. Teach clients to report any visual disturbance.	5. Corneal pigmentation occurs in most clients, but generally does not interfere with vision; if it does, dosage is decreased.
		6. Teach clients with photophobia to wear sunglasses in the daytime.	6. Photophobia may be so severe that the client cannot go outdoors in daytime.
		7. Teach clients to use barrier sunscreens.	7. Photosensitivity reactions may occur.
Class IV Drugs			
Verapamil hydrochloride (Isoptin, Calan)	5–10 mg IV slowly, 40–80 mg q 6–8 h PO	1. Monitor blood pressure and heart rate.	1. Hypotension and bradycardia are common side effects.
		2. Teach clients to remain recumbent for at least 1 h after IV administration.	2. Hypotension may occur.
		3. Teach clients receiving oral therapy to change positions slowly.	3. Orthostatic hypotension often occurs until tolerance develops.

TABLE 64 – 2   Common Antidysrhythmic Drugs *Continued*

Drug	Usual Daily Dosage	Interventions	Rationales
Other Drugs			
Digoxin (Lanoxin)	Digitalization: 0.5 mg PO or IV initially; 0.125 – 0.25 mg PO or IV q 3 – 6 h until a total of 1 – 1.25 mg is reached Maintenance: 0.125 – 0.25 mg qod or q d PO or IV	1. Assess apical heart rate for 1 min before each dose; hold dose for heart rate less than 60 beats/min. 2. Assess for sudden increase of heart rate and change of rhythm from regular to irregular, or irregular to regular. 3. Teach clients to report anorexia, nausea, vomiting, diarrhea, paresthesias, confusion, or visual disturbances. 4. Monitor serum potassium levels. 5. Monitor serum creatinine levels.	1. Decrease in heart rate is an expected response, but bradycardia may indicate toxicity. 2. Change in heart rate or rhythm may indicate toxicity. 3. These are signs of toxicity. 4. Hypokalemia increases the risk of toxicity. 5. Impaired renal function can cause toxicity; dosage is altered if this occurs.
Atropine	0.5 – 1 mg IV repeated, to maximum of 2 mg	1. Monitor heart rate and rhythm after administration. 2 Assess for chest pain after administration. 3. Assess for urinary retention and dry mouth after administration. 4. Avoid using in clients with angle-closure glaucoma.	1. Increase in rate is expected. 2 Increased heart rate may cause ischemia in client with CAD. 3. Atropine is an anticholinergic. 4. Atropine increases intraocular pressure.

the catheter tip comes in contact with the innermost lining of the heart. The catheter is lodged within the right ventricle for ventricular demand pacing. Located at the tip of the catheter is a lead that conducts an impulse from a battery-operated pulse generator (Fig. 64–23) to the cardiac muscle to stimulate contraction. If the client needs the atrial kick from atrial contractions, a temporary AV pacemaker is inserted, with one catheter tip in the right atrium and another in the right ventricle.

Temporary pacing may also be accomplished with an insulated wire looped just beneath the epicardial surface of the heart (Fig. 64–24). This type of pacing is most often used during open heart surgery and the postoperative period. The wire loop is secured to the skin externally by sutures. These wires are applied intraoperatively in the event of bradycardias or heart blocks. Pacing in this manner is referred to as temporary epicardial pacing.

Ventricular pacing is usually done in the demand mode. This means that the pacemaker is set to sense the client's own beats, and, when the client conducts his/her own beats, the pacemaker is inhibited from firing. If

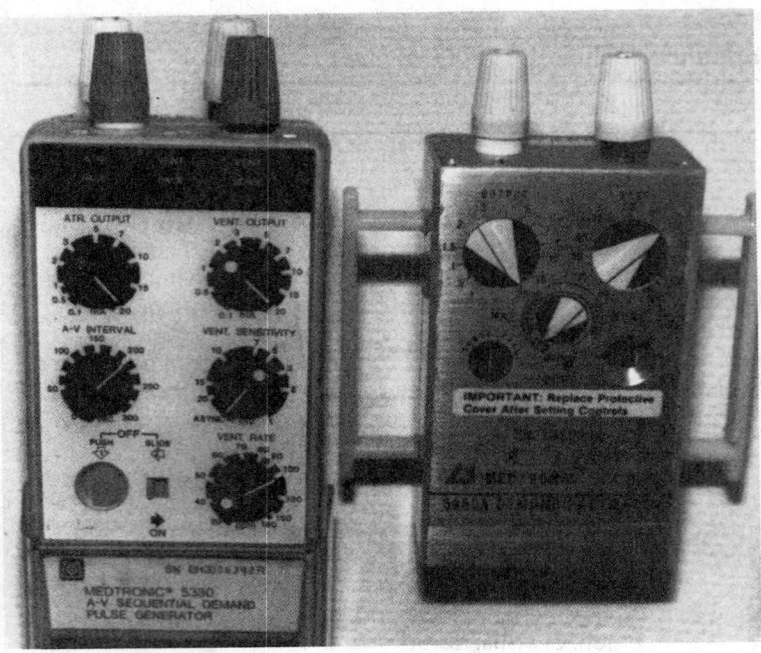

Figure 64–23

Two temporary endocardial pacemakers. Electrode placement in the right ventricle is the same as for permanent pacemakers (see Fig. 64–27). (From Schwartz, G. R., Bircher, N., Hanke, B. K., Mangelsen, M. A., Mayer, T., & Ungar, J. R. [1989]. *Emergency medicine: The essential update.* Philadelphia: W. B. Saunders.)

no beat is sensed, the pacemaker provides an electrical impulse to stimulate the heart to respond with a contraction. The client usually does not feel a pacemaker stimulus; however, occasionally, small shock-like sensations may be reported.

Electrophysiologic studies. Clients who have life-threatening dysrhythmias that occur infrequently may undergo electrophysiologic studies to reproduce the dysrhythmia and observe the response to pharmacologic treatment. In these situations, clients are given loading doses of antiarrhythmics before the studies. Studies are repeated on different days after different antiarrhythmics have been administered to assess the ideal drug for suppression of the dysrhythmia.

Catheter ablation. In cases of recurrent ventricular dysrhythmias and WPW, when atrial conduction bypasses the AV node, catheter ablation is performed after medical therapies have been proved ineffective. Catheter ablation is a technique whereby a catheter is positioned adjacent to the structure identified, during endocardial mapping, as dysrhythmogenic. A synchronized direct current shock is delivered to cause a controlled necrosis of the area. It is performed in a special laboratory equipped with emergency supplies and highly specialized personnel. Nursing care after the procedure includes recording vital signs, monitoring for dysrhythmias, and monitoring cardiac enzyme levels for MI.

Cardioversion. Elective cardioversion may be performed for hemodynamically stable ventricular or supraventricular tachycardias (such as atrial fibrillation), which are resistant to conventional medical therapies. This procedure should be performed where emergency equipment is easily accessible and back-up personnel are available if the patient experiences cardiopulmonary arrest. Because the client is conscious, sedation is absolutely imperative. Conductive pads are placed at the heart apex and just right of the sternum, and defibrillator paddles are placed over the pads. Continuous ECG monitoring is obtained at the bedside while the defibrillator is synchronized to the client's tachydysrhythmia. Synchronizing the shock to the client's rhythm avoids discharge during the vulnerable period (T wave), which

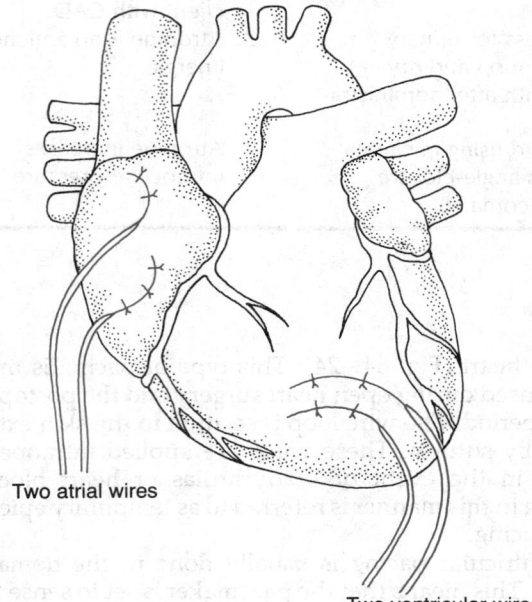

Two atrial wires

Two ventricular wires

Figure 64–24

Epicardial wire placement for temporary pacing.

may result in an even more irritable rhythm, such as ventricular fibrillation. The paddles are charged to 75 to 100 joules. The person performing the cardioversion announces for all personnel to clear contact with the client and the bed before the shock is delivered. After synchronized cardioversion, the client's response and cardiac rhythm are noted and therapy is repeated until the desired result is obtained or alternative therapies are considered. Nursing care after the procedure includes assessing and documenting the client's vital signs and level of consciousness, monitoring for dysrhythmias, and assessing for chest burns from paddle edges not protected by conductive gel pads.

Cardiopulmonary resuscitation.   Management of the client experiencing a cardiac arrest depends on prompt recognition and therapeutic interactions for successful reversal of a potentially fatal event.

When cardiac arrest occurs, cardiac output ceases. The underlying rhythm may consist of ventricular tachycardia, ventricular fibrillation, or asystole. The client is pulseless and unconscious. Loss of consciousness is evidence of inadequate tissue perfusion to the brain. Shortly after the onset of cardiac arrest, respiratory arrest develops. CPR should be initiated immediately to prevent brain damage and death (see the accompanying Emergency Care feature). At times, CPR may be ineffective in reviving the client because of the severity of the heart disease. However, every attempt must be made initially to sustain the client until others have arrived to employ advanced cardiac life-support measures.

Adjuncts to CPR, such as endotracheal intubation and supplemental oxygen, should be provided as soon as qualified personnel are available to assist. Medical and electrical therapies are ordered at this time. If cardiac arrest occurs in the field without the assistance of others, the rescuer is to perform CPR until the client is revived or the rescuer is physically unable to continue.

Complications of CPR include rib fractures, fracture of the sternum, lacerations of the liver and spleen, pneumothorax, hemothorax, lung contusions, and fat emboli.

Sustained pulseless ventricular tachycardia and ventricular fibrillation require prompt termination. Lack of blood flow to the brain for more than 5 to 10 minutes can result in permanent brain damage. Termination of the electrical chaos may be accomplished by delivering an intense electrical current (200 to 360 joules) through defibrillation paddles placed externally on the chest to both sides of the heart. With conductive gel pads at the client's heart apex and just to the right of the sternum, the defibrillator paddles are positioned over them (Fig. 64–25). The operator charges the paddles and announces to everyone to clear contact with the client and the bed in preparation for the delivery of the shock. Defibrillation causes all impulses from the heart to stop for 3 to 5 seconds, and then it is hoped that a natural impulse from the heart can resume a more therapeutic rhythm. Unless defibrillation occurs within 1 minute after onset of ventricular fibrillation, the heart is usually

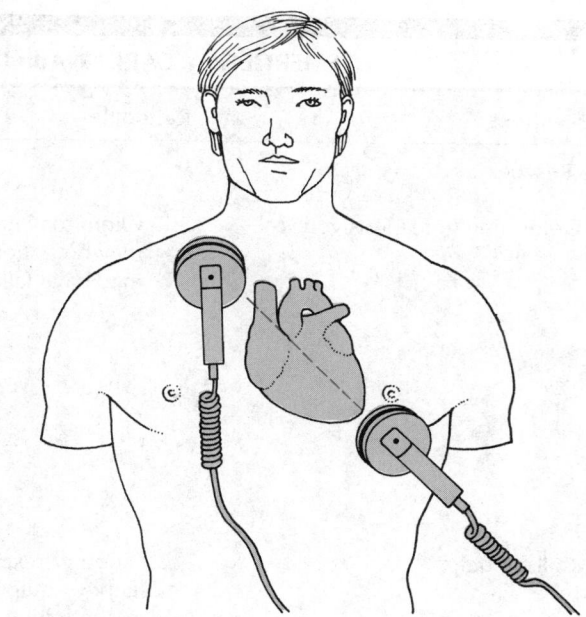

Figure 64–25

Paddle placement for defibrillation.

too weak or acidotic to be converted. This is when CPR and medical preparation of the heart, with epinephrine and sodium bicarbonate, may enhance success of defibrillation.

In the event of asystole or extreme bradycardia not responsive to medical therapies, it may be possible to pace the heart transcutaneously until qualified personnel arrive for insertion of a transvenous pacemaker. External pacing was first employed in the 1950s as a means to stimulate the heart to contract via noninvasive methods. Its use was quickly superseded by transvenous intracardiac techniques. With the expanding role of nurses in critical care units and emergency rooms, the concept of external pacing has made a comeback. With specialized training and equipment, it is possible to provide regular transcutaneous electrical stimuli to the heart when an intrinsic impulse is lacking. The stimulus from an external pacing device is delivered through two large electrodes, one placed in the posterior left subscapular area and the other in the anterior lower end of the sternum (Fig. 64–26). Rhythmic electrical stimuli passing through the heart from one electrode to another result in cardiac contractions. Pulses are checked for evidence of peripheral perfusion. The main discomfort associated with this type of pacing is related to painful cutaneous nerve stimulation and contraction of chest wall muscles. Sometimes, sedation helps to alleviate these discomforts. At times, this method of pacing the heart is unsuccessful because of the severity of cardiac disease.

Medications most commonly used during and after cardiac arrest to improve tissue perfusion include so-

Text continued on page 2144

EMERGENCY CARE ■ Adult Cardiopulmonary Resuscitation

Interventions	Rationales

One Rescuer

1. Determine unresponsiveness.

2. Call for help.

3. Position the client supine on a hard, flat surface. If the client is in bed, place a back board under the client as soon as help arrives.

4. Open the airway with a head-tilt, chin-lift maneuver. To perform this, place one hand on the client's forehead, applying firm backward pressure. Place the fingers of the other hand under the chin and lift it forward with teeth almost to occlusion.

1. Client may have fainted or may be asleep. Monitor leads may have fallen off.

2. Another rescuer and emergency equipment make resuscitation efforts more effective.

3. Firm support is necessary for external compressions to be effective.

4. This lifts the tongue away from the back of the throat to open the airway.

Are you ok?

EMERGENCY CARE ■ Adult Cardiopulmonary Resuscitation *Continued*

Interventions	Rationales
5. If neck injury is suspected, use the jaw-thrust maneuver. To perform this, grasp the angles of the client's lower jaw and lift with both hands, displacing the mandible forward while tilting the head backward.	5. Jaw thrust can be accomplished without extending the neck; it minimizes the risk of spinal injury.

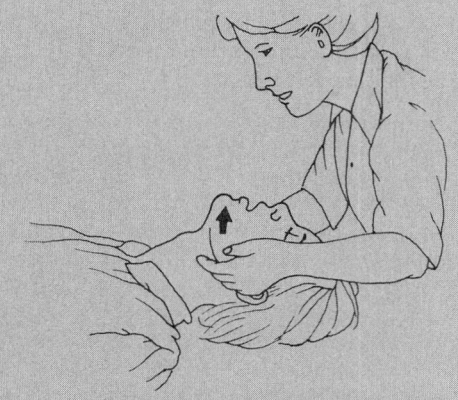

Interventions	Rationales
6. Assess for breathlessness with the airway open. Look for the chest to rise and fall, listen for air escaping, and feel for flow of air.	6. The tongue is the most common cause of obstruction in an unconscious client. Opening the airway may be all that is needed for the client to breathe spontaneously.
7. If the client is not breathing, pinch the nose with the thumb and index fingers while maintaining the head-tilt position of the client. Take a deep breath, seal the lips around the outside of the client's mouth, and give two full breaths, watching that the client's chest rises.	7. Pinching the nose prevents air from escaping through the nose. Rising of the chest validates effective ventilations.

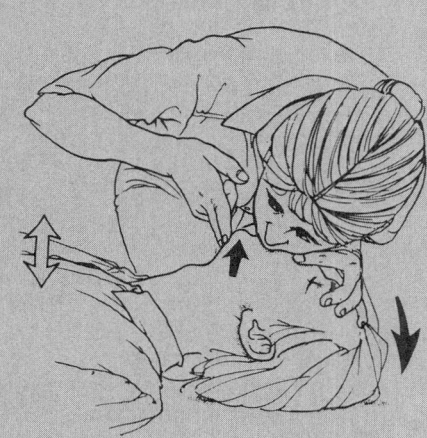

Interventions	Rationales
8. If the chest does not rise, reposition the client's head and repeat ventilations.	8. Improper positioning of the head is the most common cause of ineffective ventilation.
9. If the chest still does not rise, perform 6–10 subdiaphragmatic thrusts, perform a finger-sweep maneuver, and attempt ventilation again.	9. Foreign body obstruction may be responsible for ineffective ventilation.

Continued

EMERGENCY CARE ■ **Adult Cardiopulmonary Resuscitation** *Continued*

Interventions	Rationales
10. Assess the pulse by palpating the carotid artery on one side of the neck for 5–10 s.	10. The inability to find a palpable pulse establishes the presence of cardiac arrest and the need for external chest compressions.
11. If no pulse is palpated, determine proper hand position for chest compressions: a. Locate the notch where the rib margin meets the sternum and place the middle finger on this notch and the index finger next to it.	11. Proper hand placement is necessary for effective compressions and avoidance of complications.
b. Place the heel of the opposite hand on the lower half of the sternum, close to the index finger of the first hand.	
c. Remove the first hand and place it on top of the hand on the sternum.	

EMERGENCY CARE ■ Adult Cardiopulmonary Resuscitation *Continued*

Interventions	Rationales
12. Begin chest compressions with elbows locked, arms straightened, and shoulders positioned directly over the hands. Depress sternum 1½–2 in with each compression. Perform 15 compressions, counting "1 and 2 and 3 . . . " to 15. After 15 compressions, deliver two more ventilations.	12. This count allows for 80–100 compressions/min.
13. Perform four complete cycles of 15 compressions with two ventilations.	13. CPR should be performed for at least 1 min for client to benefit from oxygenation and circulation.
14. Reassess carotid pulse and breathing.	14. CPR may have provided sufficient oxygenation for return of heart rhythm and breathing.

Two Rescuers

1. Perform compressions at a ratio of five compressions to one ventilation.	1. With two people, you do not have to allow for time to move from chest to head.
2. The compressor counts "1 and 2 and 3 and 4 and 5," pausing 1½ s for a ventilation.	2. This allows for 80–100 compressions/min. Pause allows for adequate ventilaton volume.
3. If available, use a clear plastic face mask with a one-way valve instead of mouth-to-mouth ventilation.	3. The mask facilitates effective ventilation while protecting the rescuer from contact with the client's oral secretions. The mask also allows for administration of oxygen during artificial ventilation.

Illustrations for steps 1, 2, 7, 10, and 12 of one-rescuer CPR and for step 2 of two-rescuer CPR reproduced with permission. © *Healthcare provider's manual for basic life support*, 1988. Copyright American Heart Association.

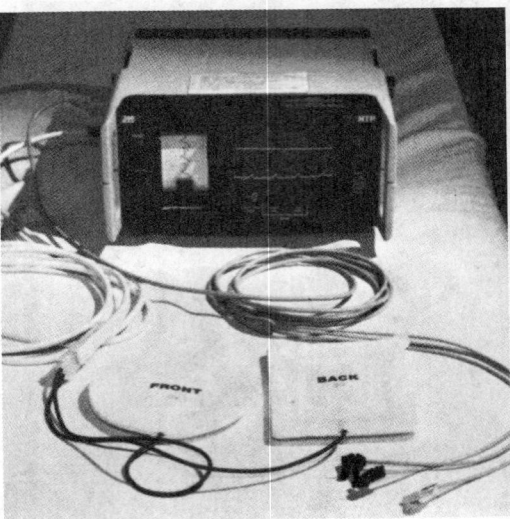 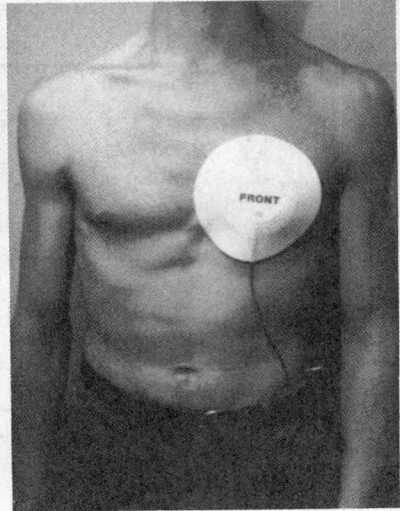 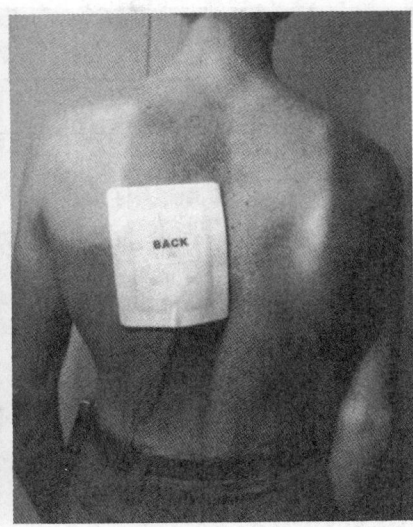

Figure 64–26

Equipment and electrode placement for transcutaneous external pacing. (From Schwartz, G. R., Bircher, N., Hanke, B. K., Mangelsen, M. A., Mayer, T., & Ungar, J. R. [1989]. *Emergency medicine: The essential update.* Philadelphia: W. B. Saunders.)

dium bicarbonate, epinephrine, norepinephrine, dopamine, dobutamine, amrinone, and isoproteronol (Table 64–3).

Surgical management. Clients who experience life-threatening dysrhythmias may require surgical treatment for long-term management. The type of treatment is dependent on the type of dysrhythmia.

Aneurysmectomy. Invasive attempts for dysrhythmia control may include *ventricular aneurysmectomy,* in which a dyskinetic or ballooning portion of the ventricular wall is surgically resected. The irregularity in the ventricular wall, damaged by MI, is usually a site that generates ventricular dysrhythmias. Resection of that area eliminates the potentially dangerous dysrhythmia. Care of the client is similar to care for clients undergoing coronary artery bypass grafting (see p. 2157).

Coronary artery bypass grafting. Coronary artery bypass graft (CABG) is performed if the cause of the dysrhythmia is coronary artery insufficiency. Care of the client undergoing CABG is described on page 2157.

TABLE 64–3 Drugs Used During Cardiac Arrest*

Drug	Usual Dosage	Interventions	Rationales
Epinephrine (Adrenalin Chloride)	IV push (1 : 10,000 concentration): 0.5 – 1.0 mg repeated q 5 min	1. Watch for return of heart rate when used for asystole. 2. Watch for tachycardia, dysrhythmias, or hypertension. 3. Watch for development of coarse ventricular fibrillation when given during fine ventricular fibrillation.	1. This is the expected response. 2. Adverse reactions can occur with a dramatic response. 3. This reaction is expected to improve response to defibrillation.
Isoproterenol hydrochloride (Isuprel)	IV drip: 1.0 mg in 500 mL of D_5W titrated for desired effect.	1. Watch for increase in heart rate. 2. Watch for hypertension, tachycardia, and dysrhythmias. 3. Assess for chest pain after resuscitation.	1. This is the expected response. 2. Adverse reactions can occur with a dramatic response. 3. Drug increases myocardial oxygen demand.

TABLE 64–3   Drugs Used During Cardiac Arrest* *Continued*

Drug	Usual Dosage	Interventions	Rationales
Dopamine hydrochloride (Intropin)	IV drip: dilute per package insert directions; 2–20 μg/kg per min increased gradually to 50 μg/kg per min	1. Watch for increase in blood pressure. 2. Monitor for tachycardia and dysrhythmias or hypertension. 3. Monitor IV site for infiltration. 4. Assess for urinary output <30 mL/h or pallor, cyanosis, pain, or numbness in the extremities.	1. This is the expected response. 2. Adverse reactions can occur. 3. Extravasation of drug can occur with necrosis. 4. Dosages >5 μg/kg per min cause vasoconstriction of renal and peripheral vessels. (Dosages of 2–5 μg/kg per min actually improve renal blood flow.)
Dobutamine (Dobutrex)	IV drip: 1000 mg in 500 mL of D_5W at 2.5–20 μg/kg per min	1. Watch for an increase in blood pressure. 2. Assess for hypertension and dysrhythmias.	1. This is the expected response. 2. Adverse reactions can occur.
Sodium bicarbonate	IV push: 1 mEq/kg	1. Assess arterial blood gas values for metabolic acidosis.	1. Administration of agent without evidence of metabolic acidosis can result in alkalosis, which can hinder resuscitation efforts.
Norepinephrine (Levophed)	IV drip: 2–12 μg/min; dilute with D_5W	1. Watch for an increase in blood pressure. 2. Monitor for bradycardia. 3. Monitor for hypertension and dysrhythmias. 4. Monitor IV site for infiltration. 5. Assess for urinary output <30 mL/h or pallor, cyanosis, pain, or numbness in the extremities. 6. Assess for chest pain after resuscitation.	1. This is the expected response. 2. Reflex bradycardia may occur with a rise in blood pressure. 3. Adverse reactions occur with a dramatic response. 4. Extravasation can occur, which necessitates immediate treatment with phentolamine. 5. Drug is a powerful vasoconstrictor. 6. Drug increases myocardial oxygen demand.

* Also see Table 64–2 for antidysrhythmic agents, many of which are given during cardiac resuscitation.

Ablation of accessory pathways.   Surgical ablation of an accessory pathway may be performed to control the pre-excitation dysrhythmia of WPW. Care of the client is similar to care given to the client undergoing CABG .

Permanent pacing.   Permanent pacemaker insertion is performed for the resolution of conduction disorders that are not temporary in nature, but require a permanent treatment (Fig. 64–27). Permanent pacemakers may be single chambered or dual chambered. With single-chambered pacemakers, a lead is positioned in the chamber to be paced, usually the ventricle. Occasionally, single-chambered atrial pacing is recommended for dysrhythmias originating from sinus node disease, when AV conduction is intact.

Dual-chambered pacemakers have leads placed in the atrium and ventricle for a more physiologic effect. A programmed AV interval, which closely relates to the

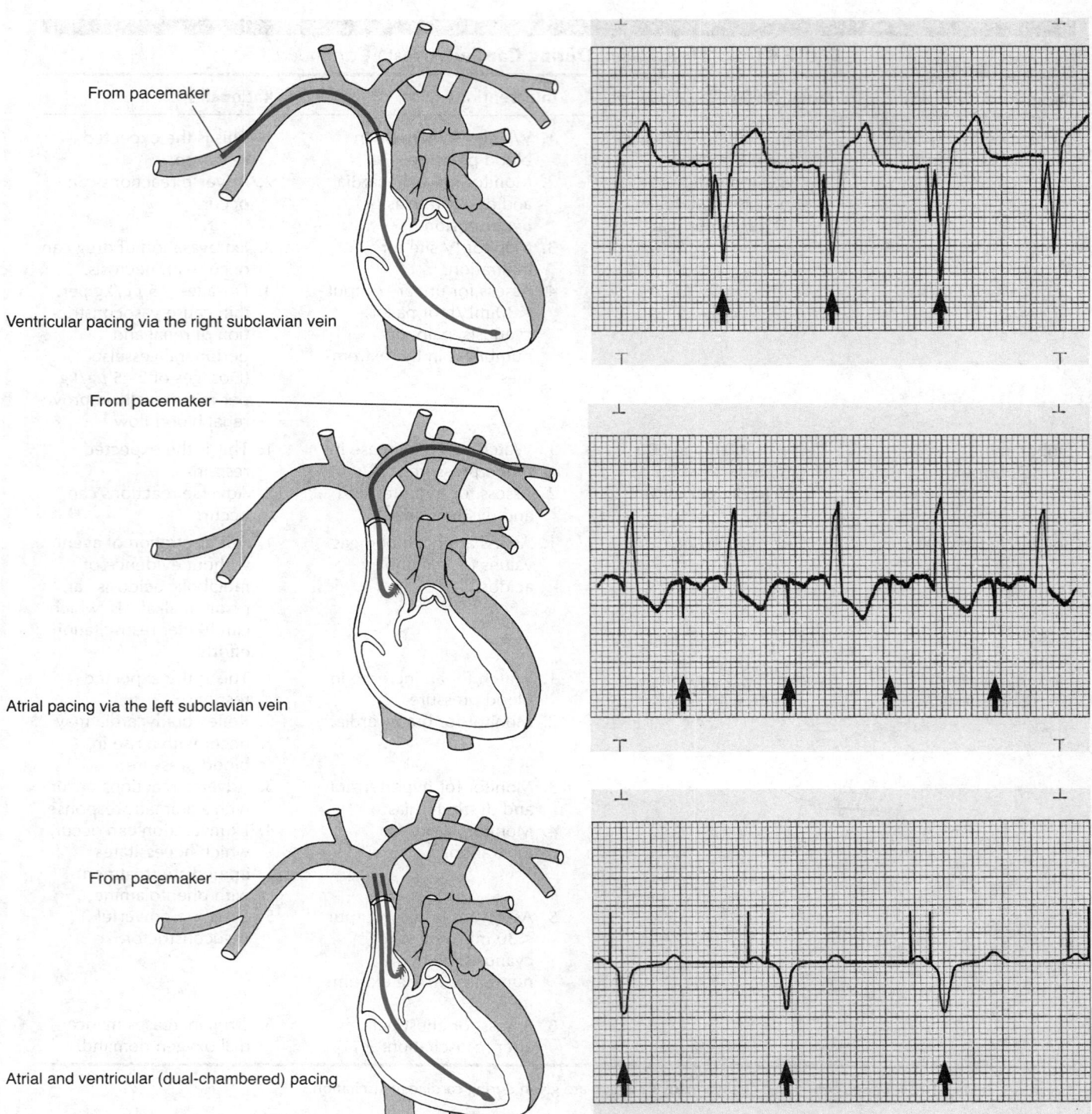

From pacemaker

Ventricular pacing via the right subclavian vein

From pacemaker

Atrial pacing via the left subclavian vein

From pacemaker

Atrial and ventricular (dual-chambered) pacing

Figure 64–27

Pacemaker placement and corresponding ECG patterns in permanent endocardial pacing. Arrows indicate pacemaker spikes. Note in the ECG showing dual-chambered pacing the pacemaker's ability to sense the client's P waves, with provision of ventricular pacing 0.16 s after the natural P wave. If the heart drops below 65 beats per minute, atrial pacing occurs.

PR interval, ensures a ventricular stimulus shortly after atrial depolarization. Dual-chambered pacemakers may also be referred to as AV sequential pacemakers.

The pulse generators of both single-chambered and dual-chambered pacemakers are implanted in a surgically made pocket at the shoulder or the abdominal area. The leads may be implanted either endocardially or epicardially. Endocardial lead placement is usually performed and necessitates a short postprocedure stay in the hospital. The client may be observed on a cardiac telemetry unit overnight and may be discharged the day after surgery, if there are no complications.

Most permanent pacemakers manufactured today are programmable with a battery-operated device provided by the pacemaker manufacturer. With certain commands, it reprograms the mode in which the pacemaker is functioning, the rate, the sensitivity, the amount of energy sent to the heart for each stimulus, and other variables. This is accomplished by placing the magnetic device over the skin where the pulse generator is located and providing the various commands (Fig. 64–28). Reprogramming is usually performed by the physician in response to pacemaker problems or concerns arising after implantation.

Insertion of an implantable defibrillator. The automatic implantable cardioverter/defibrillator (AICD) is reserved for use in clients who have experienced at least one episode of sudden death, who were successfully resuscitated, and in whom attempts to control the life-threatening dysrhythmias have not been successful by medical and surgical means. The surgical intervention for these life-threatening dysrhythmias involves the implantation of an electronic device designed to monitor and correct the disorder. The AICD is equipped with a pulse generator and leads. It weighs about ½ lb and is the size of a deck of cards. The pulse generator, consisting of a power supply and electronic circuits, is connected to one or more leads that are placed in and near the heart (Fig. 64–29). One of four surgical approaches for implanting the device may be used: thoracotomy, sternotomy, subxiphoid, or transvenous approach. If the client is scheduled for coronary artery bypass surgery, the leads and pulse generator may be implanted at that time via sternotomy.

The lead system, consisting of patches and sensing wires, sends electrical signals from the heart to the pulse generator, which continuously monitors the cardiac rhythm. When the pulse generator receives signals that the rhythm is ventricular fibrillation or ventricular tachycardia exceeding a preprogrammed rate, it sends up to four consecutive shocks to the heart to stop the abnormal rhythm.

After implantation, the client is monitored closely in the critical care unit. Care is similar to that for a client undergoing open heart surgery (see p. 2157).

■ Discharge Planning

Home Care Preparation

Clients who experience dysrhythmias that are not life-threatening may not be hospitalized. Often, these

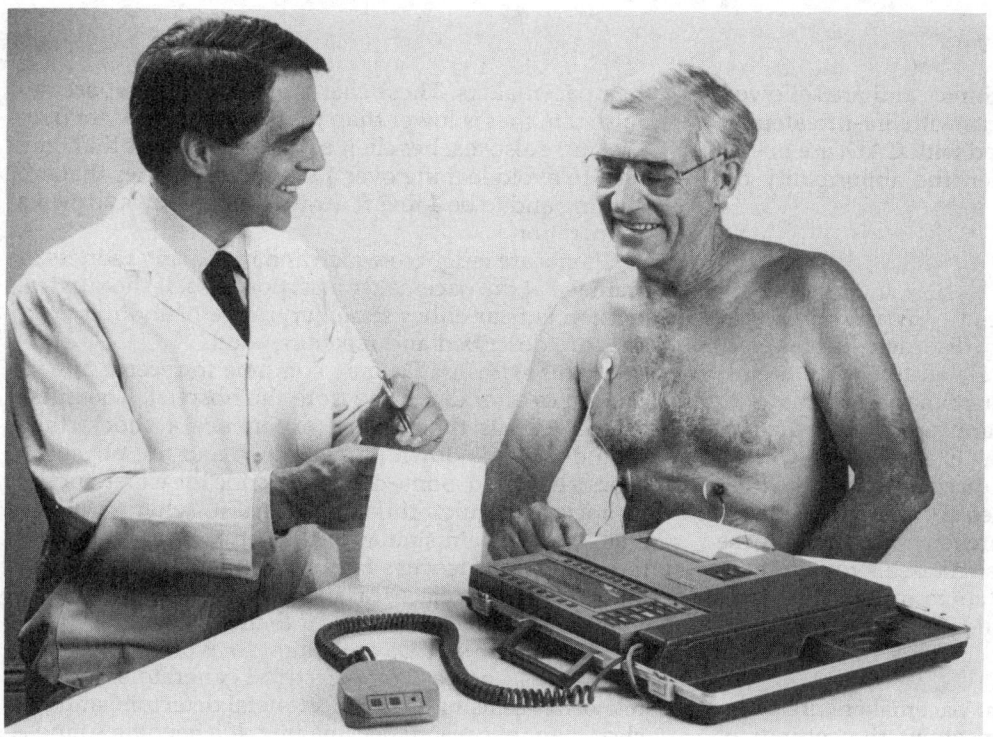

Figure 64–28

Reprogramming a pacemaker. (Courtesy of Hewlett-Packard Company.)

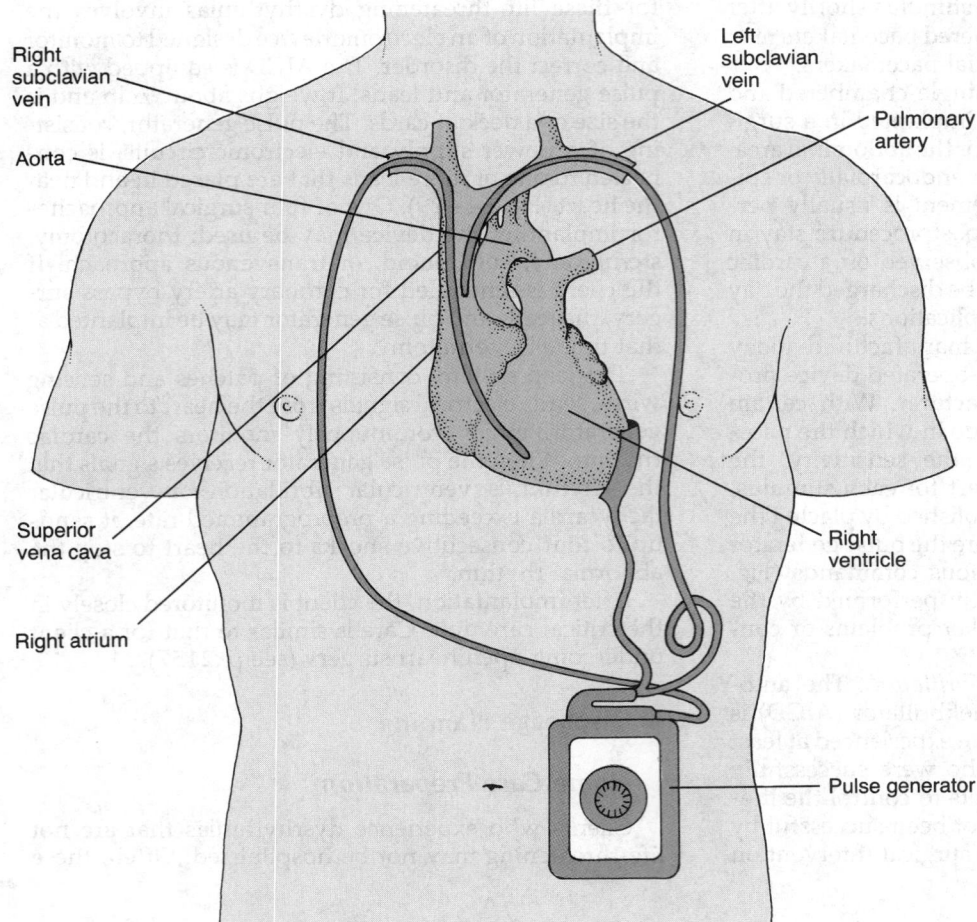

Right subclavian vein

Aorta

Superior vena cava

Right atrium

Left subclavian vein

Pulmonary artery

Right ventricle

Pulse generator

Figure 64–29

Automatic implantable cardioverter/defibrillator.

clients are first given antiarrhythmics and are followed by use of a Holter monitor. Clients with life-threatening dysrhythmias, or those associated with CAD, are hospitalized and are discharged when the abnormality responds to treatment.

Client/Family Education

Clients who have experienced a dysrhythmia that was associated with a temporary disorder, such as electrolyte imbalance or ischemia related to an MI, are instructed in how to care for their primary disorder.

The nurse teaches all clients and significant others or family members how to take the client's pulse. Clients receiving antiarrhythmics after discharge from the hospital are taught dosage schedules and common side effects (see Table 64–2). Clients are taught to report these side effects and any dizziness, nausea, vomiting, or chest discomfort. Signs of a change in heart rhythm, such as a drastic decrease in pulse, a pulse rate greater than 100 beats per minute, or increase in irregularity should also be reported.

Clients who have permanent pacemakers are given written and verbal information about the settings of their pacemakers. These clients are taught to report any pulse rate that is lower than that set on the pacemaker. The nurse also teaches clients with pacemakers that they need to avoid leaning over automobile engines that are running and to be 4 to 5 ft away from microwave ovens in operation.

Clients are taught to watch and report any redness or drainage at the pacemaker insertion sites. If the surgical incision is near either shoulder, range-of-motion exercises are described and recommended.

Clients with AICDs may continue to receive antiarrhythmics after discharge from the hospital. The nurse teaches clients that if they experience a shock, they should sit or lie down immediately, and the physician should be called. Some clients describe the experience of a shock as a quick thud in the chest, whereas others relate severe pain similar to that of external defibrillation. The nurse teaches family members that, although they may feel an electrical shock over the surface of the client's skin, this cannot harm them.

Clients with AICDs are taught to avoid strong magnetic fields, such as large electrical generators, radio or television transmitters, airport metal detectors, and nuclear magnetic resonance imaging. If a beeping sound is emitted from the pulse generator, the client should move away from the area as quickly as possible to prevent deactivation of the device.

All clients with pacemakers or AICDs are taught to carry identification cards and wear medical alert (Medic Alert) bracelets.

Psychosocial Preparation

Clients and families often fear that a life-threatening dysrhythmia may recur. The nurse provides the client and family with the opportunity to verbalize concerns and fears related to this. The nurse suggests that family or significant others consider enrolling in a basic life-support course to learn CPR. When suggesting this, the nurse emphasizes the importance of all individuals' learning CPR.

Health Care Resources

Clients may contact the local chapter of the AHA for information on dysrhythmias and basic life-support courses. Clients with pacemakers may have transtelephonic systems for transmission of their rhythms to a clinic or a health care provider's office.

Clients with AICDs should contact the local ambulance or paramedic service to inform them that they have these devices in place. Depending on the placement of the AICD patches, successful external defibrillation may be impeded if paddles are placed in the typical sternum and apex positions. The paramedics should be informed that, should the internal device fail and external defibrillation be necessary, paddles should be placed in anterior and posterior positions.

 Evaluation

On the basis of the identified nursing diagnosis, the nurse evaluates the care of the client experiencing dysrhythmias. Expected outcomes include that the client

1. Demonstrates a consistent cardiac rhythm that supports optimal cardiac output
2. States signs and symptoms of a dysrhythmia

CORONARY ARTERY DISEASE

OVERVIEW

Since 1940, CAD (coronary heart disease or ischemic heart disease) has been the leading cause of death in the United States. This disease affects the three major coronary arteries (right, left anterior descending, and left circumflex) that provide blood and nutrients to the myocardium. When blood flow through these major vessels becomes partially or completely blocked, ischemia and infarction of the myocardium may result. Ischemia occurs when the balance between oxygen supply and demand becomes disproportionate. Cellular death or infarction results when blood flow to an area of the myocardium is insufficient in meeting the oxygen and nutrient needs of the heart.

Pathophysiology

The most common cause of CAD is atherosclerosis (see Chap. 65). Atherosclerosis is characterized by the accumulation of smooth muscle cells, lipids, and connective tissue along the intimal layer of arterial vessels. A fibrous plaque is the characteristic lesion of atherosclerosis. This lesion can vary in size within the vessel wall, either partially or completely obstructing the flow. More complicated lesions consist of the fibrous plaque with calcium deposits, accompanied by thrombus formation (Fig. 64–30). Obstruction of the lumen reduces or stops blood flow to surrounding tissue.

Another cause of CAD is coronary artery spasm. Narrowing of the vessel lumen occurs when the smooth muscle fibers in the vessel wall contract. Spasm of the coronary artery may lead to actual ischemia or extension of the MI.

Other nonatherosclerotic causes that can affect the luminal diameter of the coronary vessel may be related to circulatory abnormalities; these include hypotension, anemia, hypovolemia, polycythemia, and valvular problems.

At rest, the heart extracts a large amount of oxygen (75%) from the coronary blood flow, more than any other major organ in the body. When myocardial metabolism and oxygen consumption increase, the require-

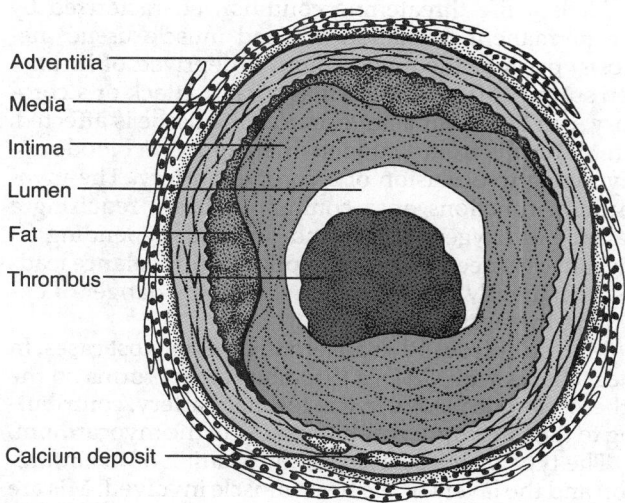

Figure 64–30

Cross-section of an atherosclerotic coronary artery.

ment of oxygen can increase manyfold. Additional oxygen is supplied by increasing coronary artery blood flow. If coronary artery blood flow is unable to supply the required amount of oxygen needed by the heart muscle, an imbalance between supply and demand occurs. Unless the ratio of supply and demand becomes balanced, the myocardial tissue develops ischemia and infarction. Around the area of infarction are two zones classified as the zone of injury and the zone of ischemia. The area of infarction continues to enlarge if blood supply remains compromised. The actual extent of the zone of infarction is dependent on three factors: collateral circulation, anaerobic metabolism, and workload demands on the myocardium. Typically, ischemia and infarction progress from endocardium to epicardium.

Angina pectoris, a name derived from a Greek word meaning "strangling of the chest," is a disorder that is most often due to atherosclerotic heart disease. The presence of angina indicates ischemia. Ischemia that occurs with angina is limited in duration, and it does not cause permanent myocardial tissue damage. However, angina is life-threatening in that it can cause a dysrhythmia or progress to MI.

Angina may be classified into three types: stable (stable exertional) angina, unstable (crescendo or preinfarction) angina, and variant (Prinzmetal's) angina. The term *stable* angina describes chest pain or discomfort that is brought on by increased physical effort or emotional stress; it is characterized by a stable onset, duration, and intensity of symptoms. *Unstable* angina refers to chest pain or discomfort that is brought about by an unpredictable degree of exertion; it is characterized by an increase in the number of attacks and the intensity of the pain. *Variant* angina describes chest pain or discomfort that is likely to happen during rest or sleep, rather than during exertion. Variant angina is thought to be related primarily to coronary artery spasm. Clients with variant angina may or may not have atherosclerosis of the coronary arteries.

MI is a life-threatening condition characterized by the permanent formation of dead muscle tissue (necrosis) because the myocardium is deprived of its oxygen supply. MI, also known as a heart attack or a coronary, can be fatal if a large area of the tissue is affected. An MI results from a sudden interruption in blood supply owing to occlusion of a coronary artery. The myocardium functions on a continuous basis, requiring a balance of oxygen supply and demand, depending on the muscle's needs. An interruption in this balance leads to permanently damaged tissue, with the danger of enlarging the necrotic area.

MI results from atherosclerotic CAD in most cases. In most clients with CAD, a thrombus or clot forms on the atherosclerotic plaque in the coronary artery, contributing to the interruption of blood flow to the myocardium.

The type of MI is based on the location of the infarction and the layers of the heart muscle involved. MIs are classified as anterior, inferior, lateral, or posterior. The infarcted area can involve the subendocardium, the epi-

cardium, or all three layers of heart muscle. When all three layers are involved, the MI is described as *transmural.*

Most MIs occur in the left ventricle because its oxygen supply is the greatest. About one-third of MIs involve the inferior surface of the left ventricle and the right ventricle. Autopsies reveal a small percentage of right ventricular infarctions. Septal infarction and atrial infarctions can occur in the left ventricle. The right atrium is involved more frequently than the left atrium.

Etiology

The exact etiology of CAD is unknown; however, numerous contributing risk factors have been identified. Risk factors have been classified as modifiable and nonmodifiable.

Nonmodifiable risk factors are personal elements that cannot be altered or controlled. These risk factors include age, sex, family history, and ethnic background. Risk of CAD increases with age. Of all clients who experience MI, almost 55% are age 65 years or older. Men have a greater risk of MI than women, and they have MIs earlier in life. Family history is a risk factor in that individuals whose parents had cardiovascular disease are more likely to experience it. Ethnic background affects the risk; for example, American Blacks have moderate hypertension twice as often as Caucasians, and severe hypertension three times as often. Consequently, their risk for CAD is also greater (AHA, 1989a).

Modifiable risk factors include elevated serum cholesterol levels, cigarette smoking, hypertension, obesity, stress, physical inactivity, and impaired glucose tolerance. The risk of CAD rises as serum cholesterol levels increase. Elevated levels of low-density lipoproteins (LDLs) with low levels of high-density lipoproteins (HDLs) increase the risks further.

Cigarette smokers have twice the risk of MI as nonsmokers and two to four times the risk of sudden cardiac death (AHA, 1989a). Hypertension increases the workload of the heart, increasing the risk of myocardial infarct. Impaired glucose tolerance (e.g., in diabetes) seriously increases the risks. Eighty per cent of individuals with diabetes die of some type of cardiovascular disease (AHA, 1989a).

Physical inactivity has not been clearly established as a risk factor for CAD. However, physical inactivity often contributes to obesity, which is an established risk factor. Stress is thought to influence CAD through its effect on other established risk factors, such as cigarette smoking and obesity. For example, when clients are under stress they may smoke more cigarettes and overeat.

Clients with several risk factors, such as hypertension, obesity, smoking, high cholesterol levels, and diabetes, have several times the risks of CAD as those without these characteristics.

Incidence

In 1987 the incidence of CAD (MI and angina) in the United States was 1,500,000. Also in 1987 513,700 Americans died of CAD, with MIs being the leading cause of death. It is estimated that 5 million persons who have experienced angina or MI are still living (AHA, 1989a).

PREVENTION

Identification and control of modifiable risk factors can retard the progress of coronary atherosclerosis, thus contributing to the prevention of CAD. Abstinence from cigarette smoking, early identification and control of hypertension, maintenance of appropriate weight, and management of stress are recommended strategies to prevent CAD. Modified fat and cholesterol diets can prevent elevation of serum cholesterol levels in many individuals. Other individuals may require anticholesterol agents to assist in prevention of CAD. In addition to following these guidelines, clients with impaired glucose tolerance can participate in treatment to control serum glucose levels to decrease their risks of CAD.

COLLABORATIVE MANAGEMENT

 Assessment

History

Identification of *chest discomfort* is the most important aspect of the history, although pain related to ischemia can also occur in the upper back, the jaw, or the arms. The client is asked to describe past experiences with chest discomfort in terms of sensation, location, radiation, and duration. For example, does the discomfort occur with exertion, or rest, and what relieves it (e.g., rest or medication, such as nitroglycerin)? The nurse also obtains information about prior hospitalizations for angina or MI.

If chest discomfort is present at the time of the interview, further collection of historical data is delayed until interventions for ischemic pain and dysrhythmias are initiated, and the discomfort resolves. When the client is pain free, the nurse obtains information about *medications, family history,* and *modifiable risk factors,* including eating habits, life style, and physical activity levels.

Physical Assessment: Clinical Manifestations

The nurse assesses for the presence of *chest, epigastric, jaw, back, or arm discomfort* and asks the client to rate the discomfort on a scale of 1 to 10. Clients often describe the discomfort as tightness, burning sensation, pressure, or indigestion. The discomfort is most often *not* described as severe, and the nurse needs to be sure that clients are reporting *any* and *all* episodes of chest

discomfort, even though it is not perceived as severe or painful. (See Nursing Research feature in Chap. 63.)

Chest discomfort related to angina is often indistinguishable from that which occurs during an MI. However, some characteristics of each assist in differentiating an anginal attack from an acute MI. Anginal chest discomfort is typically of short duration, usually 3 to 5 minutes, but can last up to 30 minutes. Chest discomfort related to angina usually occurs with exertion or stressful situations and subsides with rest or the administration of nitrates. Chest discomfort that occurs with an MI often lasts longer than 30 minutes, and symptoms often recur. Because it is frequently difficult to differentiate angina from MI during the episode of chest discomfort, clients are often hospitalized when chest pain occurs, to rule out MI.

The nurse continues the assessment of clients with CAD by identifying symptoms that commonly occur during ischemic episodes, including *nausea, vomiting, diaphoresis, dizziness, weakness, palpitations,* and *shortness of breath.* The presence of these symptoms without chest discomfort is also significant. In 15% to 25% of clients with an MI, chest pain or discomfort may be mild or absent.

A high-priority nursing assessment for the client with suspected angina or MI is to obtain a *blood pressure measurement,* auscultate the *apical pulse,* and interpret the *cardiac monitor pattern* to assess for dysrhythmias. Dysrhythmias may be present during anginal attacks or acute MIs.

The nurse next assesses all *distal peripheral pulses* and *skin temperature.* The skin should be warm, with all pulses palpable if angina or an MI is uncomplicated. In clients with complicated anginal attacks or MIs, poor cardiac output may occur, manifested by cool, diaphoretic skin.

The nurse auscultates for an S_3 gallop, which often indicates CHF, a serious and common complication of an MI. *Respiratory rate* and *breath sounds* are important to assess for signs of CHF; these include increased respiratory rate, crackles or rales, and wheezes. Auscultation of an S_4 is a common finding in clients who have had a previous MI or hypertension.

Psychosocial Assessment

Denial is a common early reaction to chest discomfort associated with angina or MI. On average, the client with an acute MI waits more than 2 hours before seeking medical attention. Clients often rationalize that their symptoms are due to indigestion or overexertion. In some situations, denial is a normal part of adapting to a stressful event. However, denial that interferes with identification of a symptom, such as chest discomfort, can be harmful to the client. The nurse explains the significance of reporting any discomfort, emphasizing that the cause of the symptoms is important to determine and reassuring the client that much can be done to control the cause.

Fear, anxiety, and anger are other common reactions that clients and families manifest. Nursing assessment focuses on assisting clients and their families in identifying these feelings. The nurse often has to assess behavioral patterns that occur because of these reactions. For example, clients may not report recurrent chest discomfort because of fear.

Laboratory Findings

No laboratory tests can confirm the diagnosis of angina. Serum enzyme determinations are not useful in assessing the presence of angina, but an absence of serum enzymes reflects that the client has not had an acute MI.

An MI can be confirmed by the presence of abnormally high levels of cardiac enzymes and isoenzymes. Of all the cardiac enzymes, creatine kinase (CK) is considered the most sensitive and reliable indicator for diagnosis of an MI. Total CK levels rise within 3 hours after the onset of chest pain and peak within 24 hours after cardiac tissue damage and death. When cardiac muscle tissue dies, CK-MB isoenzymes enter into the blood stream (normally, serum does not contain CK-MB isoenzymes), with a peak elevation occurring approximately 24 hours after the onset of chest pain. Elevated CK-MB levels are necessary to confirm the diagnosis of a transmural MI.

Serum measurement of lactate dehydrogenase (LDH) may be used to confirm an MI; however, identification of this substance is not as reliable as that of CK-MB. LDH levels start to rise within 12 to 24 hours after an MI, reach a peak between 48 and 72 hours, and fall to normal in 7 days. Serum levels of LDH_1 isoenzyme rise higher than serum levels of LDH_2 in the presence of an MI.

Other laboratory findings that are useful in diagnosing an MI are an elevated white blood cell count (10,000 to 20,000 cells/mm^3) appearing on the second day and lasting up to a week.

Radiographic Findings

Unless there is associated cardiac dysfunction (e.g., valvular disease) or heart failure, the chest x-ray film is not diagnostic for angina or for MI.

Other Diagnostic Tests

Unless the client is having an anginal episode, the ECG is usually normal. ECGs obtained during an anginal episode reveal ST depression, T wave inversion, or both, representing myocardial ischemia. Variant angina, due to coronary spasm, causes ST elevation during anginal attacks. These ST and T wave changes usually subside. During the early stages of an acute MI, ischemic changes, such as those that occur during angina, may be present. The development of abnormal Q waves with ST changes supports the diagnosis of MI (Fig. 64–31).

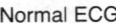
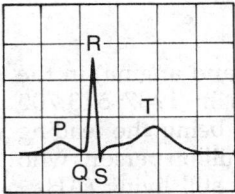
Normal ECG

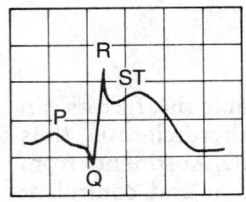
The ST segment becomes elevated during ischemia.

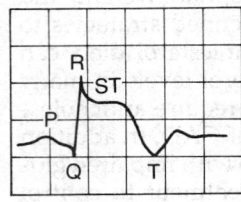
ST segment elevation is accompanied by T wave inversion and the appearance of a Q wave hours to days after acute MI.

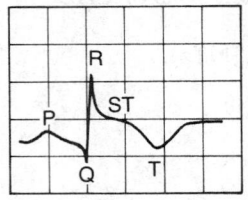
The ST segment returns to normal days to weeks after acute MI.

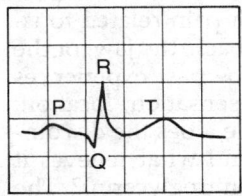
A Q wave persists as a permanent indicator of past MI.

Figure 64–31

ECG changes in ischemia leading to MI.

Thallium scans utilize radioisotope imaging to assess for ischemia or necrotic muscle tissue related to angina or MI. Areas of decreased or absent perfusion, referred to as cold spots, identify ischemia or infarction.

Cardiac catheterization is done after the acute stages of angina or MI to diagnose blocked or partially blocked coronary arteries. When cardiac catheterization is performed during the acute phase of ischemia, treatment of the obstructed lumen is usually the intent of the procedure.

An exercise tolerance test (stress test) is often done after the acute stages of an anginal episode or MI to assess for ECG changes consistent with ischemia.

Analysis: Nursing Diagnosis

The client with CAD may have either angina or MI. If an MI is suspected or cannot be completely ruled out, the client is admitted to a coronary or critical care unit for continuous monitoring.

Common Diagnoses

On the basis of the assessment data, the nurse often identifies the following common diagnoses for the client with CAD:

1. Altered (cardiopulmonary) tissue perfusion related to imbalance between myocardial oxygen supply and demand
2. Decreased cardiac output related to electrical and mechanical malfunction
3. Activity intolerance related to imbalance between myocardial oxygen supply and demand

Additional Diagnoses

Clients with CAD frequently have the following additional diagnoses:

1. Pain related to imbalance between myocardial oxygen supply and demand
2. Knowledge deficit related to unfamiliarity with the disease process, medical or surgical treatment plan, and risk factor modification
3. Anxiety related to change in health status, change in role function, or threat of death
4. Potential for noncompliance related to knowledge deficit of CAD and its affect on life style and methods for adaptation

 Planning and Implementation

Altered (Cardiopulmonary) Tissue Perfusion

Planning: client goals.   The major goal for this diagnosis is that the client will experience improved tissue perfusion as evidenced by absence of chest pain and absence of dysrhythmias.

Interventions: nonsurgical management.   The objective of treatment is to reduce the workload of the heart by decreasing myocardial oxygen demand and increasing myocardial oxygen supply.

Drug therapy.   Medications used in the treatment of angina include nitrates, beta-blockers, calcium channel blockers, and platelet antiaggregants (Table 64–4).

Nitroglycerin agents (sublingual, oral, intravenous, and topical) are vasodilators that primarily act to reduce venous return to the heart (preload) and, therefore, decrease myocardial oxygen consumption. Nitrates also increase coronary blood flow and reduce coronary spasm, thus increasing myocardial oxygen supply.

Beta-blocking agents, such as propranolol (Inderal), decrease myocardial oxygen consumption by decreasing heart rate and contractility. Calcium channel blockers' mechanism of action is to cause coronary arterial dilation and peripheral arterial dilation. Verapamil (Calan) and diltiazem (Cardizem) reduce the heart rate by slowing the sinus node discharge and conduction through the AV node. The overall effect of the calcium channel blockers is to decrease myocardial oxygen utilization. These agents can be used alone or in combination with either nitrates or beta-blockers.

Antiaggregants are drugs that modify platelet behavior. Dipyridamole (Persantine) and aspirin (acetysalicylic acid) are examples of drugs that may be used to prevent platelet adhesion in the coronary arteries.

Nitroglycerin is also used for clients with MI. The client may be given nitroglycerin sublingually, topically, or intravenously. In the acute phase of a MI, narcotic analgesics are used for chest pain that is unrelieved by nitroglycerin. Morphine sulfate intravenously is the drug of choice. Beta-blockers and calcium channel blockers are also given as previously discussed. Sedatives, such as lorazepam (Ativan), are used to decrease anxiety and promote sleep or rest.

Other interventions.   During an acute attack of angina or possible MI, the client is usually restricted to bed rest, and given supplemental oxygen to provide the ischemic heart muscle with additional oxygen. The client's heart rate and rhythm are continuously assessed on a cardiac monitor. The nurse administers medications and assesses the effect of drug therapy on the client. Clients receiving nitroglycerin or morphine should not have their heads elevated to more than 30 degrees to avoid dizziness, fainting, and hypotension, which commonly occur after administration of these medications. Vital signs are evaluated frequently to determine the hemodynamic effect of the drugs and the client's tissue perfusion.

The nurse assists in decreasing the client's myocardial oxygen needs by promoting bed rest and controlling the environment to minimize anxiety and stress. Ice and iced beverages are restricted for all clients with acute ischemia (see the Nursing Research feature on p. 2156).

Percutaneous transluminal coronary angioplasty (PTCA) is an invasive but nonsurgical technique used in the treatment of CAD that is unresponsive to medical therapy. Performed under fluoroscopy in the cardiac catheterization laboratory, PTCA is done by introducing the balloon-tipped catheter through a guidewire into a coronary vessel with a proximal, accessible, noncalcified lesion. The balloon is inflated in an attempt to reduce or eliminate the occluding lesion (Fig. 64–32). Continuous heparin therapy given intravenously is used to prevent thrombus formation, and IV nitroglycerin is given to

TABLE 64-4 Drugs Used in the Treatment of Coronary Artery Disease

Drug	Usual Daily Dosage	Interventions	Rationales
Nitrates			
Nitroglycerin (Nitrostat, Tridil)	0.3–0.4 mg q 5 min sublingually, up to three tablets	1. Instruct client to lie in semi-Fowler's position.	1. Hypotension can be dramatic, immediate, and intensified by upright position.
	5 μg in 5% D_5W IV started at 5 μg/min and titrated to keep client pain free with stable blood pressure. Transdermally started at 5 mg (10 cm² system)/24 h	2. Monitor blood pressure.	2. Decrease in blood pressure occurs with vasodilation.
		3. Instruct the client to allow the sublingual tablet to dissolve and to avoid swallowing the tablet.	3. Sublingual dose is absorbed through sublingual mucous membranes.
		4. Check expiration date on sublingual tablets. Tablets should be replaced q 3–5 mo.	4. Efficacy of tablets decreases with time.
		5. Monitor for headache.	5. Vasodilation is generalized.
Isosorbide dinitrate (Isordil, Iso-Bid)	2.5–5 mg q 4–6 h sublingually 5–30 mg qid PO 40-mg sustained-release tablet q 6–12h	1. Instruct the client taking sublingual forms to lie down before administration.	1. Hypotensive effect can be dramatic and immediate with sublingual administration.
		2. Monitor blood pressure and assess for dizziness.	2. Decrease in BP occurs with vasodilation.
Beta-Blockers			
Propranolol (Inderal)	10–80 mg bid–qid to 240 mg/day PO 1–3 mg at rate not to exceed 1 mg/min IV	1. Assess heart rate before administration.	1. Beta$_1$-blocking effects cause decrease in heart rate.
		2. Monitor blood pressure.	2. Hypotensive effect occurs owing to decrease in cardiac output, suppressed renin activity, and beta-blocking effects.
		3. Assess for shortness of breath and wheezing.	3. Beta$_2$-blocking effects in lungs can cause bronchoconstriction.
Calcium Channel Blockers			
Nifedipine (Procardia, Adalat)	10–30 mg tid PO or sublingually	1. Monitor blood pressure and assess for dizziness.	1. Vasodilation can cause dramatic hypotension, which occurs within minutes, especially after sublingual administration.
		2. Assess for headache and peripheral edema.	2. These are common side effects.

TABLE 64 – 4   Drugs Used in the Treatment of Coronary Artery Disease *Continued*

Drug	Usual Daily Dosage	Interventions	Rationales
Verapamil hydrochloride (Calan, Isoptin)	40 – 80 mg qid PO or 240-mg sustained-release tablet once a day 5 – 10 mg over 2 min IV	1. Monitor heart rate. 2. Monitor blood pressure and assess for dizziness. 3. Assess for constipation.	1. Agent slows SA node and AV conduction. 2. Vasodilation decreases blood pressure. 3. This is a common side effect.
Diltiazem hydrochloride (Cardizem)	30 – 60 mg qid PO	1. Monitor blood pressure and assess for dizziness. 2. Monitor heart rate.	1. Vasodilation decreases blood pressure. 2. Drug slows SA node and AV conduction, but decrease is not as great as that which occurs with verapamil.

prevent coronary spasm. Streptokinase infusion may also be used with PTCA. The result of the PTCA is an increase in the diameter of the lumen of the coronary vessel (as judged by angiographic findings) and improvement of myocardial blood flow.

Physicians are also treating acute MIs with thrombolytic agents that lyse or dissolve clots. Streptokinase is an example of a thrombolytic agent used to dissolve thrombi in the coronary arteries, restoring myocardial blood flow. As the clots are dissolved, the myocardium is reperfused, and the chest pain is often relieved. Streptokinase can be administered intravenously in the coro-

nary care unit or by intracoronary route, which is performed during a cardiac catheterization. Before intracoronary streptokinase infusion, the client is given IV nitroglycerin. Streptokinase therapy is most effective if administered within 1 to 4 hours of the coronary event.

Tissue-type plasminogen activator (TPA) is another thrombolytic agent; unlike streptokinase, it is clot specific and does not cause generalized lysis and problems with bleeding. Tissue-type plasminogen activator may also be administered by the IV or intracoronary routes. To maintain anticoagulation after thrombolytic therapy,

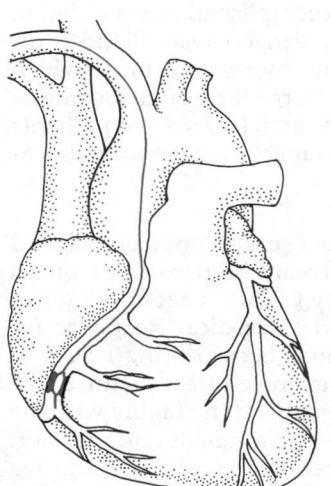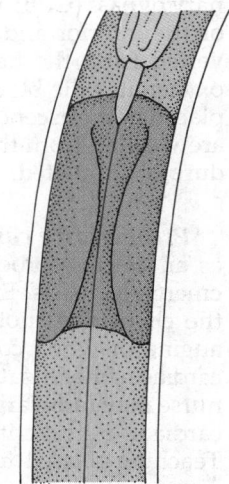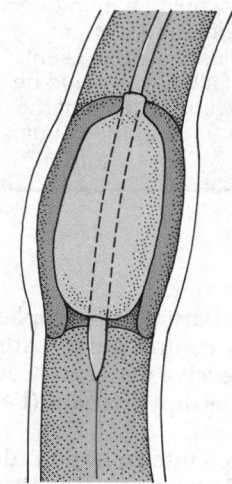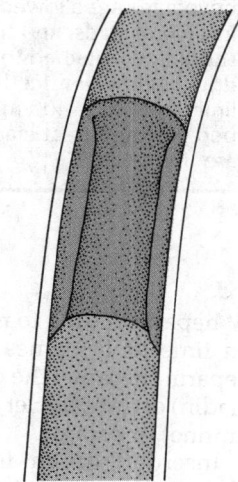

1. The balloon-tipped catheter is positioned in the artery.

2. The uninflated balloon is centered in the obstruction.

3. The balloon is inflated, which flattens plaque against the artery wall.

4. The balloon is removed, and the artery is left unoccluded.

Figure 64 – 32

Percutaneous transluminal angioplasty.

NURSING RESEARCH

Restriction of Iced Beverages Is Warranted for Clients with Ischemia.

Kirchhoff, K. T., Holm, K., Foreman, M. D., & Rebenson-Piano, M. (1990). Electrocardiographic response to ice water ingestion. *Heart and Lung, 19,* 41–48.

Iced beverages are commonly restricted for clients experiencing acute MIs. This nursing and medical intervention is based on the notion that ingestion of iced beverages causes elevation of blood pressure and ST segment and T wave changes similar to those that occur with ischemia. Statistical evidence to support this notion, however, is lacking.

This study involved 89 clients in a coronary care unit, admitted with an acute MI or to rule out MI. A 12-lead ECG was obtained 3, 10, and 25 min after ingestion of 200 or 400 mL of iced water, with clients at low-Fowler's (25 degrees) and high-Fowler's (45 degrees) positions. Multivariate analysis of variance (MANOVA) showed that mean change scores for ST segments and T wave amplitude were not clinically significant. However, three clients had ST changes of > 1 mm, two clients had T wave changes of > 10 mm, and six clients exhibited T wave inversion, which was clinically detectable on bedside monitors.

Critique. Even though the results of this study were not statistically significant, the finding that even a few clients are at risk for ECG changes is clinically important. More invasive studies are needed to assess if these ECG changes indicate actual ischemia.

Possible nursing implications. Because it is not known which clients will have ECG changes after ingestion of iced beverages, nurses should restrict iced beverages for all clients with acute ischemia. If the restriction of iced beverages is a hardship for certain clients and iced beverages are allowed, the clients should be monitored in several leads, and tracings of the monitor pattern should be obtained for up to 30 min after these clients drink iced water. Iced beverages, if allowed, should be limited to 200–400 mL and given with the head of the bed elevated to at least 25 degrees, until further studies are undertaken.

IV heparin is used to maintain the partial thromboplastin time at 1½ times the client's control value. After heparin therapy, the client may receive warfarin (Coumadin) or antiplatelet drugs, such as dipyridamole (Persantine) or aspirin.

Insertion of an intra-aortic counterpulsation device, such as the intra-aortic balloon pump (IABP), is another invasive intervention used to improve myocardial perfusion during an acute MI or during an episode of angina, when an MI is a threat. The IABP can be inserted percutaneously or through surgical cutdown. Inflation of the IABP during the client's diastole allows for improved coronary perfusion. Deflation of the balloon just before systole reduces afterload at the time of systolic contraction, facilitating emptying of the left ventricle and improving cardiac output. The balloon catheter is attached to a pump console, which is triggered by an ECG tracing and arterial waveform (Fig. 64–33).

Prevention of complications. Clients with unstable angina are at high risk for MI and sudden death. Ongoing assessment of the client during the acute anginal attack is critical. During this time, the nurse watches for development of heart failure and dysrhythmias. The nurse is prepared for possible emergency heart catheterization, PTCA, or insertion of an IABP; these measures are able to bring improved blood supply to the ischemic myocardium when symptoms cannot be controlled.

For those clients receiving thrombolytic therapy, particularly streptokinase, bleeding is a potential complication that the nurse assesses for. In addition to hemorrhage at the femoral puncture site, there may be hematuria, guaiac-positive stool, abdominal pain, or a decreased hemoglobin level. With extreme blood loss, clients may experience hypovolemic shock.

Interventions: surgical management. Clients who do not respond to treatments described may require CABG to prevent an MI if acute or chronic ischemia is present. CABG is a surgical procedure in which a saphenous vein from a leg, or the internal mammary artery, is used to bypass an occlusion or a lesion in the coronary artery (Fig. 64–34). The vein is anastomosed (sutured) proximally and distally to the coronary artery to bypass blood around the occluded artery, thus improving myocardial perfusion. The procedure is performed with the client under general anesthesia and undergoing cardiopulmonary bypass (CPB). CPB is accomplished by cannulation of the inferior and superior venae cavae. Blood is diverted from the heart to the bypass machine, which oxygenates the blood and returns it through a cannula placed in the ascending aortic arch (Fig. 64–35). Clients are weaned from the bypass machine when the procedure is completed.

Preoperative care. CABG surgery may be planned as an elective procedure or may be performed on an emergency basis. Emergency CABG is necessary when the client does not respond to medical treatment for angina or when complications occur during PTCA or cardiac catheterization. If the procedure is planned, the nurse may familiarize the client and the family with the cardiac surgical critical care environment and the staff. Teaching related to postoperative respiratory and leg exercises and measures for treatment of pain is provided by the nurse (see Chap. 18). The nurse informs the client that he/she should expect to have a sternal incision, one or two drains from the chest, a Foley catheter, and several IV fluid catheters. In describing the postoperative course, the nurse emphasizes that close monitoring and use of sophisticated equipment are standard treatment.

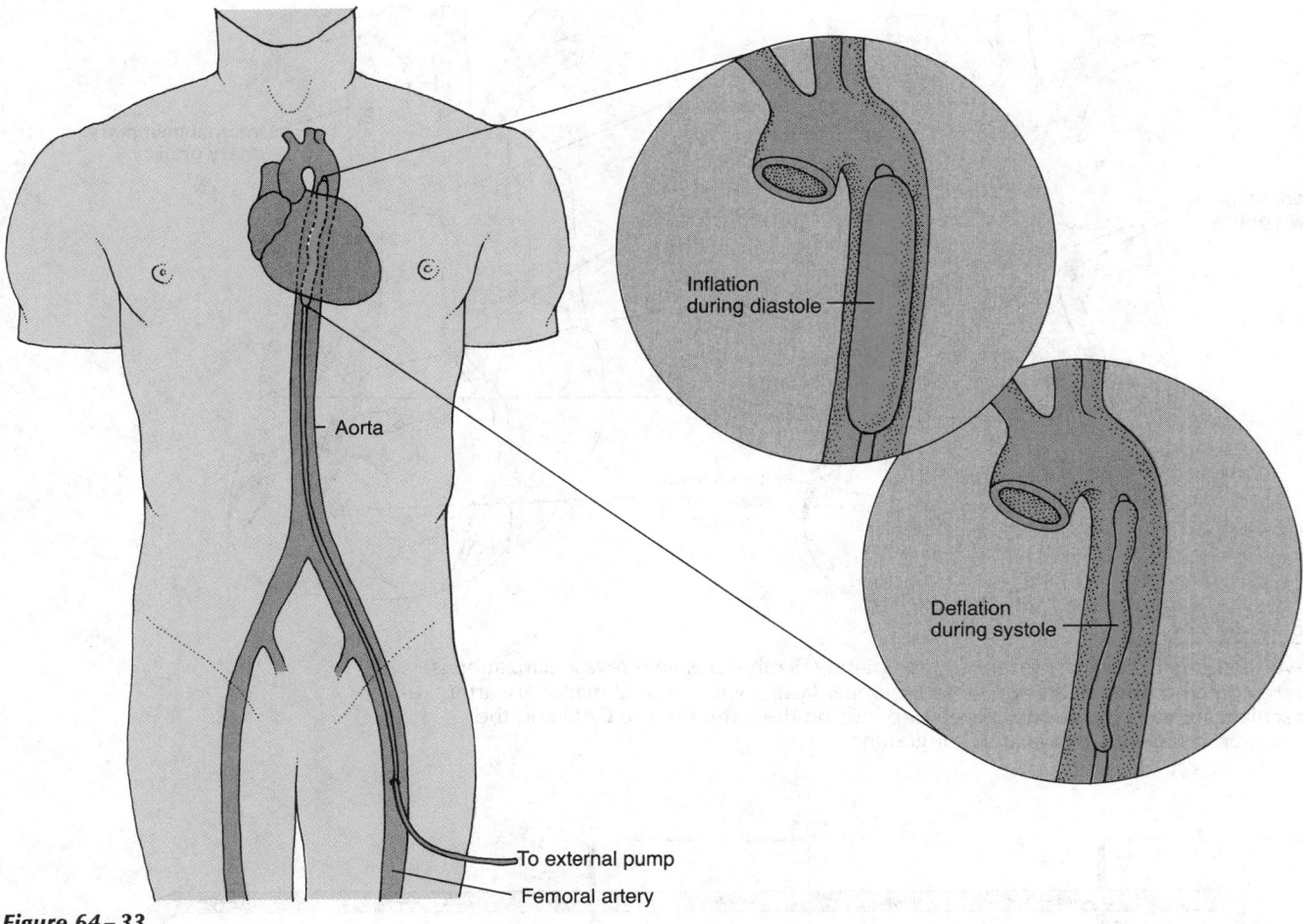

Aorta

Inflation
during diastole

Deflation
during systole

To external pump

Femoral artery

Figure 64–33

Intra-aortic balloon catheter is inserted into the femoral artery and advanced into the
descending aorta. The polyethylene balloon lies just distal to the left subclavian artery.
Immediately after it is inserted, the catheter is connected to the external pump.

The client is encouraged to keep the nursing staff informed about any discomfort that might occur postoperatively.

Postoperative care. On arrival in the cardiac surgical critical care unit, the client who has undergone CABG is usually extremely pale from CPB. The client is often intubated and undergoes mechanical ventilation for several hours, until hemodynamic measurements are stable. Mediastinal tubes are connected to water seal drainage systems, and epicardial pacer wires extend from the sternal incision and are grounded and taped to the client. Pulmonary artery and arterial catheters are connected to monitors, which also monitor the client's heart rate and rhythm. The nurse closely assesses the client for dysrhythmias, which often include ventricular ectopic rhythms or heart block. If heart block occurs, the nurse connects pacer wires to a pacemaker box and sets the appropriate rate.

Fluid and potassium replacement is a high priority in the early postoperative period, as is monitoring of hemodynamic variables and arterial blood levels. The nurse assesses these variables, watching particularly for signs and symptoms of ischemia or heart failure.

Decreased Cardiac Output

Planning: client goals. The major goal for this diagnosis is to promote circulatory function as evidenced by stable blood pressure and pulse rate, mental alertness and orientation, urinary output equal to or greater than 30 mL within a 2-hour period, and clear lung fields.

Interventions: nonsurgical management

Drug therapy. For clients with CAD, a major objective is the maintenance of cardiac output. Control of chest pain associated with a decreased cardiac output is managed by the administration of nitrates and other vasodilating agents. Another objective is the maintenance of normal sinus rhythm. An asynchronous, irregular rhythm can result with a low cardiac output. Antidysrhythmics may be instituted to restore normal sinus rhythm (see Table 64–2). If the client's cardiac output

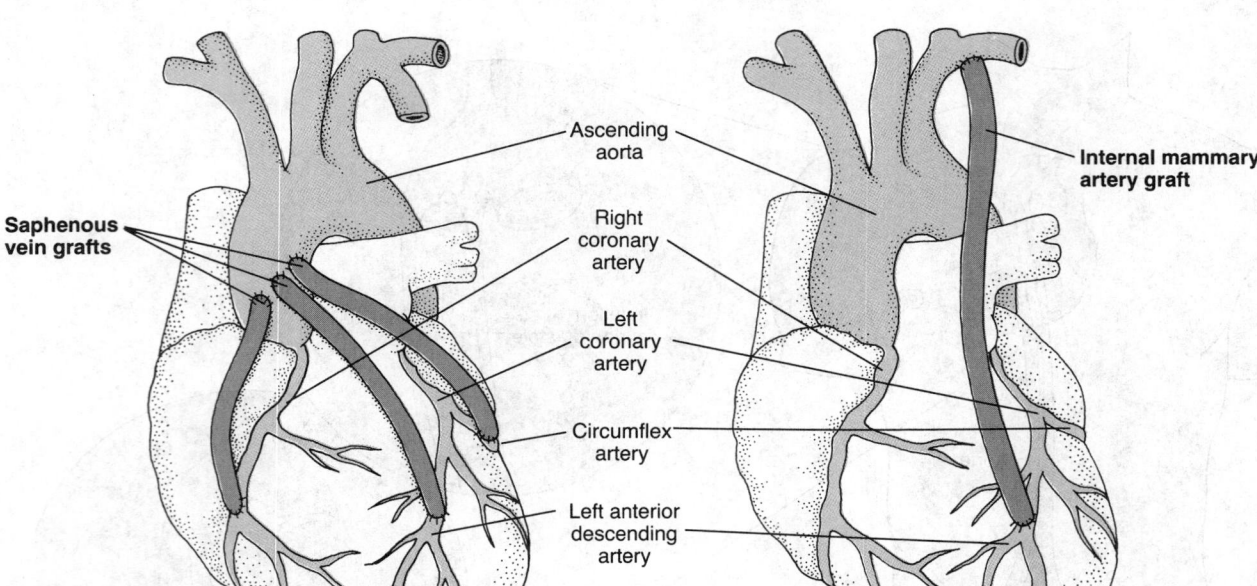

Figure 64–34

Two methods of coronary artery bypass grafting. Saphenous vein revascularization is more common, but results appear to be longer lasting with internal mammary artery revascularization. The procedure used depends on the nature of the CAD and the condition of the vessels available for grafting.

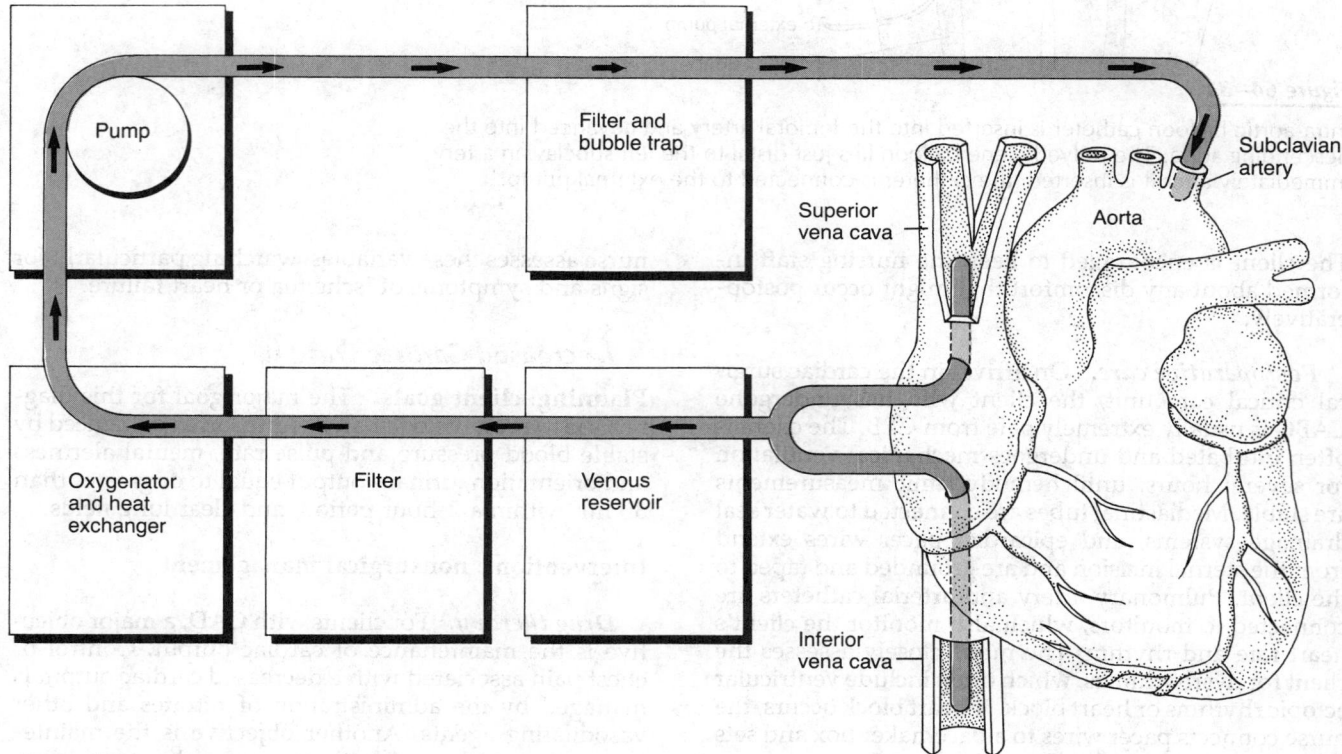

Figure 64–35

Heart-lung bypass circuitry used during cardiopulmonary bypass.

becomes critically low (less than 2 L/minute), medical therapy may include the use of inotropic medications, such as dopamine and dobutamine (Table 64–5). Caution and care are required when using these agents because of the potential risk of increasing myocardial oxygen consumption and further reducing cardiac output. Clients experiencing second-degree (Mobitz's type II) or third-degree AV block as a result of their MI most likely require at least temporary pacing. Clients who develop some types of bundle branch block may also require pacing.

Prevention of complications. Nursing care involves monitoring of the ECG and assessment of impending signs and symptoms of compromised perfusion to the peripheral tissues and organs. The nurse must be aware

TABLE 64–5   Inotropic Drugs

Drug	Usual Daily Dosage	Interventions	Rationales
Cardiac Glycosides			
Digoxin (Lanoxin, Lanoxicaps)	Loading dose of 1.0 mg divided over 24 h, then maintenance with 0.125–0.5 mg daily PO Usually 0.25–0.5 mg IV	1. Assess for previous use of digitalis glycosides before initiation of therapy, and give the preparation of digitalis as previously taken (do not substitute one preparation for another). 2. Be alert to the following factors: a. MI b. Potassium depletion c. Kidney or hepatic disorders d. Diuretic therapy e. Diarrhea f. Advancing age g. Metabolic alkalosis	1. Dosages, absorption rates, and duration of effects differ among drugs. 2. All these factors may cause an increased sensitivity to digitalis.
Digitoxin	Loading dose of 1.2–1.6 mg divided over 24 h; then 0.1 mg daily IV or PO	3. Monitor serum potassium levels and ECGs. 4. Take apical pulse before administering each dose of digitalis. 5. Monitor serum concentration of digitalis. Therapeutic levels of digoxin are 0.8–1.6 ng/mL; digitoxin, 14–26 ng/mL.	3, 4. There is a predisposition to dysrhythmias if a potassium imbalance is not corrected. 5. The incidence of digitalis toxicity is high because of the narrow margin between therapeutic and toxic doses.
Sympathomimetics			
Dopamine (Intropin)	IV only: starting dose of 2–5 μg/kg per min, titrate up to 20 μg/kg per min	1. Observe client continuously during administration. 2. Titrate dosage carefully based on heart rhythm, ECG findings, hemodynamic variables, and urinary output.	1, 2. Agent is potent activator of alpha- and beta$_1$-receptors as well as dopaminergic receptors. Dosage-dependent drug: Low dosage of 2–5 μg/kg per min

Table continued on next page

TABLE 64 – 5 Inotropic Drugs *Continued*

Drug	Usual Daily Dosage	Interventions	Rationales
			stimulates dopaminergic receptors, which promote renal and mesenteric blood flow, and beta$_1$-receptors, which increase heart rate and contractility. As dosage increases, alpha effects predominate, causing peripheral vasoconstriction. With dosage > 20 μg/kg per min, mainly alpha effects are seen.
		3. Use with caution in clients receiving monoamine oxidase inhibitors or under halothane anesthesia.	, 3. MAO inhibitors potentiate effects of dopamine. There is an increased risk of dysrhythmias with halothane anesthesia.
Dobutamine (Dobutrex)	IV only: 2.5 – 10 μg/kg per min	1. Observe client continuously during infusion. 2. Titrate drug on the basis of heart rate, ECG findings, hemodynamic measurements, and urinary output.	1, 2. Agent is a very strong beta$_1$-receptor activator and a moderately strong beta$_2$-activator.
Bipyridines			
Amrinone lactate (Inocor)	IV only: start with bolus of 0.75 mg/kg over 2 – 3 min; usual maintenance dose 5 – 10 μg/kg per min	1. Observe the client continuously during infusion. 2. Titrate drug on the basis of heart rate, ECG findings, hemodynamic measurements, and urinary output. 3. Keep the drug in light-resistant container. 4. Do not mix with dextrose solution.	1, 2. Drug is a positive inotropic agent with vasodilator activity. 3, 4. Light and dextrose solution decrease the drug's activity with time.

of the following indicators of cardiogenic shock: hypotension; urinary volume less than 30 mL/hour; cool, clammy, or cyanotic skin; restlessness; apathy; and lessening of responsiveness. Medical intervention must occur immediately or death ensues.

Heart failure occurring with MI is a common complication that can diminish cardiac output. An MI reduces the ability of the left ventricle to eject blood forward, leaving greater residual volumes, thus yielding higher left ventricular pressures with ensuing pulmonary complications. The nurse assesses for the development of left ventricular failure and pulmonary edema, manifested by shortness of breath, diffuse crackles, wheezing, tachycardia, and frothy sputum production. Hemodynamic monitoring is often instituted for the client at risk or with symptoms of heart failure to assess determinants of preload, afterload, and cardiac output. Hemodynamic monitoring requires the insertion of a pulmonary artery catheter, usually into the right subclavian or internal jugular vein (see Chap. 63). The nurse obtains and records hemodynamic measurements, which include pulmonary artery systolic and diastolic pressures, pulmonary artery wedge pressure (a measure of preload), right atrial pressure, systemic vascular resistance (a measure of afterload), and cardiac output. Values for the pressures are calculated by the nurse from printed waveforms obtained from monitoring systems (Fig. 64–36). These measurements help both the nurse and the physician in titrating fluids and vasoactive drugs used to maintain an adequate cardiac output.

Clients who do not respond to drug therapy with improved tissue perfusion, decreased workload of the heart, and increased cardiac contractility might need to have an IABP inserted (see earlier).

The nurse reports any change in vital signs, mentation, chest pain, heart sounds, or respiratory status to assist in early identification of other complications related to an MI. Complications include papillary muscle rupture, ventricular septal rupture, ventricular aneurysms, cerebral and pulmonary emboli, and pericarditis.

Activity Intolerance

Planning: client goals. The overall goal for this diagnosis is that the client will remain active within levels of tolerance.

Interventions: nonsurgical management. Cardiac rehabilitation is a process of actively assisting the client with cardiac disease to achieve and maintain a vital and productive life, while remaining within the heart's ability to respond to increases in activity and stress. Cardiac rehabilitation can be divided into three phases. The first phase begins with the acute illness and ends with discharge from the hospital. Phase 2 begins after discharge and continues through convalescence at home, and phase 3 refers to long-term conditioning.

In the acute phase, the nurse promotes rest, yet ensures some limited mobilization. The nurse assists with all activities of daily living (ADL), such as feeding, bathing, and toileting. The client progresses through various levels of activity. For example, on the first day the client may be restricted to complete bed rest with the use of bedside commode; on the second day, the client may

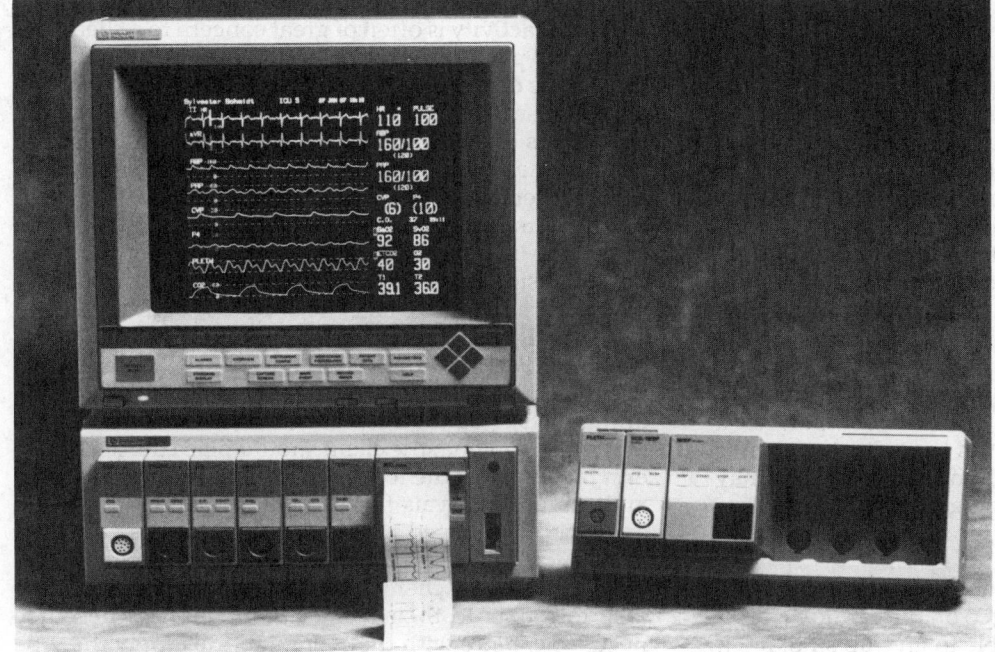

Figure 64–36

Component monitoring system monitors and records hemodynamic measurements. (Courtesy of Hewlett-Packard Company.)

dangle the legs at the side of the bed once during each nursing shift; on day 3, the client is out of bed and sits in a chair as tolerated, usually for 30 minutes three times a day. When the client is restricted to bed or chair, range-of-motion exercises are usually instituted to help prevent emboli formation and stasis ulcers and to maintain muscle strength and tone. Assessment of heart rate, blood pressure, respiratory rate, and level of fatigue is performed with each level of activity. Decreases in systolic blood pressure greater than 10 mmHg with or without an increase in pulse rate indicate cardiac intolerance to activity.

■ Discharge Planning

The client with angina is usually discharged home with pharmacologic therapy. Clients who have had an MI may or may not have intermittent angina, which requires continued treatment. All clients require treatment or avoidance of risk factors to prevent recurrent ischemia.

Home Care Preparation

Clients who recover from anginal episodes or an MI may need assistance with ADL on a temporary basis to allow for rest. Clients who have undergone CABG or are recovering from an MI complicated by heart failure or shock often require more assistance with ADL because of their limited activity tolerance. Many clients with angina or MIs greatly benefit from involvement in a structured cardiac rehabilitation program to assist clients in increasing their activity level, while being monitored.

Client/Family Education

After the nurse has determined that the client and the family are ready to learn, a teaching plan should be developed, which includes the normal anatomy and physiology of the heart, the pathophysiology of angina and MI, risk factor modification, cardiac medications, and activity and exercise protocols.

The nurse informs the client about the normal function of the heart and coronary arteries and explains what angina and MI are. Clients are taught that, after an MI, myocardial healing begins early and is usually complete in 6 to 8 weeks. Clients who have undergone CABG are told that the sternotomy heals in about 6 to 8 weeks.

Risk factor modification is a necessary part of a client's management and involves changing the client's health care patterns. Modification of risk factors may include ceasing smoking, changing dietary habits, exercising regularly, controlling high blood pressure or diabetes, and reducing stress.

For clients who smoke, the nurse explains the detrimental effects of smoking tobacco on the cardiovascular system. Many clients may be able to give up smoking if they are motivated, but others may need behavior modification and support groups to do so.

Dietary changes that need to be made include reducing total fat intake, substituting polyunsaturated fats for saturated fats, reducing sodium intake for clients with high blood pressure or heart failure, and maintaining an ideal body weight. There are many booklets and cookbooks that can assist the client in learning to cook with reduction of fats, oils, and salt. In addition, the client can be instructed to read labels with greater care, looking particularly for saturated fats, such as palm and coconut oils, in many processed foods.

Control of high blood pressure in the hypertensive client involves teaching the client to take his/her own blood pressure. Clients are instructed to take their blood pressure on a daily basis and keep a record. A blood pressure of 140/90 or greater should be reported to the primary health care provider. Clients with diabetes mellitus are assessed for their participation in efforts to control hyperglycemia. The nurse reviews the prescribed dosage of insulin or oral hypoglycemic agents and instructs the client in checking his/her blood or urine for glucose and acetone levels.

A program of physical activity has beneficial effects on cardiac performance. The client is instructed to engage in normal daily activities that do not precipitate angina and to avoid isometric activity, such as lifting or pulling heavy objects. Joining a formal exercise program is encouraged, ideally one that assists the client in monitoring her/his cardiovascular progress. The client can be instructed to take her/his pulse and to check the pulse before, halfway through, and after exercise. The fundamentals of a warm-up period before exercising and a cool-down period are also discussed. A simple walking program three times a week may provide enough motivation for the client to make exercise a lifelong habit.

Sexual activity is often of great concern to a client and the sexual partner. Sexual relations may be resumed on the advice of the physician, usually after exercise tolerance is assessed. If the client can walk briskly or climb two flights of stairs without symptoms, he/she usually can resume sexual activity. Nitroglycerin may be taken before intercourse as a prophylactic measure.

The nurse assists the client in understanding the type of cardiac drug prescribed, the benefit of the drug, the potential side effects to watch for, and the correct dosage and time of day to take the drug. Use of nitroglycerin sublingually deserves special attention. The client is instructed to carry nitroglycerin tablets at all times and to keep the tablets in a light-resistant container. Nitroglycerin tablets should be replaced every 3 months. At the first sign of angina, the client should place the nitroglycerin tablet under the tongue. The dose may be repeated at 5-minute intervals for a total of three tablets. If the angina is not relieved after taking three tablets, the client is instructed to seek emergency medical attention.

Two-thirds of clients who experience a first MI are able to return to their former occupations. The nurse needs to explore with the client and the family the type of occupation the client is engaged in and to help the client to make any adjustments necessary.

Clients who have undergone CABG require instruction on incision care for the incision over the sternum and the incision over the donor site, most often the saphenous vein of the leg. The leg of the donor site often is edematous, and the client is instructed to elevate the limb when sitting in a chair.

Psychosocial Preparation

Having angina, experiencing an acute MI, or having CABG may be the most frightening experience in a client's life. Any of these experiences may also cause an altered self-image. Common coping mechanisms are anxiety, denial, anger, regression, and depression. Clients need reassurance and an opportunity to express fears and feelings regarding their acute illness or future recovery. Teaching and counseling sessions with family members regarding the illness and preventive measures give tangible techniques to cope with CAD.

A cardiac rehabilitation program can be beneficial for clients, as they can identify with others who have experienced the same illness and receive emotional support. Methods of stress reduction, such as relaxation techniques or the use of biofeedback response, can be taught (see Chap. 6).

Health Care Resources

The AHA is a great source for booklets, films, video cassettes, cookbooks, and professional service referrals for the client with CAD. Many local affiliates have their own cardiac rehabilitation programs for clients to join.

Within the community, there may be cardiac rehabilitation programs affiliated with local hospitals, YMCAs, YWCAs, or other facilities, such as clinics. Many shopping malls open before shopping hours to allow for a measured walking program indoors. This has been particularly popular for the elderly client and also provides a good support group.

For clients who have had CABG, Mended Hearts is a nationwide program, with local chapters, that provides education and support to clients and their families. Smoking cessation programs and clinics are found within the community, as well as weight reduction programs. Many hospitals have also sponsored annual health fairs and promote blood pressure screening and risk factor modifying programs as well.

◤ Evaluation

The expected outcomes for the client with CAD include that the client

1. States that the chest pain or discomfort is alleviated
2. Takes appropriate measures to relieve chest pain
3. Demonstrates restoration and maintenance of hemodynamic stability
4. Exhibits no signs of complications, such as heart failure or life-threatening dysrhythmias

HEART FAILURE

OVERVIEW

Heart failure is a general term to describe a state in which the heart can no longer pump an adequate supply of blood or cardiac output to meet the demands of the body. Heart failure is not a diagnosis, and its etiology should be carefully sought. Whatever the cause, heart failure results in inadequate tissue perfusion and pulmonary and systemic congestion.

Pathophysiology

Basic cardiac physiologic mechanisms, such as stroke volume, heart rate, cardiac output, preload, afterload, and contractility, are altered in heart failure (see Chap. 63). Impaired cardiac function results in failure to empty venous reservoirs and reduced delivery of blood into the arterial circulation. Hemodynamically, these alterations appear as elevated ventricular end-diastolic pressures, elevated systemic and pulmonary venous pressures, and a decreased cardiac output. Clinical indicators are due to activated compensatory mechanisms, reduced cardiac reserve, impaired organ perfusion, and accumulation of extracellular fluid.

Compensatory Mechanisms

Three compensatory mechanisms attempt to maintain normal cardiac pumping function: increased sympathetic nervous system response, Frank-Starling response, and myocardial hypertrophy.

In heart failure, stimulation of the *sympathetic nervous system* represents the most immediate compensatory mechanism. Stimulation of the adrenergic receptors causes an increased heart rate, increased myocardial contractility, and venous and arterial vasoconstriction. As a result of venous vasoconstriction, there is an increased venous return to the heart, which increases the preload. Blood flow is shunted from the peripheral tissues to the large organs, and afterload increases owing to arteriolar vasoconstriction. Because of vasoconstriction on the renal arteries, renal blood flow is reduced, and the kidneys respond by retaining water and sodium.

The *Frank-Starling response* increases preload, which helps sustain cardiac output. In this response, the cardiac muscle fibers contract more forcibly the more they are stretched before contraction. By increasing the venous return to the heart, the fibers are stretched, which provides for a more forceful contraction, thus increasing stroke volume, which results in an increased cardiac output.

Myocardial hypertrophy, with or without chamber dilation, is seen as a thickening of the walls of the heart, providing more muscle mass, resulting in more effective contractility, and further increasing cardiac output.

All mechanisms of compensation act primarily to restore cardiac output to near-normal levels. However, during the course of heart failure, these cardiac and peripheral circulatory adjustments may eventually cause deleterious effects on pump function because all of them contribute to an increase in myocardial oxygen consumption. At this point, signs and symptoms of heart failure develop.

Classification of Heart Failure

Heart failure can be classified in many ways. Four main categories are discussed here.

Backward versus forward failure.   Backward failure is said to result when the ventricle is unable to pump out its volume of blood, causing blood to accumulate and raising the pressure within the ventricles, the atria, and the venous system. Forward failure is the result of the inability of the heart to maintain cardiac output, thus diminishing tissue perfusion. The effects of forward and backward failure in right and left ventricular failure are compared in the accompanying Key Features of Disease.

As the heart is a part of the closed system, backward and forward failure are always associated with each other.

Left versus right ventricular failure.   Left ventricular failure is by far the more frequent of the two instances in which only one side of the heart is affected. It is typically caused by hypertensive disease, CAD, or valvular disease (involving the mitral or aortic valve). Pulmonary congestion and edema usually signal the onset of left ventricular failure. Right ventricular failure is most often caused by left ventricular failure. Sustained pulmonary hypertension also develops into right ventricular failure, leading to systemic venous congestion and peripheral edema.

Low- versus high-output syndrome.   Low-output syndrome occurs when the heart fails as a pump, resulting in impaired peripheral circulation and peripheral vasoconstriction. The word *syndrome*, however, makes it clear that the failure represents a reaction rather than a primary pathologic change.

When cardiac output remains normal or above normal but the metabolic needs of the body are not met, high-output syndrome is present. It may be caused by increased metabolic needs, as seen in hyperthyroidism, fever, and pregnancy, or it may be triggered by hyperkinetic conditions, such as arteriovenous fistulas, beriberi, or Paget's disease.

Acute versus chronic failure.   The clinical manifestations of acute and chronic heart failure depend on how rapidly the syndrome develops. Acute heart failure re-

---

KEY FEATURES OF DISEASE ■ Effects of Forward and Backward Failure in Left and Right Ventricular Failure

Left Ventricular Failure	Right Ventricular Failure
Effects of Backward Failure	
Increased volume and pressure in left ventricle and left atrium (preload)	Increased volume in venous circulation
Pulmonary edema	Increased right atrial pressure (preload)
	Hepatomegaly and splenomegaly
	Dependent peripheral edema
Effects of Forward Failure	
Decreased cardiac output	Increased blood volume
Decreased tissue perfusion	Decreased volume to lungs
Increased secretion of sodium and water-retaining hormones	
Increased retention of sodium and water	
Increased extracellular fluid volume	

sulting from a marked decrease in left ventricular failure may be due to acute MI, acute valvular dysfunction, or hypertensive crisis. The onset of events occurs so rapidly that the compensatory mechanisms are ineffective, resulting in the rapid development of pulmonary edema and circulatory collapse (cardiogenic shock).

Chronic heart failure develops over time and is usually the end result of an increasing inability of the compensatory mechanisms to be effective. Chronic heart failure can be caused by hypertension, valvular disease, or chronic obstructive pulmonary disease.

Etiology

Heart failure may result from conditions causing volume overload, pressure overload, myocardial dysfunction, filling disorders, or increased metabolic demand (see the accompanying Key Features of Disease).

Incidence

The incidence of heart failure is difficult to determine because heart failure is a symptom, not a diagnosis. Data on this sympton usually relate to the underlying cause.

PREVENTION

Because heart failure results mainly from heart disease, preventing heart disease is the first step in preventing heart failure. Modification or prevention of heart disease states, such as CAD, infective endocarditis, constrictive pericarditis, hypertension, and rheumatic heart disease, is imperative. However, as these and other forms of heart disease cannot always be prevented, the next step is to delay the onset of heart failure. This may include dietary management, such as low-salt or low-fat diets or weight loss diets; smoking cessation programs; exercise prescription; and prompt treatment of infections.

COLLABORATIVE MANAGEMENT

 Assessment

Manifestations of heart failure depend on which ventricle fails, the duration of failure, and the underlying etiology. Pulmonary congestion and edema dominate the picture of left ventricular failure. Systemic venous congestion and peripheral edema are associated with right ventricular failure.

History

When taking a history, the nurse needs to keep in mind the many conditions that may lead to heart failure.

KEY FEATURES OF DISEASE ■ **Causes of Heart Failure**

Volume Overload

Aortic incompetence
Mitral incompetence
Tricuspid incompetence
Overtransfusion
Left-to-right shunts
Hypervolemia

Pressure Overload

Aortic stenosis
Hypertrophic cardiomyopathy
Hypertension

Myocardial Dysfunction

Cardiomyopathy
Myocarditis
CAD
Ischemia
Infarction
Dysrhythmias
Toxic disorders

Filling Disorders

Mitral stenosis
Tricuspid stenosis
Cardiac tamponade
Restrictive pericarditis

Increased Metabolic Demand

Anemias
Fever
Beriberi
Paget's disease
Arteriovenous fistula

Michaelson, C. R. (Ed.). Reproduced by permission from *Congestive heart failure* (p. 45). St. Louis, 1983, The C. V. Mosby Co.

The best means of controlling heart failure is through early detection of the predisposing factors.

The client is carefully questioned regarding *past medical history*, including a history of high blood pressure, angina, MI, rheumatic heart disease, valvular disorders, endocarditis, and pericarditis.

Subjective data are collected concerning the client's

perception of his/her *breathing pattern, fluid retention, response to activity,* and the client's *knowledge and response to heart failure.*

Left ventricular failure. *Dyspnea,* or abnormally uncomfortable breathing, is a cardinal manifestation of left ventricular failure. The failing left ventricle causes the pulmonary venous pressure to rise, which results in pulmonary congestion. The nurse carefully questions the client regarding the presence of dyspnea and the sequence in which it developed. The client may refer to dyspnea as trouble in catching one's breath, breathlessness, or difficulty in breathing.

In *exertional dyspnea,* the client becomes aware of the inability to continue previously tolerated levels of activity. Dyspnea at rest in the recumbent position is known as *orthopnea.* Clients usually use a number of pillows to sleep or may sleep in an upright position in a bed or a chair.

Clients who describe sudden awakening with a feeling of breathlessness 2 to 5 hours after falling asleep have *paroxysmal nocturnal dyspnea.* Sitting upright, dangling the feet, or walking usually relieves this condition.

Cough is another key finding associated with dyspnea. The client describes the cough as irritating, nocturnal, and usually nonproductive.

The client's *level of activity* is assessed. Can the client perform normal ADL or climb flights of stairs without dyspnea, or does the client report weakness or fatigue even at rest? Owing to decreased tissue perfusion, weakness or fatigue is precipitated and is described by the client as a feeling of heaviness in arms and legs.

Decreased cerebral perfusion due to low cardiac output leads to *changes in mental status.* The nurse assesses for a history of insomnia, memory loss, or confusion.

The client may describe palpitations, skipped beats, or a fast heart beat. An *irregular heart rhythm* resulting from premature atrial or ventricular contractions and atrial fibrillation is common in clients with heart failure.

Right ventricular failure. *Peripheral edema* is a manifestation in which edema begins in the lower legs and ascends to the thigh and abdominal walls. Clients may note that shoes fit more tightly or have marks left on their feet from the shoes or socks. Most clients report *weight gain.* An adult may retain 4 to 7 L of fluid (10 to 15 lb) before pitting edema occurs.

Gastrointestinal (GI) complaints of nausea and anorexia may be a direct consequence of the increased intra-abdominal pressure. Another finding related to fluid retention is *diuresis at rest.* The client describes frequent awakening at night to urinate. At rest, the body's metabolic requirements are decreased; cardiac function improves, decreasing systemic venous pressure. Edema fluid is thus mobilized and excreted.

Owing to various problems of fluid retention, a careful *nutritional history* is obtained. The client is carefully questioned regarding the use of salt and types of food consumed.

Physical Assessment: Clinical Manifestations

The signs and symptoms of heart failure can be considered in the context of the four components of the syndrome: failure of the left ventricle as a pump, pulmonary venous congestion, failure of the right ventricle as a pump, and systemic venous congestion.

Left ventricular failure. Associated with elevated pulmonary venous pressure and decreased cardiac output, left ventricular failure appears clinically as *breathlessness, weakness, fatigue, dizziness, confusion, pulmonary congestion, hypotension,* or *death.*

The nurse palpates the precordium. *Increased heart size* is common, with a displacement of the apical impulse to the left. The *pulse* may be *tachycardiac* or be *alternating* in strength (pulsus alternans). On auscultation, the nurse may hear an S_3 gallop, an early diastolic filling sound indicating an increase in left ventricular pressure. An S_4 can also occur, although it is not a sign of failure but a reflection of decreased ventricular compliance.

The nurse also assesses lung status. *Crackles* (rales) are produced by intra-alveolar fluid. Wheezes may also be auscultated.

Right ventricular failure. Associated with increased systemic venous pressures, right ventricular failure gives rise to the clinical signs of *jugular vein distention, hepatomegaly, dependent edema,* and *ascites.*

On inspection, the nurse assesses the neck veins for distention. The client must also be assessed for the presence of hepatomegaly (liver engorgement) or ascites. The collection of fluid in the abdomen (ascites) can reach volumes of more than 10 L. The extremities should be checked for edema caused by gravity when the client is upright.

Classification. The knowledge of the manifestations of left and right ventricular failure allows the nurse to evaluate the client's current level of involvement. A functional classification of cardiac status by the New York Heart Association summarizes clinical indicators (see Chap. 63, Table 63–1).

Psychosocial Assessment

Clients with heart failure often manifest fear of death, especially when they have difficulty with breathing. Many clients with acute heart failure continue to have chronic failure, and many have symptoms that are not well controlled. These clients may have anxiety and frustrations related to dealing with a chronic illness, which has an impact on many facets of daily life. The nurse assesses clients and their families for fears, anxieties, and frustrations and also assesses their usual methods of coping.

Laboratory Findings

Electrolyte imbalance in heart failure reflects complications of failure, as well as the use of diuretics and other drug therapies. Hyponatremia and hypokalemia are common side effects of diuretic therapy. Any impairment of kidney function may be reflected by elevated blood urea nitrogen, serum *creatinine,* and creatinine clearance levels. Urinalysis may reveal proteinuria and high specific gravity.

Radiographic Findings

Chest radiographs can be helpful in diagnosing left ventricular failure. Typically, the cardiac silhouette is enlarged, representing hypertrophy or dilation. Pleural effusions develop less often and generally reflect biventricular failure.

Other Diagnostic Tests

The ECG is not helpful in determining the presence or extent of heart failure, but demonstrates ventricular hypertrophy, dysrhythmias, and any degree of myocardial ischemia, injury, or infarction.

Echocardiography is useful in diagnosing cardiac valvular changes, pericardial effusion, chamber enlargement, and ventricular hypertrophy. Radionuclide studies (thallium imaging or technetium pyrophosphate scanning) can also provide information as to the presence and etiology of heart failure.

Pulmonary artery catheters allow for direct measurement of cardiac pressures. These measurements are often necessary for the diagnosis of heart failure. The right atrial pressure may be normal in left ventricular failure and elevated in right ventricular failure. Pulmonary artery and pulmonary artery wedge pressures are elevated in left-sided heart failure, with a concomitant decrease in cardiac output.

 Analysis: Nursing Diagnosis

Common Diagnoses

A common nursing diagnosis pertinent to the client with acute or chronic heart failure is decreased cardiac output related to reduction in stroke volume as a result of mechanical alterations.

Additional Diagnoses

The client may also have one or more of the following:

1. Impaired gas exchange related to inadequate ventilation/perfusion ratio secondary to pulmonary congestion
2. Fluid volume excess related to sodium and water retention

3. Activity intolerance related to reduced cardiac output and impaired gas exchange
4. Fear related to the diagnosis of heart failure, symptoms of shortness of breath, and death
5. Knowledge deficit related to unfamiliarity with the disease process and its treatment

 Planning and Implementation

The major approach to heart failure involves treatment of the underlying cause, such as ischemia related to an MI and treatment or control of the heart failure.

Decreased Cardiac Output

Planning: client goals. The major goal is that the client will experience the maintenance or return to an adequate cardiac output as evidenced by a heart rate within normal limits, no gallop heart sounds, no dependent edema, clear lungs, no neck vein distention, and normal blood pressure.

Interventions: nonsurgical management. Interventions for decreased cardiac output are aimed at improvement in pump performance, reduced cardiac workload, and control of excessive sodium and water retention.

Drug therapy. Improvement of pump performance or enhancement of contractility can be achieved by the use of inotropic agents (see Table 64-5). Digitalis is given to improve contractility and to slow the heart rate. This results in increased cardiac output and decreased heart size and venous pressure. In the setting of a supraventricular rhythm (e.g., atrial fibrillation), digitalis is used to slow the ventricular response.

Sympathomimetic agents such as dopamine (Intropin) and dobutamine (Dobutrex) are administered by continuous infusion to clients whose condition is severely compromised by heart failure. Amrinone (Inocor) is usually reserved for those clients who have not responded to other inotropic therapies.

Reduction of cardiac workload and control of excessive sodium and water retention can be accomplished by the use of diuretics and vasodilator therapy. Diuretics enhance renal excretion of sodium and water, reducing the circulating blood volume, decreasing preload, and reducing systemic and pulmonary congestion. The type and dosage of diuretic given depend on the degree of heart failure and renal function (see Chap. 63, Table 63-2). Loss of potassium from diuretic therapy and potential hypovolemia are complications that need to be assessed for and prevented. The nurse assesses for the signs and symptoms of hypokalemia, which include muscle weakness and irregular heart rate. Serum potassium levels should be assessed. The serum potassium level should be kept between 3.5 and 5.0 mEq/L.

Vasodilators are used to increase cardiac output by dilating the peripheral vascular vessels and reducing impedance or resistance to left ventricular outflow. By relaxing the systemic veins, vasodilators reduce ventricular filling pressure and volume (preload). By relaxing resistance vessels or arterioles, vasodilators can reduce impedance to left ventricular ejection (afterload) and improve cardiac output. Invasive hemodynamic monitoring is often used with careful monitoring of blood pressure to guide administration of the vasodilators and to avoid hypotension. Table 64–6 compares the effects of selected agents that reduce the preload, the afterload, or both.

The oxygen content of the blood in clients with heart failure is markedly reduced because of a decreased cardiac output and pulmonary congestion. The percentage of oxygen is determined by the client's arterial blood gas values.

Diet therapy. A low-sodium diet is usually suggested to clients to control water retention. Many clients with heart failure may need to omit only table salt (no added salt) from their diet, thus reducing the sodium intake to 1.6 to 2.8 g/day. If there is need for further salt reduction, the client may eliminate all salt in cooking, thus reducing sodium intake to 1.2 to 1.4 g/day. For clients with more severe heart failure, a strict low-sodium diet would limit the daily salt intake to 0.2 to 1 g of sodium per day. High- and low-sodium foods are listed in the accompanying Health Promotion/Maintenance feature. A weight reduction diet should also be considered for obese clients to decrease the workload of the heart.

Other interventions. Reduction of cardiac workload in both acute and chronic failure requires physical and emotional rest.

The nurse places the client in semi-Fowler's or high-Fowler's position. These positions reduce venous return to the heart and maximize oxygenation by permitting greater lung expansion. The nurse also encourages coughing and deep breathing exercises every 1 to 2 hours, and assists in repositioning the client who is restricted to bed rest every 2 hours to prevent atelectasis.

The nurse weighs the client daily (1 kg of weight gain equals 1 L of retained fluid) and keeps accurate records of fluid intake and output. Fluid restriction may be imposed on the hospitalized client, and the nurse adjusts oral and IV therapy accordingly.

Prevention of complications. Acute pulmonary edema is a life-threatening event that indicates severe heart failure. Rapid-acting diuretics, such as furosemide (Lasix), are given intravenously over 1 to 2 minutes, usually starting with 40 mg and repeating with another 40 mg if needed.

Oxygen is administered to the client, who is placed in high-Fowler's position. Morphine sulfate may be given intravenously, 1 to 2 mg at a time, to reduce venous return (preload), but respiratory rate and blood pressure need to be monitored closely. Aminophylline may be administered intravenously to relieve bronchospasm. Vasodilators, such as nitroglycerin (Tridil) or nitroprusside sodium (Nipride), may be administered via continuous infusion pumps, but low dosages of these drugs must be given initially and increased slowly to avoid severe hypotension.

Application of rotating tourniquets may be necessary to assist in reducing preload while waiting for the medications to be effective. Foley's catheter should be inserted by the nurse during the episode of pulmonary edema to assess the client's urinary output after diuretic administration and to minimize exertion related to voiding.

Clients often respond dramatically and quickly to these interventions, but their condition can also deteriorate quickly because of pulmonary congestion, which causes severe hypoxemia. Clients frequently require intubation and ventilation to survive the acute episode. The nurse needs to be prepared to assist with intubation.

TABLE 64–6   Effects of Vasodilators*

Drug	Preload Reduction (Vasodilates Peripheral Veins)	Afterload Reduction (Vasodilates Arterioles)
Nitrates (nitroglycerin, isosorbide dinitrate)	+++	+
Hydralazine hydrochloride (Apresoline)	0	+++
Nifedipine (Procardia)	0	++
Nitroprusside sodium (Nipride)	+++	+++
Captopril (Capoten)	+	++
Prazosin (Minipress)	++	++

* 0, no effect; +, mild effect; ++, moderate effect; +++, maximal effect.

HEALTH PROMOTION/MAINTENANCE ■ Relative Sodium Content of Foods

High-Sodium Foods	Low-Sodium Foods
Beverages	
Mineral water, club soda, tomato juice, Dutch-processed cocoa	Fresh fruit juices, coffee, tea
Breads and Cereals	
Saltines, biscuits, pretzels, pizza, commercial pancake mix, granola, instant cooked cereal	Some breads and crackers (check label), Cream of Wheat
Dairy Products	
Regular cheese, buttermilk	Skim milk, eggs, cottage cheese, ice cream
Desserts	
Commercially baked products, commercially made puddings	Sherbet, fruit ice
Fats	
Bacon fat, commercially produced salad dressings, peanut butter	Margarine, oils, shortening
Meats	
Smoked or cured products such as bacon, ham, sausage, and hot dogs; lunch meat; TV dinners; sardines; anchovies	Chicken, turkey, fresh fish, lamb, veal, tuna packed in water
Seasonings	
Salt, garlic, celery or onion salt, monosodium glutamate, meat tenderizer, soy sauce, ketchup, mustard, canned soup	Pepper, onion, garlic, dill, cinnamon, nutmeg, thyme, sage, rosemary, vanilla extract
Vegetables and Fruits	
Any canned or pickled vegetable or fruit	Fresh or frozen fruit or vegetable
Miscellaneous	
Baking soda, baking powder, salted nuts	Unsalted nuts, vinegar

Interventions: surgical management. For clients younger than age 55 years who have end-stage heart failure or cardiomyopathy, heart transplantation may be considered. A donor heart from a person younger than age 40 years with a comparable body weight and ABO compatibility is transplanted to a recipient less than 6 hours after procurement.

The surgery consists of removal of the diseased heart, leaving the posterior walls of the client's atria, followed by the anastomosis of the atria, aorta, and pulmonary arteries (Fig. 64–37). Immunosuppressive drugs, such as cyclosporine, are used to maintain natural defense mechanisms to prevent transplant rejection (see Chap. 27).

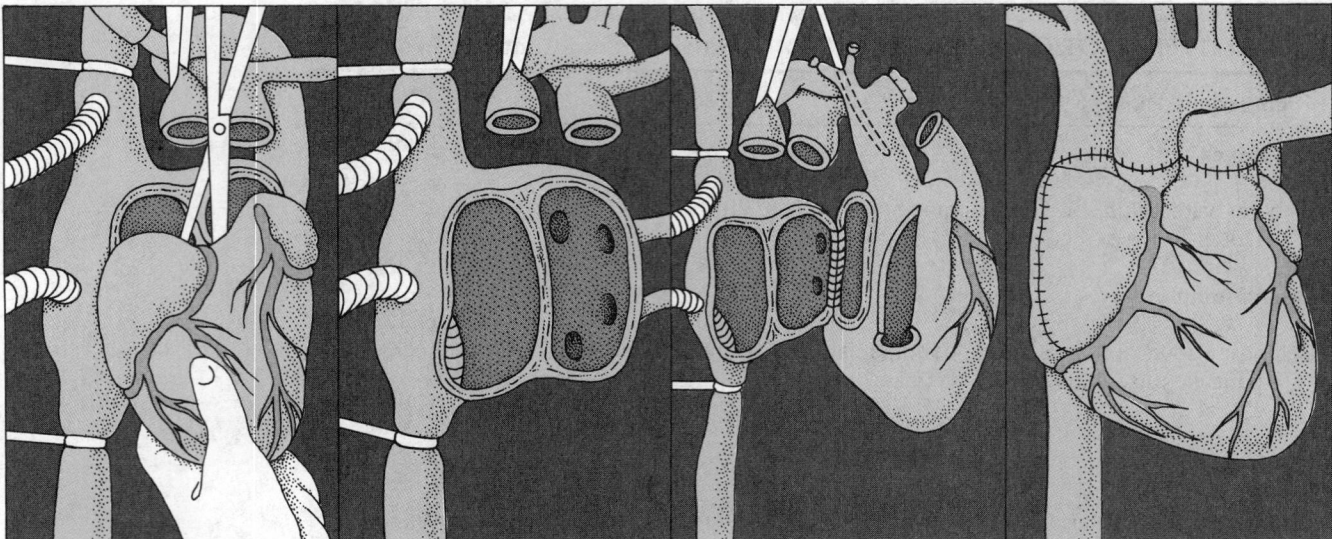

1. After the recipient is placed on cardiopulmonary bypass, the heart is removed.

2. The posterior walls of the recipient's left and right atria are left intact.

3. The left atrium of donor heart is anastomosed to the recipient's residual posterior atrial walls, and the other atrial walls, the atrial septum, and the great vessels are joined.

POSTOPERATIVE RESULT

Figure 64-37

Heart transplantation.

■ Discharge Planning

Heart failure becomes a chronic disorder for many clients. Clients are discharged to home with activity restrictions ranging from minimal (New York Heart Association functional class I) to strict (functional class IV) for clients who have symptoms with rest (see Chap. 63, Table 63-1).

Home Care Preparation

Evaluation of the home environment is done with consideration of activity restraints. The nurse determines if the client needs to climb stairs and asks about the location of the bathroom and the bedroom. Clients with strict activity restrictions should avoid stair climbing, and alternative arrangements for toileting and sleeping may be required.

Client/Family Education

The nurse assists the client in planning to reach an optimal level of functioning within the limits of his/her cardiac function. The goal for clients who have experienced heart failure is to maximize rehabilitation gains and prevent recurrent acute episodes. Activity schedules during all stages of heart failure are individualized to maintain the client in a state below symptom threshold, or as symptom free as possible. The client is instructed to increase walking and other activities gradu-

ally and to continue whatever activity level can be maintained without symptoms.

The nurse and the client identify factors that might precipitate symptoms. The nurse instructs the client to watch for and report a weight gain of more than 2 or 3 lb, swelling of the ankles and feet, a persistent cough, or frequent urination during the night. Oral and written instructions are given regarding the medication regimen. If the client is taking digoxin, the family and the client are taught how to count a pulse rate. The nurse instructs the client to take the pulse daily and record it. A dramatic decrease or increase in the pulse rate, or a change in rhythm from regular to irregular, or irregular to regular, needs to be reported to the health care provider. Other signs and symptoms of digoxin toxicity, which include anorexia, nausea, vomiting, diarrhea, and visual disturbances, are also reviewed with the client. Clients taking diuretics are advised to take them in the morning to avoid waking during the night to void. The nurse reviews the signs and symptoms of hypokalemia (see p. 2167) with clients who are taking potassium-wasting diuretics and instructs clients to report the occurrence of these effects. Written information on high-potassium foods is also supplied to these clients (see Chap. 13).

Clients with chronic heart failure are advised to restrict their dietary sodium. The nurse provides written instructions on low- or restricted-sodium diets. Clients are instructed to confer with their physician if they want to use commercial salt substitutes. This is done because most salt substitutes contain potassium, and renal status needs to be considered before recommending these products. To enhance the flavor of low-salt foods, the nurse suggests that clients use lemon, garlic, and other herbs.

Psychosocial Preparation

The client with chronic heart failure must make necessary adjustments in life style and adhere to a medical regimen that includes dietary restrictions, activity restrictions, and drug therapy. Careful, concise explanations of the treatment plan are needed. The nurse encourages the client to verbalize fears and concerns regarding his/her illness and assists the client in exploring appropriate coping skills. Clients are encouraged that their participation in treatment can help alleviate and control symptoms.

Health Care Resources

A home care nurse may be needed to assess adherence to medication and diet therapy and to assess for worsening heart failure. Clients with activity restrictions benefit from the services of a home care aide. A dietitian could be consulted to assist with menu planning and teaching.

The AHA is an excellent resource for pamphlets, books, cookbooks, and video tapes related to heart failure and heart disease, as well as a referral for various support groups in the community.

 Evaluation

On the basis of the identified nursing diagnoses, the nurse evaluates the care of the client with heart failure. Expected outcomes include that the client

1. Demonstrates restoration and maintenance of adequate cardiac output and adequate gas exchange
2. Demonstrates a decrease and control of fluid volume
3. Demonstrates tolerance to activity within her/his level of cardiac function

VALVULAR HEART DISEASE

Valvular heart disease occurs when the heart valves are unable to open fully (valvular stenosis) or fully close (valvular insufficiency or regurgitation). Acquired valvular dysfunctions most often involve the left side of the heart, especially the mitral valve. Acquired valvular dysfunctions in rank order of occurrence are mitral stenosis, mitral insufficiency, mitral valve prolapse, aortic stenosis, and aortic insufficiency. The tricuspid valve is involved infrequently, and the pulmonic valve rarely.

Often, stenosis and regurgitation occur simultaneously in a defect called a mixed lesion. The following discussion is limited to the valvular dysfunction of the mitral and aortic valves.

MITRAL STENOSIS

OVERVIEW

Pathophysiology

Rheumatic fever can cause valve thickening by fibrosis and calcification. The valve leaflets fuse together and become stiff, and the chordae tendineae contract and shorten. The valvular orifice narrows, preventing normal blood flow from the left atrium to the left ventricle.

The left atrial pressure rises, the left atrium dilates, pulmonary artery pressures increase, and the right ventricle hypertrophies. Pulmonary congestion and right-sided failure occur. The left ventricle receives insufficient end-diastolic blood volume, and thus the cardiac output is decreased.

Etiology

Rheumatic fever is most often the cause of mitral stenosis even though a history of rheumatic fever is often absent. Nonrheumatic causes of this disorder include atrial myxoma, calcium accumulation, and thrombus formation.

Incidence

Two-thirds to three-fourths of all clients with mitral stenosis are females. About two-thirds of the women with rheumatic mitral stenosis are younger than age 45 years.

MITRAL INSUFFICIENCY (REGURGITATION)

OVERVIEW

Pathophysiology

The pathologic process of mitral insufficiency is the same as for mitral stenosis, but the fibrotic and calcific changes cause the mitral valve to fail to close completely, allowing a backflow of blood. During the systolic phase, a great deal of pressure is generated within the left ventricle. Lack of closure of the mitral valve allows leakage of blood into the left atrium during ventricular systole. During the diastolic phase, regurgitant output is returned from the left atrium to the left ventricle, in addition to the normal amount of blood, increasing the volume that must be ejected during systole. This high volume forces the heart to work harder and to compensate; the left atrium and left ventricle dilate and hypertrophy.

Etiology

Rheumatic heart disease is the predominant etiologic factor. When mitral insufficiency is a result of rheumatic heart disease, it usually coexists with some degree of mitral stenosis.

Nonrheumatic etiology includes papillary muscle dysfunction or rupture secondary to ischemic heart disease, infective endocarditis, or a congenital anomaly.

Incidence

Mitral regurgitation resulting from rheumatic heart disease is more commonly seen in women than in men. When the nonrheumatic etiology is considered, the incidence of mitral regurgitation is greater in men.

MITRAL VALVE PROLAPSE

OVERVIEW

Pathophysiology

Mitral valve prolapse occurs because the valvular leaflets enlarge and prolapse into the left atrium during systole. Usually, this is a benign abnormality, but it may progress to a stage of pronounced mitral regurgitation.

Etiology

Etiology of mitral valve prolapse is variable and is associated with a number of conditions, such as endocarditis, myocarditis, and acute or chronic rheumatic heart disease. It is also present in otherwise apparently healthy individuals. Familial occurrence is well established.

Incidence

Mitral valve prolapse affects 5% to 10% of the population (Braunwald, 1988). Although present in all age groups, it is most common among women between the ages of 20 and 54 years.

AORTIC STENOSIS

OVERVIEW

Pathophysiology

The aortic valve orifice narrows, obstructing left ventricular outflow during systole. This increased resistance to

ejection or afterload results in ventricular hypertrophy. As the stenosis progresses, cardiac output decreases. The left atrium may be unable to empty completely, and thus the pulmonary system becomes congested. Eventually right-sided heart failure can result.

Etiology

Congenital valvular disease or malformation is the predominant etiologic factor in aortic stenosis. Rheumatic aortic stenosis is always concomitant with rheumatic disease of the mitral valve. The client's age when the condition manifests itself is usually suggestive of its cause. Congenital aortic stenosis with a bicuspid or a unicuspid valve occurs most frequently in persons younger than the age of 30 years. Between age 30 and 70 years, it is attributed equally to congenital malformation and to rheumatic heart disease. Atherosclerosis and degenerative calcification of the aortic valve are the predominant causative factors in individuals older than 70 years.

Incidence

Aortic stenosis has become the most common valvular disorder in countries with aging populations. Eighty per cent of clients with aortic stenosis are men (Sokolow & Massie, 1988).

AORTIC INSUFFICIENCY (REGURGITATION)

OVERVIEW

Pathophysiology

The aortic valve leaflets do not close properly during diastole, and the annulus may be dilated, loose, or deformed. This allows a regurgitation of blood from the aorta back into the left ventricle during diastole. The left ventricle, in compensation, dilates to accommodate the greater blood load and eventually hypertrophies.

Etiology

Aortic insufficiency is less frequently caused by rheumatic heart disease because antibiotics have been effective in controlling this disease. Nonrheumatic causes include infective endocarditis, congenital anatomic aortic valvular abnormalities, hypertension, and Marfan's syndrome (a generalized, systemic disease of connective tissue).

Incidence

Approximately three-fourths of the clients with aortic regurgitation are men.

PREVENTION OF VALVULAR HEART DISEASE

Rheumatic heart disease, a common cause of mitral and aortic valvular heart disease, is preventable. Nurses working in clinics, health care centers or schools, and emergency departments can often detect individuals with beta-hemolytic streptococcal infections. These individuals need to be referred for appropriate diagnosis and prophylactic antibiotic intervention. Control of atherosclerosis in affected clients also assists in preventing some valvular disorders.

COLLABORATIVE MANAGEMENT OF VALVULAR HEART DISEASE

 Assessment

History

A client with valvular disease may have become ill at an early age or may have been disabled over the course of many years.

The nurse collects information on the client's *family health history*, including occurrences of valvular or other forms of heart disease to which the client may be genetically predisposed. The client is questioned about attacks of *rheumatic fever* and the specific dates these occurred and whether *antibiotic prophylaxis* against recurrence of rheumatic fever is used. Included is a discussion of the client's *fatigue level* and the *level of activity* that is tolerated.

Physical Assessment: Clinical Manifestations

See the accompanying Key Features of Disease.

Mitral stenosis. Clients with mild mitral stenosis are usually asymptomatic. As clinical symptoms develop, the client may experience excessive *fatigue*. This fatigue may be accompanied by *dyspnea* on exertion, orthopnea, paroxysmal nocturnal dyspnea, and *dry cough*. As the pulmonary hypertension and congestion progress, *hemoptysis* and *pulmonary edema* appear. Right-sided heart failure can cause hepatomegaly, neck vein distention, and pitting edema.

The pulse may be normal on palpation, tachycardiac, or irregularly irregular, as in atrial fibrillation. On auscultation, the finding is a rumbling, apical diastolic murmur.

Mitral insufficiency. Mitral insufficiency usually progresses slowly; clients may remain symptom free for decades or their entire lives. As the cardiac output falls, the client may complain of *fatigue, dyspnea on exertion,* and *orthopnea*. Assessment may reveal normal vital signs, atrial fibrillation, or changes in heart rate and respirations characteristic of left ventricular failure.

When right-sided heart failure results from left ventricular decompensation, the *neck veins become distended,* the liver enlarges (hepatomegaly), and *pitting edema* is noted. On auscultation, the nurse hears a high-pitched holosystolic *murmur* at the apex, with radiation to the left axilla. Severe regurgitation often exhibits a third heart sound.

KEY FEATURES OF DISEASE ■ **Signs and Symptoms of Valvular Heart Disease**

Mitral Stenosis	Mitral Insufficiency	Mitral Valve Prolapse	Aortic Stenosis	Aortic Insufficiency
Fatigue	Fatigue	Atypical chest pain	Dyspnea on exertion	Palpitations
Dyspnea on exertion	Dyspnea on exertion	Dizziness, syncope	Angina	Dyspnea
Orthopnea	Orthopnea	Palpitations	Syncope on exertion	Orthopnea
Paroxysmal nocturnal dyspnea	Palpitations	Atrial tachycardia	Fatigue	Paroxysmal nocturnal dyspnea
Hemoptysis	Atrial fibrillation	Ventricular tachycardia	Orthopnea	Fatigue
Hepatomegaly	Neck vein distention	Systolic click	Paroxysmal nocturnal dyspnea	Angina
Neck vein distention	Pitting edema		Harsh, systolic crescendo-decrescendo murmur	Sinus tachycardia
Pitting edema	High-pitched holosystolic murmur			Blowing, decrescendo diastolic murmur
Atrial fibrillation				
Rumbling, apical diastolic murmur				

Mitral valve prolapse. *Atypical chest pain* is a common complaint of clients and is described as a sharp pain localized to the left side of the chest. Dizziness, syncope, and palpitations may be associated with atrial or ventricular arrhythmias.

On physical examination, the nurse usually finds the heart rate and blood pressure to be normal. On auscultation, the first heart sound may be followed by a nonejection systolic click.

Aortic stenosis. The classic symptoms of aortic stenosis are *dyspnea on exertion, angina,* and *syncope on exertion.* When cardiac output falls in the late stages of the disease, the client has marked fatigue, orthopnea, and paroxysmal nocturnal dyspnea. A diamond-shaped systolic crescendo-decrescendo murmur is characteristically noted on auscultation.

Aortic insufficiency. Clients with aortic regurgitation remain asymptomatic for many years owing to the compensatory mechanisms of the left ventricle. The symptom that the client may note is *palpitations,* especially while lying on the left side. As the disease progresses and left ventricular failure occurs, the client describes *dyspnea, orthopnea,* and *paroxysmal nocturnal dyspnea.* Many clients with aortic regurgitation develop *angina.*

On palpation, the nurse notes a *bounding arterial pulse.* The pulse pressure is usually widened, with an elevated systolic pressure and diminished diastolic pressure. The classic auscultatory finding is a high-pitched, blowing, decrescendo diastolic *murmur.*

Psychosocial Assessment

Clients with valvular disorders may fear that symptoms may become worse and their disorders may progress to the point at which they require surgery. Symptoms of shortness of breath or fatigue can interfere with ADL. The nurse assesses for fears and frustrations related to these problems, as well as coping skills of the client and the family.

Laboratory Findings

No laboratory tests confirm a diagnosis of valvular heart disease.

Radiographic Findings

For mitral stenosis, the chest x-ray film shows left atrial enlargement, prominent pulmonary arteries, and an enlarged right ventricle. In mitral regurgitation, the chest x-ray film reveals an increased cardiac shadow, indicating left ventricular and left atrial enlargement.

In the later stages of the disease process of aortic stenosis, the chest x-ray examination may show left ventricular enlargement and pulmonary congestion. Left atrial and left ventricular dilation is seen on chest radiography in aortic regurgitation. If heart failure is present, pulmonary venous congestion is evident.

Other Diagnostic Tests

In general, all clients with valvular heart disease have echocardiography, as it is an excellent tool for defining abnormal movement of the valve leaflets. Exercise tolerance testing (ETT) is sometimes performed to evaluate symptomatic response, assess functional capacity, and enhance auscultatory events.

In clients with either mitral or aortic stenosis, cardiac catheterization is frequently done to assess the severity of the stenosis and its other effects on the heart.

An ECG is done to assess abnormalities such as left ventricular hypertrophy as seen with mitral regurgitation and aortic regurgitation, or right ventricular hypertrophy as seen in severe mitral stenosis. Atrial fibrillation is a common finding in both mitral stenosis and mitral regurgitation.

 Analysis: Nursing Diagnosis

The following nursing diagnoses are derived from the assessment data collected for clients with valvular disorders.

Common Diagnoses

Clients with valvular disorders commonly have decreased cardiac output related to narrow or incompetent valves with backflow or decreased forward flow of blood.

Additional Diagnoses

Additional diagnoses may include the following:

1. Impaired gas exchange related to backflow of blood into pulmonary vessels
2. Activity intolerance related to decreased cardiac output
3. Fear related to the diagnosis of valve disease, symptoms such as shortness of breath, and the possibility of surgery
4. Altered (cardiopulmonary) tissue perfusion related to increased myocardial consumption secondary to decreased coronary blood flow

 Planning and Implementation

Decreased Cardiac Output

Planning: client goals. The major goal for this diagnosis is that the client will experience restoration and maintenance of hemodynamic status as evidenced by a stable blood pressure and pulse rate, clear lung fields, mental alertness and orientation, and adequate urinary output.

Interventions: nonsurgical management

Drug therapy. A major concern in valvular heart disease is the maintenance of cardiac output with the commonly occurring dysrhythmia atrial fibrillation. Atrial fibrillation occurs frequently in both mitral stenosis and mitral regurgitation. Heart failure can result from the loss of the atrial kick, which decreases cardiac output by 25% to 30%. Stasis of blood by ineffective atrial contraction can also lead to thrombosis in the left atrium. For these reasons, drug therapy is aimed at at-tempting to restore normal sinus rhythm or, if that is unsuccessful, slowing the ventricular rate.

If the situation is considered an emergency, digitalis is the drug of choice and is usually given intravenously. If digitalization slows the ventricular rate, but atrial fibrillation does not resolve, quinidine or procainamide (Pronestyl) may be added to the regimen. Propranolol (Inderal), a beta-blocking agent, or verapamil (Calan), a calcium channel blocker, may also be considered. If atrial fibrillation is acute and unresponsive to medical treatment, synchronized countershock is the method for

TABLE 64-7   Antibiotic Prophylaxis for Clients with Heart Disease

Procedure	Standard Regimen	For Clients Allergic to Penicillin
Dental procedures and surgery of the upper respiratory tract	Penicillin alone. Parenteral-oral combined: aqueous crystalline penicillin G (1,000,000 U IM) mixed with procaine penicillin G (600,000 U IM). Give 30 min to 1 h before procedure and then give penicillin V (formerly called phenoxymethyl penicillin) 500 mg q 6 h PO for 8 doses. Oral: penicillin V (2 g orally 30 min to 1 h before procedure PO and then 500 mg q 6 h for 8 doses PO).	Erythromycin (1 g orally 1½–2 h before procedure).
For clients with prosthetic heart valves	Penicillin plus streptomycin: aqueous crystalline penicillin G (1,000,000 U IM) mixed with procaine penicillin G (600,000 U IM) plus streptomycin (1 g IM). Give 30 min to 1 h before procedure; then penicillin V 500 mg q 6 h for 8 doses PO.	Vancomycin (1 g IV over 30 min to 1 h). Start initial vancomycin infusion ½–1 h before procedure; then erythromycin 500 mg q 6 h PO for 8 doses.
Genitourinary tract and gastrointestinal tract surgery or instrumentation*	Aqueous crystalline penicillin G (2,000,000 U IM or IV) or ampicillin (1 g IM or IV) plus gentamicin (1.5 mg/kg—not to exceed 80 mg—IM or IV) or streptomycin (1 g IM). Give initial doses 30 min to 1 h before procedure. If gentamicin is used, give a similar dose of gentamicin and penicillin (or ampicillin) q 8 h for 2 additional doses.† If streptomycin is used, then give a similar dose of streptomycin and penicillin (or ampicillin) q 12 h for 2 additional doses.†	Vancomycin (1 g IV given over 30 min to 1 h) plus streptomycin (1 g IM). A single dose of these antibiotics begun 30 min to 1 h before procedure is probably sufficient, but same dose may be repeated in 12 h.†

* In clients with significantly compromised renal function, it may be necessary to modify the dosage of antibiotics used. Some of these dosages may exceed the manufacturer's recommendations for a 24-h period. Because they are recommended only for a 24-h period in most cases, however, it is unlikely that toxicity will occur.

† During prolonged procedures, or in case of delayed healing, it may be necessary to provide additional doses of antibiotics. For brief outpatient procedures such as uncomplicated catheterization of the bladder, one dose may be sufficient.

Data from Kaplan, E. L., Anthony, B. F., Bisno, A., Durack, D., Houser, H., Millard, D., Sanford, J., Shulman, S. T., Stillerman, M., Taranta, A., & Wenger, N. (1977). Prevention of bacterial endocarditis. *Circulation 56*, 139A–143A.

cardioversion. When a client has valvular heart disease and chronic atrial fibrillation, anticoagulation with warfarin (Coumadin) is usually a part of the medical treatment plan (see Chap. 65).

Prophylactic antibiotic therapy is required for all clients with valve disease before any invasive procedure. Procedures that require antibiotic coverage include bronchoscopy, endoscopy, sigmoidoscopy, colonoscopy, genitourinary instrumentations, surgery, or dental procedures of any type (Table 64–7).

If left ventricular failure and pulmonary congestion are present in clients with valve disorders, digoxin, diuretics, vasodilating agents, and oxygen are also administered (see earlier).

Other interventions. Rest is often an important part of treatment. Activity may be limited because the client's cardiac output cannot meet increased metabolic demands, and angina or heart failure can occur as a result.

Interventions: surgical management. Surgical repair or replacement of heart valves has a major effect on the prognosis of valvular heart disease. Correct timing is crucial. Replacement of the mitral valve in mitral insufficiency is usually performed before irreversible left ventricular dysfunction occurs. Surgical therapy is the only definitive treatment for aortic stenosis and is recommended when left ventricular failure, angina, or syncope develops. After symptoms of aortic insufficiency have developed, the aortic valve should be replaced.

Reparative procedures. In selected clients, mitral valve repair can be performed with success. The aortic valve is rarely repaired in adults.

Mitral commissurotomy, the procedure of choice in pure mitral stenosis, is accomplished during cardiopulmonary bypass surgery by incising the fused commissures, widening the orifice.

Mitral annuloplasty is the reparative procedure for mitral insufficiency in those clients with a mobile, noncalcified valve. The annuloplasty is also done during cardiopulmonary bypass surgery. The leaflets and the annulus are reconstructed in such a way as to narrow the orifice.

Replacement procedures. Development of prosthetic (synthetic) and biologic (tissue) valves has improved the surgical therapy and prognosis of valvular heart disease. Prosthetic valves come in a wide variety (Fig. 64–38). Although an advantage of prosthetic valves is their durability, all clients must receive oral anticoagulation for their lifetime because of the possibility of clot formation.

Biologic valves are usually xenografts, or valves composed of other species valves, such as a porcine valve (from a pig) (Fig. 64–39) or a bovine valve (from a cow). Tissue valves have little risk of clot formation, so long-term anticoagulation is not indicated. However, biologic

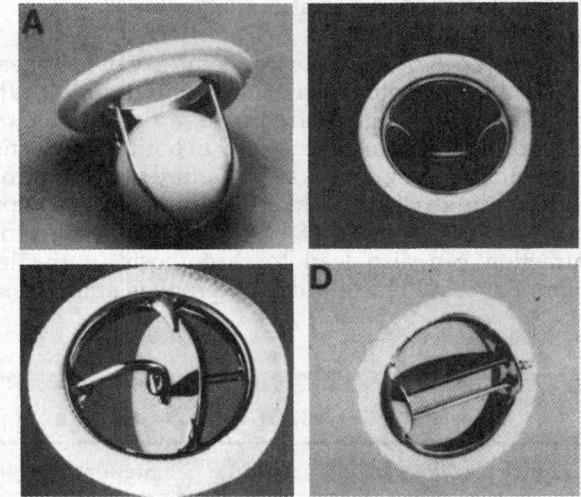

Figure 64–38

Prosthetic heart valves. *A,* Starr-Edwards. *B,* Björk-Shiley. *C,* Medtronic Hill. *D,* St. Jude Medical. (From Sabiston, D. C., Jr. [1986]. *Textbook of surgery: The biological basis of modern surgical practice* [13th ed.]. Philadelphia: W. B. Saunders.)

valves are not as durable as the prosthetic valves and are usually replaced every 7 to 10 years.

Mitral valve replacement is indicated if the leaflets are calcified and immobile. The valve is excised during cardiopulmonary bypass surgery, and the new valve, either biologic or prosthetic, is sutured into place.

Aortic valve replacement is indicated for both aortic stenosis and aortic insufficiency. As with mitral valve replacement, the aortic valve is excised during cardiopulmonary bypass surgery, and the new valve is sutured into place.

Preoperative care. Clients undergoing valve surgery have open heart surgery similar to the procedure

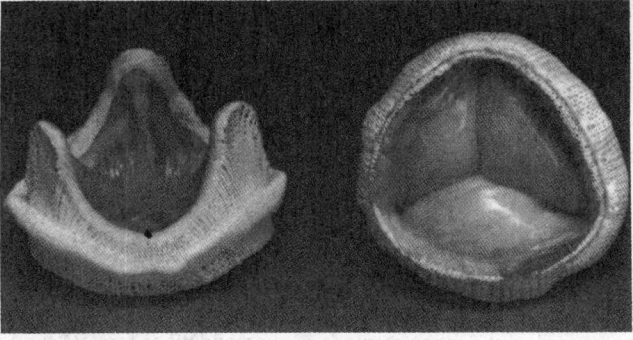

Figure 64–39

Biologic heart valve: the Carpentier-Edwards porcine xenograft. (From Sabiston, D. C., Jr., & Spencer, F. C. [1989]. *Gibbon's surgery of the chest* [5th ed.]. Philadelphia: W. B. Saunders.)

for clients undergoing a CABG (see earlier). Surgery is ideally an elective, planned procedure. Therefore, the nurse can assist in preparing the client by instructing the client and the family about treatment for postoperative pain, incision care, and strategies to prevent respiratory complications (see Chap. 18). The nurse may also introduce the client and the family to the staff and the environment of the surgical critical care unit, where the client will be transferred after surgery. Clients taking oral anticoagulants need to stop taking these medications at least 72 hours before the procedure.

Postoperative care. Nursing interventions for clients undergoing open heart surgery for valve disorders are similar to those for clients undergoing a CABG (see earlier). Clients who have had valve replacements with prosthetic valves require lifetime prophylactic anticoagulation therapy to prevent thombus formation.

■ Discharge Planning

The client with valvular heart disease may be discharged to home on medical therapy or postoperatively after annuloplasty or valve replacement.

Home Care Preparation

Because fatigue is a common problem for clients with valve disorders, the nurse assists the client and the family in assessing the home environment to see that it is conducive to providing rest. If stair climbing overexerts the client, and access to the client's bedroom or bathroom requires this, alternative arrangements for sleeping and toileting need to be made. The client may benefit from the use of a bedside commode, a reclining chair, or a wheelchair to conserve energy.

Client/Family Education

The teaching plan for the client with valvular heart disease includes teaching about the disease process; medications, including diuretics, vasodilators, cardiac glycosides, antibiotics, and anticoagulants; prophylactic use of antibiotics; good oral hygiene; a plan of work, activity, and rest to conserve energy; and the purpose and nature of surgical intervention, if appropriate. Because these clients are at risk for infective endocarditis, they are taught to perform dental care twice a day with a manual toothbrush, followed by oral rinses. The client is instructed to avoid irrigation devices, electric toothbrushes, or flossing, because these activities may cause gums to bleed, allowing bacteria to enter mucous membranes and the blood stream. Frequent check-ups by a dentist who is aware of the client's valve disorder are also advised.

The nurse instructs clients to inform all health care providers of the valvular heart disease history before receiving any treatment. They are also told that they require antibiotics before all invasive procedures and tests.

Clients taking anticoagulants must be taught how to successfully manage their drug therapy and prevent bleeding as described in Chapter 65.

Clients who have undergone valve surgery are instructed on care of the sternal incision. The nurse instructs clients to watch for and report any drainage or redness at the site or fever. Lifting of heavy objects should be avoided, and clients should exercise caution with driving, to allow for optimal healing of the sternotomy incision. Clients who have had valvular surgery should also avoid any dental procedures for 6 months after surgery.

Psychosocial Preparation

Clients with valvular heart disease may have complicated medication schedules, as well as long-term antibiotic or anticoagulant therapy. These circumstances may potentially lead to noncompliance. The nurse fosters a feeling that the client is an active participant in care and provides clear, concise instructions regarding medication schedules.

Limitations on physical activity can depress and frustrate the client. The nurse discusses the client's fears and anxieties with him/her.

The psychologic response to valve surgery is similar to that after coronary artery bypass surgery. Clients may experience an altered self-image owing to the changes required in life style or the visible medical sternotomy. In addition, clients with prosthetic valves may have to adjust to a soft but audible clicking sound of the prosthetic valve. Clients are encouraged to verbalize their feelings about the sternotomy incision and the prosthetic heart valve.

Health Care Resources

A home care nurse may be needed to assist the client with adherence to both medication and activity schedules and to detect any problems, particularly with anticoagulant therapy. Clients who have undergone surgery may also require a nurse for assistance with incisional care.

A home health care aide may be utilized to assist clients with ADL.

The AHA provides information to clients regarding valvular heart disease. A wallet-sized card can be obtained for the client, which identifies her/him as needing prophylactic antibiotics. For clients receiving anticoagulants, it may be prudent to obtain an identification bracelet stating the name of the drug they are taking.

⬙ Evaluation

The nurse evaluates the care of the client with valvular disease with reference to the expected outcomes of treatment. Expected outcomes include that the client

1. Demonstrates restoration and maintenance of cardiac output
2. Demonstrates adequate gas exchange
3. Demonstrates tolerance to activity within her/his level of cardiac reserve

INFLAMMATIONS AND INFECTIONS

Inflammations and infections of the heart frequently follow systemic infections. Recovery from these infections is often prolonged, and these clients are at great risk for future heart problems. Inflammation and infection may involve the endocardium (endocarditis) or the pericardium (pericarditis).

INFECTIVE ENDOCARDITIS

OVERVIEW

Pathophysiology

Infective endocarditis (previously called bacterial endocarditis) implies an inflammatory process involving the endocardial surface of the heart, which includes the valves. An invading organism travels in the blood stream and attaches to the endocardial lining of the normal heart or to an area of defect in a diseased heart. These lesions are called vegetations and tend to occur where blood flows through a narrow orifice, usually growing on the low-pressure side of a defect or injury. Major embolic complications may occur if these vegetations are torn away. The mitral valve is the site most frequently involved, followed by the aortic, tricuspid, and pulmonic valves.

Acute infective endocarditis causes sloughing of tissue early in its course. Erosion of a valve leaflet or myocardial damage from this may quickly give rise to heart failure. There is a greater incidence of right-sided failure in acute infective endocarditis.

Subacute infective endocarditis is much more commonly found on the left than on the right side of the heart. Left-sided heart failure and embolization are dangers posed to the untreated client.

Etiology

Infective endocarditis is currently categorized according to the virulence of the infecting organism. The organism is extremely pathogenic and virulent in acute infective endocarditis. *Staphylococcus aureus* causes most of the cases, but beta-hemolytic streptococcus is another virulent organism capable of causing acute endocarditis.

Subacute infective endocarditis is usually caused by organisms relatively low in virulence and normally present in the body. Causative organisms include *Streptococcus viridans* and *Escherichia coli.*

Conditions predisposing to endocarditis include rheumatic heart disease, congenital heart disease, mitral valve prolapse, and others (see the accompanying Key Features of Disease). Possible ports of entry for infecting organisms include the oral cavity (especially if dental procedures have been performed within the previous 3 to 6 months); rashes, lesions, or abscesses of the skin; infections (cutaneous, genitourinary, or GI); and surgery or invasive procedures, such as tonsillectomy, endoscopy, bronchoscopy, cystoscopy, and prosthetic valve replacement.

Incidence

The incidence of infective endocarditis is much lower today because of the use of antibiotics. Fewer than 1% of all clients with cardiac dysfunction have infective endocarditis. Clients between the ages of 20 and 40 years are most susceptible to this disorder.

In 50% to 60% of cases of acute infective endocarditis, clients have no previous cardiac deformities. Of the clients with subacute infective endocarditis, 75% have had rheumatic fever and an additional 10% have congenital defects.

PREVENTION

Primary prevention of infective endocarditis should focus on education of the population at risk. Included in the health care teaching program is information on the

---

KEY FEATURES OF DISEASE ■ **Conditions Predisposing to Endocarditis**

Rheumatic heart disease
Congenital heart disease
Mitral valve prolapse
Cardiac surgery
Cardiac defects
IV drug abuse
IV foreign bodies or devices, such as
   IV catheters
   Pacemaker electrodes
   Dialysis shunts
   Hyperalimentation catheters
Immunosuppression related to
   Diabetes
   Burns
   Cancer
   Hepatitis

disease process, the importance of good daily oral hygiene, and signs and symptoms to watch for.

Secondary care is the specific preventive care in the hospitalized population at risk. Clients at risk are those with a history of rheumatic or congenital heart disease, those who have had cardiac surgery, or clients with intravascular devices, such as IV catheters, hyperalimentation catheters, or pacemakers.

For the client with valvular or congenital heart disease, the AHA recommends prophylactic antibiotic treatment (see Table 64–7). Antibiotic prophylaxis should be used when such clients undergo dental procedures, surgery of the upper respiratory tract, and surgery or invasive procedures of the GI and genitourinary tracts.

COLLABORATIVE MANAGEMENT

 Assessment

History

When taking a history from a client, the nurse keeps in mind the conditions predisposing to endocarditis, such as rheumatic heart disease, congenital heart disease, and cardiac defects (see earlier). The history is particularly important in terms of duration of symptoms and pre-existing pathologic conditions.

A common finding related to subacute infective endocarditis among clients with pre-existing cardiac abnormalities is a recent history of *dental procedures*. The client is asked to recall what type of procedure was performed and if there was any bleeding from the gums. The client is also questioned as to any recent history of *respiratory, genitourinary, GI,* or *cutaneous infections* or *surgery or invasive procedures* involving these systems.

In addition, a client with a prosthetic valve can develop infective endocarditis during *cardiac surgery*, during the postoperative hospitalization, or any time after discharge. The same information regarding procedures as described earlier is needed for these clients.

Physical Assessment: Clinical Manifestations

Manifestations of infective endocarditis include *infection, cardiac involvement, embolic complications,* and *peripheral manifestations*. Acute infective endocarditis, a rapidly progressing infection, presents with *high fever, heart murmurs, embolic events,* and *splenomegaly*. Subacute infective endocarditis, a more slowly progressing infection, presents with a *continuous fever, fatigue, joint pain,* and *weight loss*.

Assessment consistently reveals fever. Clients with acute infective endocarditis usually have high-grade fever with temperatures ranging from 39.4° to 40° C (103° to 104° F), whereas clients with subacute infective endocarditis usually have temperatures from 37.2° to 38.8° C (99° to 102° F). Other symptoms of infection include chills, malaise, night sweats, and fatigue.

The client's cardiovascular status is evaluated, as some type of cardiac involvement is demonstrated in most clients. In clients with subacute infective endocarditis, 85% to 90% have heart murmurs, in contrast to clients with acute infective endocarditis who do not have murmurs in the early stages of the disease. As new murmurs may develop (usually regurgitant in nature) or changes occur in the intensity and quality of an old murmur, the nurse carefully auscultates the precordium and documents the findings.

Heart failure is the most common complication of both acute and subacute infective endocarditis. The client is assessed for right-sided heart failure, as evidenced by peripheral edema, weight gain, and anorexia, as well as left-sided heart failure, as evidenced by fatigue, shortness of breath, and crackles (rales) on auscultation of breath sounds.

Arterial embolization is a major complication in up to 50% of clients with either acute or subacute infective endocarditis. As fragments of vegetation break loose and travel through the circulation, the signs of embolization vary according to the site of occlusion. When the left side of the heart is involved, vegetation fragments are carried to the spleen, the kidneys, the GI tract, the brain, and the extremities. When the right side of the heart is involved, emboli enter the pulmonary circulation.

For splenic infarction, the client describes sudden abdominal pain with radiation to the left shoulder. When performing an abdominal assessment, the nurse notes rebound tenderness on palpation. The classic pain described by the client with renal infarction is flank pain with radiation to the groin, accompanied by hematuria or pyuria.

Emboli to the central nervous system cause either transient ischemic attacks or a cerebrovascular accident. The client may appear confused, have reduced concentration and inability to speak (aphasia), or have difficulty in swallowing (dysphagia). The reader is directed to Chapter 32 for further discussion of physical assessment of the client with neurologic dysfunction.

Pleuritic chest pain, dyspnea, and cough are often described by the client who is experiencing pulmonary infarction related to embolization (see Chap. 62).

Arising from a variety of causes, peripheral manifestations are classic findings in infective endocarditis. Petechiae occur in up to 50% of clients with endocarditis. On examination, the nurse notes petechiae around the neck, shoulders, wrists, ankles, mucous membranes, and conjunctivae. Splinter hemorrhages appear on the distal third of the nail bed as black longitudinal lines.

Psychosocial Assessment

Nursing assessment focuses on gathering data about the client's and the family's reaction to the acute illness and the ability to cope with the chronic nature of infective endocarditis. Because lengthy intervention is required, including prophylactic antibiotic treatment, the nurse assesses the client's ability to comply with prescribed treatment and the knowledge level about infective endocarditis.

Laboratory Findings

A positive blood culture is of prime diagnostic and therapeutic importance. Both aerobic and anaerobic cultures are obtained. Low hemoglobin and hematocrit levels are also found in subacute infective endocarditis.

Radiographic Findings

If heart failure is present, the chest x-ray film shows pulmonary congestion and cardiac enlargement. Echocardiography may visualize large valvular vegetations characteristic of *S. aureus* or fungi.

 Analysis: Nursing Diagnosis

The following nursing diagnoses are derived from assessment data.

Common Diagnoses

A common nursing diagnosis in clients with infective endocarditis is decreased cardiac output related to cardiac valve dysfunction.

Additional Diagnoses

The client may also have one or more of the following diagnoses:

1. Potential for injury (venous or arterial embolization) related to the presence of valvular vegetations
2. Pain related to fever and malaise
3. Knowledge deficit related to unfamiliarity with the disease process of infective endocarditis and the course of treatment
4. Impaired physical mobility related to prolonged IV therapy and activity restriction
5. Ineffective individual coping related to the chronic nature of infective endocarditis

 Planning and Implementation

Decreased Cardiac Output

Planning: client goals. The major goal for this diagnosis is that the client will experience restoration and maintenance of hemodynamic status as evidenced by stable blood pressure and pulse, mental alertness and orientation, clear lung fields, adequate urinary output (> 30 mL/hour), and no new heart murmur development.

Interventions: nonsurgical management

Drug therapy. Antibiotics are the mainstay of treatment for infective endocarditis, with the choice of antibiotics depending on the specific organism involved. Antibiotics are given in sufficiently high dosages, most often intravenously, with the course of treatment lasting 4 to 6 weeks. In most cases, the ideal antibiotic is penicillin. Until recently, clients with endocarditis were hospitalized for up to 6 weeks for IV antibiotic therapy. More recently, clients have been hospitalized for 5 to 7 days to institute IV therapy and then are discharged for continued IV therapy at home.

Anticoagulants, such as heparin, for short-term therapy in the hospital, and warfarin (Coumadin), for long-term therapy, may be prescribed prophylactically. These are prescribed to prevent arterial or venous thrombus formation, a complication of endocarditis.

Other interventions. Complete bed rest need not be enforced, unless fever or signs of heart failure develop. However, activities are carefully monitored by the nurse to allow for adequate rest. The nurse assists clients in range-of-motion exercises and frequent position changes to decrease the risk of thrombi formation. Antiembolism stockings are worn by the client to promote venous return. The nurse also promotes good oral and general body hygiene for the client and consistently uses appropriate medical and surgical aseptic technique when caring for the client to protect the client from contact with potentially infective organisms.

Nursing assessment for rapid pulse, fatigue, dyspnea, signs of heart failure, new heart murmurs, and early signs of embolization (see earlier) is ongoing.

Interventions: surgical management. Current surgical interventions for infective endocarditis include removing the infected valve (either natural or prosthetic); removing congenital shunts; repairing injured valves and chordae tendineae; and draining abscesses in the heart or elsewhere. Preoperative and postoperative care for client having surgery involving the valves is similar to that described for clients undergoing a CABG or valve replacement (see earlier).

■ Discharge Planning

Discharge planning for clients with infective endocarditis is essential for resolution of this disorder and avoidance of complications. Clients or families involved in the treatment need to be motivated and have the knowledge, physical ability, and resources to administer IV antibiotics.

Home Care Preparation

The nurse arranges for appropriate supplies to go home with the client. Supplies include IV tubing, alcohol wipes, needles, normal saline solution, and heparin lock flush solution drawn up in syringes. A heparin lock is positioned at a new venous site that is easily accessible to the client or a family member.

The nurse contacts the pharmacist who will be preparing the antibiotics and arranges for ordering of related supplies for future client use.

Client/Family Education

The teaching plan for the client with infective endocarditis includes instruction in the cause of the disease and its course, medication regimens, the technique for administering antibiotics intravenously, and practices that help avoid and identify future infections.

The nurse teaches the client how to purge the antibiotic through the IV tubing, how to attach the needle to the tubing and into the heparin lock, and how to turn off the IV infusion, disconnect the tubing, and flush the lock. The client and/or a family member demonstrates this technique before the client is discharged from the hospital.

The nurse encourages the client to maintain good hygiene, particularly oral hygiene. Clients are advised to use a soft toothbrush to brush their teeth at least twice a day and to rinse the mouth with water after brushing. Irrigation devices and flossing should be avoided.

Clients are instructed to inform their health care providers, including their dentists, of their endocarditis history, because they need to take prophylactic antibiotics before many procedures, including dental examinations. Clients taking anticoagulants are instructed in bleeding precautions and monitoring of prothrombin times as described in Chapter 65.

Self-monitoring for the manifestations of endocarditis is taught, including the complications of heart failure and embolic phenomena. The client is instructed to monitor the temperature daily and record it for up to 6 weeks. Clients are also taught to report fever, chills, malaise, weight loss, or increase in fatigue to their primary care provider.

Psychosocial Preparation

Many clients find it difficult to cope with the chronic nature of infective endocarditis, the lengthy intervention needed, and the potential financial drain of antibiotic prophylaxis. Clear, concise explanations concerning the disease process and reasons for lengthy intervention promote compliance with the intervention program. Consistent encouragement from a supportive spouse, family member, or significant other can help facilitate recovery.

Health Care Resources

A home care nurse may be needed for follow-up care in the home environment. This becomes important for those clients who self-administer IV antibiotics. The nurse in this setting can be contacted to monitor the client's progress and monitor for any complications.

The AHA provides information to clients and health care professionals regarding infective endocarditis. A wallet-sized card can be obtained for the client, which identifies him/her as needing prophylactic antibiotics and lists the recommended uses of prophylactic antibiotic therapy, as well as the specific antibiotics, dosage, and route of administration.

 Evaluation

The nurse evaluates the care of the client with infective endocarditis. Expected outcomes include that the client

1. Demonstrates restoration and maintenance of cardiac output
2. Demonstrates absence or resolution of venous or arterial embolization
3. Complies with prescribed antibiotic regimens

PERICARDITIS

OVERVIEW

Pericarditis is an inflammation or alteration of the pericardium, the membranous sac that encloses the heart. There are two general types of pericarditis: acute and chronic constrictive.

Acute pericarditis can be caused by viruses, bacteria (streptococcus, *S. aureus*, meningococcus, or *Mycobacterium tuberculosis*), trauma, uremia, post-MI syndrome (Dressler's syndrome), postpericardiotomy syndrome, metastatic tumors, lymphomas, radiation therapy, or rheumatoid arthritis, or it can be idiopathic. Acute viral pericarditis commonly follows a respiratory infection and is more common in men aged 20 to 50 years. Acute pericarditis after MI (Dressler's syndrome) occurs in less than 5% of clients who experience an MI, from 1 to 12 weeks after infarction (Sokolow & Massie, 1988).

Chronic constrictive pericarditis is caused by tuberculosis, radiation therapy, trauma, and metastatic cancer. In chronic constrictive pericarditis, the pericardium becomes rigid, preventing adequate filling of the ventricles and eventually resulting in cardiac failure.

COLLABORATIVE MANAGEMENT

Assessment findings classically include substernal precordial pain that radiates to the left neck, the shoulder, or the back. Pain is classically pleuritic and is aggravated by breathing (mainly on inspiration), coughing, and swallowing. The pain is worse when the client is in the supine position and can be relieved by the client's sitting up and leaning forward. Differentiation must be made between the pain of pericarditis and that of acute MI.

A pericardial friction rub is heard on auscultation of the heart. This is a scratchy, high-pitched sound; it is produced when the inflamed, roughened pericardial layers create friction as their surfaces rub together.

Clients with acute pericarditis may have an elevated white blood cell count and ECG changes consisting of ST-T wave elevation in all leads, with a return to baseline in few days after T wave inversion. Clients with infectious pericarditis always manifest fever. Blood cultures may be obtained to assess for possible bacterial infection.

Clients with chronic constrictive pericarditis show signs of right-sided heart failure, including dyspnea, exertional fatigue, hematomegaly, and orthopnea. These clients may have thickening of the pericardium on echocardiography or computed tomography scan. ECG changes include inverted or flat T waves. Atrial fibrillation is common.

Clients with acute pericarditis are given analgesics or anti-inflammatory agents for relief of pain. Some clients may receive corticosteroid therapy. Appropriate antibiotics are given if the etiology is a bacterial infection. Clients should rest and maintain a position of comfort, usually sitting up, leaning forward. The usual clinical course of acute pericarditis when related to acute MI, postpericardiotomy syndrome, or idiopathic, viral, or traumatic etiology is short term, from 2 to 6 weeks; however, there may be recurrent episodes.

Interventions for clients with chronic constrictive pericarditis include digoxin (Lanoxin) and diuretics for symptoms of right-sided heart failure.

Complications of pericarditis include pericardial effusion, which occurs when the space between the parietal and visceral layers of the pericardium fills with fluid. Pericardial effusion is the most significant complication of pericarditis because it puts the client at risk for cardiac tamponade. Tamponade occurs when the accumulated fluid in the pericardial cavity restricts diastolic ventricular filling, and cardiac output drops. Assessment findings and treatment of effusion and tamponade are discussed in Chapter 25.

OTHER DISORDERS OF THE HEART

CARDIOMYOPATHY

OVERVIEW

Cardiomyopathy simply means heart muscle disease. Its cause is usually unknown, and it usually leads to heart failure with a poor prognosis. Treatment is usually palliative, not curative; clients have to deal with a shortened life span with numerous changes in their life style.

Cardiomyopathies are classified into three categories on the basis of abnormalities in structure and function: dilated, hypertrophic, and restrictive (see the accompanying Key Features of Disease).

The most common type, *dilated* cardiomyopathy (DCM), involves extensive damage to the myofibrils and interference with myocardial metabolism and is characterized by dilation of both ventricles and impairment of systolic function. As a result of the inefficient contractile state, the heart ejects less than 40% of the blood in the left ventricle (compared with a normal of approximately 70%). Consequently, CHF soon follows.

The cardinal feature of *hypertrophic* cardiomyopathy (HCM) is massive ventricular hypertrophy and small ventricular cavities. The left ventricular hypertrophy leads to a hypercontractile left ventricle with rigid ventricular walls. Obstruction in the left ventricular outflow tract is seen in 75% to 80% of clients with HCM. This obstruction results from movement of the anterior leaflet of the mitral valve against the hypertrophied septum during systole, decreasing the amount of blood ejected.

Restrictive cardiomyopathy, the least common of the three cardiomyopathies, denotes restriction of filling of the ventricles. It is caused by endocardial or myocardial disease or both and produces a clinical picture similar to that with constrictive pericarditis.

Cardiomyopathies can also be broadly divided into two etiologic categories: primary (disease of the heart muscle without a known cause) and secondary (disease of the heart muscle with a known or suspected cause). Secondary causes may include infectious processes (e.g., viral and bacterial infection), metabolic disorders (e.g., thiamine deficiency and scurvy), immunologic disorders (e.g., leukemia), pregnancy and postpartum disorders, toxic processes (e.g., alcohol use and chemotherapy), and infiltrative processes (e.g., amyloidosis and cancer).

COLLABORATIVE MANAGEMENT

Assessment findings in cardiomyopathy depend on the variations in the pathophysiology. Left ventricular or biventricular failure is the outcome of the characteristic changes in DCM. Clients may be asymptomatic for months to years and still have left ventricular dilation that is found only by x-ray examination. Symptoms of left ventricular failure as described by the client are dyspnea on exertion, fatigue, and weakness. This is followed by paroxysmal nocturnal dyspnea, dyspnea at rest, fluid retention, and abdominal swelling (right ventricular failure). Clients are usually hospitalized with heart failure, dysrhythmias, and embolic phenomena.

The clinical picture of HCM results from the hypertrophied septum, which in 80% of cases causes a mechanical obstruction and thereby reduces stroke volume and cardiac output. Most clients are asymptomatic until late adolescence or early adulthood. The primary symptoms of HCM are exertional dyspnea, angina, and syncope. The chest pain is atypical in that it usually occurs at rest, is prolonged, has no relation to exertion, and is not relieved by nitrates. A high incidence of ventricular dysrhythmias is associated with HCM. Sudden death

KEY FEATURES OF DISEASE ■ Pathophysiology, Signs and Symptoms, and Treatment of Cardiomyopathies

Dilated Cardiomyopathy	Hypertrophic Cardiomyopathy		Restrictive Cardiomyopathy
	Nonobstructed	*Obstructed*	
Pathophysiology			
Fibrosis of myocardium and endocardium	Hypertrophy of all walls	Same as nonobstructed, except for obstruction of left ventricular outflow tract associated with the hypertrophied septum and mitral valve incompetence	Mimics constrictive pericarditis
Dilated chambers	Hypertrophied septum		Fibrosed walls cannot expand or contract
Mural wall thrombi prevalent	Relatively small chamber size		Chambers narrowed; emboli common
Signs and Symptoms			
Fatigue and weakness	Dyspnea	Same as for nonobstructed, except with mitral regurgitation murmur	Dyspnea and fatigue
Heart failure (left sided)	Angina	Atrial fibrillation	Heart failure (right sided)
Dysrhythmias or heart block	Fatigue, syncope, palpitations		Mild to moderate cardiomegaly
Systemic or pulmonary emboli	Mild cardiomegaly		S_3 and S_4 gallops
S_3 and S_4 gallops	S_4 gallop		Heart block
Moderate to severe cardiomegaly	Ventricular dysrhythmias		Emboli
	Sudden death common		
	Heart failure		
Treatment			
Symptomatic treatment of heart failure	For both:		Supportive treatment of symptoms
Vasodilators	Symptomatic treatment		Treatment of hypertension
Control of dysrhythmias	Beta-blockers		Conversation from dysrhythmias
Surgery: heart transplant	Conversion of atrial fibrillation		Exercise restrictions
	Surgery: ventriculomyotomy or muscle resection with mitral valve replacement		Emergency treatment of acute pulmonary edema
	Digitalis, nitrates, and other vasodilators contraindicated with the obstructed form		

Data from Wynne, J., & Braunwald, E. (1988). The cardiomyopathies and myocarditis. In E. Braunwald (Ed.), *Heart disease: A textbook of cardiovascular medicine* (3rd ed.). Philadelphia: W. B. Saunders.

occurs frequently and may be the first manifestation of the disease.

The earliest clinical finding in restrictive cardiomyopathy is exertional dyspnea. Cardiac output cannot increase during periods of exertion because of the fixed ventricular volume. The client also complains of weakness and dyspnea.

Echocardiography, radionuclide imaging, and angiocardiography during cardiac catheterization are performed to diagnose and differentiate cardiomyopathies.

Care of clients with dilated or restrictive cardiomyopathy is the same as that for clients with heart failure (see earlier). Drug therapy includes the use of diuretics, vasodilating agents, and cardiac glycosides to increase cardiac output. Combined arterial and venous vasodilators are useful in clients with symptoms of biventricular failure. Antiarrhythmics are used to control dysrhythmias, including tachycardia.

Management of HCM is similar to that of myocardial ischemia (see earlier). Prevention and treatment of dysrhythmias is the major goal. Antiarrhythmic drugs are used along with beta-adrenergic or calcium channel–blocking agents to control heart rate and decrease sympathetic stimulation.

The obstructive form of HCM is managed somewhat differently. Although beta-adrenergic agents and calcium channel blockers are used, vasodilators and cardiac glycosides are contraindicated in obstruction because vasodilating and positive inotropic effects may augment the obstruction.

Heart transplantation is the treatment of choice for clients with severe DCM. Surgical treatment of HCM includes ventriculomyotomy (area of the mitral outflow tract) or a partial septal resection in selected clients.

CARDIOGENIC SHOCK

Cardiogenic shock represents circulatory failure resulting from severe depression of myocardial contractility in which cardiac output is markedly depressed. Cardiogenic shock may be produced by any condition that causes the heart to fail. The most common cause is MI. It may also be the result of dysrhythmias, severe heart failure, cardiomyopathy, pulmonary embolism, papillary muscle rupture, and cardiac tamponade. Clients with cardiogenic shock have a mortality rate of 75% to 80% (Schroeder & Chatton, 1988).

Clinical manifestations are hypotension (systolic blood pressure <90 mmHg); urinary output less than 30 mL/hour; tachycardia; cool, moist skin; impaired state of consciousness; and metabolic acidosis.

The medical management is based on the cause of cardiogenic shock. The medical treatment is the same as for heart failure, which includes determining and eliminating the cause, treating the condition that precipitated heart failure, and improving pump performance. If the cause is mechanical, as in papillary muscle rupture, immediate surgery may be needed. As cardiogenic shock is

a severe form of heart failure, the nursing management is the same as for heart failure. The reader is referred to Chapter 17 for a discussion of shock.

SUMMARY

Cardiovascular disease is the leading cause of death in Americans, with MI being the disorder most commonly responsible for death (AHA, 1989a). Primary prevention and secondary prevention have been effective in reducing morbidity and mortality related to these disorders. Because of the prevalence of heart disease, the nurse should assess all clients for risk factors related to heart disease and teach all clients primary preventive strategies to decrease morbidity and mortality.

IMPLICATIONS FOR RESEARCH

The literature contains a great deal of nursing research related to the care of clients with heart disease. Risk factors for CAD have been identified through nursing research and research in related fields. However, controversies as to the role these risk factors play in heart disease abound. For example, elevated serum cholesterol levels and type A behavior have long been associated with the development of heart disease, but their relationship has recently been disputed. More research to assess the relationship of risk factors already identified would assist in support or revision of primary and secondary preventive strategies currently being promoted. Research questions related to risk factors and heart disease include

1. What is the effect of normal serum cholesterol levels on the development of CAD?
2. What is the effect of type A behavior on the development of CAD?
3. What is the effect of nurses' teaching primary prevention of CAD to all clients?
4. What methods of teaching primary prevention are most effective?

REFERENCES AND READINGS

American Heart Association. (1987). *Textbook of advanced cardiac life support.* Dallas, TX: Author.

American Heart Association. (1989a). *1990 heart and stroke facts.* Dallas, TX: Author.

American Heart Association. (1989b). *Heart facts.* Dallas, TX: Author.

American Heart Association. (1989c). *1989 research facts.* Dallas, TX: Author.

Aronow, W. S., Epstein, S., Schwartz, K. S., & Koenigsberg, M. (1987). Prevalence of arrhythmias detected by ambulatory electrocardiographic monitoring and of abnormal left ventricular ejection fraction in persons older than 62 years in long-term health care facility. *American Journal of Cardiology, 59,* 368–369.

Braunwald, E. (1988). *Heart disease: A textbook of cardiovascular medicine* (3rd ed.). Philadelphia: W. B. Saunders.

Brunner, L. S., & Suddarth, D. S. (1989). *The Lippincott manual of nursing practice* (5th ed.). Philadelphia: J. B. Lippincott.

Campbell, R. W. F. (1983). Treatment and prophylaxis of ventricular arrhythmias in acute myocardial infarction. *American Journal of Cardiology, 52,* 55C–59C.

Cardiac Pacemakers, Inc. (1987). Patient manual for the automatic implantable cardioverter defibrillator system. St. Paul, MN: Author.

Carrieri, V. K., Lindsey, A. M., & West, C. M. (1986). *Pathophysiological phenomena in nursing.* Philadelphia: W. B. Saunders.

Conover, M. B. (1988). *Understanding electrocardiography, arrhythmias and the 12-lead ECG.* St. Louis: C. V. Mosby.

Coodley, E. L. (1985). *Geriatric heart disease.* Littleton, MA: PSG Publishing.

Cowan M. J. (1989). Pathogenesis of atherosclerosis. In S. L. Underhill, S. L. Woods, E. S. Froelicher, & C. J. Halpenny (Eds.), *Cardiac nursing* (2nd ed., pp. 184–193). Philadelphia: J. B. Lippincott.

Elias, J. W., & Marshall, P. H. (1987). *Cardiovascular disease and behavior.* Washington, DC: Hemisphere Publishing.

Fardy, P. S., Yanowitz, F. G., & Wilson, P. K. (1988). *Cardiac rehabilitation, adult fitness, and exercise testing* (2nd ed.). Philadelphia: Lea & Febiger.

Goldberg, K. E. (Ed.). (1987). Cardiac problems. *Nurse review.* Springhouse, PA: Springhouse Corp.

Govoni, L. E., & Hayes, J. E. (1988). *Drugs and nursing implications.* Norwalk, CT: Appleton & Lange.

Guyton, A. C. (1986). *Textbook of medical physiology* (7th ed.). Philadelphia: W. B. Saunders.

Johnson, P. (Ed.). 1984. *Cardiovascular disorders.* Springhouse, PA: Springhouse Corp.

Kern, L. S. (1988). *Cardiac critical care nursing.* Rockville, MD: Aspen Publishers.

Laurent-Bopp, D. (1989). Heart failure. In S. L. Underhill, S. L. Woods, E. S. Froelicher, & C. J. Halpenny (Eds.), *Cardiac nursing* (2nd ed., pp. 220–227). Philadelphia: J. B. Lippincott.

Le Heuzey, J. Y., & Guize, L. (1988). Cardiac prognosis in hypertensive patients: Incidence of sudden death and ventricular arrhythmias. *American Journal of Medicine, 84*(1B), 65–68.

Lie, K. I., & Durrer, D. (1980). Acute and chronic aspects of conduction disturbances in acute myocardial infarction.

In B. Befeler, R. Lazzara, & B. J. Scherlag (Eds.), *Selected topics in cardiac arrhythmias* (pp. 75–93). Mt. Kisco, NY: Futura Publishing.

Mandel, W. J. (1987). *Cardiac arrhythmias: Their mechanisms, diagnosis and management.* Philadelphia: J. B. Lippincott.

Marriott, H. J. L. (1987). *ECG/PDQ.* Baltimore: Williams & Wilkins.

Messerli, F. H. (1984). *Cardiovascular disease in the elderly.* Boston: Martinus Nijhoff.

Palatini, P., Maraglino, G., Sperti, G., Calzavara, A., Libardoni, M., Pessina, A. C., & Dal Palu, C. (1985). Prevalence and possible mechanisms of ventricular arrhythmias in athletes. *American Heart Journal, 110,* 560–567.

Plotnik, G. D. (1985). *Unstable angina—a clinical approach.* Mt. Kisco, NY: Futura Publishing.

Razin, A. M., et al. (1985). *Helping cardiac patients.* San Francisco: Jossey-Bass.

Return to external cardiac pacing? (1983). *Lancet, 2,* 1346.

Reuther, M. A., & Hansen, C. B. (1984). *Cardiovascular nursing.* New Hyde Park, NY: Medical Examination Publishing.

Romhilt, D. W., Chaffin, C., Choi, S. C., & Irby, E. C. (1984). Arrhythmias on ambulatory electrocardiography monitoring in women without apparent heart disease. *American Journal of Cardiology, 54,* 582–586.

Schroeder, S.A., & Chatton, M.J. (1988). General care—symptons and disease prevention. In S.A. Schroeder, M.A. Krupp, & L.M. Tierrey (Eds.), *Current medical diagnosis & treatment* (pp. 1–16). Norwalk, CT: Appleton & Lange.

Sokolow, M., & Massie, B. (1988). Heart and great vessels. In S. Schroeder, M. A. Krupp, & L. M. Tierney (Eds.), *Current medical diagnosis and treatment* (pp. 189–265). Norwalk, CT: Appleton & Lange.

Sokolow, M., & McIlroy, M. B. (1981). *Clinical cardiology.* Los Altos, CA: Lange Medical.

Standards and guidelines for cardiopulmonary resuscitation (CPR) and emergency cardiac care (ECC). (1986). *JAMA, 255,* 2841–3044.

Surawicz, B. (1985). Ventricular fibrillation. *Journal of the American College of Cardiology, 5,* 43B.

Underhill, S. L., & Stephen, S. A. (1989). Coronary heart disease—risk factors. In S. L. Underhill, S. L. Woods, E. S. Froelicher, & C. J. Halpenny (Eds.), *Cardiac nursing* (2nd ed., pp. 194–206). Philadelphia: J. B. Lippincott.

Vander, A. J., Sherman, J. H., & Luciano, D. S. (1985). *Human physiology: The mechanisms of body function* (4th ed.). New York: McGraw-Hill.

Wallworck, J. (1989). *Heart and heart-lung transplantation.* Philadelphia: Harcourt Brace Jovanovich.

Wassertheil-Smoller, S., Alderman, M.H., & Wylie-Rosell, J. (1989). *Cardiovascular health and risk management—the role of nutrition and medication in clinical practice.* Littleton, MA: PSG Publishing.

Woods, S. L. (1982). Arrhythmias complicating, myocardial infarction. In S. L. Underhill, S. L. Woods, E. S. Sivarajan, & C. J. Halpenny (Eds.), *Cardiac nursing* (pp. 363–377). Philadelphia: J. B. Lippincott.

ADDITIONAL READINGS

Allen, J. K. (1990). Physical and psychosocial outcomes after coronary bypass graft surgery: Review of the literature. *Heart and Lung, 19,* 49–54.

This article summarizes recent studies related to the physical and psychosocial outcomes of CABG surgery. The author discusses research findings as they relate to prolongation of life, relief of angina, improvement in functional status, and return to work.

Andrews, L. K. (1989). ECG rhythms made easier with algorithms. *American Journal of Nursing, 89,* 365–372.

This article was written as a continuing education offering to assist the nurse with dysrhythmia interpretation. It discusses the relationship of ECG tracings to cardiac structure and function, identifies key concepts in interpreting ECG rhythms, and describes characteristic ECG features associated with select dysrhythmias.

Brenner, Z. R. (1987). Nursing elderly cardiac clients. *Critical Care Nurse, 7*(2), 78–88.

This article discusses age-related changes in the cardiovascular system and common nursing diagnoses related to these changes. The author also discusses learning concepts, nutritional factors, and the pharmacokinetics of medications as they relate to elderly clients. A table summarizing cardiac drugs with special considerations for the elderly is provided.

Futterman, L. G. (1988). Cardiac transplantation: A comprehensive nursing perspective, Part 1. *Heart and Lung, 17,* 499–510.

Cardiac transplantation has been established as the only therapeutic modality that can significantly prolong life in clients with end-stage heart disease. This article discusses indications and contraindications for transplantation, nursing interventions for clients awaiting a donor, and interventions for the organ donor and his/her family. The author also includes a basic description of an orthotopic heart transplant procedure.

Henderson, E. (1988). Assessment of successful reperfusion after thrombolysis. *Heart and Lung, 17*(Suppl.), 761–770.

Cardiac catheterization is the most quantitative measure of successful reperfusion in clients receiving thrombolytics for acute MI. However, because catheterization is not possible in many hospitals, clinical variables to assess reperfusion are most often used. This article reviews noninvasive markers that the nurse can use to evaluate reperfusion.

Kleven, M. R. (1988). Comparison of thrombolytic agents: Mechanism of action, efficacy, and safety. *Heart and Lung 17*(Suppl.), 750–755.

Administration of thrombolytic agents has recently become the standard treatment for clients with acute MI. This article reviews the mechanism of action, efficacy, and safety profiles of Food and Drug Administration–approved thrombolytics, which include streptokinase, urokinase, and tissue-type plasminogen activator. The author also briefly discusses investigational thrombolytics.

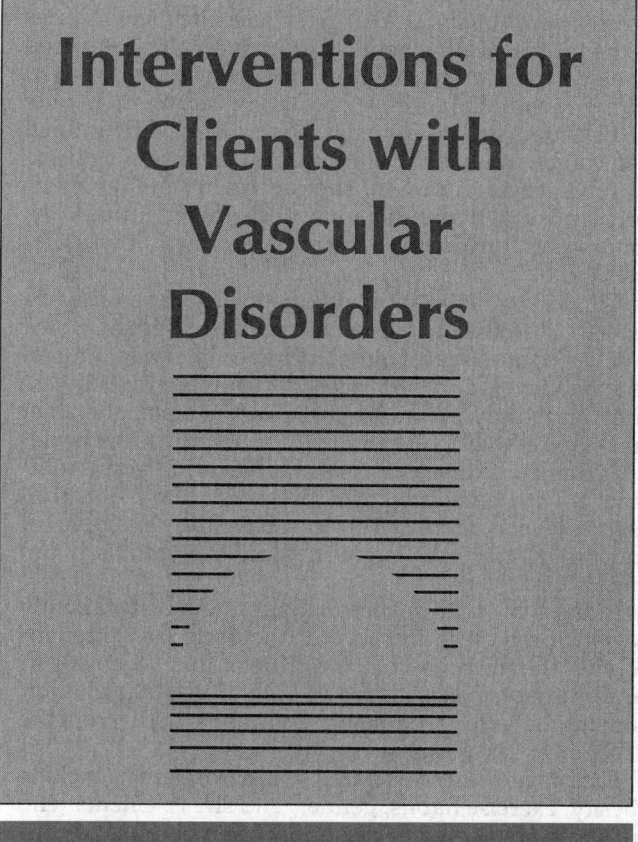

CHAPTER 65

Interventions for Clients with Vascular Disorders

The vascular system has the heart as its central organ and four categories of vessels: arteries, capillaries, veins, and lymphatics. Each vessel performs a separate function, although each function is intricately linked to the others, to provide the necessary nutrients for human tissues. Disorders of the vascular system cause many problems for the human body and may lead to complete shut-down of all body organs or eventually death. Each year, vascular disorders leave millions of people limbless, disabled, or dead and the economic considerations are overwhelming.

Although vascular diseases affect any portion of the human body, such as the heart, the brain, and the kidneys, the primary focus of this chapter is on the peripheral vascular system and its associated diseases.

ARTERIOSCLEROSIS AND ATHEROSCLEROSIS

OVERVIEW

Arteriosclerosis describes a thickening or hardening of the arterial wall. *Atherosclerosis,* a type of arteriosclerosis, involves the formation of plaque within the arterial wall. Atherosclerosis is the most common cause of arterial obstruction. The process of atherosclerosis results in coronary artery disease (CAD), cerebrovascular disease, and peripheral vascular disease (PVD). CAD is the most common cause of death in the United States (American Cancer Society, 1989), with cerebrovascular disease and PVD also contributing greatly to mortality and morbidity.

Pathophysiology

The exact pathophysiology of atherosclerosis is not known, but it is thought to occur in the following way (Fig. 65–1): It begins as a fatty streak on the intimal surface of the artery (see Chap. 63). At this stage, the fatty streak may appear flattened or elevated, but it generally does not affect the integrity of the arterial wall. The development of a fibrous plaque is the next stage of atherosclerosis. This plaque is described as a white, glistening, fibrous elevation that covers a lipid core. At this stage, the plaque is elevated enough to partially or completely occlude the blood flow of an artery. The final stage of atherosclerosis occurs when the fibrous lesions become calcified, hemorrhagic, ulcerated, or thrombosed. The rate of progression of this process is thought to be influenced by genetic factors, environmental factors, and certain diseases, such as diabetes mellitus.

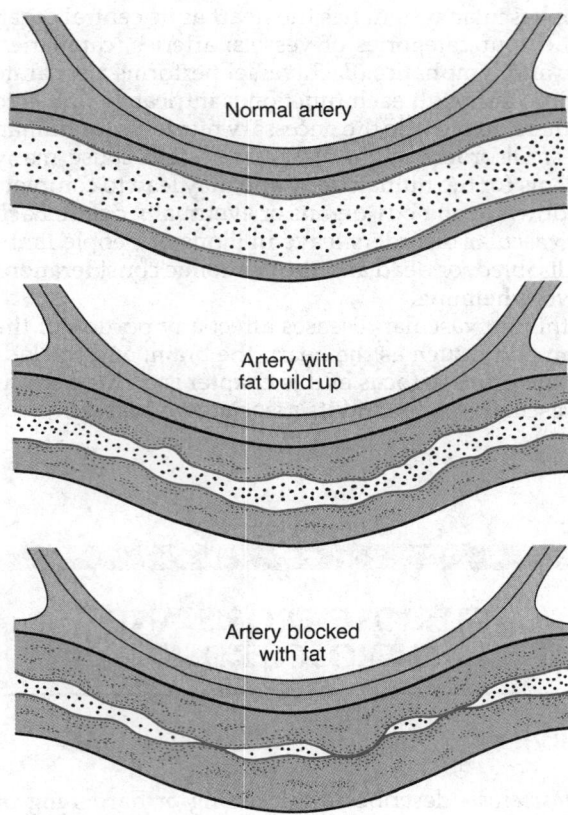

Figure 65-1
Pathophysiology of atherosclerosis.

Etiology

The exact etiology of atherosclerosis is unknown, but several theories attempt to explain its cause. It is believed that an injury to the intimal layer of the artery initiates the development of atherosclerosis. One popular theory is that after the intimal injury has occurred, platelets aggregate to the arterial wall and produce a peptide that stimulates the proliferation of the smooth muscle cells of the intima. Eventually, this proliferation can narrow the artery enough to compromise the flow of the blood or completely occlude arterial blood flow.

Another theory of origin is known as the lipid hypothesis. This theory is based on the assumption that after an intimal injury, a transudation of blood lipids (fats) accumulates. Again, this accumulation can partially or completely occlude arterial blood flow. The principal lipids related to atherosclerosis are cholesterol and triglyceride.

Many theorists believe that a combination of these two events is the most appropriate view of the atherosclerotic process and that this can occur in any arterial wall of the body. Usually, the disease affects the larger arteries, such as the coronary arterial beds, the major branches of the aorta, the visceral branches of the aorta, the terminal abdominal aorta, the carotid and vertebral arteries, or any combination of these (see Chap. 63, Fig. 63-12, left).

Intimal injury of the major arteries of the body can be attributed to many factors. Hypertension can cause a mechanical injury, whereas elevated levels of low-density lipoproteins (LDL) and decreased levels of high-density lipoproteins (HDL) can cause chemical injuries to the intimal wall. Chemical injury can also be caused by elevated levels of toxins in the blood stream, such as during renal failure, or by circulating carbon monoxide in the blood stream of a cigarette smoker. The intimal wall can be weakened by the natural process of aging or by physiologic disorders, such as diabetes. Hypertension, smoking, hyperlipidemia, and other identified risk factors also contribute to the progression of atherosclerosis.

Genetic predisposition and diabetes have a fairly direct effect on the development of atherosclerosis. Some families demonstrate inherited hyperlipidemia, an elevation in levels of blood lipids, two of which are cholesterol and triglyceride. In these individuals, the liver makes excessive cholesterol, which accounts for the development of atherosclerosis. However, in some individuals with hereditary atherosclerosis, the blood cholesterol level is normal. The reason for the development and progression of plaque in these individuals is not understood.

Individuals with severe diabetes mellitus frequently develop premature and severe atherosclerosis, often involving the microvasculature. This occurs because diabetes promotes an increase in LDL in plasma. In addition, intimal arterial damage is thought to occur from the effect of hyperglycemia.

Factors not directly related to atherosclerosis include obesity, exercise habits, gender, and stress. Clients who are obese are at greater risk, most often because of concomitant elevations in cholesterol levels. Men, individuals with sedentary life styles, and clients who demonstrate high levels of stress are thought to be at greater risk for development and progression of atherosclerosis.

Incidence

It is not known exactly how many individuals have atherosclerosis, but small plaques can almost always be found in the arteries of young adults. Generally, it is considered a disease of men older than age 45 years and women after menopause. The incidence can be better quantified by assessing disease that results from this process. Approximately 42.7 million Americans have some form of blood vessel disease (Kannel et al., 1984).

PREVENTION

Atherosclerosis is a degenerative disease that progresses for many years before clinical manifestations are evident. Although it was once considered an inevitable consequence of aging and genetic make-up, it can be viewed as a preventable disease. This is partially due to better methods of controlling hypertension and diabetes, but it is also due to early identification of individuals at high risk. Risk factors are modified as a result of client education, community education, drug therapy, and psychologic support. Methods for controlling risk factors may need to be long term and may be frustrating to implement. Most individuals with atherosclerosis have long-standing behavior habits that are difficult to change. Perhaps the hardest task is convincing the individual with atherosclerosis that decreasing risk factors is beneficial to health and may in turn halt the progression of disease.

One of the risk factors most effectively controlled through public awareness is hypertension. Hypertension cannot be cured, but, through the appropriate diet and medication regimens, it can be controlled (see later).

Another risk factor with a more subtle presentation is hypercholesterolemia (an elevation of total blood cholesterol levels). Most people are not aware of their increased cholesterol levels. Cholesterol is present in every cell and is important for building body products, such as bile salts for the digestive process and the chemical base for hormone development. However, there tends to be an overconsumption of exogenous cholesterol and fats that increase cholesterol levels in the body. Elevated cholesterol levels can be controlled or decreased if fat in the diet is limited to no more than 30% of total calories (American Heart Association Nutrition Committee, 1982). To assess what 30% of the caloric intake is, clients first need to determine their ideal daily caloric intake (see Chap. 46). Clients can then calculate their fat limit in grams (see the Health Promotion/Maintenance features, below and on pp. 2190–2192).

In addition to tracking fat intake in grams, individuals need to assess the fatty acid content of foods and to avoid saturated fats. Fat intake should further be limited to 10% or less saturated, 15% monosaturated, and 10% polyunsaturated fats. Meats and eggs have mostly saturated fats. Poultry and fish usually have a better balance between polyunsaturated and saturated fats. Oils such as safflower and sunflower oil are higher in polyunsatu-

rated fats, but this is not the case for all vegetable oils. For example, coconut and palm oils are high in saturated fat, and they should be avoided.

The diet should be supplemented with foods high in fiber. Studies indicate that water-soluble types of dietary fiber can significantly lower serum cholesterol levels (Anderson & Gustafson, 1988; Anderson & Tietyen-Clarke, 1986). Foods high in water-soluble fiber include oat bran and dried beans or legumes.

Finally, caloric intake should be adjusted to maintain an ideal body weight. (Adherence to limitation of dietary fat intake is also recommended as a weight reduction strategy for obese adults.)

Cholesterol intake should be limited to no more than 300 mg/day. Cholesterol is found in only animal products; the saturated fat content in meats and eggs is also high. Some foods with small amounts of fat may contain significant amounts of cholesterol. Clients should be taught to read the labels on foods to assess the total fat, saturated fat, and cholesterol content.

One of the most significant risk factors is cigarette smoking. Cigarette smoking is one of the most difficult behavior habits to change. Many individuals who continue to smoke are not convinced that there is a relationship between atherosclerosis and smoking. According to Doyle (1984), 98% of people who experience symptoms of PVD have a history of smoking. Nonsmokers with PVD, especially those who have had surgical revascularization, have a higher rate of 5-year survival than those individuals who smoke (Faulkner et al., 1983). A study conducted at the Mayo Clinic in 1982 documented an 11% incidence of limb amputations in clients with established PVD who continued to smoke, whereas no amputations occurred in the clients who quit smoking (Doyle, 1984).

Prevention of atherosclerosis can also be achieved through regular exercise. It is thought that exercise may lead to regression of the atherosclerotic plaque and the building of collateral circulation.

In addition to modifying risk factors, regular examinations by a health care provider when clients are older than 40 years of age should be included as part of secondary prevention efforts.

HEALTH PROMOTION/MAINTENANCE ■ How to Determine Dietary Fat Limits

Procedure	Example
1. Begin with the number of calories consumed in a day.	1800 kcal
2. Multiply the number of calories by 0.30 (30% of total calories) to determine the maximal number of calories that should be obtained from fat.	$1800 \times 0.30 = 540$ kcal/d from fat
3. Divide by 9 (1 g of fat contains 9 kcal) to determine the maximal number of grams of fat in the diet per day.	$540 \div 9 = 60$ g/d of fat. To limit fat intake to 30% of calories, the client must take in no more than 60 g of fat daily.

Adapted from Tufts University. (1989). What is a gram of fat . . . and how many should you eat? *Tufts University Diet and Nutrition Letter, 7,* 6.

Food	Fat (g)	Calories
Beef		
(3 oz with removable fat trimmed)		
Corned beef	16	213
Eye of round (roasted)	5	151
London broil, braised (choice)	12	208
T-bone steak, broiled (choice)	9	182
Luncheon Meats		
(1 slice)		
Louis Rich 96% fat-free turkey pastrami	0	25
Oscar Mayer bologna	4	50
Weaver Chicken Frank with cheese	12	140
Seafood		
(3 oz cooked unless otherwise indicated)		
Haddock	1	95
Lobster	1	83
Swordfish	4	132
Tuna, canned in oil and drained	7	158
Tuna, canned in water and drained	0	111
Shrimp	1	84
Shrimp, breaded and fried	10	206
Poultry		
(3 oz roasted unless otherwise indicated)		
Chicken breast, meat with skin	7	165
Chicken breast, meat only	3	142
Chicken drumstick, meat with skin, batter dipped and fried, 1 average	11	193
Chicken drumstick, meat only, 1 average	2	76
Turkey, light meat with skin	7	168
Turkey, light meat only	3	133
Turkey, dark meat with skin	10	188
Turkey, dark meat only	6	160
Eggs		
1 large	5	75
Fleischmann's Egg Beaters, ¼ c	0	25
Morningstar Scramblers, ¼ c	3	60
Milk and Other Dairy Products		
Milk (1 c)		
Whole	8	150
2% fat	5	120
1% fat	3	100
Skim	0	90

Food	Fat (g)	Calories
Cream (1 tbsp)		
Half and half	2	20
Heavy whipping cream	6	52
Sour cream	3	26
Cheese		
American, 1 oz	9	106
Cheddar, 1 oz	9	114
Cottage cheese, creamed, 1 c	9	217
Cottage cheese, 1% fat, 1 c	2	164
Cream cheese, 1 oz	10	99
Ricotta, ½ c	16	216
Ricotta, part-skim, ½ c	10	171
Swiss, 1 oz	8	107
Weight Watchers American Pasteurized Process Cheese Product, 1 slice	2	45
Yogurt		
Colombo, plain, 8 oz	7	150
Colombo, plain, nonfat lite, 8 oz	0	110
Breads		
Bagel, 1	1	163
English muffin, 1	1	135
Whole-wheat bread, 1 slice	1	61
Other Grains		
Pasta, 1 c cooked	1	159
White rice, 1 c cooked	1	223
Pancakes, 4-in plain	2	62
Waffles, 7-in plain	8	206
French toast, 1 slice	7	153
Fruits and Vegetables		
Apple, 1 medium	1	81
Banana, 1 medium	1	105
Orange, 1 medium	1	65
Raisins, ⅓ c	1	150
Avocado, ½ medium	15	153
Broccoli, ½ c cooked	0	23
Carrot, raw, 1 medium	0	31
Corn, canned, ½ c	1	66
Green beans, ½ c cooked	0	22
Peas, ½ c cooked	0	67

Continued

HEALTH PROMOTION/MAINTENANCE ■ Fat Content of Selected Foods *Continued*

Food	Fat (g)	Calories
Spreads and Oils		
Butter, 1 tsp	4	36
Margarine, 1 tsp	4	34
Diet margarine, 1 tsp	2	17
Vegetable oil (corn, safflower, olive, peanut, soybean, sunflower, and sesame), 1 tbsp	14	120
Vegetable oil, spray, 2.5-s spray	1	6
Salad Dressings		
Blue cheese, 1 tbsp	8	77
French, 1 tbsp	6	67
Italian, 1 tbsp	7	69
Russian, 1 tbsp	8	76
Thousand Island, 1 tbsp	6	59
Sweets		
Apple pie, ⅛	12	282
Cheesecake, ⅛	13	278
Chocolate pudding, 1 c	12	385
Chocolate syrup, 2 tbsp	1	92
Fudge topping, 2 tbsp	5	124
Ice cream, Sealtest, vanilla, chocolate, or strawberry, ½ c	6	140
Orange sherbet, ½ c	3	92
Popsicle ice pop	0	50
Snack Foods		
Lay's Bar-B-Q Flavored Potato Chips, 1 oz	9	150
Orville Redenbacher's Natural Microwave Popping Corn, 4 c popped	7	110
Popcorn, air-popped, 1 c	0	23
Pringle's Light Potato Chips, 1 oz	8	150

From Tufts University. (1989). What is a gram of fat . . . and how many should you eat? *Tufts University Diet and Nutrition Letter, 7,* 4–5.

COLLABORATIVE MANAGEMENT

 Assessment

History

The nurse considers the risk factors related to atherosclerosis while taking a complete history. Biographical data about the individual, such as *age, sex, race, weight, height, exercise habits, smoking habits,* and *diet* are obtained. Information about diseases affecting family members and the client's previous diseases, such as diabetes, hypertension, or hyperlipidemia, is also obtained. The nurse asks about previous *related vascular diseases,* such as a cerebrovascular accident (CVA), myocardial infarction (MI), or PVD. The nurse also needs specific information, such as how many MIs occurred and when the last one occurred, which side the CVA affected, and in which leg (if not both) PVD occurs. It is also helpful to know methods of control used for diabetes and hypertension.

Another important aspect of the health history is *pre-*

vious surgical procedures, such as a coronary bypass, carotid endarterectomy, or any lower-extremity revascularization. The nurse asks if the individual has received an angioplasty or thrombolytic therapy or if any *medications* are being taken.

Important information to collect is how the client describes the *present clinical manifestations.* How often does the pain occur? How long does it last? Does it have a crescendo effect? What activity exacerbates or relieves the symptoms? It is important to know if the client experiences discomfort with exertion or at rest. If a client has cerebrovascular disease, he/she may experience dizziness, numbness, tingling, visual changes, or complete paralysis unilaterally. Obtaining information about the frequency and duration of symptoms, as well as precipitating activities, enables the nurse to assess the severity of disease and to implement the initial interventions needed.

Physical Assessment: Clinical Manifestations

A typical client with vascular disease generally has *pain* or some *change in function related to a decreased oxygen supply.* The nurse inspects the client for areas of dry skin; atrophic changes, such as loss of hair, loss of muscle size, and thickened or clubbed nails; pallor around the lips and the nail beds; and rubor (red hue) of the skin. The nurse notes any reddened areas, cellulitis, distended veins, varicosities, or edema. The nurse also assesses for *ulcers;* many clients with PVD have early signs of ulcer formation, such as discoloration of lower or upper extremities. Thorough assessment of the heart is performed in clients with PVD because concomitant cardiac disease is often present (see Chap. 63).

After auscultating the heart, the nurse auscultates each large artery from the carotid to the dorsalis pedis and posterior tibial. This can be done with a stethoscope or a Doppler probe. In the larger arteries, many clients with vascular disease have a bruit. A *bruit* is described as a turbulent sound, which can be soft or loud in pitch. The mere existence of a bruit is considered abnormal, but the role it plays in indicating the severity of vascular disease is not well demonstrated. Bruits usually occur in the carotid, aortic, femoral, and popliteal arteries and usually indicate some degree of narrowing of the arterial wall. It is important for the nurse to document the location of a bruit and its pitch.

The nurse also notes the rate and intensity of the pulse in each artery during auscultation. A decrease in intensity and audibility or complete loss of a pulse as the nurse progresses distally with auscultation may indicate an arterial occlusion. The nurse notes at which point the pulse intensity changes.

The nurse palpates *pulses* at all of the major sites on the body, and notes any differences. Many clients with PVD have normal pulses in one extremity, while having no pulse in the other. The nurse palpates for temperature differences in the lower extremities and checks capillary filling. Prolonged capillary filling (>5 seconds)

generally indicates poor circulation. The affected side may be cool or cold, whereas the normal side is warm.

Psychosocial Assessment

The client with atherosclerosis may deny the need for further assessment or intervention in the disease process. This is often a problem with clients who have no symptoms of disease and thus cannot see its immediate impact. Some clients, however, may fear progression of the disease. The nurse assesses the client's perception of the disease. The nurse also assesses the client's life style with regard to stress and support from significant others, as these play a role in the progression of disease.

Laboratory Findings

Serum cholesterol levels are frequently elevated in the client with atherosclerosis. Elevated cholesterol levels must be validated by LDL and HDL determinations. Elevated LDL levels indicate an increased risk of atherosclerosis. Low or normal levels of HDL also increase the risks. As individuals age, their cholesterol levels increase. Therefore, a younger client with high levels of cholesterol is at higher risk than an older client with the same level (see the accompanying Key Features of Disease).

Triglyceride levels may also be elevated. Atherosclerosis affecting the kidneys results in elevated serum creatinine and blood urea nitrogen (BUN) concentrations.

Radiographic Findings

Radiography may be performed to assess clients with diseases associated with atherosclerosis. The lower extremities are most often evaluated via arteriography when assessing atherosclerosis in PVD. Because arteriography involves injecting contrast medium into the arterial system, the risks, which include hemorrhage, thrombosis, embolism, and death, are serious. This procedure, therefore, is not a routine examination and is performed only if there is evidence of significant disease. Angiography is most always performed before surgery for arterial disease to pinpoint the location of

---

KEY FEATURES OF DISEASE ■ Risk of Atherosclerosis by Age and Serum Cholesterol Level

Age (yr)	Serum Cholesterol Level (mg/dL)	Risk
<29	>200	Moderate
	>220	High
29–39	>220	Moderate
	>240	High
≥40	>240	Moderate
	>260	High

abnormality for the surgeon. The nurse prepares the client and carefully implements follow-up care, as described in Chapter 63.

Other Diagnostic Tests

Doppler ultrasonography is a noninvasive procedure that is often used to assess arterial obstruction in the extremities before angiography. An electrocardiogram (ECG) is obtained to assess for CAD associated with atherosclerosis. Signs of heart disease include hypertrophy of the left ventricle, MI, ischemia, and arrhythmias.

 Analysis: Nursing Diagnosis

Atherosclerosis is often diagnosed when symptoms of occlusion develop in an artery; these symptoms indicate disease resulting from atherosclerosis. Diagnoses and interventions discussed in this section refer to atherosclerosis without occlusive disease.

Common Diagnoses

A common nursing diagnosis related to atherosclerosis is potential for altered (peripheral) tissue perfusion related to obstructed arterial blood supply.

Additional Diagnoses

Nursing assessment and analysis may reveal other diagnoses, including

1. Altered nutrition: greater than body requirements related to high intake of saturated fats and cholesterol
2. Knowledge deficit related to unfamiliarity with the disease process
3. Altered health maintenance related to difficulty in changing life style

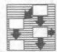 Planning and Implementation

Nursing care is planned to meet the individual needs of the client with atherosclerosis without symptomatic disease. As noted earlier, this chapter focuses on disease affecting the peripheral vascular system.

Potential for Altered (Peripheral) Tissue Perfusion

Planning: client goals. The major goal is that the client will experience no subjective or objective symptoms of PVD.

Interventions. Clients without symptoms of occlusion are treated to prevent progression of disease. Interventions are similar to those used to prevent the occurrence of disease.

Nonsurgical management. Clients are strongly encouraged to stop smoking, limit their dietary fat to 30% of a total day's calories (10% or less saturated, 15% monosaturated, and 10% polyunsaturated), and limit cholesterol intake. Clients with elevated cholesterol levels that do not respond adequately to dietary intervention are given cholesterol-lowering agents such as nicotinic acid (niacin) or lovastatin (Mevacor). Nicotinic acid is initially given in dosages of 100 mg two or three times daily with meals. Common side effects include flushing, pruritus, and gastrointestinal (GI) upset. The flushing is transient and is usually well tolerated. The nurse teaches clients to anticipate these effects. Lovastatin is started at a dosage of 20 mg once a day with the evening meal and is later increased to 40 mg/day. This drug is generally well tolerated by clients.

Routine exercise is advised for most clients with asymptomatic disease. The nurse instructs the client that, if discomfort occurs in the chest or legs with exercise, the client should stop all activity and lie down. The pain should resolve with rest, but the client should inform his/her health care provider of the pain, even if it resolves. Chest discomfort or pain in the extremities that does not resolve with rest needs to be evaluated by a physician immediately. The client with chest discomfort should be transported to the nearest medical facility by ambulance.

Surgical management. Surgery is not indicated for atherosclerosis until significant narrowing or changes such as an aneurysm occur within the artery. Changes in peripheral, coronary, or cerebral arteries usually cause symptoms when they are altered to this degree. Changes within the aorta may not be associated with symptoms. Surgical management of PVD and aortic aneurysms is discussed later. Surgical management of carotid stenosis or occlusion is discussed in Chapter 34. Surgical management of CAD is discussed in Chapter 64.

■ **Discharge Planning**

The client with atherosclerosis is hospitalized only if symptoms of occlusion occur. At that point, the diagnosis relates to the specific area of occlusion, such as PVD.

Home Care Preparation

Preparation depends on the specific symptoms and disease for which the client has recently been treated. The ability of the client to procure and prepare nutritions, low-fat foods and the availability of walking space or equipment to exercise is assessed and planned.

Client/Family Education

The nurse instructs the client and the family about the importance of maintaining a low-fat and low-cholesterol diet and exercising. Clients are taught symptoms of occlusive atherosclerotic disease. The nurse emphasizes the need for clients to report these symptoms immediately. Symptoms include discomfort in the chest, the upper back, or the jaw, which may or may not radiate down one or both arms; pain in the legs; episodes of weakness, dizziness, blurred vision, tingling, numbness, or loss of sensation in the face or extremities; or severe abdominal or back pain.

Psychosocial Preparation

The client often requires a great deal of emotional support to motivate the changes in life style habits that are often required. The nurse involves families in discussions of required changes in diet, exercise, and smoking habits and encourages the client and the family to discuss strategies to make changes.

Clients may fear future disease states related to atherosclerosis. The nurse assures the client that changes in life style can significantly decrease the risk of disease.

Health Care Resources

A nutritionist is consulted to assist the client in developing diets limited in fat and cholesterol. Physical therapists may be consulted when the client's exercise ability is compromised.

 Evaluation

On the basis of the identified nursing diagnosis, the nurse evaluates the client's ongoing response to treatment. Expected outcomes include that the client

1. Demonstrates a serum cholesterol level less than 200 mg/dL
2. Verbalizes compliance with dietary changes
3. Verbalizes that he/she does not smoke
4. Verbalizes compliance with routine exercise
5. Verbalizes absence of pain in the extremities or the chest
6. Verbalizes absence of dizziness or weak spells, blurred vision, tingling, numbness, or loss of sensation in the face or the extremities

HYPERTENSION

OVERVIEW

Hypertension is generally defined as a systolic blood pressure greater than or equal to 140 mmHg and/or a

---

KEY FEATURES OF DISEASE ■ **Classification of Hypertension in Clients 18 Years of Age and Older**

Blood Pressure Range (mmHg)	Category*
Diastolic	
<85	Normal blood pressure
85–89	High-normal blood pressure
90–104	Mild hypertension
105–114	Moderate hypertension
≥115	Severe hypertension
Systolic, When Diastolic Is <90 mmHg	
<140	Normal blood pressure
140–159	Borderline isolated systolic hypertension
≥160	Isolated systolic hypertension

* A classification of borderline isolated systolic hypertension (systolic, 140–159 mmHg) or isolated systolic hypertension (systolic, ≥160 mmHg) takes precedence over a classification of high-normal blood pressure (diastolic, 85–89 mmHg) when both occur in the same person. A classification of high-normal blood pressure (diastolic, 85–89 mmHg) takes precedence over a classification of normal blood pressure (systolic, <140 mmHg) when both occur in the same person.

From U.S. Department of Health and Human Services. (1988). *The 1988 Report of the Joint National Committee on Detection, Evaluation, and Treatment of High Blood Pressure* (NIH Publication No. 88–1088). Washington, DC: U.S. Government Printing Office.

diastolic blood pressure greater than or equal to 90 mmHg occurring in a client on at least three separate occasions. Several classifications of hypertension have been identified (see the Key Features of Disease on p. 2195).

Hypertension is a major risk factor for coronary, cerebral, renal, and peripheral vascular disease. However, control of hypertension has resulted in significant decreases in cardiovascular morbidity and mortality.

Pathophysiology

The systemic arterial pressure is a product of the cardiac output and the total peripheral resistance (Fig. 65–2). Cardiac output is determined by stroke volume and heart rate. Control of peripheral resistance is maintained by the autonomic nervous system and circulating hormones. Consequently, any factor producing an alteration in peripheral resistance, heart rate, or stroke volume affects the systemic arterial pressure.

Stabilizing mechanisms exist in the body to exert an overall regulation of systemic arterial pressure and prevent circulatory collapse. Four control systems that play a major role in maintaining blood pressure are the arterial baroreceptor system, the regulation of body fluid volume, the renin-angiotensin system, and vascular autoregulation.

The arterial baroreceptors are found primarily in the carotid sinus, but also in the aorta and the wall of the left ventricle. These baroreceptors monitor the level of arterial pressure. The baroreceptor system counteracts a rise in arterial pressure through vagally mediated cardiac slowing and vasodilation with decreased sympathetic tone. Therefore, reflex control of circulation elevates the systemic arterial pressure when it falls and lowers it when it rises. The exact reason why this control fails in hypertension is unknown. There is evidence for upward resetting of baroreceptor sensitivity, so that pressure rises are inadequately sensed, even though pressure decreases are not.

Changes in fluid volume affect the systemic arterial pressure. If the body has an excess of salt and water, the blood pressure rises through complex physiologic mechanisms that change the venous return to the heart, producing a rise in cardiac output. If the kidneys are functioning adequately, a rise in systemic arterial pressure produces diuresis and a fall in pressure. Pathologic conditions that change the pressure threshold at which the kidneys excrete salt and water alter the systemic arterial pressure.

Both renin and angiotensin play a role in blood pressure regulation (Fig. 65–3). The kidney produces renin, an enzyme that acts on a plasma protein substrate to split off angiotensin I, which is removed by a converting enzyme in the lung to form angiotensin II, then angiotensin III. Angiotensin II and III have strong vasoconstrictor action on blood vessels and are the controlling mechanism for aldosterone release. The significance of aldosterone in hypertension is most evident in primary aldosteronism. By increasing the activity of the sympathetic nervous system, angiotensin II and III also appear to have an inhibiting effect on sodium excretion, with a resultant elevation in blood pressure.

Inappropriate secretion of renin has been investigated as a cause of increased peripheral vascular resistance in essential hypertension. In high blood pressure, renin levels should be expected to fall because the increased renal arteriolar pressure should inhibit renin secretion. However, in most people with essential hypertension, renin levels are normal. Sustained blood pressure elevation in clients with essential hypertension results in damage to blood vessels in vital organs. Essential hypertension produces medial hyperplasia (thickening) of the arterioles. As the blood vessels thicken and perfusion decreases, body organs are damaged, causing MI, stroke, PVD, or renal failure.

Vascular autoregulation is another possible mechanism involved in hypertension. Vascular autoregulation is the process that keeps perfusion of tissues in the body relatively constant. If flow changes, the process of autoregulation should decrease the vascular resistance as a result of reduction in flow and should raise vascular resistance as a result of an increase. Vascular autoregulation appears to be an important mechanism in causing hypertension accompanying salt and water overload.

Malignant hypertension is a severe type of hypertension that is rapidly progressive. An individual with malignant hypertension usually has symptoms such as morning headaches, blurred vision, and dyspnea, and/or symptoms of uremia (accumulation in the blood of substances ordinarily eliminated in the urine). The client is often in the fourth, fifth, or sixth decade of life. The diastolic blood pressure is greater than 110 mmHg and frequently much higher, with diastolic pressures ranging from 130 to 170 mmHg. Malignant hypertension leads to renal failure, left ventricular failure, and stroke, unless intervention occurs promptly.

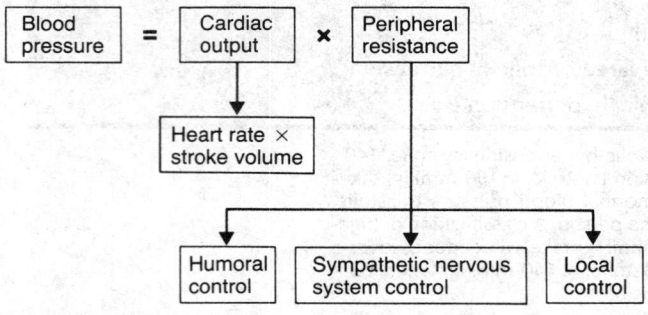

Figure 65–2

The components of blood pressure.

Etiology

Hypertension is divided into two major classifications: essential (primary or idiopathic) and secondary hypertension (see the accompanying Key Features of Disease).

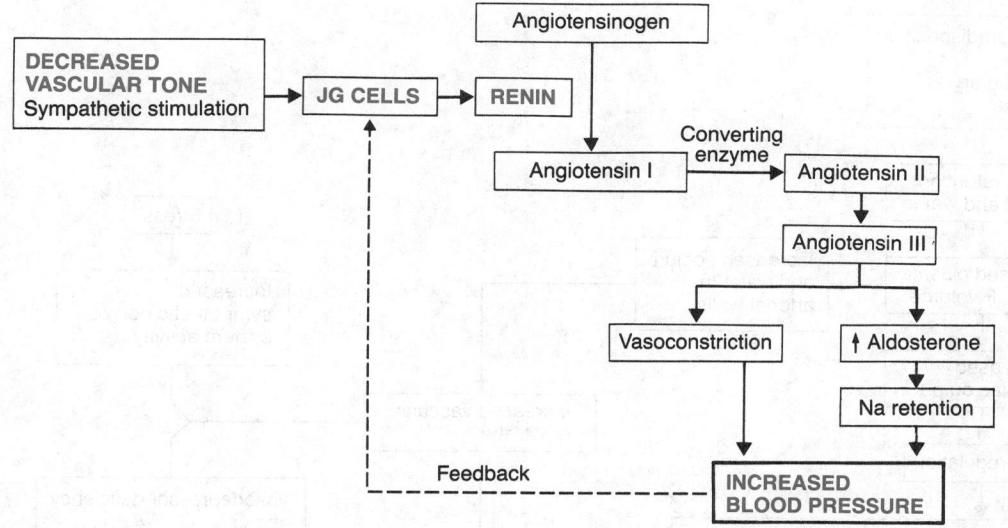

Figure 65 – 3

Effect of the renin-angiotensin system on blood pressure control. (From Cotran, R. S., Kumar, V., & Robbins, S. L. [1989]. *Robbins pathologic basis of disease* [4th ed.]. Philadelphia: W. B. Saunders.)

Essential hypertension is the most frequently encountered type, accounting for more than 95% of all cases (Oparil, 1988).

Essential Hypertension

The exact etiology of essential hypertension is unknown. However, a number of interacting homeostatic forces are likely to be involved (Fig. 65 – 4). The initial defect is thought to be the renal body fluid and pressure control mechanisms. Heredity may play an important role, if there is a genetic inability to handle normal amounts of sodium. Excessive dietary intake can increase fluid volume and cardiac output. The blood vessels respond to increasing flow through the vessel by constricting or by increasing peripheral resistance. The high blood pressure that is initially the result of an elevated cardiac output is then maintained at an elevated level by a resultant rise in peripheral resistance.

Secondary Hypertension

In secondary hypertension, the cause of the elevated blood pressure is known. A variety of specific disease states or problems are responsible. The causes of secondary hypertension are considered in order of their relative frequency.

The use of estrogen-containing oral contraceptives can cause secondary hypertension. Many women who take birth control pills have a slight rise in blood pressure, and approximately 5% develop hypertension (Oparil, 1988). The birth control pills may cause hypertension through renin-aldosterone–mediated volume expansion. For most women, when birth control pill administration is discontinued, the blood pressure returns to normal levels within several months.

Renal vascular and renal parenchymal diseases are two of the most common causes of secondary hypertension. Hypertension can develop when there is any sudden damage to the kidneys. Renovascular hypertension is associated with narrowing of one or more of the main arteries directly carrying blood to the kidneys. Approximately 90% of renal artery lesions in hypertensive individuals are caused by either atherosclerosis or fibrous dysplasia (abnormal development of fibrous tissue) (Doyle, 1985). Renal parenchymal diseases are related to infection, inflammation, and changes in the structure and function of the kidneys.

KEY FEATURES OF DISEASE ■ Etiology of Hypertension

Essential

Primary or idiopathic

Secondary

Oral contraceptive use
Renal vascular and renal parenchymal disease
Endocrine disorders
Coarctation of the aorta
Neurogenic
  Brain tumors
  Encephalitis
  Psychiatric disturbances
Pregnancy
Increased intravascular volume
Burns

Other Factors

Obesity
High saturated fat intake
High sodium intake
Cigarette smoking
Heavy alcohol intake
Stress

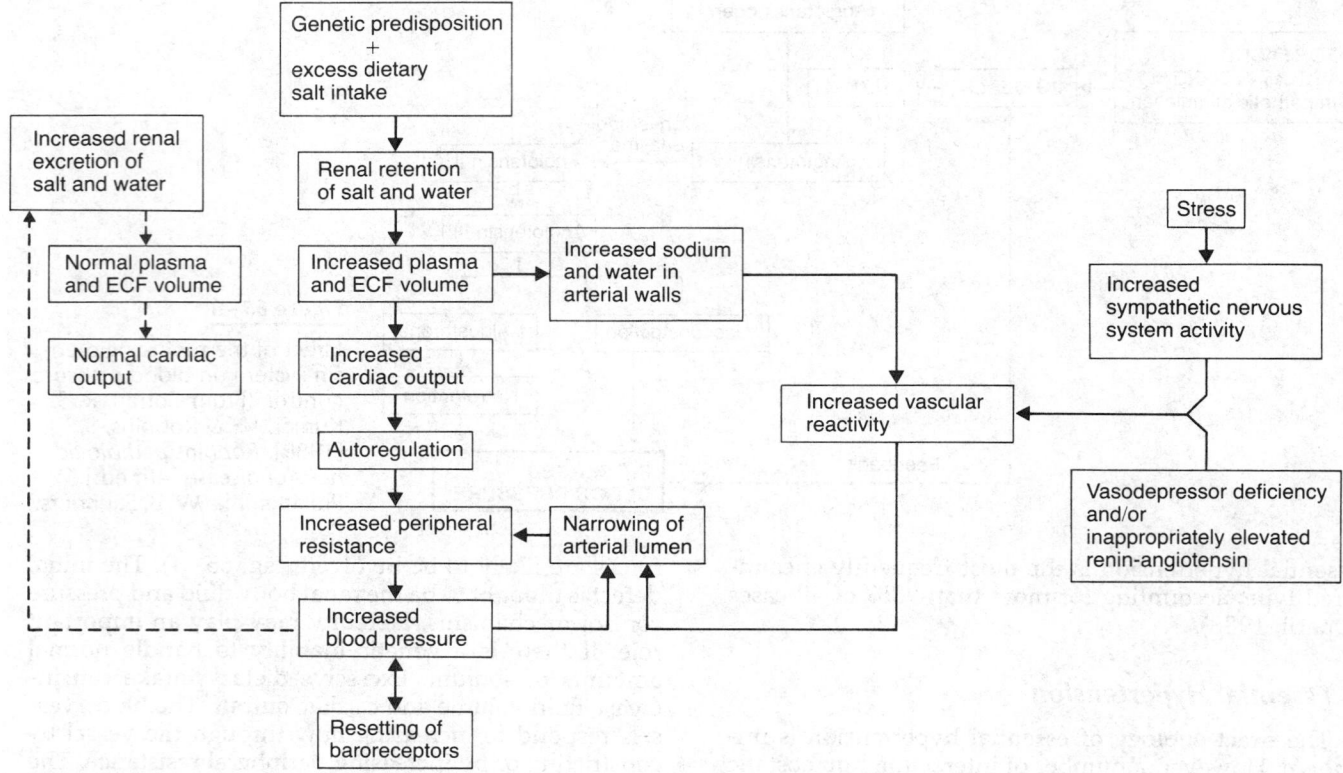

Figure 65-4

Pathogenesis of essential hypertension. (From Kaplan, N. M. *Clinical hypertension* [2nd ed.] © [1978], The Williams & Wilkins Co., Baltimore.)

Dysfunction of the adrenal medulla or the adrenal cortex can cause secondary hypertension. Adrenal-mediated hypertension is due to primary excesses of aldosterone, cortisol, and catecholamines. In primary aldosteronism, excessive aldosterone causes hypertension and hypokalemia. Primary aldosteronism usually arises from benign adenomas of the adrenal cortex. Pheochromocytomas originate most commonly in the adrenal medulla and result in excessive secretion of catecholamines. In Cushing's syndrome, excessive glucocorticoids are excreted from the adrenal cortex. The cause of Cushing's syndrome may be either adrenocortical hyperplasia or adrenocortical adenoma (see Chap. 48).

Coarctation of the aorta is a congenital narrowing of the aorta that may occur at any level of the thoracic or abdominal aorta. The narrowing restricts blood flow through the aortic arch and results in an elevated blood pressure above the constriction. The blood pressure subsides eventually after surgical repair.

Secondary hypertension is also associated with other diverse neurogenic disturbances, such as brain tumors, encephalitis, and psychiatric disturbances. A number of women also develop hypertension during pregnancy. Hypertension in pregnant women may be pregnancy induced, as in pre-eclampsia, or it may represent chronic essential hypertension.

Other Factors Affecting Hypertension

Research has found a positive correlation between body weight and blood pressure (U.S. Department of Health and Human Services, 1988). Weight reduction often results in lower blood pressure. Reduction of dietary intake of saturated fats can help minimize the risk of cardiovascular disease, but not enough evidence exists at this time to recommend it for hypertension control. High sodium intake has also been associated with hypertension in some clients.

Cigarette smoking can both elevate blood pressure and accelerate the development of atherosclerotic disease. Nicotine stimulates catecholamine release, produces myocardial irritability, increases heart rate, and causes vascular constriction, resulting in a transient rise in blood pressure. Excessive alcohol intake and stress can also elevate blood pressure. In addition, a stressful environment can result in an individual's smoking more cigarettes, overeating, and eating an improper diet.

Incidence

It is estimated that as many as 58 million Americans have elevated blood pressure. The incidence increases with age and is higher in Blacks than in Caucasians ("Hypertension prevalence," 1985).

PREVENTION

Prevention of hypertension involves modification of risk factors. Risk factors amenable to modification include obesity, alcohol intake, sodium intake, cigarette smoking, and stress.

Weight reduction and/or maintenance of ideal body weight and limitation of sodium intake can prevent hypertension in some individuals. Limiting alcohol intake to no more than 1 oz daily can help prevent hypertension and can assist in weight control. A regular exercise program can also assist in weight reduction and maintenance and control of stress. A minimal level of physical fitness for individuals without CAD is achieved through participation in one or more forms of aerobic exercise for at least 30 minutes three to five times a week. Examples of beneficial exercise include walking, jogging, bicycling, and swimming. Exercise should be increased gradually.

Clients with a single elevated blood pressure reading need to have their blood pressure reassessed a second and third time at subsequent visits before a diagnosis of hypertension can be made. The timing of re-evaluation depends on the level of blood pressure at each reading (Table 65–1).

Individuals who smoke should be encouraged to stop smoking. The importance of smoking cessation must be recognized for the individual to stop smoking.

Another method to prevent hypertension and reduce stress is biofeedback therapy. Through increased awareness of the effects of stress on the body's physiology, a client may be able to gain control of previously uncontrolled changes (see Chap. 6) Deep relaxation techniques, in conjunction with biofeedback, may assist in maintaining the blood pressure within the normal range.

COLLABORATIVE MANAGEMENT

 Assessment

History

The nurse considers risk factors for hypertension when obtaining the history. Data to collect include *age, race,* and *family history of hypertension.* The nurse also assesses the client's *alcohol intake, salt intake,* and *smoking* and *exercise habits.*

Past and present history of renal or cardiovascular disease is assessed by the nurse, as well as current use of medications, both prescribed and over the counter (OTC). A baseline sexual history is obtained from the client so that the effect of treatment, if any, on sexual function can be evaluated.

Physical Assessment: Clinical Manifestations

The nurse asks the client about any symptoms of *hypertension,* such as headache, edema, nocturia, lethargy, nosebleeds, or vision changes. The nurse obtains *blood pressure* readings in both arms. Blood pressure readings should be taken with the client in the supine and erect positions to detect changes with different positions. Two or more readings are taken at each visit, with the average blood pressure obtained used as the value for the visit.

To obtain an accurate blood pressure measurement, the nurse utilizes properly functioning equipment and the correct technique. The blood pressure is taken in a quiet environment. If possible, the client sits quietly for 5 minutes before the blood pressure reading is obtained. The cuff size should be chosen on the basis of the client's arm circumference. The cuff should encircle and cover two-thirds of the length of the upper arm.

Funduscopic examination of the eyes is done by a skilled practitioner to observe vascular changes. Hypertension can result in arteriovenous compression, hemorrhages, exudates, and papilledema of the optic fundus (edema of the optic nerve at its point of entrance into the eyeball). The appearance of the retina has been found to be a reliable index of the severity and prognosis of hypertension.

TABLE 65 – 1   Follow-Up Criteria for Blood Pressure Measurement for Clients 18 Years of Age and Older

Range (mmHg)	Recommended Follow-Up*
Diastolic	
<85	Recheck within 2 yr
85–89	Recheck within 1 yr
90–104	Confirm within 2 mo
105–114	Evaluate or refer promptly to source of care within 2 wk
≥115	Evaluate or refer immediately to source of care
Systolic, When Diastolic Is <90 mmHg	
<140	Recheck within 2 yr
140–199	Confirm within 2 mo
≥200	Evaluate or refer promptly to source of care within 2 wk

* If recommendations for follow-up of diastolic and systolic blood pressure are different, the shorter recommended time should take precedence.

From U.S. Department of Health and Human Services. (1988). *The 1988 Report of the Joint National Committee on Detection, Evaluation, and Treatment of High Blood Pressure* (NIH Publication No. 88–1088, p. 6). Washington, DC: U.S. Government Printing Office.

All pulses are palpated bilaterally, including the carotid, radial, ulnar, femoral, popliteal, dorsalis pedis, and posterior tibialis pulses. The nurse assesses the pulses for rate, rhythm, and force. The nurse auscultates for bruits (an adventitious sound of venous or arterial origin) over the carotid and abdominal arteries.

Physical assessment provides information that is helpful in diagnosing several conditions that produce *secondary hypertension.* The presence of abdominal bruits is typical of clients with renovascular disease. Tachycardia, sweating, and pallor are suggestive of pheochromocytoma or adrenal medulla tumor. Coarctation of the aorta is often characterized by delayed or absent femoral pulses.

Psychosocial Assessment

The nurse assesses for psychosocial stressors that can aggravate the client's hypertension. The client is asked to recall a typical day from the time he/she gets up through bedtime. The client is evaluated for evidence of type A behavior. Characteristics of type A behavior include competitiveness, impatience, work addiction, aggressiveness, hostility, excessive ambition, and abruptness of speech and gesture. The person who exhibits type A behavior has a twofold increased risk of CAD when compared with those with type B behavior (Kannel & Schatzkin, 1983).

The nurse assesses the client for job-related, economic, or other life stressors, as well as the client's response to these stressors.

Laboratory Findings

No laboratory test results are diagnostic of essential hypertension. Several laboratory tests can assess the severity of vascular disease and the possible causes of secondary hypertension. The presence of protein, red blood cells, pus cells, and casts in the urine and elevated levels of BUN or serum creatinine are indicative of renal disease. In clients with a pheochromocytoma, a urinary test for the presence of catecholamines has positive results. Elevation of levels of serum corticoids and 17-ketosteroids in the urine is diagnostic of Cushing's syndrome.

Radiographic Findings

Routine chest radiography may be of assistance in recognizing left ventricular hypertrophy that results from hypertension. The x-ray film serves as a baseline for assessing future complications of hypertension.

Intravenous pyelography (IVP) (excretory urography) is often the initial procedure performed when clinical features suggest renovascular hypertension. Renal arteriography is undertaken to establish the exact location and the extent of any lesions, the degree of obstruction, and the basic pathologic change in the renal arteries. Renal arteriography is diagnostic in renovascular hypertension.

Other Diagnostic Tests

An ECG is of value in determining the degree of cardiac involvement. Left atrial abnormality is the first ECG sign of cardiac involvement from hypertension.

 Analysis: Nursing Diagnosis

Common Diagnoses

Two nursing diagnoses are commonly found in clients with hypertension.

1. Knowledge deficit related to unfamiliarity with the pathophysiology of hypertension
2. Potential for noncompliance related to the treatment regimen for hypertension

Additional Diagnoses

The client may also have one or more of the following diagnoses:

1. Altered (renal, cerebral, cardiopulmonary, and peripheral) tissue perfusion related to the effects of hypertension on the body
2. Altered nutrition: more than body requirements related to overindulgence of food or an excess of salt in the individual's diet
3. Fear related to risk of complications associated with hypertension
4. Potential for sexual dysfunction related to the side effects of drugs used in the treatment of hypertension

 Planning and Implementation

Knowledge Deficit

Planning: client goals. The goal for this nursing diagnosis is that the client will verbalize an understanding of the management of hypertension.

Interventions: nonsurgical management. For the client with essential hypertension, diet therapy, weight reduction, stress management, and exercise are often recommended initially to lower and control blood pressure. If nonpharmacologic therapy is unsuccessful, the physician must consider the use of antihypertensive drugs.

Diet therapy. A high sodium intake can cause hypertension in some salt-sensitive individuals. However, there is no easy way to identify which clients will benefit from sodium restriction. All clients with hypertension are advised to avoid adding salt at the table, to avoid cooking with salt, and to avoid adding seasonings that contain sodium, and to limit eating canned, frozen, and other processed foods to achieve moderate sodium restriction. The nurse reviews a 3-day dietary recall with the client to identify those clients who may have excessive sodium intake. The nurse suggests spices, herbs, fruits, and other non–salt-containing substances, such as powdered garlic and onion, to enhance the flavor of meat, chicken, seafood, and snacks. The nurse instructs clients to read the labels on processed foods and to avoid those that are high in sodium. Salt substitutes are an alternative to salt, but their use requires a physician's order, because they are high in potassium. Hyperkalemia can occur in clients who are taking potassium-sparing diuretics and in clients with renal impairment; these individuals need to avoid using salt substitutes.

The effect of salt restriction on the client's hypertension is assessed in follow-up. Clients who respond with lowering of blood pressure should be identified, so that salt restriction can be consistently reinforced. The nurse also evaluates the client's weight and discusses the rationale for reduction or maintenance of weight. The nurse and the dietitian work with the client to plan a weight-reducing diet. Clients are instructed to limit alcohol intake to no more than 1 oz daily, because alcohol consumption may elevate arterial blood pressure and can add empty calories.

Exercise. With the physician's approval, the nurse can assist the client in developing a regular exercise program (see earlier). The client is instructed to initiate exercise gradually and to stop and notify the physician if symptoms such as severe shortness of breath, fainting, or chest pain occur.

Stress management. Various forms of behavior modification (meditation, yoga, progressive relaxation, and biofeedback) have been utilized to help individuals relax and reduce their level of stress. The nurse assists the client in identifying causes of stress and identifying ways of successfully managing the stress (see earlier discussion of biofeedback and Chap. 6).

Drug therapy. Controversy exists about treating all clients with diastolic blood pressure readings between 90 and 94 mmHg with pharmacologic therapy if other measures are unsuccessful in controlling blood pressure. Initiation of therapy in any client requires the physician's consideration of at least two factors: the severity of the blood pressure elevation and the presence of other complications or additional risk factors. Through control of hypertension, the client may be able to avoid the complications of hypertensive vascular disease.

Drug therapy for the client with hypertension can involve one or a combination of antihypertensive drugs. The goal of therapy is to arrive at a regimen that successfully reduces blood pressure without producing intolerable side effects. Several drugs or combinations of drugs may have to be tried, as well as dosage adjustments.

A wide variety of medications are available to control hypertension (Table 65–2). Diuretics can be separated into three basic types: thiazide diuretics, loop (high-ceiling) diuretics, and potassium-sparing diuretics. Thiazide diuretics, such as hydrochlorothiazide (Esidrix and HydroDIURIL), prevent sodium and water reabsorption in the distal tubules, while promoting potassium excretion. Loop diuretics, for example, furosemide (Lasix), depress sodium reabsorption in the ascending loop of Henle and promote potassium excretion. Potassium-sparing diuretics, such as spironolactone (Aldactone), act on the distal tubule to inhibit reabsorption of sodium ions in exchange for potassium, thereby retaining potassium. Diuretics are often used in combination with other drugs, for example, beta-blockers, such as propranolol (Inderal), because of the diuretic's ability to potentiate the effect of other antihypertensive drugs.

Diuretics are relatively inexpensive. Adherence to the medication regimen is enhanced because the drug can usually be prescribed on a once-a-day or, at most, a twice-a-day schedule. However, the frequent voiding that occurs after taking a diuretic may interfere with a client's daily activities. The most frequent side effect associated with diuretics is hypokalemia. The nurse monitors the client's serum potassium level and assesses for signs and symptoms of irregular pulse and muscle weakness, which may indicate hypokalemia. Clients receiving potassium-depleting diuretics are advised to eat foods high in potassium. However, a potassium supplement is often required to maintain adequate serum potassium levels (see Chap. 13). Clients taking potassium-sparing diuretics are assessed for hypokalemia and hyperkalemia. Both of these electrolyte disturbances are characterized by weakness and irregular pulse.

Beta-blocking agents, such as propranolol, lower blood pressure by blocking beta-receptors in the heart and peripheral vessels, reducing cardiac rate and output. Monitoring of heart rate is important because beta-blockers cause a decrease in heart rate, and bradycardia can occur. Beta-blockers should be avoided in clients with a history of asthma, bronchospasm, or congestive heart failure (CHF) because of their blocking effect on bronchodilation. All clients taking beta-blockers are monitored for shortness of breath and wheezing, as these symptoms indicate bronchospasm. Clients are also monitored for side effects such as fatigue and weakness. Sexual dysfunction can occur with some beta-blockers, such as propranolol.

Calcium channel blockers, such as verapamil hydrochloride (Calan), lower blood pressure by interfering with the transmembrane flux of calcium ions, resulting in reduced vasoconstriction. The nurse instructs the client taking calcium channel blockers to rise slowly from a prone or supine position to a sitting or standing position to avoid orthostatic (postural) hypotension. The nurse also monitors the client for other side effects, including headache, pedal edema, flushing, and constipation.

Captopril (Capoten) is a specific competitive inhibitor of the angiotensin I–converting enzyme (ACE). This enzyme is responsible for the conversion of angiotensin I to angiotensin II. The client receiving this drug for the first time is instructed to stay in bed for 3 hours. This is

TABLE 65–2 Drugs Used in the Treatment of Hypertension

Drug	Usual Daily Dosage	Interventions	Rationales
Diuretics			
Thiazides			
Chlorothiazide (Diuril)	500–1000 mg/d	1. Monitor potassium level. 2. Watch for muscle weakness or irregular pulse. 3. Encourage intake of foods high in potassium (e.g., bananas and orange juice).	1, 2. To detect hypokalemia. 3. To replenish depleted potassium supplies.
Hydrochlorothiazide (Esidrix, Hydro-DIURIL)	50–100 mg/d	1. Same as for chlorothiazide.	1. Same as for chlorothiazide.
Chlorthalidone (Hygroton)	25–50 mg/d	1. Same as for chlorothiazide.	1. Same as for chlorothiazide.
Loop Diuretics			
Furosemide (Lasix)	20–40 mg/d	1. Same as for chlorothiazide.	1. Same as for chlorothiazide.
Ethacrynic acid (Edecrin)	50–100 mg/d	1. Same as for chlorothiazide.	1. Same as for chlorothiazide.
Potassium-Sparing Diuretics			
Spironolactone (Aldactone)	25 mg bid	1. Monitor potassium levels.	1. To detect hyperkalemia.
Vasodilators			
Hydralazine (Apresoline)	25 mg bid	1. Monitor pulse rate. 2. Administer with food.	1. To detect tachycardia. 2. To prevent nausea and vomiting.
Minoxidil (Loniten)	10–15 mg/d	1. Same as for hydralazine.	1. Same as for hydralazine.
Drugs Acting on the Central Nervous System			
Reserpine (Serpasil)	0.1 mg/d	1. Assess for history of depression. 2. Monitor for increased appetite. 3. Administer with food and monitor for signs of peptic ulcer.	1. To detect contraindication to use of drug. 2. To detect need for caloric restrictions. 3. To prevent or detect complications of drug use.
Methyldopa (Aldomet)	250 mg bid	1. Instruct the client to sit on the side of the bed for several minutes before arising and to avoid standing suddenly. 2. Instruct the client to report any difficulty in sexual function. 3. Monitor for positive Coombs' test result.	1. To prevent injury from drug-related postural hypotension. 2. To detect impotence. 3. To detect hemolytic anemia.

TABLE 65–2   Drugs Used in the Treatment of Hypertension *Continued*

Drug	Usual Daily Dosage	Interventions	Rationales
Clonidine hydrochloride (Catapres)	0.1 mg h.s. or 0.1 mg once a week transdermally	1. Administer at bedtime. 2. Instruct the client to report any difficulty in sexual function.	1. To prevent injury from drug-related sedation and drowsiness. 2. To detect impotence.
Beta-Blockers			
Propranolol (Inderal)	10 mg bid initially, increased to 40 mg once or twice daily	1. Monitor pulse rate. 2. Watch for shortness of breath or cough.	1. To detect bradycardia. 2. To detect bronchospasm caused by blockage of beta-receptors in the lungs.
Metoprolol tartrate (Lopressor)	50 mg bid	3. Instruct the client to report any difficulty in sexual function. 4. Monitor platelet count.	3. To detect impotence. 4. To detect thrombocytopenia.
Nadolol (Corgard)	40 mg/d	1–4. Same as for propranolol.	1–4. Same as for propranolol.
Calcium Channel Blockers			
Nifedipine (Procardia)	10 mg tid, increased to 30 mg tid	1. Monitor blood pressure and pulse. 2. Observe lower extremities.	1. To detect hypotension. May also cause headache and flushing. 2. To detect pedal edema.
Verapamil (Calan)	40 mg q 8 h, increased to 80 mg q 8 h, or 240 mg SR once a day	1. Monitor blood pressure and pulse. 2. Encourage intake of foods high in fiber.	1. To detect hypotension and atrioventricular block. May also cause headache and flushing. 2. To prevent constipation.
Diltiazem hydrochloride (Cardizem)	30 mg q 8 h initially, increased to 60 mg q 8 h	1. Monitor blood pressure and pulse.	1. To detect hypotension and atrioventricular block. May also cause headache and flushing.
Angiotensin-Converting–Enzyme Inhibitor			
Captopril (Capoten)	6.25 mg tid initially, increased to 50 mg tid	1. Instruct client to stay in bed for 3 h after the first dose. 2. Monitor blood pressure.	1. To prevent severe hypotension that may follow the first dose. 2. To detect hypotension.

done to avoid symptoms resulting from the severe hypotensive effect that can occur with this medication. The nurse monitors the client's blood pressure closely after the first dose. Orthostatic hypotension may also occur with subsequent doses, but it is less severe than with the initial dose.

Drugs acting on the central nervous system (adrener-gic inhibitors), such as methyldopa (Aldomet), lower blood pressure by stimulating alpha-receptors in the brain. This stimulation leads to inhibition of the sympathetic vasomotor center and sympathetic outflow. The nurse monitors clients taking these medications for side effects, including sedation, postural hypotension, and impotence.

Vasodilators, such as minoxidil (Loniten), lower blood pressure by relaxing vascular smooth muscle tone, thus reducing total peripheral resistance. Clients are monitored for side effects, including tachycardia, flushing, and nausea.

Guanethidine monosulfate (Ismelin sulfate) is an adrenergic blocking agent; it is used rarely and only when other antihypertensives are ineffective. Clients taking this medication are instructed to rise slowly from a lying position to prevent orthostatic hypotension. The nurse assesses for this side effect and others such as sexual dysfunction, nasal congestion, and diarrhea.

A stepped-care approach has frequently been employed to treat hypertension (Table 65–3). This approach was first recommended with the intent that small doses of different types of drugs could be used to control blood pressure, with minimal side effects. In 1984, the Joint National Committee on Detection, Evaluation, and Treatment of High Blood Pressure recommended that initial therapy for hypertension include either a thiazide diuretic or a beta-blocker ("Hypertension prevalence," 1985). Since that time, calcium antagonists and ACE prohibitors have also been recommended for initial therapy. Because of changes in recommendations, and more available drug options, the nurse sees a variety of drugs protocols used to meet the individual needs of clients.

Interventions: surgical management. There is no surgical treatment of essential hypertension. Surgical treatment is often employed for certain types of secondary hypertension, such as renal vascular disease, coarctation of the aorta, and occasionally pheochromocytoma.

Potential for Noncompliance

Planning: client goals. The goal for this nursing diagnosis is that the client will adhere to the therapeutic regimen.

Interventions: nonsurgical management. Clients who require pharmacologic treatment for essential hypertension usually need to take medication to control blood pressure for the rest of their lives. Frequently, clients stop taking antihypertensive medications, assuming that because they have no symptoms, the hypertension is under control. Clients may also assume that if their blood pressure returns to normal levels with antihypertensives, they no longer need them. Clients may also stop taking antihypertensives because of adverse side effects or cost.

The nurse and the client should discuss the goals of therapy. Potential side effects of the client's individualized treatment are discussed to assist the client in identifying potential problems. The nurse then assists the client in tailoring the therapeutic regimen to the client's ADL.

■ Discharge Planning

Home Care Preparation

If possible, the client should obtain a blood pressure monitor for use at home so that blood pressure can be periodically checked. The nurse evaluates the client's ability to learn how to check his/her blood pressure. If weight reduction is a goal, the nurse suggests that the client have a scale in the home.

Client/Family Education

Clients are instructed about salt restriction, weight maintenance or reduction, alcohol restriction, stress reduction, and an individual exercise prescription (see earlier).

Clients taking medication for hypertension are provided with oral and written information about the indications, dosage, times of administration, side effects, and drug interactions of the prescribed medication (see Table 65–2). The nurse explains that when the prescription is empty, it must be renewed on a continual basis. The nurse emphasizes that clients should report unpleasant side effects, such as sexual dysfunction. A variety of alternative medications can be prescribed to minimize certain side effects.

If the client has access to equipment to measure blood pressure, the client or a family member or both are instructed in the proper technique for blood pressure measurement. The nurse instructs the client to record all blood pressure readings in a diary and to bring the diary to all medical appointments so that progress can be followed. Plans for follow-up are arranged for all clients, regardless of their therapy.

Psychosocial Preparation

Hypertension is a chronic illness, and clients may not be prepared to accept this. The nurse allows clients to verbalize feelings about this disease and its treatment. Clients are advised that their involvement in the treat-

---

TABLE 65–3   Stepped-Care Approach to Drug Therapy of Hypertension

Step 1   The physician starts with less than a full dose of a thiazide diuretic, beta-blocker, calcium channel blocker, or ACE inhibitor and adjusts the dosage as necessary.

Step 2   If blood pressure control is not obtained, the physician increases the dose of the first drug or adds a drug of a different class.

Step 3   If blood pressure control is not obtained, the physician substitutes a second drug or adds a third drug of a different class.

Step 4   If blood pressure control is not obtained, the physician adds a third or fourth drug and evaluates further.

From U.S. Department of Health and Human Services. (1988). *The 1988 Report of the Joint National Committee on Detection, Evaluation, and Treatment of High Blood Pressure* (NIH Publication No. 88–1088). Washington, DC: U.S. Government Printing Office.

ment can lead to control of this disease and can avoid complications.

Health Care Resources

A home care nurse may be needed for follow-up to monitor blood pressure. The nurse evaluates the ability of the client or the family to obtain accurate blood pressure measurements and assesses compliance with treatment. Clients may be referred to the American Heart Association or Red Cross for free blood pressure checks.

 Evaluation

On the basis of the identified nursing diagnoses, the nurse evaluates the care of the hypertensive client. The expected outcomes include that the client

1. Explains the rationale for treatment of hypertension
2. Maintains blood pressure of less than 140/90 mmHg
3. Demonstrates no signs or symptoms of target organ damage

PERIPHERAL VASCULAR DISEASE

OVERVIEW

PVD includes diseases that alter the natural flow of blood through the arteries, veins, and lymphatics of the peripheral system or the extremities. Generally, PVD affects the lower extremities. The diseases that affect each of these vessels need to be reviewed individually because the treatment differs according to the vessel involved and whether the symptoms are acute or chronic. The most frequently reported forms of PVD are arterial and venous; however, some individuals can have both arterial and venous diseases that differ in clinical manifestations and pathophysiology. These conditions are painful, disabling, and frightening for clients.

PERIPHERAL ARTERIAL DISEASE

OVERVIEW

Pathophysiology

Body tissues cannot live without an appropriate oxygen and nutrient supply. Partial or total arterial occlusion disrupts this natural process, and tissue eventually dies. Atherosclerosis is the most common cause of this altered flow. Although the true pathophysiology of atherosclerosis is unknown (see earlier), many theories have been proposed. The consensus is that intimal injury results

from some unknown process or processes; fatty substances then accumulate at the site of injury and alter or totally occlude arterial blood flow.

Tissue damage generally occurs below the arterial obstruction. The amount of damage depends on the extent of the arterial blockage, on the nature of the decreased arterial blood flow (chronic or acute), and on the location of the destruction. Tissue damage is believed to be caused by malnourishment of tissues with nutrients and oxygen.

The location of occlusion determines the location of tissue damage. Inflow disease is located above the superficial femoral artery (SFA), and outflow disease is below the SFA. Gradual inflow occlusions may not cause significant tissue damage; gradual outflow occlusions typically do.

Chronic Peripheral Arterial Disease

The clinical course of chronic peripheral arterial disease (PAD) can be divided into four stages (see the accompanying Key Features of Disease). The disease is asymptomatic in its early stages. Most clients initially seek treatment for a characteristic leg pain known as *intermittent claudication* (a term derived from a word meaning "to limp"). Clients with intermittent claudica-

---

KEY FEATURES OF DISEASE ■ Clinical Course of Chronic Peripheral Arterial Disease

Stage I: Asymptomatic

No claudication is present.
Bruit or aneurysm may be present.
Physical examination may rarely reveal decreased pulses.

Stage II: Claudication

Muscle pain, cramping, or burning is exacerbated by exercise and relieved by rest.
Symptoms are reproducible with exercise.

Stage III: Rest Pain

Pain while resting commonly wakes the client at night.
Pain is described as numbness, burning, toothache-type pain.
Pain usually occurs in the distal portion of the extremity —toes, arch, forefoot, or heel—rarely in the calf or the ankle.
Pain is sometimes relieved by placing the extremity in a dependent position.

Stage IV: Necrosis/Gangrene

Ulcers and blackened tissue occur on the toes, the forefoot, and the heel.
Distinctive gangrenous odor is present.

tion can walk only a certain distance before a cramping, burning muscle discomfort or pain forces them to stop. The pain subsides after rest. When clients resume walking, they can walk the same distance before the pain returns. The pain is thus considered reproducible. As the disease progresses, clients can walk shorter and shorter distances before pain recurs. Ultimately, pain may develop even while clients are at rest.

Rest pain, which may begin while the disease is still primarily in the stage of intermittent claudication, is a numbness or burning, often described as feeling like a toothache, that is severe enough to awaken clients at night. It is usually located in the distal portion of the extremities—in the toes, the arches, the forefeet, and the heels—and rarely in the calves or the ankles. Relief of rest pain can sometimes be achieved by keeping the limb in a dependent position. Clients with rest pain have advanced disease that may result in limb loss.

Acute Peripheral Arterial Disease

Although PAD is usually a chronic disorder that exists for many years before clinical manifestations are reported, acute obstruction by a thrombus or embolus can occur. There is usually severe, acute pain below the level of obstruction.

Etiology

Because atherosclerosis is the most common cause of chronic and acute arterial obstruction, the risk factors for atherosclerosis apply to PAD as well. These include hypertension, hyperlipidemia, diabetes mellitus, cigarette smoking, obesity, and familial predisposition.

Incidence

The true incidence of PAD is unknown. Reported data usually involve other diseases that override PAD, such as CAD, CVA, and aneurysms. However, it is estimated that more than 1 million people each year experience PAD and approximately 70,000 of those individuals undergo an amputation (Bunt & Haynes, 1984).

PAD is generally found in men older than age 45 years and in postmenopausal women. However, because genetic factors play a role, younger individuals can have severe PAD.

PREVENTION

Atherosclerosis can be controlled and prevented through education and alteration of behavior habits. Identifying high-risk individuals is one method of prevention (see earlier). Controlling risk factors and managing problems such as diabetes and hypertension decrease the chance of problems related to PAD.

Education plays a big role in disease control for indi-

viduals with PAD. Although they cannot eradicate PAD, these clients can affect how the disease progresses. A client with the diagnosis of chronic PAD must learn about the disease process, risk factors, and foot care. Educating the client provides control and can prevent complications, such as foot ulcers. An exercise program should be developed for each client individually. This helps the development of collateral circulation, which provides additional oxygen to the affected tissues. Collateral circulation is the use of alternative vessels to compensate for decreased blood flow through the diseased vessels. However, this phenomenon does not occur in everyone with chronic PAD.

COLLABORATIVE MANAGEMENT

 Assessment

History

The nature of the client's *leg pain* provides important clues to the location and severity of PAD. The nurse therefore asks the following questions: "Where does the pain occur?" "How far can you walk before your legs begin to hurt?" "What does the pain feel like?" "What relieves the pain?"

Clients with inflow disease experience discomfort in the lower back, the buttocks, or the thighs. Lower-back or buttock discomfort indicates obstruction at or above the common iliac artery or aorta. Thigh discomfort indicates obstruction at or above the profunda femoris artery. Clients with mild inflow disease experience discomfort after walking about five blocks. This discomfort is not severe, but causes the client to stop walking. It is relieved with rest. Clients with moderate inflow disease experience pain in these areas after walking about two blocks. The discomfort is described more like pain, but it subsides with rest most of the time. Severe inflow disease causes the client severe pain after walking one-half to one block. These clients usually have rest pain.

Clients with outflow disease describe burning or cramping in the calves, the ankles, the feet, and the toes. Calf discomfort usually indicates arterial obstruction at or below the SFA or popliteal artery. Instep or foot discomfort indicates an obstruction below the popliteal artery. Clients with mild outflow disease experience discomfort after walking about five blocks. This discomfort is relieved by rest. Clients with moderate outflow disease have pain after walking about two blocks, and intermittent rest pain may be present. Clients with severe outflow disease are usually unable to walk more than one-half block and usually experience rest pain. They may hang their feet off the bed at night for comfort. Clients with outflow disease complain more frequently of rest pain than do clients with inflow disease.

Clients with acute PAD usually describe acute, severe pain below the level of the obstruction, which occurs even at rest. They may describe a previous history of chronic PAD and claudication, but many clients do not have such a history.

Physical Assessment: Clinical Manifestations

Physical assessment for PAD is the same as that for atherosclerosis, but specific findings differ for PAD and depend on the severity of the disease. Inspection reveals ischemic changes that develop in chronic PAD, but not necessarily with acute PAD. These include *loss of hair* on the lower calf, the ankle, and the foot; *dry, scaly skin;* and *thickened toenails.* With severe disease, the extremity becomes cold and gray-blue. The client manifests *ascending pallor* and *descending rubor.*

Acute arterial obstruction causes the extremity to become *mottled* and *cool or cold.* The nurse observes *delayed capillary filling.* Long-term ischemic symptoms, such as hair loss and thickened toenails, may not be present, but acute gangrene can exist. If the source is embolic, minute areas of the toes may be blackened. This phenomenon is sometimes called trash foot. Emboli may be dispersed from plaques above the foot, aneurysms, or clotting factor disorders. These emboli result in gangrene of the toes.

With chronic PAD, the pulses below the level of obstruction may be decreased or absent; with acute occlusion, the pulses are most often absent. The affected extremity is cool to cold when compared with the nonaffected extremity. If both extremities are cool, the causative factor may be room temperature.

The nurse may also assess early signs of ulcer formation or complete ulcer formation. The nurse must differentiate arterial and venous stasis ulcers from diabetic ulcers, which may have a different cause (see the accompanying Key Features of Disease). *Arterial ulcers* usually are painful and develop on the toes, between the toes, or on the upper aspect of the foot. *Diabetic ulcers* develop on the plantar surface of the foot, over the metatarsal heads, and on the heel, anywhere that pressure is exerted. Diabetic ulcers may not be painful. *Venous stasis ulcers* cause minimal pain and occur in the ankle area. With venous ulcers, the foot is warm and distal pulses are palpable. The nurse notes discoloration of the lower extremity at the ulcer site.

Psychosocial Assessment

With chronic arterial disease, disabling pain can cause depression and anxiety. Pain becomes a part of the client's life. Mobility is limited, and some people may need to change or relinquish their jobs.

Many clients experience fear. The fear of losing a limb or life can cause increased anxiety and depression. The nurse assesses each client's coping mechanisms, noting symptoms of maladjusted coping, such as anxiety or depression. If limb loss occurs, the client must deal with disfigurement. Assessment of the client's feelings about prosthetics and other assistive devices can be important when developing interventions for future care. With acute arterial occlusion, the client also expresses fear of losing the limb, but severe pain is often the greatest concern.

Laboratory Findings

The laboratory findings in arterial disease are the same as those for atherosclerosis.

Radiographic Findings

The most common radiographic test for PAD is arteriography of the lower extremities (see earlier).

Other Diagnostic Tests

Noninvasive evaluation of arterial disease has recently become a popular method of diagnosing PAD. Noninvasive testing provides information about the arterial system with minimal risk to the client.

Segmental systolic blood pressure measurements of the lower extremities at the thigh, the calf, and the ankle are a noninvasive test for PAD. Normally, blood pressure readings in the thigh and the calf are higher than those in the upper extremities. With the presence of arterial disease, these pressures are decreased when compared with the brachial pressure. The ankle pressure is normally equal to or greater than the brachial pressure. With inflow disease, pressures taken at the thigh level indicate severity of disease. Mild inflow disease may cause only a 10 to 30 mmHg difference in blood pressure on the affected side when compared with the brachial pressure. Severe inflow disease can cause a pressure difference of greater than 40 to 50 mmHg.

To evaluate outflow disease, the ankle pressure is compared with the brachial pressure, which provides a ratio known as the ankle/arm index. This can be derived by dividing the ankle blood pressure by the brachial blood pressure. With mild outflow disease the client has an ankle/arm index of 0.8 to 1.0; pressures are decreased by about 10 to 30 mmHg. The client with moderate outflow disease has an ankle/arm index of 0.5 to 0.8, with pressure differences of 20 to 40 mmHg. An ankle/arm index less than 0.5 indicates severe outflow disease.

Stress testing may be informative in clients experiencing claudication without rest pain. The client has resting pulse volume recordings done and then is asked to ambulate or walk on a treadmill until the symptoms are reproduced. At the time of symptom onset or after approximately 5 minutes, even if the client does not experience symptoms, the pulse volume recording is repeated. Normally, there may be an increased waveform with minimal, if any, drop in the ankle pressures. In clients with arterial disease, the waveforms are dampened and there is a decrease in the ankle pressure of the affected limb of 40 to 60 mmHg for 20 to 30 seconds. If the return to normal temperature is delayed (longer than 10 minutes), the test result is indicative of abnormal arterial flow in the affected limb.

Plethysmography can also be performed to evaluate arterial flow in the lower extremities. This measurement provides graph or tracing readings of arterial flow in the limb. If an occlusion is present, the waveforms are

KEY FEATURES OF DISEASE ■ Differential Features of Ulcers of the Lower Extremity

Feature	Diabetic Ulcers	Arterial Ulcers	Venous Ulcers
History	Diabetes Peripheral neuropathy No complaints of claudication	Client complaints of claudication after walking approximately 1–2 blocks Rest pain usually present Pain at ulcer site Two or three risk factors present	Chronic nonhealing ulcer No claudication or rest pain Moderate ulcer discomfort Client complaints about ankle or leg swelling
Ulcer location and appearance	Plantar area of foot Metatarsal heads Pressure points on feet Deep Pale, with even edges Little granulation tissue	End of the toes Between the toes Deep Pale, with even edges Little granulation tissue	Ankle area Usually superficial, with uneven edges Granulation tissue present
Other assessment findings	Pulses usually present Cool or warm foot Painless	Cool or cold foot Decreased or absent pulses Atrophy of skin Hair loss Ascending pallor Descending rubor Possible gangrene When acute, neurologic deficits noted	Ankle discoloration and edema Full veins when legs slightly dependent No neurologic deficit Pulses present May have scarring from previous ulcers
Treatment	Rule out major arterial disease Control diabetes Client education Prevent infection	Treat underlying cause (surgical revascularization) Prevent trauma and infection Client education, stressing foot care	Long-term wound care (Unna's boot, wet-to-dry dressings) Elevate extremity Client education Prevent infection

Photograph of diabetic ulcer from Kozak, G. P., Hoar, C. S., Jr., Rowbotham, J. L., Wheelock F. C., Jr., Gibbons, G. W., & Campbell, D. (1984). *Management of diabetic foot problems.* Philadelphia: W. B. Saunders.

dampened to flattened, depending on the degree of occlusion.

 ### Analysis: Nursing Diagnosis

Common Diagnoses

The following nursing diagnoses are commonly found in clients with arterial disease:

1. Altered (peripheral) tissue perfusion related to an impaired arterial blood flow
2. Impaired skin integrity related to oxygen deficit to tissues
3. Activity intolerance related to pain of arterial obstruction

Additional Diagnoses

Additional nursing diagnoses related to arterial disease include

1. Pain related to obstruction of arterial flow
2. Potential for infection related to decreased tissue oxygenation
3. Body image disturbance related to discoloration, ulcers, or amputations
4. Fear related to possible limb loss
5. Knowledge deficit related to risk factors and actions to prevent complications

 ### Planning and Implementation

Altered Tissue Perfusion

Planning: client goals. The major goal for this diagnosis is that the client will have an increased arterial blood flow to the extremities, thereby improving the tissue oxygen balance.

Interventions. The nurse first determines if the altered tissue perfusion is of arterial or venous origin. An accurate assessment often provides this information. However, in some individuals both conditions may exist, in which case, each must be considered when developing appropriate interventions.

Nonsurgical management. Nonsurgical management is not usually appropriate for the acute phase of PAD, except for short-term management of the disease. These clients are usually surgical candidates for limb salvage. However, with chronic arterial disease, there are a few methods of increasing arterial flow to the affected limb. These involve exercise, position changes, drug therapy, and prevention of further vasoconstriction.

Exercise improves arterial blood flow to the affected limb through build-up of collateral circulation. Collateral circulation provides blood to the affected area through smaller vessels that compensate for the occluded vessels. Exercise is individualized for each client, but it should not be undertaken by individuals with severe rest pain, venous ulcers, or gangrene. Many other clients with PAD can benefit from exercise that is gradually initiated and slowly increased. An excellent exercise for these clients is walking. Clients are instructed to walk until it is impossible to continue, stop and rest, then walk a little farther. Eventually, clients are able to walk longer distances, as collateral circulation develops.

Positioning of the client to promote circulation has been somewhat controversial. Some clients have swelling in their extremities. Because swelling prevents arterial flow, these individuals should elevate their feet at rest. Clients with PAD should refrain from raising their legs above the heart level. In severe cases, these clients may sleep with the affected limb hanging from the bed or sitting upright in a chair for comfort.

An important intervention that is appropriate for these clients is to improve vasodilation and prevent vasoconstriction. One method of promoting this is by providing warmth to the affected extremity and preventing long periods of cold. The nurse encourages the client to maintain a warm environment at home and to wear socks or insulated bedroom shoes at all times. The client is cautioned *never* to apply direct heat to the limb, such as by heating pads or extremely hot water. Sensitivity is decreased in the affected limb, and the client may get burned without feeling it.

Preventing vasoconstriction is slightly more difficult to achieve. The nurse encourages clients to prevent exposure of the affected limb to the cold because cold temperatures cause vasoconstriction and therefore decrease arterial blood flow. Vasoconstriction is also caused by emotional stress, caffeine, and nicotine. The nurse educates the client about these factors (see earlier discussion of the effects of nicotine on arterial disease). Complete abstinence from smoking or chewing tobacco is the most effective method of decreasing vasoconstriction. The vasoconstrictive effects of each cigarette may last up to 1 hour after the cigarette is smoked.

Drug therapy for chronic arterial occlusion is another controversial method of treatment of PAD. Opinions vary in regard to drug therapy, which may be due to the limited effect that drugs have had on limiting progression of the disease. Some drugs may diminish symptoms, but may not actually improve circulation. Drug therapy, at present, includes vasodilators, defibrination agents, and antiplatelet therapy (Table 65-4). These may increase blood flow at rest, but no drug has been shown to increase arterial flow or oxygen exchange during exercise. Therefore, a client with claudication may not necessarily benefit from these measures.

Vasodilators either block the effect of adrenergic blockers or directly affect the wall of the blood vessels. Some of the more common vasodilators used are cyclandelate (Cyclospasmol) and isoxsuprine (Defencin).

Agents that decrease the serum fibrinogen level and in turn decrease blood viscosity have been shown to cause some clinical improvement in clients with PAD. Pentoxifylline (Trental) is currently used to decrease blood viscosity.

TABLE 65-4 Drugs Used in the Treatment of Arterial Disease

Drug	Usual Daily Dosage	Interventions	Rationales
Dipyridamole (Persantine)	25-75 mg qid PO	1. Administer 1 h before meals. 2. Assess blood pressure with the client lying and standing.	1. To promote optimal absorption. 2. To detect orthostatic hypotension.
Pentoxifylline (Trental)	400 mg tid with meals	1. Administer with meals. 2. Assess blood pressure in clients receiving antihypertensives. 3. Instruct the client to continue to take the drug as ordered, even if no change in symptoms occurs.	1. To prevent GI upset. 2. To detect hypotension. 3. To promote compliance while the drug takes effect, sometimes 6-8 wk.
Isoxsuprine hydrochloride (Defencin, Rolisox, Vasodilan)	10-20 mg tid or qid PO	1. Do not administer in the early postpartum period. 2. Assess blood pressure with the client lying and standing.	1. To prevent bleeding, which may occur at this time. 2. To detect orthostatic hypotension.
Cyclandelate (Cyclospasmol)	200-400 mg qid PO	1. Administer with antacids or food. 2. Assess and report chest pain.	1. To prevent GI distress and nausea. 2. To detect CAD, which is a contraindication to use of the drug.

Probably the most commonly used agents for clients with PAD are the antiplatelet agents, such as dipyridamole (Persantine) and aspirin (acetylsalicylic acid). These agents are more commonly used in clients with cerebrovascular disease. In acute PAD, an anticoagulant agent such as heparin is used to prevent further clot formation.

Controlling hypertension can improve tissue perfusion by maintaining pressures that are adequate to perfuse the periphery, but not vasoconstrict the vessels. Clients should be made aware of the effect that blood pressure has on their circulation and instructed in methods of control. Clients taking beta-blockers may develop drug-related claudication or experience an exacerbation of their symptoms. Clinicians must closely monitor clients with PAD receiving beta-blockers.

Another nonsurgical but invasive method of improving arterial flow is *percutaneous transluminal angioplasty* (PTA). This procedure involves dilating arteries that have been occluded or stenosed with a balloon catheter. Successful PTA opens the vessel lumen and improves arterial blood flow, creating a smooth inner vessel surface. PTA is performed for clients who have stenoses that are accessible with a balloon catheter. Many times, PTA is used for clients who are poor surgical candidates who cannot withstand general anesthesia or for whom amputation may be inevitable. This method of treatment of arterial obstructions is only available for certain types of lesions, and reocclusion may occur. The actual duration of the treatment is unknown; some clients have

been occlusion free for up to 3 to 5 years, whereas others experience reocclusion within a year of the PTA.

Another invasive procedure is laser-assisted angioplasty. Laser-assisted angioplasty is usually performed by a trained vascular surgeon or radiologist. Different types of lasers are used. The argon laser utilizes a disposable quartz laser fiber with a metal alloy tip. The heat at the tip reaches approximately 400° C and vaporizes the arteriosclerotic plaque. After a channel is formed by the laser, a PTA balloon catheter is inserted to further dilate the artery and decrease the stenosis.

Mechanical rotational abrasive atherectomy is a technique that is being investigated for improving blood flow to ischemic limbs in individuals with PAD. The rotational atherectomy device (Rotablator) is a high-speed rotary, metal bur ranging in sizes from 1.25 to 4.5 mm in diameter. The distal half of the bur is embedded with fine abrasive bits, which at rotational speeds of 100,000 to 120,000 rotations per minute result in fine-particle ablation of tissue. The Rotablator is designed to preferentially scrape harder surfaces such as plaque, while minimizing damage to the vessel surface (Zacca et al., 1989).

Preparation of the client for PTA or laser-assisted PTA is similar to the preparation of a client undergoing a diagnostic angiography. The client must receive nothing by mouth (NPO) after midnight and have the groin area scrubbed with an aseptic soap. Some clients are shaved. Post-PTA nursing care involves observing for bleeding at the puncture site, closely observing vital signs, and checking the distal pulses on the affected limb. These clients are restricted to bed rest with the limb straight for approximately 6 to 8 hours before ambulation is encouraged. Many of these clients receive anticoagulant therapy, such as heparin, for approximately 3 days and then dipyridamole for 3 to 6 months. Clients are usually given aspirin on a permanent basis.

Surgical management. Clients who experience acute peripheral artery occlusion by an embolus often undergo emergency embolectomy. Clients with acute occlusion from a thrombus usually undergo emergency surgery that involves bypass grafting. Grafting is performed in this situation because more extensive surgery is needed to correct damage from a thrombus than for damage that occurs with an embolus. Although surgery is not indicated for many clients with chronic PAD, those with severe rest pain or with claudication that interferes with the ability to work or threatens loss of limb become candidates for surgical intervention. Surgery for clients with chronic PAD is usually elective.

Arterial revascularization is the surgical procedure most commonly used to increase arterial blood flow in an affected limb. The surgical procedures can be classified as inflow or outflow procedures. Inflow procedures involve bypassing arterial occlusions above the SFAs, and outflow procedures are surgical bypassing of arterial occlusions at or below the SFAs. Clients who have both inflow and outflow problems generally have the inflow (larger arteries) procedure done before the outflow repair.

Inflow procedures include aortoiliac bypass, aortofemoral bypass, and axillofemoral bypass (Fig. 65–5). Outflow procedures include femoropopliteal bypass and femorotibial bypass. Inflow procedures have a higher incidence of success, with less chance of reocclusion or postoperative ischemia. Outflow procedures are less successful in relieving ischemic pain and are associated with a higher incidence of reocclusion.

Graft materials for the bypasses are selected on an individual basis. For outflow procedures, the preferred graft material is autogenous saphenous vein. However, these clients can experience systemic vascular disease and may need this vein for coronary artery bypass, so the saphenous vein may not be used. Femoropopliteal bypass grafts with the saphenous vein may have a 70% patency rate for 5 years, whereas the femorotibial grafts have lower patency rates (Bunt & Haynes, 1984).

When the saphenous vein is not usable, synthetic graft materials are used. Polytetrafluoroethylene material is employed as a graft and Gore-Tex grafts are commonly used. Using synthetic materials decreases the 5-year patency rate for distal or outflow grafts; but, for inflow procedures such as the aortofemoral bypass, a patency rate of 85% for a 5-year period and approximately 60% for a 10-year period has been reported (Bunt & Haynes, 1984).

Preoperative care. Preoperative preparation is similar to that described for the client having general anesthesia in Chapter 18. Documentation of vital signs and periph-

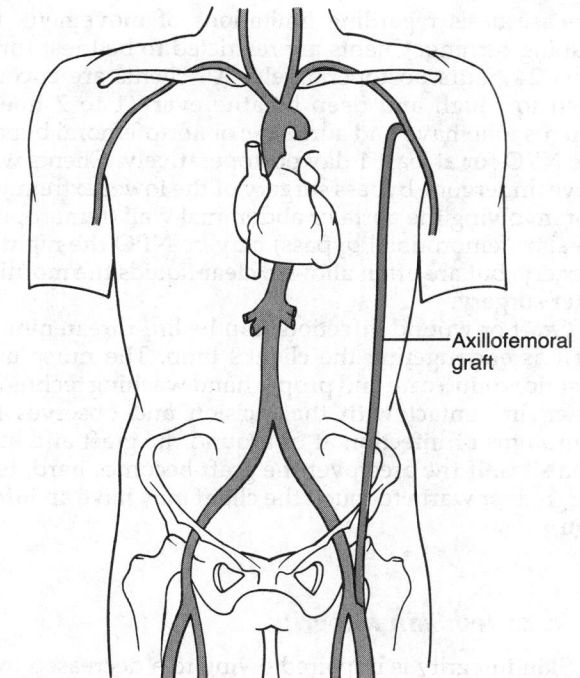

Figure 65–5

An axillofemoral bypass graft.

eral pulse checks provide a baseline of information for comparison during the postoperative phase. Depending on the surgical procedure, the client may have an IV, urinary, central venous catheter, or arterial line. To prevent postoperative infection, many clients receive antibiotic therapy for about 48 hours before the procedure.

Postoperative care. Postoperative graft occlusion often occurs within the first 24 hours. Therefore, astute nursing care is crucial. The nurse monitors the patency of the graft by checking the extremity for changes in color, temperature, and pulse intensity. Immediately postoperatively, the operating room nurse should mark the site where the distal (dorsalis pedis or posterior tibial) pulse is best palpated or heard by Doppler ultrasonography. This information needs to be communicated to the nursing staff on the unit to which the client will go.

An indicator of postoperative graft occlusion is pain experienced by the client. Many people experience a throbbing pain owing to the increased blood flow to the extremity. This pain is different from ischemic pain, and the nurse must assess the type of pain that the client experiences. If graft occlusion occurs, the client has a severe increase in ischemic pain described as similar to the pain felt before surgery.

To promote prevention of graft occlusion, the nurse monitors the client's blood pressure and notifies the surgeon if the pressure increases or decreases beyond normal limits. Range of motion of the affected limb is usually limited, with bending of hip and knee contraindicated. The nurse consults with the surgeon on a case-by-case basis regarding limitations of movement, including turning. Clients are restricted to bed rest for at least 24 hours postoperatively. All clients are encouraged to cough and deep breathe every 1 to 2 hours. Clients who have had aortoiliac or aortofemoral bypass are NPO for at least 1 day postoperatively. Clients who have undergone bypass surgery of the lower extremities not involving the aorta or abdominal wall (femoropopliteal or femorotibial bypass) may be NPO the night of surgery, but are often allowed clear liquids the morning after surgery.

Graft or wound infections can be life-threatening as well as endangering the client's limb. The nurse uses aseptic wound care and proper hand washing technique when in contact with the incision and observes for symptoms of infection at or around the graft and incision sites. If the area over the graft becomes hard, tender, red, or warm to touch the client may have an infection.

Impaired Skin Integrity

Skin integrity is impaired owing to a decreased oxygen supply to the affected limb. This impairment can range from ischemia to gangrene.

Planning: client goals. The primary goal for this nursing diagnosis is that the client will not develop an ulcer. If ulcer formation occurs, the goal is that the ulcer will heal.

Interventions: nonsurgical management. Prevention is the most important intervention associated with impairment of skin integrity or ulcer formation. The nurse educates the client about how ulcers occur. Arterial ulcers can occur because of minor trauma or poor foot care. Clients are instructed about proper foot care and protective measures to help prevent ulcer formation. An ulcer may develop despite preventive measures, necessitating wound interventions.

Managing arterial ulcers can be difficult. Some are chronic in nature, but many are acute. The underlying cause of arterial obstruction must first be determined. Arterial ulcers have minimal response to treatment if the arterial blood flow to the affected limb is not improved.

Nonsurgical treatment of the ulcer can vary. Because all ulcers are fertile ground for infection, sterile technique is used for wound care. Antibiotic therapy may be indicated, via oral, topical, or IV administration, if the ulcer is accompanied by cellulitis (reddened, inflamed area). Wet-to-dry saline dressings are commonly used with arterial ulcers. The nurse secures the dressing without tape so as not to endanger the integrity of surrounding tissue.

Arterial ulcers are commonly odorous. The nurse notes any change in odor, secretions, or redness extending up the foot or leg. Close observation can enable treatment to prevent further complications.

Interventions: surgical management. Surgical débridement is used early in the course of management of leg ulcers. Surgical débridement involves removing the dense eschar (outer) tissue so the wound can granulate, form healthier tissue, and heal. This procedure may need to be done several times before healing can occur.

Preoperative care. If the wound is superficial, débridement can be done with local anesthesia. The client needs reassurance and education about the procedure and its indications. A preoperative medication may be administered to relax the client before the procedure.

Postoperative care. Postoperatively, the nurse should observe for any bleeding at the ulcer site. Pain medication may be indicated after débridement. Aseptic dressing changes are necessary to prevent infection, and the nurse continues to observe for signs of infection.

Another surgical procedure indicated in the management of ulcers is amputation. Amputation may include the digits, a foot, or the entire limb, depending on the extensiveness of the problem. Amputations are usually indicated in clients who have compromised overall health owing to an ulcer infection (or gangrene), which may progress to septicemia or severe disabling pain. Amputation is also indicated in clients who have had unsuccessful revascularization procedures for arterial disease and in diabetics with severe diabetic ulcers.

The trend is toward distal amputations, such as transmetatarsal or below the knee instead of above the knee. These promote better postamputation rehabilitation. The goals of an amputation procedure are successful stump healing, promotion of optimal rehabilitation to ambulation, and elimination of predisposing factors. Distal amputations are not possible if the infection, gangrene, or cellulitis extends high on the limb. They are also not indicated if there is an arterial occlusion above the knee.

Physiologic amputation may occur in clients with arterial or diabetic ulcers. Usually, a digit with gangrene amputates itself after a period of time. Some clients have the extremity wrapped in dry ice for an average of 72 hours to promote physiologic amputation. For further discussion of the care of a client with an amputation, the reader is referred to Chapter 31.

Activity Intolerance

Activity intolerance is related to pain experienced by the client with PAD. The degree of activity intolerance is directly related to the severity of disease.

Planning: client goals. The goals are that the client will (1) increase activity tolerance to an optimal level of functioning through pain management and (2) participate in an exercise program that increases activity tolerance.

Interventions: nonsurgical management. Exercise and pain management are the key interventions for activity intolerance. An exercise program should be developed for each client individually. Clients with arterial disease can develop collateral circulation through exercise, whereas clients with venous disease may prevent edema through exercise.

The nurse first assesses the walking distance that each client can tolerate before claudication. The client is encouraged to begin exercise by walking on flat surfaces, avoiding hills and stairs. The client starts out slowly with walking a block or two and increases the distance each week as tolerated. With arterial disease, the client is encouraged to rest at intervals and then continue to walk. The nurse evaluates the exercise program regularly and makes adjustments as needed.

Pain management is another key in increasing activity tolerance. Clients with arterial disease can experience severe pain with ambulation. In addition to pain medications, other methods of pain management should be encouraged, such as relaxation. Pain can be chronic and difficult to manage.

■ Discharge Planning

Home Care Preparation

Clients with arterial compromise may need assistance with ADL if activity is limited by pain. Stair climbing may be limited or avoided, depending on the severity of disease. Clients who have undergone surgery have activity limits necessitating temporary assistance with ADL.

Client/Family Education

The nurse instructs all clients on methods to promote vasodilation (see earlier). Instruction about positioning

---

CLIENT/FAMILY EDUCATION ■ Foot Care Instructions for Clients with Peripheral Vascular Disease

"Keep your feet clean by washing them with a mild soap in room-temperature water."

"Keep your feet dry, especially between the toes and ankles."

"Avoid injury to your feet and ankles. Wear comfortable, well-fitting shoes. Never go without shoes."

"Keep your toenails clean and cut. Have someone cut them if you cannot see them clearly. Cut your toenails straight across."

"To prevent dry, cracked skin, apply a mild lanolin lotion to your feet."

"Prevent exposure to extreme heat or cold. Never use a heating pad on your feet."

"Avoid constricting garments."

"If a problem develops, see a podiatrist or a physician."

"Avoid extended pressure on your feet or ankles, such as occurs when you lean against something."

---

and exercise is individualized. All clients are inst. to avoid raising their legs above the level of the h. unless they have concomitant venous stasis. Wri. and oral instructions on foot care and methods to pr. vent injury and ulcer development are provided for all clients (see the accompanying Client/Family Education feature). Clients who continue to take medications after discharge from the hospital receive instructions on dosage, times of administration, and pertinent side effects. Those who have undergone surgery require additional instruction regarding incision care (see Chap. 20). All clients are encouraged to avoid smoking and limit the intake of fat in the diet to less than 30% of the total day's calories (see earlier).

Psychosocial Preparation

The client who is hospitalized with chronic arterial obstruction often fears recurrent occlusion of the artery or further narrowing. The client may fear that he/she

---

NURSING RESEARCH

Nursing Interventions for Clients with Peripheral Vascular Disease Save Money.

Ventura, M. R., Young, D. E., Feldman, M. J., Pastore, P., Pikula, S., & Yates, M. A. (1985). Cost savings as an indicator of successful nursing intervention. *Nursing Research, 34,* 50–53.

Health-promoting behaviors for clients with PVD include exercise, foot care, and reduction of or abstinence from smoking. One way of measuring the effects of these behaviors is to look at the clients' need for hospital care. This experimental study involved 86 clients with arterial insufficiency of the lower extremities, randomly assigned to an experimental (n = 44) or control group (n = 42). The experimental group participated in services focused on health-promoting behaviors for clients with PVD. A pretest and a posttest were used to assess health-related activities of both groups before and at 26 weeks after the study. Data on inpatient and outpatient hospital usage in terms of cost and staff time were also collected for both groups. Results of the data showed that the experimental group increased exercise more than control clients, but there was no difference in clinical outcomes. Data on hospital usage showed that the experimental group spent significantly less time in the hospital and had significantly lower hospitalization costs for PVD-related illness.

Critique. The study is significant in terms of its conclusive support that nursing interventions for clients with PVD are cost-effective. Reports of reliability and validity of tools and description of interventions are lacking in this article.

Possible nursing implications. Cost containment related to health care is a high priority within and outside the health care arena. Nursing interventions that can be supported as cost-effective will be more valued and better utilized.

me debilitated in other ways. s commonly get worse, espe- es mellitus. The nurse, how- their participation in prescribed pharmacologic therapy, along with r smoking, can limit further atherosclerotic que formation.

The client recovering from an acute arterial occlusion is assured that treatment of the underlying problem responsible for the occlusion often prevents recurrence of occlusion.

The client who undergoes amputation of a limb requires significant support to assist in coping with changes in gait and possible disturbance in body image.

Health Care Resources

The client with limited activity because of PAD may benefit from the assistance of a home care aide. The client who has undergone surgery may require a home care nurse to assist with incision care. Clients who have amputations usually need physical therapy to assist with ambulation.

 Evaluation

Evaluation of the client with arterial occlusive disease is based on outcome criteria for each nursing diagnosis. The expected outcomes are that the client

1. Demonstrates improved peripheral tissue perfusion, manifested by palpable or audible pedal pulses and absence of claudication

2. Does not develop arterial ulcers

3. Demonstrates improved activity tolerance as evidenced by performance of ADL and exercise

4. Verbalizes an understanding of interventions that can help prevent complications of arterial disease

By meeting these outcome criteria, the likelihood that disease progression will result in limb loss is decreased.

VENOUS DISEASE

OVERVIEW

Pathophysiology

Veins must be patent with functioning valves to function properly. Veins also require the assistance of the surrounding muscle beds to help pump blood toward the heart. If one or more of these are not operating efficiently, the veins become distended, and clinical manifestations occur. Two distinct phenomena alter the blood flow in veins: thrombus formation and defective valves. Venous thrombosis can lead to pulmonary embolism, which is a life-threatening complication (see Chap. 62). Defective valves lead to varicose veins and

venous insufficiency, which are not life-threatening, but problematic.

Thrombus formation constitutes one of medicine's greatest challenges. A *thrombus* (blood clot) is believed to result from an endothelial injury, venous stasis, and/or hypercoagulability. However, the thrombosis may not be specifically attributable to one element, or it may involve all three elements. Thrombosis is often associated with an inflammatory process. When a thrombus develops, inflammation can occur around the thrombus, thickening the vein wall and consequently leading to embolization. *Thrombophlebitis* is the term used when a thrombus is associated with inflammation, and *phlebothrombosis* is a thrombus without inflammation. Thrombophlebitis can occur in superficial veins; however, it most frequently occurs in the deep veins of the lower extremities. Deep venous thrombophlebitis, commonly referred to as deep venous thrombosis (DVT), is not only more common, but is also more serious than superficial thrombophlebitis because it presents greater risk for pulmonary embolism.

Varicose veins are dilated and tortuous superficial veins that occur primarily in the lower extremities. Their clinical significance relates mainly to their discomfort and unattractive appearance. Varicose veins are discussed later.

Venous insufficiency occurs from prolonged venous hypertension, which stretches the veins and damages the valves. This can lead to a back-up of blood and venous hypertension, resulting in edema. Edema occurs as the by-products of red blood cells break down and infiltrate the surrounding tissues. Waste products cannot be eliminated, so they accumulate within the tissues. With time, this stasis results in damaged tissue's causing venous stasis ulcers, swelling, and cellulitis. Venous stasis ulcers are discussed later.

Etiology

The efficiency of veins is altered when thrombosis occurs or when valves are not functioning correctly.

Thrombus formation has been associated with stasis of blood flow, endothelial injury, and/or hypercoagulability. Precise information about the cause of these events remains unknown; however, a few predisposing factors have been identified. Thrombosis has more commonly occurred in individuals undergoing certain surgical procedures. The highest incidence of clot formation occurs with hip surgery and open prostate surgery. Other conditions that seem to promote thrombus formation are pregnancy, ulcerative colitis, and CHF. Immobilization can be a predisposing factor for thrombosis. This can occur during prolonged bed rest and immobility, such as that which occurs during the perioperative period. Phlebitis associated with invasive procedures, such as IV therapy, can predispose clients to thrombosis. Severe infections, lupus erythematosus, polycythemia, and trauma have also been linked to thrombosis.

Defective valves can result from prolonged venous

hypertension, which stretches the veins and damages valves. This can occur in individuals who stand or sit in one position for long periods.

Pregnancy and obesity can also cause chronically distended veins, which lead to damaged valves. Thrombus formation can also cause valve destruction.

Incidence

Approximately 3% of clients who undergo major general surgery develop manifestations of thrombophlebitis. However, signs and symptoms are absent in about half of the clients who have a thrombophlebitis. Clients who undergo a surgical procedure such as total hip replacement or who have disorders that require long periods of bed rest have a higher than expected incidence of thrombophlebitis. Women who use oral contraceptives have a higher than expected incidence, especially if they are older than age 30 years and smoke.

Chronic venous insufficiency often occurs in clients who have had thrombophlebitis, although a history of this is not obtainable in 25% of these clients (Tierney & Erskine, 1988).

PREVENTION

Awareness of individuals who are at risk for thrombosis is crucial for the nurse. Close observation after surgery or during any time of immobilization assists in early detection. The nurse mobilizes asymptomatic, but high-risk clients as soon and as much as possible after surgery or other periods of immobilization. Instructing clients at risk to exercise their legs may help prevent the development of a thrombus. A prophylactic dose of an anticoagulant, such as heparin (5000 units twice daily subcutaneously), is often used postoperatively for selected clients at high risk for thrombus formation.

Venous insufficiency may be prevented in individuals prone to this problem by instructing clients to wear support stockings and to avoid immobilization. Clients who sit for long periods at work or during recreation should ambulate intermittently. Chairbound or bedridden clients should exercise their extremities as regularly as possible to provide muscle support and to facilitate pumping of blood back to the heart. If edema is present, the lower extremities should be elevated at every opportunity, or for more than 2 hours/day.

COLLABORATIVE MANAGEMENT

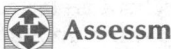 **Assessment**

History

The nurse collects a health history, which includes *age*, history of *thrombophlebitis*, and *recent medical history*, including surgery and trauma. Clients are assessed for recent *immobilization*, such as that induced by traveling in an airplane or an automobile. The nurse asks the female client if she is pregnant or receiving *estrogen therapy*, such as oral contraceptives. All clients are questioned about intermittent *leg swelling*.

Physical Assessment: Clinical Manifestations

The classic signs and symptoms of DVT are *calf or groin tenderness* and *pain*, with or without *leg swelling*. Pain in the calf on dorsiflexion of the foot (Homan's sign) is another possible indicator of DVT. The nurse examines the area that the client describes as painful, comparing this site with the contralateral limb. The nurse gently palpates the site, observing for warmth and edema. Signs and symptoms, however, are often absent with thrombophlebitis. Because there are often silent clinical findings, the nurse must have a high index of suspicion for this disorder when caring for clients at high risk.

Localized edema in one extremity suggests thrombophlebitis. Edema in both extremities is seen in clients with venous insufficiency. Edema is described by the degree of pitting that occurs (see Chap. 13). Checking the degree of pitting edema is done by pressing two fingers into the edematous area and, after a few seconds, removing the fingers. If the edema is pitting, impressions of the fingers are still visible. With edema caused by venous stasis, there may be *stasis dermatitis* or discoloration along the ankles, extending up to the calf.

In individuals with long-term venous insufficiency or stasis, *ulcer formation* often occurs. Ulcer formation can result from the edema, or it may be due to minor injury to the limb. Generally, these ulcers are chronic and difficult to heal (see Key Features of Disease: Differential Features of Ulcers of the Lower Extremity). Many of these clients live with ulcers for years, and recurrence is common. Some of these individuals may lose one or both of their limbs.

Psychosocial Assessment

Clients with thrombophlebitis are confronted with an unexpected illness, which requires significant interruption in ADL. The nurse assesses the client's usual roles (e.g., parent, caregiver, and employee) and their significance to the client. The nurse asks the client how these roles are affected by the illness and assesses for anxiety and stress related to the role change. The nurse also assesses the client with thrombophlebitis for fear related to the risk of pulmonary embolus.

Venous insufficiency is a chronic condition, and clients are required to limit the time they spend standing and to elevate their legs as much as possible. Clients with venous stasis ulcers often undergo treatment for months to years. The nurse assesses clients for anxiety and stress related to the chronicity of their illness.

Laboratory Findings

There are no specific laboratory tests to diagnose thrombophlebitis or venous insufficiency. The white blood cell count may be elevated with thrombophlebitis. Partial thromboplastin time (PTT) and prothrombin time (PT) are determined if thrombophlebitis is suspected. These tests are done to assess the client's baseline clotting capabilities before administering heparin.

Radiographic Findings

A method of evaluating the venous system is through radiopaque contrast venography. This method provides visualization of clot formation in approximately 95% of cases. Venograms were previously viewed as a diagnostic standard, but now are *not* deemed necessary for every client. The test requires venous injections of contrast medium into the affected limb. Risks of this procedure are dangerous, as the study itself can cause thrombophlebitis or clot formation. Venograms should not be performed on individuals with suspected or acute phlebitis.

Other Diagnostic Tests

One method of evaluation of the venous system is fibrinogen scanning. Fibrinogen with a radioactive iodine marker is injected into the vein of a client with suspected DVT. The substance acts similarly to the client's own fibrinogen, collecting in the clot. This collection shows up on a scintillation camera. The clot is then identified by higher counts of radioactive iodine than circulating levels in the blood. If this persists for 24 hours, the diagnosis of DVT is supported.

Some of the same tests that are used to evaluate the arterial system are used for the venous system, such as Doppler ultrasonography. Normal venous circulation has audible signals, whereas thrombosed veins produce little or no flow.

Impedance phlebography is used to evaluate DVT of the iliac or femoral veins, but it does not give information about thrombi activity in the calf, the ankle, or the toes.

The Perthes test is performed to evaluate the competency of the saphenous vein and/or to look for DVT. This test is accomplished by applying a tourniquet around the thigh of a client in the standing position. The client is asked to walk for approximately 5 minutes. After walking, the veins may appear collapsed.

 Analysis: Nursing Diagnosis

Common Diagnoses

Common nursing diagnoses for clients with venous disease include

1. Altered (peripheral) tissue perfusion related to impaired venous flow
2. Impaired skin integrity related to edema

Additional Diagnoses

Additional nursing diagnoses related to venous disease include

1. Potential for infection related to ulcer formation
2. Fear related to the threat of pulmonary embolus
3. Knowledge deficit related to unfamiliarity with venous disorders
4. Potential for impaired gas exchange related to the risk of pulmonary embolism

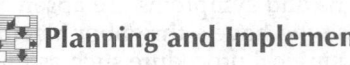 **Planning and Implementation**

Altered Tissue Perfusion (Peripheral)

Altered (peripheral) tissue perfusion occurs because the venous blood flow is impaired. Impairment is caused by incompetent valves, thrombosis, or injury of the lower extremities.

Planning: client goals. The major goal is that the client will have improved venous blood return to the heart, decreasing stasis and waste by-product interactions.

Interventions. The focus of treatment for thrombophlebitis is to prevent complications, such as pulmonary emboli, and to prevent an increase in size of the thrombus. Thrombophlebitis of the deep veins, also called deep venous thrombophlebitis, is the most common type of thrombophlebitis. Interventions discussed here relate to DVT. All clients with DVT are hospitalized for treatment.

The focus of treating venous insufficiency is to decrease edema and promote venous return from the extremity. Clients are not usually hospitalized for this condition alone, unless it is complicated by an ulcer or another disorder is occurring simultaneously.

Nonsurgical management. Thrombophlebitis and chronic venous insufficiency are most often treated medically without surgical intervention. Supportive therapy for deep venous thrombophlebitis includes bed rest and elevation of the extremity. Some physicians order intermittent or continuous warm, moist soaks. Clients are instructed on the importance of maintaining bed rest to avoid dislodgement of the thrombus. The nurse assesses all clients for signs and symptoms of pulmonary embolus, which include shortness of breath and chest pain.

As soon as the diagnosis is made, the client is started on a regimen of IV heparin therapy. Heparin is an anticoagulant agent that prevents the activation of clotting factor IX and inhibits the formation of fibrin threads. Heparin does nothing to the existing clot. It is given to prevent formation of other clots, which often develop in the presence of an existing clot. Heparin is initially given by a bolus IV dose of approximately 100 units/kg, followed by constant infusion regulated by a reliable infusion device. Concentrations of heparin (in 5% dextrose in water) and the number of units or milliliters per hour are ordered by the physician to maintain a therapeutic PTT. PTTs are obtained daily, or more frequently, and reported as soon as results are available, to allow adjustment of heparin dosage. Therapeutic levels of PTTs are usually 1½ to 2 times normal control levels. The nurse assesses clients for signs and symptoms of bleeding, which include hematuria, frank or occult blood in stool, ecchymosis, petechiae, altered level of consciousness, or pain.

After the client's signs and symptoms of thrombophlebitis have greatly resolved, the client is given warfarin sodium (Coumadin). Warfarin inhibits hepatic synthesis of the four vitamin K–dependent clotting factors. It takes 2 to 3 days before warfarin is able to exert therapeutic anticoagulation. For this reason, warfarin administration is started while the IV heparin is being infused. The heparin continues to provide therapeutic anticoagulation until this effect is achieved with warfarin. IV heparin is discontinued at that time. Therapeutic levels of warfarin are monitored by measuring PT. A therapeutic PT with warfarin administration is often 1½ times normal control levels. The initial dosage of warfarin is usually 10 to 15 mg daily for 1 to 2 days. Maintenance therapy ranges from 2.5 to 7.5 mg given once a day in the evening. Clients are usually given warfarin for 6 months after an episode of thrombophlebitis. Assessment for bleeding is similar to that described for clients receiving heparin.

Interventions for clients with chronic venous insufficiency include use of elastic stockings, which fit from the middle of the foot to just below the knee. The stockings should be worn during the day and evening. Clients are instructed to elevate their legs for at least 20 minutes four or five times per day, but to avoid long periods of sitting or standing in place. When the client is in bed, the legs should be elevated above the level of the heart.

Surgical management. Surgical removal of a deep venous thrombus is rarely performed, unless there is a massive occlusion that does not respond to medical treatment, and the thrombus is of recent (1 to 2 days') onset. Preoperative preparation and postoperative care of clients undergoing thrombectomy are similar to that for clients undergoing arterial surgery (see earlier).

Surgical intervention is most frequently indicated for clients who have recurrent thrombophlebitis and/or pulmonary emboli that are unresponsive to medical treatment. Insertion of an inferior vena cava filter is the most common surgical treatment performed for these clients. This surgery involves inserting a filter device to trap emboli in the inferior vena cava, before they progress to the lungs. Holes in the device allow blood to pass through, thus not significantly interfering with the return of blood to the heart. Preoperative care of the client having this procedure is similar to that provided for clients having local anesthesia (see Chap. 18). If clients have recently been taking anticoagulants, such as warfarin or heparin, the nurse consults with the physi-

cian about interrupting this therapy in the preoperative period to avoid hemorrhage. Postoperative nursing care involves inspecting the incision in the right side of the chest for bleeding and signs or symptoms of infection. Ligation, which involves tying off the inferior vena cava, or plication, which involves stitching the inferior vena cava to block emboli, may be performed if anticoagulant therapy is contraindicated or if filter devices cannot be placed.

Surgery for chronic venous insufficiency is usually not performed because historically it has not been successful. Attempts at transplanting vein valves have had limited success.

Impaired Skin Integrity

Skin impairment occurs because of waste product interactions and edema. Ulcer formation is common.

Planning: client goals.   The primary goal for this nursing diagnosis is that the client will not develop an ulcer. If ulcer formation occurs, the goal is that the ulcer will heal.

Interventions: nonsurgical management.   Venous stasis ulcers are slightly more manageable than ulcers due to arterial disease. They are chronic in nature, with some clients manifesting the same ulcer for years. Ulcers often heal only to reoccur at a later time in the same area. The client may have simultaneous ulcers for several years. Managing venous stasis ulcers is twofold: first to heal the ulcer and second to prevent stasis with recurrence of ulcer formation. Two types of occlusive dressings can be used on venous stasis ulcers: oxygen permeable and oxygen impermeable. Because the role of atmospheric oxygen in wound healing is controversial, opinions vary with regard to which type of dressing is preferred. Dressings include the oxygen-permeable polyethylene film (e.g., Op Site) and an oxygen-impermeable hydrocolloid dressing (e.g., DuoDerm). Whatever the choice, the dressing should be evaluated frequently and changed often to keep the ulcer clean.

If the client is ambulatory, an Unna boot may be indicated. An Unna boot is constructed of gauze that has been moistened with zinc oxide. This is applied to the affected limb from the toes to the knee after the ulcer has been cleaned appropriately. The Unna boot is then covered with an elastic wrap and hardens like a cast. This promotes venous return and prevents stasis. The Unna boot also forms a sterile environment for the ulcer. Unna's boots should be changed approximately once a week, and clients should be instructed about what to look for if arterial occlusion should occur from an Unna boot that is too tight.

Drug therapy includes topical agents for venous ulcers. Chemical débridement may be necessary to eliminate necrotic tissue and promote healing of venous ulcers. Sutilains (Travase) is a proteolytic enzyme that digests necrotic tissue and is used to débride venous ulcers. Sutilains is most effective for ulcers that are superficial limb ulcers, such as venous stasis ulcers. Fibrinolysin and desoxyribonuclease (Elase) débrides necrotic tissue and fibrinous exudates. Fibrinolysin and desoxyribonuclease is most effective after dry eschar tissue has been removed surgically.

If an infection occurs or cellulitis develops, systemic antibiotics are more effective than local ointments. Local antibiotic ointments inhibit the ulcer's healing by occluding the ulcer and prohibiting the needed interactions with air.

Interventions: surgical management. Débridement for venous ulcers is similar to that performed for arterial ulcers (see earlier).

■ Discharge Planning

Home Care Preparation

Clients recovering from thrombophlebitis are usually ambulatory when discharged from the hospital. Education related to the hazards of anticoagulation therapy is the primary focus of planning for discharge. The nurse assists the client in identifying situations and equipment that might cause trauma, such as the use of a straight-edged razor. Arrangements are made to avoid hazardous situations and to procure alternative types of equipment, such as an electric razor. Clients with venous stasis are assisted in planning for opportunities and facilities to allow for elevation of the affected extremity.

Client/Family Education

Clients recovering from thrombophlebitis are discharged from the hospital on a regimen of warfarin. The nurse instructs clients and their families to avoid potentially traumatic situations, such as participation in contact sports. All clients are provided with written and oral information about the signs and symptoms of bleeding (see earlier). Any of these manifestations must be reported to the health care provider immediately. The anticoagulant effect of warfarin may be reversed by the omission of one or two doses of the drug or by the administration of vitamin K. In case of injury, clients are directed to apply pressure to bleeding wounds and to seek medical assistance immediately. Clients are encouraged to carry an identification card or wear a medical alert (Medic Alert) bracelet that states that they are taking warfarin.

Clients are instructed to inform their dentist and other health care providers that they are taking warfarin before receiving treatment or prescriptions. PTs are affected by many prescription and OTC medications, such as antacids, antihistamines, aspirin, mineral oil, oral contraceptives, and large doses of vitamin C. The action of warfarin is also affected by high-fat and vitamin K–rich foods, such as cabbage, cauliflower, broccoli, asparagus, lettuce, turnip, spinach, kale, fish, liver, coffee, and green tea. Clients are therefore instructed to eat a well-balanced diet and to avoid taking additional medi-

cations without consulting a physician. Arrangements for clients to have PTs determined 1 to 2 weeks after discharge from the hospital also need to be made.

Clients with thrombophlebitis or venous stasis are taught to avoid standing still, to elevate their legs when sitting, to avoid crossing their legs, and to avoid wearing tight girdles, tight pants, and narrow-banded knee-high socks. Support hose or antiembolism stockings are prescribed by the physician. The nurse instructs the client to apply these stockings before getting out of bed in the morning and to remove them just before going to bed at night. Exercise is prescribed on an individual basis with the physician's input. All clients are encouraged to maintain an optimal weight. Clients with venous stasis ulcers are instructed on the care of the ulcer (see earlier).

Psychosocial Preparation

Clients who fear recurrence of thrombophlebitis are assured that participation in the prescribed treatment frequently assists in resolution of this problem. Clients with venous stasis disease, especially those with venous stasis ulcers, may require long-term emotional support to assist them in meeting their chronic care needs.

Health Care Resources

Clients who have occupations that require standing or prolonged sitting may need to consider a job change. Social services agencies and occupational therapists may be consulted to discuss these problems and to suggest alternative employment opportunities. Clients with venous stasis ulcers who cannot perform dressing changes independently may require the assistance of a home care nurse.

 Evaluation

Evaluation of the client's progress is based on outcome criteria developed for each nursing diagnosis. The expected outcomes are that the client

1. Demonstrates improved tissue perfusion manifested by absence of pain and edema
2. Has no signs or symptoms of pulmonary embolus
3. Avoids development of venous ulcers

ANEURYSMS

OVERVIEW

Aneurysms have been recognized for centuries. Galen provided the first accurate description of an arterial aneurysm in the second century, and aneurysms of the aorta were recognized by anatomists in the 16th century. The clinical course and management vary, depending on the location, the size, and the type of the aneurysm.

Pathophysiology

An *aneurysm* is an abnormal dilation of an artery as a result of localized weakness and stretching of the arterial wall. A variety of different disease processes can lead to the formation of an aneurysm. An aneurysm is formed, regardless of the etiology, when the middle layer (media) of the artery is weakened, producing a stretching effect in the inner layer (intima) and outer layers (adventitia) of the artery. The effect of blood pressure on the artery wall produces further weakness in the media of the artery and enlarges the aneurysm.

Arteriosclerosis is the most common etiology of aneurysms. With arteriosclerosis, an atheromatous plaque forms on the intimal surface of the artery. The medial coat weakens as a result of a combination of factors, including wear and tear and impaired nutrition. The destruction of the medial layer containing the elastic fibers is believed to result in formation of the aneurysm.

Arteriosclerotic aneurysms can contain mural thrombi. The development of the thrombus and the formation of fibrous tissue around the arterial wall are thought to be attempts to prevent progressive enlargement of the aneurysm. The mural thrombus can be a reservoir of emboli below the aneurysm in the distal arterial tree.

True aneurysms involve all three layers of the arterial wall. Most aneurysms are designated as true aneurysms. A false aneurysm is a pulsating hematoma. With false aneurysms, the clot is outside the arterial wall.

Types

Several types of aneurysms have been identified: *saccular* aneurysm, an outpouching from a distinct portion of the artery wall; *fusiform* aneurysm, a diffuse dilation that involves the total circumference of the artery; *dissecting* aneurysm, a cavity formed when blood separates the layers of the artery wall; and *false* aneurysm, a complete rupture of an artery with subsequent aneurysm formation.

Locations

Aneurysms tend to occur at certain anatomic sites (Fig. 65–6). The most common site for aneurysm formation is the aorta. Often, aneurysms are found at a point where the artery is not supported by skeletal muscles or on the lines of curves or lines of flexion in the arterial tree.

Abdominal aneurysms are most often the result of arteriosclerosis. Abdominal aneurysms arise below the level of the renal arteries, but above the iliac bifurcation. Abdominal aneurysms can be either saccular or fusiform, but the latter is the most common.

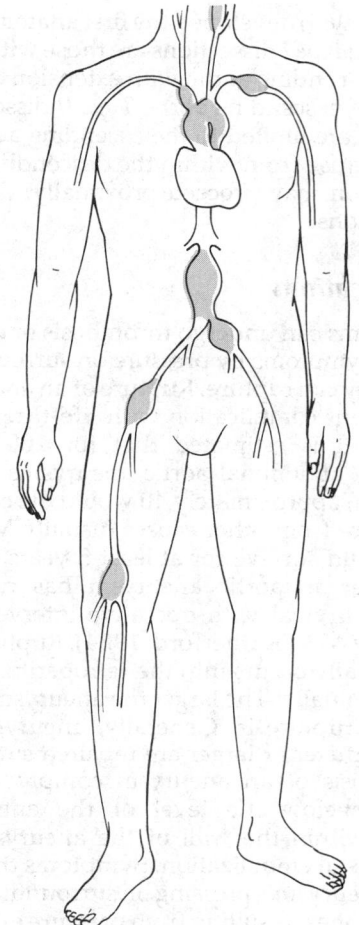

Figure 65–6

Common anatomic sites of arterial aneurysms.

Thoracic aneurysms commonly develop between the origin of the left subclavian artery and the diaphragm. Thoracic aneurysms can be seen in the descending, ascending, or transverse sections of the aorta. The thoracic aorta is the most common site for the formation of dissecting aneurysms. Arteriosclerotic aneurysms of the thoracic aorta are usually fusiform.

Femoral and popliteal aneurysms are relatively uncommon. Bilateral aneurysms are often seen in clients with popliteal or femoral aneurysms. Femoral and popliteal aneurysms result most often from arteriosclerosis and can be either fusiform or saccular. Often, these aneurysms are associated with an aneurysm in another location of the arterial tree.

Classification of Aortic Aneurysms

The basic pathophysiology of aortic dissections is not completely understood. Medial degeneration of the aorta may eventually lead to an intimal tear, followed by the propagation of a dissecting hematoma of varying depth and length along the aortic wall. DeBakey and associates (1965) developed the first anatomic classification scheme: *type I* dissections are those with the intimal tear in the ascending aorta, with extension of the dissection into the descending aorta. *Type II* dissections originate in and are limited to the ascending aorta. *Type III* dissections arise from within the descending aorta, and the dissection may proceed proximally, distally, or in both directions.

Complications

Aneurysms can undergo thrombosis or embolization and cause symptoms by pressure on surrounding structures, or they can rupture. Rupture of an aneurysm is the most frequent complication with life-threatening consequences. It is estimated that for 100 consecutive clients with abdominal aortic aneurysms that are not operated on, approximately 40 would die of rupture, 30 would expire from other causes (usually MI or stroke), and 30 would survive for at least 5 years (Rutherford, 1989). After an aortic aneurysm has ruptured, the chance of survival with operative intervention is approximately 45% (Rutherford, 1984). Rupture of the aneurysm usually occurs into the retroperitoneal space or intra-abdominally. The larger the aneurysm, the greater the risk of rupture is. Generally, aneurysms that are 4 cm in diameter or larger are repaired surgically.

Thrombosis of an aneurysm compromises arterial circulation below the level of the aneurysm. The thrombus within the wall of the aneurysm can be a source of distal embolization. Symptoms that can result from the aneurysm's pressing on surrounding structures include dyspnea, resulting from pressure on the trachea; hoarseness, resulting from pressure on the left recurrent laryngeal nerve; or dysphagia, resulting from impingement on the esophagus.

Etiology

An aneurysm is either congenital or acquired. Acquired aneurysms can result from arteriosclerosis, trauma, infection, or syphilis. Congenital aneurysms have been found to be related to Marfan's syndrome or Ehlers-Danlos syndrome. Arteriosclerosis is the most common cause of aneurysms at all locations in the body.

The aorta is subjected to approximately 3 billion pulsations during an average life span. Normally, the wall of the aorta is elastic, constantly expanding during the pulse wave of the beating heart. Hypertension is believed to cause destruction of the media of the aorta and decrease intimal adherence. Through weakening the wall of the aorta, hypertension seems to enhance aneurysm formation.

Inherited or congenital defects such as Ehlers-Danlos syndrome may lead to aneurysm formation.

Inflammation of the arteries is a late manifestation of syphilis. The spirochetes of syphilis commonly attack the aorta at the aortic arch, ascending aorta, and pulmonary artery. Syphilis produces medial necrosis by impairing nutrition of the medial coat, resulting in slow degeneration of the muscle fibers. The wall of the aorta weakens, and an aneurysm is formed. At one time, syphilis frequently resulted in thoracic aneurysms. However, because of the declining incidence of syphilis, syphilis is no longer a common cause of aneurysm formation.

Infection can also cause aneurysms. Mycotic aneurysms of the aorta can follow septicemia that seeds a pre-existing arterial lesion, whether atherosclerotic, congenital, or traumatic. A local suppuration weakens the medial layer to the point at which aneurysm formation or rupture occurs. Bacterial infections with methicillin-resistant staphylococcus organisms have been associated with popliteal aneurysms.

Trauma can result in both true and false aneurysms. False aneurysms are the most common type of aneurysm to develop after trauma. Automobile accidents can produce acute traumatic rupture of the aortic arch, at times with false aneurysm formation. Bullet wounds can tear the outer coats of an artery or cause rupture with little external bleeding. A hematoma could develop, forming a false aneurysm. True aneurysms can develop in superficial arteries, such as those in the palm of the hand, when the arteries are subjected to repeated blunt trauma.

Incidence

Arteriosclerotic abdominal aneurysms are the most common type of aneurysm. Abdominal aneurysms usually develop in clients older than age 50 years. More men than women have an abdominal aneurysm, with ratios of 2 : 1 or greater reported. The incidence of abdominal aneurysms has increased in the past 30 years from 8.7 new aneurysms diagnosed per 100,000 individuals in a year from 1951 to 1960 to 36.5 aneurysms per 100,000 individuals in a year from 1971 to 1980 (Bickerstaff, 1984).

Thoracic aneurysms occur most often in the sixth and seventh decades of life. The incidence of the disease is higher in men than women, by at least 3 : 1. Popliteal aneurysms account for approximately 70% of peripheral aneurysms, with femoral aneurysms accounting for the remainder (Rutherford, 1984). Most popliteal aneurysms are found after the sixth decade.

Aortic dissections occur in approximately 60,000 clients per year (Sabiston, 1986). Aortic dissections are about three times more frequent in men than in women. Acute dissections are usually seen in clients between the ages of 45 and 70 years. The incidence of aortic dissection seems to be higher in clients with Marfan's syndrome or congenital heart disease (Sabiston, 1986).

PREVENTION

Arteriosclerotic aneurysms are the most common type of aneurysms at almost every location. The nursing interventions are aimed at risk factor modification of the arteriosclerotic process (see earlier). Risk factors include hypertension, cigarette smoking, hypercholesterolemia, obesity, diabetes mellitus, elevated triglyceride levels, sedentary life style, stress, and familial predisposition.

COLLABORATIVE MANAGEMENT

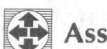 **Assessment**

History

When taking a history from a client with an aneurysm, data collection includes *age, sex,* and *race,* as aneurysms occur more frequently in middle-aged or older Caucasian males. Other risk factors to investigate include *cigarette usage, hypercholesterolemia, hypertension, obesity, stress,* and *familial predisposition.* The nurse obtains information about the client's past medical history. Clients are asked about the use of medications, including OTC drugs. Examples of OTC drugs to look for include nasal sprays and antihistamines that have vasoconstrictive properties. It is important to know if the client is being treated for hypertension, as there is a higher incidence of aneurysm rupture associated with hypertension. If the client is diabetic, the nurse inquires about measures used in diabetes control.

Physical Assessment: Clinical Manifestations

Abdominal aneurysms may be palpated by the nurse as a prominent *pulsation* in the upper abdomen, slightly to the left of the midline. Small aneurysms are approximately 5 cm in diameter, but can range in size to 20 cm or greater. Tenderness may be present on palpation; therefore, palpation should be performed gently. Percussion of the abdomen over the prominent pulsation assists in confirming the palpation findings regarding the size of the aneurysm.

Abdominal aneurysms may occur with no symptoms or with symptoms of *abdominal or lower-back pain.* The enlargement of the aneurysm can result in partial *intestinal obstruction* or, if erosion occurs, upper GI tract *bleeding.* The nurse assesses for this by palpating the abdomen for tenderness or rigidity.

Thoracic aneurysms cannot be detected by physical assessment. The clinical manifestations reported by the client commonly result from compression or obstruction of adjacent structures, dissection, or rupture. The most common symptom is *chest pain,* which is often deep and aching. Pain is usually located in the chest and may radiate to the neck, the back, or the shoulders. Less commonly, the client may complain of pain in the lower back or abdominal area. Thoracic aneurysms can cause hoarseness or coughing if there is stretching of the left recurrent laryngeal nerve. In the face of impending rupture, the pain can become severe.

Popliteal aneurysms can be detected by palpating a *pulsating mass* in the popliteal space. With a femoral aneurysm, the nurse detects a pulsatile mass over the femoral artery. Both extremities should be evaluated because more than one femoral or popliteal aneurysm may be present. The client may exhibit symptoms of limb ischemia. Pain may be present if an adjacent nerve is compressed.

Rupture of an aortic eneurysm usually is accompanied by severe abdominal or back pain, with the client going into immediate *shock.* The most common clinical manifestation of an aortic dissection is *pain of sudden onset,* which is often tearing in quality. The pain is usually located in the substernal area, but it may also be felt in the precordium, the neck, the jaw, the extremities, the epigastric region, or the back. Other physical findings include symptoms of pulmonary edema, diminished heart sounds, and a murmur of aortic insufficiency. The blood pressure readings in the client's arm may vary if compromise of the distal artery has occurred. Hypertension can occur during dissection, but hypotension would be a finding if the client has gone into shock. Neurologic changes occur if cerebral vessels are compromised.

Psychosocial Assessment

The nurse assesses each client's perception of the diagnosis of an aneurysm. Clients may see the diagnosis as a sentence of impending death or may understand that an aneurysm can be surgically corrected with relatively low risk.

The nurse assesses the client's occupational history; clients with strenuous occupations may not be able to work until several months after the aneurysm is surgically repaired or may need to alter other activities.

Laboratory Findings

No laboratory tests can confirm a diagnosis of an aneurysm. If the client is actually bleeding, as in the case of a ruptured or dissecting aneurysm, there is a rapid decrease in hemoglobin and hematocrit levels.

Radiographic Findings

X-ray films of the abdomen show the presence of an abdominal aortic aneurysm. Plain films of the abdomen or a lateral film of the abdomen (in calcified aneurysm) is ordered. The "eggshell" appearance of the aneurysm is essentially diagnostic (Fig. 65–7).

Arteriography is an invasive method that can be utilized in the diagnosis of an abdominal aortic aneurysm.

X-ray films of the chest reveal the eggshell appearance of the aneurysm in the thoracic aorta. The diagnosis is confirmed by arteriography of the aortic arch. Popliteal and femoral aneurysms are best found on arteriography. X-ray films of the chest that reveal mediastinal widening are suggestive, but not diagnostic, of aortic dissection. Diagnosis of aortic dissection is best provided by aortography.

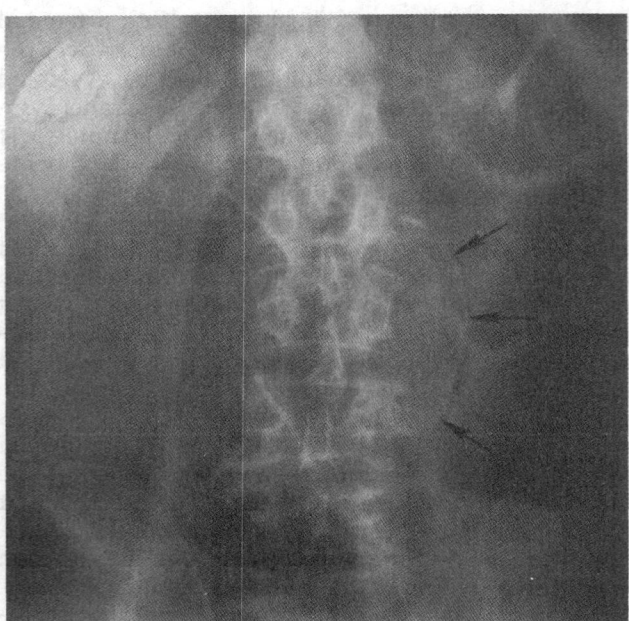

Figure 65–7
Plain x-ray film of the abdomen of a client with an abdominal aortic aneurysm (arrows). Note the "eggshell" appearance of the border of the aneurysm, caused by calcification. (From Sabiston, D. C. [1986]. *Textbook of surgery: The biological basis of modern surgical practice* [13th ed.]. Philadelphia: W. B. Saunders.)

Computed tomographic (CT) body scanning is another useful means of assessing an aortic aneurysm. Small aneurysms are followed to assess for enlargement in clients who are not ideal surgical candidates.

Other Diagnostic Tests

Ultrasonography is a noninvasive technique that provides an accurate diagnosis, as well as information about the size and location of the aneurysm. Ultrasonography is particularly useful in following the size of small aneurysms to allow for early detection of enlargement and for prompt surgical intervention when warranted.

 Analysis: Nursing Diagnosis

The client with an intact aneurysm may have no symptoms. Clients experiencing dissection or rupture are in severe pain and often in shock.

Common Diagnoses

The nursing diagnosis that is commonly noted in clients with an aneurysm is potential for altered (peripheral, cerebral, cardiopulmonary, gastrointestinal, renal) tissue perfusion related to a bleeding aneurysm.

Additional Diagnoses

The client may also have one or more of the following diagnoses:

1. Potential impaired skin integrity related to altered circulation secondary to the aneurysm
2. Activity tolerance related to chest, stomach, leg, or back pain secondary to the aneurysm
3. Knowledge deficit related to unfamiliarity with treatment
4. Potential for powerlessness related to the possibility of aneurysm rupture
5. Anxiety related to the possibility of aneurysm rupture.

 Planning and Implementation

The plan of care of the client with an aneurysm focuses on identified nursing diagnoses.

Potential for Altered (Peripheral, Cerebral, Cardiopulmonary, Gastrointestinal, Renal) Tissue Perfusion

Planning: client goals. The major goal for this nursing diagnosis is that the client will maintain adequate circulation without rupture of the aneurysm.

Interventions. Clients with an abdominal aortic aneurysm have either surgical or nonsurgical treatment, often depending on the size of the aneurysm.

Nonsurgical management. Because the client with an aneurysm usually has atherosclerosis, drug and diet therapy can be used to prevent progression of the disease process and further weakening of the aneurysm.

Diet therapy. To prevent or treat hypercholesterolemia, dietary restriction of fat to less than 30% of the total day's calories is recommended (see earlier). Cholesterol is restricted to less than 300 mg/day. Alcohol is restricted to no more than 1 oz/day.

Drug therapy. Clients with hypertension are often treated with antihypertensives (see earlier), to maintain normal blood pressure and limit stress on the aneurysm. Cholesterol-lowering agents such as nicotinic acid (niacin) or lovastatin (Mevacor) may be used for clients who are unable to maintain their cholesterol levels at 200 mg/dL or less.

Other measures. The prevention of complications, primarily rupture of the aneurysm, is essential. The nurse monitors for changes in vital signs, mentation, and pain in the back, the chest, the abdomen, or the legs. Clients who have a ruptured or dissecting aneurysm may be in shock, which is manifested by severe hypotension, cool skin or diaphoresis, and low urinary output. A dissecting or ruptured aneurysm requires immediate emergency surgery to control bleeding.

Surgical management. Surgical management of an aneurysm may be performed as an emergency or an elective procedure. The surgical technique for removal of an aneurysm involves exposure of the aneurysm; application of clamps just above the aneurysm and below it; excision of the aneurysm; and replacement of the excised segment with a woven, preclotted Dacron graft sutured in end-to-end fashion (Fig. 65–8). Operation for excision of an abdominal aneurysm is through a midline incision that extends from the xiphoid process to the symphysis pubis. Excision of a thoracic aneurysm is accomplished either through a median sternotomy incision or a thoracotomy incision, depending on the location and the extent of the aneurysm in the thoracic aorta. Surgical technique for repair of a femoral or popliteal aneurysm involves adequate exposure of the aneurysm, excision of the aneurysm, and restoration of circulation utilizing a Dacron graft or an autogenous saphenous vein graft.

Preoperative care. Preoperative care of clients with ruptured or dissecting aneurysms involves the administration of IV fluids, often in large volumes if tolerated by the client, to maintain tissue perfusion. Clients are usually transferred directly to surgery when the diagnosis is made. If elective procedures are planned, preoperative care involves interventions similar to those discussed for clients undergoing surgery with general anesthesia (Chap. 18). The nurse assesses all peripheral pulses, including radial, femoral, popliteal, posterior tibial, and dorsalis pedis, to serve as a baseline for comparison postoperatively. The nurse may mark where the pulse is palpated or heard by Doppler ultrasonography to facilitate locating the pulse postoperatively.

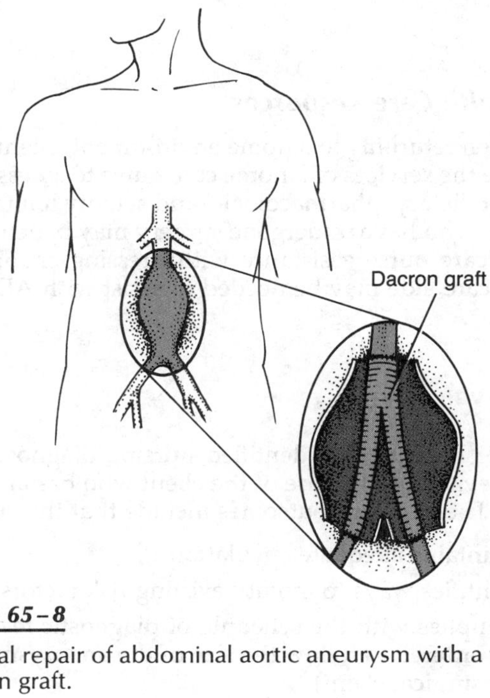

Figure 65–8
Surgical repair of abdominal aortic aneurysm with a woven Dacron graft.

Postoperative care. Postoperative care varies, depending on the type of aneurysm repair. The care of the client with abdominal aneurysm is similar to that provided for clients with other abdominal surgery. Immediately postoperatively, the client is usually admitted to a critical care setting for 24 to 48 hours. Often, the client is maintained on a ventilator at least overnight. This is done to facilitate respiratory exchange. The nurse assesses vital signs and circulation at least hourly, with assessment of pulses distal to the graft site (including posterior tibial and dorsalis pedis). Any signs of occlusion, including changes in pulses, severe pain, cool to cold extremities below the graft, and white or blue extremities, are reported to the physician immediately.

Clients undergoing aortic aneurysm repair have renal function assessed hourly, because the aorta was clamped during the repair, potentially compromising the kidneys. The nurse monitors hourly urinary output and urine color and daily BUN and creatinine levels. The client is medicated for pain as needed.

As with other abdominal surgery, the nurse monitors the client for postoperative ileus and distention. Clients normally have a nasogastric tube in place for 1 to 2 days postoperatively. The nurse auscultates the abdomen for the presence of bowel sounds. Prolonged absence of bowel sounds may indicate an ileus or a bowel infarction.

Prevention of postoperative complications is important. Frequent turning, coughing, and deep breathing or suctioning (if the client is maintained on a ventilator) is performed to assist in preventing pulmonary complications. Firm abdominal support of the incision is required during coughing to prevent incision separation. The nurse asks the client to dorsiflex and plantar flex the feet often to avoid thrombophlebitis.

The care of a client who has undergone thoracic aneurysm repair is similar to that after other chest surgery. Most dissecting aneurysms are thoracic in origin. The surgeon may repair the thoracic aneurysm utilizing either a thoracotomy or a median sternotomy approach. Most clients who have the thoracic aneurysm repaired by median sternotomy approach undergo cardiopulmonary bypass. Postoperatively, the nurse monitors vital signs until the client is stable. Any signs of shock, including a drop in blood pressure, an increase in pulse rate, rapid respirations, and diaphoresis, are reported to the physician. The nurse assesses for bleeding or separation at the graft site by noting significant increases in chest drainage from the chest tubes.

After thoracic aneurysm repair, clients are especially susceptible to development of atelectasis or pneumonia as a result of both cardiopulmonary bypass and incision discomfort that may cause shallow breathing and poor cough effort. Therefore, these clients are also often maintained on a ventilator, at least overnight after surgery. For individuals with a median sternotomy, the incision is splinted firmly to prevent separation of the sternum.

The nurse assesses all clients who are recovering from thoracic aneurysm repair for cardiac abnormalities. The stress of the thoracic surgery added to the increased incidence of arteriosclerosis in this population may predispose these clients to an MI, cardiac arrhythmias, or CHF (see Chap. 63).

In caring for clients with femoral or popliteal aneurysms, the nurse monitors for lower-limb ischemia. The nurse palpates pulses below the graft to assess graft patency. Often, Doppler ultrasonography is necessary when pulses are difficult to palpate. When using the Doppler probe, the probe is placed over the area of the artery to assess blood flow via auscultation. Sudden development of pain or discoloration of the extremity is reported immediately, because it may indicate graft occlusion.

■ Discharge Planning

The client who has an aneurysm, regardless of whether it has been surgically repaired, is usually discharged to the home environment. In rare instances, the client may be discharged to an extended (long-term) care facility for rehabilitation in the absence of family or other support systems.

Home Care Preparation

Because a fall could cause aneurysm rupture, elimination of potential hazards in the home environment is important. Clients should remove scatter rugs that could cause slipping. If the client is weak or unstable, grab bars or other devices should be installed in the bathroom to decrease the chances of a fall. Support railing can be added to the house to facilitate going up and down stairs. A walker or a cane can provide additional support when walking if needed.

Client/Family Education

The teaching plan for the client who has *not* had the aneurysm surgically repaired includes risk factor modification, avoidance of strenuous activities, prevention of falls, and compliance with the schedule of diagnostic follow-up tests.

The nurse instructs the client and the family to control modifiable risk factors. Complete cessation of smoking is strongly advised. Control of hypertension is managed through compliance with the medication regimen, diet, and frequent blood pressure checks. Hypercholesterolemia and diabetes are controlled by diet and compliance with the prescribed medication regimen. The client should maintain an ideal body weight if possible. Information is provided to the client and the family on methods of relaxation and stress reduction.

Clients who have an aneurysm are followed at regular intervals with radiography, CT, or ultrasonography to detect enlargement of the aneurysm. When an aneurysm has enlarged to an unacceptable point, prompt

surgical intervention is required. The 5-year risk of rupture for 8-cm aneurysms is more than 75%, and the chance of survival after rupture occurs varies between 17% and 66% (Hollier & Rutherford, 1989). The diagnostic tests and their importance are explained to the client and the family to facilitate compliance.

The client who *has* undergone repair of the aneurysm is taught activity restrictions, wound care, and pain management. The activity of a client who undergoes repair of an aneurysm is restricted until healing occurs. Activities that involve lifting of heavy objects, usually more than 15 to 20 lb, are not permitted for 6 to 12 weeks postoperatively. The client is advised to use discretion in activities that involve pulling, pushing, or straining. Examples of activities to restrict include vacuuming, changing bed linens, moving furniture, mopping or sweeping, raking leaves, mowing grass, and chopping wood. Examples of hobbies that should be avoided are tennis, swimming, horseback riding, and golf (putting practice is allowed). Because of postoperative weakness, the client is usually restricted from driving a car for several weeks after discharge from the hospital.

The nurse instructs the client and the family in wound care (see Chap. 20.).

Psychosocial Preparation

Clients who have not had their aneurysm repaired may fear rupture and subsequent death. The nurse assesses for clients and family perceptions related to this potential situation. Clients are assured that their involvement in risk behavior modification and close follow-up by health care providers assists in avoiding rupture.

Health Care Resources

When returning to a home environment, clients may require the services of a home care nurse to assess tolerance of dietary, pharmacologic, and activity limitations. Clients who have undergone surgery may benefit from home care nurse assistance with dressing changes. A home care aide may be needed to assist with ADL.

 Evaluation

On the basis of the identified nursing diagnoses, the nurse evaluates the care of the client who has an aneurysm. The expected outcomes include that the client

1. Maintains adequate circulation
2. Identifies ways to modify existing risk factors
3. Complies with the schedule of diagnostic tests that are ordered to follow the size of the aneurysm (for a nonsurgical client)

VASCULAR TRAUMA

OVERVIEW

Many types of trauma can result in vascular injury. Injuries to the blood vessels in the upper and lower extremities account for approximately 70% of all vascular injuries to the human body (Lim, 1987).

Vascular injuries to the blood vessels include punctures, lacerations, and transections. Acute blunt or penetrating trauma may result in true or false aneurysm formation. Arteriovenous fistulas may be seen after penetrating injuries. The more common causes of penetrating injuries to the blood vessels are gunshot or knife wounds. Blunt trauma, which is less common, can be seen after high-speed automobile accidents as a result of the shearing force of rapid deceleration. Vascular trauma can also be found after arterial puncture for arteriographic or hemodynamic studies in which there is development of dissection, false hematoma, or occlusive lesions.

COLLABORATIVE MANAGEMENT

The history and physical examination aid in establishing the diagnosis in the client with vascular injury. The nurse obtains information from the client or the family about the mechanism of injury, the site of injury, the amount of blood loss, and the symptoms present after the injury. Physical examination provides information that allows evaluation of the client for signs of circulatory, sensory, or motor impairment. The nurse takes the client's vital signs and uses these as a basis with which to compare any changes. Pulses distal to the site of injury should be evaluated, as well as other peripheral pulses.

Radiographic assessment by arteriography provides essential information about the vascular injury. Common arteriographic findings in clients with trauma include obstruction, extravasation, false aneurysm formation, wall irregularity, or arteriovenous fistula. Emergency or urgent surgical intervention is warranted for clients with ischemia to maximize successful revascularization.

Initial management of vascular injuries is often initiated in a hospital emergency room. Careful triage by the nurse is crucial. Snyder and associates (1989) suggested that vascular injuries fall into three categories: category I injuries expose clients to immediate threats of survival and are treated immediately. Examples of category I injuries are tension pneumothorax, cardiac tamponade, and exsanguinating hemorrhage. Category II injuries are serious, but not quite as severe, allowing time for more extensive evaluation before treatment is initiated. Examples of category II injuries are major fractures, abdominal trauma in clients with stable vital signs, and genitourinary trauma. Category III injuries permit man-agement of the injury at a more leisurely pace; examples are lacerations, simple lacerations, and contusions.

The most important principles in the management of vascular trauma are establishment of a patent airway, control of bleeding, and restoration of blood flow. The method of repair of vascular injuries varies with the type of injury. Methods of repair of vascular injuries include synthetic vein bypass grafting, lateral suture repair, thrombectomy (excision of blood clot), resection with end-to-end anastomosis, and vein patch grafting.

OTHER VASCULAR DISORDERS

Atherosclerosis is the foremost cause of vascular disorders; however, it is important to address the other types of arterial obstruction and other venous disorders. The unique etiology of each disorder necessitates individual attention and special therapy.

Arterial Disorders

BUERGER'S DISEASE

Buerger's disease (thromboangiitis obliterans) is a relatively uncommon occlusive disease limited to the medium and small arteries and veins in the body. The distal upper and lower limbs are the most frequently affected. Buerger's disease is typically identified in young adult males who smoke. Larger arteries, such as the femoral and brachial, become involved in the late stages of the disease. The veins are less commonly involved.

The disease often extends into the perivascular tissues, resulting in fibrosis and scarring that binds the artery, the vein, and the nerve firmly together. For individuals who have this disease, smoking cessation arrests the disease process, whereas persistence in smoking causes occlusion in the more proximal vessels.

The cause of Buerger's disease is unknown, although a strong association with tobacco smoking exists. A familial or genetic predisposition and an autoimmune etiology of the disease may also be possible.

The first clinical manifestation of Buerger's disease is usually claudication (pain in the muscles resulting from an inadequate blood supply) of the arch of the foot. Intermittent claudication may occur in the lower extremities. The pain may be ischemic, occurring in the digits while at rest. Often, the pain is aching in quality and more severe at night. Paroxysmal shock-like pain can be the result of ischemic neuropathy. Increased sensitivity to cold with complaints of coldness and numbness is often seen. On physical examination, pulses are often diminished in the distal extremities, and extremities are cool to the touch and are red or cyanotic in the dependent position.

Diagnosis of Buerger's disease is commonly based on a physical finding of peripheral ischemia, often in association with migratory superficial phlebitis. Ulcerations and gangrene may be seen in the digits. The ulcerations are usually sharply demarcated (Fig. 65–9). The gangrenous lesion could be small or affect the entire digit.

Arteriograms can be useful in delineating the degree of disease present in the arteries. Commonly, arteriography reveals multiple segmental occlusions in the smaller arteries of the forearm, the hand, the leg, and the foot.

Plethysmographic studies of the fingers or the toes may be diagnostic of the disease in the early stages. These studies can also be of use in following the progression of the disease in more proximal arteries.

Nursing interventions are directed at preventing the progression of the disease, avoiding vasoconstriction, promoting vasodilation, relieving pain, and treating ulceration and gangrene. Complete abstinence from tobacco in all forms is essential to prevent disease progression. The client is instructed to prevent extreme or prolonged exposure to cold to prevent vasoconstriction. The nurse instructs the client about medications that are prescribed for vasodilation, such as nifedipine (Procardia). The reader is referred to Chapter 7 for interventions and nursing management for pain relief. The treatment of clients with Buerger's disease is similar to that of clients with PAD (see earlier).

SUBCLAVIAN STEAL

Subclavian steal occurs in the upper extremities from a subclavian artery occlusion. It results in altered blood flow and ischemia in the arm. Subclavian steal can occur at any age, but usually is more common in individuals

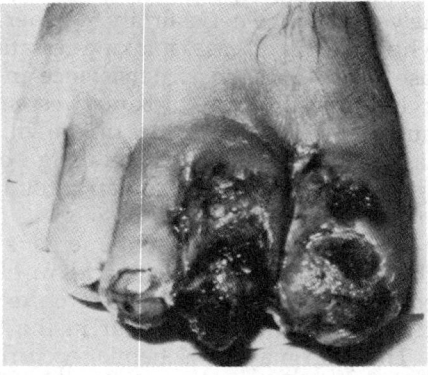

Figure 65–9

Ulceration of the foot in a client with Buerger's disease. (From Pardy, B. J., Lewis, J. D., & Eastcott, H. H. G. [1980]. Preliminary experience with prostaglandins E_1 and I_2 in peripheral vascular disease. Surgery *88*, 826. Reproduced by permission of the C. V. Mosby Company.)

with risk factors for atherosclerosis. Client symptoms include paresthesias, syncope, dizziness, headaches, and occasionally pain and discomfort.

Physical examination usually reveals a significant difference in the blood pressures between the arms. A difference greater than 20 mmHg is considered significant. Another important finding is a subclavian bruit, which can occur on the affected side. The subclavian pulse may be decreased on the occluded side when compared with the opposite side. The client may also have discoloration or cyanosis of the affected arm; however, this finding generally occurs only in severe cases.

Surgery is the recommended intervention for this disorder. Surgical intervention involves one of three procedures: endarterectomy of the subclavian artery, carotid-subclavian bypass, or dilation of the subclavian artery.

Nursing care encompasses providing general postoperative care of the client and monitoring the arterial flow in the affected arm. Frequent checks of brachial and radial pulses and observation for ischemic changes are essential. The nurse also observes the arm for edema, redness, or any other signs of problems.

THORACIC OUTLET SYNDROME

Thoracic outlet syndrome is a compression of the subclavian artery at the thoracic outlet by anatomic structures, such as a rib or muscle. Damage of the arterial wall can occur, producing thrombosis or embolization to distal arteries of the arms. The three common sites of compression in the thoracic outlet are the interscalene triangle, between the coracoid process of the scapula and the pectoralis minor tendon, and, most commonly, the costoclavicular space.

Thoracic outlet syndrome is more common in females and in individuals whose occupations require holding their arms up or leaning over. It is also more prominent in individuals with poor posture.

Clients generally complain of neck, shoulder, and arm pain that may be intermittent. The client may also have numbness and moderate edema of the extremity. The pain and numbness are worse when the arm is placed in certain positions, such as over the client's head or out to the side. The affected arm may appear cyanotic.

The treatment usually is conservative, unless there is severe pain, loss of hand function, or poor response to conservative treatment. Conservative treatment includes physical therapy, exercises, and avoiding aggravating positions, such as elevating the arms. Surgical treatment involves resection of the anatomic structure that is compressing the artery.

RAYNAUD'S PHENOMENON

Raynaud's phenomenon is caused by vasospasm of the arterioles and arteries of the upper and lower extremities, usually unilaterally. *Raynaud's disease* occurs bilaterally. The two terms are sometimes used interchangeably and, although they are related, there are some differences. Raynaud's phenomenon usually occurs in individuals older than 30 years, whereas Raynaud's disease can occur between the ages of 17 and 50 years. Raynaud's disease is more common in women, and Raynaud's phenomenon can occur in either sex.

The pathophysiology is the same for the disease and the phenomenon. The etiology is unknown. As a result of vasospasm, the cutaneous vessels are constricted and blanching of the extremity occurs, followed by cyanosis. When the vasospasm is relieved, the tissue becomes reddened or hyperemic. The client has numbness and coldness of the extremities and may complain of pain and swelling. The client may also have ulcers. These attacks are intermittent and can be aggravated by cold or stress. In severe cases, the attack lasts longer and gangrene of the digits can occur.

Treatment involves relieving or preventing the vasoconstriction by drug therapy. Common pharmaceutical agents used are reserpine (Serpasil), nifedipine (Procardia), cyclandelate (Cyclospasmol), and phenoxybenzamine (Dibenzyline). These agents may help to relieve the symptoms, but cause uncomfortable side effects, such as facial flushing, headaches, hypotension, and dizziness.

For severe symptoms that drug therapy does not alleviate, a lumbar sympathectomy can be performed. This method is effective for symptoms of the feet. For the upper extremities, a sympathetic ganglionectomy may provide relief of the symptoms. Long-term effectiveness of these treatments is questionable.

Client education plays an important role in prevention of complications. The client is taught methods to prevent vasoconstriction, which include minimizing exposure to cold and decreasing stress. The client is instructed to wear warm clothes, socks, or gloves when exposed to cool or cold temperatures. Clients should keep their homes at a comfortably warm temperature. The nurse helps the client to identify stressors and provides suggestions for reducing them.

POPLITEAL ENTRAPMENT

Popliteal entrapment causes ischemic symptoms in the affected leg or foot because of anatomic compression of the popliteal artery. Popliteal entrapment is found in young people, usually men complaining of intermittent claudication of one extremity.

Physical examination may reveal ischemic changes of the affected extremity, with normal function of the unaffected limb. At rest, the nurse may find diminished distal pulses, although this is a rare finding. Diagnosis of this disorder occurs only after an accurate history, physical examination, and arteriography.

Surgical repair of the anatomic compression is the recommended treatment. Reconstruction of the popli-

teal artery may be necessary to restore arterial blood flow to the limb. Nursing care involves preventing general postoperative complications and evaluating patency of the graft or artery postoperatively. The nurse observes for ischemic changes and evaluates distal pulses frequently postoperatively.

Venous Disorders

PHLEBITIS

Phlebitis is an inflammation of the superficial veins caused by an irritation, such as IV therapy. The client has a reddened, warm area radiating up an extremity, commonly an arm. The client may also experience pain, soreness, and swelling of the extremity.

Treatment involves application of warm, moist soaks, which dilate the vein and promote circulation. Sometimes, a heating unit is used to keep the soaks warm. Rarely, ice packs are used. Nursing care involves applying the warm soaks, making sure the temperature is not warm enough to burn the client, and assessing for complications, such as tissue necrosis, infection, or pulmonary embolus. After a few days of conservative therapy, the inflammation usually subsides.

VARICOSE VEINS

Varicose veins are distended, protruding veins that appear darkened and tortuous. They can occur in anyone, but commonly in clients older than 30 years whose occupations require prolonged standing. Varicose veins are also found in pregnant women; clients with systemic problems, such as heart disease; obese clients; and those with a family history of varicose veins.

As the vein wall weakens and dilates, venous pressure increases, and the valves become incompetent. The incompetent valves enhance the vessel dilation, and the veins become tortuous and distended.

The client may complain of pain, especially after standing, and experience a fullness in the legs. Physical examination reveals distended protruding veins. The Trendelenburg test assists with the diagnosis. The client is placed in a supine position with elevated legs. As the client sits up, the veins would normally fill from the distal end; however, with varicosities the veins fill from the proximal end.

Conservative measures are the treatment of choice. These involve the client's wearing elastic stockings and elevating the extremities as much as possible. Clients who continue to have pain or unsightly veins, despite this treatment, may opt for surgery.

Surgery most often entails ligation (tying) and stripping (removal) of affected veins with the client under general anesthesia. This procedure involves threading a long wire through an incision in the groin to an incision in the ankle. Stripping is accomplished by tying the wire onto a vein in the groin and pulling the wire out from the ankle. After this procedure, the client's legs are bandaged with firm elastic (Ace) bandages. Postoperatively, the nurse assesses the groin and entire leg for bleeding through the elastic bandage. The nurse also instructs the client to keep the legs elevated and to perform range-of-motion exercises of the legs at least hourly. Clients are ambulatory and are often discharged from the hospital by the first postoperative day. At this time, the nurse instructs clients to continue to wear elastic stockings, to walk, to limit sitting, and to avoid standing in one place. When sitting, clients should have their legs elevated.

Sclerotherapy involves the injection of a sclerosing agent into a varicose vein. This procedure may be done as primary treatment or after surgical ligation and stripping.

DISORDERS OF THE LYMPH VESSELS

LYMPHANGITIS

Lymphangitis is an inflammation of the peripheral lymphatic channels or vessels. Single attacks result in minor degrees of lymphedema, but, with repeated episodes, the edema may increase. A function of the lymphatic system is transport of lymph. Lymphatic vessels can also transport bacteria and viruses that infect the lymphatic channels, producing lymphangitis.

Usually, lymphangitis is caused by infection with beta-hemolytic streptococci. Years ago, serious epidemics of invasive streptococcal infections were seen in the form of an acutely spreading cellulitis and lymphangitis referred to as erysipelas. With the advent of antibiotics such as penicillin, epidemics are no longer seen; however, erysipelas continues to occur. Other causes of lymphangitis include influenza, tuberculosis, and septicemia.

Lymphangitis is characterized by red streaks that extend up the arm or leg, outlining the course of the lymphatics as they drain. The lymph nodes that are found along the course of the lymphatic channels enlarge, becoming red and tender. Often, the infection enters the body through a break in the skin. An ingrown nail, fungal infections, or a puncture wound can be the site of entry as well as the source of infection.

Lymphangitis is treated with rest and immobilization of the affected part. Local heat applications and elevation can be utilized. Cultures of both the wound and the blood are done to determine the causative organism. After the organism is identified, administration of the correct antibiotic is undertaken. Because the organisms are usually sensitive to the prescribed antibiotics, abscess formation is uncommon.

LYMPHEDEMA

Lymphedema is a swelling of the soft tissues attributable to an increased amount of lymph. Two types of lymphedema exist. Primary lymphedema is found as a result of abnormal development of the lymph vessels. Secondary lymphedema occurs as the result of obstruction or destruction of normal lymphatic channels. Lymphedema becomes especially marked when the affected extremity is placed in a dependent position.

Three different types of primary lymphedema are found. Lymphedema congenita is present at birth. Lymphedema praecox develops before age 35 years, whereas lymphedema tarda develops after age 35 years. Lymphedema praecox is the most common type. The incidence of lymphedema is higher in females of all age groups, accounting for 63% to 77% of cases (DePalma, 1986). Lymphedema involves both legs in about 50% of clients. Lymphangiography is utilized to diagnose primary lymphedema.

Causes of secondary lymphedema include radiation, trauma or excision of lymph pathways, inflammation, parasitic invasion, or malignant disease. The most common cause of secondary lymphedema in the United States is malignant disease and its treatment (O'Donnell, 1987). Radiation of malignant disease results in obstruction of lymphatic trunks from extensive fibrosis at the lymph node level.

Diagnosis of secondary lymphedema is often made by history and physical examination. The history reveals the presence of certain predisposing factors. Common physical examination findings include an elephantine distribution of limb swelling, a dorsal buffalo hump over the metatarsal area in the foot, and failure of the skin over the dorsum of the toes or fingers to tent when pinched. Venous plethysmography can be utilized to document the presence of obstruction of venous outflow. CT can be helpful in clients with malignant disease to rule out recurrent neoplasm as the cause of the lymphedema.

Conservative management is employed in clients with lymphedema. Treatment is aimed at decreasing edema by improving lymph drainage. To promote lymph drainage, the client may be asked to elevate the affected limb by placing blocks under the foot of the bed or, for upper-extremity lymphedema, to suspend the arm in a sling. Clients may utilize compression therapy in the form of either elastic stockings or pneumatic compression devices in an effort to reduce limb girth.

The client should be measured for properly fitting elastic stockings. The nurse instructs the client to apply the elastic stocking before arising from bed in the morning. The client should purchase at least two stockings for each limb so that one stocking can be laundered while the other is worn. Elastic stockings should be discarded if the elasticity is gone.

Surgical treatment is seldom utilized for lymphedema. Two general types of surgical procedures are employed: excisional and physiologic. Surgery that utilizes the excisional technique removes excessive skin and subcutaneous tissue. This type of operation offers a potential solution to the problem of massive limb enlargement. Physiologic techniques try to provide or enhance lymph drainage by establishing a lymphovenous shunt.

LYMPHADENOPATHY

Lymphadenopathy is a swelling or enlargement of one or more lymph nodes. Lymphadenopathy can result from infection, inflammation, or neoplasms. The common causes of bacterial infections are streptococcal or staphylococcal organisms. Viral infections can occur with influenza, measles, or infectious mononucleosis. Children may exhibit a more widespread lymph node enlargement from infection when compared with adults. Lymphadenopathy can also occur when lymph nodes are invaded by neoplastic cells. Hodgkin's disease and leukemia may produce lymphadenopathy. Diagnosis of lymphadenopathy is facilitated by lymphangiography. This radiologic technique is helpful in evaluating lymph nodes for the presence of disease. Biopsy of the lymph nodes can be utilized in obtaining the differential diagnosis.

SUMMARY

Vascular disease can be frightening and disabling, affecting people of all ages. Prevention is paramount and is an important responsibility of the professional nurse. During the past 10 years, awareness, detection, diagnosis, and early treatment of vascular disease have significantly increased. New techniques of cardiac and vascular surgery (cardiopulmonary bypass, open heart surgery, aneurysmectomy, and artificial grafts) have improved the management of vascular disease. The introduction of pharmacologic agents such as anticoagulants, antihypertensives, and cholesterol-lowering drugs has improved the success of treating previously untreatable vascular diseases.

Atherosclerosis is the leading cause of death in industrialized countries and the leading cause of vascular diseases. Risk factors such as smoking, obesity, hypercholesterolemia, and diabetes have been linked to vascular disease. Hypertension has also been found to be a major risk factor for atherosclerosis. Evidence supports the treatment of hypertension because it prolongs life, even in the atherosclerotic individual. Atherosclerosis has been found to precede the development of aneurysms. Primary prevention through risk factor modification is important in decreasing mortality and morbidity from vascular diseases.

IMPLICATIONS FOR RESEARCH

Unraveling the mystery of vascular disease will undoubtedly provide answers about diagnosis, prevention, and treatment. Future clinical research must focus on defining the pathophysiology and etiology. Currently, the emphasis is on risk factor identification and prevention.

Nursing research is aimed at promoting wellness through client education. Comprehensive education programs should include the general public and health care professionals and should address methods of detection, referral, and follow-up.

Vascular disease requires lifelong therapy to prevent devastating consequences. Specific questions that nursing research should address include

1. What methods can be used to identify individuals at risk for vascular disease?
2. How can nurses promote wellness and prevention of vascular disease?
3. What can nurses do to reach clients with undetected hypertension?
4. How do the risk factors for CAD apply to clients with vascular disease?
5. Can reliable and simple screening tests be developed to detect vascular disease in the early stages?

REFERENCES AND READINGS

Arteriosclerosis and Atherosclerosis

American Cancer Society. (1989). *Cancer facts and figures— 1989.* Atlanta: Author.

Anderson, J. W., & Gustafson, N. J. (1988). Dietary fiber and heart disease: Current management concepts and recommendations. *Topics in Clinical Nutrition, 3*(2), 21.

Anderson, J. W., & Tietyen-Clarke, J. (1986). Dietary fiber: Hyperlipidemia, hypertension, and coronary heart disease. *American Journal of Gastroenterology, 81,* 907–919.

Blackburn, H. (1980). Risk factors and cardiovascular disease. In *American Heart Association heartbook: A guide to prevention and treatment of cardiovascular disease* (pp. 2–21). New York: E. P. Dutton.

Blankenhorn, D. H., Rooney, J. A., & Curry, P. J. (1983). Noninvasive assessment of atherosclerosis. *Progress in Cardiovascular Diseases, 26*(4), 295–307.

DeBakey, M. E., Lawrie, G. M., & Glaeser, D. H. (1985). Patterns of atherosclerosis and their surgical significance. *Annals of Surgery, 2,* 115–131.

Doyle, J. E. (1984). Things the Surgeon General didn't tell us: The impact of cigarette smoking on peripheral circulation. *Society for Peripheral Vascular Nursing Journal,* 11–12.

Gotto, A. M. (1985). Some reflections on arteriosclerosis: Past, present, and future. Presidential address. *Circulation, 72,* 8–16.

Govoni L. E., & Hayes, J. E. (1988). *Drugs and nursing implications.* Norwalk, CT: Appleton & Lange.

Graham, S., & Marley, M. (1984). What foot care really means. *American Journal of Nursing, 84,* 888–890.

Grundy, S. M. (1983). Atherosclerosis: Pathology, Pathogenesis, and role of risk factors. *Disease-a-Month, 29,* 3–47.

Hazzard, W. R. (1985). Atherogenesis: Why women live longer than men. *Geriatrics, 40,* 42–51.

Kannel, W. B., Doyle, J. T., Ostfeld, A. M., Jenkins, C. D., Kuller, L., Podell, R. N., & Stamler, J. S. (1984). Optimal resources for primary prevention of atherosclerotic diseases. *Circulation, 70,* 157A–195A.

Kim, M. J., McFarland, G. K., & McLane, A. M. (1984). *Nursing diagnosis.* St. Louis: C. V. Mosby.

National Cholesterol Education Program. (1987). *Report of the Expert Panel on Detection, Evaluation, and Treatment of High Blood Cholesterol in Adults.* Bethesda, MD: National Heart, Lung, and Blood Institute.

Rutherford, R. B. (Ed.). (1989). *Vascular surgery* (3rd ed.). Philadelphia: W. B. Saunders.

Tierney, L. M., & Erskine, J. M. (1988). Blood vessels and lymphatics. In S. A. Schroeder, M. A. Krupp, & L. M. Tierney (Eds.), *Current medical diagnosis and treatment* (pp. 266–293). Norwalk, CT: Appleton & Lange.

Whitney, E. N., Cataldo, C. B., & Rolfes, S. R. (1987). *Understanding normal and clinical nutrition.* St. Paul, MN: West Publishing.

Williams, S. R. (1989). *Nutrition and diet therapy.* St. Louis: Times Mirror/Mosby College Publishing.

Hypertension

Bates, B. (1987). *A guide to physical examination* (4th ed.). Philadelphia: J. B. Lippincott.

Braithwaite, J. D., & Morton, B. G. (1981). Patient education for blood pressure control. *Nursing Clinics of North America, 16,* 321–329.

Doyle, J. E. (1985). Renovascular hypertension. *Critical Care Quarterly, 8*(2), 51–59.

Dustan, H. P. (1988). Pathophysiology of hypertension. In J. W. Hurst (Ed.), *The heart* (6th ed., pp. 1038–1048). New York: McGraw-Hill.

Fink, J. W. (1981). The challenge of high blood pressure control. *Nursing Clinics of North America, 16,* 301–308.

Frohlick, E. D. (1985). Practical management of hypertension. *Current Problems in Cardiology, 10,* 8–55.

Foster, S. B., & Kousch, D. (1981). Adherence to therapy in hypertensive patients. *Nursing Clinics of North America, 16,* 331–341.

Grim, C. M. (1981). Nursing assessment of the patient with high blood pressure. *Nursing Clinics of North America, 16,* 349–364.

Guyton, A. C. (1986). *Textbook of medical physiology* (7th ed.). Philadelphia: W. B. Saunders

Hill, M. (1981). Helping the hypertensive patient control sodium intake. *American Journal of Nursing, 79,* 906–909.

Hypertension prevalence and the status of awareness, treatment, and control in the United States: Final Report of the Subcommittee on Definition and Prevalence of 1984 Joint National Committee. (1985). *Hypertension, 7,* 457–468.

Kannel, W. B., & Schatzkin, A. (1983). Risk factor analysis. *Progress in Cardiovascular Diseases, 26,* 309–331.

Kaplan, N. M. (1988). Systemic hypertension: Mechanisms and diagnosis. In E. Braunwald (Ed.), *Heart disease: A textbook of cardiovascular medicine* (3rd ed., pp. 819–861). Philadelphia: W. B. Saunders.

Marcinek, M. B. (1980). Hypertension: What it does to the body. *American Journal of Nursing, 80,* 928–936.

Oparil, S. (1988). Arterial hypertension. In J. B. Wyngaarden & L. H. Smith Jr., (Eds.), *Cecil textbook of medicine* (18th ed., pp. 276–293). Philadelphia: W. B. Saunders.

Peterson, F. (1983). Assessing peripheral vascular disease at the bedside. *American Journal of Nursing, 83,* 1549–1551.

Rossi, L. P., & Antman, E. M. (1983). Calcium channel blockers. *American Journal of Nursing, 83,* 382–387.

U.S. Department of Health and Human Services. (1988). *The 1988 Report of the Joint National Committee on Detection, Evaluation, and Treatment of High Blood Pressure* (NIH Publication No. 88–1088). Washington, DC: U.S. Government Printing Office.

Peripheral Vascular Disease

Andros, G., Harris, R. W., Dulawa, L. B., Oblath, R. W., & Salles-Cunha, S. X. (1984). Patency of femoropopliteal and femorotibial grafts after outflow revascularization to bypass distal disease. *Surgery, 96,* 878–885.

Appleton, D. L., & LeQuaglia, J. D. (1985). Vascular disease and post-operative nursing management. *Critical Care Nurse, 5*(3), 34–42.

Baum, P. L. (1985). Heed the early warning signs of peripheral vascular disease. *Nursing '85, 15*(3), 50–57.

Benson, J. L., & Allastair, K. M. (1987). In situ artery bypass. *AORN Journal, 45,* 40–54.

Bergin, J. J., Flinn, W. R., & Yao, J. S. T. (1984). Operative therapy of peripheral vascular disease. *Progress in Cardiovascular Diseases, 26,* 273–294.

Bosiljeuac, J., & Farha, J. S. (1981). Ischemic problems following vascular reconstruction. *Journal of the Kansas Medical Society, 82,* 346–348.

Bunt, T. J., & Haynes, J. L. (1984). Lower extremity revascularization. *Journal of the South Carolina Medical Association, 2,* 285–288.

Carico, H. N. (1985). *Manual of health assessment.* Boston: Little, Brown.

Carney, W. I., Balko, A., & Barrett, M. S. (1985). In situ femoropopliteal and infrapopliteal bypass. *Archives of Surgery, 120,* 812–816.

Clyne, C. A. (1981). Non-surgical management of peripheral vascular disease: A review. *British Medical Journal, 281,* 794–798.

Cronenwett, J. L., Warner, K. G., Zelenock, G. B., White-house, W. M., Jr., Graham, L. M., Lindenauer, M., & Stanley, J. C. (1984). Intermittent claudication. *Archives of Surgery, 199,* 430–436.

Doyle, J. E. (1981). If your patient's legs hurt, the reason may be arterial insufficiency. *Nursing '81, 11*(4), 74–78.

Doyle, J. E. (1983). All leg ulcers are not alike: Managing and preventing arterial and venous ulcers. *Nursing '83, 13*(2), 58–63.

Faulkner, K. W., House, A. K., & Castleden, W. M. (1983). The effect of cessation of smoking on the accumulative survival rates of patients with symptomatic peripheral vascular disease. *Medical Journal of Australia, 1,* 217–219.

Friedman, S. J., & Daniel Su, W. P. (1984). Management of leg ulcers with hydrocolloid occlusive dressing. *Archives of Dermatology, 120,* 1329–1336.

Harris, R. W., Andros, G., Dulawa, L. B., Oblath, R. W., Salles-Cunha, S. X., & Apyan, R. (1984). Successful long-term link salvage using cephalic vein bypass grafts. *Annals of Surgery, 200,* 785–791.

Herman, J. (1986). Nursing assessment and nursing diagnosis in patients with peripheral vascular disease. *Nursing Clinics of North America, 21,* 219–231.

Huisman, M. V., Büller, H. R., ten Cate, J. W., & Vreeken, J. (1986). Serial impedance plethysmography for suspected deep venous thrombosis in out-patients. *New England Journal of Medicine, 314,* 823–828.

Johnson, A. (1984). Towards rapid tissue healing. *Nursing Times, 80*(48), 39–43.

Johnson, G., Jr., Kupper, C., Farrar, D. J., & Swallow, R. T. (1982). Graded compression stockings. *Archives of Surgery, 117,* 69–72.

Johnson, W. C., O'Hara, E. T., Corey, C., Widrich, W. C., & Nasbeth, D. C. (1985). Venous stasis ulceration: Effectiveness of subfascial ligation. *Archives of Surgery, 120,* 797–800.

Juergens, J. L., Spittell, J. A., & Fairbairn, J. F., II (1980). *Peripheral vascular diseases* (5th ed.). Philadelphia: W. B. Saunders.

Kim, M. J., McFarland, G. K., & McLane, A. M. (1984). *Nursing diagnosis.* St. Louis: C. V. Mosby.

Lamb, C. (1983). When acute ischemia threatens a limb. *Patient Care, 17,* 157–167.

Lamb, C. (1983). When chronic ischemia worsens. *Patient Care, 17,* 171–183.

McCarthy, W. J., & Williams, L. R. (1985). Femoral artery reconstruction. *Critical Care Quarterly, 8*(2), 39–48.

Newberger, G. B., & Reckling, J. B. (1985). A new look at wound care. *Nursing '85, 15*(2), 34–41.

Paskin, L. S. (1982). Percutaneous transluminal angioplasty in peripheral vascular disease. *Radiography, 48*(571), 129–133.

Prineas, R. J., Harland, W. R., Janzon, L., & Kannel, W. (1982). Recommendations for use of non-invasive methods to detect atherosclerotic peripheral arterial disease—in population studies. *Circulation, 65,* 1561A–1565A.

Smith, M. (1982). Nursing management of the leg ulcer in the community. *Nursing Times, 78*(29), 1228–1232.

Schwartz, S. (Ed.). (1984). *Principles of surgery* (4th ed.). New York: McGraw-Hill.

Taheri, S. A., Pendergast, D., Lazar, E., Pollack, L. H., Shores, R. M., McDonald, B., & Taheri, P. (1985). Continuous ambulatory venous pressure for diagnosis of venous insufficiency. *American Journal of Surgery, 150,* 202–206.

Taheri, S. A., Pendergast, D. R., Lazar, E., Pollack, L. H., Meenaghan, M. A., Shores, R. M., Budd, T., & Taheri, P. (1985). Vein valve transplantation. *American Journal of Surgery, 150,* 201–202.

Turner, J. A. (1986). Nursing interventions in patients with peripheral vascular disease. *Nursing Clinics of North America, 21,* 233–240.

Ventura, M. R. (1984). Health promotion for patients with peripheral vascular disease. *American Journal of Nursing, 38,* 800.

Zacca, N. M., Raizner, A. E., Noon, G. P., Short, D., Weillbaeder, D., Gotto A., & Roberts, R. (1989). Treatment of symptomatic peripheral atherosclerotic disease with a rotational atherectomy device. *American Journal of Cardiology, 63,* 77–80.

Aneurysms

Bates, B. (1987). *A guide to physical examination* (4th ed.). Philadelphia: J. B. Lippincott.

Benson, H. (1984). *Beyond the relaxation response.* New York: Times Books.

Bickerstaff, L. K., Hollier, L. H., Van Peenan, H. J., Melton, L. J., Pairolero, P. C., & Cherry, K. J. (1984). Abdominal aortic aneurysm: The changing natural history. *Journal of Vascular Surgery, 1,* 6–12.

Bush, H. L., Corey, C. A., & Nasbeth, D. C. (1983). Distal in-situ saphenous vein grafts for limb salvage. *American Journal of Surgery, 145,* 542–548.

Campbell, C. (1984). *Nursing diagnosis and intervention in nursing practice* (2nd ed.). New York: Wiley.

Chobanian, A. V. (1983). The influence of hypertension and other hemodynamic factors in atherogenesis. *Progress in Cardiovascular Diseases, 26,* 177–196.

Collins, J. J. (1983). Aneurysms of the descending thoracic aorta. In W. L. Glen (Ed.), *Thoracic and cardiovascular surgery* (4th ed., pp. 200–300). Norwalk, CT: Appleton-Century-Crofts.

DeBakey, M. E., Henly, W. S., Cooley, D. A., et al. (1965). Surgical management of dissecting aneurysms of the aorta. *Journal of Thoracic and Cardiovascular Surgery, 49,* 130–140.

Doyle, J. (1986). Treatment modalities of peripheral vascular disease. *Nursing Clinics of North America, 21,* 241–253.

Ekers, M. (1986). Psychosocial considerations in peripheral vascular disease. *Nursing Clinics of North America, 21,* 255–262.

Fairbairn, J. F., II, & Juergens, J. L. (1980). Principles of medical treatment. In J. L. Juergens, J. A. Spittell, & J. F.

Fairbairn, II (Eds.), *Peripheral vascular diseases* (5th ed., pp. 855–878). Philadelphia: W. B. Saunders.

Hollier, L. H., & Rutherford, R. B. (1989). Infrarenal aortic aneurysms. In R. B. Rutherford (Ed.), *Vascular Surgery* (3rd ed., pp. 909–927). Philadelphia: W. B. Saunders.

McCaffery, M. (1983). *Nursing the patient in pain.* London: Harper & Row.

Peterson, F. (1983). Assessing peripheral vascular disease at the bedside. *American Journal of Nursing, 83,* 1549–1551.

Rutherford, R. B. (Ed.). (1984). *Vascular surgery* (2nd ed.). Philadelphia: W. B. Saunders.

Sabiston, D. C. (Ed.). (1986). *Textbook of surgery: The biological basis of modern surgical practice* (13th ed.). Philadelphia: W. B. Saunders.

Saynor, R., Verel, D., & Gillot, T. (1984). The long term effect of dietary supplements with fish lipid concentrations on serum lipids, bleeding time, platelets, and angina. *Atherosclerosis, 50,* 3–10.

Thom, G., Edelund, L., Herrlin, K., Linstedt, E. L., Olin, T., & Bergentz, S. E. (1983). Renal artery aneurysms: Natural history and prognosis. *Annals of Surgery, 197,* 348–352.

Turner, J. (1986). Nursing intervention in patients with peripheral vascular disease. *Nursing Clinics of North America, 21,* 233–239.

Wagner, M. (1986). Pathophysiology related to peripheral vascular disease. *Nursing Clinics of North America, 21,* 195–205.

Vascular Trauma

Juergens, J. L., & Pluth, J. R. (1980). Trauma and peripheral vascular disease. In J. L. Juergens, J. A. Spittell, & J. F. Fairbairn, II, *Peripheral vascular diseases* (5th ed., pp. 607–628). Philadelphia: W. B. Saunders.

Lim, L. T. (1987). Extremity arterial penetrating injury. In C. B. Ernst & J. C. Stanley (Eds.), *Current therapy in vascular surgery.* Toronto: B. C. Decker.

Merzoian, J. O., Doyle, J. E., Cantelmo, N. L., LoGerfo, F. W., & Hirsch, E. (1985). A comprehensive approach to extremity vascular trauma. *Archives of Surgery, 120,* 801–805.

Snyder, W. H., Thal, E. R., & Perry, M. O. (1989). Vascular injuries of the extremities. In R. B. Rutherford (Ed.), *Vascular surgery* (3rd ed., pp. 613–637). Philadelphia: W. B. Saunders.

Watkins, L. W., & Gott, V. L. (1983). Blunt and penetrating trauma to the great vessels. In W. W. Glenn (Ed.), *Thoracic and cardiovascular surgery* (4th ed., pp. 10–250). Norwalk, CT: Appleton-Century-Crofts.

Other Vascular Disorders

Adar, R., Papa, M. Z., Halpern, Z., Mozes, M., Shoshan, S., Sofer, B., Zinger, H., Dayan, M., & Mozes, G. (1983). Cellular sensitivity to collagen in thromboangiitis obliterans. *New England Journal of Medicine, 308,* 1113–1116.

Bartolo, M., Rulli, F., & Raffi, S. (1980). Buerger's disease: Is it a rickettsiosis? *Angiology, 31,* pp. 660–665.

Craven, R. F., & Curry, T. D. (1981). When the diagnosis is Raynaud's. *American Journal of Nursing, 11,* 1007–1009.

Janoff, K. A., Phinney, E. S., & Porter, J. M. (1985). Lumbar sympathectomy for lower extremity vasospasm. *American Journal of Surgery, 150,* 147–151.

Juergens, J. L. (1980). Thromboangiitis obliterans (Buerger's disease, TAO). In J. L. Juergens, J. A. Spittell, & J. F. Fairbairn, II (Eds.), *Peripheral vascular diseases* (5th ed., pp. 469–492). Philadelphia: W. B. Saunders.

Kontos, H. A. (1988). Vascular diseases of the limbs. In J. B. Wyngaarden & L. H. Smith, Jr. (Eds.), *Cecil textbook of medicine* (18th ed., pp. 375–389). Philadelphia, W. B. Saunders.

Pollak, E. W. (1980). Surgical anatomy of the thoracic outlet syndrome. *Surgery, Gynecology and Obstetrics, 150,* 97–103.

Porter, J. M. (1984). Raynaud's syndrome and associated vasospastic conditions of the extremities. *Arteriosclerosis, 10,* 697–706.

Roos, D. B. (1984). Thoracic outlet and carpal tunnel syndrome. *Arteriosclerosis, 10,* 708–723.

Shionoya, S. (1989). Buerger's disease (thromboangiitis obliterans). In R. B. Rutherford (Ed.), *Vascular Surgery* (3rd ed., pp. 207–217). Philadelphia: W. B. Saunders.

Wheeler, H. B. (1986). Thromboangiitis obliterans (Buerger's disease). In D. C. Sabiston (Ed.), *Textbook of surgery: The biological basis of modern surgical practice* (13th ed., pp. 1922–1925). Philadelphia: W. B. Saunders.

Zweifler, A. J., & Trinkaus, P. (1984). Occlusive digital artery disease in patients with Raynaud's phenomenon. *American Journal of Medicine, 77,* 995–1001.

Disorders of the Lymph Vessels

Browse, N. L. (1987). Primary lymphedema. In C. B. Ernst & J. C. Stanley (Eds.), *Current therapy in vascular surgery* (pp. 50–150). Toronto: B. C. Decker.

DePalma, R. G. (1986). Disorders of the lymphatic system. In D. C. Sabiston (Ed.), *Textbook of surgery: The biological basis of modern surgical practice* (13th ed., pp. 1696–1708). Philadelphia: W. B. Saunders.

O'Donnell, T. F. (1987). Acquired lymphedema. In C. B. Ernst & J. C. Stanley (Eds.), *Current therapy in vascular surgery* (pp. 50–100). Toronto: B. C. Decker.

Wolfe, J. H. (1989). Diagnosis and classification of lymphedema. In R. B. Rutherford (Ed.), *Vascular surgery* (3rd ed., pp. 1656–1667). Philadelphia: W. B. Saunders.

ADDITIONAL READINGS

Becker, D. M., Larosa, J. H., & Watson, J. E. (1989). Interpreting the new guidelines. *American Journal of Nursing, 89,* 1622–1624.

This article provides an explanation of guidelines for serum cholesterol levels based on the 1988 report of the National Cholesterol Education Program. Recommended levels for total cholesterol and

HDL and LDL levels are discussed, as well as the risks and management of each level.

Cann, R. L., & Clements, F. M. (1989). Silent ischemia in patients undergoing peripheral vascular surgery: Incidence and association with perioperative cardiac morbidity and mortality. *Journal of Vascular Surgery, 9,* 583–587.

Atherosclerosis is a systemic disorder, and CAD is highly prevalent in clients treated for lower-extremity obstructive disease. MI and ischemia represent the most frequent and most clinically important complications of surgical procedures for lower-extremity revascularization. Despite attempts in several areas, no practical, sensitive, and specific method for identifying clients at highest risk for myocardial events postoperatively has been found. This study reports observations on a series of 50 consecutive clients who underwent continuous perioperative ECG monitoring with a microprocessor-based ECG ischemia monitor, which helped to identify clients at high risk for cardiac-related morbidity and death during lower-extremity revascularization.

Frohlich, E. D. (1989). Calcium antagonists for initial therapy of hypertension. *Heart and Lung, 18,* 370–376.

This article discusses the pathophysiology of hypertension and characteristics of ideal pharmacologic agents used for treatment. The focus of the article is on calcium antagonists, with a description of the pharmacologic and physiologic effects of these drugs.

Krokosky, N., & Vanscoy, G. J. (1989). Running an anticoagulation clinic. *American Journal of Nursing, 89,* 1304–1307.

This article, written by a nurse and a pharmacist, discusses the development and workings of a clinic for clients receiving warfarin therapy. In addition to describing their experiences, they provide current information on the indications and goals for anticoagulation therapy.

Miller, R. A., & Evans, W. E. (1988, July). Nurse and patient: Allies preventing amputation. *RN,* pp. 38–44.

This article provides a thorough discussion and pictorial review of assessment findings associated with PAD. Collaborative interventions to prevent further tissue damage are briefly discussed.

Stoy, D. B. (1989). Controlling cholesterol with diet. *American Journal of Nursing, 89,* 1625–1627.

This article provides an explanation of the effect of saturated fatty acids and cholesterol on serum cholesterol levels. The author emphasizes the importance of controlling high serum cholesterol levels by diet and discusses recommended restrictions to lower serum cholesterol levels.

Stoy, D. B. (1989). Controlling cholesterol with drugs. *American Journal of Nursing, 89,* 1628–1633.

This article describes the five major cholesterol-lowering drugs in terms of their pharmacology, effect on CAD, cost, and side effects. The nurse-author focuses on the issue of client compliance with each therapy, discussing common problems and possible solutions for each.

Todd, B. (1988). Newer antihypertensive agents. *Geriatric Nursing, 9,* 187–188.

This feature focuses on the pharmacologic treatment of hypertension in the elderly. The clinical effects of diuretics, beta-blockers, ACE inhibitors, and central and peripheral sympatholytic agents in elders is described. The author emphasizes common side effects of several agents and identifies new agents.

Unit 18 Resources

Nursing Resources

American Association of Critical-Care Nurses (AACN), One Civic Plaza, Suite 330, Newport Beach, CA 92660. Telephone 714-644-9310.

American Association of Critical-Care Nurses Certification Corporation, One Civic Plaza, Suite 315, Newport Beach, CA 92660. Telephone 714-644-9310.
Certifies nurses with experience in critical care.

American Thoracic Society, Section on Nursing, 1740 Broadway, New York, NY 10019. Telephone 212-315-8700.

Society for Peripheral Vascular Nursing (SPVN), 309 Winter Street, Norwood, MA 02062. Telephone 617-762-3630.

Promotes comprehensive care of clients with peripheral vascular disease, with a special focus on client education. Produces "Circulating the Facts About Peripheral Vascular Disease," which is client education material on various specialized topics. Publishes *SPVN Journal* (quarterly).

Other Resources

American Diabetes Association, National Service Center, 1660 Duke Street, Alexandria, VA 22314. Telephone 800-232-3472.

American Dietetic Association, 216 West Jackson, Suite 800, Chicago, IL 60606. Telephone 800-877-1600.

American Red Cross, 430 17th Street NW, Washington, DC 20006. Telephone 202-737-8300.

Mended Hearts, 7320 Greenville Avenue, Dallas, TX 75231. Telephone 214-373-6300, ext. 7061442.

National Center for American Heart Association, 7320 Greenville Avenue, Dallas, TX 75231. Telephone 214-373-6300.

UNIT 19

Problems of Tissue Perfusion: Management of Clients with Disruptions of the Hematologic System

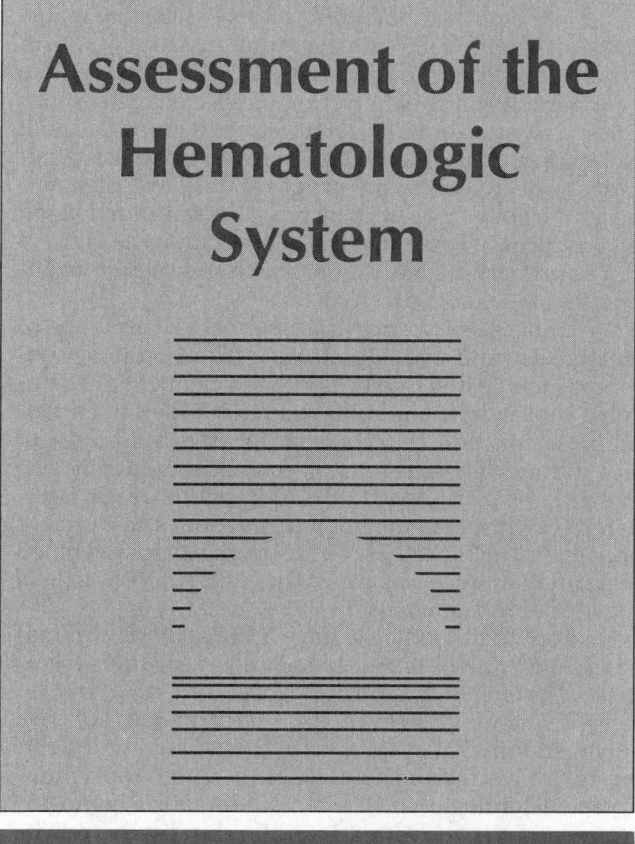

CHAPTER 66

Assessment of the Hematologic System

The incidence of hematologic disorders has been steadily increasing in recent years. Yet, hematologic assessment is often a weak area in the nurse's assessment skills. It is the purpose of this chapter to review the physiology and pathophysiology on which assessment findings in the client with hematologic disease are based and to delineate skills that are essential to a comprehensive physical assessment of these clients.

ANATOMY AND PHYSIOLOGY REVIEW

STRUCTURE AND FUNCTION

BONE MARROW

Each day, the bone marrow in the healthy adult produces and releases about 2.5 billion red blood cells, 2.5 billion platelets, and 1 billion granulocytes per kilogram of body weight. In the fetus, blood components are formed in the liver, the spleen, and, by the last trimester, the bone marrow. At birth, there is bone marrow in every bone. The flat bones, such as the sternum, the skull, and the pelvic and shoulder girdles, contain active bone marrow throughout life. In the long bones, as a person ages, the amount of functional bone marrow decreases until, by age 18 years, it is limited to the ends of these bones. In adulthood, fatty tissue replaces inactive bone marrow; in the elderly, the proportion of fatty marrow increases to occupy about one-half of the marrow that is found in the sternum and ribs. However, at a time of increased demand for blood cells, functional marrow can reappear quickly.

The bone marrow is a blood-forming, or hematopoietic, organ. It produces most of the cellular elements of the blood, including red blood cells, white blood cells, platelets, and some of the immune reactive cells such as lymphocytes and macrophages. The bone marrow is directly involved in some aspects of the immune response, including antibody-mediated and cell-mediated immunity (see Chap. 23 for further discussion of inflammation and the immune response).

As described in Chapter 23, the bone marrow produces cells via stem cells. The bone marrow contains *pluripotential stem cells,* i.e., cells that give rise to any of several lines of blood cells. The pluripotential stem cell can differentiate into a red blood cell, white blood cell, or platelet line, depending on the needs of the body (see Chap. 23, Fig. 23–3). The next stage in cell development is the *unipotential stem cell,* or the precursor cell. A unipotential stem cell has been committed to one specific maturational pathway and is capable of maturing or differentiating into only *one* cell type. Unipotential stem cells are in the active phase of the cell cycle but require a humoral poietin for further development. Erythropoietin is specific for the red blood cell line, and there is evidence of the existence of a leukopoietin and a thrombopoietin for the white blood cell and platelet lines, respectively.

BLOOD COMPONENTS

Blood is composed of cellular elements and plasma. *Plasma* is part of the extracellular fluid of the body. It is similar to interstitial fluid that is found between tissue cells, except that plasma contains about 7% protein, whereas interstitial fluid normally contains less than 2% protein. There are three major types of plasma proteins: albumin, globulins, and fibrinogen. The primary function of *albumin* is to increase osmotic pressure at the capillary membrane, thereby preventing the fluid of the plasma from leaking into the tissues. *Globulins* perform diverse functions such as transporting other substances and protecting the body against infection. Globulins are the main component of antibodies. *Fibrinogen,* when activated, is a protein molecule capable of self-association to form large polymeric structures, which are of basic importance in blood clotting.

The cellular components of the blood include red blood cells, white blood cells, and platelets. These blood components differ in their anatomic features, sites of maturation, and functional capacities.

Red blood cells, or *erythrocytes,* are the largest or greatest cellular component of the blood. The mature, anuclear cells are biconcave disks that can change their shape as they pass through capillaries. The number of cells varies according to sex and age, but the range is from 4,400,000 to 5,500,000/mm³. The stages in red blood cell development include the proerythroblast, the basophilic erythroblast, the polychromatophilic erythroblast, the orthochromatic erythroblast, the reticulocyte, and the mature red blood cell. The *reticulocyte* stage has particular clinical importance. Normally, about 2% of circulating red blood cells are reticulocytes, or immature red blood cells. Active hemoglobin synthesis occurs in these cells. The reticulocyte count is a valid parameter of the red blood cell production rate.

Red blood cells are primarily responsible for the transport of *hemoglobin,* which in turn carries oxygen from the lungs to the tissues. Red blood cells also transport carbon dioxide from the tissues to the lungs for excretion. Red blood cells contain carbonic anhydrase, which catalyzes the reaction between carbon dioxide and water (described in Chaps. 14 and 15) and increases the rate of this reaction dramatically. This rapid reaction allows the blood to combine with, and subsequently excrete, large quantities of carbon dioxide. Also, hemoglobin is an excellent acid-base buffer and thereby contributes to the buffering power of whole blood.

The most important feature of the hemoglobin molecule is its ability to combine loosely and reversibly with oxygen. With only a small drop in oxygen tension at the tissue level, there is a considerable transfer of oxygen from hemoglobin to tissues. Some pathologic conditions can alter the speed and quantity with which oxygen is released to the tissues. Acidosis, fever, and hypercapnia can all lead to increased amounts of oxygen's being released to the tissues.

The total mass of red blood cells is precisely regulated, by the process of *erythropoiesis*—selective maturation of stem cells into mature erythrocytes—to prevent overconcentration of red blood cells. The predominant control of erythropoiesis is via alterations in tissue oxygenation. *Erythropoietin* is a humoral agent that appears in the circulation in response to tissue hypoxia, or decreased tissue oxygenation. This substance causes the bone marrow to increase the rate of red blood cell production. Presently, it is believed that the kidneys are the primary organs that produce and release erythropoietin in response to hypoxia.

A number of substances are essential for formation of hemoglobin and red blood cells. These critical substances include iron, which is a component of the hemoglobin molecule; vitamin B_{12}, which is called the maturation factor and is required for the synthesis of deoxyribonucleic acid (DNA); folic acid, which is also required for synthesis of DNA; copper, which is required for normal hemoglobin formation; and pyridoxine, cobalt, and nickel, which are necessary for red blood cell formation. A lack of any of these substances can lead to maturational anemias.

Healthy red blood cells have a life span of approximately 120 days. As red blood cells age, their membranes become more fragile. These old cells are sequestered and destroyed by macrophages of the reticuloendothelial system or by the spleen and liver. The iron released from hemoglobin is reused for synthesis of new hemoglobin. The remainder of the hemoglobin molecule is converted into bilirubin by the reticuloendothelial system.

The *white blood cells,* or *leukocytes,* constitute the second most common category of blood components. There are six types of leukocytes (as described in Chap. 23, Table 23–1), which are the mobile arm of the body's protective immune system.

White blood cells are formed partially in the bone marrow (granulocytes, monocytes, and some lymphocytes) and partially in the lymphatic system (lymphocytes and plasma cells). The cells formed in the bone marrow are stored there until needed. Normally, about three times as many cells are stored in the marrow as circulate in the blood. In general, the white blood cells need essentially the same vitamins and amino acids as most of the other cells of the body for normal growth and development. Folic acid is particularly necessary to the growth of white blood cells. Chapter 23 details the development and function of the various types of leukocytes.

The *platelets* are another cellular component of the blood. They are the smallest of the formed elements of the blood, being fragments of a giant precursor cell in the bone marrow—the *megakaryocyte.*

Platelets adhere to injured blood vessel walls and

form hemostatic plugs, which stop the flow of blood from the injured site. Platelets also produce substances called *phospholipids,* which are important in coagulation. Platelets are thought to maintain the integrity of the vessels by repairing injuries of small blood vessels. They perform most of their function by *aggregation,* or clumping.

Platelet production in the bone marrow is also precisely regulated, presumably by some type of humoral poietin. After platelets leave the bone marrow, they are taken up by the spleen for storage and are released slowly according to the needs of the body. Normally, 80% of platelets are circulating and 20% are stored in the spleen. Platelets have a life span of 1 to 2 weeks, after which they are gradually consumed during normal intravascular clotting.

SPLEEN, LIVER, AND LYMPHATIC SYSTEM

The spleen and liver are both important to the hematopoietic system. The *spleen,* which is located beneath the diaphragm to the left of the stomach, contains both lymphoid and reticuloendothelial elements. It plays an active part in antibody synthesis and other defense mechanisms. There are three types of matter within the spleen: white, red, and marginal pulp. *White pulp* is filled with lymphocytes and macrophages. *Red pulp* is composed of vascular sinuses that phagocytose unwanted cells from the blood. Many arteries terminate in the *marginal pulp.* During hematopoiesis, the spleen destroys aged or imperfect red blood cells through phagocytosis; plays an important part in iron metabolism by catabolizing hemoglobin released from these destroyed cells; stores platelets; and filters antigens. Clients who have had splenectomies have a greatly increased risk of sepsis and death, particularly from *Streptococcus pneumoniae, Neisseria meningitidis,* or *Haemophilus influenzae.* Splenectomized clients cannot dispose of blood-borne pyogenic organisms because they lack the spleen-produced opsonins, which are important in defense against pyogenic organisms. *Opsonins* are substances that increase the rate of ingestion of bacteria by phagocytes by binding to the surface of the bacteria (Chap. 23). Without opsonins, the unimpeded organisms can double in number every 20 to 40 minutes.

The *liver* is important in erythropoiesis if red blood cell production in the marrow is abnormal. It is extremely important in the production of blood coagulant substances. The liver also converts bilirubin, the end product of hemoglobin catabolism, to bile, which is necessary for fat digestion, and stores iron in the form of ferritin.

The *lymphatic system* is composed of two types of tissue: central lymphoid and secondary lymphoid. *Central lymphoid tissues* (including the thymus, bone marrow, spleen, and liver) are essential for stimulating the development and differentiation of lymphocytes. *Secondary lymphoid tissues* include the spleen and the lymph nodes. Lymph fluid, often called just *lymph,* is derived from the blood through the process of filtration and has the same composition as interstitial fluid: some antibodies, lymphocytes, granulocytes, and enzymes. Lymph is the fluid that is filtered from the arterial end of the capillaries and does not get reabsorbed at the venous end of the capillaries (see Chap. 12). Without the presence of the lymphatic drainage vessels and ducts, this fluid would remain in the interstitial space to cause edema formation and contribute to a vascular fluid volume deficit.

Lymphatic vessels and ducts collect lymph, and their main function is drainage. *Lymph nodes* are bean-shaped bodies that usually occur in chain formation at frequent intervals along lymphatic vessels. The nodes remove foreign particles from the extracellular fluid. All lymph fluid passes through at least one node.

HEMOSTASIS

Hemostasis is the process in which clotting occurs to repair defects in vascular integrity, while simultaneously the fluidity of blood is maintained. It is a complex process that balances the production of clotting factors against the production of factors that dissolve clots. Extrinsic factors are involved in coagulation.

The extrinsic components in coagulation involve vascular and cellular mechanisms. *Vascular* injury activates all components of the hemostatic response. After a blood vessel is cut, the wall of the vessel constricts, resulting in a decrease in blood flow and the release of *tissue thromboplastin,* which stimulates the extrinsic coagulation system. Cellular mechanisms of hemostasis include the activities of *platelets,* which adhere to injured blood vessels and form plugs. Platelets produce adenosine diphosphate (ADP), which enhances their adherence to each other.

The *coagulation system* consists of a series of reactions that result in the formation of a *fibrin clot.* In severe trauma, the clot begins to form in 15 seconds. Fibrin forms a network of threads that traps platelets, leukocytes, and erythrocytes to form a clot. The clot occludes the lumen of the blood vessel and prevents further blood loss. Within a few minutes, the clot retracts and pulls the edges of the vessel together to ensure hemostasis. Clear *serum* is released from the clot into the blood. Serum differs from plasma because it does not contain clotting factors and fibrinogen. *Serum cannot clot; plasma can.*

The coagulation system consists of clotting proteins, or factors, that circulate in plasma in an inactive state until they are stimulated to initiate clotting through one of two pathways: the intrinsic and the extrinsic coagulation cascades. Various factors are needed by these two cascades for completion of a final common pathway that results in the formation of a fibrin clot. These factors are summarized in Table 66–1.

No direct injury is needed for activation of the *intrinsic coagulation cascade.* It can be activated by exposure to a foreign substance, such as collagen during periods of

Text continued on page 2244

TABLE 66-1 The Coagulation Factors

Factor	Amount in Circulation	Site of Synthesis	Action	Significance of Altered Levels	Comments
I: fibrinogen	200–400 mg	Synthesis occurs in liver.	Factor is converted into fibrin by thrombin; it is essential for normal platelet function and wound healing.	*Increased* levels occur in cirrhosis, nephrosis, myeloma, inflammation, and tissue necrosis, and during stress, pregnancy, and oral contraceptive use. *Decreased* levels occur in hypothyroidism, in the presence of circulating tissue thromboplastin, and in liver disease.	
II: prothrombin	100 mg	Synthesis occurs in liver.	Factor is inactive precursor of thrombin.	*Increased* levels occur during stress and in the presence of fever, infection, and gram-negative bacterial endotoxin. *Decreased* levels occur in liver disease and vitamin K deficiency and during coumarin therapy.	Vitamin K dependent.*
III: tissue thromboplastin		Factor arises from virtually any body tissue, but especially from the brain, lungs, prostate, and placenta.	Factor interacts with factor VII in the extrinsic coagulation pathway.	*Decreased* levels occur in liver disease.	

IV: calcium	9–11 mg, 50% ionized		Factor is required in many phases of blood coagulation.	*Decreased* levels occur if massive blood transfusions are done with citrated blood products because ionized calcium combines irreversibly with EDTA, which makes calcium unavailable for participation in coagulation. *Decreased* levels occur in hypergammaglobulinemia because of abnormal calcium binding.	Only extremely small quantities are required for coagulation; deficiency is rarely a cause of coagulopathy.
V: labile factor (proaccelerin)	75–125 mg	Synthesis occurs in liver.	Factor is essential in the formation of prothrombin in the final common coagulation pathway.	*Decreased* levels occur in acquired factor V deficiency (caused by severe liver disease or circulating anticoagulants). *Increased* levels occur in fibrinolysis and during pregnancy, oral contraceptive use, and inflammation.	Factor is totally consumed during the process of coagulation.
VI†					
VII: proconvertin (stable factor)	72–125 mg	Synthesis occurs in liver.	Factor is required in the extrinsic coagulation pathway.	*Decreased* levels occur in liver disease.	Factor is vitamin K dependent;* it is active only in the presence of factor III.

Table continued on following page

TABLE 66–1 The Coagulation Factors *Continued*

Factor	Amount in Circulation	Site of Synthesis	Action	Significance of Altered Levels	Comments
VIII: antihemophilic factor	75–150 mg	Synthesis occurs primarily in liver and in endothelial cells.	Factor is required for thromboplastin generation; is a procoagulant; exerts antisera actions.	*Deficiency* results in classic hemophilia. *Increased* levels occur during inflammation, pregnancy, oral contraceptive use, exercise, stress, and epinephrine infusions.	Factor is stored primarily in spleen.
von Willebrand's factor		Synthesis occurs in endothelial cells and platelets	Factor reacts with a specific receptor site on platelets.	*Deficiency* results in von Willebrand's disease.	Factor circulates in combination with factor VIII, of which it was once considered to be a part.
IX: plasma thromboplastin (Christmas factor)	75–150 mg		Factor is essential in the intrinsic coagulation pathway.	*Deficiency* results in Christmas disease. *Decreased* levels occur during coumarin therapy.	Vitamin K dependent.*
X: Stuart-Prower factor	75–125 mg	Synthesis occurs in liver.	Factor is required for intrinsic thromboplastin formation and prothrombin conversion; it forms the final common pathway.	*Decreased* levels occur in liver disease and vitamin K deficiency. *Increased* levels occur during pregnancy and oral contraceptive use.	Vitamin K dependent.*

Factor	Amount	Synthesis	Function	Clinical notes
XI: plasma thromboplastin antecedent (antihemophilic factor C)	70–130 mg	Synthesis occurs in liver.	Factor is essential in the intrinsic coagulation pathway.	*Decreased* levels occur in hemophilia C and liver disease.
XII: Hageman's factor	70–130 mg	Synthesis occurs in liver.	Factor reacts with factor XI to form active prothromboplastic substance, initiating the intrinsic coagulation pathway; it is possibly a trigger mechanism that responds to injury by initiating diverse processes associated with hemostasis and fibrinolysis, antibody-mediated and cell-mediated defense, and inflammation.	*Deficiency* does not result in a hemorrhagic state but prolongs venous clotting time and partial thromboplastin time.
XIII: fibrin-stabilizing factor	4–9 units, 50% associated with platelets	Factor may be derived from platelets.	Factor acts in the common coagulation pathway, in which it forms a stabilizing bond within fibrin strands.	*Increased* levels occur during pregnancy, oral contraceptive use, and inflammation. *Deficiency* (hereditary) causes abnormal scar formation and wound dehiscence.

* Vitamin K–dependent factors require the presence of vitamin K for synthesis. Vitamin K is not stored in the body but is synthesized by bacteria of intestinal flora. Should this flora be disturbed, especially by use of certain antibiotics, vitamin K–dependent factors decrease. Vitamin K is fat soluble: bile salts produced by the liver are required for its absorption from the intestine. Diseases that interfere with fat absorption, e.g., obstructive jaundice, impair vitamin K absorption.

† Factor VI was once thought to be an inactive form of factor V. It is no longer considered to have a role in hemostasis.

Modified from Griffin, J. P. (1986). *Hematology and immunology: Concepts for nursing.* Norwalk, CT: Appleton-Century-Crofts.

blood stasis. All factors required for the intrinsic system are present in the blood. It can also be activated by antigen-antibody reactions, circulating debris, platelet clumps on damaged vessels, and bacterial endotoxins. A chain reaction follows until factor X is activated, which leads to the final common pathway of clot formation. Figure 67–1 in Chapter 67 illustrates the steps of the coagulation cascade and the impact of various drugs on them.

The *extrinsic coagulation cascade* is activated by release of tissue thromboplastin (factor III) from damaged tissues. Damaged tissues produce and release tissue thromboplastin, which initiates the clotting cascade to form activated factor X.

Regardless of the etiologic event, the final result is the same: stimulation of prothrombin activator to convert prothrombin into thrombin. The production of thrombin leads to the formation of a fibrin clot.

To maintain a flow of blood within the vascular space, *anticoagulant forces* also operate. The *fibrinolytic system* involves the dissolution of the fibrin clot (Fig. 66–1). The central event of fibrinolysis is the conversion of plasminogen to plasmin. Plasmin then digests fibrin, fibrinogen, prothrombin, and factors V, VIII, and XII, thus breaking down the fibrin clot. The dissolution of fibrin results in the formation of *fibrin split products* (FSPs) (sometimes called fibrin degradation products [FDPs]), which are anticoagulants in and of themselves.

HEMATOLOGIC CHANGES ASSOCIATED WITH AGING

Some researchers have found that the total leukocyte count tends to be lower after age 65 years, primarily because of a decrease in the lymphocyte count. Lymphopenia can occur in the aged, with the result that the absolute number of T cells is decreased. Also, lymphocytes from aged subjects may show significantly less reactivity to antigens. Antibody levels and responses are significantly lower in the elderly compared with the young adult. The leukocyte count does not rise as high in response to infection in elderly individuals as in young people, and often the principal manifestation of a leukocyte response is an increased number of bands.

Another parameter that changes with age is hemoglobin levels. Nearly all studies have shown that hemoglobin levels fall after middle age. It is speculated that iron-deficient diets may play a role in this finding.

No age-related changes in the platelet count have been reported. The cellularity of the marrow decreases in old age, inactive bone marrow being replaced by fatty tissue. Occasionally, the red blood cell sedimentation rate may increase with age. Any other hematologic abnormalities in elderly clients are usually due to an underlying disease.

HISTORY

DEMOGRAPHIC DATA

Age and *sex* are important demographic data to obtain to accurately assess the client's hematologic status. Bone marrow and lymphoid activity appears to diminish with age. Women have lower blood cell counts than men at all ages. The exact etiology of this sex difference is unknown but may be related to a dilutional effect of female hormones, which cause increased volume of vascular fluid, differences in bone marrow activity, or sex-related increased red blood cell loss. Information on *occupation, hobbies,* and *geographic location of housing* is also important to collect because these data may reveal exposure to specific agents or chemicals that are known to affect hematologic function.

PERSONAL AND FAMILY HISTORY

The nurse obtains information about *inherited hematologic disorders, allergies, current medications* (prescribed and over the counter), and *family history.* The nurse asks if anyone in the family has suffered from frequent nose-

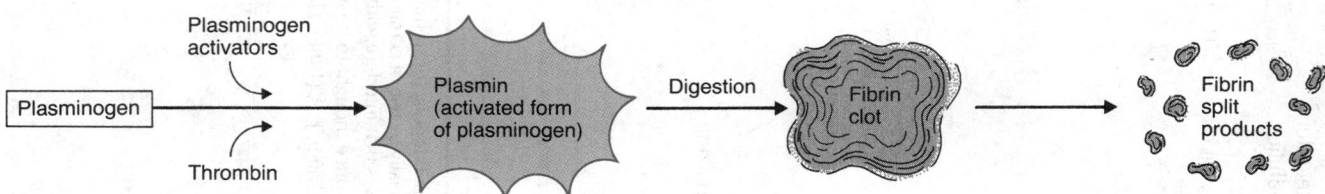

Figure 66–1

The process of fibrinolysis. Plasminogen is converted to plasmin by thrombin and plasminogen activators in the microcirculation. The active plasmin digests the components of the fibrin clot and breaks it down into fibrin split products.

bleeds, postpartum hemorrhages, or excessive bleeding after dental extractions. Questions are asked about jaundice, anemia, and gallstones in relatives.

The nurse questions the client about use of blood "thinners" such as warfarin sodium (Coumadin) or aspirin. A person who consumes large quantities of aspirin may have bleeding problems, and many over-the-counter medications contain aspirin. All medications that the client consumes at present and in the past are determined. Use of antibiotics is noted because prolonged therapy can lead to coagulopathies. Chloramphenicol is an antibiotic that can lead to serious hematologic abnormalities, such as aplastic anemia, and its use should be noted. Any past or present use of cytotoxic drugs, such as those used in chemotherapy, should be noted.

DIET HISTORY

The nurse asks the client to *record everything he or she eats for a week.* This information can be invaluable in determining etiologies of anemias. Diets high in fat and carbohydrates and low in protein, iron, and vitamins can precipitate various maturational anemias. The nurse also asks if the client has recently experienced weight loss.

SOCIOECONOMIC STATUS

The nurse determines the client's extrapersonal resources, such as finances. An individual who has a marginal income may have a diet that is low in iron and protein. The nurse asks if there are community resources available to the client and if he or she is willing to use them. The client's occupation, if the client is employed, is noted. The nurse asks if the work involves noxious or toxic agents. The nurse also assesses the social support that is available to the client: family, friends, and caregivers.

CURRENT HEALTH PROBLEM

The nurse determines whether the client has noted swelling of lymph nodes or excessive bruising or bleeding and whether the bleeding was spontaneous or induced by trauma. The nurse determines whether the client suffers from excessive fatigue, dyspnea on exertion, palpitations, frequent infections, fevers, weight loss, or diarrhea. The nurse inquires about the amount of bleeding that the client has experienced after routine dental work. The nurse assesses if the client suffers from menorrhagia, or excessive menstrual flow and if the client experiences headaches and paresthesias, which are both frequent accompaniments of hematologic dis-

ease. Inquiries are made about vertigo and tinnitus because both can be symptoms of marked anemia. Anorexia, dysphagia, and a sore tongue can be symptoms of anemia.

The nurse has the client describe the presenting health problem in terms of the following profile:

1. Date and time of onset of symptoms
2. Type of onset: gradual or abrupt
3. Course of the problem: continuous or intermittent
4. Duration of each episode
5. Frequency of episodes
6. Quality and severity of symptoms
7. Interference with usual activities
8. Associated symptoms
9. Precipitating conditions
10. Relieving factors

The nurse determines the client's perception of his or her own health status and identifies stressors as the client perceives them. The nurse notes if there is a discrepancy between the client's perception and that of the nurse. The nurse also determines whether the client has ever experienced a similar problem and how it was handled, as well as what the client anticipates for himself or herself in the future as a consequence of the present situation. The nurse discusses with the client what the client can do and what the client can expect from caregivers, family, and friends.

PHYSICAL ASSESSMENT

The physical assessment performed by the nurse is a comprehensive one, inclusive of all body systems. The comprehensive assessment is particularly necessary for the hematologic system because its dysfunction affects the body as a whole. Certain problems are specific for hematologic assessment in the aged, as noted in the accompanying Focus on the Elderly feature.

SKIN

The nurse inspects the *color* of the skin for pallor or icterus (jaundice). Mucous membranes and nail beds are observed for pallor or cyanosis. Gums, conjunctivae, and palmar creases are also useful guides to hemoglobin levels and should be assessed for pallor. Any *lesions* or *draining areas* are noted. The nurse assesses for signs of *bleeding* that may be in the form of petechiae and con-

FOCUS ON THE ELDERLY ■ **Overcoming Problems in Hematologic Assessment in the Elderly**

Assessment Area	Findings in Hematologic Disorders	Normal Changes in the Elderly	Significance/Alternatives
Nail beds (for capillary refill)	Pallor or cyanosis may indicate a hematologic disorder.	Thickened and/or discolored nails make visualization of skin color beneath the nails impossible.	Use another body area, such as the lip, to assess central capillary refill.
Hair distribution	Thin or absent hair on the trunk and/or extremities may indicate poor circulation to a particular area.	Progressive loss of body hair is a normal facet of aging.	A relatively even pattern of hair loss that has occurred over an extended period is not significant.
Skin moisture	Skin dryness may indicate any of a number of hematologic disorders.	Skin dryness is a normal facet of aging.	Skin moisture is not usually a reliable indicator of an underlying pathologic condition in the elderly.
Skin color	Skin color changes, especially pallor and jaundice, are associated with some hematologic disorders.	Pigment loss and skin yellowing are common changes associated with aging.	Pallor in an elderly person may not be a reliable indicator of anemia; laboratory testing is required. Yellow-tinged skin in an elderly person may not be a reliable indicator of increased serum bilirubin levels; laboratory testing is required.

fluent ecchymoses. Petechiae are pinpoint hemorrhagic lesions that may appear anywhere on the body. Ecchymoses, or bruises, may be confluent or clustered. Both petechiae and ecchymoses indicate bleeding disorders. For hospitalized clients, the nurse determines whether the client is bleeding from obvious sites or from covert sites, such as nasogastric tubes, endotracheal tubes, central lines, peripheral intravenous sites, or Foley's catheters. Skin *turgor* and *itching* are also noted because dry skin and hair and intense itching can indicate hematologic disease.

HEAD AND NECK

Pallor or *ulceration of the oral mucosa* is noted. The tongue may be completely smooth in pernicious anemia and iron deficiency anemia. The tongue may be smooth and red in clients with nutritional deficiencies, and these manifestations may be accompanied by fissuring at the corners of the mouth. The nurse observes for jaundice of the sclera.

All lymph node areas are inspected and palpated. Any *lymph node enlargement* is documented, along with whether palpation of the enlarged node causes pain. In addition, the nurse determines whether the enlarged node moves with palpation or is in a fixed position.

Redness and *swelling* of the skin, indicators of inflammation, are also noted.

CHEST

The nurse determines how easily the client is *fatigued*, whether the client experiences *shortness of breath* at rest or on exertion, and whether the client requires a certain number of pillows to sleep comfortably at night. Many anemias cause these symptoms.

The nurse observes for placement of the point of maximal impact in the cardiovascular system. The presence of *heaves, distended neck veins, edema,* or signs of *phlebitis* is noted. The nurse auscultates for *murmurs, gallops, irregular rhythms,* and *abnormal blood pressure.* Severe anemias can precipitate right ventricular hypertrophy and subsequent cardiac disease.

MUSCULOSKELETAL SYSTEM

Increased rib or sternal tenderness is an important sign, and the *superficial surfaces of all bones* should be examined thoroughly by applying intermittent firm pressure with the fingertips. This sign can indicate various hematologic malignancies.

GASTROINTESTINAL SYSTEM

The normal adult spleen is usually not palpable. *Enlarged spleens* may be detected by percussion, although palpation is more reliable. In examining for an enlarged spleen, it should be remembered that the organ lies just beneath the abdominal wall and is identified by its movement during respiration. During palpation, the client lies in a relaxed, supine position while the nurse, standing on the client's right, palpates the left upper quadrant.

Palpation of the edge of the liver in the right upper quadrant of the abdomen is commonly used to detect *hepatic enlargement.* The normal liver may be palpable as much as 4 to 5 cm below the right costal margin but is usually not palpable in the epigastrium. Both the liver and spleen may be enlarged in hematologic disease.

CENTRAL NERVOUS SYSTEM

A thorough examination of cranial nerves and neurologic function is necessary in many clients with hematologic disease. Vitamin B_{12} deficiency impairs cerebral, olfactory, spinal cord, and peripheral nerve function, and severe chronic deficiency may lead to irreversible neurologic degeneration. A variety of *neurologic abnormalities* may develop in clients with various hematologic malignancies as a consequence of infiltration, bleeding, or infection.

PSYCHOSOCIAL ASSESSMENT

The individual with hematologic disease may be suffering from chronic illness, such as cancer, or from an acute exacerbation of a chronic disease, such as disseminated intravascular coagulation. In either instance, each individual brings his or her own individual coping style to the illness. After developing a rapport with the client, the nurse can ascertain what coping mechanisms the client has used in the past during illness or other crises. If the client has used destructive coping mechanisms, such as overeating, drinking, or smoking, the nurse can work with the individual to develop alternative coping mechanisms.

Additional information that should be obtained from the client and family includes social support networks, community resources, and financial health. A problem in any of these areas can interfere with the client's compliance with therapy and, ultimately, recovery.

The nurse ascertains how the client views himself or herself and how the perceived role fits in the family and society. A prolonged illness, in which the client is subjected to the forced dependency of hospitalization and earning capacities may be disrupted, can lead to self-esteem difficulties in the client who is used to being independent and performing the breadwinner role.

DIAGNOSTIC ASSESSMENT

LABORATORY TESTS

In hematologic disease, the most definitive signs are often the laboratory tests. Table 66–2 summarizes pertinent laboratory data associated with hematologic function.

A *complete blood count* (CBC) includes a number of studies: a *red blood cell* (RBC) *count,* an actual count of circulating red blood cells in 1 mm³ of venous blood; *hemoglobin level* (Hb), the total amount of hemoglobin in peripheral blood; *hematocrit* (Hct), the percentage of red blood cells in the total blood volume; and *mean corpuscular volume* (MCV), a measure of the average volume or size of a single red blood cell. The MCV is useful for classifying anemias. When the MCV is elevated, the cell is said to be *macrocytic,* or abnormally large, as seen in megaloblastic anemias. When the MCV is decreased, the cell is abnormally small, or *microcytic,* as seen in iron deficiency anemia. The CBC also includes the *mean corpuscular hemoglobin* (MCH), the average amount of hemoglobin in a single red blood cell; and *mean corpuscular hemoglobin concentration* (MCHC), a measure of the average concentration of hemoglobin in a single red blood cell. When the MCHC is decreased, the cell has a deficiency of hemoglobin and is *hypochromic,* as in iron deficiency anemia. Because red blood cells cannot contain more hemoglobin than is physiologically possible, an elevated MCHC cannot occur.

The white blood cell count with differential is also part of the CBC and is a measure of the total number of white blood cells (WBCs) and the percentages of the five types. Elevations of any one type of white blood cell or a change in the percentages can indicate the presence of disease or injury (see Chaps. 23, 27, and 67).

Another hematologic test that is often helpful includes the *reticulocyte count,* which is a test for determining bone marrow function. A reticulocyte is an immature red blood cell, and an elevated reticulocyte count indicates increased red blood cell production by the bone marrow. There are situations in which an elevated reticulocyte count is desirable, such as in anemias or after hemorrhage. This elevation would indicate that the bone marrow is responding appropriately to a decrease in the total red blood cell mass.

Hemoglobin electrophoresis enables detection of abnormal forms of hemoglobin, such as Hb S in sickle cell anemia. Hb A_1 constitutes the major component of hemoglobin in the normal red blood cell.

Leukocyte alkaline phosphatase (LAP) is useful in the differentiation of chronic leukemias from hematologic reactions seen in severe infections and polycythemia vera.

Coombs' test is an important hematologic test that is used for blood typing. It exists in two forms: direct and indirect. The direct test detects antibodies against red blood cells. Certain diseases, such as erythroblastosis fetalis, systemic lupus erythematosus, mononucleosis, and lymphomas, are associated with the production of antibodies directed against the client's own red blood cells. Frequently, the production of these antibodies is not associated with any specific disease at all. The result is a hemolytic anemia. The test is performed by mixing the client's red blood cells, presumably covered with autoantibodies, with Coombs' serum (a solution containing antibodies against human blood serum). If the red blood cells are coated with autoantibodies, clumping occurs. When a transfusion with incompatible blood is given, Coombs' test can detect the antibodies coating the transfused red blood cells.

The indirect test detects the presence of circulating antibodies against red blood cells. The major purpose of this test is to determine whether the client has serum antibodies to red blood cells that she or he is about to receive by blood transfusion.

Serum ferritin (Fe) and the total iron-binding capacity (TIBC) test are measures of iron levels. Abnormal

TABLE 66–2 Normal Values and Significance of Abnormal Findings in Common Laboratory Tests Used for Hematologic Assessment

Test	Normal Values	Significance of Abnormal Findings
Tests of the Hematologic System		
RBC count	3.6–5.0 million/mm³ (women) 4.2–5.5 million/mm³ (men)	*Decreased levels* indicate possible anemia or hemorrhage. *Elevations* indicate possible chronic anoxia.
Hemoglobin (Hb)	12–15 g/dL (women) 14–16.5 g/dL (men)	Same as for RBC count.
Hematocrit (Hct)	37%–45% (women) 42%–50% (men)	Same as for RBC count.
Mean corpuscular volume (MCV)	80–95 μm³	*Elevations* indicate possible macrocytic RBCs. *Decreased levels* indicate possible microcytic RBCs.
Mean corpuscular hemoglobin (MCH)	27–31 pg	*Elevations* are associated with macrocytic anemia. *Decreased levels* are associated with microcytic anemia.
Mean corpuscular hemoglobin concentration (MCHC)	32–36 g/dL (32%–36%)	*Decreased levels* indicate possible hypochromic cells. *Elevations* are associated with spherocytosis.
White blood cell (WBC) count	4,500–11,000/mm³	*Elevations* indicate possible infection. *Decreased levels* indicate possible bone marrow failure.
Reticulocyte count	0.5%–2% of total RBC count	*Decreased levels* indicate possible inadequate RBC production. *Elevations* indicate possible polycythemia vera.
Iron (Fe)	60–90 μg/dL	*Decreased levels* indicate possible iron deficiency anemia.
Total iron-binding capacity (TIBC)	250–420 μg/dL	Same as for iron.
Serum haptoglobin	100–150 mg	*Decreased levels* indicate possible hemolytic liver disease. *Elevations* indicate possible inflammatory disease.

levels of iron and TIBC are characteristic of many diseases, including iron deficiency anemia. The *serum ferritin test* measures the direct quantity of iron bound to a substance called transferrin, which transports iron. The *TIBC test* is a measure of the amount of transferrin.

The *capillary fragility test,* or Rumpel-Leede test, measures vascular hemostatic function. The test is done by increasing intracapillary pressure in the arm by occluding venous outflow. Usually, a blood pressure cuff is inflated to a pressure halfway between the systolic and diastolic pressures, and inflation is maintained for 5 minutes. The number of petechiae that appear are then counted; normally, fewer than five appear. The clot retraction test and the capillary fragility test are rarely used for clinical evaluation of a client.

Coagulation studies that are more widely used include the bleeding time test, which is used to evaluate vascular and platelet activity during hemostasis. A small incision is made in the forearm, and the time required

for the bleeding to stop is recorded. The *prothrombin time* (PT) evaluates the adequacy of the extrinsic coagulation cascade. When factors V and VII are deficient, the PT is prolonged. With obstructive biliary disease, vitamin K is not absorbed. Factor VII depends on vitamin K, so the PT is prolonged in obstructive biliary disease. Coumarin therapy is monitored by use of PT levels. Appropriate coumarin therapy should prolong the PT by 1.5 to 2 times normal. The PT test results are given in seconds, along with a control value. A normal PT should be about equal to the control value.

The *partial thromboplastin time* (PTT) assesses the intrinsic coagulation cascade. It evaluates factors II, V, VIII, IX, XI, and XII. When any of these factors exists in deficient amounts, as in hemophilia or disseminated intravascular coagulation, the PTT is prolonged. Because factors II, IX, and X are vitamin K–dependent factors that are produced in the liver, liver disease or biliary obstruction can decrease their concentration and pro-

TABLE 66–2   Normal Values and Significance of Abnormal Findings in Common Laboratory Tests Used for Hematologic Assessment *Continued*

Test	Normal Values	Significance of Abnormal Findings
Platelet count	150,000–350,000/mm³	*Decreased levels* indicate possible bone marrow failure, hypersplenism, or accelerated consumption of platelets. *Elevations* indicate possible hemorrhage, polycythemia vera, or malignancy.
Hemoglobin electrophoresis	Hb A₁ 95%–98% Hb A₂ 2%–3% Hb F 0.8%–2% Hb S 0% Hb C 0%	*Variations* indicate hemoglobinopathies.
Direct Coombs' and indirect Coombs' tests	Negative	*Positive findings* indicate antibodies to RBCs.
Coagulation Tests		
Prothrombin time (PT)	11–12.5 s (85%–100%)	*Elevations* indicate possible deficiency of factors V and VII.
Partial thromboplastin time (PTT)	30–40 s	*Elevations* indicate possible deficiency of factors II, V, VIII, IX, XI, or XII.
Bleeding time	1–9 min	*Elevations* indicate possible thrombocytopenia, marrow infiltration, or inadequate platelet function.
Euglobulin lysis time	90 min–6 h	*Decreased levels* indicate possible fibrinolysis.
Fibrin split products (FDPs)	<10 µg/mL	*Elevations* indicate possible disseminated intravascular coagulation or fibrinolysis.

From Griffin, J. P. (1986). *Hematology and immunology: Concepts for nursing.* Norwalk, CT: Appleton-Century-Crofts.

long the PTT. Heparin therapy is monitored by use of PTT. Desired ranges for therapeutic anticoagulation are 1.5 to 2.5 times normal.

Platelet aggregation, or ability to clump, can be tested by mixing the client's platelet-poor plasma with a substance called ristocetin. The degree of aggregation can then be noted. Aggregation can be impaired in von Willebrand's disease and during intake of a variety of drugs such as aspirin, anti-inflammatory agents, and psychotropic agents.

RADIOGRAPHIC EXAMINATIONS/ NUCLEAR SCANS

Assessment of the client with a suspected hematologic abnormality occasionally includes radioisotopic imaging. The bone marrow can be evaluated via isotopes for sites of active erythropoiesis and sites of iron storage. The macrophage system within the marrow can be visualized by means of radioactive isotopes. Radioactive colloids are routinely used to determine organ size and liver and spleen function.

The client is usually given a radioactive isotope intravenously about 3 hours before the procedure. The client is then taken to the nuclear medicine department for the scan, where he or she must lie still for about an hour. There are no special client preparations or follow-up care for these tests.

OTHER DIAGNOSTIC STUDIES

BONE MARROW ASPIRATION

Bone marrow aspiration is frequently done for evaluation of the client with a possible hematologic disorder.

Client preparation. The procedure is explained to the client. The nurse tells the client that the injection of a local anesthetic will be felt, and, as the marrow is being aspirated, a sensation of pulling will be experienced. This sensation is quite painful. The client is then assisted onto an examining table, and the site of aspiration is exposed. The site is usually the iliac crest.

Procedure. A local anesthetic solution is injected around the site. The client may receive a mild tranquilizer. Sterile precautions must be observed. The skin over the site is shaved and cleaned with a disinfectant solution. The needle is inserted with a twisting motion and marrow is aspirated. Pressure is applied to the site until hemostasis is ensured.

Follow-up care. The site of the aspiration is observed closely for 24 hours for signs of bleeding and infection. A mild analgesic usually controls the discomfort.

A normal bone marrow examination reveals active

red blood cell, white blood cell, and platelet production. It is performed to fully evaluate hematopoiesis.

SUMMARY

Assessment of the client with hematologic disease is complex and often integrates knowledge and skills used in evaluation of other body systems. The nurse must also possess excellent communication techniques to determine which life style or dietary modifications are beneficial for the client.

REFERENCES AND READINGS

Berne, R., & Levy, M. (1988). *Physiology* (2nd ed.). St. Louis: C. V. Mosby.

Colman, R., Hirsch, J., Marder, V., & Salzman, E. (1987). *Hemostasis and thrombosis: Basic principles and clinical practice* (2nd ed.). Philadelphia: J. B. Lippincott.

DeVita, V., Hellman, S., & Rosenberg, S. (1990). *Cancer: Principles and practice of oncology* (3rd ed.). Philadelphia: J. B. Lippincott.

Griffin, J. P. (1986). *Hematology and immunology: Concepts for nursing.* Norwalk, CT: Appleton-Century-Crofts.

Guyton, A. C. (1987). *Human physiology and mechanisms of disease* (4th ed.). Philadelphia: W. B. Saunders.

Haeuber, D., & DiJulio, J. (1989). Hemopoietic colony stimulating factors: An overview. *Oncology Nursing Forum, 16*(2), 247–255.

McIntire, S., & Cioppa, A. (1984). *Cancer nursing: A developmental approach.* New York: Wiley.

Rapaport, S. (1987). *Introduction to hematology* (2nd ed.). Philadelphia: J. B. Lippincott.

Sieff, C. (1987). Hematopoietic growth factors. *Journal of Clinical Investigation, 79,* 1549–1557.

Simmons, A. (1989). *Hematology: A combined theoretical and technical approach.* Philadelphia: W. B. Saunders.

Williams, W., Beitler, E., Erslev, A., & Lichtman, M. (1983). *Hematology.* New York: McGraw-Hill.

ADDITIONAL READINGS

Griffin, J. P. (1985). Nursing care of the critically ill cancer patient. In G. Carlon & W. Howland (Eds.), *Critical care of the cancer patient.* Chicago: Year Book Medical.

This chapter is a comprehensive discussion of the many complications that can beset the client with cancer. Septic shock, disseminated intravascular coagulation, and adult respiratory distress syndrome occurring in the leukemic client are discussed.

Griffin, J. P. (1986). Be prepared for the bleeding patient. *Nursing '86, 16*(6), 34–42.

This article is a well-illustrated discussion of the pathophysiology and nursing care that is required for the client with disseminated intravascular coagulation.

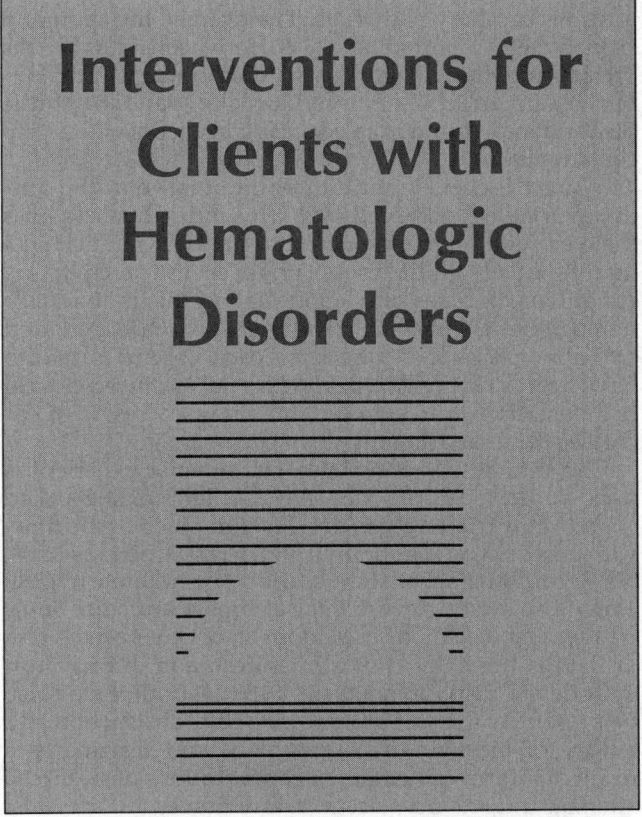

CHAPTER 67

Interventions for Clients with Hematologic Disorders

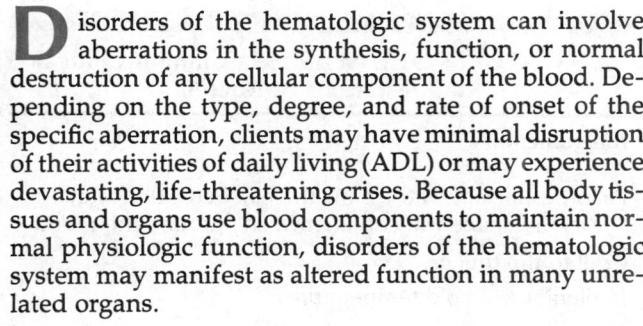

Disorders of the hematologic system can involve aberrations in the synthesis, function, or normal destruction of any cellular component of the blood. Depending on the type, degree, and rate of onset of the specific aberration, clients may have minimal disruption of their activities of daily living (ADL) or may experience devastating, life-threatening crises. Because all body tissues and organs use blood components to maintain normal physiologic function, disorders of the hematologic system may manifest as altered function in many unrelated organs.

RED BLOOD CELL DISORDERS

As discussed in Chapter 66, the major cellular component of the blood is the population of red blood cells (RBCs), or erythrocytes. Normal physiologic function is dependent on maintaining the circulating volume of erythrocytes within the normal range for the individual's age and sex and ensuring that the erythrocytes are able to perform their normal functions. RBC disorders include problems in RBC production, function, and destruction. These problems may result in an insufficient number or function of RBCs (e.g., anemia) or an excess of RBCs.

Anemia

OVERVIEW

Anemia is defined as a reduction in the number of RBCs, the quantity of hemoglobin, or the hematocrit (the volume of packed RBCs per 100 mL of blood) (Froberg, 1989a). Anemia is a clinical sign, rather than a diagnosis, because it is the principal manifestation of a number of abnormal conditions. It can result from dietary deficiency states, hereditary disorders, bone marrow disease, or bleeding states. The incidence of anemia is high, especially in underdeveloped countries where nutrition is poor.

There are many types of anemia. Some arise from decreased hemoglobin synthesis, such as iron deficiency anemia. Others develop from a deficiency state, such as vitamin B_{12} or folate deficiency and pernicious anemia. Additional causes of anemia include decreased development of the RBC line precursors, decreased erythropoiesis, and increased destruction of RBCs. Despite the varied etiologies of anemia, the effects on the client (see the accompanying Key Features of Disease) and the requisite nursing care are similar (Froberg, 1989b). Because disorders of many other organ systems can result in an

KEY FEATURES OF DISEASE ■ Common Clinical Manifestations of Anemia

Integumentary

Pallor, especially of the ears, the nail beds, the palmar creases, and the conjunctiva and around the mouth

Cool to the touch

Intolerance of cold temperatures

Cardiovascular

Tachycardia at basal activity levels, increasing with activity and during and immediately after meals

Murmurs and gallops heard on auscultation when anemia is severe

Orthostatic hypotension

Respiratory

Dyspnea on exertion

Neurologic

Increased somnolence and fatigue

Headache

anemic condition through blood loss, especially insidious but chronic blood loss, any client presenting with anemia requires a detailed assessment to determine the actual cause of the anemia.

Anemias Resulting from Increased Destruction of Red Blood Cells

Sickle Cell Anemia

Sickle cell anemia is an autosomal codominant hereditary disorder resulting from a single amino acid change in the beta chain of the hemoglobin molecule. This abnormal hemoglobin is hemoglobin S (Hb S) instead of hemoglobin A (Hb A). Hb S is sensitive to changes in the oxygen content of the RBC. Insufficient oxygen causes the abnormal beta chains to polymerize within the cell, causing severe distortion in the overall shape of the entire RBC. These cells assume a sickle shape. When the RBCs assume the sickle shape, the cells become rigid, clump together, and form clusters that obstruct capillary blood flow. This leads to further tissue hypoxia and more sickling. The result can be microscopic obstructions or large infarctions in the locally affected tissues. A number of situations can precipitate sickling, including hypoxia, vascular stasis, low environmental and/or body temperatures, acidosis, strenuous exercise, anesthesia, dehydration, and infections.

Usually, sickled cells resume a normal shape when the precipitating condition is removed and proper oxygenation occurs. However, membranes of the cells can become damaged over time, with the end result of irreversibly sickled cells. Additionally, the altered membrane of sickled cells makes them more fragile and more easily destroyed in the spleen and other organs with tortuous capillary pathways. The average life span of a sickled cell is approximately 20 days, considerably reduced from the 120-day life span of normal RBCs (Robbins & Kumar, 1987). This reduced life span is responsible for hemolytic anemia occurring in clients with sickle cell anemia.

When the client inherits one abnormal gene, the condition is called sickle cell *trait*. This individual can pass the condition on to offspring, but has only mild clinical manifestations of the disease under severe precipitating conditions, because only about half of this individual's hemoglobin is abnormal. The client who has inherited two abnormal genes (one from each parent) is said to have overt sickle cell *anemia*, with easily induced clinical manifestations and chronic anemia as a result of increased RBC destruction.

The individual with sickle cell anemia experiences periodic episodes of extensive cellular sickling called *crises*. Many clients are in good health much of the time, with crises occurring sporadically in response to precipitating conditions that stimulate local or systemic hypoxemia. The crises have a sudden onset and can be as frequent as weekly or as seldom as once a year.

Pain is the chief clinical manifestation during most episodes of crisis (Bojanowski, 1989). Jaundice may also be present as a result of increased RBC destruction and release of bilirubin. Tissue damage and scarring as a result of infarcts are common complications of sickle cell anemia. Infarcts may occur in any tissue, but are most common in organs of the chest and the abdomen. Infarctions in the spleen are so common that, after childhood, the spleen of most individuals with sickle cell anemia is small and scarred. Other clinical manifestations vary with the site of tissue damage. More common clinical manifestations associated with sickle cell anemia in adults include necrosis of the head of the femur, necrotic bone marrow with the development of infection, renal medullary ischemia with resultant diminished capacity to concentrate urine, priapism (persistently engorged penile blood vessels causing a prolonged and painful erection), pulmonary infarctions leading to repeated episodes of chest pain and pneumonia, myocardial infarctions leading to heart failure, and cerebrovascular accidents.

Management of this disease focuses on prevention and treatment of crises. Clients are taught to avoid the specific activities that lead to hypoxia and hypoxemia. In addition, clients are taught to recognize the early signs and symptoms of crisis so that medical advice can be sought and appropriate treatment can be initiated early to prevent undue pain, complications, and permanent tissue damage. Additionally, clients are counseled about the hereditary aspects of this problem and information concerning prenatal diagnosis and options is offered.

Treatment of actual crises includes pain management, fluid replacement to ensure adequate hydration and maintain blood flow, oxygen therapy, and correction of the specific condition causing or contributing to hypoxia. Transfusions usually are not administered, unless aplastic crisis is present without an accompanying vascular occlusion.

Glucose-6-Phosphate Dehydrogenase Deficiency Anemia

Many forms of congenital hemolytic anemia result from defects or deficiencies of one or more enzymes within the RBC. Most of these enzymes are essential to catalyze some critical step in intracellular energy production. More than 200 such disorders have been identified. The most common type of congenital hemolytic anemia by far is associated with a deficiency of the enzyme glucose-6-phosphate dehydrogenase (G6PD). This disease affects American Black males more frequently than any other population (Robbins & Kumar, 1987).

G6PD catalyzes critical reactions in the glycolytic pathway. Because RBCs contain no mitochondria (sites of high-efficiency production of the energy compound adenosine triphosphate [ATP] through the Krebs' cycle), active glycolysis is essential for energy metabolism. Cells that have reduced amounts of G6PD are more susceptible to hemolysis during oxidant injuries, which can be induced through exposure to specific drugs (e.g., phenacetin, sulfonamides, aspirin [acetylsalicylic acid], quinine derivatives, thiazide diuretics, and vitamin K derivatives) and toxins (Rapaport, 1987). Normal RBCs avoid injury from these agents by increasing the production of ATP and stimulating defensive metabolic processes. Newly produced RBCs from individuals with G6PD deficiency have relatively sufficient quantities of G6PD; however, as the cells age, the concentration of this enzyme diminishes drastically.

With exposure to any of the above-mentioned agents, the individual experiences acute intravascular hemolysis lasting from 7 to 12 days. During this acute phase, the client has anemia and jaundice. The hemolytic reaction is self-limited because only older erythrocytes are destroyed.

Because drugs that precipitate hemolytic reactions are common and because a G6PD deficiency has a high worldwide incidence, screening tests should be part of every public health program. It is important that individuals be screened for this deficiency before donating blood, as administration of cells deficient in the enzyme can be hazardous for the recipient. Identification and total removal of the precipitating drug or the agent responsible for the hemolytic reaction are imperative.

Management during and immediately after an episode of hemolysis focuses on maintenance of adequate hydration to prevent precipitation of cellular debris and hemoglobin in the kidney tubules, leading to acute tubular necrosis. Osmotic diuretics may assist in preventing this complication. Transfusion therapy is indicated when anemia is present and kidney function is normal.

Autoimmune Hemolytic Anemia

Increased RBC destruction through the process of hemolysis can occur in response to a variety of situations. Such situations include mechanical trauma (seen in individuals who have valvular prostheses, mechanical hearts, or significantly narrowed blood vessels), microbial infection (e.g., malarial infections with the protozoon *Plasmodium*), and autoimmune reactions directed against self blood components. All of these situations increase the rate at which RBCs are destroyed by causing internal or external lysing of the membrane. The most common types of hemolytic anemias seen in industrialized countries are the autoimmune hemolytic anemias (Simmons, 1989).

The *autoimmune hemolytic anemias* are a group of hemolytic anemias in which RBC destruction occurs because the clients' immune system components attack their own RBCs. Usually, the attacking immune components are antibodies (either immunoglobulin G [IgG] or immunoglobulin M [IgM]) or complement proteins (see Chap. 23). The exact mechanism that causes immune components to no longer recognize the client's own blood cells as self and to initiate destructive processes against the RBCs is not known. When these anemias are present without any accompanying disease or disorder, it is possible that the membrane surface of the RBC is expressing a new protein (antigen) not made elsewhere in the body and not recognized as part of the normal self, thus triggering an immune response. In such instances, the pathologic change actually resides in the RBCs. When these anemias are present with other autoimmune disorders (such as systemic lupus erythematosus) or lymphoproliferative disorders, the pathologic change may actually reside within the immune system. Whatever the defect, the RBC is viewed as nonself by the immune system and is destroyed.

Two classifications of autoimmune hemolytic anemia are the warm antibody type and the cold antibody type. The *warm antibody* type is usually associated with IgG antibody excess. These antibodies are most active at 37° C and may be induced by drugs, chemicals, or other autoimmune problems. The *cold antibody* type of hemolytic anemia is associated with fixation of complement proteins on IgM. This action occurs best at 30° C and is commonly associated with a Raynaud-like response in the distal extremities.

Treatment depends on clinical severity. Steroid therapy for mild to moderate immunosuppression is the first line of treatment and is temporarily effective in the majority of clients. Splenectomy and more intensive immunosuppressive therapy may be instituted if steroid therapy fails.

Anemias Resulting from Decreased Production of Red Blood Cells

Anemias associated with decreased production of RBCs can occur as a result of pathologic alterations in any of a variety of physiologic mechanisms. Some anemias arise from failure or inability of the bone marrow to properly synthesize RBCs. Other anemias occur because the body cannot synthesize or absorb a specific component necessary for RBC production.

Iron Deficiency Anemia

The adult body contains about 50 mg of iron per 100 mL of blood. Total body iron ranges between 2 and 6 g, depending on the size of the individual and the amount of hemoglobin the client's cells contain. Approximately two-thirds of this iron is contained in hemoglobin; the other third is stored in the bone marrow, the spleen, the liver, and muscle. If an individual has an iron deficiency, the iron stores are depleted first, followed by a reduction in hemoglobin. As a result, RBCs are small in size (microcytic) and diminished in number to the extent that the client has relatively mild manifestations of anemia, including weakness and pallor (Griffin, 1986).

Iron deficiency anemia is the most common type of anemia. It can result from blood loss, increased internal demands (e.g., with pregnancy, adolescence, infection, and high-metabolism states), malabsorption (e.g., in celiac sprue and after partial or total gastrectomy), or dietary inadequacy (e.g., as a result of chronic alcoholism or poverty). In this anemia, the basic problem is a decreased supply of iron for the developing RBC.

Iron deficiency anemia is seen frequently in underdeveloped countries, as well as in technologically advanced societies, such as in the United States. It can occur at any age, but is more frequently noted in women, children, the elderly, and those with restricted diets (e.g., as a result of low income) or unbalanced diets.

The primary treatment of iron deficiency anemia is an increase in the oral intake of iron. Iron is obtained from food. Important sources are red meats, organ meats, kidney beans, whole-wheat products, spinach, egg yolks, carrots, and raisins. An adequate diet supplies the body with about 12 to 15 mg of iron per day, of which only 5% to 10% is absorbed. The amount of iron normally absorbed daily from the diet is sufficient to meet the needs of healthy men and healthy women after the childbearing age, but is not sufficient to supply the greater needs of menstruating women and adolescents during growth spurts. Fortunately, if iron intake is inadequate or if bleeding or pregnancy occurs, the gastrointestinal (GI) tract is capable of increasing the absorption of iron to about 20% to 30% of the total daily intake. When iron deficiency anemia develops in nonmenstruating women or adult men, other possible sources of insidious blood loss should be explored (such as GI lesions).

Vitamin B$_{12}$ Deficiency Anemia

Proper production of RBCs is dependent on adequate deoxyribonucleic acid (DNA) synthesis in the precursor cells so that mitosis and further maturation into functional erythrocytes occur. All DNA synthesis requires adequate amounts of folic acid (folate) to ensure the availability of the nucleotide thymidine to stimulate DNA synthesis. One function of vitamin B$_{12}$ is to serve as an essential cofactor for the activation of the enzyme system responsible for transporting folic acid from the extracellular fluid into the cell, where DNA synthesis occurs. Thus, a deficiency of vitamin B$_{12}$ indirectly causes anemia by inhibiting folic acid transportation and limiting DNA synthesis in RBC precursor cells. As a result, these precursor cells have improper DNA synthesis that does not lead to cell division (mitosis). Instead, these immature precursor cells increase in size and only a few are released from the bone marrow. This type of anemia is called *megaloblastic,* or *macrocytic,* because of the large size of these abnormal cells (Froberg, 1989b).

A deficiency of vitamin B$_{12}$ can result from either inadequate intake of this substance (dietary deficiency) or lack of absorption of ingested vitamin B$_{12}$ from the intestinal tract. Anemia caused by failure to absorb vitamin B$_{12}$ is called *pernicious* anemia and is caused by a deficiency of intrinsic factor (normally secreted by the gastric mucosa), which is necessary for intestinal absorption.

Anemia as a result of vitamin B$_{12}$ deficiency may be mild or severe, usually develops slowly, and produces few symptoms. Clients characteristically demonstrate severe pallor and slight jaundice. Clients also have glossitis (a smooth, beefy red tongue), fatigue, and weight loss. Because vitamin B$_{12}$ is also necessary for normal nervous system functioning, especially of the peripheral nerves, individuals with this type of anemia may also manifest neurologic abnormalities, especially symmetric paresthesias in the feet and the hands, along with associated disturbances of vibratory sense and proprioception, progressing to spastic ataxia.

For clients with anemia as a result of dietary deficiency of vitamin B$_{12}$, treatment consists of increasing the dietary intake of foods rich in this vitamin (animal proteins, eggs, and dairy products). Vitamin supplements may be prescribed when anemia is severe. For clients with anemia as a result of a deficiency of intrinsic factor, vitamin B$_{12}$ must be administered parenterally on a regular schedule (usually weekly for initial treatment, then monthly for maintenance).

Folic Acid Deficiency Anemia

In addition to folic acid deficiencies produced by vitamin B$_{12}$ deficiency, primary folic acid deficiency can also cause a megaloblastic anemia. Clinical manifestations are similar to those of vitamin B$_{12}$ deficiency without the accompanying nervous system manifestations because folic acid does not appear to play a major role in neuronal function. The disease develops insidiously, and symptoms may be attributed to other coexisting diseases, such as cirrhosis. GI disturbances include dyspepsia and glossitis. The absence of neurologic problems is an important diagnostic finding because it differentiates folic acid deficiency from vitamin B$_{12}$ deficiency.

There are three common causes of folic acid deficiency. Poor nutrition, especially a diet lacking in leafy green vegetables, liver, yeast, citrus fruits, dried beans, nuts, and greens, is the most common cause. This type of diet is seen in chronic alcohol abusers and those individuals receiving parenteral alimentation lacking in folic acid supplements. Malabsorption syndromes, such as Crohn's disease, are the second most common cause of folic acid deficiency. Additionally, the ingestion of specific drugs impedes the absorption and conversion of folic acid to its active form (tetrahydrofolate) and can also lead to folic acid deficiency and anemia. Such drugs include methotrexate, some anticonvulsants, and oral contraceptives.

This type of anemia is largely preventable. Prevention is aimed at identifying high-risk clients, such as the older, debilitated alcoholic; others prone to malnutrition; and those with increased folic acid requirements. Other high-risk clients include those receiving certain medications and total parenteral nutrition (TPN). A diet high in folic acid and vitamin B_{12} also prevents a deficiency. By routinely incorporating questions about dietary habits in a health history, the nurse can determine which clients are at risk for diet-induced anemias and can provide appropriate follow-up.

Aplastic Anemia

Aplastic anemia is a deficiency of circulating erythrocytes because of arrested development of RBCs within the bone marrow. It results from an injury to the hematopoietic precursor cell, the pluripotent stem cell. Although aplastic anemia sometimes occurs alone, it is usually accompanied by agranulocytosis (a reduction in leukocytes) and thrombocytopenia (a reduction in platelets). These three problems occur simultaneously because the bone marrow produces not only RBCs but white blood cells (WBCs) and platelets as well. Consequently, if the bone marrow is abnormal for any reason or if it has been exposed to a myelotoxin (any substance that is toxic and damaging to bone marrow), production of erythrocytes, leukocytes, and thrombocytes slows greatly. Pancytopenia, or a deficiency of all three cell types, is common in aplastic anemia. The onset of aplastic anemia may be insidious or rapid. In idiopathic cases (without a known cause), the onset is usually gradual. When pancytopenia results from exposure to a myelotoxic chemical or radiation, the onset is rapid.

The development of aplastic anemia, although relatively rare, is associated with chronic exposure to a variety of myelotoxic agents, although, in about half of cases, the etiology is unknown. Specific known myelotoxins are radiation, benzene, alkylating agents, antimetabolites, chloromycetin (26% of cases), sulfonamides, anticonvulsants, and some insecticides. Some evidence exists to suggest that aplastic anemia may occur as a sequela of viral infection (e.g., Epstein-Barr virus infection, cytomegalovirus infection, and hepatitis B) (Robbins & Kumar, 1987). The mechanism by which the damage to the bone marrow occurs is unknown.

Injury to the stem cell, direct injury to the bone marrow, or suppression of hematopoiesis by immunologic events can cause aplastic anemia.

Prevention of aplastic anemia is through avoidance of exposure to toxic agents. After the condition is diagnosed, exposure to any potentially toxic agent or drug should be discontinued. Clients should have frequent hemograms while being treated therapeutically with myelotoxins.

Blood transfusions are the mainstay of treatment. Transfusions are discontinued as soon as the bone marrow begins to produce RBCs. Transfusion for anemia must only be used when the anemia causes real disability or when bleeding is life-threatening owing to thrombocytopenia. Unneeded transfusion increases the opportunity for development of immune reactions to platelets, shortens the life span of the transfused cell, and may increase the rate of rejection of transplanted marrow cells if this course of treatment is elected. Corticosteroids and androgens are sometimes given to help stimulate bone marrow function. Splenectomy is considered when the client has an enlarged spleen that is either destroying normal RBCs or suppressing their development within the marrow. Bone marrow transplantation can be performed for those clients who have a sibling with a close tissue match.

COLLABORATIVE MANAGEMENT

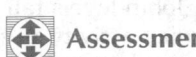 Assessment

History

The nurse collects data regarding the risk factors, as well as the causative factors, related to the anemia. Demographic data are collected because *sex* and *age* are key risk factors for some types of anemia. Information regarding *occupation* and *hobbies* may yield important clues about chronic exposure to substances that are linked to the development of some types of anemia.

The nurse determines if the client is aware of *how long he/she has been anemic*. Additionally, the nurse asks if anyone else in the family is currently anemic or if there is a positive *family history* of specific types of anemia. Clients are asked if obvious conditions of blood loss, such as trauma, melena (blood in the stool), hematemesis, hematuria, and menorrhagia (excessive menstrual flow), have occurred recently. The client is asked to attempt to quantify blood loss by any of these modes. Women are asked specific information regarding the number of pads or tampons used per day during the menstrual cycle.

Any underlying *alcohol or drug abuse* should be established, as any type of substance abuse is often associated with malnutrition. The nurse reviews exposure to *medications* and potentially harmful *industrial or household toxins*. Causative agents include thiazide diuretics, chloramphenicol, aspirin, quinine derivatives, anticonvulsants, sulfonamides, alkylating agents, benzene, and insecticides.

The nurse obtains a thorough *diet history* to determine daily caloric, protein, and vitamin intake. The client is asked to list everything consumed during the previous 24 hours. In this way, dietary deficiencies of iron, folate, or vitamin B_{12} are determined.

The client is asked about the presence of any *associated symptoms,* such as chronic fatigue and shortness of breath, increased susceptibility to infection, anorexia, weight loss, indigestion, sore mouth and tongue, bone pain and deformity, and chronic depression. The client is asked whether headaches, behavior changes, increased somnolence, decreased alertness, decreased attention span, lethargy, muscle weakness, and increased fatigue have been experienced. Having the client relate the previous 24 hours' activities may disclose additional information about *activity intolerance, changes in behavior,* and the presence of *unexplained fatigue.*

Physical Assessment: Clinical Manifestations

When the body becomes anemic, several compensatory mechanisms develop. Many of the physical findings seen in an anemic client are a result of these mechanisms.

The individual's cardiac output increases to increase tissue oxygenation. Cardiac output does not measurably increase in chronic anemia until hemoglobin levels fall to 7 g/dL. Signs of compensatory cardiac activity include *tachycardia,* a *systolic flow murmur,* and *orthostatic hypotension. Angina* and *high-output heart failure* may occur if there is pre-existing heart disease. An *increased respiratory rate* also occurs in an attempt to increase oxygenation. This accounts for symptoms of exertional dyspnea and orthopnea.

Compensation also occurs by the use of all potential capillary channels to increase tissue perfusion to vital areas, at the expense of nonvital areas. Vasoconstriction occurs in the skin, producing the characteristic *pallor.* There is also a shift of blood flow away from the kidneys. Although the kidneys are vital organs, the oxygen supply to the kidneys is in excess of its demand under normal conditions.

An increase in the rate of RBC production may result in client complaints of *bone pain* and *sternal tenderness.* Other symptoms often seen in the anemic client include chronic fatigue, shortness of breath, increased susceptibility to infection, anorexia, weight loss, indigestion, sore mouth and tongue, headaches, vertigo, and loss of consciousness. Other signs of anemia include bounding arterial pulses, vascular bruits, cardiac enlargement, murmurs, dependent edema, pallor (particularly of the mucous membranes and the nail beds), pale palm lines, delayed wound healing, jaundice, and spider angiomas. Clients with sickle cell anemia may also exhibit the following signs: growth abnormalities, bony abnormalities on x-ray film, necrosis of the femoral head, priapism, hematuria, splenomegaly, jaundice, hepatomegaly, retinal changes, and leg ulcers.

Psychosocial Assessment

Anemia is often a chronic disease, which can lead to psychosocial problems. Self-concept, including such aspects as body image and role perception, serves as a frame of reference for reality. Illness, especially when it is chronic, alters the self-concept by interfering with perceptions of self. The client may experience a feeling of loss over what has been lost or changed in her/his life as a result of chronic illness (e.g., independence or role as a provider). Chronic depression may be seen in anemic clients.

The nurse caring for this client should continuously assess for the psychologic impact of the illness and the hospital environment on the client, the family, and social and sexual roles.

Laboratory Findings

Laboratory studies useful in the diagnosis and monitoring of anemia include the following: complete blood count (CBC), mean corpuscular hemoglobin, mean corpuscular volume, mean corpuscular hemoglobin concentration, iron levels and total iron-binding capacity test, bone marrow examination, hemoglobin electrophoresis, and peripheral blood smears. Coagulation variables may also be determined.

Anemic clients usually have decreased RBC counts, hematocrit, and hemoglobin levels. Other findings may be abnormal, depending on the etiology of the anemia.

 Analysis: Nursing Diagnosis

Many clients are at risk for the development of anemia as a result of poor dietary intake, autoimmune disorders, trauma, and exposure to specific agents that suppress erythropoiesis. A typical client with anemia is a 40-year-old female with excessive bleeding during menstrual periods and a diet deficient in foods containing iron.

Common Diagnoses

1. Activity intolerance related to decreased oxygen-carrying capacity of the blood
2. Altered nutrition: less than body requirements related to inadequate dietary intake

Additional Diagnoses

Clients may also have one or more of the following diagnoses:

1. Potential impaired skin integrity related to decreased tissue perfusion
2. Altered oral mucous membrane related to decreased tissue perfusion
3. Anxiety related to chronic illness

Planning and Implementation ⟹

The plan of care for the client experiencing anemia focuses on the common nursing diagnoses and is aimed at supporting the physiologic compensatory mechanisms (Griffin, 1986).

Activity Intolerance

Planning: client goals. The major goal for this nursing diagnosis is that the client will not become excessively fatigued while carrying out ADL.

Interventions: nonsurgical management. Rest is essential for the anemic client. To lower the individual's oxygen requirements and to reduce the strain on the heart and the lungs, the client should be encouraged to rest frequently throughout the day. If possible, the working day should be shortened. Clients with severe anemia are usually hospitalized and restricted to bed rest until improvement occurs. An extremely weak client needs help in bathing, turning, eating, and providing self-care. In addition, to ensure sufficient rest, the nurse protects the client from frequent visitors, continuous telephone interruptions, and excessive noise.

Blood transfusions are sometimes indicated for some types of anemia. Blood transfusions increase the oxygen-carrying capacity of blood and replace missing RBCs and some coagulation factors. Treatment with blood components is summarized in Table 67–1. For the anemic client, whole blood or packed RBCs would usually be the blood component of choice. Whole blood, usually supplied in 500-mL bags, is generally given for volume replacement, as well as RBC replacement. Packed RBCs, supplied in 250-mL bags, are a concentrated source of RBCs. Blood transfusions are actually transplantations of tissue from one person to another. Because this donated tissue can be recognized by the immune system of the recipient as nonself, the client may have a reaction to the transfused products.

Four types of transfusion reactions can occur: hemolytic transfusion reactions, allergic reactions, febrile reactions, and bacterial reactions. The nurse must be extremely vigilant to prevent serious complications through early detection and initiation of appropriate treatment.

Hemolytic transfusion reactions are usually caused by blood type or Rh incompatibility. When blood containing antibodies against the recipient's blood is infused, antigen-antibody complexes are formed and released into the circulation. These complexes can destroy the transfused cells and initiate inflammatory responses. The ensuing reaction may be mild, with fever and chills, or severe, with disseminated intravascular coagulation (DIC) and circulatory collapse. Other clinical signs include apprehension, headache, chest pain, and a sense of impending doom. The onset of this type of reaction may be immediate or may not occur until subsequent units have been transfused.

Allergic reactions are most often seen in clients with a

TABLE 67–1 Blood Components Used in the Treatment of Anemia

Component	Comments
Whole blood	For massive blood loss, 500 mL.
Packed RBCs	For treatment of severe anemia, 250 mL. Decreases chance of circulatory overload.
Buffy coat–poor RBCs	Plasma and WBC layer removed to decrease incidence of allergic reactions.
Washed RBCs	Platelet and leukocyte antigens removed.
Fresh frozen plasma	Plasma contains coagulation factors until thawed.
Cryoprecipitate	Factors VIII, XIII, and fibrinogen for hemophilia and von Willebrand's disease.
Platelets	For thrombocytopenia, give as rapidly as possible.
WBCs	Controversial treatment for leukopenia.

From Griffin, J. P. (1986). *Hematology and immunology: Concepts for nursing*. Norwalk, CT: Appleton-Century-Crofts.

history of allergy. The client may have urticaria, itching, bronchospasm, or, occasionally, anaphylaxis. Onset of this type of reaction is usually during the transfusion or up to 24 hours after the transfusion. Clients with histories of allergy can be given buffy coat–poor or washed RBCs in which the WBCs are removed from the blood. This procedure minimizes the possibility of an allergic reaction.

Febrile reactions occur in individuals with antibodies directed against their WBCs, a situation seen after multiple transfusions. The recipient experiences sensations of cold, tachycardia, fever, hypotension, and tachypnea. Again, buffy coat–poor RBCs can be ordered by the physician.

Bacterial reactions are seen after transfusion of contaminated blood products. Usually a gram-negative organism is the source, because these bacteria grow rapidly in blood stored under refrigeration. Symptoms include tachycardia, hypotension, fever, chills, and shock. Onset is rapid.

Nursing actions during transfusions are aimed largely at prevention or early recognition of reactions. Preparation for transfusion therapy is imperative. Legally, a physician's order is needed for the administration of blood and its components. The order must specify the type of component to be delivered, the volume to be transfused, and any special conditions the physician judges to be important. The order should be verified by the nurse for accuracy and completeness and evaluated, considering both the client's clinical condition and the laboratory values. Many hospitals require that a separate consent form for the administration of blood products be obtained before a transfusion.

A blood specimen must be obtained for cross-matching (the testing of the donor's blood and the recipient's blood for compatibility). The procedure and responsibility for obtaining this specimen are specified by hospital policy. Most hospitals require a new cross-matching specimen at least every 48 hours.

Because of the viscosity of blood components, a 19-gauge or larger needle is needed for venous access. Both Y tubes and straight tubing sets are available for blood component administration. A blood filter (approximately 170 μm) is included with component administration equipment and must be used for the transfusion of all blood products. This filter removes aggregates from the stored blood products. If the client is receiving a massive transfusion, a microaggregate filter (20 to 40 μm) may be used.

Normal saline is the solution of choice for blood component therapy. Ringer's lactate and dextrose in water are contraindicated as solutions for the initiation of transfusions. Medications should never be added to blood products, as they could have a damaging effect on the blood cells.

Before initiating the transfusion, it is essential to determine that the blood component delivered is the correct one for the client. Two registered nurses simultaneously check the physician's order, the client's identity, and whether the hospital identification band name and number are identical to those on the blood component tag. The blood bag label, the attached tag, and the requisition slip are examined to ensure that the ABO and Rh types are compatible.

The client's vital signs, including temperature, are taken immediately before initiating the transfusion. Infusion of the transfusion begins slowly. If a severe reaction is to occur, it usually happens with administration of the first 50 mL of blood. A nurse remains with the client for the first 20 minutes of the transfusion. Vital signs are taken 15 minutes after initiation of the transfusion to detect signs of a transfusion reaction. If there are no signs of a reaction, the infusion rate can be increased to transfuse 1 unit in about 2 hours. The client should have vital signs taken every ½ hour during the transfusion and then hourly after it is completed for 3 hours.

Blood components without large amounts of RBCs can be infused more quickly. The identification checks are the same as for RBC transfusions. Standard filters should not be used with platelets, as the filter traps the platelet itself. Plasma and platelet concentrates can be infused as rapidly as the client can tolerate. Client monitoring is the same as for the transfusion of RBC components.

Altered Nutrition: Less Than Body Requirements

Planning: client goals. The major goals are that the client will (1) receive optimal protein, calories, vitamins, and minerals and (2) not develop iron deficiency or folic acid or vitamin B_{12} deficiency anemias.

Interventions: nonsurgical management. For anemias caused by deficiencies of vitamin B_{12}, folic acid, or iron, increased intake of these substances is therapeutic. Intake can be accomplished by drug and diet therapy.

Drug therapy. Drug therapy for vitamin B_{12} and folic acid deficiency anemias consists of vitamin supplements, which can be given parenterally or orally until symptoms abate. Both of these vitamins should routinely be added to TPN and tube feeding solutions. Medicinal iron can be administered orally or parenterally; however, the preferred route is oral (Froberg, 1989c). The drugs of choice for oral administration are ferrous sulfate and ferrous gluconate. It is important to administer iron preparations correctly. Because iron is a gastric irritant, it should always be given with meals. Undiluted liquid preparations of iron stain the teeth and so should be given well diluted and through a straw. Whenever possible, ferrous salts are given with orange juice because ascorbic acid promotes iron absorption. Clients are instructed that iron preparations change the color of stools to black. Parenteral iron therapy is given to clients who have an intolerance to oral iron preparations or who continue to experience blood loss. Iron dextran is the drug of choice. Iron dextran causes darkening and discoloration of the skin around the injection site unless administered by Z track injection technique.

Diet therapy. The client is taught which foods are high in vitamin B_{12}, folic acid, and iron. Foods high in vitamin B_{12} include animal products, such as liver, milk, and eggs. Folic acid is found in green vegetables and liver. Iron is found in red meats, liver, green vegetables, egg yolks, oysters, and whole-wheat products.

Prevention of complications. For clients with vitamin B_{12} deficiency anemia, injury as a result of neurologic alterations is possible. The client should be instructed to use caution when climbing stairs and using the bathroom. A hazard-free environment is necessary to meet this goal, and the nurse should educate the client about its importance. If the client is experiencing paresthesias of the feet, bath water should be tested before stepping into the bathtub to avoid burns. For clients with any type of anemia, syncope can occur and lead to injury. The client should be advised to rise slowly from a seated position.

■ Discharge Planning

The anemic client can usually be treated at home. Severe cases of aplastic anemia, sickle cell anemia, and other anemias may be treated in the hospital.

Home Care Preparation

Depending on the diagnosis, various factors about the home environment become important. Often, clients with sickle cell anemia are prescribed narcotic analgesics for self-management of sickle cell crises at home. The client and the family need education on correct administration of the drugs. Clients and family members are specifically instructed to keep iron supplements out of the reach of children, as an overdose can be lethal.

The environment must be assessed for potential hazards before the client is discharged from the hospital if the client is prone to falls. If the client is experiencing excessive fatigue and shortness of breath as a result of anemia, stair climbing may be a problem. The nurse should work with the social services department to identify adaptations in home life.

Client/Family Education

For any of the hereditary anemias, such as sickle cell anemia, individuals and their families should be provided with education on the genetic transmission of the disease, signs and symptoms of crises, management of crises on an outpatient basis, and indications on when to seek medical attention. For diet-induced anemias, nutritional counseling should be a part of nursing care from the time of diagnosis.

Psychosocial Preparation

Explaining the importance of proper diet and sufficient rest to the client and the family increases the likelihood of compliance. Clients who are anemic need frequent visits to health care personnel for monitoring and therapy. Involvement of the family may increase the client's motivation and ensure a complete recovery. Most clients are able to work while anemic, although they may need to take frequent rest periods. Allowing the client to ventilate his/her feelings regarding restrictions in ADL can aid the individual's coping abilities.

Health Care Resources

Before the nurse can expect a client to be compliant with a healthy diet, health care resources must be evaluated. A healthy diet is more expensive than a high-calorie, high-carbohydrate one. The client may need financial assistance, and the nurse can provide the necessary referrals to social services. For many anemic clients who are extremely weak, a home care nurse or aide may be necessary for assistance with ADL and ambulation. The hospital nurse documents the client's needs on the transfer chart and communicates these to the home care agency.

Evaluation

On the basis of the identified nursing diagnoses, the nurse evaluates the care of the anemic client. The ex-

pected outcomes for the client with anemia include that the client

1. States that she/he is not fatigued after performing ADL
2. Selects correctly from a list those foods that contain significant quantities of iron and vitamin B_{12}
3. Describes and complies with the drug therapy as needed
4. States correctly the signs and symptoms of anemia
5. States which health care resource person should be notified when symptoms of anemia occur

Polycythemia

Polycythemia is defined as a condition in which the number of RBCs in whole blood is increased to above normal levels. The problem is characterized by hyperviscosity and may be an *absolute* condition, in which the number of RBCs is increased, or a *relative* condition, in which the total number of RBCs is normal but the plasma volume of the blood is decreased. Polycythemia may be transitory, as a consequence of other conditions, or chronic.

POLYCYTHEMIA VERA

OVERVIEW

Polycythemia vera is a sustained increase in blood hemoglobin concentration to 18 g/dL, RBC count to 6 million/mm³, or hematocrit to 55% or greater. It is believed to be a form of malignancy analogous to leukemia. Three major hallmarks of this condition are the relentless, unrestrained production of massive numbers of erythrocytes; production of an excessive number of leukocytes; and an overproduction of thrombocytes.

COLLABORATIVE MANAGEMENT

Clinical features found during assessment are a result of increased blood viscosity and volume (Trotta & Knobf, 1987). These features include headaches, plethora (a ruddy complexion with redness of mucosa), dyspnea, thrombosis, splenomegaly, and paresthesias. In spite of the RBC excess, most clients with polycythemia vera are prone to bleeding problems because of an apparent associated platelet dysfunction (Rapaport, 1987). Without treatment, clients with polycythemia vera have a life expectancy of 2 years after diagnosis. The most common complication of this disorder is serious thrombus formation within vital organs.

Treatment consists of phlebotomy, or the routine collection of RBCs from the client to decrease the RBC mass and to diminish blood viscosity. Maintaining adequate hydration and promoting venous return are essential to prevent thrombus formation (Wheby, 1988). Therapies are prescribed to prevent the formation of clots and include anticoagulant drugs. The client needs education on measures to prevent blood stasis, such as elevating the feet when seated, wearing support hose and socks, and complying with medical therapy.

WHITE BLOOD CELL DISORDERS

As discussed in Chapter 23, WBCs (leukocytes) function by a variety of mechanisms to provide the individual with protection from invading nonself cells (viruses, bacteria, molds, spores, pollens, protozoa, helminths, proteins, and cells from other living organisms) and from self cells that are no longer totally normal. These protective functions are generally dependent on maintaining normal numbers and ratios of many specific mature circulating leukocytes. When any one type of WBC is present in either abnormally high or abnormally low amounts, hematopoietic function and immune function may be altered to some degree, causing the individual to be at risk for specific complications. This section discusses the pathologic changes and nursing care requirements for clients with disorders characterized by malignant overgrowth of specific cell forms of the myeloproliferative and lymphoproliferative hematopoietic systems. The pathologic alterations and care requirements for clients with leukocyte-related problems of immunodeficiency, allergy, autoimmune disorders, and diminished granulocyte function are discussed in Chapters 26 and 27.

Leukemia

OVERVIEW

The *leukemias* are a group of malignant disorders involving abnormal overproduction of a specific cell type, usually at an immature stage, in the bone marrow. Leukemia may be acute in onset and short in duration or may have an insidious onset and persist as a chronic disorder. The types of leukemia are further categorized by the specific maturational pathway from which the abnormal cells arose. Leukemias in which the abnormal cells arise from within the committed lymphoid maturational pathways (see Chap. 23, Fig. 23–3) are categorized as *lymphocytic* or *lymphoblastic*. Leukemias in which the abnormal cells arise within the committed myeloid maturational pathways are categorized as *mye-*

locytic or *myelogenous*. Several subtypes exist for each of these and are categorized by the degree of maturity of the abnormal cell and the specific cell type involved (see the accompanying Key Features of Disease).

Pathophysiology

The basic pathologic defect in leukemia is a malignant transformation of the stem cells or early committed precursor leukocyte cells, producing an abnormal proliferation of a specific type of leukocyte. The immature leukocytes, which are functionally abnormal, are produced in excessive quantities in the bone marrow, essentially shutting down normal bone marrow production of erythrocytes, platelets, and functionally mature leukocytes. This situation leads to anemia, thrombocytopenia, and leukopenia of other WBC types, even though the client has a greatly elevated number of circulating WBCs. Death usually results from infection or hemorrhage, unless treatment is instituted. For the acute leukemias, these pathologic changes occur rapidly and progress quickly to death without intervention. Chronic leukemia may be present for many years before overt pathologic changes related to the illness are manifested. Usually, chronic leukemia progresses to a blastic crisis stage, in which the leukemia becomes an acute illness closely resembling acute leukemia.

Etiology

Epidemiologic studies suggest that many different genetic and environmental factors may be involved in the development of leukemia. Although only a few of these factors have been identified as having a definite role in leukemia development, the basic mechanism appears to involve gene damage of cells, leading to transformation of those cells from the normal state to a malignant state. The processes appear to be the same as for development of solid tumors (see Chap. 24). The following conditions and factors constitute possible risk factors for development of leukemia: ionizing radiation, chemicals and drugs, marrow hypoplasia, environmental interactions, genetic factors, viral factors, immunologic factors, and interactive factors (Rubin, 1983).

Exposure to large quantities of ionizing radiation appears to be a major risk factor in the development of leukemia. Exposures ranging from therapeutic irradiation of diseases, such as ankylosing spondylitis and Hodgkin's disease, to irradiation from the atomic bomb at Hiroshima or the Chernobyl accident are associated with leukemia.

Many different chemicals and drugs have been linked to the development of leukemia. Of these chemicals, benzene is the most closely associated with development of leukemia. Phenylbutazone, arsenic, and chloramphenicol also appear to be related to later development of leukemia. Unfortunately, antineoplastic drugs, especially alkylating agents, used as treatment for other malignant conditions also are linked to leukemia development (Fraser & Tucker, 1989; Workman, 1989).

KEY FEATURES OF DISEASE ■ Differential Features of the Four Major Types of Leukemia

Leukemia Type	Age at Onset (yr)	Sex	Race	Cell of Origin	Specific Markers	Comments
ALL	<15	M	Caucasian	B cell	CALLA+	Prognosis poorer for adults than for children
					Hyperdiploidy TDT+	Prognosis better than in AML Curable in children
AML	15–39	Equal incidence		Myeloblast	TDT−	Prognosis generally poor
				Myelocyte Promyelocyte Myelomonocyte	t(9;22) t(15;17)	Heterogeneous tumor cell populations Best prognosis with bone marrow transplant
CML	>50	M		Myeloid cell	Ph¹ chromosome	Prognosis generally poor; worse if no Ph¹ chromosome No blockage of maturation of nonmalignant leukocytes Blastic crisis indicative of more acute disease
CLL	>50	M	Caucasian	B cell	Trisomy 12	Prognosis poor Long (4–10 yr) course with rare conversion to acute form Only leukemia with a possible genetic predisposition

Marrow hypoplasia can increase the risk of leukemia. A reduction or alteration in production of hematopoietic cells may predispose individuals to leukemia. Examples of conditions associated with later development of leukemia include Fanconi's anemia, paroxysmal nocturnal hemoglobinuria during its aplastic phase, and myelodysplastic syndromes (Yeomans, 1987).

Environmental factors that predispose to leukemia are difficult to identify, as they can be multiple and interactive. Exposure of children to many risk factors or prenatally is an example. Such exposures include in utero irradiation, maternal irradiation, maternal history of fetal wastage, and early childhood viral disease.

An increase in frequency of leukemia among the following populations suggests possible genetic involvement: identical twins of clients with leukemia and individuals with Down's syndrome, Bloom's syndrome, Fanconi's anemia, and Klinefelter's syndrome. Chromosomal aberration may be an important factor in the development of leukemia in these syndromes.

The ribonucleic acid (RNA) viruses have been implicated in the causation of leukemia. Retroviruses that carry the gene for reverse transcriptase are also suspected of producing leukemia.

Deficiency in the immune system may favor the development of leukemia. It has not yet been determined whether leukemia among immunodeficient individuals is a result of immunosurveillance failure or if the pathologic mechanisms that cause the immune deficiency also trigger malignant transformation of leukopoietic cells.

The interaction of multiple host and environmental factors may result in leukemia. The interaction of these factors is tolerated differently by each person, frequently making it difficult to determine the etiology of any specific leukemia.

Incidence

The incidence and frequency of leukemia depend on many factors, including the morphologic type of WBC affected, and the age, sex, race, and geographic locale of the individual (Rubin, 1983). Acute myelogenous leukemia (AML) occurs with a similar frequency in all ages and is the most common form of leukemia among adults. Acute lymphocytic leukemia (ALL) occurs more commonly as a childhood disease, although it does constitute approximately 10% of adult leukemias. Chronic myelogenous leukemia (CML) constitutes about 20% of adult leukemias and occurs more frequently in individuals older than 50 years of age. Chronic lymphocytic leukemia (CLL) is the most rare type of the major leukemia groups and occurs primarily in individuals older than 50 years of age. The leukemias account for 3% of all newly diagnosed cases of cancer, and they are responsible for 4% of all cancer deaths (American Cancer Society, 1989).

PREVENTION

Except for avoiding exposure to radiation and the chemical agents implicated in the etiology of leukemia, there is no known absolutely effective way to prevent leukemia. Because exposure to alkylating agents, especially in combination chemotherapy, appears to be associated with an increased incidence of later leukemia development, risks versus benefits must be weighed when prescribing such agents, especially for nonmalignant conditions.

COLLABORATIVE MANAGEMENT

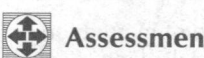 **Assessment**

History

The nurse collects data regarding risk factors, as well as causative factors, for the development of leukemia. *Age* is important because the incidence of leukemia increases with age. Demographic information regarding *occupation* and *hobbies* may reveal specific environmental exposures that increase the client's risk of leukemia. *Previous illnesses* and *medical history* may indicate exposure to ionizing radiation or medications that increase the client's risk of leukemia.

Because of leukemia-related alterations of immune function, clients with leukemia are at an increased risk for infections. Clients are asked about the frequency and severity of *infectious processes* (such as colds, influenza, pneumonia, bronchitis, and unexplained episodes of fever) experienced during the preceding 6 months. Additionally, because some of the clinical manifestations of leukemia, especially chronic leukemia, are nonspecific, the client may have thought these symptoms were related to other illnesses.

Because platelet function may be diminished with leukemia, the nurse questions the client about any overt or hidden excessive *bleeding* episodes, such as tendency to bruise easily, nosebleeds, increased menstrual flow, bleeding from the gums, rectal bleeding, hematuria, and prolonged bleeding after minor abrasions or lacerations. If such episodes have occurred, the nurse asks the client whether this type and extent of bleeding constitute the client's usual response to injury or represent a change in injury pattern.

Clients with leukemia frequently experience weakness and fatigue resulting from anemia and increased metabolic and energy demands of the leukemic cells. The client is asked whether headaches, behavior changes, increased somnolence, decreased alertness, decreased attention span, lethargy, muscle weakness, diminished appetite, weight loss, or increased fatigue has been experienced. Having the client relate the previous 24 hours' activities may disclose additional infor-

mation about *activity intolerance, changes in behavior,* and the presence of *unexplained fatigue.* The nurse determines how long the client has had any of these debilitating symptoms.

Physical Assessment: Clinical Manifestations

Leukemia involves one or more pathologic mechanisms in the bone marrow, which influence the composition and activity of various components of the blood. Because blood influences the health and functional capacity of all organs and systems, clinical manifestations of leukemia involve many areas remote from the actual site of origin of malignant cells (see the accompanying Key Features of Disease). The following clinical manifestations are associated with the acute leukemias (Cotran et al., 1989). Some of these findings may also be present in clients with chronic leukemia in the blast phase.

Skin and mucous membranes may manifest abnormalities associated with leukemia. The skin may be pale and cool to the touch as a result of the accompanying anemia. *Pallor* is especially evident on the face, around the mouth, and in the nail beds. The conjunctiva of the eye also is pale, as are the creases on the palmar surface of the hand (most evident when the skin over the palm of the hand is stretched). *Petechiae* may be present on any area of skin surface, especially the lower extremities. The petechiae may be unrelated to any obvious trauma. The nurse carefully inspects the skin for the presence of any *skin infections* or *traumatized areas* that have failed to heal. The nurse inspects the mouth for evidence of bleeding from the gums and the presence of any sore or lesion of the oral cavity indicating infection.

Cardiovascular manifestations of leukemia generally are related to anemia. *Heart rate* may be increased, with blood pressure decreased. *Murmurs* and *bruits* may be present. *Capillary filling time* is increased.

Respiratory manifestations of leukemia are primarily associated with anemia and infectious complications. *Respiratory rate increases* as the degree of anemia becomes greater. If respiratory tract infections are present, the client may experience shortness of breath; abnormal breath sounds are present on auscultation.

GI manifestations may be related to the increased bleeding tendency and to the fatigue. *Weight loss, nausea,* and *anorexia* are common. The nurse examines the rectal area for fissures and tests the stool for the presence of occult blood. Many clients with leukemia have *diminished bowel sounds* and *constipation.* Hepatosplenomegaly and abdominal tenderness also may be present from leukemic infiltration of abdominal viscera.

Central nervous system (CNS) manifestations include possible *cranial nerve disturbances, headache,* and *papilledema* as a result of leukemic infiltration of the meninges or the CNS. Seizure activity and coma may be present in advanced cases. Although fever is commonly noted, this manifestation appears to be more a response to the presence of infection, rather than to malignancy-related changes in the CNS.

KEY FEATURES OF DISEASE ■ Common Clinical Manifestations of Acute Leukemia

Integumentary

Ecchymoses
Petechiae
Open infected lesions
Pallor of the conjunctiva, the nail beds, and the palmar
    creases and around the mouth

Gastrointestinal

Bleeding gums
Anorexia
Weight loss
Enlarged liver and spleen

Renal

Hematuria

Cardiovascular

Tachycardia at basal activity levels
Orthostatic hypotension
Palpitations

Respiratory

Dyspnea on exertion

Neurologic

Fatigue
Headache
Fever

Musculoskeletal

Bone pain
Joint swelling and pain

Miscellaneous manifestations of leukemia include bone and joint tenderness as a result of marrow involvement and bone resorption. Leukemic cell growth or infiltration may produce enlarged lymph nodes or masses.

Psychosocial Assessment

The client with newly diagnosed leukemia is extremely anxious. The average lay person equates a diagnosis of any cancer with a death sentence. Current therapies have greatly improved the prognoses of most cancers, yet the public is largely unaware of these advances. The nurse spends time with the client and the family to ascertain what the diagnosis means to them

and what they expect from the future. Without knowing the client's expectations and feelings, the nurse cannot educate and support clients and family members in an individualized manner. Areas of concern for the client and the family must be determined before the nurse can develop a meaningful plan of care.

A diagnosis of leukemia has dramatic implications for a client's life style. After initial therapy, the client may be able to resume work, depending on the occupation. However, adjustments must be made to accommodate changes in the client's functional status. In addition, the client often has repeated hospitalizations. The nurse works with the social services department to facilitate the client's resumption of a normal life style.

Laboratory Findings

The client with acute leukemia usually has decreased hemoglobin and hematocrit levels, a decreased platelet count, and an altered WBC count. The WBC count may be low, normal, or elevated, but is usually quite elevated. The definitive test for leukemia includes various examinations of cells obtained as a result of bone marrow aspiration or biopsy. The bone marrow is dominated by leukemic blast phase cells. The composition of various cell surface proteins (antigens) on the leukemic cells assists in the diagnosis of the actual type of leukemia. Such markers include the presence or absence of the T-11 protein, the enzyme terminal deoxynucleotidyl transferase (TDT), and the common acute lymphoblastic leukemia antigen (CALLA). These markers also indicate prognosis.

Coagulation variables are usually abnormal for the client with acute leukemia. Hypofibrinogenemia and reduced levels of coagulation factors are typical. Whole blood clotting time (Lee-White clotting test) is increased, as is the activated partial thromboplastin time (aPTT).

Chromosomal analysis may be performed on the malignant bone marrow cells. The purpose of such studies is to determine the presence of specific marker chromosomes, which can be used to assist in the diagnosis of leukemia type, predict prognosis, and be used as a determinant of therapy effectiveness.

Radiographic Findings

Specific symptoms determine the feasibility of specific tests. For instance, a client with a symptom of dyspnea needs chest radiography to determine if leukemic infiltrates are present in the lung. Skeletal x-ray films may help to determine the degree of bone reabsorption present with subperiosteal involvement.

 Analysis: Nursing Diagnosis

A typical adult client with AML is a 28-year-old man who works in a setting where contact with industrial solvents occurs on a daily basis. The nursing diagnoses and plan of care (see the accompanying Client Care Plan) discussed are for clients with AML.

CLIENT CARE PLAN ■ The Client with Acute Myelogenous Leukemia

Goal/Outcome Criteria	Interventions	Rationales
Nursing Diagnosis 1: Potential for Infection Related to Decreased Immune Response		
Client will remain free from cross-contamination–induced infection. ■ Limits close contact with other individuals. ■ Does not experience a shifting population of WBCs. ■ Maintains a core body temperature of < 100° F (38° C). ■ Does not have pathogenic organisms in cultures of blood, urine, and wound drainage.	1. Wash hands between caring for different clients. 2. Keep supplies for the client (e.g., paper cups, straws, dressing materials, and nonsterile gloves) separate from supplies for other clients. 3. Limit the number of care personnel entering the client's room. 4. Have the client maintained in a private room. 5. Limit visitors to healthy adults. 6. Reduce exposure to environmental microorganisms by avoiding raw fruits and vegetables in the client's diet and by not having standing water in the client's room (e.g., remove vases, humidifiers, and water games). 7. Clean the client's room at least once per day.	1. To reduce the number of vector transmissible microorganisms. 2. To limit the potential for cross-contamination infection. 3. To decrease the client's exposure to nonself microorganisms. 4. To reduce traffic and exposure to nonself microorganisms. 5. To prevent transmission of microorganisms by small children, who may incubate microorganisms and inadvertently transmit them to the client by not adhering to good personal hygiene. 6. To prevent contact with some potentially harmful microorganisms. 7. To inhibit proliferation of environmental microorganisms.
Client will remain free from auto-contamination-induced infection. ■ Complies with prescribed hygiene measures. ■ Does not experience a shifting population of WBCs. ■ Maintains a core body temperature of < 100° F (38° C). ■ Does not have pathogenic organisms in cultures of blood, urine, and wound drainage.	1. Bathe the client every day and prn. 2. Touch the client gently to avoid injuring the skin. 3. Assist the client with oral hygiene at least once per nursing shift. 4. Change IV tubing each day. 5. Administer stool softeners and laxatives. 6. Change dressings on open wounds and around Hickman's catheter every day.	1. To reduce microorganisms on skin surfaces. 2. To prevent new portals of entry for microorganisms. 3. To reduce the number of oral tract microorganisms. 4. To reduce the risk of contamination. 5. To reduce intestinal stasis and bacterial overgrowth. 6. To reduce the number of colony-forming microorganisms at the site of a portal of entry and to allow inspection of the site for signs and symptoms of infection.
Client will not experience septicemia. ■ Does not experience a shifting population of WBCs. ■ Maintains a core body temperature of < 100° F (38° C). ■ Does not have pathogenic organisms in cultures of blood, urine, and wound drainage.	1. Assess the client for signs and symptoms of infection every 4 h. a. Measure oral temperature. b. Inspect wound areas for the presence of discharge or odor. c. Examine the differential WBC count for the presence of changing populations of cells and cell maturity levels.	1. To identify infectious process early, so that appropriate therapy may be instituted.

CLIENT CARE PLAN ■ The Client with Acute Myelogenous Leukemia *continued*

Goal/Outcome Criteria	Interventions	Rationales
Nursing Diagnosis 2: Potential for Injury Related to Excessive Bleeding Secondary to Thrombocytopenia		

	2. If symptoms of infection are present.
	   a. Obtain blood cultures through the venous access device and the peripheral vein before antibiotic therapy is initiated.
	   b. Obtain culture of open lesions, urine, and sputum.
	
	   c. Administer the prescribed antibiotic therapy.
		2. To institute appropriate treatment.
		   a. To determine if microorganisms are present in the blood and whether the venous access device is the site of contamination.
		   b. To determine the origin of infection and to identify the infecting organism.
		   c. To limit proliferation of microorganisms within the client.

Nursing Diagnosis 2: Potential for Injury Related to Excessive Bleeding Secondary to Thrombocytopenia		
Client will not experience injury. ■ Has intact skin and mucous membranes. ■ Manifests no bruising or petechiae. ■ Does not participate in activities that increase the risk of falls and other injuries.	1. Handle the client gently. 2. Use soft bristle toothbrush or cloth or sponge tooth cleaners. 3. Avoid intravenous, intramuscular, and subcutaneous injections. 4. Apply firm but gentle pressure to a needle stick site for at least 10 min after removal of the needle. 5. Offer mechanically soft foods that are cool to warm in temperature. 6. Permit the client to use only an electric razor for shaving. 7. Pad side rails of the bed and sharp corners. 8. Remove extra furniture from the client's room. 9. Discourage the client from engaging in activities involving the use of sharp objects (e.g., hand sewing and whittling). 10. Use soft cloths, mild soap, and light touch when bathing client. 11. Avoid dressing client in clothing that is tight or rubs. 12. Avoid taking blood pressure with a standard external, inflatable cuff. 13. Instruct the client to avoid blowing or picking the nose.	1. To avoid traumatizing sensitive tissues. 2. To prevent damage to oral mucous membranes. 3. To avoid trauma to the skin and to prevent bleeding. 4. To prevent excessive capillary blood loss. 5. To avoid mucous membrane injury. 6. To reduce the risk of abrasion or laceration injuries. 7. To reduce the risk of contusion injury. 8. To increase space and reduce the risk of the client's becoming injured by bumping into environmental objects. 9. To reduce the risk of injury. 10. To prevent abrasion injury. 11. To reduce the risk of abrasion injury. 12. To prevent skin injury from cuff pressure. 13. To reduce trauma to nasal mucous membranes.

Client will not experience significant blood loss.
■ Has normal hematocrit and hemoglobin values.
■ Has no manifestations of overt bleeding from wounds or body orifices.
	1. Examine the client every 4 h for signs and symptoms of bleeding, including
	   a. Increase in abdominal girth.
	   b. Presence of petechiae.
	   c. Oozing from mucous membranes.
	   d. Increase in bruise sizes.
	   e. Drainage on dressings and around IV sites.
		1, 2. To determine the site and extent of bleeding.

continued

CLIENT CARE PLAN ■ The Client with Acute Myelogenous Leukemia *continued*

Goal/Outcome Criteria	Interventions	Rationales
Nursing Diagnosis 2: Potential for Injury Related to Excessive Bleeding Secondary to Thrombocytopenia		

	2. Examine all body fluids and excrement for the presence of overt or occult blood.
	  a. Vomitus.
	  b. Urine.
	  c. Stools.
	3. When the client is menstruating, count the number of pads or tampons used and weigh each before and after use.
	4. Instruct the client in the signs and symptoms of overt and occult hemorrhage.
	5. Instruct the client to avoid drug products that contain aspirin and nonsteroidal anti-inflammatory agents.
		3. To determine the rate and amount of blood loss.
		
		4. To permit the client to assist in self-care and accept responsibility in health maintenance.
		5. To avoid products that further diminish the client's capacity to form clots appropriately.

Nursing Diagnosis 3: Fatigue Related to Anemia and Increased Energy Demands		
Client will be able to participate in some self-care activities without becoming overly fatigued. ■ Verbalizes symptoms of mild fatigue. ■ Performs self-care activities within limitations. ■ Identifies alternative means of performing daily activities that require less energy than normal.	1. Assist the client in selection of food items high in protein and calories. 2. Provide small meals that require little chewing. 3. Administer blood products as ordered. 4. Assist the client in turning and self-care. 5. Allow rest time between nursing interventions for the client. 6. Examine the schedule of ordered events and cancel those activities not essential to the client's immediate well-being.	1. To restore nutritional balance and increase available energy substrates. 2. To prevent the client from becoming fatigued while eating. 3. To directly replace RBCs and hemoglobin to ameliorate anemia and decrease fatigue. 4–6. To conserve the client's energy.

Common Diagnoses

The following nursing diagnoses are commonly seen among clients with AML:

1. Potential for infection related to impaired immune response

2. Potential for injury related to excessive bleeding secondary to thrombocytopenia

3. Fatigue related to anemia and increased energy demands

Additional Diagnoses

In addition, many clients with AML have one or more of the following nursing diagnoses:

1. Impaired skin integrity related to prolonged immobility

2. Altered oral mucous membrane related to effects of chemotherapy and pancytopenia

3. Total self-care deficit related to progressive debilitation and weakness

4. Altered nutrition: less than body requirements related to anorexia, nausea, and vomiting

5. Anxiety related to fear of death

6. Powerlessness related to an inability to control the progression of the disease

7. Altered family processes related to perceived inability to fulfill parental and other family roles and prolonged hospitalization

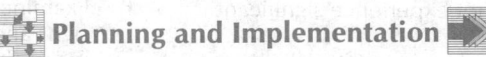 **Planning and Implementation**

Potential for Infection

Infection is a major cause of death in the immunosuppressed client, and septicemia is a common sequela. Infection of clients with leukemia occurs through auto-contamination, in which the client's normal flora overgrows and penetrates the internal environment, and through cross-contamination, in which microorganisms from another person or the environment are transmitted to the client.

Planning: client goals.   The major client goals for this diagnosis is that the client will (1) remain free from cross-contamination–induced infection and (2) not experience sepsis.

Interventions: nonsurgical management.   Interventions for this diagnosis are aimed at interrupting or halting the infection processes, controlling infection, and initiating early, effective treatment regimens for specific infections.

Drug therapy for leukemia.   Drug therapy for AML is usually divided into three distinctive phases: induction therapy, consolidation therapy, and maintenance therapy (Ziegfeld, 1987).

Induction therapy is intensive and consists of combination chemotherapy initiated at the time of diagnosis. This therapy is aimed at achieving a rapid, complete remission of all manifestations of the disease (Champlin, 1987). Different institutions and different physicians vary both the agents used and the treatment schedule. An example of a typical course of aggressive chemotherapy for induction of remission in clients with AML includes intravenous (IV) administration of cytosine arabinoside (at 200 mg/m^2 of body surface area per day) for 7 days with concomitant administration of daunorubicin (60 mg/m^2 per day) for the first 3 days. A major problem is that one side effect of these agents is severe bone marrow suppression. As a result, the client becomes even more prone to infection than before the treatment started.

Consolidation therapy usually consists of another course of either the same agents as used for induction at a different dosage level or a different combination of chemotherapeutic agents. This treatment occurs early in remission, and its intent is curative. At some institutions, consolidation therapy is a single course of chemotherapy; at other institutions, consolidation therapy consists of regularly scheduled repeated courses of chemotherapy during 1 to 2 years. Both induction and consolidation therapies are administered intravenously. Usually the client has a double-lumen external venous access device in place for this treatment.

Maintenance therapy may be prescribed for months to years after successful induction and consolidation therapies. The purpose of this treatment is to maintain the remission achieved through induction and consolidation. Agents used for maintenance are more mild, are often given orally, and may be given for 2 to 5 years. The treatment of leukemia requires facilities for the transfusion of RBCs, platelets, and granulocytes, as well as facilities for the diagnosis and management of unusual infections.

Drug therapy for infection.   Drug therapy is a primary defense against infections that tend to develop among clients undergoing therapy for AML. Agents used depend on the sensitivity of the specific organism causing the infection, as well as the extent of the infection. Agents are categorized by specificity as antibacterial, antiviral, or antifungal.

Antibiotic and antibacterial agents used for prophylaxis or treatment of infection in clients with AML usually include at least one of the aminoglycosides (amikacin, gentamicin, and tobramycin) and a systemic penicillin. Additional powerful antibiotics frequently used for clients with leukemia are vancomycin and drugs from the tetracycline and third-generation cephalosporin classes.

Antifungal agents are usually used when an actual fungal infection has been diagnosed or is strongly suggested. The major systemic antifungal agents are amphotericin B and ketoconazole.

Antiviral agents may be prescribed prophylactically or not until an actual viral infection is diagnosed. The most common systemic antiviral agent in use today is acyclovir.

These drugs, although helpful in combating severe infections, are associated with a wide range of serious adverse effects. The most significant of these effects are ototoxicity and nephrotoxicity. The nurse carefully monitors clients treated with such drugs for signs of renal insufficiency and hearing impairment.

Infection control.   A major objective for the nurse caring for leukemic clients is to protect them from infection (Konradi, 1989). Extreme care is used in all nursing procedures. Frequent, thorough hand washing is of utmost importance. A mask should be worn by any person with an upper respiratory infection who must enter the client's room. Strict procedures should be observed when performing dressing changes or inserting a central venous catheter or Hickman's catheter. Some hospitals specify that masks should be worn by both the client and the nurse when an IV line is manipulated in any way. Strict aseptic technique in the care of these catheters should be maintained at all times.

If possible, the client should be in a private room to minimize cross-contamination. Statistics show that infection in the immunosuppressed individual is derived from organisms that are normal inhabitants of the body. Therefore, protective (reverse) isolation has been deleted from the Centers for Disease Control guidelines for infection control. However, other environmental precautions still exist for clients with leukemia. No standing collections of water, such as in vases or denture cups, should be allowed in the client's room, as they are excellent breeding grounds for microorganisms. Any uncooked foods, such as raw fruit and vegetables, should be eliminated from the diet. Uncooked food contains large numbers of bacteria. Black pepper is also high in microorganisms. Whether these restrictions are clinically beneficial is highly controversial.

The nurse constantly assesses the client for the presence of infection. This task is made somewhat more difficult because clients with leukopenia do not always manifest infections in the same way that clients with normal WBC counts do. Fever development and formation of pus (both indicators of infection) are dependent on the presence of leukocytes. Therefore, leukopenic clients may have severe infections without the manifestations of either fever or pus. The nurse monitors the client's daily CBC with differential WBC count. The oral mucosa is inspected during every nursing shift for the presence of lesions indicating fungal or viral infection. Lung sounds are auscultated every 4 hours for the presence of crackles, wheezes, or diminished breath sounds. Each time the client voids, the nurse inspects the urine for odor and cloudiness. The client is asked whether any sensation of urgency, burning, or pain is present during urination.

The nurse takes the client's vital signs frequently, at least every 4 hours, to assess for the presence of fever. A temperature elevation of even 0.5° F above baseline is significant for a leukopenic client and should be regarded as indicative of the presence of an infection until proved otherwise.

Many hospital units that specialize in the care of neutropenic clients have specific protocols to be followed if infection is suspected. Physicians are notified immediately, and specific cultures are obtained. Blood for bacterial and fungal cultures is obtained from peripheral sites and from the central venous line. Urine and sputum cultures are also obtained. Any open lesion also is cultured, and chest x-ray films are obtained. After cultures are obtained, the client is started on a regimen of IV antibiotic agents.

Skin care. Skin care is important for the leukemic client. The skin may be the only intact defense that the client has. Turning is necessary every hour, if the client is immobile, and the skin should be well lubricated. Similarly, pulmonary toilet should be performed every 2 to 4 hours. Frequent assessments and promotion of coughing, deep breathing, and postural drainage are vital for prophylaxis and early detection of an infection.

Interventions: surgical management. Bone marrow transplantation is being used more frequently in the treatment of leukemia. It is the treatment of choice for younger clients who have closely matched donors and who are experiencing temporary remission with induction therapy. The concept of bone marrow transplantation is to rid the client of all leukemic cells through high-dose chemotherapy coupled with whole body irradiation (Freedman, 1988). These treatments are lethal to the bone marrow, and, without replacement of bone marrow function through transplantation, the client would die of infection or hemorrhage. The transplanted bone marrow can either be from another person (allogeneic transplant) or have been taken from the client during a period of complete remission (autologous transplant). Because the bone marrow is the actual site of production of leukemia cells and it can be difficult to be certain that all leukemic cells have been eradicated

during remission, the most successful bone marrow transplants among clients with AML are allogeneic.

Procedure. A suitable donor is selected after family members are tested for human leukocyte antigen (HLA) types. The most preferable transplants are those between HLA-identical siblings, but can also be successful between those with closely matched HLA types. After tissue typing, the donor is taken to the operating room, where marrow harvesting is accomplished through multiple aspirations to retrieve sufficient bone marrow for the transplant (Ruggiero, 1988). The client receives a large dose of chemotherapeutic agents and total body irradiation.

The harvested marrow is administered to the client by IV infusion via the Hickman catheter. The marrow stem cells circulate briefly through many parts of the body, but find their way to the medullary cavities, where subsequent growth and reconstitution of the marrow is confined.

Complications. The posttransplant period is difficult and complicated. The client remains without any natural immunity until the donor marrow begins to proliferate and the client's body accepts this graft—a minimum of 10 days. Therefore, infection is a major problem. The client also has severe thrombocytopenia during this period. The nursing care requirements for these clients are virtually identical to those required by clients undergoing aggressive induction therapy for AML.

In addition to the problems related to the period of pancytopenia, other immediate hazards associated with bone marrow transplantation include failure to engraft and the development of graft-versus-host disease (GVHD).

Failure to engraft occurs more frequently among allogeneic transplant recipients than among autologous transplant recipients. The causes of graft failure may be related to insufficient numbers of cells transplanted, attack or rejection of donor cells by residual immunologically competent recipient cells, infection of transplanted cells, and unknown biologic factors. If the transplanted bone marrow fails to engraft, the client will die unless another transplantation is attempted and is successful.

GVHD is an immunologic event that occurs in the presence of the following two conditions: (1) the recipient is *not* immunocompetent and (2) donor tissue has active leukocytes, especially effector T cells and T cell precursors. Because the recipient is totally immunosuppressed, the recipient is not able to recognize the donated bone marrow cells as foreign or nonself. Instead, the immunocompetent cells of the donated marrow recognize the host (recipient) cells, tissues, and organs as foreign and mount an immune offense against them. In this situation, the graft is actually trying to attack the host.

Although all host tissues can be attacked and harmed, the tissues that most commonly manifest symptoms of this damage are the skin, the GI tract, and the liver. Approximately 30% to 70% of all allogeneic bone marrow transplant recipients develop some degree of GVHD. The presence of this problem indicates that the transplanted cells are competent and have successfully engrafted; however, more than 15% of the individuals who develop GVHD die of complications associated with the event. GVHD is managed by administering immunosuppressive agents and supporting the tissue systems sustaining the heaviest damage. Care must be taken to avoid suppressing the new immune system to the extent that either the client becomes more prone to infection or the transplanted cells stop engrafting.

Potential for Injury

Because normal bone marrow production is severely limited in clients with AML, the number of circulating erythrocytes and platelets is severely diminished, creating a condition of thrombocytopenia. This condition puts the client with AML at a greatly increased risk for excessive bleeding in response to minimal trauma.

Planning: client goals. The goal is that the client will remain free from bleeding.

Interventions: nonsurgical management. As a result of chemotherapy-induced pancytopenia, the client's platelet count is decreased. At the height of chemotherapy's effectiveness, called the *nadir*, the platelet count may be as low as 10,000/mm³. Obviously, with such low platelet counts, the client is at great risk for bleeding. A major objective of the nurse is to protect the individual from situations that could lead to bleeding and to closely monitor the amount of bleeding that is occurring.

The nurse assesses frequently for evidence of bleeding, in the form of oozing, confluent ecchymoses, petechiae, or purpura. All stools, nasogastric drainage, and vomitus are examined visually for the appearance of blood and are tested for occult blood. The nurse measures any blood loss as accurately as possible. The client's abdominal girth is measured during every nursing shift. Increases in abdominal girth can indicate internal hemorrhage. Bleeding precautions are instituted. The precautions consist of the avoidance of injections via intramuscular and subcutaneous routes, the use of straight-edge razors, and the insertion of rectal suppositories or thermometers. Diets high in roughage or spicy food and ill-fitting dentures are also avoided in the client when bleeding precautions are instituted. Blood pressure should be checked by cuff as infrequently as possible, as blood vessels are easily ruptured in the thrombocytopenic client. Only paper or silk tape should be used, and all tubes and catheters should be well lubricated. Gentleness should be used in all nursing care, and skin care is important in this client. Aspirin should be avoided.

For the client with a platelet count less than 20,000/mm³, a platelet transfusion may be required. Platelet transfusions are usually pooled from as many as 10 donors. The platelet transfusion does not have to be of the same blood type as the client's blood; however, if a bone marrow transplant is planned or if a client receives frequent transfusions, HLA matching is done.

The transfusion must be given immediately after being brought to the client's room, as the platelet is an easily destroyed cell. The transfusion should be administered during about 10 minutes, using a special filter and Y tubing. Only about 3% of platelets are lost by passage through these filters. The client may be premedicated with meperidine or hydrocortisone to minimize the possibility of reaction. Clients can become febrile and experience rigors (severe chills) during transfusion of platelets, but these symptoms are not considered a true transfusion reaction. IV administration of amphotericin B, an antifungal agent that many clients with leukemia receive, should be discontinued during the transfusion of platelets and should not be resumed for at least 1 hour.

Fatigue

Because normal bone marrow production is severely limited in clients with AML, the number of circulating erythrocytes is severely diminished creating a condition of anemia. The decrease in erythrocyte levels diminishes the blood's capacity to carry oxygen and causes the client to be unable to meet the oxygen demands required by even basal metabolic levels. Because leukemic cells tend to have higher rates of metabolism and greater utilization of oxygen, the anemic client with leukemia is at risk for an even more severe fatigue response.

Planning: client goals. The major goals include that the client will (1) not experience an increase in fatigue and will (2) increase baseline activity.

Interventions: nonsurgical management. Interventions are aimed at decreasing the effects of anemia and conserving the client's energy expenditure.

Diet therapy. Diet therapy is indirectly related to fatigue and subsequent activity intolerance. The client must ingest enough calories to meet at least basal energy requirements. This can be difficult when the client is extremely fatigued. The nurse provides small, frequent meals that are high in protein and carbohydrate content. Food items that are liquid or easy to chew require less effort to consume.

Oxygen therapy. Oxygen therapy may be useful in ameliorating fatigue during periods of anemia. However, caution is necessary whenever oxygen is administered to clients with anemia because hypoxia is the stimulus for the kidney to synthesize and secrete erythropoietin. This factor enhances bone marrow production and maturation of erythrocytes. Thus, excessive oxygen administration can suppress this desired physiologic action.

Oxygen can be administered by mask, hood, nasal

cannula, nasopharyngeal tube, endotracheal tube, and tracheostomy tube. Most commonly, nasal cannulas are used to administer oxygen continuously. The nurse administers oxygen to the client in the amount of liters per minute (for cannula and nasopharyngeal tube administration) or concentration by percentage (for administration by mask, hood, endotracheal tube, and tracheostomy tube) specified by the physician's prescription. Whenever oxygen is administered, it should be nebulized to prevent drying of airway tissues.

Blood transfusions. Blood transfusions are sometimes indicated for treatment of fatigue. Blood transfusions increase the oxygen-carrying capacity of blood and replace missing RBCs and some coagulation factors (see Table 67–1). For the leukemic client experiencing fatigue related to anemia, whole blood or packed RBCs would usually be the blood component of choice. Nursing care actions and responsibilities during transfusions are discussed earlier under the heading Collaborative Management in the section on anemia.

Conservation of the client's energy. The nurse examines the hospitalized client's schedule of prescribed and routine activities. Those activities that do not have a directly positive effect on the client's condition are assessed in terms of their usefulness to the client. If the benefit (actual or potential) of the activity does not outweigh its actual or potential aggravation of the client's fatigue, the nurse consults with other members of the health care team about eliminating or postponing the activity. Candidates for cancellation or temporary postponement may include hair washing, obtaining rectal temperatures, undergoing physical therapy, and performing specific invasive diagnostic tests not required for the assessment or the treatment of presenting problems.

■ Discharge Planning

The leukemic client is discharged to the home setting after induction chemotherapy or bone marrow transplantation. Follow-up care is provided on an outpatient basis.

Home Care Preparation

Planning for home care for the client with leukemia begins as soon as a remission is achieved. The client may need assistance at home until the physical condition improves, and assessment should be made of the support mechanisms available. Many clients require the services of a visiting nurse to assist with dressing changes for Hickman's catheters and to answer questions.

Client/Family Education

The client and the family need to be educated about the importance of continuing therapy and appropriate medical follow-up, despite the unpleasant side effects of such therapy. Protecting the client from infection after discharge from the hospital is just as important as when the client was hospitalized. Using proper hygiene and avoiding crowds and others with infections should be stressed. Neither the client nor her/his household contacts should receive immunization with a live virus for diseases such as poliomyelitis, measles, or rubella. Mouth care regimens should be continued. Any fever, or other sign of infection, should be brought to the immediate attention of the client's physician. The client and the family need to be aware of the necessity of a healthy diet, as the immune system cannot function without adequate protein, calories, and carbohydrates.

Psychosocial Preparation

Psychosocial preparation of the client for discharge from the hospital is important. A diagnosis of leukemia is a threat to the client's self-esteem and role within the family. The client is confronted with the reality of death, and treatment causes major adjustments in the way the client views himself/herself. The client and the family experience changes in the client's body image, level of independence, and life style. Some clients feel threatened by the environment, seeing everything as potentially infectious. The nurse must help the client and the family redefine priorities, understand the illness and its treatment, and find hope. Support groups such as I Can Cope and Make Today Count can be enormously beneficial to both the client and the family, and the nurse should make referrals to such groups.

Health Care Resources

A client with limited social support may need assistance at home until strength and energy improve. A home care aide may suffice for some clients, whereas a visiting nurse may be needed for other clients to reinforce teaching. The client may need equipment to facilitate ADL and ambulation. In addition, financial resources are assessed. Treatment of cancer is extraordinarily expensive, and the nurse works closely with the social services department to ensure that insurance is adequate. If the client is without insurance, other sources must be explored. Because prolonged outpatient contact and follow-up is necessary, the client needs transportation to the outpatient facility. Many local divisions of the American Cancer Society offer free transportation to clients with any form of cancer, including leukemia.

Evaluation

On the basis of the identified nursing diagnoses, the nurse evaluates the care of the client with leukemia. The expected outcomes include that the client

1. States the signs and symptoms of infection
2. Knows whom to contact if signs and symptoms of infection are present

3. Describes the mouth care regimen
4. Has minimal or no disruptions in the oral mucous membranes
5. Remains free from episodes of bleeding
6. Maintains appropriate weight for height and body build
7. Is able to participate in ADL
8. Recognizes symptoms of fatigue and alters activity before fatigue becomes excessive
9. Verbalizes decreased feelings of fear
10. Identifies role change within the family
11. Has no evidence of skin breakdown
12. Verbalizes increasing feelings of control of the response to the disease process and treatment regimens

Malignant Lymphoma

Although malignant lymphomas reflect abnormal proliferation of one type of leukocyte (lymphocytes), they differ from the leukemias in the degree of differentiation of the affected cells and the location of the production of these cells. *Lymphomas* are malignancies characterized by a proliferation of *committed lymphocytes,* rather than the stem cell precursors (as in leukemia). In addition, this proliferation does not occur in the bone marrow, but rather in the other lymphoid tissues scattered throughout the body, especially the lymph nodes and the spleen. As such, lymphomas are actually solid-tissue masses rather than cellular suspensions within the blood and the bone marrow.

HODGKIN'S DISEASE

OVERVIEW

Hodgkin's disease is a malignancy that occurs primarily among young adults. Factors implicated as possible causes of Hodgkin's disease include viral infections and previous exposure to alkylating chemical agents. This neoplastic disorder usually originates in a single lymph node or a single chain of nodes. The lymphoid tissues within the node undergo malignant transformation and usually initiate some inflammatory processes at the same time. These nodes contain a specific transformed cell type, the Reed-Sternberg cell, which is a characteristic marker of Hodgkin's disease. This initially localized disease first metastasizes to other lymphoid structures and eventually invades nonlymphoid tissues.

COLLABORATIVE MANAGEMENT

Assessment most often reveals a greatly enlarged, but painless lymph node or nodes, usually the earliest man-

ifestation of Hodgkin's disease. General clinical manifestations include fever, malaise, and night sweats. More specific clinical manifestations are dependent on the site or sites of malignancy and the extent of the disease.

Diagnosis is established when biopsy of a node or a mass reveals the presence of Reed-Sternberg cells. Four types of Hodgkin's lymphoma have been defined on the basis of other cellular characteristics present within the malignant lymphoid tissues: lymphocytic predominance, mixed cellularity, lymphocytic depletion, and nodular sclerosis (Cotran et al., 1989). Although prognosis is determined more by the extent or the stage of disease at the time of diagnosis, the lymphocytic predominance subtype has the most favorable prognosis and the lymphocytic depletion subtype has the least favorable prognosis (Rapaport, 1987).

After diagnosis, extensive staging procedures are performed to determine accurately the exact extent of disease (see the accompanying Key Features of Disease). This staging has to be detailed and accurate because the treatment regimen is determined by the extent of disease. Typical procedures for staging of Hodgkin's disease include biopsies of distant lymph nodes, lymphangiography, computed tomography of the thorax and the abdomen, CBC, liver function studies, and bilateral bone marrow biopsies.

Such progress has been made with the treatment regimens that Hodgkin's disease is now one of the most curable of the adult malignancies. Generally, for stages I and II without mediastinal node involvement, the treatment of choice is extensive external radiation of involved lymph node regions. With more extensive disease, radiation coupled with an aggressive multiagent chemotherapy regimen is the most effective means of achieving a complete response. Chapter 25 discusses general care for clients receiving radiation and/or chemotherapy.

Specific nursing management of the client undergoing treatment for Hodgkin's disease focuses on the side effects of therapy. In addition to the drug-induced pancytopenia, which results in increased risk of infection and anemia, clients with Hodgkin's disease usually experience severe nausea and vomiting, skin irritation and breakdown at the site of radiation, and body image changes. Hepatic function may be impaired either by disease extension to the liver or by the multiagent chemotherapy. In addition, for male clients receiving radiation in an inverted Y pattern to the abdominopelvic region along with specific chemotherapeutic agents, permanent sterility can be expected. Clients should be informed of this side effect and the option of storage of sperm in a sperm bank before treatment begins.

NON-HODGKIN'S LYMPHOMA

OVERVIEW

Non-Hodgkin's lymphoma is the classification for all neoplastic disorders originating from lymphoid tissues that

KEY FEATURES OF DISEASE ▪ Staging of Hodgkin's Disease

Stage Ia	Disease confined to a single lymph node region or only one extranodal site.
Stage Ib	Disease confined to a single lymph node region or only one extranodal site. Client also experiences some or all of the following systemic symptoms: persistent fever, night sweats, and significant weight loss (>10%).
Stage IIa	Disease confined to either two or more lymph node regions on the same side of the diaphragm or contiguous extranodal sites on the same side of the diaphragm.
Stage IIb	Disease confined to either two or more lymph node regions on the same side of the diaphragm or contiguous extranodal sites on the same side of the diaphragm. Client also experiences some or all of the following systemic symptoms: persistent fever, night sweats, and significant weight loss (>10%).
Stage IIIa	Disease extends to lymph node regions on both sides of the diaphragm.
Stage IIIb	Disease extends to lymph node regions on both sides of the diaphragm. Client also experiences some or all of the following systemic symptoms: persistent fever, night sweats, and significant weight loss (>10%).
Stage IIIs	Disease extends to lymph node regions on both sides of the diaphragm. Client also experiences some or all of the following systemic symptoms: persistent fever, night sweats, and significant weight loss (>10%). Spleen also involved in disease.
Stage IV	Disease has widely disseminated foci of involvement, including one or more extranodal tissues and organs.

are not diagnosed as Hodgkin's disease. The majority of non-Hodgkin's lymphomas arise from lymph nodes, but these lymphomas can originate in virtually any tissue or organ. With the exception of a few subtypes, most non-Hodgkin's lymphomas occur among older adults. Definitive etiology is unknown, but factors such as viral infection, exposure to ionizing radiation, and exposure to toxic chemicals have been implicated.

COLLABORATIVE MANAGEMENT

Because lymphomas may arise from lymphoid cells in any tissue and because the malignancy can spread to any organ, assessment reveals no specific clinical manifestations that are common to all types of lymphoma, other than lymphadenopathy. Diagnosis is made from the histologic features apparent on biopsy specimens of any suspicious node or mass. Classification of specific lymphoma subtype is based on a complex grading of the presence or absence of surface markers, cytogenetic features, cell size, and expression of viral antigens. Staging is usually expressed in a manner similar to that for Hodgkin's disease. It may be difficult to differentiate some subtypes of non-Hodgkin's lymphoma from CLL.

Depending on the cell type, prognosis may range from excellent to poor. Overall, however, non-Hodgkin's lymphomas have a poorer prognosis than Hodgkin's disease because most non-Hodgkin's lymphomas originate within lymphoid tissue and are widely distributed in nodes, marrow, or blood by the time a diagnosis is made. Some types of non-Hodgkin's lymphoma have a protracted course, extending over many years, and are not treated in the early phases. However, for most types of non-Hodgkin's lymphoma, death ensues rapidly if treatment is not instituted.

Treatment usually consists of radiation therapy and multidrug chemotherapy. Nursing care needs are similar to those of clients with Hodgkin's disease, taking into account additional organ-specific problems when disease is widely disseminated.

COAGULATION DISORDERS

Coagulation disorders are synonymous with bleeding disorders. Such disorders are characterized by abnormal or increased bleeding as a result of defects in one or more components regulating hemostasis. Bleeding disorders may be spontaneous or traumatic, localized or generalized, and lifelong or acquired. Bleeding disorders can originate from a defect in the hemostatic processes at the vascular level, the platelet level, or the clotting factor level. Figure 67–1 outlines the blood clotting cascades and sites where specific defects and drugs disrupt the hemostatic processes.

The role of the blood vessel wall in hemostasis is less well understood than the roles of platelets and coagulation factors. Vascular disorders are a heterogeneous group of conditions with a wide spectrum of clinical manifestations. Usually, these disorders involve increased capillary fragility (innate or acquired) and are clinically characterized by cutaneous petechiae and purpura, tendency to bruise easily, and bleeding. Such

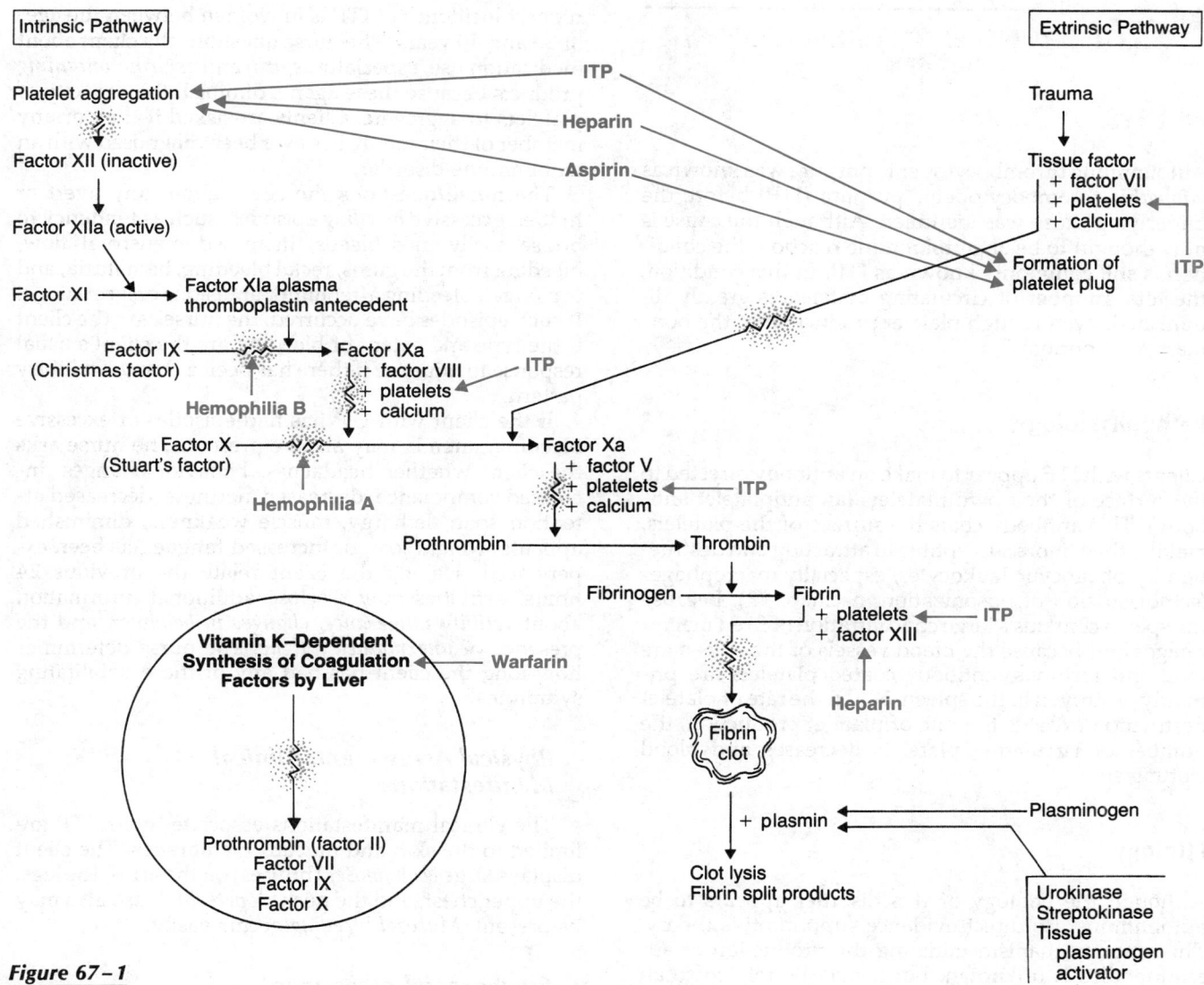

Figure 67–1

Sites of disruption of the coagulation mechanism by drugs and diseases.

disorders include purpura simplex, hereditary hemorrhagic telangiectasia, allergic purpura (Henoch-Schönlein purpura), and hypertensive vascular disease. Even though clients with these disorders have an apparent bleeding problem, the defect is not within the hematopoietic system and thus is beyond the scope of this chapter.

Platelet Disorders

The role of the platelet in hemostasis is important. For both the intrinsic and extrinsic pathways, coagulation starts with platelet adhesion and formation of a platelet

plug. Any condition that either diminishes the number of platelets or interferes with the ability of platelets to adhere (to one another, blood vessel walls, collagen, or fibrin threads) can manifest as a disorder of increased bleeding. Platelet disorders can be inherited, acquired, or temporarily induced by the ingestion of substances that limit platelet production or inhibit aggregation. When the actual number of platelets is below that which is needed for normal coagulation, the condition is called *thrombocytopenia*. Thrombocytopenia may occur as a result of other conditions or treatments that suppress general bone marrow activity. Additionally, thrombocytopenia can occur by processes that specifically limit platelet formation or increase the rate of platelet destruction. The two thrombocytopenic conditions affecting adults are autoimmune thrombocytopenic purpura and thrombotic thrombocytopenic purpura.

AUTOIMMUNE THROMBOCYTOPENIC PURPURA

OVERVIEW

Autoimmune thrombocytopenic purpura was known as *idiopathic* thrombocytopenic purpura (ITP) before the underlying cause was identified. Although the cause is now thought to be an autoimmune reaction, the condition is still commonly known as ITP. In this condition, the total number of circulating platelets is greatly diminished, even though platelet production in the bone marrow is normal.

Pathophysiology

Clients with ITP appear to make an antibody directed to the surface of their own platelets (an antiplatelet antibody). This antibody coats the surface of the platelets, making them more susceptible to attraction and destruction by phagocytic leukocytes, especially macrophages (see discussion of opsonization in Chap. 23). Because the spleen contains a large concentration of fixed macrophages and because the blood vessels of the spleen are long and tortuous, antibody-coated platelets are primarily destroyed in the spleen. When the rate of platelet destruction exceeds the rate of platelet production, the number of circulating platelets decreases and blood clotting slows.

Etiology

Although the etiology of this disorder appears to be autoimmune, no direct evidence supports this theory. The exact mechanism initiating the production of autoantibodies is unknown, but it may be related to an immune system defect resulting from viral infection (Cotran et al., 1989).

Incidence

The exact incidence of ITP is not known. The disease is most common among women between the ages of 20 and 40 years. It is also more prevalent among individuals with a pre-existing autoimmune condition, such as systemic lupus erythematosus (Cotran et al., 1989).

COLLABORATIVE MANAGEMENT

 Assessment

History

The nurse collects data about the history of the present illness. *Age* and *sex* are important because the

highest incidence of ITP is in women between the ages of 20 and 40 years. The nurse questions the client about medication use, especially *aspirin* and *aspirin-containing* products because these agents diminish the capacity of platelets to aggregate. Clients are asked if they or any member of their family has ever been diagnosed with an autoimmune disorder.

The nurse questions the client about any overt or hidden excessive *bleeding* episodes, such as tendency to bruise easily, nosebleeds, increased menstrual flow, bleeding from the gums, rectal bleeding, hematuria, and prolonged bleeding after minor abrasions or lacerations. If such episodes have occurred, the nurse asks the client if the type and extent of bleeding are the client's usual response to injury or if there has been a change in injury pattern.

If the client with ITP has had episodes of excessive bleeding, anemia may also be present. The nurse asks the client whether headaches, behavior changes, increased somnolence, decreased alertness, decreased attention span, lethargy, muscle weakness, diminished appetite, weight loss, or increased fatigue has been experienced. Having the client relate the previous 24 hours' activities may disclose additional information about *activity intolerance, changes in behavior,* and the presence of *unexplained fatigue.* The nurse determines how long the client has had any of these debilitating symptoms.

Physical Assessment: Clinical Manifestations

The clinical manifestations associated with ITP are limited to the skin and mucous membranes. The client displays large *ecchymoses* (bruises) on the arms, the legs, the upper chest, and the neck. A *petechial rash* also may be present. *Mucosal bleeding* occurs easily.

Psychosocial Assessment

The majority of clients with ITP have no associated changes in psychosocial function. Some clients experience anxiety as they encounter the health care system and learn that they have a significant illness that requires treatment.

A rare complication among clients with ITP is an intracranial bleeding–induced cerebrovascular accident. Therefore, the nurse assesses the client for neurologic function and mental status (see Chap. 32). The nurse asks family members or significant others if the client's behavior and responses to the mental status examination are typical for this client or represent a change from usual reactions.

Laboratory Findings

Diagnosis is made by noting a decreased platelet count and large numbers of megakaryocytes in the bone marrow. Antiplatelet antibodies may be present in detectable levels in peripheral blood. If the client has been experiencing any episodes of bleeding, the hematocrit and hemoglobin levels may be low.

 Analysis: Nursing Diagnosis

A typical client with ITP is a 35-year-old woman. The nursing diagnoses are identified for a typical client.

Common Diagnoses

A nursing diagnosis commonly found in hospitalized clients with ITP is potential for injury related to thrombocytopenia.

Additional Diagnoses

The client experiencing ITP may also have one or more of the following nursing diagnoses:

1. Fear related to outcomes of the disease process
2. Potential fluid volume deficit related to excessive vaginal bleeding
3. Altered family processes related to prolonged hospitalization
4. Knowledge deficit related to the disease and the treatment regimen

 Planning and Implementation

The plan of care for the client with ITP focuses on the common diagnosis. Nursing care is aimed at providing a safe environment and identifying early any episodes of bleeding.

Potential for Injury

Planning: client goals. The goal is that the client will remain free from bleeding.

Interventions: nonsurgical management. As a result of the decreased platelet count, the client is at great risk for bleeding. Interventions include therapy for the underlying condition, as well as protection of the client from trauma-induced bleeding episodes.

Drug therapy. Agents that have assisted in controlling ITP include drugs that suppress immune function to some degree. The premise for the use of these agents is to inhibit immune system synthesis of autoantibodies directed against platelets. Such agents include corticosteroids and azathioprine. More aggressive therapy can include low doses of chemotherapeutic agents, such as the vinca alkaloids and cyclophosphamide.

Transfusion therapy. For the client with a platelet count of less than 20,000/mm³ who is experiencing an acute life-threatening bleeding episode, a platelet transfusion may be required. Platelet transfusions are not

performed routinely, as the donated platelets are just as rapidly destroyed by the spleen as the client's own platelets. Platelet transfusions are usually pooled from as many as 10 donors. The platelet transfusion does not have to be of the same blood type as the client's.

The transfusion must be given immediately after being brought to the client's room, as the platelet is an easily destroyed cell. The transfusion should be administered during about 10 minutes, using a special filter and Y tubing.

Maintaining a safe environment. A major objective of the nurse is to protect the individual from situations that could lead to bleeding and to closely monitor the amount of bleeding that is occurring.

Nursing care actions for this intervention are discussed under the earlier heading Nonsurgical Management for the nursing diagnosis potential for injury in the leukemia section.

Interventions: surgical management. For clients whose ITP does not respond to drug therapy, splenectomy may be the treatment of choice. Nursing care after surgery is discussed in Chapter 20.

■ Discharge Planning

ITP is seldom an acute and self-limited disease process among adults. Individuals whose therapy includes splenectomy may be discharged to home with minimal or no bleeding problems remaining. However, most clients with ITP are managed more conservatively. For these individuals, ITP remains a chronic but controllable disease process requiring their understanding of their disease process and prescribed treatment regimen and active participation in care.

Home Care Preparation

The admission nursing history usually includes essential information regarding the family composition and the home environment. The client may require minimal assistance at home after discharge from the hospital. The major issue for clients with ITP at home is the safety of the environment. Not only does the nurse at the hospital spend time consulting with the client and the family about the need for specific safety precautions, but a home visit by a home care nurse for the purposes of identifying potential hazards is advisable.

Client/Family Education

The nurse assesses the client's understanding of the disease process and the accompanying risk of bleeding. The client is asked to identify from a list of specific daily care and home activities those that constitute a hazard to the individual with a bleeding problem. When specific activities are identified, the nurse and the client formulate a plan to decrease the risk associated with each activity when possible. The client and the family should be able to identify the signs and symptoms of decreased coagulation and internal and external hemorrhage. The nurse ascertains that the client and a family member know whom to contact if an increased bleeding tendency becomes evident. The nurse reminds the client to avoid aspirin and instructs the client to examine the labels of over-the-counter medications to determine whether aspirin or other nonsteroidal anti-inflammatory agents are included.

The nurse reinforces the prescribed treatment schedule, including the timing and dosage of all medications. The side effects of some prescribed medications, including general bone marrow suppression, can increase the client's risk of infection. The nurse reviews the signs and symptoms of infection with the client and the family. The client is taught how to use and correctly care for an oral thermometer.

 Evaluation

On the basis of the identified nursing diagnoses, the expected outcomes for the client with ITP include that the client

1. Remains free from injury
2. Lists clinical manifestations of increased bleeding
3. Identifies actions to take when signs and symptoms of increased bleeding occur
5. Lists signs and symptoms of infection
6. Identifies actions to take when signs and symptoms of infection occur
7. Describes activity limitations
8. Reduces anxiety
9. Describes and complies with the prescribed drug regimen

Clotting Factor Disorders

Bleeding disorders can result from a clotting factor defect. Defects may include inability to synthesize a specific clotting factor, synthesis of insufficient quantities of a clotting factor, or synthesis of a less active form of a clotting factor. Most clotting factor disorders are congenitally transmitted gene abnormalities of one clotting factor. The few acquired clotting factor disorders are related to the inability to synthesize many of the clotting factors at the same time as a result of liver damage or an insufficiency of clotting cofactors and precursor products. Common congenital disorders that result in defects at the clotting factor level include the hemophilias and von Willebrand's disease.

HEMOPHILIA

OVERVIEW

Hemophilia describes several hereditary bleeding disorders resulting from deficiencies of specific clotting factors. Hemophilia A (classic hemophilia) results from a deficiency of factor VIII. It accounts for 80% of the cases of hemophilia. Hemophilia B (Christmas disease) is a deficiency of factor IX and accounts for 20% of the cases.

Hemophilia has a 1 in 10,000 incidence. It is an X-linked recessive trait. Female carriers risk transmitting the gene for hemophilia to half of their daughters (who then are carriers) and to half of their sons (who develop overt hemophilia). Hemophilia A is, with rare exception, a disease of men, all of whose sons will not have the gene for hemophilia and all of whose daughters will be obligatory carriers of the trait.

The bleeding disorder associated with hemophilia A is so severe that before blood transfusions were available, hemophiliacs rarely survived past age 3 years. With the availability of blood transfusions, mean survival time increased to approximately 12 years. During the 1970s, isolation of large quantities of factor VIII from pooled human serum was possible. As a result of the widespread availability of this treatment, life expectancy for clients with hemophilia A dramatically increased, as did their quality of life, so that hemophilia was commonly seen among adult clients as well as children.

The clinical pictures of hemophilia A and B are identical. The client has abnormal bleeding in response to any trauma because of an absence or deficiency in the specific clotting factor. Hemophiliacs form platelet plugs at the bleeding site, but the clotting factor deficiency impairs the hemostatic response and the capacity to form a stable fibrin clot. This produces abnormal bleeding, which may be mild, moderate, or severe, depending on the degree of factor deficiency.

COLLABORATIVE MANAGEMENT

Assessment reveals excessive hemorrhage from minor cuts or abrasions caused by the abnormal platelet function, joint and muscle hemorrhages that lead to disabling long-term sequelae, tendency to bruise easily, and prolonged and potentially fatal postoperative hemorrhage. The laboratory test results for a true hemophiliac demonstrate a prolonged aPTT, normal bleeding time, and normal prothrombin time (Rapaport, 1987). The most common health problem associated with hemophilia is degenerating joint function resulting from chronic bleeding into the joints, especially at the hip and the knee.

The bleeding problems of hemophilia A can be well managed by either regularly scheduled IV administra-

NURSING RESEARCH

Blood Drawn from a Single-Lumen Central Venous Line May Give Inaccurate aPTT Values.

Almadrones, L., Godbold, J., Raaf, J., & Ennis, J. (1987). Accuracy of activated partial thromboplastin time drawn through central venous catheters. *Oncology Nursing Forum,* 14(2), 15–18.

Central venous catheters have many advantages over standard venipuncture access for clients who require continuous or frequent venous access for transfusions, medication administration, nutritional support, and laboratory testing of blood samples. Controversy exists as to whether venous blood specimens drawn through central venous catheters accurately reflect the status of the client's venous blood. This study sought to compare the results of a specific blood test (aPTT) from blood samples drawn through single-lumen central venous catheters, double-lumen central venous catheters, and direct venipuncture from the client's noninvolved arm.

Venous blood specimens drawn from the nonheparinized side of a double-lumen central venous catheter yielded the same aPTT values as blood drawn by direct venipuncture. Venous blood samples drawn from either single-lumen central venous catheters or the heparinized side of double-lumen central venous catheters yielded aPTT values that were significantly different from those obtained by direct venipuncture.

Critique. This study was well defined and carefully controlled.

Possible nursing implications. Because the timing and dosages of some therapies are based on the client's aPTT values, accuracy of those values is critical. Although client comfort should always be considered, accuracy should not be sacrificed for comfort. Therefore, for clients who have only a single-lumen catheter, venous blood samples for aPTT should be drawn from a direct venipuncture and not through the central venous catheter.

tion of factor VIII cryoprecipitate or intermittent administration as needed depending on activity level and injury probability. However, the cost of the drug is high and prohibitive for many individuals with hemophilia. In addition, because the factors are currently derived from pooled human serum, the risk of viral contamination is present, even with the use of heat-inactivated serum. Major complications of therapy for hemophilia during the 1980s were infection with hepatitis B virus, cytomegalovirus, and the human immunodeficiency virus. Although the use of heat-inactivated serum has reduced these risks, they have not yet been eliminated. New techniques for mass producing factor VIII may lead to uncontaminated and less expensive sources of this vital substance.

Disseminated Intravascular Coagulation

OVERVIEW

DIC occurs as an acquired, acute complication of other conditions, most commonly septicemia and septic shock. The proposed pathophysiologic mechanisms to explain the demonstrated events indicate that this coagulation disorder has at least two distinct phases.

The first phase is characterized by diffuse and abnormal formation of many minute clots within the microcirculation of all organs. The triggering event for this phase generally appears to be the release of tissue factors in response to contact with endotoxins during episodes of septicemia. These tissue factors stimulate widespread coagulation within microcirculatory areas. This widespread coagulation consumes excessive quantities of the preformed clotting factors and cofactors. During this phase, fibrinogen is degraded to form fibrin threads and an increase in the fibrin split products (fibrin degradation products). The excessive formation of fibrin and increased utilization of clotting factors are responsible for the second phase of DIC.

The second phase of DIC is characterized by an inability to form clots and the presence of overt or hidden hemorrhage. These problems occur because the first phase of the process used all available clotting factors. If the client survives initial completion of the two phases without intervention, DIC tends to become a vicious, repeating circle as the extensive clotting in the first phase causes tissue hypoxia and ischemia, which leads to necrosis and release of more tissue factors to initiate the process over again when more clotting factors have been synthesized.

COLLABORATIVE MANAGEMENT

The effectiveness of the interventions varies with the phase of the process. DIC is most effectively treated during the first phase. At this time, if the process is recognized, the appropriate treatment consists of the administration of heparin to inhibit unnecessary, harmful, excessive coagulation and to halt the consumption of vital clotting factors.

If DIC has progressed to the second phase, heparin therapy is inappropriate, as the client can no longer form clots anywhere. Treatment at this stage focuses on the administration of clotting factors and the initiation of appropriate therapy to treat the underlying triggering event.

A major management priority for DIC is prevention through identification of clients at risk for precipitating events, such as sepsis and septic shock. Clients at risk are observed carefully, and prophylaxis is initiated at the first indication of either sepsis or the first phase of DIC.

SUMMARY

Hematologic disease can range in degree of severity from no impairment to life-threatening crisis. The human suffering involved in many hematologic diseases is intense. At diagnosis, clients are suddenly confronted with a frightening-sounding diagnosis, which may have major ramifications for their health. The challenge for nurses is to anticipate the questions and crises that a client may experience and to guide the client toward an optimal health state.

IMPLICATIONS FOR RESEARCH

The gaps in knowledge in caring for the hematologically impaired client are immense. Research areas include using behavior interventions to modify the impact of disease on a client's life style, determination of optimal skin care regimens, and testing of various mouth care regimens. It is a challenge to examine nursing care practices for relevance and effectiveness and creatively modify and test new and different intervention strategies.

A few questions to stimulate nursing research in the area include

1. Does the normal skin flora of neutropenic clients differ from the normal skin flora of clients with normal granulocyte function?

2. Which cleaning techniques are effective in reducing the colony count of the skin over the site of an implanted venous access device?

3. What assessment criteria are essential in the early identification of oral infections in neutropenic clients?

4. Which mouth care regimens most effectively reduce pain in clients with stomatitis?

5. Which mouth care regimens most effectively reduce oral opportunistic infections in clients with stomatitis and neutropenia?

6. Is relaxation therapy more effective than guided imagery in controlling the nausea from chemotherapy?

7. Does a regular exercise regimen influence immune activity in clients receiving immunosuppressive agents?

8. What role does hope play in the client's coping with a potentially fatal disease?

9. Which analgesics are most effective in controlling the bone pain from lymphoma?

REFERENCES AND READINGS

American Cancer Society. (1989). *Cancer facts and figures—1989* (pp. 4–14). Atlanta: Author.

Bojanowski, C. (1989). Use of protocols for emergency department patients with sickle cell anemia. *Journal of Emergency Nursing, 15*(2), 83–87.

Champlin, R. (1987). Acute myelogenous leukemia: Current treatment approaches. *Issues in Oncology, 4,* 1–8.

Cotran, R., Kumar, V., & Robbins, S. (1989). *Robbins pathologic basis of disease* (4th ed.). Philadelphia: W. B. Saunders.

Fraser, M., & Tucker, M. (1989). Second malignancies following cancer therapy. *Seminars in Oncology Nursing, 5*(1), 43.

Freedman, S. (1988). An overview of bone marrow transplantation. *Seminars in Oncology Nursing, 4*(1), 3–8.

Froberg, J. (1989a). The anemias: Causes and courses of action, part 1. *Registered Nurse, 52*(1), 24–30.

Froberg, J. (1989b). The anemias: Causes and courses of action, part 2. *Registered Nurse, 52*(3), 52–57.

Froberg, J. (1989c). The anemias: Causes and courses of action, part 3. *Registered Nurse, 52*(5), 42–50.

Griffin, J. (1986). *Hematology and immunology: Concepts for nursing.* Norwalk, CT: Appleton-Century-Crofts.

Konradi, D. (1989). A close-up look at leukemia. *Nursing '89, 19*(6), 34–41.

Rapaport, S. (1987). *Introduction to hematology* (2nd ed.). Philadelphia: J. B. Lippincott.

Robbins, S., & Kumar, V. (1987). *Basic pathology* (4th ed.). Philadelphia: W. B. Saunders.

Rubin, P. (1983). *Clinical oncology: A multidisciplinary approach* (6th ed.). New York: American Cancer Society.

Ruggiero, M. (1988). The donor in bone marrow transplantation. *Seminars in Oncology Nursing, 4*(1), 9.

Simmons, A. (1989). *Hematology: A combined theoretical and technical approach.* Philadelphia: W. B. Saunders.

Trotta, P., & Knobf, M. (1987). Nursing assessment of symptoms associated with hyperviscosity syndrome. *Oncology Nursing Forum, 14*(1), 21–25.

Wheby, M. (1988). The high hematocrit: Managing blood flow problems. *Emergency Medicine, 20*(15), 24–28, 30–32.

Workman, M. (1989). Immunologic late effects in children and adults. *Seminars in Oncology Nursing, 5*(1), 36–42.

Yeomans, A. (1987). Myelodysplastic syndromes: A preleukemic disorder. *Cancer Nursing, 10*(1), 32–40.

Ziegfeld, C. (1987). *Core curriculum for oncology nursing.* Philadelphia: W. B. Saunders.

Unit 19 Resources

American Cancer Society, 1599 Clifton Road NE, Atlanta, GA 30329. Telephone 404-320-3333.

American Red Cross, 430 17th Street NW, Washington, DC 20006. Telephone 202-737-8300.

Center for Sickle Cell Disease, Howard University, 2121 Georgia Avenue NW, Washington, DC 20059. Telephone 202-636-7930.

Leukemia Society of America, 733 Third Avenue, New York, NY 10017. Telephone 212-573-8484.

National Association for Sickle Cell Disease, 4221 Wilshire Boulevard, Suite 360, Los Angeles, CA 90010. Telephone 213-936-7205.

National Hemophilia Foundation, 110 Greene Street, Suite 406, New York, NY 10012. Telephone 212-219-8180.

GUIDE TO
SPECIAL FEATURES

GUIDE TO SPECIAL FEATURES

FOCUS ON THE ELDERLY FEATURES

CLIENT CARE PLANS

EMERGENCY CARE FEATURES

KEY FEATURES OF DISEASE

INDEX/GLOSSARY

Note: Page numbers in *italics* refer to illustrations; page numbers followed by b refer to boxed
material; and page numbers followed by t refer to tables. Glossary terms are in boldface type.

A delta fibers, 109, 110
AACN. *See* American Association of Critical-
Care Nurses (AACN).
Abandonment, fear of, 212
Abdomen, assessment of, 1230–1232, *1231*
auscultation and, 1231
inspection and, 1231
palpation and, 1232, *1232*
percussion and, 1231–1232
Abdominal aneurysm, 2219, 2220, 2221. *See also*
entries under Aneurysm.
Abdominal breathing, 2031, *2032*
Abdominal examination, in female, 1643
Abdominal girth, measurement of, *1484*, 1484–
1485
Abdominal pain, appendicitis and, 1344–1345
Crohn's disease and, 1363
diverticulitis and, 1373
intestinal obstruction and, 1395
irritable bowel syndrome and, 1366
lupus erythematosus and, 702
pancreatic carcinoma and, 1475
Abdominal paradox, 1994
Abdominal reflex, 854
Abdominal trauma, 1400–1401
blunt, 1400
management of, 1400–1401
penetrating, 1400
Abdominal-perineal resection, colorectal cancer
and, 1383
Abducens nerve, 839t
assessment of, 851, *851*
Abduction, pillow, 682
ABGs. *See* Arterial blood gases (ABGs).
ABO blood system, 664
Abortion, 1732–1735
induced, 1734–1735
discharge instructions and, 1735b
spontaneous, 1732–1734
characteristics of, 1733b–1734b
complete, 1732, 1734
incomplete, 1732, 1733
inevitable, 1732, 1733
missed, 1732, 1734
threatened, 1732, 1733
**Abscess(es): a localized collection of pus in a
cavity, 1843.** *See also specific sites.*
anorectal, 1404–1405
management of, 1405
Bartholin's, 1715
brain, 903–905
management of, 904–905
epidural (extradural), 904
formation of, 616
intracerebral, 904
liver, 1505
lung, 2045
management of, 2045
pancreatic, 1479
perinephric, 1843
peritonsillar, 1249–1250, 1250–1254, 1960
renal, 1843
subdural, 904
Absolute granulocyte count (AGC), 533
Absolute neutrophil count (ANC), 533
Absorption, intestinal, 1219, *1220*, 1225–1226
Absorption atelectasis, 2004
Absorptive endocytosis, 538

Abstract reasoning, mental status assessment
and, 850
AC. *See* Assist-control mode (AC).
Acanthosis nigrans, gastric carcinoma and, 1331
Accelerated junctional rhythm, 2124–2125, *2125*
Acceleration injury, 924
Acceptance stage of dying, 199
Access to care, 43, 43–44
third-party payment and, 43
Accessory duct of Santorini, 1223, *1223*
Accessory pathways, ablation of, 2145
Accident(s). *See also specific injuries.*
disability and, 491
in late adulthood, 78–79
in young adulthood, 64
**Accommodation: the process by which a clear
visual image is maintained as the gaze is
shifted from a distant to a near point, 850,
997, 1001**
**Accreditation: the process by which a
nongovernmental agency approves and grants
accredited status to a health care agency
after it meets certain predetermined criteria,
46, 46t**
of home care agencies, 39
of hospitals, 38
Acetaminophen (Tylenol), for chronic pain, 134
Acetazolamide (Diamox), for ophthalmic
disorders, 1023t, 1043
Acetohexamide (Dymelor), for diabetes mellitus,
1607t
Acetylcholine (ACh), 832t, 838, 840
impulse transmission and, 829
myasthenia gravis and, 969
Acetylsalicylic acid. *See* Aspirin (acetylsalicylic
acid).
ACh. *See* Acetylcholine (ACh).
**Achalasia: a condition of progressively worsening
dysphagia that is evidenced by chronic and
sometimes vague complaints of a feeling of
food "sticking" in the esophagus, 1285–1288**
analysis: nursing diagnosis and, 1286
assessment and, 1286
diagnostic tests and, 1286
history in, 1286
physical, 1286
psychosocial, 1286
radiographic findings in, 1286
discharge planning and, 1288
client/family education and, 1288
health care resources and, 1288
home care preparation and, 1288
psychosocial preparation and, 1288
etiology of, 1285
evaluation and, 1288
incidence of, 1285
pathophysiology of, 1285
planning and implementation and, 1286–1288
**Acid(s): any substance that liberates or donates a
hydrogen ion when dissolved in water, 328.**
See also named acid.
excessive intake of, 338–339
fixed, 330
titratable, 332, *333*
Acid autodigestion, 1303
Acid deficit, 351
Acid phosphatase, as tumor marker, 572
Acid solutions, 329

Acid-base balance, 327–335
anatomy and physiology and, 327–334
chemical regulatory mechanisms and, 330–
331
compensation and, 334
definitions and, 328
free hydrogen ion concentration and pH
and, 328–329
hydrogen ion sources and, 329–330, *330*,
330t
renal regulatory mechanisms and, 332, *332*,
334
respiratory regulatory mechanisms and,
331, 331–332
anion gap and, 334
tests of, in renal failure, 1894b–1895b
Acid-base buffering pairs, 331
Acid-base imbalances. *See* Acidemia; Alkalemia.
**Acidemia: an acid-base imbalance in the body in
which there is an excess of acids compared
to bases, 336–350.** *See also* **Acidosis.**
analysis: nursing diagnosis and, 346
planning and implementation and, 346,
348–349
assessment and, 343–346
history and, 343
laboratory findings in, 344–346, 345b
physical, 343–344, 344b
psychosocial, 344
base deficit, 340
discharge planning and, 349–350
client/family education and, 349–350
health care resources and, 350
home care preparation and, 349
psychosocial preparation and, 350
etiology of, 337–343
combined metabolic and respiratory acidosis and, 343
metabolic acidosis and, 337–340
respiratory acidosis and, 340, 342
evaluation and, 350
incidence of, 343
pathophysiology of, 337
prevention of, 343
Acid-fast bacteria (AFB) isolation, 614b, 615
**Acidosis: the process that causes blood pH to
decrease, 336.** *See also* **Acidemia.**
metabolic. *See* Metabolic acidosis.
respiratory. *See* Respiratory acidosis.
Acknowledgement, body image disturbance
and, 162
**Acne vulgaris: erythematous pustular eruptions
affecting the sebaceous glands of the
epidermis, also referred to as acne, 680,
1140, 1144, 1211, color plate 71**
Acoustic nerve, assessment of, 851
Acoustic neuroma, 949, 1126–1127
management of, 1127
Acquired hypogammaglobulinemia, 647
**Acquired immunodeficiency syndrome (AIDS): an
infection caused by the human
immunodeficiency virus (HIV), 548, 632–
646, 1775**
analysis: nursing diagnosis and, 637
assessment and, 634–636
history in, 634–635
laboratory findings in, 636
physical, 635–636

INDEX / GLOSSARY

INDEX / GLOSSARY

Chronic obstructive pulmonary disease (COPD)
(*Continued*)
cigarette smoking and, 1992
family history and, 1992–1993
evaluation and, 2040
incidence of, 1993
lung cancer and, 2050
pathophysiology of, 1990–1992
asthma and, 1991–1992
bronchiectasis and, 1992
chronic bronchitis and, 1991
complications and, 1992
emphysema and, *1990*, 1990–1991
planning and implementation and, 1996–2035
impaired gas exchange and, 1996–2034
ineffective airway clearance and, 2034–2035
prevention of, 1993
**Chronic pain: pain that persists for more than six
months and has an insidious onset; is usually
diffuse, poorly localized, and often difficult
to describe, 118, 123, 134–140**
chronic pancreatitis and, 1471–1472
client care plan and, 124b–125b
degenerative joint disease and, 678–688
interventions: nonsurgical management and,
134–139
cognitive and behavioral strategies and,
137–139
drug therapy and, 134–137, 136t
interventions: surgical management and, 139–
140
planning: client goals and, 134
rheumatoid arthritis and, 697–698
Chronic pain syndrome(s), 118
therapeutic interventions for, 119–120
Chronic pancreatitis, 1469–1474
alcohol-induced, 1469
analysis: nursing diagnosis and, 1471
assessment and, 1470–1471
diagnostic tests and, 1471
history in, 1470
laboratory findings in, 1471
physical, 1470–1471
psychosocial, 1471
radiographic findings in, 1471
calcifying, 1469
discharge planning and, 1473
client/family education and, 1473
health care resources and, 1473
home care preparation and, 1473
psychosocial preparation and, 1473
etiology of, 1469
evaluation and, 1473–1474
incidence of, 1470
obstructive, 1470
pathophysiology of, 1469–1470
planning and implementation and, 1471–1473
prevention of, 1470
Chronic persistent hepatitis, 1497
Chronic rejection, 666, 1913b, 1914
**Chronic renal failure (CRF): a condition in which
the kidney ceases to remove metabolic
wastes and excessive water from the blood,
1884–1917**
analysis: nursing diagnosis and, 1897
assessment and, 1889–1897
diagnostic tests and, 1891, 1897
history in, 1889
laboratory findings in, 1891, 1892b–1897b
physical, 1889–1890, 1890b
psychosocial, 1890–1891
radiographic findings in, 1891
causes of, 1887b
discharge planning and, 1916–1917
client/family education and, 1916
health care resources and, 1917
home care preparation and, 1916
psychosocial preparation and, 1916–1917
etiology of, 1887–1888
evaluation and, 1917
incidence of, 1888
pathophysiology of, 1884–1887
cardiac alterations and, 1886–1887

Chronic renal failure (CRF) (*Continued*)
metabolic alterations and, 1885–1886
pathologic alterations and, 1885
stages and, 1884–1885
planning and implementation and, 1897–1916
altered nutrition and, 1914–1915, 1915b
anxiety and, 1915–1916
fluid volume excess and, 1897–1914
prevention of, 1888
progression toward, 1885b
urologic disorders causing, 1865b
Chronic sinusitis, 1954
Chvostek's sign, 1566, 1580
alkalemia and, 354
hypocalcemia and, 297, 299, 301
Chyme, 1222
Chymotrypsinogen, 1224
Cibalith-S (lithium citrate), for cluster headache,
875
Ciclopirox olamine (Loprox), for skin disorders,
1179t
Cigarette smoking, atherosclerosis and, 2189
cancer and, 560–561, 561t
cardiovascular system assessment and, 2088
chronic obstructive pulmonary disease and,
1992
coronary artery disease and, 2150
hypertension and, 2198
infection and, 617
Cilia, 995
Ciliary body, 994
Ciliary flush, 1053
Cimetidine (Tagamet), for anaphylaxis, 657t
for gastroesophageal reflux disease, 1275,
1276t
for peptic ulcer disease, 1314, 1315t
CIN. *See* Cervical intraepithelial neoplasia (CIN).
Cinobac pulvules (cinoxacin), for cystitis, 1837t
Cinoxacin (Cinobac pulvules), for cystitis, 1837t
Circle of Willis, 844, 845t, 879
Circulating nurse, 454–455
Circulation, cardiac, 2069, 2070, *2071*
cerebral, 843–844, *844*, 845t
determination of, 861–862
coronary, 2070, 2072, *2072*
age-related changes in, 2086b
impaired, casts and, 793
Circulatory overload. *See* Hypervolemia.
**Circumcision: surgical removal of the prepuce, or
foreskin, of the penis, *1635*, 1636, 1768**
penile carcinoma and, 1767
problems related to, 1768
Circumferential traction, 794
Circumflex coronary artery (CCA), 2070, 2072,
2072
Circumvaginal muscle (CVM) exercise,
effectiveness of, 1848b
urinary incontinence and, 1847
**Cirrhosis: a degenerative liver disease often
caused by alcoholism, 1479–1497**
alcohol-induced, 1480
analysis: nursing diagnosis and, 1486–1487
assessment and, 1484–1486
diagnostic tests and, 1486
history in, 1484
laboratory findings in, 1485–1486, 1486b
physical, *1481*, *1484*, 1484–1485, *1485*
psychosocial, 1485
radiographic findings in, 1486
biliary, 1480
etiology of, 1483
cardiac, 1480
etiology of, 1483
discharge planning and, 1496–1497
client/family education and, 1496
health care resources and, 1496–1497
home care preparation and, 1496
psychosocial preparation and, 1496
etiology of, 1483
evaluation and, 1497
incidence of, 1483
Laënnec's, 1480

Cirrhosis (*Continued*)
etiology of, 1483
macronodular, 1480
micronodular, 1480
mixed, 1480
nutritional, 1480
pathophysiology of, 1480–1483
classification and, 1480
complications and, 1480–1483, *1481*
types and, 1480
planning and implementation and, 1487–1496
fluid volume excess and, 1487–1490
potential for altered thought processes and,
1495–1496
potential for injury and, 1490–1494
portal, 1480
postnecrotic, 1480
etiology of, 1483
prevention of, 1483–1484
vascular, 1480
Cisterns, 846
CK. *See* Creatine kinase (CK).
**Claudication: an aching sensation in the legs
when performing activity such as walking
(intermittent claudication), 2205–2206**
Clavicle, fractures of, 803. *See also* Fracture(s).
CLE. *See* Centrilobular emphysema (CLE).
Client, 13
as data source, 24–25
elderly. *See* Elderly.
perception of problem, 10
Client advocate, nurse as, *18*, 18–19
**Client care plan: a display of specific
interventions to resolve the health problems
identified through assessment and analysis,
29**
client recovering from gastric surgery and,
1324b–1326b
client recovering from retroperitoneal lymph
node dissection and, 1763b
client recovering from thyroidectomy and,
1567b–1568b
client undergoing breast reconstruction and,
1684b
client undergoing cholecystectomy and,
1451b–1453b
client undergoing excision of oral cavity tumor and, 1261b–1263b
client undergoing mastectomy and, 1676b–
1679b
client undergoing orchiectomy and, 1761b
client undergoing surgery of esophagus and,
1278b–1280b
client undergoing total abdominal hysterectomy and, 1712b–1713b
client with acute myelogenous leukemia and,
2264b–2266b
client with acute pancreatitis and, 1466b–
1467b
client with AIDS and, 638b–640b
client with alteration in sexuality and, 189b
client with anorexia nervosa and, 1423b–
1428b
client with cataract and, 1040b–1042b
client with chronic obstructive pulmonary disease and, 1997b–1999b
client with fractures and, 806b–807b
client with hypovolemic shock and, 416b–
417b
client with migraine headache and, 867b–868b
client with osteoporosis and, 741b–742b
client with pain and, 124b–127b
client with partial-thickness and full-thickness
chemical burns and, 382b–384b
client with psoriasis and, 1189b–1194b
client with sensory deficit and, 152b
computer programs for, 30
Client educator, nurse as, 18
Client/family education. *See under specific
conditions.*
**Climacteric: the phase of a woman's life from
menopause to cessation of symptoms caused**

INDEX / GLOSSARY

INDEX / GLOSSARY

INDEX / GLOSSARY

INDEX / GLOSSARY

INDEX / GLOSSARY

INDEX / GLOSSARY

INDEX / GLOSSARY

Hemophilia (*Continued*)
management of, 2276–2277
Hemophilia A (classic), 2276–2277
Hemophilia B (Christmas disease), 2276–2277
Hemoptysis: bloody sputum, 1938, 2095
achalasia and, 1287
oral cavity carcinoma and, 1257
Hemorrhage, control of, in ectopic pregnancy,
1736
from reproductive tract, 1642
gastrointestinal, causes of, *1311, 1339*
head injury and, 925, *926*
increased risk for, cancer and, 570
into anterior chamber of eye, 1044, 1064–1065
of esophageal varices, cirrhosis and, 1481–
1482
postmenopausal. *See* Postmenopausal bleeding.
retinal, acquired immunodeficiency syndrome
and, 1073
subconjunctival, 1026–1027
management of, 1026–1027
ulcers and, 1310, 1312
management of, 1317, *1317,* 1319–1320,
1320
uterine. *See* Dysfunctional uterine bleeding
(DUB).
vitreous, 1052
Hemorrhagic stroke, 880, *880,* 883b
Hemorrhoid(s), *1403,* 1403–1404
external, 1403
internal, 1403
management of, 1403–1404
Hemorrhoidectomy, 1404
Hemostasis, 2239, 2240t–2243t, 2244, *2244*
Hemothorax: blood loss into the thoracic cavity
as a result of chest trauma, 2056
Hemovac drainage system, 478, *480,* 483, 1260,
1968, *1969*
Henderson-Hasselbalch equation, 328–329
Henderson's definition, of nursing, 16t
Henle, loop of, 1801
Heparin sodium (Lipo-Hepin), perioperative
effects of, 431t
Heparin therapy. *See also* Anticoagulants.
cerebrovascular accident and, 887
fractures and, 797
peritoneal dialysis and, 1909
pulmonary embolism and, 2026
thrombotic stroke and, 887
total hip replacement and, 685
venous disease and, 2216, 2217
Hepatic. *See also* Liver *entries.*
Hepatic coma, 1482
four stages of, manifestations of, 1483b
Hepatic encephalopathy, 1233, 1482
four stages of, manifestations of, 1483b
Hepatitis: inflammation of the liver, 1497
analysis: nursing diagnosis and, 1503
assessment and, 1501–1503
diagnostic tests and, 1503
history in, 1501–1502
laboratory findings in, 1502–1503
physical, 1502
psychosocial, 1502
chronic, 1497
chronic active, 1497
chronic lobar, 1497
chronic persistent, 1497
discharge planning and, 1504–1505
client/family education and, 1504
health care resources and, 1504–1505
home care preparation and, 1504
psychosocial preparation and, 1504
etiology of, 1500
evaluation and, 1505
fulminant, 1497
incidence of, 1500
management of, 1501–1505
pathophysiology of, 1497–1500
classification and, 1498–1500
pathologic changes and, 1497
sequelae and, 1497

Hepatitis (*Continued*)
planning and implementation and, 1503–1504
prevention of, 1500–1501
toxic and drug-induced, 1497, 1500, 1502
idiosyncratic, 1500
type A, 1498–1499, 1500–1501
differential features of, 1498b–1499b
type B, 1499, 1500, 1501
differential features of, 1498b–1499b
type C, 1499, 1500, 1501
differential features of, 1498b–1499b
type D, 1499–1500, 1501
differential features of, 1498b–1499b
urticaria and, 663
viral, 1497. *See also specific types.*
differential features of, 1498–1501, 1498b–
1499b
management of, 1501–1505
Hepatocellular jaundice, 1482
Hepatocytes, 1224
Hepatoma, 1506
Hepatomegaly: enlarged liver, 1484
cirrhosis and, 1484
gastric carcinoma and, 1331
lupus erythematosus and, 702
tissue transplant reactions and, 668
Hepatorenal syndrome, 1482–1483
Hernia(s): a weakness in the abdominal wall
through which a segment of the bowel or
other abdominal structure protrudes, 1368–
1371
analysis: nursing diagnosis and, 1370
assessment and, 1369–1370
history in, 1369
physical, 1369–1370
psychosocial, 1370
discharge planning and, 1371
client/family education and, 1371
health care resources and, 1371
home care preparation and, 1371
psychosocial preparation and, 1371
etiology of, 1369
evaluation and, 1371
femoral, 1368
hiatal. *See* Hiatal hernia.
incarcerated, 1369
incidence of, 1369
incisional, 1369
inguinal, direct, 1368
examination for, 1647
indirect, 1368
irreducible, 1369
pathophysiology of, 1368–1369, *1369*
planning and implementation and, 1370–1371
prevention of, 1369
reducible, 1369
strangulated, 1369
umbilical, 1369
ventral, 1369
Herniation, diverticula and, 1371. *See also*
Diverticulum(a).
head injury and, 925–926, *927*
of nucleus pulposus, 813–814, *814*
Hernioplasty: a surgical procedure in which the
weakened muscular wall of the abdomen is
reinforced with mesh, fascia, or wire to
prevent recurrence of a hernia, 1370–1371
Herniorrhaphy: a surgical procedure in which the
contents of a hernia are replaced into the
abdominal cavity and sutured into place,
1370–1371
Heroin (diacetylmorphine), for chronic pain,
136t
Herpes simplex virus (HSV): causes infections
responsible for cold sores (Type I) and
genital herpes (Type II), 1173, color plate 48
clinical manifestations of, 1175b
genital, 1777, 1779–1781
management of, 1780b, 1780–1781
skin infections and, 1173
stomatitis and, 1247–1248, *1247*
Herpes zoster virus: causes shingles; an infection
caused by reactivation of the latent varicella-

Herpes zoster virus (*Continued*)
zoster virus in individuals who previously
had chickenpox, 1173, color plate 49
clinical manifestations of, 1176b
Herpetic whitlow, 1173
Herplex (idoxuridine), for ophthalmic disorders,
1017t
Hertz unit of frequency, 1084
Hesitancy, 1810
Heterograft: application of skin from another
species (usually pigskin) to promote healing
of a burn, 389, 1165
Hex-Fix external fixation system, 797
HHNKS. *See* Hyperglycemic hyperosmolar
nonketotic syndrome (HHNKS).
Hiatal hernia: the displacement of the lower
esophagus and possibly the upper portion of
the stomach above the diaphragm, 1281–
1285
analysis: nursing diagnosis and, 1283
assessment and, 1282–1285
diagnostic tests and, 1283
history in, 1282
laboratory findings in, 1282
physical, 1282
psychosocial, 1282
radiographic findings in, 1283
discharge planning and, 1284–1285
client/family education and, 1285
health care resources and, 1285
home care preparation and, 1284–1285
psychosocial preparation and, 1285
etiology of, 1282
evaluation and, 1285
gastroesophageal reflux disease and, 1273
incidence of, 1282
paraesophageal, 1281
pathophysiology of, *1281,* 1281–1282
planning and implementation and, 1283–1284
prevention of, 1282
rolling, 1281
sliding, 1281
Hiccups (singultus), intestinal obstruction and,
1396
Hierarchy of needs, 28, *29*
self-concept and, 158
High-density lipoproteins (HDL), 2099, 2100t
atherosclerosis and, 2188
High-dose dexamethasone suppression test,
hypercortisolism and, 1551–1552
High-energy phosphate (P), 234
High-flow oxygen systems, 2007, 2008t, *2009*
High-level wellness: a dynamic attempt by an
individual to reach his or her highest
potential within the environment in which he
or she is functioning, 6
Hill-Burton Act, 36
Hill's repair, 1277, 1283
Hilum, of kidney, 1799
of lungs, 1935
Hinge joints, 720
Hip, fractures of, 803–805, *804, 805. See also*
Fracture(s).
fixation devices for, 804t
Hip replacement, degenerative joint disease
and, 681–682, *682–686,* 683t, 684–686
Hiprex (methenamine hippurate), for cystitis,
1837t
Hirsutism: excessive hairiness, especially in
women, 1148
His, bundle of, 2075
Hispanics, AIDS in, 633
diabetes mellitus in, 1593
tuberculosis in, 2042
Histamine, 612, 651, 832t
Histamine antagonists. *See* Histamine receptor-
blocking drugs.
Histamine receptor-blocking drugs, for acute
pancreatitis, 1468
for peptic ulcer disease, 1314, 1315t–1316t
gastritis and, 1305
ulcers and, 1314
History. *See under specific conditions.*

INDEX / GLOSSARY

Hypertonic dehydration *(Continued)*
  etiology of, 253
  pathophysiology of, 252, *252*
Hypertonic fluids, 232
Hypertonic overhydration. *See* Overhydration.
Hypertrophic cardiomyopathy (HCM), 2182
  features of, 2183b
  management of, 2182, 2184
Hypertrophic ungual labium, treatment of, 773b
Hyperuricemia, as oncologic emergency, 596
  burns and, 379
  chemotherapy and, 583
  gout and, 706
Hyperventilation, electroencephalography and,
    860
  head injury and, 931
  isocapnic, 2032–2033
Hyperviscosity syndrome, 669
Hypervitaminosis D, 303
**Hypervolemia: excessive fluid in the vascular
    compartment of the body, 261**
  hypotonic overhydration and, 262, *262*
  isotonic overhydration and, 261, *261*
Hyphema, 1044, 1064–1065
  management of, 1065
Hypnosis, burns and, 387
  chronic pain and, 138–139
Hypnotics, preoperative, 451t
Hypoactive reflex, 854–855
Hypoanesthesia, 457
**Hypocalcemia: inadequate amount of calcium in
    the blood, 294–301**
  analysis: nursing diagnosis and, 298–299
  anorexia nervosa and, 1419
  assessment and, 296–298
    history in, 296–297
    laboratory findings in, 298
    physical, 297b, 297–298
    psychosocial, 298
    radiographic findings in, 298
  cardiac manifestations of, 2101
  causes of, 295b
  discharge planning and, 301
  etiology of, 294–296
    conditions decreasing ionized fraction of
        calcium and, 295
    conditions inhibiting calcium absorption
        and, 294–295
    endocrine disturbances decreasing serum
        calcium levels and, 295
    miscellaneous conditions decreasing serum
        calcium levels and, 295–296
  evaluation of, 301
  hypophosphatemia and, 310
  incidence of, 296
  pathophysiology of, 294
  planning and implementation and, 299–301
  prevention of, 296
Hypochloremia, 284
**Hypochromic cells: red blood cells with a
    deficiency of hemoglobin, 2247**
Hypogammaglobulinemia, acquired, 647
Hypoglossal nerve, 839t
  assessment of, 852
**Hypoglycemia: inadequate blood glucose, 1593,
    1596**
  brain activity and, 860
  diabetes mellitus and, 1588–1589, 1594
  emergency care and, 1596–1597
  features of, 1596b
  reactive, 1588–1589
  risk of, drugs increasing, 1608t
Hypoglycemic agents, insulin preparations as,
    1608–1614, 1609t–1610t
  oral, diabetes mellitus and, 1607t, 1608, 1608t
**Hypokalemia: deficit of potassium in the blood,
    268–274**
  analysis: nursing diagnosis and, 271–272
  assessment and, 270–271
    history in, 270
    laboratory findings in, 271
    physical, 270b, 270–271
    psychosocial, 271

Hypokalemia *(Continued)*
  causes of, 269b
  discharge planning and, 273
  early recognition of, 273
  etiology of, 269
  evaluation and, 273–274
  hypotonic dehydration and, 252
  incidence of, 269
  pathophysiology of, 268–269
  planning and implementation and, 272–273
    constipation and, 273
    knowledge deficit and, 273
    potential for injury and, 272
  prevention of, 269, 273
Hypokinetic pulse, 2094
Hypomagnesemia, 312–313
  etiology of, 312
    conditions decreasing intestinal magnesium
        absorption and, 312
    conditions increasing renal magnesium ex-
        cretion and, 313
  hypoparathyroidism and, 1580
  interventions in, 313
  physical assessment of, 313
**Hyponatremia: deficit of sodium in the blood,
    279–287**
  analysis: nursing diagnosis and, 284–285
  assessment and, 281–284
    history in, 281–282
    laboratory findings in, 284
    physical, 282b, 282–284
    psychosocial, 284
  causes of, 280b
  discharge planning and, 287
  etiology of, 280
  evaluation and, 287
  hypotonic dehydration and, 252
  incidence of, 280–281
  pathophysiology of, 279–280
  planning and implementation and, 285–286
    pain (headache) and, 286–287
  prevention of, 281
**Hypoparathyroidism: a condition resulting from
    an inadequate secretion of parathormone,
    1580–1582**
  hyperphosphatemia and, 312
  hypomagnesemia and, 313
  iatrogenic, 1580
  idiopathic, 1580
  laboratory findings in, 1580, 1582, 1582b
  management of, *1579*, 1580, 1582
Hypopharynx, tumors of, TNM classification of,
    1256b
Hypophosphatemia, 309–311
  anorexia nervosa and, 1419
  etiology of, 309–310
    conditions decreasing intestinal phosphorus
        absorption and, 309–310
    conditions increasing phosphorus excretion
        and, 310
    conditions shifting extracellular fluid phos-
        phorus to intracellular space and, 310
  interventions in, 311
  physical assessment of, 310–311
**Hypophysectomy: surgical resection of the
    pituitary gland, *1537*, 1537–1538, 1553**
Hypophysis, 838
Hypopigmentation, postinflammatory, color
    plate 22
**Hypopituitarism: a condition in which there is a
    deficiency of one or more of the anterior
    pituitary hormones, 1529**
  analysis: nursing diagnosis and, 1531
  assessment and, 1529–1531
    diagnostic tests and, 1531
    history in, 1530
    laboratory findings in, 1530–1531
    physical, 1530
    psychosocial, 1530
    radiographic findings in, 1531
  discharge planning and, 1532–1533
    client/family education and, 1532–1533
    health care resources and, 1533

Hypopituitarism *(Continued)*
    home care preparation and, 1532
    psychosocial preparation and, 1533
  etiology of, 1529
  evaluation and, 1533
  idiopathic, 1529
  incidence of, 1529
  pathophysiology of, 1529
  planning and implementation and, 1531–1532
  prevention of, 1529
  primary, 1529
  secondary, 1529
Hyposensitization therapy, atopic reactions and,
    659, 661
Hyposmotic fluids, 232
Hyposthenuria, 1885
Hypotension: very low blood pressure, 255
  dehydration and, 255
  postural (orthostatic), 255
  shock and, 412
  spinal anesthesia and, 464–465
Hypothalamic-pituitary cycle, 1631, 1632, *1632*
Hypothalamic-pituitary-ovarian-uterine axis,
    1631
Hypothalamus, 838, 1513, 1514
  antidiuretic hormone and, 238
  function of, 1516
  hormones of, 1516t
  structure of, 1514
Hypothermia, anorexia nervosa and, 1419
**Hypothyroidism: a condition resulting from
    inadequate secretion of thyroid hormones,
    1569–1574**
  analysis: nursing diagnosis and, 1572–1573
  assessment and, 1572
    history in, 1572
    laboratory findings in, 1572, 1573b
    physical, 1572
    psychosocial, 1572
  congenital (cretinism), 1571, *1571*
  discharge planning and, 1574
    client/family education and, 1574
    health care resources and, 1574
    home care preparation and, 1574
    psychosocial preparation and, 1574
  etiology of, 1569, 1571, *1571*
  evaluation and, 1574
  incidence of, 1571
  myxedema coma and, emergency care and,
    1571, 1572
  pathophysiology of, 1569
  planning and implementation and, 1573–1574
  prevention of, 1571
  primary, 1571
  secondary, 1571
  signs and symptoms of, 1570b
  tertiary, 1571
Hypotonic dehydration. *See also* Dehydration.
  causes of, 253b
  etiology of, 253
  pathophysiology of, 252
**Hypotonic fluid: fluid that has a lower osmolarity
    than body fluid, 232**
  gastroenteritis and, 1342
Hypotonic overhydration. *See also*
    Overhydration.
  pathophysiology of, 262, *262*
Hypotony, 1051
Hypoventilation, oxygen-induced, oxygen
    therapy and, 2003
**Hypovolemic shock: shock that occurs due to
    inadequate amount of circulating blood
    volume, 252, 405, 407. *See also under*
    Shock.**
  client care plan for, 416b–417b
  clinical manifestations of, 406b
  craniotomy and, 954
  emergency care for, 410b
  head injury and, 928
  interventions for problems in, 415b
Hypoxemia, 2003
  asthma and, 664
  overhydration and, 267

INDEX / GLOSSARY

INDEX / GLOSSARY

Laryngoscopy, burns and, 386
  client care and, 1948b
Larynx, 1933, *1933*
  age-related changes in, 1936b
  assessment of, 1939
LAS. *See* Localized adaptation syndrome (LAS).
Laser photocoagulation: a surgical procedure in
  which thermal energy is used to obliterate
  small blood vessels and seal capillary
  leakage; treatment for diabetic retinopathy,
  1592
  diabetic retinopathy and, 1054
  pleural effusions and, 593
  ulcers and, 1320
Laser therapy, breast cancer and, 1674
  cervical cancer and, 1724
  endometriosis and, 1695
  lung cancer and, 2050–2051
  oral cavity tumors and, 1259
  peripheral vascular disease and, 2210
Laser trabeculoplasty, 1050
Lasix (furosemide), for heart failure, 2168
  for hypertension, 2202t
  for renal failure, 1900t
Late adulthood, 68–81. *See also* Elderly.
  body image in, 160–161
  economic issues in, 80–81
  health issue in, 75–80
  mortality in, causes of, 76, 76b
  physiologic changes in, 68–72
  positive health habits in, 76
  psychosocial development in, 72–75
Lateral corticospinal tract, 836
Lateralization, tuning fork tests and, 1084
Latex agglutination test, for rheumatoid
  arthritis, 695, 696t
Lavage: irrigation or washing out, e.g., gastric
  lavage, 1319, *1320*
  abdominal trauma and, 1401
  ulcers and, 1319
  variceal hemorrhage and, 1490
Laxatives, bulk-forming, for irritable bowel
  syndrome, 1367
  for bowel dysfunction, 514t–515t
  for renal failure, 1899t
  hypermagnesemia and, 313
  hypokalemia and, 273
LBB. *See* Left bundle branch (LBB).
LBP. *See* Low back pain (LBP).
LCA. *See* Left coronary artery (LCA).
LDH. *See* Lactate dehydrogenase (LDH).
LDL. *See* Low-density lipoproteins (LDL).
Left anterior descending (LAD) artery, 2070,
  2072, *2072*
Left bundle branch (LBB), 2075
Left coronary artery (LCA), 2070, *2072*
Left shift, 534
Left ventricular end-diastolic pressure (LVEDP),
  2109
Leg cast, 791, 792t
Leg exercises, postoperative, 445, 447b
Legal blindness, 1002, 1010
Legionella pneumophila pneumonia, features of,
  1980b
Legislation, burn prevention and, 370
Leiomyomas: common benign, slow growing
  tumors, 1709
  esophageal, 1288
  evaluation and, 1714
  uterine, 1709–1714
    analysis: nursing diagnosis and, 1710
    assessment and, 1710
    cervical fibroids and, 1709, *1709*
    discharge planning and, 1711–1714
    etiology of, 1709
    incidence of, 1709
    intraligamentous fibroid and, 1709, *1709*
    intramural, 1709, *1709*
    parasitic fibroids and, 1709, *1709*
    pathophysiology of, 1709, *1709*
    planning and implementation and, 1710–
      1711
    submucosal, 1709, *1709*

Leisure, in late adulthood, 75
  in middle adulthood, 68
  in young adulthood, 64
Lens, 994–995
  pathophysiology of, 1037. *See also* Cataract.
Lens implants, intraocular, 1044
Leprosy (Hansen's disease), 1211
Leukemia: a group of malignant disorders
  involving abnormal overproduction of a
  specific cell type, usually at an immature
  age, in the bone marrow, 559, 560, 2260–
  2271
  acute, clinical manifestations of, 2263b
  acute lymphocytic, 2261
  acute myelogenous, 2261
    analysis: nursing diagnosis and, 2263, 2266
    client care plan and, 2264b–2266b
    planning and implementation and, 2269–
      2270
  analysis: nursing diagnosis and, 2263, 2266
  assessment and, 2262–2263
    history in, 2262
    laboratory findings in, 2263
    physical, 2262–2263
    psychosocial, 2263
    radiographic findings in, 2263
  chronic lymphocytic, 2261
  chronic myelogenous, 2261
  differential features of, 2261b
  discharge planning and, 2270
    client/family education and, 2270
    health care resources and, 2270
    home care preparation and, 2270
    psychosocial preparation and, 2270
  etiology of, 2260–2261
  evaluation and, 2270–2271
  incidence of, 2261–2262
  lymphoblastic, 2260
  lymphocytic, 2260
  myelocytic, 2260
  myelogenous, 2260
  pathophysiology of, 2260
  planning and implementation and, 2266–2270
    fatigue and, 2269–2270
    potential for infection and, 2266–2269
    potential for injury and, 2269
  prevention of, 262
Leukocyte(s), 529, 2238. *See also* White blood
  cell(s); *named cells.*
  immune functions of, 531t
Leukocyte alkaline phosphatase (LAP), 2248
Leukocyte count, 2101
  differential, cancer and, 572
Leukopenia, burns and, 379
  Felty's syndrome and, 694
Leukoplakia: white patches or spots on the oral
  mucous membrane, 1254
  management of, 1257–1264
  vulvar, 1701
Leukotaxins, 536
Levallorphan tartrate (Lorfan), for narcotic
  overdose, 484t
Levarterenol. *See* Norepinephrine (Levophed).
LeVeen (peritoneovenous) shunt, for treatment
  of ascites, 1489, *1489*
Level of consciousness. *See also* Coma.
  mental status assessment and, 849
Level of Rehabilitation Scale (LORS), 501
Levin tube: a single lumen nasogastric tube that
  can be used for gastric decompression or
  feeding, 477, *1317*
Levo-Dromoran (levorphanol), for chronic pain,
  136t
Levophed (norepinephrine), 832t, 1519
  for anaphylaxis, 657t
  for cardiac arrest, 2145t
  for shock, 419t
  impulse transmission and, 829
Levorphanol (Levo-Dromoran), for chronic pain,
  136t
Leydig's cells, 1636
LGV. *See* Lymphogranuloma venereum (LGV).
LH. *See* Luteinizing hormone (LH).

Lice, body, 1209
  crab, 1209, 1701, 1792
  head, 1209
Licensed practical nurse (LPN), 15
  nursing homes and, 37–38
Licensure of nurses, 46, 46t
Lichen planus, 1210, 1248, color plates 37, 70
  management of, 1250–1254
  stomatitis and, 1248
Lichenification, 1141, 1155
  defined, 1145, *1145*
Lidocaine (Xylocaine), 461t
  for dysrhythmias, 2135t
  for shock, 419t
Life care facilities, 38. *See also* Continuing care
  facilities.
Life cycle, loss and, 197
  of body image, 158–161
Life style, health and, 8
Life support systems, dying and, 198
Ligament(s), 720
  broad, uterine, 1629, 1630
  cardinal, 1630
  Cooper's, 1634
  knee, injuries to, 820
  round, 1630
  uterosacral, 1630
Ligation, tubal. *See* Tubal ligation.
Ligation and stripping: surgical tying and removal
  of varicose veins, 2227
Light perception testing, 1002
Limb-girdle muscular dystrophy, 776b
Limbic lobe, 842–843
Limbic system, 838
Lincomycin, for infection, 622t
Linton tube, *1492*
Lioresal (baclofen), for bladder dysfunction, 518t
Lip(s), tumors of, TNM classification of, 1255b
Lip reading, 1099
Lipase, 1224
  serum, 1233, 1235t
Lipectomy, 1402
Lipids. *See also* Fat(s).
  serum levels of, 2099, 2100t
Lipo-Hepin (heparin sodium). *See also* Heparin
  therapy.
  perioperative effects of, 431t
Lipolytic process, 1462
Lipoproteins, high-density. *See* High-density
  lipoproteins (HDL).
  low-density. *See* Low-density lipoproteins
  (LDL).
Liquids, thermal burns and, 368
Lithium, hypercalcemia and, 303
Lithium carbonate, for hyperthyroidism, 1565t
Lithium citrate (Cibalith-S), for cluster
  headache, 875
Lithotripsy: the crushing of calculi in the
  gallbladder or urinary system via a machine
  that emits shock waves, 1458
  extracorporeal shock wave, 1458, *1459*
  urolithiasis and, 1860, 1861
Liver, 1224–1225, 2239. *See also headings*
  beginning with terms Hepatic *and* Hepato-.
  and digestive changes related to aging, 1227b
  enlargement of. *See* Hepatomegaly.
  fatty, 1505
  function of, 1224–1225
  inflammation of. *See* Hepatitis.
  structure of, 1224, *1224*
  trauma to, 1505–1506
Liver abscesses, 1505
Liver cancer, 1506
Liver disease, 1479–1507. *See also specific*
  disorders.
  abnormal laboratory findings in, significance
  of, 1486b
  hypomagnesemia and, 312
  research implications and, 1507
  sexuality and, 182
Liver flap (asterixis), 1232–1233, 1485, *1485*
Liver scan, 1233
Liver spots (actinic lentigo), color plate 10

Myasthenia gravis (MG) *(Continued)*
  psychosocial, 970
  autoimmunity and, 671b
  etiology of, 969
  factors precipitating or worsening, 971b
  impaired mobility and, 492b
  incidence of, 969
  Osserman's staging of, 970b
  pathophysiology of, 969
  planning and implementation and, 972–979
    altered nutrition and, 978–979
    body image disturbance, self-esteem distur-
      bance, and anticipatory grieving and,
      979
    impaired physical mobility and activity in-
      tolerance and, 973–977
    impaired verbal communication and, 978
    perceptual alterations and, 978
    potential for injury and, 978
    respiratory dysfunction and, 972–973
    self-care deficit and, 977–978
Myasthenic crisis, 971
  characteristics of, 976b
Mycelex (clotrimazole), for skin disorders, 1179t
Myciguent (neomycin sulfate), for burns, 394t
  for skin disorders, 1178t
Mycobacterium avium-intracellulare infection, 635
Mycobacterium leprae infection. *See* Leprosy
  (Hansen's disease).
Mycobacterium tuberculosis infection. *See*
  Tuberculosis.
Mycolog (nystatin), for skin disorders, 1179t
Mycoplasma pneumoniae pneumonia, features of,
  1979b
Mycoplasmas, 610
Mycoses. *See* Fungal infections.
Mycostatin (nystatin), for skin disorders, 1179t
Mydriacyl (tropicamide), for ophthalmic
  disorders, 1022t
Mydriatics, for ophthalmic disorders, 1021t–
  1022t
Myelinization, 828
Myelocytic leukemia, 2260. *See also* Leukemia.
Myelogenous leukemia, 2260. *See also* Leukemia.
Myelography: radiographic visualization of the
  vertebral column after instillation of a
  contrast medium, 726–727, 857
  client care and, 728b
Myeloma, multiple, 560, 669–670
Myenteric plexus, 1219
Myidone (primidone), for epilepsy, 894t
Mylanta (magnesium hydroxide with aluminum
  hydroxide), for peptic ulcer disease, 1315t,
  1316
Myocardial contractility, agents enhancing,
  shock and, 418
Myocardial hypertrophy, 2164. *See also* Heart
  failure.
Myocardial infarction (MI): a life-threatening
  condition characterized by the permanent
  formation of necrosis in the myocardium due
  to lack of oxygen, 2149, 2150–2153, 2156,
  2161–2162. *See also entries under* **Coronary**
  artery disease (CAD).
  transmural, 2150
Myocardial perfusion, agents enhancing, shock
  and, 418
Myocardial working cells, 2072–2073
Myocardium, 2069
Myochrysine (gold sodium thiomalate), for
  connective tissue disease, 679t
Myogenic ptosis, 1013
Myoglobin, burns and, 385
Myomas. *See* Leiomyomas, uterine.
Myomectomy: local surgical removal of myomas
  with preservation of the uterus, 1710–1711
Myometrium, 1630
Myopia: a type of refractive error in which the
  refracting power of the eye is too strong for
  its length and the image converges in front of
  the retina;, also known as nearsightedness,
  996, 996–997, 1060
Myotomy, 1287

Myotonia, 175
Myotonic muscular dystrophy, 776b
Myringoplasty: simple reconstruction of the
  tympanic membrane, 1113, 1121
Myringotomy: a surgically performed perforation
  of the pars tensa of the tympanic membrane,
  1111–1112, *1112*
Myxedema: advanced hypothyroidism causing an
  increase in interstitial fluid, 1569, *1571*
Myxedema coma, 1571
  emergency care and, 1571, 1572b

Nadir, 586, 2269
Nadolol (Corgard), for hypertension, 2203t
Nafcillin, for infection, 621t
Nails, 1135, *1135*
  and changes related to aging, 1139b, color
    plates 13, 15
  assessment of, 1148–1149, 1149t, 1150t
  disorders of, 1211–1212
    endocrine problems associated with, 1523
  fungal infection of, color plate 15
  pigmentation of, color plates 19, 20
  thickening of, 1212
Nalidixic acid (NegGram), for cystitis, 1837t
Nalline (nalorphine), for narcotic overdose, 484t
Nalorphine (Nalline), for narcotic overdose, 484t
Naloxone (Narcan), for narcotic overdose, 484t
NANDA. *See* North American Nursing
  Diagnosis Association (NANDA).
NAON. *See* National Association of Orthopaedic
  Nurses (NAON).
Naproxen sodium (Anaprox), for
  dysmenorrhea, 1690t
  for migraine headache, 872t
Narcan (naloxone), for narcotic overdose, 484t
Narcotic agonists, 135, 137t
Narcotic analgesics, adverse effects of, 136–137
  chronic pain and, 128t, 135–137, 136t, 137t
  general anesthesia and, 462
  pain and, 128, 128t–129t, 129–130
  postoperative pain and, 484
Narcotic antagonists, 130, 135, 137t
Narcotic overdose, drug treatment of, 484t
Narcotic potentiators, chronic pain and, 137
Narcotics, preoperative, 451t
Nardil (phenelzine), for migraine headache,
  870t–871t
Nares, anterior, 1931
  posterior, 1931
Nasal. *See also* Nose.
Nasal cannula: a small tube with two nasal
  prongs used for administration of oxygen,
  2004, 2005t, 2006, *2006*
Nasal flaring, 1938
Nasal polyps, 1938, 1956
Nasal septum, 1931
  deviated, 1954–1955
  perforated, 1938
Nasal turbinates, 1931
  hypertrophy of, 1956
Nasogastric suctioning, cholecystitis and, 1450
  diverticulitis and, 1375
  hypomagnesemia and, 312
  isotonic dehydration and, 252
Nasogastric tube, client care and, 1318b–1319b
  insertion of, 1317, *1317*, 1318b–1319b, 1490
  postoperative use of, 477
  preoperative use of, 441, 443
  testing placement of, 1319b
Nasogastric tube feeding, esophageal surgery
  and, 1293, 1296, 1300
  head injury and, *934*, 935b, 935–936
  laryngectomy and, 1968
  oral cavity tumors and, surgery for, 1264
  pancreatic carcinoma and, altered nutrition
    and, 1478
  wound healing and, 1167
Nasointestinal tube, care of, 1398b
  intestinal obstruction and, 1397
  testing placement of, 1319b

Nasopharynx, 1932
  tumors of, TNM classification of, 1256b
Nasoseptoplasty: surgical procedure performed to
  correct a deviated nasal septum, 1954–1955
National Association of Orthopaedic Nurses
  (NAON), 20
National Conference for the Classification of
  Nursing Diagnoses, First, 26
National Council on Radiation Protection
  (NCRP), 580
National Health Planning and Resource
  Development Act of 1974, 36
National Institute for Mental Health, 82
National Institute on Aging, 82
National League for Nursing (NLN), 20, 39, 46
National Student Nurses' Association (NSNA),
  20
Native American(s), cholelithiasis in, 1457
  otitis media in, 1108
  rheumatoid arthritis in, 676
Natriuretic factor, 237, 238
Natural immunity, 605–606
Natural killer (NK) cells, 531t, 546, 548
  immune surveillance and, 554
Nausea, cancer therapy and, 565
  gastroenteritis and, 1341
  gastroesophageal reflux disease and, 1274
  intestinal obstruction and, 1395
  postoperative, 466
NCRP. *See* National Council on Radiation
  Protection (NCRP).
NCT. *See* Noncontact tonometer (NCT).
Near point, 998
Nearsightedness, *996*, 996–997, 1060
Near-syncope, 2091
Neck arteries, baroreceptors in, 2081
Neck trauma, 1973–1974
Neck veins, filling of, dehydration and, 255
Necrosis: tissue destruction, 1162
  avascular, 702, 785
  caseation, 2041
  of blood vessels, 1462
  pressure, casts and, 793
Necrotizing stomatitis, 1248, *1248*
Necrotizing vasculitis, 708–709
Needle aspiration biopsy, 572
  endocrine assessment and, 1526
  of breast, 1657, *1657*
  of prostate, 1657–1658
  peritonitis and, 1349
Negative nitrogen balance, 321
Negative protein balance, 321
Negative-pressure ventilator, 2023, *2025*
NegGram (nalidixic acid), for cystitis, 1837t
Neglect syndrome, stroke and, 883, 885
Neisseria gonorrhoeae, detection of, 1652
Nelson's syndrome, 1553
Nematodes, 1407
Nembutal sodium (pentobarbital sodium),
  preoperative, 451t
Neomycin sulfate (Myciguent), for burns, 394t
  for skin disorders, 1178t
Neoplasia: growth of new or abnormal cells; may
  be benign or malignant, 550. *See also* **Cancer**
  (Ca); Malignancy; Metastasis; *specific types*
  and sites.
  benign, 551, 551b, 552b
  classification of, 552b
  malignant, 551b, 552, 552b
  middle ear, 1121
  Paget's disease and, 750
Neostigmine (Prostigmin), for myasthenia
  gravis, 973, 974t
Neo-Synephrine (phenylephrine HCl), for
  ophthalmic disorders, 1021t–1022t
Neovascularization, 1592
Nephrectomy: surgical removal of a kidney,
  1830, 1842
  partial, renal trauma and, 1879
  radical, 1867
  renal trauma and, 1879
Nephritis, granulomatous, 1843
  lupus erythematosus and, 702

INDEX / GLOSSARY

INDEX / GLOSSARY

Propranolol (Inderal) *(Continued)*
  perioperative effects of, 430t
Proptosis, 999, 1026
Propylthiouracil (PTU), for hyperthyroidism, 1565t
Prosopagnosia, 919
Prospective payment system (PPS): a payment method provided to hospitals that participate in the federal Medicare program; pays a predetermined amount based on medical diagnoses, 36, 41
  surgery and, 428
Prostacyclin, 1805
Prostaglandin(s), 1639
  acid autodigestion and, 1303
  cancer-related pain and, 118
  kidney and, 1805
Prostaglandin analogues, ulcers and, 1317
Prostaglandin synthetase inhibitor drugs. *See also* Anti-inflammatory drugs; Nonsteroidal anti-inflammatory drugs (NSAIDs).
  for dysmenorrhea, 1690t
Prostate biopsy, 1657–1658, 1752, *1752*
Prostate cancer, *1750*, 1750–1754
  management of, 1751–1754, *1752*, *1753*
  TNM classification for, 1751
Prostate gland, 1637, 1638–1639
  examination of, 1647, *1647*
  needle biopsy of, 1657–1658
Prostatectomy: surgical removal of all or part of the prostate gland; several surgical approaches commonly used, 1752–1753
  client instructions and, 1749b
  extravesical, 1747
  perineal, 1747
  radical, 1752, *1753*
  retropubic, 1747
  suprapubic, 1747
  transvesical, 1747
Prostate-specific antigen, 1752
  as tumor marker, 572
Prostatic acid phosphatase, as tumor marker, 572
Prostatic hyperplasia, 1742. *See also* Benign prostatic hypertrophy (BPH).
Prostatic hypertrophy, 1742. *See also* Benign prostatic hypertrophy (BPH).
Prostatic sinuses, 1639
Prostatic urethra, 1638–1639, 1807
Prostatism, 1744
Prostatitis: inflammation of the prostate gland, 1769, 1833
  abacterial, 1769
  bacterial, 1769
Prostatodynia, 1769
Prostheses: artificial body parts, e.g., artificial limb, breast, 813. *See also* Implant(s).
  care of, 813b
  esophageal tumors and, 1291
  Moore's, *804*
  ocular, cleaning, 1072b
    insertion and removal of, 1070b–1071b
  penile, 1755–1756, *1756*
    home care and, 1757b
  tracheoesophageal, 1969–1970, *1970*
Prosthetic heart valves, 2176, *2176*
Prostigmin (neostigmine), for myasthenia gravis, 973, 974t
Proteases, 1990
Protein(s), acid-base balance and, 331
  in urine, 1816t, 1817
    in renal failure, laboratory values of, 1896b
  nutritional support and, 320–321
  restriction of, renal failure and, 1914–1915, 1915b
  wound healing and, 1167b
Protein electrophoresis, serum, 1233, 1234t
  rheumatoid arthritis and, 695, 696t
Protein-calorie malnutrition (PCM), 646
Proteoglycans, hydrophilic, 1569
Proteolysis, 1462
Proteolytic enzymes, 1162
Protest, grieving and, 200–201

Protestantism, grieving and, 207t
Prothrombin, 2240t
Prothrombin time (PT), 1233, 1234t, 2101, 2249
  normal values and abnormal findings in, 2249t
  perioperative assessment of, 436t
Proton(s), 327. *See also* Acid-base balance.
Proton acceptors, 328
Proto-oncogenes, 553
Protozoa, 610
Proventil (albuterol), for chronic obstructive pulmonary disease, 2001t
Proximal: nearest to a point of reference, 1801
Proximal convoluted tubule (PCT), 1801
Pruritus: itching, 1141, 1156
  therapeutic baths for, 1157t
PSE. *See* Portal-systemic encephalopathy (PSE).
Pseudocysts, pancreatic, 1463, 1479
Pseudodiabetic condition, burns and, 378
Pseudogout, 710
Pseudohypoparathyroidism, 1580, *1581*
Pseudomenopause, endometriosis and, 1695
Pseudomonas aeruginosa, pneumonia caused by, features of, 391, 1981b
Pseudoparkinsonism, 911
Pseudopregnancy, endometriosis and, 1695
Psoralen and UVA (PUVA), psoriasis and, 1195, *1195*
Psoriasis: a chronic, recurrent skin disease marked by discrete red macules, papules, or patches covered with silvery scales, 1186, 1186–1197, color plates 57–60
  analysis: nursing diagnosis and, 1188
  assessment and, 1187–1188
    history in, 1187
    laboratory findings in, 1188
    physical, 1187
    psychosocial, 1187
  discharge planning and, 1196–1197
    client/family education and, 1196–1197
    health care resources and, 1197
    home care preparation and, 1196
    psychosocial preparation and, 1197
  erythrodermic, 1187
  etiology of, 1186
  evaluation and, 1197
  exfoliative, 1187, color plate 59
  guttate, 1187, color plate 58
  incidence of, 1186
  pathophysiology of, 1186
  planning and implementation and, 1188–1196
    body image disturbance and, 1194b, 1196
    impaired skin integrity and, 1188, 1189b–1192b, 1194–1195
    ineffective individual coping and, 1193b, 1195–1196
    pain related to pruritus and, 1193b
  pustular, 1187, color plate 60
Psoriasis vulgaris, 1187, color plate 57
  client care plan for, 1189b–1194b
Psoriatic arthritis, 710
PSS. *See* Progressive systemic sclerosis (PSS).
Psychogenic pain: pain experienced by the client without any detectable physical cause, 113
Psychologic assessment, rehabilitation client and, 501–502
Psychologic component, of body image, 158
Psychologic factors, grieving and, 203, 205
Psychologic shock, body image disturbance and, 161
Psychologic state, 6
Psychologic testing, anorexia nervosa and, 1421–1422
  bulimia nervosa and, 1439
Psychologic theories of aging, 61
Psychologists, on interdisciplinary rehabilitation team, 497
Psychosexual development, 174–175
  in adolescence, 175
  in adulthood, 175
  in childhood, 174–175
Psychosexual morbidity, breast cancer and, 1669b

Psychosocial assessment. *See also under specific conditions.*
  of stress, 98
Psychosocial development, in late adulthood, 72–75
  in middle adulthood, 66–68
  in young adulthood, 62–64
Psychosocial influences, on pain, 113
Psychosocial preparation. *See under specific conditions.*
Psychosomatic disease, 95
Psychosomatic pain, 113
Psychotherapy, anorexia nervosa and, ineffective individual coping and, 1432
Psyllium hydrophilic mucilloid (Metamucil; Hydrocil), for bowel dysfunction, 514t
PT. *See* Physical therapy (PT); Prothrombin time (PT).
PTA. *See* Percutaneous transluminal angioplasty.
PTCA. *See* Percutaneous transluminal coronary angioplasty (PTCA).
PTH. *See* Parathyroid hormone (PTH).
Ptosis: drooping of the eyelid, 969, 999, 1013–1014
PTT. *See* Partial thromboplastin time (PTT).
PTU (propylthiouracil), for hyperthyroidism, 1565t
Public health, 35
Public Health Service Act, Title VI of, 36
  Title XVI of, 36
Public Law (PL), 37, 100–103
PUD. *See* Peptic ulcer disease (PUD).
Pulley exercise, postmastectomy, 1680b
Pulmonary. *See also entries under* Lung.
Pulmonary artery, age-related changes in, 1936b
Pulmonary artery catheterization, heart failure and, 2167
Pulmonary artery pressure (PAP), monitoring, 2109–2111, *2111*
Pulmonary artery wedge pressure (PAWP), monitoring, 2109–2111, *2111*
Pulmonary capillary wedge pressure: intravascular pressure as measured by a Swan-Ganz catheter introduced into the pulmonary artery, 2109–2111
Pulmonary care, head injury and, 934
Pulmonary circulation, 1935
Pulmonary congestion. *See* Pulmonary edema.
Pulmonary contusion, 2057
Pulmonary edema: an effusion of serous fluid into the pulmonary interstitial tissues and alveoli, 2164–2171. *See also entries under* Edema.
Pulmonary embolism (PE), 2059–2060
  differential features of, 784b
  management of, 2059–2060
Pulmonary emphyema, 2045–2046
Pulmonary fluid overload, burns and, 374–375
Pulmonary function tests: evaluations that determine the lungs' ability to maintain ventilation and the effects of ventilation and oxygenation on the cardiopulmonary system, 1949, 1950t
Pulmonary parenchymal failure, burns and, 374, *374*
Pulmonary sarcoidosis, 2040–2041
Pulmonary system, in late adulthood, 69b–70b
Pulmonary toxicity, of chemotherapy, 582
Pulmonary tuberculosis. *See* Tuberculosis (TB).
Pulmonic valves, 2070, *2070–2071*
Pulpectomy, 1244, 1246
Pulse(s), 2094, *2096*
  effect of, on perioperative experience, 432t
  hyperkinetic, 2094
  hypokinetic, 2094
  peripheral, hypokalemia and, 270
  shock and, 411–412
Pulse deficit, 2117
Pulse oximeter, 2003
Pulse pressure: the difference between the systolic and diastolic arterial pressures, 412, 2080, 2094
  measurement of, 2094

INDEX / GLOSSARY

Index/Glossary

INDEX / GLOSSARY

COLOR PLATE CREDITS

The authors and publisher gratefully acknowledge the following sources of color illustrations:

Plates 1, 2, 4, 5, 6, 7, 8, 9, 10, 13, 15, and 17 photographs by Mr. Dave Bishop, Easton, MD.

Plate 3 courtesy of Dr. John Costin, Lorain, OH.

Plates 11, 22B, 44, 45, 46, 47, and 60 courtesy of Ms. Janice Z. Cuzzell, Woodland Hills, CA.

Plate 14 from Cuzzell, J. Z. (1990). Derm detective—Clues: Bruised, torn skin. *American Journal of Nursing, 90(3),* 16.

Plates 16, 20, 21, 22A, 24, 25, 42, 57B, and 73 courtesy of Dr. Beverly A. Johnson, Howard University Hospital, Washington, DC.

Plates 18, 19, and 23 courtesy of Dr. John A. Kenney, Jr., Howard University Hospital, Washington, DC.

Plates 26 and 28 courtesy of Dr. Robert Tomsak, Division of Neuro-ophthalmology, Case Western Reserve University, Cleveland, OH.

Plate 27 courtesy of Drs. Harry Kaplan and Lawrence P. Roach, Philadelphia, PA.

Plates 29, 30, 31, 32, 33, 34, and 35 from Swartz, M. H. (1989). *Textbook of physical diagnosis: History and examination.* Philadelphia: W. B. Saunders.

Plate 36 from Radford, J., & Thatcher, N. (1988). The toxicity of cancer chemotherapy in adults. *Cancer Care 5,* 4–7.

Plates 37 and 38 courtesy of Dr. Andrew Martof, University of Virginia Health Sciences Center, Charlottesville, VA.

Plates 12, 39, 40, 41, 43, 48, 49, 50, 51, 53, 54, 55, 56, 57A, 61, 62, 63, 64, 65, 66, 67, 68, 69, 70, and 71 from Lookingbill, D. P., & Marks, J. G., Jr. (1986). *Principles of dermatology.* Philadelphia: W. B. Saunders.

Plate 52 courtesy of the Institute for Dermatologic Communication and Education, Evanston, IL.

Plates 58, 75, and 76 from Hurwitz, S. (1981). *Clinical pediatric dermatology: A textbook of skin disorders of childhood and adolescence.* Philadelphia: W. B. Saunders.

Plate 59 from Behrman, H. T., Labow, T. A., & Rozen, J. H. (1978). *Common skin diseases: Diagnosis and treatment* (3rd ed.). New York: Grune & Stratton.

Plate 72 from the AHPA Arthritis Teaching Slide Collection, second edition, copyright 1988. Used by permission of the Arthritis Foundation, Atlanta, GA.

Plate 74 courtesy of Ms. Christine Grady, National Institutes of Health, Bethesda, MD.

Special thanks to Mildred Hazelton Gillespie and William Hill Manor, Easton, MD.

SHOWCASE ILLUSTRATIONS

Alphabetic List of Approved Nursing Diagnoses from the 9th Conference of the North American Nursing Diagnosis Association, 1990

Activity intolerance
Activity intolerance, potential
Adjustment, impaired
Airway clearance, ineffective
Anxiety
Aspiration, potential for
Body image disturbance
Body temperature, potential altered
Breastfeeding, effective*
Breastfeeding, ineffective
Breathing pattern, ineffective
Cardiac output, decreased
Communication, impaired verbal
Conflict, decisional (specify)
Conflict, parental role
Constipation
Constipation, colonic
Constipation, perceived
Coping, defensive
Coping, family, ineffective: compromised
Coping, family, ineffective: disabling
Coping, family: potential for growth
Coping, individual, ineffective
Denial, ineffective
Diarrhea
Disuse syndrome, potential for
Diversional activity deficit
Dysreflexia
Family processes, altered
Fatigue
Fear
Fluid volume deficit
Fluid volume deficit, potential
Fluid volume excess
Gas exchange, impaired
Grieving, anticipatory
Grieving, dysfunctional
Growth and development, altered
Health maintenance, altered
Health-seeking behaviors (specify)
Home maintenance management, impaired
Hopelessness
Hyperthermia
Hypothermia
Incontinence, bowel
Incontinence, functional
Incontinence, reflex
Incontinence, stress
Incontinence, total
Incontinence, urge
Infection, potential for

Injury, potential for
Knowledge deficit (specify)
Mobility, impaired physical
Noncompliance (specify)
Nutrition, altered: less than body requirements
Nutrition, altered: more than body requirements
Nutrition, altered: potential for more than body requirements
Oral mucous membrane, altered
Pain
Pain, chronic
Parenting, altered
Parenting, altered, potential
Personal identity disturbance
Poisoning, potential for
Post-trauma response
Powerlessness
Protection, altered*
Rape-trauma syndrome
Rape-trauma syndrome: compound reaction
Rape-trauma syndrome: silent reaction
Role performance, altered
Self-care deficit: bathing/hygiene
                    dressing/grooming
                    feeding
                    toileting
Self-esteem, chronic low
Self-esteem disturbance
Self-esteem, situational low
Sensory/perceptual alterations (specify) (visual, auditory, kinesthetic, gustatory, tactile, olfactory)
Sexual dysfunction
Sexuality patterns, altered
Skin integrity, impaired
Skin integrity, potential impaired
Sleep pattern disturbance
Social interaction, impaired
Social isolation
Spiritual distress
Suffocation, potential for
Swallowing, impaired
Thermoregulation, ineffective
Thought processes, altered
Tissue integrity, impaired
Tissue perfusion, altered (specify type) (renal, cerebral, cardiopulmonary, gastrointestinal, peripheral)
Trauma, potential for
Unilateral neglect
Urinary elimination, altered
Urinary retention
Violence, potential for: self-directed or directed at others

---

* New diagnoses, 1990